FAMILY-CENTERED
Nursing Care of Children

FAMILY-CENTERED
Nursing Care of Children

Second Edition

Cecily Lynn Betz, PhD, RN
Associate Director
University Affiliated Program
University of California–Los Angeles Neuropsychiatric Institute
Los Angeles, California
Editor, *Journal of Pediatric Nursing*

Mabel Metzger Hunsberger, MSN, RN
Associate Professor
McMaster University School of Nursing
Hamilton, Ontario

Stephanie Wright, PhD, RN
Assistant Professor
School of Nursing
Georgetown University
Washington, D.C.

W.B. SAUNDERS COMPANY
A Division of Harcourt Brace
& Company
Philadelphia London Toronto
Montreal Sydney Tokyo

W.B. SAUNDERS COMPANY
A Division of Harcourt Brace & Company

The Curtis Center
Independence Square West
Philadelphia, Pennsylvania 19106

Library of Congress Cataloging-in-Publication Data

Betz, Cecily Lynn.
Family-centered nursing care of children/Cecily Lynn Betz, Mabel Metzger Hunsberger, Stephanie Wright.—2nd ed.
p. cm.

Rev. ed. of.: Family-centered nursing care of children/Roxie L. Romness Foster, Mabel Metzger Hunsberger, Jo Joyce Tackett Anderson. 1989.
Includes bibliographical references and index.
ISBN 0-7216-4489-9
1. Pediatric nursing. 2. Family nursing. 3. Pediatric Nursing. I. Hunsberger, Mabel. II. Wright, Stephanie, Ph. D. III. Foster, Roxie L. Romness. Family-centered nursing care of children. IV. Title.
[DNLM: 1. Child Care—nurses' instruction. 2. Child Development—nurses' instruction. 3. Family Health—nurses' instruction. WY 159 B565f 1994]
RJ245.F67 1994
610.73'62—dc20
DNLM/DLC 93-2268

Cover photograph supplied by © COMSTOCK, INC.

Family-Centered Nursing Care of Children ISBN 0-7216-4489-9

Printed in the United States of America

Last digit is the print number: 9 8 7 6 5 4 3 2

To my husband, Robert Nini, who has been a great source of support and encouragement.

C.B.

To my husband, Merrill, for his enduring patience and encouragement, and to my son, Jason, for helping me to understand the world of adolescents.

M.H.

To my husband, Bob, for his unflagging support for my endeavors. To my children, Rob, Kate, and Debby, who have taught me so much about myself, children, and being grown up. And to my students who provide the motivation for my work.

S.W.

CONSULTING EDITOR

Sandra B. Frick-Helms, PhD, RN, RPT-S
Associate Professor, Department of Family and Community Health Nursing, College of Nursing, University of South Carolina, Columbia, South Carolina

With great appreciation, to my husband, Johnny; my three children, Danny, Lisa, and Charles; my grandchildren, Meggie and Christopher; and my friend and mentor, Maxine Loomis.

CONTRIBUTORS

Carolyn M. Byrne, MHSc, RN
Associate Professor, School of Nursing, McMaster University; Public Health Associate, Hamilton Wentworth Teaching Health Unit, Hamilton, Ontario

Nancy Carter, BScN, RN
Staff Nurse, Pediatric Surgical Unit; Part-Time Clinical Educator, Chedoke-McMaster Hospitals, Hamilton, Ontario

Denise Charron-Prochownik, PhD, MSN
Senior Research Fellow, School of Medicine; Adjunct Assistant Professor, School of Nursing, University of Pittsburgh, Pittsburgh, Pennsylvania

Pamela N. Clarke, RN, MPH, PhD
Associate Professor, College of Nursing, University of South Carolina; Consultant in Home Health Care, Columbia, South Carolina

Regina M. Cusson, RN, PhD, NNP
Assistant Professor, Maternal Child Nursing, University of Maryland School of Nursing; Neonatal Nurse Practitioner, Mercy Medical Center, Baltimore, Maryland

Elaine Daberkow-Carson, RN, MSN
Clinical Nurse Specialist, Pediatric Cardiology, Lucile Salter Packard Children's Hospital at Stanford, Stanford University, Stanford, California

Anne Davidson-Mundt, RN, MS
Clinical Faculty, University of Colorado School of Nursing, Denver, Colorado; Faculty, University of Phoenix, Phoenix, Arizona; Clinical Nurse Specialist, Children with Special Needs, Denver Health and Hospitals, Denver, Colorado

Carolyn Pedigo Delahoussaye, RN, MSN
Associate Professor, Nursing, University of Southwestern Louisiana, College of Nursing, Lafayette, Louisiana

Jennifer Disabato, MS, BSN
Clinical Faculty, University of Colorado School of Nursing; Clinical Nurse Specialist/Pediatric Nurse Practitioner for Pediatric Neurosurgery, The Children's Hospital, Denver, Colorado

Lynn Feenan, RN, MS
Clinical Assistant Professor; Pediatric Pulmonary Clinical Nurse Specialist, University of Wisconsin Children's Hospital, Madison, Wisconsin

Irving Feller, MD
Professor Emeritus of Surgery, University of Michigan Burn Center, Ann Arbor, Michigan

Kathleen Lord Feroli, RN, MS, CPNP
Instructor, Department of Maternal Child Health, University of Maryland School of Nursing; Clinical Instructor, Division of Adolescent Medicine, University of Maryland School of Medicine, Baltimore, Maryland

Roxie L. Foster, PhD, RN
Assistant Professor, School of Nursing, University of Colorado Health Sciences Center; Co-Director, Pain Consultation Service, The Children's Hospital, Denver, Colorado

Janet S. Hadley, RN, MS, CPNP
Former Head Nurse, Pediatric Clinic, Ambulatory Care Center, Denver General Hospital, Denver, Colorado

Ann Harkins, PhD, RN
Clinical Research Associate, Allergy, Immunology and Respiratory Medicine, Lucile Packard Children's Hospital at Stanford, Palo Alto, California

Marcia J. Hill, RN, MSN
Assistant Clinical Professor, Dermatology, Baylor College of Medicine; Wound Care Advisory Committee; Chair, Clinical Practice Model Task Force; Manager/Advisor, *Nursing Avenues* Editorial Board; Manager of Nursing, Methodist Hospital, Houston, Texas

Claudella Archambeau Jones, RN
Director, National Institute for Burn Medicine, Ann Arbor, Michigan

Marcia Sosnowski Leonard, RN, PNP
Clinical Nurse IV/Pediatric Nurse Practitioner, University of Michigan, Ann Arbor, Michigan

Margaret M. Mahon, PhD, RN, C
Assistant Professor, Nursing of Children, University of Pennsylvania, School of Nursing; Coordinator, Sibling Bereavement Program, Children's Hospital of Philadelphia, Philadelphia, Pennsylvania

Kimberly J. Mason, RN, MSN, ONC
Clinical Nurse Specialist, Orthopaedics, Children's Hospital of Philadelphia, Philadelphia, Pennsylvania

Linda Waite Maurano, MSN, RN
Adjunct Faculty, Catholic University of America, School of Nursing; Instructor, Georgetown University, School of Nursing; President/CEO, Visiting Nurse Association of Washington, District of Columbia

Darlene E. McCown, PhD, PNP, RN, Certified Death Educator
Associate Professor, University of Rochester, School of Nursing, Rochester, New York

Noreen Heer Nicol, RN, MS, FNC
Clinical Senior Instructor, University of Colorado School of Nursing; Clinical Specialist/Nurse Practitioner, Chair, Advanced Clinical Practice Group, National Jewish Center for Immunology and Respiratory Medicine, Denver, Colorado

Connie B. Ott, RN, MS, MN
Instructor, Associate Degree Nursing Program, Orangeburg-Calhoun Technical College, Orangeburg, South Carolina

Janet Pinelli, RN, MSN
Associate Professor, School of Nursing, McMaster University; Clinical Nurse Specialist/Neonatal Practitioner, Chedoke-McMaster Hospitals, Hamilton, Ontario

Judith A. Ruble, MS, RN, PNP
Clinical Nurse Specialist, Pediatric Endocrinology, Children's Hospital, Oakland, California

Laurie E. Scudder, RN, MS, CPNP
Instructor, Primary Care Program, University of Maryland, School of Nursing; Pediatric Nurse Practitioner, Department of Pediatrics, Mercy Medical Center, Baltimore, Maryland

Florence Simmons, RN, MSN, CCRN
Nurse Case Manager, Burn/Trauma Service, Medical University of South Carolina, Charleston, South Carolina

Patricia Smith, RN, MN
Clinical Nurse Specialist, Department of Pediatric Nursing, Pediatric Cardiology, University of Wisconsin Children's Hospital, Madison, Wisconsin

Bonnie Stevens, RN, PhD
Assistant Professor, University of Toronto; Perinatal Nursing Research Consultant, Mount Sinai Hospital, Toronto, Ontario

B. Helen Thomas, RN, MSc (Health Behaviour)
Associate Professor, School of Nursing, McMaster University; Clinical Nurse Consultant, Hamilton Wentworth Department of Public Health Services, Hamilton, Ontario

Annette Vigneux, RN, MHSc
Assistant Clinical Professor, School of Nursing, McMaster University; Clinical Nurse Specialist, Pediatric Nephrology, Children's Hospital, Chedoke-McMaster Hospitals, Hamilton, Ontario

Mary J. Waskerwitz, BSN, CPNP
Pediatric Nurse Practitioner, Division of Pediatric Hematology-Oncology, DeVos Children's Hospital at Butterworth, Grand Rapids, Michigan

John T. Wiernikowski, BScPhm, PharmD
Lecturer, Faculty of Pharmacy, University of Toronto, Toronto; Clinical Pharmacist, Pediatrics, Pediatric Haematology/Oncology, Children's Hospital at Chedoke-McMaster Hospitals, Hamilton, Ontario

Astrid Hellier Wilson, RN, DSN
Assistant Professor, Parent-Child Nursing Department, Georgia State University, Atlanta, Georgia

Elizabeth Wonnacott, BScN, MSN, RN
Tutor, University of Toronto, Faculty of Nursing, Toronto, Ontario

Lynette Wright, BSN, MN
Clinical Instructor, Nell Hodgson Woodruff School of Nursing, Emory University; Director, Clinical Services, Integrated Genetics, Atlanta Center, Atlanta, Georgia

Stephanie Wright, PhD, RN
Assistant Professor, Georgetown University School of Nursing, Washington, District of Columbia

Judy Wulf, BSN, MN, CNRN
Adjunct Faculty, University of Minnesota School of Nursing; Clinical Nurse Specialist, Department of Neurosurgery, University of Minnesota Hospital and Clinics, Minneapolis, Minnesota

Mary Jean Yablonky, CRNA, MA
Staff Nurse Anesthetist, Oakwood Hospital, Dearborn; Clinical Instructor, University of Detroit–Mercy/St. Joseph Mercy Hospital Program in Nurse Anesthesiology, Pontiac, Michigan

PREFACE

The second edition of *Family-Centered Nursing Care of Children* builds on the successful themes and organization of the first edition while incorporating the ideas and attitudes of a team of nurse authors newly working together. Each of the authors provided a unique perspective whose synergistic effect accumulated in many improvements in this edition. The basic premise of the text—*that the child is best understood and cared for within the context of the family*—remains the same. The themes of the text have been strengthened throughout:

- Growth and development chapters include both child and family development.
- Strong emphasis on anticipatory guidance is provided at each developmental stage.
- Separate chapters are devoted to the concepts of health promotion to provide the theoretical base that students need about the issues of paramount importance to the health of children—parenting, self-esteem, communication, safety, nutrition, immunizations, and play.
- Detailed up-to-date information is provided on clinical skills needed for the care of children—procedures, fluid and electrolyte management, pharmacology, and pain management.
- Disorders and diseases are organized from simple to complex by body system. Grouping together disorders relating to a body system allows the student to understand the physiology, treatments, and care more easily.

Growth and Development of Children and Families

Chapter 2, Family Theories and Assessment, has been totally updated to reflect today's family structures. Chapters 4 through 9, in Unit II, Growth and Development of Children Within Families, have been significantly revised and reorganized. Each chapter begins with a section on family development, followed by sections on physical, intellectual, and emotional-social competencies for the child's developmental level. Each chapter concludes with a section entitled Health Maintenance and Promotion. This consistently recognizable format will assist the nursing student in locating information, making comparisons between developmental stages, and preparing for clinical experiences.

Each developmental chapter emphasizes anticipatory guidance for the family, about both developmental milestones and health promotion. The health promotion sections have been expanded to address the health maintenance, protection, and promotion concerns specific to each stage of development. Discussion of the anticipatory guidance strategies will assist the nursing student in understanding health concerns at each age and in incorporating health promotion into nursing care. Examples of content covered in these sections are:

- Health screening and promotion related to the developmental stage.
- Dental care.
- Sleep behaviors.
- Nutrition.
- Elimination.
- Safety concerns.
- Sexuality.
- Appropriate play activities.

Clinical focus inserts in each of the growth and development chapters provide the student with clinical application examples of how to apply theoretical concepts of growth and development to clinical situations.

Content has been updated to reflect contemporary issues affecting children, such as gay and lesbian development and violent and aggressive behavior. Sections pertaining to faith and moral development, fears, coping mechanisms, and temperament have been added to the chapters as well. Great attention has been directed to incorporating applicable nursing research into the text discussion. Highlighting the research conducted by nurse researchers was a priority in revising the chapters not only for informative and scientific purposes but, as importantly, to socialize nursing students to the important contributions nursing research has made.

Concepts Related to Health Promotion and to Illness

Unit III, Promoting Health, and Unit IV, Concepts Related to Illness, provide the strong theoretical base that the nursing student deserves. Separate chapters on Communicating with Children and Families, Promoting Healthy Parenting, and Fostering Self-Esteem are unique to this text. Chapters on Promoting Safety, Healthy Dietary Practices, and Promoting Healthy Play provide the theory and overview that the student needs in order to apply information to various developmental levels. Chapter 18, Stress, Crisis, and Coping, and Chapter 19, Chronic Illness, prepare the student for the Physiologic Alterations chapters by discussing the management of crises and problems of chronicity that occur in a wide variety of disorders.

Nursing Interventions in Developmental-Behavioral Health Concerns and in Physiologic Alterations

Unit VI, Developmental-Behavioral Health Concerns, has been reorganized to emphasize nursing assessments and multidisciplinary management. Chapter 31, Genetic Principles and Disorders, has been rewritten to reflect the nursing role in recognition and management of genetic variations and to help the student understand the recent developments in genetic research.

The 16 chapters that make up Unit VII, Nursing Interventions in Physiologic Alterations, are consistent in format and approach and are thoroughly updated by nurses expert in specific clinical areas. Content is presented with the primary goal of showing the interrelationship among pathophysiology, medical treatments, and the application of the nursing process. Chapters begin with an overview of the age-related differences in the structure and function of the child's physiologic system. Wherever appropriate, **summarizing tables** are used to present information relating to the entire body system:

- Developmental differences in structure and function of the system.
- Assessment and nursing history guidelines.
- Diagnostic procedures; laboratory tests.
- Common medications.
- Clinical manifestations of alterations in the body system.
- Nursing procedures and interventions common to various disorders of the body system.

By using summarizing tables extensively, the text allows the student to more quickly access information in the narrative while still providing the detailed reference information needed when caring for a child with a particular disorder.

The section on application of the nursing process within each of the chapters has been expanded to provide the student with in-depth information. Nursing care is delineated using the five-step nursing process—assessment, diagnosis, planning, implementation, and evaluation. NANDA nursing diagnoses are identified, and interventions specific to each diagnosis are presented. Collaborative problems are identified when both medical and nursing interventions are required for resolution of the patient problem.

Textbook Features

- *Ethical Issues Boxes*. A new feature in this edition is the Ethical Issues boxes, written by Margaret M. Mahon. In Chapter One, a framework for the process of ethical decision making is presented, with the focus on the child and the family. In later chapters, issues such as access to and responsibility for vaccinations, infants with disabilities, refusal of treatment, adolescent compliance, and use of human growth factor are discussed.
- *Research Issues*. Nursing research findings are incorporated throughout the text. On some topics of special interest, research issues are highlighted in boxes to bring them to the student's attention. Topics include the impact of parental presence during procedures, application of EMLA cream, instruments to assess children's fears of medical events, and techniques for breastfeeding premature infants.
- *Learning Features*. Each chapter begins with learning objectives, a chapter outline, a related topics box, and an overview of the chapter, to help students organize their reading. Chapters end with a listing of the most significant concepts in the chapter, organized into three major schema: Concepts Pertaining to Basic Information, Concepts Pertaining to Nursing Assessment, and Concepts Pertaining to Nursing Interventions.
- *Family-Centered Teaching Tables*. Parent and child teaching information has been organized and identified in over 40 Family-Centered Teaching tables.
- *Growth and Development Tables*. A Summary of Growth and Development and Health Maintenance tables is provided for each developmental age chapter. In addition, Growth and Development Plans in each developmental chapter help students apply their knowledge of development to clinical situations.
- *Ancillaries Available to Educators*. The Instructor's Manual to accompany *Family-Centered Nursing Care of Children* provides ideas for clinical and classroom learning activities, audiovisual resources, and multiple-choice test questions covering the text. A computerized test bank, ExaMaster, which provides the educator with a variety of testing options, is available to qualified adopters, as is a package of 50 two-color transparencies to enhance classroom presentations.

ACKNOWLEDGMENTS

This book would not be possible without the tremendous work of many people. First and foremost, we thank the contributors, who have spent much time in writing, researching, updating, and revising. Their professional expertise and standards of excellence are reflected throughout the chapters of this edition.

We are especially appreciative of the contribution throughout the book of Sandra B. Frick-Helms, RN, PhD. Her expertise in nursing diagnoses was invaluable and adds a very important dimension to the text. We believe that the emphasis on the accurate use of nursing diagnoses and collaborative problems and the exploratory use of the Nursing Intervention Classifications is not only unique to this book but is also a needed step to further the use of nursing diagnoses in practice.

We are grateful to the cadre of reviewers who gave us their comments and insight on chapters in the first edition and on revised manuscript. It is wonderful to discover how carefully and thoughtfully reviewers will share their ideas about teaching and practice. In reading reviews, one discovers differences in the needs and perspectives of educators, making it impossible to act on each suggestion, but all are appreciated.

Cathy R. Arvidson, PhD, RN
University of Texas
Arlington, Texas

Judy A. Beal, DNSc, RN, PNP
Simmons College
Boston, Massachusetts

Helene Berman, MS, RN
University of Western Ontario
London, Ontario

M. Catherine Buffet, DME, MSc, BScN, RN
Hamilton-Wentworth Department of Health
Hamilton, Ontario

Denise Charron-Prochownik, MSN, RN, CPNP
University of Michigan Medical Center
Ann Arbor, Michigan

Roxanne Chinambu, ECE, BA, BED
Chedoke-McMaster Hospitals
McMaster University Medical Centre
Hamilton, Ontario

Diane F. Colizza, MN, RN
Duquesne University
Pittsburgh, Pennsylvania

Susan P. Colvin, MN, RN
Duquesne University
Pittsburgh, Pennsylvania

Aletha J. Cushinberry, EdD, RN
Washburn University
Topeka, Kansas

Betty Davies, PhD, RN
University of British Columbia
Vancouver, British Columbia

Janet A. Deatrick, PhD, RN
University of Pennsylvania
Philadelphia, Pennsylvania

Jane Cerruti Dellert, MSN, RNC, CPNP
Clara Maass Medical Center
Belleville, New Jersey

Marilyn M. Dickerson, MA, RN, CPNP
Missouri Baptist Medical Center
St. Louis, Missouri

Irene M. Elliott, MHSc, RN
Hospital for Sick Children
Toronto, Ontario

Jan M. Frederickson, MN, RN, CPNP
University of City of Los Angeles
Los Angeles, California

Deborah Gleason-Morgan, MSN, RN, CPNP
Children's Hospital
Los Angeles, California

Nancy Hagelgans, MSN, RN, CETN
Children's Surgical Associates, Ltd.
Philadelphia, Pennsylvania

Mary Ruth Hallum, EdD, MS, BSN, RN
Memphis State University
Memphis, Tennessee

Theresa C. Harper, MSN, RN-C, FNP
Chedoke-McMaster Hospitals
McMaster University Medical Centre
Hamilton, Ontario

Deborah P. Henderson, MA, RN, CEN, CCRN
Harbor-UCLA Medical Center
Torrance, California

Lori Jean Hendricks, MSN, RN
Shriners Burns Institute
Cincinnati, Ohio

Rosamund Hennessey, RN
Chedoke-McMaster Hospitals
McMaster University Medical Centre
Hamilton, Ontario

Julie A. Herda, MN, RN
Children's Hospital
Orange, California

Bonnie Holaday, DNS, RN
Vanderbilt University
Nashville, Tennessee

Janet T. Ihlenfeld, PhD, RN
D'Youville College
Buffalo, New York

Diane S. Jakobowski, MSN, RN, CRNP
Children's Hospital
Philadelphia, Pennsylvania

Jane A. Jedwabny, BA, RNC
Institute of the Pennsylvania Hospital
Philadelphia, Pennsylvania

Mary D. Jerrett, EdD, RN
Queen's University
Kingston, Ontario

Ann B. Johnson, MS, RN
Children's Hospital
Boston, Massachusetts

Catherine Knox-Fischer, MSN, RN
Children's Hospital
Philadelphia, Pennsylvania

Lynda L. LaMontagne, DNSc, RN
Vanderbilt University
Nashville, Tennessee

Cynthia R. Levin, RN, MACS
Children's Hospital
Boston, Massachusetts

Deborah G. Loman, PhD, MSN, BSN
St. Louis University
St. Louis, Missouri

Suzanne J. McKim, MS, RN
Monroe Community College
Rochester, New York

Roma G. Magtoto, MSN, RN
Shelby State Community College
Memphis, Tennessee

Marjorie Marine, EdD, RN
Ball State University
Muncie, Indiana

Barbara L. Marino, PhD, RN
Children's Hospital
Boston, Massachusetts

Kimberly J. Mason, MSN, RN
Children's Hospital
Philadelphia, Pennsylvania

Phyllis M. Mulholland, MS, RN, C
University of Michigan
Ann Arbor, Michigan

Mary E. Muscari, MS, RN, CRNP
Luzerne Community College
Nanticoke, Pennsylvania

Anita Norton, MSN, RN
Jefferson State Community College
Birmingham, Alabama

Cheryl Panzarella, MS, RN
Children's Hospital
Boston, Massachusetts

Susan N. Peck, MSN, RN, CPNP
Children's Hospital
Philadelphia, Pennsylvania

Alexis Bulka Perri, MSN, RN
Bloomsburg University
Bloomsburg, Pennsylvania

Diane Pirhonen, RD, CN
Chedoke-McMaster Hospitals
McMaster University Medical Centre
Hamilton, Ontario

Janet F. Pope, PhD, RD, LDN
Louisiana Technical University
Ruston, Louisiana

Sandra D. Reed, PhD, RN
University of North Carolina
Greensboro, North Carolina

Mary E. Rittling, MSN, BSN, RN
State University of New York
College of Technology
Delhi, New York

Tanya M. Sudia Robinson, MN, RN
Emory University
Atlanta, Georgia

Christine M. Rosner, MSN, RN
Holy Family College
Philadelphia, Pennsylvania

Janice Rumfelt, EdD, MSN, RNC
Southern Illinois University
Edwardsville, Illinois

Gyneth R. Sanders, MN, RN
Washburn University
Topeka, Kansas

Kathleen Scheller, MSN, BSN, RNC
University of Evansville
Evansville, Indiana

Kathryn Anne Sheppard, MSN, RN
Mobile College
Mobile, Alabama

Edith Elaine Shutt, MN, MS, RN
Baker University
Baldwin City, Kansas

Doreen B. Siegel, RNC, FNP
State University of New York
Stony Brook, New York

Janis B. Smith, MSN, RN, CCRN
Children's Hospital
Philadelphia, Pennsylvania

Lucinda Steele-Olynyk, RN
Chedoke-McMaster Hospitals
McMaster University Medical Centre
Hamilton, Ontario

Mary Jo Stralka, MSN, RN, CPNP
Barnes College
St. Louis, Missouri

Karen Uzark, PhD, RN
Mott Children's Hospital
Ann Arbor, Michigan

Melissa Vandeveer, MSN, RN, PNP
University of Southern Indiana
Evansville, Indiana

Pamela S. Verbin, MS, RD, CNSD
Children's Hospital
Philadelphia, Pennsylvania

Annette Vigneux, MHSc, RN
Chedoke-McMaster Hospitals
McMaster University Medical Centre
Hamilton, Ontario

Kristina Rociunas Volertas, MSN, BSN, RN
The Institute of Pennsylvania Hospital
Philadelphia, Pennsylvania

Janet K. Williams, PhD, RN, CPNP
University of Iowa
Iowa City, Iowa

Lucinda Williams, MSN, RN, CPNP
Children's Hospital
Boston, Massachusetts

Ronda M. Wood, MN, RNC
Children's Hospital
Los Angeles, California

We also wish to acknowledge and express our appreciation to all those who participated in the first edition of *Family-Centered Nursing Care of Children,* especially to Jo Joyce Anderson and Roxie Foster, whose careers and choices have led to different paths, but whose dedication to a family-centered approach and a solid research base for nursing care echoes on every page of this text. Revisions in this edition have built on the work of contributors to the first edition; their contributions are listed here:

S. Elizabeth Baldwin, MSN, RNC, PNP
Altered Genitourinary Function

Kathleen Underman Boggs, PhD, RN
Behavioral and Psychiatric Alterations

Maureen H. Clark, MS, RN
Principles of Genetic Inheritance

Deborah Coody, MSN, RN, CPNP
Altered Endocrine Function

Margaret C. Crandall, MSN, RN
Altered Immune Function

M. Corinne Devlin, MD, FRCS(C), FACOG, FSOGC, DABS
Pregnancy During Adolescence

Peggy J. Drapo, PhD, RN
Alterations in Development

Ruth Heyn, MD
Aberrant Cell Growth

Robert M. Issenman, MD, FRCP
Altered Digestive Function

Judith W. Maserang, PhD, RN
Family Health

Alba Mitchell, RegN, MSc, PhD Candidate
Pregnancy During Adolescence

Mary Lou Moore, PhD, RN, C, FACCE, FAAN
Infants: Variations in Development Related to Gestational Age

Eleanor G. Pask, EdD, MScN, RN
Altered Metabolic Function

Charlotte R. Patrick, MD, MEd, RN
Alterations in Development

Lynn Rew, EdD, RN, C, FAAN
Promoting Healthy Sexuality

Joan M. Rimar, MSN, BSN, RN
Fluid and Electrolyte Maintenance

Patricia Neel Scott, MSN, RN, CPNP
Families with Adolescents

Claire Smith, RN
Altered Metabolic Function

Ann Wiebmer Strang, MSN, RN
Altered Behavior

Linda L. Upton, MS, RN
Infant: Growth and Development

Susan Van Cleve, MS, RN, CPNP
Altered Genitourinary Function

Anna Frances Z. Wenger, PhD, RN
The Developing Family

Cecily Betz also thanks Sharon Fryer-Johnson, Sharon Dobeck, and Robert Nini, who provided assistance in the preparation of the manuscript, and Sandra Kaler, RN, PNP, PhD, Therapist in private practice, Los Angeles; Rhonda Sena, PhD, Psychology Training Coordinator, UCLA University Affiliated Program; and Judy Beal, RN, DNS, Professor of Nursing, Graduate School for Health Studies, Simmons College, Boston. Mabel Hunsberger expresses her thanks to colleagues for review of manuscript: Dr. Brian Steele, MRC, FRCP(C), Associate Professor of Pediatrics, Pediatric Nephrologist, Children's Hospital, Chedoke-McMaster Hospitals; Marilyn Parsons, Assistant Professor, School of Nursing, McMaster University; Nadine Cross, Consultant, Nadine L. Cross & Associates, University of Toronto; and Kris Patton and Rienne Austin, IV Team (Pediatrics), Chedoke-McMaster Hospitals, McMaster Division. For assistance in retrieving literature and manuscript preparation, Hope Schrieber, Alina Brotea, and Lee Wilson are sincerely thanked.

BRIEF CONTENTS

UNIT ONE
Perspectives on the Nursing Care of Children and Adolescents 1

UNIT TWO
Growth and Development of Children Within Families 105

UNIT THREE
Promoting Health 377

UNIT FOUR
Concepts Related to Illness 627

UNIT FIVE
Managing Illness 715

UNIT SIX
Developmental-Behavioral Health Concerns 951

UNIT SEVEN

Nursing Interventions in Physiologic Alterations 1165

DETAILED CONTENTS

CHAPTER 41
Altered Musculoskeletal Function 1815
Kimberly J. Mason and Stephanie Wright

CHAPTER 42
Neoplasms/Cancer 1874
Mary J. Waskerwitz

CHAPTER 43
Altered Endocrine Function 1938
Judith A. Ruble and Denise Charron-Prochownik

CHAPTER 44
Altered Metabolic Function 2012
Anne Davidson-Mundt

CHAPTER 45
Sensory and Communication Alterations 2042
Laurie E. Scudder

CHAPTER 46
The Injured Child 2080
Elizabeth Wonnacott

CHAPTER 47
The Child with Burns 2127
Claudella Archambeau Jones, Irving Feller, and Florence Simmons

APPENDICES
Appendix One

Appendix Two

SPECIAL FEATURES

NURSING PROCESS PLANS

GROWTH AND DEVELOPMENT TABLES AND PLANS

(continued)

GROWTH AND DEVELOPMENT TABLES AND PLANS (*Continued*)

FAMILY-CENTERED TEACHING TABLES

FAMILY-CENTERED TEACHING TABLES (*Continued*)

ETHICAL ISSUES

RESEARCH ISSUES

UNIT • ONE

Perspectives on the Nursing Care of Children and Adolescents

CHAPTER • 1

Child Health Issues, Ethics, and Nursing Process

NURSING PROCESS PLAN
Figure 1–5. Elements of the NPP

RELATED TOPICS
Nontraditional family styles, Chapter 2
Safety, Chapter 15
Legal aspects of consent, Chapter 23
Injuries, Chapter 46

LEARNING OBJECTIVES

- Identify the overall goals of pediatric nursing.
- Describe the relevance of morbidity and morbidity statistics as an indication of the health problems impacting the pediatric population.
- Discuss the effects of poverty on the pediatric population and its implication on the health care status of children.
- Review the role of the pediatric nurse in addressing the health care needs of children and families.
- Explain the historical, societal, political, and professional influences affecting the health care of children.
- Analyze the uniqueness of ethical considerations affecting professional ethics in pediatric health care.
- Synthesize information from the developmental theorists to the care of children and their families.
- Apply the nursing process to the care of children and their families.

The celebrations and rituals that mark the birth and development of a child in every culture testify to the mystery and wonder that are associated with the first two decades of life. Nurses who choose to work with children and adolescents seem drawn to that mystery—perhaps not so much to unravel it as just to experience it. They are warmed more than most by a child's smile; they are touched more than most by a

child's cry. They recognize the "personhood" of even their youngest client. They are genuinely interested in a child's opinion of what the moon is made of and in an adolescent's explanation for purple-striped hair. They are highly skilled — there is little room for error. They are gentle and kind — the spirit of a child is fragile. Pediatric nurses care not only *for* children and families, they care *about* children and families.

The Goal for Nursing Care of Children and Adolescents

The goal for nursing care of children and adolescents is best understood as it relates to the practice of nursing as a whole. Nursing has been defined by the American Nurses' Association (1980, p. 9) as "the diagnosis and treatment of human responses to actual or potential health problems." More specifically, nursing is a discipline whose focus is the well-being of persons and whose practice involves the contracting (either formally or by inference) with individual clients and/or families and communities to prevent, assess, and intervene in disease processes and to promote wellness in life and dignity in death by use of the caring and curing processes deemed morally and legally appropriate. Within the framework of that definition *the goal of pediatric nursing is to promote the healthy maturation of the child/adolescent as a physical, intellectual, and emotional-social being within the context of the family and the community.* This goal incorporates prevention and assessment of and intervention for threats to physical, intellectual, and emotional-social well-being.

Implications for Nursing Practice

The key word within the stated goal is *maturation.* It emphasizes the *uniqueness* of nursing care for children and adolescents in terms of their response to illness and their need for advocacy. The child* has developing, and, therefore, often immature physical characteristics and immature physiologic and cognitive processes. Self-concept, coping patterns, and social behaviors are also less well developed than in the adult. Because of this immaturity, the physical, cognitive, and emotional responses of the child to illness will vary with chronologic age and with achievement of developmental tasks. Also because of this immaturity, the developing child or adolescent requires adult advocacy for the maintenance and restoration of health. The overwhelming influence of the family on all aspects of the child's health and development makes the family integral to all nursing assessment, analysis, planning, intervention, and evaluation. Generally, the term "client" in this text refers to child and family.

One of the fundamental goals of nursing is to provide family-centered nursing care. This is in part based on the premise that, since the family is a system, no one individual member can be effectively cared for if that care does not consider the other members who both affect and are affected by the member seeking nursing care. Practitioners who care for the children in families must acknowledge this relationship because it is the family that is largely responsible for that child, that most significantly enhances or hinders that child's development, and to which that child must ultimately be accountable.

Where "family" once referred primarily to the traditional nuclear group of two parents and one or more children, family structure is changing so that the nuclear family is no longer the standard. Nursing must consider that modern families are often headed by single parents, may be transcultural, biracial, blended, adoptive, communal, gay, or one of several other alternative or nontraditional family styles. Each family must be approached as a unique group of individuals with particular strengths and limitations. Family assessment along with the most common types of nontraditional family styles is discussed in Chapter 2.

Desired Outcomes

The overall goal for pediatric nursing is realized when the nurse (1) recognizes developmental immaturity and distinguishes these normal characteristics from disease processes, (2) identifies threats to well-being related to physical, intellectual, and emotional-social developmental processes, (3) directs nursing strategies to support the unique response of *this* child to issues of health and illness, and (4) supports parental advocacy and initiates professional advocacy for the child within the health care system and within the community.

A Perspective on the Pediatric Population

Three major areas are discussed in this section for the purpose of gaining a perspective on the child popu-

*The word "child" is used in this chapter as a generic term to connote the developmental stages of infancy through adolescence.

lation and nursing activities within it. Morbidity and mortality are addressed because they speak to numbers and causes of diseases and death among children and adolescents. The effect of poverty on the pediatric population is included to detail a social issue that increasingly holds implications for the type of clients we see today and will see in the future. Finally, the role of the nurse is discussed as it pertains to care for children and adolescents.

Morbidity and Mortality

Morbidity refers to "sickness" or disease condition.
Mortality refers to the death rate.

The word "morbid" means diseased, unhealthy, unwholesome. "Morbidity" is the term used to denote the disease conditions seen within a population. The *morbidity rate* for a specific disease is the number of cases of that disease in a specified period of time (usually a year) within a specified unit (stated number, e.g., 10,000, 100,000) of the population.

The word "mortal" means human or subject to death. "Mortality" refers to the number of deaths within a stated population. The *mortality rate* for a given disease is the ratio of the number of deaths from that disease divided by the total number of reported cases of that disease. Together, morbidity and mortality provide a thumbnail sketch of the illness problems that bring children to the health care system and an indication of which diseases carry the highest risk of mortality within a given age group.

Morbidity by Hospital Admission. Pediatric nurses who work in acute care settings see children who have a different mix of disease conditions, depending on whether the facility is a children's hospital or a general hospital. Children are more likely to be admitted to a *general hospital* with respiratory and gastrointestinal illnesses, for surgery for tonsillectomy and adenoidectomy, and for injury-related causes. Children are more likely to be admitted to a *children's hospital* for specialized treatment for diseases such as congenital anomalies, malignancies, gastrointestinal disease, and central nervous system anomalies (Nadler & Evans, 1987). Table 1–1 details the most common diagnoses of children admitted to children's hospitals. Of course, hospital admittance depends on hospital access. If access to a local or regional children's hospital is limited by geographic or financial factors, the closest general hospital must adapt to more specialized pediatric needs.

In 1989, it was estimated that more than 4 million children under the age of 22 years were discharged from hospitals. The major cause for hospitalization for children ages 1 to 9 years was for diseases of the respiratory system. Three diagnostic categories—namely, diseases of the digestive system, diseases of the respiratory system, and unintentional injury—accounted for 54 per cent of the hospital discharges of children ages 1 to 14 years in 1989. The rates of hospitalization decrease with age until age 14, wherein the rates begin to rise during later adolescence. For adolescent girls and young women, between the ages of 15 and 21 years, pregnancy and childbirth accounted for 65 per cent of hospitalizations (National Center for Health Statistics, 1989a). The major causes of hospitalization according to age groups are listed in Figure 1–1.

Injury as a Cause of Morbidity. The importance of considering injury under the category of morbidity is emphasized by the fact that for every death attributed to injury (accident), at least 1000 other injuries occur that, although they are nonfatal, are serious enough to require treatment (Guyer & Gallagher, 1985). The most common site of injuries for children under 15 years is the home. Twenty per cent of injuries occurring to children between the ages of 5 and 9 happen in the school setting. This statistic increases to nearly 30 per cent in the 10- to 14-year-old age group (National Center for Health Statistics, 1990a).

Mortality. The majority of deaths that occur in the first year of life are attributed to the neonatal period, the first 28 days of life. Neonatal deaths significantly outrank those for the postneonatal period (after the first month of life) for both African-American and white infants (US Department of Health and Human Services, 1991). About 65 per cent of all deaths in the first year occur within the first 24 hours (Behrman,

TABLE 1-1
Top Admission Diagnoses in Children's Hospitals

Bronchitis and asthma
Esophagitis, gastroenteritis, and miscellaneous digestive disorders
Seizure and headache
Simple pneumonia and pleurisy
Chemotherapy
Nutritional and miscellaneous metabolic disorders
Viral illness
Otitis media and upper respiratory infections
Neonate, birth weight over 2499 g, without significant operating room procedures but with significant other problems
Tonsillectomy and/or adenoidectomy only

These diagnoses are compiled by the National Association of Children's Hospitals and Related Institutions, Inc., 401 Wythe Street, Alexandria, Virginia, 22314, from a total of 383,583 discharges from free-standing acute care hospitals, during the calendar year 1992.

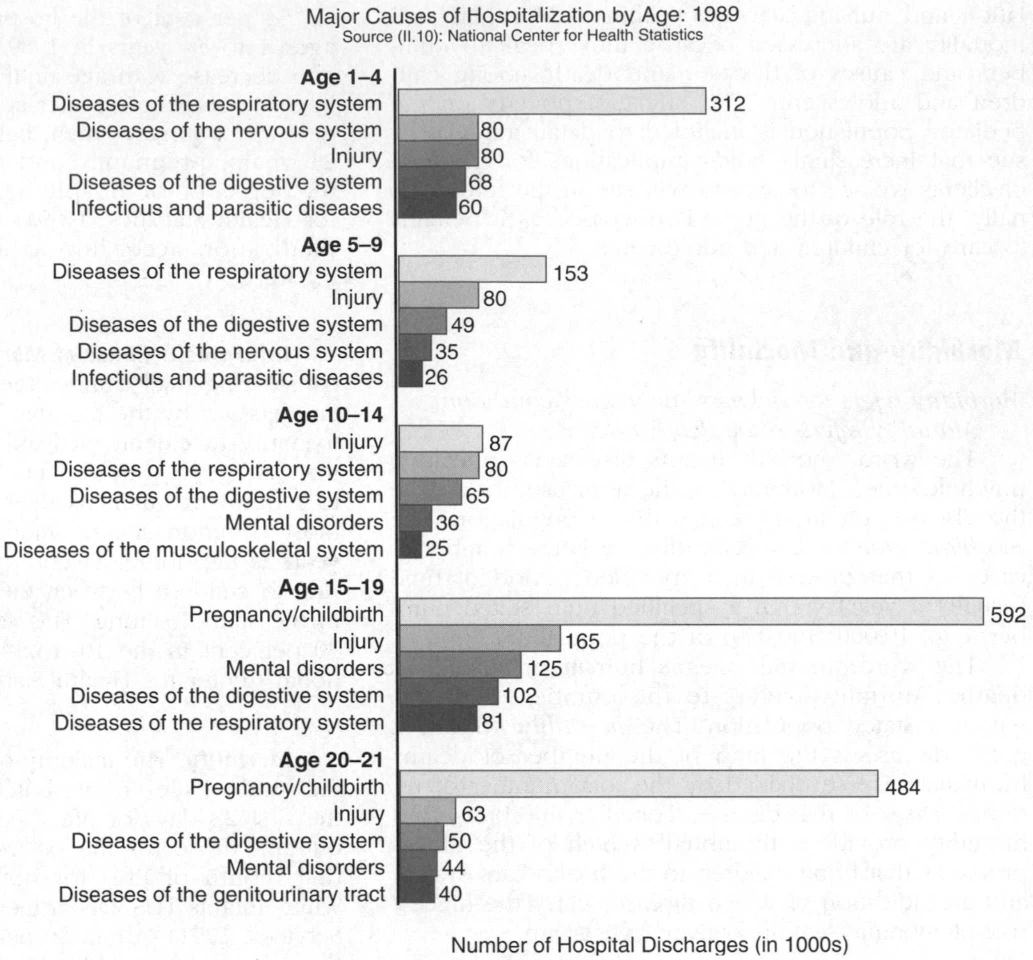

FIGURE 1 - 1. Major causes of hospitalization by age: 1989. (From U.S. Department of Health and Human Services. [1991]. *Child health USA '91*. Washington, DC: DHHS, Public Health Service, Health Resources and Services Administration, Office of Maternal and Child Health, HRS–M–CH 91–1, p 26.)

1992). The major causes of neonatal deaths are congenital anomalies and prematurity.

Although the United States has experienced a decline in infant mortality, the rate of 10 deaths per 1000 live births in 1988 was still higher than for that in 23 other nations (National Center for Health Statistics, (1991a). Mortality rates for African-American infants in the United States remain significantly higher than those for white infants (Fig. 1–2). Analysis of the National Infant Mortality Surveillance project revealed three factors contributing to the higher mortality rate for African-American infants: (1) a higher percentage of low birthweight in African-American infants, (2) a higher neonatal mortality rate for African-American infants more than 2500 g at birth compared with white infants of comparable weight, and (3) a higher postneonatal death rate for African-American infants in all birthweight categories (CDC, 1987a).

Major Causes of Death

Figure 1–3 lists causes of death for children 9 years and younger (National Center for Health Statistics, 1991c). Three of these leading causes of death—injuries, homicides, and suicides—deserve additional discussion.

Injuries/Accidents. Injuries are the leading cause of death in children 19 years and younger. Figure 1–4 details the leading causes of death attributed to injury (Fingerhut & National Center for Health Statistics, 1988). Guyer and Gallagher (1985) argued for use of the word "injury" to replace "accident." They stated, "Gradually the unscientific term accident, with its connotation of chance, fate and unexpectedness, is being replaced by the description of injuries and the physical and chemical agents that cause them." The importance of this difference in perception is that injury

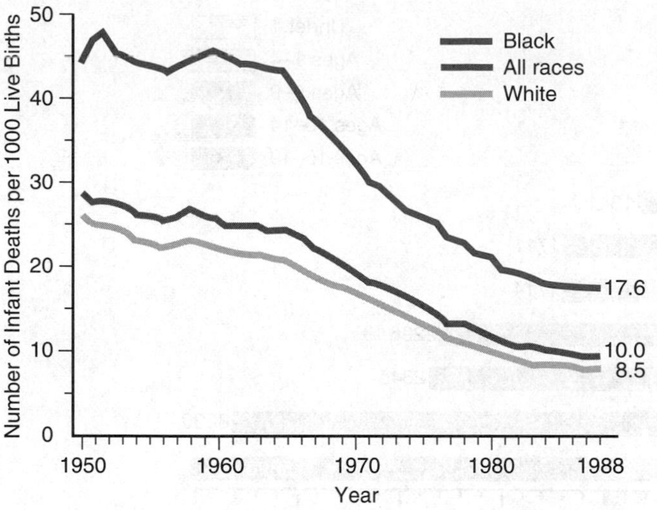

FIGURE 1-2. United States infant mortality rates by race in 1988 showed 3,909,510 babies were born in the United States, and 38,910 infants died before their first birthday. The infant mortality rate was 10.0 deaths per 1000 live births. The rapid decline in infant mortality, which began in the mid-1960s, slowed for both blacks and whites during the 1980s. The infant mortality rate for black infants remains about twice as high as that for white infants. (From U.S. Department of Health and Human Services. [1991]. *Child health USA '91*. Washington, DC: DHHS Pub. No. HRS-M-CH-91-1, p 18.)

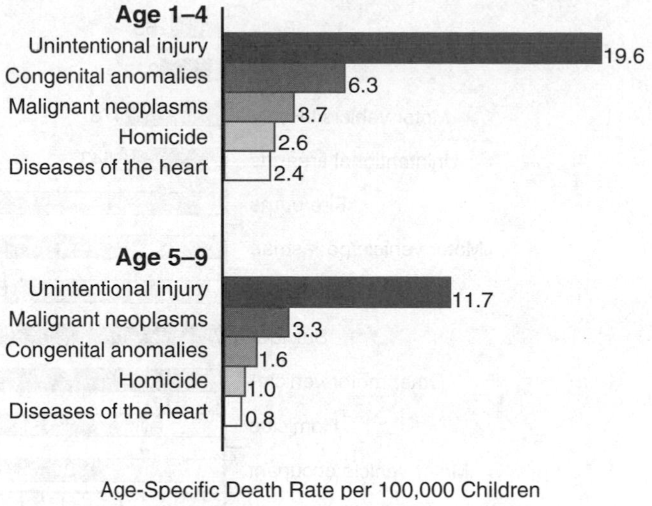

FIGURE 1-3. The leading causes of death in children ages 1 to 9 years in 1988 included unintentional injury, which claimed nearly 5000 lives among the age group in 1988. Although childhood mortality rates have substantially declined during the 1980s, the death rate due to homicide has nearly tripled since 1960. (From U.S. Department of Health and Human Services. [1991]. *Child health USA '91*. Washington, DC: DHHS Pub. No. HRS-M-CH-91-1, p 24.)

prevention may then seem a more feasible goal. Chapter 15 deals with issues of safety for children and adolescents.

Motor vehicle crashes accounted for nearly 50 per cent of the 22,411 fatal injuries involving children (CDC, 1990). It is estimated that between 15 and 30 per cent of these fatalities were associated with alcohol use. Fatality rates for males were nearly twice those for females.

Homicides. Homicides rank as the second leading cause of death in children. Homicides account for approximately 13 per cent of fatalities occurring to children. Over 60 per cent of homicides occur in the 15- to 19-year-old age group; whereas 23 per cent were among children 5 years and younger. Sixty per cent of the male homicides involved the use of firearms compared with 32 per cent of the female homicides. The homicide rate for African-American children is five times greater than that for white children. In 1987, 37 per cent of the homicides of adolescent African-American males were committed with firearms.

Suicide. Between 1970 and 1980, the suicide rate among American teen-agers and young adults (15 to 24 years) increased 40 per cent (CDC, 1987). In 1986, suicides ranked as the third leading cause of fatalities in children (CDC, 1990). The increase is due in large part to an escalation in the rate of suicide among young white men. The method of suicide also changed significantly in this 10-year reporting period. The proportion of suicides attributed to firearms increased sharply for both young men and women while intentional poisoning decreased.

The Children of Today and Tomorrow: Effects of Poverty

As we enter the last decade of the 20th century, we are faced with a major social problem that directly affects the young people of our nation: poverty. Despite our marvels of modern technology, despite the growing movement toward "holism" and "caring," despite decades of antipoverty programs, and despite the emphasis placed on the American family, *the children of the United States are currently the poorest age group in the population*. Approximately 13 million children under 18 years of age live in poverty. African-American and Hispanic children are three times more likely to live in poverty than white children (US Bureau of the Census, 1990). The following facts chronicle the status of poor children and their families in the United States:

- 12.6 million children under 18 years old live in poverty, representing 40 per cent of the nation's poor.
- The poor are not just those who are on welfare and who live in ghetto communities. The majority (about 60 per cent) of American poor who are capable of working do so but have incomes that

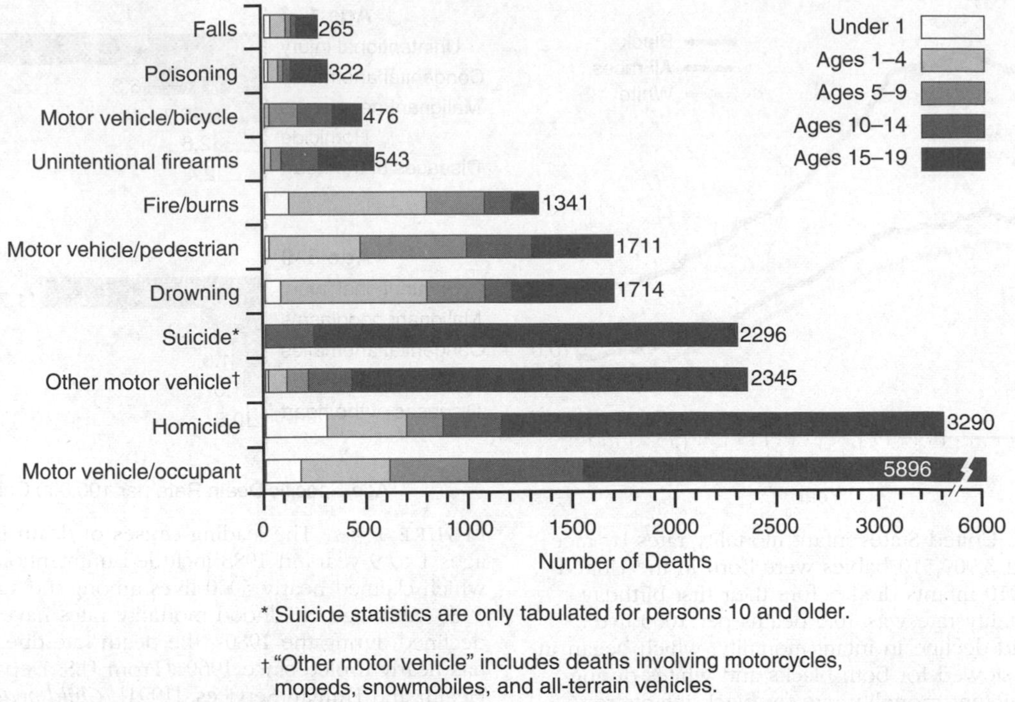

FIGURE 1-4. Number, percentage, and rate of fatal injuries for children under 19 years of age by leading cause of injury. (From Fingerhut, L., & National Center for Health Statistics [NCHS]. [1988]. [Vital statistics: Mortality statistics for ages 0–19.] Unpublished data.)

fall below the poverty line, set at $12,675 (US Bureau of the Census, 1990) in annual cash income for a family of four (US Department of Health and Human Services, 1991).

- Most poor families in which one or more members work are white, two-parent families. The "working poor" are quite evenly divided among central cities, suburbs, and rural areas (Whitman et al, 1988).
- Approximately 1 million teens become pregnant each year (Alan Guttmacher Institute, 1991). Poor and minority teens are a greater risk for teenage pregnancy: In 1988 the teen birth rate (ages 18 to 19) was 69.2 for whites and 150.5 for African-Americans (National Center for Health Statistics, 1990b).
- The number of female-headed single-parent families in America is increasing at an alarming rate. It is estimated that during the period 1980 to 2000 the number of female-headed families will increase at more than five times the rate of husband-wife families. In 1990, 40 per cent of children living with mothers only were poor (US Bureau of the Census, 1991).
- In 1989, 9.5 million children under 18 had no insurance coverage (National Center for Health Statistics, 1990b).
- In 1987, although 52 per cent of Medicaid recipients were 21 years and younger, they accounted for only 19 per cent of the expenditures. This averages out to $742 per child compared with $3362 per adult (Health Care Financing Administration, 1989).
- Between 1980 and 1988 the number of children living in poverty increased by 1 million compared with a decrease of 3.9 million for persons 65 years and older (US Bureau of the Census, 1990).
- Between 1970 and 1984 the average elderly person receiving aid from Old-Age and Survivors Insurance saw a 54 per cent increase in cash benefits. During the same period the mothers receiving aid from Aid to Families with Dependent Children (AFDC) saw dollar benefits *decline* by 34 per cent.
- For a medium-status four-person family, the average cost (i.e., not need, but actual expenditure) to raise a child from birth to 18 years is in excess of $82,000. That figure increases if the mother is also employed outside the home.
- In 1948, fully 75 per cent of median family income was exempt from taxation, providing in part for the cost of raising a family. By 1983, less than 33 per cent of median family income was tax-exempt, thus eroding protection for the rearing of American families.

Implications for Nursing Practice

What do these statistics mean to the pediatric nurse? They mean that there is likely to be a significant change in the population of children and adolescents who present themselves for treatment in the coming years. The pediatric population in America at the turn of the 21st century may well be

- Increasingly ethnically mixed (the birth rate has declined faster for white families in the United

States than for people of color, and as American birth rates decline in general, the nation will be pressed to increase immigration).
- More sickly because prenatal care and well child care are luxuries in a poverty-level environment.
- More susceptible to delays in growth due to improper nutrition and improperly treated illnesses.
- More prone to drug and alcohol abuse, depression, and suicide related to unstable and non-nurturing environments.

The Challenge for Pediatric Nursing

The challenge to the nurse who cares for children, therefore, is to provide care of such *quality* that it can offset the potential decline in *quantity* of interactions with a child and family.

On some fronts, of course, the pediatric nurse will have increasing resources to help meet this challenge. Morbidity and mortality are likely to be decreased through additional organ transplants and innovations in immunotherapy and pharmacotherapy. Computerization of hospital and agency files will eventually decrease time spent on paperwork. Employment opportunities for nurse practitioners are also expected to increase as third party payment (direct payment to nurses from insurance companies) becomes more common and as health care costs force alternatives to care solely by private physicians. Nursing research will provide nursing with an increasing base for practice that is goal-oriented rather than task-oriented; that is, it will help eliminate mundane and repetitive tasks, freeing the nurse for additional creative and therapeutic endeavors.

The effective nurse of the coming generation will base his or her practice on sound knowledge of the nursing process and the professional role. The nurse will need to understand not only where pediatric nursing is going but also the social and historical influences that have dictated practice as we know it today. Increasingly, the nurse will need to be skilled in intercultural communication and ethical decision making. The remainder of this chapter details these influences on attainment of the goal of pediatric nursing —healthy maturation of children and adolescents.

Factors Influencing the Health Care of Children

A Historical Perspective on Societal Values

It has been suggested that in the future pediatrics will become synonymous with the science of growth and development (Nadler & Evans, 1987). In many respects, that may already be the case. Viewing pediatric practice (whether medical or nursing) as a science of growth and development emphasizes a change in focus from a time when medical practices for children consisted of adult remedies administered to smaller bodies. For example, in the early 1900s bloodletting, purging, and opiates were the mainstays of medical treatment regardless of the patient's age (Brodie, 1986). For the purpose of developing a perspective on pediatric nursing, it is pertinent to understand the historical factors that have led to changing attitudes about children in the health care community and in the whole of society.

The Relative Value of a Child: Society's Indifference to Its Young

Vaughan (1987) wrote, "The caring qualities of any society may best be measured by the concerns it manifests for its aged, its disadvantaged . . . . and its young" (p 1). Historically, the young have often been among the most disadvantaged. Few historical accounts of the experience of childhood or of society's attitudes toward children exist before modern times. We can only speculate, therefore, about the reasons for what Brodie (1982) has referred to as "society's indifference to protecting and providing for its young" (p 219). Among these reasons are a shorter life span and ignorance of developmental processes.

In the 15th century it is estimated that almost 65 per cent of children died before age 5 years (Forsyth, cited in Brodie, 1986). The mortality rate had not improved by the 18th century, and it is said that even Queen Anne, who can be presumed to have had the best available care for her children, lost 18 babies in early infancy (Dolan et al, 1983). In 1900, the mortality rate in the United States remained at 23 per cent for children under 5 years of age. Today that rate has diminished to 1.3 per cent (UNICEF, 1986).

Another probable cause for the historical indifference to children is that *childhood,* as we know that concept today, was not born before the 16th century and not commonly recognized before the 18th century. Not until the 18th century did children come to be viewed as minors by the legal system and given sentences that differed from those handed down to adults (Brodie, 1986).

Although it seems strange that people of any era could have failed to recognize childhood, the idea becomes more believable when one considers that the physiologic and cognitive processes of maturation had not yet been delineated. Without an understanding of the developmental differences between children and adults, there were few conclusions one could draw other than that children were miniature adults who behaved rather badly.

The Influence of Developmental Theory on Attitudes Toward Children

Despite the beginning realization that children were distinct from adults and differed among themselves according to age, it was not until the acceptance of theories of development that the concept of *childhood* was fully realized. The delineation of physical/behavioral, psychosexual, cognitive, and psychosocial development painted an entirely new picture of childhood and irrevocably changed societal attitudes toward children and childrearing practices. The work of developmental theorists in the early 20th century remains unparalleled, although it is now common to combine several of these works to form a more integrated approach to development. These notable theorists include Arnold Gesell, Sigmund Freud, Jean Piaget, and Erik Erikson.

The Contribution of 19th Century Authors. Although theories of child development were not conceived until the early 1900s, certain authors of the mid-19th century helped prepare the American public for a change in thinking about childrearing. Lydia Sigourney's classic, *Letters to Mothers,* published in 1838, suggested that less severe tactics might better serve the parent and the child. As cited in Levine and associates (1983), she saw the primary problem of child nurture as one of "how the harp might be so tuned as not to injure its tender and intricate harmony." Catherine Beecher, a popular author of childrearing materials during the same era, echoed Sigourney's themes of valuing the child and accepting the "sacred" responsibility to guide its development to adulthood. In 1871, Jacob Abbott published *Gentle Measures in the Management and Training of the Young.* He emphasized the need to keep in mind physiologic and neurologic readiness in the moral guidance of children. This was a novel approach both in the attention to a process of development during childhood and in the assertion that "bad habits of action" were not due to inherent evil but to improper guidance of the child (Levine et al, 1983).

Health Care for Children in the 20th Century: The Effects of Increased Understanding and Advancing Technology

Advances in Nursing and Medical Care of Children. At the turn of the 20th century, the major health issues for children involved infection control and sanitation. Robert McCombs, a physician who wrote a book for nurses about the diseases of children, detailed the most frequent illnesses of infancy and childhood in the early 1900s:

> Diseases of the gastro-intestinal tract and broncho-pneumonia are seen more often than any other diseases before the second year. The other common conditions met with during this period are affections of lymph glands, tubercular meningitis, pertussis, and measles.
>
> After the second year the following diseases are most frequently seen: Disorders of nutrition, such as rickets and scurvy; bone and joint diseases, these being usually tubercular and more rarely syphilitic; diseases of the blood; organic diseases of the heart; pneumonia, typhoid fever, the acute contagious diseases, such as measles, mumps, pertussis, varicella, scarlet fever, and diphtheria. [1907, p 19]

The contamination of the milk supply presented a major health hazard. Milk was not pasteurized and often came from cows that were diseased with tuberculosis and housed in filthy sheds. These animals were fed on distillery wastes, further reducing the quality of the milk produced. Pitchers of milk were purchased from open barrels and then stored in homes without refrigeration (Brodie, 1986). In 1889, a milk distribution center opened in New York for the purpose of providing uncontaminated milk to sick infants. Although this effort was certainly a step in the right direction, it was ineffective because once the sick infant recovered contaminated milk was fed again (Dolan et al, 1983).

Nursing at this time was primarily oriented toward meeting the basic physical needs of sick children since immunization and antibiotics were not yet available and there was not yet a significant emphasis on the preventive aspects of care. Much of the care of sick children took place in isolation units within hospitals. Family visitation was discouraged because of the concern for "containing" the infectious diseases.

Training for pediatric nurses in the late 1800s and early 1900s was just that—on-the-job training in hospitals for children rather than education about children and their health. Linda Richards, who has been called America's first trained nurse, was educated at such an institution, The New England Hospital for Women and Children. Influenced by Florence Nightingale, whom she met, she distinguished herself by advocating better training of nurses. Mary Eliza Mahoney, America's first African-American nurse to graduate from a school of nursing, was also a graduate of The New England Hospital for Women and Children (Dolan et al, 1983).

The work of Lillian Wald, who has been credited with founding community health nursing, was important to the health care of children. Henry Street Settlement, which she established in 1893, was the first American institution conceived and administered by a trained nurse (Silverstein, 1985). The house on Henry Street not only provided holistic nursing care and the support of social workers for the sick (and often immigrant) poor of New York City, but also established the importance of teaching health-promoting behaviors. The Henry Street Settlement still exists as a social settlement, although the nursing component separated in 1944 to become the Visiting Nurse Service of New York (Silverstein, 1985). Wald encouraged the use of nurses in the schools of New York and initiated school lunch programs (Dolan et al, 1983). She was also largely responsible for establishment of the US Children's Bureau, which helped states create divisions of Maternal and Child Health.

Nursing care for children became more sophisticated as advances in medicine led to increasing knowledge about the physiology of childhood and increasing options for treatment. The establishment of the American Academy of Pediatrics in 1929 reflected the discoveries about the unique nature of health and illness in children. The 1940s and 1950s saw the introduction of penicillin and corticosteroids and immunization for diphtheria, tetanus, and pertussis. In addition, anticonvulsants and antihistamines were introduced. Classic research by Spitz and Robertson and others revealed the detrimental effects of maternal deprivation on institutionalized children. This led to the movement to allow increased family visitation and parental involvement in the care of hospitalized children. The play therapy (child life) programs, play rooms, and preparation visits for hospitalization, common today, were initiated as a result of this research.

Physicians increasingly began to devote time to well child care instead of just to the treatment of disease. Well child clinics provided another health maintenance/disease prevention role for nurses in the community. Testing for phenylketonuria (PKU) began in the 1950s, and in the next decade legislation made mandatory the reporting of child abuse. Immunology and clinical genetics developed as clinical specialties within medicine in the 1960s. Increasing knowledge of the physiology of the immune system and the role of genetics in predisposition to health and disease has influenced nursing assessment, analysis, planning, intervention, and evaluation of children.

In 1965 the University of Colorado introduced a nurse practitioner option within its master's program in nursing. The role of the nurse practitioner was developed in response to what was at that time a shortage of physicians, especially in rural areas. Nurse practitioners have advanced skills in physical assessment and health promotion. Today pediatric nurse practitioners work in clinics, in home care, in day care centers, and in many other areas in the community where nurses must function with greater than usual autonomy.

Major technologic advances of the 1970s included fetal monitoring, echocardiography, and computed axial tomography. Technologic advances led to increased survival of those with several previously fatal diseases, resulting in an increase in the number of children treated for chronic illnesses. Increasing emphasis was placed on the psychologic effects of illness and hospitalization during childhood. In a review of the literature on pediatric hospitalization since 1965, Thompson (1986) reported 306 research studies related to responses of children to hospitalization. Factors considered in relation to these responses were separation and rooming-in, parental anxiety, the unfamiliarity of the hospital setting (including specific activities of children during hospitalization, interactions with others, and sleep patterns when in the hospital), the effects of play during hospitalization, and the effects of preparation for hospitalization and for health care procedures.

The modern nurse who cares for children must be sensitive to the changing family structure, to the increasing number of children who live in poverty, and to the changing health care milieu wherein children are generally hospitalized only for severe and involved conditions and obtain the remainder of their care in outpatient departments, in offices of physicians and nurse practitioners, and in the home.

Social Policies to Protect Children. It was not coincidental that at the time developmental theorists were defining the concept of childhood, President Theodore Roosevelt initiated the First White House Conference on Children and Youth in 1909. In 1912 the Children's Bureau was formed, an agency that served as a national repository and resource for childhood development data, which became the current Department of Health and Human Services. In 1916 a federal law was enacted to protect children from harsh labor practices. Within a year, however, this law was repealed and not re-enacted until 1940.

Under the Social Security Act of 1935, financial aid to poor families became available through Aid to Families with Dependent Children (AFDC). Despite criticism from those who would abolish welfare programs, Moynihan (1987) has called AFDC the single most important program affecting the lives of children apart from the public schools. As cited in the previous section on poverty, recent federal cuts in AFDC are directly linked to the growing ranks of children in the United States who live below the poverty level.

The decades of the 1960s and 1970s saw the reinstatement of day care under the Economic Opportunities Act and the establishment of the National Institute of Child Health and Human Development. Project Head Start began in 1965, and the Child Nutrition Act was enacted in 1966. These and other acts under Title XX of the Social Security Act (1975) reflected an era of increased social concern for children (Wallace, 1983).

The 1980s: The Effect of Shrinking Funds. In the 1980s, escalating health costs without resultant decreases in morbidity and mortality resulted in reduced concern for equal access to health care and increased pressure to ensure that the health care delivered was both necessary and cost-effective. In 1983 the federal government instituted prospective payment for health care in the form of Diagnosis-Related Groups (DRGs). This federal mandate has had a tremendous impact on health care delivery, resulting in earlier hospital discharge and a rapidly expanding home care market. Another economic indicator for the health care industry has been the establishment of health maintenance organizations (HMOs).

The 1990s: Resource Allocation—Shifting to Prevention and Community Care

Children with Chronic Conditions. As the 21st century approaches, a shift in the health care needs in the face of limited resources has emerged. For example, many children who would have died even a decade ago are now surviving owing to advances in medical technology. Children with chronic conditions who formerly would not have survived, such as children with catastrophic illnesses, life-threatening traumatic injuries, and congenital defects, now have extended life expectancies. These children reap the benefits of changing social values, health care systems, and norms enabling them to be cared for at home in their own communities and to receive the necessary support services.

Children with highly complex health care needs are now being cared for at home. For example, the Office of Technology Assessment (OTA) estimates that there are as many as 100,000 children who are technology-dependent that receive care in the home (OTA, 1987). With the shift of care to the home setting, the parents become the health care providers, assuming the major responsibility for the complex technologic and nursing care. Now, it is customary to expect parents to manage sophisticated hospital equipment, such as ventilators and apnea monitors, and to serve as the case manager for their child's condition (Komelasky, 1990). Studies have documented the psychologic and economic benefits of home care for children with chronic and technology-dependent conditions (Smith, 1984). For example, the yearly costs of providing care to the child who is medically stable and technology-dependent in the hospital amounts to over $300,000 (Stein, 1989). Health maintenance costs for children with less complicated chronic health care needs range between $6000 and $10,000 (Perrin & Ireys, 1984).

Caring for the child with intense medical and nursing care needs can exact a heavy toll on parents. Parents must adjust their lives dramatically to meet the demands of care their child requires at home. The scenarios of this heavy responsibility may well include the need for one of the parents to give up their job to become the primary caretaker in the throes of escalating financial expenses, disruption of the parents' sleep routine resulting in sleep deprivation, and alteration of the daily routines and schedules to meet the child's constant need for assistive support and care. The parents' access to respite and burden of care at home will depend on the third party payer's policies on funding for in-home care, the medical needs of the child, and the family's ability to meet the medical care needs of their child. The range of home care services available for families can vary from 16 hours of professional nursing care each day to 30 hours per week of nursing aide/homemaker services (OTA, 1987).

The need for in-home family-centered pediatric care will continue to grow as the number of children with chronic illnesses rises. The number of children ages 1 through 19 who are limited in their daily activity owing to chronic diseases has doubled since 1960 (National Center for Health Statistics, 1990a).

Developmental Disabilities. Concepts of independence, productivity, and integration provide the foundation and vision for services and programs for children with developmental disabilities. Providers and policy makers realize the value and importance of including the child into the community early during infancy. Early intervention programs for infants at risk for or with developmental disabilities have demonstrated beneficial outcomes in the acquisition of developmental milestones (Infant Health Development Program, 1990). Children with developmental disabilities once segregated from their nonhandicapped peers are being mainstreamed and *included* into school settings, youth clubs, and activities. Given the advantage of supported inclusive environments, it is hoped that children with developmental disabilities will live more enriched, productive lives within the mainstream of society as adults, as compared with generations of the past. The deinstitutionalization of children and adults with developmental disabilities has significant economic benefits since the cost of care in home and community settings is far less expensive. Currently, it is estimated that institutionalization costs approximately $60,000 to $100,000 per year.

It is likely that the population of children with developmental disabilities will increase owing to demographic trends. As the nation's population increases so can a corresponding increase in the number of children with developmental disabilities be expected. Recent and emerging trends in health care will contribute to the increase as well. Medically fragile and technology-dependent children will change the profile of children considered to be developmentally disabled. Infants with AIDS and infants exposed to in utero substance abuse may have or be at risk for developmental delays and disabilities. Children of immigrant families who may not have had access to prevention services in this country or their country of origin will increase the number of children with developmental disabilities requiring services.

Anticipatory Guidance. Studies have demonstrated the value of anticipatory guidance activities and community-based programs in maintaining and promoting child and family health outcomes. For example, after 1 year of age, injuries account for more deaths in children than any other cause (National Center for Health Statistics, 1991c). Parent education and community prevention programs are designed as a means of decreasing injuries to alert parents to safety issues, such as use of infant car seats and seat belts and storage of poisonous and corrosive materials.

Infant Mortality. Infant mortality continues to be a major health problem in spite of significant reduction in the rate. The United States ranks 23rd among the industrialized nations in infant mortality (National Center for Health Statistics, 1991a). Approximately 40,000 infants in this country die before reaching their first birthday (National Commission to Prevent Infant Mortality, 1988). This problem is most acute in the large metropolitan areas and in the South. Eighty per cent of the largest cities in the United States reported infant mortality rates higher than the national average. Ten of the 12 states with the highest infant death rates are located in the South (National Commission to Prevent Infant Mortality, 1988). A report by the Institute of Medicine (1985) indicated the most effective strategy to reduce the infant mortality rates is to reduce the number of low birthweight (LBW) births. Efforts to achieve this goal will depend on increasing the availability, accessibility, and affordability of quality health care to women and children.

Nearly 26 per cent of women of childbearing age do not have insurance for prenatal and obstetric care.

The barriers affecting the availability and accessibility of services for underinsured and uninsured women include the perceived intimidating nature of the system of health care, social isolation, and limited resources (e.g., transportation) because of socioeconomic status. The Office of Technology Assessment estimates that every low birthweight infant born results in increased medical and health care costs between $14,000 and $30,000 (Brecht, 1989). Medical and long-term costs escalate to as high as $400,000 if the infant is born disabled (Blum, 1989).

In response to the problem of infant mortality, the National Commission to Prevent Infant Mortality (1988) has recommended that prenatal care be available to all pregnant women and that maternal-child health become a national priority. The American Nurses' Association (ANA) report (1987), "Access to prenatal care: Key to preventing low birth weight," supports the recommendations of the congressional commission as well as provides suggestions for research priorities for funding on improving outcomes for LBW infants and improving access to prenatal care.

The decade of the 1990s will continue to bring about massive changes in the health care system. The push to develop and implement programs in child health promotion and prevention services will continue. The focus of health care will not be so much on *cure* as it will be on *care*. Care and quality of life issues will emerge as pertinent questions in health care decision making affecting not only individual children but all the nation's children.

The Role of the Pediatric Nurse

Certain aspects of the pediatric nursing role are unique because of the vulnerability and developmental immaturity of children and adolescents. These aspects include the issues of advocacy and health teaching.

The Pediatric Nurse as Advocate. The advocacy role in pediatric nursing includes the responsibility to work with the family to substitute judgment for that of the child who is too young to make self-care decisions and to be a spokesperson for the child who is too young, too inexperienced, or too frightened to make care needs known. An advocate is someone who pleads in behalf of another. An effective advocate is knowledgeable of the values and beliefs of the child and family so that the "plea" truly represents the client's needs from the client's point of view. The pediatric nurse will at times be the primary advocate for a child or for an entire family, but more often will join forces with the family and other health care professionals in obtaining optimal services.

An important aspect of advocacy was brought to light by Romero (1986). Her research with school-age children revealed that many of them experienced an overwhelming lack of control in the hospital situation. Several children drew pictures of themselves as "captives" in their hospital beds. The children indicated that they not only *needed* the nurse to act as an advocate in helping them gain a sense of control within the hospital environment but also *expected* this behavior.

The Nurse as Teacher. The pediatric nurse must structure health teaching to incorporate the family's values and health beliefs. A nurse colleague tells of her experience as a nurse practitioner in an Alaskan village. She became increasingly frustrated because in the clinic mothers seemed to comprehend her instructions to use tepid water to reduce a child's fever but then repeatedly returned with febrile children and admitted they had not tried the water bath. After "time in residence" at the clinic, she learned that a family's water had to be hauled several miles across frozen tundra and that most families did not have enough "extra" water to use it for fever reduction. She recalls, with a smile, "I would have been better off to suggest they buy a can of soda pop at the local store and use it to sponge the child. Soda pop was much less costly to a family than water."

Health teaching must include both those aspects of care the child can perform alone and more complex instructions for the adult caregiver. Encouraging the parent to allow appropriate self-care will increase the child's sense of self-esteem and will increase the probability that the child will comply with the prescribed therapy. Sometimes health teaching is best carried out through role modeling. The nurse's role modeling of appropriate child care can be especially effective when parents do not understand how to care for the child and do not have the advantage of advice from extended family.

Diversity of Practice in Pediatric Nursing

Technologic advances in health care and the emphasis on wellness have dramatically increased the opportunities for varied positions within pediatric nursing. Pediatric nurses are found in clinics and doctors' offices; in schools, rehabilitation centers, summer camps, and day care centers; on cruise ships; in administrative positions related to quality assurance and control of infectious diseases; in the client's home; in acute care, intensive care, and emergency care facilities; on board flight-for-life helicopters and emergency transport craft; and virtually everywhere else there are children.

Positions vary in their requirements for educational preparation and experience. Expanded roles for nurses with master's degrees and doctorates in nursing include positions for nurse practitioners, clinical specialists, nurse administrators, nurse educators, and nurse researchers. Nursing research is a growing field with implications for nurses at all levels of practice. The current and potential influence of nursing research on nursing care of children and adolescents is covered later in this chapter.

The growing professionalism among pediatric nurses is becoming more evident. Several subspecialty associations within pediatric nursing have formed since the early 1980s, including the Association of Pediatric Endocrinology Nurses and the Association of Pediatric Oncology Nursing. Within larger nursing associations, pediatric interest groups exist to share information of mutual concern like the pediatric critical care nurses within the Association of Critical Care Nurses (ACCN). The Society of Pediatric Nurses, an organization for all pediatric nurses involved in all aspects of the care of children and their families, held its first national convention in 1991. Several professional journals exist that publish clinical and research articles in the field of pediatric nursing. These journals include the *Journal of Pediatric Nursing, Maternal-Child Nursing Journal, Pediatric Nursing,* and *Issues in Comprehensive Pediatric Nursing.*

Legal Aspects of the Pediatric Nursing Role

Clarification of legal aspects requires that the nurse be aware that legal and ethical aspects are not synonymous. In fact, an action that is legal may not always be ethical and an act that is ethical may not always be legal. Herein lies the potential for professional conflicts.

The legality of nursing practice is determined in part by the practice acts of each state and in part by the courts that pass judgment on cases involving nurses. Every nurse must be aware of the legal boundaries governing practice in the state in which she or he is licensed.

Legal aspects unique to the role of the pediatric nurse include state laws governing consent for treatment of a minor, laws pertaining to automobile restraints for children, and laws regarding child abuse. Each pediatric nurse is accountable for knowing the laws and institutional policies relating to individual practice. Chapter 23, Principles and Skills Adapted to the Care of Children, deals with legal aspects of consent and abuse. Chapter 15, Promoting Safety, addresses laws pertaining to automobile safety. Chapter 16, Child Abuse and Maltreatment, provides information on the issues and nursing care related to child abuse and maltreatment.

Research to Advance Nursing Practice

Critical to the advancement of nursing practice is nursing's ability to answer its own practice questions through research. That level of research expertise has only recently become a reality. As noted by Fawcett, "Significant progress has been made in the past several years in establishing nursing as a discipline with a corps of scholars leading its advancement. This scholarly influence is perhaps the most critical factor involved in the elimination of obstacles to nursing research . . . " (1984, p 6).

The education of a *corps of nursing scholars* has historical significance. Until the 1950s, nursing "borrowed" much of its scientific knowledge from medicine and the basic sciences. Although this provided a large, eclectic base for nursing practice, it required "modification" of research findings and theoretical explanations of phenomena to fit the unique practice of nursing. Nursing, at this time, was also limited in its ability to answer questions generated by practice. Clearly, professional advancement required that nursing define its unique subject matter (generate theories of nursing) and conduct its own research of these phenomena. The coming of age of nursing research, then, has required the education of nurses prepared in theory construction and in research methodology appropriate to nursing phenomena.

Nursing education began as training of nurses in hospitals by physicians for the purpose of providing cheap labor. It soon progressed in both the United States and Canada to in-hospital education by early nursing leaders, such as Isabel Hampton Robb and Mary Agnes Snively, and was patterned after the Nightingale system to focus on education rather than on hospital service. Isabel Hampton Robb was instrumental in establishing university education for nurses in the United States. Her efforts resulted in the establishment of a course in hospital economics for graduate nurses at Teacher's College, Columbia University, in 1907. Adelaide Nutting became the world's first professor of nursing at Columbia University (Dolan et al, 1983).

College education for nurses was furthered by the 1965 position paper of the American Nurses' Association, which called for preparation of nurses at the baccalaureate level. Another significant development at this time was the initiation of the federally funded "nurse scientist" program that provided support to nurses wishing to obtain doctoral degrees in the basic sciences. Although research in nursing was not new at this time (it had been advocated and conducted since the time of Florence Nightingale, and the journal *Nursing Research* had been circulating since the early 1950s), the nurse scientist program was notable for providing the first significant influx of doctorally prepared nurses who were interested in, committed to, and prepared to conduct research. Many of the nursing leaders responsible for the establishment, in the 1970s, of graduate programs in nursing were educated in the nurse scientist program. The emphasis within master's degree programs is primarily advancement of the practice field through the preparation of clinical specialists and nurse practitioners. Nursing theory is studied rather than generated, and the research emphasis is often more on analysis and utilization than on conduct. The conducting of nursing research and developing of theory receive major emphasis within nursing doctoral programs, and graduates of these programs are expected to provide the leadership required to advance future "scientific inquiry."

As outlined by the American Nurses' Association Commission on Research in 1981, responsibility for research within nursing is not limited to nurses with graduate degrees. Graduates of Associate Degree Nursing Programs are expected to demonstrate an awareness of the value of nursing research and to as-

TABLE 1-2
Making Research Work at the Level of Practice: Notes from a Nurse Researcher

In my role as nurse researcher at The Children's Hospital of Denver it is exciting for me to see nurses questioning the time-honored way of carrying out a particular task or performing a procedure. Staff nurses are questioning "the way it's always been done" and they use me as a sounding board for their ideas. My relationships with staff nurses are collegial because they recognize my knowledge and skills as a clinical nurse as well as a research nurse.

In conjunction with other nurse researchers on staff, I teach a workshop on the research process to encourage staff nurses to answer their own research questions. Nurses interested in research can then receive one-on-one consultation through all phases of the research process—from formulation of a researchable question, through selection or development of research tools (e.g., questionnaires), data collection, data analysis, and interpretation of results. We also encourage the nurses to share research results through hospital sponsored communication sessions and at research conferences, through a research newsletter that I edit, and through publication of articles in nursing journals.

Nursing research can have a positive effect on the public's perception of the nursing role. In my own research activities I have found that children and their families are very interested in nursing research. They are quite supportive of the nurse at the bedside looking at, "researching," a new and better way to care for children. I have found that parents are very eager to have the research findings shared with them. I keep track of these families and send them research results at the completion of the study.

Nurses in our hospital are involved in a wide variety of research. We have categorized the studies according to their focus: (1) those that study children (Human Care studies), (2) those that involve families as well as children (Family Care studies), and (3) those that study nurses (Health Care Delivery System studies). Examples of research recently completed or currently in progress include:

- A study of the effectiveness of transcutaneous electrical nerve stimulation (TENS) in reducing the pain of radial artery puncture in neonates
- A comparison of regular Pedialyte and "Pedipops" for oral rehydration ("Pedipops" was coined by the nurses who developed a Pedialyte and Kool-Aid solution of controlled molecular weight that is then frozen on a stick)
- A study of the effect of increased parental involvement on the metabolic control of a child with diabetes
- An exploration of the impact of emergency transport on the child's family
- A study of nurses' attitudes about breastfeeding versus bottlefeeding
- Development of a technique for restructuring group meetings for effectiveness

If nursing is to grow and develop with a scientific knowledge base to guide practice, we must continually evaluate what we do and how we do it. We need to be accountable for our actions, and we need to validate when those actions make a difference in the lives of our clients. Those of us in expanded roles must foster and maintain a spirit of inquiry within the profession. Providing high-quality care and support to families should be the constant challenge for all nurses. Questioning and evaluating how we practice will help us meet that challenge.

—Anne Marie Kotzer, RN, MS

sist in problem identification and data collection. Graduates of Baccalaureate Nursing Programs are expected to read, interpret, and evaluate research for its relevance to practice, identify researchable problems in clinical practice, gather research data, apply established research findings to practice, and share research findings with colleagues (American Nurse's Association, 1981).

Nursing has prepared its corps of scholars, but this alone will not ensure professional advancement. That advancement will be realized as nurses at *all levels of professional preparation work cooperatively* to reach for excellence, to think at the level of "what if," to incorporate into practice the systematic, scientific questioning and answering that is research.

Cooperative research efforts within work settings require the guidance of nurse researchers who are prepared at the graduate (both master's and doctoral) level. These researchers serve as consultants to staff nurses to teach the research process, assist with analysis of published research, promote research utilization, assist with conduct of research studies, and model the value of nursing research through conduct and application of their own studies. The vignette in Table 1–2 is an account by a master's-prepared nurse of her role as a nurse researcher at a children's hospital.

Cooperative research involves sharing results (both successes and failures) through formal and informal "networking" processes such as research conferences and journal articles. Researchers have a responsibility to communicate clearly to their audience—if the researcher is unable to articulate implications for clinical nursing, it is unlikely that the staff nurse will be able to use these results in practice.

The body of nursing research has grown rapidly in recent years as nurses have begun to realize the value of generating and answering their own practice questions and as they have had increasing access to graduate-prepared nursing research consultants. Nursing research is, however, still in its infancy.

Application of research findings requires first that something of a "critical mass" of research accumulate to help ensure the success of implemented findings. In other words, research is much like a jigsaw puzzle; it is hard to predict the total picture from one piece. This is especially true of nursing research because of the complexity of many of the phenomena pertinent to nursing, such as pain, parent-infant attachment behaviors, health concepts of children, clin-

TABLE 1-3
Nursing Practice and Ethics

Principles

Autonomy, self-determination of patients and professionals

Do good, do no harm (beneficence, nonmaleficence)

Justice, fairness (allocation of resources)

Truth telling (veracity)

Informed consent

Quality of life/sanctity of life

The Golden Rule

Ethical Rights

Right to privacy (confidentiality)

Right to decide what happens to oneself/one's body (self-determination)

Right to health care (currently debatable; some say equal access only, others say not a right at all)

Right to information (informed consent, access to records)

Right to choose whom you care for (frequently limited to physicians in nonemergency situations)

Right to live, right to die

Rights of children

Ethical Duties/Obligations

Respect persons

Be accountable for decisions/actions

Maintain competence (professionals)

Exercise informed judgment in professional practice

Implement and improve standards of profession

Participate in activities contributing to profession's knowledge base

Safeguard clients from incompetent, unethical, or illegal practice of any person

Promote efforts to meet health needs of public

Participate in the formulation of public policy

Ethical Loyalty

Professional-patient relationship (covenant fidelity, contract, seller of services)

Accountability to whom as employee

Professional-professional relationships

Professional-patient family relationships

Who decides?

Concern in Life Cycle

Contraception and sterilization

Genetic engineering and embryo transfer

Abortion (when does life begin?)

Infanticide

Adolescent sexuality

Allocation of scarce resources

Lifestyle

Euthanasia

Compiled from Thompson, J. E., & Thompson, H. O. (1985). *Bioethical decision making for nurses*. Norwalk, CT: Appleton-Century-Crofts.

ical decision making of nurses, and so on. When several pieces of research begin to fit together, one can have increased confidence in results that are congruous with those of other nurse researchers working with that same subject matter. That nursing is now achieving that critical mass of research, in at least some subject areas, is evidenced by the advent of nursing research conferences that are designed to share research ready for immediate clinical application. The ability to critique and utilize such results will become increasingly important for every professional nurse in the next decade.

Ethical Practice in the Nursing of Children and Adolescents

When determining what should or ought to be done for a client, nurses are often faced with ethical decisions. *Ethics deals with "practical problems that arise from human conduct when an individual is faced with a choice between alternative values"* (Sigman, 1986, p 26).

Ethical decisions are inescapable in nursing practice because nursing involves the moral goal of seeking good for others and involves relationships with other persons (Curtin, 1986). Many nursing decisions involve hard choices, but not all hard choices are ethical decisions. Ethical decisions may involve choosing between two equally unacceptable choices. Table 1–3 lists examples of ethical issues that arise from conflicts of principle, ethical rights, ethical duties/obligations, ethical loyalty, and concern within the life cycle. Although this grouping of issues shows extensive overlapping, the value of this classification is in listing examples of common ethical issues.

Sometimes an ethical decision is of such consequence to society as to make media headlines, such as the sensitive process for allocating scarce donor organs for transplant. Though the nurse may at some point be involved in a headline case, the types of ethical decisions that follow are more reflective of day-to-day practice. It is important that these common decisions be identified as ethical issues so that the nurse will know to employ the correct approach in their solution.

- The nurse is exhausted and is concerned about the ability to stay alert during the shift, but the unit is already short-staffed; if this nurse leaves, the patients may receive even less care.
- A 16-year-old victim of an auto accident confides in the nurse that she is sexually active and wants counseling about birth control. She says that her parents would not understand because of their religious convictions.
- An 8-year-old boy with leukemia refuses to undergo another round of chemotherapy. The parents ask the nurse whether they should respect his wishes or go ahead with the therapy.
- The foster mother leaves instructions that the young child's biologic mother is not to visit because she upsets the child. The biologic mother arrives on the unit and looks through the window at her son who begins crying "Mommy" and holding his arms out to her.
- The father of an adolescent boy with an inoperable tumor requests that his son not be told the truth about his diagnosis.

The Nurse's Unique Perspective. "Nursing ethics is different from biomedical ethics, not in process but in substance" (Sigman, 1986, p 33). Nurses have a unique perspective on the values of the client because they spend more time with the client and because clients are often less intimidated by nurses than by physicians and tend to confide in them. The nurse is also in a position of liaison between the client and other health care professionals and often can understand the rationale for differing values among all the parties involved.

The Issue of Autonomy in Pediatric Nursing. Pediatric nursing is unique in the number of ethical decisions involving autonomy. Since infants and small children do not possess the knowledge to make decisions for themselves and since children under age 18, under normal circumstances, cannot sign consent forms, the judgment of adults often must be substituted for that of the child. Issues of substituted judgment involve decisions made for the child by either the nurse or the parent(s). Sometimes these decisions must be carried out against the will of the child, such as when the nurse must administer an oral medication to a resisting toddler or give a preoperative injection to a resisting 10-year-old. Although this is not a pleasant part of the nursing role, the choice to administer the medications seems clear-cut in these two examples. What about the child in the earlier example who refused chemotherapy, however? Does the child have some rights in a decision that has such a profound bodily effect? At what age can a child make a personal decision? Should the wishes of a chronically ill or terminally ill child be given more consideration than those of an acutely ill child? There are no general answers. The ambiguity of the autonomy issue is a concern for every pediatric nurse.

Resources for Ethical Decision Making

Surely there must be rules and guidelines for making such decisions. Yes and no. Yes, there are guidelines in the form of ethical theories, codes of ethics, and various linear problem-solving procedures. No, these guidelines do not always lead to clear-cut answers. In gathering the facts about an ethical dilemma, one must consider not only the broad theoretical principles offered by various guidelines but also the facts as they relate to the unique situation. This approach is necessary because aspects of the issue that emphasize only universal principles tend to be insensitive to the unique aspects of the case, and aspects that emphasize only the unique characteristics are easily clouded by emotion.

In addition to the failure of broad principles to consider the uniqueness in a situation, there is no way to assure that the principles on which ethical theories are based are true. "The ethical principles that we develop from our philosophy are no more certain than the philosophy on which they are based, and these principles raise additional uncertainties about how to apply them to specific situations" (Quinn & Smith, 1987, p 52). That is one reason why there is no universal ethical theory on which everyone agrees. Persons tend to favor one theory or another because the tenets of the theory are more in keeping with their own value system. The best chance for making a good decision in an ethical conflict is to have an education that includes a base in the arts and humanities, an awareness of guidelines from ethical theories, an awareness of professional and personal ethics, an openness to the values and perspectives of others, and knowledge of one's professional resources.

Distinguishing Between Personal and Professional Ethics. Upon becoming a professional, one implicitly agrees to abide by the stated ethics of that profession. It behooves the nurse, therefore, to be well versed in the implications of the American Nurses' Association Code and in the ANA Standards of Clinical Nursing Practice (Tables 1–4 and 1–5).

Occasionally the nurse may be caught in a conflict between personal and professional values. Perhaps the most common example is the nurse who holds strong personal values against abortion but recognizes the professional value of allowing the client to make her own decision. In such an instance it is not just permissible but, rather, advisable for the nurse to remove herself or himself from the situation if another nurse is available and willing to help. The nurse has the right not to compromise strong personal values, and the client has the right to nursing care that is nonjudgmental.

TABLE 1-4
Code for Nurses

1. The nurse provides services with respect for human dignity and the uniqueness of the client unrestricted by considerations of social or economic status, personal attributes, or the nature of health problems.
2. The nurse safeguards the client's right to privacy by judiciously protecting information of a confidential nature.
3. The nurse acts to safeguard the client and the public when health care and safety are affected by the incompetent, unethical, or illegal practice of any person.
4. The nurse assumes responsibility and accountability for individual nursing judgments and actions.
5. The nurse maintains competence in nursing.
6. The nurse exercises informed judgment and uses individual competence and qualifications as criteria in seeking consultation, accepting responsibilities, and delegating nursing activities to others.
7. The nurse participates in activities that contribute to the ongoing development of the profession's body of knowledge.
8. The nurse participates in the profession's efforts to implement and improve standards of nursing.
9. The nurse participates in the profession's efforts to establish and maintain conditions of employment conducive to high-quality nursing care.
10. The nurse participates in the profession's effort to protect the public from misinformation and misrepresentation and to maintain the integrity of nursing.
11. The nurse collaborates with members of the health professions and other citizens in promoting community and national efforts to meet the health needs of the public.

From *Code for nurses with interpretive statements* (1985). American Nurses' Association, 600 Maryland Avenue, SW, Suite 100W, Washington, DC 20024–2521.

TABLE 1-5
ANA Standards of Care and Standards of Professional Performance

Standards of Care

Standard I. Assessment

The nurse collects client health data.

Standard II. Diagnosis

The nurse analyzes the assessment data in determining diagnosis.

Standard III. Outcome Identification

The nurse identifies expected outcomes individualized to the client.

Standard IV. Planning

The nurse develops a plan of care that prescribes interventions to attain expected outcomes.

Standard V. Implementation

The nurse implements the interventions identified in the plan of care.

Standard VI. Evaluation

The nurse evaluates the client's progress toward attainment of outcomes.

Standards of Professional Performance

Standard I. Quality of Care

The nurse systematically evaluates the quality and effectiveness of nursing practice.

Standard II. Performance Appraisal

The nurse evaluates his/her own nursing practice in relation to professional practice standards and relevant statutes and regulations.

Standard III. Education

The nurse acquires and maintains current knowledge in nursing practice.

Standard IV. Collegiality

The nurse contributes to the professional development of peers, colleagues, and others.

Standard V. Ethics

The nurse's decisions and actions on behalf of clients are determined in an ethical manner.

Standard VI. Collaboration

The nurse collaborates with the client, significant others, and health care providers in providing client care.

Standard VII. Research

The nurse uses research findings in practice.

Standard VIII. Resource Utilization

The nurse considers factors related to safety, effectiveness, and cost in planning and delivering client care.

From American Nurses' Association. (1991). *Standards of clinical nursing practice,* 600 Maryland Avenue, SW, Suite 100W, Washington, DC 20024: Author.

ETHICAL ISSUES

The Process of Ethical Decision Making

by Margaret M. Mahon, PhD, RNC

Nurses are constantly faced with situations involving ethical decision making. These issues are often thought of as life and death, the stuff of headline news, legislative efforts, and national debate. Certainly such cases do occur, but most ethical dilemmas encountered by nurses are not of this magnitude. Rather, the dilemmas are relatively smaller and can often be categorized as management issues. For example, the nurse has 14 medications to give at 4:00; how does one decide which medication to administer in what order? Why is this an ethical dilemma? Is it always an ethical dilemma? Perhaps not. What if two of the medications are pain medications for children in severe pain? The nurse's understanding of, and beliefs about, pain management will influence when, and how often, these medications are administered. If a nurse believes (albeit incorrectly) that children's pain is not as severe as that of adults, or that postoperative morphine is likely to be addictive, pain medication might be withheld. What if a child is having peaks and troughs drawn to assess the therapeutic level of gentamicin? Time is essential in administration of gentamicin and drawing the subsequent blood test for peak levels. And what if a parent of a child is there, and this parent's method of establishing control is to ensure that his or her child receives all her or his medications *precisely* when they are scheduled?

With the addition of each variable the situation becomes more complicated. This problem is often more complicated for the beginning level nurse, who is still acquiring time management skills that allow the distribution of 14 medications in a brief period of time. To consider all these needs and utilize the breadth of information necessary for planning is not easy. These same skills are required for ethical decision making. It is often assumed that anyone can make ethical decisions. In health care, the question must be, Who is qualified to make ethical decisions? Ethical decisions are not visceral responses to a perceived injustice. Rather, involvement in ethical decision making mandates the responsibility for preparedness. It is also helpful to know the resources available to help in making these decisions. As a foundation for all of this, all health care professionals must assume the personal work of awareness of their own beliefs and prejudices. How does each person's experience influence the decision they are likely to make, or their ability to implement a decision with which they disagree?

This much work also goes into professional ethical decision making as well. There are several models of ethical decision making that can guide this process. One of these (Thomasma, 1978) is explored in depth here. Models such as this provide guidelines for gathering appropriate information to be used in health care decision making. It may be helpful to identify a specific clinical encounter when beginning to apply this model. With some adaptation, the model is:

1. Identify and articulate the health care and social facts and their most likely consequences. Identify the significant human factors in the case, such as the child's age, attitudes, family situation, and behavior history, as well as values and beliefs (including religious beliefs) that may be relevant.
2. Identify all related ethical factors (medical, professional, social, or personal) present for the (a) child, (b) family, (c) health care and other professionals, and (d) relevant people involved in the case.
3. Identify major value conflicts in the case and delineate the major features of the value conflicts utilizing the analysis in steps 1 and 2.
4. Set priorities for the values that have been found to be in conflict in step 3. State the reasons that would support this priority in setting your views.
5. Develop an argument that supports the reasons advanced in step 4 by answering the following questions:
   a. What underlying ethical norms support your views? (e.g., respect for patient rights, the obligation to preserve life, benefiting the patient, avoiding harm to the patient).
   b. Why should these norms be accepted as guides for conduct in this and similar cases? Here you need to examine and defend basic ethical presuppositions—concerning values, rights, and duties that are the grounds for saying that the ethical norms in step 5a ought to characterize the relationship between health care professional and patient in this and similar cases.
6. Critique the argument you have advanced in steps 4 and 5. What is the strongest criticism that could be made of the value priority developed in step 4 and defended in step 5? How would you defend your position from this criticism?

An example can clarify the process. Tia R. is a 2-year-old female with a history of frequent otitis media. She has had six ear infections over the past 7 months, each of which has responded to antibiotic therapy, though it has taken several different drugs to clear each infection. Tia's mother, Ms. R, is frustrated with Tia's illnesses. Over the past 7 months, Tia has had to miss 4 days of day care owing to ear infections, associated upper respiratory illness, and fever. Tia is currently on antibiotics, and her current infection is responding well. At this point, the decision is whether to put Tia on prophylactic antibiotics for 4 months to attempt to prevent further infections, or to schedule surgery to insert myringotomy tubes.

Use of the model as it applies to this case demonstrates several points. First, there are several sources to which one will go to gather appropriate information. In this case, sources include the child's primary care provider, the family, sources of information about the potential advantages and disadvantages of both prophylaxis and surgery, and even information about funding. Does the family's health care mean that both are viable options? Ethical factors focus around the best interest of

ETHICAL ISSUES
The Process of Ethical Decision Making (continued)

the child, the ability to minimize harm, autonomy, and other ethical and moral considerations. And even with all this information, there may not be one, right answer. Should Ms. R. decide on one course of treatment, and complications arise, self-recrimination is likely. The fact that a decision making model was used, and an appropriate decision reached, does not mean that one will necessarily feel good about the decision that was made.

When initially using this or any other decision making model, the process can be cumbersome. With repeated use, one becomes more facile in applying the model, and in identifying factors that influence ethical decision making. There are several specifics that become clear when applying this model to issues with children. First, the patient must be interpreted as the child and the family. Furthermore, the family must be interpreted to mean whomever the family members identify as members of the family. This is an area in which many nurses find their values at odds with those of families. Some of this is a result of cultural differences. A difficult but essential skill is the ability to assess without judging, and then to use the information in a way that will be helpful to the child and the family.

Other factors influence the nurse's ability to make decisions and to intervene with children and families. These include nurse practice guidelines, hospital policy, legal considerations, the American Nurses' Association Code of Ethics, The International Congress of Nurses Code of Ethics, physicians' orders, and one's own comfort with children and their level of health or illness. In addition to these, there are other specific documents that guide the process of ethical decision making. It is becoming increasingly common for nurses to have some training in ethics. Though this information may be applied or understood differently when one has a foundation in clinical practice, an understanding of the historical factors and resulting theories provides a broader preparation for the process of decision making. An understanding of child development is necessary, because it provides a framework for analyzing not only the child's understanding of the situation but also the likely impact of various situations on children.

Usually the family is considered as a unit in nursing care of children. Legally, but also morally, parents are usually in the best position to make decisions for their children. Depending on the age and abilities of the child, the child may be a verbal partner in this process. "The best interest of the child" is the principle used to guide ethical and health care decision making. There is usually no or minimal dispute about what constitutes the best interest of the child. In applying this standard to the situation of the seriously ill newborn, the President's Commission for the Study of Ethical Problems in Medicine and Biomedical and Behavioral Research (1983) delineated more specific guidelines that are applicable to children of all ages. Situations are likely to fit one of three situations: "(1) a treatment is available that would clearly benefit the infant, (2) all treatment is expected to be futile, or (3) the probable benefits to an infant from different choices are quite uncertain" (1983, p 217). There is usually a treatment of choice or there may be a few options available, all of which are beneficial. In these cases, convenience, level of pain, or parental preference or experience is likely to influence the choice made, and this is fine. If a choice is being made, the range of viable options are being considered, and the parents are making the decision for their child.

Occasionally there are cases in which there is disagreement, either between parents or between parent(s) and health care professionals about what course to take in caring for a child. In most of these cases, *reciprocal* communication and education allow a peaceful resolution to a difficult situation. In rare cases, the disagreement continues. In these cases, the child may be removed from the hospital or pediatric practice by the parents. If, however, the health care team believes that the parents' refusal to consent to recommended treatment is life-threatening, the hospital may instigate legal intervention. In these cases, a guardian ad litem is likely to be appointed. The purpose of a guardian ad litem is to ensure that there is someone acting specifically and independently for the best interest of the child. This is an important distinction, because in most of these cases, everyone believes they are acting in the best interest of the child.

Hospital ethics committees are other avenues for help with, and perspective in, problem solving. The use of ethics committees has evolved since the early 1960s (Oddi & Cassidy, 1990). The committees were originally used in resource allocation decision making in the 1960s; committees decided which patients in renal failure had access to dialysis machines. In 1983 the President's Commission for the Study of Ethical Problems in Medicine and Biomedical and Behavioral Research recommended the use of such committees for the most difficult ethical cases. In 1984, the Congress recommended the establishment of Infant Care Review Committees to deal with ethical issues that arise with the birth of seriously ill neonates.

Ideally, ethics committees are a multidisciplinary forum for the discussion of a range of issues. In most institutions, ethics committees make recommendations about the direction of a treatment process. In some cases, ethics committees represent a forum for all involved in a case to present their impressions, opinions, and issues. This can include the child, parents, nurses, physicians, and others. Ethics committees can be consultation bodies and can provide educational programs. They are used with varying degrees of frequency within institutions. Some hospitals have regular meetings of the ethics committee, not only to discuss pertinent cases but also to develop policy for the institution. In other institutions, meetings are rare.

Despite the increasing avenues for information, support, and advice, ethics still often comes down to the understanding and action of the individual. There is not always one, right answer. Furthermore, agreement by a group of people on a course of action does not mean it is a right course of action. Integration of ethics into nursing practice is not a luxury available to those with advanced training in the discipline, rather it is a requirement for all who interact with children and families. This integration comes only with work: learning, self-awareness, and skills in communication and collaboration.

Throughout this book, several case studies are presented. Most of these do not represent life and death situations for most people to whom they would apply. They are representative of the situations facing nurses and other health care professionals on a daily basis. It is hoped that by using the framework described here, and examining your own responses to the situations, each of you will be better prepared to integrate the ethical perspective and responsibility into future interactions with children and families.

BIBLIOGRAPHY

Fry, S. T. (1982, September). Ethical principles in nursing education and practice: A missing link in the unification issue. *Nursing and Health Care, 3*(7), 363–368.

Levine, M. (1989). The ethics of nursing rhetoric. *Image: Journal of Nursing Scholarship, 21,* 4–6.

Mahon, M. (1990). The nurse's role in decision making for the child with disabilities. *Issues in Law and Medicine, 6,* 247–268.

Oddi, L. F., & Cassidy, V. R. (1990). Participation and perception of nurse members in the hospital ethics committee. *Western Journal of Nursing Research, 12,* 307–317.

President's Commission for the Study of Ethical Problems in Medicine and Biomedical and Behavioral Research. (1983). *Deciding to forego life-sustaining treatment.* Washington, DC: U.S. Government Printing Office.

Thomasma, D. C. (1978, December). Training in medical ethics: An ethical work-up. *Forum in Medicine,* pp 33–36.

Openness to the Values of Others. The nurse who has explored personal and professional values is better prepared to be open and accepting of the values of others. Conversely, the nurse who operates only from subconscious, gut-level feelings (values) of right and wrong is less likely to be aware that right and wrong are relative concepts and is likely to disagree with anyone who holds a different view. The nurse must be sincerely open to other values in order to adequately explore the perspectives of each person involved in an ethical issue. Without such exploration, the actual problem (specific value conflicts) may never be identified.

Professional Resources. The nurse has several professional resources to help with decision making: knowledge of the arts and humanities, knowledge of ethical theories, professional codes, client bills of rights, senior staff members who have had more experience with ethical decisions (e.g., shift supervisor, head nurse, assistant head nurse), and, where available, the hospital or agency ethics committee (i.e., through either a formal presentation to the committee or a consultation with a nursing representative on the committee).

Ethics and Excellence

"The willingness to enter with a patient that predicament which he cannot face alone is an expression of moral responsibility; the quality of the moral commitment is a measure of the nurse's excellence" (Levine, 1977, p 845). More recently Levine's sentiments were echoed by Bishop and Scudder: "Since nursing practice aims at the well-being of the patient, the first moral responsibility of any nurse is excellence of practice" (1987, p 36).

What Constitutes Excellence of Practice? Benner described the expert nurse as one who "with an enormous background of experience now has an intuitive grasp of each situation and zeroes in on the accurate region of the problem without wasteful consideration of a large range of unfruitful, alternative diagnoses and solutions" (1984, p 32). In light of this definition of excellence, perhaps one might amend Bishop and Scudder's statement to include the notion that the first moral responsibility of any nurse is to first *develop* excellence in practice. The novice nurse is not expected to be an expert in ethical decision making. He or she is expected, however, to be prepared to develop that expertise.

Professional Values Clarification. Because nursing depends on human relationships in every aspect of practice, and because each individual holds a unique value system, the nurse cannot escape making decisions among conflicting values in the course of providing patient care. The development of excellence in practice is contingent on the nurse's ability to identify ethical issues as such and to base decisions on facts and on professional values. The nurse's ability to discover pertinent facts and to clarify professional values is enhanced by knowledge of the arts and humanities, by knowledge of ethical theories and professional codes of conduct, and by clarification of personal and professional values.

The Nursing Process as It Relates to Children and Adolescents

The nursing process is a deliberate method of problem solving that incorporates five steps:

- Assessment.
- Analysis.
- Planning.
- Implementing.
- Evaluating.

The nursing process as it relates to children and adolescents takes into account the central role of the family. (See Chapter 2: Family Theories and Assessment.)

Domains

The nursing process is an integral part of nursing practice and includes its three domains—dependent, interdependent, and independent practice (Iyer et al, 1991).

Dependent Domain. The dependent domain of nursing practice refers to those client responses and associated nursing functions/responsibilities that require direction (orders) from physicians. Problems within the dependent domain are often referred to as medical problems.

Interdependent Domain. The interdependent domain of nursing practice refers to those client responses and associated nursing functions/responsibilities that are carried out conjointly with another discipline. Problems within the interdependent domain are often called collaborative problems.

Nurses have legal and ethical responsibilities in relation to carrying out physicians' orders. For this reason, dependent functions are also referred to as collaborative problems.

Independent Domain. The independent domain of nursing practice refers to those client responses and associated nursing functions/responsibilities that the nurse can independently, by virtue of education and experience, diagnose and treat. Problems and life processes within the independent domain are referred to as nursing diagnoses or **nursing diagnostic statements.**

Problems

The nursing process also comprises collaborative and medical problems as well as nursing diagnostic statements.

Collaborative Problems. Collaborative problems and associated **interdependent** nursing interventions can include observing for and notifying the physician of the occurrence of complications that are then legally treated by the physician.

Medical problems are diagnosed by the physician, who orders associated nursing interventions, such as administration of medications, enhanced by the nursing decisions made about these interventions.

Nursing Diagnosis

Nursing problems and life processes, referred to as nursing diagnostic statements, are diagnosed by the nurse and treated with associated **independent** nursing interventions, such as teaching the client home care required by her or his condition. Nursing diagnostic statements are "clinical judgements about individual, family, or community responses to actual and potential health problems/life processes." Nursing diagnostic statements "provide the basis for selection of nursing interventions to achieve outcomes for which the nurse is accountable" (North American Nursing Diagnosis Association [NANDA], 1992, pp 6–9).

Steps of the Nursing Process

Assessment

Nursing assessment is the first phase of the nursing process. Nursing assessment answers the question, "What do I need to find out about this client in order to provide the best care?" Data are collected in a systematic way, using a framework or guideline designed to remind the nurse of all aspects of care that must be considered for any client (just as body systems or head-to-toe framework is used in carrying out a physical assessment). Two commonly used frameworks for nursing assessment are Gordon's (1987) functional health patterns (Table 1–6) and the North American Nursing Diagnosis Association's (NANDA, 1992) human response patterns (Table 1–7). It is emphasized that an assessment framework is a guideline. It would not be practical to include data regarding each point in the guideline in every client assessment. Instead, a framework helps assure that the nurse will cover all aspects of the assessment (both subjective and objective) pertinent to the particular client. These assessments will become the defining characteristics of the Nursing Process Plan.

Subjective Assessment. Subjective information exists in the experiencer's (client's) mind and cannot be verified externally. Subjective information is obtained via interaction between the nurse and the client (child and/or family member) and includes the client's perceptions, feelings, and ideas. Figure 1–5 is an excerpt from Table 21–5: Nursing Process Plan: The Hospitalized Child. This figure shows subjective information related to physiologic function for a child being admitted to the hospital.

Subjective information for the pediatric patient often will be supplied by a combination of answers from the child, the parents, or other caregivers. The child should be allowed to answer questions whenever possible, because the parent and the child's perceptions may differ on a given issue. Often a parent may not even be aware of this difference of opinion. When the child is the focus of the assessment, his or her perceptions are vital to the entire nursing process. Acknowledgment of the child's knowledge and opinions at this point in the nursing process also allows the child a feeling of control that is so important to a sense of security, coping, and mastery.

Objective Assessment. Objective information is verifiable externally. Objective data are both observable and measurable. This information is obtained directly by the nurse via the senses—sight, smell, hearing, and touch. It includes all observable responses of the

TABLE 21-5

Nursing Process Plan: The Hospitalized Child

Analysis: Nursing Diagnostic Statement 1 3

Response and Related or Risk Factors: **Sleep pattern disturbance (child),** *related to anxiety associated with* 4

- Unfamiliar environment
- Separation from parents/family
- Discomfort of illness
- Interruptions for medication administration 5

Projected Outcome: The child will experience no disruption in sleep time. 8

Defining Characteristics 6

Subjective: 1

- Verbal complaints of difficulty falling asleep, not feeling well rested
- Awakening earlier or later than desired
- Interrupted sleep
- Changes in behavior and performance (increasing irritability, restlessness, disorientation, lethargy, listlessness)

Objective: 2

- Mild fleeting nystagmus
- Slight hand tremor
- Ptosis of eyelid
- Expressionless face
- Dark circles under eyes
- Frequent yawning
- Changes in posture
- Thick speech with mispronunciation and incorrect words

Nursing Interventions 9

Sleep Enhancement

Decrease the child's anxiety related to hospitalization. (See Diagnoses 8 and 10 of this NPP)

Determine usual sleep patterns, including naptime and bedtime routines and rituals (the younger the child, the more important these familiar activities are to promote sleep)

Provide for continuity of care. When parents cannot be present to prepare the child for sleep, the primary nurse can assume this responsibility while talking to the child about the parents so he or she will know the nurse supports his or her need for parents

Establish a record of sleep.

- If the hospital uses a flow sheet, label one column for sleep; cumulatively total hours of sleep over the 24-hr period
- Compare the child's usual sleep patterns with this guide from Chapters 4–9 and determine appropriate adjustments to meet the body's increased need for sleep and rest during illness

Neonate	20–22 hrs/24 hrs
6 wks	14–16 hrs/24 hrs
6 mos–1 yr	12–16 hrs/24 hrs
1–3 yrs	10–14 hrs/24 hrs
3–5 yrs	12–14 hrs/24 hrs
6–9 yrs	11–12 hrs/24 hrs

Evaluation Criteria 10

Child or parent verbalizes ease of child in falling asleep, sleeping as

NURSING PROCESS PLAN ELEMENTS

Assessment

1. SUBJECTIVE: Information supplied by the client (child, parent, or guardian)
2. OBJECTIVE: Information obtained directly through observation, physical examination, and interpretation of diagnostic test results

Analysis

3. NURSING DIAGNOSIS
4. RESPONSE
5. RELATED OR RISK FACTORS OR ETIOLOGY
6. DEFINING CHARACTERISTICS
7. COLLABORATIVE PROBLEMS

Planning

8. PROJECTED OUTCOME: The desired change in client condition or behavior, agreed upon by the client and nurse
9. NURSING INTERVENTIONS: The plan and actions the nurse undertakes. (The Nursing Intervention Classification label appears in ***bold italic*** type.)

Evaluation

10. CRITERIA: The observable and/or measurable indications that the client's condition or behavior has changed

FIGURE 1-5. Elements of the Nursing Process Plan.

client, results of physical examination, and results of diagnostic tests (Fig. 1–5).

Analysis

In the second step of the nursing process, the nurse identifies client responses and life processes for which nursing functions or responsibilities are implied. As stated previously, these include collaborative problems and nursing diagnoses. Discussion here focuses on nursing diagnostic statements.

Components of the Nursing Diagnostic Statement. A nursing diagnostic statement consists of three major components: the response, related or risk factors or etiology, and the list of defining characteristics.

The response is the diagnostic label. It is the actual or high-risk problem or the life process (wellness state) that the nurse (by virtue of his or her education and experience) can legally diagnose, e.g., "ineffective individual coping." *Note that in addition to actual or high-risk problems, the label can delineate a life process.* This addition to the definition of nursing diagnosis allows nurses to diagnose and treat in the wellness domain, such as "health seeking behaviors."

Problematic responses may be qualified by the words "high risk for." A high-risk problem is one that may develop unless certain preventive nursing strategies are carried out. A possible problem is one that may actually exist but that requires additional assessment data for validation. The absence of these qualifying words implies that the nurse has sufficient assessment data to validate the diagnosed response.

The related factor or etiology is the factor that can cause or maintain an *actual* or *high-risk* response. It is commonly signified in the nursing diagnostic statement of an actual problem or life process by the words, "related to," abbreviated RT (e.g., RT knowledge deficit regarding signs and symptoms of

TABLE 1-6
Use of Gordon's Functional Health Patterns as an Assessment Guide for Children and Adolescents

I. Physical Function

- A. Sleep-rest
  1. Client patterns
  2. Family patterns
- B. Nutrition-metabolism
  1. Skin integrity
  2. Nutrition
  3. Fluid balance–electrolytes
  4. Teeth
  5. Height, weight, status on growth chart
  6. Temperature
  7. Client and family eating patterns
- C. Elimination
  1. Urinary, toilet training
  2. Bowel, toilet training
  3. Client patterns
- D. Activity-exercise
  1. Pulse, respirations, blood pressure
  2. Client and family patterns
  3. Self-care/family/care deficit
  4. Airway/gas exchange/breathing
  5. Diversional/play activities
  6. Tissue perfusion/cardiac output
  7. Neuromuscular integrity
  8. Developmental level

II. Emotional-Social Function

- A. Self-perception/self-concept
  1. Self-concept
     - a. Body image
     - b. Self-esteem
     - c. Role performance
     - d. Identity
  2. Parenting patterns
     - a. Child safety
     - b. Family beliefs/values
     - c. Social behaviors and roles
     - d. Self-regulation and independence of child
- B. Sexuality
  1. Appropriate to developmental stage
  2. Related family values and beliefs
- C. Coping-stress-tolerance patterns
  1. Client patterns
  2. Family patterns
  3. Fear/anxiety
  4. Coping strategies appropriate to developmental stage
  5. Resources
- D. Spiritual health
  1. Sense of purpose
  2. Sense of hope
  3. Sense of wholeness
  4. Sense of peace

III. Intellectual-Perceptual Function

- A. Health perception/management
  1. Child's perception of illness
  2. Parent's perception of illness
  3. Health beliefs/cultural values
- B. Knowledge of illness/health management
  1. Anticipatory guidance and discharge planning related to
     - a. Disease process
     - b. Home management
     - c. Well child care
     - d. Prevention of physical injury, poisoning, trauma, suffocation
- C. Pain
- D. Sensory perceptual alterations

Adapted from Gordon, M. (1987). *Nursing diagnosis: Process and application*. New York: McGraw-Hill.

TABLE 1-7
Use of NANDA's Nine Human Response Patterns as an Assessment Guide for Children and Adolescents

Pattern 1: Exchanging	**Pattern 6: Moving**
Nutrition	Activity-exercise
Body temperature	Diversional/play activities
Bowel and urinary elimination	Home management
Fluid volume	Health maintenance/home management
Tissue perfusion/cardiac output	Self-care
Airway/gas exchange/breathing	Swallowing
Potential complications/safety problems	Breastfeeding
Skin/mucous membrane/tissue integrity	Growth and development patterns
Pattern 2: Communicating	**Pattern 7: Perceiving**
Verbal communication	Self-esteem/body image/identity disturbance
Pattern 3: Relating	Sensory perceptual patterns
Social behavior and roles	Sense of situational control
Parenting patterns	**Pattern 8: Knowing**
Sexuality	Knowledge
Family functioning	Thought processes
Pattern 4: Valuing	**Pattern 9: Feeling**
Spiritual health	Pain
Pattern 5: Choosing	Grief patterns
Coping/stress-tolerance patterns	Trauma responses
Health-related decisions	Fear/anxiety

Adapted from North American Nursing Diagnosis Association. (1992). *NANDA nursing diagnoses: Definitions and classifications 1992–1993*. Philadelphia: NANDA.

diabetic ketoacidosis [DKA]). A risk factor is anything that puts the client at risk for a *high-risk* problem. *Related or risk factors or etiologies are also determined by assessment.* Sometimes the related factor will be so complex as to require more information that can be communicated in the "related to" clause. In this case the related factor or etiology statement can be extended by using the words *associated with*. The information in the "associated with" clause further explains the "related to" statement as in the following example:

Ineffective individual coping, RT perception of helplessness in crisis of hospitalization associated with the multiple stressors of

- *Separation from parents and significant others.*
- *Unfamiliar environment.*
- *Pain.*
- *Unclear limits and expectations.*
- *Loss of self-control.*

Clearly, the information added to this nursing diagnostic statement after "crisis of hospitalization" is important to direct the nurse's plan and execution of care.

It is appropriate to list more than one related or risk factor/etiology. For example, the following response from Figure 1–5 lists four reasons for the etiology of anxiety for sleep pattern disturbances. Essentially more than one related factor/etiology exists: . . . anxiety associated with

- Unfamiliar environment.
- Separation from parents/family.
- Discomfort of illness.
- Interruptions for medication administration.

The nursing diagnostic statements in this text frequently list multiple related factors because these statements serve as guidelines and need to be as inclusive as possible. In actual care-planning the nurse would identify and list only those related factors applicable to a particular client.

Defining characteristics justify the assignment of the response. They are the cluster of cues that allow the nurse to diagnose a response. They usually include a combination of subjective and objective assessment data, as in the following example from Figure 1–5:

Defining Characteristics

Subjective: verbal complaints of difficulty falling asleep, not feeling well-rested; awakening earlier or later than desired; interrupted sleep; changes in behavior and performance (increasing irritability, restlessness, disorientation, lethargy, listlessness).

Objective: mild fleeting nystagmus; slight hand tremor; ptosis of eyelid; expressionless face; dark circles under eyes; frequent yawning; changes in posture; thick speech with mispronunciation and incorrect words.

Just as a medical diagnosis is formulated by assessing a predetermined cluster of signs and symptoms along with other diagnostic criteria, a nursing diagnostic **response** is the result of careful assessment of related and observed clusters of defining characteristics. Defining characteristics of each response, which were accepted by NANDA for clinical testing, are included in the published listing of nursing diagnoses in Appendix 1.

A nursing diagnostic statement is *not* assumed because of the existence of a medical diagnosis. It can exist independently of a medical diagnosis. This means that assessment for responses and related or risk factors or etiology does not necessarily start with the identification of a medical diagnosis. The factors that would determine the existence of a nursing diagnosis would be the predetermined cluster of NANDA accepted defining characteristics.

The nursing diagnostic statement is the result of thoughtful analysis of the particular assessment data for this specific client. *Note that the parts of a nursing diagnostic statement can be summarized in the acronym RRED—**R**esponse, **R**elated or risk factors or **E**tiology, **D**efining characteristics.* The diagnostic statement is chosen on the basis of the lowest common denominator of meaning. That is, one should strive to select the diagnostic statement that is most meaningful and the most concrete for nursing practice. It is obtained by repeatedly asking oneself, "What does this mean for the child and does it fit the assessed cues as well as the definition of nursing diagnosis?" For example, the nurse who is caring for a child whose blood values and medical findings have led to a medical diagnosis of anemia legitimately could choose any of the following responses and etiologies:

- Impaired gas exchange, RT ventilation perfusion imbalance
- Altered tissue perfusion, RT interruption of blood flow
- Impaired physical mobility, RT activity intolerance

Impairment of the oxygen-carrying components of the blood in anemia leads logically to defining characteristics of either of the first two responses, and to a response of activity intolerance. Similarly, activity intolerance can be seen as a result of ventilation perfusion imbalance and interruption of blood flow; but the question "What does this mean and does it fit the assessed cues as well as the definition of nursing diagnosis?" will further reduce the determination of the response to impaired physical mobility because it, in turn, is the result of activity intolerance. Additionally, activity intolerance is a related or risk factor/etiology that can be *independently* and legally treated by the nurse.

When choosing a response from the NANDA list, it is important to assure that the response matches the defining characteristics that most accurately describe the child or family's condition. For example, the responses *altered family processes* and *ineffective family coping* might seem quite interchangeable if one failed to consider their definitions and defining characteristics. *Altered family processes* describes a family that normally functions effectively but is challenged by a factor that has altered the family functioning. This response differs from *ineffective family coping* that describes a family that has become unable or less able to assist the client to adapt to their problem (Appendix 1). These responses also have different validating defining characteristics.

Sometimes qualifying data must be added to a NANDA response to make it more meaningful. When this occurs, the qualifying data are attached to the NANDA stem with a colon, as the following example:

Diversional activity deficit: altered play behavior

The response is more meaningful if one knows the type of diversional activity that is being addressed.

Developing a Plan of Care

In the planning phase, the nurse identifies client goals or projected outcomes, interventions that will accomplish the projected outcomes, and outcome measurements to be used in the evaluation plan. When a nursing diagnostic statement is included in a nursing process plan, each of the steps of the nursing process are associated with one component of the nursing diagnostic statement.

The projected outcome (also called goal or objective) is associated with the response. The projected outcome of the nursing process is always to cure or ameliorate the actual problem, prevent the high-risk problem from occurring, or strengthen the life process. Wording of the projected outcome is dependent on these three areas:

- The actual problem is projected to be cured or ameliorated, e.g., the client will be able to cope effectively.
- The high-risk problem is projected *not* to occur, e.g., the client will not experience ineffective coping.

- The life process is projected to continue or be maintained and/or strengthened, e.g., the client will continue coping effectively.

As demonstrated in Figure 1–5, the projected outcome is actually the desired outcome of the nursing interventions (cure, amelioration, prevention, or maintenance/strengthening of the response).

Implementing the Plan

The nursing interventions for actual problems and life processes are associated with the related or risk factor, etiology, or supporting factor that causes or maintains the problems or life processes. Removing the related factor will cure or ameliorate an actual problem. Accentuating the supporting factor will maintain the life process. The nursing interventions section should be as specific as possible since the plan is also designed to provide guidance for nurses who care for the child in the absence of the nurse who formulated the plan. Note how each intervention in Figure 1–6 is designed to remove, ameliorate, or accentuate a related or risk factor or etiology.

Designing nursing interventions should reflect the complex reasoning process used by the nurse in developing an action that is designed to accomplish a projected outcome. There are many reasons why a standardized classification for the things nurses do (interventions), as well as the responses they treat, should be developed. McCloskey and Bulechek (1992) have listed eight: to standardize nomenclature, expand nursing knowledge, develop information systems, teach decision making, cost out nursing, allocate nursing resources, communicate nursing to nonnurses, and link nursing content.

A team of nurses at the University of Iowa has been working since 1987 to develop and validate a comprehensive taxonomy of research-based interventions (Bulechek & McCloskey, 1992b; McCloskey & Bulechek, 1992). Phase one of this research has been completed, with a resulting list of 319 nursing interventions. This list includes what Bulechek and McCloskey (1992b) refer to as "nurse-initiated" and "physician-initiated" interventions. In this text, all nursing interventions included for a particular **nursing diagnostic statement** are nurse-initiated. Interventions for a particular **collaborative problem** may be nurse-initiated or physician-initiated and in the collaborative domain of nursing practice. McCloskey and Bulechek (1992) define nursing intervention as "any direct care treatment that a nurse performs on behalf of a client" (p. xvii). Nursing interventions include activities in the independent and collaborative domains of nursing practice.

In McCloskey and Bulechek's (1992) *Nursing Interventions Classification (NIC),* "each nursing intervention has three parts: the **label** or name describing the concept, the **definition** of the concept (represented by the intervention label), and a set of **defining activities** or the actions that a nurse must perform to implement the intervention concept" (p. xii). Many of the Nursing Process Plans in this text will use the *NIC* classification **labels** for nursing interventions. When an *NIC* label is used it will be in ***bold italics*** (e.g., ***Communication Enhancement***). The reader is urged to consult the *NIC* directly for *NIC* defining activities of the intervention, which are similar to the activities contained in the Nursing Process Plans.

"The need to develop standardized language to describe nursing practice has become increasingly important" (Bulechek & McCloskey, 1992a). NANDA's nursing diagnoses language has provided nurses with a standardized language to identify actual client problems, problems for which clients are at high risk, and positive (wellness) states of clients. Werley and Lang (1988) have pointed out the need to have similar standardized classifications of interventions and outcomes. The American Nurses' Association (1989) supports the development of such classifications:

> Nursing must be able to name itself and describe what it does in order to function effectively in a world where computerized information is used to establish everything from diagnosis-related groups (DRGs) to cardiac output. Until nurses can name what they do and assign a computer code to that name, we may be neither reimbursed nor recognized as a profession with unique skills and knowledge.

Several teams have been working to develop standardized taxonomies of nursing interventions. Cohen and colleagues (1991) have published a classification of interventions for low birthweight infants. Grobe (1990) has described work to develop common language for nursing interventions. Taxonomies of nursing interventions for home health care have been developed by Saba and coworkers (1991) and Verran (1981). Several textbooks of nursing interventions have been published (Bulechek & McCloskey, 1992b; Snyder, 1985), including one focusing on nursing interventions for infants and children (Craft & Denehy, 1990).

Evaluating the Success of Nursing Strategies

The evaluation plan is associated with the defining characteristics. Just as the effectiveness of medical treatment for a medical diagnosis is evaluated by determining if the cluster of signs and symptoms for that medical diagnosis is gone or alleviated, so the effectiveness of nursing treatment (interventions) for a nursing diagnostic statement is evaluated by determining if the cluster of *defining characteristics* for the **response** is gone or alleviated or, in the case of high-risk problems, does not occur. (Compare the defining characteristics [6] with the evaluation criteria [10] in Fig. 1–5.)

Since nursing diagnostic statements are in the independent domain of nursing practice, the response that is diagnosed and the strategy that is ordered must be in the independent domain. The nurse must be able to independently intervene to remove or alleviate the related or risk factor or etiology or to prevent the high-risk problem from occurring. Because nurses cannot legally "by virtue of education and experience" (Gordon, 1976) remove or alleviate (treat) medical diagnosis and pathology, these *cannot* be related or risk factors or etiologies for nursing diagnoses.

Situations When a Response Is Diagnosed for Which the Etiology Cannot Be Changed. Occasionally, a response is diagnosed for which the etiology cannot be changed. On analysis, the nurse may discover (by looking at her or his proposed strategies) that she or he has actually assessed the related factor for a yet unidentified response. For example, a nurse might consider a diagnosis of "impaired swallowing related to cleft lip." She or he knows that this is *not* a nursing diagnosis because she or he cannot legally treat cleft lip. She or he examines the interventions she or he has in mind. They include: position in a semi-upright position for feeding; use an Asepto syringe with rubber tubing directed to the side of the mouth. As the nurse considers *why* she or he is planning these interventions, she or he realizes she or he is trying to prevent aspiration from occurring. The client's diagnostic statement is ***"High risk for aspiration;** risk factor impaired swallowing."*

There *are* responses that have related or risk factors or etiology that the nurse cannot change. As previously noted, the intervention phase of the nursing process is most effective when it is directed at removing or correcting the factor that causes or maintains the problem. Sometimes this is not possible. In these cases, the response is treated symptomatically and nursing interventions are geared to defining characteristics (note that this is similar to a physician's treatment of "fever of unknown origin"). As determined previously, this does not mean that such things as medical diagnoses, pathology, and factors that a nurse cannot change must be excluded from the nursing care plan. They will be included as part of the collaborative domain (and function) of nurses—collaborative problems.

Nursing Process Plans Versus Individualized Care Plans. An important distinction exists between a nursing process plan and a care plan: a Nursing Process Plan provides general guidelines for any child with a similar condition; a Care Plan is individualized for a specific client. Both include nursing diagnostic statements *and* collaborative problems. Nursing Process Plans, such as those found throughout this text, provide standards of excellence to guide the nurse in formulating a Care Plan specific to the needs of an individual child. As previously stated, a nursing diagnostic statement is *not* assumed because of the existence of a medical diagnosis. It can exist independently of a medical diagnosis. Two children with the same medical diagnoses can have dissimilar nursing diagnostic statements. The Nursing Process Plans in this text are designed to ensure that major nursing diagnostic statements, which commonly occur in conjunction with a given condition, will be considered in designing an individual plan of care and help maintain continuity and excellence in care among unit staff. *A Nursing Process Plan is never intended to be used without modification for the individual client.* When possible and as applicable, strategies in the individualized care plan should detail what will be done along with when, where, and how.

Implementing the Plan

Implementing the plan of care is a two-step process. Before the interventions are actually implemented, they must be discussed with the client.

Discussing the Plan of Care with the Client.* The first phase of implementation is to discuss the plan with the child and at least one family member. *Failure to apprise the child and family of projected outcomes for care and proposed interventions to meet those projected outcomes communicates that their input and cooperation are unnecessary and that they have little or no control and few if any rights in the situation.* This discussion also affords the nurse the opportunity to ensure that projected outcomes and interventions are in accord with the family's values and beliefs. Projected outcomes and interventions that are attempted in ignorance of value conflicts (or in spite of them) have little chance for success.

Ideally, the plan of care should be presented to the family within a few hours of the child's admission. It need not be written in final form at this time because information gained during the interaction often results in additions or modifications. It usually takes only a few minutes to discuss the plan of care and to obtain input from the child and the family. The information gained in this exchange of ideas will save the nurse a great deal of time in implementation and usually results in a more cooperative and less frightened parent and youngster.

Implementing the Plan. The implementation of a well-conceived plan is one of the joys of the nursing of children. At this point the nurse may realize some of the greatest rewards of the nursing role: the quieting of a fussy infant who cuddles into the nurse's arms, the smile on the face of a previously distraught child as pain is relieved, the relief in a parent's face when the treatment process is explained, the satisfaction of significant reduction in an elevated body temperature. Quite frankly, isn't this the part of the nursing process that you envisioned as the whole of nursing when you first began your education? It is the "doing" phase. Every nurse must remember, however, that *doing* without adequate *planning* results, at best, in mediocrity.

*"Client" is used to convey the child/family unit or any part of that unit. Since pediatric nursing so often involves at least one family member, the word "client" provides a concise way to connote consideration of the family.

Evaluating the Success of Nursing Interventions

Evaluation is often accomplished simultaneously with implementation. At this point the linear, point-by-point discussion of the nursing process breaks down. Evaluation is the least "linear" of any of the components. Rather, it is the impetus for recycling—for going back for more assessment and analysis, further planning, additional modifications, and new strategies. Evaluation is so natural to the experienced nurse as to be an integrated and essential part of each of the other components. Evaluation answers the question, "Did the intervention work?" "Is this child making progress toward the projected outcome, and if not, why not?" "Did I obtain the necessary data?" "Can I rely upon my findings and upon my interpretation?" "Is this an appropriate projected outcome for this client?" "Are there more appropriate or more descriptive evaluation criteria for the goal?" "Did the interventions accomplish what I intended them to?" "Are there other interventions that might work better or faster?" "Is there a way to accomplish this with less stress to the child?"

Evaluation will be most effective when client input (subjective information) is elicited and used to make modifications in the plan. When a nurse is working with children, evaluation is often hindered by their lack of socialization into adult patterns of illness behavior. This factor makes it necessary to validate evaluation criteria with the child and the parent. For example, a nurse who used relaxation techniques to alleviate pain 30 minutes ago and now finds the child lying quietly, watching television, might assume the intervention was effective in reducing the pain. On questioning the child, however, the nurse might learn that "The hurt is still there, but it helps if I lie real still and try not to think about it." The action taken by the nurse in the latter instance would differ significantly from an action based on the former evaluation.

The nursing process embodies the role of the professional nurse. This text provides information about illnesses in a nursing process format and includes nursing process plans designed to be applicable across a broad span of conditions. Nursing diagnoses are incorporated throughout the text to familiarize the reader with the use of NANDA-approved diagnoses. Chapters 3 through 9 contain Growth and Development Plans detailing nursing diagnoses applicable to health promotion and related nursing outcomes and interventions.

KEY CONCEPTS

Concepts Related to Basic Information

- The family structure is changing so that the nuclear family is no longer the standard: nursing must consider that modern families are often headed by single parents, or may be transcultural, biracial, blended, adoptive, communal, gay, or one of several other nontraditional family styles.
- Morbidity rate refers to the number of cases of a specific disease in a specified period of time (usually a year) within a specified unit (stated number) of the population.
- Mortality rate refers to the ratio of the number of deaths from a given disease divided by the total number of reported cases of that disease.
- The pediatric population at the turn of the 21st century may well be increasingly ethnically mixed as the birth rate has declined faster for white families in the United States than for people from ethnically diverse groups and increased rates of immigration.
- It was not until the acceptance of theories of development that the concept of *childhood* was fully realized.
- The 1990s will be marked by a shift in health care priorities from cure to care, from treating illness and disease to preventing them, and from care provided in tertiary care settings to care provided in the community and home.
- The growing professionalism among pediatric nurses is evident in the growing number of pediatric subspecialties and the formation of the Society of Pediatric Nurses, an organization for all pediatric nurses involved in all aspects of providing care to children and families.
- Ethics addresses problems that arise when an individual must make a choice between alternative values related to human behavior.
- On becoming a professional, it is incumbent on the nurse to be well versed about implications of the American Nurses' Association Code and the ANA Standards of Maternal-Child Health Nursing Practice.

Concepts Related to Nursing Assessment

- The nurse must be open to the values of others in order to adequately explore the perspectives of each person involved in an ethical issue.
- Nursing diagnoses are "clinical judgments" about individual, family, or community responses to actual and high-risk health problems/life processes.
- Nursing assessment is the first phase of the nursing process, answering the question, "What do I need to find out about this client in order to provide the best care?"
- Subjective information exists in the client's mind and cannot be verified externally; subjective information for the pediatric client will often be supplied by a variety of sources, including the parents or other caregivers.
- Objective information is verifiable externally; objective data are both observable and measurable.
- A nursing diagnostic statement consists of three major components: the response; related or risk factors or etiology; and the list of defining characteristics.

Concepts Related to Nursing Intervention

- The goal of pediatric nursing is to promote the healthy maturation of the child/adolescent as a physical, intellectual, and emotional being within the context of the family and community.
- In light of the significant change in the population of children and adolescents, the challenge for the pediatric nurse is to provide quality care so it can offset the decline in the quantity of interactions with the child and the family.
- Studies have demonstrated the value of anticipatory guidance activities and community-based programs in maintaining and promoting child and family health outcomes.
- Advocacy and health teaching are unique aspects of the pediatric nursing role because of the vulnerability and developmental immaturity of children and adolescents.
- One of the fundamental goals of pediatric nursing is to provide family-centered care.
- The role of the pediatric nurse includes the responsibility to work with the family to substitute judgment for the child who is too young to make self-care decisions and to advocate on behalf of the child.
- If the nurse researcher is unable to articulate implications for clinical nursing, it is unlikely that the pediatric staff nurse will be able to use these results in practice.
- There are three domains of nursing practice: dependent, interdependent, and independent. Dependent and interdependent domains rely on collaborative problem-solving processes; the independent domain relies on nursing diagnoses.
- In the planning phase, the nurse identifies client goals or projected outcomes, interventions that will accomplish the projected outcomes, and outcome measures to be used in the evaluation criteria.
- Implementing the plan of care is a two-step process because, before the interventions are actually effected, they must be discussed with the client.
- Evaluation is often accomplished simultaneously with implementation.

REFERENCES

Alan Guttmacher Institute. (1991). Unpublished data. New York. Author.

American Nurses' Association. (1987). *Access to prenatal care: Key to preventing low birth weight*. Kansas City, MO: Author.

American Nurses' Association. (1989). *Classification systems for describing nursing practice: Working papers*. Kansas City, MO: Author.

American Nurses' Association. (1985). *Code for nurses with interpretive statements*. Kansas City, MO: Author.

American Nurses' Association. Commission on Nursing Research. (1981). *Guidelines for the investigative function of nurses*. Kansas City, MO: Author.

American Nurses' Association. (1980). *Standards of maternal-child health nursing practice*. Kansas City, MO: Author.

Behrman, R. (1992). *Nelson textbook of pediatrics* (14th ed.). Philadelphia: WB Saunders.

Benner, P. (1984). *From novice to expert*. Menlo Park, CA: Addison-Wesley.

Bishop, A., & Scudder, J. (1987). Nursing ethics in an age of controversy. *Advances in Nursing Science, 9*(3), 34–43.

Blum, S. (1989). Infant mortality: Stop "the trend." *Saint Raphael's Better Health*, pp 25–34.

Brecht, M. (1989). The tragedy of infant mortality. *Nursing Outlook, 37*, 18–22.

Brodie, B. (1982). Children: A glance at the past. *MCN, 7*(4), 219–220.

Brodie, B. (1986, Winter). Yesterday, today and tomorrow's pediatric world. *Children's Health Care, 14*(3), 168–173.

Bulechek, G. M., & McCloskey, J. C. (1992a). Defining and validating nursing interventions. *Nursing Clinics of North America: Nursing Interventions, 27*(2), 289–297.

Bulechek, G. M., & McCloskey, J. C. (1992b). *Nursing interventions: Essential nursing treatments*. Philadelphia: WB Saunders.

CDC. (1990). Fatal injuries to children. *Morbidity and Mortality Weekly Report, 39*(26), 443.

CDC. (1987). Youth suicide . . . United States, 1970–1980. *Morbidity and Mortality Weekly Report, 36*(6), 87–88.

Cohen, S. M., Arnold, L., Brown, L., & Brooten, D. (1991). Taxonomic classification of transitional follow-up care nursing interventions with low birthweight infants. *Clinical Nurse Specialist, 5*(1), 31–36.

Craft, M. J., & Denehy, J. A. (1990). *Nursing interventions for infants and children*. Philadelphia: WB Saunders.

Curtin, L. (1986). The nurse as advocate: A philosophical foundation for nursing. In P. Chinn (Ed.), *Ethical issues in nursing* (pp 11–20). Rockville, MD: Aspen Systems Corporation.

Dolan, J., Fitzpatrick, M., & Herrmann, E. (1983). *Nursing in society: A historical perspective* (15th ed.). Philadelphia: WB Saunders.

Fawcett, J. (1984, October). Hallmarks of success in nursing research. *Advances in Nursing Science, 7*(1), 1–11.

Fingerhut, L., & National Center for Health Statistics (NCHS). (1988). [Vital statistics: Mortality statistics for ages 0–19.] Unpublished data.

Gordon, M. (1987). *Nursing diagnosis: Process and application*. New York: McGraw-Hill.

Gordon, M. (1976). Nursing diagnosis and the diagnostic process. *American Journal of Nursing, 76*, 1276–1300.

Grobe, S. J. (1990). Nursing intervention lexicon and taxonomy unit: Language and classification methods. *Advances in Nursing Science, 13*(2), 22–33.

Guyer, B., & Gallagher, S. (1985). An approach to the epidemiology of childhood injuries. *Pediatric Clinics of North America, 32*(1), 5–15.

Halloran, M. C. (1982). Rational ethical judgments utilizing a decision-making tool. *Heart and Lung, 11*(6), 566–570.

Health Care Financing Administration. (1989). [2082 data.] Bureau of Data Management and Strategy. Unpublished data.

Infant Health Development Program. (1990). Enhancing the outcomes of low-birth-weight premature infants. *Journal of the American Medical Association, 263*(76), 3035–3042.

Institute of Medicine. (1985). *Preventing low birth weight*. Washington, DC: National Academy Press.

Iyer, P. W., Tapich, B. J., & Bernocchi-Losey, D. (1991). *Nursing process and nursing diagnosis* (2nd ed.). Philadelphia: WB Saunders.

Komelasky, A. (1990). The effect of home nursing visits on parental anxiety and PR knowledge retention of parents of apnea-monitored infants. *Journal of Pediatric Nursing, 5*(6), 387–392.

Levine, M. C., Carey, W. B., Crocker, A. C., et al. (1983). *Developmental-behavioral pediatrics*. Philadelphia: WB Saunders.

Levine, M. E. (1977). Nursing ethics and the ethical nurse. *American Journal of Nursing, 77*(5), 845.

McCloskey, J. C., & Bulechek, G. M. (1992). *Nursing interventions classification (NIC)*. St. Louis: CV Mosby.

McCombs, R. (1907). *Diseases of children for nurses*. Philadelphia: W.B. Saunders.

Moynihan, D. P. (1987). *Family and nation.* San Diego: Harcourt, Brace, Jovanovich.

Nadler, H., & Evans, W. (1987). The future of pediatrics. *American Journal of Diseases of Children, 141,* 21–27.

National Center for Health Statistics. (1991a). *Health United States, 1990.* (DHHS Pub. No. [PHS] 91–1232.) Public Health Service. Hyattsville, MD: Author.

National Center for Health Statistics. (1990a). *National Health Interview Survey, 1989.* Unpublished data.

National Center for Health Statistics, Centers for Disease Control, Public Health Service. (1989a). *Hospital discharge survey.* Unpublished data.

National Center for Health Statistics, Division of Vital Statistics. (1991b). Unpublished data.

National Center for Health Statistics, Division of Vital Statistics, Public Health Service. (1991c). Unpublished data.

National Center for Health Statistics. Public Health Service. (1989b). *Health United States.* (DHHS Publication No. PHS 89–1221.) Washington, DC: US Government Printing Office.

National Center for Health Statistics. Public Health Service. (1990c). Advance report of final mortality statistics, 1988. *Monthly Vital Statistics Report, 39* (4, Suppl.). Hyattsville, MD: Author.

National Center for Health Statistics & Ries, P. (Ed.). (1990b). *Characteristics of persons with and without health coverage: United States, 1989. Advance data from vital and health statistics;* no. 20. Hyattsville, MD: Public Health Service.

National Commission to Prevent Infant Mortality. (1988). *Infant mortality: Care of our children, care for our future.* Washington, DC: Author.

North American Nursing Diagnosis Association (NANDA). (1992). *NANDA nursing diagnoses: Definitions and classifications.* St. Louis, MO: Author.

Office of Technology Assessment (OTA). (1987). *Technology dependent children: Hospital vs. home care. A technical memorandum.* Washington, DC: Congress of the United States.

Perrin, J., & Ireys, H. (1984). The organization of services for chronically ill children and their families. *Pediatric Clinics of North America, 31,* 235–257.

Quinn, C. A., & Smith, M. D. (1987). *The professional commitment: Issues and ethics in nursing.* Philadelphia: WB Saunders.

Romero, R. (1986). Autobiographical scrapbooks: A coping tool for hospitalized school children. *Issues in Comprehensive Pediatric Nursing, 9*(4), 247–258.

Saba, V. K., O'Hare, P. A., Zuckerman, A. E., Boondas, J., Levine, E., & Oatway, D. M. (1991). A nursing intervention taxonomy for home health care. *Nursing and Health Care, 12*(6), 296–299.

Sigman, P. (1986). Ethical choice in nursing. In P. L. Chinn (Ed.), *Ethical issues in nursing.* Rockville, MD: Aspen Systems Corporation.

Silverstein, N. G. (1985, January). Lillian Wald at Henry Street, 1893–1895. *Advances in Nursing Science, 7*(2), 1–12.

Smith, J. (1984). Psychosocial aspects of infantile apnea and home monitoring. *Pediatric Annals, 13,* 219–223.

Snyder, M. (1985). *Independent nursing interventions.* New York: Wiley.

Stein, R. (1989). *Caring for children with chronic illness: Issues and strategies.* New York: Springer.

Thompson, J. E., & Thompson, H. O. (1985). *Bioethical decision making for nurses.* Norwalk, CT: Appleton-Century-Crofts.

Thompson, R. H. (1986, Spring). Where we stand: Twenty years of research on pediatric hospitalization and health care. *Child Health Care, 14*(4), 200–210.

UNICEF. (1986). *The state of the world's children.* UK: Oxford University Press.

U.S. Bureau of the Census. (1991). *Marital status and living arrangements, 1990.* Washington, DC: US Government Printing Office.

U.S. Bureau of the Census. (1990). United States population estimates by age, sex, race, and Hispanic origin: 1989. *Current Population Reports.* (Series P–25, No. 1057.) Washington, DC: US Government Printing Office.

U.S. Department of Health and Human Services. (1990). *Child health USA '90* (p 24). Washington, DC: DHHS, Public Health Service, Health Resources and Service Administration, Office of Maternal and Child Health (HRS–M–CH–90–1).

U.S. Department of Health and Human Services. (1991). *Child health USA '91.* Washington, DC: DHHS, Public Health Service, Health Resources and Service Administration, Office of Maternal and Child Health (HRS–M–CH–91–1).

Vaughn, V. C. (1987). The field of pediatrics. In R. E. Behrman & V. C. Vaughn (Eds.), *Nelson textbook of pediatrics* (13th ed., pp. 1–5). Philadelphia: WB Saunders.

Verran, J. (1981). Delineation of ambulatory care nursing practice. *Journal of Ambulatory Care Management, 4,* 1–13.

Wallace, H. (1983). Policies regarding health and social welfare of mothers and children in the United States. *Clinical Pediatrics, 22*(1), 14–21.

Werley, H. H., & Lang, N. M. (1988). *Identification of the nursing minimum data set.* New York: Springer.

Whitman, D., Thornton, J., Shapiro, J. P., et al. (1988, January 11). America's hidden poor. *U.S. News and World Report, 104*(1), 18–24.

BIBLIOGRAPHY

General

Baldwin, J., & Davis, L. (1989). Assessing parents as health educators. *Pediatric Nursing, 15,* 453–463.

Broome, M. (1990). Preparation of children for painful procedures. *Pediatric Nursing, 16*(6), 537–542.

Brooten, D., Kumar, S., Brown, L., Finkler, S., Butts, P., Bakewell-Sacks, S., Gibbons, A., & Delivoria-Papadopoulos, M. (1986). A randomized clinical trial of early hospital discharge and home followup of very low birthweight infants. *New England Journal of Medicine, 315,* 934–939.

Burr, H., Greyer, B., Todres, I., Abrahams, B., & Chiodo, T. (1983). Home care for children on respirators. *New England Journal of Medicine, 309,* 1319–1323.

Davis, B., & Steele, S. (1991). Case management for young children with special health care needs. *Pediatric Nursing, 17*(1), 15–19.

Defriese, G. H., Crossland, C. L., Pearson, C. E., & Sullivan, C. J. (Eds.). (1990). *Comprehensive school health programs: Current status and future prospects.* Kent, OH: American School Health Association.

Dryfoos, J. G. (1988). School-based health clinics: Three years of experience. *Family Planning Perspectives, 20*(4), 193–200.

Fenichel, E. S., & Eggbeer, L. (1990). *Preparing practitioners to work with infants, toddlers and their families: Issues and recommendations for education and training.* Washington, DC: National Center for Clinical Infant Programs.

Goldberg, A., Faure, A., Vaughn, C., Snarski, R., & Seleny, R. (1984). Home care for life-supported persons: An approach to program development. *Journal of Pediatrics, 104,* 785–795.

Hamburg, D. A. (1989). *Early adolescence: A critical time for interventions in education and health.* New York: Carnegie Corporation of New York.

Hoffman, A., & Greydanus, D. (Eds.). (1989). *Adolescent medicine.* Norwalk, CT: Appleton and Lange.

Holt, J., & Johnson, S. (1991). Developmental tasks: A key to reducing teenage pregnancy. *Journal of Pediatric Nursing, 6*(3), 191–196.

Irwin, C. (1990). The theoretical concept of at-risk adolescents. *Adolescent Medicine: State of the Art: Reviews, 1*(1), 1–14.

Korngrith, M. (1990). School illnesses: Who's absent and why? *Pediatric Nursing, 16,* 95–99.

Krywanio, M., & Jones, L. (1988). Developing an early intervention program for infants at risk. *Journal of Pediatric Nursing, 3*(6), 375–382.

Lankard, B. (1989). *Case management of adolescents with chronic disease.* Columbus, OH: Center on Education and Training for Employment, Ohio State University.

Mitchell, C., Rutherford, P. A. (1987). Dilemmas in practice: The fragile survivor. *American Journal of Nursing, 87*(5), 603–606.

Newacheck, P., & Halfon, N. (1986). Access to ambulatory care services for economically disadvantaged children. *Pediatrics, 78,* 813–818.

O'Brien, R., Bush, P., & Purcel, G. (1989). Stability is a measure of children's health locus of control. *Journal of School Health, 59,* 161–164.

Ooms, T., & Herendeen, L. (1989). *Integrated approaches to youth's health problems: Federal, state and community roles* and *The unique health needs of adolescents: Implications for health care insurance and financing.* Washington, DC: American Association for Marriage and Family, Therapy, Research and Education Foundation.

Sandelowski, M. (1986). The politics of parenthood. *MCN, 11*(4), 235–238.

Shulsinger, E. (1990). Needs of sheltered homeless children. *Journal of Pediatric Health Care, 4*(3), 136–140.

Wood, D. (1989). Homeless children: Their evaluation and treatment. *Journal of Pediatric Health Care, 3*(4), 194–199.

Zabin, L. S., Hirsch, M. B., Smith, E. A., Street, R., & Hardy, J. B. (1986). Evaluation of pregnancy prevention programs for urban teenagers. *Family Planning Perspectives, 18,* 119–126.

Child Health Statistics

Andrulis, D., Weslowski, V., & Gage, L. (1989). The 1987 U.S. hospital AIDS survey. *Journal of the American Medical Association, 262,* 784–794.

CDC. (1990). Homicide among young black males, United States 1978–1987. *Morbidity and Mortality Weekly Report, 39*(48), 869–873.

Davidson, L., Rosenberg, M., Mercy, J., Franklin, J., & Simmons, J. (1989). An epidemiologic study of risk factors in two teenage suicide clusters. *Journal of the American Medical Association, 262,* 2687–2692.

National Center for Health Statistics. Public Health Service. (1990). Advance report of National Center for Health Statistics, 1991. *Vital statistics of the United States.* (Vol. 2, Mortality, Part A.) Washington, DC: US Government Printing Office.

National Center for Health Statistics. Public Health Service. (1990). *Health United States, 1989.* (DHHS Publication No. PHS 90–1233.) Washington, DC: U.S. Government Printing Office.

National Center for Health Statistics. Public Health Service. (1989). Advance Report of Final Natality Statistics, 1987. *Monthly Vital Statistics Report,* 39 (3, Suppl.) (DHHS Publication No. PHS 90–1120.) Hyattsville, MD: Author.

National Center for Health Statistics, Public Health Service, & Ries, P. (1989). Characteristics of persons with and without health coverage: United States. 1988 Vital Statistics, Mortality statistics for ages 0–19. Report, *39*(4, Suppl.). Hyattsville, MD: Author.

U.S. Bureau of the Census. (1989). Poverty in the United States 1987. *Current Population Reports.* (Series P–60, No. 163.) Washington, DC: US Government Printing Office.

U.S. Department of Health and Human Services. Vital and Health Statistics. (1988). Detailed diagnosis and procedures for patients discharged from short-stay hospitals, United States, 1986. (DHHS Publication No. PHS 88–1756.)

Childhood Injuries

Agran, P., Castillo, O., & Winn, D. (1990). Childhood motor vehicle occupant injuries. *American Journal of Diseases of Children, 144,* 653–662.

American Academy of Pediatrics. Committee on Accident and Poison Prevention. (1989). Skateboard injuries. *Pediatrics, 83,* 1070–1071.

American Academy of Pediatrics. Committee on Accident and Prevention. (1990). Safe transportation of newborns discharged from the hospital. *AAP News, 6*(7), 12.

American Academy of Pediatrics. Committee on Sports Medicine and Committee on School Health. (1989). Organized athletics for preadolescent children. *Pediatrics, 84,* 583–584.

American Academy of Pediatrics. Committee on Adolescence. (1988). Suicide and suicide attempts in adolescents and young adults. *Pediatrics, 81,* 322–324.

Baker, S. (1989). Injury science comes of age. *Journal of the American Medical Association, 262*(16), 2284–2285.

Bourgrut, C., & McArtor, R. (1989). Unintentional injuries: Risk factors in preschool children. *American Journal of Diseases of Children, 143,* 556–559.

CDC. (1990). Childhood injuries in the United States. *American Journal of Diseases of Children, 144,* 627–646.

CDC. (1990). Fatal injuries to children—United States, 1986. *Morbidity and Mortality Weekly Report, 39*(26), 442–451.

Children's Safety Network. (1991). *A data book of child and adolescent injury* (p 7). Washington, DC: National Center for Education and Maternal and Child Health.

Christoffel, K. (1989). Child passenger safety. *American Journal of Diseases of Children, 143,* 1271–1272.

Dolan, M., Knapp, J., & Andres, J. (1989). Three wheel and four wheel all terrain vehicle injuries in children. *Pediatrics, 84,* 694–698.

Fingerhut, L., & Kleinman, J. (1990). International and interstate comparisons of homicides in black young males. *Journal of the American Medical Association, 263,* 3292–3295.

Gould, J., Davey, B., & LeRoy, S. (1989). Socioeconomic differentials and neonatal mortality: Racial comparison of California singletons. *Pediatrics, 83,* 181–186.

Humphrey, N. (1990). U.S. Consumer Product Safety Commission. *Journal of Pediatric Health Care, 4,* 323–324.

Keen, T. (1990). Nursing care of the pediatric multitrauma patient. *Nursing Clinics of North America, 25,* 131–141.

Lee, E., Jacobson, J., & Levanas, V. (1989). Stressful life events and accidents at school. *Pediatric Nursing, 15,* 140–142.

Pless, I., Verreault, R., & Tenina, S. (1989). A case-control study of pedestrian and bicyclist injuries in childhood. *American Journal of Public Health, 79,* 995–998.

Rice, D., MacKenzie, E., Jones, A., et al. (1989). The cost of injury in the United States: A report to Congress. San Francisco: Institute for Health and Aging. University of California, Injury Prevention Center.

Rivara, F., et al. (1989). Attitudes and practices toward children as pedestrians. *Pediatrics, 84,* 1017–1021.

U.S. Department of Health and Human Services. (1989). *Child health USA '89.* Washington, DC: U.S. Government Printing Office. (HRS–M–C11-8915).

Urtis, J., Clayton, D., & Jay, S. (1988). Infant morbidity: A measurement of severity and occurrence of illness in preterm and term infants. *Journal of Pediatric Nursing, 3,* 110–117.

Wilson, H. (1989). Preventing injury in the "middle years." *Contemporary Pediatrics, 6,* 20–54.

History of Children's Care

Cherry, B. S., & Carty, R. M. (1986). Changing concepts of childhood in society. *Pediatric Nursing, 112,* 421–424.

Gardner, M. (1989, December 20). Quest for infant day care challenges working parents. *The Christian Science Monitor,* pp. 10–11.

Hoekelman, R. A., Starfield, B., McCormick, M., et al. (1983). A profile of pediatric practice in the United States. *American Journal of Disabled Children, 137,* 1057–1060.

Nadler, H. L., & Evans, W. J. (1987). The future of pediatrics. *American Journal of Disabled Children, 141,* 21–27.

Rosenbaum, S., Hughes, D., & Johnson, K. (1988). Maternal and child health services for medically indigent children and pregnant women. *Medical Care, 26,* 315–332.

Velsor-Friedrich, B. (1993). Homeless children and their families, Part II: Federal Programs and Alternative Health Care Delivery Systems. *Journal of Pediatric Nursing, 8*(3), 190–192.

Pediatric Nursing Practice

Beal, J., Betz, C. (1992), November/December). Intervention studies in pediatric nursing research: A decade of review. Pediatric *Nursing, 18*(6), 586–590.

Carlson, J., Craft, C., McGurie, A., & Popkess-Vervter, A. (1991). *Nursing diagnosis: A case study approach.* Philadelphia: WB Saunders.

Carpenito, L. (1989). *Nursing diagnosis: Application to clinical practice* (3rd ed.). Philadelphia: JB Lippincott.
Clifford, J. (1991). The practicing nurse as leader. *MCN: American Journal of Maternal Child Nursing, 16,* 18–20.
Davies, B., & Eng, B. (1993). Survey of nursing research programs in children's hospitals. *Journal of Pediatric Nursing, 8*(3), 159–166.
Donahue, M. (1985). *Nursing: The finest art, an illustrated history*. St. Louis: Mosby Year Book.
Harris, M., & Bean, C. (1991). Changing the role of the nurse in the hematology-oncology outpatient setting. *Oncology Nursing Forum, 18,* 43–46.
Hayes, V., & Cook, K. (1991). Pediatric nursing in British Columbia. *Journal of Pediatric Nursing, 6,* 216–219.
Lane, K., & Peppe, K. (1987). Where are the standards? *Journal of Pediatric Nursing, 2,* 291–294.
McVetz, D. (1989). Old fashioned care still makes the difference. *MCN: American Journal of Maternal Child Nursing, 14,* 126–127.
Montana, J. (1988). Computers and nursing care. *Journal of Pediatric Nursing, 3,* 48–53.
Mullaly, L. (1991). Choosing to make a difference. *MCN: American Journal of Maternal Child Nursing, 16,* 21–23.
Rew, L. (1987). Nursing intuition. Too powerful—and too valuable—to ignore. *Nursing 87, 17,* 43–45.
Rimar, J. (1991). The bedside nurse: Nursing's grass-roots leader. *MCN: American Journal of Maternal Child Nursing, 16,* 27–29.
Starn, J., & Niederhausen, V. (1990). An MCN model for nursing diagnoses to focus intervention. *MCN: American Journal of Maternal Child Nursing, 15,* 180–183.
Steeves, R., Kahn, D., & Benoliel, J. (1990). Nurses' interpretation of the suffering of their patients. *Western Journal of Nursing Research, 12,* 715–728.
Styles, M. (1990). Challenges for nursing in this new decade. *MCN: American Journal of Maternal Child Nursing, 15,* 347–352.
Williams, M. (1991). Educating nurses to thrive on chaos. *Journal of Pediatric Nursing, 6,* 143–144.

Child Health Policy

American Medical Association, Healthier Youth by the Year 2000 Project. (1990). *Healthy youth 2000: National health promotion and disease prevention objectives for adolescents.* Chicago: American Medical Association.
Arnold, L., et al. (1990). Legislative issues affecting parenting: An overview of current policies. *Journal of Perinatal and Neonatal Nursing, 4,* 24–32.
Avard, D., et al. (1990). The role of the Canadian Institute of Child Health in promoting family-centered care. *Children's Health Care, 19,* 209–212.
Betz, C. (1990). Health care for all children. *Journal of Pediatric Nursing, 5,* 77.
Betz, C. (1990). Putting power into empowerment. *Journal of Pediatric Nursing, 5,* 369.
Betz, C. (1989). Clinical practice and scholarship. *Journal of Pediatric Nursing, 4,* 319.
Brazelton, T. (1986). Issues for working parents. *American Journal of Orthopsychiatry, 56,* 14–25.
Brindis, C. (1990). *Reducing adolescent pregnancy: The next steps for program, policy and research.* Santa Cruz, CA: ETR Associates/Network Publications.
CDC. (1988). CDC recommendations for a community plan for the prevention and containment of suicide clusters. *Morbidity and Mortality Weekly Report, 37*(5–6), 1–12.
CDC. (1990). HIV prevalence estimates and AIDS case projections for the United States: Reports based on a workshop. *Morbidity and Mortality Weekly Report, 39*(RR–16), 30.
Children's Defense Fund. (1990). A children's defense budget, S.O.S. America. Washington, DC: Author.
Children's Defense Fund. (1987). Child care: The time is now. Washington, DC: Author.
Chollet, D. (1988). Public and private issues in financing health care for children. *EBRI Issue Brief No. 79.*
Devney, P. (1990). Organ donation and required request legislation. *Journal of Pediatric Nursing, 5,* 288–289.
Feeg, V. (1990). The future of pediatric nursing: Anticipating the health care needs of children. *Imprint, 37,* 70, 72–73, 75.
Feeg, V. (1989). New legislative efforts to improve child health and decrease infant mortality. *Pediatric Nursing, 15,* 145–148.
Frager, B. (1991). Teenage childbearing: Part II: Program and policies. *Journal of Pediatric Nursing, 6,* 202–205.
Frager, B. (1990). A national child care crisis: Action for the 90s. *Journal of Pediatric Nursing, 5,* 229–231.
Gale, C. (1989). Inadequacy of health care for the nation's chronically ill children. *Journal of Pediatric Nursing, 3,* 20–27.
Harrington, C., & Lempert, L. (1988). Medicaid: A public program in distress. *Nursing Outlook, 36,* 6–8.
Harvey, B. (1991). Why we need a national child health policy. *Pediatrics, 87,* 1–6.
Johnson, F., Lay, P., & Wilbrandt, M. (1988). Teenage pregnancy: Issues, interventions and direction. *Journal of the National Medical Association, 80,* 145–152.
McManus, M., Greaney, A., & Newacheck, P. (1989). Health insurance status of young adults in the United States. *Pediatrics, 84,* 709–716.
Miller, C., Fine, A., & Adams-Taylor, S. (1986). Monitoring children's health: Key indicators. Washington, DC: American Public Health Association.
Miller, G. (1989). Introduction of the child investment and securities act. *Congressional Record, Proceedings and Debates of the 101st Congress, First Session.* Washington, DC.
Mitchell, F., & Brindis, C. (1989). Adolescent pregnancy: The responsibility of policy makers. *HSR: Health Services Research, 22,* 399–437.
Murphy, M. (1989). What price success: Can we afford "saved" babies? *Journal of Pediatric Health, 3,* 285–286.
National Association for the Care of Children's and Related Institutions (NACHRI). (1988). Medicare and poor children: State variation in eligibility and service coverage.
Newacheck, P. (1989). Improving access to health services for adolescents from economically disadvantaged families. *Pediatrics, 84,* 1056–1063.
Newacheck, P., & Halfon, N. (1988). Preventive care use by school-aged children. Differences by socioeconomic status. *Pediatrics, 82,* 462–468.
Newacheck, P., & McManus, M. (1989). Health insurance status of adolescents in the United States. *Pediatrics, 84,* 699–708.
Nienhuis, M. (1987). As the health care system bypasses children pressure mounts on schools to fill the gap. *Journal of School Health, 57,* 144–146.
Oberg, C. N. (1990). Medically uninsured children in the United States, a challenge to public policy. *Pediatrics, 85,* 824–833.
Oberg, C. N. (1987). Pediatrics and poverty. *Pediatrics, 79,* 567–568.
O'Conner, C., Murr, A., & Wingert, P. (1986, June 2). Affluent America's forgotten children. *Newsweek,* pp. 20–21.
Public Health Service. (1990). *Healthy people 2000: National health promotion and disease prevention objectives.* Washington, DC: US Department of Health and Human Services, Public Health Service.
Rhodes, M. (1991). Brewing issues in MCH. *MCN: American Journal of Maternal Child Nursing, 16,* 73.
Rosenbaum, S. (1989). New focus on children's health issues. *Hospitals, 63*(12), 71–72.
Rymer, M., & Adler, G. (1987). Children and Medicaid: The experience in four states. *Health Care Financing Review, 9,* 1–39.
Styles, M. (1990). Challenges for nursing in this new decade. *MCN: American Journal of Maternal Child Nursing, 15,* 347–348, 350, 352.
Swartz, M. (1990). Infant mortality: Agenda for the 1990s. *Journal of Pediatric Health Care, 4,* 169–174.
Television and teens: Health implications. (1990). *Journal of Adolescent Health Care, 11,* 86–90.
Updegrove, N. A. (1990). *Childhood obesity and cardiovascular disease: January 1985–May 1990.* (Quick biography series: QB 90–59.) Beltsville, MD: National Agricultural Library, U.S. Department of Agriculture.

van Eys, J. (1991). The impact of Medicaid on research-based care in pediatric hematology/oncology. *American Journal of Pediatric Hematology and Oncology, 13,* 91–96.

Velsor-Friedrich, B. (1991). Healthy goals for children and their families: 1991 and beyond. *Journal of Pediatric Nursing, 6,* 62–63.

Velsor-Friedrich, B. (1990, April). Medicaid: The war on child poverty: Status report. *Journal of Pediatric Nursing, 5,* 140–142.

Velsor-Friedrich, B. (1990, October). Women and children first? *Journal of Pediatric Nursing, 5,* 354–355.

Velsor-Friedrich, B., & Frager, B. (1990). The federal government and child health. *Journal of Pediatric Nursing, 5,* 56–58.

Whitman, D., Thornton, J., Shapiro, J. P., et al. (1988, January 11). America's hidden poor. *U.S. News and World Report, 104*(1), 18–24.

Young, K. T., & Zigler, E. (1986). Infant and toddler day care: Regulations and policy implications. *American Journal of Orthopsychiatry, 56,* 43–55.

Pediatric Nursing Research Issues

Beal, J. (1989). Methodological issues in conducting pediatric nursing research. *Journal of Pediatric Nursing, 4,* 2.

Brown, M., & Hellings, P. (1988). A case study of qualitative versus quantitative reviews: The maternal-infant bonding controversy. *Journal of Pediatric Nursing, 4,* 104–111.

Burke, S. & Roberts, C. (1990). Nursing research and the care of chronically ill and disabled children. *Journal of Pediatric Nursing, 5,* 316–327.

Hoskins, L. M., McFarlane, E. A., Rubenfeld, M. G., et al. (1986). Nursing diagnosis in the chronically ill: Methodology for clinical validation. *Advances in Nursing Science, 8,* 80–89.

Keefe, M. & Biester, D. (1988). Developing a research program in a clinical setting. *Journal of Pediatric Nursing, 3,* 269–272.

Kotzer, A. (1990). Creative strategies for pediatric nursing research: Data collection. *Journal of Pediatric Nursing, 5,* 50–53.

Lower, M. S., & Burton, S. (1989). Measuring the impact of nursing interventions on patient outcomes—The challenge of the 1990s. *Journal of Nursing Quality Assurance, 4,* 24–34.

Lynn, M. (1991). Gastric tube insertion length: Routine or research-ing. *Journal of Pediatric Nursing, 6,* 127–128.

Lynn, M. (1991). Money is available for that small research project if you know where to look. *Journal of Pediatric Nursing, 6,* 197–198.

Lynn, M. (1990). Don't be fooled by statistical significance. *Journal of Pediatric Nursing, 5,* 350–351.

Lynn, M. (1990). Extra! Extra! Nurse beats machine. *Journal of Pediatric Nursing, 5,* 223–224.

Lynn, M. (1990). Research commitment starts at the top. *Journal of Pediatric Nursing, 5,* 136–137.

Lynn, M. (1990). There's no such thing as free research. *Journal of Pediatric Nursing, 5,* 286–287.

Lynn, M. (1989). Readability: A critical instrumentation consideration. *Journal of Pediatric Nursing, 4,* 295–297.

Lynn, M. (1989). Research in practice: No individual's responsibility. *Journal of Pediatric Nursing, 4,* 374–376.

Lynn, M. (1987). Pediatric nurse practitioner—Patient interactions: A study of the process. *Journal of Pediatric Nursing, 2,* 268–271.

Lyons, J., & Hester, N. (1987). Research-generated nursing diagnoses for healthy school-age children. *Issues in Comprehensive Pediatric Nursing, 10,* 149–159.

Lyons, N., et al. (1990). Too busy for research? Collaboration: An answer. *MCN: American Journal of Maternal Child Nursing, 15,* 67–72.

Marino, B. (1991). Studying infant and toddler play. *Journal of Pediatric Nursing, 6,* 16–20.

Olson, R., Heater, B., & Becker, A. (1990). A meta-analysis of the effects of nursing interventions on children and parents. *MCN: American Journal of Maternal Child Nursing, 15,* 104–108.

Sidoni, S. (1991). Mentoring the novice nurse researcher. *Journal of Pediatric Nursing, 6,* 57–59.

Walsh, J. (1991). The substance-abusing family: Consideration for nursing research. *Journal of Pediatric Nursing, 6,* 49–56.

Webster-Stratton, C., Glascock, J., & McCarthy, A. M. (1986). Nurse practitioner-patient interactional analysis during well-child visits. *Nursing Research, 35,* 247–249.

Weekes, D. (1991). Application of the life-span developmental perspective to nursing research with adolescents. *Journal of Pediatric Nursing, 6,* 38–48.

Ethics

American Nurses' Association. (1985). *Human rights guidelines for nurses in clinical and other research.* Kansas City, MO: Author.

Bocchino, C. (1990). U. N. convention on the rights of children. *Pediatric Nursing, 16*(6), 600.

Chaney, E. (1986). The rights of disabled infants. *Journal of Pediatric Nursing, 1,* 409–411.

Dormire, S. L. (1989). Models for moral response in care of seriously ill children. *Journal of Nursing Scholarship, 21*(2), 81–84.

Fowler, M. (1989). Ethical decision making in clinical practice. *Nursing Clinics of North America, 24,* 955–965.

Fromer, M. J. (1986). Solving ethical dilemmas in nursing practice. In P. L. Chinn (Ed.), *Ethical issues in nursing* (pp 81–87). Rockville, MD: Aspen Systems Corporation.

Fry, S. (1989). Ethics. 1. Issues in nursing. *Nursing Clinics of North America, 24,* 461–577.

Jagla, E. (1986). The nurse's loyal duty to report changes in patient status. *Journal of Pediatric Nursing, 1,* 373–375.

Leff, E. W. (1986). Ethics and patient teaching. *MCN: American Journal of Maternal Child Nursing, 11,* 375–378.

Lynn, M. R. (1986). Children have rights too. *Journal of Pediatric Nursing, 1,* 345–348.

Mahon, N., & Yarcheski, A. (1988). Ethical concerns in research with adolescents. *Journal of Pediatric Nursing, 3,* 341–344.

McClowry, S. G. (1987). Research and treatment: Ethical distinction related to the care of children. *Journal of Pediatric Nursing, 2,* 23–29.

Rae, W. A., & Fournier, C. J. (1986). Ethical issues in pediatric research: Preserving psychosocial care in scientific inquiry. *Children's Health Care, 14,* 242–248.

Rhodes, M. (1991). Major legal initiatives in MCH. *MCN: American Journal of Maternal Child Nursing, 16,* 21–31.

Van Cleve, L. (1993). Nurses' experience in caring for anencephalic infants who are potential organ donors. *Journal of Pediatric Nursing, 8*(2), 79–84.

Veatch, R. M., & Fry, S. T. (1987). *Case studies in nursing ethics.* Philadelphia: JB Lippincott.

Weil, W. (1989). Ethical issues in pediatrics. *Current Problems in Pediatrics, 19*(12), 617–618.

CHAPTER • 2

Family Theories and Assessment

Pamela N. Clarke

RELATED TOPICS
The effects of poverty on child health, Chapter 1
The effects of increased understanding and advancing technology in health care, Chapter 1
Values clarification, Chapter 1
The effect of culture and lifestyle on development, Chapter 3
Growth and Development of Children Within Families, Unit 2, Chapters 4 through 9
Health Concepts: Children's Perceptions and Behaviors, Chapter 10
Communicating with Children and Families, Chapter 11
Assessing and promoting healthy parenting, Chapter 12
Fostering Self-Esteem, Chapter 14

LEARNING OBJECTIVES

- Define the concept of family.
- Identify the characteristics of the contemporary family.
- Compare and contrast the theories of family.
- Apply the family-centered nursing process to the care of the child and family.
- Use family assessment tools in the gathering of data on the child and family.
- Describe the dimensions of family health.
- Identify the characteristics of vulnerable families.
- Describe categories of families considered at risk for health problems.
- Apply nursing interventions to the care of families at risk.
- Discuss the primary roles of pediatric nurses working with families.

The quality of family life and the health of its members form a symbiotic relationship. No other aspect of a child's life has a more lasting impact on the child's development — physically, socially, and culturally — than the family experience.

This chapter introduces the facets of healthy family life — its structure, functions, and roles — in its many constructs.

This chapter also introduces a range of theories that can be used to assess families. An attempt is made to emphasize the nurse's role as advocate for the family, while cultural variances in the structure and

function of the family unit are recognized. Intervention is addressed, with a focus on the benefits of an interdisciplinary approach in assisting families to stay well or to cope with problems. The major goal of the chapter is to expand the nurse's understanding of various approaches to family nursing.

The family has been viewed in nursing as the unit or recipient of family-centered nursing care or as the significant nurturing environment in which ill persons recover. In child health the family is usually viewed as the essential environment; healthy families are generally a prerequisite for healthy children. Therefore, the focus of nursing care in child health must include some consideration of family needs, goals, and priorities. In each situation, understanding family health patterns is a prerequisite for nursing care and nursing intervention.

Definitions of Family

"Family" is defined as a complex organization of one or more persons with a pattern of interrelationships that have a past, present, and future. Families consist of persons who are closely related by blood, marriage, or friendship (Mallinger, 1989). The family unit is a living, open system of interacting persons who see themselves in a reciprocal relationship that provides affection and promotes development of its members. The boundaries of the contemporary family are extremely fluid, and relationships among persons who call themselves "family" are increasingly diverse and complex. The definition of family is necessarily flexible and inclusive. The term can apply to adults of either gender, single parents and their children, blended families (stepfamilies), and extended families. The term "family" is not restricted by residence and can refer to one's family of origin as well as to close friends who may actually reside elsewhere (Mallinger, 1989).

Jarrett (1992) distinguishes family membership from household composition in a study of impoverished African-American families. In many communities, single mothers and children may live independently but receive social, economic, and child care support from other households. An open definition is needed in order to understand the unique family structure and attributes for a comprehensive family assessment. The underlying question is not *if* persons are related; rather, it is *how* they are related. Persons who call themselves "family" consider themselves to be related to one another.

Whall and Fawcett (1991) summarized the following attributes of family in *Family Theory Development in Nursing: State of the Science and Art:* "The concept of family has evolved over time both in theory and in practice. The family performs a caregiving function defined as protection, nourishment, and socialization of children. Family members may or may not be related by birth, marriage or adoption and the unit may or may not contain dependent children" (p 33). It is now accepted that the family is self-defined, change and development are inherent, and commitment and attachment exist among members with some notion of future obligation.

Contemporary Families

The most commonly studied characteristics in family research have been marriage, birth, and adoption. Historically, the dominant view of the family was based on the nuclear family with two parents (breadwinner father and homemaker mother) and their children. Currently this model represents only a small portion of American families, estimated to be as small as 14 per cent. The US Census Bureau defines family as "a group of two or more persons related by birth, marriage, or adoption residing together as a household" (US Census Bureau, 1990). Given these data, which show that the majority of American households no longer "fit" a nuclear model, information in this chapter includes all family structures. That is, *all* types of families, no matter what the structure, are considered as potentially healthy families. Risk factors are presented as potentially problematic for *any* family. In theory and practice, families must be taken "as they are," not as we might like them to be.

Family: A Historical Perspective

Contemporary family life is best understood within the context of changing family forms throughout history. The family functions or tasks are similar, regardless of the form.

Historically, the family has taken the form of *extension* (an extended family pattern in which parents, children, and other related kin sustain themselves, either under the same roof or on attached or nearby homesteads, with shared daily activities) and *contraction* (a nuclear family pattern in which a couple and their children are separate from other relatives and maintain a separate routine of daily activities). These modes are affected by modification of the political order and economic conditions. Throughout time, people have continually shown imagination in constructing various styles of family living and of relating the family to the larger community; each transition has reaffirmed the family as a basic unit of human living, social stability, and health. Growth is continually in evidence, moving the family, in its hundred variations, toward more diversity and flexibility. The American family has progressed from a preindustrial (agricultural) family, housed rurally, to an industrial (traditional) family in urban residence, and, further, to a postindustrial (modern) family with a suburban or small-town abode.

The "ideal" three-generational family is an important part of American folklore. During preindustrial times, households consisted of family members living with servants, boarders, and apprentices who cared for the children. The family was not considered a private retreat; rather, it served a broad array of functions, including assisting immigrants and training young women. Early in the 20th century, apprentices generally disappeared, and children assumed a major role in household labor and in the work force.

The nuclear family form became common after World War II. Following the depression and war, great value was placed on a return to normalcy. The GI bill fostered employment opportunities for "breadwinner" fathers; women workers were replaced by men returning from the war, and the "baby boom" distanced women from paid employment. Suburbs expanded in the postwar economic boom, and media images of the happy two-parent family with children proliferated. Family forms that emerged during this era reflected the prevailing circumstances as being normal for all families (Skolnick, 1991).

The nuclear family form served a specific purpose during the 1950s, but its present value is a matter of debate (Demos, 1986; Skolnick, 1991). Some argue that the nuclear family was created as a unit of labor production and social control. The strong emphasis on this family form is reflected in popular notions of "traditional family values," which imply a nuclear family with children. Instead, the concept of family needs to be open in order that nurses and other providers involved in planning and delivering health services will include all types of families, given population projections for the year 2000 and beyond. Phenomena traditionally viewed as "family breakdown" or "family disorganization," such as the trend toward increased single-parent families, may be more appropriately conceptualized as important evolutionary transitions in family forms. Society allows more freedom, and diverse families are more visible. The positive aspects of different lifestyles are recognized. For example, research on African-American families demonstrates their strength and flexibility and the great variety of ethnic family behavior (Pinderhughes, 1982).

Family Structures

Family structures are as unique as humans are creative. Projections for the year 2000 yield an estimated 40 million "nonfamily households" (unmarried adults) and 16 million single-parent households (US Census Bureau, 1990). Together these varied family forms, which do *not* fit the Census Bureau's definition, will make up more than half of the projected total of 110 million American households by the year 2000. Over 60 per cent of American mothers of minors are currently employed. Approximately 14 per cent of the adult population is divorced; over 35 million persons are stepparents; and between 1 and 10 per cent of the population is gay or lesbian. Clearly the model of the nuclear family is not adequate for society today. It is no longer appropriate to use terms such as "nontraditional" when families representing the so-called norm are in the minority (Cody, in press).

Extensive research on families of divorce, one-parent families, dual-career families, "binuclear" families, childless families, "co-habitation," "reconstituted" or blended families, and homosexual families demonstrates an expanding typology of "new" family forms (Dornbusch & Strober, 1988). However, there is little evidence that one family form is better than another. Families of all types may experience family violence, incest, alcoholism, or child abuse. Characteristics of a healthy family, delineated later in this chapter, can be found in all types of families.

Legal policies, however, are not equally supportive of all types of families. In working families, for example, health coverage and other benefits are generally provided only to members with legal ties such as marriage, birth, or adoption. In contrast, Aid to Families of Dependent Children (AFDC) benefits tend to be provided only to single-parent families. Two married parents who are unemployed may find they must be divorced in order to qualify for assistance. Generally, such families remain supportive to each other, although the noncustodial parent "officially" resides elsewhere.

Establishing a Family System

A family system is established when members demonstrate a commitment to the family unit with the intent of some degree of permanence (regardless of whether legal sanctions such as marriage or adoption have been established). The commitment is usually based on emotional attachments among family members, and permanence primarily depends on the continuation of those attachments. Every healthy family system contains some tensions that ebb and flow along with attachments and conflict among family members. A family unit that displays extreme attachments (enmeshed) or weak attachments (disengaged) tends to be more vulnerable. Families are most vulnerable during the initial phase of becoming established. This may also be a time of financial difficulties, which create an additional strain. The birth of the first child has been described as "a bomb" for most parents unprepared for the enormity of change and restriction in their lives (Rubenstein, 1989, p 34).

Theoretical Frameworks

Nursing Frameworks

In discussing nursing perspectives for family science, Whall and Fawcett (1991) reviewed developments in some of the major nursing theories. The nursing metaparadigm concepts of person, environment, health, and nursing specify the content domain of nursing. This metaparadigm can be expanded to include family by extending the concept of "person" to include "family as the unit of care or family as the context of care" (Feetham, 1991; Leahy & Wright, 1988).

Nursing theory definitions of family vary, from focusing on the family as an important environment for the individual (Orem, 1985), to presenting a unitary perspective of each person as a human energy field that may include family (Rogers, 1988). By using Roy's (1984, 1988) definition of health, the family has been viewed as a dimension of an adapting system and subsystems. King (1981, 1992) views the family as an interpersonal system embedded in social systems (society). Nurse-family interactions provide assessment data and result in interventions that lead to goal attainment. Parse's (1981, 1992) human becoming theory focuses on the meaning of human experience with health as a "cocreated process of living value priorities" (Parse, 1981, p 31). Persons freely choose meaning in their unique unfolding processes, and the goal of nursing is a good quality of life as defined by those who call themselves family. Detailed applications of nursing theory to the family are beyond the scope of this chapter. However, additional readings that address expansion of nursing models to include the family are listed at the end of this chapter.

Family Theory

Family theory and nursing theory form the framework of nursing approaches to family health. Whall (1980) suggested that a reformulation of existing family theories in terms of nursing theory is important for nursing practice. This chapter addresses the most common family theories. Their application is framed by using concepts from the nursing metaparadigm, rather than specific nursing theories, to guide nursing assessment and the analysis of families with children.

Theories are guides for identifying significant factors related to the family's functioning and to the potential for crisis and growth. In family nursing, the theoretical framework must allow for viewing the individual and the dynamic unit, and their interrelatedness (Gillis, 1983). The goal of nursing may vary, depending on the theory, to include (1) reduction of stressors for system maintenance (systems theory), (2) improved family functioning (structural-functional theory), or (3) health promotion at different life stages (developmental theory). The family theory and the nursing theory together form the framework for assessment and analysis. For example, the family may be assessed by using the specific dimensions of Roy's adaptation framework or according to Rogers' principles. Health promotion according to Roy would focus on successful adaptation.

Systems Theory

Systems theory is a broad interdisciplinary framework that has served as the standard for the development of other theories. There are various interpretations of systems theory (Doherty & McCubbin, 1985; Bowen, 1978). The family system may be viewed as having a semipermeable boundary with the world that may be "too open" (disengaged) or "too closed" (enmeshed) (Beavers & Voeller, 1983). Boundary maintenance is an ongoing process that varies in flexibility and degree of functionality. Boundary maintenance is functional when the family can be flexibly opened or closed, depending on the needs of its members. Serious illness of a child tends to be a time when families may need to allow others to participate in the family process and offer assistance.

Behaviors and actions of family members are assessed as subsystems that process matter, energy, and information (including food and material goods as well as emotions and knowledge). The system and subsystems have the capacity to adapt and evolve. Change is inherent in family life as families configure and reconfigure; the only constant is this continual change. Persons form a family unit, have children, or take in an aging parent, knowing that the children will eventually leave home or the parent will die and the family will reconfigure. Janosik and Green (1992) refer to *expanding* families as those that are adding children or elderly dependents, and *contracting* families as those losing members through the natural transitions of independence, divorce, or death. These changes can be viewed as a time for growth, regardless of whether they are expected or unexpected.

Structural-Functional Theory

The structural-functional theory was developed in the field of sociology. Within this broad framework, the family is viewed as part of the social system, with individuals being parts of the family system. "Function" and "dysfunction" of the family refer to the utility of the system for society. A basic assumption of this view is that social systems perform functions that serve individuals as well as society. Role specialization is a focus of this theory: role structures are analyzed as being essential to function. The analysis of the family would focus on performance of its essential roles; one specialized role is child socialization. The role structure is defined as "who does what" to maintain the family and its health.

The structure of a system and subsystems is assessed in relation to role structure, value systems, communication patterns, and power structure. Family structure (the number and types of persons available to perform tasks/roles) is analyzed in relation to function. Family functions include the following: (1) the affective function, (2) socialization, (3) reproduction, (4) coping or the maintenance of order and stability, and (5) economic function. The "affective function" refers to meeting the psychologic needs of the family members for love and belonging. "Socialization" and "reproduction" refer to the function of the family in relation to society. The family is responsible for developing new members of society so that they are productive citizens. The "coping function" concerns the family's responsibility for order within itself and within the community, or society. The steady increase in violent crimes is viewed by most of society as a result of family breakdown or lack of family values. Finally, the "economic function" of the family system refers to the family's responsibility for providing adequate food, shelter, and other necessities.

The advantage of the structural-functional approach is that it provides a meaningful way of studying the family as a system and the linkages between the family and other institutions in society. It provides a comprehensive framework for the focus on the dynamics of the family, its members, and the forces in society that may affect the family. However, the approach gives the family a heavy responsibility for society's work. An increasing number of families are no longer able to provide economically for their members. Unemployment is a reality in a time when college graduates often cannot find work in their fields. It may be unrealistic, in today's world, to expect families to provide the same kind of functions for society that they did in previous generations. Communities may need to assist families to a greater degree than ever before.

Social Exchange Theory

Social exchange theory has been used to examine money, property, labor, and relationships. Persons are viewed by analyzing their choices as rewards, costs, and equity in relation to societal norms and family roles. In a marriage, the cost of "peacekeeping" has typically belonged to the woman, particularly if she did not work outside the home; the man's income and their home have been viewed as her rewards by society. This theory focuses on the relationship of the individual to society more than on the family as a unit. Social exchange theory was originally developed by drawing on works in which kinship was studied as social exchange (Levi-Strauss, 1976). Elements of social exchange theory are also used to argue for public policy (Scanzoni, 1983). In other words, behaviors are viewed as a balance of rewards and costs of differing values. Key concepts include choice, power differentials, reciprocity, conflict, obligation, and equality. In some families, the breadwinner has the financial power and may feel fewer obligations for household tasks. The family uses its resources to negotiate within family roles. For example, if the mother is the primary income provider, she may expect the father to assume the role of caregiver for the children. By using this model, the nurse can examine family behavior in terms of the rewards and costs among family members. Breadwinners may use their power to influence other members to contribute to equity in the unit. Because of its relatively narrow focus, social exchange theory is infrequently used in family nursing. This view fails to explain complex family dynamics, such as child abuse and neglect or other types of family violence. Factors in society, such as lack of day care for children, may play a key role in contributing to stress within the family. The analysis of family must inevitably include the role of community and society.

Interactional Frameworks

Interactional frameworks are narrowly focused, solely on interactions among and meanings of persons within the family unit. Norms are regarded as social creations and, thus, are contingent on the social milieu and situation. In farm families, grown children may be expected to stay on the farm and, as they mature, to assume a greater proportion of the work. Symbolic interactionism (Mead, 1934) stresses the symbolic meanings, so that the social reality, the self, and the family are seen as products of the interactions. The social influence on the symbolic environment is generally emphasized in analyzing the individual's ability to interpret events. Roles are integrated sets of social norms distinguished from individual normative behavior in other roles (Burr et al, 1979). Farm wives are expected to maintain the home and care for children and, in addition, to assist with farm work during harvest. An outsider may view the lack of communication in farm families as problematic without understanding the meaning that family members give to their lives. When such families are waiting for rain or conditions for growth, normal conversation is silenced.

Family interaction and communication patterns can be analyzed according to the meaning the members give to interactions. Nurses in the mental health field often use interactional frameworks to help families examine their dynamics. However, the role of society is not included in this framework.

Developmental Frameworks

The developmental, or family life-cycle, approach evolved from the theories already mentioned in com-

TABLE 2-1
Assessing Family Developmental Task Mastery

Tasks Common to All Developmental Stages	Assessment Factors	Nursing Interventions to Facilitate Coping
Maintaining family internal system	Communication and interaction that reflect family goals/values Respect for members' and family's needs by each member Decision making/problem solving adequate to manage crises and adapt to necessary developmental changes Mutual age-appropriate attempts by members to gratify needs and maintain family harmony Consideration of situational variables, such as fatigue, being busy, illness, and of constant variables of personality, age and experience, resources available	Be a role model of effective communication patterns Demonstrate respect for members Provide anticipatory guidance regarding age-related and situation-related needs Help members interpret feedback from members, and problem solve to make changes Provide or refer for counseling if dysfunction persists
Meeting physical needs	Basic necessities (food, clothing, shelter, health care) provided Resources recognized and used appropriately	Reinforce attempts and successes in providing basic needs Help family identify and obtain access to helpful resources
Integrating family member and group into external environment	Amount and type of involvement by each member and by family unit in church, school, work force, health care facilities, community activities Any isolated member(s) Family leisure activity patterns Extended family relationships Friendships outside family membership	Help family problem solve in identification of barriers to positive interaction with the external world Help family identify resources to aid in making opportunities for socialization outside the family and as a family within the community Reinforce attempts at external socialization
Helping members meet individual developmental tasks	How family adjusts when member moves from one developmental stage to another Degree of consistent nurturing for each member; any member not receiving/not offering nurturance; protective behavior displaced in proportion to member's abilities or need for autonomy Difficulty of toddlerhood and adolescence (seem most difficult for many families); both stages require a careful balance between nurturing and allowing autonomy Family identification of impact of developmental needs on family values, priorities, goals, relationships	Provide anticipatory guidance regarding developmental stages/tasks/needs; have family describe necessary changes to family priorities, relationships, goals Reinforce nurturing behaviors Demonstrate nurturing behaviors Help family identify support systems and resources to assist members in coping with changes required as children's developmental needs change and/or when complications in task accomplishment arise Provide or refer for counseling if dysfunctional behaviors persist

bination with theories of individual development. Critical role transitions of individuals, such as birth, retirement, and death of a spouse, are viewed as "causing" distinct change in family life patterns. Duvall and Hill's stage criteria reflect (1) changes in number of family members, (2) developmental stage of the oldest child, and finally, (3) retirement and death of one of the parents. The model is based on the assumption of a nuclear family that bears children and continues through stages until the death of the last surviving spouse (Duvall, 1977). Tasks common to all developmental stages are presented in Table 2-1. The stage concept allows the nurse to address certain aspects of health promotion and child health that may be common to all families, despite class, ethnic, or other differences. The "family life cycle" is a sequence of developmental tasks conceptualized according to the norms of the nuclear family model. The concepts of role performance, function of reproduction and socialization, and social control are used to describe the developmental tasks. Social control refers to the responsibility of the family to keep its members functioning within the norms set by society. Juvenile delinquency is viewed as a problem in which the family has failed to adequately achieve the developmental task of social control.

Developmental concepts predict movement to a higher level of functioning with transitional periods from one phase to the next. Normative and unexpected transitions create disorganization with subsequent resolution and progress to a higher level of functioning (Gillis et al, 1989). Successful achievement on a developmental task at one period is viewed as predictive of good achievement on similar transitions at subsequent periods. The problems in using family developmental theory are significant. Societal trends are such that emphasis on individual life-span issues may not fit with the model of the family lifestyle (Holman & Burr, 1980). For example, most mothers are now employed and can expect to live longer than 30 years after the last child leaves home (Skolnick, 1991). Family development issues are very different for couples without children, persons who divorce, women who have their first child earlier or later in life, families of gay persons, and blended families (Macklin, 1980). Families are unique in their capacity for change and development, and nurses must recognize that families may arrive at similar developmental levels through different processes (Gillis et al, 1989). Each family defines its own health uniquely. New family units form their family health "estate," which is a combination of health beliefs, values, behaviors, and interactions with social systems, such as the health care system (Bomar, 1990). "In addition to determining how families define their health, it is crucial for the health care professional to use a theoretical framework to understand, assess, and collaborate with families to improve or maintain their level of health" (Bomar, 1990, p 3).

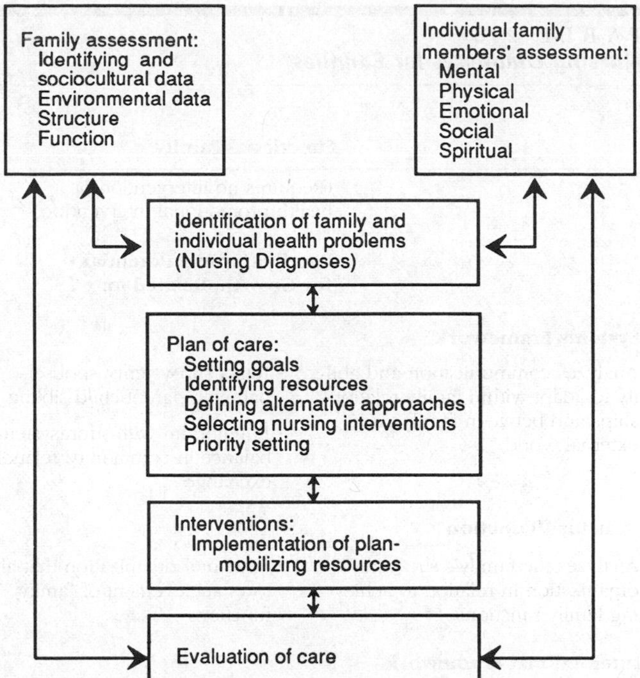

FIGURE 2-1. Steps in the family-centered nursing process. (From Friedman, M. [1992]. *Family nursing—Theory and assessment* (3rd ed.). Norwalk, CT: Appleton-Century-Crofts.)

Family-Centered Nursing Process

In family-centered nursing process, the nurse uses the same steps as in applying the nursing process to the individual (see Chapter 1). The difference is that the focus of the process is simultaneously the individual child and the family system. The duality makes the process more extensive and complex (Fig. 2-1). The critical point for the nurse is that family functioning cannot be determined from only one member; nor can a child be fully understood unless viewed within the context of the entire family.

Assessment. Assessment data come from as many sources as it is possible and feasible to include. The family is a highly complex system, and as many family members as possible (including youngest and oldest members) should be interviewed as age-appropriate. The nurse should realize that subjective appraisal is invaluable. Different members convey different information and do so at varying depths. Whenever possible, objective observation of the family's interaction in the home environment should incorporate both the *action* and the *feeling* levels. Additional information may be available from records, other team members, and referral sources.

Analysis. Analysis is ideally done with the family. Their involvement provides a useful learning opportunity for them to see themselves in an organized, objective fashion. Analysis should include identification of both individual member and family unit health states, family and member strengths and assets, and family and member deficits and limitations (Friedman, 1992). At a family level, nursing diagnoses can be derived from any of the many frameworks or available approaches indicated in Table 2-2.

Problems that involve at least two members (a subset) or the entire family are *family health problems.* There is evidence that a serious illness in one family member exerts a powerful influence on family health and that family behavior can influence individual health (Gillis et al, 1989). This presents a special challenge to pediatric nurses, because the illness of a child is likely to have a profound effect on the family. Identified real and potential problems should be assigned priorities from the family's perspective in order to achieve maximal effectiveness from interventions. Common problems in young families include

TABLE 2-2
Nursing Diagnoses for Families*

	Functional Family	Vulnerable Family: High Risk	Vulnerable Family: Actual
	(Requires no intervention or health promotional intervention)	(Requires preventive or health promotional nursing action)	(Requires resolutional, rehabilitative nursing actions)
	Family Coping: Potential for Growth, Related to:	**Altered Family Process (Actual/High Risk), Related to:**	
Systems Framework			
Analyzes communication and ability to adapt within family relationships and between family and external world	• Intact subsystems: spousal, parental, parent-child sibling • Equilibrium with suprasystem: balance in community/relational exchange	• Lack of intact subsystems: spousal, parental, parent-child, sibling • Disequilibrium with suprasystem: community/relational overinvestment; community/relational underinvestment or isolation	
Structure/Function			
Analyzes the family's structure or organization in relation to achieving family functions	• Structural organization that allows achievement of family functions	• Structural disturbance • Functional difficulties: shelter, communication, power	
Interactional Framework			
Analyzes how family members relate to each other, focusing on roles and communication	• Adaptive role transition • Role congruity or adaptive resolution of role incongruity • Open communication among members	• Role transition • Role incongruity • Communication disturbances	
Developmental Framework			
Analyzes family group adjustment at various life stages	• Congruent goal setting between members and family or family and external systems • Adequate knowledge regarding developmental tasks • Dependency-independence balance appropriate for family/member stage • Boundary maintenance that balances input exchange with external environment • Appropriate assimilation or adaptation to family task performance	• Conflicting goal setting between members and family or family and external systems • Lack of knowledge regarding developmental tasks • Inappropriate dependency or independence for family/member stage • Disturbance in boundary maintenance • Inappropriate assimilation or adaptation to family task performance	

* Utilizing NANDA categories.

abuse and violence, substance abuse, poverty, lack of day care for working families or those looking for work, and actual or potential health or environmental problems. Referral to appropriate community resources, including home care, should be made for any problems that need significant evaluation or ongoing intervention.

Planning. For change to be successfully implemented, mutual goal setting, based on diagnosis priorities, should take place. The nurse's responsibility is to see that goals (projected outcomes) are clearly stated in writing and are accepted by the family. Further, the nurse helps the family identify and mobilize its own resources (strengths and potentials of members, family group, and external support systems). The nurse also facilitates problem solving, by allowing the family members to talk through their situation and be full participants in the nursing process. Through this process the family develops its own plan toward deriving a workable approach to resolve problems that they care about. The following questions have been adapted from Friedman (1992) as key questions the nurse should consider in assisting the family's planning or problem solving:

- Will the proposed approach(es) foster child growth and development in the family, or are additional resources needed?
- What information does the family desire to have access to in order to build on their own resources?
- Are there adequate family and community resources available to carry out the plan?
- Can the plan be carried out with the available resources, or is there a need for "special" services from a voluntary agency, such as the local heart association or Parents Anonymous (child abuse)?

Once resources are identified and an approach selected, accountability is delineated, so that all involved know the nurse's responsibility, the responsibilities of the family group or its members, and what responsibilities rest elsewhere. The nurse will have to accept family decisions that may run counter to the advice given, but the family should not be rejected or support withdrawn because of the decision. Families always must select courses of action that meet their own needs (Table 2–3).

Implementing. The nurse's role during intervention can be seen as developmental, facilitative, or supplemental in nature (Friedman, 1992). Developmental roles involve teaching the family and supporting their own self-care and self-help activities, including referrals for social support through community groups. The facilitative role is necessary when the family needs assistance in removing barriers to care. These needs are generally economic, social, or related to transportation.

Implementing financial interventions may have to be performed by the nurse in situations in which no social worker is available. The nurse must be aware of the financial implications of health care in order to make appropriate referrals. The supplemental role may be necessary when the family is unable to do alone what is required for goal achievement. Family interventions that involve "doing for" should be performed only on the request of the family. For example, a teen-age parent may need to apply for Medicaid for herself and the baby but may find it too difficult to call for the appointment. The nurse can sit with this parent and demonstrate how to make the call. Any intervention that fosters overdependence will inevitably stifle the family's growth, and the nurse should be aware of what is happening to the family throughout the process.

Evaluating. Evaluation is ongoing and addresses the entire family. Interventions designed to help families achieve their goals must be evaluated in terms of the individuals and the family as a whole. Barriers to helping families achieve goals need to be assessed from a broad perspective. Lack of collaboration by health care providers, limited information, and typical family patterns for resolving problems may be involved. For example, the family with a chronically ill child may be viewed as being noncompliant with the medication regimen. In reality, reasons for failure to take medication are numerous and include financial limitations, lack of understanding, side effects of the medication, other family problems, and a multitude of other reasons. In order to improve the health of families, it is important to address health needs in all types of families, such as single-parent, poor, and multiproblem families. Specific nursing roles to assist families are discussed later in this chapter in the section on primary nursing roles.

TABLE 2-3
Family Involvement According to Child's Health Status

Child's Health Status	Family Involvement
Health Promotion and Illness Prevention	Wellness strategies of the child require involvement of family system as a whole: • Improvement in entire family lifestyle may be necessary • Wellness strategy may induce conflict because of impact on family as unit • Child's self-view and body image as either healthy and active or sickly and frail is learned in family context
Symptom Experience Stage	Family assesses child's health behavior and provides basic definition of health and illness: • Interprets symptoms by conveying to child the seriousness of symptoms, possible causes, significance, and degree of concern or attention to be given to symptoms • Protects child from health hazards to extent family unit is aware of such hazards • Family disorganization may be cause of symptoms
Care-Seeking Stage	Family decides when ailing child is really sick and needs help Family decides where child's illness should be treated (home, clinic, hospital)
Medical Contact Stage	Family serves as primary referral agent, deciding what type of intervention should be sought
Dependent Patient Stage	Family defines the patient role (to what degree advice will be followed) and patient role behaviors (how soon patient is expected to recover), ranging from making no demands on patient to forcing a prompt recovery
Rehabilitation Stage	Family determines degree of support for child's convalescence or rehabilitation; when the person's condition is serious or the person is a pivotal or crucial family member, the impact on family is more pronounced

Based on Friedman, M. (1992). Family nursing theory and assessment (3rd ed.). Norwalk, CT: Appleton-Century-Crofts.

Family Health Assessment

Just as there are several frameworks from which family assessment can be approached, a multitude of tools are available as guides to achieving that assessment. The nurse should become familiar with several and select one or more, according to the philosophy of practice and the theory that the nurse is using. In addition, assessment guides should be suited to the purpose for which the assessment is being conducted, the depth of knowledge needed, and the availability of family members. The tools presented in this chapter represent only a few of the many available. Speer and Sachs (1985) reviewed nine family assessment tools and evaluated them on ease of administration and scoring, clinical relevance, and type of family situation in which they were appropriate.

Basic Assumptions

There are several basic assumptions about families that drive family assessment and family nursing. Leahy and Wright (1988) noted the importance of the *family's* perception of its own reality. Different family members may have differing views of the truth, and the nurse must be careful to encourage the family to understand and discuss differences within the family. In addition, understanding the problem does not, by itself, lead to change. Most important, "psychosocial problems or symptoms may serve a positive family function" (Leahy & Wright, 1988, p 23). Not all problems can or should be "fixed." Finally, families must be full participants in their own care. This is increasingly recognized in health care institutions in which parents are actively involved in caring for premature infants and acutely ill children.

Assessment Process

The family assessment process itself becomes an intervention if the entire family is included as team members. As the family focuses on itself, awareness of the family's situation is enhanced. Members see their problems within a broader perspective as they identify strengths and limitations in meeting needs and coping with crises. As roles, relationships, and functions are explored within the family, members may recognize the value of interdependent responses and cooperation in problem solving. The assessment process may lead to problem solving behaviors that increase the family's capacity to set goals for themselves and for the family. It is the family's view of its own problems that necessarily drives any nursing care plan.

Assessment information may be gained through interviewing and questioning, through observing parent-child interactions, and by carefully listening to family members' comments as well as attending to what is not said. A clear picture of the family environment necessitates a visit to the home, if this is feasible in the nurse-family relationship (community health nurse, family nurse practitioner, school nurse, hospital nurse visiting a client before admission to or discharge from the hospital), or feedback from other professionals who have visited the home (social worker, mental health worker). Direct family contact is essential, although *not all* family members need to participate in the dialogue. The nurse should get a "sense" of the family from discussion with the major caregivers.

Family interviewing is a necessary skill in assessing and intervening with families. Ideally, a family assessment covers all members within the family group, including young children. At a minimum, the assessment should include the child and primary caregivers. The fullest assessment is completed entirely within the child's home environment. There the nurse can note such factors as environment, sociocultural variables, and interaction patterns of family members. These observations must be documented as assessed, as must all other components of the data base (Table 2–4).

A home visit may not be possible or desirable in every circumstance. For most children's short-term hospital stays, the family assessment can be done during history taking at admission, during observation of child and family throughout the hospital visit, and during the discharge planning procedure. However, all high-risk infants and children deserve a home visit and comprehensive family assessment prior to discharge. Low birthweight babies and children hospitalized for lead poisoning or problems with nutrition are high-risk individuals. Too frequently, infants are dis-

TABLE 2–4
Brief Family Overview

Observe and describe home and environment

Observe and describe significant sociocultural influences

Observe family members and interaction patterns

Determine family's perception of

- Child
- Goals for child/family
- Problems
- Attempted solutions
- Emotional reactions to possible solutions (i.e., special education)
- Coping responses

Assess

- Growth and development
- Health history
- Systems (skin, cardiorespiratory, gastrointestinal, musculoskeletal, neurologic)
- Child's coping responses

Review family history

- Family composition (age, sex, siblings, age of parents, extended family)
- Family members' current/previous health status
- Parent's education and work experience
- Family history milestones

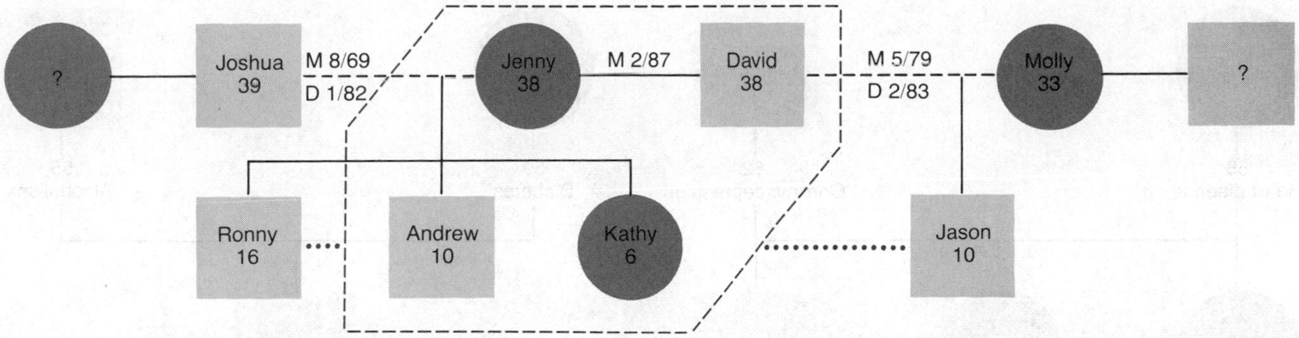

FIGURE 2-2. Example of a blended family genogram.
Key:
Vertical line indicates offspring
Circle indicates female
Square indicates male
Triangle indicates sex unknown
Circle and square connected by solid line horizontally is a marital pair
Circle and square connected by broken line horizontally is a divorced pair
M and date indicates date of marriage
D and date indicates date of divorce
Broken line encompassing several circles/squares indicates members who constitute household
Dotted line indicates persons who are occasional members of household
Types of data that can be included inside circles and squares, providing information about the individual the symbol represents, are the following:
Name
Age or birthdate
Death date (indicated by d. and followed by date of death)
Place of birth
Occupation
Health problem or cause of death (* placed after disease or accident when cause of death)
Any other data relevant to the assessment.

charged into environments that cannot support their needs. For example, an infant on an apnea monitor requires electricity and adequate electrical outlets.

Guides and Assessment Tools

Tables 2–1 through 2–7 and Figures 2–1 through 2–5 are examples of the major family assessment tools that may be used to gather data about family relationships, environment, development, and satisfaction with family functioning. Any tool is meant to be a guide for systematic data collection. However, the family needs and priorities should determine the focus of the assessment. For example, families having difficulty obtaining needed health care for their child may require concentrated assessment of the health care function and less attention given to socialization or communication patterns. Assessment data should be analyzed according to the theoretical framework of the nurse and should include family strengths and the goals perceived by the family.

Family genograms are presented in Figures 2–2 and 2–3 and provide a framework to help the nurse and family examine the family structure and history of certain diseases. The family genogram may be used to identify risk factors related to the child's health or to provide epidemiologic information of a communicable or genetic trait. The genogram is usually diagrammed by nurses while they interview family members during history taking, but it is limited to the extent of each family's knowledge and recall of disease over time. This approach can be used for specific diseases, including mental health problems and alcoholism. A family ecomap of external relationships is illustrated in Figure 2–4. This tool reveals the relationship of a family unit to its external environment. This assessment is made by interview, observation, and collaboration with other agencies involved with the family. It is particularly valuable in ascertaining the strengths of family networks and what resources, if any, the family already has to draw on during crisis or distress. It can also reflect whether those resources are supportive or disruptive to the family. Knowledge of resources is particularly valuable if a child is diagnosed as having a chronic health problem or terminal illness, or when home care is being considered.

A Comprehensive Guide to Assess Family Function is presented in Table 2–5. A family assessment guide is intended to highlight important areas of family life

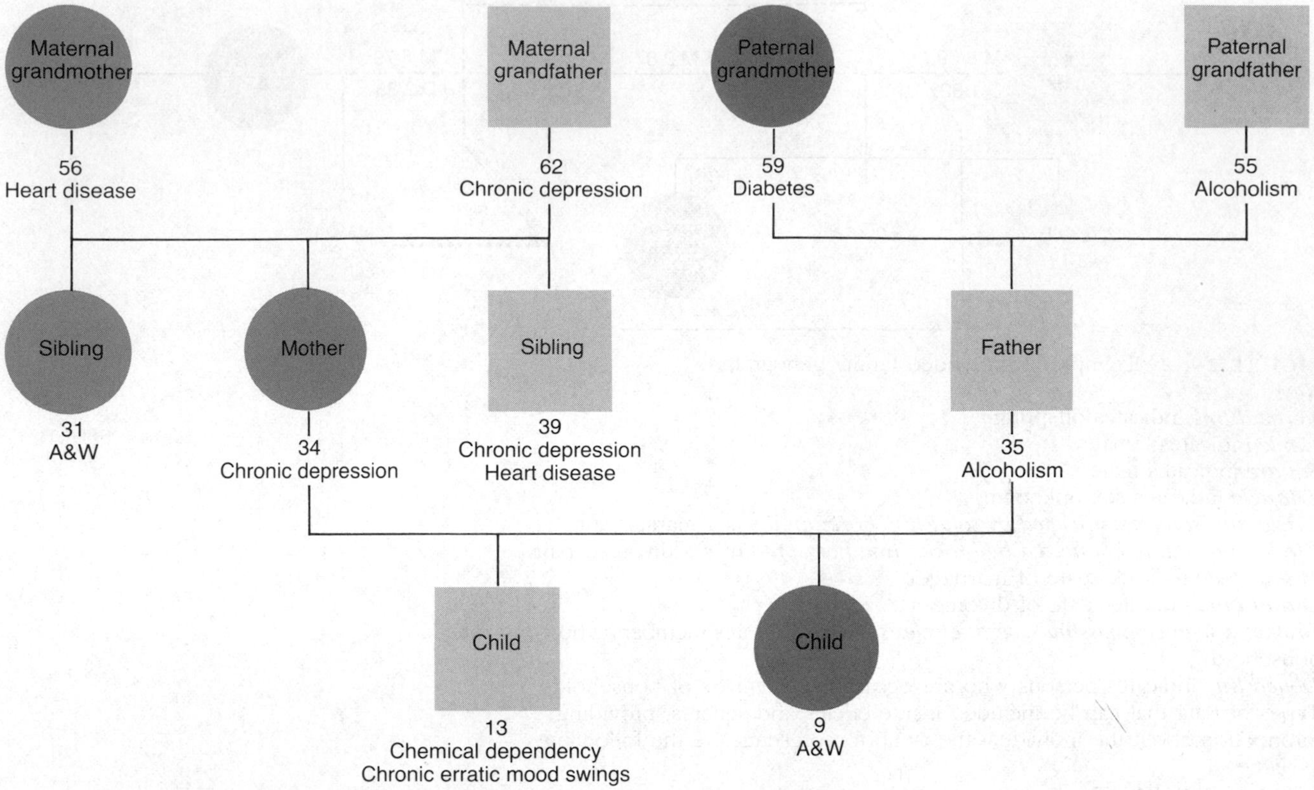

FIGURE 2-3. Family genogram of disease patterns. See Figure 2–2 for a definition of symbols. *A&W* indicates alive and well, in good health. An *arrow* indicates a specific client if the nurse is doing the assessment with regard to a particular family member. Twins are indicated by a *line joining the boxes or circles*.

and family health. The assessment guide should not serve as the interview guide. In other words, the nurse should review the guide *prior* to the visit to the family, so that the dialogue can focus on the family's concerns and priorities. The numbers of areas assessed, and to what depth, will be guided by the circumstances and purpose of the assessment. The nurse uses other assessments, those of other health professionals or agencies who have already seen the family, as a part of the total data base.

Smilkstein's Family APGAR (1984) is reproduced in Figure 2–5. This is a tool that can quickly measure a family's satisfaction with its general state of functioning and is referred to as the family's APGAR (*a*daptation, *p*artnership, *g*rowth, *a*ffection, *r*esolve). The questionnaire can be used to measure the APGAR of subsystem relationship functioning (i.e., husband-wife, parent[s]-child, sibling-sibling) as well as satisfaction with total family functioning. The questionnaire may be filled out by each family member or completed by the family collectively through the process of consensus, under the nurse's direction. The tool, of course, is not useful for obtaining very young children's input. It quickly presents a picture of the family's overall satisfaction, from which the nurse can identify areas needing more thorough assessment, or it can offer clues about risk when abuse or emotional or behavioral illness is suspected. It is also of obvious relevance when home care is being considered. If a family is already demonstrating coping problems, more intensive home care may be needed for management of a child's health state. However, a single APGAR is not meaningful. Families should participate in analysis of the APGAR in order to provide a perspective on satisfaction with family life over time. All families experience times of better functioning and more difficult periods; therefore, periodic reassessments are indicated for families that have regular contact with the nurse over time.

Otto's Family Assessment Criteria Check List, presented in Table 2–6, has 13 assessment criteria that contribute to family unity and the development of family potential. The concept of this check list is similar to Smilkstein's (1984) Family APGAR questionnaire, in that it gives the nurse a basis for determining family patterns that may need intervention. The nurse marks the check list on the basis of an assessment of each of the criteria. By using the assessment data, the nurse and health care team can apply principles of change to increase support and reinforce family strengths or to eliminate or correct family limitations. A combination of these may be needed to produce changes in knowledge, attitudes, or practices that will result in problem prevention or resolution that are necessary to foster healthier adaptation of the family unit and its members. Recognition of family strengths is imperative in order to identify family resources so as to prevent or resolve problems, as well as to plan realistic interventions. Likewise, acknowledging family limitations guides nursing diagnoses by identifying both real and potential problems. Family limitations can be seen in illness-producing, adaptation-disrupting behaviors. Families recognize their own limitations and should be full participants in establishing realistic boundaries for goal setting.

Family Goals and Values

Family goals and values must be considered on two levels: (1) goals and values of the unit and (2) the goals of each individual family member. The goals of a family satisfy the affiliation needs of each member and maintain family cohesiveness. When individual goals conflict with those of the family, there may be conflict. For example, teen-agers may find that their use of the telephone or car is viewed as excessive by other family members. Each family has individual goals and values. In some families, eating together is important for family cohesiveness. In others, family members may come home to eat, or they may not, according to their own needs and the needs of the family. How families spend their time together is extremely variable.

Nurses need to recognize that their own values, derived from their families, influence encounters with any group. The family is no exception. Nurses must be aware that their values may be communicated verbally and nonverbally to the family and can become embedded in the relationship. It is therefore important to recognize those values and to clarify them, as nurses will always encounter families whose beliefs, values, and attitudes are different from their own.

Families at Risk/Special Intervention

Family Health

The classic study of energized families (Pratt, 1976) found that the healthy family was one in which the following existed: (1) regular interaction among members, (2) active participation with the community, (3)

(Continued on Page 56)

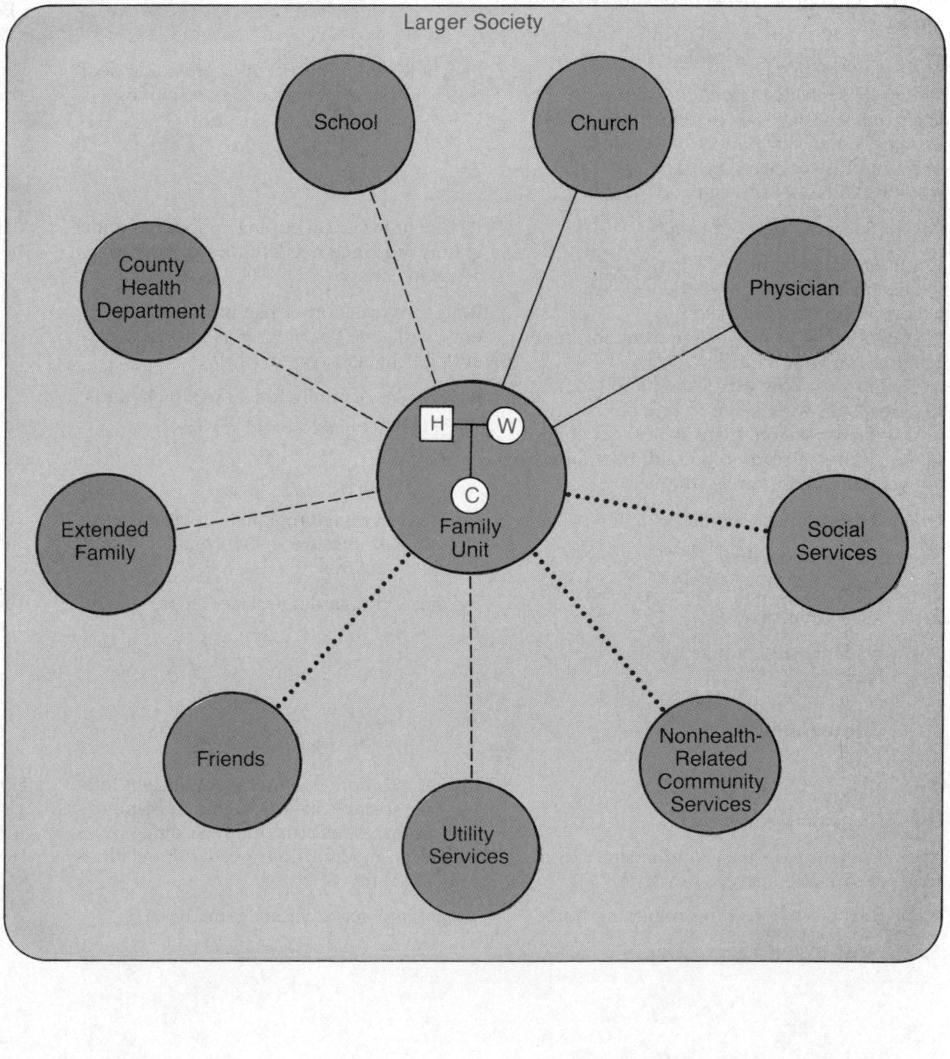

FIGURE 2-4. Family ecomap of external relationships. Pictured here are but a few of the many that could be considered.
Key:
——— Strong, supportive, positive relationship
- - - - - - Erratic, conflicted relationship, sometimes supportive and sometimes disruptive
.... Negative, disruptive, or nonexistent relationship

TABLE 2-5
A Comprehensive Guide to Assess Family Function

Elements of Assessment	Reasons or Uses	Special Considerations
Identifying Data		
Family Composition Names, birth order, occupation, education	Familiarity with family, communication of interest in whole family	The importance here is whether the family lifestyle permits health promotion and developmental nurturance of children
Risk Potential • Single parent • Teen parent • Impoverished, homeless	Capsule view of family in relation to contemporary organizational structures	
Cultural/Ethnic or Religious Orientation • Identity • Degree involved in identification, acculturation (replication in dominant culture of one's beliefs, values, practices	Understanding of family behavior, value system, perceived functions, and the priority of those functions	Must evaluate each family member, as acculturation may differ Important to assess in relation to potential family function, especially when a family has been transplanted into another cultural setting
Social Class Status Occupational status, income level/expenditures, educational level	Determination of strongest influence on lifestyle, structure/function, characteristics, and association with external environment	Variations result from different conditions of and demands placed on family by society at large
Adequacy of financial resources: *Adequate:* solely personal resources used *Marginal:* unemployment and general relief aid *Inadequate:* solely from general relief, welfare, or self, but so low cannot supply basics	Insight into resources available, values stressed, level of teaching appropriate, what are perceived as problems and priority placed on them	Greatest overall influence on family life; influences: • Early socialization • Role expectations • Values stressed • Behavior considered positive or negative • World experiences of members
Allocation adequacy: *Adequate:* realistic budget and spending *Marginal:* conflict over management of resources, unrealistic budget/expenditures *Poor:* Impulsive spending, excessive debts resulting in family's basic needs unmet	Insight regarding function of providing necessary physical and economic resources	Poor money management alone does not mean child's basic welfare is endangered
Developmental History of Family Common and unique: Each person's past experiences—how accomplished or perceived Own family of origin—present and past relationship with them Begin with how established and family of origin's responses, life in original family and ordinal position, plans when first child coming, impact/plan each child, how family spends time, daily family routines	Picture of historical coping, amount of anticipatory guidance needed, idea of how to adapt to change Better appreciation of parents during parents' formative years; insights into their parenting behaviors, potential risks Assessment of family function, which tends to be generationally perpetuated	Make sure that family is open to exploring the past and that nurse's purpose is meaningful
Family Recreational Activities Activities done together How family relaxes: diversion, self-development, social participation Subsystem activities: adults, parent-child, sibling-sibling	Information regarding family cohesiveness and stability, resources, involvement of parents with children Information regarding relationships	There is a high positive relationship between number of leisure time factors and family health There is positive correlation between outdoor recreation and family solidarity
Environmental Data		
Housing Adequacy of space, setting State of repair, adequacy, and facilities available for sanitation, sleep, privacy	Insight into home environment; insight into possible social isolation, access to community resources; information regarding environmental modifications needed in relation to home care	Home visit is best approach Family behaves most naturally at home Home has psychologic effects; influences self-perception and life satisfaction; illness-related stressors and motivation
Family's subjective feelings regarding home Safety; lead exposure	Insight into space, lifestyle, interests	

TABLE 2-5
A *Comprehensive Guide to Assess Family Function* *(Continued)*

Elements of Assessment	Reasons or Uses	Special Considerations
Neighborhood and Community Association and Interaction	Insight into family exchange with outer environment; degree of homogeneity with neighbors; level of awareness family has of community resources; degree they seek; degree of isolation/security	Homogeneity more influential than proximity in family friendships
Length of residence—degree of geographic mobility		*Urban* more impersonal; *rural* more personal
Condition of structures: house, streets, sanitation, security/safety		
Demographic characteristics: social/ethnic characteristics, occupancy, density		
Resources available for basic physical/social needs: who uses what, how often, knowledge of resources		
Family attitudes/satisfaction regarding community		
Social Support Systems	Degree of isolation	Numerous research studies have identified an association between isolation and violent/abusive behaviors
Family, friends, helping person ready to assist family	Resources to help family or share during crisis, coping, celebration	
Liabilities/relations with above; whether interactions are task-oriented or emotionally supportive		Lack of a support group is a common characteristic of multiproblem families
People with whom family interacts, and satisfaction with interaction		
Friendships established, frequency of contact		
What external resources does family have? Use? Know about? • Community based? • Formal professional services?		
Assessment questions: 1. Who has helped you when ____________________? 2. Whom would you get help from if ____________________?		
Communication Patterns		
Overt Openness and Clarity, Honesty	Evidence of acceptance of differences; permitting autonomy; fostering authenticity and self-growth; empathizing	Functional family uses communication to create and maintain mutually beneficial relationships
Can discuss personal and social issues		
Lack of total agreement not a catastrophe	This section is particularly important to assessment of vulnerable families	Cultural norms influence openness of communication in relation to modesty, privacy, sexual roles
Each listens		
Can stay focused on one issue		
Affective Communication (Physical and Verbal)	Evidence of fulfillment of family members' affectional needs and satisfying of affectional responsibility of family unit; degree of self-centeredness of members	Methods of appropriate expression are culturally defined
Express caring, spontaneity, positiveness		Degree of verbal behavior is also culturally defined
Focus on various members' needs		
Power Hierarchy and Family Rules	Insight into degree of relative cooperation vs. coercion; where decisions are made; who is consulted for planning interventions	Power relationships are culturally influenced
Is distribution of power based on family members' developmental needs and ability, resources of members?		
Use of cooperative vs. coercive statements		
Tone used in conversation		
Conflict Resolution	Insight into family's ability to reach consensus and ability to problem solve, manage conflict	
Open discussion with problem solving interventions evolved from group discussion employed		

Table continued on following page

TABLE 2-5
A Comprehensive Guide to Assess Family Function *(Continued)*

Elements of Assessment	Reasons or Uses	Special Considerations
Appropriate use of authority to make decisions as necessary		
Family Power Structure	Insight into family's underlying value system	Contemporary family changes have steadily improved sharing of decision making (a measure of family power and individual power)
Who makes what kinds of decisions regarding • Finances • Social plans • Major decisions, e.g., job changes, residence change • Childrearing?	Understanding of family interpersonal relations and family relations with health professionals and outside agencies Knowledge and appreciation critical to provide effective care, especially in areas of health regimen compliance and motivation to seek/use health services; knowledge of who in family to consult and acknowledge to obtain family cooperation with health care or other diagnosis-related issues	Best way to assess is combined observation of marital, parent-child, sibling, and family subgroup interactions, coupled with self-reporting by all members if possible
What is the approach to decision making: consensus; accommodation (bargaining, compromising, coercion); de facto, i.e., no decision making?	Insight into how family makes decisions	
Who makes decisions and how?	Insight into how authority and power of individuals in family are derived	Power and authority are not always reflected in same individual; a person can have power but not receive the recognized authority to employ it; conversely, a person in authority may not employ the associated power
Are there any intermediaries (go-betweens) in the family communication network?		Cultural differences will exist relative to how power is derived
Who enforces/implements decisions once made?	Important information for nurse relative to whom to work with once decision is made to accept interventions prescribed	Power and authority in family are frequently role assigned
Where does the family rest on the family power continuum? If dominance, who is the dominant person? To find this out, a good question is "Who usually has the last say about important family issues?" or "Who runs the family?" or "Who wins if there is disagreement?"		
Are members satisfied with the present power structure: "Are you satisfied with how decisions are made and with who makes them?"	Insight into conflicts or confusion children may experience in home, causing mental stress and physical illness	
Family Role Structure Are formal positions and roles fulfilled?	Determination of family strengths and resources necessary to plan interventions Determination of whether role changes or problems exist, as these can create substantial disequilibrium and tension within family, compromising family and individual members' level of wellness. To understand roles/relationships of child within family and responsibility assumed by each parent in child care Important component of assessment when family dysfunction is suspected or demonstrated (see discussion under Assessing Dysfunction in this chapter)	Important for teaching and therapy purposes; use as information/demonstration of role to family in therapy or teaching in order to determine support, help or counseling needed and to assist members in adapting to new roles Gives evidence of any role strain, conflict, or confusion Cannot assume certain roles accompany certain positions as this is very individual in families, especially in contemporary society Applicable to assessment of interactional framework described earlier in this chapter
Are family members satisfied with who holds each role and with the way they carry out the role?		

TABLE 2-5
A Comprehensive Guide to Assess Family Function *(Continued)*

Elements of Assessment	Reasons or Uses	Special Considerations
Is there flexibility in roles where needed?	Insight into adaptive quality of family relationships and ability of members to collaborate and adjust during crisis (e.g., during illness of a member)—especially important to nurse dealing with situations that add stress to roles and relationships, such as terminal illness of a child	A strong social class and cultural impact on roles exists; the nurse needs to be acquainted with social class and culture of family to determine whether role behaviors and role assignments are appropriate; critical issue, however, is member satisfaction with roles and role performance
What informal or covert roles exist in the family, who plays them, and how frequently?	Insight into adequacy and character of subsystem dyad relationships	Need to determine whether the informal role, if it exists, is permanently assigned one member or is transferred
Are these covert roles consistent with the formal roles family members hold? Are they appropriate to the age, competency, and personality of individual members?	Insight into emotional climate/needs of family and its members as these roles are played out to meet those emotional needs	
What purpose does each covert role serve?		
Are any members labeled, thereby encouraging self-fulfilling prophecy behavior?		If informal role assumed as a result of labeling (i.e., self-fulfilling prophecy), must ascertain if having negative effect and thus interfering with that and/or other members' healthy emotional development Informal roles are necessary to fulfill the integrative and adaptive requirements of a family group; these informal roles include • *Encourager:* draws out family members so they feel important • *Harmonizer:* mediator during conflict • *Intermediary:* censors and transmits information between two persons with blocked communication; confidant • *Initiator:* creative, encourages problem-solving ideas • *Compromiser:* yields in conflict to resolve it • *Blocker:* negative, illogical • *Follower:* passive cooperation, serves as audience in family interaction • *Dominator:* tries to assert authority by manipulating and flaunting of member with power • *Recognition seeker:* strives to be center of attention • *Martyr:* sacrifices for family's sake continually • *Stone face:* lectures continually on "right" way to do things • *Pal:* playmate to family • *Self-indulger:* stays peripheral to family interaction, doing own thing These informal roles are learned through role models, the emotional responses the behavior receives, imitation of adults (usually selects ones comfortable to age and personality to imitate) Member may accept role to fill a vacuum not being filled by members in the formal roles
In parents' early lives, who were role models of parenting and adult relationship?	Information useful to help family members see how past models influence their present expectations and behavior Important assessment when role problems exist	

Table continued on following page

TABLE 2-5
A *Comprehensive Guide to Assess Family Function* (*Continued*)

Elements of Assessment	Reasons or Uses	Special Considerations
Family Values		
Compare family values with those of the dominant American culture (or of the specific ethnic culture if assessor is knowledgeable of these)	Degree of conformity or divergence is important in understanding family and family members' responses to health care delivery system and to establishing acceptable interventions	Values and norms cannot be observed directly but are inferred from observation and assessment of family roles, power structure, communication, as these are strongly influenced by underlying family values
Family Values Evaluate the following with family: • Value conflicts evident in family? • How do family values affect health status or family?		
Health issues created by value conflicts		
Affective Function		
Family Need—Response Patterns Awareness of each family member of needs (physical, emotional, mental) of other individuals in family	Understand degree of mutual nurturance and identity; where teaching, support, counseling are needed for one or more members	Fulfillment of this function is critical to healthy growth and development of family members and central base for formation and continuation of family unit
Are each member's needs, differences, interests respected by other family members?	Important area to assess when family dysfunction is suspected or demonstrated. (See discussion of Relationship Disturbances under Assessing Dysfunction in this chapter)	
Are rights of parents and children recognized and valued?		
Are recognized needs of family members met by family? To what extent?		
Mutual Nurturance, Closeness, and Understanding How much do family members support each other?	Casefinding regarding intimacy problems in relationships	
How well do family members get along with each other? Expressions of affection evident?		
Who are resources for nurturance available to individual members during illness, rehabilitation?		
Are mutual understanding and bonding apparent as evidenced by empathetic statements, concern for other members' feelings and problems, interest in other members' experiences?		
Separateness and Connectedness How does family help members who want to be together and be cohesive?	Understanding impact of separation/loss on family unit and members	Family connectedness essential to development of sense of belonging
Opportunity for developing separateness encouraged appropriately?	Insight into inappropriate opportunity for mastery and freedom, over/underdependency	Age and development affect the degree of connectedness and separateness members need or feel—for example, the infant is very connected to the main caregiver and only gradually experiences separateness; conversely, the adolescent expends much energy developing separateness and focuses on connectedness mostly during particularly stressful times or during family rituals
Are behaviors indicative of enmeshment (subsystem boundaries are continually violated) present? In enmeshment members are too engrossed in each other. Family members speak for other members, not allowing them to speak for themselves, and there is supersensitivity when a member sends out messages for help		
Are behaviors indicating disengagement present, as demonstrated by • Insensitivity toward other family members • Underinvestment of members in each other		

TABLE 2-5
A Comprehensive Guide to Assess Family Function *(Continued)*

Elements of Assessment	Reasons or Uses	Special Considerations
• Rigid or closed boundaries between subsystems • Little or no interest or concern for member's messages for assistance?		
Socialization Function		
What are family's childrearing practices in these areas: • Discipline • Rewards/punishment • Autonomy and independence • Giving and receiving love • Age appropriateness of behavior expected and training offered?	Casefinding in unhealthy parenting styles Understanding anticipatory guidance needed and approach to be taken in teaching and other socialization-related interventions Important assessment when child abuse is suspected	Nurse must be aware of own attitudes/biases and not interject them into the assessment or analysis process; must also evaluate reasonableness of own expectations for parents and children; good balancing question for assessment is "How functional is this family's approach to socialization for them in their own situation?"; be aware of compliance expectations in regard to teaching—was teaching realistic or ideal?
Are family's childrearing practices realistic and adaptive for their situation?	Helps nurse temper the "idealistic with the realistic" in planning interventions	
Who assumes responsibility for child care and socialization?; if shared, how is that managed—is the message to children consistent?	Knowing who to address about anticipatory guidance and teaching regarding parenting	
How are children regarded in family—what cultural beliefs are apparent in childrearing approach?	Essential for planning realistic interventions in relation to the child to enhance compliance	
Health Care Function		
How does family decide who's sick? Clues used? Who decides? Family's general level of knowledge regarding health, disease, hazards to health? Can family observe and report significant symptoms and changes? To what health problems does family perceive they are vulnerable or susceptible and what do they think they can do to reduce that risk? Do they carry these actions out? Adequacy of family practices (age appropriate) in health promotion: • *Diet:* The function of mealtime for the family; adequacy of diet; shopping practices; adequacy of storage/refrigeration; way food is prepared; who is responsible for planning, shopping, preparing meals? • *Sleep:* Age-appropriateness of habits; who decides when children go to bed; where they sleep; who naps; who decides how members relax? • *Exercise/recreation:* Family attitudes regarding regular exercise/recreation; daily work activities permit exercise?; how manage stress release? • *Family drug habits:* Use of alcohol, tobacco, caffeine, stimulants: by whom, how much; is use perceived as problem?; does use interfere with ADL performance?; use of over-the-counter and prescription drugs: how long keep/reuse?; properly labeled and stored safely?	Critical in determining when discharge from hospital is appropriate and in determining whether home care is an option (also how much teaching and supervision will be necessary); guideline for teaching Casefinding regarding health problems; actual/potential; epidemiologic information regarding contributing health practice deficits Insight into receptivity to teaching/counseling of health promoters and of how realistically family identifies needs Establishing reasonableness of health service prescribed/needed, information on resources available/used by family, especially in relation to acute/chronic care	Four primary components to health care function are *Lifestyle practices:* diet, sleep, exercise, self-care, drug habits, stress management *Environmental practices:* cleanliness, safety *Medical-based preventive practices:* physical examinations, eye/hearing examinations, immunizations, record-keeping *Dental health* (Refer to chapters in text that discuss these in detail)

Table continued on following page

TABLE 2-5
A Comprehensive Guide to Assess Family Function *(Continued)*

Elements of Assessment	Reasons or Uses	Special Considerations
Family Health Maintenance Measures		
Who are health leaders for family? Health decision makers? Amount of self-care assumed by members?		
Adequacy of environmental practices; exposure to pollutants (air, noise, water, etc.)		
Attention to hygiene and cleanliness		
Medically based preventive measures: age/sex/health state–appropriate actions; physical health surveillance and dental checkups; family attitudes regarding examination and immunization status; family medical history (genogram); attitudes toward health services; satisfaction regarding care and relationships with health care personnel (ecomap)		
What is the health care provider coverage for an emergency? If none, does family know nearest ER services available? Know how to call an ambulance service?		
What arrangements exist for paying for health services?		
Private or group plan, Medicare or Medicaid? An amount family must pay? Receive any free services? Knowledge of what services are covered by payment sources?		
Distance of health care services from home? Transportation to get to them? If public transportation, what problems, i.e., travel time or hourly service?		Cost affects use of health care
Family Coping Function		
What stressors are impinging (long and short-term) on family? What strengths does family perceive it has to counterbalance these? Is family able to make realistic, objective appraisal of situation and from there make decisions? Problem-solving abilities of each member? Typical family reaction to stress situation?	Insight to know what resources family has to deal with health issues, what can be enhanced and supported, what stressors can be decreased, how weaknesses can be diminished or reverted to strengths Knowledge of how well family does at helping itself achieve/maintain wellness	All families have strengths *and* weaknesses Constantly faced with need (from within and outside) to modify perceptions and lives, forcing families to cope or adapt
Functional Strategies		
Family group relies on each other more when under stress by providing greater organization and structure until the stressor is resolved, closing family boundaries temporarily?		
Use of sense of humor?		
Sharing of feelings, thoughts, actions?		
Strong subsystem support?		
Control management of problems?		
Draw on external resources for support?		

Families at Risk Information drawn from Leahy, K. M., Cobb, M. M., & Jones, M. C. (1982). *Community Health Family Inventories—Inventories in the National Survey of Families Across the Family Life Cycle*. St. Paul: University of Minnesota Press; Roberts, C., & Feetham, S. (1982, April). Assessing family functioning across three areas of relationships. *Nursing Research*, pp 231–235; Wright, L. M., & Leahy, M. (1984). *Nurses and families: A guide to family assessment and intervention*. Philadelphia: FA Davis. Speer, J., & Sachs, B. (1985, September–October). *Selecting the appropriate family assessment tool. Pediatric Nursing*, pp 349–355; and Friedman, M. (1992). *Family nursing theory and assessment* (3rd ed.). Norwalk, CT: Appleton-Century-Crofts.

The Family APGAR Questionnaire

	Almost always	Some of the time	Hardly ever
I am satisfied with the help that I receive from my family* when something is troubling me.	____	____	____
I am satisfied with the way my family discusses items of common interest and shares problem solving with me.	____	____	____
I find that my family accepts my wishes to take on new activities or make changes in my lifestyle.	____	____	____
I am satisfied with the way my family expresses affection and responds to my feelings such as anger, sorrow, and love.	____	____	____
I am satisfied with the way my family and I spend time together.	____	____	____

SCORING

Scoring: The patient checks one of three choices, which are scored as follows: 2 points for "Almost always," 1 point for "Some of the time," and 0 for "Hardly ever." The scores for each of the five questions are then totaled. A score of 7 to 10 suggests a highly functional family. A score of 4 to 6 suggests a moderately dysfunctional family. A score of 0 to 3 suggests a severely dysfunctional family.

* According to which member of the family is being interviewed, the nurse may substitute for the word "family" either spouse, significant other, parents, or children.

WHAT IS MEASURED

Adaptation	How resources are shared, or the member's satisfaction with the assistance received when family resources are needed.
Partnership	How decisions are shared, or the member's satisfaction with mutuality in family communication and problem solving.
Growth	How nurturing is shared, or the member's satisfaction with the freedom available within the family to change roles and attain physical and emotional growth or maturation.
Affection	How emotional experiences are shared, or the member's satisfaction with the intimacy and emotional interaction within the family.
Resolve	How time* is shared, or the member's satisfaction with the time commitment that has been made to the family by its members.

* Besides sharing time, family members usually have a commitment to share space and money. Because of its primacy, time was the only item included in the Family APGAR; however, the nurse who is concerned with family function will enlarge understanding of the family's resolve by requiring about family member's satisfaction with shared space and money.

FIGURE 2-5. The Family APGAR Questionnaire. (Adapted from Smilkstein, G. [1984, Fall]. The physician and family function assessment. *Family Systems Medicine,* 263–279.)

TABLE 2-6
Otto's Family Assessment Criteria Check List*

Assessment Criteria for Behaviors	Degree of Family Strength, Behavior Demonstrated as Family Strength: Most of the Time	Occasionally	Rarely
1. Able to meet members' physical, emotional, and spiritual needs.	______	______	______
2. Parents have joint responsibility and are comfortable in childrearing.	______	______	______
3. Effective communication among members.	______	______	______
4. Able to provide support, security, and encouragement to members.	______	______	______
5. Able to initiate and maintain growth-producing relationships within and outside the family.	______	______	______
6. Demonstrates responsible community relationships.	______	______	______
7. Home used as matrix for growth of adult and child members.	______	______	______
8. Able to help themselves and to accept help when needed.	______	______	______
9. Flexible in performing functions and roles.	______	______	______
10. Demonstrates mutual respect for individuality of each member.	______	______	______
11. Uses crisis as a means of growth.	______	______	______
12. Concern for family unit, loyalty, cooperation by members.	______	______	______
13. Flexible in initiating and using family strengths.	______	______	______

From Otto, H. (1968, September). Criteria for assessing family strength. *Family Process*, p 329.
*Ethnic and cultural variance must be considered.

a high degree of autonomy and individuality, and creative problem solving and active coping. Other studies have supported this general structure for healthy families (Curran, 1983; Hanson, 1991). Loveland-Cherry (1989) expanded on Smith's dimensions of health to describe four models of family health illustrated in Table 2–7. In the most basic clinical model, health is viewed as the absence of symptoms or lack of evidence of deterioration of the family system. The highest level of family health is the eudaimonistic (exuberant well-being) model, which promotes the view of maximal well-being and support within the unit and with the community throughout the family's life span.

Studies have typically examined single-parent families to observe pathology. In contrast, Hanson (1991) investigated characteristics of healthy single-parent families and found good physical and mental health of the parents and children. Differences in health of parents and children were related to gender and custody. For example, boys living with their mothers had the best overall health, whereas girls living with their fathers were least healthy. Fathers with sole custody of boys reported the highest mental health, whereas mothers with sole custody of boys had the lowest mental health. The study reveals important findings for clinical practice. Single-parent families are as variable as any other family type and may be more healthy or less healthy, depending on individual circumstances.

Vulnerable Families

It is important to identify families in need of support services. Families with special needs that may require nursing intervention are presented here. Most texts refer to these families as "dysfunctional families." It is

TABLE 2-7
Four Models of Family Health

Family Health: Clinical Model	Lack of evidence of physical, mental, or social disease or deterioration or dysfunction of family system
Family Health: Role-Performance Model	Ability of the family system to carry on family functions effectively and to achieve family developmental tasks
Family Health: Adaptive Model	Family patterns of interaction with the environment characterized by flexible, effective adaptation or ability to change and grow
Family Health: Eudaimonistic Model	Ongoing provision of resources, guidance, and support for realization of family's maximum well-being and potential throughout the family life span

From Bomar, P. J. (ed.). (1989). *Nurses and family health promotion*. Philadelphia: WB Saunders.

the perspective of this author that all families, at some time, exhibit behaviors that might be considered dysfunctional. These so-called dysfunctional patterns may be functional for a particular family in a particular circumstance. Conflict and crisis are natural occurrences in life, just as it is natural for families to resolve crises in their own way — they adapt and change. Families with specific problems that may place the child at risk for illness or injury (child abuse and neglect) need direct intervention and sensitivity. (See Chapter 28 for more information on child abuse and maltreatment.) The label "dysfunctional" tends to be overused and often does not illustrate the unique needs of families at risk. Therefore, the term "vulnerable families" is used to identify families likely to need special intervention.

Risk Factors

Risk factors for *all* families include multiple factors such as significant economic constraints (unemployment, interruption in AFDC payments), lack of social support, alcohol or drug problems, multiple family illness, and chronic illness or disability with a child. When families experience more than one problem at a time, they may become what is often termed "families in crisis." Families in crisis often experience disorganized daily living patterns (see "Health Care Function" section of Table 2–5 for assessment factors). Often food is not provided for family members, meals are not prepared, and sleeping arrangements are erratic or crowded, or the children's sleep needs are disregarded in favor of adult activities. Noise may disturb rest and sleep schedules of parents and children alike. General environmental disorder is visible. Children may have disturbed behavior, such as nightmares, somnambulism, compulsive solitary rocking or head banging, and despairing crying, whining, or wailing. These children may be ignored and their needs discounted by the parents.

These families are often disoriented as to time, space, sequence, and social obligations, which is evident to the nurse by their missing appointments or coming on the wrong day or at the wrong time, or both. They move frequently; they may give relatives' addresses and telephone numbers and cannot be located or reached by telephone. They are often trying to avoid creditors and bill collectors; they may view health professionals with suspicion.

Children in Jeopardy

The most extreme characteristic seen in multiproblem families is children in jeopardy. Infant morbidity and mortality are a national problem, and early casefinding is the responsibility of all nurses. Often, multiproblem families neglect or cannot manage the fulfillment of basic human needs for food, shelter, body protection from the elements; for security and protection from harm; for rest and stimulation; and for recognition and self-identity (see "Health Care Function" section of Table 2–5 for assessment factors). Nurses may be the crucial persons in the health care field who advocate the understanding of children. They can help break the chains of miscommunication that bind generations together with missed signals, anguish, and despair. Behaviors that the nurse may discover during child appraisal or from school referral, and that indicate the need for a family appraisal for risk status, are listed in Table 2–8.

TABLE 2-8
Behaviors of Children That Warrant a Comprehensive Family Assessment

Inattentiveness
Frequent tiredness, chronic fatigue
Poor nourishment (below 3rd percentile on growth chart)
Inappropriate attire for weather conditions
Few friendships, watches TV most of time
Unsupervised for large blocks of time or left in care of strangers
School difficulties/truancy
Difficulty recognizing or expressing own or others' feelings; marginal communication skills
Sadness or depression prevalent
Affection sought from unfamiliar or inappropriate sources
Timid or evasive toward adults, as if fearful of being struck or yelled at
Despairing cry or whining
Compulsive, repetitive behaviors, such as solitary rocking or head banging
Preoccupation (fear of loss, hunger, abandonment, harm)
Developmental delays
Poor physical health, frequent infections
Arriving early and staying late at school
Precocious sexual behavior
Behaviors indicative of drug or alcohol abuse
Aggressive destructive behaviors
Cruelty toward animals
Physical or behavioral signs of sexual abuse
Age-inappropriate behaviors or concerns
Persistent, excessive behaviors such as enuresis, encopresis, fire-setting

Data from Arent, R. (1980). *The child in stress: Strategies for support.* Littleton, CO: Arent and Associates; Friedman, M. (1992). *Family nursing theory and assessment* (3rd ed.). Norwalk, CT: Appleton-Century-Crofts; and Leatherland, J. (1986, November). Do you know child abuse when you see it? *RN,* 28–36.

Families at Risk

Specific categories of families known to be at risk for health problems are presented, with a focus on families, such as adolescent families and homeless families, who are likely to need special nursing care. Many families are young (adolescents), single, and homeless. In addition, families in crisis or multiproblem families are those with multiple social, economic, legal, and health problems. These families tend to be known for chronicity and repeated major crises (Kaplan, 1986). Health is a secondary concern that becomes primary only when it interferes with daily activities. These families may repeatedly miss appointments because of lack of child care or transportation (Lynch & Tiedje, 1991). Multiproblem families often "clash" with a health care system that is unresponsive to their needs. The middle-class value system of nurses is a major factor contributing to ineffectiveness with multiproblem families (Carey, 1989). Each family must be recognized within its unique environment and lifestyle. The most important thing that the nurse can do for a family in crisis is to attempt to understand what life may be like for that family. A receptive provider may make the difference between bringing the child back for the follow-up examination or "moving on" to yet another emergency room.

Identifying Families at Risk

A family can be considered "at risk" through consideration of a number of complex factors. The nurse must recognize that families may exhibit risk factors without being in crisis. Being at risk indicates a greater potential for disruption in family function; however, many families in risk categories cope very effectively and are able to meet the needs of members adequately. Obviously, the more risk factors a family accumulates, or the more severe or chronic a risk factor is, the greater is the likelihood of major crisis. Significant structural and environmental stressors are identified in Table 2–9.

There is a tendency to think of single-parent families as at risk for health and developmental problems. However, the single-parent family is one of the most common family forms, and single-parent status is not, by itself, a major risk factor. In fact, single-parent families are a diverse group and include never-married women with children (biologic or adopted), divorced persons (custodial fathers or mothers), widows and widowers with children, and married persons with an absent spouse. Studies reveal that divorce often means drastically lower (78 per cent) living standards for women, yet a 42 per cent gain in income for men (3000 cases reviewed) (Weitzman, 1985). Female single-parent families may be vulnerable, unless there are contributing adults who assist economically and help with socializing the children.

TABLE 2–9
Indicators of Families at Risk

Family Structure
Any family with inadequate supports
Teen-age family
Young family with several children close in age
Single parent with changing live-in partner
Family with peripheral spouse—viewed by spouse as unreliable, incompetent, tyrannical
Parental separation
Family Environment
Impoverished family
Multiproblem family
Immature parents
Member(s) with disabling, chronic, or fatal disease
Migrant or highly mobile family
Employment instability of key family members
Violence-prone family
Chemically dependent family member(s)
Chronic marital discord

Data from Clark, J. (1986, August 6–12). Supporting the family: Heading off a breakdown. *Nursing Times*, pp. 33–34; Friedman, M. (1992). *Family nursing theory and assessment* (3rd ed.). Norwalk, CT: Appleton-Century-Crofts; and Leatherland, J. (1986, November). Do you know child abuse when you see it? *RN*, 28–36.

Adolescent Parents

Teen-age parents and their children are one of the highest-risk groups that should be targeted for special attention from service providers and nurses. Incredibly, 84 per cent of adolescents who become pregnant each year did not intend to become pregnant (US Department of Health and Human Services, 1991). Negative health outcomes of teen-age pregnancy include low birthweight infants, unemployment for the teen-age mother, and lack of parenting skills. Poor pregnancy outcomes, including prematurity, low birthweight, birth defects, and infant death, are linked to low income, teen-age pregnancy, little or no prenatal care, and low pregnancy weight gain, smoking, and other substance abuse (Jones et al, 1986). Mothers in the 15- to 19-year-old age group are more likely than women in other age groups to have poor nutrition and weight gain; to smoke, drink, and use other drugs; and to lack prenatal care. Consistently, the infants of teen-age mothers are at the highest risk for infant death and disability. Parenting problems tend to be compounded when the young mother has the added responsibility of an infant with a disability.

Van Cleve and Sadler (1990) described the shared developmental issues with adolescent parents and their toddlers. For example, the toddler is striving for independence at the same time that the adolescent seeks emancipation from her family. Teen-agers who have toddlers find that conflict arises when both must participate in limit testing and negativism or rebellion as part of their developmental phases.

Homeless Families

Homeless families are the fastest-growing group of homeless people in the United States in the 1990s. Many homeless families are mothers with small children who have been victims of abuse. Homeless women tend to report that they have been abused as children and that they experienced violence in previous or current relationships with men (Bassuk & Rosenberg, 1988). McChesney (1992) found four basic types of homeless families who were seeking shelter:

1. Unemployed couples.
2. Mothers leaving relationships.
3. AFDC mothers.
4. Mothers who had been homeless teen-agers.

Unemployed couples were traditional families in which the employed father had lost his job and the wife's job was to care for the children. Mothers leaving relationships were women who had lived with male partners who were supporting them. Their entry into poverty was sudden and simultaneous with the separation from their male partners. Many of these women had some education and would have been able to work if they had been able to find child care. AFDC mothers were generally single parents with two or more children who had been receiving aid in the year prior to becoming homeless. The difficulty saving sufficient money for the first and last month's rent was a primary factor precipitating homelessness. Mothers who had been homeless teen-agers often had a history of severe abuse, foster home placement, and further abuse from which they ran away. Living on the streets by subsistence prostitution became their main source of support.

Patterns of Poverty

Theories of poverty tend to explain *who* the poor are and *why* they are poor (Handler, 1992). The oldest and dominant view is the pathology theory of poverty. Poverty has been viewed as caused by individual or family defects. If one worked and lived a decent life, being poor was not considered a sin. If one was able to work and did not, however, the individual was considered morally blameworthy. Nurses tend to make value judgments about families who are indigent, on Medicaid, or homeless. One must understand who the homeless are in order to gain insight into the range of circumstances in which families find themselves. Many homeless families are middle-class unemployed persons who do not know how to obtain necessary aid for themselves and their children.

Socioeconomic disadvantage is a primary factor affecting health and longevity in almost every category of disease, disability, and traumatic injury in every age group. Poor children experience more trauma, physical and mental retardation, environmental exposure to lead, and infectious disease than the total population (US Department of Health and Human Services, 1991). Friedman (1992) refers to the importance of sociocultural interventions and health information that is designed to be culturally sensitive. Indeed, ethnic differences are critically important in nutrition teaching and home care. However, the devastating effects of poverty on young people is more significant than any other factor. Nurses and other health care providers can do more to promote child health by being sensitive to the effects of poverty on family health than by any other intervention. Most important, nurses need to ensure that all children have a source of primary care when they leave the hospital, clinic, or other pediatric setting. Health departments, ambulatory care clinics, and some health maintenance organizations (HMOs) are potential sources of primary care for children. In some areas, private physicians or pediatric nurse practitioners (PNPs) will accept Medicaid and provide primary care. Pediatric nurses working in school health and other community settings should know the names of physicians and PNPs who will accept indigent clients in order to make knowledgeable referrals. Indigent families tend to become frustrated when referred for follow-up care, only to be told that the provider does not accept Medicaid.

Assessing Families at Risk

All families have times when they function well and other periods when they function poorly, even to the extent of "disintegration" or transition to another family form. However, families that are not able to provide for the physical and emotional needs of their members may place their children in jeopardy—physically, emotionally, socially, and intellectually. Such families need to be identified and referred for "high-risk" services available in most communities. The potential for child abuse or neglect is always present in high-risk families (see Chapter 28), and it is important to do early intervention for health promotion and prevention.

Difficult Communication Patterns

Members of families with difficult communication patterns tend to respond in a seemingly inappropriate way to others and to situations. One woman laughed and giggled as she talked about the loss of her first baby and the severe illness of her newborn son. As a child, she had not been allowed to express her feelings or needs, especially sadness. Her parents expected her to cope on her own and not to bother adults. Laughter at seemingly inappropriate moments may cover fear. Anger may also be used to camouflage fear or sadness, and vice versa. In understanding the nature of communication patterns within the family, it is important to note that many families come with traumatic histories and live in communities that are increasingly violent.

Communication Through Violence

Patterns of violence affect every aspect of family life and reflect patterns learned in childhood. Risk factors vary, but they include financial stressors and the influence of drugs and alcohol. *Healthy People 2000* states objectives that address the need for reduction of violence and abusive behavior as a priority for the nation (US Department of Health and Human Services, 1991). Studies of families who communicate through violent behavior find that both men and women who were victims of or who witnessed abuse as children tend to find themselves in violent relationships as adults (Bullock et al, 1989). Communication through violence originates with the adults in the family system. Moss (1991) proposes two categories of violence-prone marriages. The first involves a man with a violence-prone character. He initiates the violence that occurs early in the marriage. The violence is not limited to his wife but also involves any children. This type of family constitutes the majority of domestic violence cases involving law enforcement agencies. The second category involves partners with psychologic conflicts arising from the relationship itself. In both cases, child abuse is a natural companion to spouse abuse. The violence may encompass and has the potential to consume the whole family in communication patterns that result in at least one member feeling, or being, abused. Paradoxically, the abuser struggles with issues of control and may suffer remorse with loss of control that ends in an abusive episode. Abusers frequently promise "this will never happen again." Such well-intentioned promises may be important in making families more receptive to referrals for counseling following abusive episodes than at other times.

Families who participate in patterns of violence tend to experience difficult communication in their family activities. Ernest (1991) states that the issue is that of taking and maintaining control, not just venting anger. Abusers may appear to be loving, charismatic figures who are successful in the workplace and who never lose control in front of their colleagues. At home, such parents may respond to their children with irritation and anger, which tends to destroy creativity and problem solving. Other families have hidden "rules" that inhibit expression of feelings. Relationships between children and their parents in these families tend to be apathetic, revealing little affection or feeling. The child from such an environment often seeks inappropriate affection (usually in excess) from casual acquaintances or strangers and does not portray the "stranger anxiety" that usually is characteristic of the child's developmental age. For example, a 2-year-old's clinging to the nurse during the examination or home visit would be considered uncharacteristic of that age category (see section on "Communication Patterns" in Table 2–5 for assessment factors). It is necessary to assess families for a history of violence whenever a psychosocial history is taken. Sensitive but direct questions about the safety of the mother and children must be asked. Finally, as an underpinning of any nursing approach, nurses must be aware of state laws related to abuse and the availability of community resources (Brendtro & Bowker, 1989).

Perpetuation of Patterns

Although the extended family can be supportive when a young family undertakes its parenting tasks, sometimes the family members develop difficult interaction patterns. For example, well-meaning grandparents may take over the care of a newborn baby and not allow the parents to establish an attachment with the child or to re-establish their marital relationship in a new way following the birth or adoption. Relatives and friends are often unaware of how they may be compounding distress in the family by their efforts to be helpful.

Unhealthful parenting practices may be the parents' own unsuccessful solution to a developmental hurdle. Young parents may themselves have gone through a difficult period at a particular age. When their own children reach that age, or stage, the parents have a difficult time nurturing the children. Instead, they react more as siblings than as parents. Unwed teen-age mothers are often caught in this situation with their own mothers.

A woman who had a turbulent adolescence may discover that her parents had a similar upset at the same age. One mother expressed terror as her children approached their teen-age years, not because she herself had a hard time, but because her sister did. Her sister acted out and caused much disruption in the family. This mother had been extra "good" as a teen-ager in order to compensate for her sister's "badness." Reliving or compensating behavior re-created pain for her as her children entered adolescence.

Parental guilt may be perpetuated in the next generation. When parents feel guilty, they may be overly nurturing to their children. Parents who work hard to give their children advantages that they may have missed can become overly invested in their child's achievements. The children in these families may feel overwhelmed by expectations, or "swallowed up."

Intervening with Families at Risk

From a review of the literature, Anderson and Tomlinson (1992) identified five realms of family experience that direct nursing practice:

- Interactive process.
- Development.
- Coping.
- Integrity
- Health processes.

Based on the family health literature the interactive process refers to communication, nurturance, and social support. Developmental phases include family transitions and individual developmental tasks. Coping processes include problem-solving and adaptation to stress and crisis. Integrity is the family's sense of self and meaning, values, and rituals—identity. Health processes are defined as family health beliefs, health promotion behaviors, and health care during health and illness.

The five realms constitute a holistic view of the family health system such that the family's well-being is more than just the health of all the individuals (Anderson & Tomlinson, 1992). Pediatric nursing necessarily influences the family as a whole, and an assessment of family caregiving is an essential component. Family involvement varies according to the child's health status, as indicated in Table 2–3. High-risk families need special attention and intervention to assist with coping in multiple crises.

Two important concepts in Zerwekh's (1991) family caregiving model include fostering family understanding and resolving crises. Fostering family understanding is accomplished by working through emotions related to parenting. Zerwekh identifies the need for exploration of feelings related to pregnancy, children, and relationships; grief work following the death of a child; and focus on reality rather than denial. Resolving crises includes assistance with problem solving and encouraging self-help.

Building trust involves getting the family to feel accepted and understood. Trust is an essential element of interventions with complex families (Lynch & Tiedje, 1991; Zerwekh, 1992). Scolding and blaming the family results in alienation and isolation. Neglecting behavior that is so serious that the child's health is threatened should be reported as child neglect. Less serious "noncompliance," or failure to follow through, must be addressed from within the client's value system. People who feel threatened by health care providers may withdraw if they sense that they are being blamed or attacked. The nurse must spend time building a trusting relationship so that the family members feel free to share their values and hopes. Understanding and trust are essential underpinnings of a therapeutic relationship.

Social support may serve to mediate the effects of other risk factors. Support networks serve to assist families during times of stress and illness. Support persons may include family members, friends and neighbors, colleagues, and self-help groups. Extended family networks play a major role in the ability of the family to provide respite for the primary caregiver. For example, families with an infant on an apnea monitor may have difficulty doing normal chores such as grocery shopping. It would be important to include all potential support persons (grandparents, uncles, or aunts) in teaching cardiopulmonary resuscitation (CPR) and management of the monitor, so that mother or father can feel free to take time away from the infant. The family ecomap (see Fig. 2–4) is designed as a useful tool for determining significant relationships and potential sources of support in the life of a family. McCubbin and colleagues (1983) found single parents to be "at risk" in caring for a chronically ill child when there was no other available adult with coping skills; the single parent had sole responsibility for the child with cystic fibrosis. Families with limited income also had difficulty coping with the combined family hardship. The authors concluded that support services should be targeted for primary prevention (before a problem is manifest). The family without strong connections is potentially vulnerable.

Adolescent Parents

Healthy growth and development of young parents and children require an extensive support system. Teen-agers with toddlers are at risk for conflict, because they tend to be struggling with similar issues of independence and limit testing. Van Cleve and Sadler (1990) suggest that these families need advice about parenting and interacting with the health care system. For example, the teen-age parent may not understand return appointments or how to obtain medications for the child but may be reluctant to ask questions. The pediatric nurse can use role playing to show how to ask questions and can include anticipatory guidance for typical toddler behaviors that may be particularly difficult for teen-age parents. Referral to a teen-age parent support group is an essential component of nursing intervention for adolescent parents. Sharing and peer advice on problems encountered in raising children is especially important for this group, because teen-agers tend to listen to advice from peers more than that from health providers. Ensuring that the teen-age parent has an ongoing source of health care for herself and her child is essential.

Homeless Families

Homeless families need direct intervention. Young families are the fastest-growing group among the homeless. The primary interventions include reconnecting the family to a home, to an adequate source of income, to health care services, and to schools (Francis, 1991). Many of these families have become alienated from their family of origin and their friends. The nurse should consider exploring relationships to assist the family in evaluating potential sources of social support. Nurses working with homeless families may want to develop a "help line" or referral system, so that homeless families with hospitalized children can be quickly connected to shelters, social work services, and a family advocate who can provide assistance in reconnecting the family to a home. McChesney (1992) emphasized the need for shelter, referral, rehabilitation, and education plus income support. Shelter and health care are primary needs of homeless families. Families with hospitalized children have an opportunity for advocacy that can potentially provide comprehensive services; these children would have been "lost" to health care, if not for the acute illness that brought them into the system. Children from homeless families are likely to go "unnoticed," until severe developmental delays or physical symptoms make medical care necessary.

An integrated nursing approach for families in poverty requires addressing issues of priorities and power. For lasting change, nurses must concentrate their efforts on the social factors first. "Health and illness and nursing interventions become experiences within a social context" (Moccia & Mason, 1986). Health teaching for a child who is sleeping on the street is unlikely to be meaningful. Interventions that include helping people to develop the skills necessary to exercise collective power are more likely to contribute to social and community change for the greater good.

A Multidisciplinary Team Approach

The multidisciplinary approach has numerous advantages. First, families receive several resource alternatives from which to choose. This also prevents any one resource from becoming depleted in efforts to help the family with all its needs. Professional burnout with multiproblem families is high, because progress is slow or sometimes not visible. A multidisciplinary team allows professionals collegial support to help offset the possible burnout risk. A team approach also adds creative alternatives that professionals working separately might not consider. Community resources frequently needed to intervene in multiproblem families are listed in Table 2–10.

In establishing the team members, the initial intervener should first identify with the family their needs. Next, resources currently used by the family and the degree of family involvement and satisfaction should be listed. Team members may be individually contacted by the coordinator, or team planning evaluation meetings may be scheduled. The family should not be overlooked as team members, for success is extremely unlikely without them. The schools of the children should be considered key resources in interventions with multiproblem families. Teachers should be educated and encouraged to identify children whose behaviors indicate family problems and families who may not be able to provide nurturance.

Obviously, the critical element in successful intervention is casefinding at the primary and secondary levels. If nurses, teachers, and other professionals who have regular contact with children and families are alert to the subtle indicators (risk factors, family characteristics, early behavioral signs) that a family is experiencing repeated crises or multiple problems, interventions can be initiated before the family becomes embedded in a problematic life pattern and before problems become too complex. The costs of families in crisis to family and community certainly attest to the fiscal soundness of preventive and early intervention programs.

As part of the intervention team, the nurse should be familiar with the rules of approach in interacting with families at risk. A genuine, warm, and sensitive approach is fundamental. Families who are usually mistrustful have low esteem levels and may not be skilled enough to be able to clearly state their needs. An aggressive approach will result in family withdrawal and rejection of team efforts. Services or resources need to be presented positively; for example, the nurse might describe a program as being designed to foster and support parenting, rather than to prevent child abuse. Agencies keep this concept in mind when they establish their organizational titles and when they describe their services on printed and advertising media. A title such as "The Nurturing Center" is used in many communities for parenting centers. This positive presentation fosters interest, rather than causing families to be defensive and further diminishing their already-weak self-esteem and motivation.

Primary Nursing Roles in Working with Families

Caring is the foundational underpinning of any therapeutic nursing intervention. Pepin (1992) describes the two primary dimensions of caring as (1) the affective, nurturing, or compassionate aspect and (2) the work or service aspect. Nurses have stated that the affective aspect of caring is their primary motivation for entering nursing practice, in relation to the quality of the nurse-client relationship and their style of nursing (Morse et al, 1991). The humanistic qualities of caring cannot be separated from scientific nursing actions (Koldjeski, 1990). Pepin's (1992) analysis noted that the affective aspect of caring, previously relegated to the family, is now a major focus in the *professional* caregiving literature. In contrast, the burden of caring activities is currently addressed in the *family* caregiving literature.

Casefinder

The nurse is often the first health professional to have direct contact with families at risk. In clinic settings,

TABLE 2-10
Community Resources Commonly Needed for Interventions with Families with Children*

Counseling/Legal Services	**Support/Self-Help Groups**
Legal assistance services	Religious-affiliated groups
Juvenile authority	Singles clubs
Tough love group and hot line	Friendly Visitor program
Family and/or marital counseling	Parents Anonymous
Mental health centers	Alcoholics Anonymous, Al-Anon, Ala-Teen, Ala-Tot, Narcotics Anonymous, Gamblers Anonymous
Financial Resources	**Development/Rehabilitation**
Housing authorities	Vocational rehabilitation, employment services
Fuel assistance agencies	WIC program
Free or sliding scale medical and dental care	Child development clinics
Aid to Families with Dependent Children (AFDC)	Child guidance centers
Medicaid or other health financial assistance	**Parenting Assistance**
Food stamps	Single parent clubs
Welfare	Foster grandparent program
Public housing	Big Brothers/Big Sisters program
Budget and financial incentives counseling	Surrogate parent program
Emergency shelters	Subsidized or sliding scale child care
Health Care Services	Division of Child and Youth Services (DCYS)
Home health services	Foster care
School health programs	Parent aid programs (nurturance to parents)
Occupational health settings	
Ambulatory care settings	
Visiting Nurse Association	
Family planning services	
Homemaker services	

*The system of resources varies from state to state and community to community. Many communities develop reference books of community resources that describe services rendered, eligibility requirements, how to gain access to services, fee basis, and so on, which are available in public libraries, county health departments, or chambers of commerce. The yellow pages in phone books list local agencies and resources by title.

the nurse may perform initial assessments, well child examinations, immunizations, and teaching and referral functions. In hospitals, the nurse's sensitivity to potential risk factors during history taking can "set the stage" for a positive encounter with the health care system. Identification of high-risk families, such as homeless families or teen-age parents, is an important step that must occur prior to referral to special programs that assist high-risk families with children. Hospital and clinic pediatric nurses should be alert for potentially vulnerable families that may need referral for additional services. Most communities provide some type of pediatric home care or support services, such as a "mother's helper" for vulnerable families. The purpose of such services is to prevent infant morbidity and mortality through the prevention of child abuse and neglect. Such programs are useless to families who do not receive the referral or who do not receive follow-up in the home.

Families with children who "slip through the cracks" can face devastating consequences. For example, in the following case study Ms. Hardin was "found" too late; early casefinding and referral might have provided earlier intervention.

Ms. Hardin was a young mother with two little girls (toddlers) when she gave birth to a 6-pound boy. The mother was not identified as high risk, even though she was a single parent and had three children under the age of 3 years. At the time of the infant's first visit to the child health clinic at 6 weeks of age, he had gained only 8 ounces. The family was then referred for a home visit; however, it was not designated as a priority, the file was misplaced, and the visit was never made. Six months later, a community health nurse visiting another family in the apartment complex stopped to see Ms.

Hardin and her two girls. One of the girls seemed to have a severe upper respiratory infection (URI) and was referred by the nurse for medical care. Ms. Hardin gave no indication that there was a baby in the family. A week later the nurse made a second home visit. The child had been taken for medical care, but the nurse now observed that both toddlers had coughs. Chronic URIs are often indicators of other problems.

The nurse began a comprehensive family assessment. In the investigation of family structure, the mother stated the baby boy was upstairs in the bedroom because "he cried all the time." At 8 months of age, this infant was the size of a newborn infant and weighed 7 1/2 pounds. The nurse immediately contacted Protective Services and helped Ms. Hardin to understand the need for the referral. The mother cried and said she knew that something was wrong with the baby, but she did not know what to do with him. She had taken him to the emergency room twice for "crying," but no diagnosis was made and the family was not identified as needing home follow-up. Eventual "casefinding" by the nurse in this situation enabled the child to be placed in foster care while the family received counseling and health teaching. Sadly, the growth and development of the child were permanently delayed because of the lack of early identification and referral for family and home assessment.

Advocate

Findings from a recent study illustrate how families acted as negotiators to advocate for their adoptive children (Lightburn, 1992). The nurse serves an important role as advocate in supporting families in their efforts to obtain needed care for their children.

Mrs. Nolan believed two of her children would not be alive had she not negotiated for needed portable medical equipment. Mrs. Nolan saw herself as co-worker with the doctors. She often negotiated from this self-ascribed position. She said, "Mothers are head doctors," a designation doctors did not recognize. . . . Her effectiveness as a mediator depended upon her conviction of her authority to mediate her children's care. She had expert knowledge from her years of experience as their mother. [Lightburn, 1992]

The role of nurse as advocate is especially important for families with chronically ill or disabled children. Poyadue (1988) discussed the need for parent-to-parent contact through a formal support group for parents of children with special needs. Pediatric nurses should be prepared with current information on parent support groups for children with different diagnoses. For example, there are chapters throughout the country for families of children with cystic fibrosis, sickle cell anemia, and Down syndrome. Again, Poyadue, a nurse and parent of a child with Down syndrome, makes the point, "While parents may not be experts on their children's illness, they are experts on their children" (1988, p 84).

Educator

The supportive-educative function of the nurse is well documented in the nursing literature (Orem, 1985; Neuman, 1989). Families with children have special needs for information about their children's condition. Such information must be provided with the understanding that the family is the expert on the child's personality and environment and on the context of his or her family life. In addition, other factors such as the family's health beliefs are important in the initiation of any health action (Pender, 1987).

Parent education consists of (1) anticipatory guidance (health promotion or health protection) and (2) health supervision (management of a health problem). Health promotion education is teaching focused on promoting overall growth and development of the child. Anticipatory guidance that is health-protective focuses on information on protection from specific diseases or injury. Teaching about immunizations or safety car seats is health-protective education. In addition, pediatric nurses often need to focus on the health supervision of an acute or chronic diagnosed health problem. Assessing the readiness for learning and the family's perception of what they need to know is a prerequisite for any parent education.

Parents often learn better if they ask questions and the nurse responds. Teaching high-risk parents requires role modeling and demonstration at a concrete level (Zerwekh, 1991). Showing parents how to hug and play with their baby may be the "key" for inexperienced families or family members. Some families may not respond to traditional pamphlets or books about their child's condition. Lynch and Tiedje (1991) discussed the problems in client-caregiver relationships with families in crisis. Health may be secondary to the problems of daily living, and information is not used in the same way with multiproblem families. Placing blame on the family who does not use health information results inevitably in withdrawal. Nurses need to develop ways of being with families that help them to feel empowered, regardless of their situations.

Collaborator

The nurse as collaborator works with the family on its own goals. The nurse must be absolutely committed to family goals and family values. High-risk families often have difficulty trusting others. Not judging but rather accepting people as they are was found to be critical to building trust between nurses and families in the community (Zerwekh, 1992).

In current family therapy theory, the focus of therapy is the story that the family members tell about their lives. Fine and Turner (1991, p 307) reject the view of therapist as "privileged, objective management-consultant" in favor of the family therapist as one who collaborates with clients in constructing new realities. It is what the family decides to do with its life and health that will make a difference in the future. The nurse's role as consultant allows the family and nurse to be full and equal participants in the plan for the family's care. In discharge planning, it is important to collaborate with the family to design a plan that fits the family situation, while understanding that further modification may be needed once the child is home.

Summary

The principles, assessment guides, and tools in this chapter are presented with an over-riding perspective that families are both unique and similar in their needs and situations. No family form is better than another; rather any family may develop multiple risk factors that contribute to family crises. The family must be viewed as full participants in promoting health for their family. Ultimately, the family members are "in charge" of their health and the care of their child or children.

KEY CONCEPTS

Concepts Related to Basic Information

- Family is defined as a complex organization of one or more persons with a pattern of interrelationships that have a past, present, and future.
- Currently, the nuclear family represents only a small portion of American families, estimated to be as low as 14 per cent.
- It is estimated that by the year 2000 more than half of the projected American households will be composed of "nonfamily households" and single-family households.
- A family system is established when members demonstrate a commitment to the family unit with the intent of some degree of permanence.
- Family and nursing theories serve as a guide for identification of significant factors related to family functioning and potential for crisis and growth.
- Several family theories have been developed for viewing the individual, the dynamic unit and their interrelatedness: systems, structural-functional, social exchange, interactional, and developmental theories.
- The goals of a family satisfy the affiliation needs of each member and maintain family cohesiveness; when individual goals are different from those of the family there may be conflict.
- Vulnerable families are those families likely to need special intervention.
- Risk factors for all families include significant economic constraints, lack of social support, alcohol or drug problems, multiple family illness, and a child with a chronic illness or disability.
- The most extreme characteristic seen in multiproblem families is children in jeopardy.
- Homeless families are the fastest-growing group of homeless people in the United States in the 1990s.

Concepts Related to Nursing Assessment

- The family is a highly complex system, and as many family members as possible should be interviewed as age-appropriate.
- Family members' views of the "truth" may vary, and the nurse must be careful to encourage the family to understand and discuss differences within the family.
- Family genograms provide a framework for the nurse and family to examine the family structure and history of certain diseases.
- *Smilkstein's Family APGAR* is a tool that can quickly measure a family's satisfaction with their general state of functioning.
- *Otto's Family Assessment Criteria Check List* has 13 assessment criteria that contribute to family unity and the development of family potential.

Concepts Related to Nursing Intervention

- The goal of nursing may include (1) reduction of stressors for system maintenance, (2) improved family functioning, and (3) health promotion at different life stages.
- The nurse's role during intervention can be seen as developmental, facilitative, or supplemental in nature.
- The family assessment process itself becomes an intervention, if the entire family is included as team members.
- Five realms of family experience that direct nursing practice are the interactive process, development, coping, integrity, and family process.
- A critical element in successful intervention with multiproblem families is casefinding at the primary and secondary levels.
- The primary nursing roles in working with families are casefinder, advocate, educator, and collaborator.

REFERENCES

Anderson, K. H., & Tomlinson, P. S. (1992). The family health system as an emerging paradigmatic view for nursing. *Image: Journal of Nursing Scholarship, 24*(1), 57–63.

Arent, R. (1980). *The child in stress: Strategies for support.* Littleton, CO: Arent and Associates.

Bassuk, E. L., & Rosenberg, L. (1988). Why does family homelessness occur? A case-controlled study. *American Journal of Public Health, 78,* 783–788.

Beavers, W., & Voeller, M. (1983). Family models: Comparing and contrasting the Olson circumplex model with the Beavers systems model. *Family Process, 22*(3), 71.

Bomar, P. J. (ed.). (1989). *Nurses and family health promotion.* Philadelphia, WB Saunders.

Bomar, P. J. (1990). Perspectives on family health promotion. *Family Community Health, 12*(4), 1–11.

Bowen, M. (1978). *Family theory in clinical practice.* New York: Jason Aronson.

Brendtro, M., & Bowker, L. H. (1989). Battered women: How can nurses help? *Issues in Mental Health Nursing, 10,* 169–180.

Bullock, L. F. C., Sandella, J. A., & McFarlane, J. (1989). Breaking the cycle of abuse: How nurses can intervene. *Journal of Psychosocial Nursing, 27,* 11–13.

Burr, W. R., Leigh, G., Day, R., & Constantine, J. (1979). Symbolic interaction and the family. In W. R. Burr, R. Hill, F. I. Nye, & I. L. Reiss (Eds.), *Contemporary theories about the family* (Vol. 2, pp. 42–111). New York: Free Press.

Carey, R. (1989). How values affect the mutual goal setting process with multiproblem families. *Journal of Community Health Nursing, 6*(1), 7–14.

Clark, J. (1986, August 6–12). Supporting the family: Heading off a breakdown. *Nursing Times,* pp. 33–34.

Cody, W. K. (in press). Human values and the notion of normality: The use of power/knowledge in practice. *Nursing Science Quarterly.*

Curran, D. (1983). *Traits of a healthy family.* New York: Ballantine Books.

Demos, J. (1986). *Past, present, and personal: The family and the life course in American history.* New York: Oxford University Press.

Doherty, W., & McCubbin, H. (1985). Families and health care: An emerging arena of theory, research, and clinical intervention. *Family Relations, 34,* 5–11.

Dornbusch, S. M., & Strober, M. (Eds.). (1988). *Feminism, children, and the new families.* New York: Guilford Press.

Duvall, E. M. (1977). *Family development* (5th ed.). Philadelphia: JB Lippincott.

Ernest, V. (1991, October). *Domestic violence.* Presentation conducted at St. Francis Women's Hospital, Greenville.

Feetham, S. L. (1991). Conceptual and methodological issues in research of families. In A. L. Whall & J. Fawcett (Eds.), *Family theory development in nursing: Sociological science and art.* Philadelphia: FA Davis.

Fine, M., & Turner, J. (1991). Tyranny and freedom: Looking at ideas in the practice of family therapy. *Family Process, 30,* 307–320.

Francis, M. B. (1991). Homeless families: Rebuilding connections. *Public Health Nursing, 8*(2), 90–96.

Friedman, M. (1992). *Family nursing theory and assessment* (3rd ed.). Norwalk, CT: Appleton-Century-Crofts.

Gillis, C. L. (1989). Family research in nursing. In C. L. Gillis, B. L. Highley, B. M. Roberts, & I. M. Martinson (Eds.), *Toward a science of family nursing* (pp. 37–63). Menlo Park, CA: Addison-Wesley.

Gillis, C. L. (1983). The family as a unit of analysis: Strategies for the nurse researcher. *Advances in Nursing Science, 5*(3), 50–59.

Gillis, C. L., Highley, B. L., Roberts, B. M., & Martinson, I. M. (Eds.). (1989). *Toward a science of family nursing.* Menlo Park, CA: Addison-Wesley.

Handler, J. (1992). The modern pauper: The homeless in welfare history. In M. J. Toberson & M. Greenblatt (Eds.), *Homelessness: A national perspective.* New York: Plenum Press.

Hanson, S. M. H. (1991). Healthy single parent families. In A. L. Whall & J. Fawcett (Eds.), *Family theory development in nursing.* Philadelphia: FA Davis.

Holman, T. B., & Burr, W. R. (1980). Beyond the beyond: The growth of family theories in the 1970's. *Journal of Marriage and the Family, 42,* 729–741.

Janosik, E., & Green, E. (1992). *Family life: Process and practice.* Boston: Jones & Bartlett.

Jarrett, R. L. (1992). A family case study: An examination of the underclass debate. In J. F. Gilgun, K. Daly, & G. Handel (Eds.), *Qualitative methods in family research* (pp. 172–197). Newbury Park, CA: Sage Publications.

Jones, E. F., Forrest, J. D., Goldman, N., Henshaw, S., Lincoln, R., Rosoff, J. I., Westoff, C. F., & Wulf, D. (1986). *Teenage pregnancy in industrialized countries: A study sponsored by the Alan Guttmacher Institute.* New Haven: Yale University Press.

Kaplan, L. (1986). *Working with multiproblem families.* Lexington, MA: Lexington Books.

King, I. M. (1992). King's theory of goal attainment. *Nursing Science Quarterly, 5*(1), 19–26.

King, I. M. (1981). *A theory for nursing: Systems, concepts, process.* New York: John Wiley & Sons.

Koldjeski, D. (1990). Toward a theory of professional nursing caring: A unifying perspective. In M. Leininger & J. Watson (Eds.), *The caring imperative in education* (pp. 45–57). New York: National League for Nursing.

Leahy, K. M., Cobb, M. M., & Jones, M. C. (1982). *Community health nursing.* New York: McGraw-Hill.

Leahy, M., & Wright, L. M. (1988). Families and psychosocial problems. Springhouse, PA: Springhouse Corporation.

Leatherland, J. (1986, November). Do you know child abuse when you see it? *RN,* 28–36.

Levi-Strauss, C. (1976). Reflections on the atom of kinship. In C. Levi-Strauss (Ed.). *Structural anthropology.* (M. Layton, Trans.; Volume 2, pp 82–112). New York: Basic Books.

Lightburn, A. (1992). Participant observation in special needs adoptive families: The mediation of chronic illness and handicap. In J. F. Gilgun, K. Daly, & G. Handel (Eds.), *Qualitative methods in family research* (pp. 217–235). Newbury Park, CA: Sage Publications.

Loveland-Cherry, C. J. (1989). Family health promotion and protection. In P. J. Bomar (Ed.), *Nurses and family health promotion: Concepts, assessments and interventions.* Baltimore: Williams & Wilkins.

Lynch, I., & Tiedje, L. B. (1991). Working with multiproblem families: An intervention model for community health nurses. *Public Health Nursing, 8*(3), 147–153.

Macklin, E. D. (1980). Nontraditional family forms: A decade of research. *Journal of Marriage and the Family, 42,* 905–922.

Mallinger, K. M. (1989). The American family: History and development. In P. J. Bomar (Ed.), *Nurses and family health promotion: Concepts, assessment, and interventions.* Baltimore: Williams & Wilkins.

McChesney, K. (1992). Homeless families. In M. J. Roberson & M. Greenblatt (Eds.), *Homelessness: A national perspective.* New York: Plenum Press.

McCubbin, H. I., McCubbin, M. A., Patterson, J. M., Cauble, A. E., Wilson, L. R., & Warwick, W. (1983). CHIP—coping health inventory for parents: An assessment of parental coping patterns in the care of the chronically ill child. *Journal of Marriage and the Family, 45*(2), 359–370.

Mead, G. H. (1934). *Mind, self, and society.* Chicago: University of Chicago Press.

Moccia, P., & Mason, D. J. (1986). Poverty trends: Implications for nursing. *Nursing Outlook, 34*(1), 20–24.

Morse, J. M., Bottorff, J., Neander, W., & Solberg, S. (1991). Comparative analysis of conceptualizations and theories of caring. *Image: Journal of Nursing Scholarship, 23*(2), 119–126.

Moss, Y. A. (1991). Battered women and the myth of masochism. *Journal of Psychological Nursing, 29*(7), 19–23.

Neuman, B. (1989). *The Neuman systems model—application to nursing education and practice* (2nd ed.). Norwalk, CT: Appleton & Lange.

Olson, D., et al. (1982). *Family inventories—Inventories in the national survey of families across the family life cycle.* St. Paul: University of Minnesota Press.

Orem, D. E. (1985). *Nursing: Concepts of practice* (3rd ed.). New York: McGraw-Hill.

Otto, H. (1968, September). Criteria for assessing family strength. *Family Process,* p 329.

Parse, R. R. (1992). Human becoming: Parse's theory of nursing. *Nursing Science Quarterly, 5*(1), 35–42.

Parse, R. R. (1981). *Man-living-health: A theory of nursing.* New York: John Wiley & Sons.

Pender, N. J. (1987). *Health promotion in nursing* (2nd ed.). Norwalk, CT: Appleton & Lange.

Pepin, J. I. (1992). Family caring and caring in nursing. *Image: Journal of Nursing Scholarship, 24*(2), 127–131.

Pinderhughes, E. (1982). Afro-American families and the victim system. In M. McGoldrick, J. K. Pearce, & J. Giordano (Eds.), *Ethnicity and family therapy.* New York: Guilford Press.

Poyadue, F. S. (1988). In my opinion . . . Parents as teachers of health care professionals. *Community Health Care, 17*(2), 82–84.

Pratt, L. (1976). *Family structure and effective health behavior.* Boston: Houghton-Mifflin.

Roberts, C., & Feetham, S. (1982, April). Assessing family functioning across three areas of relationships. *Nursing Research,* pp. 231–235.

Robertson, M. J., & Greenblatt, M. (1992). *Homelessness: A national perspective.* New York: Plenum Press.

Rogers, M. E. (1988). Nursing science and art: A perspective. *Nursing Science Quarterly, 1*(2), 99–102.

Roy, C. (1988). An explication of the philosophical assumptions of the Roy adaptation model. *Nursing Science Quarterly, 1*(1), 26–34.

Roy, C. (1984). *Introduction to nursing: An adaptation model* (2nd ed.). Englewood Cliffs, NJ: Prentice-Hall.

Rubenstein, C. (1989, October 8). The Baby Bomb. *New York Times Good Health Magazine,* pp 34–41.

Scanzoni, J. H. (1983). *Shaping tomorrow's family: Theory and policy for the 21st century.* Beverly Hills, CA: Sage Publications.

Skolnick, A. (1991). *Embattled paradise: The American family in an age of uncertainty.* New York: Basic Books.

Smilkstein, G. (1984, Fall). The physician and family function assessment. *Family Systems Medicine,* pp 263–279.

Speer, J., & Sachs, B. (1985, September-October). Selecting the appropriate family assessment tool. *Pediatric Nursing, 11*(5), 349–355.

U. S. Census Bureau. (1990). *Statistical abstract of the United States.* U. S. Department of Commerce.

U. S. Department of Health and Human Services: Public Health Service. (1991). *Healthy people 2000: National health promotion and disease prevention objectives.* (DHHS Publication No. [PHS] 91–50213). Washington, DC: U. S. Government Printing Office.

Van Cleve, S. N., & Sadler, L. S. (1990). Adolescent parents and toddlers: Strategies for intervention. *Public Health Nursing, 7*(1), 22–27.

Weitzman, L. J. (1985). *The divorce revolution.* New York: Free Press.

Whall, A. L. (1980). Congruence between existing theories of family functioning and nursing theories. *Advances in Nursing Science, 2*(2), 59–67.

Whall, A. L., & Fawcett, J. (1991). *Family theory development in nursing: State of the science and art.* Philadelphia: FA Davis.

Wright, L. M., & Leahy, M. (1984). *Nurses and families: A guide to family assessment and intervention.* Philadelphia: FA Davis.

Zerwekh, J. V. (1991). A family caregiving model for public health nursing. *Nursing Outlook, 39*(5), 213–217.

Zerwekh, J. V. (1992). Laying the groundwork for family self-help: Locating families, building trust, and building strength. *Public Health Nursing, 9*(1), 15–21.

BIBLIOGRAPHY

Gilgun, J. F., Daly, K., & Handel, G. (Eds.). (1992). *Qualitative methods in family research.* Newbury Park, CA: Sage Publications.

Institute of Medicine. (1985). *Preventing low birthweight.* Washington, DC: National Academy Press.

Leonard, B., Brust, J., & Nelson, R. (1993). Parental distress: Caring for medically fragile children at home. *Journal of Pediatric Nursing, 8*(1), 22–30.

NANDA Nursing Diagnoses: Definitions and classifications. (1992). St. Louis: North American Nursing Diagnosis Association.

Neuman, B. (1989). The Neuman nursing process format: Family. In J. P. Riehl-Sisca (Ed.), *Conceptual models for nursing practice* (3rd ed., pp 49–62). Norwalk, CT: Appleton & Lange.

Nightingale, F. (1858). *Notes on matters affecting the health, efficiency, and hospital administration of the British army.* London: Harrison & Sons.

Orem, D. E. (1983). The family coping with a medical illness. Analysis and application of Orem's theory. In I. W. Clements & F. B. Roberts (Eds.), *Family health. A theoretical approach to nursing care* (pp 385–386). New York: John Wiley & Sons.

Perkins, M. (1993). Parent-Nurse Collaboration: Using the Caregiver Identity Emergence Phases to Assist Parents of Hospitalized Children with Disabilities. *Journal of Pediatric Nursing, 8*(1), 2–9.

Reed, K. S. (1989). Family theory related to the Neuman Systems Model. In B. Neuman (Ed.), *The Neuman Systems Model. Application to nursing education and practice* (2nd ed., pp 385–395). Norwalk, CT: Appleton & Lange.

Reed, P. G. (1986). The developmental conceptual framework: Nursing reformulations and applications for family therapy. In A. L. Whall (Ed.), *Family therapy theory for nursing. Four approaches* (pp 69–91). Norwalk, CT: Appleton-Century-Crofts.

Rogers, M. E. (1970). *Introduction to the theoretical basis of nursing.* Philadelphia: FA Davis.

Rogers, M. E. (1980). Nursing: A science of unitary man. In J. P. Riehl & C. Roy (Eds.), *Conceptual models for nursing practice* (2nd ed., pp 329–337). New York: Appleton-Century-Crofts.

Roy, C. (1976). *Introduction to nursing. An adaptation model.* Englewood Cliffs, NJ: Prentice-Hall.

Roy, C. (1983). Roy adaptation model. In I. W. Clements & F. B. Roberts (Eds.), *Family health. A theoretical approach to nursing care* (pp 255–278). New York: John Wiley & Sons.

Velsor-Friedrich, B. (1993). Homeless children and their families, Part I: The changing picture. *Journal of Pediatric Nursing, 8*(2), 122–123.

Velsor-Friedrich, B. (1993). Homeless children and their families, Part II: Federal programs and alternative health care delivery systems. *Journal of Pediatric Nursing 8*(3), 190–192.

CHAPTER • 3

Development of Children

RELATED TOPICS

Expanded discussion of the influences of poverty, Chapter 1
Expanded discussion of culture, family lifestyles, Chapter 2
Religious influences, Chapter 2
Development of health concepts, Chapter 10
Development of self-esteem, Chapter 14
Nutritional influences on growth, Chapter 16
Play, Chapter 17
Concepts of stress and coping in childhood, Chapter 18
Genetic influences on development, Chapter 31

LEARNING OBJECTIVES

- **Describe the major competencies that are affected by the child's growth and development.**
- **Define the terminology used by various theorists to describe and explain the child's growth and development.**
- **Identify the major human responses (nursing diagnoses/collaborative problems) the nurse may identify in caring for the child and family.**
- **Explain the major tenets of the following developmental theorists: Piaget, Freud, Gesell, Erikson, Fowler, and Kohlberg.**
- **Describe the principles evident in growth and development.**
- **Identify the factors influencing the child's development.**
- **Apply theoretical perspectives of growth and development to the care of the child and family.**

Growth and development are the words that succinctly describe the process of maturation from childhood to adulthood. This chapter builds the foundation for all the specific growth and development chapters in the next unit. Theories are introduced to help explain and predict physical, intellectual, and emotional-social development. Growth, development, and maturation are defined and specific principles examined. Development is considered as a process of maturation, learning, conflict resolution, cognitive change, and cultural adaptation. Various factors within the child's environment are explored for their influence on growth and development: culture and family lifestyle, school, socioeconomic status, neighborhood, mass media, and certain physical aspects, varying from intrauterine environment to climate. Genetic influences are discussed in Chapter 31.

Why Study Growth and Develoment? Nursing Implications

Anyone who has watched a sleeping infant, studied closely the determined way toddlers force their whole body into mobility, listened to the imaginative conversation of two preschoolers at play, tolerated the teasing of an active school-age child, or cried over the tense struggle of an identity-seeking adolescent cannot deny the miraculous fascination of the young human being. Researchers and professionals in the helping arts attest to the intricacies and complexities that interplay to create a whole being who is unique and yet shares a core of commonalities with all others of the species.

By studying these commonalities in our existence, we can better understand how we grow, develop, and mature into unique individuals who seek to achieve our full potential. Nurses who work with children use their knowledge of the commonalities of development as a basis for recognizing potential and actual deviations from or alterations in growth and development. Also, as health professionals, nurses must sometimes intervene in this growth and development relationship in order to deal with disease, abnormality, or other factors threatening health; we ought to know with what we are intervening (Craft & Denehy, 1990).

The nurse needs such knowledge to develop and deliver a plan of care that is developmentally appropriate and relevant to the needs of the client. Nurses working with childbearing and childrearing families require developmental knowledge to provide anticipatory guidance to parents, enhancing the parental contribution and encouraging parents' contribution to their children's attainment of optimal growth and development.

Altered growth and development is a key nursing diagnosis for the nurse who works with children. A clear problem statement usually requires that this diagnosis be further explained by one or more of the three competency categories of growth and development: physical, intellectual, or emotional-social. Any factors enhancing or altering the development of those competencies become essential aspects of the nursing assessment and contribute to the nursing diagnosis and plan of care. For example, a diagnosis might be *altered growth and development: physical related to inadequate oxygen transport associated with a congenital heart defect*.

The growth and development plan for developing children presents the nursing diagnosis: *high risk for altered growth and development* (Table 3–1). It describes the components of nursing care needed to achieve the projected outcome of an increase in the acquisition of behaviors appropriate to the level of development.

When assessing the impact of a disorder or situation on the child's growth and development, the nurse must consider (1) that "growth" and "development" are not synonymous terms (see discussion under "Defining Growth, Development, and Maturation") and (2) that the family's development may also be altered by the child's illness. Altered family development can be defined through diagnoses such as *altered family process, ineffective family coping: compromised,* and *ineffective family coping: disabling*.

Using Chronologic and Competency Approaches to Study Growth and Development

As the previous discussion implies, a child's development is a complicated process with intertwined aspects. To facilitate learning, the chapters on growth and development are divided according to widely recognized chronologic divisions. Although any chronologic division is somewhat arbitrary, the list of stages that follows is based on the performance or competency criteria that signal change or that progress from one developmental stage to another. It must be remembered that these chronologic divisions and associated developmental stages are not such obvious divisions in the real child's life. *The nurse in practice would do well to assign developmental norms to an individual child that are based on behaviors of the child, rather than on the chronologic age of the child.*

TABLE 3-1

Growth and Development Plan: Developing Children

Analysis: Nursing Diagnostic Statement

Response and Related or Risk Factors: *High risk for altered growth and development; risk factors*

- Illness
- Treatment-related procedures
  - Isolation
  - Injection
  - Traction
  - Casts
  - Bed rest
- Separation from caregiver(s) (parent[s] and significant others)
- Inadequate, inappropriate caregiver(s) support (abuse and neglect)
- Change in environment
- Inadequate sensory stimulation
- Caregiver(s) anxiety
- Caregiver(s) knowledge deficit about age-appropriate development
- Knowledge deficit (child/adolescent)
- Dependency status in health care situations
- Perceived/actual threats to body image/integrity
- Inadequate/deviant coping mechanisms
- Lack of privacy

Projected Outcome: *The child/adolescent will demonstrate acquisition of developmentally appropriate behaviors in the physical, intellectual, and emotional-social domains*

Defining Characteristics

Subjective:

- Child demonstrates inability to keep up with peers in motor and cognitive skills
- Child demonstrates mistrust, shame/doubt, guilt, inferiority, role diffusion
- Child appears to "be a loner, not to need anyone"
- Child senses caregivers' expectations, parental feelings concerning parenting
- Child uses deprecating humor to describe self/others, expressions and behaviors indicating low self-esteem

Objective:

- Flat affect
- Listlessness
- Decreased responses
- Slow social responses
- Limited signs of satisfaction to caregiver

Nursing Interventions

Health Screening

- **Assess factors that can identify altered growth and development** (evidence of infant/child/adolescent's behavior deviating from age-appropriate levels will be observed and documented based on theoretical basis of growth and development; altered peer support and parent-child relationships; inadequate social support; inadequate knowledge of physiologic effects of disease on the child and family)
- **Assess child/adolescent's level of development using developmental norms and specific assessment tools** (refer to Chapter 13, Assessing Child Health, and Appendices 2 through 6)

Evaluation Criteria

- **Any developmental delays will be identified as evidenced by**
- Charted assessment of screening for physical, intellectual, and emotional/social development
- Referral for deviations from the norm detected during screening
- The child/adolescent will achieve age-appropriate developmental tasks at a level appropriate to him/her
- Referrals to community resources will be made as needed

TABLE 3-1 (continued)

Growth and Development Plan: Developing Children

Defining Characteristics	Nursing Interventions	Evaluation Criteria
Objective: • Limited eye contact • Difficulty feeding, decreased appetite • Lethargy • Irritability • Negative mood • Regressive behaviors • Interrupted sleep pattern • Delay in language skills • Delay in gross and fine motor skills • Delay in bowel and bladder control • Failure of infant and parent to display social-affective play activity • Excessive/inappropriate use of defense mechanisms • Decline in school performance • Avoidance of age-appropriate social activities • Isolation of self from others	*Anticipatory guidance; Parent education: Childrearing family* • **Provide anticipatory guidance to caregivers regarding acquisition of knowledge and ability to interact with the child/adolescent, and provide opportunities to support/enhance age-appropriate developmental tasks** (refer to information on developmental norms in each chapter related to specific age groups). • **Provide opportunities for the child/adolescent (including acutely and chronically ill) to meet age-related developmental tasks** (refer to information on nursing interventions and anticipatory guidance in each chapter related to specific age groups and in Chapter 17). *Support system enhancement* • **Refer child/adolescent and family to appropriate community resources as needed:** • Appropriate agency for counseling for child and family treatment • Appropriate agency for supportive services (i.e., occupational therapy, physical therapy, home care services) • Community programs specific to factors affecting the child's altered growth and development (e.g., child protection services, early intervention services, WIC, educational and social services) • Provide information on community self-help groups, parent and sibling support groups, advocacy groups (e.g., Epilepsy Foundation of America, American Heart Association, Association of Retarded Citizens)	

The terms used to describe the chronology of development are

- **Prenatal life**—period of life from conception to birth.
- **Newborn or neonatal life**—period extending from birth through the first month of life.
- **Infancy**—period beginning at the end of the first month of life and ending at 1 year of age.
- **Toddlerhood**—period extending from age 1 year through the 36th month of life.
- **Preschool years**—period extending from the beginning of the 3rd year to the end of the 5th year of life.
- **School-age years or middle childhood**—period from the start of the 6th to the end of the 11th year.
- **Adolescence and young adulthood**—period from the beginning of the 12th to the end of the 21st year of life.

Furthermore, since the whole person is more easily understood if described in terms of broad categories, this book describes the child's development as involving three facets of the self called *competencies: physical, intellectual,* and *emotional-social.* Again, the division is arbitrary and often not clear-cut, since change in each developmental competency affects development in the other spheres as well.

The three competency areas described in this book are defined as follows:

- *Physical competency* involves the child's ability to apply various motor, neurologic, and biologic capacities to steadily achieve more mature self-care abilities requiring mobility and manipulative skills. Aspects of this competency include physical health; body build and configuration; size; strength; rate of motor, neurologic, and biologic maturation; and motor skill performance.
- *Intellectual competency* involves the development of language and reasoning to the point of mature abstract thought and the development of perceptions and communication skills. Some aspects of intellectual competency are perceptual level, memory, problem solving and reasoning ability, language skills, academic achievement, and IQ.
- *Emotional-social competency* concerns development of an inner sense of security that is supported by self-awareness and acceptance and evidenced by the capacity to form productive interpersonal relationships with individuals and groups. Temperament, interpersonal relations skills, emotional adjustment, and development of sexuality and morality are measures of this competency.

Description of the whole person and his or her competencies—physical, intellectual, and emotional-social—is often facilitated when facts or data about the person are organized according to a conceptual framework. Theories of human growth and development provide conceptual frameworks that allow child health care professionals to describe typical behaviors of different-age children, explain the significance of these behaviors, predict behaviors that might occur in a given situation, or control behavioral manifestations. Since human growth and development is highly complex and multifaceted, many developmental theories deal only with one aspect or domain of development.

Understanding of development can be enhanced by the study of several theories. This text emphasizes two major theories, Piaget's theory of intellectual (cognitive) development and Erikson's theory of emotional-social (psychosocial) development, and incorporates other theories as they are applicable. It is useful to analyze different theories of growth and development to determine their utility in guiding nursing practice. Table 3–2 provides a comparison of major theories of human growth and development.

Developmental Theories

Physical Competency

Intellectual and emotional-social competencies are both deeply rooted in and influenced by the capacities and needs of one's physical competency. Underlying each developmental advance is a physical maturational or functional change. Likewise, a child's feelings and behavior are directly affected by both physical and emotional states and current physical needs. An example of this is the peak period of misbehavior that is typical just prior to a child's usual mealtimes, when there is a physical need for food or there is less attention from a parent during meal preparation.

Because physical development is mostly quantitative, it is easily measured. Physical development also displays some conspicuous age uniformities, so it is a useful means of evaluating the relative health status of a child (see Chapter 13, Assessing Child Health, for examples of methods of evaluating physical competency). The level of physical competency achieved by a given child is compared with established norms or averages. These norms are derived from the mathematical average obtained by measuring a given trait in many children of similar ages. The norm is more truly representative when the children measured are drawn from varying social and cultural groups. However, if a group of children digress significantly from the norm for a given trait, many of them should be measured for that trait to establish an appropriate average.

Growth charts for height and weight represent an example of norms established to determine physical competency. These grids are especially helpful when a pattern is obtained over a period of time for the child and compared for consistency in height and

TABLE 3-2
Comparison of Theories of Human Growth and Development

Underlying Theoretical Motivation for Behavior	Theoretical Assumptions	Use	Nursing Interventions
Theorist: GESELL. Description of typical physical and mental characteristics of infants, children, and adolescents. Focus: motor skills and hygiene, language skills, and personal-social skills, including play and past-times, school, emotional expression, fears, dreams, self and sex, ethical sense, and philosophical outlook			
Development is genetically programmed. Cycles of behavioral stages influenced by genetic inheritance alternate between equilibrium (in which the child is in harmony with the environment) and disequilibrium (or periods of disharmony). Environment has little effect on development. Individual differences are explained in relation to genetically determined body types (somatotype)	Behavioral cycles tend to occur at specified chronologic ages in all children. Prior practice or training does not influence age at which behaviors occur. Readiness for developmental progression of behaviors is genetically preprogrammed.	Primarily descriptive; explains prior behaviors; predicts future development	Allows for comparisons of individual child with average behaviors for age to assess developmental level; can be used in parent teaching and anticipatory guidance of parents to help them understand their child in relation to other children of same age; does not allow for control of future development
Theorist: HAVIGHURST. Description of physical, cognitive, affective, and social developmental tasks			
Heredity and environment interact to produce biologic, psychologic, and cultural tasks that the child strives to accomplish. Accomplishment leads to happiness and future success. Failure to accomplish leads to unhappiness, lack of future success, and lack of approval from society	Critical periods are assumed for some tasks, whereas other tasks tend to recur in successive stages. Theory implies optimal age range for teaching to facilitate achievement of critical period tasks	Primarily descriptive, does not explain; describes how child is and was, does not explain why; can be used to predict future development	Allows for comparison of individual child with average behaviors for age to assess developmental level; can be used in parent teaching and anticipatory guidance of parents to suggest ways environment can be structured to facilitate task achievement; also assists parents in ability to predict readiness for future tasks
Theorist: FREUD. Psychosocial; emphasis on development of personality			
Developing child is essentially a passive recipient of two internal, biologic forces or instinctual urges: the urge to survive and procreate (libido) and a death urge that governs aggressive or destructive acts. Libido or life force is predominant. Satisfaction of urges results in tension reduction or pleasure; frustration of urges results in increased tension or pain. Motivation for behavior, simply stated, is to achieve pleasure and avoid pain	Invariable sequence of four stages (oral, anal, phallic, latency) is assumed, in which pleasure is invested in a different erogenous zone or modality. Sensual pleasure is derived from use of this zone. Three personality components (id, ego, superego) develop sequentially during birth, toddlerhood, and preschool years, respectively. Id is raw libido seeking pleasure. Ego is reality component, which mediates conflicts occurring when id urges are frustrated by environmental realities. Defense mechanisms are ego creations, which allow for tension reduction when urges are frustrated. Superego (conscience) arises from the ego and puts good or bad labels on behavior. According to Freud, psychosexual development is essentially complete at approximately 6 years of age	Allows for explanation of past and present behaviors; not useful in predicting specific future behaviors; limited control of behavior is implied in pleasure motive	Can be used in parent teaching and anticipatory guidance of parents to explain basis for past and present behaviors, guide parenting behaviors to facilitate healthy development; care of the infant focuses on provision of pleasurable sensory experiences and protection from unnecessary frustration of pleasure motive; as child enters toddlerhood, care will include careful guidance for learning of environmental realities and appropriate problem solving to attain pleasurable goals. Care in preschool years includes setting reasonable standards of right and wrong and appropriate limits to enforce these standards. Awareness of sensory zone or modality for age and stage allows nurses to avoid painful or intrusive procedures involving that modality if possible (e.g., axillary rather than rectal temperatures when anal zone is predominant)

Table continued on following page

TABLE 3-2
Comparison of Theories of Human Growth and Development *(Continued)*

Underlying Theoretical Motivation for Behavior	Theoretical Assumptions	Use	Nursing Interventions
Theorist: ERIKSON. Psychosocial development			
Forces within the individual interact with societal and cultural forces to produce a series of eight tasks, conflicts, or crises, which the individual strives to successfully resolve. Each stage's task is represented by opposite extremes between a positive and a negative aspect. The individual strives and is impelled by social and cultural forces to establish equilibrium between these opposite aspects, ideally with a predominance of the qualities of the positive aspect. Successful resolution of the conflict or task of one stage produces in the individual the attributes necessary for meeting the task of the next stage	Stages are invariant, with each stage being built on and dependent on the preceding stages (epigenesis). Critical periods exist during which resolution of the central crisis must occur in order for optimal future development to occur. Each new stage requires that important aspects of the previous stage must be relinquished, at least in part. For example, in order to achieve a sense of autonomy, the dependence of trust must be relinquished. Prior practice and teaching do not facilitate passage through stages. Psychologic and social readiness must be present for this to occur	Little attention to individual differences decreases ability to use in describing development in relation to other children; explains past and present development; predicts what might occur in future development	Provides a useful framework for helping parents understand behaviors and development of their child; useful in anticipatory guidance of parents in helping them to structure the environment and to use parenting skills that will facilitate healthy development; highly useful as a theoretical framework for nursing interaction with and provision of nursing care to children. Awareness of the current development characteristics allows for interventions that would promote achievement at the positive extreme for the crisis of that stage and avoid imposition of negative aspects of that stage. It is especially useful in the structuring of dramatic play sessions to assist the child in working through his or her feelings; can be used to provide nursing care in a way that will ensure maximum compliance
Theorist: PIAGET. Cognitive development			
Heredity, or innate biologic structure, and environment (physical and social) interact. Individuals are seen as active organisms who initiate acts that result in development. All individuals have a tendency to organize their mental activities in order to be able to deal with their environment (adaptation). Adaptation involves the attempt to maintain a balance (equilibration) between the taking in of new information that fits existing mental structures (assimilation) and the changing of mental structures to allow contrary information to fit these structures (accommodation)	Cognitive development proceeds in an invariant sequence of four stages for all children. Each stage has substages. Prior practice or teaching has little effect on development of new cognitive skills and progression to the next stage, until suitable cognitive maturity or readiness for that stage has occurred	Little attention to individual differences decreases ability to use in describing development in relation to other children; explains past and present; predicts patterns of future cognitive development	Useful in parent teaching and anticipatory guidance of parents to help explain to them the nature of their child's understanding of the environment at different stages; of high practical utility in structuring of patient teaching; implies definite guidelines for the kinds and amount of information that the child will require; allows nurses to know types of misperceptions that can occur as a result of the level of mental operations that occur at different stages and to assess and intervene in relation to these perceptions
Theorist: KOHLBERG. Moral development			
Extends Piaget's theory and theorizes same or similar behavioral motivation. Standards of the social environment and social rewards play a major role in motivation for movement to higher levels of moral reasoning. Urges within the child beginning with premoral urge to satisfy own needs also interact with societal standards. Modeling is also recognized as influential in development of moral standards	Moral development proceeds in an invariant sequence of six stages. Theory is heavily tied to Piagetian cognitive stages; acquisition of higher levels of moral reasoning cannot occur until appropriate cognitive development has occurred	Little attention to individual differences decreases ability to use in describing development in relation to other children; explains past and present; predicts what can occur within appropriate societal context in future	Main utility is in parental guidance and in counseling of adolescents. Higher levels of moral reasoning can be facilitated by setting realistic standards of right and wrong, teaching the child ways to avoid misbehavior, emphasizing the rights and need of others, and providing multiple opportunities to explore the elements of moral problems and their possible solutions

TABLE 3-2
Comparison of Theories of Human Growth and Development *(Continued)*

Underlying Theoretical Motivation for Behavior	Theoretical Assumptions	Use	Nursing Interventions
Theorist: SKINNER, WATSON (Learning Theory; Behaviorism). Focus entirely on behavior; internal processes such as thoughts and feelings, while sometimes acknowledged, are not dealt with			
Behavior is determined (conditioned) by environmental events or experiences or consequences. Behaviors that are rewarded (reinforced) are repeated. Behaviors that are not rewarded or are punished are not repeated	A previously neutral stimulus can be paired with a response that elicits a behavior so that the behavior is elicited by the neutral stimulus (classic conditioning). Making a reward contingent on the emission of a certain behavior increases the strength of that behavior's occurrence (operant or instrumental conditioning). Development does not occur in stages but is recurrent throughout the life span	Allows for prediction and control of behavior	High practical utility; childrearing and nursing care can be focused on ways to encourage desired behaviors; extremely useful in discipline issues and in compliance issues related to medical and nursing treatment regimens; not suited to in-depth explanations of internal processes, such as thinking, feeling
Theorist: BANDURA, BANDURA, AND WALTERS (Social Learning or Observational Learning Theories). Focuses on how behaviors that are appropriate to age, sex, and social class are learned			
Motivation is primarily environmental. Child will imitate or model behaviors that he or she observes, especially if those behaviors are perceived as being rewarded. These imitated behaviors are then reinforced when performed by the child. If the individual modeling a behavior is a significant individual in the life of the child, the behavior may be imitated, even if no reward is perceived (vicarious reinforcement)	Theory is heavily dependent on operant conditioning model. It accepts internal mental processes as an aspect of behavior. Memory is acknowledged, in that behaviors may not be emitted until long after they are observed. Idea of free choice is incorporated, in that individuals are seen as being able to deliberate on the consequences of observed behaviors. Modeling as a motivator of behavior and behavioral change is seen as recurrent throughout the life span	Explains past development; does not predict future; allows for control of behaviors instrumental in development	Great practical utility, especially in guidance of parents regarding childrearing. Parents can be taught to model as well as preach those behaviors that they desire in their children and to encourage association with positive models. This would involve the "do as I do" approach to parenting. It includes useful nursing implications, in that exposure of children to others who successfully and appropriately cope with procedures and treatment regimens would provide a model for their coping behaviors
Theorist: SEARS. Social learning theory applied to socialization; focus on overt behaviors			
As in observational learning, child imitates observed or modeled behaviors, which are rewarded or emitted by significant others. A secondary source of reward is intrinsic to the act of imitation itself, in that the child experiences a pleasurable sense of closeness to the significant other whose behavior is emitted. Internal and external motivational sources interact, in that reduction of anxiety and psychic tension is seen as significant in reward system for imitated behaviors	Modeling as a motivator of behavior and behavioral change is recurrent throughout the life span. New behaviors that are then rewarded can become the basis for learning even newer behaviors	Explains past development; does not predict future; allows for control of behaviors instrumental in development	Great practical utility, especially in guidance of parents regarding childrearing. Parents can be taught to model as well as preach behaviors that they desire in their children and to encourage association with positive models. Specific implications for child discipline are included. Physical punishment is viewed as modeling of aggressive behavior. This would involve "do as I do" approach to parenting. It includes useful nursing implications, in that exposure of children to others who successfully and appropriately cope with procedures and treatment regimens would provide a model for their coping behaviors

Table continued on following page

TABLE 3-2
Comparison of Theories of Human Growth and Development *(Continued)*

Underlying Theoretical Motivation for Behavior	Theoretical Assumptions	Use	Nursing Interventions
Theorist: MASLOW (Humanistic Theory). Focuses on attributes or characteristics that contribute to healthy personality development and are not traditionally dealt with in other theories, e.g., love, creativity, self			
Humans are motivated by two need systems. Basic or deficiency needs such as food, water, and shelter are imposed and rewarded by the environment. Growth needs or metaneeds such as the needs for beauty and self-fulfillment are internally motivated and reinforced. These need systems are hierarchically arranged with lower level needs assuming dominance or prepotency over higher level needs. When one need level is satisfied, the next becomes prepotent	Theory does not address developmental stages or shaping of human behaviors; is concerned with the uniqueness and the potential of individuals	Not intended for use in describing individuals or groups of individuals; explains behavior only in reference to need systems; cannot be used to predict or control development, except as this is related to ability to meet individual needs	Primary utility lies in awareness of needs hierarchy. Parenting and nursing care practices that meet basic needs will assist the individual in reaching the next need state
Theorist: FOWLER. Faith development			
The theory is an extension of developmental theories of developmentalists Piaget, Erikson, Levinson, Kohlberg, and Gilligan. Faith beliefs are understood as a system of order and activities, rather than as an inner spiritual process and presence in the world	Faith development proceeds in an invariant sequence of seven stages. It is strongly tied to Piagetian cognitive stages; acquisition of higher levels of faith development cannot occur, unless appropriate cognitive development has occurred	Little attention to individual differences; decreases ability to use in describing development to other children; explains past and present, predicts patterns of future faith development	Provides a useful framework for parental guidance and for counseling children and adolescents; implies definite guidelines for the kinds and amount of information that the child will require; allows nurses to know types of perceptions the child has, as a result of mental operations manifested at different stages, and to assess and intervene in relation to these perceptions

By Sandra B. Frick-Helms, PhD, RN.

weight gains. Growth charts are now available that allow for consideration of parental size in evaluating a child's growth. The influence of parental size on these evaluations is shown in Figure 3–1.

Body weight has proved to be a useful index of nutritional status and correlates positively with height increases. For example, a child at 4 to 6 months is considered to have adequate caloric intake if the birthweight has doubled. Beyond that age, weight increases usually correspond closely to height increases.

Head circumference also is used to monitor physical development. Growth charts for head circumference are available for evaluating a child in relation to established norms. Head circumference is usually a part of the physical appraisal until about age 4 or 5 years. This is because a composite of these measurements provides an estimate of the rate of brain growth. The normal range is narrow for each age group. Brain and nerve cell growth specialization are most rapid from birth to approximately 4 years of age, at which point there should be a significant slowing. Thus, this age span is considered a *critical period* for protein and caloric intake and for intellectual development. A critical period in growth or development, or both, is one in which optimal growth must occur. If it is delayed, growth will not occur or will be delayed significantly. There are critical periods in all domains of development. If growth does not occur during a critical period, catch-up growth can be facilitated in some instances. Figure 3–2 shows some organ tissues for which critical growth periods exist. Brain growth is almost complete by 2 years of age, when 80 per cent of the adult head size has been attained. These first 2 years, then, represent the most critical period for brain growth. Factors that interfere significantly with brain growth during the first 2 years of life can mean lifelong problems. The most readily available method of assessing brain growth is measuring head circumference. See Chapter 13 for further explanation of this measurement.

Another measurement of physical development is skeletal growth or bone age. Skeletal growth is most rapid during infancy and adolescence. Norms have also been established for dental development and vi-

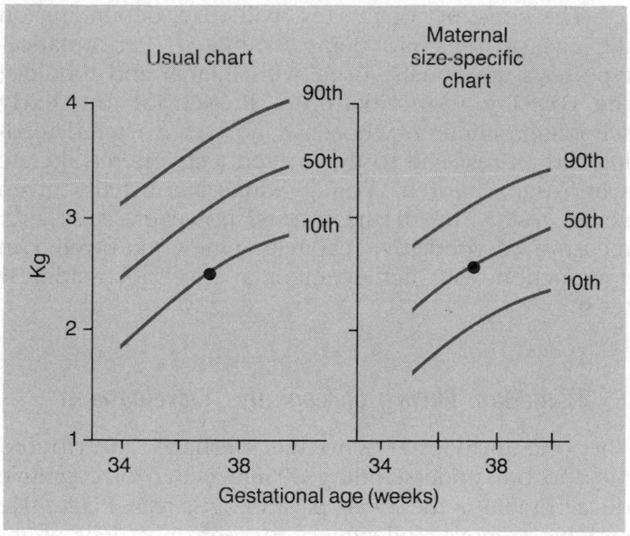

FIGURE 3-1. The weight of a 5-pound newborn baby, born of a 4-foot, 11-inch, 88-pound mother, plotted on a usual growth grid *(left)* and on one that is specific for the maternal size *(right)*. (*Left,* Redrawn from Winick, M. [1970]. Biological correlations. *American Journal of Diseases of Children,* 120, 416. *Right,* Redrawn from Thomson, A. M., et al. [1968]. The assessment of fetal growth. *Journal of Obstetrics and Gynecology of the British Commonwealth, 75,* 903. By permission of Blackwell Scientific Publications.)

tal signs (temperature, pulse, respirations, and blood pressure) for children at various ages, which are also measures of physical competency. Likewise, laboratory determinations important to routine health appraisal have established normative values for children at different ages. Normative ranges for vision and hearing performance at different ages also exist.

Nutritional patterns and intake needs at different ages also have been determined through averages. An estimation of the child's nutritional adequacy is an important aspect of the evaluation of physical competency.

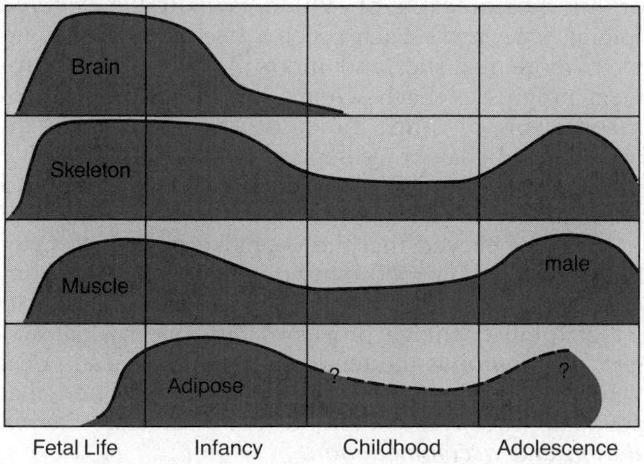

FIGURE 3-2. Critical periods of increasing cell numbers for several organ tissues. (Redrawn from Smith, D. W., & Bierman, F. L. [1973]. *The biologic age of man.* Philadelphia: WB Saunders.)

Physical activity patterns associated with sleep, rest, exercise, and elimination also are significant features of physical competency for which normative ranges exist. However, these must be evaluated in context with the typical patterns of the family unit.

In evaluating physical competency in areas for which norms are not measurable, such as motor skills, screening tools are useful. The Denver Developmental Screening Test revised (DDST-R), which evaluates fine and gross motor development, is an example. (Frankenburg et al, 1992).

Specific norms of physical competency are presented in Chapter 13, in the age-related chapters on growth and development, and in the appendices.

Keen observation is required by the nurse assessing a child's physical development and physical needs. Children, especially those under 5 or 6 years of age,* have difficulty identifying and describing their physical discomforts or needs in ways adults can understand. Also, physical changes in children often occur suddenly and without any accompanying warning signs.

The nurse caring for children should always keep in mind that the physical care offered is not only supportive to the child's physical needs and development but is also a means of communicating support for emotional-social and intellectual needs. The nurse's understanding of physical development and recognition of the alterations to physical development caused by stress—whether accidental (illness), maturational (change in structure or function), or environmental (inadequate diet related to poor socioeconomic status of family unit)—will give direction for nursing strategies to prevent, minimize, or remedy those stresses and for interventions to enhance the child's environment in ways that support healthy physical development.

Intellectual Competency

Intellect is a composite of skills, behaviors, and adaptive abilities that make it possible for an individual to adjust to new situations, to think abstractly, and to profit from his or her experiences. Although only ambiguous measures of intellect exist, it is demonstrable in the way a person solves problems and in the appropriateness of his or her response in any given situation.

Intelligence, once believed to be genetically fixed, has been found, in longitudinal studies, to be fluctuating (Vaughan & Litt, 1990; Hetherington & Parke, 1975). This finding illustrates the effect of environment on intellectual development and function.

*Language and intellectual development have not progressed enough before this age to allow clarity in verbalization of mental processes.

Findings of environmental effects on intellect have resulted in a rising concern for the provision of primary or early learning opportunities (Fig. 3–3). Evidence of this concern has been exemplified in the movements for development of Head Start or Get Set programs, early intervention programs, preschool or kindergarten education, nursery schools, play programs for children during confinement, and similar social structures whose aim is to counteract any sensory deprivations that a child might experience because of any sociocultural or physical limitations in the child's early life. Other programs that have arisen out of a recognition of the importance of early motor and sensory stimulation are early intervention for immature babies and infant-stimulation programs for any infants with signs of developmental lag.

Knowledge of intellectual development and intellectual needs of children at various ages is extremely valuable to the nurse who interacts with children. *Understanding the child's level of intellectual thought and function helps the nurse to decipher more meaningfully a child's communications, to interpret more accurately the behaviors and the processes that motivate them, and to realize more emphatically the meaning various experiences have for the child.* This understanding should be demonstrated in the nursing interventions planned, the approach with which those interventions are offered, and the age-appropriateness of nurse-child communication.

Although most tests available for measuring predictive intellectual capacity or estimating level of intellectual function are done by personnel in other health-related professions, the nurse should be familiar with existing tests and the caution with which they must be interpreted. The nurse should also be aware of the variability of test results in young children and of the limited correlation between results of these early tests and of tests conducted later in the child's life, although more consistency usually exists after age 5.

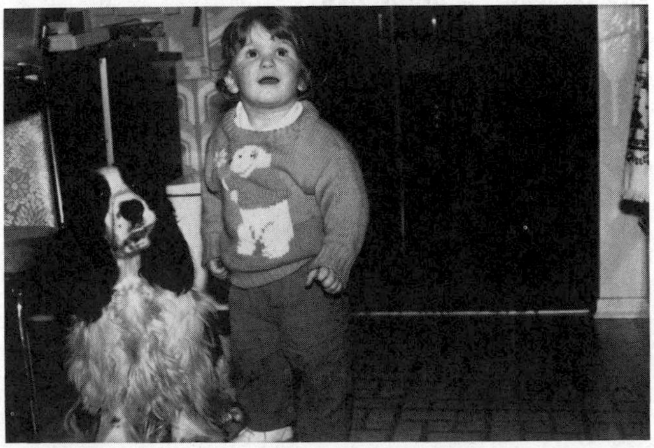

FIGURE 3-3. The child's growing capacity to take in the world is the source of individuality.

The construct of the test will vary, depending on the age of the child being evaluated. Performance-type tests are usually used with infants and toddlers; the DDST-R is an example. Preschool and early school-age children who have not yet mastered reading cannot respond to the written tests offered literate school-age children. Young adults are usually given verbal tests. Any of these tests, however, is a fairer measure of predictive capacity when interpreted in conjunction with achievement and school readiness tests.

Piagetian Theory of Cognitive Development

The one individual who has perhaps contributed most to our understanding of intellectual or cognitive development is the Swiss psychologist Jean Piaget. He and his Geneva colleagues, through a variety of ingenious studies, derived the stage theory about children's intellectual activity and how it undergoes qualitative changes over the span of childhood.

According to Piaget (1952, 1970) and Piaget and Inhelder (1969), there are four major stages of cognitive development: sensorimotor, preoperational, concrete operational, and formal operational. Each stage has its own substages or phases. Each of the major stages of cognitive development represents a qualitative change in the way the individual thinks or behaves. All individuals progress through the stages of cognitive development in the same order, and no stage of development is skipped. (This idea of invariance of occurrence of stages of cognitive development has been supported by research.) Each of the stages is built on what occurred in the previous stage, and each stage provides the basis for the next stage. In the following overview of Piaget's theory, the terminology of the theory, summarized in Table 3–3, is used.

At each stage of development, the individual has mental representations or cognitive structures of her or his world, each of which is called a *schema* (plural, *schemata*). Each schema becomes more complex, more realistic, and more abstract as development progresses. Each schema involves a mental representation of some facet of the world and an observable behavior. Schemata become more highly developed through the processes of assimilation and accommodation.

Piaget believed that the cognitive development of individuals is governed by two major organizing principles. *Organization* is the tendency of all species to integrate all cognitive processes into one overall system. *Adaptation* is the tendency for all species to deal with their environment. Piaget further asserted that adaptation involves continuous twin processes, *assimilation* and *accommodation*.

Accommodation is a process involving the changing of mental representations in order to include new information that does not fit the existing schema. In

TABLE 3-3
Definition of Piagetian Terms

Schema (Plural, Schemata)	Mental representation or cognitive structure representing objects, events, ideas; known by its observable behavior
Assimilation	Mental process that involves the taking in of new sensory information that fits or matches existing schemata
Accommodation	Mental process that involves the changing of schemata in order to include new information that does not fit the existing schemata
Adaptation	Tendency for all species to adapt to (or deal with) their environment; an equilibrium between assimilation and accommodation
Organization	Tendency of all species to integrate all cognitive processes into one overall system; the proper interrelationship among schemata
Equilibrium	Cognitive balance between assimilation and accommodation
Equilibration	Process involved in equilibrium
Operations	Mental activities that develop from manipulation of objects

By Sandra B. Frick-Helms, RN, PhD.

life a baby obtains food by crying and subsequently sucking on the nipple that is offered. The baby's schema for obtaining food changes when solids are offered from a spoon. The baby must accommodate his or her schema for obtaining food by changing the way in which it is ingested and the sensory qualities of what is ingested. Later the baby will again accommodate when self-feeding begins.

Assimilation is the process of incorporating new information into one's current activity or way of thinking (making the unfamiliar seem familiar). New information is assimilated via all of the senses. Therefore, one's schema for an object or event can consist of multiple types of sensory information. For example, a child will form a schema for dog by assimilating visual information (two ears, a tail, four legs), auditory information (bark), and tactile information (texture of fur, the feel of a wet tongue). As different dogs are encountered, they can be assimilated into the existing dog schema as long as no change in mental representation occurs.

Assimilation allows for the addition of new perceptions to a schema with existing capabilities; accommodation requires that existing schema be changed to fit more complex circumstances. Assimilation and accommodation function together to bring about a cognitive balance called *equilibrium*. The process of equilibrium allows the individual to form a mental representation of the world that is suitable to existing capabilities and that allows for growth and change. As the individual grows and capabilities increase, the balance or equilibrium between assimilation and accommodation is threatened. The individual is thereby motivated to maintain equilibrium by altering old ways of thinking to solve new problems. Figure 3-4 illustrates the flow of the intellectual processes for adaptation.

The following is an outline of Piaget's theorized sequence of the development of intellect.

Sensorimotor Period—First 2 Years of Life

During the sensorimotor period, the child moves from neonatal birth reflexes to the construction of symbolic images. (Fig. 3-5). The task involved is mastery of coordinating simple sensorimotor activity. During this stage, children are dependent on their bodies for self-expression and communication. They work to create an organized world that links their desires for physical satisfaction to their sensory experiences.

There are six substages in the sensorimotor period, which are listed in Table 3-4 and discussed in Chapter 5.

Preoperational Period—2 to 7 Years

The major qualitative change in cognitive function from the sensorimotor period to the preoperational period involves the ability to use symbols. This period continues to be characterized by egocentric* thought that is expressed in animism,† artificialism,†† realism,§ and magic omnipotence.** The child at this state continues to seem illogical to adults. The child's task is to use language and memory to begin to understand the past, present, and immediate future. These children display progressively more socialized behavior in this period as they move steadily away from egocentric thought. The irreversibility of this stage evolves into a conception of reversibility in the concrete state. If a preschooler is asked whether he has a brother, he will say "yes." If asked whether his brother has a brother, he will say "no." The preoperational period is composed of two stages: preconceptual and intuitive (Table 3-5).

*The child sees things only from his or her own point of view.
†The child attributes lifelike qualities to inanimate objects.
††The child perceives that all things are designed by human beings.
§Everything is considered real by a child in this stage—even dreams.
**The child believes that things can be made to happen just by thinking them and that the world exists for the child alone.

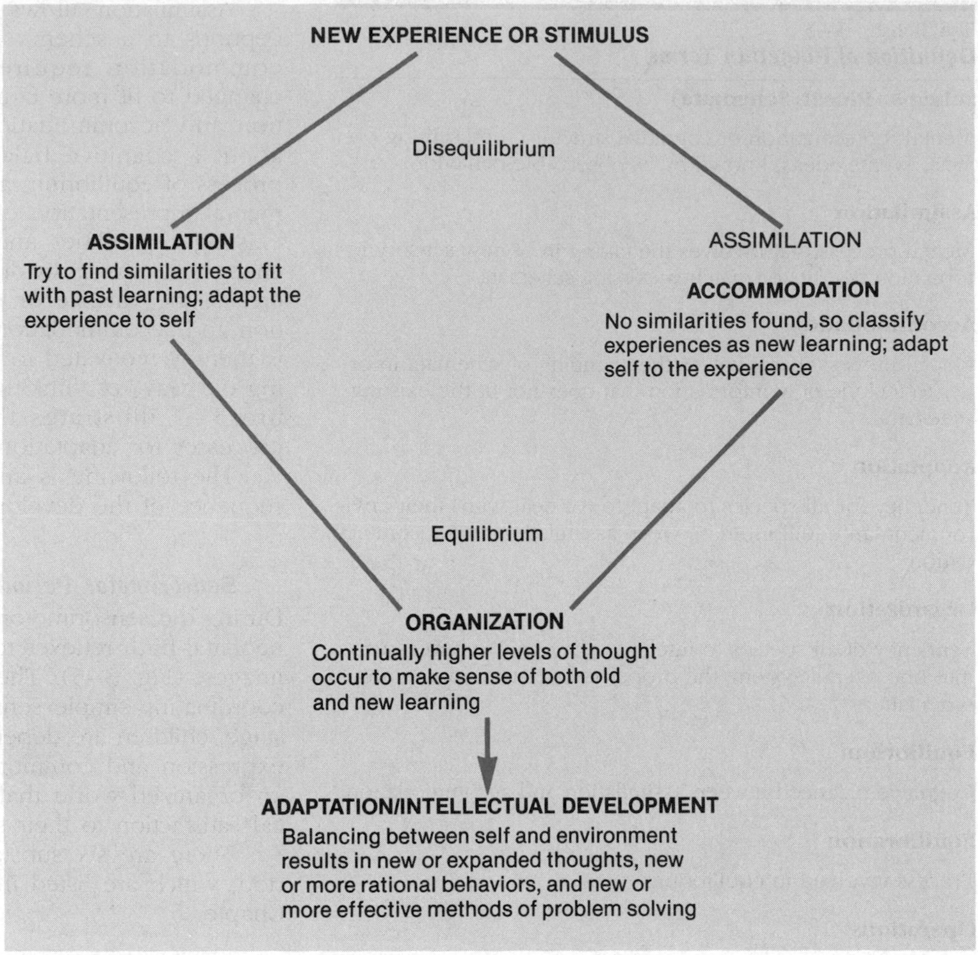
NEW EXPERIENCE OR STIMULUS
Disequilibrium
ASSIMILATION
Try to find similarities to fit with past learning; adapt the experience to self
ASSIMILATION
ACCOMMODATION
No similarities found, so classify experiences as new learning; adapt self to the experience
Equilibrium
ORGANIZATION
Continually higher levels of thought occur to make sense of both old and new learning
ADAPTATION/INTELLECTUAL DEVELOPMENT
Balancing between self and environment results in new or expanded thoughts, new or more rational behaviors, and new or more effective methods of problem solving

FIGURE 3-4. Intellectual process in adaptation (a diagrammatic presentation of Piaget's theory of intellectual development as an adaptive process).

Stage 1 (Preconceptual Stage)—2 to 4 Years. Children now form mental images to stand for things they cannot see (symbolic thought), including their various properties. These concepts are reinforced through drawings, language, dreams, and "make believe" and "imitative" play. Play involving language, action, and symbolic imitation is this child's primary tool for adaptation and consumes most of his or her waking hours. A child uses symbolic thought in play that focuses on deferred imitation of previously viewed activities, such as Mommy washing dishes or Daddy fixing the car. Symbolic thought is also evident in play in which one object is made to stand for something else. For the preoperational child, a packing carton has endless possibilities as a car, a spaceship, a house, a swimming pool, and so on. Most play at this stage is parallel. Because of children's egocentrism, they are engrossed in their own thoughts, feelings, and experiences and so are not able to give attention to what someone else is doing or may want. This egocentrism is also operational in their perception of objects and events. For example, these children cannot visualize the other side of a box or the other side

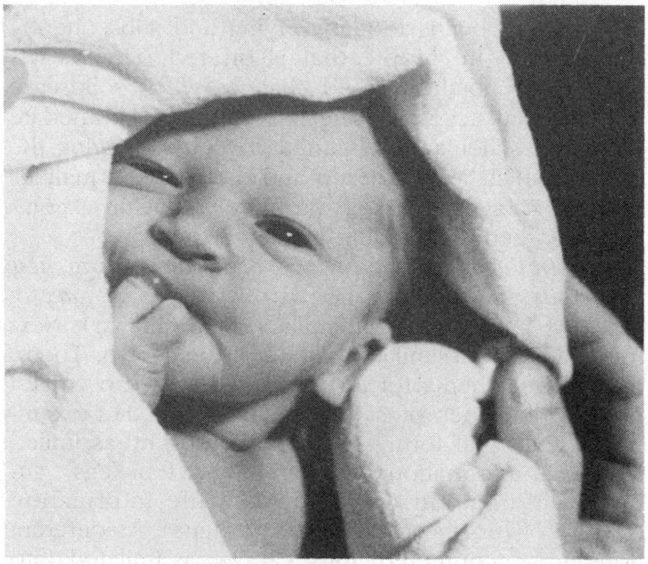

FIGURE 3-5. Primitive reflexes, accidentally produced (stage 1), are repeated for pleasure (stage 2) during the sensorimotor period.

TABLE 3-4
Six Substages: Sensorimotor Period (Birth to 2 Yrs)

Substage 1: Use of Reflexes (Birth to 1 Mo)

- Reflex responses to external stimuli
- Random body movements
- Genuinely intelligent behavior absent

Substage 2: Primary Circular Reactions (1–4 Mos)

- Active effort to reproduce behavior that was first performed by chance
- Accidentally acquired behavior becomes a new sensorimotor habit

Substage 3: Secondary Circular Reactions (4–8 Mos)

- Greater awareness of environment
- Increasing interest in results of actions
- First notion of causality emerges with recognition that certain actions have certain results
- Dim awareness of *before* and *after*
- Achievement of eye-hand coordination
- Beginning development of object permanence

Substage 4: Coordination of Secondary Circular Reactions (8–12 Mos)

- Solution of simple problems
- Demonstration of anticipatory behavior
- More highly developed object permanence

Substage 5: Tertiary Circular Reactions (12–18 Mos)

- Rudimentary trial and error
- Beginning of reasoning
- Evident object permanence

Substage 6: Invention of New Means Through Deduction (18–24 Mos)

- Well-developed understanding of the nature of objects
- Basic concept of causality
- Well-developed object permanence
- View of self as separate from others in environment
- Ability to use symbols mentally

Based on Piaget, J. (1952). *The origins of intelligence in children*. New York: International Universities Press.

TABLE 3-5
Preoperational Period (2–7 Years)

Stage 1: Preconceptual Stage (2–4 Yrs)

- Forms symbolic thought
- Is egocentric in thoughts, feelings, and experiences
- Is egocentric in perception of objects and events
- Displays deferred imitation
- Understands instructions literally

Stage 2: Perceptual or Intuitive Stage (4–7 Yrs)

- Prelogical reasoning appears
- Experiences and objects are judged by outside appearances and results
- Can concentrate only upon one characteristic of an object at a time (centration)
- Uses words to express thoughts
- Demonstrates illogical reasoning (transductive reasoning)
- Play becomes more socialized

Based on Piaget, J. (1952). *The origins of intelligence in children*. New York: International Universities Press.

of a profile of a face (Fig. 3–6). They wonder if ocean waves stop at night when they are asleep (i.e., all else in the world sleeps when they sleep). Children comprehend "doing what they are told" and relate it causally to pleasing their parents. They take their instructions literally, therefore needing specific instruction in behaviors to be carried out; "be good" is not specific enough for children in this stage to enact.

Stage 2 (Perceptual or Intuitive Stage)—4 to 7 Years. Prelogical reasoning appears and is based on perceptions that do not acknowledge intrinsic aspects. Experiences and objects are judged by outside appearances and results. For example, given an equal number each of toothpicks and pencils, a child may insist there are more pencils because they are bigger or they take up more space. Nor can the child accept that two differently shaped 4-ounce glasses contain the same amount of water if one is short and wide and the other tall and narrow. Selective attention is also present in that the child can concentrate only on one characteristic of an object at a time. For example, red balls cannot at the same time be rubber balls, even though the child's image of the object attributes to it multiple properties. This focus on only one aspect of a situation at a time is called *centration*. Not until the next period of cognitive development will the child be capable of decentration. Children at this stage begin to use words to express their thoughts, but during the first couple of years in this stage, some thoughts are still acted out. During the first half of

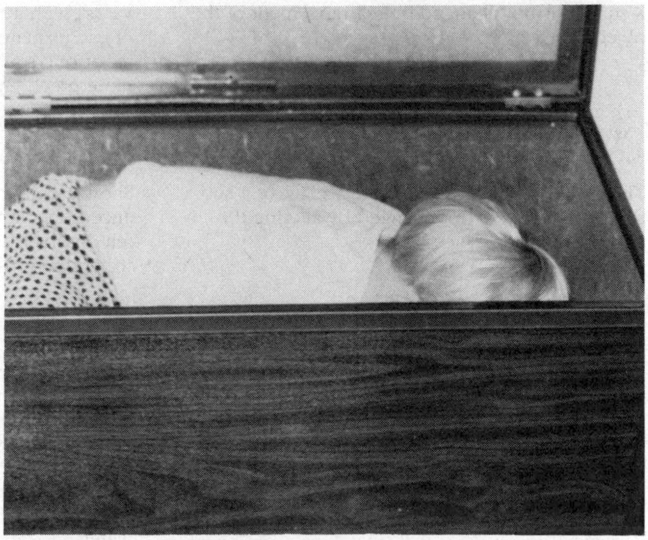

FIGURE 3-6. During the preoperational stage, children see things only from their own point of view. Children of age 2½ think that because they cannot see anyone, they cannot be seen.

TABLE 3-6
Conservation Abilities and Tasks Used to Detect Their Existence

Conservation Ability	Conservation Task	Conserving Response
Number		
The ability to recognize that number is not changed if arrangement or physical properties of items changes	Arrange five pennies in a row close together and another five pennies in a row but spaced at a distance from one another; ask the child which row has more pennies	Both have the same number of pennies
	Show the child four blue marbles and two red marbles; ask whether there are more red marbles or more blue marbles	There are more blue marbles
Length		
The ability to recognize that length is not changed if configuration changes	Show a child two straight strings of identical length; curve one string into an S curve; ask the child which string is longer	Both strings are the same length
Liquid Amount		
The ability to recognize that the amount of liquid is not changed by the shape of the container into which it is poured	Show a child a short, wide container filled to the brim with colored water; pour the colored water into a tall narrow container that holds the same amount of liquid as the first container; ask the child which glass holds the most water	They both hold the same amount of water
Solid Amount (Substance)		
The ability to recognize that the amount of a solid substance is not changed by altering the shape of the substance	Show a child two identical balls of clay; roll one ball into a "snake"; ask the child which ball has more clay	They both hold the same amount of clay
	Show the child two identical bags of potato chips; smash one bag so that the chips are broken into crumbs; ask the child which bag has more potato chips	They both have the same amount of potato chips
Space (Area)		
The ability to recognize that the amount of area on a surface is not changed by rearrangement of the objects on it	Show a child two identical green square "farmyards" with a farm building placed on each corner of each square; move all four buildings to the center of one square; ask the child which farmyard has more green grassy space	They both have the same amount of grassy space
Weight		
The ability to recognize that the weight of a substance or object is not changed by altering the shape of the substance	Show a child two identical balls of clay evenly balanced on a scale; remove them from the scale; flatten one ball; ask the child which ball will now weigh the most	They both still weigh the same
Volume		
The ability to recognize that displacement of liquids results from the volume of an object and will not be changed by altering the shape of the object	Show a child two containers of water; drop identical balls of clay into the water and tell the child to watch how high the water rises; remove one ball of clay from its container and alter its shape by flattening or elongating it or dividing into several separate balls of clay; ask the child which water will be higher when the clay is again dropped into the water	The water level will be the same in both containers

By Sandra B. Frick-Helms, RN, PhD.

this stage, the child still perceives anything that moves or is active as being alive. Play becomes gradually more social, demanding collective rules, organized games, and fantasy enactments of the rules and values of the child's elders. An additional limitation of preoperational thought is *transductive reasoning*. There are two kinds of logical reasoning: deductive reasoning goes from general to particular; inductive reasoning goes from particular to general. The preoperational child goes from particular to particular without considering the general situation. This type of illogical thinking can result in the child's assuming the existence of a cause-and-effect relationship between two unrelated events: "I was a bad boy, so I got sick."

Concrete Operational Period—7 to 11 Years

The child at the beginning of this stage thinks and reasons with inductive logic, but by the end of this stage the thinking is deductive and the child's world shifts from "one of mythology to one of science," in which objects and events have explanations (Maier, 1969). These children can mentally perform tasks that previously they actually had to carry out. They learn to comprehend *conservation* and *reversibility*. Conservation, the ability to recognize that two equal quantities of matter remain equal regardless of the transformation they undergo, may be the most important contribution of Piaget's theory to our understanding of cognitive development. Children develop the ability to conserve for different qualities of matter at different times. The abilities to conserve for length and number occur early in the period, while the abilities to conserve for space and volume do not occur until the end of the period. Examples of different types of conservation and the tasks through which they are demonstrated are shown in Table 3–6. Learning about one kind of conservation cannot be transferred to another kind of conservation. Each kind is learned separately through manipulation of the different qualities of matter. (This is an example of just how concrete mental operations are during this period.)

The concrete operational child is capable of *decentration,* the ability to focus on multiple aspects of an object, event, or situation at the same time. These children understand that most actions can be reversed. They also understand the value of rules, and they base judgments on reason (Fig. 3–7). The future and the abstract are still beyond comprehension. Concrete operational children invest much energy into efforts to order and classify the objects and experiences in their lives, as evidenced by their endless collections and scrapbooks.* By the end of this stage children can comprehend that they belong to a family, a city, and a country simultaneously. Play and conversation now serve to establish progressive mutuality and equality in their relationships. Notions of animism and artificialism continue during this period but gradually decrease.

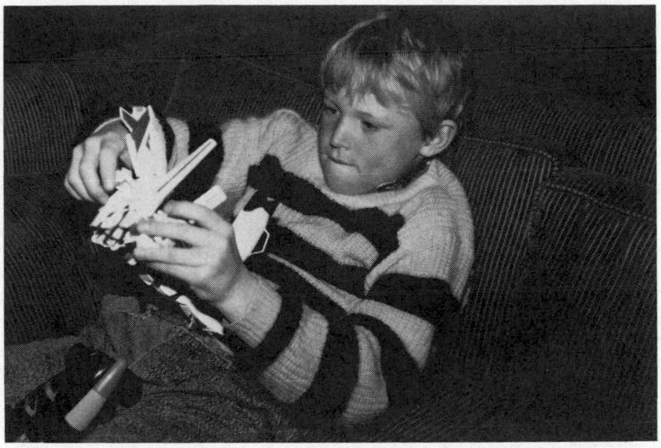

FIGURE 3-7. Children in the stage of concrete operations develop an increasing capacity for problem solving.

Formal Operational Period—11 Years On

This stage is characterized by logical reasoning and the ability to think about the hypothetical and abstract. It is no longer necessary for mental problems to involve concrete objects. Children in this period can systematically analyze abstract problems and arrive at their possible solutions. Relative realism exists, by means of which they can separate what is thought from what is of the real world. Thought patterns incorporate the past, present, and future.

Piaget's theories can help nurses better understand children's concepts about their bodies and their world and about health care experiences. Not all of Piaget's concepts are universally accepted. Research evidence is accumulating that suggests the need to reject or revise some of Piaget's concepts. A large body of research has been carried out (and continues), however, that provides empirical validation of many of Piaget's concepts (Halford et al, 1986; Kruger & Tomasello, 1986; Madden, 1986; Miller, 1986).

Developmental assessment of a child should always include a focus on cognitive development. In addition to gaining data that might contribute to a nursing diagnosis of altered growth and development, information about the child's level of cognitive development will help the nurse to know how to structure the provision of information to the child. For example, research has been carried out that explains children's understanding of the computed tomographic scan procedure, using Piaget's concepts as a framework (Hellier et al, 1986).

Behavioral Learning Theory

Another developmental focus that should be included in the nurse's consideration of a child's intellectual

*These children are able to sort objects into categories according to characteristics such as color or shape, an act also referred to as *seriation*.

development (as well as other domains of development) is behavioral learning theory. Learning theories, in contrast to stage theories (Piaget), see development as not necessarily sequential or fixed. Stage theories focus on different processes (e.g., centration, irreversibility) that occur at various stages of development. Learning theories focus on the same processes (e.g., conditioning, social imitation) throughout the life cycle. Stage theorists stress changes in internal structures that impel development, while learning theorists stress the influence of environmental forces on behavior.

Learning, defined as a change in behavior, is seen as occurring through the process of classic conditioning, operant conditioning, and imitation of social models.

Classic conditioning, a method of using environmental stimuli to bring about a change in behavior, was demonstrated by the Russian psychologist Ivan Pavlov. Classic conditioning involves a process of stimulus substitution in which a new, previously neutral stimulus is substituted for the stimulus that originally elicited the response. In classic conditioning, the stimulus elicits the response. Pavlov rang a bell whenever food was presented to a dog; soon the stimulus of ringing the bell was all that was needed to elicit the response of salivation.

Benjamin F. Skinner extended the concept of classic conditioning to *operant conditioning,* a type of conditioning in which a behavior or response is altered by the stimuli or consequences that follow the response. There are two types of consequences, *reinforcers* and *punishers.* A punisher is a consequence that follows a response that has the effect of decreasing the frequency of the response it follows. A reinforcer is a consequence that follows a response that has the effect of increasing the frequency of the response it follows. *Behavior modification* involves the use of reinforcement and punishment to alter behavior.

Social learning theory, also called observational learning theory and modeling theory as formulated by Albert Bandura (1977) builds on the principles of classic and operant conditioning. Social learning theory posits that one does not have to have the opportunity of actually making a particular new response in order to learn the new response. Social learning theory says that new responses can be learned by watching the behavior of socially competent people (models).

Learning theories are useful to nurses in their interactions with children and families. Nurses can use behavior modification techniques to help shape desired behaviors in children and can teach parents these strategies. Nurses often learn novel parenting strategies from some parents that can be shared with other families. For example, one young couple taught their infant son to look straight ahead and open his mouth for the spoonful of solid food by only putting the food in his mouth in response to that behavior. Anyone who has ever "chased" a little mouth in an effort to feed an infant solid food can appreciate the logic in the strategies used by these parents.

Role modeling is another important teaching strategy for showing parents how to care for their well or ill children and for demonstrating to children appropriate self-care (Sears, 1957, 1958). These learning theory strategies are detailed for specific situations throughout this text.

Development of Language

Language is an important aspect of intellectual development that has only recently gained much attention by researcher and health professionals. Language development involves an increasingly complex expansion of receptive (comprehension of language) and expressive (speaking of language) skills over time. Language efforts that are rewarded with approval from parents and other adults in the child's environment (socially reinforced) seem to result in more effective language skills. Nurses should apply this knowledge in their own verbal interactions with children and in their child guidance instruction to parents.

It is also known that receptive language skills are achieved earlier than expressive language skills, as is evidenced in the early toddler's ability to follow an instruction before he or she has learned the vocabulary skills to acknowledge that instruction. Nurses can apply this fact in their nursing care, too. *Even infants have a less stressful response to nursing procedures if they are spoken to before, during, and for a brief interval after the procedure.*

Children's interaction with adults stimulates their language development, so when that interaction is diminished, language skills take longer to develop. Females show evidence of earlier language acquisition than males. It has been speculated that parents' interactions with their daughters may be more verbal, whereas their interactions with their sons may more often be physical in nature.

Twins usually are slower in language achievement than are children born singly. This may be because there is less conversation between each of them and their mother, most likely because of the fact that they are so close with each other that the mother often addresses them as one.

Socioeconomic influences on language also exist, with language mastery occurring earlier in children from middle and upper class homes. Children from bilingual backgrounds may have difficulty with mastery of one or both languages. When children are expected to learn two languages at once with differing rules and letter pronunciation, they become confused. Learning a second language is usually easier once one language has been mastered well enough for the child to be comfortable with it. However, the single most influential factor in learning a second language is whether the child is being reprimanded for trying to use one of the languages. Dialects (language variations) are structured by professional association (incorporation by professional jargon-terminology into language), age (adolescent slang is usually unique to that generation alone), geographic location (usually different inflections or pronunciations of the same words, called colloquialisms, from one locale to another), and socioeconomic class (more complex word forms are used in upper classes).

Theories of Language Development

Three theories of language development seem equally viable to our current knowledge of language development (Evans & McCandless, 1978; Helms & Turner, 1978; Vaughan & Litt, 1990). Noam Chomsky's research supports an *innate theory* in which he depicts language development as genetically determined. Through this innate capacity of brain cells to act on linguistic input, triggered by a system known as a *language acquisition device* (LAD), native language learning occurs. LAD enables the child to select and fit together properties of language and concrete experiences, eventually synthesizing them into language competency.

B. F. Skinner has applied *reinforcement theory,* also called behavior modification theory and stimulus-response theory, to language development. He supports the concept that language, as all behavior, is acquired or learned as a result of one's environmental interactions through which behaviors that produce language are reinforced.

Social learning theory describes the development of language as a modeling process resulting from the child's imitation of adult remarks and from caretakers' expansion of her or his utterances.

All three theories are most likely functioning in language development, each being a description of one facet of yet another complex component of human development.

TABLE 3-7
Age Ranges of Language Developmental Stages

Cooing stage	0–2 mos
Babbling stage	2–6 mos
First word, usually imitated	12–18 mos
Rapid vocabulary acquisition	18 mos–3 yrs
Open and pivot words Telegraphic sentences	
Steady word acquisition	3–5 yrs
Multiword sentences Basic mastery of language by end	
Progressively complex sentences	6–11+ yrs
Use of pronouns, proper nouns, prepositions	
Basic grammatic mastery by end	

Moreover, all three theories are in accord as to the approximate age range during which various stages of language acquisition occur. The progression of language development is seen in Table 3–7.

Emotional-Social Competency

A child's personality is the integration of feelings, attitudes, and relationships as expressed by behavior patterns. The measure of a healthy adult personality (e.g., the goal of emotional-social development) is one's capacity to love, to achieve, and to become interdependent in function. Yet emotional-social development is not something that has been mastered by adulthood. It is, rather, a process that unfolds throughout the individual's life, with each stage of life having its own tasks to be mastered and the leftover tasks of other stages to be re-resolved.

Psychosocial Development

Erikson's theory on the psychosocial development of human beings illustrates this lifelong struggle for emotional-social equilibrium. Erikson's theory is unique in that it describes psychosocial development throughout the entire life span. Psychoanalyst Erik Homburger Erikson (1963, 1965, 1968) extended Sigmund Freud's theory of psychosexual development. Freud emphasized the id and biosexual connotations of human behavior. Erikson's theory emphasizes the ego and social connotations of human behavior.

According to Erikson, individual development occurs within the context of the social and cultural environment. Social and cultural factors influence or impinge on development at all stages, and only when these factors are taken into account can psychosocial (or emotional-social) development be understood. External social and cultural factors do not operate alone. Each individual possesses within himself or herself an internal or innate capacity to interact with the environment.

In Erikson's theory there are eight stages of psychosocial development (Erikson's eight ages of man). During each stage of development, the individual is presented with a basic developmental task (also referred to as a dominant central problem or crisis). This task, problem, or crisis requires the individual to resolve a conflict between two opposing forces (one positive and one negative). The individual cannot progress to the next stage until the conflict of the previous stage is resolved. Ideal resolution results in a greater predominance of the positive psychologic attribute (ego qualities) for the stage. Many individuals misinterpret the meaning of crisis resolution. Erikson was adamant that healthy psychologic development does *not* mean that the individual develops all characteristics of the positive psychologic attributes (e.g., trust, autonomy, initiative) and no characteristics of the negative psychologic attributes (e.g., mistrust, shame and doubt, guilt). Rather, development of these attributes should be viewed as occurring on a continuum. Ideal development would involve more positive than negative attributes, but some of the negative should be present. For example, an individual who develops all trust and no mistrust would be at risk for danger and discomfort. Similar statements can be made about the negative attributes of later stages. The individual who develops all autonomy and no shame and doubt, all initiative and no guilt will have difficulty coping in society. Optimal resolution of the first developmental crisis is diagrammed in Figure 3–8.

Each succeeding task, therefore, is built on what occurred in the previous stage of development. Table 3–8 illustrates Erikson's eight stages, the approximate age at which each task or crisis is experienced, the negative counterpart of unsuccessful task mastery, and the significant interpersonal relationships and experiences in the environment of the person needed to support him or her in task accomplishment. To show the relationship between Erikson's theory and that of Freud, Freud's stages (Freud, 1950, 1957) are shown in parentheses after the appropriate Erikson stage.

Illness or accident can compound the problems confronting a child who is already at the peak of a psychologic crisis. The nurse who is a part of the child's environment can support development if he or she knows the task being faced. Regression to a previous task level, or reversion in the direction of the negative counterpart of a task level currently confronting the child, is common in children (and parents) during extreme or continued stress. The nurse should respect the individual's need to regress, help the child and his parents to accept that fact and the accompanying increased dependency, support them as they rework those tasks, and provide an environment that fosters a return to their age-appropriate tasks. It is helpful to the parents that the nurse be cognizant of their developmental needs in planning care for the child and family.

Sexual Development

Another component of a child's emotional-social development is his or her sexual development. Although sex is determined genetically at conception, a child's total sexuality is influenced by his or her developmental progress in all three competency areas (physical, intellectual, emotional-social). Sexuality also affects the development of those competencies. The summary of stages in sexual development is listed in Table 3–9. The nurse can assist the child and family with promoting healthy sexuality and preventing the nursing diagnosis *altered sexuality patterns* from being necessary (Table 3–10).

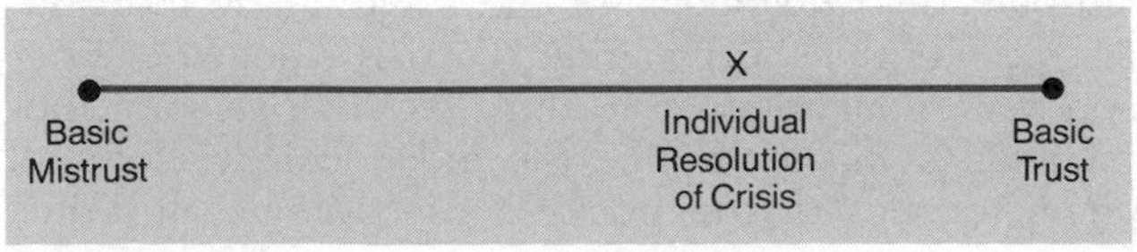

FIGURE 3-8. Example of positive resolution of Erikson's first developmental crisis.

Moral Development

A third component of emotional-social development is moral development. Morality is composed of developmental tasks in two areas. Children must achieve a realistic acceptance of their social responsibility. They must also integrate personal principles of justice and reciprocity that are based on empathy, mutual respect, and regard for the integrity and rights of others (Castiglia, 1991).

One of the leading theorists in the area of moral development is Lawrence Kohlberg. He states that moral development is prefaced by the child's ability to reason; thus, moral development follows a sequence that corresponds to the development of intellect. Kohlberg's model describes three phases of moral development. In the first phase, *preconventional* or *premoral morality* (4 to 7 years), children perceive rules as absolute and unalterable. This perception is congruent with the intellectual egocentrism and realism of children this age. A punishment and obedience orientation prompts acceptable moral behavior at this phase. This "do what's right or be punished" attitude, coupled with a naive instrumental hedonism (doing right earns one favor or rewards), makes the child in this phase fairly compliant to adult-set rules.

The *conventional morality* phase (7 to 11 years) is based on the child's perception of rules as existing for the good of all, to preserve order and to protect people. Children in this phase comply with rules because of their desire to please or help others and to maintain approval as a "good" child, which helps them to avoid the feelings of guilt they experience by not "being good."

Principled morality (12 years on), the last phase in Kohlberg's schema, is the period during which individuals accept rules on the basis of their own judgments of what is universally ethical and on the basis of personal conscience. Their moral conduct is prompted by (1) a sense of obligation to social contract and democratic law and (2) a desire to avoid loss of respect among peers and in the wider community.

Kohlberg's theory has been criticized as biased. Kohlberg's longitudinal study of moral development was based on data from 84 boys (Kohlberg, 1968, 1981). Gilligan's (1982) research of moral development in females noted significant differences compared with Kohlberg's findings. In examining the process of moral decision making, Gilligan found that females expressed greater concern for the interdependence of relationships involved, compared with the emphasis on a system of rules reported in Kohlberg's work.

TABLE 3-8
An Expansion Chart of the Eight Stages in the Human Life Cycle

Task and Subtasks	Task's Negative Counterpart	Significant Persons	Significant Supporting Experiences
Infancy (Oral)* (0–1 Yr)			
Sense of trust: realization of hope Getting; tolerating frustration in small doses; recognizing mother as distinct from others and self	Mistrust	Primary caregiver	Consistency and quality in the care received
Toddler (Anal) (1–3 Yrs)			
Sense of autonomy: realization of will Child will try out new powers of speech; beginning acceptance of reality vs. pleasure principle	Shame and doubt	Parent(s)	Opportunity to attain some self-control based on a feeling of self-esteem rather than fear
Preschool (Oedipal) (3–6 Yrs)			
Sense of initiative; realization of purpose Questioning; exploring own body and environment; differentiation of sexes	Guilt	Basic family	Opportunity to do for self with a balance between imaginative exploration and set limits
School Age (Latent) (6–12 Yrs)			
Sense of industry; realization of competence Learning to win recognition by producing things; exploring, collecting; learning to relate to own sex	Inferiority	Neighborhood; school; same-sex peers; adult, nonparent idols	Opportunity to achieve success and recognition by engaging in manageable tasks in the child's social world so he or she can learn responsibility, social and work skills, cooperation, and fair play
Adolescence (Mature) (12–? Yrs)			
Sense of identity: realization of fidelity Moving toward heterosexuality; selecting vocation; beginning separation from family; integrating personality (e.g., altruism)	Identity diffusion	Peer groups and out groups; models of leadership	Opportunity to establish who the child is and what her or his purpose in society is to be through both private and social experiences that build self-esteem, foster increased need for independence, and cushion periods of feeling of not belonging
Late Adolescence and Young Adulthood			
Sense of intimacy and solidarity: realization of love Becoming capable of establishing a lasting relationship with a member of the opposite sex; learning to be creative and productive	Isolation	Partner in friendship, sex, competition, cooperation	Opportunity to experience close, shared relationships with individuals of own and opposite sex in which the child's identity is verified and accepted and he or she accepts the identity of others
Adulthood			
Sense of generativity: realization of care Learning effective skills in communicating with and managing children; developing active interest in the next generation	Self-absorption and stagnation	Spouse; children; friends and work associates	Opportunity for involvement in activities that arouse concern for and advocacy for the next generation
Late Adulthood			
Sense of integrity: realization of wisdom Reconciling life accomplishments; learning to accept death; putting life in order; accepting retirement without quitting life	Despair	Spouse; children and grandchildren; friends	Opportunity to be acknowledged for life accomplishments by self, children, peers in a manner that emphasizes what was achieved, rather than what was not, so that end of life can be dealt with gracefully and peaceably

Based on Erikson, E.H. (1963). *Childhood and society* (2nd ed.), New York: WW Norton; and Maier, H. (1969). *Three theories of child development*. New York: Harper & Row.

*The corresponding stage in Freud's theory of development is listed in parentheses.

TABLE 3-9
Summary of Stages in Sexual Development of Children

Factors Affecting Attitude Development	Behaviors	Learning Needs
Prenatal		
Parental expectations	Genetic determination Differentiation	Anticipated role change of parents and siblings
Infancy (0–1 Yr)		
Tone of voice, touch Caregiver's acceptance	Sucking Random self-discovery Pelvic rocking Erection, lubrication	Language Trust Physical and emotional well-being
Toddler (1–3 Yrs)		
Parental reactions Freedom to explore	Names body parts Draws body parts Games such as "house" Gender roles Explores body orifices	Language (correct terminology) Social appropriateness Assertive rights Facts of reproduction
Preschooler (3–5 Yrs)		
Approaches to nudity and privacy in the home Increasing influence outside home	Masturbation, orgasm Name calling Curious manipulation of other child's genitalia Games with sex roles	Social appropriateness Respect of privacy Assertive rights Facts of reproduction repeated with more detail
School-Age (6–12 Yrs)		
Interaction with peers, school authorities Influence from mass media	Sex-linked play—role modeling Kissing, hugging, dancing with opposite sex Close friendships Voyeurism	Re-explanation about facts of reproduction and clarification of terminology heard at school Preparation for changes of adolescence Decision making about sex behaviors Basic information about consequences of sexual activity
Adolescent (13–18 Yrs)		
Audience of peers Pressure to belong by conforming	Adjustment to changing body Purposeful masturbation Experimentation with others	Express feelings Values clarification Decision making Contraception STD/AIDS

STD, sexually transmitted disease; AIDS, acquired immunodeficiency syndrome.

TABLE 3-10

Analysis: Nursing Diagnostic Statement

Response and Related or Risk Factors:

Altered sexuality patterns, related to

- Development of negative attitudes about sexuality associated with early childhood experiences
- Lack of information about sexuality

Nursing Interventions

Development of healthy sexual behavior by child and family

- Help child develop self-awareness of feelings about sexuality
- Permit normal developmental expressions of sexuality
- Foster development of healthy attitudes about sexuality by open discussion with child at appropriate level of age
- Use correct anatomic terminology when referring to sex organs and sex-related topics
- Avoid reprimand for age-appropriate sexual exploration, such as masturbation and toddler or preschool sex play
- Teach child to protect self from sexual abuse
- Assess child's and family's needs and knowledge deficit
- Encourage children and families to discuss sexuality openly at a level appropriate for age
- Provide age-appropriate information about reproduction
- Prepare school-age child for physical and emotional maturational changes during adolescence
- Provide information about contraception, pregnancy, and sexually transmitted diseases to late school-age children and adolescents
- Develop or implement teaching programs for school and community organizations

Gilligan (1982) noted that moral decision making by girls was influenced by an "ethic of care," compared with the "logic of justice" as expressed by the boys in Kohlberg's study. The work of Gilligan (1982) demonstrates the need to expand the theory of moral development to incorporate the perspectives not only of gender but also of diverse cultures.

Faith Development

Another component of emotional-social development is faith development. The work of James Fowler (1980, 1984) provides a framework for describing the stage-related process of faith development from infancy to adulthood. Particular emphasis is placed on the changes of knowing and valuing that are involved in developing faith beliefs. Fowler's theory draws heavily on the work of other developmentalists such as Piaget (1952), Erikson (1963), Levinson and colleagues (1978), Kohlberg (1981), and Gilligan (1982). Parallels in the developmental patterns of faith beliefs can be found in the domains of cognitive (Piaget), moral (Kohlberg), and psychosocial (Erikson) development. Table 3–11 outlines the stages of faith development. Further discussion of the developmentally related issues can be found in each of the development chapters.

Temperament

Temperament is yet another facet of emotional-social development that needs to be discussed. Temperament is a behavioral style that makes unique one's approach to people and situations. The characteristics of one's temperament are evidenced from birth and are predictive of one's adult personality. Whether the behaviors typical of a given temperamental characteristic will present in acceptable or aberrant ways depends largely on how the significant others in one's life respond to those characteristics. Additionally, any situation* or demand that strongly conflicts with one's

*Such situations might include inconsistent care, inappropriate performance expectations, a series of traumatic events, imitations of aberrant behavior in other member(s) at home.

TABLE 3-11
Stages of Faith Development

Stage	Age	Characteristics
Primal (undifferentiated)	Infancy	Primary caregivers provide first experiences with superordinate presence; feelings of trust, nurturance, and attachment provide foundation for developing faith beliefs
Intuitive/projective	2–6 yrs	Images, feelings, and symbols provide the basis of faith beliefs; influenced by the meaning derived from exposure to caretaker behaviors, religious practices, and stories; egocentric thinking pervades; misconceptions likely
Mythic/literal	7–12 yrs	Faith beliefs become concrete and literal; rigidity in thinking exists; faith beliefs are understood as a system of order and activities, rather than as an inner spiritual process and presence in the world
Synthetic convention	Preadolescence (13 to adolescence years)	Synthesis of ideas about spiritual matters derived from significant others and life experiences; strong reliance on authority figures emerges; self-reflection and insight emerge
Individualize/reflexive	Young adulthood (early mid-twenties) to mid-thirties	Solidification of faith beliefs occurs as an outcome of examining them; a self-conscious spiritual identity emerges
Conjunctive/faith	Mid-life (35 yrs) and beyond	Integration and acceptance of various dimensions of faith beliefs; leads to sincere openness to other religious traditions and communities
Universalizing faith	45 yrs and older	Acquisition of a detached yet concerned attitude toward living; unconditional regard and love for others emerges

Based on Fowler, J. (1980). Moral stages and the development of faith. In B. Munsey (Ed.), *Moral education and Kohlberg*. Birmingham, AL: Religious Education Press.

temperament produces severe stress, during which time signs and symptoms of behavior problems may arise (Vaughan & Litt, 1990).

Although temperament has been found to have a genetic origin,† it has been shown that one's environment can heighten, diminish, or otherwise modify temperamental characteristics but not abolish them. In fact, some research suggests that these apparent changes are only fronts enacted to gain social acceptance (Thomas et al, 1968). This tendency of temperament to remain basically unchanged despite environmental pressures is called *persistence in personality and self-concept.* If any modifications are possible in these genetically transmitted traits and the associated self-concept, they are more likely to occur in early childhood than at any other time in one's life—thus the importance of an environment that fosters these traits as assets and that positively reinforces self-concept from the beginning of life.

Extensive research conducted by Thomas and coworkers (1968) indicated nine clearly recognizable characteristics, or traits, of temperament. They are categorized according to reactivity.

1. Motor activity—the intensity and frequency of activity or motility.
2. Rhythmicity—regularity of repetitive biologic functions, such as sleep and wakefulness, eating patterns, bowel and bladder patterns.
3. Approach to the new—withdrawal from or acceptance of it—the child's initial reaction to a new stimulus.
4. Adaptability—the ease or difficulty with which initial responses to new stimuli can be modified.
5. Intensity of response—degree or amount of energy invested in reactions to stimuli.
6. Threshold of responsiveness—level of external stimulation necessary to evoke an overt response.
7. Quality of mood—general cheerfulness or unhappiness, amount of pleasant and friendly behavior as opposed to unpleasant and unfriendly behavior.
8. Distractibility—effectiveness of extraneous environmental stimuli in altering the direction of ongoing behavior.
9. Attention span and persistence—length of time an activity is pursued, whether self-initiated or planned or structured, and the amount of frustration tolerated in activity despite obstacles.

These traits tend to combine to form three clearly different personality structures.* Table 3–12 describes the incidence and traits of these three personalities.

The nurse who is able to recognize these three personality structures or temperaments is able to make a more reasoned judgment about the child's behavior and about the approach that will be most ef-

†Similar research studies carried out in Norway by Ann Torgurson and in America by Thomas and others resulted in remarkably similar findings. The same distribution of temperament types was found, despite marked differences in culture, parenting style, socioeconomic status, and racial factors.

*Approximately one third of the population cannot be fit neatly into these three categories but instead consists of blends that are not clearly separable.

TABLE 3-12
Incidence and Characteristics of the Three Personality Types

Easy Child (Sanguine, Endomorph)

Well adjusted psychologically and physically; adapts rapidly

Friendly, likes company

Seeks people during stress

May need urging to complete ambitions

Sleeps and eats well; highly regular biologic rhythm, good candidate for demand feeding as infant; easily toilet trained

Displays low to mild intensity of response

Positive mood predominates; smiles and laughs much more than he or she cries; caregiver can usually be sure something is amiss when he or she does cry; tends to find good in any situation, even disappointing ones

Incidence: 40% of all children; 18% develop maladjustments

Difficult Child (Choleric, Mesomorph)

Slow to adapt to any new situation, but can function well once she or he "learns rules" of situation

Likes people but is not dependent on them and sometimes functions better alone—a natural leader

Seeks activity during stress; needs acceptable outlets for her or his vigor and aggressive motor drive; competitive

Seems to be constantly moving and highly destructive; intense in reactions; needs unbreakable, well-constructed toys and clothing

Displays mostly negative withdrawal responses to new situations; frustration expressed in tantrums or destruction; pleasure expressed loudly and boisterously, but these outbursts do not necessarily reflect the value of the situation to child—his or her responses simply have an "all or nothing" quality

Has irregular biologic functioning; sleeps poorly and lightly and requires less sleep; erratic in appetite and frequency of hunger; not a good candidate for demand feeding as an infant, and much patience and time are required for toilet training, with more frequent accidents

Negative mood predominates; seems to fuss or cry constantly; finds reasons to be unhappy; tends to be an "I can't" person; seldom a good scholar

Incidence: 10% of all children;* 70% develop maladjustments

Slow-to-Warm-Up Child (Phlegmatic, Ectomorph)

Slow adaptive capacity; usually quietly withdraws, but is watchful and contemplative all the while

Primarily a loner; usually prefers only one or two close friends; socially shy

Seeks to be alone during stress; avid reader

Often matures late; oversensitive and immature, compared with most peers

Poor relaxer; frequently experiences disturbed sleep and eating patterns

Displays low intensity of reaction

Fairly high frequency of negative mood, although it sometimes is not immediately noticeable because of low intensity with which it is expressed

Incidence: 15% of all children; 40% develop maladjustments

*Research by Someroff and Zax at the University of Rochester showed that women who were highly anxious or who had a psychologic disorder during the prenatal period have a higher incidence of difficult children.

Compiled from Thomas, A., Chess, S., & Birch, H. (1968). *Temperament and behavior disorders in children.* New York: New York University Press; Gesell, A., Ilg, F., & Bates-Ames, L. (1974). *Infant and child in the culture of today.* New York: Harper & Row; and Segal, J., & Yahroes, H. (1978). *A child's journey: Forces that shape the lives of our young.* New York: McGraw-Hill.

fective (Table 3–13). Knowledge of temperament is especially helpful to parents. Knowing that some aspects of their child's behavior are due to his or her nature helps to relieve many parents of guilt feelings and of undue pressure caused by their belief that their parenting methods are creating the behavior. Understanding the parenting methods most effective with the various personality types can aid parents in adopting the method most appropriate for each of their children. (See Chapter 12 for further discussion of temperament and parenting style.)

Defining Growth, Development, and Maturation

Growth and development are not synonymous terms, but in the healthy child these two processes do parallel each other and are interdependent in function. The ways in which the whole child changes over time are both *quantitative* and *qualitative* in nature.

Growth refers to *quantitative* change, involving an increase in size of the whole child or in size and number of any body parts. The change is measurable—usually either in centimeters or inches (height), kilograms or pounds (increased organ mass, weight), or numbers (increased vocabulary, increased number of relationships with others, increased number of physical skills able to perform)—and is easily observed or studied.

Qualitative changes are the "leaps" (increased skill or capacity) in function that result from mastering a series of smaller steps.* The qualitative component, called *development,* is more complex and less easily measured or studied.

*Piaget's steps of progressive intelligence, Erikson's stages of progressive sociability, Kohlberg's steps to adult morality, Freud's steps of sexuality formation illustrate qualitative change.

TABLE 3-13
Family-Centered Teaching: Temperament

- Every child's temperament is unique: the way your child behaves will depend primarily on his/her innate characteristics of reaction (Thomas, 1968); understanding his/her traits allows you to structure care with less conflict and reactivity; this knowledge also will help you encourage your child to learn to use these traits to his/her best advantage
- A child's deviation from culturally desirable behavior *does not* indicate bad parenting or a pathologic problem in the child
- When you approach changes in care patterns such as weaning and toilet training, consider your child's characteristics of temperament (i.e., adaptability, rhythmicity, distractibility).
- When your child is ill, changes in behavior may reflect the severity of illness (i.e., quality of mood—withdrawn or cantankerous; motor activity—quiet, listless)
- Consider your child's temperament when caring for specific symptoms, such as colic, night awakenings, or hyperactivity
- Your child's adjustment to nursery school or a day care center will be influenced by reactions to new situations and ease of adaptability
- Your child's ease or difficulty in establishing peer relations will affect adjustment to school
- Persistence and distractibility will influence your child's ability to function at school with classwork and homework

The timing of these quantitative and qualitative changes is, to some extent, controlled by a maturational process that involves the child's biologic (genetic) ability and environmental opportunity to relinquish previous functions and learning or to integrate new functions and learning into his or her existing structure for more mature performance, or to perform both these actions. For example, the child relinquishes the palmar grasp in favor of the more manipulative pincer grasp that will allow better investigation of the environment, but not until he or she has developed the biologic structures—increased muscle cells and nerve cell specialization—necessary to perform this action.

Principles Evident in Growth and Development

Development Is Complex

Human development is a continuous, irreversible, and complex process that is lifelong. Inherent in this developmental process is aging, which, interestingly enough, is most rapid during the fetal stage, and is also lifelong.

Development Has Direction

Human development is progressive and orderly (i.e., follows a sequence). It proceeds as follows:

1. *From simple to complex.* This is exemplified in the child's ability to make basic "cooing" sounds before learning to refine those sounds into speech.

2. *From general to specific.* Illustrative of this principle is the infant's acquisition of palmar grasp before learning the finer control of pincer grasp.

3. *From head to toe (cephalocaudally).* An example is the fact that an infant gains neck and head control before being able to control the movements of trunk and limbs (Fig. 3-9).

4. *From inner to outer (proximodistally).* This principle is similar to the cephalocaudal principle in that the child learns control of the near structures before control of the structures farther away from the body center. The ability to coordinate the arms to reach for an object occurs before learning the hand and finger coordination necessary to grasp it (see Fig. 3-9).

Development Is Predictable

The orderly sequence of development is invariable, and although the precise age for the sequential steps to occur varies for each child, there is a general chronology that involves wide norm ranges to allow

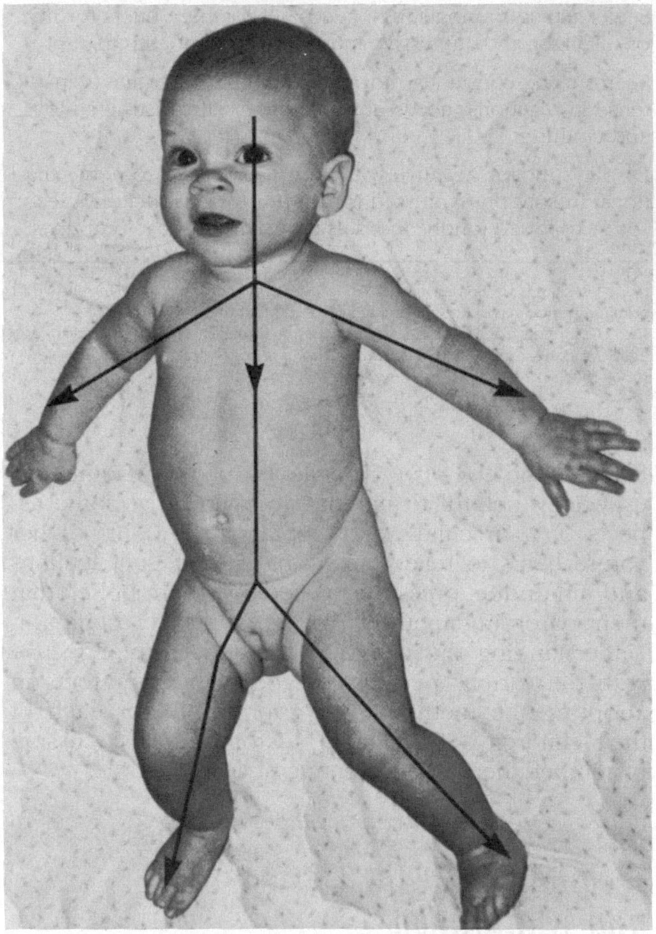

FIGURE 3-9. The development of muscular control proceeds from head to tail (cephalocaudal), and from the center of the body to its periphery (proximodistal).

for these individual differences. For example, the age range for learning to walk is usually given as 9 to 15 months, with the average age being 12 months. Walking can occur as late as 28 months and still be considered normal.

A child usually follows a consistent pattern with respect to either an early or a late rate of development. Therefore, *deviation from the child's own pattern may be more indicative of a problem than lack of conformance to the norm.*

Children Develop Uniquely

Each child has his or her own genetic potential for growth and development that cannot be exceeded but may be deterred or modified at any stage in the sequence. For example, although intellect is primarily set by genetic inheritance, a child's experiences during the critical periods will either stimulate or discourage intellectual achievement. If affected by poor nutrition, confined to the crib or playpen, and offered few interactions with the people in the environment, the child may not achieve intellectually, regardless of genetic potential. Conversely, offered opportunities to experience the world from a number of positions (crib, playpen, floor, shoulder, tabletop), sustained on a nutritionally balanced diet, and provided with regular opportunities to interact (to be spoken to, played with, cuddled) with the important people and objects in the environment, the child is on the way to achieving intellectual potential.

Knowledge of growth and development principles is as important to the nurse as knowledge of discrete norms for growth and development skills and behaviors and knowledge of theoretical assumptions that assist in the description, explanation, prediction, and control of behaviors. The nurse can use these principles as a kind of basic yardstick in assessment for possible alterations in growth and development. They are also invaluable in anticipatory guidance of parents (see Table 3–2). Parents should know that the norms for developmental attainments exist in a wide range, and any comparisons with other children should be made in the context of these ranges.

Theoretical Perspectives on Development

Developmental research has led to several points of view or theoretical conceptualizations of how children reach adulthood (see Table 3–2). Each is an attempt to describe systematically the phenomenon of human growth and development. A collective view that incorporates all these perspectives probably gives the most holistic view of how children proceed to adulthood (refer to Table 3–14).

Development as Maturation: Critical Periods

This perspective holds that the development of human behavior and physiologic growth occurs in predictable patterns as the child ages, i.e., reaches a new level of maturity. The child's increasing age results in the behavioral and physiologic changes. Human variations in the maturational process are the result of genetic and temperamental differences. Thus, development as maturation means that a child develops at an individual but predictable pace, according to an inherited biologic schedule for maturation. Within this maturational process are critical periods. A critical period is a specific time frame during which certain environmental events or stimuli have their greatest impact on a child's development. The time frame involved is either the point at which maximum capacity for a particular aspect of development is first present or the point at which the structures to be developed are undergoing their most rapid growth.

During these critical periods some form of minimal sensory stimulation is necessary for normal progression in development. If the stimuli are not introduced during this critical period, the task in question cannot be mastered, at least not without much difficulty (Craft & Denehy, 1990). After this critical period, the child can be either totally unaffected by certain stimuli or resistant to them. For example, a fetus is not affected by maternally contracted rubella virus after the critical first 3 months of fetal development. Deficits of appropriate sensory stimulation during the critical periods are cumulative and can progressively interfere with future development of other competencies besides the one competency involved during the critical period (Erikson, 1963). Figure 3–10 illustrates this relationship.

Conversely, sensory stimuli that are necessary to the development of a particular skill or task and are exerted on a child before the critical period will have a negligible, if any, effect. For example, infants cannot learn to read, regardless of how often they are exposed to the media that would produce reading skills, whereas children at the right age and stage in their development have a "readiness" to read; that is, during their critical period they acquire reading skills fairly rapidly.

Development as Learning: Reinforcements

Researchers holding the perspective of development as learning attempt to understand development by studying the child's personal history and environmental and social interactions. According to this view, the child is shaped by the environment while reacting to the events in that environment. The child chooses various ways of behaving, depending on the consequences (rewards or punishment). A given behavior or practice is repeated because some factor in the external environment prompts or reinforces that action,

TABLE 3-14
Common Developmental Perspectives

Critical Periods	Periods during which developing structures are undergoing their most rapid growth Minimal level of sensory stimulation is necessary for normal progression in development Deficits of appropriate sensory stimulation during critical periods are cumulative and progressively interfere with development, i.e., nonorganic failure to thrive
Behavior Reinforcements	Child's behavior is shaped by the environment while child is reacting to the events in that environment Behavior is repeated because some factor in the external environment reinforces the action Behavior modification programs are based on this premise
Resolving Conflicts/ Adapting to Challenges	Child is continually torn between natural instincts (physiologic impulses) and social constraints while moving from one maturational stage to another A physical task of the toddler is learning to walk without aid; a school-age child's task is the ability to use symbols and concepts they represent
Cognitive Change Requiring Practice and Energy	Developmental energy flow is invested most heavily in certain competency areas at any given time, depending on child's current level of comprehension Toddler's energy concentration is invested in selfhood and body control; the adolescent directs energy into development of sexual and social identity and capacity for intimacy
Cultural Adaptation	Mastery of developmental tasks occurs within the context of the cultural and ethnic group characteristics of the child's primary care providers In contemporary society, the majority of young children are socialized with other children much earlier in various day care settings, compared with a decade ago

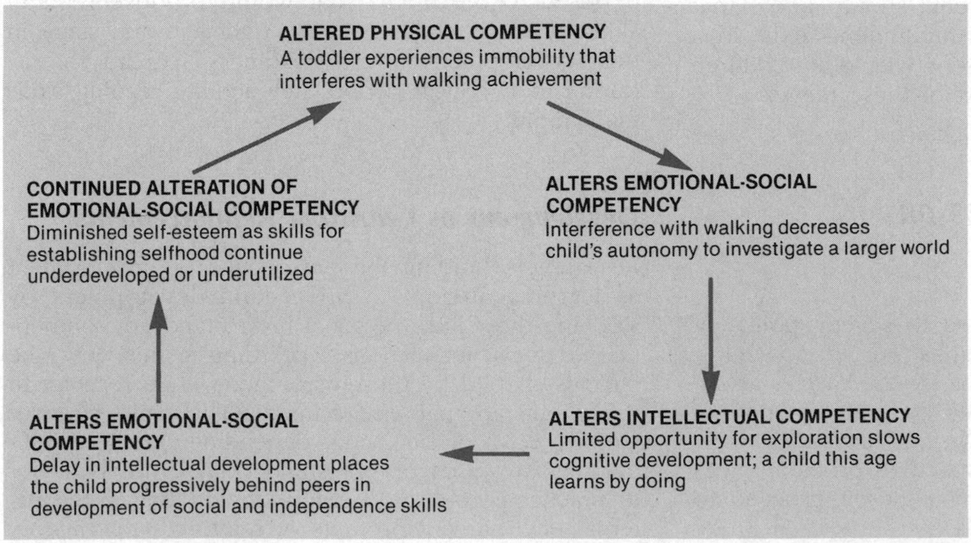

FIGURE 3-10. Alteration of one competency interferes with development of other competencies.

or does both. Pavlov, Watson, Skinner, and Bandura's (1977) writings reflect this theoretical position.

Development as Resolution of Conflict: Adapting to Challenges

Social expectations for each developmental or maturational stage exist; these are called developmental tasks. The task of each stage is to overcome the problem or challenge that confronts a child because of his or her age. Delay or failure in task achievement makes further development more difficult. Examples of developmental tasks are as follows: (1) Erikson defines the infant's emotional-social task as resolving inner and environmental conflicts so as to develop more trust than mistrust; (2) Piaget defines the school-age child's intellectual task as learning to use symbols and the concepts they represent; (3) a physical task of the toddler is learning to walk without aid.

Conflict arises out of children's motivation to master their environment and their lack of competency needed for that mastery. Equilibrium exists before the new environmental or maturational stimulus occurs that demands adaptation by the child, and after the child has developed the necessary competence to adapt to the stimulus. Disequilibrium exists in the interval between recognition of and desire to master (adapt to) the new stimulus and mastery of the stimulus. Growing children repeatedly evidence their strength and competence to adapt and achieve, if their environment gives them at least some support.

Development as Cognitive Change: Practice and Energy Investment

Developmental energy is invested most heavily in certain competency areas at any given time, depending on the child's current level of comprehension, so that different aspects of development progress at different rates. Earlier achievements in one competency area may even regress temporarily while some other aspect of that or another competency area is being stimulated, because a strong preoccupation exists to practice and perfect the skill required for mastery of the newly confronted stimulus. For example, during infancy the central focus of energy is on sensorimotor and physical growth.

Development as Cultural Adaptation

Research into the cultural variations in development is relatively recent. Only since the 1960s have ethnic variations and social class variations been considered in accounting for the nonuniform and unusual. Although there is now increased sensitivity to the child's assimilation of his or her culture, the research on the actual impact on development is incomplete. It is clear that mastery of developmental tasks occurs within the context of the cultural and ethnic group characteristics of the child's primary care provider(s). This influence is second only to gender socialization in shaping the child's developing attitudes and behaviors (Craft & Denehy, 1990; Gillis et al, 1989).

In summary, human development, although complex, is continuous, follows an orderly sequence and general chronologic pattern that may vary slightly among different cultures, involves task mastery, and requires concentration of energy on the task confronting the child at that particular time. However, task achievement in one competency area is not accomplished in isolation but interacts simultaneously with skills in other competency areas to result in characteristic ways of behaving.

Factors Influencing Child Development

It is generally accepted that nature sets the limits on potential development, whereas nurturing forces present the realm of opportunities or possibilities for attaining that potential. Research has demonstrated that physical development is primarily influenced by natural forces and that long-term deprivation in nurturing is required to interfere with physical development. However, research to date has also shown that intellectual and emotional-social development, although controlled by nature with regard to ultimate capacity for development, is much more influenced by nurturing forces (i.e., environmental stimuli); individuals may either maximize their genetic (natural) potential or to allow it to depreciate. These are examples of the interrelationship between heredity and environment.

Social Milieu and Physical Environment as Forces in Development

Culture and Lifestyle as Milieu

A child's developmental task mastery, although dependent on biologic potential and maturation, occurs "within the context of the cultural and ethnic group characteristics of the child's primary care providers" (Eiduson, 1983). Cultural input* is second only to gender socialization, which itself is culturally affected, in its impact on a child's development (Alexander & Blank, 1988; Sobralske, 1985). That input may contribute either constructively or deleteriously to development. See Chapters 2 and 11 for a more detailed discussion of cultural and ethnic factors affecting individual and family development.

---

*Cultural input refers to ethnicity, demographic setting, socioeconomic class, parental occupation, and family structure.

Family lifestyle is also a part of the milieu that shapes a child's development. During the late 1970s and early 1980s, there was a growing recognition of the existence of family structures other than the two-parent nuclear family. Hanson and Sporakowski (1986) listed the possible types of families as traditional (two parents, father working, mother at home); dual-earner; stepparent; single-parent; househusband; communal; and gay. An additional family type—the black extended family—was described by Wilson (1986). See Chapter 2 for a more comprehensive discussion of the impact of alternative family lifestyles on the child's development.

Family Environment as Milieu

Family interaction, especially parenting (see Chapter 12 for a detailed discussion of parenting), is a source of influence on particular facets of child development. There is a definite reciprocal dependency between family development and the individual child's development (Gillis et al, 1989). Other family relationships affect and are affected by the dyadic (parent-child) relationship. Likewise, the dyadic relationship changes over time, primarily as a function of the child's developmental changes. Most parents are not equally adept at parenting at all the different developmental stages; thus, the quality of parenting is also likely to change as the child develops, fostering either positive or negative consequences in the child's developmental progress.

Birth order and family size are aspects of family interaction that have also demonstrated their effect on a child's development. The middle child's exposure to older siblings fosters earlier and easier learning, particularly of motor, social, and language skills.

School as Milieu

As children grow older, their siblings, and later their peers, have an increasingly greater impact. The school milieu contributes to their development in the form of skill training, cultural transmission, and self-actualization. Again, the relationship between school progression and the child's development is reciprocal. As the child develops and matures, the curriculum content and form also change, presumably to reflect different developmental needs. Table 3–15 describes the five major transitions within the school milieu, which are intended to foster progressive intellectual and social development and problem areas likely to arise when there is a mismatch of developmental tasks at each transition. Whether each transition affects development positively depends on the particular school system and its approach to facilitating the child's adaptation to each transition and on the particular child. If the child's individual maturation is not consistent with the norm, a misfit may occur between the child's developmental readiness and the school-

TABLE 3-15
Developmental Transitions of the School Milieu

School-Critical Developmental Tasks	*Potential Conflicts*
School Entry (Age 3–5 Yrs*)	
Peer interactions—sharing, taking turns	Demands do not match motor or mental capabilities
Social development—basic self-care skills	No previous exposure to other children
Following directions Developing language skills	No previous experience with separation from parent(s)
Academic Reading Instruction (Age 5–7 Yrs)	
Learning fundamentals of reading	Neurologic or cognitive unreadiness; success interferences, such as moving, family upsets, poor self-concept
Reading to Learn (2nd–3rd Grade)	
Content of reading becomes important	Poor mastery of reading fundamentals results in poor reading skills with resultant behavior or attendance problems Learning deficits associated with neurologic immaturity or experiential naivety
Start Middle School (Junior High)	
Subject-oriented emphasis Change to multiteacher and multiclass experience Often change in school building and administrative personnel	Output failure is greatest potential problem because of • Difficulty for child in having a relationship with a single caring adult • Risk of losing sight of child's specific or special needs • Troublesome nature of organizational structure for child with more rigid personality
Start High School (9th or 10th Grade)	
Change building and administrative personnel Student selection of courses to coincide with career goals Student responsible for balancing academic and social obligations	Removes familiar supportive adults and records/information about child's specific/special needs Student may not have identified any career goals yet Diminished special education focus and of special education resources Vocational education now available but too late for failure-prone child whose academic problems began at junior high level or earlier Serious mismatch of developmental rate and school expectations has greatest likelihood in this transition

*Earlier if disabled.

critical developmental tasks that the transition requires of the student.

Likewise, if the child's temperament is one that adapts to changes slowly or with difficulty, each new transition is likely to pose some developmental conflict. Wesley and Wesley (1977), among others, have documented that boys generally lag behind girls by about 12 months in neurologic development during the early school years, which helps explain why more boys experience reading failure in those early school years.

Although these mismatches between child and school expectations do occur, more often the problem is one in which parents' expectations of their child's school performance are unrealistic for that child, either developmentally or relative to that child's personality. Rutter's (1979, 1980) extensive studies of school outcomes for children reflected that those facets of the school milieu that most obviously influence school problems are (1) increased expectations that do not fit with the child's developmental/emotional status, (2) changes in important personnel, such as teachers or principal, (3) repeated incidences of intimidation by peers or a teacher, and (4) a coercive, unstable teacher.

Neighborhood as Milieu

A child's neighborhood is the child's first and most impressionable exposure to the world outside the home. To foster healthy development, that environment should be protective, friendly, and familiar (Bronfenbrenner, 1979). The neighborhood ideally offers the child an opportunity to experience the world outside home as accepting, supportive of a child's physical and psychosocial needs, and reinforcing of the child's self-confidence and safety. The availability of such neighborhood experiences today, however, is rapidly diminishing. Zill (1982) found, when he surveyed children from communities of various sizes and socioeconomic levels of affluence, that an overwhelming majority of children, regardless of the neighborhood they resided in, perceived that neighborhood as dangerous and unsupportive of children. Some of the fear is admittedly stimulated from media exposure to the vandalism, violence, and abuse occurring within the community rather than from direct experience of these things. However, the effect is the same, in that most children perceive the world outside home negatively. This perception breeds fear; inhibits learning, socialization, and recreational activities; and disturbs children's development of trust and confidence.

Socioeconomic Status as Milieu

Poverty can be an obvious deterrent to healthy development. The Census Bureau has specified the poverty line at the lowest level of family income that should be sufficient to provide an adequate diet. The line is defined in relation to the number of family members and is adjusted each year to the cost-of-living index.

Poor families tend to be characterized by lack of education, high unemployment rates, larger families headed by women, residential crowding, and lack of adequate bathroom facilities. In 1989, 32.5 per cent of children living in poverty had no health coverage (US Department of Health and Human Services, 1991). The poor are five times more likely than the nonpoor to perceive their health status as only fair or poor. Poverty and minority status are inversely related to life expectancy. Residents in poverty areas show higher crude death rates for tuberculosis and homicide than residents in nonpoverty areas. Infant mortality rates among African-Americans remain significantly higher than the rates for whites, despite an overall decrease in infant mortality rates in past years (US Department of Health and Human Services, 1991).

Learning disabilities, language delays, and mental retardation (50 to 80 per cent of all cases are from low income homes) are disproportionately present in the poverty-level population (Levine et al, 1983). Behavior problems are much more common than in the general population, probably associated with the greater exposure to antisocial behaviors in adults. There is also a higher incidence of accidents, mostly related to structural deficiencies in the environment.

Significant national policy changes are necessary to go beyond the health care system and its professionals to reverse the deleterious effects of poverty on children's development. Some measures can be taken, however, to help offset these deficits, such as the availability of preventive health services in areas accessible to these families and the mobilization of community support groups to affect local and regional services.

Affluence, too, can adversely affect children's development. Parent-child relationships are often lacking as a result of long or frequent absences by the parents or general inattentiveness to their children's needs as they respond to social and business pressures. As a result, substitute caretakers often replace parents, further disrupting parent-child bonds. Parents may also fail to set sufficient standards or goals beyond material success, thereby placing extraordinary pressure on their children to measure up to a relatively narrow definition of success. These children also experience little opportunity to learn how to delay gratification of their wants, to "do without," or to learn to make choices. Drug abuse and accidents, particularly from automobiles, are higher among affluent children because of the easier access.

Mass Media as Milieu

Television is said to be the most pervasive force in United States society. It is the primary source of socializing for children and is their major source of information about the world. There is at least one television set in 98 per cent of homes, and many homes have several sets. By the time of high school graduation, the average child in the United States will have spent more time in front of the television (15,000 to 18,000 hours) than in school (12,000 hours) (Harris et al, 1988; Strasburger, 1989). Children are estimated to spend 21 to 28 hours per week watching television instead of engaging in other activities (Strasburger, 1992). A child from a home in which television is not available will often watch at the home of a friend. Television is described as the dominant diversional activity of hospitalized children (Bordeaux, 1986). The financial importance of children's television is demonstrated by the fact that advertisers spend $600 million a year on children's shows.

The effect of television viewing on family life is a subject of concern. Many parents and children argue over what to watch, and there is speculation that mass communication may be replacing interpersonal communication. It may be difficult to carry on other activities, such as reading, conversing, telephoning, or sleeping, in proximity to the television set. If living quarters are cramped, this problem is intensified, since alternative space for other activities may not be available. The second problem that television creates for the family lies in its use as a coping mechanism that allows escape from family problems. The family may use the television to avoid tension-laden interactions and to provide an outlet for anger and aggression.

Recent research has demonstrated that young children spend much of their time co-viewing television with their parents. Five-year-olds were found to spend 85 per cent of their time viewing television in the presence of parents and siblings (Field, 1987). School-age children reported spending up to 66 per cent of their television viewing with parents (Carpenter et al, 1989). One study found that young children are more likely to be exposed to crime shows, soap operas, and news programs because of co-viewing television with parents rather than according to the presumed stereotype, being left alone to watch these programs (St. Peters et al, 1991).

There is an average of six times more violence during 1 hour of children's television than there is in 1 hour of adult television. By high school graduation, the average child will have witnessed approximately 18,000 murders, most of them bloodless and painless (Fosarelli, 1986), and numerous episodes of violence, such as beating, robbery, and arson (Rothenberg, 1985). Over 1000 studies and reviews suggest that aggressive and antisocial tendencies are stimulated by viewing television violence (Comstock & Strasburger, 1990). Others suggest that effects of viewing violence on TV can result in acceptance of aggressive behavior, blunting sensitivity to violence, and adopting a negative worldview (Gadnon & Sprafkin, 1989).

Another consideration raised by viewing many of the cartoons that children watch is the unrealistic portrayal of the physical and moral consequences of violence and aggression. Cartoon characters are virtually indestructible. Humans and animals are beaten, shot, bombed, knifed, thrown from windows, pushed over cliffs, smashed with jackhammers, squashed by falling boulders, and subjected to any number of other traumas; yet—after a brief period of looking frazzled and a bit foolish—they are always completely restored to their former condition. The character perpetrating this mayhem is often the hero of the episode. What does this teach the child about the result of violent behavior? It certainly does not show that it is harmful in an immediate or long-range sense. Nor does it teach the child that there is anything morally wrong with the infliction of pain and harm to others. The child is stimulated to perform actions without having accurate information about the results.

Television has other documented effects as well. One study found that children who spent more time watching TV were more likely to have stereotypical sex role attitudes (Strasburger, 1989). Television programming is dominated by Caucasian males and shows little cultural diversity of characters. Women, even when depicted in professional roles, are not portrayed as autonomous, independent adults. Most characters seen on TV have high-level professional or managerial roles.

TV programs and rock music videos convey unhealthy and irresponsible messages about sex and sexuality. For example, daytime soap operas, which are extremely popular with adolescents, portray sex between unmarried couples 24 more times than sex between married couples, with rare references to responsible and safer sexual activity (Lowry & Towles, 1989). A content analysis of rock videos revealed that 75 per cent contain sexually suggestive material and 56 per cent portray violence (Baxter et al, 1985; Sherman & Dominick, 1986).

Alcohol consumption as portrayed in advertisements suggests that alcohol and youth are synonymous with "a good time." Many of the commercials portray youthful characters at an appealing location, such as at the beach or at a sports bar having a good time drinking. In the United States, the per capita alcohol consumption has increased 50 per cent (nearly $1 billion a year is spent on advertising, compared with a decrease of 20 per cent in Sweden, where alcohol advertisements on TV are banned).

Food products account for 71 per cent of network advertisements; of this proportion, 30 per cent advertise breakfast cereals, and 34 per cent account for cookie, candy, and snack advertisements (Cotunga, 1988). These commercials promote unhealthy nutritional practices and consumption of high-calorie, minimally nutritious foods. Findings of one study suggest that the number of TV viewing hours is a strong predictor of adolescent obesity (Dietz & Gortmaker, 1985). Criticism has also been directed at the advertising of "junk food" during children's TV on Saturday morning programs.

Commercialism in television is another point of

contention for advocates. Young children cannot distinguish between commercials and TV programs. This fact is further complicated by the commercial promoting format of children's TV programs. There are more than 70 program-length commercials that serve to promote a specific toy (Committee on Communications, 1992; Strasburger, 1992).

Several questions have been raised regarding the effects of television viewing on children. What role does television play in the development of role models and value systems? Does the enforced passivity brought about by television decrease the child's opportunities to observe and imitate the behavior of meaningful adults in order to learn appropriate patterns of social and emotional interaction? Does television viewing result in a decrease in the normal physical activity that is one of the hallmarks of childhood? Does television produce a passive attitude to life, blunt the imagination, or inhibit the child's ability to engage in creative play? Do "flashy" educational programs, such as "Sesame Street" or "3-2-1 Contact," cause lack of interest in the more mundane, regimented, and difficult world of classroom learning? Does television, by occupying the child's leisure time, discourage personal emotional discoveries that the child could be making? These are questions to which we have no answers at present, but certainly parents should be made aware of these issues as they make decisions about television for their children. The facts do exist that while a child is watching television, he or she is not playing, sleeping, conversing, reading, or participating in outdoor or social recreational activities. Whatever the child may be learning is happening vicariously (and not necessarily with information reflective of the real world), rather than through direct experience. Table 3–16 lists some effects of heavy television watching that have been derived from studies conducted.

TABLE 3–16
Effects of Heavy Television Viewing

- Increased aggressive behavior and acceptance of violence
- Difficulty in distinguishing between fantasy and reality
- Distorted perception of reality in relation to importance of consumption of products and services; extent of violence and role of minorities
- Trivialization of sex and sexuality
- Increased passivity and disengagement
- Negative effects on academic performance, especially reading performance
- Potential to inform, teach, and promote "prosocial" behavior not fully realized
- Promotion of unhealthy nutritional practices resulting in overweightness, obesity, and energy imbalance
- Naive and misinformed commercialism
- Development of stereotypical attitudes toward women and minorities
- Glamorization of guns and criminals

Nursing Implications

What are the nursing implications related to the effects of television on the child? If comprehensive family care is a nursing goal, the nurse must critically evaluate the often contradictory findings of research in the area and present accurate information to families. Here are a few recommendations that may help guide the nurse during counseling:

1. Parents should be in control of the use of television. They have the responsibility to guide their children in making wise choices.
2. Parents need to spend time with their children, both when they are watching television and when they are engaged in other activities.
3. Television watching must not be allowed to occupy completely the time individuals and families need for exercise, reading, talking together, and pursuing other activities.
4. Television should not be used as a reward or a punishment.
5. Television should not be used as a babysitter.
6. Parents should be able to inculcate their own values and attitudes; if television interferes with this process, they must re-evaluate its use.
7. As they develop, children should be learning progressively to appreciate the difference between reality and unreality. Parents must be careful that use of television does not impede this process.

Nurses can ask about the type and amount of television watching as a part of the history taking phase of child assessment. An obvious way that nurses can become familiar enough with children's programming to make evaluative judgments about it is to watch the programs children watch (Strasburger, 1992). This is especially important in families with communication problems or in those in which children have behavioral problems. Parents can be asked if any problematic behaviors, such as fears or heightened aggression, customarily follow their child's television viewing (Fosarelli, 1986). Nurses can teach parents to use television selectively and creatively.

Physical Environment as Milieu

Research is increasingly supporting the idea that the physical environment has a significant effect on one's overall development. In the fetal stage, certain intrauterine conditions may jeopardize development. A few obvious examples are nutritional deficits; malposition; maternal metabolic or endocrine imbalances; the impact of teratogenic agents, such as maternal exposure to radiation, smoking, or drug use during pregnancy; and Rh incompatibility.

Climate and season also affect development. Climatic influences are secondarily related to sanitary problems posed by warm or temperate climates. Growth spurts are seasonally correlated; for example, height gains correlate positively with the coming of spring.

One's state of general health also has an impact on developmental progression. Illness or injury with associated disability, nutritional impairment, immobility, and energy diversion for recovery rather than learning all hamper progress in some facets of development.

In summary, there is substantial evidence to support the interactional theory that biologic environment, social milieu, and physical environment affect any individual child's developmental progress. The implication for assessing and affecting that environment by health professionals is of obvious importance in promoting and maintaining the healthy development of human beings at all ages.

KEY CONCEPTS

Concepts Related to Basic Information

- Physical competency involves the child's ability to apply various motor, neurologic, and biologic capacities to achieve steadily more mature self-care activities requiring mobility and manipulative skills.
- Intellectual competency involves the development of reasoning to the point of mature abstract thought and the development of perceptions and communication skills.
- Emotional-social competency concerns development of an inner sense of security that is supported by self-awareness and self-acceptance, as evidenced by the capacity to form productive interpersonal relationships with individuals and groups.
- Growth charts for height and weight represent an example of norms established to determine physical competency.
- According to Piaget, there are four major stages of cognitive development: sensorimotor, preoperational, concrete operational, and formal operational.
- Three theories of language development appear equally viable to the current knowledge of language development: language acquisition, reinforcement theory, and social learning theory.
- According to Erikson, individual development occurs within the context of the social and cultural environment.
- According to Kohlberg, moral development follows a sequence that corresponds with the development of intellect.
- Extensive research conducted by Thomas and Chess indicate nine clearly recognizable characteristics or traits of temperament.
- Growth refers to quantitative change, involving an increase in size of the whole child or in size and number of body parts.
- Development refers to changes in function that result from mastering a series of smaller steps.
- Deviation from a child's own pattern may be more indicative of a problem than is lack of conformity to the norm.
- Developmental research has led to several points of view or theoretical conceptualizations of how children reach adulthood.
- Cultural impact is second only to gender socialization, which itself has a culturally affected impact on a child's development.
- Fowler's framework describes the stage-related process of faith development from infancy to adulthood.

Concepts Related to Nursing Assessment

- *Altered growth and development* is a key nursing diagnosis for the nurse who works with children.
- Altered family development can be defined through diagnoses such as *altered family process, ineffective family coping: compromised,* and *ineffective family coping: disabling*.
- The nurse in practice assigns developmental norms to an individual child on the basis of behaviors of the child, rather than on the chronologic age of the child.
- Understanding the child's level of intellectual thought and function helps the nurse to decipher more meaningfully a child's communications, to interpret behaviors and their motivations.
- The nurse can use developmental tools to assess the child's level of development as it relates to a particular area of competency.
- Assessment of the child's developmental level is an essential preliminary step in identifying potential or actual nursing diagnoses, their defining characteristics and etiologies, and planning for care.

Concepts Related to Nursing Intervention

- Application of nursing care based on developmental theories is essential as a scientific basis for care of children and families and understanding the meaning of the child's behavior.
- Application of research findings into clinical practice enables the nurse to utilize nursing care approaches that have been empirically tested.
- Infants demonstrate a less stressful response to a nursing procedure if spoken to before, during, and for a brief period after the procedure.
- The nurse should respect the child's need to regress, assist the child and family to accept it, and support them to provide an environment that fosters a return to age-appropriate tasks.
- The nurse can assist the child and family with promoting healthy sexuality and preventing the nursing diagnosis *altered sexuality patterns* from being necessary.
- Understanding the parenting methods most effective with various personality types can assist par-

ents in adopting the method most appropriate for each function for each of their children.

- Nurses can teach parents to use television selectively and creatively.
- Understanding the child's level of cognitive ability enables the nurse to plan care that is individualized to the needs of the child.
- Knowledge of the psychosocial needs of the child at a particular developmental level is necessary in planning and implementing care that is appropriate to the needs of the child.

REFERENCES

Alexander, M., & Blank, J. (1988). Factors related to obesity in Mexican-American preschool children. *Image: Journal of Nursing Scholarship, 20*(2), 79–82.

Bandura, A. (1977). *A social learning theory.* Englewood Cliffs, NJ: Prentice-Hall.

Baxter, R., DeRiemer, C., Landini, A., et al. (1985). A content analysis of music videos. *Journal of Broadcasting and Electronic Media, 29,* 333–340.

Bordeaux, B. R. (1986). Television viewing patterns of hospitalized school-age children and adolescents. *Child Health Care, 15,* 70–75.

Bronfenbrenner, U. (1979). *The ecology of human development.* Cambridge, MA: Harvard University Press.

Carpenter, J., Huston, A., & Spera, L. (1989). Children's use of time in their everyday activities during middle childhood. In M. Brock & A. Pellegrini (Eds.), *The ecological context of children's play* (pp. 165–190). Norwood, NJ: Ablex.

Castiglia, P. (1991). Moral development. *Journal of Pediatric Health Care, 5*(1), 324–326.

Committee on Communications. (1992). The commercialization of children's television. *Pediatrics, 89*(2), 343–344.

Comstock, G., & Strasburger, V. (1990). Deceptive appearances: Television, violence and aggressive behavior. *Journal of Adolescent Health Care, 11,* 31–44.

Cotunga, N. (1988). TV ads on Saturday morning children's programming: What's new? *Journal of Nutrition Education, 20,* 125–127.

Craft, M., & Denehy, J. (1990). *Nursing interventions for infants and children.* Philadelphia: W. B. Saunders.

Dietz, W., & Gortmaker, S. (1985). Do we fatten our children at the television set? Obesity and television viewing in children and adolescents. *Pediatrics, 75,* 807–812.

Eiduson, B. (1983). Culture and ethnicity. In M. Levine et al. (Eds.), *Developmental-behavioral pediatrics.* Philadelphia: WB Saunders.

Erikson, E. (1965). *The challenge of youth.* New York: Doubleday Anchor.

Erikson, E. H. (1963). *Childhood and society* (2nd ed.). New York: WW Norton.

Erikson, E. (1968). *Identity, youth and crisis.* New York: WW Norton.

Evans, E., & McCandless, B. (1978). *Children and youth: Psychological development.* New York: Holt, Rinehart, & Winston.

Field, D. (1987). Child and parent coviewing of television: Its extent and its relationship to cognitive performance. *Dissertation Abstracts International, 48,* 2799B–2800B. (University Microfilms No. 8727045, 149).

Fosarelli, P. (1986). In my opinion . . . Advocacy for children's appropriate viewing of television: What can we do? *Children's Health Care, 15,* 79–81.

Fowler, J. (1984). *Becoming adult, becoming Christian.* San Francisco: Harper & Row.

Fowler, J. (1980). Moral stages and the development of faith. In B. Munsey (Ed.), *Moral education and Kohlberg.* Birmingham, AL: Religious Education Press.

Frankenburg, W., Dodds, J., Archer, P., Shapiro, H., & Bresnick, B. (1992). The Denver III: A major revision and restandardization of the Denver Developmental Screening Test. *Pediatrics, 89*(1), 91–97.

Freud, S. (1957). Beyond the pleasure principle. In J. Strachey (Ed.), *The standard edition of the complete psychological works of Sigmund Freud* (Vol. 18). London: Hogarth.

Freud, S. (1950). Some psychological consequences of the anatomical distinction between the sexes. In *Collected papers* (Vol. 5). London: Hogarth.

Gadnon, K., & Sprafkin, J. (1989). Field experiments of television violence: Evidence for an environmental hazard? *Pediatrics, 83,* 399–405.

Gesell, A., Ilg, F., & Bates-Ames, L. (1974). *Infant and child in the culture of today.* New York: Harper & Row.

Gilligan, C. (1982). *In a different voice: Toward a psychology of the life cycle.* New York: Jason Aronson.

Gillis, C., Highley, B., Roberts, B., & Martinson, I. (1989). *Toward a science of family nursing.* Reading, MA: Addison-Wesley.

Halford, G., Brown, C., & Thompson, R. (1986). Children's concept of volume and flotation. *Developmental Psychology, 22,* 218–222.

Hanson, S. M. H., & Sporakowski, M. S. (1986). Single parent families. *Family Relations, 35,* 3–8.

Harris, L., et al. (1988). *Sexual material on American network television during the 1987–1988 season.* New York: Planned Parenthood Federation of America.

Hellier, A., Ptak, H., & Cerreto, M. (1986). CATS inside my brain: Children's understanding of the cerebral computed tomography scan process. *Children's Health Care, 14,* 211–221.

Helms, D., & Turner, J. (1978). *Exploring child behavior: Basic principles.* Philadelphia: WB Saunders.

Hetherington, E., & Parke, R. (1975). *Child psychology: A contemporary viewpoint* (pp. 279–306). New York: McGraw-Hill.

Kohlberg, L. (1968). Moral development. In D. Sills (Ed.), *International encyclopedia of social science.* New York: Macmillan.

Kohlberg, L. (1981). *The philosophy of moral development.* San Francisco: Harper & Row.

Kruger, A., & Tomasello, M. (1986). Transactive discussions with peers and adults. *Developmental Psychology, 22,* 681–677.

Levine, M., et al. (1983). *Developmental-behavioral pediatrics.* Philadelphia: WB Saunders.

Levinson, D., et al. (1978). *The seasons of a man's life.* New York: Knopf.

Lowry, D., & Towles, D. (1989). Soap opera portrayals of sex, contraception and sexually transmitted disease. *Journal of Communication, 39,* 76–83.

Madden, J. (1986). The effects of schemes on children's drawings and the results of transformation. *Child Development, 57,* 924–933.

Maier, H. (1969). *Three theories of child development.* New York: Harper & Row.

Miller, S. (1986). Certainty and necessity in the understanding of Piagetian concepts. *Developmental Psychology, 22,* 3–18.

Piaget, J. (1952). *The origins of intelligence in children.* New York: International Universities Press.

Piaget, J. (1970). Piaget's theory. In P. Mussen (Ed.), *Carmichael's manual of child psychology* (Vol. 1). New York: John Wiley.

Piaget, J., & Inhelder, B. (1969). *The psychology of the child.* New York: Basic Books.

Rothenberg, M. B. (1985). In my opinion . . . Role of television in shaping the attitudes of children. *Children's Health Care, 13,* 148–149.

Rutter, M. (1979). *Fifteen thousand hours.* Cambridge, MA: Harvard University Press.

Rutter, M. (1980). *Scientific foundations of developmental psychiatry.* London: Heinemann Medical.

Sears, R. (1957). Identification as a form of behavioral development. In D. Harris (Ed.), *The concept of development.* Minneapolis: University of Minnesota Press.

Sears, R. (1958). Personality development in the family. In J. Seedman (Ed.), *The child: Handbook of readings.* New York: Holt, Rinehart, & Winston.

Segal, J., & Yahroes, H. (1978). *A child's journey: Forces that shape the lives of our young.* New York: McGraw-Hill.

Sherman, B., & Dominick, J. (1986). Violence and sex in music video: TV rock 'n roll. *Journal of Communication, 36,* 79–93.

Smith, D. W., & Bierman, F. L. (1973). *The biologic age of man.* Philadelphia: WB Saunders.

Sobralske, M. (1985, October). Perceptions of health: Navajo indians. *Topics in Clinical Nursing, 7*(3), 32–39.

St. Peters, M., Fitch, M., Huston, A., Wright, J., & Enkins, E. (1991). Television and families: What do young children watch with their parents? *Child Development, 62,* 1409–1423.

Strasburger, V. (1989). Adolescent sexuality and the media. *Pediatric Clinics of North America, 36,* 747–773.

Strasburger, V. (1992). Children, adolescents and television. *Pediatrics in Review, 13*(4), 144–151.

Thomas, A., Chess, S., & Birch, H. (1968). *Temperament and behavior disorders in children.* New York: New York University Press.

Thomson, A. M., et al. (1968). The assessment of fetal growth. *Journal of Obstetrics and Gynecology of the British Commonwealth, 75,* 903.

U. S. Department of Health and Human Services. (1991). *Child health USA '91.* Washington, DC: Author.

Vaughan, V., & Litt, I. (1990). *Child and adolescent development: Clinical implications.* Philadelphia: WB Saunders.

Wesley, F., & Wesley, C. (1977). *Sex-role psychology.* New York: Human Sciences Press.

Wilson, M. N. (1986). The black extended family: An analytical consideration. *Developmental Psychology, 22,* 246–258.

Winick, M. (1970). Biological correlations. *American Journal of Diseases of Children, 120,* 416.

Zill, N. (1982). *American children: Happy, healthy and insecure.* New York: Doubleday.

BIBLIOGRAPHY

Arnett, J. (1989). Caregivers in day care centers. Does training matter? *Journal of Applied Developmental Psychology, 10,* 541–552.

Arnold, L., et al. (1990). Legislative issues affecting parenting: An overview of current policies. *Journal of Perinatal and Neonatal Nursing, 4*(2), 24–32.

Avard, D., et al. (1990). The role of the Canadian Institute of Child Health in promoting family centered care. *Children's Health Care, 19*(4), 209–212.

Bandura, A. (1967). The role of modeling processes in personality development. In W. Hartup & N. Smothergill (Eds.), *The young child review of research* (pp. 42–58). Washington, DC: National Association for the Education of Young Children.

Bandura, A., & Walters, R. (1963). *Social learning and personality development.* New York: Holt, Rinehart, & Winston.

Barnes, L. (1991). Teaching self care to children. *MCN: American Journal of Maternal Child Nursing, 16*(2), 101.

Basch, C., et al. (1990). Validation of mother's reports of dietary intake by four to seven year old children. *American Journal of Public Health, 80*(11), 1314–1317.

Belsky, J. (1988). The "effects" of infant day care reconsidered. *Early Childhood Research Quarterly, 3,* 235–272.

Betz, C. (1980). Faith development in children. *Pediatric Nursing, 7*(2), 22–24.

Biro, F., Lucky, A., Huster, G., & Morrison, J. (1990). Hormonal studies and physical maturation in adolescent gynecomastia. *Journal of Pediatrics, 116*(3), 450–455.

Bocchino, C. (1990). U. N. Convention on the Rights of Children. *Pediatric Nursing, 16*(6), 600.

Bowlby, J. (1980). *Attachment and loss: Loss* (Vol. 3). New York: Basic Books.

Bowman, O., & Wallace, B. (1990). The effects of socioeconomic status on hand size and strength, vestibular function, visuomotor integration and praxis in preschool children. *American Journal of Occupational Therapy, 44*(7), 610–621.

Brabeck, M. (1983). Moral judgment: Theory and research in differences between males and females. *Developmental Review, 3*(3), 274–291.

Bretz, A., et al. (1990). Occurrence of infectious symptoms in children in day care homes. *American Journal of Infection Control, 18*(6), 347–353.

Brown, M., & Tanner, C. (1990). Measurement of type A behavior in preschoolers. *Nursing Research, 39*(4), 207–211.

Burns, E., et al. (1990). Value of health incidence of depression and level of self esteem in low income mothers of preschool children. *Issues in Comprehensive Pediatric Nursing, 13*(2), 141–153.

Carpenito, L. (1989). *Nursing diagnosis: Application to clinical practice* (3rd ed.). Philadelphia: JB Lippincott.

Caty, S., Ritchie, J., & Ellerton, M. (1989). Helping hospitalized preschoolers manage stressful situations: The mother's role. *Children's Health Care, 18*(4), 202–209.

Caty, S., Ritchie, J., & Ellerton, M. (1989). Mother's perceptions of coping behaviors in hospitalized preschool children. *Journal of Pediatric Nursing, 4*(6), 403–410.

Chess, S., & Thomas, A. (1977). *Temperament and development.* New York: Brunner and Mazel.

Clarke-Stewart, A. (1993). Day care. (Rev. ed.) Cambridge, MA: Harvard University Press.

Cowell, J., et al. (1991). School health services: A hub of services to children and their families. *Pediatric Nursing, 17*(1), 86–88.

Crowley, A. (1988). The child care dilemma: Expanding nurse. *Early Childhood Research Quarterly, 3,* 293–318.

Davis, R., & Truesdale, M. (1993). Creative approaches to promoting parent-infant bonding. *Journal of Pediatric Nursing, 8*(3), 201–202.

Feeg, V. (1990). The future of pediatric nursing: Anticipating the health care needs of children. *Imprint, 37*(4), 70, 72–73, 75.

Frankenburg, W., Sciarillo, W., & Burgess, D. (1981). The newly abbreviated and revised Denver Developmental Screening Test. *Journal of Pediatrics, 99*(6), 995–999.

Gillis, A. (1990). Nurse's knowledge of growth and developmental principles in meeting psychosocial needs of hospitalized children. *Journal of Pediatric Nursing, 5*(2), 78–87.

Goetting, A. (1986). The developmental tasks of siblings over the life cycle. *Journal of Marriage and the Family, 48,* 703–714.

Grey, M. (1993). Stressors and children's health. *Journal of Pediatric Nursing, 8*(2), 85–91.

Grimes, D., & Woolbert, L. (1989). Measles outbreak: Who are at risk and why. *Journal of Pediatric Health Care, 3*(4), 187–193.

Gross, D. (1989). Implications for the development of children. *Image: Journal of Nursing Scholarship, 4*(2), 103–107.

Haley, S., & Baryza, M. (1990). A hierarchy of motor outcome assessment: Self initiated movements through adaptive motor function. *Infants and Young Children, 3*(2), 1–14.

Hamburg, D. (1989). Preparing for life: The critical transition of adolescence. *Crisis, 10,* 1–15.

Hanson, M. (1990). Growing pains: Helping children deal with everyday problems through reading. *Journal of Pediatric Health Care, 4*(5), 268–269.

Harrison, M. (1990). A comparison of interactions with term and preterm infants. *Research in Nursing and Health, 13*(3), 173–179.

Hauck, M. (1991). Cognitive abilities of preschool children: Implications for nurses working with young children. *Journal of Pediatric Nursing, 6*(4), 1–6.

Hausman, A., Spivak, H., Roeher, J., & Prothrow-Stith, D. (1989). Adolescent interpersonal assault injury admissions in an urban municipal hospital. *Pediatric Emergency Care, 5*(4), 275–280.

Havighurst, R. J. (1972). *Developmental tasks and education* (3rd ed.). New York: David McKay.

Hoffman, A., & Greydanus, D. (Eds). (1989). *Adolescent medicine.* Norwalk, CT: Appleton & Lange.

Holaday, B., et al. (1990). Patterns of fecal coliform contamination in day care centers. *Public Health Nursing, 7*(4), 224–228.

Holloway, S., & Reichart-Erickson, M. (1988). The relationship of day care quality to children's free play behavior and social problem solving skills. *Early Childhood Research Quarterly, 3,* 39–54.

Howes, C. (1989). Pressuring children to learn versus developmentally appropriate education. *Journal of Pediatric Health Care, 3*(4), 181–186.

Humphrey, N. (1990). U. S. Consumer Product Safety Commission. *Journal of Pediatric Health Care, 4*(6), 323–324.

Irwin, C. (1989). Risk taking behaviors in the adolescent patient: Are they impulsive? *Pediatric Annals, 18*(2), 122–133.

Irwin, C. (1990). The theoretical concept of at-risk adolescents. *Adolescent Medicine: State of the Art: Reviews, 1*(1), 1–14.

Irwin, C., & Varyhan, E. (1988). Psychosocial context of adolescent development: Study group report. *Journal of Adolescent Health Care, 9,* 115–195.

Johnson, B. (1990). Children's drawing as a projective technique. *Pediatric Nursing, 16*(1), 11–17, 34–35.

Johnson, M., Jay, M., Shoup, B., & Rickert, V. (1989). Anabolic steroid use by adolescents. *Pediatrics, 83*(6), 921–924.

Kohlberg, L. (1975). The cognitive-developmental approach to moral education. *Phi Delta Kappan, 46,* 670–677.

Kohlberg, L. (1963). Moral development and identification. In H. Stevenson (Ed.), *Child psychology* (Sixty-second Yearbook of the National Society for the Study of Education. Part 1). Chicago: University of Chicago Press.

Langley, M. (1990). A developmental approach to the use of toys for facilitation of environmental control. *Physical and Occupational Therapy in Pediatrics, 10*(2), 69–91.

Macoby, E. (1980). *Social development: Psychological growth and the parent-child relationships.* New York: Harcourt Brace Jovanovich.

Macoby, E., & Jacklin, C. (1974). *The psychology of sex difference.* Stanford, CA: Stanford University Press.

Maslow, A. (1970). *Motivation and personality.* New York: Harper & Row.

McManus, M., Greaney, A., & Newacheck, P. (1989). Health insurance status of young adults in the United States. *Pediatrics, 84*(4), 709–716.

Meagher, D., et al. (1990). The effect of an educational program on knowledge and attitudes about blood pressure by junior high school students: A pilot project. *Canadian Journal of Cardiovascular Nursing, 1*(5), 15–22.

Moynihan, D. (1987). *Family and nation.* San Diego: Harcourt Brace Jovanovich.

National Association of Pediatric Nurse Associates and Practitioners. (1988). *Policy statement on child care.* Cherry Hill, NJ: Jannetti Publications, Inc.

Newacheck, P. (1989). Improving access to health services for adolescents from economically disadvantaged families. *Pediatrics, 84*(6), 1056–1063.

Newacheck, P., & McManus, M. (1989). Health insurance status of adolescents in the United States. *Pediatrics, 84*(4), 699–708.

Nugent, K. (1989). Routine care: Promoting development in hospitalized infants. *MCN: American Journal of Maternal Child Nursing, 14*(5), 318–321.

Phuphaibul, R. (1993). Concepts of illness of school-age children in rural and urban Thailand. *Journal of Pediatric Nursing, 8*(1), 61–65.

Romanczuk, A. (1987). Helping the stepparent parent. *MCN: American Journal of Maternal Child Nursing, 12,* 106–110.

Schepp, K. (1991). Factors influencing the coping effort of mothers of hospitalized children. *Nursing Research, 40*(1), 42–46.

Schraeder, B., Heverly, M., & Rappaport, J. (1990). Temperament behavior problems and learning skills in very low birth weight preschoolers. *Research in Nursing and Health, 13*(1), 27–34.

Shafer, M., & Sweet, R. (1989). Pelvic inflammatory disease in adolescent females. *Pediatric Clinics of North America, 36*(3), 513–532.

Sieving, R., & Zirbel-Donisch, S. (1990). Development and enhancement of self-esteem in children. *Journal of Pediatric Health Care, 4*(6), 290–296.

Skinner, B. (1938). *The behavior of organisms.* New York: Appleton.

Stark, L., Spirito, A., Williams, C., & Guevermont, D. (1989). Common problems and coping strategies 1: Findings with normal adolescents. *Journal of Abnormal Child Psychology, 17,* 203–212.

Stevens, M. (1989). Coping strategies of hospitalized adolescents. *Children's Health Care, 18*(3), 163–169.

Styles, M. (1990). Challenges for nursing in this new decade. *MCN: American Journal of Maternal-Child Nursing, 15*(6), 347–348, 350, 352.

Television and teens: Health implications. (1990). *Journal of Adolescent Health Care, 11*(1).

Tiedeman, M. E., & Clatworthy, S. (1990). Anxiety of 5- to 11-year-old children during and after hospitalization. *Journal of Pediatric Nursing, 5,* 334–343.

Tobey, G., & Schraeder, B. (1990). Impact of caretaker stress on behavioral adjustment of very low birth weight preschool children. *Nursing Research, 39*(2), 84–89.

U. S. Department of Health and Human Services, Office of Maternal Child Health. (1990). *Child health USA '90.* (HRS–M–CH–90–1). Washington, DC: Author.

Van Cleve, S., & Sadler, L. (1990). Adolescent parents and toddlers: Strategies for intervention. *Public Health Nursing, 7*(1), 22–27.

Vandell, D., Henderson, V. K., & Wilson, K. S. (1988). A longitudinal study of children with day care experiences of varying quality. *Child Development, 59,* 1286–1292.

Vessey, J., & Mahon, M. (1990). Therapeutic play and the hospitalized child. *Journal of Pediatric Nursing, 5*(5), 328–333.

Vessey, J. A., Braithwait, K. B., & Weidmann, M. C. (1990). Teaching children about their internal bodies. *Pediatric Nursing, 16,* 29–35.

Wasserman, G., Brunelli, S., & Rauh, V. (1990). Social supports and living arrangements of adolescent and adult mothers. *Journal of Adolescent Research, 5*(1), 54–66.

Watson, J. B. (1914). *Behavior: An introduction to comparative psychology.* New York: Holt.

Wenger, J., et al. (1990). Day care characteristics associated with *Haemophilus influenzae* disease. *American Journal of Public Health, 80*(12), 1455–1458.

Whitebrooks, M., Howes, C., & Phillips, D. (1989). *Who cares? Child care teachers and the quality of care in America: Executive summary of the national child care staffing study.* Oakland, CA: Child Care Employee Project.

Wilson, D., & Ratekin, C. (1990). An introduction to using children's drawings as an assessmental tool. *Nurse Practitioner: American Journal of Primary Health Care, 15*(3), 23–24, 27, 30–32.

Woollacott, M., & Shermeong-Cook, A. (1990). Changes in posture control across the life span—A systems approach. *Physical Therapy, 70*(12), 799–807.

UNIT • TWO

Growth and Development of Children Within Families

CHAPTER • 4

Families with Neonates

Carolyn Pedigo Delahoussaye

RELATED TOPICS
Family theories and assessment, Chapter 2
Development of children, Chapter 3
Families with Infants, Chapter 5
Promoting Healthy Parenting, Chapter 12
Promoting healthy dietary practices, Chapter 16
The High-Risk Infant, Chapter 30
Genetic inheritance, Chapter 31

LEARNING OBJECTIVES

- Describe the major concerns of the family with a neonate.
- Identify instruments used in the assessment of the neonate.
- Identify the physiologic norms of the neonate's neurologic and sensory conditions.
- Apply the major considerations in provision of nursing care to the normal neonate.
- Discuss the prominent anticipatory guidance concerns for parents during the neonatal period.

The newborn period is defined as the first month of life. The beginning of this chapter discusses the adaptational and developmental processes parents undergo in attaching and adjusting to their newborn. Nursing strategies to promote family members' attachment to the infant are described.

The remaining portion of the chapter presents content on the growth and development of the neonate. Physical assessment of the normal neonate is discussed at length, including the use of assessment measurements. The health promotion and maintenance concerns of neonates are reviewed in detail as the nurse plays an important role in providing anticipatory guidance to parents. These anticipatory concerns include thermoregulation, bathing, cord care, circumcision care, clothing, feeding, sleeping, and safety concerns.

Development and Adaptation of the Family with a Neonate

Prenatal Attachment

Health professionals have begun to realize the valuable experiences families can have prenatally to facilitate bonding to the yet unborn child. These experiences can help the family to be more receptive to the infant from birth. Scientific advances such as the Doppler device that permits early audibility of the fetus' heartbeat, ultrasound that permits visualization of the fetus and sometimes even identification of its sex, as well as greater awareness of the effects of external environment on fetal movement, have all intensified parents' and siblings' awareness of the baby's realness and existence even before birth. Preliminary research has been carried out that suggests that nursing interventions to promote prenatal maternal-infant bonding increase the frequency of maternal attachment behaviors (Beal, 1991). Such interaction with the fetus facilitates the family internalization of the infant's existence by the time it is born (Glover, 1989).

Despite the scant amount of research in prenatal attachment, it seems likely that parents can be helped to prepare for their infant's birth by nursing interventions designed to help them perceive the baby as a real, growing person. The nurse can ask questions such as "Do you ever think about what your baby looks like?" "Do you have a pet name for the baby?" "What do you think your baby's personality will be like, judging from the way he or she moves inside you?"

Parents who seem the least attached to their unborn fetus will require the most intense and innovative nursing care to help them prepare for the reality of their child. Although it has been speculated that a high-risk pregnancy (i.e., one involving significant danger to the fetus or the mother) might affect prenatal attachment to the fetus, one study (Kemp & Page, 1987) found no difference between the prenatal attachment scores of women in the normal and the high-risk groups. In addition, this study found no significant relationships between the attachment scores and any of the following demographic variables: educational level, age, race, whether the pregnancy was planned, whether the women had a sonogram, or the ordinal position of the infant in the family.

Identification: Attachment after Birth

The identification and claiming process is an important first step in the family's incorporation of the "real" baby into their family. According to Beal (1991), after the baby's birth, the mother establishes a realistic image of her infant and absorbs the infant into her self and her social systems through an acquaintance-attachment process. Rubin (1963) has described the typical manner in which a mother identifies and claims her infant. She examines the baby's soft and tiny features first by touching them with her fingertips and then with her palms and finally she enfolds the baby in her arms and looks directly into the baby's eyes—an en face position. Klaus and Kennell (1976) define "en face" as the position in which the mother's face is rotated so that her eyes and those of the infant meet fully in the same vertical plane of rotation.

Whether a mother touches her newborn infant along this orderly pattern, however, should not be used as a single measure of the quality of the beginning relationship. Reaching is another indication of identification at work. At first, the mother may receive her baby passively, but over the next few days most mothers progress toward active reaching for the baby. Active reaching indicates a desire to take the infant into the mother's personal body space and to get closer.

The father of a newborn infant also must identify the infant as a real person joining his family. Opportunities to be with his infant will increase his involvement with the baby and the mother; he becomes part of the family unit. The nurse must recognize the importance of the father and include him in the assessment and plan of care (Beal, 1989).

Model methods of interacting with the baby by pointing out characteristics of the baby that resemble the family, encouraging the unwrapping and examination of the whole baby, and talking to the baby and responding to his or her behavior. This gives permission and endorsement to the family to proceed with their developmental task of identifying and claiming the infant as their own.

Forming a Bond

The term "bonding," introduced by Klaus and Kennell (1976), and the term "attachment" are sometimes used interchangeably, but have different meanings. "Bonding" generally refers to a parent's tie to a child and is thought of as a fairly rapid process that occurs immediately after birth (Vaughan & Litt, 1990). Bonding is unidirectional from parent to child. "Attachment" is somewhat different, referring to an affectional tie between parents and infants that is a two-way process. Attachment develops gradually during the first year of an infant's life (Beal, 1991).

Theories of bonding and attachment have their roots in studies of animal behavior. Highly predictable behavior can be elicited in a certain species by specific stimuli at a time when the organism is in a state of readiness (Pressler, 1990).

Brief experimental separation of certain animals (rats, goats, monkeys) from their mothers has resulted in disturbed maternal caretaking following the separation. Such animal experiments gave rise to the speculation that for humans also an especially sensitive period, known as a "critical period," may exist, during which time optimal mother-infant bonding could take place. Based on these findings from animal studies, Klaus and Kennell (1976) suggested that a *sensitive period* exists immediately after birth during which the maternal-infant bond was most likely to be established.

Klaus and Kennell published articles in the early 1970s reporting on studies in which early and extended contact was provided between mother and infant dyads. These infants were followed to study the effect of such early contact on later parent-infant relationships and child development.

These early studies reported some positive outcomes in their experimental groups, such as mothers being more attentive, exhibiting more soothing and fondling behavior, and more en face positioning (Klaus et al, 1972). Research studies proliferated that further examined whether a sensitive period exists and, if it does, whether maternal-infant contact during that time would have a lasting effect on subsequent parent-child relationships and child development. Table 4–1 summarizes the findings of some of the major research studies.

Reviews and critiques of the bonding/attachment literature are also listed in this table. Most reviewers conclude that there is insufficient evidence to support the idea that a human sensitive period exists during which time optimal parent-infant bonding takes place. Some of the studies have shown that early mother-infant contact may have a positive effect on maternal-infant bonding, but long-term effects have been difficult to demonstrate. In addition, confusion exists about a valid measure of maternal-infant bonding, and populations used in the studies have varied widely in racial and cultural backgrounds; in general, the results from bonding studies have not been clearly positive.

Although there is consensus that early contact between mother and infant has been overrated, few would disagree that the studies of Klaus and Kennell have influenced modern maternal-infant care in a positive way and have humanized hospital procedures. The trend today is to encourage early mother-infant contact, which sets into motion the ongoing process of developing an affectional tie. At the same time, many parents miss the early moments of being with their infant, and it is important for health care professionals to recognize that parents can form strong emotional bonds to their infants despite this. Mothers may require anesthesia for obstetric reasons, or the infant may be whisked away to an intensive care unit. Mothers who are fatigued and prefer to rest rather than spend extra time with their infants should not be made to feel less worthwhile. Adoptive parents and fathers who missed their infant's birth also form emotional bonds with their infants and should not be made to feel that they have missed the crucial moment of beginning a relationship.

Mother-Infant Bond

A healthy mother-child relationship does not spontaneously occur at the birth of a child but has to develop as the mother and child learn to respond to each other. A mother may not always feel the enormous happiness that she expected to feel at the birth of her baby. Instead, she often feels disoriented and tired.

Brazelton (1973) has researched mother-infant interactions by studying videotape recordings. He found that infants exhibit a cycle that is characterized by eight stages of interaction:

- Initiation: The infant's attention is attracted by the mother and the infant looks back at her.
- Orientation: The infant orients body to face the mother.
- State of Attention: The infant alternately sends and receives cues.
- Acceleration: There are fewer oscillations of attention and inattention.
- Vocalizing: Cooing.
- Peak of Excitement: The infant whirls arms and kicks legs, exhibits jerky activity.

TABLE 4-1
A Summary of Major Research on Maternal and Infant Bonding

Author and Date of Study	Brief Description	Findings
Klaus et al, 1972	A group of mothers and infants experienced early contact and were compared with a control group who received routine care	Mothers with early contact exhibited more attentive, soothing, and fondling behaviors at 1 mo postexperiment
Kennell et al, 1974	Same group of mothers (as above) were examined at 1 yr postexperiment	Mothers with early contact reported missing baby to a greater extent when they returned to work than routine care group
Hales et al, 1977 (first study to look at *timing* of extra contact)	Twenty mothers had 45 min of early contact, compared with 20 who had a 45-min contact at 12 hrs	Early contact group engaged in more kissing, smiling, talking, and en face; no differences in proximity or caregiving
De Chateau and Wiberg, 1977	Fifteen mins of skin-to-skin contact immediately after delivery; mother, father, and infant together 2 hrs in delivery; compared with routine care: contact 1 of every 4 hrs for first 2 days then daytime rooming-in; evaluated at 36 hrs, 3 mos, and 1 yr	Contact group at 30 hrs showed more en face, kissing, baby smiles; by 3 mos, contact group reported more breastfeeding problems. By 1 yr of age, contact group breastfed for 175 days versus 108 days for controls
Craig et al, 1982 (controls in this study had more early contact [≤10 min] than most controls in other studies)	Twenty-six mothers given 1 hr of skin-to-skin contact after delivery were compared with ≤10-min contact (baby wrapped)	At 1 mo of age no difference was noted between groups on any measures
Svejda et al, 1980	Contact given for 15–25 min after birth + 45 min in own room and an extra hour at each feed. Control group given 5 mins at delivery and 30 mins every 4 hrs	No differences in any discrete behaviors or in categories of behaviors
Grossman et al, 1981	Mothers assigned to one of four groups: (a) yearly contact; (b) extended contact; (c) early and extended contact; and (d) control groups	Mothers in early contact group showed more tender touch and cuddling behaviors than mothers in control group; differences disappeared after first week
Taylor et al, 1985	Seventy-eight middle income women assigned to either regular contact group (nursery care) or extended contact (maternal contact) within 10 mins of birth	No difference found on outcome measures
Siegal et al, 1990	Three-hundred and twenty-one low income women assigned to one of four groups: (a) early hospital contact; (b) early and extended hospital contact; (c) home visits only; and (d) control group	Early and extended contacts did not make a significant difference; differences between groups attributed to maternal background variables

Some critiques and reviews of the bonding literature can be found in Campbell & Taylor, 1980; Chess & Thomas, 1982; Goldberg, 1983; Klaus & Kennell, 1982; Lamb & Hwang, 1982; Mitchell & Mills, 1983; Svejda et al, 1982; and Brown & Hellings, 1988.

- Deceleration: Activity, eye contact, and vocalization gradually decrease.
- Withdrawal: The infant withdraws from looking and interacting.

The infant's overtures must be perceived and reciprocated by the mother for their interrelationship. It is clear that both mother and baby are active participants in the attachment process.

The term "maternicity" has been used to mean the characteristic quality of a woman's personality that supplies her with the emotional energy for feeling that her infant occupies an essential part of her life as determined by bonds of affection. These bonds include feelings of warmth, devotion, and protectiveness toward the infant, concern for the infant's well-being, and pleasant anticipation of continuing contact. Maternicity develops as the mother and infant are in close contact and indicates a high probability for the successful development of a healthy mother and child relationship.

The mother's style of feeding and bathing her infant is also an indicator of maternal behavior. Parameters to observe in mothers for the development of maternicity are (Luddington-Hoe, 1977; Pressler, 1990):

- Initial identifying behaviors prior to and after delivery.
- Active and passive reaching behavior.
- Touch progression: Fingertip to palm or to hand; hand-to-arm embrace.
- Positioning of the infant to the left of mother's sternum, en face positioning (in right-handed mothers).
- Eye-to-eye contact.
- Verbal identifying behaviors: Association and pronoun identification.

- Developmental phases: Taking-in phase of dependency; taking-hold phase of task execution; letting go of predelivery expectations.
- Rhythm-reciprocity patterns.*
- Cooing behaviors.

Absence of these behaviors suggests further evaluation of the mother-infant attachment.

Assessment of deviations and early therapeutic intervention when maladaptive maternal behaviors exist may prevent child abuse, mental illness, and many psychosomatic and learning disorders. This type of assessment may be compromised by the current trend toward early discharge of mothers and babies. The nurse should be alert to the need for home follow-up to prevent future problems.

Father-Infant Bond

Although mothers require a period of time to separate from the image they have developed of the baby as an integral part of themselves, the father's image of his baby is one of separateness. Before the early 1970s, very little was known about father-infant attachment. Bowen and Miller (1980) found that bonding may be stronger in fathers present at the delivery of their infant.

One reason early father-infant bonding is important today is because the extended family is seldom available for new parents as it was in the past and the role of fathers, by necessity, has changed. Thus, fathers need and want to contribute to the early emotional and physical care of new infants in the nuclear family (Novak & Novak, 1990).

Sibling-Infant Bond

The attachment between infant and siblings has been explored and documented far less than has parent-infant attachment. When older children are prepared to expect a new baby in the family, they will be able to handle their jealous feelings at displacement with less stress. Even though a young child cannot verbalize these feelings, it is logical that she or he might be thinking, "Where have I failed? Mommy and Daddy wanted to have another baby. They must not have been satisfied with me." A child's excitement at meeting a new brother or sister is often tempered by these negative feelings.

With these factors in mind, some hospitals are providing prenatal classes for siblings and allowing siblings in the delivery room to view the birth of their brother or sister. The older child's attachment to a new sibling seems to be facilitated when parents help the child understand what is happening, explain that this is the child's baby as well as theirs, and reassure her or him of their continuing love by verbal expression and by demonstration. The infant's responses to the older sibling will also be influential in establishing a bond between them. As children have an opportunity to examine, touch, and interact with their new sibling, their negative feelings can be altered and finally replaced by feelings of protectiveness and love.

* That is, the rhythm and reciprocity of the behaviors and responses between mother and infant, resulting in a cyclic exchange indicating mutual satisfaction.

Accepting Responsibility for the Infant

Another task that is a part of internalizing the infant's existence is the acceptance of new or added responsibilities associated with the infant (Duvall & Miller, 1985). For some people, having a baby may satisfy a need for purpose and responsibility. For others, the responsibility for another's survival is overwhelming.

One of the most crucial needs often felt by an infant's parents is based on their sense of insufficient knowledge. Nurses who work with such parents should include in their care plan an ongoing assessment of parental knowledge of basic infant care. This assessment will allow them to recognize when a diagnosis of *knowledge deficit* is appropriate and needs intervention.

Assuming the Parent Role

The new responsibilities associated with the infant require that all members in the infant's family assume some new roles. The addition of parental or sibling roles creates critical role transition periods while each family member works out an accommodation among new and old roles. Making a transition to parenthood requires development of several new interrelated roles. What these new roles are perceived to be and how they are internalized varies according to the individual's own experiences, feelings, and needs. A parent who has been an only child or the youngest child in a family has had fewer opportunities for exposure to infant and child care responsibilities and may be unprepared for what to expect of infant behaviors.

Any situation that involves a change in roles or in which new roles are perceived as conflicting with existing roles has the high risk for a resulting *disturbance in self-concept: role performance*. Nursing assessment must include consideration of the defining characteristics of this nursing diagnosis. Awareness of the facets of the roles of mother, father, and sibling contributes to the nursing assessment.

Mother Role

The mother in the family of an infant usually experiences the greatest change in her position. Her maternal role usually requires at least temporary interruption of her occupational role and often most of her other extrafamilial responsibilities.

Nursing interventions incorporate recognizing the mother's dependency needs. During this time the new mother is overloaded. It is an especially hard time for the educated, career woman who is used to being in control. Support groups for new mothers in this category can be particularly helpful for dealing with feelings of frustration and anxiety that can arise when the employed woman perceives herself to be less competent in the mothering role than in her professional role. Adolescent mothers will be faced with complex emotional challenges as they attempt to adjust to and meet the needs of their newborn yet try to satisfy their own unresolved developmental needs. For more in-depth discussion about the issues and nursing care needs of pregnant adolescents and adolescent parents, refer to "Adolescent Pregnancy" in Chapter 9.

Single, separated, and divorced women make up a growing segment of parents with infants. This group of parents presents with unique needs as they lack the social and, many times, financial support that mothers with husbands have. According to the United States Bureau of the Census (1991), single-parent families have increased from 11.9 to 24.7 per cent owing to the rise in the divorce rate and number of unmarried parents. Forty per cent of children living in single-parent families live in poverty. This group of mothers is likely to need additional support from interdisciplinary professionals and referral to community agencies that can provide assistance in areas of education, job training, housing, and food.

The nurse's reassurance of the mother will help build her self-confidence. At no time should a nurse's behavior communicate that she or he is better able to care for the baby than the mother; instead the nurse must use every opportunity to foster feelings of adequacy in the mother.

Father Role

Fathers are not only able to be involved with their infants, many also want to have this involvement as a parent. Their involvement makes a difference to the baby's well-being. Nurses in contact with the families of infants can promote opportunities for fathers to be with their infants in the hospital and to encourage their family involvement at home. The changes in attitudes regarding a father's involvement are evident in the changing policies within hospitals. In the 1970s barely one fourth of hospitals allowed fathers in the delivery room. Now nearly all do, even during cesarean births; many hospitals accommodate the presence of siblings as well.

The father's involvement in the home may call for the development of sociocultural support systems such as paternity leaves from employment after the birth of a baby. This type of social change may be hastened by nurses who recognize the importance of the father-infant involvement to the baby, the father, and the total family. Such nurses can seek opportunities to increase community awareness of this and make contacts with persons in positions of power to help bring about changes in policies.

The foregoing discussion about the assumption of parental roles may lead one to think that the responses of parents to each child as she or he is born are similar. This is not so. The baby actually molds or triggers adult behavior. It is the individual characteristics of the child that set up specific parental responses and influence their feelings and nurturing. The mother's and father's orientation to their parental roles surely will be influenced by this particular baby as they learn to communicate and to stimulate the baby's further development.

Sibling Role

Just as parents must assume new roles in relation to the neonate, older children in the family have the sibling role thrust on them by the baby's arrival (Andenberg, 1988). The need to assume this developmental task comes at a time when support structures are not as available and predictable as usual. If the birth occurs at a hospital, the older children likely will be separated from their mother for one or more days and nights. As the father tries to establish an early relationship with his infant, he too may be separated from the older child for extended periods of time. Some hospital maternity units are attempting to reduce the older child's stress at being separated from the mother by promoting sibling visitation at the hospital.

Some changes have been observed in the nature of the relationship between the mother and the older child when a new baby arrives. A new baby's arrival seems to stimulate higher expectations by the mother for her older children, as she pressures them to master additional developmental tasks without as much maternal encouragement. The children may resent the family newcomer whose presence seems to have prompted these changes in their mother's behaviors.

Older children will be able to assume the sibling role in a healthier way if they can express to an understanding person—preferably the parents—their honest feelings about the changes they are experiencing and also can have their personal needs for affection and security met.

Nursing Care and Guidance

Facilitating Identification

Nurses can assist families to identify with and become attached to the infant. The nurse present at the birth and afterward can provide opportunities for all family members to relate to the neonate. Nursing interventions in this early stage can assist in the prevention of the nursing diagnosis *alteration in parenting*.

Traditional hospital practices often interfere with the process of identification and claiming by isolating the baby from some family members. Fortunately, these practices have changed in many places. Within the confines of the setting, the nurse minimizes or prevents interruption of contact between the infant and the family members.

Facilitating Mother-Infant Bond

In assessing the development of maternicity in the mother of an infant, the nurse should remember that observation of eye-to-eye contact (en face position) between mother and infant is of primary importance. Other behaviors of maternicity assessed by the nurse have been discussed previously under the heading "Mother-Infant Bond."

Facilitating Father-Infant Bond

The following are important elements in the assessment of father-infant attachment:

Inspection: Does the father look at the infant, assume an en face position, smile at the infant, express awareness of distinct characteristics of the infant, or turn away from the infant?

Verbalization: Does the father vocalize to the infant? Does he call the baby by name? Does he use affectionate terms for the infant?

Tactile contact: Does the father touch the baby with fingertips and whole hand? Does he rock, kiss, or hold the infant? Does he refuse to hold the infant?

Caretaking: Does the father feed the infant? Does he burp, clean, or diaper the infant? Does he respond to the infant's cues and demands for attention?

The infant's state of activity during interactions with the father may also indicate father-infant attachment. Is the infant active and alert or inactive and passive? Has the father been with the infant only during periods of sleeping or crying? What is the behavior of the father when he is alone with the infant? Is there a change when the mother, infant, and father are together (Weiser & Castiglia, 1984; Novak & Novak, 1990)?

Facilitating Sibling-Infant Bond

Supporting parents and siblings during the early infant acquaintance is an important nursing function. For this, the nurse observes the quality and progress of interactions between parents and children and offers reinforcement when they observe their infant, talk to the baby, and comment about her or his behaviors. The nurse can also teach family members to interpret their infant's behaviors appropriately.

Accepting Responsibility

The need for parenting education has become ever more acute with early discharge of mothers and babies from maternity units (within 24 to 72 hours after birth for most healthy neonates). Just as nurses have led in the development of childbirth education classes for expectant families, community parenting support offers many professional opportunities for the nurse.

If the criteria for making a nursing diagnosis are followed, the nurse will include in the diagnostic process the factors related to the etiology of knowledge deficit. Interventions can then be directed toward these factors, and, if the factor is a matter of lack of exposure to information, nursing interventions will focus on client-appropriate teaching of the necessary information.

Basic infant care is taught before and after the baby is born, prenatally in classes and postnatally in the hospital or home. However, two factors make this teaching less effective than it might be at a different time. The teaching of baby care in a prenatal class occurs before the baby is born, and parents tend to forget this information because they cannot relate it to their baby until they can see and hold her or him. The teaching done in the hospital following the birth comes at a time when the mother feels very dependent and is not yet ready to think in terms of caring for her baby. She has a need for care herself. Much of what a mother is taught in the first days after the birth of her baby is not retained after discharge.

The effectiveness of in-hospital teaching cannot be discounted, however. A study of 140 postpartum mothers found that in-hospital teaching significantly increased perceptions of competence for infant feeding and care (Rutledge & Pridham, 1987).

Other factors influencing the etiology of *knowledge deficit* include anxiety, lack of interest or motivation, and cultural-language differences that interfere with the use of learning resources. Teaching infant care skills would be an inappropriate intervention for these etiologic factors. Therefore, subjective and objective assessment of parents and accurate use of the etiology *knowledge deficit* are important.

Knowledge deficit as an etiologic factor for the nursing diagnoses of *ineffective individual coping: parent; fear; disturbance in self-concept: self-esteem; powerlessness;* and *disturbance in self-concept: role performance* has been traditionally recognized; well-developed interventions to remedy knowledge deficit are available. Nurses must be aware that the problem area may not be knowledge deficit and must be prepared to include interventions that are appropriate to other problems in their plan of care.

A nurse who suspects that the family is experiencing feelings of being overwhelmed should consider a possible diagnosis of *ineffective family coping*.

The feeling of being overwhelmed by the new responsibilities is emphasized when parents first realize that the parent role is irrevocable.

When the parental stresses of insecurity, fear, and low self-esteem exist, the nurse's major intervention is one of reassurance and of identification of the parents' strengths. The parental need for reassurance is poignant even in those families in which the knowledge base is strong; frequent questions are, "What am I doing wrong?" "Do other mothers feel this way?" "Do bottlefed babies cry this much?"

Fostering Role Adaptation

Nurses can do much to provide extensive opportunities for parent-infant interaction. One group of nurses planned, carried out, and evaluated a highly structured intervention session designed to facilitate the bonding process (Dean et al, 1982). Each neonate was individually assessed by a nurse before the intervention session. During the session, the baby's identifying characteristics were explained to the mother; the individuality and uniqueness of the infant were emphasized. Any variations from expected neonate characteristics were thoroughly discussed. The infant's hearing, sight, and reflexes were demonstrated and explained. The atmosphere was deliberately kept warm, gentle, and interactive. At the end of the session, each mother received a written record of material covered to reinforce what had been learned. Mothers who participated had lower anxiety scores than mothers who did not. In every contact nurses can reinforce parents' strengths and capacity to cope, thereby improving parents' self-images and increasing the self-confidence they pass on to their babies.

However, the nurse should realize that attachment is a multifactorial process and should intervene at all periods of development to strengthen parent-child relationships (Mitchell & Mills, 1983). Any practices that humanize or enrich the childbearing and childrearing experiences for the family should be encouraged as a means of enhancing parental satisfaction and self-esteem, which correlate directly with healthy parent-child attachments and contribute to healthy parenting. One researcher reported greater numbers of feelings of attachment with guided fetal visualization by the nurse during ultrasound (Glover, 1989).

The nurse can also offer reassurances to parents who, for whatever reason, are not afforded the early contact with their infant. These parents need reassurance that this does not automatically mean there will be deficits in their relationships with that child. The bonding process, in most instances, has already begun prenatally. Nursing actions that help foster parental satisfaction and self-esteem despite limited opportunity for direct contact with the infant will facilitate the maintenance and building of the bonding process when direct contact does become possible.

Growth and Development of the Neonate

This section focuses on the appraisal and care of the normal full-term neonate. "Normal" refers to the absence of problematic physiologic, pathologic, or neuromuscular conditions, or any combination of these three. Minor deviations are common and considered normal; therefore, they are included in this section. "Full-term" refers to gestational age. The full-term neonate is one born following 38 to 42 weeks of gestation in utero.

Nursing assessment and care are best learned first with the normal full-term neonate. Working from a normal base, the nurse can begin to recognize deviations from normal as minor or major, formulate an appropriate nursing diagnosis, and carry out appropriate nursing interventions. Nurses providing care to the neonate in the hospital, birthing center, or other community setting will consider the nursing diagnosis *high risk for altered growth and development* as an integral component of care. Other nursing diagnoses that may be considered when providing care for the neonate and family are *high risk for altered parenting*, and *high risk for alterations in family processes* (Table 4–2).

"It's a girl!" "It's a boy!" A baby has been born. The gamut of emotional responses might be compressed into this exclamation. After 9 months of waiting, the momentous event has occurred. Parental adaptation to the birth may be influenced by many factors: whether the pregnancy was planned, whether the pregnancy was normal, the length of time and degree of difficulty in labor and delivery; the medications administered during labor and delivery; and the sex and appearance of the newborn infant. Nursing interventions are geared toward identifying those factors—parental or neonatal, or both—that might interfere with a positive adaptation.

The birth transition from intrauterine to extrauterine existence may enhance or interfere with neonatal adaptation. In the neonate born at term, all systems are considered mature enough to adapt and support life outside the uterus. Following a 9-month existence in an environment that is totally protected and nur-

TABLE 4-2
Growth and Development Plan: Families with Neonates

Analysis: Nursing diagnostic statement

Response and related or risk factors: *High risk for altered growth and development; risk factors*

- Pathophysiologic conditions
- Treatment-related factors
  - Hospitalization
  - Painful treatments
- Environmental sound level, chaotic environmental stimulation
- Disruption of sleep-wake cycle
- Multiple caretakers
- Separation from caretaking figure(s)
- Neurologic immaturity, thermoregulation
- Caregiver knowledge deficit about neonate development
- Caregiver anxiety
- Inadequate sensory stimulation
- Gestational age
- Need for oral gratification is interfered with

Projected outcome: *The neonate will demonstrate acquisition of developmentally appropriate behaviors in the physical, intellectual, and emotional-social domains*

Defining Characteristics *(Actual Response)*	**Nursing Interventions**	**Evaluation Criteria**
Subjective: • Parents express anxiety about ability to parent with statements such as "I'm afraid I'm going to hurt her/him"; "He looks like he is going to break!"; "She is so little"; parents acknowledge lack of skill and information in caretaking and stimulation activities with statements such as "How do I give her a bath?" or "How do I breastfeed him?" or "How do I respond to his smile?" • Lack of attachment behaviors between parent and neonate	*Health Screening* • **Assess factors that can identify altered growth and development.** The neonate's physical maturity as measured by assessment tools will be documented; this assessment includes: • The Apgar score done at 1 minute and 5 minutes following birth • The Dubowitz Assessment for estimation of gestational age, length, weight and head circumference, initial and 24-hour physical assessments that include neurologic and sensory examination	• **Developmental delays will be identified as evidenced by:** • Charted assessment of screening for physical, intellectual, and emotional-social development • Referral for deviations detected during screening • Caregiver(s) demonstrates knowledge and ability to develop an attachment with neonate and provide appropriate stimulation activities
Objective: • Altered physical maturity and growth • Below normal values on Apgar scores	• Social support and attachment behaviors will be observed and noted	• Neonate demonstrates behavior within developmental norms • Neonate demonstrates attachment behaviors with caregivers

(continued)

TABLE 4-2 (continued)

Defining Characteristics (Actual Response)	*Nursing Interventions*	*Evaluation Criteria*
• Dubowitz assessment and placement on growth charts	*Anticipatory guidance; Parent education: Childrearing family; Attachment promotion* • **Provide anticipatory guidance to caregivers regarding the neonate's developmental needs.** • Information provided to parents will be based on findings from Apgar scores, Dubowitz assessment, length, weight, head circumference, and physical examination • Health promotion concerns include thermal management, bathing, cord care, circumcision care, clothing, feeding, sleep behaviors, and safety concerns • **Assist parents to provide appropriate stimulation to meet developmental needs of neonate.** Refer to information on nursing interventions and anticipatory guidance related to neonate's developmental needs in Chapter 4 and in Chapters 15 and 17. • **Create an environment that promotes trust and security.** • Schedule activities to promote natural rhythm of sleep-wake cycle • Provide consistent caregiver(s) • Encourage parental participation in care • Encourage and support parent(s) in providing care *Support system enhancement* • **Refer neonate and family to appropriate community resources as needed:** • Appropriate agency for supportive services (e.g., occupational therapy, physical therapy)	

TABLE 4-2 *(continued)*

Defining Characteristics *(Actual Response)*	**Nursing Interventions**	**Evaluation Criteria**
	• Community programs (e.g., early intervention services, infant stimulation programs, Women, Infants, and Children [WIC] • Provide information on community self-help groups, family support groups, advocacy groups • Follow through with referrals made and assure that families participate in programs with treatment regimen	

turing, the fetus is suddenly and sometimes painfully propelled through a narrow, constricted passage into the bright, cold, and noisy environment of the delivery room. To facilitate extrauterine adaptation, the neonate's nose and mouth are suctioned with a bulb syringe to remove mucus, which may obstruct respiratory passages. Once the umbilical cord is clamped and cut, the child is forced to establish independent life-sustaining functions. At no other time in an individual's life are greater physiologic adjustments required than during the first hour after birth.

Initial Assessment of the Neonate

Assessment of the neonate includes the initial Apgar scoring and comprehensive physical assessment, including gestational age and size (weight and length), and assessment of behavioral characteristics. Assessment is done to determine how satisfactorily the neonate is adapting to extrauterine life and to rule out any risk factors that might compromise growth or life, or both.

Apgar Score

Dr. Virginia Apgar (1953) developed this tool for evaluating the infant's condition at birth. Assessment is done at 1 minute and again at 5 minutes, using five standardized observations (heart rate, respiratory effort, reflex irritability, muscle tone, and color). The 1-minute assessment is valuable because it provides a rapid method of determining the infant's ability to adapt to extrauterine life. With the 1-minute Apgar score, one can specifically identify the resuscitative measures that should be taken. The purpose of the 5-minute score is to re-evaluate the newborn's condition, particularly the response to resuscitative measures.

As soon as delivery is complete, a timer is started, so that the neonate can be assessed at exactly 1 minute. The *heart rate* is the first and most important observation made, providing the most useful diagnostic and prognostic information. It should be counted for a full minute through either auscultation of the precordium or palpation of the umbilical cord pulse located at the junction of the umbilical cord and the abdominal wall.

The second most important observation is *respiratory effort.* Only the neonate's unassisted respiratory rate is counted. Respiratory rate should be assessed by counting the number of inspirations within 1 full minute in order to note any delays in inspiratory effort. The rate may be determined by auscultation of the chest or observation of chest wall excursions.

Reflex irritability is assessed by stimulating the newborn infant in order to evoke a response. Suctioning the nares, gently rubbing the back, or lightly flicking the sole of the foot are examples of stimuli used. The more alert the neonate, the more easily one can evoke a response.

Muscle tone is assessed by observing the infant's spontaneous return to a state of flexion; that is, when limbs are extended, they should return rapidly to their original position when released. The examiner should attempt to extend the extremities, noting the presence or absence of resistance and the rapidness of return to flexion. The infant's appearance in flexion is discussed later under the heading "General Appearance."

Color is the last observation and, according to Dr. Apgar, of least significance. All babies are cyanotic at birth. With the onset of respirations the skin becomes

TABLE 4-3
Apgar Score Chart

Observation	Score 0	Score 1	Score 2
Heart rate	Absent	Slow (below 100)	Over 100
Respiratory effort	Absent (apneic)	Slow, irregular, shallow	Good, sustained cry; regular respirations
Reflex irritability	No response	Grimace, frown	Sneeze, cough, cry
Muscle tone	Limp, completely flaccid	Some flexion of extremities; some resistance to extension of extremities	Active motion, good muscle tone, spontaneous flexion
Color	Cyanotic, pale	Body pink, extremities pale	Completely pink

From Apgar, V. (1953). A proposal for a new method of evaluating the newborn infant. *Current Research in Anesthesia and Analgesia, 32*, 260.

pink, except for the extremities, which may remain slightly cyanotic *(acrocyanosis)* for the first few hours of life. Acrocyanosis is due to insufficient circulation to the extremities, a condition that becomes reversed with adaptation to extrauterine life.

The Apgar Scoring Chart is found in Table 4–3. Each of the five observation areas should receive a score of 0, 1, or 2, according to the descriptions found in the score chart. When each of the five areas is scored, the sum total equals the Apgar score. A score of 10 is the highest possible, 0 the lowest. An infant who has a score of 7 to 10 is in good condition and will only need suction of the nose and mouth and routine care and observation. A score of 3 to 6 indicates a moderately depressed infant who will need some form of resuscitation along with close observation during the first 24 hours of life. An infant who receives a score of 0, 1, or 2 is considered severely depressed and will need ventilatory assistance and intensive care as part of resuscitative measures.

Gross physical assessment is performed immediately after delivery to identify risk factors that could potentially interfere with life or growth. Within the first 24 hours of life, a thorough physical examination, including assessment of physical, neurologic, and behavioral characteristics, should be performed to provide a normal data base for comparison as the newborn baby progresses through life.

Dubowitz Assessment for Estimation of Gestational Age

A standard set of criteria should be used for estimation of gestational age (GA) as an indicator of maturity. GA is defined as the number of weeks spent in utero to the time of birth. Dr. Lillian Dubowitz and colleagues (1970) developed a standardized tool, using 11 external signs and 10 neurologic signs for estimating the GA of the neonate.

External physical characteristics should be assessed as soon as possible after birth. These physical characteristics are external signs of progressive tissue development. They provide data for evaluating the degree of physical maturity of the neonate.

The neurologic signs provide data for evaluating neurologic development and maturity through passive and active muscle tone. The infant should be alert and quiet during the neurologic testing to obtain valid results. Any signs that deviate from normal should be reassessed within 24 hours. The GA of the neonate is estimated by combining the score from the physical maturity chart (see Table 4–4) and the score from the neurologic maturity chart (Fig. 4–1). The final score

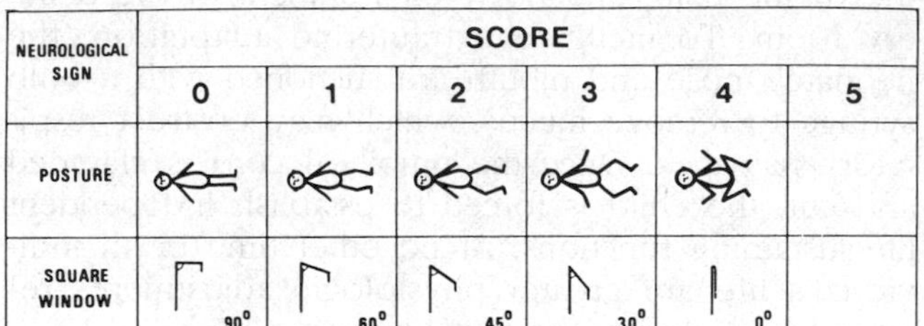

FIGURE 4-1. Score sheet for neurologic characteristics. (From Dubowitz, L., et al. [1970, July]. Clinical assessment of gestational age in the newborn infant. *Journal of Pediatrics*, p. 1.)

TABLE 4-4
Score Sheet for External Physical Characteristics

	Points					
External Sign	**0**	**1**	**2**	**3**	**4**	**Score**
Edema	Obvious edema of hands and feet; pitting over tibia	No obvious edema of hands and feet; pitting over tibia	No edema			
Skin texture	Very thin, gelatinous	Thin and smooth	Smooth; medium thickness; rash or superficial peeling	Slight thickening and peeling especially of hands and feet	Thick and parchment-like; superficial or deep cracking	
Skin color	Dark red	Uniformly pink	Pale pink; variable over body	Pale; only pink over ears, lips, palms, or soles		
Skin opacity (trunk)	Numerous veins and venules clearly seen, especially over abdomen	Veins and tributaries seen	A few large vessels clearly seen over abdomen	A few large vessels seen indistinctly over abdomen	No blood vessels seen	
Lanugo (over back)	No lanugo	Abundant; long and thick over whole back	Hair thinning, especially over lower back	Small amount of lanugo and bald areas	At least half of back devoid of lanugo	
Plantar creases	No skin creases	Faint red marks over anterior half of sole	Definite red marks over > anterior half, indentations over < third	Indentations over > anterior third	Definite deep indentations over > anterior third	
Nipple formation	Nipple barely visible; no areola	Nipple well defined; areola smooth and flat, diameter < 0.75 cm	Areola stippled, edge not raised, diameter <0.75 cm	Areola stippled, edge raised, diameter >0.75 cm		
Breast size	No breast tissue palpable	Breast tissue on one or both sides, <0.5 cm diameter	Breast tissue both sides; one or both 0.5–1.0 cm	Breast tissue both sides; one or both >1 cm		
Ear form	Pinna flat and shapeless, little or no incurving of edge	Incurving of part of edge of pinna	Partial incurving whole of upper pinna	Well-defined incurving whole of upper pinna		
Ear firmness	Pinna soft, easily folded, no recoil	Pinna soft, easily folded, slow recoil	Cartilage to edge of pinna, but soft in places, ready recoil	Pinna firm, cartilage to edge; instant recoil		
Genitals						
Male	Neither testis in scrotum	At least one testis high in scrotum	At least one testis right down			
Female (with hips half abducted)	Labia majora widely separated, labia minora protruding	Labia majora almost cover labia minora	Labia majora completely cover labia minora			
						EXTERNAL TOTAL:

From Dubowitz, L., et al. (1970). Clinical assessment of gestational age in the newborn infant. *Journal of Pediatrics, 77,* 1.

is then compared with the maturity rating scale (Table 4–5) to determine estimated GA. The full-term infant is 38 to 42 weeks of gestation.

The sections following are designed to provide experience in actual evaluation of an infant.

Physical Maturity. With the neonate on an examining surface and using the scale in Table 4–4, assess each of the following physical characteristics: edema, skin texture, skin color, skin opacity, lanugo, plantar creases, nipple formation, breast size, ear formation, ear firmness, and genitalia. The descriptions for each area range from 0 to 4, beginning with less mature development and progressing to mature tissue. After assessing the presence or absence of edema, find the description in the scale that best describes your observation and give the neonate the appropriate score. Proceed in the same manner with each characteristic until you have completed the assessment, then add all the scores for a sum total of physical maturity.

TABLE 4-5
Dubowitz Score Sheet of Gestational Age

Total Score	Gestational Age (in wks)
0–9	26
10–12	27
13–16	28
17–20	29
21–24	30
25–27	31
28–31	32
32–35	33
36–39	34
40–43	35
44–46	36
47–50	37
51–54	38
55–58	39
59–62	40
63–65	41
66–69	42

From Dubowitz, L., et al. (1970). Clinical assessment of gestational age in the newborn infant. *Journal of Pediatrics, 77*, 1.

Neuromuscular Maturity. Using the scale in Figure 4–1, assess each of the neuromuscular signs using the following guide and assign the score that is closest to your observation.

Posture—With the infant quiet and in a supine position, observe the degree of flexion in the arms and legs. Muscle tone and degree of flexion increase with maturity. Full flexion of the arms and the legs = 4.

Square window—Without rotating the wrist, flex the hand with enough pressure to get as great a degree of flexion as possible. Measure the angle between the base of the thumb and the anterior aspect of the forearm. Full flexion = 4.

Ankle dorsiflexion—At the ankle, flex the foot onto the shin with sufficient pressure to provide maximal flexion ability. Measure the angle between the dorsum of the foot and the anterior aspect of the leg. A 20-degree angle = 3.

Arm recoil—With the baby in a supine position, fully flex both arms, hold for 5 seconds, fully extend, and rapidly release arms. Recoil to a state of flexion should occur instantly. A brisk return to full flexion = 2.

Leg recoil—With the baby in a supine position, fully flex both legs without lifting the hips up from the surface. Hold flexed for 5 seconds, fully extend, and rapidly release. Recoil to a state of flexion should occur instantaneously. A brisk return to full flexion (less than 90 degrees at knees and hips) = 2.

Popliteal angle—With the neonate in a supine position, flex one thigh on the abdomen. Be certain to keep body alignment straight and hips flat on the surface. While maintaining flexion of the thigh, attempt to straighten the leg toward the head until resistance is met. Measure the popliteal angle and score. Less than 90 degrees = 5.

Heel to ear—With the neonate supine, pelvis flat on examining surface, attempt to pull the feet toward the head. When resistance is met, determine the distance between the heels and the ears and score according to distance.

Scarf sign—With the neonate in a supine position, place the arm across the chest so that the hand touches the opposite shoulder. The elbow may be lifted across the body (Fig. 4–2). The score is determined by the location of the elbow. If the elbow does not reach the midline of the thorax, the score = 3.

Head lag—With the neonate supine, grasp both arms and slowly pull the infant up to a sitting position. Observe the relationship of the head to the trunk during the procedure. If the neonate has sufficient muscle tone to hold the head slightly forward of the body, the score = 3.

Ventral suspension—With the neonate prone, place the palm of your hand supporting the chest. Raise the infant off the examining surface and observe the infant's independent postural change. Straightening of the back with slight hyperextension of the head = 4.

The sum total of these observations will yield the score for neuromuscular maturity. Find the sum total of the physical maturity scale and the neuromuscular maturity scale. Using Table 4–5, compare the score with the maturity rating scale to determine the neonate's estimated GA. This score is accurate within 2 weeks of the neonate's actual GA. After 5 days of life, the scoring becomes less accurate owing to neurologic and tissue maturation.

Appropriateness of Size for Gestational Age

Once the GA has been determined, the examiner can assess the neonate's size in relation to the estimated gestational age (EGA). In their research, Dr. Lula Lubchenco and co-workers (1963; 1966) developed standardized tools for assessing weight, length, and head circumference related to GA in order to determine whether the neonate is appropriate for gestational age (AGA), small for gestational age (SGA), or large for gestational age (LGA). According to Figure 4–3, the AGA newborn has an average gestation of

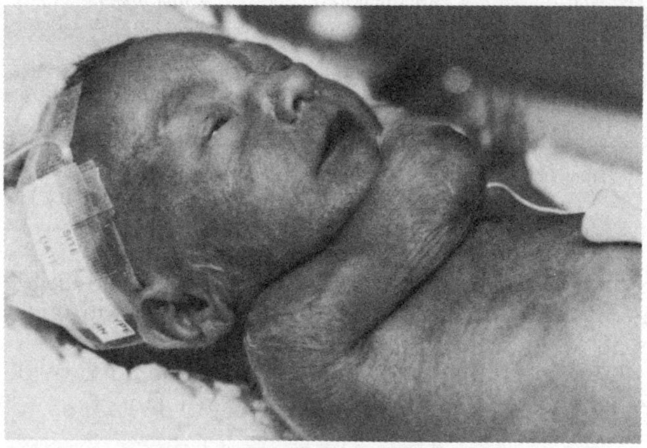

FIGURE 4-2. Scarf sign. A neonate born at 28 weeks' gestation. On assessment, elbow can be brought to midline without resistance. As the infant matures, this movement is resisted.

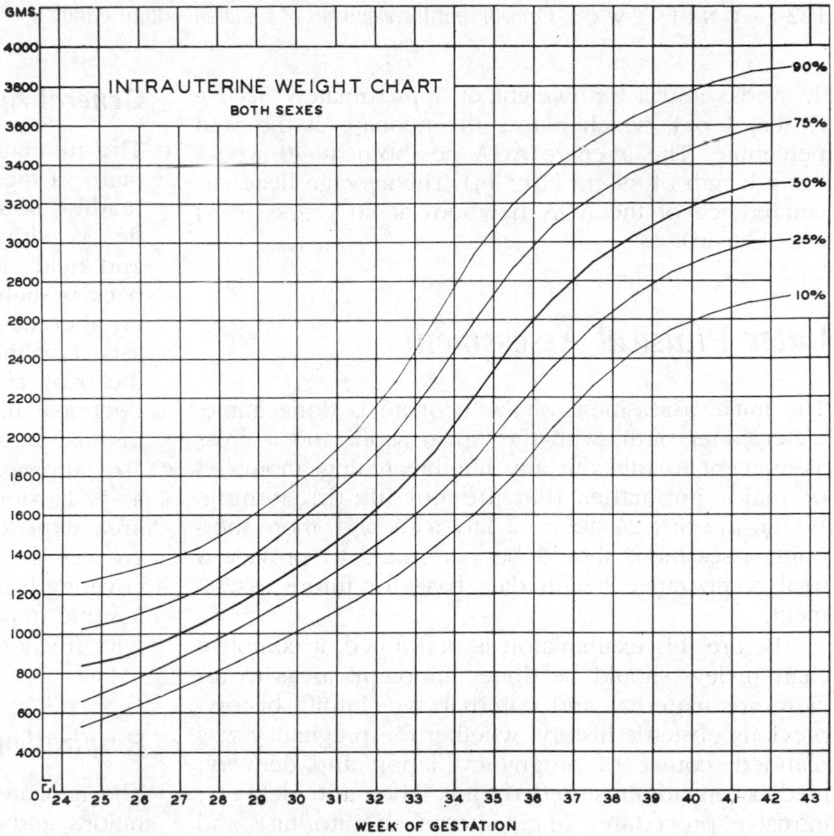

FIGURE 4 - 3. Intrauterine length, weight, and head circumference charts. (From Lubchenco, L., et al. [1963, October]. Intrauterine growth as estimated from liveborn birth-weight data at 24 to 42 weeks of gestation. Reproduced by permission of *Pediatrics,* Vol 32, p. 793, copyright 1963; and Lubchenco, L., et al. [1966, March]. Intrauterine growth in length and head circumference as estimated from live births at gestational ages from 26–42 weeks. Reproduced by permission of *Pediatrics,* Vol 37, p. 603, copyright 1966.)

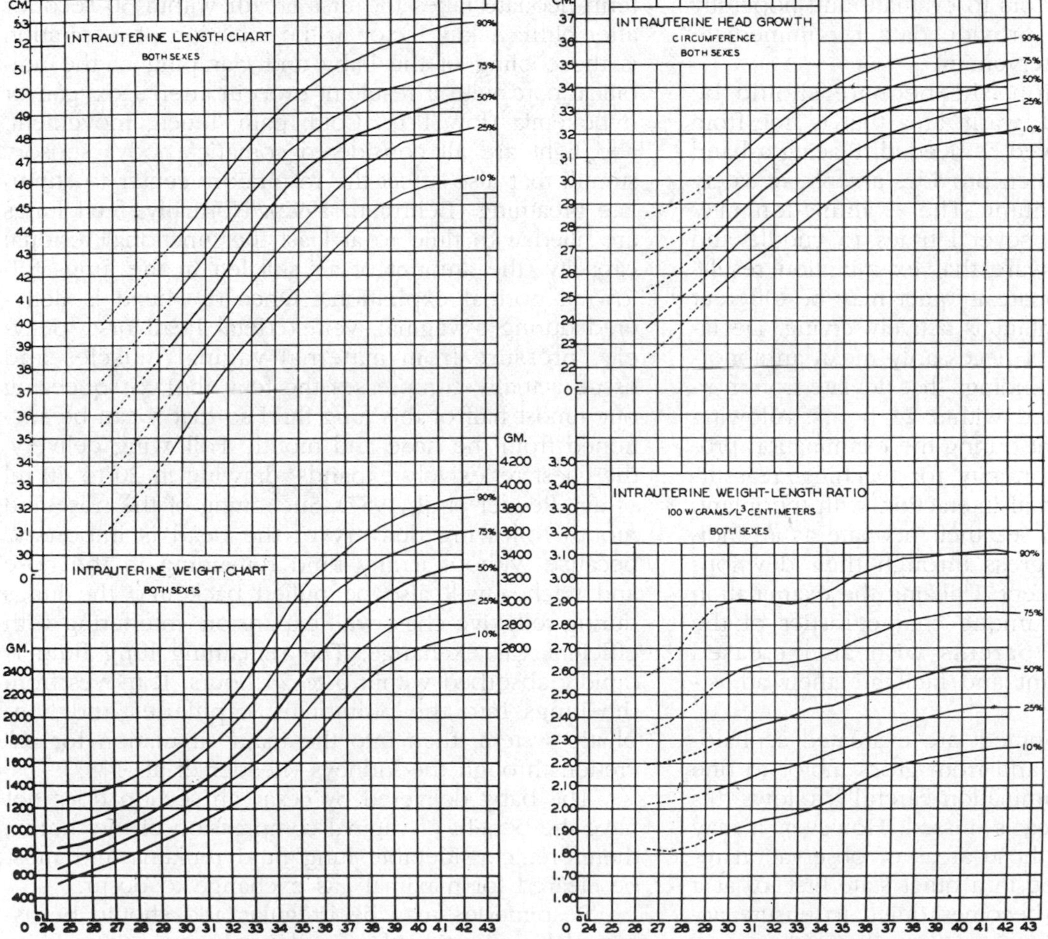

40 weeks and a birthweight of approximately 3200 g (7 lbs, 1 oz), which places the neonate at the 50th percentile. The average AGA newborn at 40 weeks has a length of 49 cm (19.3 in). The average head circumference of the AGA newborn at 40 weeks is 34 cm (13.5 in).

Later Physical Assessment

The initial assessment of the neonate is done immediately after birth, with the Apgar score and a gross assessment to rule out any life-threatening anomalies or major anomalies that are not life-threatening. Within the first 24 hours of life, a second, more thorough assessment should be performed to provide a total comparative health data base for future assessment.

Before this examination is performed, a complete chart review should be done. Important areas to review are maternal and paternal age; family history; previous obstetric history; whether the pregnancy was planned; course of pregnancy, labor, and delivery; medication administered during labor and delivery; intrusive procedures (e.g., internal monitoring); and Apgar scores with appropriate resuscitative measures. Identification of any deviations from normal gives the examiner specific indicators to evaluate and hopefully rule out anomalies or provide data for immediate medical and nursing intervention.

For the examination, the neonate should be placed in a well-lighted, warm area that is free from drafts. Clothing is removed as needed. Placing a hand on the newborn's abdomen provides a sense of safety and security for the infant. The examination may need to be interrupted several times to cuddle and soothe the baby. Be aware that examination results obtained when the neonate is quiet may be different from those when the infant is actively crying. Deviations from normal do not necessarily mean an abnormality exists; therefore, findings that deviate from normal should be reassessed within 24 hours. Allowing the parents to be present during the examination provides an excellent opportunity for teaching, reassuring, and assessing parental interaction with the infant. Parents must be able to see their neonate as an individual in order to progress through their developmental stages of adjustment. Utilizing the examination time to point out the unique characteristics of the neonate will provide parents with an increased awareness of their infant and facilitate their adjustment to their new role.

Growth and development are evaluated cephalocaudally (head to foot) and from gross motor to fine motor. A systematic examination carefully follows this sequence so that no area is missed. However, it may be necessary to assess those areas of observation requiring that the infant be in a quiet state first, or at a point when he or she becomes quiet, to ensure accurate findings.

General Appearance

The neonate assumes a posture similar to that in utero. If the fetus was in a vertex position, the infant readily assumes a posture of flexion. The head is flexed with the chin on the chest, arms are flexed and held close to the chest with hands fisted, the back is slightly bent, the knees are flexed with thighs on abdomen and feet are dorsiflexed on the anterior aspect of the leg. This is the position of comfort for the baby and is indicative of normal muscle tone. A decrease in muscle tone may be associated with trauma, sedation, or preterm gestation. The neonate's size appropriateness for GA is as outlined in Table 4–5. Flexion decreases the amount of body surface area exposed to the environment and thereby decreases the rate of heat loss. Swaddling loosely or covering lightly with a blanket will allow the infant to assume a position of flexion, yet will not interfere with freedom of movement.

Respirations

The neonate must rapidly initiate and maintain inspirations and expirations of sufficient depth and regularity to replace the terminated placental source of oxygen and carbon dioxide exchange. The normal-term neonate takes the first breath within 30 seconds after birth. A key factor in the initiation of respiration is the cooling of the baby and clamping of the umbilical cord with a resultant drop in arterial oxygen or hypoxemia (low Po_2). Cold, pain, touch, movement, and light are all considered somatic (body) sensory stimuli that also affect the respiratory center to stimulate breathing (Behrman, 1992). Normally, fetal lungs are filled with fluid to at least the functional residual capacity (the amount of air still left in the lungs following normal expiration). Once the head is delivered during a vaginal, vertex (fetal head first) delivery, pressure from maternal vaginal muscles and tissue actually compresses the fetal thorax, squeezing out almost half of this lung fluid so that it can be suctioned from the nose and mouth. Following delivery, the chest reflexively expands, drawing in 20 to 40 ml of air (Reeder et al, 1987). Suctioning of the nose and mouth following delivery of the head is important, because without it any fluid remaining in the nose and trachea will also be pulled back into the lungs during reflexive chest wall expansion, interfering with efficient gas exchange. The remaining lung fluid is rapidly absorbed within 6 to 24 hours. It moves from the lungs into the pulmonary capillaries and lymphatic system, then into the main circulation for excretion through the kidneys (Reeder et al, 1987).

The baby delivered by cesarean section does not have the benefit of vaginal compression of the thorax; therefore, considerable lung fluid remains and must be cleared for maximal gas exchange to occur.

Respirations may be irregular and should be assessed by counting the number of inspirations for a full minute. The normal respiratory rate following successful adaptation to extrauterine life is 40 to 60 breaths per minute. After the first 24 hours, the rate drops to 30 to 50 breaths per minute (Behrman, 1992).

Circulatory Changes

Fetal circulation and the changes that occur after birth are shown in detail in Chapter 33.

The peripheral circulation may be somewhat sluggish, accounting for transient cyanosis of the hands and feet *(acrocyanosis)* and around the mouth *(circumoral cyanosis)*.

At the time of birth, if the cord is allowed to cease pulsating before being clamped and cut, the baby will receive an additional 50 to 100 ml of blood from the placenta. The appropriate time to cut the cord is debatable. Some authorities think that the neonate can benefit from the additional volume of iron-rich oxygenated blood. Others believe that the additional volume is an overload for the infant's system.

Assessment of the heart is done by auscultating the apical pulse. The first and second heart sounds should be clearly distinct. The rate may be rapid but should be regular, between 120 and 150 beats per minute during the quiet, alert state. During crying periods, the heart rate may increase to 190 beats per minute and, during sleep, may decrease to 70 to 90 beats per minute (Behrman, 1992). Since activity influences the heart rate, the baby should be quiet for an accurate assessment.

Skin Assessment

The skin of the neonate provides an index of growth. Well-nourished neonates have well-defined layers of subcutaneous fat over their bodies, which provide thermoregulation and a barrier against infection. Lack of subcutaneous fat may indicate prematurity or malnutrition. The skin should be observed closely for breaks as this may be a portal of entry for bacteria.

Skin Color. Immediately after birth the term neonate's skin is erythematous (beefy red), then fades to its normal color within a few hours. Acrocyanosis is a normal transient phenomenon caused by vasomotor instability, capillary stasis, and high hemoglobin. Persistent generalized cyanosis indicates underlying distress.

Cyanosis is assessed in the white neonate by looking at the skin and by inspection of the mucous membranes of the mouth, eyes, and nailbeds of the hands and feet. In assessment of the infant with darker skin color, the mucous membranes and nailbeds are the most reliable indicators of cyanosis.

Harlequin Color Change. When the neonate is placed in a side-lying position, the side next to the mattress will turn pink while the upper side remains pale. This is known as "harlequin color change" and has no known significance. However, color distribution should remain even, in supine or prone position.

Telangiectatic Nevi (Stork Bites). These are common on the upper eyelids, back of the neck, and occiput. They are flat, localized, reddened areas created by capillary dilatation and should disappear during the first year of life.

Strawberry Hemangiomas. These may be present at birth or appear up to 2 weeks following birth. They resemble strawberry clusters and consist of dilated capillaries in the dermal and subdermal layers (Fig. 4–4). They are elevated and may continue to grow up to 1 year of age. Absorption and shrinkage takes place slowly and usually requires 7 to 10 years for completion. Although hemangiomas are unsightly and may be disturbing to parents, they are best left untreated. However, large or multiple hemangiomas may signal the presence of internal involvement. These children should be referred for evaluation of this possibility.

Mongolian Spots. Bluish-gray or purple patches of pigmentation are sometimes seen across the sacrum or buttocks (Fig. 4–5). Known as "mongolian spots," the pigmentation begins at birth in the basal layer of the epidermis and is prevalent among children of Asian, southern European, and African descent. These spots disappear by school age without treatment.

Port-Wine Stain. This is reddish discoloration of the skin of the face or neck. This vascular birthmark usually involves serious deformity because of the large skin area that is typically involved.

Lanugo. These are fine, downy hairs that cover the neonate's body. They are often concentrated over

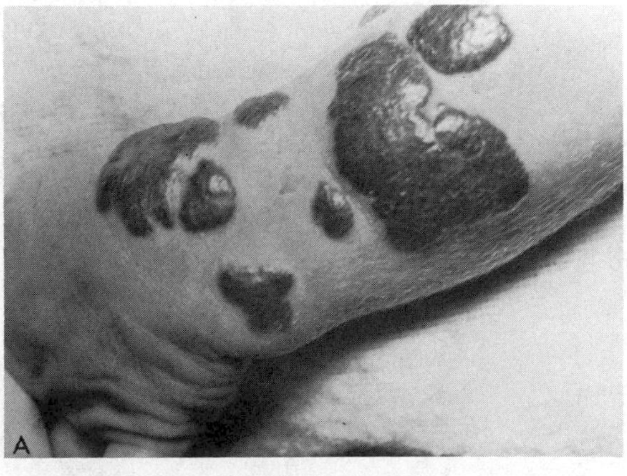

FIGURE 4-4. Strawberry hemangioma. (Courtesy of Mary Lou Moore.)

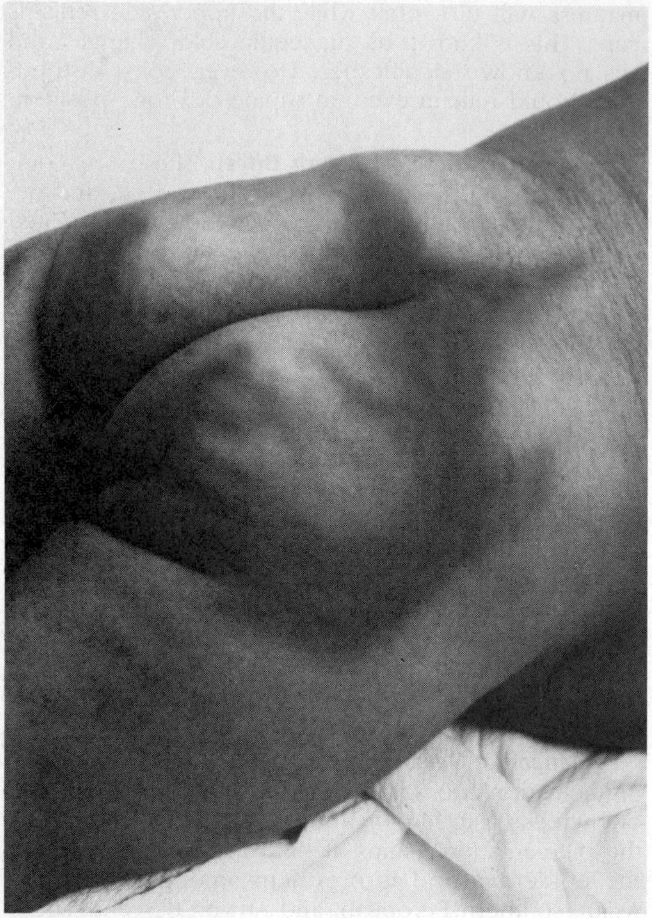

FIGURE 4-5. Mongolian spots. (Courtesy of Mead Johnson and Company, Nutritional Division.)

the shoulders and back. These hairs disappear without treatment.

Milia. The small, shiny, whitish nodules beneath the skin, found on the nose and chin, are called "milia." They are caused by retention of sebaceous gland secretions. They disappear spontaneously.

Skin Turgor. Turgor is related to tissue hydration and is present in the normal neonate. Transient edema may also be present around the eyes and dorsal aspects of the extremities due to birth trauma. Lack of skin turgor may indicate malnutrition in utero or metabolic disorders. To assess turgor, grasp the skin with thumb and forefinger and gently turn. The skin should feel elastic and return to a smooth surface when released.

Head and Neck Assessment

The head of the neonate is proportionately large (approximately one fourth the total length of the newborn infant). The forehead is prominent and the chin recedes.

Head circumference is measured by placing the tape above the eyebrows and around the most prominent aspect of the occiput. Measurement may need to be repeated several times for accuracy. Accurate assessment of circumference provides a baseline for future assessment of cephalic development.

Molding. With a vaginal, vertex delivery, the neonate's head molds to fit the birth canal more easily by gradual overlapping of the calvarium bones and narrowing or overriding of the sutures. Molding is usually not present following a cesarean birth. Parents may be anxious about the presence of molding; they need reassurance that it will disappear in a few days.

Fontanels and Suture Lines. The fontanels are soft membranous spaces where the skull bones join (Fig. 4–6). The anterior fontanel (soft spot) is diamond-shaped and lies between the sagittal and the coronal sutures. It is approximately 2 to 3 cm wide and 3 to 4 cm long. It closes at 12 to 18 months of age. The posterior fontanel is triangular and lies between the sagittal and the lambdoidal sutures. It is approximately 1 cm long and closes at about 2 months. The

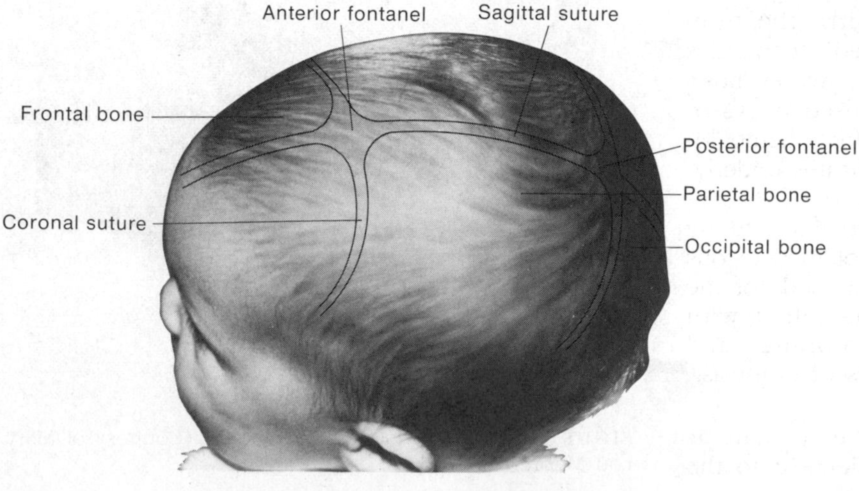

FIGURE 4-6. Location of the anterior and posterior fontanels.

nurse should feel and measure the fontanels. Bulging fontanels are indicative of increased intracranial pressure and depressed or sunken fontanels of dehydration. Parents are sometimes afraid to touch the "soft spot" for fear of causing brain damage. Actually it is as tough as canvas and needs the same amount of stimulation as the rest of the scalp. The suture lines denote the separation of the cranial bones and are either closely approximated or overriding. They should never appear or feel separated; this is indicative of increased intracranial pressure.

Caput Succedaneum. This is the result of diffuse edema (margins of swelling are indistinct) of the soft tissues of the scalp that may extend across suture lines (Fig. 4–7). It is caused by continuous pressure on the scalp during labor and is most pronounced following prolonged labor. It is gradually absorbed and disappears within a few days. Ecchymotic coloration (black and blue bruises) may be present; this may cause feelings of guilt and anxiety in parents. Nursing intervention should be directed toward helping parents resolve these feelings.

Cephalhematoma. In this condition, a collection of blood from ruptured blood vessels forms between the skull bone and the periosteum because of trauma to the head during the birth process (Fig. 4–8). It does not cross suture lines because it is confined to one bone. Obvious swelling develops within 24 to 48 hours after birth. The area may be ecchymotic owing to the presence of coagulated blood. Absorption of a cephalhematoma may take 2 to 3 weeks or longer. As with caput succedaneum, parents may experience guilt. The nurse should help absolve them of this feeling.

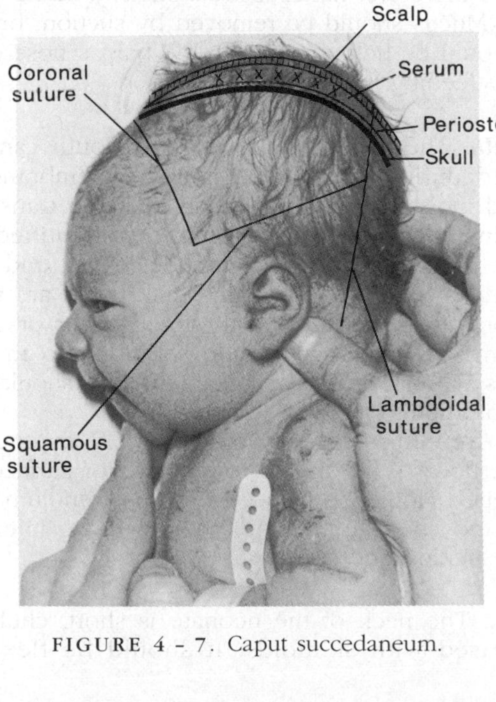

FIGURE 4-7. Caput succedaneum.

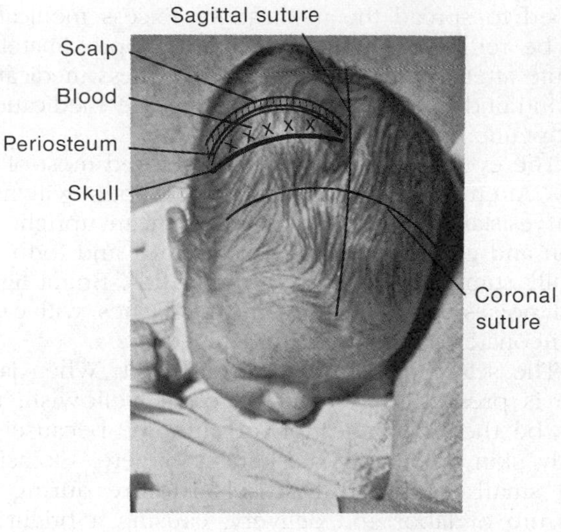

FIGURE 4-8. Cephalhematoma.

Scalp. The nurse should palpate and inspect the scalp for lesions, bleeding, or coarse, brittle hair. If an internal monitor was used during labor, the neonate will have a small puncture wound in the occipital area of the scalp. This area should be kept clean and dry and inspected for signs of infection.

Face. The face should be inspected for symmetry of parts and symmetry between the left and the right sides. Some asymmetry may be due to position—that is, resuming a position that was maintained in utero. This will disappear within a few weeks or months. Facial asymmetry may indicate facial nerve palsy due to birth trauma.

Eyes. The eyes should appear clear without redness or purulent discharge. Occasionally, the eyelids are puffy with a purulent discharge during the first 24 hours. This is a transient chemical conjunctivitis due to silver nitrate ($AgNO_3$) drops administered to prevent ophthalmia neonatorum (gonorrheal conjunctivitis). Topical 1 per cent silver nitrate, 0.5 per cent erythromycin, and 1 per cent tetracycline are all considered to be effective as prophylaxis of ocular gonorrheal infection in neonates. Silver nitrate is considered to be the most effective agent in the treatment of penicillinase-producing *Neisseria gonorrhoeae* (PPNG). Neonatal chlamydial ophthalmia, caused by *Chlamydia trachomatis,* although not as severe as gonococcal ophthalmia, equals or surpasses the frequency of gonococcal ophthalmia. Currently no topical regimen has demonstrated effectiveness in the prevention of chlamydial ophthalmia (American Academy of Pediatrics [AAP], 1991).

Before the nurse administers the prophylaxis medication, the neonate's eyes are wiped clean. Two drops of 1 per cent silver nitrate solution or a 1- to 2-cm strip of 0.5 per cent erythromycin, or 1 per cent tetracycline ointment is instilled in each of the lower conjunctival sacs. The neonate's eyelids are gently rubbed to spread the medication. Excess medication can be removed with sterile cotton approximately 1 minute after instillation. Flushing of excess medication is contraindicated, as it may reduce the medication's therapeutic effectiveness.

The eyelids of the neonate are closed most of the time. Attempts to force the eyelids open will meet with resistance. Holding the infant in an upright position and gently rocking the head back and forth will usually stimulate opening of the eyelids. Bright lights, loud noises, and touching the eyelashes will cause the neonate to promptly close the eyes.

The sclera has a slightly bluish tint. When jaundice is present, the sclera becomes yellowish; this may be the first indication of jaundice because the ruddy skin color may mask it elsewhere. Occasionally, small conjunctival vessels rupture during the pressure of labor and delivery, causing a bright-red streak near the iris. This is a subconjunctival hemorrhage and will disappear spontaneously within 2 to 3 weeks.

The iris is usually dark or grayish-blue in most neonates. Final eye color is present by 6 to 12 months of age.

Lacrimal gland ducts are immature at birth. Parents should be told not to expect tears with crying until 1 to 3 months of age.

Dacryostenosis is a congenital lacrimal stenosis that creates an obstruction of the lacrimal duct and is often accompanied by dacryocystitis. This condition is relatively common in infancy. It is suspected in infants with purulent discharge (dacryocystitis) but without any conjunctival injection or irritation. It is also suspected in infants who have prompt recurrence of purulent discharge after cessation of ophthalmic antibiotics. If pressure over the lacrimal sac produces an outpouring of mucopurulent material, diagnosis is confirmed. Excessive lacrimation (tearing) during the second month of life is a sign that suggests dacryostenosis that may be readily noticed by the nurse during infant examinations.

Nonsurgical correction involves forcing the fluid collected in the affected lacrimal sac through the obstructed duct by placing the tip of one thumb over the sac at the medial angle of the eye and slowly, steadily rolling the thumb toward the duct opening, thereby increasing pressure on the stenosis to gradually open it (Fig. 4–9). This is done four times daily for a month. The parents should be instructed in the procedure and should satisfactorily demonstrate its use. If this procedure does not open the duct within a month, an ophthalmologist can open the duct by probing the lacrimal tract. An ophthalmic antibiotic may be prescribed to control infection until the obstruction is cleared.

The pupils should be observed for any whiteness or opacities that indicate congenital cataracts. This is particularly important if the mother had rubella during pregnancy.

Incoordinate eye movements, "setting sun" eyes, and the doll's eye phenomenon are transient reflections of neuromuscular immaturity. They usually disappear after 10 days. However, setting sun eyes may also be indicative of hydrocephaly.

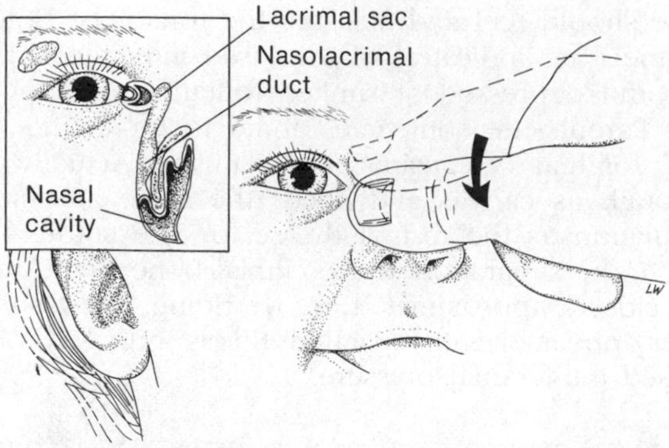

FIGURE 4-9. Massage of the lacrimal drainage tract to force fluid in the lacrimal sac through the obstructed drainage tract. The tip of the thumb is placed above the sac at the medial angle of the eye. Slowly and steadily, the thumb is rolled downward.

Ears. Cartilage formation is present in the ears, although not complete. This allows the pinna to bend easily, but it should rebound. It is important to assess the position of the ears. The top of the external ear should be slightly above the level of the eyes. Low-set ears are seen in infants with chromosomal abnormalities; these abnormalities include other physical defects and mental retardation. Low-set ears may also be associated with renal disorders.

Nose. The neonate's nose may appear large or slightly flattened. This discrepancy will disappear as the face grows. Remember that neonates are nose breathers; therefore, nasal obstructions should be prevented. (Mucus should be removed by suction; breast tissue should be held away from the baby's nose during breastfeeding.)

Mouth. The inside of the infant's mouth can be visualized during crying. The mucous membrane is pink and moist. Thrush, a candida infection transmitted during the birth process, may be identified as white or gray patches on the tongue, gums, and entire buccal mucosa. Occasionally, milk curds are mistaken for thrush. Irrigating with sterile water or gently wiping with a tongue blade should help in the diagnosis. Thrush is highly contagious and should be treated promptly (see also Chapter 39).

The frenulum linguae (mucous fold extending from the floor of the mouth to the interior surface of the tongue) should be inspected. If the frenulum linguae is too short (tongue-tie) there will be interference in sucking and speech.

Neck. The neck of the neonate is short, chubby, and creased with skinfolds. It should be flexible enough to rotate from side to side and from flexion to extension. The nurse should closely examine the folds by raising the shoulders and hyperextending the neck. Excessive folds (webbing) may be associated with pathologic conditions.

Although the neck is not strong enough to support the head, some degree of head control should be evident. Hyperextension (opisthotonus) may be associated with neurologic disease. Decreased muscle tone (hypotonia) is manifested by inability to lift the head. This may be indicative of prematurity, pathology, or hypoxia.

Torso and Extremities

Chest. The overall appearance of the chest should be symmetric. Breast engorgement may occur in both boys and girls owing to circulating maternal hormones. Occasionally, a thin, watery fluid may be secreted from the nipples. Engorgement and fluid will disappear within 2 weeks. Fluid should not be expressed from the breasts.

Abdomen. The abdomen of the neonate is slightly protuberant. The nurse should observe for signs of distention such as tight skin that makes subcutaneous vessels visible.

The umbilical stump is bluish, moist, and shiny. It should contain two arteries and one vein. An umbilical cord containing only one artery may be associated with congenital anomalies. The cord stump begins to dry, darken, and slough off by the sixth to tenth day.

The cord stump should be inspected for bleeding and signs of infection. Swabbing the cord stump with alcohol facilitates the drying process. Bellybands should not be used, since they interfere with drying and provide a dark, warm, moist environment conducive to bacterial growth.

Anogenital Area. The anus should be inspected for patency. An imperforate (closed) anus interferes with the passage of stools. The first stool should be passed within 24 hours. This condition may also be diagnosed when it is impossible to insert a rectal thermometer.

The female genitals consist of the *labia majora,* the *labia minora,* the *clitoris,* and the *vaginal opening*. The labia majora covers the labia minora. The hymenal tag is a fleshy pink tag protruding from the base of the vagina. It is present in nearly all female neonates, but gradually atrophies and disappears by the end of the fourth week. The labia may be engorged owing to the influence of circulating maternal hormones. Hormones are also responsible for a milky vaginal discharge tinged with mucus or blood, or both. Both the edema and the discharge should disappear as soon as the hormones have cleared from the neonate's system. The urinary meatus is difficult to visualize; therefore, the number of voidings should be observed and recorded.

In male neonates, the scrotum is edematous and covered with rugae. Both testes can be palpated in the sac. Occasionally, one or both testicles may recede temporarily into the body cavity through the inguinal ring when the baby is exposed to cold. *Cryptorchidism* is a condition in which one or both testes have not descended. This condition requires referral to determine the cause and treatment.

The *glans penis* (head of the penis) is covered by the *prepuce* (foreskin). The foreskin is not retractable and cannot be displaced until 4 to 6 months of age. The foreskin should never be forcefully retracted, not even for cleansing purposes. The prepuce should be examined to rule out stenosis. The external *urinary meatus* (a small slit) is located near the tip of the glans penis and should be easily visualized. Occasionally, the meatal opening is located on the ventral portion of the glans penis *(hypospadias)* or dorsal portion *(epispadias)*.

Circumcision (surgical removal of the prepuce) continues to be a common practice. For Jews, circumcision is a religious practice and takes place in a ceremony on the male infant's eighth day of life. The medical indications for routine circumcision are nonexistent (AAP, 1989b). Only rarely is it required to correct a defect, as when the foreskin is so constricted that it interferes with voiding or circulation *(phimosis)*. Circumcision is contraindicated in the presence of hypospadias because the foreskin will be used during surgical reconstruction of the meatal opening at a later time (Behrman, 1992).

Extremities. The arms and legs of the neonate appear short. They should be symmetric in shape and movement. The nurse should observe the position (flexion) assumed at rest and inspect fingers and toes for extra digits, clubbing of fingers, fusion, or webbing. The hands are examined for palmar creases. A simian crease (single line crease across the palm) is associated with Down syndrome. The feet are inspected for sole creases and clubbing.

Hip dislocation is determined by placing the neonate in a supine position and testing for Ortolani sign. Both legs are flexed and abducted (away from the body) to nearly touch the examining surface. A click may be felt or heard if a dislocation is present. With the infant in a prone position, the nurse should note the creases of the buttocks and thighs. They should be symmetric and the legs should be the same length. Movement should be noted, as fine tremors of the extremities may indicate hypoglycemia.

Back. The back is examined and palpated for spinal defects and curvature. Tufts of hair may indicate *spina bifida*. The coccygeal area (base of the spine) should be examined for pilonidal dimples or cysts.

ETHICAL ISSUES

Circumcision

by Margaret M. Mahon, PhD, RNC

Evan is a 1-day-old male, the second child and first son born to Ms. Casey. Prior to his birth, no definite plans had been made about whether or not Evan would be circumcised. When the nurse came into Ms. Casey's room to do neonatal teaching, Ms. Casey asked, "Do you think I should have my son circumcised? What would you do if you had a son?"

Routine circumcision continues to be extremely common in the United States, though it is the exception rather than the rule in most other countries. In the United States, 60 to 90 per cent of newborn males are circumcised. Of these, about 20 per cent are done for religious reasons. In 1971 and again in 1975, the AAP made public recommendations against routine neonatal circumcision; there were no medical indications for the procedure. In 1978, the American College of Obstetrics issued a similar statement (Brown & Brown, 1987). In 1989, the AAP revised its earlier position when it issued a paper that recognized some medical benefits to neonatal circumcision.

Two areas of information contribute to the answer that the nurse might give in the above scenario: health care information and personal preference. The circumcision decision draws more on preferences of the parent(s) than many other health care decisions, which often rely more heavily on the health care information.

The primary medical indication for neonatal circumcision is the prevention of urinary tract infection (UTI), which does occur more commonly in boys who have not been circumcised; however, other factors must be considered. Chessare (1992) constructed a decision tree that used the possibility of complication at each level of the circumcision/no circumcision decision. For example, either Evan will be circumcised or he will not be circumcised. There are knowns and unknowns with either decision. If Evan is not circumcised, the likelihood of UTI is about 4.1 per cent; if Evan is circumcised, that risk drops to about 0.2 per cent. Therefore, the risk of UTI is greater without circumcision. There are other factors that must also be considered. No medical procedure is without risk, and the risk of complications from circumcision was set at 21.8 per cent, though the vast majority of these complications would be minor. Another factor of circumcision is that it is painful, and most practitioners use no analgesia when performing the procedure. If Evan were circumcised, he would definitely experience pain and might experience complications. If Evan were not circumcised, he would not experience the pain or complications of surgery but could be one out of approximately 2000 males who experience urinary tract complications. Chessare completed the decision tree, and concluded that the expected benefits were higher for no circumcision than for circumcision.

The health care decision about circumcision is made in the context of a personal and social structure. Parents deciding about circumcision most often decide to circumcise based on whether the father is circumcised or what they believe people will think. Parents often say something like, "I don't want him to be different from other boys in the locker room."

Is the fear of how others will react the valid basis for a decision about whether to operate? What weight should the social concerns be given relative to the weight of the health care information? If the health care facts indicate no circumcision is a healthier option than circumcision, should the options of circumcision be given? Is circumcision similar to other cosmetic surgeries? If this is the case, should the decision be postponed until the child is old enough to make the decision for himself?

Cost-benefit ratios are often used in deciding whether to undergo a certain procedure. In doing such an analysis, Ganiats and associates (1991) concluded that the fiscal and health advantages and disadvantages of routine neonatal circumcision cancel each other. They recommend that, in the absence of conclusive cost-benefit information, social factors would be the primary considerations when deciding about neonatal circumcision. Currently, most third party payers pay for circumcision. If parents had to pay for the procedure themselves, what would likely happen to the prevalence of circumcision? Is it ever acceptable to recommend a painful procedure over a nonpainful procedure? Under what circumstances? How does this fit with "the best interest of the child" standard?

It is likely that information about circumcision and the possible complications of each option will continue to accrue. It is only by keeping abreast of this information that the nurse can continue to answer questions posed by parents and others.

REFERENCES

American Academy of Pediatrics, Committee on Fetus and Newborn. (1971). *Hospital care of the newborn infant* (5th ed., p. 110). Evanston, IL: Author.

American Academy of Pediatrics, Committee on Fetus and Newborn. (1975). Report on fetus and newborn. Report of the ad hoc task force on circumcision. *Pediatrics, 56,* 610–611.

American Academy of Pediatrics, Task Force on Circumcision. (1989). Report of the task force on circumcision. Newborn circumcision has potential medical benefits and advantages as well as disadvantages and risks. *AAP News, 5,* 7–8.

Brown, M. S., & Brown, C. A. (1987). Circumcision decision: Prominence of social concerns. *Pediatrics, 80,* 215–219.

Chessare, J. B. (1992, February). Circumcision: Is urinary tract infection really the pivotal issue? *Clinical Pediatrics,* 100–104.

Ganiats, T. G., Humphrey, J. B. C., Taras, H. L., & Kaplan, R. M. (1991). Routine neonatal circumcision: A cost-utility analysis. *Medical Decision Making, 11,* 282–293.

Lund, M. M. (1990). Perspective on newborn male circumcision. *Neonatal Network, 9*(3), 3–12.

Spinelli, T. (1988). The circumcision decision: A plea for informed consent. *Henry Ford Hospital Medical Journal, 36,* 209–211.

Neurologic and Sensory Examination

Reflexes

Reflex responses provide important data on the status of neurologic functioning. Abnormal signs that are present in the first days or weeks of life may disappear and be followed by abnormal findings months or years later. Therefore, every physical examination should include assessment of reflexes. Since this may be a tedious, tiring experience for the neonate, the total examination may have to be performed in stages. Also remember that neonatal central nervous system (CNS) function may be decreased by narcotics administered to the mother during labor.

Rooting Reflex. Lightly stroking the cheek at the side of the mouth will stimulate the newborn infant to turn the head in that direction in order to find food. The rooting reflex disappears at 9 to 12 weeks, when it is no longer needed. If the mother grasps both cheeks in an effort to turn the neonate's head in the direction of breast or bottle, she creates confusion with this double stimulus. Absence, weakness, or asymmetry of responses may indicate CNS depression or dysfunction.

Sucking Reflex. The sucking reflex is stimulated by touching the baby's lips or placing an object in the mouth. Sucking should be rhythmic and strong enough to obtain nourishment from breast or bottle. If the sucking reflex is unstimulated, it will disappear rapidly.

Swallowing Reflex. The swallowing reflex is stimulated by food on the posterior portion of the tongue. Swallowing is spontaneous, but the neonate may need a little time to coordinate sucking and swallowing effectively. Gag, cough, and sneeze reflexes are protective methods of maintaining a clear airway. These are particularly evident during early feedings when the baby has to handle mucus in addition to nursing.

Grasp Reflexes: Palmar and Plantar. Exerting pressure on the palmar surface of the hand will stimulate curling or grasping of the fingers (Fig. 4–10). The grasp is so strong that the neonate can be raised momentarily by the examiner's finger. This reflex disappears at 6 weeks to 3 months of age.

Placing an object on the plantar surface (sole) of the foot will stimulate curling or grasping of the toes (Fig. 4–11). This reflex disappears at about 8 to 9 months of age.

Traction Response. This response is elicited by placing the neonate in a supine position and slowly pulling her or him to a sitting position by holding the wrists. Response should be extension of the arms with some degree of head control.

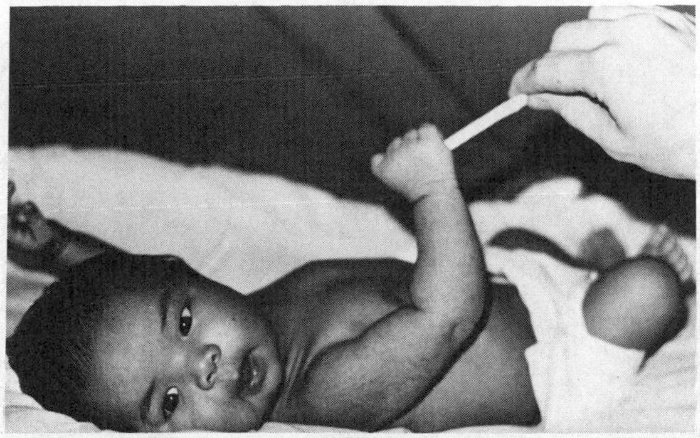

FIGURE 4-10. Palmar grasp reflex.

Moro Reflex (Startle Response). *The Moro reflex is the single most significant response denoting CNS status.* This response can be elicited by startling the baby with a loud noise or by bumping the crib. The nurse can place the neonate in a supine position, grasp both arms, allow the head to remain on the examination surface, and raise the shoulders by gentle traction on the arms; then release arms, allowing shoulders to drop to the surface, and observe the response. A normal response includes two phases: (1) quick flexion at elbows is followed by abduction (away from the body) of the upper limbs at the shoulders, extension of the forearms at the elbows and extension of the fingers and legs; (2) subsequent adduction (toward the body) of the arms at the shoulders and the legs against the abdomen (Fig. 4–12). Observe the completeness and symmetry of the response and the degree of difficulty in eliciting it.

The Moro reflex is strong during the first 8 weeks of life and fades by the end of the second or third month.

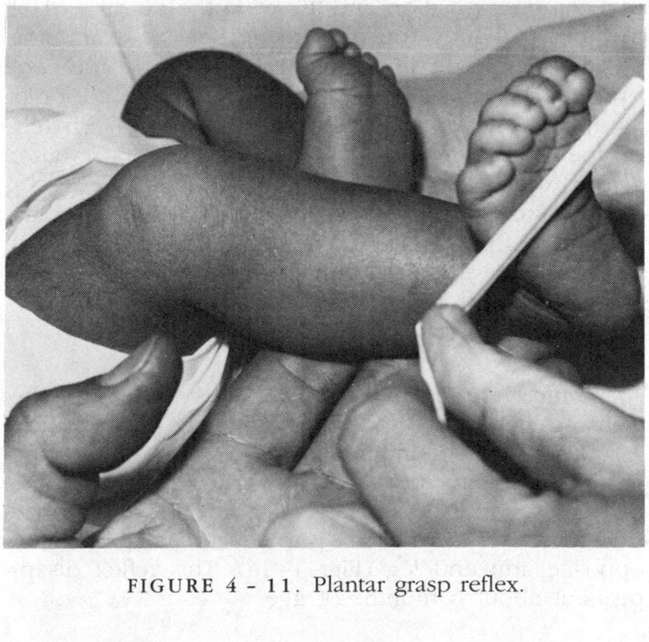

FIGURE 4-11. Plantar grasp reflex.

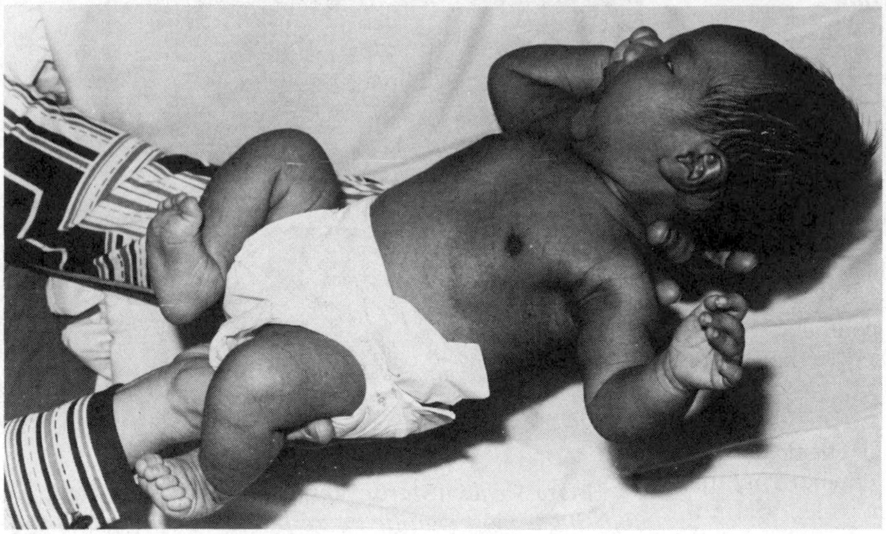

FIGURE 4-12. Moro reflex (startle response).

Yawn, Stretch, and Hiccough Reflexes. These reflexes are demonstrated spontaneously by the neonate and have been related to increasing oxygen intake and elimination of gas. Parents generally express concern and want to know how to intervene when the baby develops hiccoughs. The nurse can reassure them that this hiccoughing is normal. However, increased yawning, sneezing, and hiccoughing are frequently observed in infants of heroin-addicted mothers as they experience withdrawal syndrome.

Trunk Incurvation Reflex. With the neonate in a prone position, touching along one side of the vertebral column will elicit curvature of the spine toward the stimulated side. This is a good test of spinal cord integrity.

Placing and Stepping Reflexes. Holding the infant in an upright position and allowing the dorsal part of the foot to lightly touch one edge of the examining surface will result in spontaneous lifting of the foot by flexion of the knees and hips. The neonate looks as though she or he is *placing* each foot alternately on the examining surface. This reflex disappears after 4 to 6 weeks.

The stepping reflex is stimulated with the neonate in an upright position. When the soles of the feet touch a hard surface, the infant will take a few quick alternating steps (Fig. 4–13). The stepping reflex disappears by 3 months.

Tonic Neck Reflex (TNR). TNR is known as the "fencing position" because it simulates the position assumed by someone preparing to fence. Place the baby in a supine position and turn the head to one side. Observe extension of the arm and leg on the side to which the head is turned and flexion of the opposite arm and leg (Fig. 4–14). This reflex disappears at about 6 months of age.

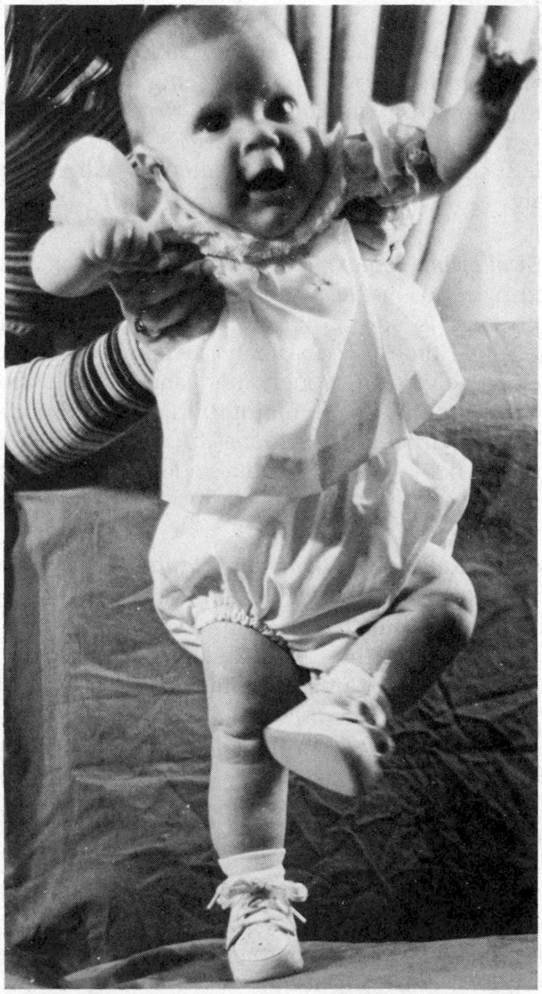

FIGURE 4-13. Stepping reflex (dancing).

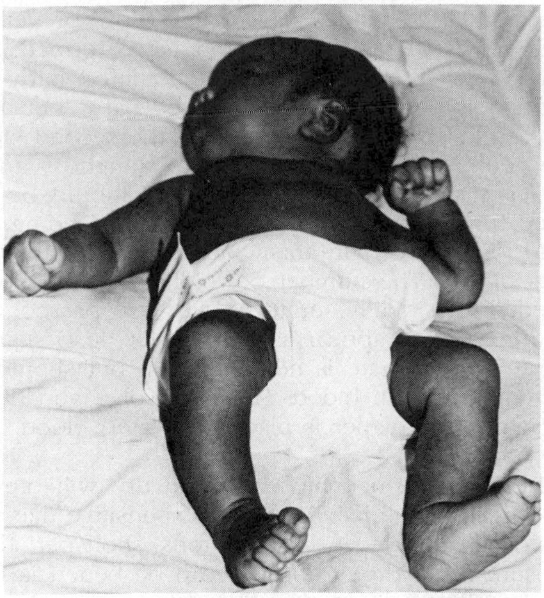

FIGURE 4 - 14. Tonic neck reflex (fencing position).

Babinski Reflex. The reflex is stimulated by stroking the sole of the foot from heel to toe. The response is dorsiflexion of the big toe and fanning or spreading of the other toes (Fig. 4–15). The Babinski reflex is present until 3 months of age but may persist until the child walks, at which time an adult response of flexion is elicited.

There are many other reflexes to include in a thorough neurologic examination; however, the ones discussed here are of greatest importance in performing a nursing assessment of the CNS of the neonate.

Senses

Vision. Visual abilities of the infant are better developed than once thought. Neonates can *fixate* (look at the same point with both eyes) for up to 10 seconds at a time and can refixate at intervals of every 1 to 1.5 seconds (Behrman, 1992). They are able to

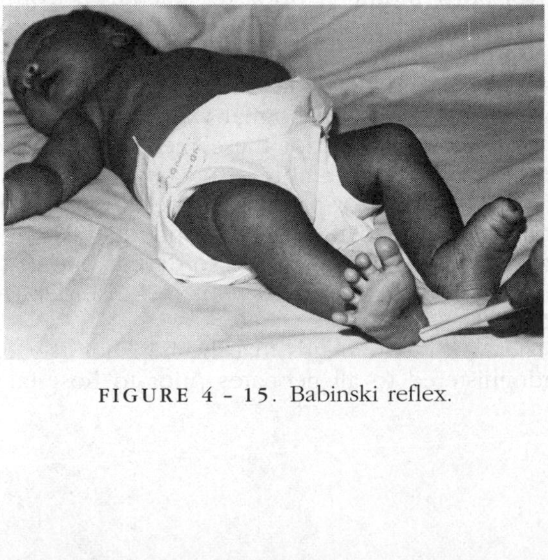

FIGURE 4 - 15. Babinski reflex.

discriminate between sizes, shapes, colors, and patterns. *Conjugation* (the ability to use both eyes together) is nearly on a par with the adult, except that newborn infants must refixate more frequently and may take longer to "find" the object after looking away. *Scanning* is defined as the ability to move across the visual field in an attempt to locate the most satisfying object. Neonates have the ability to scan and prefer areas of sharp dark-light contrast; they also show a preference for the human face over inanimate objects. Neonates, however, are unable to *accommodate* to distance (requiring flattening or thickening of the lens in response to action of the ciliary muscle). This means that during the first month of life objects are in perfect focus at only one point in space; this distance is about 8 inches, or the distance between the mother's face and her breast when she is feeding the infant. Accommodation reaches the adult level by 4 months of age.

The eyes are sensitive to light, and the neonate will blink or squint in response to light. Parents need to be informed of the baby's visual capabilities and preferences so that they can provide appropriate visual stimulation such as appropriate mobiles and changes in the infant's environment.

Hearing. Hearing is present at birth, although temporarily hindered by amniotic fluid in the middle ear. Within a few hours after birth, the fluid is absorbed and replaced by air. Behavioral manifestations of hearing include *alerting* (seems to stop and listen), eye movements, startle reaction, and crying. The neonate's ability to determine the cause and direction of sound does not develop until weeks later.

The infant will respond to various sounds in a reflexive manner (Moro, blink). An actively crying infant will respond to a soothing voice by abruptly ceasing all activity as though alerting to the sound. From 3 to 14 weeks of age, eye response to noise includes opening the eyes or squinting. Some head movement may also occur.

Taste. The neonate can differentiate between bitter and sweet tastes. Pleasurable flavors will elicit active sucking, whereas bitter or unpleasant flavors will cause tongue protrusion and active turning away.

Smell. The sense of smell is present as soon as the nose is clear of amniotic fluid and mucus, although the degree of development is unclear. Some researchers speculate that the neonate learns to differentiate his or her mother by recognizing her own particular body scent.

Touch. Tactile sensation is well developed at birth, particularly in the facial area (rooting, sucking). Sensitivity to pain and extreme temperatures seems to be present, but not distinct, at first. By the tenth day, a definite reaction to painful stimuli is observed.

Body Composition

Seventy-five per cent of body weight in the newborn infant is composed of water. The normal weight loss of up to 10 per cent of body weight after birth represents fluid loss. Parents can be assured that this weight loss is not harmful to the infant.

Fat constitutes about 12 per cent of the body weight, giving the neonate a somewhat thin appearance. The total protein is similar to that of other ages. The neonate has a high hematocrit and hemoglobin concentration, plus large stores of iron in the liver. This provides an iron concentration that is approximately double that of the adult. Calcium and phosphorus are present in low concentrations. The infant's bones are relatively flexible and poorly mineralized; this facilitates the birth process. Both fat-soluble and water-soluble vitamins are present in adequate amounts.

The supply of vitamin K (fat-soluble) is commonly less than adequate. Vitamin K deficiency may cause uncontrollable bleeding; therefore, an injection of vitamin K (AquaMEPHYTON) is routinely given shortly after birth. Bacterial synthesis in the intestinal tract leads to the production of vitamin K. However, at birth, the intestinal tract of the newborn is sterile. Breastfed babies experience more vitamin K deficiency because human milk has only one fourth as much vitamin K as cow's milk does.

The digestive tract is somewhat immature, with a scant production of saliva. "Spitting up" is common until the digestive system matures. This needs to be differentiated from vomiting, which indicates that pyloric stenosis (stricture of the pyloric sphincter between the esophagus and the stomach) or other illness may be present.

Owing to immaturity of the kidneys, production of concentrated urine is limited. Therefore, in order to excrete solutes (urea, uric acid, creatinine, minerals), a large volume of water must be excreted. Improper formula preparation, excess sweating, diarrhea, or insufficient fluid intake may cause dehydration.

Elimination

The first stools of the neonate are called "meconium." They are dark-greenish to black, sticky, and odorless. Meconium stools are present during the first 3 days of life. Then the stools change to greenish-brown, becoming greenish-yellow about the third or fourth day. This is called "transitional stool." Subsequent stool patterns are dependent on the type of food the baby receives.

Breastfed babies have bright, golden-yellow stools that are soft (mushy) and unformed but not watery. They are sometimes a light-greenish color. Their odor is sweet-smelling. Initially, a breastfed baby will have one to two stools per day, increasing to more than four per day by the second week.

Formula-fed babies have pale-yellow or yellow-white stools that are firmer and more formed. The odor is foul-smelling. Initially, a bottlefed baby has more stools per day than a breastfed baby, but these decrease to about three per day by the second week.

Green, watery stools indicate diarrhea, and a physician should be notified. Stools should be observed for blood indicative of intestinal bleeding.

Most newborn infants void during the first 12 hours of life. The number of voidings should be assessed. Occasionally, urate crystals are passed with the urine. These appear as pink (brick dust) staining on the diaper. Urate is not significant but should be differentiated from blood. Urates dissolve and disappear when the diaper is placed in water; blood does not.

Keeping the neonate clean and dry will prevent diaper rash. If the baby's skin is so sensitive that rash does occur in spite of diligent efforts, short periods of exposure to air during the day can be beneficial. Petroleum jelly applied to the clean skin can serve as a protective barrier against skin breakdown from urine and stool.

Health Maintenance and Promotion

Newborn Screening

The AAP has issued a series of fact sheets that provide information on the scope of tests available for newborn screening (AAP, 1989a). Currently, phenylketonuria (PKU) and congenital hypothyroidism (CH) are screened for in all states (for additional information on newborn screening tests refer to Chapters 31 and 44). The importance of neonatal screening as a preventive measure is highlighted by the prediction that 13 children with PKU and 40 children with CH would not be identified if 5 per cent of the neonatal population were not screened for 1 year (AAP, 1992).

Anticipatory Guidance: Newborn Infant Screening

The optimal time to obtain a blood specimen from the newborn infant is prior to discharge from the nursery or no later than 7 days of life. Cord blood is not appropriate for testing because plasma concentrations of PKU and other disorders are metabolized by the mother, resulting in normal values at birth. A period of time is needed for these metabolites to accumulate and be detectable. In cases wherein the neonate is sick and/or premature, the blood specimen is obtained prior to transfusions and dialysis. Infants are also screened for specific disorders if one of their siblings has been diagnosed with the disorder (AAP, 1992).

The AAP recommends that the hepatitis B vaccine be administered to all neonates prior to hospital discharge, with a second dose at 1 to 2 months of age and a third dose at 6 to 18 months.

Thermoregulation

Thermal balance is maintained by regulation of heat loss and heat production. The environment plays a major role in heat loss; therefore, maintenance of an optimal thermal environment is one of the most important aspects of neonatal care. Heat exchange (loss) between the body and the environment occurs by evaporation, conduction, convection, and radiation.

Heat Loss

Evaporation. Immediately after delivery, the neonate is covered with amniotic fluid (liquid), which is converted to a vapor utilizing thermal energy. Evaporation with heat loss is increased when the environmental humidity is low. Drying the neonate thoroughly with warm towels will interfere with heat loss through evaporation. Bathing the neonate may also contribute to evaporative heat loss. Therefore, bathing should not be performed until the body temperature is normal and stable. In many institutions vital signs (especially temperature) are taken before a bath is given. This is a good way to determine the appropriateness of the planned bath.

Conduction. Loss of body heat through conduction occurs when the skin is in direct contact with a cooler surface. Body heat rapidly moves to the cooler surface to equalize the different temperatures. The naked neonate should always be placed on a padded, warm surface to prevent conductive heat loss. This is important to remember when bathing and examining the infant.

Convection. Loss of body heat via convection occurs when the surrounding air is cool. Heat moves from the body surface to the cooler surrounding air. Temperature, air movement, and humidity all contribute to the rate of convection. Convective heat loss can be reduced by maintaining an ideal environmental temperature and humidity (72 to 76° F; 40 to 60 per cent humidity); however, air temperature will have no significant effect on heat loss by radiation or evaporation.

Radiation. Radiant heat loss occurs by transfer of body heat to a cooler solid object that is not in direct contact with the neonate. If the warmer or incubator has a warm padded surface, the environmental temperature is warm, and the infant is dry, then heat loss may still occur if the newborn unit is placed in close proximity to a cold window or wall or other source of coldness. The amount of heat loss through radiation is directly related to the distance from a cold surface. The implications are obvious for placement of the neonate in the delivery room, neonatal nursery, and home nursery.

Heat Production

Discussion of the four modalities of exchange of heat between the body and the environment has focused on heat loss for the neonate. However, body heat gains may occur in the same manner from external sources. Precautions should be taken to prevent excess heat loss or heat gain when caring for the neonate.

The neonate who is exposed to a heat-loss environment will compensate by increasing heat production through increased metabolic activity. The full-term infant who is exposed to cold can increase the thermogenic rate 2½ times over the resting state to a level that almost equals that of the adult (Behrman, 1992).

The neonate exposed to cold stress increases heat production through a mechanism called "nonshivering thermogenesis." This refers to heat that is produced by an increased metabolic rate in a cold environment. This in turn requires increased oxygen consumption. The type of body fat known as brown fat seems to be the major source of heat that is produced by nonshivering thermogenesis. Brown fat composes 2 to 6 per cent of the neonate's body weight. It usually disappears some weeks after birth when it is no longer needed. Exposure to cold will deplete stores of brown fat. If the depletion is severe, as with prolonged cold stress, it is hypothesized that effective thermogenic capacity is eliminated (Behrman, 1992). The cold-stressed neonate is also at risk for developing hypoxemia, metabolic acidosis, rapid depletion of glycogen stores, and reduction of blood glucose levels *(hypoglycemia)*.

Nursing Interventions: Thermal Management

All neonates lose some body heat immediately after delivery. Physiologically, cold stimuli are probably essential to the initiation of extrauterine respirations; however, too much is hazardous. The temperature of the infant's skin signals the presence of a metabolic response to heat loss. A drop in skin temperature indicates a heat-loss environment that requires warming. The metabolic responses to cold stress will be triggered before core (deep tissue) temperature changes occur. Rectal temperature may be normal in the cold-stressed newborn infant in the beginning. Axillary temperatures may be falsely high owing to the presence of brown fat padding. During the first few hours after birth, when the neonate has difficulty regulating and maintaining body temperature, a heat-sensitive probe taped to the abdomen is the most accurate method of continually assessing the body temperature status. The probe should remain uncovered to assure accuracy of skin temperature recordings. Once the infant's temperature has stabilized, rectal temperature readings are sufficiently accurate.

Anticipatory Guidance: Thermal Management

Parents should be taught how to use a rectal thermometer on their baby: lubricate the tip with petroleum jelly and gently insert the tip (about ¼ inch) into the rectum. The thermometer can be held in place with one hand while the infant's legs are grasped at the ankles with the other hand. This prevents kicking, which may cause the thermometer to be inserted deeper. If a glass thermometer is used, hold it in place for 3 minutes before reading.

Bathing

The purpose of bathing is to provide skin stimulation and maintain cleanliness while allowing inspection. Because neonates do not perspire, they do not need to be bathed daily. The face, chin, and neck should be cleansed after each feeding, and the entire diaper area cleansed with each diaper change. The condition of the skin and the environmental temperature are good guidelines in assessing the need for a bath. During the summer when it is hot and humid a daily bath may be refreshing, whereas during the winter, bathing the infant three to four times per week is sufficient.

During the first few days after birth, the vernix gradually disappears and the skin becomes dry and scaly. There may even be slight bleeding where the skin becomes cracked around the hands and feet. This is normal, but to bathe the infant daily can increase this drying process. Parents express concern about dryness and generally wish to apply lotion to the dry skin. The use of lotion benefits only the parents; however, it will cause no harm if the excess lotion is removed and the area washed before reapplication of lotion. Allowing layers of lotion to remain on the skin provides a warm, moist environment for bacteria to breed and grow. A neonate should not be immersed in a tub of water until the umbilical cord has dropped off and the stump has healed (approximately 10 days maximum). During that time, sponge bathing is appropriate.

Anticipatory Guidance: Bathing

Bath time should be planned some time before a meal and when the baby is not fussy. Bathing right after a feeding may cause the newborn infant to spit up. Bath time should be fun for the parents and the baby. Infant-bathing instruction that occurs during the hospital stay is an important part of discharge preparation.

The neonate can be bathed in a baby bathtub or while placed on the kitchen table or a bed. The bath area should be warm, draft-free, and at a comfortable height to prevent the parent from becoming overly tired (stretching and bending). The area should also be big enough to work comfortably. Some parents enjoy using the kitchen sink. If the sink is used, a few safety factors must be kept in mind:

- Clean the sink thoroughly.
- Place a folded towel in the bottom of the sink for padding.
- Prepare the water and then turn the faucet away from the baby before placing the baby in the water. Accidental burns could occur if the temperature should change while water is allowed to flow directly over the newborn infant.
- If the sink has a window over it, the window should be closed to prevent drafts.

The bath water should be comfortably warm. Feeling the water with the inner aspect of the forearm is a good way to test the temperature. The elbow is not sufficiently sensitive to temperature to detect water that would be too hot for the infant. Other articles needed are a clean towel and washcloth, a bar of mild soap, a comb or soft brush, and a clean diaper and clothing. The use of lotions, creams, or powders is unnecessary. Baby powder has a tendency to "pill" where skin surfaces rub together and can thus produce skin irritation. It can also be aspirated by the infant. Everything should be arranged in the bathing area before beginning. Once the procedure is begun, the neonate must not be left unattended for any reason. *One hand should be kept on the baby at all times.* This is an important safety rule to be applied in all areas of infant care.

Place the neonate on a padded surface and wash the eyes and face gently with clear water. Use a different portion of the washcloth for each eye and clean by wiping from the edge of the nose outward (inner canthus to outer canthus). Two cotton balls wrung out in clear water will also cleanse the eyes rapidly and safely. Some babies do not like to have their faces covered. Gentle, soothing touch and speaking or singing quietly will help the neonate learn to enjoy the experience. The ears and nose should be cleaned with a wisp of cotton or the tip of a washcloth. A cotton swab should never be inserted into these areas; damage to the delicate tissues may result.

The head should be lathered lightly and the fontanel area (soft spot) should be washed as well. There is no need for parents to be afraid to touch this area.

Cradle cap, a desquamation that may occur on the scalp (particularly over the fontanel area), can be prevented by daily washing and rinsing. If scales do occur, they can be softened with baby oil and removed with a fine-tooth comb or brush after washing. The infant should be picked up and the soap rinsed off the head. The "football carry" is a comfortable and safe way to hold the neonate. This also gives good face-to-face contact during the procedure.

Further instructions for the parent bathing the baby include placing the infant on the back on the padded surface and drying the head. Proceed to undress the infant and gently lather the baby's front; turn her or him on the abdomen and lather the back. It feels nice to lather the infant's head and skin with the hands; the skin-to-skin contact can be very satisfying to parents and baby. After lathering, remember that the baby is very slippery. Pick the neonate up gently, supporting head and back, and gradually lower into the water. Supporting the baby's head out of the water with one hand, use the other hand to gently swirl the water over the body. As the baby learns to enjoy the water, she or he will enjoy kicking and splashing. Allow enough time for this form of play.

Cord Care

The cord should be kept dry until it falls off and the stump has healed. The process of healing generally requires 5 to 10 days. There should be no active bleeding at the site during this time. However, a few drops of blood are not uncommon when the cord begins to separate. The parents should inspect the area for signs of infection (redness, edema, drainage).

Anticipatory Guidance: Cord Care

A drying agent may be used on the cord. Some physicians recommend applying triple dye once a day or swabbing the cord and base with alcohol at each diaper change. The use of belly bands is contraindicated: they do not prevent umbilical hernias and may cause infection by delaying or preventing the drying process. Diapers and rubber pants should be folded down to keep the cord area dry.

Circumcision Care

"Circumcision" is the surgical removal of the foreskin of the penis. Care following a circumcision is based on general principles of postoperative care: keep the wound clean and dry, and observe for signs of bleeding or infection, or both.

The neonate may be fussy. Crying is due to the restrained position during the procedure and to the pain caused by the procedure. Taking the baby out to the mother as soon as possible for nursing, comforting, and cuddling is reassuring for both.

Anticipatory Guidance: Circumcision Care

Following the circumcision, a sterile dressing with petroleum jelly is applied to the area. This should be changed with each voiding unless the physician wishes it to remain securely in place to serve as a pressure dressing for 24 hours. Keep the neonate off the abdomen for the first 12 hours to eliminate discomfort, pressure, or friction rubbing. The penis should be observed for bleeding at least every hour during the first 6 hours postoperatively (AAP, 1989b).

Clothing

Parents tend to overdress the neonate. They mistakenly conclude that cool, slightly bluish hands and feet mean that the baby is cold. The infant who is overheated must activate heat-loss physiologic mechanisms. Conversely, room temperatures that are comfortable for the adult may cause the neonate to initiate heat production.

Anticipatory Guidance: Clothing

The nurse should explain to parents the importance of sufficient, but not excessive, clothing. Generally, the neonate will be comfortable when dressed in the same amount of clothing as the adult, plus one additional layer. The extremities will feel slightly cool, and the trunk will be warm to touch.

Feeding

Feeding is one of the first tasks the new parents must accomplish in learning to care for their baby. The method of feeding (breast or bottle) is a choice that must be made with guidance and without undue pressure. Information should be provided as needed and the decision supported rather than judged. Information on the advantages and disadvantages can be provided. For example, a nurse researcher found that breastfed infants had fewer illnesses during infancy, which were associated with fewer toddler illnesses (Gulick, 1986). Parents must learn not only to successfully feed their infant but also to assess his or her hunger. Readiness for feeding can be determined by observing the infant's behavior. Rooting and sucking, hand-to-mouth activity, crying, and alertness are clues that the baby is hungry.

Anticipatory Guidance: Feeding

The nurse can ensure a happy, satisfying feeding time for baby and parent by showing the parent how to hold, feed, and burp the infant successfully and by providing positive feedback to strengthen healthy interaction and feeding activity.

Parents should be urged to hold their baby for feedings and to spend a few minutes talking with and stroking the infant before feeding to facilitate both their own and the baby's relaxation. Prefeeding relaxation reduces the incidence of vomiting and colic and encourages attachment.

TABLE 4-6
Breastfeeding: Proper Latch-On and Positioning

Signs of Correct Latch-On

- Mother states "It feels right"
- No nipple pain is experienced
- Noisy swallowing is heard once let-down occurs
- Deep jaw movements are seen and the ears may wiggle; the whole head will also move

Signs of Incorrect Latch-On

- Baby's cheeks are sucked in when feeding
- The nipple may appear flattened when removed from baby's mouth
- Painful, cracked, bleeding, or blistered nipples
- Baby may fuss at breast, pulling on and off
- A loud clicking sound may be heard

Wide Mouth

Before pulling baby onto the breast, the mouth must be *open wide*. The mother can facilitate this by tickling baby's lips with the nipple. For stubborn babies, put gentle downward pressure on baby's lower jaw; this will encourage baby to open the mouth wide. Now the nipple should be well back in the baby's mouth. This prevents nipple chewing, which causes pain, blisters, and cracked and bleeding nipples.

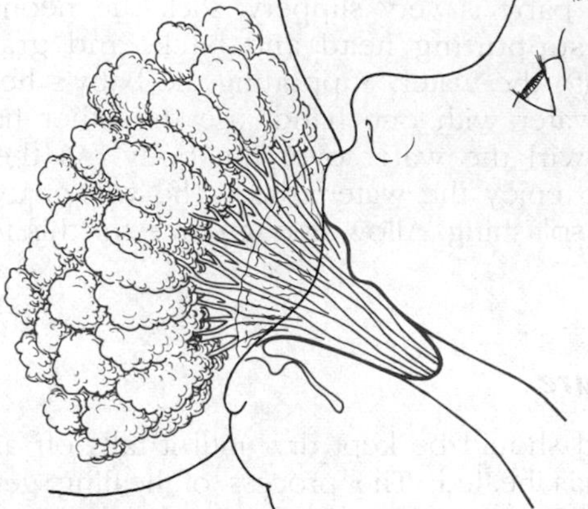

Proper position of head, lips, mouth, and tongue during breastfeeding.

Lips Curved Back

When properly latched on, the lips should be curved back almost as though they were turned inside out, rather than the pursed lips of a bottlefed baby. The lower lip should be aimed to cover more of the lower portion of the areola. The tongue will now be in place *below* the nipple. The mother may not be able to see this looking down at her baby. If the position of the mouth is not correct, the mother should break the suction by inserting her finger gently into the corner of the mouth and reposition again.

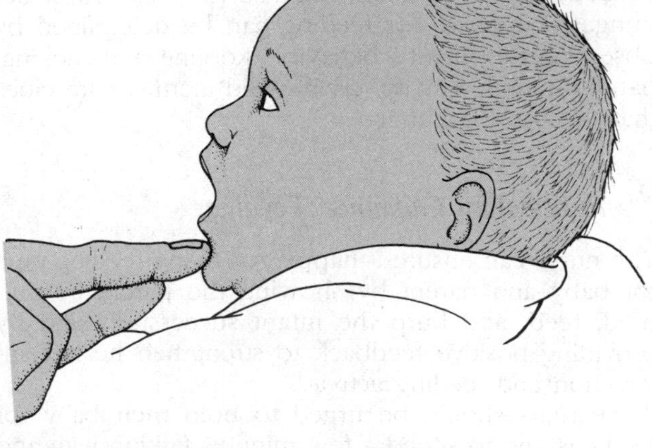

Baby can be encouraged to open mouth wide by putting gentle pressure on the lower jaw.

Head Slightly Extended

The baby's head should be extended slightly. The chin is thus pressed into the mother's breast and the nostrils are free from occlusion. Swallowing is easier in this position. The lower jaw will "milk" the breast more effectively.

Baby Close to Breast

The baby must be held as close to the mother's breast as possible. Unwrap the baby and have arms hugging the mother with one of baby's arms under the mother's arm and one arm resting on top of the breast. This helps prevent the baby from flexing the head. The nipple will not slip out of the mouth as easily, and the baby will not have to exert excess suction to keep the nipple in its mouth, thus causing nipple damage and pain.

Body Aligned

In any hold, the baby's stomach should be against the mother's body, with the mouth at the level of nipple. Pillows can be helpful here. The body should be well supported so the head and body are in straight alignment. This eases swallowing and keeps the baby close to mother. It is difficult to swallow with your head turned to the side.

TABLE 4-6
Breastfeeding: Proper Latch-On and Positioning *(Continued)*

Breast Supported

To support the breast, the mother should cup her breast with her fingers and let her thumb rest on top. The hand should be positioned well away from the areola so as not to get in the way of the latch-on. The scissor hold (nipple between index and middle finger) can obstruct milk flow and prevent a good grasp of the nipple and areola. A supported breast prevents the weight of the breast from pushing on the baby's chin, which can tire an infant when nursing.

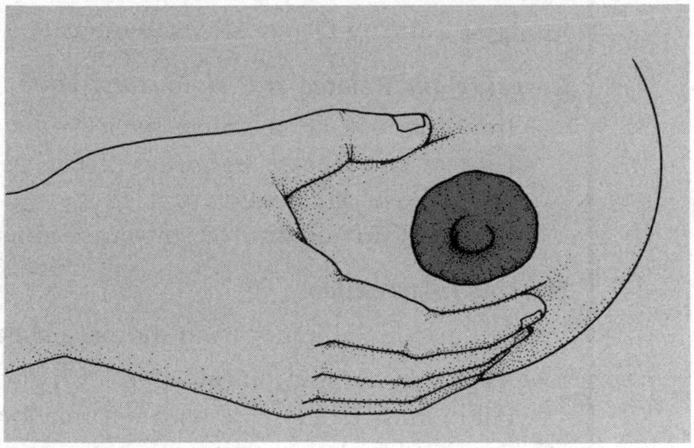

Hand is positioned well away from the areola.

Text prepared by Ruta Valaitis, BScN, BA, MHSc, Clinical Nursing Consultant, and Lecturer, McMaster University School of Nursing, Hamilton, Ontario.

Nutritional Needs

Unless the mother or infant develops health problems, breastfeeding is often begun immediately after birth, during the first period of reactivity. Findings from a nursing study suggest that neonates can feed successfully at 1 to 2 hours after birth rather than at 4 hours (Anderson et al, 1982). This can be a very meaningful experience, since the neonate is alert and interested in sucking at this time. Breastfeeding after delivery is not done to supply nutritional intake but to promote closeness and attachment. This is also an opportunity for mother and baby to practice the proper "latch-on" and positioning for breastfeeding (Table 4–6).

For bottlefed infants, the first milk intake usually occurs within 4 hours after delivery. Neonates require 100 to 120 cal per kg of body weight every 24 hours. Approximately 3 to 4 minutes sucking time at the breast, or 30 to 50 ml of formula per feeding, will meet this requirement for the first 3 to 4 days of life. A nursing research study provides support for giving the initial feeding 1 to 2 hours after birth when the neonate is much more alert compared with the 4-hour interval (Pete, 1989). Findings suggest that newborn infants prefer 5 per cent glucose and water over sterile water for feedings. Conventional practice has advocated use of sterile water because aspirated glucose water would be more irritating to lungs than sterile water. In contrast to initiating breastfeeding immediately, analysis of colostrum reveals it is more viscous and richer in protein and minerals than glucose water or milk, which provides support for early feeding of glucose water (Holmes & Magiera, 1987).

As the baby gains weight, formula amounts will increase. The nurse can calculate the child's 24-hour caloric intake to ensure that caloric requirements are met. (Most commercially prepared infant formulas contain 20 cal per ounce.) The neonate averages six to eight feedings per day.

Anticipatory Guidance: Nutritional Needs

Parents should be informed of the importance of placing their baby in a position that reduces the likelihood of regurgitation or aspiration of food after feeding. Placement in an infant seat or laying the infant on the side or on the back are all acceptable positions for 30 minutes to 1 hour after each feeding. Parents may have questions regarding the type of formula to use. Direct advertising to consumers often leaves parents in a quandary as to formula choice (Barness, 1991). The nurse can provide parents with the facts about formulas available so they can make informed choices.

Sleep Behaviors

Neonates sleep between 20 and 22 hours each day, which includes seven to eight naps. The sleep cycle consists of a high proportion of rapid eye movement (REM, active) sleep. Wrapping the neonate snugly in a blanket promotes sleep.

Anticipatory Guidance: Sleep Behaviors

The expectations that parents have for their neonates related to sleep should be realistic. Recognizing some of the common variations that exist within the range

TABLE 4-7
Promoting Safety

Analysis: Nursing Diagnostic Statement 1

Response and Related or Risk Factors: *High risk for injury: motor vehicle accidents; risk factors*

- Improper use of car safety devices
- Lack of knowledge regarding proper use of car safety devices
- Lack of use of car safety devices
- Impaired driving and/or substance abuse or alcohol/drug use

Nursing Interventions

Prevent accidental injury from motor vehicle accidents

- Assess the family's knowledge level about use of car seat
- Fill in knowledge gaps with information about safe use of car safety devices
- Support legislative actions to promote safety standards

Analysis: Nursing Diagnostic Statement 2

Response and Related or Risk Factors: *High risk for injury: suffocation; risk factor— neonate's lack of awareness of environmental hazards associated with developmental level*

Nursing Interventions

Prevent injury by suffocation

- Provide anticipatory guidance to prepare parents for neonate's developmental changes and the potential environmental hazards that could endanger his or her life

Teach parents to:

- Avoid propping a baby's bottle
- Keep plastic bags away from and out of baby's reach at all times
- Never leave baby unattended while bathing her or him
- Avoid use of pillows in baby's crib
- Never hang a pacifier around baby's head/neck
- Purchase crib that meets safety specifications

Analysis: Nursing Diagnostic Statement 3

Response and Related or Risk Factors: *High risk for injury: trauma; risk factor— neonate's lack of awareness of environmental hazard associated with developmental level*

Nursing Interventions

Prevent accidental injury resulting from falls, burns, near drowning, and foreign body aspiration

- Provide anticipatory guidance for parents to prepare them for the expected changes that increase neonate's potential for injury

of normal can provide comfort and solace to those parents having difficulty. Although not all neonates have similar sleep behaviors, an understanding of the various sleep needs and age-related behaviors can provide important guidelines when counseling parents.

Sleeping conditions provided for neonates vary according to parental values and cultural differences. Common environmental conditions used to promote restful, safe sleep are a firm mattress, no pillow during infancy, a safe bed or crib, a night light as needed, a warm bath before bed, an environment free from excessive noise, and, for some parents, a separate room. These standards are commonly encouraged in an effort to provide the maximal opportunity for restful sleep. A firm mattress provides the needed support for comfort; avoiding a pillow prevents suffocation; cribs with slats no farther than 6 cm ($2\frac{3}{8}$ in) apart are used to prevent strangulation; and a warm bath promotes rest and relaxation.

Safety Concerns

Everyone caring for a newborn infant should wash hands before and after handling the baby. Safe handling techniques should be demonstrated, taught, and practiced by all who handle the baby. These include firmly supporting all body parts, especially the head; keeping a controlling hand on the infant during weighing or giving care on any surface without protective straps; placing a hand between the baby's skin and the diaper if pins are used; placing the infant on the side or back for at least 30 minutes after feeding to prevent aspiration of regurgitated fluids; and carrying the infant in a protected, secure manner. Table 4–7 lists potential accidents and prevention strategies for neonates and infants.

Anticipatory Guidance: Safety Concerns

The nurse should discuss with parents the use of infant car seats before the neonate leaves the hospital (AAP, 1990). If an infant car seat has not been purchased, the nurse should encourage the family to do so. In many states the use of a car seat for children is mandated by law. If the family feels that a car seat costs too much, the nurse can suggest options such as borrowing or renting a used seat. Many hospitals now operate their own rental programs, offering car seats for the neonate and exchanging them for larger ones as the child grows. All health care personnel should recognize their responsibility to encourage the use of proper infant and child car restraints, because automobile accidents are a prime cause of injury and death in children. Chapter 15 discusses in detail the reasons parents do or do not use car seats and nursing interventions to promote proper use.

KEY CONCEPTS

Concepts Related to Basic Information

- Concerns of the family with a neonate include forming a bond, accepting responsibility for the infant, and assuming the parental role.
- The process of attachment begins with and grows out of bonding; the terms "bonding" and "attachment" are sometimes used interchangeably but have different meanings.
- The newborn period is defined as from birth to 1 month of age.
- Reflex responses of the neonate provide important data on the status of neurologic functioning.
- The Moro reflex is the single most significant response denoting CNS status of the neonate; the Moro reflex is strong during the first 8 weeks of life and fades by the end of the second or third month.
- Visual abilities of the neonate are better developed than once thought; neonates can fixate; discriminate between sizes, shapes, colors, and patterns; conjugate; scan the visual field; and accommodate to distance.
- Behavioral manifestations of hearing in the neonate include alerting, eye movements, startle reaction, and crying.
- Seventy-five per cent of body weight in the newborn infant is composed of water; normal weight loss of up to 10 per cent of body weight after birth represents fluid loss.
- The neonate exposed to cold stress increases heat production through a mechanism called "nonshivering thermogenesis" referring to heat that is produced by an increased metabolic rate in a cold environment that requires increased oxygen consumption. Brown fat, the neonate's body fat, is the major source of heat produced by nonshivering thermogenesis.

Concepts Related to Nursing Assessment

- The development of maternicity can be assessed by evaluating mother-infant behaviors.
- Assessment of the neonate includes the initial Apgar scoring, Dubowitz assessment, and comprehensive physical assessment.
- Awareness of the facets of the roles of mother, father, and sibling contributes to the development of the nursing diagnosis *high risk for altered role performance.*
- In assessing maternicity in the mother, the nurse should remember that observation of eye-to-eye contact (en face position) between mother and infant is of primary importance.
- Factors related to the etiology of *knowledge deficit* for families with a neonate include anxiety, lack of interest or motivation, and cultural-language differences.
- Knowledge deficit may be identified as an etiologic factor for the nursing diagnoses of *ineffective individual coping: parent; fear; disturbance in self-concept: self-esteem; powerlessness; and disturbance in self-concept: role performance* in families with a neonate.
- The nurse who suspects the family with a neonate is experiencing feelings of being overwhelmed should consider a possible nursing diagnosis of *ineffective family coping.*
- Nurses providing care to the neonate in the hospital, birthing center, or other community setting will consider the nursing diagnosis *high risk for altered growth and development.*
- The initial assessment of the neonate is done immediately after birth, with the Apgar score and a gross assessment to rule out any life-threatening anomalies or major anomalies that are not life-threatening.
- Within the first 24 hours of life, a second, more thorough assessment should be performed to provide a total comparative health data base for future assessment.

Concepts Related to Nursing Intervention

- Nursing interventions to assist the family with a neonate can assist in the prevention of actual *alterations in parenting*.
- The nurse can facilitate identification with the neonate by modeling methods of interacting with the baby by pointing out characteristics of the baby, encouraging examination of the baby by family members, talking to the baby, and responding to the baby's behavior.
- When the parental stresses of insecurity, fear, and low self-esteem exist, the nurse's major intervention is one of reassurance and of identification of the parents' strengths.
- Nurses should realize that attachment is a multifactorial process and they should intervene at all periods of development to strengthen parent-child relationships.
- Anticipatory guidance for cord care includes keeping the cord area dry, applying a drying agent such as alcohol, and avoiding the use of belly bands.
- The nurse should explain to parents the importance of sufficient, but not excessive, clothing because parents tend to overdress the neonate.
- Feeding is one of the first tasks the new parents must accomplish; parents need information about the method of feeding, whether it be breastfeeding or bottlefeeding, and must be supported rather than judged in that decision.
- The nurse can instruct parents on common environmental conditions to promote sleep that include use of a firm mattress, no pillow during infancy, a safe bed or crib, a night light, a warm bath before bed, no excessive noise, and, if possible, a separate room.
- The nurse should discuss with parents the use of infant car seats before the neonate leaves the hospital because automobile accidents are a prime cause of injury and death in children.

REFERENCES

American Academy of Pediatrics, Committee on Accident and Prevention. (1990). Safe transportation of newborns discharged from the hospital. *APP News, 6*(7), 12.

American Academy of Pediatrics, Committee on Genetics. (1992). Issues in newborn screening. *Pediatrics, 89*(2), 345–349.

American Academy of Pediatrics, Committee on Genetics. (1989a). Newborn screening fact sheets. *Pediatrics, 83*(3), 449–464.

American Academy of Pediatrics, Committee on Infectious Diseases. (1991). *Report of the committee on infectious diseases* (22nd ed.). Elk Grove Village, IL: Author.

American Academy of Pediatrics, Task Force on Circumcision. (1989b). Report of the task force on circumcision. *Pediatrics, 84*(4), 388–391.

Andenberg, G. (1988). Initial acquaintance and attachment behavior of siblings with the newborn. *Journal of Obstetric, Gynecologic, and Neonatal Nursing, 17,* 49–54.

Anderson, G., McBride, M., Dahm, J., Ellis, M., & Vidyasagar, D. (1982). Development of sucking in term infants from birth to four hours postbirth. *Research in Nursing and Health, 5,* 21–27.

Apgar, V. (1953). A proposal for a new method of evaluating the newborn infant. *Current Research in Anesthesia and Analgesia, 32,* 260.

Barness, L. (1991). Brief history of infant nutrition and view to the future. *Pediatrics, 88*(5), 1054–1056.

Beal, J. (1989). The effect on father-infant interaction of demonstrating the neonatal behavioral assessment scale. *Birth, 16*(1), 18–22.

Beal, J. (1991). Methodological issues in conducting research on parent-infant attachment. *Journal of Pediatric Nursing, 6*(1), 11–15.

Behrman, R. (1992). *Nelson textbook of pediatrics.* Philadelphia: WB Saunders.

Bowen, S., & Miller, B. (1980). Paternal attachment behavior as related to presence at delivery and preparenthood classes: A pilot study. *Nursing Research, 29,* 307–311.

Brazelton, T. (1973). *The neonatal behavioral assessment scale.* Philadelphia: JB Lippincott.

Campbell, S., & Taylor, P. M. (1980). Bonding and attachments: Theoretical issues. *Seminars in Perinatology, 3,* 3–14.

Chess, S., & Thomas, A. (1982, April). Infant bonding: Mystique and reality. *American Journal of Orthopsychiatry, 52,* 213–222.

Craig, S., et al. (1982). The effect of early contact on maternal perception of infant behavior. *Early Human Development, 6,* 197–204.

Dean, P., Morgan, P., & Towle, J. (1982). Making baby's acquaintance: A unique attachment strategy. *MCN: American Journal of Maternal Child Nursing, 7,* 37–41.

De Chateau, P., & Wiberg, J. (1977). Long-term effect on mother-infant behavior of extra contact during the first hour post-partum. I: First observations at 36 hours. II: A follow-up at three months. *Acta Paediatrica Scandinavia, 66,* 137–151.

Dubowitz, L., et al. (1970). Clinical assessment of gestational age in the newborn infant. *Journal of Pediatrics, 77,* 1.

Duvall, E., & Miller, B. (1985). *Marriage and family development* (6th ed.). New York: Harper & Row.

Glover, L. (1989). Parental-fetal attachment. *Nursing Scan in Research, 2*(4), 1–4.

Goldberg, S. (1983). Parent-infant bonding: Another look. *Child Development, 54,* 1355–1382.

Grossman, K., Thane, K., & Grossman, K. (1981). Maternal tactile contact of the newborn after various postpartum conditions of mother-infant contact. *Developmental Psychology, 17,* 159.

Gulick, E. (1986). The effects of breast feeding on toddler health. *Pediatric Nursing, 12*(1), 51–54.

Hales, D. J., et al. (1977). Defining the limits of the maternal sensitive period. *Developmental Medicine and Child Neurology, 19,* 454–461.

Holmes, J., & Magiera, L. (1987). Nursing management of the normal neonate. In J. Holmes & L. Magiera (Eds.), *Maternity nursing.* New York: Macmillan.

Kemp, V., & Page, C. (1987, May/June). Maternal prenatal attachment in normal and high-risk pregnancies. *Journal of Obstetric, Gynecologic, and Neonatal Nursing, 16,* 179–184.

Kennell, J. H., et al. (1974). Maternal behavior one year after early and extended postpartum contact. *Developmental Medicine and Child Neurology, 16,* 172–179.

Klaus, M. H., et al. (1972). Maternal attachment: Importance of the first postpartum days. *New England Journal of Medicine, 286,* 460–463.

Klaus, M. H., & Fanaroff, A. A. (1986). *Care of the high-risk neonate* (3rd ed.). Philadelphia: WB Saunders.

Klaus, M., & Kennell, J. (1976). *Maternal-infant bonding.* St. Louis: CV Mosby.

Klaus, M., & Kennell, J. (1982). *Parent-infant bonding* (2nd ed.). St. Louis: CV Mosby.

Lamb, M. E., & Hwang, C. P. (1982). Maternal attachment and mother neonatal bonding: A critical review. In M. E. Lamb & A. L. Brown (Eds.), *Advances in developmental psychology.* Hillsdale, NJ: Erlbaum.

Lubchenco, L., et al. (1963, October). Intrauterine growth as estimated from liveborn birth-weight data at 24 to 42 weeks of gestation. *Pediatrics,* 793.

Lubchenco, L., et al. (1966, March). Intrauterine growth in length and head circumference as estimated from live births at gestational ages from 26–42 weeks. *Pediatrics,* 603.

Luddington-Hoe, S. (1977). Postpartum: Development of maternity. *American Journal of Nursing, 17,* 1170–1174.

Mitchell, K., & Mills, N. (1983, March/April). Is the sensitive period in parent-infant bonding overrated? *Pediatric Nursing,* 91–94.

Novak, J., & Novak, R. (1990). Facilitating fathering. In M. Craft & J. Denehy, *Nursing interventions for infants and children.* Philadelphia: WB Saunders.

Pete, J. (1989). Newborn infants' preference for sterile water versus five percent glucose and water. *Journal of Pediatric Nursing, 4*(4), 263–267.

Pressler, J. (1990). Promoting attachment. In M. Craft & J. Denehy, *Nursing interventions for infants and children.* Philadelphia: WB Saunders.

Reeder, S., et al. (1987). *Maternity nursing.* Philadelphia: JB Lippincott.

Rubin, R. (1963). Maternal touch. *Nursing Outlook, 11,* 828–831.

Rutledge, D., & Pridham, K. (1987, May/June). Postpartum mothers' perceptions of competence for infant care. *Journal of Obstetric, Gynecologic, and Neonatal Nursing, 16,* 185–194.

Siegal, E., Bauman, K., Schaefer, E., Saunders, M., & Ingram, D. (1990). Hospital and home support during infancy: Impact on matenal attachment, child abuse and neglect, and health care utilization. *Pediatrics, 66,* 183.

Svejda, M. J., et al. (1980). Mother-infant bonding: Failure to generalize. *Child Development, 51,* 775–779.

Svejda, M. J., et al. (1982). Parent-to-infant attachment: A critique of the early "bonding" model. In R. N. Emde & R. J. Harmon (Eds.), *Attachment and affiliative systems.* New York: Plenum Press.

Taylor, P., Taylor, F., Campbell, S., Meloni, J., & Cannon, M. (1985). Effects of early mother infant contractual attitudes, perceptions and behaviors. *Acta Paediatrica Scandinavia, 316,* 3–14.

U.S. Bureau of the Census. (1991). *Marital status and living arrangement,* 1990. (Current Population Reports Series P–20, No. 450.) Washington, DC: US Government Printing Office.

Vaughan, V., & Litt, I. (1990). *Child and adolescent development: Clinical implications.* Philadelphia: WB Saunders.

Weiser, M., & Castiglia, P. (1984). Assessing early father-infant attachment. *MCN: American Journal of Maternal Child Nursing, 9,* 104–105.

BIBLIOGRAPHY

American Academy of Pediatrics, Committee on Fetus and Newborn. (1985). Home phototherapy. *Pediatrics, 76,* 136.

American Academy of Pediatrics, Committee on Fetus and Newborn. (1988). *Guidelines for perinatal care* (2nd Ed.). Elk Grove Village, IL: AAP.

Beal, J. (1989). The effects of demonstration of the Brazelton neonatal behavioral assessment scale on the paternal-infant relationship. *Issues in Perinatology, 16*(1), 18–22.

Bernard-Bonnin, A. C., et al. (1989). Hospital practices and breast feeding duration: A meta-analysis of controlled trials. *Birth, 16*(2), 64–66.

Bliss-Houtz, J. (1989). Comparison of rectal, auxillary and inguinal temperatures in full-term newborn infants. *Nursing Research, 38*(2), 85–87.

Boyer, D. (1987). Serum indirect bilirubin levels and meconium passage in early fed normal newborn. *Nursing Research, 36,* 176.

Brazelton, T. (1984). Neonatal behavior and its significance. In M. Avery & H. Taesch (Eds.), *Schaeffer's diseases of the newborn.* Philadelphia: WB Saunders.

Brown, M., & Hellings, P. (1988). A case study of qualitative versus quantitative reviews: The maternal-infant bonding controversy. *Journal of Pediatric Nursing, 4*(2), 104–111.

Budreau, G. (1987). Postnatal cranial molding and infant attractiveness: Implications for nursing. *Neonatal Nursing, 5,* 13.

Campbell, R., et al. (1988). Effects of diaper types on diaper dermatitis associated with diarrhea and antibiotic use in children in day care centers. *Pediatric Dermatology, 5*(2), 83–87.

D'Apolito, K. (1991). What is an organized infant? *Neonatal Network, 10*(1), 23–29.

Davis, R., & Truesdale, M. (1993). Creative approaches to promoting parent-infant bonding. *Journal of Pediatric Nursing, 8*(3), 201–202.

De Chateau, P. (1976). The influence of early contract on maternal and infant behavior in primiparas. *Birth and Family Journal, 3,* 149.

Dubowitz, L., & Dubowitz, V. (1977). *Gestational age of the newborn.* Menlo Park, CA: Addison-Wesley.

Erikson, E. H. (1963). *Childhood and society* (2nd ed.). New York: WW Norton.

Fond, K., & Webster, R. (1988). NAPNAP policy statement on breast feeding. *Journal of Pediatric Health Care, 2*(66), 314.

Freud, S. (1957). In J. Strachey (Ed.), *The standard edition of the complete psychological works of Sigmund Freud* (vol. 18). London: Hogarth.

Gammage, D., & Yarandi, H. (1993). The effects of diaper brands, urine volume, and time on specific gravity measurement. *Journal of Pediatric Nursing, 8*(1), 10–14.

Gladstone, I., et al. (1988). Randomized study of six umbilical cord care regimens. *Clinical Medicine, 27*(3), 127–129.

Haddock, V. P., & Merow, D. (1986). Axillary and rectal temperatures of full term neonates: Are they different? *Neonatal Network, 5*(1), 36.

Hammerschlag, M., et al. (1989). Efficacy of neonatal ocular prophylaxis for the prevention of chlamydial and gonococcal conjunctivitis. *New England Journal of Medicine, 320*(12), 769–772.

Keefe, M., et al. (1989). Development of a system for monitoring infant state behavior. *Nursing Research, 38*(6), 344–347.

Larsen, G., & Williams, S. (1990). Postneonatal circumcision: Population profile. *Pediatrics, 85*(5), 808–811.

Lascari, A. (1986). "Early" breast feeding jaundice: Clinical significance. *Journal of Pediatrics, 108,* 156.

Long, M. H. (1992). The role of the CNM in newborn management. *Journal of Nurse Midwifery, 37*(2), 8S–17S.

Lubchenco, L., et al. (1972, March). Long-term follow-up studies of prematurely born infants. II. Influence of birth weight and gestational age on sequelae. *Journal of Pediatrics,* 509.

Lund, M. M. (1990). Perspectives on newborn male circumcision. *Neonatal Network, 9*(3), 7–12.

Medoff-Cooper, B., Weininger, S., & Zukowsky, K. (1989). Neonatal sucking as a clinical assessment tool: Preliminary findings. *Nursing Research, 38*(3), 162–165.

NAACOG. (1992, January). Neonatal skin care. *OGN Nursing Practice Resource.*

NAACOG. (1991, August). Physical assessment of the neonate. *OGN Nursing Practice Resource.*

NAACOG. (1991, April). Prevention, recognition, and management of neonatal pain. *OGN Nursing Practice Resource.*

Park, M., & Lee, D. (1989). Normative arm and calf blood pressure values in the newborn. *Pediatrics, 83*(2), 240–243.

Pinyerd, B. J. (1992). Assessment of infant growth. *Journal of Pediatric Health Care, 6*(5, pt 2), 302–308.

Pitzer, M., & Hock, E. (1989). Employed mothers' concerns about separation from the first- and second-born child. *Research in Nursing and Health, 12,* 123–128.

Poland, R. (1990). The question of routine neonatal circumcision. *New England Journal of Medicine, 322*(18), 1312–1315.

Regucci, L. M. (1992). Neonatal nursing assessment by functional health patterns. *Critical Care Nursing Clinics of North America, 4*(3), 471–480.

Schoen, E. (1990). The status of circumcision of newborns. *New England Journal of Medicine, 322*(18), 1308–1312.

Sollid, D., et al. (1989). Breast feeding multiples. *Journal of Perinatal and Neonatal Nursing, 3*(1), 46–65.

Stephen, S., & Sexton, P. (1987). Neonatal axillary temperatures: Increases in reading over time. *Neonatal Network, 5*(6), 25.

Templeton, J., Edgil, A., & Douglas, A. (1988). Reva Rubin revisited. *Journal of Obstetric, Gynecologic, and Neonatal Nursing, 8*(6), 394–399.

Zachman, R., et al. (1986). Neonatal blood pressure at birth by the Doppler method. *American Heart Journal, 111,* 189.

CHAPTER • 5

Families with Infants

RELATED TOPICS
Developmental theories, Chapter 3
Promoting healthy parenting, Chapter 12
Child health assessment, Chapter 13
Infant nutrition, Chapter 16
Gavage feedings, Chapter 23
Bronchopulmonary dysplasia, Chapter 32
Oxygen administration, Chapter 32
Neonatal sepsis, Chapter 34
Retinopathy of prematurity, Chapter 45

LEARNING OBJECTIVES

- Identify the major development tasks of the family with an infant.
- Identify the milestones of the infant's physical growth and development.
- Identify the milestones of gross and fine motor development and their significance for nursing care.
- Apply knowledge of the infant's cognitive development to clinical practice.
- Identify milestones of language development in the infant.
- Discuss the importance of trust and attachment to the infant's development of emotional-social competency.
- Describe the essential components of the infant's health screening examination.
- Identify the prominent anticipatory guidance concerns for parents during infancy.

The birth of an infant is an event filled with wonder and joy for most families. Adjustments in personal and family roles are required, however, to incorporate the new family member. The first section of this chapter discusses the developmental and adaptational processes associated with assuming the parent role. The remaining sections involve health concerns and strategies for health promotion in the first year of life.

Development and Adaptation of the Family with an Infant

A major task of the family with an infant is to incorporate the child into the existing family. The addition of an infant to a family unit can strain family resources. This kind of strain on family resources can result in *impaired home maintenance management*. This nursing diagnostic response should be considered especially when several of the following defining characteristics of the response are detected in the nursing assessment (Gordon, 1987):

- Household members express difficulty in maintaining their home in a comfortable fashion. Basic needs such as heat in winter or running water may not be met, if finances are a problem.
- Household members describe outstanding debts or financial crisis.
- Unwashed or unavailable cooking equipment, clothes, or linen.
- Overtaxed family members (e.g., exhausted, anxious parents).
- Household members request assistance with home maintenance.
- Accumulation of dirt, food wastes, or hygienic wastes.
- Offensive odors.
- Lack of necessary equipment or aids.

Nontraditional families experience role stress as well. A single mother who lives with her family of origin must determine how much of the parenting role she will assume and how much she will relinquish to *her* parents. In some families cultural traditions will be influential in these role determinations. The nurse can enhance problem solving by encouraging the expectant mother to discuss these role issues before the infant's birth with the significant others with whom she lives.

Stresses on nontraditional families are often different from those for the nuclear family. The single mother who does not live with extended family or in a communal arrangement may be the only person available to meet the demands of the new infant as well as those of older siblings. This fatiguing role can be compounded by early hospital discharge. If this is the mother's first child, she may not realize how much time is required to care for a newborn (Broom, 1984) or just how much her sleep will be disrupted. The nurse can be instrumental in helping this single parent realize the need to call upon extended family or friends for help in the first days and weeks. If the woman does not have such resources, follow-up home visits are advisable.

Assuming New Family Roles

The new responsibilities associated with the infant require that all members in the infant's family assume some new roles. The addition of parental or sibling roles creates critical role transition periods while each family member works out an accommodation among new and old roles. Making a transition from husband-wife to father-mother requires development of several new interrelated roles. What these new roles are perceived to be and how they are internalized vary according to the individual's own experiences, feelings, and needs. A parent who has been an only child or the youngest child in a family has had less exposure to infant and child care responsibilities and may be unprepared for what to expect of infant behaviors.

The assumption of parental roles may lead one to think that the responses of parents to each child as it is born are similar. This is not so. The baby actually molds or triggers adult behavior. It is the individual characteristics of the child that set up specific parental responses and influence their feelings and nurturing. The orientation of the mother and father to their parental roles surely will be influenced by their particular baby as they learn to communicate and stimulate the baby's further development.

Any situation that involves a change in roles or in which new roles are perceived as conflicting with existing ones has the high risk for altered self-concept and role performance. Nursing assessment must include consideration of the defining characteristics of this nursing diagnostic response. Awareness of the facets of the roles of mother, father, and sibling contributes to the nursing assessment.

Mother Role

The economic realities facing families have created dramatic shifts in the mother's role. Over 50 per cent of mothers with children under 6 years of age are employed, an increase of 75 per cent since 1970 (US Department of Health and Human Services, 1990). The demands of being a mother and a member of the work force create role strain that, depending on the woman's individual situation, can result in any variety of outcomes. Research findings have reported negative effects of role strain that include depression, interpersonal conflicts, and increased smoking. In contrast, other studies have found that positive effects include improved self-esteem. A nursing study found that lower role strain scores were associated with positive feelings about being a mother, job satisfaction, the presence of social support, and satisfaction with child care arrangements (Hemmelgarn & Laing, 1991).

The mother in the family of an infant usually experiences the greatest change in her position. Her maternal roles usually require at least temporary interruptions of her occupational role and often most of her other extrafamilial responsibilities. Some questions that the new mother might explore, ideally with her partner, during this period of transition are:

Am I doing important things as a mother?

What is my fantasy mother (concept of what a mother ought to be and ought to do) asking me to do?

Is it possible and helpful to me and my family to do them?

If I'm important, then how can I get some sleep and eat better?

Does my fantasy mother have fun?

Do I want to be like her?

What can I do for fun everyday? Can I dance alone, listen to music, sing while I nurse?

What did I decide to give up for "fourth trimester": ironing, working on a business at home, cleaning rooms that are seldom used?

What did I decide I wouldn't give up for "fourth trimester": employment, playing the piano, reading to my 2-year-old?

How can I feel better now with my dirty house and demanding baby?

For the employed mother who returns to work outside the home 6 to 8 weeks after the birth of the child, these questions must be modified and some additional ones asked. This mother's tasks include devising viable ways to meet her role responsibilities as wife and mother while attending to responsibilities in the workplace. If she has already established a workable child care arrangement for her older children, this task may be relatively simple. However, the employed mother will have to add to her list of questions those that focus on her feelings about leaving the new baby in the care of others. Some of the mother's self-imposed demands may be the results of guilt that she is feeling about leaving her baby in someone else's care. Some research has shown that babies of employed mothers are at greater risk for emotional-social problems (Barglow, Vaughn, and Molitor, 1987). However, a growing body of evidence indicates that the mother's feelings about employment and her relationship with her baby are more important influences than is the fact that she is working outside the home. In mothers who preferred outside work to staying home, anxiety about separation from their first-born infants decreased sooner and to a greater extent than in mothers who preferred staying home (DeMeis, McBride, and Hock, 1986). More importantly, mothers who had warm, accepting relationships toward and with their infant sons demonstrated secure attachment with their babies, and neither the form nor the stability of the child care arrangements was associated with the quality of that attachment (Benn, 1986).

Nursing interventions incorporate recognizing mother's dependency needs. During this time the new mother is overloaded. It is an especially hard time for the educated career woman who is used to being in control. Support groups for new mothers in this category can be particularly helpful for dealing with feelings of frustration and anxiety that can arise when the employed woman perceives herself as less competent in the mothering role than in her professional role.

The nurse's reassurance of the mother will help build her self-confidence. At no time should a nurse's behavior communicate that she or he is better able to care for the baby than the mother; instead the nurse must use every opportunity to foster feelings of adequacy in the mother.

Father Role

Not only are fathers able to be involved with their infants, many also want to have this involvement as a parent. Their participation makes a difference to the baby's well-being. Nurses in contact with the families of infants can promote opportunities for fathers to be with their infants in the hospital and to encourage their family involvement at home. The change in attitudes regarding a father's role are evident in the evolving policies within hospitals. In the 1970s barely one fourth of hospitals allowed fathers in the delivery room. Now nearly all do, even during cesarean births; many hospitals accommodate the presence of siblings as well. A nursing study of fathers' activities with first-born infants found that fathers spent more time with play and social interaction than with caregiving. The caregiving activities that fathers most often fulfilled were changing clothes, feeding, and putting the infant down for a nap. Measures of fathers' participation in care revealed limited interactions (Tomlinson, 1987). These findings suggest that traditional roles persist in actual caregiving activities although expressed attitudes have changed.

The father's participation in the home may call for the development of sociocultural support systems such as paternity leaves from employment after the birth of a baby. This type of social change may be hastened by nurses who recognize the importance of the father-infant bond to the baby, the father, and the total family. Such nurses can seek opportunities to increase community awareness of this and make contacts with persons in positions of power to help bring about changes in policies.

Sibling Role

The arrival of a new baby sister or brother thrusts the siblings in the family into new roles and interactions (Table 5–1). Previous theoretical perspectives have emphasized concepts of sibling rivalry and negative behaviors in response to the newborn infant. Since the 1970s, research on sibling relationships has encompassed broader views, incorporating ecologic and developmental perspectives. More recent research findings have demonstrated that sibling relationships are complex, evolving, and composed of both positive and negative attributes (Stewart, 1990). Positive sibling behaviors noted include participation in sibling care, empathy toward infant needs and feelings, and sensitivity to infant cues. A nurse researcher describes the pattern of sensitive and empathetic sibling behaviors toward the neonate as *sibling mutuality* (Murphy, 1993). Research has also suggested that positive sibling behaviors are influenced by parental support and communication (Gottlieb & Mendelson, 1990).

TABLE 5-1
Family-Centered Teaching: Preparing the Young Child for a New Baby

- Begin preparation 1 to 2 mos ahead of time
- Maintain child's rituals
- Stress how things will remain the same
- Tell the child what babies are like and visit a family with an infant if possible
- Introduce the child to a new bed early in this period, before the new baby arrives
- *Do not* toilet train late in the pregnancy
- Allow the child to help prepare the baby's things
- Introduce the child to the substitute caregiver early

Nurses can assist families in adjusting to the baby's arrival. Parents can be instructed by the nurse to recognize that sibling-infant relationships take time to develop. Parents can be counseled about strategies to promote positive sibling-infant interactions (Murphy, 1993).

Family Morale

It is important to note that new coping mechanisms are needed to maintain the family's morale.

Duvall and Miller (1985) list five attitudes or behaviors that help families in the childbearing stage to cope and maintain good morale with the arrival of the infant:

1. Seeing beyond the drudgeries to the fundamental satisfactions of parenthood.
2. Valuing persons above things.
3. Resolving the conflicts inherent in the contradictory developmental tasks of parents and young children, and of fathers and mothers.
4. Establishing healthy independence as a married couple.
5. Accepting help in a spirit of appreciation and growth.

These attitudes and behaviors help to keep priorities in proper perspective for the family.

Nursing Care and Guidance

The pediatric nurse working with the new family can do much to foster healthy adaptation by being personally aware of potential stressors and, when indicated, by educating family members as to what to expect, offering reassurance regarding the "normality" of these stressors, and helping them problem solve preventively to minimize the number and intensity of stressors actually experienced. Many of the stressors that are encountered by new parents are also the defining characteristics or risk factors for the nursing diagnostic response: *caregiver role strain*. "Adjustment to parenting in general is a normal maturational process that elicits nursing behaviors of prevention of potential problems and health promotion" (NANDA, 1992). The nurse should include these defining characteristics in the assessment of all prospective parents to identify families that may need special help with caring for their infant (Table 5–2).

Follow-Up Care

Some hospitals, birthing centers, and community health agencies offer telephone follow-up or home visits to provide support during the transition to parenthood.

TABLE 5-2
Concerns Confronting New Parents

Practical

Family Income

- Baby clothing and equipment expenses
- Fewer shared decisions on economic issues
- Less money available to spend on "couple" activities
- Loss of income due to spouse's leave from work
- Economic responsibility imposed by arrival of baby
- Child care expenses

Household Tasks

- Conflict over amount of sharing in household tasks
- Conflict over amount of sharing in child care tasks
- Balancing demands of spouse, housework/job, and child
- Feeling too busy, having too much to do
- Amount of time and energy required to care for baby

Personal

Physical Affection

- Having sexual play
- Concern that sexual intercourse will never be the same due to physical changes resulting from the birth process
- Reduced spontaneity of sexual relationships
- Reduced leisureliness of sexual relations
- Beginning sexual intercourse again
- Return of my/my wife's figure
- Discomfort from stitches (episiotomy) will interfere with sexual pleasure
- Methods of birth control
- Breast soreness will interfere with sexual pleasure

Empathy

- Spouse will not understand my moodiness, depression, tension
- Emotional tension
- Feeling tied down
- Husband will feel excluded from family life due to breastfeeding
- Husband will feel excluded from family life due to work schedule
- Feeling "blue," "depressed," "down"
- Conflict (about baby) with in-laws will cause conflict with spouse

Companionship

- Less time for shared leisure activity with spouse
- Level of social activity (as a couple) will change
- Less communication with spouse
- Less time to be alone with spouse
- Activities will have to be worked around baby's schedule
- Communication with spouse will be centered on baby
- Little time/energy to devote to giving special attention to spouse
- Spouse will be less stimulating intellectually

From Broom, B. L. (1984). Consensus about the marital relationship during transition to parenthood. Copyright 1984 The American Journal of Nursing Company. Reprinted from *Nursing Research*, July/August, 1984, *33*, 223–228. Used with permission. All rights reserved.

When nurses make the initial follow-up phone call, they have the maternal and infant Kardex care plans, plus the postpartum follow-up care plan, in front of them. They assess the mother's psychosocial adjustment; knowledge of health concepts including nutrition, hygiene, sexual matters, rest, and activity; understanding of basic infant care, feeding, hygiene, safety, growth, and nurturing; maternal attachment; paternal engrossment (process of father identifying and claiming the infant as his, focusing attention and investing emotionally in the baby); and the nature of parental expectations for this baby.

During the home visit, the nurse typically performs physical examinations of the mother and infant, weighs and measures the infant, draws blood samples and obtains laboratory specimens if indicated, assesses parenting skill, and encourages questions about infant care and the mother's self-care. Nurses also discuss family role adjustments associated with the birth of the new infant. Discussion with the mother about the defining characteristics that contribute to her role strain and use of appropriate coping responses can be of assistance. Information on contacting and assessing child care arrangements can be provided. Discussion of strategies to utilize available social support resources, if not used already, can assist in alleviating role strain. During follow-up the nurse is committed to promoting confidence, competence, and independence among families. This is done by nurturing their growth and strengths. This type of program provides much support and professional help to new parents.

Nurses should be aware of professional and community sources of support to which they can refer clients. An informed referral should be based on an assessment of needs and an evaluation of the service offered (Gosha & Brucker, 1986). Nurses can systematically obtain data from clients regarding the value of services received and keep those data on file to use in future referrals.

Providing Support

Nurses in contact with families with an infant may find themselves in a good position to fulfill a strong nurturing, supportive role. The beginning goal should be to establish a helping relationship with the mother and concentrate on her needs. Identifying observed family strengths rather than focusing on problems will contribute to the support the family members feel. Parents' strengths are the qualities that can be relied on as they cope and for which they do not need the professional's help. What the professional health care worker can offer is support and encouragement for their strengths.

One of the nurse's greatest contributions to relieving stress related to the family's division of labor is the promotion of open communication. If the family members are not able to discuss their feelings on this topic, the nurse can help by asking questions, interpreting feelings, and facilitating decision making.

Accommodating the Infant

The adaptation of resources to accommodate the infant cannot be prescribed generally because the resources available to families vary extensively. However, some basic considerations in the decision making include individuals' needs for privacy, personal attention, and finances, as well as the need for family planning.

Providing Space for Individual and Couple Privacy. Providing space for privacy may be difficult in some settings. During the early days at home with an infant, parents often find it convenient to keep the infant's bed near their own because of the baby's need for care at night. However, when the baby begins to sleep through the night, it is advisable for parents to get some distance from the infant. Physically, distance means that parents are not disturbed by normal baby noises and movement and the baby is not disturbed by parental voices and movements. Psychologically, the distance provided by moving the baby's bed outside the parents' room gives the parents a sense of privacy for intimacy and for a respite from the demands of the family. When separate rooms are not possible, portable screens or dividers may be useful.

Each family member should be allowed to have some space that is his or her own to arrange, keep "treasures" in, and go to for time alone. Although this may not necessarily be an entire room, even some section of a room can be useful.

For the mother who regularly is at home caring for the infant and possibly other children, the greatest sense of privacy may come when she is relieved of all household and child care responsibilities for a period of time to go outside the home and do what she pleases. Time away from home may also be the best arrangement for the couple to have some privacy if someone can provide child care. Recognizing the need for time alone and a place for each individual to call his or her own can stimulate creative planning and be one factor in establishing a stable family unit.

Providing for Individual Attention. Finding a time and place for each family member's privacy may be difficult, but equally difficult is finding time to give attention to each family member. The importance of maintenance of existing family relationships has been discussed previously. Ways parents can maintain loving relationships with their children, and wives or husbands with their mates, have also been presented.

Adapting Financial Resources. Another significant adjustment that many families face upon the birth of an infant is in the financial realm. Few young families can escape the burden of needing to plan very carefully for adequate funds for their needs. The many expenses that accompany the birth experience and the needs of the infant can often strain the family budget.

Financial management is always a challenge that requires self-discipline and some maturity to handle successfully. The family that experienced financial problems before the birth (e.g., poverty; unemployment; mismanagement due to gambling, or alcohol or substance abuse) may be at special risk. *Although nurses cannot provide financial security for any family, they should be aware of and sensitive to the importance of financial resources as a family or single mother adapts to a new infant.* If the neonate has been born with problems that require hospitalization or other medical care at home, the cost of care is another stress on the family.

For additional information on families refer to Chapters 2 and 11.

Growth and Development of the Infant

Perhaps no single event in human growth and development requires the number of adjustments that the birth of a baby requires in the life of a family. The new responsibilities associated with the infant require that all members in the infant's family adopt some new roles. The addition of parental or sibling roles creates critical role transition periods while each family member works out an accommodation among new and old roles. What these new roles are perceived to be and how they are internalized varies according to the individual's own experiences, feelings, and needs.

The nurse must incorporate many interrelated aspects of growth and development while promoting the health of the infant within the family. The nurse provides information to parents and reinforces their self-confidence in caring for their infants. Table 5–3 contains a summary of infant growth and development.

Nurses providing care to the infant, whether in the hospital or community setting, will consider the nursing diagnosis *high risk for altered growth and development* an integral component of care (Table 5–4).

TABLE 5-3
Summary of Infant Growth, Development, and Health Maintenance

Physical Competency	Emotional-Social Competency	Intellectual Competency
1 to 2 Mos		
Holds head in alignment when prone; Moro reflex to loud sound; follows objects; smiles	Gratification through sucking and basic needs being promptly met; smiles at people	Reflex activity; vowel sounds produced
2 to 4 Mos		
Turns back to side; raises head and chest 45–90° off bed and supports weight on arms; reaches for objects; follows object through midline; drools; begins to localize sounds; prefers configuration of face	Social responsiveness; awareness of those who are not primary caregiver; smiles in response to familiar face	Reproduces behavior initially achieved by random activity; imitates behavior previously done. Visually studies objects; locates sounds; makes cooing sounds; does not look for objects removed from presence
4 to 6 Mos		
Birthweight doubled; teeth eruption may begin; sits with stable head and back control; rolls from abdomen to back; picks up object with palmar grasp	Prefers primary caregiver; sucking needs decrease; laughs in pleasure	Some intentional actions; some sense of object permanence, looks on same path for vanished object; recognizes partially hidden objects; more systematic in imitative behavior; babbles
6 to 8 Mos		
Turns back to stomach; sits alone; crawls; transfers objects from hand to hand; turns to sound behind	Differentiated response to nonprimary caretakers; evidence of "stranger" or "separation" anxiety	Continued development as in 4–6 mos
8 to 10 Mos		
Creeps; pulls to stand; pincer grasp	Attachment process complete	Actions more goal-directed; able to solve simple problems by using previously mastered responses. Actively searches for an object that disappears
10 to 12 Mos		
Birthweight tripled; cruises; stands by self; may use spoon	Begins to explore and separate briefly from parent	Begins to imitate behavior done before but not seen self do. Understands words being said; may say one to four words. Intentionality is present.

TABLE 5-3
Summary of Infant Growth, Development, and Health Maintenance *(Continued)*

Nutrition	Play	Safety
1 to 2 Mos		
Breastfed or fortified formula	Variety of positions. Caretaker should hold and talk to infant; large; brightly colored objects	Car carrier; proper use of infant seat
2 to 4 Mos		
As for 1–2 mos	Talk to and hold. Musical toys; rattle, mobile. Variety of objects of different color, size and texture; mirror, crib toys, variety of settings	Do not leave unattended on couch, bed, etc. Remove any small objects that infant could choke on
4 to 6 Mos		
Introduction of solids; initial store of iron depleted	Talk to and hold. Provide open space to move and objects to grasp	Keep environment free of safety hazards; check toys for sharp edges and small pieces that might break
6 to 8 Mos		
Introduce finger foods; begin use of cup	Provide place to explore. Stack toys, blocks; nursery rhymes	Check infant's expanding environment for hazards
8 to 10 Mos		
As for 6–8 mos	Games: hide-and-seek, peek-a-boo, pat-a-cake, looking at pictures in a book	Keep: electrical outlets plugged, cords out of reach, stairs blocked, coffee and end tables cleared of hazards Do not leave alone in a bathtub Keep poisons out of reach and locked Continue use of safety seat in car
10 to 12 Mos		
More solids than liquids; increasing use of cup; begin to wean	Increase space; read to infant. Name and point to body parts. Water; sand play; ball	As for 8–10 mos

Other diagnoses the nurse may consider when caring for the infant and family are *high risk for altered parenting* and *high risk for injury and disturbance in self-concept: role performance*. The nurse will continually assess the infant and family members for the etiology of the actual response, the risk factors associated with potential problems, and the defining characteristics of nursing diagnoses.

Physical Competency

The development of physical competency in the infant covers many aspects of his or her life. It is this competency that many people use to judge the infant's health and, indirectly, the competence of the family as caregivers. Although competency is not the only measure of health, it is useful to explore this competency in some depth, because it does significantly affect the infant's total functioning.

Height and Weight

From birth through the first year of the infant's life, one of the first questions asked is "How much does the baby weigh?" The rate of growth of the infant is usually more important than the actual height and weight (see height and weight charts, Appendices 2 and 3). Birth weight is generally doubled by 4 to 6 months and tripled by 1 year of age. Height increases about 50 per cent in the first year of life. No accurate predictions can be made about the infant's ultimate height and weight from the absolute or percentile height and weight figures of infancy.

TABLE 5-4

Growth and Development Plan: Families with Infants

Analysis: Nursing Diagnostic Statement

Response and Related or Risk Factors: *High risk for altered growth and development; risk factors*

- Illness/physical impairment
- Treatment-related procedures (isolation, injections, painful intrusive procedures)
- Prolonged pain
- Separation from caregiver(s)/(parents and significant others)
- Inadequate, inappropriate caregiver support (abuse and neglect)
- Restriction of activity
- Change in environment
- Inability to trust
- Inadequate sensory stimulation
- Caregiver anxiety
- Multiple caregivers
- Caregiver knowledge deficit
- Sleep deprivation

Projected Outcome: The infant will demonstrate acquisition of developmentally appropriate behaviors in the physical, intellectual, and emotional-social domains

Defining Characteristics

Subjective:

- Child demonstrates language delays in cooing, babbling and utterance of two-syllable words

Objective:

- Flat affect
- Listlessness
- Decreased responses
- Slow in social responses
- Alters gaze
- Holds body stiffly when held
- Shows limited signs of satisfaction to caregiver(s)
- Difficulty in feeding
- Decreased appetite
- Lethargic
- Irritable
- Interrupted sleep pattern
- Watchfulness
- Disturbed parent-infant attachment
- Caregiver inability to provide appropriate stimulation

Nursing Interventions

Health Screening

- **Assess factors that can identify altered growth and development.** Evidence of infant's behavior deviation from age-appropriate levels will be observed and documented according to theoretical basis of growth and development, and parent-infant attachment
- **Assess infant's level of development using developmental norms and specific assessment tools.** Refer to Chapter 13, Assessing Child Health, and Appendices 2 through 6

Parent Education: Childrearing Family

- Provide consistent, predictable care to foster trust

Anticipatory Guidance; Attachment Promotion; Family Involvement

- **Provide anticipatory guidance to caregiver(s) regarding acquisition of age-appropriate developmental tasks.** Refer to information on developmental norms in Chapter 5

Evaluation Criteria

- **Any developmental delays will be identified as evidenced by:**
  - Charted assessment of screening for developmental progress
  - Referral for deviation from the norm detected during screening
- Infant will achieve developmental milestones
- Caregivers will demonstrate an ability to foster attachment with the infant
- Caregivers will provide appropriate levels of stimulation
- Referral to community agencies will be made

TABLE 5-4 (continued)

Growth and Development Plan: Families with Infants

Defining Characteristics	Nursing Interventions	Evaluation Criteria
	Anticipatory Guidance; Attachment Promotion: Family Involvement • **Encourage parents to participate in infant's care (i.e., bathing, feeding, holding, cuddling)** • Assist parents to provide ongoing, appropriate levels and types of sensory stimulation *Support System Enhancement* • **Refer infant and family to appropriate community agencies as needed** • Refer to appropriate agency for supportive services • Refer to community programs specific to factors affecting the infant's altered growth and development (early intervention services, Women, Infants, and Children [WIC]) Food Supplemental Program	

Anticipatory Guidance: Height and Weight

Sharing information from growth charts with the family can be a useful teaching tool in pointing out some of the factors affecting growth. The nurse can clearly identify the infant's pattern of growth as well as the actual height and weight. Reassurance that the infant is growing at an appropriate rate, if such is the case, is an important nursing intervention. Further assessment is indicated if there has been significant change in the usual weight percentile or a slower consistent change upward or downward. An infant who is consistently above the 97th percentile in weight or below the 3rd percentile needs to be assessed more fully.

General Appearance and Skeletal Growth

The body proportions of the infant are also changing. The head is most developed at birth. The trunk and legs are not as fully developed as the head but begin to slowly catch up with head growth during the first year. By 6 months of age, the thorax circumference may be larger than the head circumference, although there is great variability in this ratio.

Head Circumference

The brain grows faster than do other tissues and organs during infancy. Rapid brain growth results from an increase in both cell number and cell size. Because the cranial bones have not completely fused, fontanels and cranial sutures are still open. This allows for growth of the skull as the brain expands. In fact, the growth rate of the skull is mainly determined by the growth rate of the brain. Growth of the skull, as determined by increasing head circumference, is a much more accurate index of brain growth than is the presence or size of fontanels (Behrman, 1992). The anterior fontanel normally closes by 12 to 18 months and the posterior fontanel by 2 months. The size and shape of the fontanel may be affected by conditions other than the rate of brain growth, such as hydration and intracranial pressure.

The head circumference is an important measurement in the physical assessment of the infant. The circumference of the head increases from an average of 35 cm at birth to 47 cm at 1 year (Vaughan & Litt, 1990). The use of head circumference charts is valuable in determining the absolute growth as well as the rate of growth of the skull. Deviations from the normal pattern need to be assessed in detail by a physician.

Anticipatory Guidance: Head Circumference

While measuring the head circumference the nurse has an opportunity to point out to the family why this measurement is being taken. This is also a good time to reiterate the information that the fontanel, which may be referred to as the "soft spot," is covered by a very strong membrane, so there is no substance to the common belief that the brain can be damaged by touching the area. Since the young infant's skull is pliable, the skull may be flattened if the infant spends a great deal of time in the same position. This flattening does not cause brain damage and usually is gradually corrected as the skull continues to grow and the infant spends more and more time with the head erect. If the infant's head has become flattened and the hair rubbed off in one spot, the nurse should explore in more detail the infant's daily routine: these signs may be a clue that the infant is spending a majority of the day in the same position. This, in turn, *might* suggest a lack of parental attention to the infant. The nurse should offer suggestions about positioning the infant on the back, on the side, and in a sitting position. Placement of colorful stimuli in a variety of locations can stimulate infants to turn themselves at the age of 5 to 6 months.

Oral Maturation

Mature sucking, which occurs at about 16 weeks of age, is an acquired function of the orofacial muscles with the tongue moving back and forth. The oral cavity is growing larger so that the tongue no longer fills the mouth. The tongue is growing differentially at the tip. These two features allow the tongue more mobility. The longer tongue can be protruded to receive and pass food between the gum pads and erupting teeth, allowing mastication (Pipes, 1985). Around 24 to 28 weeks the up-and-down movement of the jaw occurs.

Motor Development

The rapid development of neuromuscular control is an extremely important aspect of physical competency. The maturation of the central nervous system provides progressively better control and integration of muscular movements throughout the first year of life.

The infant's motor development is inextricably interrelated with cognitive and emotional-social competencies. The infant learns about and interacts with the world through increasing motor abilities. The two major motor tasks that the infant must learn are upright postural control or locomotion, and fine motor manipulation, including prehension or grasping. Even though the age when each motor skill is attained may differ among babies, all will follow the same sequence.

Upright Postural Control or Locomotion

The sequence of motor skills involved in the achievement of upright postural control or locomotion is a visible example of the principle that states that growth and development proceed in a cephalocaudal direction. (See Fig. 3–9.)

Head Control. One of the major motor tasks of early infancy is head control, which is necessary for the infant to sit and eventually to walk. Head control develops in the following order:

Birth	Turns head when prone.
↓	Holds head up momentarily while prone.
	Holds head 45 to 95 degrees while prone.
	Holds head in fairly good control in a variety of positions.
	No head lag when pulled to sit.
4 months	Sits with stable head and back control.

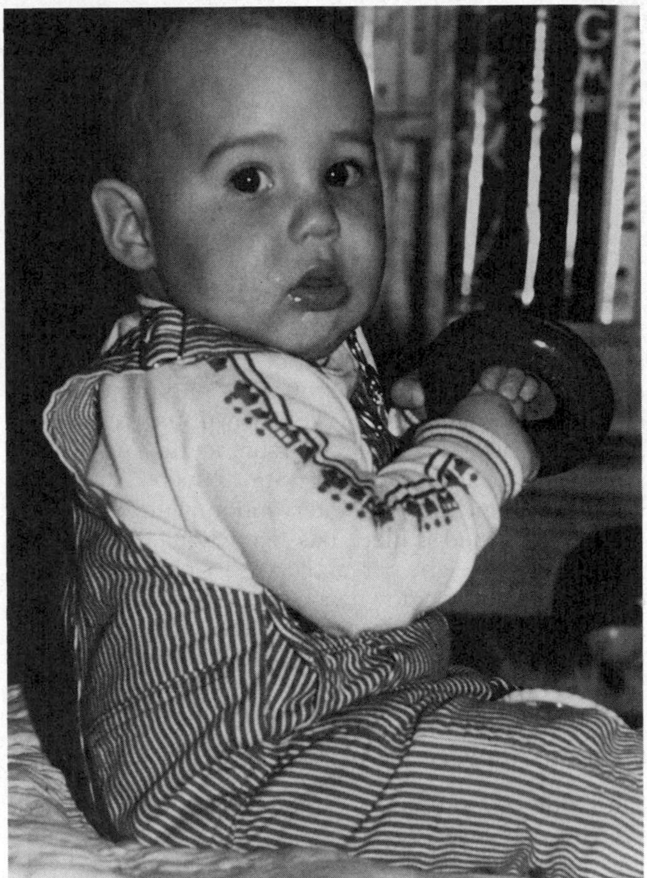

FIGURE 5 - 1. At 7 to 8 mos, the infant can sit alone without support. To do so, the infant must be able to sit with the back straight.

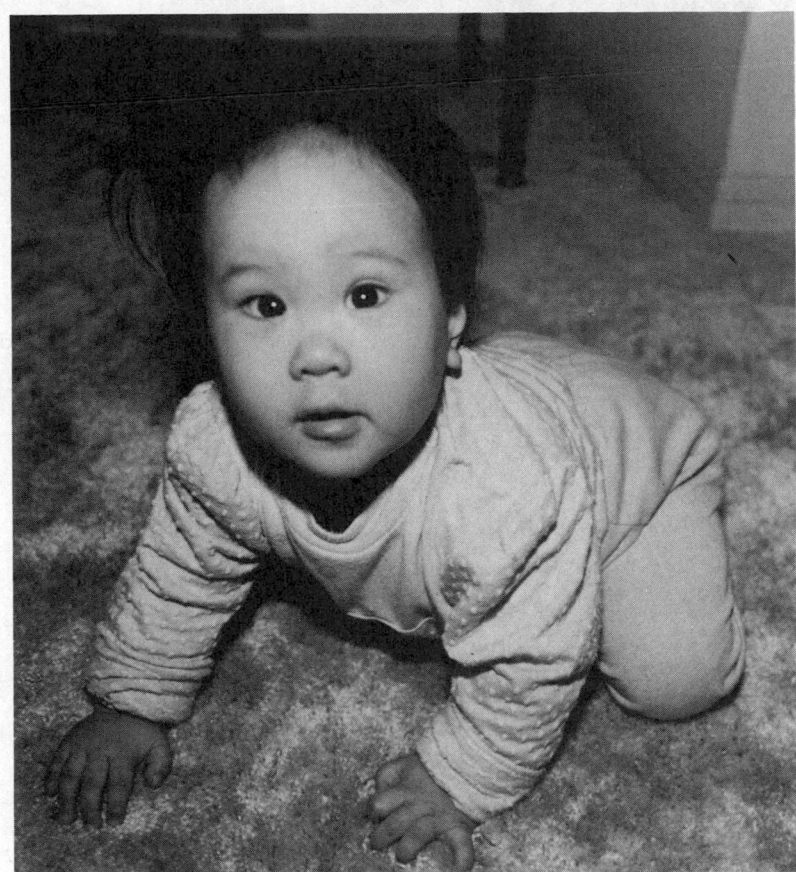

FIGURE 5-2. Creeping is one of the incremental steps that the infant masters in learning to walk.

Sitting. Another important skill is sitting alone. Infants must achieve head control before they can sit alone. The ability to sit alone develops gradually from 4 to 8 months (Fig. 5–1):

4 months	Sits with support.
6 months	Sits alone momentarily with own hand for support.
7 months	Sits alone briefly.
8 months	Sits without support.

Locomotion. During this same period infants are learning a variety of locomotion skills that will prepare them for walking. The ability to roll over develops from approximately 2 to 6 or 7 months:

2 months	Rolls from side to back.
4 months	Rolls from back to side.
5 to 6 months	Rolls from abdomen to side.
6 to 7 months	Rolls from back to stomach.

Many infants use this rolling ability to get from one place to another, and may be able to move about much farther than the parent or nurse expects.

Another means of locomotion is hitching or scooting (moving along while sitting up), which appears at about 6 months. Crawling (wriggling on abdomen, pulling with arms) usually appears by 8 months. Creeping (on hands, knees, with trunk off floor) usually appears by 9 months (Fig. 5–2). Some infants may use hitching or crawling as a substitute for creeping and progress to walking without creeping. At about 10 months of age infants begin to pull themselves to a standing position (Fig. 5–3) and soon stand with assistance. They then begin to cruise around furniture (walking sideways while holding onto supporting object).

Once the infant is able to stand alone it is usually not long (about 1 month) before he or she attempts to walk unassisted. The average infant can walk alone well by 15 months. Throughout the first year of life the infant has mastered many incremental steps in learning to walk (Fig. 5–4).

Fine Motor Manipulation

The infant is also rapidly developing fine motor skills that greatly assist in manipulating her or his environment. Fine motor development is complex and involves eye-to-hand coordination. Fine motor skills, as with other aspects of physical competency, seem to occur in an orderly sequence.

Prehension or Grasping. One of the fine motor skills to be developed is that of grasping an object. The sequence of skills involved in the development

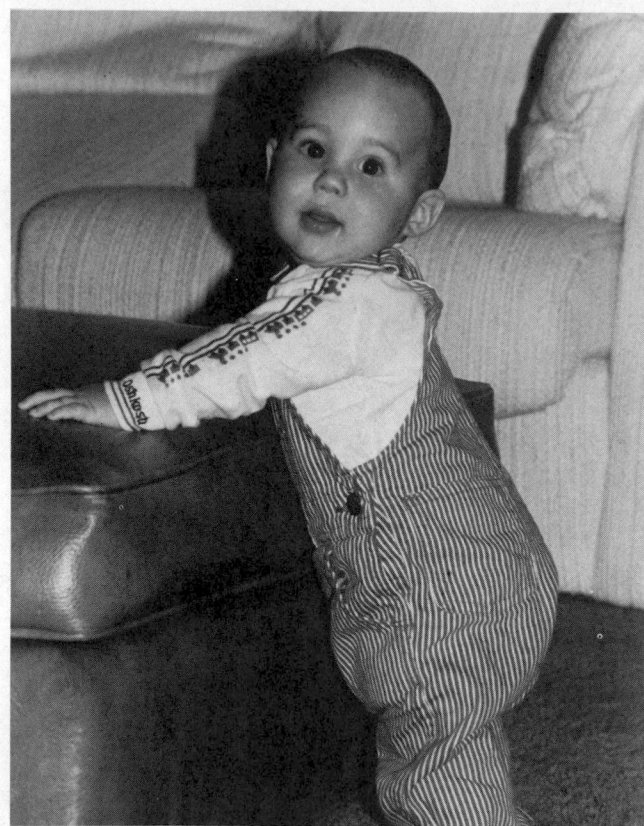

FIGURE 5 - 3. The infant of 7 to 8 mos can stand for short periods with support.

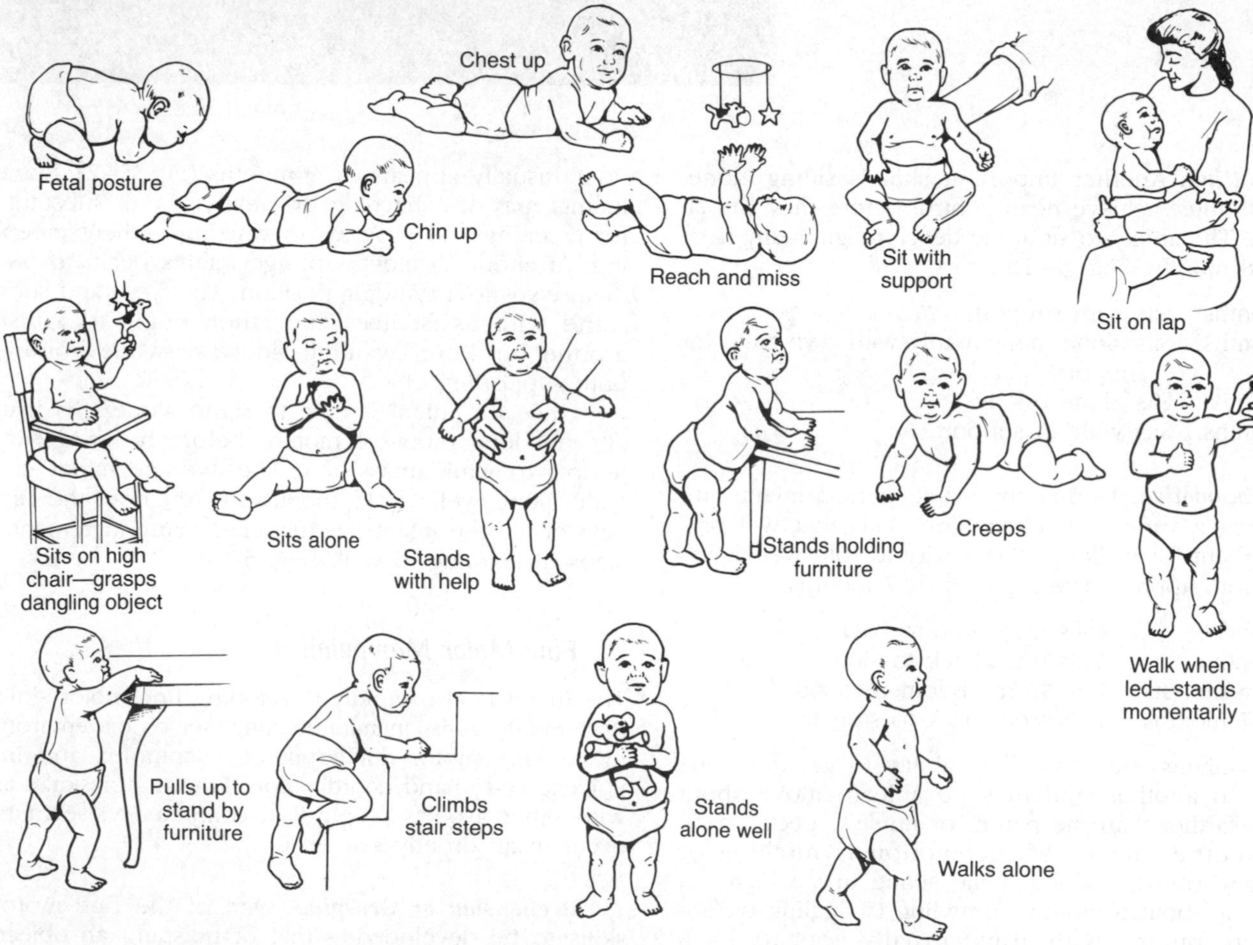

FIGURE 5 - 4. The sequence of motor skill development from initial reflexes to independent walking. Although timing varies from one child to another (in the age range from 9 mos to 15 mos), the sequence of development is always the same.

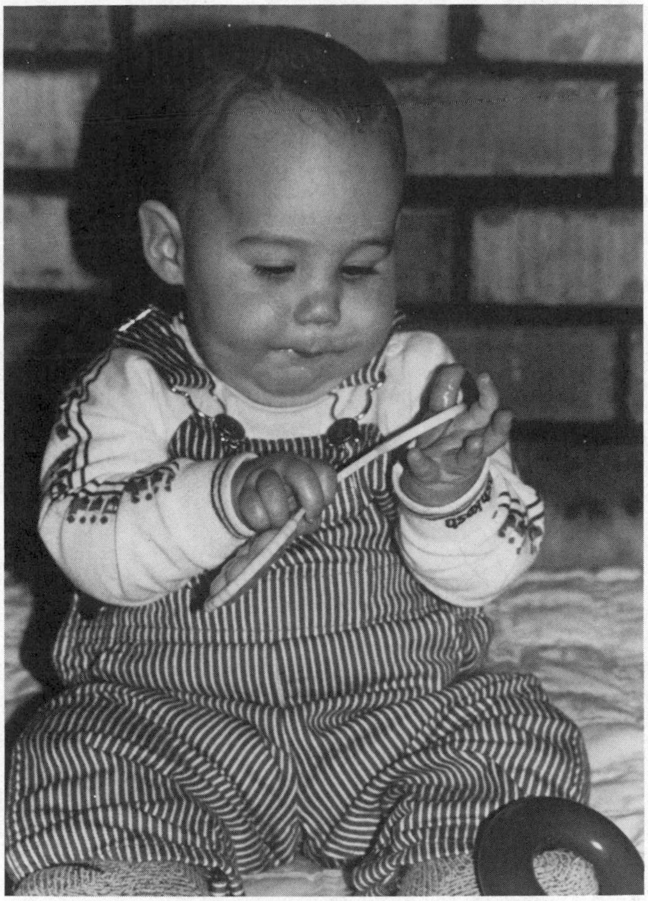

FIGURE 5-5. The infant of 6 to 7 mos can transfer objects between hands.

of the ability to grasp provides an example of the general to specific and proximal to distal principles of growth and development.

The neonate has a grasp reflex that gradually gives way to an intentional grasp. Before this skill has developed it may appear to the parents that the infant actually has lost a skill she or he once had. Alerting parents to the normal sequence of this developmental task can be reassuring to them.

The sequence of events in development of the infant's ability to grasp is as follows:

3 months	Object placed in hands retained briefly.
4 months	Reaches for objects and picks them up with raking action of fingers.
6 months	Picks up objects deftly with palmar grasp.
6 to 7 months	Transfers objects from hand to hand. Bangs objects together. (Fig. 5–5).
8 to 9 months	Pincer grasp developed.

The infant develops the visual skill to follow objects past midline by 2 or 3 months of age. She or he is usually able to follow objects through 180 degrees by the age of 3 to 4 months. This skill, in combination with the neonate's increasing skill of grasping objects, gives the infant ever-increasing ability to manipulate the environment (Fig. 5–6).

Nursing Interventions: Motor Development

Nurses who work with children in health care settings include consideration of all aspects of development in their plan of care. Safety factors in relation to the child's motor development will influence decisions regarding positioning. The nurse who is aware of the importance of motor development will be more likely to provide for supervised removal of restraints whenever possible and allow for motor movement of extremities.

If locomotion will be restricted for extended periods because of treatment devices such as casts and braces, the nurse can encourage exploration of the environment by placing the child in a wagon or cart and by moving the crib to other areas such as the playroom.

Anticipatory Guidance: Motor Development

Nurses can help parents explore ways to promote the motor development of their infant.

Specific suggestions can be made as to how to promote head control. The infant can be periodically placed in a prone position; he or she will be able to lift the head more easily in this position. This assists development of the necessary muscles for head control.

The infant also needs to have an opportunity to be placed in a sitting position and to practice holding the head erect. Once the head is fairly steady in the sitting position, pulling the infant to a sitting position will promote further development of head control and the ability to sit. In order to further develop the ability to sit alone, the infant needs the opportunity to practice with gradually decreasing support as he or she becomes more stable.

As locomotion is developing, the infant again needs the opportunity to try out and practice these skills. Placing the infant on the floor and allowing space to move will promote development of the various locomotion skills. Keeping the infant confined to a playpen or walker does not allow sufficient opportunity for turning, rolling, and eventually creeping. As the infant progresses in readiness to pull to a standing position he or she needs opportunities to do so. The playpen can provide this opportunity, as can safe, sturdy pieces of furniture that have no sharp edges. The infant needs the opportunity to practice the skills of cruising around items and eventually walking. There is some controversy over the use of "walkers" in this period. Used for short periods several times a day, the walker may assist the infant in some skills, such as use of leg muscles and balance. However, walkers can limit the developing locomotion and exploratory skills of infants if used in place

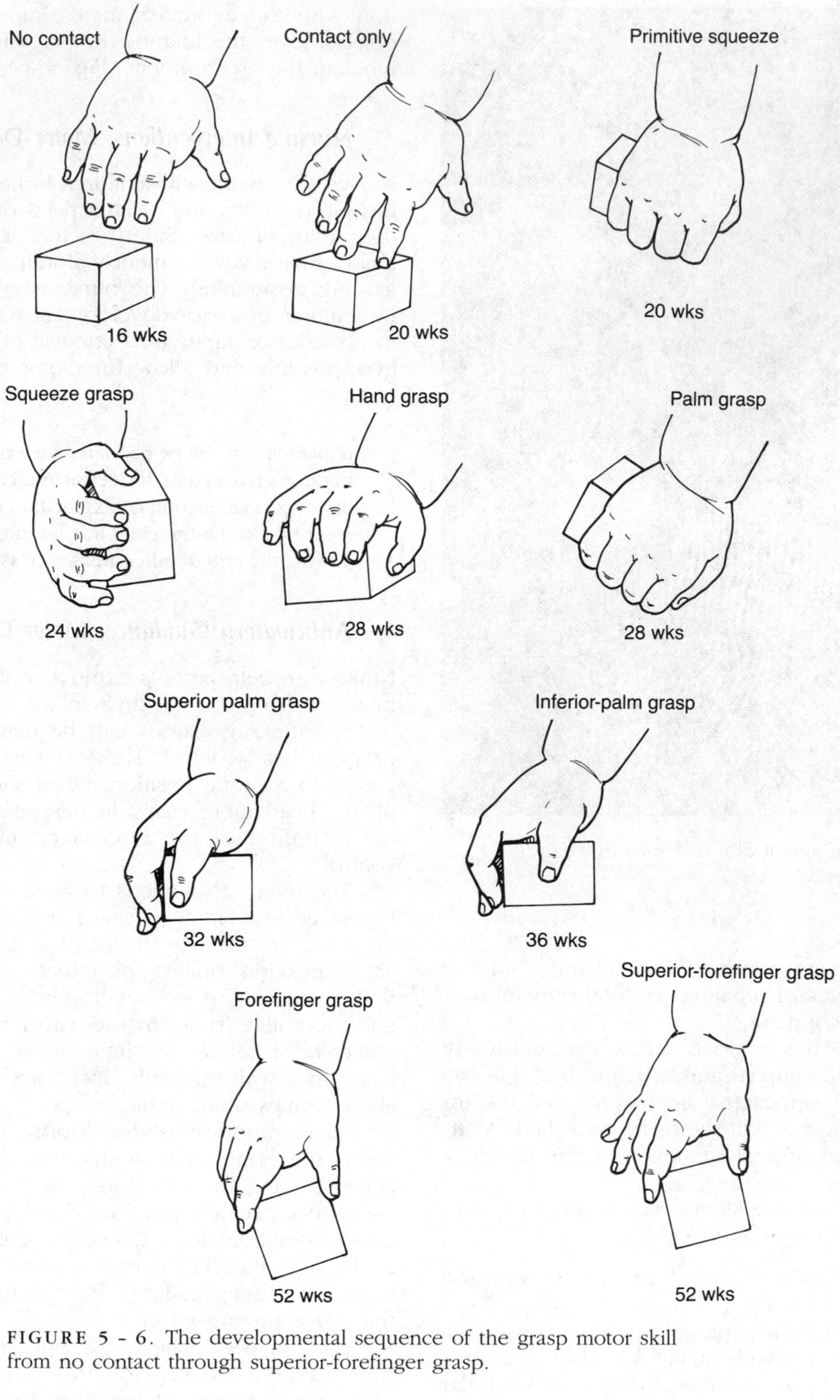

FIGURE 5 - 6. The developmental sequence of the grasp motor skill from no contact through superior-forefinger grasp.

of opportunities for crawling, cruising, and walking on their own. In addition, the use of walkers is accompanied by hazards such as tipping over, rolling down stairs, and so forth.

There are a variety of ways that parents can promote their infant's fine motor development. In order to develop the infant's grasp, attractive objects can be presented within reach by 3 to 4 months. Chapter 17 describes age-appropriate objects for infant stimulation. These objects also encourage the infant to develop the skill of banging objects together and transferring them from hand to hand. To encourage the pincer grasp as the infant approaches 9 months, smaller objects need to be provided, but with supervision to prevent aspiration. Giving the infant dry cereals for self-feeding can be one mechanism to promote the pincer grasp.

At the same time, the infant can be given activities to stimulate development of the ability to follow objects and further increase eye-hand coordination. The placement of mobiles and brightly colored objects within the infant's range of vision is useful. Many of the same objects that promote grasp also can be used to promote hand-eye coordination. Placing the infant in a variety of settings and positions stimulates him or her to look at and reach for new objects. Expensive toys are not necessary; items commonly found in the home can be used such as colorful plastic cups.

Intellectual Competency

Another major competency area that undergoes rapid change in the infancy period is intellectual development. There are a number of factors in intellectual development that are essential for the nurse to be aware of while assessing the growth, development, and total health status of the infant.

Intelligence

Questions are often raised about the feasibility of measuring infant intelligence. Intelligence is a difficult concept to define and measure, especially for infants. Since infants do not have command of language, they cannot be tested for thinking or reasoning. Their range of behaviors is limited. In addition, their motivation cannot be controlled. There is almost no predictability between an infant's score on various infant intelligence tests and scores on intelligence tests given later. This may be because tests for infants measure behavior and tests for older children can measure additional cognitive processes. Tests such as the Bayley Scale of Infant Development (1965) are useful in finding deviations from normal development.

Cognitive Development: Sensorimotor Period

The infant is in the sensorimotor stage as described by Piaget (1952, 1970). The infant progresses from responding primarily through reflex activity to beginning to organize sensorimotor activities in relation to the environment. Piaget used the term *sensorimotor period* to describe the processes by which the infant learns during this period of time, namely through gross and fine motor movement and the use of senses.

The concept of *object permanence* is an important achievement of the sensorimotor period. The permanent object has a reality of its own and continues to exist even though the infant cannot see, hear, feel, taste, or smell it. Within the sensorimotor stage Piaget outlines six substages in the development of the concept of object permanency. Four of these substages are usually developed in the first year of life (Table 5–5). The first substage (0 to 1 month), *use of reflexes,* is a period basically consisting of reflex activity that allows the infant to adapt and survive. Learning occurs in this substage but is confined to the sphere of reflexes. The second substage (1 to 4 months) is characterized as that of *primary circular reactions.* At this time the infant makes an active effort to reproduce a behavior that is initially achieved by random activity. The behavior must have some value to the baby, such as the pleasure produced by placing her or his thumb in the mouth. Another example is when the infant accidentally shakes a toy, producing an interesting sound; the infant can then be observed actively trying to reproduce both of these behaviors. Infants study objects, including faces, during this period. They begin to develop hand-eye coordination. As activities of looking and grasping begin to extend infants' environments, they are attracted to objects that are moderately novel. Piaget believes that the curiosity of infants at this stage is stimulated by objects that are not too familiar to them. However, an object that is completely foreign to infants does not seem to attract them as readily, perhaps because they cannot relate it to anything with which they are familiar, and therefore it has little meaning to them. Piaget called this phenomenon the principle of *moderate novelty.* Infants (1 to 4 months) have not developed a true concept of object permanence. When an object is removed from their presence they do not look for it; it is as if the object no longer exists. This can be seen clearly when the infant is being held and is attracted to the eyeglasses of the adult. If the adult removes the glasses and places them behind a book on the table the infant does not look for the glasses but moves on to some other activity.

More recent research has revealed that infants demonstrate rudimentary awareness of object permanence as early as 3.5 months of age (Baillargeon, 1987; Baillargeon & DeVos, 1991). The infants demonstrated awareness that an object was hidden, indicating their ability to both represent and reason about the hidden object. Several months later the infants were capable of accurately searching for the hidden object. These findings reveal that the infant has far more advanced cognitive capabilities than was previously acknowledged.

The third substage (4 to 8 months) is described as that of *secondary circular reactions.* Infants are now beginning to show evidence of intentional action. Their horizons are expanding and their reactions involve events in the external environment. Infants are becoming interested in the results of their actions. They have perceived an interesting external result from an accidental movement, and, connecting the results to their actions, they want to repeat the result. One can note this particular sequence as the infant accidentally knocks over a tower of blocks, expresses

TABLE 5-5
Summary of Cognitive Achievements During Infancy

	Causality	*Object Permanence*	*Imitation*	*Object in Space*
Substage 1: Use of reflexes; reflex activity				
Substage 2: Primary circular reactions	Makes active effort to repeat pleasurable activity (e.g., sucks thumb)	"Out of sight out of mind," moderate novelty	Imitates actions that have been spontaneously performed before (e.g., cooing)	Begins to develop hand-eye coordination
Substage 3: Secondary circular reactions	Evidence of intentional action Interested in results of actions Begins to differentiate means from ends	Under special circumstances, will look for missing object Recognizes and seeks partially hidden objects	Imitates those acts that he or she has been able to watch himself or herself do (e.g., clap hands)	
Substage 4: Coordination of secondary schema	Goal-directed activity; can apply previously learned behavior to new situations; can coordinate two behaviors to achieve a desired outcome (push and grab)	Realizes object exists even though visual perception of it changes; will search for object that disappears	Imitates actions that he or she has done before but has never watched himself or herself do (e.g., form facial expression)	

pleasure, and repeats the action over and over. Given the opportunity, infants learn to prolong an interesting activity. They have become interested in their external environment and are beginning to have an impact on it. They are gradually differentiating between means and ends. Secondary circular reactions do have limitations in that they are not fully intentional; with them, infants do not attempt to invent new behaviors. For instance, in the block episode, the infant does not build the tower initially for the purpose of knocking it over.

During this substage (4 to 8 months), the infant makes progress in the formation of the concept of object permanence, but it is far from the mature concept. Infants indicate by various behaviors that they have some sense of object permanence. They begin to look for objects that have disappeared, but only under special conditions. The searching behavior must lead to early discovery of the lost object, or it ceases. Infants do not pause and renew the search for the object. This behavior seems to relate to the infant's own actions rather than to the independent individual existence of the object. Another indication of some progress in the concept of object permanence is the infant's ability to recognize and seek objects that are partially hidden. A favorite toy partially covered by a blanket will now attract the infant's attention.

Substage four (8 to 12 months) is that *of coordination of secondary circular reactions* and their application to new situations. Infants' actions now are becoming increasingly goal-directed. They can solve simple problems by using responses they have previously mastered. If an obstacle arises that prevents the infant from attaining his or her goals, new means for removing the obstacle must be developed in order to achieve the desired end. The new means developed by the infant have limitations. The infant can generalize patterns of previously learned behavior, modify them slightly, and coordinate two secondary behaviors to achieve the desired ends by removing the obstacle. An example of this kind of activity is seen when an older sibling grabs a toy away from the infant. The infant may initially just try to grab randomly for the object. Soon, however, he or she will first push aside the sibling's hand and then grab the toy. The infant has not invented new means (behaviors) but has coordinated two previously learned behaviors: those of pushing aside a hand and grasping a toy. The infant has removed an obstacle (the hand) to achieve the end (holding the toy).

A number of types of learning are a part of the infant's developing intellectual competency. *Imitative learning* seems to be one of the most important types during infancy. A number of investigators, including Piaget and Uzgiris, have explored the steps in the development of imitative behavior and have arrived at similar sequences. By about 3 months old, infants imitate certain behaviors, but only those that they have previously spontaneously performed themselves (such as cooing). Around 4 to 8 months, infants become more systematic in their imitative behavior. They are more interested in the action of others. As they develop more behaviors of their own, they are capable of imitating more behaviors. Infants still imitate only those acts they have previously been able to watch themselves do (such as clapping their hands). At times, it appears as if they will imitate only enough

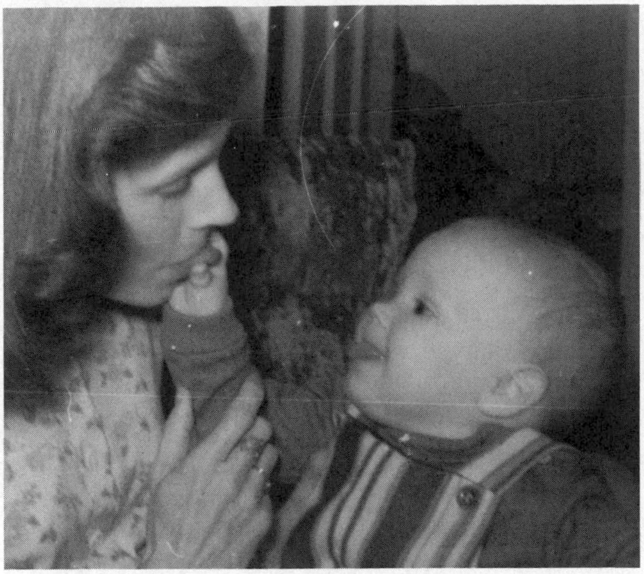

FIGURE 5-7. By 10 mos, the infant can imitate facial expressions. (Photograph by David Trainor.)

of the behavior to get the other person to repeat the behavior.

By 10 to 12 months, infants have made progress in their use of imitation. They begin to imitate actions that they have done before but never watched themselves do (such as forming facial expressions, Fig. 5–7). They can make a connection between what they see and the corresponding movement of their own body parts. They may begin to imitate new actions. There are limitations in the accuracy of the infants' imitations and their ability to imitate new actions.

Since the late 1960s, there has been a proliferation of research evidence regarding the intellectual competencies of infants. Whereas little was known previously, infant development, including cognitive development, is now a field that supports several specialty journals, textbooks, whole college courses, and other courses of study. For example, very young babies are capable of discriminating between tastes and smells as well as between visual sensory stimuli (Meltzoff, 1985). Babies are able to recognize facial expressions signifying emotions (Nelson, 1987), tend to prefer complex visual stimuli over simple ones, can differentiate between shapes and colors, prefer female voices to male, and have a beginning ability to categorize (Friedrich, 1983). Many of the sensory and cognitive capabilities of the infant have been demonstrated to exist in the fetus (Bernhardt, 1987).

Nursing Interventions: Cognitive Development

Nursing interventions to promote cognitive development must be individually designed to meet the developmental needs of the infant. Using developmental assessment tools, the nurse will assess the infant as a means of identifying the etiologic and risk factors and defining characteristics of the nursing diagnostic response *altered growth and development*. Developmentally appropriate activities and play materials as identified in Table 5–6 and in the anticipatory guidance section will be used to intervene to promote the infant's developmental progress. Additional suggestions for promoting cognitive development can be found in Chapter 17.

Anticipatory Guidance: Cognitive Development

In working with parents, it is appropriate to first assess what parents do know about their infant's development. This baseline of knowledge can be used as the starting point for anticipatory guidance. Research

TABLE 5-6

Promoting Cognitive Development

Annabelle, aged 6 mos, has been hospitalized for several days with RSV infection. She has responded to the medical regimen and her condition has continued to steadily improve. Activities to promote cognitive development found on the nursing care plan include:

Promote and Support Cognitive Development

- Set aside 10–15 mins/day and evening shift to play
- Offer toys to grasp
- Clap hands
- Play hide and seek with object in front of her, under blanket
- Provide rattle/squeeze toy

Encourage Verbalization

- Talk to infant during bath, treatment, and feeding
- Repeat sounds made
- Talk directly in front of infant
- Point to objects and name them
- Read age-appropriate stories
- Encourage mother to also perform these activities

has demonstrated that parents tend to be more accurate in identifying language, social, and motor milestones than in identifying sensory milestones because the former can be more easily recognized by parents (Miller, 1988). Additionally, the nurse must also consider that parents may overestimate their infant's age of mastery, perceiving their own child to be more competent than the "average" child.

1 *to* 4 *Months*. Many of the activities that stimulate development of the infant's physical competency also promote intellectual competency, since this is the sensorimotor period. The infant of 1 to 4 months needs a variety of objects to study. Studies have shown that a positive relationship exists between measures of cognitive competence and the availability of objects for exploration in the home (Power & Chapieski, 1986). Parents need to know that they should introduce new objects into the environment to stimulate this curiosity. Infants need objects to manipulate in order to associate their random activities with specific results. Infants need the opportunity to explore objects fully. These activities will promote development of their sense of object permanence. Infants also need the opportunity to explore and get to know their environment.

4 *to* 8 *Months*. Parents can initiate games with infants to help them develop the concept of object permanence. Hiding and recovering objects, dropping and recovering objects, and hide-and-seek with people are all appropriate activities.

8 *to* 12 *Months*. As infants progress to the next stage, their actions become more goal-directed. Stacking, nesting, and ring games are interesting and challenging to infants. This allows them to perceive connections between events, such as placing a certain block on top of another and building a tower. Toys or household items that can be placed in containers and taken out easily also contribute to infants' goal-directed abilities and development of the concept of object permanence. By this time, because infants do imitate new actions, demonstration by the parents may assist them to learn activities. Infants enjoy imitating facial expressions and body movements. Throughout discussion with parents the nurse should include the rationale for the suggested activities.

In recent years, a controversy has arisen regarding programs to develop infant intellectual competencies early. Programs and centers have been developed to teach reading, math skills, music appreciation, and other topics to babies and very young children. Many parents see these programs as a desirable way to produce an exceptional child. Opponents of these programs argue that overstimulation occurring too early might have an adverse effect on long-term developmental abilities. Parents need guidance to help them to see the drawbacks as well as the benefits of any program. They need to consider whether the program under consideration allows the baby time and opportunity to experience and explore the environment spontaneously, as well as rest periods from intense stimulation. Additionally, even though many skills may be gained through reinforcement, the baby is not truly aware of the meaning of what has been acquired.

Language Development

Language development is an important aspect of intellectual competency. It has been repeatedly noted that children throughout the world go through the same basic stages of language acquisition. Language development is affected by intellectual development, maturation of the central nervous system, development of the organs of speech, and exposure to human language. Receptive language (what a person understands) and expressive language (what a person says) are both important to consider. The infant appears to be especially attuned to the types of sound needed for language development. It can be observed that by about 10 months of age infants understand some of the words being said to them, such as "bye-bye" and "peek-a-boo."

Vocalization in infancy follows a definite sequence. During the first 2 months, most of the sounds produced are vowels (Vaughan & Litt, 1990) and are made mostly in the front part of the mouth. Crying is a means of communication during this period. Cooing sounds are noted at about 2 to 3 months; they consist of a variety of simple vowel-like sounds. These sounds are usually produced when the infant is happy and is responding to an adult's social smiling and vocalizing. Around 4 to 6 months, babbling appears, which consists of sounds of vowels and consonants resembling syllables. The most common sounds are "ma," "mu," "da," "di." By 9 to 10 months, these sounds are repeated as two syllables. The infant is attempting to imitate sounds at this point. Sounds are mixed with play such as bubble-blowing or gurgling. By 12 months, words such as "Mama" and "Dada" are emerging. All normal children learn their native language and show similarities in this learning.

Nursing *Interventions*: Language Development

The nurse, in order to promote language development most effectively, needs to make sure parents understand the process of language development in the infant. A number of activities are appropriate to promote language development in the infant. The strategies described in the anticipatory section for parents can be applied by the nurse as well.

Anticipatory Guidance: Language Development

Keeping in mind the receptive abilities of even the very young infant, parents can be encouraged to talk to infants while holding or handling them. They can be encouraged to observe the response of the infant to adult vocalization. Incorporating smiling and eye-to-eye contact while talking with the infant can make this type of interaction positive for both adult and infant. As the infant starts making sounds, the parents can imitate the sounds and vocalize in response to the infant. Infants seem to enjoy vocalization during activities such as eating, bathing, and dressing. Toys and household items that produce sounds also elicit responses from the infant. As the infant approaches 9 to 10 months of age, it is helpful to accompany simple verbal directions with gestures, to repeat the directions, and to have the infant participate in the activity. Repeating the names of familiar objects to the infant is also helpful. Continued vocalizing with the infant during activities remains important (Fig. 5–8). Parents can make sounds such as tongue-clicking or lip-smacking that the infant can imitate.

Infants at 1 year of age have made enormous strides in their intellectual competency that are consistently influencing and being influenced by the development of competence in other areas.

Emotional-Social Competency

Emotional-social competency is another essential and rapidly changing area during infancy. A number of theories have been devised to explain this phase of infant development. No one theory adequately explains all that is happening in the emotional-social areas.

Psychosocial Development: Development of Trust

According to Erik Erikson's theory (1963), the central task, conflict, or crisis for the infant is that of *basic trust versus basic mistrust*. Infants have innate capacities that facilitate their interaction with the environment as they strive to develop more trust than mistrust. Infants must learn to trust individuals in their environment in order to be able to achieve a sense of trust in themselves. Erikson sees the feeding situation as central to resolution of the trust-mistrust conflict.

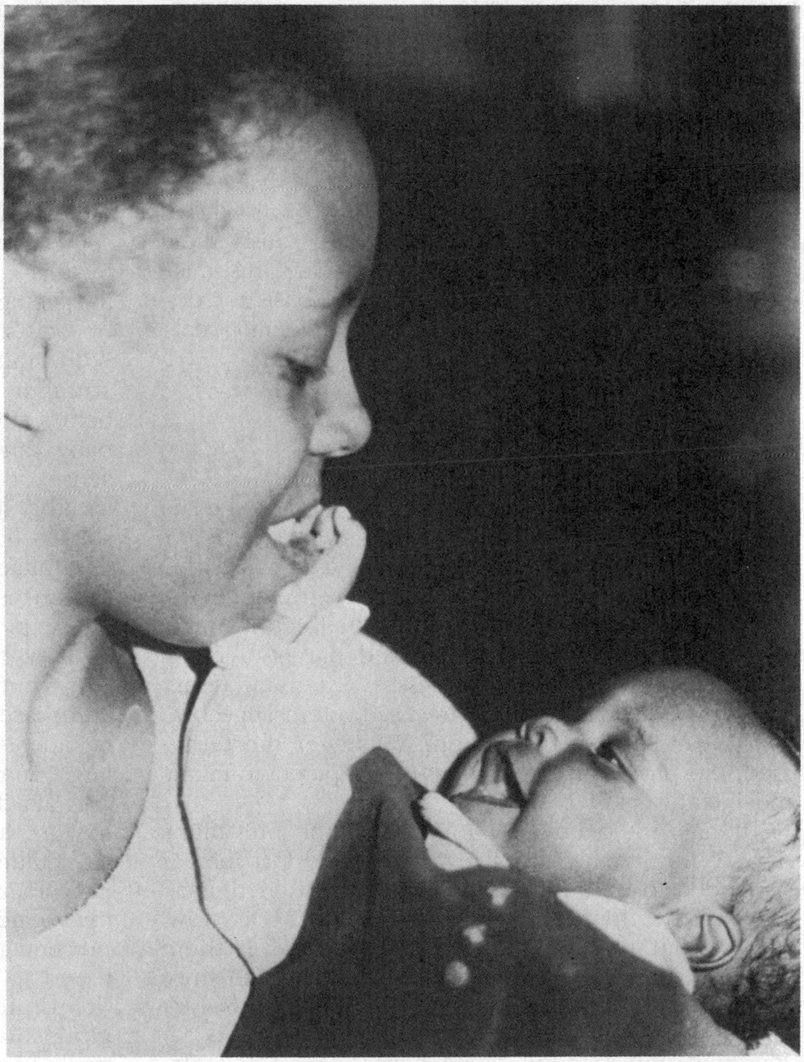

FIGURE 5-8. Talking to the infant encourages vocalizations that lead to the first words.

The very young infant cannot tolerate much frustration when hungry. The quality of the mother's/caregiver's interaction when providing the breast or bottle is crucial to the development of trust. Eventually, infants begin to develop self-trust as feelings of hunger are consistently rewarded. They can rely on their own behaviors to obtain food and are therefore able to tolerate some delay. Other interactions between the infant and mother/caregiver are also seen as contributing to the development of a sense of trust. Trust results from being held, talked to, cuddled, warmed, changed, rocked, and so on. Erikson sees "sense of" as having three components: a conscious experience that is felt within oneself, a way of behaving that is observable by others, and an inner state that can only be verified by psychoanalytic interpretation. A sense of trust therefore would involve, for infants, feelings within themselves of comfort and security. Trusting infants could also be recognized by their behaviors. Erikson states that a trusting baby is one who eats well, sleeps deeply, and enjoys bowel relaxation. This view exemplifies one criticism of Erikson's theory—that it does not take into account individual differences. It is possible that babies with different temperaments may demonstrate trust in different ways. There are also differences in caregivers, and behaviors differ at different times. A tired baby is less likely to fit Erikson's picture of trust than is a rested baby.

Erikson believes, however, that the actual skill used in handling and caring for the infant is of little importance when compared with the underlying motivation of the caregiver. Infants must learn that those who care for them can be relied on to satisfy their basic needs for survival and comfort. The trust-mistrust crisis provides a useful conceptual basis for describing, explaining, and predicting infant emotional-social behaviors.

Attachment

Bonding of parents to their infant and beginning attachment of infants to their parents were discussed earlier in Chapter 4. These processes continue to be an important component of the developing emotional-social competency of the infant. Keep in mind that infant-to-parent attachment and parent-to-infant bonding are two different processes. Often, the terms "attachment" and "bonding" are used interchangeably, which can lead to confusion. Whatever the terms used, the process is a two-way one—parent-to-infant and infant-to-parent.

It has not been very long since the prevailing view of the infant's social responses held that infants responded to all humans with little or no discrimination for the first 3 to 4 months of life. It is now known that newborns prefer the sound of their mother's voice over those of other females (Roberts, 1987). Infants also display social responsiveness earlier than was once thought. Babies as young as 12 days will imitate adult facial expressions (Meltzoff, 1985). Social responses of infants are important to the process involved in the infant becoming attached to parents. By the time their infant is 6 to 8 weeks of age, most parents have identified and are responding to at least two social responses of their baby. They notice that the baby follows them (and other objects) visually when they are within the direct line of vision and that the baby smiles in response to social stimuli. By 2 to 4 months of age, the baby will smile spontaneously at a human face.

Ainsworth (1973) characterized the initial phase of infant attachment to the parents as nondiscriminating because the babies did not appear to discriminate between their parents and other humans in these social responses. In the second phase infants progress to discrimination in their social responsiveness. By 6 months, their responses clearly indicate that the primary caregiver is preferred. By the third phase, at 9 to 10 months of age, most authorities believe infants are truly attached. They actively initiate proximity-seeking, contact-seeking behaviors and maintain contact with their parent(s) or other primary caregivers. They may relate easily to others, but with discrimination. The attachment behaviors of smiling, gazing, vocalization, and motor approach are of a different quality and intensity toward people to whom infants are attached. They do not seek the same kind of contact with people to whom they are not attached.

A new set of behaviors that occurs around 8 to 9 months of age can be seen as evidence of the infants' attachment to their parents. The 9-month-old baby will tend to respond to strangers with a serious, sometimes wary expression. "Stranger anxiety" occurs by this age and is manifested in overt distress when the stranger attempts to approach the baby. This can be devastating to grandparents who were welcomed with smiles and coos when they last visited. This stranger anxiety can be seen as evidence of the baby's strong attachment to the familiar parents. (The baby can also be said to be demonstrating a strong sense of trust in the familiar—the parents—and a healthy sense of mistrust in the unfamiliar.) Several studies have clearly indicated that formation of a secure attachment to at least one parent (or caregiving person) is necessary before 9- to 12-month-old infants will explore and start to separate from their parents, as they begin the process of developing autonomy (Ainsworth, 1973). A strong attachment serves as a secure base from which to explore. Infants do form attachments to more than one person, although not to large numbers. Once the infant is attached to a parent, attachment behaviors, rather than autonomy behaviors, are likely to increase following separation.

Cultural factors have been demonstrated to affect attachment relationships between the infant and primary caregivers. For example, in Japan and Israel the percentages of secure attachment relationships were found to be significantly lower than those found in the United States. Intracultural variation between groups in the United States is significantly different as well. Secure attachment relationships were found more frequently among middle class professionals as compared with low-income, economically disadvantaged and maritally unstable families (Ijzendoorn & Kroonenberg, 1988).

Nursing Interventions: Trust and Attachment Needs

Nurses can employ a variety of interventions to promote parent-infant attachment. Parents are included in all aspects of care as the child's condition permits. Parents can bathe, feed, cuddle, and hold the infant and, in selected instances, perform some of the nursing procedures. For example, parents who care for medically fragile infants at home are well qualified to continue to perform those procedures in the hospital, provided hospital policy and liability allow such practices and *the parents want to continue caring for their infant while hospitalized*. Parents *should not be expected* to care for their child as they may need the respite from child care demands that the hospitalization may offer.

Parents can be valuable experts concerning the needs of their infant. Consultation with parents regarding the infant's behavior, personality characteristics, daily routine, and medical care needs will serve to individualize care that meets the unique needs of the infant. Parents can be encouraged to room-in with their child, providing the infant with a constant source of love and security so as to minimize the traumatic effects of hospitalization. The infant's sense of security and trust can be fostered with the assignment of consistent nursing personnel so as to minimize the number of caretakers the infant must deal with during hospitalization (Table 5–7).

Most of parental anticipatory guidance will be done in community settings. The nurse in the hospital setting can coordinate follow-up care in the community with nurses in a variety of settings such as the clinics and early intervention and infant stimulation programs. Nurses in hospital settings can develop instructional material such as booklets, newsletters, and videos to educate parents on the needs of their infants. Many parents benefit from referrals to community-based parent support and educational groups (Turley, 1985).

Anticipatory Guidance: Trust and Attachment Needs

The nurse can help parents to understand the developing emotional-social competency of their infant and their role in promoting his or her sense of trust and attachment. The nurse can give support to the parents as they respond to the needs of their infant and can discuss the reciprocity between bonding of the parents to their infant and the infant's attachment to them. Parents generally bond earlier and more quickly to their infant; later the infant becomes attached to the parents. In addition, the nurse can point

TABLE 5–7

Promoting and Fostering Trust

The following aspects of a nursing care plan were developed to meet 3-month-old Anna's need for trust during hospitalization. Her parents both work and are able to visit twice during the week and on weekends. Anna is expected to be hospitalized for at least 3 more weeks.

Promote Trust

- Assign consistent caretakers
- Post daily schedule of care at bedside
- Cuddle in arms for 10–15 mins 2 times/shift
- Comfort, soothe after painful procedure
- Minimize disruptions in disturbing infant's sleep periods
- Reduce volume of loud, sudden noise
- Decrease glare of bright lights
- Patch eyes to attain day/night cycle

Promote Infant-Parent Attachment

- Schedule daily call from parents to describe condition and behavior; emphasize normalcy of behaviors (i.e., eating, sleeping, activity level)
- Encourage parents to take home pictures of infant
- Have parents tape-record voices and play for infant during their absence; leave scented handkerchief at bedside
- Encourage parents to participate in infant care activities (i.e., feeding, bathing)
- Encourage parents to ventilate concerns and fears about infant
- Encourage parents to bring in clothing and objects to personalize infant's crib

out the specific attachment behaviors of the infant to the parents and stress the importance of promptly responding to these behaviors. The parents should be given reinforcement for responding to attachment behaviors of their infant. The nurse can encourage parents to provide periods of close contact with their infant. The infant needs to be held, cuddled, and carried. The use of infant carriers that allow the infant contact with the parents could be encouraged.

A nursing review of studies designed to measure the effect of providing information to mothers concerning their infant's perceptual and sensory capabilities to promote maternal-infant interaction found characteristics that were associated with optimal outcomes. Providing information to mothers had the most beneficial effect compared with other interventions. The most beneficial site was the home, and 4 weeks following discharge was identified as the optimal time for teaching (Turley, 1985).

Another nursing research study found that after parents were taught infant exercises and massage, those who had used these techniques for longer periods had infants who were more alert and advanced with motor skills (Booth et al, 1985). Researchers suggest that infant exercise and massage can have beneficial effects for the infant's development and enhance the mother-infant relationship.

Discussion about meeting the basic needs of the infant for survival and comfort is appropriate. The prompt meeting of the infant's basic needs in a consistent manner helps to give the infant a secure and trusting view of the environment. The technical skill of the parents is not the key factor in meeting these needs. It is the manner (warm, consistent, caring) in which these needs are met that is the key factor. The infant is not concerned with how neatly the diaper is secured or how few wasted motions the parents use in giving the bath. What is important in these interactions is the fact that the parents respond to the infant's need to be clean and dry in a social, caring manner. *Parents need to feel confident about their ability to meet the needs of their infant.*

Parents may want to discuss coping with the changing needs of the infant as she or he progresses in the stages of attachment. In the first few months of life, the infant needs opportunity to interact with the parents; some parents express the idea that it does not seem to matter to the infant who takes care of her or him. Infants seem to respond in the same way to all caregivers. These parents need assistance in understanding that discrimination in response and ultimate attachment is a process that is enhanced by these early opportunities for interaction.

Parents often ask how much time is actually necessary to allow attachment to occur, or what effect there is on the infant if both parents work outside the home. The nurse must realize that there are no specific answers. In light of what is known about attachment, the nurse can assist parents to arrive at a satisfactory plan to promote attachment of their infant as well as meet the family's needs. It is certainly clear that there is flexibility in the amount of time needed for interaction between parents and infant and that quality of interaction is more important than quantity.

Parents need assistance in anticipating that as infants become attached to one or both parents, they will respond differently to other family members and friends and caretakers. Parents can then help others (such as grandparents) not to feel rejected. It may help to suggest a little distance in these persons' interaction with infants until the infants give clues they are ready for more interaction with them.

Parents need opportunities to discuss their feelings as the infant begins to demonstrate exploratory and independent behaviors. All of a sudden, their infant seems not to want them as much or to be as close to them. In reality, of course, the infant needs them as much as ever, but in a slightly different way. As infants explore, they need parents as a secure, consistent base to come back to for support. In this period, if infants have been separated from their parents for even a few hours, they may demonstrate more contact-seeking attachment behaviors, such as clinging and wishing to be held. Parents need to understand that this is not regressive or spoiled behavior. Infants still need close contact with their parents and are not capable of functioning independently. They use attachment behaviors to maintain the support from their parents and to build on their developing sense of trust. This period can be confusing to parents as they try to meet the attachment needs of their infant as well as her or his beginning needs for independence.

Sexuality

Psychosexual Development

Freud's theory (1957) postulated the development of three facets of personality: the id, ego, and superego. The newborn infant was seen as being governed by id impulses. The id was the driving force of personality, operating to obtain pleasure and avoid pain.

A frequent explanation of id motivation is worded, "I want what I want when I want it." Pleasure (gratification of id impulses or tension reduction) is centered in different body areas or zones. In the infant, this body area is the mouth. Through sucking, the infant derives pleasure. Freud's theory focuses mainly on forces (or tensions) within the individual as motivators of development. Freud identified the period of infancy as the *oral stage* of psychosexual development. According to Freud, the infant's mouth is the primary source of pleasure and satisfaction. Within this stage, the infant undergoes two phases of development: the *passive phase,* wherein the infant takes in the food and pacifier given, and the *active phase,* during which the infant gets food and has the need to bite because of teething.

Developing a Positive Sexual Attitude

Attitudes about sexuality begin to develop in the first few hours of life. Tone of voice and touch communicate the psychosocial makeup of the delivery. Touching the skin is the basic communication from which the infant learns about self and others. As the mother strokes and cuddles the nude baby, feelings of closeness and intimacy develop. This intimate contact between parent and child fosters the development of trust and is the framework for further relationships among the infant and others. Although this first skin-to-skin contact is not sexual in the sense of adult eroticism, it is comforting and sensual to the infant and is basic to the development of positive attitudes about sexuality.

The attitude of parents and other family members or caregivers toward the infant influences development of the infant's attitude. When parents and caregivers respond openly and acceptingly to the infant's self-exploration, a positive attitude is expressed and learned. The American attitude toward nudity in the infant affirms acceptance of the body as beautiful and sensual and is an important step in developing sexuality. As the infant experiences physical care and love, the first linkage between sensuality and affection is learned.

Sexual Behaviors

Many natural behaviors in infancy with parents or other caregivers are sexual in nature. Nursing at the mother's breast provides skin-to-skin contact with another person. The mother who relaxes with her infant provides emotional and physical gratification for the child as well as herself. The father, as observing participant in the feeding process, adds to a family experience of loving sexuality.

Other pleasurable sensations in the infant's body occur as parents kiss, fondle, tickle, feed, bathe, diaper, and dress the baby. As the baby's needs are met by others, trust develops. This trust undergirds the child's expectation that good sensations can come from interactions with other people, a necessary component of mature and satisfying sexuality.

Exploration of the infant's own body begins soon after birth. When parents are accepting of this behavior, it becomes the foundation for knowledge and acceptance of sexual feelings, which are crucial to sexual identity and satisfaction throughout the life cycle (Constantine & Martinson, 1981). Differences in the behavior of boys and girls are apparent in infancy. Obvious physical characteristics of external genitalia lead to differences in self-discovery as the little boy discovers his penis and the pleasurable sensation that accompanies touch before the little girl finds similar sensations upon discovery of her genitalia.

Masters and Johnson (1966) documented the fact that baby boys are often born with erections and baby girls with vaginal lubrication. Female infants have the potential for lubrication and orgasm, and male infants can have erections (Vaughan & Litt, 1990).

Nursing Strategies: Sexual Development

The nurse should be alert for signs of possible abuse of the child, including direct sexual abuse. Parents who express considerable concern about the gender of the child may be at risk for abuse. For more in-depth information about the phenomenon of sexual abuse and nursing care issues, consult Chapter 28.

Anticipatory Guidance: Sexual Development

The nurse can intervene in several ways to assist parents in facilitating their infant's sexual development. Nurses can remind parents that sensual pleasure observed in their infant is not to be confused with similar behaviors that may be explicitly sexual in the adolescent or adult. An infant lacks the experience and ability to make decisions associated with matured sexual expression but needs these early opportunities to learn attitudes and behaviors that will later be part of a healthy repertoire of sexuality.

Temperament

As in all areas of infant development, infant temperament has been studied in a variety of ways since the early 1980s. Previous research had sometimes looked at infant temperament without taking into account its interrelationship with other variables. It is now generally accepted that temperament is interrelated with many other variables and that negative effects of temperament can be mediated by other psychosocial variables. Current thinking also holds that it is more likely that infant temperament affects the mode of expression of security or insecurity than whether these feelings actually develop (Belsky & Rovine, 1987). A promising measure of infant temperament, the Infant Behavior Questionnaire, or IBQ (Rothbart, 1986), can be used by the nurse while working with parents to promote optimal well-being of the infant. The tool is useful in a general discussion of the differences in infant temperament. It can assist the nurse and family to better understand and meet individual infant needs.

Other research has examined the relationship between the mother's perceptions and behaviors and the infant's temperament (Bates & Bayles, 1984; Ventura, 1982). Findings have demonstrated that maternal perception is influenced by the infant's behavior. A nursing research study (Houldin, 1987) found that the mother's perceptions of the infant's behavior was associated with the quality of the childrearing environment. More responsive home environments were associated with mothers who perceived their infants more favorably. In contrast, mothers who rated their infant's temperament more negatively had home environments that were rated as less responsive to their infant's needs.

Seminal research examining the association between maternal type-A behavior and neonatal behavior has revealed findings that warrant further investigation (Parker & Barrett, 1992). Findings showed that a measure of maternal type-A behavior was related to more significant crying during neonatal examination at 2 days of age. Type-A mothers described their infants at 3 months of age differently, as responding more intensely and unpredictably. Women were less likely to be breast feeding at 3 months when they exhibited type-A behavior. These findings provide beginning evidence that measures of maternal type-A behavior may be antecedents of behavioral differences in infants.

Anticipatory Guidance: Temperament

The nurse has to take into account the effect the infant's temperament has on the family, friends, and health care providers. In order to understand an infant's behavior more fully, the parents and nurse need to be aware of the specific characteristics of the infant. If the family and nurse are aware that some infants have intense reactions and slow adaptation to change in the environment, they will approach the issue of changing the sleeping location in a different way for such infants than they would for infants who have low-intensity reactions and who readily adapt. This does not mean the parents cannot change the infant's place of sleep; rather, the best or least disturbing approach can be sought. Families need assistance in recognizing that infants, even within the same family, may have very different temperaments. The infant's temperament characteristics will affect how family members and others respond to him or her. The characteristics and responses do not indicate that either the infant or parent is good or bad. The nurse can help the family look at approaches to childrearing, taking into account the temperament of this infant and their response to his or her temperament.

Emotions

There has been much controversy over when emotions appear in the infant. Infants do not seem to have a range of emotions from an early age. They do not express emotions as adults do, nor are infant emotions likely to be exactly like those of adults. The smiles and cries of infants seem to give evidence of differentiation at an early age and are definite means of communication. Parents and professionals must be cautious about interpreting these clues (cries and smiles) in the same way they would adult cries and smiles.

The smile of the infant is considered an important developmental milestone. Many emotional connotations are placed in the powerful smile of the infant. It certainly plays an important role in promoting contact between the infant and adults. Initially the smile of the infant is spontaneous, but, by 1 month of age, the infant directs the smile toward people. By 2 to 3 months, the smile is in response to the appearance of a familiar person. The smile often occurs in conjunction with the gratification and comfort associated with these interaction experiences. These experiences help the infant to develop the association between pleasure and smiling.

Optimal emotional development in infants depends on interaction with individuals around them, particularly the mother (Fig. 5–9). There is evidence that the young infant can recognize facial expressions of emotion, although this recognition develops slowly and is still rudimentary at the end of the first 2 years of life (Nelson, 1987). This ability to recognize facial expressions influences emotional-social development during infancy. When faced with an unfamiliar situation, the infant will look to the mother's facial expression and behave in a way that demonstrates that the baby was influenced by that facial expression (Hornick et al, 1987; Klinner et al, 1986).

More evidence of the developing differentiation of emotions is seen in the temperamental characteristics of the infant, as discussed earlier. The overall regularity in patterns of functioning of the infant also influences how adults view the baby's emotions. For example, an infant with a slow-to-warm temperament might be viewed as displaying the emotion of fear. Physiologically, the infant may not have progressed to regularity in sleep, elimination, and so forth, and this unpredictability might be interpreted as emotions of anger or unhappiness.

Wolff (1969) has identified a variety of infant cries: (1) basic rhythmic cry, (2) mad or angry cry, (3) pain cry, and (4) cry of frustration. Infants do develop certain individual crying patterns. Parents need assistance in understanding crying as one of the methods

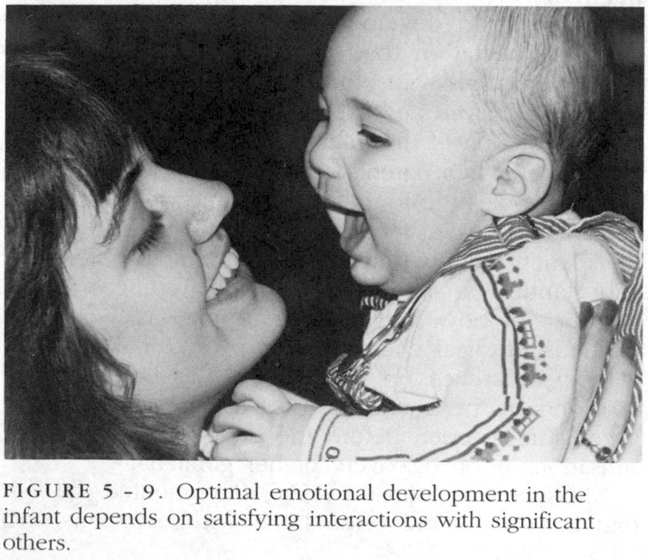

FIGURE 5 - 9. Optimal emotional development in the infant depends on satisfying interactions with significant others.

of communication available to the infant. Although there are no scientific bases for saying that certain amounts of crying are "good" for the infant, families may have strong opinions on this subject. At times, crying does seem to allow the infant to release some tension.

Anticipatory Guidance: Emotions

Nurses need to assist parents to understand behaviors of infants and our limited ability to assess adequately the emotional state of the infant. Infants do show different behaviors that indicate a range of emotions, but we do not know if the emotions differ in degree or substance, or both, from adult emotional responses. Parents need opportunities to discuss their particular infant and her or his behaviors that have emotional connotations.

It is helpful for parents to know that their baby's responses are influenced by the parents' facial expressions and emotions. This information can assist them to modulate their own expression if they believe this is appropriate in a situation. It is important to respond promptly to an infant's behavior (smiling or crying). The nurse can help parents try to understand their infant and their responses to her or him.

Fears

Infants react fearfully to stimuli that affect their sensorimotor state. For example, an infant will cry with sudden change of positions and loud noises. Fears observed in infants parallel their cognitive and psychologic development. Predominant fears of infants are listed in Table 5–8. By the end of the first year, the infant's fear response becomes more differentiated and specific.

Coping Mechanisms

The infant uses sensorimotor behaviors as coping mechanisms. Sucking, tactile needs, and motor behaviors provide the infant with rudimentary yet effective means of dealing with his or her environment. For example, the infant will cry when hungry, wet, or otherwise uncomfortable. Small or ill infants may be too tired to get their needs met.

Infants vary in their need to be held and cuddled as well as in their need for sensory stimulation. Their need can be assessed through observation of their distress and nondistressed behaviors in the hospital and clinic settings. Information gathered from parents can provide valuable insights into understanding the infant's behavior and intervening appropriately to assist the infant in coping with painful and distressing situations. Infant coping behaviors include staring, kicking, crying, fussy behavior, listlessness, thumb-sucking, rejection of primary caregiver, increased motor or decreased motor behavior, anorexia, clutching a blanket or toy, and sucking a pacifier.

TABLE 5-8
Predominant Fears in Infants

First 6 Mos	8–10 Mos	12 Mos
Sudden movements	Fear of strangers	Fear of strangers
Loud noises		Strange objects
Loss of support		Heights
Lights and flashes		Anticipated fearful/painful situations (e.g., physicians/nurses)

Moral and Faith Development

The concept of moral development becomes operative in the child's life when rudimentary cognitive functioning is evident. Knowledge of acceptable and unacceptable behavior begins during toddlerhood.

The infant's stage of faith development is described as *undifferentiated.* This is due to the infant's inability to formulate or communicate any ideas of religion or of God. The earliest feeling that the infant develops about caregivers and the environment sets the foundation for subsequent development of faith beliefs. That is, feelings of warmth, trust, and security about caregivers will be projected to religious ideas as well.

Health Maintenance and Promotion

The parents will be the people providing most of the health care for the infant. The nurse should assist parents as they care for their infant to promote her or his optimal growth and development without neglecting their own developmental needs. Throughout this chapter, growth and development issues have been discussed, which are pertinent to nurses as they provide assistance to parents through education, discussion of concerns, guidance, and counseling on the needs of their developing infants. If parents know what to expect in the process of healthy growth and development of their infant, they will be better prepared to meet these needs and feel more capable as parents. In addition to providing anticipatory guidance on the developing competencies of the infant, the nurse can help parents focus on their infant's needs in the areas of nutrition, play, safety, and immunizations. An emphasis on the individual differences between infants should be included. Nurses can use their knowledge of growth and development theories as a basis for describing and explaining the baby's behaviors and for predicting outcomes of interactions between the baby and parents.

Health Screening

Monitoring the infant's growth and development is the foremost concern of health screening. The infant's acquisition of developmental milestones in the areas of physical, intellectual, and emotional-social competencies will be carefully evaluated. Delays detected in any of these competency areas warrant close observation and monitoring. It may be necessary to refer the infant to a specialist for further assessment.

Infants may need to be screened for phenylketonuria and hypothyroidism if born at home or at a birth center. Infants from populations at risk should be screened for inborn errors of metabolism such as Tay-Sachs disease.

Infants' health status is monitored closely because infectious disease such as respiratory syncytial virus (RSV) infection is a major cause of morbidity requiring hospitalization more often than for older children. Minor conditions such as cradle cap and diaper dermatitis are observed for and treated.

Between 9 and 12 months of age, infants are screened for iron deficiency anemia, as this coincides with the depletion of fetal iron stores. Research data suggest that lead intoxication in infants may be more common than previously thought, warranting lead screening beginning at 6 months of age (Shannon & Graef, 1992). According to these data, sources of plumbism in infancy were household renovation (49 per cent), paint chip ingestion (24 per cent), and formula preparation (24 per cent). Venous lead measurements prove more accurate than erythrocyte protoporphyrin screening.

Chapter 10 provides a detailed discussion of the various facets of immunization and the currently recommended immunization schedule. The following time frame (see Table 10–6) is recommended during infancy:

2 months—DTP*, OPV†, HbCV‡.

4 months—DTP, OPV, HbCV.

6 months—DTP, OPV (optional), HbCV.

An infant may receive measles, mumps, and rubella (MMR) vaccine as early as 6 months if the child lives in a high-risk area where there has been an outbreak. If the child has received MMR vaccine before that first birthday then revaccination is needed at 15 months (American Academy of Pediatrics [AAP], 1989).

Variations to the infants' immunization schedule occur in selected clinical situations such as preterm birth, human immunodeficiency virus (HIV) infection, asplenia, presence of a chronic disease, and individual or family history of seizures (AAP, 1991). Again, the infant's primary physician or specialist will determine the need and scheduling of immunizations.

Anticipatory Guidance: Health Screening

Immunization is an important component of anticipatory guidance. Parents need to be informed about the benefits of immunization procedures and the rationale for the procedure. Parents must be informed of the risks as well as of the benefits of immunizations. The Committee on Infectious Disease of the AAP recommends immunization schedules. These are revised periodically as new information arises. The nurses should consult current resources such as latest editions of AAP's *Report of the Committee on Infectious Disease (Redbook)* (1991) for detailed information about immunizations. The nurse also needs to help prepare parents for the possible reactions by the infant to certain immunizations and related interventions. Parents may ask questions about the safety of vaccinations. There have been strong views expressed about reactions to pertussis and rubella vaccines. The Institute of Medicine (IOM) study found no or insufficient evidence to suggest that pertussis can cause neurologic damage, autism, seizures, sudden infant death syndrome (SIDS), Reye syndrome, or other disorders (Howson and Fineberg, 1992). Further, the IOM found insufficient evidence to suggest that rubella vaccine causes peripheral neuritis.

Vision and Hearing

The senses of vision and hearing are another aspect of physical competency that significantly affect the infant's growth and development. Much research has been done recently that shows that the neonate has greater development in these areas than was once thought (Behrman, 1992). The neonate's auditory system is functioning and developed well enough to detect differences in sound. If both visual and auditory cues are presented, there are no age-related differences in localization of sound. If only auditory cues are presented, the ability to localize sound develops gradually over the first 1½ years of life (Morrongiello & Ricca, 1987). Chapters 13 and 45 discuss assessment of vision and hearing in the infant.

Anticipatory Guidance: Vision and Hearing

The nurse can point out to parents the infant's visual and auditory capabilities and fascination with human faces. The infant needs to be exposed to a variety of visual and auditory stimuli. The importance of a variety of colors and shapes in the baby's environment can be stressed. The young infant responds well to black-white contrast (Slusher, 1992).

The human voice is an important and readily available sound stimulus. Infants prefer the sound of their mother's voice over that of other individuals

*DTP = diphtheria and tetanus toxoids with pertussis vaccine.
†OPV = oral, attenuated, or weakened poliovirus vaccine.
‡HbCV = *Haemophilus influenzae* b conjugate vaccine.

(Roberts, 1987). The infant also responds well to musical toys and toys that make different sounds. Stimulation needs of individual babies will vary, but periods of rest, when they are not bombarded by visual and auditory stimuli, are needed.

Dental Care

Dental development during childhood involves the eruption of two sets of teeth, deciduous and permanent (Fig. 5–10). There are 20 deciduous teeth, also called "primary" or "baby teeth." These are gradually replaced by 32 permanent teeth.

Tooth eruption varies among children. Genetic factors are the major sources of differences between individuals in tooth development and eruption. For example, siblings tend to resemble each other more in the timing of eruption than do unrelated individuals. Tooth development in females is slightly ahead of that in males, as is that of African-Americans when compared with whites in the United States.

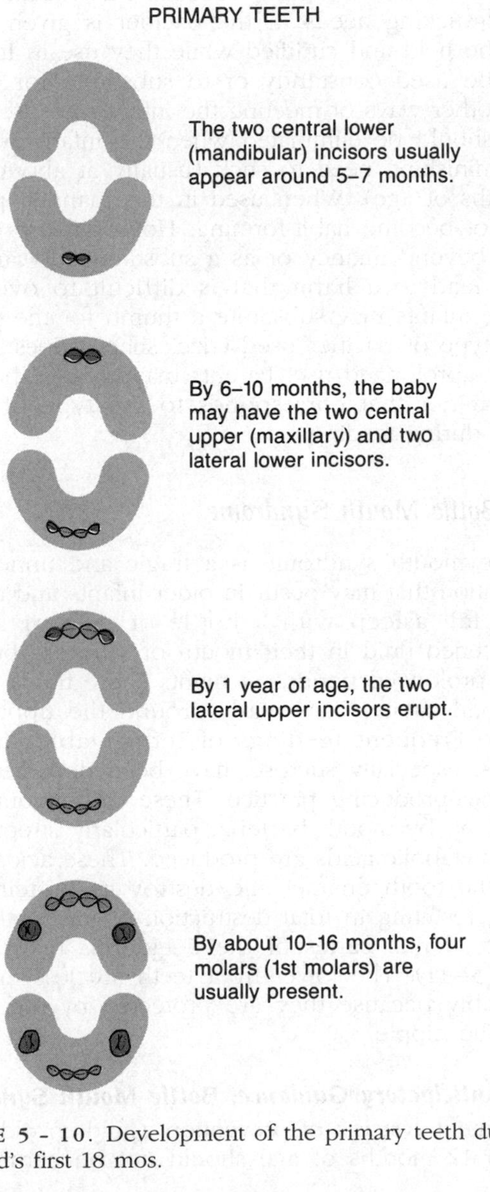
PRIMARY TEETH
The two central lower (mandibular) incisors usually appear around 5–7 months.
By 6–10 months, the baby may have the two central upper (maxillary) and two lateral lower incisors.
By 1 year of age, the two lateral upper incisors erupt.
By about 10–16 months, four molars (1st molars) are usually present.

FIGURE 5-10. Development of the primary teeth during the child's first 18 mos.

Although variation in eruption is normal, the sequence of shedding of primary teeth and emergence of permanent teeth is important to proper *occlusion* —that is, the alignment of the chewing surface of the maxillary (upper) teeth to the mandibular (lower) teeth when the jaws are closed. In the normal sequence, symmetry is evident in the eruption of permanent teeth on the right and left sides of the jaw, but slight asymmetry is evident for the maxillary and mandibular teeth (Fig. 5–10).

Deciduous tooth eruption begins around 4 to 6 months of age, although the time of the first tooth eruption varies. It is not unusual for the first tooth not to appear until the end of the first year. At 1 year of age, a child usually has six to eight teeth. Usually one tooth erupts for each month of age past 6 months up to 26 to 30 months of age. The age of a toddler in months minus 6 is used as an approximate guide to assess the expected number of teeth at a specific age.

Dentists' views vary regarding the frequency of routine dental visits. Decisions about when a child's initial visit should occur and how often asymptomatic children need visits should be based on the child's overall health status, the family dental history, and the availability of systemic fluorides. Most dentists agree, however, that the first visit to the dentist should be made by 2 years of age, preferably before any dental work needs to be done. A first visit no later than 12 months of age is recommended by some authorities to initiate preventive measures and intercept potential problems (Goepferd, 1986). The AAP encourages the initiation of dental visits 6 months after the first primary tooth erupts if the infant's history reflects any of the following: (1) a high-risk factor in any aspect of the child's health status since birth, (2) no systemic fluoride being ingested, or (3) a family history of dental disease. Unless at high risk for dental disease, asymptomatic children may be sufficiently monitored with dental visits annually and at any time the parents notice a problem.

Fluoride supplementation should begin in the first 2 weeks after birth (AAP, 1986). In communities where water is not fluoridated, a daily supplement of sodium fluoride should be given for healthy development of the permanent teeth buds in the gums. If fluoride concentration in the local water supply is less than 0.3 ppm, then the infant should receive 0.25 mg of fluoride supplement. Fluoride supplement is not needed for fluoride concentration greater than 0.3 ppm in the local water supply.

Anticipatory Guidance: Dental Care

To protect the first teeth, the gums and teeth can be massaged with a soft, moist, clean cloth after each feeding. A fluoride toothpaste (an amount about the size of a small pea) is applied to the cloth, and all sides of each tooth are wiped. Tooth brushing is recommended by 18 months of age when gingival tissue is no longer so easily damaged and a considerable number of teeth are usually present.

Anticipatory Guidance: Teething

Parents have many questions about teething. The nurse should discuss the general pattern of tooth eruption with the family when the infant is about 3 months old. Drooling occurs at about this time. Saliva is now being produced, but the infant has not yet learned to swallow it. This drooling at 3 months is not directly associated with teething. There are many myths about the supposed responses of the body to eruption of the teeth (e.g., fever, diarrhea, vomiting). However, a cause-and-effect relationship between teething and these symptoms has not been established. Since teething usually extends over quite a long period and infants have frequent minor illnesses, teething has perhaps been unjustly blamed for at least some of these. Parents need to be encouraged to consult with health care providers about any signs and symptoms that would cause concern if the infant were not teething. "The greatest danger of inaccurately ascribing the cause of such signs and symptoms to teething is that parents will delay medical treatment for a serious illness" (Bradshaw, 1981).

Teething does cause discomfort to many infants. They often are irritable, rub at their gums, and display a desire to bite. Their gums are often red and swollen. Chewing on hard, clean objects such as teething rings, hard rubber toys, or zwieback toast may bring some relief. Preparations containing alcohol should be avoided. Nurses and parents need to be aware that some teething lotions contain a high percentage of alcohol. Alcohol-containing products are potentially toxic to infants and could have systemic effects.

Bradshaw (1981) provided the following guidelines for nurses who are working with parents of teething infants:

- Do not belittle the parents for their beliefs and concerns about teething. Attacking firm ethnic, cultural, or socioeconomic group beliefs about teething runs the risk of alienating the family.
- Do not discourage home remedies for teething unless they are definitely harmful.
- Acetaminophen (10 to 15 mg/kg every 3 to 4 hours) can help relieve teething pain that does not respond to nonpharmacologic comfort measures.
- The practice of placing an aspirin tablet against the painful area should be avoided. An aspirin tablet can erode gingival tissues and can be easily aspirated.

Anticipatory Guidance: Use of Pacifiers

The importance of the oral sense to the infant should be discussed with parents. Sucking is an important way for the infant to meet nutritional needs. The mouth is also used as an organ for touch. In addition, sucking in itself seems to be an important need for the infant. Some infants have greater sucking needs than other infants. Parents may need assistance in determining if their infant is hungry or has a non-nutritive sucking need. Overfeeding can result if sucking needs are interpreted as hunger needs. Non-nutritive sucking need is greatest in the first 4 to 6 months of life. Satisfying the need for sucking provides comfort to the infant and does not lead to dependency on sucking.

Many parents, professionals, family members, and friends have strong positive or negative feelings about the use of a pacifier. The nurse can provide information about its appropriate use and can help parents determine if their infant requires this mechanism to meet sucking needs. If the pacifier is given, infants can be held and cuddled while they use it. It should not be used constantly or to substitute for holding and other ways of meeting the infant's needs. Pacifier use should be eliminated when the infant evidences a diminishing need to suck (usually at about 4 to 5 months of age). When used in this manner, pacifiers do not become habit-forming. However, use of pacifiers beyond infancy or as a substitute for caregiving may lead to a habit that is difficult to overcome. Some infants may substitute a thumb for the pacifier. The type of pacifier used (size, shape) does not justify its prolonged use. Parents may choose the shape of pacifier that corresponds to the type of nipple used during feeding.

Bottle Mouth Syndrome

Bottle mouth syndrome is a tragic and unnecessary condition that may occur in older infants and toddlers who fall asleep with a bottle of milk or another sweetened fluid in their mouth or who are breastfed over prolonged periods at night. These fluids pool in the oral cavity, particularly around the upper front teeth. Frequent feedings of fermentable carbohydrates, especially sucrose, have been documented as a caries-producing practice. These carbohydrates are acted on by mouth bacteria, particularly streptococci, and metabolic acids are produced. These acids decalcify the tooth enamel and destroy its protein structures, resulting in total destruction of the tooth. Early severe dental caries of the deciduous teeth results (Fig. 5–11). The lower front teeth are less involved, probably because they are protected by the tongue and the nipple.

Anticipatory Guidance: Bottle Mouth Syndrome

Treatment consists of prevention. Children older than 10 to 12 months of age should not be permitted to

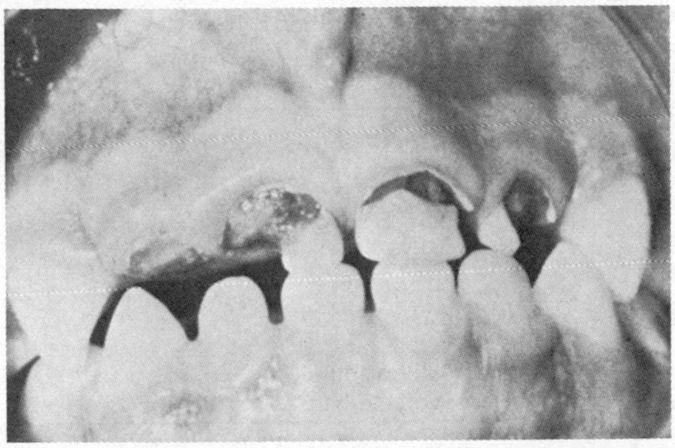

FIGURE 5 - 11. Clinical photograph of a 3-year-old suffering from "baby bottle syndrome." The four upper anterior teeth are severely decayed; the rest of the mouth is caries free. This child always went to sleep at night with a bottle containing Kool-Aid. (From Caldwell, R. C., & Stallard, R. E. [1977]. *Textbook of preventive dentistry.* Philadelphia: WB Saunders.)

sleep with a bottle in their mouth. If the older infant is accustomed to going to sleep with a bottle, plain water may be substituted for the milk or sugar-containing liquids. It should be noted that allowing a child to fall asleep unattended with a bottle in his or her mouth (as in the practice of bottle propping) could result in aspiration of formula and resultant pneumonia or even asphyxia. Following each bottle or meal with water will help to prevent prolonged contact of food sugars with teeth. The baby's teeth can also be lightly rubbed with a gauze-wrapped finger.

Sleep Behaviors

Sleep is of special interest to parents. The developmental changes in sleep in the first year involve length and timing of the sleep periods, as well as the type of sleep. Individual differences in sleep patterns for infants are significant. All too often a long sleep pattern becomes equated with "a good infant."

From birth the human organism alternates between awake and sleep states. Both these states are active physiologic and biochemical processes. A complex interaction of neural regulation (nerve cells in the brain stem and diencephalon), biochemical regulation (involving serotonin, norepinephrine, dopamine, acetylcholine, amino acids, and peptides), and the ascending reticular activating system (ARAS) results in the sleep-wake cycle. When we sleep and when we are awake is determined by our circadian rhythm (circadian rhythm is the phenomenon of rhythmic repetitions of certain processes in living organisms at about the same time during a period of approximately 24 hours each day). As the circadian rhythm of an infant matures, the sleep pattern evolves into a pattern of being awake during the day and asleep at night. This mechanism is thought to be controlled by the hypothalamus. A light impulse from the optic tract is delivered to the hypothalamus, resetting the rhythm each day (Hobson, 1982).

Wakefulness

The awake cycle depends on intact cerebral hemispheres interacting with the thalamus, hypothalamus, and brain stem. Stimulation of the ARAS results in arousal, whereas destruction of the ARAS results in coma. However, decreased activity of the ARAS alone does not initiate sleep, therefore it is postulated that sleep is an active process involving the deactivation of the ARAS and the activation of sleep centers in the brain (Weissbluth, 1987). Furthermore, according to Jouvet (1969), catecholaminergic neuron activity is involved in arousal, wakefulness, and rapid eye movement (REM) sleep, whereas serotonergic mechanisms appear to be involved with sleep initiation.

The electroencephalogram (EEG) of an awake person is characterized by spontaneous, low-voltage, fast electrical activity, and the pattern is desynchronized (Chuman, 1983). A high level of muscle activity is present, and the individual is alert and responsive.

Sleep States

Current understanding of sleep states dates from the observations in the 1950s by Aserinsky and Kleitman (1953), who noted rapid eye movements under the closed eyelids of sleeping infants. Before these findings, sleep was thought to be a single state of lowered central nervous system arousal. Sleep is now recognized to be an active rather than passive state and is composed of two distinct states of physiologic activity in the central nervous system. A state of sleep in which REM occurs and one in which there are no rapid eye movements (NREM) follow each other in a regular fashion to make up the sleep cycle (Table 5–9).

REM sleep is sometimes referred to as paradoxic sleep because of the presence of a fast-frequency EEG pattern (characteristic of wakefulness) co-existing with a diminished muscle tone (associated with a sleep state). The REM sleep state has two components: the *tonic or continuous* event, which refers to the overall inhibition of spinal neurons and reduced deep tendon reflexes, and the *phasic or intermittent* component, during which there are bursts of REM, muscle twitching, and variation in vital signs and oxygen consumption (Chuman, 1983). The REM sleep state has also been called the *active sleep state.*

NREM sleep is characterized by four stages of EEG activity numbered I through IV (see Table 5–9). Some notable physiologic differences are characteristic of the NREM phase. In normal states of wakefulness, carbon dioxide has a vasodilator effect. During NREM sleep, there appears to be a decreased cerebral vasomotor carbon dioxide responsiveness. Regional

TABLE 5-9
Characteristics of REM and NREM Sleep States

Characteristics	REM Sleep State	NREM Sleep State
General state	Highly activated	Highly regulated
Eye movements	Rapid eye movements present under closed lids	Lacks rapid eye movements
EEG characteristics	Low voltage, asynchronous, fast, cortical activity	*Stage I:* Low voltage, fast pattern *Stage II**: Sleep spindles with low-voltage background *Stages III and IV**: Slow, high-voltage waves called slow-wave sleep (SWS)
Brain activity	Marked. Most dreams occur during REM sleep	Resting phase
Muscle activity	Suppression except for bursts of twitching	Muscle tone and muscle activity are diminished
Vital signs	Pulse, respiratory rate, and blood pressure are faster and more irregular than in NREM sleep	Decrease in pulse rate, respiratory rate, blood pressure, and body temperature

*Stages II, III, and IV do not begin to appear until after the 2nd month of life.

cerebral blood flow thus decreases, especially during short wave sleep (SWS), in spite of a slight elevation in P_{CO_2} (Chuman, 1983).

The speculation that sleep enhances tissue restoration is associated with the pattern of growth hormone secretion. Growth hormone is secreted during NREM sleep, with the peak occurring during SWS (shortly after the onset of nocturnal sleep) (Takahashi, 1979). Growth hormone enhances amino acid transport into cells and stimulates synthesis of RNA, resulting in stimulation of protein synthesis; this explains the importance of sleep during periods of growth and recuperation from illness or injury.

Sleep behavior in infants differs from that of adults. These differences are summarized in Table 5–10. The proportion of REM sleep diminishes as the central nervous system (CNS) matures. Roffwarg and associates (1966) proposed that the large proportion of REM sleep and its reduction with maturation occur because (1) the immature nervous system lacks inhibitory control; therefore, a reduced amount of REM sleep reflects maturation of the CNS, and (2) REM sleep serves to stimulate the CNS, thus facilitates growth and maturation. The larger quantities of REM sleep are thought to occur because of the need for more stimulation of the cortex than can be provided by sensory stimulation from external sources during the short awake periods. The REM sleep thus provides an endogenous source of stimulation that is important for development (Roffwarg et al, 1966).

Two notable changes occur with maturation: *(1) a gradual reduction in the total number of required hours of sleep, and (2) development of consolidated sleep and awake periods into a day/night cycle.* Consolidation of sleep (sleep condensed into fewer periods of longer duration) and a diurnal cycle (sleeping through the night with alternating daytime wakefulness) develop over time. The ability to prolong periods of sleep and wakefulness depends on CNS maturation (Weissbluth, 1991). Although sleep has begun to consolidate and follow a diurnal pattern by 6 weeks of age, it has been reported that sleep onset time at approximately 8:00 P.M. does not become stable until age 4.5 months. By 6 months, the longest sleep period follows the longest wake period, and the time of day at which the wake-to-sleep transition occurs is relatively fixed. Refer to Table 5–11 for developmental characteristics of sleep-related behavior.

Patterns of sleep behaviors in infants have been reported to be influenced by a variety of environmental factors (Bronfenbrenner, 1989). These environmental factors include characteristics of parents affecting caretaking behaviors, quality of the home environment, social support, and family values and beliefs including ethnicity and social class. Research has demonstrated that sleep problems have been associated with maternal depression, parental stress, level of social support, and parental response to the infant's night waking (Crockenberg & McCluskey, 1986; Zuckerman et al, 1987).

A nursing research study found that infant sleep behavior at 4 and 12 months was influenced by environmental factors (Becker et al, 1991). Infants whose mothers reported lower levels of stress slept longer at night. These findings suggest that mothers experiencing higher levels of stress appear to interact with their infants in a way that is disruptive to infant sleeping patterns.

TABLE 5-10
Comparison of Infant and Adult Sleep Patterns

Characteristic	Infant	Adult
Proportion of REM:NREM	50:50 REM:NREM. By age 5 or 6 yrs, REM:NREM proportions are similar to those of adult. Infants spend more relative and absolute time in REM state	20:80 REM:NREM
Length of REM–NREM cycles	50–60 mins	90–100 mins; adult pattern is achieved by adolescence
Sleep onset	Sleep is entered through an initial REM period. During the latter half of the first year, sleep onset resembles that in adulthood	NREM sleep precedes REM sleep. REM sleep period is entered approximately 90 mins after sleep onset
Timing (temporal organization) of REM–NREM states during a night of sleep	Length of REM period is as long in the early part of sleep as it is in the latter part. By 6 wks of age, the diurnal pattern emerges, resulting in shortened REM periods during the early part of the night; longer REM periods (such as in the adult) begin to appear during the latter part of the night	NREM (stages III and IV) predominate in the first third of the night and the REM state predominates in the last third of the night

Other nursing research studies found that breastfed infants slept less than nonbreastfed infants, although the number of night wakings did not differ (Alley & Rogers, 1986; Osterholm et al, 1983). This difference was attributed to the possible positive reinforcement that breastfed infants derived from the skin-to-skin physical contact, but another study reported no differences.

Anticipatory Guidance: Sleep Behaviors

The nurse's assessment of an infant's sleep-related behaviors is part of any developmental assessment or parental concern raised with the nurse. Asking parents to describe their concerns about their infant's sleep can yield important information. The nurse should elicit the following information:

- History of sleep problems in the infant.
- Description of the daily sleep duration of the infant (bedtime and awaking times).
- Where the infant sleeps (bed, crib, separate room, lighting, noise level).
- Interaction of the infant and parent.
- Parental stress.
- Presence of maternal depression.
- Type and schedule of feedings.
- Level and nature of social support.
- Parental response to nightwaking.

Parents can be assisted to understand sleep patterns and the individual needs of their infant. The nurse can point out that sleep patterns (longer periods of sleep and diurnal cycles) are signs of maturation in the infant. Parents need not be left with only the general impression that infants sleep a lot.

Table 5–11 shows infant developmental characteristics of sleep and offers strategies to promote healthy sleep. The infant's temperament is an important factor to discuss with parents. An infant with an "easy" temperament will have less difficulty in falling asleep compared with an infant with a "difficult" temperament (Weissbluth, 1991). Parents can be advised to use soothing strategies that will promote sleep in infants with "difficult" temperaments.

It has also been suggested that parental expectations and parity will affect parent's ability to promote sleep. First-time parents may be unsure how to interpret their infant's sleep pattern and behaviors and thereby may intervene inappropriately. The nurse, through anticipatory guidance, can provide information and support to promote sleep learning (Table 5–12).

Sleeping arrangements for the infant vary from family to family. The nurse should ascertain common cultural practices in order to assist parents realistically. In some Asian cultures, for example, children typically sleep with parents.

Co-Sleeping

Sleeping in a room and bed separate from parents is encouraged by many to avoid later problems of adjusting to a separate bed, to promote the develop-

TABLE 5-11
Infant Developmental Characteristics of Sleep-Related Behavior

Characteristic Sleep-Related Behaviors	Promote Sleep-Related Health
6 Wks	
• Diurnal pattern emerges (sleeps more of the night and is awake for longer periods during the day) • Period of fussiness, crying, wakefulness at peak • *14–16 hrs of sleep per 24 hrs*	• Release into sleep varies with infants; some are more tense than others • The safest position during infancy (before child is able to roll) is on the right side or back after feeding • A light-weight cover is used to prevent chilling because metabolic rate decreases during sleep; thus, production of body heat is reduced
12–16 Wks	
• Day sleeping patterns emerge (napping)	• Intervals of wakefulness should be kept short; after 1 hr awake begin soothing process. Soothing may include breastfeeding or bottlefeeding • May place infant in crib to fall asleep or hold infant until falls asleep before putting in crib • Naps should be stationary site (crib) rather than during car ride to promote sleep • Period of wakefulness and soothing should not exceed 2 hrs or infant may become overtired and begin crying
6 Mos	
• Nightwaking begins in the latter half of the first year; infant begins to resist separation • Has two to three naps per day • *12–16 hrs of sleep per 24 hrs*	• See text for management of nightwaking • An established routine facilitates getting infant to sleep
1 Yr	
• Usually has morning and afternoon naps • *12–14 hrs of sleep per 24 hrs*	• Avoid putting child to bed with bottle (with milk, juice, or other sugar-containing liquid), to prevent nursing bottle-mouth syndrome

TABLE 5-12
Family-Centered Teaching: Healthy Sleep Patterns in Infants

- Infants sleep 12–16 hrs per day
- Infants spend most of their sleeping time in REM (highly activated or light) sleep
- A diurnal pattern (more night sleep; awake for longer periods during the day) emerges after 6 wks
- Quiet, relaxed periods help prepare the infant for rest. Nursing/feeding or rocking sometimes accomplishes this goal for the infant
- Infants need a comfortable and safe place to sleep
- The sleeping area should be free of excessive noise; avoid sudden loud noises
- Maintain a comfortable room temperature
- Low levels of room lighting allow easy access for child care; avoid sudden changes between dark and bright lighting

ment of independence, and to prevent parents from being awakened by every movement of their child. However, whether a child sleeps in the same bed as the parents is largely influenced by personal attitudes and cultural variations. Co-sleeping (parents and children in the same bed) is a common practice in many cultures and was routine in American culture until the 20th century (Thevenin, 1976). Although pediatric health professionals commonly advise against co-sleeping, a growing number of people (including parents) are questioning this advice (Thevenin, 1976; Brazelton, 1979; Hymovich & Chamberlin, 1980) and studying the practice of co-sleeping (Lozoff et al, 1984).

How prevalent the practice of co-sleeping is and the extent of ill effects (if any) are unknown. In a study by Lozoff and associates (1984), co-sleeping in white families was found to be more common in high school educated and nonprofessional parents and when family stress, maternal ambivalence, and disruptive sleep problems were present. Although the findings of this study support an association between co-sleeping and sleep problems, the explanation for the association is not obvious. Co-sleeping may *contribute* to sleep problems through reinforcement. Furthermore, delaying resolution of the underlying cause of a problem and not giving children the opportunity to regulate their own sleep patterns may contribute to sleep problems. Conversely, co-sleeping may occur primarily in response to an existing sleep disturbance, and it is conceivable that a sleep problem could be compounded by not permitting co-sleeping (Lozoff et al, 1984).

Nursing interventions to change practices that are rooted in cultural and individual values must be particularly sensitive and insightful. Brazelton (1979) reported on what parents think about their children sleeping alone (expressed in a thousand letters in response to a previous article). These parents did not agree that children should be left in their cribs alone, nor did they view nightwaking as a problem. On the contrary, separation from the child at night was cited by these parents as a possible contributor to the problem of nightwaking. If co-sleeping creates a problem for parents or their children, or if co-sleeping is found to be part of a more general pattern of overprotection, then intervention by the nurse may be indicated. If, on the other hand, a family chooses to experience closeness in this way and it is comforting to all family members, then the values of the health care professional cannot be the decisive factor.

Nightwaking

Sleeping through the night, or "settling in," is a developmental milestone that parents welcome with relief. This indicates to them that their infant is maturing and that they have provided the appropriate nurturing.

What comes as a surprise to many parents is that nightwaking resumes during the latter part of the first year and during the second year of life. It can occur as early as 1 month after sleeping through the night has been achieved. The reported frequency of nightwaking ranges from 25 per cent (Carey, 1974) to 50 per cent (Moore and Ucko, 1957).

Episodes of nightwaking occur without an identifiable cause, although temperamental, environmental, and maturational factors are thought to be relevant variables. Introducing solid foods has been found not to be associated with sleeping through the night.

Nightwaking has been reported to be associated with temperaments characterized by low sensory thresholds (determined by the Carey Infant Temperament Scale) (Carey, 1974; Weissbluth, 1981). Breastfeeding beyond 6 months of age is reported to be associated with nightwaking by some (Carey, 1975) but not others (Weissbluth, 1981). Osterholm and colleagues (1983) found breastfeeding, sleeping in the same room as parents, and tooth eruption to be more prevalent in infants (6 to 12 months) who did not sleep through the night. Healy (1972) reported nightwaking to be associated with sleeping in the parents' room, strained parent-child relationships, and maternal overprotection.

Several developmental factors may be associated with nightwaking. During the first several years of life, diurnal regulation and transitions between REM and NREM sleep states mature. The mechanisms responsible for the maturation of sleep states may be associated with nightwaking (Anders & Keener, 1983). In the early months, infants may awaken and console themselves and return to sleep on their own. During the latter part of the first year, separation from parents begins to be resisted, therefore infants cry out when they awaken rather than getting back to sleep on their own. Furthermore, it has been suggested that infants who have rarely been placed into their crib awake expect to be rocked back to sleep if they awaken in the night. The high prevalence of nightwaking in breastfed infants may be related to a difference in comforting practices. The breastfeeding mother may be more likely to comfort her fussing baby by offering the breast; therefore, the baby learns to expect this response (Schmitt, 1981).

Anticipatory Guidance: Nightwaking

Management options for nightwaking depend on the way parents respond to the situation. The parents who seek alternatives to getting up at night require intervention by the nurse. If parents are satisfied with their approach to handling nightwaking, then suggested options may not be welcomed. Parents need to be highly motivated to break the cycle of night crying.

Nightwaking has been described by Schmitt (1986) as "trained night crying." Trained night crying is thought to occur because of a reinforcing response to an infant's cry. Consistently responding to awake infants by holding and rocking them at night "trains" them to expect comforting. Crying is reinforced by the secondary gain of being held. If parents are seeking to break this cycle of crying and holding each night, they will need to decrease the secondary reinforcers gradually.

Schmitt (1981, 1986), on the other hand, suggests that parents have great difficulty letting their baby cry. It is therefore suggested that parents wait for 5 minutes before going to their baby's room and then go for a very brief time (1 minute or less). They should try to refrain from holding and cuddling the infant but rather give pats and make a few reassuring remarks.

Similarly, Ferber (1985) recommends that each night the parents can let their infant cry slightly longer before intervening, and the parent should stay with the infant only briefly to reassure. Asking parents to simply let a child cry for long periods until he or she falls asleep is also discouraged by Jones and Verduyn (1983) because it emphasizes the crying. What is important is that the child have practice falling asleep alone rather than while being held and rocked. Most children do not cry longer than 15 to 20 minutes unless something is wrong or unless longer crying periods have been reinforced. (Letting a baby cry for a long period of time and then holding or rocking the infant reinforces the behavior so that next time the child will cry equally long, expecting the same comfort.)

Nightwaking is usually a transient developmental phase but has the potential to result in strained parent-child relationships. Sedation is generally not recommended for nightwaking.

Nutrition

Nutritional Requirements

There have been many opinions expressed about the nutritional needs of the infant. As research in this area continues, recommendations and opinions will change; however, some basic facts about nutritional requirements remain fairly consistent. Infant nutritional requirements are based on what is considered necessary to support life, to provide for growth, and to maintain health. Components to meet the nutritional needs of the infant include water, nutrients (protein, fat, carbohydrates), vitamins, and minerals. Since the first year of life is a period of rapid change, the nutritional requirements of this period also change.

Water

The percentage of body weight provided by water is greater in the newborn infant than after a year of age, going from 75 per cent at birth to 60 per cent at 1 year (Pipes, 1985). Infants have a relatively greater need for water than do children and adults, and they are therefore more vulnerable to water imbalance. Water lost by evaporation in infancy is 60 per cent of that needed to maintain homeostasis compared with 40 to 50 per cent in the adult (Pipes, 1985). The young infant has functionally immature kidneys. The faster rate of the infant's metabolism is a factor in the need for relatively more fluid than is needed by the adult. Also, young infants are unable to let adults know when they are thirsty. The usual diets of most infants meet this basic water requirement.

The sources of water are fluids (mostly milk) and food. Most strained foods are 75 to 85 per cent water. Difficulties may occur in meeting the water requirements if formulas are improperly prepared, if infants ingest a limited amount of milk (especially with illness), if fever exists during hot weather, or if diarrhea and vomiting are present. Dehydration results much more rapidly from these difficulties in the infant because of the factors previously outlined.

Nutrients

Infants must take in adequate nutrients to promote growth as well as to provide fuel. The infant's body size and composition, physical activity, and rate of growth all affect the amount of energy expended to maintain life. The energy requirement for infants is much greater per unit of body weight than for adults. There is a gradual decrease in energy requirements per unit of body weight throughout the first year of life from 120 kcal/kg/day at birth to 100 kcal/kg/day at 1 year. There are several reasons for these changes in energy requirements of infants. The higher basal metabolic demand in early infancy is thought to be due to a larger loss of heat because of relatively greater body surface and a larger proportion of metabolic tissue (Pipes, 1985). Decreasing rate of growth throughout the first year results in decreasing energy requirements per unit of body weight.

For the infant, milk (human or fortified formula) meets most or all of the nutritional needs through most of the first year of life if consumed in appropriate quantities. Especially in the first 6 months of life, there have been no data to support the theory that solid foods are needed in order to meet the nutritional needs of the infant. Breast milk provides necessary nutrients, except possibly for vitamin D, iron, and fluoride, although there is no consensus on this point. Formula-fed infants may need no supplements, depending on the formula used. Labels on formula need to be checked carefully for information on its nutritional adequacy. The American Academy of Pediatrics (AAP, Committee on Nutrition, 1983) does not recommend vitamin D supplements for breastfed infants, unless the mother's vitamin D nutrition is inadequate. A water-soluble form of vitamin D has been found in human milk.

Normal infants of well-nourished mothers are born with adequate stores of iron to meet their needs for 4 to 6 months. Small and preterm infants' neonatal iron stores meet their needs for 2 months. In the past, iron supplements have been recommended for the breastfed infant and are still recommended by some professionals (Foman, 1977). It has been discovered that the trace quantities of iron found in breast milk are extremely absorbable, so that iron supplementation is not believed to be needed by term infants until their weight triples (Chow et al, 1984). Iron-fortified formulas are recommended for the bottlefed infant in the first year of life.

Introduction of Solids

Current information supports the view that the infant does not need solid foods for adequate nutrition until 4 to 6 months of age.

Those persons advocating later introduction of foods do so primarily on the basis of the following assumptions: (1) young infants do not require solids for adequate nutrition; (2) in allergy-prone infants, food allergies are more likely to occur early because of the incomplete digestion of food; (3) the tendency to give too many calories, producing an overweight infant; (4) the danger of choking; and (5) carbohydrates are not adequately digested because of low amylase activity. All these assumptions have some research data to support them. However, the association between an overweight infant and later obesity has not been strongly supported (Wells & Copeland, 1985). The predictability of later obesity from an actual overweight state occurs between 6 and 9 years (Peck & Ullrich, 1985).

Developmental skills give some guidance for the introduction of solids. Maturation of the CNS controls motor skills that influence the infant's ability to eat and drink. Illingsworth and Listen (cited in Pipes, 1985) point out that an infant learns to chew at about 6 to 7 months of age and therefore is ready developmentally to consume food. The sucking pattern of the infant changes in the first year as maturation alters both the form of the oral structure and the way the infant takes liquid from a nipple. Swallowing movements facilitating the ingestion of solid foods occur by 4 to 6 months (Castiglia, 1990). By 4 to 6 months, the oral cavity has grown, mature sucking and jaw motion have developed, and these indicate the readiness of the infant to start solid foods. At the same time, the infant has achieved other developmental skills that affect feeding: ability to grasp, hand-to-mouth movements, and ability to sit. The infant is truly ready to handle solid foods, including finger foods. At this age the tongue is still better able to handle spoon-feeding than drinking from a cup.

Simultaneously, the infant is developing cognitive abilities that assist with the introduction of solid foods (Pridham, 1990). The infant's sense of control becomes evident and a disinterest in sucking occurs between 7 and 12 months.

***Anticipatory Guidance*: Introduction of Solids.** The nurse can assist parents by relaying information about the nutritional requirements of infants and developmental skills that aid feeding, and the rationale for current recommendations about introduction of solids. Parents often have many questions about the sequence and methods of introducing solids. No one sequence is consistently recommended. However, some concepts that will aid the nurse in helping parents establish the pattern they will use in introduction of solids can be identified. The addition of food to the diet should be individualized to the infant and should never be forced. The infant will need some practice as she or he learns the new skill of eating solids, changing gradually from a sucking to a chewing motion. One new food should be introduced at a time, and a number of days (2 to 7) should intervene before another new food is introduced, so that an allergic response could be more easily identified.

It has been generally recommended that the first food offered to the infant be rice cereal, as it is considered to be the least allergenic of the cereal grains and because most cereals are fortified with iron. Parents should give only cereals that are fortified with iron. Labels on the numerous cereal products available need to be read carefully. These products vary significantly in their nutritional value. Parents are instructed to introduce cereal by spoon rather than by adding it to the bottle. In a study of feeding practices of low-income women, nurse researchers found that most mothers introduced cereal to their infants through bottle feeding (Solem et al, 1992). They lacked the understanding that, by feeding their infant cereal in the bottle, they were really introducing solid food too early. Fruits are often the next solid introduced. It is thought that infants find fruits better tasting than some other foods; this may be an adult bias. Vegetables are introduced next, followed by meats and eggs.

Frequently parents ask about the merits of using commercially prepared strained food as opposed to making their own strained foods. Either method can safely meet the nutritional needs of the infant. Some parents prefer to use a combination of these methods. If using commercially prepared foods, the parents should be encouraged to read the labels carefully. An item to look for is the amount of sugar and salt contained in the product; foods containing less of these are preferred. A number of companies in the last few years have altered or removed the additives in their baby food products. The nurse should also point out that the mixed dinner labels should be examined with care. There is usually substantially less meat in the dinner labeled "vegetable and meat" than in the "meat and vegetable" dinners. Even the latter type of dinner may not contain an adequate amount of meat relative to cost. Many of the commercial dessert items have a high content of starch filler and add little to the diet other than calories. If parents are preparing the strained food themselves, they must be sure to prepare a well-balanced diet. If baby foods are prepared at home, parents should remove the baby's portion before salt, sugar, or other spices or condiments are added. They may prepare just enough food to be fed immediately. If they prepare extra food, it can be mixed with a little water or milk, frozen in ice cube trays, placed in storage bags, and kept frozen until immediately before use.

At about the same time or soon after strained foods are introduced, table (finger) foods also may be given. Chewing can be done with the gums, so teeth are not necessary. Infants can feed themselves such items as Melba toast, crackers, and zwieback. As the infant gains skill in chewing, other bite-sized finger foods may be gradually added, including cereals, chicken, vegetables, cheese, and canned fruits. Finger foods should be cut to a size that is easily handled in the infant's mouth to prevent choking. Foods that are small and hard and easily aspirated, such as nuts, popcorn, kernels of corn, and chunks of meat, should not be given to infants.

Parents need to be aware that feeding time can become quite messy (Fig. 5–12). However, this is

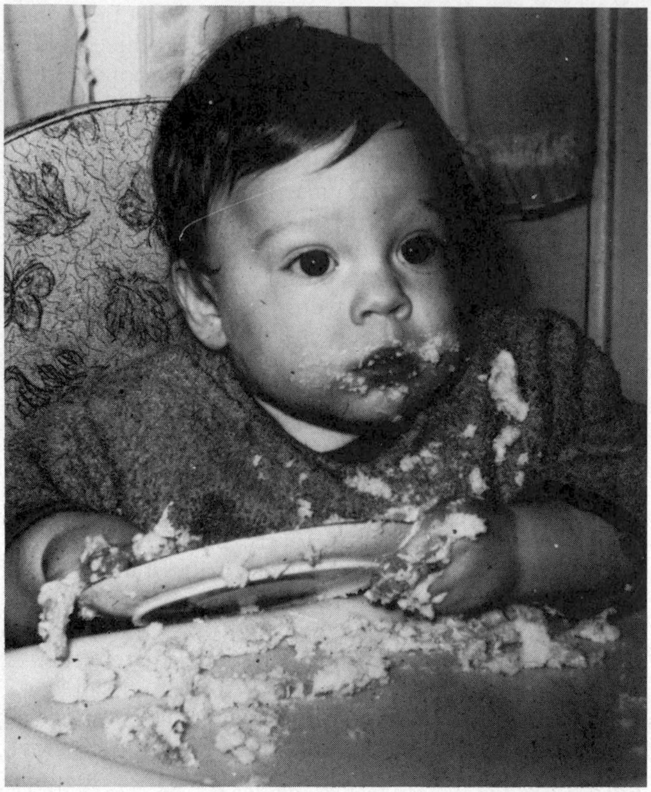

FIGURE 5 - 12. Feeding time can become messy as the infant's drive to explore includes food. (Photograph by David Trainor.)

normal as the infant explores food as well as everything else. Coordination of skills needed to finger-feed themselves eventually becomes transferred to skill in using utensils. By the end of the first year, infants have begun to feed themselves and in the next year will perfect the skills.

Use of Cup. Along with learning the skills associated with feeding herself or himself, the infant is also developing the ability to drink from a cup. As indicated by the earlier discussion related to developmental skills achieved because of neuromuscular maturation, the infant can begin to drink from the cup by 6 months of age. Most infants can drink from a cup by 12 months.

Weaning occurs as infants move from a primarily liquid diet to a more solid diet. As they increase their solid intake and begin to drink from a cup, they will need less from the bottle or breast. The issue of when to wean a particular infant fully often arises when the baby is 6 to 12 months of age. There is no one right time or way to wean an infant. Several behaviors have been identified as indicators of weaning readiness: taking food from a spoon, drinking from a bottle without assistance, the ability to feed self with fingers or spoon, and the ability to take foods that require chewing (Pridham, 1990). A danger of weaning the infant too early is iron deficiency anemia (Castiglia, 1990).

Anticipatory Guidance: Weaning. The nurse must assist parents in their individual approach to weaning their infant. Factors to be considered as this process is discussed with the parents include developmental readiness of the infant, the baby's sucking needs, parents' beliefs and feelings, environmental pressures (family, job), finances, nutritional requirements, and past experiences of family.

Elimination

Another area of physical competency that becomes somewhat regular in the first year is the timing of elimination. Both breastfed and bottlefed infants progress to a pattern of fewer number of stools per day after the first month or two. Stools of breastfed infants remain less formed than those of bottlefed infants. Stool color varies, especially with the introduction of solid food. The timing and number of stools per day tends to be stable by 6 months of age, although a large number of infants remain unpredictable. The kidneys are continuing to mature. Rectal and urethral sphincters are not mature enough for control in most infants until after a year of age.

Anticipatory Guidance: Elimination

Parents often need help to understand that even though the infant's voiding and stooling patterns have become more regular, he or she is not developmentally ready to achieve self-control. The infant must be cognitively aware of elimination before true readiness exists. Also, the young infant often strains during a bowel movement, and some parents assume that this straining means the infant is constipated. This straining may be due to the immaturity of muscle coordination rather than to constipation. If the bowel movement pattern is regular for that infant (may range from several per day to one every 4 to 5 days) and the stool is not hard, no intervention is necessary.

Diaper Choice

The choice to use cloth versus disposable diapers has become a controversial environmental issue. Disposable diapers account for 85 per cent of the diapers used (Mehta, 1990). This calculates to roughly 16 to 18 billion single-use diapers added to landfills annually. Disposable diapers account for nearly 2 per cent of municipal solid waste (MSW), and 3.5 to 4.5 per cent of household solid waste (Lehrburger, 1988). However, other categories of solid waste constitute larger percentages of MSW: newspapers 7.4 per cent, yard waste 17.6 per cent, books and magazines 3 per cent, and direct mail advertisements 2.3 per cent (US Environmental Protection Agency, 1990). It appears that issues of waste management need to be addressed from a comprehensive approach, with consideration given to variables of ease of recyclability and landfill space proportions.

Environmental concerns raised regarding the use of cloth diapers are increased consumption of water (two to six times more water) and energy in laundering (Tryens, 1990). The use of cloth diapers have been cited as causing more water and air pollution (Franklin Associates, 1990; Lehrburger et al, 1991). It is important to note that several of the studies cited were funded by special interest groups and criticized for potential bias in the assumptions made (Tryens, 1990).

Certainly other considerations must be examined in the debate of diaper choice. Cost, infection control, time, and specimen collection are other considerations. The arguments are inconclusive as to which diaper ultimately is least costly (Rockney et al, 1991). Disposable diapers have demonstrated superiority over cloth diapers in preventing environmental contamination. Comparisons of extra-absorbent diapers containing absorbent gelling material (AGM) with disposable and cloth diapers have indicated that diapers with AGM are more effective in reducing skin wetness and produce less diaper dermatitis (Lane et al, 1990; Wilson & Dalles, 1990). Measurement of urine (i.e., specific gravity weight) has been found to be more accurate using disposable rather than cloth diapers (Wong et al, 1992). Findings from a nursing research study found that urine specific gravity results were affected by the following factors: diaper brand, urine volume in the diaper, and method of measuring specific gravity (Gammage & Yarandi, 1993).

Arguments for and against the use of disposable or cloth diapers can be made. Examples of decision-making regarding the choice of diapers by hospitals influenced by environmental concerns have been reported in the literature (Anonymous, 1990; Lehrburger, 1988; Newman, 1990; Taravella, 1990). This is an issue that will warrant further study to assess the environmental, health, and social implications.

Anticipatory Guidance: Diaper Choice

The nurse can assist parents in choosing diaper type. Advantages and disadvantages of cloth and disposable diapers can be presented to parents to help in making an informed decision. Findings from one study reported that most mothers have established diaper preference before the infant is born, suggesting that information be provided during the prenatal period (Rockney et al, 1991).

Play

The needs of the infant for play are implicit throughout the discussion of promotion of infant growth and development. Play provides opportunities for the infant to learn and develop many skills. The importance of a variety of play opportunities can be pointed out to parents. Play is not just an extra activity that serves no purpose (see Chapter 17), but rather the way infants learn about themselves and their environment. As the reader reflects on the discussion of the activities that promote development of physical and intellectual competencies, it becomes clear that many of these activities are usually classified as play activities. Expensive toys are not necessary for play; articles commonly found in the home are perfectly adequate. The nurse can assist the family to creatively use the resources available to them. Play activities promote cognitive and emotional-social development of infants as they separate themselves from their environment. Many such activities foster interaction of the infant with other people. Play can stimulate the attachment of the infant to parents and the eventual ability of the infant to separate. It can provide many pleasurable experiences for infants as they learn to trust and adapt to their world (Fig. 5–13). See Table 5–13 for developmentally appropriate activities and materials for the infant.

Safety Concerns

Safety is another key issue implicit in the discussion of infant growth and development. While discussing the developing competencies of the infant, the nurse can help parents look at the environment in terms of the hazards these developing skills may introduce. The nurse can use the nursing diagnoses of *high risk for injury: falls; high risk for injury: poisoning;* and *high risk for injury: suffocation/aspiration* as a framework for discussing hazards to the safety of the infant.

Parents need to recognize that even very young infants soon will be turning and rolling over. Thus, it is not safe to leave infants unrestrained on any sur-

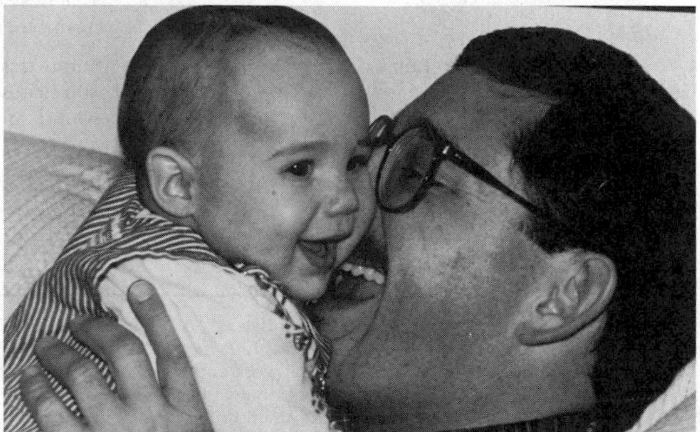

FIGURE 5-13. Social interactions with parents are a significant part of "play" for the infant.

TABLE 5-13
Toys and Play Activities

Toy or Play Activity	Development Promoted	Selection Criteria
Infants from 0 to 6 Mos of Age		
• Music boxes • Radio • Lullaby tapes, records, and CDs	• Stimulates hearing (P)* • Promotes sleep (P) • Sensory novelty (P)	• Volume control • Pleasant sounds
• Mobiles	• Stimulates sight (P) • Sensory novelty • Enhances perception (C)	• Colorful • Safe construction with secure fastener • No sharp edges
• Rattles	• Stimulates repetitive and reflexive motor skills (P) • Stimulates hearing (C) • Promotes rudimentary sense of causality (C)	• No sharp edges • Nontoxic • Unbreakable
• Crib gym and dangling toys	• Stimulates hand-eye coordination (C) • Promotes causality (C) • Stimulates hearing (C) • Stimulates repetitive and reflexive motor skills (P)	• Unbreakable • Nontoxic • No sharp edges • Safe construction with secure fasteners
Infants from 7 to 12 Mos of Age		
• Bath tub toys	• Stimulates fine and gross motor coordination (P) • Encourages mobility (P) • Stimulates balance (P) • Teaches repetitive experimentation and anticipation of events (P, C, and S)	• Unbreakable • No sharp edges
• Pots and pans • Drinking cup	• Stimulates gross motor skills (P) • Associates causal relationship with sound (C)	• Unbreakable • No sharp edges
• Large crayons	• Stimulates creativity (C) • Stimulates fine and gross motor skills (P)	• Nontoxic
• Soft blocks • Cloth books	• Stimulates observation (C) • Stimulates touch (P) • Teaches separation of self from others (P, C, and E)	• Nontoxic • No removable parts
• Busyboard	• Stimulates experimentation (C) • Stimulates sight, touch, sound, and causality (P and C)	• No removable parts
• "Peek-a-boo"	• Stimulates social development (S) • Fosters understanding of object permanence (C)	

Adapted from Betz, C., & Poster, E. (1984). Incorporating play into the care of the hospitalized child. *Issues in Comprehensive Pediatric Nursing, 7,* 343–354; Lee, J., & Fowler, M. (1986). Merely child's play and developmental work and playthings. *Journal of Pediatric Nursing, 1,* 260–269; and An approach to play and play development by Florey, L. *American Journal of Occupational Therapy, 25,* 275–280. Copyright 1971 by the American Occupational Therapy Association, Inc. Reprinted with permission.

* *Key:* C—Cognitive development; P—physical development; E—emotional development; S—social development.

face they might roll off of, such as a bed or changing table. As the infant becomes able to reach items and grasp and bring them to the mouth, parents must be even more alert to what is within reach. Small objects such as coins, buttons, and pins must be removed from the baby's territory. Nothing should be tied around the infant's neck, including pacifiers on strings.

As the infant becomes mobile, the parents or caretaker must learn to anticipate this ability to creep and crawl farther and faster than they think she or he can. An infant's ability to explore the environment increases every day. The parents must anticipate that the baby will soon be able to pull up to a standing position and begin to walk around objects.

Infants can be the victims of drowning if left unattended in the bathtub. A lapse of parental supervision in rushing to answer the phone or doorbell can have disastrous results. It is essential that parents understand their infant should *never* be considered water-safe and left unattended or out of eyesight if in the tub, *ever*. See Chapter 15 for additional information on drowning. Parents can be encouraged to attend cardiopulmonary resuscitation (CPR) and Baby Saver classes.

Car seats have reduced dramatically the potential for death and serious injury from auto accidents. According to the National Highway Traffic Safety Administration the use of safety seats saved the lives of over 200 children (4 years and younger) and prevented 280,000 injuries (NHTSA, 1991). In spite of the fact that child safety seat laws have been enacted in every state, there is great variance in what each law states, and there are problems in strictly enforcing the law. NHTSA (1991) reports that 336 unrestrained children were killed in traffic accidents in 1989.

Incorrect use of car seats has been identified as a factor contributing to death and serious injury. The areas of misuse include improper positioning and misapplication of restraining devices (seat belt, harness straps, and unapproved child restraints) (Gunnip et al, 1987). Refer to Chapter 15 for more in-depth information on child car seats. See Table 5–14 for listing of safety issues and prevention strategies during infancy.

Sex Education

Learning is important for sexual development in the infant. The sex or gender of the child is assigned at birth, and soon afterward the child hears sounds and names that are socially appropriate for sex-rearing. As the child develops an understanding of language, gender of self is gradually associated with the appropriate words. Ability to use the language follows, and body parts are categorized. As language develops, the names of parts of the body, including the genitals, can be used to establish comfortable communication concerning sexuality.

Anticipatory Guidance: Sex Education

Parents frequently ask questions about infant behavior. The nurse who carefully reviews attitudes, behaviors, and knowledge appropriate for each stage of development of the child and is comfortable with her or his own sexuality can intervene in these ways:

1. Correct misinformation about anatomic names or physiologic functions of the body. Direct and clear information enhances the parents' ability to guide the child.
2. Be alert for signs of abuse, including sexual abuse.
3. Provide an opportunity for parents to discuss their feelings about sexual behaviors, such as masturbation.
4. Educate parents/caregivers about the nature of the infant's sexual experience and how it differs from mature sexual expression.

KEY CONCEPTS

Concepts Related to Basic Information

- The major task of a family with an infant is the healthy incorporation of a new person into the existing family.
- The three major motor tasks the infants must learn are gross motor activity, locomotion, and fine motor manipulation.
- *Object permanence* is an important achievement of the sensorimotor period.
- Optimal emotional development in infants depends on interaction with individuals around them, particularly the mother.
- The central issue for the infant is that of basic trust versus basic mistrust.
- The infant uses sensorimotor behavior such as kicking as coping mechanisms.
- Until 6 months of age, breast milk or formula provides adequate nutrition for the infant.
- Birth weight is generally doubled by 4 to 6 months and tripled by 1 year of age.
- The brain grows faster than do other tissues and organs during infancy.
- The smile of the infant is considered an important developmental milestone.
- Infants demonstrate a range of emotions but it is not known if emotions differ in degree or substance or both from adult emotional responses.
- The infant's stage of faith development is termed *undifferentiated* because of the infant's inability to formulate or communicate any ideas of religion or of God.
- Variations in the infant's immunization schedule occur in selected clinical situations such as

TABLE 5-14
Safety Issues and Prevention Strategies

Prevention Strategies Requiring Repeated Monitoring Across Various Ages	
Automobile:	Use of child-restraint device in automobile (check at *each* visit) Never leave child alone in car
Burns:	Reduce hot water temperature Purchase and install smoke alarm Use nonflammable clothing and toys
Poisonings:	Safe storage of drugs, corrosives, and chemicals Use child-resistant caps on drugs Syrup of ipecac in the home Poison Control Number placed at telephone
Play:	Monitor safety of toys and activities
Drowning:	Supervise children around water
Developmental Landmarks	**Examples of Interventions**
Infant (0 to 4 Mos)	
Can roll, reach, grasp, and mouth objects	**Motor Vehicle Accidents** Child-restraint device **Falls** Protect from falls during dressing, etc. Keep one hand on baby **Suffocation/Aspiration** Avoid use of plastic bags in and near crib and playing area Avoid bottle propping Check crib safety Do not tie pacifier around neck Keep small objects and toys with removable parts out of crib Do not use pillows or excess blankets **Burns** Water temperature of bath should be checked with wrist or back of hand Avoid handling hot foods or liquids near baby **Drowning** Nonskid bottom in tub Keep hand on baby in tub at all times

preterm birth, HIV infection, asplenia, presence of chronic illness, and individual or family history of seizure disorder.

- Several behaviors have been identified as indicators of weaning readiness: taking food from a spoon, drinking from a bottle without assistance, ability to take foods requiring chewing, and self-feeding with fingers and spoon.
- An area of physical competency that becomes somewhat regular in the first year is the timing of elimination.
- The choice to use cloth versus disposable diapers has become a controversial environmental issue.

Concepts Related to Nursing Assessment

- Adjustment to a new family member has the high risk for a resulting nursing diagnostic response of *altered role performance*. Nursing assessment must include consideration of the defining characteristics of this diagnosis.
- *Knowledge deficit* regarding the development of attachment between the infant and caregiver has

TABLE 5-14
Safety Issues and Prevention Strategies *(Continued)*

Developmental Landmarks	Examples of Interventions
Infant (4 to 6 Mos)	
Is mobile and is developing some fine motor skills Can roll over Touches, reaches, and grasps to learn about environment Begins to understand off-limit areas (e.g., stove)	**Motor Vehicle Accidents** Continue use of child-restraint device **Falls** Discourage use of walkers Use gates at stairs Highchair safety **Suffocation, Aspiration, Strangulation** Keep drapery cords and mobiles out of reach Avoid hard foods, such as raw vegetables, peanuts, popcorn Avoid use of toys with small parts **Ingestions, Poisonings** Place all harmful products out of reach Remove poisonous plants from child's reach **Burns** Begin to teach meaning of "hot" and off-limit areas **Drowning** Never leave child alone in tub
Infant (6 to 12 Mos)	
Creeps, crawls, is inquisitive Pincer grasp has developed by 8 months Pulls self up and other things down May begin table foods around 8–9 months Holds own bottle and begins to drink from cup Teeth are developing Has the capability to chew a teething biscuit and soft cooked foods	**Motor Vehicle Accidents** Continue use of child-restraint device **Falls** (from windows, down stairs, and from outdoor play equipment) Keep crib away from window Constant supervision is required to prevent falls **Suffocation, Aspiration, Strangulation** Child should sit when eating to prevent aspiration Continue to avoid hard foods Cut foods into small pieces

the high risk for a resulting nursing diagnostic response of *caregiver role strain*.

- Factors to be considered in weaning the infant include developmental readiness, baby's sucking needs, parents' beliefs and feelings, environmental pressures, and past experiences.
- The addition of an infant to the family unit can strain family resources, resulting in the nursing diagnostic response of *impaired home maintenance management*.
- A change in family roles associated with the arrival of a new baby has the high risk for resulting in the nursing diagnostic response of *altered role performance*.
- Nurses providing care to the infant, whether in the hospital or community setting, will consider the nursing diagnostic response of *high risk for altered growth and development; high risk for caregiver role strain; high risk for injury*.
- The head circumference is an important measurement in the physical assessment of the infant; it is helpful in determining absolute growth as well as rate of growth of the skull.
- A useful measurement of infant temperament, the Infant Behavior Questionnaire (IBQ), can be used by the nurse while working with parents to promote optimal well-being of the infant.
- Assessment of the infant's sleep-related behaviors

includes obtaining the following data: history of sleep problems, where the infant sleeps, and interaction of the infant and parent.
- The nurse can use the nursing diagnostic responses of ***high risk for injury: falls; high risk for injury: poisoning;*** and ***high risk for injury: suffocation/aspiration*** as a framework for discussing hazards to the safety of the infant.

Concepts Related to Nursing Intervention

- Nurses can assist in relieving stress related to the family's division of labor by promoting open communication.
- Sharing information from growth charts with the family can be a useful teaching tool in discussing factors affecting growth.
- Placement of mobiles and brightly colored objects within the infant's range of vision can promote hand-eye coordination.
- Activities that stimulate development of the infant's physical competency also promote intellectual competency.
- Nurses can use their knowledge of theories of growth and development as a basis for describing and explaining the baby's behaviors and for predicting outcomes of interactions between the baby and parents.
- The nurse can do much to foster healthy adaptation by being aware of potential stressors and by educating family members as to what to expect by providing support and assisting with problem-solving to minimize the effect of stressors.
- If infant locomotion is restricted for extended periods because of treatment, the nurse can encourage exploration of the environment by placing the child in a wagon or moving the crib to other areas such as the playroom.
- Monitoring the infant's growth and development is the foremost concern of health screening.
- To protect first teeth, gums and teeth can be massaged with a soft, moist, clean cloth after each feeding.

REFERENCES

Ainsworth, M. (1973). The development of the infant-mother attachment. In B. M. Caldwell & H. N. Ricuiti (Eds.), *Review of child development research (Vol. 3).* Chicago: University of Chicago Press.

Alley, J., & Rogers, C. (1986). Sleep patterns of breast fed and non-breast fed infants. *Pediatric Nursing, 12,* 349–351.

American Academy of Pediatrics, Committee on Nutrition (1983, January). Toward a prudent diet for children. *Pediatrics, 71,* 78–80.

American Academy of Pediatrics. (1991). *Report of the committee on infectious disease (red book)* (22nd ed.). Elk Grove Village, IL: American Academy of Pediatrics.

American Academy of Pediatrics, Committee on Infectious Diseases. (1989). Measles: Reassessment of the current immunization policy. *Pediatrics, 84,* 1110–1113.

American Academy of Pediatrics, Committee on Nutrition: Fluoride Supplementation. (1986). *Pediatrics, 77,* 758–761.

Anders, T. F., & Keener, M. A. (1983). Sleep-wake state development and disorders of sleep in infants, children, and adolescents. In M. D. Levine, et al (Eds.), *Developmental behavioral pediatrics.* Philadelphia: WB Saunders.

Anonymous. (1990). Hospital's diaper experiment aimed at helping environment. *Canadian Medical Association Journal, 143,* 900.

Aserinsky, E., & Kleitman, H. (1953, September 4). Regularly occurring periods of eye motility and concomitant phenomena during sleep. *Science, 118,* 273–274.

Baillargeon, R. (1987). Object permanence in 3.5 and 4.5 month old infants. *Developmental Psychology, 23,* 655–664.

Baillargeon, R., & DeVos, J. (1991). Object permanence in young infants: Further evidence. *Child Development, 62,* 1227–1246.

Barglow, P., Vaughn, B. E., & Molitor, N. (1987). Effects of maternal absence due to employment on the quality of infant-mother attachment in a low-risk sample. *Child Development, 58,* 945–954.

Bates, J., & Bayles, K. (1984). Objective and subjective components in mother's perceptions of their children from age 6 months to 3 years. *Merrill-Palmer Quarterly, 30,* 111–130.

Bayley, N. (1965, June). Comparisons of mental and motor test scores for 1–15 months by sex, birth order, race, geographical location and education of parents. *Child Development,* 379.

Becker, P., Chang, A., Samishima, S., & Bloch, M. (1991). Correlates of diurnal sleep patterns in infants of adolescent and adult single mothers. *Research in Nursing and Health, 14,* 97–108.

Behrman, R. E. (Ed.) (1992). *Nelson's textbook of pediatrics* (14th ed.). Philadelphia: WB Saunders.

Belsky, J., & Rovine, M. (1987). Temperament and attachment security in the strange situation: An empirical rapprochement. *Child Development, 58,* 787–795.

Benn, R. K. (1986). Factors promoting secure attachment relationships between employed mothers and their sons. *Child Development, 57,* 1224–1231.

Bernhardt, J. (1987). Sensory capabilities of the fetus. *MCN: American Journal of Maternal Child Nursing, 12,* 44–46.

Betz, C., & Poster, E. (1984). Incorporating play into the care of the hospitalized child. *Issues in Comprehensive Pediatric Nursing, 7,* 343–354.

Booth, C., Johnson-Crowley, N., & Barnard, K. (1985). Infant massage and exercise: Worth the effort? *Maternal Child Nursing Journal, 10,* 184–189.

Bradshaw, T. W. (1981, May/June). Teething. *Pediatric Nursing,* 41–42.

Brazelton, T. B. (1979, June). What parents told me about handling children's sleep problems. *Redbook,* 51–54.

Bronfenbrenner, U. (1989). Ecological systems theory. In R. Vasta (Ed.), *Six theories of child development: Revised formulations and current issues.* Greenwich, CT: JAI Press.

Broom, B. L. (1984). Consensus about the marital relationship during transition to parenthood. *Nursing Research, 33,* 223–228.

Carey, W. (1974). Night waking and temperament in infancy. *Journal of Pediatrics, 84,* 756–758.

Caldwell, R. C., & Stallard, R. E. (1977). *Textbook of preventive dentistry.* Philadelphia: WB Saunders.

Castiglia, P. (1990). Weaning. *Journal of Pediatric Health Care, 4,* 38–39.

Chow, M., et al. (1984). *Handbook of pediatric primary care* (2nd ed.). New York: Wiley Medical.

Chuman, M. (1983). The neurological basis of sleep. *Heart Lung, 12,* 178–181.

Constantine, L. L., & Martinson, F. M. (1981). *Children and sex: New findings, new perspectives.* Boston: Little, Brown.

Crockenberg, S., & McCluskey, K. (1986). Changes in maternal behavior during the baby's first year. *Child Development, 57,* 746–753.

DeMeis, D., McBridge, S., & Hock, E. (1986). The balance of employment and motherhood: Longitudinal study of mothers' feelings about separation from their first-born infants. *Developmental Psychology, 22,* 627–632.

Duvall, E., & Miller, B. (1985). *Marriage and family development.* New York: Harper & Row.

Erikson, E. H. (1963). *Childhood and society* (2nd ed.). New York: WW Norton.

Ferber, R. (1985). *Solve your child's sleep problems.* New York: Simon & Schuster.

Florey, L. (1971). An approach to play and play development. *American Journal of Occupational Therapy, 25,* 275–280.

Foman, S. (1977). *Nutritional disorders of children.* Washington, DC: US Department of Health, Education, and Welfare. Publication No. (HSA) 77–5105.

Franklin Associates. (1990). *Report, energy and environmental profile analysis of children's disposable and cloth diapers.* Prairie Village, KS: Franklin Associates, Ltd.

Freud, S. (1957). In J. Strachey (Ed.). *The standard edition of the complete psychological works of Sigmund Freud* (Vol. 18). London: Hogarth.

Friedrich, O. (1983, August 15). What do babies know? *Time,* 52–59.

Gammage, D., & Yarandi, H. (1993). The effects of diaper brands, urine volume, and time on specific gravity measurement. *Journal of Pediatric Nursing, 8*(1), 10–14.

Goepferd, S. (1986). Infant oral health: A protocol. *ASDC Journal of Dentistry for Children, 53*(4), 261–266.

Gordon, M. (1987). *Manual of nursing diagnosis.* New York: McGraw-Hill.

Gosha, J., & Brucker, M. (1986). A self-help group for new mothers: An evaluation. *MCN: American Journal of Maternal Child Nursing, 11,* 20–23.

Gottlieb, L., & Mendelson, M. (1990). Parental support and firstborn girls' adaptation to the birth of a sibling. *Journal of Applied Developmental Psychology, 11,* 29–48.

Gunnip, A., Robertson, C., Meredith, J., Bell, M., Stroup, K., & Branson, M. (1987). Car seats: Helping parents do it right! *Journal of Pediatric Health Care, 1,* 190–195.

Halverson, H. M. (1931). An experimental study of prehension in infants by means of systematic cinema records. *Genetic Psychology Monographs, 10,* 107–286.

Healy, A. (1972). The sleep patterns of preschool children: General principles and current knowledge. *Clinical Pediatrics, 11,* 174–177.

Hemmelgarn, B., & Laing, G. (1991). The relationship between situational factors and perceived role strain in employed mothers. *Family and Community Health, 14,* 8–15.

Hobson, J. A. (1982). Sleep and its disorders. In J. B. Wyngaarden & L. H. Smith (Eds.), *Cecil textbook of medicine* (16th ed.). Philadelphia: WB Saunders.

Hornick, R., Risenhover, N., & Gunnar, M. (1987). The effects of maternal positive, neutral and negative affective communications on infant responses to new toys. *Child Development, 58,* 937–944.

Houldin, A. (1987). Infant temperament and the quality of the childrearing environment. *Maternal-Child Nursing Journal, 16,* 131–143.

Howson, C., & Fineberg, H. (1992). The ricochet of magic bullets: Summary of the Institute of Medicine report, adverse effects of pertussis and rubella vaccines. *Pediatrics, 89,* 318–324.

Hymovich, D. P., & Chamberlin, R. W. (1980). *Child and family development: Implications for primary health care* (p. 298). New York: McGraw-Hill.

Ijzendoorn, M., & Kroonenberg, P. (1988). Cross cultural patterns of attachment: A meta-analysis of the stranger situation. *Child Development, 59,* 147–156.

Jones, D. P. H., & Verduyn, C. M. (1983). Behavioral management of sleep problems. *Archives of Disease in Children (London), 58,* 442–444.

Jouvet, M. (1969). Biogenic amines and the state of sleep. *Science, 163,* 32–41.

Klinner, M. D., Emde, R. N., Butterfield, P., et al. (1986). Social referencing: The infant's use of emotional signals from a friendly adult with mother present. *Developmental Psychology, 22,* 427–432.

Lane, A., Rehder, P., & Helm, K. (1990). Evaluation of diapers containing absorbent gelling material with conventional disposable diapers in newborn infants. *American Journal of Diseases of Children, 144,* 315–318.

Lee, J., & Fowler, M. (1986). Merely child's play and developmental work and playthings. *Journal of Pediatric Nursing, 1,* 260–269.

Lehrburger, C. (1988). *Diapers in the waste stream: A review of waste management and public issues.* Sheffield, MA: National Association of Diaper Services.

Lehrburger, C., Mullen, S., & Jones, C. (1991). Diapers: Environmental impacts and lifecycle analysis. In *Report for the National Association of Diaper Services.* Great Barrington, MA: Authors.

Lozoff, B., et al. (1984). Co-sleeping in urban families with young children in the United States. *Pediatrics, 74,* 171–182.

Masters, W. M., & Johnson, V. E. (1966). *Human sexual response.* Boston: Little, Brown.

Mehta, N. (1990, April 19). Are you ready for diaper change? *Time,* 66.

Meltzoff, A. N. (1985). An immediate and deferred imitation in 14 and 24 month old infants. *Child Development, 56,* 62–72.

Miller, S. (1988). Parent's beliefs about children's cognitive development. *Child Development, 59,* 259–285.

Moore, T., & Ucko, C. (1957). Night waking in early infancy: Part I. *Archives of Disease in Childhood (London), 32,* 333–343.

Morrongiello, B. A., & Rocca, P. T. (1987). Infant's localization of sounds in the horizontal plane: Effects of auditory and visual cues. *Child Development, 58,* 918–927.

Murphy, S. (1993). Siblings and the new baby: Changing perspectives. *Journal of Pediatric Nursing, 8*(5), 1–12.

National Highway Traffic Safety Administration. (1991). *Idea sampler: Buckle up America.* Washington, DC: US Department of Transportation, National Highway Traffic Safety Administration.

Nelson, C. A. (1987). The recognition of facial expressions in the first two years of life. *Child Development, 58,* 889–909.

Newman, A. (1990). Environmental residency issues were hot topics at American Association of Pediatrics forum. *Pediatric News,* 3.

North American Nursing Diagnosis Association (NANDA). (1992). *NANDA nursing diagnoses: Definitions and classifications.* St. Louis: Author.

Osterholm, P., Lindeke, L., & Smidon, D. (1983). Sleep disturbance in infants aged 6 to 12 months. *Pediatric Nursing, 9,* 269–271, 301.

Parker, S., & Barrett, D. (1992). Maternal type A behavior during pregnancy, neonatal crying and early infant temperament: Do type A women have type A babies? *Pediatrics, 89,* 474–479.

Peck, E., & Ullrich, H. (1985, January). *Children and weight: A changing perspective.* Ad hoc interdisciplinary committee on children and weight. Pp. 2–18.

Piaget, J. (1952). *The origins of intelligence in children.* New York: International Universities Press.

Piaget, J. (1970). Piaget's theory. In P. H. Mussen (Ed.), *Carmichael's manual of child psychology* (Vol. 1). New York: John Wiley.

Pipes, P. (1985). *Nutrition in infancy and childhood* (2nd ed.). St. Louis: CV Mosby.

Power, T. G., & Chapieske, M. L. (1986). Childrearing and impulse control in toddlers: A naturalistic investigation. *Developmental Psychology, 22,* 271–275.

Pridham, K. (1990). Feeding behavior of 6 to 12 month old infants: Assessment and sources of parental information. *Journal of Pediatrics, 117,* S174–S180.

Roberts, M. (1987). Class before birth. *Psychology Today, May,* 41.

Rockney, R., Culpepper, L., Figueira, G., & Mize, W. (1991). Diaper choice: Too costly to bury. *Clinical Pediatrics, 30,* 472–477.

Roffwarg, H., et al. (1966, April 29). Ontogenic development of human sleep-dream cycle. *Science, 152,* 604–618.

Rothbart, M. K. (1986). Longitudinal observation of infant temperament. *Developmental Psychology, 22,* 356–365.

Schmitt, B. D. (1981). Infants who do not sleep through the night. *Journal of Developmental and Behavioral Pediatrics, 21,* 20–23.

Schmitt, B. D. (1986). The prevention of sleep problems and colic. *Pediatric Clinics of North America, 33,* 763–744.

Shannon, M., & Graef, J. (1992). Lead intoxication in infancy. *Pediatrics, 89,* 87–90.

Shirley, M. A. (1933). *Intellectual development:* Vol. 2. *The first two years.* Minneapolis: University of Minnesota Press.

Slusher, I. L., & McClure, M. J. (1992). Infant stimulation during hospitalization. *Journal of Pediatric Nursing, 7,* 276–279.

Solem, B., Norr, K., & Gallo, A. (1992). Infant feeding practices of low-income mothers. *Journal of Pediatric Health Care, 6,* 54–59.

Stewart, R. (1990). *The second child: Family transition and adjustment.* Newbury Park, CA: Sage.

Takahashi, Y. (1979). Growth hormone secretion related to the sleep and waking rhythm. In R. Drucker-Colin, et al. (Eds.), *The function of sleep* (p. 113). New York: Academic Press.

Taravella, S. (1990, December 24–31). Disposable diapers get dumped. *Modern Health Care,* 32–33.

Thevenin, T. (1976). *The family bed: An age old concept in childrearing.* Minneapolis: Author.

Tomlinson, P. (1987). Father involvement with first-born infants: Interpersonal and situational factors. *Pediatric Nursing, 13,* 101–105, 139.

Tryens, J. (1990). *Review of Arthur D. Little Inc's disposable versus reusable diapers.* Washington, DC: Center for Policy Alternatives.

Turley, M. (1985). A meta-analysis of informing mothers concerning the sensory and perceptual capabilities of their infants: The effects of maternal-infant interaction. *Maternal-Child Nursing Journal, 14,* 183–197.

US Department of Health and Human Services. (1990). *Child health,* 1990. HRS–M–CH 90–1.

US Environmental Protection Agency. (1990). *Characterization of municipal solid waste in the United States: 1990 Update.* Washington, DC: EPA 530–SW–90–042.

Vaughan, V., & Litt, I. (1990). *Child and adolescent development: Clinical implications.* Philadelphia: WB Saunders.

Ventura, J. (1982). Parent coping behaviors, parent functioning and infant temperament characteristics. *Nursing Research, 31,* 269–273.

Weissbluth, M. (1981). Sleep duration and infant temperament. *Journal of Pediatrics, 99,* 817–819.

Weissbluth, M. (1987). *Healthy sleep habits, healthy child.* New York: Fawcett Book Group.

Weissbluth, M. (1991). Sleep learning: The first four months. *Pediatric Annals, 20,* 228–238.

Wells, K., & Copeland, B. (1985). Childhood and adolescent obesity: Progress in behavioral assessment and treatment. *Progress in Behavior Modification, 19,* 145–176.

Wilson, A. (1990). Standards in maternal and child oral health. *Journal of Public Health Dentistry, 50,* 432–438.

Wilson, P., & Dalles, M. (1990). Diaper performance: Maintenance of healthy skin. *Pediatric Dermatology, 7,* 179–184.

Wolff, P. (1969). The natural history of crying and other vocalizations in early infancy. In F. Foss (Ed.), *Determinants of infant behaviors.* New York: Methuen & Company, Ltd.

Wong, D., Brantly, D., Clutter, T., Simone, D., Lammert, D., Nix, K., Perry, K., Smith, D., & White, K. (1992). Diapering choice: A critical review of the issues. *Pediatric Nursing, 18,* 41–49, 52–54.

Zuckerman, B., Stevenson, J., & Bailey, V. (1987). Sleep problems in early childhood: Continuities, predictive factors and behavioral correlates. *Pediatrics, 80,* 664–671.

BIBLIOGRAPHY

AAP, Committee on Nutrition. (1989). Iron-fortified infant formulas. *Pediatrics, 84,* 1114–1115.

Anderson, E. (1987, March/April). Enhancing reciprocity between mother and neonate. *Nursing Research,* 89–93.

Archenbach, T. M., Phares, V., Howell, C. T., Rauh, V. A., & Nurcombe, B. (1990). Seven-year outcome of the Vermont Intervention Program for low-birthweight infants. *Child Development, 61,* 1672–1678.

Arnett, J. (1989). Caregivers in day care centers. Does training matter? *Journal of Applied Developmental Psychology, 10,* 541–552.

Arnold, L., et al. (1990). Legislative issues affecting parenting: An overview of current policies. *Journal of Perinatal and Neonatal Nursing, 4,* 24–32.

Avard, D., et al. (1990). The role of the Canadian Institute of Child Health in promoting family centered care. *Children's Health Care, 19,* 209–212.

Beal, J. (1991). Methodological issues in conducting research on parent-infant attachment. *Journal of Pediatric Nursing, 6,* 11–15.

Beal, J. (1989). The effects of demonstration of the Brazelton Neonatal Behavioral Assessment scale on the paternal-infant relationship. *Issues in Perinatology, 16,* 18–22.

Belsky, J. (1988). The "effects" of infant day care reconsidered. *Early Childhood Research Quarterly, 3,* 235–272.

Bocchino, C. (1990). U.N. Convention on the Rights of Children. *Pediatric Nursing, 16,* 600.

Bower, T. (1982). *Development in Infancy* (2nd ed.). New York: WH Freeman.

Bowlby, J. (1980). *Attachment and Loss:* (Vol. 3). New York: Basic Books.

Brimhall, C., & Esterly, N. (1990). Uninvited guest: Skin infestations of childhood. *Contemporary Pediatrics, 7,* 30–36.

Brodish, M. (1982, July/August). Relationship of early bonding to initial infant feeding patterns in bottle-fed newborns. *Journal of Obstetric, Gynecologic, and Neonatal Nursing,* 248–252.

Brody, S. (1981, April). The concepts of attachment and bonding. *Journal of American Psychological Association,* 815–829.

Brown, M. & Hellings, P. (1988). A case study of qualitative versus quantitative reviews: The maternal-infant bonding controversy. *Journal of Pediatric Nursing, 4,* 104–111.

Brown, P., Rustia, J., & Schappert, P. (1991). A comparison of fathers of high-risk newborns and fathers of healthy newborns. *Journal of Pediatric Nursing, 6,* 269–273.

Budreau, G., et al. (1991). Clinical indicators of infant irritability. *Neonatal Network, 9,* 23–30.

Carver, C. S., Scheier, M. F., & Weintraub, J. K. (1989). Assessment coping strategies: A theoretically based approach. *Journalof Personality and Social Psychology, 56,* 267–283.

Castiglia, P. (1989). Sibling rivalry. *Journal of Pediatric Health Care, 3,* 52–54.

Centers for Disease Control. (1993). Standards for pediatric immunization practices. *Morbidity and Mortality Weekly Report, 42,* 1–9.

Chess, S., & Thomas, A. (1982, April). Infant bonding: Mystique and reality. *American Journal of Orthopsychiatry,* 213–222.

Christoffel, K. (1989). Child passenger safety. *American Journal of Diseases of Childhood, 143,* 1271–1272.

Coffman, S. (1991). Parent education for drowning prevention. *Journal of Pediatric Health Care, 5,* 141–146.

Coffman, S., Levitt, M., & Guacci-Franco, N. (1993). Mothers' stress and close relationships: Correlates with infant health status. *Pediatric Nursing, 19*(2), 135–142.

Cole, J. (1985). Infant stimulation reexamined: An environmental and behavioral bases approach. *Neonatal Network, 3,* 24–31.

Colombo, J. (1982, February). The critical period concept: Research, methodology and theoretical issues. *Psychological Bulletin,* 260–275.

Craig, S., et al. (1982). The effect of early contact on maternal perception of infant behavior. *Early Human Development, 6,* 197–204.

Crnic, K., Greenberg, M., Ragozin, A., et al. (1983). Effects of stress and social support on mothers and premature full term infants. *Child Development, 54,* 209–217.

Davis, M., & Akridge, K. (1987, November/December). The effect of promoting intrauterine attachment in primiparas on postdelivery attachment. *Journal of Obstetric, Gynecologic, and Neonatal Nursing,* 430–437.

Davis, R., & Truesdale, M. (1993). Creative approaches to promoting parent-infant bonding. *Journal of Pediatric Nursing, 8*(3), 201–202.

Dean, P., Morgan, P., & Towle, J. (1982). Making baby's acquaintance: A unique attachment strategy. *MCN: American Journal of Maternal Child Nursing, 7,* 37–41.

DeAngelis, C. (1984). *Pediatric Primary Care* (3rd ed.). Boston: Little, Brown.

Faller, H. S., & Ratcliff, L. (1993). Sibling visitation: How far should the pendulum swing? *Journal of Pediatric Nursing, 8*(2), 92–99.

Feeg, V. (1990). The future of pediatric nursing: Anticipating the health care needs of children. *Imprint, 37,* 70, 72–73, 75.

Fortier, J., et al. (1991). Adjustment to a newborn: Sibling preparation makes a difference. *Journal of Obstetric, Gynecologic, and Neonatal Nursing, 2,* 73–79.

Fulginiti, V. (1992). How safe are pertussis and rubella vaccines? A commentary on the Institute of Medicine report. *Pediatrics, 89,* 334–336.

Gillis, A. (1990). Nurse's knowledge of growth and developmental principles in meeting psychosocial needs of hospitalized children. *Journal of Pediatric Nursing, 5,* 78–87.

Ginsberg, H., & Opper, S. (1969). *Piaget's Theory of Intellectual Development.* Englewood Cliffs, NJ: Prentice-Hall.

Glover, L. (1989). Parental-fetal attachment. *Nursing Scan in Research, 2,* 1–4.

Goetting, A. (1986). The developmental tasks of siblings over the life cycle. *Journal of Marriage and the Family, 48,* 703–714.

Goldberg, S. (1983). Parent-infant bonding: Another look. *Child Development, 54,* 1355–1382.

Gordan, B. (1988). A conceptual model for tracking high risk infants and making early service decisions. *Journal of Developmental and Behavioral Pediatrics, 9,* 279–286.

Gordin, P. (1990). Assessing and managing agitation in a critically ill infant. *MCN: American Journal of Maternal Child Nursing, 15,* 26–32.

Gorski, P. (1985). Behavioral and environmental care: New frontiers in neonatal nursing. *Neonatal Network, 3,* 8–11.

Grace, J. (1984, January/February). Does a mother's knowledge of fetal gender affect attachment? *MCN: American Journal of Maternal Child Nursing,* 42–45.

Grossman, K., Thane, K., & Grossman, K. (1981). Maternal tactile contact of the newborn after various postpartum conditions of mother-infant contact. *Developmental Psychology, 17,* 159.

Halpern, J. (1990). How safe are child safety seats? *Journal of Emergency Nursing, 16,* 151–155.

Hanglesben, K. (1983, July/August). Transition to fatherhood: An explanatory study. *Journal of Obstetric, Gynecologic, and Neonatal Nursing,* 265.

Harms, D., & Giordano, J. (1990). Ethical issues in high-risk infant care. *Issues in Comprehensive Pediatric Nursing, 13,* 1–14.

Hogue, E. (1993). Care in the absence of primary caregivers. *Pediatric Nursing, 19*(1), 49–55.

Holaday, B. (1989). The family with a chronically ill child. In C. Gilliss, et al. (Eds.). *Toward a science of family nursing.* Reading, MA: Addison-Wesley.

Honig, J. (1986). Preparing preschool-aged children to be siblings. *MCN: American Journal of Maternal Child Nursing, 11,* 37–43.

Humphry, R. (1991). Impact of feeding problems on the parent-infant relationship. *Infants and Young Children, 3,* 30–38.

Illingsworth, R. (1983). *The Development of the Infant and Young Child* (8th ed.). New York: Churchill Livingstone.

Katz, I. T., Pokorni, J., & Long, T. (1989). *Chronically ill and at risk infants.* Palo Alto, CA: VORT.

Kemp, V. H., & Page, C. K. (1987, May/June). Maternal prenatal attachment in normal and high-risk pregnancies. *Journal of Obstetric, Gynecologic, and Neonatal Nursing,* 179–184.

Klaus, M., & Kennell, J. (1982). *Parent-Infant Bonding* (2nd ed.). St. Louis: CV Mosby.

Komelasky, A., & Bond, B. (1993). The effect of two forms of learning reinforcement upon parental retention of CPR skills. *Pediatric Nursing, 19*(1), 96–101.

Korsch, B. (1983). More on parent-infant bonding. *Journal of Pediatrics, 102,* 249–250.

Kotagal, U. (1993). Newborn consequences of teenage pregnancy. *Pediatric Annals, 22*(2), 127–132.

Krenz, M., Karlik, B., & Kiniry, S. (1989). A nursing diagnosis based model: Guiding nursing practice. *Journal of Nursing Administration, 19,* 32–36.

Kuller, J. M. (1984). Skin development and function—Part I. *Neonatal Network, 3,* 18–23.

Levitt, M., Weber, R., & Clark, M. (1986). Social network relationships as sources of maternal support and well being. *Developmental Psychology, 22,* 310–316.

Lijeberg, B. (1991). Dietary consultation for lactating women. *Journal of Pediatric Health Care, 5,* 40–43.

Lott, J. W. (1989). Developmental care of the preterm infant. *Neonatal Network, 7,* 21–28.

Lower, M. S., & Burton, S. (1989). Measuring the impact of nursing interventions on patient outcomes—The challenge of the 1990s. *Journal of Nursing Quality Assurance, 4,* 24–34.

Luddington-Hoe, S. (1983, September). What can newborns really see? *American Journal of Nursing,* 1286–1289.

Maisels, M., et al. (1983, March). Circumcision: The effect of information on parental decision making. *Pediatrics,* 453.

Marino, B. (1988). Assessments of infant play: Applications to research and practice. *Issues in Comprehensive Pediatric Nursing, 11,* 227–240.

Marino, B. (1991). Studying infant and toddler. *Journal of Pediatric Nursing, 6,* 16–20.

Minnick, S., et al. (1991). Effect of oxyquinoline ointment on diaper dermatitis. *Dermatology Nursing, 3,* 25–28.

Mitchell, K., & Mills, N. (1983, March/April). Is the sensitive period in parent-infant bonding over-rated? *Pediatric Nursing,* 91–94.

Newton, L. (1983, May/June). Helping parents cope with infant crying. *Journal of Obstetric, Gynecologic, and Neonatal Nursing,* 179.

Nugent, K. (1989). Routine care: Promoting development in hospitalized infants. *MCN: American Journal of Maternal Child Nursing, 14,* 318–321.

O'Connor, S., et al. (1980). Reduced incidence of parenting inadequacy following rooming. *Pediatrics, 66,* 176–180.

Oski, F. (1990). Whole cow milk feeding between 6 and 12 months of age? Go back to 1976. *Pediatrics, 12,* 187–189.

Parmelee, A. (1985). Sensory stimulation in the nursery: How much and when? *Developmental Behavioral Psychology, 6,* 242–243.

Pipes, P. (1989). *Nutrition in infancy and childhood* (4th ed.). St. Louis: CV Mosby.

Porter, R., Cernoch, J., & Perry, S. (1983, Fall). The importance of odors in mother-infant interactions. *Maternal-Child Nursing Journal,* 147–154.

Pridham, L., et al. (1991). Early postpartum transition: Progress in maternal identity and role attainment. *Research in Nursing and Health, 14,* 21–31.

Putnam, C., & Reynolds, M. (1989). Mupirocin: A new topical therapy for impetigo. *Journal of Pediatric Health Care, 3,* 224–227.

Ramey, C., Bryant, D., & Suarez, T. (1990). Early intervention: Why, for whom, how, and at what cost? *Clinics in Perinatology, 17,* 47–55.

Rhodes, M. (1991). Major legal initiatives in MCH. *MCN: American Journal of Maternal Child Nursing, 16,* 21–31.

Rhodes, M. (1991). Brewing issues in MCH. *MCN: American Journal of Maternal Child Nursing, 16,* 73.

Righi, F., & Krozy, R. (1983, October). The child in the car: What every nurse should know about safety. *American Journal of Nursing,* 1421.

Rutledge, D. L., & Pridham, K. F. (1987, May/June). Postpartum mothers' perceptions of competence for infant care. *Journal of Obstetric, Gynecologic, and Neonatal Nursing,* 185–194.

Schmitt, B. (1990). Sibling rivalry toward a new baby. *Contemporary Pediatrics, 7,* 111–112.

Siegal, E. (1982). A critical examination of studies of parent-infant bonding. In M. Klaus & M. Robertson (Eds.), *Birth, interaction and attachment* (pp 51–61). Edison, NJ: Johnson & Johnson.

Snyder, H. (1991). To circumcise or not. *Hospital Practice, 26,* 201–207.

Sorenson, C. (1990). Children's coping responses. *Journal of Pediatric Nursing, 5,* 259–267.

Tiedeman, M., Simon, K., & Clatworthy, S. (1990). Communication through therapeutic play. In M. Craft & J. Deneby (Eds.), *Nursing intervention for infants and children* (pp 93–110). Philadelphia: WB Saunders.

Tomlinson, P. S. (1987). Spousal differences in marital satisfaction during transition to parenthood. *Nursing Research, 36,* 239–243.

Weider, S., Drachman, R., & DeLeo, T. (1989). A developmental/relationship in-service training model for public health nurses serving multirisk infants and families. *Zero to Three, 10,* 16–20.

Weigley, E. (1990). Changing patterns in offering solids to infants. *Pediatric Nursing, 16,* 439–452.

Weiser, M. A., & Castiglia, P. T. (1984). Assessing early father-infant attachment. *MCN: American Journal of Maternal Child Nursing, 9,* 104–105.

CHAPTER • 6

Families with Toddlers

RELATED TOPICS
Developmental theories, Chapter 3
Child health assessment, Chapter 13
Promoting safety, childproofing the home, Chapter 15
Promoting healthy play for toddlers, Chapter 17

Development and Adaptation of the Family with a Toddler

Adapting Resources
Childproofing
Re-Establishing Relationships
Participating in Social, Community Activities
Promoting Healthy Independence
Resolving Developmental Task Conflicts
Accepting Help
Finding Satisfaction in Parenthood

Nursing Care and Guidance

Adapting Resources
Re-Establishing Relationships
Resolving Conflicts
Accepting Help

Growth and Development of the Toddler

Physical Competency

Height and Weight
Head and Chest Circumference
Organ Maturation
General Appearance and Skeletal Growth
Motor Development

Intellectual Competency

Cognitive Development: Sensorimotor Period
Preoperational Period
Language Development

Emotional-Social Competency

Psychosocial Development: Development of Autonomy
Sexuality
Temperament
Emotions
Fears
Coping Mechanisms
Moral and Faith Development
Peer Relationships

Health Maintenance and Promotion

Health Screening
Vision and Hearing
Dental Care
Sleep Behaviors
Nutrition
Toilet Training
Play
Safety Concerns
Sex Education

LEARNING OBJECTIVES

- Identify the major concerns in the family with a toddler.
- Describe the developmental milestones acquired during toddlerhood in the areas of physical, intellectual, and emotional-social competencies.
- Explain the coping mechanisms used by the toddler and interventions the nurse can employ to foster their use.
- Apply the nursing process to the psychosocial concerns of the toddler and the family.
- Identify the nursing diagnoses the nurse might consider in providing care to the toddler and the family.
- Discuss the anticipatory concerns related to the developmental needs of the toddler and the use of nursing interventions to foster their use.
- Identify the safety developmental concerns and describe prevention interventions used during toddlerhood.

- Identify the milestones of the toddler's physical growth and development.
- Apply understanding of the toddler's gross and fine motor development.
- Apply knowledge of the toddler's cognitive development to clinical practice.
- Identify characteristics of the toddler's speech and language.
- Discuss the importance of temperament in providing care to the toddler.
- Identify the most common coping strategies used by toddlers.
- Identify the essential components of the toddler's health screening examination.
- Identify the prominent anticipatory guidance concerns for parents during the toddlerhood.

The parents in the childbearing stage of the life cycle who now have a toddler rambling through their home, perhaps along with older children, find themselves faced with a revised set of family developmental tasks. The overall task of the family with a toddler is the establishment and maintenance of a stable home that values each member's contributions and responds to the changing needs of each. To accomplish this task the family must (1) successfully adapt its resources to accommodate an active child or children, (2) reorganize relationships within and outside the home to include the child without disrupting intimate marital bonds, and (3) continue to derive satisfaction from parenthood. This section looks at those tasks and their impact on each member, as well as each member's responsibility in accomplishing those tasks. The nurse's role in assisting families to adapt in healthy ways to these task demands is described, with consideration given to common stressors of the family with a toddler. The following section details toddler growth and development, including anticipatory guidance for the parent(s).

Development and Adaptation of the Family with a Toddler

Most commonly encountered stresses in families with toddlers are those related to parenting and either the threat of or the actual breakdown in family relationships (husband and wife, parent and child, child and sibling). The family with a toddler is ripe for stress or crisis because of several developmentally associated factors. Toddlers, in their unique developmental crises or transitional states are in disequilibrium much of the time between dependence and striving for independence; this puts extra stress on their relationship with family members. Siblings must now learn the lessons of sharing not only their mother and father but also their toys, play space, and perhaps even their bedrooms or beds as a sibling moves into toddlerhood. Or if toddlers are presented with a new baby sister or brother, they will find the demands on their immature coping skills quite draining.

Knowing about the potential stresses to families with toddlers is extremely valuable to the nurse who will interact frequently, and perhaps regularly, with

TABLE 6-1
Summary of Toddler Growth and Development and Health Maintenance

Physical Competency	Intellectual Competency	Emotional-Social Competency
General: From 1 to 3 Yrs		
Gains 5 kg (11 lb) Grows 20.3 cm (8 in) 12 teeth erupt Nutritional requirements Energy 100 Kcal/kg/day Fluid 115–125 ml/kg/day Protein 1.8 g/kg/day See Chapter 16 for vitamins and minerals	Learns by exploring and experimenting. Learns by imitating. Progresses from a vocabulary of 3–4 words at 12 mos to about 900 words at 36 mos	Central crisis: to gain a sense of autonomy vs doubt and shame. Demonstrates independent behaviors. Exhibits attachment behavior strongly and regularly until third birthday. Fears persist of strange people, objects, and places and of aloneness and being abandoned. Egocentric in play (parallel play). Imitation of parents in household tasks and activities of daily living
15 Mos		
Legs appear bowed. Walks alone, climbs, slides down stairs backward. Stacks two blocks. Scribbles spontaneously. Grasps spoon but rotates it, holds cup with both hands. Takes off socks and shoes	Trial-and-error method of learning. Experiments to see what will happen. Says at least 3 words. Uses expressive jargon	Shows independence by trying to feed self and helps in undressing
18 Mos		
Runs but still falls. Walks upstairs with help. Slides down stairs backward. Stacks three to four blocks. Clumsily throws a ball. Unzips a large zipper. Takes off simple garments	Begins to retain a mental image of an absent object. Concept of object permanence fully develops. Has vocabulary of 10 or more words. Holophrastic speech (one word used to communicate whole ideas)	Fears the water. Temper tantrums may begin. Negativism and dawdling predominate. Bedtime rituals begin. Awareness of gender identity begins. Helps with undressing
24 Mos		
Runs quickly and with fewer falls. Pulls toys and walks sideways. Walks downstairs hanging on a rail (does not alternate feet). Stacks six blocks. Turns pages of a book. Imitates vertical and circular strokes. Uses spoon with little spilling. Can feed self. Puts on simple garments. Can turn door knobs	Enters into preconceptual phase of preoperational period: Symbolic thinking and symbolic play. Egocentric thinking, imagination, and pretending are common. Has vocabulary of about 300 words. Uses 2-word sentences (telegraphic speech). Engages in monologue	Fears the dark and animals. Temper tantrums may continue. Negativism and dawdling continue. Bedtime rituals continue. Sleep resisted overtly. Usually shows readiness to begin bowel and bladder control. Explores genitalia. Brushes teeth with help. Helps with dressing and undressing
36 Mos		
Has set of deciduous teeth at about 30 mos. Walks downstairs alternating feet. Rides tricycle. Walks with balance and runs well. Stacks eight to ten blocks. Can pour from a pitcher. Feeds self completely. Dresses self almost completely (does not know front from back). Cannot tie shoes	Preconceptual phase of preoperational period as for 24 mos. Uses around 900 words. Constructs complete sentences and uses all parts of speech	Temper tantrums subside. Negativism and dawdling subside. Bedtime rituals subside. Self-care in feeding, elimination, and dressing enhances self-esteem

this family. The nurse can be involved in helping the toddler and his or her family manage stress in ways that will continue to foster healthy development both of the family as a unit and of the individuals in it.

The primary goal for the nurse working with the toddler is to promote optimal competencies within the child and to assist the child and parents to appreciate the importance of and the interrelationships between physical, intellectual, emotional, and social competencies (Table 6–1). Nursing diagnostic responses that may be applied to the care of the toddler include *high risk for altered growth and development, and high risk for impaired physical mobility and fear.* The nurse will continuously assess the child for the etiology of the actual response, the risk factors associated with the potential and actual problems, and defining characteristics. Refer to Table 6–2 for a description of nursing care for the nursing diagnostic response *high risk for altered growth and development.*

TABLE 6-1
Summary of Toddler Growth and Development and Health Maintenance *(Continued)*

Nutrition	Play	Safety
General: From 1 to 3 Yrs		
Milk 16–24 oz. Appetite decreases. Wants to feed self. Has food jags. Never force food; give nutritious snacks. Give iron and vitamin supplementation only if intake is poor	Books at all ages. Needs physical and quiet activities, does not need expensive toys	Never leave alone in tub. Keep poisons, including detergents and cleaning products, out of reach. Use car seat. Have ipecac in house
15 Mos		
Vulnerable to iron deficiency anemia. Give table foods except for tough meat and hard vegetables. Wants to feed self	Stuffed animals, dolls, music toys. Peek-a-boo, hide and seek. Water and sand play. Stacking toys. Roll ball on floor. Push toys on floor. Read to toddler	Keep small items off floor (pins, buttons, clips). Child may choke on hard food. Cords and table cloths are a danger. Keep electrical outlets plugged and poisons locked away. Risk of kitchen accidents with toddler under foot
18 Mos		
Negativism may interfere with eating. Encourage self-feeding. Is easily distracted while eating. May play with food. High activity level interferes with eating	Rocking horse. Nesting toys. Shape-sorting cube. Pencil or crayon. Pull toys. Four-wheeled toy to ride. Throw ball. Running and chasing games. Rough-housing. Puzzles. Blocks. Hammer and peg board	Falls: From riding toy In bathtub From running too fast Climbs up to get dangerous objects. Keep dangerous things out of wastebasket
24 Mos		
Requests certain foods, therefore snacks should be controlled. Imitates eating habits of others. May still play with food and especially with utensils and dish (pouring, stacking)	Clay and Play-Doh. Finger paint. Brush paint. Record player with record and story book and songs to sing along. Toys to take apart. Toy tea sets. Puppets. Puzzles	May fall from outdoor large play equipment. Can reach farther than expected (knives, razors, and matches must be kept out of reach)
36 Mos		
Sits in booster seat rather than high chair. Verbal about likes and dislikes	Likes playing with other children, building toys, drawing and painting, doing puzzles. Imitation household objects for doll play. Nurse and doctor kits. Carpenter kits	Protect from: Turning on hot water Falling from tricycle Striking matches

Adapting Resources

The American norm is to provide children with some space of their own, separate from that of their parents, by the time the children approach toddlerhood. If the family's socioeconomic situation and values about privacy make it feasible, this means that each child has her or his own bedroom or at least one that is shared with a same-sex sibling. If budget or values do not support such an arrangement, the toddler's private retreat may be a large closet renovated into play and sleep areas or a section of a room that can be closed off with folding doors or pull-around drapes. Privacy, not the size of the area, is the important consideration.

The modern family with a developmental orientation that places greater value on persons is motivated to provide whatever space is needed to help the child grow and develop at her or his best. Either approach can allow the toddler opportunities to move about, explore, and manipulate; but the modern family approach tends to grant the toddler the range of the home. The traditional approach usually means confinement of toys and explorative activities to certain rooms or certain areas in rooms within the home.

Another change that families with expressive toddlers must make is with emotional space. Toddlers' caregivers will foster their development of self-control by allowing them space for making choices and for emotional expression. For example, toddlers might choose the toys they will take to bed with them or which pajamas to wear. As long as the choices and emotional expressions are healthy, are conducive to their development, and will cause no one harm, as much choice as their ages warrant should be given.

TABLE 6-2

Growth and Development Plan: Families with Toddlers

Analysis: Nursing Diagnostic Statement

Response and Related or Risk Factors: *High risk for altered growth and development: risk factors*

- Illness/physical impairment
- Treatment-related procedures
  - Isolation
  - Injections,
  - Painful treatments
- Separation from caretaking figures
- Inadequate, inappropriate caregiver's support
- Interruption/alteration of daily routine
- Inadequate sensory stimulation
- Caregiver knowledge deficit
- Developmental characteristics (immature coping mechanisms, fear, limited language)
- Maturational factors (motor skills affecting eating, self-care activities)

Projected Outcome: The toddler will demonstrate acquisition of developmentally appropriate behaviors in the physical, intellectual, and emotional-social domains.

Defining Characteristics

Subjective:

- Child verbalizes mistrust, fear
- Caregiver expresses unrealistic expectations about toddler's behavior, negative/ambivalent feelings concerning parenting

Objective:

- Flat affect
- Listlessness
- Decreased responses
- Shows limited signs of satisfaction to caregiver
- Shows limited eye contact
- Decreased appetite
- Lethargic
- Irritable
- Regression in self-toileting
- Regression in self-feeding

Nursing Interventions

Health Screening

- **Assess factors that can identify altered growth and development.** (Evidence of child's behavior deviating from age-appropriate levels will be observed and documented based on theoretical basis of growth and development; parent-child relationships; social support; knowledge of physiologic effects of disease on the child and family)
- **Assess child's level of development using developmental norms and specific assessment tools.** (Refer to Chapter 13, Assessing Child Health, and Appendices 2 through 6)

Evaluation Criteria

- **Any developmental delays will be identified as evidenced by:**
  - Charted assessment of screening for physical, intellectual, and emotional-social development
  - Referral for deviations from the norm detected during screening
- Caregiver will demonstrate knowledge and ability to interact with the child in an age-appropriate manner and provide activities to support/enhance the developmental needs of the child.
- The child will achieve age-appropriate developmental tasks
- Referrals to community resources will be made as needed

When their choices or emotional expression breach these considerations, limits must be imposed.

If limits exist in relation to the space provided parents must make those limits realistic and clearly understood by the toddler.* Consistent enforcement of these limits is important so that toddlers know where the boundaries are and need not worry about whether they are inside or outside their limits "this time."

Childproofing

This is the time for parents to make a careful study of the home for environmental hazards and possible relocation of precious possessions. They need to become aware that special vigilance and firm discipline can prevent accidental injury to their child.

Although some families choose to leave the home

*Toddlers live in the present, having not yet developed the ability to recall the past or anticipate the future conceptually. They need frequent reminders in simple terms, not a one-time discussion.

TABLE 6-2 (continued)

Defining Characteristics	Nursing Interventions	Evaluation Criteria
• Interrupted sleep pattern • Delay in language skills • Delay in gross and fine motor skills • Failure of toddler and parent to display social-affective play activity	*Anticipatory Guidance; Parent Education: Childrearing Family* • **Provide anticipatory guidance to caregivers regarding acquisition of age-appropriate developmental tasks.** (Refer to information on developmental norms in sections on intellectual and emotional-social competencies) • **Assist parents to provide opportunities for the child (including acutely and chronically ill) to meet age-related developmental tasks.** (Refer to information on nursing interventions and anticipatory guidance in sections on intellectual and emotional-social competencies, health maintenance and promotion) *Support System Enhancement* • **Refer child and family to appropriate community resources as needed.** • Appropriate agency for counseling for child and family treatment • Appropriate agency for supportive services (e.g., occupational therapy, physical therapy, home care services) • Community programs specific to factors affecting the child's altered growth and development (e.g., child protection services, day care centers, educational services and social services), provide information on community self-help groups, parent and sibling support groups, advocacy groups (e.g., Parents Without Partners)	

unaltered and teach their toddler what he or she may handle and what must be left alone, most families opt for at least minimal childproofing. Ideally, every home with a toddler is childproofed at least to the extent that medicines and poisonous or corrosive items are not available to the child. The less childproofing there is, the more continuous watchful surveillance is necessary to ensure the toddler's safety (Fig. 6–1).

The need to include vigilance for defining characteristics of the nursing diagnostic responses *high risk for injury: falls; high risk for injury: poisoning;* and *high risk for injury: suffocation/aspiration* as the child grows and develops was introduced in the previous chapter. This need becomes critical in the toddler group. In this age group, more deaths occur from accidents than from any other cause. Nurses can use their assessment data to assist parents in childproofing the home.

Re-Establishing Relationships

The family with a toddler is at particular risk for energy depletion in one or more of its members. (The mother or primary caregiver is by far the most fre-

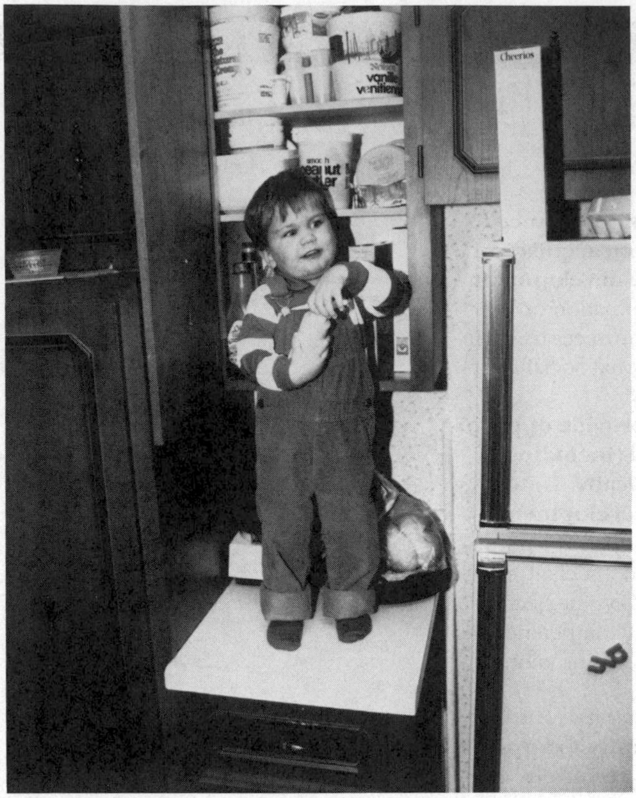

FIGURE 6 - 1. Toddlers' ability to climb places a new emphasis on childproofing the home.

quent recipient.) Any combination of circumstances can cause energy depletion.

For example, the division of labor may not be equalized among the spouses and older siblings. The mother may be pregnant again and/or employed outside the home.

If the family has not developed coping mechanisms that allow healthy adaptation to changing circumstances, some member(s) of the family will eventually become chronically fatigued. When physical or emotional energy is depleted, family relationships will inevitably suffer, with potentially serious long-term results.

All these factors that contribute to energy depletion are also factors that can lead to ineffective coping. If one family member is unable to cope because of excessive demands resulting from this family developmental crisis, the result can be *ineffective family coping: compromised or disabling*. The nurse who is vigilant for defining characteristics of these diagnostic responses can plan interventions that will result instead in the positive nursing diagnostic response of *family coping: potential for growth*.

Participating in Social, Community Activities

Parents of an infant tend to temporarily withdraw from activities involving social interactions away from home. But by the time these parents have a toddler, they are rediscovering the need to maintain relationships and involvements beyond their child and family. However, retaining some satisfying contacts with friends and personal interests away from home can be a rather complicated matter when there are small children. External activities, once spontaneously followed, now must be planned ahead and arrangements made. The trouble associated with getting the child cared for and paying for this service is so difficult for many parents that they tend to give up and stay home.

Some innovative parents have found numerous options available to them, with a little cooperation from others in the same circumstance as they. One option is to develop social relationships with other parents who have young children and take turns entertaining in one another's homes. These same parents might arrange a reciprocal child care agreement, whereby one parent watches the other's child or children so that parent can do something special and then the favor is exchanged at another time. Mothers (or fathers) who are full-time caregivers may arrange to "take turns" watching each other's child or children so that each can get away regularly to pursue personal interests or just enjoy a quiet morning at home alone. Such breaks in child care are refreshing, renewing energy for continued child care and for other significant relationships.

Some churches and synagogues provide nurseries for small children during services and social events. In those that do not, many parents have gotten together and agreed to take turns managing a children's nursery for those times, so that the other parents can participate without the interruptions of their infant or toddler.

Promoting Healthy Independence

Living together with enough harmony to allow expression of a variety of feelings, enough cooperation to permit each individual self-fulfillment in her or his development tasks, and enough open communication to condone each member's assertion of independence and self-hood or uniqueness requires a family to be in a continuous adaptive state. Having established itself as a unit that can incorporate children and having accepted the entailed responsibilities, the family group with a toddler is now faced with the task of finding parenting patterns that meet the needs of both parents and active, mobile children and of establishing enough freedom for each member so that age-appropriate independence is possible.

This freedom for independent development in a family finds its origin in the parental relationship. Spouses who are mature enough to allow each other independent social and recreational or hobby pursuits are much more likely to recognize and permit the individual endeavors of their children. Trust in the family member's motives is at the heart of such freedom.

This trust provides the security necessary to "let go" of the family member and allow him or her to develop uniqueness. The same factor undoubtedly holds true in husband-wife independence. A spouse who knows she or he can count on a partner's affection is more likely to grant freedom in the relationship for pursuit of personal happiness.

In conveying their respect for toddlers' self-hood or fulfillment activities, parents certainly want to let them be as grown up as they can be without pushing them too quickly out of babyhood. Parental respect for the developing toddler's individual efforts must be focused on three aspects of this activity: (1) the child's need to explore; (2) the child's need to learn self-control of body functions and emotional expression; and (3) the child's need to develop an identity that will accommodate childhood rather than infancy. Refer to the section "Psychosocial Development: Development of Autonomy" later in this chapter for further discussion of the balances between dependence and independence and the impact of separation on the toddler and family unit.

Resolving Developmental Task Conflicts

This stage in the family life cycle seems full of paradoxes. Having just become settled in and comfortable as parents, the spouses find that new and more difficult roles now emerge—those of limit setter, guide, and teacher. These new parental roles involve much patience; the parent must accept the child's individual pace, let him or her make mistakes and learn from them, and accept a role as assistant to rather than director of the child's activities. Some of the decisions to be made now are clear-cut, but most are not. When there are two parents, they must agree on a form of discipline that is logical, consistent, and comfortable without causing damage to the child's physical, intellectual, or emotional-social development. Daily family rituals are also invaluable means of providing a workable daily routine that eases conflict while giving family members a sense of order, security, and satisfaction in living together.

Accepting Help

The tasks of the family with a toddler are not easily achieved, and, owing to the rapidity with which the toddler develops, most families find themselves in an atmosphere of urgency, during which time they feel a need for increased support and guidance, whether from relatives and neighbors (grandparents become important resources again), from health and child care professionals, or from all these sources. The nursing diagnosis *altered family process* is defined as "inability of family system (household members) to meet needs of members, carry out family functions, or maintain communications for mutual growth and maturation" (Gordon, 1987). The family with a toddler is in a developmental phase with a high risk for the occurrence of altered family process. Often this problem can be resolved by assisting family members to explore and accept outside help in dealing with their situation.* Most parents are willing to make use of any outside help that will enrich what they have to offer their child or the family group, but only if they are allowed to retain their parenting responsibilities throughout the helping situation. The acceptance of help is made easier if a family's philosophy recognizes the basic interdependence of all people.

The first step in accepting help is to acknowledge those areas of family life in which limitations exist. Then the family can draw on those outside resources that enhance existing strengths and those that will help strengthen weak spots (lack of knowledge, communication breakdown, chronic illness). Utilizing outside support systems such as relatives, helping professionals, self-help support groups, or government aid programs can help build and maintain internal support systems (members themselves, their skills, their caring), making life as a family with a toddler a happy, growth-producing experience.

Finding Satisfaction in Parenthood

The parents' satisfaction or frustration during this period depends largely on their confidence and the love, care, and attention they can give the child. Children can be a ticket back to fantasy and wonder, if their parents pause and enjoy their children's new exploits. The child can now offer parents a reciprocal relationship of shared love and pleasure, bringing satisfaction in being together.

But the parental task of realistically balancing the needs and demands of this active child with the expectations of a spouse or significant other and commitments to their own personhood can leave the best-intentioned parent with some bouts of ambivalence toward parenthood. Some of the ambivalent feelings experienced by parents stem not from the fact that they sometimes do not like their child or children so much, but, rather, from not knowing how to cope with either the child or the whole juggling act just described. One study demonstrated that mothers who had been rejected as children and who received little support from the father after the birth of a child were more likely to parent their toddlers in angry, punitive ways (Crockenberg, 1987). Unfortunately, this kind of parenting seems more likely to be associated with angry, noncompliant behavior in the child. During this exciting but critical period of development, parents need all the help, reinforcement, and information available so that their relationship

*Inability to accept and receive help is a defining characteristic of *alteration in family process.*

with their toddler will be mutually satisfying and rewarding.

Nursing Care and Guidance

Adapting Resources

Because the behaviors and developmental skills of the toddler are so drastically different from those of the infant, family members may need guidance in understanding their toddlers. As in all nurse-family interactions, nurses should include in their ongoing assessment awareness of cues suggesting a nursing diagnosis of *altered role performance (parental related to) knowledge deficit*. If the nurse determines that a knowledge deficit exists, he or she must establish the reason for the knowledge deficit before planning interventions (Frankel, 1993). As in all situations in which knowledge is lacking, interventions must be directed toward the reason. If the reason is a simple lack of familiarity with necessary information, the nursing intervention will focus on education.

One of the most critical aspects of teaching with the family of a toddler is related to providing information regarding the toddler's rapid (almost daily) developmental advances. Because development is still occurring at such a rapid pace, parent education will involve anticipatory guidance in relation to the multiple issues with which they will be presented. Safety risks associated with that rapid development, especially motor development, must be emphasized. The nurse may also be a useful resource to families in helping them assess their space needs (physical, emotional, and social) and in facilitating innovative problem solving that is realistic for the family budget. Acquainting the family with community resources to assist them in adapting their own resources to the needs of their toddler and family life is often needed.

Parents must see that childproofing plans are carried out and periodically re-evaluated in light of their toddler's progressive motor skills (eventually they will climb, unscrew caps, open latches, and unlock doors). Whatever limits are to exist must be communicated to all family members and to any of the toddler's caregivers during parental absences. Enforcement of limits should be consistently enacted, especially because the child's safety may be at stake.

Re-Establishing Relationships

Nurses whose focus is on the child and her or his family will see the significance of identifying families at risk for energy depletion of one or more members. They are motivated to help members of that family build their confidence and coping capacity by praising them in their healthy efforts and backing them in the options they choose. These nurses will initiate a plan of care that has as its goal helping the family learn to solve problems by focusing on their actual or potential stress, to recognize that options exist to resolve or minimize that stress, to select that option with which they are most comfortable, and to carry it through.

All parents should be helped to realize that there will surely be bad days, even in the most smooth-running household, when there is a busy toddler around. And they should be helped to see that they have a number of options available to them from which they can select without guilt when the bad days occur. For instance, when the mother is at her wits' end, she could opt for any one of these solutions that best suit her situation and resources. She can get a sitter and leave for a time; or forget about any tasks she planned to accomplish that day and indulge herself and her toddler in some unwinding, just-for-fun activities, such as take a walk with her toddler. Or she can call a friend to come support her and share her day, or select from any other options that will relieve boredom, change the scene, or put embattled relationships into a different perspective.

Resolving Conflicts

The ways in which the parents resolve their conflicts and the ways they interact with each other are imitated by toddlers, who use these observations in a hundred ways to cope with their personal processes of self-development. Parents best handle the conflicts of this stage when they

- Remember that their child's rebellion, expressed by contrariness, is temporary and normal and that what often appears to be destructive behavior is simply the child's curiosity in action.
- Agree on democratic, shared parenting.
- Support each other in their role shifts.
- Work out realistic ways for each to fulfill some personal career interests.
- Learn to approach each other and their child or children positively, encouraging desirable actions through compliments and rewards for well-intentioned efforts.

Accepting Help

The nurse can assist the family to find ways to successfully accomplish the tasks that cause difficulty by offering them useful information that will help them move forward, by referring them to resources or support systems that can help them correct limitations to task achievement, and by reinforcing the efforts they are making to grow and develop as a family unit through praise, encouragement, and advocacy of their needs and rights.

The nurse should reinforce those routines, parenting methods, affectional demonstrations, and self-care expectations that the child is accustomed to from the parents. Knowledge of these factors should be learned from the nurse's assessment and integrated into the plan of care.

Growth and Development of the Toddler

The developmental changes that occur in a child from 12 to 36 months of age engage the entire family in a life full of drama. Of the years between birth and adolescence, no period is as unsettled or tumultuous as the period of toddlerhood. The newly acquired abilities of locomotion give them access to an expanded world. Their developing intellectual and language abilities enable them to attach meaning to their discoveries.

Because they have had only limited experience with people and objects, toddlers are dependent on their families to rescue them from conflicts and protect them from danger. Their physical, intellectual, and emotional-social development require mutually adaptive behaviors between toddlers and their families. Nurses use themselves, their knowledge, and their skills to promote healthy family functioning that allows each member to realize her or his full potential as the toddler grows and develops.

Nursing diagnoses are influenced by a variety of variables including treatment-related situational and maturational factors. Defining characteristics will need to be considered as well in formulating high risk or actual nursing diagnoses (see Table 6–2).

Physical Competency

In this chapter, assessment parameters that reflect physical growth and development during the toddler years are discussed, with emphasis on the nurse's role with parents in promoting physical competency of their toddler. Table 6–1 summarizes growth and development of toddlers.

Height and Weight

From 2 years of age through the preschool years, growth remains relatively stable. A toddler gains about 2.5 kg (5.5 lb) a year and usually quadruples his or her birthweight by 2 to 2½ years of age. At 2 years, a toddler's height represents approximately 50 per cent of his or her eventual adult height. During the 2 years of toddlerhood, a child grows approximately 20.3 cm (8 in) compared with 25.4 cm (10 in) during the first 12 months of life.

Head and Chest Circumference

Head circumference reflects the growth of the brain and is an important parameter to be assessed until at least 2 years of age. At 2 years of age, the brain attains approximately 90 per cent of adult size. The posterior fontanel usually closes by 2 months of age and the anterior fontanel by 18 months, but there is a wide range of normalcy. Head circumference increases approximately 3.5 cm (1.8 in) during the toddler years, compared with a growth of 12 cm (4.7 in) during the first year of life. At birth, the head circumference exceeds the chest circumference, but during the second year of life, the head and chest circumference usually become equal. The chest circumference continues to gradually increase and during childhood exceeds head circumference.

Organ Maturation

During early childhood the lymphatic tissue increases in size, accounting for the presence of peripheral nodes, enlargement of tonsils and adenoids, and a spleen tip that is more likely to be palpable (Smith, 1977). Hyperplasia of lymphoid tissues is a phenomenon of normal physiologic growth and is thought to occur as a response to the numerous infections of childhood. The excessive swelling and hyperplasia of lymphoid tissue in a normal child may persist long after the primary infection has resolved. Lymphatic tissue shows progressive growth during the toddler years and attains maximal size by 10 to 11 years of age. Parents are better able to cope with the stress of repeated visits to the practitioner's office if they understand that the hypertrophied tonsils and adenoids are thought to be a protective response to infection and a phenomenon of normal growth. Parents should also know that lymphatic tissue serves a protective response in the body throughout life.

General Appearance and Skeletal Growth

The general appearance of the toddler changes markedly between 12 and 36 months of age. When toddlers first begin to walk, the trunk is long, the legs and arms are short, and the head is proportionately large, giving them a top-heavy appearance. They walk with their feet spread apart to create a broad base (toddling gait) that helps to compensate for their weight distribution and immature musculoskeletal system.

During the toddler years, muscle tissue begins to replace the high proportion of adipose tissue characteristic of an infant, and bone ossification takes place. With increased ambulation and maturation, a toddler's legs and arms lengthen, the body straightens, and the pot-bellied appearance disappears. The lordosis resolves as ambulation increases and muscle and bone develop. The legs retain a slightly bowed appearance until around 18 months of age. The toddler's unsteady gait disappears as muscle and bone develop (Fig. 6–2).

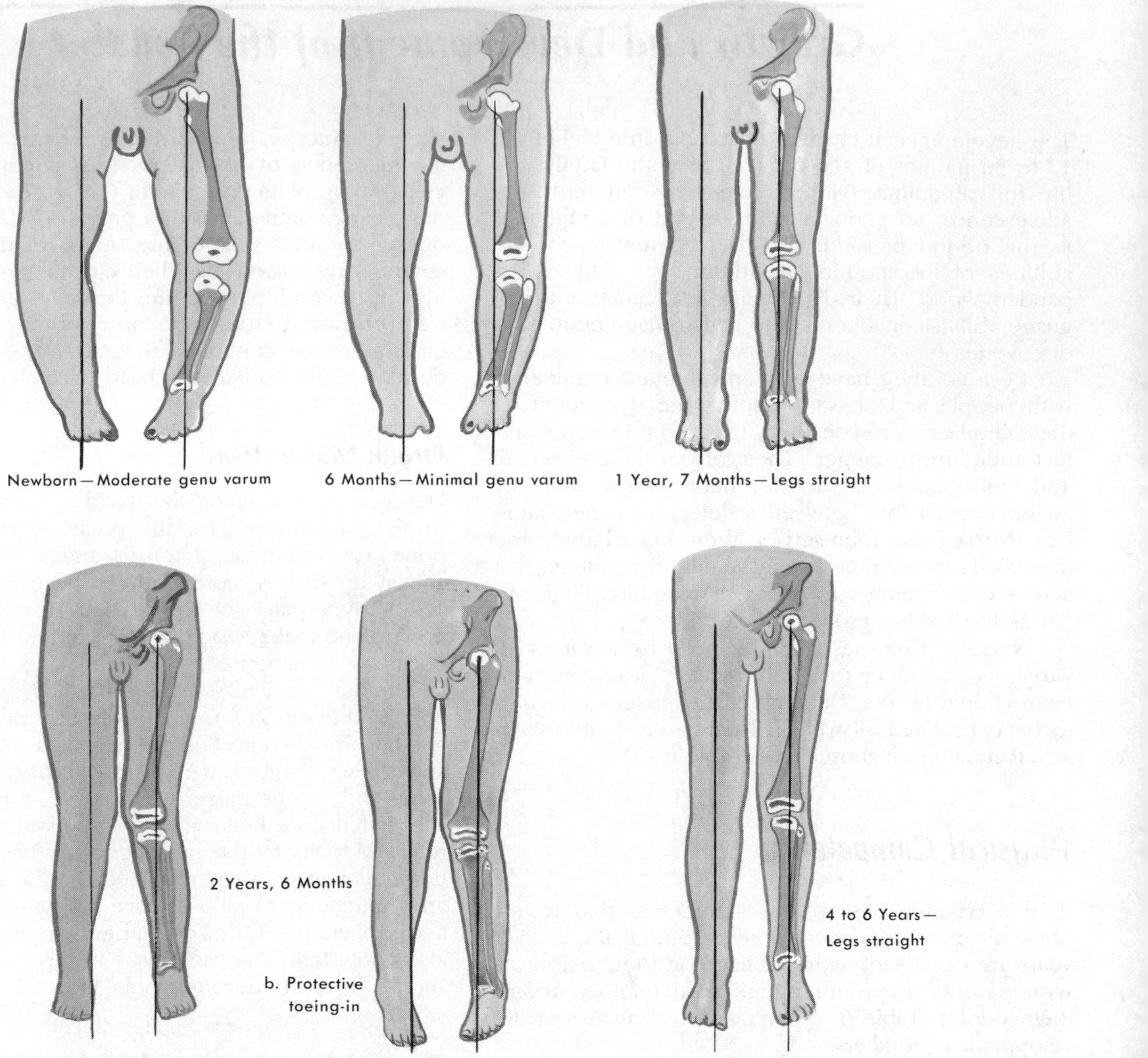

FIGURE 6 - 2. Physiologic evolution of the alignment of the lower limbs at various ages in infancy and childhood. (From Tachdjian, M. O. [1972]. *Pediatric orthopedics* [Vol. 2, p. 1463]. Philadelphia: WB Saunders.)

Anticipatory Guidance: Physical Growth

Parents continue to have a keen interest in the physical growth of their child during the toddler years. Also a parent may be comparing the child with a friend's child or with an older sibling. An explanation of their child's *growth trajectory* will provide parents with information regarding the tracking of growth patterns. The child's growth trajectory in height and weight is plotted on the growth charts and compared with other children's height and weight trajectories over time. Explanations offered to parents regarding their child's physical growth will provide them not only with needed information but also with assurance of what is developmentally appropriate.

Motor Development

The significant advances in motor development during the toddler years affect the child's physical, mental, and emotional-social development. Physical maturation coupled with opportunities for practice fosters mastery of increasingly complex skills.

Gross Motor Skills

Important gross motor skills that are perfected during the toddler years are the ability to walk and run. The age at which these skills are perfected varies from one child to another and particularly from one culture

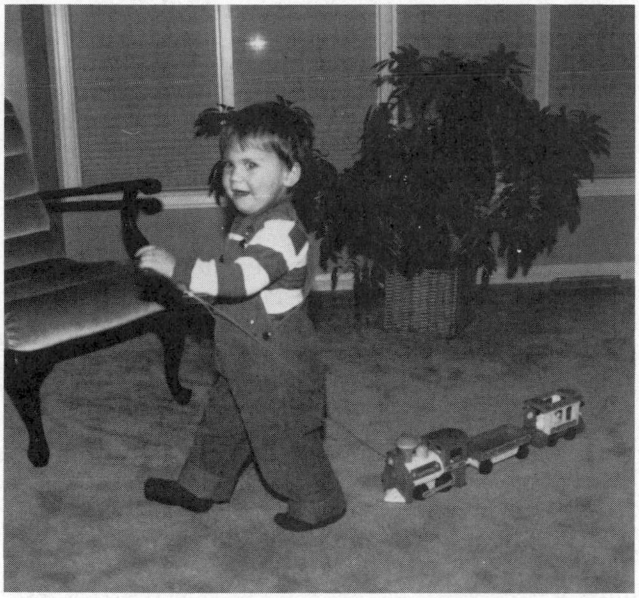

FIGURE 6 - 3. Toddlers like to pull things while they walk.

to another. Ethnic differences in locomotion observed during the first year are thus generally not as observable during the toddler years.

Most children are able to walk alone by the age of 15 months, although some normal children walk as late as 21 months and others as early as 10 months. The 15-month-old is an avid climber, climbing onto chairs, sofas, and low tables, and may climb out of a crib, high chair, or stroller. At this age a toddler can quickly disappear by climbing up a staircase on hands and knees. She or he can get down stairs by going backward and sliding from one step to the next, but an occasional accident may still occur as the child slips down the stairs too quickly.

At 18 months of age, toddlers walk well. If they fall, it is usually because they try to run too quickly. They now push chairs to cupboards and tables so they can climb to higher, more intriguing destinations. They can walk up stairs one step at a time if someone holds onto one hand, but they still slide down the stairs backward. They like to push and pull things while they walk and can even walk sideways while pulling a toy, making this an ideal age for pull toys (Fig. 6–3).

At 2 years of age, toddlers have acquired a more steady gait and generally run well with fewer falls but are not able to stop quickly. They can now go up and down stairs alone by holding onto a handrail but do so by putting both feet on each step rather than the more advanced method of alternating feet. By 3 years of age, they can walk downstairs alternating feet, can run and walk skillfully, and can ride a tricycle. Their skills of locomotion have progressed from the characteristic toddling gait to one of balance and control.

Fine Motor Skills

Small muscle coordination shows steady improvement. At 15 months, toddlers are still highly engaged in gross motor activities, but they also enjoy the challenge of fine motor control. At this age, toddlers stack two blocks, put objects into a container and pour them out, and scribble spontaneously if they are ingenious enough to get possession of a pencil.

At 18 months of age, toddlers can build a tower of three to four blocks, which gives evidence of improving hand-eye coordination (Fig. 6–4). They can also manipulate a pounding bench, although rather crudely. They will try to assist with turning the pages of a book but do so by turning two or three at a time. Although they cannot effectively kick a ball, they are able to clumsily catch and throw one without falling.

By 24 months, toddlers can build a tower of six blocks and can line them horizontally to make a train. They now can turn the pages of a book one at a time and imitate vertical and circular strokes, but they still hold the crayon or pencil with a fist. By 30 months, they can use their fingers to hold a pencil or a crayon, and by age 3, their hands are steady enough to build a bridge, an 8- to 10-block tower, and a structure that resembles a house. See Chapter 17 for further discussion of play.

Motor Skills Affecting Eating

At 15 months of age, the spoon is grasped, but because toddlers rotate the spoon, they frequently lose its contents on the way to their mouth. At this age, they spend a great deal of time practicing the skill of

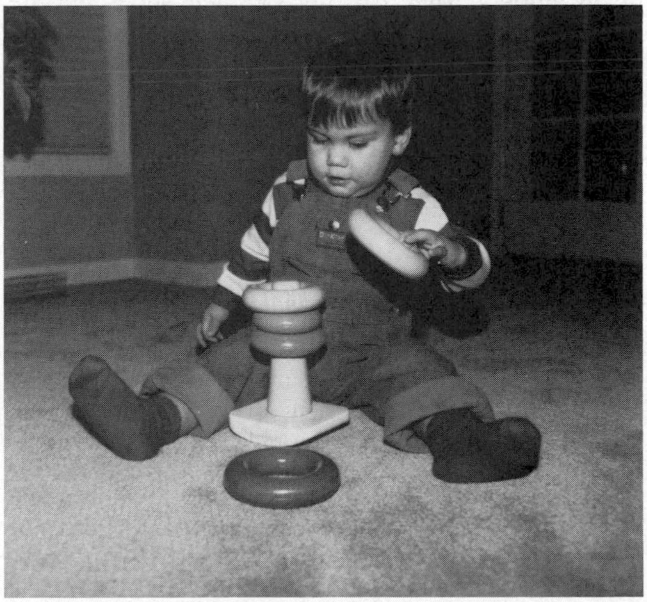

FIGURE 6 - 4. Toddlers gain increasing hand-eye coordination.

stirring their food during mealtime. They enjoy and are able to pick up pieces of food with their fingers. They can also hold a cup by grasping it rather clumsily with both hands, and, as with the spoon, they spill the contents frequently because they tilt the cup before it reaches their mouth.

From 15 months to 2 years of age, toddlers demonstrate remarkable advances in their eating skills. At 18 months of age, they can use a spoon and drink from a cup or glass. They are able to partially feed themselves but need adult supervision because they easily get engrossed in playing with their food. By 2 years of age, they can feed themselves, hold a cup with one hand, and set it down after drinking without spilling. By 2 years, they have mastered the use of the spoon and spill little.

By 3 years of age, toddlers can pour from a pitcher and prepare their own dishes of milk and cold cereal. They feed themselves completely and have only occasional accidents of spilling.

Motor Skills Affecting Self-Care Activities

At 15 months of age, toddlers are dependent on their caregivers for most of their physical care. Toddlers at this age have the fine motor skills to take off their socks and shoes and do so as a playful, experimental activity. By 18 months, they assist in undressing more than dressing and may not necessarily be undressing when it is time for bed. They can unzip a large zipper and take off simple garments. They will also try to brush teeth at this age but have not acquired sufficient fine motor skill to perform this task. By 2 years of age, they are able to assist in self-care by putting on simple garments but do not differentiate front from back. They are now able to zip and unzip zippers. They can put on their shoes but are not able to buckle or tie them. They wash and dry their hands, brush teeth crudely, and, if helped to reach the sink, can turn on a water faucet. They can also turn doorknobs and open doors without assistance. By 3 years, toddlers dress themselves almost completely but still do not know front from back and cannot tie their shoes.

Nursing Interventions: Motor Skills

In many instances, the toddler's motor abilities will be affected or restricted owing to the effects of illness and hospitalization. It is then up to the nurse to encourage simpler activities the child can perform until the child feels better able to perform at a developmentally appropriate level. Table 6–3 provides a clinical example for illustration. Initially, parents may be alarmed by this regression; however, the nurse can reassure parents that this is another effect of the illness on the toddler. Assurance that this regression is temporary will help to relieve their concern.

Anticipatory Guidance: Motor Skills

Parents may need suggestions in how they can provide a safe environment without detracting from the toddler's opportunity to practice her or his motor skills. A toddler can be given the opportunity to practice stair climbing under supervision and to practice running outdoors on the grass, where a fall is less dangerous. The nurse should also encourage parents to allow their toddler to practice fine motor skills by permitting self-feeding, assistance in dressing, and participation in other self-care activities.

If parents can regard the practice of motor skills as an essential component of their toddler's developing self-esteem as well as physical development, the frustrations that eager toddlers pose to parents may be more tolerable. Encouraging parents to provide opportunities for the development of motor skills without undue emphasis on premature perfection builds an environment within which the toddler thrives.

Intellectual Competency

Stages of cognitive development identified by Piaget (1952, 1970) provide a theory base that the nurse can use to assess cognitive growth and development.

Cognitive Development: Sensorimotor Period

Infants enter toddlerhood with a beginning understanding of spoken words and engage in prelinguistic formation of sounds. Things learned in the first four substages during infancy continue to be practiced, and new learning emerges between their 12th and their 36th month. *Substage 5* (12 to 18 months) is characterized by what Piaget has called *tertiary circular reactions* that differ from the other two (primary and secondary) circular reactions. In this stage, children knock down a tower of blocks, help to rebuild it, and knock it down again, not for the sake of repetition (primary circular) and not only to observe the results (secondary circular). Now they are searching for new ways to bring about the same results or experimenting to see if they can produce new results, or both. They may therefore push the blocks over gently one time, and the next time stand up and swing their arms to see if something new will happen. It is this "experimenting to see" that brings about new behaviors and results in trial and error as a predominant method of learning. Deliberate manipulating to find out what will happen fills the day of a busy toddler during this phase of development.

Substage 6 (18 to 24 months) marks the transition from predominantly trial-and-error behavior to thinking about solutions and consequences before carrying them out. Piaget describes this as the stage of *inventing new means through mental combinations*.

TABLE 6-3

Promoting Motor Development During Hospitalization

Stacy (age 20 mos) was hospitalized with diagnosis of bacterial meningitis. Her activity was limited owing to her acute illness and administration of IV antibiotics. Stacy's nursing care plan included the following problems and interventions to promote motor development:

Encourage Fine Motor Activity	• Notice Stacy's reaction with handling toys in bed • Ability to self-feed • Ability to pull self to standing position
Encourage Fine Motor Activity as Tolerated	• Ask Stacy which of her favorite activities she would like to do • Play with building blocks • Hug stuffed animal • Turn pages of books • Play with crayon and paper • Refer to Child Life Specialist for additional play activities
Encourage Parents to Foster Motor Activities	• Have parents bring in favorite toys when isolation is discontinued • Encourage parents/siblings to play with Stacy • Blocks • Crayons • Observe child's gait when walking and ability to bear weight
Encourage Walking When Condition Permits	• Accompany child when ambulating • Let sit in stroller for meals • Take to playroom

This stage is characterized by a beginning ability to use mental images and words when referring to absent objects. Toddlers can also anticipate what will happen to the object as a result of a certain action, and, therefore, they solve problems by thinking about the results rather than always having to carry them out by trial and error. For example, during this stage children are less fascinated with throwing a variety of objects from the high chair than they were earlier. They remember, without doing it every day, that an object falls and makes a noise. By 20 months of age, the toddler demonstrates a rudimentary sense of volitional behavior. That is, the child begins to recognize a linkage between her or his action on an object and the outcome. The toddler will express pleasure in producing an outcome as seen during play activities. For example a toddler shows pleasure when playing with stacking blocks or push-pull toys (Bullock & Lutkenhaus, 1988).

This ability to retain mental images is demonstrated when a toddler imitates a past event in the absence of the original stimuli. For example, when a child pretends he is shaving in front of the mirror hours after his father has gone to work, he is engaging in what has been described by Piaget as *deferred imitation.* During this stage, children imitate a model in their environment that has significance and meaning to them. The process of *identification* takes place as they take on the behavior and values of those in their environment (Fig. 6–5).

The concept of *object permanence* is now fully developed. If a ball rolls under the sofa, toddlers have a concept of the ball continuing to move even though they cannot see the movement. If they cannot find the ball under the sofa, they will conclude that the ball has moved through to the other side and they will go around the sofa to look for the ball. It is the child's ability to retain a mental image of the ball and to think about the property of the ball that brings about this level of behavior.

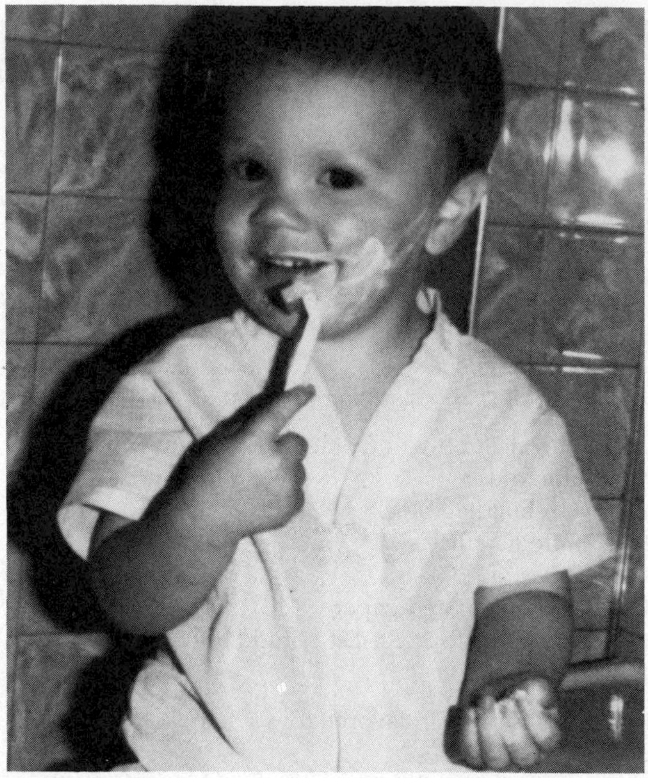

FIGURE 6-5. The toddler portrays deferred imitation when he pretends to be shaving with a toy razor after father has gone off to work. (Photograph by David Trainor.)

Preoperational Period

Entrance to the *preoperational period* (2 to 7 years) is characterized by an increase in *internal representation* of objects and the ability to engage in symbolic thought. The ability to retain mental images allows children to internalize what they see and experience in their world. However, these concepts are not as complete and logical as those of an adult; thus, the term *preconceptual*. For example, all dogs will be called by the name of the child's dog. He or she is not able to comprehend that all objects within a class are not one and the same object. The child is not capable of comprehending these types of differences. Therefore, the child's attempts at generalization result in cognitive errors. Symbolic play is at peak in children from 2 to 4 years of age. *Symbolization* is greatly enhanced by rapidly developing language ability during this period. *Egocentric thought* also facilitates symbolic play.

The child is capable of thinking only about her or his own perspective and not that of another (egocentrism) (Flavell, 1988). The child's play is characterized by vivid imagination and pretending. Children create their own reality as they both see and want it. At times, the distortion between the actual and the child's reality can be great. The child believes that inanimate objects have a life of their own, which Piaget identifies as *animism*, a characteristic of thinking during this age. For example, the child will pretend an object has human feelings such as the child getting angry at an injection for causing pain.

The child has difficulty comprehending past mental states. The child may be able to recall a past action but not his or her previous beliefs. Children have difficulty recalling their past desires and intentions, especially if these have changed. These discrepancies in remembering earlier mental states are characteristic of the child's representational ability (Gopnik & Slaughter, 1991).

By 3 years of age, volitional behavior becomes evident. The child is seen regulating her or his own behavior in order to produce a desired outcome. For example, the child will correct the placement of blocks in order to stack them. This behavior reflects the early beginnings of performing according to a "standard." The child will attempt to correct an action in order to achieve the desired outcome (Bullock & Lutkenhaus, 1988). Table 6–4 reviews the characteristics of a toddler's thought process illustrated by clinical examples.

Nursing Interventions: Cognitive Development

Knowledge of the child's cognitive stage will assist the nurse in understanding both the behavior and the conversations of the toddler, which will allow the nurse to interact with the child in a more therapeutic manner (McClowry, 1993).

Just as nurses encourage understanding of the toddler's cognitive development by the parents, they must keep it in mind when working with the hospitalized toddler. Cognitive development can be encouraged through carefully planned play programs in hospitals. For example, an immobilized toddler will need play activities adapted to her or his current physical status and abilities. Activities that encourage sensory or intellectual capabilities instead of physical skills would be appropriate as play activities for the hospitalized toddler (Table 6–5). The nurse can work with the child life specialist to assure that the child is prepared for procedures in developmentally appropriate ways. Further information about the child's level of development can be shared with parents to assist them in providing support to their child during the particularly stressful times of illness and hospitalization.

Anticipatory Guidance: Cognitive Development

Parents should be helped to understand that a toddler's intense examination and incessant manipulation of anything new is the way he or she learns. Toys and games that allow practice of cognitive skills should be encouraged. Besides being fun, playing "peek-a-boo" helps that toddler to gain the concept of object permanence. A jack-in-the-box serves a similar purpose as well as teaching cause (turn the crank)

TABLE 6-4

Characteristics of the Toddler's Thinking

Characteristic	Definition	Clinical Example
Internal Representation	Able to create a mental image	Toddler begins to cry when told going to the doctor's office for a visit. Toddler replies, "I don't want a shot." At the last visit the child received an immunization shot
Preconceptual	Forms inaccurate or illogical conclusions or concepts	Toddler is visibly upset and begins to whimper as nurse enters the room. The child believes the nurse is going to give him or her a shot. (A nurse gave him or her a shot, therefore, all nurses give shots.) Toddler has to be assured that he or she will not receive shot in order to feel comforted
Symbolism	Ability to create ideas or play with vivid imagination	Toddler is in hospital playroom. Takes cup and begins to give "medicine" to the stuffed animal who is "sick" to make it "all better"
Egocentrism	Able to think only about themselves. Cannot take into account that another might feel, act or think differently	Toddlers become very upset seeing another child undergoing a painful treatment as they fear it *is going to* and *can* happen to them
Deferred Imitation	Able to think about activities or presence of another	In the hospital playroom, the toddler "pretends" he or she is the "doctor" with the doll he or she is playing with

TABLE 6-5

Promoting Cognitive Development

Jamie, age 3, is brought to the day surgery center by his mother for repair of an inguinal hernia. The nurse knows that Jamie's preparation must be geared to his level of cognitive understanding. The following vignette illustrates the play preparation he received:

Interaction	**Rationale**
Nurse: Points to teddy bear's tummy and says: "You know that Freddy has a bump right there just like you have?" Toddler: Reacts timidly; nods hesitantly	***Identification*** "Relates" to the bear's situation as it is like his own
Nurse: Freddy is going to have his "bump" fixed just like you, too!	***Symbolism*** Use object to represent the medical and surgical situation in an understandable and less threatening manner
Toddler: Remains quiet and stares at teddy bear	***Animism*** Believes teddy bear has feelings and thoughts
Nurse: Freddy is going to the room where the doctor is so he can have it fixed just like you	***Egocentrism*** Thinks the teddy bear responds in the same way he does

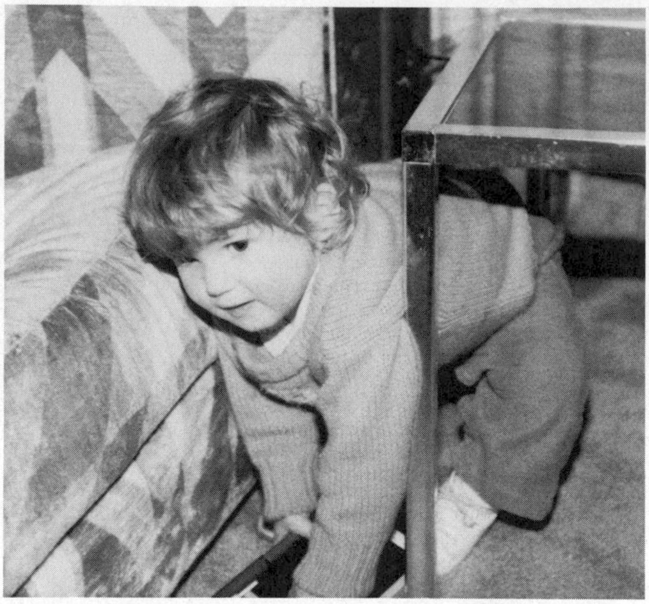

FIGURE 6-6. During the trial-and-error stage, toddlers need the opportunity to solve problems on their own. This toddler is trying to get both herself and her storybook out of a tight place.

and effect (jack pops up). Toddlers are growing intellectually when they insist on examining the contents of cupboards, drawers, boxes, and anything they can reach. If a nurse will take the time to explain the meaning of such toddler behavior, a family is more likely to feel a sense of pride and even intrigue in their toddler's fascination with and scrutiny of everything and everybody he or she encounters.

During the trial-and-error stage, toddlers need parents who can patiently stand by and watch their countless attempts to complete a task without reaching in and making the final move just as they are about to accomplish it on their own (Fig. 6–6). The limit-setting and constant surveillance that are required by a family with a toddler are exhausting and often stressful. It is important for a nurse to explore with the family ways that encourage the development of their toddler without exhausting and immobilizing the rest of family life. Nurturing home environments during toddlerhood have been associated with improved school performance during middle childhood (Bradley et al, 1988).

As a child enters the preoperational period (around 2 years of age) parents need to be prepared for the symbolic play that emerges. A nurse can explain to them that games of pretending and creation of imaginary playmates are normal behaviors for a toddler from 24 to 36 months and continue through the preschool years. Nurses can encourage parents to listen to their toddlers as they describe the contents of a box that has become a truck or the qualities of a plastic container that has become a rocket. It is appropriate for parents to carry on a conversation with toddlers about their imagined play and inappropriate to discourage the child's imagination with "But that is a box, not a truck." Research has demonstrated that children benefit from having parents read stories to them before they can read themselves. Storytelling contributes to what experts have described as "emergent literacy." This term refers to the precursor skills the child develops prior to the ability to read. Parents who spend more time describing meanings of words and illustrations appear to contribute to their child's development of reading skills (Bus & van Ijzendoorn, 1988).

Language Development

It is the nurse's role to assess the appropriateness of the toddler's language ability and help families to provide an environment conducive to language development. Nurses must therefore be knowledgeable about (1) stages of language acquisition, (2) characteristics of toddler language, and (3) factors that contribute to language development.

Stages of Language Acquisition

From 15 to 18 months of age, an *expressive jargon* emerges that has rhythmic intonations, but no real words can be recognized. Although expressive jargon does not seem to contain real words, toddlers use it in conjunction with pointing and movement toward the object or person they are "talking" about, thereby communicating their wants (Table 6–6).

Between 18 and 24 months of age, one-word utterances are commonly used to communicate increasingly complex ideas. When one-word sentences are used to express whole ideas, the accompanying gestures give clues to the meaning. For example, saying "Bye-bye" while standing at the door and hitting on it after playing indoors for several hours may mean "I want to go bye-bye," whereas standing at the door quietly as father is leaving for work and saying "Bye-bye" probably means "Da-da is going bye-bye." If, however, hitting the door again accompanies the ut-

TABLE 6-6
Language Milestones

15–18 mos	Expressive jargon Names familiar pictures/objects
18–24 mos	Holophrastic speech Knows 10 words Phrases composed of nouns/verbs
24 mos	300-word vocabulary 2-word utterances Uses pivot words Telegraphic sentences
30 mos	900-word vocabulary 3-word sentences
36 mos	Uses complete sentences Uses all parts of speech

terance "Bye-bye" as Daddy leaves, it now clearly means "I want to go bye-bye with Da-da." These one-word utterances that carry whole ideas are referred to as *holophrastic speech*. Giving careful attention to the situation surrounding one-word utterances and the accompanying gestures becomes an integral part of successful communication with a toddler.

From 18 months to 3 years of age, vocabulary growth and complexity of sentence structure progress rapidly and constantly. Although there is a wide variation in the number of words a toddler is able to say, a typical vocabulary at 18 months of age is 10 or more words; by 2 years of age, the child may easily progress to a phenomenal 300-word vocabulary; and by 3 years, she or he uses around 900 words. At about 2 years of age, two-word utterances become increasingly common; by 2½ years of age, an average sentence contains three words; and by 3 years, complete sentences are constructed, using all parts of speech. Children's expressive language has been found to increase with positive reinforcement. These findings suggest that actively intervening in stimulating acquisition of language can accelerate the child's learning (Whitehurst & Valdez-Menchaca, 1988).

Characteristics of Toddler Speech

Around 2 years of age, a characteristic pattern of speech emerges. There are a few words that seem to be used repeatedly, and other, less frequently used, words are attached to them. The frequently used words have been described as *pivot* words, and the less frequently used words as *open*. For example, "down" may emerge as a pivot word in "sit down," "put down," "go down." "Sit," "put," and "go" (open words) are used less frequently than "down." Another characteristic is that when words are combined, it is usually a noun and verb. For example, "me do" is a grammatically incorrect sentence containing only the words that carry meaning. Articles, prepositions, and adjectives are generally lacking, as is typical in a telegram, which accounts for the use of the term *telegraphic sentences* to describe these phrases.

The egocentric thinking of the toddler influences the style and content of speech. Toddlers in this stage engage in a monologue with little regard for a response of another child or adult who happens to be present. The function of this *egocentric speech* is that it meets the toddler's need to practice speech. As toddlers mature and are able to consider another's view, their speech becomes more socialized and they engage in increasingly more conversation with one another and less monologue. Children raised in bilingual environments may have difficulty learning two languages simultaneously. The child's language development may be slightly delayed. Two- and 3-year-olds were found to perform better in learning a second language when reinforced compared with children who were not. The findings suggest that positive reinforcement can influence the rate of acquisition of expressive language (Whitehurst & Valdez-Menchaca, 1988).

Nursing Interventions: Language Development

Toddlers have limited abilities to express their feelings and communicate their wants and needs. Each child and family come into the hospital with a unique system and repertoire of words for communication. There, it is essential during the admission procedure for the nurse to gather information about what words are used for elimination, transitional objects, and favorite foods, to name a few.

Names used for significant others in the toddler's family are obtained, especially for those who will be serving as caretakers during the toddler's hospitalization. "Morfa," "Nini," and "Tutu" are examples of names used by children to call their grandmother. Words used for elimination vary considerably as well. "Pee," "titi," and "number 1" are terms the toddler is likely to use to indicate the need to urinate.

Parents are also asked to provide the words used by their toddler to indicate pain, discomfort, and anxiety. Again, the family may or may not use specific terms to indicate these discomforts. It is necessary, though, for the nurse to observe the nonverbal behavior of the toddler, as this is a primary channel of communication for the child. Crying, having tantrums, and pushing the nurse away are examples of the toddler's communicating some form of discomfort. The toddler's pain responses are discussed in further detail in Chapter 25.

Anticipatory Guidance: Language Development

When parents have a concern that their toddler's language is not developing as rapidly as that of a sibling or other playmates, the nurse can help parents to understand the wide range of normal language acquisition and can explain the impact of other areas of their child's development. For example, pointing out that a toddler's language development is often delayed by her or his absorption in learning motor skills during the second year of life is reassuring to parents.

The nurse can also offer some practical suggestions on how parents can facilitate language development. A nurse can encourage parents to respond to their toddler's speech by using correct communication and by expanding and rephrasing what she or he says in a grammatically correct statement. They should not, however, correct the child's language by saying "No, it's not wa-wa, it's water." If the parents avoid responding with "baby-talk," correct language is learned. Parents may need help in understanding that the repetition of favorite words is a toddler's way of practicing language and is not necessarily a request or true expression of her or his desires. At all stages of language development, toddlers need a family whose members talk to them and respond to their language efforts. It is important for the nurse to stress that toddlers understand a great deal of what they hear.

The American Speech and Language Association estimates that 2 to 30 per cent of 3-year-olds are language-impaired (Leske, 1981). This figure does not include language delays reported in children with developmental disabilities. The prevalence rate of language delays in this group of children is estimated to be significantly higher. Experts have noted that the referral rate of younger children is low owing to inaccurate assessment of the language ability or failure of the screening tool to identify problems (Borowitzs & Glascoe, 1986).

Emotional-Social Competency

The emotional-social development of a toddler is dramatic. Toddlers are now able to differentiate the responses of those around them. They try to curb those behaviors that result in disapproval and repeat performances that are given attention and approval. As they become increasingly aware of themselves and the world around them, they experiment with a variety of ways to gain control over what happens to them without losing the approval of their parents and significant others.

Psychosocial Development: Development of Autonomy

The Eriksonian task, conflict, or crisis for the toddler is *autonomy versus shame and doubt* (1963). To be autonomous is to see oneself as a separate being with a will of one's own. Once infants have learned to trust their own body, their mothers, and the world, they begin to discover that they can exert a predictable effect on others. They learn that they can control. To control is synonymous with autonomy and autonomy is synonymous with independence and self-governance. Therefore, autonomy requires children to relinquish some of their dependence on or trust in others. This produces conflict in the toddler in a number of ways. Some of the child's physical venturing out into his or her environment inevitably results in falls and physical hurts. These physical hurts provide toddlers with a realization of their own limits and a resulting possibility of doubt in their ability to be autonomous. Three major struggles during this stage—toilet training, limit setting and discipline, and sibling rivalry—all involve the conflict between autonomy and shame and doubt. Toddlers are in conflict because they wish to exercise their own will but fear situations that exceed their coping capacity.

Nursing Interventions: Fostering Autonomy

Hospitalization and illness impose significant restrictions on the toddler's need for autonomy, control, and independence. Several interventions can be used to address the toddler's needs in these areas of psychosocial concerns. Incorporating the child's usual rituals and routines from home into the hospitalization experience will provide the toddler some sense of control and security and help to alleviate feelings of helplessness and fear. Bedtime routines and rituals associated with mealtimes can be easily incorporated into the toddler's plan of care (Table 6–7).

Opportunities for choices, although limited, can be provided to the toddler. Choices can be creatively offered. For example, choices can be offered pertaining to selection of food and fluids and playful activities such as selection of a story to read. Choices involving treatment and medications can be made available as well. The nurse might offer the child selection of location of where the medicine is administered. Another nursing action might include selection of liquids for medication.

Anticipatory Guidance: Fostering Autonomy

This crisis of autonomy versus doubt and shame is largely affected by how the family responds to the child's assertive behavior. If toddlers feel secure in their families, they are likely to venture farther in their exploration and take on unfamiliar tasks and territory. The family can further assist the development of healthy autonomy and avoid shame and doubt by encouraging activities that are age-appropriate. If a family encourages and rewards age-appropriate expressions of expanding cognitive and motor development, the child gains a sense of mastery and positive self-esteem. If a toddler's explorative behaviors are discouraged and repeatedly punished, the strivings for autonomy are thwarted. However, in the life of every toddler, some punishment and interruption of intent must take place to ensure his or her physical safety, to maintain the integrity of personal belongings, and to set limits that help the child gain self-control and feel secure.

Attachment and Separation

During the toddler years, attachment behavior (seeking and maintaining proximity) is neither less intense nor less frequent than at the end of the first year. Typical toddler attachment behaviors are watching, smiling, following, calling, and listening. Beginning in the latter half of the first year of life, children express distress when separated from their mothers and or other individuals who are emotionally significant to them. This phenomenon is referred to as *separation anxiety* (Table 6–8). As with stranger anxiety, separation anxiety demonstrates a cognitive developmental ability. Separation anxiety also has emotional-social significance. It demonstrates the child's achievement of *object permanence*. The child's distress at being separated from her or his mother

TABLE 6-7

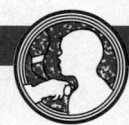

Promoting Security in the Hospitalized Toddler

Maria, age 2, has been hospitalized for a series of tests and possible surgery. Her nurse understands the need to foster and promote Maria's sense of control and security during this period and has obtained information concerning the rituals and routines that Maria is accustomed to at home. Incorporation of this knowledge in the nursing care plan will provide some familiar structure to Maria's days and thus promote her sense of security.

Routine	***Home Ritual***
Bathing and hygiene	Maria takes a morning shower with her mother. Maria washes her tummy; her mother washes the rest of her. Teeth are brushed twice each day and flossed by her mother at the bedtime brushing.
Eating	Maria likes many foods. Meals are served family-style and dinner menus are Yucatan/Mexican. Grace is said before dinner. Maria uses a booster seat and feeds herself.
Bedtime and sleeping	Maria goes to bed at 7:30 P.M. and rises at 6:30 A.M. She shares a room with her two sisters, ages 4 and 6 yrs. Maria knows her bedtime prayers (Our Father and special intentions for the family). She sleeps soundly with a "blankie," sucks her thumb, and has a night light in the wall socket.

TABLE 6-8

Phases of Separation Anxiety

Protest

Crying
Temper tantrums
Flails arms and legs
Pushes substitute caretaker away
Refuses to be comforted
Ignores parent on return
Feelings of abandonment
Anorexia
Nightwaking/terrors

Despair

Listless
Anorexia
Withdrawn
Not interested in toys
Depressed
Sleeps excessively
Feels abandoned

Depression

Appears "cheerful," "recovered"
Overly affectionate with strangers, hospital personnel
Labeled everyone's "favorite"
Friendly, outgoing with strangers

demonstrates the strength of the mother-infant bond. It is a behavioral indication that a sense of basic trust has been developed.

Nursing Interventions: Attachment and Separation

Toddlers will become extremely upset on the departure of significant caretakers during hospitalization. It is important, therefore, that the nurse discuss with the parent the child's behavioral response to separation as well as methods to deal with it. A planned coordinated approach will help alleviate the distress the toddler will feel. Interventions include toddler observation of nurse-caretaker interaction suggesting to the child the nurse is a trusted individual. Parents can be encouraged to bring from home pictures, scented handkerchiefs, and tape recordings of family members. The toddler's own toys and use of clothing (when appropriate) are therapeutic as well. A nursing care plan to alleviate toddler *separation anxiety* is listed in Table 6–9.

Toddlers who are separated for prolonged periods of time will manifest detrimental effects. Prolonged separation can be due to a variety of factors, such as distant geographic location of home from hospital, demanding family needs at home, and mul-

TABLE 6-9
Alleviating Separation Anxiety During Hospitalization

Isaiah is 22 mos old and was admitted to the hospital for pneumonia. Isaiah's mother rooms-in but leaves every afternoon for several hours to see other children at home and cook for them. She returns to the hospital after Isaiah is asleep. In collaboration with his mother, the nurse formulates the following plan of care to alleviate Isaiah's separation anxiety.

Action	Results
Mother and nurse will interact in front of Isaiah. Mother will refer to nurses by name and talk to Isaiah about them	Gives Isaiah the message that nurses can be trusted, as his mother demonstrates she trusts them
Mother will bring in following items from home: • Picture of his brothers and sisters • Picture of the family dog, "Daisy" • Pillow from his bed • One of his mother's old purses • A few favorite toys	Provides a sense of security by having items from home
Isaiah's bedtime routine: • Goes to bed at 8 P.M. • Sleeps on tummy • Mother reads a story in bed • Sleeps with "special pillow"	Routines from home provide sense of security and comfort
Provide support and comfort when Isaiah protests mother's leaving • Acknowledge OK to be upset but Mommie will return after he goes to bed (mother arrives at 9 P.M. to spend the night with Isaiah) • Sit in chair and hold to comfort with pillow/purse • As calms down, begin to play one of favorite activities	Help to alleviate the pain of separation and promote mastery of anxiety

tifaceted responsibilities of working single parents. Unfortunately, prolonged separation can result in serious problems with the child-and-parent relationship.

Toddlers who manifest the effects of prolonged separation demonstrate behaviors that can be misperceived as adapted. Initially, the toddler will be depressed, withdrawn, and seemingly uninterested in the environment. This is called the *despair* phase. If this separation continues, the child will appear to have adjusted and "get better." The child is playful and affectionate with everyone. The child can be seen hugging and shadowing nursing and hospital staff. This behavior suggests a maladaptive response to prolonged separation and a sign that the toddler may have difficulty forming an attachment to anyone.

Anticipatory Guidance: Attachment and Separation

The nurse needs to be aware of the particular lifestyle within a family, which will affect the toddler's ongoing development of attachment. If parents can be encouraged to take an interest in what has happened during the day—what their toddler has said, how he or she played, what he or she ate, and what discipline was required—they can feel more integrally a part of the child's development and experience an ongoing attachment. The nurse might suggest that frequent conversations be held with the substitute caregiver so that parents will feel more in control. Findings from a nursing study revealed that mothers of very young children wanted to provide care during hospitalizations. The implications of this study suggest that nurses can ameliorate the effects of hospitalization on the toddler by encouraging parents to assume caregiving responsibilities while their child is in the hospital (Schepp, 1992).

The nurse can also provide some guidance in helping parents understand how a toddler perceives and responds to separation. If parents understand the kinds of behavior that brief separation causes, their coping ability is enhanced. For example, a toddler, after being left with a babysitter, may become more clingy and show an increase in attachment behaviors. Conversely, she or he may ignore the parents and demonstrate an ostentatious interest in the substitute caregiver. Parents need to respond to such behaviors by providing extra attention and affection and need to guard against demanding the level of independence that their toddler exhibited before the babysitting experience.

These kinds of understanding must also be facilitated in parents of the hospitalized toddler. One mother, who had been hospitalized after an automobile accident, when finally reunited with her toddler, who had also been hospitalized, was devastated when the child turned her back on her. This mother was assisted by the nurse in understanding and responding to the child's behavior as expected and normal.

Sexuality

According to Freud's theory, the body area or zone in which pleasurable feelings or tension reduction is centered in the toddler is the bowels. Freud stated that pleasurable sensations are derived from moving the bowels and therefore called this *anal stage of development*. Freud further believed that a conflict occurred in toddlers between the desire for the physical satisfaction of involuntarily relaxing the bowel sphincter and the emotional gratification of receiving their mother's loving approval when they did not. The process of toilet training was seen by Freud as a way of resolving this conflict and improper toilet training as a way of producing lifelong psychologic trauma. Freud's theory (1957), although recognized for its contribution to understanding human nature, is considered to be somewhat outdated.

Gender Identity

Awareness of gender identity (subjective sense of being male or female) begins around 18 months and is fully established by 5 years of age (Armstrong, 1978). Although 2-year-olds are not aware of anatomic differences, they can distinguish between males and females by general appearance. Most toddlers know whether they are boys or girls by 3 years of age and have some notion of sex-appropriate behaviors.

During the toddler years, gender identity and sex-role identification are primarily influenced by experiences within the family. When a toddler is consistently treated as being of a particular sex, the child internalizes that gender identity. For example, repeated expression to him as a "big boy" or to her as a "sweet girl" help a child learn this identity. Rewards for proper self-identification as male or female also help the child develop normal gender identity.

Developing Sex-Role Identification

Sex-role identification during the toddler years is learned through imitation and involves differences in the way parents interact with girls and boys. A toddler imitates both parents but particularly the same-sex parent, adopting appropriate roles, attitudes, and values. From the child's birth, parents generally behave differently toward girls and boys, resulting in early socialization into female and male roles. Some of the differences are that mothers talk and respond more to infant girls than to boys; boys may be handled more roughly in play, and more aggressive behavior is tolerated in boys than in girls.

Developing a Positive Sexual Attitude

The toddler as a curious and independent creature develops more awareness of self as a sexual being. Mastery of gender identity begins to some extent at this age, as evidenced by the 3-year-old child who can identify self or others as girl or boy. Through interaction with others, toddlers learn attitudes about the acceptability of their gender. Adults reinforce identity through tone of voice when encouraging specific types of play; by providing sex-linked toys, clothing, and room decor; and by linking socially approved behavior with being girl or boy.

Parental reactions to their child's play and self-exploration affect the toddler's developing attitude toward sexuality. The parent who reacts with alarm or disgust when discovering sex play among children contributes destructive negativism to attitude development. Likewise, the adult who fears that a child will be harmed by masturbation and slaps the child's hand and threatens that blindness will result conveys an attitude that sexual feelings and expressions are harmful or bad. Some parents are less obvious about their feelings. They may themselves fear that masturbation is harmful but express their feelings by avoiding *any* discussion with their child. Without explanation, a toddler is repeatedly told not to touch the genital area. Such behaviors also introduce negative feelings that the child associates with sexuality. If parents can be tolerant of sex play among toddlers, with gradual limit-setting as the child matures, positive attitudes can develop. Sometimes sex play among children is unsafe and requires limit-setting by parents. Providing safety and maintaining a sense of humor about the child's exploration of the world communicates a positive attitude.

Sexual Behaviors

Sexual behavior in the toddler reflects the curiosity and independence of this developmental stage. Toddlers learn new words and find new categories for their experiences. With delight the toddler shares these with others, as did the 2-year-old sitting in her highchair pointing to her cheeks and then to her chest, singing "dimples, nipples, dimples, nipples." Parents and caregivers who accept this as natural will contribute to healthy sexuality in the young child.

During the toddler years, a major developmental task children strive to achieve is toilet training. Because the urinary and anal orifices are in close proximity to the genitalia, it is important that achieving bowel and bladder control not be confused with sexuality. The attitudes of disapproval, anger, and impatience that parents so easily convey when a child is not progressing according to parental expectations may become associated with sexuality. Parents who are sensitive to the readiness of the child to learn, considering the child's interest, mastery of language, and muscle coordination, will avoid power conflicts and separate toilet training from sexual issues.

Other sexual behaviors of the toddler include a variety of types of sex play. It is not uncommon to find that toddlers place small objects into ears, nostrils, anuses, or vaginas. For example, a 3-year-old in the bath is enjoying a new plastic toy boat that has a flag on top of a pole. He discovers that the flag can be removed from the pole and is just the right size to hide in his rectum. However, in a short while the flag is gone and cannot be retrieved. The child may not tell the parent what happened. Parents and health professionals need to be aware that this type of natural behavior may happen so that they are alert to the possibility of injury or infection.

Sex play with other children is natural and a part of normal development. Many games of "doctor" and "house" have sexual overtones and at times contain overtly sexual behaviors. Describing the play of toddlers, Pitcher and Schultz (1983) found that girls frequently assumed child care roles, whereas boys exhibited this role play much less. Girls were also more likely to play both traditionally male and traditionally female roles (e.g., "mommy" or "firefighter") than were boys. This sex-linked play is part of the practice for *gender role* typical of the toddler. Gender role is learned behavior that is undifferentiated or neutral at birth. With the acquisition of language, such roles become unique to each sex as toddlers model the roles of significant others. Gender roles do not represent opposite ends of a spectrum but are identifiable along a continuum (Sears, 1974). For example, aggressive play may be seen more in boys than in girls at this age but is not limited to boys.

Anticipatory Guidance: Sexual Development

The nurse can facilitate normal development of gender identity by encouraging parents to develop a close relationship with their toddler. Parents should be assisted to plan their responsibilities so that both can spend time with the child. If only one parent is present, the nurse should explore with the parent ways in which a substitute mother or father figure can be established. Often a relationship with a relative, friend, or neighbor can play a significant role in a toddler's life and warrants the extra time and effort that a parent puts into providing such an opportunity.

It is during the toddler years that parents become aware of more deliberate genital self-exploration in their child. Also, parents begin to have concerns about their own nudity in the presence of a toddler of the opposite sex. The nurse should encourage parents to deal with these issues in a way that is comfortable for them, but they should not shame or punish a toddler for exploring his or her genitals. The way parents respond to those early sexual behaviors and interests forms the beginning of the child's own sexuality. The question of choice of toys may be brought to the nurse because parents disagree or because parents have read about the advantages of teaching all children the sex-role behaviors of both sexes. The nurse can be most helpful by encouraging parents to make traditionally sex-typed toys equally available to female and male children if this approach is consistent with their own philosophy. The nurse's role is to provide information so parents can make their own decisions according to their personal and cultural orientation.

Children at this age are not particularly concerned about privacy, but they should be taught that older children and adults are not to be allowed to touch their genitals.

Temperament

The temperament (behavior style) apparent during infancy tends to persist through toddlerhood and throughout later years, but it is changeable. The environment has a powerful effect on the child's temperament. A goodness-of-fit occurs if the environments provide appropriate nurturing, expectations, and demands in relation to the toddler's characteristics and style of behaving. If this does not occur, then developmental delays and maladaptive behavior can result (Carey, 1992).

This view has particular meaning for the toddler years because of the numerous demands for socialization that are encountered. These demands include: (1) establishment of regular sleep and feeding patterns; (2) mastery of self-care (feeding, dressing, toilet training); (3) compliance to family expectations; (4) response to masturbatory experiences; and (5) the emergence and growth of interpersonal relationships within the family. The way the developmental tasks are handled by parents may indeed bring about adaptations in the basic behavioral style. The environmental influences that children experience within their families may accentuate, modify, or alter traits of temperament (Thomas & Chess, 1977). The basic temperament types a child may have are listed in Table 3–12 (Thomas & Chess, 1977).

Regardless of the temperament of the child and the expectations of parents, there is likely to be some stress and conflict between parent and toddler.

Nursing Interventions: Temperament

Knowledge of the child's temperament can be incorporated into the nursing care plan. Information on the child's temperament can be best obtained by interviewing parents and observing the child's behavior (Johnson, 1992). For example, children with a low activity level would prefer quiet play activities such as looking at a picture book and watching TV.

TABLE 6-10

Promoting Temperament: Appropriate Care and Activities

Activity Level	
High	*Low*
• Refer to Table 6–16 for toys and play activities that promote physical and social development	• Refer to Table 6–16 for toys and play activities that promote quiet activities
Mood Level	
Negative	*Positive*
• Provide frequent rest periods • Provide "time-outs" when child gets upset • Encourage therapeutic play to ventilate feelings • Use rewards for behavior management	• Encourage play with favorite activities
Activity and Noise Threshold	
Low	*High*
• Limit unnecessary intrusions into room • Should avoid having child in wardroom • Admit child to single room as condition warrants (e.g., being away from noisy nurse's station)	• Child can be admitted to wardroom
Approach	
Withdrawn	*Approachable*
• Assign to small and consistent number of nurses • Do not force child to go to playroom; may need time to "warm up" to other children • Nurse or parent can initially accompany child to playroom	• Encourage child's going to playroom

Children who are easily distracted can best be prepared immediately prior to a procedure and in a quiet setting. Nursing care that incorporates temperament-appropriate activities is listed in Table 6–10.

Anticipatory Guidance: Temperament

Parents need assistance to understand that these temperamental variations do not constitute bad or good behavior but that toddlers of certain temperaments need responses from their families that are suited to their particular temperaments.

The nurse can be of assistance by encouraging parents to identify those behaviors that are most stressful and then helping them develop approaches that are congruent with their own temperament as well as their toddler's.

Emotions

The emotions expressed by a toddler become socially more obvious than they were during infancy. Young babies show discomfort and displeasure by crying or screaming, whereas toddlers add to their repertoire by throwing, biting, hitting, stamping their feet, and pushing or pulling (Fig. 6–7). Their pleasant emotions are also now expressed overtly. If they feel a need to be close to their parents, they have the physical ability to pull on them and to hug them, and the verbal ability to say "love Ma-ma" or "love Da-da." Expressions of both pleasant and unpleasant emo-

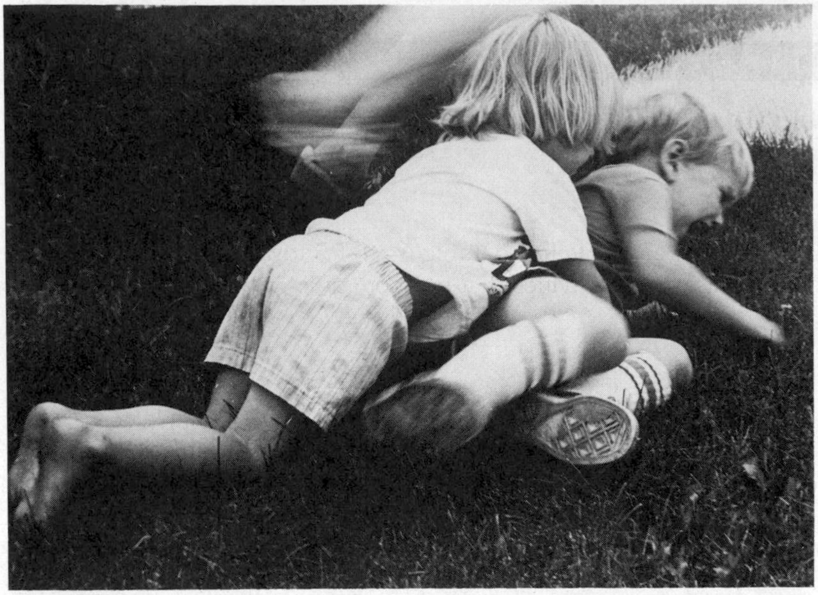

FIGURE 6 - 7. Toddlers express emotions physically through biting, hitting, or pulling. (Photograph by Jim Tackett.)

tions elicit various responses from those in their environment. That which children experience tends to encourage or discourage certain behaviors, and in this way they begin to adapt to the social demands of their families and society. If toddlers can feel loved and accepted, with some sense of control over their own destiny, they are likely to develop a sense of worth and high self-esteem. As toddlers strive to master developmental tasks, their experiences within the family to a large degree shape their emotional and social development. Each family interprets the confines of acceptable behavior and has its own ideals and expectations for its developing toddler.

Fears

Each age seems to bring with it typical or characteristic *fears*. An increasing perception of their environment makes toddlers more alert to auditory, spatial, and visual changes. The types of fears that result are fear of noise, sudden movement, an approaching object, and unusual sensations (height, water). Fear of the water develops most frequently around 18 to 24 months of age in relationship to being bathed. Children typically suddenly refuse to take baths and scream each time someone attempts to wash their face. Fear of strange people and strange objects and places and of aloneness persists from the latter part of the first year until the third year, then tends to diminish (Bowlby, 1973). The toddler's greatest fear is separation from caretakers. Fear of the dark and of animals runs somewhat parallel and is not common before the age of 2 years.

Nursing Interventions: Fears

Parents whose toddler is hospitalized need to be encouraged to be sensitive to the fears their child may develop in response to the foreign environment of a hospital. The toddler's limited cognitive abilities make her or him particularly vulnerable to imagined and real fears about the hospital environment and personnel.

The nurse can alleviate both the imagined and the real fears of hospitalization by providing developmentally appropriate explanations of hospital equipment and procedures (McClowry, 1993). Unfamiliar terminology used in hospital settings, such as "tid," "prn," or "stat," can be explained to the toddler so as to demystify the power of these new words and phrases. Use of hospital play programs and activities enables the toddler to participate in individual and group activities that promote development and reduce hospital-related fears.

Anticipatory Guidance: Fears

The fears of children under the age of 3 years are usually not a problem. If parents can be sensitive to the normal fears of their toddlers and provide the security they need, children are likely to progress through this period experiencing only the normal fears. When children are consistently fearful and clinging, however, and when fears restrict normal activities, this is a signal that pressures are too great and special effort may be needed to disclose the basic cause of insecurity. In some cases, further diagnostic evaluation may be necessary to rule out the possibility of a more serious problem.

Coping Mechanisms

During the toddler years, *anger* is commonly expressed through physical means. For a toddler, the obstacles encountered within a day are more frequent than many adults realize. Not only do adults interfere with a toddler's goals but the child's own ineptness leads to one predicament after another. Toys get stuck, ice cream cones fall, and balloons break, resulting in disappointment and frustration. They must learn to cope with their situations with little realization of the cause.

Anger (Temper Tantrums)

As toddlers develop in language and cognitive abilities, they have other options for dealing with their feelings (Table 6–11). However, for most of the toddler years, their modes of expression of anger include varied degrees of screaming, kicking, throwing things, and even hurting themselves by banging their head or biting themselves. Sometimes toddlers will hold their breath when overcome with intense anger. When a display of anger reaches an uncontrollable level, it is typically referred to as a *temper tantrum*. The most common age for temper tantrums is 18 months to 3 years—the age of negativism and resistive behavior. This developmental stage makes toddlers particularly vulnerable to physical demonstrations of anger.

Anticipatory Guidance: Temper Tantrums

Although it is the nurse's role to help parents understand that temper tantrums are normal for this age, he or she should also assist the family to make every attempt to alter those circumstances that predictably result in a tantrum. The frequency, duration, and intensity of tantrums can be reduced if situational factors are controlled.

During the toddler years, the most effective method of handling temper tantrums is to avoid rewarding the behavior. If a tantrum is to achieve nothing, parents are obliged to give nothing in response to it. If the temper tantrum is accompanied by breath holding, the parents need to know that ignoring this behavior will not result in harm. The child will resume breathing as a reflex when he or she needs to.

Nurses must realize that there is no foolproof method to handle temper tantrums. The counsel they offer must be given with an attitude of suggestions and options rather than solutions. Whenever temper tantrums become the pattern of behavior, the nurse should assist parents to carefully evaluate the circumstances surrounding the tantrums and correct any that predictably bring on a tantrum.

Negativism and Dawdling

Negativism and dawdling are manifestations of the noncompliant spirit that pervades the personality of a toddler. *Negativism* is the resistance a toddler displays around 18 months that lasts to about 3 years of age.

TABLE 6-11
Toddler's Coping Mechanisms

Mechanism	Example
Temper Tantrums	
Uncontrollable expressions of anger, including screaming, kicking, and throwing things	Maria begins kicking and screaming as the nurse approaches to give her an injection
Negativism	
Resistance to behaving in a requested manner	George answers "no" when the nurse offers suggestions of play activities
Dawdling	
Resists responding as requested by doing something else	Angela continues to play with doll as nurse tries to coax her to get in wheelchair to go to x-ray
Regression	
A return to an earlier stage of development in thought, feeling, or behavior	Ginny, who hasn't sucked her thumb for months, begins again while hospitalized
Withdrawal	
A physical and/or emotional removal from a situation that is stressful	Tung has stopped playing with toys and appears disinterested in environment during his prolonged hospitalization
Projection	
Attributing one's own thoughts or impulses to another person	Lucy hit her doll in the leg in the same location where she has just received an injection

This stage is characterized by a seeming delight in doing the opposite of what she or he is asked to do. *Dawdling* is a form of controlling others by responding to demands in a self-determined way. If children sense that they are being hurried to perform or are asked to do something specifically, they may do it but prolong the activity unmercifully. Dawdling then controls to what degree they can be manipulated by others, whereas negativism is a decided resistance to being controlled by others.

The "no, no" toddlers proclaim tells more about their ego development than it does about their desired course of action. Most of the time the firm assertion "no" is little more than an affirmation of their power to decide their own course. The telltale feature of toddler's "no" that means "yes" is that, while repeating "no, no, no," they simultaneously carry out the very thing they are resisting, as if their words had no relationship to their actions. Dawdling is an expression of feelings similar to those reflected in the use of "no, no"; that is, toddlers have the need to assert their power to control. There is no better way for toddlers to be in control.

Anticipatory Guidance: Negativism and Dawdling

Family members can learn to cope with negativism and dawdling if the nurse informs them about the developmental significance of these behaviors, gives them an opportunity to express their own frustrations, and gives suggestions to manage the behaviors. There are a number of consolations for parents with toddlers; these behaviors are normal, it is a stage that will eventually resolve, and other parents feel similar frustrations.

The following suggestions may be helpful if parents find their toddler's negativism and dawdling particularly stressful:

- Avoid questions that can be answered by "no."
- Do not phrase a request as a choice if no choice is really available to the child.
- Avoid requesting completion of tasks when the toddler is tired or hungry.
- Help the child finish when he or she dawdles (at the toddler's own pace).
- Pay special attention to the child when there is excessive stimulation caused by the presence of many people.
- Avoid drawing attention to negativistic and dawdling behaviors.

Forewarning a family of the activities that are potential battleground is a preventive nursing function. Other toddler coping mechanisms are listed in Table 6–11.

Moral and Faith Development

The toddler's understanding of what constitutes right and wrong is limited. Their understanding of what is prohibited is derived from their parents. The repeated warnings from parents about what is/is not permissible is eventually incorporated into the toddler's behavior, but only after considerable frustration and effort from the parents. This is due in large measure to the child's limited cognitive ability, shortened attention span, and limited memory capacity. This accounts in considerable measure for a toddler's supposed intentional transgressions after having just been warned not to do something. For example, a toddler will repeatedly take cookies from the cookie jar despite parental warning not to do so. These repeated acts of misbehavior are not necessarily deliberate. Limited memory capacity and cognitive ability of the toddler result in the repetition of a forbidden act until it is comprehended. Eventually, the toddler differentiates between acceptable and nonacceptable behavior according to parental standards. This type of moral behavior is referred to as the *preconventional level of development* (Kohlberg, 1981). That is, the toddler is reliant on external sources for determining what is right or wrong. As with everything else that the toddler experiments with, parental guidelines are needed in order to understand what is and is not acceptable.

The earlier manifestations of conscience development can be observed as early as 18 months. The toddler demonstrates distress behaviors with minor mishaps and transgressions. Research has shown that toddlers with temperaments more vulnerable to anxiety and parents with less controlling childrearing practices were found to be contributory to the development of conscience in school-age children (Kochanska, 1991).

The toddler is in the *intuitive-projective stage* of faith development according to Fowler (1974, 1984). The faith beliefs the toddler learns are primarily from the parents. The toddler learns to imitate the parents' religious practices and behaviors. As an example, the child will imitate the parents' prayer gestures without realizing what they mean. Since the child is egocentric, misconceptions about religious beliefs are likely to occur. The child does not understand the concept of supernatural. The toddler's idea of God can be described in human terms, as that reflects their level of cognition.

Peer Relationships

Friendships among toddlers are limited. "Friendship" is best described as having a playmate. That is, whoever the toddler is playing with at the time is considered to be a "friend." Children are limited in terms of developing friendships, as they have an egocentric orientation and lack social skills. The toddler is unable to take another child's feelings into consideration. In addition, owing to limited cognitive abilities, the child is not able to distinguish accurately what is the reality of the situation. Children will have fights over the use of toys or whether there has been an intrusion into their space.

Toddlers play *beside* peers (parallel play) but not *with* them, since true cooperation is not yet possible. Toddlers will say "mine" in word or gestures and hold toys away from any other child who approaches. If they want the cookie the youngster beside them is munching contentedly, they will snatch it and consume it greedily.

Early speech during play is also egocentric; a little later it may resemble a monologue, taking no consideration of playmates' interests or answers. At times, they push, poke, hit, bite, and scratch without reference to the hurt they are inflicting, since they do not themselves feel the pain. They are unable to comprehend the feelings and pain of another.

Anticipatory Guidance: Peer Relationships

The nurse can assist parents in understanding their child's behavior with age mates by providing information about what is developmentally appropriate. Understanding of their child's behavior will prevent parents from misinterpreting and judging it and possibly punishing the child for misbehaving. Children can be assisted by parents, however, to learn to interact in considerate ways with their friends by role modeling and guidance.

Health Maintenance and Promotion

Health Screening

The toddler continues with the immunization schedule, receiving measles, mumps, rubella (MMR), and *Haemophilus influenzae* b conjugate vaccine (HbCV) at 15 months. Diphtheria and tetanus toxoids with pertussis vaccine (DTP) is given 6 to 12 months after the third dose, somewhere between 15 and 18 months of age. It can be administered simultaneously with MMR at 15 months. The oral poliovirus vaccine (OPV) can be given with the MMR and HbCV at 15 months or between 12 and 24 months of age (American Academy of Pediatrics [AAP], 1991; see Table 10–6). Routine tuberculin skin testing can be done at 15 months with the MMR. The AAP recommends the use of the Mantoux skin test, as it has greater specificity for *Mycobacterium tuberculosis* (Richardson et al, 1991).

Infants as young as 6 months may receive the MMR vaccination during an outbreak in a high-risk area. Children who receive MMR vaccines before their first birthday should receive a repeat vaccination at 15 months (AAP, 1989b). For further discussion of immunizations, see Chapter 10.

Well child visits include health screening for hypertension, iron deficiency anemia, and elevated cholesterol and triglycerides. Annual blood pressure screening for children begins at 3 years. Blood pressures above the 95th percentile are checked on three separate occasions. A thorough family and medical history and physical examination are then done to determine the cause of hypertension. Although not routinely done, initial screening for elevated cholesterol and triglyceride levels is performed when the child is between 2 to 5 years of age. Indications for screening include a positive family history for elevated cholesterol levels, hypertension, obesity, and early heart attack or cerebrovascular accident.

Follow-up screening for iron deficiency anemia done initially during infancy is performed again at 3 years, prior to the child's entering preschool. Iron deficiency anemia ranks first as the most common hematologic problem seen in young children between the ages of 9 to 24 months. Screening for anemia is not a reliable method for detecting lead poisoning. Venous lead measurements are recommended for lead screening in toddlers (Shannon & Graef, 1992).

The growth trajectory is monitored for significant alterations in pattern as indicated on the growth chart. Normally, after the first year of life until adolescence, the growth pattern parallels the percentile lines on the growth chart. A drop off or crossing of lines may be an early indicator of a medical, emotional, or social problem.

Children who immigrate from third world countries in Asia, Africa, or Central or South America present with unique health care needs. The influence of culture and lifestyle must be considered in assessing health care needs. Growth charts that are commonly used are problematic when applied to children from third world countries. Studies of immigrant children 2 to 5 years old from Asia reveal 30 to 40 per cent of them to be 2 standard deviations below the National Center for Health Statistics (NCHS) height median and within normal range for weight (Baldwin & Sutherland, 1988), suggesting that the child's size is due to genetic factors rather than to malnutrition.

Immunization is a serious health problem. Children from migrant families are at higher risk for not being immunized. The AAP has developed recommendations for children with delayed and/or incomplete immunization records (AAP, 1991). Tuberculosis screening is recommended for children at age 1 year and again at 4 to 6 years from high-risk groups from the areas previously mentioned and from the Middle East and Caribbean.

Given the lifestyle of poverty often associated with migrant families, these children are at greater risk for respiratory and ear infections, gastroenteritis, parasitic diseases, skin infections, poor nutrition, and anemia (AAP, 1989a). Awareness of the unique health care needs these children present will require prompt identification, treatment, and referral. Nurses working in various community settings, such as the school and public health clinics, can develop collaborative relationships with leaders and members from culturally diverse communities to promote improved access to health care.

Vision and Hearing

Impaired hearing is difficult to detect if there is unilateral or minimal hearing loss. Hearing loss can inhibit language development. For example, a hearing-impaired infant may babble at 6 months and then show a marked decrease in vocalization, eventually producing no sounds. The reports of parents can give the first clue to vision and hearing problems (Rapin, 1993).

Hyperopia (farsightedness) is normal during toddlerhood. Distance fixation is not well developed; an object must be within a 6-foot range for clear vision. Before the age of 3 years, vision can be assessed by observing the child's eye-hand coordination and her or his response to bright lights and objects. After age 3, the child can cooperate sufficiently for the Snellen illiterate E chart. For additional information on ophthalmic examinations refer to Chapter 45.

Anticipatory Guidance: Vision and Hearing

The nurse should explain the relationship between hearing and language development. Parents should be taught the normal progression of language development (see Table 6–6) as a preventive measure to detect hearing impairment. Parents should be encouraged to assess hearing and vision by observing their toddler's response to stimuli. The reports of parents can give the first clue to vision and hearing problems. A recent study found that parents were the first to suspect their child's hearing loss (Thompson & Thompson, 1991). Should a hearing loss be detected, the toddler can be referred for audiometric testing. There are procedures both electrophysiologic and behavioral that can be conducted.

Dental Care

At 1 year of age, a child usually has 6 to 8 teeth. Usually one tooth erupts for each month of age past 6 months up to 26 to 30 months of age. The age of a toddler in months minus 6 is used as an approximate guide to assess the expected number of teeth at a specific age. During the toddler years, 4 first molars, 4 cuspids, and 4 second molars erupt to complete the set of 20 deciduous teeth by about 30 months of age.

Anticipatory Guidance: Dental Care

Toothbrushing is recommended by 18 months of age, when gingival tissue is no longer so easily damaged and a considerable number of teeth are usually present. A toddler's teeth should be brushed twice a day, and parents should continue to assist with toothbrushing after the child begins to brush his or her own teeth. Toddlers will want to brush their own teeth by the age of 2 years, but they need supervision. Short back-and-forth or simple up-and-down motion (Fig. 6–8) is used to clean teeth. A survey of

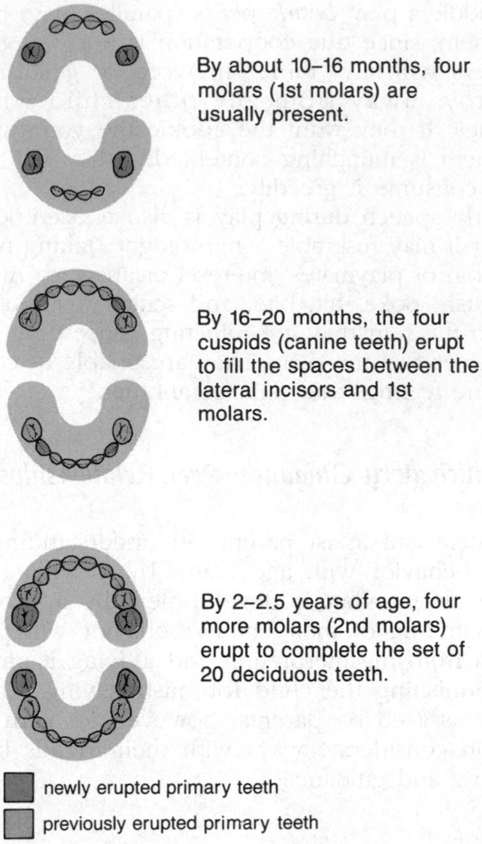

By about 10–16 months, four molars (1st molars) are usually present.
By 16–20 months, the four cuspids (canine teeth) erupt to fill the spaces between the lateral incisors and 1st molars.
By 2–2.5 years of age, four more molars (2nd molars) erupt to complete the set of 20 deciduous teeth.
newly erupted primary teeth
previously erupted primary teeth

FIGURE 6-8. Development of teeth. A combination of primary and secondary teeth is present in the child's mouth simultaneously during the process of eruption and shedding.

toddler's dental care practices found that children ingested substantial amounts of fluoride from toothpaste. This source of fluoride, combined with dietary sources and water fluoride concentration, may result in a total fluoride intake higher than recommended. Although not harmful, mild to moderate dental fluorosis has been associated with higher thresholds of fluoride (Simard et al, 1991). Parents can be instructed to delay the use of toothpaste with fluoride and use very small amounts until the child is older than 2 years. The use of fluoride supplements should be carefully considered in view of the child's total consumption of fluoride.

Sleep Behaviors

A toddler requires approximately 10 to 13 hours of sleep. Nurse researchers found the range of nighttime sleep to vary from 7½ to 10½ hours (Edgil et al, 1985). Most toddlers take an afternoon nap, and before 2 years of age, some may need a morning and an afternoon nap. Keeping toddlers on a relatively consistent sleeping schedule reduces the frequency of irritable and cranky periods. They cannot tolerate losing sleep without showing changes in their behavior (Table 6–12).

TABLE 6-12
Toddler Developmental Characteristics of Sleep-Related Behavior (1–3 Yrs)

Characteristic Sleep-Related Behaviors	Promote Sleep-Related Health
• May need morning and afternoon nap but usually by 1½–2 yrs one nap is sufficient • Dawdling and delay tactics are used to resist sleep • Child resists sleep because cannot tolerate the separation • As child approaches 3 yrs of age, may also fear the dark; also may find it difficult to "unwind" because of high motor activity during the day • 10–14 hrs of sleep per 24 hrs	• Don't insist that child sleep during nap time, but a quiet time in the crib after lunch is encouraged • Following a routine at bedtime is essential • A few minutes of warning that bedtime is approaching, a warm bath, and a bedtime story help promote sleep • A special blanket, doll, or toy gives comfort to alleviate the pain of separation • This is usually the period when a hall light, night light, or small table light must be left on • Usually, advance from crib to bed by the end of the toddler period

Developmental characteristics that are displayed in sleep behaviors of toddlers are ritualism, separation anxiety, and autonomy (they resist sleep). Beginning at 18 to 21 months and continuing until 3 years, they prepare for bed by performing several activities in a precise order (washing, brushing teeth, turning a light switch, putting shoes into a certain place, and a variety of other time-consuming tasks). Rituals can be viewed as a form of dawdling, in which toddlers go to bed after they have done what they want to and when they are ready to do so. These rituals give toddlers a sense of security that they need when they are learning to separate themselves from their attachment figures. At this stage, it is also common to have a favorite toy or blanket (transitional object), which is taken to bed for security. A nurse researcher found differences in the temperament of toddlers with sleep problems compared with those who did not (Jimmerson, 1991). Toddlers with sleep problems were identified as having more "difficult" temperaments compared with toddlers with no sleep problems who were described as having "easy" temperaments. Toddlers with sleep problems were less adaptable and more likely to withdraw or resist new situations.

Sleep is also resisted by more obvious behaviors, especially as toddlers approach their second birthday. Toddlers may resist so violently that they have temper tantrums or they may stand in the crib and cry for their parents. Such behaviors are eventually given up as toddlers overcome separation anxiety and as their intense need to control lessens.

Anticipatory Guidance: Sleep Behaviors

Parents should be advised to keep bedtime activities as simple as possible. Once a routine has been established, a toddler will insist on following it; therefore, it is easier to avoid adding additional rituals than it is to omit them after they have been started. It does not work to tell a toddler, "Just tonight you may turn the light switch off and on."

Bedtime can be a pleasant time if parents allow extra time for the rituals rather than altering them against the toddler's wishes. Once the usual rituals have been carried out, it is most effective if the parent says "good night" and does not return to the room. If a toddler can manipulate a parent to repeatedly return for minor requests, the behavior is likely to be repeated. If the child has a legitimate request, it is only reasonable to grant it, but repeated requests are the toddler's way of postponing separation, and this is a form of sleep resistance. If a child stands in the crib and cries after the usual routines have been completed, it is better to leave and usually the child goes to sleep. She or he may cry until falling asleep, but eventually the child learns that the parents are in control of the sleep routine. It is not uncommon for toddlers to have particular difficulty separating from their mother at bedtime, in which case the fathers may have more success in getting them in bed.

A toddler's resistance to sleep can be exasperating to parents. It is helpful to point out that many of a toddler's fears are encountered at bedtime. Children's fear of separation, of the dark, and of noises, such as flushing the toilet and water rushing out of the tub, all happen in relation to going to bed. Although fear of the dark is more common after 3 years of age, some toddlers show signs of such fear earlier. It is important for the nurse to help parents recognize that the child's fear is real and should not be ridiculed and that most bedtime fear can be dispelled with help and patience from parents. Although sleeping practices vary in cultures, it is generally recommended that children not sleep in their parents' bed. For further information, refer to the section on "Fears."

Anticipatory guidance can assist the parent to be sensitive to the temperamental characteristics of the child. Assessment of the mother, the toddler, and the sleeping environment will provide information about the defining characteristics affecting the nursing diagnosis *sleep pattern disturbance*. Children with "difficult" temperaments will need particular attention directed to the falling asleep period. This can be a period of quiet activity such as reading a bedtime story. Further information on promoting healthy sleep is found in Table 6–12.

Nutrition

Nutritional Requirements

A toddler needs a greater number of total calories (1000 to 1500 kcal/day) than during infancy owing to an increase in body size, but the requirements *per unit of body weight* decrease as the growth rate decreases (Table 6–13).

Although physical growth rate slows during the toddler years, protein requirements remain relatively high because of the rapid growth of muscle tissue. In spite of a decrease in appetite, under normal circumstances, the toddler's protein requirements are met if a balanced diet is consumed.

By about 2 years of age, the percentage of total body water is similar to that of an adult, i.e., approximately 60 per cent of total body weight. Metabolic rate remains relatively high; therefore, a toddler's fluid requirement is 115 to 125 ml/kg/day. A balanced diet including 16 to 24 ounces of milk supplies vitamin D, calcium, and phosphorus in recommended amounts.

Eating Behaviors

By 1 year of age, many children have been weaned from the bottle, with the exception of a nighttime bottle. The eruption of additional teeth during the

TABLE 6–13
Recommended Food Intake for Good Nutrition According to Food Groups and Daily Dietary Allowances (Toddlers, 1–3 Yrs)

Food Groups	**Servings Per Day**	**Serving Size** **1 yr**	**2–3 yrs**
Bread Group	At least 4	½ slice	1 slice
• Bread		½ oz	¾ oz
• Cereal		¼ C	⅓ C
• Rice and pasta			
Vegetable Group	At least 3 total	2 tbsp	3 tbsp
• Green-yellow vegetables (vitamin A source)	1 or more	⅓ C	½ C
• Other vegetables	2		
Fruit Group	At least 3 total	⅓ C	½ C
• Citrus fruits, berries, tomato, cabbage, cantaloupe	1 or more (twice as much tomato as citrus)		
(vitamin C source)		¼ C	⅓ C
• Other fruits (apple, banana	2	½ C	½–¾ C
Milk Group	3		
• Milk/yogurt			
• Cheese		1½ oz cheese = 1 C milk	
Meat Group	2 (6 oz total)		
• Cooked lean meat, poultry, fish		2 tbsp	2 tbsp
• Dry beans		2 tbsp	3 tbsp
• Egg		1	1
• Peanut butter			1 tbsp
Fats, oils, and sweets—USE SPARINGLY			

Recommended Daily Dietary Allowances

Protein	**Fat-Soluble Vitamins**		**Water-Soluble Vitamins**		**Minerals**		**Energy Needs**
16 g	Vitamin A	400 μg RE	Vitamin C	40 mg	Calcium	800 mg	1300 kcal
	Vitamin D	10 μg	Thiamine	0.7 mg	Phosphorus	800 mg	
	Vitamin E	6 mg α—TE	Riboflavin	0.8 mg	Magnesium	80 mg	
	Vitamin K	15 μg	Niacin	9 mg NE	Iron	10 mg	
			Vitamin B_6	1.0 mg	Zinc	10 mg	
			Folate	50 μg	Iodine	70 μg	
			Vitamin B_{12}	0.7 μg	Selenium	20 μg	

Adapted with permission from *Recommended Dietary Allowances:* 10th Edition. Copyright 1989 by the National Academy of Sciences. Published by the National Academy Press, Washington, D.C.; and US Department of Agriculture, Human Nutrition Information Service. (1992). *Food guide pyramid.* (Leaflet No. 572). Washington, DC: Author.

Key: RE, retinol equivalent; TE, tocopherol equivalent; NE, niacin equivalent.

second year makes it possible for toddlers to eat most adult foods. Their slowed growth decreases their requirement for food and is reflected in a decreased appetite. Their increased motor abilities enhance their eating skills, and their emotional-social development markedly influences the eating behavior. Parents who know of and are prepared for these changes can more effectively prevent or cope with the stress involving eating during these years. Nutritional practices established during these early years will have an impact on weight gain during childhood. Identification of risk factors for obesity provides the basis for early intervention. These risk factors include overweight or obese family members, mother's preference for a chubby baby, low socioeconomic status, and involvement of several caretakers in childrearing activities (Sherman & Alexander, 1990).

Anticipatory Guidance: Nutrition

Parents should be told that a decrease in appetite is common, and that they can expect a pattern of fluctuation in the amount and type of food their toddlers eat. It is difficult for parents to cope with toddlers who one day eat their meals eagerly and the next refuse to eat anything. Toddlers may insist on certain foods (food jags), which can make it difficult for parents to ensure that they have a balanced diet. These food jags cannot be easily altered but often last for only a few days. During such time, toddlers may refuse to eat anything if they are not given at least a small portion of the preferred food. Other foods can be offered in small portions and within a few days, the toddler will likely request a different food as the favorite. If the nurse can adequately inform a family and offer suggestions to handle normal developmental behaviors, mealtime and eating can be associated with pleasure and satisfaction in these early impressionable years (Table 6–14). A toddler eats approximately half as much food as an adult and should be served foods from the basic food groups. Vitamin and iron supplementation is unnecessary unless a well-balanced diet is not consumed.

The nurse should also discuss nutritional concerns involving dentition, iron deficiency anemia, and obesity. The major points to discuss with parents regarding nutrition and dentition are that sweets should be avoided as between-meal snacks, that 16 to 24 ounces of milk be consumed daily, and that a bedtime bottle, if offered, not contain juice or milk. Iron deficiency anemia is prevented if adequate iron-rich foods are consumed and milk is limited to 24 ounces daily. This is recommended because toddlers may drink too much milk. This causes satiation that, in turn, decreases intake of solid foods rich in iron (liver, dark green vegetables, iron-enriched cereals, egg yolk). Obesity can be prevented by using skim or low-fat milk and by offering limited sweets (especially candy and sodas). Snacks should consist of small amounts of nutritious foods. Obesity in toddlerhood is also prevented by providing opportunities for physical exercise. The nurse should pay particular attention to how food is used by the parents. The practice of using food as a reward or to pacify may establish patterns that lead to obesity later. Familial values toward weight control warrant exploration, particularly in families with overweight members or wherein the primary caretaker expresses preference for a "chubby infant." Long-term nutritional counseling and support may be needed to facilitate changes in family eating behaviors (Sherman & Alexander, 1990).

Toilet Training

Physical maturation of the sphincter muscles and myelination of the spinal cord are biologic requirements for the control of elimination. By the time toddlers sit and walk well (12 to 18 months), their nerve pathways have developed to the extent that they can physically control their bowel and bladder sphincters. The regularity of bowel movements is usually better established by 18 months than it was in infancy. Bowel movements are often associated with meals, with one after breakfast or one after supper or at both times. However, there is a wide variation in when toddlers develop regularity and in the pattern of regularity.

In addition to the physical ability of sphincter control, the child must have cognitive awareness of elimination and the ability to communicate this awareness to the parent or caregiver. It is generally agreed that by 18 months of age toddlers have some awareness that a bowel movement is occurring and that some children even indicate by gestures that they know it is coming; however, it is usually not until closer to 2 years of age that they can give enough advance warning to be helped to the toilet. Children must also possess psychologic readiness, a desire to please their parent by holding on and letting go at appropriate times. The child must also exhibit the desire to be autonomous and to control impulses. Waiting until closer to 2 years or 30 months of age to begin toilet training increases the success rate considerably (Fig. 6–9).

Some children attain bowel control before bladder control. If training is not achieved by age 5 or later, the child should be referred for further evaluation.

Nursing Interventions: Toilet Training

Parents will understand that their toddler's need to use diapers when hospitalized, after having been toilet trained, is not unexpected. This is the child's response to dealing with an overly stressful situation. The toddler's regression is likely to be temporary. The toddler will resume the previous level of elimination control acquired prior to hospitalization once the crisis of the illness experience has passed.

TABLE 6-14

Promoting Socialized Eating Behavior

Principles	Examples
To develop skill in manipulating utensils, toddlers need the opportunity to practice but may need some assistance. They will often refuse assistance even though they need it	At 15 mos: help by feeding with a second spoon, provide finger foods. At 18–24 mos: be supportive by helping the child get food onto spoon to mouth. Continue finger foods
At mealtime, a toddler should learn to associate mastery, pleasure, and acceptance with the experience of eating	Avoid forcing of food. Allow self-feeding but assist on toddler's terms; avoid punishment for spills and messiness. Praise attempts at self-feeding even though many spills occur
A toddler needs total concentration to accomplish the skills of self-feeding	Provide a quiet place with minimal distraction; no loud music or television. Once the meal has begun, getting up from the table and returning by parents and siblings distract a toddler
Food intake is likely to decrease if toddlers have been involved in vigorous physical activity immediately prior to a meal, or if they have had to wait a significant time past regular mealtime. They also take less interest in food if they are overtired (lacking sleep) or overfatigued (too much physical activity)	A time of quiet before meals and regularity in mealtimes is conducive to a toddler's appetite. Keeping children on a balanced schedule of rest and activity improves their dispositions and general eating behavior
A toddler imitates eating behaviors of her or his family	Parents need to provide appropriate role modeling and to discipline siblings in table manners
A toddler finds security in following certain routines and rituals	Use the same plate, cup, and utensils and consistency in the order of preparing the toddler for eating (washing hands, sitting in chair, serving food)
Toddlers' appetites fluctuate, as do their moods. Variation from dependence to independence is prevalent in toddlers' eating behaviors, as is a strong need to have their own way. A toddler cannot be forced to eat	Do not try to force a child to eat. When toddlers refuse to eat and insist they want to get out of the high chair or down from the table, let them miss a meal. Avoid snacks and they will probably eat the next scheduled meal. Over a period of a week, intake is usually adequate

Anticipatory Guidance: Toilet Training

The nurse should explain that there are no precise rules or schedules that can be applied to guarantee successful toilet training. From the beginning, parents need to feel relaxed and confident that their toddler will achieve that task of toilet training without undue pressure and control from them. Some useful suggestions that the nurse can offer are listed in Table 6–15.

In a nursing study of mothers' descriptions of the toilet training process, five recurrent themes were identified: timing, trajectory of successes and failures, approaches to toileting, factors influencing the mother, and traits and skills of the child (Hauck, 1991). Although each mother interviewed shared unique perspectives about the toilet training process, the findings of the study indicated there were commonalities of experiences. This study highlights the need for nurses to be sensitive to the complexity of factors affecting the toileting training process when providing anticipatory guidance.

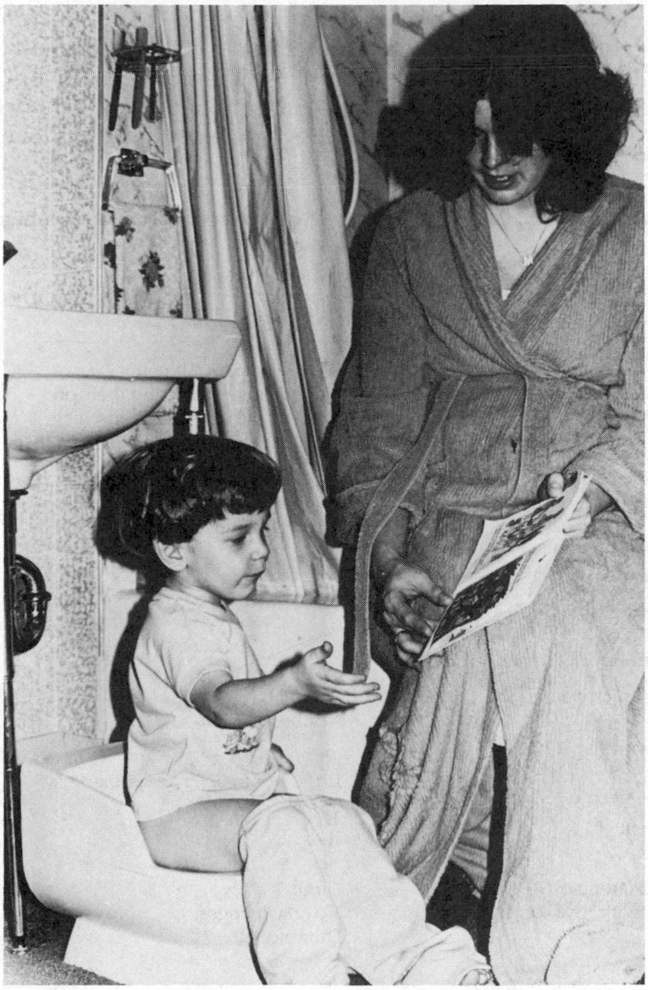

FIGURE 6-9. In a positive, reinforcing environment, toddlers actually train themselves. (Photograph by Jim Tackett.)

Play

The characteristics of toddlers' play are determined by their developmental level. They remain primarily egocentric in play activities, showing little regard for the feelings of others. Egocentrism in play is characterized by a predominance of behaviors that prove children's own power and central position. This is how they build their self-image, which contributes to their rapidly developing awareness of themselves as persons. The type of play coming out of these needs is *parallel play,* in which children engage in similar activities while playing beside one another but not together.

During this period, children learn a great deal by imitating their caregivers. They particularly enjoy helping with household tasks (Fig. 6–10). The classic example is the toddler's fascination with emptying a cupboard of pots and pans. To a toddler, manipulation of pots and pans is a form of helping by imita-

TABLE 6-15
Family-Centered Teaching: Strategies for Successful Toilet Training

- Observe the time of day that child has bowel movement and place her or him on the potty prior to that time
- The potty should be comfortable and feel secure to the child
- Use acceptable and simple, easy-to-understand words and gestures to indicate to the child what is expected of him or her
- Encouraging the child to play with toys may distract from the purpose of toilet training; use distraction judiciously, if at all
- Ten to 15 mins is long enough for the child to sit on the potty
- Reinforce success with verbal praise and physical affection
- Do not punish lack of success or noncompliance

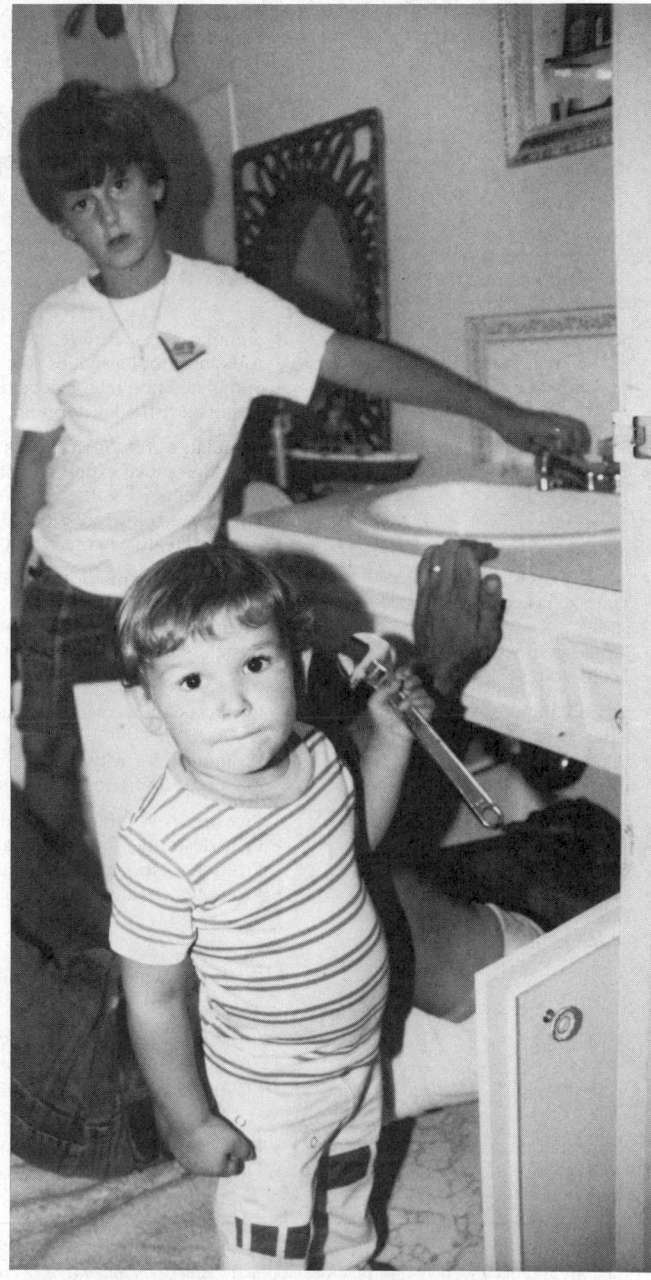

FIGURE 6-10. Toddlers enjoy playing with real items used by parents.

tion. Although the help toddlers give usually creates work for their parents, these imitative behaviors are an important step in development.

Another characteristic of a toddler's play is the love of active play and manipulation of objects. Exercise of both large and small muscles is necessary for toddlers to develop a sense of control over their bodies and their environments. Toddlers' needs to explore are facilitated by their gross and fine motor abilities that give them access to almost anything that

TABLE 6-16
Toys and Play Activities for Toddlers

Toy or Play Activity	Development Promoted	Selection Criteria
• Pull toys	• Simulates gross motor skill and strengths (P) • Stimulates awareness of object when not seen (C)	• Wooden with pull cords • Makes noise indicating their presence (noise may be offensive)
• Picture books	• Teaches page manipulation (P) • Stimulates guided language development (C) • Teaches remembered properties of objects (forms and objects) (C) • Provides social experiences when assisted (S) • Stimulates knowledge and aids in school activities (C)	• Cloth or washable • Nontearable • Facilitates creativity and development of language
• Book of rhymes	• Provides fine distinctions in hearing (P & C) • Social experience and humor (E & S) • Stimulates language development (C & S)	
• Toys as symbols of adult activities • Dress-up kits • Nurse/doctor kits	• Symbols represent actions (e.g., lunch pail equals going to work) (C & S)	• Durable • Nonbreakable
• Scribbling on paper	• Stimulates creativity (C) • Aids in school activities (C) • Stimulates fine motor development (P) • Fosters artistic development (E & C)	• Large nontoxic crayons/markers
• Small push-pull toys • Cars and trucks	• Stimulates gross motor skills and strength (P) • Provides active experimentation with toys, objects, and movements (C & P) • Stimulates self-expression (E) • Aids in creative expression (C)	• Large • No sharp edges • Durable
• Large, crawl-in box • Trapeze set • Slides • Jungle gym • Teeter-totter	• Teaches gross motor skills (P) • Stimulates creativity (C) • Creates own environment (P & C) • Fosters social development (S)	• Durable • Adult supervision with trapeze, jungle gym equipment, and slides
• Stuffed animals • Dolls • Blanket • Blanket surrogate	• Comforts and provides security through familiarity (C, E, & S) • Promotes creativity (C) • Promotes imitative behaviors (C & S)	• No pieces that can be removed and swallowed
• Filling and emptying toys • Take-apart toys • Large size Legos • Loc-blocks • Block set • Hammer and nail sets	• Provides self satisfaction with repetition (P, C, & E) • Provides outlet for emotional expression (E) • Promotes gross motor skill and strength (P) • Promotes creativity (C)	• Durable • Nonbreakable
• Puzzles • Tinker Toys	• Provides awareness of simple shapes (C)	
• Balls • Sandbox • Wagons • Hobbyhorse	• Provides awareness of shapes/textures (C) • Promotes gross/fine motor development (P) • Promotes social development (S)	
• Finger paints • Drums • Modeling clay	• Promotes awareness of textures, colors, shapes (C) • Promotes artistic development (E & C)	• Nontoxic substances • No sharp edges

Adapted from Lee, J., & Fowler, M. (1986). Merely child's play and developmental work and playthings. *Journal of Pediatric Nursing, 1*(4), 260–269; Florey, L. (1971). An approach to play and play development. *American Journal of Occupational Therapy, 25*(6), 275–280; Betz, C. (1983). Teaching children through play therapy. *Journal of Association of Operating Room Nurses, 88*(4), 709, 712–713, 716–717; and Betz, C., & Poster, E. (1984). Incorporating play into the care of the hospitalized child. *Issues in Comprehensive Pediatric Nursing, 7*(6), 343–355.

Key: C, cognitive development; P, physical development; E, emotional development; S, social development.

intrigues them. Toddlers enjoy activities of motion such as a ride on a tricycle, stroller, wagon, or swing (Table 6–16).

Toddlers also learn about their environment through their sensory experiences. Anyone who observes toddlers at play will note that much of what they do provides sensory benefits. Toddlers touch objects to see how they feel, run their fingers over them, and still explore with their lips and tongue, although mouthing objects is now less frequent than during infancy. They are also fascinated by the various sounds they can make and experiment using voice, tongue, and lips to create new sounds or to imitate the sounds they hear.

Some quiet, sedentary activities are also appropriate for the toddler and are especially useful before bedtime. Much of a toddler's encounter with books during the period from 12 to 24 months involves identification of objects, turning pages, and imitating familiar sounds of animals and objects such as trains, cars, and trucks. Toddlers also enjoy having parents read to them and repeat nursery rhymes. From 2 to 3 years of age, as their attention spans increase, they become increasingly interested in listening to and imitating nursery rhymes and hearing short stories illustrated by pictures. Children develop language through their play. Their play experiences increase their encounters with the world, requiring them to attach labels to what they sense and do.

The frustrations that toddlers experience because of their struggles with developing autonomy can be directed into suitable play activities. Simple activities of running, throwing a ball, and hammering on a pegboard are ways to dissipate excess energy safely. Many sensory experiences have the added benefit of providing a means for expression of aggressive behavior. Pounding, splashing, or hitting is harmless when directed at sand, water, or soap bubbles.

Anticipatory Guidance: Play

The nurse can increase a family's awareness and understanding of how play enhances the toddler's development. The motor skills that affect play (see Chapter 17 for a discussion on skills affecting play) can be discussed with parents, along with the characteristics of a toddler's play, his or her developmental needs for play, and appropriate activities to meet these needs. The nurse should encourage parents to play with their toddler. Toddlers will play alone or beside another toddler for short periods, but they also enjoy the attention and interaction that play with adults affords.

There are certain circumstances that require special effort on the part of parents to provide adequate play opportunities. When a toddler is an only child, some provision should be made for play with another child or children about the same age. When there are siblings close in age, parents also have problems, such as arguments and fighting during play. Each family develops its own pattern of handling conflicts between children, but a basic rule is to let children solve their own problems as much as possible. The nurse should stress that a toddler needs a variety of play opportunities; however, it is unnecessary to buy expensive toys.

Safety Concerns

Accident prevention is one of the greatest challenges that face health professionals who care for children (Allshouse et al, 1993). The stages of childhood development can be used to predict the type of accidents most likely to occur. By 1 year of age, toddlers are very mobile, and as they pull themselves to standing position, they pull at whatever is within reach. Hanging tablecloths, dangling cords, and unstable furniture are hazards. From 1 to 2 years, the child's curiosity without a sense of danger makes her or him vulnerable to accidents. By the time children are 2 years old, their speed of mobility adds still another danger to which parents must be alerted (Fig. 6–11). Types of accidents that parents should guard against as common hazards to toddlers are: (1) accidents while riding in a car, (2) being hit by a moving vehicle, (3) drowning, (4) ingesting harmful substances,

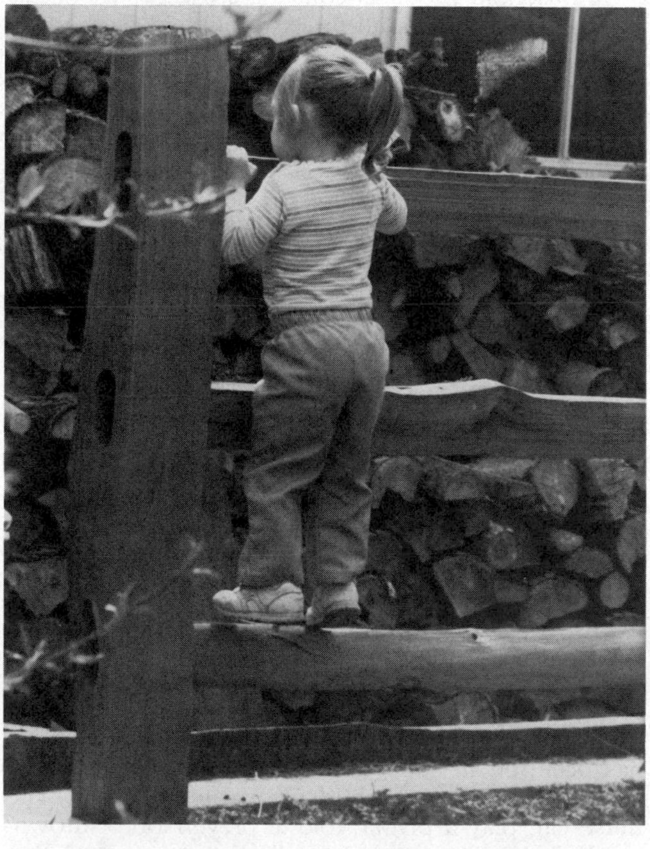

FIGURE 6 - 11. The need to explore and the climbing ability extend to objects outdoors, calling for caregiver vigilance.

(5) burns, (6) aspiration of a foreign body, (7) suffocation, (8) falls, and (9) toy accidents.

Burns. The peak incidence for burns occurs during toddlerhood (1- to 2-year-old group). Burns occur more frequently with boys than with girls (Uchiyama & German, 1987). Scalding burns from hot liquids are the leading cause of burns in children, accounting for 56 per cent. This burn injury can occur with the spillage of hot liquids from the stovetop and immersion into hot water in the tub.

Toddlers are also prone to burn injury from hot objects, such as curling irons and toasters, contact with electrical outlets, and playing with matches.

Ingestions. The toddler is vulnerable to ingestion of a multitude of toxic substances. These substances include lead, pesticides, and household products. For further information on lead poisoning, refer to the section "Health Screening," earlier in this chapter. Toddlers are at risk for pesticide poisoning because children may ingest improperly washed fruits and vegetables and pesticides used in the home and garden. Symptoms of acute pesticide poisoning include excitation or coma, bradycardia, hypotension, headache, mental confusion, nausea, vomiting, and diarrhea. Pesticide exposure is thought to increase lifetime carcinogenic risk.

Household products containing organic chemicals pose a significant health threat if ingested by the toddler. These products include toilet bowel cleaners, air fresheners, and oven cleaners. Other equally dangerous products are varnishes and paint thinners. Acute or chronic effects may be seen in the nervous system, in the respiratory tract, or on the skin.

Toddlers whose parents smoke are exposed to environmental tobacco smoke (ETS). Forty-two per cent of children are exposed to ETS from parents. Effects of ETS on children reported are diminished lung growth, increased incidence of respiratory infections and some types of cancer, and worsening of asthma.

Drowning. Drowning accounts for more deaths between the ages 1 and 4 years than those caused by motor vehicles. Children between the ages of 1 and 4 years most often drown in freshwater bodies, such as pools, lakes, or ponds. Between 50 and 90 per cent of drownings occur in residential swimming pools (Flood et al, 1990; Wintemeute et al, 1987; Wintemeute & Wright, 1991). The economic costs calculated from drowning are estimated to be somewhere between $450 and $650 million annually (Zamula, 1987).

Submersion accidents usually result when a lapse has occurred in supervision, the swimming barrier is ineffective, and the child is unable to swim. The nurse can play a pivotal role in prevention of drowning by educating parents on the levels of protection from this injury.

Anticipatory Guidance: Safety Concerns

A familiarity with what toddlers are likely to do is a parent's best defense. Safety should be discussed at each health care visit to keep the parents abreast of the rapid development that takes place during the toddler years. Parents need frequent reminders that toddlers are compelled by a constant drive to see "what would happen if . . ." but do not comprehend the danger involved. It is the preventive measures of their parents that keep toddlers safe, and it is the nurse's responsibility to provide the motivation and guidance required to help parents meet that obligation. Table 6–17 summarizes some of the prevention interventions the nurse can share with parents and caregivers.

Parents will require thorough teaching and support to manage burns at home after the child has been treated in the hospital. Information will need to be provided on procedures for dressing changes, importance of nutrition to facilitate wound healing, and pain management. Parents will be instructed to have the child wear mittens should itching occur to prevent scratching of the healing skin. Home instructions will also include protection of the healed skin from the sun to prevent hypertrophic scar formation.

Homeproofing is an essential component of anticipatory guidance. Instruction sheets for parents can be obtained from the local poison prevention center or child advocacy organizations. Parents can be referred to professionals in the community who conduct safeproofing home visits. These specialists go through the home with a "fine-toothed comb" to identify sources of potential and actual dangers to the child and to provide safety suggestions.

Parents can be apprised of the hazards their smoking causes their child. It is likely parents may not be aware of the effects of ETS on their child. Areas of designated smoking minimizing the inhalation of secondhand smoke can be discussed with the parent.

Prevention of drowning and near-drowning involves a threefold approach: supervision, use of effective barriers (e.g., fencing around the pool), and emergency procedures (Coffman, 1991). These safety tips are highlighted in Table 6–18. Refer to Chapter 15 for additional information on drowning.

Sex Education

The toddler spends much time learning names and categories for things and experiences, practicing new terms until they are mastered. Names that are socially acceptable and easily understood by others are necessary for the toddler to continue mastering the world. Terms are not always understood by a young toddler, but an attempt is made to use them to be acceptable. A mother explained that the proper word for "going potty" is to "urinate." The child understood this as "your nate." The toddler tried to use the ap-

TABLE 6-17
Safety Developmental Concerns and Prevention Strategies

Developmental Stage: Toddler (1–3 Yrs)	Prevention Strategies: Teach Child All Aspects of Safety
Walks, runs quickly, and often darts onto the street More independent and developing autonomy Will stray farther from a parent Not aware of dangers but is intent on exploration	Motor vehicle accidents (as a passenger, cyclist, and pedestrian) • Reaffirm importance of car seat even if toddler resists • Ride in center of back seat (restrained) • Stay off streets with riding toys and tricycle • Supervise because cannot be trusted • Provide a fenced-in play area if possible
Has unsteady gait	Falls • Instruct child not to run with popsicle sticks or lollipops in mouth
By 3 yrs, has full set of deciduous teeth	Aspiration • Table foods can be given, but avoid nuts and other small, hard foods
Can reach higher, climb, open lids, turn doorknobs	Open windows from the top • Remove objects from crib that child could stand on to climb out window Suffocation • Show the danger of plastic bags and similar objects Burns • Expand on teaching about hot things; especially about hot water, the stove, and hot food on the stove Ingestion, poisoning, trauma • Re-evaluate placement of poisons and medicines • Discuss meaning of poison with child
May be learning to swim but continues to need supervision	Drowning • Provide close supervision around water • Instruct not to run around pools or other bodies of water • Supervise in tub

propriate term but continued to say "I have to do 'my nate.'"

Self-exploration and the innocent exploration of another toddler's body may be appropriate playful behavior among toddlers and should not be punished. However, sexual games and behavior are not appropriate when playing with older children or adults. Because young children are vulnerable, they need to learn to say "NO" to older children or adults who may try to take advantage of them.

Frequently, toddlers ask questions about reproduction and hear stories that may confuse them. Bernstein (1978) found that a group of toddlers thought babies came from a duck because the book used for their sex education showed baby ducks and then baby people. Although using animals in teaching is common and not inappropriate, this example shows that the stories read to young children must be carefully interpreted.

Anticipatory Guidance: Sex Education

The nurse working with the toddler and family should remind parents that positive attitudes toward one's body and sexuality are learned responses. The use of correct terminology, tolerance of innocent sex play and masturbation during toddlerhood, and the teaching of correct hygiene should all contribute to healthy sexuality. Table 6–19 offers some helpful guidelines.

TABLE 6-18
Family-Centered Teaching: Safety Tips for Drowning Prevention

Supervision

Never leave a young child alone, out of eye contact supervision, in or near the pool, spa, or bathtub—*not even for a minute*

Keep toys, tricycles, and other children's playthings away from the pool or spa

Young children should never be considered water-safe, despite their swimming skills, previous instruction, or experience

Do not go inside to answer the telephone; let it ring or provide outside phone facilities

Do not allow fences or other barriers to give you a false sense of security; *there is no substitute for adult supervision*

Barriers

Provide layered security based on the ages of your children. *The younger the child, the more layers of security you will need*

Install nonclimbable fencing to prevent access to the pool area

Make sure that all entrances to the pool are self-closing and self-locking and that these are kept locked at all times when the pool area is not in use

Always drain standing water from a pool or spa cover

Emergency Procedures

If your child is missing, look in the pool first; go to the edge and look the entire pool over completely

Learn how to administer CPR and think through how you would institute it in an emergency

Know how to contact local emergency medical services; *post the emergency number 911 in an easy-to-see place*

TABLE 6-19
Family-Centered Teaching: Guidelines for Sex Education

Use correct terms for anatomy and physiology

Provide information that is consistent with the toddler's ability to understand

Avoid confusing terms known by the toddler for toileting with those for genitalia

Tolerate innocent sex play between toddlers but provide limits; provide adequate supervision and alternative activities to limit sex play

Plan for safety; avoid giving toddlers toys with small parts that might be placed in body openings

Show positive attitudes toward the child and the characteristics that are gender-related

Accept masturbation as a natural, but private, behavior; teach toddlers that touching private body parts is done in private

Teach hygiene with toileting, preventing urinary infections by wiping the female's vulva from front to back and keeping fingernails short and clean

KEY CONCEPTS

Concepts Related to Basic Information

- The most commonly encountered stresses in families with toddlers are those related to parenting and either the threat of or the actual breakdown in the family relationship.
- The concerns of the family during toddlerhood are adapting resources, re-establishing relationships, and working on family philosophy.
- The concept of object permanence is fully developed during toddlerhood.
- Entrance into preoperational period is characterized by beginning ability to engage in symbolic thought.
- Toddlers have limited ability to express their feelings and communicate their wants and needs.
- Of the years between birth and adolescence, no period is as unsettled or tumultuous as the period of toddlerhood.

- Three major struggles during toddlerhood—toilet training, limit-setting and discipline, and sibling rivalry all involve the conflict between autonomy and shame and doubt.
- During early childhood, the lymphatic tissue increases in size, accounting for the presence of peripheral nodes, enlargement of tonsils and adenoids, and a spleen tip that is likely to be palpable.
- The toddler is capable of thinking only about her or his own perspective and not about another.
- Between 18 and 24 months of age, one-word utterances are commonly used to communicate increasingly complex ideas.
- Awareness of gender identity begins around 18 months and is fully established by 5 years of age.
- Sex-role identification during the toddler years is learned through imitation and involves differences in the way parents interact with boys and girls.
- The Eriksonian task, conflict, or crisis for the toddler is *autonomy versus shame and doubt.*
- The primary fear of the toddler is separation from caretakers.
- The toddler differentiates between acceptable and nonacceptable behavior according to parental standards during the *preconventional level of development.*
- According to Fowler, the toddler is in the *intuitive-projective stage* of faith development.
- Children who immigrate from third world countries in Asia, Africa, or Central or South America present unique health care needs.
- Toddlers require approximately 10 to 13 hours of sleep.
- A toddler needs a greater number of total calories than during infancy, owing to an increase in body size, but the requirements per unit of body weight decrease as the growth rate decreases.
- By the time toddlers sit and walk, their nerve pathways have developed to the extent that they can physically control their bowel and bladder sphincters.
- The toddler's play remains primarily egocentric, showing little regard for the feelings of others.

Concepts Related to Nursing Assessment

- The family with a toddler is in a developmental phase with a high risk for the occurrence of altered family process.
- The nurse can assist parents to identify those behaviors that are most stressful and develop approaches congruent with their toddler's temperament.
- Well child visits include health screening for hypertension, iron deficiency anemia, and elevated cholesterol and triglycerides.
- Assessment of defining characteristics of the nursing diagnostic responses *ineffective family coping: compromised or disabling* can plan intervention that will result in the positive nursing diagnostic response of *family coping: potential for growth.*
- Stages of cognitive development identified by Piaget provide a theory base that the nurse can use to assess cognitive growth and development.
- Nursing diagnoses that may be applied to the care of the toddler include *high risk for altered growth and development; high risk for impaired physical mobility and fear.*
- The nurse will continuously assess the child for the etiology of the actual response, the risk factors associated with the high risk and actual problems, and defining characteristics.
- The need for vigilance for defining characteristics of the nursing diagnoses *high risk for injury: falls; high risk for injury: poisoning;* and *high risk for injury: suffocation/aspirations* is necessary as the child grows and develops.
- Assessment of the mother, toddler, and sleeping environment will provide information about the defining characteristics affecting the nursing diagnosis *sleep pattern disturbance.*

Concepts Related to Nursing Intervention

- An explanation of their child's growth trajectory will provide parents with information regarding the tracking of growth patterns.
- Parents should be helped to understand that a toddler's intense examination and incessant manipulation of anything is the way he or she learns.
- Nurses can assist the family to encourage and reward age-appropriate expressions of expanding development, thereby enhancing the child's sense of mastery and positive self-esteem.
- Interventions to alleviate the toddler's separation anxiety include bringing pictures, scented handkerchiefs, and tape recordings of family members.
- The nurse should explain that there are no precise rules or schedules that can be applied to guarantee successful toilet training.
- Incorporating the child's usual rituals and routines from home into nursing care activities will provide the toddler with some sense of control and security, helping to alleviate feelings of helplessness and fear.
- The nurse can assist parents in understanding their child's behaviors by providing information about what is developmentally appropriate.

- Parents should be taught the normal preventive measure to detect hearing impairment.
- A toddler's teeth should be brushed twice a day, and parents should continue to assist with toothbrushing after the child begins to brush her or his own teeth.
- Homeproofing is an essential component of anticipatory guidance.

REFERENCES

Allshouse, M., Rouse, T., & Eichelberger, M. (1993). Childhood injury: A current perspective. *Pediatric Emergency Care, 9*(3), 159–164.

American Academy of Pediatrics. (1991). *Report of the Committee on Infectious Diseases* (22nd ed.). Elk Grove Village, IL: Author.

American Academy of Pediatrics, Committee on Community Health Services. (1989a). Health care for children of migrant families. *Pediatrics, 84*(4), 739–740.

American Academy of Pediatrics, Committee on Infectious Diseases. (1989b). Measles: Reassessment of the current immunization policy. *Pediatrics, 84*(6), 1110–1113.

Armstrong, J. (1978). Development of sexual identity. In R. A. Hoekelman, et al. (Ed.), *Principles of pediatrics*. New York: McGraw-Hill.

Baldwin, L., & Sutherland, S. (1988). Growth patterns of first-generation Southeast Asian infants. *American Journal of Diseases of Children, 142,* 526–531.

Bernstein, A. (1978). *The flight of the stork*. New York: Delacorte Press.

Betz, C. (1983). Teaching children through play therapy. *Journal of Association of Operating Room Nurses, 88*(4), 709, 712–713, 716–717.

Betz, C., & Poster, E. (1984). Incorporating play into the care of the hospitalized child. *Issues in Comprehensive Pediatric Nursing, 7*(6), 343–355.

Borowitzs, K., & Glascoe, F. (1986). Sensitivity of the Denver developmental screening test. *Journal of Pediatrics, 78,* 1075–1078.

Bowlby, J. (1973). *Attachment and loss series: Separation: Anxiety and anger*. (Vol. 3). New York: Basic Books.

Bradley, R., Caldwell, B., & Rock, S. (1988). Home environment and school performance: A ten-year follow-up and examination of three models of environmental action. *Child Development, 59,* 852–867.

Bullock, M., & Lutkenhaus, P. (1988). The development of volitional behavior in the toddler years. *Child Development, 59,* 664–674.

Bus, A., & van Ijzendoorn, M. (1988). Mother-child interactions, attachment and emergent literacy: A cross-sectional study. *Child Development, 59,* 1262–1272.

Carey, W. (1992). Temperamental issues in the school age child. *Pediatric Clinics of North America, 39*(3), 569–583.

Coffman, S. (1991). Parent education for drowning prevention. *Journal of Pediatric Health Care, 5*(3), 141–146.

Crockenberg, S. (1987). Predictors and correlates of anger toward and punitive control of toddlers by adolescent mothers. *Child Development, 58,* 964–975.

Edgil, A., Wood, K., & Smith, D. (1985). Sleep problems of older in fants and preschool children. *Pediatric Nursing, 11,* 87–89.

Erikson, E. H. (1963). *Childhood and society* (2nd ed.). New York: WW Norton.

Flavell, J. (1988). The development of children's knowledge about the mind: From cognitive connections to mental representations. In J. Astington, P. Harris, & D. Olson (Eds.), *Developing theories of mind* (pp 244–271). Cambridge: Cambridge University Press.

Flood, T., Aickin, M., Englender, S., & Tucker, D. (1990). Child drownings and near-drownings associated with swimming pools: Maricopa County, Arizona, 1988 and 1989. *Morbidity and Mortality Weekly Report, 39,* 441–442.

Florey, L. (1971). An approach to play and play development. *American Journal of Occupational Therapy, 25*(6), 275–280.

Fowler, J. (1984). *Becoming adult, becoming Christian* (pp 6–64). San Francisco: Harper & Row.

Fowler, J. (1974). Toward a developmental perspective on faith. *Religious Education, 69,* 207–219.

Frankel, I. (1993). Sources of family annoyance (SOFA): Development, reliability, and validity. *Journal of Pediatric Nursing, 8*(3), 177–184.

Freud, S. (1957). In J. Strachey (Ed.), *The standard edition of the complete psychological works of Sigmund Freud* (Vol. 18). London: Hogarth.

Gopnik, A., & Slaughter, V. (1991). Young children's understanding of changes in their mental states. *Child Development, 62,* 98–110.

Gordon, M. (1987). *Manual of nursing diagnosis*. New York: McGraw-Hill.

Hauck, M. (1991). Mother's descriptions of the toilet-training process: A phenomenologic study. *Journal of Pediatric Nursing, 6*(2), 80–85.

Jimmerson, K. (1991). Maternal environmental and temperamental characteristics of toddlers with and toddlers without sleep problems. *Journal of Pediatric Health Care, 5,* 71–77.

Johnson, J. (1992). The tendency for temperament to be "temperamental": Conceptual and methodological considerations. *Journal of Pediatric Nursing, 7*(5), 347–353.

Kochanska, G. (1991). Socialization and temperament in the development of guilt and conscience. *Child Development, 62,* 1379–1392.

Kohlberg, L. (1981). *The philosophy of moral development*. San Francisco: Harper & Row.

Lee, J., & Fowler, M. (1986). Merely child's play and developmental work and playthings. *Journal of Pediatric Nursing, 1*(4), 260–269.

Leske, M. (1981). Prevalence estimates of communicative disorders in the US: Language, hearing and vestibular disorders. *ASHA: Journal of the American Speech and Hearing Association, 23,* 229–236.

McClowry, S. (1993). Pediatric nursing psychosocial care: A vision beyond hospitalization. *Pediatric Nursing, 19*(2), 146–149.

National Academy of Sciences. (1989). *Recommended dietary allowances* (10th ed.). Washington, DC: National Academy Press.

Piaget, J. (1952). *The origins of intelligence in children*. New York: International University Press.

Piaget, J. (1970). Piaget's theory. In P. H. Mussen (Ed.), *Carmichael's manual of child psychology* (Vol. 1). New York: John Wiley & Sons.

Pitcher, E. G., & Schultz, L. H. (1983). *Boys and girls at play—The development of sex roles*. South Hadley, MA: Bergin & Garvey.

Rapin, I. (1993). Hearing disorders. *Pediatrics in Review, 14*(2), 43–49.

Richardson, V., Zickler, C., & Wheat, L. (1991). Tuberculosis screening and treatment in children. *Journal of Pediatric Health Care, 5*(1), 11–17.

Schepp, K. (1992). Correlates of mothers who prefer control over their hospitalized children's care. *Journal of Pediatric Nursing, 7*(2), 83–89.

Sears, R. R. (1974). Development of gender role. In F. A. Beach (Ed.), *Sex and behavior*. New York: Robert E. Krieger.

Shannon, M., & Graef, J. (1992). Lead intoxication in infancy. *Pediatrics, 89*(1), 87–90.

Sherman, J., & Alexander, M. (1990). Obesity in childhood: A research update. *Journal of Pediatric Nursing, 5*(3), 161–167.

Simard, P., Naccache, H., Lachapelle, D., & Brodeur, J. (1991). Ingestion of fluoride from dentifrices by children aged 12 to 24 months. *Clinical Pediatrics, 30*(11), 614–617.

Smith, D. W. (1977). *Introduction to clinical pediatrics*. Philadelphia: WB Saunders.

Stewart, R., Mobley, L., VanTuyl, S., & Salvador, M. (1987). The first-born's adjustment to the birth of a sibling: A longitudinal assessment. *Child Development, 58*(2), 341–355.

Tachdjian, M. O. (1972). *Pediatric orthopedics* (Vol. 2). Philadelphia: WB Saunders.

Thomas, A., & Chess, S. (1977). *Temperament and development*. New York: Brunner/Mazel.

Thompson, M., & Thompson, G. (1991). Early identification of hearing loss: Listen to parents. *Clinical Pediatrics, 30*(2), 77–80.

Uchiyama, N., & German, J. (1987). Pediatric considerations. In B. Achauer (Ed.), *Management of the burned patient* (pp 223–241). Norwalk, CT: Appleton & Lange.

US Department of Agriculture, Human Nutrition Information Service (1992). *Food guide pyramid.* (Leaflet No. 572). Washington, DC: Author.

Whitehurst, G., & Valdez-Menchaca, M. (1988). What is the role of reinforcement in early language acquisition? *Child Development, 59,* 430–440.

Wintemeute, G., Kraus, J., Tiret, S., & Wright, M. (1987). Drowning in childhood and adolescence: A population-based study. *American Journal of Public Health, 77,* 830–832.

Wintemeute, G., & Wright, M. (1991). The attitude practice gap revisited: Risk reduction beliefs and behaviors among owners of residential swimming pools. *Pediatrics, 88*(6), 1168–1171.

Zamula, W. (1987). *Social costs of drowning and near-drownings from submersion accidents occurring to children under five in residential swimming pools.* Washington, DC: Directorate for Economic Analysis, US Consumer Product Safety Commission.

BIBLIOGRAPHY

Berk, L., & Friman, P. (1990). Epidemiologic aspects of toilet training. *Clinical Pediatrics, 29*(5), 278–282.

Bowlby, J. (1969). *Attachment.* New York: Basic.

Brazelton, T. (1976). *Toddlers and parents.* New York: Dell.

Busen, N. (1988). Societal values: A cause of stress in children. *Journal of Pediatric Health Care, 2*(6), 300–306.

Castiglia, P. (1989). Sibling rivalry. *Journal of Pediatric Health Care, 3*(1), 52–54.

Castiglia, P. (1988). Temper tantrums. *Journal of Pediatric Health Care, 2*(5), 267–268.

Centers for Disease Control. (1993). Standards for pediatric immunization practices. *Morbidity and Mortality Weekly Report, 42,* 1–9.

Christophersen, E. (1982). Incorporating behavioral pediatrics into primary care. *Pediatric Clinics of North America, 29*(2), 261–296.

Clark-Stewart, A. (1988). The "effects of infant day care reconsidered": Risks for parents, children and researchers. *Early Childhood Research Quarterly, 3,* 293–318.

Erikson, E. (1950). *Childhood and society.* New York: WW Norton.

Fraiberg, S. (1959). *The magic years.* New York: Scribner's.

Gross, D. (1988). Implications for the development of children. *Image: Journal of Nursing Scholarship, 4*(2), 103–107.

Gulick, E. (1986). The effects of breastfeeding on toddler's health. *Pediatric Nursing, 12*(1), 51–54.

Halpern, J. (1990). How safe are child safety seats? *Journal of Emergency Nursing, 16*(3), 151–155.

Hoekelman, R., et al. (1987). *Primary pediatric care.* New York: McGraw-Hill.

Hoff-Ginsberg, F. (1986). Function and structure in maternal speech: Their relation to the child's development of syntax. *Developmental Psychology 22*(2), 155–163.

Honig, J. (1986). Preparing preschool-aged children to be sibling. *MCN: American Journal of Maternal-Child Nursing, 11,* 37–43.

Horner, M., & McClellan, M. (1981, July). Toilet training: Ready or not? *Pediatric Nursing,* 12–18.

Howard, B. (1990). Growing together: The toddler years need not be turbulent. *Contemporary Pediatrics, 7*(6), 21–40.

Howes, C. (1988). Pressuring children to learn versus developmentally appropriate education. *Journal of Pediatric Health Care, 3*(4), 181–186.

Hymovich, D., & Barnard, M. (1979). *Family health care: Development situational crises* (Vol. II). New York: McGraw-Hill.

Marino, B. (1991). Studying infant and toddler play. *Journal of Pediatric Nursing, 6*(1), 16–20.

Martinez, S. (1992). Ambulatory management of burns in children. *Journal of Pediatric Health Care, 6*(1), 32–37.

Oberklaid, F., et al. (1990). Assessment of temperament in the toddler age group. *Pediatrics, 85*(4), 559–566.

Phillips, J. (1969). *Origins of intellect: Piaget's theory.* New York: WH Freeman.

Piaget, J., & Inhelder, B. (1969). *The psychology of the child.* New York: Basic Books.

Pipes, P. (1989). Nutrition in infancy and childhood (4th ed.). St. Louis: CV Mosby.

Prugh, D. (1985). *The psycho-social aspects of pediatrics.* Philadelphia: Lea & Febiger.

Pulaski, M. (1971). *Understanding Piaget.* New York: Harper & Row.

Rivara, F., & Kemper, K. (1991). Health supervision for the high risk pre-schooler. *Pediatrics in Review, 12*(6), 181–186.

Sande, D. (1985). Language development in infants and toddlers. *Nurse Practitioner, 10*(9), 39–41.

Schmitt, B. (1990). The stubborn toddler who just says "No." *Contemporary Pediatrics, 7*(4), 71–72.

Schmitt, B. (1990). Sibling rivalry toward a new baby. *Contemporary Pediatrics, 7*(3), 111–112.

Schmitt, B. (1989). When your toddler or preschooler won't eat. *Contemporary Pediatrics, 6*(9), 127–128.

Shiller, V., Izard, C., & Hembree, E. (1986). Patterns of emotions expression during separation in the strange-situation procedure. *Developmental Psychology, 22*(3), 378–382.

Slade, A. (1987). A longitudinal study of maternal involvement and symbolic play during the toddler period. *Child Development, 58,* 367–375.

Sorenson, C. (1990). Children's coping responses. *Journal of Pediatric Nursing, 5*(2), 259–267.

Van Cleve, S. (1990). Adolescent parents and toddlers: Strategies for intervention. *Public Health Nursing, 7*(1), 22–27.

CHAPTER • 7

Families with Preschoolers

RELATED TOPICS
Theories of moral development, Chapter 3
Promoting Healthy Parenting, Chapter 12
Vision and hearing assessments, Chapter 13
Fostering Self-Esteem, Chapter 14
Coping with stress, Chapter 18
Alterations in development of speech and language, Chapter 45

LEARNING OBJECTIVES

- Identify the milestones of physical development.
- Identify and apply the concepts of cognitive development to the care of the ill and hospitalized child.
- Identify and apply the principles of psychosocial development to the care of the ill and hospitalized child.
- Identify the major concerns of health promotion during the preschool years.
- Identify and provide anticipatory guidance information for parents on the selection of appropriate day care options.

The world of the preschool child is rapidly expanding both within and beyond the confines of the family unit. All family members are changing cognitively, physically, emotionally, and socially, and those changes affect every family member's functioning. New relationships are forming within the family structure as parents and siblings relate to a preschool child. The nurse needs an awareness of these family interrelationships to give guidance effectively to families with a preschooler.

Development and Adaptation of the Family with a Preschooler

The preschool years find the family reorienting their activities to meet the demands of their preschooler. Children of this age seek expanding activities and opportunities to meet their needs that are an outgrowth of their developing physical, intellectual, and emotional-social competencies. This section will explore the issues the family must deal with during the preschool years. For additional discussion of families, refer to Chapter 2.

Supplying Adequate Space and Equipment

Preschool children, through their initiative, are becoming active members of their existing world. New developmental attainments and expanding interests put new demands on available family resources. A rapidly expanding interest in drawing, coloring, painting, cutting, and pasting necessitates more supplies and space.

The need for larger play equipment to enhance large muscle development and the need for added space to house toys, crafts, and projects of the preschooler are a concern to parents (Duvall & Miller, 1985). The child needs a larger bed; additional bedrooms and a larger dining table may be needed as the preschooler grows and matures. For families on a strict budget, these requirements demand reallocation of funds as well as innovative methods of using household materials to make play equipment (making paste and modeling dough; saving partially used paper for the preschooler to draw or paint on; saving safe, empty containers to utilize as building blocks or imaginative play items).

For the financially secure, employed parent, toys and equipment can be enjoyable to supply, but for the poor family, the suddenly unemployed family, or the family whose income is strained through medical expenses or other family crises, supplying the preschooler's play needs may have a low priority.

Promoting Family Communication

Adult family members should be encouraged to have private conversations that are not child-related and that stimulate and satisfy mutual intellectual needs, interests, and goals.

The preschool child's questioning can disrupt family unity and test parental patience. When a child first begins the "why" questions, parents view it as a challenge to respond appropriately. However, as the "why" questions increase in frequency, often with no logical progression, parents can become frustrated with this behavior, even though the majority of parents realize the child is learning about the world through the torrent of questions. Because of the cognition level, the child may be unable to assimilate an answer given by the parent and may require repeated explanations for the same question. This cycle of events frustrates busy, tired, overworked parents!

Apportioning Responsibilities

As preschoolers develop, increased capabilities change their behavior as well as the expectations for their behavior that are held by parents, peers, siblings, and relatives. Preschoolers may enjoy "helping" with household activities, such as sweeping, dusting, and outside chores.

Sharing Parental Responsibilities

Parents are also changing their roles to encompass the duties and responsibilities that correlate with expanding family needs as related to active play, crafts, reading time, formal learning activities, quiet individual times, and family group activities. The constant supervision of children's activities is mentally and physically exhausting to parents. In single-parent families, the parent is especially vulnerable to physical and mental exhaustion without a network of social support. Grandparents, sisters or brothers of the parent, other single parents, or formal support groups can provide shared caregiving and respite for the single parent. The nurse can help by "giving permission" to the single parent to ask for assistance and by offering realistic suggestions to prevent social isolation.

In two-parent families, both parents can be active in planning and supervising their child(ren)'s routine tasks. This joint parenting process allows children to see parents as a team and also frees one parent to complete household tasks, to rest, or to pursue individual interests while the other is helping the preschooler perform activities of daily living and diversional or craft projects. Tension between spouses may accompany role changes within the family if these changes have not been anticipated or clearly delineated. Tension may be evidenced by frequent verbal or physical abuse or emotional isolation between spouses. Nurses can help parents by anticipating these possible role changes and by helping parents identify their unique response to these changes.

Rearing Children

Parents may find themselves in a continual dilemma as their preschool child develops initiative and self-confidence. Parents do not want to stifle the initiative that both they and their preschooler enjoy, yet specific limits need to be applied to the aggressive tendencies of the preschooler. Even though the preschooler's cognition remains preoperational (lack of ability to make appropriate generalizations or to reason deductively), cause-and-effect reasoning is advancing, so that parents can utilize natural consequences of inappropriate actions as a disciplinary approach with their preschooler. The parenting approach can also consider the preschooler's developing ability to put off immediate need gratification to enjoy a future event more fully. For example, the preschooler who demands to finger-paint immediately will agree to postpone this when mother explains that the child's friend will arrive later that day with paints and so provide a better selection of equipment.

Cultivating Relationships with Relatives

Relatives of the preschool child fulfill various roles for the child, depending on the physical distance between family and relatives. Grandparents, cousins, and other relatives represent roles such as censor, educator (they show the preschooler different viewpoints on subjects), authority figure, baby sitter, and playmate to the child and the family. By cultivating fuller relationships with relatives, the parents and the child can utilize them as resource persons to enhance their understanding of the family heritage and values. Also, parenting skills can improve by learning through the experience of relatives. As the social circle expands, the preschooler learns to share people, starting with mother and father. The preschooler who belongs to an extended family has many opportunities to share with and learn from a large variety of family members (Wilson, 1986).

Expanding Contacts Outside Home

Community activities—group play, gymnastics, crafts, religious activities—add more dimensions to the preschooler's world. Parents may notice new behaviors as a result of their preschooler's exposure to influences outside the home. The entire family can also attend events together (zoo, children's theater, and sports events).

Socialization with other families changes for the family with a preschooler. The preschooler can now play alone or can play with peers for longer periods of time without direct supervision. Parents' socializing can therefore be more relaxed and enjoyable. In addition, parents may be more relaxed in visiting friends because the friends' home need not be as childproof as during toddlerhood.

Nursing Care and Guidance

Nurses knowledgeable about the stressors that can potentially affect families with a preschooler can assist family members to manage stress adaptively. The goal of nursing care is to foster the development of the family as a unit and as individual members.

Promoting Health

Preschool years are active years during which accidents are not uncommon. Accidents increase financial demands on the already-strained family budget. Nursing priorities are (1) continuing to assess for the defining characteristics of the nursing diagnostic response *high risk for injury* and (2) stressing the importance of safety measures to minimize the probability of accidents. Teaching families how to determine when medical care is needed and teaching basic first aid measures to eliminate frequent emergency room visits may significantly decrease the medical costs of many families.

The preschooler comes into contact with many individuals beyond the nuclear family, which increases the exposure to upper respiratory infections and communicable diseases. The applicable nursing diagnostic response is ***high risk for infection.*** Health maintenance costs for families with a preschooler may increase because of these frequent illnesses. When the preschooler contracts a communicable illness, other family members may become ill. Some of the expenses incurred (throat cultures, medication) may be included in insurance plans for the family. A nurse can increase the family's awareness of insurance coverage to which they are entitled or can assist them in locating other sources of assistance for the costs of health maintenance, including dental care and immunizations.

Promoting Sibling Interactions

Siblings will relate differently to the preschooler than they did to the toddler, and parents need to accept this relationship change as a natural, developmentally healthy event. Older siblings may now see the child who has become a preschooler as a nuisance—no longer a plaything but an individual with his or her own desires and needs. Verbal battles and physical aggression between siblings are common as the preschooler becomes increasingly capable of self-preservation. Parents need to be alert to problems of physical abuse and dominance by the older sibling, so that the fragile self-concept of the preschooler is not damaged. At the same time, they must avoid overprotection of the younger child.

Jealousy between siblings may cause behavioral acting out by the preschooler or sibling. Each child needs time alone with each parent to enhance individual identity and security as well as to decrease the feelings of jealousy toward siblings or parents. There is perhaps no remedy more effective for behavioral acting out than increased quality time with the parents. Family unit play, special times for each child to discuss pertinent matters with parents or all family members, and quiet times for children to pursue individual interests may also help the family respect each member.

Imitating Sex Roles

The preschooler may begin to imitate the sex roles personified within the family structure. Developmentally, the child is coping with feelings of intense affection toward the parent of the opposite sex and rivalry with the parent of the same sex. This oedipal phase (Oedipus or Electra complex) (see discussion "Developing Sex-Role Identification" under "Emotional-Social Competency: Sexuality") may cause feelings of rejection and frustration for the unsuspecting same-sex parent.

Understanding Developmental Concerns

Nurses can help parents understand the developmental struggle with which the child is coping, thereby relieving undue parental stress caused by the competitive preschooler. It is helpful for the parents of the preschooler to know that they do not have to give in to every affectional demand made by the preschooler. Setting limits on these demands, coupled with the preschooler's observations of displays of affection between the parents, aids in resolving the feelings of the oedipal phase.

The preschooler's curiosity is far-reaching and includes questions about sex ("Where did I come from?"), death ("Where is heaven?" "What happens to people when they die?"), and common, everyday events. Often the questions about sex cause parents discomfort. Communication and attitudinal patterns within each family dictate how parents respond to these questions. The responses range from openness to refusal to discuss sex, or to giving erroneous answers to a child's probing questions.

Developing Appropriate Expectations

Parents need an awareness of age-appropriate expectations for the child. For example, realistically the 5-year-old child could be responsible for dressing and tidying the room, whereas the 3-year-old may not be able to perform these tasks in their entirety. Role prescriptions may change from month to month, and setbacks in behaviors are not uncommon. The use of rewards (stars pasted on a clearly designed daily worksheet or additional privileges) may be suggested to parents who have difficulty maintaining the preschooler as a contributing family member with increasing responsibilities.

Expanding the Child's World

Nurses should encourage families to interact with relatives and friends, as these interactions may renew and positively influence learning for both the preschooler and parents.

Encouraging parents to utilize as teaching tools the many educational children's magazines *(Ranger Rick's Nature Magazine, Humpty Dumpty,* or *World)* can greatly expand the preschooler's learning about the world as well as provide an opportunity for intense interaction, learning, and enjoyment among all family members through reading and discussion.

Growth and Development of the Preschooler

Between 3 and 5 years of age, the child is very active, progressing rapidly in motor abilities, cognitive function, and language development. The constant practice of these abilities and skills brings amazing changes in personality development: an individual appears. Some preschoolers are boisterous, outgoing, active, curious, and constantly exploring, whereas others are quiet, shy, passive, and withdrawing. One child is aggressive; another appears totally nonaggressive. Each child develops a "self"; some children become leaders, and others are content to be followers. A refinement of gross motor skills and a progressive mastery of fine motor abilities evolve during this period. Having discovered themselves as separate people by the end of their toddler years, their performance now directly affects their developing self-esteem. Competencies related to the growth, development, and health maintenance of the preschooler are listed in Table 7–1.

Nurses working with preschoolers in a variety of settings such as the preschool, hospital, or clinic will consider the nursing diagnostic response *high risk for altered growth and development* as a component of the nursing care provided (Table 7–2). Other nursing diagnostic responses that may be applied to the care of the preschool child include *fear, high risk for injury,* and *ineffective individual coping.* The nurse will continually assess the preschool child and family for the etiology of the actual response, the risk factors associated with potential problems, and the defining characteristics in formulating the nursing diagnostic responses.

Physical Competency

Height and Weight

The preschooler's growth continues to be slow and steady, as in the toddler years. On average, the preschooler grows about 2 to 3 inches (5 to 7.5 cm) a year and gains 4 to 5 pounds (1.8 to 2.3 kg) a year. The child's weight at 1 year of age is doubled by the end of the preschool period.

General Appearance and Skeletal Growth

In general, the preschooler is tall and thin, compared with the toddler, and looks sturdy yet graceful and agile. The baby fat of infancy becomes muscle tissue, so that the posture is erect. By age 6 years, 45 per cent of the child's height is in the legs. Increased tone in abdominal muscles results in disappearance of the pot-bellied shape. The chest becomes more developed and prominent.

At age 3 years, the head circumference for boys ranges from 47.9 to 52.7 cm with the 50th percentile at 50.4 cm, whereas the range for girls is 46.8 to 52.0 cm with the 50th percentile at 49.3. Head circumference is not usually measured after 3 years of age. By age 6 years, the head has achieved 90 per cent of its growth and nears adult size.

Many 3-year-olds appear to have flat feet because of the fat pad that normally exists under the medial arch until the child has walked for a couple of years. Flat feet, even in 4- and 5-year-old children, is not a problem unless it causes some specific symptoms.

One of the best methods of evaluating the structure and function of the foot is to look at the child's shoe. Lateral wear on the heel and sole of the shoe indicates a well-functioning foot. Fair function is seen with even wearing of the heel and sole, and poor functioning is evident when the sole has become worn on the medial aspects (Trainex Corporation, 1980).

Nursing Interventions: General Appearance and Skeletal Growth

Assessment guidelines that characterize the preschooler's physical development are presented in Table 7–1. The nurse's role is to help parents stimulate their preschooler's physical competency. Nurses should provide information on the achievement of developmental tasks when undertaking anticipatory guidance with parents of preschoolers. The nurse should spend time playing with and talking with the child to gain the child's cooperation and trust, especially before attempting any procedures. During health care procedures, a preschooler is usually more cooperative than a toddler. When the parent is allowed to remain close, separation anxiety is minimal.

Anticipatory Guidance: General Appearance and Skeletal Growth

Once the height and weight have been measured and plotted on a graph, it is important to discuss the significance of these findings with the parent. Parents should be reassured that there is wide variance in size and stature among preschoolers. As with all age groups, the size of the parents can affect the child's placement on the graph.

Parents should be informed of the normal changes that will occur in their preschooler's appearance. Information and reassurance that knock-kneed, flat-footed characteristics of their child are normal at this age can save parents the needless expense of correc-

TABLE 7-1
Summary of Preschooler Growth and Development and Health Maintenance

Physical Competency	Intellectual Competency	Emotional-Social Competency
General Summary, 3 to 5 Yrs		
Gains 4.5 kg (10 lb)	Becomes increasingly aware of self and others	Freud's phallic stage Oedipus complex—boy Electra complex—girl
Grows 15 cm (6 in)	Vocabulary increases from 900 to 2100 words	Erikson's stage of initiative vs. guilt
20 teeth present	Piaget's preoperational/intuitive period	Fowler's intuitive-projective stage
Nutritional requirements Energy 1250–1600 cal/day (or 90–100 kcal/kg/day) Fluid: 100–125 ml/kg/day Protein: 30 g/day (or 3 g/kg/day) Iron: 10 mg/day		Kohlberg's preconceptual stage
3 Yrs		
Runs, stops suddenly	Knows own sex	Shifts between reality and imagination
Walks backward	Desires to please	Engages in bedtime rituals
Climbs steps	Has sense of humor	Negativism decreases
Jumps	Language—900 words	Animism and realism: anything that moves is alive
Pedals tricycle	Follows simple direction	
Undresses self	Uses plurals	
Unbuttons front buttons	Names figure in picture	
Feeds self well	Uses adjectives/adverbs	
4 Yrs		
Runs well, skips clumsily	Is more aware of others	Focuses on present
Hops on one foot	Uses alibis to excuse behavior	Egocentrism: unable to see the viewpoint of others, unable to understand another's inability to see own viewpoint
Heel-toe walks	Is bossy	Does not comprehend anticipatory explanation
Goes up and down steps without holding rail	Language—knows 1500 words	Has sexual curiosity
Jumps well	Talks in sentences	Shows evidence of Oedipus complex
Dresses and undresses	Knows nursery rhymes	Shows evidence of Electra complex
Buttons well, needs help with zippers, bows	Counts to 5	
Brushes teeth	Is highly imaginative	
Bathes self	Uses name calling	
Draws with some form and meaning		
5 Yrs		
Runs skillfully	Is aware of cultural differences	Continues in egocentrism
Jumps three or four steps	Knows name and address	Has fantasy and daydreams
Jumps rope, hops, skips	Is more independent	Resolves Oedipus/Electra complex: girls identify with mother, boys with father
Begins to dance	Is more sensible/less imaginative	Body image and body boundary are especially important in illness
Roller skates	Copies triangle, draws rectangle	Shows tension in nail biting, nose picking, whining, snuffling
Dresses without assistance	Knows four or more colors	
Ties shoelaces	Language—knows 2100 words, meaningful sentences	
Hits nail on head with hammer	Understands kinship	
Draws person—six parts	Counts to 10	
Prints first name		

(continued)

TABLE 7-1
Summary of Preschooler Growth and Development and Health Maintenance *(Continued)*

Nutrition	Play	Safety
General Summary, 3 to 5 Yrs		
Carbohydrate intake is approximately 40–50% of calories	Reading books is important at all ages	Never leave alone in bath or swimming pool
Good food sources of essential vitamins and minerals are necessary	Balance highly physical activities with quiet times	Keep poisons in locked cupboard; learn what household items are poisonous
Regular toothbrushing should be done	Quiet rest period takes the place of nap time	Use car seats and seat belts
Parents are seen as examples; if parent does not eat it, child will not	Sturdy play materials should be provided	Never leave child alone in car
		Remove doors from abandoned freezers and refrigerators
3 Yrs		
1250 cal/day	Participates in simple games	Teach safety habits early
Because of increased sex identity and imitation, child copies parents at table and will eat what they eat	Cooperates, takes turns	Let water out of bathtub, do not stand in tub
Different colors and shapes of foods can increase interest	Plays with group	Caution against climbing in unsafe areas, onto or under cars, in unsafe buildings, in drainage pipes
	Uses scissors, paper	Insist on seat belts being worn at all times in cars
	Likes crayons, coloring books	
	Enjoys being read to and "reading"	
	Plays "dress-up" and "house"	
	Likes fire engines	
4 Yrs		
Good nutrition	Has longer attention span with group activities	Teach to stay out of streets, alleys
1400 cal/day	Plays "dress-up" with more drama	Continually teach safety; child understands
Nutritious between meal snacks are essential	Draws, pounds, paints	Teach how to handle scissors
Emphasis is on quality not quantity of food eaten	Likes to make paper chains, sewing cards, scrapbooks	Teach what items are poisons and why to avoid them
Mealtime should be enjoyable, not for criticism	Likes being read to, records, and rhythmic play	Never allow to stand in moving car
As dexterity improves, neatness increases	"Helps" adults	
5 Yrs		
Good nutrition	Plays with trucks, cars, soldiers, dolls	Teach how to cross streets safely
1600 cal/day	Likes simple games with letters or numbers	Teach not to speak to strangers or get into cars of strangers
Encourage regular toothbrushing	Engages in much gross motor activity: plays with water, mud, snow, leaves, rocks	Insist on seat belts being worn
Encourage quiet time before meals	Plays matching picture games	Teach to swim
Child can learn to cut own meat		
Frequent illnesses from increased exposure increase nutritional needs		

tive shoes. If extreme variations in these normal preschool skeletal features exist, the nurse should refer the child for further evaluation.

During this period, children develop an image of their bodies as attractive or unattractive, and normal or "different," as a reflection of the opinions of others, particularly those of parents. When any type of physical defect or disability is present, the manner in which parents respond to it will color the child's sense of self and body image for a lifetime. This is true even for normal variations of strength, stature, body weight, and other characteristics. These normal variations can have a tremendous influence on how children view their bodies.

TABLE 7-2

Growth and Development Plan: Families with Preschoolers

Analysis: Nursing Diagnostic Statement

Response and Related or Risk Factors: *High risk for altered growth and development; risk factors*

- Illness/physical impairment
- Treatment-related procedures
  - Isolation
  - Injections
  - Immobilization
- Separation from caregivers (parents, siblings, peers)
- Loss of independence
- Change in environment
- Inadequate sensory stimulation, isolation
- Caregiver anxiety
- Caregiver knowledge deficit
- Fear of bodily harm
- Maturational factors
  - Preoperational period
  - Initiative vs. guilt

Projected Outcome: The preschool child will demonstrate acquisition of developmentally appropriate behaviors in the physical, intellectual, and emotional-social domains

Defining Characteristics	Nursing Interventions	Evaluation Criteria

Subjective:
• Child expresses fear/anxieties such as "What are you gonna do?" or "I don't wanna do that."
• Child verbalizes feelings of mistrust such as "Are you gonna hurt me?" "Is that gonna hurt?"
• Caregiver expresses unrealistic expectations about child's behavior, negative/ambivalent feelings concerning parenting
 	
Objective:
• Is depressed
• Is withdrawn
• Cries
• Is irritable
• Sucks thumb
	Health Screening
	• **Assess factors that can identify altered growth and development.** (Evidence of child's behavior deviating from age-appropriate levels will be observed and documented on the basis of theory of growth and development; parent-child relationships; social support; knowledge of physiologic effects of disease on the child and family)
	• **Assess child's level of development using developmental norms and specific assessment tools.** (Refer to Chapter 13, Assessing Child Health, and Appendices 2 through 6)
		• **Any developmental delays will be identified as evidenced by**
		  • Charted assessment of screening for physical, intellectual, and emotional-social development
		  • Referral for deviations from the norm detected during screening
		• Caregiver will demonstrate knowledge and ability to interact in an age-appropriate manner with the child and provide activities to support/enhance the developmental needs of the child
		• The child will achieve age-appropriate developmental tasks
		• Referrals to community resources will be made as needed

(continued)

Motor Development

By the time a child reaches 3 years of age, gross and fine motor skills have reached considerable maturation because of increased nerve myelinization (development of an insulating myelin sheath around the nerve fibers) and the separation of nerve fibers as the central nervous system matures. Additionally, the brain has increased in size. This allows the child greater coordination and enables such abilities as running, going up and down stairs easily, jumping up and down, jumping over objects, and throwing a ball with some accuracy. Preschoolers are able to pedal a tricycle and balance on one foot for brief periods of time. They can undress themselves and, with some assistance, dress themselves. They can do some sim-

TABLE 7-2 *(continued)*

Defining Characteristics	*Nursing Interventions*	*Evaluation Criteria*

• Does not perform self-care/self-control activities for age (e.g., bowel/bladder control)
• Bites nails
• Pulls hair
• Does not function at expected developmental level in one or more domains, such as
  • Gross and fine motor skills
  • Psychosocial abilities
  • Language abilities
  • Cognitive abilities
  • Aggressive behavior
	Anticipatory Guidance; Parent Education: Childrearing Family
	• **Provide anticipatory guidance to caregivers regarding acquisition of age-appropriate developmental tasks** (refer to information on developmental norms in this chapter)
	• **Assist parents to provide opportunities for the child (including acutely and chronically ill) to meet age-related developmental tasks** (refer to information on nursing interventions and anticipatory guidance in this chapter and in Chapter 19)
	
	Support System Enhancement
	• **Refer child and family to appropriate community resources as needed:**
	  • Appropriate agency for counseling for child and family treatment
	  • Appropriate agency for supportive services (e.g., occupational therapy, physical therapy, home care services)
	  • Community programs specific to factors affecting the child's altered growth and development (e.g., child protection services, early intervention services, Women, Infants, and Children [WIC], supplemental food program, educational services, and social services)
	  • Provide information on community self-help groups, parent and sibling support groups, advocacy groups (e.g., Epilepsy Foundation of America, American Heart Association, Association of Retarded Citizens)	

ple buttoning on the front of clothing (Fig. 7–1). The 3-year-old is able to put large beads on a string, copy a circle, stack eight blocks on top of each other, draw a vertical line parallel to another, and cut with scissors (Fig. 7–2).

By the age of 4 years, they can run easily, hop on one foot, and sometimes skip clumsily. They can balance on one foot for up to 10 seconds, heel-toe walk forward, and climb steps without holding onto a rail; their movements are more graceful and rhythmic. They sit well balanced, even while reaching forward and twisting, and they are able to touch the nose with a finger when asked. They generally can dress without supervision, button well, and can distinguish the front and back of clothing.

Children at this age can cut out pictures. They

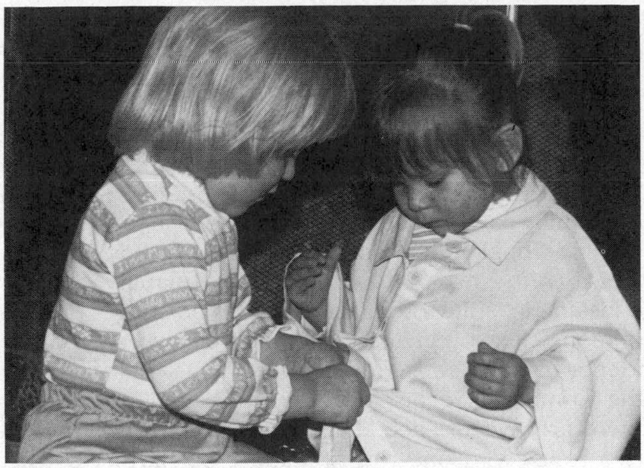

FIGURE 7 - 1. Buttoning is mastered during the preschool years.

can copy a cross and imitate the drawing of a square. They can draw a person with three parts and build a bridge with blocks.

By the age of 5 years, the preschooler has developed the skill to run with speed and agility, and to play games with others. Coordination increases. Preschoolers can balance on their toes and begin to dance with rhythm, roller skate, hop and skip well, jump rope, and climb on a jungle gym. They can dress without supervision and tie their own shoelaces, if they have had practice with shoes that have laces instead of Velcro.

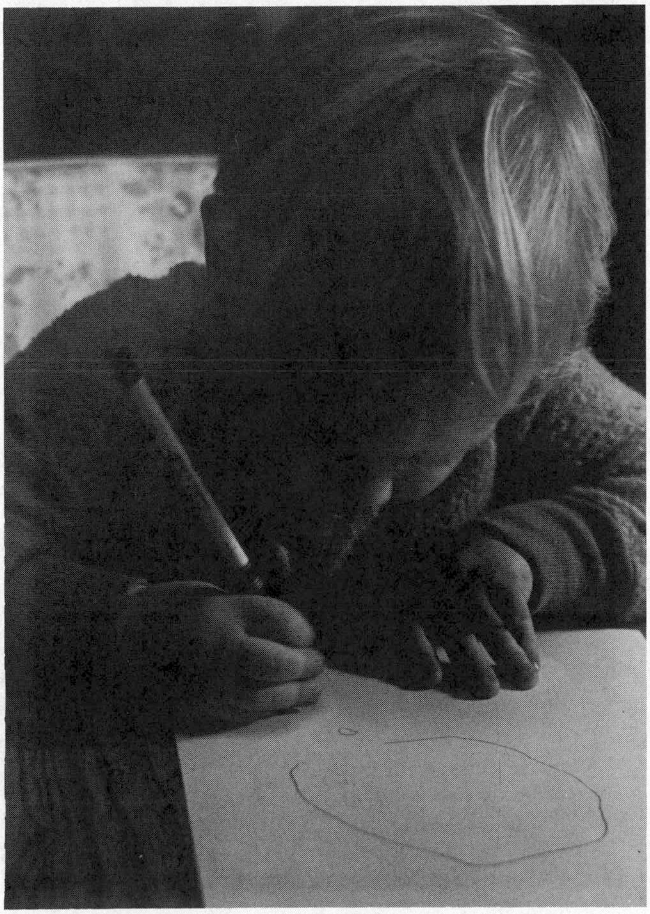

FIGURE 7 - 2. Mastery of fine motor skills requires eye-hand coordination. The 3-year-old can copy a circle.

These children can draw a square without assistance, a six-part person, and other recognizable objects. They can hit a nail with a hammer.

Nursing Interventions: Motor Skills

Knowledge of the preschooler's motor development can assist the nurse in assessing and intervening to promote developmentally appropriate motor activities. Illness and hospitalization can have adverse effects on the child's normal range of motor skills. For example, a child's arm may be restrained because of intravenous therapy or immobilized because of traction. Children on respirators or other forms of life support are significantly restricted. The nurse can encourage activities that are simpler to perform until the child's condition improves and the former abilities are regained. Parents' concerns are understandable. Explanations of their child's behavior will alleviate parental concerns. Parents themselves will then be able to support their child more appropriately.

Anticipatory Guidance: Motor Skills

Knowledge of developmental milestones will assist parents in promoting an environment appropriate to their child's needs. Encouraging parents to provide opportunities for motor skills development without placing undue pressure on the child creates a supportive environment for the preschooler.

However, safety is of utmost importance, because accidents constitute the most common cause of death among preschoolers. Nursing assessment must continue to focus on the defining characteristics of the *high risk for injury* nursing diagnostic response. Safety rules must be clear-cut, consistent, and simply explained to preschoolers. Children should be given praise as a reinforcement for safe behavior. Frequent punishment and constant threats eventually will be ignored, and children become resentful and rebellious.

Children must have access to paper, pencils, and crayons and be encouraged to use them. They must have clothes that need buttoning and shoes that need tying to learn those skills. The parent who does everything for a child does not help her or him to learn and mature.

Intellectual Competency

Generally, the 3-year-old child has an attention span of 10 to 15 minutes and has a beginning comprehension of the past and the future but is primarily con-

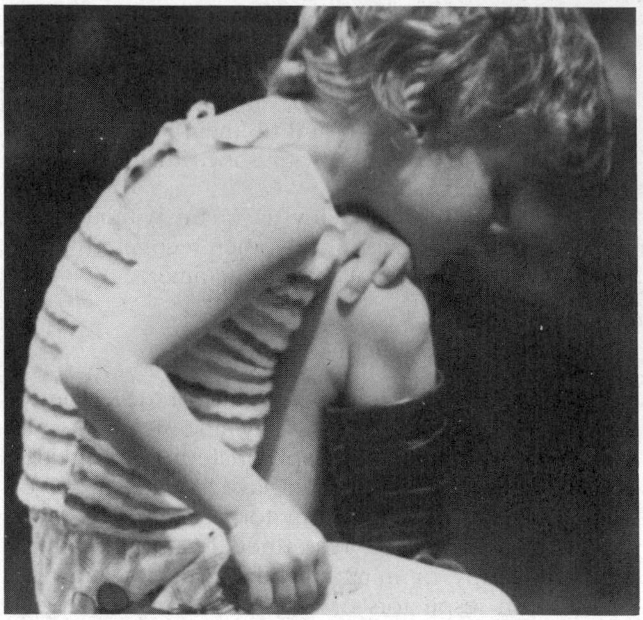

FIGURE 7-3. Preschoolers begin to ponder their expanding environment.

cerned with today. Although children at this age are frequently characterized as having a short attention span, it is probably more correct to describe them as easily distractible. They know their own age and can understand simple directions. They are imaginative, can organize their thoughts, and can be bargained with.

By the age of 4 years, the attention span has increased to 20 minutes, and a concept of time has developed. They know what day of the week it is, how old they are, when the next birthday will come, and that birthdays and holidays are particular time units and are related to parties. They can count to five and understand the concepts of one, two, and so on.

Children at age 5 years have become less imaginative than at age 4, and they are interested in detail and the definition of words. They can be reasoned with logically, become more practical and sensible, and have some understanding of money. They are beginning to understand the meaning of being related to another person. The attention span is now 30 minutes, memory is good. Five-year-olds have a good sense of time, including months, years, and weeks. In addition, they should be able to solve some problems without assistance, to start and complete activities of interest, and to play without continuous supervision (Fig. 7–3).

Cognitive Development: Preoperational Period

Preschoolers fall into Piaget's stage of preoperational thought. During this stage, they treat objects as symbolic of things other than what they are. For example, a block of wood becomes a car, and the child will move it around like a car, making a noise as it travels. Preschoolers cannot take into account another's point of view; they cannot imagine that the way they see something might not be the way another might see it. Piaget calls this *egocentrism*. Preschoolers seem to feel that their experiences are universal and that the world revolves around them. This becomes obvious in their speech, in which everything is centered on self.

Preschoolers have not yet learned the principle of *conservation,* that is, that a certain quantity remains constant in spite of transformation of shape. This is demonstrated by giving these children two sets of five identical coins and counting for them, or with them, the number of coins in each set, so that they know there are five in each. The coins are then laid out in two rows, with one row spreading out farther so that it is longer. The preschooler will tell you that there are more coins in the longer row than in the shorter row (Fig. 7–4). The same phenomenon is shown by pouring a specific amount of water from a short fat glass into a tall thin glass; the child will tell you that there is more water in the tall thin glass because it appears higher.

Another aspect of the preoperational stage is the limited ability of the child to classify or sort objects in any order. For example, the child given a group of small toys would be able to sort according to one attribute at a time, usually by color or shape (Stiles et al, 1991).

Piaget described another characteristic of preoperational thought, called *centration*. Because of this characteristic, the child is able to focus or center attention on only one aspect or characteristic of a situation at a time. Nurses aware of this characteristic will realize that explanations of procedures that focus on the benefit of wellness will probably be blocked by the child's more immediate centration on such aspects as fear of the procedure.

Animism is another characteristic of preoperational thought described by Piaget. Animism involves

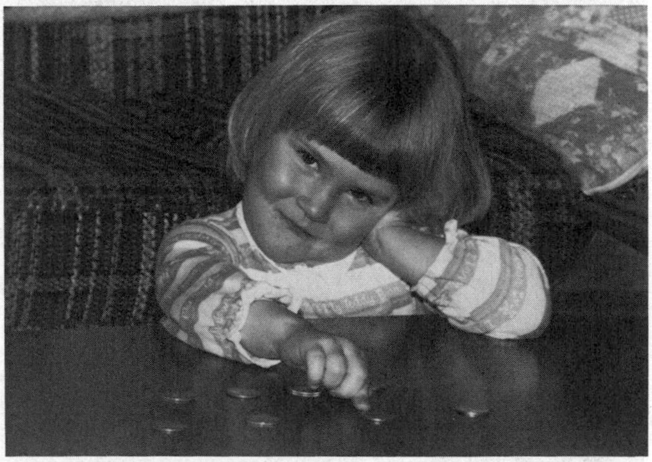

FIGURE 7-4. Preschoolers have not yet mastered the principle of conservation. A preschooler will indicate that there are more coins in the row that is longer.

endowing inanimate objects with human powers and abilities. Piaget saw animism as an example of cognitive immaturity. Recent research has demonstrated that this may not be the case. One study revealed that children personified inanimate objects selectively, indicating that animism may just be a comfortable way for the child to describe the environment (Inagaki & Hatano, 1987). Large pieces of equipment used in the hospital, such as the x-ray machine and electrocardiography machine, may be viewed as frightening or capable of attack. (One can only imagine what animism would mean in the child's perceptions of the CT scanner!)

An additional characteristic of preoperational thought is *transductive reasoning* (see Chapter 3). Transductive reasoning proceeds from particular to particular without taking the general situation into account. This can cause the child to assume cause and effect where none exists ("I wished Mommy were dead; now she's sick; it's my fault.").

Preschoolers do not have the ability to reverse or reconstruct their thinking. This characteristic of thinking is called *irreversibility*. For example, a child taken to the hospital playroom for the first time is unlikely to retrace steps back to his or her room. Characteristics of the preschooler's thinking are listed in Table 7–3.

Some children at this age have imaginary friends. The child believes this imagined friend really exists. *Fantasm* refers to the child's perception of objects that have no physical reality. *Artificialism* refers to the child's belief that all objects and events in the world are made and controlled by humans. For example, the child will believe that the sun appears after a rainfall so that it is possible to play outdoors.

Preschoolers do not have a well-conceived view of past events. Children have difficulty locating a past event earlier than the preceding day. Up to about 5 years of age, the child does not understand the meaning of days of the week, seasons, and months of the year. A child is capable of remembering selected aspects of a past event. For example, a preschooler would be able to describe a few salient features of a past event but without associating it with a particular point in time (Friedman, 1991).

More recently, researchers investigating preschoolers' cognitive abilities have offered perspectives differing from those of Piaget (Menig-Peterson, 1975; Siegler, 1986). This body of research suggests that preschoolers have more cognitive competencies than reported by Piaget (1950, 1952, 1954). Several studies have demonstrated that preschoolers are not egocentric but are capable of attending to another's perspective (Borke, 1975; Menig-Peterson, 1975). Illustrative of this concept are bilingual children who know when to speak their mother tongue and when to speak the second language. Research by Bullock and Gelman (1977) demonstrated that preschool children understand the concept of numbers, such as differences in numbers, concepts of "more" and "less," and difference between adding and subtracting.

Unlike Piaget's explanation of cognitive development that suggests an innate approach, other child developmentalists have suggested that children learn on the basis of their experiences what is useful. For example, children who have been hospitalized will learn to distinguish the meanings of different treatments. Mention of a bone marrow aspiration will create fear in the child who has undergone one, compared with the child who has had a less intrusive procedure.

Nursing Interventions: Cognitive Development

Health care personnel, especially the nurses and the child life worker, can help a preschooler deal with and master fears by means of dramatic play. Many hospitals have tours for children who are scheduled for hospital admission to acquaint them with the hospital and some of its equipment. (The practice of providing hospital tours for kindergarten groups and other preschoolers not scheduled for hospitalization may produce unnecessary fears in those children and is therefore not recommended.) Explanations of procedures and other hospital-related events and equipment need to be developmentally appropriate. Children at this age have limited understanding of their internal anatomy (Jones et al, 1992). Understanding of the preschooler's characteristics of thinking will enable the nurse to use terminology and provide explanations that are understandable to the child. A sample preprocedural explanation is provided in Table 7–4.

On the basis of the premise that children acquire knowledge through practical experience, nurses can assist children in understanding and assimilating their hospital experience by listening to how they recall it (Hauck, 1991). The nurse can correct misconceptions and provide emotional support, thereby enabling the child to integrate the experience to promote a sense of mastery. In addition, the child's recounting will assist the nurse in individualizing the child's care to meet both emotional and cognitive needs.

Anticipatory Guidance: Cognitive Development

Developing the skills that are evidence of intelligence is essential to children's enjoyment and learning in the school environment. Parents should be encouraged to help their children achieve these skills by exposing them to the concepts of time, money, and memory tasks (see Table 7–1). Much of that exposure can be achieved merely by encouraging and assisting preschoolers to become independent. They should be allowed to participate in their own care, and they should have some items of their own.

Much of preschoolers' mastery of cognitive tasks results from their discoveries during play investigation. Parents can help their child learn to classify objects by naming the object groups that the child encounters in activities of daily life. For example, while

TABLE 7-3
Characteristics of the Preschooler's Thinking

Characteristic	Definition	Clinical Example
Egocentrism	World revolves around self; does not understand that another's perspective exists	Child expects that nurse will understand a need without having to express it
Centration	Focuses on one aspect of a situation	Child repeatedly asks parent when the "shot" will be given, after being prepared by the nurse for surgery
Animism	Endows an inanimate object with human powers and abilities	Child begins to cry when wheeled into room for a CT scan and says, "I don't want an x-ray, I'm scared. I don't want that [referring to CT scanner] to hurt me."
Transductive reasoning	Reasoning focuses on particular aspects of situation, rather than the general situation	Child's grandmother usually visits hospital after lunchtime; when finished with lunch, child wants to wait at elevator for grandma
Fantasm	Perceives objects that have no physical presence	Child scolds imaginary friend for crying when the nurse brings medicine; child tells friend, "Don't be silly, taking medicine [referring to pills] doesn't hurt."
Artificialism	Objects/events are made and controlled by humans	Child believes elevator doors open just for him/her as nurse pushes gurney toward door on their way to radiography
Irreversibility	Inability to reverse or reconstruct thinking	During play session, nurse asks child to apply dressing to doll's arm, which was removed; child is confused and does not know correct order for reapplying bandages
Relations	Cannot order objects; has no overall scheme for arranging objects in order	If asked to arrange objects from smallest to largest, child can only do so after much trial and error
Classification	Classifies objects in one of several different ways: size, shape, and color	If asked to arrange a set of small cars, child may do so according to type of car
Conservation	Unable to conserve objects/liquids in terms of weight, volume, and mass	Child was not able to finish ice cream on the way to chest radiography; on returning, child finds the melted ice cream and asks, "Where is my ice cream?"
Relationship of part to whole	Incapable of seeing the relationship of part to whole (e.g., father and husband are same person)	Uncle visits child in hospital; one of the nurses brings a lunch tray into the room and addresses him as Dr. Pedersen, as he is an attending pediatrician at the hospital; child looks surprised

TABLE 7-4
Promoting Cognitive Development: Surgical Preparation

The following is an excerpt of the preparation session the nurse has with Angelica, age 4. The vignette illustrates the concepts of cognitive developments integrated into the teaching session.

Interaction	***Rationale***
Nurse: The teddy bear's name is Teddy. He has a dressing on his tummy just like you're going to have after your operation.	*Animism* Children at this age believe inanimate objects have human qualities.
Angelica: (Remains silent.)	
Nurse: He had an operation just like you're going to have.	
Nurse: Yes, and he feels much better now, even though his dressing feels sticky and funny on his tummy. Do you want to feel it? (Nurse points to dressing.)	*Transductive Reasoning* By providing simplistic explanations of the upcoming surgery, misconceptions the child has will be corrected.
Angelica: (Reaches out to feel dressing.)	
Nurse: Now can I tell you a little more about Teddy's trip to the operating room?	*Centration* Children tend to focus on only one aspect of a situation.
Angelica: (Shakes her head yes.)	

The nurse continues with a basic explanation of the operating room procedure. The nurse covers content that includes description of sequence of events, use of equipment, and sensations Angelica would feel.

selecting the shirt the preschooler is going to wear, the parent might say, "These are all shirts. Which do you want to wear: the blue shirt that buttons, the red shirt that zips, the green shirt that goes over your head, or the brown shirt that snaps?"

Parents may need assistance to understand the fears and misconceptions of their preschooler as a natural developmental phenomenon resulting from the cognitive processes characteristic of this period. When parents can anticipate that, because of these cognitive processes, objects or experiences may elicit fear in their preschooler, they can prepare the child; this can be done by means of appropriate books, by gradually exposing the child to the feared situation through pretend play opportunities, and by being present and supportive during the experience.

Reassurances should be based on knowledge of the characteristics of preoperational thought. Considering egocentrism, the parent would begin a reassuring statement with, "Nothing *you* did [or said, or thought] caused . . . " Similarly, explanations of cause would deny the products of the child's transductive reasoning. Recognizing that the child's fears are real and finding ways to help the child master those fears are probably more helpful than insisting that the child is imagining things.

Active parent participation is essential to fostering optimal outcomes for the child. Parental knowledge is associated with positive parenting behaviors. The importance of providing parents with information about developmental milestones, characteristics, concerns, and interventions to foster them cannot be emphasized enough. The nurse serves a valuable role as an educator and can be a role model for parents who have questions about their preschooler. There are numerous other resources to which parents can be referred that can provide support and information. These resources include the preschool teacher, librarian, parks and recreations specialists, child development experts, and even retail merchants. Many excellent books and newsletters are available to assist parents in providing current information and access to valuable resources.

Research has demonstrated positive associations between parental beliefs and behavior and the child's development (Miller, 1988). That is, parental beliefs will be manifested in their childrearing activities. Parents who value their child's intellectual curiosity and need for experimentation will provide the home environment to support that belief. Appreciation and respect for the child's need to learn and develop will influence every decision the parent makes, from purchasing food and selecting child care arrangements to establishing lifestyle priorities. Parental knowledge and involvement in the child's development are essential.

Language Development

"Where does the sun go at night? Why can't I go outdoors? Where did baby Susie come from? Why is it wrong? Why can't I see Grandma? Why? What? Where? When? How?" This is the language of the preschooler. This is the way to learn, to get information and gain attention, and to gain social experience and understanding. Others' responses to these questions are essential for the child to relate to others and to solve problems. Without response, the preschooler will attempt to find refuge in a fantasy world and neglect the verbal communication that is necessary for the period of growth from infancy to school age.

At 3 years of age, preschoolers have a vocabulary of about 900 words and are using plurals. They use language more fluently than previously, and they sing simple songs. They can make up a phrase and repeat it, not seeming to care whether anyone is listening. They talk to themselves or to imaginary playmates.

By 4 years, the vocabulary has increased to 1500 words, and preschoolers understand prepositions. They use "I," talk in sentences, ask many questions, and want detailed explanations. They exaggerate, tattle, and tell family problems outside the home. They are starting to know one or more colors, if they have been exposed to them.

By age 5 years, preschoolers have a vocabulary of 2100 words and use language correctly with meaningful sentences. They talk constantly, ask questions (about the meaning of words and how things work), and can tell a story accurately, sometimes adding a little fantasy to make it "better." They can sing fairly well, count to 10, and know some colors, again depending on exposure.

During the preschool years, children gradually master vowel and consonant sounds. Table 7-5 shows ages at which the various sounds are usually mastered. Nonfluency typifies the preschoolers' language. Probably because of their incomplete mastery of sounds, their speech lacks the smoothness and rhythm of fluent speech. Egocentric speech typical of the toddler and early preschooler yields more to social speech by the end of the preschool stage as the child learns how both to listen and to initiate conversation, is able both to ask and to answer questions, and is able to offer as well as understand commands, requests, or threats.

TABLE 7-5
Approximate Ages for the Mastery of Vowels and Consonants

Age 3–4 yrs	Most vowel sounds and *p, b, m, h, w*
Age 4–5 yrs	*k, g, f, d, m, ng* as in "sing," *ya* as in "yellow"
Age 5–6 yrs	*F, v, sh, l, th, s, z, r, ch, jah* as in "jar"

Nursing Interventions: Language Development

Children's use of words for body parts and functions is dictated by family custom. A preschooler's hospitalization will be made less threatening if the nurses caring for the child can speak in familiar terms and with expressions used in the home.

Preschoolers are particularly inquisitive. They ask questions about everything. Their questions can be answered and anticipated by providing information and explanations about the hospital experience. Because most aspects of the hospitalization are unfamiliar to the preschooler, explanations are needed for practically everything the child will encounter, including hospital equipment, procedures, and terminology.

In some cases, the child's language and speech problems indicate a more serious language delay. Speech and language delays affect 1.5 million children (Coplan, 1985). Psychosocial and school problems can ensue if language and speech problems are not identified early. Generally, parents are fairly accurate in their identification of their child's language and speech problems (Capute et al, 1987). Although language screening tools are available for nurses to administer, practicality, reliability, and validity are significant factors to consider before using them (Walker et al, 1989). One study indicated that the Denver Developmental Screening Test (DDST) did not identify 47 per cent of children with delayed expressive language (Borowitz & Glascoe, 1986). Referral to a speech and language specialist is appropriate for further evaluation when language and speech delays are suspected (Kilmon et al, 1991).

Anticipatory Guidance: Language Development

The nurse is often approached by parents about the speech of their preschooler. Parents become particularly concerned when their child mispronounces sounds or hesitates in speech. Parents should be encouraged not to expect or demand perfection in the preschooler's speech. The child should not be criticized or forced to repeat correctly the mispronounced sounds or words, as such measures only serve to create speech disturbances such as stuttering. Parents *can* help their preschooler master correct pronunciation by modeling the proper pronunciation of sounds in their own speech, giving special clarity to the particular sounds that the preschooler is learning at the time (Table 7-6). Bringing to children's attention the

TABLE 7-6
Language Milestones

3 Yrs	
Has 900-word vocabulary	
Uses complete sentences	
Uses all parts of speech	
Masters vowel sounds and *p, b, m, h, w*	
4 Yrs	
Has 1500-word vocabulary	
Understands use of prepositions	
Uses first person in sentences	
Learns to count	
Masters *k, g, l, d, m, ng* as in "sing," *ya* as in "yellow"	
5 Yrs	
Has 2100-word vocabulary	
Can print name/simple familiar words	
Masters *f, v, sh, l, th, s, z, r, ch, jah* as in "jar"	

sounds that are present in the environment (engines running, wind blowing) and talking with them about what makes the sounds helps them learn to listen and to understand what they hear. Obscure or curse words should be ignored. The more attention is given to this type of language, the more it is reinforced.

In addition to an adult's response to the child's attempts at communication, language is developed from reading to the child and making reading materials available. Stories should be simple at first, and colorfully illustrated to interest the child. Content should fit into the child's world of fantasy and reality, such as animals that talk as well as inanimate objects that act like humans.

Emotional-Social Competency

As preschoolers' environment broadens and their interests expand, they become more social beings. At 3 years of age, they are friendly but still self-centered; by 4 years, they are not as pleasant and have become noisy; at 5, they are becoming more sociable (see Table 7–1). They become companions, rather than individuals to care for, and their company can be a pleasure. Their imaginations assist them in learning about others. They learn to get along with both children and adults, and they behave in a more grown-up manner. In their play, they imitate adults, mimic their conversations and manner of speaking, and love to pretend by "dressing up" in their old clothes.

Psychosocial Development: Initiative and Self-Esteem

The preschooler is in the stage of *initiative versus guilt,* which is the third Eriksonian (Erikson, 1963) stage of development. The central task, crisis, or problem of this stage is for the child to develop a sense of initiative that outweighs any sense of guilt. Initiative may be defined as active beginning of a task, readiness to begin, or enterprise. Preschoolers now are ready to try new activities and experiences. Their curiosity and inventiveness are part of their innate capacity for developing a sense of initiative. At the same time, the environment presents them with opportunities to develop initiative, either formalized ones (e.g., preschool) or simply new areas for play and self-care in the home. Excursions into fantasy may have an important purpose in the development of a sense of initiative. Children may find it easier to tolerate the frustrations and prohibitions of the real world if they can periodically retreat into a fantasy world in which those frustrations and prohibitions are mastered. However, their fantasies can also result in a sense of guilt if preschoolers know they would be unacceptable to parents (e.g., "Daddy's mean; I wish he was dead").

Guilt is possible because much of what preschoolers would like to do is either forbidden or they are physically or mentally unable to do it. Guilt also occurs when those they wish to please are not pleased or when they themselves are not happy with what they have done (Stipek & DeCotis, 1988). Because preschoolers have a rigid conscience, they frequently have unwarranted guilt feelings over obvious or secret wrongs. As in the previous developmental stages, some guilt is desirable. The individual who develops no sense of guilt is amoral (typically referred to as sociopathic). Preschoolers must learn what actions are inappropriate or wrong and should feel guilty when they commit them. At the same time, they must learn to feel a sense of initiative for developmentally appropriate acts and thoughts.

Preschoolers' developing sense of self gives a feeling of belonging, which provides security and a sense of competence. The feeling of competence, in turn, motivates them to perform tasks that develop initiative. During the preschool years, children judge self-worth on the basis of this competence with things, competence with parents and other adults, and competence with peers. If they have not developed a sense of belonging and self-worth, they will be hindered in the ability to move out into the bigger world of school and community.

Nursing Interventions: Fostering Initiative and Self-Esteem

The preschooler is particularly vulnerable to interpreting illness and hospitalization as punishment for misdeed. Several interventions can be used to allevi-

TABLE 7-7
Promoting Initiative in the Hospitalized Child

Christie, a 4-year-old preschooler, was hospitalized following an automobile accident. These excerpts from her nursing care plan are specifically designed to promote her needs for developing a sense of initiative after a traumatic experience

Encourage Christie to ask questions
- Allow time and encourage questions
- Always explain why you are in room and what you are going to do
- Be direct and honest
- Encourage expression of feelings

Provide opportunities to direct care
- Allow to have some say in scheduling activities, e.g., bath
- Allow to select which fluids to take with medicine
- Allow to select own menu

Promote expression of creative activities
- Encourage favorite diversional activities
- Encourage wearing own clothing/articles of clothing (hair clip, bracelet, pin)
- Encourage use of therapeutic play to express feelings
- Provide opportunity for child to choose age-appropriate toys and games and use them in manner chosen, as long as it is not destructive

ate feelings of guilt. Preschoolers need constant reassurance that they are not being punished. To avoid the guilt reaction, the actual causes of illnesses need to be discussed in terms that the child can understand. Storytelling or puppet play with the child can uncover misconceptions and fantasies about their illness. This is an excellent opportunity for the nurse to improve the child's understanding and provide reassurance that the illness did not occur because of a misdeed or omission on the part of the child.

Projective play techniques, such as drawing and storytelling, are useful in eliciting the child's feelings. The feelings of wrongdoing and guilt exhibited through these techniques can be clarified and dealt with. Opportunities for creative expression by, for example, drawing and making paper cutouts do much to enhance the child's sense of initiative. Encouraging preschoolers to make choices when possible enhances their self-worth. For example, the preschooler can participate in meal selection. Facilitating the hospitalized child's developmental needs is exemplified in Table 7–7.

Anticipatory Guidance: Fostering Initiative and Self-Esteem

Adults, especially parents, should use praise and affection, rather than scolding and threats, in their relationships with preschoolers. Guidelines for discipline continue to apply to the preschooler. Punishment of unacceptable behaviors by physical means, verbal threatening, attacks on the child as a person, or threats of consequences to the child (especially loss of parental approval) all can produce a child who is anxious and fearful about loss of parental love and in whom guilt predominates over initiative. When the child misbehaves, discipline should focus on the behavior, not the child. Examples of interventions that should be avoided when disciplining the preschooler include the following:

> "Nice boys [or girls] don't do that."
>
> "You're a bad [or terrible] person."
>
> "If you do that, Mommy won't like you."
>
> "Mommy [or Daddy] doesn't like boys [or girls] who . . ."

Parents should refrain from comparing their preschooler with siblings or other preschoolers. Children develop at different rates, and comparing makes it difficult for the child to develop a sense of competence and self-worth. Parents who are warm and accepting of their children, although not necessarily always of their behavior, will help them develop a high level of initiative.

Observation of parent-child interactions will provide important information concerning parenting skills.

Sexuality

Psychosexual Development

According to Freud's theory of psychosexual development, in the preschooler the phallic zone is the body zone in which pleasurable sensations or tension reduction is centered. Freud referred to this period as the *phallic (urethral) stage.* This designation indicates that Freud was more definitive in his description of psychosexual development of little boys than of little girls. According to Freud, little boys develop sexual strivings (or id impulses) toward their mothers, whom they wish to have all to themselves. They perceive their fathers as rivals and wish to replace them. These wishes bring about conflict, as the little boys fear retribution from the father in the form of castration. This conflict is referred to as the *Oedipus complex.* The little boy resolves the oedipal conflict by suppressing his sexual feelings toward his mother and developing feelings of identification with his father. Freud described a phenomenon in little girls called the *Electra complex,* in which they note the absence of a penis and presume the mother is responsible for its loss. Freud attributed penis envy in little girls to the Electra complex. According to Freudian theory, the alliance with the same-sex parent that occurs at this age results in role modeling not only daily tasks and behaviors but also the parent's standards, ethics, and morals. Freud believed that the superego, or conscience, developed as a result of the Oedipus and Electra complexes. (See the discussion of conscience development later in this chapter.)

Most child development experts currently do not see the Oedipus and Electra complexes as entirely valid explanations of preschool-age children's behaviors or motivations for behaviors. In evaluating Freud's theory, it is often helpful to examine it in a historical context. Children *do* show castration anxiety and penis envy. Their motivation is probably quite different from that which Freud hypothesized during the Victorian age.

Developing a Positive Sexual Attitude

The attitude of the young child develops as new feelings are experienced in association with life events. Issues that emerge at this stage of development include nudity and privacy. Although most parents are comfortable with their own nudity and that of their infant or toddler, they express concern as the child gets older. Some parents fear that their own nudity may be provocative to children. Nudity within a healthy family actually has little impact other than validation of the similarities and differences between children and adults. Privacy is needed for sexual expression between parents. At this stage, parents are often concerned about the preschooler unexpectedly finding them during sexual intercourse. The interruption handled in a matter-of-fact way is not harmful to the child. Parents are cautioned that young children may be frightened or confused by explicit sexual acts, which they may confuse with violence. Explanations should be given to the preschooler by the parents together to help the child understand that both parents agree on what is explained. If a preschooler is treated with acceptance and respect, the experience is not likely to cause any difficulty.

Sexual Behaviors

As an extension of the toddler's experience, the preschooler continues self-exploratory behavior, engaging in masturbation or sex play with siblings or peers. Reports from parents suggest that children at this age engage in purposeful behavior leading to orgasm. This play may be solitary or with other children and in most instances is part of the normal sequence of development. The Study Group of New York (1983) cited many examples, such as the following:

> Penelope described an incident in which her own daughter and the daughter of a friend were riding a Brahma bull statue at the local library. "My child said to my girlfriend's child, 'If you ride real fast it feels really good when it rubs your vagina.' They continued riding until my daughter got a very delirious expression on her face" (p 122).

As experience and ability increase, the preschooler continues to engage in self-manipulation of the genitalia when bathing or curiously manipulating the genitalia of another child sharing a bath or shower. Experimentation with body parts and orifices continues as a natural behavior but requires some supervision. A 5-year-old boy was brought to the emergency room after allegedly falling out of his wagon and injuring his penis, which was red and swollen. Being unable to urinate, he had made up the story about falling, rather than telling his parents that he had put his older sister's tiny rubber band (from her braces) around the glans of his penis. Fortunately a nurse discovered the band prior to a catheterization procedure and removed it.

Other types of play include pretending to give birth to dolls or stuffed animals, playing house with mommy and daddy sleeping together, or other imitations of the expanded roles in which they now see their parents. They enjoy calling each other names, sometimes using vocabulary that is associated with their genitalia and bodily functions, such as "peenose," "pooh-head," and the like.

Developing Sex-Role Identification

Preschoolers' sense of self is further defined by developing sexual curiosity and an awareness of how they differ from others. They are learning about their body, what it looks like, and what it can do; all of this helps them form a sense of sex-role identification. Sex-role identification in the child includes the ability to apply correctly a gender label—male or female—to oneself. The development of sex-role identity is explained in different ways by various theories of development. Freud's psychosexual theory sees sex-role identification as the result of the Oedipus complex. Cognitive developmental theory sees it as a function of cognitive development. Children hear and learn the labels "boy" or "girl" as symbols that stand for gender classifications. Social learning theory says that children observe that certain (sex-appropriate) behaviors are rewarded and other (inappropriate) behaviors are not rewarded.

Sex-role identity begins at birth. Baby clothes and other items (sheets, blankets, furniture) are color-coded by sex: pink for girls and blue for boys. Infant girls and boys are also treated in different ways. Fathers tend to be more physical with male infants than with female infants. Such attitudes convey subtle messages regarding sex-role identity. From infancy onward, the types of toys given to a child tend to be sex-typed. A male infant is more likely to receive a rattle shaped like a boxing glove than is a female infant.

Toddlers and preschoolers are influenced by our culture, which tends to sex-type them. Many parents have definite ideas of how boys should behave, such as "fighting back" and not crying when unhappy, whereas girls are punished for fighting back, although tears are acceptable. Parents may also buy toys that help endorse those cultural sex-type expectations: war games for boys and dolls for girls. Boys are pressured to develop characteristics of their fathers, and girls model themselves after their mothers. By the late preschool age, children identify themselves and others by the correct gender.

Children learn and acquire behaviors that are culturally accepted as sex-appropriate through imitation of behaviors that they see rewarded. Television plays a primary role in the modeling of sex-appropriate behaviors. Television—including commercials—tells the child what to eat, what toys to desire, and how to dress and act.

Changing family lifestyles and the numerous families in which both parents work have tended to decrease sex-role stereotyping. Children are more likely to be exposed to many examples of appropriate sex-role behavior. To decrease the amount of sex typing in the family, it is important for children to observe parents doing activities together, such as housework and yardwork. Parents can provide a variety of toys and encourage preschoolers to play with toys that interest them, regardless of the sex-typing connotations traditional culture imposes on them.

The child in a single-parent family needs substitute experiences with a relative or family friend of the opposite sex to provide the relationship of a missing parent. In some two-parent families, one parent is too busy, not interested, or out of town a great deal; the same need is present and can be filled by an interested relative, neighbor, or family friend.

Anticipatory Guidance: Sex-Role Identification

Sexual exploration, masturbation, or sex play in preschool children is fairly common. Preschoolers learn by exploration; they should not be punished for attempting to satisfy their curiosity. Children should not be made to feel guilty about this very natural response to their inquisitiveness and developing sexual identity.

The way in which some parents verbally respond to their preschooler's masturbation can create guilt in the child, such as, "Don't touch *it*," or "Stop doing *that*." Limits on sexual expression could be expressed in statements such as, "Touching your penis is a private thing, like going pee-pee," or, "Just like you don't have a bowel movement in front of people, you don't touch your vulva in front of people." Additional guidance is to advise the parents to ignore the behavior whenever possible. Focusing attention on the behavior may be reinforcing to the child. Often the child can be distracted to another pleasurable but more socially acceptable activity. Most preschoolers gradually decrease the frequency of genital manipulation. The nurse should be aware, however, that some religious groups condemn masturbation. Sensitivity to family values is an essential characteristic for the nurse who counsels families about child behavior. It is often a good idea to preface advice with further assessment of parental values, for example, "Some parents have religious or cultural beliefs about masturbation being wrong or harmful. Do you have concerns such as these?"

The preschooler also needs to learn to say "No" to adults or older children whose intention may be to exploit the child.

Fears

It is difficult to distinguish between fear and anxiety in preschool children. Preschoolers cannot sufficiently differentiate between what is inside and outside their control and between real and imagined dangers. Because preschool children do not yet have a realistic sense of causality, they may fear many phenomena in the natural world and fantasize causes that are self-related (Table 7–8). Their world now extends beyond the home, and they may be exposed to many situations and experiences that are potential sources of fear and anxiety.

Fear does have a protective value, and it often is evoked by parents and other adults with protection in mind. Fear of crossing the street, fear of automobiles, and fear of dangerous animals, for example, are induced as a safety precaution. Fears may also have value in motivating curiosity and learning. For example, a fear of wild animals, thunderstorms, and other aspects of nature may stimulate a child's curiosity in natural science.

Fear of strangers and strange situations, so intense during the toddler period, decreases by the preschool age. Because of increased cognitive capac-

TABLE 7-8
Common Fears of Preschoolers

Home and Community
Dark
Bad people
Bodily injury
Bedtime
Close/confining places
Pain
Natural World
Animals
Thunderstorms
Water
Earthquakes
Disasters
Fantasy World
Nightmares
Ghosts/bogeyman
Monsters
Being alone

ity and greater ability in symbolic representation and imagination, however, many fears of supernatural or imaginary dangers increase, as does the range of possibilities for threats, such as that of inadequacy. Furthermore, preschool children also incorporate parental fears during this period—fear of storms, insects, certain animals, and so on.

Nursing Interventions: Dealing with Fears

The preschooler's parents need to be sensitive to their child's imagined and real fears about hospitalization. Because of an increased ability to imagine the range of possible threats, preschoolers are vulnerable to particular sensitivity about the hospital environment.

Developmentally appropriate explanations given prior to procedures and use of therapeutic play can alleviate the preschooler's concerns. Explanations of what and how procedures will be done, no matter how seemingly insignificant, such as taking a temperature, will satisfy the preschooler's inquisitiveness and fears.

Anticipatory Guidance: Dealing with Fears

Fear may unwittingly be stimulated by parents, other adults, and the mass media in order to achieve compliance with adult wishes. For example, in American society, witches, bogeymen, or goblins are still occasionally cited as instruments of retribution. Unfortunately, helpful personnel, including policemen, physicians, and nurses, whom the child may later encounter, may also be used as threats.

Parents can benefit from discussion about the detrimental effects of evoking fears to generate compliant behavior. Other more productive interventions can be taught to parents, such as ignoring behavior, rational explanations, or behavior modification techniques.

Coping Mechanisms

The preschooler's use of coping mechanisms is directly related to level of development. These children rely heavily on motor behaviors, such as kicking and hitting, to express aggressive feelings. Temper tantrums and protest behaviors are other examples of aggressive responses. Most preschool children, however, have more defenses at their command than do toddlers. Defense mechanisms such as repression, projection, and identification are used by children to alleviate stress and anxiety. Preschoolers are less physical than toddlers, because it is easier for them to express themselves verbally. Their comments "I hate you" or "I think you're ugly" or the use of scatologic terms, such as "poop-head" and "nerd" largely replace toddler behaviors of kicking, screaming, and temper tantrums.

Research studies have identified several factors that influence the preschooler's response to distress. Parenting interventions used in helping the child cope are important. The manner in which a child is taught to respond to a situation and to handle emotions affects the child's development. The child's unique personality characteristics, such as assertiveness and sociability; acquisition of cognitive skill, and understanding of another's perspective are components that contribute to the child's individualized response (Denham, 1986).

To a great degree, young children appraise a situation through the eyes of their parents. Parents and significant adult figures play a role mediating between the child and the larger world. They act as a filter, interpreting the stressful situation and giving it meaning for the child.

Children learn these lessons through observations of their family interactions as well. Children monitor closely and with intense interest the character and consequences of interactions between their parents and siblings as further evidence for interpretation (Dunn et al, 1991). A sensitive child quickly perceives the adult's level of ease or anxiety in a stressful situation. Coping strategies used during the toddler and preschool years are listed in Table 7-9.

Nursing Interventions: Coping Mechanisms

Through observation and parental interview, the nurse learns about the child's coping mechanisms.

TABLE 7-9
Preschooler Coping Mechanisms

Cognitive/Intellectual	Behavioral	Defense Mechanisms
Asking questions (why)	Motor activity	Aggression
Use of rituals/routines	Play	Denial
Experimentation—trial and error	Temper tantrums	Withdrawal
Transitional object/favorite toy	Aggressive behavior (fighting)	Repression
Use of scatology, e.g., calling peer "poop-head"	Experimentation—trial and error	Projection
	Thumb sucking	Identification
	Hair twisting	Masturbation
	Nailbiting	

Understanding the child's behavior enables the nurse to support the child more effectively during the periods of stress. Interventions based on an understanding of each child's behavior will enhance the ability to achieve mastery of the situation and of the accompanying feelings.

Anticipatory Guidance: Coping Mechanisms

Family members can support the needs of the preschooler if the nurse informs them of the developmental significance of these behaviors, gives them an opportunity to express their own frustrations, and provides suggestions for managing the behaviors. Explaining the child's behavior is an important first step for parents in understanding their child's underlying needs.

Moral and Faith Development

By the time they enter school, most children know the basic moral rules and conventions of our society and are functioning at the *preconceptual stage of moral development.*

During the preschool and early school years, children view rules as fixed, absolute, and passed down by their parents, who are all-knowing and perfect. Young children tend to judge actions as "bad" mainly in terms of their consequences. For instance, a girl may state that five cups broken while helping her mother is worse than one cup broken while stealing jam. Children also view an act as totally right or totally wrong and believe that the adult's view is always the right one. During the preschool years, punishment is usually seen as deserved. Misfortune is also seen as occurring after misdeeds because it was willed by God or parents as retribution. As children's experience increases, their moral judgment progresses toward more internal and subjective values, and there is less concern for immediate external physical consequences.

The preschooler's understanding of spiritual matters continues to be determined by perceptions, feelings, and fantasy. Misunderstandings of the supernatural persist as the preschooler progresses through the *intuitive-projective* stage of faith development. Religious symbols, customs, and practices begin to have more realistic meaning for the child. The preschooler begins to understand that death is not simply a separation but rather has qualities of permanence associated with it. Imagined fears of bad and evil can take on frightening dimensions (e.g., the devil will come and get me). The concept of God can be described in either human terms (e.g., God is mad at me) or with animistic qualities (i.e., God is everywhere; God is in the trees, sky, and ocean).

Developing a Conscience (Superego)

The development of conscience, or superego, is the acquisition of moral beliefs. Conscience begins developing during the preschool years as children learn what behavior is acceptable to their parents. When children's behavior is not acceptable, they feel guilty. The moral behavior they develop is adopted from that of the parents, because they are the judges. During these preschool years, rules are absolute and passed by parents who are "perfect;" actions are totally right or totally wrong, and the parent is always right. Parents and nurses should realize the preschooler often believes that sickness, accidents, and hospitalization are punishment for some real or imagined transgression.

Likewise, preschoolers cannot comprehend the rationale that makes some behaviors acceptable and others unacceptable. Nevertheless, to facilitate cognitive development they need opportunities to question or disagree, even if they do not comprehend.

Anticipatory Guidance: Developing a Conscience

Parents need to be aware of the role models they provide for their child. The nurse can help parents to identify what values and attitudes they want to instill in their child and then help them to recognize their behaviors or practices that either foster or hinder their preschooler's acquisition of those values and attitudes. The nurse may encourage parents to participate actively and regularly in religious or ethnic activities that will provide their preschooler with the needed role models, if they identify these as important in their child's development.

Parents also may require assistance to understand that their child is not ready to adopt acceptable behaviors or avoid inappropriate behaviors only on the basis of discussions or explanations of why these behaviors are correct or not correct.

Peer Relationships

Preschool children continue their egocentric orientation toward playmates. However, they have a beginning capacity to understand that their playmates and friends in preschool or in their neighborhood can and do perceive and react differently in similar situations. In one study, the way in which preschoolers who were friends managed conflicts was different from the method of those who were not friends. Preschool friends' conflicts were less intense than nonfriends' conflicts. Strategies to terminate conflicts also differed between groups; friends turned away from each other, whereas nonfriends continued to assert their positions. Friends continued to have social contacts following conflicts (Hartup et al, 1988).

The preschooler will continue to insist that play activities proceed in the manner that means "Do it my way." Reciprocity or give-and-take in the child's relationships is mainly limited to sharing their possessions. Being a friend at this age means playing together and being with each other to share similar interests. The preschooler does not tolerate differences in other children who are friends. This child has the emerging recognition that individuality exists by virtue of actions, thoughts, and feelings.

Health Maintenance and Promotion

Health Screening

Basic immunizations should be complete by the preschool age. Tuberculin skin testing, however, may be done before school entry, and diphtheria, pertussis, and tetanus (DPT) and polio boosters will be given at that time (Williams, 1990).

Physical growth and development are monitored. Should a pattern of deviation become evident, such as the child's placement on the growth curve dropping off, further evaluation and referral are indicated. Children can be screened for anemia, particularly preschoolers from disadvantaged homes in which the diet may be insufficient for nutritional daily requirements because of limited finances.

Data on the child's health status are obtained from parents. The frequency and types of illness are noted, because they may indicate an underlying, chronic problem. For example, the child who has frequent ear infections may have chronic serous otitis media. Information gathered during the health assessment provides the opportunity for the nurse to provide anticipatory guidance in areas of parental concern. For example, the parents may express concerns about their child's occasional bed wetting. This provides the opportunity for the nurse to explore the concern more fully and provide management interventions for the parents.

Cardiovascular risk factors should be assessed, as research data have demonstrated possible precursors of cardiovascular disease to be evident as early as the preschool years (Rosenbaum et al, 1987). Dietary intake of cholesterol and saturated fats is assessed. Total serum cholesterol levels of 160 to 170 mg/dl may be excessive. Obesity is considered a risk factor, as is elevated blood pressure (persistent elevated blood pressure over 6 to 12 months that is not associated with other hypertensive cardiovascular disease) (Berenson et al, 1988). The potential risk of secondhand parental smoking is not known. The relationship of environmental stress and exercise to cardiovascular disease is speculative at this time (Howard et al, 1991; Jenkins, 1988). Finally, information on family history is obtained, because history of cardiovascular disease is a predictor. The American Academy of Pediatrics (1989) recommends regular serum cholesterol testing in children older than 2 years of age with positive family history of hyperlipidemia or premature myocardial infarction. Some experts recommend both a serum total cholesterol and a high-density lipoprotein HDL–cholesterol measurement. Referral to a nutritionist is made for values exceeding 200 mg/dl on more than one occasion (DeClue & Shocken, 1991).

School nurses in day care and preschool settings can play an important role in screening children (Carmon et al, 1990). In one preschool setting, nurses started a school-based clinic (Honig, 1991). A multitude of services were offered to preschoolers, including complete physical examinations, primary/episodic care, and immunizations. The benefits of this clinic enabled children who otherwise would not have had access to care to receive services and be followed closely, thereby enhancing the identification of developmental problems and early intervention.

Vision and Hearing

Sensory function is highly developed by the time a child becomes a preschooler. Because a child at this age who has a visual problem is unaware of it and because amblyopia (lazy eye) becomes an irreversible condition usually by the age of 6 years, preschool vision screening is essential.

Vision screening is done for the preschool child

with the use of the E chart, which is similar to the standard Snellen chart except that the letter E replaces the alphabet, or with the Denver Eye Screening Test (DEST, 1973). Visual acuity may reach 20/20 as early as 6 months of age.

Preschool hearing testing should be done at the same time that preschool vision testing is done. Because the development of speech depends on the child's ability to hear, the nonhearing child is generally diagnosed before the preschool period (Thompson & Thompson, 1991). Occasionally a child of this age who has been treated for retardation will be found to have severe hearing loss.

An otoscopic examination is an important part of each health appraisal during the preschool years. Preschoolers are particularly prone to upper respiratory infections and secondary ear infections. After a few ear infections, the tympanic membrane may become stretched or perforated so that the child no longer expresses discomfort when infections do occur; therefore, the condition of the internal ear should be monitored regularly.

Anticipatory Guidance: Vision and Hearing

Although the Snellen E test or the DEST (1973) for visual acuity can identify many visual problems while they are still treatable, parents should be informed that these tests in no way replace an ophthalmic examination. This examination should be conducted at each health appraisal or whenever the parents notice any behaviors in their preschooler that suggest visual problems (frequent eye rubbing, squinting, attention span deficit).

Parents should be encouraged to take advantage of organized preschool vision screening programs. A nursing research study conducted to evaluate the effectiveness of preschool vision, hearing, and developmental screening found that performance was significantly improved at school age (Sullivan, 1988). These findings provide support for screening programs as a means of early intervention and remediation of problems. These programs, however, are far from reaching all the children in this age group who need to be screened. Nurses can help make these programs available in areas where they do not exist and can make parents aware of those that do exist. Home test kits are also available to parents, especially those who live in areas where this screening does not exist. These kits can be obtained from the National Society for the Prevention of Blindness.

Eye safety should be taught to preschoolers and their parents. Most eye injuries are preventable, and they can cause blindness. Usually they are caused when children throw small objects at their siblings or friends. Children should be taught to use silverware for eating, not as weapons, and preschoolers should never play with knives, darts, or sticks. At this age they should be well supervised during play activities. Toys should be inspected: those with small removable parts and those that can become dangerous weapons should not be allowed.

Parents should be instructed to report promptly any behaviors suggestive of hearing loss in their preschooler, such as playing alone despite the availability of peers for cooperative play, delays in speech development, or lack of response to repeated requests made in normal voice tones. Some experts suggest that excessive noise levels, such as generated by firecrackers, can cause hearing loss (Eavey, 1992).

Dental Care

Preschoolers have all their primary teeth. For most children, permanent teeth do not begin erupting until early school age. Toothbrushing should be a regular activity. Maintenance of primary teeth is the major emphasis of anticipatory guidance during the preschool years, including the first dental visit at age 3 years.

Thumb sucking, begun in infancy, sometimes persists during preschool years. Dentists usually do not express concern about thumb sucking until the permanent teeth begin erupting. The older preschooler can usually be reasoned with to attempt abandoning this habit, if it has persisted to this time.

Anticipatory Guidance: Dental Care

Because preschoolers enjoy imitating others, it is good for them to observe adults toothbrushing. A nursing research study (Hitchens-Serota, 1986) assessing parental knowledge of dental care revealed the following results. Most parents of preschoolers had not received information on dental care. Tooth care and toothbrushing were initiated later than American Dental Association recommendations, and bedtime bottles contained fluids other than water. The results of this study support the need for nurses to provide preventive dental care as a component of anticipatory guidance for parents of preschoolers.

Parents should monitor the child's toothbrushing and assist the preschooler in brushing at least once a day. Most dentists encourage the use of dental floss to clean between the teeth once the spacing between the teeth that exists in young children has disappeared. Usually flossing must be completed by the parent, since a great deal of manual dexterity is required. Nursing diagnostic responses and interventions to promote dental health are identified in Table 7–10.

Sleep Behaviors

The preschooler seems to have an endless supply of energy and may be "on the go" continually. Parents need to be aware of this and initiate rest periods or periods of quiet activity, such as reading. The 3-year-olds need from 10 to 14 hours of sleep daily. They

TABLE 7-10
Promoting Dental Health

Analysis: Nursing Diagnostic Statement

Response and Related or Risk Factors: *Altered health maintenance: risk factor knowledge deficit: care of deciduous teeth; associated risks*

- Lack of exposure to information
- Lack of recall
- Information misinterpretation
- Cognitive limitation
- Lack of motivation to learn

Nursing Interventions

- Provide information about the importance of the child's teeth
- Teach basics of dental care to parents and child as appropriate
  - Limit intake of foods with high sugar content
  - Supplement with fluoride as necessary
  - Take child to dentist by 2 yrs of age (some recommend 1 yr of age)
- Provide information to child as appropriate for age and setting (use teaching opportunities in school, camp, or other settings)
- Explain relationship of healthy deciduous teeth to later dental health
- Reinforce information on each subsequent visit

Analysis: Nursing Diagnostic Statement

Response and Related or Risk Factors: *High risk for self-care deficit: dental care; risk factors*

- Lack of necessary developmental skills to perform care
- Lack of opportunity to practice skills
- Lack of knowledge
- Lack of appropriate equipment and supplies

Nursing Interventions

- Promote self-care of teeth as appropriate for age
- Encourage parents to
  - Monitor toothbrushing by preschoolers
  - Use disclosing tablets to show children whether toothbrushing is adequate
  - Teach 8- to 9-year-olds to floss teeth
  - Role model regular dental care
  - Foster child's independence in dental care, beginning in the toddler years
  - Have appropriate-size brush, dental floss, and mirror available for child to use
  - Give fluoride supplement as required
  - If sweet snacks are permitted, offer them *with* meals, rather than between meals
- Provide assistance with equipment and teaching for children with physical or developmental disabilities

Analysis: Nursing Diagnostic Statement

Response and Related or Risk Factors: *High risk for fear: dental visit; risk factors*

- Learned response as modeled by parents or siblings
- Separation from support systems
- Knowledge deficit
- Forbidding appearance of equipment
- Lack of preparation

(continued)

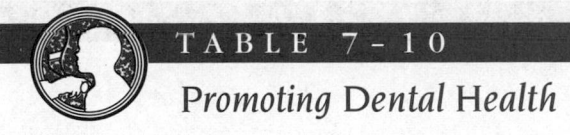

TABLE 7-10 *(continued)*

Nursing Interventions

- Allay child's fears of visiting the dentist
- Encourage parents to
  - Permit child to accompany parents on a dental visit to observe
  - Provide factual and sensory information about the environment and painful stimuli
  - Stay with child during the dental examination

Analysis: Nursing Diagnostic Statement

Response and Related or Risk Factors: *High risk for impaired skin integrity: gums and mouth; risk factors*

- Inadequate brushing and flossing of teeth

Nursing Interventions

- Maintain skin integrity of gums and mouth
- Teach family to
  - Teach child proper toothbrushing techniques
  - Monitor and periodically supervise child's toothbrushing and flossing techniques
  - Provide healthy diet
  - Restrict child's sugar intake
  - Maintain regular dental appointments

may still nap during the day or at least rest quietly for 1 to 2 hours. By 5 years of age, the sleep requirement is down to 9 to 13 hours, and the child seldom naps. Ritualistic bedtime routines continue during the preschool years and can be used as a means to postpone bedtime (Table 7–11).

Many preschoolers fear the dark, and this fear is exaggerated when they are exposed to ghost stories, scary television programs, or very active play before bedtime. In addition, the child of this age has a vivid imagination, and at night in the dark, stuffed animals, designs on wallpaper, rustling leaves, and blowing branches become frightening objects. Many preschoolers have dreams and nightmares that wake them during the night.

Nightmares and Night Terrors

Night terrors must be differentiated from the more common nightmare (Table 7–12 describes each). Sleep problems, particularly night terrors, peak during the preschool years, whereas nightmares are seen more frequently in older children (Wender, 1984). Dreams are an essential part of sleep and nightly average five or more in number (Herbert, 1975). Young children confuse waking and dreaming experiences easily, and their dreams are extremely vivid and real; thus, a dream may frighten a child, regardless of whether it is pleasant or scary, simply because it looms as being so real. The fright is heightened by the fact that dreams usually focus on the dreamer as

TABLE 7-11
Preschooler Developmental Characteristics of Sleep-Related Behavior (3 to 5 Years)

Characteristic Sleep-Related Behaviors	Promotion of Sleep-Related Health
Some children continue to need an afternoon nap (1–2 hrs), whereas others do not	A rest period after lunch should be encouraged, even though child does not sleep
Imagination and fantasies result in dreaming and increasing fears of the dark	Bedtime stories should not contain scary themes
Nightmares and night terrors are characteristic of this age; fear of going to sleep may be related to fear of having a bad dream	Some form of lighting is often required
12–14 hrs of sleep per 24 hrs	

TABLE 7-12
Family-Centered Teaching: Characteristics and Management of Sleep Disturbances

Nightmares		
Psychologic motivation: anxiety expressed, worked through in negative theme; occurs during rapid-eye-movement (REM) sleep; if child awakens, can recall all or most of dream—no recall if not awakened	Moves around restlessly in bed, may whimper or cry but not hysterically; may or may not wake; face may show facial grimace or expression of fear	Do not overreact. If child cries, parent who wishes to respond should satisfy self that nothing is wrong (not caught in blankets, not fallen out of bed, no fever) then leave without waking child. If child awakens, give reassurance that it was only a dream and child can safely go back to sleep. Then leave; making a fuss over the child only reinforces the behavior
Night Terrors		
Psychologic motivation: result of immature CNS function; psychologic factors determine theme. Occurs during non–rapid-eye-movement (NREM) sleep. Child usually can recall only a single frightening image, if anything; usually repetitive	Sits up in bed screaming, or assumes bizarre crouching posture; pulse and respirations increase, pupils dilate; senses doom, intensely anxious and agitated; appears to be staring at something with eyes wide open; is disoriented; does not recognize persons who respond to the distress but will gradually respond to a soothing voice	Although the child does not recognize the adult who responds to the shrieks, reassurance and cuddling do eventually calm the child, allowing return to sleep. One can do little to alter the course of events during the episode

From Herbert, M. (1975). *Problems of childhood*. Baltimore, MD: Paul Brooks, Ltd.; Wender, E. (1984). Common behavior problems in preschool children. In P. Shelov, et al. (Eds.), *Primary care pediatrics: A symptomatic approach* (pp. 265–282). Norwalk, CT: Appleton-Century-Crofts; Ferber, R. (1985). Sleep disorders in infants and children. In T. Riley (Ed.), *Clinical aspects of sleep and sleep disturbance*. Stoneham, MA: Butterworth; and Anders, T. (1987). Nightmares and other sleep disturbances. *In* R. Hoekelman et al (eds.), *Primary pediatric care* (pp 744–748). St. Louis: CV Mosby.

the active participant or central figure, rather than as a passive observer.

A young child's dream life is influenced by life experiences and circumstances. Dreams are more likely to be negative during periods of poor health or family stress. A negative-theme dream life is also more likely to occur in children who display exaggerated fear of the dark. Most children express some fear of the dark during the preschool years, but those exposed to significant others (parents, siblings, peers) who show apprehension of the dark, those for whom darkness has been used as a punishment, and those for whom death has been equated with sleep are most at risk of developing fear of the dark. The fear of darkness expressed by a child is best acknowledged as real and should be combined with a program of positive reinforcement and weaning from the fear. Two weaning programs that have been successful with preschoolers are described in Table 7–13.

Disturbed Psychodynamics and Clinical Manifestations

Normal sleep disturbances in young children are basically temporary and show a variety of themes. A recurrent negative theme that exists over time is symptomatic of some underlying emotional disturbance

TABLE 7-13
Family-Centered Teaching: Managing Fear of the Dark

Program 1

Leave a lamp on in the child's room, on the floor near the bed. Gradually move it farther from the bed and eventually out of the room. How quickly this can be done will vary with the child. (The average is to move it farther away every two or three nights.) If the lamp is moved and the child reacts negatively, move it back to its former position for a few more nights, then try again. Once the lamp is out of the room for a few nights, turn it off after the child is asleep. Then, a few nights later, try not turning it on at all. The child who tolerates that for several nights has been weaned from fear, and the lamp can be removed completely. If the child regresses during illness or other upset, go to the room and give comfort but without holding her or him or turning on the light, and the child will overcome the fear.

Program 2

Place the child in bed with the room light on, but turn it off once the child is asleep, keeping the door of the room open and a hall light on. During the daytime, teach the child how to turn the light on during the night. Once the child knows how to do it, the parent praises the child as a big boy or girl who can be responsible to turn it on as wanted at night, and enforces that expectation. Each time the child turns on the light, the parent turns it off again after the child returns to sleep. The child will eventually tire of getting up to turn on the light and will just go back to sleep.

that needs intervention. Fortunately, children express their feelings simply and clearly in their dream life, seldom with the distortion of symbolism typical of adult dreams. Therefore the problem is usually identifiable within the child's description of the dream. Nightmares may be stimulated by disturbing or overly exciting experiences or by repressed unacceptable feelings of rivalry, hostility, or sexual attraction to the parent (Prugh, 1983). Nightmares arise out of rapid-eye-movement (REM) sleep and involve imagery occurring over time and as a story (Ferber, 1985). The child is fully awake after a nightmare and can usually recall parts of it.

Night terrors differ from nightmares in pathology. The child is not fully awake, appears to be hallucinating, and is difficult to awaken and comfort. They occur at the moment of arousal from slow-wave sleep and are associated with little or no imagery. Usually, the child has no memory of the experience. Table 7–12 describes the characteristics of these dream patterns and how each is most effectively managed.

Anticipatory Guidance: Nightmares and Night Terrors

The definitive action to be taken in alleviating nightmares is to identify the underlying cause and eliminate it. This requires an evaluation of the child's reactions to various situations, coupled with consideration of the content of the nightmares (again, children do not dream symbolically). Parents may need assistance with this process, or they may require a psychology expert's input.

Intervention to diminish night terrors is less easily accomplished. Because central nervous system immaturity is a primary factor, terrors cannot be completely eliminated until the central nervous system becomes more mature. Actions can be taken to eliminate environmental or psychologic stresses that may be intensifying or increasing the frequency of the night terrors. This is done as for nightmares, although professional assistance to decipher the dream may be needed, since the child often recalls only a single image.

Anticipatory Guidance: Sleep Behaviors

Parents may need guidance in the management of sleep behaviors common to preschoolers. The preschooler's wish to postpone bedtime can be dealt with in various ways. Usually a consistent, regular routine, such as taking a favorite toy or blanket to bed followed by a story and prayers of a specified time limit, encourages readiness for bed. The endless "drink of water" and "go to the bathroom" tactics can be minimized by incorporating these two activities into the bedtime routine. Solutions to the problem of bedtime fears include monitoring television, keeping play quiet before bedtime, removing objects that can appear scary at night, and leaving a night light on.

Preparing a child for bed by following the same routine each night promotes more successful bedtime experiences for parents and children. Bedtime routines become particularly important during the preschool age, when the struggle for autonomy and self-control influences behavior. Routines of the necessary activities of bath, toothbrushing, toileting, and undressing are established and maintained. Young children cooperate when they are not asked to adapt to new situations. Particularly at this developmental level, routines provide an element of security at a time when children resist being separated from their parents.

Maintaining a positive attitude promotes successful bedtime experiences. Parents should be encouraged to avoid reprimand and discussion of unpleasant happenings of the day. Pleasant experiences and positive feelings should be reinforced to provide the child with a feeling of contentment and acceptance.

Bedtime could become a time of conflict and frustration. Limit setting is essential to preventing unreasonable requests and expectations from a child. Preparing a child for bedtime and following through with the stated bedtime is important. A child who resists bedtime should not be granted a later hour for bedtime because of the degree of insistence. This practice promotes additional resisting efforts, because the behavior is reinforced. After the usual reading time, bedtime snack, and drink of water have been provided, additional requests should be handled firmly, without, however, becoming insensitively rigid and missing the special needs that children have at bedtime.

Regardless of the child's sleep problem and its frequency, parents should be cautioned by the nurse not to overreact to the child's behavior, or the child will learn to use the sleep disturbance to manipulate them. Discussion of family tensions and conflicts may be appropriate when the problem is marked or persistent. Occasionally, the child and family may need referral for psychotherapy.

When terrifying nightmares wake preschoolers, they need reassurance that they are safe and that the dream only seemed to be real. An understanding parent sitting with the child and placing a light to reassure the child of her or his safety is much preferable to taking the child into the parent's bed, which can easily become a habit that is very difficult to break. When these measures do not effectively manage the sleep disturbances or fears, additional evaluation and counseling are appropriate.

Nutrition

Nutritional Requirements

Nutrition for preschool children includes the same basic five groups of food needed by adults. Their growth remains stable throughout the preschool years. Their curiosity about what is happening around them persists, so they may have little interest in eating.

Calories from proteins and carbohydrates are essential for muscle growth in the preschooler. The child in the 3- to 5-year-old range requires from 90 to 100 kcal/kg of body weight per day. Water, an essential element for life, constitutes approximately 60 per cent of the child's body weight. The principal source of water in the diet is fluids, although many fruits and vegetables that children eat are up to 90 per cent water. The average daily requirement of water for the child of 3 to 5 years is 100 to 125 ml/kg (1.5 to 2.0 oz/lb) of body weight. Protein requirements for the preschool age child are 2 to 3 g/kg (0.9 to 1.35 g/lb) of body weight. See Table 7–14 for vitamin, mineral, and other dietary requirements during the preschool years.

Childhood obesity is a serious health problem. It is estimated that 5 to 15 per cent of children are obese, and this number is growing (National Institutes of Health Consensus Development Conference Statement, 1985). Predictors of adult obesity have been correlated with childhood obesity from as early as 4 years of age (Garn & La Velle, 1985). During childhood the child learns and establishes eating patterns that can last a lifetime. Parents and other caregivers serve as influential nutritional role models for the child.

It is from their adult models that children learn what to eat, how to eat, and how much to eat. Other risk factors for obesity identified by nurse researchers (Alexander & Blank, 1988) include parental nutritional knowledge, feeding practices, and parental values. Additional risk factors identified were select demographic variables, such as lower socioeconomic status, presence of a male in the household, mother's mari-

TABLE 7-14

Recommended Food Intake for Good Nutrition According to Food Groups and Daily Dietary Allowances: Preschool (4 to 6 Years)

Food Groups	Servings Per Day	Serving Size: 4–5 yrs	Serving Size: 6 yrs
Bread Group	4–6		
• Bread		1½ slice	1–2 slices
• Cereal		1 oz	1 oz
• Rice and pasta		½ C	½ C
Vegetable Group	3–5 total		
• Green-yellow vegetables (vitamin A source)	1 or more	4 tbsp	4 tbsp
• Other vegetables	2 or more	4 tbsp	⅓ C
Fruit Group	At least 3 total		
• Citrus fruits, berries, tomato, cabbage, cantaloupe (vitamin C source)	1 or more	½ C	1 medium
• Other fruits (apple, banana)	2	¼ C	⅓ C
Milk Group	2–3		
• Milk/yogurt		½–¾ C	½–1 C
• Cheese		(1.5 oz cheese = 1 C milk)	
Meat Group	2		
• Cooked lean meat, poultry, fish		4 tbsp	4–6 tbsp
• Dry beans		½ C	½ C
• Egg		1	1
• Peanut butter		2 tbsp	2–3 tbsp
Fats, oils, and sweets—USE SPARINGLY			

Recommended Daily Dietary Allowances

Protein	Fat-Soluble Vitamins		Water-Soluble Vitamins		Minerals		Energy Needs
24 g	Vitamin A	500 μg RE	Vitamin C	45 mg	Calcium	800 mg	1800 kcal
	Vitamin D	10 μg	Thiamine	0.9 mg	Phosphorus	800 mg	
	Vitamin E	7 mg α—TE	Riboflavin	1.1 mg	Magnesium	120 mg	
	Vitamin K	20 μg	Niacin	12 mg NE	Iron	10 mg	
			Vitamin B_6	1.1 mg	Zinc	10 mg	
			Folate	75 μg	Iodine	90 μg	
			Vitamin B_{12}	1.0 μg	Selenium	20 μg	

Data reprinted with permission from *Recommended dietary allowances: 10th edition*. Copyright 1989 by the National Academy of Sciences. Published by the National Academy Press, Washington, D.C.; and U.S. Department of Agriculture, Human Nutrition Information Service. (1992). *Food guide pyramid* (Leaflet No. 572). Washington, DC: Author.

Key: RE, retinol equivalent; TE, tocopherol equivalent; NE, niacin equivalent.

tal status, maternal body mass index, and weight status of siblings. This period of childhood is the key to establishing a healthy approach to nutrition and physical activity.

Eating Behaviors

Mealtime for the preschooler should be a happy time within a warm atmosphere. It should be regular and should include all present family members. A planned quiet period for the preschooler and siblings may be necessary before the mealtime. Conversation should include the preschooler.

Table manners at this age are best learned from observation and should not be stressed. Parents should not expect the child to use better table manners than they use. Mealtime spills should be accepted, cleaned up, and forgotten.

Because preschoolers grow at a relatively slow rate, they have a small appetite. Serving small portions with "seconds" allowed or allowing children to serve themselves is preferable to serving more food than the child can eat. It is normal for the child to want more food on some days than on others (this occurs in adults), but some parents tend to think that children should always eat a specific amount of food each day.

All preschoolers still enjoy finger foods; these should be offered in some form at mealtime. By the age of 4 years, most children can use a fork and can spread with a knife. Many 5-year-olds are able to cut their meat with a knife. All food should be served in small amounts so that children can handle it easily. As they learn colors, they become more aware of food colors and may prefer brightly colored foods to dull ones.

Nursing Interventions: Nutrition

Awareness of the risk factors for childhood obesity can alert the nurse to assess for these factors. The nurse assesses the child and family for the following: fat or chubby child, overweight siblings, maternal obesity, multiple caregivers, nutritional knowledge, feeding/dietary practices, family values, and low socioeconomic status (Sherman & Alexander, 1990). Prevention efforts by the nurse, in the hospital or in community settings, may reduce the rise in numbers of obese children (Jonides, 1990).

Anticipatory Guidance: Nutrition

Attitudes about foods and eating habits formed during early childhood will last throughout life. One should introduce children to new and different foods so that they can learn more about the world around them. A variety of foods increases the child's ability to select and accept foods that contribute to a well-balanced diet. New foods should be introduced gradually and include a variety of tastes, colors, and consistencies. It is essential that foods introduced to the preschooler be accepted by adults in the home and eaten by them at mealtimes. Most preschoolers will try new foods, owing to their initiative, but will refuse them if other family members make disparaging remarks.

Parents exert tremendous control over what their preschool child eats, because they are responsible for the planning, preparing, and serving of meals. It therefore is essential that parents understand the concepts of the basic five food groups, the child's daily nutritional requirements, and their influential role in shaping their child's eating behavior. To enhance family involvement, anticipatory guidance should address the cultural preference and economic considerations affecting the family.

Between-meal snacks should be planned at appropriate intervals and should consist of juice, fresh fruits or raw vegetables, cheese, peanut butter on crackers, and other similar foods. Sweet foods should be offered infrequently, as they tend to contribute to dental caries, malnutrition, and obesity. Snack time should be supervised. Snacks should not be given just before mealtimes.

If the child is growing in accordance with height and weight charts for age and is happy and healthy, plays well, and has healthy teeth, parents should be advised that "not eating a thing" is probably a result of the normal decrease in appetite for the age. It is important for the nurse to go over proper diet with the parent(s) and explain the role of junk food in decreasing appetite. If the diet seems adequate, it usually is not necessary for the child to be taking supplemental vitamins.

Bowel and Bladder Control

The preschooler has bowel control and daytime bladder control, as these skills usually have been learned during the toddler period. Some young preschoolers may have accidents if they become absorbed in play, so they need to be reminded to take time to go to the bathroom. Nighttime bladder control is usually accomplished between 3 and 4 years of age. By 4 years of age, children can usually manage their own clothing at elimination, and by 5 years they are completely responsible for the entire process (Fig. 7–5).

The average urinary output in a 24-hour period for the preschooler is 500 to 780 ml. The 5-year-old voids about four to six times a day while awake and generally sleeps through the night without waking up to void.

Anticipatory Guidance: Bowel and Bladder Control

The nurse should help parents understand that the occasional bowel or bladder accidents, or both, are to be expected during the preschool years and that punishment will not alter this fact. Children are old enough to take responsibility for cleaning themselves and changing clothing at such times with only minimal parental assistance. Periodic reminders and

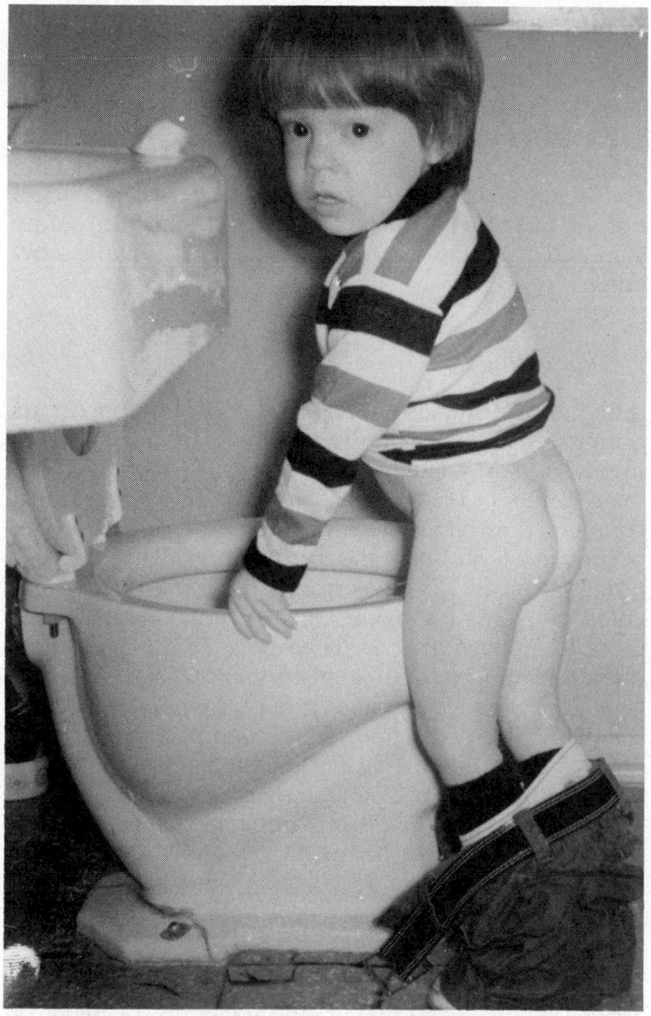

FIGURE 7-5. By 4 yr of age, preschoolers may be independent in using the toilet. (Photograph by David Trainor.)

checks on the child's use of hygienic measures during elimination, especially girl's use of front to back wiping, are appropriate during the preschool period.

Play

Imaginary play is a predominant form of preschool play activity. Preschoolers play house using what they observe at home, and if there are older siblings in the home, they play school (Fig. 7–6). As toddlers they played alone, even if side by side with another toddler (parallel play). This play time was spent learning to use fingers and manipulate objects. The preschooler is more coordinated and is experienced in manipulation, so these activities take up much less time.

Young preschoolers start to play with at least one other preschooler *(cooperative play)*. They still remain somewhat selfish but are more interested in what is going on around them. By the age of 4 years, they have a long attention span and play with groups of children. Much of this play is noisy, aggressive, and

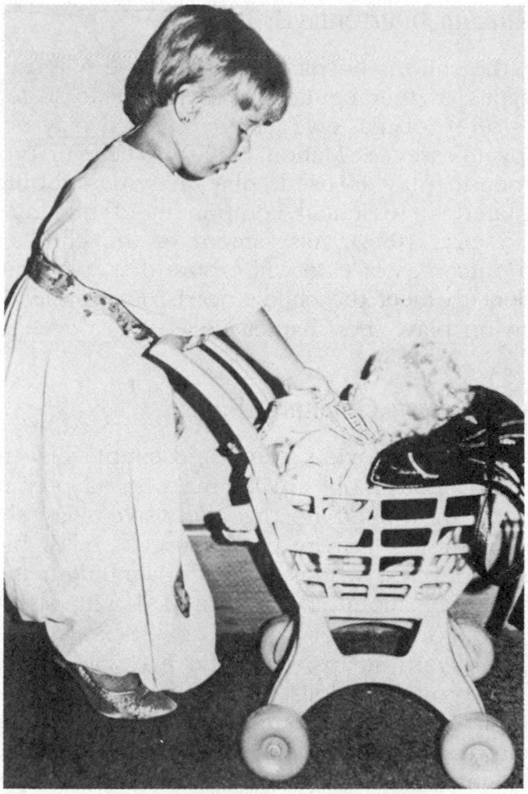

FIGURE 7-6. The preschooler loves to pretend.

dramatic. When children reach 5 years of age, they can play simple games with other children and can share with them. All preschoolers like quiet times involving such activities as coloring, pasting, cutting, and being read to. They also like noisy, boisterous activities, active games, riding tricycles, playing with cars and trucks, playing with water, mud, snow, leaves, and other outdoor activities. Preschoolers enjoy getting wet and getting dirty and frequently do so (Fig. 7–7).

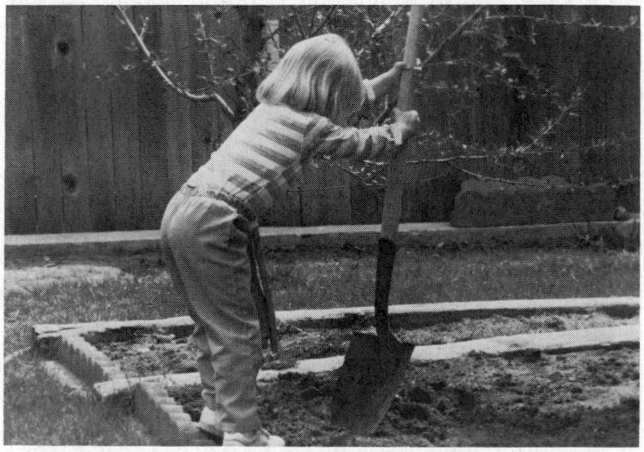

FIGURE 7-7. Increased coordination and strength of large-muscle groups allow preschoolers to attempt increasingly difficult tasks. This preschooler is helping plant a garden.

Nursing Interventions: Play

While the child is hospitalized, the nurse will use several types of therapeutic play activities to foster the child's sense of mastery, such as medical play or play therapy (Vessey & Mahon, 1990). Whatever type of therapeutic play is used, play activities should be considered an essential component of nursing care (McClowery, 1993). Assessment of the child's projected outcomes of care will ensure that "play care" is sufficient to meet the child's needs. For further information on play, see Chapter 17.

Anticipatory Guidance: Play

Parents should provide sturdy and simple play materials. Many household articles make good play materials, and they need not be expensive. Play should provide physical activity by the use of balls, blocks, wagons, tricycles, swings, and safe climbing materials. Creative play should be encouraged with sheets of paper, crayons, finger paints, clay, scissors, boxes, cloth, and yarn scraps. Dramatic play can be stimulated by providing dolls, cars, and dress-up clothes. Quiet play can be encouraged with books, records, and puzzles. Parents should provide opportunity, equipment, space, and safety during play, but they should avoid attempting to structure the child's play (Table 7–15).

Safety Concerns

The most frequently occurring accidents that occur during the preschool years are motor vehicle accidents, drowning, burns, poisonings, falls, and bodily damage (Table 7–16).

Motor vehicle accidents are the leading cause of accident mortality of children 1 year and older. They are the cause of 33 per cent of all accidental deaths in preschool boys and 40 per cent among girls. Motor vehicle accidents involving preschoolers were most often due to pedestrian traffic accidents. Generally, the preschooler has gained proficiency in walking and running but lacks awareness of the potential danger in carelessly crossing the street. Annually, over 48,000 children are seriously injured in motor vehicle accidents.

Drowning ranks as the second leading cause of death for preschool boys and third as the cause of death for preschool girls. Preschool children have a natural curiosity that leads them to explore. They lack both the experience and the knowledge to assess a hazardous situation accurately. Even after a child has had swimming classes, the child should not be considered water safe. Parental supervision is necessary (Coffman, 1991).

Children must be supervised closely when near bodies of water such as lakes, pools, and rivers. They should be wearing a life preserver at all times when playing on the shore of the ocean or river. Ideally, children are instructed on how to swim and on water safety. The preschooler should not be allowed to play with toys near the pool or to leave play items, such as the tricycle, at poolside. See Chapter 6 and Table 6–18 for additional information on prevention of drownings. Pool safety includes secured fencing and being locked. The pool should be covered when not in use. Some pool coverings include a safety alarm that is activated if someone falls on the covering.

Poisonings

Although the highest prevalence of poisoning occurs during toddlerhood, large numbers of preschoolers ingest poisonous materials. Ingestion of lead and toxic amounts of vitamins and aspirin are the most common poisonings in preschoolers. Lead poisoning occurs most often in the preschooler. This child is usually a pica eater (eats nonfood substances). A few chips of paint, for example, may contain 200 times the safe amount of lead. Lead poisoning occurs most often in families with a history of pica eaters and from lower socioeconomic groups. Aspirin poisoning is one of the most frequently occurring poisonings. One of the problems is that children's aspirin has an appealing taste, which encourages the child to eat it. The vitamins that manifest symptoms when ingested in toxic amounts are A and D.

Anticipatory Guidance: Safety

The preschooler is old enough to start learning about safety. The desire to imitate and the sense of initiative assist in the ability to learn safety measures. Parents should take advantage of this readiness and teach the rationale for safety rules. For example, preschoolers can comprehend why it is dangerous to cross the street. They are old enough to learn to look both ways before crossing streets and to cross busy streets only with a green light, if available, or with an adult.

Pedestrian injuries are higher across all age groups, except for male adolescents and for African-American children, compared with white children (Children's Safety Network, 1991). It is speculated that the higher injury rate for African-American children may reflect fewer off-street play areas (Malek et al, 1990). Also children have limited ability to judge the speed of the moving vehicle and its actual distance from them. Most pedestrian accidents occur as the child attempts to dart out from parked cars into the street.

A school training program to educate preschoolers about street-crossing skills was demonstrated to be effective (Rivara et al, 1991). The school nurse can assume a leading role in developing and implementing a pedestrian accident prevention program.

Car accidents are still a leading cause of injury to preschoolers, and parents need to explain the rationale for use of car seats and seat belts. It is estimated that 72 per cent of 4-year-olds routinely use seat belts

TABLE 7-15
Toys and Play Activities for Preschooler

Toy or Play Activity	Development Promoted	Selection Criteria
Jungle gym	Fosters active play (P)	Adult supervision
Teeter ball	Fosters gross and fine motor strength and skill (P)	
Mallet and peg set	Fosters fine motor strength and skill (P)	Durable
Tool bench	Provides outlet for aggression (E)	Nonbreakable
Beanbag game	Fosters fine and gross motor strength and skill (P)	Durable
Ringtoss game	Stimulates sharing (S)	Low fulcrum with handle near seat area
Croquet sets	Stimulates group participation (S)	
Seesaw		
Jump rope		
Construction sets	Stimulates creative play (C)	Large pieces
Legg-O	Stimulates problem solving (C)	
Simple crafts	Causes preoccupation with parts, not the whole (C)	
Simple jigsaw puzzles	Fosters artistic development (C)	
Scissors and paste		Blunt, unbreakable
Modeling clay		Nontoxic
Painting sets		
Tricycle and transport toys	Teaches motor skills and coordination (P)	Low center of balance; rounded edges
Skates		Safety helmet properly equipped
		Use in safe-designed areas
Toy theater	Fosters creativity (C)	Durable
Medical kits	Provides outlet for emotional expression (E)	Rounded edges
Toy musical instruments	Stimulates imagination (C)	Stable; does not tip easily
Puppets	Stimulates imitation (C)	
Playhouse		
Make-believe stores		
Dolls		
Costumes		
Stamps and albums	Fosters cognitive skills (C)	Basic shapes
Map puzzles	Fosters interest and knowledge of environment (C/S)	Large and easily recognized objects/subjects
Counting games	Aids in school activities (C)	Durable
Collection books (birds and animals)	Encourages responsibility (E)	
"Dress-up"	Provides opportunity for role play (S)	
Playing cowboys, family roles	Stimulates interaction with others (E, S)	
Housekeeping toys	Aids in development of gender identification (S)	
Occupational clothing, fireman/ nurse costumes		
Small pet	Encourages responsibility and social interaction with animal (E, S)	Vaccinated
		Gentle
	Encourages attachment (E)	Does not bite/chew
Excursions	Helps build self-confidence (E)	Supervision
Outdoor trips	Stimulates social interaction and participation in group activities (C)	
	Aids in school activities (C)	
Balls	Stimulates hand-eye coordination (C)	Rubber/soft material
	Fosters fine and gross motor development (P)	
Magic games	Stimulates problem solving (C)	May need to limit use
Computer games	Stimulates peer interactions (S)	
Hide and seek	Stimulates group interaction (S)	Unable to follow rules consistently
Four-square	Promotes organized thinking (C)	
Simple races		

Adapted from Betz, C., & Posler, E. (1984). Incorporating play into the care of the hospitalized child. *Issues in Comprehensive Pediatric Nursing, 7,* 343–354; Florey, L. (1971). An approach to play and play development. *American Journal of Occupational Therapy, 25,* 275–280; Lee, J., & Fowler, M. (1986). Merely child's play and developmental work and playthings. *Journal of Pediatric Nursing, 1,* 260–269; and Betz, C. (1983). Teaching children through play therapy. *Journal of the Association of Operating Room Nurses, 88*(4), 709, 712–713, 716–717.

Key: C = cognitive development; P = physical development; E = emotional development; S = social development.

TABLE 7-16
Safety Developmental Concerns and Prevention Interventions

Developmental Stage: Preschool (3 to 5 Yrs)	**Prevention Interventions: Teach Child All Aspects of Safety**
Eager to learn and capable of understanding simple explanations Has the motor and coordination skills to ride a tricycle and is learning to ride a bicycle Curious and explorative, particularly outdoors Active in playground and outdoor play Motor abilities exceed cognitive skills; therefore, child engages in physical activities without foreseeing danger Is more independent and may walk or ride bike in the neighborhood with less supervision than when a toddler Engages in sex play Engages in dramatic play	Motor vehicle, pedestrian, cycle accidents • Begin to teach how to cross street safely • Teach rules of the road • Teach purpose of car seats and seat belts Falls, trauma • Caution against climbing into unsafe areas, marshy lands, drainage pipes, unsafe building • Teach child how to handle scissors Suffocation, aspiration • Teach child not to run while eating • Teach child not to crawl into areas where he or she could be entrapped (refrigerators, drainage pipes, excavation areas) Burns • Teach fire escape rules • Caution child against playing with matches • Keep matches out of reach Drowning • Begin organized swimming lessons • Never leave alone in bath or while swimming Street safety • Teach child not to accept rides or foods without permission of parents Bodily injury • Teach child not to insert objects into body orifices Ingestion, inhalation • Expand on teaching about poisons and medicines • Include teaching about cosmetics and sprays, which child may use in playing house

(Nation's Health, 1988). However, of this number, approximately two-thirds are using seat belts improperly (NAACOG, 1987). Nurse researchers Arneson and Triplett (1990) found that preschool children's knowledge of automobile safety, but not their use of seat belts, improved significantly following an education program. The researchers concluded that preschool children can learn self-care skills but require parental involvement to use seat belts. If children observe their parents wearing seat belts consistently, they will be more likely to comply. When the child is too short to see out of the car window, a car seat causes less resistance than does restraint by a seat belt.

The nurse should counsel parents *never to leave a child alone in a car, even for a few minutes,* awake or asleep. A preschooler can quickly set a car into motion while imitating the parent driving. The child could also climb out of the car and be injured by other cars or might get lost. Although it takes longer to unbuckle a child and take him or her into the store for a moment, the safety of the child is ensured by doing so. The preschooler is not mature enough to be left alone at home or to be responsible for self or siblings.

Preschoolers sometimes get into trouble while playing outside and hiding from others. Poor judgment and lack of experience may lead preschoolers into dangerous hiding places, such as under cars or in abandoned refrigerators, freezers, and buildings. They should be taught to refuse to talk to strangers and to refuse rides and gifts from them. Preschoolers should also know their own names, addresses, and telephone numbers and how to approach a police officer for help.

Sun Protection

Children are vulnerable to acute and chronic injury to the skin caused by exposure to the sun. Children spend far more time outdoors in the sun, compared with adults. It is estimated that by age 18 years, one receives most of one's lifetime radiation dose from exposure to the sun (Nicol, 1989). In spite of this fact, sunscreen for children and other protective measures are not widely used (Stern et al, 1986). For further information on sun protection, refer to Chapter 38.

Anticipatory Guidance: Sun Protection

Nurses can educate parents about the potential risks of skin overexposure to the sun. Parents can be educated about the type of sunscreen to use, method of application, and limits on sun exposure. Parents can be instructed on methods of sun avoidance and physical protection. The child should avoid playing in the intense sunlight between 10 A.M. and 3 P.M. Wearing protective clothing, such as long-sleeved shirts and brimmed headgear, is helpful.

Sex Education

The preschooler needs to learn what behaviors, including language, are socially acceptable and appropriate. The use of sexual terms for name calling may occur as children repeat words they overhear. The parents' value system determines what language is considered acceptable. Parents can control the use of such language by not overreacting but by matter-of-factly stating that these are not words their family uses.

The preschooler learns to respect the privacy of others using the bathroom and the need of parents to retreat to their own bedroom. Finding that others have times when and places in which they wish to be alone allows the child to learn to value privacy.

The sex education of the preschooler is a continuation of information given in earlier years. Even though a toddler was given correct terms and accurate explanations of how babies are born, this information may need to be repeated when the child is older, with more detail given as time and experience allow. Questions can be answered simply and directly.

The preschooler also needs to learn to say "No" to adults or older children whose intention may be to exploit the child sexually. Although this should not be stressed to children to the extent that they become suspicious of all adults, sexual abuse of young children by adults whom they have trusted does occur, and it is necessary to teach children assertiveness while minimizing fear. (Recognition of sexual abuse and interventions are discussed in Chapter 28.)

Sex education is influenced for good or ill by the quality of a child's interpersonal relationships. Before children have reached 3 years of age, some of the most important lessons in sex education have already been assimilated. For the first 5 years, parents transmit to their children information and a sense of values about sexuality (Aquilino & Ely, 1985). Early bodily care in an atmosphere of affection makes it possible for children to discover, love, and respect themselves. Later, it teaches them to receive and give love and to develop an interest in assuming responsibility for themselves and, eventually, for others.

Anticipatory Guidance: Sex Education

Children's questions indicate that they have been pondering the subject of sex and are now ready to learn about it. However, they can assimilate only one idea at a time. This means that they may require repeated explanations before they can use facts to solve their problems. Because children persist in asking questions, adults should not conclude that they are obsessed with the subject. They are merely trying to piece together observations to gain some understanding of themselves in a two-gender world. Their quick transition from questions about sex to queries about other subjects proves that they have a myriad of accessory interests. The experiences of children are limited, and the conclusions they draw are usually highly colored by imagination. Before answering a question, it is wise to encourage children to relate their own versions of the subject. This can be done simply: "I'd like to hear the story you've told yourself about that. You tell me yours, and I'll tell you mine."

To hear children out first is valuable for several reasons:

- It reassures the children that adults are interested in everything that is of importance to them.
- It brings fantasies with their emotional meaning to the surface, where they can be managed constructively.
- It prevents imagination from distorting the facts when they are given.
- It encourages further questioning.

A child who has repressed misconceptions because they were too frightening to think about has a difficult time gaining emotional understanding of truths at a later time.

Other guidelines for parents include the following:

- Determine the level of vocabulary used by the child to refer to body parts and functions, clarifying or providing correct terms when necessary.
- Guide parents in anticipating how they would handle an invasion of privacy by a curious preschooler.
- When intrusive procedures are required (e.g., catheterization or pelvic examination), explain them to the child, realizing that the young child may feel embarrassed or exploited.

- Be firm and matter-of-fact in setting limits about where and with whom the child sleeps outside of the family. Sometimes, brothers and sisters, and children and parents, sleep together at this age.
- On discovering a child masturbating in private, ignore the behavior and proceed with the task. If repetitive masturbating is done in the parent's presence, it is appropriate to ask the child to wait until he or she can do so in privacy. Excessive masturbation can be handled by providing additional opportunities for social interaction and play.

A study by nurse researchers (Aquilino & Ely, 1985) found that parents benefited from discussion of preschool sexual matters, because it helped parents to answer questions and provided suggestions for interventions that were not available in printed material on the topic.

Television Viewing

The toddler and preschooler are highly vulnerable to the messages and stereotypes conveyed by television (Rothenberg, 1985). This is because the child has limited exposure to the world as well as limited ability to interpret accurately the distortions and meanings communicated by television. Therefore, it becomes imperative that parents as well as nurses monitor the amount and type of television a child views. This applies to all types of television programming, even cartoons. Some cartoons are inappropriate for the young viewer, because they are too sophisticated in plot and portrayal of characters.

Television has discernible beneficial effects, too. Children can learn much about music, art, history, and literature that would not have been available to them without television. In addition, television has made children more aware of world affairs. Celebrations, scientific discoveries, conflicts, and an assortment of events from all over the world are within the child's grasp. A variety of children's programs provide the young audience with stimulating content that makes learning fun.

In summary, television has both positive and negative effects on children. Nurses can do much in health teaching about television viewing to maximize its potential for beneficial use with children. For anticipatory guidance strategies, refer to Chapter 3.

Day Care

Many parents do not have the luxury of making a choice between staying home and placing their child in day care. More mothers are working outside the home, more women are delaying childbearing until their careers are established, and the number of single mothers who must work to support their children is increasing. In 1988, national data revealed that 57.1 per cent of women with children under 6 years of age and 50.8 per cent of women with infants less than 1 year old were employed (US Department of Commerce, 1990; US Department of Labor, 1989). Translated into actual numbers, nearly 9 million children have mothers in the work force. The three factors mentioned all contribute to the increased number of children who are cared for outside the home.

When a day care or preschool program is chosen, parents should explain to the preschooler what the preschool program is and why it is necessary that the child spend some time there each day. Appropriate preparation will help the preschooler avoid feeling abandoned or rejected. School should be discussed at home, and a visit should be made to the preschool to see what it looks like and to meet the teacher (ideally, several visits are made). Friends or siblings already attending school can offer the preschool child positive reactions. Parents should have confidence in the preschool and convey that feeling to their child. If possible, a parent should transport the child each day and assure the child of his or her return at the end of the day, rather than entrust this task to someone whom the child does not know well.

Day Care Homes

In the family day care home, the child's immediate needs (nutrition, safety, supervised play, nap time) are satisfactorily met. In this setting, generally, no activities are related to long-term plans to enhance the child's development. Care is given for one to six children, from infancy to school age.

Day care homes are of three general types: (1) several children in a caretaker's home (with or without the caretaker's own children), (2) a nonfamily member caretaker in the family's residence, and (3) a care situation in which the children (sometimes including the caretaker's own children) are cared for by more than one caregiver. Day care homes are a popular choice of formal day care for preschoolers in the United States and worldwide. These homes are usually located relatively close to the family's residence or to the place of employment of one parent.

Home day care provides the opportunity for children to be in a home setting for the hours during which they are not with their parent(s). Although caregivers in a day care home are less likely to have special preparation or education, this arrangement does tend to provide a stable, warm, and stimulating environment, especially for the younger preschooler (Clarke-Stewart, 1982). In many states, day care homes are not required to be licensed.

Day Care Center

Day care center programs are generally located in their own facility and provide daily care for children of from 2 or 3 to 6 years of age. Over 50 per cent of day care centers are business enterprises, run for profit, that provide mostly for the physical needs of the children (Clarke-Stewart, 1982). Many now have extended services to provide transportation to and from school and make available the supervision of school-age children (age 12 years) for the nonschool hours during which parents are working. However, the long-term goal of the day care center includes careful attention to planning and structuring environments for learning to provide for the physical, social, cognitive, and emotional needs of the children who attend (Fig. 7–8). The day care plan includes physical care of children, supervised play activities, rest periods, health supervision, and crafts. The parent may sometimes be included in the center's activities.

Although the quality varies, each state has established minimum standards for day care centers. The staff is generally composed of trained caretakers. Public centers administered by a unit of the state or local government and some voluntary centers administered by social agencies, settlements, or churches may receive federal monies for operation. This subsidy permits parents to pay according to their income level.

Nursery School

The nursery school operates 2 to 5 days a week for either 2 or 2½ hours a day and as morning or afternoon sessions. Groups can be composed of children of the same age or different ages (as 3- to 5-year-olds). Various types of nursery schools exist: guided observation schools (laboratory to study growth and development, often associated with colleges and universities); cooperative nursery schools (parents are utilized as teacher-helpers, thereby decreasing tuition costs as well as including parents in their preschooler's learning world); schools with full-time teachers and no daily solicitation of parent help (private schools such as Montessori schools); child development centers (governmental Head Start program for disadvantaged children); and schools for exceptional children (US Department of Health and Human Services, 1984). Nursery school can be nonprofit or profit enterprises, but all exist to enrich the world of the preschooler.

The nursery school will afford the preschooler socialization opportunities and enhance learning about the physical environment. Opportunities to expand language and visual acuity, develop fine and large motor coordination, and participate in school readiness activities (familiarization with numbers and letters and identification of like objects) may be a part of the curriculum. Free self-expression through various means allows the preschooler to develop a positive self-concept and encourages cognitive growth (Fig. 7–9). A good nursery school should afford parents the opportunity to participate in some aspect(s) of the program.

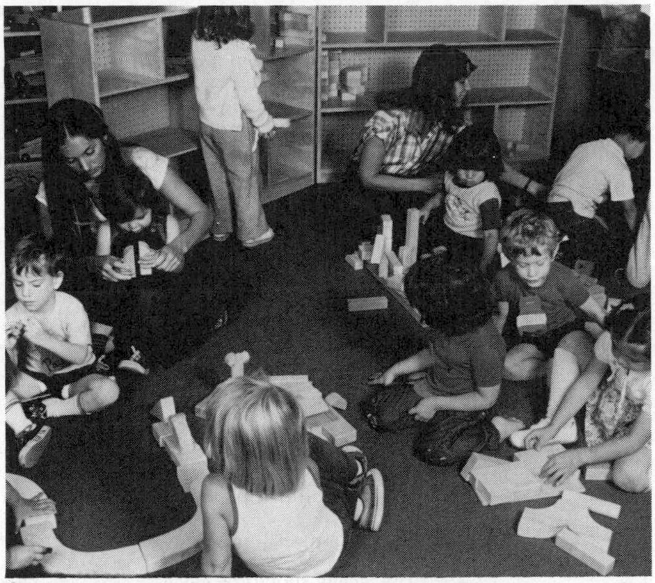

FIGURE 7 - 9. Under the supervision of skilled, competent caregivers, the preschooler has opportunities for socialization and self-expression. Note how blocks are used to develop motor skills (manipulating the blocks), social skills (working together to construct towers), and intellectual skills (identifying and matching shapes). Thus, three important skill areas are practiced in what seems at first glance only to be play. (Photograph by Brian Leatart.)

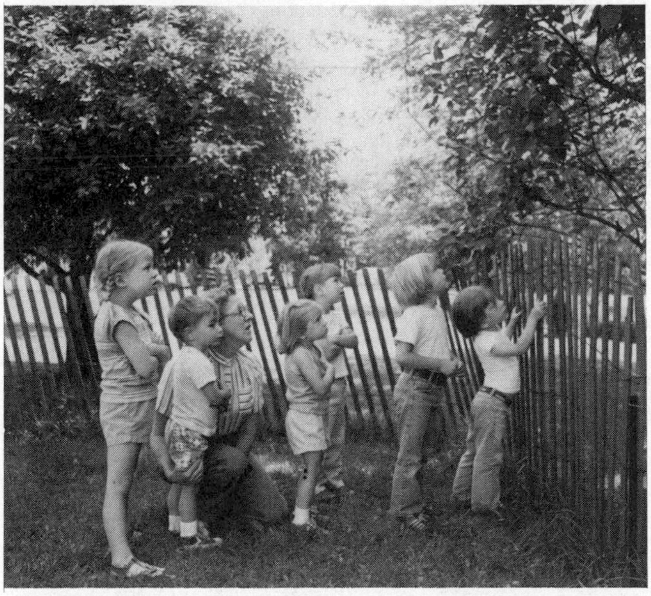

FIGURE 7 - 8. The day care center program has planned activities that are structured to stimulate children cognitively as well as care for their physical and emotional needs. Day care homes are a popular choice of formal day care for preschoolers. These children learn about nature in the back yard.

Play Schools

Local play schools or neighborhood play sessions are child care alternatives that many parents find helpful for occasional use. Voluntary organizations (churches

TABLE 7-17
Family-Centered Teaching: Selecting a Day Care Facility

What is the Purpose(s) of the Program?

Focus should foster development of the child.

How is the Program Structured?

Children should be able to pursue their individual interests. Organized, continuous experiences should be suited to the children attending. What are the cultural expectations? These expectations should be realistic in relation to, and supportive of, the preschooler's developmental tasks.

Observe and Interview Personnel

The ratio of children to caretaker/teacher should be realistic for the ages and needs of the children attending. The teachers should be professionally competent. The personnel and facility should be certified. Aides should supplement the child-to-teacher ratio. What training and qualifications do they have? The general emotional climate should be warm and nurturing. How do staff discipline children? How do staff spend most of their time?

Observe the Facilities

The facility should be easily accessible to home or employment. The space (indoor and outdoors) should be adequate for the needs of active preschoolers. Appropriate materials and equipment should be provided. Are the fees and manner of payment manageable?

What Are the Health and Safety Provisions?

Nutritious meals and snacks should be provided and in sufficient quantity. Health records should be kept on employees and children. What are the entry requirements regarding health status? Does the facility have an established plan for ill children? Is the health status of children identified daily? Is adequate provision made for first aid and emergency care? Is there adherence to public health codes? Have the staff been tested for tuberculosis? Do staff practice good hand washing habits? Is the staff certified in cardiopulmonary resuscitation? Are fire/earthquake/tornado drills practiced? Unprotected chemicals/drugs should be out of reach and locked. Electrical receptacles should be covered. Fire extinguishers should be visible. The yard should be fenced. Toys should be safe and in good repair.

What Special Services Are Offered?

Special services provided to parents may include help for children with special needs or financial adjustments (e.g., more than one child, payment plans). Consider what expectations you have of the facility and inquire about them. Ask for documentation of the expectations that the facility has for parents and children.

Adapted from Rassin, G., Beach, P., McCormick, D., Niebuhr, B., & Weller, S. (1991). Health and safety in day care: Parental knowledge. *Clinical Pediatrics, 30*(6), 344–349; American Academy of Pediatrics. Committee on Early Childhood Adoption and Dependent Care. (1987). *Health in day care: A manual for health professionals.* Elk Grove Village, IL: Author; Skolnick, A. (1989). Health and safety standards being developed for child care programs. *Journal of the American Medical Association, 262,* 3387–3388; Davis, W., & McCarthy, P. (1988). Safety in day care centers. *American Journal of Diseases in Children, 142,* 386; and Lee, E., & Bass, C. (1990). Survey of accidents in a university day care center. *Journal of Pediatric Health Care, 4*(1), 18–23.

or groups of neighborhood mothers) may provide play sessions. These are short-term arrangements with no planned curriculum—only baby sitting, because the population served varies daily. These alternatives are used most often by the family that has a parent in the home full time.

Other Day Care Alternatives

An innovative concept of day care that has the added benefit of exposing children and the elderly to each other is the provision of child day care services within nursing homes. Vujovich (1984) describes one such project, called GrandKids. The children and nursing home residents share numerous activities during the day, such as exercise time, crafts, story and music hours, play time, field trips, and pet times. This concept has increased the alertness and orientation of residents while enhancing the children's conceptions of and respect for the elderly. The arrangement provides the child with a homelike atmosphere and a richness of cultural and historical exposure not available in other day care settings (Sugarman & Brown, 1983).

Some employers are also establishing day care facilities at the workplace. Companies that have initiated such programs report decreases in employee turnover, tardiness, and absenteeism and increases in productivity, morale, and work schedule flexibility.

Such programs also improve the company's image and facilitate employee recruitment (Burud et al, 1983).

Another relatively new day care alternative is the day care center for sick children. These centers are designed to provide safe, competent day care to children with minor illnesses. They are staffed with nurses as well as other day care workers. Some of these centers are free standing, and some are run by hospitals. Guidelines are available for the care of ill children in traditional day care centers (Aronson, 1987).

Anticipatory Guidance: Day Care Evaluation

Tables 7–17 and 7–18 list factors that nurses should encourage parents to review when contemplating any type of day care for their preschooler (Rassin et al, 1991; American Academy of Pediatrics, 1987). The nurse should urge parents to trust their own feelings and impressions about the best arrangement and the best setting for their child. Nurses can help parents realize the value of preparing the child for day care, help the parents and child adjust to school (separation from each other), help parents provide continuity between the experiences of day care and life at home, and screen for safety measures employed by the center. A research study found that 75 per cent of preschool injuries were preventable. Over 50 per cent of the injuries involved a consumer product, such as playground equipment or bicycles (Chang et al, 1989).

TABLE 7-18
Characteristics of Good Day Care

Stable Caretakers

Low turnover rates

Educational and experiential background

Assignment to specific children or specific groups of children

Small Groups

Centers	*Homes*
1:3 infants*	1:5 children 2 yrs and under
1:4 children under 3 yrs	1:6 children 3 to 6 yrs
1:8 children 3 to 6 yrs	

Right Kind of Attention

Under 3 yrs—frequent direct contact with a few adults; informal learning experiences

Over 3 yrs—adult supervision and periodic direct contact; some formal instruction

Right Activities

More emphasis on learning about themselves, their neighborhood, and the world than on academics (e.g., math, reading)

Parental Involvement

Parental involvement welcomed, invited, and planned

Child development and other educational workshops for children

From *Mother care/other care* by Sandra Scarr. © 1984 by Basic Books, Inc. Reprinted by permission of BasicBooks, a division of HarperCollins Publishers, Inc.

*That is, one caretaker for every three infants.

Infection Control

Infection control is a major health issue for children in day care settings. The major pathogens and infections that can be transmitted in day care settings are listed in Table 7–19. There are several factors that affect the spread of infection in these settings. Risk of infection declines significantly with age. Recent enrollment of children into the center increases the risk. However, the primary factor in infection transmission is the caregiver's practice of personal hygiene and environmental sanitation (Morrow et al, 1991). In a nursing research study, Birchfield (1986) found the most common illnesses reported in a preschool setting were, in order of frequency, respiratory infections, fevers, gastrointestinal symptoms, and skin changes.

Anticipatory Guidance: Infection Control

The nurse can advise parents to obtain information on the center's infection control procedures and conduct physical inspection of the facility before selecting a day care center (see Table 7–17) (Shapiro & Hadler, 1991; Skolnick, 1989). Once the child has been admitted to a program, continuous monitoring of infection outbreaks is warranted.

Kindergarten

Kindergarten is a structured learning environment available to most preschool children through local public school systems. It is generally a half-day experience for 5 days a week that provides a gradual transition from home to school. Kindergarten affords an opportunity for children to develop positive attitudes toward school; to complete learning of the alphabet, numbers, and application of letter sounds and combinations to form words; and to develop abilities to think, discover, reason, and concentrate on one activity for a period of time. A professional is responsible for teaching the classes. Emphasis is placed on easing the transition into formal learning activities of the low elementary grades.

Anticipatory Guidance: School Readiness

In the United States, it is generally believed that children should begin their formal education sometime between ages 4½ and 6 years. However, children dif-

TABLE 7-19
Pathogens and Infections That Can Be Transmitted in Day Care

Mode of Transmission	Bacteria	Viruses	Parasites
Fecal-oral	*Campylobacter* *Escherichia coli* *Salmonella* *Shigella*	Enteroviruses Hepatitis A Rotaviruses	*Cryptosporidium* *Entamoeba histolytica* *Enterobius vermicularis* *Giardia lamblia*
Respiratory	*Haemophilus influenzae* type b *Neisseria meningitidis* Pertussis Tuberculosis	Adenovirus Influenza A & B Measles Parainfluenza Parvovirus B19 Respiratory syncytial virus Rhinoviruses Varicella	
Person-to-person via skin contact	Group A streptococci *Staphylococcus aureus*	Herpes simplex	Pediculosis Scabies
Contact with blood, urine, or saliva		Cytomegalovirus Hepatitis B Herpes simplex	Tinea capitis Tinea corporis

Used with permission of the American Academy of Pediatrics, *Report of the Committee on Infectious Diseases* (22nd ed.). Elk Grove Village, IL: Author, 1991.

fer in their readiness for school, just as they differ in other ways. There are no specific rules, but parents can generally identify when their child has the maturity for school. The nurse can offer parents guidance as they evaluate their child's readiness and help them recognize that school can be more complicated and threatening to children than adults realize. Reassure parents that they need not push their child into school at the earliest age the community allows. Table 7–20 lists the areas of maturity needed by a child to be ready for the school experience.

More recent research has revealed that pushing academics too soon on young children can have detrimental effects. Early and pressured learning can result in psychosomatic illnesses and behavioral problems. Children who are overly pressured and stimulated are likely to manifest signs of "burnout" in the elementary school years. These symptoms include headaches, stomach aches, and sleeping disorders. In extreme cases, young children have reported chest pains!

Parents should be encouraged to respond to the cues their child provides, rather than force academics. For example, if a 3-year-old wants to read, the child will spontaneously begin to read things such as street signs and labels on toys. Furthermore, parents should be encouraged to examine their own motivations for pushing academics on their child at this early age. Feelings of inadequacy as a parent, guilt, and zealous desire for their child's success are some of the motivators of parental pressure.

KEY CONCEPTS

Concepts Related to Basic Information

- The issues the family must address include supplying adequate space, maintaining communication, rearing children, and apportioning realistic responsibilities.
- Preschoolers are in Piaget's stage of preoperational thought, wherein they treat objects as symbols of other things.
- The central task of the third Eriksonian stage is for the child to develop a sense of initiative that outweighs any sense of guilt.
- Preschoolers tend to judge actions in terms of their consequences.
- Conscience begins to develop during the preschool years as children learn what behavior is acceptable.
- Sleep problems, particularly night terrors, peak during the preschool years.
- More recently, researchers have suggested that preschoolers have more cognitive competencies than previously reported by Piaget.
- Sexual exploration, masturbation, or sex play in preschool children is fairly common.
- Preschoolers are particularly vulnerable to interpreting illness and hospitalization as punishment for misdeeds.

TABLE 7-20
Check List for School Readiness

Characteristic	Preparatory Experiences
Physically healthy and strong	Balanced diet
	Adequate rest and sleep
	Opportunities for exercise
	Positive reinforcement for skill mastery
Capable of separating from parent	Experiences with substitute caregivers in caregiver's home
	Day care or nursery school a few hours a day or a couple of days a week
	Social activities away from home, such as Sunday school, play at a friend's home, supervised play with unfamiliar children at park
Long enough attention span	Listening to rather long stories
	Experiences working through activities that take a while, such as large puzzles, weaving mats
	Sitting through a full-length television program, movie, circus show
Able to tolerate frustration	Parent should not always respond to requests immediately; help child learn to wait until the activity of parent is finished or at a good stopping point
	If siblings, enforce rules about taking turns
	Experiences with small groups of children and a single caregiver
Has some basic hand-eye skills	Practice with child and provision of toys that stimulate recognizing shapes and colors
	Books in which child has to turn pages
	Experiences with a pencil and crayons
	Craft experiences; cutting with blunt-end scissors, pasting, painting, molding clay
	Exposure to simple computer games, to television shows that reinforce learning word sounds, alphabet letters, shapes, and colors

- The preschooler's use of coping mechanisms is directly related to level of development.
- The preschooler's understanding of spiritual matters continues to be based on perceptions, feelings, and fantasy; this stage of faith development is described as *intuitive-projective*.
- Preschool children have a beginning capacity to understand that the reactions of their friends and playmates are different from theirs.
- Normal sleep disturbances in young children are basically temporary and show a variety of themes.
- Childhood obesity is a serious health problem: it is estimated that 5 to 15 per cent of children are obese, and this number is growing.
- Car accidents are a leading cause of injury to preschoolers.

Concepts Related to Nursing Assessment

- Nurses providing care for the preschooler will consider the following diagnostic responses: *altered growth and development, fear, high risk for injury,* and *ineffective individual coping*.
- Knowledge of the preschooler's motor development can assist the nurse in assessing and intervening to promote developmentally appropriate motor activities.
- Although language screening tools are available for nurses to administer, their practicality, reliability, and validity should first be considered.
- Cardiovascular risk factors should be assessed, as research has shown evidence of precursors of cardiovascular disease during the preschool years.
- It is difficult to distinguish between fear and anxiety in preschool children, as they cannot distinguish between real and imagined dangers.
- Guidelines used in the selection of a day care facility include type and structure of program, personnel, facilities, health and safety, and special services.
- Children differ in their readiness for school, and children need to be assessed for their readiness.

Concepts Related to Nursing Intervention

- On the basis of the premise that children acquire knowledge through practical experience, nurses can assist children to understand and assimilate their hospital experience by listening to them recount it.

- The use of developmentally appropriate explanations prior to procedures and the use of therapeutic play can alleviate the preschooler's concerns.
- Parents should be cautioned by the nurse not to overreact to the child's sleep problems, or the child will learn to use the sleep disturbance to manipulate them.
- The nurse will use several types of therapeutic play activities to foster the hospitalized child's sense of mastery, such as emotional outlet play, instructional play, and physiologic enhancement.
- Parents should be reassured that there is a wide variance of size and stature among preschoolers.
- Several interventions can be used to alleviate feelings of guilt, including reassurances, projective techniques, and creative activities.
- It is imperative that parents monitor the amount and type of television a child watches.

REFERENCES

Alexander, M., & Blank, J. (1988). Factors related to obesity in Mexican-American preschool children. *Image: Journal of Nursing Scholarship, 20*(2), 70–82.

American Academy of Pediatrics. Committee on Early Childhood Adoption and Dependent Care. (1987). *Health in day care: A manual for health professionals.* Elk Grove Village, IL: Author.

American Academy of Pediatrics. Committee on Nutrition. (1989). Indications for cholesterol testing in children. *Pediatrics, 83*(1), 141–142.

American Academy of Pediatrics. Committee on Infectious Diseases. (1991). *Report of the committee on infectious diseases* (22nd ed.). Elk Grove Village, IL: Author.

Aquilino, M., & Ely, J. (1985). Parents and the sexuality of preschool children. *Pediatric Nursing, 11*(1), 41–46.

Arneson, S., & Triplett, J. (1990). Riding with Bucklebear: An automobile safety program for preschoolers. *Journal of Pediatric Nursing, 5*(2), 115–122.

Aronson, S. (1987). Care of ill children in child care programs. *Child Care Information Exchange, 56,* 34–38.

Berenson, G., Ingelfinger, J., & Jesse, M. (1988). Identifying the young hypertensive. *Patient Care, 22,* 105–130.

Betz, C. (1983). Teaching children through play therapy. *Journal of the Association of Operating Room Nurses, 88*(4), 709, 712–713, 716–717.

Betz, C., & Posler, E. (1984). Incorporating play into the care of the hospitalized child. *Issues in Comprehensive Pediatric Nursing, 7,* 343–354.

Birchfield, M. (1986). Illness and children in a preschool center. *Maternal-Child Nursing Journal, 15,* 187–197.

Borke, R. (1975). Three mountain task revisited. *Developmental Psychology, 11,* 375–382.

Borowitz, K., & Glascoe, F. (1986). Sensitivity of the Denver Developmental Screening Test in speech and language screening. *Pediatrics, 78,* 1075–1078.

Bullock, M., & Gelman, R. (1977). Numerical reasoning in children: The ordering principle. *Child Development, 48,* 427–434.

Burud, S., Collin, R., & Divine-Hawkins, P. (1983, May/June). Employee supported child care: Everyone benefits. *Children Today.*

Capute, A., Shapiro, B., & Palmer, E. (1987). Marking the milestones of language development. *Contemporary Pediatrics, 4,* 24–41.

Carmon, M., Hauber, R., Howell, C., & Rice, M. (1990). Cardiovascular screening programs: Implications for school nurses. *Pediatric Nursing, 16*(5), 509–511.

Chang, A., Lugg, M., & Nebedum, A. (1989). Injuries among preschool children enrolled in day care centers. *Pediatrics, 83*(2), 272–277.

Children's Safety Network. (1991). *A data book of child and adolescent injury.* Washington, DC: National Center for Education in Maternal and Child Health.

Clarke-Stewart, A. (1982). *Day care.* Cambridge, MA: Harvard University Press.

Coffman, S. (1991). Parent education for drowning prevention. *Journal of Pediatric Health Care, 5*(3), 141–146.

Coplan, J. (1985). Evaluation of the child with delayed speech or language. *Pediatric Annals, 14,* 202–208.

Davis, W., & McCarthy, P. (1988). Safety in day care centers. *American Journal of Diseases of Children, 142,* 386.

DeClue, T., & Shocken, D. (1991). Cholesterol screening management of Florida's pediatric population. *Clinical Pediatrics, 30*(6), 340–342.

Denham, S. (1986). Social cognition, prosocial behavior and emotion in preschoolers: Contextual validation. *Child Development, 57,* 194–201.

DEST. (1973). Denver, CO: University of Colorado Medical Center.

Dunn, J., Brown, J., Slomskowske, C., Lesla, C., & Youngblade, L. (1991). Young children's understanding of other people's feelings and beliefs: Individual differences and their antecedents. *Child Development, 62,* 1352–1366.

Duvall, E., & Miller, B. (1985). *Marriage and family development* (6th ed.). New York: Harper & Row.

Eavey, R. (1992). New concepts in the care of the pediatric ear and related structures. *Clinical Pediatrics, 31*(1), 4–9.

Erikson, E. H. (1963). *Childhood and society* (2nd ed.). New York: W. W. Norton.

Ferber, R. (1985). Sleep disorders in infants and children. In T. Riley (Ed.), *Clinical aspects of sleep and sleep disturbance.* Stoneham, MA: Butterworth.

Florey, L. (1971). An approach to play and play development. *American Journal of Occupational Therapy, 25,* 275–280.

Friedman, W. (1991). The development of children's memory for the time of past events. *Child Development, 62,* 139–155.

Garn, S., & La Velle, M. (1985). Two decade follow-up of fathers in early childhood. *American Journal of Diseases of Childhood, 139*(2), 181–185.

Hartup, W., Laursen, B., Stewart, M., & Eastenson, A. (1988). Conflict and the friendship relations of young children. *Child Development, 59,* 1590–1600.

Hauck, M. (1991). Cognitive abilities of preschool children: Implications for nurses working with young children. *Journal of Pediatric Nursing, 6*(4), 230–235.

Herbert, M. (1975). *Problems of childhood.* Baltimore, MD: Paul Brooks, Ltd.

Hitchens-Serota, J. (1986). Assessing parent's knowledge of pediatric dental disease. *Pediatric Nursing, 12*(6), 435–438.

Honig, J. (1991). A school-based clinic in a preschool. *Journal of Pediatric Health Care, 5*(1), 34–39.

Howard, J., Bindler, R., Dimico, G., Norwood, S., Nottingham, J., Synoground, G., Tulling, J., Gemert, F., Kirk, M., Newkirk, G., Leaf, D., & Cleveland, P. (1991). Cardiovascular risk factors in children: A Bloomsday research report. *Journal of Pediatric Nursing, 6*(4), 222–229.

Inagaki, K., & Hatano, G. (1987). Young children's spontaneous personification as analogy. *Child Development, 58,* 1013–1020.

Jenkins, C. (1988). Epidemiology of cardiovascular disease. *Journal of Consulting and Clinical Psychology, 56*(3), 324–332.

Jones, E., Badger, T., & Moore, I. (1992). Children's knowledge of internal anatomy: Conceptual orientation and review of research. *Journal of Pediatric Nursing, 7*(4), 262–268.

Jonides, L. (1990). Child obesity: An update. *Journal of Pediatric Health Care, 4*(5), 242–251.

Kilmon, C., Barber, N., & Chapman, K. (1991). Instruments for the screening of speech/language development in children. *Journal of Pediatric Health Care, 5*(2), 61–70.

Lee, E., & Bass, C. (1990). Survey of accidents in a university day care center. *Journal of Pediatric Health Care, 4*(1), 18–23.

Lee, J., & Fowler, M. (1986). Merely child's play and developmental work and playthings. *Journal of Pediatric Nursing, 1,* 260–269.

Malek, M., Guyer, B., & Lescohier, I. (1990). The epidemiology and prevention of child pedestrian injury. *Accident Analysis and Prevention, 22*(4), 301–313.

McClowry, S. (1993). Pediatric nursing psychosocial care: A vision beyond hospitalization. *Pediatric Nursing, 19*(2), 146–149.

Menig-Peterson, C. (1975). The modification of communicative behavior in preschool-aged child as a function of the listeners' perspective. *Child Development, 46,* 1015–1018.

Miller, S. (1988). Parents' beliefs about children's cognitive development. *Child Development, 59,* 259–285.

Morrow, A., Townsend, I., & Pickering, L. (1991). Risk of enteric infection associated with child day care. *Pediatric Annals, 20*(8), 427–433.

NAACOG. (1987). National awareness week targets child passenger safety. *NAACOG Newsletter, 14,* 5.

Nation's Health. (1988, April). Health interview survey shows gaps in prevention behavior. *Nation's Health,* p. 10.

National Academy of Sciences. (1989). *Recommended dietary allowances* (10th ed.). Washington, DC: National Academy Press.

National Institutes of Health Consensus Development Conference Statement. (1985). Health implications of obesity. *Annals of Internal Medicine, 103*(6), 1073–1077.

Nicol, N. (1989). What's new with sunscreens? Choices-choices-choices. *Pediatric Nursing, 15*(4), 417–418.

Piaget, J. (1950). *The psychology of intelligence.* New York: Harcourt Brace.

Piaget, J. (1952). *The origins of intelligence in children.* New York: Basic Books.

Piaget, J. (1954). *The construction of reality in the child.* New York: Basic Books.

Prugh, D. (1983). *The psychological aspects of pediatrics.* Philadelphia: Lea & Febiger.

Rassin, G., Beach, P., McCormick, D., Niebuhr, B., & Weller, S. (1991). Health and safety in day care: Parental knowledge. *Clinical Pediatrics, 30*(6), 344–349.

Rivara, F., Booth, C., Bergman, A., Rogers, L., & Weiss, J. (1991). Prevention of pedestrian injuries to children: Effectiveness school training program. *Pediatrics, 88*(4), 770–775.

Rosenbaum, P., Elston, R., Scrinivasan, S., Webber, L., & Berenson, G. (1987). Predictive values of parenteral measures in determining cardiovascular risk factor variables in early life. *Pediatrics, 80*(5, Pt. 2), 807–816.

Rothenberg, M. (1985). Role of television in shaping the attitudes of children. *Children's Health Care, 13,* 148–149.

Scarr, S. (1984). *Mother care/other care.* New York: Basic Books.

Shapiro, L., & Hadler, S. (1991). Hepatitis A and hepatitis B virus infection in day care settings. *Pediatric Annals, 20*(8), 435–441.

Sherman, J., & Alexander, M. (1990). Obesity in children: A research update. *Journal of Pediatric Nursing, 5*(3), 161–167.

Siegler, R. (1986). *Children's thinking.* Englewood Cliffs, NJ: Prentice-Hall.

Skolnick, A. (1989). Health and safety standards being developed for child care programs. *JAMA, 262,* 3387–3388.

Stern, R., Weinstein, M., & Baker, S. (1986). Risk reduction for non-melanoma skin cancer with childhood sunscreen use. *Archives of Dermatology, 122,* 537–544.

Stiles, J., Delis, D., Tada, W. (1991). Global-local processing in preschool children. *Child Development, 62,* 1258–1275.

Stipek, D., & DeCotis, K. (1988). Children's understanding of the implications of causal attributions for emotional experiences. *Child Development, 59,* 1601–1616.

Study Group of New York. (1983). *Children and sex: The parents speak.* New York: Facts on File.

Sugarman, J., & Brown, P. (1983, November/December). Child care centers in long-term care facilities. *Nursing Homes,* pp. 4–7.

Sullivan, L. (1988). How effective is preschool vision, hearing and developmental screening? *Pediatric Nursing, 14*(3), 181–183.

Thompson, M. D., & Thompson, G. (1991). Early identification of hearing loss: Listen to parents. *Clinical Pediatrics, 30*(2), 77–80.

Trainex Corporation. (1980). *Physical examination of the school age child: The musculoskeletal system* [Filmstrip]. Los Angeles: Undergraduate Dietetic Program and the Department of Nursing, California State University at Los Angeles.

U. S. Department of Agriculture, Human Nutrition Information Service. (1992). *Food guide pyramid* (Leaflet No. 572). Washington, DC: Author.

U. S. Department of Labor Women's Bureau. (1989). *Facts on working women, 89,* 1–2. Washington, DC: Author.

U. S. Department of Commerce, Bureau of the Census. (1990). U. S. Statistics in Brief. A Statistical Abstract Supplement.

Vessey, J., & Mahon, M. (1990). Therapeutic play and the hospitalized child. *Journal of Pediatric Nursing, 5*(5), 328–332.

Vujovich, J. (1984, January/February). Child day care livens a nursing home. *Geriatric Nursing.*

Walker, D., Gugenheim, S., Downs, M., & Northern, J. (1989). Early language milestone scale and language screening of young children. *Pediatrics, 83*(2), 284–288.

Wender, E. (1984). Common behavior problems in preschool children. In P. Shelov et al. (Eds.), *Primary care pediatrics: A symptomatic approach* (pp. 265–282). Norwalk, CT: Appleton-Century-Crofts.

Williams, B. (1990). Immunization coverage among preschool children: The United States and selected European countries. *Pediatrics, 82,* 1052–1055.

Wilson, E. (1986). The black extended family: An analytical consideration. *Developmental Psychology, 22*(2), 246–258.

BIBLIOGRAPHY

Advisory Committee of Immunization Practices. (1989). Measles prevention: Recommendation of the Immunization Practices Advisory Committee. *Morbidity and Mortality Weekly Report, 38*(9), 1–17.

Ada, G. (1990). The immunological principles of vaccination. *Lancet, 335*(8687), 523–526.

Agran, P., Wian, D., & Dunkle, D. (1989). Injuries among 4 to 9 year old restrained motor vehicle occupants by seat location and crash impact site. *American Journal of Diseases of Children, 143,* 1317–1321.

Anderson, R., & Anderson, K. (1984, June). Day care: Social, emotional and intellectual effect. *Occupational Health Nursing,* pp. 301–306.

Bausell, R. (1985). A national survey assessing pediatric preventive behaviors. *Pediatric Nursing, 116,* 438–442.

Bellanti, J. (Ed.) (1990). Pediatrics vaccination: update 1990. *Pediatric Clinics of North America, 37*(3), 513–784.

Betz, C. (1981). Faith development in children. *Pediatric Nursing, 7*(2), 22–25.

Biro, P., & Thompson, M. (1984). Screening young children for communication disorders. *MCN: American Journal of Maternal Child Nursing, 9*(6), 410–413.

Brown, M., & Haylor, M. (1989). Nursing research with preoperational age children: The use of standardized tests. *Journal of Pediatric Nursing, 4*(1), 19–25.

Brown, M., & Tanner, C. (1988). Type A behavior and cardiovascular responsivity in preschoolers. *Nursing Research, 37,* 152–155.

Bull, M., et al. (1990). Establishing special needs car seat loan program. *Pediatrics, 85*(4), 540–547.

Butler, J. (1983, November). A walk-in unit for pre-school children and their mothers. *Health Visitor,* pp. 411–412.

Castiglia, P. (1989). Sibling rivalry. *Journal of Pediatric Health Care, 3*(1), 52–54.

Castillo, N. (1982, July/December). Framework skills for nursing day care and early childhood education managership. *Pediatric Nursing,* pp. 29–30.

Centers for Disease Control. (1990, April 6). Measles—United States. *Morbidity and Mortality Weekly Report, 39*(13), 211–212.

Centers for Disease Control. (1993). Standards for pediatric immunization practices. *Morbidity and Mortality Weekly Report, 42,* 1–9.

Children's Defense Fund. (1982). *The child care handbook: Needs, programs and responsibilities.* Washington, DC: Author.

Committee on Communications. (1992). The commercialization of children's television. *Pediatrics, 89*(2), 343–344.

Crowley, A. (1990). Health services in child day-care center: A survey. *Journal of Pediatric Health Care, 4*(5), 252–259.

Current Status of *Hemophilus influenzae* type b—conjugate vaccines. *Pediatrics, 85*(Suppl. 4, Pt. 2), 631–704.

Dateline Child Care. (1987). *Child Care Information Exchange, 56,* 9–10.

Dunne, R., Asher, K., & Rivara, F. (1992). Behavior and parental expectations of child pedestrians. *Pediatrics, 89*(3), 486–490.

Engel, N. (1990). The National Vaccine Injury Compensation Program. *MCN: American Journal of Maternal Child Nursing, 15,* 109.

Fish, L. (1985). Identifying gifted preschoolers. *Pediatric Nursing, 11*(2), 125–127.

Food and Nutrition Board, National Research Council. (1989). *Recommended dietary allowance* (10th ed.). Washington DC: National Academy Press.

Fowler, J. (1984). *Becoming adult, becoming Christian.* San Francisco: Harper & Row.

Frank, J., & Loh, J. (1991). SSPE: But we thought measles was gone. *Journal of Pediatric Nursing, 6*(2), 87–92.

Freud, S. (1957). In J. Strachey (Ed.), *The standard edition of the complete psychological works of Sigmund Freud* (Vol. 18). London: Hogarth Press.

Fuchs, S., et al. (1989). Cervical spine fractures sustained by young children in forward facing car seats. *Pediatrics, 84*(2), 348–354.

Gadnow, K., & Sprafkin, J. (1989). Field experiments of television violence with children: Evidence for an environmental hazard? *Pediatrics, 83*(3), 399–415.

Gates, D., & Morwessel, N. (1989). Night terrors: strategies for family coping. *Journal of Pediatric Nursing, 4*(1), 48–53.

Gedaly-Duff, V. (1988). Preparing young children for painful procedures. *Journal of Pediatric Nursing, 3,* 169–179.

Gilligan, C. (1982). *In a different voice: Toward a psychology of the life cycle.* New York: Jason Aronson.

Gilliss, C., et al. (1989). A health-education program for day-care centers. *MCN: American Journal of Maternal Child Nursing, 14,* 266–268.

Grey, M. (1993). Stressors and children's health care. *Journal of Pediatric Nursing, 8*(2), 85–91.

Griffin, M., et al. (1990). Risk of seizures and encephalopathy after immunization with diphtheria-tetanus-pertussis vaccine. *JAMA, 263*(12), 1641–1645.

Grimes, D., & Woolbert, L. (1989). Measles outbreaks: Who are at risk and why. *Journal of Pediatric Health Care, 3*(4), 187–193.

Hayden, G., et al. (1989). Progress in world wide control and elimination of disease through immunization. *Journal of Pediatrics, 114*(4), 520–527.

Hobbie, C. (1989). Choosing quality child care programs. *Journal of Pediatric Health Care, 3*(5), 270–271.

Howes, C. (1989). Pressuring children to learn versus developmentally appropriate education. *Journal of Pediatric Health Care, 3*(4), 181–186.

Kohlberg, L. (1981). *The philosophy of moral development.* San Francisco: Harper & Row.

LaMontagne, L. (1993). Bolstering personal control in child patients through coping interventions. *Pediatric Nursing, 19*(3), 235–237.

Linley, J. (1984). Mothers' attitudes regarding health care for their children. *MCN: American Journal of Maternal Child Nursing,* (1), 37–41.

Long, T. (1989). Falls from pickup trucks during childhood. *American Journal of Diseases of Children, 143,* 997–998.

Lynn, M. (1989). Siblings' responses in illness situations. *Journal of Pediatric Nursing, 4*(2), 127–129.

Lyons, J., & Hester, N. (1987). Research-generated nursing diagnoses for healthy school-age children. *Issues in Comprehensive Pediatric Nursing, 10*(3), 149–159.

Maheady, D. (1986). Health concepts of preschool children. *Pediatric Nursing, 12*(3), 195–197.

Markowitz, L., et al. (1989). Patterns of transmission in measles outbreaks in the United States, 1985–1986. *New England Journal of Medicine, 325*(2), 75–81.

McMenamy, C., & Katz, R. (1989). Brief parent assisted treatment for children's nighttime fears. *Journal of Developmental and Behavioral Pediatrics, 10*(3), 145–148.

Moxon, E. (1990). The scope of immunization. *Lancet, 335*(8687), 448–451.

Novak, J., & Pecoraro, N. (1989). Policy and position statement: Child care. *Journal of Pediatric Health Care, 3*(3), 158–159.

Pagel, J. (1989). Nightmares. *American Family Physician, 39*(3), 145–148.

Parks, B., & Smith, D. (1989). Treatment of head lice and scabies infestations. *Pediatric Nursing, 15*(5), 522–523.

Pass, R. (1991). Day care centers and the spread of cytomegalovirus and parvovirus B19. *Pediatric Annals, 20*(8), 427–433.

Pipes, P. (1989). *Nutrition in infancy and childhood* (4th ed.). St. Louis: Mosby.

Rapin, I. (1993). Hearing disorders. *Pediatrics in Review, 14*(2), 43–49.

Recommendations of the Immunization Practices Advisory Committee (ACIP). (1989). Prevention and control of influenza 1 vaccines. *Morbidity and Mortality Weekly Report, 38*(17), 297–309.

Recommendations of the Immunization Practices Advisory Committee (ACIP). (1990). Protection against viral hepatitis. *Morbidity and Mortality Weekly Report, 39*(Suppl. 2), 1–26.

Recommendations of the Immunization Practices Advisory Committee (1989). Pneumococcal polysaccharide vaccine. *Morbidity and Mortality Weekly Report, 38*(5), 64–76.

Risser, W. (1992). The acute management of minor soft tissue injuries. *Pediatric Annals, 21*(3), 170–173.

Ritchie, J., Caty, S., & Ellerton, M. (1984). Concerns of acutely ill, chronically ill and healthy preschool children. *Research in Nursing & Health, 7,* 265–274.

Rivara, F., et al. (1989). Risk of injury to children less than 5 years of age in day-care versus home care settings. *Pediatrics, 84*(6), 1011–1016.

Roberts, M., & Broadbent, M. (1989). Increasing preschoolers' use of care safety devices: An effective program for day care staff. *Children's Health Care, 18*(3), 157–162.

Rose, M. (1989). Development and use of the preschool behavior inventory. *Journal of Pediatric Nursing, 4*(1), 9–17.

Rubella and congenital rubella syndrome. United States 1985–1988. *Morbidity and Mortality Weekly Report, 38*(11), 173–182.

Ruddy-Wallace, M. (1987). Temperament: Assessing individual differences in hospitalized children. *Journal of Pediatric Nursing, 2*(1), 30–36.

Schmitt, B. (1990). Sibling rivalry toward a new baby. *Contemporary Pediatrics, 7*(3), 111–112.

Schmitt, B. (1989). When your toddler or preschooler won't eat. *Contemporary Pediatrics, 6*(9), 127–128.

Schraeder, B., & Tobey, G. (1989). Preschool temperament of very low birth weight infants. *Journal of Pediatric Nursing, 4*(2), 119–126.

Sherman, J., & Alexander, M. (1990). Obesity in children: A research update. *Journal of Pediatric Nursing, 5*(3), 161–167.

Smith, D. (1986). Common day-care disease: Patterns and prevention. *Pediatric Nursing, 12*(3), 195–197.

Smith, K., Shellam, P., & Zimmerman, F. (1989). Standards and criteria: Group child care for sick children. *Pediatric Nursing, 15*(6), 600–602.

Sommers, K. (1985). The generation mix: Child care in the nursing home. *Nursing Homes, 34*(4), 27–30.

Sorensen, E. (1990). Children's coping responses. *Journal of Pediatric Nursing, 5*(4), 259–267.

Standiford, D., Ahlrichs, J., Carmicle, C., & Wells, P. (1993). Extended day program: Bringing preschool to the hospital. *Pediatric Nursing, 19*(3), 238–241.

Starr, S. (1989). Status of varicella vaccine for healthy children. *Pediatrics, 84*(6), 1097–1099.

Stiehm, E. (1990). Skin testing prior to measles vaccination for egg sensitive patients. *American Journal of Diseases of Children, 114*(1), 32.

Thompson, C., & Stroud, S. (1987). The motorized tricycle: An accident waiting to happen. *Journal of Pediatric Nursing, 2*(2), 120–125.

U. S. Department of Health and Human Services. (1984). *A parent's guide to day care.* Washington, DC: U. S. Government Printing Office.

Van Cleve, L., & Savedra, M. (1993). Pain location: Validity and reliability of body outline markings by 4- to 7-year-old children who are hospitalized. *Pediatric Nursing, 19*(3), 217–220.

Washing out day-care infection. (1983). *Emergency Medicine, 15,* 220–222.

Wasserman, R., et al. (1989). Injury hazards in home day care. *Journal of Pediatrics, 114*(1, Pt. 1), 591.

Weiss, B. (1992). Trends in bicycle helmet use by children: 1985 to 1990. *Pediatrics, 89*(1), 78–80.

Werner, E. (1983, September/October). Alternate caregivers for children: A perspective. *Children Today,* pp. 22–27.

Wilson, A. (1990). Standards in maternal and child oral health. *Journal of Public Health Dentistry, 5*(6), 432–438.

Woodward, G., & Botte, R. (1990). Children riding in the back of pickup trucks: A neglected safety issue. *Pediatrics, 86*(5), 683–691.

CHAPTER • 8

Families with School-Age Children

RELATED TOPICS
Family assessment, Chapter 2
Theories of cognitive and moral development, Chapter 3
Children's health perceptions and health behaviors, Chapter 10
Promoting Healthy Parenting, Chapter 12
Fostering Self-Esteem, Chapter 14
Promoting healthy nutrition, Chapter 16
Substance use and abuse, Chapter 29
Common childhood infectious diseases, Chapter 39
Common childhood injuries, Chapter 46

LEARNING OBJECTIVES

- Identify major areas of concern of families with school-age children.
- Describe changes of physical maturation in the school-age child.
- Identify the age-specific gross and fine motor abilities of the school-age child.
- Discuss characteristics of the school-age child's level of thinking and its application to nursing practice.
- Identify the major developmental milestones of the school-age child's level of emotional-social competency.
- Explain the essential components of the school-age child's health examination.
- Consider the prominent anticipatory guidance concerns for parents during the child's school-age years.

Second only to the family, the school is a major socializing agency available for transmitting values as well as knowledge to children. This chapter describes common needs of families with school-age children, presents the developmental tasks of families with children in the age group of 6 to 12 years, and considers methods of adapting to life changes encountered. Available support systems are discussed. Interventions aimed at promoting the well-being of the child and family are described.

Development and Adaptation of the Family with School-Age Children

The family with school-age children is confronted with major areas of change. These are (1) reorganizing to adapt family living to the child's expanding world as the child moves into school and the world of teachers and peers, (2) expanding family communications and activities to recognize the school-ager's readiness for independent thinking and greater responsibility both within and outside the family unit, and (3) maintaining financial solvency as family costs escalate to meet the needs of school and extracurricular activities (Duvall & Miller, 1985).

Reorganizing to Adapt Family Life

One changing characteristic of all school-age children and their families is the need to adjust to a world no longer totally controlled by parents and the home environment. The school environment takes over many social functions and provides new models for children to imitate. They are faced with the need to master basic skills in reading, writing, and arithmetic. By second grade, educational experiences expand beyond these basic skills to the natural sciences. The timing is congruent with the developing cognitive ability, which leads children to be curious about the natural sciences.

As children begin school, the family must adjust to the new parameters presented by school and peers. Children may, for the first time, experience labels (e.g., "Fatso," "Skinny," "the kid from Becker Street") and prejudice. With exposure to different moral attitudes and beliefs, both children and parents must now contend with the incongruities between family beliefs and expectations and those of school peers. In addition, children beginning to handle sibling rivalry are faced with a new peer rivalry as they compete with other children for the teacher's attention and approval.

As children begin to absorb the values of the peer group and school, conflicts often arise. Home becomes a testing ground for new ideas and behaviors—parents are sometimes nonjudiciously compared with teachers and cooperative preschool "darlings" can become relentlessly sassy school-age teases. The inevitable consequence of this, even in the best-adjusted families, is some degree of conflict, particularly between parent and child; between home and school; or between home and peer groups, especially with the older school-age child. Some parents perceive the decrease in control over their child's life as threatening; they sense a progressive impotence as parents. They may respond with alarm or anger directed toward the child or the school (usually the teacher). Sometimes parents overreact as their child expresses new ideas or imitates peer behaviors. Parents may impose overly strict rules or punishment in response to the experimentation. Other parents give up and refuse to set any limits on these experimental ideas and behaviors. However, many parents find comfort from sharing concerns and frustrations (not to mention the humor created by some of their children's experimental antics) with parents in similar situations. These parents, although they sometimes feel like packing their bags and running away or hiding out for a day, usually set realistic limits on their children's experimental activities.

The rapidity and extent of adaptation by the child and family primarily depend on the degree of congruence that exists among home, peer, and school values. Research has demonstrated an association between the familial environment and the child's social competence and acceptance by peers. Positive parental support has been associated with better social competence and more positive peer interactions (Putallaz, 1987). In one study, children rejected by their school-age peers were found to be raised in homes with fewer positive interactions with parents and in which parents used physical aggression (Pettit et al, 1988).

Teachers

As the child strives to achieve and master new knowledge or skills to develop talents, the teacher can be a vital supporter. Teachers can also set standards that are realistic. Many children do not realize that some goals are best met by gradually increasing the level of the standard against which performance is measured. In their attempt to predict outcomes, children strive to master unknown situations. School-agers try to predict what will happen in school, how well they will perform on a test, or how many hits they will score in the afternoon baseball game. In the learning environment, the teacher can promote optimal predictability by structuring situations in such a way that children can confirm their predictions at least part of the time.

In a similar fashion, the teacher can play an important part in preventing the development of feelings of inferiority in the child. Besides structuring the learning situation so that a child can experience relative success, the teacher can contribute toward the maturing of positive feelings toward self and others. School-age children still greatly depend on the opinion and attitudes of significant adults as an aspect of their own self-esteem. The implications of this for teachers go beyond merely providing a warm and accepting climate. Teachers must have knowledge of childhood developmental processes in psychodynamic terms. The teacher who understands that conflicts occur naturally in development will be able to convey to children that doubts, fears, problems, and backsliding are acceptable parts of being a person.

Peers

Peers can also become important members of the child's support system. From their peers, children learn how to cooperate, compete, and learn the meaning and importance of following rules. They are also forced to consider situations from perspectives other than their own. An extra feature of these "supporters" is that there is a greater likelihood of forming enduring relationships with them, because children normally progress through their school years with the same peers, in contrast to the yearly exposure to different teachers. In response to the need to develop a sense of industry, to feel good about one's products, and to compete with others for recognition, the peer group watches and judges each child's performance and lets the individual know how well he or she has done. Typically, the latter process is conveyed through inclusion or exclusion from group activities. Essentially, children look to their peers to measure their own skills and worth (Fig. 8–1). According to Maier (1969), "A sense of accomplishment for having done well, being the strongest, best, wittiest, or fastest is the success toward which he strives. The child wards off failure at almost any price." Thus, children look to others for approval of themselves as worthwhile people (Fig. 8–2).

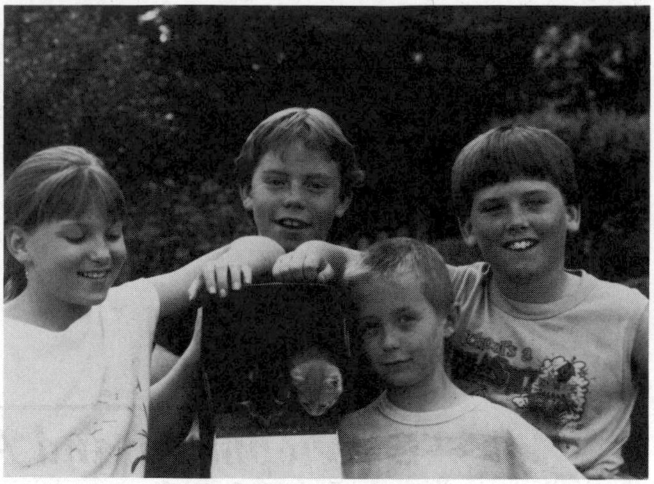

FIGURE 8-1. Peer groups are important to children's feelings of acceptance and self-esteem. Often, children have one group of friends at school and another group of friends who live nearby and are available for play after school and on weekends. Neighborhood groups more often involve members of the opposite sex.

The structure of childhood social groups progresses roughly through three stages—from a global or undifferentiated group of children to a highly differentiated group with an exaggerated structure, and finally to an articulated functional unit. Stages of children's social groups are listed in Table 8–1.

The major challenges for the school-age child, parents, and teachers working to achieve adequate school adjustment are summarized in Table 8–2. Nursing interventions to facilitate the child's and family's adjustment are also listed. Family experiences serve as the training arena for later expanded social interactions. Preventive interventions can be employed to facilitate more positive parent-child interactions, peer interactions, and non-kin adult and authority interactions (Pettit et al, 1988).

Utilizing Effective Family Communication

Letting children "go" is one of the hardest tasks parents must undertake. Letting go requires that parents free their children to make increasingly more of their own decisions, learn from their own choices and experiences, and take progressively more responsibility for themselves and their actions. Letting go also involves allowing children to experience hurt and humiliation when choices were unwise, to feel the exuberance of having done something "all alone," and to know the satisfaction that comes from working with others because of personal choice. Parents grant this

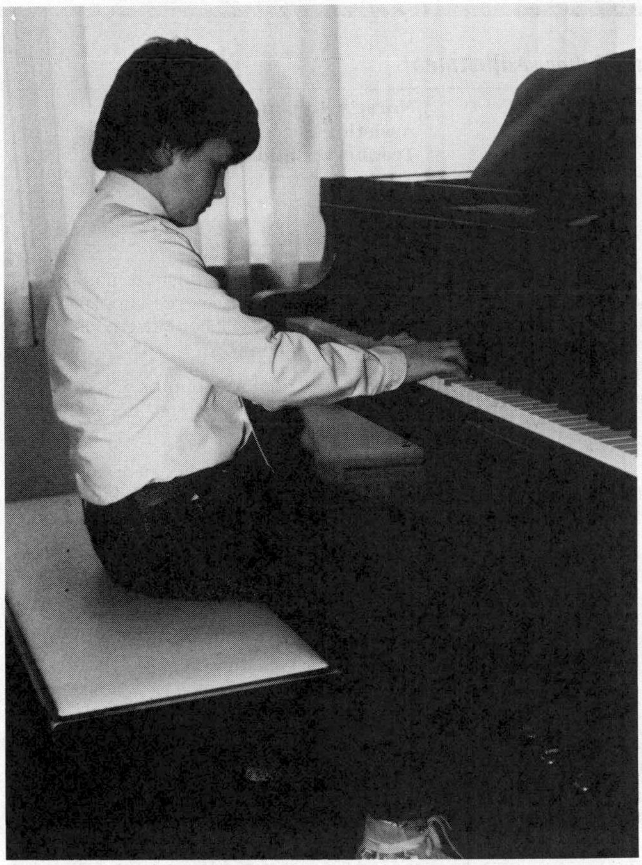

FIGURE 8-2. School-age children need to develop one relatively superior skill that they can be proud of.

freedom by keeping their mouths closed and hands at their sides when they are tempted to give instructions, assist in tasks, or baby the child. Giving in to these temptations often alienates the child and impairs the development of independence and responsibility.

Along with this spirit of allowing freedom, parents need to communicate faith in the child's competence and resilience. Children who know that their parents believe in them and are proud of them have fewer failures and bounce back more quickly when they do fail. Children who experience belittling of ideas and efforts and whose parents communicate doubt in their abilities usually comply with these expectations for failure. Keeping an open door requires giving the child room to make mistakes and offering support or comfort during recuperation from the lapses in self-confidence and self-esteem that mistakes or failures create.

Parents also need to understand the "angel at school, hellion at home" syndrome of childhood. If they recognize that the family unit is the resource to the school-age child for security and stability as the child attempts to integrate and adapt to a new world of people, ideas, and experiences, the dichotomous behavior is met with better understanding. In order to meet the social expectations outside the home, the school-ager needs to be able to come home and express all the fears, disappointments, and self-doubts imposed by the new world. These feelings are generally expressed through misbehaving, whining, or demanding behaviors. Within this dichotomy, the child goes through a process of self-evaluation to achieve self-acceptance within a new framework of multiple roles and values.

Nursing Care and Guidance

The nurse who assists the family in recognizing the phenomenon of development fosters healthy relationships, despite the stress that is a consequence of increased independence for the child. The nurse can assist parents in targeting the sources of their stress and implement interventions that reduce their stress (Frankel, 1993). Urging parents to enforce a wide set of rules consistently, to continue to set limits, and to provide positive feedback as their child struggles to adapt is important, because such actions foster the child's developing sense of reality and self-confidence in decision making.

TABLE 8-1
School-Age Children's Social Groups

6 to 8 Yrs
Activities organized around playful games
Little formality or organization to groups
Group membership collects by chance
Not allowed to be part of group/gang; allowed to perform tasks for members, such as "fetch and carry"
8 to 9 Yrs
Same-sex grouping
Mixed sexual groups common
Strong affiliation and loyalty develop among group members
Cross-sex interactions taboo
Secret languages/codes
Formal rites
Leaders becoming well established
Secret club forms
Group/gang becomes social support
Membership depends on ability to keep secret and not tell mom everything
10 to 12 Yrs
"Secret" groups not seen as enticing
Activities of group organized around particular activity/or function
Same-sex best friends evident

TABLE 8-2
Tasks of Children, Parents, Teachers, and Nurses in Facilitating School Adjustment

Child's Tasks	Parents' and Teacher's Role in Facilitating Task Achievement	Nurse's Role in Assisting Parents, Teachers, Child
Diffusion into Larger World (5 or 6 to 8 Yrs)		
Must adapt to differences in teacher's and parents' disciplinary approach and behavioral expectations	Parents and teacher should communicate their respective expectations to identify extreme differences; they should work out compromises that permit the child to meet expectations of each so that parents and teachers can mutually reinforce their expectations	School nurse can help organize parent-teacher interaction (e.g., preschool roundups; parent-teacher-nurse conferences) or mediate in conflicts During preschool roundup or school physical, learn child's and parents' expectations for school
Must compete with peers for teacher's attention and approval as teacher replaces parent for large portion of day	Teachers should avoid obvious favoritism in classroom, give individual attention and praise to each child, and avoid comparisons of achievement	School nurse can offer guidance to teacher and intervene in unhealthy child-teacher relationships During preschool registration or school physical, evaluate parent-child relationship for problems, as these often carry over to teacher-child relationships
Must learn to handle blatant, hurtful honesty and downright rudeness of peers without damage to self-concept	Peer activities and behaviors need close adult supervision	Nurse in well-child facilities or schools can provide this guidance to parents and teachers
Needs to test out new ideas and behaviors in security of home environment	Parents need to recognize developmental function of "trying on" ideas and behaviors incongruent with family's but set reasonable limits on how much and what type of "trying on" are allowed	Nurse in well-child facilities or schools may offer this anticipatory guidance
Disorganization Created by Disparities Between Home and School or Peers (8 to 10 Yrs)		
Must learn to concentrate on cognitive achievements in school life	Parents and teachers need open communication about cognitive tasks that are being focused on at any one time and which skills the child finds difficult so that both parties can support the mastery of those skills	School nurse's observations in classroom will help identify children having difficulty with this task. Investigation of state of health, sensory organ function, and neurologic, physical, and emotional function should follow to determine source of problem in achieving task
Must learn to integrate peer values in a manner that does not deny family values and to transfer family values into larger world in socially acceptable ways	Parents and teachers must understand that just as children fall as they learn to walk, so will they fall as they learn to think. These falls during school age are typically boasting, teasing, fighting, lying, cheating, sassing, and whining. Teachers and parents need to develop the art of overlooking minor "falls" and feel comfortable seeking help for more serious or persistent ones. Children left alone with their peer group often overcome problems with peer assistance, rather than adult intervention	School nurses should regularly monitor playground and classroom activities to identify extricated children and then set the task force (parents, teachers, nurses, other pertinent school or health personnel) in motion to uncover source of problem and offer help. Well-child facility and school nurse should evaluate child's behavior patterns and self-concept at each contact, to pick up clues that all is not well in child's emotional and social relationships. Nurse in clinic or school should offer parent/teacher anticipatory guidance regarding handling of behavior problems

Recognizing and Rewarding Achievements

Parents may need to be encouraged to invite school-age children to participate in family projects and outings that are appropriate to their interests, talents, and developmental level. The freedom to become involved in or help organize family activities and the parents' respect for the contribution to the cooperative endeavor can reinforce the school child's self-worth and convey feelings of belonging that could provide a positive frame of reference for addressing group activities outside the family. The nurse should encourage parents to speak of the unique contributions made by their children. In this manner, individ-

TABLE 8-2
Tasks of Children, Parents, Teachers, and Nurses in Facilitating School Adjustment *(Continued)*

Child's Tasks	Parents' and Teacher's Role in Facilitating Task Achievement	Nurse's Role in Assisting Parents, Teachers, Child
Disposition of Compromise Between Home and Larger World (10 to 12 Yrs)		
Must take increasing responsibility for initiating and carrying out own learning activities at school and home; find internal satisfaction in performance	Family and teacher must acknowledge child's ability to manage responsibility and allocate responsibilities, in which child can take pride and feel success	Nurse in any setting in contact with parents and teachers may offer this anticipatory guidance. Nurse may role model such interactions in dealing with child
Must take interest in organized school and peer activities to be accepted as a group member	Parents need to see developmental advantage of child's involvement in organized activities and plan with child how to get to these—how to financially handle the expenses involved and still manage home and school responsibilities. Teachers should understand the need for such involvement and assign homework reasonably	Same as above. Nurse may help family learn about community activities available to children this age and about financial assistance available through schools, community clubs, churches
Must become capable of maintaining appropriate personal conduct (control impulses, resist temptation) with little or no adult supervision	Child should be given increasing opportunity to go to school and to religious and peer functions unattended by parents and be praised for reports of good conduct. Digression from appropriate conduct should be dealt with in accordance with the seriousness of digression. Parents need to communicate faith in child's ability to handle himself or herself adequately	Same as first entry under this heading, above

ual differences that contribute to identity formation will be encouraged. In addition to being involved in family activities, children need separate time with their parents. The nurse involved in counseling parents can bring this to their attention.

Keeping Financially Solvent

Families with school-age children are expected to continue to provide for the physical safety and economic needs of their members and to obtain enough goods, services, and resources to survive. Because financial and social pressures heighten as children enter school and participate in extracurricular activities and parents' free time increases as their children attend school for longer periods of time, mothers who previously did not work outside the home may now become employed.

The single parent will experience unique pressures to maintain financial solvency. In 1990, 15.9 million children lived in single-parent families (US Department of Health and Human Services, 1991). The majority of these families are headed by mothers. Typically, single mothers are particularly hard-hit when faced with the reality of becoming the head of household, because usually the woman's income is less than that of her male partner. It is estimated that 40 per cent of single-parent families live in poverty (US Department of Health and Human Services, 1991). The mother's problems with finances are further compounded if the father does not contribute child support.

Both fathers and mothers may "moonlight," work overtime, or seek promotion to positions of greater responsibility and stress. The demands of employment will require some shifting of roles and responsibilities of some or all family members. The school nurse, community health nurse, and clinic nurse frequently see the effects of financial problems in the health and behavior of children. Health promotion for children is not adequate unless it includes participation in the political process as an advocate for children.

Adapting Resources to Growing Family Needs

The family of the school-age child is frequently faced with changes in composition by the addition of a new child; the moving in of an elderly grandparent; the death of a parent; career changes, which often involve geographic moves; a parent who goes to work or loses a job; or the separation or divorce of parents who have not been able to cope with all the stresses.

Because of the increased risk of family stress during school-age years, the nurse should take some time at each opportunity to evaluate parents' needs and to assist them, as necessary, through counseling, teaching, or referral to support sources. For this age group, the school nurse may be in a position to offer the most assistance. Assessment data would include a determination of whether the child has medical, dental, hearing, or vision problems that have not been corrected because the family cannot afford care. Most schools have established programs of screening for such problems; however, it does no good to notify parents that their child needs dental work or glasses if the family cannot afford such assistance. The nurse should also be aware that family members may not be able to read, or may not read English, and thus may not be able to understand referrals for medical attention. Any system of health screening in schools should have a strong follow-up program and reflect consideration of the financial inability of some families to provide care (Igoe, 1993).

Growth and Development of the School-Age Child

The school-age period, 6 to 12 years of age, is characterized by slow but steady physical growth, refinement of neuromuscular skills, and rapid expansion of cognitive and social skills. It is a time for "doing" and mastering the ever-expanding world of things and people. During this period, the foundations are laid for future adult roles in the world of work, recreation, and social interaction.

Statistically, the school-age child has the lowest rates of mortality and serious morbidity of any age group. In a health interview survey conducted in the United States, 95 per cent of this age group was reported to be in good or excellent physical health (US Department of Health and Human Services, 1984).

The primary goal of the nurse working with this age group is to promote optimal competencies within the child and to assist the child and parents to appreciate the importance of and the interrelationship of physical, intellectual, emotional, and social competencies (Table 8–3).

Nursing diagnostic responses that may be applied to the care of the school-age child include *high risk for altered growth and development, ineffective individual coping, high risk for sensory-perceptual alteration, high risk for impaired physical mobility,* and *high risk for alteration in health maintenance.* The nurse will continuously assess the child for the etiology of the actual response and the risk factors associated with the high risk problems and defining characteristics. Refer to Table 8–4 for a description of nursing care for the nursing diagnostic response *high risk for altered growth and development.*

Physical Competency

To assess the physical competency of a school-age child, the nurse must be aware that each child has a unique growth pattern although the most obvious measures of physical growth are increases in height and weight (Fig. 8–3). Other indicators of normal development, such as neuromuscular ability, sensory organ development, tooth eruption, and other measures are included in a complete assessment of physical competency (see Table 8–3).

Height and Weight

During the early school-age period, the child's progress in height and weight is relatively slow and steady at approximately 5.5 cm (2 inches) per year for height and 2.5 kg (5.5 pounds) per year for weight. Boys are an average of 1 inch taller and 2 pounds heavier than girls in the early school-age period. The average weight in early school-age years is 40 to 50 pounds, and the average height is 44 to 48 inches.

The yearly increment in height and weight is comparable for boys and girls through age 9 years, when it begins to increase more rapidly for girls than for boys. By age 12 years, girls are 1 inch taller and 2 pounds heavier than boys. This preadolescent growth spurt for girls, beginning between 10 and 12 years, is an initial sign of pubertal maturation. Boys typically have to wait another 2 years for the acceleration in growth; that is, between 12 and 14 years.

Growth is not constant. Periods of acceleration occur at different times in any group of children, with the overall pattern evening out over time. Often children experience an acceleration in height during the spring and an acceleration in weight during the fall of the year.

General Appearance and Skeletal Growth

Body composition changes little during the school-age period. Body fat remains at approximately 15 per cent of total body weight in the school-age child. Muscle mass and extracellular fluid increase by 1 to 2 per cent at this age, whereas organ weight decreases by 1 to 2 per cent. Until the adolescent growth spurt, body composition of boys is comparable to that of girls.

TABLE 8-3
Summary of School-Age Child Growth and Development and Health Maintenance

Physical Competency	Intellectual Competency	Emotional-Social Competency
General: (6 to 12 Yrs)		
Gains an average of 2.5–3.2 kg/yr (5½–7 lbs/yr); overall height gains of 5.5 cm (2 in) per year; growth occurs in spurts and is mainly in trunk and extremities. Loses deciduous teeth, most of permanent teeth erupt. Is progressively more coordinated in both gross and fine motor skills; caloric needs increase with growth spurts	Masters concrete operations. Moves from egocentrism; learns he or she is not always right. Learns grammar and expression of emotions and thoughts. Has vocabulary of 3000 words or more; handles complex sentences	Central crisis; industry vs. inferiority; wants to do and make things. Progressive sex education needed. Wants to be like friends; competition important. Fears body mutilation, alterations in body image; earlier phobias may recur, also nightmares; fears death. Nervous habits common Engages in constant activity. Enjoys group activities but no cooperative play. Temper tantrums used to express anger; is restless and indecisive
6 to 7 Yrs		
Gross motor skill exceeds fine motor coordination. Balance and rhythm are good—child runs, skips, jumps, climbs, gallops; throws and catches ball; dresses self with little or no help	Has vocabulary of 2500 words. Is learning to read and print; begins concrete concepts of numbers, general classification of items. Knows concepts of right and left; morning, afternoon, and evening; coinage. Has intuitive thought process. Is verbally aggressive, bossy, opinionated, argumentative. Likes simple games with basic rules. Has simple understanding of money	Boisterous, outgoing, a know-it-all, whiney; parents should sidestep power struggles, offer choices. Becomes quiet and reflective during seventh year; very sensitive. Can use telephone. Likes to make things: starts many, finishes few. Give some responsibility for household duties. Uses words rather than physical means to express anger
8 to 10 Yrs		
Myopia may appear. Secondary sex characteristics begin in girls. Hand-eye coordination and fine motor skills are well established. Movements are graceful, coordinated. Child cares for own physical needs completely; is constantly on move; plays and works hard. Enforce balance in rest and activity	Is learning correct grammar and to express feelings in words. Likes books he or she can read alone; will read funny papers, scan newspaper. Enjoys making detailed drawings. Is mastering classification, seriation, spatial and temporal, numerical concepts. Uses language as a tool; likes riddles, jokes, chants, word games. Rules are guiding force in life now. Very interested in how things work, what and how weather, seasons, etc., are made	Strong preference for same-sex peers; antagonizes opposite-sex peers. Self-assured and pragmatic at home; questions parental values and ideas. Has a strong sense of humor. Enjoys clubs, group projects, outings, large groups, camp. Modesty about own body increases over time; is sex-conscious. Works diligently to perfect skills he or she does best. Is happy, cooperative, relaxed, and casual in relationships, increasingly courteous and well-mannered with adults. Gang stage at a peak; secret codes and rituals prevail. Responds better to suggestion than dictatorial approach
11 to 12 Yrs		
Vital signs approximate adult norms. Growth spurt occurs for girls. Inequalities between sexes are increasingly noticeable; boys have greater physical strength. Eruption of permanent teeth is complete except for third molars. Secondary sex characteristics begin in boys. Menstruation may begin	Able to think about social problems and prejudices; sees others' points of view. Enjoys reading mysteries, love stories. Begins playing with abstract ideas. Interested in "whys" of health measures and understands human reproduction. Very moralistic; religious commitment often made during this time	Intense team loyalty; boys begin teasing girls and girls flirt with boys for attention; best friend period. Wants unreasonable independence. Rebellious about routines; wide mood swings; needs some time daily for privacy. Very critical of own work. Hero worship prevails. "Facts of life" chats with friends prevail; masturbation increases. Appears under constant tension

(continued)

TABLE 8-3
Summary of School-Age Child Growth and Development and Health Maintenance *(Continued)*

Nutrition	Play	Safety
General: (6 to 12 Yrs)		
Fluctuations in appetite due to uneven growth pattern and tendency to get involved in activities. Tendency to neglect breakfast owing to rush to get to school. Although school lunch is provided in most schools, child does not always eat it	Plays in groups, mostly of same sex; "gang" activities predominate. Books read, all ages. Bicycles important, also sports equipment, cards, board and table games. Most of play is active games requiring little or no equipment	Enforce continued use of seat belts during car travel. Bicycle safety must be taught and enforced. Enforce use of bicycle helmets. Teach safety related to hobbies, handicrafts, mechanical equipment
6 to 7 Yrs		
Preschool food dislikes persist. Tendency for deficiencies in iron, vitamin A, and riboflavin. Needs 100 ml/kg of water per day; 3 g/kg protein daily	Still enjoys dolls, cars, and trucks. Plays well alone but enjoys small groups of both sexes; begins to prefer same-sex peer during 7th year. Is ready to learn how to ride a bicycle. Prefers imaginary, dramatic play with real costumes. Begins collecting for quantity, not quality. Enjoys active games such as hide-and-seek, tag, jump rope, roller skating, kickball. Ready for lessons in dancing, gymnastics, music. Restrict television time to 1–2 hrs/day	Teach and reinforce traffic safety. Still needs adult supervision of play. Teach to avoid strangers, never take anything from strangers. Teach illness prevention and reinforce continued practice of other health habits. Restrict bicycle use to home ground; no traffic areas; teach bicycle safety. Enforce use of bicycle helmets. Teach and set examples to prevent harmful use of drugs, alcohol, smoking
8 to 10 Yrs		
Needs about 2100 calories/day; nutritious snacks. Tends to be too busy to bother to eat. Tendency for deficiencies in calcium, iron, and thiamine. Problem of obesity may begin now. Has good table manners. Is able to help with food preparation	Likes hiking, sports. Enjoys cooking, woodworking, crafts. Enjoys cards and table games. Likes radio and records. Begins qualitative collecting now. Continue restriction on television time	Stress safety with firearms. Keep them out of reach and allow use only with adult supervision. Know who the child's friends are; parents should still have some control over friend selection. Teach water safety; swimming should be supervised by an adult
11 to 12 Yrs		
Male needs 2500 calories per day; female needs 2250 (70 cal/kg/day). Needs 75 ml/kg of water per day. 2 g/kg protein daily	Enjoys projects and working with hands. Likes to do errands and jobs to earn money. Is very involved in sports, dancing, talking on phone. Enjoys all aspects of acting and drama	Continue monitoring friends; stress bicycle safety on streets and in traffic

TABLE 8-4

Growth and Development Plan: Families with School-Age Children

Analysis: Nursing Diagnostic Statement

Response and Related or Risk Factors: *High risk for altered growth and development; risk factors*

- Illness/physical impairment
- Treatment-related procedures
  - Isolation
  - Injections
  - Tractions
  - Casts
  - Bed rest
- Separation from caregivers and peers (parents and significant others)
- Change in environment
- Inadequate sensory stimulation
- Caregiver anxiety
- Caregiver knowledge deficit
- Perceived/actual threats to body image/integrity

Projected Outcome: The school-age child will demonstrate acquisition of developmentally appropriate behaviors in the physical, intellectual, and emotional-social domains

Defining Characteristics	Nursing Interventions	Evaluation Criteria

Subjective:
• Child verbalizes inability to keep up with peers in motor and cognitive skills
• Child verbalizes mistrust, shame/doubt, guilt, inferiority, role diffusion
• Child professes to "be a loner, not to need any one"
• Child senses caregivers' expectations, parental feelings concerning parenting
• Caregiver expresses unrealistic expectations about child's behavior, negative/ambivalent feelings concerning parenting
	Health Screening
	• **Assess factors that can identify altered growth and development.** (Evidence of child's behavior deviating from age-appropriate levels will be observed and documented on the basis of theory of growth and development; parent-child relationships; social support; knowledge of physiologic effects of disease on the child and family)
	• **Assess child's level of development using developmental norms and specific assessment tools.** (Refer to Chapter 13, Assessing Child Health, and Appendices 2 through 6)
		• **Any developmental delays will be identified, as evidenced by**
		  • Charted assessment of screening for physical, intellectual, and emotional/social development
		  • Referral for deviations from the norm detected during screening
		• Caregiver will demonstrate knowledge and ability to interact in an age-appropriate manner with the child and provide activities to support/enhance the developmental needs of the child
		• The child will achieve age-appropriate developmental tasks
		• Referrals to community resources will be made as needed

(continued)

The rate of growth of the trunk and extremities continues to exceed that of the head during the school-age period. Although head circumference increases little, remodeling of facial bones occurs. Because of facial bone remodeling, the eustachian tube gradually assumes a more downward, forward, and inward direction than previously. This structural change is associated with a decrease in the frequency of ear infections as the child grows older.

By age 10 or 11 years, the distance from the crown of the head to the symphysis pubis is approximately equal to the distance from the symphysis pubis to the sole of the foot, and it remains so thereafter. Because of these variations in the rate of growth of the head, trunk, and extremities, the center of gravity of the body with erect posture moves from a point just below the umbilicus at age 5 years to below the crest of the ileum by age 13 years. Improved

TABLE 8-4 (continued)

Defining Characteristics	Nursing Interventions	Evaluation Criteria
Objective: • Flat affect • Listlessness • Decreased responses • Slow social responses • Limited signs of satisfaction to caregivers • Limited eye contact • Decreased appetite • Lethargy • Irritability • Negative mood • Regression in coping skills • School failure • Interruption of sleep pattern • Withdrawal from peers and usual activities	*Anticipatory Guidance; Parent Education: Childrearing Family* • **Provide anticipatory guidance to caregivers regarding acquisition of age-appropriate developmental tasks.** (Refer to information on developmental norms in Chapter 8) • **Assist parents to provide opportunities for the child (including acutely and chronically ill) to meet age-related developmental tasks.** (Refer to information on nursing interventions and anticipatory guidance in Chapter 8 and in Chapter 30) *Support System Enhancement* • **Refer child and family to appropriate community resources as needed** • Appropriate agency for counseling for child and family treatment • Appropriate agency for supportive services (e.g., occupational therapy, physical therapy, home care services) • Community programs specific to factors affecting the child's altered growth and development (e.g., child protection services, educational services, and social services) • Provide information on community self-help groups, parent and sibling support groups, advocacy groups (e.g., Epilepsy Foundation of America, American Heart Association, Association of Retarded Citizens)	

balance of the older school-age child is attributed to this lower center of gravity.

The overall bodily appearance of school-age children also changes—they tend to look thinner than preschool children and adolescents. As skeletal growth progresses, the "rounded" shoulders, slight lordosis, and prominent abdomen of the early school years gradually gives way, by the end of the period, to a more erect posture as the spine becomes straighter. The mild knock-knees or flat feet seen during the earlier years appear to correct themselves during the school-age years (Fig. 8–4).

Organ Maturation

The lymphatic tissues such as tonsils and adenoids grow rapidly during the school-age period, with growth reaching a peak toward the end of the period. Thereafter, involution of lymphatic tissue occurs. School-age children may have as many as six illnesses a year; their response to infection has greater similarity to that of an adult than to a younger child (Behrman, 1992).

Nearly 75 per cent of ocular development is completed during the first 3 years of life. The final growth

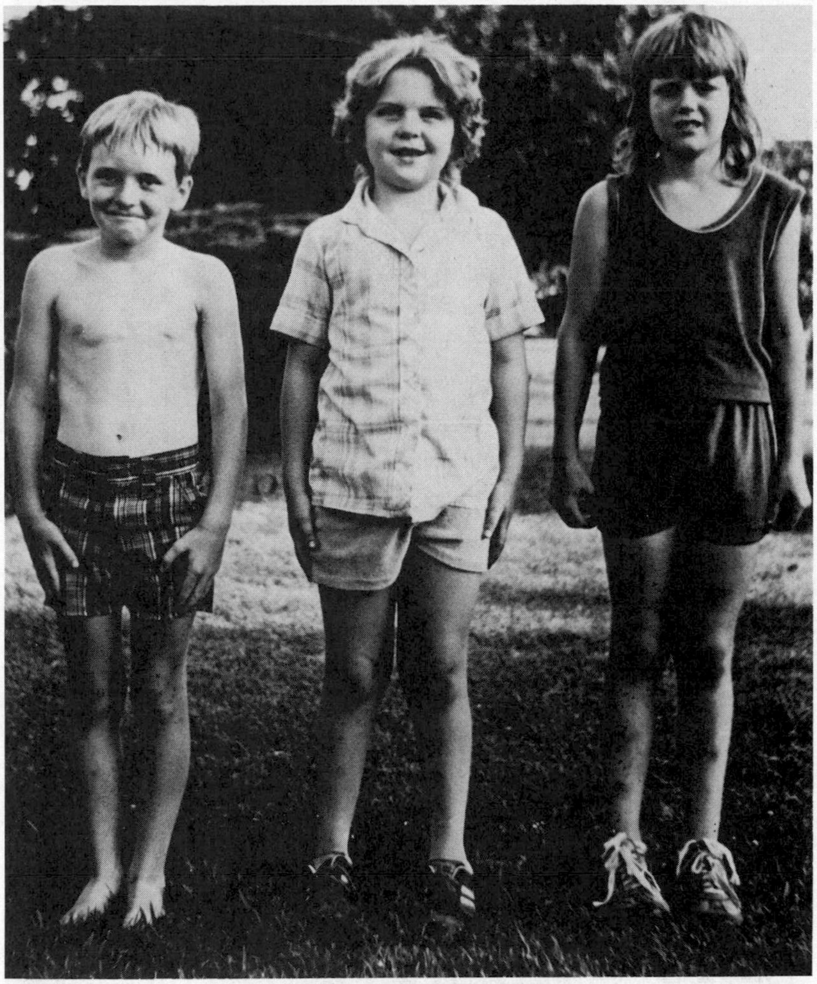

FIGURE 8 - 3. These three 9-year-olds exemplify the typical variations in size of children of the same age during the school years.

phase, affecting only the posterior segment of the eye, proceeds at a very slight and steady pace until approximately 15 years of age. The crystalline lens is the only component of the eye that continues to grow throughout life. Its growth, associated with alterations in its shape, pliability, and refractive index, has important implications for visual acuity.

The normal hyperopia of the young child gradually diminishes during the early school-age period, owing to the growth of the posterior segment of the eye globe. If the eye axis grows to be longer than average, myopia results. This refractive error, which tends to manifest itself between 8 to 10 years of age, usually increases until ocular and body growth are completed.

Anticipatory Guidance: Physical Growth

Comparisons of oneself to others are inevitable. Children and parents should be helped to understand that genetic endowment, nutrition, and exercise are major issues for the healthy child. Parents can be taught how to weigh and measure the child accurately so that together they can plot the child's growth between health assessment visits.

Knowledge of body composition and skeletal growth can help the nurse guide parents and children in handling selected health problems that might occur during this age period. If enlarged tonsils and adenoids or susceptibility to ear infections is of concern, simple explanations about the growth patterns of lymphoid tissue and the direction in which the eustachian tube lies are helpful.

Excessive exercise to develop a specific skill that places undue strain on a bone or joint should be avoided. Because the bones are still ossifying, they cannot tolerate pressure and muscle pull as well as mature bones can. In addition, growth of bone, muscle, tendon, and support tissues may not be synchronous, especially during the preadolescent growth spurt. For these reasons, children are more prone than adults to injury from excessive exercise. Caution also needs to be exercised in carrying heavy loads. Heavy loads, such as books or a pack of newspapers, should be shifted periodically.

Adults (parents or teachers) may become unduly concerned about the posture of an early school-age child, even though normal growth will eventually alleviate the "rounded" shoulders, lordosis, and prominent abdomen of that age group. Posture should be

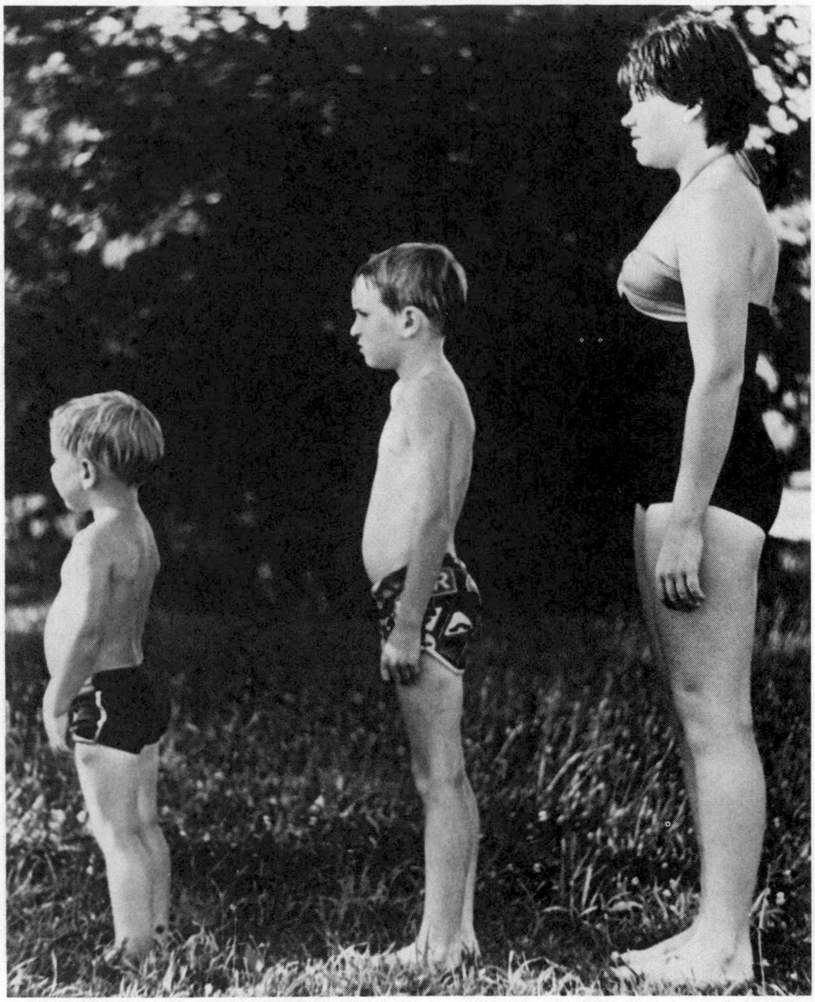

FIGURE 8-4. Note the changes in posture from preschool to school age and to adolescence.

considered satisfactory if a straight line can be visualized to pass from the front of the ear through the shoulder and the greater trochanter to the anterior part of the longitudinal arch of the foot (Fig. 8–5). Ensuring that the child has regular physical activity and regular changes in position when sedentary is more effective in promoting good posture than are exhortations to stand straight. A healthy, rested child typically assumes a balanced, comfortable posture.

Motor Development

The word that best describes the neuromuscular development of the school-age period is *refinement*. The basic mechanisms involved in neuromuscular skills already have been acquired; however, they are rudimentary. The school-age period is the time for refinement and expansion of those skills.

Gross Motor Skills

The six basic gross motor skills that are refined during this age period are running, jumping, sequencing foot movements, balancing, throwing, and catching. Steady improvement in all six basic skills is seen in school-age children, if they are given the opportunity to practice them. The games of childhood, which seem to pass from generation to generation, provide experience in the basic gross motor skills. Examples include running in tag, hide-and-seek, and red rover; jumping, sequencing foot movements, and balancing in skipping, jump rope, hopscotch, bicycling, skating, skateboarding, scrimmaging, and tug of war; and throwing and catching in many games (Fig. 8–6). In most games that school-age children play, coordination of the basic skills is required, and complex movements evolve.

Play of a child changes over time, in keeping with the development of motor skills. The 6-year-old has boundless energy and rudimentary skills. Consequently, play is active, is somewhat disorganized, and requires rather simple skills, such as running, jumping, throwing, and skipping. The 7-year-old seems more cautious, quiet, and intent on acquiring skills such as sequencing foot movements, balancing on a bicycle, throwing, and catching. The 8-year-old has greater smoothness in movements and becomes more

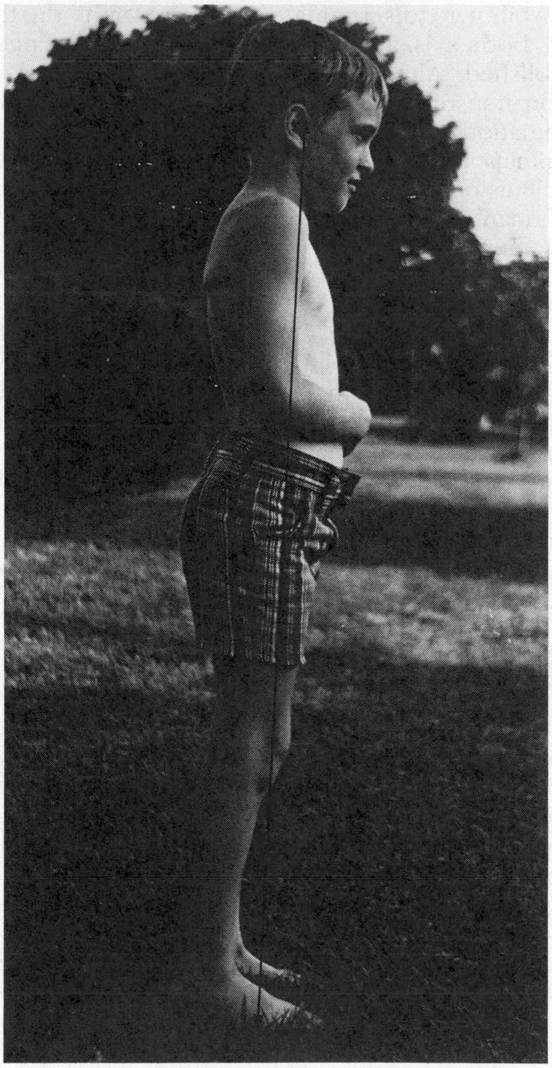

FIGURE 8-5. A straight line that passes from the front of the ear through the shoulder and the greater trochanter to the anterior part of the longitudinal arch of the foot indicates satisfactory posture during the school-age period. (Photograph by Jim Tackett.)

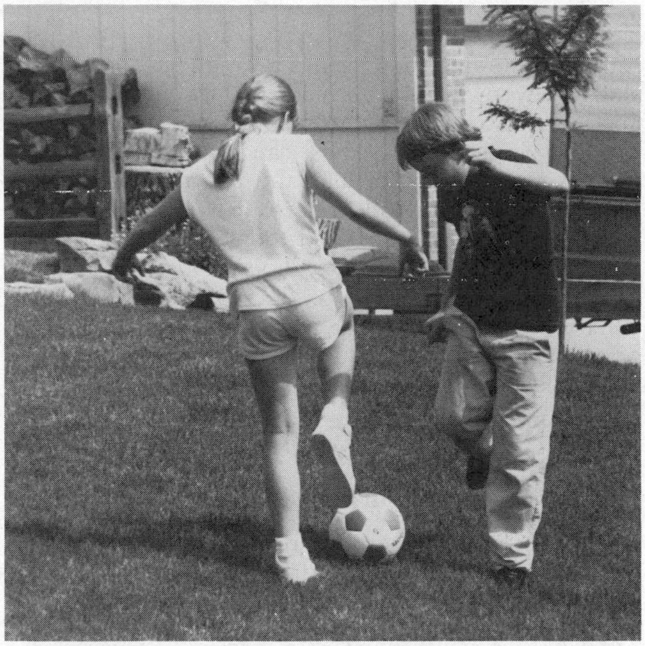

FIGURE 8-6. A game of soccer demonstrates the gross motor skills of running, sequencing foot movements, and balancing.

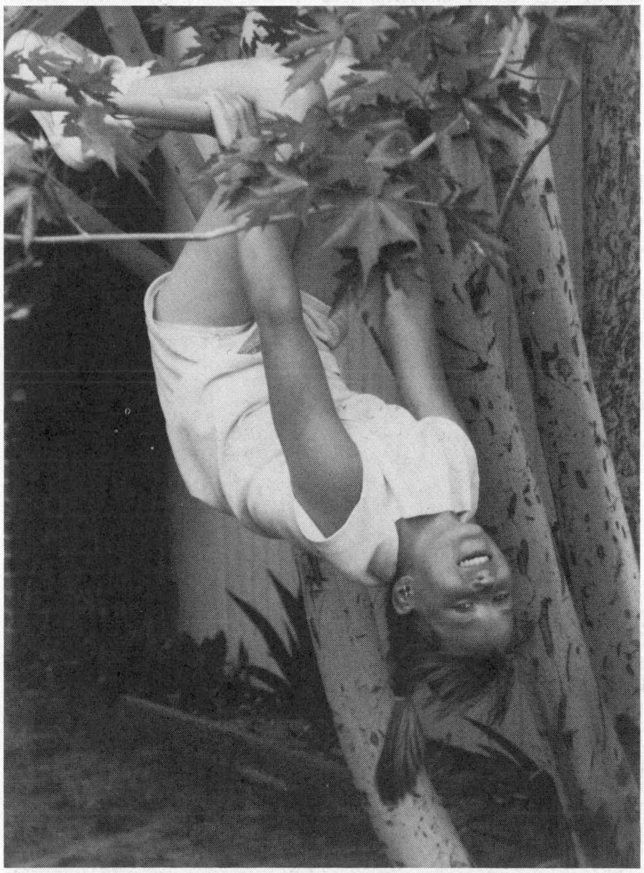

FIGURE 8-7. Gymnastic activities demonstrate the increased coordination of large muscle groups in school-age children. A tree becomes a jungle gym for this 11-year-old.

involved in group activities than a younger child. The 9-year-old works intently on and takes great pride in demonstrating motor skills and strength. Competitive team sports are of interest, and disparity between the skills of individuals becomes more apparent than previously. During the tenth through twelfth years, muscular control and skills in all gross motor areas are established. Just as the school-age period was ushered in for a child experiencing a great need for physical activity, it ends on the same note. The 11- to 12-year-old is energetic, although sporadically, and is very active physically (Fig. 8–7). Because of the preadolescent growth spurt, this increased physical activity may appear more clumsy than the activity of a year or so earlier.

Fine Motor Skills

Although the fine motor skills lag behind gross motor skills, they progress approximately at the same rate. Six-year-olds can cut with scissors, can paste, can button and zipper their clothes, can copy a triangle, can draw a man with 12 details, and can use a pencil for printing. However, skill in these activities tends to be uneven in development, and they may be performed clumsily. The 7-year-old ties shoes, copies a diamond, and draws a man with 16 details. At 8 years old, cursive writing begins. The 9-year-old has well-developed eye-hand coordination. The child can manipulate objects skillfully enough to benefit from hand crafts.

Eye-Hand Coordination

The development of eye-hand coordination is related to development of gross and fine motor skills. By the age of 9 years, the child works well with both hands concurrently on large and small motor tasks but shows preference for either the right or the left hand (Fig. 8–8). *Lateral preference* for using the left or right hand and foot is established during the late preschool or early school-age period. Preference is determined by asking the child to perform a task such as throwing a ball, writing, or kicking a ball. Eye dominance typically occurs by 2 years of age. The child with a dominant right eye will tend to be right-handed (Behrman, 1992).

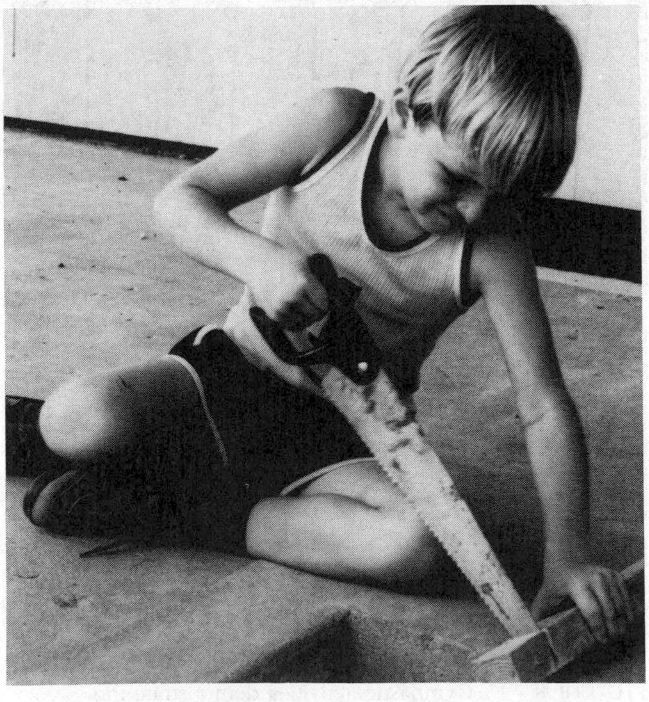

FIGURE 8-8. The 9-year-old has coordination of eye and hand that allows manipulation of objects and the benefits of a variety of projects and crafts.

Ability to discriminate left from right on their own bodies is achieved after hand preference is established. Almost all children can make this discrimination on their own bodies by age 7 years. Discrimination of left and right on others follows self-discrimination. Children with visual-spatial perception problems often have delays in left-right discrimination (Behrman, 1992). The perceptual ability to imitate the movements of another person standing facing the child, however, is a more difficult task, and the skill may not be acquired until adolescence.

The reaction time or speed in performing fine motor skills, such as tapping, turning small objects, and removing and placing pegs, increases rapidly from 6 to 9 or 10 years of age, after which the rate of improvement gradually slows. Accuracy of movement improves markedly from 5 to 9 years and then less rapidly to adolescence. Girls tend to have better dexterity of hands and fingers than boys and tend to perform fine motor skills at a greater speed and more accurately than boys.

Nursing Interventions: Motor Skills

Knowledge of the school-ager's motor development can assist the nurse to assess and intervene to promote developmentally appropriate activities. Nursing diagnostic responses related to motor skills development are ***high risk for altered growth and development*** and ***high risk for impaired physical mobility***. The ill and/or hospitalized school-ager's motor abilities can be affected or restricted. The nurse who recognizes these developmental effects can encourage activities that are more appropriate to the child's level of current abilities. A clinical illustration is presented in Table 8–5. Parents may be alarmed by their child's loss of functioning. The nurse can reassure parents that this is another effect of the illness/hospitalization.

Anticipatory Guidance: Motor Skills

The healthy school-age child will pursue gross and fine motor activities if provided with the opportunity. Parents should be encouraged to provide these opportunities for a variety of reasons. The benefits of physical activity are numerous, including the promotion of bone growth, enhancement of learning, and promotion of fitness and a physically active lifestyle.

Physical fitness is almost synonymous with *physical activity*. A physically fit child who finds pleasure in gross motor activity usually carries this fitness and pleasure into adulthood. Childhood provides a unique opportunity for promoting healthful exercise habits, because of the child's propensity for delighting in gross motor activity. The opportunities parents provide for gross and fine motor activities need not be elaborate or expensive. Many gross physical activities can take place in a relatively small space. Walking or

TABLE 8-5

Promoting Motor Development in the Hospitalized Child

Jake, age 9 years, has been hospitalized for 2 days and is on bed rest. He will be on bed rest for at least 7 more days until his course of antibiotic therapy for osteomyelitis is completed. Jake's nursing care plan included the following problems and interventions to promote motor development

Encourage fine motor activity as tolerated: Ask Jake which of his favorite activities he would like to do:

- Play computer games
- Build airplane model
- Work on stamp collection
- Work on baseball card collection

Encourage activities with age-appropriate peers

- Play cards
- Play Trivial Pursuit
- Watch television programs: teen-age dance program (4–5 P.M.) and news (6–6:30 P.M.)

Allot time for school activities (for fine motor skills)

- Schedule time with hospital teacher
- Set aside time to complete homework

jogging can be a family affair. Advantage can be taken of community programs and parks. For fine motor activities, paper, pencils, crayons, water colors, scissors, string, beads, empty food cartons, and so forth can be implements for creative activities.

Periods of physical activity also enhance academic learning. Schools have long recognized this phenomenon and have provided recess periods for gross motor activity. Research also has demonstrated the positive influence of such motor activity on learning. One of the largest and most notable studies showed that in a school in which classroom time was decreased by one third and the gained time was devoted to physical education, children performed better academically than their counterparts whose school maintained the regular schedule. Even though the time of instruction was decreased by a third, the children did as well or better on scholastic tests than the "regular" counterparts (Bailey, 1978).

Limits may need to be set on television viewing if it interferes with more productive pursuits. Increased competency in skills should be rewarded by praise that is deserved but not exaggerated.

Intellectual Competency

Although physical development during the school-age period is characterized as slow and steady, cognitive development is characterized as rapid and expanding. It is as though physical development in general is held somewhat in abeyance, so that all the child's energies can be directed toward cognitive development. That is not to say that physical development decreases; it continues and contributes much to cognitive development. Neurologic development, including refinement of the corpus callosum of the brain at age 7 or 8 years, promotes the expansion of cognitive competency.

Intelligence

Intelligence is generally considered to be the ability to learn, or acquire and retain knowledge. Intelligence is assessed by various tests. The Stanford-Binet test and the Wechsler Intelligence Scale for Children are widely used to test intelligence.

Results of intelligence tests must be interpreted with caution, especially the results of group testing, which is the usual testing method. These tests are encumbered by the problem common to any paper-and-pencil test—their results depend on the motivation to do well on the test and on the well-being of the child at the time the test is given. The results of the test can be affected by a variety of other factors, including reading skills and luck in guessing correctly.

Since the 1960s, intelligence tests have been the subject of controversy, primarily because of the misuse of test results to label and track children educationally. African-Americans, Hispanics, and other children not exposed to mainstream middle class experiences are at a disadvantage in taking the tests.

Much effort has been devoted to developing tests that are valid and reliable across the range of culture and experience.

Anticipatory Guidance: Intelligence

Intelligence tests should be considered only as screening tools to help the child reach full potential. IQ can and does change. If used appropriately, the tests can help the parent and child recognize the child's strengths and weaknesses and set realistic goals and expectations.

Parents can promote intellectual competency by stimulating the child's desire for achievement and by offering a variety of experiences that foster mental development. The extent to which families value intellectual pursuits profoundly affects their children's achievement orientation, as well as the experiences to which they are exposed. Certainly a child who is exposed to books and magazines in the home and sees parents reading with interest will have an orientation to intellectual achievement different from that of a child who is exposed to neither situation.

Cognitive Development: Preoperational Period

During the school-age period, the child's thought processes undergo dramatic shifts. According to Piaget (1966), at the beginning of the school-age period these thought processes are characterized as *intuitive thought;* they move into *concrete operations* at about 7 or 8 years of age and from there into *formal operations* at about 11 to 12 years (refer to Table 8–6 for characteristics of the school-age child's thinking).

Intuitive Stage

With intuitive thought (6 to 7 years), thinking is based on an immediate, unanalyzed relationship between any particular environmental phenomenon and the child's own viewpoint. For example, this child believes that anything moving is alive *(animism)*. Conversations tend to be monologues, because children believe that others think as they do *(egocentrism)* and can even read their minds.

Children focus their attention on one aspect of an object or a situation *(centration)*. They cannot consider more than one aspect. The following vignette illustrates this concept:

A boy was upset that the pair of running shoes he received were not similar to the pair he wanted that his father wore. His mother pointed out that they were exactly the same; the same brand and style only a smaller version. Jeremy pointed to the difference in color of the pin striping along the edge of the sole of the shoe. His was blue, compared to the red color of his father's running shoe. This small difference indicated to Jeremy that the shoes were not the same but vastly different.

These characteristics of intuitive thought lead the child to make gross misinterpretations of phenomena. They do not provide the cognitive tools for organizing the world of people, places, and things into systems. Those cognitive tools are provided through "operations"—first, concrete operations for dealing with people, places, and things that can be experienced through the senses and then formal operations for dealing with abstracts and for playing with ideas.

Significant improvements are observed between 5 and 12 years in the child's capacity for remembering past events. Between 6 and 8 years of age the child learns a great deal about the days of the week, months, and seasons of the year. At this time, a child can locate a past event in terms of these specific times. For example, a child will remember an event as occurring on Saturday as he was watching cartoons on TV in the morning. The child's ability to develop a chronologic sense of the past can be enhanced by teaching these concepts both at school and in the home (Friedman, 1991).

Concrete Operations Stage

During the stage of *concrete operations* (approximately 7 to 11 years), children step outside their own thought processes and realize that their way of thinking is not the only way. Real conversation and information sharing become possible. Gradually, the egocentric and fluctuating rules for games and behavior give way to democratically derived rules for games and reasonable expectations for behavior.

The children can now decenter, or consider more than one characteristic or attribute of an object or environmental phenomenon at the same time. They can consider the various parts of a whole while maintaining the concept of the whole. An important characteristic of the thought process is retracing the steps taken mentally to arrive at a conclusion. Piaget referred to this ability as *reversibility*. At this stage, children realize that there may be more than one way of arriving at the same conclusion. They can mentally perform tasks that previously had to be actually carried out. *Conservation* is learned. They achieve the ability to recognize that two equal quantities of matter remain equal, regardless of the transformation they undergo. They are capable of using various mathematical calculations such as addition, subtraction, multiplication, and division. *Numbering* also refers to the child's ability to order and classify objects. That is, a child can order objects according to various properties of objects, such as size—smallest to largest. The school-ager can classify entities, such as pets—dogs, cats, birds, and so forth.

Prior to age 8 or 9 years, the concept of chance is lacking. Everything has a reason—often based on immediate, unanalyzed relationships between environmental events. For example, falling down and skinning a knee may be attributed to disobeying

TABLE 8-6
Characteristics of the School-Age Child's Thinking

Characteristic	Definition	Clinical Example
Preoperational Period—Intuitive Phase		
Animism	Inanimate objects have existence	Child cries when sees equipment; exclaims "It will hurt me!"
Egocentrism	Cannot separate self from others; believes others think as child does	Child sees another child receive an injection and begins to cry when the child does
Centration	Can focus on only one aspect of a situation	Child states does not want to go to the hospital, since that is where "people die"—grandfather died in the hospital 3 mos earlier
Concrete Operations		
Decentration	Can consider more than one characteristic of object/situation	During preoperative teaching, child asks several questions
Reversibility	Realizes more than one way of arriving at some conclusion—mentally performs tasks	Child tells nurse he cannot take pill form; asks nurse to crush pills and put in applesauce
Conservation	Equal qualities of matter remain equal regardless of transformation they undergo	Child is on strict fluid limit, but wants some watermelon for lunch; understands the reasons nurse gives for having to measure amount first before eating
Numbering	Capable of counting and other mathematical calculation; can order and classify objects	Child wants to look at his/her incision and wants to count the number of "sticks" from the stitches
Concept of Chance	Realizes not everything occurs because of egocentric predetermined cause	Child assures nurse that he/she understands illness was not caused by behavior (e.g., being "bad")
Physical/Psychologic Causality	Learns and seeks physical and psychologic reasons for events	Child understands that infections are caused by microorganisms

mother an hour earlier. Not only does everything have a reason, but because of the young child's egocentric thought patterns, the reason often centers on the self. For example, the child may think a parent has become ill because the child angrily wished it so. With the realization at age 8 or 9 years of the concept of *chance,* life becomes much more benevolent than it was previously.

Children during this stage rely less on their own reality for explanations of the world around them. Animistic and artificialistic ideas are disappearing. Children learn and seek the physical and psychologic reasons for the events they observe around them. Piaget refers to the acquisition of these cognitive skills as *physical and psychologic causality.*

After age 7 or 8 years, games are characterized by increasing structure, with common observance of rules and mutual surveillance to make sure all players observe the rules. The spirit of the game is honest competition; some players win and others lose, according to the rules. True communication, cooperative play, and mutual respect are now possible. After age 10 or 11 years, handicaps are even added to games when appropriate, because to win over a less-skilled opponent is not to win at all.

From ages 8 or 9 years, the behavior of children also evidences an increased perceptual ability, with attendant self-criticism of activities such as drawing. Drawings consequently seem less creative and imaginative as the child tries to replicate reality. In everyday life, the age of 9 years is known as the age of erasures, in which children demonstrate increased dissatisfaction with their efforts if the drawing does not appear realistic.

When children enter the stage of concrete operations, all characteristics of the stage are not necessarily available in all situations. For example, children discover the conservation of substance at 7 or 8 years by realizing that changes in shape do not change the quantity of such substances as clay. However, they do not discover the conservation of weight until they are about 9 or 10 years old and do not discover the conservation of volume until 11 or 12 years (measured by displacement of water when an object is immersed).

During the stage of concrete operations (7 to 11 years), children work hard to discover how the world of people, places, and things—which they can experience through their senses—functions. The concrete operational child is not yet able to work with the abstractions, hypotheses, and propositions that are removed from the concrete and present observation; that is, the child is still unable to play with ideas. That ability will begin to develop at age 11 or 12 years as the child moves into adolescence and the stage of formal operations.

Nursing Interventions: Cognitive Development

The nurse who has a thorough knowledge of Piaget's theory will be better able to recognize the defining characteristics of *high risk or actual altered growth and development.* If either of these nursing diagnostic responses is verified, interventions will often involve guidance for the parents. During periods of illness and hospitalization, developmentally appropriate activities can be planned for the school-ager. For example, board games, video or electronic games, and books can be used to stimulate cognitive processes. As the child's condition permits, continuing with school activities is a priority. Parents can make arrangements with the child's teacher to continue with classroom assignments. In some cases, referral to the hospital's school teacher is made (see Tables 8–7 and 8–8). Children's understanding of bodily functions improves significantly during the period of concrete operations. Children develop rudimentary notions of the brain, heart, bones, and stomach. Knowledge of other bodily functions and organs remains limited. Recognition of the child's deficits of understanding of internal bodily functions must be incorporated in explanations to the child (Jones et al, 1992).

The child's ability to accurately recall past events is not dependable until approximately 8 years of age (Friedman, 1991). The nurse must gather information from the child regarding the perception of past events, because it will provide insights as to how the child has incorporated them. Interventions may be warranted to correct the child's misperceptions and to alleviate fears and anxieties.

Anticipatory Guidance: Cognitive Development

During the intuitive stage, parents and teachers may utilize a variety of "think games" to nurture the development of concrete operations. For example, several cups of different colors and progressive sizes may be used to help learn ranking and arrangement of objects by common characteristics; a variety of pictures of objects may be used to help learn to compare, contrast, and classify items that are alike and different in some way, such as baseball or football cards. Similarly, games can be used with other children to help them master temporal and numeric concepts.

Parents should be encouraged to have patience and allow school-age children to do some of their own problem solving. Parents may need to be reminded that trial and error is a valuable part of learning problem solving. Parents should not expect the school-age child to handle more than one big problem at a time, and they should be cautioned to expect some fluctuation in the child's skill.

Play continues to be a necessary main activity if the school-age child is to progress cognitively. Through play, group games, and peer interaction the child learns the cognitive concepts necessary to cooperation, compromise, persuasion, and productivity. Parents may need help from the nurse to understand this valuable function.

Language Development

As might be expected from the profound changes in cognitive development, language development progresses rapidly during the school-age period. An assessment of the progress in language development includes examination of the three interactive components of language itself: *phonics,* or speech sound; *syntax,* or grammar; and *semantics,* or meaning in language forms such as words and sentences. The assessment is not complete, however, without considering the child's personal and social uses of language.

Usually, speech is fluent and the voice well-modulated in the 6-year-old. Also, *articulation,* or phonetically correct speech, is usually good, with the possible exceptions of *thr, shr, sk, sh, ch, s, j,* and *z* sounds. By 7 or 8 years, however, these sounds should be pronounced correctly (Smart & Smart, 1978). Articulation difficulties may result from physical problems, such as cleft palate or hearing losses, or from true cultural factors. Apparent speech defects may be a consequence of the child's imitating the speech patterns of the home or neighborhood environment.

Syntax grammar is usually correct by 6 years of age, and the child can form five- or six-word sentences. Semantically, the 6-year-old has a vocabulary of 2500 to 3000 words, can carry out commands involving three or four actions, and comprehends "if," "because," and "why" (Lowery, 1978). Complex and compound sentences are used increasingly after age 7. Nuances of word meaning, of words standing alone or included in a sentence, are comprehended increasingly. In addition to increasing the vocabulary, the child learns new meaning and more subtle connotations for old words. Whereas younger school-age children typically define words by offering descriptions of the thing signified or examples of its functions, the older school-age child tends to employ explanations or synonyms. At the end of the school-age period, word meanings increasingly approximate those of adults.

The function of chants, rituals, and superstition in the culture of school-age children is an example of how the many aspects of development are inextricably interrelated. Although they are expressed in language and thus are important in language development, chants, rituals, and superstitions are also important aspects of emotional-social development. The countless

TABLE 8-7

Promoting Cognitive Development: Continued Educational Experiences During Hospitalization

Arturo is expected to be in the hospital for at least 3 weeks. The clinical nurse specialist anticipates his need to continue school assignments and includes the following entries on his nursing care plan

Refer to school teacher

- Schedule time for school and homework into daily activities
- No IVs in right hand
- Limit use of television (parents do not encourage television watching; watches two programs during the week)

Encourage parents to bring materials/activities that Arturo normally does

- Bring in desktop computer
- Bring in favorite books
- Bring in writing materials
- Encourage and make available games that can be played alone or with nurse or peer, such as solitaire, crossword puzzles, electronic games, and brain teasers

TABLE 8-8

Promoting Cognitive Development: Discharge Teaching

Miguel, age 11, is about to be discharged from the hospital. He will continue taking certain medications. To prepare him for assuming this responsibility, his nurse demonstrates the proper procedure for taking his antibiotics

Interaction	***Rationale***
Nurse: Which way do you want to take your medicine . . . the liquid or pill form? Miguel: Pills	***Conservation*** Understands that different forms of matter can be equal
Nurse: The doctor has ordered the medicine to be taken four times a day for 10 days. Here is a chart that you can use to check off the times you take the medicine.	***Numbering*** Is able to understand notion of counting
Miguel: What time am I supposed to take them?	***Concrete Operations*** May indicate comprehension of abstract concept, yet does not; graphic demonstration enhances comprehension
Nurse: It depends on what works best for your daily schedule. It is best to take the pills before meals, and you'll probably not want to take more than one pill at school.	***Decenter*** Is able to consider more than one factor of a situation

chants and magic-making words of school-age children provide a sense of control in a sometimes frightening and bewildering world. Chants accompany many ancient games, such as London Bridge, ring-around-the-rosy, jump rope, and ball bouncing. Some are saved for special occasions: "Ladybug, ladybug, fly away home" and "It's raining, it's pouring, the old man is snoring." Some have special powers to grant wishes or protect from unseen harm: "Star light, star bright, first star I see tonight," "Cross my heart and hope to die," and "Knock on wood." Some may be verbalized or just acted out: "Hold your breath crossing a bridge," "Lift your feet crossing a railroad track," and "Cross your fingers." These words tend to have a magical quality for school-age children, as well as being fun to say.

Illustrative of the expansion in mental processes involved in language are the typical questions the child asks during the school-age period. As children advance in age, their questions become less global (Why?), more specific (What? Who? Where? Which?), and finally, more definitive (How?).

The language of school-age children has a distinctive quality and unique personal and social functions. This language is a part of the culture of childhood—a culture that is learned, shared, and transmitted among children but that is shaped by the adult world around them. Children teach other children the rhymes, chants, and rituals of childhood. Language enables school-age children to meet their abiding need to master and control their expanding world and to acquire a social identity with peers.

Humor is also expressed through language. Verbal humor can function just for the sheer joy of demonstrating mastery over language. This delight in language mastery is seen in "knock knock" jokes, puns, tongue twisters, and riddles. The verbal humor of early school-age children is often expressed in riddles. Riddles can provide children with a sense of authority or power. So much of what adults say is incomprehensible or difficult to understand; a riddle can create a situation in which the child is the authority with the answer. Likewise, jokes, which become more common around ages 8 or 9, often tend to disparage adults and thus release tensions children may experience about their inadequacy in knowledge and power in relation to adults. Jokes can serve as a way of releasing anger, aggression, or frustration in a socially acceptable manner—for example, expressing hostility toward a sibling.

Language during the school-age period is the vehicle for expanding knowledge as well as personal and social growth of children.

Nursing Interventions: Language Development

School-agers are far more adept with language, which enables greater verbal communication with the nurse. Children can express their needs to the nurse, for example, when they are in pain or when they are afraid. However, it is important not to assume, because of the school-ager's growing competencies, that the child will communicate openly with the nurse. Feelings of trust, familial customs regarding communications, and anxieties and fears surrounding hospitalization affect the child's willingness and ability to communicate with the nurse.

The nurse must give school-agers the opportunity to explain what they know about their treatment, medications, and pathology of their disease. The school-age child derives satisfaction from incorporating medical terminology and the hospital jargon into conversations. Acknowledgment of the child's sharing of information serves to reinforce the satisfaction of being able to speak in this fashion.

There may be a tendency for the nurse to assume that children understand more than they actually do. This is especially true for explanations of medically related procedures, tests, and diseases. Unfamiliarity with medical terminology and disease-related information necessitates the use of drawings, pictures, and replications of medical and hospital paraphernalia. Repeated explanations are necessary, because the anxieties the child experiences and the unfamiliarity with the hospital will interfere with the acquisition of information.

Anticipatory Guidance: Language Development

As with other aspects of development, children need to be provided with opportunities to exercise and expand their language skills. They should be exposed to the pronunciation and usage of society's mainstream language and to reading.

Parents can facilitate language development in the expression of feelings and thoughts by regularly encouraging discussion of their child's ideas, plans, and reactions. Likewise, parents can be urged to express their own feelings, observations, and ideas to their children, so that they learn the appropriate words to describe feelings and thoughts. Such discussion opportunities not only help the child develop vocabulary and learn correct grammar (provided proper grammar is used by the parents), but such activity helps keep communication lines open as the child approaches adolescence.

Anticipatory guidance about the personal and social uses of childhood language helps parents conjure up at least hazy memories of the chants, rituals, and secret languages they used as children, which facilitates their acceptance of these language forms as a part of growing up.

Emotional-Social Competency

The major focus of emotional-social development in the school-age period is the introduction of the child into society. This development is related to and runs parallel with physical and intellectual development and language development. Separating them is somewhat artificial, but doing so provides a more coherent picture of development than considering all three facets together. Included in the discussion of emotional-social development are psychosocial development, sexuality, temperament, emotions, culture, and the developing person.

Psychosocial Development: Industry and Self-Esteem

The major purpose of psychosocial development in the school-age period is the establishment of the ego quality of industry versus inferiority, Erikson's fourth stage. As Erikson (1967) stated:

> One might say that personality at the first stage crystallizes around the conviction "I am what I am given," and that of the second, "I am what I will." The third can be characterized by "I am what I can imagine I will be." We must now approach the fourth stage: "I am what I learn." The child now wants to be shown how to get busy with something and how to be busy with others.

Erikson continued to describe what he meant by the term "sense of industry":

> Children become dissatisfied and disgruntled without a sense of being useful, without a sense of being able to make things and make them well and even perfectly: this is what I call the *sense of industry*.

The child becomes involved in production of things, work completion, division of labor, equality of opportunity, and positive identification with those who *know* things and know how to *do things* (Fig. 8–9). The child's social world is continually expanding to include school, clubs, physical activities, and sports. Through interactions with peers, the child works on becoming an equal and accepted member of the group. This may mean directing extra time and effort into doing school work or improving an athletic skill.

As is clear from Erikson's words, the ego quality of industry versus inferiority has personal and social implications. On the personal level, the focus is on the competency of the individual, especially in physical and cognitive skills. Previous discussion of these skills demonstrates the progress the normal child makes in these areas. The child's psychic energies are directed toward the acquisition and perfection of these skills. "Industrious" is an apt description of school-age children. This age group's sense of self or self-concept is heavily influenced by interactions with the expanding world of social contacts: family, friends, classmates, and authority figures (Winklestein, 1989). These feelings about self will influence the child's activities and behaviors. For example, research has shown that children with positive self-concepts do better academically than children with negative self-concepts (Leonardson, 1986).

The danger of this stage is that children will find their physical and cognitive skills wanting and will develop a sense of inadequacy and inferiority, rather than of industry and competence. Most children, however, are capable of developing competence in some area of activity. However, few are capable of developing competence in all areas of activity. For example, self-destructive health behaviors in children, such as alcoholism and drug abuse, have been associated with negative self-concepts. Successful completion of this stage, then, means that children come to recognize their abilities as well as their liabilities and develop a sense of competence, pride, and self-esteem for what they can do (Fig. 8–10). Competition among individuals is very much a part of this stage. Through competition with peers, youngsters gain recognition of personal assets and liabilities.

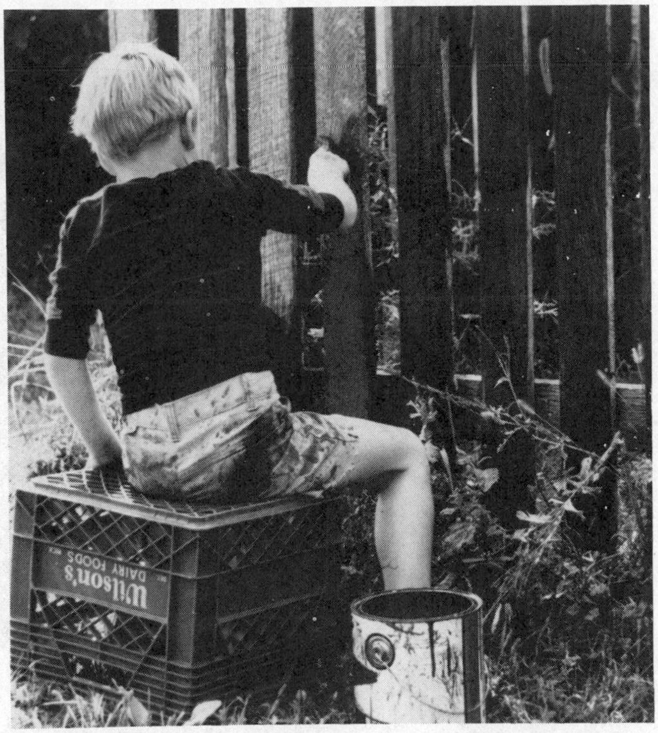

FIGURE 8-9. The school-age child is industrious.

A sense of inferiority in some areas of activity is inevitable for the vast majority of children. As Erikson points out, the "versus" in the stage designations does not mean that the negative component is not present; it only means that for successful completion of the stage, the positive component must outweigh the negative one in the equation. School-age children, therefore, need to recognize their limitations and to accept them without a diminution of self-esteem. Not everyone has artistic talent, but just because an individual does not have artistic talent does not mean the individual is less of a person than one who has such ability. The same holds true for any type of activity. This major achievement of a personal and social identity as an industrious and competent individual and group member occurs rather slowly over the entire span of the school-age period. The characteristic be-

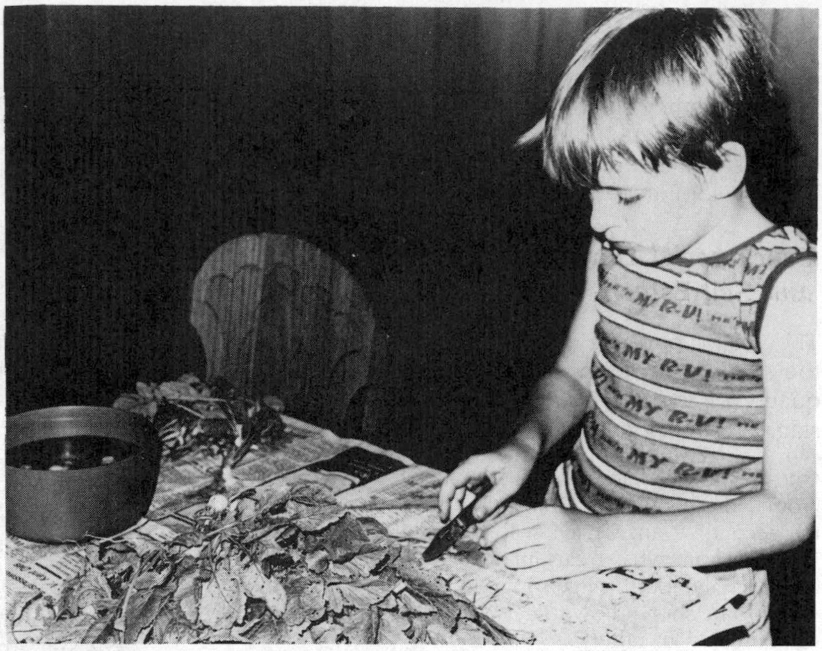

FIGURE 8-10. By 9 years, the child can assume responsibility for assisting with meal preparation and cleanup.

haviors of the child at each age from 6 to 12 years illustrate this gradual progression.

Nursing Interventions: Fostering Industry and Self-Esteem

Hospitalization and illness can impose significant restrictions on the school-age child's need to be an industrious and competent individual. For example, one youngster may worry that she cannot keep up with school work because of absences from school. Another child who is diabetic may feel inadequate compared with his classmates because of the treatment-related activities and monitoring needed to manage his condition. Nursing care needs to focus on *what* the child can do and *adjustment to* activities that are restricted temporarily or on a long-term basis. The child can be encouraged to maintain contact with his circle of friends as a means of enhancing his sense of self (Winklestein, 1989). If friends are not available, then activities with other children on the unit can be encouraged. Table 8–9 specifies the nursing care that addresses these unique school-age needs.

Nurses in a variety of community settings can develop programs to foster the child's self-concept, which is essential to maintaining health-promoting behavior. For example, a school nurse developed an instructional program to encourage positive self-concept (Winklestein, 1989). Through a variety of group learning activities, the students began to understand what kinds of remarks and actions promoted a positive self-concept. During these activities, the nurse identified the risk factors or defining characteristics of the children with the nursing diagnosis of *self-esteem*.

Anticipatory Guidance: Industry and Self-Esteem

School-age children need to recognize and accept their limitations without a decrease in self-esteem. Parents can assist youngsters in learning to respect the abilities of others and take pride in the accomplishments attained in group activities. They learn that the strengths and weaknesses of individuals, including their own, can be counterbalanced by the group. Children also learn perhaps the hardest lesson of all, that the accomplishments of others do not diminish their own achievements. These are not easy years for either the child or parents. The parents' understanding of the typical behavior of the child, however, will help provide the support the child needs for progress in the long struggle for a sense of industry and competency, rather than inferiority and inadequacy.

Sexuality

The child of 6 to 12 years of age continues to develop sexual awareness and purposeful sexual behaviors. The psychoanalytic term *latency* used by Freud to describe this state of psychosexual development is now considered a myth.

Developing a Positive Sexual Attitude

The attitude of the school-age child continues to form in response to increasing influence from outside the family. Interaction with peers, school authorities, and the mass media shapes expanding views.

TABLE 8-9

Promoting Industry and Self-Esteem in the Hospitalized Child

Jacob was recently admitted to the hospital for second- and third-degree burns on his right forearm and hand. The following nursing care plan was formulated to promote Jacob's self-esteem and encourage independent action. Information obtained from the nursing assessment provided the basis for the individualized nursing care plan

Encourage continuation of school activities

- In hospital, initiate a school teacher referral
- Schedule bedside teaching and homework times into daily activities
- Contact volunteer to assist Jacob in completing assignments (right hand is writing hand)

Substitute passive activities for favorite interests (e.g., baseball, football)

- Watch baseball games on television
- Obtain sports videos from lounge
- Generate interest in sports trivia/knowledge via newspapers/magazines
- Take to adolescent lounge to play with video games

Encourage socialization with peers

- Age-appropriate roommate
- Schedule daily visits to lounge
- Encourage phone calls, visits, and letters from peers
- Inform parents to encourage friends to visit

Encourage self-care and responsibility

- Assist in accurate recording of intake/output
- Assist in helping with dressing changes
- Assist in calculating protein and calorie intake

Sexual identity, although not well differentiated at 5 years of age, gradually develops during the school-age years. Girls show more consistent and rapid development of sexual identity than do boys. This parallels their more rapid physical growth and development. Many studies show that parental attitudes and values have a significant effect on the child's developing sexual identity. However, peer influence is more important in this age group than among younger children.

Sexual Behaviors

Children in lower grades (ages 5 and 6 years) may engage in sex play such as "house" and "doctor," each of which may include direct physical contact of a sexual nature. At this age, play becomes more explicit as girls experiment with wearing makeup, placing pillows under their skirts to mimic pregnancy, and kissing little boys. Boys play at fighting to show their prowess, and they tease little girls by trying to peek under their skirts.

Children in the second and third grades (ages 7 to 9) behave with greater sophistication. More interest is shown in sex role–related objects, such as clothing and perfume. Both sexes are interested in peeking at the bodies of members of the opposite sex, and boys begin to practice street-wise sexual vocabulary (Janus & Bess, 1981).

From fourth grade through junior high school, preadolescent behavior includes both same-sex and opposite-sex contacts. The formation of close friendships with the same-sex groups is necessary for confirming sexual identity. Increasing physical contact with members of the opposite sex prepares the individual for mature heterosexual relationships. Sexual activity gradually progresses to hugging, kissing, and dancing with members of the opposite sex. Voyeurism continues, gradually being replaced by explicit magazines, movies, and drawings. By the end of fifth grade (age 11), some boys and many girls already begin to acquire mature sexual characteristics with development of breast and hip tissue and growth of pubic, underarm, and facial hair.

Masturbation and orgasm often occur during the sixth grade year (ages 11 and 12) and most frequently are normal expressions of sexuality for both sexes. Self-stimulation of the genitals may be direct or indirect. Although some girls may give up masturbation during the school years, they continue to engage in activities like sliding down ropes and banisters, gymnastics, and horseback riding, which they report as providing pleasurable sensations in the genitalia. Both boys and girls engage in sex-related fantasies; girls enjoy those related to romance, and boys are more directly concerned with specific sexual acts, such as intercourse.

Temperament

Because of their awareness of the individual differences among children that could not be accounted for by developmental theories, health professionals who deal with children have welcomed the work of Thomas and Chess (1977) on temperamental styles. Although innate characteristics of temperament seem to be relatively stable, their expressions may vary over time, being influenced by environment and intrinsic developmental factors. Factors affecting childhood temperament include hormonal changes, changes in sleep patterns and diet, substance abuse, and rigorous athletic training (Carey, 1992). Therefore, an understanding of the nine major categories of temperament provides a means of seeing how the individual child approaches learning tasks and interacts with peers and adults. The factors involved in temperament are activity level, approachability, adaptability, intensity of reaction, threshold for stimulus, mood, distractibility, attention span, and persistence. These are discussed in greater depth in Chapter 3. During the school years, persistence, attention span, and distractibility assume greater importance.

A child's innate *activity level* is not likely to present problems in the adjustment to school if it is average or low. However, a high activity level may make it difficult for the child to settle down to sedentary activities in the classroom. Opportunities for regular motor activity are important, especially for the child with a high activity level, as is patience on the part of the teacher and parent.

The child who has a personality characterized by high *approachability* responds well to new situations, people, places, and learning demands and usually is a joy for a teacher. The child who initially withdraws from new situations and is "slow to warm" may be misjudged by teachers and adults as being mentally slow or noncooperative. This child needs extra time or repeated exposures to new materials to function optimally and to maintain a sense of dignity and self-worth.

The quality of high *adaptability* helps counteract the effects of high withdrawal in new situations. With extra time or repeated exposures, the child with high withdrawal and high adaptability will function well in new learning situations. However, if the child has high withdrawal and low adaptability, new learning situations will create great difficulty for both the child and the teacher. Much patience and individualized attention are needed to prevent failure in academic achievement for this type of child. Early successes in overcoming difficulties with new learning situations will help motivate the child to persist despite high withdrawal and low adaptability in subsequent new situations.

With many children, one can judge their interest, moods, likes, and dislikes with great accuracy merely by observing their reactions to situations or people. These are children with moderate to high *intensity of reaction*. However, for those with a mild intensity of reaction, simple observations of their responses will not give an accurate evaluation. For these children, the teacher or other adult must be alert for more subtle cues in order to assess their reactions accurately and respond to them appropriately.

Children vary greatly in their ability to discern visual, auditory, and tactile stimuli. The hypersensitive child with a low *threshold for stimuli* may be easily distracted in a classroom situation, whereas the child with a high threshold may be oblivious to distracting stimuli. The child with a low threshold is likely to pick up small nuances in voice and behavior that go unnoticed by the child with a high threshold. Consequently, the child with a high threshold may need more detailed instructions to carry out a task than the child with a low threshold.

The quality of *mood* also varies among children. The good-natured child with a typically positive mood is likely to be treated more positively than the ill-natured child with a negative mood. Responses to both types of children are likely to reinforce their prevailing quality of mood. Children with a negative mood may feel "picked on" and find confirmation for the feeling that a negative response is appropriate to the predominantly negative world in which they live.

A child who is highly *distractible* may be aware of extraneous visual and auditory stimuli in the environment, whereas the child with low distractibility will be able to concentrate on the task at hand with only peripheral awareness of extraneous stimuli. The latter child usually has the advantage in the classroom situation. However, in social situations, the child who is highly distractible often has capacities for social sensitivity, empathy, and constructive behavior that are lost to the child with low distractibility.

In the classroom situation, long attention span and marked persistence are assets, whereas short attention span and low persistence are usually liabilities (Carey, 1992). However, unusually long attention span and marked persistence can lead to stubborn insistence on completing a task, even if another activity is called for.

Nursing Interventions: Temperament

The reactions of children to illness, injury, and hospitalization vary according to temperament characteristics. The nurse must assess the temperament characteristics of the child, if nursing care is to meet the child's needs (Johnson, 1992). For example, the child with a low threshold for stimuli will respond best to preoperational teaching if it is conducted in a quiet setting. In order to benefit from a preparation program, the child may require an environment that is free of interruptions from hospital personnel and of distractions caused by the usual activity of a hospital atmosphere. What works with one child will not work with another of a different temperament. A "canned" preoperative teaching program may be ideal for one child but may alienate another who has a different temperament.

Anticipatory Guidance: Temperament

The key to ensuring an optimal response for slow-to-warm children is giving them time to adapt at their own pace. If they are pressured, their reactions tend to be exaggerated. Difficult children are most vulnerable to the demands of socialization, that is, the altering of spontaneous responses and patterns to conform to the social rules of living with family, schoolmates, and peers. However, once these children do learn the rules they function easily, consistently, and energetically (Schor, 1985). The parents may not know about temperaments and how the concept applies to their own child. The nurse may be placed in the position of providing information on the topic to the parents for the first time. Obviously, there are parents who will be extremely well informed about their child's unique needs as influenced by temperament, and they will likely serve as the experts for the nurse. There is abundant lay literature for parents on the subject of parenting children with various types of temperaments. Parents can also be referred to community agencies and parent support groups that provide education and emotional support in raising a child with a temperament that requires special consideration.

Emotions

The emotional-social development of the school-age child is related to and runs parallel with physical, intellectual, and language development. Separating them is somewhat artificial but provides a more coherent picture of development than considering all three facets together. If properly used, emotions contribute to total personality patterns and enrich life. By age 6, the major emotions of anger and aggression, fear and worry, jealousy, and love and affection are fairly well established. At this age, children also begin to understand that emotional responses can be influenced by their own efforts and abilities. For example, a child begins to identify feelings of guilt, shame, and pride that are associated with achievement (Stipek & DeCotis, 1988). During the school-age period, emotional expression becomes more organized and controlled. The major movement is from primarily physical expression to verbal expression of emotion. The intensity of emotional expression, of course, depends on the temperamental characteristics of the child.

The major task of the maturing child is to control and express emotions in a manner acceptable to the society in which the child lives. The acceptable expression, however, varies among the subcultural groups within that society. Some subcultural groups are more demonstrative in emotional expression than others. What may be acceptable at home may not be acceptable at school or with a peer group. Consequently, the child must learn not only to control the expression of emotion but also to learn acceptable means of expression in different environments. Usually, if the home is a safe haven in which the child can count on abiding love, emotions can be expressed more openly there than in other environments.

Research has shown that children's knowledge of how and when to control emotional displays improves between the first and fifth grades and then levels off (Gnepp & Hess, 1986). That research demonstrated that children can understand and regulate spoken expressions of emotion better than facial expressions of emotion. This may happen because adults hold children more responsible for words than for nonverbal communication.

Anger

Anger is a natural emotion of childhood. The usual cause of children's anger is being in situations in which they are not able to do what they want. The situation may be one in which the child is restrained or inhibited by adults or peers who enforce limits on behavior, by circumstances such as stormy weather, by objects such as defective tools, or by the child's own lack of skill. Any of these situations may precipitate an outburst of anger. Physical states such as hunger or fatigue may cause an otherwise benign situation to be anger-provoking. Also, if expressions of anger are rewarded by giving in to the child or if parents are overly concerned about expressions of anger, the child may use this expression inordinately.

As children become better able to control motor skills, to use words more glibly, and to understand rules for behavior, life becomes more reasonable and children are able to bring anger under control. Verbal rather than physical expressions of anger increase with age. The self-centered anger of the school-age years increasingly gives way to anger triggered by social injustices to others. However, such anger is more typical of the adolescent than of the school-age child. Such anger can be and is used constructively as the energizing force for social action (Fig. 8–11).

As verbal expressions of anger become more available to the child, so do more covert or devious methods of expression, such as sassing, sulkiness, sneering, belittling, plotting, arguing, or scapegoating. At about 8 or 9 years of age, children tend to tease and criticize each other excessively.

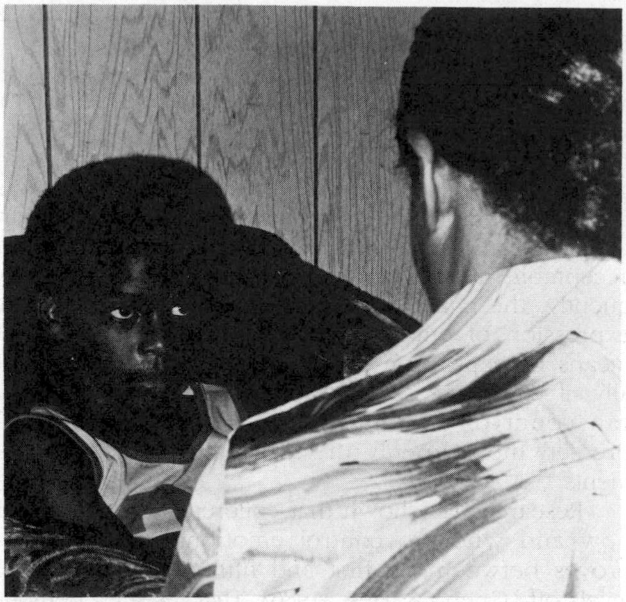

FIGURE 8-11. The school-age child needs help learning to verbalize anger and to examine the circumstances that triggered the anger in order to learn to use the anger constructively.

Aggression

Aggressive behavior usually is a result of anger but is different from simple expressions of anger. It often involves intentional injury to an animal or human or destruction of an inanimate object. Behavior such as hitting another person is fairly common in the young school-age child. However, from age 10 years on, when aggressive tendencies are better controlled, it occurs rarely. In the younger school-age group, boys are involved in interpersonal conflict more often than are girls, and boys respond to conflicts with physical force more often than do girls (Miller et al, 1986). Society tends to be more tolerant of aggression in boys than in girls. The same methods of helping the child control anger apply to controlling aggression. In a longitudinal study, aggressive behaviors observed between ages 7 and 12 were predictive of adjustment problems in adolescence. These findings suggest that children who manifest negative emotional behaviors early in childhood are more likely to manifest them later. This finding suggests that aggressive behavior observed in children may be an indication of more serious emotional problems later in life (Lerner et al, 1988).

Peers play a major role in the emotional well-being of school-age children. Some children are more popular than others with their peers. Children who are popular and well liked by their peers tend to be physically attractive, self-confident, energetic, and considerate. The well-being of children who are not well accepted by their peers can be negatively affected, which leads to feelings of decreased self-worth and inferiority.

Children develop their basic emotional patterns and characters during the school-age period. Character traits are stabilized, as is the fundamental manner of responding to people and things. With proper guidance and models to emulate, the pattern will be healthy and successfully carry the child through adolescence and adulthood.

Nursing Intervention: Emotions

Nursing assessment of the school-ager must focus on the defining characteristics of nursing diagnostic responses that describe the child's perceptions of self and pattern of role relationships. The following responses should be considered if problems are suspected: *fear, anxiety, disturbance, chronic low self-esteem, situational low self-esteem, personal identity disturbance, social isolation,* and *altered growth and development.* During the nursing admission, the nurse gathers information from the child and caregiver about their emotional well-being and emotional patterns. This information provides the basis of the nursing care plan. For example, in several Asian cultures, it is not acceptable to express feelings of pain or fear. In working with such an Asian family, the nurse would adapt communication techniques out of respect for the culture.

Probably the best way to help children learn to use anger constructively is to help them verbalize the anger, examine honestly the circumstances that triggered the anger, and figure out how those circumstances can be changed or what can be done about them. For example, a parent reported an episode in which her daughter and son began hitting each other. The mother interrupted the fight and sought to determine the reasons for it by talking to both children. After the children offered their explanations for the fight, the mother discussed alternate ways of displaying and expressing anger with the children and gave them what she thought were just consequences for their behavior. Providing models of acceptable expressions of anger is also important. As with adults, physical activity can take the edge off the anger. Also, role playing, either puppetry or doll play, can help a child express and resolve anger and aggression. Children need to learn and accept the fact that anger is an acceptable feeling.

Anticipatory Guidance: Emotions

Nurses can assist parents in supporting their child's expressions of emotion. If properly channeled, even negative emotions can lead to positive outcomes. Anger that is just can lead to social concern and reform. Fear and worry can be motivators for positive action and cautions for avoiding negative action. Jealousy can promote empathy and identity. The positive emotions of affection and joy give meaning to life.

Fears

As the world of school-age children expands, so do their worries and fears. Although fears and worries are learned, they are not necessarily related to actual experiences. During the early school years, *fears and worries* tend to be related to family and school. Children worry about such things as parental illness or death, not being liked, getting into trouble and getting hurt, and being harmed by supernatural beings or monsters, wild animals, or the dark. With age, children's fears and worries become more generalized in many respects, as well as more personalized and realistic than they were previously.

Bodily injury becomes a prominent fear during middle childhood. Children increasingly worry about themselves and their possible failures and about scolding or embarrassment related to specific situations. The mass media opens the door to more generalized fears, such as those involving cancer, air pollution, cigarette smoke, war, and civil disorder. Fear of such supernatural beings as monsters is abandoned at around age 10. Consequently, horror stories and films may be fun or therapeutic for the child of 10 or older, although they are very frightening for the younger child. Less overt, but demonstrable, signs of anxiety in the school-age children are nailbiting and hair pulling or twisting. These behaviors are often seen in the school-ager who is less vocal or who has a more sensitive self-concept.

Nurse researchers have explored school-age children's fears pertaining to health care experiences. One study of healthy school-age children's fears of health care experiences found that the predominant ones were fears of having an operation, having a shot, receiving a finger stick, and being separated from family (Broom, 1986).

Anticipatory Guidance: Fears

Parents concerned with anxious behaviors such as nailbiting should be urged to encourage their child to verbalize fearful or anxious feelings and to role model such expressions of feelings themselves. Hounding the child to stop the behavior serves only to increase anxiety and, most likely, to increase the frequency of the behavior. Socially acceptable alternative behaviors, such as doodling or pounding a punching bag and physical activity, may be suggested until the child develops the ability to verbalize feelings of anxiety.

Fear or worry can be of value, if it is not excessive. It warns children of danger and can motivate learning or healthful behavior. Excessive fear, however, can narrow a child's field of experience and damage self-concept. *A positive self-concept is a powerful deterrent to excessive fears and worries.* Frank discussion of fears and worries, successful experiences in overcoming specific fears, and role models who display mastery over fears can help children master their own fears and worries.

Coping Mechanisms

The school-age child utilizes a variety of coping mechanisms to handle stressors and problems (Table 8–10). During the school years, a wider range of defense mechanisms are used as experience and cognitive skills increase. Social support and avoidant emotional and distracting behaviors were found to be used most frequently in a study of 8- to 10-year-olds (Ryan, 1988). Several research studies have revealed that children who experience more stressful events are more likely to become ill, be hospitalized, and use health services (Grey, 1993).

During the early school years, the child develops a conscience (superego). The value system of rights and wrongs learned from the child's environment become internalized. The child's conscience is most punitive at the time, which causes the child to easily feel guilt and shame for wrongdoings. For example, the school-ager may feel unduly guilty about not achieving the grades expected by parents. Fortunately, as the child grows, the sense of self (ego) strengthens to balance the restrictive effects of the conscience. The child learns to become more rational and make reasonable judgments. With successful experiences in school, however, their defenses become strengthened.

Nurse researchers have studied the coping mechanisms of hospitalized school-age children. Information-seeking and controlling behaviors were the most predominant coping strategies used by hospitalized school-age children (Caty et al, 1984; Savedra et al, 1981). LaMontagne (1984) found a relationship between preoperative coping and locus of control. Children with a higher degree of internal locus of control were more likely to use active coping strategies, compared with children with a higher degree of external locus of control who used more avoidant coping strategies.

Nursing Interventions: Coping Mechanisms

During the hospital admission, the nurse can gather information about the school-ager's responses to stressful situations. This information can then be incorporated into the child's care. Nursing interventions are designed to bolster the child's sense of control. For example, viewing a film of a peer successfully coping with a surgical procedure assists the child to understand the procedure and deal with it more effectively (LaMontagne, 1993). For example, the nurse would help the child count during the insertion of an intravenous needle, if this is what the child normally

TABLE 8-10
Coping Mechanisms of the School-Age Child

Fantasy	Used as an escape when anxious, frustrated, worried, angry, or bored; creates imaginary scenarios as an outlet for emotional needs or tensions
Use of support systems	Shares privileged information or confidences with intimate peers as a means of receiving validation, trust, and intimacy
Obsessive/compulsive behavior	Exerts much energy in the performance and completion of tasks; great attention is paid to detail; seen most often in academic activities
Competitiveness	Attempts to "outdo" peers in performance as a means of supporting self-esteem; observed most often in sports and school activities
Compliance	Adheres to the norms of peer group/adult authority, although feelings and behavior of child are not in complete accord, for fear of negative/unwanted consequence
Use of defense mechanisms: displacement, projection, denial, sublimation, repression, regression	Used to protect the child's ego from real or perceived emotional threats
Cognitive strategies	The range of cognitive skills (logical thinking), such as decentration, enables child to solve problems and communicate needs, feelings, and desires more effectively
Aggression	Provides an outlet for release of emotional tension
"Rough-and-tumble" play	Provides opportunity for high-pitched, aggressive, and physical activity as a release for tension

TABLE 8-11

Promoting Coping Skills in the Hospitalized Child

The following interventions.were incorporated into Gina's nursing care plan to foster her mastery of the experiences faced during hospitalization

Prepare prior to all painful and intrusive procedures

- Provide information on the *sequence* of *events* and types of *sensations* she will feel
- Needs encouragement to ask questions; is shy; tends to act as "good girl" and wants "to please"

Support during procedure

- Prefers to squeeze nurse's hand during procedure; if not possible, will hit surface with pounding motion
- Needs to know "how much longer" procedure takes
- Stay with Gina following procedures, as she is "a little shaky" afterwards; responds to touching/hugging

Provide closure after procedure and support during hospitalization

- Provide opportunity to ventilate feelings; have to ask how she feels to elicit response
- Keeps a diary; inquire whether she's recording her experience
- Ask if there was anything unexpected that occurred with treatment and procedures; correct any misconceptions

does in stressful situations. Table 8–11 illustrates the incorporation of coping mechanisms into a plan of care.

Anticipatory Guidance: Coping Mechanisms

Parents can be assisted in fostering their child's use of a broad range of productive coping mechanisms. Furthermore, an understanding of their child's vulnerability to feelings of guilt and shame can enable them to correct their child's misperceptions as situations arise. Parents can be referred to child guidance materials that can provide them with additional information on the subject.

Moral and Faith Development

The changes in moral feelings and judgments make life more benevolent during the period of concrete operations than during the intuitive stage. According to Kohlberg, the child's moral development can be described as being at the *conventional level*. The child basically relies on the rules and regulations made by others for moral judgments. The motivation for acting correctly is primarily to earn the approval or respect of others. The child's behavior is not yet guided by an individual's internal sense of right and wrong. At this time, the school-ager's participation in clubs at school, organized sports, and unorganized play with peers greatly influences behaviors. Contact with authority figures shapes the child's moral behavior by means of modeling reinforcement, punishment, and disciplinary practices.

For the 6- or 7-year-old, the many rules of behavior are immutable. Rules are based on adult directions and are taken literally. These children are likely to judge an act in a unidirectional way, as being absolutely right or absolutely wrong. They are likely to consider that an act is bad if it elicits punishment, and they tend to be harsh in the punishment they prescribe for another child who has broken a rule.

As concrete operations become available to the child, the absolutes become tempered by the realization that the same act may be viewed in many different ways by different individuals. The intentions that prompted an act are now taken into consideration. Through interaction and cooperative endeavors with peers, the child develops respect for them and for self and realizes that rules evolve through mutual consent and the democratic process of consensus. Rules are no longer absolute and immutable but can be changed by either mutual consent or extenuating circumstances. Punishment the child now recommends is less harsh, more specific to the infraction, and no longer considered absolutely necessary. Children become increasingly more independent of adults in making moral judgments as the solidarity between peer groups grows and a morality based on cooperation develops. The importance of peers in the development of moral reasoning was demonstrated in the research findings of Kruger and Tomasello (1986). They found that moral discussions between school-age peers were characterized by a more spontaneous use of reasoning than were similar discussions between school-age children and adults.

The conscience, or moral judgment, of the 6-year-old is strict, literal, and unreliable. Cheating is common but goes against the child's conscience. The child's behavior at home may be very different from that at school. This is not an easy age for child or parent. Seven-year-olds assume responsibility more readily than 6-year-olds and are deeply concerned about what is right and wrong, even though they may take items that do not belong to them. The 8-year-olds begin to see themselves in relation to others and have a beginning capacity for self-evaluation. Their conscience is less rigid than previously, and they begin to resent parental authority and to look more often to the group for support. Behavior is likely to improve away from home.

The 9-year-old is self-sufficient, self-critical, and somewhat of a perfectionist. A strong sense of fairness and of right and wrong, along with being mature enough to accept blame for wrongdoing, develops at this age. However, these children do not like to be "talked down to." For the 10-year-old, interests in the world of people, places, and things continue to expand, and a strong moral sense of good and bad is often expressed.

Several factors are thought to influence the development of the child's conscience. These factors include the child's temperament and the parent's childrearing strategies. Toddlerhood precursors of conscience development in school-age children were toddlers' vulnerability to anxiety and parents' childrearing practices that de-emphasized the use of control (Kochanska, 1991). More recent research suggests that environmental factors and unique characteristics of the child need to be considered in discussions of moral development.

The school-age child is in the *mythical literal* stage of faith development. At this stage, the child learns to distinguish religious fact from fantasy. Children rely heavily on authority figures, such as parents, priest, minister, or rabbi, for information. The opinions and information gathered from peers is subordinated to that learned from authority figures. These children continue to have misperceptions about religious beliefs because of their level of reasoning. The child is learning to distinguish between the natural and supernatural. However, abstract concepts such as grace and heaven need to be presented in concrete terms in order to be understood. God is conceived of as a human being having a body and feelings.

Research studies of school-age children's understanding of God reveal their multifaceted perceptions. God is seen as both a protector watching over them with love and support and as a punisher and avenger of misdeeds. One nurse researcher found that children experiencing acute illness referred to God as benevolent, loving, and a source of comfort (Ebmeier et al, 1991). Negative feelings regarding guilt and punishment were not as prevalent a theme in children's responses as previously reported. Findings have suggested that school-age children aged 9 to 13 have personal religious experiences, especially in times of distress (Klingberg, 1959). God is seen as a source of protection in these situations.

Peer Relationships

For the first time, school-age children are able to consider the needs and concerns of their friends. They are able to see their friend's point of view, not their own only. A "give-and-take" exists between children and their friends. They are now able to share their feelings and thoughts, not only their play activities, with another. However, the school-ager is likely to end contact with his friend over an argument. Children are not able to maintain contacts with their friends after they have a disagreement. Sharing feelings means total agreement with one another at this age. Hence, the term "fair-weather friend" can be applied to the abrupt turnabout that may occur in friendships at this age.

Social Relationships

Through wider social relationships, children have the opportunity to become sensitive to the feelings of others. As children reach middle childhood, they become capable of true cooperation. They can now see themselves in the place of another, appreciate various opinions, and value and respect both their personal autonomy and the viewpoints of others. This development allows for true friendship, for collaboration in group work, for real discussion and exchange of ideas, and for the capacity to share a common goal (see Table 8–1).

During the early part of this period, peer groups are rather loosely organized, with much shifting of members within and between groups. However, by age 11 the organization of peer groups becomes separated by sex, with much tighter cooperation within and competition between groups (Fig. 8–12). Peer groups coalesce through shared goals and group norms. They may form for a particular purpose, such as sports or scouting, or they may be composed of friendship subgroupings that come together over time as a result of strong common motivations.

Many of these groups are considered "clubs" by their members, with the use of a special insignia, shared dress norms, and rules for governing activities. Members compete for election of officers; vote on passwords, secrets, and meeting places; and formulate means of controlling themselves and others. Such activities give children the thrill of governing themselves and prepare them for membership in teen-age and adult organizations.

Purpose of Peer Groups

The peer group serves many purposes for children and is of great significance for further personality development. Children learn social skills and how to live with others. The peer group is also a valuable testing ground for the worth of ideas, for self-actualization, and for self-expression in a nonthreatening environment. In play with a group, children are able to test reality and to try out various roles. It is a new field for acquiring status and self-esteem, earned through their own efforts.

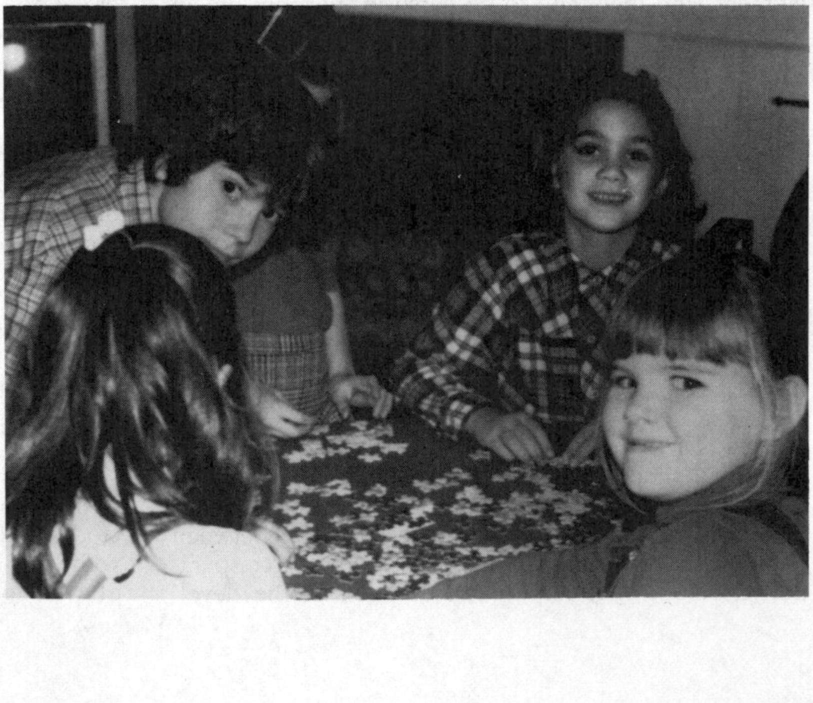

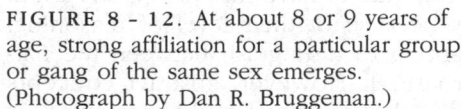

FIGURE 8-12. At about 8 or 9 years of age, strong affiliation for a particular group or gang of the same sex emerges. (Photograph by Dan R. Bruggeman.)

Much new learning takes place within the group, in which members act as powerful models for each other. Slightly older children, in particular, become highly influential with the younger members of the group. The peer group provides many direct rewards and satisfies needs for belonging and security, which parents can no longer entirely meet. It also promotes the beginning of distancing from parents and provides an identity that is no longer totally dependent on the family identification with persons of equal status (Fig. 8–13).

Just as a child's self-concept influences acceptance by peers, so does peer acceptance affect self-concept. Rejected children and those less popular than their agemates generally consider themselves to be inferior and withdraw even further from social overtures, whereas the self-esteem of popular children becomes more positive.

The 6-year-old enters group activities with excitement but is not yet ready for cooperative play. Often these children will leave a game if they do not get their way or are distracted. Seven-year-olds are sensitive to the feelings and attitudes of both peers and adults, and they want to be liked by them. Group activity assumes increasing importance, and the child seeks it out actively, disliking to be alone. Segregation by the sexes is obvious, and the child chooses a best friend of the same sex. However, these friendships tend to be unstable, and the child may have several best friends in sequence during the year. The same-sex groups or gangs of childhood are all-important. Conformity within the group is accentuated, and the group may leave out a child who is different in any way. New forms of independence from adults are attained through the peer group.

A stable and lasting friendship with the same sex is formed by the 10-year-old. A separation through a move to a distant new home by either child may be traumatic. The same-sex cleavage is often intensified in 11- and 12-year-olds, and frequent expressions of resentment and disgust toward the opposite sex are common. Girls are the first to close the cleavage by becoming "boy crazy." Memberships in groups and clubs that are organized around a specific function are of increasing importance. The need for peer activities must be respected.

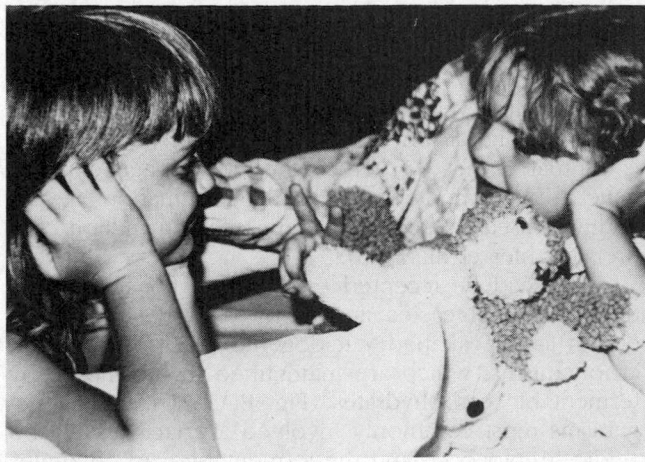

FIGURE 8 - 13. Spending the night at a best friend's home is typical of the school-age period.

Health Maintenance and Promotion

The school-age period is a relatively healthy one for children. Morbidity and mortality are lower than at any other time during childhood.

Acute illnesses, especially respiratory illnesses, are fairly common with this age group. Over one half the acute illnesses reported are due to respiratory conditions. The average number of days of restricted activity for illness per child in the 6 through 16 age group is approximately 10, with approximately 5 school days lost because of illness (US Department of Health and Human Services, 1984). Although acute illnesses are to be expected as a normal part of life, this information about the incidence of acute conditions indicates that prevention of respiratory conditions should be included in health promotion efforts for this age group.

Health Screening

School-agers should continue to be screened for blood pressures (Jung & Ingelfinger, 1993). Screening audiograms are done every 2 years, usually as part of the school health program. Many school districts have scoliosis screening programs. Five per cent of students with scoliosis require further management (an at-risk group is girls diagnosed with scoliosis at early age, with family history of scoliosis and no growth spurt). The school-age child and siblings may require revaccination if a measles outbreak at the school occurs. Two criteria are necessary for revaccination: (1) the student and siblings were born after January 1, 1957, and (2) they did not receive two measles vaccinations after the first birthday (American Academy of Pediatrics, 1991). See Chapter 10 for further information on immunizations.

Over 10 per cent of the children in the United States have blood cholesterols of 200 mg/dl or higher (Davidson et al, 1989). Children with elevated blood cholesterol levels are at higher risk for coronary artery disease and atherosclerotic disease. Although the American Academy of Pediatrics (Committee on Nutrition, 1989) recommends that screening for blood cholesterol be done with a positive family history of hyperlipidemia or early myocardial infarction, other experts recommend that all school-age children be screened, because a significant number of children with blood cholesterol levels exceeding 200 mg/dl would be missed using the American Academy of Pediatrics guidelines (Merz, 1989).

Portable desktop screening analyzers make cholesterol screening possible in school settings. Initial high readings of total blood cholesterol (TBC) are repeated to ensure the accuracy of the level reported. If the repeated TBC remains elevated, a lipid and lipoprotein panel are ordered. Children with elevated cholesterol levels are referred to the preventive cardiology department for dietary and, if needed, pharmacologic management (Davidson et al, 1990).

The following concerns need to be included in a health promotion program: nutrition, play safety, immunizations, sex education, and values clarification. These components are discussed further on.

Vision and Hearing

No assessment of the school-age child is complete without a careful examination of the eyes and ears. The ear and the sense of hearing are well developed by school age. Overall mild hearing losses (not exceeding 25 decibels) usually do not produce communication problems for the school-age child. Chapter 45 discusses hearing and visual losses in detail. The normal hyperopia of the young child gradually diminishes during the early school-age period, owing to the growth of the posterior segment of the eye globe.

Anticipatory Guidance: Hearing and Vision

Parents need to be aware of the symptoms of visual problems and should be encouraged to have them corrected. If corrective lenses are prescribed, every effort should be made to help the child view them positively and to wear them as directed.

Eyestrain should be avoided for the general well-being of the child. Causes of eyestrain include using poor lighting (either too little or glaring) and poor posture while reading; reading too-small print; reading in a moving vehicle; doing close work; or watching television, films, or a computer screen for prolonged periods without rest or change of focus.

To prevent hearing problems, parents need to be aware that middle ear infections require prompt treatment and that consistent follow-up and regular hearing tests are indicated for recurrent otitis media. Immunizations also should be encouraged as the primary method of prevention for complications of the communicable diseases that may cause neural (perceptual) hearing losses. The parents and child should be informed that trying to remove wax from the ear canal with a hairpin or similar implement probably will only impact the wax more firmly against the tympanic membrane and may even damage the membrane.

Dental Care

In most children, permanent teeth do not erupt before the early school-age years. One of the most obvious developmental milestones to occur during the school-age period is the loss of all 20 primary teeth and their "replacement" by 28 of the 32 permanent teeth. All permanent teeth (except the third molars) start calcification between birth and 3 years but are not completely calcified until about age 16. The first permanent teeth to complete root development are the central incisors at ages 9 to 10 years (Fig. 8–14).

The major emphasis of dental health during school-age years is dental hygiene, which helps to preserve the primary teeth until all are lost and protects the secondary teeth as they erupt. Frequency of dental checkups will vary depending on the general state of health of the child's mouth and teeth and on how well the child complies with dental health practices.

A cooperative dentist lets the young child look around the office, ride up and down in the dental chair, and become familiar with the instruments. The dentist's approach to the child can greatly influence future visits. Many children's books are available to help prepare children for routine dental visits as well as for specific dental procedures. Books should be evaluated for accuracy before they are shared with the child.

The 6- to 8-year-old usually does not possess the fine motor skills to be totally responsible for flossing the teeth. Children of this age lack the cognitive skills and are not sufficiently future-oriented to appreciate the reasons for performing preventive measures. From the age of 9 years on, the child has sufficient motor and cognitive skills and is future-oriented enough not only to assume total responsibility for dental health practices but also to understand simple explanations and appreciate the rationale for preventive dental help practices.

Dental Caries

By far, the most important and prevalent dental problem is caries, affecting 98 per cent of the population. During the last decade, there has been a progressive increase in the number of children with reported visits to the dentist. Seventy per cent of children between 5 and 17 years of age had visited a dentist in the preceding year (Waldman, 1991). Rates for dental caries are higher among ethnically diverse children. It is estimated that 92 per cent of school-age children have mild to moderate gingival inflammation. Severe gingival disease affects approximately 1.4 million children (Kohler et al, 1983).

The widely accepted explanation for the formation of dental caries is that the tooth enamel and dentin are decalcified γ-acidogenic (acid-forming) microorganisms, which are maintained in the mouth by fermentable carbohydrates (Fig. 8–15). The microorganisms most commonly involved are lactobacilli and acidic streptococci, and the fermentable carbohydrates most commonly involved are sugars. The tooth surfaces most susceptible to attack are located where the

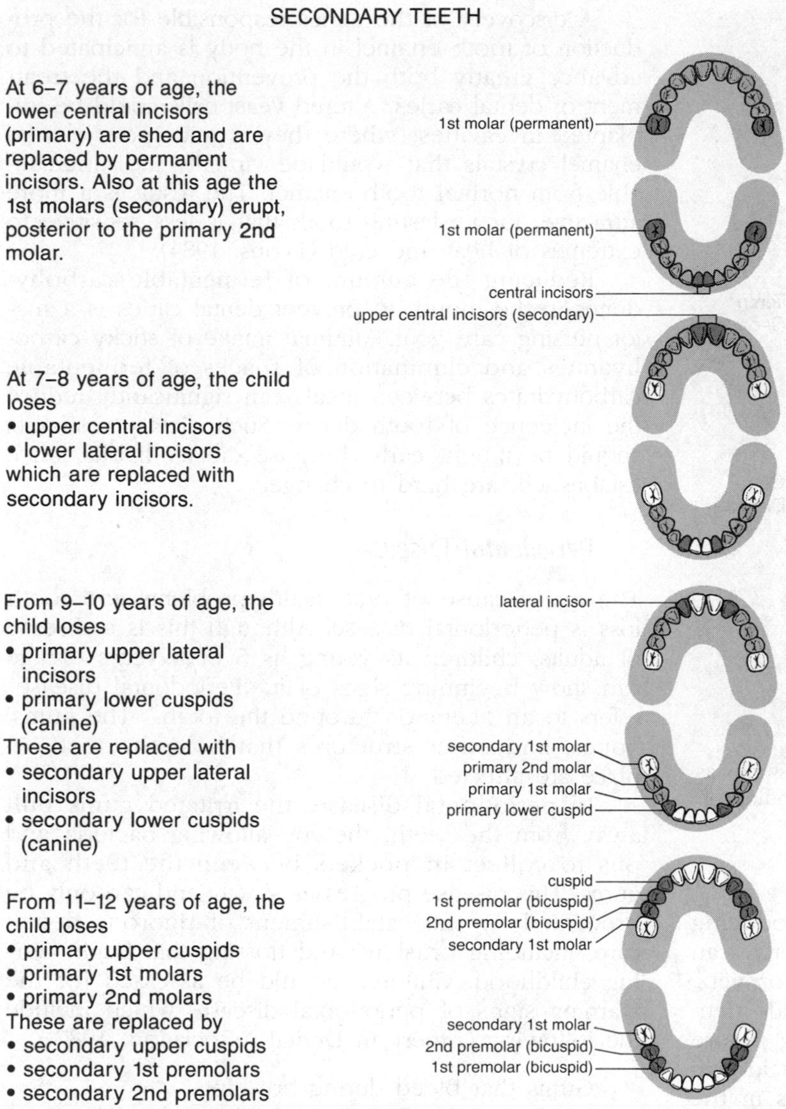
SECONDARY TEETH
At 6–7 years of age, the lower central incisors (primary) are shed and are replaced by permanent incisors. Also at this age the 1st molars (secondary) erupt, posterior to the primary 2nd molar.
1st molar (permanent)
1st molar (permanent)
central incisors
upper central incisors (secondary)
At 7–8 years of age, the child loses
• upper central incisors
• lower lateral incisors
which are replaced with secondary incisors.
From 9–10 years of age, the child loses
• primary upper lateral incisors
• primary lower cuspids (canine)
These are replaced with
• secondary upper lateral incisors
• secondary lower cuspids (canine)
lateral incisor
secondary 1st molar
primary 2nd molar
primary 1st molar
primary lower cuspid
From 11–12 years of age, the child loses
• primary upper cuspids
• primary 1st molars
• primary 2nd molars
These are replaced by
• secondary upper cuspids
• secondary 1st premolars
• secondary 2nd premolars
cuspid
1st premolar (bicuspid)
2nd premolar (bicuspid)
secondary 1st molar
secondary 1st molar
2nd premolar (bicuspid)
1st premolar (bicuspid)

FIGURE 8 - 14. Development of teeth. Primary and secondary teeth are simultaneously present in the child's mouth during the process of eruption and shedding.

fermentable carbohydrates and bacteria are prone to accumulate: that is, the contact area between the teeth and grooves or fissures on the chewing surface of teeth. This accumulation takes the form of plaque, a sticky transparent coating that becomes firmly attached to the tooth surface.

This explanation for dental caries leads to a three-pronged approach to a prevention program: (1) increase the tooth's resistance to acids, (2) reduce the activity of microorganisms, and (3) reduce the amount of fermentable carbohydrates in the mouth.

An adequate supply of fluoride is needed to help prevent cavities. Fluoride is provided in most communities through the water system at a concentration of 1 part per million (ppm). Some schools add fluoride to their drinking water in areas where the local water lacks fluoride. In communities in which water is not fluoridated, a daily supplement of sodium fluoride should be given orally for healthy development of the permanent teeth buds in the gums. The fluoride concentration in the local water supply is 1 mg for less than 0.3 ppm; 0.50 mg for 0.30 to 0.07 ppm; and no fluoride supplementation for greater than 0.07 ppm (American Academy of Pediatrics, 1986).

Topical application of stannous fluoride is available from the dentist, in tooth dentifrices, and in fluoride mouth rinses. Because of its mottling effect if taken in excessive amounts, parents should be cautioned against using more than the prescribed dose of fluoride. The nurse should be prepared to discuss up-to-date findings pertaining to the use of fluoride. Recommendations are periodically provided by the American Academy of Pediatrics (1986) and the American Dental Association (1987).

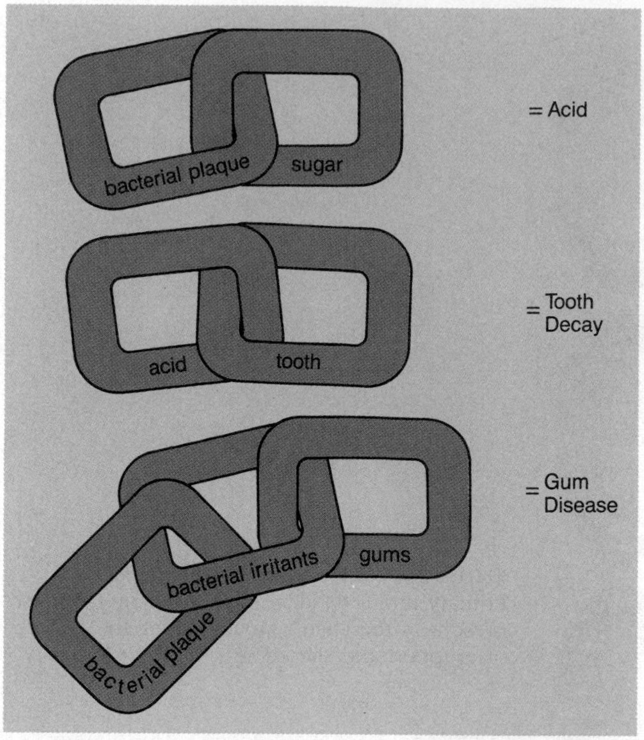

FIGURE 8-15. Showing the results of "poor brushing" as simple line drawings increases the child's understanding of abstract ideas.

Brushing and flossing remove caries-producing bacteria from the mouth and, if done properly, can contribute to the prevention of gum disease (Horowitz, 1984). Teeth should be brushed with a fluoride dentifrice after each meal, if possible. Brushing before bedtime is especially important, because the acid-producing activity of bacteria normally increases in the environment of the mouth during sleep. If brushing is not possible after eating, the mouth should be rinsed with water or an antimicrobial mouth rinse. To cleanse between the teeth, where bacteria and plaque are likely to accumulate, dental floss or a water jet should be used at least once a day. A fluoride-containing mouth rinse swished through the mouth has the advantage of getting some fluoride into the spaces between teeth.

The restoration of deep developmental grooves and fissures in the teeth and the repair of cavities also reduce bacterial activity. The advent of dental sealants, applied to the pits and fissures of the grinding surfaces of molars, can diminish the likelihood of tooth decay on the chewing surfaces, which is not completely prevented by fluoridation. Most studies indicate that if the sealant remains intact until the child is 6 years old, it is likely to remain for a number of years (Starr & Gravitz, 1985). The use of dental sealants on permanent or primary posterior teeth depends on the child's susceptibility to dental caries, timing of tooth eruption, and tooth morphology (Wilson, 1990).

A discovery of the genes responsible for the production of tooth enamel in the body is anticipated to advance greatly both the prevention and the treatment of dental caries. Altered yeast cells could be implanted in cavities, where they would grow cloned enamel crystals that would be virtually indistinguishable from normal tooth enamel. The result is a more attractive, longer-lasting tooth that is less sensitive to extremes of heat and cold (Lyons, 1984).

Reducing the amount of fermentable carbohydrates in the mouth to prevent dental caries is a major nursing care goal. Minimal intake of sticky carbohydrates and elimination of snacks of fermentable carbohydrates between meals can significantly reduce the incidence of tooth decay. Such dietary restraints should be taught early, because dietary habits, once established, are hard to change.

Periodontal Disease

The major cause of oral health problems and tooth loss is periodontal disease. Although this is a disease of adults, children as young as 5 or 6 years of age can show beginning signs of it. "Periodontal disease" refers to an alteration "around the tooth." The gums, bones, and other structures that hold the teeth in place are affected.

In periodontal disease, the irritated gums pull away from the teeth, thereby allowing bacteria and pus to collect in pockets between the teeth and gums. This disease progresses slowly and can only be prevented by the establishment of rigorous dental care, including brushing and flossing that begin during childhood. Children should be assessed for the warning signs of periodontal disease, which include the following (American Dental Association, 1987):

- Gums that bleed during brushing.
- Gums that are pulled away from the teeth.
- Loose permanent teeth.
- Changes in the way teeth fit while biting.
- Bad breath.
- Pus that can be pushed out between teeth and gums when gums are pressed.

Malocclusion

Dental orthodontia is a specialized area in dentistry in which malocclusions are treated. "Malocclusion" is a term used to describe the condition in which the teeth of the upper and lower dental arches are not in proper alignment. If a severe malocclusion is present, the child may experience speech dysfluency, mastication problems, facial deformities, and eventual loss of teeth in adulthood. Significant psychologic problems often occur in the child with an untreated malocclusion (Klima et al, 1979). Peer or sibling rejection will perpetuate the child's poor body image.

Malocclusions are skeletal deformities of the mandible and maxilla and usually are genetically caused (Klima et al, 1979). Skeletal facial development may predispose an individual to develop malocclusion: jaw bone size may not correspond to tooth size, the mandible may deviate posteriorly or may be hypertrophic, or the face may be asymmetric. The child with premature loss or prolonged retention of primary teeth, or tooth loss that interferes with the normal chewing position, may also develop a bite problem. Nurses are often asked by concerned parents if their child's teeth will be damaged by thumb or finger sucking. The likelihood of long-term effects from thumb sucking remains an area of controversy. Modier and colleagues (1982) noted various occlusion problems in children who used a pacifier or bottle or who sucked their thumb after 2 years of age, and they reported problems in 30 per cent of 4-year-old children who continued to suck a digit or a pacifier. If children continue the habit beyond the age of 6 years and into the period of mixed and permanent dentition, the prognosis worsens (Berkowitz & Johnson, 1987; Grossman, 1987).

Early recognition of malocclusion allows intervention at the appropriate time and prevents the psychologic and dentition problems that commonly follow. Although nurses are not experts on occlusions, assessment of the overall dentition should be a part of every child's health maintenance visits. Many children do not routinely have dental care, and the nurse is often the person who first recognizes a potential problem. Jumbled, crossed, or missing teeth should also alert the nurse to the possibility of an occlusion problem.

Dental Emergencies

Dental emergencies are rare, but they can happen. Parents should learn how their child's dentist can be reached if the unexpected happens. If a dentist is not accessible in an emergency, parents should be instructed to go to a hospital or clinic emergency room. When a child completely knocks out a secondary tooth, the chances of implanting it are excellent if the child gets care within 30 minutes. Few teeth reimplanted after 2 hours survive (Krasner, 1990). The dislodged tooth should be rinsed gently, while any scraping of the root is carefully avoided. The tooth should then be placed back in the socket and held in place by having the child bite on a washcloth until emergency care is received. Such care should be sought immediately. If the tooth cannot be put back in place, it should be placed in milk and emergency care sought immediately. *Time is crucial!* If a primary tooth is avulsed, it is not reimplanted, because it could damage the underlying secondary tooth. A dentist is consulted, because it may be necessary to provide treatment that maintains the space properly (Baker, 1987; Krasner, 1990).

Dental emergencies are most often the result of sports injuries and children's rough-housing. Children who play contact sports such as football or soccer should wear mouth protectors. A catcher's mask should be worn by children who play catcher in softball or baseball. Children should be taught the consequences of pushing and shoving in general, and particularly around play equipment and at the water fountain.

Anticipatory Guidance: Dental Care

The major emphasis of dental health during school-age years is dental hygiene, which helps preserve the primary teeth until they all are lost and protect the secondary teeth as they erupt. Although 5- to 8-year-olds usually do not possess the fine motor skills necessary to be totally responsible for flossing their teeth, they should be able to do a fairly adequate job of brushing them. Children of this age lack the cognitive skills to understand the reasons for performing the preventive measures and are not future-oriented enough to appreciate these practices. These children are still dependent on adults for guidance. From the age of 9 years on, the child has sufficient fine motor and cognitive skills and is future-oriented enough to assume total responsibility for dental health practices.

Frequency of dental checkups will vary, depending on the general state of health of the child's mouth and teeth and how well the child complies with dental health practices. The schedule recommended by the child's dentist should be followed. Parents may need information about the normal pattern of eruption of the secondary teeth. This usually occurs during the school-age years. The 5- to 8-year-olds are still highly dependent on adults and look to parents and teachers for guidance. Good dental health practices instituted at this age will be followed, because they are the "thing to do," or the "rules." Parents should check the adequacy of the child's technique. From 9 years old on, the child is able to employ the rotary-motor brushing technique.

Convincing parents that a pedodontic or orthodontic referral is needed may be difficult, especially if the parent has not formerly recognized the problem or is not a firm believer in the necessity of dental care. An explanation of eventual long-term problems should be provided. Orthodontic treatment is expensive, and many families cannot afford to receive treatment. Nurses may be able to help the family obtain financial assistance from community service groups or refer the child to a dental college that may provide treatment for a reduced fee. Diagnosis should be made by a specialist in orthodontics or children's dentistry (pedodontist). Skull radiographs will be needed in order to establish the extent of the problem.

Children's acceptance of the need for treatment will depend on their prior experiences with dentists and their current awareness of the problem. Children need a thorough explanation of the problem, including why treatment is necessary, although children who have been teased about their teeth will usually accept treatment.

Removable acrylic appliances require much cooperation from the child, because the child is responsible for wearing the device and may see the dentist only every 6 months. Children with fixed appliances are seen every 2 to 3 weeks. Headgear that provides cervical traction may be used to reduce the treatment time and aid in a more permanent occlusion correction. Appliances require conscientious oral hygiene measures. Proper toothbrushing after meals is necessary in order to prevent the development of caries beneath the appliance. School nurses can be helpful in encouraging the child to follow through on brushing and in reinforcing the need for a nutritious diet.

Sleep and Rest

At the beginning of the school-age period, the child usually averages 11 to 12 hours sleep per night. The amount of sleep per night gradually diminishes to an average of 9 to 10 hours per night at age 12. Ordinarily, a healthy child naturally seeks the amount of sleep required to meet health needs (Table 8–12).

Sleeptalking and Sleepwalking

Sleeptalking (somniloquy) and sleepwalking (somnambulism) occur most commonly during the school-age years. Approximately 15 per cent of children between the ages of 5 and 12 years have walked in their sleep at least once. Persistent sleepwalking occurs in only 1 to 6 per cent of children.

Sleeptalking and sleepwalking are associated with neurologic immaturity and occur during the transition from stages III and IV of non–rapid-eye-movement (NREM) sleep to the first rapid-eye-movement (REM) period (approximately 1 to 2 hours after sleep onset). Sleeptalkers are not revealing their deep secrets, and most children outgrow this problem. Sleepwalking, similarly, resolves spontaneously. Adults with persistent sleepwalking have usually begun it in adolescence, rather than during the school-age years. Table 8–13 summarizes characteristics and management of sleeptalking and sleepwalking.

If children who usually sleep well experience sleep problems without apparent reason, they may be upset or worried about some aspect of school or home life. This cue should be followed up with the child, and efforts made to alleviate the problem.

Anticipatory Guidance: Sleep Behaviors

If a school-age child has developed the habit of retiring for sleep at a late hour and sleeping late in the morning, difficulties can be anticipated with the start of regular school attendance. Parents can be advised that this difficulty can be resolved by making the retirement hour earlier and earlier over a period of several months before the start of school. To promote sleep, a period of quiet activity just prior to bedtime is advised. An exciting or stimulating television program is not included in the category "quiet activity." Overstimulation—physical, mental, or emotional—can have an adverse effect on the restful sleep that is the norm for the school-age child. Sleepwalking and sleeptalking are common events during these years.

The school-age child's bedtime routine varies depending on family habits. In some families, bedtime prayers, reading of inspirational material or favorite stories, quiet discussions about the day's events, or "tucking in" continue to be cherished rituals through early adolescence.

Nutrition

As has been noted previously, the school-age years are characterized as a period of relatively slow and steady growth. The exception is the preadolescent growth spurt at about 10 to 12 years for girls and 12 to 14 years for boys.

Until the adolescent growth spurt begins, the nutritional needs of the child are relatively stable. There

TABLE 8-12
School-Age Child Developmental Characteristics of Sleep-Related Behavior: 6 to 12 Years

Characteristic Sleep-Related Behaviors	Promote Sleep-Related Health
Child no longer takes naps or rest periods	Continue with a bedtime routine
Verbalizes many excuses to not go to bed	Avoid sending to bed as a punishment
Bargains for special privileges to stay up; watches the clock concerning bedtime	Maintain a positive attitude about bedtime by keeping conversations pleasant
May try to begin a project close to bedtime	Introduce more responsibility for the child for getting ready for bed and performing all the related tasks without being reminded
Sleepwalking and sleeptalking are common during these years (discussed in this chapter)	Regular bedtime and sufficient sleep are necessary for school achievement
11–12 hrs of sleep per 24 hrs for 6- to 9-year-olds	
9–12 hrs of sleep per 24 hrs for 10- to 12-year-olds	

TABLE 8-13
Family-Centered Teaching: Characteristics and Management of Sleep Disturbances

Description	Behavior Manifested	Management During Episode
Sleepwalking (Somnambulism)		
More common in boys; onset is usually before age 10 yrs and usually resolves by age 15 yrs; one to four episodes per week may occur	Sits upright abruptly for 15–30 seconds, climbs out of bed, and wanders around room or house, from a few minutes to as long as 30 mins; unconscious of environment—although eyes are open, child is not awake; movements are rigid, repetitive, and not purposeful; child answers in monosyllables if spoken to; speech is slurred and mumbled	Do not attempt to wake child but protect from injury; keep doors to basement, outdoors, and other areas of potential danger locked; allow child's own return to bed; if guided back to bed before ready, child usually will get up again anyway; medication may be considered for child with severe, intractable sleepwalking
Sleeptalking (Somniloquy)		
Occurs on occasion in the sleep of most children and adults; is thought by some to reflect anxiety-provoking daytime experiences	Speech is usually monosyllabic and incomprehensible; sometimes the sound of one's own voice causes individual to awaken	One should not try to awaken the child; should not be cause for alarm

Data from Wender, E. (1984). Common behavior problems in preschool children. In P. Shelov, et al. (Eds.), *Primary care pediatrics: A symptomatic approach* (pp. 265–282). Norwalk, CT: Appleton-Century-Crofts; Ferber, R. (1985). Sleep disorders in infants and children. In T. Riley (Ed.), *Clinical aspects of sleep and sleep disturbance*. Stoneham, MA: Butterworth; and Anders, T. F. (1987). Nightmares and other sleep disturbances. In R. H. Hoekelman, et al. (Eds.). *Primary pediatric care* (pp. 744–748). St. Louis: CV Mosby.

is a slightly increased need for quantity (to accommodate the increases in height and weight) rather than quality.

Proportionately, however, in calculating the daily needs for calories, protein, and water per kilogram of body weight, a slight and steady decrease in requirements is seen. Table 8–14 describes nutrient and caloric needs specific to the school-age child. For additional nutritional information, see Chapter 16.

Just as the school-age period is noted for being probably the healthiest of any age period, it also is one with relatively few nutritional problems. Information about eating habits as well as kind and amount of food eaten is essential to the total evaluation of nutritional status. Snacks for school-age children are common and often consist of empty-calorie foods that can interfere with proper nutrition. Snack foods can have other unintended effects as well. A study found that the purchase of candy cigarettes may facilitate the development of a positive attitude toward cigarette smoking (Klein et al, 1992). Children who frequently purchased candy cigarettes were three times more likely to report having smoked a cigarette in junior high school, compared with children who had not.

Various forms of interviews are used to assess nutritional status (see Chapters 13 and 16). On the basis of the interviews, an assessment can be made of a child's diet. The results should be compared with the recommended food intake and average size of servings for a child of that age (see Chapter 16 for recommendations). This comparison should disclose possible deficiencies that should be included in anticipatory guidance.

Obesity may be a problem in the school-age population as well as other populations. Obesity is a growing health problem among children. It is estimated that 5 to 15 per cent of American children are obese (Dietz, 1986). There is a strong association between childhood obesity and obesity later in adulthood, because eating patterns become firmly established in the early years (Sherman & Alexander, 1990).

As school-age children become absorbed in school or play activities, meals may be forgotten or ignored. When children become hungry, they are often likely to fill up with nutritionally poor, calorie-laden junk foods. These foods are made desirable in the television commercials to which the child is exposed daily. The pace of life in our society has resulted in a generation of individuals who do not eat at home. Much of this eating is done in fast-food restaurants, where calorie levels and fat content are quite high. In addition to eating excessively, obese children often do not exercise as much as children of average weight. A vicious circle may ensue; the more obese the child is, the more difficult it is to keep up with the other children in physical activity, and eating becomes a consolation (Jonides, 1990).

The nurse should be alert to the defining characteristics of this nursing diagnostic response for several reasons. For children, obesity is both an emotional-social risk factor and a physiologic problem. In one study, obese children reported lower self-concept, were more depressed, and were rejected more and

TABLE 8-14
Recommended Food Intake for Good Nutrition According to Food Groups and Daily Dietary Allowances: School-Age (7 to 10 Years)

Food Groups	Servings Per Day	Serving Size
Bread Group	6–9	
• Bread		2 slices
• Cereal		1 oz.
• Rice and pasta		½ C–¾ C
Vegetable Group	3–5 total	
• Green-yellow vegetables (vitamin A source)	1 or more	4 tbsp
• Other vegetables	2 or more	⅓ C
Fruit Group	3–4 total	
• Citrus fruits, berries, tomato, cabbage, cantaloupe (vitamin C source)	1 or more	1 medium orange
• Other fruits (apple, banana)	2 or more	1 medium
Milk Group	2–3	
• Milk/yogurt		½–1 C
• Cheese		(1.5 oz cheese = 1 C milk)
Meat Group		
• Cooked lean meat, poultry, fish	3 or more	4–6 tbsp
• Dry beans		½ C
• Egg		1
• Peanut butter		2–3 tbsp
Fats, oils, and sweets—USE SPARINGLY		

Recommended Daily Dietary Allowances

Protein	Fat-Soluble Vitamins		Water-Soluble Vitamins		Minerals		Energy Needs
28 g	Vitamin A	700 μg RE	Vitamin C	45 mg	Calcium	800 mg	2000 kcal
	Vitamin D	10 μg	Thiamine	1.0 mg	Phosphorus	800 mg	
	Vitamin E	7 mg α—TE	Riboflavin	1.2 mg	Magnesium	170 mg	
	Vitamin K	30 μg	Niacin	13 mg NE	Iron	10 mg	
			Vitamin B_6	1.4 mg	Zinc	10 mg	
			Folate	100 μg	Iodine	120 μg	
			Vitamin B_{12}	1.4 μg	Selenium	30 μg	

Adapted with permission from *Recommended dietary allowances: 10th edition*. Copyright 1989 by the National Academy of Sciences. Published by the National Academy Press, Washington, D.C.; and U. S. Department of Agriculture, Human Nutrition Information Service (1992). *Food guide pyramid* (Leaflet No. 572). Washington, DC: Author.

Key: RE, retinal equivalent; TE, tocopherol equivalent; NE, nicotinic acid equivalent.

liked less by their non-obese peers (Strauss et al, 1985). These findings suggest that the obese school-age child may also be at risk for the development of behavior problems.

Eating Behaviors

The 6- or 7-year-old may find it difficult to sit through a meal and may need to be excused early. By 9 years, the child's table manners are good and responsibilities for assisting with meal preparation and cleanup can be assumed. The younger child can help, too, but may be somewhat erratic in carrying through on assigned tasks. Tasks for the younger child need to be simple, such as putting the napkins on the table or clearing away the dishes.

Anticipatory Guidance: Nutrition

As a child enters school and moves from the confines of the home and its immediate environment, other influences become increasingly important to the child's health practices. These influences can be both positive and negative. Ideally, the teacher, the school nurse, and perhaps peers will have a positive influence on health practices, including eating habits.

High-risk home environments for childhood obesity include family members who are obese themselves, multiple caretakers who assume childrearing responsibilities, and families from low socioeconomic levels (Sherman & Alexander, 1990).

Health education is an important and integral part of a school curriculum. The American Academy of Pediatrics has repeatedly affirmed its support for health education in the schools. Although school nurses can contribute directly to the health education program by teaching selected content, a more effective role is to serve as a consultant and resource person for teachers. Health education, to be truly effective, must be a consistent and integral part of daily classroom instruction—something no school nurse could possibly accomplish or schedule alone.

Because school-age children do not have control over meal preparation at home, nutrition education should extend into the community to include the parents. However, school-age children do have control over intake at meals, and they need to have sufficient knowledge to select appropriate types and quantities of available foods. Breakfasts and snacks need special emphasis, because they are often deficient in quantity or quality.

Education in nutrition, dental health, and physical activity overlaps, and therefore instruction for these areas is combined. An example is the fact that nutritious snacks also promote dental health. Suggestions about anticipatory guidance for dental health, discussed previously, apply equally to nutrition education. Children and their families can be instructed about the importance of physical activity to basal metabolism and to the cardiovascular and musculoskeletal systems. Children can be encouraged to be physically active in group sports or individual activities. For some children, participation in group sports may be unappealing because they do not perform as well as their peers, for example, children with weight problems (Jonides, 1990). An exercise program will be of greatest benefit for children who are able to integrate it comfortably into their lifestyle.

In health education about nutrition, cultural factors play a greater role than in most other topics of health education. Children need to learn that a great variety of foods, eaten in proper quantities, will meet their daily nutritional requirements. Respect for their own cultural heritage and for that of others can be an indirect benefit of well-planned nutrition education.

Proper nutrition, discussed previously and in Chapter 16, is essential for the health and well-being of children. A properly nourished child is less susceptible to acute illnesses and is better able to develop the physical, intellectual, emotional, and social competencies so important to this age group.

One problem area in nutrition for this age group is that children may become too busy and too involved in activities to eat properly. Children like structure and rituals, and adults can use this fact to the advantage of both themselves and their children. Regularity of mealtimes and snack times gives children the structure they need around which to plan activities. Mealtimes should also be pleasant occasions to look forward to and should provide opportunities for social interaction with the family.

Bowel and Bladder Control

Most healthy school-age children experience no difficulties with elimination. Bowel and bladder control are usually well established. However, when a child is under undue stress, temporary lapses are not unusual. For discussions of problems with bowel control (encopresis) and bladder control (enuresis), see Chapters 35 and 36.

Play

It has often been said that play is the work of children. When consideration is given to what play does for the development of physical, cognitive, and social competence, this might even be considered an understatement (see Chapter 17).

Play is of vital importance to the acquisition of the ego quality of industry versus inferiority. Children acquire physical competence and skills through play involving gross and fine motor activity. Active involvement in play promotes cognitive development, and by means of playful experiments on the environment, the child discovers much new knowledge and many new cognitive skills. Socialization to the peer group is acquired primarily through the play of children. Peer group and team activities are important to the school-age child's developing peer identity, not just during the school year but also during the summer months. The value of play in the promotion of a healthy childhood cannot be overestimated (Table 8–15).

A 6-year-old is noted for almost constant activity; the whole body seems to be involved in almost anything and everything being done. Throwing a ball involves the entire body; telling a story involves gesturing with the arms and face. Much spontaneous dramatization is evident during this year. The child tends to be restless and indecisive and needs activities that require use of the large muscles. Rudeness is common, especially at home and at play.

Seven-year-olds are full of vitality and energy but are more cautious in exercising it in play than are 6-year-olds. They enjoy songs, rhymes, fairy tales, myths, nature stories, comics, television, and movies.

Eight-year-olds are eager to do things and perform activities with more smoothness and poise than previously. Play outdoors may be vigorous, but quiet activities are important, and dramatic play is popular. Collections of miscellaneous objects are common and are treasured. The child is eager to learn and usually enjoys school. Areas of interest expand beyond the immediate environment.

The 9-year-old is fairly responsible, reasonable, and dependable. Individual differences in abilities and

TABLE 8-15
Toys and Play Activities for School-Age Children

Toy or Play Activity	Development Promoted	Selection Criteria
Team games	Fosters fine and gross motor strength and skill (P)	Protective equipment fitted properly
	Teaches rules, fair play, and team effort (S)	
	Play becomes more intellectual (C)	
	Learn rules (C & S)	
	Learn to lose (E & S)	
	Learn to cooperate as team member (E & S)	
Model kits	Fosters creativity (C)	Nontoxic materials
Construction sets	Promotes artistic development (E & C)	Cost may be a limitation
Woodburning/woodcarving	Stimulates problem solving (C)	Equipment in good working order
Swimming	Enhances large muscle development (P)	Safety rules
Archery		
Aerobics	Enhances sense of accomplishment (C & E)	
Running		
Rock climbing	Enhances use of problem solving (C)	
Parties/social activities	Provides interactions with others (S)	Supervision
	Decreases tension, but may be difficult for shy children (E)	
Electronic games	Enhances problem solving (C)	Monitor for age-appropriate content
	Enhances decision making skills (C)	May require limits on frequency of use
Movies	Enhances ability to concentrate (C)	Monitor for age-appropriate content
Videos		
Television watching	Fosters peer activity (S)	May require limits on frequency of use
Special artistic/musical interests	Promotes self-esteem (E)	Cost may be a limiting factor
Sewing	Enhances creativity (C)	
Painting	Promotes self-expression (E)	
Pottery	Teaches classification of objects and similarities and differences (C)	
Crafts		
Collections		
Board games	Play becomes more intellectual (C)	
Chess	Rules become variable and complex (C)	
Cards	Teaches fairness and adhering to standard (S)	

Data from Betz, C., & Poster, E. (1984). Incorporating play into the care of the hospitalized child. *Issues in Comprehensive Pediatric Nursing, 7,* 343–354; Florey, L. (1971). An approach to play and play development. *American Journal of Occupational Therapy, 25,* 275–280; Lee, J., & Fowler, M. (1986). Merely child's play and developmental work and playthings. *Journal of Pediatric Nursing, 1,* 260–269; and Betz, C. (1983). Teaching children through play therapy. *Journal of the Association of Operating Room Nurses, 88*(4), 709, 712–713, 716–717.

C = cognitive development; P = physical development; E = emotional development; S = social development.

skills among children become more distinct and clearer both to adults and to the children themselves. There is less interest in fairy tales and fantasy and more interest in the community, country, and other countries and people. The scope of interest in the world around them expands. The 9-year-old is interested in learning about the origin of babies and how they grow.

Team sports and cooperative activities are prominent, and the child readily submits to the rules of the game. Collections are no longer miscellaneous but are very distinct and organized and may lead to a lifelong hobby. An increase in curiosity and physical activity in both sexes is seen. Team games and sports are very popular with 11- and 12-year-olds.

Anticipatory Guidance: Play

As the child enters school, the issue of organized sports becomes a central concern. The nurse can assist parents in assessing whether their child's participation in sports and recreational activity is an enjoyable experience or whether it is placing undue pressure on the child. For example, the 6-year-old child who misses the ball in Little League baseball and turns to a parent who is watching on the sideline to convey "Sorry, Dad" or "Sorry, Mom" exemplifies how play can be abused. Placing excessive pressure on children to perform is inappropriate.

A child's maturity should be considered in determining appropriateness of a particular sport. Recommended chronologic guidelines according to Belkengren and Sapala (1982) are as follows:

Age 6—noncontact sports, including swimming, gymnastics, track and field, martial arts, tennis, and skating.

Age 8—with trained supervision: basketball, volleyball, softball, soccer, and wrestling.

Age 12—collision sports: football, rugby, and hockey.

In seeking information about sports injuries, parents can be assured that the overall rate of injury to children participating in sports is low (Landry, 1992). As a rule of thumb, the risk for sports injury increases as the young athlete grows and develops. For example, rate of injury was found to increase in football players of ages 9 to 14 years who were heavier (100 to 130 pounds), compared with players who weighed less (80 to 115 pounds). The rate of injury was reported to be 23.9 per cent and 12.7 per cent, respectively (Goldberg et al, 1984). Football has been identified most often as having the highest injury rate, followed by gymnastics and wrestling (McLain & Reynolds, 1989).

The two most common types of sport injuries are acute lesions (sprains, strains, and, to a lesser extent, fractures) and overuse. A special problem in children is injury of the epiphyseal plate resulting in altered growth potential (Greene, 1983). The younger the child is at the time of injury, the more serious will be the growth disturbance. Another exercise-related injury in the young child is heat-induced illness. Children do not tolerate climate extremes as well as adults do. Precautions taken include monitoring and limiting strenuous periods of activity, suitable hydration during strenuous activity (150 ml of cold tap water each 30 minutes for a child weighing 40 kg), and light-weight clothing.

Some parents may require assistance in meeting the continuing need of the school-age child for ample playtime. Parents may need information about community facilities, programs, and camps that provide opportunities for play experiences. A childhood without ample opportunities for play is no childhood at all (see Table 8–15 for age-appropriate play materials and activities).

Safety Concerns

Safety education is of primary importance in health maintenance efforts for the school-age group. Accidents are, by far, the leading cause of death (Allshouse et al, 1993). Because motor vehicle accidents account for nearly one half of those deaths, automobile safety should be stressed (US Department of Health and Human Services, 1989). Children like rituals, and one ritual that should be automatic is buckling the seat belt. Children can learn the rules of the road, and the rules include proper behavior in the automobile, so that the driver is not distracted from the primary task of driving the car.

Children can incur serious injury by riding in the back of pickup trucks, open or enclosed. Unfortunately, only 17 states have restrictions for passengers riding in the back of pickup trucks (Woodward & Bolte, 1990). Injuries and fatalities occur with ride-on mowers, lawn tractors, and other types of farm equipment (American Academy of Pediatrics. Committee on Accident and Poison Prevention, 1990; Salmi et al, 1989).

Although motor vehicle accidents are a major cause of death, the most common site for accidents of this age group is the home or an adjacent property (National Center for Health Statistics, 1989). Therefore, home safety measures also are of major significance, and high risk for injury continues to be a diagnostic response of importance to the nurse. Of injuries in children between the ages of 5 to 9, 20 per cent occur in school.

Boys are twice as likely as girls to have accidents. According to one study, the most common commercial products involved in these accidents were bicycles, glass, swings, skateboards, and nails.

School-age children may be victims of drowning because of overestimating their swimming ability. For example, children may ignore the lifeguard's warnings of riptides and may attempt to ride waves that can easily overpower them. Reckless and daredevil behavior creates a potential danger as well. The need to impress peers with bravado can lead the child to take dangerous chances, such as swimming in rough water and jumping from steep precipices. Drownings can also be attributed to boating accidents and suicide (Suncoast Drowning Prevention Committee, 1989).

Anticipatory Guidance: Safety Concerns

Children benefit from instructional programs that are aimed at teaching safety behavior. Programs directed at teaching school-age children pedestrian safety, wearing of helmets with bicycles, and wearing of safety gear with skateboarding and horseback riding have demonstrated positive changes in behavior (Weiss, 1992).

Caution in play and other activities needs to be stressed. However, caution should not be overly stressed, because excessive caution or fear can inhibit normal development. A certain number of skinned knees and bruises seem inevitable in the normally developing child. Typical accidents, listed according to developmental age and prevention strategies, are specified in Table 8–16.

TABLE 8-16
Safety Developmental Concerns and Prevention Interventions

Developmental Stage: School-Age (6 to 12 Yrs)	**Prevention Strategies: Teach Child All Aspects of Safety**
More coordination in motor skills; runs, skips, jumps, climbs, constantly on the move Active in sports Increasing independence and need for peer acceptance Curiosity about sexuality	Motor vehicle, pedestrian, bicycle accidents • Pedestrian safety needs to be repeated • Bicycle safety must be emphasized Bodily injury, fractures • Teach how to prevent injury from cold • Teach safety related to hobbies, handicrafts, sports, mechanical equipment Drowning • Teach water safety • Supervise water sports Burns • Teach appropriate use of matches and campfires Firearms • Teach respect for firearms • Avoid keeping a loaded weapon in house Bodily harm and trauma • Reinforce to avoid accepting things from strangers or getting into a car with anyone without parents' knowledge • Teach child about harmful use of drugs, alcohol, and cigarettes Sex education • Make child aware of "good touching" and "bad touching" to prevent sexual abuse

The school-age child is able to learn rules of water safety. These rules include the prohibition of running, jumping, shoving, or diving into shallow water. Screaming and mimicked pleas for help should be discouraged. Junior lifeguard programs provide the child with additional knowledge and skills about water safety. Ocean swimming should be done only on beaches with lifeguard protection. Swimming in the ocean should only be done under safe conditions, as indicated by the lifeguard's flag. Finally, the school-age child should not be permitted to swim alone.

Sex Education

Sex education is a value-laden topic, and many adults are uncomfortable talking about it. Ideally, a child should receive information about sex and sexuality from parents. However, many parents avoid discussing sexual issues with their child and rely on other sources to provide this information. More and more commonly, sex education is provided in the school setting. Nurses who have experience teaching human sexuality can be valuable resources to school faculty responsible for teaching sex education.

Regardless of whether sex education occurs in the home or school, or in both, concerned adults should be available to respond to children's questions appropriately and to provide values clarification. Otherwise, questions will be answered and values clarified with peer group only, and this situation is often one of "the blind leading the blind."

The older school-age child can assimilate factual knowledge about menstruation, nocturnal emissions, and reproduction if he or she has information about the anatomy and physiology of the human body. If sex education is given in isolation, learning is more difficult; undue emphasis is placed on sexual function as the only bodily function of importance. If presented in context with a study of the wonders of the human body, it becomes a natural process to be respected, as are all other natural processes of the body. If given in this context, certainly the 11-year-old can assimilate the information, and the 9-year-old can handle introductory information. Serious health problems, such as acquired immunodeficiency syndrome (AIDS) and sexually transmitted diseases, and teen-age pregnancy warrant particular concern in sex education programs.

Anticipatory Guidance: Sex Education

Results obtained 2 years following an elementary school sexuality program taught by a nurse revealed that participating students' knowledge of sexual information was significantly higher than that of those who had not participated. Nurses can serve as important resources for school-age children and parents in a variety of settings—clinics, schools, and hospitals.

Sex education for the child is a major concern that parents need to face during the school-age period. The older school-age child must acquire factual knowledge and values about sex. The younger school-age child needs to have questions answered in terms appropriate to cognitive development, but the older child needs more specific information and clarification of values.

The following principles provide guidelines for the nurse to use with the school-age child and family:

1. Stress to parents that maintaining a comfortable, open home atmosphere encourages a school-ager to discuss questions about sex and sexuality.
2. Encourage parents to provide re-explanations about the process of reproduction. Scientific understanding is often sought at this age, but parents frequently need to take the initiative to discuss it.
3. Because of the prevalence of sex-related conversations among peers, parents are encouraged to use and explain correct terms.
4. A school-age child may wish to speak to a nurse in private.
5. The nurse provides the child and the parents with information about bodily changes that occur during preadolescence and adolescence.
6. As a school-ager's television viewing expands to include movies that have sexual implications, parents are encouraged to view television shows with their child to provide opportunities for discussion.
7. School-age children are exposed to conversation about sex preferences at school; therefore, parents are encouraged to discuss a child's understanding of what is heard at school.
8. Consequences of sexual activity may be difficult for parents to discuss, but such discussions should be encouraged to make their children aware of pregnancy, sexually transmitted diseases, and AIDS. The nurse can provide parents and children with accurate information and help them find appropriate community resources, as needed.

Sun Protection

School-age children spend much time outdoors. Evidence strongly suggests that children not adequately protected from excessive sun exposure are at risk for skin cancer in childhood (Truhan, 1991). However, the practice of applying sunscreen regularly (sun protection factor [SPF] of 15) during childhood and adolescence could reduce the incidence of skin cancer (excluding melanoma) by 78 per cent (Stern et al, 1986). For additional information on sun protection, see Chapter 38.

Anticipatory Guidance: Sun Protection

Parents can be informed about the use of effective sun protection methods. Sun protection measures include use of sunscreen, wearing of protective clothing such as long sleeve shirts, and sun avoidance. Instruction on application of sunscreen includes applying it 30 to 60 minutes prior to sun exposure for maximum skin penetration, followed by repeated applications with sweating, after swimming, and after toweling. Caution parents that repeated application should not exceed the period of protection stated in the product instructions. Nurses in all settings, in the hospital or in community sites such as schools, can emphasize the importance of using sun protection measures (Nicol, 1989).

Substance Use and Abuse

Substance use may occur in school-age children. If it does, it usually denotes significant problems in the child or family, or in both. Unstable family situations increase the risk for substance abuse. Children of alcoholics, for example, are known to be at risk for alcoholism. It has not been determined whether this fact is explained by genetics, personality factors, or a combination thereof (Bloch et al, 1988; Carey, 1992).

Drug education is a major concern pertaining to the child that needs to be faced by parents during the school-age period. The older school-age child must acquire factual knowledge and values about drugs. The younger school-age child needs to have questions answered in terms appropriate to cognitive development, but the older child needs more specific information and clarification of values.

Anticipatory Guidance: Substance Abuse

With the increasing availability of drugs to younger children, all children need to be made aware of their harmful effects. Rather than use scare tactics, it is more effective to emphasize how drugs hinder the ability to accomplish all the feats so important to the age group. Nurses can educate teachers about how to identify students at risk for drug abuse and how to manage drug emergencies at school.

School Adjustment

The school environment takes over many social functions and provides new models for children to imitate. They are faced with the need to master basic skills in reading, writing, and arithmetic. By second grade, educational experiences expand beyond these basic skills to include the natural sciences. The timing is congruent with the developing cognitive ability that leads children to be curious about the natural sciences. Beginning school is an event that creates anxiety in some children; this situation can be mitigated by anticipating potential sources of difficulty.

The school nurse may be in a more advantageous position than the teacher to manage crisis situations arising from school performance, because school performance is associated with teachers' evaluations. In any family, the child's learning problems may impinge on the goals and aspirations of the parents. A child may be perceived as a psychologic extension of the parents, the bearer of their genetic traits, and the product of their childrearing efforts. If the child fails in school, the parents may see themselves as failures. Feelings of guilt, doubt, and anxiety may turn into anger, which is projected onto the school. Principals, teachers, learning disabilities specialists, and remedial instructors may not be able to obtain the trust and confidence of the parents, because these educators are often the conveyors of bad news about the child's achievements. In situations such as these, the school nurse may be more successful in engaging the family in counseling and may be more effective in any therapy efforts. Thus, such actions may relieve some of the tension between school personnel and individual children.

Factors that seem to foster school adjustment are a positive regard for a child's individuality by parents, teachers, and peers; a willingness among these support groups to respond appropriately to signals of need; an atmosphere within the family and school that is conducive to growth; and the availability of effective support systems. By assessing the family unit and classroom routinely for psychosocial dysfunctions, the school nurse can identify "stressors" and develop appropriate methods of intervention. Table 8–2 summarizes the major challenges to the school-age child, parents, and teachers to achieve adequate school adjustment. Nursing interventions to facilitate the child's and family's adjustment are also listed.

Afterschool care has become both a financial and a social concern for families. Unfortunately, there is a widespread lack of afterschool programs available for children. Coupled with the dearth of afterschool programs and financial constraints, many children return home unattended until their parents, or parent, return from work. Concerns have been raised about the well-being and potential consequences of these "latchkey" children. Most studies have reported no adverse effects. No differences have been found between latchkey children and those attending afterschool programs in measures of academics, peer approval, self-esteem, or conduct (Vandell & Corasaniti, 1988; Steinberg, 1986).

KEY CONCEPTS

Concepts Related to Basic Information

- Areas of concern for the family with school-age children are reorganizing family living to child's expanding world, expanding family communications, and maintaining financial solvency.
- During the early school-age period, the child's progress in height and weight is relatively slow and steady at approximately 5.5 cm (2 inches) per year for height and 2.5 kg (5.5 pounds) per year for weight.
- Body composition changes little during the school-age period.
- The lymphatic tissues, such as tonsils and adenoids, grow rapidly during the school-age period; the school-ager may have as many as six illnesses a year.
- The word that best describes the neuromuscular development of the school-age period is *refinement; the six basic gross motor skills that are refined during this time are running, jumping, sequencing foot movement, balancing, throwing, and catching.*
- During the school-age period, the child's thought processes undergo dramatic shifts; Piaget characterizes thought processes at the beginning of the school-age period as *intuitive thought;* they move into *concrete operations* at about 7 or 8 years of age, and from there into *formal operations* at about 11 to 12 years.
- The child of 6 to 12 years of age continues to develop sexual awareness and purposeful sexual behaviors; the psychoanalytic term *latency* used by Freud to describe this state of development is now considered a myth.
- The major thrust in psychosocial development in the school-age period is the establishment of the ego quality of *industry versus inferiority*—Erickson's fourth stage.
- Although innate characteristics of temperament seem to be relatively stable, their expressions may vary over time, being influenced by environmental and intrinsic developmental factors.
- The major task for the maturing child is to control and express emotions in a manner acceptable to the society in which the child lives.
- Bodily injury becomes a prominent fear during middle childhood. The child worries about self and possible failures and about scolding and embarrassment related to specific situations.
- During the school years, a wider range of defense mechanisms are used, as experience and cognitive skills increase, to cope with stressful situations.
- According to Kohlberg, the child's moral development can be described as being at the *conventional level.*
- The child is in the *mythical literal* stage of faith development, in which the child learns to distinguish religious fact from fantasy.
- One of the most obvious developmental milestones to occur during the school-age period is

the loss of all 20 primary teeth and "replacement" by 28 of the 32 permanent teeth.

- Play is of vital importance to the acquisition of the ego quality of industry versus inferiority.

Concepts Related to Nursing Assessment

- Nursing diagnostic responses that can be applied to the school-age child include *high risk for altered growth and development, ineffective individual coping, high risk for sensory-perceptual alteration, high risk for impaired physical mobility,* and *high risk for alteration in health maintenance.*
- The nurse will continuously assess the child for the etiology of the actual response, the risk factors associated with the potential problems, and defining characteristics.
- In order to assess the physical competency of the school-age child, the nurse must be aware that each child has a unique growth pattern.
- Nursing diagnostic responses related to motor skills development are *high risk for altered growth and development* and *high risk for impaired physical mobility.*
- The nurse who has a thorough knowledge of Piaget's theory will be better able to recognize the defining characteristics of *high risk for actual altered growth and development.*
- An assessment of the progress in language development includes examination of the three interactive components of language itself: phonics, syntax, and semantics.
- The nurse must assess the temperament characteristics of the child, if nursing care is to meet the child's needs, because the reactions of children to illness, injury, and hospitalization will vary according to temperament characteristics.
- Nursing assessment of the school-age child's emotions must focus on the defining characteristics of nursing diagnostic responses that describe the child's perceptions of self and pattern of role engagement and relationships.
- Children can be assessed for the warning signs of periodontal disease, which include the following: gums that bleed during brushing, gums that are pulled away from the teeth, loose permanent teeth, changes in the way teeth fit while biting, bad breath, and pus from the gums when pressed.
- By routinely assessing the family unit and classroom for psychosocial dysfunctions, the school nurse can identify stressors and develop appropriate methods of instruction.

Concepts Related to Nursing Intervention

- The nurse can assist parents in enforcing a wide variety of rules, setting limits, and providing positive feedback, because such actions foster the child's sense of reality and self-confidence.
- The nurse should give school-agers the opportunity to explain what they know about their treatment, their medications, and the pathology of the disease and/or medical condition.
- Parents can facilitate language development in the expression of feelings and thoughts by encouraging regular discussion of their child's ideas, plans, and reactions.
- Nursing care needs to focus on *what* the child can do and *adjustment of* activities that are restricted temporarily or on a long-term basis.
- Parents concerned with anxious behaviors, such as nailbiting, should be urged to encourage their child to verbalize fearful or anxious feelings and to role model such expressions of feelings themselves.
- The major emphasis of dental health during school-age years is dental hygiene, which helps preserve the primary teeth until they all are lost and protect the secondary teeth as they erupt.
- To prevent hearing problems, parents need to be aware that middle ear infections require prompt treatment and that consistent follow-up and hearing tests are indicated for recurrent otitis media.
- As the child enters school, the issue of organized sports becomes a central concern; the nurse can assist parents in assessing whether their child's participation in sports and recreational activity is an enjoyable experience or whether it is placing undue pressure on the child.
- Children benefit from instructional programs that are aimed at teaching safety behavior, such as teaching children pedestrian safety, wearing of helmets with bicycles, and wearing of safety gear with skateboarding and horseback riding.
- Parents can be informed on the use of effective sun protection methods, such as use of sunscreen, wearing of protective clothing, and sun avoidance.

REFERENCES

Allshouse, M., Rouse, T., Eichelberger, M. (1993). Childhood injury: A current perspective. *Pediatric Emergency Care, 9*(3), 159–164.

American Academy of Pediatrics. Committee on Accident and Poison Prevention. (1990). Ride-on mower injuries in children. *Pediatrics, 86*(1), 141–143.

American Academy of Pediatrics. Committee on Infectious Diseases. (1991). *Report of the committee on infectious diseases* (22nd ed.). Elk Grove Village, IL: Author.

American Academy of Pediatrics. Committee on Nutrition. (1986). Fluoride supplementation. *Pediatrics, 77,* 758–761.

American Academy of Pediatrics. Committee on Nutrition. (1989). Indications for cholesterol testing in children. *Pediatrics, 83*(1), 141–142.

American Dental Association. (1987). Guide to dental health. *Journal of the American Dental Association* (Special issue).

Anders, T. F. (1987). Nightmares and other sleep disturbances. In

R. H. Hoekelman, et al. (Eds.), *Primary pediatric care* (pp. 744–748). St. Louis: CV Mosby.

Bailey, D., et al. (1978). The influence of exercise, physical activity and athletic performance on the dynamics of human growth. In F. Falkner & J. Tanner (Eds.), *Human growth: Vol. 2: Postnatal growth*. New York: Plenum Publications.

Baker, B. (1987). Emergency dental treatment for the family physician. *Canadian Family Physician, 33,* 1521–1524.

Behrman, R. E. (1992). *Nelson textbook of pediatrics*. Philadelphia: WB Saunders.

Belkengren, R., & Sapala, S. (1982, July/August). Physical fitness from infancy through adolescence. *Pediatric Nursing,* 249–257.

Berkowitz, R. J., & Johnson, D. C. (1987). Malocclusion. In R. E. Behrman & V. C. Vaughan (Eds.), *Nelson textbook of pediatrics* (13th ed.). Philadelphia: WB Saunders.

Bloch, J., Bloch, J., & Keyes, S. (1988). Longitudinally foretelling drug usage in adolescence: Early childhood personality and environmental precursors. *Child Development, 59,* 336–355.

Broom, M. (1986). The relationship between children's fears and behavior during a painful event. *Children's Health Care, 14*(3), 142–145.

Carey, W. (1992). Temperament issues in the school-aged child. *Pediatric Clinics of North America, 39*(3), 569–585.

Caty, S., Ellerton, M., & Ritchie, T. (1984). Coping in children: An analysis of published case studies. *Nursing Research, 33,* 277–282.

Davidson, D., Bradley, B., Landry, S., Iftner, C., & Bramblett, S. (1989). School-based cholesterol screening. *Journal of Pediatric Health Care, 3*(1), 3–8.

Davidson, D., Smith, R., & Iaqundah, P. (1990). Cholesterol screening in children during office visits. *Journal of Pediatric Health Care, 4*(1), 11–17.

Dietz, W. (1986). Prevention of childhood obesity. *Pediatric Clinics of North America, 33*(4), 823–833.

Duvall, E., & Miller, B. (1985). *Marriage and family development* (6th ed.). New York: Harper & Row.

Ebmeier, C., Lough, M., Huth, M., & Autio, L. (1991). Hospitalized school-age children express ideas, feelings and behaviors toward God. *Journal of Pediatric Nursing, 6*(5), 337–349.

Erikson, E. (1967, January). Identity and the life cycle: Selected papers. *Psychological Issues Monograph*.

Ferber, R. (1985). Sleep disorders in infants and children. In T. Riley (Ed.), *Clinical aspects of sleep and sleep disturbance*. Stoneham, MA: Butterworth.

Frankel, F. (1993). Sources of family annoyance (SOFA): Reliability and validity. *Journal of Pediatric Nursing, 8*(3), 177–184.

Friedman, W. (1991). The development of children's memory for the time of past events. *Child Development, 62,* 139–155.

Gnepp, J., & Hess, D. (1986). Children's understanding of verbal and facial display rules. *Developmental Psychology, 22,* 103–108.

Goldberg, B., Rosenthal, P., & Nicholas, J. (1984). Injuries in youth football. *Physical Sports Medicine, 12,* 122–130.

Greene, J. C. (1983, November/December). Prevention and treatment of sports injuries. *Nurse Practice,* pp. 39–44.

Grey, M. (1993). Stressors and children's health. *Journal of Pediatric Nursing, 8*(2), 85–91.

Grossman, L. K. (1987). Malocclusion. In R. A. Hoekelman, et al. (Eds.), *Primary pediatric care*. St. Louis: CV Mosby.

Horowitz, A. M. (1984, January/February). Community oriented preventive dental programs that work. *Health Values,* pp. 21–29.

Igoe, J. (1993). School-linked family health centers in health care reform. *Pediatric Nursing, 19*(1), 67–70.

Janus, S. S., & Bess, B. E. (1981). Latency: fact or fiction? In L. L. Constantine & F. M. Martinson (Eds.), *Children and sex: New findings, new perspectives*. Boston: Little, Brown.

Johnson, J. (1992). The tendency for temperament to be "temperamental": Conceptual and methodological considerations. *Journal of Pediatric Nursing, 7*(5), 347–353.

Jones, E., Badger, T. & Moore, I. (1992). Children's knowledge of internal anatomy: Conceptual orientation and review of research. *Journal of Pediatric Nursing, 7*(4), 262–268.

Jonides, L. (1990). Childhood obesity: An update. *Journal of Pediatric Health Care, 4*(5), 244–251.

Jung, F., & Ingelfinger, J. (1993). Hypertension in childhood and adolescence. *Pediatrics in Review, 14*(5), 169–179.

Klein, J., Forehand, B., Oliver, J., Patterson, C., Kupersmidt, J., & Strecher, V. (1992). Candy cigarettes: Do they encourage children's smoking? *Pediatrics, 89*(1), 27–31.

Klima, R., et al. (1979, May). Body image, self concept, and the orthodontic patient. *American Journal of Orthodontics,* p. 507.

Klingberg, G. (1959). A study of religious experience in children from 9–13 years of age. *Religious Education, 54*(3), 211–261.

Kochanska, G. (1991). Socialization and temperament in the development of guilt and conscience. *Child Development, 62,* 1379–1392.

Kohler, B., Bratthall, D., & Krasse, B. (1983). Preventive measures in mothers influence the establishment of the bacterium *Streptococcus mutans* in their infants. *Archives of Oral Biology, 28,* 225–231.

Krasner, P. (1990). The treatment of avulsed teeth. *Journal of Pediatric Health Care, 4,* 186–190.

Kruger, A. C., & Tomasello, M. (1986). Transactive discussions with peers and adults. *Developmental Psychology, 22,* 681–685.

Landry, G. (1992). Sports injuries in childhood. *Pediatric Annals, 21*(3), 165–168.

LaMontagne, L. (1993). Bolstering personal control in child patients through coping mechanisms. *Pediatric Nursing, 19*(3), 235–237.

LaMontagne, L. (1984). Three coping strategies used by school-age children. *Pediatric Nursing, 10,* 25–28.

Leonardson, G. (1986). The relationship between self concept and selected academic and personal factors. *Adolescence, 21,* 474.

Lerner, J., Hertzog, C., Hooker, K., Hassibi, N., & Thomas, A. (1988). A longitudinal study of negative emotional status and adjustment from early childhood through adolescence. *Childhood Development, 59,* 356–366.

Lowery, G. (1978). *Growth and development of children*. Chicago: Year Book Medical Publishers.

Lyons, R. (1984, March 25). Look Ma, no cavities. *St. Louis Post Dispatch,* p. 7.

Maier, H. (1969). *Three theories of child development*. New York: Harper & Row.

McLain, L., & Reynolds, S. (1989). Sports injuries in a high school. *Pediatrics, 84,* 446–450.

Merz, B. (1989). New studies fuel controversy over universal cholesterol screening during childhood. *Journal of the American Medical Association, 261,* 814.

Miller, P. M., Danaher, D. L., & Forbes, D. (1986). Sex-related strategies for coping with interpersonal conflict in children aged five and seven. *Developmental Psychology, 22,* 543–548.

Modier, T., et al. (1982). Sucking habits and their relation to posterior crossbite in four-year-old children. *Scandinavian Journal of Dental Research, 90,* 323–330.

National Academy of Sciences (1989). *Recommended dietary allowances* (10th ed.). Washington, DC: Author.

National Center for Health Statistics (1989). *Health United States—1988*. (DHHS Publication No. [PHS] 89–1221). Washington, DC: US Government Printing Office.

Nicol, N. (1989). What's new with sunscreens? Choices-choices-choices. *Pediatric Nursing, 15*(4), 417–418.

Pettit, G., Dodge, K., & Brown, M. (1988). Early family experience, social problem solving patterns and children's social competence. *Child Development, 59,* 107–120.

Piaget, J. (1966). *The psychology of intelligence*. Totowa, NJ: Little field, Adams & Company.

Putallaz, M. (1987). Maternal behavior and children's sociometric status. *Child Development, 58,* 324–340.

Ryan, N. (1988). The stress-coping process in school-age children: Gaps in the knowledge needed for health promotion. *Advances in Nursing Science, 11,* 1–12.

Salmi, L., Weiss, H., Peterson, P., Spengler, R., Sattin, A., & Anderson, H. (1989). Fatal farm injuries among young children. *Pediatrics, 83*(2), 267–271.

Savedra, L., Tesler, M., Ward, J., et al. (1981). Description of the pain experience: A study of school-age children. *Issues in Comprehensive Pediatric Nursing, 5,* 373–380.

Schor, D. (1985). Temperament and the initial school experience. *Children's Health Care, 13,* 129–134.

Sherman, J., & Alexander, A. (1990). Obesity in children: A research update. *Journal of Pediatric Nursing, 5*(3), 161–167.

Smart, M., & Smart, R. (1978). *School-age children—Development and relationships*. New York: Macmillan.
Starr, R. M., & Gravitz, R. F. (1985). Pit and fissure sealants in the prevention of tooth decay. *Pediatric Nursing, 11,* 289–290.
Steinberg, L. (1986). Latchkey children and susceptibility to peer pressure: An ecological analysis. *Developmental Psychology, 22,* 433–439.
Stern, R., Weinstein, M., & Baker, S. (1986). Risk reduction for non melanoma skin cancer with childhood sunscreen use. *Archives of Dermatology, 122,* 537–544.
Stipek, D., & DeCotis, K. (1988). Children's understanding of the implications of causal attributions for emotional experiences. *Child Development, 59,* 1601–1616.
Strauss, C., Smith, K., Frame, C., et al. (1985). Personal and interpersonal characteristics associated with childhood obesity. *Journal of Pediatric Psychology, 10,* 337–343.
Suncoast Drowning Prevention Committee. (1989). *We need your help—Don't let the kids down*. Clearwater, FL: Author.
Thomas, A., & Chess, S. (1977). *Temperament and development*. New York: Brunner and Mazel.
Truhan, A. (1991). Sun protection in childhood. *Clinical Pediatrics, 30*(12), 676–681.
U. S. Department of Agriculture, Human Nutrition Information Service (1992). *Food guide pyramid* (Leaflet No. 572). Washington, DC: Author.
U. S. Department of Health and Human Services. (1991). *Child health policy '91*. Washington, DC: Author.
U. S. Department of Health and Human Services. (1984). *Health United States—1984*. (DHHS Publication No. [PHS] 84–1232). Washington, DC: Author.
U. S. Department of Health and Human Services (1989). *Health United States—1989*. Washington, DC: Author.
Vandell, D., & Corasaniti, M. (1988). The relation between third graders' after-school care and social, academic and emotional functioning. *Child Development, 59,* 868–875.
Waldman, H. (1991). Oral health status of women and children in the United States. *Journal of Public Health Dentistry, 50*(6), 379–389.
Wender, E. (1984). Common behavior problems in preschool children. In P. Shelov, et al. (Eds.), *Primary care pediatrics: A symptomatic approach* (pp. 265–282). Norwalk, CT: Appleton-Century-Crofts.
Weiss, B. (1992). Trends in bicycle helmet use by children: 1985–1990. *Pediatrics, 89*(1), 78–80.
Wilson, A. (1990). Standards in maternal and child oral health. *Journal of Public Health Dentistry, 50*(6), 432–438.
Winklestein, M. (1989). Fostering positive self concept in the school age child. *Pediatric Nursing, 15*(3), 229–233.
Woodward, G., & Bolte, R. (1990). Children riding in back of pickup trucks: A neglected safety issue. *Pediatrics, 86*(5), 683–691.

BIBLIOGRAPHY

Alex, M., & Ritchie, J. (1992). School-aged children's interpretation of their experience with acute surgical pain. *Journal of Pediatric Nursing, 7*(3), 181–188.
American Academy of Pediatrics. Committee on Infectious Diseases. (1989). Measles: Reassessment of the current immunization policy. *Pediatrics, 84*(6), 1110–1113.
American Academy of Pediatrics. Committee on Sports Medicine and Fitness. (1992). Horseback riding and head injuries. *Pediatrics, 89*(3), 512.
Baker, M. (1989). Bites and scratches: When pets fight back. *Contemporary Pediatrics, 6*(6), 76–84.
Chapman, M., Longonia, J., & Parcel, G. (1989). An ecological approach to the prevention of injuries due to drinking and driving. *Health Education Quarterly, 16*(3), 397–411.
Chauvin, V. (1989). Common skin rashes in children and adolescents. *School Nurse, 5*(1), 23–38.
Christoffel, K. (1989). Child passenger safety. *American Journal of Diseases of Children, 143,* 1271–1272.
Clore, E. (1989). Dispelling the common myths about pediculosis. *Journal of Pediatric Health Care, 3,* 28–33.
Coffman, S. (1991). Parent education for drowning prevention. *Journal of Pediatric Health Care, 5*(3), 141–146.
DeAngelis, C. (1984). *Pediatric primary care* (3rd ed.). Boston: Little, Brown.
Erikson, E. (1968). *Identity, youth and crisis*. New York: WW Norton.
Feeg, V. (1990). The future of pediatric nursing: Anticipating the health care needs of children. *Imprint, 37*(4), 70, 72–73.
Fortier, J., et al. (1991). Adjustment to a newborn: Sibling preparation makes a difference. *Journal of Obstetric, Gynecologic, and Neonatal Nursing, 2*(1), 73–79.
Fowler, J. (1980). Moral stages and the development of faith. In B. Munsey (Ed.), *Moral development, moral education and Kohlberg*. Birmingham, AL: Religious Education Press.
Freud, S. (1957). In J. Strachey (Ed.), *The standard edition of the complete psychological works of Sigmund Freud* (Vol. 18). London: Hogarth Press.
Galli, N., Greenberg, J., & Tobin, F. (1987). Health education and sensitivity to cultural, religious and ethnic beliefs. *Journal of School Health, 57*(5), 177–180.
Gibson, L. (1989). Bedwetting: A family recurrent nightmare. *MCN: American Journal of Maternal Child Nursing, 14,* 270–272.
Gillis, A. (1990). Nurse's knowledge of growth and developmental principles in meeting psychosocial needs of hospitalized children. *Journal of Pediatric Nursing, 5*(2), 78–87.
Ginsberg, H., & Opper, S. (1969). *Piaget's theory of intellectual development*. Englewood Cliffs, NJ: Prentice-Hall.
Goetting, A. (1986). The developmental tasks of siblings over the life cycle. *Journal of Marriage and the Family, 48,* 703.
Hitchens-Serota, J. (1986). Assessing parent's knowledge of pediatric dental disease. *Pediatric Nursing, 12*(6), 435–438.
Jose, N. (1987). The silent gift: A project for spiritual health. *Journal of School Health, 47*(2), 72–73.
Kohlberg, L. (1981). *The philosophy of moral development*. San Francisco: Harper & Row.
Miller, J., & Janosik, E. (1980). *Family focused care*. New York: McGraw-Hill.
Pendergrast, R. (1990). Skateboard injuries in children and adolescents. *Journal of Adolescent Health Care, 11*(5), 408–412.
Pless, I., Verreault, R., & Tenina, S. (1989). A case-control study of pedestrian and bicyclist injuries in childhood. *American Journal of Public Health, 79,* 995–998.
Rivara, F., et al. (1989). Attitudes and practices toward children as pedestrians. *Pediatrics, 84,* 1017–1021.
Rivara, F., Booth, C., Bergman, A., Rogers, L., & Weiss, J. (1991). Prevention of pedestrian injuries to children: Effectiveness of a school training program. *Pediatrics, 88*(4), 770–775.
Ruddy-Wallace, M. (1987). Temperament: Assessing individual differences in hospitalized children. *Journal of Pediatric Nursing, 2*(1), 30–36.
Rushton, H. (1989). Nocturnal enuresis: Epidemiology, evaluation and currently available treatment options. *Journal of Pediatrics, 114*(Suppl.), 691–696.
Shaw, L., & Glenwright, H. (1989). The role of medications in dental caries formation: Need for sugar free medication. *Pediatrician, 16,* 153–155.
Simons-Morton, B., Brink, S., Simons-Morton, D., McIntyre, R., & Sorenson, C. (1990). Children's coping responses. *Journal of Pediatric Nursing, 5*(4), 259–267.
Stadtler, A. (1989). Preventing encopresis. *Pediatric Nursing, 5,* 282–284.
Strasburger, V. (1992). Children, adolescents and television. *Pediatrics in Review, 13*(4), 144–151.
Thompson, C., & Stroud, S. (1987). The motorized tricycle: An accident waiting to happen. *Journal of Pediatric Nursing, 2*(2), 120–125.
Tiedeman, M., Simon, K., & Clatworthy, S. (1990). Communication through therapeutic play. In M. Craft & J. Deneby (Eds.), *Nursing intervention for infants and children* (pp. 93–110). Philadelphia: WB Saunders.
U. S. Department of Health and Human Services (1991). *Healthy children 2000*. (DHHS Publication No. HRSA–M–CH 91). Washington, DC: Author.
Wilson, H. (1989). Preventing injury in the "middle years." *Contemporary Pediatrics, 6*(6), 20–54.

CHAPTER • 9

Families with Adolescents

NURSING PROCESS PLAN
NPP: Care of Pregnant Adolescent, Table 9–19.

GROWTH AND DEVELOPMENT PLAN
NPP: Families with Adolescents, Table 9–2.

RELATED TOPICS
Developmental theories, Chapter 3
Adolescents' concepts of health, Chapter 10
Health assessment, Chapter 13
Fostering Self-Esteem, Chapter 14
Promoting Safety, Chapter 15
Promoting healthy nutrition, Chapter 16
Anorexia nervosa, bulimia, Chapter 29
Substance abuse, Chapter 29

LEARNING OBJECTIVES

- Describe the issues the family will deal with during the period of adolescence.
- Identify the milestones of the adolescent's physical growth and development.
- Apply knowledge of the adolescent's cognitive development to clinical practice.
- Apply knowledge of the adolescent's social-emotional competencies to clinical practice.
- Demonstrate ability to apply the nursing process to the care of the adolescent and family to promote their development and adaptation.
- Identify the essential components of the adolescent's health screening exam.
- Apply the prominent anticipatory guidance concerns for parents and adolescents to nursing care.

The adolescent period is defined as beginning with the appearance of secondary sex characteristics at approximately 12 years of age, and ending with the completion of somatic growth at about age 19. However, adolescence must also be considered within the context of psychosocial and cognitive development, rather than just as a chronologic or physical event.

As the adolescent develops, the family develops as well, and adolescent development and family development have a reciprocal relationship. Changes during adolescence influence the family and relationships within. Normal adolescent developmental events may potentially stress the family. The nurse can play a pivotal role in working with adolescents and their families, not only by aiding them during stressful times but also by helping them to maintain health. This chapter will cover growth and development of families with adolescents, potential stresses of families with adolescents, adolescent growth and development, and health care of adolescents.

Development and Adaptation of the Family with an Adolescent

The family with an adolescent begins when the oldest child is 12 years of age and ends when that child is independent. The period may be brief, as for a family whose adolescent joins the military at age 18, or may last longer, as for a family whose adolescent remains at home throughout graduate school. The overall family goal is to prepare for impending separation by promoting adolescent responsibility and by gradually loosening ties. Further discussion about families is found in Chapter 2.

Providing Facilities for Widely Different Needs

Parents need to understand their adolescent's desire to spend time away from the family and to be involved in outside activities. Parents should be encouraged to support activities in which the teen-ager is interested, within their financial and time limitations. Some parents may need to be reminded not to push a teen-ager into an activity in order to meet their own spoken or unspoken needs.

Adolescents need privacy to think and dream. It is often difficult for younger siblings to understand their older brother's or sister's need to be alone.

Although parents may not be able actually to increase the space available to their adolescent, they may rearrange home furnishings to include special interest areas more acceptable to the teen-ager. They should allow the youth the opportunity to organize and decorate her or his own room to satisfy adolescent tastes (Duvall & Miller, 1985).

Assigning Greater Responsibility

The adolescent can assume greater household responsibilities than the younger child. Adolescents are forming their sense of identity. Encouraging their participation in household responsibilities helps them to incorporate into their identity a sense of being a useful and participating member of a family unit (Fig. 9–1). Adolescents should be given creative as well as routine tasks. Responsibilities should be increased as the adolescent matures. It is important for parents to recognize and comment on teen-agers' efforts. Another reason adolescents may be given a greater share of household responsibilities is because their help is needed as both parents work.

Re-Establishing Relationships

In families with both partners living at home, the adolescent period provides more time for the couple to be alone. This is true for the traditional as well as the nontraditional couple, with the possible exception of large communal or extended families. The couple may enjoy activities they used to do or re-establish

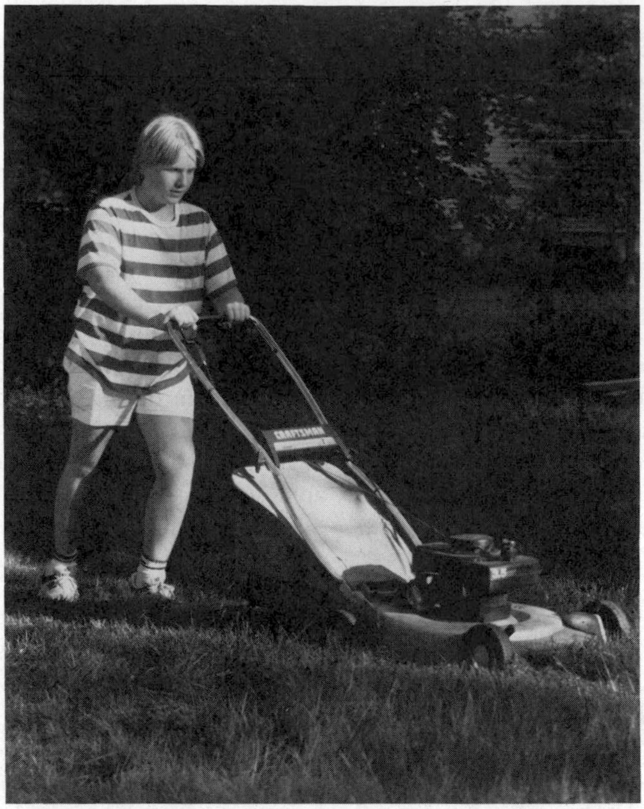

FIGURE 9-1. Sharing the tasks and responsibilities of family living. (Photograph by Ken Kasper.)

old friendships. They often begin to consider their own future together with an "empty nest." Couples may rediscover one another and the characteristics that brought them together. Physical and emotional intimacy may be rekindled. On the other hand, more time together may mean facing problems in their relationship. A loving relationship between partners provides a good model for a teen-ager's future relationships.

Promoting Communication

Open communication is a necessary aspect of living with an adolescent who may be loquacious, argumentative, or moody. It requires attentiveness as well as acceptance of the youth as an individual. Many parents find it trying to listen to adolescents as they talk at length about personal discoveries that they consider of universal significance or as they discuss matters that may seem trivial to adults. Listening attentively lets teen-agers know that they have something worthwhile to say (Fig. 9–2). Teen-agers also need to listen to themselves and to get feedback from adults to aid in establishing opinions and values. Talking also helps develop communication and social skills.

Parents often feel threatened when teen-agers disagree with them. Negativism is typical of young adolescents especially, as they attempt to express autonomy. Disagreements are natural in all families and should not be suppressed but rather expressed as rationally and respectfully as possible. Parents should insist that opposing views be expressed respectfully and should express their own views respectfully. Consciously humiliating an adolescent does nothing to improve the reasoning skills and can be detrimental to her or his self-esteem. Humor may help in arguments but adolescents like to be taken seriously, so the humor should be directed at the situation and not the youth.

Family harmony has been associated with positive personality characteristics in adolescents. Research findings revealed that adolescent girls from harmonious family environments described themselves as more socially competent; adolescent boys were described as more intellectually competent. These findings support the importance of a supportive family environment to promote positive outcomes in children (Vaughn et al, 1988).

Developing Peer Relationships

Adolescence is a time when a person seeks friends to fulfill the needs to be liked, to be accepted, and to belong to a group. The adolescent moves away from the family, and friends become the bearers of his or her ideals and standards. Making friends is an important developmental task. As adolescents become more and more resistive to parental admonitions about behavior acceptable for them, they double their efforts to act like and dress like their selected friends of the moment.

Many times the adolescent's selection of friends and allegiance to them produces a stressful situation for the family. Parents may need help to understand that this exaggerated conformity to peer groups is a manifestation of the adolescent's process of achieving identity and independence from the parents. Adoles-

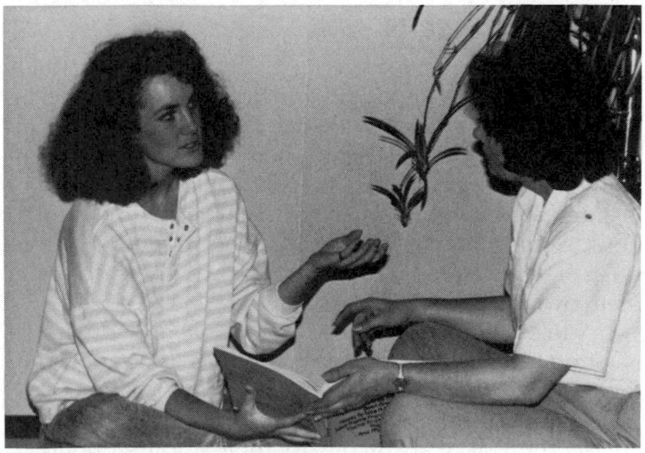

FIGURE 9-2. Listening attentively is one of the most important requirements for successful communication, particularly with teen-agers.

cents desperately need approval, and, since they are moving away from dependence on their parents, they need the support that approval from friends provides. Once parents recognize the adolescent's desire and need to make friends, their attention becomes focused on the "desirability" of the friends selected. For additional discussion on peer relationships, refer to discussion later in the chapter under "Emotional-Social Competency."

Understanding the Need for Independence

Issues of independence and rebellion are probably the primary sources of family stress during adolescence. Impending independence is often met with ambivalence by both parents and teen-agers. Parents look forward to the freedom, but dread letting go. Adolescents want to be treated like adults, yet expect complete financial support.

To begin the process of separation, adolescents create psychologic and physical distance between themselves and their parents. They prefer to spend time with their peers and no longer idealize parents (Buhrmester & Furman, 1987). Not all adolescents can create the necessary distance and still demonstrate love and respect. Not all parents understand the separation process; even if they can intellectualize the process, they still often feel rejected by their teen-agers. Parents who are lonely and dependent on their teen-agers often feel more rejection than parents who have an adult source of support, such as a spouse. Conflicts heighten with the anger and guilt that may result. The nurse can help by listening to the parents, explaining the adolescent's behavior, and assuring them that their teen still needs them very much. Rebellion is a natural part of seeking independence and identity (Erikson, 1959). It generally involves defiance of limits and argumentiveness. Rebellion is not usually intended to hurt the family, but many families see it as such. Parents may feel that the teen-ager is selfish and unappreciative. Siblings may resent the attention the teen-ager receives by "being bad."

Single-Parent Families

The preceding section has described stresses that occur in the family with an adolescent. The proportion of single-parent families continues to rise dramatically. In 1990, 25 per cent of all family groups were headed by one parent, and most of those were headed by a divorced mother (US Bureau of the Census, 1991). The effects of divorce and its byproducts on family and child development have been studied extensively. Much of that research has revealed that children of divorced parents are more likely to engage in problem behaviors and to develop emotional disorders (Kaltar et al, 1984; Zill, 1984; Hetherington et al, 1985; Steinberg, 1987) than are children from intact two-parent families. The potential for problem behaviors in the adolescent is greater in single-parent families headed by the mother (Dornbusch et al, 1985), and mother-son conflicts are more likely than mother-daughter conflicts (Gjerde, 1986). A nursing study revealed that adolescents from single-parent families viewed the future as less predictable, structured, and controlled compared with adolescents from two-parent families. Previous studies have demonstrated associations between an ill-defined future perspective and decreased academic motivation, difficulty delaying gratification, irresponsible behavior, and difficulty formulating life goals. In extreme cases, it has been associated as a variable in adolescents with delinquency problems, drug addiction, and emotional disturbances (Yarcheski & Mahon, 1986).

Nursing Care and Guidance

Assessing Families

The nurse should always obtain information regarding the family structure of the clients. Awareness of the presence of such risk factors as imminent or recent divorce or the presence of a divorced female head of family will allow the nurse to assess in greater depth for the existence of problems. A number of guides to interventions have been reported in the literature, and the nurse with education and experience in individual and family counseling should be aware of those interventions. Divorced parents who have high self-esteem, who show respect for each other, who are able to empathize with their child and the other parent, and who are flexible and open to receiving help have families with fewer difficulties (Steinman et al, 1985). School-based counseling groups have assisted children of divorced families to adjust to the new stresses confronting them (Kaltar et al, 1984). Intensive counseling and therapy, as well as vocational and peer support groups, are options that may be of benefit to the adolescent (Yarcheski & Mahon, 1986). One study found that the provision of information via newsletter assisted single parents in coping with stress (Nelson, 1986). Of particular interest is a study by Hanson (1986) that demonstrated that social support and good parent-child communication predict physical and mental health of single parents, whereas social support, good communication, and religiousness predict physical and mental health of their children. This focus on wellness allows for the identification of specific defining characteristics of positive individual coping and *family coping: potential for growth*. The nurse can intervene in a wellness-oriented way to identify and enhance those attributes that contribute to healthy family functioning. The stresses that have been discussed can all represent risk factors for the occurrence of *ineffective family coping: compromised*. Since developmental crises, family role changes, and temporary family disorganization are all etiologic factors for this nursing diagnostic response (Gordon, 1987), the nurse should be alert to the possibility that it exists.

Facilitating Change

The nurse may consider the nursing diagnostic response *ineffective family coping: compromised* since there are a variety of circumstances that can create disequilibrium in the family. These circumstances could include family situations such as parental career changes requiring moving to a new community, parental separation and/or divorce, death of a family member, and changes in the developmental needs of family members. In addition to assessing for the defining characteristics of that nursing diagnostic response, the nurse can assist the family in adapting to this change in the family unit. The nurse may help the family to understand the effects of changes on family members and recognize their positive and constructive aspects, as they are not necessarily unsatisfactory. The family must agree on what is expected of each member and work together to continue to function adaptively.

Dealing with Rebellion

After defining with the family the extent of the rebellion, the nurse can help the family to deal with it. If the rebellion is causing harm to the teen-ager or to others, as in vandalism or drug abuse, for example, the family will require more intensive counseling. For milder forms of rebellion, such as staying out past curfew, parents can be assured that this is not unusual and that it does not usually indicate rejection or lack of appreciation. Parents should be advised to set reasonable and specific limits and to explain the reasons for the limits (Friedman & Sarles, 1980). Both parents should be consistent in expectations and in discipline. Limits are necessary, for ignoring rebellious behavior can cause an adolescent to feel ignored and rejected, and may possibly cause more extreme rebelliousness in order to receive parental attention and demonstration of concern (Sedgwick & Hildebrand, 1980). Limits as well as privileges will need to be revised as the teen-ager matures.

Facilitating Communication

One of the more difficult aspects affecting communication with the adolescent is the fluctuating emotional state. Parents may need assistance in recognizing their child's behavior as a form of communication. In dealing with this moodiness during adolescence, parents may be most helpful by making themselves available to comfort, advise, or listen during a low mood; understand during a quiet mood; and share the fun during a happy mood. Sometimes parents' attempts to keep the lines of communication open are perceived by adolescents as "picking" on them. The most destructive effect of fault-finding on the adolescent is the lowering of self-concept. This reduces confidence in the youth's ability to solve problems and in her or his interpersonal relationships.

Growth and Development of the Adolescent

Adolescence is characterized by physical, intellectual, and emotional-social development changes. The changes interact and are multidimensional in the complete process. Goals for adolescent development are linked to the developmental changes. The goals are to accept one's body, to achieve the capacity for formal operational thought, to form a sense of identity, to become independent, to attain a workable value system, and to establish mutually giving relationships with others. This section covers the physical, intellectual, and emotional-social changes of adolescents with these developmental goals in mind. Growth, development, and health promotion stages and competency levels are listed in Table 9–1.

Nurses working with adolescents in a variety of settings such as the school, hospital, and clinic will consider the nursing diagnostic response *high risk for altered growth and development* as a component of the nursing care provided (Table 9–2). Other diagnostic responses that may be applied to the holistic care of the adolescent include *high risk for impaired adjustment, alteration in health maintenance,* and *ineffective individual coping*. The nurse will continually assess the adolescent for the etiology of the actual response, the risk factors associated with high-risk problems, and the defining characteristics in formulating the nursing diagnostic response.

Physical Competency

Height and Weight

Adolescence is the only time after birth that the velocity of growth significantly increases. During puberty, both males and females attain the final 20 per cent of their mature height. Most of this growth occurs as a "growth spurt" that lasts 2 to 3 years. This spurt usually occurs 2 years earlier for females than for males. The beginning age is variable, from 9.5 to 14.5 years for girls and 10.5 to 16 years for boys.

During the growth spurt, boys average an 8-inch height gain, with 4 inches attained during the peak year (around age 14). During the growth spurt, a girl's average gain is over 3 inches per year. At age 18, more than 99 per cent of growth has occurred and only about 1 inch in height remains to be gained.

The adolescent's weight varies according to pubertal maturation, the degree of adiposity, and size of muscle mass. Boys have greater weight increases than girls. During the pubertal growth spurt, weight increases 50 per cent.

General Appearance and Skeletal Growth

Growth follows a pattern, with almost every part of the body being affected. The legs usually lengthen first, causing the youth to appear lanky and awkward, then the thighs become wider. Next the shoulders broaden, followed by trunk growth. Facial bones change, particularly the mandible and maxilla. The maxilla grows forward and the ramus of the mandible lengthens. Coordination is often affected during this time of uneven growth, and the adolescent may go through periods of clumsiness.

Skeletal changes are dramatic during adolescence. Skeletal mass doubles, contributing significantly to weight gain in puberty.

Muscle or lean body mass and nonlean body mass (principally fat) double during puberty. In males, muscles increase both in number of individual cells and in size, whereas, in females, muscles increase only in size. This probably accounts for greater male strength, but the cause is unclear. At the time of physical maturation, females average twice as much body fat as males. Total body fat in males actually decreases during puberty.

Nursing Intervention: Promoting Physical Growth

The physical assessment provides a good time to discuss physical development. Changes may be pointed out and discussed in a casual, matter-of-fact manner. Adolescents should be assured that their growth and development are normal. Because most adolescents do not ask questions they may have about their body changes or lack thereof, adults around them must anticipate questions.

Anticipatory Guidance: Promoting Physical Development

Dramatic physical changes require adolescents to adjust to their new appearance and to develop a feeling of comfort inside their maturing body. Furthermore, the adolescent must cope with the emotional and social pressures that accompany these physical changes. These changes may overwhelm the adolescent or they can be used as the foundation for learning adaptation mechanisms useful later in life. The understanding of young people by parents and other adults is crucial to smooth progression through adolescence.

Both girls and boys observe their peers, see variations in development, and compare themselves with those around them. These variations produce anxiety in those who develop slightly earlier or later than their peers. A high degree of error was found in young adolescents' (ages 11 to 14 years) self-reports of pubertal maturation when compared with physicians' and nurse practitioners' evaluations. Adolescents tended to overestimate their development early in puberty and underestimate it later in puberty (Schlossberger et al, 1992). The physical assessment presents the opportunity to provide anticipatory guidance regarding physical maturation and to correct misconceptions causing discomfort or anxiety in the adolescent.

Maturation of Organs

The heart, lungs, liver, spleen, kidneys, pancreas, thyroid, adrenals, gonads, phallus, and uterus double in size during puberty. It is also thought that the digestive tract enlarges. In contrast, the tissues of the lymphatic system (thymus, tonsils, adenoids, and portions of the spleen) decrease in size. Reasons for this decrease and its relationship to antibody production remain to be investigated.

Sexual Maturation

Sexual maturation involves the development of primary and secondary sexual characteristics. The total process is not considered complete until about 20 to 21 years of age. Primary sex characteristics involve the physical and hormonal changes necessary for reproduction. Secondary sex characteristics, although not necessary to reproduction, are the characteristics that externally differentiate male from female.

Regulation of this onset of puberty is a complicated and not fully understood process. Trophic hormones are produced in the pituitary gland but are thought to be the result of a "feedback" mechanism. The hypothalamus becomes less sensitive to negative feedback with increasing age and begins to produce releasing factors. These gonadotropic-releasing hormones then signal the pituitary to secrete gonadotropic hormones such as follicle-stimulating hormone (FSH). FSH in turn stimulates both the growth of ova in the female ovary and the growth of sperm-producing cells in the male testes. Cells in the ovary and testicle produce female and male sex hormones, respectively. Estrogen (female hormone) is produced by the ovary, and testosterone (male hormone) is produced by the testes. These hormones are responsible for development of the secondary sex character-

TABLE 9-1
Summary of Adolescent Growth and Development and Health Maintenance

Physical Competency	Intellectual Competency	Emotional-Social Competency
General Summary: 12 to 21 Yrs		
Puberty begins 2 yrs earlier for girls than boys; girls stop growing sooner and have smaller increases in height and weight than boys During pubertal growth spurt, weight increases 50%; varies according to pubertal maturation, degree of adiposity, and size of muscle mass During puberty, growth spurt results in 15–20% increase in height *Early Maturer:* About 80th percentile for weight for height at 12 yrs *Late Maturer:* Below 20th percentile at 12 yrs	Marked by Piaget's formal operations period, which includes hypotheticodeductive, combinational thinking, relativity, and objectivity	Exhibits characteristics of Freud's genital stage, Erickson's stage of identity versus role confusion, Kohlberg's postconventional level, and Fowler's state of individuation reflexive
Early Adolescence (12–14 Yrs)		
Secondary sex characteristics develop. Testicular enlargement occurs first in 98% of boys (ejaculation occurs approximately 1 yr later with appearance of pubic hair). Breast budding occurs first in 84% of girls; menarche begins. There is an increase in body fat associated with each stage of pubertal development in females. Males become more muscular rather than fatter during puberty. Neurodevelopmental maturity is seen	Has difficulty solving problems; thinks in present; cannot use past experience to control behavior. Exhibits a strong sense of invulnerability—society's rules don't apply to him or her. Becomes comfortable with own body: egocentric	Struggle between dependent and independent behavior is obvious; begins forming peer alliances
Middle Adolescence (15–16 Yrs)		
Growth spurt is evident (females: 8 cm/yr; males: 10 cm/yr). Sex patterns evident in growth, arms and legs of males are longer. Secondary sex characteristics are seen in females—menarche has begun; breast and areola enlarges; pubic hair coarsens, darkens, and covers the mons. The penis elongates and widens, testes enlarge, and scrotum pigment becomes evident in males. Both axillary and facial hair increase, along with body odor. No apparent neurodevelopmental growth.	Begins to solve problems through analysis and abstract thinking. Peak turmoil in child-family relations; able to debate issues and use some logic, but not continuously	"Tries out" adultlike behavior. Establishes peer group alliance with associated risk-taking behavior
Late Adolescence (17–21 Yrs)		
Most of linear growth is achieved, secondary sex development completed, and adult genitalia attained. The male voice deepens. No neurodevelopmental changes are apparent	Able to verbalize conceptually, deals with abstract moral concepts, makes decisions about future	Aware of own strengths and limitations; establishes own values system. Peer group diminishes in importance; may develop first intimate relationship. Turbulence subsides. May move away from home. More adultlike friendship with parents

TABLE 9-1
Summary of Adolescent Growth and Development and Health Maintenance *(Continued)*

Nutrition	Recreation	Safety
General Summary: 12 to 21 Yrs		
Caloric needs increase with size; growth can be influenced by dietary fads, diets, and drugs. Protein requirement is 12–14% of daily total caloric intake. Zinc, calcium, and iron are three essential minerals needed during this period	Romantic friendships emerge. Special talents and interests influence selection of activities. Social outings to the mall or beach are heavily influenced by desire to meet members of the opposite sex. Participation in group and individual competition can enhance social stature	Educational programs for teens are vital. They should stress: • Prevention of substance abuse • Sex education including prevention of sexually transmitted diseases (STDs) • Sports injury prevention • Driver safety • Personal safety • Anti-gang programs
Early Adolescence (12–14 Yrs)		
Male needs 2500 cal/day; female needs 2200 cal. Protein requirement for both is 0.29 g/cm of height	Enjoys physical activity—bicycling, skateboarding, team/competitive sports, swimming. Quiet time focuses on books, computer games/videos	Fact-based information should focus on prevention of: • Alcohol/drug abuse • STDs/teen pregnancy Safe use should be stressed with • Bicycles, skateboards, skates • Automobile—seat belts, speed • Athletic equipment Physical conditioning should be emphasized in relation to all intense physical activity (e.g., team sports)
Middle Adolescence (15–16 Yrs)		
Male needs 3000 cal; female needs 2200 cal. Protein requirement for males is 0.32 g/cm of height; 0.28 g/cm of height for females	Enjoys dressing up, parties, and makeovers. Is preoccupied by computer games, videos, movies, and music. Likes outings to the mall, beach, or park. Driving and dancing are important pastimes	Preventive education continues concerning: • Substance abuse • Use of seat belts • Use of safety equipment with bicycles, motorized scooter, motorcycles, and automobiles • Physical conditioning related to sports injuries • Athletic safety equipment • Students Against Drunk Drivers (SADD) • Date rape prevention
Late Adolescence (17–21 Yrs)		
Male needs 2900 cal; female needs 2200 cal. Protein requirement for males is 0.32 g/cm of height; 0.28 g/cm of height for females	Continues to enjoy computer games and videos. Dating increases in importance. Other activities include athletic competition and sports, trips to the mall and beach, movies, dancing, teen nightclubs, and rock concerts	Preventive education continues concerning: • Substance abuse • Use of seat belts • Driver safety • Athletic safety equipment • SADD • Preseason physical conditioning • Sex education • Date rape prevention

TABLE 9-2

Growth and Development Plan: Families with Adolescents

Analysis: Nursing Diagnostic Statement

Response and Related or Risk Factors: *High risk for altered growth and development; risk factors*

- Illness/physical impairment
- Treatment-related procedures
- Separation from family and peers
- Lack of privacy
- Perceived/actual threats to body image/integrity
- Dependency status in health care situations
- Caregiver has unrealistic expectations about adolescent's behavior; negative/ambivalent feelings about parenting
- Inadequate/deviant coping mechanisms

Projected Outcome: The adolescent will demonstrate acquisition of developmentally appropriate behaviors in the physical, intellectual, and emotional-social domains

Defining Characteristics (Actual Response)	Nursing Interventions	Evaluation Criteria

Subjective:
• Delay or difficulty in performing skills typical of age group, often seen as feelings of low self-esteem such as:
  • "Why would he choose me as his friend?"
  • "I'm no good."
  • "I'm stupid."
  • "I'm fat."
• Uses deprecating humor to describe self/others
• Caregiver expresses unrealistic expectations about adolescent's behavior, negative/ambivalent feelings concerning parenting
	Health Screening
	• **Assess factors that can identify altered growth and development.** (Evidence of the adolescent behavior deviating from age-appropriate levels will be observed and documented based on theoretical basis of growth and development; parent-child relationships; peer relationships; social support; knowledge of physiologic effects of disease on the child and family)
	• **Assess adolescent's level of development using developmental norms and specific assessment tools.** (Refer to Chapter 13 and Appendices 2 through 6)
		• **Developmental alterations will be identified as evidenced by**
		  • Charted assessment of screening for physical, intellectual, and emotional/social development
		  • Referral for deviations from the norm detected during screening
		• **Caregiver will demonstrate knowledge and ability to interact in an age-appropriate manner with the adolescent and provide activities to support/enhance the developmental needs of the adolescent**
		• **Adolescent will demonstrate age-appropriate developmental tasks**
		• **Referrals to community resources will be made as needed**

istics. Sex hormones are also produced by the adrenal gland so that both sexes have some of both male and female hormones.

Many practitioners and investigators have observed the more or less orderly (although widely variable) progression of sexual development in both sexes. The description and labeling of these stages by Tanner (1962) are generally accepted as guidelines to normal development (Tables 9–3 and 9–4). These tables enable an examiner to determine the stage of development, to detect abnormalities, and to guide the adolescent as to changes to expect next.

Female secondary sexual development during puberty involves increase in size of the ovaries, uterus, vagina, labia, and breasts. Body hair appears in the pubic area and under the arms; menarche occurs. The first visible signs of sexual maturity are pubic hair or breast buds, or both. These developments occur in orderly fashion but do not necessarily occur together. Each aspect of development (growth, pubic hair,

TABLE 9-2 (continued)

Defining Characteristics	Nursing Interventions	Evaluation Criteria

Objective:
• Flat affect
• Limited eye contact
• Anorexia
• Excessive eating
• "Acting out" behaviors
• Self-destructive behaviors
• Delinquent behaviors
• Weeping
• Angry outbursts
• Limited social interactions
• Lethargy
• Decline in school performance
• Regressive behavior (behavior inappropriate for age)
• Listlessness
• Excessive/inappropriate use of defense mechanisms
• Hostile relationships with family and peers
• Avoidance of social gatherings/group sports
• Isolates self from others
	Anticipatory Guidance; Parent Education: Childrearing Family
	• **Provide anticipatory guidance to caregivers regarding acquisition of age-appropriate developmental tasks.** (Refer to information on developmental norms in sections on physical, intellectual, and emotional-social competencies.)
	• **Provide opportunities for the adolescent (including acutely and chronically ill) to meet age-related developmental tasks.** (Refer to information on nursing interventions and anticipatory guidance in sections on growth and development and health maintenance and promotion.)
	Support System Enhancement
	• **Refer adolescent and family to appropriate community resources as needed:**
	  • Appropriate agency for counseling for adolescent and family treatment
	  • Appropriate agency for supportive services (e.g., occupational therapy, physical therapy, home care services)
	  • Community programs specific to factors affecting the adolescent's altered growth and development (e.g., remedial program for educational skills, drug treatment program, job training program, neighborhood/personal safety, prenatal classes)
	  • Provide information on community self-help groups, parent and sibling support groups, advocacy groups (e.g., MADD, SADD, Candlelighters)
	Teaching: Preoperative; Procedure/Treatment; Safe Sex
	• **Provide explanation in concrete, graphic and understandable terms** (e.g., preprocedural/preoperative teaching; sex education)	

breast appearance) must be evaluated to determine if the young woman is developing normally. For example, it is rare for a girl to reach pubic hair stage 3 or 4 without breast development. In this case, the girl should be evaluated for the presence of hypothalamic, pituitary, or gonadal dysfunction. The vast majority of girls will achieve adult breast size by age 19.

Menarche (the appearance of menstruation) has occurred earlier each generation; present-day adolescent females begin menstruating at an average age of 12 years and 3 months compared with age 17 a century ago. Reasons for these changes are unclear, but effects of environment, nutrition, and better health care are most likely responsible. Menarche occurs at

TABLE 9-3
Classification of Sex Maturity Stages in Boys

Stage	Pubic Hair	Penis	Testes
1	None	Preadolescent	Preadolescent
2	Scanty, long, slightly pigmented	Slight enlargement	Enlarged scrotum, pink texture altered
3	Darker, starts to curl, small amount	Longer	Larger
4	Resembles adult type, but less in quantity; coarse, curly	Larger; glans and breadth increase in size	Larger, scrotum dark
5	Adult distribution, spread to medial surface of thighs	Adult	Adult

From Behrman, R. (Ed.). (1992). *Nelson textbook of pediatrics* (14th ed.). Philadelphia: WB Saunders.

about the time the growth spurt slows. About 99 per cent of girls will reach menarche within 5 years after beginning breast development. If no evidence of puberty can be seen by age 13, a medical assessment should be done. Menarche usually occurs at stage 4.

Male secondary sexual development consists of genital growth and the appearance of pubic and body hair. The first event is usually enlargement of the testes. During puberty the testes, epididymides, and prostate will increase their prepuberty size seven times. As the testes enlarge, so does the scrotum; the scrotum develops rugae and becomes darker in color. The next sign is growth of the penis and a few tufts of long, straight, and slightly pigmented pubic hair. The genitals progress to near-adult size before more pubic hair appears. The final stage of hair growth is to adult type, with hair extending to the medial thigh areas.

Ejaculation has usually occurred in boys by stage 3 and probably earlier. Spermatozoa are almost always present. Stage 4 must be reached before the full adult number of sperm are present.

The male growth spurt occurs at about the same time as penile growth and about a year after the increase in testicular size. If growth has not begun by sexual development stage 4, the boy should be evaluated for thyroid dysfunction, growth hormone adequacy, or chronic disease. Generally, a boy who is short at stage 4 will continue to grow but will be shorter than average as an adult.

Males normally experience an increase in size of breast areola. About 30 per cent or more will also experience some bilateral, nontender increase in size of the breasts. Transient breast tenderness is also common. Facial and axillary hair appear at about stage 5. Breaking and deepening of the voice also occur at this stage (Behrman, 1992).

Anticipatory Guidance: Female Sexual Maturation

Menarche is a rather late occurrence in female sexual development. Therefore, when a girl who has neither begun the growth spurt nor developed breast buds by 13.2 years is anxious about not menstruating, the nurse can inform her that sexual characteristics have a wide range of rate of development. Statistically, the adolescent girl should begin menstruation by age 13.2 years (or 5 years after breast budding begins); if she has not, medical evaluation is indicated (Rosenfield, 1990). A complete history and physical examination are done to assess for pathologic causes of delayed sexual maturation. If no underlying physical cause is

TABLE 9-4
Classification of Sex Maturity Stages in Girls

Stage	Pubic Hair	Breasts
1	Preadolescent	Preadolescent
2	Sparse, lightly pigmented, straight, medial border of labia	Breast and papilla elevated as small mound; areolar diameter increased
3	Darker, beginning to curl, increased amount	Breast and areola enlarged, no contour separation
4	Coarse, curly, abundant but amount less than in adult	Areola and papilla form secondary mound
5	Adult feminine triangle, spread to medial surface of thighs	Mature, nipple projects, areola part of general breast contour

From Behrman, R. (Ed.). (1992). *Nelson textbook of pediatrics* (14th ed.). Philadelphia: WB Saunders.

found, then the girl with delayed puberty may be started on anabolic steroid therapy and low-dose estrogen (Castiglia, 1991b).

It is also normal for a young woman to experience irregularity in the amount of menstrual flow and in the spacing of periods. She can be reassured that for the first year or more her periods will be unpredictable (Tuttle, 1991). What is more, emotional changes affect the menstrual cycle; the teen-age girl may find that her period is delayed during times of stress, such as final examinations.

The school-age or prepubertal adolescent girl should be prepared for the onset of menstruation. Parents should be advised to obtain menstrual supplies for the girl long before she will need them. Their use should be explained and the girl allowed to become familiar with them. Myths that baths and physical exercise should be avoided during menstruation can be dispelled. Menstruation is a normal physiologic process that requires additional attention to hygiene but generally does not interrupt normal activities of the adolescent girl. If menstrual discomfort does occur, it usually does not happen until several months after menarche (after periods become ovulatory).

Toxic shock syndrome (TSS) frequently affects adolescent females between the ages of 15 and 19 who use tampons (Farley, 1990). As a component of anticipatory guidance, the signs and symptoms of TSS can be discussed with the adolescent, which include the following:

- Abrupt spiking temperature
- Vomiting
- Diarrhea
- Dizziness
- Desquamation of the skin, especially the palms and soles
- Hypotension
- Severe myalgia
- Inflamed mucous membranes (oropharyngeal, conjunctival, or vaginal)
- Central nervous system (CNS) disorders (alteration in consciousness, disorientation, and coma)

The teen-ager can be instructed in the proper use of tampons. Instructions would include information on reviewing the manufacturer's instruction for use, storage in a clean dry place, hand washing before and after insertion and removal of the tampon, and selection of the appropriate absorbency range.

Between 18 and 21 years, normal gynecologic care is instituted. If the adolescent is sexually active, or has a pelvic or menstrual disorder, such care should be started earlier (Castiglia, 1991b). The Society for Adolescent Medicine (1992b) does not recommend breast self-examination under the age of 20, since the risk factors are not a health concern until the mid-30s.

Anticipatory Guidance: Male Sexual Maturation

One of the major concerns of boys is their height; most want to be tall. If a boy's growth spurt has not occurred by the time his genitals are at stage 4, he should be medically evaluated. After an examination is done, and if no abnormalities are found, the nurse should provide an opportunity for the boy to express his feelings about being short. In 85 per cent of males who are shorter than average, the cause is familial. Health professionals should concentrate on helping the boy who will not be tall to feel good about himself. If underlying physical causes are ruled out as causes for delayed bone age, adolescent growth spurt, and sexual development, then *constitutional delay in growth and development (CDGD)* may be the diagnosis. CDGD is a variation of normal growth, but will likely still cause the adolescent distress since he feels inadequate because of delayed sexual maturation and smaller physical size. Depending on the boy's circumstances, he may be started on oxandrolone or low-dose testosterone (Castiglia, 1991b).

Size of penis is also a major concern for adolescent boys and adult men. If this concern exists, the boy should be reassured that penile size is not the determining factor in being able to satisfy one's sexual partner.

Erections and nocturnal emissions (wet dreams) are signs of sexual development; however, these are often sources of great embarrassment for the young man. He should be reassured that they are normal and that the frequency of the unwanted erections will gradually decrease.

Uncircumcised boys need to be taught to retract the foreskin and carefully cleanse the glans, if they have not already learned to do so. Infections can result if this is not done. Also, the foreskin should be returned to its normal position over the glans to avoid constriction and edema of the glans.

Boys should be educated to seek medical help if they experience testicular pain. There are several conditions, some serious, that can occur in males, including injury, torsion of the testicle, and epididymitis. In addition, young men should be taught self-examination of the testicles. The best time to examine the testes is right after a hot bath. The fingers are placed under each testis and the testicle is gently rolled between the thumb and fingers. The testes are oval, measuring about 4 × 3 cm. The epididymis on the back of the testicle should not be confused with an abnormal lump. Lumps should be examined immediately by a doctor, as testicular cancers detected early have an excellent prognosis.

Intellectual Competency

Adolescents are able to think about thinking. They think about their own thoughts and become introspective. Physical changes and introspection stimulate the self-preoccupation so typical of adolescents. They can also think about the thoughts of others.

On entering the formal operational stage, young people are for the first time able to think about their values and reasoning processes. Often this new ability leads adolescents to idealism. They are able to question their own and their family's values.

Cognitive Development: Formal Operations

Concrete operations provide the substance and pave the way for formal operations. Piaget sees *formal operations* as a reconstruction of concrete operations to a new level (Table 9–5) (Piaget & Inhelder, 1958).

A formal operational youth can imagine possibilities and make suppositions before acting. When solving a problem, young people can form a hypothesis, draw deductions from the hypothesis, formulate a plan to test the hypothesis, test it systematically, and then interpret the results. Unexpected results are not as confusing to an adolescent as to a school-age child, because the teen-ager has considered several possibilities (Ginsberg & Opper, 1979).

Adolescents are able mentally to reverse a sequence of events so that they can better understand why something occurred. Because of the ability to form hypotheses and to reason deductively, Piaget refers to adolescent thought as *hypotheticodeductive*. Also, thought processes become flexible and previous learning can be applied to new problems (Piaget, 1976). The adolescent is capable of considering many factors that affect an outcome. This is referred to as *combinational thinking*.

Use of implication refers to the adolescent's ability to deduce relationships on the basis of shared similarities and differences. These acquired capabilities denote the adolescent's use of a much more systematic approach to problem-solving.

Formal operational youths can understand *symbolism*. Metaphors or figures of speech take on new meanings. An adolescent will recognize the symbolism in verse and realize that the image conjured is a representation of something more intangible.

Adolescents become able to understand abstract and theoretical concepts such as existentialism. They can also attach emotion to abstractions (Ginsberg & Opper, 1979). For example, a school-age child can love a puppy and hate spiders, but a teen-ager can love peace and hate bigotry.

Future becomes a possibility (reality versus possibility). The notion of future plus the ability to make suppositions enables adolescents to construct ideals. They can think of how things "could be." In exercising this newfound ability, teen-agers often become intolerant of people, conventional establishments, and the status quo.

Adolescents are capable of analyzing their own thinking process. This ability to engage in reflective

TABLE 9–5
Characteristics of the Adolescent's Thinking

Characteristic	Definition	Clinical Example
Reality vs. possibility	Able to consider future possibilities	"I want to be a nurse so I can help others."
Adolescent egocentrism	Often cannot differentiate others' concerns from their own	Adolescent is horrified by an acne breakout the day of the prom. Parents spend much time consoling—"Everything is NOT ruined."
Propositional thinking	Capable of analyzing their own thinking	"I get nervous when the doctor comes in the room because I don't know what she wants to do next."
Symbolism	Comprehends abstract and theoretical concepts	Adolescent requests visit from chaplain in order to pray for strength in preparation for surgery
Combinational thinking	Considers many factors affecting outcome	Adolescent discusses medication scheduling with nurse to fit in with daily regimen
Hypotheticodeductive thinking	Able to reason deductively	Adolescent discusses the pros and cons of surgical versus medical management of his or her condition with his or her physician
Use of implication	Deduces relationships on basis of similarities and differences	Uses a peer to serve as a role model and support in relating shared experiences about being diabetic
Objectivity	Objectively assesses a situation	Adolescent asks nurse many questions about surgery
Relativity	Takes into account another's perspective	Adolescent volunteers as a candy striper at local pediatric hospital

thought enables the adolescent to construct theories. This cognitive ability is referred to as *propositional thinking*.

Objectivity and *relativity* are other cognitive abilities the adolescent develops. Objectivity refers to the adolescent's ability to objectively assess a situation. This ability enables the adolescent to discern similarities and differences in situations. Furthermore, an adolescent is able to take into account another's perspective. This acquired capacity enables the adolescent to think and reason beyond his or her own realistic world and beliefs.

Young teen-agers often cannot differentiate others' concerns from their own. Therefore, they erroneously believe that others are equally as interested in their behaviors, weaknesses, assets, and appearances. This is known as *adolescent egocentrism* and accounts for the characteristic self-consciousness of adolescents over things younger children and adults find insignificant. They are reacting to an *imaginary audience*. Thus, the hours and attending to every detail of appearance are spent in anticipation of the audience's reaction.

Adolescent egocentrism engenders feelings of uniqueness. Teen-agers cannot imagine that anyone has even been through what they have, loved as much, or suffered as much. They believe that their life events are of universal significance and that no one will even understand them or their complex thoughts. Elkind (1970) refers to this as the *personal fable*. The feelings of uniqueness may lead to the idea that "it can never happen to me." The personal fable thus helps to explain some of the risk-taking during adolescence. By late adolescence, egocentrism diminishes.

Progression to formal operations is not universal. Some people may never attain that level of thinking; or an individual may use formal operations in a task that has personal relevance but not in another task. For example, an adolescent may use formal operations in understanding the symbolism in a play but not in solving an algebra problem. A variety of factors can affect use of formal thinking, such as fatigue, aptitude, boredom, or wealth of knowledge. Furthermore, an adolescent's vocational and professional interests can limit the attainment of formalized thinking.

Nursing Interventions: Cognitive Development

Application of the principles of cognitive development will enable the nurse to intervene more effectively with the adolescent. Explanations regarding the adolescent's condition and medical procedures need not rely as heavily on concrete illustrations and simpler terminology. The effect of stress on cognitive perceptions must be taken into account. Adolescents may be able to repeat information that was provided to them but still may not be able to assimilate it and act on it because they cannot cope with the stress it imposes.

Adolescents will be especially sensitive to the perceived threats that illness and hospitalization may cause them. Acknowledgment of their anxieties and support of productive coping strategies will help alleviate their stresses. Examples of incorporating principles of cognitive development into the nursing care plan are described in Tables 9–6 and 9–7.

Anticipatory Guidance: Cognitive Development

How can the foregoing knowledge help the nurse help adolescents and their parents? Sachs (1987) stresses the need to assess the cognitive developmental level of adolescent clients. Before the entry into formal operational thinking, adolescents may discuss problems with parents, but often the adolescents' arguments are critical of the parents and related to what could be or might have been. Parents' viewpoints are not easily understood or tolerated. These handicaps, combined with the adolescent's limited ability to discern the emotions of other people, make it important to explain one's point of view and feelings to the young adolescent patiently instead of assuming that she or he has an adult's ability to "pick up vibes."

Being unable to abstractly perceive a situation or pattern that is not immediately evident causes many young adolescents to be criticized. If an adolescent member of a family seems repeatedly to attempt a task and is unable to complete it in a mature manner, parents need to realize that the reason may be the youth's developmental stage rather than laziness or disobedience.

Poor school performance is a problem experienced by some adolescents and is often a problem of cognitive development that is troublesome to parents. The process of learning is complex; after a complete history and physical examination, the school is usually the best source of advice and referral for such problems. Learning disabilities can and do lead to emotional problems and often result in the child's dropping out of school and other behavioral problems. Parents need to show interest in school work, assist with homework, and keep in close contact with teachers to be able to spot correctable problems.

Piaget's beliefs about formal operational thinking can be supplemented with the inclusion of other concepts. Some researchers see Piaget's formulations as descriptions of competencies that were never meant to allow for understanding of how particular adolescents respond to real problems in real-life situations. They believe that the effect of stress and environment on cognitive perceptions must be taken into account.

Emotional-Social Competency

"The tension between freedom and attachment and attempts to achieve the impossible union of the two" may be, as Bloom (1987) stated, "the permanent con-

TABLE 9-6
Promoting Cognitive Development: Surgical Preparation

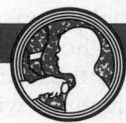

Sheila, age 15, has been admitted to the hospital's adolescent unit for a spinal fusion procedure. The nurse meets with Sheila to discuss the procedure and the postoperative care. The following vignette illustrates the preparation given

Interaction	*Rationale*
Nurse: Shows Sheila an anatomic drawing of the spine and drawing of the procedure	Explanations given are of same character given to adults. Use of visual aids assists with understanding of anatomic and physiologic information
Nurse: Answers Sheila's questions regarding pain, level of physical activity following surgery, and appearance of incision	Explanations about surgery and postoperative course given openly and in terms of same nature given to adults. Explanations are given for medical and physiologic terminology if not understood
Nurse: Asks Sheila to ring call light when parents arrive so she can provide explanations to them	Explanations about procedure given to adolescent first. Presence of parents will depend on physical and emotional status of adolescent. This acknowledges the adolescent's need for independence
Nurse: Encourages Sheila to ask nurses on evening and night shifts questions should she have need for clarification	Timing of explanations needs to be sensitive to emotional and physical status of adolescent. The adolescent's sense of time and memory capacity are fully developed, but preoperative anxiety will inhibit Sheila's processing of information

dition of man" (p. 113). Certainly, however, this tension is prevalent in the adolescent. Struggling to become a functional, stable entity independent of one's family while still maintaining needed bonds of love and support; risking one's self-esteem in forming heterosexual attachments; enduring the pain of broken relationships—such is the turbulence of this period. Add to this adolescent dilemma the fact that young people making the transition from childhood to adulthood today find themselves in a flux of societal values and traditions in which right and wrong have become relative, "situational" conditions. The struggle for identity within such ambiguous boundaries may contribute to the escalating rates of pregnancy, substance abuse, violence, and suicide among teen-agers (Jessor, 1982). (Suicide is discussed in Chapter 29.)

Psychosocial Development: Development of Identity

Formal operations enable adolescents to have an internal representation of themselves, a self-concept or *identity*. Identity may even be a kind of cognition about the self (Ellis & Davis, 1982). Identity is displayed by one's personality. Erikson (1963) refers to the central task, crisis, or problem of the adolescent period as *identity versus role confusion*. An adolescent either develops a stable identity or remains confused, complicating adulthood with old struggles or settling on a negative identity, such as "dummy." Identity formation may be more problematic for adolescents from culturally diverse populations. The adolescent must learn to integrate an identity based not only on personality, but also on one's "racial identity" (Gibbs & Mokowitz-Sweet, 1991). The socialization process of culturally diverse adolescents differs from that of adolescents from the dominant culture as it relates to social norms and values, conceptual style, problem-solving skills, speech and language, and physical appearance. These differences contribute to misunderstandings and prejudice. Negative societal attitudes can be internalized and can create psychologic conflicts.

Erikson (1963) believes that confusion during adolescence has several sources: the body is chang-

TABLE 9-7
Promoting Cognitive Development: Career Counseling

Jane, a 17-year-old senior, approaches the nurse at the adolescent clinic on her high school campus. Jane is in the process of applying to several nursing schools and has previously sought the advice of the school nurse about entering the nursing profession

Interaction	Rationale
Jane: What attracted you to nursing?	*Relativistic Thinking.* Jane demonstrates ability to take another's perspective into account
Nurse: Lots of things. I wanted to do something that helped others . . . be self-supporting, have career flexibility	*Combinational Thinking.* Nurse is aware Jane has ability to consider the many factors that affect outcome
Jane (interrupts): What do you mean by career flexibility? Changing jobs, working with different groups of people? Can you move to another state and still be a nurse?	*Objectivity.* Jane demonstrates ability to gather information and objectively assess a situation
Nurse: There are numerous possibilities for professional growth. First you have to figure out what you want to do, what you want to achieve, and go for it	*Reality versus Possibility.* Nurse is aware of Jane's ability to consider future possibilities. She can imagine how things "could be"
Jane: I'm not sure what I want. I've just always thought it would be neat to be a nurse. I haven't thought much beyond that	*Reality versus Possibility.* Jane expresses her capacity to consider future possibilities
Nurse: Well, you have plenty of time to figure out what you want. In the meantime, pay attention to what you think is interesting and talk to other nurses about what they do. The more information you get, the better	*Propositional Thinking.* Nurse's response acknowledges Jane's capacity of analyzing her own thinking
Jane: That sounds like a good idea . . . what do you like about being a school nurse?	*Relativistic/Combinational Thinking.* Jane demonstrates ability to take another's perspective into account and consider the factors affecting an outcome

ing rapidly and the adolescent must come to terms with skeletal growth, development of secondary sex characteristics, and libidinal urges. The future and the responsibilities of adulthood become real. Therefore, the sense of familiarity felt during childhood is intensely disturbed. Coming to terms with the perceived successes and failures of childhood and with the loss of the security of earlier years is a process that requires a great deal of time and emotional energy for the adolescent (Table 9–8 offers one view). Adolescents have various means of alleviating identity confusion and of discovering their identities, including learning about their bodies and accepting the changes, experimenting with roles, seeking independence from families, rebelling and arguing, identifying with a peer group, and becoming idealistic.

Body Image

Body image is an intricate aspect of identity. It is "the picture of our own body which we form in our own mind, that is to say, the way in which our body appears to ourselves" (Schilder, 1935, p. 104). Body changes and adolescent egocentrism evoke preoccupation with the body. Adolescents are acutely aware of every change. They scrutinize their bodies and compare their bodies with those of others. Preoccu-

TABLE 9-8
Teen-age Crisis

As a teen you reach an overlook point
Where your fondest memories
And your worst fears of the past
Are put before you,
As if to test your strength.

For the past must be conquered
Before you are ready to move on.

And as you reach back through your childhood
You are forced to realize
All that you've left behind
Is now beyond your grasp.

Learning to cope with the loss
Of the you that you used to be
Is the "mid-life crisis" of a teenager.

—*Andrea Foster, 1988*
Age 16

pation may aid in understanding and becoming familiar with one's body, and thus in gaining a clear body image (Fig. 9–3).

Role Experimentation

An adolescent's search for identity involves experimenting with a variety of roles. A youth's earlier identification and the roles and skills that have been learned must now be integrated (Erikson, 1963). The adolescent faces countless alternatives and combinations of choices. Adolescents' choices of roles with which to experiment are influenced by many factors such as family expectations, societal norms, and past roles that have proved effective. They must try a role and verify its effectiveness and its consequences. This explains the changes often seen in young adolescents, such as changes in dress, academic achievement, manner of speaking, and groups of friends. Older adolescents continue some role experimentation through work or volunteer activities. For some young men and women, education and apprenticeships are still a part of role experimentation. For instance, college freshmen may change majors several times before finding a major that "fits."

Independence

Adult responsibilities and careers become tangible to adolescents. They are able to make plans for becoming independent and can suppose how independence will be. Independence from parents contributes to an adolescent's sense of individuality, and thus to her or his sense of self.

Early adolescents usually use parents for role models and accept their authority. As adolescence progresses the teen-ager continually tests the parents, and more and more freedom is demanded. By mid-adolescence a typical complaint is that parents give too little freedom and do not trust the adolescent. This is in conflict with the parents' views: parents feel that both the freedom and the trust they do offer is abused.

Peer Group Identification

School and the peer group divisions that the school environment affords become the teen-ager's social "mini world." Banned from participation in adult society and insulted by the society of childhood, teen-agers are forced to shape their own subculture or group identity to preserve their sense of belonging.

Belonging to a peer group helps an adolescent avoid role confusion (Erikson, 1963). Membership in a particular group provides an adolescent with a focus of identity through the clique's attitudes, behaviors, dress, and interests. Teen-agers begin to rely on peers rather than solely on parents for sources of ideals, values, and behavior. The peer group is a kind of "social laboratory" where teen-agers can experiment with roles and behavior (Nicholson, 1980).

As adolescents mature, they rely less on their peer group to clarify normal and accepted behavior. A clear identity enables teen-agers to be what they want even if peers are different.

Rebellion

The process of identity formation often results in rebellious behavior. Rebellion is a way of saying, "I am different from the adults around me. I am special." Rebellion against parental authority may be a means of affirming maturity, or an adolescent's perception of maturity. For example, a teen-ager may think, "Chil-

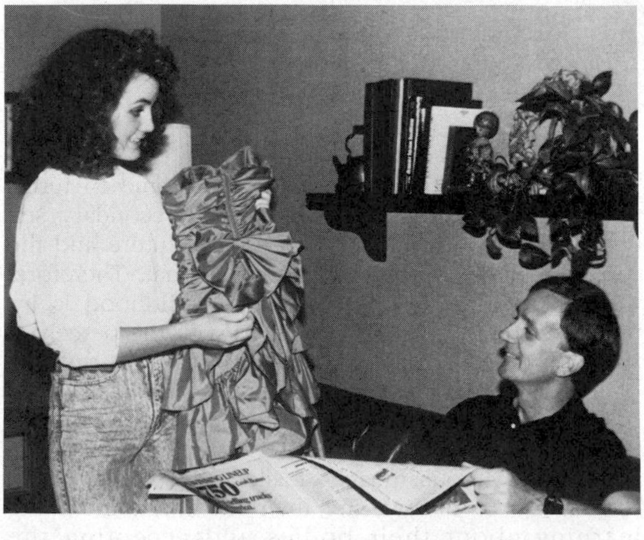

FIGURE 9-3. "Do you like it, Dad?" Parental support and approval can help promote development of a healthy body image.

TABLE 9-9
Promoting Identity

Roberto, age 17, is scheduled for an ileostomy at the end of the week. He has been hospitalized for several weeks for exacerbation of Crohn's disease. Pharmacologic and nutritional management have not been successful in alleviating symptoms. The clinical nurse specialist has formulated a plan of care to address his psychosocial needs and provide emotional support

Intervention	*Rationale*
Encourage ventilation of feelings regarding the impact of physical changes, being seriously ill, and cessation of normal lifestyle activities	· Provides sense of acceptance for feelings · Clarifies misconceptions regarding body image · Fosters sense of identity by acknowledging *validity* and *importance* of feelings
Encourage continuation of usual activities (e.g., recreational, educational, avocational, and vocational)	· Fosters acknowledgment of the importance of factors contributing to the adolescent's identity
Stomal therapist to consult	· Answers questions regarding surgery and postoperative management · Uses role-playing to simulate experience after hospitalization · Discusses anxieties, fears, and concerns associated with changes in body image · Reinforces positive aspects of body image · Discusses methods for dressing that are in style and acceptable to adolescent's taste
Schedule visit with peer who has ileostomy	· Facilitates expression of feelings through sharing mutual concerns · Encourages symbolic role experimentation as living with ileostomy is shared · Facilitates adjustment and acceptance through positive role modeling

dren are nondrinkers. Adults are drinkers. If I drink, I can be more grown-up." Rebellion is harmful when it interferes with school, interpersonal relationships, or physical or emotional health, or when it is harmful to others (vandalism or truancy, for example).

Once adolescents are more confident with their own identities, they are less threatened by parental controls, philosophies, and perceived interferences. Although they may not conform and be like their parents, the nonconformity will be due to personal convictions, not rebellion.

Idealism

To alleviate uncertainty, adolescents search for something enduring. The ability to imagine how things "could be" enables them to develop ideals. Ideals such as sincerity and genuineness become important, as they seem solid in a time of confusion. Teen-agers become intolerant of things they see as being phony or hypocritical. They may not be able to understand when others do not share their ideals and often become disillusioned with people or establishments. It is very common for adolescents to devote themselves to causes such as fund-raising for the needy, ecology, or antinuclear movements. Idealism not only helps adolescents feel as if there are some enduring things in the world but also paves the way for development of adult values and convictions (Erikson, 1963).

Nursing Interventions: Fostering Identity

The nurse incorporates the developmental needs for autonomy and identity that the adolescent has into the plan of care. The nurse designs interventions that will be sensitive to the adolescent's need to do it for oneself and be treated as an "adult." Table 9–9, Promoting Identity, provides an example of how the nurse incorporates these developmental considerations into the nursing care plan.

Anticipatory Guidance: Fostering Identity

Parents play a critical role in increasing and maintaining their adolescent's self-esteem. First, the success and self-esteem of the parents is influential in establishing self-esteem in the adolescent. Parents should pay attention to their own needs and growth. Second, parents should accept an adolescent for just *being* and express often that she or he is liked. Third, parents and teachers can emphasize positive aspects of the adolescent and not magnify negative aspects or failures. Assistance in developing strengths builds self-confidence (Fig. 9–4).

One help to developing a secure identity is investigation of vocational opportunities and the making of career plans. Parents should discuss future plans with their son or daughter. Parents cannot choose an identity for their child, however. Who or what he or she becomes must be the young person's personal choice; but parents can offer advice from their own experience when it is solicited. Open communication lines help the young person seek advice and bounce ideas off the adult without fearing ridicule or criticism.

Teen-agers are old enough to get part-time, after-school, and summer jobs and should be encouraged to do so. Teen-agers should also be able to manage their own checking and savings accounts and assist in family budgeting.

Teen-agers need opportunities to contribute to others. Volunteer work, running errands for an elderly neighbor, taking food to a sick friend, or any other unpaid good deed will help the teen-ager develop a positive self-image. Organizations such as Boy and Girl Scouts and Four-H Clubs help adolescents learn and develop a sense of pride and accomplishment.

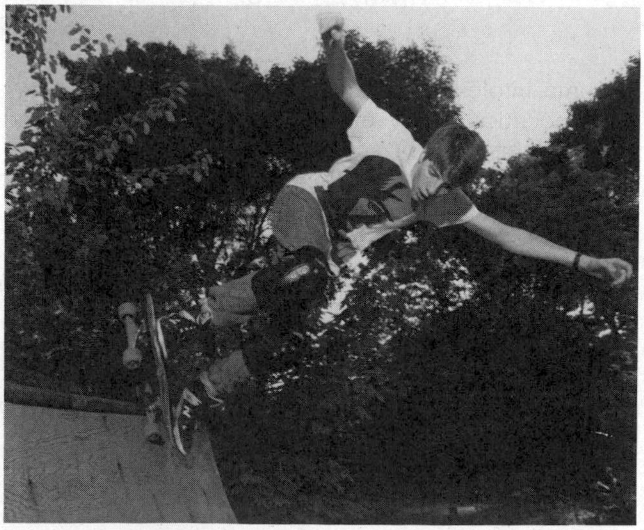

FIGURE 9 - 4. Risk-taking behavior is characteristic of teen-agers. It can be channeled into constructive pursuits like sports rather than into antisocial behavior. (Photograph by Ken Kasper.)

Sexuality

Psychosexual Development

The transition from child to adult occurs gradually or suddenly between the ages of 13 and 18 years. Changes in body characteristics and functions are accompanied by shifting moods and behaviors that alternate between instability and maturity. Freud (1957) refers to this period of adolescence as the *genital stage* of psychosexual development.

Developing a Positive Sexual Attitude

Often before physical changes are apparent, hormonal changes occur in both boys and girls, accounting for some rapid alterations in mood and attitude. With physical changes that render the individual capable of reproduction come social responsibilities for behaviors associated with increased libido. Identity formation is a major task in an adolescent's development. During this stage, an adolescent's primary influential group changes from family to peers. Developmental tasks are now achieved in the context of society in general rather than primarily in one's family. In our society, strong sexual messages through films, advertising, and popular music are part of society's input. Adolescents are pushed into early intimate relationships in our society. If early sexual contact precedes formation of a sense of self, an adolescent may have difficulty resolving other developmental tasks into a firm identity (Howe, 1986).

The young adolescent is preoccupied with self, easily embarrassed, and frequently unsure. The attitude toward a body that is changing, sexual urges, and social responsibilities can be overwhelming. Encouragement and affirmation from significant others, such as family and peers, influence positive attitudes.

Sexual Behavior

Although no longer engaged in the fantasy play of childhood, the adolescent begins to live as though responding to an imaginary audience of peers (Elkind, 1978). Consistent with development of a mature identity is the need to conform with peers in matters of dress and behavior. The need for approval drives the adolescent to experiment in a variety of ways. Equipped with a changed body capable of mature sexual behavior, the adolescent may feel peer pressure to have sexual intercourse.

Both girls and boys adopt specific behaviors related to the changes in their bodies. Girls engage in new hygienic measures and altered clothing as they adjust to menstruation and breast development, which begins between ages 8 and 18 years. Boys adjust to unpredictable erections and nocturnal emissions. Preoccupation with the size of the penis is a frequent subject of locker room comparisons. Penis size depends on stage of development; eventual mature size cannot be known at this time.

Masturbation continues in adolescence. Boys typically increase this activity as a way to relieve sexual tension, whereas girls may increase it to minimize feelings of loneliness. Fantasies of boys tend to focus on performance, whereas those of girls focus on romance.

Homosexual and heterosexual attraction lead to specific behaviors that may vary from minimal mutual exploration to mutual masturbation, intercourse, or oral-genital contact. Sexually transmitted diseases (STDs), including acquired immunodeficiency syndrome (AIDS), and pregnancy are consequences that adolescents may be aware of but not sufficiently informed about to act responsibly.

Early in adolescence, relationships are based on close friendships with members of the same sex. In mid-adolescence, direct contact is sought with members of the opposite sex in group situations. Such contacts may be sexually arousing and give the individuals opportunities to experiment with a variety of identities. The final stage of adolescence consists of explicit sexual behaviors of a transitory or permanent nature.

Nursing Interventions: Sexual Development

The nurse can assist young people in making decisions about sexuality. First, it is important to help teen-agers explore their own values. Often teen-agers' values contradict peers' values or their perception of peers' values. It sometimes helps to remind adolescents that they are unique individuals who can make their own choices. In other words, it is fine if they do not want to have sexual intercourse.

Nurses can also help the adolescent with problem solving. Formal operational thinking will enable many adolescents to think through their alternatives and consider the consequences of intercourse. The nurse should teach about reproduction if gaps in the adolescent's knowledge are discerned. Misconceptions must be dispelled. As knowledgeable as adolescents may be about some aspects of sex, they often believe such myths as, "You can't get pregnant the first time." Because of a teen-ager's lack of experience in decision making, the nurse may need to assist by applying an everyday process of decision making.

Many schools now incorporate family living classes as curriculum requisites. Formal curriculum packages for use in schools, as courses in church youth programs or social agencies for youth (e.g., YM/YWCAs, ROTC, youth camps), or as college electives have also been developed, many from government grants. An example of counseling about sexual maturation is presented in Table 9–10.

Anticipatory Guidance: Sexual Development

For the teen-ager to hold positive attitudes about sex, it is essential for her or him to observe interactions of emotionally mature adults, to have a positive relationship with the parent of the opposite sex, and to see discipline used to foster growth and not to control family members. The adolescent who learns that sexual contact is most fulfilling when it involves caring, commitment, and sensitivity to the best interest of others does not generally resort to indiscriminate sexual experimentation, which can lead to devastating consequences.

Parents may help their children to think through some difficult situations in advance and consider the consequences of their actions. Such anticipatory guidance may help the adolescent handle difficult situations and not become caught up in the situation or the intensity of emotion. Kastner (1984) found that contraceptive use was increased among teen-agers who had positive communication with parents about sexuality. Adolescents who may be most at risk for unplanned pregnancy are those affected by an inadequate education, poverty, social isolation, and a perceived lack of control over life situations (Burke, 1987). Additional information on adolescent pregnancy can be found later under "Health Maintenance and Promotion."

Nurses should always encourage parents to be involved in educating their children about sex well before adolescence as well as during adolescence. Parental discussions with children before the age of 12½ years have been shown to be very important in delaying sexual activity and its consequences.

Gay and Lesbian Adolescents

It is estimated that 10 per cent of adolescents are gay or lesbian (Sanford, 1989). For most adolescents, coming to grips with one's homosexuality is difficult at best. The adolescent must face feelings of anxiety, alienation, loneliness, and perceived forthcoming rejection. Often, the adolescent who begins to acknowledge his or her homosexuality does not find the needed support to cope with this identity crisis in the home, in school, or with peers.

Troiden (1988) has described how adolescents proceed through stages in developing identities as gay and lesbian individuals. These stages are *sensitization, identity confusion, identity assumption, and commitment*. During the first stage of *sensitization,* which usually occurs during puberty, the child perceives himself or herself as feeling "different" from peers. The girls report not being attracted to or interested in boys and viewing themselves as less feminine and more masculine than their heterosexual peers. Gay boys report they did not share the same heterosexual interest as do other boys their age. They report having no interest in girls and sports and being subjected to deprecating name calling by classmates.

TABLE 9-10
Promoting Sexual Maturation

Mervat, age 12, comes to the school nurse's office for the third time in 2 wks complaining of a headache. The timing of her headaches coincides with her physical education class. The nurse gently explores with Mervat the association between headaches and physical education. Mervat soon begins to cry, saying, "I can't stand going to gym anymore. Everyone looks at me because I'm the only one who doesn't have a bra." The following interventions were used to allay Mervat's distress over the progression of her sexual maturation

Intervention	*Rationale*
Actively listen to Mervat's concern	· Promotes expression of feelings · Facilitates Mervat's understanding of her feelings · Assists Mervat to identify her feelings · Conveys feelings of empathy and support for Mervat
Explore psychosocial history including evaluation of suicidal thoughts or depression	· Psychologic turmoil of adolescence can create psychosomatic complaints · Provides information useful in evaluating symptoms
Provide information on sexual maturation · Normalcy of differences	· Information and understanding can help reduce concern
Explore family attitudes towards sexuality Identify possible cultural influences affecting family attitudes and behaviors	· Gains understanding of family attitudes and cultural influences shaping them
Role-play with Mervat the situation of approaching parent about age-appropriate undergarments	· Fosters communication between adolescent and parent · Fosters sense of identity (independence) · Fosters sense of self-care

During the second stage, *identity confusion,* the gay or lesbian adolescent develops the awareness that perhaps he or she is homosexual. According to Troiden, the adolescent boy's realization of this fact occurs around age 17, whereas, for lesbian girls, it occurs at approximately 18 years. In a recent survey of high school students, more than 10 per cent were unsure of their sexual orientation (Blum et al, 1989). In spite of their disinterest in opposite-sex peers and their attraction to same-sex peers, a profound struggle to deny their feelings ensues. This denial is created by their fear of the truth and the resulting consequences of admitting their homosexuality.

Reactions vary as to dealing with this emerging truth. Some gay and lesbian adolescents may seek out support and counseling to accept comfortably their homosexuality. Others may engage in extreme forms of behavior to deny their homosexuality, such as substance abuse and adolescent pregnancy. For other adolescents, the process of soul-searching is short-lived and they comfortably accept their homosexuality (Remafedi, 1987).

Identity assumption is the third stage of development for gay and lesbian identities. According to Troiden, the gay identity is assumed between ages 19 and 21, and the lesbian identity between ages 21 and 23. Relationships are made with same-sex friends and partners based on homosexual interests. The need to protect oneself against social disapproval continues by hiding one's homosexuality or pretending to be heterosexual. This need to conceal results in the leading of "double lives" (Sanford, 1989).

The last stage of *commitment* occurs when the individual commits fully to the identity of being gay or lesbian. Disclosure of sexual preference is variable depending on the perceived social consequences.

Anticipatory Guidance: Gay and Lesbian Adolescents

Gay and lesbian adolescents need to feel that their concerns are important and that they are safe from judgment and ridicule. Information on sex education needs to include the particular risks that homosexual youths may be exposed to, including STDs. Gay males are at higher risk for STDs than are lesbians, especially for gonorrhea, syphilis, hepatitis, and AIDS (Bidewell & Deisher, 1991). Information on "safe" and "safer" sex needs to be provided. Human immunodeficiency virus (HIV) testing can be recommended for those who are sexually active.

For homosexual adolescents, the developmental concerns are intensified. Gay and lesbian adolescents need to be assessed for emotional concerns and trauma. The incidence of suicide, substance abuse, and emotional problems is high among this group of adolescents. Referrals can be made to community organizations and hot lines that provide gay and lesbian services. Parents can be referred to the Federation of Parents and Friends of Lesbians and Gays, Inc.,* for assistance to deal with their son's or daughter's homosexuality.

Fears

Adolescent fears become more abstract and individualized than they were during the school-age years. The most significant fears identified by adolescents concern economic and political events, social relations, and personal conduct. Unlike anxiety, fears are evoked by particular situations and life or world events. For example, an adolescent may be fearful that conflict in a particular area of the world may escalate into war. The adolescent may experience a fear reaction in arriving home past curfew in anticipation of parental response. Fear responses normally do not debilitate the adolescent, nor do they significantly interfere in her or his life. An apprehensive overreaction is a phobia and is an abnormal response to an external event.

Coping Mechanisms

The period of adolescence poses challenges and choices for the youth unlike any other stages of childhood. The challenges of integrating one's identity, adjusting to one's developing sexuality, and establishing one's place in society pose heavy demands on adolescents.

A variety of factors influence the adolescent's ability to cope. Age, temperament, ability to communicate, and family support are some of the factors that affect the adolescent's coping ability. Other variables influencing the adolescent's ability to cope include previous and current patterns of coping, intelligence, and sex (Garmezy & Rutter, 1984).

TABLE 9-11
Adolescent Coping Mechanisms

- Acting-out
- Aggression
- Anger
- Asceticism
- Attention-seeking
- Avoidance/withdrawal from persons
- Avoidance/withdrawal from tasks
- Compulsive opposition to parents
- Conformity
- Controlling behaviors
- Daydreaming
- Defense mechanisms
  - Denial
  - Disassociation
  - Displacement
  - Intellectualization
  - Projection
  - Rationalization
  - Reaction formation
  - Regression
  - Repression
- Eating disorders
- Fantasizing
- Information-seeking
- Introspection
- Motor activity
- Overly compliant
- Perfectionism
- Risk-taking behavior (high-speed driving)
- Substance abuse

The adolescent has more intrapersonal resources available, such as the ability to solve problems and think abstractly, when coping with problems. More highly developed cognitive capabilities and social skills enable them to use new means of coping. Further, adolescents have learned to develop skills of monitoring their own thought processes and performances, and problem-solving strategies are utilized more often. Other adolescent coping mechanisms are listed in Table 9–11.

Peers can help the adolescent cope with stress more effectively. Peer relationships as a support network changes from activity-oriented to emotionally supportive systems. This is because adolescents become increasingly more sensitive and understanding of their peers.

In the extreme, delinquent adolescents choose more self-destructive behaviors as a means of responding to stress. In this context, crimes such as robbery, drug involvement, rape, and offenses including excessive truancy can be viewed as extreme and deviant forms of coping. It is suggested that marginal social status, cultural background, racial factors, perceived social alienation, and economic need are significantly associated with delinquent behavior (Dolin et al, 1992).

Moral and Faith Development

Kohlberg (1969) refers to this last stage of moral development as the *postconventional* level. Preteenagers and young teen-agers would approach a situa-

* Friends of Lesbians and Gays, P.O. Box 28009, Washington, DC 20038.

tion requiring moral judgment differently than would older adolescents and young adults. As an example, if presented with a story about a poor woman who must steal food in order to feed her starving children, a child in the conventional level would likely say "Stealing is bad, but the mother's duty is to provide food for her children. She should eventually pay for the food or be punished in some way." Youths at the postconventional level would discuss the story in terms of the higher principle of saving hungry children. They may conclude that the mother is morally right to steal. As with formal operations, the ability to make postconventional moral judgments is not universally attained, nor are postconventional moral judgments used exclusively.

Adolescents become more introspective and reflexive regarding their faith beliefs, attaining the fourth stage of faith belief *individuating reflexive* (Fowler, 1980). During this period of time, the adolescent may adopt one of many options as a means of resolving conflicts related to faith beliefs. The adolescent may become overly zealous or adopt an opposite attitude of "devil may care" toward the sectarian group he or she was previously associated with. The adolescent may grow and develop in a religious sense. Some adolescents regress to a previous stage of growth when religious beliefs were a particular source of comfort.

Peer Relationships

Adolescents become capable of sharing themselves on a deeper level with others. Feelings and commonality of experiences are shared. The adolescent seeks out friendships that are mutually supportive. Through these relationships, the adolescent learns and grows in knowledge of self and others. Networks among friends are established for specific purposes or centered around mutual interests (e.g., self-help groups, sports interest).

Adolescence is a time when a person seeks friends to fulfill the needs to be liked, to be accepted, and to belong to a group. It is during adolescence that the need for emotional support extends beyond the familial confines to peers and non-kin adults in the community (Cauce & Strebnik, 1989). The adolescent moves away from the family; friends become the bearers of his or her ideals and standards. Making friends is an important developmental task. As adolescents become more and more resistive to parental admonitions about behavior acceptable for them, they double their efforts to act like and dress like their selected friends of the moment.

Many times, the adolescent's selection of friends and allegiance to them produce a stressful situation for the family. Parents may need help to understand that this exaggerated conformity to peer groups is a manifestation of the adolescent's process of achieving identity and independence from the parents. Adolescents desperately need approval, and, since they are moving away from dependence on their parents, they need the support that approval from friends provides. Once parents recognize the adolescent's desire and need to make friends, their attention becomes focused on the "desirability" of the friends selected.

Romantic friendships become an area of concern for the adolescent. A romantic relationship exemplifies the adolescent's need to care for and be cared for by a significant other (Fig. 9–5). Social status of the adolescent is often measured by their social desirability, perceived physical attractiveness, and effectiveness (Thornton & Ryckman, 1991). Research has demonstrated lower levels of self-esteem among adolescents who were not able to establish romantic friendships (Silberstein & Noack, 1990).

The confidence an adolescent feels with her or his physical attractiveness carries over to interpersonal relationships. More attractive adolescents were found to be more popular with their peers. Physical effectiveness has been found to enhance the adolescent's level of popularity with peers. Physically effective teens, both boys and girls, have been found to be more self-confident and less self-conscious, contributing to their level of greater popularity and reflecting the changing social values regarding sex roles for males and females (Thornton & Ryckman, 1991).

Leisure activities of adolescents will change in order to achieve the goal of starting new relationships. Visits to developmentally enhancing locations such as malls, beaches, and discotheques are often done for the express purpose of meeting the opposite sex (Silberstein et al, 1992). Research focusing on peer influences on adolescent behaviors indicates that this can be a problem area. Boys tend to be more susceptible than girls to peer influences to engage in antisocial acts and misconduct (Clasen & Eicher, 1986). In one study, girls were more susceptible than boys to peer influences to abuse substances (Huba & Bentler, 1980). As one would expect, adolescents who are left without adult supervision are more susceptible to peer pressures to engage in antisocial activities than are adolescents who are supervised (Steinberg, 1986). Peer pressure is seen by adolescents as more effective

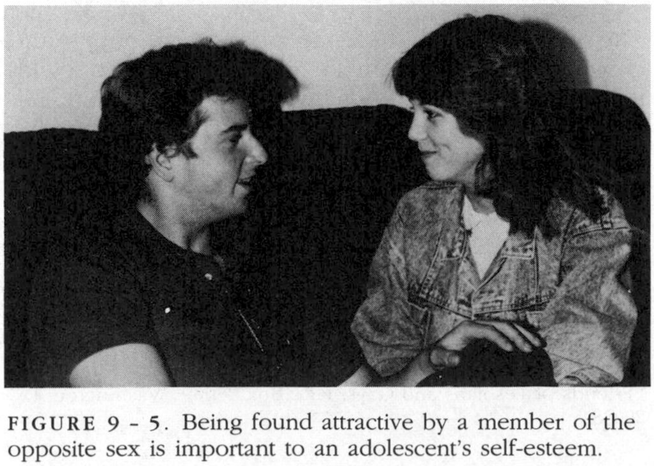

FIGURE 9-5. Being found attractive by a member of the opposite sex is important to an adolescent's self-esteem.

in relation to issues of socialization than in relation to the commission of antisocial acts.

Anticipatory Guidance: Peer Relationships

The nurse may assist the family to understand that the adolescent needs to test a wide variety of friendships that may include those adolescents from differing cultural, social, and economic backgrounds, and those whose values are quite different. It is helpful for these parents to know that continuing parental support can make a difference in the adolescent's behaviors. One finding of a study investigating the influences on adolescents to smoke was that adolescents with higher levels of parental support were less likely to smoke (Chassin et al, 1986). The choice of lasting friends can be influenced by parents making themselves available to discuss family value systems, to participate in activities of interest to the child and her or his group, and to foster strong kinship and generational ties.

Health Maintenance and Promotion

Health Screening

Adolescents should be seen by a physician or other primary care provider at least every 2 years, even if no problems arise. During routine health visits, the health professional should provide guidance and counseling based on the individual needs of the adolescent. Anticipatory guidance is basic to adolescent health maintenance, as it is at any age (Igoe, 1993). The health care provider working with adolescents requires knowledge in such areas as personal care, dental care, nutrition, STDs, birth control, substance abuse, smoking, and accidents.

Indications for health screening of adolescents are listed in Table 9–12 (Cromer et al, 1992). Additional screenings may be indicated if the adolescent is a member of a particular population, as indicated in Table 9–13 (Cromer et al, 1992). The level of sexual maturity is assessed using the Tanner staging method (see Tables 9–3 and 9–4).

During the pubertal growth spurt, it is not uncommon to observe wide variations in height and weight among adolescents. The adolescent's chronologic age may not accurately reflect the biologic maturation. Based on this variation, adolescents are categorized as early, middle, and late maturers. Acceleration of growth corresponds to the development of secondary sex characteristics. When direct measurements of height and weight are not available, the reliance on the adolescent's self-report of height and weight may be questionable. A study of adolescents' self-reports found weights were understated and heights overstated by both adolescent girls and boys. Underreporting of weight is greatest for adolescents who are heavier (Fortenberry, 1992).

TABLE 9–12
Adolescent Health Screening: General Population

Screening	Method
Annual	
Growth	Height/weight measurements Sexual maturity rating
Vision	Snellen chart
Iron status	Complete blood count, transferrin saturation ratio or free erythrocyte protoporphyrin
Dental status	Dental history and oral examination
Scoliosis	Adam's test
Blood pressure	Sphygmomanometer
Thyroid disease	Thyroid gland examination
Behavior	Psychosocial history
School performance, attendance	
Substance use	
Affective state	
Sexual activity/abuse	
Somatoform symptoms	
Once During Adolescence	
Immunity to measles, mumps, rubella	Booster dose of MMR vaccine upon entrance to secondary school
Immunity to poliovirus infection	Record review; booster dose of OPV with foreign travel
Tetanus (diphtheria) immunity	Record review; Td every 10 yrs

Reprinted by permission of Elsevier Science Publishing Co., Inc. From A critical review of critical health screening in adolescents by Cromer, B., McLean, C., & Heald, F. *Journal of Adolescent Health, 13,* 35–65. Copyright 1992 by the Society for Adolescent Medicine.

Key: MMR = measles, mumps, rubella; OPV = oral polio vaccine; Td = tetanus toxoid and diphtheria toxoid (reduced dose) in combination.

Laboratory evaluation may include screening for elevated cholesterol and triglycerides (Davidson et al, 1990). The American Heart Association recommends testing for cholesterol at least once during the school years. The American Academy of Pediatrics (AAP) recommends a fasting lipoprotein profile if there are first-degree relatives with early cardiovascular disease (AAP, 1989b).

Adolescents should also be screened for iron deficiency. This age group is particularly susceptible to iron deficiency because of increased growth, poor dietary intake, and, in females, menstrual blood loss. Screening for STDs such as gonorrhea, herpes, and chlamydia is done if the adolescent is sexually active. Papanicolaou smears are done in sexually active females and those whose mother received diethylstilbestrol (DES).

TABLE 9-13
Adolescent Health Screening: Selected Populations of Adolescents

	Population	Method
Tuberculosis	Hispanic, African-American, Asian-American, Alaskan, American Indian populations, or communities where prevalence exceeds 1%	Mantoux test
Sickle cell trait	African-American or Mediterranean heritage who give informed consent	Sickledex/Sickle prep
Thalassemia conditions	As above (sickle cell trait) and Southeast Asian heritage	Mean corpuscular volume (MCV)
Urine culture	Previous urinary tract infection or structural anomaly	Clean voided specimen for culture
Testicular self-examination	All 18-year-olds or those with history of cryptorchidism	Instruction beginning at onset of puberty
Hypercholesterolemia	Family history of early myocardial infarction or hyperlipidemia	Random cholesterol
Hearing testing	Family or personal history of hearing loss or chronic exposure to firearms or loud farm machinery	Pure-tone audiometry
Iron status	Competitive athletes	Ferritin

Anticipatory Guidance: Health Screening

Actual health concerns of adolescents may be vastly different from what is perceived by professions. A nursing study surveyed adolescent concerns and found them to be vastly different (Smith et al, 1987). The adolescent reported two major areas of health concern: psychosocial concerns and concerns about physical appearance. Adolescents expressing psychosocial concerns stated they were worried about their future, feelings, and relationships with family members.

Concerns about physical appearance centered on the weight, musculature, skin, and hair. Gender differences were evident. Health concerns of boys were, in order of importance: future, weight, vision, body build, height, acne, and school relationships. The girls identified their health concerns in the following order: weight, hair, family relationships, emotions, feelings, future, skin, figure, and acne. These findings would suggest that the nurse needs to listen carefully to what is actually important to the adolescent in terms of health concerns.

Skin care is a major concern of adolescents. Acne affects 70 per cent of all adolescents (Novotny, 1989). The psychologic consequences may be a far greater concern to the teen-ager than the actual physical problem itself. Although the teen-ager is referred to a dermatologist or nurse practitioner for further evaluation and treatment, the nurse can correct misconceptions about the causes of acne. It is an excellent time to provide information on the factors that exacerbate acne, such as particular foods, stress, fatigue, medications, and cosmetic products. For more in-depth information on acne vulgaris, see Chapter 38.

Sun protection measures can be discussed with adolescents. Experts state that the risk of developing a nonmelanoma skin cancer using sunscreen with a sun protective factor of 15 for the first 18 years can be reduced by 78 per cent (Stern et al, 1986). A survey on attitudes toward sun exposure and sunscreen use found that 81 per cent of adolescents spent weekend time or more in the sun and that over 60 per cent reported using sunscreen 25 per cent or less of the time. This study found that adolescents were more inclined to use sunscreen when one of their friends did. Anticipatory guidance on the use of sun protection measures would include warnings about use of tanning salons. Experts have suggested that frequent use of tanning salons should be considered a "risk-taking behavior" (Banks et al, 1992).

Testicular self-examination should be taught to adolescent males since they are at far greater risk for testicular cancer than are adolescent females for breast cancer. Testicular cancer is the third most common malignancy affecting males between 15 and 19 years, occurring at an incidence rate of 2.2 per 100,000 (Friman & Finney, 1990). Risk factors cited for testicular cancer are mumps orchitis, testicular trauma, and history of cryptorchidism, which is the highest risk factor (Brown et al, 1987). In comparison, an adolescent female does not enter a risk category for breast cancer until 20 years later. The Society for Adolescent Medicine recommends routine instruction in testicular self-examination during annual health visits (Society for Adolescent Medicine, 1992b). Breast self-examination or mammography is not recommended in women younger than 20 years of age.

Headaches are a common complaint of adolescents, and tension headaches are the most common recurrent form. The school nurse is usually the health care provider to whom complaints of headaches are taken. The nursing management of the adolescent with a headache should include a complete assessment embracing history and measures to decrease the effects of stressors that may precipitate the headache.

Adolescent smoking is a major health problem. Each year, 1 million youths begin smoking cigarettes. It is estimated that approximately 28 per cent of adolescents are smokers (US Department of Health and Human Services, 1988). A variety of biopsychosocial factors have been identified as influencing the adolescent's decision to smoke. These factors include addictive properties of nicotine, peer pressure, parent who smokes, decreased self-esteem, increased stress, and inadequate coping skills (Winkelstein, 1992). Successful nursing interventions will be directed to assessing the factors that influence the adolescent to initiate and continue smoking and devising a plan of care to address the adolescent's situation specifically and directly. For example, the nurse would counsel parents who smoke to alter their behavior by ceasing to smoke, removing cigarettes from accessible locations, and admonishing their children not to smoke.

Depending on when initial childhood immunizations were completed, diphtheria and tetanus (DT) boosters as well as periodic tuberculin testing will be necessary sometime during the adolescent years (AAP, 1991). Adolescents should be informed they need to be revaccinated with measles-mumps-rubella (MMR) if there is an outbreak of measles in their school. This revaccination applies to all students and their siblings born after January 1, 1957, who did not receive the two doses of the measles vaccine after their first birthday (AAP, 1991).

In a study by nurse researchers of the relationship of demographic, lifestyle, and stress variables to blood pressure in adolescents, differing patterns were found according to gender (Thomas & Groer, 1986). Males had higher mean systolic pressures than females did. In males, body mass index was the strongest predictor of diastolic and systolic pressures. For females, living in the city was the strongest predictor for systolic pressure, smoking for the diastolic pressure. Findings of this study need to be investigated further to understand the relationship between selected variables and elevated blood pressure in adolescents. Although further research is needed, the implications for the nursing clinician suggest that a comprehensive nursing assessment is needed when adolescents with elevated blood pressures are detected during health screenings.

Vision and Hearing

Adult visual levels were attained in early childhood. Adolescents have normal adult hearing, although they are sometimes accused of selective deafness or hearing only what they want to hear.

Dental Care

A full set of permanent teeth, with the exception of the wisdom teeth, is expected by 13 to 14 years of age (Fig. 9–6). These last four permanent teeth (third molars) lag behind the other teeth by an average of 8 or more years, not erupting until early adulthood when the person is in the early 20s.

The eruption or appearance of a tooth, however, is but one aspect of tooth development, albeit the most obvious. For each of the 52 teeth (20 primary and 32 permanent), development of the tooth matrix and its calcification proceeds in the same orderly manner from crown to roots. The time lag between the start of the calcification and the eruption of each permanent tooth is 6 to 9 years, depending on the particular tooth. Full development of the root structure takes another 2 to 4 years after eruption. Calcification of the first molar (permanent) begins at birth, but the tooth does not erupt until 6 years of age and is not completely calcified until 9 to 10 years of age. All permanent teeth (except the third molars) start calcification between birth and 3 years but are not completely calcified until about age 16. The first permanent teeth to complete root development are the

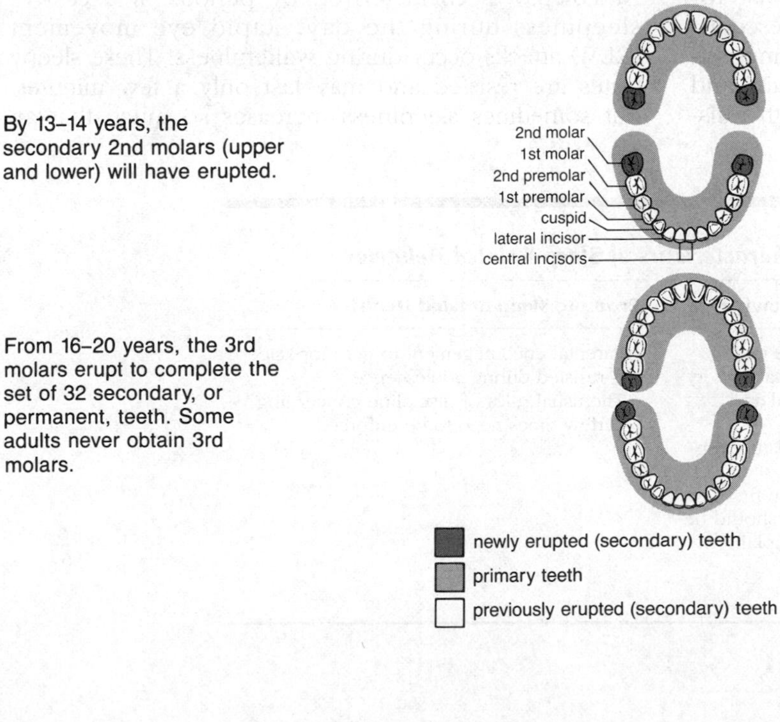
By 13–14 years, the secondary 2nd molars (upper and lower) will have erupted.
2nd molar
1st molar
2nd premolar
1st premolar
cuspid
lateral incisor
central incisors
From 16–20 years, the 3rd molars erupt to complete the set of 32 secondary, or permanent, teeth. Some adults never obtain 3rd molars.
newly erupted (secondary) teeth
primary teeth
previously erupted (secondary) teeth

FIGURE 9-6. Development of teeth. A combination of primary and secondary teeth is present in the child's mouth simultaneously during the process of eruption and shedding.

central incisors at age 9 to 10 years, and the last to complete root development are the third molars at 18 to 25 years.

Because of the length of time between the initiation of calcification and the actual emergence of a tooth, its soundness at eruption is not as dependent on current health and nutritional status as on previous health status. Because teeth and bones are of different embryologic origins, there is little correlation between stature or onset of puberty with tooth development. Tooth development, therefore, seems relatively independent of other body systems.

Canker Sores

A canker sore is a small, painful, craterlike ulcer on the mucous membranes of the oral cavity, appearing singly or in groups. These ulcerations occur most often in the 10- to 20-year-old. Some people are more prone to develop the ulcers than others. Most children will call their parents' attention to a canker sore. There is no known cause of canker sores, although various etiologies are suspected, including food hypersensitivity, allergies, toxic drug reactions, endocrine factors, emotional stress, and trauma. It has also been suggested that an autoimmune reaction of the oral epithelium may cause ulcer formation. There is no specific treatment and the ulcers will heal spontaneously within a week or two. Viscous lidocaine (Xylocaine) or topical steroids may decrease the discomfort or shorten the course.

Anticipatory Guidance: Dental Care

Adolescent years are peak years for dental caries, and yet preventive and therapeutic treatment by dental professionals is one of the most neglected needs of teen-agers. Dental care is often a low financial priority of families. Several important reasons exist for making the repair and maintenance of adolescents' teeth a priority. Adequate nutrition is nearly impossible when teeth hurt or are missing. Fresh fruits and vegetables, for example, are difficult to eat with pulsing, aching, or decayed teeth. Appearance is extremely important to teen-agers. Teen-agers with decayed teeth usually have problems with self-esteem, whereas healthy white teeth help the teen-ager to develop positive self-concept.

Adequate dental maintenance includes proper brushing with a fluoride-containing dentrifice at least twice a day. Daily flossing and regular dental visits are recommended. An adequate supply of fluoride is needed to help prevent cavities and can be obtained from drinking water (1 ppm), from topical application annually or semi-annually in the dentist's office, or from oral fluoride tablets if the drinking supply has no fluoride.

If the adolescent is active in competitive sports, especially contact or collision sports, she or he should be encouraged to wear a mouthguard and protective oral-facial equipment. Anticipatory guidance should also include discussion of avoidance of foods high in sugar, such as candy bars, and the risks associated with tobacco and alcohol use (Wilson, 1990).

Sleep Behaviors

Adolescents may be known both for sleeping "all the time" and for chronically "burning the candle at both ends." The actual amount of sleep required by an adolescent covers a wide range. Rather than state a specific number of hours, it is wiser to advise parents to be cognizant of their adolescent's sleep patterns and symptoms of fatigue. Many other effects can result from a lack of adequate sleep, such as crankiness, accidents, and frustration. If the sleep pattern changes suddenly, a call or visit to a primary care provider is in order (Table 9–14).

Narcolepsy

Narcolepsy is characterized by periods of excessive sleepiness during the day. Rapid eye movement (REM) attacks occur during wakefulness. These sleepy states are resisted and may last only a few minutes, but sometimes sleepiness increases so much that an

TABLE 9-14
Adolescent Developmental Characteristics of Sleep-Related Behavior

Characteristic Sleep-Related Behaviors	Promote Sleep-Related Health
• Sleep is important because of the increased growth, strenuous physical activity (if in sports), and increased social and emotional demands • Loss of sleep typically results in late sleeping and daytime sleepiness • Symptoms of narcolepsy are often first recognized during adolescence and should be differentiated from the usual complaint of tiredness • *8–10 hrs of sleep per 24 hrs*	• Parental encouragement to get more sleep is resisted during adolescence • The usual rules of discipline concerning curfew times need to be enforced

REM nap takes place. Daytime sleepiness begins 3 to 4 hours after waking and may occur repeatedly throughout the day. Narcolepsy can be differentiated from similar episodes of sleepiness that can normally occur during driving or lectures. Narcoleptic attacks are often accompanied by cataplexy (loss of muscle tone precipitated by surprise or emotion, which may cause knees to weaken, resulting in a fall), sleep paralysis (an inability to move voluntary muscles when falling asleep), and hypnagogic hallucinations (vivid visual hallucinations at sleep onset). These symptoms often result in an intense fear of falling asleep. The peak onset of narcolepsy is between 15 and 25 years of age.

Daytime sleepiness may be counteracted by excessive activity in an attempt to stay awake. Learning difficulties may arise and be the first indication of a problem. Narcolepsy is thought to be a genetic disorder. The incidence in families with narcolepsy has been found to be 60 times greater than in the general population (Anders & Keener, 1983).

Treatment for narcolepsy remains inadequate. The adolescent, parents, and teacher require information about the disorder to help them understand the nature of the problem. Narcolepsy does not indicate an increased need for nocturnal sleep or daytime naps. Drug therapy may reduce attacks to some extent. Medications may be prescribed to reduce the sleep attacks and to alleviate the symptoms of sleep paralysis, cataplexy, and hypnagogic hallucinations.

Anticipatory Guidance: Sleep Behaviors

Parental encouragement to get more sleep is resisted during adolescence. The adolescent may resist for a variety of reasons, including the need to assert oneself as independent of parental concerns. The adolescent may be sleep-deprived from trying to cram during examination time, last-minute "catch-up" to get school assignments completed on time, or staying up late to watch favorite TV programs. Obviously, the student who does not get adequate sleep is going to be tired and fatigued, resulting in diminished academic performance. On weekends during the summer, the adolescent may have developed a pattern of late-night activity that interferes with adequate sleep.

Parents can assist their adolescent in better organizing study habits to avoid encountering these periods of sleep deprivation. The nurse can provide suggestions to parents on limit setting and rules of curfew to meet both health and social needs of the adolescent. Parents need to be encouraged to remain consistent in enforcing curfew.

Nutrition

Nutritional Requirements

Total nutritional needs are greater during adolescence than at any other time (Society for Adolescent Medicine, 1992a) (see Table 9–15 and Chapter 16). Caloric and protein requirements increase for boys from ages 11 to 18. Girls at this age have a slightly increased protein need, but caloric needs decrease. The iron needed by the adolescent is almost double that needed by the adult male or the postmenopausal woman. Iodine is necessary for proper thyroid function, and the need rises sharply during this growth spurt; the amount of calcium and zinc required for skeletal and dental growth also increases. Niacin and thiamine needs increase during adolescence in males. Most of these nutrient needs drop after adolescence. Adolescents are generally ill-informed about appropriate nutritional intake. Their diet is characterized by intake in high-calorie, low-nutritional-value "junk food" and foods high in fat and carbohydrates. Fruits and vegetables are low on their list of food preferences.

An adolescent's eating pattern is erratic. It is characterized by skipping of meals such as breakfast and lunch, with the bulk of calories consumed in the late afternoon and evening (Jonides, 1990). Studies of adolescent girls show that their perceptions of nutrition, dieting, and weight include an exaggerated fear of becoming obese, regardless of weight. Bingeing and vomiting were used by students to regulate weight (Moses et al, 1989).

Anticipatory Guidance: Nutrition

Nutritional counseling should focus on the five basic food groups and should be done with the adolescent's likes and dislikes and cultural influences in mind. Relating nutrition and appearance is an effective way to obtain a teen-ager's interest in nutrition. Adolescents like snacking, which is a part of most social events. The nurse can teach teen-agers about healthy snacking and about avoidance of high-fat, high-carbohydrate "fast foods." Fad diets and overzealous dieting should be highly discouraged, although some experts have indicated that adolescents may seek nutritional counseling to achieve an inappropriate weight goal (Moses et al, 1989). (See Chapter 29 for a discussion of anorexia and obesity in adolescents.)

Nurses are often asked to advise athletes on nutrition needs. No special formulas or supplements are necessary, with the exception of the young female athlete, for whom it is recommended to take 30 to 60 mg of iron per day. The best diet for athletes includes the basic food groups outlined in Chapter 16. The number of servings from each group will depend on the energy requirement of the individual and the sport. Cold water is the best hydrating beverage (AAP, 1983). Nutritional counseling can be combined with information on physical activity and exercise. Adolescents who are concerned about weight management will need to know about the importance of physical activity to elevate the basal metabolic rate to counteract the decrease caused by dieting (Wells &

TABLE 9-15
Recommended Food Intake for Good Nutrition According to Food Groups and Daily Dietary Allowances

Adolescent (11–18 yrs)

Food Groups	*Servings Per Day* Male	*Servings Per Day* Female	*Serving Size*
Bread Group	11	9	
• Bread			1 slice
• Cereal			1 C
• Rice and pasta			1 oz ⅓ C
Vegetable Group	5	4	
• Green-yellow vegetables (vitamin A source)	1 or more	1 or more	¾ C
• Other vegetables	3 or more	3 or more	¾ C
Fruit Group	4	3	
• Citrus fruits, berries, tomato, cabbage, cantaloupe (vitamin C source)	1 or more	1 or more	1 C or 1 medium orange
• Other fruits (apple, banana)	2 or more	2 or more	1 medium
Milk Group	3	3	
• Milk/yogurt			1 C
• Cheese			(1.5 oz cheese = 1 C milk)
Meat Group	3	2	
• Cooked lean meat, poultry, fish			3 oz
• Dry beans			1 C
• Egg			1–2
• Peanut butter			2 Tbsp
Fats, oils, and sweets—USE SPARINGLY			

Recommended Daily Dietary Allowances

Male (11 - 14 Yrs)

Protein	*Fat-Soluble Vitamins*		*Water-Soluble Vitamins*		*Minerals*		*Energy Needs*
45 g	Vitamin A	1000 μg RE*	Vitamin C	50 mg	Calcium	1200 mg	2500 kcal
	D	10 μg	Thiamine	1.3 mg	Phosphorus	1200 mg	
	E	10 mg α-TE	Riboflavin	1.5 mg	Magnesium	270 mg	
	K	45 μg	Niacin	17 mg NE	Iron	12 mg	
			Vitamin B_6	1.7 mg	Zinc	15 mg	
			Folate	150 μg	Iodine	150 μg	
			Vitamin B_{12}	2.0 μg	Selenium	40 μg	

Copeland, 1985). An exercise program is likely to be successful if it can be easily incorporated into the adolescent's lifestyle. For example, suggestions to walk, ride a bicycle, or swim may sound more appealing to the adolescent instead of group sports wherein skill proficiency becomes an issue.

Recreation

Adolescents exhibit a wide range of recreational interests depending on their personal abilities and preferences, peer and familial influences, and economic and environmental circumstances. This range of activities of interest to adolescents is listed in Table 9–16. Pressure felt by adolescents in trying to "keep up" with their peers can result in unrealistic demands on parents to purchase expensive athletic equipment or casual clothing. For example, "high-top" shoes, which are extremely popular with adolescents, are a high-priced item for families whether they can or cannot afford them. Conflicts may ensue between the adolescent and the parents when demands for recreational expenses are not met.

The adolescent may feel "deprived" or believe that parents purposely refuse expenses in order to "punish" them. Adolescents can learn valuable lessons

TABLE 9-15
Recommended Food Intake for Good Nutrition According to Food Groups and Daily Dietary Allowances *(Continued)*

Recommended Daily Dietary Allowances

Male (15–18 Yrs)

Protein	*Fat-Soluble Vitamins*		*Water-Soluble Vitamins*		*Minerals*		*Energy Needs*
59 g	Vitamin A	1000 μg RE*	Vitamin C	60 mg	Calcium	1200 mg	3000 kcal
	D	10 μg	Thiamine	1.5 mg	Phosphorus	1200 mg	
	E	10 mg α-TE	Riboflavin	1.8 mg	Magnesium	400 mg	
	K	65 μg	Niacin	20 mg NE	Iron	12 mg	
			Vitamin B_6	2.0 mg	Zinc	15 mg	
			Folate	200 μg	Iodine	150 μg	
			Vitamin B_{12}	2.0 μg	Selenium	50 μg	

Recommended Daily Dietary Allowances

Female (11–14 Yrs)

Protein	*Fat-Soluble Vitamins*		*Water-Soluble Vitamins*		*Minerals*		*Energy Needs*
46 g	Vitamin A	800 μg RE*	Vitamin C	50 mg	Calcium	1200 mg	2200 kcal
	D	10 μg	Thiamine	1.1 mg	Phosphorus	1200 mg	
	E	8 mg α-TE	Riboflavin	1.3 mg	Magnesium	280 mg	
	K	45 μg	Niacin	15 mg NE	Iron	15 mg	
			Vitamin B_6	1.4 mg	Zinc	12 mg	
			Folate	150 μg	Iodine	150 μg	
			Vitamin B_{12}	2.0 μg	Selenium	45 μg	

Recommended Daily Dietary Allowances

Female (15–18 Yrs)

Protein	*Fat-Soluble Vitamins*		*Water-Soluble Vitamins*		*Minerals*		*Energy Needs*
44 g	Vitamin A	800 μg RE*	Vitamin C	60 mg	Calcium	1200 mg	2200 kcal
	D	10 μg	Thiamine	1.1 mg	Phosphorus	1200 mg	
	E	8 mg α-TE	Riboflavin	1.3 mg	Magnesium	300 mg	
	K	45 μg	Niacin	15 mg NE	Iron	15 mg	
			Vitamin B_6	1.5 mg	Zinc	12 mg	
			Folate	180 μg	Iodine	150 μg	
			Vitamin B_{12}	2.0 μg	Selenium	50 μg	

Adapted with permission from *Recommended dietary allowances: 10th edition.* Copyright 1989 by the National Academy of Sciences. Published by the National Academy Press, Washington, DC; and US Department of Agriculture, Human Nutrition Information Service. (1992). *Food guide pyramid.* (Leaflet No. 572). Washington, DC: Author.

Key: R = retinol equivalent; TE = tocopherol equivalent; NE = niacin equivalent.

about pursuing various recreational interests by earning part or all of the money needed. Situations like these provide the opportunity for parents and other non-kin adults in the adolescent's life to work on issues such as delay of gratification, seeking different yet acceptable and enjoyable alternatives, the strength of individuality, the true meaning of friendship, and the reality of economic constraints.

It is estimated that 20 million youths between the ages of 8 and 16 participate in organized sporting activities (Rowland, 1986). Approved high school organized sports number more than 39 for boys and 27 for girls. Participation in organized sports can foster the adolescent's development. The adolescent learns rules of social conduct and the importance of peer support, group dynamics, and an awareness of self as

TABLE 9-16
Recreation Activities for Adolescents

Activity	Development Promoted	Selection Criteria
Bicycling Skateboarding	Promotes gross/fine motor development (P) Provides awareness of environment (C) Provides outlet for emotional expression (E)	Knows rules of the road Uses safety helmet, protective padding Equipment in good working order
Team sports/activities • Volleyball • Football • Basketball • Running • Baseball	Promotes gross/fine motor development (P) Fosters social development (S) Stimulates self-expression (E) Provides outlet for emotional expression (E) Teaches fair play and team effort (S) Teaches about adherence to rules (S)	Athletic/running shoes fit properly Avoid hard surfaces for practice (e.g., concrete, asphalt)
Hobbies/crafts	Enhances creativity (C) Enhances ability to concentrate (C) Enhances self-expression, accomplishment, and imagination (C) Enhances fine-motor skills (P)	Cost of items may be a consideration Age-appropriate content
Swimming	Enhances large-muscle development (P)	Safety rules
Books	Increases reading and language ability (C) Teaches implications of sentence structure versus individual words (C)	Age-appropriate content
Movies/plays	Enhances ability to concentrate (C) Enhances peer activity (S)	Movie rating appropriate for age
Rock concerts	Provide outlet for emotional expression (E) Enhances peer activity (S) Enhances ability to concentrate (C)	Concert cost may be limitation Concert location may be too distant Music/performers' behavior may be controversial
Dating	Enhances interactions with opposite sex (S) Develops notion of social position and role (S) May reduce tension (E) May create tension (E)	Requires supervision
Cooking	Teaches creativity and self-expression (E, S)	Safety rules
Sewing	Teaches creativity and self-expression (E, S) Teaches self-care (E)	Safety rules
Electronic games Computers	Enhances problem-solving and decision making skills	Age-appropriate content May require limit on frequency of use
Outings to beach, amusement parks, etc.	Provides interaction with others (S) Can reduce tension (E) Stimulates exploration of the environment (S)	May require supervision
Mall shopping	Stimulates exploration of the environment (S) Stimulates social communication and language skills (C, S) Teaches lessons about consumerism (E) Teaches concepts of delayed gratification, satisfaction of desires (E)	May need supervision Cost may serve as a limitation

TABLE 9-16
Recreation Activities for Adolescents (Continued)

Activity	Development Promoted	Selection Criteria
Television/video watching	Stimulates creativity and imagination (C)	Not all parents want to encourage TV watching because of subject matter and level of passivity created
Radio/music listening	Teaches illusion versus reality (C)	
		Age-appropriate content
		Limits on frequency of use
Make-overs	Stimulates creativity and imagination (C)	Product ingredients may cause allergic/toxic reaction
Dress-up	Fosters self-care activities (E)	Cost of items may be a consideration
	Teaches self-expression (E)	
	Provides emotional outlet (E)	

Key: C = Cognitive development; P = physical development; E = emotional development; S = social development.

a competitor and as a member of a team. Team participation provides the opportunity for developing values of tolerance, acceptance, empathy, a sense of fairness, and a sense of right and wrong. Students can be encouraged to participate in organized sporting activities that match their physical abilities and interest; there is a range in competitive sports from contact/collision to nonstrenuous activities (Table 9–17). Athletes should undergo annual physical examinations prior to the training season as a means of identifying actual or potential problems.

There have been greater numbers of youths participating in track and field sports. Long distance running has become a popular choice. Long distance

TABLE 9-17
Classification of Sport Activities

		Noncontact		
Contact/Collision	**Contact/Impact**	**Strenuous**	**Moderately Strenuous**	**Nonstrenuous**
Boxing	Baseball	Aerobic dancing	Badminton	Archery
Field hockey	Basketball	Crew	Curling	Golf
Football	Bicycling	Fencing	Table tennis	Riflery
Ice hockey	Diving	Field		
Lacrosse	Field	Discus		
Martial arts	High jump	Javelin		
Rodeo	Pole vault	Shotput		
Soccer	Gymnastics	Running		
Wrestling	Horseback riding	Swimming		
	Skating	Tennis		
	Ice	Track		
	Roller	Weight lifting		
	Skiing			
	Cross-country			
	Downhill			
	Water			
	Softball			
	Squash, handball			
	Volleyball			

Reproduced by permission of *Pediatrics:* A.A.P. Committee on Sports Medicine: Recommendations for participation in competitive sports. *Pediatrics, 81,* 737, Copyright 1988.

running may result in a variety of injuries and health problems, however. Common musculoskeletal problems include overuse injuries (e.g., stress fractures, tendonitis) that can lead to chronic disability. For females, delayed menarche or amenorrhea can occur. Other problems include iron depletion, heat stroke, or hypothermia due to inefficient thermal homeostasis and psychosocial difficulties (AAP, 1988).

Injury in youth sports is infrequent. Injury rates increase with age and with skill level. For example, in a study of injuries to juvenile hockey players, the rate was 2.4 per cent for school-age children; 20 per cent for high schoolers, and 120 per cent for college students (Sutherland, 1976). In a study by Garrick and Requa (1978), injury rates to high school and college students in the following sports were football (81 per cent), wrestling (75 per cent), and girl's gymnastics (40 per cent).

Anticipatory Guidance: Recreation

It may be difficult to encourage the adolescent to voluntarily wear safety equipment such as helmets and knee pads. Instruction in the use of safety equipment needs to be reinforced with a discussion of injury statistics and advocacy group recommendations (e.g., AAP, US Consumer Product Safety Commission).

A preseason sports assessment should be performed on all adolescent athletes who participate in competitive sports. The assessment focuses on the cardiovascular, neurologic, and musculoskeletal systems. Health problems detected during the physical, such as hypertension, abnormal murmur, presence of arrhythmias at rest, and orthopedic problems, such as joint instability or asymmetry of muscular strength, require further evaluation.

Other conditions requiring additional evaluation and management are hernias, cryptorchidism, and organomegaly. Students will be disqualified from collision/contact sports with heritable cardiac conditions such as valvular stenosis, hemorrhagic disease, and absence of an organ. Students with poorly controlled seizures should be counseled not to participate in gymnastics and to never swim without supervision (AAP, 1988).

The nurse can provide the adolescent and parents with information on the associated health risks in pursuing particular athletic activities. Certainly adolescents should be encouraged to participate fully in athletics of their choice if no symptoms are present. If problems arise, however, the adolescent needs to be referred for appropriate treatment.

Safety Concerns

Peer pressure, high energy, intoxication, and feelings of being indestructible cause recklessness in adolescents. Accidents are the leading cause of adolescent mortality. Motor vehicle accidents are the leading cause of death and are often intoxicant-related, with adolescents being passengers or drivers. Adolescents aged 15 to 19 accounted for 65 per cent of the 10,428 motor vehicle deaths to children in 1988 (Fingerhut & NCHS, 1988). The death rate for adolescents aged 15 to 19 is five times greater than that for any other pediatric age group. One of three adolescents involved in a fatal crash had a blood-alcohol concentration greater than the legal limit (Centers for Disease Control, 1991).

Adolescent occupants are among the highest risk groups for injury from motor vehicles (Guyer & Gallagher, 1988). Adolescents continue to wear seat belts less often than other age groups. For example, 44 per cent of adolescents reported wearing a seat belt the last time they rode in a car (American School Health Association, 1989).

Following motor vehicle accidents, the primary accidents causing death in teen-agers are those caused by drowning, firearms, and poisoning (Children's Safety Network, 1991). Male adolescents are among the highest risk group for drowning (Baker & Waller, 1989). Drowning in adolescents may be due to the use of drugs and alcohol. Other causes of adolescent drowning are boating and automobile accidents, lack of supervision, and suicide (Coffman, 1991).

Homicides have become the second leading cause of injury death among children and adolescents. In 1988, over 3200 children and adolescents were victims of homicide. Males are at far greater risk than females: 7 out of 10 homicides involve males (Children's Safety Network, 1991). Homicides of adolescents are caused by arguments and crimes involving peers and gangs (Christoffel, 1990). Recent studies have reported alarming findings on the use of weapons in school settings. One study reported that 20 per cent of students had carried a weapon to school the previous month. Five per cent of the adolescents indicated that they had carried a firearm to school (Centers for Disease Control, 1991). It is understandable, therefore, to see how male adolescents aged 10 to 19 are at particular risk for unintentional firearm injuries.

Adolescents aged 15 to 19 are also at highest risk for unintentional poisoning. Accidental poisonings in adolescents are most often by psychoactive substances, usually barbiturates. Excess ingestion occurs in a teen-ager who is already intoxicated, or in one who thinks that more is better; fatal accidental overdose may also be caused by addiction. Adolescent boys are 2.5 times more likely than girls to die from unintentional poisoning. A significant number of these deaths are thought to be unidentified suicide (Kozak, 1991). Table 9–18 lists the major safety concerns during adolescence.

Injuries occurring in school have been surveyed as well. Nurse researchers examined the profile of accidents in several high schools (Lee & Jacobson, 1987). They found that 55 per cent of the accidents occurred during supervised athletic activity. The majority of injuries were sustained in lower (32 per cent)

TABLE 9-18
Safety Developmental Concerns and Prevention Strategies

Developmental Stage: Adolescent (13–18 Yrs)	**Prevention Strategies: Teach Adolescent All Aspects of Safety**
• Drive motor vehicles (cars, motorcycles) • Peer pressure and their acceptance predominates • Risk-taking to establish self with peers is common • Activities in work and sports involve dangerous equipment • Independence in all activities	Motor Vehicle Accidents • Re-emphasize use of seat belts • Emphasize the danger of alcohol and drug use (especially related to motor vehicle accidents) Bodily Injury and Trauma • Teach proper use of equipment and maintenance of equipment Drowning • Teach water safety • Instruct in the use of emergency care equipment • Teach cardiopulmonary resuscitation (CPR) Firearms • Close supervision regarding firearms is required • No loaded weapon in house Street Safety • Use buddy system; don't go out alone after dark

and upper (23 per cent) extremities. Sprains, fractures, and dislocations accounted for 44 per cent of the injuries reported. Nearly 75 per cent of the injuries resulted in major first-aid treatment, and 73 per cent of them were treated by nurses. In another nursing study, high school students with highest stressful life events scores reported a higher number of accidents compared to noninjured students (Lee et al, 1989). These findings suggest a potential relationship between stress and injuries.

Anticipatory Guidance: Safety

Nurses play an instrumental role in accident prevention. They should work toward stricter drinking and driving laws and support organizations that promote more responsible behavior such as Mothers Against Drunk Driving (MADD) and Students Against Drunk Driving (SADD) in the United States and in Canada. In states where the drinking age was raised, there was a 29 per cent decrease in motor vehicle accidents (Wagnaar, 1981). If a teen-ager has made the choice to drink alcohol, smoke marijuana, or snort cocaine, the nurse should present alternatives to driving while intoxicated. Such options include taking public transportation or calling friends or family for a ride home or appointing a designated driver who abstains from substance use. Many parents would rather pick their teen-ager up after a party than allow drunken driving.

Nurses must advise their adolescent patients to take swimming and water safety classes, and never to swim while intoxicated. Nonswimmers can take swimming classes during the winter so that they can join friends in summer swimming without taking risks. If adolescents drive or sail boats, then participation in navigation safety classes is a must.

Stricter gun control laws would very likely decrease the incidence of accidental shootings. Nurses should encourage gun control regulations. If parents insist on having guns at home, for hunting, for example, the guns must never be kept loaded at home and parents must teach their teen-agers gun safety and proper handling. The Child Safety Network (CSN) provides information to professionals and parents to develop programs in the community and in the schools to decrease the incidence of unintentional injuries and violence.*

Nurses in school settings can be watchful of the events that occur in student lives and the potential risk for injury that can ensue. Also, monitoring of school accident records will provide data the school nurse can use in the planning and implementation of school safety programs.

Sex Education

The need to learn about sexuality increases rapidly in adolescence. In one study of adolescents aged 11 to 14, 21 per cent reported that they were sexually active. Fifty-one per cent reported having sex without contraceptives; 37 per cent reported not taking precautions against STDs. Thirty-six per cent reported having had casual sex at least on one occasion. Ado-

*Child Safety Network: National Center for Education in National and Child Health, 38th and R Sts., NW, Washington, DC 20057; 202–625–8400.

lescents who reported themselves as being sexually active were more likely to be involved in other risk behaviors, such as using tobacco, alcohol, and illicit drugs and driving under the influence (Millstein et al, 1992). By age 14, 10 to 20 per cent of boys and 5 to 10 per cent of girls have had sexual intercourse (AAP, 1990).

Recent statistics indicate that 52 per cent of adolescents aged 15 to 19 are sexually active (Forrest & Singh, 1990). Every year, 1 in 10 adolescent girls becomes pregnant (Shearin & Boehlke, 1989). This rate has remained constant since the mid-1970s because of the increase in pregnancy rates for younger adolescents with the concurrent decline for older adolescents.

Learning to express feelings and resolve conflicts is essential to formation of sexual identity. Clarification of values about sexual behavior is essential for the adolescent. Sexual values depend on one's religious, family, social, and cultural context. The development of responsibility for one's own behavior must be stressed for both girls and boys. Increased peer pressure may generate internal conflict, making values clarification counseling beneficial for adolescents.

Exploring alternatives is essential to the decisions the adolescent must make with regard to sexual behaviors. The choice of whether to be sexually active, with whom, for what purpose, and in what context of responsibility is a critical issue at this age (Stout & Kirby, 1993).

Anticipatory Guidance: Sex Education

In addition to clarifying personal attitudes and values toward sexuality, the following interventions are appropriate for the nurse working with adolescents:

1. Review anatomy and reproductive processes, clarifying terms.
2. Provide reliable information about menstruation, physical development, pregnancy, contraception, and STDs.
3. Clarify values regarding orientation and responsibility.
4. Explore alternatives in the decision making process.
5. Reflect feelings and support during crises.
6. Encourage involvement of parents with adolescents.
7. Support community projects to educate the sexually active adolescent.

See Chapter 37 for prevention of AIDS, and Chapter 39 for prevention of STDs.

Sexually Transmitted Diseases (STDs)

The evidence of STDs is very high among adolescents in the United States (Gittes & Irwin, 1993). Approximately one million cases of gonorrhea are reported annually, and nearly 25 per cent of those cases involve adolescents. In a study of sexually active young adolescents (grades 6 through 8), 5 per cent reported acquiring an STD (Millstein et al, 1992). It is estimated that 29 per cent of the newly diagnosed persons with AIDS became infected during the adolescent or young adult years. It is therefore imperative that sexually active adolescents be screened for STDs, even when they are asymptomatic. Recommended tests for sexually active adolescents are as follows (see Table 39–8 for additional information on STDs):

Females: Annual or semi-annual in high-risk group; Pap smear, cervical gonorrhea culture, cervical chlamydia culture, syphilis serology, and vaginal wet-mount.

Males: Annual syphilis serologic, and, in high-risk groups, annual urethral cultures for gonorrhea and chlamydia. Homosexual males will also need rectal and pharyngeal cultures for gonorrhea.

Educating adolescents about "safe" and protected sex will be a challenge for the pediatric nurse. Several studies have indicated that health concerns do not have a significant effect on the adolescent's decision to use a condom (Kegeles et al, 1989; Pendergrast et al, 1992). Adolescents indicated that more immediate concerns such as degree of hassle, confidence in using devices correctly, and partner's attitude had far greater effect on the choice to use a condom.

More recent studies have reported alarming percentages of adolescents engaging in the high-risk behavior of anal intercourse. Percentages of sexually active adolescents reporting the practice of anal intercourse varies from 25 to approximately 15 per cent (Pendergrast et al, 1992; McDonald et al, 1990; Jaffe et al, 1988).

Anticipatory Guidance: STDs

Adolescents at risk for AIDS and those who have had partners who were at risk for AIDS should be tested for HIV. Pre- and post-test counseling by a skilled professional is an important part of AIDS screening (Heins, 1989). See Chapter 37 for further information about AIDS.

The nurse can counsel adolescent males about the use of a condom to lessen the risk of transmitting an STD. The boy needs to be instructed regarding proper condom use. Only latex condoms that are packaged for "disease prevention" should be used. Lambskin condoms are not considered effective in preventing STDs. Adolescents should be advised not to purchase condoms from vending machines since exposure to extreme temperatures or direct sunlight can change the composition of the latex condom to make it gummy or brittle and thereby ineffective. Nor should condoms be stored in wallets, purses, or glove compartments of cars, for the same reasons. The spermicide *nonoxynol-9* has been found effective with STDs. Additional spermicide can be added inside the condom at the tip and outside after it has been applied to the penis.

Birth Control

The prevalence of sexual intercourse in American adolescents is high, and studies have confirmed that the rate is increasing. Most adolescents are sexually active 6 to 12 months prior to seeking birth control (White, 1987). Some 1.2 million teen-agers become pregnant annually (Williams & Pratt, 1990). The costs of teen-age pregnancy are significant for teens, their families, and for society. As noted by Edelman (1987):

- Only 50 per cent of the teen-agers who become parents graduate from high school.
- Teen-age mothers are twice as likely as older mothers to be poor.
- Infants born to teen-age mothers are at a significantly greater risk of low birthweight and other health problems because pregnant adolescents frequently fail to obtain adequate prenatal care.
- Special hospital care for low birthweight babies averages $1000 per day.
- Medicaid pays for 30 per cent of hospital deliveries for adolescents, at an annual cost of about $200 million.
- The public cost for babies born to teen-age girls in 1985 was $16.6 billion.

For teen-agers who choose to be sexually active, the nurse has a primary role in making birth control accessible and in helping teen-agers to make informed decisions about birth control methods.

Withdrawal is a method of birth control used by many teen-agers, usually early in the sexual relationship. It is free, involves no devices, and is always available. The couple has intercourse until just before ejaculation. Then the penis is removed from the vagina and the sperm is deposited at a distance from the vagina. The biggest problem with this method is its low rate of effectiveness. The reasons for this are that some sperm escape even before ejaculation, and timing of withdrawal before the moment of ejaculation is very difficult to control. Therefore, withdrawal is not recommended as a form of birth control.

The *condom,* or "rubber," is another common birth control device used by teen-agers. Condoms are relatively cheap, are available without the need to visit a health care professional, and allow a male to control his fertility. Many clinics and schools provide condoms at no charge. They prevent pregnancy by providing a barrier between the penis and the cervix and prevent the spread of STDs. When used properly, the condom is very effective. When used with spermicide foam, the effectiveness rate approaches that of oral contraceptives. *All* sexually active adolescents should be encouraged to use condoms every time they have intercourse, even if they are using another form of birth control. Condoms are a mechanical barrier that prevents the spread of STDs including *Chlamydia trachomatis, Neisseria gonorrhoeae, Treponema pallidum,* HIV, herpes simplex virus, *Trichomonas vaginalis, Mycoplasma hominis, Ureaplasma urealyticum,* human papilloma virus, hepatitis B, and cytomegalovirus (AAP, 1990). Some precautions for the young client using condoms are:

- Use only latex condoms.
- Keep condoms away from heat (such as body heat from storing in a wallet).
- Be sure to put the condom on an erect penis (uncircumcised men should pull foreskin back before placing condom on penis) and before the penis gets anywhere near the vagina.
- Leave a half-inch space at the end of the condom.
- Use intravaginal spermicide *nonoxynol 9 with condom* and with *each act of intercourse.*
- Penis must be withdrawn from vagina before it becomes flaccid.
- Be sure to hold on to the condom when the penis is withdrawn from the vagina.
- If the rubber breaks or tears, insert spermicide foam into the vagina immediately.

Condoms are very effective in preventing the spread of STDs. See Chapter 37 for a discussion of AIDS.

Spermicides may also be used alone. The spermicide is placed in the vagina before intercourse. It comes as foam, jelly, cream, or tablets. The spermicide then blocks entry across or through the cervix and immobilizes or kills the sperm. Use with condoms greatly increases effectiveness of the spermicide, which also serves as a lubricant. The user must remember to do the following:

- Shake the can well before dispensing (when using foam).
- Fill the applicator completely full (when using foam).
- Insert the spermicide just before intercourse.
- Insert more spermicide if intercourse occurs again.
- Insert as far as comfortably possible so the spermicide will cover the cervix.
- Avoid douching for at least 8 hours after intercourse.
- Wash the applicator with soap and warm water.

Spermicides decrease the incidence of STDs (Mishell, 1989).

The *diaphragm* is a dome-shaped latex cup with a flexible rim that is inserted into the vagina. It must be fitted, for both size and type, by a health professional. Of the three types of diaphragms, the coil spring is the diaphragm of choice for teen-agers (Bullough & Bullough, 1991). The diaphragm is always used with a spermicidal cream, foam, or jelly and serves to hold the spermicidal agent against the cervical os.

TABLE 9-19

Nursing Process Plan: Care of Pregnant Adolescent

Analysis: Nursing Diagnostic Statement 1

Response and Related or Risk Factors: *High risk for altered nutrition; less than body requirements; risk factors*

- Lack of adequate financial resources
- Lack of information about nutritional requirements for fetal growth

Projected Outcome: The adolescent will maintain an intake of nutrients sufficient to meet own bodily needs and those of fetus.

Defining Characteristics (Actual Response)	Nursing Interventions	Evaluation Criteria
Subjective: • Reported food intake less than recommended daily allowance (adolescent states she likes to eat junk food!) • Does not know how to respond to questions about diet. Responds "no" or "I dunno" to questions asked *Objective*: • Delayed/slow fetal growth • Deficient weight gain • Signs and symptoms of preeclampsia/toxemia	*Nutritional Monitoring; Nutritional Counseling; Nutritional Therapy* **Assess height and weight accurately at first visit to provide baseline from which to monitor weight gain at subsequent visits** **Establish and try to maintain caloric intake that allows for adequate fetal growth.** Encourage foods high in nutrient value; and stress the importance of eating foods high in dietary iron to avoid anemia **Refer those adolescents with inadequate intake for ongoing nutritional counseling.** Nutritional counseling should be appropriate in relation to their socioeconomic status and cultural patterns Collaborate when the physician prescribes vitamins and/or iron, to assure that the adolescent: • Understands how they will affect her health • Understands dose, frequency of administration, and side effects • Has money/drug plan to cover their cost • Continue to monitor to assure that prenatal supplements are being taken as prescribed	Appropriate weight gain during pregnancy evidenced by a 16kg weight gain for the adolescent under 16 yrs; 17–25 yrs, 11 kg weight gain Fetal growth within normal limits Uses nutritional information to improve dietary status Explains rationale for dietary concern, vitamin/iron supplements. Takes supplements as prescribed Absence of symptoms of preeclampsia/toxemia

TABLE 9-19 (continued)

Analysis: Nursing Diagnostic Statement 2

Response and Related or Risk Factors: *High risk for injury (of self and fetus); risk factors—chemical effects of drug use and abuse (including tobacco and alcohol)*

Projected Outcome: The adolescent will not use drugs during pregnancy.

Defining Characteristics (Actual Response)	Nursing Interventions	Evaluation Criteria
Subjective: • Adolescent admits to drug use and abuse including tobacco and alcohol *Objective*: • Misses appointments • Is not adhering to prenatal care regime • Positive toxic screen • Detect odor of alcohol/smoking on breath • Demonstrates signs/symptoms of drug abuse (see Chapter 29)	*Substance Use Prevention* **Explain the effect of drug use/abuse on the adolescent, as well as the fetus.** Information can be used by the adolescent to determine risk of continued behavior. Accurate information can sometimes motivate behavior change if the risk is serious enough *Support System Enhancement; Support Group* **Assess social supports available to assist the adolescent in decreasing or stopping drug use** **Provide ways to access community support groups for decreasing drug use**	Adolescent identifies desire and method for behavior change Adolescent begins program for decreasing drug use and continues in program throughout pregnancy

Analysis: Nursing Diagnostic Statement 3

Response and Related or Risk Factors: *Fear, related to*

- Potential for pain upon physical examination (internal)
- Separation from support systems during a threatening procedure
- Unfamiliarity with procedure
- Unfamiliarity with health professional

Projected Outcome: The teen will be relaxed and free of fear during procedures.

Defining Characteristics	Nursing Interventions	Evaluation Criteria
Subjective: • Asks questions such as "What are you going to do?" "Will that hurt?" • States she is "afraid it will hurt" and "tired of all of this stuff." *Objective*: • Misses appointments • Is late for appointments	*Teaching: Procedure/Treatment; Truth Telling* **Provide clear, honest explanation before doing procedures.** The adolescent is able to understand the explanation **Make sure the same person does the history, physical, and internal examination.** This reassures the teen and decreases embarrassment	Teen verbalizes comfort and decrease in or absence of fear

(continued)

TABLE 9-19 (continued)

Analysis: Nursing Diagnostic Statement 4

Response and Related or Risk Factors: *High risk for altered health maintenance; risk factor/knowledge deficit about:*

- Body changes during pregnancy
- Fetal growth
- Process of labor

Projected Outcome: The adolescent will be able to identify, manage, and seek out help to maintain health during pregnancy and in relation to signs of possible complications and the process of labor.

Defining Characteristics (Actual Response)	Nursing Interventions	Evaluation Criteria
Subjective: · Asks questions "What is happening to me now?" "What is the baby doing?" "When will the baby begin to move?" · Asks questions about physical changes she has noticed · Asks questions such as "Will being in labor hurt?" "How long will it take?" *Objective*: · Body changes during pregnancy; fetal growth	*Prenatal Care; Teaching: Procedure/Treatment* **Explain changes and fetal growth using plastic models and charts.** Have adolescent summarize content of discussion **Clarify understanding of normal changes, and explain signs of complications** **Assess adolescent's current knowledge about the process of labor and delivery.** Determine learning needs to establish an appropriate educational plan more likely to meet the needs of the adolescent. Dispel myths **Encourage teen to participate in prenatal classes in which techniques for use during labor are taught, preferably a session of adolescents only, so it can be tailored to their level of development**	**Is able to identify, manage, and/or seek out help to maintain health during pregnancy as evidenced by:** · Adolescent describes and uses techniques previously taught when in labor and during delivery · Relevant questions · Notification of nurse/physician of possible complications when signs/symptoms appear

Effectiveness is directly correlated with proper use of the diaphragm and motivation. The diaphragm can be inserted up to 6 hours before intercourse by folding and inserting it, jelly side up, into the vagina, or by use of an applicator. It *must* be checked by inserting a finger into the vagina to feel for the cervix inside the dome's rim. If it has been inserted for more than 2 hours, additional spermicide is needed.

The wearer must be sure to leave the diaphragm in place at least 6 hours after the last intercourse, and should not douche. It should be in place no more than 24 hours because of risk of TSS. The diaphragm should be washed and dried carefully, dusted with cornstarch, and kept in its case. A return visit is necessary to have the fit checked after 1 to 2 weeks of use and after pregnancy, pelvic surgery, or weight gain or loss of 10 to 20 pounds, or if any discomfort is experienced. One diaphragm should last about 2 years but should be checked regularly near a light for holes or tears.

Oral contraceptives, or birth control pills, are used by 10 to 15 million women in the United States. The oral contraceptives containing a combination of estrogen and progestogen suppress ovulation by inhibiting the secretion of hypothalamic gonadotropin-releasing hormone and may also act directly on the pituitary to inhibit release of gonadotropins. The combination pill also causes development of "hostile cer-

TABLE 9-19 *(continued)*

Analysis: Nursing Diagnostic Statement 5

Response and Related or Risk Factors: *High risk for injury, self and contacts; risk factors*

- Presence of sexually transmitted disease (STD)
- Unwillingness of adolescent (diagnosed to have STD) to provide names and addresses of sexual contacts because of fear that contact will know source of report
- Lack of knowledge regarding availability of STD treatment for self and others

Projected Outcome: The adolescent will comply with treatment for STD and will provide names and addresses of sexual contacts so they can receive treatment

Defining Characteristics (Actual Response)	*Nursing Interventions*	*Evaluation Criteria*
Subjective: • Admits she is sexually active *Objective:* • Positive laboratory results for STD	*Teaching: Safe Sex* **Explain and initiate ordered treatment.** Clarify treatment requirements. Encourage compliance with treatment **Help adolescent to understand that source of contact information is held confidential and that reason for obtaining information about contacts is to provide treatment of other infected individuals to prevent further spread of disease** **Explain methods to prevent/minimize future STD** (e.g., consistent use of condoms during sexual intercourse)	Adolescent completes prescribed course of treatment for STD Adolescent provides names and addresses of sexual contacts so they can receive treatment

(continued)

vical mucus," which decreases the chance of sperm penetration.

Contraindications to using the pill include cardiovascular disorders, migraine headaches, liver problems, malignancy, and pregnancy. A low-dose pill containing 30 to 35 U of estrogen and 0.15 to 1.5 mg of progestin is preferred for adolescents (AAP, 1990).

The pills are taken once a day for 21 days, followed by a 7-day "off" period before another 21-day cycle is resumed. The 28-day cycle of pills (containing 7 days' worth of inert pills) is recommended for the adolescent because with it she simply takes a pill every morning instead of having to interrupt and resume the sequence.

To be given a prescription for oral contraceptives, a girl must have a complete gynecologic examination, including a Pap smear, hematocrit, blood pressure, and tests for STDs. Minor side effects of taking the pill are mid-cycle bleeding, weight gain, headache, irritability, breast tenderness, depression, acne, and dysmenorrhea.

The nurse can be helpful in counseling the young woman in the importance of taking her pill every day. Since doses are lower, if a pill is missed or taken more than 4 hours later, the girl should avoid intercourse until menses occurs or use another contraceptive method in addition to completing the rest of the pill cycle. Any side effects such as spotting, nausea, or weight gain should be reported to a doctor or nurse practitioner.

The practitioner is contacted immediately with complaints of severe abdominal pain, severe chest pain, severe headaches, visual loss or blurring, severe depression, or severe leg pain (Woods, 1991). Questions should be encouraged. The girl's nutritional requirements for folic acid and vitamins C, B_6, and B_{12} are increased by taking oral contraceptives. The nurse should assess the teen-ager's diet and recommend foods that are high in B-complex vitamins and vitamin C.

The *intrauterine device (IUD)* is a contraceptive method that is not recommended for adolescents because of increased pelvic infection and expulsion rate (Woods, 1991).

The *periodic abstinence method,* formerly known as the "rhythm method," is also used by some ado-

TABLE 9-19 *(continued)*

Analysis: Nursing Diagnostic Statement 6

Response and Related or Risk Factors: *Decisional conflict about whether to keep baby and how to prepare for its arrival related to knowledge deficit about*

- Lifestyle options for care of the baby
- Items needed for the baby

Projected Outcome: The adolescent will choose a course of action to be taken when baby arrives.

Defining Characteristics	*Nursing Interventions*	*Evaluation Criteria*
Subjective: • Verbalizes uncertainty about choices, e.g., shares concerns about keeping the baby such as "I don't know if I would be a good mother." "I don't know what to do." "I don't want to give the baby up." • Vacillation between alternative choices, e.g., expresses ambivalence about impending motherhood; states she feels pressure from family, boyfriend, and friends to "give baby up" or "keep it." • Verbalization of undesired consequences of alternative actions being considered, e.g., states she is afraid she can't give baby what it needs; alternated with fear of guilt feelings if she "gives baby up."	*Decision Making Support* **Provide opportunity for the adolescent to hear the fetal heart, feel the fetus.** This introduces reality set about the infant, and encourages bonding **Review of rationale for lifestyle option after delivery and assessment of support for choice.** Assist adolescents in clarifying their choice	Adolescent verbalizes understanding of the lifestyle choices possible after pregnancy Demonstrates awareness of the lifestyle changes needed following the baby's birth Adolescent verbalizes confidence in choice and uses information taught to arrive at choice

lescents. Unfortunately, many are grossly misinformed about this method. Its use requires knowledge, skill, and motivation to be successful; however, even when used properly, it is not very effective. The periodic abstinence method is based on the fact that ovulation usually occurs 14 days before the onset of menstruation. In a regular 28-day cycle, ovulation can be identified by a slight rise in temperature (0.2 to 0.4°C or 0.4 to 0.8°F) and change in cervical mucus (thick and sparse to thin and viscous).

Sperm live for 2 to 3 days, and the ovum survives about 24 hours. The woman must chart her cycles for at least 8 months, then subtract 18 days from her shortest cycle and 11 days from her longest cycle; the period of time between those days is her fertile time. For example, if her longest cycle (space between the first days of two periods) was 30 days and her shortest was 25 days, she should abstain from sexual intercourse between days 7 and 19 of each cycle.

A central problem with this method is that adolescent girls have irregular menstrual cycles. It is also not a preferred method of adolescents because it requires abstinence for a period of time each month, and time calculations are complicated.

Adolescents are known to be poor contraceptors, even after they secure a birth control method. There is no way to ensure compliance, but it may be helpful to assure confidentiality, to explain the birth control method simply and completely, to discuss the risks of pregnancy versus the risks of contraception, and to schedule frequent follow-up visits.

Substance Use and Abuse

Abuse of psychoactive substances is a growing concern to individuals providing health care services to adolescents. Adolescents may turn to drugs and alcohol for many reasons. For some teen-agers, these sub-

TABLE 9-19 *(continued)*

Analysis: Nursing Diagnostic Statement 7

Response and Related or Risk Factors: *High risk for altered role performance; risk factors*

- Unrealistic estimate of short- and long-term implications of being a mother
- Multiple life changes associated with the care of a newborn baby

Projected Outcome: The adolescent will understand behaviors required for parenting role.

Defining Characteristics	*Nursing Interventions*	*Evaluation Criteria*
Subjective: · Denial of role, e.g., states she is planning to resume activities with friends as soon as baby is born, states her mother would "help her a lot" with taking care of the baby · Lack of knowledge of role behaviors, e.g., asks questions about baby care such as "When can the baby begin to eat baby food?" "When will the baby begin to sleep through the night?" "When can I take the baby to the mall with me?" · Change in usual patterns of responsibility, e.g., parenting behaviors will be added to what is expected of her prenatally	*Childbirth Preparation* **Assess adolescent's knowledge and acceptance of parenting role behaviors** **Facilitate understanding of realistic expectations for role changes after delivery;** e.g., identify items needed for care of a newborn baby and suggest ways to acquire them. Help adolescent recognize need to prepare for baby's birth. This will aid in adjustment to motherhood by giving the adolescent a sense of control over her life **Refer adolescent to the services of appropriate community agencies or programs** **Use techniques to assist adolescent to meet expectations of new role;** e.g., role taking and role making, role clarification, role supplementation	Correctly verbalizes expected role behaviors. Can role-play these behaviors Verbalizes a practical plan for meeting role expectations of parenting role

(continued)

stances provide "false courage" in threatening social situations or "make the world seem more bearable" when social anxiety causes withdrawal from peer interactions (Windle et al, 1991). Substance abuse may be subconsciously encouraged by parents, or the adolescent may use substance abuse to divert parental attention from marital problems. Some teen-agers use alcohol or drugs because they believe this makes them seem grown up (see Chapter 29 for a complete discussion of substance abuse).

Studies reveal experimentation with alcohol and illicit drugs to be common. In one study, age of initiation for alcohol and drug use occurred prior to the sixth grade (Millstein et al, 1992). Another report indicates that 11 is the average age for the first alcoholic drink. The three most frequently used drugs by adolescents are alcohol, marijuana, and cocaine (National Institute on Drug Abuse, 1986). The prevalence of alcohol use among adolescents has been reported to be 66 per cent, marijuana 26 per cent, and cocaine 6.7 per cent (Johnston et al, 1985).

The adolescent substance abuser demonstrates a different profile of characteristics from the adult user. An adolescent reaches a crisis point seven times faster than an adult, meaning the adolescent is no longer able to function adequately in school and behavior problems become evident. Also, the adolescent may not have the capacity to understand his or her behavior and treatment goals as compared with adults. Lastly, an adolescent's participation in a treatment program is highly dependent on the parents' support. If parents do not recognize their teen-ager's problem or cannot afford to pay for a recovery program and do not participate in the process, the prospects for recovery of the adolescent are lessened (Myers & Anderson, 1991).

TABLE 9-19 (continued)

Analysis: Nursing Diagnostic Statement 8

Response and Related or Risk Factors: *High risk for ineffective management of therapeutic regimen: failure to use appropriate contraceptives; risk factors*

- Lack of knowledge about contraceptive options and their benefits
- Belief system that adolescent use of contraceptives is unnecessary or improper
- Cultural values that oppose use of contraceptives
- Economic difficulties related to paying for contraceptives
- Perceived powerlessness regarding ability to prevent "getting pregnant"

Projected Outcome: The adolescent will regulate and integrate into her daily living a program for use of contraceptives to prevent future unplanned pregnancy.

Defining Characteristics (Actual Response)	***Nursing Interventions***	***Evaluation Criteria***
Subjective: • Choices of daily living ineffective for meeting the goals of a prevention program, e.g., states she is sexually active and engages in unsafe and unprotected sex • Verbalizes difficulty with regulation of prescribed regimen for prevention of another pregnancy, e.g., indicates ambivalence about using contraceptives; states using contraceptives is a "bother" or she "forgets to use them." *Objective:* • Pregnancy	*Family Planning: Contraception* **Assess adolescent for knowledge, attitudes, feelings, values about use of contraceptives after delivery** **Introduce information about contraceptives and the topic of responsible sexual behavior early in pregnancy** **Provide adolescent with the opportunity to explore the idea of being responsible for her sexual behavior and fecundity** **Assist the adolescent in clarifying values around use of contraception in general and specific methods in particular** **Explain advantages, disadvantages, and the effectiveness of the various methods of contraception**	**Demonstrates knowledge of contraceptive use as evidenced by description of appropriate use** **Obtains chosen contraceptive and uses it correctly as evidenced by absence of pregnancy**

Anticipatory Guidance: Substance Abuse

The nurse can assist the adolescent in seeking treatment for substance abuse by providing support and information for referral. For additional information on treatment of substance abuse, see Chapter 29. The school nurse will be active in teaching and serving as a resource to students, teachers, and parents on the prevention of substance abuse. Prevention programs should be initiated during the elementary school years *before* substance abuse typically begins.

Use of Steroids

A major problem affecting competitive professional and amateur sports is the use of anabolic steroids. These steroids are used by athletes to increase muscle strength and size as a means of enhancing athletic performance. There are no scientific data to support the belief that steroids will enhance performance. Yet, steroid use is widespread at all levels of athletic competition (Dyment, 1990). Recent surveys of high school students indicated that 6 to 11 per cent of boys admitted to current or past steroid use. One fourth of the boys admitted using steroids as a means to improve appearance, not athletic performance. One per cent of high school girls admitted to steroid use (Buckley et al, 1988; Johnson et al, 1989).

Anabolic steroids have potential toxic effects, many of which are not reversible after use has been discontinued. These toxic effects are listed in Table

TABLE 9-20
Anabolic Steroid Use: Toxic Side Effects

Cardiovascular	Endocrinologic	Skeletal
• Hypertension • Increased low-density-lipoprotein cholesterol • Decreased high-density-lipoprotein cholesterol • Increased total cholesterol	• Acne • Male-pattern baldness • Testicular atrophy • Priapism • Impotence • Gynecomastia • Oligospermia • Decreased sperm motility • Masculinization (in females)	• Epiphyseal closure **Hepatic** • Hepatoma • Cholestatic jaundice • Toxic hepatitis • Peliosis **Behavioral** • Aggressiveness • Increased libido • Increased energy • Irritability

From Dyment, P. (1990). Steroids: Breakfast of champions. *Pediatrics in Review, 12,* 104. Reproduced by permission of Pediatrics, copyright 1990.

9-20. Both the American College of Sports Medicine (1987) and the AAP (1989c) have strongly condemned the use of anabolic steroids.

Anticipatory Guidance: Use of Steroids. The nurse needs to assess adolescents, particularly those in whom a weight gain and muscular bulk have been observed. Athletes participating in power sports such as weight lifting and football need to be assessed for steroid use. Anticipatory guidance regarding effects of steroid use are warranted even if the adolescent denies such use. The school nurse may be asked by the high school coach to instruct athletes on the effects of steroid use. An instructional program providing objective information without using "scare tactics" has been shown to be most effective in instructing adolescents about the dangers of using steroids (Goldberg et al, 1991).

Adolescent Pregnancy

Over 1.1 million teens become pregnant each year (Johnson et al, 1988). Births to unwed teen-agers increased 67 per cent from 1969 to 1987 (Children's Defense Fund [CDF], 1990). The greatest risk of teen-age pregnancy occurs in poor and minority groups. The teen-age birth rate in 1980 per 1000 was 41.2 for whites, 105.1 for African-Americans, and 82.2 for Latinos (Mitchell & Brindis, 1987). In 1987, 51 per cent of white teen-age births occurred to unmarried women as compared with 91 per cent for African-American women (CDF, 1990).

Based on a study of teen-age reproductive behavior in six developed countries, researchers reported that pregnancy rates (abortions plus live births) among adolescents 15 to 19 years of age vary from 96 per 1000 to 14 per 1000 for the United States and the Netherlands, respectively. The rates for England, France, Canada, and Sweden fall between the two extremes and range from 45 per 1000 to 35 per 1000 (Jones et al, 1985).

It is clear that the financial and resource costs of adolescent pregnancy to society are very high. Many adolescent mothers require long-term public assistance. Their lack of knowledge about infant development and care, coupled with sometimes limited social support, makes this group of mothers and children frequent users of the health and social systems (Frager, 1991). The Center for Population Options estimated the single-year cost of teen-age childbearing to be staggering.

The 1985 single-year cost of teen-age births was estimated at $16.65 billion. This included Medicaid, food stamps, Aid to Families with Dependent Children (AFDC), and direct payments to care providers (Burr & Haffner, 1986). The facts that the earlier teen-agers conceive the more children they are likely to bear, and that pregnancy in early adolescence occurs more frequently among offspring of mothers who were also pregnant very young, suggest that without effective primary prevention, adolescent pregnancy will continue to be a major health and social problem in our society (Cooley & Unger, 1991).

Health and Social Consequences

When carried to term, adolescent pregnancy has significant short-term and long-term health and social consequences for the pregnant teen-ager, her partner, their families, their offspring, and society at large. There is general agreement that teen-agers 16 years of age and older who receive early, thorough prenatal care are at no greater risk for physical complications than women 20 years of age. Low birthweight is the only major complication that has been associated with age (AAP, 1989a). Some researchers have attributed this to the biologic immaturity of these adolescents (McAnarney, 1987).

Others believe that the increased rate of complications is a result of young teen-agers not seeking prenatal care until late in the pregnancy and other unhealthy lifestyle habits. The controversy is complicated by the fact that behaviors such as unprotected sexual intercourse (and resulting pregnancy) in early adolescence; the use of alcohol, tobacco, and psychoactive drugs; poor diet; and poor compliance with health care are highly interrelated (Loris et al, 1985).

Furthermore, socioeconomic status (SES) and race appear to influence the development of complications even when age is taken into account. Complications of pregnancy occur more frequently at all ages in those of lower SES (Zuckerman et al, 1984). Hypertension during pregnancy is much more common in African-Americans than in those of other races.

Maternal mortality among teen-agers is approximately 40 per cent greater than for 20- to 25-year-olds, largely because of the increased incidence of preeclamptic toxemia (hypertension, edema, proteinuria) (Society of Obstetricians and Gynecologists of Canada [SOGC], 1986). Cephalopelvic disproportion (CPD) is more common in young adolescents than in older women. This results in an increased rate of cesarean births for this age group, with the increased and attendant risks of anesthesia and major surgery.

The Adolescent Mother

Adolescence is a period of rapid growth, yet many adolescents have poor eating habits and subscribe to fad diets. Low weight gain and anemia during pregnancy may result from inadequate nutritional and caloric intake (Table 9–21). Adolescents with a gynecologic age (age at conception minus age at menarche) of 2 years or less, who are most likely to still be growing fairly rapidly, are at increased risk for nutritional problems (Piecchnik & Corbett, 1985).

In addition to the effects on physical development and physical health hazards, adolescent pregnancy can profoundly influence normal psychosocial development of girls in this age group (Cooley & Unger, 1991). The major task of adolescence, establishing an individual identity, is made more difficult by the fact that the teen-ager must learn to accept her pregnant state and incorporate it into her personal self-concept. The pregnant teen-ager is at high risk for the nursing diagnostic response of *altered role performance*. At this time, many teen-agers have trouble accepting normal body changes. Incorporating additional changes caused by pregnancy can be overwhelming. These changes are not "normal" and are a major difference between the pregnant teen-ager and her peer group (Castiglia, 1991a).

Pregnancy can lead to *social isolation*. This isolation can be self-imposed or a result of peer rejection. Regardless of the cause, it hinders normal psychosocial development. Being isolated from peers not only retards the development of interpersonal social skills but also reduces the opportunities to discuss important issues with same-aged males and females—an important exercise in the process of values clarification. Rejection by the peer group can lead to a decreased sense of self-worth, which in turn may lead to a host of poor lifestyle choices that have long-term negative effects on the adult life of the adolescent.

Pregnancy and motherhood may interrupt or alter educational goals and career choice. Increasing numbers of adolescents are choosing to remain single and keep their offspring (Castiglia, 1991a). Pregnancy is the most common reason girls fail to complete high school in the United States: 50 to 67 per cent of all female dropouts are pregnant or already parents (Spivak & Weitzman, 1987). Lack of a high school diploma increases the probability that earning power will be lost or reduced and increases the likelihood of a future life of poverty. The younger the mother at the time of birth, the greater the likelihood she will live in poverty and subsist on long-term public assistance (Castiglia, 1991a).

In contrast, a nurse researcher found that pregnant adolescents indicated that they perceived motherhood as a viable career choice (Pass, 1986). Furthermore, measures of self-esteem and locus of control did not reveal significant differences between pregnant and nonpregnant adolescents. Cultural values and beliefs have been found to influence both positively and negatively the mother's adjustment to pregnancy. Adolescent Hispanic mothers were found to adjust more positively than African-American adolescents to their pregnancy (Dore & Dumois, 1990).

Heterosexual relationships will also be influenced by unintended pregnancy. The pregnant teen-ager's relationship with the father of the child may suddenly change. On learning about the pregnancy, teen-age males are often frightened and unprepared to accept any responsibility. These young men may terminate the relationship. One study reported that approximately half of the biologic fathers were no longer involved with the situation 8 months post birth (Unger & Wandersman, 1988). Others may wish to remain actively involved with the adolescent and infant and may or may not wish to live with or marry the mother.

TABLE 9-21
Family-Centered Teaching: Suggested Daily Diet for the Pregnant Adolescent

Your daily diet should include:

- Six slices of whole-grain bread, pancakes, tortillas, cornbread, or a serving of whole-grain cereal, or pasta. Use wheat germ and brewers' yeast to fortify other foods
- A serving of fresh, leafy green vegetables—spinach; dark, looseleaf lettuce; broccoli; cabbage; Swiss chard; kale; collard, mustard, or beet greens; alfalfa sprouts
- A yellow or orange vegetable or fruit
- One or two vitamin C–rich foods—whole potato, grapefruit, orange, melon, green pepper, cabbage, strawberries, fruit, orange juice
- A quart of milk (whole, skim, buttermilk) or milk equivalents (cheese, yogurt, cottage cheese). If you are allergic to dairy products, take calcium lactate. Seaweed, sesame seeds, butter, molasses, and shellfish contain calcium; some tofu is also made with calcium lactate
- Two to three protein servings of meat, fish, poultry, cheese, tofu, eggs, or nut-grain-bean-dairy combination. A pregnant teen needs approximately 100 g of protein each day
- Six to eight glasses of liquid—fruit and vegetable juices, water, and herb teas. Avoid sugar-sweetened juices and colas
- For snacks, dried fruits, nuts, pumpkin and sunflower seeds, popcorn
- Since fats, oils, and sweets provide calories but few vitamins and minerals, they should be used SPARINGLY. Salt lightly; avoid foods and drinks with needless sodium

Don't fixate on weight gain. Every metabolism is different; when you eat a well-balanced diet, your weight will take care of itself. An adolescent under 16 yrs old should expect to gain 35 pounds to guarantee proper nutrition for herself and her baby. Pregnancy is no time to diet!

Adapted from The Boston Women's Health Book Collective. (1992). *The new our bodies, ourselves: Updated and expanded for the 1990s.* New York: Simon & Schuster.

The Adolescent Father

Until recently, the role of the father had been largely ignored in adolescent pregnancy. Stereotypic images of the father as irresponsible, uncaring, immature, physically absent, and psychologically unavailable have contributed to this negative view (Freeman, 1988). Findings currently reveal that the involvement of the father enhances the adolescent mother's self-worth and attachment to the infant. Involvement of the father has been shown to enhance a child's cognitive and social skills (Public/Private Ventures, 1990).

The extent to which the father remains involved with his child and mother appears to be influenced by several factors. A preexisting committed relationship with the mother will enhance the likelihood of the father remaining involved. The social norms, cultural beliefs, and acceptance and support of family and friends will play a role in the father's response to the pregnancy. Young fathers who can see beyond the immediate crisis of the pregnancy to the educational, vocational, or professional opportunities available will be able to cope more positively.

Most important of all is the reaction of the mother's family to the father. The mother's family plays a significant role in determining the father's relationship with both the mother and the child. Some families may react protectively and attempt to exclude the father from the situation as the pregnancy actually creates greater family harmony and closeness than previously existed (Cereva, 1989). It becomes incumbent for the nurse to assess the father's role in the pregnancy and subsequent relationships with the mother and child and provide needed support to promote optimal outcomes.

The Adolescent's Parents

Although many families of pregnant adolescents are supportive, initial reactions of guilt for having failed the teen-ager, anger at their daughter and/or the father, disappointment that former ambitions for the girl may not be fulfilled, and embarrassment within the extended family and among social peers are not uncommon. Teen-age pregnancy may be perceived more positively, depending on the cultural norms of the family (Dore & Dumois, 1991).

As parents learn to live with the reality, they may become active in planning the future care of the unborn child. Particularly with young adolescents, parents may take over all the decision making about the future for the adolescent and the infant. If the teen-ager is not involved in these decisions, long-term resentment and feelings of inadequacy may result.

Family support is associated with the teen-age mother's overall well-being. Teens who live with parents express fewer concerns about matters of daily living and finances (Unger & Wandersman, 1988). Teen-age mothers are more likely to continue with their education when they live with parents. However, later problems may emerge if confusion regarding the boundaries of parenting occurs between the grandmother and the mother. The grandmother's role may influence the teen-ager mother to be less involved with her infant (Cooley & Unger, 1991).

The Adolescent's Infant

Being a "child-of-a-child" has numerous risks. Low birthweight and prematurity are much more common in offspring of young adolescents than in women aged 20 to 25 years (AAP, 1989a).

Low birthweight appears to be related broadly to sociodemographic factors and to inadequate nutrition and other unsound health practices. Low socioeconomic status may account for inadequate nutrition in that the long-term diet of adolescents in this group is often missing essential nutrients because of lack of knowledge or money, or both. Weight prior to pregnancy, weight gain during pregnancy, infant gestational age, and use of tobacco, alcohol, or other illicit drugs primarily account for infants with low birthweight (Zuckerman et al, 1983). The gynecologic age of the mother is also important in that optimal prebirth weight gain for adolescents is 13 to 16 kg (35 lbs) as opposed to an 11 kg (24 lbs) weight gain for mothers aged 17 to 25 years (Frisancho et al, 1984).

The precise reasons for higher rates of premature births among this group of mothers are unclear. Some factors that have been suggested include frequent illicit drug use, the presence of STDs (particularly gonorrhea), intercourse during the later part of pregnancy, poor nutrition, and an immature reproductive system. Many of these risk factors for the infants of adolescents can be dramatically decreased through early, effective prenatal care.

Long-term effects on the child of a young adolescent have also been documented. In comparison with children of the older mothers, children of the adolescent mothers were performing less well academically and had repeated a school grade more frequently. Others have also noted that behavior problems, school problems, low intellectual functioning, lower educational attainment, and lower overall lifetime income are more common among children of adolescent parents (Davis, 1988).

The frequency of drug use and abuse among these teen-agers also has devastating effects on their offspring. The incidence of fetal alcohol syndrome (FAS) (see Chapter 30), newborn drug addiction, and congenital STDs is more common among infants of adolescent mothers than among those of mothers in other age groups. Although child abuse appears more frequently with adolescent parents, the relationship of one to the other is unclear.

Nursing Interventions: Adolescent Pregnancy

The factors influencing adolescent pregnancy are multiple. Their interactions are indeed complex and not fully understood. In order to systematically develop therapeutic interventions, it is necessary to recognize how adolescent development and behavior influence nursing interventions and to place the problem within a framework (Holt & Johnson, 1991; Howard & Mitchell, 1993). The factors that influence adolescent pregnancy are summarized in Table 9–22.

The first step in effectively caring for a pregnant adolescent is to establish a therapeutic relationship based on trust. This will increase the probability that the adolescent will be honest and open about her problems and work at setting and meeting reasonable expectations for her health. It is important for the nurse to understand the adolescent's normal developmental needs and related nursing implications, as outlined in Table 9–23, to establish a relationship with a pregnant adolescent. Common nursing diagnostic responses for pregnant adolescents, relevant nursing strategies, rationales, and expected outcomes are summarized in Table 9–19. The stresses that have been discussed can all represent risk factors for the occurrence of *ineffective family coping: compromised.* Since developmental crises, family role changes, and temporary family disorganization are all etiologic factors for this nursing diagnostic response (Gordon, 1987), the nurse should be alert to the possibility that it exists.

In assisting the adolescent and her significant others to explore the possible alternatives, keep in mind the implications for nursing interventions found in Table 9–23. Nursing care of the pregnant adolescent is described in Table 9–19. Effective prevention of adolescent pregnancy is a multifaceted, challenging, sometimes frustrating activity. Nurses who choose to develop the knowledge and skills to intervene with not-yet-pregnant or pregnant adolescents, their partners, their offspring, or their other family members will be vital members of health care teams that are improving the health, in the broadest sense, of not only the target group but also society at large. One group of nurses is currently testing nursing protocols of care designed to assess and foster the decision making and parenting skills of adolescent mothers (Clarke & Strauss, 1992).

TABLE 9–22
Factors Influencing the Incidence of Adolescent Pregnancy

Developmental Factors
Early physical sexual maturation
Gender role confusion
Egocentrism
Personal fable (feeling that "it won't happen to me")
Responsiveness to peers' sexual activity
Independence from family
Lack of future orientation
Concrete thinking
Denial of personal sexuality
Frustration in achieving independence
Societal Factors
Variety of adult sexual behavior values
Implied acceptance of intercourse outside of marriage
Importance of involvement in heterosexual relationships stressed by the media
Inadequate access to contraception
Access to public financial support for teen parents and offspring
Appropriate and congruent with familial lifestyles and values
Family and Friends
Difficult mother-daughter relationship
Lack of religious affiliation
Sexually permissive behavior norms of the larger peer group
Sexual permissive values and behavior of close friends
Inadequate communication in heterosexual relationships

KEY CONCEPTS

Concepts Related to Basic Information

- Some of the tasks the family must deal with during adolescence are providing facilities to meet needs, assuming greater responsibility, re-establishing relationships, promoting communication, developing peer relationships, and understanding the need for independence.
- Nursing diagnostic responses that the nurse may consider for holistic care of the adolescent are *high risk for impaired adjustment, alteration in health maintenance, ineffective individual coping, altered role performance, altered growth and development,* and *body image disturbance.*
- The adolescent's weight varies according to pubertal maturation, degree of adiposity, and size of muscle mass; weight increases by 50 per cent during puberty.
- Sexual maturation, the process involving the development of primary and secondary sexual characteristics, is not complete until about 20 to 21 years of age.
- During *formal operations,* the adolescent becomes capable of thinking about her or his own thoughts and becomes introspective.
- The physical changes that occur in adolescence account for the alterations in mood and attitude.
- It is estimated that 10 per cent of adolescents are gay or lesbian.
- Erikson refers to the central task of adolescence as identity versus role confusion.
- Identity formation may be more problematic for adolescents from culturally diverse populations.
- *Body image* is an intricate aspect of identity.

TABLE 9-23
Adolescent Development: Implications for Nursing Interventions with the Pregnant Adolescent

Normal Adolescent Behavior	Implications for Nursing Interventions
Task: Increasing Independence from Family	
Rebellion against family rules and behavior norms	Adolescents may view the nurse as another authority figure and may be suspicious initially. This is normal behavior and should be treated as such
Secretive about personal life	Nurse must establish the limits of confidentiality from the outset. Limits are influenced by • State laws about providing contraception/abortion to adolescents without parental consent • Practice setting regulations about confidentiality • Clarification of personal values about adolescent sexual activity and pregnancy, so they do not interfere with professional therapeutic relationships
Seek out adult role models	Adolescents do not come to nurses for peer support; they want a competent professional in whom they can have confidence. Consequently, nurses should adopt this demeanor
Critical of family/social values	The nurse should appreciate this and allow the adolescent to verbalize these feelings. Adolescents are very aware of hypocrisy. To be effective, the nurse needs to like and respect adolescents and demonstrate this in a nonjudgmental, caring approach
Ambivalent about independent decision making	The adolescent may ask the nurse to make decisions for her related to telling significant others about the pregnancy and/or options for pregnancy outcome. It is more therapeutic for the nurse to: • Provide clear, understandable information required for decision making • Assist in exploring possible solutions and consequences • Assist in implementing the decision selected by the teen-age client
Task: Establishing an Individual Identity **1. Physical**	
Denial of normal physical changes by dressing to hide them	Adolescents require: • Reassurance that there is a broad range of normal development and honest appraisal of whether theirs is normal • Accurate information about the normal sequence of physical development • Accurate information about the fertility cycle and their ability to reproduce
Fad diets to "improve" physical appearance	For pregnant adolescents, adequate nutritional and caloric intake is essential
Decreasing intake to reduce weight gain so pregnancy will not be obvious to others	Careful assessment of dietary habits, explanation of an adequate diet, and rationale, particularly in relation to adolescent health, are important Services of a nutritionist to plan intake that is both adequate and within the adolescent's lifestyle can be very valuable
2. Sexual	
Experimenting with different sexual behaviors	Nonjudgmental approach that assists adolescents to clarify behavior with which they are comfortable. Nurses are sometimes the "other adults" adolescents seek out
Discussing values/feelings, clarifying myths about sexuality with peers, parents, and other adults	A nonjudgmental approach that assists adolescents in: • Expressing values/feelings about sexuality • Understanding that they have a choice about sexual behavior • Understanding the risks of sexual activity • Dispelling myths about fertility and fecundity • Problem solving about responsible sexual behavior

(continued)

TABLE 9-23
Adolescent Development: Implications for Nursing Interventions with the Pregnant Adolescent *(Continued)*

Normal Adolescent Behavior	Implications for Nursing Interventions
3. Social/Emotional	
Behavior strongly influenced by peers (e.g., style, dress, academic attitude/success, extracurricular activities, drug use/abuse, sexual activity)	Nurse requires a thorough social history to assess risk factors applicable to each client and to determine their strengths, which will facilitate treatment. Because peer approval is so important for adolescents, the use of peer groups in learning and decision making can be very valuable
Development of skills valued by peers (e.g., hobbies, sports, other activities, constructive communication skills), which enhances self-esteem Negative behaviors learned for peer approval include drug use/abuse and exploitation of others	Knowledge of these positive and negative attributes is essential to understand adolescent strengths and to assess those factors that will impede compliance with treatment plans. As well, it will clarify areas to be discussed with the adolescent in relation to desired methods for change
Need for intimacy fulfilled by experimenting with behavior and one-to-one relationships in order to begin to identify the desirable characteristics in a future mate	Need to know the methods of communication used in these relationships, as well as the intensity of the relationship as perceived by both partners, to assess the potential role of the partner related to sexual activity, decisions about the pregnancy, and parenting
Ambivalent about roles of significant others	Assess the values and beliefs of the adolescent/significant others toward pregnancy and mother-child relationship • Father's level of involvement during pregnancy • Mother's family level of communication, closeness and opinions toward father • Mother's pre-existing relationship with father and opinions regarding continued involvement with pregnancy Assist in mediating father's involvement with baby if mother's family present obstacles Refer for individual/conjoint family therapy
4. Cognitive	
Career planning and academic/apprentice work necessary	Future plans are important for the nurse to know about, in order to assist the pregnant adolescent in long-term planning
Egocentrism: concern of the pregnant adolescent may be only for herself and not include the fetus	Recognize that this is normal for adolescents and not react judgmentally. Support her concerns for herself. Encourage the adolescent to plan for the baby. Indicate the value of healthy behaviors to her personally as opposed to the value for the infant
Idealism	Assess the level of this by asking where the adolescent expects to be in 5 yrs and how she will care for an infant, if that is her choice
Concrete thinking as opposed to use of abstractions	When introducing a treatment plan, ensure the adolescent understands her role by having her demonstrate the expected behavior
Peer counseling for psychosocial support	Age-appropriate teen (who has gone through experience of pregnancy) serves as role model and support Encourages expression of feelings and relates personally to teen's experiences Assists in solving problems confronted

- Fears in adolescence become more abstract and individualized than they were during the school-age years.
- The adolescent has more highly developed cognitive capabilities and social skills that enable her or him to use new means of coping.
- The ability to attain the postconventional level of moral development is not universally achieved.
- During the *individuating reflexive* stage of faith belief, the adolescent becomes more introspective and reflexive.
- Romantic friendships become an area of concern for the adolescent, exemplifying the adolescent's need to care for and be cared for by a significant other.
- A full set of permanent teeth is expected by age 13, with the exception of wisdom teeth, which erupt by 23 years.

- It is estimated that 20 million youths between the ages of 8 and 16 participate in organized sports.
- Accidents are the leading cause of adolescent mortality.
- It is estimated that 52 per cent of adolescents aged 15 to 19 are sexually active.
- Most adolescents are sexually active 6 to 12 months prior to seeking birth control.
- Research reveals that experimentation with alcohol and illicit drugs is common among adolescents.
- Over 1.1 million teen-agers become pregnant each year; the financial and resource costs to society are high, amounting to more than $16 billion each year.

Concepts Related to Nursing Assessment

- The nurse assesses the adolescent's level of cognitive development as a means of structuring interventions that are appropriate for the adolescent.
- Assessment of factors affecting the adolescent's ability to cope include temperament, family support, intelligence, and ability to communicate.
- The adolescent should have a health assessment every 2 years.
- Screening for STDs is done if the adolescent is sexually active.
- Findings of the adolescent's physical assessments will indicate whether the adolescent is an early, a middle, or a late maturer.
- A preseason sports assessment should be performed on all adolescent athletes who participate in competitive sports.

Concepts Related to Nursing Intervention

- The physical assessment provides the opportunity to provide anticipatory guidance regarding physical maturation and to correct the adolescent's misconceptions.
- The prepubertal adolescent girl should be prepared for the onset of menstruation as a normal physiologic process that requires additional attention but generally does not interrupt everyday activities.
- Application of the principles of cognitive development will enable the nurse to intervene more effectively with the adolescent.
- The nurse can assist young people in making decisions about sexuality by helping teen-agers explore their own values and with problem solving.
- The nurse designs interventions that are sensitive to the adolescent's need to be independent and autonomous.
- The nurse can assist the family to understand the adolescent's need to test a wide variety of friendships.
- The adolescent and family need encouragement to seek dental care during adolescence, since these are the peak years for dental caries.
- Anticipatory guidance on nutrition and eating behaviors should focus on providing accurate information on the five food groups, since adolescents are generally ill-informed about appropriate nutritional intake.
- Nurses in school settings can be watchful of the events that occur in the student's life and the potential risk for injury that can ensue.
- The adolescent's personal attitudes and values need to be clarified in order to provide counseling appropriate for the adolescent.
- The nurse can assist the adolescent in seeking treatment for substance abuse by providing support and information for referral.
- The first step in effectively caring for a pregnant adolescent is to establish a therapeutic relationship based on trust.

REFERENCES

American Academy of Pediatrics, Committee on Adolescence. (1990). Contraception and adolescents. *Pediatrics, 86,* 131–138.

American Academy of Pediatrics, Committee on Adolescence. (1989a). Counseling the adolescent about pregnancy. *Pediatrics, 83,* 132–134.

American Academy of Pediatrics, Committee on Infectious Diseases. (1991). *Report of the committee on infectious diseases. 1991 Red-book.* Elk Grove Village, IL: Author.

American Academy of Pediatrics, Committee on Nutrition. (1989b). Indications for cholesterol testing in children. *Pediatrics, 83,* 141–142.

American Academy of Pediatrics, Committee on Sports Medicine. (1989c). Anabolic steroids and the adolescent athlete. *Pediatrics, 83,* 127–128.

American Academy of Pediatrics, Committee on Sports Medicine. (1983). Nutrition and athletic performance. In N. Smith (Ed.), *Sports medicine: Health care for young athletes.* Evanston, IL: AAP, pp 161–175.

American Academy of Pediatrics, Committee on Sports Medicine. (1988). Recommendations for participation in competitive sports. *Pediatrics, 81,* 737–740.

American College of Sports Medicine. (1987). Position statement on the use and abuse of anabolic/androgenic steroids in sports. *Medicine Science Sports, 19,* 534–539.

American School Health Association (ASHA). Association for the Advancement of Health Education, and Society for Public Health Education, Inc. (1989). *The national adolescent student health survey: A report on the health of America's youth.* Oakland, CA: Third Party Publishing Company.

Anders, T. F., & Keener, M. A. (1983). Sleep-wake state development and disorders of sleeping infants, children, and adolescents. In M. D. Levine, et al (Eds.), *Developmental-behavioral pediatrics* (pp 596–606). Philadelphia: WB Saunders.

Baker, S., & Waller, A. (1989). Childhood injury state-by-state mortality facts. Baltimore: The Johns Hopkins Injury Prevention Center.

Banks, B., Silverman, R., Schwartz, R., & Tunnessen, W. (1992). Attitudes of teenagers toward sun exposure and sunscreen use. *Pediatrics, 89,* 40–42.

Behrman, R. (Ed.). (1992). *Nelson textbook of pediatrics* (14th ed.). Philadelphia: WB Saunders.

Bidwell, R., & Deisher, R. (1991). Adolescent sexuality: Current issues. *Pediatric Annals, 20,* 293–302.

Bloom, A. (1987). *The closing of the American mind: How higher education has failed democracy and impoverished the souls of today's students.* New York: Simon & Schuster.

Blum, R., McKay, C., & Rasnick, M. (1989). *The state of adolescent health in Minnesota.* Minneapolis: Minnesota Department of Health and University of Minnesota Adolescent Health Program. Adolescent Health Database Project.

Boston Women's Health Book Collective. (1992). *The new our bodies, our selves: Updated and expanded for the 1990s.* New York: Simon & Schuster.

Brown, L., Pottern, L., & Hoover, D. (1987). Testicular cancer in young men: The search for causes of epidemic increase in the United States. *Journal of Epidemiology and Community Health, 41,* 349–350.

Buckley, W., Yesalis, C., Friend, K., et al. (1988). Estimated prevalence of anabolic steroid use among male high school seniors. *Journal of the American Medical Association, 260,* 3441–3445.

Buhrmester, S., & Furman, W. (1987). The development of companionship and intimacy. *Child Development, 58,* 1101–1113.

Bullough, B., & Bullough, V. (1991). Contraceptives for teenagers. *Journal of Pediatric Health Care, 5,* 237–244.

Burke, P. (1987). Adolescents' motivation for sexual activity and pregnancy prevention. *Issues in Comprehensive Pediatric Nursing, 10,* 161–171.

Burr, M., & Haffner, D. (1986). *Public costs for teenage childbearing: Executive summary.* Washington, DC: Center for Population Options.

Castiglia, P. (1991a). Adolescent mothers. *Journal of Pediatric Health Care, 4,* 262–264.

Castiglia, P. (1991b). Delayed sexual development. *Journal of Pediatric Health Care, 5,* 213–214.

Cauce, A., & Strebnik, D. (1989). Peer networks and social support: A focus for preventive efforts with youths. In L. Bond & B. Lompas (Eds.), *Primary prevention and promotion in the schools* (pp. 235–256). Beverly Hills, CA: Sage.

Centers for Disease Control. (1991, June 21). Quarterly table reporting alcohol involvement in fatal motor-vehicle crashes. *Maternal and Child Health Practices* (3rd ed.). Oakland, CA: Third Party Publishing.

Cereva, N. (1989). Unwed teenage pregnancy: Family relationships with the father of the baby. *The Journal of Contemporary Human Services, 72,* 29–37.

Chassin, L., et al. (1986). Changes in peer and parent influence during adolescence: Longitudinal versus cross sectional perspectives on smoking initiation. *Developmental Psychology, 86,* 327–334.

Children's Defense Fund. (1990). *S.O.S. American! A children's defense budget.* Washington, DC: Author.

Children's Safety Network. (1991). *A data book of child and adolescent injury.* Washington, DC: National Center for Education in Maternal and Child Health.

Christoffel, K. (1990). Violent death and injury in U.S. children and adolescents. *American Journal of Diseases of Children, 144,* 677–706.

Clarke, B., & Strauss, S. (1992). Nursing role supplementation for adolescent parents: Prescriptive nursing practice. *Journal of Pediatric Nursing, 7*(5), 312–318.

Clasen, D., & Eicher, S. (1986). Perceptions of peer pressure, peer conformity dispositions, and self-reported behavior among adolescents. *Developmental Psychology, 22,* 521–530.

Coffman, S. (1991). Parent education for drowning prevention. *Journal of Pediatric Health Care, 5,* 141–146.

Cooley, M., & Unger, D. (1991). The role of family support in determining developmental outcomes in children of teen mothers. *Child Psychiatry and Human Development, 21,* 217–234.

Cromer, B., McLean, C., & Heald, F. (1992). A critical review of critical health screening in adolescents. *Journal of Adolescent Health, 13,* 35–65.

Davidson, D., Smith, R., & Quaqundah, P. (1990). Cholesterol screening in children during office visits. *Journal of Pediatric Health Care, 4,* 11–17.

Davis, R. (1988). Adolescent pregnancy and infant mortality: Isolating the effects of race. *Adolescence, 23,* 899–908.

Dolin, I., Kelly, D., & Beasley, M. (1992). Chronic self-destructive behavior in normative and delinquent adolescents. *Journal of Adolescence, 15,* 57–66.

Dore, M., & Dumois, A. (1990). Cultural differences in the meaning of adolescent pregnancy. *Journal of Contemporary Human Services, 71,* 93–101.

Dornbusch, S., et al. (1985). Single parents, extended households, and the control of adolescents. *Child Development, 56,* 326–341.

Duvall, E., & Miller, B. (1985). *Marriage and family development.* New York: Harper & Row.

Dyment, P. (1990). Steroids: Breakfast of champions. *Pediatrics in Review, 12,* 103–106.

Edelman, M. (1987). Teenage pregnancy: An epidemic takes its toll. In A. Cohn & L. Leach (Eds.), *Generations.* New York: Pantheon Books.

Ellis, D., & Davis, L. (1982). The development of self-concept boundaries across the adolescent years. *Adolescence, 17,* 695–710.

Elkind, D. (1970). *Children and adolescents, interpretive essays on Jean Piaget.* New York: Oxford University Press.

Elkind, D. (1978). Understanding the young adolescent. *Adolescence, 12,* 126–134.

Erikson, E. H. (1959). *Identity and the life cycle: Selected papers, psychological issues.* (Monograph, Vol. 1, No. 1). New York: International Press.

Erikson, E. (1963). *Childhood and society* (2nd ed.). New York: WW Norton.

Farley, D. (1990, February). Preventing toxic shock syndrome: New tampon labeling lets women compare absorbencies. *EDA Consumer, 24,* 6–9.

Fingerhut, L., & National Center for Health Statistics (NCHS) (Unpublished). (1988). Vital statistics: Mortality statistics for ages 0–19.

Forrest, J., & Singh, S. (1990). The sexual and reproductive behavior of American women 1982–1988. *Family Planning Perspectives, 22,* 206–214.

Fortenberry, J. (1992). Reliability of adolescents' report of height and weight. *Journal of Adolescent Health, 13,* 114–117.

Fowler, J. (1980). Moral stages and the development of faith. In B. Munsey (Ed.), *Moral development, moral education and Kohlberg.* Birmingham, AL: Religious Education Press.

Frager, B. (1991). Teenager child-bearing: Part 1, the problem hasn't gone away. *Journal of Pediatric Nursing, 6,* 131–133.

Freeman, E. (1988). Teenage fathers and the problems of teenage pregnancy. *Social Work in Education, 10,* 36–53.

Freud, S. (1957). In J. Strachey (Ed.), *The standard edition of the complete psychological works of Sigmund Freud* (Vol. 18). London: Hogarth.

Friedman, S. V., & Sarles, R. M. (1980). "Out of control" behavior in adolescents. *Pediatric Clinics of North America, 27,* 99–107.

Friman, P., & Finney, J. (1990). Health education for testicular cancer. *Health Education Quarterly, 17,* 443–453.

Frisancho, A., et al. (1984). Influence of growth status and placental function on birth weight of infants born to young still growing teenagers. *American Journal of Clinical Nutrition, 40,* 801–807.

Garmezy, N., & Rutter, M. (1984). *Stress, coping, and development in children.* Baltimore: Johns Hopkins University Press.

Garrick, J., & Requa, R. (1978). Injuries in high school sports. *Pediatrics, 61,* 645–649.

Gibbs, J., & Mokowitz-Sweet, G. (1991). Clinical and cultural issues in the treatment of biracial and bicultural adolescents. *Journal of Contemporary Human Services, 72,* 579–591.

Ginsberg, H., & Opper, S. (1979). *Piaget's theory of intellectual development* (2nd ed.). Englewood Cliffs, NJ: Prentice-Hall.

Gittes, E., & Irwin, C. (1993). Sexually transmitted diseases in adolescents. *Pediatrics in Review, 14*(5), 180–190.

Gjerde, P. (1986). The interpersonal structure of family interaction settings: Parent-adolescent relations in dyads and triads. *Developmental Psychology, 22,* 297–304.

Goldberg, L., Bents, R., Bosworth, E., Trevisan, L., & Elliot, D. (1991). Anabolic steroid education and adolescents: Do scare tactics work? *Pediatrics, 87,* 283–286.

Gordon, M. (1987). *Manual of nursing diagnosis.* New York: McGraw-Hill.

Guyer, B., & Gallagher, S. (1988). Childhood injuries and their prevention. In H. Wallace, G. Ryan, & A. Oglesby (Eds.), *Material and child health practices* (3rd ed.). Oakland, CA: Third Party Publishing.

Hanson, S. (1986). Healthy single parent families. *Family Relations, 35,* 125–132.

Heins, K. (1989). Commentary on adolescent acquired immunodeficiency syndrome: The next wave of the human immunodeficiency virus epidemic? *Journal of Pediatrics, 114,* 144–149.

Hetherington, E., Cox, M., & Cos, R. (1985). Long-term effects of divorce and remarriage on the adjustment of children. *Journal of the American Academy of Child Psychiatry, 24,* 518–530.

Holt, J., & Johnson, S. (1991). Developmental tasks: A key to reducing teenage pregnancy. *Journal of Pediatric Nursing, 6,* 191–196.

Howard, M., & Mitchell, M. (1993). Preventing teenage pregnancy: Some questions to be answered and some answers to be questioned. *Pediatric Annals, 22*(2), 109–119.

Howe, C. (1986, February). Developmental theory and adolescent sexual behavior. *Nurse Practitioner,* 65–71.

Huba, G., & Bentler, P. (1980). The role of peer and adult models for drug taking at different stages in adolescence. *Journal of Youth and Adolescence, 9,* 449–465.

Igoe, J. (1993). School-linked family health centers in health care reform. *Pediatric Nursing, 19*(1), 67–70.

Jaffe, L., Seahaus, M., & Wagner, C. (1988). Anal intercourse and knowledge of acquired immunodeficiency syndrome among minority group female adolescents. *Journal of Pediatrics, 112,* 1005–1007.

Jessor, R. (1982). Problem behavior and developmental transition in adolescence. *Journal of School Health, 52,* 295–300.

Johnson, M., Jay, M., Schoup, B., & Rickert, V. I. (1989). Anabolic steroid use by adolescent males. *Pediatrics, 83,* 921–924.

Johnson, F., Lay, P., & Wilbrandt, M. (1988). Teenage pregnancy: Issues, interventions and directions. *Journal of the National Medical Association, 80,* 145–152.

Johnston, L., O'Malley, P., & Bachman, J. (1985). *Use of licit and illicit drugs in America's high school students: 1975–1984.* Rockville, MD: National Institute on Drug Abuse.

Jones, E., et al. (1985). Teenage pregnancy in developed countries: Determinants and policy implications. *Family Planning Perspective, 17,* 53–63.

Jonides, L. (1990). Childhood obesity: An update. *Journal of Pediatric Health Care, 4,* 224–251.

Kaltar, N., Pickar, J., & Lesowitz, M. (1984). School-based development facilitation groups for children of divorce: A preventive intervention. *American Journal of Orthopsychiatry, 54,* 613–623.

Kastner, L. (1984). Ecological factors predicting adolescent contraceptive use: Implications for interventions. *Journal of Adolescent Health Care, 5,* 79–86.

Kegeles, S., Adler, N., & Irwin, C. (1989). Sexually active adolescents and condoms: Changes over the year in knowledge, attitudes and use. *American Journal of Public Health, 78,* 460–461.

Kohlberg, L. (1969). *Stages in the development of moral thought and action.* New York: Holt, Rinehart & Winston.

Kozak, J. (1991). Estimated discharges of patients under 20 years of age discharged from short-stay nonfederal hospitals with a first-line diagnosis of injury or poisoning: United States, 1989. [Unpublished data.]

Lee, E., & Jacobson, J. (1987). Accident reports: Survey of high school injuries. *Pediatric Nursing, 13,* 151–154.

Lee, E., Jacobson, J., & Levanas, V. (1989). Stressful life events and accidents at school. *Pediatric Nursing, 15,* 140–142.

Loris, P., et al. (1985). Weight gain and dietary intake of pregnant teenagers. *Journal of American Dietician Association, 85,* 1296–1305.

McAnarney, E. R. (1987). Young maternal age and adverse neonatal outcome. *American Journal of Diseases in Children, 141,* 1053–1059.

McDonald, N., et al. (1990). High-risk STD/HIV behavior among college students. *JAMA, 263,* 3155–3159.

Meyers, D., & Anderson, A. (1991). Adolescent addiction: Assessment and identification. *Journal of Pediatric Health Care, 5,* 86–93.

Millstein, S., Irwin, C., Adler, Cohn, L., Kegeles, S., & Dolcini, M. (1992). Health risk behaviors and health concerns among young adolescents. *Pediatrics, 89,* 422–428.

Mishell, D. (1989). Medical progress: Contraception. *New England Journal of Medicine, 320,* 777–787.

Mitchell, F., & Brindis, C. (1987). Adolescent pregnancy: The responsibility of policy makers. *HSR: Health Services Research, 22,* 399–437.

Moses, N., Banilivy, M., & Lefshitz, F. (1989). Fear of obesity among adolescent girls. *Pediatrics, 83,* 393–398.

National Institute on Drug Abuse. (1986). *(NIDA0919860 Cocaine use in America) (DHHS Publication No. ADM: 86–143).* Washington, DC: US Government Printing Office.

Nelson, P. (1986). Newsletters: An effective delivery mode for providing educational information and emotional support to single-parent families? *Family Relations, 35,* 183–188.

Nicholson, S. (1980). Growth and development. In J. Howe (Ed.), *Nursing care of adolescents* (pp 246–280). New York: McGraw-Hill.

Novotny, J. (1989). Adolescents, acne and the side effects of accutane. *Pediatric Nursing, 15,* 247–248.

Pass, C. (1986). Psychological factors, childbearing and black female adolescents. *Journal of Pediatric Nursing, 6,* 191–196.

Pendergrast, R., DuRant, R., & Gaillard, G. (1992). Attitudinal and behavioral correlates of condom use in adolescent males. *Journal of Adolescent Health, 13,* 133–139.

Piaget, J., & Inhelder, B. (1958). *The growth of logical thinking from children to adolescence.* New York: Basic Books.

Piaget, J. (1976). *The psychology of intelligence.* Towota, NJ: Littlefield, Adams & Company.

Piecchnik, S., & Corbett, M. (1985). Reducing low birth weight among socioeconomically high-risk adolescent pregnancies. *Journal of Nurse-Midwifery, 30,* 88–98.

Public/Private Ventures. (1990). Serving unwed teen fathers: A new demonstration. *Public/Private Ventures, 15,* 1.

Remafedi, G. (1987). Male homosexuality: The adolescent's perspective. *Pediatrics, 79,* 326–330.

Rosenfield, R. (1990). Clinical review, diagnosis and management of delayed puberty. *Journal of Clinical Endocrinology and Metabolism, 70,* 559–562.

Rowland, T. (1986). Preparticipation sports examination of the child and adolescent athlete: Changing views of an old ritual. *Pediatrician, 13,* 3–9.

Sachs, B. (1987). Cognitive screening for adolescent health education. *Journal of Pediatric Nursing, 2,* 113–119.

Sanford, N. (1989). Providing sensitive health care to gay and lesbian youth. *Nurse Practitioner, 14,* 30–37; 42, 47.

Schilder, P. (1935). *The image and appearance of the human body.* London: Kegan Paul.

Schlossberger, N., Turner, R., & Irwin, C. (1992). Validity of self report of pubertal maturation in early adolescents. *Journal of Adolescent Health, 13,* 109–113.

Sedgwick, R., & Hildebrand, S. (1980). The adolescent at risk: Crisis, the delicate balance. In J. Howe (Ed.), *Nursing care of adolescents* (pp 281–304). New York: McGraw-Hill.

Shearin, R., & Boehlke, J. (1989). Hormonal contraception. *Pediatric Clinics of North America, 36,* 697–715.

Silberstein, R., & Noack, P. (1990). Adolescents' orientations for development. In S. Jackson & A. Bosma (Eds.), *Coping and self concept in adolescence* (pp 112–127). Berlin and New York: Springer-Verlag.

Silberstein, R., Noack, P., & Van Eye, A. (1992). Adolescent development of romantic friendship and change in favorite leisure contexts. *Journal of Adolescent Research, 7,* 80–93.

Smith, K., Turner, J., & Jacobsen, R. (1987). Health concerns of adolescents. *Pediatric Nursing, 13,* 311–314.

Society for Adolescent Medicine. (1992a). Preparticipation sports evaluation. *Journal of Adolescent Medicine, 13,* 615–655.

Society for Adolescent Medicine. (1992b). Self screening. *Journal of Adolescent Medicine, 13,* 585–605.

Society of Obstetricians and Gynecologists of Canada, *Bulletin 2.* (1986, March/April). 15–16.

Spivak, H., & Weitzman, M. (1987, September 18). Social barriers faced by adolescent parents and their children. *Journal of the American Medical Association, 258,* 1500–1504.

Steinberg, L. (1986). Latchkey children and susceptibility to peer pressure: An ecological analysis. *Developmental Psychology, 22,* 433–439.

Steinberg, L. (1987). Single parents, stepparents, and the susceptibility of adolescents to antisocial peer pressure. *Child Development, 58,* 269–275.

Steinman, S., Zemmelman, S., & Knoblauch, T. (1985). A study of parents who sought joint custody following divorce: Who reaches agreement and sustains joint custody and who returns to court. *Journal of American Child Psychiatry, 24,* 554–562.

Stern, R., Weinstein, M., & Baker, S. (1986). Risk reduction for non melanoma skin cancer with childhood sunscreen use. *Archives of Dermatology, 122,* 537–544.

Stout, J., & Kirby, D. (1993). The effects of sexuality education on adolescent sexual activity. *Pediatric Annals, 22*(2), 120–126.

Sutherland, G. (1976). Fire on ice. *American Journal of Sports Medicine, 4,* 264–269.

Tanner, J. (1962). *Growth at adolescence.* Oxford: Blackwell Scientific Publications.

Thomas, S., & Groer, M. (1986). Relationship of demographics: Lifestyle and stress variables to blood pressure in adolescents. *Nursing Research, 35,* 169–171.

Thornton, B., & Ryckman, R. (1991). Relationship between physical attractiveness, physical effectiveness, and self-esteem: A cross sectional analysis among adolescents. *Journal of Adolescence, 14,* 85–98.

Troiden, R. (1988). Homosexual identity development. *Journal of Adolescent Health Care, 9,* 105–113.

Tuttle, J. (1991). Menstrual disorders during adolescence. *Journal of Pediatric Health Care, 5,* 197–203.

Unger, D., & Wandersman, L. (1988). The relation of family and partner support to the adjustment of adolescent mothers. *Child Development, 59,* 1056–1060.

US Bureau of the Census (1991). Marital status and living arrangements, 1990. Current Populations Reports, Series P–20, No. 450. Washington, DC: US Government Printing Office.

US Department of Agriculture, Human Nutrition Information Service. (1992). *Food guide pyramid* (Leaflet No. 572). Washington, DC: Author.

US Department of Health and Human Services (1988). *The health consequences of smoking, nicotine addiction.* (DHHS Publication No. CDC 88–8406). A Report of the Surgeon General. Rockville, MD: Author.

Vaughn, B., Block, J., & Block, J. (1988). Parental agreement on child rearing during early childhood and the psychological characteristics of adolescents. *Child Development, 59,* 1020–1033.

Wagnaar, A. (1981). *The raising of the legal drinking age in Michigan and Maine.* Rockville, MD: National Institute on Alcohol and Alcoholism.

Wells, K., & Copeland, B. (1985). Childhood and adolescent obesity: Progress in behavioral assessment and treatment. *Progress in Behavior Modification, 19,* 145–176.

White, J. (1987). Influence of parents, peers and problem-solving on contraceptive use. *Pediatric Nursing, 13,* 317–321.

Williams, L., & Pratt, W. (1990). *Wanted and unwanted childbearing in the United States: 1973–88. Advance Data from Vital Health Statistics.* Hyattsville, MD: US Department of Health and Human Services, Public Health Service, Centers for Disease Control, National Center for Health Statistics.

Wilson, A. (1990). Standards in maternal and oral health. *Journal of Public Health Dentistry, 5,* 432–438.

Windle, M., Miller-Tutzauer, C., Barnes, G., & Welte, J. (1991). Adolescent perspectives of help-seeking resources for substance abuse. *Child Development, 62,* 179–189.

Winkelstein, M. (1992). Adolescent smoking: Influential factors, past preventive efforts and future nursing implications. *Journal of Pediatric Nursing, 7*(2), 120–127.

Woods, E. (1991). Contraceptive choices for adolescents. *Pediatric Annuals, 20,* 313–321.

Yarcheski, A., & Mahon, N. (1986). Future time perspective and loneliness: A comparison between adolescents from father-absent and two parent families. *Journal of Pediatric Nursing, 1,* 102–110.

Zill, M. (1984). *Happy, healthy and insecure.* New York: Doubleday.

Zuckerman, B., et al. (1983). Neonatal outcome: Is adolescent pregnancy a risk factor? *Pediatrics, 71,* 489–493.

Zuckerman, B. S., Walker, D. K., Frank, D. A., Chase, C., & Hamburg, B. (1984). Adolescent pregnancy: Biobehavioral determinants of outcome. *Journal of Pediatrics, 105,* 857–863.

BIBLIOGRAPHY

Alan Guttmacher Institute. (1986). *Teenage pregnancy: The problem hasn't gone away.* New York: Author.

Alexander, C., & Guyer, B. (1993). Adolescent pregnancy: Occurrence and consequences. *Pediatric Annals, 22*(2), 85–89.

American Academy of Pediatrics, Committee on Adolescence. (1983). Homosexuality and adolescence. *Pediatrics, 72,* 249–250.

American Academy of Pediatrics, Committee on Infectious Diseases. (1989). Measles: Reassessment of the current immunizations policy. *Pediatrics, 84,* 1110–1113.

Aro, H., Hanniren, V., & Paronen, O. (1989). Social support, life events and psychosomatic symptoms among 14–16-year-old adolescents. *Social Science and Medicine, 29,* 1051–1056.

Baker, S., & Waller, A. (1989). *Childhood injury state-by-state mortality facts.* Baltimore: The Johns Hopkins Injury Prevention Center.

Bakkala, C. (1990). The role of the school nurse in suicide prevention. *School Nurse, 6,* 13–15.

Barry, M., Shirley, L., Grady, M., Etkind, S., Almeida, C., Bernardo, J., & Lamb, G. (1990). Tuberculosis infections in urban adolescents: Results of a school-based testing program. *American Journal of Public Health, 80,* 439–441.

Bearinger, L. (1990). Study group report on the impact of television on adolescent views of sexuality. *Journal of Adolescent Health Care, 11,* 71–75.

Bearinger, L. (1987). Priorities for adolescent health: Recommendations of a national conference. *MCN: American Journal of Maternal Child Nursing, 12,* 161–164.

Berlin, I. (1990). The role of community mental health center in prevention of infant, child and adolescent disorders: Retrospect and prospect. *Community Mental Health Journal, 26,* 89–106.

Boggio, N., & Cohall, A. (1990). Evaluating the adolescent: The search for the hidden agenda. *Emergency Medicine, 22,* 18–22, 27–32, 34.

Brindis, C., & Lee, P. (1990). Public policy issues affecting the health care delivery system of adolescents. *Journal of Adolescent Health Care, 11,* 387–392.

Brown, J., Childers, K., & Waszak, C. (1990). Television and adolescent sexuality. *Journal of Adolescent Health Care 11,* 62–70.

Browne, C., & Urback, P. (1989). Pregnant adolescents: Expectation vs. reality. *Canadian Journal of Public Health, 80,* 227–229.

Castiglia, P. (1990). Suicide in adolescents. *Journal of Pediatric Health Care, 4,* 149–151.

Castro, O. (1990). Adolescents and AIDS: A special population. *NAACOG's Clinical Issues in Perinatal and Women's Health Nursing, 1,* 99–114.

Chestnut, C. (1989, September/October). Is osteoporosis a pediatric disease? Peak bone mars attainment in the adolescent female. *Public Health Report Supplement,* 50–54.

Church, J. (1987). Examination of the adolescent: A practical guide. *Journal of Pediatric Health Care 2,* 3–12.

Craft, M. (1987). Health care preference of rural adolescents: Types of services and companion choices. *Journal of Pediatric Nursing, 2,* 3–12.

Davis, B. (1990). Loneliness in children and adolescents. *Issues in Comprehensive Pediatric Nursing, 13,* 59–69.

Deatrick, J. (1990). Developing self regulation in adolescents with chronic conditions. *Holistic Nursing Practice, 5,* 17–24.

Denholm, C. (1989). Reactions of adolescents following hospitalization for acute conditions. *Children's Health Care, 18,* 210–217.

Desmond, S., Price, J., Lock, R., Smith, D., & Steward, P. (1990). Urban black and white adolescents' physical fitness status and perceptions of exercise. *Journal of School Health, 60,* 220–226.

Diaz, A., Jaffe, L., Leadbetter, B., & Levin, L. (1990). Frequency of use, knowledge and attitudes toward the contraceptive sponge among inner-city Black and Hispanic adolescent females. *Journal of Adolescent Health Care, 11,* 125–127.

Domino, G., & Leenaars, A. (1989). Attitudes toward suicide: A comparison of college students. *Suicide and Life-Threatening Behavior, 19,* 160–173.

Dryfoos, J. G. (1988). School-based health clinics: Three years of experience. *Family Planning Perspectives, 20,* 193–200.

Dunne-Maxim, K., McIntosh, J., & Dunne, E. (1988). *The Aftermath of Suicide.* Norton.

Duvall, E. (1985). *Family development* (5th ed.). New York: JB Lippincott.

Frager, B. (1991). Teenage childbearing: Part II, program and policies. *Journal of Pediatric Nursing, 6,* 202–205.

Garrison (1989). Studying suicidal behavior in the schools. *Suicide and Life-Threatening Behavior, 19,* 120–131.

Gattuso, J., Hinds, P., & Weekes, P. (1990). Why longitudinal research with adolescents who have cancer? *Journal of Pediatric-Oncology Nursing, 7,* 158–160.

Gibbs, J. T. (1988). Issues in black youth suicide. *Suicide and Life-Threatening Behavior. 18,* 73–90.

Gortmaker, A., Walker, D., Weitzman, M., & Sobol, A. (1990). Chronic conditions, socioeconomic risks and behavioral problems in children and adolescents. *Pediatrics, 85,* 267–276.

Greydonus, D., & Shearin, R. (1990). *Adolescent sexuality and gynecology.* Philadelphia: Lea & Febiger.

Gutierrez, Y., & King, J. (1993). Nutrition during teenage pregnancy. *Pediatric Annals, 22*(2), 99–108.

Hayes, C. (1987). *Risking the future: Adolescent sexuality, pregnancy and childbearing.* Washington, DC: National Academy Press.

Heiney, S., Wells, L., Sweggert, E., & Coleman, B. (1990). Psychosocial support programs for adolescents with cancer and their parents. *Journal of Pediatric Oncology Nursing, 7,* 75–76.

Heiney, S., Wells, L., Coleman, B., Sweggert, E., & Ruffin, J. (1990). Lasting impressions: A psychosocial support program for adolescents with cancer and their parents. *Cancer Nursing, 13,* 13–20.

Herrman, C. (1989). A descriptive study of daily activities and role conflict in single adolescent mothers. *Occupational Therapy in Health Care, 6,* 53–68.

Hinds, P. (1990). Quality of life in children and adolescents with cancer. *Seminars in Oncology Nursing, 6,* 285–291.

Hinds, P., Scholes, S., Gattuso, J., Roggins, M., & Heffner, B. (1990). Adaptation to illness in adolescents with cancer. *Journal of Pediatric Oncology Nursing, 7,* 64–65.

Hinds, P. (1988). The relationship of nurses' caring behaviors with hopefulness and health care outcomes in adolescents. *Archives of Psychiatric Nursing, 2,* 21–29.

Hingson, R., Struain, L., Berlin, B., & Heeren, T. (1993). Beliefs about AIDS, use of alcohol and drugs and unprotected sex among Massachusetts adolescents. *American Journal of Public Health, 80,* 295–299.

Hobbie, C. (1990). Sex education for children and adolescents. *Journal of Pediatric Health Care, 4,* 98–99.

Hosltey, S., Gussard, R., Hassler, C., & Linden, P. (1989). Adolescent autonomy project: Transition skills for adolescents with physical disability. *Children's Health Care, 18,* 12–18.

Inland, D. (1990). New attitude/new look: An African American adolescent health education program. *Pediatric Nursing, 16,* 175–178, 205.

Jacks, M. (1989). Personal fable: A potential explanation for risk taking behavior in adolescents. *Journal of Pediatric Nursing, 4,* 334–338.

Janke, J. (1989). Dealing with AIDS and the adolescent population. *Nurse Practitioner: American Journal of Primary Health Care, 14,* 35–36, 38, 41.

Jones, M., & Mondy, L. (1990). Prenatal education outcomes for pregnant adolescents and their infants. *Journal of Adolescent Health Care, 11,* 437–444.

Jones, M., & Bonte, C. (1990). Conceptualizing community interventions in social service needs of pregnant adolescents. *Journal of Pediatric Health Care, 4,* 193–201.

Jung, F., & Ingelfinger, J. (1993). Hypertension in childhood and adolescence. *Pediatrics in Review, 14*(5), 169–179.

Kalmuss, D. (1986). Contraceptive use: A comparison between ever-and-never-pregnant adolescents. *Journal of Adolescent Health Care, 7,* 3332–3337.

Kegles, S., Adler, N., & Irwin, C. (1989). Adolescents and condoms: Association of beliefs with intentions to use. *American Journal of Disease of Children, 143,* 911–915.

Klein, J., Berry, C., & Felice, M. (1990). The development of testicular self examination instructional booklet for adolescents. *Journal of Adolescent Health Care, 1,* 235–239.

Kotagal, U. (1993). Newborn consequences of teenage pregnancy. *Pediatric Annals, 22*(2), 127–132.

Koval, J. (1989). Violence in dating relationships. *Journal of Pediatric Health Care, 3,* 298–304.

Lachapelle, D., Desaulneers, G., & Bujold, N. (1989). Dental health education for adolescents: Assessing attitude and knowledge following two educational approaches. *Canadian Journal of Public Health, 80,* 339–344.

Lamb, J. (1990). The suicidal adolescent: How you can be of help. *Nursing, 20,* 72–73, 75–76.

Liese, L., Swoden, L., & Ford, L. (1989). Partner status, social support and psychological adjustment during pregnancy. *Family Relations, 38,* 311–316.

Magilvy, J. (1987). The health of teenagers: A focused ethnographic study. *Public Health Nursing, 4,* 35–42.

Manning, M. (1990). Health assessment of the early adolescent: Challenges and clinical issues. *Nursing Clinics of North America, 25,* 823–831.

McBride, A. (1987). *The secret of a good life with your teenager: Thriving in the second decade of parenthood.* New York: New York Times Books.

National Academy of Sciences. (1989). *Recommended dietary allowances* (10th ed.). Washington, DC: National Academy Press.

Nelson, P. (1990). Repeat pregnancy among adolescent mothers: A review of the literature. *Journal of National Black Nurses Association, 4,* 28–34.

Newacheck, P. (1989). Adolescents with special health needs: Prevalence, severity and access to health services. *Pediatrics, 84,* 872–881.

Newacheck, P. (1989). Improving access to health services for adolescents from economically disadvantaged families. *Pediatrics, 84,* 1056–1063.

Newacheck, P., & McManus, M. (1989). Health Insurance Status of Adolescents in the United States. *Pediatrics, 84,* 699–708.

Newacheck, P., McMouers, M., & Brindis, C. (1990). Financing health care for adolescents: Problems, prospects and proposals. *Journal of Adolescent Health Care, 11,* 398–403.

Ohanian, V. (1990). Informational needs of child and adolescent cancer patients and their parents. *Journal of Pediatric Oncology Nursing, 7,* 63–64.

Paperny, D., Aono, J., Lehman, R., Hammar, S., & Risser, J. (1990). Computer-assisted detection and intervention in adolescent high risk behaviors. *Journal of Pediatrics, 116,* 456–462.

Pendergrast, R. (1990). Skateboard injuries in children and adolescents. *Journal of Adolescent Health Care, 11,* 408–412.

Pete, J. (1990). Self-concept: Younger vs older black, pregnant adolescents. *Journal of National Black Nurses Association, 4,* 35–44.

Pfeffer, C. (1989). Suicidal preadolecents and adolescent inpatients. *Suicide and Life-Threatening Behavior, 19,* 58–78.

Pidgeon, V. (1989). Compliance with chronic illness regimens: School-aged children and adolescents. *Journal of Pediatric Nursing, 4,* 36–47.

Porter, L., & Sobong, L. (1990). Differences in maternal perception of the newborn among adolescents. *Pediatric Nursing, 16,* 101–104.

Preskar, K., Lamb, J., & Norton, M. (1990). Adolescent mental health: collaboration among psychiatric mental health nurses and school nurses. *Journal of School Health, 60,* 69–71.

Proctor, S. (1986). A developmental approach to pregnancy prevention with early adolescent females. *Journal of School Health, 56,* 313–316.

Providing medical services through school-based health programs . . . to adolescents. *Journal of School Health, 60,* 87–91.

Quine, S., & Stephenson, J. (1990). Predicting smoking and drinking intentions and behaviors of pre-adolescents: The influence of parents, siblings and peers. *Family Systems Medicine, 8,* 191–200.

Rimsza, M. (1989). An illustrated guide to adolescent gynecology. *Pediatric Clinics of North America, 36,* 639–663.

Saunders, J. M., & Buckingham, S. (1988). When depression turns deadly. *Nursing '88, 7,* 59–64.

Schneck, M., Sideresk, Fox, R., & Dupuis, L. (1990). Low income pregnant adolescents and their infants: Dietary findings and health outcomes. *Journal of the American Dietetic Association. 90,* 555–558.

Simons-Morton, B., Brink, S., Simons-Morton, D., McIntyre, R., Chapman, M., Longonia, J., & Parcel, G. (1989). An ecological approach to the prevention of injuries due to drinking and driving. *Health Education Quarterly, 16,* 397–411.

Slap, G., Vorters, D., Chadhuri, S., & Centor, M. (1989). Risk factors for attempted suicide during adolescence. *Pediatrics, 84,* 762–772.

Stanley, S. (1990). Review of the Institute of Medicine report on children and adolescents. *Journal of Child and Adolescent Psychiatric and Mental Health Nursing, 3,* 62–64.

Stevens-Simon, C., Fullor, S., & McAnarney, E. (1989). Teenage pregnancy: Caring for adolescent mothers with their infants in pediatric settings. *Clinical Pediatrics, 28,* 282–283.

Stiffman, A., & Carls, F. (1990). Behavioral risks for human immunodeficiency virus infection in adolescent medical patients. *Pediatrics, 85,* 303–310.

Story, M. (1990). Study group report on the impact of television on adolescent nutritional status. *Journal of Adolescent Health Care, 11,* 82–85.

Stout, J. W., & Rivara, F. (1989). Schools and sex education: Does it work? *Pediatrics, 83,* 375–378.

Tucker, S. (1990). Adolescent patterns of communication about the menstrual cycle, sex and contraception. *Journal of Pediatric Nursing, 5,* 393–400.

US Department of Agriculture, Human Nutrition Information Service. (1992). *Food guide pyramid* (Leaflet no. 572). Washington, DC: Author.

Valente, S. M. (1989). Adolescent suicide: Assessment and intervention. *Journal of Adolescent Psychiatric Mental Health Nursing, 2,* 33–39.

Valente, S. M., Saunders, J. M., & Street, R. (1988). Adolescent bereavement after suicide. *Journal of Counseling and Development, 67,* 174.

Van Cleve, S., & Sadler, L. (1990). Adolescent parents and toddlers: Strategies for intervention. *Public Health Nursing, 7,* 22–27.

Wasserman, G., Brunelli, S., & Rauh, V. (1990). Social supports and living arrangements of adolescent and adult mothers. *Journal of Adolescent Research, 5,* 54–66.

Yarcheski, A., & Mahon, N. (1989). A causal model of positive health practices: The relationship between approach and replication. *Nursing Research, 38,* 88–93.

Zabin, L. S., Hirsch, M. B., Smith, E. A., Street, R., & Hardy, J. B. (1986). Evaluation of pregnancy prevention programs for urban teenagers. *Family Planning Perspectives, 18,* 119–126.

UNIT • THREE

Promoting Health

CHAPTER • 10

Health Concepts: Children's Perceptions and Behaviors

Mabel Hunsberger

RELATED TOPICS
Children and poverty, Chapter 1
Promoting Healthy Parenting, Chapter 12
History and physical assessment, Chapter 13
Fostering Self-Esteem, Chapter 14
Children's concepts of illness, Chapter 18
Principles of administering medications, Chapter 24
The immune response, Chapter 37
Childhood infectious disease, Chapter 39

LEARNING OBJECTIVES

- **Identify major themes or subconcepts that are reflected in common definitions of health.**
- **Discuss alternate theoretical approaches used to explain how children view health and are motivated to perform healthy behaviors.**
- **Differentiate the clinical application of the terms "prevention," "health maintenance," and "health promotion."**
- **Differentiate between a child's role as an active and as a passive participant in achieving health.**
- **Discuss the nurse's role in promoting self-care behavior in children and their families.**

- Describe the impact of family, school, and peers on the health behaviors of children.
- Identify the nurse's role in health supervision, managing minor illness, and immunizing children.
- Define routine immunization schedules.
- Identify adjustments in immunization schedules made in special circumstances.

To a large extent, children's adoption of healthy behaviors is influenced by role models and environmental factors. Children's beliefs about how people stay healthy and how they get sick also influence their health practices. Because children model the behavior of others, health promotion of children necessarily focuses on the entire family. Self-responsibility of each family member for maintaining and improving health is the nurse's ultimate goal.

This chapter examines definitions of health, identifies health subconcepts that are important to pediatric nursing, and discusses the development of children's health attitudes and behaviors. Finally, health care management, including child health visits and childhood immunizations, is presented, with an emphasis on the nurse's role in health promotion.

The overall goal of pediatric nurses in child health promotion is to provide all children with the best possible environment in which to develop. This means that nurses facilitate families to create a health promoting environment for children and assist them to access health care resources needed to maximize the health of children and families. The underlying philosophy is that nurses facilitate parents and children to take responsibility for their own health.

Health care supervision involves a broad view of the concept of health, with the recognition that a child's home, school, and community have an impact on the child's opportunity to achieve health. Nurses have opportunities to promote children's health through counseling and teaching parents about children's health and preparing them for growth and developmental changes. Health promotion is a component of patient care in acute care as well as primary health care settings. Additionally, children with chronic conditions present a unique challenge and are in particular need of health promotion services because of the inherent difficulties and susceptibilities they face in just "growing up" and "staying healthy." As health promotion becomes a primary goal in all settings, nurses need to expand their knowledge and skills in this area of practice. Availability of health care is fundamental to this goal.

A Concern for Our Children's Health

Child health cannot be addressed without giving recognition to the growing problem of poor and underserved children (Haggerty, 1991; Maurer, 1991; Harvey, 1991). Children, especially young children, continue to be the single largest poverty group in the United States and are inadequately insured (Maurer, 1991). Even those who are insured do not necessarily receive care that focuses on health promotion. Health insurance coverage frequently provides for major medical and catastrophic coverage, but not health promotion and particularly routine immunizations (Oberg, 1990). These issues are further addressed in Chapter 1. These dilemmas exist amid a seemingly new health consciousness as evidenced by officially established goals and strategies that include: the World Health Organization (WHO) global strategy for "health for all by the year 2000"; health promotion and disease prevention objectives for the United States, as identified in the report "Healthy People 2000" by the US Department of Health and Human Services (1990); and in Canada, "Achieving Health for All: A Framework for Health Promotion" (Epp, 1986).

There is an ongoing concern for the welfare of our children (Frager, 1990; Igoe, 1990; Velsor-

Friedrich, 1991) with the recognition that "major changes in social, political, and environmental conditions of living . . . of large segments of society are necessary if significant improvements in health are to occur during the next century" (Pender, 1990). In addition to the pediatric nurse's focus on health promotion in clinical practice, there is an urgent need for political involvement of health care professionals to advocate for health promotion in child care.

Translation of the goals of health promotion into clinical nursing is complicated by the diversity of beliefs about two key questions: (1) What is health? and (2) What motivates healthy behavior? These questions are the subject of considerable debate because health is a concept that is individually interpreted. When applied to children, these questions are even more perplexing. Fundamental to promoting health of children is an understanding of the meaning of health and its related concepts. Following is an overview of the concept of health and its related themes.

A Definition of Health

No universal norms of the concept of health exist. Health is perceived differently across individuals and cultures, and varies over time. By simplest definition, "health" means being sound in body, mind, and spirit (Hales, 1992). In 1947, WHO defined health as "a state of complete physical, mental, and social well-being, not merely the absence of disease or infirmity." The traditional view of health prior to this time had been that health is the absence of any overt disease. The WHO definition has one short-coming: it does not allow for the various *degrees* of health states individuals can attain. However, three characteristics of the WHO definition that are essential to a conceptualization of health are:

- The individual is viewed as a total person rather than the sum of his or her parts.
- Health is presented in the context of internal and external environments.
- Health is equated with predictive and creative living (Pender, 1990).

Although health is not a universally agreed-on concept, the WHO definition, despite criticism, has endured.

Can health and illness be viewed as a continuum, with health and illness at opposite poles? This view is criticized because it suggests that in the absence of illness a person is automatically healthy and that health cannot be achieved by someone with an illness or disability. In contrast, current nursing theories view health as a dynamic process; it is also described as a functional state, as personal and subjective and a life span process (King, 1990; Pender, 1990). A "health within illness" perspective focuses on "getting in touch with the illness" rather than viewing it as an enemy and "getting rid of" the illness (Moch, 1989). All of these interpretations support the view that a pathologic condition does not preclude achievement of health and well-being. Across the many definitions of health, some common themes are noted. Following is a discussion of the most common themes reflected in definitions of health: *adaptation and stability, actualization, effectiveness, and responsibility for one's own health.*

Adaptation and Stability

The themes of adaptation and stability reflect the view that health exists when a person effectively interacts with the physical and social environments. These concepts are based on the writings of Dubos (1959, 1965) and Selye (1976), who view health as a state dependent on one's ability to adjust to the various internal and external environmental tensions. According to this view, disease occurs when there is failure to cope with changes in the environment.

Adaptation and stability are common themes in theoretical models of nursing (Levine, 1971; King, 1981; Roy, 1976). The focus of nursing care from this perspective is to facilitate adaptive behavior or reduce the impact of the environment when unusual stressors or weakened coping mechanisms threaten to alter one's state of health. From a framework of adaptation, the nurse caring for children and families is concerned with environmental stressors and developmental crises of the child as well as of the family. If achievement of optimal growth and development is the goal, then one must go beyond merely surviving crises. Health promotion is a proactive process in which anticipatory guidance, teaching, counseling, and health care supervision support ongoing adaptation and stability.

Self-Actualization and Wellness

The concept of wellness is similar to that of health, but not identical. To understand the relationships, the concepts of *illness, health,* and *wellness* have been described as follows: comparing these concepts to a car, having a disease (illness) is like going in reverse; absence of disease (health) is like being in neutral; positive health changes (wellness) is like being in drive-forward motion (Hales, 1992). Good health has also been described as a *state of being at one point* along the health continuum, whereas wellness is a process of *reaching a higher level of being* in which the individual actively participates to achieve self-actualization (Bruhn & Cordova, 1977). Wellness is related to learning and development with cumulative results, in contrast to a state of homeostasis in which there is freedom from illness. No one level of wellness exists; each person has the potential to reach a level of wellness that is optimal for that person (Dunn, 1961). Optimal health for each individual is different because it is determined by past experiences, genetic potential, and environmental circumstances (Bedworth & Bedworth, 1982).

Application of these concepts to a clinical situation means that the presence of a disease does not equate to illness. An individual with a chronic illness or disability may in fact function at maximal capacity (wellness); on the other hand, a person without an illness may function at a level below her or his potential (illness). This concept has particular relevance to the care of children and families. The variations in how developing children interact within a growing family are infinite. The opportunities available to children have a long-lasting impact on their health behaviors. The nurse strives to advocate for children so that they can reach their maximal potential. Recognition of the individual nature of what constitutes wellness for each child in a particular family is the foundation of pediatric nursing practice.

Effectiveness

Health can be thought of in terms of effectiveness. Health is "the quality of our physical, psychological, and sociological functioning that enables us to deal adequately with self and others in a variety of situations" (Bedworth & Bedworth, 1982). A similar theme is reflected by Bruhn and Cordova (1977), who include the idea of competence in their definition of wellness, describing it as "the social ability to master one's self and one's situation in life" (active coping). The ideas of effectiveness and competence are also inherent in the role-performance model (Smith, 1981), which views health as effective performance of one's roles. To promote competence and effectiveness in the developing child, the scope of nursing care must broaden to include strategies that foster a child's self-esteem and support the development of a good self-concept. (See Chapter 14 for discussion of development of self-esteem.)

Self-Responsibility

That a healthy person has the capacity for self-responsibility in health care is a theme reflected in the holistic view of health. The idea of holism originates from gestalt theory, which implies a "state of feeling complete and balanced" (Payne, 1983). It is based on the concept that each individual is an integrated whole with constant interaction of the biologic, psychologic, and sociologic dimensions.

Self-care is a predominant theme in Orem's model (1991) and is viewed as a learned behavior relative to beliefs, habits, and practices within the cultural group of an individual. It is defined as a deliberate activity and is one's personal, ongoing contribution to one's own health and well-being.

Self-responsibility for one's own health is an important concept to incorporate into nursing practice with children and families. Children are taught to take responsibility for their health; as well, parents must be encouraged in self-responsibility so that they model positive health behavior to their children. Children adopt many of their parents' health-related habits and practices; therefore, nursing interventions necessarily include the parents.

Children's Health Beliefs and Behaviors: Theoretical Approaches

An important role of the nurse is to teach children to become active in health-promoting activities. Self-empowerment of children by teaching them decision making, coping, and skills in community participation is required to move children out of a passive role into one of action (Hart-Zeldin et al, 1990). To increasingly involve children in their own health care, nurses need to understand how children view health and recognize factors that motivate behavior. Some theoretical approaches used to explain children's concepts of health and health behaviors include: (1) the cognitive developmental view based on Piagetian theory, (2) the expectancy model based on social psychology or social learning theory, (3) locus of control, and (4) motivation.

Cognitive-Developmental Model

Children's concepts of health change qualitatively as cognitive skills develop, advancing from preoperational through concrete and formal operations (Natapoff, 1978; Kalnins & Love, 1982; Mickalide, 1986). This progression is summarized in Table 10–1. In a comparison of handicapped and able-bodied children, Natapoff and Essoka (1989) found that, in children 6 to 14 years of age, ideas about health were influenced more by age than by handicap. Children at 10 to 11 years of age, in particular, define health as the ability to do things they want to do, an enabling concept, and older children (12 to 14 years of age) tend to define health as not being sick. Equating health with a state of physical fitness, a view commonly held by children, increases with age and is a reflection of society's emphasis on physical fitness (Natapoff & Essoka, 1989).

An important practical implication of how cognition affects health behavior is the child's immaturity in understanding causality. Causality is not well understood until formal thought processes are acquired (after age 11 years). The notion of prevention, therefore, is not grasped until this time because it requires an understanding that a specific action or lack of action at present can bring about a changed state in the future. Children's concepts of illness are also related to cognitive development (Bibace & Walsh, 1980; Campbell, 1991) and are discussed in Chapter 18.

TABLE 10-1
Health Concepts, Cognitive Skills, and Self-Responsibility by Age, with Teaching Approaches to Them

Cognitive Level	Health Concept	Responsibility for Self-Initiated Care	Age-Related Teaching Approach
0–23 Mos			
Sensorimotor	No concept, learns to value needs on basis of how well and how consistently they are met	Child moves from total dependence on caregiver to performance of simple tasks	Basic needs are generally met by caregiver
24–47 Mos			
Preoperational (preconceptual)	Children merely imitate behavior of role models that are satisfying and/or earn reward; health concepts in children at this age have not been sufficiently studied	Some capacity to carry out tasks to promote own health if taught skills and allowed opportunity to take responsibility; likes to practice wellness behaviors	Continue meeting basic needs but steadily demand that child master skills of daily living; role model wellness behaviors; reward imitation. Play with child to learn the child's perceptions since they are not verbalized adequately
4–7 Yrs			
Preoperational (perceptual or intuitive) Egocentric, cannot consider whole and part simultaneously. Cannot conserve, i.e., cannot keep the original in mind and simultaneously consider a change	Health involves a series of health practices (eat right, brush teeth, stay clean), and health is apparent when one is able to perform usual activities. Does not consider cause and effect, cannot be part healthy and part not healthy at the same time. Sickness is unrelated to health status at another time	Can carry out many tasks to promote own health, seeks responsibility; practice important. Can take independent action to identify many health needs and can identify some realistic solutions	Encourage any account of what the health need is, what caused it, what the child might do to resolve that need. Correct misperceptions. Use teaching techniques that provide tactile, visual, auditory, and motor experience. Teaching should be related to child's own experiences
7–11 Yrs			
Concrete operational Cause and effect are considered. Gradual increase in causal reasoning. Decentralization but still favors concrete reality. Able to conserve (consider original and changed state). Can classify objects and concrete ideas	Concept of health as sense of physical well-being, evidenced by "feeling good or being in shape." Believes can be part healthy and part not healthy	Can plan for and take initiative to carry out most health needs if has learned trust and autonomy. Can actively participate in managing own health needs. Acute interest in health education. Can consider possible risks and benefits of health behaviors if allowed to participate in problem solving	Share assessment and/or findings, to allow child to perceive changes in health status. Allow time for child to validate perceptions of needs and what actions should be taken; respect views and opinions. Give simple rationale for health practices/procedures. Make the invisible processes of health real with diagrams, models. Teach the skill/procedure (tangible, concrete) then give the rationale (abstract) in simple terms

(continued)

Expectancy Theory

According to expectancy theory, a behavior is performed if one expects that the behavior will bring about a desired outcome. This theory is based on the social psychology of Lewin (1935), from which the social learning theories of Rotter (1954) and Bandura* (1977) and the health belief model (Becker, 1974; Rosenstock, 1974) are derived. Social learning theory is based on concepts similar to the health belief model with the addition of the concept of self-efficacy, the conviction that one can successfully perform the behavior required to produce the expected outcome. According to the health belief model, the likelihood of taking preventive actions is determined by *perceived benefits of preventive action* minus *perceived barriers to preventive action* (Rosenstock et al, 1988).

*Bandura's theory has now been relabeled as social cognitive theory (Bandura, 1986).

TABLE 10-1
Health Concepts, Cognitive Skills, and Self-Responsibility by Age, with Teaching Approaches to Them *(Continued)*

Cognitive Level	Health Concept	Responsibility for Self-Initiated Care	Age-Related Teaching Approach
Above 11 Yrs			
Formal operational Realizes realm of possible and hypothetical as well as the real. Develops theories. Craves details for egocentric purposes primarily. Can consider abstractions; deductive reason develops	Concept of health as long-term physical, emotional, social stability though superimposed brief illness may cause temporary instability. Evidenced by feeling good, being in control of self, being able to participate in desired activities. Future health is considered	Can assume full responsibility to identify health needs, determine possible resolutions, and carry them out. Can experientially apply wellness to life choices	Significant other role models of wellness behavior crucial to overcoming peer pressures. Inform of realities of health problems and the possible outcomes; honesty imperative to child's cooperation. Present all details, relate them to child personally. Especially likes theoretical explanations and discussions. Discuss the effects of health problems and health behaviors on the future. Let child determine the possible resolutions to health needs and collaborate to determine management. Begin by presenting rationale for a skill/procedure, then give details of performing it

Data from Bruhn and Cordova, 1977; Pidgeon, 1977; Natapoff, 1978, 1982; Flaherty, 1986; Logsdon, 1991; Chiloh & Waiser, 1991.

The perceived benefits of preventive action are modified by the person's perceived susceptibility* and threat of the disease. The greater the sense of vulnerability* and the more serious the threat, the more likely a preventive action will be taken. If it is expected that the behavior can effect a positive outcome, the likelihood of action is even greater. This theory is related to the nurse's work of motivating parents to follow through on health care for their children. Although increased perceived vulnerability has been found to influence adult health behaviors positively, the same relationships have not been observed in children. Children have been found *not* to be highly motivated by health goals and *not* to perceive themselves as particularly vulnerable to health problems (Gochman & Saucier, 1982).

A sense of vulnerability seems to be related to a child's self-concept and anxietylike states. Children with lower self-concepts and greater anxiety have been found to perceive themselves to be more vulnerable to health problems compared with children with higher self-concepts and less anxiety (Gochman & Saucier, 1982). Furthermore, children seem to *decrease* healthy behaviors as their sense of vulnerability is *increased*. Thus, children with a lower self-concept and higher anxiety states demonstrate fewer healthy behaviors. These findings suggest that perceived vulnerability is an anxietylike state that makes an individual feel incapable of coping and causes a person to see oneself in a basically negative way. Perceived vulnerability is, therefore, viewed as a personality characteristic and part of a child's cognitive makeup (Gochman & Saucier, 1982). The finding that children's reported vulnerability was generally consistent across health problems and over time further substantiates the belief that it is a component of the basic nature of a child. This has particular relevance for the teaching of children, in that recognizing that children's responses to educational programs may be affected by differences in self-concept.

*The term "vulnerability" refers to a likelihood of encountering a variety of health problems, in contrast to "susceptibility," which is concerned with a certain isolated problem (Gochman & Saucier, 1982).

Locus of Control

The way children think about influencing their health varies. Some may feel they can significantly affect their own health (internal control), whereas others may feel helpless and view forces outside of themselves as affecting their health (external control). The degree of internal control felt by children increases with socioeconomic status as well as with age (Bush & Iannotti, 1988). Scales to measure this concept and its usefulness continue to be evaluated (Bush & Iannotti, 1988; Hearne & Klockars, 1988; Parcel, 1988; O'Brien et al, 1989). There is increasing support for the belief that individuals are not either externally or internally controlled but rather the locus of control is a continuous variable that changes over time (La Montagne & Hepworth, 1991). This variable in healthy behavior is closely related to the concept of motivation, both of which deal with stimuli as a factor in health behavior.

Motivation

Children's motivation in health behavior is described as intrinsic or extrinsic. For intrinsically motivated children, accomplishment of health behaviors and experiencing positive outcomes reinforces their own sense of competency and self-determination (Cox et al, 1990). The nurse then helps the child to make the logical connection between the desired health outcomes and the chosen behavior. This process of feedback not only reinforces the child's sense of competency but also sustains the behavior. A simple example is the cavity-free dental visit that occurs in response to a school-age child's regular brushing and flossing of teeth. However, younger children are more extrinsically motivated and may require concrete rewards to establish a behavior. To plan nursing interventions according to a particular child's learning needs, it may be useful to assess a child's motivational state. The Health Self-Determination Index for Children is a tool that has been developed to measure intrinsic motivation. This tool needs to be subjected to further testing across a variety of populations, but it has the potential to assist nurses in the tailoring of interventions to a particular child's motivational state (Cox et al, 1990).

Nursing Roles in Health Promotion

Not only is there diversity in the way health is defined, but terminology used to describe how to achieve health is used inconsistently. "Prevention" and "health protection" are often used interchangeably but, according to Pender (1987), should be differentiated from "health promotion." To "prevent" is to keep something from occurring, whereas "to promote" is to help or encourage something to be or to develop. Health care includes prevention and promotion as well as curative and rehabilitative interventions. The difficulty in separating these terms lies in the fact that a single activity may be carried out for numerous reasons. For example, an exercise program may be carried out to cure a health problem, to prevent a problem from developing, to maintain one's current health status, or to promote one's sense of well-being.

"Prevention" traditionally has been defined to exist at three levels: primary, secondary, and tertiary (Shamansky & Clausen, 1980), which are defined as follows:

1. "Primary prevention" is health promotion as well as protection against health problems.
2. "Secondary prevention" is the early identification of a health problem and prompt intervention to alleviate the problem, resulting in shortened duration and reduced severity, with a return to normal function at the earliest possible time.
3. "Tertiary prevention" is the process of rehabilitation once the effect of a problem is fixed or irreversible. It is the process of restoring an individual to an optimal level of function within the constraints of the disability.

Conceptual differences between prevention (or health protection) and health promotion are clearly described by Stachtchenko and Jenicek (1990). The basis of preventive programs is described as a focus on risk reduction that is targeted at a specific population. Health promotion, on the other hand, has a broad scope, involving not only lifestyle modification of individuals but also a process of enabling individuals and communities to have more control over the determinants of health through a broad range of political, legislative, fiscal, and administrative means (Stachtchenko & Jenicek, 1990). Basic to any health promotion program is the philosophy that children can be powerful, lifelong learners (Cowell et al, 1991) and that they can be empowered to care for themselves (Lewis & Lewis, 1990). The various ways that nurses intervene to promote health are discussed next.

Monitoring Well Child Visits

The appropriate use of periodic health visits has been studied collaboratively by the United States Preventive Services Task Force and the Canadian Task Force. Table 10–2 provides the guidelines for health supervision set forth by the Committee on Practice and Ambulatory Medicine and the American Academy of Pediatrics (AAP).

Although schedules for health supervision and the content of each health visit vary from one clinical setting to another, all have common general goals:

- To promote healthy self-care behaviors.
- To promote general health through teaching and anticipatory guidance (discussion of child health and child development issues before they arise on an age-related basis).
- To provide counseling and make referrals as appropriate.
- To prevent illness through immunizations.
- To detect illness early through history, physical assessment, and screening.
- To provide prompt treatment for identified health problems (major and minor problems).
- To prevent complications and unnecessary disability with effective management of chronic disease.

Teaching and Anticipatory Guidance

Assessment of a child and family for the purposes of teaching is presented in Chapter 23, including assess-

TABLE 10-2
Recommendations for Preventive Pediatric Health Care

Each child and family is unique; therefore these **Recommendations for Preventive Pediatric Health Care** are designed for the care of children who are receiving competent parenting, have no manifestations of any important health problems, and are growing and developing in satisfactory fashion. **Additional visits may become necessary** if circumstances suggest variations from normal. These guidelines represent a consensus by the Committee on Practice and Ambulatory Medicine in consultation with the membership of the American Academy of Pediatrics through the Chapter Presidents. The Committee emphasizes the great importance of **continuity of care** in comprehensive health supervision and the need to avoid **fragmentation of care.**

A **prenatal visit** by the parents for anticipatory guidance and pertinent medical history is strongly recommended.

Health supervision should begin with medical care of the neonate in the hospital.

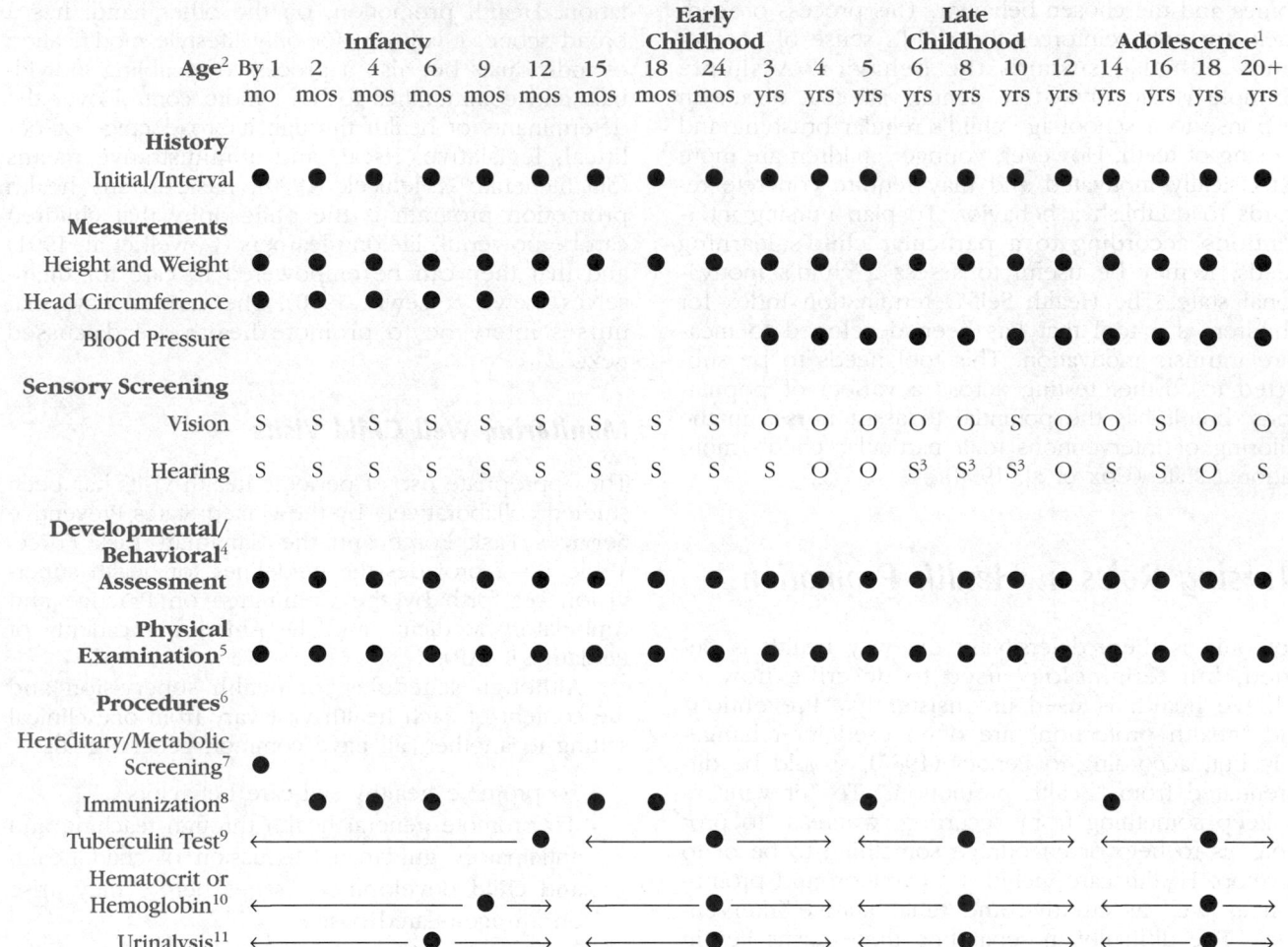

	Infancy								**Early Childhood**				**Late Childhood**				**Adolescence**[1]			
Age[2]	By 1 mo	2 mos	4 mos	6 mos	9 mos	12 mos	15 mos	18 mos	24 mos	3 yrs	4 yrs	5 yrs	6 yrs	8 yrs	10 yrs	12 yrs	14 yrs	16 yrs	18 yrs	20+ yrs
History																				
Initial/Interval	●	●	●	●	●	●	●	●	●	●	●	●	●	●	●	●	●	●	●	●
Measurements																				
Height and Weight	●	●	●	●	●	●	●	●	●	●	●	●	●	●	●	●	●	●	●	●
Head Circumference	●	●	●	●	●	●														
Blood Pressure										●	●	●	●	●	●	●	●	●	●	●
Sensory Screening																				
Vision	S	S	S	S	S	S	S	S	S	O	O	O	O	O	S	O	O	S	O	O
Hearing	S	S	S	S	S	S	S	S	S	S	O	O	S[3]	S[3]	S[3]	O	S	S	O	S
Developmental/ Behavioral[4] **Assessment**	●	●	●	●	●	●	●	●	●	●	●	●	●	●	●	●	●	●	●	●
Physical Examination[5]	●	●	●	●	●	●	●	●	●	●	●	●	●	●	●	●	●	●	●	●
Procedures[6]																				
Hereditary/Metabolic Screening[7]	●																			
Immunization[8]		●	●	●			●	●				●					●			
Tuberculin Test[9]	←	—	—	—	—	●	←	—	●	—	→	←	—	●	—	→	←	—	●	→
Hematocrit or Hemoglobin[10]	←	—	—	—	●	→	←	—	●	—	→	←	—	●	—	→	←	—	●	→
Urinalysis[11]	←	—	—	●	—	→	←	—	●	—	→	←	—	●	—	→	←	—	●	→

ment of learning needs, child and family personal resources, anxiety level of the child and parent, family relationships, lifestyle and cultural patterns, coping styles, and the developmental level of the child. Educational interventions according to the age of the child are summarized in Table 23–1. In this section, the nurse's teaching role is addressed as it pertains to health promotion. Through teaching, the nurse attempts to help families gain information to competently initiate their own problem solving and overcome the barriers to healthy change in their lives. Teaching may be done formally in a planned situation, such as a parent education or school health class. More often, teaching is informal or incidental, occurring at any opportune moment and prompted by immediately identified knowledge deficit.

Parents expect health professionals to be sources of information and education. The process should be one in which an atmosphere is created for an exchange of information rather than a prescriptive "giving information and directives." With the problem solving approach, the knowledge and skills of both the client and the professional are used collaboratively to define the problem, goals, and solutions. The

TABLE 10-2
Recommendations for Preventive Pediatric Health Care *(Continued)*

	Infancy							**Early Childhood**					**Late Childhood**				**Adolescence**[1]			
Age[2]	By 1 mo	2 mos	4 mos	6 mos	9 mos	12 mos	15 mos	18 mos	24 mos	3 yrs	4 yrs	5 yrs	6 yrs	8 yrs	10 yrs	12 yrs	14 yrs	16 yrs	18 yrs	20+ yrs
Anticipatory Guidance[12]	●	●	●	●	●	●	●	●	●	●	●	●	●	●	●	●	●	●	●	●
Initial Dental Referral[13]										●										

From American Academy of Pediatrics, Committee on Psychosocial Aspects of Child and Family Health, 1985–88. (1988). *Guidelines for health supervision II.* Elk Grove Village, IL. Used with permission of the American Academy of Pediatrics.

Key: ● = to be performed: S = subjective, by history; O = objective, by a standard testing method.

N.B.: Special chemical, immunologic, and endocrine testing are usually carried out upon specific indications. Testing other than on newborn infants (e.g., inborn errors of metabolism, sickle cell disease, lead) are discretionary with the physician.

[1]Adolescent-related issues (e.g., psychosocial, emotional, substance usage, and reproductive health) may necessitate more frequent health supervision.

[2]If a child comes under care for the first time at any point on the schedule, or if any items are not accomplished at the suggested age, the schedule should be brought up to date at the earliest possible time.

[3]At these points, history may suffice; if a problem is suggested, a standard testing method should be employed.

[4]By history and appropriate physical examination; if suspicious, by specific objective developmental testing.

[5]At each visit, a complete physical examination is essential, with infant totally unclothed, older child undressed and suitably draped.

[6]These may be modified, depending on entry point into schedule and individual need.

[7]Metabolic screening (e.g., thyroid, phenylketonuria [PKU], galactosemia) should be done according to state law.

[8]Schedule(s) per Report of Committee on Infectious Disease, *1986 Red Book.*

[9]For low-risk groups, the Committee on Infectious Diseases recommends the following options: (1) no routine testing or (2) testing at three times—infancy, preschool, and adolescence. For high-risk groups, annual TB skin testing is recommended.

[10]Present medical evidence suggests the need for re-evaluation of the frequency and timing of hemoglobin or hematocrit tests. One determination is therefore suggested during each time period. Performance of additional tests is left to the individual practice experience.

[11]Present medical evidence suggests the need for re-evaluation of the frequency and timing of urinalysis. One determination is therefore suggested during each time period. Performance of additional tests is left to the individual practice experience.

[12]Appropriate discussion and counseling should be an integral part of each visit for care.

[13]Subsequent examinations as prescribed by dentist.

teaching that the nurse does concerning future events and circumstances has been called *anticipatory guidance.*

Anticipatory guidance is teaching parents what to expect before it happens. The focus is on events to be expected as children grow and develop. The primary goal of anticipatory guidance is to facilitate parents' capabilities to promote their children's well-being. The effectiveness of health care for children is largely dependent on the assistance parents receive in increasing their own competence and confidence to meet their children's needs. As children grow, parental tasks change. Anticipatory guidance helps parents to plan in advance for these developmental changes and the associated alterations in their own parenting role. The nurse attempts to promote mutual love and respect and a relaxed atmosphere within the parent-child relationship throughout the various phases of development. Development of the child, as well as of the parents and other siblings, is taken into consideration.

Counseling Role

A counseling relationship, whether with child or parent, is a two-way interaction involving both verbal and nonverbal communication. Its purposes are (1) to realistically define or resolve a problem, (2) to increase the client's awareness of self and needs, and (3) to get a broader understanding of a situation causing conflict for the client. Many times counseling is initiated during developmental or situational crises. Developmental and situational crises requiring counseling in families are infinite. Changes in family constellation, experiences of loss or change, and family conflicts occur to varying degrees in many families and are often not verbalized openly by family members. Creating an environment in which children and families feel accepted and supported is the first step to a counseling relationship. Developmental and health care issues at each age level are discussed in Chapters 4 through 9.

The nurse counselor, to be successful, must develop skills of astute observation, tactful questioning, objective listening, and, foremost, allowing the client to choose alternatives and solutions. In determining the family members who should be included in counseling, a general rule is that all who will be affected by the situation or its resolution should participate in the decision making. This mutual participation is most successful because it allows each involved family member to gain perspective on the problem and his or her particular role in its management. An indirect effect is that this approach motivates a cooperative partnership among all members of the counseling relationship, including the nurse counselor.

The environment can be a valuable adjunct in promoting the counseling relationship and the desired problem solving. The decor, furniture arrangement, and opportunity provided for the client to initiate contact with the nurse all have significant impact. Colors, style, and texture of furniture and play equipment and lighting help convey that the client is welcome, that comfort and privacy (not isolation) are the nurse's concern, and that the client's needs as well as those of the staff have been considered. The decor should emphasize living and health rather than illness and morbidity. Decor and furnishings can also be effective in reminding staff of the needs of the children and families they serve. Any room arrangements or approaches to clients should encourage eye-to-eye contact and conversation; an "assembly line" approach must be avoided. When choices are feasible (which nurse to confer with, which room to have the meeting in), they should be offered, since choices permit the client some sense of control.

The nurse's responsibility as a counselor is to help the family attain the counseling goals by evoking their sense of security and self-confidence in handling problems, by offering health information that will help them solve problems, and by guiding them in the decision making process. However, the nurse is not to be a decision maker for them.

The Nurse's Role in Referrals

Health promotion is a multiposition, interdisciplinary responsibility that requires a sharing of skills and cooperative division of labor. The nurse alone cannot possibly manage the complexity of the needs that can exist in a family. When the nurse is unable to provide the needed assistance, the appropriate action is to refer family members to resources that can help. This does not absolve the nurse of responsibility for the family, but rather adds to the helping role. To refer appropriately, the nurse must become acquainted with the many potential health team members on a local, regional, and statewide or provincial basis. Nurses must know what each resource offers, what its capabilities are (its record of success in handling the problems it professes to be able to manage), and how the family can obtain those services. When a family is to be referred to the resource, the nurse is responsible for informing the family. To attain or maintain the needed services, the nurse may be called on to act as an advocate for the client or as a liaison (negotiator, mediator) between the client and the resource provider. If several resources are needed by the family, the nurse is often the team member selected to coordinate the various services in a manner that does not overwhelm the family.

Application of the Nursing Process: Health Promotion

Assessment

The nurse's role in health promotion begins with a thorough assessment of the child and the family. Assessments are made through history taking, physical assessment, developmental and behavioral assessment, and appropriate screening tests.

The family is an interactive system through which all members influence one another's behaviors: parent-child, child-parent, and sibling-sibling. A direct relationship exists between health behaviors of children and those of their parents (Bush & Iannotti, 1988; Dielman et al, 1982; Blecke, 1990). The extent to which the family influences a child's behavior varies with the age of the child, with the greatest influence being exerted during early childhood. By early adolescence, peers become the dominant influence. In today's society, the potential influence of parents even on the young child may be decreasing as the childrearing patterns in families change. As young children spend more time in day care, preschools, and after-school care facilities and in front of TV sets, the relative influence of parents on young children may be altered. Under these circumstances, it becomes even more important that whatever influence the family has is a positive one.

Some dimensions of family functioning that the nurse should assess are (1) the kind of behaviors that are modeled; (2) interaction patterns within a family; (3) the way reinforcement is used to encourage certain behaviors; (4) the opportunities provided to learn and practice health behaviors; and (5) the constraints that are put on certain behaviors (Bruhn & Parcel, 1982). These dimensions involve both the physical and the mental health of children. Children not only learn principles about hygiene, diet, and sleep but also are exposed to patterns of coping and attitudes toward others.

Gaps in our knowledge about families and children's health are:

1. What are the long-term effects of family influences?
2. What type of communication patterns within families have an impact (negative or positive) on health behaviors?
3. What are the desirable patterns for family interactions that promote children's health behavior? (Bruhn & Parcel, 1982).

Factors outside the family that influence a child's development of healthy behaviors are predominantly school- and peer-related. As the child matures, school and peers increasingly have an impact on health behaviors. Schools exert their influence through formal classroom instruction, a climate of support and appropriate discipline, physical education activities, and school health services. The influence of peers peaks as a child approaches the teen-age years. Acceptance by a valued group is of primary importance; therefore, an adolescent mimics the behavior of peers to ensure a source of social support. An assessment of positive and negative influencing factors within the child or adolescent's life activities is made.

The *health history and physical assessment* (see Chapter 15) provide the data needed to identify asymptomatic or symptomatic illness and to monitor the control of chronic illness. Any marked increase or decrease in growth usually indicates the presence of an illness of a chronic nature. This aspect of health supervision also provides an opportunity to talk to the child and parent to pick up clues about insidious or overt psychologic problems.

A *developmental and behavioral assessment* provides data about neurologic development as well as specific areas such as self-esteem (see Chapter 14). This assessment may be accomplished through observation, structured testing (e.g., Denver Developmental Screening Test, Appendix 4) and/or asking questions about daily living activities and parental satisfaction with the child's progress, and the child's relationships.

As major organic illness in children has been contained by medical advances, a "new morbidity" has received epidemiologic attention. This new morbidity —acting out behaviors and behavior problems, failure to thrive, alcohol and drug abuse, family violence and abuse, school failure, accidents, delinquency, and other manifestations of adjustment difficulties—needs the serious attention of health professionals. Astute behavioral assessments and appropriate counseling can help prevent or diminish these childhood disabilities that are of acute concern to parents.

Screening tests, both clinical (e.g., vision testing) and laboratory (e.g., hemoglobin testing), provide data to complement the physical and behavioral assessments in identifying altered health states.

Nursing Diagnostic Statements

High risk for altered health maintenance; risk factors:

- Child's immature understanding of health associated with developmental level.
- Lack of opportunity for child to participate in managing own health needs.
- Ineffective role modeling of health promoting behaviors demonstrated by parents to child.
- Inadequate support of caregivers in the health care of children, secondary to feelings of inadequacy, lack of access to information.

Health seeking behaviors (child and parent) related to:

- Desire to achieve optimal well-being.

Planning and Implementation

Health teaching aimed at children takes into account the child's thinking ability at various ages, the concept of health that is characteristic of the age, and the degree of independent action that a child is realistically capable of at each stage of development. Table 10–1 describes such characteristics for children in the various age groups and their relevance in selecting an appropriate teaching approach. Realistic health behaviors at various ages are presented in Table 10–3.

TABLE 10-3
Examples of Realistic Health Behaviors Children Have Identified at Various Ages

Early Childhood
I will brush my teeth after breakfast and at bedtime
I will cover my coughs and sneezes with my hand or a tissue
I will drink a glass of milk at breakfast, lunch, and supper
Middle Childhood
I will try to remember to wash my hands after using the toilet and before eating
Whenever possible I will change wet shoes and socks or stockings for dry ones
I know what a good breakfast is, and I will try to eat one every day
I will go to bed willingly when I am told to do so
Late Childhood and Preadolescence
I will try to learn to eat some foods that are new to me or that have been prepared in a new way
I will listen to the morning weather report and dress accordingly
I will try to cooperate with my parents and other adults who help to keep me well
I will keep my hands clean and will also keep them away from my face, especially from my eyes, nose, and mouth, and away from any sores
Adolescence and Young Adulthood
I will study my own posture and try to do the things that will improve it
I know about the food pyramid, and I will try to eat foods according to its guidelines every day
I will take frequent baths and wash my hair at least once each week
I will listen to my parents' point of view in areas in which we disagree and seriously evaluate their points

Promote Effective Health Maintenance by the Child; and Support Health Seeking Behaviors in the Child and Parents

Too often health teaching about children is directed only toward their parents.

> **If we expect children to assume more responsibility for their own health as they grow, we need to teach them how to make decisions about health and what is involved in staying healthy. To carry out a behavior requires knowledge of how it is performed and the ability to resolve any barriers that interfere with enacting it. For example, to maintain dental hygiene when a child has braces, the special techniques required must be learned.**

Youngsters can learn ways to reduce stress in their environments, acquire effective coping skills, and develop attitudes that are oriented toward health rather than illness. All of these would result in health maintenance by the child and would encourage continued health seeking behaviors. Knowledge deficit is a frequent etiology for nursing diagnostic statement responses such as altered health maintenance, altered role performance, ineffective coping, impaired adjustment, and decisional conflict. Health seeking behaviors often imply that *knowledge* is being sought. Children need information about their own development and health issues to make good decisions about health behavior. And if they are to initiate their own health care, they must learn how to approach health care providers and be assertive with them.

Interventions: Teaching: Individual, *and* Teaching: Group

Acquisition and maintenance of healthy behavior by children involves four processes. They must develop an *awareness* of health from their role models. They must be exposed to developmentally appropriate *information* about wellness and health practices. If they are to learn responsibility, they must be included as *active participants* (as early in life as possible) in making health choices so that they can master the problem solving required to make healthy decisions about life. And finally, they must be *reinforced* for their attempts and their successes in practicing wellness behaviors.

When a child needs support and encouragement to develop health behaviors, the nurse begins by eliciting the child's perception of a problem or situation and its cause. This helps the nurse to understand how much health information the child needs. After historical information and assessment data are gathered from the child and the family, findings are interpreted for the child to understand. The child is encouraged to offer an opinion and list alternative actions with reasons as to why each would help. In this way, the child learns problem solving skills. The next step is to ask the child to select one of the alternatives and identify whether it will be carried out alone or with assistance. Finally, the child is asked to identify the resources (personal or in the external environment) that will be needed to accomplish the alternative. This approach involves the child actively in identifying health needs, finding viable solutions, and carrying them out. The nurse supports the child by reinforcing the child and giving support for decisions made. If decisions are inappropriate, the nurse provides additional information to clarify the issue.

Support Caregiver to Promote Child's Health: Support System Enhancement *and* Parent Education

The support system available to a family is assessed for its adequacy. Barriers to using support systems are identified and referrals are made to community-based programs as needed. A self-help parent group may be an appropriate resource to consider.

The nurse's assistance with early parental tasks can enhance the number of successes that parents experience from the beginning. It is critical for the nurse to share professional knowledge and skills in a manner that enhances parental self-esteem.

Areas of child care and parenting that are commonly discussed are:

1. Expectations about child development and how parents can support it (fostering self-esteem, development through play, and socialization activities).
2. Providing healthy diet.
3. Injury prevention at all levels of development.
4. How to manage child behavior (home, school, community).
5. Balancing the needs, care, and problems of all family members.
6. How to access and relate to health professionals and other community resources.
7. Family relationships related to personal and interpersonal crises, illness, divorce or separation, single parenting, and extended family issues.

Underlying these many expectations brought to the health professional is the parents' desire to succeed in the care of their child and to receive encouragement in parenting. Age-specific discussions of safety, nutrition, sleep, play and exercise, development, and discipline can be found in Unit 2: Growth and Development of Children Within Families (see Chapters 4 through 9).

Evaluation

Evaluation of the child's health status and ability to acquire and maintain healthy behavior is an ongoing process adapted according to the child's age. As the child matures, the degree of self-responsibility increases. An evaluation of this progress is made by asking children to report on their own perception of their health care behaviors.

Childhood Immunizations

Immunizations are administered during child health care visits by the primary care nurse or physician or through a local public health department. Children not immunized because of irregular attendance at a clinic or their physician's office may be identified during a visit for an acute illness.

Making Immunizations a Priority in Health Promotion

Health professionals in all settings must keep accurate records to facilitate identification of inadequately immunized children and adolescents and search for ways to help parents and children access available care. Contact with child patients in any setting presents an opportunity to assess their immunization status and to make the appropriate vaccine available. In particular, those children from families who fail to return for routine immunizations need to be assessed, and, if possible, immunizations are brought up to date prior to discharge from a hospital or outpatient facility. In these circumstances, parent recall should be accepted as sufficient documentation if records are unavailable. Premature infants and children with chronic conditions require special attention because their immunizations may have been delayed and inadvertently missed.

Routine immunization of children has dramatically reduced the incidence and prevalence of infectious diseases since the 1950s. In spite of the widespread, major, positive impact that vaccines have had on the reduction of communicable diseases, nurses and other health professionals must continue to make immunizations a priority in order to protect children from preventable diseases. In recent years, the incidence of vaccine-preventable diseases, such as mumps, rubella, pertussis, and measles, have increased (Arnold & Schlenker, 1992).

Recommendations for childhood immunizations have recently undergone significant revisions, and additional changes are likely to occur as new data are evaluated and new vaccines become licensed. Knowing where to find the most recent information and consulting such resources are essential because of the rapidly expanding knowledge in this area. Organizations and committees that make recommendations for immunization policies and procedures are as follows. In the United States:

- Advisory Committee on Immunization Practices (ACIP) of the Public Health Service.
- Committee on Infectious Diseases of the AAP

In Canada:

- National Advisory Committee on Immunization is a group that operates under the authority of the Minister of National Health and Welfare.

Types of Agents Used for Immunization

Immunity is a state in which the host is resistant to specific diseases. Resistance to disease is developed naturally or artificially, and the mechanism is either passive or active. Table 10–4 presents definitions of natural, artificial, passive, and active. Following are examples of the various types of immunity:

Natural Passive

Transfer of plasma proteins from mother to fetus via placenta—temporary.

TABLE 10-4
Types of Immunity

Natural Immunity:
is an innate immunity or resistance that is developed by natural processes versus artificial ones. It develops when the host is exposed to organisms of low virulence over time or by contracting the actual disease. It can be passive or active.

Artificial Immunity:
develops when an antigen (vaccine) is introduced into the host artificially. It can be passive or active.

Passive Immunity:
is acquired when ready-made antibody or complement is transferred to the host. The host's body does not develop its own antibodies. It can be natural or artificial.

Active Immunity:
develops when immune bodies are actively formed by the host against specific antigens. It can be natural or artificial.

Natural Active

Host develops immune bodies in response to contracting the disease (clinical), e.g., chickenpox, or by being exposed over time to organisms of low virulence (subclinical). For example, some adults have never had chickenpox but have been exposed through contact with children who have the disease.

Artificial Passive

Produced by injection of the host with plasma proteins (antibodies) that have been produced by another actively immunized human or animal, e.g., human immune serum globulin or animal antiserum (antitoxin)—temporary.

Artificial Active

Immunity produced by the injection of the host with various vaccines and toxoids, resulting in the development of antibodies; this is the most common form of childhood immunizations. Types of agents used are presented in Table 10–5. The purpose of immunizations is to protect the host against a specific group of known microbes that have the potential to cause serious illness.

Current Issues

Childhood immunizations is a changing field of practice as new discoveries are made and outbreaks of disease call for new practices. Current issues and recent changes have received significant attention in the literature and are summarized here to provide a basis for understanding updated immunization schedules.

Vaccinations—Access and Responsibility

by Margaret M. Mahon, MSN, RN

Case 1. *Dyane is a 3-year-old brought to the Community Health Center by her mother with a "fever and a runny nose." Dyane has never been to the Center before. Prior health care has been obtained in two emergency rooms, each time for treatment of a minor illness. A history revealed that Dyane has received none of her required immunizations. A 26-month-old brother is also present.*

Case 2. *Early in the 1990 measles epidemic, two children from the same neighborhood contracted measles and died. Several more children from the same area of the city also had measles. During interviews with the families, public health nurses learned that several of the families belonged to the same church, and that one of the teachings of this church prohibited immunization. Subsequently, two more children who were members of the church died from measles, and three others were critically ill.*

During 1989 and 1990, there was a resurgence of measles cases in this county; in 1989, 41 people died from measles; in 1990, more than 60 people died. Of the tens of thousands affected with the disease during this time, many were left with short-term or even permanent complications. Public reaction was an admixture of incredulity, shock, and anger. How could a presumably preventable disease have killed so many people? The question for nurses and other health care professionals becomes: Is there a responsibility to ensure adequate vaccination for all children? If there is such a responsibility, how does it translate to action for each health care professional?

Before examining the ethical issues regarding immunization, a foundation of facts is necessary. The measles vaccine first became available in 1963. With the epidemics of 1989 and 1990, the recommendation for administration was expanded. In addition to an MMR (measles, mumps, rubella) vaccination at 15 months of age, a second dose at 4 to 6 years of age is now required. Many practitioners choose routinely to administer this second dose at the time of the child's 4-year checkup.

A combination of factors resulted in the 1989 and 1990 outbreaks. The initial challenge is to understand these factors so that modifications can be made to prevent recurrences of this tragedy of preventable morbidity and mortality. Understanding what contributed to the measles epidemics is an opportunity to understand broader and contributory problems to inadequate vaccinations. These problems can be understood from two perspectives: the child and family and the health care system. Inadequacies in both systems contribute to the magnitude of the problem of undervaccination.

About 95 per cent of school-aged children are immunized appropriately for their ages; this represents an all-time high. The population of undervaccinated children is primarily preschoolers. Almost all school districts and day care centers require documentation of up-to-date vaccination before a child is enrolled at the school. Many families use this deadline to obtain a full complement of vaccinations. Children who are not vaccinated are therefore likely to be those who have not yet begun to attend a licensed day care center or grade school.

Cost is an oft-cited factor for people not receiving vaccinations. Certainly vaccinations are not cheap; however, the cost of vaccination is much less than the cost of the morbidity or mortality of the diseases prevented by vaccination. Cost of immunizations received in the public sector was about $95 per child (Hinman, 1991), although the cost to the family is likely to be nothing or a small fee for administrative expenses. For a child in the private sector to receive all immunizations, the cost is about $305, although this is reimbursed or paid by many insurance carriers. Even when the cost of vaccinations are completely covered, however, the rate of immunization remains low among populations of children for whom documentation of vaccination is not required.

Other family reasons for lack of immunizations include fear of side effects. This fear has had multiple repercussions. One implication is that fewer pharmaceutical companies make immunizations, and, for those companies who continue to provide this service, the cost of insurance has skyrocketed. The other implication of the fear of side effects is that some families have just refused to have their children immunized. While ethics should never be reduced to a numbers comparison, it is sometimes necessary to have accurate numbers to understand the magnitude of a problem. For example, the chance of death from immunization is minute compared with the chance of death from many of the diseases against which children (and adults) are immunized. The success of immunizations has been a part of the result of underimmunization. Because, for example, polio is so rare in the United States, parents are unaware of how devastating polio can be. There is a resulting lack of understanding of the necessity for immunizations.

Although it is rare, cases such as case #2 did occur in several places during the measles epidemics. The question in this case is similar to that of children who need blood, but to receive blood is against the family's religion. In the case of blood transfusion, there are sometimes options; for example, children may be able to receive volume expanders without receiving blood. There are also rare cases in which families are assured that their child will not receive blood in the operating room, blood is given, and the family is merely not notified. In these cases, the rationale is often that the blood is necessary to save the child's life, and this is easier than going through the legal maneuvering necessary to administer blood without parental consent. Immunization is different, however, in that there are not options, such as volume expanders. To prevent disease, immunization is required. In some cases like this one, cities or other local governments have intervened to require immunization. Some argue that this is acceptable because children this young have not chosen the religion, it is the parents'.

ETHICAL ISSUES

Vaccinations—Access and Responsibility (continued)

Low immunization is not just a problem of families; there are many barriers within the health care system. Probably foremost among these barriers is the inflexibility of scheduling relative to immunizing. For example, a complete physical examination is often required before an immunization is given. In addition, the following restrictions frequently exist: immunizations may only be given during certain office hours, or during a visit in which immunizations are a preplanned component; registration with a different agency may be required; and/or payment of an administration fee is necessary.

If more complete immunization coverage is to be achieved, all children's appointments with health care professionals must be considered potential opportunities for immunizations. For example, Dyane's emergency room visits and her clinic visit today are all viable options for immunization. Certainly, fever is a contraindication to some immunizations; however, contraindications used in deferring immunization are often too broad. Clinicians have the responsibility to apply such standards judiciously. The scope of each encounter must be broadened in the minds of nurses and physicians.

There is an additional responsibility for those who actually administer immunizations. In addition to underimmunization, some of those who have contracted measles and other communicable diseases had documentation to prove that they had been immunized. No immunization is effective all the time; however, some of the reason for the lack of efficacy of immunizations in the past may be the result of improper administration. As with all medications, the right route is essential in administering immunizations. A medication that is to be administered subcutaneously may be ineffective if given intramuscularly.

What other factors contribute to the process of inadequacy of immunization? What can be done within different practice areas to improve the percentage of children who are immunized, especially those not currently enrolled in school? Is it possible to address this issue on inpatient units?

BIBLIOGRAPHY

Hinman, A. R. (1991). What will it take to fully protect all American children with vaccines? *American Journal of Diseases of Children, 145,* 559–562.

The National Vaccine Advisory Committee. (1991). The measles epidemic: The problems, barriers, and recommendations. *Journal of the American Medical Association, 266,* 1547–1552.

Orenstein, W. A., Atkinson, W., Mason, D., & Bernier, R. H. (1990). Barriers to vaccinating preschool children. *Journal of Health Care for the Poor and Underserved, 1,* 315–330.

United States Department of Health and Human Services. (1990). *Healthy people 2000: National health promotion and dis-ease prevention objectives.* (DHHS Publication No. [PHS] 91–50213). Washington, DC: US Government Printing Office.

1. *Haemophilus influenzae* b conjugate vaccine (HbCV) is recommended for infants beginning at 2 months of age. This change has occurred as a result of the development of new vaccines.

2. It has recently been recognized that children must be reimmunized against measles with a second dose of vaccine. The American Academy of Pediatrics recommends a second dose of MMR at 5 years and the United States Public Health Service at 12 years of age.

3. An enhanced-potency killed (inactivated) polio vaccine (e-IPV) has been developed to reduce the risk of vaccine-induced paralysis from live attenuated vaccine. Routine use of the killed vaccine for the first two immunizations at 2 and 4 months and live vaccine for booster doses at 18 months and 4 to 6 years is being considered but is not yet recommended (Phillips, 1991). It continues to be used for immunocompromised children.

4. The threat of neurologic damage from pertussis vaccine is being reassessed. *Whole cellular* pertussis vaccine has been associated with some neurologic risks, which has led to a search for another vaccine. An *acellular* pertussis (ACP) vaccine holds promise for reduction of the incidence of side effects.

5. A live, attenuated varicella vaccine has been developed and tested in Japan; however, routine immunization has not been recommended in the United States and Canada.

6. It is now recommended that all newborn infants be immunized with hepatitis B vaccine.

7. WHO is proposing a "super vaccine," containing as many as 14 immunogens, that would be administered to infants in a single dose to prevent a variety of infectious illnesses, a goal for the year 2000 (Pichichero et al, 1990).

Immunizing Agents and Schedules

Many of the vaccines are administered in combination to reduce the number of injections required. The two major examples are DTP (diphtheria, tetanus, and pertussis) and MMR (measles, mumps, and rubella). A combination of tetanus and diphtheria (Td), instead of DTP, is used at 7 years of age and thereafter. These combinations along with polio, *Haemophilus influenzae* B, and hepatitis B make up the commonly

TABLE 10-5
Types of Agents Used in Immunization

Live Vaccines

The objective is to induce protective immunity without producing the actual, full-blown, clinical illness. To accomplish this, the organisms are attenuated, which means the virulence has been diminished to a level at which immunity is achieved, but the clinical illness is avoided. Measles, mumps, rubella, varicella, and polio (Sabin) vaccines are examples of live attenuated viruses. Bacillus Calmette-Guérin (BCG) vaccine is an example of live attenuated bacteria.

Killed Vaccines

Immunity is stimulated by the host's reaction to the killed microbe. Polio (Salk) and influenza vaccines are examples of killed viruses. Pertussis vaccine is an example of a killed bacteria.

Toxoids

A toxoid is a bacterial toxin that has been treated by heat or by chemicals to destroy its toxic properties, but to retain its antigenic quality (i.e., ability to stimulate antibody production). Tetanus toxoid and diphtheria toxoid are examples of treated toxins.

Adsorbed Agents and Fluid Agents

Adsorbed agents (vaccines and toxoids) have substances added to the immunizing agent to enhance its antigenic effect. Antigens are therefore released more slowly, enhancing the response by prolonged contact. Adsorbed agents must be given intramuscularly.

Fluid agents are more rapidly absorbed and produce a more rapid secondary response. Fluid tetanus toxoid is used at the time of an injury if the victim has had the initial series of tetanus immunization.

Human Immune Serum Globulin

Human immune serum globulin may be prepared from pooled plasma and is used to reduce the severity of diseases or to prevent diseases such as measles, viral hepatitis A, and viral hepatitis B (if specific hepatitis B immune globulin is not available). Specific human immune serum globulin is also available. This is prepared from the plasma of patients recuperating from specific illnesses such as tetanus, pertussis, hepatitis B, mumps, and varicella-zoster (chickenpox). Plasma of a recuperating patient contains the antibody for that specific illness.

Animal Antiserum (Antitoxin)

Animal antiserum is prepared from animal serum (horses, cows) in which the antibody has been actively produced. Because reactions to the foreign serum may occur, the individual is first pretested to determine hypersensitivity. Examples of this method of passive immunity are tetanus antitoxin and diphtheria antitoxin.

used immunizations (see Tables 10–6 and 10–7 for routine schedules in the United States and Canada, respectively).

DTP (*Diphtheria Toxoid, Tetanus Toxoid, and Pertussis Vaccine*)

DTP is given by intramuscular injection starting at 2 months of age in a series of three doses 2 months apart, followed by a booster 6 to 12 months after the third dose, and another booster on entry into school. A preparation of diphtheria and tetanus toxoid only (Td) is given to children under 7 years of age in whom pertussis vaccine is contraindicated. Children 7 years of age and older are routinely given Td. The small "d" indicates a reduced diphtheria dose containing only 20 per cent of that in DTP. It is recommended that the adult form (Td) is given at 10-year intervals.

Diphtheria toxoid is a safe vaccine with a low incidence of fever and only minor local pain at the site of injection. The primary series of DTP is greater than 90 per cent effective in the prevention of serious cases of diphtheria.

Tetanus toxoid is the form of tetanus that is administered in routine immunizations. Other forms of tetanus vaccine include tetanus immune globulin (TIG) and tetanus antitoxin (usually horse serum). Tetanus toxoid is administered routinely in the form of DTP, as described earlier. In addition to the routine immunizations, a form of tetanus immunization is sometimes required in the event of injury. A child with a minor clean wound who has received the primary immunization and a booster within 10 years prior to the injury does not require a booster of tetanus toxoid. In the event of a more serious wound to a previously appropriately immunized child, a booster is given if tetanus toxoid has not been received in the preceding 5 years. If the three primary injections have not been received, then a child under 7 years of age receives DTP and a child over 7 receives Td (even in the event of a minor wound). Serious wounds are treated with TIG to provide passive protection if the three primary injections were not received. In this event, Td is also administered. When both TIG and Td are administered, separate syringes and sites are used (AAP, 1991).

Reactions to DTP vaccinations are largely due to the *pertussis* portion of the vaccine. Reactions are of three types:

1. Local swelling and tenderness at site of injection, a slight fever, and irritability.
2. Excessive tiredness, inconsolable crying that lasts 4 hours or longer, and a shocklike syndrome also lasting for several hours.
3. Neurologic reactions, including occasional convulsions and, in rare occasions, encephalopathy with brain damage or even death.

TABLE 10-6
Recommended Schedule for Immunization of Healthy Infants and Children (United States)*

Recommended Age†	Immunizations‡	Comments
2 mos	DTP, HbCV,§ OPV	DTP and OPV can be initiated as early as 4 wks after birth in areas of high endemicity or during epidemics
4 mos	DTP, HbCV,§ OPV	2–mo interval (minimum of 6 wks) desired for OPV to avoid interference from previous dose
6 mos	DTP, HbCV§	Third dose of OPV is not indicated in the US but is desirable in other geographic areas where polio is endemic
15 mos	MMR,‖ HbCV¶	Tuberculin testing may be done at the same visit
15–18 mos	DTP,**†† OPV#	(See footnotes)
4–6 yrs	DTP,§§ OPV	At or before school entry
11–12 yrs	MMR	At entry to middle school or junior high school unless second dose previously given
14–16 yrs	Td	Repeat every 10 yrs throughout life

From American Academy of Pediatrics, Committee on Infectious Diseases. (1991). Report of the Committee on Infectious Diseases. *The redbook.* (22nd ed.). Elk Grove Village, IL. Used with permission of the American Academy of Pediatrics.

*For all products used, consult manufacturer's package insert for instructions for storage, handling, dosage, and administration. Biologics prepared by different manufacturers may vary, and package inserts of the same manufacturer may change from time to time. Therefore, the physician should be aware of the contents of the current package insert.

†These recommended ages should not be construed as absolute. For example, 2 mos can be 6–10 wks. However, MMR usually should not be given to children younger than 12 mos. (If measles vaccination is indicated, monovalent measles vaccine is recommended, and MMR should be given subsequently, at 15 mos.)

‡DTP = diphtheria and tetanus toxoids with pertussis vaccine; HbCV = *Haemophilus influenzae* b conjugate vaccine; OPV = oral poliovirus vaccine containing attenuated poliovirus types 1, 2, and 3; MMR = live measles, mumps, and rubella viruses in a combined vaccine; Td = adult tetanus toxoid (full dose) and diphtheria toxoid (reduced dose) for adult use.

§As of October 1990, only one HbCV is approved for use in children younger than 15 mos.

‖May be given at 12 mos of age in areas with recurrent measles transmission.

¶Any licensed HbCV may be given.

**Should be given 6–12 mos after the third dose.

††May be given simultaneously with MMR at 15 mos.

#May be given simultaneously with MMR and HbCV at 15 mos or at any time between 12 and 24 mos; priority should be given to administering MMR at the recommended age.

§§Can be given up to the 7th birthday.

Note: Since 1991, it is also recommended that all infants are immunized for hepatitis B (HB) at birth, and at 1 mo and 6 mos after the first dose.

Pertussis vaccine is recommended except in the following circumstances. Current absolute contraindications to further vaccination include:

1. Convulsions with or without fever occurring within 3 days following immunization.
2. Encephalopathy occurring within 7 days after immunization.
3. Anaphylaxis associated with the administration of pertussis vaccine.
4. Hyporesponsive or hypotensive episodes associated with pertussis vaccine administration.
5. A fever greater than 105°F (40.5°C).
6. Persistent and high-pitched crying for more than 3 hours (Frenkel, 1990).

Pertussis vaccinations are also deferred in infants with an unstable or developing neurologic problem (new onset of seizures or muscle weakness). The nurse must also be alert to the fact that even though the first DTP did not result in unusual side effects, the second immunization may produce problems. Continuation of diphtheria and tetanus immunization can be provided by administering DT (diphtheria and tetanus) in a child under 7 years of age in the event of a reaction to pertussis.

The risk of death from pertussis in the unimmunized child is estimated to be 30 times greater than in the immunized child (Phillips, 1991). Pertussis continues to be the most controversial immunizing agent, yet numerous studies have concluded that brain damage resulting from the pertussis vaccine is an extremely rare event (Griffin et al, 1990; Long et al, 1990). Concern about serious side effects has led some professionals to reduce the dose of DTP to less than 0.5 ml per dose. This practice is not approved by the ACIP and AAP, and current recommendations

TABLE 10-7
Immunization Schedules for Infants and Children (Canada)

Age	Immunization Against				
2 mos	Diphtheria	Pertussis	Tetanus	Poliomyelitis	*Hemophilus influenzae* B (HIB) vaccine
4 mos	Diphtheria	Pertussis	Tetanus	Poliomyelitis	*Hemophilus influenzae* B (HIB) vaccine
6 mos	Diphtheria	Pertussis	Tetanus	Poliomyelitis[1]	*Hemophilus influenzae* B (HIB) vaccine
12–15 mos	Measles	Mumps	Rubella[2]		
18 mos	Diphtheria	Pertussis	Tetanus	Poliomyelitis	*Hemophilus influenzae* B (HIB) vaccine
4–6 yrs	Diphtheria	Pertussis	Tetanus	Poliomyelitis	
14–16 yrs	Diphtheria[3]		Tetanus[3]	Poliomyelitis	

[1]This dose may be omitted if live (oral) polio vaccine is being used exclusively.

[2]Rubella vaccine is also indicated for all girls and women of childbearing age who lack proof of immunity. At all medical visits, the opportunity should be taken to check whether girls and women need rubella vaccine.

[3]Diphtheria and tetanus toxoid (Td), a combined adsorbed "adult type" preparation for use in persons 7 yrs of age or more, contains less diphtheria toxoid than preparations given to younger children and is less likely to cause reactions in older persons.

Note: The *Canadian immunization guide.* (4th ed.) was not available at time of publication. This schedule is based on current practice in Ontario and the most recent publication: National Advisory Committee on Immunization. (1989). *Canadian immunization guide.* (3rd ed.). (Cat. No. H49–8/1989E). Ottawa: Ministry of National Health and Welfare.

are to give the full dose (AAP, 1991). It has even been suggested that small doses could sensitize a child and increase the chances of adverse reactions (Garber & Mortimer, 1992). Even if pertussis is not found to cause brain damage, the usual side effects of fever, irritability, and local reactions continue to provide an impetus for the development of a new vaccine. An acellular vaccine has been developed and used in Japan, but large-scale studies are required before the vaccine will be licensed for routine use in infants (AAP, 1991) in the United States and Canada.

Polio Vaccine

Polio vaccine is a trivalent vaccine that produces immune titers against the three main strains of poliovirus. Three types of vaccines are available:

- Oral polio vaccine (OPV), a live, attenuated trivalent polio vaccine (Sabin).
- Inactivated polio vaccine (IPV), a killed trivalent polio vaccine given subcutaneously (Salk) (used in Canada).
- Enhanced inactivated polio vaccine (e-IPV); used in the United States for immunocompromised and in Canada for routine immunizations.

OPV is the recommended drug for routine immunization in the United States, and IPV is used in Canada. A properly timed combination of OPV and IPV is an alternative that has been used in some countries and is thought to have some advantages (Phillips, 1991). The current acceptance of OPV is due to (1) oral preparation and ease of administration, (2) rapid and lasting immunity, and (3) infection of the gastrointestinal tract that provides systemic and local immunity (Frenkel, 1990). See Table 10–8 for further explanations about poliovirus vaccine.

Trivalent oral polio vaccine (TOPV) is started at the 2-month visit, with a second dose at 4 months. A third dose at 6 months is optional. Booster doses are recommended at 18 months of age and at school entry. The risk of paralysis following receipt of OPV is greater in immunocompromised children than in healthy children; therefore, it is not used in immunocompromised children. An enhanced-potency, killed (inactivated) vaccine (e-IPV) has been available since 1988 and is the recommended vaccine for immunocompromised children and for children who have a family member that is immunocompromised. In Canada, IPV is used in these circumstances.

MMR (*Measles, Mumps, and Rubella Vaccine*)

A single dose of MMR vaccine was once thought to give lifelong immunity. However, since the mid-1980s, there has been a steady increase in the number of measles outbreaks in the United States and Canada. It is now recommended that two doses are administered routinely and, in high-risk populations, three doses.

MMR is a triple vaccine and is administered subcutaneously. The first dose is given at 15 months of age in the United States and at 12 or 15 months in

TABLE 10-8
Understanding Poliovirus Vaccines

The advantage of oral poliovirus vaccine (OPV) is that it is more effective in preventing spread of *wild polio viruses* (viruses that occur in nature versus vaccine-associated shedding of the virus) than enhanced inactivated polio vaccine (e-IPV) or inactivated poliovirus vaccine (IPV). The increased protection against wild polio virus by OPV occurs because this vaccine immunizes the gastrointestinal tract, protecting it from later replication of wild polio viruses.

On extremely rare occasions, OPV results in vaccine-related paralysis in recipients or their close contacts. Reported incidences are 1:520,000 following the first dose and 1:10 million following subsequent doses. The critical role of nurses in this regard is to explain to parents that the risk of *not* being vaccinated far exceeds the risk associated with receiving the vaccine. Only those infants and contacts who are immunocompromised or contacts who have not been immunized are at risk. The degree of risk to unimmunized contacts is not known because it can vary according to their exposure to OPV recipients over time. It is thought that some immunity may be developed by repeated exposure to OPV vaccines because of poliovirus shedding from the gastrointestinal tract; this is often referred to as "herd immunity."

If infants or their contacts are immunocompromised, the IPV is given. Even if a close contact is not immunocompromised but has not been immunized, then that person should be simultaneously immunized rather than assume that "herd immunity" has taken place. In the case of an infant in a premature nursery with other sick infants, OPV is given on discharge to avoid exposing other vulnerable infants in the same hospital unit to gastrointestinal shedding of the poliovirus.

Summary:

- All infants must be vaccinated for polio with OPV or e-IPV/IPV as indicated.
- Shedding of the OPV in the stool is only a danger to contacts who are immunocompromised or unimmunized.
- Immunocompromised infants should receive e-IPV (US) or IPV (Canada).
- If a close contact of an OPV recipient has not been vaccinated, they should be vaccinated simultaneously.
- Infants of immunocompromised close contacts should receive e-IPV (used in US) or IPV (used in Canada) so as not to endanger their caretakers.
- OPV is given on discharge in a premature nursery.

From Kimpen, J. L. L., & Ogra, L. L. (1990). Poliovirus vaccines: A continuing challenge. *Pediatric Clinics of North America, 37*(3), 627–649; and Phillips, C. G. (1991). Keeping up with the changing immunization schedule. *Contemporary Pediatrics, 8,* 20–46.

Canada. The younger a child is the more likely that maternal antibodies can interfere with antibody production and inhibit immunity. On the other hand, delaying immunization puts the child at greater risk for contracting the disease. Revaccination is recommended by the AAP at 11 or 12 years of age; in some states, this dose is required at 4 to 6 years of age, if the particular public health jurisdiction is following the guidelines set by the ACIP of the Public Health Service.

In the event of a measles epidemic, measles vaccine can be given to children as young as 6 months of age. In these cases, it is recommended that the immunization be repeated at 15 months of age. Contraindications to the measles vaccine are (1) pregnancy, (2) documented immunosuppression or immunodeficiency disease, and (3) anaphylactic reactions to eggs (Frenkel, 1990). Anaphylaxis to eggs is only a relative contraindication because these children can receive MMR by following a desensitization protocol.

The routine schedule and changes in timing for administration of mumps are as described for measles vaccine. There have been recent outbreaks in 10- to 19-year-old children and adolescents. This is thought to reflect the fact that routine mumps immunization did not become a recommendation until 1977. With the second universal dose of MMR, there should be a reduction in the incidence of the disease of mumps. Mumps vaccine is one of the safest vaccines available. There are no contraindications to the administration of the vaccine. Even though the live mumps vaccine has the potential to cause adverse reactions in those who are allergic to eggs, there has not been a well-documented case of anaphylaxis with mumps vaccine (Frenkel, 1990).

Rubella is a disease that has the potential to affect the developing fetus. Since the disease presents as a mild infection in children but can seriously damage the unborn child, the target population is women likely to become pregnant. Rubella vaccine is administered in combination as MMR according to the routine and updated schedules described. Rubella vaccine has prevented large epidemics, but small epidemics still occur regularly in high schools, colleges, and places of employment where large numbers of young people work. It is important to vaccinate all unimmunized prepubertal children and susceptible adolescents if epidemics are to be reduced.

Certain precautions must be taken when vaccinating women (including adolescents) of childbearing age. Women in their first trimester of pregnancy should not receive the vaccine because the live attenuated virus may cross the placenta and present a risk to the developing fetus. When the vaccine is given to women in childbearing age, it must first be established that the woman is not pregnant; for 3 months following vaccine administration, birth control is necessary if the woman is likely to become pregnant during that time if not protected. All pregnant women should be screened for rubella immunity, and, if not immune, should be immunized immediately after delivery. Although vaccination of pregnant women is to be avoided, in cases in which it has inadvertently occurred, deleterious effects to the fetus have not been reported (AAP, 1991; Rubella, 1989).

Haemophilus Influenzae Type B (HIB) Vaccine

Haemophilus influenzae type B (HIB) is the leading cause of meningitis and septic arthritis in infants. About 75 per cent of all serious HIB infections occur in children under 18 months of age. The difficulty with eradicating this disease is that the first vaccines developed did not reliably stimulate protective antibodies in children under 2 years of age; therefore, those at greatest risk were not protected. A variety of vaccines have now been developed that are *conjugated* (coupled or joined to a protein), making them more immunogenic (able to induce antibody production). Three conjugated vaccines were licensed in the United States prior to May 1990: these vaccines were effective in children as young as 15 months of age. In the early 1990s, the AAP recommended that any one of these licensed HIB conjugated vaccines should be administered to all children at 15 months of age (AAP, 1990). More recently, newer conjugated vaccines have been licensed with the first dose given at 2 months of age. It can be given simultaneously with DTP, MMR, OPT/IPV if different injection sites are used (AAP, 1991). Since the fall of 1992, this vaccine has also been made available in Canada, with the first dose being given at 2 months of age.

Hepatitis B (HB) *Vaccine*

Universal immunization of infants for hepatitis B (HB) has been endorsed by the AAP and the Immunization Practices Advisory Committee of the US Public Health Services since 1991 to be given at birth and at 1 month and 6 months after the first dose. Those who are at high risk for infection with the hepatitis B (HB) virus should also be vaccinated. Groups at risk for contracting hepatitis include: (1) clients and staff of institutions for the developmentally disabled, (2) recipients of frequent blood transfusions and blood products and dialysis patients, (3) close contacts of HB virus carriers and/or those with an acute HB virus infections, e.g., sexual, household, especially mother-child contact, (4) children from countries and localities of high HB virus endemicity, (5) heterosexually active persons with multiple partners, (6) homosexually active men, (7) intravenous drug abusers, (8) international travelers, (9) infants born to mothers who are HB surface antigen (HBsAg)–positive, and (10) health care workers who are exposed to blood, e.g., operating rooms, intensive care units, emergency rooms, laboratories, and those who care for dental patients. Possible transmission of HB virus in the child care setting is an increasing concern to public health authorities. Children who are HB virus carriers can transmit the virus if they have generalized dermatitis, bleeding problems, and scratches or if they bite others.

A recombinant DNA HB vaccine was licensed in 1986. Prior to 1986, a plasma-derived HB vaccine was the only one available. Babies born to HBsAg-positive mothers should receive HB immune globulin (HBIG) in addition to HB vaccine at birth, with additional doses of the vaccine at 1 month and 6 months of age. All adolescents with a sexually transmitted disease should receive a full course of vaccine. As well, all children under 7 years of age in refugee families from endemic areas and children in a family with a carrier of HB should be immunized.

Pneumococcal Polysaccharide Vaccine

A pneumococcal vaccine containing the polysaccharides of 23 types of streptococcus pneumonia (pneumococci) is licensed, but not recommended for routine immunizations. Responsiveness to the vaccine is unpredictable in children under 2 years of age. Vaccination is indicated for children at risk because of asplenia, sickle cell disease, nephrotic syndrome, or other immunodeficiency syndromes. Children with Hodgkin disease should be immunized before beginning therapy.

Meningococcal Polysaccharide Vaccine

Meningococcal vaccine protects against *Neisseria meningitidis* stereotypes A, C, Y, and W135. Meningococcal vaccine is currently recommended for use only under the circumstance of epidemic outbreaks; protection lasts for 1 to 3 years.

Varicella Vaccine

A live, attenuated, varicella vaccine, developed and tested in Japan, has been found to be safe and immunogenic in children. However, questions remain about the duration of immunity and the effect of vaccination on varicella epidemiology. In 1985, the vaccine was licensed in five European countries for use in persons with leukemia. Studies have shown that the vaccine is safe, immunogenic, and highly protective in both healthy and immunocompromised children (Gershon, 1990). Specific recommendations regarding the use of this vaccine have not yet been developed in the United States. Licensure of varicella vaccine in healthy children is likely to occur soon; however, children with leukemia should be vaccinated cautiously and under controlled circumstances. In the future, children about to undergo an organ transplant may be vaccinated against varicella. Its use with children with acquired immunodeficiency syndrome (AIDS) continues to be debated. This vaccine has not been used widely because varicella is generally a mild disease in normal, healthy children.

Yellow Fever, Cholera, Typhoid Fever, and Rabies Vaccines

Yellow fever, cholera, typhoid fever, and rabies vaccines are not recommended as a part of the routine immunization schedule in the United States. However, they are given routinely in some parts of the world and to Western world children traveling to those countries. All of these vaccines have side effects and, for some individuals, receiving the vaccine is inadvisable. In such cases, travel to countries where these diseases are epidemic is discouraged.

BCG (Bacillus Calmette-Guérin) Vaccine

BCG vaccine is a preparation of an attenuated strain of *Mycobacterium tuberculosis* (bacillus Calmette-Guérin). BCG vaccine is not given routinely against tuberculosis in the United States; rather, those who have been exposed, are at high risk, or are especially susceptible are given regular skin testing and treated prophylactically if the skin test results are positive.

Tuberculosis (TB) Testing

TB testing, while not an immunization, has historically been part of the immunization schedule recommended by the AAP. In recent years, there has been some controversy because of the potential for false-positive results. An alternative to no skin testing recommended by the AAP is that skin tests be performed at (1) 12 to 15 months of age (before or on the same day as MMR is given); (2) before school entry (4 to 6 years of age); and (3) in adolescence (14 to 16 years of age). Annual TB skin testing is highly recommended for individuals in high-risk groups.

Alterations of Immunization Schedules

Circumstances that may make it difficult to follow routine immunization schedules include (1) interrupted schedules, (2) unimmunized children, (3) immunocompromised children, and (4) immunization of premature infants.

Interrupted Schedule

Interruption of the recommended schedule does not require starting over in the schedule (AAP, 1991). The immunization is continued as if the usual time interval had elapsed.

Unimmunized Children

Children not immunized in the first year of life may be started on a schedule of primary immunization any time before the age of 7 years, according to Table 10–9 in the United States or according to Table 10–10 in Canada. The goal is to provide protection as efficiently as possible.

Children who start or continue immunization after 7 years of age should use the adult form of tetanus diphtheria (Td) vaccine. The schedule to follow for unimmunized children 7 years of age or older is also presented in Tables 10–9 and 10–10. When immunizations are not obtained as prescribed, further assessment is required to identify those factors that are interfering with the family's response to this aspect of health care. Strategies to facilitate the achievement of adequate immunization status are instituted by the health care team.

Immunization of Immunocompromised Children

Children may be immunocompromised because of an underlying disease or as the result of therapy that suppresses the immune response. Generally, live virus vaccines are contraindicated in children with congenital disorders of immune function. Other modes of management include use of inactivated vaccines and monthly administration of immune globulin.

After immunosuppressive therapy has been discontinued, the normal immunologic response does not resume until 3 months to 1 year later. Live virus vaccines can be given to patients with leukemia in remission if chemotherapy has been terminated for 3 months (Garber & Mortimer, 1992). Immunocompromised children need special consideration with respect to poliovirus and varicella vaccines.

Immunization of Premature Infants

It is recommended that premature infants receive routine immunizations according to their chronologic age, and that vaccine doses are not reduced (AAP, 1991). If an infant is still in the hospital at the age of 2 months when the first immunization is received, the OPV is postponed until discharge. This is done to prevent cross-infection of poliovirus to the other infants in the nursery. Inactivated polio vaccine (IPV) can be given to an infant still in the hospital. Preterm infants should be routinely immunized with HB vaccine, as are all other infants. As for all neonates, they should also receive HBIG if exposed to a mother who is HBsAG-positive.

Application of the Nursing Process: Immunization

Assessment

A child's immunization status is reviewed with the parent(s) to determine whether the child has received the appropriate vaccines. An assessment is made to identify the occurrence of severe reactions to previously received vaccines. If a family has missed appointments, an assessment is made to determine reasons for the irregularity of health visits such as family demands, forgetting appointment, too long a waiting period in clinic, lack of transportation, or health beliefs that run counter to immunization recommenda-

TABLE 10-9
Recommended Immunization Schedules for Children Not Immunized in First Year of Life (United States)

Recommended Time/Age	Immunizations*	Comments
Younger Than 7 Yrs		
First visit	DTP, OPV, MMR	MMR if child ≤ 15 mos old; tuberculin testing may be done at same visit
	HbCV†	For children aged 15–59 mos, can be given simultaneously with DTP and other vaccines (at separate sites)‡
Interval after first visit		
2 mos	DTP, OPV (HbCV)	Second dose of HbCV is indicated only in children whose first dose was received when younger than 15 mos
4 mos	DTP	Third dose of OPV is not indicated in the US but is desirable in other geographic areas where polio is endemic
10–16 mos	DTP, OPV	OPV is not given if third dose was given earlier
4–6 yrs (at or before school entry)	DTP, OPV	DTP is not necessary if the fourth dose was given after the 4th birthday; OPV is not necessary if third dose was given after the 4th birthday
11–12 yrs	MMR	At entry to middle school or junior high
10 yrs later	Td	Repeat every 10 yrs throughout life
7 Yrs and Older§, ‖		
First visit	Td, OPV, MMR	
Interval after first visit		
2 mos	Td, OPV	
8–14 mos	Td, OPV	
11–12 yrs	MMR	At entry to middle school or junior high
10 yrs later	Td	Repeat every 10 yrs throughout life

From American Academy of Pediatrics, Committee on Infectious Diseases. (1991). Report of the Committee on Infectious Diseases. *The redbook.* (22nd ed.). Elk Grove Village, IL. Used with permission of the American Academy of Pediatrics.

*DTP = diphtheria and tetanus toxoids with pertussis vaccine; HbCV = *Haemophilus influenzae* B conjugate vaccine; OPV = oral poliovirus vaccine containing attenuated poliovirus types 1, 2, and 3; MMR = live measles, mumps, and rubella viruses in a combined vaccine; Td = adult tetanus toxoid (full dose) and diphtheria toxoid (reduced dose) for adult use.

†If child is younger than 15 mos, only one HbCV (HbOC), as of October 1990, is approved for use.

‡The initial three doses of DTP can be given at 1- to 2-mo intervals; hence, for the child in whom immunization is initiated at age 15 mos or older, one visit could be eliminated by giving DTP, OPV, and MMR at the first visit; DTP and HbCV at the second visit (1 mo later); and DTP and OPV at the third visit (2 mos after the first visit). Subsequent doses of DTP and OPV 10–16 mos after the first visit are still indicated. HbCV, MMR, DTP, and OPV can be given simultaneously at separate sites if failure of the patient to return for future immunizations is a concern.

§If person is ≥18 yrs old, routine poliovirus vaccination is not indicated in the US.

‖ Minimal interval between doses of MMR is 1 mo.

TABLE 10–10
Immunization Schedules for Children Not Immunized in Early Infancy (Canada)

Timing	Immunization Against				
For Children 1–6 Yrs of Age					
First visit[3, 5]	Diphtheria	Pertussis	Tetanus	Poliomyelitis	*Haemophilus influenzae* B (HIB)[3]
Interval after 1st visit					
1 mo	Measles	Mumps	Rubella[2]		
2 mos	Diphtheria	Pertussis	Tetanus	Poliomyelitis	
4 mos	Diphtheria	Pertussis	Tetanus	Poliomyelitis[1]	
16 mos	Diphtheria	Pertussis	Tetanus	Poliomyelitis	
Preschool[6]	Diphtheria	Pertussis	Tetanus	Poliomyelitis	
At age 14–16 yrs	Diphtheria[4]	Tetanus[4]	Poliomyelitis[1]		

Timing	Immunization Against			
For Children 7 Yrs of Age and Over				
First visit[5]	Diphtheria[4]		Tetanus[4]	Poliomyelitis
Interval after 1st visit				
1 mo	Measles	Mumps	Rubella[2]	
2 mos	Diphtheria		Tetanus	Poliomyelitis
14 mos	Diphtheria		Tetanus	Poliomyelitis
10 yrs	Diphtheria		Tetanus	Poliomyelitis[1]

[1]This dose may be omitted if live (oral) polio vaccine is being used exclusively.

[2]Rubella vaccine is also indicated for all girls and women of childbearing age who lack proof of immunity. At all medical visits, the opportunity should be taken to check whether girls and women need rubella vaccine.

[3]Children beginning their series at age 12–14 mos require one dose followed by a booster at age 18 mos. Unimmunized children aged 15–59 mos require only a single dose.

[4]Diphtheria and tetanus toxoid (Td), a combined adsorbed "adult type" preparation for use in persons 7 yrs of age or more, contains less diphtheria toxoid than preparations given to younger children and is less likely to cause reactions in older persons.

[5]Measles, mumps, and rubella vaccines may also be given at the first visit if it is considered likely that a child will not return for further immunization.

[6]If the last dose of the primary series for diphtheria, tetanus, pertussis, and polio is given after the 4th birthday, this dose may be omitted.

Note: The *Canadian immunization guide* (4th ed.) was not available at time of publication. This schedule is based on current practice in Ontario and the most recent publication: National Advisory Committee on Immunization. (1989). *Canadian immunization guide.* (3rd ed.). (Cat. No. H49–8/1989E). Ottawa: Ministry of National Health and Welfare.

tions. Misinformation about vaccines and misinterpretation of the child's reaction to a vaccine may introduce anxiety and reveal family teaching needs.

Prior to administering a vaccine, the child is assessed for signs of physical illness, and the nurse elicits from the parent(s) whether their child has been healthy. If the child is described to have an illness, an assessment is made about the severity. The child's illness is assessed with respect to the particular vaccine that the child is scheduled to receive. The decision to give or not to give a vaccine is a decision made in collaboration with a physician and the family.

Nursing Diagnostic Statements

High risk for injury (chemical); risk factor: unsafe vaccine immunization practices associated with:

- Lack of preparation of child and parent.
- Inappropriate decision related to a child's illness.

Ineffective management of therapeutic regimen (parents): failure to follow routine immunization schedule related to:

- Fear of serious side effects.
- The child's illness.
- Conflict of religious beliefs.
- Inadequate knowledge.
- Lack of transportation.
- Ineffective support for caregiver.

Planning and Implementation

Preventing Chemical Injury to the Child: Immunization/Vaccination Administration

Nurses must be prepared to give the immunization safely and with as little pain infliction as possible. Additionally, nurses are called on to answer the many questions associated with immunization and follow-up care. Important aspects of safe administration include child and parent preparation; safe administration with respect to appropriate site, route, and administration of multiple vaccines; appropriate decisions with respect to a child's illness; and safe handling and storage of vaccines.

Preparation of Child and Parents: Teaching: Procedure/Treatment

Children are prepared for the procedure according to their developmental age. Principles of preparing children for procedures are discussed in Chapter 23. Giving parents information about vaccines has received public attention because of the proliferation of lawsuits associated with vaccinations. Lawsuits have been brought against vaccine producers because of incidents of serious sequelae following certain vaccines. In response to the public's concern, a National Childhood Vaccine Injury Act was passed and became effective March 21, 1988 (National Childhood Vaccine Injury Act, 1988). It requires health care professionals to report specific adverse reactions that occur following immunizations. Records are kept and the patient should receive a copy. Recorded information includes name of vaccine, site, manufacture lot number, expiration date, and the names and title of person administering the vaccine.

As of April 15, 1992, provision of information to parents became a government mandate. Immunization brochures, prepared by the United States Centers for Disease Control, must now be distributed to the parents of children who are to receive any of three vaccines, DTP, MMR, and polio. These brochures are required under the Federal Vaccine Injury Compensation Act of 1986, and anyone who administers these vaccines must ensure that parents read and understand the brochures. Unfounded fears need to be dispelled and the importance of return visits stressed in an attempt to reduce the numbers of unimmunized children.

Site and Route. The recommended site and route of administration varies with the type of vaccine and size of the child. The preferred sites for intramuscular injection are vastus lateralis and ventrogulteal muscle; the deltoid can be used for children 18 months or older (Ipp et al, 1989). The gluteus muscle should not be used for immunizations, especially in infants and young children, because the gluteal region consists mostly of fat until the child has been walking for some time and because there is a danger of damaging the sciatic nerve (AAP, 1991).

Needles used for intramuscular injection should be of sufficient length to actually reach the muscle. A 1-inch needle is usually required to penetrate the muscle in a normal 4-month-old infant. The amount of fat present, rather than the age of the child, determines the length of needle required. Adsorbed vaccines must be injected deep into the muscle mass to reduce the risk of local reactions. Shorter needles specifically designed for subcutaneous injections are used for MMR. Types of agents and route of administration are summarized in Table 10–11. For further discussion of general principles of giving injections, see Chapter 24.

Administration of Multiple Vaccines. Administration of multiple vaccines is standard practice. Protective responses and side effects of vaccines administered simultaneously have been found to be similar to those that are administered separately (Frenkel, 1990). It is sometimes advisable to administer vaccines simultaneously, especially if it is unlikely that a child will be brought back for additional immunizations. A disadvantage of multiple immunizations is that adverse reactions are more confusing to decipher (Pichichero et al, 1990).

There are a few circumstances that require special attention. If immunoglobulin is required at the same

TABLE 10-11
Type of Immunization Agent, Side Effects, and Route of Administration

Route and Side Effects	Comments*
Diphtheria Toxoid	
Administration: Intramuscularly (if *fluid vaccine* rather than an *adsorbed vaccine* is used then it is given subcutaneously) Low incidence of fever and local soreness, redness, and swelling at injection site	Usually given in combination with tetanus and pertussis (DPT) or just DT (for the child < 7 yrs old who has reacted to pertussis). Td is an adult vaccine (used for children ≥ 7 yrs). It contains the standard amount of tetanus toxoid but only 20% of the diphtheria toxoid supplied by DTP or DT *Contraindications:* (1) An acute febrile illness; (2) an evolving or suspected neurologic disease; (3) a prior severe reaction.
Tetanus Toxoid	
Administration: Intramuscularly (if *fluid vaccine* rather than an *adsorbed vaccine* is used then it is given subcutaneously) Low incidence of fever and mild local tenderness, redness, and swelling at injection site. Antipyretics are used for fever postinjection. Prophylactic use of antipyretics is often recommended if fever occurred following previous immunizations	Usually administered in combination with diphtheria and pertussis (DPT) to children < 7 yrs old and Td to children ≥ 7 yrs and to adults
Pertussis Vaccine	
Administration: Intramuscularly (if *fluid vaccine* rather than an *adsorbed vaccine* is used then it is given subcutaneously) Over 50% have temporary local tenderness. A swelling or lump may remain at injection site for a few weeks or even months but gradually disappears. Approximately 50% of the children have fever, irritability, or lethargy. More serious reactions can occur on rare occasions. Antipyretics used for fever. Warm soaks on involved area for comfort (or warm bath)	Usually given in combination with tetanus and diphtheria toxoids (DPT). Parents need clear explanations about risks and benefits of the vaccine (see discussion in this chapter). Nurse should ask about reactions to previous pertussis vaccine before administering vaccine
Polio† (Trivalent Oral Poliovaccine, TOPV)	
Administration: Orally Virtually no side effects. A few cases of vaccine-associated paralytic disease have been reported in the primary vaccinee (person vaccinated): 1:10 million. In the primary vaccinee plus close contacts: 1:4 million incidents of paralysis have been reported	Not administered to family members of immunodeficient child. Although antibodies in breast milk can neutralize the vaccine, it does not interfere with development of immunity. Not given to premature infants until discharged from hospital, because of dissemination to other prematures (because OPV produces secretory antibodies within the intestinal tract, infection of close contact may occur). Such indirect immunization can also be beneficial to contacts
Measles	
Administration: Subcutaneously Approximately 5% of vaccinees develop fever between 6 and 10 days after vaccination, lasting up to 5 days. Transient rashes reported in 3–5%. Antipyretics used for fever; warm soaks or warm bath and antihistamine for rash if pruritic	Given in combination with mumps and rubella vaccines *Contraindications:* Pregnancy, immunodeficiency, therapeutic immunosuppression, or an acute febrile illness (see text for each vaccine)
Mumps	
Administration: Subcutaneously Rarely fever and rash	Given in combination with measles and rubella vaccines Same as for Measles
Rubella	
Administration: Subcutaneously Approximately 30% of vaccinees have transient rash, lymphadenopathy, or arthralgia. Approximately 1% have self-limited arthritis (occurs about 2 wks after the immunization). More common in women than in children. Mild analgesic may be used for pain	Given in combination with measles and mumps vaccines Same as for Measles

(continued)

TABLE 10–11
Type of Immunization Agent, Side Effects, and Route of Administration *(Continued)*

Route and Side Effects	Comments*
***Haemophilus influenzae* Type B, A Polysaccharide**	
Administration: Intramuscularly or subcutaneously Approximately 50% of children have fever and mild local reactions at vaccination site. Significant fever occurs in only 1% of children. Antipyretics used for fever	When this vaccine is given simultaneously with DPT, the incidence of reactions is not increased more than if DPT is given alone
Hepatitis B (Plasma-Derived) and Hepatitis B (Recombinant DNA) Vaccines	
Administration: Intramuscularly Approximately 15% of vaccinees have mild local tenderness at injection site Anterolateral thigh for infants and deltoid for older children (over 18 mos). Immunogenicity is diminished when given in buttocks	Indications for use of plasma-derived and recombinant DNA are similar, except plasma-derived vaccine is used for hemodialysis patients and the immunosuppressed Universal vaccinations of infants is now recommended, using a three-dose regimen
Pneumococcal Vaccine	
Administration: Intramuscularly or subcutaneously Local redness and mild soreness occurs in 50% of cases	Children under 2 yrs old do not respond to the vaccine with protective antibody titers. Reimmunization is not recommended
Influenza Vaccine	
Administration: Intramuscularly preferred (also subcutaneously) Approximately one third of vaccinees develop mild local redness and swelling at injection site. Systemic reactions of fever and malaise are infrequent. In 1976, a temporal association was noted between administration of the "swine flu" vaccine and Guillain-Barré syndrome in adults	Individuals with egg allergies should not receive the vaccine, because it is made from egg-grown viruses. November is generally accepted as the optimal time for organized vaccination campaigns. Routine immunization is not recommended for children. Inactivated influenza viral vaccines are safe; live vaccines have been successfully used in adults, but insufficient studies have been done in child populations

From American Academy of Pediatrics, Committee on Infectious Diseases. (1991). Report of the Committee on Infectious Diseases. *The redbook.* (22nd ed.). Elk Grove Village, IL. Used with permission of the American Academy of Pediatrics and National Advisory Committee on Immunization. (1989). *Canadian immunization guide.* (3rd ed.). (Cat. No. H49–8/1989E). Ottawa: Ministry of National Health and Welfare.

*All vaccines must be stored according to manufacturer's recommendations.

†Inactivated polio virus (IPV) is administered subcutaneously; DPT polio, a combined vaccine, is given intramuscularly.

visit as a vaccine, the vaccine-induced immunity (especially that of measles) may be compromised. The MMR immunization should be administered at a site remote from the immunoglobulin (Edwards & Karzon, 1990). Also, live virus vaccines can interfere with a tuberculin test. Tuberculin testing should be done on the same day as the live virus vaccine is given or approximately 2 months thereafter.

In all circumstances of multiple vaccine administration, each injection is given at a different site. A different needle and syringe must be used for each injection. A charting system must document which vaccine was given in each site for follow-up of any reactions.

Illness and Vaccination. It is not uncommon for a child to present with a febrile or acute illness on the day immunizations are scheduled. Minor illnesses (e.g., mild upper respiratory tract infections, allergic rhinitis, or a mild episode of diarrhea) should not preclude routine vaccination. Deferring the immunization of children with minor illnesses too frequently results in children remaining unimmunized for too long; thereby subjecting them to the danger of contracting a preventable disease. However, children with a fever and moderate-to-severe illness should not be immunized. Parents are asked to bring their child for immunization as soon as the febrile illness has subsided. See Table 10–11 for summary of contraindications with respect to illness.

Handling and Storage. Appropriate handling and storing of vaccines is the responsibility of anyone who administers the vaccine. Recent evidence indicates that more attention needs to be given to storage practices (Casto & Brunnell, 1991). Vaccines should be stored according to product information directions. It is the nurse's responsibility to ensure that vaccines are not left on the counter at room temperature unsafely. Also, when multidose vials are used, bacterial contamination must be prevented by adherence to sterile technique.

Promoting Effective Management of Therapeutic Regimen: Teaching: Parent

Parents sometimes question or do not understand the purpose of immunizations or how the immunization works to protect the body from the particular disease. Parents need explanations to help them understand that the body's immune system does not provide perfect protection from all diseases and that immunity does not occur unless the individual either experiences the disease (natural immunity) or receives an agent (by injection or orally) to stimulate the body into producing antibodies (acquired immunity). The immunizing agent is a strain of the infection-causing virus or bacteria, in either a dead or attenuated state that is incapable of causing the full-blown disease. These dead or attenuated strains serve as antigens to the body, resulting in the production of antibodies making the individual resistant to the disease when exposed to the specific live virus or bacteria. See Chapter 37 for further discussion of the immune response in relation to disease.

Once the parents understand how a child becomes immunized, a few explanations about the consequences of not being immunized should be given. The most obvious rationale for immunizing all children is to prevent unnecessary discomfort, disability, and potential mortality that can result when children get communicable diseases. It seems unreasonable to place a child's health at risk of sterility, as a consequence of mumps, or of paralysis, as a result of poliomyelitis.

Another rationale to stress to parents and older children and adolescents is the threat that the presence of such diseases causes to others in society. Risks include (1) congenital malformations of the fetus if an unimmunized pregnant woman is exposed to a child with rubella; (2) more severe side effects to unimmunized adults who might contract these infectious diseases from children; (3) infants coming in contact with the disease who are too young to be immunized but too old to still have neonatal immunity; (4) the potentially fatal consequence for those children with diseases that do not permit them the privilege of receiving immunizations; and (5) the hazardous effects to elderly persons with already compromised health states.

It must also be stressed to family members that, although immunizations begin during infancy, boosters are required in later life. For some infections, boosters are necessary periodically throughout life to keep antibody titers effectively high. It is helpful and important to keep an immunization record for each family member to aid in keeping immunizations current.

Some children do experience reactions to particular immunization vaccines. These reactions may be relatively immediate and short-term or, rarely, long-term in the form of residual effects (usually related to central nervous system function). The reaction may be localized at the injection site or result in systemic responses. It must be emphasized that rarely are reactions serious in nature. If the child is acutely ill, it may be necessary to defer the immunization. Parents are cautioned that the child must be brought back as soon as the child has recuperated because of the child's need for the vaccine.

If parents have fears or misconceptions about reactions to the vaccine, the nurse can reassure them that simple measures can be used to reduce their child's discomfort. Increased publicity about adverse effects of routine childhood immunizations and concern about litigation have prompted the use of written information and consents prior to immunizations.

Questions that children and parents have must be clarified before the vaccine is given. Some families may not understand the importance of immunization because of a language barrier. Informed consent is an essential before vaccines are given; therefore, an interpreter should be accessed to ensure full understanding.

Evaluation

The child's response to the vaccines is evaluated at the time the immunization is given and by asking parents about the child's previous response. The return visits are monitored and parents are asked to keep records of their child's immunization. These records should be compared so that no immunizations are missed.

Legislative and Societal Actions

Governmental involvement in the issue of mass immunization has existed in varying degrees since the first vaccine was discovered. The United States Food and Drug Administration approves and regulates the vaccines available for use on human beings. The government budget continues to include financial support for research into the development, refinement, and effectiveness of various vaccines. WHO continually studies the issue of immunizable diseases around the world, developing and recommending policies for countries to adopt and enforce.

The current need is to focus on the preschool and infant populations, in which immunization levels are substantially lower. Some measures are not being taken in which pediatric nurses can be actively involved: (1) increasing the number of health care provider–based immunization programs (independent nursing practices, pediatrician practices, health maintenance organizations, walk-in clinics, and so on) rather than continual dependence on government-organized programs; (2) increasing hospital, prenatal, and well baby clinic–based education programs for parents of neonates and infants; and (3) acquiring cooperation of day care, nursery school, and preschool programs to enforce proof of immunization as a prerequisite for attendance, similar to the policy in the school system.

Although society as a whole supports immunizations of all children, each individual family is still responsible for ensuring that immunizations are obtained by its members. Noncompliance tends most often to be associated with ignorance or misunderstandings regarding the rationale for immunizations and the potentially serious consequences of not taking such preventive actions. Many families are unaware of the immunizations that are needed, when they should be received, or where they may be obtained. With so many dual-career and single, working-parent family units, the problem is sometimes a lack of accessibility during evening or weekend hours when parents are not at work. This is especially true in smaller and rural communities that do not have access to the multiplicity of health care services or to the 24-hour availability of services that exists in large cities.

Families cannot be held totally accountable for the underimmunization of infant and preschool children, however. All health care providers have not taken seriously their part of the responsibility of promoting preventive immunizations among their patients. Assessment and education regarding immunizations need to become an automatic part of every contact with a pediatric patient, regardless of the reason for that particular contact.

Immunizations are one of the miracles of this century that can prevent a tremendous amount of discomfort and grief. An immunization program that is right for one population is not necessarily the most preferred for another at all times. For each immunization available, the cost and the benefits must be considered. Those responsible for establishing recommended schedules consider carefully: (1) whether the costs involved in immunizing can be repaid monetarily or in social terms, or both; (2) how seriously and with what frequency the disease occurs in unimmunized populations; (3) what protection the immunization offers and for how long; and (4) what the risks of the vaccine itself are. All these factors are balanced against the benefits of eliminating the specific infection from the world population. The nurse has a role in all facets of these decisions, from the collection of epidemiologic data to the education of the public and the administration of immunizations to patients.

Management of Minor Health Problems

The nurse's interaction with children and families during a minor illness may take place on the phone, in a clinic, in a hospital, or at home. The interaction begins with a health assessment of the child's condition; then, the problem and its etiology are identified, and, in collaboration with the parents and other professionals, interventions are planned and carried out. Since knowledge deficit is often a risk factor of the high risk for altered health maintenance, a primary role in the care of a child with minor illness is to teach the family how to assess and evaluate the condition of their child and how to care for their child at home. Most minor illness causes a disruption in the child's usual activities and routines. Family members may experience sleep pattern disturbance when called on to soothe their irritable, uncomfortable, or sleepless child or to administer the necessary symptomatic treatments. Particularly while symptoms are most acute, parental anxiety exists about whether to seek help from a health professional, whether their judgment is adequate to determine if the child is improving or getting worse, and what measures they should take to relieve their child's discomfort.

Since care is usually administered at home, the caregiver who works away from home must either miss work or secure an adequate substitute caretaker for the sick child at home during work hours. The question of who will stay home from work may cause some antagonism between the parents. The rearrangements of work schedules and conflicts concerning roles can upset the child and family even in the face of minor illness.

Anticipatory guidance early in parenthood should provide some basic information that will be useful to parents when their child becomes ill. This information should include: (1) when to seek nurse or physician assistance, (2) facts to gather before calling for assistance, (3) what to do during the office or clinic visit, (4) symptom assessment (temperature taking, throat inspection), and (5) instruction and practice in basic treatment of common symptoms (measures to reduce fever, evaluating respirations). The nurse also plays an active part in offering education and health services that can *prevent* many of the minor illnesses.

When to Seek Assistance

Parents need to know the early signs of illness if they are to make judgments about intervention. Illness is

TABLE 10-12
Family-Centered Teaching: When to Seek Health Care

You should seek health care for your child when he or she:

- Is under 6 mos of age and has a fever of 37.8°C (100°F) or above
- Has persistent high fever of 39.2°C (102°F) or above
- Is irritable or lethargic
- Has received a serious blow to the head or other serious injury
- Has any signs of respiratory difficulty
- Has persistent vomiting or diarrhea
- Has pain
- When you recognize a combination of changes in your child (e.g., does not eat, play, or sleep as usual)

TABLE 10-13
Information Parents Should Be Prepared to Provide Before Seeking Assistance*

Child's Age

(Symptoms may change suddenly in children under 6 mos; age may affect treatment prescribed.)

When Child Last Well

(If symptoms are mild and recent, physician or nurse will probably follow by phone. If symptoms worsen or have lasted several days, child should be seen.)

Behavior

Is the child irritable? Lost interest in play? Decreased appetite? For how long has this been the case? (Child acting sick more than 24 hrs should be seen by doctor or nurse even if symptoms are minor.)

Fever

What is child's temperature? Rectally or orally? How long has the fever existed? What has been done for it—results? (Consult physician if fever is high, longer than 3 days, if infant under 6 mos, if accompanied by a stiff neck, and if child is dehydrated).

Pain

Difficulty swallowing? Stiff neck? Pulling or holding ear—which one? Headache? Stomach ache—where? Pain when extremities moved? Hurt to breathe? (Consult physician immediately for acute, persistent pain; physician or nurse if child presents with no other symptoms or if minor injury is associated.)

Breathing

Slow or fast? Any noise? Coughing? Stuffy or runny nose? Unable to eat or drink? Any extra effort made to breathe? Any blueness around mouth? (See physician immediately if any distress or noise! See physician or nurse if breathing difficulty interferes with feeding, or if cough interrupts sleep.)

Skin

Cool or hot? Dry or moist? Blotchy? Any rash—flat or raised, color, location, single or several together, itchy? (See physician or nurse if child's neck is also stiff, has swollen glands, or if child looks very sick.)

Any Vomiting/Diarrhea

How many times today? How long has it been occurring? Any mucus? What does it look like? (See physician or nurse if frequent or constant, blood present, dehydration exists, possible poison or drug ingestion.)

Eyes

Dull? Tearing? Discharge—amount and color? Partly closed? (See physician or nurse if discharge present or if, coupled with other symptoms, dehydration suggested.)

Other

Any other family members ill presently or recently (past 2 wks)? Any similar illness in neighborhood or school? Any major changes in routines? Any recent family crises? Child have any chronic conditions? (A chronically ill child should be seen by physician even if symptoms are mild.)

What Has Been Tried

Any medicines given? Have any of the things tried helped? (Gives some clue to caregiver's judgement re: interventions. If questionable, child should be seen, as other observations may be inaccurate.)

What Caregiver Is Most Worried About

(If other family situations are being affected by the illness [party, trip, work] it may be important to the family for the child to be seen even if symptoms are mild.)

*The material in parentheses is a guide to the nurse in determining whether the child should be seen and by whom.

usually preceded by a change in the child's normal behavior, especially related to play and eating.

A sudden or dramatic decrease in appetite and unusual irritability and lassitude, as well as fever and pain, are definite signs that all is not well.

Fever and pain are also common precursors to illness. Although there is some variation in management of minor illness, parents are usually given guidelines about when to seek professional advice. Generally, parents are advised to call if they "think something is wrong." Parents know their children, and their observations are very important and should be taken seriously. Parents should be taught when to seek a professional (Table 10–12).

Facts to Gather

Before parents seek assistance, they should look over their child for symptoms, take the temperature, and take note of the child's behavior so that the nurse's or doctor's questions can be answered. Prior to seeking assistance, whether by telephone or a visit, there are observations that a parent or caregiver should be taught to make and write down in preparation (Table 10–13). From this information, the health professional can decide how urgent the problem is and how it should be managed (e.g., over the phone, in the office, in the hospital, or at home).

Teaching Parents Symptomatic Care

The ultimate success of the family's involvement in home treatment is largely determined by their ability and preparation to participate in it. Evaluating signs of illness, including knowing how to take rectal and oral temperatures, is an important aspect of home care to teach parents. Additional home health care management to teach parents includes fever control, dietary measures for mild vomiting or diarrhea, emergency first-aid procedures (including those for bleeding and choking and artificial respiration and circulation), aseptic measures, including the management of contagious illnesses, and how to measure and administer medicines according to the child's age. Obviously, caregivers cannot absorb all this information at one time. Therefore, information is introduced gradually and supplemented with written materials. Knowledge deficit is a risk factor for high risk of altered health maintenance. An ongoing assessment is required to determine the child's and the parent's knowledge about the symptomatic care required.

Caregivers may also need assistance in developing convalescent activities for their recuperating child. A potential diversional activity deficit can occur during an illness. The key elements of successful convalescent activities is that age-appropriate motor development is encouraged. Keep the child involved in an activity that is enjoyable and promotes cognitive development. Many household items can be used for creative play and help to pass the time. Macaroni, paper plates, paper bags, old magazines or catalogues, or fabric scraps (the possibilities are almost endless) coupled with scissors, paste, watercolor paints, and crayons can occupy many hours. Have children create stories based on a name, a character, or a situation, or, perhaps, write their own life story. If they are too young to write, they can dictate the story into a tape recorder or draw pictures. See Chapter 17 for other age-appropriate play activities. Children are also helped through their convalescence if they are allowed to get at least partly dressed every day and occasionally to be on the living room couch, if possible. If the child cannot join the family at meal times, each member (except those susceptible to the disease if it is contagious) can take turns having dinner with the ill child.

KEY CONCEPTS

Concepts Related to Basic Information

- Common themes of health that provide a frame work for promoting health care are:
  - Adaptation and stability.
  - Actualization.
  - Effectiveness.
  - Taking responsibility for one's own health.
- Children with lower self-concepts and greater anxiety perceive themselves to be more vulnerable to health problems.
- Children's concepts of health change qualitatively as cognitive skills develop.
- A primary need in our society is to enhance current levels of children's immunization status.
- Active immunization involves administration of a microorganism (live vaccine) or a modified product of an organism (toxoid).
- Vaccines that contain a microorganism may be live, attenuated, or killed.
- An immunologic response following a vaccine mimics a natural infection, but presents little or no risk to the child.
- Even minor illness can cause considerable disruption to a family.

Concepts Related to Nursing Assessment

- Health needs as identified by the child and family determine nursing intervention.
- Assessment of the child's thinking ability and concept of health and degree of independent action determines choice of teaching approach.
- The nurse's primary role in the assessment of an ill child is to teach the family how to gather data and evaluate their child's condition at home.
- A child's illness is usually preceded by changes in normal behavior and activities.
- Although fever per se is not a contraindication to receiving a vaccine, if it is associated with other clinical manifestations suggesting a more serious illness, vaccination is postponed.
- Prior to vaccination, an assessment is made to determine the presence of contraindications for the particular vaccine being administered.

Concepts Related to Nursing Intervention

- Health promotion is a goal of nursing care in acute care as well as primary health care settings.
- Nursing care must include interventions that foster a child's self-esteem as well as physical health.
- The goal of nursing care is to promote competence in developing children so that they move from passive into active roles to achieve health.
- Provision of written information for parents of children receiving vaccines is a government mandate requiring nurses and all health professionals to ensure that the client reads and understands the brochure.
- Teaching parents the importance of return visits is a priority.
- Preparing parents for normal reactions to vaccines and how to manage their child's minor discomfort may reduce the fear and anxiety associated with immunization.
- Teaching parents how to assess an ill child, the facts to gather, and when to seek assistance is essential to minor health problem management.

REFERENCES

American Academy of Pediatrics, Committee on Infectious Diseases. (1990). *Haemophilus influenzae* type b conjugate vaccines: Immunization of children at 15 months of age. *Pediatrics, 86,* 794–796.

American Academy of Pediatrics, Committee on Infectious Diseases. (1991). Report of the Committee on Infectious Diseases. *The Redbook* (22nd Ed.). Elk Grove Village, IL: Author.

American Academy of Pediatrics, Committee on Psychosocial Aspects of Child and Family Health 1985–88. (1988). *Guidelines for health supervision II.* Elk Grove Village, IL: Author.

Arnold, P. J., & Schlenker, T. L. (1992). The impact of health care financing on childhood immunization practices. *American Journal of Diseases of Children, 146,* 728–732.

Bandura, A. (1986). *Social foundations of thought and action: A social cognitive theory.* Englewood Cliffs, NJ: Prentice-Hall.

Bandura, A. (1977). *Social learning theory.* Englewood Cliffs, NJ: Prentice-Hall.

Becker, M. H. (1974). The health belief model and personal health behavior. *Health Education Monographs, 2,* 324–473.

Bedworth, A. E., & Bedworth, D. A. (1982). *Health for human effectiveness.* Englewood Cliffs, NJ: Prentice-Hall.

Bibace, R., & Walsh, M. E. (1980). Development of children's concepts of illness. *Pediatrics, 66,* 912–917.

Blecke, J. (1990). Exploration of children's health and self-care behavior within a family context through qualitative research. *Family Relations, 39,* 284–291.

Bruhn, J. G., & Cordova, F. (1977). A developmental approach to learning wellness behavior. Part 1: Infancy to early adolescence. *Health Values, 1,* 246–254.

Bruhn, J. G., & Parcel, G. S. (1982). Current knowledge about the health behavior of young children: A conference summary. *Health Education, 9,* 142, 165–238, 261.

Bush, P. J., Iannotti, R. J. (1988). Origins and stability of children's health beliefs relative to medicine use. *Social Science and Medicine, 27,* 345–352.

Campbell, D. W. (1991). Family paradigm theory and family rituals: Implications for child and family health. *Nurse Practitioner, 16,* 22–31.

Casto, D. T., & Brunnell, P. A. (1991). Safe handling of vaccines. *Pediatrics, 87,* 108–112.

Chiloh, S., & Waiser, R. (1991). Adolescents' concepts of health and illness. *International Journal of Adolescent Medicine and Health, 5,* 69–87.

Cowell, J. M., Mosley, E., Pelt, P., & Mootry, P. (1991). School health services: A hub of services to children and their families. *Pediatric Nursing, 17,* 86–88.

Cox, C. L., Cowell, J. M., Marion, L. N., & Miller, E. H. (1990). The health self-determinism index for children. *Research in Nursing and Health, 13,* 237–246.

Dielman, T. E., et al. (1982). Parental and child health beliefs and behavior. *Health Education Quarterly, 9,* 60, 156.

Dubos, R. (1965). *Man adapting.* New Haven, CT: Yale University Press.

Dubos, R. (1959). *Mirage of health.* Garden City, NY: Doubleday.

Dunn, H. L. (1961). *High level wellness.* Arlington, VA: RW Beatty.

Edwards, K. M., & Karzon, D. T. (1990). The search for an improved pertussis vaccine. *Pediatric Annals, 19,* 695–701.

Epp, J. (1986). *Achieving health for all: A framework for health promotion.* Ottawa, Canada: Development of National Health and Welfare.

Flaherty, M. (1986). Preschool children's conceptions of health and health behaviors. *Maternal-Child Nursing Journal, 15,* 205–265.

Frager, B. (1990). A national child care crisis: Action for the 90s. *Journal of Pediatric Nursing, 5,* 229–231.

Frenkel, L. D. (1990). Routine immunizations for American children in the 1990s. *Pediatric Clinics of North America, 37,* 531–548.

Garber, R. M., & Mortimer, E. A. (1992). Immunizations: Beyond the basics. *Pediatrics in Review, 13,* 98–106.

Gershon, A. A. (1990). Immunization practices in children. *Hospital Practice, 25,* 91–107.

Gochman, D. S., & Saucier, J. F. (1982). Perceived vulnerability in children and adolescents. *Health Education Quarterly, 9,* 46, 58–142, 154.

Griffin, M., Ray, W., Mortimer, E., Fenichel, G., & Schaffner, W. (1990). Risk of seizures and encephalopathy after immunization with the diphtheria-tetanus-pertussis vaccine. *Journal of the American Medical Association, 263,* 1641–1645.

Haggerty, R. J. (1991). Care of the poor and undeserved in America. *American Journal of Diseases of Children, 145,* 569–571.

Hales, D. (1992). *An invitation to health: Taking charge of your life.* Redwood City, CA: Benjamin/Cummings Publishing.

Hart-Zeldin, C., Kalnins, I., Pollack, P., & Love, R. (1990). Children in the context of "Achieving health for all: A framework for health promotion." *Canadian Journal of Public Health, 81,* 196–198.

Harvey, B. (1991). Why we need a national child health policy. *Pediatrics, 87,* 1–6.

Hearne, J., & Klockars, A. J. (1988). Applicability of the Parcel-Meyer children's locus of control scale. *Journal of School Health, 58,* 16–19.

Igoe, J. (1990). A blueprint for health promotion: Children's rights and community action. *Pediatric Nursing, 16,* 410–411.

Ipp, M. M., Gold, R., Goldbach, M., et al. (1989). Adverse reactions to diphtheria, tetanus, pertussis-polio vaccination at 18 months of age: Effect of injection site and needle length. *Pediatrics, 83,* 687–692.

Kalnins, I., & Love, R. (1982). Children's concepts of health and illness and implications for health education: An overview. *Health Education Quarterly, 9,* 8, 9–104, 115.

Kimpen, J. L. L., & Ogra, L. L. (1990). Poliovirus vaccines: A continuing challenge. *Pediatric Clinics of North America, 37,* 627–649.

King, I. M. (1990). Health as the goal for nursing. *Nursing Sciences Quarterly, 13,* 123–128.

King, I. M. (1981). *A theory for nursing: Systems, concepts, process.* New York: John Wiley.

La Montagne, L. L., & Hepworth, T. (1991). Issues in the measurement of children's locus of control. *Western Journal of Nursing Research, 13*(1), 67–83.

Levine, M. E. (1971). Holistic nursing. *Nursing Clinics of North America, 6,* 253–264.

Lewin, K. (1935). *A dynamic theory of personality.* New York: McGraw-Hill.

Lewis, M. A., & Lewis, C. E. (1990). Consequences of empowering children to care for themselves. *Pediatrician, 17,* 63–67.

Logsdon, D. A. (1991). Conceptions of health and health behaviors of preschool children. *Journal of Pediatric Nursing, 6,* 396–406.

Long, S. S., DeForest, A., Smith, D. G., Lazaro, C., & Wassilak, S. G. F. (1990). Longitudinal study of adverse reactions following diphtheria-tetanus-pertussus vaccine in infancy. *Pediatrics, 85,* 294–302.

Maurer, H. M. (1991). The growing neglect of American children. *American Journal of Diseases of Children, 145,* 540–541.

Mickalide, A. D. (1986). Children's understanding of health and illness: Implications for health promotion. *Health Values, 10,* 5–21.

Moch, S. (1989). Health within illness: Conceptual evolution and practice possibilities. *Advances in Nursing Science, 11,* 23–31.

Natapoff, J. (1978). Childrens' views of health: A developmental study. *American Journal of Public Health,* 995–999.

Natapoff, J. (1982, Summer/Fall). A developmental analysis of children's ideas of health. *Health Education Quarterly,* 130–140.

Natapoff, J., & Essoka, G. C. (1989). Handicapped and able-bodied children's ideas of health. *Journal of School Health, 59,* 436–440.

National Advisory Committee on Immunization (1989). *Canadian Immunization Guide* (3rd ed.). (Cat. No. H49–8/1989E). Ottawa: Ministry of National Health and Welfare.

National Childhood Vaccine Injury Act. (1988). National Childhood Vaccine Injury Act: Requirements for permanent vaccinations records and for reporting of selected events after vaccination. *Morbidity and Mortality Weekly Report, 37,* 197–200.

Oberg, C. N. (1990). Medically uninsured children in the United States: A challenge to public policy. *Pediatrics, 85,* 824–833.

O'Brien, R. W., Bush, P. J., & Parcel, G. S. (1989). Stability in a measure of children's health locus of control. *Journal of School Health, 59,* 161–164.

Orem, D. E. (1991). *Nursing: Concepts of practice.* St. Louis: Mosby Year Book.

Parcel, G. S. (1988). CHLC scale developer comments on applicability. *Journal of School Health, 58,* 19–20.

Payne, L. (1983). Health: A basic concept in nursing theory. *Advances in Nursing Science, 3,* 393–395.

Pender, N. (1990). Expressing health through lifestyle patterns. *Nursing Science Quarterly, 13,* 115–122.

Pender, N. (1987). *Health promotion in nursing practice* (2nd ed.). Norwalk, CT: Appleton & Lange.

Phillips, C. G. (1991). Keeping up with the changing immunization schedule. *Contemporary Pediatrics, 8,* 20–46.

Pichichero, M. E., Green, J. L., Francis, A. B., Marsocci, S. M., & Disney, F. A. (1990). New vaccines and vaccination policies. *Pediatric Annals, 19,* 686–694.

Pidgeon, V. (1977, Spring). Characteristics of children's thinking and implications of health teaching. *Maternal Child Nursing Journal,* 1.

Rosenstock, I. M. (1974). Historical origins of the health belief model. *Health Education Monographs, 2,* 328–335.

Rosenstock, I. M., Strecher, V. J., & Becker, M. H. (1988). Social learning theory and the health belief model. *Health Education Quarterly, 15,* 175–183.

Rotter, J. B. (1954). *Social learning and clinical psychology.* Englewood Cliffs, NJ: Prentice-Hall.

Roy, C. (1976). *Introduction to nursing: An adaptation model.* Englewood Cliffs, NJ: Prentice-Hall.

Rubella vaccination during pregnancy—United States, 1971–1988. (1989). *Morbidity and Mortality Weekly Report, 38,* 289–293.

Selye, H. (1976). *The stress of life.* New York: McGraw-Hill.

Shamansky, S. L., & Clausen, C. L. (1980). Levels of prevention: Examination of the concept. *Nursing Outlook, 28,* 104–108.

Smith, J. A. (1981). The idea of health: A philosophical inquiry. *Advances in Nursing Science, 3,* 43–50.

Stachtchenko, S., & Jenicek, M. (1990). Conceptual differences between prevention and health promotion: Research implications for community health programs. *Canadian Journal of Public Health, 81,* 53–59.

US Department of Health and Human Services (1990). *Healthy people 2000: National health promotion and disease prevention objectives.* Washington, DC: US Public Health Service Publication.

Velsor-Friedrich, B. (1991). Health goals for children and their families: 1991 and beyond. *Journal of Pediatric Nursing, 6,* 62–63.

World Health Organization (1947). *Constitution of the World Health Organization: Chronicle of the World Health Organization.* Geneva: Author.

BIBLIOGRAPHY

Baldwin, J. A., & Davis, L. L. (1989). Assessing parents as health educators. *Pediatric Nursing, 15,* 453–457.

Biester, D. J. (1992). Childhood immunization: Nursing's role and responsibility. *Journal of Pediatric Nursing, 7,* 65–66.

Brandon, L. J., & Fillingim, J. (1990). Health fitness training responses of normotensive and elevated normotensive children. *American Journal of Health Promotion, 5,* 30–35.

Burns, E. I., Doremus, P. C., & Potter, M. B. (1990). Value of health, incidence of depression, and level of self-esteem in low-income mothers of pre-school children. *Issues in Comprehensive Pediatric Nursing, 13,* 141–154.

Coppens, N. (1985). Cognitive development and locus of control as predictors of preschoolers' understanding of safety and prevention. *Journal of Applied Developmental Psychology, 6,* 43–55.

Hansen, M., & Aradine, C. (1974). The changing face of primary pediatrics. *Pediatric Clinics of North America, 21,* 245.

Honig, J. C. (1991). A school-based clinic in a preschool. *Journal of Pediatric Health Care, 5,* 34–39.

Igoe, J. B. (1992). Health promotion, health protection and disease prevention in childhood. *Pediatric Nursing, 18,* 291–292.

Igoe, J. B. (1990). Healthy people 2000. *Pediatric Nursing, 16,* 584–588.

Ireland, D. I. (1990). New attitudes/new look: An African-American adolescent health education program. *Pediatric Nursing, 16,* 175–178.

Jones, R. T., McDonald, D. W., Fiore, M. F., Arrington, T., & Randall, J. (1990). A primary preventive approach to children's drug refusal behavior: The impact of rehearsal-plus. *Journal of Pediatric Psychology, 15,* 211–224.

Levine, B. E., & Lavi, S. (1991). Perils of childhood immunization against measles, mumps, and rubella. *Pediatric Nursing, 17,* 159–161.

Kenny, T., Gaes, G., Saylor, W., Grossman, L., Kappelman, M., Chernoff, R., Toler, S., & Majer, L. (1990). The pediatric early elementary examination: Sensitivity and specificity. *Journal of Pediatric Psychology, 15,* 21–26.

Lutz, M. E. (1990). The effects of family structure and regular places of care on preventive health care for children. *Health Values, 14,* 38–45.

O'Brien, R. W., Smith, S. A., Bush, P. J., & Peleg, E. (1990). Obesity, self-esteem, and health locus of control in black youths during transition to adolescence. *American Journal of Health Promotion, 5,* 133–139.

Osborn, L. (1982). Group well-child care: An option for today's children. *Pediatric Nursing,* 306–308.

Sevel, F. (1990). Designing effective health promotion and disease prevention programs: A course model. *Health Values, 14,* 32–37.

Velsor-Freidrich, B., & Frager, B. (1990). The federal government and child health. *Journal of Pediatric Nursing, 5,* 56–58.

Vessey, J. A., Braithwaite, K., & Weidmann, M. (1990). Teaching children about their internal bodies. *Pediatric Nursing, 16,* 29–33.

Weingarten, C. T., & Gomberg, S. M. (1992). Measles: Again and epidemic. *Pediatric Nursing, 18,* 369–371.

West, D. J., Calandra, G. B., & Ellis, R. W. (1990). Vaccination of infants and children against hepatitis B. *Pediatric Clinics of North America, 37,* 585–601.

Whatley, J. H. (1991). Effects of health locus of control and social network on adolescent risk taking. *Pediatric Nursing, 17,* 145–152.

CHAPTER • 11

Communicating with Children and Families

Mabel Hunsberger

RELATED TOPICS
Promoting Healthy Parenting, Chapter 12
Interviewing children and families, Chapter 13
Promoting Healthy Play, Chapter 17
Therapeutic play, Chapter 17
Preparation of children for procedures, Chapter 21
Teaching Children, Chapter 23

LEARNING OBJECTIVES

- Explain the process of communication.
- Describe how communication is affected by culturally diverse participants.
- Describe the four elements of the Social Model for Intercultural Communication.
- Differentiate between verbal and nonverbal communication.
- Describe three skills of communication.
- Relate communication characteristics to the developmental level of the infant, toddler, school-ager, and adolescent.
- Explain how the concepts *respect, acceptance,* and *empathy* are used to establish a parent-child-nurse relationship.
- Differentiate among a therapeutic, a professional, and an intense, overinvolved relationship.
- List and give examples of the basic principles of communicating with children.
- Explain how to respond to two developmental linguistic characteristics in a child's conversation.
- Explain the direct and indirect communication techniques that can be utilized with children in order to encourage conversation.

Whether we are aware of it or not, we are always communicating something. Thoughts, feelings, and opinions are exchanged consciously or unconsciously, by verbal and nonverbal means. Interpersonal communication is the avenue through which we achieve our humanity. From infancy, a person becomes oriented to the physical and social worlds through a continuous exchange of behaviors and responses. It is the interactions within a family that primarily determine a child's communication style.

Talking to a child differs from talking to another adult. Children's language has characteristics that adults must learn to understand in order to communicate effectively. Children do not necessarily understand what they appear to have comprehended, and the questions they ask are often less complex than adults interpret them to be. Also, children cannot express their feelings in adult-type conversations, so a variety of alternative techniques can be used to help children express their thoughts and feelings. The health of children is promoted through the nurse's own communication with parents and children and through interventions to support high-quality relationships between parents and children in the home. This chapter discusses principles of communicating with children and families, with emphasis on developmental differences that affect how children think and respond.

Communication can be simply defined as the sending and receiving of messages. The actual process, however, is a complex one. Communicating involves a composite of verbal and nonverbal behaviors that establish human-to-human relationships. To a great extent, the quality of interpersonal relationships provides the basis of one's sense of self. The childhood years are particularly influential in this process.

Children's communication skills and use of techniques vary according to their ability to process cognitive information and their level of emotional-social development. Furthermore, experiences within a particular family with a unique communication style affect the child's capabilities. It is useful to have some background information about a particular child and family prior to an encounter. However, in many instances, a nurse must begin a relationship with children and their families while having very little information.

Effective communication with children is a skill that adults, both parents and professionals, learn over time; it requires knowledge about the development of children, sensitivity about children's feelings and experiences, and skill in listening and responding. Nurses who are new to the field of pediatrics need to appreciate that these skills are developed by means of accumulated experience. Although the dynamics of a parent-child-nurse relationship can be studied and principles and skills of communication can be explained, the art can be acquired only by working among children and their families.

The Process of Communication

In the communication process, a stimulus causes an individual to form a message that is transmitted to another person, the receiver. The way in which messages are formed (coded) and interpreted (decoded) is subject to the context within which the exchange occurs. If a parent sends a message to the nurse in the presence of children, the nurse must decode that message with the realization that parents may not feel free to speak openly in front of their children. For example, the question "Do you have concerns in the area of discipline?" may not bring an accurate response if the child is present. When children talk in the presence of their parents, the nurse must recognize that communication is influenced by the parent-child relationship. Furthermore, the specific meaning attributed to the setting in which the encounter takes place and the child's relationship to the nurse influence the outcome (Garbarino & Stott, 1989).

Communication has not been accomplished until a message is received in the context within which it is sent. Receiving a message involves decoding both the verbal and nonverbal content of the communication. Aside from the relationship that exists between communicants, each person's biases and life experiences always affect communication. In the case of children and parents, the family within which they live greatly influences their communication with each other and with those outside the family unit. These family experiences and the cultural influences that govern families are covered in the following discussion, which details how cultural differences across identity groups affect communication.

Understanding Culture as the Context for Communication

Culture provides the pattern for living; it has to do with how people interpret their experiences. It gives meaning to life and affects the system of values and lifestyle that is adopted. Formally defined, *culture* is "the deposit of knowledge, experiences, beliefs, values, attitudes, meanings, hierarchies, religion, timing, roles, spatial relations, concepts of the universe, and material objects and possessions acquired by a large group of people in the course of generations through individual and group striving" (Porter & Samovar, 1985, p 19). Culture includes socioeconomic, ethnic, and religious factors and other characteristics that qualify an individual for membership in various identity groups.

The ideas and feelings of people within a defined group are influenced by culture, because "people learn to think, feel, believe, and strive for what their culture considers proper" (Porter & Samovar, 1985, p 19). Cultural orientation determines how messages are encoded. Culturally determined symbols in the form of words and gestures are sent along channels considered culturally appropriate. The message may be a hug, a symbol that encodes affection and is delivered tactilely. A hug may be more appropriate among members of some identity groups than among others. These differences are acknowledged when nurses relate to families of many different cultures. Less obvious in health care delivery are the cultural differences that exist among different identity groups. For example, childhood is a subgroup with an identity of its own, as is adolescence. Intercultural communication, therefore, includes relating to people from distinctively different cultures but also to those who are members of the same dominant culture but from different subcultures or subgroups (Porter & Samovar, 1985). Given the diversity between the identity group adulthood and the identity group childhood, it is safe to say that *the majority of interactions in pediatric nursing involve intercultural communications,* regardless of whether there are differences in ethnicity or nationality.

Childhood as an Identity Group

Childhood is a culture (for our purposes, an identity group) in itself. It is pertinent for child health nurses to consider the characteristics and implications of such a group. Perhaps more than members of any other subgroup within our culture, children have an identity unto themselves. By virtue of their stature, behavior, and youthful appearance, children and adolescents are easily identified as children or "nonadults." Their language differs from that of the adult population: first in the attempts at "baby talk," then in the school-age struggle with mastery of grammar, and later in the adolescent "stylization" of language that renders it unintelligible to many adults.

Behavior also identifies the members of the childhood group. Whether it be the clumsy curiosity of the toddler, the exuberance of mid-childhood, or the yo-yo–like behavior of the adolescent who is tenuously balancing between childhood and adulthood, the actions are different from those of an adult. Perceptions also vary between children and adults. Who among us fails to remember the "monsters" in our childhood closets, the "bigness" of our fathers, the unlimited "power" of the doctor and nurse to do anything they pleased to us, the "length" of one childhood hour, or the sheer delight of a chocolate milkshake? Socially, the child is characterized by immature blunders and occasionally by endearing attempts to make amends for them. Even the adolescent struggles with social graces and with the transitions in behavior that must continually be made between the social world of peers and the social world of parents. These are but a few of the many disparities between the perceptions of children and those of adults. It is necessary to recognize the identity group of childhood, because the differences in perceptions can lead to distortion in nurse-child communications. The resulting challenge is one that pediatric nurses can ill afford to ignore.

A Social Model for Intercultural Communication

Intercultural communication occurs whenever a message encoded by someone in culture "A" is received and decoded by someone in culture "B." The goal of an intercultural discussion is to achieve the highest level of mutual understanding between culturally different communicators (Sloat & Matsuura, 1990). The following is a discussion of the various components of intercultural communication as they affect nurse-parent-child communications.

Preparing for the Initial Encounter with a Child and Family

The purpose of preparing to meet the child and family is to clear the mind of distractions and prejudicial thoughts that could limit the nurse's ability to begin to know this child and this family as unique individuals. This step is often overlooked, although it takes only a few moments of the nurse's time and can dramatically affect the tone of the encounter. Such preparation is necessary because of the distraction of other job-related details and because of the human tendency to categorize this child as being like others with the same race, age, disease process, and so on.

Values clarification is a critical part of the preparation process that begins long before the nurse considers a particular encounter. Personal values must be identified as they relate to the meaning of life; to illness, pain, and death in children; and to various cultural characteristics. See Chapter 1 for further discussion of values clarification and ethics.

Preparation at the time of the initial encounter may take only a few moments. It involves only the nurse's brief awareness of mind set and a conscious effort to be open and genuine. The effect of this moment of preparation before entering the room, however, is often vividly communicated in the nurse's nonverbal behavior and can set the tone for all future encounters with this client.

Searching for Similarities in Identity Groups

Just as one searches for similarities on which to base a social conversation, one must identify commonalities on which to base the nurse-client relationship. Communication tends to be easiest among those who identify most closely with each other and to be most difficult among individuals whose perceptions are dissimilar (Singer, 1985).

Nursing assessment for cultural similarities is most effective when conducted in an informal manner. Although the strategies are almost identical to those used in a social situation, the nurse is constantly aware that a nurse-client relationship has a goal. Although in a social context it is often desirable to share as much about oneself as the other shares, in a professional situation the nurse's goal is simply to establish the existence of similarities without elaborating on them. For example, during the course of the admission interview, a nurse shares with a rural family that she or he lived on a farm as a child, or shares with the child an understanding of what it is like to be an only child. The nurse then continues the interview, focusing on the client. If the client asks additional details about the nurse's experiences, of course, answers are appropriate. Rarely, however, does the client become confused about the goal of the conversation, and the client rarely fails to recognize the identified similarities as a basis for trust and support. Often the child or parent seizes the opportunity "to talk with someone who must understand how I feel."

The more identity groups two people share, the more similar their perceptions will be in a given situation. It follows that the more dissimilar they are, the greater is the probability for misunderstandings. Dissimilarities such as race, religion, or geographic origin can often be offset by similarities in other areas, for example, age, occupation, marital and parenting status. What if dissimilarities between the nurse and client remain significant? As discussed, culture is significant to the extent that it affects communication. If progress toward the goal of communication is unimpeded by cultural differences, they are unimportant. If, however, communication suffers to the extent that it affects progress toward the therapeutic goal, it is the professional responsibility of the nurse to recognize this fact and to adjust nursing assignments cooperatively to achieve a better nurse-client "match."

Appreciating Differences in Nurse-Client Experiences and Perceptions

Differences in nurse-client experiences and perceptions can be the impetus for innovations in the nursing process and for individualization of care. To appreciate these differences, however, the nurse first must possess enough self-esteem to view differences as nonthreatening. The nurse who values the self is prepared to value the other person.

Differences are *appreciated* when they are identified and met with openness and genuineness. Appreciating differences, therefore, requires (1) a genuine attempt to discern the client's perspective of the situation, (2) identification of ways in which that perspective is similar and dissimilar to the nurse's perspective, and (3) exploration of the reasons for differences in attitudes and perceptions. When these differences are the result of misunderstanding on the part of the nurse or client, further discussion can alleviate potential problems. When these differences result from dissimilar experiences and differing world views, the nurse can base further nursing interactions on one of two premises. First, the nurse may conclude that the client's view is wrong and/or old-fashioned because it differs from the nurse's perspective. In this case, the nurse's nonverbal behavior usually communicates intolerance of different views and blocks therapeutic communication with the client. Second, the more informed nurse may view the identified difference as an opportunity to explore another viewpoint and as having the potential for discovering other viable approaches to a problem. Determination of health and childrearing beliefs and practices through research (Lenart et al, 1991) and efforts to give attention to cultural differences in practice (Niederhauser, 1989; Rosenburg, 1986) are becoming more significant as the number of immigrants increases. If nurses approach differences in experience or perception by trying to understand other cultures, they communicate that their clients are valued members of the "treatment team." Clients then feel freer to express preferences and ideas about health care practices and to ask questions about other aspects of treatment. This is the basis of therapeutic communication. *Appreciating differences means recognizing the potential of every interpersonal encounter to expand and enrich existing knowledge.*

Validating Perceptions

Validating perceptions is integral to the three preceding elements of this model for intercultural communication. Because it is essential to the success of this model, however, it warrants inclusion as a separate topic. It involves determining whether the message sent was the message received and incorporates the communication elements of receiver response and feedback.

It is often more important to validate nonverbal response than verbal response. This is especially true when a language barrier exists, such as between a child and a nurse or between an English-speaking nurse and a non–English-speaking client. The importance of nonverbal communication within our culture in general is emphasized by Hall's (1984) estimate that only 10 per cent of communication is accomplished verbally. This cultural propensity for nonverbal communication benefits the pediatric nurse, because it means one enters the profession with some expertise in reading nonverbal signals. Child health nurses who refine these observations will greatly enhance their professional communication skills.

Perceptions must be validated almost continuously when there are great disparities between the cultural identities of persons involved. For example, when a language barrier exists, validation by means of nonverbal gestures and the help of an interpreter may be necessary. We must also be sure to validate perceptions with the client who seems "more like" us. We have but to reflect on miscommunications within our own families to remember that perceptions can never be taken for granted.

Culture has a complex and pervasive influence on every child and parent. The nurse and client come together as products of culture to attempt understanding through communication, which is also culturally patterned. This means that nurse-client interactions often involve intercultural communication. This section has proposed a model for intercultural communication, one that

- Prepares the nurse to meet the client nonjudgmentally, with openness and genuineness.
- Establishes similarities for the purposes of building a trusting relationship and assessing whether the client's values and beliefs are in keeping with the goals and strategies of care.
- Encourages exploration of value differences to enrich the nurse's awareness and appreciation of other ideas.
- Evaluates the effectiveness of communication through continual validation of perceptions.

Types of Communication

Nonverbal

For nurses to communicate effectively, they must learn how to use and be responsive to verbal and nonverbal communication. Invariably gestures, facial expressions, and tone of voice add important dimensions to what is said. Nonverbal communication is less easily governed by conscious control than is verbal communication, and it is therefore more reliable. Children, particularly, show with their actions how they feel, even before they have the language to express such feelings. Nonverbal communication is a child's natural mode of expression (Fig. 11–1). Crying, staying close to a caregiver, and becoming very quiet or overactive are ways that young children express their needs. Older children may be able to express feelings verbally to adults when encouraged, but they often prefer to share feelings with peers. Behavioral changes are often due to their feelings and concerns. A change in mood, activity, or eating may signal an important message. See Table 11–1 for a listing of nonverbal cues used by children and adolescents.

Adults exercise more control over their nonverbal messages than do children, but tone of voice, facial expression, and body language are hard to control, even for an adult. Parents may conceal their true feelings because they believe they must play a certain role, or they may say whatever they think the nurse wants to hear. An incongruity between verbal and nonverbal communication may be the nurse's only indication that parents hold feelings they hesitate to verbalize.

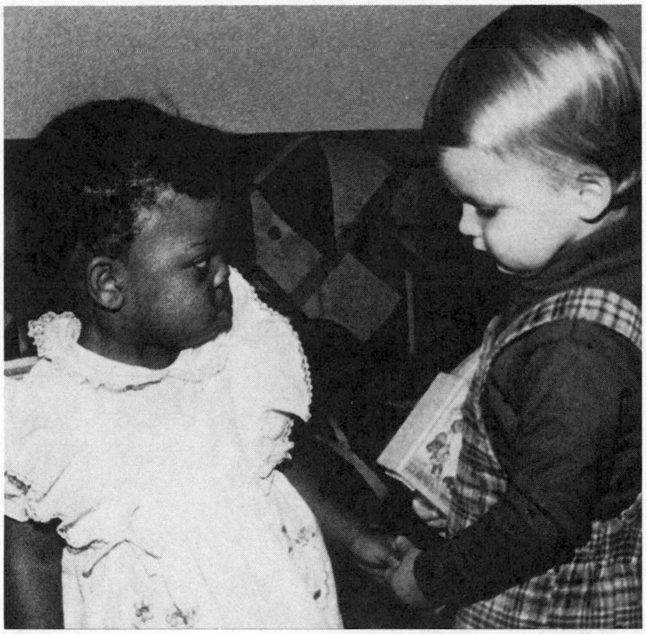

FIGURE 11 - 1. Relationships are formed as thoughts and feelings are communicated.

Verbal

The spoken word is the most obvious expression of thoughts and feelings, but it is not necessarily the most accurate one. Nurses should be aware of the many possible etiologies for impaired verbal communication. Individuals vary in their ability to use language as a way to communicate; the person who is reluctant to talk may be telling the listener something about limitation in self-expression, rather than about mood. The nurse must also recognize that minimal verbal expression has cultural significance.

If verbal communication is hampered by language barriers, the nurse must be sensitive enough to recognize when a nod of the head and lack of verbal communication really mean that the client does not understand. When a language barrier is the reason for reduced verbal expression, the nurse should search for interpreters and make an effort to communicate by speaking slowly and softly, using gestures, and having bilingual dictionaries available. In today's multicultural society, institutions should have established systems through which to contact interpreters.

Even with adults, words are subject to misunderstanding. Children may pose additional barriers to effective communication. Although children may be honest and straightforward, sometimes embarrassingly

TABLE 11-1
Cues to Nonverbal Communication

Body Language
Facial Expression
Tense/relaxed
Smiling/frowning
Eye contact/avoidance
Mouth open/closed
Body Movements
Motionless
Nodding of head
Kicking, flailing
Biting
Shaking
Twitching
Banging fist
Body Posture
Orientation: turned away or toward another
Body stiff/relaxed
Open or closed body position
Vocal Cues
Crying
Whining
Humming
Silence
Tone of voice
Proximity
Staying close or moving away
Moving away, but looking back
General Actions/Responses
Holding still/resisting
Following instructions/ignoring instructions
Refusing to eat/overeating
External Environment
Banging doors
Ripping paper
Kicking furniture
Racing an engine

so, their abilities to understand what is spoken and to express their ideas have some developmental limitations. Nurses' interactions with children and their roles in supporting parent-child communications can be enhanced by an understanding of these developmental characteristics (see discussion under "Communicating with Children" later in this chapter).

Skills of Communication

Observation

Observation of nonverbal communication provides meaningful clues to what the child and parent are saying to each other and to the nurse. Children communicate with us by *how* they do things as well as by *what* they do: observing their eyes, quality of voice, facial expression, and body posture and movement tells us how they feel about situations and people. Do children say, "I feel disappointed," or do they show us this by their sad eyes, quiet mood, or sobbing cry?

The interaction between parent and child is a constant and integral part of communication and should be the focal point of the nurse's observations. The nurse should observe how the parents respond to their child's requests for attention. Does the child receive rewards for good behavior, or is attention granted only when unacceptable behavior ensues? The way a parent physically handles a child, the way questions are answered (or whether they are answered at all), and the manner in which the parent elicits cooperation from the child demonstrate how parents relate to their children. Effective communication strategies that respect the nature of their relationship can then be formulated.

Listening

To listen carefully, one must give attention to the words, the tone of voice, and the predominant theme of a conversation. Listening to communication between a parent and child makes it apparent whether the child is encouraged to speak out or whether the parent completes the sentence, corrects the child, and shows little regard for the child's ideas. Children should be supported in their attempt to engage in the conversation, especially when the conversation concerns them. Addressing children by name and responding to their concerns is a necessary part of listening to children.

Listening to concerns of parents and children requires special skills of openness and acceptance by the nurse, because parent-child relationships are often highly charged with emotion, and parents frequently have difficulty acknowledging problems. The concerns that parents verbalize about themselves, their children, and each other may therefore be distorted because they do not wish to be regarded as incompetent parents or to reveal difficulties in a marriage. By sensitively assessing what is heard and seen, the nurse can develop a true understanding of how parents feel. In receiving messages from parents, the nurse should realize that they may be under much stress in trying to conform to the model of "good parenting."

When listening to children, an understanding of their level of language development and cognition is fundamental. Listening to the cry of an infant and trying to interpret it are the beginnings of sensitive communication with children. When children begin to talk, one must take time to listen to what they say to adults and other children.

For adults, perhaps the greatest problem is not so much when children cannot use language, but rather when they can speak. Children speak early in life, and it is easy to assume that the thought underlying their speech is the same as that of adults. Children's thinking changes as they develop, and adults' responses to children should be based on each child's level of development. For example, a child may ask for a drink of water, ask to see the stethoscope, or ask to listen to the nurse's watch. What the child is asking may involve more than the obvious request. The child may be thirsty or curious; alternatively, the child may be trying to delay the nurse because of fear of what is coming next, or may be asking for company because of fear or loneliness.

The greatest disservice we can do to a child is not to listen at all. Ignoring a request without any explanation not only cuts off communication, but it interferes with trust. If one does not have time to listen, one must explain why and establish another time to talk. Rules and limits can be set to regulate when it is appropriate to talk, but they should be clear to both parties. Just as a child can accept that others have the right to speak, adults must accept a child's right to be heard.

Silence

Silence is a common medium of communication for parents and children. Children may be quiet because they are afraid, angry, or shy or because they are busy. Therefore, silence cannot be understood without taking into account the individual child and the surrounding stimuli. The age of the child, the usual behavior of the child, and the nature of the situation are important elements of the meaning of silence. Perhaps the parent or the child does not wish to speak about a certain topic in front of the other, or maybe the topic is a point of conflict within the family. When silence is used to block communication, the nurse must be sensitive to the unreadiness of the child or the parent to discuss the problem. The role is to resume conversation at a level that is more comfortable, thereby allowing the child or parent to regain composure.

Silence can be used positively by the nurse to encourage communication. Silence is needed for the processing of thoughts and feelings; during silence, people seek to understand the content of what has been said. An inability to understand the meaning of what has been said results in a puzzled silence. For a child, thoughtful silence may primarily be filled with fear of the unknown and the inability to express that fear. Often, words do not dispel fear in a child, but the nurse's presence brings comfort. The nurse's silent presence can be one of the most effective ways to share the difficulties and fears of another's thoughtful silence.

Developmental Factors Affecting Communication with Children

Each child develops within a unique family and set of circumstances that affect communication. In addition, the child's developmental level (cognitive and linguistic) is to be considered.

The Child as a Member of a Family

Each child reacts to a unique set of stimuli, which combine to form the child's personality. What has happened to a child within the family creates the most important force in development, and within the family a child develops a style of communication. According to Satir (1975), all communication is learned. From the family, a child develops ideas about self (self-concept), has experiences of interacting with others, and learns how to engage with the world. The child who is encouraged to participate in decision making at home is likely to take an active role in doing so outside the home. A more dependent role is to be expected when the child comes from an adult-centered home in which children are expected to be submissive and are allowed little opportunity to make a contribution in family matters.

Communication patterns are further affected by the relationships between siblings. When sibling rivalry predominates, the internal family relationship may deteriorate. Friction develops between husband and wife as well as between parent and child when blame is attributed to various family members. A child who comes from a family in which relationships are strained often has difficulty developing relationships outside the home.

Cognitive and Developmental Level

In communicating with children, it is also recommended to *consider their cognitive and developmental level.* The following is a discussion of how children at various ages communicate.

Infant

During infancy, nonverbal methods are the primary mode of communication. However, adults speak to infants long before they expect their words to be understood, because speech is a means of communicating love and attention. Although they may have no comprehension of words spoken to them, infants attend to the human voice and face, synchronizing their movements with the adult's pauses and segments of speech. Pleasure and displeasure are associated with certain voice tones because of simultaneous experiences. For example, an adult speaking in a soft voice while rocking and feeding a baby is how the infant learns to experience pleasure in response to a soft-spoken voice. Furthermore, the common stroking and patting of infants communicates feelings of attachment. The reciprocal system between parent and child develops a sense of competence in the infant and is rewarding for the parent.

By 6 months of age, vocalizations become a major form of communication between infants and their caregivers. Different pitches of sound are used in response to the tone of the caregiver's voice. Crying is another forceful way in which an infant communicates various needs; different qualities of cries represent hunger, anger, tiredness, pain, and stranger anxiety (Fig. 11–2). An infant's arm-waving and leg-kicking behavior is also a stimulus that elicits caring; therefore, it is a way of communicating. When a parent soothes and settles a thrashing infant, the responsiveness of the infant, in turn, gives the parent a sense of being needed. Rhythmic sound or motion is comforting and soothing to the infant and provides further sensations of love.

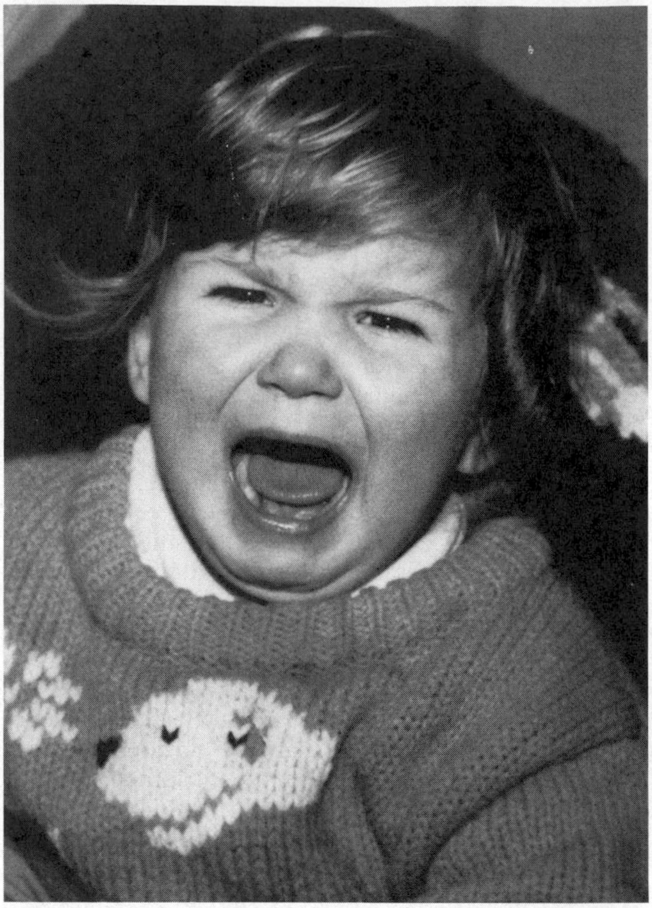

FIGURE 11 - 2. Crying is a forceful way to communicate a need. The pitch of the cry, the facial expression, and the tenseness of the child's body communicate the power of the message.

Toddler and Preschooler

As children begin to understand and use words, one needs to recognize the thought processes that affect their communication. According to Piaget (1967), between 2 and 7 years of age (preoperational thought), children are egocentric; they see things from their own points of view and in reference to themselves.

Dealing with Egocentric Thinking

It is difficult for children to understand why they cannot have a drink of water before a diagnostic test, because they can only comprehend the sensation of thirst and want to have the need met. They cannot understand how not taking a drink affects the test. They also make causal errors by thinking that events that happen in proximity to each other are related. To give an injection immediately after a child has been reprimanded for some unacceptable behavior causes the child to think that the behavior resulted in the shot.

Even though children do not completely understand verbal explanations of the relationship between treatments and a child's state of health, one should explain in simple terms how and why the procedure will be done. Although the full implication of words may not be understood, children's ability to understand (receptive language) is more advanced than their speech (expressive language). In addition, verbal communication should be accompanied by touch to communicate a caring and supportive attitude.

Role of Imaginary Thought

During the preoperational stage, a child engages in pretending; this form of communication is often difficult for adults to understand. Children's natural tendency to act out their feelings and experiences helps them cope with the real world and can provide information to others. Allowing children to act out that which is about to happen is frequently more beneficial than a verbal explanation. If they can see and imagine with dolls, puppets, or conversations, they have an acceptable and bearable perception and are able to defuse some of the emotions pertaining to the event.

Imaginary play is frequently accompanied by talk in the form of a monologue. During this stage, play is sustained by talking. In other words, children have to say what they are doing in order to do it. During this phase of language learning, children do not necessarily expect or seek responses to their utterances. Especially when involved in imaginative play, children do not want the interruption of a real conversation.

Responding to "Why?"

One of the most challenging aspects of communication with children at this stage of development is answering the *Why?* question. Answering this question is difficult because of the difference between children's and adults' interpretations of "why." According to Piaget (1967), an adult perceives "why" to have two distinct meanings: the goal ("Why are you going?") and the cause ("Why is the car moving?"). A child's "why" implies both meanings at the same time but does not appear to differentiate between the goal and cause (Piaget, 1967). Children often ask questions pertaining to phenomena, even when there is no "because." They are also thought to use why questions to learn the meaning of "why." Concrete objects are easily labeled with words, but children of this age have difficulty understanding the abstract concept of such words as "why" and "how."

When answering why and how questions, it is recommended not to read too much into the questions and to avoid explanations that require abstract thinking. For example, "Why is that wagon in my room?" is most simply answered with "Because Danny is being taken out for a ride." A child of this age often responds with "But why?" Additional information such as "Because he can't walk" may be sufficient to satisfy the child, but sometimes the answers stimulate further questions. Providing simple, concrete answers helps the child understand relationships and satisfies curiosity. If explanations are not offered when questions are asked, a child does not learn to seek answers. Answering questions is a way of showing interest and fostering the relationship. Children may ask questions to satisfy curiosity or to gain information, or for other reasons. Children sometimes practice language and make social contacts by asking questions without expecting an answer. For example, a young child who sees his mother returning from the grocery store with obvious purchases of food may ask, "Why did you go to the store?" This may be an effort to make his presence known, rather than to discuss the activity of shopping. On some occasions, it is apparent that children ask questions to gain attention or as a request for help with a problem. Persistent questioning also may be an indication of fear, insecurity, or unresolved concern. By attempting to answer a child's questions, we gain insight into what is motivating the question.

Explanations need to be given in concrete terms and with reference to familiar happenings in the child's life experience. For example, time is understood when it is explained in relation to "after you wake up, have your breakfast, and brush your teeth." Explanations such as "There will be bright lights, the room will be cool, and they will take your picture with a large camera" give the child concrete facts to think about and do not leave thoughts to an imagination capable of visualizing an event as being far more injurious than it really is. One should also avoid words such as "cut" or "bleed" when giving explanations. Because of a child's difficulty in separating fact from fantasy, a painful procedure should be explained just prior to its occurrence and followed with physical comfort. Whenever possible, explanations should also be accompanied by pictures or dramatization with dolls or puppets. See Chapter 17 for further discussion of how play is used to prepare young children for procedures.

School-Age Child

During the stage of concrete operations (7 to 11 years), the child makes major cognitive advancements that affect communication. At around age 7 years, children are better able to cooperate, because they begin to comprehend viewpoints other than their own. They are now able to engage in discussions about events, because they are able to focus on more than one aspect of an experience. They can comprehend explanations that describe an event, although they still are bound to concrete thought. For example, they can understand that it is not painful to have a chest radiograph but cannot comprehend how taking repeated x-ray films may be harmful to the body.

Their cognitive ability enables them to explore and consider many alternatives to a problem. School-age children need to be given the opportunity to question and explore what is being said and what will happen to them. An increased understanding of their body and environment requires that details be painstakingly explained in the description of an event that pertains to the body. It is essential to encourage the expression of fears when the child's body integrity is threatened by invasive procedures. School-age children's increased use of word symbols makes it possible for them to make language express their concerns and to understand more complex explanations (Fig. 11–3).

Children of this age also use language as a means of gaining control. As children become socially experienced, they discover that others seek to control them by talking and that they can control the behavior of others by their increased facility with words. At this stage, parents begin to see themselves reflected in the way children apply communication patterns to cope with and solve problems.

Preadolescent and Adolescent

The period of formal operations (11 to 15 years) is when abstract thinking begins so that hypothetic situations can be created. During this stage, there is an

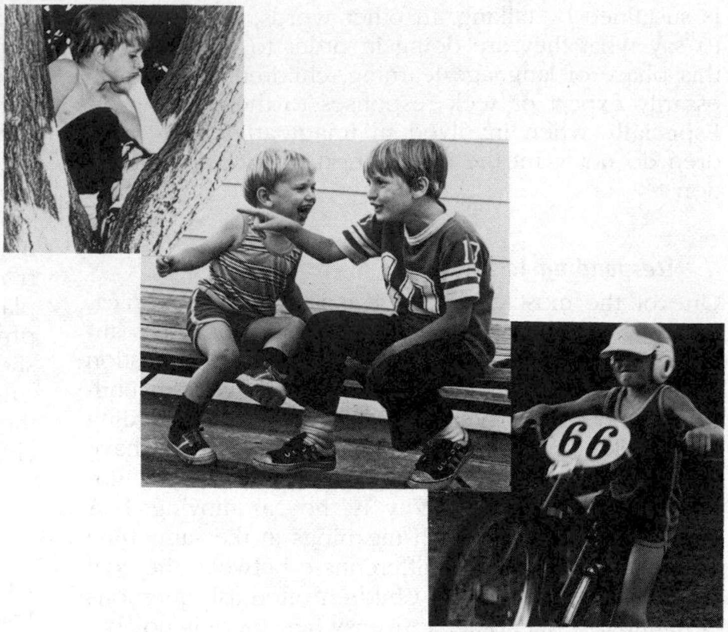

FIGURE 11-3. School-age children express feelings when they are quiet, when they talk, and especially when they play. Their increased cognitive ability helps them use language successfully.

increased need to express feelings verbally. Adolescents, no longer bound to concrete phenomena, wish to discuss their values and ideals. They now can hypothesize about how things should be done, especially when the issues involve their own destinies. They do not wish to be told what to do and are much more cooperative if included in making the decisions that affect them. For example, their responsibilities in the home can be discussed and negotiated, then committed to writing. By clarifying the task and involving an adolescent in deciding what is expected, one can thwart daily hassles.

A major difficulty during adolescence is the confusion between an *ideal* world and the *real* world. This preoccupation with what "could be" characterizes the thinking during the stage of formal operations and sometimes produces conflict with other people. Adolescents need to have the opportunity to express their thoughts about how the world should operate in order to help them evaluate their own ideas. They formulate their ideas more precisely by putting them into words, and eventually they resolve the confusion between the real and ideal.

Adolescent thinking is characterized by egocentricity, as was thinking early in life. Adolescents often wrongly imagine that other people have certain thoughts and feelings, which are really their own. They have the need to engage in egocentric thinking and need the privacy to do so. A special respect for their private thoughts should be communicated by not prying into personal matters. Because of their egocentricity, they often misinterpret the meaning of someone else's communication by not differentiating their own thoughts from the thoughts of others. They are highly sensitive to nonverbal communication and need an environment of acceptance within which they will feel the freedom to express personal views, if they so desire.

The Parent-Child-Nurse Relationship

Because communication is the heart of human relationships, it is the most valuable skill a nurse can have in relating to children and their families. Much of what a nurse can accomplish depends on the ability to make parents and children feel accepted and comfortable in the relationship (Fig. 11–4).

Elements of the Relationship

Respect for the individuality of each person within the relationship has particular relevance in relationships with parents and children. The way an individual thinks and feels, and therefore responds to a message, is a reflection of that person's total life experience, including values of family, friends, community, and society.

Acceptance of the total person is another essential attitude to communicate. It can be difficult to convey acceptance of a person when one does not condone a behavior. For example, to be accepting of a parent, a nurse must understand that a child's temper tantrums produce intolerable frustration in the parent. The nurse does not have to agree with the method of discipline to be accepting of the parent. The nurse accepts the need that motivates the behavior and does not condemn the parent for the behavior. The nurse can help a parent to express feelings about stresses impinging on the family and to identify alternate means of expression. Communication with chil-

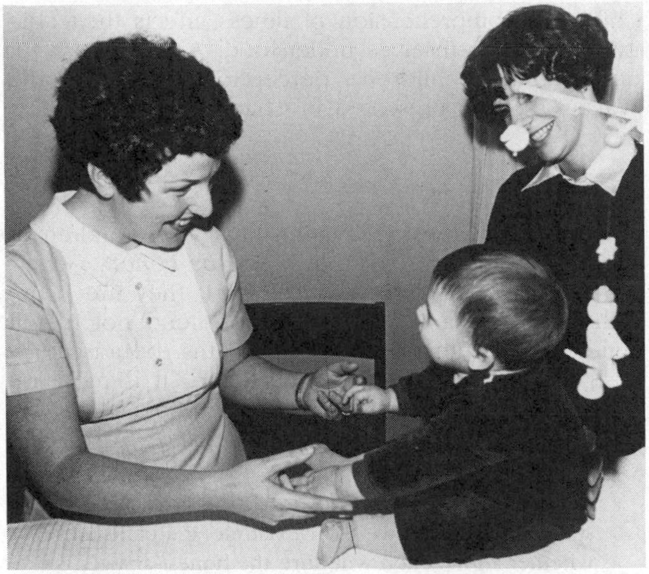

FIGURE 11-4. The nurse who is skilled in communication can make parents and children feel accepted and comfortable in a relationship.

dren involves a similar approach. The behavior of the child does not have to be condoned, even though the need of the child is accepted.

Empathy is an essential element of the parent-child-nurse relationship. Nurses are empathic when they can make parents and children feel that the meanings of their life experiences are being understood. The significant feature of empathy is that the recipient feels it. In communicating with children, empathy means that one has to be able to see the world through a child's eyes. Children express how they feel when they are quiet, when they talk, and especially when they play. To grasp how children feel, one must pay attention to all aspects of their behavior, because children are often unable to verbalize how they feel. If a nurse is able to "tune in" and "be with" a child as private thoughts and feelings are explored, loneliness and alienation are less likely. Providing this comfort is one of the most valuable things a nurse can do for a child.

Parents also respond to the concern and caring of an empathic nurse. The goal is to assist parents in clarifying their own thinking and to engage them in problem solving to enhance self-care abilities. To effectively achieve this goal, the parents' beliefs and biases, which are rooted in their family and cultural experiences, must be honored. An empathic response does not necessarily result in agreement, but it is an attempt to recognize another's point of view (Wexler, 1991).

Developing a Relationship

A relationship is established for the purpose of supporting children and families in their quest for health care. It is a collaborative process that may last a few hours, months, or years. The length of time as well as the setting determine the content and the nature of the interactions. See Chapter 10 for a discussion of the various roles of the pediatric nurse in health care settings.

For a parent-child-nurse relationship to develop in any setting, an atmosphere of trust and security must be established. Respect is communicated by recognizing that parents need to feel accepted and that children, in particular, need to be included in the interaction. Children are sensitive to lack of recognition when adults talk to one another. One must seek their viewpoint and give them an opportunity to express their fears and concerns. Even though children may initially seem to be too reserved or too shy to speak out, the nurse maintains sensitivity to the child's readiness for involvement (Fig. 11–5). Children also

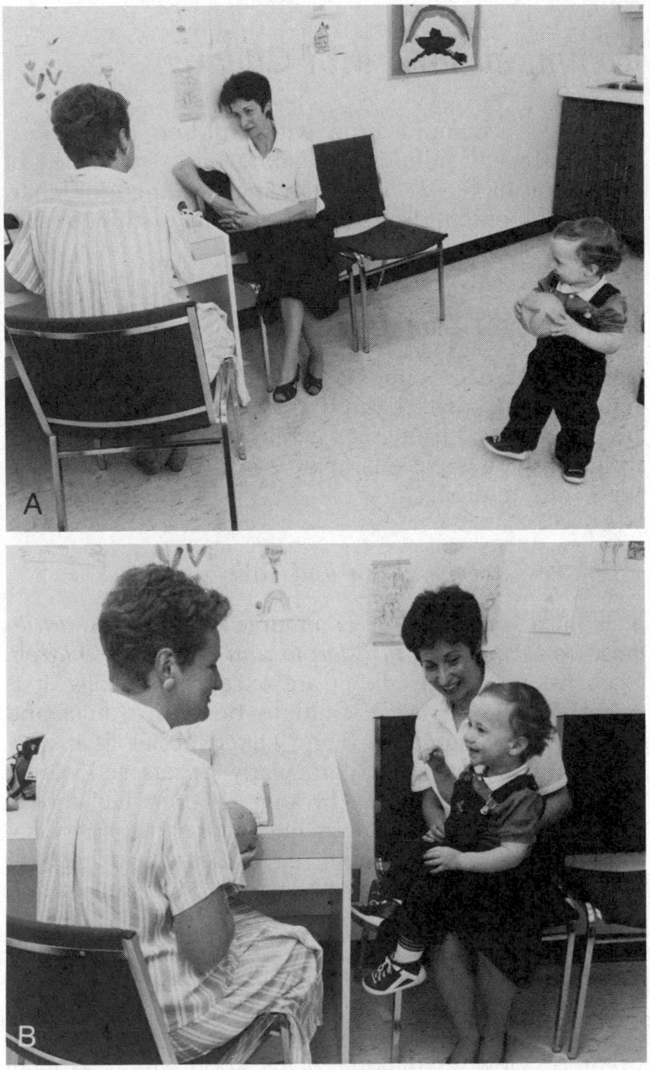

FIGURE 11-5. *A,* Approaching a fearful child by first speaking to the parent gives a child time to accept a stranger. A child looks to a parent for the cue that "it's OK." *B,* A parent's lap is a good place from which to begin a relationship.

respond to touch, play, and eye contact, even though they may choose not to express themselves verbally.

A therapeutic relationship contains identifiable phases that involve both the child and parents: contact phase, contract phase, associative phase, working phase, and termination phase. A therapeutic relationship has boundaries that are positive, professional, and contribute to the family's ability to manage their child's health care. Especially in chronic and terminal illness, nurses are vulnerable to the development of intense relationships in which overly involved behavior may appear. A therapeutic relationship is one that empowers the family and the nurse and maintains an open, clear channel of communication. In this type of relationship, one is "meaningfully related to a patient and family, yet separate enough to distinguish one's own feelings and needs"; a level of professional objectivity is maintained and self is preserved (Barnsteiner & Gillis-Donovan, 1990).

Communicating with Children

A nurse's communication with children can be enhanced by (1) adhering to some basic principles of communication, (2) understanding the linguistic characteristics of children, and (3) using techniques to promote communication.

Principles of Communication

The attitude that underlies all the principles of communication is that children are valued. The nurse adheres to these principles while relating to children and encourages parents to do so in their relationships with the children.

Take Time to Listen and Talk

The basic principle of communication is that *adults need to take time and listen to and talk with children*. Both listening and talking are exceptional skills. It is most distressing for a child to be with adults and shown no recognition. Being talked about as if they were not in the room particularly upsets school-age children and adolescents; young children feel threatened, because they cannot understand the conversations. Children are people, have ideas, and need to feel important. Involving them in conversations and considering their point of view encourage further conversation.

Children should be involved in making decisions that affect them. Recognizing children as an "identity group" is necessary to "hearing" and considering their point of view in making plans about them. Not all wishes can or need to be granted to give a sense of well-being; the significant element is being given the opportunity to talk and to be heard.

A child's view about health needs to be heard and considered when health care is being planned. Children's comprehension of illness affects their ability to make themselves understood. A framework for understanding children's perception by Bibace and Walsh (1980) is presented in Chapter 18.

Be Honest

For nurses to develop relationships with children in which they are trusted, they must *be honest*. Generally, adults do not consciously think they are being dishonest with a child; rather, they tend not to tell children the truth or to tell half truths, because they wish to protect them from being hurt. It is more reassuring for children to be told when something will hurt and to offer the support they need.

A fair approach to a child's question is an honest, straightforward answer. For example, if a child asks whether an injection will hurt, the honest answer is "Yes," but this is coupled with a reassuring statement such as "Yes, a needle hurts, but only for a little while, and I am going to stay right here with you."

Touch, facial expression, and a few words of simple explanation and encouragement can make a hurt tolerable. A child can accept the truth, even if it means discomfort, as long as the nurse communicates a sense of caring and stays with the child.

Be Reliable

An adult must *be reliable* in a relationship with a child, so that an environment of trust is created in which the child feels secure. Promises that cannot be kept are a great disappointment to children and make them feel deceived. If you tell a child you will be back to play a game, it does not matter so much when you return, but you must do so to fulfill the promise. Should it be absolutely impossible to return, the broken promise must be explained. Another potential deception is offering a choice when there are no options. However, in many instances, small choices can be offered to a child to give a sense of importance and some control. For example, asking whether a child wishes to take the pink medicine or the orange medicine first is a significant way to give a child some control.

Set Limits

To *set limits* is to demonstrate respect and care to a child, whereas setting no limits produces feelings of insecurity within a child. Children feel isolated and left out of communication when those responsible for their care are unaware of the child's activities. The "testing" of adults by children should be recognized as a normal part of how children receive feedback. Trying to crawl up on a forbidden table one more time and being prevented from doing so may be a test of whether that child can feel confidence in adults. The school-ager who dawdles to extend bedtime curfew is likewise testing parents. Consistency and fairness in limit setting provide security in child-adult relationships and are beneficial to the child.

Communicate Through Touch

Communication by touch is a sensitive dimension of care. Touch is a powerful tool of communication that is increasingly recognized for its benefits (Molsberry & Shogan, 1990; Kramer, 1990). Touch is used in routine caregiving in the care of infants and children through holding, rubbing, stroking, swaddling, massaging, or hand-holding. Additionally, the use of therapeutic touch is a conscious, intentional act involving the art of interpersonal energy transfer to promote healing (Molsberry & Shogan, 1990). Nevertheless, inappropriate touching of children is now such a prevalent offense in our society that it is imperative for nurses to make astute assessments (see Chapter 28 for discussion of assessment for child abuse).

Even when touching does not have sexual overtones, adults are often unaware of the intrusion that touching can cause. Treating children as objects to be indiscriminately patted, kissed, and picked up without being given a choice can be interpreted as disrespect for them as persons. A child may be engaged in planning an important course of action, only to be abruptly picked up by an adult. When adults meet their own needs by holding and cuddling with little regard for where the child was going or what the child was about to do, touch has been used indiscriminately. A sensitive adult will observe what a child is doing and will use touch in response to the child's needs and as a way to communicate affection. This approach shows respect for the child and simultaneously teaches a child self-respect and self-esteem.

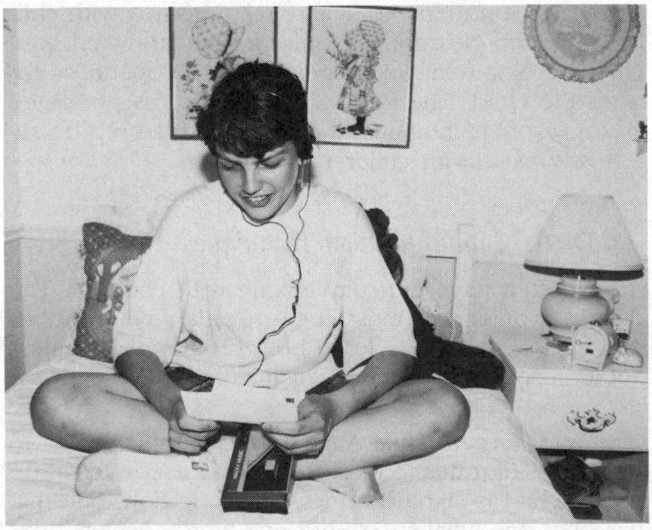

FIGURE 11-6. To have privacy is a child's right. Respect and confidence cannot be forced—they are won.

Acknowledge Right of Privacy

While recognizing that a child needs stimulation and communication from adults, the *right of privacy* must also be preserved. Even at a young age, a child's private thoughts should not be interrupted. Children need a private world for many reasons. They need safe retreats in which to fantasize or quiet times in which to sort out stormy emotions. When the big world outside becomes too confusing, they may need a psychologic refuge (Fig. 11-6). To the question "What were you talking to your sister about?" a child may express the need for privacy with a retort such as "Oh, we were just talking." Taking an interest in an adolescent's relationships by saying "How do you feel about Dave moving?" provides an opening for discussion, but does not pry into specific information about the relationship.

Respect Emotions

In relating to children effectively, it is essential to *respect their emotions*. Children gradually become socialized and learn to control their emotions and translate their feelings into actions as well as words. To communicate with children, it is necessary to realize that emotions change rapidly; hate exists one moment, and love the next. Respecting emotions means that a child is allowed to cry when hurt and to become angry when thwarted. It does not mean that the child is allowed to be destructive or cause injury. If aggressive acting out becomes a pattern of behavior, action is taken to channel the aggression into constructive play and exercise or into positive verbal communication and problem solving. The goal is to help the child learn to control emotions, rather than have the emotions control the child (Davis, 1984).

Avoid Rushing a Relationship

The fears of a child make it imperative to *avoid rushing a child into a relationship*. Children need time to become acquainted with and investigate a new environment. An infant or a toddler may be frightened if approached and spoken to directly.

For a child who fears strangers, it is effective to speak first to the parent in the presence of the child and gradually become acquainted with the child through the parent. The approach can be made by first glancing at the child while speaking to the parent and gradually moving closer to the child while making reference to him or her. It is important not to block the child's view of the parent, so that the child will not fear the parent has disappeared.

Young children can often be approached through the medium of play by letting the child use medical instruments on an imaginary patient, such as a doll or favorite stuffed animal.

Meet Child at Eye Level

A child's lack of height is a disadvantage to her or his ability to feel any sense of power. Consequently, to make children feel that they have something valuable to say about the discussion at hand, every attempt should be made to *meet them at eye level* (Fig. 11–7). Because children are highly sensitive to nonverbal communication, they need to be able to see the speaker's face for additional clues. Meeting children on their level gives them a greater sense of equality. In this way, the exchange from child to adult and from adult to child is facilitated.

Characteristics of Children's Language

Maintaining a conversation within the linguistic and cognitive boundaries of the developmental level is necessary in order to retain children's attention. If their part in a conversation requires speech and thinking ability beyond their level, they will soon become disinterested and frustrated. Children maintain conversations with adults by using some identifiable techniques when they do not understand adult conversation.

Ambiguous Answers to Questions

Children aged 5 to 11 years often use ambiguous terms to answer questions not understood. For example, in answer to the question "How does a doctor know how to mend your bone?" a 6-year-old child answered, "Because he's special" (Pickert & Furth, 1980). Further clarification is needed to bring a child to an understanding of the question. "How does a doctor get to know?" leads the child to answer, "By learning, like a nurse." Ambiguity in a child's answer may indicate that the question requires further clarification. Additionally, the use of qualifiers in an answer, such as "partly," "sort of," and "sometimes," is another technique that children use to maintain a conversation, even though they do not fully understand the question. These qualified responses permit children to maintain the topic of conversation without committing themselves to a definite answer.

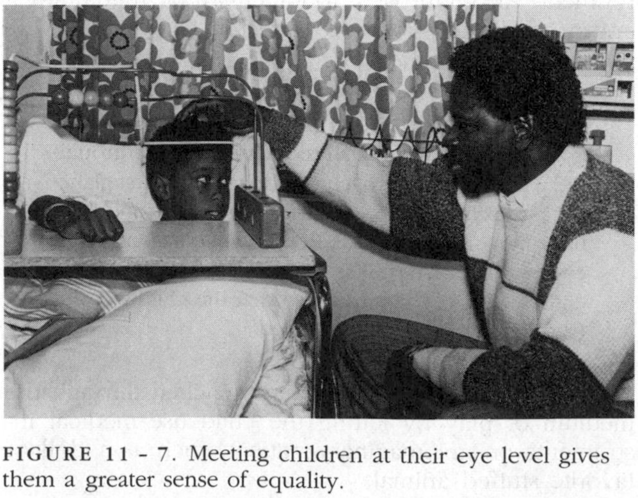

FIGURE 11 - 7. Meeting children at their eye level gives them a greater sense of equality.

Responses to Vague Messages

Children's responses to vague messages differ from those of adults. One cannot always be sure that children understand. They may briefly show behavioral signs of uncertainty but not request clarification for a vague message they have received. On the contrary, they resolve uncertainties by making guesses at the speaker's intended meaning. Very young children are thought to have such trust in the person sending the communication that they would be unaware that such a trusted individual could make a vague or ambiguous statement. It has also been noted that kindergarten children seem to persist in relying on nonverbal cues to determine a speaker's intent. When children rely on the physical context and the speaker's gesture to determine intent, misinterpretation can easily occur. Eventually, children learn to seek clarification. Recognition of these factors points out the need for adults to explain carefully what will happen to a child and, more important, to determine a young child's understanding after the explanation.

Communication Techniques

Developmental level, experiences, and personality account for the notable variations in how children communicate. Some children readily engage in conversation, whereas others remain reticent. Various techniques can be used to engage children in communication. Especially when children are experiencing stress, no one technique is likely to help children express themselves.

Rigid adherence to a set of communication techniques does not ensure quality relationships with children. Techniques are used along with knowledge of child development, experience, and an openness toward the child. The following discussion is presented as suggested techniques (direct and indirect) to be selectively used with children.

Direct Communication Techniques

Adults often have difficulty talking with children. The diverse worlds that must come together when adults and children talk may leave both disinterested, unless adults respond with sustained interest.

Questions in Child-Adult Conversation

The type of question used to initiate conversation with a child is significant. A closed question, one that has only one answer (often a one-word answer) does little other than supply a label for an object or action. Open questions, however, provide an opportunity for the child to communicate more ideas; sometimes conversation is not stimulated by open questions, but other fears and feelings may be revealed by their response.

Questions can be useful and are often necessary to help gather information. Even in an interview situation, however, it should be recognized that successive questions make demands on the child. Questions are a form of power through which the child's thoughts, attention, memories, and ideas are directed and controlled (Wood, 1982).

An open question, one that invites a range of possible answers, stimulates a child to think and express ideas and thoughts. For example, "What do you think will happen next?" offers the opportunity for a child to share ideas, because there is no one right answer. It must be recognized that an "I don't know" answer or shrug of the shoulders means that a child may lack confidence to answer, may not understand the question, or may not have had experience considering alternative answers.

Continued questioning can result in the suppression of a child's spontaneous volunteering of information.

Children's responses to questions are also affected by what is suggested by the particular setting. The surrounding circumstances of an interview can affect how a child responds. For example, a child brought to an outpatient clinic because of the exacerbation of a chronic illness, might be asked to describe the symptoms; in these circumstances, the child may under-report the symptoms and give only a partial list in order to avoid being admitted to the hospital.

Humor

Humor is increasingly being recognized as an appropriate effective way to relate to children who are experiencing illness, hospitalization, and pain. If used constructively, humor can create change in behavior, values, and relationships (Robinson, 1986). A series of tapes using humor to help children cope with hospitalization have been reported to be effective (Grimm & Pefley, 1990).

Dialogue Techniques

Five strategies to encourage conversation have been identified by Tough (1979) and are summarized in Table 11–2. They are labeled according to the function they have in conversation: orienting, enabling, informing, sustaining, and concluding. They are effective regardless of whether a conversation is at a simple reporting level, such as about a trip to the museum, or in a more advanced problem solving situation. Four examples of conversational processes are summarized in Tables 11–3 to 11–6, including reporting, logical reasoning, predicting, and projecting, respectively. Each table gives examples of questions reflecting the five strategies of orienting, enabling, informing, sustaining, and concluding.

Simple *reporting on a present or past experience* (Table 11–3) is a common form of language use. To encourage dialogue under these circumstances, the goals are

- Label the components of the scene.
- Refer to detail.
- Refer to incidents and the sequence of events.
- Identify the central meaning.

TABLE 11–2
Dialogue Strategies to Promote Conversation with Children

Orienting Strategies

Comments and questions that direct the child's thinking toward a particular topic and to think in a particular way (i.e., predicting, reasoning)

Enabling Strategies

Utterances that enable a child to move toward an extended interpretation (extend meaning that a situation has for a child as far as is possible)

a. *Follow-through strategies:*
Statements that help child give further detail explanations, and justifications; they follow up the child's response and help extend a description or interpretation
b. *Focusing strategies:*
A deliberate focusing of child's attention on essential features to promote a fuller interpretation of a picture, event, or experience
c. *Checking strategies:*
To help the child reconsider the statements, giving an opportunity to provide omitted information; for example, "Did you really mean . . . ?"

Informing Strategies

Providing information when a child seems ready to receive it or when additional information is needed to complete an idea or solve a problem

Sustaining Strategies

Supportive comments encourage the child to say more and indicate that she or he has the attention of the listener; strategies may be verbal, e.g., "Really?" "Good!" "What else?" or nonverbal (gestures and facial expressions); comments also may be repetitions of what the child has said, using intonation and a pause that encourages the child to go on

Concluding Strategies

Comments that indicate intention to bring a particular topic of discussion to a close; it is important to leave the child with a sense of satisfaction because efforts have been recognized or difficulties understood

Adapted from Tough, J. (1977). *Talking and learning.* London, Ward Lock Educational, 1977, © School Curriculum Development Committee.

TABLE 11-3
Reporting on Present: Talking About a Toddler's Experience with an Abdominal Ultrasound

Goals

Label the components of the event

Refer to detail (machine/people)

Refer to incidents and the sequence of events

Identify central meaning

Reflect on the meaning of the experience (include feelings)

Orienting

I'd like you to tell me what is . . .

What is being done to you right now?

What is this machine?

Who are the people around you?

Enabling

Follow-through/focusing/checking . . .

What will the machine do?

How does lying very still help?

How does the room feel to you?

Informing

The test will take a picture of your tummy; it will not hurt and it will take about 15 minutes

Your mom is here with you

To take the picture of your tummy, you will need some jelly on your tummy; the jelly will feel cold just for a minute

You will need to lie still for the test

You will be able to see on the TV what is happening in your tummy

Sustaining

The nurse is watching for the picture on the TV

It's really good when you lie still; it really helps

So you want to go back to your room—you want it to be finished

You say the jelly felt really cold?

What else did you feel?

Concluding

I enjoyed being with you for your test

I'm sure they got a good picture because you held so still

By Nadine Cross, R.N., M.H.Sc., C.N.S., & Annette Vigneux, R.N., M.H.Sc., C.N.S., Children's Hospital, Chedoke-McMaster Hospitals, Hamilton, Ontario.

- Reflect on the meaning of the experience (include feelings).

More complex ways of thinking are employed when language is used to engage a child in reasoning processes (Table 11–4). Adults can foster movement toward logical reasoning by encouraging a child to

- Explain a process.
- Identify causal and dependent relationships.
- Recognize problems and their solutions.
- Justify decisions and actions.
- Reflect on events and draw conclusions.
- Recognize principles.

Even though a child's thinking is prelogical, a reasoning mode is used by some young children and can be fostered in conversation.

Encouraging the use of language *to predict or describe anticipated events* is another way to foster communication with children (Table 11–5). In such a conversation one attempts to

- Anticipate and forecast events.
- Anticipate the detail and sequence of events.
- Anticipate problems and possible solutions.
- Anticipate and recognize alternative courses of action.
- Predict the consequence of actions and events.

This process is particularly useful to the child who is anticipating a painful procedure. These strategies can be employed by engaging the child in conversation or by using play. As the child communicates understanding of the anticipated event, misconceptions can be clarified.

Using language to *project into the feelings of others* is not easily done by the young child (Table 11–6). However, to teach children to appreciate another's point of view, they can be encouraged to

- Project into the experiences, feelings, and reactions of others.
- Project into situations never experienced.

These various processes of reporting, reasoning, predicting, and projecting can be employed when talking to children. Encouraging the application of language to these purposes prompts children to engage in more complex thinking than the mere labeling of events and experiences. Regardless of the type of conversation in which the child is being engaged, the five dialogue strategies listed in Table 11–2 facilitate achievement of the goals in each of these processes.

Indirect Communication Techniques

Children tell about their thoughts and feelings indirectly through their usual patterns of self-expression

TABLE 11-4
Toward Logical Reasoning: Talking with a 9-Year Old about Taking Oral Prednisone

Goals

Explain a process

Identify casual and dependent relationships

Recognize problems and their solutions

Justify decisions and actions

Reflect on events and draw conclusions

Orienting

What do you know about how the medicine works?

It is important to understand why you are taking prednisone (the white pills)

Enabling

Follow-through . . .

What are some of the side effects to watch for?

It is important to take the medicine exactly as your doctor told you

Focusing . . .

Can you tell me how the medicine helps you to get better?

Checking . . .

Did you say you sometimes feel like not taking it?

You said you are taking a little bit less medicine now than a few weeks ago—tell me why that is

Informing

If you reduce the drug rapidly, it may make you feel sick

This medicine might make you feel hungry

You should wear a necklace or bracelet indicating that you need prednisone

Sustaining

What else might you want to know about the medicine?

It's great that you know so much about taking this medicine

Concluding

You seem to know a lot about the medicine already

If you think about any other questions, we can talk about them

By Nadine Cross, R.N., M.H.Sc., C.N.S., & Annette Vigneux, R.N., M.H.Sc., C.N.S., Children's Hospital, Chedoke-McMaster Hospitals, Hamilton, Ontario.

(stories, drawing, play) more readily than by means of a formal interview. An interview depends on language for communication, and it may be misinterpreted by a young child. Furthermore, it is often too direct and confronting for children. The following indirect approaches can promote self-expression in children and can help determine the need for additional therapy.

Third-Person Technique

In the third-person technique, feelings are explored through a statement such as "Lots of times kids feel

TABLE 11-5
Predicting: Talking with a 4-Year Old about a Visit to the Nurse Practitioner's Office

Goals

Anticipate and forecast events

Anticipate the detail and sequence of events

Anticipate problems and possible solutions

Anticipate and recognize alternative courses of action

Predict the consequences of actions and events

Orienting

Do you know why your mommy and daddy brought you here today?

Enabling

Follow-through . . .

Do you know what I am going to check you for?

Do you remember what we did the last time you were here?

Focusing . . .

Let's look at a few pictures about going for a checkup

Is there anything in these pictures you would like to ask about?

Checking . . .

Tell me again what you are expecting me to do

Did you say you would like to listen to your own heart?

Did you say you don't like when I look in your ears—what is it that makes it unpleasant for you?

Informing

Now I will measure how tall you are and check how much you weigh

Now I will listen to your heart

Now I will look in your mouth and ears

Sustaining

What did you hear when you listened to your own heart?

Concluding

You had some good questions today; it is good that you are interested in being healthy

By Nadine Cross, R.N., M.H.Sc., C.N.S., & Annette Vigneux, R.N., M.H.Sc., C.N.S., Children's Hospital, Chedoke-McMaster Hospitals, Hamilton, Ontario.

TABLE 11-6
Projecting: Projecting into an Imagined Scene with a 15-Year Old About Impending Surgery for Scoliosis

Goals

Project into experiences, feelings, and reactions of others

Project into situations never experienced

Orienting

Your surgery has been scheduled for 9 A.M. tomorrow—what do you think that you will need to do to prepare for surgery?

Enabling

Follow-through . . .

Let's talk about the events that will happen from now until tomorrow when you have your surgery

Focusing . . .

Have you had surgery before?

Have you spoken to anyone who has had this surgery?

Checking . . .

You said you talked with your parents about the surgery—did you understand everything?

You had some questions about the laboratory work before surgery?

Informing

Your parents can stay with you until you go to the operating room

You will need a blood test before the surgery

Sustaining

You seem to be interested in exactly what the doctor will do

Yes, you will have medication for pain

Concluding

You know a lot about what will happen over the next few days

I will be back later if you want to talk more about how you feel about the surgery

By Nadine Cross, R.N., M.H.Sc., C.N.S., & Annette Vigneux, R.N., M.H.Sc., C.N.S., Children's Hospital, Chedoke-McMaster Hospitals, Hamilton, Ontario.

afraid or lonely in the hospital." A discussion about how "other children" feel may eventually encourage the child's own expression of feelings.

Sentence Completion Technique

The sentence completion technique is particularly valuable with school-age children and can be introduced as a game. Nonthreatening topics are described by incomplete sentences, such as "The thing I like best about summer is. . . ." Gradually personal statements can appear, such as "The thing I like least about being in the hospital is. . . ." This approach can be expanded into having children list as many "good things" and as many "bad things" as they can generate about a certain event or topic.

Story-Telling

Engaging the child in *story-telling,* either verbal or in conjunction with drawing and writing, provides a natural medium through which children express themselves. A child can simply be asked to tell a story about being in the hospital or about a specific event the child has experienced. The technique of writing a story or drawing a picture and telling a story to accompany it is a common method of teaching in the elementary schools and is familiar to school-age children. Feelings can also be explored by showing a child predrawn pictures or a comic strip. The child can be asked either to tell or write a story to go with the pictures.

Mutual Story-Telling

The mutual *story-telling technique* is a technique that works well with children. This psychotherapeutic approach is designed to elicit the child's thinking, but it also introduces new ways of thinking (Gardner, 1971). This technique involves asking a child to tell a story for a make-believe television program. The child is instructed to tell the moral of the story. The therapist then tells a story about the same characters but with healthier adaptations and ways of thinking. Anxiety-provoking confrontations are avoided in this method. This is not an easy technique, and proficiency may require months or even years of practice.

Bibliotherapy

Another way to use stories is to have *books on the topics and events* that are similar to what a child is experiencing or is about to experience (bibliotherapy). Life events such as moving, starting school, birth of a sibling, adoption, divorce, illness, hospitalization, and other new or stressful experiences can be introduced through books. A child can learn about the nature of an event and is given the opportunity to express feelings and concerns about a personal situation. This technique can be combined with *story-telling, drawing, and writing stories* by introducing a topic with a book and then encouraging a child to relate personal ideas in response to it.

Communication Through Play

Play as an avenue for communication and its developmental characteristics are discussed in Chapter 17. Play is believed to be an important activity through which children and adolescents can maximize their coping skills when encountering the stress of hospitalization and illness. Children placed into stressful circumstances are less likely to play spontaneously. Play and its role in the hospital are discussed in

Chapter 17. It should be recognized that even in less threatening places, such as a clinic, office, elementary school, and home, play should be introduced as a way of facilitating communication. For example, taking an interest in the child's normal play activity, using puppets and miniature versions of office equipment, handling unfamiliar equipment, and using stories and drawings in these less threatening environments are important supportive nursing measures.

Drawings

Another technique frequently employed to help children express how they feel is drawing (Johnson, 1990). The medium of drawing is especially valuable for children who cannot talk about anxiety-producing events. Children can be encouraged to draw a picture and to talk about it. Although drawings express children's feelings and can open a door to communication, a full interpretation of drawings should not be attempted without specialized preparation. The technique of drawing as an assessment tool for children has been reviewed by Wilson and Ratekin (1990).

Communication with Parents

The nurse who hopes to relate to parents in a beneficial way must begin from the premise that parents are individuals. In communicating with parents, nurses must recognize that the way parents perceive their role will affect the communication process. Parents may think that they are expected to have certain feelings and to respond in prescribed ways because they are parents. The nurse can dispel some of these erroneous ideas by acknowledging that their frustrations with parenting are normal reactions.

Established family communication patterns affect the way in which parents and nurses relate to each other. The openness of a family and the level at which communication takes place must be respected. When the usual communication within a family remains at a level at which little self-disclosure and no sharing of personal feelings takes place, nurses cannot expect parents to suddenly engage in an open, self-revealing conversation. Over time, parents may develop new levels of comfort in expressing their feelings and concerns, but the relationship cannot be forced. It is the nurse's responsibility to determine the comfort level and needs of parents. The need for information, support, and a listening ear can be determined by means of effective approaches.

The goal is to establish an atmosphere that encourages communication and leads to independent family functioning and problem-solving (Fig. 11–8). The nurse uses the skills of silence, listening, and observation in conjunction with personal characteristics of acceptance of, respect for, and empathy with others. A nondirective approach (with open-ended questions) often creates an environment within which a parent feels accepted and is able to think about a problem and consider new ways of approaching it. The nurse's role is to reflect the parent's thinking, so that the issues can be more easily clarified and decision making by the parent can be facilitated. The goals parents set for themselves are more likely to be reached and to bring beneficial results to the family than are those the nurse can establish for the parents.

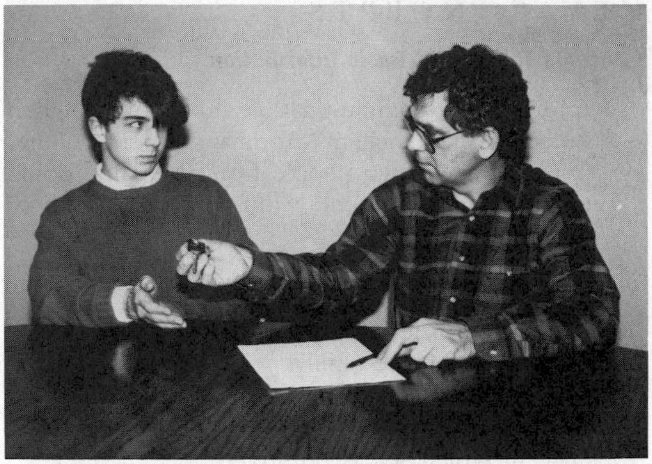

FIGURE 11-8. Communication between parents and adolescents involves fair negotiation in which the teenager's views are respected. Here an agreement is made between father and son about use of the family car.

The degree of comfort parent(s) have in their own role also affects how a nurse communicates with parents. It is recommended that nurses establish a role that does not compete with parents and one in which parents are encouraged to help care for their child. How parents think and feel about their role in their child's care is an individual matter. The parental role is a manifestation of each person's total life experiences, including cultural, moral, and ethical dimensions. This accounts for phenomena that nurses may find troublesome: parents may disagree with each other regarding decisions related to their child's care. The nurse should acknowledge the uniqueness of each parent by encouraging individual expression and giving equal recognition. The nurse's acceptance of and respect for the opinions of each can also teach parents to respect each other's individuality. As the nurse seeks to empower the family, defined professional boundaries can be established in a caring, positive environment (Barnsteiner & Gillis-Donovan, 1990). To help families in this process of empowerment, dependence on the health care provider is decreased, and families take responsibility for their own health care. Specific comments to parents about their parental role can provide them with a significant source of encouragement.

The nurse who acknowledges effective parenting gives the parents needed reassurance. Most parents need to hear that their children are growing and developing normally, but it is equally important for the nurse to attribute the health of children to the care and nurturing of the parents.

KEY CONCEPTS

Concepts Related to Basic Information

- Intercultural communication takes place when nurses relate to clients from a different culture, but also when two people from the same dominant culture represent a different subculture or identity group.
- A child's communication ability parallels cognitive and developmental stages.
- A child's style of communication has been learned within the family.
- A therapeutic relationship has boundaries that bring one into a meaningful interactive experience in which self is preserved.
- The underlying principle of communicating with children is that *children are valued*.

Concepts Related to Nursing Assessment

- When data are gathered in a parent-child-nurse setting, it should be recognized that the context of communication can affect the content; children may not speak accurately in front of parents, and vice versa.
- Nonverbal communication accurately represents how children feel, because they do not conceal true feelings as adults do.
- Observing the interaction between parents and children can help a nurse understand established patterns of communication within a specific family.

Concepts Related to Nursing Intervention

- Direct communication techniques used to facilitate conversation include
  - Use of questions.
  - Use of humor.
  - Special dialogue techniques that orient, enable, inform, sustain, and conclude.
- Indirect communication techniques that help children express themselves include
  - Third-person technique.
  - Story-telling.
  - Mutual story-telling.
  - Bibliotherapy.
  - Play.
  - Drawing.

REFERENCES

Barnsteiner, J. H., & Gillis-Donovan, J. (1990). Being related and separate: A standard for therapeutic relationships. *MCN: American Journal of Maternal Child Nursing, 15,* 223–228.

Bibace, R., & Walsh, M. E. (1980). Development of children's concepts of illness. *Pediatrics, 66*(6), 912–917.

Davis, A. (1984). *Listening and responding*. St. Louis: C. V. Mosby.

Garbarino, J., & Stott, F. M. (1989). *What children can tell us: Eliciting, interpreting, and evaluating information from children*. San Francisco: Jossey-Bass.

Gardner, R. A. (1971). *Therapeutic communication with children: The mutual storytelling technique*. New York: Science House.

Grimm, D. L., & Pefley, P. T. (1990). Opening doors for the child "inside." *Pediatric Nursing, 16*(4), 368–369.

Hall, E. T. (1984). *The dance of life*. New York: Anchor Books.

Johnson, B. H. (1990). Children's drawings as a projective technique. *Pediatric Nursing, 16*(1), 11–17.

Kramer, N. A. (1990). Comparison of therapeutic touch and casual touch in stress reduction of hospitalized children. *Pediatric Nursing, 16*(5), 483–485.

Lenart, J. C., St. Clair, P. A., & Bell, M. A. (1991). Childrearing knowledge, beliefs, and practice of Cambodian refugees. *Journal of Pediatric Health Care, 5*(6), 299–305.

Molsberry, D., & Shogan, M. G. (1990). Communicating through touch. In M. J. Craft & J. A. Denehy (Eds.), *Nursing interventions for infants and children* (pp. 127–150). Philadelphia: W. B. Saunders.

Niederhauser, V. P. (1989). Health care of immigrant children: Incorporating culture into practice. *Pediatric Nursing, 15,* 569–574.

Piaget, J. (1967). *Six psychological studies*. New York: Random House.

Pickert, S. M., & Furth, G. (1980). How children maintain a conversation with adults. *Human Development, 23,* 162–176.

Porter, R. E., & Samovar, L. A. (1985). Approaching intercultural communication. In L. A. Samovar & R. E. Porter (Eds.), *Intercultural communication: A reader* (pp. 15–39). Belmont, CA: Wadsworth.

Robinson, V. M. (1986). Humor is a serious business. *Dimensions of Critical Nursing, 5*(3), 132–133.

Rosenberg, J. A. (1986). Health care for Cambodian children: Integrating treatment plans. *Pediatric Nursing, 12,* 118–125.

Satir, V. (1975). *Peoplemaking*. Palo Alto, CA: Science and Behavior Books.

Singer, M. R. (1985). Culture: A perceptual approach. In L. A. Samovar & R. E. Porter (Eds.), *Intercultural communication: A reader*. Belmont, CA: Wadsworth.

Sloat, A. R., & Matsuura, W. (1990). Intercultural communication. In M. J. Craft & J. A. Denehy (Eds.), *Nursing interventions for infants and children* (pp. 166–180). Philadelphia: W. B. Saunders.

Tough, J. (1979). *Talking and learning*. London: Ward Lock Educational.

Wexler, D. B. (1991). *The adolescent self*. New York: W. W. Norton.

Wilson, D., & Ratekin, C. (1990). An introduction to using children's drawings as an assessment tool. *Nurse Practitioner, 15*(3), 23–35.

Wood, D. J. (1982). Talking to young children. *Developmental Medicine and Child Neurology, 24*(6), 856–859.

BIBLIOGRAPHY

Arnold, E., & Boggs, K. (1989). *Interpersonal relationships: Professional communication skills for nurses*. Philadelphia: W. B. Saunders.

Azarnoff, P. (1990). Teaching materials for pediatric health professionals. *Journal of Pediatric Health Care, 4*(6), 282–289.

Beal, C. R. (1987). Repairing the message: Children's monitoring and revision skills. *Child Development, 58,* 401–408.

Beal, C. R., & Flavell, J. M. (1984). Development of the ability to distinguish communicative intention and literal message meaning. *Child Development, 55,* 920–928.

Bretherton, I. (1990). Communication patterns, internal working models, and the intergenerational transmission of attachment relationships. *Infant Mental Health Journal, 11*(3), 237–252.

Claflin, C. J., & Barbarin, O. A. (1991). Does "telling" less protect more? Relationships among age, information disclosure, and what children with cancer see and feel. *Journal of Pediatric Psychology, 6*(2), 169–192.

Faber, A., & Mazlish, E. (1980). *How to talk so kids will listen and listen so kids will talk.* New York: Avon Books.

Fosson, A., & deQuan, M. M. (1984). Reassuring and talking with hospitalized children. *Children's Health Care, 13*(1), 37–44.

Garvey, C. (1984). *Children's talk.* Cambridge, MA: Harvard University Press.

Green, M. (1986). Interviewing children and adolescents. *Patient Care, 20*(15), 76–78.

Greenspan, S. I. (1981). *The clinical interview of the child.* New York: McGraw-Hill.

Hoffer, J. (1989). Family communication. In P. J. Bomar (Ed.), *Nurses and family health promotion: Concepts, assessment, and interventions* (pp. 78–89). Baltimore: Williams & Wilkins.

Kopp, C. B. (1989). Regulation of distress and negative emotions: A developmental view. *Developmental Psychology, 25*(3), 343–354.

Lloyd, P. (1990). Children's communication. In R. Grieve & M. Hughes (Eds.), *Understanding children.* Cambridge, MA: Basil Blackwell.

Lytton, H. (1980). *Parent-child interaction.* New York: Plenum Press.

Murphy, K. A. (1990). Interactional styles of parents following the birth of a high-risk infant. *Journal of Pediatric Nursing, 5*(1), 33–41.

Penner, S. G. (1987). Parental responses to grammatical and ungrammatical child utterances. *Child Development, 58,* 376–384.

Rice, M. (1984). *Child language and cognition: Contemporary issues.* Baltimore: University Park Press.

Sundeen, S. J., Stuart, G. W., Rankin, E. A. D., & Cohen, S. A. (1989). *Nurse-client interaction.* St. Louis: C. V. Mosby.

Thayer, M. (1990). Touching with intent: Using therapeutic touch. *Pediatric Nursing, 16*(1), 70–72.

Thompson, S. W. (1991). Communication techniques for allaying anxiety and providing support for hospitalized children. *Journal of Child and Adolescent Psychiatric and Mental Health Nursing, 4*(3), 119–122.

Tronick, E. Z. (1989). Emotions and emotional communication in infants. *American Psychologist, 44*(2), 112–119.

Walters, J., & Walter, L. (1980). Parent-child relationships: A review 1970–1979. *Journal of Marriage and the Family, 42,* 807–822.

Wilson, C. J. (1991). Use of children's art work to evaluate the effectiveness of a hospital preparation program. *Children's Health Care, 20*(2), 120–121.

Winkelstein, M. (1989). Fostering positive self-concept in the school-age child. *Pediatric Nursing, 15*(3), 247–249.

CHAPTER • 12

Promoting Healthy Parenting

Mabel Hunsberger

RELATED TOPICS
Alternative family lifestyles, Chapter 2
Theory of developing children and families, Chapters 2 and 3
Adolescent parenting, Chapter 9
The relationships between parenting style and development of self-esteem, Chapter 14
Parenting in behavioral problems, Chapter 29

LEARNING OBJECTIVES

- Describe the role that effective discipline plays in a child's development.
- State the five essential elements of parenting and their role in socializing the child.
- Compare and contrast positive and negative reinforcement methods, and give examples of the use of each in promoting acceptable child behavior.
- Apply the guidelines and principles of effective parenting to developing a care plan for working with parents.
- Describe the sociocultural influences on parenting style.
- Describe the problems related to parenting that may be experienced by dual-earner parents, and apply appropriate nursing measures.
- List the major areas of concern for *home-alone children* and measures for minimizing them.
- Describe factors that contribute to difficulties in integration within blended families, and apply appropriate nursing interventions.
- Describe nursing interventions used to support the role of parents.

Fundamental to pediatric nursing is helping parents to be the best parents they can be. An understanding of what parents experience in raising their children is as critical as a knowledge of growth and

development. Each family is unique, making it difficult for nurses to fully understand the dynamics within a particular family. A basic principle to understand is that the relationship between parent and child is reciprocal; the development of one has a dynamic impact on the development of the other. Therefore, the needs of parents within each family differ according to the relationships that develop among its members.

Nurses have the opportunity to support and encourage parents during the normal developmental transitions as well as through conflict situations. An important function of the nurse is to recognize when families require counselling or could benefit from a parenting program.

The intent of this chapter is to acquaint the nurse with principles of parenting and describe the role of the nurse in assessment, teaching, anticipatory guidance, and making referrals. Emphasis is placed on nursing interventions that can be used to guide a person's transition in the role of parent.

Parenting: A *Changing Concept*

Few experiences in life demand as much patience, time, and energy as parenting. Raising children is one of the most challenging tasks to be performed by family and society, and it compares with no other in consequence. The task encompasses facilitating the development of a child into an adult who is capable of functioning in our society. Central to this process is the perpetuation, through generations, of values, skills, knowledge, beliefs, and activities deemed useful for happy, healthy living.

In the past, society exerted great pressure on couples to become parents—often before they were ready to take on the responsibility. Today, alternative lifestyles and scientific advances make more options available; young people can delay parenting, and older couples can have children after other goals have been achieved. Adoption, artificial insemination, and surrogate parenting present a myriad of options to infertile couples or singles who wish to have children. Some couples, however, choose to have no children.

Regardless of the family constellation, parenting is a task for which most are ill-prepared. An emerging awareness of parents' needs has led to the availability of parenting programs such as Systematic Training for Effective Parenting (STEP) (Dinkmeyer & McKay, 1989) and Parent Effectiveness Training (PET) (Gordon, 1975; Gordon, 1989) and others in many communities. Education for parenting is increasing in high schools; some regions have kindergarten through grade 12 curricula that include topics in parenting. In spite of the increase in programs in family life education, the actual benefits of these programs have not been documented, and there is a need to evaluate their effectiveness (Small, 1990) if policymakers and agencies are to give them priority for funding.

The economic circumstances of many families has propelled parenting arrangements into a new era. Because both mothers and fathers are in the work force, the need for high-quality child care programs is escalating. Some large corporations are providing day care centers and accommodating part-time and split-shift schedules, especially for parents of young children. More commonly, families with young children struggle to find economical, good care for their children while they are working outside the home.

The stress that securing and retaining jobs causes parents can leave a family exhausted with little energy and patience available for the task of nurturing children.

Socialization of Children

Socialization is a process of learning societal rules. Expectations for a child's behavior depend on the child's developmental stage, physical and cognitive capacities, culture and society, and values and beliefs of home and school environments. Health behaviors valued by one society may be insignificant in another, and considered vices in a third. The same is true for the behaviors family units consider desirable or important. The particular cultural beliefs held by a family to a large degree determine the nurse's role in supporting parents.

Most of a child's learning is internally motivated by the desire to grow up. Discipline, then, is something children do for themselves, with adult help. The goal of parenting is to foster the child's developing self-control. Initially, during infancy and early childhood, parents provide external controls for the child. Eventually and steadily, the child, properly guided and simultaneously "released" by the adult caregivers, takes responsibility for that control, and behavior becomes more internally driven.

If caregivers give consistent messages, children are able to learn from these role models the basic principles of behavior. The daily "do's and don'ts" simply reinforce those principles. Through this process, the child learns the culturally and societally approved behaviors by example. The responsibility of parents, teachers, and other role models is to demonstrate consistent, appropriate behaviors for the child to emulate (Fig. 12–1).

Parental Role in the Socialization of Children

Four goals that most directly motivate parenting activities are as follows:

- Keep the child safe.
- Instill familial beliefs and standards.
- Teach social behaviors and roles.
- Help the child become self-regulating and independent.

Of these goals, some are more important than others. The strength of these goals as motivating forces varies with the child's age, the parents' intellectual and social levels, the parents' interests and individual personalities, the child's temperament, and familial attitudes about parenting. These same factors determine which parenting methods are selected and influence the degree of their effectiveness (see discussion of methods later in this chapter).

Discipline organizes the child's world. Limits and rules consistently enforced make the world predictable and give the child boundaries within which to grow and develop. Predictability and boundaries increase the child's security and reinforce the development of trust of others and self. Feelings of security and trust help a child to achieve self-confidence and contribute to a child's ability to cope with difficult situations and solve problems. As children progressively master the rules and roles of living, they experience a sense of accomplishment and acceptance that builds self-esteem. Positive self-esteem encourages children to make their own decisions on the basis of their own good judgment and inner convictions, rather than peer suggestion or impulse, thereby readying them for healthy adult independence (see Chapter 14 for further discussion of self-esteem).

Rules, consistency, punishment and reward, role modeling, and use of a child's imagination are essential elements of parenting. The following is a discussion of how these elements operate in the socialization of children. Table 12–1 defines these elements and summarizes the major function of each in this socialization. The nurse's assessment of parenting skills requires an evaluation of each of these five elements.

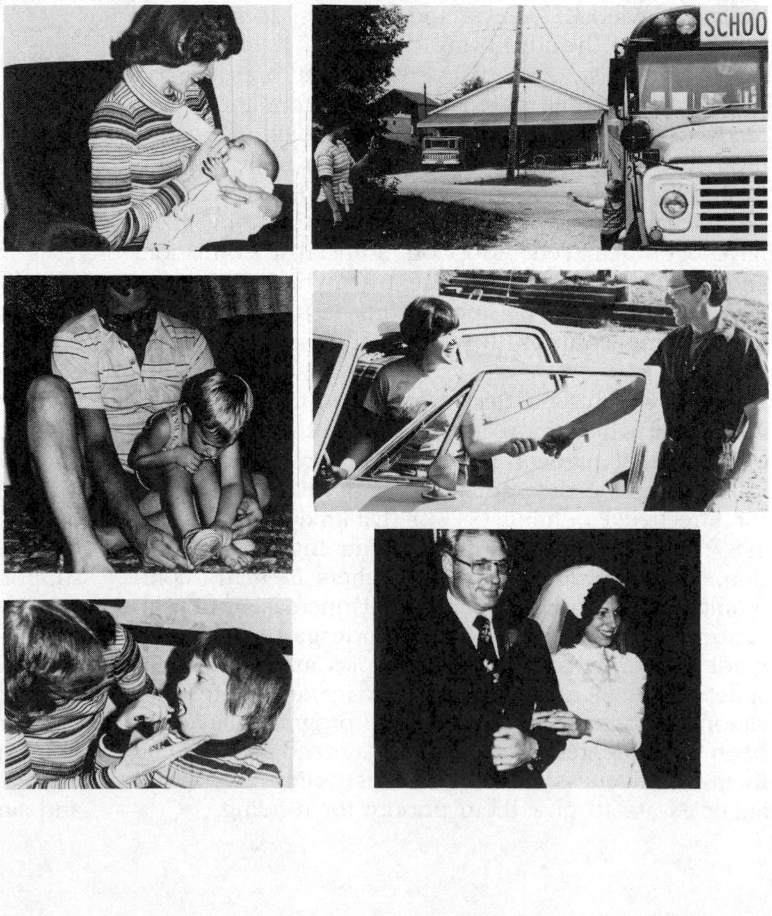

FIGURE 12 - 1. Socialization begins in and is sustained by the family but ultimately propels the child beyond the family. This series portrays the changing parent-child relationship in that socialization life cycle.

TABLE 12-1
Essential Elements of Parenting and Their Function in Socialization

Element	Definition	Functions in Socialization
Rules	Guidelines for behavior; may differ, depending on setting and situation; establish what is and is not permitted	Educates child by identifying behaviors acceptable to cultural and social milieu; restrains misbehavior by placing limits or boundaries on behavior; develops moral conscience
Consistency • In rules • In required compliance • Between parents in parenting methods	Maintaining uniformity or persisting in expectations for child; enforcing rules; retaining authority by using parenting methods congruent with rules, child's unique character, and situation	Speeds learning process by regular reinforcement and repetition; provides security, since child knows what is expected and what to expect from person in authority; fosters respect for rules and authority (essential to social survival)
Reinforcement	Negative consequences, natural or artificial, of breaking rule (misbehavior)	Educates by emphasizing which behaviors are not acceptable and that consequence follows misbehavior; restricts repetition of unacceptable behavior, at least temporarily; motivates appropriate behavior following misconduct, at least temporarily
	Positive reinforcement of behavior by physical, emotional, social, or material means that the child finds pleasurable or satisfying	Powerful motivator for acceptable behavior; stimulates repetition of desirable behavior after such behavior has occurred
Role modeling (observation)	Imitation of actions, attitudes, emotional expression of persons child perceives as competent and as possessing behaviors the child desires	Extremely effective way to educate child about acceptable behaviors and probable consequences of behaviors, especially if model provides cues to child to imitate and behavior is frequently demonstrated; reward for imitation stimulates repetition of the behavior
Using child's imagination	Try out or rehearse behaviors through role play, free play, talking to self, stories, and children's television shows that demonstrate problem solving and behavior/consequences	Speeds learning process through experimentation and practice; educates about problem solving and self-control behaviors while building self-confidence, without risk of negative consequence

Rules

Rules are essential to the child's moral development. Consistency in enforcing rules across a variety of circumstances makes it easier for children to integrate principles of conduct into their general moral code. For example, "Be kind to others" is a rule that can be applied often and is therefore internalized at a fairly early age (e.g., a toddler can learn to share and not to bite or hit). However, "Tell the truth" varies in its application, depending on the situation, and the child needs many years to learn which degree of truth is appropriate for any given situation. As children mature, they learn when to use the absolute truth and when to avoid and modify absolute truth. One does not tell the lady at the grocery store that she is fat.

Learning rules advances the child toward greater freedom and more mastery of the environment. It is expected that in the process of learning rules, a degree of frustration is unavoidable. Ultimately, rule mastery makes it easier to get along in the world as one assumes more responsibility for one's own behavior. This process of learning rules leads to self-regulation and a developing moral code.

Clearly established rules (i.e., limit setting) give children guidelines as to what is acceptable and what is not acceptable. They learn that some actions are never acceptable because they are dangerous, illegal, unethical, or antisocial. Conversely, they learn that some behaviors are always acceptable. They also gradually learn that a gray area exists in which some behaviors are acceptable at certain ages or in some circumstances and are unacceptable at other times.

Rules can be conveyed in a number of ways. The method most frequently used with infants and young toddlers is environmental control to ensure their safety. Confinements in space, restrictions on play materials, and childproofing are measures taken to convey rules by environmental control. Direct verbal communication is increasingly used as a child masters language. Even though this is the most common method of teaching rules, it is the least effective. Younger children respond to a tone of voice when reprimands and explanations are given; however, direct verbal methods are not effective until children reach an age (usually school age) at which they can comprehend simple explanations.

The nurse's assessment of parents' childrearing skills should include observation and discussion of the rules being communicated by the parents. Areas to address are as follows:

- Are the parents aware of the rules they are currently teaching their child? Are they able to establish rules? To say "No" when appropriate?

- Are the rules they verbalize consistent with their own behaviors?
- Are the number and type of rules they are currently working on realistic for the child's age, temperament, and mental capacity? For example, some children may not comply to rules because of memory or organizational deficits, rather than disobedience.
- Are the parents using age-appropriate methods to communicate the rules? Are rules being clearly communicated?
- Are the rules logical and enforceable?
- Is the child showing evidence of rule mastery? If so, is the child being given the opportunity for self-regulation in that area of living?

For areas in which parents answer negatively or express difficulty, intervention strategies can be instituted by the nurse; for more severe difficulties, a referral is made for in-depth counseling.

Consistency

Consistency, meaning holding to the same principles or practices throughout childrearing, is a difficult goal to achieve for many parents. Nurses can help parents identify the principles they are striving to uphold and assist them in devising strategies acceptable to both parents. Although the goal is to achieve consistency, it is even more important to maintain a nurturing environment through open parent-parent communications and parent-child communications.

Consistency in Rules

The learning of rules is facilitated when they are consistently applied to all family members. Some breaches of limits may be tolerated by parents when rules are first being learned by a child or in certain stressful circumstances; relapses can be anticipated during illness or fatigue. It is easier to be consistent when only a few rules are to be maintained.

Of particular significance is the consistency of messages children receive from fathers, mothers, and other caregivers. Parents need to strive toward agreement on rules. Any differences between parents should be resolved in privacy. Parental or family rules should be conveyed to other caregivers, along with the expectation that such rules will be enforced and modeled while they are caring for the children. For example, if a rule has been established that children cannot say "shut up," parents and caregivers must model the behavior by refraining from using this terminology.

Rules must be consistently modeled and applied by all caregivers; for example, if children are taught not to say "shut up," parents and other caregivers need to refrain from saying this.

Consistency in Enforcement

Children usually respond more favorably to situations in which they can predict the outcome. Rules or limits should be enforced consistently and to the same degree each time. Restrictions should not be set that parents cannot or do not intend to enforce. However, consistency in enforcement does not mean refusal to consider the circumstances involved; that would be rigidity, not consistency. Breaches of limits or rules should be dealt with immediately, first with a warning and then, if the behavior does not stop, by applying either natural or prescribed negative consequences. *Warnings ideally state what should be done, rather than what should not be done.* Rules should be enforced without obvious anger and with a minimum of words. Explanations of "why" should follow the consequence, provided the child is old enough to understand. Even then, explanations should be simple and brief. By means of consistently enforced rules, the child slowly learns to connect the act with the consequence and changes the behavior to avoid discomfort.

Consistency in Parenting Methods

Parenting methods should acknowledge children's individual temperaments. Some temperaments thrive better on firmness and consistency, whereas other temperaments make children relatively adaptable with less dependency on consistency of method. Fair parenting adapted to the individual helps children to develop respect for rules and authority.

Some couples develop a comprehensive parenting "master plan" when they have children. Such a plan is established by consensus of family members and takes into account the mutual rights, privileges, and responsibilities of every family member. Such a plan establishes the disciplinary methods allowable in the family and identifies those who will take responsibility for parenting. Agreement about these issues may not be easy to achieve, especially if the parents have difficulty in communicating with each other. In a study based on preschoolers and their parents, parental agreement on childrearing was positively related to effective parenting (Deal et al., 1989). It has also been shown that mothers of conduct-problem preschoolers act inconsistently during conflict episodes (Gardner, 1989). A nurse's assistance in developing a parenting plan to achieve consistency can be a major contribution to the well-being of the whole family.

Agreement in parenting is a process that evolves by means of open communication between parents. The child very quickly learns how to play one parent against the other, and consequently, family members may experience a high level of anxiety. The child ends up in the middle of a parental struggle that results in stress for the child and loss of respect for the parents. Single parents experience similar struggles as they try to achieve consistency from one day to the next and among other adults involved in the care of their children.

The nurse's assessment in this area of potential stress in families is especially crucial, because parents often do not seek professional help on their own. When nurses identify a family unit that is either at high risk for or currently displays conflicts related to childrearing attitudes, they can help parents to express their difficulties honestly and privately. In two-parent families, the couple should be encouraged to try to understand each other's views and to work toward a satisfactory compromise in areas of opposition. Nurses should also attempt to expand the parents' understanding of their children's differences (developmental, temperamental), so that a comfortable parenting schema can be selected for their situation. Nurses may make appropriate reading materials available, teach individually, or involve the parents in parent groups or may assist them in changing by using other appropriate resources in the community.

Reinforcement

Reinforcement is a method used to encourage acceptable behavior.

Positive Reinforcement

Positive reinforcement is a means of enforcing rules or setting limits by rewarding desired behaviors. All of us, but especially children, need praise, encouragement, and rewards to reinforce positive behavior. The positive reinforcement is given spontaneously during or after the act. Rewards should be differentiated from *bribes*. Children are bribed when they are either told beforehand that they will be rewarded or are actually rewarded in advance for a promise to avoid misbehavior.

Positive reinforcement increases the likelihood that a child will repeat a desired behavior. It also communicates to the child what the desired behavior is, without a confusing verbal exchange. Positive reinforcers fall into five general categories. Table 12–2 describes the advantages and disadvantages of each type.

To be effective, a positive reinforcer must meet certain criteria: (1) it must be something the child finds satisfying and desirable; (2) it must be readily available; and (3) it must be offered to the child in response to the desired behavior. When and how frequently the reinforcer is offered also determine its effectiveness. Whatever its form, the reinforcer or reward should be given while the child is still engaged in the desired action or immediately after it ends. Initially, the behavior must be reinforced regularly, preferably each time it occurs. Gradually, the reward can be given only occasionally, and eventually, the desired behavior should become a habit that requires no external reward.

Accentuating the positive aspects of behavior (i.e., "catching" the child during the appropriate behavior) can reduce parent-child conflicts. A child who perceives the parent as a supporter of the growing self is more apt to imitate that parent's values and beliefs. However, the psychology laboratory has produced evidence that both rewards (positive reinforcement) and punishment have strong motivational effects on socializing behavior (Fisher & Fisher, 1986). Unfortunately, scientific investigation has not determined when to use each; that is still left to parents' intuition and judgment. The following are suggested topics for discussion of positive reinforcement with parents:

TABLE 12–2
Advantages and Disadvantages of Rewards

Reward Category	Advantages	Disadvantages
Objects (food, toys, trinkets, clothing)	Since object is visible, reinforcement continues each time object seen or used; stimulates several sense modalities	Can be costly; if food is used, calories involved; cannot always be given immediately after the desired behavior
Activities (television, theater, roller skating, whatever activity the child finds rewarding and parents approve)	Usually inexpensive; perceived as desirable by most children May be contingent on earning so many tokens or points	What appeals can change rapidly; avoid problem somewhat by giving child choices or by letting child suggest activities
Social (hugs, kisses, pats, smiles, praise)	Can use lavishly without any cost	Needs to be combined with tangible rewards occasionally to retain effectiveness
Token (stars, check marks, points)	Good for all ages, can be promptly given	Reward finally earned by accumulated tokens can be expensive
Personal (self-satisfaction, feeling good)	Most desirable; fosters self-regulation	Must be learned, cannot be given by another; seldom effective in child with poor self-concept

- Do parents offer rewards or bribes? Do they know the difference?
- What type of positive reinforcers do the parents employ? Are they appropriate to the child's developmental level?
- Are the rewards realistic and given only when merited?
- Do the parents know how and when to wean the child from external rewards?

Negative Reinforcement

Negative reinforcement is a method that uses *removal* of undesirable or aversive stimuli to enforce rules, set limits, and increase the frequency of a desired behavior. When a mother says to her child, "You can get off the chair as soon as you're ready to say 'you're sorry'," she is using negative reinforcement. By removing the aversive condition of having to sit quietly in a chair, she increases the possibility that her child will follow rules regarding politeness.

Methods Used to Decrease Undesirable Behavior

Punishment

Punishment is a method used to reduce the frequency of undesirable behavior. Punishment is the "fine," or price, for not adhering to established rules. It is essential that a child understand two things: (1) the consequence of misconduct and (2) the reason for punishment. Punishment may be given in the form of disapproval, withdrawal of privileges, isolation, or substitution. Physical punishment has too many undesirable consequences to be included as a recommended option.

Disapproval may be verbal or nonverbal. Tone of voice often conveys the parent's disapproval. Numerous facial expressions and gestures can be used; their meanings are quickly learned, even by young children.

Privilege withdrawal is often effective with older children. Something they would like to do or have is withheld. The privilege withheld should be reasonable, not something critical, such as a birthday party, or long-anticipated, such as a prom, and should occur fairly soon after the misdeed. When possible, the withheld privilege should be something associated with the misconduct.

Isolation works with some children. By isolating the child from stimuli, the parent assures that undesired behavior will not be inadvertently *reinforced.* As a general rule, isolation periods of longer than 1 hour breed contempt for the parent rather than redirecting the offender's behavior. Usually, this method is not easily carried out before preschool age. *Time-out* is a form of isolation.

Substitution is a form of environmental control generally used with infants and young toddlers. The parent bodily removes the child from the situation that is prompting inappropriate behavior or diverts the child's attention with another activity or toy. When it is coupled with a message of disapproval, it becomes punishment.

Physical punishment is a punitive act that is more a vent for parental feelings than a tool for teaching. The term itself reflects a philosophy of "getting back" (punishing) rather than teaching and correcting behavior (discipline). There is no evidence that spanking and hitting children are effective disciplinary measures. Furthermore, physical punishment puts the child at risk for physical and psychologic harm. Especially for parents with poor impulse control, physical punishment sets up a situation in which a potential outcome is the serious injury of children. Some believe spanking cancels the crime for the child, freeing the child to repeat the act. Many parents feel disappointed in themselves when they resort to physical punishment (Osborne, 1989). Nurses have a valuable role in assisting families who resort to physical punishment. New patterns of discipline need to be established through counseling and parenting programs to protect the children in our society. See Chapter 28 on child abuse for further discussion of the nurse's role in protecting children from abuse.

Physical punishment has too many undesirable consequences for nurses to recommend it as an option for decreasing undesired behaviors. It is not a coping strategy that parents wish to model, and it instills frustration and anger in the child. For example, the child who has just been spanked is likely to turn to a doll and spank the doll while repeating the words uttered by the parent and using the same tone of voice.

Actually, punishment seldom works; withdrawal of any response stimuli tends to be the preferred method of decreasing undesired behavior.

Natural Consequences

Natural consequence may also be used to decrease undesirable behavior and is probably most effective in helping the child see self-regulation as a personal responsibility. For example, refusal to eat at mealtime results in extreme hunger before the next meal at which the child can have food. This approach requires restraint from intervening by the parents, but it allows the natural consequence to occur. It is usually most successful with preschool and early school-age children.

Positive Practices

Having the child use *positive practices* (apologizing for behavior, repairing the results of the misdeed, correcting inappropriate behavior, practicing correct behavior several times) as a way of decreasing undesired behavior is often realistic and has the double advantage of also reinforcing desirable behavior. However, this often takes time. Although encouraging the child to make amends can pave the way for reconciliation, parents should be advised that *forcing* an apology can suppress feelings (Osborne, 1989).

Parents' use of methods to decrease undesired behaviors can be assessed by addressing the following areas:

- Is the parents' goal to educate or motivate desirable behavior, or to impart revenge?
- Is the reason for the action explained to the child?
- What forms of punishment are usually employed?
- Is the method age-appropriate and developmentally appropriate?
- Is the method realistic in relation to the misdeed?
- Are misdeeds immediately followed by punishers or withdrawal of stimuli?
- Are the parents usually able to apply punishment without emotional display?
- If a rule is broken, does the child express, through words or behaviors, an understanding of the consequence?

Learning by Observation: Role Modeling

Children naturally imitate as a way of learning. Through imitation, they learn to perform specific actions; they learn attitudes and emotional expression. Parents, older siblings, and other caregivers provide cues that influence children's behavior. Psychologists stress that most of what we learn about our world comes from our observations of other people. Children who are inexperienced or unsure of how to behave in a situation are likely to observe and imitate someone they respect and perceive as behaving appropriately.

Children vary in how much they rely on role models to learn behaviors, however. Those who have established some appropriate behaviors in familiar situations are more likely to handle new situations on their own, rather than to imitate others. Parents can usually encourage imitation, regardless of how children perceive their parents' competencies or their own capabilities by making sure rewards are provided for imitative behavior. Parents' conscious use of role modeling can be assessed by addressing the following:

- Can parents identify instances when their child has imitated them? Of these instances, how often was the parent aware that the child was observing?
- Do the parents consciously role model behaviors they specifically want the child to learn or with which the child is having difficulty?
- Do parents reward the child for imitated behavior?
- If other caregivers are involved, have parents discussed with them examples of behaviors to which they wish to have the child exposed? Likewise, have they discussed specific behaviors to which they do not want the child exposed (e.g., smoking, drinking, foul language)?

Using the Child's Imagination for Socialization

Much of a child's world is imaginative. Children experiment imaginatively, trying out new behaviors. They rehearse and refine behaviors and practice problem solving to overcome problems or fears and to learn new or better ways of interacting with the world (Fig. 12–2). Parents can utilize this natural activity to teach desirable behavior. Parents also can use children's tendency to talk to themselves to help them master the problem solving process. Children talk to themselves more than adults do because they are less capable of the private communication adults call "thinking." For example, a child expresses frustration over a task, saying, "I can't do it." The parent can teach problem solving by saying, "I'll show you." As parents demonstrate, they can talk aloud to themselves, enumerating what must be done first and why, what is done second, and so on until the task is completed. By describing each of the necessary steps of the task and why it is done, occasionally questioning whether it is correct and evaluating and praising the results aloud, the child learns not only the motor action required and how to handle any complications, but also how to "think through" a problem.

Many well-designed children's television programs and story-telling can be useful in teaching children

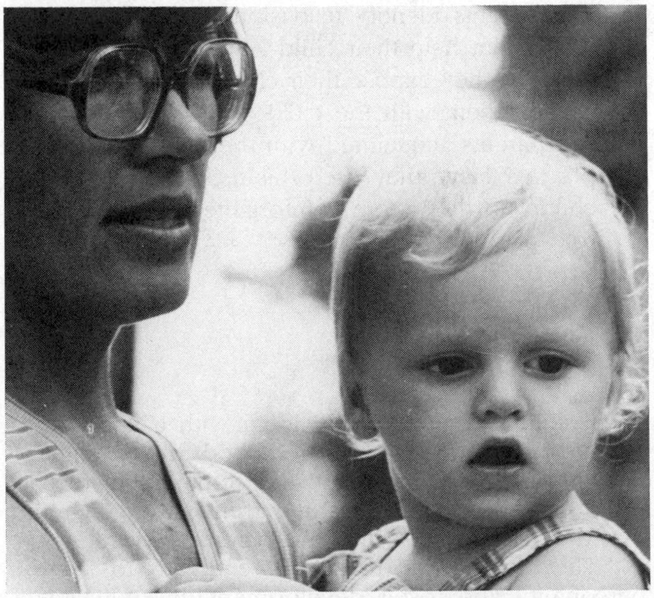

FIGURE 12 - 2. "Deep are the thoughts of a child."

appropriate behavior. These stories and televised programs are structured to capture the child's attention, center on a particular problem faced by children, and provide a convenient way of solving the problem, with rewards being given to the successful problem-solver hero or heroine. Parents can fabricate their own stories to fit a particular problem or behavior facing their child, while following these same guidelines and being careful not to focus so intently on the moral that the entertaining aspect of the story is lost. All these approaches to learning behavior are enhanced if followed by discussion between the parent and child about the intended theme and how the child might apply the information learned to a life situation.

An enjoyable teaching method for some that is similar to story participation is parent and child role playing. This is especially successful with older children. The parent and child then discuss how each felt in the new role, reinforcing for the child the fact that people do not all think or feel alike in a given situation. Discussion also reveals the reasons behind each person's behavior. Role playing themselves in various problem situations can also aid children in improving their behavior. Once the parent sees what is provoking the problem behavior and the responses it is receiving, the parent or nurse observer can help the child practice more desirable alternative behaviors by modeling another role. Practicing the behavior increases the child's confidence and the likelihood that it will be carried out. Additionally, the child can receive immediate feedback. To assess whether parents use their child's imagination to teach behaviors, the following areas can be addressed:

- Do parents "talk through" the steps of tasks with their child to aid problem solving?
- Are parents conscious of the behaviors of their child that illustrate learning through imagination?
- Can parents identify television programs or story books that help their child learn desirable behaviors? Do they expose their child to these? Do they discuss them with the child?
- Are parents acquainted with the technique of role playing? Have they used this technique with their child? Do they seem comfortable doing a sample role play with the nurse?

Parental Roles

Each child is a unique individual with a special potential; that factor makes parenthood an exciting endeavor for those who make the commitment to parenting. However, successful parents keep in mind that they are persons first and parents second.

The most crucial role of parenting is to *nurture* personality and foster development in a climate of *love and security*. The paradox of parenting is that *we live with our children so we can teach them to live without us*. This nurturing begins before the child's birth as the parent prepares emotionally and intellectually for the parenting role.

Parents are their children's first teachers (Fig. 12–3). They teach the most valuable lesson of living: how to interact with other humans. Parents teach children to be happy and loving by providing them with happiness and love. Expressions of love can be woven into all that parents do for or with their child.

An effective parent cannot be passive but must participate in the child's learning process. How a parent participates in the learning process will change as the child grows and develops. Table 12–3 describes the primary parental roles at each developmental stage of childhood. Changing parental roles are discussed later in this chapter, namely dual-career families, blended families, and single parenting.

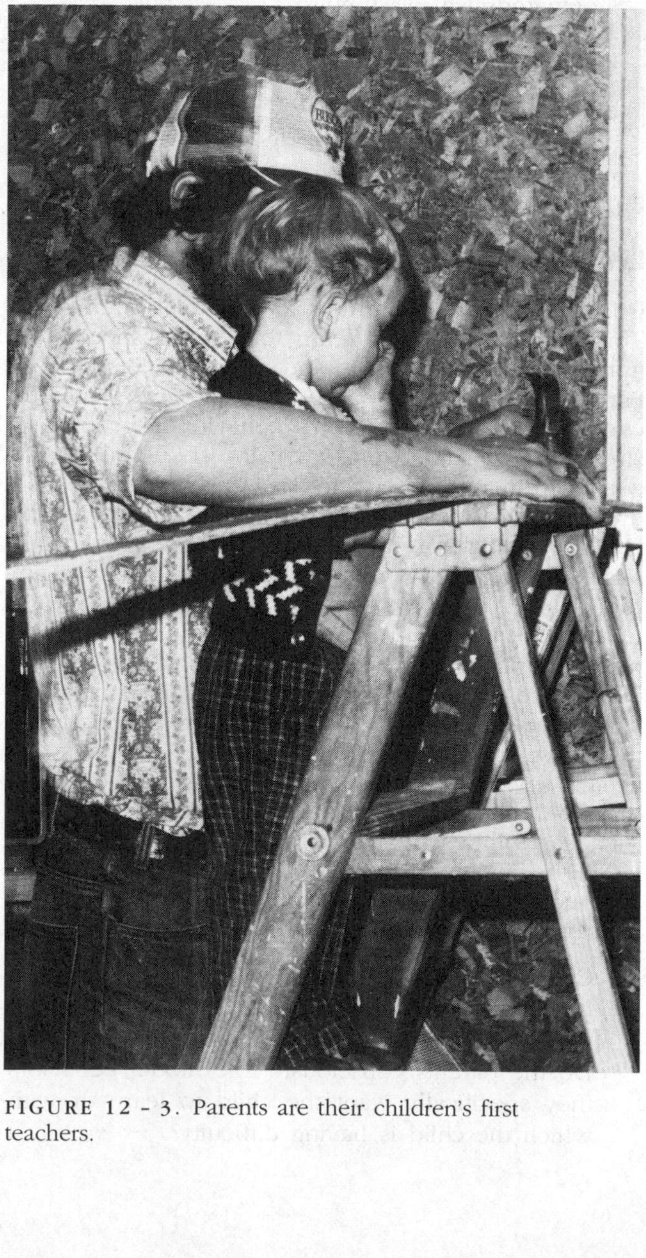

FIGURE 12-3. Parents are their children's first teachers.

TABLE 12-3
Development-Related Parental Tasks and Nursing Considerations

Nursing Diagnostic Statement: *Altered parenting or ineffective parenting related to:*

- Knowledge deficit regarding appropriate behaviors and skills for the child's stage of development
- History of ineffective relationship with own parents (therefore lack of an appropriate model for parenting skills)
- Knowledge deficit (of first-time parents) regarding basic parenting skills associated with lack of access to information and desire to learn
- Parental perceptions of inadequacy in being able to meet the child's needs

Parental Task/Role	Nursing Strategies
Infancy	
Learning infant's cues and interpreting infant's needs, so that attachment can occur Physical caregiver—affirming love and acceptance; stimulating all aspects of development; building trust by being predictable and consistent Learning to balance needs of infant with other demands	Provide parenting and child care education Empathize with parent's sense of immense responsibility and offer support and reassurance that parent can learn child's needs Provide positive reinforcement for appropriate behavior Teach parents the importance of balance between infant's needs and needs of other family members, including themselves—self-sacrifice not healthy Help family identify and utilize personal and community resources Provide positive reinforcement for appropriate behaviors
Early Childhood (Toddler)	
Learning to accept child's growth and development and accompanying acceptance of some loss of control while maintaining reasonable limits Learning to understand and appreciate child's refusals and negativism as a positive aspect of development Physical helper—affirming developing selfhood; stimulating self-regulatory body functioning Facilitating exploration within set limits	Teach parents about normalcy of child's behavior, including negativity, for developmental stage Reassure parents that child still loves them and needs them, despite negative outbursts or refusals of parental assistance Provide information that children develop individual personalities by asserting themselves with people they trust Help family identify and obtain assistance from personal and community resources Provide positive reinforcement for appropriate parenting behaviors and attempts at same Teach parents how to relax and enjoy their child(ren) Teach parents how to manage rebellious behaviors
Middle Childhood (Preschooler and Early School-Age Child)	
Learning to become separate from child, allowing independent development while demonstrating appropriate standards through role modeling Learning how to give child verbal instructions that are congruent with what is role modeled Becoming comfortable with endless questions of child Providing opportunities for child to initiate activities with a sense of purpose Physical-psychologic helper—affirming creative efforts; facilitating emotional self-control, moral and sexual development; stimulating self-care skills and limits	Teach parents about normal development and associated behaviors, including increased independence, of child of this age Provide parenting education Provide positive reinforcement for appropriate parenting behaviors and attempts at same Provide reassurance that child still loves them and is not being disrespectful just because of questioning everything Help family identify and utilize personal and community resources

(Continued)

TABLE 12-3
Development-Related Parental Tasks and Nursing Considerations *(Continued)*

Parental Task/Role	Nursing Strategies
Late Childhood (School-Age Child and Early Adolescent)	
Learning to accept rejection without abandoning the child at a time when the child is assuming greater self-sufficiency	Provide parenting and child development education
Allowing child to pursue acceptable activities that are of interest to her or him, even when contrary to what the parent wants for the child	Make referral to parent support groups
Encouraging child's involvement in appropriate activities and interests outside the family circle	Provide reassurance that the child still needs them but is shifting from a need for physical support to a need for psychologic support
Psychologic helper—affirming capacity to be productive; stimulating mental, social, ongoing moral development; facilitating acceptance of changing skills and body image; progressive freedom-giving with reasoned limit-setting that allows child to assume greater self-	Encourage setting of special time each day with child, but allowing child to pursue own interests and friendships as well
	Help full-time caregivers to assess skills/interests and develop them as caregiver role decreases
Later Adolescence and Early Adulthood	
Learning to build a new life by adjusting to altered family roles and relationships during teen-ager's identity crisis; understanding and assisting teen-ager (when appropriate) with social and sexual issues	Provide parenting and child development education—relate to parents' developmental stage
Providing security and reliability through clear, reasonable limits and communication of expectations for acceptable behavior	Reassure parents that it is OK to admit when they make bad decisions and that their critical teen-ager still loves and needs them
Psychologic supporter—affirming developing adult image; facilitating open communication; freedom-giver—reinforcing moral limits	Prepare parents that upheavals are a normal part of this stage, and stress the importance of being objective and communicating
	Provide positive reinforcement for appropriate parenting and attempts at same
	Refer to community resources

Parenting Styles

No one method of parenting has proved more effective than another, as long as the method is not carried to extremes. No method will work until a child respects the parents and their authority.

Three parenting styles can be derived from the parenting behaviors within families. Any one of them, if extreme, can result in incomplete or unhealthy socialization of children. Conversely, any of them, if conducted in an atmosphere of love that positively reinforces desired behavior, can support the healthy socialization of children. Table 12–4 summarizes these three styles.

Factors Influencing Selection of Parenting Style

Each child has a unique response to all of life's experiences and challenges. Parents also vary with regard to the parenting styles they can effectively and comfortably employ. There is no one right or wrong parenting style; nor can a given parenting style be successful with all children.

A child's temperament and developmental stage as well as parental interests and sociocultural values are factors that influence the effectiveness of the various parenting styles. The discussion that follows is intended to offer some guidelines for counseling parents in their efforts to socialize their children.

Temperament or Basic Personality

Temperament is used to describe differences in a child's way of relating to the world. Parents have known for centuries that children in the same family act in different ways. Temperament is discussed in Chapter 6, which describes the easy child, slow-to-warm child, and difficult child. These different temperaments of children can cause parents to become confused and frustrated. Some basic techniques that the nurse can encourage parents to try include the following:

- Make demands and expectations realistic for children.
- Encourage children to function at their potential; do not foster complacency or underachievement.
- Accept that some temperaments reinforce more

TABLE 12-4
Three Parenting Styles

Main Theme	Predominant Approach to Teaching Socialization	Primary Teaching Methods	Comments
Autocratic or Authoritarian			
Obedience, respect	Favors punitive measures to curb self-will when child does not comply with code of conduct	State rules; declare expectations; assert parental values; apply negative reinforcement for noncompliance; occasionally grant privileges or increased responsibility for compliance	Behavior evaluated in accord with a set standard of conduct, often theologically based; tends to employ primarily negative reinforcement
Democratic or Authoritative			
Autonomous problem solving based on self-regulation and disciplined conformity; rational, issue-related approach	Shares rationale for desired behavior with child; affirms child's efforts to comply but sets limits or boundaries for acceptable behavior; shows flexibility in rules	Describe problem or explain rules; help child find own solutions to problem or way to comply with rule based on uniqueness; reinforce positively for compliance, negatively for noncompliance	Least likely to be carried to extremes; encourages development of child's own inner controls over behavior, self-reliance; more verbal exchanges; employs both positive and negative reinforcement; respects opinion and right to disagree; however, parent retains ultimate control
Permissive			
Absence of restraints; child free of parental input	Uses reason; punitive measures seldom (if ever) used to teach socialization	Suggest rules, giving reasons for them; give child choice of complying or not complying; sometimes positively reinforce compliance, usually ignore or tolerate noncompliance	Does not foster development of inner controls; makes few demands for responsibility, unless child chooses to have it; tends to leave child on own, reinforcing neither positively or negatively

tolerance than others; some children are more at risk for behavior problems.

- Try to accept the nature of each child and to channel negative features in a desirable direction. Occasional frustration is normal, but seek help if it is prolonged or chronic.
- Professional help should be sought early; therefore, identify problems as soon as they appear.

Parenting methods affect whether children's traits develop into assets or problems. See Table 12–5 for a description of how the various temperaments can be managed to derive the most positive functioning of the child.

Age and Developmental Stage

Parents will need to adapt their basic parenting plan for each child as the child grows and matures. The need for external (parent-initiated) reinforcements diminishes as a child gets older; the external reinforcements that are provided can gradually become less action-oriented and more reason-oriented as the child develops intellectually. Keeping a child's developmental tasks in mind at each age helps parents determine what adaptations to the basic parenting approach are needed. Parental expectations at each level of development are summarized in Table 12–6.

Issues Related to Parenting

A profound influence on families is the economic circumstances in which they live. High rates of poverty, declining earnings, underemployment, and single parenting have affected families and how they care for children (Select Committee on Children, Youth, and Families, US House of Representatives, 1989). The difficulty in providing high-quality child care has escalated to ever-increasing numbers of crises. Traditional family structures, in which mothers cared for children at home, have been largely replaced with dual-earner

TABLE 12-5
Family-Centered Teaching: Adapting Parenting to the Child's Temperament

Easy Child

Provides realistic parenting that will not be incongruent with what child finds in the world outside. If these children develop behavior problems, they are most often due to a conflict between home-taught values and those of the outside world

Do not initiate any practice or ritual that is undesirable to continue over time, as the child will quickly incorporate that practice into his or her living pattern

Slow-to-Warm Child

Use a patient, relaxed, persevering approach. Present new situations or rules gradually, but repeatedly, without much pressure. Because of some common elements in the traits of difficult and slow-to-warm personality types, some management guidelines apply to both. The remaining items in this section apply to both

Refuse to compete with the child or to force adherence to every rule of the home to its more rigid interpretation. Such action only increases a negative display of behavior

Try not to explode at the child, as such fury only exaggerates the inappropriate behavior

Clearly identify on a regular basis what behaviors will be accepted and what behaviors are unacceptable. (A picture chart or check list posted in rooms where the child spends much time are creative ways to reinforce expectations regularly.) Help the child identify what behaviors are contingent on the situation at hand; do this clarifying at times when the child is not misbehaving, because if tense, the child may not "hear" the rules. Then carry through consistently in enforcing established limits. (A democratic approach is least overwhelming to this child. However, an autocratic approach also suits the difficult child, as long as it is not extreme)

Since this child learns slowly, repeat the rules often

Build in daily successes for this child

Maintain established routines while child is mastering a rule or behavioral expectation

Remember the key words to management:

- Firmness
- Repeated exposure
- Consistent reinforcement
- Patience

Difficult Child

Use firm, consistent approach that emphasizes the positive. Aspects of a child's temperament that may have undesirable consequences if allowed unrestricted expression should be controlled and limited in a calm but firm and consistent manner

Patience is essential. Active effort is necessary to avert negative parent-child relationships from arising out of the child's constant stressful behaviors

Parents of this "testy" child do best if they take turns coping with the child's behavior and give each other a daily chance to get away

In activities that predictably cause negative behavior, parents are wise to take turns handling the child; it is important to persist in introducing the child to this situation or expectation, however, so that the child can eventually learn control

Provide gradual and repeated reinforcement (positive and negative) of expected behaviors so the child can internalize them. (Problems in behavior usually arise from conflict between the children and almost any aspect of their environment—parents, new situations, or the world outside)

Give only one to three rules at a time. The rules need to be straightforward and unencumbered by explanations or choices

Provide constructive avenues for excess emotions and energy

Mixed-Temperament Child

Respond to whichever of the other three personality types seems to predominate in this child

Data from Thomas, A., & Chess, S. (1977). *Temperament and development*. New York: Brunner-Mazel. With permission from the publisher.

and single-parent families, phenomena that have brought with them "home-alone" children.

In over 50 per cent of two-parent families in America today, both parents work. Single-parent families constitute about 40 per cent of American homes at any given time. In families who suffer a parental loss through death or divorce, 80 per cent will be a blended family an average of 2 to 3 years later (Select Committee on Children, Youth, and Families, US House of Representatives, 1989). A blended family results from a marriage in which one or both spouses had offspring prior to the marriage who become family unit members after the marriage. These alternate family structures have changed many aspects of family life that potentially influence parenting.

Parenting and Dual-Earner Families*

Over the last 2 decades, the proportion of children with mothers in the labor force increased dramatically. Fifty-one per cent of children under 6 years of age and 60 per cent of these from 6 to 17 years of age have mothers in the work force. Women with

*"Dual-earner family" is defined here to mean that both heads of household pursue employment and at the same time maintain a family life together. The literature uses many terms. "Dual careers" usually implies that the employment is a professional career that both partners hold by choice and that both careers are taken seriously. Some refer to an arrangement in which both partners work but one partner's "job" is dispensable or secondary to the other partner's as a "two-job" family. "Dual-earner" encompasses both possibilities.

TABLE 12-6
Age and Developmental Stage as a Factor in Parenting

Parenting Goals	**Infant (0 to 1 Yr)**	**Toddler (1 to 3 Yrs)**	**Preschooler (3 to 5 Yrs)**	**School-Age Child (6 to 12 Yrs)**	**Adolescent/Young Adult (13 to 21 Yrs)**
Safety	Needs protection from falls, injuries, etc., as motor skills increase	Place limits on investigations and mobility; childproof home	Assist in protecting self; teach safety rules	Allow unassisted activities but with safe limits, as riding bike on road but not on heavily traveled streets	Self-responsible for safety
Family beliefs and values	Learns to adjust to family routines, but needs security of stable routines	Child can begin integrating religious and cultural values through practice and participation in rituals	Child can conform to home routines, take responsibility for helping with some; is able to learn manners, feel guilt; increases participation in family practices and rituals	Is ready to comprehend reasons, explanations behind values, beliefs, practices; ready for involvement in group activities and practices	Is ready to decide or choose for self what beliefs and values to accept—time to "let go" and allow that choice; enforce morality rules of family until child learns to trust own moral judgment
Social behavior and role	Recognizes disapproval and approval in voice and facial expression	Expect obedience most of the time; child is able to learn respect for other's belongings, and to accept substitute caregivers	Is able to cooperate, learning to share; can increasingly control anger and aggression; tries many roles during play; needs sexual questions answered; will investigate	Can have regular responsibility for some home chores; needs guidance on friend selections; expect acceptable school behaviors, peer tolerance	Needs limits on sexual expressions; do not expect mature judgments; avoid overreacting to typical teen crises; expect acceptable social behavior
Self-regulation and independence	Depends on others to meet needs; no self-control	Can take increasing responsibility for regulation of body functions; needs to learn proper language for body and its functions; learns to accept, respect limits; "Do it myself" really means "Let me do what I can, then help me"	Can accomplish most self-care in activities of daily living; will need help in more complex tasks	Is able to accomplish ADL increasingly without aid—anticipate occasional regression; increasingly socialized (internal enforcement) in behaviors, but still heavily guided by imitating significant others	Has internalized most rules of living; is able to maintain own ADL and many of home chores if given opportunity; needs faith in abilities reinforced and support during failures—otherwise, independent, self-regulating

children under 6 years of age make up the fastest-growing group; since 1970 there has been nearly an 80 per cent increase (Select Committee on Children, Youth, and Families, US House of Representatives, 1989).

A number of factors affect the decision that both parents will work. In today's society, financial necessity is a common reason that women enter the work force. Unanticipated medical expenses, inflationary costs of housing and food, and expenses of raising children, as well as family desires (music lessons, attendance at entertainment and sports events), necessitate larger incomes for families. Personal fulfillment of goals, career opportunities, or a sincere enjoyment of the challenge may also influence the decision to seek outside employment.

Unlike in most other industrialized countries, in the United States the freedom to work is accompanied by the challenge that each family must arrange its own child care and home maintenance, usually without economic or social support from either the employer or the government. The extent to which child care and home maintenance needs can be adequately satisfied influences parents' ability to fulfill work responsibilities successfully. Although the availability of early and extended day care and afterschool programs is increasing, these options are unaffordable to many parents. In addition, many programs do not accommodate parents whose work schedules do not fall within normal business hours or who are not in close proximity to either home or work. A few sick care programs are beginning to appear; these provide care to ill children, either in the home or in a special area of child care facilities for working parents, but they are still scarce and unaffordable to many parents.

The number of women employed outside of the home has increased, but working women continue to carry the primary responsibility for child care as well as for housekeeping and home management. Dual-career fathers experience "inter-role conflict" associated with wanting to support their spouse's career and to participate in family and home care, yet wanting to give priority to personal goals. Dual-career men and women with children in the home have been found to cope by adjusting work responsibilities in order to meet family needs (Schnittger & Bird, 1990). There is also some indication that investment in work does not occur at the expense of investment in children (Greenberger & Goldberg, 1989). These

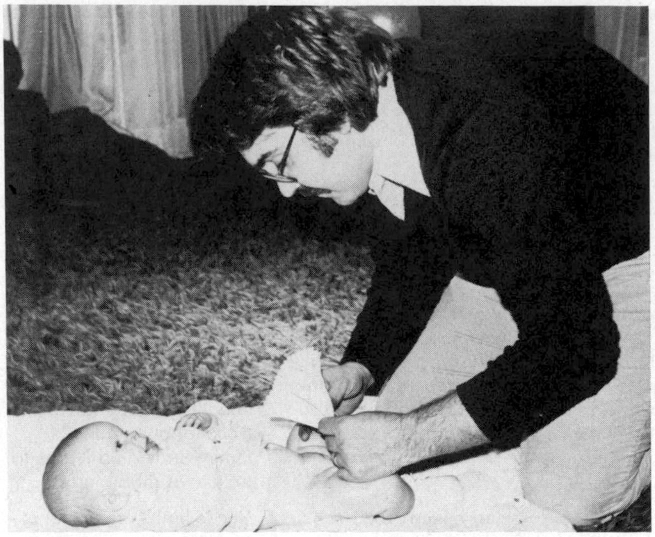

FIGURE 12-4. Many fathers, even in traditional homes, enjoy the closeness that helping care for their children allows them.

studies indicate that the *intention* of parents is to provide high-quality care for their children (Fig. 12–4). How children are actually affected is not agreed on.

There is strong support by some for the belief that "high-quality" care by someone other than the child's parent does not put a child at risk (Scarr et al., 1989; Goldsmith, 1990). However, Hojat (1990) argues that a child's sense of security is less likely to develop with working than with nonworking mothers. A review of the research concerning the relationship of early adolescent adjustment and parental employment shows "mixed or no associations for academic, emotional, social, or cognitive well-being" (Orthner, 1990). Although the full impact of dual-career families on children is not known, nurses can facilitate families in assessing their own situations. The nurse working with dual-earner parents should explore whether specific role expectations have been discussed, to avoid assumptions by one or both spouses. Important issues for families to discuss include the following list developed by Kutzner & Toussic-Weingarten (1984):

- What are each parent's reasons for working? Are they congruent with the other parent's reasons?
- If conflicts exist, how can they be resolved? Do the jobs demand more than the parents are willing or able to give?
- What are the benefits? What problems are expected at work and at home?
- How will responsibilities be assigned or shared concerning child care, household routines, and other day-to-day decision making? Who will transport children?
- How will family integrity be maintained in the mornings as parents prepare themselves and their children for departure?
- Can child care and other community resources be found that are compatible with parental values and philosophies?
- Does each parent feel comfortable with the child care arrangements?
- Who have the parents identified as back-up child care providers for unexpected situations? What will be done if a child is ill? Who will handle any emergencies?
- Have work schedules been planned so that there is time for family activities together? Is there conscious planning for open communication channels for all family members?

The child who is a member of a dual-earner family can be encouraged to help the parents in tasks that are part of daily living activities for the family. This helps the child develop skills and feelings of self-worth. It also helps distribute family tasks. Most children develop pride in their parents' accomplishments and benefit from the increased exposure to multiple role models (Scott, 1984). The dual-earner family can provide an egalitarian parental role model for children, and provide the child with enriching experiences with both mother and father.

Parenting and Single-Parent Families

Single-parent families are created by a spouse's death, divorce, an unmarried single person keeping a child, a single person adopting a child, or a single individual choosing to have a child by any of various technologic means of reproduction. With respect to employment, most single parents are confronted with the same parenting dilemmas as are dual-earner families. The major difference is that instead of spousal support, the single parent must seek out other adult support systems (e.g., friends, relatives, Parents Without Partners groups).

In the event of divorce, the nurse must understand its effect on the parenting capabilities of both parents. Financial necessity forces most divorced parents to retain, regain, or obtain employment. Unless co-parenting is arranged, the parent with custody bears the major responsibility for childrearing. The visiting parent becomes primarily a "playtime" parent, experiencing only brief or periodic intervals with the children. The feelings that can be engendered by both parents and by the children—guilt, jealousy, anger, a sense of being overwhelmed—become obvious in such situations. There is a tendency for divorced parents to neglect or even exploit their children's emotional needs during the first weeks or even months of loss. These parents usually love their children, but they are emotionally, and sometimes physically, drained by the stresses of their marital battles and, finally, by the loss of a partner. Children sometimes temporarily take on roles as mini-parents of the real parent, or older children may so serve younger siblings. Fortunate children have other significant persons (grandparents, teachers, neighbors) who can help them deal with their own despair until their parent regains control and resumes appropriate parenting.

Home-Alone Children

Millions of children in the United States are responsible for their own care after school. About 10 million children between the ages of 5 and 12 years and another 5 to 10 million between ages 12 and 16 years are home alone for several hours a day while their parents are at work (Robinson et al., 1989). The term "latchkey kids" surfaced during the 1980s, making reference to the key around the child's neck. During the 1940s, keys around a child's neck signaled poverty, neglect, and lack of parental care. The negative connotation of the term has made parents feel guilty and distressed, even though they have taught their children how to be self-sufficient and safely care for themselves. The fear that home-alone children will suffer psychologic harm has been based primarily on reports in popular magazines. Commonly held stereotypes are that these children have more fears and anxieties, that they get into more trouble, and that they suffer from serious social and emotional damage.

There seem to be no clear-cut negative or positive consequences that apply to all home-alone children. Three significant factors that affect how well home-alone children adjust seem to be family social status, sex of the child, and type of community or neighborhood in which the child resides. An increased risk for accidents or injuries and delinquent behavior seems to be associated with a lower social class and more densely populated communities. Lower class girls seem to be the only group who show diminished academic achievement. This group is also more likely to clean the house, do laundry, care for younger children, and possibly even prepare dinner when they come home from school. The children frequently are not permitted to "waste time" in activities considered by the parents to be unimportant. Consequently, they may not participate in school activities; they may not have friends or appear to enjoy life. The excessive demands made on them by their parents has been thought by some to result in a passive attitude toward life (McClellan, 1984). On the other hand, Padilla and Landreth (1989) report both negative and positive effects of the home-alone experience. Potential benefits include increased maturity, self-reliance, decision making ability, and responsibility. Negative effects include a feeling of neglect or actually being neglected, feeling isolated, or being at medical risk. An analysis of health states reported by Williams and Boyce (1989) indicates that children in self-care are not more obese, do not miss more school days, and do not make more visits to the school health office. When former latchkey children were studied at university age for personality and academic achievement differences, no differences were reported (Messer et al, 1989). Although not all children seem to be affected in the same way, the nurse can assist parents in preparing children to be home alone as described in Table 12–7.

Parents may need some assistance from a nurse in making the decision to leave children in self-care arrangements. Parents need to recognize that this decision is an individual matter for each child, before entering into self-care arrangements. Recommendations for parents who are considering leaving children home alone are as follows:

- Examine their own feelings.
- Consider their child's age.
- Observe their child's maturity level.
- Prepare their child for the basis of self-care.
- Examine the safety of their neighborhood.
- Check their community resources.
- Determine the length of time their child will be alone.
- Decide on some type of checking system in their absence.

Children should not be left alone without first establishing that they are ready for it. They should be able to manage all daily self-care activities, know how to use the telephone—especially for emergencies, and be able to anticipate possible problem situations and describe how to manage them, and preferably demonstrate this with some trial runs. A parent or back-up person should be available by telephone (important numbers should be in plain view near the telephone). A neighbor, relative, or adult friend who is usually available should be established as a resource for emergencies. Parents should be urged to utilize an afterschool program as an alternative, if one is available. Many schools are now providing such services, and some day care facilities are providing extended-school day care.

Parenting and the Blended Family*

Statistics show that most people remarry 2 to 3 years after a spouse's death or departure. Of all married couple families with children under the age of 18, 17.4 per cent are stepfamilies, and 40 per cent are expected to become stepfamilies before their youngest child reaches 18 years of age (Glick, 1989). Research on children who have lost a parent to death or divorce shows that these children fare no worse than those who are raised entirely in nuclear family units (Stern, 1984). However, these children do retain the mind set that they have only one mother and one father, no matter how undesirable the lost parent may have been and no matter whether the lost parent ever makes contact with the child again. A second charac-

*Other names are "reconstituted family," "stepfamily," "combined family," and "remarriage."

TABLE 12–7
Family-Centered Teaching: Protecting the Home-Alone Child

Safety

Teach children not to display keys and always to lock doors; keep a spare key at a neighbor's house

*Tell children not to go into the house after school if the door is ajar, a window is open, or if anything looks unusual; teach child not to open the door to anyone unless the person has been approved by you

*Walk through the afterschool routine with the child; some children have keys but cannot reach the locks; teach child not to get in cars with strangers

*Consult with fire and police officials about burglar-proofing and fire-proofing the home; teach child what to do if a burglary attempt occurs

Teach children first-aid procedures

*Prepare a safety kit

Teach safety rules to children who are expected to cook; microwave ovens are the safest

Fire safety:

- Teach child to leave the house and not return if a fire starts
- Practice fire drills and evacuation at home, including a safe place to meet outside the home

Prevent traffic accidents

- Children are often not ready to cross streets alone until age 7 yrs
- Do not allow children to ride bicycles in the street without adult supervision

Be alert to the dangers of garage door openers; children have been fatally injured when they have activated the doors and the doors closed on them

Teach children about weather-related safety

- Stay in the house in an electrical storm; do not take a bath during an electrical storm
- Stay in the storm cellar or in the safest part of the house during a tornado warning. Practice tornado drills with children
- Keep a flashlight handy to child in case of power failures

Prevent drowning

- Instruct children that they should never swim without adult supervision
- Teach older children caring for infants and toddlers about safe bathing methods
- Keep toilet lid down; older infants and toddlers have drowned by falling headfirst into toilets

Use locked storage for firearms. Instruct children that firearms are to be handled by adults only

Telephone Use

Teach children to tell callers that their parents are "busy," rather than saying "They're not here"

*Keep police, fire department, and other important telephone numbers by the phone; be sure child knows how to report emergencies

*Investigate the neighborhood for families who will be at home and available for help with emergencies

Ask police and fire officials to offer classes about when and how to call them

If a "telephone hotline" for latchkey children exists, teach children how to use it

Be sure children know their own telephone numbers, addresses, and parents' names

Afterschool Activities

*Arrange for the child to spend some afternoons with friends

*Provide structured activities, such as art projects

*Have the child go to a public library–sponsored activity, rather than watch television at home

Establish clear rules with child as to what may/may not be done until parent gets home

*Offer children a choice of activities

Teach children that independence and resourcefulness are virtues, but do not demand too much

Help children feel successful in taking care of themselves

*Do not allow older children (who are not developmentally ready) to care for younger ones

Loneliness

Talk to children about their experiences of being alone after school

*Consider getting a pet to help comfort the child

*Be punctual; children's anxiety escalates when parents do not return home as promised

*Call the child when you will be late

*Leave a tape-recorded message for children to play when they arrive home

*Form a group of parents with flex-time so that their children can be cared for by one of the group after school

*Items specifically for parents.
Refer to McClellan, (1984); McKnight & Shelsby, (1984); Dennis (1986), and Robinson et al. (1989) for further information.

teristic is that these children fantasize that someday Mom and Dad will somehow get back together. Therefore, a stepparent, no matter how loving and kind, is going to be perceived as an intruder.

The blended family can assume many different, complex forms, depending on whether one or both parents were previously married and/or have had children, whether the children are living with them, and whether there are children from their own union. In a study by Pill (1990), almost one third of the couples in stepfamilies expressed the sentiment that "living in a stepfamily requires continual and deliberate effort." Table 12–8 identifies the most common barriers to blended family integration and suggests mea-

TABLE 12-8
Common Barriers to Blended Family Integration and Nursing Interventions

Barriers to Family Integration	Nursing Interventions
Role Confusion	
Custodial parent after death or divorce (usually mother) has ambivalence about what role he or she wants the stepparent to take with regard to their children and with family decision making Stepparent shares the same ambivalence and uncertainty about options and responsibility toward the spouse's children Feelings of jealousy, confusion, resentment, and inadequacy experienced by some or all members of new family unit	Empathize with each member's feelings, and help each anticipate and deal with the complex issues involved in blended family development through anticipatory guidance and counseling Provide reassurance of the normality of the feelings members are experiencing and that growth and time will support healthy family and member development Be an advocate for the blended family in the community and state Assist spouses to recognize their ambivalence and to openly discuss it and arrive at a comfortable role description, stressing that they should not attempt to emulate either primary family but rather formulate their own role definitions that suit the needs and strengths of members Encourage creativity in roles and emphasize that the stepparent role may differ with each child depending on the child's age, willingness to bond, and nature of the relationship with the custodial parent (i.e., allow natural relationships to develop) Foster marital bonding by helping family look at ways spouses can have time alone together and develop their own romance and friendship Refer family to self-help support groups for stepfamilies within the community
Conflicting Family Cultures	
At the individual family cultural level, rules are established as to where silverware goes, the things children may or may not do during meals or when adults are present, and general rules about how mothers, fathers, and children should act When blended family develops, individual family cultural rules are brought to the union from two primary families, which produces power struggles and conflict (culture shock) during early cohabitation. Compromise gradually occurs in some areas, usually taking 2–7 yrs for the infinite differences to be negotiated and resolved, resulting in development of a new individual family culture. New conflicts will emerge at various developmental stages	Facilitate open communication between family members (fear of confrontation is common because of a previous marriage failure) Refer to community self-help support group for stepfamilies or, if conflicts are serious, to family group therapy Provide education on crisis management, culture shock, and communication skills Support and reinforce members as they take steps toward conflict resolution
Discipline of Children	
Discipline involves a series of lessons designed to develop behaviors that can be tolerated by adults and move children toward healthy adulthood. Obviously rules will be in conflict from the differences each primary family brings to the blended unit Research repeatedly shows the discipline of children as a major stumbling block to integration of the blended unit. Dangers to watch for are (1) the custodial parent feels a need to monitor the stepparent's interactions with children, tends to interpret stepparent's behavior to children and vice versa, preventing stepparent and children from establishing their own relationships; or (2) stepparent insists on early assumption of co-management privileges and spouse agrees, but children respond with shock, resentment, and resistance or even display behavior problems because they have not had time to adjust to and learn to trust the new stepparent first	Refer family to community self-help support group for stepfamilies or to family group therapy if serious conflict exists Educate and assist stepparent to carry out "befriending/affiliating" behaviors, i.e., make friends with each stepchild before making new rules and enforcing them (single most important action to achieve success in stepparenting) Strategies: 1. Spend time with each stepchild, being sensitive to the timing of interactions 2. Spend some money on stepchildren—will not buy love, but does earn stepparent favorable attention from children 3. Role model being a kind, friendly person 4. Come through for the child in times of trouble 5. Use clear communication, i.e., leveling, encouraging children to respond in kind 6. Accept each child for who and what she or he is 7. Have tolerance for children's inconsistent responses—remember that trust takes time to develop Reinforce positive efforts of the stepparent and encourage open communication between spouses

(Continued)

TABLE 12-8
Common Barriers to Blended Family Integration and Nursing Interventions *(Continued)*

Barriers to Family Integration	Nursing Interventions
Semipermeable Boundaries (Dual-Family Membership)	
A multitude of persons are attached to former relationships, which continually surface in the blended family's life, particularly the children's other parent and children of one or both blended family spouses who do not live in the blended unit Potential problems to watch for: 1. A tendency for any conflicts between ex-spouses and/or new spouses to be fought through the children, instead of through direct confrontation between the adults 2. A spouse who has not been around children is likely not to have realistic expectations about the behavior of children 3. A frequent conflict is that children who do not live with a parent are favored or given exceptions to family rules during their visits to the blended family unit The nearer the remarriage is to the time the original family unit lost its intactness, the more resistant the single parent unit is to blending	Educate the family about stress management, the importance of open communication, and the potential problems of relationships beyond the blended unit Refer the family to a community self-help support group for stepfamilies or to family group therapy if serious problems exist in the family's ability to be creative and flexible Provide parenting and growth and development education if one parent has not had experience with children Support family through periods of crisis
Unresolved Grief	
Unresolved grief over past failed relationships may be repressed and acted out in disguised ways by members of family Children often have unresolved grief because of their unrelenting hope that their parents will get back together some day, and often the grief is compounded by their egocentric belief that they are responsible for the family break-up. They may extend this egocentric "power," thinking they can also break up the new marriage, if they are not offered assistance to handle their grief Unresolved grief is a more common problem when a blended family unit is formed within a short time frame after the primary family break-up (sources vary in the time required to resolve that grief, usually 1 to 3 yrs) The grief related to divorce is somewhat different from other grief in that it results from a change in the nature of relationships, not a separation or loss Feelings of vulnerability to loss, since one marriage failed, may inhibit the open dialogue necessary to resolve conflicts and to bond the blended family together Remarriage shatters the child's hopes of a reunion of the original family unit. Children may also feel stepparents are dislodging them from the close relationship with the custodial parent developed during the single-parent stage	Refer for individual or family group counseling Foster open family communication through education, role modeling, positive reinforcement, or communication efforts Apply usual interventions to facilitate resolution of grief (refer to any one of the many excellent references available on this subject) Educate the family about the grief process and how members or other family resources can assist and support the grieving member(s)

Data from Stern, P. (1984). Stepfather family dynamics: An overview for therapists. *Issues in Mental Health Nursing,* 89–103; and copyright 1986 The American Journal of Nursing Company. Reprinted from MCN; American Journal of Maternal-Child Nursing, July/August, 1986, Vol. 11, No. 4. Used with permission.

sures to help the family organize its own cultural unit in time.

A prospective stepparent should not be introduced to children until the couple has dated each other exclusively for some time or until they have decided to marry. If children are introduced to their parents' dates repeatedly, they develop a pattern of keeping distant so as not to have to experience grief and loss each time Mom or Dad changes "friends." Once a decision to marry is made, the couple should take time to consider how they feel about sharing the parenting responsibility. They must face the fact that they will not have the luxury to be alone to adjust to each other and to establish living patterns as a couple, because the children's needs must also be met from the beginning.

Prospective stepparents should understand the value of just being themselves—efforts to "win" the children by forcing "fun" on them or trying to be the "perfect stepparent" are perceived by the children as artificial and lead to strained relationships. Stepparents who expect jealousy, resentment, and rejection will not be surprised or destroyed by its appearance; children make friends slowly with unfamiliar adults.

Another issue to discuss is discipline. The couple should privately discuss the limits and controls and the roles of each parent in disciplining, so that a consistent approach is presented to the children. Just as school teachers and many other authority figures guide children, so too should stepparents take an active role in discipline.

The couple entering a remarriage should be encouraged to learn (or review) the developmental stage characteristics of childhood. Knowing the usual struggles and behavioral characteristics helps keep children's actions in perspective and avoids blaming every misbehavior on the blended family situation. Parenting teen-agers is particularly difficult. Stepparents need to remember that all teen-agers are challenging to parents, even those in first-marriage families.

The nurse should regularly assess the parents' knowledge of developmental behavior and the family's awareness of problems in adapting. Education, counseling, or referral should be offered as indicated. Support of each member is continuously needed. The nurse can use role playing to determine whether the couple is developing or maintaining open communication and sharing parenting responsibilities. Information regarding community support groups for blended families can be provided. The nurse can be an objective confidante with whom children can express fears, hostility, or anxiety that they do not feel ready to express at home.

The nurse should assist the family in maintaining the perspective that the integration into a new family cultural unit takes *time* and *tolerance,* both role ambiguities and reactions of family members. Reassurance that their feelings are normal and that the stressors are surmountable is important feedback for the blended family.

Supporting Parents in Parenting Goals

Raising a family should not be approached as an exercise in perfection. Parenting will be affected not only by parents' strengths and flaws but also by their children's strengths and weaknesses. No family is perfect, and yet the great majority of parents do a more-than-adequate job of raising their children to be successful adults—sometimes against tremendous odds. Health professionals have a responsibility (1) to help parents free themselves from unjustified guilt when their child does not always measure up to expectations; (2) to help parents develop self-confidence and trust in their parenting instincts, enhanced by accurate information and professional guidance; and (3) to help parents find a compromise between what they expect of themselves and their children and what is realistic.

Reassuring Parents

Health professionals can help parents accept three reassurances:

1. It's OK not to be perfect.
2. It's OK to exert authority.
3. It's OK not to be rich.

It's OK Not to Be Perfect

Parents who are able to accept that neither they nor their children are perfect can feel comfortable accepting that their parenting actions will not always be perfect either, and that this is all right. Although there are certain minimal elements parents must provide for satisfactory parenting—rules, consistency, positive and negative reinforcements, all based on love—there is no single formula for providing those ingredients. Parents should periodically evaluate the impact their approach is having on their child, to see whether unpleasant feelings, increased misconduct, or an atmosphere of family tension is building up.

It's OK to Exert Authority

To raise children takes enormous energy and ingenuity and is rarely a peaceful endeavor, but parents who feel comfortable setting limits for themselves and their children make the tasks of learning and growing easier. A sense of humor is also helpful. A smile or laugh can lighten serious moments, ease tension, reduce anger, and restore perspective. To nurture their children effectively, parents sometimes need to exert authority. Relationships that are loving and caring readily withstand acts of authority, with the end result being respect and cooperation: two desirable characteristics to be developed as children grow into adults. It is essential that parents and children realize that parents can use different reactions and parenting styles with each child and still be loving. Effective parenting does not require equal or identical parenting behaviors for all children in a family.

Expert advice from professionals can be helpful and even life-saving, but children are not all alike, and the expert does not know a child as the parents do. Parents should not be condemned if their approach does not match the recommendations in the latest manual or the beliefs of the professional. The professional's obligation is to ascertain objectively that the parental approach is not having a negative impact on the child or family. If it is not, the parents' approach should be reinforced. If a negative effect exists, parents need to be provided insight into the conflict, to be offered information that will give them broader parenting options to choose from, and to be supported in their efforts to change.

It's OK Not to Be Rich

The conflict between children's desires and the realities of the budget is a common frustration to most families. It is important for parents to recognize the influence of finances on their parenting decisions.

Parents need to realize and be reassured that children do not need everything they request; in fact, they are often better off without most things the glamorous ads make them believe they need. Every family's budget has a limit. Parents who recognize that fact are able to set priorities and to focus on doing things *with* their children rather than buying things *for* them. These positive actions establish values that will be important to the children's ability to handle money as adults. Children can be told honestly that a certain item is not affordable. These facts assist children in developing realistic approaches to the economics of living.

Maximizing Strengths and Identifying Problems

As with any aspect of living, problems in parenting can and do arise. Each family has a unique style of interacting, and each has certain strengths and difficulties. Encouraging parents to discuss these areas openly can lead to maximizing their strengths and resolving problems. Parents should be asked to identify their own strengths, a process that provides an opportunity for acknowledgment and attention to positive attributes in both the parents and children. Labeling the joys and positive experiences in a family is a therapeutic process that should not be overlooked. It is a morale-building process that parents often need.

Table 12–9 lists four categories of parenting problems and symptomatic behaviors. Nurses and other professionals who work with children and families should be watchful for these symptomatic behaviors each time they observe and interact with their clients.

The child's overt behavior can also be a direct barometer of the state of health of parenting. A knowledge of normal development and temperament helps nurses distinguish temporary deviant behavior from that which is indicative of a long-term problem. Nurses should offer guidance or help parents and children obtain guidance from appropriate sources whenever they observe or receive parental reports of the following persisting behaviors:

1. A child who continually does not behave at the expected level for children of same age and temperament.
2. Bizarre behavior or speech that persists or receives frequent negative social response.
3. Prolonged adverse reactions to common situations or experiences.
4. An accumulation of several related or unrelated troubling behaviors—unhappy, confused, rebellious, "ornery" without regard for others' responses, stubborn beyond reason, lazy, oversensitive, aggressive, delinquent—that seem to be lingering, worsening, or steadily involving more of the child's time.

TABLE 12-9
Parenting Problems and Symptomatic Parental Behavior

Unrealistic Expectations

Parent requires more self-control from child than age, development, or circumstances make reasonable

Parent expects immediate obedience

Parent enforces too many rules at once or provides no rules (children need rules for behavior and will seek them elsewhere, often in gangs)

Parents request social skills of the child that they do not model, owing to lack of knowledge or experience

Inconsistency

Family disharmony

Parents lack a united front in goals, values, parenting philosophy, or moral stance about right and wrong

Parents model behaviors and values incongruent with what they teach verbally and in rules established

Enforcement is not consistently carried out

Distortions in communication—too vague, too long, contradictory, or void

Extremes in Style, Methods

No limits established or no guidance and reinforcements to help child comply with limits; overpermissive

Lack of firmness; parent not respected as authority

Limits too rigid; power replaces authority and fear or anger replaces respect

Reinforcements (positive or negative) do not match deed; too excessive, too long, teach wrong lesson

Primary disciplinary methods employed are bribes, promises, threats, sarcasm

Disturbed Relationships

Parent is too close to child to permit growth—intrusive control, dominance; exemplified by parent who always (1) wants to change child, (2) demands to know child's activities and conversation, (3) interferes in child's problem solving or decision making, (4) reminds child of misdeeds

Basically unfriendly or ambivalent interaction

Interaction inappropriate for child's age, stage, or temperament

Parent is too distant for child to develop respect: (1) parent preoccupied with self and own activities or wishes, (2) child feels isolated or unwanted

Seeking professional help should be a first-aid measure rather than a last resort; this often requires alertness and initiative on the professional's part to help the family acknowledge that the problem potentially exists or is developing. See Chapter 29 for a full discussion of children with behavior problems.

Another preventive measure is for the nurse to be alert to family situations that place the parents at high risk for ineffective parenting. Situational crises in the family overlying the parenting responsibility are always of concern and require preventive intervention by the nurse. See Chapter 2 on family assessment and Chapter 28 on child abuse for further guidelines in identifying problems.

Counseling Parents

Parenting is a topic that should be approached with the parent(s) early in the parenting relationship. Ideally, parents would have sought and been offered information before deciding to have children. However, very few parents discuss such things before their infant arrives.

The parenting process begins when the infant is born, so parents need information by this time, at least, and additional information can be added as the nurse and parents together anticipate the child's changing needs throughout the developing years.

As nurses counsel parents through their child's developing years, they should bear in mind that within a loving, secure home with routines, parents can try any style of parenting with which they feel confident and comfortable, and most children will respond favorably as long as extremes are avoided. Occasional "mistakes" do not destroy a child for life.

In early counseling, the nurse should listen sensitively, observe the parent-child relationship and the individual temperaments involved, and then help the parents find the style they can live with and feel comfortable with on a daily basis. Ongoing assessment of the parenting process and its impact on the child should occur at each contact, with particular attention given to symptoms in the four categories summarized in Table 12–9.

If symptoms are suggested either by the nurse's own observations, parental report, or the child's deviant behavior, the nurse should intervene early to reverse unhealthy parenting patterns. Intervention may involve helping the family see the problem area and referring its members to a competent resource for assistance. Problems that are minor, that are identified early, or that the nurse is competent to intervene in directly should be promptly managed.

When teaching or helping parents to modify their approaches, the nurse should always work with and emphasize the strengths of the parents and child. In addition, the nurse is responsible for locating appropriate resources to help offset their deficiencies. It is impossible to predict or teach all the skills involved in parenting. However, if nurses can help parents develop an ability to sort out problems, look at options, and negotiate suitable interventions, they have progressed a long way toward effective preparation for the challenge. Table 12–10 highlights the main issues or guidelines that the nurse and parents can use as a base for developing successful parenting behaviors. As children grow, so should their parents, for all life experiences—positive and negative—can be growth experiences.

Parenting the Adolescent

Although most of the principles discussed in this chapter apply to adolescents, the serious consequences that result when parents and teen-agers do not get along warrant a separate discussion. When communication between parent and teen-ager concerning rules and discipline breaks down, the results are often drastic. Teen-agers leave home before they are prepared to support themselves; they drop out of school, get involved in street life, and are estranged from their family—sometimes permanently. The stress, sorrow, and loss that result for both the family and the teen-ager are immeasurable.

The teen-ager changes so rapidly that it is a challenge for parents to adapt to their child's changing body, needs, moods, and friends. Teen-agers, meanwhile, have difficulty understanding why parents continue to set curfews and monitor their activities, and why parents want to know where they are. As teen-agers struggle for more freedom, parents may need help in letting their teen-agers separate from them. Some parents may have difficulty establishing and enforcing any limits because of the excessive and continuous resistance from their teen-agers. The nurse's role is to assess what kind of help is needed by parents and adolescents to establish rules that result in a positive relationship between parents and their teen-agers.

At this stage of development, patterns of communication and rule setting have long been established. Both parents and teen-agers need to discover that a modification of past approaches and responses is necessary if communication and problem solving are to be successful. The ability of the teen-ager to retort with well-thought-out logical arguments makes resolution tedious. For the teen-ager, the rule must be examined and argued according to the teen-ager's point of view. Furthermore, the teen-ager's idealism can result in strong opinions that are not easily modified. If parents are unwilling or unable to listen to their teen-ager's point of view and make harsh demands without rationale, a teen will eventually not express views but simply do what she or he wants to do and stop communicating with parents. Once the teen-ager becomes noncommunicative and does not engage in problem solving with parents, the parenting role becomes one of reprimanding for unacceptable behaviors in a struggle of wills. If nurses can identify early signs of a communication breakdown between par-

TABLE 12-10
***Family-Centered Teaching*: Fostering Open Parent-Child Communication**

Listen Actively

- Accept that your child has something worthwhile to communicate and identify with the child's feelings, perceptions, and thoughts, recognizing that they are real
- Try not to ask questions or interrupt while the child is speaking
- Avoid presenting an opinion about what the child is saying; instead, share your feelings when the child is finished
- Do not interpret the child's speech or try to restate what you think the child was REALLY trying to say; such behavior suggests to children that their opinions are inferior
- Do not recommend solutions or changes in view; rather, redirect the child to identify possible resolutions and the associated likely consequences
- Let the child continue to the end, then seek an evaluation of the situation, rather than interrupting to interject your own evaluation or judgment

Express Thoughts and Feelings Clearly and Honestly

- Use "I messages" rather than "you messages" (see example), subjectively stating your own needs or feelings (gets a cooperative response) rather than placing judgment on the child's behavior (gets a defensive response of hostility or a power struggle). I messages also avoid overgeneralizations or character criticisms. Adding feelings to the I message allows the child to participate in relieving the situation and to be aware of your feelings too

You Message:	"You are too noisy! Stop turning the TV louder!"
I Message:	"I need to have quiet right now so I can get this reading done. Please turn down the TV."
I Message: (feelings described):	"I feel angry because I have so little time to read and no quiet in which to do it. I have a right to some quiet just as you do. I need some quiet time right now."

- Express basic positive feelings about the child in association with requests for behavior change. (For example, "I feel you really tried harder last evening to help me have quiet, but I am still frustrated that I cannot have a quiet time every evening. I will feel more like talking or watching television with you if I have some quiet time for a half-hour after dinner each evening.") Messages that express the parent's needs by describing the behavior that needs to be changed without character criticisms allow the child to correct the behavior or offer alternative solutions without diminished self-esteem
- Empathize with the child while expressing your feelings or expectations. This shows the child that you understand the reason for the undesirable behavior, but that it must stop. (For example, "You must want to go play with your friends right now, but you will have to wait till you have finished clearing the table.")

Minimize Unacceptable Behaviors

Modify the Environment to Encourage Age-Appropriate Independence and Opportunities for Learning and Recreation

- Age-appropriate toys/resources available to child at home
- Specified areas reserved as each child's private place for own pursuits
- Quiet, sedate activities available for child when needed to "wind down," such as before meals or bedtime
- Opportunities in home or related to home functioning that allow self-care responsibility and contribution to family living
- Childproof home surroundings and set limits to extent that safety is ensured and all members can relax. Must be based on development and temperament of members

Set Limits

- Firm, consistent limits foster competence and reduce anxiety in children
- Strive for agreement and support among adult members regarding major expectations of child. These expectations change as members grow and develop
- Provide reasons for the limits and explain consequences for violations of limits. Child may participate in establishing limits and consequences
- Separate disapproval of behavior from acceptance of child by conveying love but explaining unacceptable behavior. DISAPPROVE OF THE BEHAVIOR, NOT THE CHILD. "I messages" help accomplish this

Avoid Win-Lose Conflicts

- Accept that conflicts are likely to be frequent and are a part of "growing" for all members
- Allowing child as much self-care responsibility as possible eliminates the source of many parent-child power struggles
- Strive for a "no lose" mind set that involves mutual discussion and compromise (once child has mastered basic language skills). Parent and child identify problem and discuss possible solutions. Seeking cooperation eliminates power struggles

Spend Time Together as a Family and with Each Child

- Establish some time each day that is exclusively with children. Does not have to be scheduled or a certain time span but appropriate to family situation. If time occurs regularly, children can take the occasional exception in stride. Children will also have less need to compete by acting out to get time with parent(s)
- Make time together enjoyable for all involved
- Communicate to child you are available to talk or share concerns whenever the child feels a need and you are able

(Continued)

TABLE 12-10
Family-Centered Teaching: Fostering Open Parent-Child Communication *Continued*

Utilize a Disciplinary Approach That "Fits" the Parent and Child

- Never hesitate to seek assistance in evaluating management approaches and their appropriateness to your situation and values. Nurses should convey that they are available to help parents with parenting concerns. Assistance includes helping them clarify key issues about their child and delineate specific target behaviors needing intervention
- Recognize that good parenting can be accomplished in different ways
- If physical punishment is used, seek alternative methods of discipline
- Recognize each child's need for privacy as well as one's own privacy needs and provide for this
- Utilize the child's creativity for discipline through expressive play activities, fantasy play activities, parallel story telling (tell a story that depicts the child's situation and reveal how the story child felt and responded; follow story with problem-solving questions to child)
- Allow children to learn discipline through the experiencing of natural results of their misbehavior as long as their safety is not threatened by doing so and no moral judgment is involved. This involves allowing the child to choose between acceptable/unacceptable behavior
- Utilize behavior modification to reduce repetitious unacceptable behaviors and/or to increase repetition of desirable behaviors
- Use "time out" for stopping behaviors that cannot be allowed to simply decrease over time. Key is an environment that is unstimulating and unpleasant for a reasonably brief period.
- Interject lots of humor into both pleasurable and stressful interactions with your child(ren)

Summary: Give your child all the courtesies you would offer any adult or nonfamily member, and you will get a positive return for your effort

Based on Gordon, T. (1975). *Parent-effectiveness training.* New York: New American Library; Humenick, S., et al. (1987, January/February). Expectations versus reality. *MCN: American Journal of Maternal Child Nursing,* pp. 36–39; Osborne, P. (1989). *Parenting for the '90s.* Intercourse, PA: Good Books; and Dinkmeyer, D., & McKay, G. D. (1989). The parent's handbook: STEP (systematic training for effective parenting) (3rd ed.). Circle Pines, MN: American Guidance Service.

ents and teen-agers and intervene to restore it, parenting of teens can be effective and rewarding. (See Chapter 11 for further discussion of communication.)

KEY CONCEPTS

Concepts Related to Basic Information

- The relationship between parent and child is reciprocal, which means that as the parent develops the child is affected, and as the child develops the parent is affected.
- Central to the process of parenting is the generational perpetuation of values, skills, knowledge, beliefs, and activities that contribute to happy, healthy living.
- Four goals of parenting are to keep the child safe, to instill family values, to teach social behaviors, and to help the child become self-regulating and independent.
- The most important role of parenting is the nurturing of personality and fostering of development in a climate of love and security.
- Three parenting styles are autocratic, democratic, and permissive.
- Limits and rules, consistently enforced, give the child boundaries that lead to security and trust.
- Essential elements of parenting include rules, consistency, reinforcement, role modeling, and use of the child's imagination.
- Temperament refers to the particular way in which a child relates to the world (see Chapter 3).
- In today's society, financial necessity is a common reason for women entering the work force.
- There is considerable support for the belief that high-quality care of children by someone other than the child's parent does not put a child at risk.
- "Latchkey children" refers to children at home alone, usually school-age children.
- Both positive and negative effects of being at home alone have been reported.

Concepts Related to Nursing Assessment

- Assessment of parenting effectiveness is important, because parents often do not seek professional help in this area.
- The nurse should assess the child's temperament and developmental stage as well as parental interests and sociocultural values in assessing the effectiveness of parenting.
- The nurse should regularly assess the parents' knowledge of developmental behavior and the family's awareness of problems in their children's adaptation following the blending of families.

Concepts Related to Nursing Intervention

- An understanding of cultural beliefs held by a family is fundamental to the nurse's role in supporting parents.

- Physical punishment is not a recommended option for negative reinforcement, because it has many undesirable consequences.
- The nurse should assist families in establishing new patterns of discipline, if they have resorted to physical punishment.
- The nurse can assist parents in making the decision to leave their children alone at home and in selecting areas of teaching directed at keeping the children safe.
- Nurses should support parents by reassuring them, identifying parenting problems and making referrals as necessary, and counseling them.

REFERENCES

Deal, J. E., Halverson, C. F., & Wampler, K. S. (1989). Parental agreement on child-rearing orientations: Relations to parental, marital, family, and child characteristics. *Child Development, 60,* 1025–1034.

Dennis, L. A. (1986, July/August). A comparison of family characteristics and attitudes toward afterschool care for latchkey children. *Pediatric Nursing,* pp. 215–225.

Dinkmeyer, D., & McKay, G. D. (1989). *The parent's handbook: STEP (systematic training for effective parenting)* (3rd ed.) Circle Pines, MN: American Guidance Service.

Erickson, E. (1986). *Childhood and society.* New York: W. W. Norton.

Fisher, S., & Fisher, R. (1986). *What we really know about childrearing.* New York: Aronson.

Gardner, F. E. M. (1989). Inconsistent parenting: Is there evidence for a link with children's conduct problems? *Journal of Abnormal Child Psychology, 17*(2), 223–233.

Glick, P. C. (1989). Remarried families, stepfamilies, and stepchildren: A brief demographic profile. *Family Relations, 38,* 24–27.

Goldsmith, E. B. (1990). In support of working parents and their children: Response to commentary on Scarr et al. article. *Journal of Social Behavior & Personality, 5*(6), 517–520.

Gordon, T. (1975). *Parent-effectiveness training.* New York: New American Library.

Gordon, T. (1989). *Teaching children self-discipline at home and at school.* New York: New York Times Books.

Greenberger, E., & Goldberg, W. A. (1989). Work, parenting, and the socialization of children. *Developmental Psychology, 25*(1), 22–35.

Hojat, M. (1990). Can affectional ties be purchased? Comments on working mothers and their families. *Journal of Social Behavior & Personality, 5*(6), 493–502.

Humenick, S., et al. (1987, January/February). Parenting roles: Expectations versus reality. *MCN: American Journal of Maternal Child Nursing,* pp. 36–39.

Kutzner, S., & Toussic-Weingarten, C. (1984). Working parents: The dilemma of child rearing and career. *Topics in Clinical Nursing, 6*(3), 30–37.

McClellan, M. (1984). On their own: Latchkey children. *Pediatric Nursing, 10*(3), 198–202.

McKnight, J., & Shelsby, B. (1984, May/June). Checking in: An alternative for latchkey kids. *Children Today,* pp. 198–202.

Messer, S. C., Wuensch, K. L., & Diamond, J. M. (1989). Former latchkey children: Personality and academic correlates. *Journal of Genetic Psychology, 150*(3), 301–309.

Orthner, D. K. (1990). Parental work and early adolescence: Issues for research and practice. *Journal of Early Adolescence, 10*(3), 246–259.

Osborne, P. (1989). *Parenting for the '90s.* Intercourse, PA: Good Books.

Padilla, M. L., & Landreth, G. L. (1989). Latchkey children: A review of the literature. *Child Welfare, 68*(4), 445–454.

Pill, C. J. (1990). Stepfamilies: Redefining the family. *Family Relations, 39,* 186–193.

Reutter, L., et al. (1986, July/August). Yours, mine, and ours: Stepparents and their children. *MCN: American Journal of Maternal Child Nursing,* pp. 264–266.

Robinson, B. E., Rowland, B. H., & Coleman, M. (1989). *Home-alone kids: The working parent's complete guide to providing the best care for your child.* Lexington, MA: Lexington Books, D. C. Heath and Company.

Scarr, S., Phillips, D., & McCartney, K. (1989). Working mothers and their families. *American Psychologist, 44*(11), 1402–1409.

Schnittger, M. H., & Bird, G. W. (1990). Coping among dual-career men and women across the family life cycle. *Family Relations, 39,* 199–205.

Scott, P. (1984). What is happening to the dual-career family? *Nursing Economics, 2*(5), 351–355.

Select Committee on Children, Youth, and Families, U. S. House of Representatives (1989). *U. S. children and their families: Current conditions and recent trends.* Washington, DC: U.S. Government Printing Office.

Small, S. A. (1990). Some issues regarding the evaluation of family life education programs. *Family Relations, 39,* 132–135.

Stern, P. (1984). Stepfather family dynamics: An overview for therapists. *Issues in Mental Health Nursing, 6,* 89–103.

Thomas, A., & Chess, S. (1977). *Temperament and development.* New York: Brunner-Mazel.

Williams, R. L., & Boyce, W. T. (1989). Health status of children in self-care. *American Journal of Diseases of Children, 183,* 112–115.

BIBLIOGRAPHY

Arditti, J. A. (1990). Noncustodial fathers: An overview of policy and resources. *Family Relations, 39,* 460–465.

Barnard, K. E., Magyary, D., Sumner, G., Booth, C. L., & Mitchell, S. K. (1988). Prevention of parenting alterations for women with low social support. *Psychiatry, 51*(3), 248–253.

Bernstein, J. (1990). Parenting after infertility. *Journal of Perinatal and Neonatal Nursing, 4*(2), 11–23.

Bozett, F. W. (1989). Gay fathers: A review of the literature. *Journal of Homosexuality, 18*(1/2), 137–162.

Burns, L. H. (1990). An exploratory study of perceptions of parenting after infertility. *Family Systems Medicine, 8*(2), 177–189.

Campbell, D. W. (1991). Family paradigm theory and family rituals: Implications for child and family health. *Nurse Practitioner, 16*(2), 22–31.

Cooke, B. (1991). Thinking and knowledge underlying expertise in parenting: Comparisons between expert and novice mothers. *Family Relations, 40,* 3–13.

Cox, M. J., Owen, M. T., Lewis, J. M., & Henderson, V. K. (1989). Marriage, adult adjustment, and early parenting. *Child Development, 60,* 1015–1024.

Dawson, D. A., & Cain, V. S. (1990). *Child care arrangements: Health of our nation's children, United States; 1988* (Advance data from vital and health statistics, No. 187). Hyattsville, MD: National Center for Health Statistics.

Dormire, S. L., Strauss, S. S., & Clarke, B. A. (1989). Social support and adaptation to the parent role in first-time adolescent mothers. *Journal of Obstetric, Gynecologic, and Neonatal Nursing, 18*(4), 327–337.

Fassinger, P. (1989). Becoming the breadwinner: Single mothers' reactions to changes in their paid work lives. *Family Relations, 38,* 404–411.

Guerney, B. (1979). Fortifying family ties. In *Families Today.* (DHEW Publication No. 79-815). Washington, DC: U. S. Department of Health, Education, and Welfare.

Hanson, S. M. H., & Bozett, F. W. (1986). The changing nature of fatherhood: The nurse and social policy. *Journal of Advanced Nursing, 11*(6), 719–727.

Huggins, S. (1989). A comparative study of self-esteem of adolescent children of divorced lesbian mothers and divorced heterosexual mothers. *Journal of Homosexuality, 18*(1/2), 123–135.

Johnson, C. (1988). Postdivorce reorganization of relationships between divorcing children and their parents. *Journal of Marriage and the Family, 50,* 221–231.
King, D., & MacKinnon, C. (1988). Making difficult choices easier: A review of research on day care and children's development. *Family Relations, 37,* 392–398.
Knafl, K. A., & Deatrick, J. A. (1990). Family management style: Concept analysis and development. *Journal of Pediatric Nursing, 5*(1), 4–14.
McBride, B. A. (1990). The effects of a parent education/play group program on father involvement in childrearing. *Family Relations, 39,* 250–256.
Quinn, P., & Allen, K. (1989). Facing challenges and making compromises: How single mothers endure. *Family Relations, 38,* 390–395.
Rawlins, P. S., Rawlins, T. D., & Horner, M. (1990). Development of the family needs assessment tool. *Western Journal of Nursing Research, 12*(2), 215–228.
Richards, L. (1990). The precarious survival and hard-won satisfaction of white single-parent families. *Family Relations, 38,* 396–403.
Roberts, T. W., & Price, S. J. (1989). Adjustment in remarriage: Communication, cohesion, marital and parental roles. *Journal of Divorce, 13*(1), 17–43.
Spitzke, G. (1988). Women's employment and family relations: A review. *Journal of Marriage and the Family, 50*(3), 595–618.
Statistics Canada (1990). *Canada year book.* Ottawa: Author.
Williams, R. L., & Boyce, T. (1989). Health status of children in self-care. *American Journal of Diseases of Children, 143,* 112–115.
Wismont, J. M., & Reame, N. E. (1989). The lesbian childbearing experience: Assessing developmental tasks. *Image: Journal of Nursing Scholarship, 21*(3), 137–141.

Parenting Handbooks

Brooks, A. A. (1989). *Children of fast-track parents: Raising self-sufficient children in an achievement-oriented world.* New York: Viking.
Clarke, J. I., & Davison, C. (1989). *Parenting ourselves, parenting our children.* San Francisco: Harper & Row.
DeSisto, M. (1991). *Decoding your teenager: How to understand each other during the turbulent years.* New York: William Morrow.
Ehrensaft, D. (1987). *Parenting together: Men and women sharing the care of their children.* New York: Collier Macmillan.
Einon, D. (1988). *Parenthood: The whole story.* London: Bloomsburg.
Fisher, J., & Grenoble, P. B. (1988). *How to be a good role model for your child.* Chicago: Contemporary Books.
Fitzpatrick, J. G. (1988). *The superbaby syndrome: Escaping the dangers of hurrying your child.* New York: Harcourt Brace Jovanovich.
Greven, P. (1991). *Spare the child: The religious roots of punishment and the psychological impact of physical abuse.* New York: Knopf.
Ives, S. B., Fassler, D., & Lash, M. (1989). *The divorce workbook: A guide for kids and parents.* Burlington, VT: Waterfront Books.
Kimball, G. (1988). *50-50 parenting: Sharing family rewards and responsibilities.* Lexington, MA: Lexington Books, D.C. Heath and Company.
Lansky, V. (1989). *Vicki Lansky's divorce book for parents: Helping your children cope with divorce.* New York: New American Library.
Lash, M., Loughridge, S. I., & Fassler, D. (1990). *My kind of family: A book for kids in single-parent homes.* Burlington, VT: Waterfront Books.
Levant, R. F., & Kelly, J. (1989). *Between father and child: How to become the kind of father you want to be.* New York: Viking.
McBride, A. B. (1987). *The secret of a good life with your teenager.* New York: New York Times Books.
McBride, K. (1989). *Tips for working parents: Creative solutions to everyday problems.* Rownal, VT: Storey Communications.
McKay, S. E. (1990). *The new parent survival handbook.* Toronto: Macmillan of Canada.
Olds, S. W. (1989). *The working parents' survival guide.* Rocklin, CA: Prima Publishing & Communications.
Rosin, M. B. (1987). *Stepfathering: Stepfathers' advice on creating a new family.* New York: Simon & Schuster.
Samalin, N., & Jablow, M. M. (1989). *Loving your child is not enough: Positive discipline that works.* New York: Viking.
Siegel, S. E. (1989). *Parenting your adopted child: A complete and loving guide.* Englewood Cliffs, NJ: Prentice-Hall.
Somers, L., & Somers, B. (1989). *Talking to your children about love and sex.* New York: New American Library.
Wassil-Grimm, C. (1990). *How to avoid your parents' mistakes when you raise your children.* New York: Pocket Books.
Williamson, P. A. (1990). Good kids, bad behavior: Helping children learn self-discipline. New York: Simon & Schuster.
Wylie, B. J. (1988). *All in the family: A survival guide for family living and loving in a changing world.* Toronto: Key Porter Books.
Yarrow, A. L. (1991). *Latecomers: Children of parents over 35.* New York: Maxwell Macmillan International.
Yellin, A., & Grenoble, P. B. (1988). *When your child grows too fast.* Chicago: Contemporary Books.

CHAPTER • 13

Assessing Child Health

Janet S. Hadley

RELATED TOPICS
Child growth and development, Unit 2
Immunization schedule, Chapter 10
Dietary health and nutritional requirements, Chapter 16
Family genogram, Chapter 31
Development of visual acuity, Chapter 45

LEARNING OBJECTIVES

- **Identify the five components of the nursing process.**
- **Identify the five major categories included in a comprehensive child health assessment.**
- **Describe a developmentally appropriate sequence for a physical examination of a child in each age group.**
- **Describe the four physical assessment techniques.**
- **Identify the physical assessment techniques and equipment used for each physiologic system evaluated.**
- **Identify the vital components of assessment for children with irregular patterns of health care.**
- **Identify for each examination component two findings that would require a timely referral for in-depth assessment.**
- **Describe the purpose and value of developmental screening.**

A vital component of the nursing process is the nursing assessment, which consists of evaluating the quality of current health status. This is done by gathering data from the interview and physical assessment and from diagnostic and developmental testing. The assessment must be multifocal to be complete and should include an evaluation of family dynamics as well as any cultural, sociologic, environmental, and religious variables that may affect the child's development overall.

During a routine well-child visit, a thorough history combined with physical assessment and appropriate diagnostic and developmental testing provides an avenue for early identification of health deficits. The gathered data also provide an opportunity for health teaching: reinforcing healthful practices and providing anticipatory guidance in other areas.

The comprehensive quality of a well-child assessment will vary depending on the health setting, the time allotted for the evaluation, and the role of the nurse in that setting. Regardless of these variables, the goal of the assessment is to evaluate a child's physical, intellectual, and emotional-social competence and to promote the health of the child and family.

Documentation of Nursing Assessment

The information gathered by the nurse is the data base. This data base must be recorded in a systematic way so that other members of the health care team can use it. Although each work setting has its own system for recording information, the following components are universally accepted as those needing to be documented:

- Assessment.
  - Subjective data.
  - Objective data.
- Nursing diagnosis.
  - Analysis of data.
  - Identification of nursing diagnostic statement(s) or collaborative problem(s).
- Development of a plan of care.
- Nursing interventions.
- Evaluation of patient outcomes.

Taking a History

Historical information is gathered from two sources—the existing medical record and the interview of parent and child. These data allow the nurse to decide what components of physical assessment must be completed. Then, from both the history and the physical assessment, the nurse decides what diagnostic and developmental screenings need to be completed.

Interviewing

The interview is a time for the nurse to establish a trusting relationship with both the child and the parent. It should be conducted in a private, quiet, comfortable room. For younger children, all evidence of invasive, potentially painful equipment should be concealed until it is necessary for examination. The interview should not begin until the nurse has been introduced and explains what is about to happen.

Types of Interviews

There are several kinds of interviews, each devised to meet different needs and situations. The two types of interviews discussed here are the well-child interview and the interim health history.

The *well-child interview* is commonly done in ambulatory care settings. Initially, it includes a complete history, which is updated on subsequent visits. After completing the health history and the physical examination, the care provider offers the child and family guidance pertaining to health promotion and growth and development issues.

The *interim health history* focuses on an immediate physical, social, or emotional problem that has been identified by the family, child, or the health care provider. Although the interview focuses on a specific problem, sufficient data are collected to determine the general health status of the child. The thoroughness of this interview varies with the visiting pattern of the family. If a child is seen for regular well-child visits, the interview may be relatively problem-focused. If the family generally seeks health care only when problems arise, the nurse is responsible for obtaining as full a history as possible with emphasis on the following:

- Significant past medical history.
- Immunization status.
- Sensory screening.
- Dental care.
- Access to health care.

Once a problem has been identified and management begun, a follow-up assessment may be required. Information is obtained about how a problem—especially one that is persistent, complex, or long-term—is responding to the planned intervention.

Principles of Interviewing

Interviewing is complex and requires attention to specific points. Some principles to follow include the following:

- Using clear and concise language.
- Avoiding jargon and medical terminology.
- Using open-ended questions.
- Avoiding closed questions.

- Using indirect questions to elicit more elaborate responses.
- Using double questions to give children choices.
- Being an active listener.

Types of Questions

Following are descriptions of the types of questions:

Open-ended questions allow the child or parent the opportunity to express views, opinions, thoughts, and feelings.
Example: "What do you think makes Jane's breathing become more difficult?"

Closed questions, instead of developing rapport, make the interview clinical and concise.
Example: "Do you like school?"

Direct questions are stated in a manner that generally requires a yes or no answer.
Example: "How old are you?"

Indirect questions do not sound like questions. They permit the client to select or elaborate on information.
Example: "You must have some thoughts about discipline," or "It must be difficult to have twins." They do not end in question marks but obviously invite a response. Such questions express the interviewer's interest in the child and family and offer another way to gather information. The response to such questions gives the nurse an opportunity to learn more about a client's perception of a situation as well as information about the client's communication style.

Double questions are a type of question that is particularly helpful when the nurse needs to gain the cooperation of a child for a physical examination. They provide the child with the opportunity to choose between two alternatives.
Example: "Do you want me to examine your ears or your nose first?" Such questions enable the child to control part of the examination, thus providing a sense of security and lessening the anxiety (Fig. 13–1).

Almost every interview will contain a variety of these questions. The style of questioning will depend on the type of information that is needed by the interviewer. Certain kinds of data lend themselves to particular techniques. For example, direct questions may be used when collecting data in the review of body systems, whereas an open-ended question may be better when collecting data about family or social relationships. When an indirect, open-ended approach does not produce the information desired, more direct or close-ended questions may be more successful.

To conduct a successful interview, the nurse must listen carefully for what is said, what is implied, and what is omitted. Throughout the interview, the nurse will need to ask for clarification of client answers. At the end of the interview, the nurse should present the child and family with a summary of perceptions based on the information gathered. This will allow the interviewee to clear up any misinterpreted statements.

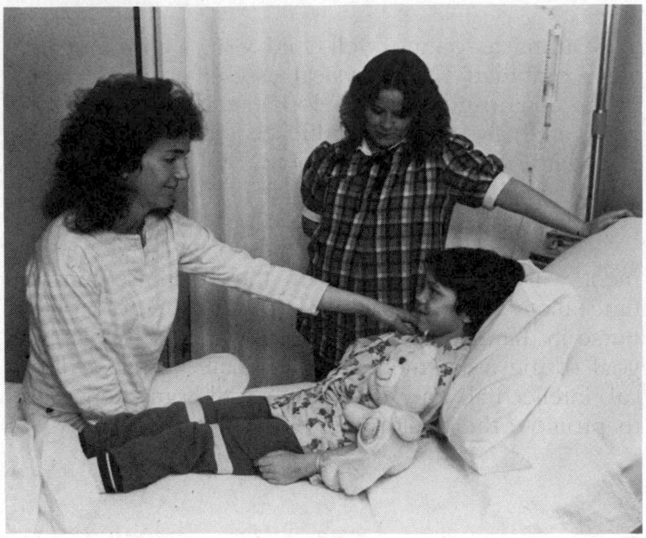

FIGURE 13-1. "Do you want me to examine your ears or your nose first?"

Developmental Considerations for Interviewing

The developmental stage and age of a child as well as the competency of the parents are additional considerations in interviewing. Language and cultural barriers, sensory impairment, and cognitive alterations will all have an impact on the ability of involved parties to understand.

Children can participate in an interview to varying degrees according to age, personality, and developmental level. The *pre-schooler* is verbal enough to tell the nurse about daily routines if questions are put in terms that can be understood. The preschooler may also be able to locate discomforts or sensations if they are being experienced during the interview or examination (e.g., stomachache); however, an accurate recall of past sensations may be vague at this age. Optimal cooperation can be more easily obtained when parents remain present throughout the interview and examination of preschoolers.

School-age children can provide the majority of current information about themselves and their family, school, and daily lives. The older school-age child can be a significant informant about health history and systems review. Encouraging an older school-age child to participate in the interview conveys to the child a sense of competence and reliability as a health care consumer. Parents can remain present during most of the interview; however, the school-age child should have some time alone with the nurse so that concerns that may not be expressed comfortably in front of a parent may be expressed to the nurse. Whether the parent is present during the physical examination should be decided during the child's time alone with the nurse. The child's decision should not be influenced by the parent's presence.

Generally, the *adolescent* can be independent in contributing the necessary information to the interview. Once the interview is complete and the examination is done, the clinical summary and planned management should be shared first with the youth and then with the youth and parent together.

Finally, the interviewer must be attuned to the nonverbal component of the interview. While actively listening to the parent and the child, the nurse should be aware of clients' body postures and facial expressions. The nurse should specifically watch to see how well the verbal message matches the nonverbal cue.

In summary, the successful interview requires multiple skills and techniques. The interviewer must first establish appropriate environmental conditions and a rapport with the parent and child. Next, the nurse must use a sound knowledge of growth and development, a variety of direct and indirect question techniques, and appropriate verbal and nonverbal communication skills. By using all of these skills and techniques, the nurse can glean from the family the information necessary to assess overall health status.

Health History

The discussion here focuses on the type of information obtained in each category of a pediatric history. See Table 13–1 for an example of history format. It is one approach for gathering data in an organized manner. Titles may vary in different settings, although the format is similar.

TABLE 13–1
Pediatric History-Taking Outline

Demographic Data

Date of interview

Name (nickname or preferred name)

Address

Telephone number

Date and place of birth

Sex

Age

Race/nationality

Religion

Primary language spoken

First names of parents

Source and reliability of informant(s)

Reason for Contact (Chief Complaint)

Statement in child's or informant's own words of the reason health care is presently being sought—well-child care, problem, or symptom

Present Illness (Analysis of Chief Complaint)

1. Onset—events coincident with onset, sudden or gradual, previous episodes, when began
2. Characteristics of chief complaint (analysis)
   a. Type, or *character*, of complaint (pain: dull, sharp, aching, burning, radiating, itching, tickling)
   b. *Location* (if applicable). Should be anatomically precise (ask child to point to affected area)
   c. *Severity* (annoying, uncomfortable, incapacitating) and effect on normal daily activities (eating, sleeping, elimination, playing mood)
   d. *Duration* (intermittent, persistent or continuous, interval between if intermittent)
   e. *Influencing factors* (precipitating, aggravating, relieving, ameliorating, recent illness exposure)
   f. *Past treatment* or evaluation of complaint (when, where, and by whom, what studies were performed in the past and what were the results [blood studies, x-ray, etc.], results of past treatment, past diagnosis)
   g. *Current treatment* or evaluation of the complaint (treatment, medications, tests) and response of condition to these measures
3. Present status of complaint (getting worse, better, unchanged)
4. Reason for seeking care now

Family Profile

1. Family members—list or diagram
2. Familial and hereditary diseases
   a. Glaucoma, cataracts, other eye disorders
   b. Tuberculosis, asthma, heart disease, hypertension
   c. Ulcers, colitis
   d. Kidney disease
   e. Arthritis, muscular dystrophy
   f. Mental disorder, epilepsy, learning disorders
   g. Allergies, diabetes, sickle cell disease, cancer, congenital anomalies
3. Family social history (see Table 13–2)
   a. Family relationships
   b. Residence
   c. Finances
   d. Resources
   e. Health attitudes and practices

(continued)

TABLE 13-1
Pediatric History-Taking Outline *(Continued)*

Past Health History

Birth History (Prenatal)

1. Mother's state of health during pregnancy
   a. Illnesses (fever, rash, vomiting, infection); month in pregnancy when occurred; treatment prescribed
   b. Hospitalizations; month in pregnancy when hospitalized; treatment prescribed
   c. X-rays; month in pregnancy when taken
   d. Medications taken (over-the-counter or prescribed); month in pregnancy when taken; reason(s) taken
   e. Use of tobacco, alcohol, or illicit drugs
   f. Diet during pregnancy; amount of weight gained
2. Previous obstetric history
   a. Gravida including this pregnancy
   b. Para including this pregnancy
   c. How long before this pregnancy were there any stillbirths, abortions or miscarriages and their causes, if known?
   d. Have any live-born children died? How long before this pregnancy and cause if known?
   e. Length of this pregnancy
3. Prenatal factors
   a. Mother's age with this pregnancy
   b. When was prenatal care initiated and for how much of pregnancy was it maintained?
   c. Bleeding or complications (toxemia) during this pregnancy and blood type of both parents
4. Attitude toward this pregnancy
   a. Mother describes as easy or difficult pregnancy
   b. Planned or unplanned pregnancy
   c. Child wanted by either or both parents

Birth History (Natal)

1. Circumstances of birth
   a. Where was baby born (e.g., home, birthing room, hospital)?
   b. Natural or induced labor; length of labor; any problems during labor
   c. Was fetal monitoring used? Why?
   d. Any drugs given during labor?
2. Characteristics of delivery
   a. Natural, assisted (forceps used) or cesarean section delivery
   b. Was the father present?
   c. Was the mother awake during delivery?
   d. Was baby in normal position? Breech?
3. Condition of baby at birth
   a. Birthweight
   b. APGAR score
   c. Did baby cry immediately?
   d. Was mechanical suctioning or oxygen required? Was baby intubated?
   e. Was neonatal intensive care or special care nursery needed?
   f. Any abnormalities noted at birth?

Birth History (Postnatal)

1. Weight loss or gains and amount during hospital stay
2. Any difficulties during stay in nursery (feeding or sucking problems; cyanosis, jaundice, rashes)?
3. Length of baby's hospital stay? Nursery or rooming in? Baby and Mother went home together?
4. Feeding method
5. If male, circumcised?

Past Illnesses

Accidents

1. Age at each injury
2. Circumstances surrounding injury (cause, where occurred)
3. Facts regarding injury

   Extent of injury

   Treatment received

   Complications or residual problems

   Child's reaction
4. Any current problems associated with injuries?

Illnesses

1. Illnesses or infections
2. Age
3. Severity
4. Treatment received
5. Complications or sequelae

Operations

1. Date and age at each operation
2. Why was surgery done?
3. Outcome of surgery
4. Child's reaction to each operation
5. Any follow-up or complications?

Hospitalizations

1. Reason for each hospitalization
2. Dates and child's age at each
3. Length of each
4. Child's reaction to hospitalization(s)
5. Outcome
6. Complications

Allergies

1. Untoward response to medications, foods, animals, insect bites
2. Type of reaction (hives, rash, swelling, rhinitis, nausea)
3. Do symptoms occur seasonally?

TABLE 13-1
Pediatric History-Taking Outline *(Continued)*

4. Do symptoms occur immediately or a few to several hours after exposure?

Immunizations

1. Type received
2. Dates received
3. Untoward reactions

Developmental History

1. Motor development milestones
2. Language development milestones
3. Intellectual development
4. Social development milestones
5. Current developmental status with regard to activities of daily living
   a. Nutrition

Infant:	How is child's appetite?
	Bottlefed? Breastfed?
	If breastfed, mother's diet and fluid intake? If bottle, what kind, how much, how formula mixed? Amount in 24 hrs? Number of feedings in 24 hrs, length of each feeding, how progressing? If taking solids, what kind, portion size, how often?
Older child:	What kinds of food and what portions? How well does child feed self? Cup use? Does child eat alone or with family?
	Does child take vitamins (kind, how often, with or without iron)?
	Food dislikes, food likes, food jags?

   b. Elimination

   What are child's bowel patterns? Consistency? Discomfort?

   Is child toilet trained?

   Any associated stresses with elimination habits? Enuresis?

   c. Sleep

   Does child sleep through night?

   Difficulties with putting the child to bed?

   How many hours does child sleep in 24 hrs?

   Naps (when, how long)? Difficulty falling asleep?

   Where does child sleep? Does child have own bed?

   Any change in sleep patterns? Nightmares, night terrors?

   d. Play

   What kinds of games does child like to play? Describe types of play between parent and child. How does child play with peers?

   e. Safety

   Safety of environment (drugs, corrosives, pot handles, electrical outlets). Availability of syrup of ipecac. Poison Control telephone number. Supervision of children (water, matches, stoves, guns). Street safety (seat belts, helmets, street crossings). Sports safety

   f. Dental health

   Brushing properly? Regular dental visits? Fluoride? Orthodontics?

   g. Personality/school performance

   How does parent describe child's personality?

   What are child's school interests? Grades?

   School performance?

   How does child interact with teachers, classmates?

   How does child get along with family members?

   What chores does child do?

   What does child do when mad, sad, glad, scared?

   h. Discipline

   How is the child disciplined (verbal, physical)? When is child disciplined? How often?

   i. Sexuality

   What questions is child asking?

   What are parent's responses?

   What does child or adolescent know about secondary sexual development, sexuality, menstruation, sexual exploration?

   Is child's/adolescent's information about sexually transmitted disease and HIV/AIDS accurate?

   Is adolescent sexually active? Using birth control (type, frequency of use, problems)?

   Does the adolescent female know how to examine her breasts?

Child Review of Systems (see Table 13–3)

1. General appearance
2. Skin and lymphatics
3. Eyes, ears, nose, and throat
4. Cardiopulmonary system
5. Gastrointestinal system
6. Genitourinary system
7. Musculoskeletal system
8. Neurologic status

Demographic Data

These are the data that identify the patient. Usually, such data are found in the chart and need only be verified by the interviewer. Both the informant and the informant's reliability should be noted. If the child is one of the historians, note that also.

Reason for Contact (Chief Complaint)

This is the specific reason for the visit to the office, clinic, or hospital. It is a brief statement recorded in the child's or parent's own words. Generally, the purpose of the visit is routine health assessment or investigation of health problems. If the visit is for well-child care, an opportunity for the parent to express any specific concerns should precede history taking.

Present Illness

This portion of the history is obtained if the child presents with a specific problem. The problem may be physical, intellectual, or emotional-social. This portion of the history may be omitted if there is not a specific complaint. The present illness history consists of four components:

- A description of the onset and progression of the problem.
- Identification of the characteristics of the problem.
- Present status of the problem.
- Reason for seeking health care at this time.

If more than one problem exists, they must be investigated in order of occurrence. See Table 13–1 for a summary of the type of information to be gathered for these components of the present illness.

Family Profile

The primary purpose for obtaining a family health history is to discover potential hereditary or familial diseases that could affect the health of the child. The second purpose for a family health history is to identify possible stress factors that could affect the child and the family. A recent death or chronic illness of one of the family members may interfere with the normal function and developmental progress of the child. The family health history may be represented in written form or pictorially by a genogram.

Family Members

A list or diagram (genogram) of family members, including age, sex, and state of health, should be made. If a genogram is used, symbols represent relationships and gender. See Figure 13–2 for an example of a family genogram and a description of symbols used.

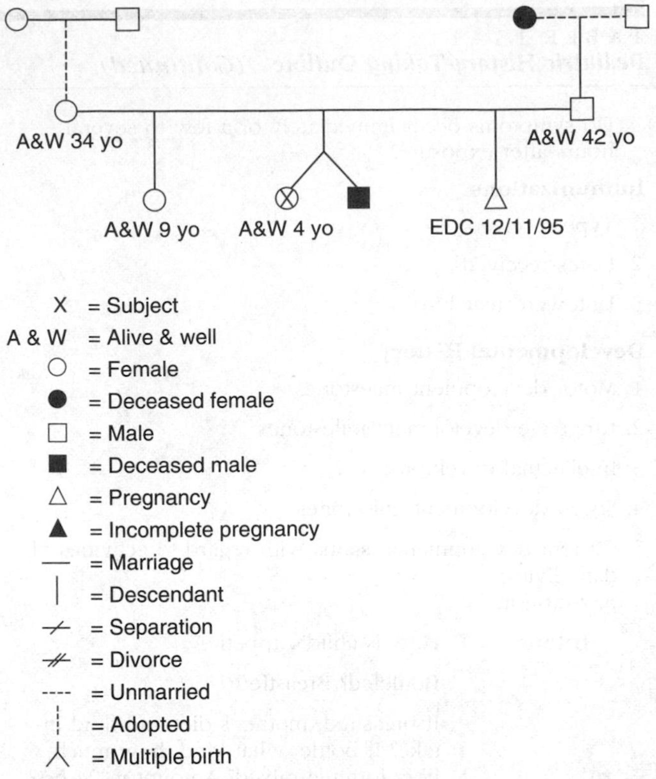

FIGURE 13-2. Genogram depicting a history of family members.

Familial or Hereditary Diseases

Information on existing or past conditions that are of a familial or hereditary nature in parents, grandparents, first aunts and uncles, and siblings should be obtained. A review of the specific problems noted in Table 13–1 will enable the nurse to identify the significant problems.

Family Social History

This portion of the history includes information on environmental, economic, personal, and social factors that influence the child's and family's overall development and health. Often in a multidisciplinary setting, the nurse may have access to data collected by the social worker or psychologist to gain an understanding of the family's circumstances. Much of the information requested in this section is of a sensitive and personal nature. Therefore, if these data are not already documented, it is important to recognize that an accurate family social history may be gathered only after the family has established a trusting relationship with the nurse. Table 13–2 summarizes the pertinent data in this area.

Past Health History

Birth History

A thorough birth history includes data concerning the prenatal, natal, and postnatal periods. The extent of

TABLE 13-2
Family Social History

Finances

1. Who is employed? Where? Occupation?
2. Does the family have enough money to do the things that are important to its members?
3. Are they receiving financial assistance (welfare, food stamps)?
4. Do they have health insurance?

External Resources

1. What schools, day care, or preschool facilities are being used?
2. Are there babysitters? How often used?
3. Training, primary language, child's response?

Family Relationships

1. Who lives at home (parents, grandparents, significant others)?
2. What are the family interrelationships?
3. What is the marital status?
4. What is the home atmosphere like (happy, sad, cooperative, antagonistic, chaotic)?
5. Who shares in household chores?
6. Who within the family shares in caring for the children?
7. What is the level of education?
8. What are some of the family activities?
9. How were the parents disciplined as children?

Residence

1. Type of housing (house, apartment, room)?
2. Is there a yard and is it fenced?
3. Is there a pool and is it fenced?
4. Are there stairs?
5. Is a busy street nearby?
6. What is the proximity to transportation, shopping, playground, schools, health care facilities?
7. Is it a safe neighborhood?
8. What is the source of water? Is it fluoridated?

Health Attitudes and Practices

1. How does the family regard health services and personnel?
2. How is the family's role as health consumer perceived?
3. Who makes decisions about health issues, management of illness, when to seek health care?
4. What cultural or religious traditions exist that affect health care or childrearing practices?
5. What are the family's attitudes and participation in preventive health practices?
6. How is safety stressed in home and family living?
7. Are seat belts, infant car seats, and bicycle helmets used?

history taken, however, varies according to the age of the child and the current health status. The older the child the less need there is for a detailed birth history unless it is indicated by a presenting problem. Table 13–1 lists questions that should be covered in a comprehensive birth history.

Past Illnesses

The past health history includes a summary of any diseases, injuries, operations, or hospitalizations that the child has experienced. Table 13–1 summarizes the areas to question to document these experiences.

Immunizations

The types and dates of the child's immunizations should be noted. Children who need special attention paid to their immunization records include immigrants, premature infants whose immunizations may have been omitted or delayed, and those children with erratic well-child care: homeless families, foster care situations, and transient families (AAP, 1986). Any reactions to the immunizations and the treatment that followed should also be noted. A record of tuberculin skin testing is included with the immunizations. If a child has not been immunized for a specific reason (e.g., chronic illness, immunodeficiency, religious beliefs), it should also be noted in this section. Chapter 10 summarizes the recommended schedule of immunizations for infants and children.

Developmental History

Documentation of the age at which the child mastered developmental milestones is included in the health history. Although parental recall may be hazy, such information may give insight into a current abnormality. Milestones recorded include motor, language, intellectual, and social development. These vary according to age and are reviewed in the growth and development chapters, 4 through 9, in Unit 2.

Additionally, the child's developmental status may be assessed by exploring the activities of daily living:

- Nutrition patterns and skills.
- Elimination patterns.

TABLE 13-3
Outline of Review of Systems

General

Overall state of health? Fatigue? Growth patterns? Recent or unexplained weight loss or weight gain? Contributing factors (illness, dieting, change in appetite)? Exercise tolerance? General ability to perform normal daily functions?

Skin and Lymph

Skin problem such as excessive dryness, pruritus, skin sensitivity? Rashes? Acne? Skin color changes? Tendency for bruising? Petechiae? Abnormalities of nail color, nail growth? Hair loss? Hair color change? Use of hair dyes, chemicals for hair straightening? Swollen lymph glands?

Eyes

Known visual problems? Behaviors that may indicate visual problems: turning head to one side, sitting close to the television set,* squinting, rubbing the eyes, bumping into objects? Crossed eyes (strabismus)? Lazy eye (amblyopia)? Wears glasses or contact lenses? Eye infections? Excessive tearing or absence of tears? Burning? Edema of eyelids? Redness?

Ears

Earaches, ear infections, ear discharge? Hearing loss? Behaviors that may indicate this: turning radio, stereo, or television very loud, frequent use of headphones, requests to repeat in conversation, loud speech, inattentive behavior, decreased or no response to loud noises?

Nose

Nosebleeds (episodic, recurrent, severe)? Frequent nasal congestion or runny nose? Nasal obstruction or difficulty with breathing? Seasonal or frequent sneezing, sinus pain, sinus infections?

Throat

Mouth breathing? Bleeding gums? Toothaches? Teething? Sore throats, infections, strep throats? Hoarseness? Difficulty swallowing?

Cardiorespiratory

Trouble breathing, choking, turning blue? Difficulty feeding, tires easily, difficulty running or playing? Cough (where, when, position, wet, dry)? Wheezing? Keeps up with other children? Number of colds per year? Heart murmur? Anemia? Date and result of last blood count? Blood type? Blood transfusion? Rheumatic fever?

Gastrointestinal

Bowel patterns, frequency, color, discomfort? Abdominal pain, diarrhea, constipation? Flatulence, bloody stools, bleeding, fissures, nausea, vomiting?

Genitourinary

Urinary stream, frequency, pain on urination, urgency, periods of dryness (as opposed to dribbling or constant wetness), bleeding, enuresis? Menstruation (when started, how often, amount, length of each menses, discomfort, problems)? Vaginal discharge, pruritus? Pain or discharge from penis? Swelling or pain of testicles? Change in testicular or penile size? Pubic hair?

Musculoskeletal

Weakness, history of fractures, strains, sprains? Painful joints, swelling, redness of joints? Clumsiness, lack of coordination, tremors, abnormal gait, restricted or painful movement?

Neurologic

Convulsions, febrile seizures? Fainting, tremors, twitches, blackouts, dizziness, frequent headaches? Learning problems, clumsiness, coordination problems? Numbness, memory loss, speech problems, unusual habits? Taste, tactile sense? Sees, hears, smells?

* Young children tend to sit close to TV even though no visual problem exists. In school-age or older children, it may indicate a visual problem.

- Sleep habits and patterns.
- Developmental progress.
- Personality and school performance.
- Discipline.
- Sexuality.

Review of Systems

The review of systems is done for a complete data base for a well child as well as for a child who presents with an illness or specific complaint. It focuses attention on any deviations from health, thus allowing the nurse a more comprehensive picture of the child's health status and potential need for interventions. The information received in this part of the history is invaluable even when it may appear unrelated to the problem at hand. Table 13-3 is an outline of suggested areas for review of each body system. The nurse should use terms that are easily understood by the parent and child. The questions will vary depending on the age and developmental level of the child.

Physical Assessment

Approaching the Child

There are seven key issues in approaching a child for a physical assessment:

- Atmosphere must be comfortable.
- Examination must be done quickly.
- Child's modesty must be respected.
- Examiner must take advantage of opportunities for assessment as they arise.
- Procedures must be explained before they are done.
- Examination must be done systematically.
- Examiner must be skilled in the assessment techniques and have a good knowledge base in anatomy as well as child development.

Incorporating all of these components into the examination routine comes about after much practice. However, paying attention to all seven points should help minimize the child's anxiety about the examination.

Providing a comfortable environment will vary for each age group. An infant needs a warm room; a preschooler needs some toys with which to play. A school-age child may need some books to read.

Doing an examination quickly requires preparation. Before beginning the examination, the nurse should develop a mental outline of the steps of the examination and prepare a mental list of significant findings for that system. The examination can then be conducted very quickly.

For example, if a child presents with a complaint of an earache the nurse would mentally outline the following check list before beginning with the examination:

- Is the external ear normal in appearance?
- Is the ear canal patent?
- Is the tympanic membrane normal in appearance?
- Is the tympanic membrane mobile?
- Is the examination painful for the child?
- Are the lymph nodes of the neck swollen?
- Is there any redness or swelling at the mastoid process?

By preparing such a check list for each system, the nurse can more quickly evaluate normality versus abnormality while proceeding systematically with the examination.

Children at any age may exhibit modesty that must be respected. Beginning in the preschool years, all children should be offered cover gowns to wear during the examination. School-age children and adolescents will need the opportunity to dress and undress in privacy. A helpful technique with young children is to have them remove one article of clothing at a time. For example, most children will readily remove shoes and socks. The nurse can then examine the feet. Next, the child could remove pants or skirt and then be examined from the waist down. Cooperation may be extended by allowing the child to replace pants or skirt before removing shirt or blouse. Finally, children ranging in age from toddlers to adolescents usually dislike being without underwear. Often, an adequate examination of buttocks, anus, and genitalia can be done by merely pulling the undergarment to the side while inspecting the perineum.

It is helpful to take full advantage of opportunities as they arise. For example, because the infant or young child may cry during the examination, the nurse could auscultate heart and lungs first while the child lies quietly in the parent's arms. Other examples would be to observe the child's neurologic and developmental status while the child plays with toys in the examination room. The nurse may also listen to speech and articulation as the child converses with siblings or parents.

Many children like to be involved in the health examination. This interest offers the nurse the opportunity to explain the examination to the child. The explanation given will vary with the child's ability to understand. The message needs to be simple, concise, and honest. Examples of appropriate statements may be "I need to check your teeth to see if you are taking good care of them," or "I need to look inside your ears so I can learn about your hearing. It will not hurt, but it will feel a little funny when I give you a tiny puff of air." In addition to a verbal explanation, a child may be more cooperative if allowed to handle the equipment that will be used for the examination (Fig. 13–3).

Very young children may be more cooperative if the examination is presented as a game. The toddler may enjoy playing "this little piggy went to market"

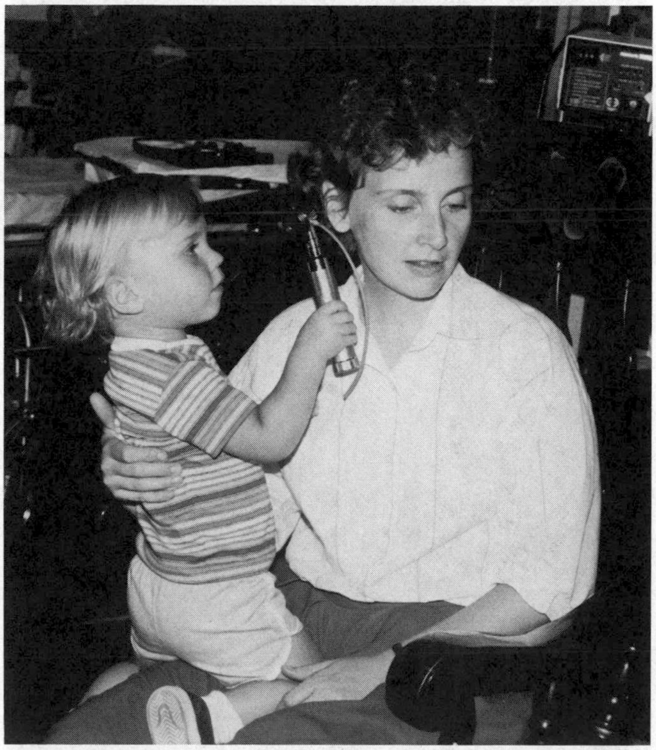

FIGURE 13 - 3. The young child may enjoy handling the equipment used for the examination and may become more confident and cooperative if allowed to examine an adult.

when the feet are examined. When palpating the abdomen, the nurse may say, "See if I can guess what you had for breakfast." If the right food is guessed, the child is delighted and generally enthralled with the process of the guessing game.

The younger school-age child may like to listen to the heart sounds. The young child may enjoy handling the equipment that will be used for the examination and may become more confident and cooperative if allowed to examine a doll or an adult. Other techniques that are sometimes helpful include the use of dolls, puppets, and stories. Sometimes pretending to examine the mother or a sibling first will also help a child to gain the necessary trust and to become cooperative.

Finally, despite multiple efforts to facilitate cooperation, the child may have to be restrained or positioned for the examination to take place. The child may be held in the nurse's or a parent's lap for the abdominal and musculoskeletal examination. The parent may also need to hold the child's head against his or her shoulder for the ear examination. The ear examination can also be conducted with the child supine on the examination table while the parent restrains the knees and an assistant holds the child's arms extended straight up beside the head. The examiner then has only to control the head and otoscope. No child should be restrained without an explanation, and the child should never be scolded for resisting restraint. See Figures 13–4 and 13–5 for examples of restraint.

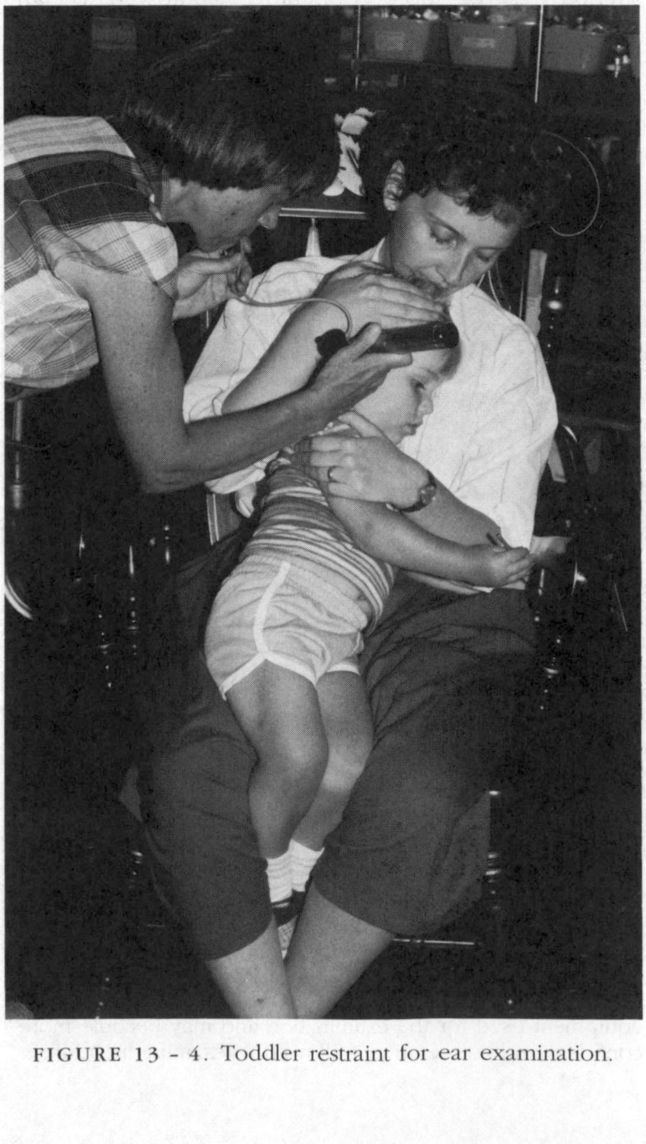

FIGURE 13 - 4. Toddler restraint for ear examination.

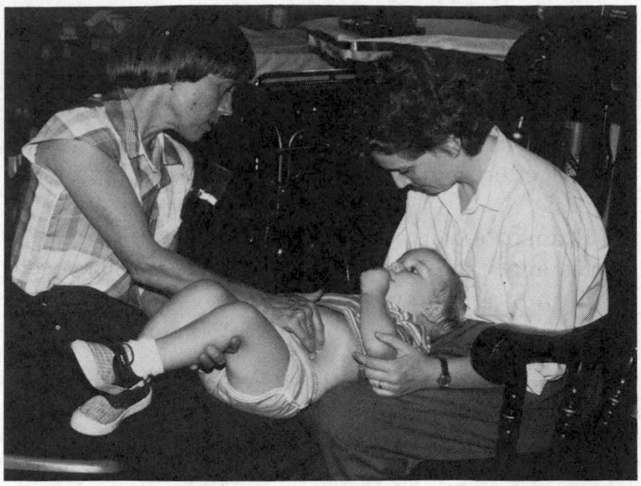

FIGURE 13 - 5. Toddler restraint for abdominal examination.

The nurse may be able to anticipate the child's ability to cooperate by merely asking the child where the examination should take place—in the parent's lap or on the examination table. In a study, Moss (1983) found that children between the ages of 2 and 3 years who chose to be examined on the examination table were always cooperative, whereas children who chose to be examined in the parent's lap were cooperative 50 per cent of the time.

The final issue in physical assessment is for the nurse to develop a systematic approach to the examination. Although opportunities may present themselves for some physical evaluation (e.g., examining the child's heart and lungs while she or he is quiet in the mother's arms), the nurse should develop a routine that is adhered to for every examination. This may be a head-to-toe or toe-to-head examination or examination in another order. This systematic approach minimizes the chance of missing parts of the examination because of distraction of the child's behavior or the parent's questions.

Measurements

Height and Weight

For the child, the measurements of height and weight should be obtained and plotted on a standardized anthropometric chart at each physical examination. This is usually done at all well-child visits—approximately five times during the first year of life and once or twice a year thereafter through adolescence. Height and weight measurements reflect overall growth of the child. (See Appendices 2 and 3 for height and weight charts.)

The method of measuring the child's height varies with age. The preferred method for the infant or young child is to place the child in a supine position with the knees extended and to use a special device for measuring length. These devices vary in each setting. When a measuring device is not available, an infant or young child can be placed in the supine position, and the nurse can mark on the examination table paper where the child's head and feet are and then measure the distance between the two points. The older child (after 2 years of age) can stand on a standard balanced scale with a movable rod or be measured against a wall-mounted measuring device.

Weight is also an important index of the child's growth and should be measured with every examination whether the child is well or ill. It is an easily obtainable measurement. *Of primary importance is the need to ensure that a scale has been balanced before a child is weighed.* Infants are weighed naked or wearing only a diaper on a balanced infant scale. A child who is able to stand independently may be weighed on a balanced adult scale. When weight gain or loss is of great clinical significance (as with premature infants, children with growth problems, and children with cardiac or gastrointestinal disorders), it is imperative that the same scale be used for subsequent weighings. The exact scale should be identified and noted in the medical record.

For the child who is afraid, unwilling to cooperate, or physically unable to stand on a scale, the nurse may have the parent hold the child while the parent stands on the scale. After the combined weight of the parent and child is noted, the nurse then has the parent stand on the scale alone. The parent's weight is then subtracted from the combined weight to give the child's weight.

Whenever there are unusual conditions existing during weighing or measuring, the nurse should note such on the child's record (e.g., child weighed with shoes on).

Once measurements have been taken, they can be compared with past measurements by plotting them on a growth grid according to the child's age. Usually health care facilities use standardized percentile charts. These charts use percentiles to show the distribution of height, weight, and head circumference for a typical series of 100 children born at term. For example, the 25th percentile indicates that 75 children are taller and 25 children are shorter than the child being measured. In general, a child in the 25th percentile will continue at about this percentile throughout life. A child who suddenly has an increase to a higher or lower percentile requires further investigation. *If a measurement differs greatly from previous visits, the nurse should check the technique and reevaluate the measurement.* Often the measurement has been taken incorrectly or plotted on the graph incorrectly.

Some general rules exist regarding height and weight:

- Height and weight measurements provide important information, but a single measurement is of less importance than a series of measurements.
- The relationship between height and weight is significant. For example, a child who falls at a high percentile for height and at a much lower percentile for weight requires a more detailed assessment.
- Children should constantly progress in height and weight. Any persistent plateauing or weight loss needs a more detailed assessment.

Head Circumference

The brain achieves 80 per cent of its adult size by 2 years of age. More than half of total head growth occurs during the first year of life. Therefore, the head circumference should be taken at each well-child visit during the first 3 years.

A reliable reading of head circumference is obtained by using a metal or paper tape measure around the broadest part of the head. The tape is placed over the widest diameter of the head, the occipital protuberance and the frontal bones (Fig. 13–6). If an accurate measurement is difficult to obtain, it is best to take three measurements and use the largest. Head circumference increases 4 inches (approximately 10 cm) in the first year and only 2 inches (approximately 5 cm) between the ages of 1 and 7.

The head circumference is also plotted on a growth chart (see Appendices 2 and 3). As with height and weight, serial measurements provide more information than a single measurement, and marked differences should be investigated.

Vital Signs

As in other areas of the physical examination of children, it is important to reduce anxiety and gain cooperation when vital signs are being obtained. The same techniques to gain cooperation previously described may be employed while taking the vital signs.

The order in which vital signs are measured will depend on the age of the child and the child's ability to understand and cooperate. A rule of thumb is to proceed from the least intrusive procedure to the most intrusive procedure. For very young children, vital signs should be taken in the following order: pulse and respirations, blood pressure, and temperature. Following this order increases cooperation and produces more accurate results, since temperature taking can produce sufficient anxiety to alter the respiratory and pulse rates.

Temperature

Normal temperature values will depend on the route by which the temperature is measured. Generally the

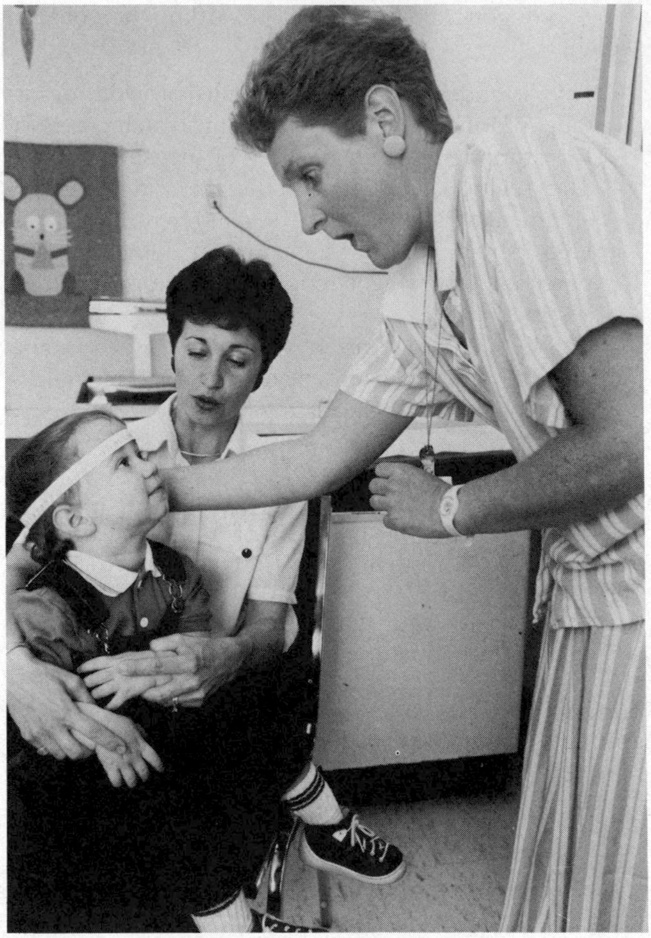

FIGURE 13 - 6. Head circumference is measured around the broadest part of the head over the occipital protuberance and the frontal bones.

accepted values are between 35.5° C and 38° C (96° F and 100.4° F) for oral temperatures. There is no consensus about how much rectal and axillary temperatures differ from an oral temperature. Rectal temperatures are thought to be slightly higher than oral temperatures, and axillary slightly lower than oral, but the difference is not believed to be a full degree Fahrenheit as was traditionally assumed. When temperatures are recorded, the route of measurement should be noted and the same route of measurement should always be used for a particular child.

The route of temperature taking and the length of time allowed for accurate measurement depends in part on custom in each setting. With increasing frequency, care providers recognize the anxiety produced by taking rectal temperatures. Some settings use the less traumatic axillary temperature as the preferred route of measure.

There are three instruments for temperature measurement: glass and mercury thermometers, electronic thermometers, and, most recently, the introduction of infrared devices that measure temperature via the tympanic membrane. All are accurate. The first is inexpensive, common, and breakable. The electronic thermometers are rapid, unbreakable, and require the use of special probes (Barrus, 1983). The infrared device, although rapid and painless, is sometimes associated with an uncomfortable otoscopic examination (Rogers et al, 1991). This device is gaining wider use.

Heart Rate and Respiration

Both heart rate and respirations should be counted for a full minute in infants and young children because of the variability in both rates. In older children, the pulse may be palpated. Table 13–4 describes average pulse rates and respiratory rates.

Blood Pressure

Figure 13–7 displays blood pressure readings at various ages. *The single most common cause for inaccurate documentation of blood pressure is the use of a blood pressure cuff of the wrong size.* Therefore, it is imperative that the nurse be familiar with the correct technique for obtaining all vital signs. Chapter 23 describes in more detail some of the special techniques used in assessing vital signs in children.

Physical Examination

Physical examination utilizes four basic assessment techniques:

- Inspection.
- Palpation.
- Percussion.
- Auscultation.

Table 13–5 describes these techniques. The examination is usually conducted from head to toe. When a body part is examined, it is usually inspected generally and then more specifically. For example, when examining the head, the general appearance is

TABLE 13 - 4
Normal Pulse and Respiratory Rates for Specific Ages*

Age	Pulse (Beats per Minute)	Average Pulse	Respirations (Breaths per Minute)
Neonate	70–170	120	30–40
2 yrs	80–130	110	25–32
4 yrs	80–120	100	23–30
6 yrs	75–115	100	21–26
8 yrs	70–110	90	20–26
10 yrs	70–110	90	20–26
12 yrs	70–110	85	18–22
14 yrs	65–105	85	18–22
16 yrs	60–100	85	16–20
18 yrs	50–90	80	12–24

* These are averages and vary with the sex of the child.

noted first, followed by the skin of the face and head. Finally, a more detailed examination of the parts of the face (e.g., nose and mouth) is carried out.

General Appearance

The examination should begin with an overall impression of the child. Observation of the child is made to formulate an impression that can be verified or disproved following a more extensive examination. Examples of some areas used to develop a general appearance statement are physical appearance (ill or well); nutritional status; behavior and degree of activity; facial expression; interactions with parents or nurse; developmental status; consciousness level; speech or nature of cry; gait; coordination; and posture. The general appearance focuses on physical characteristics or behaviors of the child and should be a brief summary statement. An example of a general appearance statement is as follows: alert, smiling, well-developed, well-nourished toddler playing on mother's lap and in no acute distress.

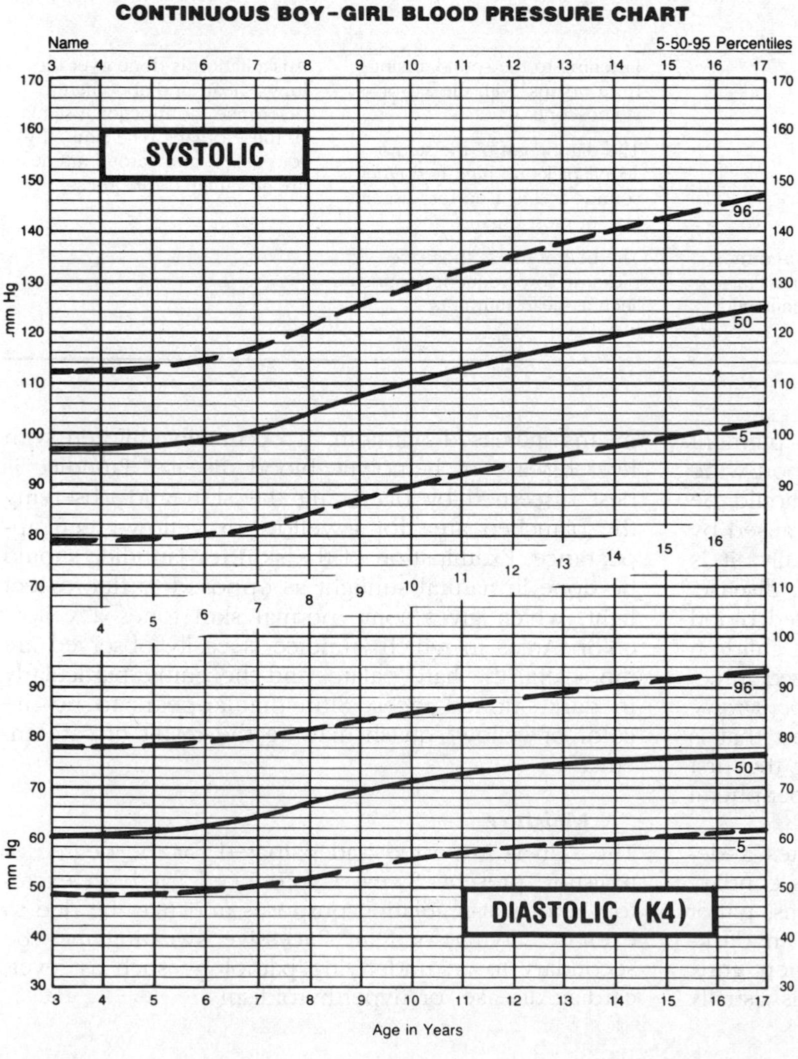

FIGURE 13-7. Children's blood pressure chart. (From Jaworski, A. [1978, September]. New boy-girl blood pressure chart for pediatric office use: A single sheet graph for all children. *Clinical Pediatrics,* 699. Reproduced with permission of The Cortlandt Group, Inc., publisher.)

Skin

Techniques	**Equipment**
Inspection	Natural lighting
Palpation	

Examine for

Color	Temperature
Moisture	Lesions/rashes
Texture	Hair
Turgor	Nails
Edema	

The skin is examined as a whole to determine its overall condition and then more specifically as each body part is assessed.

Color

Normal skin color varies depending on race. The skin should be inspected for areas of increased or de-

TABLE 13-5
Techniques Utilized in Physical Assessment

Purpose	Comments
Inspection	
Evaluation of visible characteristics	Adequate exposure of area being visualized and good direct lighting necessary
Palpation	
Use of hands to touch or feel area being assessed for temperature, texture, vibration, size or position	Temperature (e.g., of the skin) is assessed best with the dorsum of the fingers
Light palpation is gentle pressure applied with the fingertips or palms	Texture, size or position (e.g., texture of the hair, size or position of an organ or mass) is best assessed with the fingertips
Deep palpation is firm pressure applied with the fingertips to evaluate organs within the abdomen. Deeper palpation is achieved by placing the fingers of one hand over the fingers of the hand that is palpating	Vibration (e.g., of air or sound moving through the lungs) is assessed best with the palms
Ballottement is application of pressure by tapping or bouncing of several fingers to note pressure within an organ (e.g., ocular pressure) or rebound tenderness (e.g., of the abdomen or a specific organ)	
Percussion	
A rapping motion utilized to determine the density of an area being assessed or the borders of a specific organ	Direct percussion is used most often to percuss the nasal sinuses or tendons or inflamed organs
Blunt or direct percussion is done by striking the surface being assessed with a partially flexed finger (usually the middle finger)	Indirect percussion may be used to percuss any area of the body. Percussion sounds include:
Bimanual or indirect percussion is accomplished by placing the middle finger of one hand on the surface to be percussed. The other fingers should not rest on the surface to be percussed as this will diminish the sound created by percussion. The middle finger or index and middle fingers of the other hand strike the middle finger resting on the body surface on the upper phalange. Only the very tip of the striking finger is used	*Tympany* (drumlike) such as is heard over the stomach or abdomen normally *Hyperresonance* (hollow sound with air interference) as is heard in pneumothorax *Resonance* (hollow sound without air interference) as is heard normally over the lung *Impaired resonance* (diminished hollow sound) as is heard when fluid has accumulated in a hollow cavity such as the lung *Dullness* is heard normally over muscle or a thick or solid tissue organ such as the liver *Flatness* is heard normally over bone
Auscultation	
Listening to the sound arising from organs, with the aid of a stethoscope	Auscultation is done over the lungs, heart and abdomen to determine the functional status of these organs. The skull, thyroid gland, and carotid arteries are auscultated for bruits
The diaphragm of the stethoscope picks up high-frequency sounds and is used for auscultation of most organs	
The bell of the stethoscope picks up low-frequency sounds such as heart murmurs	

creased pigmentation. Normal variations in pigment include birthmarks, café-au-lait spots, and port-wine stains. Signs of generalized color change should be noted. *Cyanosis,* a bluish tint to the skin, is caused by reduced hemoglobin in the capillaries. Usually, it is seen in children with respiratory or cardiac disease. *Erythema,* an increased amount of oxygenated blood in the vasculature of the dermis, is found in children who are febrile, have a sunburn or a localized infection, or have been exposed to the cold. *Acrocyanosis,* the bluish discoloration of the hands and feet that is frequently seen in newborns, is normal for the first few days of life. It is caused by inadequate peripheral vasculature.

Skin that is *markedly pallid* demonstrates a decrease in hemoglobin content, often seen secondary to anemia or shock. In white-skinned persons, pallor is noted by a loss of pink skin coloring; in dark-skinned persons, the skin becomes an ashen gray. *Jaundice* is seen as a yellow-green hue; this usually means increased bilirubin. It occurs in children with liver disease or hemolytic blood disease. Jaundice is best discerned by blanching the skin and observing the blanched area for a yellow or yellow-green appearance. Examination of the skin for jaundice should be done in natural sunlight as opposed to fluorescent light, which gives some normal skin tones a yellow color. Areas in which jaundice is easily observed are the sclera, the hard palate, and the gums, particularly in dark-skinned races. Skin that appears to be the color of yellow squash may be the result of carotenemia.

Moisture

The skin is inspected and palpated for the degree of moisture present. Sweat is produced for both excretory and heat-regulating purposes and may be due to exercise, crying, or fear. Excessive sweating may be secondary to an underlying pathology such as fever, cardiac disease, or hyperthyroidism.

Texture

Inspection and palpation of the quality and character of the skin surface is necessary for the evaluation of skin texture. Normal skin is smooth, soft, and pliable. Skin that is rough and dry often indicates an endocrine problem; it is also seen in children who bathe very frequently or who are exposed to cold weather. Rough, dry skin is also seen with vitamin A deficiencies. If *scaling* is found, the extent and location should be described. Scaling present only between fingers and toes could be a sign of a fungal infection. Scaling of the palms and soles might be associated with scarlet fever. Eczema often causes scaling of the cheeks and behind the ears, knees, and elbows. Thick, yellow, oily scales on the scalp may indicate *seborrhea,* which can spread into a red maculopapular rash on the face and trunk.

Turgor

One of the best indicators of nutrition and hydration is skin turgor. Normal skin turgor is elastic and taut. Turgor is evaluated by pinching the skin between thumb and forefinger, usually of the lower abdomen, and noting the reaction of the pinched skin. If the skin returns promptly to the normal position, it is assessed as elastic. Skin that does not promptly return may indicate a loss of turgor due to dehydration or excessive exposure to ultraviolet rays. Skin that stays pinched or tented for a few seconds after the skin is released is considered flabby or decreased in turgor and may indicate chronic disease and muscle disorders.

Edema

An excess of water that is stored in the skin in the form of edema is evaluated as "pitting" or "nonpitting." The nurse's thumb is firmly pressed over the medial aspect of the child's malleoli for at least 5 seconds. After releasing the skin, any sign of indentation that lasts several seconds indicates pitting edema. Puffiness or edema that does not remain indented is nonpitting edema. Any body surface areas can be edematous and should be evaluated using the technique just described. Generalized edema, however, is often evaluated by examining the lower extremities. Edema is seen in children who have allergies, kidney or heart anomalies, or malnutrition.

Temperature

Palpation of the skin to determine its temperature is best completed by comparing body parts. Skin temperature is not an accurate reflection of the internal temperature of the body but may reflect a maladjustment in the thermoregulating mechanism of the body. Localized hyperthermia, an indication of increased blood flow, may be secondary to a burn or cellulitis. Generalized hyperthermia may be the result of generalized sunburn, fever, or hyperthyroidism. Children in shock may exhibit generalized hypothermia.

Lesions

Examination of the skin is not complete unless the skin has been inspected and palpated for lesions. Any lesions or markings on the skin should be noted and described in detail as follows: size, color, shape, location, surface characteristics, anatomic distribution, configuration, and morphology.

Primary lesions include macules, papules, wheals, vesicles, petechiae, pustules, and bullae. Examples of secondary lesions are scales, crusts, striae, excoriations, erosion, ulcers, and fissures. Plaques may be either primary or secondary lesions. Comedones and milia are examples of special lesions.

Many skin lesions can be normal, such as capillary hemangiomas, freckles, nevi, and mongolian spots. Mongolian spots are often seen in children of African-American, South American, or Asian descent and usually appear on the buttocks or coccygeal area. Mongolian spots can also be differentiated from bruises in two other ways: color and appearance over time. Mongolian spots are usually slate-blue overall, and they do not change in color or size from day to day as do bruises.

Other skin lesions such as cysts, port-wine stains, and large, hairy moles require further evaluation and possible referral. Lesions in the form of a skin rash are seen frequently in children of all ages. Heat rash and diaper rash are common in infants and young children. Another common condition is acne. It generally begins during adolescence and can range from mild to severe. Newborns often contract a skin rash that is frequently labeled *"neonatal acne."*

Hair

Hair is examined for color, length, distribution, cleanliness, amount, and texture. Scalp hair should be examined to determine whether it is clean and shiny and whether it covers the entire head. Hair texture is noted as being thick or thin, fine or coarse, soft or brittle. Nutritional and endocrine disturbances may affect hair texture. Facial, axillary, or pubic hair that has appeared prematurely may be an indication of precocious puberty or could signify an endocrine problem. The spine is inspected and palpated for hair tufts of the sacral area, which are seen in children with spina bifida.

Nails

Nails are examined as part of the integumentary system. Nails are inspected and palpated for their size, shape (convex or concave), and color (pink, cyanotic, pale). Characteristics such as smoothness, pitting, ridging, and clubbing are carefully noted. Clubbing is generally a sign of chronic lack of oxygen and is often seen in children with congenital heart disease or chronic pulmonary disease. It can also be a normal familial trait. Any change in color should be noted. Adolescents and children who smoke heavily may have yellow nail tips. The cuticles should be assessed for intactness, smoothness, and any splitting or hangnails.

Lymphatic System

Techniques	Equipment
Inspection	None
Palpation	

Examine lymph nodes for	
Size	Redness
Mobility	Distribution
Tenderness	Consistency
Warmth	

The lymphatic system provides important information about the child's health status. A large lymph node or generalized lymphadenopathy may be the first sign of disease. Lymph nodes are inspected and palpated during the examination of the part of the body in which they are located. Palpable lymph nodes in children may be normal but should be evaluated carefully. It should be noted whether lymphadenopathy is localized or generalized. The physical examination should include evaluation of these major lymph node areas: head, neck, axillae, and inguinal (Figs. 13–8 through 13–11).

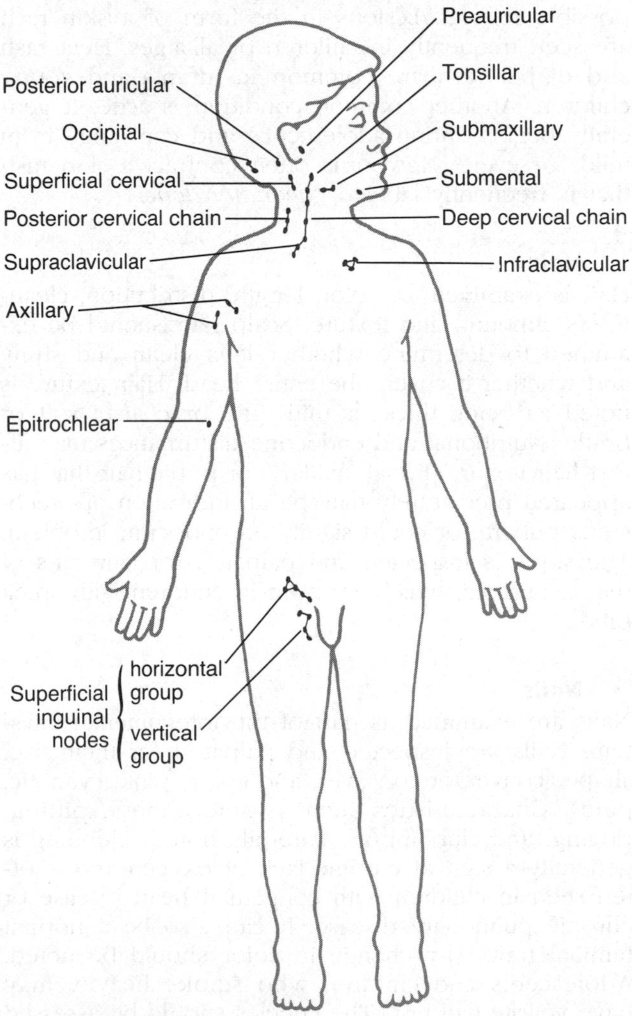

FIGURE 13 - 8. Lymph nodes of the body.

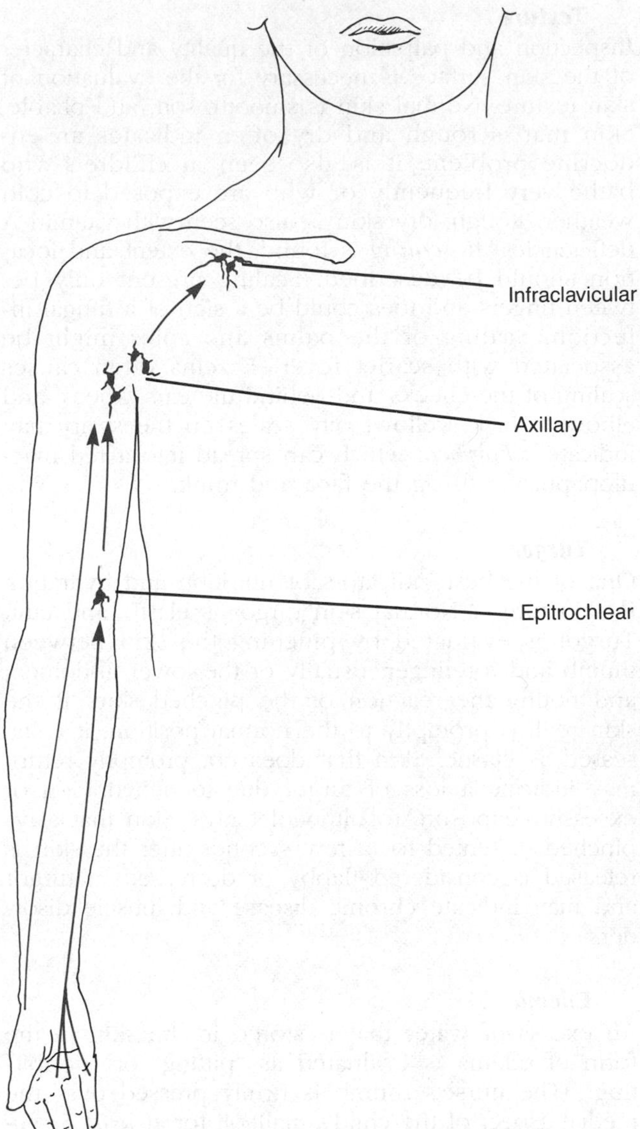

FIGURE 13 - 9. Direction of lymph draining in the arm.

Lymph nodes are palpated using the finger pads and gently but firmly pressing in a circular motion along the regions in which the nodes are normally present. It is easiest to palpate the nodes of the head and neck by positioning the child's head in an upward tilt. Axillary nodes are palpated with the arms relaxed and slightly adducted, with the child's forearm resting on the examiner's forearm to eliminate pull and tension on the axillae. Often this area is very ticklish and the child may need to be distracted. Inguinal nodes are palpated when the child is supine.

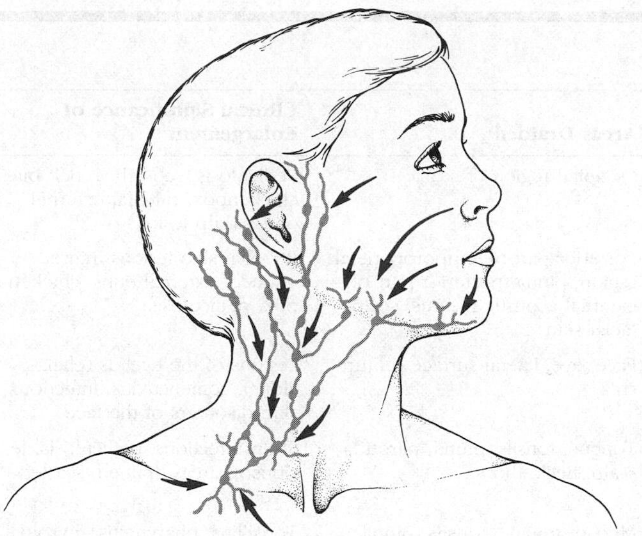

FIGURE 13-10. Lymphatic drainage of the head and neck.

Shotty (small and pelletlike), movable, cool, nontender, discrete nodes up to 3 mm in diameter are normal in all of these areas; however, cervical and inguinal nodes may normally be as large as 1 cm. Lymph nodes that are large, tender, warm, or red are usually an indication of infection, and the source should be determined. Lymphadenopathy distribution can be characteristic of certain infections (Table 13–6). Generalized lymphadenopathy can be seen in systemic illnesses such as leukemia, salmonellosis, syphilis, mononucleosis, and measles.

Head, Face, and Neck (Excluding Ear, Eye, Nose, and Mouth)

Techniques	**Equipment**
Inspection	Tape measure
Palpation	Flashlight

Examine for

Appearance	Mobility
Size	Paralysis
Shape	Weakness
Symmetry	

Head

Inspection from all angles is necessary to determine the size, shape, and symmetry of the head. The shape of the skull is generally round but may be long or broad. Newborn infants frequently have asymmetric heads owing to intrauterine positioning and to molding, which may occur during the birth process. Size is best determined by obtaining a measurement of head circumference.

Suture lines and fontanels are inspected and palpated during examination of the infant's and young child's head. The head should be carefully palpated to determine whether the suture lines are closed, overriding, or separated at birth. Premature closure of suture lines can vary the shape of the head depending on which sutures are closed. The first 2 years of a child's life are important for brain growth; any sign of premature closure of a suture should be thoroughly investigated.

There are six fontanels, but, generally, only two, the anterior and the posterior, are of clinical significance. Fontanels are inspected and palpated for size, shape, number, and location. They are also palpated and inspected for bulging, tenseness, pulsation, or depression. Occasionally, a third fontanel is also found. It should be evaluated in the same way the anterior and posterior fontanels are. A fontanel that is depressed may indicate malnutrition and dehydration. Children who have a bulging fontanel may have hydrocephaly, meningitis, lead poisoning, vitamin A poisoning, or a subdural hematoma.

Children under 6 months of age may normally have an anterior fontanel over 4 to 5 cm in diameter, but such a size may also be diagnostic of increased intracranial pressure, subdural hematoma, rickets, hypothyroidism, or osteogenesis imperfecta. Small, anterior fontanels should be checked closely for premature closure.

Fontanels are generally diamond-shaped and should be measured in two dimensions: anterior-posterior and horizontal. The examiner uses a tape measure to measure these two dimensions.

The average anterior fontanel may be very small or absent at birth but generally enlarges to an average size of 2.5 cm by 2.5 cm. It should remain open for at least 9 to 10 months to allow for adequate head growth. Approximately 97 per cent of all anterior fontanels close between 9 and 19 months of age. Very large fontanels may not close until 2 years of

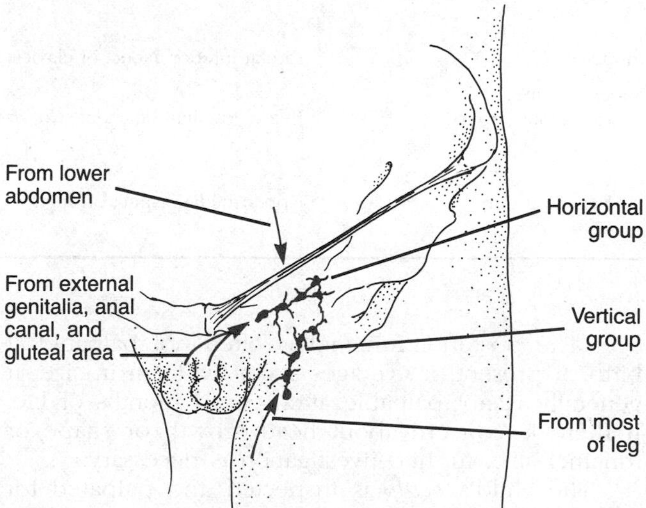

FIGURE 13-11. Lymphatic drainage of the lower torso and leg.

TABLE 13-6
Lymphatic System

Chain	Location	Areas Drained	Clinical Significance of Enlargement
Occipital	At nape (lower occipital bone)	Occipital region of scalp	Pediculosis, seborrhea, tick bites, chickenpox, rubella, external otitis, scalp lesions
Posterior auricular	Mastoid, posterior to pinna	Posterior part of temporoparietal region, pinna, posterior part of external acoustic meatus, scalp, facial skin	Rubella, skin lesions in area drained, external otitis, chickenpox, pediculosis
Preauricular	Directly in front of ear (anterior to tragus), temporal	Face, eye, lateral surface of auricula	Lesions of the eyelids (chalazions), conjunctivitis, infectious skin disorders of the face
Superficial cervical	Chain over sternocleidomastoid muscle at upper section of neck superficially	Tongue, tonsils, pinna, parotid, scalp, neck, thorax	Scalp infections, pediculosis, lesions in areas drained, scarlet fever
Deep cervical (jugular)	Begins with *tonsillar* node at the angle of jaw and continues under sternocleidomastoid muscle, ending posterior to this muscle in supraclavicular chain	Most of tongue, tonsils, pinna, parotid, oropharynx, nose, paranasal sinuses, palate, larynx, trachea, esophagus, middle ear	Tonsillitis, pharyngitis, thyroid disease, inflammatory process of areas drained, scarlet fever
Submaxillary (submandibular)	Beneath body of mandible midway between chin and ear	Medial conjunctiva, cheek, side of nose, upper lip, lateral part of lower lip, gums, submaxillary gland, anterior margin of tonge	Stomatitis, conjunctivitis
Submental	Beneath chin	Central portions of lower lip, floor of mouth, apex of tongue	Dental infections
Tonsillar	The first of the deep cervical chains at angle between ear and jaw	Mouth, pharynx, principal node for tonsil	Tonsillitis, pharyngitis
Parotid	Parotid gland; lateral wall of pharynx at junction of mandible and maxilla; occasionally in subcutaneous tissue over parotid gland	Parotid gland, tissues of face, root of nose, tympanic cavity, eyelids, frontotemporal region, external auditory canal	Parotitis, mumps, tumors
Supraclavicular	Directly over medial area of clavicle	Head, abdomen, breast, thorax, arm, lung	Infection of drained areas
Axillary	Center of axilla	Breast, arm, hand	Infection of breast, arm, or hand
Epitrochlear	Medial surface above elbow	3rd, 4th, and 5th fingers	Congenital syphilis, cat-scratch disease, localized infection of 3rd, 4th, or 5th finger
Infraclavicular	Lateral inferior aspect of clavicle	Hands, arms, chest	Infection of drained areas
Superficial inguinal			
Horizontal group	Below inguinal ligament	Skin of lower abdominal wall, external genitalia except testes, anal canal, gluteal area	Infection of drained area
Vertical group	Upper medial aspect of thigh	Most of leg excluding heel and outer aspect of thigh	Infection of drained area

age. The posterior fontanel is often not palpable at birth. If present, it averages 1 cm by 1 cm in size. It generally is not palpable after 1 to 2 months of life. If there is concern about head growth or shape or fontanel size, further investigation is necessary.

The child's *scalp* is inspected and palpated for scaliness, infections, and hair. Inspect the scalp closely for signs of cradle cap. This can be done by scraping the scalp lightly with a fingertip.

Examine the *hair* as discussed in the section on skin examination. Scalp hair should be examined closely for signs of alopecia, nits, and lice. Excessive hair and low-set hairlines are noted, since they may be indicative of congenital anomalies. The head should be inspected and palpated for any bulges or swellings. Cephalohematomas and caput succedaneum may be seen in the neonatal period (see Chapter 4).

Control, movement, and position of the head are also observed. An infant may be observed for head lag when pulled from a supine to a sitting position. Little or no head lag should be evident after 3 months of age. The position in which the child holds his or her head may also indicate abnormalities. Persistent positioning at an angle may indicate torticollis or visual problems. The head should also be evaluated for full range of motion. The examiner must rotate the head of the neonate for passive range of motion, but, for the older child, the nurse can elicit active range of motion by having the child follow a toy or a bright light. The head should move smoothly from an extended or flexed position and from side to side. Jerky or limited movement warrants further investigation.

Face

The face should be inspected for shape, symmetry, paralysis, placement of features, distribution of hair, and skin color and texture. Symmetry and placement of features should be evaluated from the front and from each side. The eyes should be set at the same level and not set wide apart or close together.

The nose should be midline with symmetric nares; the mouth should be symmetric, and the ears set at the same level on both sides of the head. The top of the pinna (external ear) should meet or cross an imaginary line that extends from the lateral corner of the eye to the most protuberant part of the occiput. This is the eye-occiput line. Ears that do not cross this line are low-set and may indicate hydrocephalus or one of many syndromes, including Potter; trisomy 13, 18, or 21; Turner; DiGeorge; Pierre Robin; and others.

Facial mobility and symmetry of facial movement should be closely observed. This is easily done when an infant cries or yawns. Older children can smile and wrinkle their foreheads so that the examiner can check for paralysis. The skin and underlying tissue should be palpated for edema. Twitchings and tics should also be looked for and noted. Facial coloring is observed, and any evidence of pallor, jaundice, cyanosis, or any unusual marking is noted.

Neck

Following examination of the head and face, the neck is inspected for control, mobility, pulsations, symmetry, size, and shape. Palpation of the neck is used to determine strength, pulsations, and position of structures such as the thyroid and the trachea. The sternocleidomastoid and trapezius muscles are palpated for tone and presence of any masses or hematomas. Strength of these muscles is evaluated by having the child move them against the resistance of the nurse's hands. Range of motion should also be determined. A child with any nuchal rigidity (neck stiffness) should be referred for evaluation. Enlarged veins or excessive pulsations can indicate cardiac problems.

The *trachea* is inspected and palpated to determine whether it is midline. The examiner inspects the neck hyperextended and then palpates the trachea, beginning at the suprasternal notch and moving upward. The thumb is placed on one side of the tracheal rings and the index and middle fingers on the other side to evaluate the tracheal rings and determine whether the trachea is deviated. A shift from the midline could indicate a serious problem.

Palpation of the *thyroid gland* requires instruction and practice. For assessment, the thyroid is inspected and palpated. Inspection takes place in the hyperextended position. The examiner looks for bulges, asymmetry, or enlargement. With the neck tilted slightly forward, the examiner palpates for the hyoid bone, cricoid and thyroid cartilages, thyroid isthmus, and finally lobes of the thyroid gland (Fig. 13–12). The thyroid is palpated with the child in a supine or sitting position. The thumb is placed on one side of the thyroid and the index and middle fingers on the opposite side. In the older child, the examiner may stand behind the seated child and place the index and middle fingers of each hand on the sides of the thyroid. Having the child swallow some water moves the thyroid upward and allows for better palpation. Any nodules, enlargement, or tenderness of the thyroid gland should be considered abnormal; these signs warrant further evaluation.

Examination of the *lymph nodes* is done during the examination of the neck. The examiner generally begins with palpation of the occipital nodes and progresses to the posterior auricular and preauricular lymph nodes. The examiner then continues to the anterior and posterior cervical triangles. See Figure 13–8 for locations of these nodes.

Finally, any hoarseness or stridor of the *voice* is noted. An infant's cry is evaluated for its quality. A

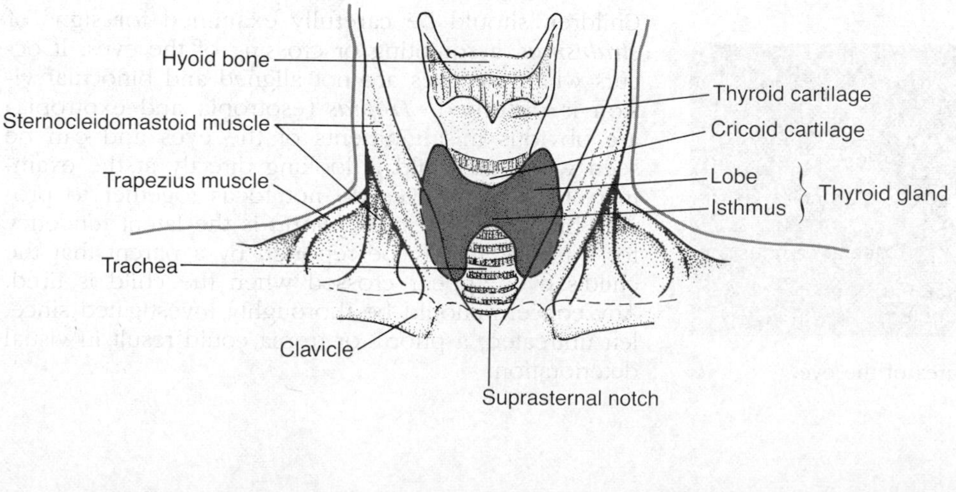

FIGURE 13 - 12. Structures of the neck.

high-pitched cry, a catlike cry, or a low, hoarse cry is an indication of abnormalities. The older child is evaluated for voice quality and speech.

Eye

Techniques	Equipment
Inspection	Ophthalmoscope
Palpation	Flashlight
	Tool for testing vision

Examine for	
Appearance	Color
Size	Mobility
Shape	Function

Examination of the eye (Fig. 13–13) begins with the *eyelids,* which are inspected for ptosis, edema, redness, or epicanthal folds. They should also be inspected for any lesions. Edema of the lids may indicate serious problems such as renal failure, or it may be caused by allergies, injuries, drugs, or infection.

Presence or absence of eyelashes is determined, as are their color and texture. The nasolacrimal duct should be inspected for patency, position, redness, and swelling. Eyes that tear excessively or have any discharge should be investigated further. Excessive tearing before the age of 3 months may be due to a blocked nasolacrimal duct. It may also result from infections, a foreign body, allergies, or exophthalmos.

Next, the *conjunctivae* (Fig. 13–14) are examined for color, moisture, and integrity. The *palpebral conjunctivae,* which line the upper and lower lids, are easily inspected. To examine the lower conjunctiva, the lower lid is pulled down while the child looks up. The upper lid is examined by gently pulling the eyelashes down and forward while the child looks up. The *bulbar conjunctiva* covers the surface of the eye up to the corneal circumference. Normally it is transparent but it can appear red when its blood vessels are dilated secondary to inflammation or irritation. Overall, the conjunctivae are examined for pallor, inflammation, injection, and abnormal lesions or growth.

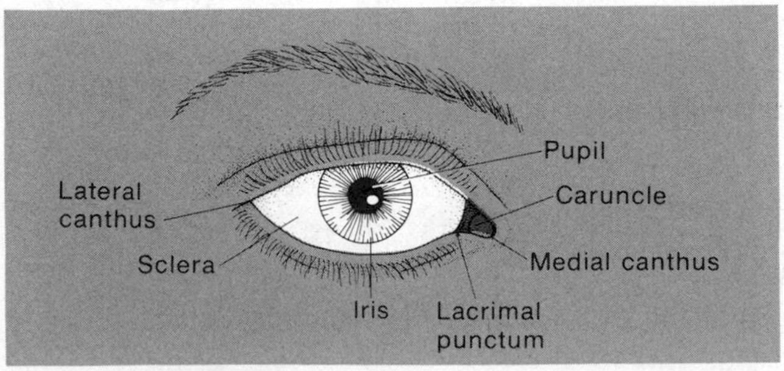

FIGURE 13 - 13. Structures of the eye.

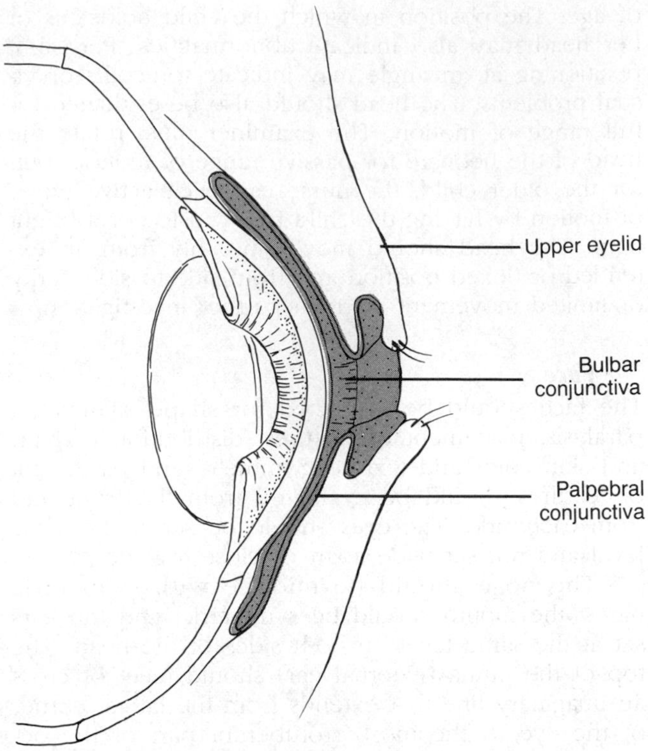

FIGURE 13 - 14. Examine the *palpebral* and *bulbar conjunctivae* for color, moisture, and integrity.

The *orbit of the eye* is also assessed. Children with sunken, blank eyes may be severely ill or malnourished. Small orbits usually indicate underlying pathology. Inspection of the eye orbits also determines hypotelorism or hypertelorism (abnormal width between the eyes). The globe of the eye and the ridges are palpated for tenderness, turgor, and swelling. Exophthalmos, bulging of the eye, and endophthalmos, sunken eyes, are significant findings and should be referred for evaluation.

The *full range of motion* of the extraocular muscles is evaluated by having the child follow an object to each of the six visual fields (Fig. 13–15). The eyes are observed closely for smooth, symmetric tracking and any sign of nystagmus.

Strabismus Screening

Children should be carefully examined for signs of *strabismus,* a squinting or crossing of the eyes. It occurs when the eyes are not aligned and binocular vision is disturbed. *Tropias* (esotropia and exotropia) are obvious misalignments of the eyes and can be seen when the child is looking directly at the examiner. The child's eyes do not focus together to provide binocular vision. A *phoria* is the latent tendency for a tropia. It may be reported by a parent that the child's eyes appear crossed when the child is tired. Any concern should be thoroughly investigated since, left untreated, a phoria or tropia could result in visual deterioration.

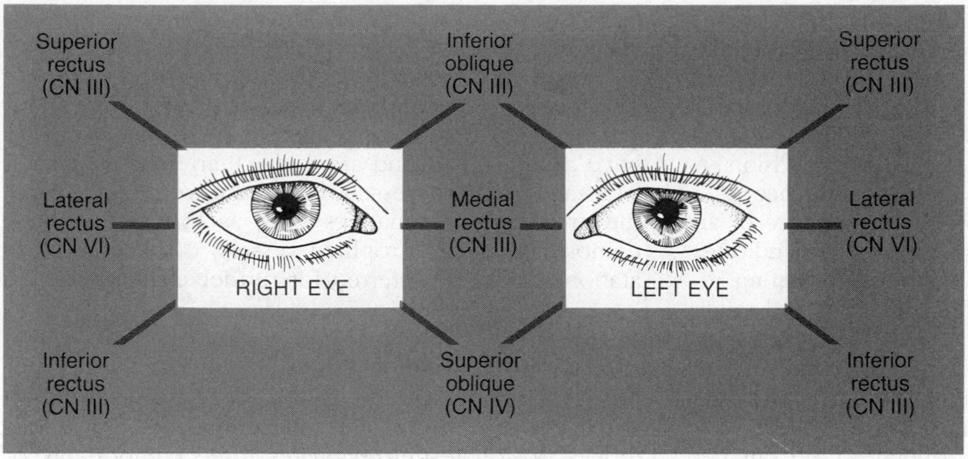

FIGURE 13 - 15. The visual fields of extraocular movement. If the child's eye is unable to move to any one of the positions, dysfunction of either that muscle or the cranial nerve (CN) is suspected. (A young child may not be able to follow instructions to move only the eyes; the nurse then should hold the child's head still.)

Two tests are commonly used to detect strabismus. The corneal light reflex (Hirschberg test) is one of the most important screening tests to determine a tropia. The cover test is another screening test to help rule out a tropia or a phoria. The *symmetry of the corneal light reflex (Hirschberg test)* is determined by shining a penlight at the bridge of the nose while the child looks straight ahead. Inspection of the child's eyes should then be done to determine whether the reflection of light falls at the same point on each pupil. Any deviation indicates strabismus or trophia.

A *cover test* can also be done by holding a light 12 inches from the child's eyes and asking the child to focus on the light. The examiner occludes one of the child's eyes, making sure that both eyes remain open, and observes the uncovered eye for movement inward or outward. The occluder is then moved quickly over the other eye, and the eye that had been covered is inspected for any inward or outward deviation. The test is then done on the other eye and rechecked a number of times at each examination. Normally, no deviation occurs in either eye. The cover test is repeated having the child focus on a distant object. A cover test can be done on even the youngest child by having a bright, flashing object to attract attention. Older children can focus on the examiner's finger or on a picture placed on the wall.

Children having a wide nasal bridge or epicanthal folds may appear to have strabismus. This is referred to as *pseudostrabismus*. A negative cover test and an equal corneal light reflex rule out actual strabismus. If, however, there is any question of the possibility of strabismus, the child must be referred for evaluation.

The *cornea, sclera, iris, and pupil* are considered to compose the eye proper and are examined next. The cornea is inspected for clouding, enlargement, abrasions, lesions, or change in color. Abrasions or lesions are best observed by shining a light from the side across the eye. The sclera is observed for color, hemorrhage, or discoloration. The sclera of neonates is often light blue because of its thinness, but a dark blue sclera can indicate osteogenesis imperfecta or glaucoma. A yellow sclera is often the first clinical sign of jaundice.

The iris and pupil are examined together. The size, shape, and color of the irises are noted. Any freckles, spots, or other irregularities should be noted. Pupils are examined for size, shape, equality, reaction to light, and accommodation. A difference in pupil size may be normal but can also be caused by central nervous system damage. The pupillary reaction to light can be performed by shining a light directly in the eye and noting the response—whether the pupil constricts. Additionally, the nurse should shine a light in one eye and note whether the opposite pupil also constricts. Accommodation—a change in dilatation and medial movements of both pupils—can be tested even in the young child by having the child focus on a brightly colored object at a distance and then quickly bringing the object toward the eyes. The pupils constrict as the object is brought close to the eyes and dilate when the child focuses on the object at a distance. The eyes are accommodating from far to near vision. An older child can be asked to look far off into the distance, then to focus on an object 12 to 14 inches from the eyes.

Funduscopic Examination

The remaining parts of the examination of the eye are done on older, cooperative children. Skill in the use of an ophthalmoscope to examine the fundus requires instruction and practice. Once that skill is achieved, the nurse may examine the eyegrounds.

Examinations of the lens, cornea, and retina are done in a semidark room. An explanation for the dimming of the lights will help put the child at ease. The examiner holds the ophthalmoscope in the right hand and looks into the right eye of the child. Examination of the left eye is accomplished by reversing the process. The child should be instructed to focus on a fixed object such as a fluorescent sticker on the wall.

The remainder of the examination begins with observation of the lens. The *lens* is examined by shining a light on the eyes and inspecting the lens for opacities. Next comes the examination of the retina. The ophthalmoscope is dialed to 0. The examination begins by focusing the light into the child's eyes at a distance of about 12 inches from a position that is about 15 degrees to the side of the line of vision. A *red reflex* is obtained at this time. An absence of a complete, circular red reflex or the appearance of an opaque density surrounded by a red reflex indicates a cataract or other pathologic condition requiring referral to a physician. In nonwhite races the red reflex is normally paler and may have a pink or salmon appearance. Examination of the fundus of the eye (Fig. 13–16) requires a child who is cooperative and able to hold the eyes still and focused on an object for a short period. If the child can cooperate, the examiner approaches from 12 inches (used to obtain a red reflex) to within 3 inches of the child. As the examiner approaches the child, each layer of the eye is inspected, beginning with the cornea, progressing to the lens, and then on to the vitreous. As the examiner moves in, the dial of the ophthalmoscope is turned to smaller numbers until red minus numbers are reached. The exact number will depend on the refractive ability of the examiner's eyes and the child's eyes.

During the internal examination of the fundus, the *optic disk* is located and observed for size, shape, color, margins, and physiologic depression. The disk is usually round but may, occasionally, be vertically oval. The disk is creamy pink or pale yellow and has a depression slightly temporal of the center that is the physiologic cup. The margins should be smooth and slightly darker than the rest of the disk.

The *macula* is a small circular area located 2 disk diameters temporal to the optic disk with the *fovea centralis* seen as a gleaming light in its center. The *fundus* is normally orange-red and should be uniform throughout. Lightness and darkness in color varies

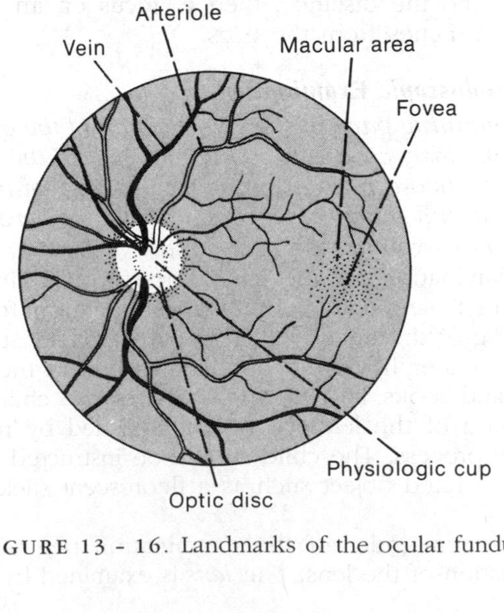

FIGURE 13-16. Landmarks of the ocular fundus.

from one race to another. The fundus should be inspected for signs of hemorrhage or papilledema.

The *arteries and veins* should also be examined. The arteries are narrower than the veins and exhibit a light reflex from their center. Veins do not normally have a light reflex and are wider than arteries, with a 3:2 ratio. As the vessels cross, the veins are under the arteries. Abnormalities such as tortuous vessels, hemorrhages, hypertrophied vessels, or excessive dilatation should be referred for further evaluation.

Assessing Visual Acuity

Finally, visual capacity is tested. Vision screening should begin early in life and continue at regular intervals. Vision testing evaluates three components of vision: light perception, visual acuity, and color perception. Light perception is tested generally in the newborn infant by shining a light into the eyes and noting responses such as blinking, following the light, and increased alertness. A rotating black-and-white–striped drum placed in front of the neonate's face should cause nystagmus if vision is present. The nurse should be aware of signs that may indicate visual loss, such as fixed pupils, marked strabismus, constant nystagmus, and "setting-sun" sign (this sign is characterized by the white of the eye showing between the iris and the edge of the upper eyelid).

Visual acuity is defined as the ability to see near and far objects clearly. There are a variety of tools that can be used to test visual acuity (Table 13–7). Figure 13–17 gives examples of two types of visual acuity charts.

Whatever test is employed, appropriate test techniques should always be used. These items are essential for reliable testing:

- There should be adequate illumination and no glare on the eye chart.
- The chart should be at the child's eye level.
- Children should be tested individually so they do not memorize the chart while they are waiting to be examined.
- Children should be preeducated for the vision test: have children stand a few feet away from the chart and explain what they should do.
- Learn the names the children use for symbols if a picture chart is being used.
- Cover the nontest eye with an occluder or a paper cup. Prevent the child from closing that eye during the examination.
- Begin the test with an easily read line and move on to a more difficult one.
- Use two examiners if necessary: one to point to the chart and one to occlude the child's nontesting eye.
- Expose one line of letters, Es, or symbols at a time.

TABLE 13-7
Tools for Testing Visual Activity

Tool	Use	Comments
Snellen Alphabet Chart (8 lines of letters in decreasing sizes)	Children and adolescents who are familiar with the alphabet	Person being examined stands with heels 20 ft from chart. Examiner asks child, who has one eye covered, to read one line at a time. Reading the majority of letters in the line being tested constitutes a passing score. Visual acuity is noted as the line value (line 7–10 ft, line 8–15 ft) over a denominator of 20
Snellen E Chart (8 lines of Es pointing in four different directions. Es decrease in size)	Clients unfamiliar with alphabet; or non–English-speaking clients. Often too difficult for children <6 yrs	Same as Snellen Alphabet Chart. Sometimes helpful to refer to the E as a table and ask child to indicate which direction table legs point
Titmus Vision Tester (machine that has Snellen Alphabet Chart and Snellen E Chart as well as a tool used to test for amblyopia)	Same candidate as eligible for Snellen Alphabet and Snellen E	Advantages of using it are (a) light source is controlled, (b) less distracting than testing in a room or hallway, and (c) can be used in a small area
STYCAR Chart (the nine letters H, C, O, L, U, T, X, V, A are on a chart. The child has a card with the same nine letters. The child points to the letter which matches the one being pointed to on the chart)	For preschoolers	Children can easily recognize these letters
Allen Cards (a series of cards with simple black-and-white pictures of familiar objects —e.g., telephone, Christmas tree, car, birthday cake)	Older toddlers and preschool children	Examiner starts examination approximately 20 ft from child. If child cannot identify the symbols, examiner moves to 15 ft distance and so forth. The distance in feet at which the child is able to recognize three of the pictures determines the numerator over the denominator of 30. A child who has a visual acuity difference of 5 ft between eyes should be referred
Picture charts—e.g., Kindergarten Chart, California Clown Test, Osterberg Chart (lines of symbols with which young child should be familiar [e.g. heart, circle, star, sailboat]. Symbols decrease in size. These charts are not as well standardized as the Snellen Charts)	Preschoolers and kindergarteners. May be used with non–English-speaking children if someone can interpret their labels for the items	Same as Snellen Alphabet. Children may identify a symbol by an unusual name—e.g., circle may be a "tire," a "doughnut," or a "hole." Examiner need only know what the child's label is

Visual acuity becomes increasingly organized as the child develops. Most infants are able to see objects clearly at close range, usually 10 to 14 inches, roughly the distance between a mother's breast and her face. Binocular vision is clearly established between 4 and 7 months of age, and mature function of the eye muscles is generally developed by 1 year of age. The infant's vision can be evaluated by watching the child's ability to focus and follow brightly colored objects or a light. The infant should be followed closely for any signs of developmental delay or an obvious lack of response to the environment, which could indicate visual problems.

Children have better vision than was previously believed. See Table 45–3 for visual acuity at various ages. Any child who does not have the visual acuity expected for his or her age should be referred. Also, any child who has a two-line difference between eyes should have further evaluation (e.g., OD 20/20, OS 20/40). This may indicate poorer vision in the one eye, which may be compensated for, resulting in eventual loss of vision in the deficient eye if this is not corrected.

Finally, color vision is assessed in every child, usually at preschool age. Although color vision deficit is rare in females, it is important to determine the child's ability to determine colors. The child who has a color vision deficit will need counseling for safety purposes such as interpreting traffic signals and, later, regarding occupational choices. This child will also need assistance in developing the ability to coordinate colors of wearing apparel so that ridicule by peers does not become a problem. The Ishihara Plates have figures composed of dots hidden in a background of similar dots. The figure is a different color so that the only way to distinguish the figure is by color. These plates are useful for children who have the skills to discriminate figure ground, letters, numbers, and geometric figures. The younger child may not be able to do this. Other tests such as match-

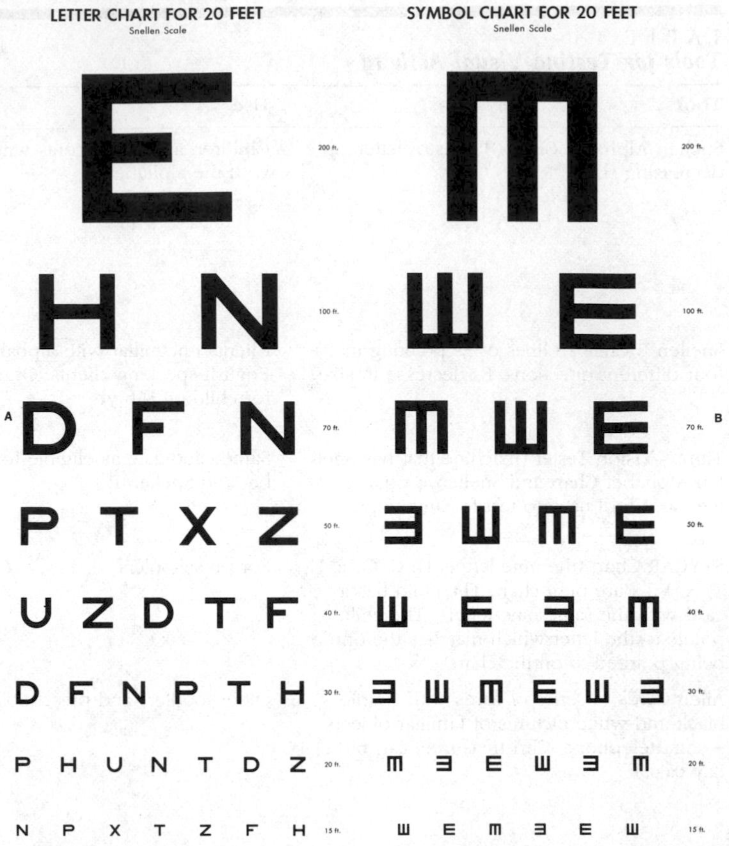

FIGURE 13 - 17. Two types of visual acuity charts. The standard Snellen alphabet chart (left) can be used as early as the child's ability to name letters allows. The Snellen "E" chart can be used with younger children. The child is asked to point with hand or fingers in the direction the E points. (Courtesy of Prevent Blindness America [formerly National Society to Prevent Blindness].)

ing colored yarns or putting colored tennis balls in similarly colored muffin-tin compartments can be used; however, the Ishihara test is a standardized color vision test.

Ear

Techniques	Equipment
Inspection	Otoscope
Palpation	Cerumen spoon
Examine for	
Appearance	Placement
Shape	Condition of the tympanic membrane
Position	

Examination of the ears begins with inspection for shape, position, and placement of the *external ears*. The pinna should cross the eye-occiput line and should be within a 10-degree angle of a perpendicular line drawn from the eye-occiput line to the lobe (Fig. 13–18). The pinna is also inspected for color and structural anomalies. Mumps, mastoiditis, cellulitis, or congenital anomalies may cause the auricle to stand out. The pinna is palpated for cartilage formation, masses, tenderness, and cysts.

The bony prominence located immediately posterior to the ear lobe is the *mastoid process*. This area is inspected and palpated for erythema, swelling, and tenderness. The outer canal of the ear is then inspected for discharge. Bloody discharge is seen with a perforated tympanic membrane, foreign body in the canal, irritation or scratching of the canal, or basilar skull fracture. Purulent drainage commonly denotes a fungal or bacterial infection.

Otoscopic Examination

Internal structures are examined with the aid of an otoscope. Use of an otoscope requires instruction and supervision until the skill is mastered.

The procedure is usually painless unless an infection or furuncle exists in the ear canal or the otoscope touches the bony part of the ear canal. Children may become anxious during this part of the examination, but giving adequate explanations and allowing time for the child to become familiar with the instrument often alleviate anxiety.

Restraining a Child. A child who is not able to cooperate should be adequately restrained. The young infant can be placed on the examining table prone with the head to one side. The examiner can retract the pinna with the left hand and keep the head still while holding the otoscope in the right hand. The

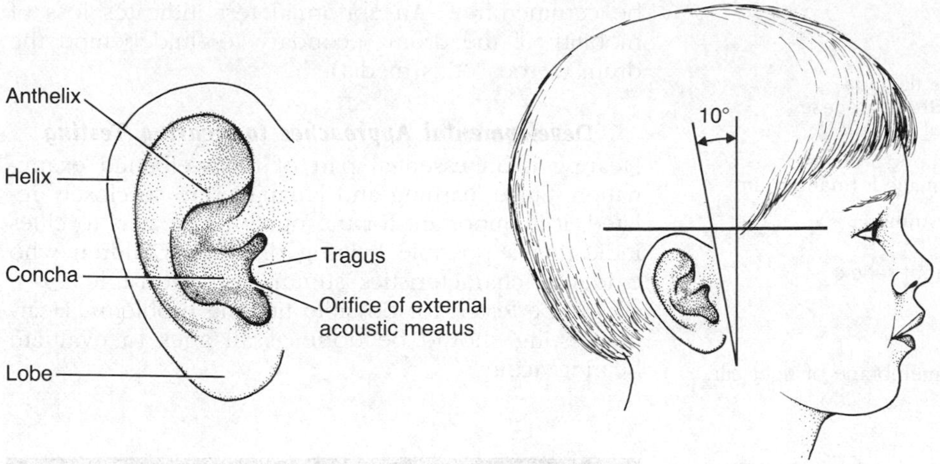

FIGURE 13-18. The parts of the external ear, and its normal placement on the head. The pinna should cross the eye-occiput line and be within a 10-degree angle of a perpendicular line drawn from the lobe to the eye-occiput line.

otoscope is held like a pencil with the right side of the hand and fifth finger resting on the child's head to cushion the otoscope if the child's head should move. The toddler or preschool child can sit on the parent's lap with the legs held firmly between the parent's legs. The parent places an arm firmly across the child's trunk and arms, and the other arm is used to hold the child's head firmly against the parent's chest (see Fig. 13–4). A child of this age can also be restrained while lying supine on an examination table with the arms extended above the head and held firmly by the parent. The examiner then leans over the child's trunk and restrains the head to one side. The examiner should be careful not to put weight on the child's chest; this could frighten the child and cause respiratory distress. Children who will sit on the examination table need only to tilt their heads to one side to allow for better visualization.

Examination. Once the child has been appropriately restrained, the ear canal may be examined. The ear canal is normally curved and must be straightened before the nurse can visualize the *canal and tympanic membrane.* In infants and toddlers, the auricle is pulled down, and in the child over 3 years of age, the auricle is pulled up and back to straighten the ear canal (Fig. 13–19). The canal is then examined internally for erythema, lesions, furuncles, or discharge. The amount and consistency of cerumen are also noted and described. If the cerumen obscures the view of the tympanic membrane, it can be removed using a cerumen spoon. *This should be done only after the examiner has been instructed in the proper technique.*

Once the canal has been inspected, the examiner proceeds to the tympanic membrane. The tympanic membrane is assessed for color, landmarks, and mobility. A normal tympanic membrane is a light, pearly-gray color. An erythematous membrane may be seen in the child who has been crying or the child with otitis media. A dull gray or yellowish color is often seen with serous otitis, and a vivid red in suppurative

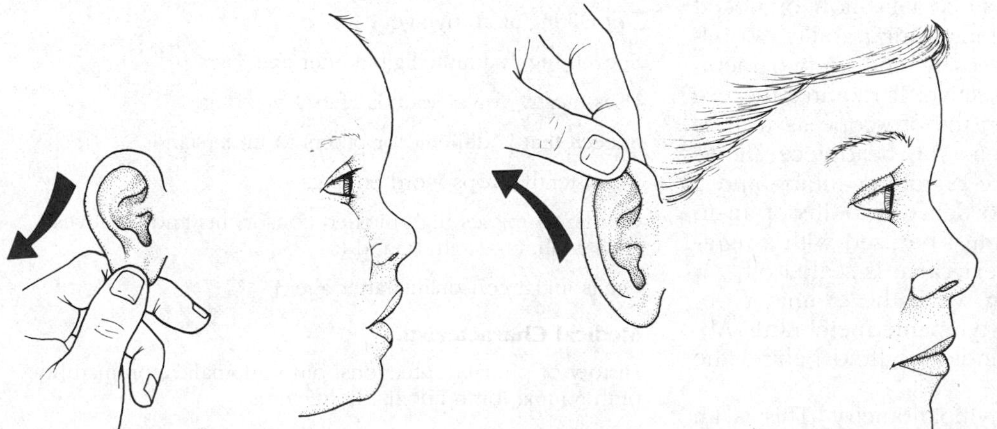

FIGURE 13-19. To straighten the ear canal, the auricle is pulled down in infants and children less than 3 years of age. In the older child, it is pulled up and back.

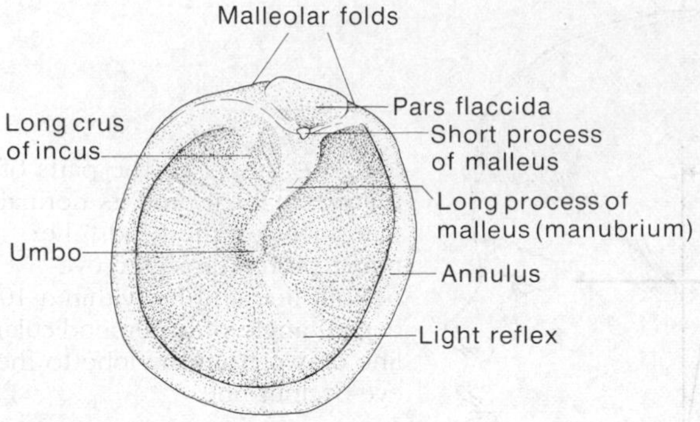

FIGURE 13-20. Normal tympanic membrane of right ear.

otitis. The landmarks are the umbo, light reflex, long process, short process, pars flaccida, annulus, and the anterior and posterior malleolar folds (Fig. 13–20).

The *light reflex* is a small, triangular cone of light that is seen at the anterior inferior quadrant. It is located directly below the umbo. A diffuse, spotty, or absent cone of light may indicate infection or fluid in the middle ear. The umbo, found at the top of the cone of light, appears as a round, white fibrous area. The long process (handle of malleus) can be seen above and nasally of the umbo. The short process of the malleus looks like a sharp, white, protuberant bone through the membrane. When the membrane is retracted, the landmarks appear more pronounced; bulging makes them more obscure. A bulging or retracted tympanic membrane requires further investigation.

The *annulus* is a white fibrous ring surrounding the periphery of the eardrum. The three small bones or ossicles (malleus, incus, and stapes) lie directly behind the membrane. The incus and stapes may be seen only if the drum is very translucent or is retracted.

Evaluating the *mobility of the tympanic membrane* is useful in determining the presence or absence of fluid in the middle ear. Fluid will cause the membrane to move in a restricted fashion or not at all, thus decreasing conduction hearing ability. Mobility of the eardrum is assessed by one of two methods. The first method is subjective. It requires the use of a pneumatic headpiece on the otoscope as well as an ear canal free of cerumen. The headpiece allows for the attachment of a piece of rubber tubing and a bulb that can be squeezed to deliver a bolus of air to the tympanic membrane. It must be used with a tight-fitting speculum so that the ear canal is sealed off. Air is puffed through the tubing while the examiner observes the movement of the tympanic membrane. Absent or decreased mobility indicates fluid behind the membrane.

The second method is tympanometry. This is an objective test that uses a specialized piece of equipment call a *tympanometer*. The tympanometer measures the mobility of the eardrum (see Table 45–16). The test is painless and the canal does not have to be cerumen-free. An abnormal test indicates loss of mobility of the drum secondary to fluid behind the drum (serous otitis media).

Developmental Approaches to Hearing Testing

Hearing is an essential part of the well-child examination. Since learning and language are so closely related, it is important for the nurse to be alert to clues indicating a possible hearing disorder. Children who evidence characteristics summarized in Table 13–8 should be tested for possible hearing problems. Hearing testing should be done at all ages to evaluate hearing acuity.

TABLE 13-8
Characteristics of Children Who May Have Hearing or Language Deficits

Response to Auditory Stimuli
(See Table 13–9 for normal development of hearing responses
Inattentive to speech
Does not react with a startle to loud noises during first year
Does not react to name or commands by 6–9 mos
Does not turn to source of sound by 4 mos
Does not understand commands or instructions by 18 mos
Inconsistent responses to environmental sounds during first 2 years of life
Turns up volume on radio or TV
Voice Characteristics
Voice quality is poor
Voice is loud or monotone
Speech Characteristics
Babbles normally until 6 mos then gradually decreases sound production
Not talking at all by age 2 yrs
Speech highly unintelligible after age 3 yrs
Uses mostly vowel sounds after 1 yr of age
Speech that is difficult for others to understand
Consistently drops word endings
Constantly misses high-pitched consonants and fricatives such as th, ch, s, sh, b, and k
Omits initial consonants after age 3
Medical Characteristics
History of prenatal infections, birth anomalies, prematurity, birth trauma, birth anoxia, kernicterus
History of treatment with ototoxic drugs during infancy
Familial history of congenital hearing impairment
History of frequent upper respiratory or ear infections

TABLE 13-9
Development of Hearing Responses

Age	Hearing Response
Birth	Startle reflex; blinking of eyes; attends to voice
12 wks	Eye movement toward sound when prone
12–18 wks	Eye movement toward sound when upright
4 mos	Widening of eyes; quieting; listening posture; slight head turning; looks in same direction as sound
6 mos	Turns head to source of sound; may have beginning localization; downward localization occurs before upward localization
8–12 mos	Turns head 45 degrees or more in direction of sound; localizes sound source above and below; rapid automatic response to sound by one year
12–36 mos	Rapid speech development and language patterns based on hearing input

For *young infants and toddlers,* testing is often accomplished by using a noisemaker. The child is seated on the parent's lap and distracted visually from the front. A noisemaker is then used to one side. The child should be distracted visually by one examiner while another examiner produces the sound to one side at 18 to 24 inches from the child. The first examiner observes for the response. Table 13–9 summarizes the characteristic responses of infants who can hear.

The sounds produced should be of high, medium, and low frequency and should be repeated on each side. The examiner should reproduce the sound approximately 8 to 12 inches above and below the level of the ear to determine whether the child can localize the sound.

Toddlers and preschoolers are difficult to examine for hearing, but it is important that adequate hearing testing is done since hearing is critical to appropriate speech development. Play audiometry is used for children over 15 months of age. The child can be tested with or without earphones; however, more specific information about each ear is gathered if the child will allow earphone testing. The child is conditioned through a play technique to respond to sound stimuli. Once the child has been conditioned to respond to the sound, by dropping the block in a box or putting a ring on a peg, the examiner can test the child with the earphones in place. Often the examiner puts several toys in front of the child, places the earphones on the child, and then requests that the child pick up a certain toy. This is done at certain frequencies and decibels. The child's responses are then recorded. By 3 to 4 years of age, the child can frequently have routine pure-tone audiometric testing with a minimum of preparation. Hearing and hearing loss are further discussed in Chapter 45.

Tuning forks can also be used to identify conductive or neurosensory hearing loss. This can be done only on an older child (at least 5 years of age) who can follow directions and give appropriate responses. The Weber test is performed by placing an activated tuning fork on the midline of the skull. The child should indicate whether the sound can be heard equally in both ears or if it is localized to one ear. If the sound is lateralized to one ear, that ear may have a conductive hearing loss. Room noise is blocked out because of the impairment; therefore vibrations are detected better than normally. In unilateral sensorineural loss, the lateralization is to the unimpaired ear. The inner ear or nerve is affected; therefore, vibrations are not as well detected from the bone. The sound is heard better in the unaffected ear.

The Rinne test is performed by striking the tuning fork and placing the stem on the mastoid process until the child indicates that the sound can no longer be heard. The tuning fork, still vibrating, is then placed 1 to 2 inches from the ear opening. The child is asked if the sound can still be heard. The vibrations should be heard in the air longer than the vibration on the bone because air conduction is two times longer than bone conduction. Any child who cannot hear the sound via air conduction longer than via bone conduction should be referred to a physician.

Audiometric Testing

Although the information received from using tuning forks is very helpful, it is not a precise assessment of the child's hearing. Audiometric hearing testing is the most reliable method to evaluate hearing. Pure-tone audiometry is done by presenting electronically generated pure tones of various frequencies and intensities to a child through earphones. Children are instructed to raise their hands as soon as they hear the sound. For children younger than 5 years of age, a play activity should be substituted for raising the hand. The child should not be able to see the audiometer controls. The usual procedure is to present the various frequencies at an intensity of 20 to 25 dB; however, a 15- to 20-dB tone is required to identify minor hearing loss caused by otitis media. Testing at 15 dB is often not done because it requires a more soundproof room than can be created in an unspecialized clinical setting. Various methods of testing are used. Downs (1981) recommends this procedure:

- Present a pure tone of 50 dB at 1000 Hz; this acquaints the child with the procedure. Praise the child for correctly raising a hand.
- Set the dial to 15 dB and present tones at 1000, 2000, and 4000 Hz to one ear.
- Switch ears; present tones in reverse sequence: 4000, 2000, and 1000 Hz.

Test results are marked on a standardized graph for each frequency. A child who fails to respond to any of the tones at 15 dB in either ear fails the test. The child should be retested later in the same day; if failure occurs again, referral is necessary.

Nose

Techniques	Equipment
Inspection	Otoscope with nasal speculum
Palpation	
Percussion	
Auscultation	
Examine for	
Appearance	Condition of mucosa
Shape	Secretions
Patency of nares	Sinus discomfort

Determining whether the child is breathing through the nose or through the mouth is the first step in the examination of the nose. *Patency of the nares* of the newborn is assessed by placing the diaphragm of the stethoscope against one naris while blocking the other naris and listening for breath sounds. Since infants are nose-breathers, an infant who does not have patent nasal passages may experience respiratory distress. Flaring of the nares also indicates respiratory distress and can be caused by obstruction, pneumonia, and fever. A child who mouth-breathes may have nasal polyps, allergies, enlarged adenoids, or a deviated septum.

The *shape* of the nose is inspected. A flat or saddle-shaped nose is seen in some races. It may also be indicative of congenital anomalies. A crease across the nose may be a result of the allergic salute, in which a child frequently pushes against the tip of the nose because of rhinitis or itching. The nose is also palpated for tenderness and stability.

Internal examination of the nose requires a penlight or an otoscope with a nasal speculum. The otoscope provides a better visualization of the internal structures. The examiner gently pushes the tip of the nose up and places the speculum at the opening of the naris to inspect the *nasal mucosa*. Normal mucosa is pink and moist. Inflamed mucosa indicates irritation or infection. Pale, boggy mucosa is seen in children with allergies, and swollen, gray mucosa indicates chronic rhinitis.

The examiner also determines the type and amount of *nasal secretions*. Thin, watery secretions are seen in children with allergies, upper respiratory infections, or foreign bodies high in the nose. Purulent discharge is commonly seen with nasal and sinus infections or foreign bodies that have been lodged for a time. Nasal bleeding occurs at the Kesselbach plexus, which is located at the anterior tip of the septum. Trauma, allergies, dry climate, or blood dyscrasias will cause epistaxis from this point.

The *septum* should be inspected for deviations or perforations. Septal deviations are seen rarely in children. The examiner should also inspect the turbinates and meatal openings. Any swelling, color change, or discharge should be noted.

Finally, *palpation and percussion of the sinuses* are performed. The maxillary and ethmoid sinuses are developed in infancy. The frontal sinuses develop around 7 to 8 years of age, whereas the sphenoid sinuses do not develop until after puberty. Firm pressure is applied along the supraorbital ridge and maxillary area, and on the infraorbital ridge nasally (Fig. 13–21). Any indication of tenderness with percussion or palpation may indicate a sinus infection.

Mouth and Throat

Techniques	Equipment
Inspection	Otoscope or penlight
Palpation	Tongue depressor
Percussion	Disposable glove
Examine for	
Color	Number and condition of teeth
Moisture	Condition of gums
Clefts	Condition and mobility of uvula
Lesions	Condition and mobility of tongue
Odor	
Edema	
Bleeding	

Examination of the mouth (Fig. 13–22) is often difficult and traumatic for the child. This part of the examination, along with the otoscopic examination, may be done last. An attempt is always made to gain the cooperation of a child of any age. An uncooperative child should be adequately restrained to allow for a safe examination. The infant can be examined while in the supine position, arms held above the head. The young child can sit on the parent's lap and be restrained in the same way as was described for otoscopic examination. The older child generally needs no restraint if time is taken to explain the procedure and acquaint the child with the equipment. A tongue depressor and a good light source are essential for this portion of the examination.

Examination begins with *inspection of the lips* for color, moisture, size, shape, asymmetry, drooping, fissures, clefts, edema, or lesions. In addition, the lips and the surrounding area are inspected for pallor or cyanosis. Cherry-red lips are seen in children with acidosis or carbon monoxide poisoning. Unusual mouth odors should be noted, because they can be clinically significant. Unusual odors are present in children with poor oral hygiene, dental caries, sinusitis, allergies, diabetic acidosis, and malnutrition.

Teeth are inspected for number, type, position, caries, malocclusions, color, and hygiene. Children have two sets of teeth; the first teeth, or deciduous teeth, begin to erupt around 6 months of age. All 20 of the deciduous teeth usually have erupted by 2½ to

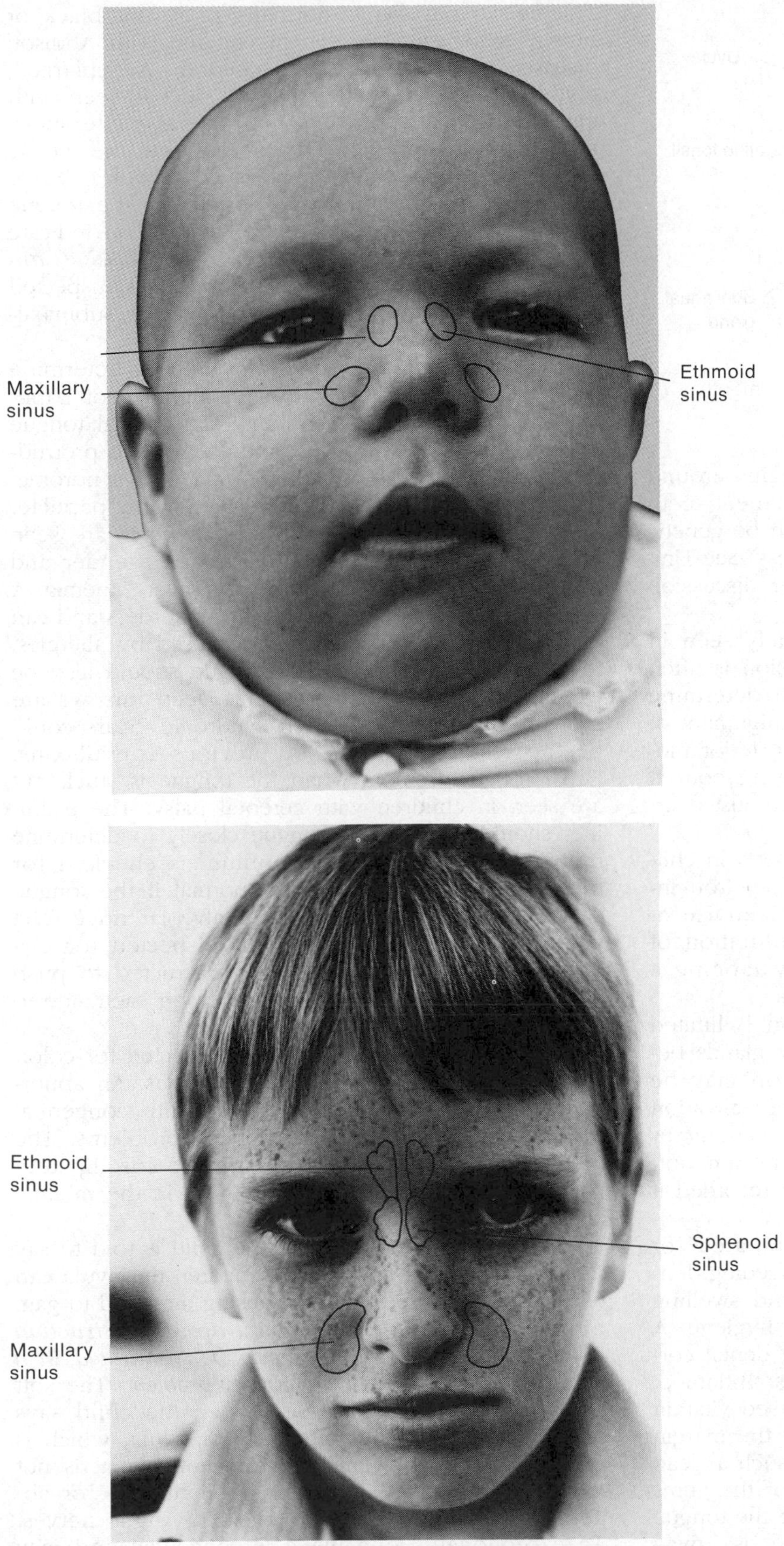

FIGURE 13 - 21. Facial sinuses indicated on an infant and a child.

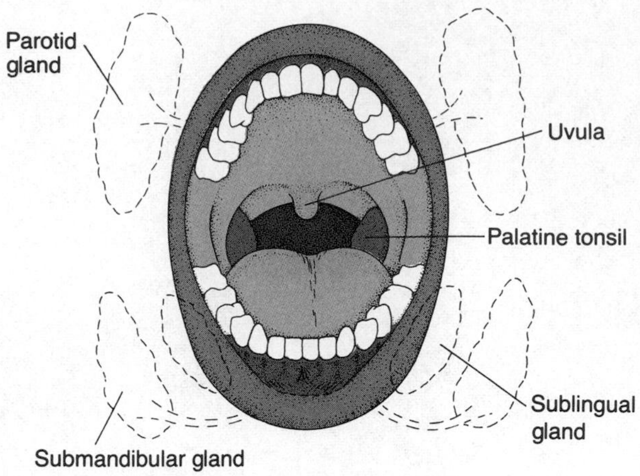

FIGURE 13 - 22. Structures of the child's mouth.

3 years of age. Permanent dentition begins around age 6 and progresses until all 32 permanent teeth have erupted. Delay in tooth eruption can be genetic or significant of underlying disease process. See Unit 2—Growth and Development for further discussion of teeth eruption.

Teeth with flattened edges are usually seen in children who grind their teeth. Malocclusion is often caused by persistent thumbsucking. To determine malocclusion, the examiner inspects the alignment of the teeth. In normal occlusion the top posterior molars meet and rest snugly on the opposing bottom molars, and then the upper central incisors just overlap and touch the lower incisors.

Teeth that are mottled or pitted are seen in children who have ingested excessive fluoride. Iron ingestion, antibiotic ingestion, or severe jaundice at birth can cause a green or black discoloration of teeth. A tooth should be percussed by tapping a tongue depressor on the crown and sides.

Salivation is noted. Salivary secretion is limited until 3 months of age, when the salivary glands become more active. Absence of salivation may be caused by fever or dehydration. Excessive salivation is frequently seen in children who are teething or who have caries or mouth infections. The amount, color, consistency, and odor of saliva are recorded if they are abnormal.

Gums should be inspected and palpated for color, moisture, inflammation, swelling, bleeding, tenderness, and ulcerations. Inflammation and swelling are secondary to infection or poor oral hygiene. A herpesvirus infection or improperly fitting dental corrective appliances may cause ulcerations. Inflamed, bleeding gums may be a result of decreased vitamin C intake or infection. A black line along the margin of the gum may signify metal poisoning, such as lead poisoning. Any raised or receding areas of the gums should be identified. It is important to use the tongue depressor gently to move the buccal mucosa away from the gums to allow adequate inspection of upper and lower gums.

The *buccal mucosa* is inspected and palpated for color, moisture, lesions, parotid ducts, and masses. The buccal mucosa is normally pink, but black or brown areas may be seen in children with Addison disease and in dark-skinned children. An enlarged, erythematous, or swollen parotid duct is seen with parotitis. Koplik spots, a group of gray-white spots, are seen on the buccal mucosa opposite the molars in the prodromal stage of measles (rubeola). White patches on the oral mucosa—especially the tongue and hard palate—that cannot be scraped off indicate a yeast infection called "thrush" or "moniliasis" *(Candida albicans)*. The floor of the mouth is inspected and palpated for cysts, masses, calculi, or submaxillary glands.

Inspection of the *tongue* is done to determine color, moisture, size, tremors, coating, size of papillae, and the presence of lesions. The normal tongue is pink and should fit in the mouth. A large protruding tongue is seen in children with Down syndrome. Normally, the tongue has conical filiform papillae; large red papillae resembling a strawberry are seen with scarlet fever. The tongue becomes tender and red in some vitamin deficiencies or severe anemia. A geographic tongue has gray, irregular borders and can be considered normal or can be caused by allergies, fever, or drug ingestion. The tongue should also be examined for furrows and scars. Deep furrows are seen in children with Down syndrome. Scars could be the result of trauma or previous convulsions. Gross tongue tremors when the tongue is stuck out are seen in children with cerebral palsy. The examiner should observe the tongue closely to determine mobility. In infants, the frenulum is checked for tongue-tie and is considered abnormal if the tongue cannot extend beyond the lower alveolar ridge. The ventral surface of the tongue is inspected for distended veins. The older child is instructed to push against the tongue depressor laterally on each side to determine the tongue's strength.

The hard and soft palates are inspected for color, shape, clefts, and the presence of lesions. An abnormally high arch may be associated with congenital disorders and may result in speech problems. The palates are usually a striated pink color. Epstein pearls are seen as firm white nodules in the midline and are of no significance.

The *uvula* is inspected as the child is told to say "ahh." In crying or cooperative children the uvula can usually be visualized without causing the child to gag. *Because the possibility of instant airway obstruction exists, a gag reflex should never be stimulated in a child who presents with an airway problem.* The soft palate and uvula should rise when the child says "ahh." Paralysis of the soft palate or uvula, which is indicated by no movement or movement that is not midline, may signify diphtheria, poliomyelitis, or abnormality of the glossopharyngeal or vagus nerves. An exceptionally long uvula is congenital and may cause gagging or coughing.

Tonsils are inspected for color, size, symmetry, inflammation or exudate, and possible lesions. Tonsils are much larger during childhood and begin to shrink between the ages of 8 and 12 years. Tonsillar crypts usually indicate past infection.

The *posterior pharynx* is checked for color, drainage, edema, and abnormal lesions or growth. Lymphoid hyperplasia and inflammation are seen in infection. A pale, puffy mucosa usually denotes edema. Ulcers and vesicles are seen in children with viral infections. Postnasal drainage may indicate either allergy or infection of the nasopharynx or sinuses, depending on the type of discharge seen.

Chest and Lungs

Techniques	Equipment
Inspection	Stethoscope
Palpation	
Auscultation	
Percussion	

Examine for

Condition of cartilage

Condition of bones

Quality of breath sounds

Respiratory function

Location and condition of nipples

Condition of breasts

Condition of muscles

Skillful inspection, palpation, percussion, and auscultation are needed to examine the thorax, breast, and lungs (Fig. 13–23). The chest is inspected for size, shape, symmetry, and movement. The shape of the chest is round in the newborn. With growth, the chest shape becomes more oval, with the transverse diameter being greater than the anteroposterior diameter. Pigeon breast, barrel chest, funnel breast, and Harrison groove are examples of abnormal chest structure (Table 13–10). Asymmetry, such as precor-

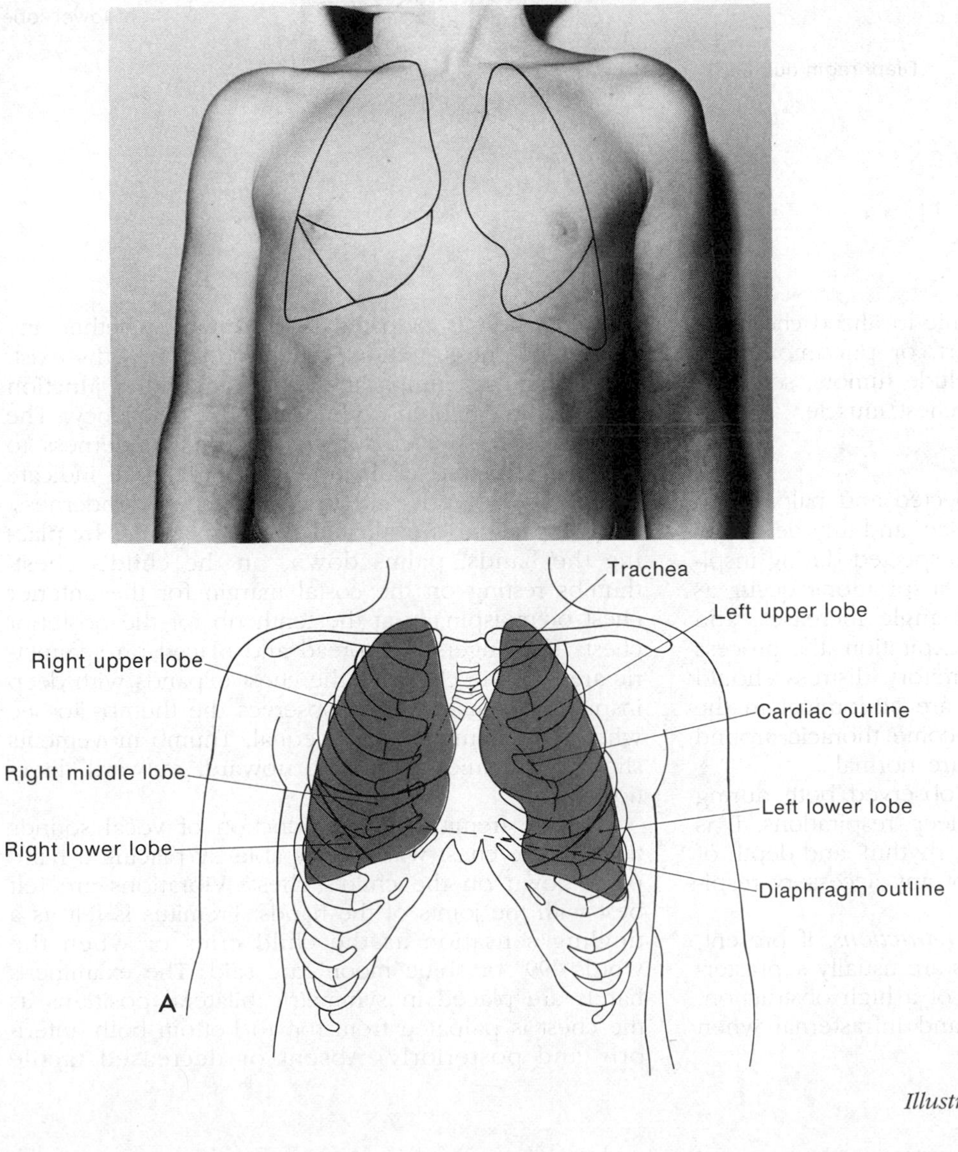

FIGURE 13 - 23. The four parts of the lung within the chest. *A*, Anterior thorax; *B*, posterior thorax; *C*, left lateral thorax; and *D*, right lateral thorax.

Illustration continued on following page

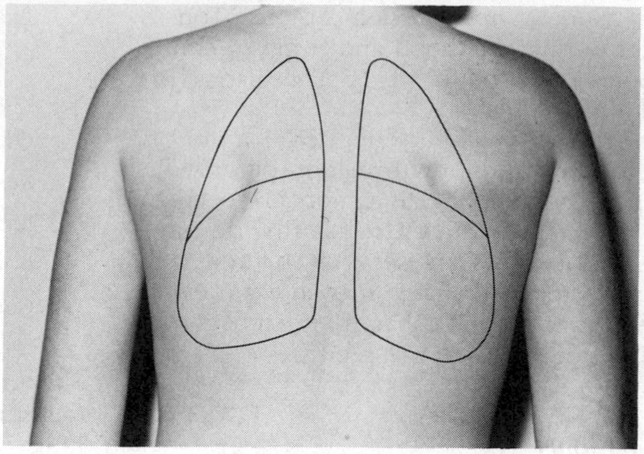

FIGURE 13 - 23 *Continued*

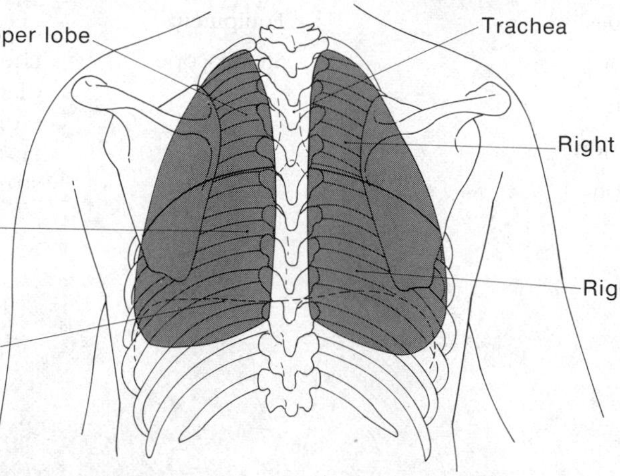

dial bulging, may indicate chronic localized chest disease, enlargement of the heart, or pneumothorax. Other causes of asymmetry include tumors, scoliosis, and congenital absence of the chest muscle.

Inspection and Palpation

The *posterior chest wall* is inspected and palpated to determine equality of the scapulae, and any deformity is noted. The chest should be inspected during inspiration and expiration. Normal inspirations occur as the chest expands, the sternal angle increases, and the diaphragm descends. With expiration, the process is reversed. Any signs of respiratory distress should be noted. Normal respirations are abdominal in the infant and young child and become thoracic around 7 years of age, although both are normal.

Respiratory motion is also observed both during quiet respirations and during sleep respirations. It is important to note the type, rate, rhythm, and depth of respiration as well as the use of any accessory respiratory muscles.

The *location and depth of retractions,* if present, should be described. Retractions are usually suprasternal and severe in the presence of a high obstruction. They are usually less intense and infrasternal when there is low obstruction.

The chest is palpated to determine whether any cysts, tenderness, tumors, or abnormal growths exist. Sharp angular bumps at the costochondral junction are seen in children with vitamin D deficiency. The clavicles are palpated for crepitus and tenderness to rule out a fracture. Palpation of the ribs will indicate the number of ribs and the presence of tenderness. Lung expansion is evaluated by the examiner by placing the hands, palms down, on the child's chest, thumbs resting on the costal margin for the anterior chest or midspinally at the tenth rib for the posterior chest. The fingers are spread and placed on symmetric areas of the chest. As the chest expands with deep inspiration, the examiner observes the thumbs to see whether their movement is equal. Thumb movements should be equidistant in an upward, outward direction.

Tactile fremitus, the conduction of vocal sounds through the chest wall, is palpable by placing a hand palm down on the child's chest. Vibrations are felt best with the joints of the hands. Fremitus is felt as a tingling sensation as the child cries or when the words "99" or "blue moon" are said. The examiner's hands are placed in symmetric bilateral positions as the chest is palpated from top to bottom both anteriorly and posteriorly. Absent or decreased tactile

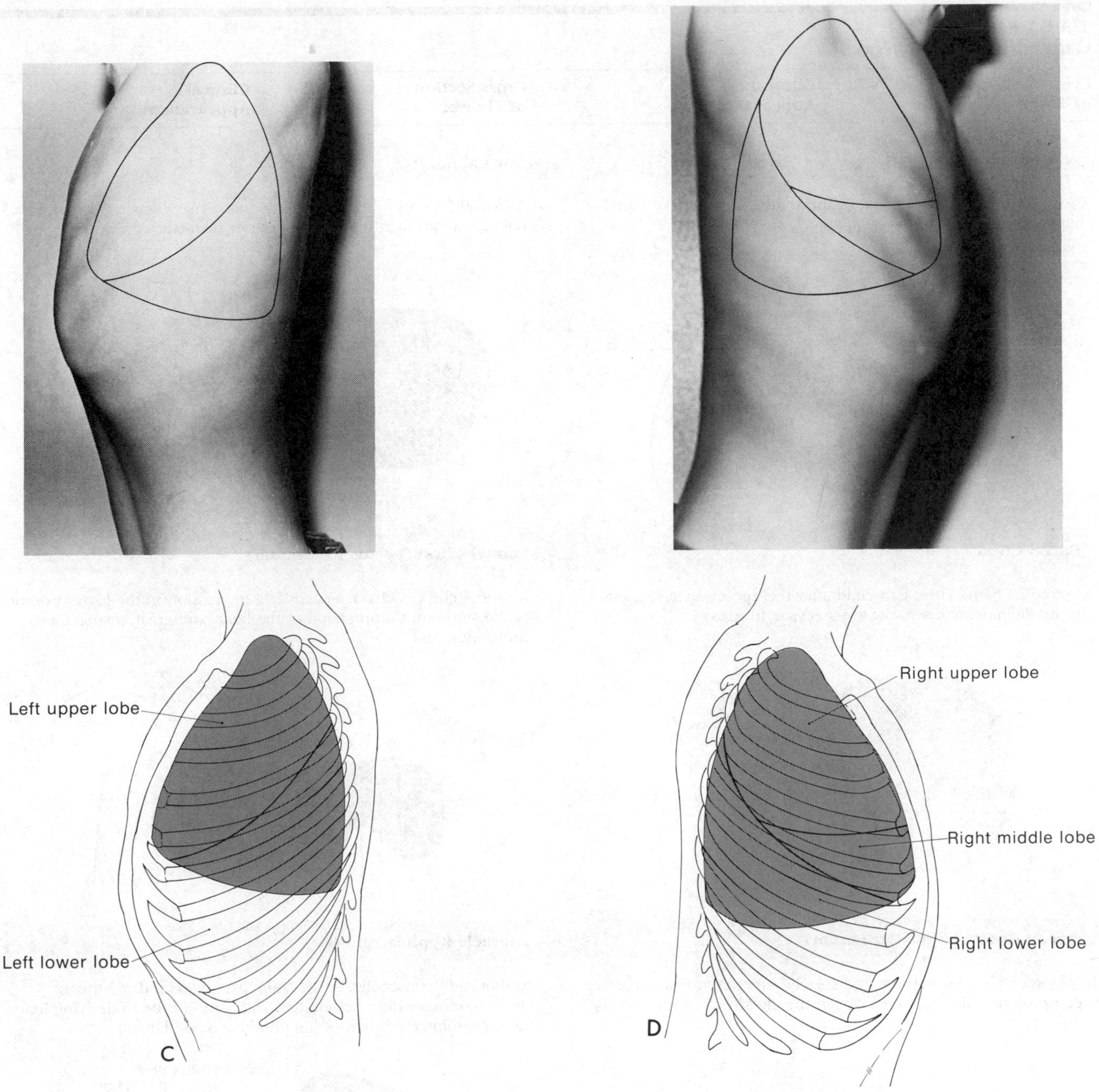

FIGURE 13 - 23 *Continued*

fremitus is seen with bronchial blockages, asthma, pleural effusion, and pneumothorax. Increased vibrations are seen with consolidation, such as pneumonia or atelectasis. The chest should also be palpated for pleural crepitus, which is felt as a coarse, crackling sensation when pressure is applied.

Percussion

The indirect method is used to percuss the chest. Percussion proceeds symmetrically from side to side and downward to determine the presence, size, and density of underlying structures. Percussion should be done in the intercostal space, not on the rib, and should be just lateral to the sternum anteriorly and the spine posteriorly. Percussion starts in the supraclavicular area on the anterior chest. Dullness is percussed over the diaphragm, liver, and heart and tympany over the stomach. The liver is percussed beginning at the right fifth or sixth intercostal space in the midclavicular line. Percussion from this point downward to a point where the sound changes indicates the size of the liver. Beginning as resonant sounds, percussion sounds change to dullness over the liver, then return to resonance beyond the liver border.

TABLE 13-10
Deformities of the Thorax

Cross-Section of Thorax	Clinical Appearance	Cross-Section of Thorax	Clinical Appearance
Normal Infant		**Normal Adult**	
The chest of the normal infant is approximately round or barrel-shaped in cross-section		As a child grows to adulthood, the transverse diameter of the thorax enlarges more than the anteroposterior diameter	
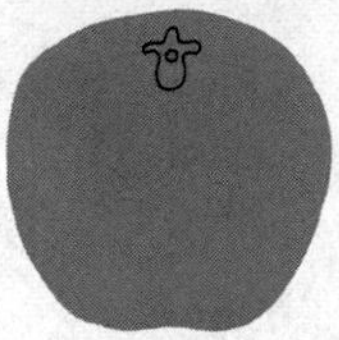	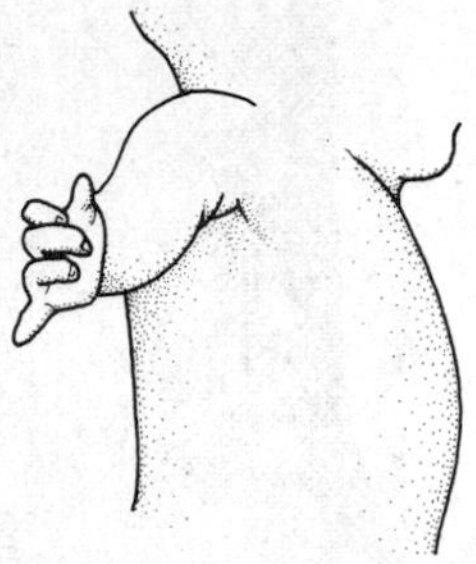		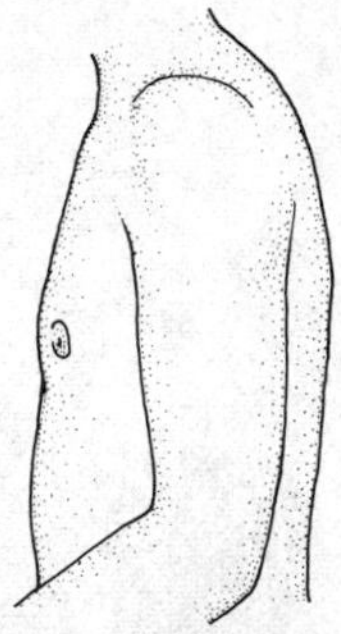
Barrel Chest		**Funnel Chest (Pectus Excavatum)**	
A round or barrel chest in a child after the age of 6 yrs suggests a chronic pulmonary disease (asthma, cystic fibrosis)		A funnel chest is characterized by a depression in the lower portion of the sternum. Compression of the heart and great vessels may cause murmurs	
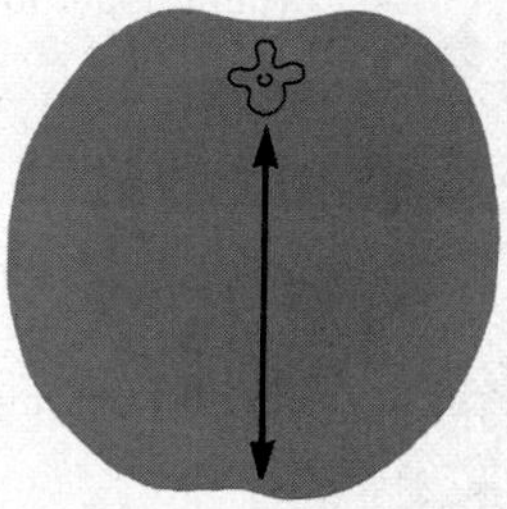	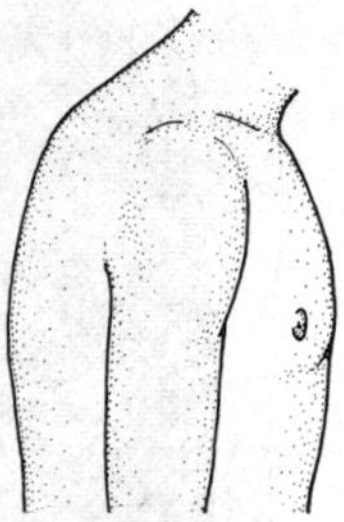	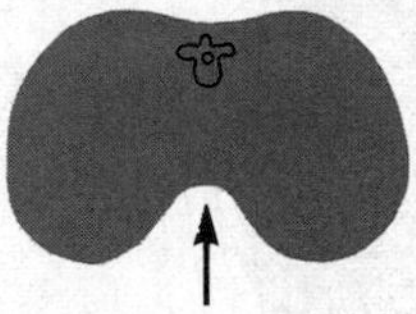	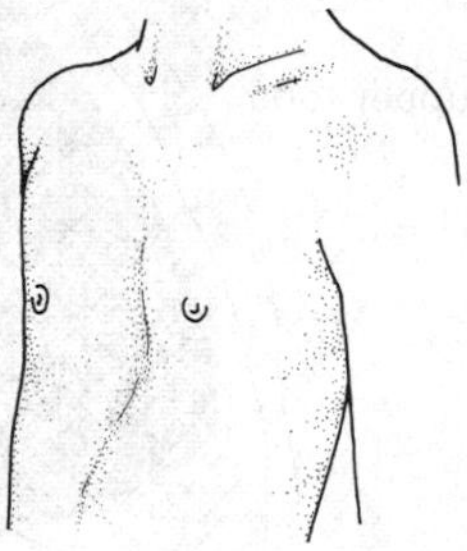
Pigeon Chest (Pectus Carinatum)		**Thoracic Kyphoscoliosis**	
In pigeon chest, the sternum is displaced anteriorly, increasing the anteroposterior diameter. Grooves in the chest wall accentuate the deformity		In thoracic kyphoscoliosis, the spine is curved, and the thorax shows corresponding deformities. Distortion of the underlying lungs may make interpretation of lung findings very difficult	
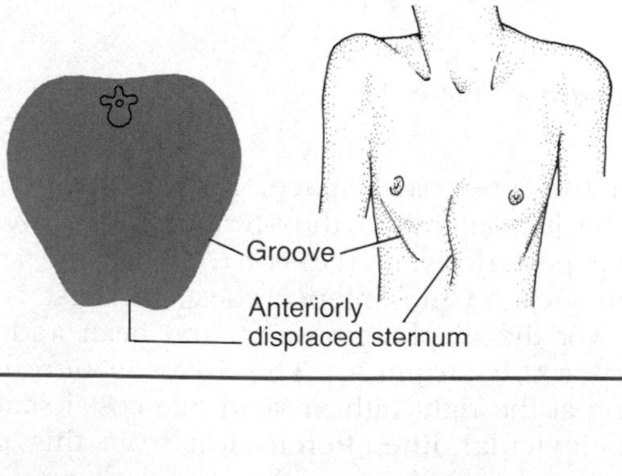		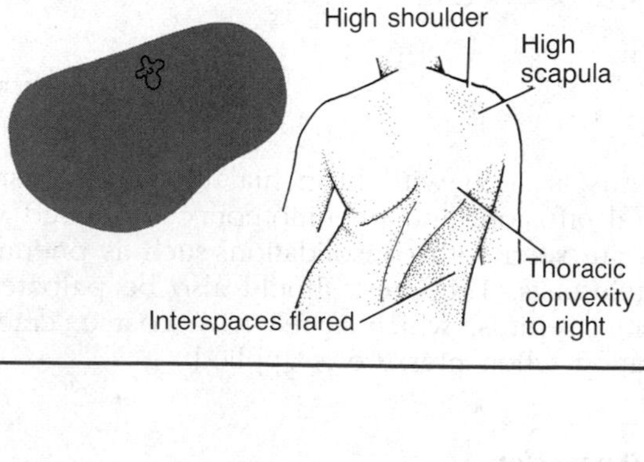	

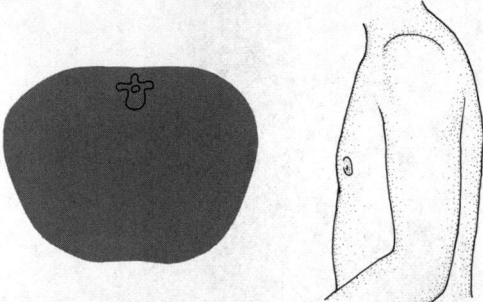

Posterior percussion begins at the shoulder level. The diaphragm is percussed posteriorly at the level of the eighth to tenth ribs. The lateral chest is percussed in symmetric areas, moving from the top of the axillae downward. Percussion of the lung fields should be heard as resonant. Hyper-resonance or dullness in unexpected areas should be considered abnormal. Hyper-resonant lung sounds are normal in the newborn, however, because of the thin chest wall. The examiner should listen for obvious respiratory sounds, such as grunting or wheezing, before auscultating the chest.

Auscultation

Auscultation is done using the diaphragm of the stethoscope. The chest is auscultated in a systematic fashion from side to side moving from top to bottom, including the anterior and posterior and the lateral aspects. Respiratory rate and depth are recorded. Table 13–4 summarizes average respiratory rates by age. These can be obtained by observing thoracic or abdominal movement, placing a hand on the thorax or abdomen, and observing the movement of the examiner's hand, or auscultating the breath sounds for rate, rhythm, and depth.

Breath sounds are evaluated for type, quality, pitch, duration, and intensity. Breath sounds are normally louder in children under 6 years of age because of the thin chest wall. There are three types of breath sounds: vesicular, bronchial, and bronchovesicular. Table 13–11 summarizes the characteristics of each. *Vesicular breath sounds* are louder, longer, and higher-pitched in inspiration and are shorter, softer, and lower-pitched in expiration. This type of breath sound is normally found all over the chest except in the areas of the sternum anteriorly and scapulae posteriorly. The ratio of the length of inspiration to the length of expiration is about 5:2. Vesicular sounds are exaggerated in the late stages of pneumonia, emphysema, and tuberculosis. In the early stages of pneumonia, vesicular breath sounds are diminished.

Bronchial breath sounds are shorter on inspiration than on expiration. They are usually louder than the other types of breath sounds. This type of breath sound is normally heard over the trachea. If heard in other areas, it may indicate atelectasis or consolidation. *Bronchovesicular breath sounds* are equal on inspiration and expiration and are louder and higher-pitched than vesicular sounds. They are heard over the sternum and upper intrascapular area.

Additional respiratory sounds not normally heard are *adventitious sounds.* These sounds are superimposed on normal breath sounds when air being exchanged passes through secretions or through a narrowed lumen or when the pleura loses its normal lubrication. See Table 13–12 for a description of these sounds. Crackles and wheezes, traditionally called "rales" and "rhonchi," can be heard while auscultating the chest anteriorly and posteriorly as described. A pleural friction rub is best heard by placing the stethoscope at the base of the lungs on each lateral chest wall. Adventitious sounds are often dynamic in nature. Crackles and wheezes heard on auscultation may disappear or change location after a child coughs or changes position. A description of the sound and whether it occurs during inspiration or expiration, or both, should be noted. Children with adventitious breath sounds should have further evaluation.

Decreased or absent breath sounds are abnormal. Breath sounds are absent or decreased when the flow of air is obstructed and the sound of air exchange is not transmitted. Obstruction of air flow can be caused by a foreign object or mucus, pneumothorax, or pleural effusion. Often in children with a partially obstructed airway, respiratory efforts will be observed but no air movement can be auscultated. To avoid overlooking these conditions, the chest should be symmetrically auscultated from side to side with careful comparison of breath sounds from one side to the other.

Breast Examination

Breasts should be examined in both males and females. During inspection of the anterior chest, the nipples should be checked for color, spacing, placement, symmetry, fissures, inversions, secretions, scaling, and lumps. In the female, breast bud formation usually begins around 10 to 14 years of age. One breast may begin to develop before the other and is often tender. Precocious breast development may be normal but can also indicate diethylstilbesterol inges-

TABLE 13-11
Characteristics of Breath Sounds

Type	Length of Inspiration and Expiration	Quality and Intensity	Normal Location
Vesicular	Loud Soft	Softest; swishing sound	Throughout lung fields except over sternum and scapulae
Bronchial	Soft Loud	Loudest; blowing, hollow sound	Trachea
Bronchovesicular	Same	Louder and higher pitched sound than vesicular; tubular quality	Sternum, upper intrascapular area

TABLE 13-12
Adventitious Lung Sounds

Type	Cause	Description
*Rales** (Crackles: A crackling or bubbling sound produced by air flow through secretions)		
Fine	Watery secretions in the alveoli	Fine, minute crackling. It is a sound similar to that of several strands of hair being held up to your ear and rubbed together through your fingers. Heard at end of inspiration
Medium	Watery secretions extending from the alveoli pathway up the tracheobronchial tree	A loose, crackling sound heard in mid and late inspiration
Coarse	Secretions in the trachea and bronchi	Low, rumbling bubbling sound on early inspiration and part of expiration
*Rhonchi** (Wheezes: Sounds heard as air passes through the trachea, the bronchi, or bronchioles in which the lumen has been narrowed, irrespective of cause)		
Sibilant	(1) Anatomic narrowing of trachea, bronchi, or bronchioles or (2) bronchospasm	High-pitched wheezing or musical sound primarily in mid or late expiration but may be present throughout respiratory cycle
Sonorous	Originates in larger bronchi and the trachea. The flow of air continuously vibrates thick secretions along the airway	Loud low-pitched gurgling sound throughout the respiratory cycle that can be cleared by coughing or suctioning
Friction rub	Inflamed pleural surface with diminished lubricating fluid	A grating sound, as if leather is being bent or rubbed together. It is heard near the end of inspiration at the lower anterolateral chest wall

* The terms "rales" and "rhonchi" are gradually being replaced by "crackles" and "wheezes," respectively. Both sets of terms are retained here for clarity. Crackles generally include the categories of fine and coarse, whereas rales traditionally have been classifed as fine, medium, and coarse.

tion or ovarian tumors. The breasts are inspected and palpated for redness, heat, tenderness, and masses. For palpation, the child or adolescent lies in a supine position with the right arm extended above the head. The examiner lightly palpates the right breast with the fingertips in a rolling circular motion. Examination is begun at the center of the nipple and progresses in a counterclockwise manner in concentric rings until the entire breast and area surrounding the breast has been examined. Alternative methods of examination may be used as long as the method is systematic to ensure complete assessment of breast tissue. The axilla is also palpated for swelling, tenderness, and lymphadenopathy. The procedure is repeated on the left breast.

The breast should be examined with the female child in various positions: (1) in a sitting position with hands raised above the head, (2) leaning forward, and (3) with the hands resting on the hips, pressing the elbows back and toward the midline. Inspection for dimpling, asymmetry, discharge, and color takes place in each of these positions. While examining the breasts, the nurse may educate the female adolescent about self-examination techniques and the importance of routine examination.

The male breast should also be inspected and palpated for abnormalities. Any increased size should be noted, since it may be indicative of endocrine problems. The adolescent male also normally has some breast development during puberty.

Heart

Techniques	Equipment
Inspection	Stethoscope
Palpation	
Auscultation	
Percussion	

Examine for

Precordial abnormalities

Size and shape of the heart

Quality, rate, rhythm of heart sounds

Abnormal heart sounds

Inspection and Palpation

Inspection and palpation of the precordium is done to detect precordial bulging, thrills, lifts or heaves, precordial friction rubs, and the apical impulse. Traditionally, this has been called "point of maximal impulse" (PMI), but the more common term now used is "apical impulse." The apical impulse is palpable in the fourth or fifth intercostal space at or just medial to the midclavicular line in older children and adults. In infants, it is palpable in the fifth intercostal space (or slightly below), lateral to the midclavicular line. In thin children, the apical pulse may be visible.

A *lift or heave* is seen and felt when the cardiac action is abnormally forceful, actually lifting the ribs

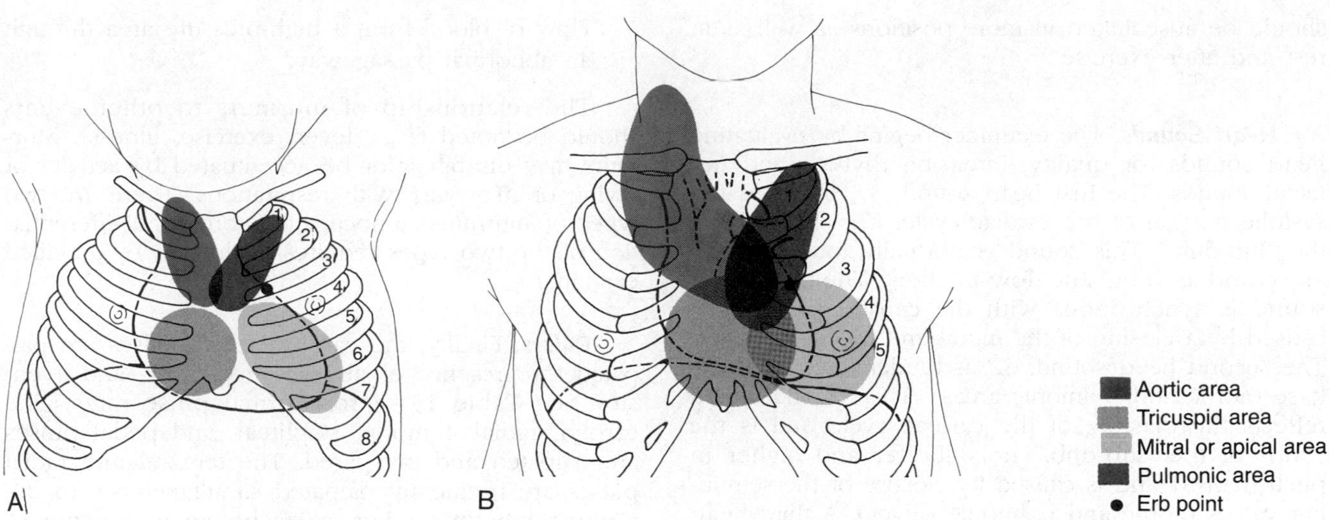

FIGURE 13-24. Position of heart in chest, illustrating areas of auscultation for the infant *(A)* and adult *(B)*. In an infant, the heart lies more horizontally in the chest because the diaphragm is higher and the rib cage is shorter than in an older child. This tends to displace the point of maximal impulse (PMI) more laterally, but it usually remains in the 5th intercostal space (or slightly below). The PMI in an infant is not higher in relation to the rib cage (i.e., it is not at the 3rd or 4th intercostal space); rather, it is the rib cage that is shorter compared with that of an older child. As the rib cage elongates and the diaphragm lowers with growth, the heart assumes a more vertical position; the PMI is then at the left midclavicular line in the 5th intercostal space.

The central point of each shaded area represents the most accurate area for auscultation. The perimeter of each shaded area represents the extent of radiation from each auscultation area. The location of the nipple varies considerably in both neonates and older children.

(Courtesy of Dr. R. C. Way, Director of Pediatric Cardiology, Chedoke-McMaster Hospitals, McMaster University Medical Centre Division, Hamilton, Ontario.)

and sternum with each heartbeat. A *thrill* is a palpable heart murmur. It is a vibration and is often described as similar to the feel of a cat purring. Other observations related to the examination of the heart include respiratory distress, finger clubbing, edema, and cyanosis.

Percussion

Percussion of the heart may be done using the direct or indirect percussion technique. Percussion of the heart outlines its size and shape. The heart normally is in the shape of an inverted triangle, with the right border extending along the right side of the sternum from the second to the fifth ribs and from the right sternum at the fifth rib to the left midclavicular line at the fifth rib. The hypotenuse of the triangle is extended along the right side of the sternum at the second rib to the left midclavicular line at the fifth rib (Fig. 13–24). The heart in an infant lies slightly more horizontally, with the apex to the left of the nipple line. Percussion dullness that is located other than in the expected area could mean cardiac enlargement or heart displacement. This technique is frequently omitted during examination.

Auscultation

Auscultation is the most informative method of assessing cardiac function. It is used to evaluate the quality, rate, and rhythm of the heart and to detect abnormal heart sounds. There are five areas of the heart to examine when evaluating function (Fig. 13–24). They are:

1. Aortic.
2. Pulmonic.
3. Erb point.
4. Apical (mitral).
5. Tricuspid (epigastric).

First, the apical pulse rate, intensity, and rhythm are noted. Rapid or decreased pulse rates may be normal or may indicate pathology. The heart is auscultated with both the bell and the diaphragm of the stethoscope. The bell picks up low frequencies, and the diaphragm picks up high frequencies. The heart may be examined with the child in several positions: standing, sitting, leaning forward, supine, or left-lateral lying. For a routine examination, the heart should be auscultated in both the supine and the sitting positions. If there is a suspicion of a problem, the heart should be auscultated in more positions as well as at rest and after exercise.

Heart Sounds. The examiner begins by evaluating heart sounds for quality, intensity, rhythm, and unusual sounds. The first heart sound, *S1,* indicates the systolic portion of the cardiac cycle; it is the "lub" of the "lub-dub." This sound is normally louder at the apex and is long and low-pitched. The first heart sound is synchronous with the carotid pulse. It is caused by a closing of the mitral and tricuspid valves. The second heart sound, *S2,* is louder than S1 at the base (aortic and pulmonic areas). This second sound reflects the diastole of the cardiac cycle and is the "dub" of the "lub-dub." It is shorter and higher in pitch than S1 and is caused by closure of the semilunar valves (aortic and pulmonic valves). A third heart sound, *S3,* is occasionally heard because of blood rushing through the mitral valve and rapidly filling the ventricle. The third heart sound is low-pitched and occurs early in diastole. It is heard best at the apex. It can be normal in a child but is almost always abnormal in an adult. A fourth heart sound, *S4,* may exist but is seldom normal. It is caused by an inaudible atrial contraction at the end of diastole and is heard best at the apex.

The *heart sounds* are evaluated for quality, intensity, and splitting. The first and second sounds should be clear and distinct. Any muffling or indistinctness may indicate pathology. *Intensity* refers to where each heart sound is heard best. S1 should be heard best at the apex and S2 heard best at the base of the heart. If this is not the case, the heart should be evaluated in more depth for a possible abnormality.

The *rhythm of the heart* is evaluated by listening carefully to determine whether any irregularity exists. If an irregular rhythm is present, the examiner should attempt to determine a specific pattern. Sinus arrhythmia is a common irregularity in which the heart speeds up with inspiration and slows down with expiration. It should disappear when the child holds his or her breath and is considered normal in children.

Murmurs. One classification of unusual or abnormal heart sounds is heart murmurs. Heart murmurs are described in Chapter 33 in the section on heart anomalies. A heart murmur originates within the heart or its great vessels. The flow of blood is altered, causing an abnormal sound that is audible on auscultation. Murmurs are usually caused by the following:

- Flow across a partial obstruction.
- Flow across an irregularity within the heart or vessel.
- An increased amount of blood flow through a normal passageway.
- Flow from a normal passageway into a dilated area.
- Regurgitation (backward) flow through a valve or defect.
- Flow of blood from a high-pressure area through an abnormal passageway.

The relationship of murmurs to other events should be noted (e.g., fever, exercise, illness). Murmurs may disappear or be accentuated by activity or crying or may vary with respirations. There are two types of murmurs: innocent and organic. Differentiation of the two types requires evaluation by a skilled examiner.

Pulses. Finally, the cardiovascular pulses are palpated for presence or absence, regularity, and intensity. See Table 13–4 for normal pulse rates. The carotid, radial, femoral, popliteal, and pedal pulses are palpated and compared. The femoral and radial pulses are frequently palpated simultaneously to determine whether a lag exists between the two. A femoral-radial lag (the femoral pulse and radial pulse are not felt simultaneously when being palpated simultaneously) or absent or diminished femoral pulses are characteristic of coarctation of the aorta. Temperature and color of the extremities should also be assessed. Cold, pale, or cyanotic extremities suggest cardiac disease or peripheral vascular disease.

A thorough examination of the heart should include blood pressure (see Fig. 13–7 for normal values) and observation of the child before and after exercise or, in the infant, eating. Any color changes or fatigue should be noted.

Abdomen

Techniques	Equipment
Inspection	Stethoscope
Auscultation	
Palpation	
Percussion	
Examine for	
Abdominal movement	Peristalsis
Abdominal shape	Muscle tone
Condition of umbilicus	Organomegaly
Herniations	Tenderness

Examination of the abdomen requires inspection, auscultation, palpation, and percussion of its four major divisions:

1. Right upper quadrant (RUQ).
2. Right lower quadrant (RLQ).
3. Left upper quadrant (LUQ).
4. Left lower quadrant (LLQ).

It is essential that the child be quiet and cooperative if the examiner is to evaluate this system thoroughly. The abdominal muscles are relaxed by flexing the child's knees slightly. Infants can be distracted or quieted by giving them a bottle in order to help relax the abdominal wall for examination. Before beginning the examination, the examiner's hands should be warmed.

Inspection

Inspection allows the examiner to determine *shape and contour,* movement and peristalsis, distention, bulges, and condition of the rectus muscle. Children normally have a pot belly that should begin to disappear by 4 or 5 years of age. The abdominal wall moves with respiration until 6 or 7 years of age; failure to do so may indicate appendicitis, peritonitis, paralytic ileus, diaphragmatic paralysis, or a large amount of air in the abdominal cavity.

Peristalsis is not generally visible in children. Visible peristaltic waves usually indicate an obstruction in the gastrointestinal tract. Pyloric stenosis is suspected if peristaltic waves occur from left to right.

Abdominal distention may be a sign of pregnancy, feces, organomegaly, ovarian cysts, ascites, or air in the abdominal cavity. The abdomen should be inspected from the front and from the sides to determine the extent of the distention; it is then palpated and percussed. Diastasis (splitting) of the rectus muscle is a protrusion in the midline from the xiphoid to the umbilicus and can be inspected and palpated. The split can be part way or the entire length between these two points. The width of the bulging can be ½ to 2 inches and still be considered normal. However, it may also be caused by a congenital weakness of the muscle or a chronically distended abdomen. Close follow-up with measurement of the length and width should be done.

The *umbilicus* is inspected closely for bulging, color, and discharge. A bluish umbilicus can be caused by intra-abdominal hemorrhage. At birth, the umbilical cord should be inspected for the presence of one vein and two arteries. During follow-up examinations, the neonate's umbilical cord should be inspected for bleeding and signs of infection. Protrusion of the umbilicus usually indicates a hernia. Palpation of the hernia should be done to confirm a hernia after auscultation of the abdomen has been completed. Hernias are seen commonly in children up to the age of 2 or 3 years. They persist longer in African-American children, being seen until 7 or 8 years of age. Drainage from the umbilicus should be checked for color, odor, amount, and consistency. If infection is suspected, the fluid may be cultured. In addition to infection, a patent urachus, a remnant of fetal development, or a urachal cyst may be the cause of umbilical drainage.

Finally, the abdomen is inspected for distended veins and obvious pulsations. The skin is examined thoroughly as discussed earlier in this chapter.

Auscultation

Auscultation follows inspection of the abdomen so that peristaltic sounds are not disturbed by palpation or percussion. The diaphragm of the stethoscope is placed firmly over the abdomen, and the examiner listens in all four quadrants for peristaltic sounds. These are metallic, short, tinkling sounds. Normally, an average of 15 to 34 bowel sounds per minute is audible. High-pitched, frequent, or hyperactive sounds are heard in children with diarrhea, gastroenteritis, and intestinal obstruction. Absence of peristaltic sounds may indicate a paralytic ileus or early peritonitis. Peristaltic sounds are very irregular; before concluding that they are absent, the examiner must listen for at least 5 or 10 minutes.

Vascular sounds may be detected by auscultation of the abdomen. A venous hum may indicate abnormality of the umbilical vein or portal obstruction. Murmurs may indicate coarctation of the aorta or a renal artery defect. Friction rubs and bruits heard in the abdomen are also abnormal and should be referred.

Percussion

Percussion follows auscultation and is done with the child supine, either on the parent's lap or on the examination table. Percussion should be used to outline the border and size of underlying structures. The examiner begins at the child's thorax at the left midaxillary line. The diaphragm is percussed above the spleen. Occasionally, tympany under the left diaphragm is percussed if a stomach bubble is present. This procedure is then repeated at the right side, where liver dullness is expected at the sixth interspace anteriorly and at the ninth rib posteriorly. The lower edge of the liver should be percussed at the right costal margin or, occasionally, 2 to 3 cm lower. With respiration, the liver descends about two finger breadths. Ask the child to take a deep breath and hold it to facilitate percussion. The remainder of the abdomen is then percussed. Dullness encountered elsewhere may indicate a full bladder, feces, or a mass. Tympany usually indicates air in the stomach and may be more pronounced in children who swallow air excessively or who have a gastrointestinal obstruction.

Palpation

The final method of examination is palpation. Light palpation begins the examination and should proceed in a systematic fashion. If, however, the child is presenting with a complaint of abdominal discomfort, palpate the nonaffected areas first and the painful area last. Using the fingertips, the examiner gently and superficially palpates the quadrants in the following order: left lower, left upper, right upper, and right lower. Initially, the examiner notes whether the abdomen is soft or hard, tender, or distended.

After completing light palpation, the examiner proceeds in the same systematic way, using deep palpation. Deep palpation is accomplished best during deep inspiration and deep expiration. The examiner may wish to place one hand on top of the other to provide firmer pressure for this examination technique. Deep palpation is useful in discovering masses, tenderness, deep vessels, and palpable organs. A pyloric tumor would be palpable at the right costal margin just to the right of the midline of the abdomen. Wilm tumor may be palpated adjacent to the vertebral column in the kidney area.

The *liver,* if palpable, is felt for size, consistency, and tenderness. Any liver palpable below the costal margin should be percussed for size and evaluated for possible pathology.

The *spleen* can be palpated more easily if the child lies on the right side and takes a deep breath. The examiner lightly places the fingers just below the left costal margin at the midaxillary line and palpates the tip of the spleen. If more than the tip of the spleen is palpable, it is considered abnormal. In some children, the tip is not normally palpated.

To palpate the *kidneys,* the examiner must use very deep palpation. They are adjacent to the vertebral column and will descend slightly with inspiration. The lower pole may be felt particularly on the right, since this kidney is lower than the left. The child's flank should be firmly supported with the examiner's left hand while the right hand palpates the abdomen deeply. Normal kidneys are rarely palpable, except in the neonate immediately following birth. However, palpation of the kidneys should always be attempted, since enlargement indicates significant pathology.

In early childhood, it is possible to palpate the full bladder. The intestines may also be palpable, and, in intussusception, a telescoping of the bowel on itself, a sausage-shaped tumor may be found.

Palpation is not complete until the child is checked closely for *hernias*. Umbilical hernias may be located and inspected with palpation. The examiner places a finger into the umbilicus and palpates for protrusion of intestines. The size of the opening through which the intestine protrudes should be noted. Hernias vary in size and should be measured at each visit to see whether they are resolving. Occasionally, epigastric hernias are palpated, since a small nodule protruding between the fibers of the linea alba is often felt best when the child is standing. Examination for a femoral hernia is done by placing the right index finger on the child's femoral artery. The next finger then lies atop the femoral vein, and the ring finger is placed directly over the femoral canal. The standing child is then asked to strain as if having a bowel movement or to cough in order to elicit the hernia if one exists. The femoral hernia is felt or seen as a small bulge that results from a weakness in the musculature at the femoral canal (Fig. 13–25). A femoral hernia is more common in females. The technique for palpating inguinal hernias is described with assessment of male genitalia.

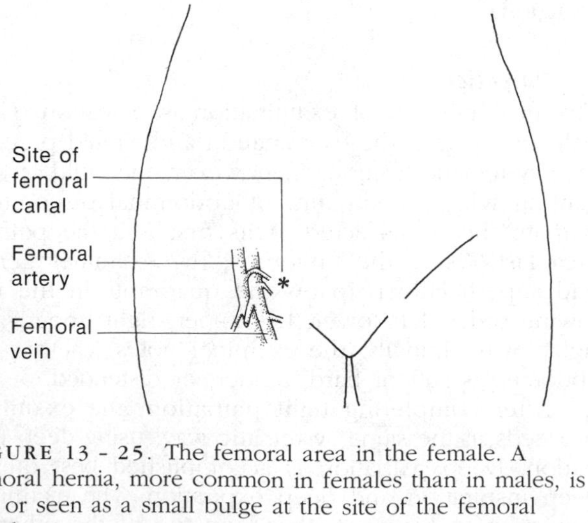

FIGURE 13 - 25. The femoral area in the female. A femoral hernia, more common in females than in males, is felt or seen as a small bulge at the site of the femoral canal.

Female Genitalia

Techniques	Equipment
Inspection	Gloves
Palpation	

Examine for	
General appearance of anatomic structures	Lesions
	Adhesions
Masses	Size of vaginal opening

Every child should have a thorough examination of the genitalia. The examiner can complete this portion of the examination last if the child or adolescent is shy or embarrassed. This should be accomplished in a matter-of-fact manner that will put the child at ease. The extent of the examination will be determined by the presenting problem, age, and sexual activity of the child. If indicated, a pelvic examination should be done. However, this text discusses simply the examination of external structures.

Inspection and Palpation

With gloved hands, one inspects the female genitalia and palpates for presence or absence and symmetry of the external structures (Fig. 13–26). Evidence of edema, color changes, moisture, lesions, and masses should be identified and recorded. The examiner begins by inspecting the mons pubis for any masses or abnormalities. The presence or absence of pubic hair should be noted. Hair should be described according to color, quantity, texture, and distribution. It should also be inspected for lice.

The *vulva* is inspected for erythema, swelling, masses, and varicosities. The labia minora are normally quite large in the infant and may protrude from behind the labia majora. Swelling of the vulva could be a sign of sexual molestation, infection, a foreign body, trauma, or lymphedema.

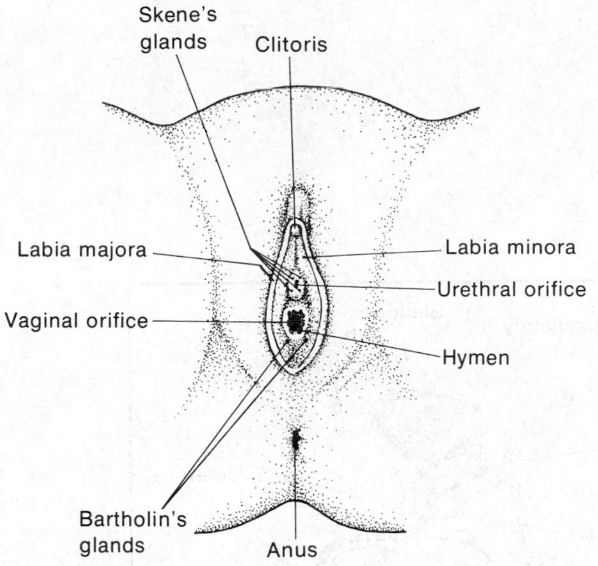

FIGURE 13-26. The female genitalia.

Next, inspect and palpate the Bartholin and Skene glands. They are not normally seen or felt. If visible or palpable, enlargement exists and is due to infection, usually gonorrhea.

The *clitoris* is inspected carefully to determine whether its size is abnormal. It may normally be large in the newborn, whereas a hypertrophied clitoris in an older child may indicate labioscrotal fusion or pseudohermaphroditism. Because of its sensitivity, the clitoris should not be palpated unless there is a specific reason for doing so.

The *vestibule* is inspected and palpated for lesions and masses. There will be few abnormal findings here until the child is older, when the examiner may find ulcerated venereal lesions. It is also important to examine the urethral meatal opening for inflammation, erythema, and discharge. Location of the meatus should be noted for possible epispadias. Finally, the vaginal opening and hymen are checked for congenital absence of the vagina or imperforate hymen. The care provider should note the size of the vaginal opening; an enlarged opening in a young female may be indicative of sexual abuse. Newborn infants may have a small amount of bloody vaginal discharge until 1 month of age as a result of absorption of the maternal hormones during fetal life. Foul-smelling discharge may be due to infection, the presence of a foreign body, or pinworms.

Male Genitalia

Techniques	**Equipment**
Inspection	Good lighting
Palpation	Penlight

Examine for	
Structural anomalies	Lesions
Abnormal discharge	Hernias

The male genitalia (Fig. 13–27) are also examined thoroughly in a matter-of-fact, efficient manner.

Inspection and Palpation

The examiner should begin by first inspecting and palpating the *penis* for size and consistency. An enlarged penis may be due to precocious puberty, central nervous system lesions, or testicular tumors. It should be noted whether the child has been circumcised; if not, it should be noted whether the foreskin is retractable or whether adhesions are present. Normally, the foreskin does not retract easily for the first 2 to 3 months because of a thin membrane that connects it to the surface of the glans. At 4 months, the foreskin is more easily retracted, and, by 4 years, it is usually fully retractable. If, by 4 years of age, the foreskin has not gradually become retractable, the boy may be considered to have phimosis, an abnormal narrowing at the opening of the foreskin that prohibits retraction. Phimosis should be referred for evaluation.

The *meatal opening* is inspected for size, position, and any discharge. Hypospadias or epispadias is present if the opening is on either the ventral or the dorsal surface of the glans penis. These conditions require medical evaluation. A pinpoint meatal opening may cause urinary obstruction. If possible, the child's urinary stream should be observed or information should be obtained from the child or parent during the history. A urinary stream that dribbles or is not steady and strong may be seen with meatal stenosis or other anomalies. The glans is also inspected for lesions, swelling, or venereal warts.

The *shaft of the penis* is examined for size, varicosities, and masses. The infantile penis is approximately 2 to 3 cm long when nonerect. Any penis smaller than this should be examined for the possibility of hermaphroditism. During puberty, the penile shaft lengthens and widens. Pubic hair, if present, should be described in the same way as the female pubic hair. Assessment of pubertal changes is very important in both the male and the female child. See Chapter 9 for illustrations and discussion of staging in secondary sex characteristics development.

The *scrotum* is inspected and palpated for edema, inflammation, masses, and color. The rugae are inspected also. A smooth, shiny scrotum without rugae may indicate undescended testes, which requires referral. The scrotal sac should be palpated for the presence or absence of *testes* and for their size and any masses or tenderness. Testes reflexively retract up out of the scrotal sac. To keep the testes from becoming stimulated and retracting into the inguinal canal, the examiner occludes the inguinal canals by finger pressure before beginning the examination of the scrotum. If the testes are not palpable in the scrotum, they may be milked back into the scrotum for palpation. If they are not palpable at all, the child should be referred for further evaluation.

Next, the *spermatic cord* can be palpated and fol-

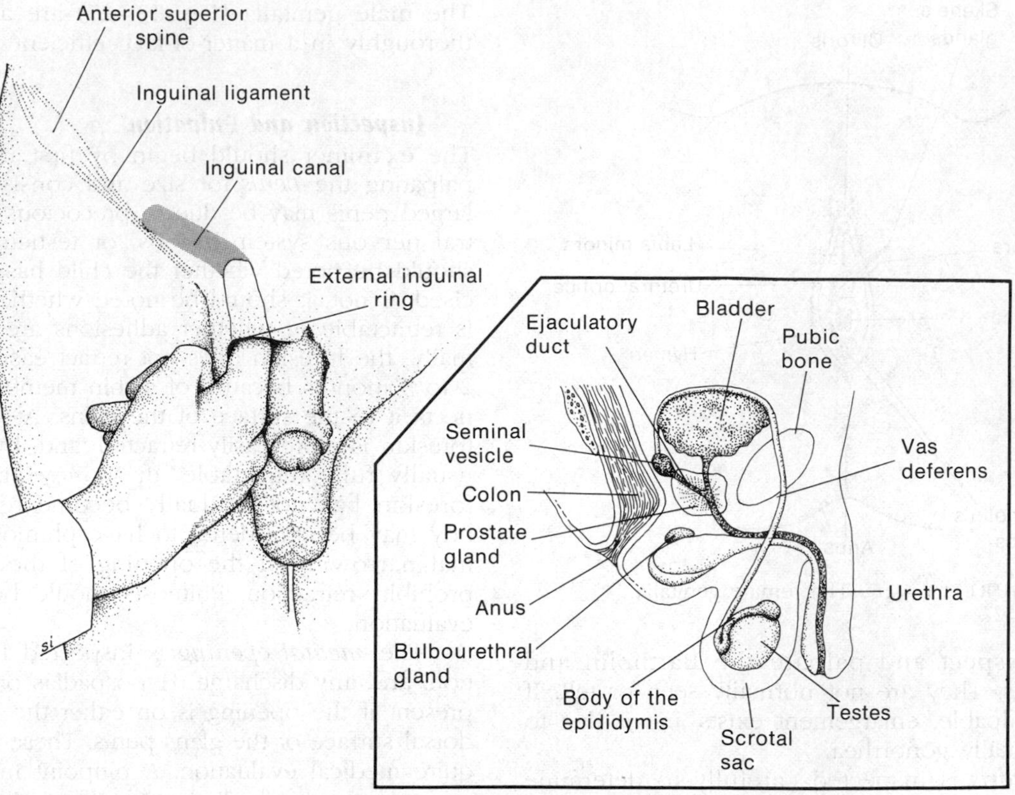

FIGURE 13 - 27. The male genitalia. The inguinal canal is palpated to check for a possible hernia. In a younger child, the little (fifth) finger is used.

lowed to the testes. Any swelling, thickening, or the presence of nodules should be noted. An enlarged or pendulous scrotum should be transilluminated to determine whether a hydrocele, hernia, or mass is present. This is accomplished by placing a penlight behind the scrotal sac. Illumination occurs in a hydrocele but not in a hernia or masses. Swelling and discoloration of the scrotum that has developed suddenly may be a sign of spermatic cord torsion, which requires immediate medical attention.

The *inguinal canal* is palpated to rule out a possible hernia (Fig. 13–27). A hernia of this type is indirect and may be congenital. It is seen in males nine times more frequently than in females and occurs most commonly on the right side. The examiner should place a finger (in a young child, the fifth little finger should be used) in the scrotal sac and gently approach the inguinal canal, following the spermatic cord. The finger tip should not be able to enter the canal through the external inguinal ring unless the ring is abnormally dilated. Weakness of the ring may signal a potential hernia. This weakness is tested by having the child cough or strain. The external ring is palpated for tone. The examiner also palpates the inguinal canal, noting (by pressing through the side of the abdominal wall) whether any abdominal contents can be felt pressing down into the inguinal canal or whether the bulge is palpable. These findings would indicate a hernia. Regional lymph nodes and the femoral canal and pulses should also be examined at this time if they were not during the abdominal survey.

Rectum and Anus

Techniques	Equipment
Inspection	Glove
Palpation	Lubricant
Examine for	
Patency	Masses
Sphincter tone	Lesions
Fecal consistency	

Routinely, examination of the rectum and anus is limited to inspection. If, however, history indicates the need for a digital examination, it should be done.

The *anal sphincter* is best viewed with the child in a knee-chest position. The sphincter area is inspected for fissures, bleeding, inflammation, rashes, and lesions. Fissures, the most common problem, are usually the result of constipation. When the child passes hard stools, the mucosa tears slightly. This is often accompanied by a history of stool with blood streaks. Occasionally, this will lead to further constipation as the child refrains from stooling in order to avoid painful defecation. Treatment to soften the stool consistency is necessary to break this cycle.

Signs of scratching or irritation may be due to diaper rash or pinworms. Pinworms may be suspected if there is a history of nocturnal perianal itching. Testing for pinworms is simple and should be conducted, if necessary.

If there are concerns regarding rectal patency, sphincter tone, stricture, or stool quality, a digital examination is necessary. The tone of the external anal sphincter is evaluated by eliciting the anal reflex. This is done by pin-pricking or scratching the perianal area and noting the presence or absence of a quick contraction. The internal examination is done by inserting a gloved, lubricated finger slowly into the rectum and gently palpating the walls of the rectum. The presence or absence of stool should be noted. Sphincter tone and the character, amount, and consistency of feces should be identified. Presence of masses, tenderness, or a lack of sensation should be investigated further. Fecal masses are present in children with mental deficiency, anal stenosis, psychologic difficulties, and chronic constipation. Complete absence of feces in the rectum may indicate ileus, peritonitis, or obstruction.

Musculoskeletal System

Techniques	Equipment
Inspection	None
Palpation	
Examine for	
Structural anomalies	Function of extremities
Posture	Spinal deformities
Range of motion	

A general inspection of the skeletal system begins with observation as the child walks into the examination room. The child is also observed during play activities and while performing tasks such as undressing. Symmetry of movement, position, general alignment, deformities, gait, extra digits, and unusual posture are observable while the child is unaware of the examiner's scrutiny.

During the formal examination, soft tissues and muscles are inspected and palpated for symmetry, contractures, erythema, swelling, and tenderness. Muscles are inspected and palpated for symmetry, mass, tone, strength, and paralysis. The bones are palpated for shape, outline, thickening, abnormal prominence, or indentation. The examiner should determine whether the temperature of one extremity seems higher than that of the others. All joints should be inspected and palpated for swelling, redness, or tenderness and should be actively and passively placed through full range of motion.

The extremities are compared for equality of strength, length, and symmetry of movement. To evaluate the strength of the *arms,* the examiner applies pressure to the child's arms while they are held in the following positions: raised above the head, out to the sides, and straight out in front. The child should be able to maintain each of these positions while the examiner tries to force the arms in the opposite direction. The child can also stand with arms flexed across the chest while the examiner tries to straighten them, and, in reverse, the child can extend the arms while the examiner tries to flex them.

The *hands* are checked closely for extra digits, webbing, missing digits, or abnormally short or long digits. Creases of the hands are inspected closely. Evidence of a simian crease may indicate Down syndrome but is also normal in some individuals. The knuckles should be inspected for their presence and any anomalies. Examination of the extremities should incorporate examination of the regional lymph nodes, skin, nails, hair, and pulses.

The *lower extremities* are observed for shape. Genu varum (bowlegs) is present when the medial malleoli are touching and the knees are more than 1 inch apart. Genu valgum is normally seen in the child between 2½ and 3½ years of age. A child has genu valgum (knock-knees) if the knees are together and the medial malleoli are more than 1 inch apart. Genu varum is often seen in a child until walking has been established for a year. See Figure 6–2 for diagrams of lower limb development. The tibia should be inspected and palpated for torsion. See Chapter 41 for torsional assessment technique.

The lower extremities are checked for equality in length. The child should lie supine and with legs extended. The four malleoli should be in the same plane (Fig. 13–28). The child may also be requested

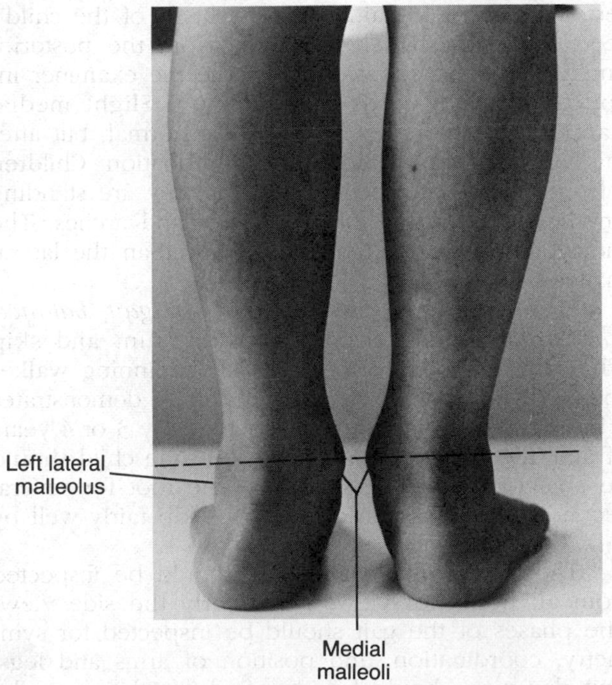

FIGURE 13-28. Check lower extremities for equality in length and alignment of the four malleoli in a straight line.

to stand while the examiner inspects the patellae and the crease in the popliteal fossas for symmetry. This should be done when the child is standing straight with the knees and feet together.

Strength of the legs is checked in much the same way as strength in the upper extremities is. The legs are flexed, and the examiner tries to straighten them. This process is reversed by having the legs extended while the examiner exerts pressure in trying to prevent the child from flexing the legs.

Range of motion of the hips, knees, ankles, and toes should also be checked. It is particularly important to evaluate hip rotation in the infant to rule out congenital hip dislocation. See Chapter 41 for detailed assessment for a congenitally dislocated hip.

The *feet* are inspected for equality of size and shape and for position. If possible, the feet should be examined with the child standing. The arch is examined for unusual height or a flatness. Children have a fat pad under their medial arch until they have been walking 1 to 2 years, which gives them the appearance of having flat feet. The examiner should be able to fit at least one finger under the medial arch. An arch that allows more than one finger is high. An arch that does not allow at least one finger is considered flat. Wetting both feet and then having the child stand on a piece of paper will yield an outline of the arches.

The position of the feet should be noted. Pes valgus (toeing out) and pes varus (toeing in) refer to the entire foot turning either out or in and are caused by structural anomalies. In metatarsus varus (forefoot in) and metatarsus valgus (forefoot out), the heel is straight and midline. These conditions should be referred for further evaluation. The heels of the child's feet should be closely observed from the posterior angle. The child should stand while the examiner inspects the heel cords for deviation. Slight medial slanting before the age of 5 or 6 is normal, but after this age may be an indication of pronation. Children who have pronated feet look as if they are standing on the inner aspects of their heels and arches. The medial malleoli are frequently lower than the lateral malleoli.

Finally, children are observed for *gait, balance, and stance.* Children should walk, run, and skip while the examiner observes. The beginning walker (between 12 and 18 months) generally demonstrates a broad-based gait with poor balance. By 3 or 4 years of age, the gait is narrow-based, and the child should be able to maintain balance on one foot for several seconds. Most children are able to skip fairly well by 5 or 6 years of age.

The child's gait and stance should be inspected from all points of view, particularly the side view. The phases of the gait should be inspected for symmetry, coordination, and position of arms and legs. Any deviation should be identified in relation to the appropriate phase and stage.

Spine

At birth, the spinal curve is in the shape of a "C" rather than the double "S" seen later in life. The curves present in the neonate are the thoracic and pelvic curves. Around 3 to 4 months of age, the cervical curve develops. This is the time when children begin to hold their heads upright. The lumbar curve appears between 12 to 18 months, when the child begins to walk. The four curves then are the cervical (a convex line), the thoracic (concave), the lumbar (ventrally convex), and, finally, the pelvic curve (concave, directed caudally and ventrally). The cervical and lumbar curves are secondary or compensatory curves because they do not develop until after birth. It is important to remember this evolution of spinal curvatures when examining the spine in a young child.

Inspection and palpation of the spine should be done with the child standing if possible. The examiner checks for symmetry of bony landmarks, alignment, and other skin manifestations such as dimples, cysts, and tufts of hair. The spine is inspected and palpated for the presence or absence of each spinous process and for masses and tenderness. The child's posture is examined from the front, back, and side and when the child is in a flexed position. A child with an exaggerated concave curve in the thoracic region has kyphosis. On the other hand, an exaggerated convex curve in the lumbar region indicates lordosis, which may be normal in some children. Poor posture, commonly seen in adolescence, may appear as kyphosis but is usually not a permanent skeletal deformity. Scoliosis is a lateral curvature of the spine that requires medical evaluation. Positional evaluation of scoliosis is described in Chapter 41.

Neurologic System

Techniques	**Equipment**
Observation	Reflex hammer
Interview	Familiar odors in test tubes
	Safety pin
Examine for	
Cerebral function	Tuning fork
Cranial nerves	Ophthalmoscope
Cerebeller function	Small, easily recognizable objects (coin, bottlecap)
Motor system function	Audiometer for hearing testing
Sensory capacity Reflex action	Developmental screening tools

A complete neurologic examination requires an in-depth knowledge of nervous system function, expertise in the performance of the examination, and an extended time period. Rarely is a complete neurologic examination performed as part of a routine physical examination. More often, the nurse uses selective tests, such as developmental testing, and observations from the physical examination to evaluate the baseline function of the child's nervous system. Any abnormal results would then require further evaluation.

The neurologic examination involves testing of function within six major areas: the cerebrum, the cranial nerves, the cerebellum, the motor system, the sensory system, and reflex action.

Cerebral Function

This area is evaluated by history taking as well as sensory and developmental tests. The nurse should begin by noting general behavior, level of consciousness, intellectual performance, and emotional state. In addition, the child's posture, facial expression, gestures, movement, level of activity, attention span, and speech should be noted. Observations about specific behavior should be verified with the parent.

Memory is part of general cerebral function; immediate, recent, and remote memory should be evaluated. "Immediate recall" refers to the retention of an idea or thought for a brief time; this is tested by having a child repeat numbers. A child of 4 years can usually repeat three numbers, a child of 5 years can repeat four numbers, and a child of 6 can usually repeat five numbers correctly. Memory of an idea that lasts slightly longer is "recent memory." The child can be shown an object and told to remember the object. Later, the child is asked to tell what the object was. "Remote memory" refers to memory for longer periods. Children can be asked what they ate for dinner last night or their address or birthday.

Evaluation of specific cerebral function includes testing three functional areas:

- *Cortical sensory interpretation*—the ability to recognize objects through the use of senses: visual, tactile, auditory, somatic.
- *Cortical motor integration*—the ability to perform purposeful acts.
- *Language*—expressive, receptive.

Evaluation of *visual sensory capacity* can be accomplished by playing the "find it" game. The examiner places several objects on a table and then instructs the child to pick up the objects as they are named. *Tactile integration* (stereognosis) is evaluated by placing one of several objects in the child's hands while the child's eyes are closed and asking the child to identify the object. Familiar objects such as coins, bottlecaps, and buttons should be used. Graphesthesia is the ability to identify shapes traced in the palm or on the back of the hand. School-age children can usually identify the numbers 0, 1, 3, 7, and 8. Younger children usually identify geometric forms, parallel lines, or crossing lines. If the child cannot identify the shape, the examiner does the tracing twice and asks the child if the two are the same or different.

Evaluation of *auditory sensory capacity* is done by having the child listen with closed eyes and identify different common sounds such as a whistle or a hand clap.

Body part perception, or *somatic sensory perception,* can be accomplished by observing the child's response to tactile stimuli. The child's eyes are occluded. With the child's hands held out in front, the examiner touches one or two fingers and the child is asked to show which finger(s) were touched. By the age of 6, children may still occasionally confuse the third and fourth fingers, especially if two fingers were touched.

Kinesthesia, the ability to perceive direction of movement or weight, is evaluated in children over 5 years of age by manipulating the child's finger to either an up or a down position. The child's eyes should be closed for this test and the examiner should be careful to handle only the sides of the child's fingers so that the weight of the examiner's fingers does not give the child a clue to the direction. Texture discrimination can be done by having the child feel different textured items while the eyes are closed and tell whether the items are smooth or rough. *Visual motor integration and cortical motor integration* can be tested by having the child copy various designs that are drawn or shown. A child of 3 years of age can usually draw a circle; by the age of 4 years, a square can be drawn, and, by 5 years, the child can draw a triangle. Children 6 years of age can draw a diamond.

The last specific cerebral function to be tested is the child's *ability to communicate and understand both spoken and written language.* Screening tests for articulation and speech may be used and are described later in this chapter. Having the child repeat numbers or nonsense syllables, testing the ability to follow directions, and testing language discrimination are other ways of evaluating language ability. An inability to repeat may indicate that the child has poor ability to perceive what is heard. Discrimination is evaluated by saying two familiar words, such as "fright" and "flight." The child is then asked if they are the same or different words.

Part of the neurologic examination of the infant is an evaluation of its cry. A high-pitched shrill cry may indicate intracranial damage, whereas a high-pitched screeching cry may indicate a syndrome of genetic congenital defects, especially if associated with microcephaly, low-set ears, or micrognathia (small chin).

Cranial Nerves

Evaluation of the 12 pairs of cranial nerves is easily integrated into the nurse's physical examination. Children and adolescents enjoy the active participation required for testing cranial nerve functions. Difficulty is encountered in the assessment of cranial nerves in infants and young children, owing to the child's developmental level. Specific nerves and procedures for testing are indicated in Table 13–13.

TABLE 13-13
Assessment of Cranial Nerves

Cranial	Test for Function
I Olfactory (S)*	
Olfactory nerve, mucous membrane of nasal passages and turbinates	With eyes closed child is asked to identify familiar odors such as peanut butter, orange, peppermint. Test each nostril separately
II Optic (S)	
Optic nerve, retinal rods and cones	Check visual acuity, peripheral vision, color vision, perception of light in infants, funduscopic examination for normal optic disk
III Oculomotor (M)*	
Muscles of the eye (superior rectus, inferior rectus, medial rectus, inferior oblique)	Have child follow an object or light with the eyes (EOM)* while head remains stationary. Check symmetry of corneal light reflex. Check for nystagmus (direction elicited: vertical, horizontal, rotary). Check cover-uncover test
Muscles of iris and ciliary body	Reaction of pupils to light, both direct and consensual, accommodation
Levator palpebral muscle	Check for symmetric movement of upper eyelids. Note ptosis
IV Trochlear (M)	
Muscles of eye (superior oblique)	Check the range of motion of the eyes downward (EOM). Check for nystagmus
V Trigeminal (M, S)	
Muscles of mastication (M)	Have child clamp the jaws and palpate jaw muscles and temporal muscles for strength and symmetry. Ask child to move lower jaw from side to side against resistance of the examiner's hand
Sensory innervation of face (S)	Test child for sensation using a wisp of cotton; warm and cold water in test tubes; a sharp object on the forehead, cheeks, jaw. Check corneal reflex by touching a wisp of cotton to each cornea. The normal response is blink
VI Abducens (M)	
Muscles of eye (lateral rectus)	Have child look to each side (EOM)
VII Facial (M, S)	
Muscles for facial expression (M)	Have child make faces: look at the ceiling, frown, wrinkle forehead, blow out cheeks, smile. Check for strength, asymmetry, paralysis
Sense of taste on anterior ⅔ of tongue. Sensation of external ear canal, lacrimal, submaxillary and sublingual glands	Have child identify salt, sugar, bitter (flavoring extract) and sour substances by placing substance on anterior sides of tongue. Keep tongue out until substance is identified. Rinse mouth between substances
VIII Acoustic (S)	
Equilibrium (vestibular nerve)	Note equilibrium or presence of vertigo (Romberg sign)
Auditory acuity (cochlear nerve)	Test hearing. Use a tuning fork for the Weber and Rinne tests. Test by whispering and use of a watch
IX Glossopharyngeal (M, S)	
Pharynx, tongue (M)	Check elevation of palate with "ah" or crying. Check for movement and symmetry. Stimulate posterior pharynx for gag reflex
Sense of taste posterior third of the tongue (S)	Test sense of taste on posterior portion of tongue
X Vagus (M, S)	
Mucous membrane of pharynx, larynx, bronchi, lungs, heart, esophagus, stomach, kidneys Posterior surface of external ear, external auditory meatus	Note same as for glossopharyngeal. Note any hoarseness, stridor. Check uvula for midline position, movement with phonation. Stimulate uvula on each side with tongue depressor—should rise and deviate to stimulated side. Check gag reflex. Observe ability to swallow
XI Accessory (M)	
Sternocleidomastoid and upper trapezius muscles	Have child shrug shoulders against mild resistance. Have child turn head to one side against resistance of examiner's hand. Repeat on the other side. Inspect and palpate muscle strength, symmetry for both maneuvers
XII Hypoglossal (M)	
Muscles of tongue	Have child move the tongue in all directions, then stick out tongue as far as possible; check for tremors or deviations. Test strength by having child push tongue against inside cheek against resistance on outer cheek. Note strength, movement, symmetry

* S = sensory, M = motor, EOM = extraocular movement.

Cerebellar Function

Tests for cerebellar function primarily involve assessment of balance and coordination. Developmental screening tools provide an accessible, standardized method of assessing fine and gross motor balance and coordination skills. General cerebellar examination begins with observing gait, watching the child walk heel to toe, and checking the ability to dress and undress, button, stack blocks, throw, kick, and so on. Balance is specifically evaluated by observing the gait and having the child stand with the eyes both open and closed. This test of sensory equilibrium (Romberg test) is positive if the child loses balance.

Examples of coordination tests are finger-to-nose, heel-to-shin, and various activities that involve alternating motion. For the finger-to-nose test, the child stands erect with arms extended at the sides and then touches index fingers alternately to the nose. This test is repeated with the eyes closed. An abnormal response would be "past pointing," in which the child completely misses touching the nose. In the heel-to-shin test, the child lies supine on the examination table and places one heel rapidly down the shin from the knee to the ankle. This is repeated using the other heel. Uncoordinated or inaccurate movements suggest a cerebellar dysfunction.

Rapid alternating motion is tested by having the child rapidly alternate pronation and supination of the hands on the knees. One hand should be tested and the other observed for mirroring movements. Slow and inaccurate movements are considered abnormal. Additional information can be obtained by having the child stand erect and balance on one foot. By the age of 4 years, a child should be able to balance for about 5 seconds; by the age of 6, the child should be able to balance on one foot with arms folded across the chest. The child should balance on the right and then the left leg to evaluate symmetry. Another test would be to have the child touch each finger to the thumb of the same hand in rapid succession. This should be done with each hand to check for symmetry. The hand not performing the task should also be observed for mirroring. The cerebellar function of the infant may be grossly assessed by observing coordination in sucking, swallowing, reaching, and grasping.

Motor System

Examination of the motor system includes evaluation of muscle size, muscle tone, muscle strength, and abnormal muscle movements. Most of the motor system evaluation is accomplished through the examination of the extremities and spine and developmental screening tools. Muscles should be checked for hypertrophy, atrophy, and asymmetry. Any abnormality or asymmetry should be referred.

Muscle strength is discussed in the section on examination of the extremities in this chapter. Involuntary movements are assessed by observing a child in a stationary state with hands resting on the knees or stretched out in front.

Sensory System

Both primary and discriminatory sensation are evaluated as part of the assessment of the neurologic system. Many of the tests already discussed will give the examiner sufficient information about the sensory system for the routine examination. However, further evaluation may include an assessment of the primary, symmetric sensation of the face, trunk, arms, and legs. See Table 13–14 for the types of sensations to be evaluated and the procedures for testing.

Reflex Action

The infant has an array of protective reflexes that are present at birth and gradually fade as the child matures neurologically. Evaluation of these is covered in Chapter 4. The reflexes evaluated in the older child and adult fall into two categories: superficial and deep. Table 13–15 provides a description of the reflex and procedures employed in testing. Although superficial reflexes may not always be elicited as part of the neurologic examination, deep tendon reflexes usually are.

Deep tendon reflexes (DTRs) are illustrated and described in Table 13–16. DTR responses are usually graded using the following scoring system: 0 = absent; +1 = sluggish; +2 = active; +3 = hyperactive; +4 = transient clonus; +5 = permanent clonus.

Deep reflexes are evaluated for strength and symmetry from side to side and from upper to lower extremities. The tendon should be slightly stretched and briefly tapped with a reflex hammer. The expected response is contraction of the muscle. Pathologic reflexes are particularly significant in identifying neuro-

TABLE 13-14
Evaluating the Sensory System

Sensations	Procedure
Superficial tactile sensation	Brush body part with a wisp of cotton
Superficial pain	Evaluate ability to sense sharpness or dullness. Use both ends of a safety pin or a broken tongue depressor
Temperature	Have child identify the temperature of test tubes filled with both warm and cold water
Vibration	Assess the child's ability to feel a vibrating tuning fork on sternum, elbows, iliac crests, knees, and toes
Deep pressure pain	Never evaluated unless indicated by a decreased level of consciousness. Tested by applying strong pressure on eyeballs, sternum, calf or forearm muscles, or testicles
Motion and position	Tested as part of the evaluation of cerebellar function (see Chapter 40)
Discriminatory sensation	With the child's eyes closed, examiner touches a body part, then asks child to identify part touched

TABLE 13-15
Evaluating Superficial Reflexes

Procedure for Eliciting	Normal Response	Comments
Abdominal Reflex		
Using a sharp point, the examiner strokes the four quadrants of the abdomen in a diamond or square pattern	The umbilicus moves toward the stimulus	Present after the first 2 days of life. Absence or asymmetry of response may not be significant but should be noted
Cremasteric Reflex		
Stroke the inner aspect of the thigh with a fingernail; test both sides	Testis on the stimulated side recedes into inguinal canal	Often occurs spontaneously during examination. Abnormality could indicate pathology
Gluteal (Anal Wink)		
Examiner separates the buttocks and strokes the perianal area with a wisp of cotton	A brisk contraction of the anal sphincter	

logic abnormality. Clonus is abnormal in the older child but can be normal in the newborn infant if it is mild. The child's ankle is grasped and firm pressure is exerted on the ball of the foot, quickly dorsiflexing the foot. Clonus is present when the foot alternately moves up and down. Sustained clonus is significantly abnormal and requires further investigation.

The Babinski reflex is one of the most significant neurologic signs. It is elicited by stimulating the lateral aspect of the sole with a blunt point or fingernail. The stimulus begins at the midpoint of the heel and moves upward on the lateral aspect of the sole and across the ball of the foot toward the great toe. A Babinski response consists of fanning of the toes and dorsiflexion of the great toe. This is accompanied by dorsiflexion of the foot at the ankle and flexion at the knee and hip. A Babinski response is normal only in the neonate and infant until approximately 18 months of age.

Soft Signs

Neurologic "soft" signs are frequently discussed in pediatric neurology. There is controversy, however, regarding the existence, definition, interpretation, and significance of such signs. In general, this term is applied to subtle behaviors or signs whose significance is viewed differently. Examples of "soft" neurologic signs are:

Clumsiness	Hyperactivity
Perceptual difficulties	Short attention span
Language/articulation problems	Mirroring movements
Confused laterality	Difficulty with balance

Many clinicians believe that "soft" neurologic signs are significant and as such should be given careful consideration. A child with any significant neurologic finding should be referred for appropriate medical follow-up.

Developmental Screening

Assessing the Child

Developmental screening is an absolutely vital component of child health assessment. Unfortunately, it is often omitted during routine health assessment. Without the use of formal developmental screening tools, children with developmental disabilities can remain unidentified. However, if, through screening, problems are identified early in the developmental process, intervention is more likely to be successful (Roberts, 1983; Castiglia & Petrini, 1985; Fandal et al, 1978).

Denver II

Many tools are available for developmental screening. One of the most widely used tools was the Denver Developmental Screening Test (DDST). It has recently been replaced by its designers with the Denver II, shown in Appendix 4. This tool is still used to assess the child from birth to 6 years in four skill areas: personal-social, fine motor–adaptive, language, and gross motor. The changes in the test include the following:

- Increase in language items.
- Items for the evaluation of articulation.
- Age scale that corresponds to that used by the American Academy of Pediatrics (AAP) for well-child evaluations.

TABLE 13-16
Evaluating Deep Tendon Reflexes (DTR)

Name	Procedure for Eliciting	Normal Response	Comments
Triceps 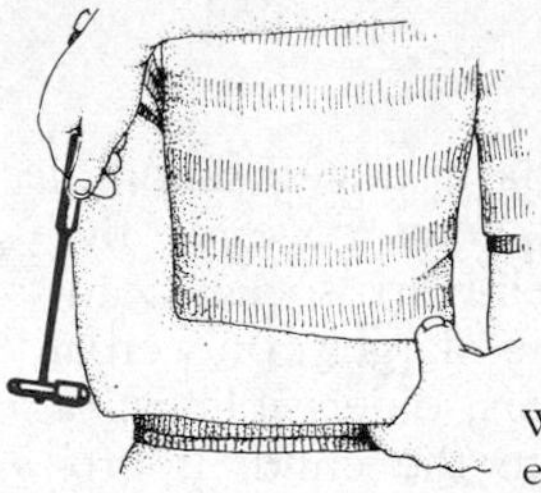	With the child's arm flexed at the elbow, the tendon is struck just above olecranon process	Muscles of the forearm contract	Grade response, evaluate symmetry
Biceps 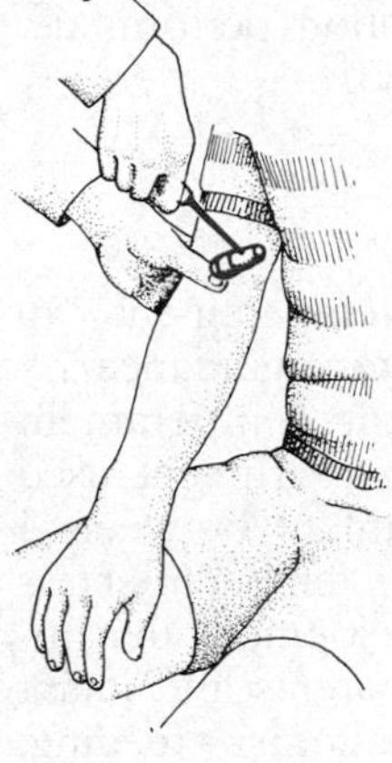	With the child's arm semiflexed at the elbow, slightly pronated, and with the elbow resting on the examiner's arm, the examiner places a thumb over the tendon and strikes the thumb	Contraction of biceps and forearm	Grade response, evaluate symmetry
Brachioradialis reflex 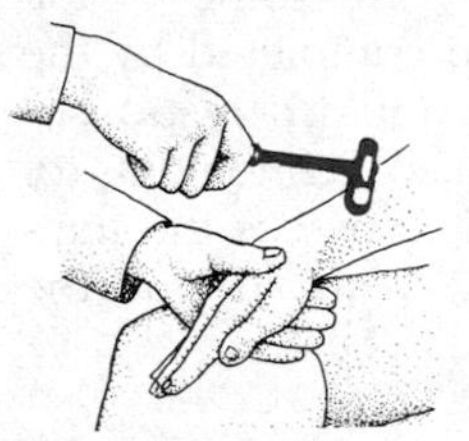	The styloid process of the radius is tapped sharply with the reflex hammer	Elbow flexion and forearm pronation	Grade response, evaluate symmetry
Patellar reflex 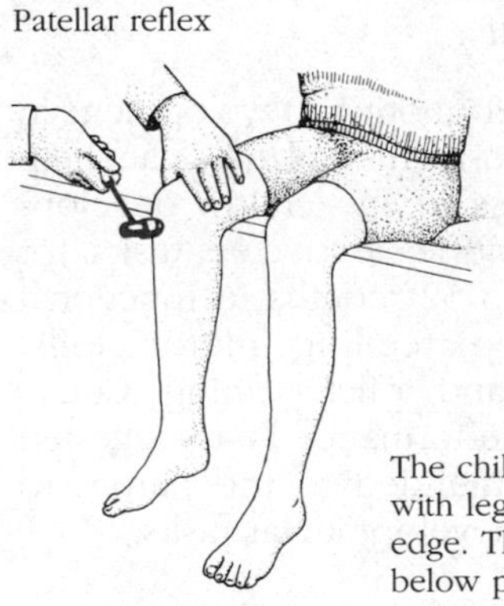	The child is in a sitting position with legs dangling freely over table edge. The patellar tendon—just below patella—is struck	Contraction of quadriceps, and extension of lower leg	Grade response, evaluate symmetry
Achilles reflex 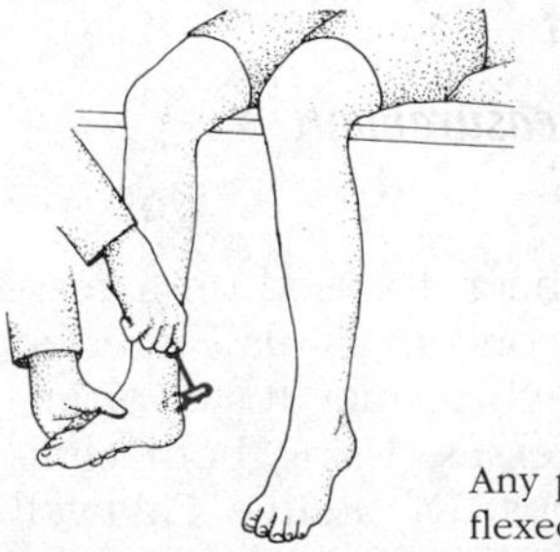	Any position in which foot can be flexed to stretch tendon	Plantar flexion of foot	Grade response, evaluate symmetry

- Scale for noting the child's behavior during examination.
- More detailed written and video training materials.

The Denver II has been found to be reliable and valid. The authors describe it as a tool that simply identifies children who, for whatever reasons—biologic or environmental—are unable to perform at a level comparable to their age mates. Children with questionable or abnormal scores are at risk for developing school problems despite intelligence (Frankenburg et al, 1992).

Nurses working with a large population of a specific ethnic group may find that consistent failures of specific items on the Denver II may be related to cultural practices. For example, Southeast Asian groups routinely place infants in the supine position and rarely in the prone position in the early months of life. These children, not often being in the prone position, are not offered the opportunity to practice some of the early gross motor skills (e.g., holding head upright, chest and head up with arm support) and may, therefore, fail that portion of the Denver II. These children do catch up with their peers on these gross motor skills within the first year of life. Understanding the reasons for failure of portions of a developmental screening allows the nurse to develop an informal standard of development for a particular ethnic group.

It is important to carry out developmental screening accurately. The Denver II Screening Manual has information calculating ages for premature children, scoring criteria for each item, general information on scoring, and symbols used for proper scoring. Numerous pointers on preparation, administration, scoring, and interpretation are also provided. Video training material is also available.

Each item is designated as a bar that represents the ages at which 25, 50, 70, and 90 per cent of the tested population could perform the particular item. Scoring is based on the number of delays found in the test. A delay is defined as the failure to perform an item that 90 per cent of children the same age can perform or failure in any item to the left of any age line. These items are those that could be performed by younger children.

Before beginning the test, the nurse must be sure to adequately explain to parents the purpose of the test and how it is performed. The Denver II is not an intelligence test, and this should be clearly stated to the parent. The parent should also understand that the child will be asked to perform tasks below and above the expected performance so that the best possible performance is obtained. Denver II results should be completely explained to the parent, reinforcing the child's satisfactory performance. Children with abnormal or questionable results should be rescreened before referral for diagnostic testing.

The child's performance is affected by factors such as fatigue, anxiety, illness, shyness, or separation from the parent. Also, undetected visual or hearing problems or neurologic or developmental problems may influence the child's performance and should be considered.

Developmental Profile II

The Developmental Profile II is a developmental screening tool consisting of 168 items covering five developmental areas: physical, self-help, social, academic, and communication. It relies largely on verbal responses from the parent, teachers, older siblings, or other individuals acquainted with the child. It provides an individual profile that can be compared with data on what is normal for specific ages at which children in the standardized population perform developmental skills (Alpern et al, 1986).

Profile of Temperament

Obtaining a profile of the child's temperament can also be useful in planning anticipatory guidance regarding parenting. The Carey Infant Temperament Questionnaire is a clinical screening instrument used to study the temperament of the infant between 4 and 8 months of age. Carey identifies temperament as an important variable in infant development that influences the relationships between parents and infant and other caregivers. The child's patterns—feeding, sleeping, eliminating, and playing—are some of the areas identified in the questionnaire completed by the parent. The items also look at the infant's responses to different situations. There are also refinements of this questionnaire that can be used to assess the temperament of the toddler, the 3- to 7-year-old, and the 8- to 12-year-old.

Promoting Development

The Washington Guide to Promoting Development in the Young Child is an assessment tool that can help in an evaluation of progress in the child's development. This instrument identifies expected tasks for age groups from 1 month to 52 months in functional activity areas such as sleep, feeding, motor skills, play, language, discipline, and toilet training. Corresponding to the expected performance is a suggested activity that can be recommended to the parent to help the child accomplish developmental tasks.

Environmental Assessment

Home Observation for Measurement of the Environment

Although much attention has been focused on assessing the child's development, concern is also directed at assessing the environment, which may foster or impede the developmental processes. Using both clinical and home visit observations, Dr. Bettye Caldwell developed an assessment tool designed to identify characteristics of the environment of children from birth to 3 years and from 3 to 6 years (Bradley & Caldwell, 1988). The instrument is the Home Observation for Measurement of the Environment (HOME) (see Appendix 5 for these forms). The birth-to-3-years inventory measures six subscales: emotional and verbal responsiveness of the mother, avoidance of restriction and punishment, organization of physical and temporal environment, provision of appropriate play materials, maternal involvement with the child, and opportunities for variety in daily stimulation.

The inventory for 3- to 6-year-olds measures seven subscales: provision of stimulation through equipment, toys, and experiences; stimulation of mature behavior; provision of stimulating physical and language environment; avoidance of restriction and punishment; pride, affection, and thoughtfulness; masculine stimulation; and independence from parental control. The purpose for both scales is to identify certain aspects of the quantity and quality of the social, emotional, and cognitive environmental supports available to the young child in her or his home.

This tool must be administered by a person who goes into the home and observes the child when awake during the normal daily routine. It takes approximately an hour to obtain the data. The parent should be notified of the forthcoming visit. The HOME can be used in combination with other screening tools to assist parents to solve current problems and prevent development of other problems by providing anticipatory guidance for appropriate parenting.

Speech Screening

No developmental screening would be complete without a speech evaluation (Kilmon et al, 1991). One easily administered test for children who speak English is the Denver Articulation Screening Examination (DASE), which is a word-imitative procedure. The child repeats 22 different words while the examiner listens for errors in the articulation of 30 different sound elements. See Appendix 6 for a copy of the examination with instructions for its use.

Intelligibility is also scored by selection of one of four categories ranging from "easy to understand" to "cannot evaluate." The DASE is designed to pinpoint significant speech delays and normal variations in the acquisition of speech sounds. Abnormal conditions such as tongue thrust, lisp, hypernasality, and hyponasality can also be detected. Speech and language development is also evaluated by direct observation of the child's verbal skills, in addition to speech patterns and history of speech patterns and development.

Nutritional Assessment

Nutrition is a significant factor that influences and is influenced by growth and development. Physical competency is especially affected by nutritional status. Nutritional requirements are based on what is considered necessary to support life, to provide for growth, and to maintain health. Nutritional assessment is discussed in Chapter 16, with specific requirements according to age presented in Chapters 5 through 9 on growth and development.

The nurse should learn basic principles of nutritional assessment and counseling applicable at all ages. There are four major purposes for assessing food intake:

- Identify dietary practices of the family.
- Obtain baseline data on caloric and nutrient intake and appropriate anthropometric measurements from which progress can be measured.
- Promote healthful dietary practices through counseling and teaching.
- Provide parents with the opportunity to ask questions about nutrition and feeding behaviors.

Before obtaining a nutritional history, the nurse must be prepared to ask questions in a nonjudgmental way. Food and feeding practices can be extremely sensitive issues, especially for parents whose children are having problems involving body weight. Also, it is important to listen carefully to what parents are saying and what it appears they are practicing. Parents of young children can recite an appropriate diet and deny the consumption of junk food while their child is found to be mildly obese. The nurse must also be prepared to accept some unfamiliar cultural food practices. For example, some cultures may not give any solids for the first year of life, whereas another may give an infant food that has first been chewed by the mother to make it an appropriate consistency.

The details of a nutritional assessment are discussed in Chapter 16, including the use of a 24-hour intake and other approaches such as a 3-day or 7-day food diary (see Tables 16–11 and 16–12). Recommended Dietary Allowances (RDAs) are presented in Table 16–1, and physical indicators of nutritional status in Table 16–13.

Eating patterns and exercise/activity patterns that contribute to a healthy child should be reinforced. If necessary, the parents and child should be counseled regarding modification of the child's and family's food choices. It is important to include both the parents and the child in the plans for change. It is also important that they know the reasons for change and how their beliefs, attitudes, and actions are affecting the nutrition of the child. The parents and the child may need support and help in dealing not only with their own feelings and behaviors but also with those of friends and relatives. See Chapter 16 for further discussion of nutritional counseling and related concerns and issues.

Laboratory Screening

Laboratory tests are used as diagnostic or screening aids; when combined with subjective and objective findings, they provide a complete data base. Many of the laboratory specimens needed for diagnostic examination of children are obtained by the same methods used for adults. The young child usually requires restraint. The older child is often able to cooperate and follow directions adequately to assist in obtaining the laboratory specimens. Appendix 8 gives normal laboratory values for children.

Blood Specimens

Most blood samples are obtained by laboratory staff. The nurse is often responsible for making certain that the parent and child understand the procedure, assisting in restraint, and making sure the child is comforted and rewarded after the traumatic procedure. In some settings, however, such as intensive care units, offices, and clinics, the nurse is also responsible for collecting specimens needed. Since all traumatic procedures are best completed swiftly, it is imperative that all necessary preparation be done in advance and out of the child's view.

Most blood screening tests can be performed on either venous or capillary blood specimens. Whatever method is used to collect the blood specimen, it is essential that the parent and child be adequately prepared for the procedure and adequate restraint be provided if the child is unable to cooperate. See Chapter 23 for discussion of specific techniques used to collect blood and the preparation of children for procedures.

As after any painful procedure, the child should be comforted by the parent. The infant should be cuddled, the toddler held and praised, the preschooler and early school-age child should be rewarded with praise and perhaps a small token (e.g., a sticker).

Hematocrit

One of the most frequently used laboratory screening tests is the hematocrit. The hematocrit is a comparison of packed red blood cell volume to whole blood. This is generally a screening test used for anemia. Using the procedure described in Chapter 23 for obtaining capillary blood, two capillary tubes of blood are filled to be centrifuged. Normal hematocrit values at sea level vary according to the age of the child. See Appendix 8 for normal ranges listed according to age.

Hemoglobin

A hemoglobin refers to the measurement of hemoglobin within each blood cell. Since the hematocrit measures the volume of red blood cells and the hemoglobin measures the hemoglobin within each cell, it is frequently important to measure both to determine whether anemia is present. Depending on the method used to determine the hemoglobin, either capillary or venous blood is obtained. Hemoglobin values are expressed in g/dl of blood or mmol/L of blood (the latter expression is in international units).

The hemoglobin and hematocrit are always done if there is a suggestion of possible anemia by history or physical findings. The child should be screened at 6 to 9 months of age, between 12 and 18 months, and again during adolescence. These are the ages at which the child is most frequently at risk for developing iron-deficiency anemia. The test at 6 to 9 months may be omitted if the child is still drinking iron-fortified formula.

Sickledex

A simple screening procedure for sickle cell anemia is the Sickledex. This disease is a defect in the structure of the red blood cell, which loses its round shape and becomes sickled by stress or lack of oxygen. Approximately 10 per cent of the African-American population has this condition. The test is done only on African-American children over 6 months of age because of the amount of fetal hemoglobin present before that age. The Sickledex is a screening test, and any positive test should be referred for more specific diagnostic testing.

Phenylketonuria

Phenylketonuria (PKU), a disorder of amino acid metabolism, causes an abnormal accumulation of the amino acid phenylalanine in the blood, resulting in brain damage. Testing for PKU has become mandatory on all newborns in most states (AAP, 1982, 1992; Doherty et al, 1991). Hospital discharges sooner after birth have led to changes in the timing of the test. When examining a neonate or very young infant, the nurse should carefully review the medical record to be sure that the initial PKU screening was completed and that the results have been documented. Chapter 44 describes the details of this test.

Lead

Screening for lead toxicity is done by both blood and urine testing. Blood testing requires venous blood. Screening varies according to whether a child is considered to be at risk. Blood lead concentration and erythrocyte-protoporphyrin (EP) level are the commonly used tests. See Chapter 46 for a further discussion of screening for lead toxicity.

Urine Specimens

One of the most painless and effective ways to evaluate the functioning of the entire body is examination of the urine. The various techniques for collecting urine specimens are described in Chapter 23. Older children and adolescents can readily provide a specimen with correct instructions but may be embarrassed by carrying specimens through hallways. If this is the case, a paper bag should be provided or the specimen may be retrieved discreetly. Adolescent females who are menstruating should delay providing a specimen, or a notation should be made on the laboratory slip to explain the presence of red blood cells.

School-age children are cooperative but, like adolescents, are very curious and concerned regarding the reasons for obtaining the specimen. Explanations of the method and reasons for obtaining a urine sample will greatly expedite the procedure.

Preschoolers and toddlers are less able to cooperate. Before trying to obtain a specimen, the nurse should offer liquids and wait 20 to 30 minutes. Fluids are not given in excessively large amounts since this may distort the results of the test. The parent should be questioned as to the child's terminology for this bodily function, and these words should be used. Children who have difficulty voiding in an unfamiliar receptacle may be provided with a clean or sterilized potty chair or bed pan placed on the toilet. Toddlers, in particular, may have difficulty voiding in unfamiliar surroundings since they have undoubtedly been admonished for urinating in places not approved by parents during the toilet training phase. The parents may need to reassure the child it is all right to void in the bed pan.

A standard urinalysis includes an examination for the color, pH, and specific gravity; testing for glucose, ketones, and protein; and a microscopic determination for cells, bacteria, and crystalline content. Simple qualitative screening tests can be done for pH, glucose, protein, blood, and other substances by using reagent-covered test strips that are dipped directly into the urine or pressed between two urine-saturated surfaces of a diaper. The presence of the test substance causes a color change on the strip, which is then compared with the colors identified on a chart or on the test strip bottle. The odor should also be noted, because it can indicate an abnormality. Microscopic examination of the urine is done by an experienced laboratory clinician. Further information on collection of urine specimens is presented in Chapter 23.

Urine cultures are done for children who are suspected of having a urinary tract infection and for children whose routine urinalysis indicates abnormal microscopic findings. Techniques for obtaining urine specimens for culture are described in Chapter 23.

KEY CONCEPTS

Concepts Related to Basic Information

- The purpose of a complete history, physical examination, and developmental assessment is to identify any findings that fall outside the normal parameters and that will need a more detailed assessment.
- Assessments must be multifocal to be complete and include an evolution of family dynamics as well as cultural, social, environmental, and religious variables that may affect the child's overall development.
- Interviewing is a complex process that includes information from direct and indirect questions as well as observation of nonverbal cues.
- Children who have irregular patterns of health care are at increased risk for familial, school, social, and health problems. These children require special assessment when they appear in the health care system.

Concepts Related to Nursing Assessment

- The five components of the nursing process are:
  1. Assessment.
  2. Nursing diagnosis.
  3. Development of a plan of care.
  4. Nursing interventions.
  5. Evaluation of patient outcomes.
- The five major categories included in a comprehensive child health assessment are:
  - Taking a history.
  - Performing a physical assessment.
  - Completing developmental screening.
  - Completing a nutritional assessment.
  - Performing necessary laboratory screening.
- The sequencing of a physical examination is usually done in a head-to-toe pattern. However, the pattern may be altered depending on the physical, emotional, and developmental capacities of the child.
- The four physical assessment techniques are:
  - Inspection.
  - Palpation.
  - Auscultation.
  - Percussion.

Concepts Related to Nursing Intervention

- Physical examination includes general appearance plus close scrutiny of all body systems.
- Key issues in approaching a child for physical assessment include comfortable atmosphere; quick and systematic examination; respect for child's modesty; flexibility relating to examination opportunities; explanation of all procedures before they are done; skill in all assessment techniques; and a good knowledge base in anatomy as well as in child development.
- Height, weight, head circumference, and vital signs are significant indicators, particularly when viewed in a continued series of examinations.

- Diagnostic tools help assess the child through developmental screening, nutritional assessment, and laboratory screening.
- Abnormal findings during examinations will require further evaluation. The finding, the system affected, and the severity of the problem will dictate the rapidity with which referral will be sought.

REFERENCES

Alpern, G., Boll, T., & Shearer, M. (1986). *The developmental profile II.* Los Angeles: Western Psychological Services (12031 Wilshire Blvd., Los Angeles, 90025).

American Academy of Pediatrics. (1986). *Report of the Committee on Infectious Diseases* (20th ed.). Elk Grove Village, IL: Author.

American Academy of Pediatrics, Committee on Genetics. (1992). Issues in newborn screening. *Pediatrics, 89,* 345–349.

American Academy of Pediatrics, Committee on Genetics. (1982). New issues in newborn screening for phenylketonuria and congenital hypothyroidism. *Pediatrics, 69,* 104–106.

Barrus, D. H. (1983). A comparison of rectal and axillary temperatures by electronic thermometer measurement in preschool children. *Pediatric Nursing, 9,* 424-425.

Bradley, R. H., & Caldwell, B. M. (1988). Using the HOME inventory to assess the family environment. *Pediatric Nursing, 14,* 97–102.

Castiglia, P. T., & Petrini, M. A. (1985). Selecting a developmental screening tool. *Pediatric Nursing, 11,* 8–17.

Doherty, L. B., Rohr, F. J., & Levy, H. L. (1991). Detection of phenylketonuria in the very early newborn blood specimen. *Pediatrics, 87,* 240–244.

Downs, M. P. (1981). Early identification of hearing loss. In N. Lass, et al (Eds.). *Speech, language, and hearing.* Philadelphia: WB Saunders.

Fandal, A. W., Kemper, M. B., & Frankenburg, W. K. (1978). Needed: Routine developmental screening for all children. *Pediatric Basics* (Issue 24). Freemont, MI: Gerber Products Company.

Frankenburg, W. K., et al. (1992). The Denver II: A major revision and restandardization of the Denver Developmental Screening Test. *Pediatrics, 89,* 91–97.

Jaworski, A. (1978, September). A new boy-girl blood pressure chart for pediatric office use: A single-sheet graph for all children. *Clinical Pediatrics,* 699.

Kilmon, C. A., Barber, N., & Chapman, K. (1991). Instruments for the screening of speech/language development in children. *Journal of Pediatric Health Care, 5,* 61–70.

Moss, J. R. (1983). Predicting young children's cooperation with the physical examination. *Pediatric Nursing, 9,* 188–190.

Roberts, P. H. (1983). Nursing assessment: Screening for developmental problems. In M. Krajicek & A. T. Tomlinson (Eds.). *Detection of developmental problems in children* (2nd ed., pp 9–40). Baltimore: University Park Press.

Rogers, J., et al. (1991). Evaluation of tympanic membrane thermometer for use with pediatric patients. *Pediatric Nursing, 17,* 376–378.

BIBLIOGRAPHY

Athreya, B. (1985). *Pediatric physical diagnosis.* Norwalk, CT: Appleton-Century-Crofts.

Barnes, L. S. A. (1981). *Manual of pediatric physical diagnosis* (5th ed.). Chicago: Year Book.

Brown, M. S., & Murphy, M. A. (1981). *Ambulatory pediatrics for nurses* (2nd ed.). New York: McGraw-Hill.

Cadman, D., et al. (1984). The usefulness of the DDST to predict kindergarten problems in a general community population. *American Journal of Public Health, 74,* 1093–1097.

Eiliman, A. M., et al. (1985). Denver developmental screening tests and preterm infants. *Archives of Disease in Childhood, 60,* 20–24.

Frankenburg, W. K., et al. (1975). Development of preschool-aged children of different social and ethnic groups: Implications for developmental screening. *Journal of Pediatrics, 87,* 125–132.

Fung, K., & Lau, S. (1985). Denver developmental screening test: Cultural variables. *Journal of Pediatrics, 106,* 343.

Green, M., & Haggerty, R. J. (1984). *Ambulatory pediatrics III.* Philadelphia: WB Saunders.

Hall, D. M. B., & Baird, G. (1986). Developmental tests and scales. *Archives of Disease in Childhood, 61,* 213–215.

Hancock, L. (1987). First temp. *Journal of Pediatric Health Care, 1,* 163–164.

Hoekelman, R. A. (1991). The physical examination of infants and children. In B. Bates (Ed.). *A guide to physical examination and history taking* (5th ed.). Philadelphia: JB Lippincott.

Jarvis, C. (1992). *Physical examination and health assessment.* Philadelphia: WB Saunders.

Kempe, C. H., Silver, H. K., & O'Brien, D. (1984). *Current pediatric diagnosis and treatment* (8th ed.). Los Altos, CA: Lange Medical Publications.

Kotzer, A. M., & McCabe, E. R. B. (1988). Newborn screening for inherited metabolic disease: Principles and practice. *Neonatal Network, 6,* 15–19.

O'Flynn, M. (1992, April). Newborn screening for phenylketonuria: Thirty years of progress. *Current Problems in Pediatrics, April,* 159–165.

Powell, M. L. (1981). *Assessment and management of developmental changes and problems in children* (2nd ed.). St. Louis: CV Mosby.

Sturner, R. A., et al. (1982). Adaptation of the DDST: A study of preschool screening. *Pediatrics, 69,* 346–350.

Tudor, M. (1977). Developmental screening. *Issues in Comprehensive Pediatric Nursing 2,* 1–13.

CHAPTER • 14

Fostering Self-Esteem

Mabel Hunsberger

RELATED TOPICS
Family structures and systems, Chapter 2
Concepts of child development, Chapter 3
Development of children at different stages, Unit 2, Chapters 4 through 9
Communication, a significant component of self-esteem development, Chapter 11
Self-esteem and altered behavior patterns, Chapter 27

LEARNING OBJECTIVES

- Define the terms "self-concept" and "self-system."
- Describe the factors that contribute to the development of the *self-system.*
- Identify the ages or events most crucial to development of the *self-system.*
- Describe the parental characteristics that promote or deter positive development of the *self-system.*
- Explain ways that the nurse can foster self-esteem in children and adolescents.
- Describe the various methods for obtaining an assessment of *self-concept.*
- Illustrate the types of experiences that help children adopt positive attitudes in the areas of sense of security, sense of identity, sense of belonging, sense of purpose, and sense of personal competence.

Self-esteem development is perhaps one of the most crucial elements of an individual's growth process. Nurses are in a key position to promote the healthy development of a child's self-esteem because of the opportunity to support children, as well as to influence parents in how they parent. Through support, counseling, and teaching, nurses can help to prevent the occurrence of self-esteem disturbance or low self-esteem. Nurses need to know how self-esteem develops, how that development is influenced by people and experiences, and how self-esteem contributes to attaining an adaptive lifestyle. Assessment tools that can be used in the practice setting are identified and measures to build and maintain a healthy self-esteem are presented.

Achievement of healthy adaptation skills in childhood provides the foundation for self-actualization in adulthood. Coping strategies are learned that help a child to achieve equilibrium as maturational and situational stressors are encountered. A child instinctively experiments with and adopts behaviors that help to reduce the anxiety associated with the problems and challenges of living. The behaviors learned are influenced by the child's previous experiences, the developmental stage, temperament, environmental demands, and the behaviors role-modeled by the significant people in the child's world. If the learned behaviors are adaptive, they will service the child successfully in later experiences. If maladaptive, the behaviors will increase the child's stress, disrupt learning potential, and may result in dysfunctional behavior patterns.

A key element influencing acquisition of adaptive or maladaptive behavior is the child's self-perceptions. Self-esteem is an extremely important component of healthy living, preceded only by satisfaction of physiologic and safety needs and one's need to be loved. According to Maslow's hierarchy of needs, the need for self-esteem includes: *self-respect, others' respect, self-confidence, and feelings of competence, independence, success, and recognition from others* (Maslow, 1968).

Defining the Self-System

The self-system develops gradually as a child matures. It begins to develop during the first year of life and becomes more differentiated as the child matures (Battle, 1989). The self-system accounts for the uniqueness of a person. *Although some aspects of the self-system may change over time, the central core of this system appears to remain intact and to endure over time* (Eder, 1990; Cairns et al, 1990). Self-esteem, a component of the self-system, temporarily fluctuates like a barometer that rises and falls as a function of one's experiences (Heatherton & Polivy, 1991), but returns to a level that is fairly stable and resistant to change (Battle, 1989).

Although self-concept and self-esteem are differentiated in this chapter, the terms "self-system" and "self-concept" are used synonymously. "Self-concept" and "self-system" are generic terms that encompass many smaller constructs (e.g., self-image, self-esteem, self-ideal). Constructs of the self-system are presented in Figure 14–1. This broad concept comprises both a *physical self* and a *personal self* (Fig. 14–2). The process of self-definition and self-evaluation takes place through interpersonal interactions; the self is seen through the reactions of others.

The belief that development of the self-system has its origin in interpersonal relationships is based on Sullivan (1953). It is through these "reflected" appraisals that the self-system develops. As children receive feedback from their interactions, they evaluate whether they are a "good person" or a "bad person." Those behaviors that generate extremely negative feedback and, thus, extreme anxiety are rejected as "not me" and denied. "Good person" perceptions result from consistent approval or positive feedback from significant others. "Bad person" perceptions are derived from consistent disapproval or negative feedback from significant others. Characteristics of children with high and low self-regard are presented in Table 14–1. Once this core of self-regard is established in the young child, it becomes an important factor in the adaptive strategies chosen, task mastery accomplished, and social competence achieved in later developmental stages.

Influences on Self-System Development

Children are not born with an identity or self-concept. The self-system is developed gradually, with different parts of the system receiving emphasis and maturing at differing times. Acquisition is somewhat predictable, as is cognitive, moral, and psychosocial development. Several elements of experience seem especially pertinent to development of the self-system: (1) developmental psychosocial crises, (2) expectations of significant others, (3) social role expectations and cultural factors, (4) physical health status, and (5) temperamental coping style. Development of the self-system, and of self-esteem in particular, forms the basis for trying out new skills and relationships at each new developmental stage.

Developmental Psychosocial Crises

Early childhood is identified by many theorists as a crucial time for the healthy development of the core component of the self-system. A supportive, responsive environment during infancy fosters the attainment of developmental milestones that form the foundation for a healthy self-esteem. Typically, in the first year of life, infants (1) develop an awareness of separateness from another, (2) develop a sense that they can have an effect on people and objects, and, (3) through experience, learn that the world is basically responsive or nonresponsive to their needs (Sieving & Zirbel-Donisch, 1990). With sufficient and positive interpersonal interactions during the phases of development, these experiences produce an individual with a positive self-concept and a high level of self-actualization during adulthood, as depicted in Figure 14–3.

Some believe the experiences that contribute to a person's eventual self-esteem may begin even before birth, suggesting "there never is tabula rasa" (Hattie, 1992, p 120). The developmental progress of the self-

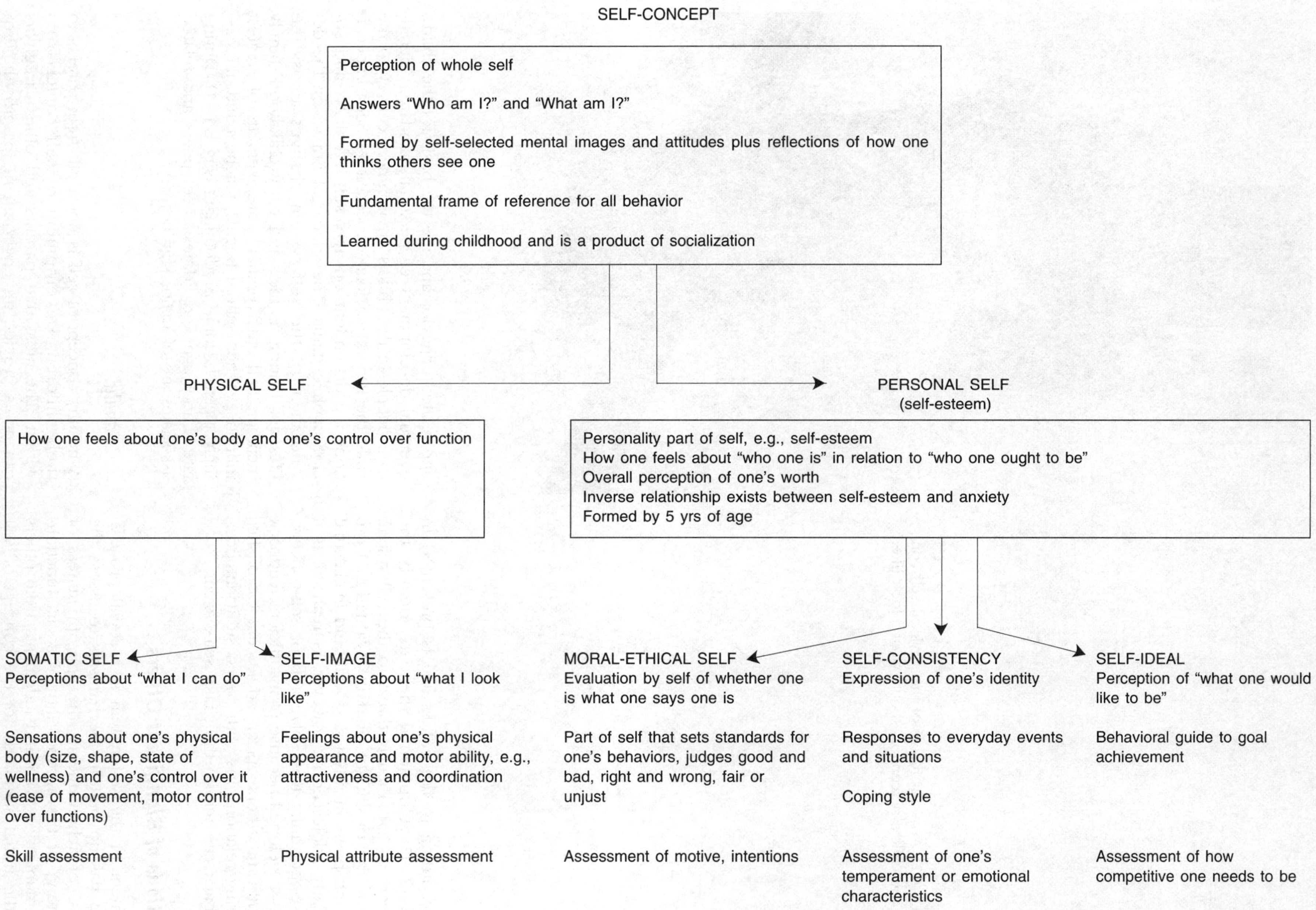
SELF-CONCEPT
Perception of whole self
Answers "Who am I?" and "What am I?"
Formed by self-selected mental images and attitudes plus reflections of how one thinks others see one
Fundamental frame of reference for all behavior
Learned during childhood and is a product of socialization
PHYSICAL SELF
How one feels about one's body and one's control over function
PERSONAL SELF
(self-esteem)
Personality part of self, e.g., self-esteem
How one feels about "who one is" in relation to "who one ought to be"
Overall perception of one's worth
Inverse relationship exists between self-esteem and anxiety
Formed by 5 yrs of age
SOMATIC SELF
Perceptions about "what I can do"
Sensations about one's physical body (size, shape, state of wellness) and one's control over it (ease of movement, motor control over functions)
Skill assessment
SELF-IMAGE
Perceptions about "what I look like"
Feelings about one's physical appearance and motor ability, e.g., attractiveness and coordination
Physical attribute assessment
MORAL-ETHICAL SELF
Evaluation by self of whether one is what one says one is
Part of self that sets standards for one's behaviors, judges good and bad, right and wrong, fair or unjust
Assessment of motive, intentions
SELF-CONSISTENCY
Expression of one's identity
Responses to everyday events and situations
Coping style
Assessment of one's temperament or emotional characteristics
SELF-IDEAL
Perception of "what one would like to be"
Behavioral guide to goal achievement
Assessment of how competitive one needs to be

FIGURE 14 - 1. Constructs of the self-system. (Data from Harter, S. [1982]. Developmental perspectives on the self-system. In E. Hetherington [ed]: *Carmichael's manual of child psychology* (Vol. 4). New York: John Wiley & Sons; Rambo, B. [1984]. *Adaptation nursing*. Philadelphia: WB Saunders; Roy, C. [1984]. *Introduction to nursing: An adaptation model*. Englewood Cliffs, NJ: Prentice-Hall; and Battle, J. [1989]. *Enhancing self-esteem and achievement*. Edmonton, Alberta: James Battle & Associates.)

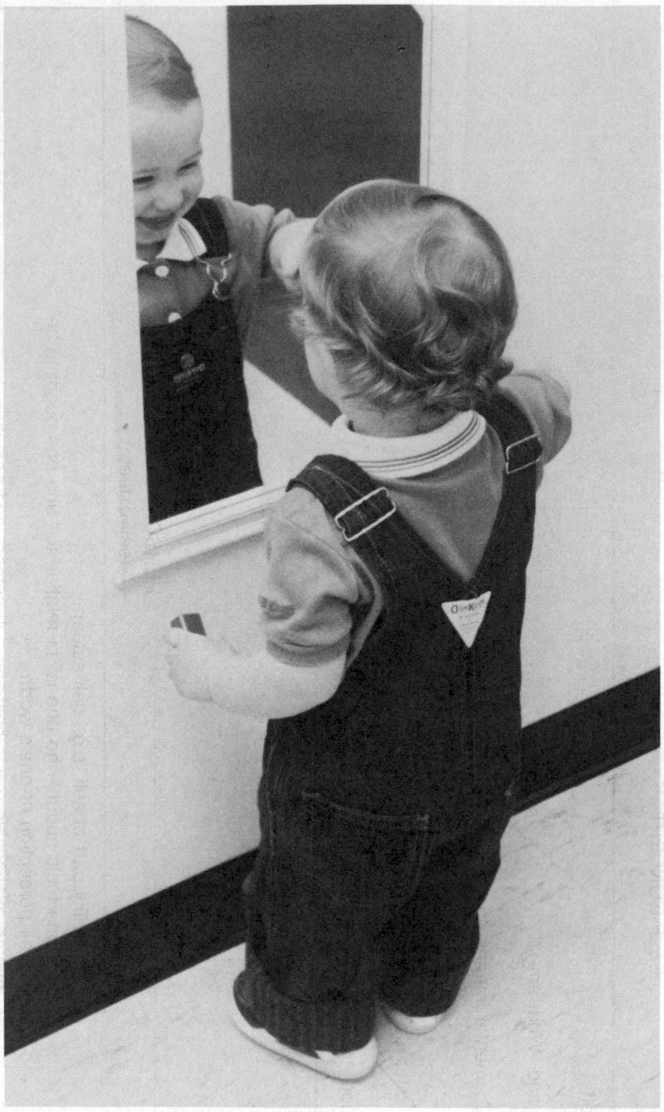

FIGURE 14 - 2. A mirror image of the physical self contributes to the child's perception about "what I look like."

system according to the child's age is presented in Table 14–2. Developmental theorists identify the school years as a particular threat to the self-system because of the onslaught of daily evaluation from teachers and peers in physical, social, and intellectual realms. Early adolescence, however, is realized as a potential opportunity to resolve a poor self-concept, which has developed because of insufficient feedback from significant others. As an adolescent establishes close, caring relationships with peers, sufficient positive feedback can reform the shaky self-system.

Expectations of Significant Others

Development of the self-system is a social process. The child has no built-in mechanisms to assess the worthiness of achievements, the appropriateness of task mastery, or the acceptability of social functioning. Communication with and judgments from others provide the initial standards for the concept of self and related behavior and are the basis for the child's eventual development of personal standards. Significant people in the child's environment convey to the child the general societal expectations. Such expectations are dependent on age, sex, ethnicity, and socioeconomic status. The source of impact on the development of the self-system changes across the lifespan. During infancy and early childhood, family members and other primary caregivers are of greatest influence. When school begins, teachers and, increasingly, peers become predominant (Fig. 14–4). During late school age and adolescence, peers and related associates are of major significance.

Family

A healthy concept of self is not a gift from parents to their children. Development of self comes from within. The most that parents and other caregivers can do is provide an environment for growth. Pro-

TABLE 14-1
Characteristics of Children with High and Low Self-Regard

Behaviors Demonstrating High Self-Regard	Behaviors Demonstrating Low Self-Regard
More active—seek activities and new experiences	Hesitant to participate in activities and anxiety is provoked by new experiences
Self-confidence. Inner assuredness of success and of positive responses from people	Feel inferior. Assume others will respond negatively. Pessimistic
Demonstrate leadership skills in groups, independence	Tend to follow or watch others achieve. Unable to function in groups
Recognize self as more skillful in some areas than in others and this is OK (self-coping)	Easily discouraged. Inner pressure to resort to self-defeating behaviors rather than coping directly (defensive coping), e.g., rebellious, acting-out behaviors
Handle criticism, hold realistic worldview	Cannot stand losing, not being first. Self-centered and egotistic
Express feelings of being likable, worthwhile, important	Express feelings of being unlikable, unacceptable, undesirable, insignificant
Behaviors reflect self-respect, pride in self and achievements	Doubt own ability to do well or have friends. Boast to cover up fragile sense of worth
Steadily increase and willingly assume self-control (internal locus of control), effectiveness in solving problems	Hesitate or refuse to assume self-control (external locus of control). Dependent on acceptance for control
Expressive, happy, optimistic, enjoy interpersonal interaction	Depressed, timid, poor social interactions

Data from Coopersmith, S. (1967). *The antecedents of self-esteem.* San Francisco: WH Freeman; Harter, S. (1982). Developmental perspectives on the self-system. In E. Hetherington (Ed.): *Carmichael's manual of child psychology* (Vol. 4). New York: John Wiley & Sons; and Sieving, R. E., & Zirbel-Donisch, S. T. (1990). Development and enhancement of self-esteem in children. *Journal of Pediatric Health Care, 4(6),* 290–296.

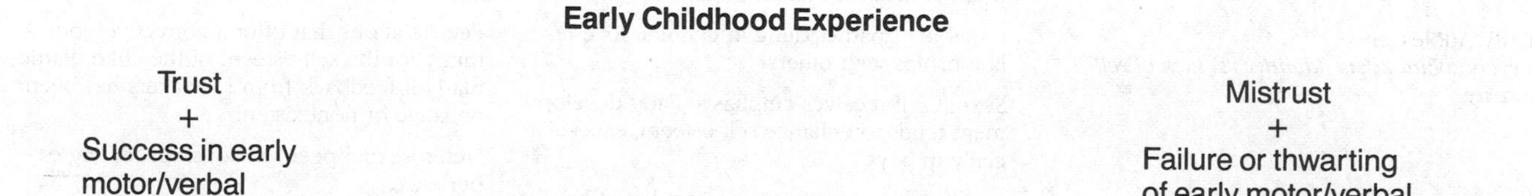

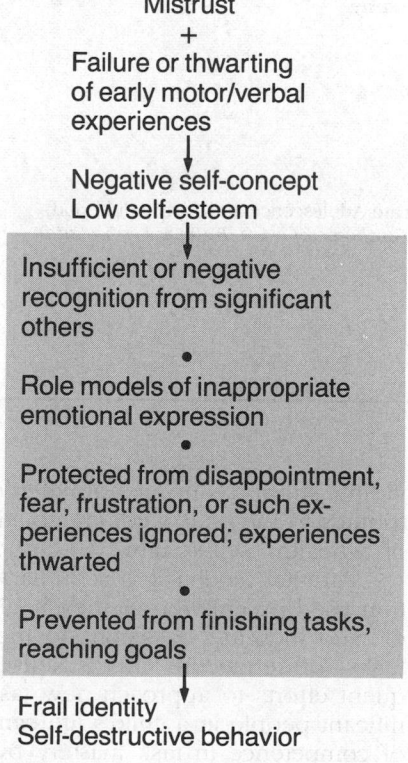

Success in early motor/verbal experiences

Permitted to experience disappointment, fear, frustration and given empathetic support
Encouraged and permitted to finish tasks and reach goals
Sturdy identity

Failure or thwarting of early motor/verbal experiences

Protected from disappointment, fear, frustration, or such experiences ignored; experiences thwarted
Prevented from finishing tasks, reaching goals
Frail identity

FIGURE 14-3. Requisites of childhood self-system development to support adult self-actualization.

TABLE 14-2
Stages of Healthy Self-System Development During the Childhood Years

Phase	Level of Self-Mastery	Critical Experiences
Infancy *Psychosocial crisis: Trust vs. mistrust*	Learns to trust others to gratify needs. This provides basis for confidence or hesitancy in child's approach to tasks or self-responsibility later in life	Prompt, consistent responses to needs
	Sensitive to anxiety or contentment of caretakers; struggles to feel secure and avoid anxiety	Tenderness from caretakers. Relative freedom from caretaker's anxieties
	Learns that certain behaviors result in certain responses or consequences	Realistic responses to behaviors; not uncritical or overcritical
Early Childhood *Psychosocial crisis: Autonomy vs. shame or doubt*	Self-recognition (self-concept and -identity) and self-pride (self-esteem) evolve. "I" can produce changes in my environment. "I" can accomplish this task (mostly motor tasks)	Develop autonomy. Consistent, realistic limits; not uncritical nor overcritical. Experience delays in gratification—opportunity to cope with interference with wish fulfillment
	Modifies actions to suit social role expectations (sex roles, peer roles, family member roles). Has developed personal view of world and place and value in it	Role models that give appropriate emotional expression
	Uses movement and language to avoid anxiety and to build self-competence. Develops general strategy for dealing with world	Reasonable opportunities to master skills without assistance, but with encouragement and affirmation. Avoid too little or too much freedom
Middle Childhood *Psychosocial crisis; Industry or mastery vs. inferiority*	Learns to accept subordination to authority figures outside family	Teachers who hold realistic, but not underestimated expectations for child
	Develops intellectual competence, initiative, achievement	Opportunity to explore and change own world. Follow through on projects to closure
	Self-status and role stabilized. Develops consideration and concerns outside the self	Peer relationships with mutual caring and acceptance
	Comparisons made of real self and ideal self. Internal locus of control begins forming	Be confronted with challenges, set goals, and carry them out
Early Adolescence *Psychosocial crisis: Identity vs. lack of self-clarity*	Capable of participating in genuine love relationships with others	Peer relations that offer a corrective opportunity for the self-esteem of the child. Particularly if feedback from caretakers has been negative or nonexistent
	Sexual self receives emphasis. Early development tends to enhance self-esteem, especially in boys	Heterosexual peer relationships, dating experiences
	Learns to cope with interpersonal relationships that are anxiety-producing. Learns to master adult level independence and satisfactory relations with the opposite sex	Realistic expansion of opportunities to assume adult tasks and responsibilities. Social opportunities outside family events
Late Adolescence and Early Adulthood *Psychosocial crisis: Intimacy vs. isolation*	Establishes durable, responsible relationships. Sense of self as an integrated person and sexual being	Opportunity for intimate relationships. Movement toward establishment of own residence or college attendance or moving away from family of origin
	Uses communication skills to protect self from conflicts with others. Behaviors based on internal locus of control; moral self established	Many social and personal relationships outside family. Job or career relations

viding support during normal life experiences contributes to the child's coping abilities and the building of a healthy self-system.

Parental feedback is a primary source of information used by children as they begin to form an image of who they are. Reactions to the child's attempts at tasks influence the child's self-concept and subsequent efforts to approach new tasks (Fig. 14–5). Significant people in a child's life can help foster a sense of competence in task mastery by gently challenging a child to cope with developmental tasks. Expectations are adhered to even when the child insists she or he cannot do the task, thereby demonstrating interest and support. Criticism and messages of disapproval in these instances contribute to a poor sense of self. Reasonable expectations, adhered to kindly but firmly until the child sees the way through the task, require parental patience and persistence.

Parenting styles and the amount, type, and consistency of control exerted by parents can have an impact on a child's development of self. When there is consistent enforcement of demands and rules com-

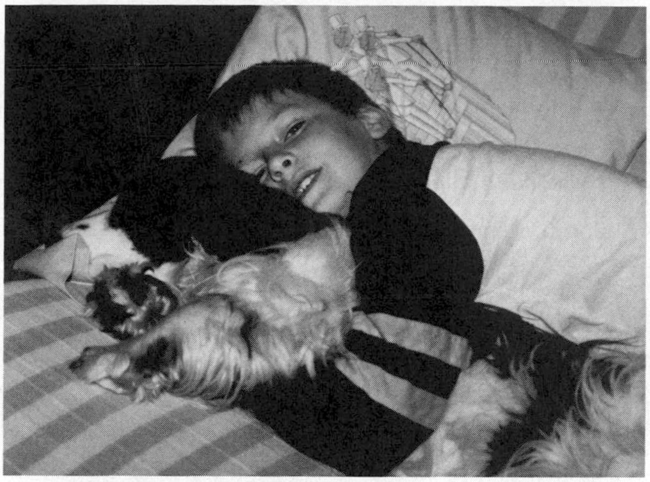

FIGURE 14-4. Pets give unconditional love and can be a "significant other." As a child cares for a pet, feelings of closeness and acceptance are experienced.

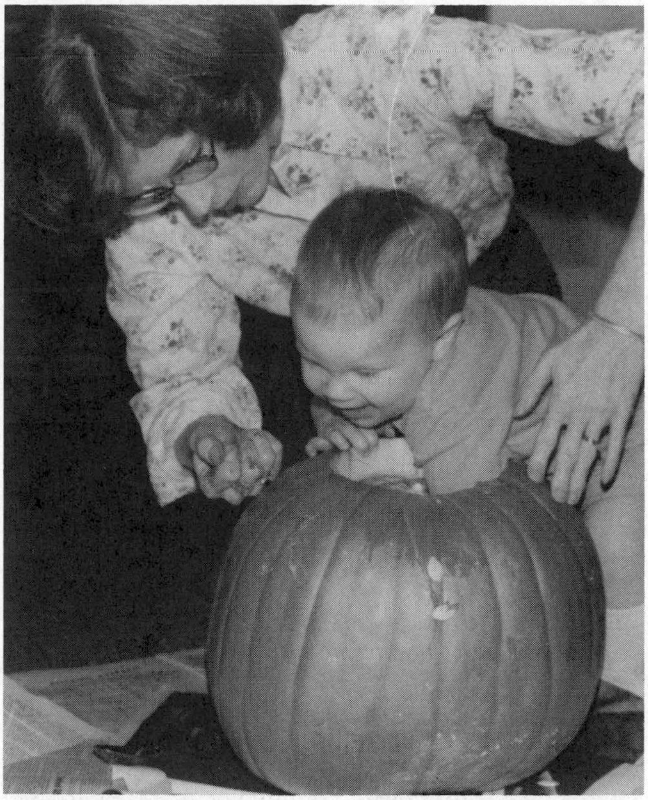

FIGURE 14-5. Reactions to the child's first attempts at tasks influence the child's self-concept and subsequent efforts to approach new tasks.

bined with warmth, acceptance, respect, and open communication, children grow up to be self-controlled and are able to approach new situations with confidence and to initiate and complete tasks. A summary of the three parenting styles discussed in Chapter 12 and their impact on self-concept development is provided in Table 14–3. It should be recognized that these findings relate to North American children; childrearing practices from different cultures and socioeconomic backgrounds vary.

The environment provided within the family is critical to the development of a healthy self-system. Three elements of the home environment that appear critical to development of a healthy self-system are (1) acceptance of the child, (2) clearly defined limits, and (3) respectful treatment (Coopersmith, 1967). Feelings and attitudes that exist within the home have a powerful influence. If there is a "mismatch" between parent and child with respect to achievement expectations, children may feel they have disappointed their parents. When parents are achievement-

TABLE 14-3
Three Parenting Styles: Impact on Self-Concept Development

Parenting Style	Main Theme	Predominant Approach	Impact on Child's Self-Concept
Democratic or authoritative (most effective)	Autonomous problem solving based on self-regulation and disciplined conformity	Shares rationale for desired behavior with child: affirms child's efforts to comply but sets limits or boundaries for acceptable behavior	High in self-esteem (Coopersmith, 1967). Competent self-controlled, independent (Baumrind, 1967, 1971)
Autocratic or authoritarian	Obedience: respect	Favors punitive measures to curb self-will when child does not comply with code of conduct	Low in self-esteem (Coopersmith, 1967). Poor internalization of moral standards and seeks external rewards and punishment (Baldwin, 1948). Lacking in independence (Baumrind, 1971)
Permissive or low level of demands	Provide minimal direction to child's behavior	Uses reason; punitive measures seldom (if ever) used to teach socialization	High level of aggression (Sears et al, 1957). Impulses poorly controlled. Immaturity (Baumrind, 1967)

oriented, frustrations and anger can result unless they can modify expectations in a direction that is more in accord with their child's performance (Brooks, 1992).

Siblings

In a family of two or more children, the children tend to turn to each other for interaction (Fig. 14–6). Thus, siblings may more strongly affect development of a child's self-system than do parents, particularly prior to exposure to peers in school. Siblings close in age, in particular, have the potential to influence one another's self-concept development.

Teachers and Peers

Entering school poses a substantial challenge to autonomous behavior. Many new teacher- and peer-imposed rules are encountered, and virtually every behavior is subject to evaluation. These experiences pose a threat to self-concept, particularly for the child with a primarily external locus of control. If teacher and peer evaluations and the child's self-image agree, that image is confirmed; if they do not, self-esteem may be adjusted toward the majority of evaluations. Children with a high internal locus of control do not need others' appraisals continually in order to feel good about themselves. These children will accept only those evaluations consistent with their self-esteem, rejecting or ignoring all other evaluations. Children with low self-esteem tend to set unrealistically high or low goals for their school performance so that consequent positive evaluation is either impossible or meaningless. Children with high self-esteem tend to use more adaptive coping strategies, leading to growth and mastery. Children with low self-esteem rely on coping behaviors that are self-defeating and retreat from problems, adding to the child's plight (Brooks, 1992). This demonstrates what is known as a "self-fulfilling prophecy."

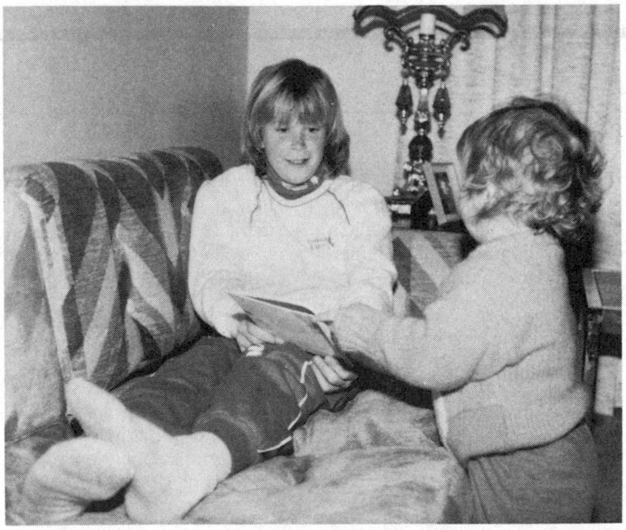

FIGURE 14 - 6. In a family of two or more children, the children tend to turn to each other for interaction. Siblings strongly affect the development of a child's self-system.

Modeling Significant Others' Behavior

Children imitate the prominent coping and behavioral strategies of significant others. Modeled behaviors that are even temporarily functional are repeated and become patterned (Stanwyck, 1983). Modeled behaviors that encourage autonomy and independence enhance self-esteem. Conversely, modeled behaviors that encourage strict conformity and dependence are costly and disruptive to healthy esteem development.

Social Roles and Culture

Socialization experiences take place in the context of one's gender role, culture, and ethnicity. Since the definition of self and the development of personal identity evolve within social experiences, these same factors—gender role, culture, and ethnicity—are influential. Social status appears to be only weakly related to self-esteem, with those in the higher social class having greater self-esteem (Battle, 1989). The effects of social status variables on self-concept are thought to be indirect through family psychologic characteristics (Hattie, 1992). Culture and ethnicity provide clues to the children about their affiliation with the rest of the world. They serve as a frame of reference as children define their worth, make judgments, and set standards for the self-system.

Discriminatory experiences have an impact on the development of self-concept (Thomas & Chess, 1980). Many children are able to recognize the source of the threat to their self-system's integrity, develop appropriate anger toward the injustice, and reject the prejudiced judgments. On the other hand, some children are overwhelmed and suffer serious damage to their self-system. *Self-attitudes develop in response to how children think others see them.* When those in the majority project depreciating attitudes on minority members, development of a healthy self-concept can be threatened.

There is an increasing body of literature that demonstrates differences in self-concept and self-esteem development across cultures. Findings from one study of Israeli-born children indicated that Jewishness is an important component of self-definition and that children are affected differently at different ages (Dor-Shav, 1990). A cross-cultural study on adolescents from India and Bangladesh also demonstrated that cultural differences have a profound affect on the personally and socially perceived self (Karim, 1990). Also, when cultural differences cause conflict and there is a dissonant social situation, there is a potential for negative effects on the self-concept (Lazarus et al, 1985). For example, a Native American boy who enters an Anglo-American school may begin to compare himself to the child of the dominant culture, and these comparisons may have a detrimental effect on his developing self-system. If, however, a Native American girl goes to school on a tribal reservation, her self-concept is not threatened because she compares herself with peers of the same culture (Lazarus et al, 1985). The development of self-concept is affected by the children's perception of their living conditions and the views that they believe others hold of them.

State of Physical Health

A child's attitude toward the body influences self-concept development (Watson & Johnson, 1985). Illness may impose any number of coping problems that affect the physical self-concept. Diseases or injuries related to sexual identity and task performance affect the body image; the extent depends primarily on how much the physical problem impedes normal functioning and on the feedback received from significant others. A substantial change in weight also requires adjustments in body image. Losses of body parts or of function can be battering to the child's body image. Although such persons may appear to accept and adjust to these body changes, they tend to retain an image of an intact body (Levine et al, 1992). The physically or mentally handicapped child experiences special stress in the struggle to achieve mastery and competence, making a positive self-concept harder but not impossible to accomplish. In one adolescent group of athletes, the self-concept of able-bodied youth was found to be similar to that of disabled youth (Sherrill et al, 1990). High self-esteem is thought to insulate the individual from certain debilitating physical problems. An association between low self-esteem and poor adjustment during illness and greater severity of symptoms has also been suggested (Antonucci & Jackson, 1983).

Temperamental Coping Style

Temperament* seems to influence the child's tolerance or coping level when confronted with tasks or challenges. Children of easy temperament are stimulated and respond positively, reflecting characteristics typical of the individual with high self-regard. The more characteristically difficult the temperament, the less the child seems able to display qualities indicating high self-regard. Research investigating the correlational nature of self-concept with temperament is substantially lacking. However, most parents who have children of both temperaments will insist that some correlation surely exists. Children with difficult temperaments seem to have fragile coping systems that leave them vulnerable to less adaptive perceptions about themselves and their experiences. Adults will be faced with the task of conscientiously providing the environmental conditions known to foster healthy self-system development when their child has a difficult temperament. To achieve success with these children, it is important to recognize that a different kind of parenting style may be necessary compared with that used in parenting an easy-to-raise child (Brooks, 1992; Turecki, 1989).

* Refer to Chapter 3 for a review of temperament as a characteristic of personality.

Nurse's Role in Fostering Self-Esteem

The nurse working with children and families has opportunities to foster the self-esteem of developing children both directly and indirectly. In the role of counseling, health teaching, and giving anticipatory guidance, nurses can direct the attention of parents to their child's needs for an environment of positive, affirming interactions. A child's self-concept can be assessed in a variety of ways.

Self-Concept Assessment

Although self-concept and self-esteem scales of measurement are used, the validity of these scales is an enduring problem (Hattie, 1992), nor do they differentiate self-concept and self-esteem. A child's self-concept cannot be observed directly, but it can be inferred from behavior (see Table 14–1). Self-concept can be measured by statements that reflect self-worth, by personal competence, and by the achievement aspirations of the child (Gilberts, 1983). Self-ratings and ratings of observed behavior complement each other and the use of both is preferred over either method alone (Coopersmith, 1967).

Self-Ratings as Measures of Self-Concept

One of the major difficulties with self-ratings is children's tendency to give information about themselves that they perceive to be socially desirable or that will gain them approval, rather than to disclose their true thoughts and feelings. Coopersmith found children below grade 4 to display significant social desirability response bias. Second, children's ability to apply the necessary symbolic thinking to represent real feelings of self-worth is not well established. Verbal self-ratings, therefore, are not recommended for children before grade 6. Observational scales and draw-a-person tests are preferred for estimating the self-concept of preschool and primary grade children to circumvent these difficulties.

Draw-a-person tests are most useful in demonstrating young children's perceived body images and self-esteem. The child is asked to draw a picture of herself or himself and of one other child on the same sheet of paper. Children with poor body image or low self-esteem portray themselves smaller than the other child. Typically, the child's self-picture bears a sad expression, shows distortion of one or more body parts or of the entire body, and, frequently, depicts the child in some antisocial behavior.

Self-esteem inventories can be used with children in grades 4 through 12. Coopersmith's inventory (a widely used instrument) contains groups of statements about family, school, peers, self, and general social activities. The responses reflect the degree to which children rate themselves as capable, significant, successful, and worthwhile. The statements are followed by columns in which the child checks whether the statement describes a frequent feeling as being *Like Me or Not Like Me*. The total score reflects the child's level of self-esteem as high, medium, or low. General guidelines for assessing components of the self-system are presented in Table 14–4.

Observational Measures of Self-Concept

The question of whether one person can adequately infer another person's self-concept presents philosophic dilemmas. Observational methods assume that the self-concept is demonstrated in observable behaviors and relates to some criterion such as health, social adaptability, or evidences of success. Such observation scales must carefully depict pertinent behaviors that presumably measure self-esteem. Observational methods generally are more valid if children do not know they are being observed and if they are being observed in their usual environment.

Building and Maintaining a Healthy Self-System

Human interaction, decision making, and growth and development (the elements of living) are all based on a healthy self-concept. The nurse's role(s) in building and maintaining a child's self-system will depend largely on the context of interactions with the child and family unit. When only occasional, short-duration interaction occurs (e.g., pediatric clinic, short-term hospitalization), the nurse's major roles are likely to be to assess the stability of the child's developing self-concept and family members' understanding of their part in guiding and fostering healthy self-system development.

In home care nursing, long-term hospitalization, and school nursery, there are more regular and extended periods of contact. In these settings, nurses can become more involved in setting up long-term programs.

Building and Maintenance Strategies (External Resources)

Researchers and psychologists generally agree on some basic attitudes apparent in persons who develop healthy, motivated self-systems: a sense of security, a sense of identity, a sense of belonging, a sense of purpose, and a sense of personal competence (Coopersmith, 1967; Maslow, 1968; Holden et al, 1990; Sugarman & Jaffe, 1990). Further, environmental conditions that foster these attitudes are crucial, generating feelings within the child of self-confidence, personal competence, and independence, which are the significant elements of a healthy self-system. Adults must provide these environmental con-

TABLE 14-4
Guidelines for Self-Concept Assessment

Throughout the interview, note general mood, emotional response, affect

I. *Physical Self* (Problem: Loss)
   A. Let's pretend that I'm blind and can't see you—describe yourself to me
   B. Draw a picture of yourself for me (up to 6 yrs of age)
   C. Are you satisfied with your physical appearance? What is it that you are not satisfied with?
   D. What concerns do you have now about your body or physical function?
   E. How are you feeling physically now (strong, weak, tired, sexually responsive, etc.)?
   F. Think of a time in your life when you lost something or someone you valued. Describe that experience for me
   G. What concerns you now about experiencing a loss? What might you do if you experience a loss again?

II. *Personal Self*
   A. *Self-Consistency* (Problem: Anxiety)
      1. What kind of person are you? Tell me about yourself. (Pick up on cues to facilitate description.)
      2. What makes you happy? What do you do to show it?
      3. What makes you irritated? What do you do to show it? Or, when you are irritated, what do you do to show it?
      4. What if your whole day is organized and something happens to alter your plans, what happens then? (May need situation for child to relate to in order to get elaboratation.)
      5. What are your feelings right now?
      6. Note verbal and nonverbal cues related to the level of anxiety
   B. *Self-Ideal* (Problem: Powerlessness)
      1. Often people dream about things or engage in wishful thinking or have hopes for the future. What are your wishes and hopes for the future?
      2. What is your most important plan or goal today? In a few years from now? In many years from now?
      3. When are some times you feel you have control over your life?
      4. When are some times you feel you do not have control over your life?
   C. *Moral-Ethical Self* (Problem: Guilt)
      1. Complete the sentences: "I believe in . . ." "I believe that I can . . ." "I believe that one should . . ."
      2. Who or what helps you know what is right or wrong? (See behavioral cues regarding guilt.)

Data from Roy, C. (1984). *Introduction to nursing: An adaptation model.* Englewood Cliffs, NJ: Prentice-Hall.

ditions by recognizing that children need to be treated as important individuals and guided to assume steadily greater responsibility for their own lives.

Building a Sense of Security

Children develop security through honest interactions with significant others, so that they can learn to trust and be confident in the adults responsible for them (Fig. 14–7). A firm but kind approach that defines clear, reasonable limits, consistently enforced, offers the child security. Children's lives also need routine. Established patterns of living tend to reduce conflicts and assist children to meet expectations adding to a sense of security. Check lists, charts (pictures can be used for young children who cannot read), and calendars or tally sheets serve as reminders and reinforcers of limits while enabling children to monitor their own adherence. Self-monitoring builds positive images and encourages responsibility for self-care. Use of logical consequences and realistic rewards encourages children to take responsibility for their behavior and its consequences.

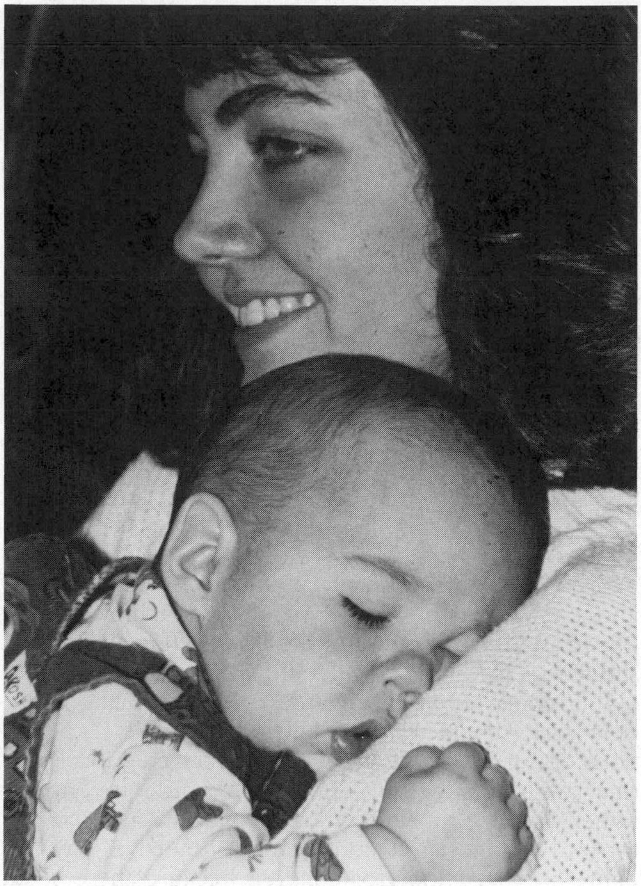

FIGURE 14 - 7. Children develop security through loving relationships with significant others.

Building a Sense of Identity

The foundation for a sense of identity is love and acceptance. Identity is built through positive feedback, providing recognition to children for their strengths and demonstrating respect for their uniqueness. Children behave in ways that are consistent with the picture they hold of themselves. Thus, a child's sense of identity is an important key to understanding behavior. Children who receive positive feedback from tasks accomplished acquire a realistic view of what they can and cannot do. Feedback should include a steady supply of appreciation of traits children possess, as well as identification of skills observed. Too often adults have a tendency to pay undue attention to shortcomings of children and to overlook their achievements. Whether children see themselves as primarily successful or as lacking important qualities is largely determined by feedback.

Feedback and recognition from adults should be generated from a sense of love and respect for the child as a thinking, feeling individual. Touching and active listening combined with appropriate verbal expressions of love and affection convey warmth and sensitivity to children. Verbal expression alone does not provide the support children need and does not compensate for a general lack of acceptance of the child.

Part of a sense of identity is self-confidence in one's own decisions and intuitions. Thus, feedback from others, although extremely important, should be coupled with encouragement for the child to judge self-performance and find ways to confirm self-assessments. The educational system has many built-in opportunities for such confirmations if children have been taught to consider their own performance as part of the feedback system that contributes to their identity.

Building a Sense of Belonging

The need to feel accepted is important to children, peaking during adolescence. A sense of belonging is developed as individual differences and similarities are recognized. The development of uniqueness as an individual occurs simultaneously with the realization that being a team or group member is a rewarding experience (Fig. 14–8).

Through family and group activities, children experience the process of functioning in a group while still being an individual. Through a balance of the feelings of wanting their own way and giving in, they learn the responsibility of belonging, of group membership, and the necessity of compromise. When children are encouraged to express empathy and to find ways to help others, they learn social concern and how to reduce feelings of alienation.

Building a Sense of Purpose

A sense of purpose can be created by setting reasonable expectations for children, by helping them set

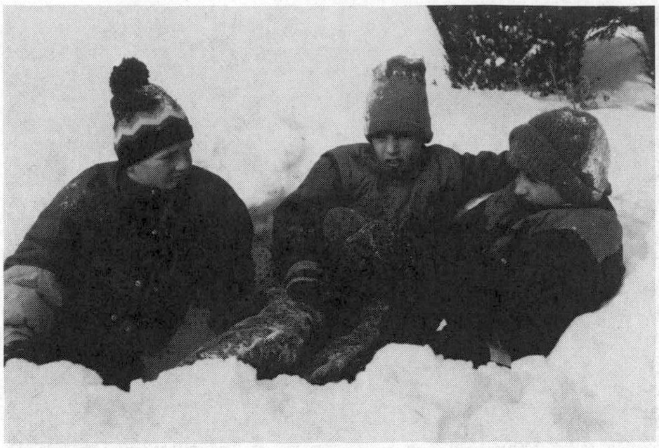

FIGURE 14-8. The foundation of a sense of identity for the school-age child is acceptance by peers.

realistic goals for themselves, and by exhibiting faith and confidence in their capability to achieve goals. Expectations are communicated by setting behavioral standards and limits, by identifying achievement levels as goals to work toward, and by labeling those personality characteristics that are desirable. Expectations above or below children's perceived capacity or that are too specific (e.g., an A grade in English rather than to improve writing skills) are not motivators. Challenges and contracts are effective ways to express expectations for children because these seem to reduce the perceived risk of penalty or failure.

Exposing children to new experiences can help them identify goals, especially if the experiences are congruent with their unique interests or abilities. Adults need to realize that, although children's interests may be short-lived, each interest expands their body of knowledge. Once a child's goal or interest is expressed, it is the responsibility of the parent, teacher, or other adult to convey belief in the child's ability to succeed and to give assistance as needed to achieve the goal.

Building a Sense of Personal Competence

Personal competence is the feeling of being able to cope with problems or accomplish goals. A sense of competence develops from experiencing success and completing tasks (Fig. 14–9). Adults can help children by providing feedback about their progress and helping them look at options when there are blocks to success or task completion. It is critical that adults not prescribe how children go about achieving their goals; telling children how to do something tends to build dependency, not confidence. Keeping children in dependency roles fosters feelings of helplessness, worthlessness, frustration, and anger (Sieving & Zirbel-Donisch, 1990).

A better approach is to discuss options with children, permitting them to make the final decision on how they will proceed. Once the child has decided on the process and resources needed, the adult's role is to monitor progress, praising both effort and accomplishment. Reward or recognition should not always be offered when the goal or task is accomplished, since the aim is to encourage self-motivation and self-satisfaction in success. The growth of self and success in achievements is cyclic. As one feels more self-assured, more tasks are attempted, and their successful completion, in turn, instills confidence.

Self-System Enhancement (Internal Resources)

Self-concept development, positive feedback, and success in tasks are positively correlated. However, whereas adults can and should act to increase children's self-concepts, an equally important role is to teach children to enhance their own self-concepts so that self-concept enhancement, like decision making, becomes a lifetime skill rather than a transitory state.

Keeping Successes and Failures in Perspective

Children must also be taught to accept love and praise and to receive compliments in a manner that

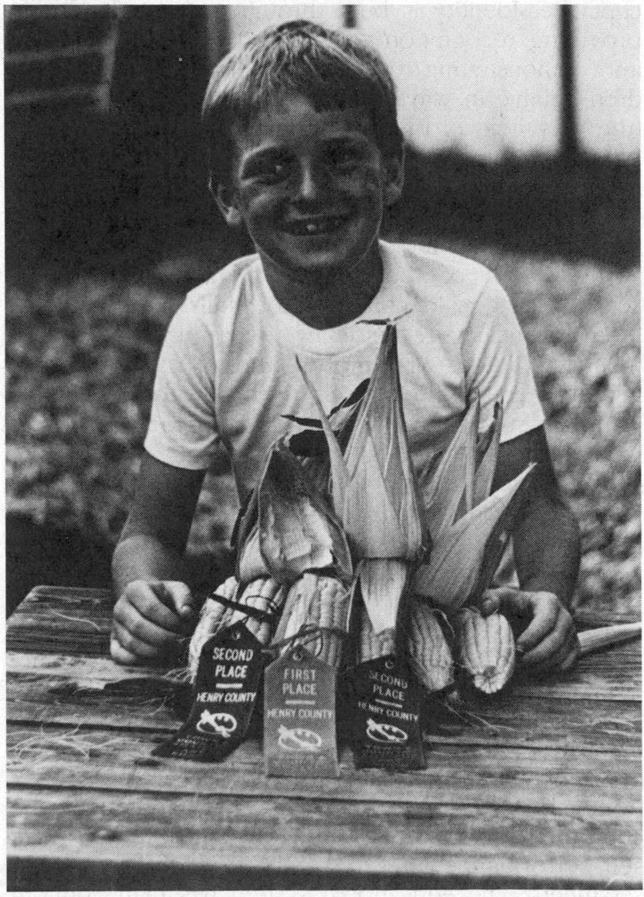

FIGURE 14-9. The school-age child builds self-esteem through accomplishments and evidence of competency.

enhances rather than diminishes self. Simply teaching children by example that saying, "Thank you, I'm good at that" or "Thank you, that is one of my stronger points," is a healthy response that will give them another tool valuable to self-concept enhancement. Another method to foster self-esteem is to deal with failure. Children need to learn that everyone "comes up short" sometimes, but that such shortcomings are to be used as opportunities to learn from mistakes, as well as to accept occasional failure, as part of a healthy existence rather than as times to diminish self.

Self-Care as Enhancement

Children should be encouraged and provided opportunities to steadily increase personal responsibility for maintaining and making decisions about their own health and daily care. As more responsibility is taken and successes are achieved, more confidence is developed.

KEY CONCEPTS

Concepts Related to Basic Information

- The self-system/self-concept develops through feedback that takes place in interpersonal relationships.
- As children progress through the various ages and stages attaining development tasks, the experiences they have influence the development of their self-system.
- The self-system/self-concept develops in response to societal expectations that are conveyed by the family, siblings, teachers, peers, and significant others.
- Socialization experiences take place in the context of one's gender role, culture, and ethnicity.
- Illness can affect how a child perceives his or her body and makes it more difficult, but not impossible, to develop a positive self-concept.
- A child's temperament seems to affect the tolerance and coping levels, which, in turn, influence their experiences and self-perceptions.

Concepts Related to Nursing Assessment

- A child's self-concept cannot be observed directly, but it can be inferred from behavior.
- Self-ratings and ratings of observed behavior complement each other and the use of both is preferred over either method alone.
- One of the major difficulties with assessing children's self-concept by their own statements about themselves is that they tend to give responses about themselves that they think are socially desirable or will gain approval or reward.
- Preschool and primary grade children do not have the cognitive skills to represent their self-perceptions verbally; therefore, observational scales and draw-a-person tests are preferred.

Concepts Related to Nursing Intervention

- The role of nursing is to assist families to develop the environmental context that fosters the development of a positive self-system in their children.
- Implementations are focused on helping families to provide both the internal and the external resources that foster the development of a positive self-system in their children.
- Nurses assist families to provide environments within which children can build a sense of security, identity, purpose, and personal competence.
- Parents are taught to help their children develop internal resources so that self-concept enhancement becomes a lifetime skill rather than a transitory state.

REFERENCES

Antonucci, T., & Jackson, J. (1983). Physical health and self-esteem. *Family Community Health,* pp 1–9.

Baldwin, A. L. (1948). Socialization and the parent-child relationship. *Child Development, 19,* 127–136.

Battle, J. (1989). *Enhancing self-esteem and achievement.* Edmonton, Alberta: James Battle and Associates.

Baumrind, D. (1967). Child care practices anteceding three patterns of preschool behavior. *Genetic Psychology Monographs, 75,* 43–88.

Baumrind, D. (1971). Current patterns of parental authority. *Developmental Psychology Monographs, 4*(1) Part 2.

Brooks, R. B. (1992). Self-esteem during the school years: Its normal development and hazardous decline. *Pediatric Clinics of North America, 39*(3), 537–550.

Cairns, E., McWhirter, L., Duffy, U., & Barry, R. (1990). The stability of self-concept in late adolescence: Gender and situational effects. *Personality and Individual Differences, 11*(9), 937–944.

Coopersmith, S. (1967). *The antecedents of self-esteem.* San Francisco: WH Freeman.

Dor-Shav, Z. (1990). Development of an ethnic self-definition: The ethnic self-concept "Jew" among Israeli children. *International Journal of Behavioral Development, 13*(3), 317–332.

Eder, R. A. (1990). Uncovering young children's psychological selves: Individual and developmental differences. *Child Development, 61,* 849–863.

Gilberts, R. (1983). The evaluation of self-esteem. *Family and Community Health,* pp 29–37.

Harter, S. (1982). Developmental perspectives on the self-system. In E. Hetherington (Ed.): *Carmichael's manual of child psychology* (Vol. 4). New York: John Wiley & Sons.

Hattie, J. (1992). Corollaries of the facet model. In J. Hattie (Ed.). *Self-concept.* Hillsdale, NJ: Hove & London.

Heatherton, T. F., & Polivy, J. (1991). Development and validation of a scale for measuring state self-esteem. *Journal of Personality and Social Psychology, 60*(6), 895–910.

Holden, G., Moncher, M. S., Schinke, S. P., & Barker, K. M. (1990). Self-efficacy of children and adolescents: A metanalysis. *Psychological Reports, 66*(3, pt. 1), 1044–1046.

Karim, S. F. (1990). Self-concept: A cross-cultural study on adolescents. *Psychological Studies, 35*(2), 118–123.

Lazarus, P. J., et al. (1985). Multicultural influences on the development of the young child (pp. 183–217). In C. S. McLoughlin, & D. F. Guilo (Eds.): *Young children in context: Impact of self, family, and society on development.* Springfield, IL: Charles C Thomas.

Levine, M., et al (1992). *Developmental-behavioral pediatrics.* Philadelphia: WB Saunders.

Maslow, A. (1968). *Toward a psychology of being.* Princeton, NJ: Van Nostrand.

Rambo, B. (1984). *Adaptation nursing.* Philadelphia: WB Saunders.

Roy, C. (1984). *Introduction to nursing: An adaptation model.* Englewood Cliffs, NJ: Prentice-Hall.

Sears, R. R., Maccoby, E., & Levin, H. (1957). *Patterns of child rearing.* Evanston, IL: Row Peterson.

Sherrill, C., Hinson, M., Gench, B., & Kennedy, S. O. (1990). Self-concepts of disabled youth athletes. *Perceptual and Motor Skills, 70*(3), 1093–1098.

Sieving, R. E., & Zirbel-Donisch, S. T. (1990). Development and enhancement of self-esteem in children. *Journal of Pediatric Health Care, 4*(6), 290–296.

Stanwyck, D. J. (1983). Self-esteem through the life span. *Family and Community Health, 6*(2), 11–28.

Sugarman, A., & Jaffe, L. S. (1990). Toward a developmental understanding of the self schema. *Psychoanalysis and Contemporary Thought, 13*(1), 117–138.

Sullivan, H. (1953). *The interpersonal theory of psychiatry.* New York: WW Norton.

Thomas, A., & Chess, S. (1980). *Dynamics of psychological development.* New York: Brunner-Mazel.

Turecki, S. (1989). *The difficult child.* New York: Bantam.

Watson, E., & Johnson, A. (1985). The emotional significance of acquired physical disfigurement in children. *American Journal of Orthopsychiatry, 28,* 85–97.

BIBLIOGRAPHY

Amato, P. R., & Ochiltree, G. (1986). Family resources and the development of child competence. *Journal of Marriage and the Family, 48,* 47–56.

Bandura, A. (1982). Self-efficacy mechanisms in human agency. *American Psychologist, 37,* 122–147.

Brown, B., & Lohr, M. (1987). Peer group affiliation and adolescent self-esteem: An integration of ego-identity and symbolic-interaction theories. *Journal of Personality and Social Psychology, 52,* 47–55.

Burns, E. I., Doremus, P. C., & Potter, M. B. (1990). Value of health, incidence of depression, and level of self-esteem in low-income mothers of pre-school children. *Issues in Comprehensive Pediatric Nursing, 13*(2), 141–154.

Bybee, J., Glick, M., & Zigler, E. (1990). Differences across gender, grade level, and academic track in the content of the ideal self-image. *Sex Roles, 22*(5/6), 349–358.

Folsom-Meek, S. (1991). Relationships among attributes, physical fitness, and self-concept development of elementary school children. *Perceptual and Motor Skills, 73*(2), 379–383.

Gecas, V., & Schwalbe, M. L. (1986). Parental behavior and adolescent self-esteem. *Journal of Marriage and the Family, 48,* 37–46.

Harter, S., & Connell, J. (1982). *A model of children's achievement and related self-perceptions of competence, control, and motivational orientation.* Greenwich, CT: JAI Press.

Harter, S., & Pike, R. (1984). The pictorial scale of perceived competence and social acceptance for young children. *Child Development, 55,* 1969–1982.

Hayes, D. M., & Fors, S. W. (1990). Self-esteem and health instruction: Challenges for curriculum development. *Journal of School Health, 60*(5), 208–211.

Huggins, S. (1989). A comparative study of self-esteem of adolescent children of divorced lesbian mothers and divorced heterosexual mothers. *Journal of Homosexuality, 18*(1/2), 123–135.

Jackson, P. L., & Ott, M. J. (1990). Perceived self-esteem among children diagnosed with precocious puberty. *Journal of Pediatric Nursing, 5*(3), 190–203.

Kegan, R. (1982). *The evolving self.* Cambridge, MA: Harvard University Press.

Meisenhelder, J. B. (1985). Self-esteem: A closer look at clinical interventions. *International Journal of Nursing Studies, 22*(2), 127–135.

O'Brien, E. J. (1991). Sex differences in components of self-esteem. *Psychological Reports, 68,* 241–242.

O'Brien, R. W., Smith, S. A., Bush, P. J., & Peleg, E. (1990). Obesity, self-esteem, and health locus of control in black youths during transition to adolescence. *American Journal of Health Promotion, 5*(2), 133–139.

Pardeck, J. A., & Pardeck, J. T. (1990). Family factors related to adolescent autonomy. *Adolescence, 25*(98), 311–319.

Pulkkinen, L. (1982). *Self control and continuity from childhood to adolescence.* New York: Academic Press.

Raskin, R., Novacek, J., & Hogan, R. (1991). Narcissistic self-esteem management. *Journal of Personality and Social Psychology, 60*(6), 911–918.

Reasoner, R. W. (1983). Enhancement of self-esteem in children and adolescents. *Family and Community Health, 6*(2), 51–64.

Riffee, D. M. (1981). Self-esteem changes of hospitalized school-age children. *Nursing Research, 30,* 94–97.

Stipek, D. J., Gralinski, J. H., & Kopp, C. B. (1990). Self-concept development in the toddler years. *Developmental Psychology, 26*(6), 972–977.

Winkelstein, M. (1989). Fostering positive self-concept in the school-age child. *Pediatric Nursing, 15*(3), 229–233.

CHAPTER • 15

Promoting Safety

Mabel Hunsberger

RELATED TOPICS
Safety Concerns, Chapters 4 through 9
Play/recreation, Chapters 4 through 9
Description and use of Heimlich maneuver, Chapter 46
Care of the child with injuries, Chapter 46
Care of the child with burns, Chapter 47

LEARNING OBJECTIVES

- **Identify the variables in a host, an agent, and the environment that interact to increase the risk of injury in children and adolescents.**
- **Differentiate between active and passive approaches in injury prevention programs.**
- **Give an example of how developmental characteristics increase the risk of injury in a child.**
- **Identify three factors that continue to put children at risk while riding in a car.**
- **Discuss three approaches that are used to prevent motor vehicle injuries.**
- **Describe the pattern of incidence and types of violence in homicide involving children and adolescents.**
- **Identify populations most at risk for drowning.**
- **Explain the common barriers to effective safety education and the measures nurses can use to decrease these barriers.**

Safety of children is of concern to every nurse, parent, school, and community. Despite the movement toward various forms of legislation and the commitment of community organizations to promote the safety of children, injury is the leading cause of death in children age 1 year to young adulthood. One may ask, how can such a major preventable health problem persist? The event of becoming injured has a multifactorial etiologic basis, including variations in the *host,* the *agent* (or vector), and the *environment.* The solution is not one of isolating a causative agent against which immunity can be developed, but rather involves effecting changes in human behavior through education, consumer product regulation, and legislation. This chapter addresses the epidemiology of injuries with reference to host, agent, and environmental variables and provides a review of the common types of injuries and their related nursing interventions for prevention. Age-related safety concerns are discussed in Chapters 4 through 9.

Definitions of Terms

Fundamental to increasing the safety of children are the beliefs that injuries have causes and that these causes can be altered to prevent or modify an injury. For this reason, the terms "injury" and "injured child" are used in this chapter rather than "accident." The term "accident" suggests that an event happened by chance and implies that every member of the population has the same probability of being affected. An epidemiologic approach of identifying variables in the host, agent, and environment offers a framework that gives some predictability to injuries and, therefore, serves as a guide for prevention.

Scope of the Problem

Injury is the leading cause of death in children aged 1 to 19 years, accounting for more deaths than all diseases combined (Division of Injury Control, 1990). Under 1 year of age, conditions associated with birth and congenital abnormalities are the leading causes of death. The causes of injury in children 0 to 19 years of age resulting in death are as follows (Division of Injury Control, 1990):

1. Motor vehicle–related injuries: 47 per cent (includes occupant, bicycle, pedestrian, and motorcycle).
2. Homicide: 12.8 per cent.
3. Suicide: 9.6 per cent.
4. Drowning: 9.2 per cent.
5. Fire and burns: 7.2 per cent.
6. Falls: 1.4 per cent.
7. Other injuries: 12.8 per cent.

The use of antibiotics, immunizations, and chemotherapy has had a major impact on reducing mortality due to disease. For example, since the 1930s, deaths due to infectious diseases declined 90 per cent, whereas those resulting from injuries declined only 40 per cent. Injuries in children are probably the most underrecognized child health problem that exists today—with long-lasting effects that go far beyond that which mortality statistics represent. There are no national data available to estimate the cost of childhood morbidity and disability resulting from injury. Estimates based on data in a single state are that for every child that dies from injury 45 children are hospitalized and 1300 require treatment in an emergency department (Guyer & Ellers, 1990).

Analysis of an Injury

Childhood injuries should be viewed as events that are predictable and controllable. A study of the causes of injuries and the identification of high-risk groups is the first step to intervening. Following is an epidemiologic framework for the analysis of an injury based on a discussion of host factors, agent characteristics, and the environment. Interaction of these variables leads to injury.

Characteristics of the Child (Host)

Age-related physical and cognitive skills of children and their psychosocial needs are strong determinants of whether an injury is likely to happen and which type of injury is most likely to occur. Immaturity in motor skills and inexperience in how to safely explore the environment increase the chance of falls and suffocation during infancy. When curiosity is paramount and locomotion improves during late infancy, a child can no longer be kept from dangers in the environment. At this stage, *the environment must be modified to protect the child.* Advancing skills make older infants, toddlers, and preschoolers vulnerable to falls and new agents, such as poisons, bodies of water, and sources of heat. During the school years, children are less supervised by their parents and they become more competitive in many of their activities. They are now trusted to participate in new activities, such as crossing the street, playing on larger playground equipment, and riding a bicycle on the street.

As adolescence is approached, a need for independence and emancipation from childhood introduces yet more dangerous sources for injury, including motor vehicles.

Injury prevention takes into consideration the combined physiologic and psychologic characteristics of the host that influence the likelihood and the degree of injury at the various stages. For example, children's cognitive immaturity combined with their capacity for mobility and their curiosity may lead them to pull hot water on themselves. Furthermore, a child's skin is less mature and, therefore, is a less effective barrier to damage compared with that of an adult. These factors combined predispose children to more severe scalding than a similar injury in an adult. Strategies to prevent childhood injuries need to be adapted as the child's body grows and new activities emerge in response to a developing social being.

A long-standing myth is that some people are "accident-prone." This term refers to the notion that some individuals possess certain psychologic characteristics that predispose them to relatively high accident rates. Boys at all ages do suffer more injuries than girls, but this is more likely to be associated with activity type and participation level than with personality characteristics. There has been no consistent identification of personality characteristics as direct causes of injury (Langley, 1982). Even when traits have been identified that were thought to typify the "accident-prone" individual, the same traits are found in those without a history of repeated injuries (Nyman, 1987).

Agent (Vector) Characteristics

The specific vehicle causing the injury is the "agent" or "vector." The characteristics of the agent determine the degree of potential for injury. For example, the design of toys, the temperature of hot water in a home, the packaging of medicine, and the toxicity of poisons influence the occurrence and nature of the event. Interventions have been directed at agents through regulation of fireworks, packaging of drugs in child-resistant containers, and manufacturing of flame-retardant children's clothing. These are called "passive" because no further action is required by the host. Regulation of speed limits and seat belt laws are examples of interventions that potentially alter the causative agent, but require change in human behavior. These are called "active" because they require an action by the host. Strategies such as putting on a seat belt require repeated behaviors and, therefore, may meet with more resistance than one-time actions, such as turning down the thermostat that regulates water temperature in a home or buying syrup of ipecac for use when poison is ingested. Prevention strategies that modify the agent do not necessarily prevent the event, but the *extent* of injury can be modified (e.g., water temperature reduction, seat belt wearing).

Environment (Physical and Sociocultural)

Physical and sociocultural environmental factors play an important role in the initiation of injury. Time of day, type of equipment, and physical arrangements can contribute to injury. Environmental factors such as traffic patterns and road systems leading to playgrounds and schools affect injury potential. The influence of sociocultural factors on injuries is difficult to study and findings are varied. Injuries in childhood are reported to disproportionately affect African-American and non–African-American minority children (Division of Injury Control, 1990). Children who live in rural areas and work on farms are also at risk for certain kinds of injuries because of their work environment, which contains machinery (Cummings, 1991).

Socioeconomic factors that are stress producers play a significant role in injury risk. Examples include unemployment or change in employment, death in the family, move to a new residence, birth of a sibling, single parent, limited education, and drug or alcohol dependence (Simon, 1992). There are cultural differences in reported death rates. Injury death rates are highest for Native Americans, followed by African-Americans, whites, and Asian-Americans (Jones, 1992).

The creation of organizations to protect the consumer (United States [US] Consumer Product Safety Commission) and legislative actions to improve safety standards (building codes, car manufacturing standards) are examples of modification of the environment. Community organizations and local governments can also act to improve safety through provision of crossing guards, development of bike paths, and placement of signs such as "Children Playing."

Prevention of Common Injuries: Nursing Interventions

Approaches used to reduce injuries are *passive:* providing external control (e.g., automatic air bags, safe design of products and environment); or *active:* requiring specific behaviors or adherence to laws and regulations (e.g., putting on a seat belt and driving within the speed limit). Guidelines for state and local health care professionals developed by the National Committee for Injury Prevention and Control (1989) identify three general preventive approaches:

- Persuade at-risk persons to change behavior.
- Require the general population to change behavior or the environment by law.
- Safely design products and environment to protect the public.

Recommendations for injury control established at the Third National Injury Control Conference (Centers for Disease Control [CDC], 1992a) include:

- Increase public awareness of injuries and injury control.
- Increase attention and support from the Office of the Assistant Secretary for Health to coordinate multiagency and multidepartment efforts.
- Increase resources for injury surveillance, research, control programs (state capacity), intervention evaluation, training, and health services.
- Allow cooperative industry/government research and development projects.
- Require E-codes (i.e., external causes) for all hospital discharges as part of a national surveillance system at CDC.
- Establish a Center for Injury Control with CDC to provide national leadership.
- With CDC playing a key role, develop a national applied injury control research laboratory to study both human and engineering factors.

Most injuries occur as the result of complex interactions of a host, an agent, and the environment. A major determinant in the type of injury that is likely to occur in children is the child's age. No single method of prevention is effective; a combination of approaches is required, as outlined at the injury control conference. Types of injuries and related preventive strategies according to the child's development can be found in Chapters 4 through 9 for neonates, infants, toddlers, preschoolers, school-agers, and adolescents. Following is a review of common injuries that happen during childhood and adolescence, including strategies directed at the host, agent, and environment.

High Risk for Injury: Motor Vehicle Accidents

Motor vehicle injuries are the leading cause of death in children (after 1 year of age) and adolescents. Motor vehicle–related fatalities include vehicle occupants, bicyclists, pedestrians, and individuals receiving other injuries associated with motorcycles and off-road vehicles. Children left in vehicles unattended is another source of injury that has been identified through a hospital surveillance system (Agran et al, 1991).

The majority of motor vehicle–related fatalities are motor vehicle occupants. This includes child and adolescent passengers as well as adolescent drivers. Deaths of motor vehicle occupants are most common among 15- to 19-year-olds, with a fatality rate of almost 10 times that of children under 10 years of age (Division of Injury Control, 1990).

Special circumstances require specific strategies and precautions to prevent injuries. The disabled child needs to have special attention given to support and protection while riding in a car (Shaw, 1987), and premature infants need to be positioned in a way that keeps the head from falling forward to minimize the risk of respiratory compromise while being protected in the event of a crash or sudden stop (AAP, 1991). For some disabled children, a special restraint device may be required to provide protection in a prone position.

Characteristics of the host supply important information in the study of motor vehicle accidents. The younger the child, the greater the risk of injury or fatality as a result of a collision. Infants have been found to be especially vulnerable to injury in a crash; they have a high center of gravity because of their proportionately large heads. This "top heaviness" makes a child especially prone to being propelled head first through a windshield. This difference in body weight distribution, coupled with the softness of a child's skull and immaturity of the spinal cord, increases the risk for serious injury.

Another factor that contributes to a higher mortality rate in young infants is the cradling of an infant in the arms of another person while riding in a vehicle. This is considered to be the most dangerous method of traveling with a child. Parents often do this because they erroneously believe it provides additional protection. On the contrary, the impact of injury on the child is affected by the weight of the parent if she or he is not restrained. The forcefulness of the impact is frequently expressed by the 10–30–300 rule (Table 15–1).

Seat belt laws have contributed immensely to altering the characteristics of the agent (i.e., the vehicle in which the child rides). Although the number of children who are restrained has increased, several factors continue to put children at risk while riding in a car: improper restraint; seat belts may not work as well as hoped for older children (Christoffel, 1989); and lack of use in older children and adolescents still persists. Improper restraint involves not fastening the seat belt around the car seat, improper positioning, not using certain devices when required, such as tether strap or shield, and the wrong type of seat for age of child. Seat belts used by older children have been reported to prevent ejection, but serious injuries still result when a car is struck on the side in a crash (Agran et al, 1990).

Prevention Strategies

Three main approaches have been used to prevent motor vehicle injuries, including: (1) consumer education, (2) legislation, and (3) vehicle improvements.

TABLE 15–1
The 10–30–300 Rule

The 10–30–300 rule means that a 10-pound baby riding in an automobile going 30 miles per hour is propelled forward with a force of 300 pounds. This is analogous to falling from the third story of a building. If an adult is *not* restrained, the infant risks being crushed by a force equal to the weight of the adult times the same speed factor of 30 miles per hour.

TABLE 15-2
Family-Centered Teaching: Tips on Proper Use of Child-Restraint Devices and Seat Belts

- Try the seat in family car and try buckling child into seat before purchase
- Read and follow manufacturer's instructions for installation
- Whenever possible, put children in the back seat; an exception is when riding alone with an infant because easy visualization of an infant is desirable
- Place young infants in seat with face toward rear of car
- Insist that all adults use seat belts because an unrestrained adult can be thrown onto a child passenger

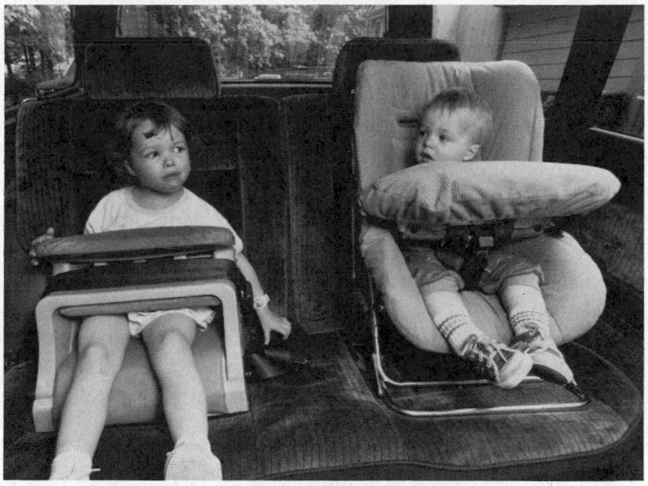

FIGURE 15-1. The safest place for a child to ride is in the back seat of a car, in the center. In a family with two young children, two car seats are placed in the back seat, one on each side. Manufacturer's instructions to secure the seat into the car vary according to the type of seat construction; some must be secured by a strap into the trunk of the car.

Consumer Education

Nurses have the opportunity to teach parents and children how to protect themselves from motor vehicle–related accidents, including use of child-restraint devices and seat belts, safe practices for cyclists and pedestrians, and education to prevent impaired driving (Fig. 15–1). Assessment and teaching to prevent these injuries should be included in all child care settings. In hospitals, clinics, and schools and on home visits, nurses should make motor vehicle safety a priority.

In any of these settings, nurses should be able to provide basic counseling about child restraint devices and seat belts and, when possible, provide an opportunity for parents to demonstrate their use. The three basic types are: (1) infants only, (2) convertible models for infants or toddlers, and (3) boosters. Rearward-facing seats are the accepted practice for infants up to 1 year of age. In Scandinavia, the benefits of these seats have been demonstrated for children up to 4 years of age (Carlsson et al, 1991). Tips on proper use of child-restraint devices and seat belts are listed in Table 15–2.

It is important for the nurse to make some attempt to understand the reasons for the lack of use of child-restraint devices. Parents report a variety of reasons for not using seat belts and restraint devices, of which the most common ones include: (1) too expensive, (2) difficult and inconvenient, (3) forgetfulness, and (4) restrictive and uncomfortable for the child. There may be other reasons that parents express, and each of these should be addressed by the nurse. Some basic ideas that the nurse should share with parents to encourage the proper use of a child-restraint device are summarized in Table 15–3. The literacy level of a particular family must also be considered. Greater than 20 per cent of the population is illiterate and unable to read installation instructions provided by manufacturers. Preventive strategies for

TABLE 15-3
Educative-Counseling Issues Concerning Use of Seat Belts and Child-Restraint Devices

Reason for Not Using	Educational Strategy
Prohibitive in cost	Nurse can refer client to community organizations. Many programs are available that provide a child-restraint device for a nominal fee. In most cases, a deposit is required, which is returned when the seat is returned
Difficult and inconvenient to use	Young children accept rituals and routines and will resist less if consistently used. Some seats are more difficult to use than others; therefore, before purchasing, it should be tried in the car and parents should practice buckling
Fear of entrapment and increased injury	Ejection from a vehicle increases the risk of death
Forgetfulness	Parents should be encouraged to use their own seat belts as an example. Developing a habit of buckling up for every ride, regardless of the distance, is the best defense against forgetfulness
Restrictive and uncomfortable (many parents do not wish to face the hassle of getting their child into a restraint and interpret resistance as discomfort)	Disruptive children have actually either directly caused or been a contributing factor in collisions. It has been found that children who are restrained exhibit less disruptive behavior (Christophersen, 1977)

the safety of cyclists and pedestrians is discussed later in this chapter. Prevention of impaired driving is discussed in Chapter 9.

Legislation

Laws now exist in all states that require young children to be properly restrained while riding in a motor vehicle. More uniformity among state laws would reduce confusion and facilitate enforcement. In Canada, most provinces require that individuals, regardless of age, wear a seat belt or use a child restraint device. Nurses can lobby for support of mandatory child restraint legislation at the state and national levels and enforcement at the local level.

Vehicle Improvements

Ongoing research to improve automobile safety is required. Air bags designed to inflate on collision to protect the passengers are becoming standard equipment in new cars. Other devices that reduce injury are automatic occupant restraints and antilock brakes. Improved vehicle side protection is required to reduce injuries that result from side crashes (Division of Injury Control, 1990). Motor vehicle injury prevention requires a multidisciplinary approach with widespread public support.

High Risk for Injury: Homicide, Assault, and Abuse

Homicide is now the second leading cause of death by injury among children. Homicide rates are high during the first 3 years of life, low from ages 5 to 10 years, after which they rise, with a dramatic increase at 15 years of age (Division of Injury Control, 1990). Homicide is the leading cause of injury death in infants under 1 year of age (Waller et al, 1989). Childhood homicides thus fall into two patterns: infantile and adolescent. In children from ages 0 to 4 years, about 50 per cent of the homicides are inflicted with blows and about 10 per cent by firearms. After 12 years of age, the leading method of homicide is by firearms. Homicide rates for African-American children are about five times as high as those for white children, and overall homicide rates among male children are about twice that for females (CDC, 1990b).

The problems of violence in families and child abuse reflect national trends. (See Chapter 28.) Interpersonal violence is a major public health issue that must be addressed by all health care professionals. Programs to support families in parenting and conflict resolution are preventive approaches that are necessary for risk reduction in homicide among children and adolescents. Programs directed at prevention of violence require close collaboration of an interdisciplinary team comprised of social service, mental health, education, and health care professionals, and public health and criminal justice officials. The heavy toll that violence has on the health of children and adolescents calls for research directed at understanding its origins and preventive strategies. Efforts to improve data on nonfatal violence are also needed (Fig. 15–2).

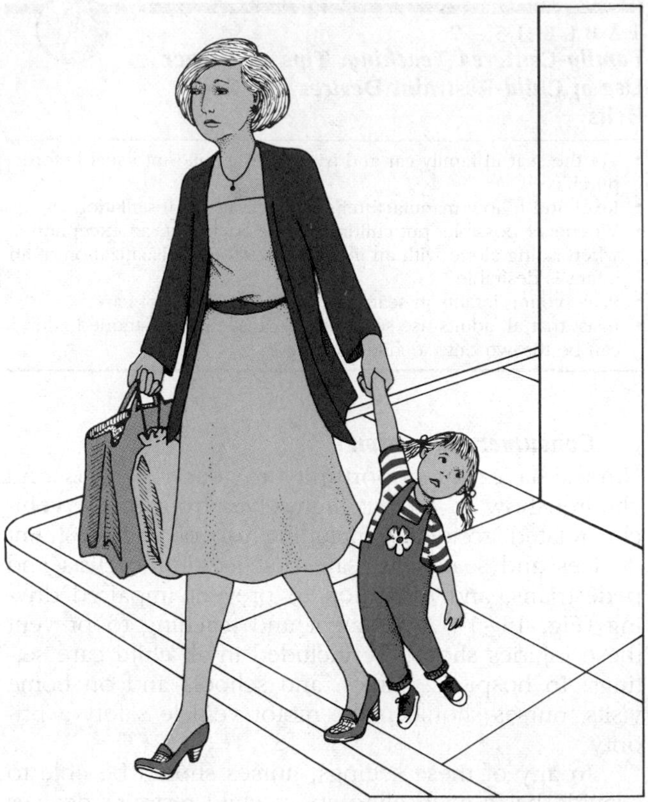

FIGURE 15 - 2. A hard upward pull or jerk on a child's arm can cause injury to tendons and muscles.

Finally, the issue of availability of firearms is an issue that parents must face. There is a trend in the United States to hold the adult owner of the gun responsible for preventing childhood tragedies (CDC, 1992b). Education about gun safety should become a common type of prevention, as is education about poisoning and other injuries (Crawley & Velsor-Friedrich, 1991).

High Risk for Injury: Suicide

Suicide is the third leading cause of death by injury among children and adolescents aged 0 to 19 years. Suicide is rare before the age of 10 years (Christoffel, 1990).

High Risk for Injury: Water-Related Accidents

Drowning* occurs at all ages in diverse environmental settings and involves different socioeconomic

* "Drowning" is defined as suffocation by immersion in a liquid medium; "near-drowning" refers to survival for more than 24 hours (with or without aspiration); "secondary drowning" means delayed death (Greensher, 1984).

groups. Drowning is the fourth leading cause of injury among children aged 0 to 19 years. The group at highest risk is toddlers from 1 to 3 years of age; therefore, for children aged 0 to 4 years, drowning is the third leading cause. In California, Arizona, and Florida, drowning is the leading cause of death from injury among this age group (Wintemute, 1990). Sixty to 70 per cent of drownings occur in fresh water. Other children drown when left unattended in a bathtub, from falls into private lakes or swimming pools, or during water-related sports. Drownings also occur when children play on ice over bodies of water that are not solidly frozen.

Prevention Strategies

Strict supervision of children when in and near bodies of water is the single most important preventive strategy. Young children should not be left in the care of child siblings around water. For infants, even a bucket of water can present a hazard if they fall into it. Inflated arm bands cannot be considered protection against drowning. Only approved life jackets should be used. Parents should be encouraged to teach children and adolescents water safety rules that are strictly enforced (Table 15–4).

Nurses should also advise parents concerning swimming lessons. Organized swimming lessons should be encouraged for children after 3 years of age. If infant swimming lessons are provided, parents should be cautioned about their infant's safety. There is a potential for parents to feel overly secure about the abilities of their infants and toddlers who have "learned to swim." It should be stressed that, even though infants are taught to swim, they cannot be taught water safety; therefore, they should be supervised, as should any nonswimming child. For school-age children and adolescents, water safety and lifesaving courses are recommended approaches to prevent drowning. All children should be taught the proper use of any water equipment they purchase (e.g., boogey boards, snorkeling equipment).

Children with seizures require special attention regarding safety in water. Such children account for up to 15 per cent of the drownings and are considered to be at risk for drowning at a rate four times higher than that for other children. To prevent drowning in this high-risk group, the following counsel is recommended:

- Encourage showering rather than bathing, as many of the drownings occur during a child's bath.
- Encourage jogging and other sports rather than swimming.
- If water activities are done
  - Ensure that child's condition is well controlled with anticonvulsants (child should be seizure-free for 2 years).
  - Supervision is facilitated by ensuring high visibility of child (e.g., distinctive bathing caps or luminescent swimming suits have been suggested).

The nurse's involvement in counseling about water safety should begin when the infant bath is discussed. A continued emphasis on water safety appropriate for the child's age is warranted, considering the number of deaths from drowning. It is essential that parents are cautioned to know where their children are in the neighborhood and who is supervising them. One half of all home swimming pool drownings occur in a neighbor's pool.

An awareness of neighborhood and community safety concerning water is also a responsibility of health care professionals, especially public health nurses. Unsafe practices in neighborhood pools and recreational areas with water should be investigated and appropriate authorities notified. Identification and reporting of inadequate fencing or riverbank railings should be the concern of every citizen but especially of a health care professional, whose concern is the health and safety of children.

TABLE 15-4
Family-Centered Teaching: Swimming and Boat Safety

- Teach children:
  - Never to swim alone
  - Not to swim during electrical storms
  - Not to run in pool areas
  - Not to dive into a shallow pool or lake
  - Not to swim after a heavy meal, drinking, or taking medicine
  - Never to issue a false alarm (call for help)
- Pools must be fenced (4–6 ft in height)
- Keep electrical appliances away from the water to avoid shock and electrocution hazards
- Make sure all nonswimmers and children under the age of 3 yrs wear life jackets when near water *(nonswimmers wearing life jackets in the water must be accompanied by an adult because a child can easily float into deep water)*
- Keep rescue devices and first-aid equipment easily accessible and teach all swimmers how to use them
- On a boat, one adult swimmer should be present for each nonswimming child
- Do not stand and do not allow children to stand in small boats
- Have children under 12 yrs of age wear life jackets in a boat whether or not they can swim
- Teach all children over the age of 12 yrs the techniques of mouth-to-mouth resuscitation

High Risk for Injury: Burns and Fires

Death caused by burns ranks second only to motor vehicle accidents in the 1- to 4-year-old age group and is the fifth leading cause of death for children aged 0 to 19 years. Fire and burn injuries often cause disfigurement, pain, emotional strain, and enormous financial cost. Costs for burned children have been estimated at $3.6 billion per year (McLoughlin & McGuire, 1990). The causes of burn injuries include thermal (flame and scald), chemical, electrical, and radiation. Children less than 5 years of age are most prone to thermal injury (Finkelstein et al, 1992). The type of burn accident that is likely to occur is highly related to characteristics of the child. For example, capabilities in locomotion and small motor skills without the cognitive reasoning skill required to protect oneself are involved in the events that lead to scalding. For example, a child may crawl into a tub, turn on the faucet, but not understand that the water will get hotter and that, to stop the burning, it must be turned off.

Of all the areas in the house, the kitchen is the most hazardous with respect to burns in young children, especially young children. A child's curiosity coupled with the parent(s) busyness in the kitchen seem to compound the likelihood of an injury occurring (Fig. 15–3). As children get older, they become more active in the kitchen and can be injured if proper supervision is lacking—for example, lifting kettles that are too heavy, touching things when they have just been removed from the oven, or reaching across torrents of steam. Microwave ovens can also be hazardous because the temperature of the liquid is significantly higher than that of the surface of the container.

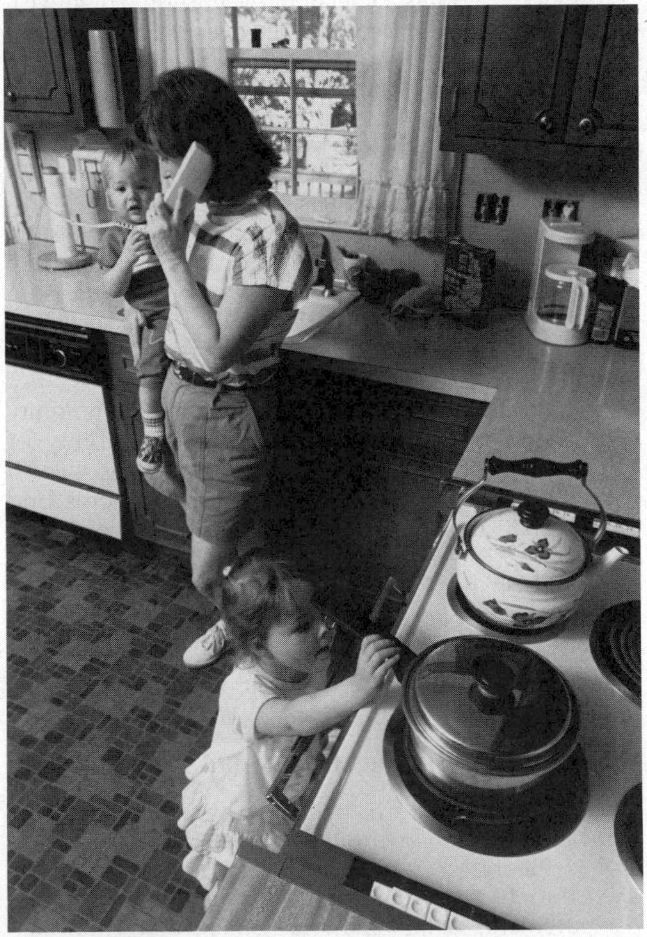

FIGURE 15-3. It takes only moments for the handle of a pan on the stove to be noticed by mobile, curious young children. In their attempt to see if they can reach it or see what is in it, a disaster and injury can occur.

The prevalence of flame burns in children after 5 years of age is related to host characteristics. Children at this age are fascinated with matches and have the fine motor skills to strike a match. A relative easing off by parents in the extent of supervision provided (environment) during this stage increases the child's risk for flame burns by matches and other agents, such as campfires or gasoline.

A serious hazard is the use of firecrackers by children. Firecrackers should not be viewed as toys, not even the sparklers, and require adult supervision, if used at all.

Prevention Strategies

Two preventive strategies that require the nurse's priority are to convince parents to (1) lower hot water temperatures to between 120° and 130° F and (2) buy a smoke detector (preferably one for each level in the house).

Reducing the hazard of the agent (heat of the water) is a simple action; yet, motivating parents to do so is not an easy task. The reasons for laxity have not been defined, although the concern of not having water hot enough for dishwashers has been a drawback for some.

Smoke detectors should be installed on each level of a house for the best protection. They should be placed on the ceiling (or high on the wall) where smoke and heat are most likely to accumulate first. They should be near the bedrooms so that the alarm can be heard even if the doors are closed. In case of a home fire, children should know how to proceed; therefore, an escape plan should be discussed and practiced in the home.

A major role of the nurse is to assist families in childproofing their homes and to teach children basic fire prevention strategies. Although many of the measures to be offered seem to be commonsense suggestions, a summary of these has been provided in Table 15–5 to use as a reference when teaching caregivers burn prevention.

High Risk for Injury: Poisonings

A "poison" is any substance that can harm one's body when exposed to it. A poisoning can occur through ingestion, inhalation, skin exposure, or eye contact or through any other mode that causes untoward effects.

Poisoning is the fourth leading cause of death in children ages 1 to 4 years. Peak incidence occurs in 1- and 2-year-olds, a time when children become increasingly mobile, are intense explorers, and have the need to demonstrate some autonomous behavior. Although the incidence of poisonings has declined in recent years (due to childproof packaging), continued efforts and strategies are required to reduce the mor-

TABLE 15-5
Family-Centered Teaching: Prevention of Burns

General Care Tips

Shelter infants from burning sun rays

Install one smoke detector on each level of the home

Teach children 5 yrs old and older the proper use of matches

Follow the recommendations of the local fire department for house checks and exit procedures, and teach these to children

Place guards around sources of heat and fires

Place guards over unused electrical outlets

From infancy, teach child the meaning of "hot"

Supervise campfires and barbeques

Adjust water heaters to a temperature between 49 and 54.4°C (120 and 130°F)

Do not store gasoline or other lighter fluids in open containers. Store these in proper, legal receptacles locked away so children cannot reach them

Do not store matches and lighters where children can reach them. Remember that purses may have matches or lighters in them

Do not allow candles to burn unattended

Do not store cleaning chemicals where children can reach them

Do not misuse extension cords or allow electrical appliances near water taps. Teach child not to chew on cords

Do not leave children unattended while a fireplace is burning

In the Kitchen

Never leave children unattended when you are cooking. By age 7 or 8, children can use toaster and do simple cooking with supervision. Older children can use microwave oven but must be taught that foods and dishes get very hot without appearing to be

Do not leave hot pans or food or liquids unattended on stove, countertops, or tables. Do not leave handles extending over the edge of a stove or countertop

Do not leave cords to electrical cooking appliances dangling. Children can grab them and receive severe burns from the spilled hot liquids and solids

Do not let young children pour or serve hot food or liquids. Do not pour hot coffee or soup at the table and leave them unattended

Do not drink coffee, tea, soup, or other hot liquids with a child on your lap. One slip or a sudden darting hand is all it takes to cause a serious scald

In the Bathroom

Check the temperature in a tub of water before you place a child in it. The skin of a 1- or 2-year-old is tender and vulnerable to scalds. Use the back of your hand to check the temperature. The water should feel warm, not hot

Do not leave a child in the tub unattended. Many scalds occur when the child or a sister or brother turns on the hot water while playing

Teach older children to keep hair dryers and other appliances away from water

In the Bedroom

Do not leave a hot steam vaporizer close enough to a child's crib or bed that it might be tipped or pulled over

Do not leave hair dryers, curling irons, or other appliances plugged in with young children around

Do not smoke in bed

bidity and mortality that results from this preventable cause (Fig. 15-4).

Some epidemiologic observations concerning poisonings give some guidance for planning of prevention strategies. At least 85 per cent of all poisonings reported to poison control centers involve ingestion. Medications are responsible for approximately 50 per cent of all poisonings, commonly involving aspirin, acetaminophen, vitamins, and minerals. Household products are common offenders, and many of these are extremely caustic.

Plants are common agents that are ingested by children, but, fortunately, a relatively small portion of plant ingestions produces severe toxic symptoms (Fig. 15-5). The few plants that produce severe symptoms are extremely toxic if eaten. Highly toxic plants include rosary pea, castor bean, rhododendron, spurge laurel, tree tobacco, water hemlock, and yew. Toxic plants most frequently ingested (in order of frequency) include philodendron, dieffenbachia, jade plant, holly berries, yew, pokeweed, poinsettia, Swedish ivy, woody nightshade, black elder, and African violets. Other causes of poisonings include inhalation of toxic substances and exposure of the skin and eyes.

Lead poisoning is another type of poisoning that

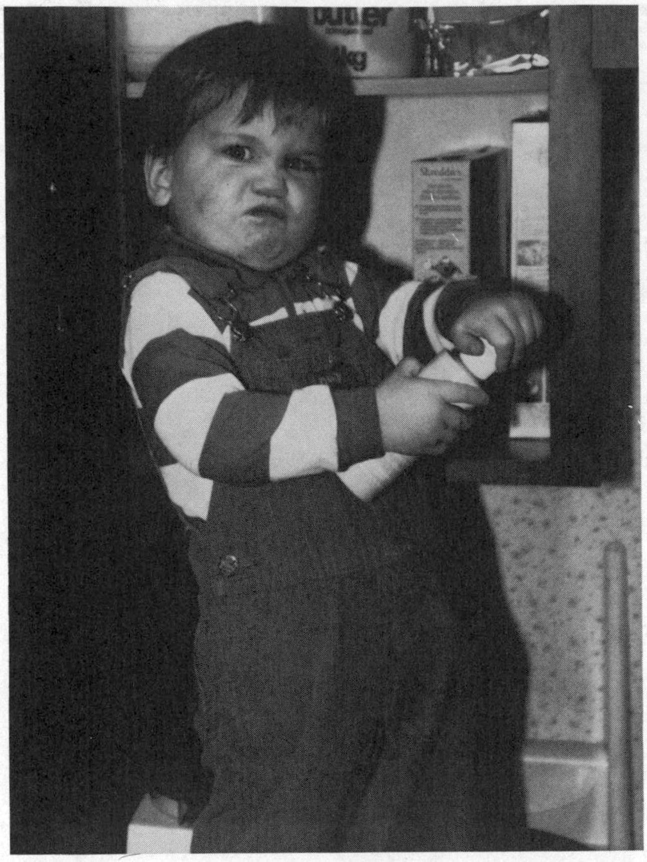

FIGURE 15-4. Mobility, curiosity, and manual dexterity lead a toddler to forbidden areas and dangerous substances if unsupervised. A determination to "get what I want" further endangers a toddler.

has been called a "silent epidemic" (Landrigan & Graef, 1987). The current attitude is that "there is essentially no safe threshold of lead exposure" (Barker & Lewis, 1990). Chronically elevated lead levels can affect children in any locality. It is particularly a problem of children in the inner cities, where lead-based paint continues to be the main source of high-dose exposure. (See Chapter 46 for further discussion of lead poisoning).

Prevention Strategies

Although legislation has had a notable impact on poison control, nurses must continue to stress the importance of teaching families to poisonproof their homes. Basic objectives in poison prevention include the following: (1) reducing the number of poisonings and (2) reducing the severity of the effects of the poisoning. Guidelines that can be followed to meet these objectives are summarized in Table 15–6.

An important aspect of counseling to prevent poisoning is to increase parents' awareness of potential poisoning dangers that emerge as their child develops. For example, as a child becomes more mobile and manual dexterity is increased, medicines in a

TABLE 15-6
Family-Centered Teaching: Poison-Proofing a Home and Poison Management

Reduce Access to Poisons:

- Keep poisonous substances in their original containers (never place near food, in food containers, or in pop bottles)
- Ensure that all harmful products and all medicines have child-resistant caps
- Store harmful products out of reach (use safety locks on cabinets)
- Know where child is and what he or she is doing at all times
- Do not refer to medicine as "candy"
- Discard outdated medicines by flushing down the toilet (not by discarding in a wastebasket)
- Avoid taking medicine in front of small children
- Avoid storing medicine in a purse (If medicine must be carried, purse must be kept out of reach at all times)
- Keep alcoholic beverages out of reach
- Use lead-free paint and do not let child chew on outdoor surfaces; ensure that toys are not coated with lead-containing paint
- Teach child not to chew on plants and shrubs

Reduce Severity of Poison's Effects:

- Purchase a 30-ml bottle of syrup of ipecac
- Post the phone number of the nearest poison control center
- Administer first aid (see Chapter 46)

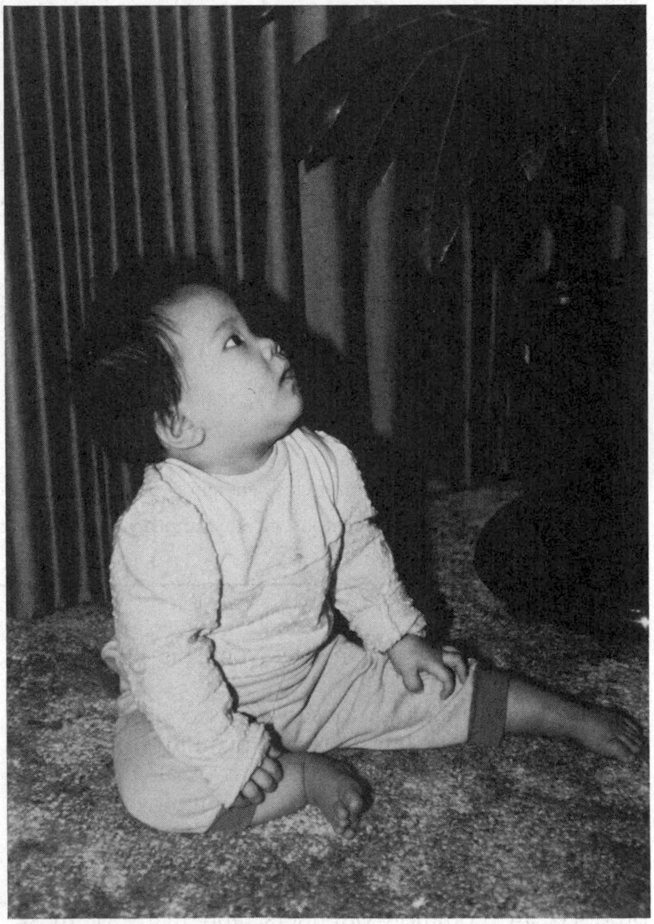

FIGURE 15-5. Young children are fascinated by everything they can see and reach. Plants can be a hazard if children are not properly supervised.

mother's purse become potentially lethal to a child. The role of anticipatory guidance is to facilitate protection of the child by modifying the environment *before* the child accomplishes the next skill (e.g., crawling, climbing, opening containers). It is advised that all poison-proofing is done before the infant crawls to ensure that a new skill is not achieved when the parent least expects it. Care of the child who has ingested a poison or been exposed to lead is presented in Chapter 46.

High Risk for Injury: Suffocation

Suffocation is a particular threat to infants under 1 year of age because of their ability to wriggle and move but an inability to untangle or dislodge themselves from a constricting object. Plastic used to cover a mattress, blankets, and anything with a string (bib, pacifier on string) can strangle and suffocate an infant if left in the crib or near the baby's reach. Mobiles strung across cribs are not recommended once an infant begins to sit up because the child can become entangled in them. Crib and playpen slats must be no more than 2⅜ inches (6 cm) apart, and the mattress should fit the crib snugly to prevent the infant's head from getting caught between two surfaces. Decorative corner posts should not be present because the infant's head can get caught in them. As an infant becomes mobile and is able to reach, the surroundings of the crib and playpen must be carefully examined. Drapery cords are a particular hazard to an infant, who could become strangled while playing on the floor or while in the crib nearby. Placing an infant on a large cushion is another hazard causing suffocation when an infant rolls face downward into the cushion and cannot move. An infant's face thus gets buried in the cushion. As a child approaches toddlerhood, abandoned refrigerators and trunks become attractive hiding places. A toddler is capable of crawling inside but does not foresee the problem of becoming entrapped. Abandoned equipment poses a danger to even the school-age child. Doors must be removed from such equipment, and children of this age should be taught the dangers of playing in deserted buildings and near excavations.

High Risk for Injury: Aspiration of a Foreign Body

Asphyxiation resulting from aspiration of a foreign body into the respiratory tract is the leading cause of accidental death *in the home* in children under 6 years of age. Safety pins are the most frequently aspirated object by infants from 0 to 1 year of age; hard foods, especially peanuts and corn, are commonly aspirated by 2- to 4-year-olds (Fig. 15–6). Infants and toddlers can find the smallest object on a thickly carpeted floor. Objects such as nails, pins, paper clips, staples, and any number of household items may be swallowed, aspirated, or stuffed into a body orifice.

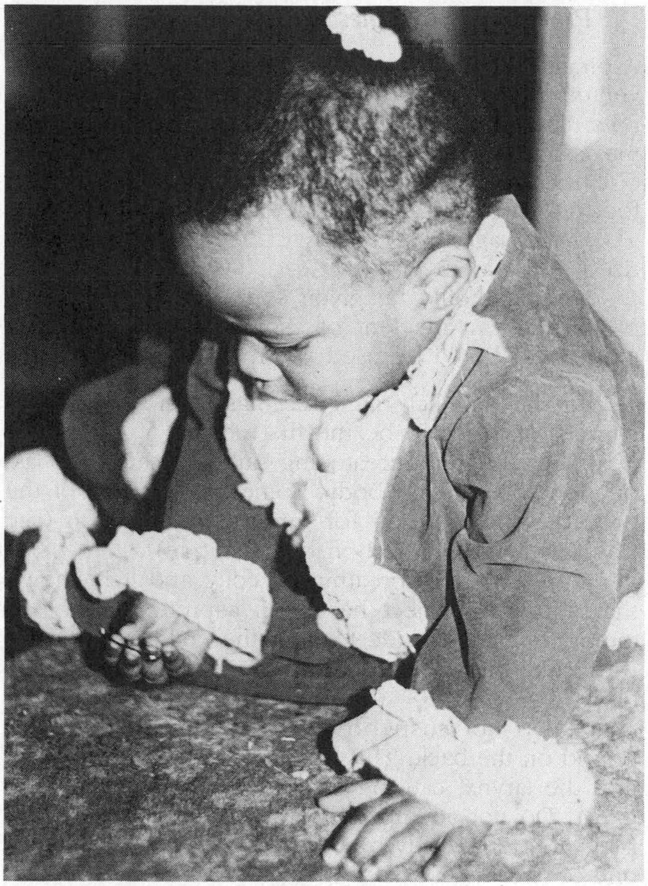

FIGURE 15 - 6. The infant's developing mobility makes childproofing mandatory. This infant has discovered an open safety pin lying in the carpet.

Coins are attractive to young children but are frequently swallowed or aspirated and *should not be treated as toys.* Toys need to be inspected for removable parts that could be swallowed or aspirated. Children not only put things into the mouth but also place things into the nose, ears, or any body orifice. Dangerous objects must not be put into an accessible wastebasket, as a young child will discover even the most obscure item.

The actions of parents can actually contribute to the aspiration of a foreign body. For example, propping an infant's bottle is potentially dangerous and should be avoided. Also, during early infancy, the ingestion of baby powder can occur quite readily. Directly shaking powder onto the baby's skin can create a puff of particles that can be inhaled; therefore, it is recommended that powder should be applied to the caregiver's hands by shaking it onto the hands while holding the can away from the baby's head, then smoothing it on the infant's skin (Wagner & Hindi-Alexander, 1984). It is not uncommon to see parents permit their infant to play with the can of powder while changing a diaper. However, the top can easily come off and allow powder to spill freely into the child's mouth and face.

Prevention Strategies

Aspiration of food particles while eating can be prevented by refraining from giving hard foods, such as nuts, Life Savers, small hard candies, corn, and tough meats, to infants and toddlers. Even though a 2-year-old has some molars, the ability to thoroughly chew food is not mastered until the preschool years (about 4 years of age). Prevention of aspiration is summarized in Table 15–7.

Parents should be given some basic guidance to prepare for an incident of aspiration. The following guidelines should be used when counseling parents:

1. The Heimlich maneuver has been successful in all ages and should be the first choice of emergency treatment for a life-threatening situation caused by aspiration of a foreign body. Some modification of the procedure is required for infants and children (see Chapter 46 for description of technique).
2. If a child is breathing quietly and it is known that a foreign object has been aspirated, every attempt should be made to rush the child to the nearest facility for treatment without disturbing the foreign body.
3. Do not suspend the child by the feet and pound on the back. This may dislodge a foreign body into the larynx, causing fatal obstruction.
4. Do not attempt to extract a pharyngeal or laryngeal foreign body by reaching into the mouth with one or two fingers. This is dangerous because the foreign body may be forced into the larynx more tightly, causing a partial obstruction to become a complete obstruction.

Foreign body aspiration can cause panic and incorrect treatment by parents in the home. It is the nurse's responsibility to reduce the number of fatalities and injuries from foreign body aspiration by teaching parents how to prevent its occurrence and how to correctly apply first-aid measures.

***High Risk for Injury*: Falls**

Falls occur as children achieve new developmental tasks (e.g., rolling over, crawling, standing, walking) and increased supervision is not provided accordingly. Falls occur when a new skill is used to satisfy an overwhelming curiosity or simply when body movements cause something to slip or fall (e.g., a plastic infant carrier placed on a smooth counter).

Prevention Strategies

The many devices that are used for children should be checked for stability and exposed parts that could cause injury. Baby walkers in particular have been reported to cause injuries, especially from falls down a flight of stairs. In spite of manufacturing regulations to improve their safety, walkers continue to cause injuries from falls. The type and number of injuries from walkers warrant that health care professionals strongly recommend that they not be used and inform parents that they do not help babies to walk sooner.

An injury not caused by a fall, but one that is associated with mobility, is injury to the arm and shoul-

TABLE 15-7
***Family-Centered Teaching*: Prevention of Foreign Body Aspiration**

Food
Place infant on side (usually the right side to facilitate digestion of food) after feedings
Avoid hard foods such as peanuts until chewing is well established, around 4 yrs of age
Cut and break food into bite-size pieces for infants and toddlers. Encourage children to chew their food and avoid putting large pieces of food into their mouths
Insist that children sit down to eat their food. Running and walking around the house (or on family outings) while eating predisposes to aspiration of particles
Do not permit eating and drinking while in a lying-down position
Objects
Do not permit young children to play with small objects (e.g., coins, buttons, marbles)
Balloons should be kept from infants and toddlers whether inflated or not. An uninflated balloon may be sucked into the posterior pharynx, larynx, or trachea
Safety pins should be kept closed and not placed near the child
Older children should not be permitted to hold objects, such as a Lego piece, a marble, or a button, in their mouths
Pacifiers should meet safety standards (mouthguard of adequate diameter—i.e., slightly under 2 ins; two ventilation holes in a mouthguard; nipple portion should not separate from mouthguard; and the handle should be easily grasped). Pacifiers should not have ribbon or string attached to place around child's neck
Do not permit infants and young children to play with baby powder

TABLE 15-8
Typical Agents Causing Falls During Infancy and Childhood: Prevention Strategies

Crib Accidents

Most falls occur while children are climbing out. Side rails should be up at all times when the infant is in the crib. Child should be moved to a bed when the height of side rail is less than three quarters of the child's height (or when the child's height is 35 ins). If a younger child is a climber and insists on crawling out, a bed with a short side rail is recommended earlier

Highchairs

Child should be secured into chair and not allowed to stand in chair. Chair should be placed away from any object that can be used from which to push off. Children in highchairs should not be left unattended

Falls During Infant Care (Dressing Tables, Crib Surface)

Fasten dressing table straps when the infant is on the table. Keep one hand on the child at all times when working at crib side or dressing table. If an article is required *away* from working area, pick the baby up or hold the baby with one hand and reach. *Do not turn your back on the baby without holding firmly*

Stairs

Place safety gate at top and bottom of any stairs to which the child has access

Infant Seats

Do not place an infant on a smooth elevated surface

Walkers

Serious falls occur; therefore, the use of walkers is not recommended

der caused by a sudden jerk. This practice should be discouraged by nurses in their contacts with parents during health care visits. See Table 15-8 for a summary of typical falls and strategies for prevention.

High Risk for Injuries: Bicycle Injuries

Bicycle riding is a favorite activity for many children and adolescents. Unfortunately, the number of bicycle-related injuries and deaths is increasing. Almost one fourth of all significant head injuries in children aged 14 years and younger are bicycle-related (Thompson et al, 1990).

The most common time for bicycle injuries to occur is from 5 to 14 years of age, with the greatest number occurring in boys. Factors associated with bicycle accidents are multiple. Mechanical or structural defects and inappropriate frame size reduce the ability to control the bike and, therefore, can increase the risk of injury. The majority of accidents occur during daylight hours, when a child is close to home and at a time when a bicycle is used for recreational purposes rather than riding to and from school.

Injuries vary from mild abrasions, contusions, and lacerations requiring minimal first aid to multiple injuries of the head, trunk, and limbs. The seriousness of the injury is determined by the type of accident. Collisions with automobiles account for a high percentage of deaths due to serious head injury. Simple falls are associated with high risk for trunk injuries caused by the impact against the handlebars.

Prevention Strategies

Teaching strategies should be directed at increasing parents' and children's awareness of the simple ways that bicycle safety can be increased. The bicycle, the child, and the environment must be considered in bicycle accident prevention. Selecting a safe and appropriate-sized bike requires the assistance of parents. A bike should allow the child to place the balls of the bottom of the feet on the ground when seated on the bicycle for easy control and safe riding. The most compelling preventive strategy to work toward is the wearing of bicycle helmets (Fig. 15-7). Safety helmets have been shown to reduce the risk of head injury by 85 per cent and brain injury by 88 per cent (Thompson et al, 1989), yet the idea of wearing helmets has not become common practice. Generally, less than 5 per cent of the population at risk wear helmets, although this varies with age and locality (Pendergrast et al, 1992). Reasons suggested for the low rates of helmet use by children are discomfort, lack of awareness, peer pressure, and cost (DiGiuseppi et al, 1990). Strong predictors reported for helmet use

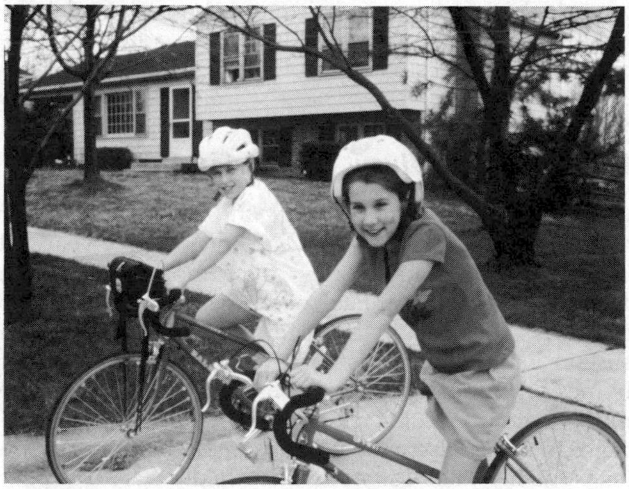

FIGURE 15-7. The wearing of a bicycle helmet can dramatically reduce the risk of serious injury if the child is involved in a bicycle accident. A few jurisdictions within the United States have passed legislation to require the wearing of bicycle helmets by children.

in the elementary school–age child are family patterns of helmet use and beliefs about helmet use (Pendergrast et al, 1992).

The child's role in preventing a bicycle accident is primary. Children start riding bicycles during the preschool or school-age years, and, therefore, they are old enough to learn bicycle rules. The nurse should direct teaching to the child, but also impress the caregiver with the need to review the rules repeatedly. It is especially important to recognize that, as children get older, they may take more risks, and, as they pattern their behavior after peers, rules that were respected at a younger age may gradually be dishonored. Also, as children grow older, they will travel farther from home and on more dangerous roads. Competitiveness with peers in performing bicycle stunts increases during school-age and early adolescent years. As children develop, they become less receptive to restrictions and rules imposed by parents. Teaching bicycle safety, therefore, must be done repeatedly and adapted to the growing independence of the child. Information on bicycle safety can be obtained from:

American Academy of Pediatrics
Educational Materials and Publications
Publication Department
1801 Hinman Avenue
Evanston, Illinois
U.S.A. 60204

Physicians for Automotive Safety
P.O. Box 208
Rye, New York
U.S.A. 10580

Information can also be obtained from local motor vehicle and license registration bureaus and from police departments. Some basic rules concerning bicycle safety are listed in Table 15–9.

TABLE 15-9
Family-Centered Teaching: Bicycle Safety Rules

Wear an approved helmet
Do not ride bike with bare feet
Inspect bike for mechanical safety regularly
Travel in the same direction as traffic
Ride as close as possible to the side of the road
Walk the bike across busy intersections
Watch for cars backing out of driveways
Watch the road for bumps and potholes
Stop and look all ways before entering the street from a driveway or lane
Don't carry parcels in hands while driving
Don't wear stereo headsets—a child needs to *hear* when a car approaches
Don't ride two on a bicycle
If riding at night, have appropriate lights and reflectors
Use hand signals appropriately (arm out for left turn, up for right turn, and down for slow)

High Risk for Injury: Pedestrian Injuries

Pedestrian injuries are a significant cause of death for all children aged 0 to 19 years; in 5- to 9-year-old children, pedestrian injuries cause more deaths than any other injury. Non-fatal pedestrian injuries are also the most common in the same age group. Children sustain injuries as pedestrians while at play near their homes, and the "dart-out" type of circumstance is the most common (Malek et al, 1990). Sex and socioeconomic factors also affect the rate of this type of injury. Fatality rates for nonwhite children are 15 times as high as for white children, and male pedestrian fatality rates are almost twice as high as for females. Pedestrian–motor vehicle collisions differ from other motor vehicle–related injuries in that few victims escape injury.

Prevention Strategies

Pedestrian injuries have not received as much attention as have those involving motor vehicle occupants. Prevention is not amenable to single interventions, such as use of seat belts, helmets, or air bags. A multifaceted approach should include teaching children basic safety rules, educating parents, enacting legislation, modifying environmental factors (e.g., with street crossing aids and improved walkways), and making design changes to the exterior of vehicles (Rivara, 1990; Division of Injury Control, 1990). An important aspect to not overlook is that prevention must include education of the *driver* as well as of the *pedestrian*.

High Risk for Injury: Animal Bites

As the number of pets increases in communities, so does the potential for animal-related injuries. It is estimated that the pet population in the United States includes more than 110 million cats and dogs. More than 60,000 animal bites result in loss of sight, facial disfigurement, or other serious injury (Mofensen & Greensher, 1987). Most animal bites occur when the animal is young. Transmissible diseases also are more common among young animals. Guidelines to use when teaching children how to interact safely with animals are summarized in Table 15–10.

High Risk for Injury: Human Bites

Human bites occur in children either through roughhousing or during fights among children or as a re-

TABLE 15-10
What to Teach Children about Animals

Avoid strange animals, especially wild, sick, or injured ones. Parents or older child should notify health department or police of wild, sick, or injured animals
Under parental supervision and with the permission and presence of pet's owner, have children make friends with pets in the child's immediate neighborhood
Alert children to dangerous or nervous animals in the neighborhood. Do not let children enter yards or houses where such animals live
Avoid riding bicycles or tricycles in areas where dogs are known to chase vehicles. Parents should notify authorities about any dog that habitually chases vehicles
Never disturb an animal that is *eating* or *sleeping*—even an animal a child is familiar with may bite
Teach children that pets are not toys. Pets are not to be mistreated or teased. An animal that is frightened, annoyed, teased, or mistreated may scratch, bite, or attack
A pet should not be purchased for a child until he or she is mature enough to handle and care for the animal, around 7 or 8 yrs old. Parents should realize that it is *their* responsibility to teach care of the pet to the child and must not let an animal suffer because of a child's immaturity

sult of child abuse. Human saliva contains a high level of bacteria; therefore, immediate treatment is required. Children should be taught not to bite and should be forewarned that if they are bitten, immediate care of the wound is required (see Chapter 46 for further discussion of care of children with a human bite).

High Risk for Injury: Farm Injuries

Farm injuries account for 300 deaths and over 20,000 significant injuries in children per year. On the farm, children work with their parents at a young age and assist with tasks around dangerous equipment. As technology advances on the farm, more and more machines are used, exposing farm children to increasing dangers. Children in rural areas should be exposed to safety programs in their school curriculum, and nurses can make both children and parents aware of the potential dangers and encourage appropriate supervision of children.

High Risk for Injury: Unsafe Toys

The United States Consumer Product Safety Commission (CPSC) has legislative power to ban any toy that presents a risk for injury through normal use. Also, the Toy Manufacturers Association (TMA) cooperates with the government to set toy safety standards. Despite the attempts at regulation, unsafe toys appear in the marketplace, leaving the final responsibility to parents.

Prevention Strategies

The safety of toys and play equipment should be brought to the attention of parents, with reference to size of the toys, sharp edges, removable parts, and supervision and safety teaching in the use of chemistry sets, scissors, and electrical toys (see Chapters 4 through 9 for discussion of age-appropriate toys).

High Risk for Injury: Child Abduction

As children grow and develop, the amount of protection that is afforded to them through direct surveillance decreases, and the amount of education required for self-protection correspondingly increases. Education is provided early, and its scope must encompass the dangers of places and *people*. "Streetproofing" is a term used to describe the process of preparing children for the potential dangers that threaten children when they embark "on the street." Streetproofing encompasses different elements according to the circumstances of the child. "The street" expands as the child grows, and, according to Gossage and Gunton (1981), it is "defined by your child's travels."

The goal to protect children from the dangers of the streets should take into consideration the host (the child), the agent or vector (those who might harm the child), and the physical and emotional environments. The nurse's role begins early by encouraging parents to teach very young children about dangers associated with walking and riding on the street, play and sports activities, and being in public places. With appropriate teaching, a child is not restricted from play and freedom in a neighborhood but can acquire some skills to detect danger and cope with threatening situations.

Prevention Strategies

Prevention of injury to children while playing and traveling in their neighborhoods is focused on: (1)

controlling the environment and (2) teaching self-protective behaviors. Control of the environment is accomplished through appropriate supervision of children and increasing the resources available. Off-limits areas need to be identified and safe routes to school established. Organized resources, such as Block Parents, are explained to children so they know who they are and how to use them.

Although children vary considerably in the type of teaching they require, the following strategies are basic and should be brought to the attention of all children:

- Never accept a ride from a stranger or any individual that has not been arranged and approved by a parent or caregiver (even if they say they are taking you home or to wherever your parent is).
- Never accept candy or gifts from a stranger.
- Do not let strangers into the house when you are alone.
- If you are asked to give directions to a stranger, do not stand near the car.
- Stay with older children or adults on the street or in public places whenever possible.
- Enter only those homes that parents have approved.
- Call home as soon as you arrive at a friend's house to inform parents of your location.
- Do not stray across the agreed-on boundaries without asking permission from parents or a designated caregiver.

Children need instructions about actions to take in the event of approach or attack. The following basic principles should be explained:

- If a child is approached or attacked, he or she should make as much noise as possible (e.g., knocking over a garbage can, screaming, or using an electronic noisemaker).
- The three basic rules are *say no, get away,* and *tell someone.*
- Try to remember what the person looks like, and check the license number (write in the snow or in the dirt).
- Children must know where they can get help (e.g., Block Parents, police, teachers).

One of the most serious crimes against children in our society today is sexual abuse. Many child molesters are individuals who are known to the family. Children must be taught about inappropriate behavior of others concerning their bodies, and anyone who wants to spend excessive amounts of time with a child should be held in suspicion. When a child expresses fear of spending time alone with anyone, whether a friend, a relative, or a parent, further investigations is indicated. (See Chapter 28 for further discussion of sexual abuse.)

Barriers to Preventive Strategies: Nurse's Role

Strategies to prevent common childhood injuries have been presented. To offer meaningful intervention for any of these problems, it should be recognized that, despite employment of the best of methods to teach and motivate parents and children to take safety precautions, the benefits of educational strategies are inconsistent. Furthermore, efforts to increase product safety through regulation and enforcement of safety behaviors through legislation, although known to be effective, are encumbered with diversity in public opinion and various degrees of governmental bureaucracy. There is no established set of phenomena that has been isolated as underlying the inability of health professionals to bring about significant reductions in the morbidity and mortality that result from childhood injury. There are, however, some basic attitudinal stances that have been proposed as forceful deterrents to successful educational programs and legislative actions.

Barriers to Safety Education and Counseling

It is recognized that educational strategies to increase health behaviors have not demonstrated consistent effectiveness. Three major attitudinal approaches that exist are: (1) a low level of perceived vulnerability (it won't happen to my child); (2) a fatalistic attitude (an "accident" cannot be prevented); and (3) "accidents" are to be expected during the growing-up years (children will be children).

Perceived Vulnerability

Perceived vulnerability is the degree to which people expect that a certain event will happen to them. Fortunately, most people do not suffer injuries; therefore, it is reasonable to believe "it won't happen to me." Furthermore, if the effort that is required to perform a safety behavior is extensive, the inconvenience is quickly perceived to outweigh the risk.

The overall goal of nursing is to give factual information about the prevalence of childhood accidents and reduce the perceived difficulty of performing safety behaviors known to reduce injury.

Attitudes and Fatalism

If the nurse is confronted with a deep-rooted attitude of fatalism, the usual methods of providing pamphlets and verbal instructions may result in colossal failures. Personalizing instructions to the family's situation, their income, and their attitudes requires an assessment of the family to determine what the family is willing and able to attempt. Strategies that require only one-time actions and that modify the agent or have the potential to reduce the severity of the injury may be more acceptable (purchase of a smoke alarm, purchase of syrup of ipecac, reduction of hot water temperature).

Children Will Be Children

The desire to permit a child the "freedom to grow" can be perceived to be in conflict with the priority of safety. The conflict that arises emerges out of the wish to provide an environment that maximizes development but ensures safety. Teaching children limits with explanations why they are important (e.g., off-limits for a toddler, bicycle rules for a school-age child, and use of the family car for an adolescent) is the best way to resolve this. The attitude that children will be children with their share of injuries is too costly. Limit-setting provides experiences from which a child learns some inner controls, self-preservation, and respect for rules of society.

Barriers to Product Regulation and Legislation

It is recognized that strategies that do *not* require any action by the consumer (passive intervention) are more effective than those requiring repeated behaviors by the consumer (active intervention). It is also recognized that *limiting* behaviors, such as speed limit enforcement, is more easily accomplished than legislating an *action* behavior (e.g., wearing a seat belt).

The barriers concerning product regulation and government legislation of health behaviors are as varied as is public opinion. Reluctance to support legal methods of accident prevention evolves from the deep-seated resistance to governmental interference of individual freedom and private enterprise. To even consider legislation as an option, there needs to be a high level of evidence that the intervention will work, and, as the amount of restriction on freedom increases, stronger evidence is required. Furthermore, if legislation is instituted, the costs, inconvenience, or undesirable effects that are introduced are reasons for resistance. For example, false alarms of a smoke detector, discomfort of a bicycle helmet, the cost of child-resistant devices, are reasons why people resist legislation.

Following are some guidelines to use when assisting children and parents to adopt healthy behavioral change:

- Find out what the individual knows and wants to know.
- Assess for attitudinal barriers and correct misinformation.
- Individualize instruction according to the client's home, the particular child, and the family income.
- Recognize the degree of effort that a behavior requires and suggest options that can reduce the difficulty of performing actions.
- Promote the teaching of children by parents and in the schools, and teach children during health supervision contacts.
- Give readable (to the level of the clients) written instructions to supplement verbal ones.
- Maintain a nonpunitive and nonjudgmental attitude but impress clients with the scope of the problem honestly and unequivocally.

The public hardly realizes that in the United States over 20,000 children die each year of injury, and a much larger number become permanently impaired annually (CDC, 1990a). It is apparent from the information presented in this chapter that nurses must become increasingly involved in designing studies to evaluate the effectiveness of current preventive strategies and to search for new, more effective approaches.

KEY CONCEPTS

Concepts Related to Basic Information

- Injury is the leading cause of death in the 1- to 19-year-old age group.
- The leading cause of injury resulting in death is motor vehicle–related injuries.
- Homicide is now the second leading cause of injury resulting in death.
- *Improper* restraint is a risk factor for children riding in a car.
- There is essentially no safe threshold of lead exposure.

Concepts Related to Nursing Assessment

- Developmental characteristics of the child largely determine the degree of risk associated with the various types of injuries that are common in children.
- Barriers to preventive strategies affect education and counseling as well as product regulation and legislation.

Concepts Related to Nursing Intervention

- Preventive strategies should be directed at altering characteristics of: the host, the agent, and the environment.
- Approaches used to reduce the incidence of injury are passive (provision of external control) and active (adherence to specific behaviors).
- All levels of intervention need to be included: education and counseling, product improvement, environmental controls, and legislation.

REFERENCES

Agran, P., Castillo, D., & Winn, D. (1990). Childhood motor vehicle occupant injuries. *American Journal of Diseases of Children, 144,* 653–662.

Agran, P., Winn, D., & Castillo, D. (1991). Unsupervised children in vehicles: A risk for pediatric trauma. *Pediatrics, 87,* 70.

American Academy of Pediatrics, Committee on Injury and Poison Prevention and Committee of Fetus and Newborn. (1991). Safe transportation of premature infants. *Pediatrics, 87*(1), 120–122.

Barker, P. O., & Lewis, D. A. (1990). The management of lead exposure in pediatric populations. *Nurse Practitioner, 15*(12), 8–16.

Carlsson, G., Norin, H., & Ysander, L. (1991). Rearward-facing child seats—The safest car restraint for children? *Accident Analysis and Prevention, 23,* 175–182.

Centers for Disease Control (1990a). Fatal injuries to children—United States, 1986. *Morbidity and Mortality Weekly Report, 39*(26), 442–445, 451.

Centers for Disease Control. (1990b). Homicides among young black males—United States 1978–1987. *Morbidity and Mortality Weekly Report, 39*(48), 869–873.

Centers for Disease Control. (1992a). Position papers from the third national injury control conference: Setting the national agenda for injury control in the 1990s: Motor vehicle injury prevention. *Morbidity and Mortality Weekly Report, 41*(RR6), 1–4.

Centers for Disease Control. (1992b). Unintentional firearm-related fatalities among children and teenagers—United States 1982–1988. *Morbidity and Mortality Weekly Report, 41*(25), 442–445.

Christoffel, K. K. (1989). Child passenger safety. *American Journal of Diseases of Children, 143,* 1271–1272.

Christoffel, K. K. (1990). Violent death and injury in U.S. children and adolescents. *American Journal of Diseases of Children, 144,* 697–706.

Crawley, T., & Velsor-Friedrich, B. (1991). The cost to our children: The issue of gun control. *Journal of Pediatric Nursing, 6*(5), 350–351.

Cummings, P. H. (1991). Farm accidents and injuries among farm families and workers. *American Association of Occupational Health Nurses Journal, 34*(9), 407–414.

DiGuiseppi, C. G., Rivara, F. P., & Koepsell, T. D. (1990). Attitudes toward bicycle helmet ownership and use by school-age children. *American Journal of Diseases of Children, 144,* 83–86.

Division of Injury Control, Center for Environmental Health and Injury, Centers for Disease Control. (1990). Childhood injuries in the United States. *American Journal of Diseases of Children, 144,* 625–646.

Finkelstein, J. L., Schwartz, S. B., Madden, M. R., Marano, M. A., & Goodwin, C. W. (1992). Pediatric burns: An overview. *Pediatric Clinics of North America, 39*(5), 1145–1163.

Gossage, R. C., & Gunton, M. J. (1981). *A parent's guide to street-proofing children*. New York: Bantam Books.

Greensher, J. (1984). Prevention of childhood injuries. *Pediatrics* (Supplement, 74), 970–975.

Guyer, B., & Ellers, B. (1990). Childhood injuries in the United States. *American Journal of Diseases of Children, 144,* 649–652.

Jones, N. E. (1992). Childhood injuries: An epidemiologic approach. *Pediatric Nursing, 18*(3), 235–239.

Landrigan, P. J., & Graef, J. W. (1987). Pediatric lead poisoning in 1987: The silent epidemic continues. *Pediatrics, 79,* 582–583.

Langley, J. (1987). The "accident-prone child"—The perpetration of a myth. *Australian Pediatric Journal, 18*(4), 243–246.

Malek, M., Guyer, B., & Lescochier, I. (1990). The epidemiology and prevention of child pedestrian injury. *Accident Analysis and Prevention, 22*(4), 301–313.

McLoughlin, E., & McGuire, A. (1990). The causes, impact, and preventability of childhood injuries in the United States: Childhood burn injuries in the United States. *American Journal of Diseases of Children, 144,* 677–683.

Mofensen, H. C., & Greensher, J. (1992). Accident prevention. In R. A. Hoekelman, et al. (Eds.). *Primary pediatric care* (pp 234–259). St. Louis: CV Mosby.

National Committee for Injury Prevention and Control. (1989). *Preventing injuries: Meeting the challenge*. New York: Oxford University Press.

Nyman, G. (1987). Infant temperament: Childhood accidents and hospitalization. *Clinical Pediatrics, 26,* 398–404.

Pendergrast, R. A., Ashworth, C. S., DuRant, R. H., & Litaker, M. (1992). Correlates of children's bicycle helmet use and short-term failure of school-level interventions. *Pediatrics, 90*(3), 354–358.

Rivara, F. P. (1990). Child pedestrian injuries in the United States. *American Journal of Diseases of Children, 144,* 692–696.

Shaw, G. (1987). Vehicular transport safety for the child with disabilities. *American Journal of Occupational Therapy, 41*(1), 35–42.

Simon, J. (1992). Accidental injury and emergency medical services for children. In R. E. Behrman (Ed.). *Nelson textbook of pediatrics* (14th ed., pp 216–224). Philadelphia: WB Saunders.

Szilagyi, P. (1992). Animal bites. In R. A. Hoekelman, N. M. Nelson, S. B. Friedman, & H. M. Seidel (Eds.). *Primary pediatric care* (pp 1129–1131). St. Louis: CV Mosby.

Thompson, D. C., Thompson, R. S., & Rivara, F. P. (1990). Incidence of bicycle-related injuries in a defined population. American Journal of Public Health, *80,* 1388–1389.

Thompson, R. S., Rivara, F. P., & Thompson, D. C. (1989). Case-control study of the effectiveness of bicycle safety helmets. *New England Journal of Medicine, 320,* 1361–1367.

Wagner, T. J., & Hindi-Alexander, M. (1984). Hazards of baby powder? *Pediatric Nursing, 10*(2), 124–125.

Waller, A. E., Baker, S. P., & Szoka, A. (1989). Childhood injury deaths: National analysis and geographic variations. *American Journal of Public Health, 79,* 310–315.

Wintemute, G. J. (1990). Childhood drowning and near-drowning in the United States. *American Journal of Diseases of Children, 144,* 663–669.

BIBLIOGRAPHY

Bellinger, D., Sloman, J., Leviton, A., Rabinowitz, M., Needleman, H. L., & Waternaux, C. (1991). Low-level lead exposure and children's cognitive function in the preschool years. *Pediatrics, 87*(2), 219–227.

Bodenhorn, K. A. (1991). Lead poisoning: The foremost preventable disease of childhood. *Journal of Pediatric Health Care, 5*(3), 156–159.

Brennen, S. R., Rhodes, K. H., & Peterson, H. A. (1990). Infection after farm machine–related injuries in children and adolescents. *American Journal of Diseases of Children, 144,* 710–713.

Christophersen, E. R. (1977). Children's behavior during automobile rides: Do car seats make a difference? *Pediatrics, 60*(1), 69–74.

Coffman, S. P. (1991). Parent education for drowning prevention. *Journal of Pediatric Health Care, 5*(3), 141–146.

Coppens, N. (1986). Cognitive characteristics as predictors of children's understanding of safety and prevention. *Journal of Pediatric Psychology, 11,* 189–202.

Coppens, N. (1985). Cognitive development and locus of control as predictors of preschoolers' understanding of safety and prevention. *Journal of Applied Developmental Psychology, 6,* 43–55.

Coppens, N. M. (1990). Parental responses to children in unsafe situations. *Pediatric Nursing, 16*(6), 571–574.

Eichelberger, M. R., Gotschall, C. S., Feely, H. B., Harstad, P., & Bowman, L. M. (1990). Parental attitudes and knowledge of child safety: A national survey. *American Journal of Diseases of Children, 144,* 714–720.

Ellerby, P., & Ward, P. M. (1989). Development of a pediatric injury prevention program for emergency departments. *Journal of Emergency Nursing, 15*(3), 584–586.

Federal Bureau of Investigation. (1986). *Uniform Crime Reports for the United States*. Washington, DC: US Department of Justice.

Holinger, P. C. (1990). The causes, impact, and preventability of childhood injuries in the United States: Childhood suicide in the United States. *American Journal of Diseases of Children, 144,* 670–676.

Jones, N. E. (1992). Injury prevention: A survey of clinical practice. *Journal of Pediatric Health Care, 6*(4), 182–186.

Kelly, B., Sein, C., & McCarthy, P. (1987). Safety education in a pediatric primary care setting. *Pediatrics, 79,* 818–824.

Kraus, J. F., Rock, A., & Hemyari, P. (1990). Brain injuries among infants, children, adolescents, and young adults. *American Journal of Diseases of Children, 144,* 684–691.

Lee, E. J., & Bass, C. (1990). Survey of accidents in a university day-care center. *Journal of Pediatric Health Care, 4*(1), 18–23.

Mandelbaum, J. K. (1992). Child survival: What are the issues? *Journal of Pediatric Health Care, 6*(3), 132–137.

Matheny, A. (1987). Psychological characteristics of childhood accidents. *Journal of Social Issues, 43,* 45–60.

McLoughlin, E. (1990). The causes, cost, and prevention of childhood burn injuries. *American Journal of Diseases of Children, 144,* 677–683.

Pless, I., & Arsenault, L. (1987). The role of health education in the prevention of injuries to children. *Journal of Social Issues, 43,* 87–103.

Schor, I. (1987). Unintentional injuries: Patterns within families. *American Journal of Diseases of Children, 141,* 1280–1284.

Selbst, S. M., Baker, M. D., & Shames, M. (1990). Bunk bed injuries. *American Journal of Diseases of Children, 144,* 721–723.

Schoettle, B. M. (1990). Car seat update. *Journal of Pediatric Health Care, 5*(3), 160–162.

Swartz, M. K. (1990). Infant mortality: Agenda for the 1990s. *Journal of Pediatric Health Care, 4*(4), 169–174.

Simm, J. E. (1992). Accidental injury and emergency medical services for children. In R. E. Behrman (Ed.). *Nelson textbook of pediatrics* (pp 216–224). Philadelphia: WB Saunders.

Valsiner, J., & Lightfoot, C. (1987). Process structure of parent-child-environment relations and the prevention of children's injuries. *Journal of Social Issues, 43,* 61–72.

Waller, A., Baker, S., & Szocka, A. (1989). Childhood injury deaths: National analysis and geographic variations. *American Journal of Public Health, 79,* 310–315.

Whatley, J. H. (1991). Effects of health locus of control and social network on adolescent risk taking. *Pediatric Nursing, 17*(2), 145–152.

Wiley, J. F. (1991). Mammalian bites. *Journal of Pediatric Health Care, 5*(1), 50.

Wintemute, G. J. (1990). The causes, impact, and prevention of childhood injuries in the United States: Childhood drowning injuries in the United States. *American Journal of Diseases of Children, 144,* 663–669.

CHAPTER • 16

Healthy Dietary Practices

Connie B. Ott

NURSING PROCESS PLANS

NPP: Care of Children on Home Parenteral Nutrition, Table 16–23

RELATED TOPICS

Maternal infant attachment, Chapter 4
Families with Infants, Chapter 5
Families with Toddlers, Chapter 6
Families with Preschoolers, Chapter 7
Families with School-Age Children, Chapter 8
Fluoride supplementation, Chapter 8
Families with Adolescents, Chapter 9
Promoting Healthy Parenting, Chapter 12
Obesity, bulimia, and anorexia, Chapter 29
Lactose intolerance, Chapter 35
Altered Digestive Function, Chapter 35

LEARNING OBJECTIVES

- Describe the nutritional status of children in North America.
- Discuss the impact of nutrition on growth and development of the child/adolescent.
- Discuss the nutritional requirements of the child/adolescent.
- Identify potential consequences relating to the excessive or deficient intake of nutrients during childhood/adolescence.
- Identify the role of the nurse within the area of nutritional assessment and counseling.
- Identify and discuss common nutritional concerns, issues, and nutritional alterations during childhood/adolescence.
- Identify appropriate nursing interventions used to promote the optimal nutritional status of the child/adolescent.

Health at all ages is enhanced by a diet that contains sufficient quantities of the essential nutrients and avoids excessive consumption. For the young, nutrition is a primary concern because food is required not only for all maintenance and energy but also for growth. The way a child grows and develops is the result of an interplay of the genetic constitution of the individual and a multitude of environmental variables. Of all the environmental factors that affect growth and development, food is one of the most influential. Both the physiologic parameters (height, weight, brain growth, and immunity) and the psychologic implications of food and feeding practices shape the growing years. The nutritional practices developed during these early years will usually continue throughout life. It is suspected that early nutrition is associated with the development of chronic disease in adulthood (hypertension, heart disease, and some cancers), although a cause-and-effect relationship has not been established. The effectiveness of nurses in promoting a healthy diet depends on their own knowledge about nutrition and also on their understanding of the beliefs and habits, cultural variations, lifestyles, and family customs in which dietary practices are based.

This chapter begins with an overview of the scope of the problem, followed by a discussion of the impact of nutrition on growth and development. A review of the nutritional requirements during childhood and adolescence is included to provide the necessary background information on which assessments are based. The assessment process and nursing interventions are reviewed, followed by a discussion of dietary issues and nutritional problems common during the developing years. The nurse's role in the promotion of a healthful diet is addressed in this chapter; those feeding issues that arise out of specific age-related changes are discussed in the respective chapters on normal growth and development (see Chapters 4 through 9).

Nutritional Status of Children in North America

Lifestyle undoubtedly affects how people eat and how their children eat. In the developed countries, there generally is access to adequate nutrients and nutritional messages bombard the consumer from all sides. With societal changes that have taken women into the workplace, young children to day care and baby sitters, and school-age children to the after-school activities of the season, consumers' versions of good nutrition are becoming whatever can fit into their lifestyle. In industrialized countries, the trend toward malnutrition is on the side of excessive intake of kilocalories, macronutrients (particularly refined carbohydrates and fat), inappropriate use of vitamin/mineral supplements, "health foods," and the use of fad diets during childhood/adolescence.

"Undernutrition" and "hunger" are terms that are used interchangeably in the context of assessing the prevalence of malnutrition in the United States (Solomons & Allen, 1983). Hunger is increasingly prevalent where children live in poverty and in environments that do not provide sufficient nutrients. In these groups, children not only suffer from inadequate diets but may actually be at risk for obesity (Golden et al, 1983) because of dietary practices. A common definition of hunger is a chronic shortage of nutrients necessary for growth and good health. By that definition, 12 million children and 8 million adults, or about 9 per cent of the United States population, are hungry (Brown, 1987). Thus, whether people are rich or poor, nutritional problems of various types prevail.

Evaluation of nutritional status is a complex task. The Ten-State Nutrition Survey of 1968–1970, a landmark comprehensive study conducted by the US Department of Health, Education, and Welfare, was the first survey of nutritional status across the ages. This study focused on populations of low income and on racial and ethnic groups most likely to be undernourished. This study evolved out of a concern during the late 1960s that Americans were suffering from hunger and malnutrition. Findings of this survey, summarized by Garn and Clark (1975), include the following:

- Acute or severe malnutrition even in the lowest income groups was not demonstrated.
- Socioeconomic status affects size, growth, and development of children. (Children of the poor grow less well.) See Figure 16–1.
- The presently used "norms" are not appropriate for use with various races. Race-specific standards for size during growth are recommended.

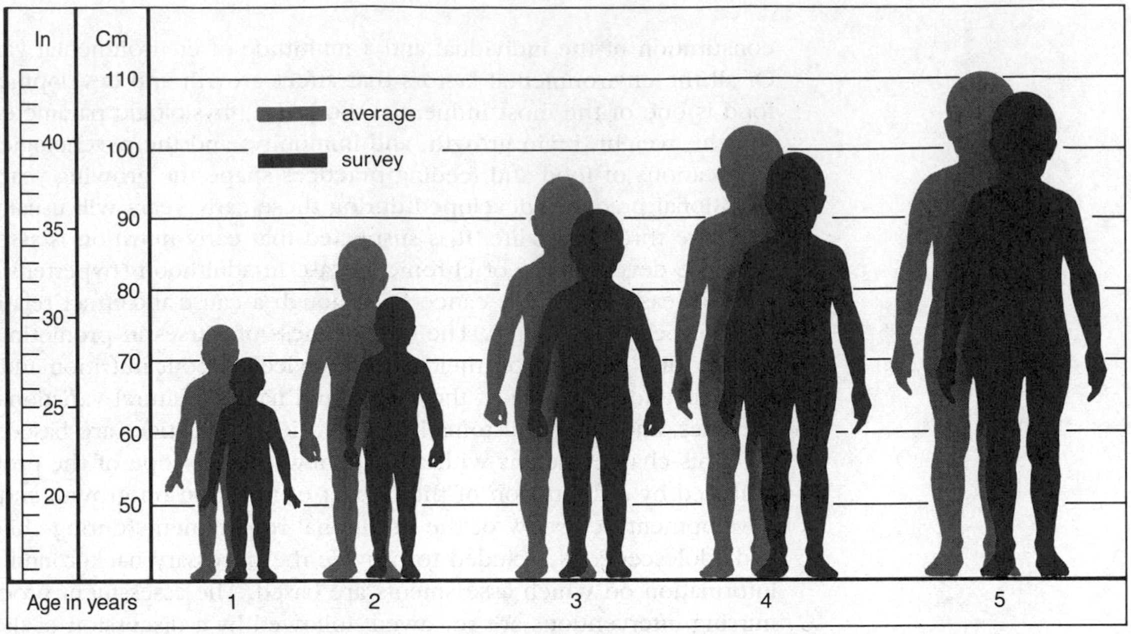

FIGURE 16 - 1. Relationship of height to age for boys 5 years of age and under, from low income households included in the National Nutrition Survey, 1968, compared with average heights for boys.

The trends identified in this survey are that existing nutritional problems are related to inadequate total energy intake (quantity) rather than improper selection of nutrient intake (quality). Anemia was a common finding across all ages and was not related to income. Obesity was found to be growth-promoting (auxogenic). Those children who were obese were further developed on ossification, had larger skeletal mass, were taller, and had higher hemoglobin levels. For both sexes, the poor were found to be leaner, but adolescent girls from lower income families were fatter and those from higher incomes were leaner (Garn & Clark, 1975). According to National Health and Nutrition Examination Surveys I and II, prevalence of obesity among adolescent girls of lower income levels still exists (Jones et al, 1985).

Another survey, the Preschool Nutrition Survey (1968–1970), included a cross-section of children representing white, African-American, Hispanic, and Native American children between the ages of 1 and 6 (Owen et al, 1974). As was found in the Ten-State survey, low economic status was correlated with smaller size. Anemia was reported at the rate of 12 per cent in African-American, 10 per cent in Hispanic, and 7 per cent in white children. In this survey, all children seemed to have adequate protein intake (it averaged 1 to $1^1/_2$ times the Recommended Dietary Allowances), but 10 to 15 per cent of the children had low intake of vitamin C, a finding that correlated with socioeconomic status. As socioeconomic status improved, intake of vitamin C improved.

The Health and Nutrition Examination Survey (HANES) of 1971–1974 was the first survey carried out under the national surveillance system established by the US Department of Health, Education, and Welfare. Under the direction of the National Center for Health Statistics, this survey analyzed adequacy of intake and use of nutrients. The following findings of the 1971–1974 HANES were based on a 24-hour dietary intake recall.

1. In some population groups, the mean intakes of protein, calcium, vitamin A, and ascorbic acid (vitamin C) were lower than the Recommended Dietary Allowances (RDAs).

2. The mean intakes of thiamin (vitamin B_1) and riboflavin (vitamin B_2) were adequate or more than adequate in all population groups.

3. For all population subgroups (except adult white men), the mean for iron intake was below the RDA (Mahan & Arlin, 1992).

The difficulties of establishing incidence and prevalence of nutritional problems are many. The impact of dietary intake on nutritional status in lower socioeconomic groups is difficult to distinguish from the impact of other factors that are associated with a low socioeconomic environment (e.g., poor housing and sanitation and a high prevalence of illness and infections). Also, surveys that use the 24-hour recall method of evaluation have potential error because of the uncertainty that it is representative of usual dietary intake. It would be expected that inadequate intake of nutrients would show deficient biochemical values, yet the biochemical data are not shown to correlate with the level of intake indicated by some food consumption surveys. Inconsistent findings of this nature may be related to individuals' inabilities to remember what they ate, difficulty in approximating portion sizes, and individuals simply telling the surveyor what they think the surveyor wants to hear (Mahan & Arlin, 1992).

Malnutrition as a consequence of famine and severe food shortages is a form of nutritional inadequacy that does not exist in the industrialized world; however, nutrition-related problems prevail. Following the reduction and modification of supplemental feeding programs in the 1980s, 20 national studies have documented the extent of hunger in the United States. Among these reporting groups are the US Conference of Mayors, the National Council of Churches, the US Department of Agriculture, and the Physician Task Force on Hunger in America (based at the Harvard School of Public Health) (Brown, 1987). Heart disease, hypertension, obesity, anemia, dental caries, and less than optimal nutritional intake are problems that nurses encounter. The challenge is to recognize, assess, and manage problems that arise from uniquely different circumstances across families and populations. For the pediatric nurse, nutrition is particularly important because of the impact that it has on the growing child. At all ages and across all populations, nutrition and dietary practices affect the child's physical, intellectual, emotional, and social development.

Impact of Nutrition on Growth and Development

A child's growth and development are affected by physiologic factors such as genetic makeup, hormonal regulation (growth hormone, thyroid hormone, and insulin), and the nutrients consumed. Environmental, socioeconomic, and behavioral factors, however, determine the availability of food and the emotional climate within which food is consumed. It is the interplay of all these factors that affects the child's growth and development. Food intake and the feeding experience influence the physiologic and psychologic development of humans from birth.

Psychologic Development

The experience of eating can be viewed from various theoretical perspectives, each of which provides a unique approach to studying human development. The psychodynamic view of Sigmund Freud shows early oral experiences to be fundamental to personality development in that it is through the mouth (oral stage) that feelings (pleasurable or hostile) are expressed. Gratification of oral needs through feeding thus is viewed as an integral component of personality development. Erickson's stages of developmental crises also begin with nutrition-related activities. A sense of trust versus mistrust is developed during infancy through consistent satisfaction of hunger and sucking needs. From a behaviorist's viewpoint, feeding is seen as a stimulus-response experience. The discomfort of hunger is felt and the relief of hunger through feeding is experienced as pleasurable. According to Piaget's organic-maturation approach to development, it is through feeding that sensations of taste, smell, motion, and touch are experienced. Feeding provides an arena for mastery and learning. Increasingly complex skills are mastered so that eventually the infant can hold his or her own bottle, drink from a cup, and eat from a spoon.

According to these various theories, food and eating, especially during infancy, play a primary role in the development of the child. The experiences that are associated with feeding are a powerful component to the healthy development of children. Through feeding, the process of attachment in infancy is fostered by a rhythmic give-and-take between the caregiver and the infant. Brazelton and colleagues (1974) noted that the rhythm was fostered when mothers were sensitive to their infants' capacity for attention, as well as their need to withdraw. Synchrony between infant and caregiver develops when the caregiver is sensitive and attentive to the infant's cues. A lack of synchrony and lack of attachment between the infant and the caregiver can result in numerous feeding problems and cause disturbances in parent-child relationships, such as the development of nonorganic failure-to-thrive (Klein, 1990).

As the child grows and strives for independence, mealtime continues to be an experience at which positive relationships can be fostered or during which struggle and conflict emerge as the predominant feelings. Beginning from infancy, children should learn to rely on their own cues for satiety rather than being forced to finish a bottle. Mealtime is an arena in which children develop confidence and a sense of well-being in their ability to function in an increasingly social role. When maladaptive responses to feeding occur, long-standing nutritional problems such as bulimia, anorexia nervosa, and obesity can result (see Chapter 29).

Physiologic Development

The influence of nutrition on the physiologic state of the human body is a complex science. Although it is widely recognized that *severe* nutritional deficits have serious consequences, the impact of marginal nutritional imbalances is less well understood. An important phase of development that is believed to be affected by nutrition is the intrauterine period of growth. Although many questions remain concerning the impact of nutrition on fetal development, the following have been reported.

- Poor nutrition of the mother during pregnancy (especially during the last trimester) is associated with low birthweight infants.
- Poor prepregnancy nutritional status of the mother is associated with low birthweight infants (the effect is compounded when the mother is

undernourished at the beginning of the pregnancy and has poor nutrition during pregnancy).

- When nutritional status is poor during pregnancy, provision of supplemental nutritious foods increases the infant's birthweight.
- Previously well-nourished women will have infants of reduced birthweight if their diets are severely limited during pregnancy (Stanfield, 1982; Creasy & Resnik, 1984).

A healthy diet during pregnancy and early childhood is particularly significant when it is recognized that the brain growth spurt begins in mid-pregnancy and continues well into the second postnatal year (Dobbing, 1984; Allen, 1990). Also, severe nutritional deficits during childhood result in reduced height and weight, a delay in puberty, and a delay in epiphyseal closure (Pipes, 1989).

The impact of nutrition during growth and later achievement remains controversial. Although many undernourished children may achieve poorly in later life, the dilemma remains whether nutrition plays a discrete role or whether the interplay of associated environmental factors determines achievement. According to Allen (1990), even though more research is needed to delineate a clear relationship between cognition and malnutrition, "iron deficiency anemia provides one of the clearest examples of a link between malnutrition and cognitive performance."

Because brain growth is linked to body growth and because there is no known method to promote brain growth, consumption of a balanced, healthful diet to promote *optimal* growth is the best solution. This raises yet another problem: infant obesity. Although infant obesity is a health concern, from the point of brain growth it has been suggested that a slight excess of intake is preferred to infant undernutrition (Dobbing, 1984).

A recent area of study is the effects of dietary intake on immune competence. It has long been recognized in the developing countries that malnutrition increases susceptibility to infection. It appears that malnutrition primarily affects cell-mediated immunity* rather than humoral immunity. As a consequence, children in underdeveloped countries with a profound nutritional deficiency readily become afflicted with viral disease (measles can be fatal in a malnourished child).

In the United States, it has been observed through experience that malnourished children may actually be more resistant to colds than their better nourished siblings (Krieger, 1982). Data from animal experiments showing that chronic malnutrition improves cell-mediated immunity offer some explanation, although this phenomenon has not been directly studied. Thus, the degree of malnutrition may play a role in its effect on immunity. For example, in animal experiments, protein restriction of 5 per cent has been reported to enhance cell-mediated immunity, whereas further restriction had an adverse effect (Krieger, 1982). Furthermore, obesity has been associated with higher frequency of infection owing to impairment of cell-mediated immunity and neutrophil function (Chandra, 1981). Continued research is required to further define the effects of dietary deficiency on the nature and degree of impairment in the development of immunity. Identification of the effects of specific nutrient deficiencies and information on how to reverse the immunologic deficit once it has occurred are required.

The relationship of nutrition to health and disease is of high priority to many consumers of health care, but it is of particular interest to parents who are concerned about the growth and development of their children. Nurses can promote children's health through nutritional assessment, education, and counseling in acute and ambulatory care, school nursing, and community nursing. Early attention given to the assessment of physical growth, as well as parent-infant relationships and psychosocial environment, provides the nurse with important data on which to base subsequent health promotion activities.

The components of promoting a healthful diet include knowledge concerning requirements, an awareness of the factors that affect dietary practices, and familiarity with measurement criteria used to assess nutritional status (Tables 16–1 and 16–2).

Nutritional Requirements

The two basic nutritional guidelines that have been established are the RDAs (Committee on Dietary Allowances, 1989) and the Food Guide Pyramid. The Food Guide Pyramid replaced the former basic four food groups. It suggests a range of daily servings from each of the major food groups: (1) bread, cereal, rice, and pasta, (2) vegetables, (3) fruit, (4) milk, yogurt, and cheese, and (5) meat, poultry, fish, dry beans, eggs, and nuts (see Table 16–2). In addition, the food guide should communicate three major concepts: (1) moderation—avoiding too much of certain food components linked to the development of chronic disease such as fat, saturated fat, cholesterol, sugars, sodium, and alcohol; (2) proportionality—eating different amounts of food from the major food groups; and (3) variety—eating a selection of foods from the major food groups (US Department of Agriculture, 1992).

During periods of rapid growth, such as in infancy and again during the adolescent years, assessment of the level of nutrition with respect to adequacy is particularly important. During these periods of growth, there is an increased risk of nutritional de-

*T-lymphocytes (thymus-derived) function in cell-mediated immunity by becoming sensitized to the invading antigen and releasing enzymes to destroy it. B-lymphocytes (bone marrow-derived) function in humoral immunity by transforming into plasma cells, which subsequently produce antibodies.

TABLE 16-1
Food and Nutrition Board, National Academy of Sciences—National Research Council Recommended Dietary Allowances,*† Revised 1989

Category	Age (Yrs) or Condition	Weight‡ (kg)	Weight‡ (lb)	Height‡ (cm)	Height‡ (in)	Protein (g)	Fat-Soluble Vitamins: Vitamin A (μg RE)§	Vitamin D (μg)‖	Vitamin E (mg α-TE)¶	Vitamin K (μg)
Infants	0.0–0.5	6	13	60	24	13	375	7.5	3	5
	0.5–1.0	9	20	71	28	14	375	10	4	10
Children	1–3	13	29	90	35	16	400	10	6	15
	4–6	20	44	112	44	24	500	10	7	20
	7–10	28	62	132	52	28	700	10	7	30
Adolescent males	11–14	45	99	157	62	45	1000	10	10	45
	15–18	66	145	176	69	59	1000	10	10	65
Adolescent females	11–14	46	101	157	62	46	800	10	8	45
	15–18	55	120	163	64	44	800	10	8	55
Pregnant						60	800	10	10	65
Lactating	1st 6 mos					65	1300	10	12	65
	2nd 6 mos					62	1200	10	11	65

Category	Age (Yrs) or Condition	Water-Soluble Vitamins: Vitamin C (mg)	Thiamin (mg)	Riboflavin (mg)	Niacin (mg NE)#	Vitamin B_6 (mg)	Folate (μg)	Vitamin B_{12} (μg)	Minerals: Calcium (mg)	Phosphorus (mg)	Magnesium (mg)	Iron (mg)	Zinc (mg)	Iodine (μg)	Selenium (μg)	Energy Needs (Kcal)
Infants	0.0–0.5	30	0.3	0.4	5	0.3	25	0.3	400	300	40	6	5	40	10	kg × 108
	0.5–1.0	35	0.4	0.5	6	0.6	35	0.5	600	500	60	10	5	50	15	kg × 98
Children	1–3	40	0.7	0.8	9	1.0	50	0.7	800	800	80	10	10	70	20	1300
	4–6	45	0.9	1.1	12	1.1	75	1.0	800	800	120	10	10	90	20	1800
	7–10	45	1.0	1.2	13	1.4	100	1.4	800	800	170	10	10	120	30	2000
Adolescent males	11–14	50	1.3	1.5	17	1.7	150	2.0	1200	1200	270	12	15	150	40	2500
	15–18	60	1.5	1.8	20	2.0	200	2.0	1200	1200	400	12	15	150	50	3000
Adolescent females	11–14	50	1.1	1.3	15	1.4	150	2.0	1200	1200	280	15	12	150	45	2200
	15–18	60	1.1	1.3	15	1.5	180	2.0	1200	1200	300	15	12	150	50	2200
Pregnant		70	1.5	1.6	17	2.2	400	2.2	1200	1200	300	30	15	175	65	+300
Lactating	1st 6 mos	95	1.6	1.8	20	2.1	280	2.6	1200	1200	355	15	19	200	75	+500
	2nd 6 mos	90	1.6	1.7	20	2.1	260	2.6	1200	1200	340	15	16	200	75	+500

* Designed for the maintenance of good nutrition of practically all healthy people in the United States.

† The allowances, expressed as average daily intakes over time, are intended to provide for individual variations among most normal persons as they live in the United States under usual environmental stresses. Diets should be based on a variety of common foods to provide other nutrients for which human requirements have been less well defined. See text for detailed discussion of allowances and of nutrients not tabulated.

‡ Weights and heights of Reference Adults are actual medians for the United States populations of the designated age, as reported by NHANES II. The median weights and heights of those under 19 yrs of age were taken from Hamill, P. V. V., et al. (1979). Physical growth: National Center for Health Statistics percentiles. *American Journal of Clinical Nutrition, 32,* 607–629. The use of these figures does not imply that the height-to-weight ratios are ideal.

§ Retinol equivalents. 1 retinol equivalent = 1 μg retinol or 6 μg β-carotene.

‖ As cholecalciferol. 10 μg cholecalciferol = 400 IU of vitamin D.

¶ α-Tocopherol equivalents. 1 mg d-α tocopherol = 1 α-TE.

\# 1 NE (niacin equivalent) is equal to 1 mg of niacin or 60 mg of dietary tryptophan.

ficiency of all nutrients, especially vitamins and minerals. There is a wide variation in nutrient requirements according to age, sex, activity level, disease, growth rate, and genetic and environmental variables. Although optimal dietary intake is desirable, the range of food intake that provides *adequate* nutrition is not as narrow as many may think it might be (MacLean & Graham, 1982). Use of the RDAs is universally accepted as the standard of nutritional intake for healthy individuals (Table 16–1). It is intended that these standards are met by a *variety* of foods. It should be recognized that these standards represent a high estimate of nutrients (except for energy) to ensure that individual variations are met, reducing the risk for deficiency diseases (Table 16–3). Consequently, an individual whose diet does not fully meet

TABLE 16-2
Food Guide Pyramid

Food Guide Pyramid
A Guide to Daily Food Choices

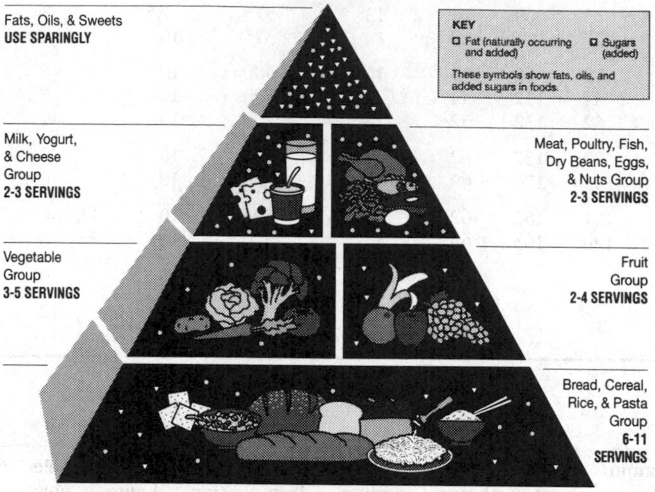

How many servings do you need each day?

	Women & some older adults	Children, teen girls, active women, most men	Teen boys & active men
Calorie level*	about 1,600	about 2,200	about 2,800
Bread group	6	9	11
Vegetable group	3	4	5
Fruit group	2	3	4
Milk group	**2-3	**2-3	**2-3
Meat group	2, for a total of 5 ounces	2, for a total of 6 ounces	3 for a total of 7 ounces

*These are the calorie levels if you choose lowfat, lean foods from the 5 major food groups and use foods from the fats, oils, and sweets group sparingly.

**Women who are pregnant or breastfeeding, teen-agers, and young adults to age 24 need 3 servings.

How to Use The Daily Food Guide

What counts as one serving?

Breads, Cereals, Rice, and Pasta
1 slice of bread
1/2 cup of cooked rice or pasta
1/2 cup of cooked cereal
1 ounce of ready-to-eat cereal

Vegetables
1/2 cup of chopped raw or cooked vegetables
1 cup of leafy raw vegetables

Fruits
1 piece of fruit or melon wedge
3/4 cup of juice
1/2 cup of canned fruit
1/4 cup of dried fruit

Milk, Yogurt, and Cheese
1 cup of milk or yogurt
1-1/2 to 2 ounces of cheese

Meat, Poultry, Fish, Dry Beans, Eggs, and Nuts
2-1/2 to 3 ounces of cooked lean meat, poultry, or fish
Count 1/2 cup of cooked beans, or 1 egg, or 2 tablespoons of peanut butter as 1 ounce of lean meat (about 1/3 serving)

Fats, Oils, and Sweets
LIMIT CALORIES FROM THESE especially if you need to lose weight

The amount you eat may be more than one serving. For example, a dinner portion of spaghetti would count as two or three servings of pasta.

A Closer Look at Fat and Added Sugars

The small tip of the Pyramid shows fats, oils, and sweets. These are foods such as salad dressings, cream, butter, margarine, sugars, soft drinks, candies, and sweet desserts. Alcoholic beverages are also part of this group. These foods provide calories but few vitamins and minerals. Most people should go easy on foods from this group.

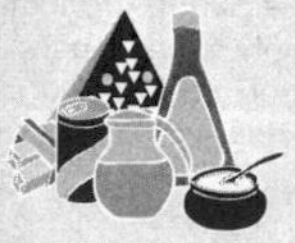

Some fat or sugar symbols are shown in the other food groups. That's to remind you that some foods in these groups can also be high in fat and added sugars, such as cheese or ice cream from the milk group, or french fries from the vegetable group. When choosing foods for a healthful diet, consider the fat and added sugars in your choices from all the food groups, not just fats, oils, and sweets from the Pyramid tip.

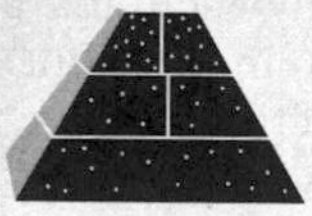

From US Department of Agriculture. (1992, August). *Food guide pyramid.* Human Nutrition Information Service. (Leaflet No. 572). Pueblo, CO, 81009: Consumer Information Center, Department 159-Y.

TABLE 16-3
Recommended Dietary Allowances

Recommended Dietary Allowances (RDAs) are the levels of intake of essential nutrients considered, in the judgment of the Committee on Dietary Allowances of the Food and Nutrition Board on the basis of available scientific knowledge, to be adequate to meet the known nutritional needs of practically all healthy persons

the RDA is not necessarily undernourished. The RDAs are guidelines for healthy populations and do not account for special nutrient needs related to premature birth, infectious disease, or chronic illness.

Children should consume a healthy diet that supports and maintains cells, provides for growth, and promotes an optimal level of nutritional status. Following is a discussion of the components of a healthy diet, including energy (calories), water, and nutrients (protein, fat, carbohydrates, vitamins, and minerals).

Energy

The energy content of food is expressed in kilocalories (the large calorie) or in kilojoules (Tables 16–4 and 16–5). Energy is required to support basal metabolism, physical activity, growth, and the thermic effect* of food (Whitney et al, 1991). Body size and composition, rate of growth, and degree of activity all affect the amount of energy expended. The energy requirements due to physical activity are as variable in infants as in other age groups since some infants are much more active than others. A negligible fuel for energy is lost in stools. Thus, precise requirements are difficult to predict for a specific child. However, the recommended energy amounts meet the needs of the average child and can be used as a basis for adjustments for a specific child.

*The thermic effect of food, also known as diet-induced thermogenesis, refers to the energy required to metabolize food (normally 10 per cent of the energy output). The thermic effect of food is sometimes called specific dynamic effect (SDE) or specific dynamic activity (SDA).

TABLE 16-4
Calorie and Kilocalorie

The calorie, or small calorie, is a standard unit for measuring heat; it is the amount of heat energy required to raise the temperature of 1 g of water by 1° Celsius (C or centigrade)

The kilocalorie (or large Calorie) is equal to 1000 small calories, or the amount of heat energy required to raise the temperature of 1 kilogram of water by 1° Celsius (C or centigrade)

1 Cal = 1 kcal = 1000 cal

TABLE 16-5
Kilocalorie and Kilojoule

The International Organization for Standardization (ISO) recommended the adoption of the joule (j) as the prefered unit of energy measurements, which was adopted by the US National Bureau of Standards in 1964.

1. The kilocalorie is a measure of thermal energy and cannot be as precise as the joule, which is a measure of mechanical energy
2. The conversion factor to convert kilocalories to kilojoules is 4.184, or approximately 4.2 (1 kilocalorie = 4.2 kilojoules)
3. The energy provided by the nutrients are:
   4 kcal or 17 kj/g of carbohydrates
   4 kcal or 17 kj/g of protein
   9 kcal or 38 kj/g of fat
4. Currently tables use both kcal and kj, but, in popular usage, kcal is most often heard

The variation in expenditure of calories at various ages is shown in Figure 16–2. Compared with adults, infants have a higher basal metabolic rate (55 kcal/kg/24 hrs) owing to a proportionately larger surface area and a larger proportion of lean body mass. Thus, energy requirements are greatest per unit of size during the first year of life (98 to 108 kcal/kg/24 hrs) and decrease about 10 kcal/kg/24 hrs for each succeeding 3-year period to adolescence. Consequently, as children grow, they require a greater number of absolute calories but the requirement per unit of size decreases (see Table 16–1). During periods of rapid growth and development, such as puberty, increased caloric intake is required.

The distribution of calories in an infant's diet of predominantly breast milk or formula provides 7 to 18 per cent of the calories from protein, 30 to 55 per cent from fat, and 35 to 50 per cent from carbohydrates (Whitney et al, 1991). This distribution differs from that recommended for older children and adults because of the higher percentage of fat and lower percentage of carbohydrates.

Water

Water is the most essential element in the diet. Water is part of every cell and is an important solvent. It is necessary for digestion, nutrient transport to the cells, and the removal of body wastes. The percentage of body weight provided by water is greater in the newborn infant than after 1 year of age. Body weight attributed to water ranges from 75 to 80 per cent at birth to 65 per cent at 1 year and remains at 55 to 60 per cent throughout childhood and the adult years. Daily consumption of fluid by an infant approximates 15 per cent of body weight, whereas it constitutes only 5 per cent in an older child and 2 to 4 per cent in an adult.

The infant has a relatively greater need for water

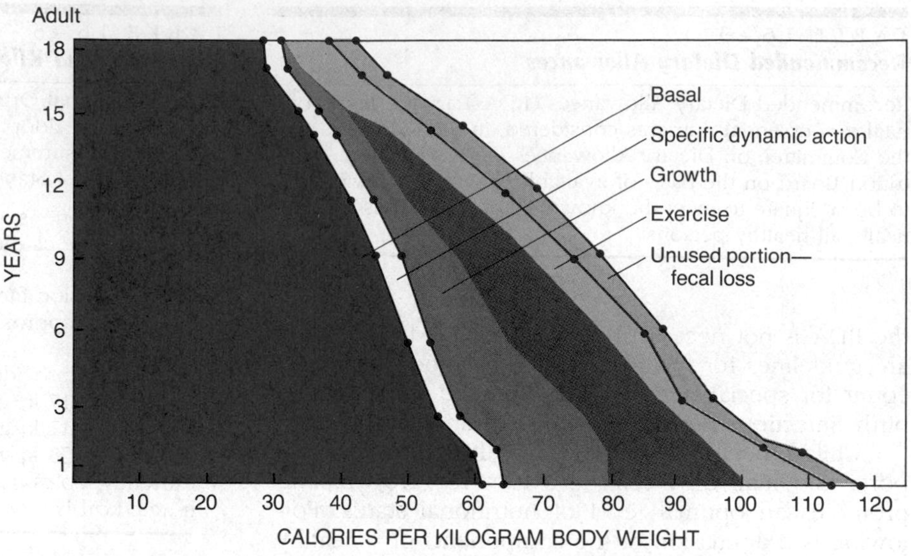

FIGURE 16-2. Total daily expenditure of calories with approximate distribution among individual factors in relation to age and weight. (Calorie = large calorie = 1 kcal = 1 cal.) (From Behrman, R. E. [1992]. *Nelson textbook of pediatrics* (14th ed.). Philadelphia: WB Saunders.)

than do children and adults (Table 16–6) and is therefore more vulnerable to water imbalance. Water lost by evaporation in infancy is 60 per cent of that needed to maintain homeostasis, compared with 40 to 50 per cent in adulthood (Pipes, 1989). The young infant also has functionally immature kidneys and produces a more dilute urine. The faster rate of the infant's metabolism is another factor that increases the need for relatively more fluid than is needed by the adult. Also, young infants are unable to let adults know when they are thirsty. The usual diets of most infants meet this basic water requirement.

The sources of water are fluids (mostly milk for infants) and food. Most strained foods are 75 to 85 per cent water. Difficulties may occur in meeting the water requirements if formulas are improperly prepared; if infants ingest a limited amount of milk (especially with illness); if fever exists, during hot weather; or if diarrhea and vomiting are present. Dehydration results much more rapidly from these difficulties in the infant because of the factors previously outlined. In contrast, water intoxication can result in hyponatremia, restlessness, nausea, vomiting, diarrhea, and polyuria or oliguria, as well as convulsions. Water toxicity can occur if water is given in place of formula feedings or if formulas are excessively diluted owing to inadequate supply or lack of knowledge regarding formula preparation (Excess water administration and hyponatraemic convulsions in infancy, 1992; Mahan & Arlin, 1992). See Chapter 26 for additional discussion on fluid balance in infants and children.

TABLE 16-6
Range of Average Water Requirements of Children under Ordinary Conditions

Age	Average Body Weight (kg)	Total Water in 24 Hrs (ml)	Water per kg Body Wt in 24 Hrs (ml)
3 days	3.0	250–300	80–100
10 days	3.2	400–500	125–150
3 mos	5.4	750–850	140–160
6 mos	7.3	950–1100	130–155
9 mos	8.6	1100–1250	125–145
1 yr	9.5	1150–1300	120–135
2 yrs	11.8	1350–1500	115–125
4 yrs	16.2	1600–1800	100–110
6 yrs	20.0	1800–2000	90–100
10 yrs	28.7	2000–2500	70–85
14 yrs	45.0	2200–2700	50–60
18 yrs	54.0	2200–2700	40–50

From Behrman, R. E., & Vaughan, V. C. (1987). *Nelson textbook of pediatrics* (13th ed.). Philadelphia: WB Saunders.

Protein

Proteins are necessary as a source of amino acids. Large protein molecules are broken down into individual amino acids, which are required for growth and tissue repair and for the production of enzymes, antibodies, and hormones. Amino acids are classified as essential and nonessential (Table 16–7). The absence of any one of these essential amino acids leads to negative nitrogen balance, weight loss, impaired growth in infants and children, and other clinical symptoms (Mahan & Arlin, 1992). Excess amino acids are broken down (catabolized) in the liver, where the nitrogen component is converted to urea and sent to the kidneys for excretion in the urine. The remainder or non-nitrogenous component will act either as a carbohydrate and provide energy or as a fat and be stored as energy reserve (Nieman et al, 1992; Pellet, 1990). During the first month of life, excess protein may not be broken down and eliminated effectively. Therefore, excessive intake may result in neurologic damage (Hughes & Griffith, 1984).

TABLE 16-7
Essential Amino Acids

Essential amino acids must be provided in the diet because the body cannot synthesize them. Absence or deficiency of one such amino acid results in negative nitrogen balance. *Nonessential amino acids* can be synthesized by the body; therefore, they are not essential in the diet

Essential Amino Acids

Threonine	Tryptophan
Valine	Phenylalanine
Leucine	Methionine
Isoleucine	Histidine
Lysine	

In addition, low birthweight infants need:
Arginine
Cystine
Taurine

From Behrman, R. E., & Vaughan, V. C. (1987). *Nelson textbook of pediatrics* (13th ed.). Philadelphia: WB Saunders.

Recommended daily intakes of protein are shown in Table 16-1. During growth, a proportionately higher amount of protein per unit of body weight is required. During the first 2 months of life, 50 per cent of the RDA of protein is required for growth; by 2 to 3 years, only 11 per cent is required; and, after the adolescent growth spurt, 0 per cent is needed for growth.

Proteins do not all have the same nutritive value. "Protein quality" is a term used to describe the ability of protein to meet the body's requirements for *essential* amino acids. Requirements for essential amino acids are higher in the infant and small child than in the older child or adult (MacLean & Graham, 1982). Low birthweight infants require additional essential amino acids because enzymes are missing to synthesize them (Table 16-7). The predominant protein in cow's milk is casein, which is low in cystine and taurine. In contrast, proteins in human milk and the whey of cow's milk provide these amino acids. Consequently, now many infant formulas have been adjusted to be closer in composition to breast milk—i.e., a whey/casein ratio of 60:40 (in breast milk the whey/casein ratio is 80:20 and 18:82 in cow's milk) (DeBruyne & Rolfes, 1989). Animal proteins in general provide all the essential amino acids in sufficient amounts after the first year of life. In contrast, vegetable proteins are somewhat deficient in at least one of the essential amino acids, and they are substantially less digestible. Protein adequacy of vegetarian diets for the growing child is, therefore, important to consider (see later discussion in this chapter on vegetarianism).

Most children in developed countries consume sufficient protein; however, protein deficiency does exist in cases in which milk has been withheld indiscriminantly, or in the case of poorly planned vegetarian diets. It is important to understand that sufficient calories in the form of fats and carbohydrates must also be provided in the diet; otherwise, protein will be deaminated and used for energy. Excessive protein intake may lead to the acceleration of the processes leading to renal glomerular sclerosis (a common phenomenon of aging) and potentially influence the development of osteoporosis (Committee on Dietary Allowances, 1989). Protein intakes greater than 20 per cent of total calories increase water requirements because of the renal solute load and may result in dehydration in infants (Hughes & Griffith, 1984). The Committee on Nutrition of the American Academy of Pediatrics (AAP) has set the minimal standard for infant formula at 1.8 g of protein per 100 kcal (AAP, 1976).

Carbohydrates

Carbohydrates provide the greatest source of energy but are not considered a dietary essential because they can be synthesized from amino acids. There are no specific recommendations for intake, but a minimal intake of 50 to 100 g/day has been suggested, or approximately 40 to 50 per cent of total calorie intake (Pipes, 1989). However, the recommended daily intake of carbohydrate depends on the age of the child.

Carbohydrates are broken down by a series of enzymic and chemical reactions into simple sugars and are stored as glycogen in the liver and muscles. Carbohydrate that is not oxidized or stored as glycogen is converted to fat. The infant's liver is 10 per cent the size of the adult's and the muscle only 2 per cent; consequently, the infant has a smaller glycogen reserve than older children and adults and requires large carbohydrate intake for immediate energy. Ingestion of less than 5 per cent of the daily caloric needs may result in breakdown of protein necessary for growth and repair of tissue (Hughes & Griffith, 1984).

During infancy, the primary source of carbohydrate is lactose (a disaccharide), found in human and cow's milk. Intestinal amylase is present in reduced amounts during the first 4 months of life, therefore the introduction of large quantities of starch (polysaccharides) may result in diarrhea. At 4 to 6 months, the time when solid foods are typically added, amylase is present and starches become the major source of carbohydrates. High intake of refined sugars should be discouraged because they are cariogenic, dull the appetite for other nutritious foods, and thus may replace the intake of more nutritious foods in the diet.

Fats

In the infant diet, calories from fats provide 40 to 50 per cent of the energy requirements, whereas in older children, approximately 35 per cent of the energy requirements is provided by fat. Fats have a high caloric density; thus, they are protein-sparing. Fat consumption is essential during growth when tissue synthesis is primary. Fats are a source of essential fatty acids in cellular structure, serve as carriers for fat-soluble vitamins (A, D, E, and K), and make food more palatable.

Polyunsaturated linoleic acid is an essential fatty acid for children and adults. Linoleic and arachidonic* acids may also be essential fatty acids. The AAP suggests that 3 per cent of total energy in the diet should be derived from *essential* fatty acids (AAP, 1985). Essential fatty acids play a key role in growth and development, platelet function, normal skin and hair, reproduction, and synthesis of prostaglandins. The fatty acids that are essential for the human body are abundant in human milk and in commercially prepared formulas. Approximately 4 per cent of calories are derived from linoleic acid in human milk, compared with 1 per cent in cow's milk. Commercially prepared formulas, however, contain vegetable oils and provide appreciably greater amounts of linoleic acid than even human milk.

The effectiveness of substituting polyunsaturated fats for saturated fats in the diet in an effort to reduce atheromatous changes has not been established (see later discussion).

Vitamins

Vitamins are nutrients that the body requires in small amounts to catalyze cellular metabolism essential for maintenance and growth. Most vitamins cannot be synthesized by the body; therefore, they must be supplied by dietary intake. Vitamins are classified into two groups: (1) fat-soluble (A, D, E, and K) and (2) water-soluble (the B vitamins and ascorbic acid [vitamin C]). Any fat malabsorption illness may also result in malabsorption of vitamins A, D, E, or K because these four are absorbed and transported in a manner similar to that of lipids (Committee on Dietary Allowances, 1989). The specific vitamins, including their function, source, and effects of excess or deficiency, are summarized in Table 16–8.

The best way to make vitamins available to the body is through the consumption of a balanced diet. Vitamin supplementation during infancy and childhood has given rise to considerable controversy. The major issues concerning vitamin supplementation are summarized in Table 16–8. Fat-soluble vitamins can be stored and cause toxicity. For example, hypervitaminoses A and D have been well documented. Toxicity of water-soluble vitamins is also possible, although it is less likely to occur (Alhadeff et al, 1984). Vitamins that are most often lacking are vitamins A and C. Persons who are most at risk for vitamin deficiencies include the following:

- Children from deprived families.
- Children who have poor eating habits or are dieting.
- Pregnant teen-agers.
- Children who consume a vegan diet (Pipes, 1989).

*Arachidonic acid can be synthesized from linoleic acid.

Minerals

The Food and Nutrition Board of the National Research Council has established recommended allowances for seven minerals (calcium, phosphorus, magnesium, iron, zinc, iodine, and selenium). Additional minerals that are relatively abundant include sodium, chloride, potassium, and sulfur. The minerals in which diets are most likely to be lacking are calcium, iron, iodine, and possibly zinc in early infancy (Mahan & Arlin, 1992). Important minerals and their functions, sources, and effects of excess or deficiency are summarized in Table 16–9. Zinc deficiency may result from diets that are high in phytate and fiber. Any illness that causes intestinal malabsorption may result in zinc deficiency. Zinc plays an important role in cell growth; therefore, its deficiency is manifested in growth failure and delayed sexual maturation (Diplock, 1987). The major issues concerning mineral supplementation are summarized in Table 16–9.

Assessment and Counseling

There are four major purposes for doing a nutritional assessment: (1) to identify dietary practices of the family; (2) to obtain baseline data concerning calorie and nutrient intake and appropriate anthropometric measurements; (3) to promote healthful dietary practices through counseling and teaching; and (4) to provide parents with the opportunity to express concerns and to ask questions about nutrition and feeding behaviors.

Assessment of Dietary Practices

Variations in food consumption occur because of individual physical differences (stage of growth, exercise, genetic, and hormonal) and because of environmental and sociocultural variations. Cultural differences, family relationships and lifestyle, peers and social influences (including television), and economic status are some of the nonphysiologic variants that predominantly affect the development of food habits (Fig. 16–3).

Cultural variations, which dictate the kinds of foods that are preferred, must be respected by the nurse. It is usually desirable to maintain the basic food pattern and employ the use of *supplementation* rather than changing the staple foods. Milk and milk product use is limited in many cultures; therefore, substitutes may be necessary. The types of vegetables used may be unfamiliar to the nurse, and the use of certain staples varies from one culture to another. Beans, rice, ground corn, and soybean products are staples in many ethnic diets and are preferred over

TABLE 16–8
Vitamins: Functions, Sources, and Supplementation

Significance in Development and Function	Deficiency Symptoms	Toxicity Symptoms	Important Sources	Supplementation
Fat-Soluble Vitamins				
		Vitamin A		
Formation of retinal pigments (rhodopsin and iodopsin) for cone (color) vision and vision in dim light Bone and tooth development Formation and maturation of epithelial tissue (skin, mucous membranes, lining of digestive tract) therefore increase resistance to infection Bile is necessary for vitamin A absorption and mineral oil interferes with its absorption	Night and glare blindness Inflammation of the eye Rough, scaly skin Dry mucous membranes, causing a general lowered resistance to microbe invasion Poor tooth formation	Anorexia Fatigue Weight loss Irritability Skin lesions—dry, scaly, itching Joint and bone pains Spleen and liver enlargement Loss of hair Increased intracranial pressure and headache	Liver and liver sausage Butter, cream, whole milk Egg yolks Green and yellow vegetables Yellow fruits Ripe tomatoes Fortified margarine Fish liver oils	Prophylactic: 2000–5000 IU daily Hypervitaminosis A can occur when doses in excess of 10 times the prophylactic dose are given Supplementation should be considered if there are not sufficient fruits and vegetables in the diet
		Vitamin D		
Regulates absorption and deposition of calcium and phosphorus (likely by affecting permeability of intestinal membrane) Reabsorption of phosphate and maintenance of serum calcium level (in conjunction with parathyroid hormone)	Soft bones Bowed legs Poor tooth development Lowered amount of calcium and phosphorus in the blood Poor posture, protruding abdomen	Anorexia Fatigue Weight loss Nausea and vomiting Diarrhea and polyuria Weakness Headache Renal damage Calcification in the soft tissues of the heart, blood vessels, lungs, stomach, renal tubules	Vitamin D milk Small amounts in butter, egg yolk, liver, saltwater fish Fish liver oils	Prophylactic: 400–800 IU Vitamin D supplementation is not usually necessary except in the following circumstances: • A breastfed infant if mother's intake of vitamin D is inadequate and if infant does not benefit from sunlight (e.g., dark skin or little exposure) • If commercial cow's milk formula is *not* used for bottlefed infant (e.g., goat's milk, evaporated milk, if not fortified with vitamin D)
		Vitamin E		
Mechanism of action unknown Vitamin E may protect erythrocytes from hemolysis Vitamin E may protect vitamin A and polyunsaturated fats from oxidation			Vegetable oils Green leafy vegetables Margarine Egg yolk Milk fat Nuts Wheat germ oil	Premature infants requiring high concentrations of oxygen at high pressures are prone to develop retrolental fibroplasia Vitamin E is currently being used in clinical trials to reduce severity of retrolental fibroplasia in prematurity Dosage varies with amount of unsaturated fats in formula

(continued)

TABLE 16–8
Vitamins: Functions, Sources, and Supplementation *(Continued)*

Significance in Development and Function	Deficiency Symptoms	Toxicity Symptoms	Important Sources	Supplementation
		Vitamin K		
Important in the formation of factor II (prothrombin) and other clotting factors (VII, IX, X)	Prolonged clotting time of the blood Hemorrhagic disease in newborn	Hyperbilirubinemia In infants: Jaundice Kernicterus Mild hemolytic anemia	Green leafy vegetables Liver Cauliflower Cabbage Soybean oil	A single intramuscular dose of 0.5–1 mg or an oral dose of 1.0–2.0 mg is given to all newborns
Water-Soluble Vitamins				
		Vitamin C		
Maintains intracellular substance preserving capillary walls; promotes healing of wounds and fractures and reduces potential for infection Aids in absorption of iron Essential for collagen formation (basic substance in connective tissue)	Sore mouth Stiff, aching joints Weak-walled capillaries (hemorrhages in joints, muscles, subcutaneous tissue, gums) Lassitude Impaired wound healing Improper bone and cartilage development	Nephrolithiasis (kidney stones) Hemolysis of red blood cells Gastrointestinal disturbances (diarrhea) Rebound scurvy (scurvy in an infant born of a mother consuming high doses of vitamin C)	Fresh fruits, especially citrus, strawberries, cantaloupe Canned fruit juices Tomatoes, fresh or canned Raw vegetables, especially greens, cabbage, broccoli, peppers Potatoes	Prophylactic: 35 mg for children up to 11 years of age 60 mg/day for children after 11 years of age (½ cup of orange juice provides 60 mg of vitamin C) May be necessary in home-prepared formula
		Vitamin B_1 (Thiamin)		
Functions as part of co-carboxylase (co-enzyme) during oxidation of carbohydrates Important for growth, normal appetite, digestion, and nervous system function	Anorexia Fatigue Constipation, atonic Depression Irritability Tenderness of the leg calf with some loss of muscular coordination Abnormal carbohydrate metabolism	Headache Irritability Insomnia Rapid pulse Weakness	Meat, especially pork Whole grain and enriched cereals Organs, especially liver Nuts and peanut butter Legumes, especially soybeans Milk, dairy foods Eggs Brewer's yeast and wheat germ	No supplementation necessary in usual diet
		Vitamin B_2 (Riboflavin)		
Essential for growth Functions in tissue oxidation-reduction processes to produce energy Essential for healthy eyes and skin	Burning and itching eyes Blurred and dim vision Eyes sensitive to light Inflammation of the lips and the tongue Lesions in the angles of the mouth Digestive disturbances Greasy, scaly skin	Yellow discoloration of urine Inhibits uptake of methotrexate by neoplastic cells	Milk, dairy foods Organs, especially liver Meat, legumes Eggs Enriched and whole grain cereals and breads Green leafy vegetables Brewer's yeast, liver concentrates	Supplementation not common If milk is avoided, such as in some vegetarian diets, a food equivalent can be used

TABLE 16-8
Vitamins: Functions, Sources, and Supplementation *(Continued)*

Significance in Development and Function	Deficiency Symptoms	Toxicity Symptoms	Important Sources	Supplementation
		Niacin		
Acts in metabolism of carbohydrates and amino acids Involved in glycolysis, fat synthesis, and tissue respiration Prevents nervous depression Promotes healthy skin, nerves, and digestion	Fatigue and lassitude Dermatitis Sore mouth, especially the tongue Gastrointestinal disturbances (diarrhea and vomiting) Nervous disturbances Mental depression Weakness Anorexia	Niacin flush (flushing of the face) Hepatotoxicity Gastrointestinal disturbances (stomach pain, nausea, diarrhea, aggravation of peptic ulcer disease) Cholestatic jaundice Increased serum uric acid levels (gouty arthritis) Cardiac arrhythmias Dermatologic pruritus, rash, and hyperkeratosis Hyperglycemia	Meat, especially liver Fish Poultry Whole grain and enriched cereals Nuts Legumes, peanuts Brewer's yeast, liver concentrates	Supplementation not common

Data from Howe, P. S. (1981). *Basic nutrition in health and disease (including selection and care of food).* Philadelphia: WB Saunders.

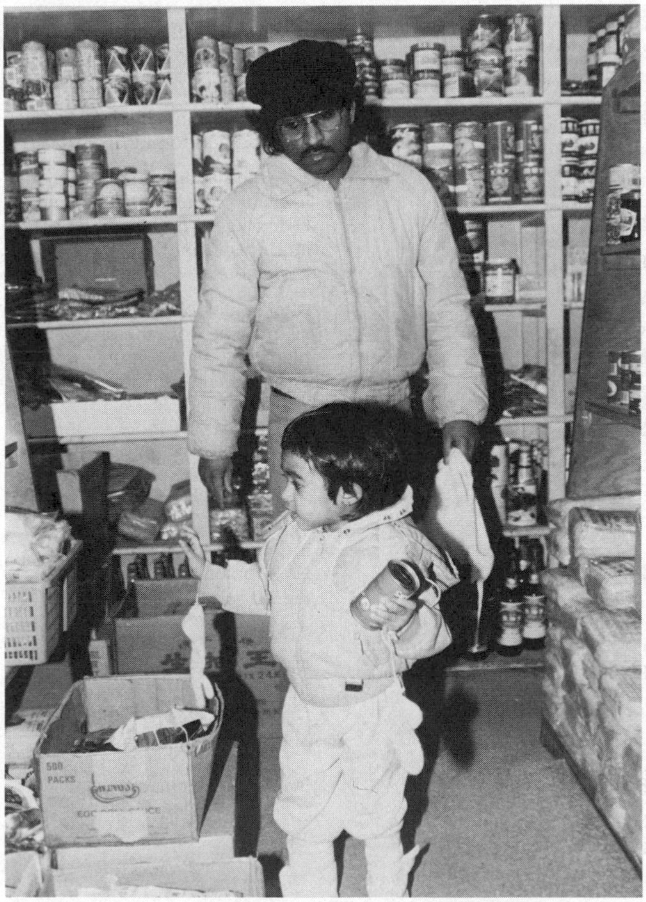

FIGURE 16-3. The availability of specialty foods increases the likelihood that children will be introduced to the preferences of a particular ethnic group.

the bread products typical of the North American diet. Making generalizations about a child's or a family's food preferences related to culture can be misleading. Burtis and colleagues identify cultural groups that may have characteristic food preferences, but warn that "individuals from any culture have different tastes and preferences; therefore, it is important not to stereotype cultural groups" (Burtis et al, 1987, p 332). Within the United States, regional preferences and specialties are strong in some families and not in others. School-age children who immigrate with their families may become acculturated quickly and may prefer fast-food style eating to traditional family foods. In hospital, school, or camp settings, children may dislike an unfamiliar method of preparation more than the actual food selections. Table 16–10 lists various cultural groups and some food traditions. How closely a family follows a cultural food tradition depends on several factors, including:

1. Whether it is an immigrant family or a first-, second-, or third-generation family.
2. How prevalent the particular group is in the community and how available specialty foods are.
3. The economic status of the family.

It is important, however, for the nurse to understand the nutritional adequacy of various diets and recommend only those changes that are necessary to maintain a healthy diet and to avoid making suggestions that are inconsistent with an individual's particular situation. For example, absence of the enzyme lactose in some persons makes milk digestion a problem. Thus, recommending an increased milk intake would be inappropriate. Suggesting the use of raw

TABLE 16-9
Minerals: Functions, Sources and Supplementation

Function	Deficiency Symptoms	Sources	Supplementation
Calcium			
Development of strong bones and teeth Helps muscles contract and relax normally Use of iron Normal blood clotting Maintenance of body neutrality Normal action of heart muscle	Rickets Porous bones Bowed legs Stunted growth Slow blood clotting Poor tooth formation Tetany	Milk, cheese Mustard, turnip greens Clams, oysters Broccoli, cauliflower, cabbage Molasses Small amount in egg, carrot, celery, orange, grapefruit, figs, and bread made with milk	No supplementation except for premature infants Dosage varies with type of milk feeding and growth rate
Phosphorus			
Development of bones and teeth Multiplication of cells Activation of some enzymes and vitamins Maintenance of body neutrality Participates in carbohydrate metabolism	Rickets Porous bone Bowed legs Stunted growth Poor tooth formation	Milk Cheese Meat Egg yolk Fish Nuts Whole grain cereals Legumes	No supplementation except for premature infants Dosage varies with type of milk feeding and growth rate
Iron			
Constituent of hemoglobin, which carries oxygen to the tissues	Nutritional anemia Pallor Weight loss Fatigue Weakness Retarded growth	Red meats, especially liver Green vegetables Yellow fruits Prunes Raisins Legumes Whole grain and enriched cereals Molasses Egg yolk Potatoes	Bottlefed infant should receive iron-fortified formula Breastfed infant should receive iron supplementation at 4 mos (1 mg/kg/24 hrs) if full term and at 2 mos (2 mg/kg/24 hrs) if premature After 6 mos of age fortified cereals provide iron, therefore supplementation is not necessary if dietary intake is sufficient
Iodine			
Constituent of thyroxin, which is a regulator of metabolism	Enlarged thyroid gland Low metabolic rate Stunted growth Retarded mental growth	Iodized salt Sea foods Food grown in nongoiterous regions	No supplementation
Sodium			
Constituent of extracellular fluid Maintenance of body neutrality Osmotic pressure Muscle and nerve irritability	Muscle cramps Weakness Headache Nausea Anorexia Vascular collapse	Sodium chloride (table salt) Sodium bicarbonate (baking powder, baking soda) Monosodium glutamate (Accent) Milk, cheese Meat, egg white	No supplementation

TABLE 16-9
Minerals: Functions, Sources and Supplementation *(Continued)*

Function	Deficiency Symptoms	Sources	Supplementation
Fluorine			
Resistance to dental caries	Tendency to have dental caries	Water supply containing 1 ppm	Formula-fed infants need no supplement
Deposition of bone calcium		Small amount in many foods	Supplementation is controversial
			If breastfed, initiate at 2 wks of age
			Dosage varies with concentration of fluoride in the local water supply (see Chapter 8)
Potassium			
Acid-base balance	Apathy	Whole grains	No supplementation
Carbohydrate metabolism	Muscular weakness	Meat	
Conduction of nerve impulses	Poor gastrointestinal tone	Legumes	
Contraction of muscle fibers	Respiratory muscle failure	Some fruit and vegetables	
	Tachychardia		
	Cardiac arrest		

vegetables to someone who has been reared in a culture in which all vegetables are boiled for sanitary reasons is also unlikely to be effective.

Family relationships and lifestyle affect children's mealtime experience. Children and parents seem to be highly susceptible to conflicts and outright battles at mealtime. The underlying relationship and method of discipline largely determine the outcome of these battles. The emotional environment at mealtime should be such that children and parents feel relaxed and positive toward one another. Children of parents who use nagging to show their concern about eating habits soon learn how much control they have by refusing to eat. Parents frequently need to be reassured that a healthy, hungry child *will* eat if a calm atmosphere is provided.

The family's degree of concern in insisting on a time when the family "eats together" affects the amount of experience children have in associating eating with positive socialization within the family. The hurried lifestyle of the modern family with high time demands on individual family members works against the goal of a calm, unhurried mealtime experience (Fig. 16–4). The potentially negative impact of a continued pattern of hurried-up meals and tension-related eating experiences should be considered when assessing nutritional status of children. Additionally, the tendency for families to rely on fast foods should be recognized as a pattern that can potentially lead to an imbalance of nutrients if fast foods are not varied and representative of a balanced diet.

Peers and social influences increasingly affect dietary habits as children become older, especially during the school-age years. Birch has found that even within the preschool setting, peers have an influence on each other's eating habits (Birch, 1987). Permission to ride a bike to a "corner store" where peers congregate enhances a child's sense of belonging and acceptance. The consumption of junk food thus becomes a socially related activity. Parents, therefore, must be supported in their effort to curtail activities that grossly interfere with a balanced diet.

Television has also been shown to have an impact on children's eating habits. Advertisements for foods low in nutrition tend to increase total calorie consumption (for boys more than girls), yet pronutrition advertisements have not been shown to be effective in promoting healthy food consumption (Dietz & Gortmaker, 1985).

Socioeconomic factors account for a high degree of inequity between and within societies. Ability to purchase food, distribution of food, and access to health care services are common variables across populations. Consequently, when assessing nutritional adequacy, it is important to distinguish between resource issues and knowledge about nutrition as a cause of an unhealthy diet. The reasons for poor dietary intake vary according to socioeconomic variables. Malnutrition in developing countries is generally the result of a chronic marginal deficit of food quality and/or quantity and is often associated with a high frequency of illness, whereas malnutrition in industrialized countries has its roots in psychosocial causes (Allen, 1990).

Developmental level of the child affects the child's feeding experience and significance of food. As chil-

TABLE 16-10
Some Food Traditions from Various Cultural Groups

African-American

Food choices are not significantly different from others in same geographic area. Southern African-American and white cooking tradition includes greens (collard, turnip, etc.), okra, pork products, cornbread, hominy grits

Native American

Traditional foods vary among tribes. Corn, beans, squashes, and chili peppers are common. Availability and cost of fresh fruits, vegetables, and meat are major problems for those living on reservations

Mexican-American

Mexican food includes influences from Spanish and Native American food. In some areas of the United States, persons of a Mexican-Hispanic background constitute 25 per cent or more of the population, and food preferences are part of the mainstream eating patterns. Characteristic foods include tortillas (the bread of Mexican culture), tamales, tacos, enchiladas. Beans, rice, tomatoes, carrots, onions, and chili peppers are used in traditional cooking. Milk drinking is low; cheese is used

Puerto Rican and Cuban

Spanish and Native American heritages are seen in use of rice and red and white beans. In Caribbean areas, a wide range of fruits and vegetables is used—plantain, sweet potato, green bananas, cassava, breadfruit, guava, acerola, mango, avocado, okra, and citrus fruits. In mainland cities, diets may suffer because these are not available or are too expensive

Chinese

Depending on area of China family is from, there is a wide range of cooking traditions. Cooking style emphasizes foods being cut into very small pieces and cooked quickly. Rice is a staple in some regions, wheat flour noodles or dumplings in others. Soybean products (bean curd, also called tofu, oil, sauce) are used widely; there is a wide range of cooked vegetables, including bok choy, bean sprouts, bamboo shoots, greens, mushrooms, snow peas, and gourds

Japanese

Fish, soybean products, rice, noodles, and vegetables (seaweed, bamboo shoots, broccoli, cauliflower) are prevalent. Traditional Japanese diets include little meat but raw fish is common; second- and third-generation families in United States often adopt Westernized diets. Green tea is the traditional beverage

Middle Eastern

The countries around the eastern Mediterranean (Greece, Turkey, Lebanon, Syria, Iraq, Iran, Israel, Jordan, and Egypt) share certain food traditions. However, religious dietary differences among Moslems, Jews, and Christians are important. Lamb and goat are staple meats; beef is rare. Ground meat mixed with rice and spices and wrapped with leaves or stuffed in vegetables is a common dish. Bread, rice, beans, lentils, chick peas, olives, and eggplant are staples. Moslems and Jews avoid pork products; Moslems also avoid animal shortenings. Milk is used little in some groups; yogurt is popular in most.

Ethiopian

Ethiopian food is an example of a highly individualized cuisine brought to the United States by recent immigration. The Ethiopian staple is injera, a thick fluffy pancakelike bread. The basic meal consists of a meat or lentil stew (wat) eaten with injera. Wat is very highly spiced by a number of ground peppers and spices. In native Ethiopian meals, the amount of meat is usually small. In US-adapted cooking, meat increases and injera becomes an accompaniment

dren develop cognitively, their understanding of the meaning and importance of food changes. Developmental issues concerning food and eating that arise at the various ages are discussed in the respective normal growth and development chapters (Chapters 5 through 9).

Baseline Data Gathering

During the process of gathering baseline data for a nutritional assessment, the nurse may request the expertise of qualified health care professionals within other disciplines, commonly known as the multidisciplinary team approach. This approach is recommended to treat childhood nutritional problems. Members of the multidisciplinary team include a physician, a dietitian, a nurse, and a pharmacist. Each of these professionals can assist the nurse in using the nursing process to care for the nutritional needs of the child/adolescent. Even though other health care professionals are members of the team, the primary participants in direct contact with the child/adolescent and the family are the nurse and the dietitian. Although the registered nurse has knowledge and skills for intervention in the area of some nutritional problems, the registered dietitian/nutritionist has extensive training in the science of nutrition and should be consulted when the scope of the problem is beyond the level of the nurse's abilities. Hence, the multidisciplinary approach is beneficial to perform a nutrition assessment and subsequently to develop an appropriate care plan.

A nutritional history is obtained for a 24-hour period of intake. For recall, questions about when the child got up and activities that took place at different times during the day can be asked. If more specific information is needed, a 3-day or 7-day food diary is kept. A food diary is helpful in establishing food intake. The most helpful diaries include the time of day and type of food consumed, as well as the emotional

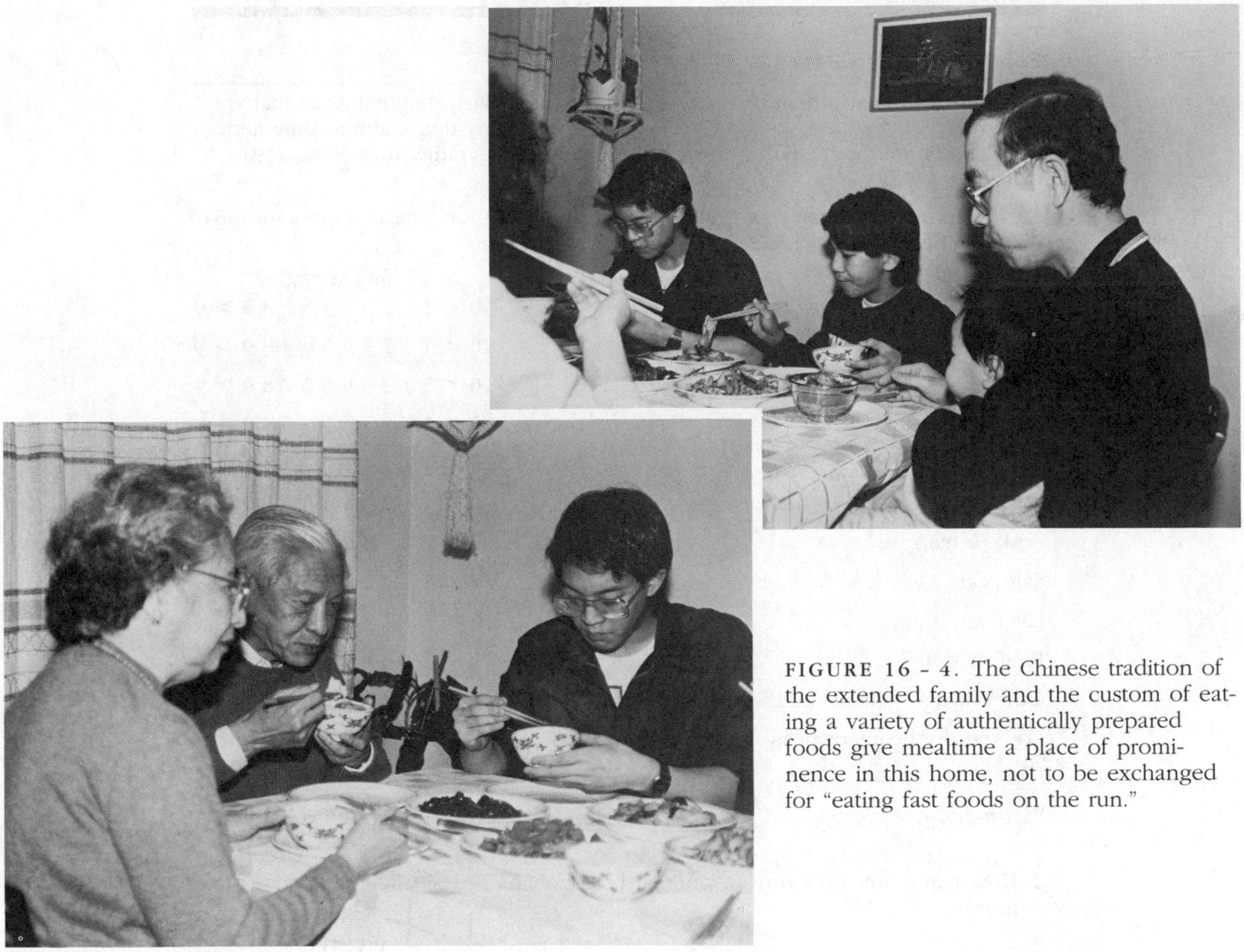

FIGURE 16-4. The Chinese tradition of the extended family and the custom of eating a variety of authentically prepared foods give mealtime a place of prominence in this home, not to be exchanged for "eating fast foods on the run."

feelings experienced prior to food consumption. Methods of preparation and household measures (cup, teaspoon) of amounts of food consumed are recorded. Mixed dishes should have the recipe or ingredients included. Additional supplements such as vitamins or minerals should also be recorded. Although this method provides comprehensive information, it is time-consuming and requires much cooperation and motivation on the part of the child and parents. It is especially helpful, however, in working with obese children to help them see exactly how much they consume. Another interview method is the food frequency check list. Specific foods are grouped in the major categories and the child and/or primary caregiver is asked to respond to whether the foods are rarely eaten (less than once a week), sometimes eaten (once a week), or eaten every day (Table 16–11).

A total assessment of the child's nutritional status includes historical data (diet history, medical history, socioeconomic history, drug history), a clinical evaluation, and biochemical evaluation of nutrients within the body. Table 16–12 identifies information that a nutrition history would include. It is essential that this information be obtained in a nonjudgmental manner. It is important to remember that parents have been exposed to many ideas about nutrition and may be confused by the conflicting information available. Direct questions should be avoided if possible. Open questions should be asked instead, such as, "What do you add to the cereal?" This approach avoids suggestion, criticism, or judgmental statements. The interviewer's attitude and nonverbal cues are frequently helpful in alleviating parental anxiety. A calm, accepting attitude helps parents provide accurate data without feeling defensive.

Additional information can be obtained by observing the parent-child interaction during feeding. Observing a mother breastfeeding or bottlefeeding may provide useful information from which an assessment may be made and counseling provided. Feeding behaviors frequently reflect the child's development; delays in feeding behaviors may also indicate delays in other areas. Also, children may not be provided the opportunity to develop certain skills, such as using a cup or spoon, and the parent may need counseling in this area.

The nurse also determines nutritional status through *objective examination*. A thorough physical examination should identify areas of concern if un-

TABLE 16–11
Food Frequency Check List

This information will help us to understand your regular eating habits so that we may offer you the best service possible. If you have any doubt about some items, be sure to underestimate the "goodness" of your habits rather than to overestimate.

1. How many times *per week* do you eat the following foods? Circle the appropriate number:

	PER WEEK
Poultry	0 < 1 1 2 3 4 5 6 7 8 9 > 9
Fish	0 < 1 1 2 3 4 5 6 7 8 9 > 9
Hot dogs	0 < 1 1 2 3 4 5 6 7 8 9 > 9
Bacon	0 < 1 1 2 3 4 5 6 7 8 9 > 9
Lunch meat	0 < 1 1 2 3 4 5 6 7 8 9 > 9
Sausage	0 < 1 1 2 3 4 5 6 7 8 9 > 9
Pork or ham	0 < 1 1 2 3 4 5 6 7 8 9 > 9
Salt pork	0 < 1 1 2 3 4 5 6 7 8 9 > 9
Liver	0 < 1 1 2 3 4 5 6 7 8 9 > 9
Beef or veal	0 < 1 1 2 3 4 5 6 7 8 9 > 9
Other meats (which?) ________	0 < 1 1 2 3 4 5 6 7 8 9 > 9
Cooked dry beans or peas	0 < 1 1 2 3 4 5 6 7 8 9 > 9
Eggs	0 < 1 1 2 3 4 5 6 7 8 9 > 9
Fast foods	0 < 1 1 2 3 4 5 6 7 8 9 > 9

2. How many times *per day* do you eat the following foods? Circle the appropriate number:

	PER DAY
Bread, toast, rolls, muffins	0 < 1 1 2 3 4 5 6 7 8 9 > 9
Milk (including on cereal)	0 < 1 1 2 3 4 5 6 7 8 9 > 9
Yogurt or tofu	0 < 1 1 2 3 4 5 6 7 8 9 > 9
Cheese or cheese dishes	0 < 1 1 2 3 4 5 6 7 8 9 > 9
Sugar, jam, jelly, syrup, honey	0 < 1 1 2 3 4 5 6 7 8 9 > 9
Butter or margarine	0 < 1 1 2 3 4 5 6 7 8 9 > 9

3. How many times *per week* do you eat the following foods? Circle the appropriate number:

	PER WEEK
Fruits or fruit juices	0 < 1 1 2 3 4 5 6 7 8 9 > 9
Vegetables other than potatoes	0 < 1 1 2 3 4 5 6 7 8 9 > 9
Potatoes and other starchy vegetables	0 < 1 1 2 3 4 5 6 7 8 9 > 9
Salads or raw vegetables	0 < 1 1 2 3 4 5 6 7 8 9 > 9
Cereal (which kind?) ________	0 < 1 1 2 3 4 5 6 7 8 9 > 9
Pancakes or waffles	0 < 1 1 2 3 4 5 6 7 8 9 > 9

TABLE 16-11
Food Frequency Check List *(Continued)*

	PER WEEK
Rice or other cooked grains	0 < 1 1 2 3 4 5 6 7 8 9 > 9
Noodles (macaroni, spaghetti)	0 < 1 1 2 3 4 5 6 7 8 9 > 9
Crackers or pretzels	0 < 1 1 2 3 4 5 6 7 8 9 > 9
Sweet rolls or doughnuts	0 < 1 1 2 3 4 5 6 7 8 9 > 9
Peanut butter or nuts	0 < 1 1 2 3 4 5 6 7 8 9 > 9
Milk or milk products	0 < 1 1 2 3 4 5 6 7 8 9 > 9
TV dinners, pot pies, other prepared meals	0 < 1 1 2 3 4 5 6 7 8 9 > 9
Sweet bakery goods (cake, cookies)	0 < 1 1 2 3 4 5 6 7 8 9 > 9
Snack foods (potato or corn chips)	0 < 1 1 2 3 4 5 6 7 8 9 > 9
Candy	0 < 1 1 2 3 4 5 6 7 8 9 > 9
Soft drinks (which?) ________	0 < 1 1 2 3 4 5 6 7 8 9 > 9
Coffee or tea	0 < 1 1 2 3 4 5 6 7 8 9 > 9
Frozen sweets (which?) ________	0 < 1 1 2 3 4 5 6 7 8 9 > 9
Instant meals such as breakfast bars or diet meal beverages (which?) ________	0 < 1 1 2 3 4 5 6 7 8 9 > 9
Wine	0 < 1 1 2 3 4 5 6 7 8 9 > 9
Beer	0 < 1 1 2 3 4 5 6 7 8 9 > 9
Whiskey, vodka, rum, etc.	0 < 1 1 2 3 4 5 6 7 8 9 > 9

4. What specific kinds of the following foods do you eat most often? Include the name of the food; whether it is fresh, canned, or frozen; and how it is prepared.

   Fruits and fruit juices ________________________________

   Vegetables ________________________________

   Milk and milk products ________________________________

   Meats and meat alternatives ________________________________

   Breads and cereals ________________________________

   Desserts ________________________________

   Snack foods ________________________________

5. Please list the names of any liquid, powder, or pill forms of vitamin or mineral products you take, and state how often you take them. Please list also any diet supplement you use (such as protein milkshakes or brewer's yeast), how much you use, and how often you use it. ________________________________

   ____

6. Is there anything else we should know about your food/nutrient intake? ________

   ____

Reprinted by permission from *Understanding normal and clinical nutrition* (3rd ed.) by Whitney, E. N., Cataldo, C. B., & Rolfes, S. R.;

TABLE 16-12
Format of a Nutritional History

I. Age

II. Concerns of parents or child about current nutrition or feeding behaviors

III. Infant history (used when client is an infant)
- A. Type of feeding method (bottle, breast)
- B. Formula feeding
  - 1. Type used
  - 2. How prepared
  - 3. When formula was started
  - 4. Other formulas used
  - 5. Number of bottles and ounces consumed in 24 hrs
  - 6. Frequency of feedings and number of ounces at each feeding
  - 7. Amount of time required for feeding
  - 8. Approach to feeding (propped bottle, held in arms, etc.)
- C. Breastfeeding
  - 1. Number of times nursed in 24-hr period
  - 2. Length of time nursed at each breast, at each feeding
  - 3. Problems with breasts (cracked nipples, swollen breasts)
  - 4. Diet, medications, and fluid intake history of mother
  - 5. Notice of milk letdown reflex by mother
  - 6. History of stress, fatigue in mother
- D. Additional intake
  - 1. Vitamins, iron, fluoride supplements
  - 2. Solid foods
    - a. Type
    - b. Frequency
    - c. Amounts
    - d. When started and how introduced
    - e. How fed (feeds crackers, solids in bottle)
  - 3. Other fluids (juices, water, sugar water)
- E. Feeding behaviors/habits
  - 1. Satisfaction of child following feeding
  - 2. Use of pacifier or thumbsucking
  - 3. Nighttime nutrition
  - 4. Sleeping through night
  - 5. Elimination patterns
  - 6. Vomiting, spitting up
  - 7. Response to foods (spitting, colic, diarrhea, rash)
  - 8. Activity and personality (crying, irritable, sleeping) after feeding
- F. Family involvement with feeding
  - 1. Family attitudes/beliefs of food, feeding practices (how food is used)
  - 2. Participation in feeding (father, siblings)
  - 3. Response of family to feeding
    - a. Breastfeeding
    - b. Self-feeding by infant and inevitable mess
    - c. Response of parent/child to new foods when introduced

IV. Toddler, preschooler, school-age, and adolescent history
- A. Number of meals eaten per day
- B. Where meals are eaten (school, fast-food chain, home)
- C. Method of feeding (fingers, utensils used)
- D. Amount of milk intake in 24 hrs
- E. Snacking
  - 1. Type of foods
  - 2. Amounts
  - 3. Where snacks eaten
  - 4. Frequency and nearness to mealtimes
- F. Food preferences and dislikes
- G. Who plans, buys, and cooks food
- H. Finances
  - 1. Amount of money available for food
  - 2. Food programs (food stamps, Head Start Breakfast, school lunch)
- I. Dietary recall for past 24 hrs
- J. Developmental behavior of eating (utensils, chewing)
- K. Habits (same as infant)
- L. Response of family to eating behavior of child
- M. Last dental visit

V. Past medical history
- A. Prenatal nutrition of mother
- B. Birthweight
- C. PKU results
- D. Developmental history
  - 1. Feeding behaviors (use of cup, spoon, fingerfeeding)
  - 2. Age of weaning
  - 3. Pica
- E. Allergies
- F. Chronic problems
- G. Medication history
  - 1. Medications currently taking
    - a. Name of medication
    - b. Dosage
    - c. Reason for taking
    - d. Reason for stopping
    - e. Duration of intake
  - 2. Previous medications
    - a. Name of medication
    - b. Dosage
    - c. Reason for taking
    - d. Reason for stopping
    - e. Duration of intake

VI. Family history
- A. Hypertension
- B. Obesity
- C. Stroke
- D. Diabetes
- E. Heart problems
- F. Allergies
- G. Hyperlipidemias
- H. Anorexia nervosa

VII. Weight history
- A. History of weight loss
- B. History of weight gain

Adapted from Fox, J., & Elsberry, C. (1980). *Primary health care of the young*. New York: McGraw-Hill.

dernourishment or overnourishment exists. Anthropometric measurements including height (or recumbent length of children <2 years of age), weight, and head circumference (for children <3 years of age) provide essential information for evaluation of nutritional status. In some instances, measurement of skin-folds using a caliper may be beneficial.* Physical indications of nutritional status are shown in Table 16–13. One or more of the signs of malnutrition indicate the need for a careful interview about food intake and eating habits. Additional data about nutritional status may be obtained from various laboratory studies: (1) hemoglobin and/or hematocrit tests to detect anemia; (2) blood albumin and total lymphocyte count to evaluate protein status; (3) nitrogen balance studies to detect nitrogen imbalances; (4) transferrin levels to assess protein and iron status; and (5) various vitamin/mineral tests to evaluate vitamin/mineral status.

Promotion of a Healthful Diet

The goal for each child is that nutrition be of the quality to support optimal growth and development. Equal attention is given to nutrition whether a child is well or has a nutritional problem. Positive reinforcement for healthful dietary practices is encouragement that parents and children need. Identification of deficits in nutrient intake and dietary practices that interfere with health should be explored. Nutritional deficits are identified by comparing collected data with standards such as RDAs, the Food Pyramid, height and weight charts, and normal ranges for biochemical laboratory data.

The nutrition history helps uncover long-standing nutritional problems and provides information about the family's knowledge and beliefs concerning nutrition. The 24-hour intake recall provides more precise information regarding adequacy of intake, and a 3- to 7-day intake record gives the necessary data to learn about variety in the child's diet. The physical examination and clinical signs of nutritional problems are evaluated. Anthropometric measures must be evaluated by plotting a series of readings on pertinent growth charts. See Appendices 2 and 3 for examples of growth charts.

The medical history can provide information to help determine whether the child is at risk for nutritional deficiencies or excesses and may be indicative of whether normal growth can be expected. The nurse should be aware of social programs to which the family may be referred (Women, Infants, and Children program). Appropriate referral should be carried out to alleviate possible long-term effects of malnutrition or overnutrition (Allen, 1990).

Obvious changes or deficits in the growth pattern may require adjustments in the diet. Parents are the decision makers for the young child, but the older child has practical decision making powers regarding nutrition. The parent and child should be counseled regarding modification of the child's diet if necessary. It is important to include both parent and child in the plans for change, so that they know the reasons why change is needed and how their beliefs, attitudes, and actions are affecting the nutrition of the child. Conditions that indicate nutritional counseling may be necessary are: the child's growth is below the 10th percentile or greater than the 90th percentile, the child is underweight or overweight for height, a certain nutrient is deficient in the diet (Pipes, 1989), or the parent identifies a concern.

*It is important that the person using a caliper be trained and competent/proficient or the information gathered may be invalid (Marshall et al, 1990).

Common Concerns and Issues: Nursing Interventions

Nutrition is a rapidly developing science. Many cause-and-effect relationships have not been established concerning nutrition and disease. These uncertainties give rise to considerable confusion and differences of opinion concerning nutrition. Common issues and concerns that the nurse should be prepared to address are discussed next.

Eating Behaviors, Limit Setting, and Socialization

Children adopt the eating behaviors of those they observe. They also learn by repeated reinforcement those behaviors that are acceptable and unacceptable. *Appropriate supervision* and *management by parents* are required to instill healthy dietary habits. Clear establishment of rules concerning food highlights important family values and attitudes. Parents should be encouraged to exercise their authority concerning behavior at the table, consumption of sweets and junk foods, and variety in their child's diet. Refusal to eat a varied diet of nutritious foods and excessive consumption of sweets and junk foods can only continue if parents purchase the food and do not monitor their child's intake. Monitoring intake of junk foods becomes increasingly difficult as the child approaches late school-age; however, parents have the responsibility to teach their children and set limits concerning food intake.

During mealtime, the dessert crisis is not always easily resolved. Each family must develop its own rules, which should be understood by the child. For example, a nutritionally adequate first course should be eaten before dessert is permitted. Dessert should never be used as a reward (e.g., "you can have dessert if you eat your vegetables"). This communicates to the child: (1) vegetables are so awful that the parent must bribe her or him to consume them, (2) dessert is especially desirable, and (3) food is a reward. If limits are not put on desserts and snacks, ex-

TABLE 16-13
Physical Indications of Nutritional Status of the Child

Well-Nourished Child	Malnourished Child	Deficiency
Height and Weight		
Within growth norms—steady gain and increase from year to year	Above or below growth norms—failure to gain or excessive weight gain each year	Protein, calorie, other essential nutrients
Skin		
Clear, smooth, elastic and firm	Rough, dry, scaly, xerosis	Vitamin A
Reddish-pink mucous membranes	Petechiae, ecchymoses, poor wound healing	Vitamin C
	Depigmentation of skin	Protein, calorie
	Lesions	Riboflavin
	Dermatitis, sensitivity of skin to sunlight	Niacin
	Pallor	Vitamin B_{12}, iron, folacin
Musculoskeletal		
Well-developed, erect posture	Head sags, winged scapula, bowed legs, costochondral beading, cranial bossing	Calcium, vitamin D
Shoulder blades flat		
Arms and legs straight		
Skull and jaw well-developed	Epiphyseal enlargement of wrists	Vitamins D, C
Firm muscles with good tonus	Small flabby muscles, muscle weakness	Phosphorus, protein
Moderate amount of fat	Faulty epiphyseal bone formation	Vitamin A
	Pretibial edema bilateral	Protein, calorie, thiamin
Head		
Hair—smooth, good amount, lustrous	Dull, dry, depigmented, abnormal texture, easily pluckable, thin	Protein, calorie
Eyes—clear and bright	Dull with dark circles and hollows; Bitot's spots, conjunctivitis, xerosis, night blindness (nyctalopia), light sensitivity (photophobia)	Vitamin A, riboflavin
Mouth—pink, moist lips; pink, firm gums; full set of teeth	Cracking and scaling lips, cheilosis, fissuring of mouth corners	Riboflavin
	Spongy, swollen gums, bleed easily (gingiva)	Vitamin C
	Irregular or missing teeth with cavities: defective tooth enamel	Vitamin D, A
	Glossitis	Folacin, vitamin B_{12}, niacin, iron
	Tongue fissuring	Niacin
Neck		
Normal size	Enlarged thyroid	Iodine
	Enlarged parotids	Protein, calorie
Neurologic		
	Listless	Protein, calorie
	Loss of ankle-jerk and knee-jerk reflexes, motor weakness, sensory loss	Thiamin
	Headache	Niacin, thiamin
	Polyneuritis, motor weakness	Thiamin
Abdomen		
Flat	Distended, protrudes, hepatomegaly	Protein, calorie
Cardiac		
Normal heart size and sounds	Cardiac enlargement and tachycardia	Thiamin, potassium
	Murmur	Iron

From Pearson, G. A. (1977). Nutrition in the middle years of childhood. Reprinted from *MCN: American Journal of Maternal Child Nursing, July/August, 1977, 2*(6), 378–384.

cessive intake of sugar can interfere with adequate dietary intake. Parents should teach their children how to snack and appropriate foods to consume for snacks. Snacks should incorporate food items that are nutritious, easy to prepare, and readily available to children/adolescents who return home after school without parental supervision (Whitney et al, 1991).

The effect maturational changes have on appetite is important for parents to understand. The frustration of "getting children to eat" is a common problem experienced by parents. It should be stressed that if sweets are curtailed and excessive milk intake is not permitted, a healthy child will eat when hungry without coercion. Strategies to gain a child's cooperation at mealtime should be employed. Children can be given some control and autonomy by letting them place food on their own plates (with some supervision depending on age and maturity of child), giving some choices, and not insisting on an empty plate if the child is satiated. A child who persistently does not eat should be further evaluated. In some cases, children control their parents by not eating, in which case parents should be counseled to put less emphasis on food intake. Lack of sufficient exercise, inadequate sleep and rest, and an underlying illness should also be considered when a child persistently does not eat.

The normal changes in appetite and food intake, however, should be recognized as factors that affect a child's intake (e.g., toddlers and some preschoolers are notorious for being picky eaters). Frequently, toddlers experience physiologic anorexia, in which their intake of or appetite for food is curtailed. This is to be expected since this age group of children is prone to "food jags" and decreased food consumption. Usually, the child will overcome this on his or her own; therefore, parents should not overreact. However, parents must remember that the provision of an assortment of nutritious foods is essential to maintain dietary adequacy during this time period (Story & Brown, 1987).

A nonconducive environment for mealtime can detract from optimal nutritional intake. Mealtime should be a pleasant, social experience. Parents are encouraged to avoid tension-producing topics and should plan for sufficient time to eat an unhurried meal. The physical aspects, such as comfortable seating, appropriate utensils, and attractive serving of food, are also amenities that children deserve.

Another concern that parents frequently express is their children's resistance to trying new foods or eating certain foods, such as vegetables. Young children normally exhibit a neophobic response when presented with a new food. Parents should be informed that this is a normal and adaptive response exhibited by a child to a new food. It is important to recognize that children have likes and dislikes but that learning to eat new foods requires work; it does not just happen. Children learn to like food by tasting it time after time; therefore, even though a food is refused, the process of taking a small bite each time can eventually change the child's response. Allowing exposure (even without eating—through the senses of smell, touch, or sight) may also increase the likelihood of future acceptance. When preschoolers observe adults consuming a new food, it is more likely that they will begin to consume the food (Sigman-Grant, 1992). According to Dietz (1986), parents should serve as role models during meals since parenteral influences on food patterns are critical.

New foods are better accepted if they are offered when the child is hungry (at the beginning of a meal) so that a pleasant sensation is associated with that particular food. Also, not permitting a second helping of a desired food (e.g., bread, potatoes) before the vegetables have been consumed allows consumption of the less desired food at a time when the child is not satiated. Always leaving the least desired food until last reduces the likelihood that a pleasant sensation is associated with that food.

When introducing new foods, remember that young children tend to reject highly seasoned foods and food mixtures in which they are unable to identify individual components of the food item. In general, children prefer foods lukewarm. Finger foods or foods that are easy to handle are also more desired by the young child. Brightly colored foods also tend to increase children's sensory appeal to certain foods (Sparkman et al, 1988). If foods such as mashed potatoes or creamed soups are served, they should be of a smooth consistency (without lumps) or a child may think there is something else in the food (Whitney et al, 1991).

Nutrition and Disease

The potential association between childhood nutrition and the risk of development of adult disease is a concept that has generated much discussion. Common areas of concern are the effects of intake of refined sugar, salt, fat, and cholesterol. Additionally, recent emphasis has been given to the benefits of a high fiber diet. The AAP Committee on Nutrition cautions that the safety of diets that (1) decrease caloric intake; (2) increase consumption of complex carbohydrates (fiber); (3) decrease consumption of fat and cholesterol; and (4) limit sodium intake has *not* been established in children and pregnant women (AAP, 1983, 1986). Although restrictive diets are not recommended in children, it is useful for nurses to have current information concerning these issues so that they can counsel parents and children appropriately. Sugar consumption as a factor in the development of coronary heart disease, hyperactivity in children, and the increasing incidence of obesity has not been documented with scientific data (Mahan & Arlin, 1992). The major offending characteristic of sugar on children's health is its cariogenic property (see Chapter 8).

In recent years, the potential protective role of fiber in the diet has been studied. A reduced fiber intake has been implicated in the development of cancer of the colon and has been identified as a factor contributing to high blood pressure (Anderson, 1983). Diets for children that contain fiber at the expense of animal protein may, however, result in deficits in vitamins and minerals. Fiber also promotes a laxative effect, which is beneficial but should be avoided in excess. With respect to fiber, a balanced diet according to the Food Guide Pyramid (see Table 16–2) is recommended.

A continuing area of study is the diet–heart disease relationship. The focus of recent research is the advisability of reducing the fat and cholesterol content of diets for infants and children. Atherosclerosis is a disease process that begins with the appearance of fatty streaks in the aorta during childhood. By age 10, virtually all children, regardless of their dietary intake and the incidence of coronary heart disease, have fatty streaks in their aortas (Roy & Galeano, 1985). Dietary recommendations have been made for adults to consume low-fat and low-cholesterol diets to reduce the risk factors for development of atherosclerosis. However, limiting fat and cholesterol intake has been questioned with respect to children because of their needs for growth and because the effect of altering fat and cholesterol intake during the early years has not been proved to reduce adult atherosclerosis. Breast milk, which contains cholesterol, is considered an ideal food for infants; it has been suggested that cholesterol may be necessary and important during the entire growing period for the formation of bile acids, hormones, and special tissues (AAP, 1983). Parents must be taught that severely decreasing the fat content of the diet of a young child who is already a "picky" eater can rob the child of calories that are essential for growth (Schifman & Hannaman, 1989). Also, low-cholesterol diets may adversely affect the myelinization of the central nervous system in infants, possibly causing the development of neurologic disorders (Glueck et al, 1978).

The amount of sodium in infant foods became a public concern in the middle 1960s. Since that time, there has been a gradual decrease in the sodium concentration of infant foods, and, since 1977, the addition of salt to infant foods has been discontinued. The hypothesis that the sodium content of infant foods contributes to hypertension in later life has not been confirmed (AAP, 1981b). The level of sodium intake (in the form of salt) during childhood is sufficiently high to prompt The Second Task Force on Blood Pressure Control in Children to issue the following statement: "It is apparent that the sodium intake of children is far in excess of that required for optimal growth and development. Thus the potential benefit of dietary sodium reduction in hypertension appears to outweigh any potential risk from this form of therapy" (Horan et al, 1987). The important aspect to consider is that it is thought that salt preference is learned and that reduction of dietary sodium can cause taste preference to shift to lower levels of salt in food (Beauchamp et al, 1983). The overall recommendation that nurses can make for children is to eat a well-balanced diet and avoid excesses. The recommendation of the AAP Committee on Nutrition (1983) is that "current dietary trends in the United States toward a decreased consumption of saturated fats, cholesterol and salt, and an increased intake of polyunsaturated fats should be followed with moderation. Diets that avoid extremes are safe for children."

Nutritional counseling is a major responsibility of the nurse. The relationship of nutrition and disease is an area of health care that is subject to misinformation and misinterpretation. A major source of information that can be used to guide the nurse in counseling is the *Pediatric Nutrition Handbook* published by the AAP (1985). The nurse may also use the assistance of a dietitian in counseling the child and/or primary caretaker regarding recommended nutritional intake.

The nurse's role is to listen to the opinions of the clients (parent, child, or adolescent) and seek to understand any inaccuracies that might be harmful to their health. Some differences in opinion may actually not require intervention if there is no potential for actual harm. The basic principles used for management are (1) *generally discourage restrictive diets for children* and (2) *maintain a balanced diet.*

Another role of the nurse in health maintenance is identification of early signs of illness. Detection of obesity by measuring height, weight, head circumference, and skin fold thickness and detection of hypertension by measuring blood pressure are nursing responsibilities.

Screening of children more than 2 years of age who are at risk for hypercholesterolemia because of family history should consist of at least two serum cholesterol measurements. Although universal cholesterol testing is not recommended by the AAP, when a reliable family history is unobtainable, the most effective approach is to screen the child for elevated cholesterol and triglyceride levels. According to the AAP (1988), children with cholesterol levels persistently above the 75th percentile (at or above 170 mg/dl) should be considered for dietary counseling. High-density lipoprotein cholesterol should be measured when levels are above the 95th percentile (at or above 200 mg/dl) (AAP, 1983, 1985).

Food Additives

Many consumers believe that some food additives may cause cancer and that childhood hyperactivity is associated with intake of additives. An increased use of convenience foods and the transportation and storage of food in industrialized nations makes the use of food additives necessary. The demand of the consumer for attractive foods with reduced perishability continues to promote acceptability of additives in spite of the potential disadvantages.

A food additive is a substance that is added to

food for the purpose of enhancing its quality and shelf life. The purposes of food additives vary, including (1) addition of nutritional value, (2) preservation of food, (3) aid in processing and preparation, and (4) improvement of the flavor, color, odor, and texture (Mahan & Arlin, 1992).

Food additives in common use have been subjected to extensive study through large doses in animals by the US Food and Drug Administration (FDA). The FDA has enforced the "Delaney Clause," which makes it necessary for any additive to be removed from the market if it has been found to induce cancer in humans or animals. The use of saccharin (a sugar substitute) has been controversial; however, it is still available as a nonprescription drug. A newer acceptable sweetener is aspartame, which was approved for use by the FDA in 1981; however, *because it is made from the amino acid phenylalanine,* people with phenylketonuria need to consult with their physicians or dietitians before including aspartame in their diets (Whitney et al, 1991).

Nitrites and nitrates used to cure meat and poultry products have also come under attack because of their potential carcinogenic qualities. Nitrate, however, is also a normal constituent of many vegetables, especially lettuce, beets, celery, and spinach (Green & Harry, 1981), and the intake through additives is considerably less than through dietary sources.

Although the claim by Feingold (1975) that chemicals added to food cause hyperactivity received wide attention, scientific research has not consistently demonstrated a relationship. A conclusion was reached by the National Institutes of Health in 1982 that (1) a few children may be helped by the Feingold (additive-free) diet and (2) a few children respond adversely to synthetic food dyes (AAP, 1985). Lipton and Mayo (1983) provide further support for the position that some hyperactive children may benefit from the additive-free diet, but that there is no support for the breadth of Feingold's original claims (see Chapter 29 for further discussion of management of the hyperactive child). The nurse's ongoing awareness of developments in research findings concerning food additives is information required to counsel parents.

Fast Foods

The largest proportion of meals served in the United States today is through fast-food industries. The popularity of fast-food restaurants matches the fast pace of modern life. The family with young children finds avoiding meal preparation and clean-up a joy and an outing to a restaurant fun. Equally so, fast-food restaurants appeal to adolescents who congregate in groups for a meal or snack that is relatively inexpensive.

The food served in fast-food restaurants is severely criticized by some nutritionists. The generalization that these foods are junk foods,* however, needs to be put into perspective. As many fast foods are consumed by teen-agers, so-called junk food intake has the potential to become the source of conflict between adolescents and parents. Because fast-food consumption has reached such high proportions, the nurse who cares for children and families requires some knowledge to distinguish between legitimate concerns and those that can be dispelled.

Some fast-food chains now make nutrition analyses available to the consumer. Nutrition data are also estimated from standard food composition tables. Independent food testing by a laboratory has been done for some industries; however, it is reasonable to believe that estimates made from the accepted standard food tables are sufficiently accurate. Concerns expressed about nutritional value of fast foods include: high fat/cholesterol content, sodium content, and calorie content; inadequate protein, calcium, vitamin A, and vitamin C content; and low fiber or roughage content. These concerns and comments about actual nutritional values with suggestions of how to alter a diet to compensate for these potential problems are summarized in Table 16–14. The overall concern that some express is that there is not a sufficient variety of foods offered. Some fast-food chains have introduced salad bars; however, since adolescents often have a narrow range of preferences, salads can be as high or higher in fat than a sandwich. Therefore, availability of salads does not necessarily improve diet (DeBruyne & Rolfes, 1989). Consuming several meals a week in a fast-food restaurant should present no nutritional problems if a few guidelines are followed in food selection and if meals consumed elsewhere consist of a balanced diet.

Vegetarianism

Throughout history, people of various religions and cultures have adhered to a vegetarian diet. In North American society, since the mid 1960s, there has been an emergence of vegetarians from new religious, philosophic, or counterculture groups. Vegetarian diets can be compatible with nutritional balance if they are based on established nutritional principles.

The term "vegetarianism" is used to describe a diet that consists primarily of plant foods and excludes the consumption of meat, fowl, and fish, with or without eggs and dairy foods. The four most common vegetarian diets are (1) *lacto-ovo-vegetarian,* which includes eggs and dairy products with plant foods; (2) *lacto-vegetarian,* which includes plant foods and dairy products but excludes eggs; (3) *ovo-*

*"Junk food" has served as the terminology referring to foods low in nutrient density. A nutrient-dense food or a food high in nutrient density provides a high quantity (relative to need) of one or (preferably) several essential nutrients, with a small quantity (relative to need) of kilocalories (Whitney et al, 1991).

TABLE 16-14
Concerns Related to Fast-Food Consumption

	Nutrient Availability	Suggested Diet Alterations
High caloric intake	A typical fast-food meal (large hamburger, french fries and milkshake) contains approximately 1000 calories; this caloric level is too high for all individuals except perhaps a teen-age male	Choosing a smaller hamburger or low-fat milk instead of a milkshake can reduce the calories significantly
Protein	Protein is abundant in fast foods	Protein may even be excessive; therefore, a smaller hamburger is sufficient
Vitamin A	Vitamin A is usually present in low quantities (pizza and tacos are an exception)	Food from a salad bar will compensate for this deficiency
Vitamin C	Vitamin C is generally present in low quantities, but inclusion of french fries is beneficial	Food from a salad bar will compensate for this deficiency
Fiber/roughage	The fiber content is usually low; the only fiber is present in the slice of tomato and the lettuce on a sandwich	Include a salad if available
Sodium content	Sodium content is generally high	Refrain from adding salt
Calcium content	Calcium content is generally low	Include milk/milkshake or frozen yogurt

TABLE 16-15
Types of Vegetarians

Traditional Vegetarians

Many vegetarians have been raised within cultural or religious groups with long-standing customs of vegetarianism (e.g., Seventh Day Adventist). Among these groups, there is adherence to some degree of animal food exclusion but less emphasis on the use of unrefined or naturally occurring food sources

New Vegetarians

Since 1960, there has been a heavy influence of Eastern thought in the Western world, resulting in various philosophic, quasi-religious, or religious groups who have adopted some form of vegetarianism. It is these groups that avoid animal food but in addition avoid other foods that are refined, are processed, or are not organic or natural. Health food stores are the primary suppliers of such foods in the market. These groups vary considerably, and include:

- *Yogi Vegetarians* (lacto-ovo-vegetarian with a stress on "natural foods")
- *Hare Krishnas* (lacto-vegetarian with a stress on "natural foods")
- *Macrobiotics* (vegan diets with strict avoidance of animal fat sources and extensive use of "natural foods")

Personal Choice

Individuals who for a variety of reasons choose to eat a diet primarily composed of vegetables, without affiliation with a specific religious or quasi-religious group. (See possible reasons in Table 16-16)

Economic Circumstances

A segment of the population within developed countries and large numbers of individuals in underdeveloped countries consume diets that exclude animal foods because of inadequate income

vegetarian, which includes plant foods and eggs but excludes dairy products; and (4) *vegan,* which includes plant food only and excludes both dairy products and eggs. The main types of vegetarians are described in Table 16-15. In today's culture, the term "vegetarian" is used in a variety of ways; some people use it loosely to indicate only that red meat is avoided. Therefore, it is important to establish from the outset what a client means by being a "vegetarian."

Understanding the reasons a person chooses to be a vegetarian is useful in establishing a working relationship (see Table 16-16). Frequently, the reasons for choosing vegetarianism determine the degree of

TABLE 16-16
Reasons Why People Choose to Be Vegetarians

Ecologic

Consumption of foods that are "lower" on the food chain (i.e., those fed to livestock) is thought to be a way to reduce world hunger

Economic

Vegetables and grains are cheaper than animal products

Religious or philosophic beliefs

Reasons are many, combining ideas concerning violence (killing of animals) and health issues

Health

Foods are lower in fat and lower in cholesterol, higher in complex carbohydrates, and perhaps lower in sugar strictness with which the diet is observed. Since vegetarians may lack confidence in or be suspicious of those who hold or advocate traditional views of nutrition, it is important to communicate an attitude of support.

The American Dietetic Association has put forth a position paper on a vegetarian approach to eating which states that "well-planned vegetarian diets are consistent with good nutritional status" (American Dietetic Association, 1988). However, it is important to recognize that *poorly planned vegetarian diets* can increase the risk of diet-related nutritional disorders, especially during the growing years.

The increasing concern for health and nutrition and the benefits of predominantly vegetarian diets have led to increases in their popularity. It has been substantially documented that vegetarians have lower serum cholesterol levels and a lower incidence of obesity, both of which are thought to be related to coronary artery disease. The possibility that vegetarian diets may reduce the risk for cancer has not been proved. There is some evidence to support the hypothesis that dietary fat and cholesterol affect the concentration and activity of bacteria in the colon. The altered bacterial activity is thought to produce tumorigenic compounds from bile acids and cholesterol metabolites (Reddy, 1976; McBurney et al, 1987). Colon cancer has also been studied in relation to fiber intake (with high fiber leading to reduced risk), although firm experimental data are lacking to support this relationship. However, because a vegetarian diet is composed of high fiber and contains reduced fat and cholesterol content, it has gained increasing acceptance as a preventive measure against cancer. The potential reduction in risk for developing disease later in life is one major reason why families make the personal choice to raise their children as vegetarians.

Successful support of children on vegetarian diets depends on the nurse's acceptance of the clients' preference. The goal thus becomes one of working out a diet suitable to the parents and child within the family's preferred dietary practices. An understanding of the potential problems must be acquired to provide appropriate and relevant counsel. Although experienced vegetarian parents have a reasonable knowledge of what constitutes a healthful vegetarian diet for themselves, they may not be fully aware of the increased potential for deficiencies that exists with respect to the growing child. Potential problems and information to use in planning interventions are summarized in Table 16–17. Adolescents who choose to become vegetarians against the wishes of their parents also need basic nutritional counseling.

A vegetarian diet can be nutritionally sound if a few guidelines are followed:

- Combine legumes with grains or nuts and seeds to ensure a proper balance of dietary protein.
- Vitamin B_{12} is not contained in plant foods; therefore, if possible, supplement the diet with dairy products and eggs, or use fortified soy milk, or take a vitamin B_{12} supplement.
- Encourage breastfeeding (with attention to mother's vitamin B_{12} intake); infants on breast milk should receive iron, fluoride, and vitamin D supplementation, and vitamin B_{12} (if mother's intake is not adequate).
- Consume a variety of foods.
- Provide a dietary source of vitamin C (it enhances nonheme iron absorption).
- Reduce amount of vegetables consumed that contain oxalate and phytate (they impair iron and calcium absorption; phytates impair zinc absorption).

When planning a vegetarian diet, the principles of the Food Guide Pyramid (see Table 16–2) should be followed daily:

- Bread group (bread, cereal, rice, or pasta)—6 to 11 servings.
- Vegetable group (including the dark green leafy)—3 to 5 servings.
- Fruit group (including one rich in vitamin C)—2 to 4 servings.
- Milk group (vitamin B_{12}–fortified vegetable protein or soy milk)—2 to 3 servings.
- Meat group (dry beans, nuts, or seeds)—2 to 3 servings.

The goals of a complete protein obtained by a combination of grains and legumes at each meal and generally a wide variety of food intake should be stressed.

Nutritional Alterations

Nutritional alterations discussed in this chapter are infant obesity, severe protein-calorie malnutrition, and vitamin D–deficiency rickets, and failure-to-thrive.

Infant and Childhood Obesity

Wide variations exist in infant feeding practices. The consequences of various feeding practices are not clearly established; therefore, recommendations regarding infant nutrition are speculative and must be considered tentative (Turkewitz and Bastian, 1986). Infants fed in a variety of ways may appear equally healthy either because the consequences of a poor diet are too subtle or because differences can be verified only by long-term observations (Turkewitz and Bastian, 1986). Some of the questions about the long-term consequences of early eating habits that remain unanswered are the following: (1) What is the relationship of intake of cholesterol during infancy to the

TABLE 16-17
***Vegetarianism*: Potential Nutritional Problems and Nursing Interventions**

Explanation of the Problem	Suggested Interventions with Explanation
Protein Deficit	
Vegetable proteins have a lower percentage of total nitrogen in the form of amino acids and all are relatively deficient in one or more of the essential amino acids (e.g., lysine is low in cereal grains and methionine is low in legumes)	Complementation of proteins compensates for this deficit Complementation of proteins is the combining of certain foods to ensure intake of quality protein (e.g., methionine-deficient legumes that have an adequate lysine content (beans, peas) should be complemented by methionine-adequate but lysine-deficient grains (rice, corn, oats) or nuts Other examples are peanut butter on whole wheat bread, bean and corn salad, corn and lima beans
Energy	
It is difficult to supply adequate energy sources because: • Bulkiness of the foods cause children to feel satiated; their consumption of sufficient quantities presents a problem • Some vegetables are poorly digested • Vegetarian diets are lower in fat Energy is more potentially a problem during the growth periods of infancy and adolescence	This problem can be overcome if sufficient fats are eaten The greater the variety of food, the more likely it is that energy requirements are met
Vitamins	
Vitamin B_{12}	
Currently there is no known plant food that contains Vitamin B_{12} This is particularly a problem for the breastfed infant whose mother is on a strict vegetarian diet and does not take a Vitamin B_{12} supplement	Vitamin B_{12} can be provided by a supplement or by fortified foods such as soybean milk or meat analogues It is also contained in yeast grown on vitamin B_{12}-enriched media, seaweed, or fermented soy If eggs and milk are included in the diet, vitamin B_{12} is usually adequate
Vitamin D	
Vitamin D is not found in foods of plant origin; therefore, it must be supplemented in the vegan diet Risk of nutritional rickets in certain populations of vegetarian children persists (Dwyer J. T. et al. [1979]. Risk of nutritional rickets among vegetarian children. *American Journal of Diseases of Children, 133*(2), 133–140; Hellebostad T., et al. [1985]. Vitamin D deficiency rickets and vitamin B_{12} deficiency in vegetarian children. *Acta Paediatrica Scandinavica, 74,* 191–195)	Vitamin D can be supplied by exposure of skin to sunlight but this is not a reliable source A supplementary source of vitamin D, such as cod-liver oil, is required if fortified soybean milk or cow's milk is excluded Egg yolks, which are also excluded in a vegan diet, are a good source of vitamin D

later development of atherosclerosis? (2) How does salt intake in infancy affect blood pressure in later life? (3) Are faulty eating habits of infancy and infant obesity an important determinant of obesity in later childhood and adulthood? The fat cell theory that the critical period for the development of obesity is during the first year or two of life has been challenged and is no longer widely supported (Rolfes & DeBruyne, 1992). It has also been suggested that onset of obesity in later childhood is more predictive of adult obesity than obesity of infantile onset. While we wait for conclusive studies regarding the effects of infant obesity, infants at risk must be identified and families assisted to establish healthful feeding practices.

Nursing Assessment

Carrying out a thorough nutritional assessment will assist the nurse in identifying those infants at risk for obesity. Intake is evaluated in terms of the total caloric intake, amount of fluid intake, calories expended for physical activity, and balance of nutrients.

Epidemiologic factors associated with obesity should be recognized in an effort to identify high-risk infants. Parental obesity, older or single parents, single children, or children in small families are epidemiologic categories that are associated with childhood obesity. Obesity in parents in particular is a risk factor. According to a 10-state nutritional survey, a child of obese parents is three times more likely to be obese than if the parents are not obese; if one child is obese, there is a 40 per cent chance that a sibling will also be obese (US Department of Health, Education, and Welfare, 1972). The similarity of obesity patterns between parents and children cannot, however, be interpreted as having only a genetic base because there is considerable similarity between spouses in terms of obesity (Garn & Clark, 1975). Family eating patterns and values placed on food are important fac-

TABLE 16-17
Vegetarianism: Potential Nutritional Problems and Nursing Interventions *(Continued)*

Explanation of the Problem	Suggested Interventions with Explanation
Riboflavin	
Riboflavin is adequate in vegetarian diets that include dairy products but marginal if such products are excluded	Large amounts of dark green vegetables, legumes, and whole grains must be consumed to achieve riboflavin in amounts equivalent to 1 cup of milk High intake of these plant foods is not without consequence in that they inhibit calcium and zinc absorption (see below)
Minerals	
Calcium	
Milk and milk products are the most common source of calcium; therefore, when these are excluded, other sources must be provided	Dark green leafy vegetables, legumes, fortified soybean milk, nuts, and seeds are sources of calcium Vegetables with high oxalic acid content (spinach, chard, beet greens) interfere with calcium absorption Oxalic acid combines with calcium oxalate (bound calcium) and therefore inhibits calcium absorption Whole grains and nuts that contain phytates can also interfere with calcium use The most reliable source of calcium is fortified soybean milk
Zinc	
The bioavailability of zinc in plant foods is questionable The phytates in whole grains and nuts tend to form zinc-phytate complexes inhibiting zinc	Yeast fermentation of whole wheat flour (i.e., as occurs in bread-making) reduces phytates, increasing zinc availability; thus, if bread with yeast is included in the diet, the problem is reduced
Iron	
Iron is absorbed form heme iron, which is animal in origin, and from nonheme iron, which is from plant foods Absorption of heme iron is higher than that of nonheme iron Also, nonheme iron is decreased by phytates and vegetable fiber	Nonheme iron absorption is enhanced by the presence of animal protein and vitamin C in the diet It should be recommended that *each meal* contain a food source of vitamin C to enhance availability of nonheme iron

Data from American Dietetic Association. (1993, November). Position of the American Dietetic Association: Vegetarian diets. *Journal of the American Dietetic Association, 93,* 1317–1319; and Rudy, D. A. (1984). Vegetarian diets for children. *Pediatric Nursing,* 10(5), 329–333.

tors to assess when parents and siblings of an infant are obese.

Obesity is an "excessive ratio of fat to fat-free body mass" (Fomon & Ziegler, 1976). A general definition of obesity in children is a triceps skinfold thickness greater than or equal to the 85th percentile, and weight for height, age, and sex greater than or equal to the 85th percentile (Sherman & Alexander, 1990). According to the National Institutes of Health Consensus Development Conference Statement (1985), the 85th percentile corresponds approximately to 120 per cent of ideal body weight and depicts the accepted definition of obesity.

Height and weight measurements made at each health visit are the nurse's primary method of detecting infants and children at risk for obesity. Height and weight are plotted on a percentile chart to identify rapid or disproportionate weight gain. (See Appendices 2 and 3 for percentile growth charts.) In some instances, bone and muscle structure may give the erroneous clinical impression that an infant or child is obese. An evaluation of fat disposition also can be obtained by measuring skinfold thickness of the triceps and subscapular area. The triceps muscle, the most widely advocated site for testing, is also the easiest site to use (Marshall et al, 1990). Use of calipers has some disadvantage in that, when measurements are taken by various personnel, a certain amount of error occurs owing to varying techniques and subjective readings.

Nursing Interventions: Prevention and Counseling

During infancy the goal in managing obesity is not to *reduce* the infant's weight but rather to *slow the rate* of weight gain or weight maintenance in an older child. Prevention and management of obesity involve two approaches: an increase in exercise and a reduction in caloric intake. During infancy, certain boundaries determine the types of interventions that are appropriate. The infant's developmental capabilities may limit the type of physical activity to only kicking, creeping, crawling, rolling, and reaching.

Exercises appropriate for the preschooler and early elementary child may include (1) walking, skipping, or jumping from carpet square to carpet square; (2) walking or skipping with a pull toy; (3) pushing a stroller; (4) jumping on a minitrampoline; (5) pushing or kicking a large ball around the room; (6) riding a tricycle or bicycle; (7) swimming or gymnastics; (8) jogging (depending on age and stamina); (9) roller skating; and (10) exercising with a parent as a part of playtime. The older elementary child and middle school child may be encouraged to participate in activities such as (1) soccer, basketball, volleyball, swimming laps; (2) stationary or outdoor bicycling; (3) gymnastics; (4) dance; (5) walking briskly; (6) jumping rope; (7) jogging; (8) roller skating; and (9) exercising with a parent (Schifman & Hannaman, 1989). Parents should be made aware of the importance of providing adequate space and opportunity to engage in such developmentally appropriate exercise. Also, the infant's or young child's high nutritional requirements cannot be overlooked. It is necessary to maintain a level of caloric intake that supports growth and daily energy needs.

Obesity in childhood can adversely affect a child's developing body image and self-esteem. The nurse can make an important contribution in the prevention and management of obesity by helping parents to (1) avoid feeding practices that could contribute to childhood obesity and (2) recognize and correct those patterns of interaction with their child that potentiate the tendency to become obese.

Feeding Practices That Contribute to Infant Obesity

The advantages of breastfeeding to infants are sufficiently established to warrant active encouragement of mothers to breastfeed (Cunningham, 1979, 1986). Although studies do not consistently show that bottlefed infants tend to become more obese than breastfed infants, it has been observed that bottlefed infants gain weight more rapidly (Cunningham, 1979; Fomon, 1974). It has been suggested that bottlefeeding invites the problem of obesity by a caregiver's tendency to encourage an infant to suck until the bottle is empty, whereas in breastfeeding the mother no longer offers the breast when an infant stops sucking (Filer, 1978). Thus, a preventive role of the nurse is to counsel parents who bottlefeed to avoid forcing their infant to empty the bottle at each feeding. Although the protective effects of breastfeeding with respect to obesity have not been proved, breastfeeding should be supported and encouraged. It is not justified, however, to say that breastfeeding prevents obesity.

Introduction of solid foods before 4 to 6 months of age adds extra calories. However, it has not been demonstrated that early introduction of solid foods causes obesity (AAP, 1981a). Parents should be assured that infants before the age of 4 to 6 months do not need the additional calories that solid foods supply. Infants are not developmentally ready for solids until they can sit alone, move their head away, experience a disappearance of the protrusion reflex, and establish lip control, which usually occurs between 4 and 6 months (see Chapter 5). They should particularly be advised against the addition of sugar and other sweets to the infant's diet. In counseling parents about solid foods for their infant, the nurse must recognize that parents start solid foods early for various reasons. Common reasons include a belief that milk does not supply adequate nutrition, social pressure exerted by family and friends, and a belief that giving solid food will cause the infant to sleep through the night (Sherman & Alexander, 1990). Many mothers receive information from their mothers or grandmothers; however, infant feeding guidelines have changed over time. Infant feeding beliefs and practices that were considered true in the 1920s to 1940s may not be currently recommended. The nurse can help families to understand what constitutes normal infant nutrition and assist them to establish healthful feeding practices.

Parental Responses That Contribute to Infant Obesity

The stereotype that a fat baby is a healthy baby is a myth that has been transmitted from one generation to another. These beliefs are deeply rooted in some families and are not easily altered. Overfeeding babies thus can stem from a cultural or familial orientation on the part of parents to "fatten" their babies because it is believed that this is a sign of good parenting. The nurse can work with parents over a period of time, pointing out sufficient positive aspects of their parenting; eventually they can give up the need to overfeed their baby.

The use of food to quiet and satisfy the infant can lead to obesity. To always offer additional breastfeedings or bottlefeedings or solid food to quiet the baby can establish a pattern whereby food is used by the child in response to anxiety rather than in response to hunger. This practice teaches an infant that internal needs can be satisfied by food and institutes a behavior pattern in which all internal tensions are interpreted as indicative of the need for food. Since other parental behaviors also have a significant impact on inappropriate weight gain in early childhood, the nurse must assist the parents to explore other interpretations of their infant's behavior to deter the establishment of an overfeeding pattern (Venter & Mullis, 1984). According to Sherman and Alexander (1990), "bottle propping" is a common practice that adds unneeded calories and reinforces the use of food as a comfort measure. The nurse can suggest alternative methods of responding when the baby cries. Visual stimulation, cuddling, change of position, exercise, or a drink of water may quiet the baby.

Counseling Role of the Nurse

It is believed that the important variable affecting risk of persistence of obesity in infancy is the *severity* of the problem. Weight in excess of 120 per cent of ideal weight in infants who appear fat requires further investigation. This is especially true when obesity is associated with epidemiologic risk factors such as parental obesity, older or single parents, or only children (Dietz, 1984).

Severe dietary restrictions are not recommended for children, but the family may need assistance to calculate recommended dietary intake. If weight is a problem, a closely supervised weight management (pediatric) program under the direction of a doctor or registered dietitian would be recommended. Infants are particularly prone to become obese during the period from 6 months to 1 year of age. As solid foods are added, the nurse should teach parents to check the labels for caloric content and help them to feed according to the caloric needs of their infant. If the daily milk and food intake exceeds the required caloric amount,* water feedings can be used to replace excess caloric intake. Skim milk is not recommended in the diet of an infant under 1 year of age. It has been recommended by some nutritionists that 2 per cent fat milk may be used in the case of severe obesity in older infants (Turkewitz & Bastian, 1986).

The question of whether frequent small feedings are better than three meals a day is not clearly answered. In adults, widely spaced large meals lead to increased serum concentrations of cholesterol and impaired glucose tolerance; the effects of feeding frequency have not been studied as they pertain to infants. The dilution of formula to increase volume intake without increasing caloric intake may not be the correct approach. Moreover, Fomon (1974) suggests that regular consumption of enormous volumes of calorically dilute food is not likely to achieve the goal of developing the habit of eating in moderation.

Although many questions regarding infant obesity remain unanswered, the nurse can play an important role in prevention by using the information that is available. Assisting families to establish healthy feeding practices for their infants and children is a primary role of the nurse. If a family tends to overfeed an infant, the nurse must carefully assess the parents' values and cultural orientation to food, instituting a gradual teaching program whereby parents can learn to relate to their child in a way that fosters eating in moderation.

Severe Protein and Calorie Malnutrition

Marasmus and kwashiorkor are two serious forms of protein and calorie malnutrition. Both are rare in the United States and common in developing countries. However, since 1981, a reduction and modification of supplemental feeding programs has occurred, which has resulted in hunger becoming more widespread in the United States (Brown, 1987). Although substantial improvements have been made regarding children's health in this century, not all groups have benefited equally. Undernutrition and inadequate food intake still exist among low income and several minority populations (Splett & Story, 1991). According to the US Department of Health and Human Services (1989), one of five United States children under 18 years of age lives in poverty. Furthermore, national surveys found that children from low income families are considerably shorter than children from higher income families (Splett & Story, 1991).

A large proportion of children in the world do not get enough to eat, are subjected to poor hygienic conditions, and have inadequate health care; these factors produce malnourishment. The incidence of protein and calorie malnutrition is markedly increased in these areas as a result of repeated bouts of gastroenteritis. Severe protein and calorie malnutrition typically results after an infant is weaned to a grossly inadequate diet. Malnutrition can also result under other circumstances, including metabolic disturbances, chronic renal insufficiency, and maladaptive parent-child relations (nonorganic failure-to-thrive). There have also been reports of malnutrition occurring as a result of a prolonged clear liquid diet in the face of infantile diarrhea (Kaplowitz & Isley, 1979). The nurse has a primary role in teaching families proper and safe administration of fluids typically prescribed for diarrhea to assist in the prevention of such an occurrence.

"Marasmus" is a condition of gradual wasting in the presence of grossly inadequate calories and protein. The caloric deficit is so severe that there is a marked reduction of subcutaneous fat, causing the skin to become wrinkled and loose. This results in an "old man" and "wasted" appearance. The marasmic infant is retarded in growth and development and appears restless, is fretful, and eventually becomes apathetic and listless. A starvation type of diarrhea may further complicate the dehydrated and undernourished state of the infant.

"Kwashiorkor" is primarily a deficiency of protein resulting in severe muscle wasting. It means "deposed child" (i.e., the child who no longer is breastfed because a younger sibling is born). There is also a deficit in calories, but it is the protein deficit that accounts for the principal symptoms (Barness, 1987). The child is usually edematous; this varies in degree from a slight localized edema (primarily eyelids and feet) to a marked generalized edema. When edema is generalized, it may mask the muscle atrophy. Skin changes occur, beginning with erythema and progressing through a sequence of hyperpigmentation, desquamation (peeling), and finally depigmentation (loss of color). During the peeling stage, the skin readily becomes infected; the risk of infection is increased by picking off the desquamating skin (Rudolph, 1982). Another characteristic symptom is the fine, sparse, reddish-tinted hair. Alternating periods of adequate and inadequate dietary intake are mirrored in the streaked hair that results. When dietary intake is adequate, hair is pigmented, and when

*Daily requirements of calories: 1 to 6 months = 108 kcal/kg; 6 to 12 months = 98 kcal/kg.

it is inadequate, it is depigmented. The general depleted nutritional state is frequently further compromised by infections. Most commonly, acute diarrhea, measles, or parasitic infestations precede or accompany kwashiorkor in underdeveloped countries. Children suffering from kwashiorkor become irritable and apathetic and are typically sullen and withdrawn.

Therapeutic Management

These children are in a severe state of nutritional imbalance. The replacement of fluids, electrolytes, and nutrients requires a highly specialized therapeutic approach. Furthermore, many infections either precede the undernourished state or occur as a result of it. Treatment consists of administration of fluids and electrolytes, antibiotic therapy to treat infections, and a gradual dietary rehabilitation.

Nursing Interventions

The nurse has a responsibility to care for the infant and to become actively involved in the process of identifying those factors that led to development of the condition. The nurse must try to prevent infection or reinfection of an already debilitated child, provide meticulous skin care in the presence of edema or skin desquamation, and carefully monitor dietary and fluid intake. Although physical care of the infant is immediate, the nurse must simultaneously begin a careful collection of data and establish a relationship of sensitive interaction with the family to assist in identifying the cause of the malnutrition.

The nurse who cares for infants and families should also make every effort to identify those children with more moderate forms of malnutrition and especially evaluate the nutritional status of those children who show growth retardation and a developmental lag. Although many factors contribute to the problem of malnutrition, the one consistent finding is poverty. The nurse's efforts to educate families in adequate nutritional intake can be most effective if equal importance is given toward increasing availability of food. Studies show a clear relationship between poverty and malnutrition so that it is safe to say "malnutrition when looked for will be found in the poor of every community" (Mauer, 1975; Splett & Story, 1991).

One of the most important roles of the nurse is to participate in the prevention of malnutrition in developed countries.

Carefully managing fluid administration, avoiding prolonged clear fluids, teaching correct preparation of formula, and counseling teen-agers regarding fad diets are areas in which the nurse becomes involved in various settings. Particularly, the management of infant diarrhea at home is an area that requires careful telephone advice and follow-up.

Vitamin D–Deficiency Rickets

Vitamin D deficiency results in poor mineralization of the growing parts of the skeleton, leading to the disease of rickets. Vitamin D–deficiency rickets is most common in children from 4 months to 2 years of age. Vitamin D is required for (1) absorption of dietary calcium and phosphorus from the intestines, (2) conservation of phosphorus by the renal tubular cells, and (3) mobilization of calcium from bone to maintain serum calcium levels when oral intake is inadequate.

The vitamin is supplied by ingestion or through ultraviolet radiation. Sunlight converts a hormone (7-dehydrocholesterol) in the skin to vitamin D_3 (cholecalciferol). Vitamin D_3, whether ingested or synthesized in the skin, must be metabolized into an active form of vitamin D. Biochemical alterations called hydroxylation first occur in the liver, then in the kidneys.

Rickets may be caused by a poor dietary intake of vitamin D or because of lack of exposure to sunlight. African-American children are particularly susceptible to rickets either due to their skin pigmentation or because of inadequate penetration of sunlight (Barness, 1987). Other circumstances that may produce rickets include (1) disorders of absorption in which vitamin D or calcium, or both, are not absorbed; (2) hepatic disease, which may decrease absorption of vitamin D or calcium or interfere with hydroxylation of vitamin D_3; (3) kidney disease, which interferes in the production of active vitamin D; (4) genetic factors, as in familial vitamin D–resistant rickets with hypophosphatemia (discussed in Chapter 44); (5) anticonvulsant therapy (the complication of rickets is a rare occurrence); (6) administration of glucocorticoids (glucocorticoids appear to be antagonistic to vitamin D in calcium transport); or (7) prolonged breastfeeding without vitamin D supplementation or omission of fortified formula (Barness, 1987; Mahan & Arlin, 1992).

Premature infants are especially prone to disturbances in vitamin D metabolism, primarily owing to a lack of sufficient phosphorus and calcium to adequately mineralize the rapidly growing bones. This occurs because, during the last trimester, significant amounts of calcium and phosphorus are transferred daily from mother to fetus. Even with formula feedings, preterm infants receive much less calcium and phosphorus than they would have received in utero (Koo & Tsang, 1987). However, preterm infant formulas have been specially developed to provide more calcium and phosphorus than formulas intended for full-term infants.

Laboratory Findings

A series of physiologic processes account for the typical laboratory findings in rickets. Whether from faulty intake, faulty absorption, or inadequate sunlight, the vitamin D deficiency leads to impaired absorption of calcium and phosphorus, so that these minerals are lost in increasing amounts through urine and feces. Consequently, serum phosphorus concentration is usually lowered; serum calcium level is usually normal* or slightly reduced. Children with rickets also have elevated serum alkaline phosphatase levels. Elevation of this enzyme reflects increased osteoblastic activity. These laboratory findings are apparent before any histologic bone changes are noted.

Clinical Manifestations

An early clinical manifestation of rickets in an infant under 6 months of age is craniotabes. Craniotabes results from a thinning or softening of the skull, usually in the occipitoparietal area. The thin skull bone can be indented by pressing it with a finger, and, on the release of pressure, it rebounds with a crackle like that of a Ping-Pong ball. After the first 6 months, it is more common to see frontal bossing (prominence of frontal and parietal bones) and delayed closure of the fontanels. Rachitic rosary (enlarged costochondral junction) may be palpable in the early stages of rickets and, in later stages, may be seen as well as felt (Barness, 1987).

In later stages of rickets, softening of the bones causes additional skeletal changes. The chest is pigeon-shaped (the sternum protrudes) and a depression is apparent along the lower border of the chest (Harrison groove). This groove is produced by the pull of the diaphragm on the pliable rib structure (Rudolph, 1982). Deformities of the spinal column, including scoliosis, kyphosis, and lordosis, also occur in advanced stages of rickets. In children with lordosis, deformities of the pelvis frequently occur; in the past, such deformities caused dystocia (difficult labor) in women who had had rickets in infancy (Barness, 1987). Also, epiphyseal enlargements at the wrists and ankles can be seen or palpated as a "thickening" in these areas in the early phase of rickets, and later this enlargement becomes even more apparent. The enlarged epiphyses consist of cartilage and uncalcified bone tissue; therefore, they are not visible on an x-ray (Barness, 1987). With weight-bearing, bending of the femur, tibia, and fibula results in bowlegs (genu varum) or knock knees (genu valgum). During development of the legs in infancy and early childhood, a degree of genu varum and genu valgum is normal and should not be mistaken for rickets (see Chapter 6 for further discussion on assessment of the stages of normal development of the legs).

*The serum calcium level may be normal because as serum calcium level is lowered, parathyroid hormone is secreted. Parathyroid hormone mobilizes calcium and phosphorus from the bone, but it increases renal tubular calcium reabsorption. Thus, the serum calcium concentration may ultimately be maintained at a normal level.

Severe vitamin D deficiency can result in certain delays in growth and development. The appearance of the deciduous teeth may be delayed and out of normal progression. The quality of both the deciduous and the permanent teeth may be affected, especially that of the enamel. Poorly developed muscles may be cause for the persisting potbelly (usually a child slims after toddler years) and delayed development in skills such as standing and walking.

Therapeutic Management

Vitamin D–deficiency rickets is treated with the oral administration of vitamin D (1500 to 5000 IU/day). Healing can be demonstrated on x-rays in 2 to 4 weeks after the beginning of treatment (except in vitamin D–resistant rickets) (Barness, 1987). Another method of treatment is to give a beginning single dose of 60,000 IU or 1500 μg of vitamin D. This results in more rapid healing, and the differentiation between vitamin D–deficiency rickets and vitamin D–resistant rickets can be made more rapidly. If no healing occurs, the rickets is probably resistant to vitamin D (Barness, 1987). Once healing is complete, 400 IU or 10 μg (normal daily requirement) of vitamin D is administered daily.

Nursing Interventions: Early Identification Strategies

The nurse has an important role in the assessment of infants and children by contributing to the prevention and early detection of vitamin D deficiency. Although vitamin D deficiency may begin to have biochemical effects in the infant in the first few months of life, visible skeletal changes may not be identified until months later. Also, a newborn infant has some reserves of vitamin D that act as a temporary protection in the event of dietary deficiency, but a history of the early diet is essential to identify those children at risk. The nurse can play a preventive role by recommending vitamin D supplementation for premature infants, artificially fed infants who do not receive vitamin D–fortified formula, and infants who are breastfed. The Committee on Nutrition of the AAP (1980) has recommended that, when the mother's vitamin intake is deficient and the infant's exposure to sunlight is inadequate, infants should receive vitamin D supplementation. The recommended requirement is 10 μg or 400 IU/day. The nurse should particularly assess for vitamin D deficiency in African-American children, who are more vulnerable to development of rickets than are non–African-Americans. It has also been reported that Asian-Americans required longer exposure to ultraviolet radiation to produce a response in vitamin D production that is similar to that of white children (Belton, 1986). Environmental conditions also need to be assessed. Those children who live in heavy smog areas and who have limited opportunity to play outdoors and those living in temperate zones are more prone to vitamin D deficiency.

Complications and Prognosis

The nurse who cares for a child being treated for rickets must be on guard for various complications. Hypocalcemic tetany is a complication of rickets that requires the nurse to make provisions for the occurrence of seizures. If the large-dose (60,000 IU or 1500 μg) vitamin D therapy regimen is used, calcium balance in the body is restored more quickly than when vitamin D is given in moderate daily doses. In any event, if hypocalcemic tetany does occur, it is treated with 5 to 10 ml of 10 per cent calcium gluconate administered intravenously. The nurse involved in such therapy assists in the careful monitoring of the heart rate to prevent bradycardia and cardiac arrest, which can result from too rapid an elevation of serum calcium level. Also, children with rickets are more prone to respiratory infections such as bronchitis or bronchopneumonia, pulmonary atelectasis due to chest deformities, and chronic gastrointestinal disturbances of diarrhea or constipation (Barness, 1987). These potential complications, identified early by the nurse, are important observations that can contribute to early treatment.

Some of the osseous changes that result from rickets may take months or years to disappear. In advanced cases, some permanent alterations may persist. The nurse's role during recovery thus varies according to the severity of the disease but continues to be one of attempting to prevent those complications to which the child is vulnerable, assisting the child and family to a healthy recovery, and preventing a repetition of circumstances that make the child vulnerable to rickets.

Failure-to-Thrive (FTT)

There is no unanimously agreed on definition for "failure-to-thrive" (FTT). The term is used to describe infants and children who fail to gain weight (or even lose weight). It results from the failure to obtain or use the necessary calories required to permit the expected velocity of growth. A parent may be offering insufficient calories because of a knowledge deficit or neglect, or the infant may be rejecting the food or not absorbing it. A weight persistently below the 3rd percentile or 2 standard deviations below the mean on a standard growth chart characterizes the FTT child. However, the National Center for Health Statistics growth charts include only those children above the 5th percentile as being characteristic of the FTT child (NIH Consensus Development Conference on Infantile Apnea and Home Monitoring, 1987).

Failure-to-thrive is a common disorder of infancy; it accounts for 2 to 3 per cent of pediatric tertiary hospital admissions. Its occurrence in the general population is not known. FTT is not actually a diagnosis but the term for a cluster of symptoms occurring concurrently.

Etiology

FTT has traditionally been classified into two categories: organic and nonorganic. A third category, mixed FTT, is now recognized as an entity caused by a combination of organic and nonorganic factors. The three categories used to describe FTT are:

- *Organic FTT* is caused by physical factors such as congenital heart defects, gastrointestinal disorders, renal disease, central nervous system abnormalities, chronic infections, endocrine disorders, chromosomal alterations, or metabolic disorders.
- *Nonorganic FTT* is an absence of history, physical, or laboratory findings that indicate organic disease capable of causing FTT. It is caused by environmental factors that affect the child's intake or use of calories. The problem usually is due to a complex set of interactive patterns between the infant and the caregivers.
- *Mixed FTT* is caused by a combination of organic and nonorganic factors. For example, a child with a cleft lip is unable to suck adequately because of a physical deformity (organic cause). The inability to suck, in turn, can interfere with the mother's feelings of adequacy. She may then stimulate and caress the infant less. The interplay of positive messages and reciprocal play associated with feeding is, therefore, blocked to a degree.

Although FTT may be due to an organic disease, it is most often the result of a disturbance in the relationship between the primary caregiver and the child. The precipitating factors underlying the disturbance are varied (Lobo et al, 1992). Parents may lack information about infant development or nutritional requirements. They may expect responses that conflict with the child's needs, development, and abilities. For example, some young parents are disappointed to discover their baby does not "love" them, as they expected, but instead demands a lot of time and attention that they are unprepared to give. The infant may be the product of an unwanted, unplanned, or stressful pregnancy. The child's birth may have been a difficult natural one or by cesarean section. The infant's appearance or temperament may be displeasing to the parents. The baby may have been premature or have some birth-associated illness or congenital defect. The parents, especially the mother, may have been separated from the infant after delivery for a period complicated by anxiety and uncertainty about the infant's prognosis.

Historically, FTT has been classified as a form of child neglect caused by maternal deprivation. Recently, it has been suggested that FTT is a separate pediatric illness and that the traditional view of FTT, as exclusively parentally induced, must be abandoned (Bithoney & Newberger, 1987). It is now recognized that the phenomenon of nonorganic FTT is a complex interplay of multiple constitutional and environmental factors involving the caregivers, the infant, and their interactions (Lobo et al, 1992). Thus, FTT could be explained within the human ecologic model of child maltreatment. Explanations that identify factors in the infant, the caregiver, and the family supersede the earlier view that FTT is caused by either medical illness or psychologic deprivation. According to Lieberman and Birch (1984), FTT is "rooted in a specific transactional impasse between the infant and caregiver." Caregivers and the infant contribute to the impasse.

The term "maternal deprivation" has been interpreted by some professionals as unloving intentional neglect. It is now understood that a mother's inability to provide the nurture required by an infant may occur because the mother has been deprived (Gagan, 1984). Mothers may be depressed or anxious because of overconcern for the child. A husband's lack of support exacerbates mother's feeling of being overwhelmed (Gagan, 1984; Karl, 1991). Furthermore, either parent may come from a background in which supportive communication patterns were undeveloped. The support of one another during the stress of child care demands is lacking within the family. A family with poor communication skills and weak social supports may be further compromised by job instability and poor living conditions. Although FTT in middle class families is well documented, it is more common in lower economic status families. Feelings of helplessness experienced by these families are often grounded in overwhelming socioeconomic conditions (Gagan, 1984).

Certain infant personalities also contribute to the impasse. They appear to fall into two extreme categories. They are described as irritable, fussy, and colicky or as passive and unresponsive. Either of these two temperaments can create negative relationships between the infant and the caregiver. The dynamics between a particular dyad (i.e., "the fit") affects the success of the relationship. The failure in the dyad is not caused by one person; rather, it develops because of the characteristics of each person. For example, an irritable infant and a tense parent reinforce each other's behavior, resulting in a negative, tense relationship devoid of a positive interactive style. Similarly, a lethargic child interacting with a depressed parent results in a deficient interaction. On the other hand, an interactive infant can engage a depressed parent and an apathetic infant can be engaged by a more active parent.

Clinical Manifestations and Diagnostic Assessment

The clinical manifestations of an infant or child with FTT can range from extreme cachexia and developmental delay to an apparently healthy-appearing infant. If weight and height are proportionately delayed, FTT may not be apparent unless a growth chart is used to evaluate the child's progress. What appears to be a healthy 9-month-old infant may be a 15-month-old child failing to thrive. Physical and behavioral indicators of potential FTT are listed in Table 16–18.

FTT is a complex problem. Diagnosis is usually made by a multidisciplinary team, involving a nurse, physician, social worker, nutritionist, psychologist, and occupational therapist. In the past, diagnostic assessment focused on a search for an organic cause of FTT. This approach is "diagnosis by exclusion." Another approach is to make a "diagnosis by response," in which the infant is fed and nurtured. If weight gain occurs, the cause is considered to be nonorganic (Powell, 1987). Currently, research is being done to identify specific behaviors that could distinguish nonorganic FTT from organic FTT infants. Specific behaviors identified by Powell (1987) that differentiate organic FTT from nonorganic FTT were (1) lack of motor activity in response to stimuli, (2) lack of smile in response to stimuli, (3) general inactivity, and (4) abnormal gaze.

Nursing Care

Data collection should include the prenatal history (including the circumstances of the pregnancy), perinatal course, feeding history, and the child's growth and development. Assessment of family functioning, including communication patterns, is essential. Since

TABLE 16–18
Indicators of Potential Failure-to-Thrive

Physical Indicators
Weight below the 3rd percentile
Sudden or rapid deceleration in the growth rate
Delay in developmental milestones
Muscular hypotonia
Decreased muscle mass
Generalized weakness
Abdominal distention
Behavioral Indicators
Avoiding eye contact
Intense watchfulness
Avoidance of physical contact with other people
Repetitive self-stimulating behaviors (e.g., rocking, head banging, head rolling, and intense sucking)
Disturbed affect (e.g., excessive irritability, apathy, or extreme compliance)
Sleep disturbances
Lack of age-appropriate stranger anxiety
Inappropriate lack of preference for parents

TABLE 16–19
Diagnostic Approaches to Rule Out Organic Disease in Failure-to-Thrive Children

Diagnostic	Purpose/Rule Out
Initial Screening	
Physical examination	R/O congenital defects; data base and measurements on admission
Denver Developmental Screening Test (DDST) (see Appendix XX)	Establish relation to developmental milestones
Tuberculin test	R/O tuberculosis
Bone survey radiographs of long bones, joints, skull	R/O old or recent fractures; establish bone age; check epiphyseal development
Anterior/posterior and lateral chest film	R/O pulmonary disease
Urinalysis	R/O urinary tract infection (UTI); diabetes
CBC and differential	R/O anemia, chronic or systemic infection
Sweat test	R/O cystic fibrosis
Stool testing;	R/O mono- and disaccharide deficiency
Reducing substance and pH	R/O milk intolerance
Occult blood	R/O internal bleeding
Ova and parasites	R/O parasitic infestation
Further Studies (When Indicated, Based on History or Failure to Gain in Hospital)	
Repeat DDST; Bayley or psychometrics	R/O mental retardation; prescribe activities for development
Detailed urinalysis: culture, 24 hr catecholamines	R/O UTI; metabolic defects
Stool testing:	
72-hr fecal fat	Malabsorption
D-xylose test culture	Infection
PBI and T4	Hypothyroidism
Electrocardiogram; cardiac catheterization	R/O cardiac anomalies; circulatory defects
Upper and/or lower GI radiography	R/O dysphagia; anatomic abnormalities; internal injuries
Intravenous pyelogram	R/O urinary tract abnormalities; internal injuries
Biopsy: bowel, muscle	R/O Hirschsprung disease; congenital muscular dystrophy; celiac disease

parents of FTT infants often feel inadequate, the nurse must use sensitivity and empathetic interviewing skills to elicit the assessment data. The nurse should remember that a thorough history may eliminate unnecessary laboratory testing. However, environmental FTT should not be assumed without sufficient data. Table 16–19 describes tests commonly performed to identify organic causes. Care should be taken not to order laboratory tests that would deprive the child of food for a period of time.

Special assessment is made of the infant's sucking technique. FTT may be caused by an actual deficit in nutrient intake because of ineffective sucking at the breast or bottle. (See Table 4–6 for a summary of principles related to a proper latch-on and positioning for breastfeeding.) If breastfeeding or bottlefeeding is not successful, the mother, infant, and dyad are assessed to determine the cause (Tables 16–20 and 16–21).

The infant should be observed interacting with her or his primary caregiver in feeding situations and in play situations, as well as observed interacting with a stranger, such as the nurse (Bithoney & Rathbun, 1983). Rosenn and colleagues (1980) developed a behavioral scale to quantify brief social interactions between the infant and the examiner. They found that the approach-withdrawal behaviors of infants between 6 and 16 months of age were useful in distinguishing organic and nonorganic FTT. This scale needs further testing in the clinical area. Within 24 hours of admission, a Denver Developmental Screening Test should be done to determine the child's level of development. Ongoing documentation of the child's activity level and the infant-parent dyad is required to make a diagnosis.

The nurse's documentation of ongoing assessment is essential and should be done regularly and thoroughly. Important aspects to document about the infant-parent interaction include:

- The ways in which the child is held and fed and how eye contact is initiated by the primary caregiver(s); the facial expressions of the child and caregiver during interactions.
- What the caregiver does with the child—play, talk, hold, stroke—and the child's response.

TABLE 16-20
Factors That Interfere with Effective Breastfeeding

Factors	Significance
The Mother	
Inadequate diet, owing to dieting or inadequate intake	A marginal diet may affect the ability to nourish an infant and the quantity of milk supply
Fatigue	Most common cause of reduced milk production May inhibit letdown
Lack of confidence, stress Husband or relative disapproves of breastfeeding Stress of other life events, i.e., demands of job, family	Known to inhibit letdown reflex Lack of confidence in adequate milk supply can lead to introduction of formula and early introduction of solids
Pain, owing to episiotomy, incision, sore nipples	Inhibits the letdown reflex
Difficult birth	May lead to delay in initial early feeding and limited length and frequency of feeds An exhausted mother may mean an exhausted infant and poor sucking
Pain medication given in labor and delivery	May suppress infant, reducing effective sucking and early initiation to breastfeeding
Medications	
Oral contraceptives	Combined estrogen and progestin and high estrogen dose formulations appear to be associated with decreased milk production
Some diuretics	May decrease milk production
Ergot derivative (Bromocriptine)	Inhibits prolactin secretion
Pyridoxine (vitamin B_6)	Some evidence that excessive doses may have inhibiting effect on lactation
Diazepam (Valium)	Excreted into breastmilk and associated with infant weight loss, lethargy, prolonged hyperbilirubinemia
Decongestants and antihistamines	May decrease milk production
Nicotine	May interfere with letdown May inhibit milk production by reducing prolactin levels
Alcohol	Large doses may partially inhibit the letdown reflex
Caffeine	Large doses may inhibit lactation
Breast surgery, which severs ducts or nerves in the periareolar region or 5 o'clock (left) or 7 o'clock (right breast) position	Reduces the stimulation to the hypothalamus, which reduces milk production and inhibits letdown reflex
Pregnancy	A reduced milk supply has been reported anecdotally
Hormonal deficiencies, such as hypothyroidism, antepartum estrogen deficiencies	Can result in reduced milk production
The Baby	
Poor sucking, owing to lethargic or medicated infant, Down syndrome, anoxia, hyper- or hypotonic infant	Leads to ineffective nipple stimulation and poor milk extraction
Illness, such as congenital heart disease, jaundice, infection, cystic fibrosis, otitis media, urinary infection, hypothyroidism	Leads to lethargy and fatigue and ineffective and less frequent sucking
Oral-facial deformities Cleft lip and palate Tongue tie (rare) Tumors of mouth	Ineffective sucking reduces nipple stimulation and ability of baby to "milk" the breast for adequate nourishment
Pacifiers	May cause nipple confusion. Delay use if possible until lactation is well established

(continued)

TABLE 16-20
Factors That Interfere with Effective Breastfeeding *(Continued)*

Factors	Significance
The Dyad	
Limited length of feeding, particularly short feedings in first days postpartum	Reduces amount of nipple stimulation Reduces emptying of milk from glands required to reduce the pressure from milk in the glands and encourage production of more milk. Neonates need 30–40 min feeds
Reduced frequency of feeding such as 4-hr feeds, lack of rooming-in facilities	Reduces amount of nipple stimulation and emptying of milk
Improper positioning	Decreased *effective* nipple stimulation; decreased extraction of milk; causes pain, bleeding, cracked nipples
Formula or water supplements, including formula samples distributed in hospital	Reduces thirst or hunger in infant, therefore reducing amount and frequency of effective nipple stimulation May cause nipple confusion in infant, leading to ineffective sucking at breast Reduces mother's confidence in her ability to supply milk Gives mixed message from health professionals regarding the importance of breastfeeding
Extended separation from mother, such as baby in NICU, baby not brought to mother at night for feedings, ill mother, etc.	Reduces length and frequency of feedings
Feeding from one breast	May be inadequate nipple stimulation

Prepared by Ruta Valaitis, BScN, BA, MHSc, Clinical Nursing Consultant and Lecturer, School of Nursing, McMaster University, Hamilton, Ontario

- Whether the caregiver talks about the child at all, and, if so, how the child is referred to. This is an indicator to others of how the caregiver perceives the child.
- The responses of the caregiver to the child's cues. For example, what is the mother's response when the child looks at her, cries, reaches toward her?
- The response of the child to the caregiver's overtures, the child's reaction to the mother's feeding rate and the way the child is being held. What the nurse should be looking for is synchrony or disharmony and, specifically, how this occurs.

The basic care is the same as for any child of similar age but it may take more time, especially for feeding, with extra attention given to holding the child, cuddling, eliciting eye contact, and helping parents feed their infant.

Special attention must also be given to monitoring the child's physical status. The nurse records the number, character, color, and consistency of the stools; the stools may be tested for occult blood and for reducing substances. (If the infant is malabsorbing, sugar will be present in the stool.) The pH of the stool is checked. (Less than 5.5 means that acid is present, which results when sugar breaks down into acids.) The child is weighed at the same time each day, under similar conditions. An accurate record of intake and output, including weighing the diapers, is kept. The nurse is responsible for monitoring the intake and keeping a calorie count of the food actually ingested. Calorie intake is increased above the usual recommended amounts. A referral is made to the nutritionist to plan the diet so that the child will have an optimal intake for "catch-up growth" without overfeeding.

Developmental activities appropriate for age are provided, with special attention given to motor and social deficits. The nurse may be responsible for such developmental programs or involve other team members, such as a child life worker and occupational therapist.

The caregiver may need "re-parenting" in those areas in which there is dysfunction. The nurse "mothers the mother" by providing emotional nurturing. This is often done most effectively through role modeling, demonstration, and positive reinforcement of the caregiver's mothering efforts by the infant's primary nurse. This re-parenting can sometimes be done even better by a foster grandmother, who may be less threatening than the nurse and nearer to the age of the mother's own mother. The parent who is not functioning well may be referred to a psychiatric social worker or psychiatrist for more intensive intervention. Social service benefits may also be required and should be explored by a social worker, according to the family's needs.

TABLE 16-21
Factors That Interfere with Effective Bottlefeeding

Factors	Significance
The Mother	
Anxiety related to care of infant or to other life stresses	Baby picks up anxious feelings from tensions in mother's approach, arms, and movements and becomes uncomfortable
Fatigue	May not provide sufficient attention or time to allow for infant to receive adequate intake
The Baby	
Poor sucking related to lethargy, medication, Down syndrome, anoxia, hyper- or hypotonic infant illness	Infant gets tired and stops sucking before an adequate amount of milk has been received
Oral-facial deformities	Inefficient sucking may occur, making it impossible for baby to get sufficient calories
Cleft lip and palate, tongue tie (rare)	
Lack of molding of infant's body to mother's body	A baby who does not cuddle readily makes it difficult to position the bottle to provide adequate intake
Technique	
Characteristics of the nipple	Hard nipples with small openings require a stronger infant suck to get the milk; the baby may become tired or frustrated and give up; soft nipples with large openings may make the infant gag or choke because the milk is received too quickly
Opening too large or small, nipple too hard or soft	
Fluid level in the bottle	As the fluid level decreases, the angle of the bottle must be decreased to prevent air from being sucked into the stomach, which causes discomfort for the infant
Temperature of formula or milk	Infants drink best if the fluid is at the same temperature at each feeding
	Fluid that is too hot may burn the mouth or esophagus
	Room temperature or slightly above is best (if heating, test on inside of wrist before beginning to feed)
The Dyad	
Lack of reciprocal messages of pleasure and comfort	Sounds, touch, and eye contact make the feeding experience pleasurable for both mother and infant; if these do not accompany the feeding, less pleasure is associated with eating and infants may stop because of boredom
Tensions between the infant and caregiver	A cycle of tension is created, and if the feeding is not completed, the mother does not encourage the infant to do so

In spite of all the nurse's anticipatory guidance and tact, parents may feel threatened, particularly if the child improves during hospitalization when no treatment other than feeding, nurturing, and stimulation has been provided. They need to have their insecurity alleviated and their self-esteem built up as they succeed in caring for the child. The nurse can point out their healthy behaviors specifically and the responses by the child. The parents can learn playfulness, joy, and laughter responses to their child.

The nurse can listen to the mother and help her work through her negative feelings that have disrupted healthy interactions with the child. The nurse can help allay her feeling of guilt regarding the diagnosis and reinforce healthful changes for the present and future. The mother's partner or spouse and relatives also may need guidance in relating to the child in ways that support the mother's self-esteem as an individual and as a parent. The Nursing Process Plan for the care of an infant with FTT (Table 16–22) provides specific nursing interventions.

The most frequently diagnosed human *response* in the child with FTT is *altered growth and development*. Among the *related factors or etiologies* are insufficient intake of calories, incomplete absorption of nutrients, other organic conditions that interfere with growth, and problematic child/caregiver interactions. Others are listed in Table 16–22. The defining characteristics include delay or difficulty in performing skills (motor, social, or expressive) typical of age group; altered physical growth; inability to perform self-care or self-control activities appropriate for age; flat affect; listlessness; and decreased responses.

TABLE 16-22

Nursing Care for the Child with Failure-to-Thrive (FTT)

Analysis: Nursing Diagnostic Statement

Response and Related or Risk Factors: *Altered growth and development: failure to thrive, related to*

- Insufficient intake of calories
- Incomplete absorption of nutrients
- Other organic condition that interferes with growth
- Problematic child/caregiver interactions associated with poor "fit" between child/caregiver temperaments
- Inadequate caregiving
- Knowledge deficit about development/child care needs
- Environmental and stimulation deficiencies
- Family stress in excess of family strengths and available support
- Multiple caregivers

Projected Outcome: The child will experience normal growth and development for age and sex.

Nursing Interventions

Nutritional Monitoring

Help to identify exact cause of failure-to-thrive

- Assess for physical alterations. Conduct baseline physical examination upon admission; continue to assesss for additional manifestations and changes in baseline assessment. Note especially changes in physical status related to feeding (e.g., fatigue, respiratory distress, colic-type behavior). Note character of body secretions (vomitus, stool, urine). Conduct tests as appropriate (e.g., Hematest, Clinitest, pH)
- Assess parent child/interactions. Note eye contact, facial expressions, whether interactions seem comfortable and pleasurable for child and parent or appear awkward and mechanical, interactions between parents, between parents and other family members or extended family. Document behaviors, not interpretation of behaviors, e.g., "Mother reads a book while feeding child," not "Mother does not seem interested in child." Determine primary caregiver (may be extended family member, not a parent). Encourage caregiver to talk about life with the child, major stresses, personal strengths, social support. Give permission to voice negative, as well as positive, feelings by such comments as, "This must be very difficult for you." "Sometimes parents feel they are being blamed for their child's failure to grow. Do you feel this way?" "Tell me what you enjoy most about your child." "Being a parent can be very stressful; what things have been most difficult since your child was born?" "Does parenthood feel like you thought it would?"
- Assess child's feeding patterns. Note sucking, food preferences, attention to eating, avoidance behaviors

Nutritional Management

Increase caloric intake

- Initially assess tolerance to age-appropriate food (i.e., ability to retain/absorb nutrients)
- If organic cause determined, institute appropriate alterations in feeding as indicated and as ordered. Prepare discharge plan; support family in adjusting to the diagnosis and teach them appropriate care for the child at home
- If cause undetermined or nonorganic, increase intake as tolerated (diagnosis by response). Feed on demand or at least every 3–4 hrs for infant. For toddler or older child, offer nutritious high-protein snacks between meals and small portions of a variety of foods at mealtime

TABLE 16-22 (continued)

- Steadily increase amount ingested per feeding (this may take several days; the child's stomach capacity may be small at first). Encourage the infant to take more than a few sucks or the child to eat more than a few bites. Gradually increase intake with each feeding
- Teach child healthy mealtime behaviors. With fingers on cheeks and under chin, gently but firmly help infant with poor suck obtain better suction on the nipple. Decrease distraction during mealtime; close door to room, turn off television, discourage interruptions by other health care professionals by posting sign outside door. Make mealtime an unhurried, pleasant experience. Provide consistent nursing care whenever possible. (Lack of consistency will confuse and frustrate the child who is trying to learn new behaviors)
- Ensure that caloric intake is greater than caloric expenditure. Plan for and facilitate naps. Intervene for crying, fretfulness. Avoid tiring infant or small child with successive interventions or therapies
- Monitor intake and weight gain. Record intake and output. Record calories ingested if appropriate. Weigh at same time each day on same scale with the same clothing (e.g., nude, diaper, or underwear)

Parent Education: Childbearing Family

Provide opportunities to practice developmental tasks

- Provide social stimulation. Talk to child during caregiving activities, attempt to elicit smile and other age-appropriate responses. Approach children with respect for their mistrust of or lack of enthusiasm for adult interactions (allow them to view you from outside their personal space). Document responses to social interactions.
- Provide opportunities to practice motor tasks. (Interesting surroundings and the opportunity for gross motor activities are usually sufficient to elicit progress in the child who has been previously deprived.) Head control and upper arm strength can be improved by placing the infant on the abdomen. If this is an unfamiliar position, the child may protest; in this case, introduce the position gradually with the distraction of toys or with the child closely attended. Strength of lower limbs can be enhanced by a walker and by placing a mobile at a level in the crib to encourage kicking. Provide play experiences for the toddler and preschooler to enhance developmental skills. Consult with the child life worker so he or she will be involved in the child's care

Role model appropriate adult/child interactions

- Talk to infant or child, initiate playful interactions. Let parent see that nurse finds the child attractive and enjoys the interactions. (Parent may also need to see that the nurse finds it appropriate to talk to an infant or young child and that the child can respond)
- Role model feeding behaviors and activities to promote motor development

Provide instruction to address identified knowledge deficit

- Include instructions with role modeling, e.g., "Babies learn to talk by listening to the people in their family. Johnnie's cooing is the first step in learning to say a word."
- Explain the developmental crisis of that age child in lay terms, giving examples of the difficulties persons might have if they did not develop a greater sense of trust than of mistrust or a greater sense of autonomy than of shame and doubt. Provide information about development in small segments, talking only about that which is pertinent for this child. (Initially, this information may seem too theoretical to apply.) Use as many different forms of materials as are available, e.g, videotapes, written brochures (to accommodate various learning styles)
- It is helpful to adopt the attitude that this parent has not had the *opportunity* to learn healthy parenting behaviors, rather than to assume the parent's behavior is willful. (Nurses' attitudes will be displayed in nonverbal, if not in verbal, ways. Belittling the parent will close communications and thwart all future teaching attempts)

(continued)

TABLE 16-22 *(continued)*

Shape parental behavior by concentrating on the positive

- Praise (appropriately and sincerely) any positive bonding or caring behaviors. Praising the positive can illustrate for the parent the desired behavior while increasing parental self-esteem. A parent with increased self-esteem has additional strength to deal with life stress, including the tasks of parenting
- Praise the parent in the presence of the spouse, significant other(s), and extended family members. The primary caretaker may use the nurse's validating comment to support self-esteem or the new parenting behavior in the presence of criticism from others

Encourage as much parental involvement in care as is practical. (This will enhance the caregiver's self-confidence and provide a means for evaluation.) Some units have policies that state that the primary caregiver must stay with and care for the child for a specified length of time before discharge. Enlist the help of the physician and the social services department in ensuring follow-up home visits for this family

Nursing interventions for the child with FTT should be directed to the etiology, if possible. For example, if the child's FTT is due to inadequate caregiving, the nurse will focus interventions on how to assure that the caregiver is able to give optimal care to the child. Nursing interventions that would be appropriate for most children with FTT are found in Table 16–22. Because the cause of FTT is often unclear initially, these interventions will deal with undifferentiated FTT (i.e., not diagnosed as either organic or nonorganic).

The evaluation plan for determining whether the interventions have been successful in meeting the projected outcome, "normal growth and development for age and sex," would be evidenced by a decrease or absence of the defining characteristics.

Parenteral Nutrition (Hyperalimentation)

Adequate nutrition in hospitalized patients is an important factor in prompt recovery from injury or illness. When nutritional integrity cannot be maintained by oral or tube feedings, parenteral nutrition (or hyperalimentation) is indicated. This therapy provides part or all of the necessary nutrients by the intravenous route. When all necessary nutrients are provided by the parenteral route, this is referred to as total parenteral nutrition (TPN). To administer parenteral nutrition safely, the nurse must be aware of the child's nutritional requirements, the composition of the solution, the indications for parenteral nutrition, the implications for nursing care, and the potential complications of the therapy.

Nutritional Requirements

Under normal conditions, children ingest enough calories and protein to meet the body's needs for energy and growth. However, the spontaneous oral intake of a sick child may be inadequate to meet the body's demands, and the child may enter a catabolic state. This destructive process can be halted by the administration of carefully prescribed parenteral nutrition. The parenteral nutrition infusate (the solution being administered) can supply the child with protein (as crystalline amino acids), carbohydrate (as glucose), electrolytes, vitamins, and minerals. Fat, or lipid emulsions, that can be administered along with the parenteral nutrition solution supplies necessary fatty acids. Fat is very important as an energy source; without it, energy requirements in the young child on peripheral parenteral nutrition cannot be met. Estimation of metabolic (energy) requirements includes the calculation of basal metabolic rate (kcal/day) and the allotment of additional calories for the child's specific condition. For example, simple trauma entails a 20 per cent increment in metabolic rate, and burns may increase the rate by as much as 50 to 100 per cent, depending on the extent of thermal injury (Seashore, 1984). Other conditions that increase energy requirements include surgery, sepsis, and fever. Average energy requirements for parenterally fed infants and children are as follows (Zlotkin et al, 1985):

Premature neonates: 90 kcal/kg/day.
Infants 0 to 1 year: 80 to 95 kcal/kg/day.
Children 2 to 9 years: 60 to 70 kcal/kg/day.
10 to 13 years: 50 to 60 kcal/kg/day.
Adolescents: 40 kcal/kg/day.

Amino acid requirements for the same group are (Zlotkin et al, 1985):

Premature neonates: 3.0 g/kg/day.
Infants 0 to 1 year: 2.5 g/kg/day.
Children 2 to 9 years: 1.5 to 2.0 g/kg/day.
10 to 13 years: 1.5 to 2.0 g/kg/day.
Adolescents: 1.0 to 1.5 g/kg/day.

Infants, children, and adults need 4, 3, and 2 g/kg/day of fat, respectively (Seashore, 1984).

Composition of Parenteral Nutrition Solutions

Amino acid solutions contain the eight known essential amino acids plus histidine, which is known to be essential for children. Dextrose (glucose) is the most important nonprotein energy source used in parenteral solutions. Trace minerals, vitamins, and electrolytes are added to base solutions. The concentration of any constituent can be changed to meet individual needs.

Parenteral nutrition may be administered through a peripheral vein or a central vein, often the superior vena cava. The amount of dextrose to be infused is limited by the location of the intravenous catheter and the tolerance of the child and the vein to the solution. The child's tolerance is measured by serum and urine glucose levels. Hypertonic parenteral nutrition is initiated slowly, and the rate and concentration of dextrose are gradually increased to allow the pancreas to respond to the increased demand for insulin (Testerman, 1989). Solutions with dextrose concentrations greater than 12.5 per cent must be infused centrally, where the rapid blood flow can dilute the solution and thereby decrease vein irritation (Testerman, 1989). A child with a central venous catheter can receive up to 25 to 47 per cent dextrose, although these high percentages are rarely necessary if lipids can also be used. The maximal final concentration of dextrose administered through a peripheral vein is 12.5 per cent; however, adequate calories cannot be obtained with solutions of 12.5 per cent dextrose or less that are administered at conventional rates. Therefore, the calories provided by fat emulsions are especially important to those receiving peripheral parenteral nutrition.

Fat or liquid emulsions are manufactured from either soybean or safflower oil, stabilized with egg phospholipid, and made isotonic with glycerol. A 10 per cent solution yields 1.1 kcal/ml, and a 20 per cent solution yields 2.0 kcal/ml (Haas-Beckert, 1987). The development of lipid emulsions makes possible adequate caloric intake in a small volume of fluid. The fat emulsion is nearly isotonic, having minimal osmotic pressure; therefore, it may be infused in either peripheral or central veins. By infusing the fat emulsion simultaneously with the dextrose and amino acid solution, the osmolality of the total infusate is decreased. Fat emulsions are also given to prevent essential fatty acid deficiency.

Electrolytes, vitamins, and trace elements are also included in the parenteral nutrition infusate. Electrolytes include potassium, sodium, chloride, calcium, phosphorus, and magnesium. Electrolyte requirements are determined by the serum levels. Daily basic electrolyte requirements must be met, along with the additional needs resulting from such factors as the particular disease process or surgery. Water- and fat-soluble vitamins are given to the child routinely. Some of these vitamins may be added to the infusate. Trace element requirements for infants are still being determined; school-age children and adolescents usually receive trace elements in the solution two or more times a week. The trace elements that may be added to parenteral nutrition are zinc, copper, iodide, chromium, selenium, and manganese (Testerman, 1989).

The dextrose, amino acids, electrolytes, vitamins, and trace elements are mixed in one container by a pharmacist. This is done under a laminar air flow hood to decrease the risk of contamination. The fat emulsion is administered from a separate container because the addition of any other solution could disrupt the stability of the emulsion.

Indications for Parenteral Nutrition Administration

Parenteral nutrition is indicated when nourishment by mouth is inadequate. A child may be malnourished, or a prolonged period without enteral feedings may be anticipated. Before parenteral nutrition is chosen, the indications for each child must be weighed against the potentially life-threatening complications related to parenteral nutrition. The child's age, current nutritional status, and clinical status also should be considered. For example, the neonate, especially the premature neonate, has minimal nutritional reserves, so parenteral nutrition may be necessary sooner than in the older child.

Clinical conditions in the neonate and infant that may necessitate the use of parenteral nutrition include major anomalies of the gastrointestinal tract, intractable diarrhea, necrotizing enterocolitis, immune deficiency, very low birthweight (less than 1000 g), and severe respiratory problems that interfere with ingestion. Indications for toddlers and older children are similar to those for adults: inflammatory bowel disease, short bowel syndrome, Crohn disease, prolonged ileus, fistulas, severe burns, major trauma, acute pancreatitis, acquired immunodeficiency syndrome (AIDS), renal failure, hepatic failure, and oncologic conditions.

Nursing Responsibilities in the Administration of Parenteral Nutrition

Nursing care to prevent complications of parenteral nutrition includes careful administration and monitoring of the solution and meticulous care of the catheter.

Administration

The parenteral nutrition solution must be administered at a constant rate to avoid potential metabolic complications. The infusion rate is never adjusted to "catch up." An infusion pump is essential for administration with hourly monitoring of the infusion. Abrupt cessation of 25 per cent glucose infusion may lead to profound hypoglycemia and seizures (Seashore, 1984). To prevent this occurrence, the nurse must assure the patency of the catheter, maintain secure connections in the line, and assure an adequate supply of the parenteral nutrition solution.

The bag, IV administration tubing, and filter (if used) must be changed every 24 hours to prevent infection. Frequently, the practice is to place the sterile extension tubing partly under the dressing so it is changed only with the dressing change. Prior to opening connections in the tubing system, they must be cleansed with an antiseptic solution to prevent yeast and bacterial growth. After reconnecting the joints, they are taped to prevent accidental separation.

Whenever a fat emulsion is being infused, it must be added aseptically below the filter because the fat particles are too large to pass through the filter. It should be added as close to the intravenous site as possible so there is minimal mixture of the two infusates. The practice of administration of fat emulsions varies. Some administer fat and parenteral nutrition into the same central or peripheral line, whereas others administer fat emulsions into a separate peripheral line.

Some drugs are compatible with the amino acid/dextrose/mineral component of parenteral nutrition solutions, but not with the lipid emulsion (Zlotkin et al, 1985). The practice of administering drugs, other IV fluids, and blood products into the same intravenous site as parenteral nutrition varies but is generally limited to patients in whom venous access is severely limited. Even in necessary cases, these interruptions compound the problem of inadequate nutrition. See Chapter 26 for a discussion of central venous access insertion, catheter types, and related nursing care.

Monitoring

The nurse must carefully monitor the child receiving parenteral nutrition. General appearance, level of activity, sense of well-being, and skin turgor are noted (Seashore, 1984). Blood pressure, pulse, respirations, and temperature must be recorded at least every 4 hours. Temperature is especially important since an increase is one of the first signs of catheter-related sepsis. An accurate daily intake and output record must be maintained to assess fluid balance. The record should indicate the type of intake and output, so that calorie and nitrogen intake and output can be determined. A diaper count may suffice for the urine output after the neonate or infant is stable on parenteral nutrition. Urine sugar/acetone fractional levels and specific gravity are checked at least every 6 to 8 hours. Glucosuria of 2^+ or greater must be corrected to prevent eventual development of hyperosmotic nonketotic coma. Dextrostix or Chemstix should be used to check the blood sugar every 4 to 8 hours upon initiation of parenteral nutrition and whenever the infusion is suddenly decreased or stopped. Daily weights are obtained, and the length and head circumference of infants are measured once a week.

Laboratory assessment includes complete blood count, blood urea nitrogen (BUN), glucose, and electrolytes daily for the first 3 or 4 days, then once or twice a week. Bilirubin, serum glutamic-oxaloacetic transaminase (SGOT), alkaline phosphatase, and ammonia levels are measured once a week (Seashore & Hoffman, 1983). Determination of serum lipid concentration should be performed frequently in children receiving fat emulsions.

Oral Hygiene

Oral hygiene is a very important but often forgotten part of nursing care. Oral hygiene must be performed at least three times a day to prevent such complications as oral lesions and parotitis and to promote comfort. Brushing teeth to prevent tooth decay is important for all children and especially for those children who are allowed to eat hard candy during parenteral nutrition administration. Different-flavored mouthwashes may be offered to the child to provide some taste sensations.

Exercise

Exercise is important to maintain or regain muscle strength. Unless contraindicated, the child should be encouraged to move freely with proper protection for the peripheral or central IV line. Physical or occupational therapists can recommend appropriate exercises for bedridden children.

Emotional Needs

Depriving a child of food can have a significant emotional impact on the child and the family. The necessity and importance of parenteral nutrition therapy must be carefully explained to everyone. The reasons for the monitoring done by the nurses and physicians and the importance of avoiding dislodgement of the IV catheter must be explained to both the child and the family. The explanation given to the child depends on the age and level of understanding. The neonate who receives nothing by mouth (NPO) needs a pacifier so that sucking needs are met. Also, the infant should be held at regular intervals because of not being held routinely for meals.

Older children also need special care during the administration of parenteral nutrition. Since some children still feel hungry even when receiving adequate parenteral nutrition, they need extra attention or distraction during mealtimes and when they see food or food advertisements. Many of these children have chronic illnesses, and, consequently, they are hospitalized for a long time. Family members are not always able to be present, so these children need extra attention from the nursing staff.

Home Parenteral Nutrition

Since nutritional support is often required over a long time, home nutritional support services have been instituted. The need for long-term therapy, experience with the technique of parenteral nutrition, and improvements in equipment contributed to the transition of using parenteral nutrition at home.

A key factor in the institution of home parenteral nutrition was the development of a Silastic catheter in the early 1970s (Broviac et al, 1974; Riella & Scribner, 1976). This catheter was very flexible and did not harden with extended use; theoretically, it could be used indefinitely (Vargas et al, 1987). A Luer-Lok at the end of the catheter made it possible to fill it with heparin and cap it when not in use. A cuff at midpoint was used to anchor the catheter to the subcutaneous tissue, preventing its dislodgement—an important feature for home use. A variety of catheters are now on the market, and they all have these key features.

A final important step contributing to sending a child home on parenteral nutrition was the realization that a child's complete nutritional needs could be administered over an 8- to 12-hour infusion period if the patient was gradually introduced to such a routine (Vargas et al, 1987). This practice enables children to attend school and other daytime activities. The daily nighttime infusion is often stressful to parents because of the daily commitment at a specific time that is required of the family.

Home parenteral nutrition is used either as a temporary measure or as a means of lifelong nutritional support. Vargas and colleagues (1987), in a report on 102 patients, stated that the average patient received home parenteral nutrition for nearly 2 years, 8 received home parenteral nutrition for more than 5 years, and 4 for a decade. The nutritional status of children on home parenteral nutrition and the numerous associated complications are areas of ongoing research (Dahlstrom et al, 1985; Merritt, 1986; Vargas et al, 1987). It is speculated that bowel transplantation may be a technique to eventually obviate the need for lifelong use of home parenteral nutrition (Vargas et al, 1987).

In some cases, parenteral nutrition is the *only* source of nutrition, that is, total parenteral nutrition (TPN), whereas in others, parenteral nutrition is supplemented with enteral nutrition. It is believed that enteral intake stimulates bile flow, therefore, it reduces the risk of cholestasis, gallstone formation, and liver disease (Postuma & Trevenen, 1979; Farrell & Balistreri, 1986).

Even small enteral feedings to interrupt the complications associated with fasting have been suggested, particularly in the care of low birthweight infants (Merritt, 1986). The nutritional value of enteral feedings, however, is affected by the amount of absorption that takes place in a particular child. The actual amount of absorption is often overestimated (Vargas et al, 1987). Consequently, long-term weight gain and growth have been reported to be best in children who receive 90 per cent or more of their nutrition parenterally (Dahlstrom et al, 1985).

Nursing Interventions: Support of Children on Home Parenteral Nutrition

Home assessment and management of a child on parenteral nutrition is a role often assumed by nurses. Nurses in acute care centers, outpatient clinics, or agencies may be called upon to provide consultation to the family with a child on home parenteral nutrition. A Nursing Process Plan of potential problems and issues that families encounter is presented in Table 16–23.

Enteral Nutrition

"Enteral nutrition" refers to the provision of food intake via the digestive tract, whether by mouth or by tube (Eschieman, 1991). Frequently, enteral nutrition is used synonymously with tube feedings. Oral feedings are the most palatable method of meeting nutritional needs of the pediatric client. However, certain medical conditions may warrant dietary modifications to meet the nutritional needs of the child. Dietary modifications of the amounts of the nutrients within the diet may be adjusted to meet the requirements of the pediatric client with special needs (e.g., diabetes, hypertension, and phenylketonuria). It is imperative that the adjustments of these nutrients be monitored carefully so that growth and development can be promoted.

Enteral Oral Feedings

Energy and protein intake may be increased by increasing food portions and adding extra snacks of high caloric density. For some pediatric clients, it may be easier to drink liquids than to chew solid foods. Specially prepared high-protein milkshakes, beverages, and puddings may be used to add more protein and kilocalories. Medium-chain triglyceride (MCT) oil may be added to the diet to replace additional kilocalories if fat malabsorption is present. Some commercially prepared formulas, such as Pregestimil, are available containing MCT oil (Whitney et al, 1991). Oral vitamin and mineral supplements may also be required for certain conditions. Usually, it is recommended that these vitamin and mineral supplements be mixed with an isotonic formula prior to administration to the infant because of the risk of adverse ef-

TABLE 16-23

Nursing Process Plan: Care of Children on Home Parenteral Nutrition

Analysis: Collaborative Problem 1

Response and Related or Risk Factors: *High risk for injury: physiologic, hyperglycemia or hypoglycemia; risk factors*

- Excessive administration of glucose

Projected Outcome: The child's nutrient intake will be appropriate for metabolic needs

Defining Characteristics *(Actual Response)*	Nursing Interventions	Evaluation Criteria
Hyperglycemia *Subjective:* • Nausea • Weakness • Headache • Increased thirst • Polyuria • Increased frequency of urination **Hypoglycemia** *Subjective:* • Sweating • Acute fatigue • Restlessness • Seizure activity • Irritability **Hyperglycemia and Hypoglycemia** *Objective:* • Urine positive for glucose	*Total Parenteral Nutrition (TPN) Administration* Administer the correct amount of glucose for the individual child *Teaching: Procedure Treatment* Instruct family: • How to infuse the correct solution at the correct rate • To maintain a constant flow rate • To avoid rapid increases in the rate of delivery of parenteral nutrition solution even if the solution is behind the prescribed rate • Give family an instruction manual containing the correct procedure and rate required to maintain a correct balance of glucose • Teach family to recognize signs and symptoms of hyperglycemia and hypoglycemia (this will reduce potential for complications from hyperglycemia or hypoglycemia) • Instruct family that if signs and symptoms of hyperglycemia or hypoglycemia occur, the physician or home health nurse should be notified immediately • Obtain feedback and return demonstrations from family member(s) caring for parenteral nutrition to assure what was learned is correct and safe • Refer family to home health nurse for regular monitoring of techniques and concerns	**Child does not experience** nausea, headache, weakness, or increased thirst, remains generally active, has normal urinary output, and does not exceed renal threshold for glucose **Child does not experience** sweating, acute fatigue or irritability, and remains calm

TABLE 16-23 (continued)

Analysis: Nursing Diagnostic Statement 1

Response and Related or Risk Factors: *High risk for infection; risk factor*

- Presence of intravenous parenteral infusion

Projected Outcome: Child will not experience infection as a result of parenteral nutrition

Defining Characteristics *(Actual Response)*	Nursing Interventions	Evaluation Criteria
Subjective: • Chills • Diaphoresis • Lethargy and weakness in the child *Objective:* • Pyrexia of >38.5°C or 101.3°F • Redness, drainage, or odor at the catheter exit site	*Teaching: Prescribed Procedure/Treatment* **Provide an instruction manual for family** **Instruct child and parents in** • Aseptic techniques • Catheter care • Dressing change • Capping of catheter when not in use • Handling and storage of parenteral nutrition solution and tubing • Preparing total parenteral nutrition infusion system • Attachment of infusion system to catheter • Proper disposal of equipment, solutions, and sharps **Reduce potential for complications from an infection** • Instruct parents and child about early signs and symptoms that indicate an early infection (see Defining Characteristics)	**Child's skin is warm and dry with a body temperature above 38.5°C** **Child will:** • Be active and energetic • Remain free from infection at the site of catheter as evidenced by no redness, drainage or odor at the exit site of catheter

(continued)

TABLE 16-23 *(continued)*

Analysis: Nursing Diagnostic Statement 2

Response and Related or Risk Factors: *High risk for ineffective family coping, (compromised); risk factors*

- Ineffective support or encouragement in the face of care demands. Resultant fatigue associated with home parenteral nutrition

Projected Outcome: Child and family will experience adaptation to the challenging tasks associated with home parenteral nutrition

Defining Characteristics *(Actual Response)*	***Nursing Interventions***	***Evaluation Criteria***
Subjective: • Child's expression of concern or complaint that parent is preoccupied and does not respond helpfully to the child's situation *Objective*: • Parents display protective behavior disproportionate to the child/family's abilities and need for autonomy • Parents withdraw, entering into limited or temporary personal communication with the child at the time of need • Parents describe or confirm an inadequate understanding or knowledge base, which interferes with effective assistive or supportive behaviors • Parents attempt assistive or supportive behaviors with less than satisfactory results	*Coping Enhancement* • Try to understand the perspective of the family members who are having difficulty coping • Acknowledge the family's experience of fatigue as an expected normal process (acceptance encourages further discussion of problem) • Explore the individual's usual methods of coping and teach additional coping strategies if indicated • Suggest to the family that another significant person learn the correct procedure of home parenteral nutrition to give the family occasional relief (other than one who is preoccupied) • Refer the parents to a parent support group if one is available • Encourage parents to take time for their own relationship • Identify and/or refer parents to groups that can assist in the care of their child while they take time for themselves • Help family members to identify changes in relationships that are a result of the demands of the child's care • Encourage family members to seek seek help in adjustment to change in family process and roles of family members that results when child requires home parenteral nutrition. Be prepared to make appropriate referrals • Use *role enhancement* to assist family members to adapt to changes in roles	**Child/family receive support from significant other as evidenced by mastery of tasks and skills**

TABLE 16-23 *(continued)*

Analysis: Nursing Diagnostic Statement 3

Response and Related or Risk Factors: *High risk for altered growth and development; risk factors*

- Multiple caretakers
- Restrictions dependency
- Reduced stimuli prescribed by chronic illness and hospitalization

Projected Outcome: Reduce risk for child to deviate in growth and development norms for age

Defining Characteristics *(Actual Response)*	Nursing Interventions	Evaluation Criteria
Subjective: • Delay in skill performance (motor, social, or expressive) compared with age group: altered physical growth; altered self-care and self-control abilities; altered social responses (flat affect, listlessness, and reduced response) *Objective:* • Physical growth below the 50th percentile • Inability to achieve skills according to age level • Altered social responses showing lack of emotion, energy, and alertness	*Teaching: Prescribed Activity/Exercise* • Explain and show child and family what activities he or she can or cannot participate in with PN catheter in place (often families believe restrictions on activity are more severe than they really are) *Parent Education: Childrearing Family* • Assist parents to provide developmentally appropriate activities for child • Assist parents to recognize and deal with typical coping mechanisms used most by children in the child's developmental stage • Refer to occupational therapy and physiotherapy for assistance as appropriate • Provide consistent school programs during hospitalization or home-bound period to maintain school performance	**Growth and development is maintained within normal limits compared to age group as evidenced by:** • Achievement of skills according to age level • Physical growth at or above 50th percentile • Social responses evidencing emotion, energy, and alertness

fects such as increased gastric residuals and regurgitation (Mahan & Arlin, 1992).

Enteral Tube Feedings

When the nutritional needs of the pediatric client are unable to be met by oral intake alone, enteral tube feeding may be required. Enteral tube feedings are preferred over parenteral feedings whenever the digestive and absorptive capabilities of the gastrointestinal tract are still functional. Fewer complications are associated with enteral tube feedings than with parenteral alimentation. In addition, enteral feedings are more cost-effective than parenteral nutrition. Furthermore, gastrointestinal immunologic and physiologic functions are maintained with enteral nutrition (Mahan & Arlin, 1992).

Characteristics of Formulas

Occasionally, commercial formulas are recommended for the pediatric client. These formulas may be consumed orally or via tube feedings. Enteral formulas are classified into two basic categories: incomplete and complete. "Incomplete formulas" may also be referred to as "modular formulas"; they contain specific nutrients and are used as supplements. "Complete formulas" are those that provide all of the nutrients necessary to meet the client's needs when given in sufficient quantities. Formulas can also be classified as intact or hydrolyzed. "Intact formulas" are those that contain complete molecules of carbohydrates, protein, and fats. Intact formulas are given to the pediatric client who is able to digest and absorb nutrients without difficulty. "Hydrolyzed formulas" are composed of broken down molecules of carbohydrates, proteins, and fats. Hydrolyzed formulas are referred to as being "predigested," and they therefore require "minimal" further digestion. Formulas containing hydrolysates are used with those pediatric clients who have limited digestive capabilities or a smaller-than-normal surface area for absorption (Whitney et al, 1991).

When selecting a formula for the pediatric client, it is important to consider the osmolality or concentration of the formula. A formula whose osmolality is close to the concentration of blood serum is known as an "isotonic formula." If a formula is more concentrated than the blood serum, this formula is referred to as "hypertonic." When this type of formula is present in the intestinal lumen, water tends to be drawn from the surrounding capillaries into the intestine, leading to fluid losses. This occurrence is of particular importance when working with the infant. Therefore, it is essential to consider the relative fluid intake and fluid losses in relation to the renal solute load of the concentrated feeding to ensure that positive water balance is maintained (Mahan & Arlin, 1992).

Method of Enteral Tube Feeding

One method of enteral tube feeding is nighttime supplementation. This type of tube feeding allows children to obtain nutrients by continuous infusion without interfering with the child's daily activity. These feedings are usually regulated with a pump and are given over a 4- to 8-hour period (Mahan & Arlin, 1992). Nasogastric or gastrostomy tube feedings are a frequent method of tube feedings used with children. Oral gastric gavage feedings are frequently used with infants, since infants are obligatory nose-breathers. A newer device known as the "gastrostomy button" may also be used with the pediatric client. This newer method of enteral tube feeding has proved to be more beneficial than conventional methods of enteral tube feedings (Huddleston & Palmer, 1990) (see Chapter 35).

Intermittent bolus feedings may also be used with the pediatric client. The intermittent feedings should infuse over a minimum of 20 minutes. The amount of formula to infuse varies in accordance with the size of the infant or child. The type of feeding method used depends on the rationale for which the feeding tube is needed, the functional capability of the gastrointestinal tract, and the age of the pediatric client (see Chapter 35 for nursing care of the child/infant with gastric tube feedings).

KEY CONCEPTS

Concepts Related to Basic Information

- Health status is enhanced by lifelong adequate nutritional intake.
- Nutritional practices developed during early childhood and adolescence will usually continue throughout life.

Concepts Related to Nursing Assessment

- The nurse is an active participant in the ongoing assessment of nutritional status of the child/adolescent and the family.
- The nurse's skills in the process of nutritional assessment and counseling are critical since the nurse may, in many instances, be the primary or sole caregiver for the child/adolescent and the family.

Concepts Related to Nursing Intervention

- Implementation of nutritional interventions during childhood should incorporate the use of a multidisciplinary team approach.
- The nurse's role in the multidisciplinary team approach is critical since the primary participant in direct contact with the child/adolescent and their family may be the nurse.
- The responsibility of the nurse includes the promotion of healthful dietary practices through counseling and teaching.

REFERENCES

Alhadeff, L., Gualtier, C. T., & Lipton, M. (1984). Toxic effects of water-soluble vitamins. *Nutrition Reviews, 42*(2), 33–40.

Allen, L. H. (1990). Functional indicators and outcomes of undernutrition. *Journal of Nutrition, 120,* 924–932.

American Academy of Pediatrics, Committee on Nutrition. (1976). Commentary on breastfeeding and infant formula. *Pediatrics, 57,* 278–285.

American Academy of Pediatrics, Committee on Nutrition. (1988). Indications for cholesterol testing in children. *AAP News, 4,* 7.

American Academy of Pediatrics, Committee on Nutrition. (1981a). Nutritional aspects of obesity in infancy and childhood. *Pediatrics, 68,* 880–883.

American Academy of Pediatrics, Committee on Nutrition. (1985). *Pediatric nutrition handbook* (2nd ed.). Elk Grove Village, IL: Author.

American Academy of Pediatrics, Committee on Nutrition. (1986). Prudent lifestyle for children: Dietary fat and cholesterol. *Pediatrics, 78*(3), 521.

American Academy of Pediatrics, Committee on Nutrition. (1981b). Sodium intake of infants in the United States. *Pediatrics, 68,* 444–445.

American Academy of Pediatrics, Committee on Nutrition. (1983). Toward a prudent diet for children. *Pediatrics, 71,* 78–80.

American Academy of Pediatrics, Committee on Nutrition. (1980). Vitamin and mineral supplementation needs in normal children in the United States. *Pediatrics, 66,* 1015.

American Dietetic Association. (1988, July). Position paper on the vegetarian approach to eating. *Journal of the American Dietetic Association,* 61–68.

Anderson, J. W. (1983). Plant fiber and blood pressure. *Annals of Internal Medicine, 98,* 842–846.

Barness, L. A. (1987). Nutrition and nutritional disorders. In R. E. Behrman, & V. C. Vaughn (Eds.). *Nelson textbook of pediatrics* (13th ed.). Philadelphia: WB Saunders.

Beauchamp, G. K., et al. (1983). Modification of salt and taste. *Annals of Internal Medicine, 98,* 763–769.

Behrman, R. E. (1992). *Nelson textbook of pediatrics* (14th ed.). Philadelphia: WB Saunders.

Belton, N. R. (1986). Rickets—not only the "English disease." *Acta Paediatrica Scandinavica* (Suppl), *323,* 68–75.

Birch, L. (1987). The role of experience in children's food acceptance patterns. *Journal of the American Dietetic Association, 87*(9, Suppl), 536–540.

Bithoney, W. G., & Newberger, E. H. (1987, February). Child and family attributes of failure-to-thrive. *Journal of Developmental and Behavioral Pediatrics, 8,* 32–36.

Bithoney, W. G., & Rathbun, J. M. (1983). Failure to thrive. In W. B. Levine, et al (Eds.). *Developmental-behavioral pediatrics.* Philadelphia, WB Saunders.

Brazelton, T. B., et al. (1974). The origins of reciprocity. In M. Lewis & L. Rosenbaum (Eds.). *The effects of the infant on its caregiver.* New York: Ivan Wille and Sons.

Broviac, V. W., et al. (1974). A silicone rubber atrial catheter for prolonged parenteral nutrition. *Surgery, Gynecology, and Obstetrics, 136,* 602–608.

Brown, J. L. (1987, February). Hunger in the U.S. *Scientific American, 256*(2), 37–41.

Burtis, G., Davis, J., & Martin, S. (1987). *Applied nutrition and diet therapy.* Philadelphia: WB Saunders.

Chandra, R. K. (1981). Nutritional deficiency, immune function and susceptibility to infection. In D. L. Yeung (Ed.). *Essays on pediatric nutrition* (pp 137–153). Ottawa: Canadian Public Health Association.

Committee on Dietary Allowances, Food and Nutrition Board, National Research Council. (1989). *Recommended dietary allowances* (10th ed.). Washington, DC: National Academy of Sciences.

Creasy, R. K., & Resnik, R. (1984). *Maternal-fetal medicine; principles and practice.* Philadelphia: WB Saunders.

Cunningham, A. S. (1979). Morbidity in breast-fed and artificially fed infants II. *Journal of Pediatrics, 95,* 685–689.

Cunningham, A. S. (1986). Breast-feeding and health. *Journal of Pediatrics, 110,* 658–659.

Dahlstrom, K. A., et al. (1985). Nutritional status in children receiving home parenteral nutrition. *Pediatrics, 107,* 219–223.

DeBruyne, L. K., & Rolfes, S. R. (1989). *Life cycle nutrition: Conception through adolescence.* St. Paul: West Publishing.

Dietz, W. H. (1984). Obesity in infancy. In R. B. Howard, & H. S. Winter (Eds.). *Nutrition and feeding of infants and toddlers* (pp 297–307). Boston: Little, Brown.

Dietz, W. H. (1986). Prevention of childhood obesity. *Pediatric Clinics of North America, 33,* 823–833.

Dietz, W. H., & Gortmaker, S. L. (1985). Do we fatten our children at the TV set?: Obesity and television viewing in children and adolescents. *Pediatrics, 75,* 807.

Diplock, A. T. (1987). Trace elements in human health with special reference to selenium. *American Journal of Clinical Nutrition, 45,* 1313–1322.

Dobbing, J. (1984). Infant nutrition and later achievement. *Nutrition Reviews, 42*(1), 1–7.

Eschieman, M. M. (1991). *Introductory nutrition and diet therapy* (2nd ed.). Philadelphia: JB Lippincott.

Excess water administration and hyponatraemic convulsions in infancy. (1992, January 18). *Lancet, 339,* 153–154.

Farrell, M. K., & Balistreri, W. F. (1986). Parenteral nutrition and hepatobiliary dysfunction. *Clinics in Perinatology, 13,* 197–212.

Feingold, B. F. (1975). *Why your child is hyperactive.* New York: Random House.

Filer, L. J. (1978). Early nutrition: Its long-term role. *Hospital Practice, 13*(2), 87–95.

Fomon, S. J. (1974). *Infant nutrition* (2nd ed.). Philadelphia: WB Saunders.

Fomon, S. J., & Ziegler, E. E. (1976). Prevention of obesity. In *Nutritional disorders of children* (No. [HSA] 78–5104). Washington, DC: US Department of Health, Education, and Welfare.

Fox, J., & Elsberry, C. (1980). *Primary health care of the young.* New York: McGraw-Hill.

Gagan, R. J. (1984). The families of children who fail to thrive: Preliminary investigations of parental deprivation among organic and non-organic cases. *Child Abuse and Neglect, 8,* 93–103.

Garn, S. M., & Clark, D. C. (1975). Nutrition, growth, development, and maturation: Findings from the Ten-State Nutrition Survey of 1968–1970. *Pediatrics, 56,* 306–319.

Glueck, C. J., et al. (1978). Value and safety of diet modification to control hyperlipidemia in childhood and adolescence. *Circulation, 58*(2), 381a–384a.

Golden, M. P., et al. (1983). Obesity and socioeconomic class in children and their mothers. *Journal of Developmental and Behavioral Pediatrics, 4*(2), 113–118.

Green, M. L., & Harry, J. (1981). *Nutrition in contemporary nursing practice.* New York: John Wiley & Sons.

Haas-Beckert, B. (1987). Removing the mysteries of parenteral nutrition. *Pediatric Nursing, 13,* 237–241.

Hellebostad, T., et al. (1985). Vitamin D deficiency rickets and vitamin B_{12} deficiency in vegetarian children. *Acta Paediatrica Scandinavica, 74,* 191–195.

Horan, M. J., et al. (1987). Report of the Second Task Force on Blood Pressure Control in Children. *Pediatrics, 79,* 1–25.

Howe, P. S. (1981). *Basic nutrition in health and disease (including selection and care of food).* Philadelphia: WB Saunders.

Huddleston, K. C., & Palmer, K. L. (1990). A button for gastrostomy feedings. *MCN: American Journal of Maternal Child Nursing, 15*(5), 315–319.

Hughes, J. G., & Griffith, J. F. (1984). *Synopsis of pediatrics* (6th ed.). St. Louis: CV Mosby.

Jones, D. Y., Neshelm, M. C., & Hableht, J. P. (1985). Influences in child growth associated with poverty in the 1970's: An examination of HanesI and HanesII cross-sectional US national surveys. *American Journal of Clinical Nutrition, 42,* 714–724.

Kaplowitz, P., & Isley, R. B. (1979, September). Marasmus-kwashiorkor in an 8-week-old infant with prolonged clear liquids for diarrhea. *Clinical Pediatrics, 18,* 5–75.

Karl, D. (1991). The consequences of maternal depression for early mother-infant interaction: A nursing issue. *Journal of Pediatric Nursing, 6*(6), 384–390.

Klein, M. J. (1990). The home health nurse clinician's role in prevention of nonorganic failure to thrive. *Journal of Pediatric Nursing, 5*(2), 129–135.

Koo, W. W. K., & Tsang, R. C. (1987). Calcium and magnesium homeostasis in the newborn. In G. B. Avery (Ed.). *Neonatology: Pathophysiology and management of the newborn* (3rd ed.). Philadelphia: JB Lippincott.

Krieger, I. (1982). *Pediatric disorders of feeding, nutrition and metabolism.* New York: John Wiley & Sons.

Lieberman, A. F., & Birch, M. (1984). The etiology of failure to thrive: An interactional developmental approach. In D. Drotari (Ed.). *New directions in failure to thrive: Implications for research and practice.* New York: Plenum Press.

Lipton, M. A., & Mayo, J. P. (1983). Diet and hyperkinesis—An update. *Journal of the American Dietetic Association, 83,* 132.

Lobo, M. L., Banard, K. E., & Coombs, J. B. (1992). Failure to thrive: A parent-infant interaction perspective. *Journal of Pediatric Nursing, 7*(4), 251–261.

MacLean, W. C., & Graham, G. (1982). *Pediatric nutrition in clinical practice.* Reading, MA: Addison-Wesley.

Mahan, L. K., & Arlin, M. (1992). *Krause's food, nutrition and diet therapy* (8th ed.). Philadelphia: WB Saunders.

Marshall, J. P., et al. (1990). Comparison of convenient indicators of obesity. *American Journal of Clinical Nutrition, 51,* 22–28.

Mauer, A. M. (1975). Malnutrition—still a common problem for children in the United States. *Clinical Pediatrics, 14*(1), 23–24.

McBurney, M. I., et al. (1987). Colonic carcinogenesis: The microbial feast or famine mechanism. *Nutrition and Cancer, 10,* 23–28.

Merritt, R. J. (1986). Cholestasis associated with total parenteral nutrition. *Journal of Pediatric Gastroenterology and Nutrition, 5,* 9–22.

National Academy of Sciences. (1989). *Recommended dietary allowances* (10th ed.). Washington, DC: National Academy Press.

National Institutes of Health Consensus Development Conference on Infantile Apnea and Home Monitoring. (1987). *Pediatrics, 79*(2), 292–299.

National Institutes of Health Consensus Development Conference Statement. (1985). Health implications of obesity. *Annals of Internal Medicine, 103*(6), 1073–1077.

Nieman, D. C., Butterworth, D. E., & Nieman, C. N. (1992). *Nutrition* (rev. 1st ed.). Dubois, IA: William C. Brown.

Owen, G. M., et al. (1974). A study of nutritional status of preschool children in the United States, 1968–1970. *Pediatrics, 53,* 597–646.

Pearson, G. A. (1977, November/December). Nutrition in the middle years of childhood. *MCN: American Journal of Maternal Child Nursing, 2*(6), 378–384.

Pellet, P. L. (1990). Protein requirements in humans. *American Journal of Clinical Nutrition, 51,* 723–737.

Pipes, P. L. (1989). *Nutrition in infancy and childhood* (4th ed.). St. Louis: CV Mosby.

Postuma, R., & Trevenen, C. L. (1979). Liver disease in infants receiving total parenteral nutrition. *Pediatrics, 63,* 110–115.

Powell, G. F. (1987, February). Behavior as a diagnostic aid in failure to thrive. *Journal of Developmental and Behavioral Pediatrics, 8*(1), 18–24.

Reddy, B. S. (1976). Dietary factors and cancer of the large bowel. *Seminars in Oncology, 3,* 351.

Riella, M. C., & Scribner, B. H. (1976). Five years' experience with a right atrial catheter for prolonged parenteral nutrition at home. *Surgery, 143,* 295–301.

Rolfes, S. R., & DeBruyne, L. K. (1992). *Life-span nutrition: Conception through life.* St. Paul: West Publishing.

Rosenn, D. W., et al. (1980). Differentiation of organic from non-organic failure to thrive syndrome in infancy. *Pediatrics, 66,* 38, 42, 689–704.

Roy, C. C., & Galeano, N. (1985, April). Childhood antecedents of adult degenerative disease. *Pediatric Clinics of North America, 32,* 517–533.

Rudolph, A. (1982). *Pediatrics.* New York: Appleton-Century-Crofts.

Rudy, D. A. (1984, September/October). Vegetarian diets for children. *Pediatric Nursing, 10*(5), 329–333.

Schifman, V., & Hannaman, K. N. (1989). Cholesterol; A practical teaching plan for children and adolescents. *Issues in Comprehensive Pediatric Nursing, 12,* 359–369.

Seashore, J. H. (1984, May). Nutritional support of children in the intensive care unit. *Yale Journal of Biology and Medicine, 57*(2), 111–134.

Seashore, J. H., & Hoffman, M. (1983, October). Use and abuse of peripheral parenteral nutrition in children. *Nutritional Support Services, 3*(10), 8–13.

Sherman, J. B., & Alexander, M. A. (1990). Obesity in children: A research update. *Journal of Pediatric Nursing, 5*(3), 161–167.

Sigman-Grant, M. (1992). Feeding preschoolers: Balancing nutritional and developmental needs. *Nutrition Today, 27,* 13–17.

Solomons, N. W., & Allen, L. A. (1983). Functional assessment of nutritional status: Principles, practice, and potential. *Nutrition Reviews, 41,* 33–50.

Sparkman, A. F., et al. (1988). Tools to measure sensory appeal of menus planned for children. *Journal of the American Dietetic Association, 88*(4), 488–491.

Splett, P. L., & Story, M. (1991). Child nutrition: Objectives for the decade. *Journal of the American Dietetic Association, 91*(6), 665–668.

Stanfield, J. P. (1982). The influence of malnutrition on development. *Practitioner, 226,* 1929–1940.

Story, M., & Brown, J. E. (1987). Sounding board: Do young children instinctively know what to eat? *New England Journal of Medicine, 316*(2), 103–106.

Testerman, E. J. (1989). Current trends in pediatric total parenteral nutrition. *Journal of Intravenous Nursing, 12*(3), 152–162.

Turkewitz, D., & Bastian, C. (1986). Infant and child nutrition: Controversies and recommendations. *Nutrition, 79*(2), 151–164.

US Department of Agriculture, Human nutrition information service. (1992, August) Leaflet No. 572.

US Department of Health and Human Services. (1989). *Child health USA '89.* Washington, DC: Bureau of Maternal and Child Health and Resources Department.

US Department of Health, Education, and Welfare. (1972). *Ten-State nutrition survey* 1968–1970. (DHEW Publication No. [HSM] 72–8130). Washington, DC: Centers for Disease Control.

Vargas, J. H., et al. (1987). Long-term home parenteral nutrition in pediatrics: Ten years of experience in 102 patients. *Journal of Pediatric Gastroenterology and Nutrition, 6,* 24–32.

Venter, M., & Mullis, R. (1984). Family-oriented nutrition education and preschool obesity. *Journal of Nutrition Education, 16*(4), 159–161.

Whitney, E. N., Cataldo, C. B., & Rolfes, S. R. (1991). *Understanding normal and clinical nutrition* (3rd ed.). St. Paul: West Publishing.

Zlotkin, S. H., Stallings, V. A., & Pencharz, P. B. (1985, April). Total parenteral nutrition in children. *Pediatric Clinics of North America, 32*(2), 381–400.

BIBLIOGRAPHY

Ament, M. E., & O'Connor, M. J. (1985). Long-term cognitive development of children raised on home total parenteral nutrition. *Clinical Research, 32,* 96A.

American Academy of Pediatrics, Committee on Nutrition. (1986). Fluoride supplementation. *Pediatrics, 77,* 758–761.

Arnold, W. C. (1990). Parenteral nutrition, and fluid and electrolyte therapy. *Pediatric Clinics of North America, 37*(2), 449–461.

Berg, C. L., Swanson, D. J., & Juhl, N. (1992). Total blood cholesterol and contributory risk factors in an adolescent population. *Journal of School Health, 62*(2), 64–66.

Berger, R., & Adams, L. (1989). Nutritional support in the critical care setting (Pt. 1). *Chest, 96*(1), 139–150.

Berger, R., & Adams, L. (1989). Nutritional support in the critical care setting (Pt. 2). *Chest, 96*(2), 372–380.

Berry, R. K., & Jorgensen, S. (1988). Growing with home parenteral nutrition: Maintaining a safe environment. *Pediatric Nursing, 14*(2), 155–157.

Birch, L. L. (1992). Children's preferences for high-fat foods. *Nutrition Reviews, 50*(9), 249–255.

Birch, L. L., et al. (1991). The variability of young children's energy intake. *New England Journal of Medicine, 324*(4), 232–235.

Bithoney, W. G. (1986). Elevated lead levels in children with nonorganic failure to thrive. *Pediatrics, 78*(5), 891–895.

Blatz, S., & Paes, B. A. (1990). Intravenous infusion by superficial vein in the neonate. *Journal of Intravenous Nursing, 13*(2), 122–128.

Buckner, M. M. (1990). Perioperative nutrition problems. *Critical Care Nursing Clinics of North America, 2*(4), 559–566.

Bull, N. L. (1992). Dietary habits, food consumption, and nutrient intake during adolescence. *Journal of Adolescent Health, 13,* 384–388.

Burson, J. Z., & Brannigan, N. (1984). The use of play in the nutritional support of hospitalized children. *Issues in Comprehensive Pediatric Nursing, 7,* 283–289.

Burt, B. A., & Ismail, A. I. (1986, December). Diet, nutrition, and food cariogenicity. *Journal of Dental Research,* [Special issue], *65,* 1475–1484.

Cady, C., & Yoshioka, R. S. (1991). Using a learning contract to successfully discharge an infant on home total parenteral nutrition. *Pediatric Nursing, 17*(1), 67–71.

Carlin, A., & Walker, W. A. (1991). Rapid development of vitamin K deficiency in an adolescent boy receiving total parenteral nutrition following bone marrow transplantation. *Nutrition Reviews, 49*(6), 179–183.

Chandra, R. K. (1987, June). Nutrition and immunity: Practical applications of research findings. *Canadian Family Physician, 33,* 1417–1420.

Contento, M. (1981). Children's thinking about food and eating—a Piagetian-based study. *Journal of Nutrition Education* (Suppl.), *13*(1), 86–90.

Cooper, A. (1982). Nutritional assessment of the pediatric patient. *American Journal of Clinical Nutrition* (Suppl), *35,* 1132–1141.

Curtis, J. A., et al. (1983, January 15). Nutritional rickets in vegetarian children. *Canadian Medical Association Journal, 128,* 150–152.

Dagnelle, P. C., et al. (1989). Increased risk of vitamin B-12 and iron deficiency in infants on macrobiotic diets. *American Journal of Clinical Nutrition, 50,* 818–824.

Davis, S. S. (1983, March). A nutritional education program for preschool children. *Journal of Nutrition Education, 15*(1), 4–5.

Drotar, D., & Sturm, L. (1988). Prediction of intellectual development in young children with early histories of nonorganic failure-to-thrive. *Journal of Pediatrics, 13*(2), 281–296.

Edwards, L. D., & Saunders, R. B. (1990). Symbolic interactionism: A framework for the care of parents of preterm infants. *Journal of Pediatric Nursing, 5*(2), 123–128.

Ellerstein, N. S., & Ostrov, B. E. (1985, February). Growth patterns in children hospitalized because of caloric-deprivation failure to thrive. *American Journal of Diseases of Children, 139,* 164–166.

Farris, R. P., et al. (1992). Nutrient contribution of the school lunch program: Implications for Healthy People 2000. *Journal of School Health, 62*(5), 180–184.

Ferraro, A. R., & Huddleston, K. C. (1991). Safe administration of small-volume enteral feedings: An alternative to intravenous pumps. *Journal of Pediatric Nursing, 6*(5), 352–354.

Finberg, L. (1990). Modified fat diets: Do they apply to infancy? *Journal of Pediatrics, 117,* S132–133.

Foltin, R. W., et al. (1990). Caloric compensation of lunches varying in fat and carbohydrate content by humans in a residential laboratory. *American Journal of Clinical Nutrition, 52,* 969–980.

Fomon, S. J., et al. (1979). Recommendations for feeding normal infants. *Pediatrics, 63,* 52–59.

Forsyth, B. W. C., et al. (1985, March). Mother's perception of problems of feeding and crying behaviors. *American Journal of Diseases of Children, 139,* 269–272.

Frank, D., & Zeisel, S. (1988). Failure to thrive. *Pediatric Clinics of North America, 35*(6), 1187–1206.

Frappier, P. A., Marino, B. L., & Shishmanian, E. (1987). Nursing assessment of infant feeding problems. *Journal of Pediatric Nursing, 2*(1), 37–44.

Fredrickson, J. M. (1990). Overview of advanced life support for pediatric patients. *Journal of Emergency Nursing, 16*(1), 17–24.

Galler, J. R., et al. (1984). The influence of early malnutrition on subsequent behavioral development. IV. Soft neurologic signs. *Pediatric Research, 18,* 826–832.

Gans, D. A. (1991, May/June). Sucrose and unusual childhood behavior. *Nutrition Today,* 8–14.

Gardner, S. L., & Hagedorn, M. I. (1991). Physiologic sequelae of prematurity: The nurse practitioner's role. Part V. Feeding difficulties and growth failure. *Journal of Pediatric Health Care, 5,* 122–134.

Gates, D. M., & McClure, M. J. (1989). Forestalling the progress of heart disease. *MCN: American Journal of Maternal Child Nursing, 14,* 174–178.

Gortmaker, S. L., Dietz, W. H., & Cheung, L. W. Y. (1990). Inactivity, diet, and the fattening of America. *Journal of American Dietetic Association, 90*(9), 1247–1252.

Greene, H. L., et al. (1988). Guidelines for the use of vitamins, trace elements, calcium, magnesium, and phosphorus in infants and children receiving total parenteral nutrition: Report of the Subcommittee on Pediatric Parenteral Nutrient Requirements from the Committee on Clinical Practice Issues of The American Society for Clinical Nutrition. *American Journal of Clinical Nutrition, 48,* 1324–1342.

Gutcher, G., & Cutz, E. (1986). Complications of parenteral nutrition. *Seminars in Perinatology, 10,* 196–207.

Haas-Beckert, B. (1987). Removing the mysteries of parenteral nutrition. *Pediatric Nursing, 13,* 237–241.

Halperin, M. L., et al. (1986). Acid-base, fluid and electrolyte aspects of parenteral nutrition. In J. P. Kokko, & R. L. Tannen (Eds.). *Fluids and electrolytes* (pp 817–831). Philadelphia: WB Saunders.

Hanning, R. M., & Zlotkin, S. H. (1985, April). Unconventional eating practices and their health implications. *Pediatric Clinics of North America, 32*(2), 429–445.

Hazinski, M. F. (1988). Understanding fluid balance in the seriously ill child. *Pediatric Nursing, 14*(3), 231–236.

Heald, F. P. (1992). Fast food and snack food: Beneficial or deleterious. *Journal of Adolescent Health, 13,* 380–383.

Huddleston, K., Vitarelli, R., Goodmundson, J., et al. (1989). MIC or foley: Comparing gastrostomy tubes. *MCN: American Journal of Maternal Child Nursing, 14*(1), 20–23.

Jacobs, C., & Dwyer, J. T. (1988). Vegetarian children: Appropriate and inappropriate diets. *American Journal of Clinical Nutrition, 48,* 811–818.

Kandt, K. A. (1991). An implantable venous access device for children. *MCN: American Journal of Maternal Child Nursing, 16,* 88–91.

Keusch, G. T. (1992, December). Immune function in the malnourished host. *Pediatric Annals, 11*(2), 1004–1014.

Klein, G. L., et al. (1991). Parenteral drug products containing aluminum as an ingredient or a contaminant: Response to FDA notice of intent. *American Journal of Clinical Nutrition, 53,* 399–402.

Kramer, M. S. (1981, June). Do breast-feeding and delayed introduction of solid foods protect against subsequent obesity? *Journal of Pediatrics, 98*(6), 883–887.

Laing, I. A., Glass, E. J., Hendry, G. M. A., et al. (1985). Rickets of prematurity: calcium and phosphorus supplementation. *Journal of Pediatrics, 106,* 265–268.

Larchet, M., et al. (1991). Calcium metabolism in children during long-term total parenteral nutrition: The influence of calcium, phosphorus, and vitamin D intakes. *Journal of Pediatric Gastroenterology, 13*(4), 367–375.

Larson-Brown, L. B. (1983, January/February). Nutritional education: How to get students to eat it up. *Health Education, 14*(1), 38–41.

Lechky, O. (1990). If children are developing poorly, ask what they had for breakfast. *Canadian Medical Association, 143*(3), 210–213.

Lewis, C. J., et al. (1990). Relationship between age and serum vitamin A in children aged 4–11 y. *American Journal of Clinical Nutrition, 52,* 353–360.

Lobo, M. L. (1992). Parent-infant interaction during feeding when the infant has congenital heart disease. *Journal of Pediatric Nursing, 7*(2), 97–105.

Lowe, C. U., et al. (1975, August). Reflections of dietary studies with children in the ten-state survey of 1968–1970. *Pediatrics, 56*(2), 306–326.

MacLean, W. C., & Graham, G. G. (1980, May). Vegetarianism in children. *American Journal of Diseases of Children, 134*(5), 513–519.

Marsh, A. G., et al. (1980). Cortical bone density of adult lacto-ovo-vegetarian and omnivorous women. *Journal of the American Dietetic Association, 76,* 148–151.

Mellin, L. M., & Frost, L. (1992). Child and adolescent obesity: The nurse practitioner's use of the SHAPEDOWN Method. *Journal of Pediatric Health Care, 6*(4), 187–193.

Mila, P. J. (1986). The weanling's gut. *Acta Paediatrica Scandinavica* (Suppl), *323,* 5–13.

Moore, M. C. (1988). Taurine supplementation: Theoretical and practical considerations. *Pediatric Nursing, 14*(6), 489–491.

Muecke, L., et al. (1992). Is childhood obesity associated with high-fat foods and low physical activity? *Journal of School Health, 62*(1), 19–23.

Neal, J., & Slayton, D. (1992). Neonatal and pediatric PEG tubes. *MCN: American Journal of Maternal Child Nursing, 17*(4), 184–191.

Pineault, M., et al. (1988). Total parenteral nutrition in the newborn: Impact of the quality of infused energy on nitrogen metabolism. *American Journal of Clinical Nutrition, 47,* 298–304.

Position of the American Dietetic Association. (1988). Vegetarian diets. *Journal of the American Dietetic Association, 88,* 351–355.

Rees, J. M. (1992). The overall impact of recently developed foods on the dietary habits of adolescents. *Journal of Adolescent Health, 13,* 389–391.

Register, U. D., & Sonnenberg, L. M. (1973, March). The vegetarian diet. *Journal of the American Dietetic Association, 62*(3), 253–260.

Rocchini, A. P. (1992). Adolescent obesity and cardiovascular risk. *Pediatric Annals, 21*(4), 235–240.

Rossouw, J. (1989). Kwashiorkor in North America. *American Journal of Clinical Nutrition, 49,* 588–592.

Santos, J. I., et al. (1983, March). Nutrition, infection and immunity. *Pediatric Annals, 12*(3), 182–194.

Seashore, J. H., & Hoffman, M. (1983, October). Use and abuse of peripheral parenteral nutrition in children. *Nutritional Support Services, 3*(10), 8–13.

Shamberger, R. (1984). The subtle signs of chronic vitamin undernutrition: Fat-soluble vitamins. *Diagnostic Medicine, 7*(3), 75–78, 80, 82.

Sherman, J. B. (1992). Intervention program for obese school children. *Journal of Community Health Nursing, 9*(3), 183–190.

Sherry, B., et al. (1992). Short, thin, or obese? Comparing growth indexes of children from high- and low-poverty areas. *92*(9), 1092–1095.

Simeon, P. S., & Gottesman, M. M. (1991). Neonatal continuous insulin infusion: A survey of ten level III nurseries in Los Angeles County. *Neonatal Network, 9*(7), 19–25.

Simopoulos, A. P. (1991). Omega-3 fatty acids in health and disease and in growth and development. *American Journal of Clinical Nutrition, 54,* 438–463.

Snetselaar, L., & Lauer, R. M. (1992, January/February). Childhood, diet and the atherosclerotic process. *Nutrition Today,* 22–28.

Snyder, P., Story, M., & Trenkner, L. L. (1992). Reducing fat and sodium in school lunch programs: The LUNCHPOWER! Intervention Study. *Journal of the American Dietetic Association, 92*(9), 1087–1091.

Solem, B. J., Norr, K. F., & Gallo, A. M. (1992). Infant feeding practices of low-income mothers. *Journal of Pediatric Health Care, 6,* 54–59.

Sullivan, B. (1991). Growth-enhancing interventions for nonorganic failure to thrive. *Journal of Pediatric Nursing, 6*(4), 236–242.

Vander, A. J., et al. (1980). *Human physiology—The mechanisms of body function.* New York: McGraw-Hill.

Weinberg, A. D., et al. (1992). Cholesterol screening using the school as a worksite. *Journal of School Health, 62*(2), 45–49.

West, K. P., et al. (1988). Vitamin A supplementation and growth: A randomized community trial. *American Journal of Clinical Nutrition, 48,* 1257–1264.

Zahr, L. (1991). Correlates of mother-infant interaction in premature infants from low socioeconomic backgrounds. *Pediatric Nursing, 17*(3), 259–263.

Zlotkin, S. H., Stallings, V. A., & Pencharz, P. B. (1985, April). Total parenteral nutrition in children. *Pediatric Clinics of North America, 32*(2), 381–400.

CHAPTER • 17

Promoting Healthy Play

Sandra B. Frick-Helms

RELATED TOPICS
Developing children, Chapters 3–9
Assessing Child Health, Chapter 13
Nursing Care During Hospitalization, Chapter 21
Preparation and support of children requiring procedures, Chapter 23
Preoperative and postoperative nursing care, Chapter 23

LEARNING OBJECTIVES

- List and discuss commonly accepted characteristics of play.
- Define "practice play," "constructive play," "symbolic or sociodramatic" play, "social play and games," and "rough-and-tumble play."
- Discuss the major categories of play and identify the stage of development at which these most commonly occur.
- Describe the interrelationships between play and the following domains of development: physical, cognitive, language, emotional, social, and moral, and gender/sex role.
- Discuss positive and negative aspects of computers and computer and video games.
- Discuss how parents can be assisted to facilitate their child's development through the use of play and play materials.
- Discuss the nurse's role in the use of play as an assessment tool, in planning play environments, and to facilitate skill development in children who are mentally retarded, developmentally delayed, emotionally disturbed, and/or have a sensory impairment.
- Differentiate among therapeutic play, play therapy, medical play, and preparation play.
- Give examples of symbolic responses of children to health care events.
- Identify and discuss the independent and collaborative roles of the nurse in applying the nursing process to children in health care settings.

Play is an intrinsic part of all aspects of the development of children. "Play has been considered to affect almost every human achievement and to be the basic foundation of human culture" (Huizinga, 1950).

The play of children has been examined by theorists for centuries. The most enduring interpretation is that children play to have fun. The character of play changes as a child matures, but children at all ages play. Play contributes to and is an expression of development. As children play, physical, emotional, social, and cognitive skills are developed. Children who develop in an environment in which appropriate play is encouraged have a greater chance to achieve their maximal potential than those in homes in which play opportunities are lacking.

A special benefit of play is its use during a health care encounter. Play can be used to assess a child's level of development. When children are hospitalized, play is used as recreation, as a diversion from thoughts about the hospital, and in therapeutic play and play therapy to help a child cope with a stressful or painful experience.

This chapter reviews theories of play as a framework for understanding the elements of play. The contributions of play to the development of children and the character of play at the various stages of development are discussed. The nurse's role in fostering the child's development through direct play with children and anticipatory guidance of parents is presented. Play as an assessment method and therapeutic intervention is also discussed.

Definitions of Play

A discussion of play usually begins with a *definition* (or definitions). A completely satisfactory definition of play has not been established. "Definitions range from any and all activities in which children engage to . . . activities in which children are intrinsically motivated, process-focused, pleasurably involved, and in an 'as if' or pretend state" (Bolig, 1988, p 132). Robert McCall (cited in Chance, 1979, p 1) said, "Defining play isn't important. After all, psychologists can't define intelligence, but that hasn't kept them from studying it."

Some sources have said that play is whatever work is not. Mark Twain said, "Work is whatever a body has to do; play is whatever a body wants to do." If a "not work" criterion is used to judge whether an activity is play, the activity would meet the following characteristics: the child retains control of the activity; the motivation for the activity, the degree or constraints of reality, and whether the setting imposes consequences or choices on the activity are left to the child. These criteria are very close to the characteristics of play that have been agreed on by most experts.

Characteristics of Play

Play includes both observable and nonobservable behaviors or activities. Characteristics that can be used to differentiate *play* activities from activities that are *not* play are useful to define and describe play. The following eight criteria are typically included in any list of characteristics that must be present in order for an activity to be considered *play*.

1. **Play is intrinsically motivated.** "Intrinsic motivation" refers to an activity done for its own sake. The motivation to play comes from within the child and involves the satisfaction of the activity itself. Play behaviors occur for their own sake, rather than as the result of external social demands or rewards. Children set their own goals and supply their own meaning to play activities. They control the activity themselves.
2. **Play is oriented toward means rather than ends.** Players are concerned with the play activities themselves more than with outcomes or goals of their play.
3. **There is an element of nonliterality in play.** Nonliteral play, often called "pretend" play, is often described by saying the child acts in an "as if" manner.
4. **Play is pleasurable.** In play, the child displays positive affect. Children at play show joy in what they are doing. Often, play is marked by evidence of a developing sense of humor.
5. **Play is marked by flexibility.** Shifts in play themes and materials occur easily and harmoniously.
6. **Play is often voluntary and spontaneous.**
7. **When children play, they are actively involved**—motorically, cognitively, and emotionally.

8. **Play involves a concept known as "flow."** Flow involves a centering of attention in which action and awareness merge and a loss of self-consciousness occurs in the sense that the child is paying more attention to the task than to her or his own body state.

Developmental Stages and Content of Play

The kind of play in which children engage is largely determined by their developmental stage. Children progress through stages of play that reflect a range of thoughts and abilities. As children grow and develop, their environment changes and so do their needs.

Categories of Play

There are several types or categories of play. In 1932, Parten (cited in Bergen, 1988) identified different types of play that are still commonly referred to today. Parten's categories of play are shown in Table 17–1. A more commonly used listing includes the following categories of play: exploratory, functional, or repetitious play; constructive or building play; symbolic, sociodramatic, fantasy, or pretend play; social play and games with rules; and rough-and-tumble play (Pellegrini & Perlmutter, 1988; Smilansky, 1968; van der Kooij, 1989). Whereas most types are seen in children at all developmental stages, one type tends to be the predominant form in each stage.

Infant and Toddler Play (Birth to 3 Years Old)

Infants spend more than 50 per cent of their time in exploratory or practice play, and practice play with objects is the most common type (Sponseller & Jaworski, cited in Bergen, 1988). "Exploratory play" is also referred to as repetition, practice, or functional play. (The term "practice play" derives from Piaget, who saw the repetitive nature of the infant's play as evidence of the existence of the six stages of sensorimotor development.) Rubin (1985) referred to the play of the infant as "functional" because the repetition of the same movements with or without objects appears to serve the "function" of providing pleasure to the infant. For the first 5 months, play primarily involves visual "exploration" of the environment. Significant visual exploration is seen by 2 months. By 4 months, the infant responds to the meaning of visual stimuli. For instance, infants show a preference for photos of the human face over photos of other visual stimuli (Fenson, 1985; Gottfried, 1985; Marino, 1988). By 5 months, eye-hand coordination allows for visually guided exploration and manipulation of objects. Manipulation includes mouthing and touching. By 7 months, the infant's manipulation involves precise fine motor skills. The 7-month-old infant has discovered the unique properties of toys and is most likely to manipulate objects that provide feedback, such as a "busy box" (Marino, 1988). By 9 months, novel objects are preferred. By 12 months, the infant shows interest in "how things work," such as fascination with light switches, push buttons, and hinged lids on boxes. By 13 months, the infant has awareness of the

TABLE 17-1
Parten's Categories of Play

Unoccupied Behavior—Child does not appear to be playing but focuses on anything that happens to be of momentary interest. Common in toddlers and young preschoolers but occurs at all ages
Onlooker Behavior—Child watches other children play and may talk to the children being watched, may ask questions or give suggestions, but does not join in the play. Differs from unoccupied behavior in that the onlooker is observing the play of other children rather than any event in the environment. Child often takes up a position close to the group to see and hear everything that takes place. Most typical of toddlers but seen in older children when they are in strange environments
Solitary Independent Play—Child plays alone with toys that are different from those used by the children in the same territory. Child may be within speaking distance of other children but may make no effort to get close to them. These children pursue their own activity without reference to what others are doing. Most common in toddlers but occurs in older children if the environment is unfamiliar
Parallel Activity—Child plays independently, but the activity chosen naturally brings him or her among other children. Child plays with toys that are similar to those of the children around him or her but does not try to influence or modify the activity of the children nearby. Children play beside rather than with each other; and seem to be aware of each other but make no attempt to control one another. Typically occurs during the toddler years
Associative Play—Children play with each other and talk about what they are doing. They borrow and lend play materials and follow one another with similar play things. No division of labor and no organization of the activity into a common group goal. Instead of subordinating individual interest to that of the group, each child acts as she or he wishes, but they play together with similar playthings or in similar activities. More common in preschool and early school years
Cooperative or Organized Supplementary Play—Children play in a group that is organized for the purpose of attaining a group goal. They work together to make something or play in a formal game. Marked sense of belonging or of not belonging to the group. Control of the group situation is in the hands of one or two of the members. The children work together with a division of labor; different roles are taken by the various group members; and activity is organized so that the efforts of one child are supplemented by those of another. This type of play is typical of school-age children

Modified from information in Bergen, D. (1988). *Play as a medium for learning and development.* Portsmouth, NH: Heinemann.

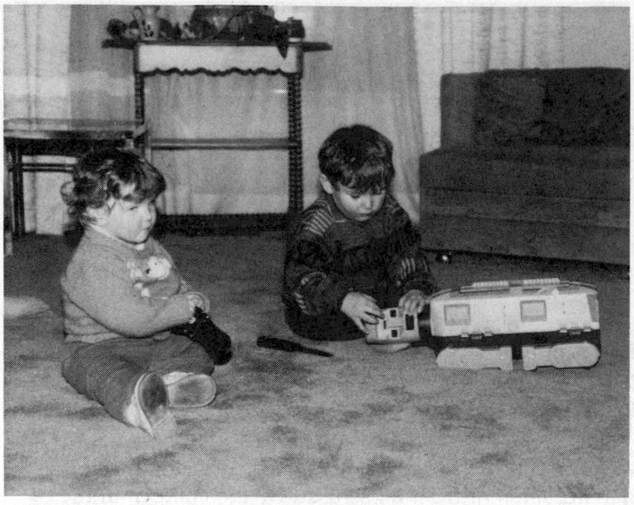

FIGURE 17 - 1. Parallel play. Toddlers play in close proximity in similar activities but do not try to influence or modify the activity of other children nearby.

function or meaning of objects. He or she will try behaviors such as putting a key in a lock, throwing a ball, or hugging a doll (Fenson, 1985).

"Solitary" or "parallel," "pretend" or "symbolic" play occurs around 9 months (Fig. 17–1). The symbolic use of objects can be seen when the infant pretends to eat pictures of food or "play" food. By 12 months, she or he "plays out" details of real life with realistic objects, such as feeding a toy nursing bottle to a doll. Gradually, the infant becomes able to substitute nonrealistic objects in pretend play, such as feeding a doll with a cylindrical block (Bergen, 1988).

"Social" play and "games" begin around 6 months. From 2 to 7 months, the infant explores his or her social influence through playful interactions, especially with the mother. At 13 months, the infant deliberately elicits social responses through play. By 21 months, symbolic social play is seen (Bergen, 1988).

Preschool and Kindergarten Play (3 to 5 Years Old)

The practice play of the infant and toddler is gradually replaced by "constructive" play. The preschool-age child moves from handling and exploring materials to using them to construct or create something that remains after the child has finished playing (Rubin, 1985). "Constructive" play is the most common activity (40 to 50 per cent) among preschool and kindergarten children (Bergen, 1988).

"Symbolic," "pretend," or "sociodramatic" play is at its peak between 4 and 5 years. Solitary pretend play is still important; but now "group" or "cooperative pretend" play becomes more popular (Fenson, 1985). A child this age can use imaginary objects with great diversity. He or she can take on roles in pretend play, including those of the narrator and the actor. Role-taking abilities increase with age (Bergen, 1988).

In the area of "social" play and "games," rough-and-tumble games and rudimentary games with rules appear. Rough-and-tumble play facilitates differentiation of play from aggression. Games have *simple* rules and are not truly competitive. Strict adherence to rules is not required. The purpose of games at this age is for everyone to enjoy the game, not to win (Bergen, 1988).

"Rough-and-tumble" play tends to appear in preschoolers, who spend 5 per cent of their free time in this activity, which is described by Pellegrini and Perlmutter (1988, pp 162–163) as "playful, nonaggressive gross motor activities that do not typically result in injury to participants or in the separation of playmates and involve positive affect." Rough-and-tumble play behaviors include laughing, play noises, running, jumping, wrestling/tumbling, chasing, and fleeing. Rough-and-tumble play serves the purposes of providing practice in social interaction skills and "blowing off excess activity" (Pellegrini & Perlmutter, 1988, p 163).

Elementary School–Age Play (6 to 12 Years Old)

"Practice" play continues in the play of school-age children. However, it now is done deliberately to enhance motor skills. "Constructive" play is still the most common form. This may be because it is encouraged and allowed in elementary school classrooms (Bergen, 1988).

There is a gradual decline in overtly manifested "symbolic" play. Symbolic content is now integrated into games with rules and in modern computer games, such as Dungeons & Dragons. Much of symbolic play becomes abstract. What was previously acted out overtly is now transformed into vicarious mental forms such as daydreaming, reading, and watching television and movies. Language play, referred to by Bergen (1988) as "verbal invention," is another form of symbolic play. It peaks around 8 to 9 years of age and includes secret codes, riddles, puns, tongue twisters, jokes, including "knock-knock" jokes, insults, chants, and rhymes. Symbolic play can also be seen in formalized (and socially acceptable) forms such as school plays and "secret" clubs. The popularity of miniature toys for this age group suggests that symbolic and fantasy play probably occur more privately (in the child's room).

The highest incidence of "social" play and "games with rules" occurs between 10 and 12 years of age (Fig. 17–2); after age 12, interests tend to shift to organized sports (Bergen, 1988). Games played by children in this age group must have some sort of challenge, and children must be able to accept division of labor and a set of prearranged rules (Rubin, 1985).

"Rough-and-tumble" play reaches a high point at age 7, when it accounts for 13.3 per cent of activities

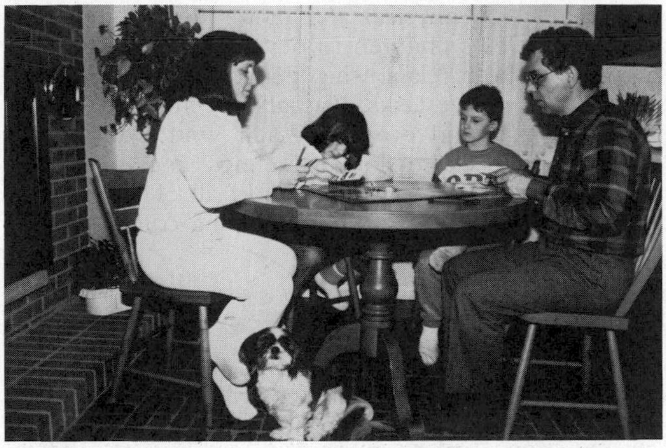

FIGURE 17 - 2. The highest incidence of social play and games with rules occurs between 10 and 12 years of age.

in the child's free time. It then declines at 9 years to 9.3 per cent, and at 11 years to 4.6 per cent.

Play of the school-age child also involves play with academic skills and problem solving. This is the age for discovery learning, and "playful" approaches to learning are frequently used in the elementary school classroom (Bergen, 1988).

Adolescence (13 to 19 Years Old)

Theorists have argued regarding whether "true" play exists in adolescents and adults. Bergen (1988, p 59) says that "the tendency to *playfulness* seems to be inherent in human beings, but its manifestations vary not only because of changes in behavior that come with various developmental stages but also because of cultural expectations." The types of play in some of the previously defined categories ("exploratory," "functional," "constructive," "sociodramatic") are not typically seen in adolescents unless it is in a culturally approved "helping" (as with a younger sibling) or "structured" role, such as babysitter, Sunday School leader, or camp counselor. If, as some experts assert, play can take place on a mental level without being overtly "acted out," adolescents engage in what can be referred to as "sociodramatic" or "fantasy" play when they imagine, for instance, having a date with someone they find attractive, being the star of a team or editor of the newspaper. Sociodramatic or fantasy play also occurs with the viewing of music videos or the playing of fantasy games. This kind of "playing around" with ideas, or mental rehearsal, occurs throughout adulthood. "Adults do participate in role simulation exercises, belong to community theater groups, hold brain storming sessions, join liars clubs, attend political conventions, and engage in work roles requiring sociodramatic-like behaviors" (Bergen, 1988, p 59). Adolescents engage in these same kinds of activities, usually as a part of school or extracurricular offerings.

Adolescents continue to engage in "games with rules." Board games symbolic of events in the real world, such as chess (simulated battle) and Monopoly (real estate transactions), begin to be preferred (Bergen, 1988). Games with rules are also seen in organized team sports at school or in a youth group. Rough-and-tumble play or "horsing around" tends to be a culturally approved way for adolescent males to *touch* and may be a rehearsal for relationships with other males in adulthood. Rough-and-tumble activities also serve as nonthreatening ways for males and females to have physical contact. If the philosophy of the local school board includes it, adolescents continue the playful approaches to learning and problem solving that began in elementary school.

Csikzentmihayli (1979) said that adults' (and we can include adolescents') play behavior is better characterized as "flow" (defined under "Characteristics of Play" in this chapter) rather than play, and that the elements of flow are similar to those of play, but they are not necessarily voluntary. He saw play as a "training ground for a more adequate adult life of flow in any kind of experience—work or play (p 275). So, the debate over whether adolescents and adults engage in "true" play continues. It would seem, though, that play in childhood serves a very valuable function for the capability and well-being of the adolescent and adult.

Developmental progression of play behaviors is summarized in Table 17–2.

Children's Art

Although not included in the cited listings of categories of play, children's art is part of their play and progresses in a developmental and universal fashion throughout childhood (Fig. 17–3). From the graphic scribbles of the young toddler, later forms of art emerge. For young children, art serves as an educational and explorational activity through which they can experiment with various colors, forms, and textures. Creation of a tangible finished product arouses feelings of accomplishment from the praise of others and simply by seeing the artwork displayed. It is a creative means through which their own thoughts, perceptions, and feelings can be communicated. Art can provide insight into the thoughts of children who may have difficulty expressing them verbally. Interpretation of art is beyond the scope of this text; however, an understanding of the developmental characteristics of art can complement other assessment tools in the care of children.

Contributions of Play to Development

Play serves many functions for the child (Fig. 17–4). Play facilitates the development of physical and motor skills, including manipulative skills involved in fine motor development. Play is the primary modality

TABLE 17-2
Developmental Progression of Play Behaviors

Infants and Toddlers
Exploratory or Practice Play
Most common activity
4 mos—responds to meaning of visual stimuli
5 mos—visually guided exploration and manipulation of objects
7 mos—manipulates objects that provide feedback; fine motor skills
9 mos—novel objects preferred
12 mos—interest in "how things work"
13 mos—awareness of the function or meaning of objects
Pretend or Symbolic Play
Solitary or parallel around 9 mos
12 mos—"plays out" details of real life with realistic objects; gradually substitutes nonrealistic objects
Social Play and Games
Begin around 6 mos
2 to 7 mos—exploration of influence through playful interactions
13 mos—deliberately elicits social responses through play
21 mos—symbolic social play
Preschool and Kindergarten Age (3–5 Yrs)
Constructive Play
Gradually replaces practice play and is the most common activity (40–50%)
Symbolic, Pretend, or Sociodramatic Play
Peaks at 4 and 5 yrs. Now *group* or *cooperative pretend play*. Diversity in use of imaginary objects. Role-taking abilities that increase with age
Social Play and Games
Rough-and-tumble games and rudimentary games with rules appear. Strict adherence to rules not required. Games not truly competitive
Elementary School Age
Practice play continues; now used deliberately to enhance motor skills
Constructive play still the most common form of play
Symbolic, Pretend, or Sociodramatic Play
Gradual decline in overtly manifested *symbolic play*. Symbolic content integrated into games with rules and computer games. Much of symbolic play transformed into vicarious mental forms, e.g., daydreaming, reading, and watching television and movies. Language play, another form of symbolic play, peaks at 8 to 9 yrs. Also in formalized and socially acceptable forms, e.g., school plays, clubs, play with miniature toys more privately
Social Play and Games
Highest incidence between 10 and 12 yrs of age. Games involve challenge and ability to accept division of labor and prearranged rules. Play also involves academic skills and problem solving.

through which physical and motor development occur. Play allows children to develop creatively. There appears to be a relationship between playfulness and ability on creative tasks. Play allows children to learn about objects and events in their world; to practice and learn the expression of feelings; and to develop social relationships (Fig. 17–5). In all of these ways, play facilitates the child in developing competence in negotiating her or his world.

Physical Development

The physical activity of play contributes to the development and coordination of the body throughout the life span (Fig. 17–6). Children's play varies from one developmental stage to the next in part because of the physical maturation of their bodies. During infancy, play is dominated by sensorimotor activities such as looking, tasting, touching, and manipulating the environment. Through reaching, grasping, and mouthing objects repetitively, the senses are developed and muscles are coordinated. Hand-eye coordination is a competency that requires practice through play and maturation through growth. Through play, children develop control of their bodies as they practice creeping, crawling, and walking. The skillful movements and coordination required to take them to new territories for exploration are practiced incessantly. As children grow older, they continue to increase their physical competency by engaging in activities that demand more precision, such as athletics, bicycle riding, swimming, dancing, and skating. Thus, through play, a person progresses from a randomly reflexive repertoire of behavior in infancy to skillfully coordinated movement in adulthood.

There is theoretical support for a direct relationship between play and physical/motor development. Erikson's (cited in Kaplan-Sanoff et al, 1988) view was that development is influenced by both biologic and environmental factors. He believed that children needed both movement experiences and mastery-oriented play to successfully achieve the psychosocial task of each Eriksonian period. "For example, trust involves being able to move closer, reach for and grasp objects in the environment and predict what actions will cause various reactions. Erikson's theory implies that play assists mastery of movement-related concepts such as laterality, directionality, and spatial awareness" (Kaplan-Sanoff et al, 1988). Havighurst (cited in Kaplan-Sanoff et al, 1988) believed that achievement of developmental tasks not only leads to feelings of pleasure but also increases possibilities of success with later tasks, whereas task failure leads to frustration and difficulty in achieving later tasks. Havighurst included in the tasks of middle childhood developing a wholesome attitude toward one's physical growth and achieving the ability to care for and enjoy using one's body, both of which are also influenced by early motor competence.

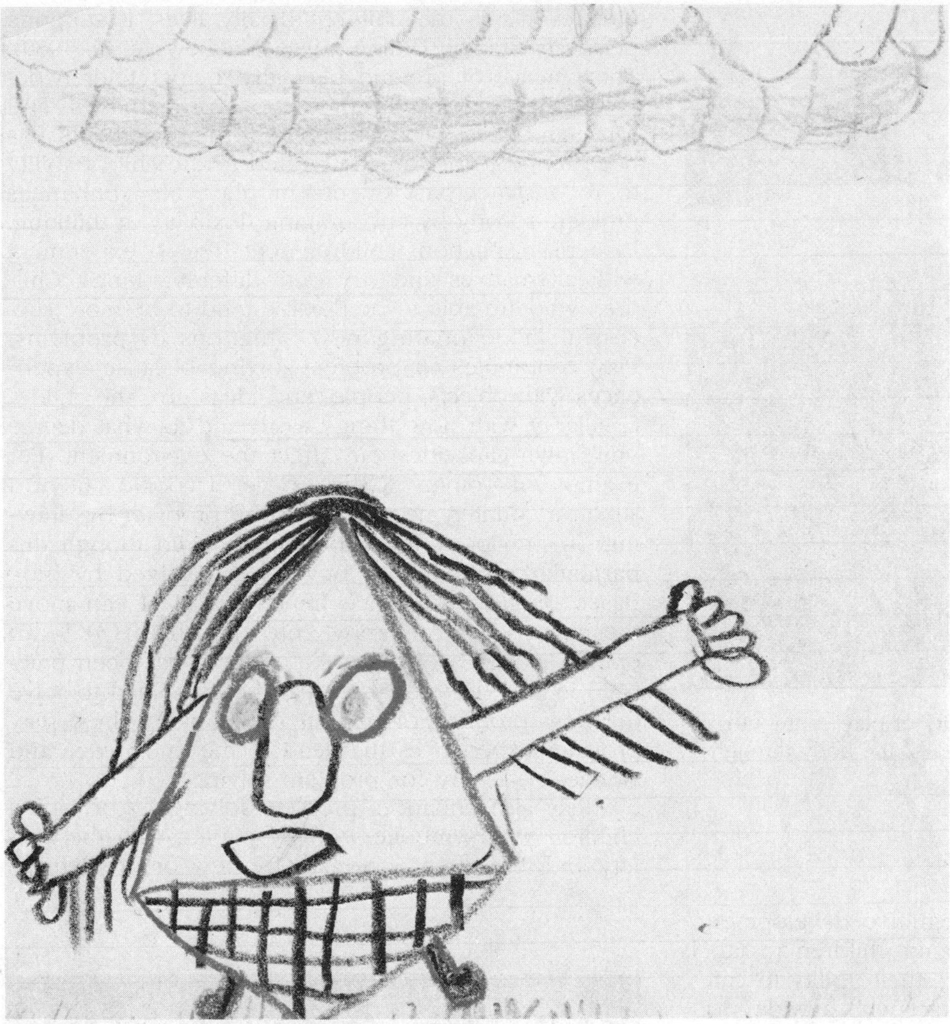

FIGURE 17 - 3. Children's art is part of their play and progresses in a developmental and universal fashion throughout childhood.

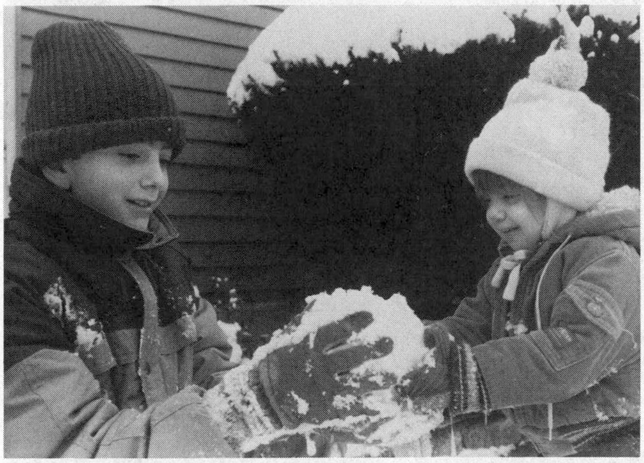

FIGURE 17 - 4. Play serves many functions for the child. While having fun, these children are learning about the environment, developing social skills, increasing their manual dexterity, and having an opportunity to create whatever they choose.

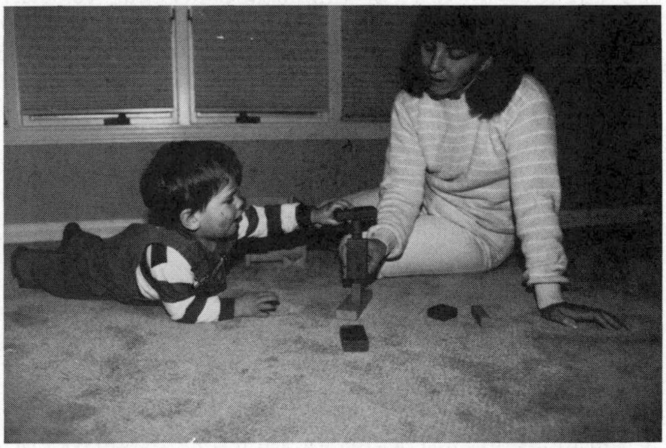

FIGURE 17 - 5. Play allows children to learn about objects and events in their world.

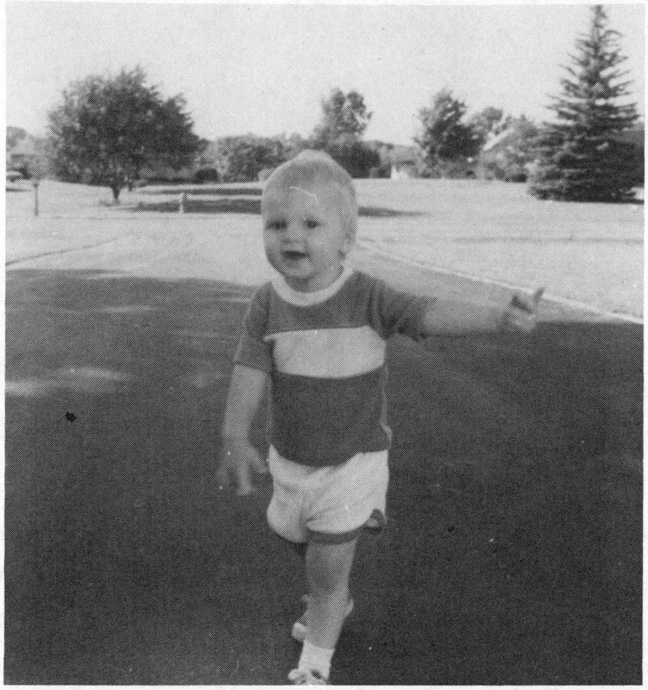

FIGURE 17-6. The physical activity of play contributes to the development and coordination of the body throughout life.

Cognitive Development

Play is critical in the child's cognitive development. Play increases the ability of young children to label objects and events and enhances their ability to categorize by bringing them in contact with a wide variety of stimuli which they can manipulate and sort (Bettleheim, 1987; DeLoache et al, 1985). Through play, a child gathers information about his or her world and compares this information with what he or she already "knows" or thinks and accepts, rejects, expands, or modifies his or her thinking accordingly (Fig. 17–7). Piaget described this as a way of assimilating and accommodating elements from the outside world and manipulating them so that they fit the child's existing mental representation of the world (Bergen, 1988, p 15). The interrelationship between play and cognitive development begins in infancy. In more securely attached infants, there is more exploration of the environment and play behaviors that are judged more sophisticated. Coates and Lewis (1984) observed mother-infant interactions and found that mothers' sensitivity to the cues for play by their 3-month-old infants predicted the children's intelligence at age 6.

Abilities in and levels of pretend, imaginary, or fantasy play are significantly interrelated with children's cognitive development and capabilities. Fantasy play cannot take place unless the child has the cognitive skills to take on the perspective of others. This requires an understanding of the played-out role behaviors. Since pretend play is usually based on common events in the children's daily lives, it supports perspective-taking (Rubin, 1988; Matthews et al, 1980). The practice of pretend play also helps children develop the concepts of prediction, probabilities, and cause-and-effect. The ability to form hypotheses has been found to be directly related to the child's ability to reconstruct past events in play. Play enhances problem-solving by encouraging flexibility in thinking. In a play situation, children feel free to experiment with alternatives and "try out" different things. Children who are able to be flexible tend to be more successful in negotiating new situations or problems. Play contributes to problem-solving because experiences with objects, people, and ideas give the child a familiarity with how things work and to what degree one's own capacities can affect the environment. For example, if Tommy wishes to get a cookie out of a jar on a counter, he can solve the problem by drawing on previous play experiences, even though this particular problem has never been solved by him. Based on his experience he knows (1) I can move the chair, (2) I can crawl into the chair, (3) I can open a jar. Each of these experiences has been practiced in play, but now they can be combined to solve the new problem of getting the cookie. Thus, play provides experiences that lead to the knowledge and abilities necessary for problem-solving.

Play also enhances problem-solving by providing children with symbolic ways of coping with the anxiety and fear often generated by new or problematic

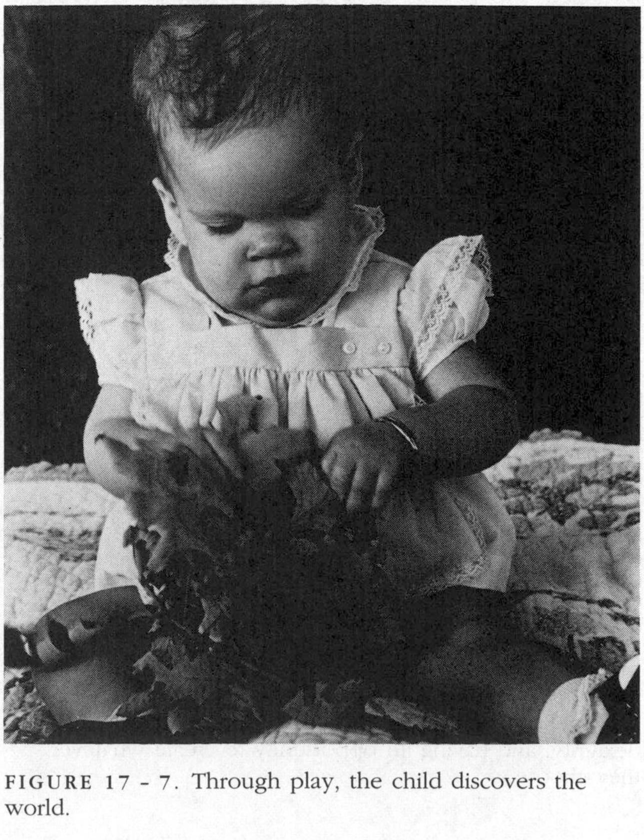

FIGURE 17-7. Through play, the child discovers the world.

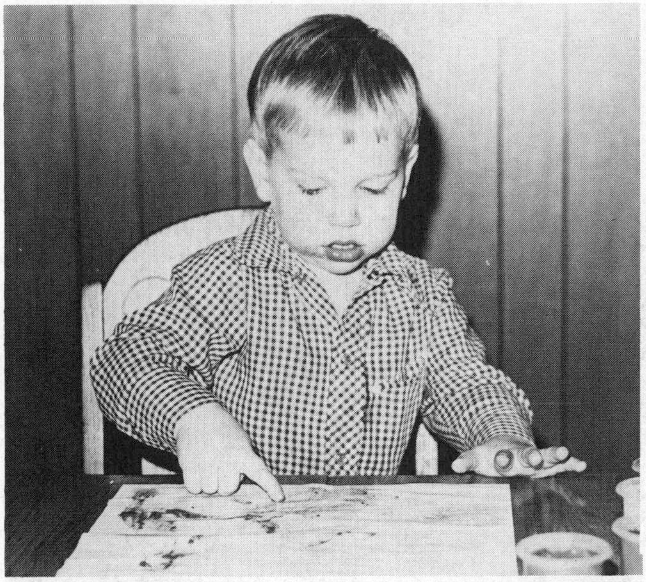

FIGURE 17-8. Play can be a natural avenue for creative expression.

situations. Play serves this anxiety-decreasing function in much the same way that talking or thinking through a problem does for adults (Vygotsky, 1962; Curry & Arnaud, 1974). It is very likely that this anxiety-decreasing function accounts for children's propensity to play "scary" games. Children can often be seen playing out problems or "scary" events such as the birth of a new sibling, potty training, disciplinary measures, violence they have witnessed or experienced. The fact that children "play out" observed or endured violence has been documented (Eisen, 1988; Malchiodi, 1990) and can now be seen on the nightly news as worldwide violence and children's reactions to it are brought into the family living room via television.

Cognitive development and creativity are often considered together. Play can be a natural avenue for creative expression (Fig. 17–8). Through play, children can experiment with new combinations of materials and ideas to create something they have never produced before. Children can be creative with very simple materials if left to their own imagination. Play opportunities provide many possibilities for creativity, some of which are object manipulation, dramatic play, drawing, painting, and daydreaming.

Another factor that has been found to be important in the interrelationship of play and cognitive and creative development involves the availability of toys and playthings in the child's environment. Availability of appropriate toys and books has been found to be a consistent predictor of cognition from late infancy through early school-age (Marino, 1988).

Language Development

Play, especially pretend play, is also closely interrelated with language development (Marino, 1988; Pellegrini, 1981; Sachs, 1980; Vygotsky, 1962). Through play, a child engages in extensive experimentation with sounds and words to enhance language development. The earliest form of language play occurs when infants attempt to repeat their parents' verbalizations, causing the parents to repeat them in a playful way. Nonsense syllables (sound play) and word substitutions are commonly observed in young children. Even before children are able to use words to describe what they see, their experiences with space, sound, color, and relationships help form impressions about the environment. Experimentation with objects provides an opportunity to discover the physical characteristics of the objects before children have the words to describe these perceptions. Play situations promote the use of words and phrases. In the toddler and preschooler, pretend play shows an underlying knowledge of an actual event. The ability to pretend actions with objects, for example, to feed a doll, shows knowledge of parts and functions (bottle is used to feed). This is equivalent to the use of a word that shows knowledge of the event (McCune, 1985). In middle childhood, much of play is with words. This is the age in which children delight in jokes, puns, riddles, and tongue-twisters.

Social, Emotional, and Moral Development

The value of play in the social and emotional development of the child can be seen from the time the child is an infant (Christie & Johnsen, 1983). Play allows children to experiment with thoughts, feelings, and actions and learn to adapt their emotions in a socially acceptable manner. According to Hay and colleagues (1979) and Bergen (1988), infant games have the following qualities of all social interactions: mutual involvement and alternation of turns, or reciprocity and cooperation, and repetition of sequences. Infant games may be the earliest examples of and the basis for all later social interactions (Fig. 17–9). Games such as "peek-a-boo," hiding objects, and "where's baby?" give infants opportunities to master tension-producing experiences and other social situations (Beckwith, 1985; Johnsen, 1991). When a baby pulls a blanket over her head and her parent responds with, "Where's baby?" allowing her to laugh delightedly, the baby quickly learns that she can influence the behavior of others. Additionally, since her gestures and actions are responded to in a predictable way, these actions soon acquire social meaning.

There is an apparent relationship between infant play and *attachment*. Marino (1988) found that quality of attachment between an infant and its mother affects the infant's play performance. Infants who have more fun with their mothers tend to become securely attached (Blehar et al, 1977). The more playful the mother, and the more positive affect she displays with her infant, the more socially responsive the infant will be to her, and the more positive affect the infant will show (Beckwith, 1985). Securely attached

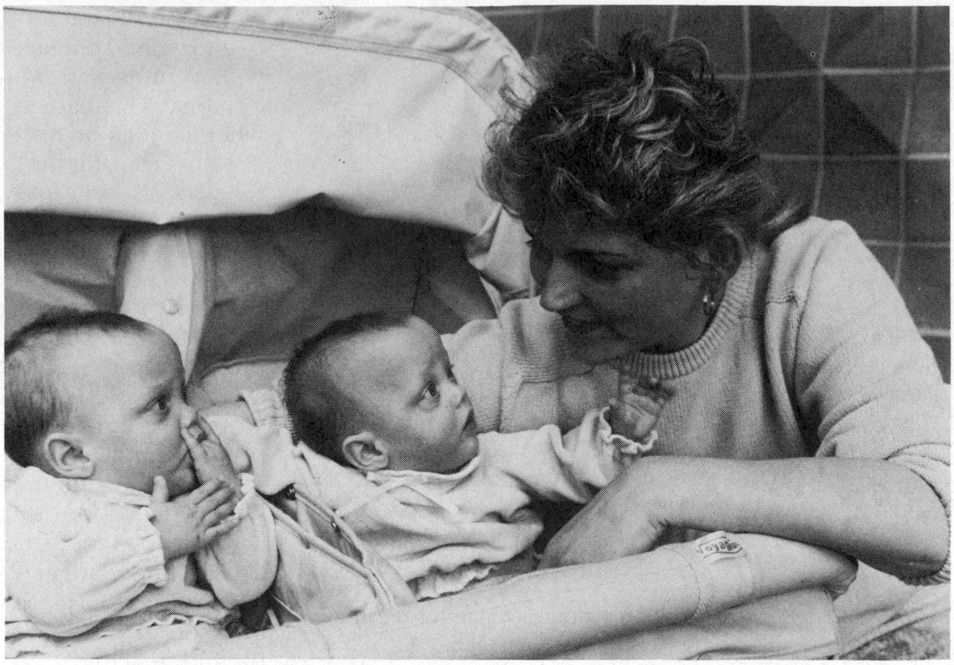

FIGURE 17-9. Infant games may be the earliest examples of and basis for all later social interaction. These 6-month-old twins readily respond to their mother's attempt to engage them in interactive play.

infants later have more fun in tasks and are more persistent (Main, 1983; Slade, 1987). Securely attached infants also tend to be more sociable with adult strangers and with peers and more socially competent with both peers and adults (Rubenstein & Howes, 1976; Cohen & Tomlinson-Keasey, 1980; Belsky & Most, 1981; Belsky et al, 1984). "Infants whose attachments to their parents provide a secure base from which to explore, experience more freedom to attend to the environment and are thus more able to not only engage in cognitively sophisticated exploration, but to spontaneously deploy their cognitive competencies in free play—even in a low stress situation" (Belsky et al, 1984, pp 415–416). Here we can see the interrelationship between play and cognitive and social development.

The importance of play to *social development* continues throughout childhood. In the preschool-age child, sociodramatic play (or "pretend play") has been found to be extremely important to the child's social development, social capabilities, and popularity with others. According to Rubin (1988), "sociodramatic play allows young children to practice persuasion, negotiation, cooperation, and even assertion/defense . . . all within a nonliteral framework." It is the "means by which children learn to communicate, negotiate, create, problem-solve, and understand social roles, rules, and perspectives" (p 69).

When children engage in dramatic play with their peers, they are exposed to differing points of view and must learn how to adapt so they can accommodate them. Therefore, they learn to respond to the feelings of others, to be patient, to wait for a turn, to be cooperative, to share, and to obtain satisfaction when others like them (Bergen, 1988; Bretherton, 1985). Children learn right from wrong in play because of the positive and negative reinforcement they receive from their family, peers, and society. Some play is rewarded and some is punished. The ability to take into account the feelings, needs, and desires of others is necessary to the *moral development* of children. Ambron (1981) suggests that ethical behavior entails "understanding that the needs of others are as valid as our own." During play, rules are enforced by peers, and cheaters are ostracized. The interaction patterns developed through these play experiences contribute significantly to the moral development of children.

Infant games assist in the *development of a sense of self*. This involves knowing what is part of self and what is outside the self. When parents alter play behavior in accordance with their infants' signals regarding emotional expectations, they facilitate the development of social responses such as surprise, anticipation, excitement, and climax.

Sociodramatic play contributes to the developing sense of self by allowing the child to experience a variety of emotions. Gould (1972) found that children who had consistently positive experiences with nurturance tend to play out more nurturant roles in pretend play. Even in aggressive play, these children tend to identify with the rescuing aspect (or "good guy"). Those children who have had negative nurturing experiences tend to play either the aggressor or the victim in their pretend play. The contributions of play to the development of a sense of self continues in school-age children. Now they begin to try out how they fit into the world in staged dramas and plays and through storytelling.

Rubin (1988) believes there is an interaction between sociodramatic play and *popularity*. "Young children who engage in high frequencies of sociodramatic play are more popular among their peers, more creative, more intelligent, better social cognizers and perspective takers than their age mates" (p 69). However, if their sociodramatic play is primarily solitary or parallel, they tend to be disliked by peers and perceived by teachers as socially incompetent. Rubin's findings also showed that these less popular children tended to be less able to understand other persons' perspectives and performed poorly on measures of social problem-solving. Additionally, it has been found that high-status children can join ongoing sociodramatic play without problem; low-status children have to ask permission. Roles played by children in sociodramatic play tend to suggest an authority structure in the group, with most popular children playing high-status roles, such as mothers and fathers, and less popular children often playing lower-status roles, such as family pets. These findings indicate that not all forms of dramatic play have the positive developmental outcomes that have been described. Positive results seem to accrue from *cooperative* rather than solitary or parallel pretend play. There seems to be ample evidence of the importance of pretend or sociodramatic play to positive developmental outcomes in children. Some authorities have said that there is a trend toward decline of such play (Mergen, 1991; Postman, 1982). Kline and Pentecost (1990) have carried out research refuting this contention. They say that sociodramatic play is on the increase owing to marketing strategies used by toy companies. Children are now exposed to mass media advertisements for fantasy figures; and, in these advertisements, the sociodramatic or fantasy play value is emphasized.

Play is also important in the development of the child's ability to master and express emotions. *Expression of emotions* is a life-long learning process. During the developmental process, children engage in fantasy play to explore feelings, lessen fears, and work through conflicts. In games of pretending, imaginary playmates or toys are safe recipients of aggressive impulses. Experiences that have frightened or excited a child may be re-enacted in play with imaginary participants. Through such play activities, a child can remember a difficult or emotionally painful event or experience and express feelings about the experience that they may not have been able to handle at the time of the experience in ways that may not be perceived as acceptable forms of behavior in the "real world." Through play, children can "play out personally painful experiences and by mastering pain in fantasy play, come to grips with their pain in reality" (Bergen, 1988, p 14).

Independence and self-care skills are learned and practiced in a child's play. The delight children experience in seeing their own accomplishments during play gives them confidence to begin doing things for themselves in other aspects of living. As children realize that they can stack their own blocks, they also demand that they be given control over their own bodies. In everyday activities of living, such as eating, dressing, bathing, and preparation for sleep, play continues as children experiment with their own skills and become increasingly more independent.

Gender/Sex Role Development

Play and the way it is encouraged and reinforced by adults and peers is important to gender or sex role development (Bergen, 1988; Carvalho et al, 1990; Fagot, 1984; Ignico, 1990). Adults differentially reinforce the play of children of different genders. Siblings and peers further this sex role differentiation of play behaviors by modeling and reinforcing what they consider gender-acceptable play. Boys tend to receive more criticism for and are discouraged from play that is considered more appropriate for girls. Bettleheim (1987) notes that because doll play has typically not been available to boys, boys do not get the same opportunity as girls to "visualize, act out, and deal with" typical problems of learning to be part of a family. Although there has been a growing trend toward similarity of play between the sexes (Mergen, 1991; Sutton-Smith, 1985), the gender gap in play activities is being fostered by mass media marketing by toy manufacturers in television ads for fantasy figures (Kline & Pentecost, 1990). Television does seem to be a factor associated with a decrease in frequency and complexity of pretend play. Children who are rated as heavy viewers of television have fewer opportunities for self-initiated themes in pretend play, show less imagination in their play, and tend to show less general ability to organize and comprehend new material (Singer & Singer, 1988).

Anticipatory Guidance: Promoting Development Through Play

Computers, Computer Games, and Video Games. Another type of activity, considered by many to be a form of children's play but not included in cited listings of categories of children's play, is computers and computer and video games. Some experts argue that computers and computer and video games do not meet the criteria for an activity to be considered "true" play and that they take children away from activities that are necessary to meet appropriate developmental tasks. They argue that "the constant distractibility provided by toys, game simulations and television programs acts as an opiate for child consumers, who learn to move incessantly from one activity to the next without real thought or questioning" (Sutton-Smith, 1985).

"Others dispute this view and believe that the young child's access to multiple modes of information leads to enormous personal development" (Sutton-Smith, 1985). Sutton-Smith (1985) also said, "Play itself is neither good nor bad. Like language or music, it is a form of expression and communication. What makes it good or bad is what we do with it." Since the use of computers and computer and video games is so pervasive in the activities of children, a discussion of these technologies in relation to play and development is included here.

Porter (1988) stated that the ultimate impact of computers in the play environment of children is as yet unknown. He pointed out that children's experiences with computers are "primarily dependent on programs written by adults," and continued, "adults who write, sell, and purchase computer programs may have theoretical views that could lead them to use the computer to teach drill and practice exercises or alternatively to promote playful experiences fostering higher levels of thought, creativity, fantasy, and sociability" (p 271). Sutton-Smith (1985) warned of the tendency of adults in the child's environment to "be so afraid of unstructured play" that a trend exists to suppress any activity that could not be called "game simulation," "adjustment," "cognition," or "problem solving." Nurses in many situations will find themselves in a position to advise parents about their child's use of computer and video games. They can guide parents by helping them to appreciate that the impact of computers, just as that of any other toy, is influenced by the way in which they are introduced to and used in the child's daily life. "In a social environment that encourages child initiative and choice of activities, the computer is seen as just another play choice in that environment" (Porter, 1988, p 272).

The computer can facilitate interaction among the different domains of development (physical, cognitive, and emotional-social). Computer game play involves manipulation of ideas and active use of the child's imagination, helping to develop the "as if" or nonliteral characteristic of play. Computer games allow object-event probabilities to be discovered and learned and then manipulated and tested in competition (Malone, 1981). There are computer games that emphasize strategic planning and problem-solving; games based on first-person perspectives of real world environments; games that allow the player to take an "alter ego" through a storyline or series of events; adventure games that are based on character development; simulations of historical or futuristic warfare from a command perspective; and games that emphasize hand-eye coordination and reflexes (Myers, 1990). "A game in any one of these six categories might be used to achieve multiple and simultaneous player goals—education, entertainment, or social integration" (Myers, 1990). This active imagining can lead to the development of deeper understandings of concepts and greater flexibility of thought (Porter, 1988). Children may also use computer games as a social mediator. According to Myers (1990), well-designed computer games give the player an infinite number of probabilities and are therefore highly interactive and entertaining. When groups of children engage in this sort of computer game, social skills such as cooperation and reciprocative turn-taking are fostered (Swigger et al, 1983). Because computer and video games allow the player to try out skills, try on pretend roles, and gain practice in playing by the rules; children and adolescents learn a great deal about themselves from these games (Porter, 1988). According to Silvern and associates (1985), video games may provide catharsis for aggressive feelings.

Physical and motor development are areas in which computer and video games seem to have potential for negative developmental outcomes. Although many writers have stressed the importance of play opportunities for motor skill development during the early childhood years (Kaplan-Sanoff et al, 1988), very little research has been carried out to determine the relationship of play to physical/motor development. It is generally accepted that "optimum physical growth of the child depends on good nutrition, sufficient rest, consistent access to health care, and opportunities for active play" (Kaplan-Sanoff et al, 1988).

Because play is a primary medium through which physical and motor development are promoted, providing opportunities for gross and fine motor play has always been important. Such opportunities include the provision of equipment that encourages motor skill development. Computer technology, when included in the play environment, provides enjoyable and challenging opportunities for fine motor development. It is important to balance the play environment with equally enjoyable and challenging opportunities for *gross* motor development. Encouragement of such balance by significant adults in the environment is critical.

> Voluntary and coordinated movements such as jumping and running, pulling and stretching, and throwing and kicking involve coordinating patterns of movement. They are not totally maturationally determined. Environmental factors such as the child's play habits, opportunities to practice, and **environmental elicitors** influence their development. Sport related movements begin around age seven (an age when many children receive their first computer game) and continue throughout life. The level of development of these complex coordinated movement skills is highly related to **movement** opportunities. [Kaplan-Sanoff, et al, 1988]

According to Gallahue (1982), children who have not had opportunities and encouragement for these voluntary and coordinated movements by age 6 will continue to have difficulty learning complex skills for games and sports throughout life. Sutton-Smith (1985) stated:

> Modern children spend an increasingly large part of their lives alone with their toys. Childhood was once a part of village life. Children didn't play separately. Play is becoming steadily less physical, more computerized, and most of all more isolated. The shift in play has been steady: a taming of most (pretend) violence; mechanization of toys, increasingly electronic in character; symbolization in games of language, information and strategy, which have largely replaced rough physical play; decreasing differentiation between play of boys and girls; increasing remoteness from **direct** experience through fantasy; and most significantly isolation.

Nursing Involvement in Promotion of Play. The importance of social play to physical, cognitive, language, social, and moral development has previously been pointed out in this chapter. Unfortunately, too

TABLE 17-3
Promoting Healthy Play

Analysis: Nursing Diagnostic Statement 1

Response and Related or Risk Factors: *High risk for altered growth and development; risk factors*

- Lack of knowledge or ability of parents to facilitate developmentally appropriate play
- Lack of resources (economic) to provide children with developmentally appropriate play materials

Nursing Interventions

Provide play opportunities that promote development

- Provide anticipatory guidance for parents about appropriate play at the various developmental levels (see Table 17–3)
- Encourage parents to play with their children
- Role model to parents how to engage in interact-play
- Compliment parents on their interactions, choice of toys, and time given to play
- Assess resources in home (space, time, finances)
- Assist parents to find household items that can be used for developmentally appropriate activities

Analysis: Nursing Diagnostic Statement 2

Response and Related or Risk Factors: *Self-care deficit related to delayed skill development associated with motor, social, and language problems, emotional disturbances, mental retardation, or learning disability*

Nursing Interventions

Use play modalities in teaching skill development to allow the child to have a sense of control over his/her skill learning

Analysis: Collaborative Problem 1

High risk for altered growth and development, social; risk factor: sensory impairment, visual or hearing, of child along with parental knowledge deficit regarding ways to respond to the child with sensory impairments

(continued)

many parents and other individuals involved with the play of children find it easier to allow children to spend most or all of their time in computer play, which is often solitary, than to become involved with children in games that facilitate gross motor development (and also have the advantage of lending themselves to group play, which assists in the development of necessary social skills).

When one is aware of how many functions play serves for the child and of the interrelationship of play with all aspects of child development, it becomes obvious that adults who work with children should have knowledge and skill in ways to promote developmentally appropriate play behaviors in children. One example of a relevant *nursing diagnostic statement* would be ineffective individual coping related to inability to play. The characteristics of optimal play, which have been described previously, then become part of the **evaluation criteria** for evaluating the effectiveness of interventions. Inability to play might also be the **related or risk factor or etiology** for a number of other actual or potential responses in nursing diagnostic statements related to different domains of development. These might include impaired physical mobility and motor skill development, if physical and motor development have not been facilitated; altered thought processes, if parents have not supplied and facilitated opportunities to learn about characteristics of the child's environment; self-esteem disturbance, if a healthy sense of self has not developed; ineffective individual coping, when adequate opportunities to play out solutions to problems have not been available; impaired verbal communication; and others. Nursing interventions would focus on promoting optimal play behaviors and activities. Nursing diagnostic statements and collaborative problems with accompanying interventions are found in Table 17–3.

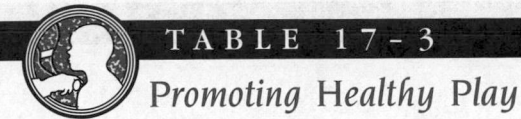

TABLE 17-3 (continued)

Nursing Interventions

Make referral to and collaborate with appropriate specialist

- Provide anticipatory guidance for parents to help them recognize and create alternative cues for interactive play, using unimpaired senses

Facilitate creation of an environment with an appropriate degree of stimulation

- Assist parents to choose a variety of stimuli (shapes, colors, textures, sounds, human touch, human voice)

Analysis: Collaborative Problem 2

High risk for altered growth and development, social and language; risk factor: emotional disturbance, mental retardation, or learning disability in child

Nursing Interventions

Make referral to and collaborate with developmental-behavioral pediatrician, speech therapist, child psychologist

- Encourage and work with parents to promote sociodramatic play
- Provide children with social rather than isolate toys

Analysis: Collaborative Problem 3

Post-trauma response

Nursing Interventions

Make referral to and collaborate with play therapist

Analysis: Nursing Diagnostic Statement 3

Ineffective individual coping related to inability to play associated with fear and anxiety regarding medical procedures including surgery

Nursing Interventions

- Implement medical play and/or psychologic preparation
- Arrange environment to encourage play
- Collaborate with child life specialist

Parents are an excellent resource to the nurse. To counsel effectively, the nurse first gains an understanding of the home situation and the availability of resources, including space, time, and playthings. It is important to adapt what is told to parents to the parameters that are feasible for the individual's family situation. Focusing part of each health care visit on play gives it the appropriate priority. From infancy, an appreciation of play can be fostered by identifying the sensorimotor activities that the infant displays.

There are certain conditions and attitudes that are necessary for play to occur. These include adequate time, space, equipment (toys and materials), peers with whom to interact, and adults who are warm and trusting and who can facilitate children's play activities (Bolig, 1990). Choosing safe, durable toys and encouraging activities suitable to their child's developmental level are tasks in which parents may need guidance. In addition to personal guidance from the nurse, there are many excellent books available to parents to assist them in choosing toys and play activities for each stage of their child's development. One such book is *Understanding Your Child Through Play* by Maggie Jones (1989). A summary of toys and activities geared to a child's age and partially adapted from Jones' (1989) book is found in Table 17–4. Jones also provides a list of the "top twenty toys" for children from birth through 5 years (pp 90–93). These are shown in Table 17–5. It is not necessary to buy expensive toys. Excellent opportunities for a child's progress are provided by common household equipment and the sounds and textures of the outdoors.

As previously noted, parents who engage in play involving exchange of facial expressions with their infant can help her or him to understand the nature and permanence of objects and separateness of iden-

TABLE 17-4
Promoting Growth and Development Through Toys and Activities

Activity or Toy	Developmental Aspects Promoted
0–3 mos	
Mobiles, crib bumpers, baby gym—brightly colored, strong patterns (especially the pattern of the human face), 8–10 inches from baby's face	Visual stimulation, awareness of environment, introduction to a variety of colors and shapes
Talking and singing, lullaby tapes, rattles, squeaky toys, musical toys, or music boxes. (Mittens with a bell sewed to each—*while attended*)	Auditory stimulation, cause-and-effect relationships, promote social relationships, promote attachment, facilitate language development
Tickling, "blowing raspberries" on her stomach, counting her toes, "bicycling her legs," providing a tactile surface to lie on and touch (sheepskin, velvet, satin, and corduroy ball), undressing her in the sun or wind, bouncing cradle, baby carriage or stroller rides, carrying her in a sling, rocking	Tactile stimulation, awareness of own body, promote attachment, promote trust and security
3–12 mos	
Things to grab and hold (that can be put in the mouth), e.g., rattles, teething rings; varying textures, e.g., wood, metal, sponge, cloth, "feely" board or blanket, mirrors, squeaky toys, and toys with moving parts, e.g., busy box, toy telephone; toys with a surprise, e.g., jack-in-the-box, household objects	Auditory and visual stimulation, safely tactile stimulation, promote hand-to-mouth activity, promote gross and fine motor skills, promote development of purposeful activity
Toys to promote exploration, e.g., containers to fill and empty (milk bottle and clothespin toy); and pour (water or sand), e.g., pitcher, teapot, sieve, old pocketbook, or suitcase and a selection of familiar items	Cause-and-effect relationships, gross (crawling) and fine motor skills, discover properties of objects, emotional development, facilitate learning of anticipation of action, stimulate size discrimination, language development, awareness of self and environment as separate, object permanence, encourage social interaction, enhance fine motor skills, teach about objects in the environment, foster social interaction
Shape sorter and stacking toys; push and go toys, stacking rings on pole, rattles on suction pads with flexible stems; toys that roll and move; games involving introduction to colors, shapes, and naming of objects; rolling, bouncing, kicking, reaching, and dancing; finger games, books, hide-and-seek games, peek-a-boo, naming body parts	
1–2 yrs	
Push and pull toys, toys to ride, rocking horse, water and sand play, small playground equipment, e.g., miniature sliding board, wading pool	Stimulate gross motor development, develop balance, promote sense of accomplishment
Imitative toys, e.g., tea set, play house, toy crib and baby, toy telephone, dolls, and soft toys	Learn roles, provide outlet for feelings and work through problems of real life, encourage language skills, provide comfort
Stacking and fitting toys, toys that unscrew, sorting toys, simple puzzles, peg and hole toys, messy play, e.g., clay, play dough, sand and water play	Fine motor skills, seeing how different shapes and sizes relate to each other, learning that objects have properties that are similar and different
Books and rhymes	Language development, learning about world, social development
Crayons and paints	Fine motor skills, stimulate creativity and self-expression, enhance eye-hand coordination, develop sense of accomplishment
2–3 yrs	
Blocks, stacking, and construction toys, large beads or empty spools, and sturdy string, toy tools, assortment of miniature objects, puppets, punching bag, dress-up props, plays with other children	Large and fine motor skills, promote imaginative play, provide outlet for handling own fears and aggressive feelings, encourage cooperative play
Puzzles, counting games, sorting and matching toys, picture lotto, simple card and board games	Facilitate understanding of how things are ordered and grouped, understanding numbers, symbol formation, learn cooperation
Trampoline or old mattress, ramp to roll things down, raised board for playing "tightrope," tunnels, sit and ride toys, ball games	Increase confidence in physical skill, discovery of properties of moving objects, promote sense of exploration
Books and storytelling, going to the library, talking about the world, word games	Language development, learning about the world, social development, increasing vocabulary
Musical instruments and singing games, art activities	Skill development, sense of rhythm, social development, learning to associate hearing with doing, encourage listening skills, fine motor skills, encourage creativity, encourage cooperative play

(continued)

TABLE 17-4
Promoting Growth and Development Through Toys and Activities (Continued)

Activity or Toy	Developmental Aspects Promoted
3–5 Yrs	
Increase opportunities for pretend play with toys, e.g., stethoscope, hats for different occupations, toy appliances, tractors, racing cars, masks, and puppets	Promote imaginative play, provide outlet for handling and learning feelings, promote cooperative pretend play
Building toys, e.g., Lego, blocks, train and highway sets and accessories, jigsaw puzzles	Increase manipulative skills, promote cooperative pretend play, sense of accomplishment, provide activities that promote thinking and planning
Art activities with safety or plastic scissors, e.g., collage, making greeting cards and posters, scrapbooks	Fine motor development will now allow coordination required for cutting
Simple board or card games, e.g., snap, snakes and ladders, dice games, counting games, memory games, magnetic letters, alphabet games, "writing" and "mailing" letters	Begin to learn rules, tolerate losing, number and letter recognition, learn concentration skills, encourage social skills
Books, stories, and songs—singing familiar songs as rounds, using percussion instruments while singing	To prepare for major events in life, deal with problems or fears, fairy tales, books to develop prereading skills. Assist to familiarize with world and address and overcome fears, encourage sense of rhythm and timing, and develop social skills
Active games, e.g., jungle gym and other playground equipment, tricycle, swimming, ball games	Development of coordination, balance, and strength, facilitate judgment of own physical capabilities and limitations, hand-eye coordination

Adapted in part from *Understanding your child through play* by Maggie Jones © 1989. Used by permission of the publisher, Prentice Hall Press/a Division of Simon & Schuster.

tity. Encouraging parents to reciprocate with sounds, movements, and facial expressions is how the beginnings of play are appreciated and encouraged. Role modeling interactive play with an infant during a health care visit is an influential aspect of promoting the beginning of healthy play behavior. As the child develops, parents need support and guidance to provide the variety of opportunities that children need. A supportive play environment for the infant would include toys that allow for learning of cause and effect and self as cause (such as busy boxes and crib gyms).

TABLE 17-5
Jones' (1989) Top 20 Toys

1. Rattles	12. Sit-and-ride toy
2. Soft toys	13. Tea set
3. Activity center	14. Dolls
4. Telephone	15. Puzzles
5. Stacking cups	16. Modeling materials
6. Shape sorter	17. Crayons, pens, and chalk
7. Pull-along toy	18. Construction toy
8. Balls	19. Practical toy, e.g., tool set or lacing cards
9. Music toy	20. Miniature toys
10. Books	
11. Pushcart—and blocks	

Data from Jones, M. (1989). *Understanding your child through play*. Englewood Cliffs, NJ: Prentice-Hall.

Since it has been demonstrated that more securely attached babies demonstrate healthier play patterns and have more advanced cognitive skills at age 6, the nurse would also carry out interventions to promote attachment.

Because it is so closely and critically related to children's development, encouragement of appropriate sociodramatic play activities is of paramount importance. Smilansky (1971) described ways in which parents can *indirectly* and *directly* facilitate their child's sociodramatic play abilities (Table 17–6).

Smilansky's influences provide a framework for looking at factors associated with the promotion of children's play by adults (Table 17–7).

Play and the Child with Problematic Human Responses

Up to this point, the discussion has focused on the child who is functioning well physically, emotionally, and psychologically. The following section focuses on play and the child who has an actual problem or is at high risk for a problem (see Table 17–3). The play of children with problems does not follow the same timetable as the play of children who do not have problems. For mentally retarded, developmentally delayed, and emotionally disturbed children and for children with a sensory impairment, play seems to follow a developmental sequence according to mental, not chronologic age. The severity of handicaps

TABLE 17–6
Smilansky's Framework for Facilitation of Children's Play

Indirect Influences

1. Providing for normal emotional relationships, essential for healthy identification
2. Providing for conceptual, informational, and verbal means essential for the understanding of human behavior and social relationships
3. Developing the power of abstraction and imagination, the ability to rise above the concretely present toward verbally described hypothetical existences
4. Encouragement of positive social relationships of the child with both parents and peers based on tolerance and self-discipline

Direct Influences

1. Providing for conditions that encourage sociodramatic play; friends to play with, toys, place, time, and so on
2. Teaching the child directly to imitate different behavior patterns in a playful manner and reinforcing this
3. Teaching the child to use make-believe in action and verbal expression

From Smilansky, S. (1971). "Can adults facilitate play in children? Theoretical and practical considerations." In Curry, N. E., & Arnaud, S. (Eds.). *Play: The child strives toward self-realization* (pp 39–50). © Copyright 1971 by the National Association for the Education of Young Children. Used by permission.

greatly affects the children's levels of exploratory and functional play (Bergen, 1988, p 147).

According to Bolig (1990, p 230), "children with intrapersonal problems (emotional or behavioral) or under threat of external events (hospitalization) are less likely to play at all or less rapidly engage in play." Some of the problems associated with the play of children who are physically or emotionally handicapped and general suggestions for their management are summarized in Table 17–8. These problems result from the interplay of factors related to the child and factors related to the parents. For instance, it is known that adults interact differently with impaired children than they do with unimpaired children.

Implications for Interventions

Assessment. Play can be used as a way to informally assess handicapped children's level of functioning, their ability to compensate for their handicap, and ways in which the environment helps or hinders their development (Bergen, 1988). This kind of assessment can provide important information regarding patterns that emerge that can be compared with other assessments and used to plan interventions (Frick, 1987). Observing children's play can provide valid insight into children's present and future levels of functioning, especially their social-cognitive functioning (Pellegrini & Perlmutter, 1988). Play patterns may give evidence of stress that children have encountered and their coping devices (Simon & Larson, 1985): themes of separation, aggression, power, need for orderliness, hypervigilance, divorce; and boundary problems (McDermott, 1968; Wallerstein & Kelly, 1981).

Environmental Design. The design of a play environment influences play frequency and abilities. "Children, especially when at play, seem to be exquisitely sensitive to *all* the qualitative aspects of their world (Bergen et al, 1988). When illness and trauma diminish essential life opportunities, the environment can make a difference" (Olds, 1988, p 218). Many children under stress cannot play and are distracted by social interactions around them. They can be helped by giving them quiet play spaces with low but defined boundaries that allow eye contact with adults. "Well-designed environments may both compensate for the child's imbalances and spark the natural potential to be as alive as possible. In particular by acknowledging the child's motivation for wholeness, the setting helps call forth latent powers to nurture self to well-being. Such an environment then acts as a healing agent" (Olds, 1988, p 218). Data from research designed to facilitate play in physically handicapped, hospitalized children suggest that a carefully designed environment led to increases in the amount of time spent in partial play, symbolic play, and total play, with a concomitant decrease in unoccupied wandering and nonplay activities (Eisert et al, 1988). There are resources from which health care facilities can obtain assistance in creating an environment that optimizes the potential of children who use it. One such resource is the Association for the Care of Children's Health Design Resource Center and *Resource Catalog* (7910 Woodmont Avenue, Suite 300, Bethesda, MD, 20814).

Skill Development. Play can be used as a way to facilitate skill development in children with special problems. Specific motor and/or self-care skills needing development or strengthening can be practiced in a play situation. A child who is learning to feed herself can begin by feeding a doll. Speech and language therapy are frequently accompanied by games. Teaching within the context of play tends to give children a greater sense of control over their learning. In play, a child can make choices and is allowed to make mistakes in a relaxed and "fun" atmosphere. Play can also be major means of acquiring coping skills. Children engage in fantasy play to deal with issues that are important to them at the time. (This can be as simple as the 2-year-old, whose mother was pregnant, who played out scenes in which the "mommy vomited the baby in the toilet.") Children who are preoccupied with serious problems often display less mature play (Hetherington et al, 1979). The role of the adult may simply be to allow play to occur so that some sense of mastery over stress is experienced.

TABLE 17-7
The Use of Smilansky's Framework in Considering the Ways in Which Parents and Other Adults Can Promote Optimal Children's Play Behaviors and Activities

Indirect Influences

1. **Providing for normal emotional relationships, essential for healthy identification**

   "The less threatened children are either by intra-personal demands or external events, the more likely and rapidly they are to engage in play" (Bolig et al, 1986). "Constructive parental interaction as well as ample opportunities for practice . . . of make-believe games leads to greater control over aggression and restlessness and to evidence of the positive emotions of interest, excitement, and joy" (Singer & Singer, 1988)

2. **Providing for conceptual, informational, and verbal means essential for the understanding of human behavior and social relationships**

   Children whose parents interact with them by labeling and explaining aspects of their environment, telling them stories, and showing tolerance of imaginary play and overt verbalizations tend to be more capable of control in waiting situations, show less overt aggressive behavior, show better ability to assimilate knowledge from the environment, and tend to be less susceptible to some of the more negative effects of watching television (Singer & Singer, 1988)

   Children need to be able to rid themselves of aggressive feelings and urges. They can do so through symbolic play. Parents can give "permission" for aggressive pretend play by providing appropriate toys for the expression of aggressive feelings and urges (Bettleheim, 1987). Games and toys such as cops and robbers, war and Ninja turtles allow children to experience how good and evil (or bad) feel. Children want and need to believe that good wins out

3. **Developing the power of abstraction and imagination, the ability to rise above the concretely present toward verbally described hypothetical existences**

   "Children's ability to use their own imaginative skills and make-believe for effective assimilation functions and schema formation depends in part on the extent to which adults interact with them" (Singer & Singer, 1988). There are constructive ways in which parents can interact with their children to assist them to develop their abilities to conceptualize. One of the most important is to make sure their child has ample opportunities for pretend or fantasy play. When parents are interacting with their children, they should take advantage of opportunities to discuss inner state and feelings of people, such as pain, sadness, cold, and hunger. There are also books available for children that allow them to explore the idea of feelings. (One excellent example is *Feelings* by J. B. Murphy, Black Moss Press)

4. **Encouragement of positive social relationships of the child with both parents and peers based on tolerance and self-discipline**

   Children need plenty of time and freedom to play. Much of children's play in today's culture is adult-directed and adult-dominated (e.g., Little League). Adults can facilitate healthy play in children by leaving them alone. Children who are left alone to play games have the freedom to argue over what to play, how to play, and the rules for playing. This kind of freedom in play helps with the development of reasoning activities and social interaction that would not occur in adult-directed play (Bettleheim, 1987, p 38).

Direct Influences

1. **Providing for conditions that encourage sociodramatic play; friends to play with, toys, place, time, and so on**

   By the time they are toddler age, children need friends to play with. The presence of a peer during play time results in more "high-level" and less "low-level" play with toys than occurs in the absence of a peer (Rubinstein & Howes, 1976; Cohen & Tomlinson-Keasey, 1980)

   Involving preschool-age children in a short planning period before play assists the children to anticipate what they will do in their play. Adults can add or delete materials from play area to stimulate new uses of existing materials and suggest new ways of "playing the game." Parents can also ask children to think about what they need to continue a story being played out or suggest new roles ("What if there was a handsome prince next door?") to be added to the story (Bergen, 1988)

   The child's physical environment, including his or her playthings, should be set up in such a way that they give permission and time to play. The child should have sufficient play materials and equipment. Toys should be easily manipulated and visually detailed

2. **Teaching the child directly to imitate different behavior patterns in a playful manner and reinforcing this**

   Given previous findings regarding gender-specific play, parents probably need to foster cross-gender play experiences. The play environments of children can be purposefully structured to be gender-free. Play groups should be mixed-gender, attempts should be made to provide children with female and male role models across gender activities (Ignico, 1990)

3. **Teaching the child to use make-believe in action and verbal expression**

   It is estimated that preschool-age children spend 25% of their waking time, or approximately 4 hrs, playing and that they usually play with manufactured toys, most of which are realistic-looking with apparent and conventional functions—almost three times as much time as is spent with materials not specifically intended for play. Detail and realism of high-realism replicas can hinder free creative play. (Toddlers need toys that are highly representative of the actual referent object.) Low-realism toys are play materials that can be used in a variety of ways, and these are more conducive to creative and rich fantasy play in older preschoolers than high-realism toys. Another problem with high-realism toys is that they do not tend to facilitate cooperative play but are more likely to produce solitary and parallel play (McLoyd, 1986)

TABLE 17-8
Factors Associated with the Play of Children with Problems

Children Who Are Abused or Neglected
Appear to lack energy for play or do not play at all—as if all of their energy is being used to meet the demands of their situation (Bergen, 1988)
Kempe and Kempe describe "the frozen watchfulness of abused children who expect punishment, are unable to play or explore, move from one toy to another in haphazard, impulsive manner, and make little use of spontaneous language to promote relationships"
Playful parent-child interactions do not occur. Abusive parents negatively perceive the noise and clutter that children create and often regard it as a reason for further abuse (Bergen, 1988)
Play therapy is the preferred method of treatment, especially for very young abused children (Chan & Leff, 1988; Gil, 1991; James, 1989; Webb, 1991)
Special techniques for using play with abused children, while they are hospitalized, are described by Chan and Leff (1988)
Children Who Are Mentally Retarded
In infants, delayed exploratory play, less use of language, less social interaction, and more time in nonplay activities (Bergen, 1988)
Later, "emotionally and mentally disturbed children show lack of self-control, more external rather than intrinsic motivation for their play, high rigidity, lack of mutuality, and infringement of rules and norms" (Marino, 1988, p 230)
Mentally retarded children with a mental age of 7 yrs prefer more structure, more concreteness, and more constructive materials than do nonretarded children, possibly owing to a greater sense of helplessness and dependency seen in retarded children as they grow older (Bergen, 1988, p 148)
When mentally retarded children were taught play forms that involved intensive interaction between adult and child, they showed improved behavioral control in play situations (van der Kooij, 1989, p 328)
Children Who Have Sensory and Language Impairments
Visually impaired preschool-age children use their hands more in functional and exploratory play (Bergen, 1988, p 147)
Levels of exploratory play increase with time spent in a school program that facilitates such play (Olson, 1983)
Toy preferences of visually impaired preschoolers are similar to those of nonimpaired preschoolers (Olson, 1983)
Visually impaired preschoolers engage in more functional play and less symbolic and social play than do nonimpaired preschoolers (Bergen, 1988, p 148)
Hearing-impaired preschool-age children and language-impaired children also show lower levels of symbolic play and spend more time in noninteractive constuctive play than in social and symbolic play. When they do engage in symbolic play, there is less play with objects (Bergen, 1988, p 148)
Autistic Children
Very low levels of pretense play (if any), even when it is modeled for them (Marino, 1988)

One of the most important areas in which skill development is indicated is the child's *social play.* It is possible that, because visually and hearing impaired and retarded infants show lower levels of responsiveness to interactions with their parents, parents' play styles are different than they would be if the child were unimpaired. The nurse should assess for the presence of the collaborative problem, ***high risk for altered growth and development; risk factors: parental knowledge deficit regarding ways to playfully respond to the child with sensory impairments.*** Anticipatory guidance for parents to help them recognize and create alternative cues (often involving unimpaired senses) that they can use with their infants to foster social play behaviors that will increase later social play (Bergen, 1988). This will usually involve consultation and referral with other health care professionals such as speech and hearing therapists.

Lack of social and language skills is one of the most stressful aspects of handicaps for emotionally disturbed, learning disabled, and retarded children (Bergen, 1988). Social and language skills can be enhanced through sociodramatic play. Marino (1988) found that pretend play can be significantly increased in a program that emphasizes the use of symbols. An intervention in which teachers planned and directed sociodramatic play increased social play levels in handicapped preschoolers (Strain, 1975; Strain & Wiegerink, 1976). Providing children with "social" rather than "isolate" toys also tends to encourage more social play (Beckman & Kohl, 1984). Social toys are those that involve play by several children at a time—a game as simple as slap-jack would be appropriate. Collaboration with other health care professionals is also useful here. The nurse can work collaboratively with a developmental disabilities specialist or a behavioral pediatrician.

Children in Health Care Settings

Entry into the health care system occurs under a variety of circumstances. There is an element of mystery and fear of the unknown for a child who faces even minimally intrusive encounters. An x-ray machine, a blood pressure cuff, or a thermometer is a potential threat to a child. It has been known for at least 40 years that hospitalization and the treatments and procedures that accompany it can be traumatic to a child (Prugh et al, 1953; Thompson, 1985; Vernon et al, 1965). Reactions to hospitalization and illness are influenced by many factors, including the child's gender, age and developmental stage, what happens during the hospitalization, past experiences, his or her personality before hospitalization, and his or her coping style. Children between the ages of 6 months and 3 years have been shown to be the "most vulnerable to persistent emotional sequelae of hospitalization" (Goldberger, 1988). Children under the age of 7 continue to show high levels of anxiety about procedures for longer periods (up to 2 years) than do older children; and girls tend to exhibit higher levels of anxiety about procedures than do boys (Katz et al, 1980).

Hospitalization does not necessarily have to be a negative experience. If the child is properly supported, hospitalization can be a period of positive growth in which the child learns new coping abilities or strengthens previous ones. This is especially true of a one-time, time-limited hospitalization for an acute condition. The benefits of play are reflected in the general acceptance of play programs and use of play in the home, physician's office, and inpatient and outpatient settings to help a child cope with stress and understand a procedure.

Therapeutic Play

Therapeutic play has been demonstrated to be a primary way to assist children to cope with problems and traumas including hospitalization. All children's hospitals and some general hospital pediatric units have separate space devoted to provision of play activities for the child client. These playrooms represent "safe" places for the child to engage in diversional or therapeutic play activities. It is important that nurses and other health care professionals do not violate that safety by performing procedures in the playroom. "Play has long been viewed as a primary means of ameliorating the negative psychosocial effects of illness and hospitalization on children" (Bolig, 1988, p 132). There is a *redundancy* of data indicating the value of therapeutic play for hospitalized children (Perrin, 1992). Even play in a hospital waiting room has been shown to have positive benefits for the child and parent (Ispa et al, 1988; Meer, 1985). With the advent of the philosophy that children should be cared for at home or through outpatient facilities, the play programs that are now established in inpatient settings are already being adapted for transfer to the community.

"Therapeutic play" is defined as the use of play specifically as a language for children to communicate their thoughts and feelings. It is goal-directed with a specific purpose established by the nurse following input from the child (Tiedemann et al, 1990, p 95). The therapeutic value of such play lies partially in the fact that it allows the child to express her or his feelings in an environment conducive to the expression of such feelings (Bergen, 1988). Unfortunately, the extent to which play is encouraged in hospital settings is highly variable. Playrooms tend to be open for shorter periods and staff often have very little time for sociodramatic play (Bolig, 1990; Bolig et al, 1986). This is one of the unfortunate results of the necessity of cost-cutting measures in hospitals. Specific functions of therapeutic play for children in health care settings, especially hospitals, are shown in Table 17–9.

Therapeutic play cannot be assumed to be an automatic panacea for all children who have problematic responses related to hospitalization and/or procedures. Factors known to inhibit play include immobility, dull or repetitive environments, overstimulating environments, and fear (Crocker, 1978). Under circumstances of severe stress, children have been observed not to play at all (Gottlieb & Portnoy, 1988; Petrillo & Sanger, 1980). Special efforts to provide play experiences have been noted to have a positive effect on the psychologic problems of sensory deprivation, time and space disorientation, boredom, passivity, anxiety, and depression that are seen in children isolated in a protective environment (e.g., for bone marrow transplant) (O'Connell, 1984; Pearson et al, 1980).

TABLE 17–9
Functions of Play for Children in Health Care Settings

1. Assessment and diagnosis of the child's feelings and perceptions regarding hospital experiences
2. Preparation for procedures and hospital experiences to allow the child to "relive and make sense of painful experiences"
3. Provide the child with a means to achieve mastery of feelings and facilitate the child's ability to cope with hospital experiences
4. Provide for emotional support, stress reduction, and tension release through facilitated expression of emotions
5. Provide a link with the child's life outside the hospital
6. Provide a temporary escape . . . into a diversional activity

Data from Bergen, 1988; Del Po & Frick, 1988; Frick & Del Po, 1987; Walker, 1989; Wilson, 1985

All therapeutic play is conducted by professionals educated in normal childhood growth and development (Garot, 1986). In most health care settings, nurses and child life specialists (CLS) collaborate in carrying out a therapeutic play program (Kuhn, 1989). A CLS is a member of the health care team who focuses on the emotional and developmental needs of hospitalized children, using play and other forms of communication to reduce stress for children and their families (Wilson, 1985). Nurses should facilitate children's *need* to play by accepting the need, providing play opportunities, encouraging emotional expressions through play, and providing times for therapeutic play (Walker, 1989). Garot (1986) emphasized the importance of the nurse's involvement in therapeutic play: "When the professional nurse incorporates therapeutic play in the care of the pediatric patient, recovery and positive outcomes are facilitated" (p 111). The use of a therapeutic play plan in conjunction with the nursing process can greatly reduce stress and the related anxiety of problems and traumas including hospitalization (Frick, 1987).

Inclusion of parents in the child's play plan is as important as their inclusion in other aspects of medical and nursing treatment. Parents who are properly prepared to participate in therapeutic play feel more comfortable and experience a greater sense of well-being than parents who do not have this opportunity (Wilson, 1985). These feelings arc passed on to their children. If parents are assessed as able, they should be supported in efforts to continue therapeutic play after discharge. Types of therapeutic play include play therapy and medical play.

Play Therapy

"Play therapy" is most commonly used with children who have *serious* emotional/psychologic problems, such as severely traumatized children. Because of the high incidence of long-term and often catastrophic illnesses (such as cancer and cystic fibrosis) in children who access the health care system today, play therapy is used with many of these children. There are many definitions of play therapy, most of which agree that it is a form of psychotherapy carried out by a professional who has been educated in play therapy methods. Play therapy has been used since the early 1900s and is based on the premise that play "serves as a window to children's emotional lives" (Bergen, 1988), just as the adult's verbalizations serve as a means to understanding his or her inner processes. Play therapy consists of a wide variety of treatment modalities with varying theoretical orientations and technical strategies. "Play therapy uses games and toys as the primary method through which the therapist and patient can process the patient's disturbing psychologic problems in order to overcome obstacles to mental and emotional growth" (Hartman & Hanson, 1986). "Play therapy is a relationship between the child and therapist . . . where the child is encouraged to express himself freely, to release pent-up emotions and repressed feelings, and to work through his fear and anger so that he comes to be himself and functions in terms of his real potentials and abilities" (Moustakas, 1959, p 227). Play therapy may be directive, in that the therapist assumes responsibility for guidance and interpretation, or it may be nondirective, in which case the therapist leaves responsibility and direction to the child (Del Po & Frick, 1988).

In play therapy, children express, work through, and master psychologic difficulties (Fig. 17–10). "So valuable is play in this connection that play therapy has become the main avenue for helping young children with emotional difficulties" (Bettleheim, 1987, p 35). What a child plays is motivated by inner processes, such as recent learning, desires, problems, anxieties. Even the most "normal" children have problems that seem overwhelming. Play gives them the opportunity to cope/practice in relation to present and past concerns. Erikson (1950) said, "to play it out" is one of the most natural self-healing measures childhood affords.

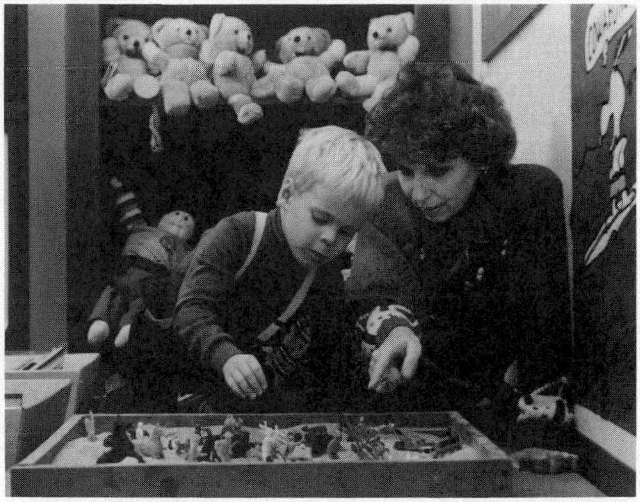

FIGURE 17 - 10. A play therapist works with the child, using games and toys to allow the child to express, work through, and master psychologic difficulties. (Photograph courtesy of University of South Carolina—University Publications, Columbia, South Carolina 29208.)

Medical Play

"Medical play" is a type of play that focuses on concrete events in health care settings (especially hospitals), such as surgery, injections, and intrusive or traumatic procedures, and that allows the child to play out these events (with toys and actual medical equipment) and the accompanying feelings in the presence of a supportive adult (Wilson, 1985). Medical play has four characteristics (McCue, 1988, p 158):

1. It always has as part of its content medical themes and/or the use of medical equipment.
2. It may be offered or initiated by an adult but is voluntarily maintained by the child.
3. It is usually enjoyable for the child and is often accompanied by laughter and relaxation; however, the process of the play can sometimes be intense and aggressive.
4. Medical play and psychologic preparation are not synonymous. When an adult attempts to prepare a child psychologically for a medical event by demonstrating a procedure or familiarizing a child with equipment, education may occur, but not necessarily play. Play may follow familiarization if play opportunities are made available.

Psychologic Preparation for Medical Events. Preparation for hospitalization, procedures, or surgery is a purposeful educative process in which a nurse and/or CLS prepares the child and parents, cognitively and psychologically, for what will happen to them. When this preparation involves the use of dolls and/or puppets and actual medical equipment in a "play" rehearsal, it is called "preparation play." If the process involves only demonstration by the health care worker, it is not preparation *play;* it is psychologic preparation without play. In preparation play, the health care worker has control over the setting and theme of the play. It is now believed by many that excessive control was maintained in the past (Bolig et al, 1986; McCue, 1988). Even in preparation play, the child should control the direction taken by the play and when it is terminated. Spontaneity must be allowed and the child must be a full participant.

Psychologic preparation focuses on three major themes: provision of information; encouragement of emotional expression; and establishment of trusting relationships between child and health care worker (Manion, 1990). Several types of information are provided to the child—information about the procedure itself, information about the sensations the child will experience during the procedure, and information regarding specific coping skills. Research has convincingly demonstrated that preparation has resulted in increased knowledge about procedures by children and in decreased anxiety and levels of behavioral upset (Manion, 1990; Perrin, 1992). When *sensory information* was added to procedural information, children's anxiety and behavioral upset scores were even lower (Johnson et al, 1975, 1976). Sensory information involves the provision of information to the child regarding how things will feel (cold, stinging, numb, etc), sound, look, or smell. Provision of information regarding coping skills has resulted in less anxiety and behavioral upset and greater skill in use of alternative coping measures (Manion, 1990). When psychologic preparation focused on provision of emotional support, children receiving the support interventions suffered lower levels of anxiety and behavioral upset and were more cooperative than children who did not receive the support. It is desirable that psychologic preparation of children for medical events be followed or accompanied by opportunities for the child to "play out" what was taught. This is *preparation play.* Recent research has indicated that preparation play should be accompanied by postprocedural play to allow the child to master the feelings that accompany the experience for which she or he was prepared (Betz, 1982; Frick & Del Po, 1987; Oremland, 1988).

Types of Medical Play Activities. Medical play "can be adult directed, child directed, or anywhere along that continuum. The more the adult takes control of the activity the more likely it is that the child will be forced to confront anxiety arousing issues (possibly) without resolution" (McCue, 1988, p 160). It was previously noted that preparation play tends to be more under the control of the adult. When the play is structured so that the adult has *minimal* control of structure and content the child is more likely to proceed at a "safe" (for him or her) pace. Medical play activities should be under the child's control as much as possible, and a variety of play equipment and opportunities should be made available. By doing so, the nurse allows the child choice and avoids the possibility of overwhelming the child with a play modality that is psychologically threatening.

McCue (1988) has described four types of medical play. In *role rehearsal/role reversal play,* children take the roles of health care professionals and (using actual medical equipment) re-enact actual medical events they have experienced (especially those that are ongoing or were intrusive or traumatic) with dolls, puppets, or stuffed animals. Burstein and Meichenbaum (1979) and McTigue and Pinkham (1978) found that children who were able to play with stress-related (surgery, dental procedures) toys react better and tend to show less anxiety after procedures. Role rehearsal/role reversal play can occur as part of preparation play or it can be a spontaneous activity on the part of the child. As was previously stated, the child should maintain control over the content and process of the play.

In *medical fantasy play,* children do not use actual medical equipment. Instead they use objects such as blocks, doll houses, play animals, and so forth to symbolically re-enact actual medical events they have experienced. This allows the fearful or anxious child to avoid contact with anxiety-producing objects while still working through the medical event. Such play is more likely to occur spontaneously and reiterates the need for having a wide variety of play materials available to the child (Fig. 17–11).

Indirect medical play is characterized by the structured use of activities such as puzzles, coloring books, music, and games with a hospital theme to provide opportunities for familiarization, exploration,

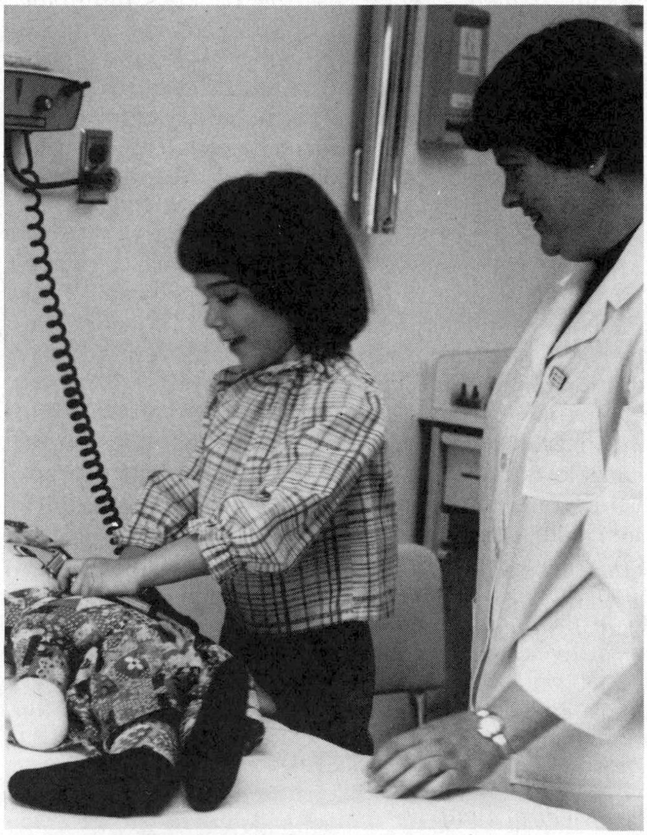

FIGURE 17 - 11. The child will benefit from therapeutic play. A girl gives her doll an examination just after she herself has undergone one. (Photograph by Cynthia Stewart.)

and education related to medical experiences. Although this can occur spontaneously, it is usually adult-structured to the extent that the game or coloring book is made available to the child by the adult. Another form of indirect medical play is the use of medical equipment in nonfantasy, nonmedical ways (such as syringes for squirt guns, medical tubing as a giant drinking straw). This form of indirect medical activity is more likely to be a spontaneous activity initiated by the child. It *can* be initiated by the adult who knows the child well enough to suggest a "game" in which "we see how many different ways we can use these things." Both of these indirect medical play activities allow desensitization of the child to the feared objects.

A fourth form of medical play is *medical art*. This involves making art materials available and allowing the child to use them in whatever way he or she chooses, including art activities that express feelings and perceptions regarding medical events.

There are many excellent resources available to the nurse who wishes to incorporate therapeutic play activities into the care of children in health care settings. Several of these are shown in Table 17–10.

Symbolic Play Responses to Health Care Events

As in the play of children without problems, the play of hospitalized children is often symbolic. This means that the nurse must observe the child's play carefully and try to understand it in relation to a previously assessed knowledge of the child's current situation and past experiences, including accompanying perceptions, play patterns, and coping methods. Only when this is done can the nurse offer support and enable the child in efforts to master experiences. Clues to the special significance of play behaviors often lie in their intensity, inflexibility, and/or repetitiveness. The child may not be aware of the meaning of her or his play behaviors. The nurse can assist her or him by following the child's lead by verbalizing what is happening, including accompanying feelings, and implications of feelings. The nurse should *never attempt to interpret what is happening, but just reflect*.

Play has an assessment value similar to that which was mentioned previously for the child with problematic human responses. Medical play also reveals important information regarding the child. There is known to be a developmental sequence in the understanding of illness and hospitalization (Brewster, 1982). Additionally, children who are hospitalized often regress to an earlier play stage. Children's misunderstandings are often reflected in their play. Nurses should assess the child to determine and provide play opportunities appropriate to the play stage and level of development to which they have regressed. Play during or after preparation often reveals fears and/or misperceptions that are held by the child. Oremland (1988) described a child who had been prepared for the schedule of turning that would occur after his spica cast was applied. He drew a hamster in a cage running in a turning wheel. Another child, newly diagnosed with diabetes mellitus, drew a map with countries labeled "Insulin," "Urinalysis," "Sugar Level," and so forth, and one small "land-locked" nation called "Scared" (Oremland, 1988). Another child who had recently been placed in bilateral Buck's traction, put Plastic Man in a toy bed and stretched his legs as far as they would go. A child who had had both feet amputated drew numerous pictures of ghosts and repeatedly requested that "Casper the Friendly Ghost" be read to her.

Some play will reveal themes suggesting a need for control. One 8-year-old, who was hospitalized with frequent episodes of status asthmaticus and who controlled his mother with the threat of asthma attacks, drew himself as a magician with a top hat and magic wand. Oremland (1988) describes a child, who desperately wanted to go home, who repeatedly allowed a jack-in-box to "get out." Efforts to maintain a sense of control can also be seen in the child who repeatedly asks for the same story, such as the child with leukemic alopecia who requested "Rapunzel" (Oremland, 1988). Children after surgery for hypospadias show repetitive, almost compulsive water play, squirting water through squirt guns and syringes and playing out crises with firetrucks and firehoses (Oremland, 1988; Petrillo & Sanger, 1980). Another way to obtain a sense of control over events and accompanying feelings is to reconstruct them in such a way as to change what originally occurred. Emma Plank (1971) described her work with burned children and their repetitive play with water to repair the damage done by fire.

Some children do not achieve control or resolution in their play. Oremland (1988) describes a board game resembling Monopoly that was created by a child with terminal leukemia. The game board included squares with smiles labeled "Remission" and frowns labeled "Exacerbations." In repeated playing of the game, the child never revealed the outcome. Such play may alert the nurse to the need to assess for the existence of problematic human responses such as anxiety, fear, anticipatory grief, powerlessness, hopelessness, spiritual distress, ineffective individual coping, and impaired adjustment. If such a response is found, the nurse can assess for the etiology and, using the assessed etiology as a guide, facilitate the child's ability to work through the response.

TABLE 17-10
Resources for Therapeutic Play Activities

Association for the Care of Children's Health (1990). *Psychosocial care of children in hospitals: A clinical practice manual*. Washington, DC: Author.
Hart, R., Mather, P. L., Slack, J. F., & Powell, M. A. (1992). *Therapeutic play activities for hospitalized children*. St. Louis: CV Mosby.

Rather than "acting out" problematic themes in dramatic play, older children often reveal such content in stories, poems, and artwork. Krietemeyer and Heiney (1992) showed the value of storytelling as a therapeutic technique in a group for school-aged oncology patients. They found storytelling useful for helping older children resolve psychologic conflicts related to their illness.

The play of children has been examined by theorists for centuries. The most enduring interpretation is that children play to have fun. The character of play changes as a child matures, but children at all ages play if they are able to. Play contributes to and is an expression of development. As children play, physical, emotional, social, and cognitive skills are developed. Children who develop in an environment in which play is encouraged have a greater chance to achieve their maximal potential than those in environments in which play opportunities are lacking. Nurses who work with children and their families can assist parents and other caretakers to encourage play that is developmentally appropriate.

A child who has a special health care or developmental problem or who has been traumatized in some way may be unable to play; or his or her play may reveal serious emotional and developmental problems. Again, the nurse who works with these children and their families can provide direct assistance through therapeutic play or by collaborating with professionals trained to provide play therapy.

KEY CONCEPTS

Concepts Related to Basic Information

- There are many definitions of play. Many include that it is self-directed and pleasurable.
- The kind of play engaged in is largely determined by developmental stage.
- Categories of play include: exploratory, functional, or repetition play; constructive or building play; symbolic sociodramatic, fantasy, or pretend play; social play and games with rules; and rough-and-tumble play.
- Infants and toddlers spend a great deal of time in exploratory or practice play.
- Pretend or sociodramatic play reaches its peak in the preschool years.
- Preschoolers also begin constructive play and rough-and-tumble play.
- Symbolic or pretend play is incorporated into games with rules and language play in the school-age years.
- Adolescents engage in fantasy or symbolic play through mental activity or fantasy games.
- Games with rules, either board or computer games, or games of physical activity (including organized athletics) are a predominant form of adolescent play.
- All areas of development have the potential for being furthered by appropriate play activities.
- Computer games can encourage the development of fine motor coordination and cognitive development and problem-solving. Computer games must be balanced with physically active play.

Concepts Related to Nursing Assessment

- Observation of play activities allows the nurse to assess many areas of development.

Concepts Related to Nursing Intervention

- Selecting or helping parents select developmentally appropriate play activities or activities that will enhance development in problem areas is a nursing role.
- Nurses can serve as role models of interactive play for parents.
- Therapeutic play assists children in coping with stressful situations.
- Play areas in hospitals and clinics should be "safe" areas from physical interventions.
- Play is an important medium through which children can be prepared for medical encounters.

REFERENCES

Ambron, S. (1981). *Child development* (2nd ed.). New York: Holt, Rinehart and Winston.

Beckman, P. J., & Kohl, F. L. (1984). The effects of social and isolate toys on the interactions and play of integrated and nonintegrated groups of preschoolers. *Education and Training of the Mentally Retarded, 19*(3), 169–174.

Beckwith, L. (1985). Parent-child interaction and social-emotional development. In C. C. Brown & A. W. Gottfried (Eds.). *Play interaction: The role of toys and parental involvement in children's development* (pp 152–159). Skillman, NJ: Johnson & Johnson.

Belsky, J., Garduque, L., & Hrncir, E. (1984). Assessing performance, competence, and executive capacity in infant play: Relations to home environment and security of attachment. *Developmental Psychology, 20*(3), 406–417.

Belsky, J., & Most, R. K. (1981). From exploration to play: A cross-sectional study of infant free behavior. *Developmental Psychology, 17,* 630–639.

Bergen, D. (1988). *Play as a medium for learning and development.* Portsmouth, NH: Heinemann.

Bergen, D., Gaynard, L., & Mousslein, E. (1988). Designing special play environments. In D. Bergen (Ed.). *Play as a medium for learning and development* (pp 275–297). Portsmouth, NH: Heinemann.

Bettleheim, B. (1987). The importance of play. *The Atlantic Monthly, 259,* 35–46.

Betz, C. L. (1982). After the operation: Postprocedural sessions to allay anxiety. *MCN: American Journal of Maternal Child Nursing, 7,* 260–263.

Blehar, M. C., Lieberman, A. F., & Ainsworth, M. D. S. (1977). Early face-to-face interaction and its relation to later infant-mother attachment. *Child Development, 48,* 182–194.

Bolig, R. (1988). Guest editorial. The diversity and complexity of play in health care settings. *Children's Health Care, 16*(3), 132–133.

Bolig, R. (1990). Play in health care settings: A challenge for the 1990s. *Children's Health Care, 19*(4), 229–233.

Bolig, R., Fernie, D. E., & Klein, E. L. (1986). Unstructured play in

hospital settings: An internal locus of control rationale. *Children's Health Care, 15*(2), 101–107.
Bretherton, I. (1985). Pretense: Practicing and playing with social understanding. In C. C. Brown & A. W. Gottfried (Eds.). *Play interaction: The role of toys and parental involvement in children's development* (pp 69–79). Skillman, NJ: Johnson & Johnson.
Brewster, A. (1982). The chronically ill child's conception of illness. *Pediatrics, 69*(3), 355–362.
Burstein, S., & Meichenbaum, D. (1979). The work of worrying in children undergoing surgery. *Journal of Abnormal Child Psychiatry, 7*(2), 121–132.
Carvalho, A. M. A., Smith, P. K., Hunter, T., & Costabile, A. (1990). Playground activities for boys and girls: Developmental and cultural trends in children's perceptions of gender differences. *Play & Culture, 3,* 343–347.
Chan, J. M., & Leff, P. T. (1988). Play and the abused child: Implications for acute pediatric care. *Children's Health Care, 16*(3), 169–176.
Chance, P. (1979). *Learning through play.* New York: Johnson & Johnson.
Christie, J., & Johnsen, P. (1983). The role of play in social-intellectual development. *Review of Educational Research, 53,* 93–116.
Coates, D. L., & Lewis, M. (1984). Early mother-infant interaction and infant cognitive status as predictors of school performance and cognitive behavior in six-year-olds. *Child Development, 55,* 1219–1230.
Cohen, N. L., & Tomlinson-Keasey, C. (1980). The effects of peers and mothers on toddler's play. *Child Development, 51,* 921–924.
Crocker, E. (1978). Play programs in pediatric settings. In E. Gellert (Ed.). *Psychosocial aspects of pediatric care* (pp 95–110). New York: Grune & Stratton.
Csikzentmihayli, M. (1979). The concept of flow. In B. Sutton-Smith (Ed.). *Play and learning* (pp 257–274). New York: Gardner.
Curry, N., & Arnaud, S. H. (1974). Cognitive implications in children's spontaneous role play. *Theory and Practice, 13*(4), 273–277.
DeLoache, J. S., Sugarman, S., & Brown, A. W. (1985). The development of error correction strategies in young children's manipulative play. *Child Development, 56,* 928–939.
Del Po, E. G., & Frick, S. B. (1988). Directed and nondirected play as therapeutic modalities. *Children's Health Care, 16,* 261–267.
Eisen, G. (1988). *Children and play in the holocaust.* Amherst: The University of Massachusetts Press.
Eisert, D., Kulka, L., & Moore, K. (1988). Facilitating play in hospitalized handicapped children: The design of a therapeutic play environment. *Children's Health Care, 16*(3), 201–208.
Erikson, E. H. (1950). *Childhood and society.* New York: WW Norton.
Fagot, B. I. (1984). Teacher and peer reactions to boys and girls play styles. *Sex Roles, 11,* 691–702.
Fenson, L. (1985). The developmental progression of exploration and play. In C. C. Brown & A. W. Gottfried (Eds.). *Play interactions* (pp 31–38). Skillman, NJ: Johnson & Johnson.
Frick, S. B. (1987). Integrating growth and development content into practice: A nursing process framework. *Nurse Educator, 12*(1), 30–33.
Frick, S. B., & Del Po, E. (1987). Play behaviors of children undergoing bone marrow aspiration. *Journal of Psychosocial Oncology, 4*(4), 69–77.
Gallahue, D. L. (1982). *Understanding motor development in children.* New York: Wiley.
Garot, P. A. (1986). Therapeutic play: Work of both child and nurse. *Journal of Pediatric Nursing, 1*(2), 111–116.
Gil, E. (1991). *The healing power of play.* New York: Guilford.
Goldberger, J. (1988). Issue-specific play with infants and toddlers in hospitals: Rationale and intervention. *Children's Health Care, 16*(3), 134–141.
Gottfried, A. W. (1985). Introduction. In C. C. Brown & A. W. Gottfried (Eds.). *Play interactions.* (pp xvii–xx). Skillman, NJ: Johnson & Johnson.
Gottlieb, S. E., & Portnoy, S. (1988). The role of play in a pediatric bone marrow transplantation unit. *Children's Health Care, 16*(3), 177–181.
Gould, R. (1972). *Child studies through fantasy.* New York: Quadrangle Books.
Hartman, L., & Hanson, G. (1986). Child psychotherapy. *Current Psychiatric Therapy, 23,* 29–43.
Hay, D. F., Ross, H. S., & Goldman, B. D. (1979). Social games in infancy. In B. Sutton-Smith (Ed.). *Play and learning* (pp 83–107). New York: Gardner Press.
Hetherington, E. M., Cox, M., & Cox, R. (1979). Play and social interaction in children following divorce. *Journal of Social Issues, 35*(4), 26–49.
Huizinga, J. (1950). *Homo ludens: A study of the play element in culture.* London: Routledge & Kegan Paul.
Ignico, A. A. (1990). The influence of gender-role perception on activity preferences of children. *Play and Culture, 3,* 302–310.
Ispa, J., Barrett, B., & Kim, Y. (1988). Effects of supervised play in a hospital waiting room. *Children's Health Care, 16*(3), 195–200.
James, B. (1989). *Treating traumatized children.* Lexington, MA: Lexington Books.
Johnsen, E. P. (1991). Searching for the social and cognitive outcomes of children's play: A selective second look. *Play and Culture, 4,* 201–213.
Johnson, J. E., Kirchoff, K. T., & Endress, M. P. (1975). Altering children's stress behavior during orthopedic cast removal. *Nursing Research, 24,* 404–410.
Johnson, J. E., Kirchoff, K. T., & Endress, M. P. (1976, July/August). Easing children's fright during health care procedures. *American Journal of Maternal Child Nursing,* 206.
Jones, M. (1989). *Understanding your child through play.* Englewood Cliffs, NJ: Prentice-Hall.
Kaplan-Sanoff, M., Brewster, A., Stillwell, J., & Bergen, D. (1988). The relationship of play to physical/motor development and to children with special needs. In D. Bergen (Ed.). *Play as a medium for learning and development* (pp 137–162). Portsmouth, NH: Heinemann.
Katz, E., Kellerman, J., & Siegel, S. (1980). Behavioral distress in children with cancer undergoing medical procedures: Developmental considerations. *Journal of Counseling and Clinical Psychology, 48*(3), 356–365.
Kline, S., & Pentecost, D. (1990). The characterization of play: Marketing children's toys. *Play and Culture, 3*(3), 235–255.
Krietemeyer, B. C., & Heiney, S. P. (1992). Storytelling as a therapeutic technique in a group for school-aged oncology patients. *Children's Health Care, 21*(1), 14–20.
Kuhn, C. L. (1989). The hospital play room: An enriching clinical experience for nursing students. *Children's Health Care, 18*(3), 153–156.
Main, M. (1983). Exploration play and cognitive functioning related to infant-mother attachment. *Infant Behavior, 6,* 167–174.
Malchiodi, C. (1990). *Breaking the silence: Art therapy with children from violent homes.* New York: Brunner/Mazel.
Malone, T. W. (1981). Toward a theory of intrinsically motivating instruction. *Cognitive Science, 4,* 333–369.
Manion, J. (1990). Preparing children for hospitalization, procedures, or surgery. In M. J. Craft & J. A. Denehy (Eds.). *Nursing interventions for infants and children* (pp 74–92). Philadelphia: WB Saunders.
Marino, B. L. (1988). Assessments of infant play: Applications of research to practice. *Issues in Comprehensive Pediatric Nursing, 11,* 227–240.
Matthews, W. S., Beebe, S., & Bopp, M. (1980). Spatial perspective-taking and pretend play. *Perceptual and Motor Skills, 5*(1), 49–50.
McCue, K. (1988). Medical play: An expanded perspective. *Children's Health Care, 16*(3), 157–161.
McCune, L. (1985). Play-language relationships and symbolic development. In C. C. Brown & A. W. Gottfried (Eds.). *Play interactions* (pp 38–45), Skillman, NJ: Johnson & Johnson.
McDermott, J. (1968). Parental divorce in early childhood. *American Journal of Psychiatry, 124,* 118–126.
McLoyd, V. (1986). Scaffolds or shackles? The role of toys in preschool children's pretend play. In G. Fein & M. Rivkin (Eds.). *The young child at play* (pp 63–77). Washington, DC: National Association for the Education of Young Children.
McTigue, D. J., & Pinkham, J. (1978). Association between children's dental behavior and play behavior. *ASDC Journal of Dentistry for Children, 45*(3), 218–226.

Meer, P. A. (1985). Using play in outpatient settings. *MCN: American Journal of Maternal Child Nursing, 10,* 378–380.

Mergen, B. (1991). Ninety-five years of historical change in the game preferences of American children. *Play and Culture, 4,* 272–283.

Moustakas, C. E. (1959). *Psychotherapy with children.* New York: Harper & Row.

Myers, D. (1990). Computer game genres. *Play and Culture, 3,* 286–301.

O'Connell, S. (1984). Recreation therapy: Reducing the effects of isolation for the patient in the protected environment. *Children's Health Care, 12,* 118–121.

Olds, A. R. (1988). In my opinion. Designing for play: Beautiful spaces are playful places. *Children's Health Care, 16*(3), 218–222.

Olson, M. R. (1983). A study of the exploratory behavior of legally blind and sighted preschoolers. *Exceptional Children, 50*(2), 130–138.

Oremland, E. K. (1988). Mastering developmental and critical experiences through play and other expressive behaviors in childhood. *Children's Health Care, 16*(3), 150–156.

Parten, M. (1932). Social participation among preschool children. *Journal of Abnormal and Social Psychology,* p 243.

Pearson, J. E. R., Cataldo, M., Turemann, A., Bessman, C., & Rogers, M. C. (1980). Pediatric intensive care unit patients: Effects of play intervention on behavior. *Critical Care Medicine, 8,* 64–67.

Pellegrini, A. D. (1981). Speech play and language development in young children. *Journal of Research and Development in Education, 14,* 75–81.

Pellegrini, A. D., & Perlmutter, J. C. (1988). The diagnostic and therapeutic roles of children's rough-and-tumble play. *Children's Health Care, 16*(3), 162–168.

Perrin, E. C. (1992). Hospitalization, surgery, and medical procedures. In M. D. Levine, W. B. Carey, & A. C. Crocker (Eds.). *Developmental-behavioral pediatrics* (pp 297–300). Philadelphia: WB Saunders.

Petrillo, M., & Sanger, S. (1980). *Emotional care of hospitalized children.* Philadelphia: JB Lippincott.

Plank, E. (1971). *Working with children.* Cleveland: Western Reserve University Press.

Porter, A. E. (1988). The computer in the play environment. In D. Bergen (Ed.). *Play as a medium for learning and development* (pp 271–273). Portsmouth, NH: Heinemann.

Postman, N. (1982). *The disappearance of childhood.* New York: Dell.

Prugh, D. G., Staub, E. M., Sands, H. H., Kirchbaum, R. M., & Leniham, E. (1953). A study of the emotional reactions of children and families to hospitalization and illness. *American Journal of Orthopsychiatry, 23,* 70–106.

Ross, H. S., & Kay, D. A. (1980). The origins of social games. In K. H. Rubin (Ed.). *New directions for child development: Children's play* (No. 9, pp 17–31), San Francisco: Jossey-Bass.

Rubin, K. H. (1985). Play, peer interaction and social development. In C. C. Brown & A. W. Gottfried (Eds.). *Play interaction: The role of toys and parental involvement in children's development* (pp 88–96). Skillman, NJ: Johnson & Johnson.

Rubin, K. H. (1988). Some "good news" and some "not-so-good" news about dramatic play. In D. Bergen (Ed.). *Play as a medium for learning and development* (pp 67–71). Portsmouth, NH: Heinemann.

Rubinstein, J., & Howes, C. (1976). The effect of peers on toddler interaction with mother and toys. *Child Development, 47,* 597–605.

Sachs, J. (1980). The role of adult-child play in language development. In K. H. Rubin (Ed.). *New directions in child development: Children's play* (No. 9, pp 33–48). San Francisco: Jossey-Bass.

Silvern, S. B., Williamson, P. A., & Countermine, T. A. (1985). Videogame play and social behavior: Preliminary findings. In J. L. Frost & S. Sunderlin (Eds.). *When children play* (pp. 279–282). Wheaton, MD: Association for Childhood Education.

Simon, J., & Larson, C. (1985). Detecting experience with violence: The uses of play interviews. *Beginnings, 2*(3), 12–15.

Singer, J. L., & Singer, D. G. (1988). Imaginative play and human development: Schemas, scripts, and possibilities. In D. Bergen (Ed.). *Play as a medium for learning and development* (pp 75–79). Portsmouth, NH: Heinemann.

Slade, A. (1987). Quality of attachment and early symbolic play. *Psychology, 23,* 78–85.

Smilansky, S. (1971). Can adults facilitate play in children?: Theoretical and practical considerations. In N. E. Curry & S. Arnaud (Eds.). *Play: The child strives toward self-realization* (pp 39–50). Washington DC: National Association for the Education of Young Children.

Smilansky, S. (1968). *The effects of sociodramatic play on disadvantaged preschool children.* New York: Wiley, 1968.

Stillwell, J. L. (1987). *Making and using creative play equipment.* Champaign, IL: Human Kinetics.

Strain, P. S. (1975). Increasing social play of severely retarded preschoolers with sociodramatic activities. *Mental Retardation, 13,* 7–9.

Strain, P. S., & Wiegerink, R. (1976). The effects of sociodramatic activities on social interaction among behaviorally disordered preschool children. *Journal of Special Education, 10*(1), 71–75.

Sutton-Smith, B. (1985, October). The child at play. *Psychology Today,* pp 64–65.

Sutton-Smith, B. (1988). The struggle between sacred play and festive play. In D. Bergen (Ed.). *Play as a medium for learning and development* (pp 45–47). Portsmouth, NH: Heinemann.

Swigger, K. M., Campbell, J., & Swigger, B. K. (1983). Preschool children's preferences for different types of CAI programs. *Educational Computer Magazine,* 38–40.

Thompson, R. H. (1985). *Psychosocial research on pediatric hospitalization and health care: A review of the literature.* Springfield, IL: Charles C Thomas.

Tiedemann, M. E., Simon, K. A., & Clatworthy, S. (1990). Communication through therapeutic play. In M. J. Craft & J. A. Denehy (Eds.). *Nursing interventions for infants and children* (pp 93–110). Philadelphia: WB Saunders.

van der Kooij, R. (1989). Play and behavioral disorders in schoolchildren. *Play and Culture, 2,* 328–339.

Vernon, D. T. A., Foley, J. M., Sipowicz, R. R., & Schulman, J. L. (1965). *The psychological responses of children to hospitalization and illness.* Springfield, IL: Charles C Thomas.

Vygotsky, L. (1962). *Thought and language.* Cambridge, MA: MIT Press.

Walker, C. (1989). Use of art and play therapy in pediatric oncology. *Journal of Pediatric Oncology Nursing, 6*(4), 121–126.

Wallerstein, J. S., & Kelly, J. B. (1981). *Surviving the breakup: How children and parents cope with divorce.* New York: Basic Books.

Webb, N. B. (1991). *Play therapy with children in crisis.* New York: Guilford.

Wilson, J. M. (1985). Play in the hospital. In C. C. Brown & A. J. Gottfried. (Eds.). *Play interactions* (pp 115–121). Skillman, NJ: Johnson & Johnson.

UNIT • FOUR

Concepts Related to Illness

CHAPTER • 18

Stress, Crisis, and Coping

Carolyn M. Byrne
Mabel Hunsberger

RELATED TOPICS

Perspectives on nursing assessment of family and health, Chapter 2
Perspectives on development of children and adolescents, Chapter 3
Promoting child health: Health concepts and principles of practice, Chapter 10
Impact of chronic illness, Chapter 19
Impact of death and dying, Chapter 20
Nursing Care During Hospitalization, Chapter 21

LEARNING OBJECTIVES

- **Understand the physiologic response to stress.**
- **Identify ways to measure stress in children.**
- **Enumerate the factors that protect children from stress.**
- **Identify stages of intervening in a crisis situation.**
- **Explain the process of coping.**
- **Identify strategies used by children to cope.**
- **Relate the perceptions of illness to the developmental stages of the child.**
- **Identify sources of stress facing families with ill children.**

A certain amount of stress is healthy, motivating, and supportive to the well-being of a child or family. It is when stress is excessive or prolonged or when it is imposed on those who are most vulnerable that negative effects result. Developing children face a series of challenges that potentially bring stress into their lives. The process of maturation itself makes demands on children, placing them into a position of vulnerability. Not only are children coping with the usual developmental crises (e.g., achieving autonomy, formulating an identity) but they encounter other situational stress to varying degrees, depending on their life circumstances. These stresses can include such events as illness, pain, hospitalization, parent separation or divorce, abuse or neglect, or their own death — all at a time when they are only beginning to develop the inner resources available to adults.

The various stresses that children face are discussed throughout this text in the chapters listed under Related Topics. This chapter presents an overview of the concepts of stress, crises, and coping and then relates

these concepts to children and families who have experienced illness. Coping with specific degrees of illness are discussed in the chapters that follow.

The Nature of Stress

"Stress" is a word that has no agreed-on definition. It encompasses the idea of a *stimulus* and the person's *response* to that stimulus. The word "stress" is used so broadly that it carries the meaning of a form of stimulus (or stressor), a force requiring the host to change or adapt (strain), a mental state (distress), or a bodily reaction (Rutter, 1978a, 1987b; Garmezy, 1983).

Hans Selye (1976), a noted stress researcher, defined stress as "the non-specific response of the body to any demand." This nonspecific response is always the same; it is the degree of the response that changes. Selye viewed the response as a process that enabled the body to resist the stimulus (or stressor) in the best possible way, by enhancing the functioning of the organ or system best able to respond to it. Through Selye's research with animals, he identified three stages that occur in adapting to stress. This is referred to as the "general adaptation syndrome" (GAS).

The first stage is the *alarm reaction stage,* in which the body shows generalized arousal (increased adrenocorticotropic hormone [ACTH] secretion) but with no specific system being affected. The second stage, the *stage of resistance,* is characterized by a specific system dealing with the stimulus (stressor). At this stage, there is a decrease in the body's ability to respond to other stimuli. The final stage is one of *exhaustion,* whereby the stimulus (or stressor) is sufficiently severe and prolonged that the system dealing with it becomes exhausted and is unable to adapt to the stress (Selye, 1980).

The Body's Response to Stress

Although every system of the body is involved at some point in the stress response, the nervous and endocrine systems are central to the stress response.

Figure 18–1 illustrates how the body responds to stress. A stimulus is perceived and interpreted by the cerebral cortex (1) to be a stressor. The cortex then

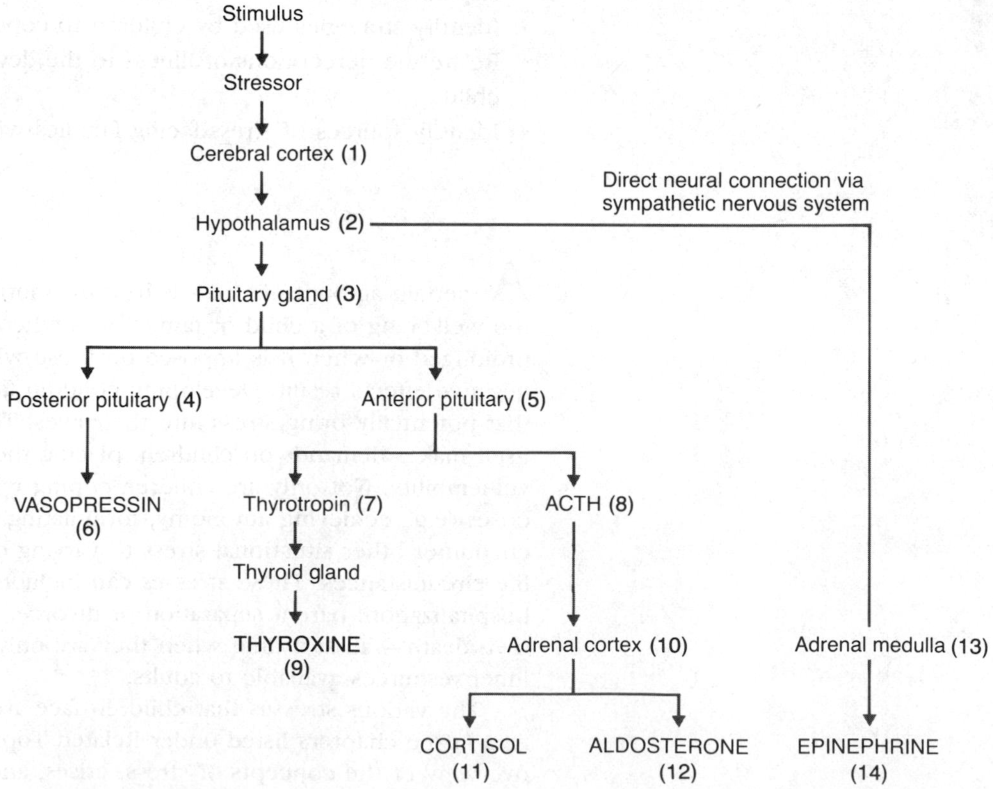

FIGURE 18 - 1. How the body reacts to stress.

triggers the hypothalamus (2). The hypothalamus is one of the major areas of the brain that regulates the activities of the autonomic nervous system. It prepares the body for action by increasing the discharge of hormones. The hypothalamus' intimate relationship to the pituitary gland (3) provides the link between the nervous and the endocrine systems.

The hypothalamus then triggers the two lobes of the pituitary gland—the posterior (4) and anterior (5) pituitary gland. The posterior lobe is mostly neural tissue, and, when stimulated, it releases the hormone vasopressin (6). Contraction of the arteries and a rise in blood pressure are due to vasopressin.

The anterior pituitary gland (5) is responsible for six of the major hormones. Two of these are involved in the stress response: thyrotropin (7) and ACTH (8).

Thyrotropin (7) stimulates the thyroid gland, which secretes thyroxine (9). Thyroxine raises the metabolic rate to prepare the body to take action. The heart rate increases and breathing becomes deep and rapid.

ACTH (8) triggers the adrenal cortex (10) of the adrenal gland. The adrenal cortex is stimulated and, in turn, secretes hormones into the blood. The two primary secretions of the adrenal cortex are the glucocorticoids—primarily cortisol (11)—and the mineral corticoids—primarily aldosterone (12).

Cortisol (11) increases the metabolic process of the liver (gluconeogenesis) and forms glucose, the most efficient source of energy, during an accelerated period of activity. Through the process of gluconeogenesis, cortisol mobilizes both fats and proteins in the blood. The mobilization of protein reduces the stores of protein in body cells. If this process is maintained because of a prolonged stress response, there may not be enough protein available for the formation of mature white blood cells and antibodies.

The increase in aldosterone (12) helps the body prepare itself for increased muscular activity and better dissipation of heat and waste products. The body retains extra sodium, which results in increased water retention, blood volume, and blood pressure.

The adrenal medulla (13) is the other part of the adrenal gland that is involved with the stress response. The adrenal medulla is connected to the hypothalamus (2) by sympathetic nerves. When the hypothalamus is stimulated, the impulse is carried to the medulla, and the hormone epinephrine (14) is released. The effects of this hormone are primarily cardiovascular: increased heart rate, increased cardiac output, and increased blood pressure (Guyton, 1991).

Stress also demands psychologic adaptation and adjustment. Not only are physiologic functions affected by stress but psychologic and behavioral responses also occur. Selye's ideas have been criticized for focusing on the biology of stress and ignoring psychologic aspects and ramifications. Others believe that the psychologic response is secondary and occurs only after the event is perceived to be threatening and the individual has responded behaviorally (Antonovsky, 1987; Monat & Lazarus, 1991). Regardless of which type of response occurs first, both physiologic and psychologic responses to stress do occur. Table 18–1 identifies the common signs and symptoms of stress.

TABLE 18–1
Signs and Symptoms of Stress

Physical	Emotional	Intellectual
Increased heart rate	Irritability, overreaction to some relatively minor situation	Forgetfulness, preoccupation
Elevated blood pressure	Angry outbursts, short-tempered reactions, hostility	Blocking
Tightness of chest	Lack of interest, withdrawn, apathetic, cannot get up in the morning	Increased fantasy life
Breathing difficulty	Crying tendencies	Decreased concentration, especially on complicated jobs
Headaches, migraine	Blaming others, suspicious attitude	Inattention to detail
Fatigue, exhaustion	Diminished initiative	Past-oriented rather than present-oriented
Insomnia	Reduction of personal involvement with others	Decreased creativity
Gastrointestinal problems: nausea, diarrhea, vomiting, intestinal disturbances, ulcers, colitis, stomachaches	Depression, worrying	Slower thinking, slower reactions, difficulty learning subjects
Restlessness, hyperactivity	Negative attitude, cynical	"Couldn't care less" attitude, mentally lazy, inclined to path of least resistance
Vague somatic complaints, feeling run down, minor ailments, psychosomatic complaints	General dissatisfaction	
Frequent or prolonged colds or flu		
Urinary frequency		
Weight gain or weight loss of more than 10 pounds		

Stress and Illness

Stress is a phenomenon that is universally experienced by all persons and groups of persons. There is no anticipated or common response to stress, since all persons respond in a highly individualistic manner (Fig. 18–2). An individual child copes with stress in his or her own way, as does a family group. What is stress for one child or family may not be for another. Although it is true that all children and families experience stress from day to day, excessive stress can be damaging.

One particular type of stress that has received considerable attention in both children and adults is the number of stressful life events and their relationship to anxiety and disease. Holmes and Rahe (1967) provided the major impetus to the scaling of life events in developing the Social Readjustment Rating Scale. This scale, developed for adults, ranks important life events and assigns a specific value to each one on the basis of the amount of coping behavior needed by the individual to deal with the event. As the score increases, the likelihood of illness occurring is thought to increase.

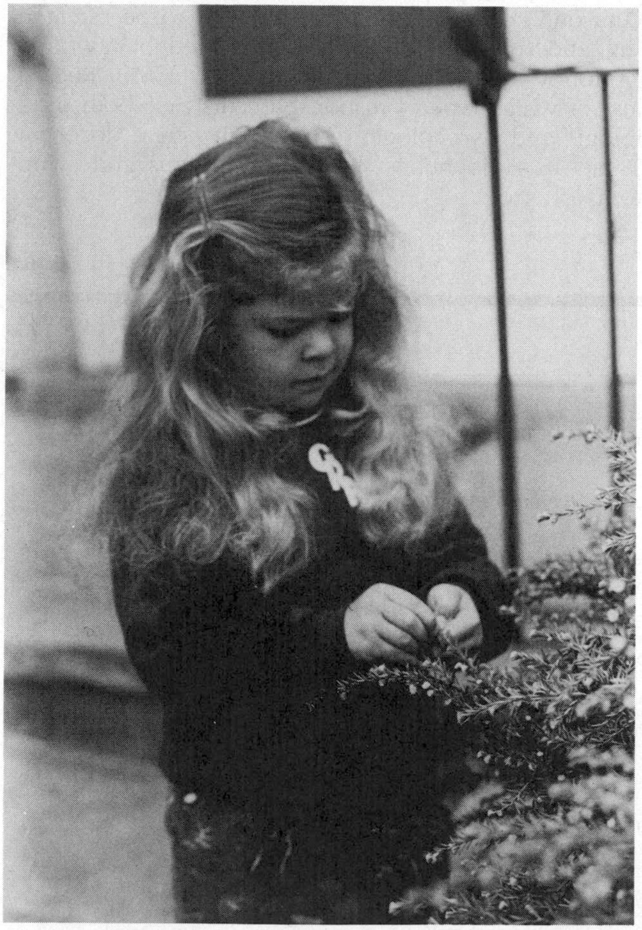

FIGURE 18-2. Persons respond in a highly individualistic manner to stress. Even young children may need just to be alone and think for a while.

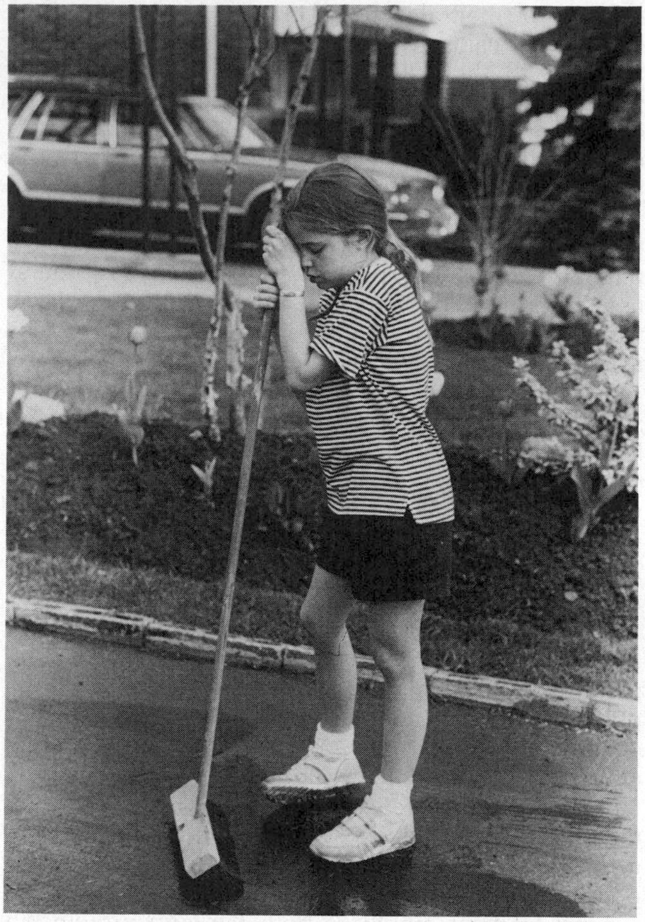

FIGURE 18-3. Too much stress can lead to exhaustion, interference with task completion, and, eventually, illness.

Coddington (1972) was the first to develop a life event scale for children based on Holmes and Rahe's work. He asked professionals working with children to judge the intensity of change required by each of the events and assigned a numeric value to each event. Each life event was assigned a weighting of the degree of change required to manage the event. The rationale behind these life event scales is that many changes, either positive or negative, occurring in a short space of time will disrupt the stability in an individual's life. It is felt that too many changes can cause a state of sustained arousal that can lead to exhaustion, interference with task completion, and illness (Fig. 18–3).

Unfortunately, conclusions regarding the impact of life events on the health of a child are far from definite. Investigators studying life events and illness-onset report that illness occurs after stressful life events more often than can be accounted for by chance (Creed, 1985; Reale, 1987). However, this research has been the subject of much criticism (Minter & Kimball, 1980; Dohrenwend & Shrout, 1985). Solely using life event scales to measure stress has been met with some criticism. First, the scales often do not consider that individuals perceive events differently. What

TABLE 18-2
Examples of Major Life Events Versus Daily Hassles

Major Life Events	Daily Hassles
Beginning school	Being late for school
Birth of a sibling	Parents in a bad mood
Death of parents	Getting into a fight at school
Divorce of parents	Having a difficult test at school
Failure of a grade at school	Losing at a sports game
Parent going to jail	Being punished

is perceived by one child to be extremely stressful may not be perceived as such by another. Second, these scales alone do not consider other factors that may influence stress, such as the type of supports available and the temperament of the child. Third, they do not measure whether the events have been anticipated. Some evidence suggests that anticipated events are less stressful than those that are not (Streiner et al, 1981). Fourth, the measurement of life events does not give an indication of "daily hassles," which are thought by some to be more stressful than the major life events and may be critical mediators in the relationship between life events and health. Table 18–2 gives some examples of major life events and daily hassles (Kanner et al, 1981; Lazarus, 1984; Oppenheimer, 1987; Zautra et al, 1988). Finally, the life event scales for children under the age of 12 years are completed by parents, and, consequently, parents are reporting events *they* remember, not necessarily what the *child* remembers as a life event.

More recent work on life event scales for children has led to the development of scales that school-age children can complete themselves (Lewis et al, 1984; Elwood, 1987). In response to criticism, recent scales have also attempted to examine both major life events and daily hassles and also to allow for individual responses to indicate the degree of stress experienced (Compas et al, 1987; Elwood, 1987; Dise-Lewis, 1988). Table 18–3 lists scales that can be used to measure stress in a child's life.

TABLE 18-3
Scales for Measuring Stress in Children

Scale Name and Author	Age of Child Appropriate For	Type of Scale; Number of Items/Questions	Focus of Questions
Life Event Scale (LES-C)	5–12 yrs	Self-administered check list that parents complete 30–35 items	Major life events
Life Event Scales (LES-A) Coddington, 1972	13–18 yrs	Self-administered check list 40–42 items	
Stressful Experiences Scale Yamamoto, 1979	7–11 yrs	Interviewer-assisted questionnaire 20 items	Major life events
Feel Bad Scale Lewis et al, 1984	6–11 yrs	Self-administered check list 20 items	Major life events
Life Events Check List (LEC) Johnson & McCutcheon, 1980	12–18 yrs	Self-administered check list 46 items	Major life events Some items reflect events that the youth has no control over Other items reflect events that the youth has control over
Daily Hassles Scale Kanner et al, 1981	15–20 yrs	Self-administered check list 117 items	Minor problems encountered in everyday life
Adolescent Perceived Events Scale (APES) Compas et al, 1987	3 versions: 12–14 yrs 15–17 yrs 18–20 yrs	Self-administered check list 164–210 items, depending on version	Both major life events and daily hassles
Stressor and Coping Response Inventories Elwood, 1987	2 versions: 8–11 yrs 12–14 yrs	*8–11 version:* Interviewer-assisted check list/questionnaire 24 stress items 14 coping items *12–14 version:* self-administered check list/questionnaire 29 stress items 16 coping items	Both major life events and daily hassles and ways of coping
Life Events and Coping Inventory Dise-Lewis, 1988	12–14 yrs	Self-administered check list 125 stress items 48 coping items	Both major life events and daily hassles and ways of coping

Nursing Implications for Assessing Stress

Despite the controversy over life event scales, they can be used very effectively by the nurse to assess stress in children and their families. It is important to recognize the signs and symptoms of stress and then to identify the source of stress. Frequently, what appears to be stressful may be compounded by many other events. Evaluating stressful changes in the child's or parent's life may assist in understanding the ways they have tried to cope. New alternatives to deal with the stress can then be developed.

The following example illustrates how understanding stressful events assists in managing stress.

> Gillian, an active 8-year-old in grade 3, had been a bright and happy child who enjoyed school until this past month. Recently, every morning she would be very difficult to get out of bed and would state she did not want to go to school because she was tired. As she had not altered her bedtime, her mother checked with the school to see whether there were changes there. The teacher at school reported no change in Gillian's performance or activities but did notice she was more quiet than she had been when she joined the class 4 months ago. The teacher, however, was not concerned. The mother took Gillian to the family doctor for a check-up and found she was physically healthy. In talking with the nurse about events at home, the following became apparent.
>
> Eight months ago, Gillian's father had received a promotion at work that would keep him away from home more. To reduce his time away from home as much as possible, the family moved closer to the father's business. This move necessitated a change in school for Gillian. The family moved during the summer, and, in the fall, Gillian settled into her new school very well. In the fall, after having settled from the move, Gillian's mother, who had been wanting to return to work for several years, found a job. She returned to work 2 months ago. With the mother's return to work, family members had to take on new responsibilities around the home. Despite a few arguments, the mother felt the family adjusted well to her return to work.
>
> In viewing the events that had occurred in the past 8 months, it became clear that Gillian had to adjust to several changes: father away from home more, a move, change in school, mother returning to work, and increased responsibility at home. Understanding this, the mother talked with Gillian about the changes. This discussion revealed that, although Gillian liked her new home and school, she did not yet feel she had a good friend to talk to. Her father was busy, and, now, so was her mother. She wanted to stay home from school with her mother so they could spend some time together.
>
> Once this was recognized, both the mother and the father began spending their own "special" time with Gillian and the difficulties in the morning disappeared.

The nurse, in assessing for stress, was able to assist the mother in identifying and understanding the stress the child was experiencing. The parents were able to find ways of reducing the stress and altering potentially problematic behavior.

Invulnerability to Stress

Nurses frequently work with individual children who seem to encounter high amounts of stress or come from disadvantaged environments, yet do not appear to suffer any physical, emotional, or psychologic ill effects. These children seem invulnerable to stress, and their behavior is marked by adaptation and competence (Fig. 18–4). This is often noted in the self-sufficient way children handle day-to-day stresses.

A beginning understanding of invulnerability or resilience to stress has come from research investigating factors that place children at risk for poor out-

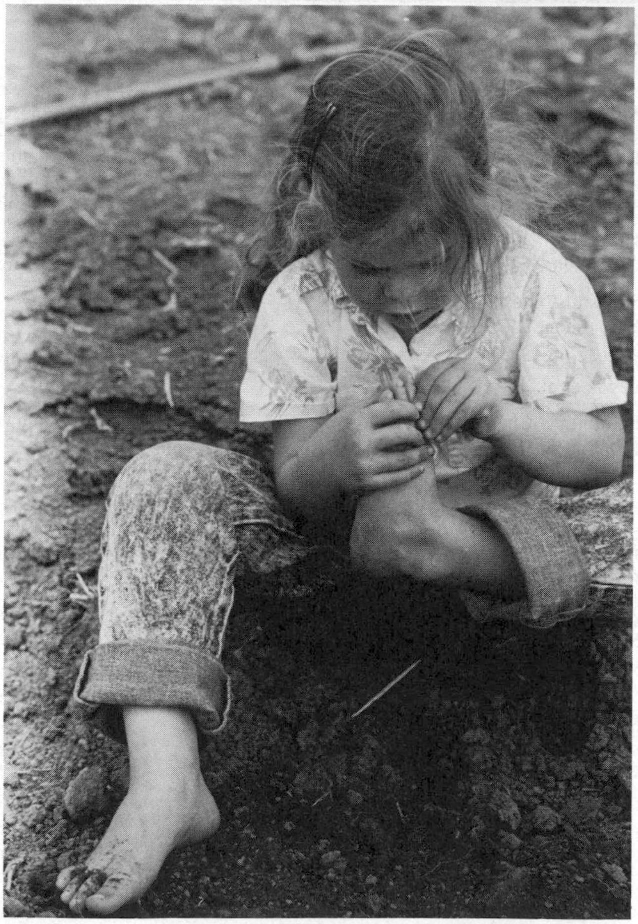

FIGURE 18-4. Invulnerability, or resilience to stress, is observed in the self-sufficient way children handle day-to-day stresses.

comes. This research has identified that a portion of children thought to be at risk for problems do remarkably well (Garmezy, 1983; Burke & Wiskin, 1984; Luthar & Zigler, 1991). This has led to an interest in determining the factors that protect children from responding negatively to stress.

Rutter (1985) has defined protective factors as "those factors that modify, ameliorate, or alter a person's response to some environmental hazard that predisposes to a maladaptive outcome." Three models used to explain why some children seem protected from stress are: (1) a "compensatory model," in which stress lowers the level of adjustment, and various personal attributes of the child work to improve the level of adjustment; personal attributes then counteract the stress; (2) a "protective model," which suggests that certain protective factors buffer stressors by improving coping; and (3) a "challenge model," which suggests a relationship between stress and adjustment so that stressors actually enhance competence as long as the stress is not excessive (Garmezy et al, 1984). Protective factors that have been identified through research can be classified to be within the child, within the family, or within the community at large (Garmezy, 1985, 1991; Rae-Grant et al, 1989; Werner, 1989; Pellegrini, 1990; Dahlin et al, 1990). They are illustrated in Figure 18–5. The move toward identifying the factors that contribute to healthy functioning is a positive one. In the future, these factors may well be used in preventive programs aimed at equipping children with resources to manage stress.

Crisis

Stress is necessary for survival, and certain degrees of it can assist the individual to grow in new ways. However, too much stress that is inappropriately timed can place excessive demands on the individual and a crisis situation can ensue.

Stress is present during a crisis but, in itself, does not constitute a crisis event. Stress produces a crisis state when the usual coping mechanisms fail. Crisis is defined as occurring "when a person faces an obstacle to important life goals that is, for a time, insurmountable through the utilization of customary methods of problem solving. A period of disorganization ensues, a period of upset, during which many abortive attempts at solution are made" (Caplan, 1961).

Phases of Crisis

Caplan (1964), the theorist most widely known in the development of crisis theory, has identified four phases of a crisis. In the *first phase,* the anxiety stimulates one's usual methods of coping into action. If,

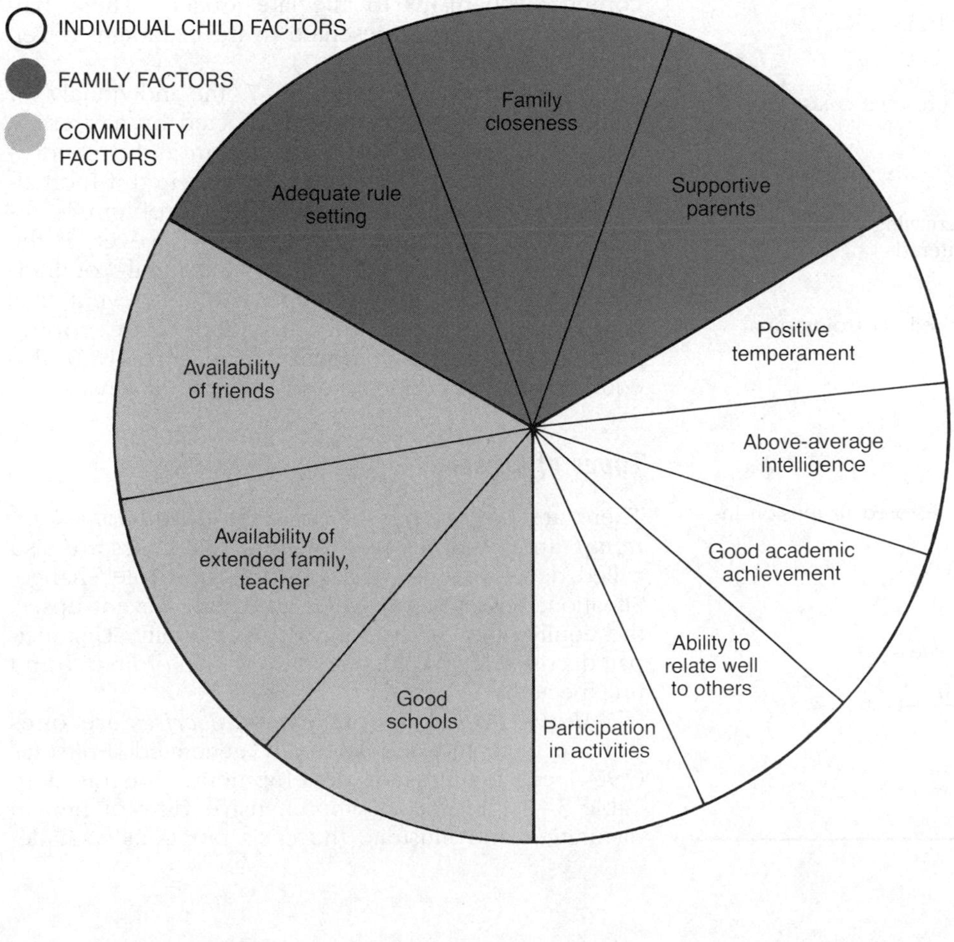

FIGURE 18 - 5. Factors found to contribute to invulnerability in children.

however, these do not bring relief and there is no support, the individual moves into the *second phase,* in which she or he becomes even more anxious as a result of the failure of the coping mechanisms. In the *third phase,* the individual tries out new coping mechanisms or redefines the threat so that old ones can work; resolution can occur at this point. If resolution does not occur, the *fourth phase* brings about severe levels of anxiety. Table 18–4 illustrates the phases of a crisis and the physical, emotional, and cognitive symptoms that are associated with each stage.

Many factors influence how individuals and families react to and cope with crisis situations. Aguilera (1994) has identified balancing factors that affect the equilibrium of individuals and families. The balancing factors are the *perception of the event,* the *available situational supports,* and *coping mechanisms.* They feel that successful resolution of the crisis is more likely if the individual's perception of the events is more realistic than distorted; if there are available supports so that others can assist in dealing with the crisis (Fig. 18–6); and if the individual has adequate coping mechanisms to alleviate anxiety. These balancing factors are represented in the paradigm developed by Aguilera (Fig. 18–7).

TABLE 18-4
Phases of Crises: Individual Responses

Physical, Emotional, and Cognitive Symptoms
Phase One: Initial Impact; Crisis Event; Usual Methods of Coping Fail
Somatic distress, shortness of breath, hyperventilation, weakness, fatigue
Anxiety, feeling overwhelmed, panicky
Hyperactivity or inability to carry out activities
Disorganized thinking
Phase Two: Increased Anxiety
Often a denial of any physical complaints
Increased tenseness and anxiety
May try different coping strategies to resolve crisis
Withdrawal or hyperactivity
Disorganized behavior
Problem-solving abilities become increasingly more disorganized—thinking appears scattered
Phase Three: Resolution or Defeat
Recurrence of physical complaints (tired, gastrointestinal upsets)
Tension and anxiety rise
Attempts to redefine problem
Try new ways to cope
Crisis can be resolved—equilibrium restored *or* tension increases
Phase Four: Severe Levels of Anxiety
Many somatic complaints
Feelings of helplessness and hopelessness
Confused—problem-solving impaired
Disorganized thinking
Withdrawal
Depression

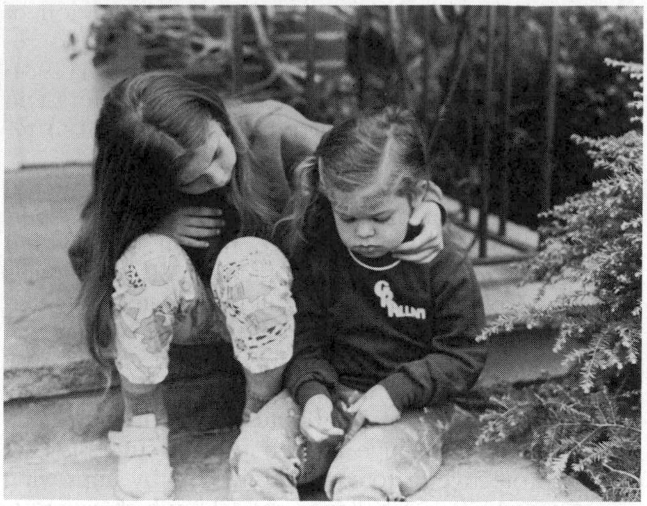

FIGURE 18-6. Available supports, such as siblings, serve as an important balancing factor that affects how a child will cope with stress.

As illustrated in Figure 18–7, the individual's or family's state of equilibrium is affected by a stressful event. This then causes disequilibrium and a need to return to the steady state. A crisis is averted if the balancing factors (*A*) are present; the problem is resolved and equilibrium is regained. However, if the balancing factors are absent (*B*), the family or individual has a distorted perception of the event, has few or no supports, and has inadequate coping mechanisms, the problem will remain unresolved, disequilibrium will continue, and a crisis will ensue.

Types of Crisis

There are three types of crisis: *maturational, situational,* and *unanticipated.* Maturational crises are also called developmental crises and require role change. Situational crises occur when an external event upsets the equilibrium of the individual or family. Unanticipated crises are accidental, out of the ordinary, and unexpected.

Maturational or developmental crises are ones that are expected and internally generated. Erikson's (1964) eight stages of development, illustrated in Table 3–8, present a comprehensive view of human maturation and illustrate the crisis points at each de-

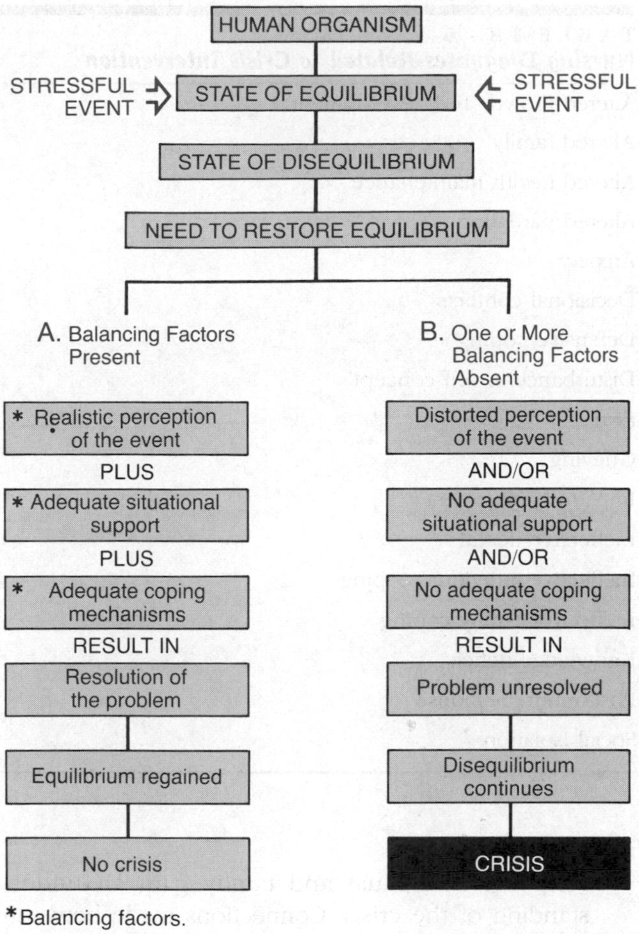

FIGURE 18-7. The effect of balancing factors is a stressful event. (From Aguilera, D. C. [1994]. *Crisis intervention* [7th ed.]. New York: CV Mosby.)

velopmental stage. Transitional periods from early childhood to middle childhood, adolescence to young adulthood, and so on are the periods of maturational crisis for the individual. The family too moves through developmental stages.

Situational crises occur when unanticipated events threaten an individual's or family's biologic, social, or psychologic integrity (Hoff, 1984). Examples of situational crises include illness, the loss of a parent's job, the death of a loved one, failure at school, divorce of parents—all situations that result in role changes and adjustments in ways of relating to others. These adjustments are similar to those occurring during maturational stages, but, unlike the maturational crises, not everyone experiences all of them.

Unanticipated crises do not occur in the lives of everyone. Examples of unanticipated crises are natural disasters such as fires, tornados, floods, earthquakes, and other tragedies; kidnappings, hostage takings, nuclear disasters, and hijackings. In this type of crisis, disaster-precipitated emotional problems can surface weeks or months after the initial crisis period (Hargreaves, 1980; Palmer, 1980).

Crisis Intervention

In reviewing the phases of crisis (see Table 18–4), it becomes apparent that the individual or family experiencing a crisis is less psychologically defended and, because of this, is perhaps more amenable to change. In addition, the distress experienced during a crisis may serve as a motivating factor to examine new ways of dealing with the crisis. Intervention during this crisis period is to help resolve the crisis and restore the individual or family to the previous level of functioning or better (Aguilera, 1994).

There are four steps in crisis intervention: assessment, planning, intervention, and evaluation (Morley et al, 1967). These steps parallel those of the nursing process.

Assessment

This phase consists of obtaining a clear understanding of the problem. During this phase, rapport is established with the individual or family. Understanding the balancing factors outlined in Figure 18–7 is helpful in the assessment phase. Table 18–5 identifies questions to ask in assessing whether the balancing factors are present.

Determine the Precipitating Event. The individual or family may be aware of being under stress but not aware of the event that caused the stress. At times, it is useful to review when the symptoms began and what events were occurring when the symptoms were first noticed. Reviewing the life events discussed ear-

TABLE 18-5
Crisis Intervention: Questions to Ask in Assessment Phase

Determine the Precipitating Event

- What event or events in your life have contributed to your feeling upset/anxious?
- What has happened in your life that is different?

Determine the Perception of the Event

- How does this event affect your life now?
- How will it affect your future?
- How does this event affect others around you?

Determine the Presence or Absence of Situational Support

- Who do you have in your life to support you?
- Who do you have to talk to about this?

Determine Coping Mechanisms

- Has anything like this happened before?
- How did you handle it?
- Have you had other stressful times in your life?
- What did you do to manage?

lier can assist in clarifying stressors. It is also important to determine how the event has affected the individual's or family's life. The nurse needs to assess the individual's or family's ability to meet basic needs as well as to assess how the problem is affecting life at the present.

Determine the Perception of the Event. Events can be interpreted in different ways by different people. It is important to gain an understanding of what meaning the event is given by the individual or family (Lazarus & Folkman, 1982). Does the individual or family view the event as a harm, loss, threat, or challenge? How do they feel it will affect or change their life? Since most crises involve some type of loss or a potential loss, it may be useful for the nurse to keep this in mind when exploring the perceptions of the event.

Determine the Presence or Absence of Situational Support. Information regarding the present and potential sources of support is useful in determining whether supports are adequate. When dealing with an individual: Whom does the person live with? With whom is she or he close? Who understands? When dealing with a family: Who supports whom in the family? What outside supports does the family have?

Determine Coping Mechanisms. The nurse needs to assess and understand the individual's or family's previous coping strategies. How did they handle previous crises? It is useful to have an understanding of the previous coping styles, as they may be strengths that could be built on in the present crisis.

Nursing Diagnosis. The final step in the assessment phase is the formulation of nursing diagnoses. This then will guide the planning and interventions. Table 18–6 identifies possible nursing diagnoses related to crisis intervention.

TABLE 18-6
Nursing Diagnoses Related to Crisis Intervention

Altered growth and development
Altered family processes
Altered health maintenance
Altered parenting
Anxiety
Decisional conflicts
Defensive coping
Disturbance in self-concept
Fear
Grieving
Impaired adjustment
Ineffective denial
Ineffective individual coping
Ineffective family coping
Knowledge deficit
Post-trauma response
Social isolation

Planning

In the planning phase, the data collected in the assessment are reviewed with the individual and family to establish goals and planning action. The nature of the crisis and the individual's and family's precrisis functioning need to be considered when planning ways to facilitate coping. Interventions should be planned that are realistic, clear, time-limited, and flexible.

Intervention

Interventions will vary depending on the individual or family and the nature of the crisis. Several guidelines can be applied to any crisis intervention:

- Help the individual and family gain an understanding of the crisis. Connections made between the meaning of the event and the crisis allow for an understanding and appreciation of why this is a crisis.
- Involve those concerned in decision making. This allows the individual or family some control and say on the approach to be taken to deal with the crisis.
- Allow time to discuss feelings. Often solutions are sought before individuals or family members have had a chance to identify normal feelings.
- Utilize the individual's or family's strengths. The use of previous successful coping strategies can give the individual or family some sense of control or mastery and assist them in having the confidence to try new ways to cope.
- Involve support systems. Using previous supports or establishing new supports can help in client assistance and gratification and establish outlets for tension (Fig. 18–8).

Evaluation

Crisis resolution and anticipatory planning are the final steps in crisis intervention. The nurse and individual or family review the coping mechanisms that have been used successfully to reduce the crisis. The

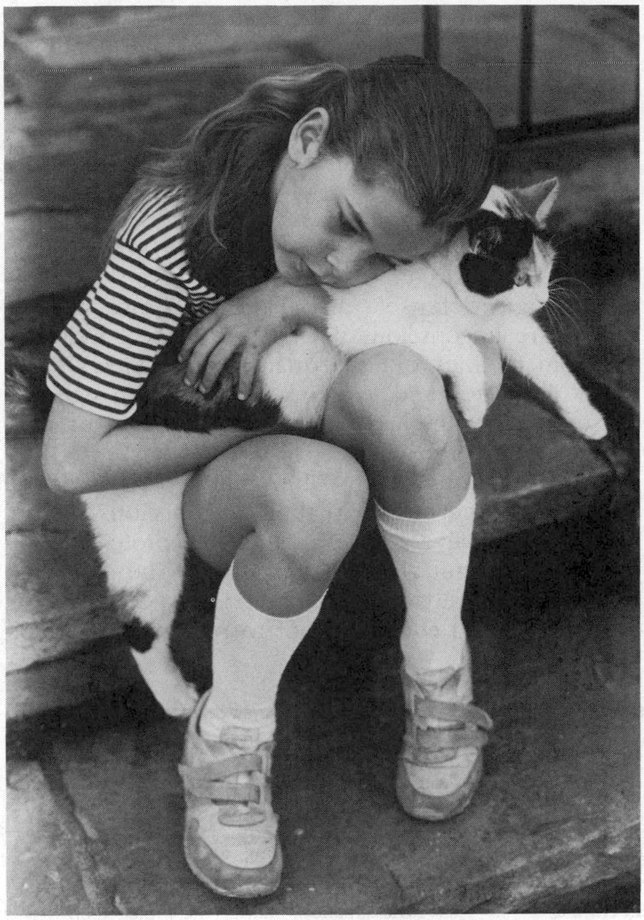

FIGURE 18-8. Children can be resourceful in finding meaningful ways to reduce tension.

present management of the crisis is used to focus on ways of managing future crises.

Coping

Coping refers to "efforts to master conditions of harm, threat, or challenge when a routine automatic response is not readily available" (Monat & Lazarus, 1985).

Lazarus and Folkman (1984) define coping as changing those cognitive and behavioral approaches used to manage specific external and/or internal demands that are viewed as taxing and excessive of the person's resources. The individual's effort to manage and shape the stress experience involves two interacting processes, appraisal and coping (Lazarus, 1966; Lazarus & Folkman, 1982). Although much of the work on appraisal and coping has been done with adults, the Lazarus and Folkman model can assist in providing a framework for understanding the process of coping in children. This is not to say that children use the same coping strategies as adults, or appraise events in the same way, but rather a process occurs that is affected by the developmental stage of the child. This process is illustrated in Figure 18–9.

Process of Coping

Lazarus and Folkman view the individual's perception or appraisal of a stressful event as a critical factor in the process of coping. They identify two types of appraisal, primary and secondary.

Primary appraisal is the evaluation of the significance of an event by individuals when they evaluate a stressful situation as damaging or potentially damaging. Lazarus identifies three ways that individuals perceive stress. The first is that the stress is viewed *as a harm or a loss;* the damage has already been done. Second, the stress is perceived *as a threat;* future damage is anticipated. Third, the stress is viewed *as a challenge;* the perception is that the stress will result in positive growth or mastery.

Secondary appraisal is the individual's evaluation of personal coping resources or mechanisms to assist in dealing with the stressful event (Holroyd & Lazarus, 1982). It is thought that more effective coping results when there is a match between primary and secondary appraisal. These appraisals give rise to physiologic responses discussed at the beginning of this chapter, coping strategies, and psychologic defenses.

Coping Strategies

Coping strategies are methods that the individual uses to assist in managing stress or anxiety. Lazarus and Folkman (1984) broadly define two types of coping strategies: problem-focused, which are behavioral efforts at acting on the source of stress to change it; and emotion-focused, which are cognitive efforts at

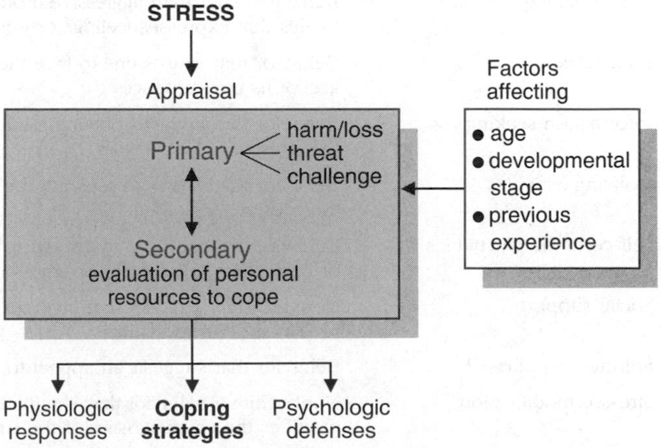

FIGURE 18-9. The process of coping.

regulating the emotional states associated with the stress. Several nurse researchers have attempted to provide empirical support for coping strategies used by children in various situations (LaMontagne, 1987; Walker, 1988; Atkins, 1991) and in population-based samples (Ryan, 1989; Shaw-Sorenson, 1990). Research to date suggests the following:

1. Children use both behavioral (e.g., go for a bike ride) and cognitive (e.g., problem-solving) strategies to cope with stress (Ryan, 1989).
2. Children are able to appraise the type of stress (think about it) and appraise their own resources (think about what to do) (Ryan, 1989).
3. Boys and girls use different types of coping strategies: boys use more physical behaviors; girls use more emotional strategies (Ryan, 1989; Shaw-Sorensen, 1990; Frydenberg & Lewis, 1991).

Recent work by Nancy Ryan-Wenger (1992) has identified 15 emotional or behavioral categories of coping strategies that children use. These categories, their definition, and examples are listed in Table 18–7. In reviewing these strategies, it becomes apparent that some will be used more frequently by the older child rather than by the younger (e.g., cognitive problem-solving, spiritual support). It is important that the nurse determine, through talking with the child and parents, the typical coping strategies that the child may use.

Psychologic Defenses

Psychologic defenses (also called defense mechanisms) are unconscious defenses to protect individuals from feelings of inadequacy and anxiety. Table 18–8 illustrates and explains the common ego defenses, with examples of how they are used by children and adults.

These strategies are often viewed as negative ways of coping owing to their unconscious nature. They can, however, serve as an initial protection following a stressful event (Elliott, 1980). The degree to which the defense mechanism is used to impair progress toward equilibrium or to protect the individ-

TABLE 18-7
Children's Coping Strategies: Coping Categories, Definitions, and Examples

Category	Definition	Examples
Aggressive activities	Verbal or motor activities that may be hurtful to persons, animals, or objects	Display of anger, yelling, arguing, hitting
Behavioral avoidance	Behavior other than isolating that is a deliberate attempt to keep oneself away from a stressor	Leave the situation; change the topic; sleep
Behavioral distraction	Behavior other than isolating or avoidance that delays the need to deal with a stressor	Do something else; play; watch TV
Cognitive avoidance	Deliberate cognitive attempts to avoid acknowledging the existence of a stressor	Deny situation exists; don't think about it; thought stopping
Cognitive distraction	Deliberate cognitive attempts to keep thoughts away from a stressor	Think about something else; fantasy; humor
Cognitive problem solving	Thoughts focused on ways to modify, prevent, or eliminate the stressor	Focus on situation; process; analyze; think; reason
Cognitive restructuring	Thoughts that alter one's perception of the characteristics of the stressor	Emphasize the positive; tell self it's OK
Emotional expression	Behavior other than aggressive motor and verbal activities that expresses feelings or emotions	Ventilate feelings; cry
Endurance	Behavior that causes one to face the stressor and accept its consequences	Expose self to fear; comply/cooperate; relinquish control
Information seeking	Behavior that involves obtaining information about the stressor	Questioning; clarifying
Isolating activities	Behavior that serves to separate the individual from the presence of others	Time out; go to a special place; isolate self
Self-controlling activities	Behavior or cognitions that serve to reduce tension or control one's behavior or emotions	Think about relaxing; eating; drinking
Social support	Nonagressive behavior that involves seeking the presence of an individual	Talk to peers, parents; tell someone how you feel
Spiritual support	Behavior that suggests an appeal to a higher being	Pray
Stressor modification	Noncognitive behavior that eliminates the stressor or modifies the characteristics of the stressor	Propose a compromise

From Ryan-Wenger, N. (1992). A taxonomy of children's coping strategies: A step toward theory development. *American Journal of Orthopsychiatry, 62*(2), 256–263. Reprinted with permission, from the *American Journal of Orthopsychiatry*. Copyright 1992 by the American Orthopsychiatric Association, Inc.

TABLE 18-8
A Description of Defense Mechanisms with Examples of Their Use by Children

Description	Example
Regression	
A return to an earlier stage of development in thought, feeling, or behavior	*Child:* A 4-year-old, Jillian, who has been toilet trained for over a year, begins to wet her pants when she is admitted into hospital for surgery *Adult:* Jillian's father has a temper tantrum when he is frustrated with the admission procedure
Denial	
A failure to acknowledge a stressful reality	*Child:* Jillian, who has been told she will be staying in the hospital for a few days, tells the child in the bed next to her she is going home with her mother *Adult:* Jillian's mother keeps forgetting her appointment for a Pap smear
Displacement	
Placing ideas, emotions, or feelings on a subject other than the one to which the feelings rightly belong	*Child:* Matthew, 5 yrs old, is angry: he has just been punished for eating a popsicle without permission before supper. He goes up to his room and plays war with his Transformers *Adult:* Matthew's mother has had a difficult day at work. She has heard she did not get the promotion she wanted. She begins yelling at her husband, Matthew, and the other children
Repression	
Painful experiences are barred from consciousness, awareness	*Child:* Jenny, age 18, does not remember spending 4 mos in a body cast at the age of 5 *Adult:* Mrs. B. does not remember her father's death when she was 7 yrs old
Projection	
Attributing one's own thoughts or impulses to another person	*Child:* John, who is envious of his sister's high academic achievements, accuses her of being envious of him *Adult:* Wife accuses husband of infidelity when she is sexually attracted to a male co-worker
Sublimation	
Transformation of unpleasant or blocked expressions into socially acceptable pursuits	*Child:* Rick, 13 yrs old, would like to walk home every day with the attractive girl who sits next to him in math class. Instead, he works out in the school gym *Adult:* Halina's husband has just left her for a younger woman. She spends much of her time reading murder mysteries
Identification	
Process by which a person becomes like something or someone else by taking on thoughts or mannerisms	*Child:* Two 15-year-olds walking to school are dressed and have hair styles exactly like the rock star on the billboard *Adult:* The new aspiring mayor of a small town dresses and acts like Bill Clinton
Reaction Formation	
Development of behavior that is exactly the opposite to what one would like to do	*Child:* Jean is angry at her mother for not letting her watch television. She goes into the kitchen to help with supper preparations *Adult:* Cathy is furious with one of her co-workers who has left a considerable amount of work to be completed. She goes out of her way to be pleasant to this person

(continued)

TABLE 18-8
A Description of Defense Mechanisms with Examples of Their Use by Children *(Continued)*

Description	Example
Rationalization	
A logical, socially acceptable explanation to make something acceptable that would be otherwise unacceptable	*Child:* A 14-year-old not picked for the hockey team explains to his friends that the coach felt he should try out for a more senior team *Adult:* A young woman fails her driving test after going through a stop sign and says that the driving instructor was biased against women drivers
Intellectualization	
Excessive reasoning is used to allay disturbing feelings	*Child:* A 17-year-old, Jackie, is fearful of dating. She tells her friends she does not wish to date because it would interfere with her school work, and she has yet to meet anyone with enough intelligence to interest her *Adult:* Jane becomes anxious in large crowded areas and explains her reasons for never going into shopping malls as a distaste for the crass consumerism of American society

ual from being responsive to the reality of the stressful situation needs evaluation. For example, it can be adaptive for a family to deny the implications of their child's having acute myelogenous leukemia when the child is in remission and doing well. This assists in coping and managing life from day to day. It could be detrimental to the family and child to continue using this defense if the child relapses.

The overview of concepts of stress, crisis, and coping should provide a basic knowledge for examining in more depth stress, crisis, and coping in children, parents, and families during illness.

Childhood Stress, Crisis, and Coping

Children are expected to adapt to increasingly complex situations in a rapidly changing world. Children are being pressured to grow up faster, fewer adults now live with children, and child abuse in all forms is increasing (Brenner, 1984; Elkind, 1986; Grey, 1990).

Sources of Stress and Crisis for Children

The source of tension for a child can arise from the microsystem, exosystem, and macrosystem within which the child lives (Brenner, 1984). The three systems can be visualized as concentric circles and are described by Brenner (1984) as follows.

The *microsystem* can cause stress to the child through the demands of growing and developing. The processes of maturing physically, intellectually, emotionally, and socially are stressors for a child. Increasing expectations to obey rules and to become more responsible for self and others requires continuous learning, role change, and adjustment of a child. As new family members are added to the system, stress is brought to the entire family as a whole and to individual children within the family. These types of stresses may be viewed as potential maturational crises for the child.

The *exosystem* produces stress when changes are made that affect the family's social connections (for example: when a family moves, joins or leaves religious groups, or makes changes in employment status). These types of stresses may be viewed as potential situational crises for the child.

The *macrosystem* brings stress to a child and family when established cultural norms are not adhered to. In addition, stressful events occurring within the community at large, such as floods, tornados, environmental disasters, or war, can bring stress to the child and family. These types of stress are unanticipated crises for the child.

The three systems interact to affect the way a child experiences individual stressors (e.g., starting school). Whenever a major stress compounds the usual stresses, a child is extremely vulnerable and may be in crisis. Illness is an example of a major stress that has the potential to cause a crisis for the child or the entire family.

Several studies have explored the types, degrees, and frequency of stress experienced by children. Children report the highest sources of stress for them are being viewed negatively by peers or adults, having conflict with teachers or parents, moving and changing schools, being excluded by peers, and having parents fight and/or separate. Most frequently occurring sources of stress are feeling ill, having nothing to do, pressure to achieve good grades, and feeling left out (Lewis et al, 1984; Dickey & Henderson, 1989; Dibrell & Yamamoto, 1986).

Reviewing the body's stress response at the beginning of this chapter should provide a basis for understanding the physiologic response to stress in the child. The major physiologic indicators of both acute and chronic stress in children are summarized in Table 18–9. Physiologic manifestations are generally diverse and nonspecific. Data on behavioral and cognitive coping strategies are also assessed to determine the well-being of children. An important understanding for nurses is that children view illness differently than adults do. The way illness is perceived has an impact on how children handle the stress associated with illness (Grey & Hayman, 1987). Table 18–10 identifies the cognitive and behavioral responses children at different developmental stages may use to cope with stress associated with illness.

Stress and Perceptions of Illness

The way children respond to illness and cope with the discomfort and unpleasant sensations can be affected by their age. How effectively one communicates with an ill child is dependent on one's understanding of the child's fears and misunderstandings that arise out of cognitive limitations. The nurse's lack

TABLE 18-9
Physiologic Indicators of Acute and Chronic Stress in Children

Acute Stress
Vital signs increase
Blood glucose increases
Glucose may be found in urine if renal threshold exceeded
Dilated pupils
Decreased gastrointestinal function
Cold, perspiring skin
Tense back muscles
Increased basal metabolic rate (BMR)
Increased temperature
Alterations in hunger/satiety
Alteration in alertness/arousal
Chronic Stress
Weight may increase or decrease
Height may fail to maintain percentile rank
Developmental milestones may be delayed
Blood glucose may increase or decrease
Changes in the immune response may occur
Increase in free fatty acids and amino acids in blood

TABLE 18-10
Coping Strategies Used by Various Age Groups

Infant
Movement
Restlessness
Rocking body
Playing with toys
Crying
Thumb/finger sucking
Sleeping
Toddler/Preschooler
Cognitive
Asking questions (why)
Wanting order (routine)
Has favorite toy
Learning—trial and error
Behavioral
Motor activity
Play
Temper tantrums
Aggression
Practicing—trial and error
Thumb sucking
Withdrawal
Psychologic Defenses
Regression
Denial
Repression
Projection
School-Age Child
Cognitive
Tries problem solving
Communicates (talkative)
Asks questions
Wants to be boss/controlling
Active fantasy life
Behavioral
Play—acts out situations
Friendships, play aggression
Withdrawal, quiet
Psychologic Defenses
Regression
Denial
Repression

(continued)

TABLE 18-10
***Coping Strategies Used by Various Age Groups** (Continued)*

Projection
Sublimation
Reaction formation
Adolescent
Cognitive
Problem solving
Reasoning through
Philosophic discussions
Abstract ideas
Behavioral
Conforms with peers
Activities
Personal interests
Asserts control
Acting out
Use of drugs/alcohol
Withdrawal
Psychologic Defenses
Regression
Denial
Repression
Projection
Sublimation
Reaction formation
Rationalization
Intellectualization

of understanding not only leads to a disregard of the child's actual experience but also can cause the nurse to unknowingly increase the child's fears and fantasies by using inappropriate word choices when giving explanations (e.g., telling a young child a "dye will be used" for a test may indeed arouse the fear of dying in a preoperational child).

Children's conceptualization of the causes, preventive measures, and treatments of illness influences their ability to cooperate and participate in illness management. For example, the young child who cannot cognitively understand that medicine (especially a shot) will speed recovery is likely to kick and scream in resistance (Fig. 18-10). Likewise, the older school-age child and adolescent who has the cognitive ability to understand cause and effect relationships suffers equally if explanations are *not* provided. In a study of school-age children and adolescents, younger children were found to lack knowledge about what does *not* cause disease. For example, they inferred that risk factors for one disease, especially AIDS, caused other diseases (Sigelman et al, 1993).

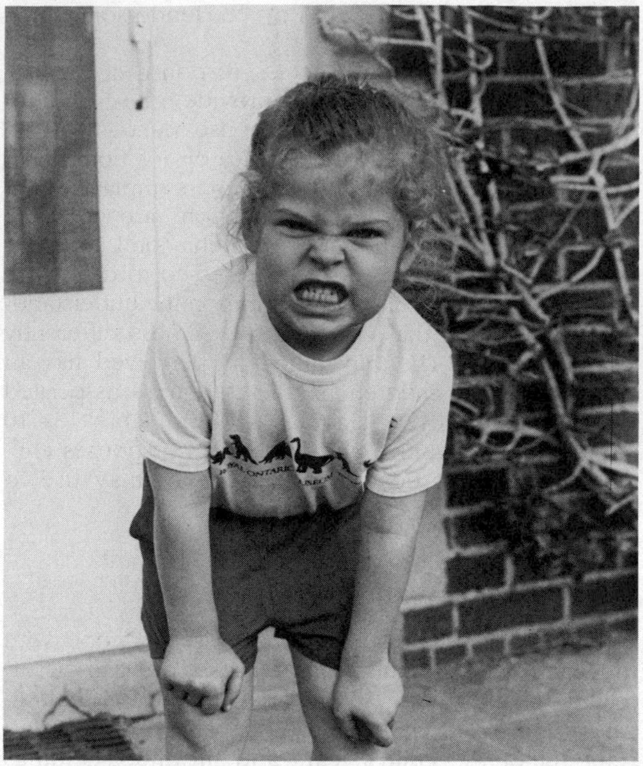

FIGURE 18-10. During toddler and preschool years, children use active behavioral coping styles, including motoric expression of anger.

It has been demonstrated that the conceptualization of illness advances through stages consistent with a Piagetian theoretical framework (Bibace & Walsh, 1980). This cognitive progression begins with magical/fantasy viewpoints advancing to increasingly more abstract thinking and reasoning ability. Bibace and Walsh (1980) identified stages of illness concept development, including:

- Incomprehension.
- Phenomenism.
- Contagion.
- Contamination.
- Internalization.
- Physiologic comprehension.
- Psychophysiologic comprehension.

Each of these illness concepts develops at corresponding developmental stages.

Infant

Bibace and Walsh (1980) used the term "incomprehension" to describe those children who were too young to explain illness. Owing to the immaturity of the child's communication ability, little is known about a child's perception of illness before 2 years of age.

Toddler and Preschooler

According to Piaget (1958), prelogical thinking is typical of children from 2 to 6 years of age. A salient characteristic of the preoperational child is that cause-and-effect relationships are explained in terms of immediate temporal and/or spatial cues (Blos, 1978; Bibace & Walsh, 1980). Concepts of illness in this prelogical stage have been described by some as global and undifferentiated (Perrin & Gerrity, 1981; Simeonsson, et al, 1979). Two types of prelogical explanations of illness identified by Bibace and Walsh (1980) are phenomenism and contagion.

"Phenomenism" is the most developmentally immature explanation of illness. The cause of illness is an external phenomenon (usually sensory) that is spatially remote and inappropriate. The relationships between the phenomenon and the illness cannot be explained; the causal link is one of magic or merely that the illness and the phenomenon occur at the same time. For example, in response to a question about how someone got a certain illness, a preschooler might say "from the sun" or "from the wind." A 4-year-old's explanation of illness as quoted by Bibace and Walsh (1980) follows: How do people get colds? "From the sun." How does the sun give you a cold? "It just does, that's all." How do people get measles? "From God." How does God give people measles? "God does it in the sky."

These examples reflect the preschooler's centering on a concrete, single phenomenon of his or her own experience and without any specification of the causal link.

"Contagion" is an explanation offered by more mature prelogical children. The child defines illness in terms of external persons, objects, or events, but the source is *near* to the ill person, or the causative event occurred *before* the illness. A child who perceives illness in this way still cannot explain the causal link; illness, if explained, is done so merely in terms of spatial or temporal proximity or magic. An example of this from the study by Bibace and Walsh (1980) follows:

> How do people get colds? "From outside." How do they get them from outside? "They just do that's all. They come when someone else gets near you." How? "I don't know—by magic I think."

The connection between the source of illness (or cure) and the actual illness is not explained; however, compared with phenomenism, the identified source is closer to the person and generally more appropriate.

A recent review of research on preschoolers' cognitive ability has suggested that they are more cognitively competent than Piaget had originally theorized. A preschooler's ability to remember and form mental representations of things warrants careful watching and listening to for cues about their understanding (Hauck, 1991).

School-Age Child

The school-age child (7 to 10 years of age) is in the concrete logical stage of development (Piaget, 1958). The major developmental advancement that characterizes this stage is differentiation of self from nonself. This enables a child to distinguish between that which is inside and that which is outside oneself. Multiple causes of illness are now stated, including the child's actions (Brewster, 1982; Carandang et al, 1979). Rule violations are often given as the reason for illness without identifying a causal link to the illness (Perrin & Gerrity, 1981).

The concept of contamination is an explanation used by younger children in the concrete logical stage. These children do not differentiate between the mind and the body; therefore, illness in their minds can be caused by bad behavior or by contact with germs. The cause or source is still external, but the bad behavior or germs are seen as being able to affect the body through surface contact. The concept of contamination is evident in the following example (Bibace & Walsh, 1980).

> How do people get a cold? "You're outside without a hat and you start sneezing. Your head would get cold, the cold would touch it, and then it would go all over your body."

The beginning of concrete operational thinking is evident in that the child begins to explain a connection between the source of the illness and the illness itself.

Older children in the concrete logical stage of development define illness in terms of an internal body part; hence, the term "internalization." The source of illness is still an external object or person (e.g., dirt, germs) or an unhealthy condition (e.g., obesity, old age), but it is seen as being able to have a direct effect on internal organs. At this stage, the process of internalization (e.g., swallowing or inhaling) can be explained, but the effect that it has on the internal body is vague and undifferentiated:

> How do people get colds? "From germs in the air, you breathe them in." How does this give you a cold? "The germs, they get in your blood." And? "They give you a cold I guess."

At this stage the primary focus is not on what happens physiologically but on the process of internalization (e.g., inhaling or swallowing). The ability to understand reversibility enables a child in this stage to realize that a person who becomes sick can become well and that illness prevention is possible through proper care.

Adolescent

According to Piaget (1958), the formal-logical stage of development occurs around 11 years of age. Children can then apply logic to abstract concepts because they are no longer bound by concrete reality. Thinking now extends into thoughts about what might be and generation of hypotheses.

The "physiologic stage" is used for younger children in the formal-logical stage of development, who describe illness to be a malfunctioning of specific internal body parts or processes. Although the cause is triggered by external events, a child at this stage is more concerned with describing the internal functions. For example, explaining the effect of an infected organism in the lungs is foremost compared with how the organism was acquired. A child senses increased control over the onset and cure of illness and has a clearer perception that personal actions can contribute to outcome.

The most mature understanding of illness is when the child can describe internal physiologic processes but can also include psychologic factors as alternative causes of illness. This is the "psychophysiologic stage." The young adolescent is now aware that a person's thoughts and feelings can cause illness; however, the cure is still viewed to be in the realm of biologic remedies, such as medicine.

These stages of illness concept development, as described by Bibace and Walsh (1980), reflect a progression in the degree of control that children sense as they mature. In the very early phase (phenomenism), children perceive objects over which they have no control, such as the sun or wind, as causing illness, whereas by early school age (contamination), illness is viewed as punishment. This, at least, brings illness into a more controllable perspective. Being good can thus also help one get better. By later school age (internalization), even greater control is evident, and a child is now able to understand that illness can be prevented by certain health behaviors.

A child's concept of illness is affected by factors other than the developmental level. Studies have shown that healthy children view illness differently than do ill, hospitalized children. Although a significant number of healthy children believed they "had to be good in order to get better," they rejected the idea that illness is a punishment; whereas ill, hospitalized children do believe that illness is a punishment for wrongdoing. Children who were found to be generally anxious (but not ill) also believed that illness was a form of punishment. In families in which a sibling has been ill, Carandang and colleagues (1979) found that the well siblings, especially those in the formal, logical stage of development, demonstrated a lower level conceptualization of illness than did children with healthy siblings. Coddington (1972) reported that sibling illness ranked among the most stressful of 42 life events for children; thus, a plausible explanation is that the stress of illness in the family is intrusive and may affect the perception of stress of healthy siblings. It has been suggested that the effect on adolescents, in particular, may be related to the fact that they, for the first time, may understand their own vulnerability to their sibling's disease. Thus, the nurse's interventions should take into account not only the child's developmental level but also individual factors such as experience with illness and general anxiety of the child.

Parental Stress and Coping with Childhood Illness

In this highly technological, fast-paced world, parents face a variety of different potential stressors arising from their personal, work, or family life. The functions, tasks, and responsibilities of parenting discussed in Chapter 12 highlight the complexity of the parenting role. The next several chapters in this section focus on the child who is ill. The illness of a child, whether acute or chronic, places the parents under stress. Sources of parental stress in the intensive care unit have been studied by Miles and Carter (1982). These include the sights and sounds of the general physical environment; the child's appearance and behavior; the child's emotional responses of fear, anger, sadness, and depression; communication or lack thereof from the caregivers; staff behaviors; and parental role deprivation. Chesler and Yoak (1984) have categorized the types of different stresses parents undergo when their child has a chronic illness. They identify the stress as being intellectual, instrumental, interpersonal, emotional, and existential.

"Intellectual stress" requires the parents to understand their child's illness: what it is and the treatment implications. For the parents of a child with a minor illness, this may require information about the type of antibiotic the child is on. Parents with a child with a more serious illness may need to know more detailed information about the disease progress, symptoms, danger signals and treatment options. The process of obtaining this information can add to this stress, as often the parents are met with health professionals who vary in their degree of giving information.

"Instrumental stress" involves the parents' concrete ways of arranging their day-to-day functioning to manage the child's illness. In families in which both parents work, it may mean one parent staying home or finding a baby sitter. If the child is hospitalized, it may mean new role allocations, caring for the child in the hospital, caring for other family members, and maintaining household and job-related tasks.

"Interpersonal stress" arises as the allocation of roles changes. Additionally, the parents are having to form new relationships in relation to their child's illness (nurses, physicians, family, friends) (Hymovich, 1976). Other children in the family may need or demand more time. As the parents encounter or change their role with each person, that person becomes a potential stressor.

TABLE 18-11
Coping Strategies for Parents with an Ill Child

Type of Stress	Positive Coping Strategies	Nursing Interventions to Promote Coping
Intellectual	***Behavioral***	Be available to answer questions
Lack of knowledge regarding illness	Seeks out others	Provide information—through books/pamphlets, etc.
	Cognitive	Teach (e.g., illness, treatment)
	Requests information	Assess for information overload by asking parents if they have been told too much, too little
	Interprets medical terms	Be available in future to answer further questions
	Protects against getting too much information (overload)	Be aware of other resources if needed—physicians, other parents, films
Instrumental	***Behavioral***	Assist parents in understanding that they may need to rearrange or alter tasks and functions
Day-to-day tasks	Arranges to help at home—baby sitters/cleaners	Assist parents in identifying resources to help them: family, friends, neighbors, colleagues at work, community resources
	Rearranges work time, extra help	
	Cares for sick child	
Interpersonal	***Behavioral***	Assist parents in understanding the changes in their particular situation (i.e., things that all new parents have to deal with)
Alteration in relationships	Seeks out others to help	Be available to listen
	Maintains relationships with family	Assist parents in understanding how others may want to avoid problem
	Discusses and shares with others	
	Avoids others who are not supportive	
	Cognitive	
	Becomes aware of how others perceive the problem	
Emotional	***Behavioral***	Assist in identifying how the stress is manifested in individual
Personal stress	Seeks help (counseling)	Assess ways of coping with stress in past
	Cares for sick child	Clarify feelings
	Cares for self (sleep, eat, etc.)	
	Takes time to be by self, away from others	
	Cognitive	
	Deals with feelings of hope, anger, fear	
Existential	***Behavioral***	Assist parents in understanding that child's illness has forced them into examining life
Challenge to previous commitments	Seeks out other's ideas and opinions; reading	
	Goes to place of worship or seeks other ways of support, groups	
	Cognitive	
	Seeks meaning and explanations for illness	
	Seeks new meaning of personal life	

"Emotional stress" is the personal stress each parent individually experiences when their child is ill. This is a very individual experience and can depend on many factors, one of which is the severity of the child's illness.

"Existential stress" forces parents to question and challenge their previous commitments and life goals. It is often experienced in more serious illness when the normal order of life and death is being questioned. Often parents will question the importance of their life and try to make sense out of this experience.

The way parents experience these stressors depends on many of the factors discussed earlier in the chapter. Table 18-11 identifies the types of stress, some task-oriented coping strategies to manage the stress, and nursing strategies to enhance coping during these periods.

Family Stress, Crisis, and Coping with Illness

The family as a system is made up of persons who are interdependent. Each member has a role to fulfill and others rely on that person to fulfill her or his role. The clarity of roles for each member is necessary and useful so that the family system can function effectively. The clarity of roles contributes to the family's maintaining a steady state as a system.

Families that are functioning effectively are able to problem solve, communicate, respond, and involve themselves together to determine roles, set rules, and care for each other. These activities contribute to the success and strength of the family unit.

When stress is introduced into the family system, significant changes and reactions occur. Within the communication network, stress affects the transfer of information. Inadequate message transmission and reception occur as stress is increased. Ineffective transmission of messages results in communication network breakdown.

Other types of stress situations that bring about dysfunction in the family system are lack of role clarity, vagueness of expectation, unresolved conflict, and conflict between the family system and other systems, such as church, school, police (Shonkoff et al, 1987; Tomlinson, 1986). The lack of role clarity results in family members being unable to identify their positions within the family structure. For younger family members, if there is a vagueness of what is expected from them, individual stress levels can increase and result in dysfunctional interpersonal relationships. Conflicts that are unresolved add to the dysfunctional quality of interaction. The continued elevation of stress levels in unresolved conflicts draws enormous amounts of energy from the family system that could otherwise be used in problem solving. Within the family system, when one member experiences stress, all members experience stress. It must be remembered that stress does not automatically lead to crisis. It is only when the family's balancing factors are inadequate that a crisis occurs. Because a family is a system, a crisis for one member will have an indirect or "ripple" effect on all other members of that family system. A crisis directly experienced by one member of a family will unsettle the equilibrium of the family system.

It makes logical sense, then, that the illness of a child will have an effect on all parts of the family system. A family's response to the illness of the child will depend on the perceived severity of the illness, the supports available to the family and the individual child, and sibling and parental coping responses to the illness. The importance of working with families, approaches to understanding them, and ways of assessing families have been discussed in detail in Chapter 2. The next chapter on chronic illness in children identifies the effects on family life and ways families cope with illness.

KEY CONCEPTS

Concepts Related to Basic Information

- The three stages of stress include: (1) alarm reaction stage, (2) stage of resistance, and (3) exhaustion.
- The nervous and endocrine systems are central to the stress response.
- The stress response results in two reactions from the hypothalamus: (1) it has a direct effect on the adrenal medulla via the sympathetic nervous system and (2) it triggers the two lobes of the pituitary gland.
- The end result of the stress response is the production of (1) vasopressin; (2) thyroxine; (3) cortisol; (4) aldosterone; and (5) epinephrine.
- Some children seem to be invulnerable to stress.
- Factors found to contribute to invulnerability in children include: (1) individual child factors; (2) family factors; and (3) community factors.
- Three different types of crises have been identified; namely, maturational, situational, and unanticipated.
- The process of coping is affected by the ability to appraise a stressful situation and to appraise resources needed to cope with the event. Age, developmental state, and previous experience affect these appraisals.

Concepts Related to Nursing Assessment

- The measurement of stress in a child's life is not easily accomplished by a single type of scale; recent approaches are to use scales that examine both major life events and daily hassles.
- There are alternate ways of assessing children who seem to be protected from stress including use of a (1) compensatory model; (2) protective model; or (3) challenge model.
- To obtain an understanding of the problem causing a crisis, the nurse should determine the precipitating event, perception of the event, presence or absence of situational support, and type of coping mechanisms usually used.
- The defense mechanisms being used to deal with crises should be assessed to determine whether they are functioning to impair or facilitate its resolution.

Concepts Related to Nursing Intervention

- Children use both behavioral and cognitive strategies to cope with stress.

- Children are able to think about the stress they are trying to cope with and can think about what to do about it.
- Boys and girls use different types of coping strategies.
- A child's concept of illness should be taken into consideration to determine the degree of cooperation and amount of participation that can be expected from the child with respect to illness management.
- Interventions with families under stress are based on the premise that a family is a system.
- A major response to stress in a family is a breakdown of communication systems.

REFERENCES

Aguilera, D. (1994). *Crisis intervention theory and methodology* (7th ed.). St. Louis: CV Mosby.

Antonovsky, A. (1987). *Unravelling the mystery of health*. San Francisco: Jossey-Bass.

Atkins, F. D. (1991). Children's perspective of stress and coping: An integrative review. *Issues in Mental Health Nursing, 12,* 171–178.

Bibace, R., & Walsh, M. E. (1980, December). Development of children's concepts of illness. *Pediatrics, 66*(6), 912–917.

Blos, P. (1978). Children think about illness: Their concepts and beliefs. In E. Gellert (Ed.). *Psychosocial aspects of pediatric care*. New York: Grune & Stratton.

Brenner, A. (1984). *Helping children cope with stress*. New York: DC Heath.

Brewster, A. B. (1982). Chronically ill hospitalized children's concepts of their illness. *Pediatrics, 69,* 355–362.

Burke, S. O., & Wiskin, N. (1984). Invulnerable handicapped children: Clinician validation of characteristic amenability to change. In M. Kravitz, & J. Lauren (Eds.). Nursing Papers; Proceedings of National Nursing Research Conference (Suppl), 50–61.

Caplan, G. (1961). *An approach to community mental health*. New York: Grune & Stratton.

Caplan, G. (1964). *Principles of preventive psychiatry*. New York: Basic Books.

Carandang, M. L., et al. (1979, July). The role of cognitive level and sibling illness in children's conceptualizations of illness. *American Journal of Orthopsychiatry, 49*(3), 474–481.

Chesler, M., & Yoak, M. (1984). Self-help group for parents of children with cancer. In H. B. Roback (Ed.). *Helping patients and their families cope with medical problems*. San Francisco: Jossey-Bass Publishers.

Coddington, R. D. (1972). The significance of life events as etiologic factors in the diseases of children. I: A survey of professional workers. II: A study of a normal population. *Journal of Psychosomatic Research, 16,* 7–18, 205–213.

Compas, B. E., Davis, G. F., Forsythe, C. J., & Wagner, B. M. (1987). Assessment of major and daily stressful events during adolescence: The Adolescent Perceived Events Scale. *Journal of Consulting and Clinical Psychology, 55*(4), 534–541.

Creed, F. (1985). Life events and physical illness. *Journal of Psychosomatic Research, 29,* 113–116.

Dahlin, L., Cederblad, M., Antonovsky, A., & Hagnell, O. (1990). Childhood vulnerability and adult invincibility. *Acta Psychiatrica Scandinavica, 82,* 228–232.

Dibrell, L., & Yamamoto, K. (1986). In their own words: Concerns of young children. *Child Psychiatry and Human Development, 19*(1), 14–25.

Dickey, J., & Henderson, P. (1989). What young children say about stress and coping in school. *Health Education, 2,* 14–17.

Dise-Lewis, J. E. (1988). The Life Events and Coping Inventory: An assessment of stress in children. *Psychosomatic Medicine,* 484–499.

Dohrenwend, B. P., & Shrout, P. E. (1985). Hassles in the conceptualization of measurement of life stress variables. *American Psychologist, 40,* 780–785.

Elkind, D. (1986). Parental pressures. *Pediatric Nursing, 12*(6), 417–418.

Elliott, S. (1980). Denial as an effective mechanism to allay anxiety following a stressful event. *Journal of Psychiatric Nursing, 18,* 11–14.

Elwood, S. W. (1987). Stressor and coping response: Inventories for children. *Psychological Reports, 60,* 931–947.

Erikson, E. H. (1964). *Childhood and society*. New York: WW Norton.

Frydenberg, E., & Lewis, R. (1991). Adolescent coping: The different ways in which boys and girls cope. *Journal of Adolescence, 14,* 119–133.

Garmezy, N. (1991). Reliance in children's adaptation to negative life events and stressed environments. *Pediatric Annals, 20*(9), 459–466.

Garmezy, N. (1983). Stressors of childhood. In N. Garmezy, & M. Rutter (Eds.). *Stress, coping, and development in children* (pp 43–84). New York: McGraw-Hill.

Garmezy, N. (1985). Stress-resistant children: The search for protective factors. In J. E. Stevenson (Ed.). *Aspects of current child psychiatry research. Journal of Child Psychology and Psychiatry,* Book Suppl No. 4. Oxford: Pergamon.

Garmezy, N., Masten, A., & Tellegen, A. (1984). The study of stress and competence in children. *Child Development, 55,* 97–111.

Grey, M. (1990). Helping children cope with stress. *Journal of Pediatric Health Care, 4*(6), 309–310.

Grey, M., & Hayman, L. (1987). Assessing stress in children: Research and clinical implications. *Journal of Pediatric Nursing, 2*(5), 316–327.

Guyton, A. C. (1991). *Human physiology and mechanisms of disease* (5th ed.). Philadelphia: WB Saunders.

Hargreaves, A. (1980). Coping with disaster. *American Journal of Nursing, 80*(4), 683.

Hauck, M. R. (1991). Cognitive abilities of preschool children: Implications for nurses working with young children. *Journal of Pediatric Nursing, 6*(4), 230–235.

Hoff, L. A. (1984). *People in crisis: Understanding and helping* (2nd ed.). Menlo Park, CA: Addison-Wesley.

Holmes, T. H., & Rahe, R. H. (1967). The social readjustment rating scale. *Journal of Psychosomatic Research, 11,* 213–218.

Holroyd, K. A., & Lazarus, R. S. (1982). Stress, coping and somatic adaptation. In C. Goldberger, & S. Brenznitz (Eds.). *Handbook of stress: Theoretical and clinical aspects*. New York: Free Press.

Hymovich, D. (1976). Parents of sick children: Their needs and tasks. *Pediatric Clinics of North America, 23,* 225–232.

Johnson, J. H., & McCutcheon, S. M. (1980). Assessing life stress in older children and adolescents: Preliminary findings with the life events checklist. In I. G. Sarason, & C. D. Speilberger (Eds.). *Stress and anxiety* (Vol. 7, pp 111–125). Washington, DC: Hemisphere.

Kanner, A. D., Coyne, J. C., Schaefer C., & Lazarus, R. (1981). Comparison of two models of stress measurement: Daily hassles and uplifts versus major life events. *Journal of Behavioral Medicine, 4,* 1–39.

LaMontagne, L. L. (1987). Children's preoperative coping: Replication and extension. *Nursing Research, 36,* 163–167.

Lazarus, R. S. (1966). *Psychological stress and the coping process*. New York: McGraw-Hill.

Lazarus, R. S. (1984). Puzzles in the study of daily hassles. *Journal of Behavioral Medicine, 7,* 375–389.

Lazarus, R. S., & Folkman, S. (1982). Coping and adaptation. In W. D. Gentry (Ed.). *The handbook of behavioral medicine*. New York: Guilford.

Lazarus, R. S., & Folkman, S. (1984). *Stress, appraisal, and coping*. New York: Springer.

Lewis, C., Siegel, J., & Lewis, M. (1984). Feeling bad: Exploring sources of distress among preadolescent children. *American Journal of Public Health, 74*(2), 117–122.

Luthar, S., & Zigler, E. (1991). Vulnerability and competence: A review of research on resilience in childhood. *American Journal of Orthopsychiatry, 61*(1), 6–22.

Miles, M. S., & Carter, M. C. (1982, Fall). Sources of parental stress in pediatric intensive care units. *Children's Health Care, 11*(2), 65–69.

Minter, R. E., & Kimball, C. P. (1980). Life events, personality traits and illness. In I. C. Kutash, & L. B. Schlesinger (Eds.). *Handbook on stress and anxiety* (pp 189–206). New York: Jossey-Bass.

Monat, A., & Lazarus, R. S. (Eds.). (1991). *Stress and coping* (3rd ed.). New York: Columbia University Press.

Morley, W. E., et al. (1967). Crisis: Paradigms of intervention. *Journal of Psychiatric Nursing, 5,* 537–544.

Oppenheimer, K. (1987). The impact of daily stressors on women's adjustment to marital separation. *Journal of Family Practice, 24*(5), 507–511.

Palmer, E. (1980). Student reactions to disaster. *American Journal of Nursing, 80*(4), 680–682.

Pellegrini, D. (1990). Psychosocial risk and protective factors in childhood. *Developmental and Behavioral Pediatrics, 11*(4), 201–209.

Perrin, E., & Gerrity, S. (1981). There's a demand in your belly: Children's understanding of illness. *Pediatrics, 67*(6), 841–849.

Piaget, J. (1958). *The growth of logical thinking from childhood to adolescence.* (A. Parson, & S. Seagren, Trans.). New York: Basic Books.

Rae-Grant, N., Thomas, H., Offord, D., & Boyle, M. (1989). Protective factors and the prevalence of behavioral and emotional disorders in children and adolescents. *Journal of the American Academy of Child and Adolescent Psychiatry, 28*(2), 262–268.

Reale, J. (1987). Life changes: Can they cause disease? *Nursing, 17*(7), 52–55.

Rutter, M. (1978a). Early sources of security and competence. In J. S. Bruner, & A. Garton (Eds.). *Human growth and development.* London: Oxford University Press.

Rutter, M. (1985). Resilience in the face of adversity: Protective factors and resistance to psychiatric disorder. *British Journal of Psychiatry, 147,* 598–611.

Rutter, M. (1978b). Stress, coping, and development: Some issues and some questions. In N. Garmezy, & M. Rutter (Eds.). *Stress, coping and development in children* (pp 1–41). New York: McGraw-Hill.

Ryan, N. M. (1989). Stress and coping strategies identified from school age children's perspective. *Research in Nursing and Health, 12*(2), 111–122.

Ryan-Wenger, N. (1992). A taxonomy of children's coping strategies: A step toward theory development. *American Journal of Orthopsychiatry, 62*(2), 256–263.

Selye, H. (1980). The stress concept today. In I. C. Kutash, & L. B. Schlesinger (Eds.). *Handbook on stress and anxiety* (pp 127–144). New York: Jossey-Bass.

Selye, H. (1976). *The stress of life* (2nd ed.). New York: McGraw-Hill.

Shaw-Sorensen, E. (1990). Children's coping responses. *Journal of Pediatric Nursing, 5*(4), 259–267.

Shonkoff, J., Jarman, F., & Kohlenberg, I. (1987). Family transitions, crises and adaptations. *Current Problems in Pediatrics, 17*(9), 501–553.

Sigelman, C., Maddock, A., Epstein, J., & Carpenter, W. (1993). Age differences in understanding of disease causality: AIDS, colds, and cancer. *Child Development,* 64, 277–284.

Simeonsson, R., Buckley, L., & Manson, L. (1979). Conceptions of illness causality in hospitalized children. *Journal of Pediatric Psychology, 4,* 77.

Streiner, D. L., et al. (1981). Quality of life events and their relationship to strain. *Schizophrenia Bulletin, 7*(1), 34–42.

Tomlinson, P. S. (1986). Applying family stress theory to nursing practice. *Nurse Practitioner, 11*(10), 78–81.

Walker, C. L. (1988). Stress and coping in siblings of childhood cancer patients. *Nursing Research, 37*(4), 208–212.

Werner, E. (1989). High-risk children in young adulthood: A longitudinal study from birth to 32 years. *American Journal of Orthopsychiatry, 59,* 72–81.

Yamamoto, K. (1979). Children's ratings of the stressfulness of experiences. *Developmental Psychology, 15,* 581–582.

Zautra, A. J., Guarnaccia, C. A., Reich, J. W., & Dohrenwend, B. P. (1988). The contribution of small events to stress and distress. In L. H. Cohen (Ed.). *Life events and psychological functioning: Theoretical and methodological issues* (pp 123–148). Newbury Park, CA: Sage.

BIBLIOGRAPHY

Brodie, B. (1974, December). Views of healthy children toward illness. *American Journal of Public Health, 64*(12), 1156–1159.

Busen, N. (1988). Societal values: A cause of stress in children. *Journal of Pediatric Health Care, 2*(6), 300–306.

Byrne, C. (1986). The social competence of children following a burn injury. *Burn Care Rehabilitation, 7*(3), 247–252.

Caplan, G. (1987). Guidance for divorcing parents. *Archives of Disease in Childhood, 62,* 752–753.

Clubb, R. L. (1991). Chronic sorrow: Adaptation patterns of parents with chronically ill children. *Pediatric Nursing, 17*(5), 461–466.

Grey, M. (1993). Stressors and children's health. *Journal of Pediatric Nursing, 8*(2), 85–91.

Leff, P. T., Chan, J. M., & Walizer, E. M. (1991). Self-understanding and reaching out to sick children and their families: An ongoing professional challenge. *Children's Health Care, 20*(4), 230–239.

Mechanic, D. (1978). *Studies under stress: A study in the social psychology of adaptation.* Madison: University of Wisconsin Press.

Mechanic, D. (1977). Illness behavior, social adaptation and the management of illness. *Journal of Nervous and Mental Disorders, 165*(2), 79–83.

Nugent, K., Hughes, R., Ball, B., & Davis, K. (1992). A practice model for a parent support group. *Pediatric Nursing, 18*(1), 11–16, 28–29.

Steffman, A. R., et al. (1986). A multivariate risk model for child behavioral problems. *American Journal of Orthopsychiatry, 56*(2), 204–211.

Walker, L. S., & Zeman, J. L. (1992). Parental response to child illness behavior. *Journal of Pediatric Psychology, 17*(1), 49–70.

Whyte, D. A. (1992). A family nursing approach to the care of a child with a chronic illness. *Journal of Advanced Nursing, 17*(3), 317–327.

CHAPTER • 19

Chronic Illness

Ann Harkins

RELATED TOPICS
Children's concepts of health, Chapter 10
Children's concepts of illness, Chapter 19
Children's perceptions of death, Chapter 20
Nursing care of a child during hospitalization, Chapter 21
Home care, Chapter 22
Supporting children during procedures, Chapter 23
Nursing management of the child in pain, Chapter 25
Principles of genetic inheritance, Chapter 31
The family in need of genetic counseling, Chapter 31
The child with an identified sensory impairment, Chapter 31

Definition, Terminology, and Classification

Incidence and Prevalence

Roles and Behaviors in Health/Illness
Health and Wellness Behavior
Sick Role
Illness Behavior
At-Risk Role

Cultural Implications of Childhood Chronic Illness

Impact of Chronic Illness on the Child and Family
Impact of Chronic Illness on the Child
Impact of Chronic Illness on the Family

Impact of Chronic Illness on Roles and Relationships
Maternal Role
Paternal Role
Marital Relationship
Siblings
Grandparents

Coping with Chronic Illness
Methods of Childhood Coping
Family Coping Strategies
Ineffective Coping Patterns
Effective Coping Patterns for Positive Adjustment

Role of the Nurse in Chronic Illness
Promoting Psychosocial Adaptation and Well-Being
Promoting Optimal Potential for Growth and Development

Utilization of Resources

LEARNING OBJECTIVES

- Identify the various definitions, terms, and means of classifying chronic illness.
- Compare and contrast the roles and behaviors of health and wellness, sick, illness, and at-risk roles.
- Explain the cultural and ethnic patterns that influence how chronic illness is perceived and defined by the child and family.
- Describe the impact of chronic illness on the child related to his or her level of development.
- Describe the impact of chronic illness on the roles and relationships of family members.
- Identify effective and ineffective coping strategies used by children and families to manage the stresses of chronic illness.
- Describe the role of the nurse in facilitating psychosocial adaptation, promoting optimal family and child development, and effectively using resources.

The knowledge that a child has a chronic illness may come suddenly, or it may be feared over a period of time with a gradual realization that a child requires special care. Even when the news comes suddenly, the impact of what the illness means to the child and family takes a lifetime to understand. Although remarkable advances in science and technology have made it possible to normalize the life of a child who has a chronic illness, the adjustment required by the child and the entire family is immense.

Some children adapt more easily than others, as do some families. The challenge to health care professionals is to recognize the uniqueness of each child in his or her situation. Optimal adaptation can be promoted only by examining the *individual* child's personal and family strengths and vulnerabilities. This chapter examines the concept of chronic illness, with a description of the nurse's role in supporting the child and family in making a lifelong adaptation to chronic illness.

The population of children and adults with chronic illness is steadily increasing. Improved health care and scientific discovery have lengthened the life expectancy of children with severe and life-threatening illnesses. These scientific and technologic advancements combined with a social climate supportive of a life-oriented value system have resulted in larger numbers of individuals living with a chronic illness (Blackburn, 1982; Ketterick, 1982; Burr et al, 1983; Hobbs et al, 1983; Hobbs & Perrin, 1985). Although the main health burdens in developing countries are still related to acute illness, chronic illness is one of the leading health problems in the industrialized world.

Definition, Terminology, and Classification

Many definitions of chronic illness exist. An early definition evolved from the keynote address in 1956 of L. Mayo, who was then chairman of the influential National Commission on Chronic Illness. This definition of chronic illness is often still used today.

All impairments or deviations from normal which have one or more of the following characteristics: are permanent, leave residual disability, are caused by non-reversible pathological alteration, require special training of the individual for rehabilitation, and may be expected to require a long period of supervision, observation or care.

Another definition of chronic illness, by Mattsson (1972), is also popular: "A disorder with a protracted course which can be progressive and fatal, or associated with a relatively normal life span despite impaired physical or mental functioning."

Terms that are similar to chronic illness are often used interchangeably and include "chronic disease," "chronic condition," and "long-term illness." Thomas (1983) describes a chronic condition as any anatomic or physiologic impairment that interferes with the individual's ability to function fully in the environment. Chronic conditions often have stable periods that are characteristically interrupted by acute episodes requiring medical intervention. Chronic conditions are managed by individual and family efforts.

A child can be identified as being a "chronically ill child" or a "child with a chronic condition." As Thomas (1987) notes, if the child is labeled as a "chronically ill child," no aspect of the child is identified other than the illness. However, when the child is perceived as having a condition, it is easier to think of the total child with ordinary developmentally appropriate behaviors as opposed to focusing entirely on the illness.

In addition to a variety of definitions, several terms describe an illness or condition that is long-term and incurable and imposes limitations on the individual. Commonly used alternative labels in the literature include "impairment," "handicap," and "disability." Researchers who use this alternative terminology tend to focus on a particular aspect of chronic illness. For example, "impairment" generally refers to physiologic or anatomic abnormalities, such as diabetes or asthma. "Handicap" describes the social consequences of the impairment resulting in an inability to attain satisfactory role fulfillment, especially the social response of others in the individual's environment. "Disability" has been widely defined and generally has some reference to functional limitations and the psychologic response resulting from the specific disease. More recent, and more positive, terms include "differently able" or "physically challenged."

Although the use of some of these alternative terms is thought to be declining, they still continue to be invoked either consciously or unconsciously. Such labels have the potential to influence the response of the individual, family, health care provider, and society at large (Diamond & Jones, 1983). This often negative response to individuals who are physically different or not fully functional is also known as the process of stigmatization. The individual who deviates from the social norm is devalued. The child and/or family may in some ways be held responsible or blamed for the child's differences.

Chronic illnesses can also be classified into various categories according to their severity or visibility to others. Categories may include life-threatening illnesses (e.g., leukemia or brain tumors) or non–life-threatening illnesses (e.g., epilepsy, cerebral palsy) and/or illnesses visible to others (e.g., blindness, mental retardation) or invisible to others (e.g., diabetes, colitis). However, these categories are neither exhaustive nor mutually exclusive. A child with a brain tumor, for example, may have a life-threatening but invisible chronic illness. The categories of chronic illness have also been subject to change over time. The cancers were previously classified as terminal illnesses. However, as a result of medical technology and increased survival rates, many childhood cancers are no longer considered life-threatening.

Incidence and Prevalence

The incidence of childhood chronic illness has been a subject of both interest and concern, particularly over the last 2 decades. Currently, there is no national data bank that supplies statistics or precise figures on how many children are affected by health conditions that require long-term monitoring and care, or ongoing treatment. Attempts to quantify the occurrence of childhood chronic illness have yielded a range of estimates, from a low of 5 per cent to a high of nearly one third of all children. The figures are dependent on how chronic illness is defined and the methods by which the information is collected (Stein, 1989; Newacheck et al, 1986). However, estimates have been advanced suggesting that numbers and severity of condition are increasing in this population.

In 1975, Pless and Pinkerton posited that 5 to 10 per cent of the population under 16 years of age were affected by chronic illness or disability. Ireys (1981) and Perrin (1985) estimated that 7.2 to 10.8 million (i.e., 10 to 15 per cent) of American children under the age of 18 years had a chronic condition. These figures are comparable to those reported in the 1988 National Health Statistics. Disagreeing with suggestions that the numbers of children with chronic health conditions had reached a plateau, Stein (1989) stated that "continued development of life sustaining technologies, improvements in early detection and treatment of premorbid conditions, and the change in the gene pool" (p. xxv) will further increase the number of affected children and their families.

When considering the incidence of chronic health conditions in children, there are new diagnostic classifications that must also be incorporated. These include acquired immunodeficiency syndrome (AIDS), drug-addicted infants, and children who suffer closed-head injuries. Added to the increasing number of children previously included, the numbers may be significantly greater.

Roles and Behaviors in Health/Illness

As providers of care to children with chronic illness and their families, nurses need to develop an understanding of the factors that influence an individual's responses to chronic illness. To this end, the roles and behaviors in chronic illness are discussed, including: (1) health and wellness behavior, (2) sick role, (3) illness behavior, and (4) at-risk role.

Health and Wellness Behavior

Children usually define "health" as the absence of illness. However, children who have chronic conditions are not likely to meet routinely the "absence of illness" criteria. Accordingly, the goal of health care for these children and their families generally focuses on promotion of optimal well-being and quality of life.

Children understand illness (especially its consequences) more easily than they comprehend the nebulous concept "health." Moreover, conceptualization of illness is associated with the child's level of cognitive development (Bibace & Walsh, 1980; Brewster, 1982; Perrin & Gerrity, 1981; Potter & Roberts, 1984; Harkins, 1990). Healthy children can easily identify with sensations such as the pain of a scraped knee or a needle. Children with a chronic illness can also usually relate to painful procedures such as blood tests and lumbar punctures. Illness is more threatening to their well-being and often interrupts the activities (such as play and school) that are central to childhood. A hypoglycemic reaction or a seizure is an event that causes fear and disruption among affected children and those around them. Illness and its consequences make an impression because they are unusual in a child's normally healthy world. It may be reasonable to expect that children with a chronic illness have a concept of illness but not necessarily of health.

In addition to differences in understanding that are based on developmental level, two major reasons may exist for children's poorly developed concept of health. First, children tend not to receive reinforcement for health behaviors (such as feeling good, energetic, or rested), whereas they do receive extra attention for illness symptoms (especially if the child is known to have a chronic illness). The child with chronic bowel disease who complains of stomach cramps will certainly receive more immediate attention than the healthy child who complains of the same symptoms. The child with Crohn disease may be rushed off to the doctor, whereas the well child may receive little attention. The urgency of the attention may heighten the sense of being sick in this child, whereas the lack of attention may decrease the healthy child's personal perception of being ill.

Second, children receive diffuse and often contradictory messages about health and illness from a variety of sources including the family, school, media, and peers. Children are taught either to engage in or refrain from certain behaviors to stay healthy. Most children view television commercials that promote alcohol; yet these same children are often taught by parents and teachers that drinking is detrimental to their health. As a result, there may be some sense of personal irresponsibility if the child experiences health problems related to drinking alcohol or to the use of other addictive products (Lewis & Lewis, 1974). Children with chronic respiratory illness, such as asthma, may feel guilt if the illness is exacerbated by even minimal contact with products or environmental situations deemed to be detrimental to their health.

Children with chronic illness can function at their optimal level. *Optimal-level functioning* is an attempt to achieve and/or balance physical, mental, and social well-being (Wilkinson, 1988). The related behaviors may be described as *wellness behaviors*. Wellness behavior can be learned at either home or school, but the child's behavior is ultimately influenced by the value the parents place on health and wellness. Parents who care for their own health (e.g., regular dental practices, sound nutritional practices, and abstinence from smoking and consuming alcohol and drugs) function as role models for their children's self-care habits.

Children also learn wellness behavior by increasing their knowledge, by being active participants, and by receiving reinforcement for practicing such behavior. For example, children suffering from chronic obesity during adolescence can increase their knowledge of nutrition and assume some of the responsibility for their own food preparation and intake. If these children can manage to adhere to their diets and receive positive reinforcement for their behavior from their parents and peers, the goal of practicing wellness behavior will have been achieved.

See Chapter 10 for further discussion of health and wellness and children's health attitudes and behaviors.

Sick Role

When a child is diagnosed with a chronic illness, subsequent behavioral changes are partly due to characteristics of illness, partly due to the family and others' reactions to the illness, and partly due to the maturity and coping ability of the child and family. A sequela that often follows the diagnosis of a child with a chronic illness is the "sick role."

In Parson's (1951) classic model of the sick role, an individual is (1) not responsible for the illness condition, (2) exempt from social role obligations, (3) obligated to get well, and (4) obligated to seek and accept professional care. Many health professionals and families with children with chronic illness function according to this model. A basic problem with Parson's model is that it reflects acute illness rather than chronic illness, in which time or length of illness is a contributing factor. In a child, exemption from normal social obligations or friends and schooling cannot be justified indefinitely. Eventually, the child will need to resume part or all of these responsibilities or will suffer from peer isolation and poor grades.

A second aspect of this sick role that may not apply to children with chronic illness is the obligation of children or their parents to seek treatment. Parents almost always seek initial treatment for sick children. However, if the treatment involves painful procedures, unpleasant side effects from drugs, or impingement on acceptable lifestyle, parents may balance the benefits of the medical help against the child's quality of life in deciding whether to return for follow-up visits.

Many factors affect parents' cooperativeness or compliance with the prescribed medical regimen. In chronic illness, parents or children are, in essence, the direct managers of day-to-day care. They often modify the treatment plan to fit their lifestyles and eliminate the symptoms most distressing to them, rather than comply with a regimen that does not always seem to make sense. If a child with diabetes screams continuously when undergoing finger sticks for blood glucose tests, parents may abandon this component of the regimen in favor of much less distressing urine tests or no testing procedure at all.

In childhood chronic illness, the care of the family and other nonprofessional supports is essential. Whole families, including nuclear and extended family members, may need to adapt to the demands of the child with chronic illness.

Fraser (1980) has expanded on Parson's (1951) model and views the sick role as one of a number of factors that handicap a child with a chronic condition. Fraser (1980) has categorized these factors into three distinct types, including the following:

- Handicapping factors A, which are structural or functional deficits.
- Handicapping factors B, which are restrictions on the child's experiences resulting from the physical and social environment.
- Handicapping factors C, which result from the attitudes toward the child's impairment in the social environment (including the social role of sickness, preconceived notions of abilities and expectation, and overprotective behaviors).

Fraser (1980) considers that the sick role does free the individual from certain responsibilities and obligations. In children with chronic conditions, this may lead to exclusion from learning experiences, because they may not be encouraged to develop skills and abilities normally demanded of healthy children. This exclusion also results in misunderstanding and exclusion by peers from play and social interactions. Lack of normal peer interaction, mitigated by the sick role, can compromise the child's emotional maturation and profoundly affect personal and social development (Isaacs & McElroy, 1980; Bullard & Dohnal, 1984).

Illness Behavior

Illness behavior during chronic illness refers to the way individuals perceive, evaluate, and take action on the symptoms of their diseases (Mechanic, 1962). In chronic illness, the goal may not be to eliminate certain symptoms but to manage the existing symptoms successfully in order to keep them from interfering with one's activities.

Illness behavior (or managing symptoms) depends on several factors, including the following:

- The nature of the child's symptoms (e.g., severity, frequency).
- The meaning of the symptoms to the child and family.
- The age and level of development of the child.
- Coping ability of the child and family.
- Degree of interference with the child's normal activities.
- Response from others.
- Nature of the child's illness (e.g., prognosis, imposed limitations).

For example, a teen-ager with cystic fibrosis may suffer from repeated bouts of difficult breathing. If the child knows how to manage the symptoms of these episodes and has coped well in the past, she or he is apt to manage the present situation well. A reasonable self-concept and acceptance of the illness by peers also promote the adolescent's participation in activities and peer relationships. However, if the symptoms have been uncontrolled or required timely attention from parents and peers, a child may not cope well with ongoing symptoms. Poor coping with symptoms of a chronic condition often leads to restricted or curtailed activities and a lowered self-esteem.

At-Risk Role

"Risk" can be defined as any factor (physical, environmental, or psychologic) that has the potential to affect an individual negatively. Recent attention has been given to identifying factors that contribute to risk in the environment (such as noise, sanitation, or pollution) and factors that protect or promote health. For the child with chronic illness, a factor that promotes health may be the social support provided by parents, peers, or caretakers in the environment. Several authors have suggested that social support has a direct and positive effect on the health status and on the physical and psychosocial level of stress in the individual (Cassel, 1976; Cobb, 1976; Kaplan et al, 1977). Accordingly, children who have the support of their parents and peers will benefit from attachment, social integration, feelings of worth, and opportunities for nurturance and guidance.

"Vulnerability" is a term that is often interchanged with "risk." Although many definitions exist, there seems to be agreement that vulnerability is related to personal components and is characterized by both constitutional and acquired factors. Constitutional factors are characteristics that are inherited and are reflected in the neuroanatomy of the organism; acquired factors result from a variety of life events that enhance or inhibit subsequent disorders. Risk appears to be primarily associated with environmental factors such as pollution, bacteria, and viruses. Risk and vulnerability appear to affect one another in a dynamic way (Murphy & Moriarty, 1976; Rose & Killien, 1983).

By definition, children with a chronic illness have inherited and/or acquired characteristics that cause them to be vulnerable. Anthony (1974) describes the vulnerable child as one who is susceptible to a variety of forces in the environment. Families of children with chronic illnesses can also be considered psychologically vulnerable when affected by such factors as stigma.

When children have chronic illnesses, the major task is to maintain control of the symptoms in order to reduce risk and vulnerability. A control of symptoms may mean that a child is not presently ill but is at risk for an exacerbation of illness if a treatment plan is not followed. This at-risk role entails duties but gives no privileges as the sick role does.

In chronic illness, levels of risk or vulnerability are not static. To illustrate this point, consider the child born with a heart defect requiring surgical repair. At birth, the child was vulnerable because of the pathophysiology that caused physical distress. However, following the surgical repair, this primary vulnerability may decrease or even disappear while secondary vulnerabilities, such as emotional and social lags in development, are created (Murphy & Moriarity, 1976). Secondary vulnerabilities often develop when concerned parents or health professionals create an overprotective and restrictive atmosphere, rather than one that promotes the total development of the child.

Because chronic illness is often characterized by long periods of time, active management by the child and family, and the necessity to comply with an often cumbersome medical regimen, the "at-risk" role may be a more appropriate framework than the sick role.

Health professionals need to understand these models and how to modify both risk and vulnerability factors in order to improve the state of health or to prevent deterioration in illness.

Cultural Implications of Childhood Chronic Illness

"Despite the 'melting pot' myth, America has one of the most heterogeneous populations of any Western

TABLE 19-1
Cultural and Ethnic Considerations in Caring for Children with Chronic Conditions

Cultural Identification	Characteristics	Implications for Care
Native Americans: Navajo Indians (beliefs, attitudes, and practices vary depending on tribal affiliations; the Navajo are one example of Native American cultures)	"Family" includes all members of extended family, all of whom may accompany a sick child to health care facilities	Understanding roles and responsibilities of the members of a large family support system is essential in management of acute and long-term care needs
	Language reflects concept of "universe in motion"; use of word "good" denotes promotion of prosperity and happiness; value is relative to definitions of respected individuals	Communication may be compromised by unshared definitions, interpretations, or implications of words/phrases or behaviors; therefore, terminology, rationale for care regimens, and projected long-term outcome may require regular clarification
	Massage of an infant is part of the bonding experience between mother and child	
	Eye contact is a sign of disrespect	Failure to establish or maintain eye contact should not be interpreted as disinterest, lack of understanding, or unwillingness/inability to participate in care regimen
	Living space is often shared by both nuclear and extended families; if a death occurs within the hogan (Navajo dwelling), tradition may require sealing, abandoning, or even burning the dwelling	Care should be planned to recognize and incorporate attitudes relative to congruence of physical and environmental elements
	Concept of health encompasses the physical body and congruence with family, environment, livestock, supernatural forces, and the community as well as harmony with supernatural forces	Housing facilities may be unable to accommodate care modalities deemed important/imperative by conventional care providers
		The possible death of a child at home may contribute to a family's concerns for security of the home or living environment
	Tribal healers often work collaboratively with conventional Western health care providers; sacred myths and legends portraying supernatural beings are often blended into religious and healing practices	Traditional tribal healing practices and measures that are neutral or beneficial should be incorporated into acute and long-term care plans
African-Americans	Personal and social space may be close and more dense, with multiple activity involvements	Children and families may benefit from discussion (possibly repeated) of structuring space or prioritizing activities for prudent care management
	In African-American families, wives/mothers often assume strong leadership roles	Understanding of family structure and patterns of decision making is necessary for determining treatment and disseminating information
	Large networks of "close family friends" as well as nuclear and extended family members often offer advice and physical and emotional support during times of crisis or illness	Problem solving tends to be action oriented (i.e., progress in alleviating the problem must be apparent)
		All components of the family system should be included in developing the care plan
	Perceptions of illness range from: (a) a natural occurrence resulting from disharmony and conflict in an individual's life; (b) everything has an opposite (e.g., for every birth there must be a death); or (c) trouble and pain are God's will, requiring acceptance and stoicism	Explanations about sources of illness and measures for both prevention and treatment are essential in clarifying and reinforcing the individual or family's role/responsibility in illness management

culture" (Wright & Leahey, 1987, p 79). This heterogeneity is reflected in geography of origin, religious beliefs, and/or regional variations. The attitudes, values, beliefs, and behaviors of different cultures and ethnicities can have profound effects on how chronic illness is perceived and defined. These factors influence how an individual and the family unit respond to the chronically ill family member, and, similarly, how the surrounding community responds. Therefore, health care providers must neither have uniform expectations nor apply common or universal interventions for families that include a child with a chronic illness. For example, the prevalent notion of individual or parent and child autonomy in decision making about health care and health care practices may seem inaccurate, perhaps foreign, to some ethnic or cultural groups in America. These issues may have to be discussed and ultimately decided by extended family

TABLE 19-1
Cultural and Ethnic Considerations in Caring for Children with Chronic Conditions *(Continued)*

Cultural Identification	Characteristics	Implications for Care
Mexican-Americans	The nuclear family with specified roles is the foundation of the Mexican community; the father usually has the dominant role as decision maker	Identification of family values and roles is essential (e.g., consultation with the father regarding treatment modalities and regimens may be essential for cooperation/compliance)
	Mexican-American families will likely not seek outside help to meet needs or solve problems	Physical examinations may be very threatening
	Mexican-Americans may be characterized as tactile in their relationships; however, there is discomfort with touch or exposure of intimate body parts	Touching the child when talking to or about him/her as well as when giving care is valued and often believed to prevent and/or treat illness
	Looking at a child when talking to or about him/her without touching the child may be believed to cause illness	Areas of disagreement must be elicited in order to promote open discussion and subsequent compliance with health care regimens
	Self-disclosure in conversation is reserved for close friends	Unusual efforts may be required to secure and retain parental and family commitment to regimens of care of the chronically ill child
	Direct confrontation or argument is thought to be rude or disrespectful	
	Behaviors often reflect belief that the outcome of circumstances is controlled by external forces (i.e., individuals have little control over their lives)	
Chinese-Americans	Communication often encompasses periods of silence. Self-control is valued while disagreement or criticism is avoided	Nonverbal cues must be noted and their implied meaning clarified to identify needs as well as understanding of, agreement with, or commitment to a regimen of care (e.g., Chinese-American children may be more stoic when experiencing pain, reflecting the cultural value and practice of self-control)
	Touching may be considered a breach of etiquette, loss of self-control, impolite, or disrespectful	To convey respect and sensitivity, the purpose and importance of touching in providing care needs to explained
	Loyalty to family, devotion to tradition, and de-emphasized individual feelings are characteristic of Chinese-Americans	The hierarchical structure of the Chinese-American family should be recognized; however, decision making and care plans need also to incorporate the personal sense of responsibility and commitment to family members
	Respect and deference are shown to older and/or family members with authority; however, decision making occurs through consensus of family members	Assessment of how families integrate culturally defined health practices into regimens for the chronically ill child is important (e.g., food/dietary interventions used as health-restoration measures may require adjustment for the child with juvenile diabetes).
	Health care may include both Western medical services and traditional oriental modalities and/or practices; the concepts of yin and yang may often be integrated into management of illness; these represent the power that regulates the body as part of the universe	

Data from Giger, J. N., & Davidhizar, R. E. (1991). *Transculture nursing: Assessment and intervention*. St. Louis: CV Mosby.

groups, if health care goals are to be reached—especially when the family member with a chronic illness is a child.

Health care providers should exercise caution when tempted to generalize a specific trait or characteristic attributed to a given culture, race, or ethnic population. Cultural and ethnic patterns may govern symptom identification and interpretation, "acceptability" of the chronic condition, and the pattern of family and individual interaction with the health care providers and the health care system. However, to varying extents, individuals or families are likely to have modified their traditional attitudes, beliefs, or practices to include some of those of the society in which they live. In spite of this caveat, Table 19-1 broadly describes some attitudes, beliefs, and practices that may be observed in four representative American groups.

Impact of Chronic Illness on the Child and Family

Each chronic illness has its own symptoms, etiology, treatments, and prognosis. However, chronic illnesses share common features that produce stress for children and their families. The family's central role in managing the child's illness throughout his or her lifetime contributes greatly to the impact of the illness on the child.

Chronic illness can occur at any age or stage of a child's development. The effect of the illness and the response to it vary considerably, depending on the stage of growth and development of both the child and the family. The various theories of physical, cognitive, and psychosocial development of the child are reviewed in Chapter 3. The child's perception of illness at various ages and cognitive stages is discussed in Chapter 18.

Impact of Chronic Illness on the Child

The child's response to chronic illness is often based on a number of factors that either separately or in combination are present throughout an illness. Some general characteristics that are of primary importance to the child include: (1) the nature and course of the illness; (2) separation caused by hospitalization; (3) sensory impairment, physical restriction, and social isolation; (4) dependency; (5) fear of treatments and procedures and the pain they may cause; (6) concern about death; and (7) the effect of the illness on mobility/immobility.

Chronic illness influences the child's physical, cognitive, social, and emotional development. The degree to which children perceive themselves as different from other children depends largely on the nature of the chronic illness (i.e., symptoms, treatment, and prognosis). For example, certain types of brain dysfunction may not limit physical functioning but may cause poor attention span, hyperactivity, or aggressive behavior, thus limiting perception and learning in a normally intelligent child. Conversely, the child with spina bifida may have normal cognitive functioning but may be severely affected in mobility and self-concept because of physical limitations.

Frequent and/or long-distance hospitalization (including medical specialty consultation) may contribute to separation of children with a chronic illness and their parents, families, and peer groups. The emotional impact of separation can vary, depending on the age of the child.

Bowlby (1973) described three stages of the child's reaction to separation, including the following: protest—crying and resistant behavior and frequent demands for parents; despair—withdrawal, lack of interest in the surroundings, and loss of hope for the parents' return; and detachment—regaining appetite and activities but avoiding attachment to any particular individual and avoiding the parents when they visit. These are responses to separation seen in children in general. The behaviors may be exaggerated in children with chronic health conditions who feel threatened and/or who may experience more frequent or prolonged separations. The vulnerability of a child to separation during hospitalization depends on many factors, including previous hospital experiences.

Childhood chronic illness is a family affair that disrupts the lives of individual family members and the family as a unit as well as the life of the affected child. A more in-depth discussion of the effects of separation due to hospitalization can be found in Chapter 21.

Impact of Chronic Illness on the Family

Many authors have described the stresses imposed on the child and family when a child is diagnosed with a chronic illness (Cohen, 1989; Harkins, 1991; Holaday, 1989; Mattson, 1972; Featherstone, 1980; Gliedman & Roth, 1980; Figley & McCubbin, 1983). Understanding the impact of a child's chronic illness on the family is a difficult task. To assess accurately the effect that a child's illness has on the family system, we also need to know how the family functioned before the diagnosis.

Gathering retrospective information requires shifting the focus to the family instead of focusing on the child. One approach to compiling this type of background is the genogram (Wright & Leahey, 1984). A family genogram is a technique that encourages discussion of family members' roles and interactive relationships, including physical relationships.

Family functioning is not only a matter of normal roles and routines. It is also influenced by how families individually and collectively define and respond to challenge. Access to social support is also crucial to the family's ability to maintain relative "normalcy." Several nurse researchers (e.g., Feetham, 1982; Feetham & Roberts, 1983; McCubbin, 1986) have led the development of instruments for assessing relationships within families and families' relationships to their social environments.

Chronic illness can affect many spheres of family life—financial, social, emotional, behavioral, and cognitive. Although specific chronic conditions vary in the stresses they impose, any chronic illness brings more tasks, time commitments, and financial burdens to the family. Often, the child's illness strains the family's financial resources because of hospitalization, treatment, and medication costs. Few insurance plans cover *all* health care services in the hospital, and even fewer cover home care expenses for long-term chronic conditions. Families who live outside metropolitan areas may spend a sizeable sum on transportation to and from health care centers. Some families even find it necessary to move to be closer to a facility that provides the necessary specialized care.

At least one parent may have to give up working

or reduce his or her time in the work force, which may result in significant income reduction. The economic impact of care and management can be substantial when families cannot maintain the employment status that preceded the child's diagnosis of chronic illness.

A chronic condition may reduce the child's and family's potential for healthy socialization. Children with chronic illnesses may evoke fear, anxiety, confusion, and embarrassment in the social environment. These responses may cause more distress than the chronic condition itself (Gliedman & Roth, 1980). Difficulty in finding caretakers for the child or problems in transporting a child with a disability may lead to social isolation. Other parents and children often do not know how to interact with children with a chronic illness; they may be embarrassed or uncomfortable. The ill child and the family often feel rejected and devalued.

Social support can be a mediator for families under such stress. Support from peers, family, and the health care system can often reduce feelings of social isolation. However, parents still struggle with child care guidance and problem solving related to the child's special needs. Extended family members provide the most consistent support (Featherstone, 1980), as the strain of chronicity tends to "burn out" nonfamily networks (Neill, 1979; Featherstone, 1980).

Emotionally, the family is faced with stresses due to the child's physical vulnerability, personal grief reactions, and feelings of guilt and blame. The grieving process is continual and is often reactivated with each new development in the child's condition (Sargent & Liebman, 1985) in what has been described as "chronic sorrow" (Damrosch & Perry, 1989; Warda, 1992; Wikler et al, 1981). Family members in their understandings of and responses to the diagnosis will likely vary. If these understandings and responses greatly contrast (whether because of wide variances in developmental stages of family members or because of role and responsibility within the family, or both) so that there is perpetual conflict, all family members are at risk for altered self-concept and esteem over time.

These changes require skilled management on the part of family members and health professionals to ensure that children can accept their differences as well as their similarities when compared with other children. The family must continually aim for a balance between normal functioning and sensitivity to their child's special needs.

Cognitively, the family needs to understand the nature of the illness, the treatment procedures, predictable and unpredictable complications, and the expected course of events. All members need to be aware of the rationale behind the various aspects of treatment. They must also understand the impact the illness and its consequences have on the social and emotional well-being of the child.

The developmental stage of each family member, the family unit, and the affected child contributes greatly to the effect of the illness on the family's behavioral, cognitive, and emotional well-being and on developmental tasks. Moreover, understanding the affected child's developmental stage enhances our insight into the problems shared by children with chronic conditions at a specific stage (Table 19–2). Each stage is therefore discussed in more detail.

The family also face the challenge of adapting behavior patterns and activities to accommodate treatment regimens in their daily lives. The family's and child's developmental needs, the age of the parents, the time the family has been established as a unit, and the family's previous coping abilities all are factors that influence the family's reaction to the illness and their ability to maintain normal functioning.

Infant

The main developmental task for the infant is to develop a sense of basic trust in self (Erikson, 1964) and in the caring adults in the environment. A long-term illness or congenital defect may affect the relationship between parents and infant and impair the development of trust.

Specific limitations of the chronic illness may limit the infant's normal growth and development. The mobility of an infant with a physical disability is often restricted; he or she is unable to explore the environment through touching, manipulating, and mouthing objects. Lags in physical and cognitive development may result. Infants also need to experience events for themselves in order to begin to develop a frame of reference. Very young children, although able to feel pain, do not understand their discomfort because they have no other experiences with which to compare it. They have no prior expectations and do not comprehend that the often painful procedures, anxious parents, or physical restrictions are related to or result from their chronic illness.

To a great extent, the way in which infants experience and adapt to their chronic illnesses depends on the degree to which their parents accept the condition. All pregnant couples dream of the ideal, perfect, healthy baby. When a baby is born or diagnosed with a chronic illness, the parents feel a great sense of loss and sorrow and grieve for the healthy baby that they feel they had the right to expect. To the parents, a child is an extension of themselves; therefore, producing an unhealthy child or a child with a disability leads to a loss of self-esteem and positive self-concept.

Chronic illness during infancy can potentially disrupt the parent/child attachment and adaptation (Mercer, 1974; Richards, 1986) as well as the smooth transition into parenthood and family life. Parents take pride in the growth and development of their baby. However, if the child is irritable or listless and does not grow at the expected rate, parents may feel less adequate in their parenting role and less gratified for their efforts. Also, the contented infant who can be

TABLE 19-2
Common Problems Experienced by Children with Chronic Health Conditions

Infants	Toddlers	Preschoolers	School-Age	Adolescents
Physical or Environmental Restrictions				
If most energy is utilized for survival, there is limited ability to assimilate environmental input. Sensory deficits (e.g., blindness, deafness) can also negatively affect infant's ability to assimilate/accommodate to environmental factors. Parent-infant interaction, synchrony, and attachment processes are potentially disrupted	Environmental limitation affects developmental aspects, including sensory, motor, and social input or interaction: e.g., physical skills (walking, running, eye-hand coordination); cognitive ("experimentation" with familiar objects, full object permanence, early mental combinations and symbolic thought); and psychosocial (early pretending, beginning preference for playing with peers, social interactions that include both positive and negative exchange)	Physical and/or environmental limits may restrict child's ability to engage in active physical and social activities, thus also limiting the growing sense of mastery	Teachers and peers are large contributors to the social development of middle childhood; physical or environmental restrictions that interfere with school attendance may hinder developing independence, social development in the context of peer groups, academic achievement, self-image, and confidence	Significant physical and social transitions may be compromised or constrained by frequent or prolonged hospitalizations. Similarly, diminished stamina may restrict physical or social activities in which the adolescent is able to participate. Environmental limitations may include educational access as a result of building or program design
Mobility/Immobility				
Restricted mobility may interfere with exploration of environment and development of motor skills	The evolving of sense of autonomy and developing independence may be impeded by immobility, whether a result of the chronic condition, environment, or enforced dependence by caretaker-person(s); both child and parents may experience frustration (and anger) with limitation in locomotion or other mobility	Motor and social competence may be compromised by mobility limitations; these may be associated with physical restrictions, limited physical strength, or pain from disease or treatment. Mobility restrictions may affect ability and will to participate in goal-directed play; inability to participate actively in play may limit child's sense of mastery	Physical activity is an integral component of middle childhood interactional behaviors; restricted or limited mobility may have a negative effect on social relationships, interactions, self-perception, and self-esteem	May experience barriers to age-appropriate activities (e.g., participation in competitive sports); immobility may interfere with participation in social activities; occupational objectives must accommodate mobility limitations
Course of Illness				
Course of illness may be affected by immature immune system and/or inadequate physical reserves; deficits (physical or mental) may be present and obvious vs. suspected, may be static and/or progressive	Social and physical development limited by chronic illness may affect cognitive and language development	Irregularities associated with bodily function (e.g., eating, toileting) may be perceived as highly disruptive in a family in which high value is placed on regularity and behaviorally scheduled patterns	School attendance and progress are a central expectation for these children; course of illness may affect school attendance and participation and role development in peer group	Course of illness may be directly influenced by degree to which the adolescent accepts responsibility for care and is compliant with associated regimens. Exacerbations of illness may interrupt the adolescent's progress in developing independence, goal-development and attainment, and managing a fragile self-esteem and sexual identity

TABLE 19-2
Common Problems Experienced by Children with Chronic Health Conditions *(Continued)*

Infants	Toddlers	Preschoolers	School-Age	Adolescents
Visibility/Invisibility of Disease				
Visible physical evidence of condition may contribute to parental feelings of guilt, grief, and embarrassment and influence their interactions with/about their infant. Even if condition is not apparent, parents may feel compelled to protect infant against perceived potential illnesses	Delays in normal development become more apparent and may lead to chronic sorrow over loss of the "normal child"	Parental sensitivity to visibility of chronic health condition may be heightened as interactions outside home and family increase	Child with a visible condition may experience derision, ridicule, and perhaps rejection from peer group; child with condition that is not visible may require special consideration that is misunderstood by peer group and may also be teased (e.g., singled out as "teacher's pet") and rejected	Visibility of condition may adversely affect social interaction when emphasis is on social conformity and appearance (e.g., delayed sexual development may contribute to anxiety and embarrassment). Invisibility of a condition may promote risky behaviors to achieve conformity while simultaneously jeopardizing short-term (and perhaps long-term) health
Dependency				
Infant generally dependent on parents and other family members for meeting basic needs (e.g., food, warmth, cleanliness) as well as stimulation and social development; others (i.e., health care providers) may be required to meet these needs	Limited mobility and protective parenting may continue to foster dependency and reduced effort or ability to develop independence, including locomotion. Child may have increased difficulty with separation, impulse control, and poor self-image; this may require more reassurance from adults	The intensity of physical care may increase as the child gets older and larger; child may be more dependent on immediate (and perhaps extended) family for social as well as physical care. Parents may attempt to protect the child in interactions with peers, thus inhibiting initiative and development of effective coping strategies	As the child begins school (initially and at the beginning of each new school year), sharing of the responsibility for the child's care with school personnel may be frightening and threatening for both the child and parents	There may be significant conflict between health needs and associated relationship between parents and health care providers. Developing sexuality, the desire for physical and social independence, and the assumption of responsibility for health care may lead to ongoing confrontation as dependence/independence issues are resolved or accepted
Interdisciplinary Care Requirements				
Coordination of numerous components of health care team needed to provide physical care for child, emotional and psychologic support for family. Educational needs of family must be determined and strategies for ongoing learning devised. Community resources must be identified and assistance provided for obtaining and coordinating services	Respite care must become a regular component of the interdisciplinary planning and support for families of toddlers with chronic conditions. Early integrated planning and intervention is essential for promoting optimal developmental progress; this includes social, health care, and governmental services	Continued evaluation, program planning, and interventions of a broad-based interdisciplinary team are necessary for maintenance of a supportive program for promoting ongoing child and family development and well-being	The school teacher and administrator become essential members of the health care team; they must be educated regarding the child's chronic condition and supported through the evolution (exacerbations or periods of quiescence) of the condition	The developing adolescent is an equal (and essential) partner in the health care team. Areas of focus include physical, social, psychologic, educational, occupational, and financial resource identification, acquisition and management

held, fed, and fondled is much more socially responsive and provides tremendous reinforcement for the family. Infants who are socially less responsive because of the constraints of their illnesses or other physical problems (such as a cleft lip or hydrocephalus) provide less social gratification.

The parents of an infant with long-term illness experience the grieving process but also have to contend with the day-to-day reality of their child's chronic condition. Such "chronic sorrow" (Olshansky, 1962) imposes stress on family functioning long after the diagnostic crisis is resolved. The family may feel that there is no escape from this situation, and it will be a lifelong stress. If the prognosis does not include a normal life span, the parents may feel even more intense sorrow, alienation, and powerlessness. The resulting disequilibrium may cause distortions in family relationships that ultimately necessitate a permanent alteration in family roles and goals. However, many families do resolve these initial grief feelings and are able both to meet the needs of their infants with special health care needs and to receive satisfaction from them.

Toddler

The toddler's developmental task is to acquire a sense of autonomy and self-control. Erikson (1964) describes the child from 18 months to 3 years as striving to conquer the maturational crisis of autonomy. Healthy children of this age rapidly develop motor and communication skills, which allow them to explore their environment more fully and to tell the world about it. If children do not accomplish this task, they may feel shame and doubt because they feel they are not in control of either themselves or their world. Toddlers develop confidence in their abilities and a sense of social competence. Toddlers want to do "everything" for themselves and take great pride in controlling and manipulating their world. Thinking in imaginative and magical ways allows toddlers to be egocentric and omnipotent enough to believe that they can make things happen. They do not understand causality through logic but rather through magic.

When long-term illness is either present or diagnosed at this stage, there is potential for a major upset in this struggle for autonomy. Cognitively, if children are restricted in their activities and movements, they will have difficulty developing a sense of self and seeing themselves as separate and intact human beings. Immobilization may also seem intolerable and very frustrating to toddlers who desire to be on the move. Frequently, toddlers with a chronic condition develop increased dependency, difficulty with separation during hospitalizations, an uncertain self-image, and poor impulse control. Some studies (Sibinga & Friedman, 1971; Dowd et al, 1977) even suggest that there is potential for delay in physical, psychosocial, and language skills as a result of physical restraint during these early formative years.

As children progress beyond the dependent stage of infancy, parents need to begin to relinquish some of the supervision and total care that they assumed when the child was younger. When children have a chronic illness and may be suffering from repeated episodes of pain, immobility, loss of control, and separation, releasing parental control may be difficult. Children who are not allowed to make some choices in their lives or have some control over them may become apathetic, passive, and clinging. These behaviors tend to induce overprotectiveness and restrictiveness from the parents. Such compensating behaviors may affect the child's abilities to master autonomy and become more independent. If toddlers have decreased energy for activity, the caretakers are faced with the challenge of assisting their children to reach their maximum potential without compromising their physical health.

Parents are also confronted with attempting to deal with the ill child's behavior, which may lead to conflict about discipline. In toddlers, the opportunity to control their activities and lives may be sharply diminished when they are diagnosed with a chronic illness. Therefore, the situations that a toddler can control take on new and exaggerated importance. Control of feeding and elimination may, for example, be characteristic of assertiveness. Refusing to eat, playing with food, or throwing food and eating utensils in the kitchen may be behaviors typical of the toddler's negativistic nature. Young children may choose to control or not to control their elimination or smear their stool all over their environment. Their choice to behave in certain ways is strongly influenced by the parents' response to the illness as well as by the child's natural desire to please them. In these situations, parents may also be reluctant to set appropriate limits or take disciplinary action for fear they might interfere with the child's normal development of impulse control. The capacity of the child with a chronic health condition is likely to be the same as that of a healthy toddler; that is, excessive permissiveness or strictness may promote feelings of shame and doubt.

During toddlerhood, children normally experience great anxiety when separated from parents, even for a short period of time. With the potential for multiple hospitalizations or medical procedures in chronic illness, children are particularly vulnerable to separation anxiety. They need their family to protect them from fears of the unknown; they are often unable to cope without them. Parents will also feel guilty and see themselves, rather than the situation, as being directly responsible for this behavior.

A toddler diagnosed with chronic illness can have tremendous effects on family relationships. The family is often young, and the parents are striving to develop a marital relationship and financial stability. The diagnosis of an ill child can either cement relationships or completely sever them. In addition, an ill child will make increased demands on the parents' personal energy and finances. The parents may find it difficult to separate themselves for even brief amounts of time from the clinging, often emotional child and feel guilty when they do so. However, occasional or regular "time-outs" for the parents may be their only means of coping with this difficult situation.

Preschooler

Children from 4 to 6 years old are increasingly active, are intent on mastering new skills, and have a need to be productive. Preschoolers win approval by mastering new tasks and taking responsibility for themselves, other things, and other people in their world. These are the building blocks for identity development and for how they will interact with their peers and all individuals in their environment. They need to attain desired goals and receive approval for this attainment, particularly from their parents and peers. Children who successfully complete this stage develop a sense of purpose, competence, and self-confidence in their own abilities. Unsuccessful completion of developmental tasks may result in a sense of defeat, guilt, and reluctance to attempt the accomplishment of new goals.

Cognitively, the preschooler is in Piaget's (1969) preoperational stage, which is characterized by illogical and egocentric thought and the inability to generalize from isolated concrete experiences. Preschoolers are beginning to develop an awareness of the course of events, but they fail to understand the multiple complexities of causal relationships. Children of this age often describe phenomena by overt perceptual characteristics.

The diagnosis of chronic illness may limit the child's ability to achieve motor and social competence. Physical limitations may subdue energy and enthusiasm for pursuing goal-directed efforts. Parents often limit their ill children in order to protect them. Because these preschoolers often cannot accomplish their desired goals and therefore receive less social approval, they may become fearful, irritable, demanding, and excessively dependent on adults.

Most preschool children can function within the limitations imposed by their disability, if they can find a different route to accomplish tasks of development according to their capacity. Also, children at this stage may require assistance in identifying and accepting their limitations. The attitudes of others, especially their parents, determine how preschoolers perceive themselves and their potentials. They are particularly inquisitive about their illnesses, including the inherent restrictions, procedures, and treatments. However, developmentally, preschoolers will probably interpret their illnesses as punishments for their actions or thoughts. Children in this age group need positive family and social interaction to help them obtain a realistic picture of their assets and limitations.

The reaction of the family to the chronic illness of the preschooler depends on whether the child has been diagnosed with chronic illness during the preschool years. If the child has been healthy until age 4 to 6 years, the family has experienced the child as normal. When these parents learn of their child's diagnosis, they experience an acute sense of loss, because they must alter expectations and hopes for the child's potential.

Normally, during the preschool years, children develop self-care skills that give them independence and give the parents freedom to pursue their own personal and career activities. However, preschoolers with a chronic illness may not master these self-care skills, and their parents may be restricted in the pursuit of their own interests and personal and career goals. Children with disabilities often make ongoing demands on the parents' time and may cause the parents to feel guilty and resentful. To compensate for these feelings, parents may reject or misplace the burden of the child's care on siblings or significant others.

The chronically ill preschooler may require early remedial education, which, coupled with dependency demands, presents a separation conflict for the parents. This conflict fosters the parents' anxiety that the child cannot function without them. Overprotective parents who have not provided their preschooler with opportunities to develop self-sufficiency within the limitations of the disability have an even greater difficulty separating from the child.

School-Age Child

The "school-age" years of childhood, generally between 6 and 12 years old, is a time when the child's focus shifts beyond the immediate family into the social environment of school and extended interactions with peers. The world of relationships widens, and the expectation for academic achievement and social competence increases. The child's ability to acquire a sense of adequacy, competence, and self-esteem is an interactive process, molded by both the child's self-perception and the several "environments" in which the child lives, works, and plays. If the child is unable to accomplish the task Erikson (1964) ascribes to this period (acquiring a sense of industry) in these environments, the child's self-perception may be that of incompetence, inferiority, and/or inadequacy.

The school-age child's progressive cognitive development also contributes to these aspects of psychosocial development. School-age children are no longer guided by superficial perceptions, because they are able to generalize rules and principles from one experience to another. In fact, at this age children are often rule-bound; these new rules add stability to previously unstable concepts, such as time and causality. However, since the child is still thinking in a very concrete manner, the rules are viewed in highly inflexible and absolute terms.

Given these developmental characteristics, chronic illness at this age may interfere with the transition from parental to peer approval. Research (Ray, 1985; Adams & Weaver, 1986; Brown & Gordon, 1987) suggests that the child's differences may become more visible to the child, peers, teachers, and others in the child's environment. For example, the child with diabetes may be seen as always eating differently, and the child with juvenile arthritis may be characterized by the inability to participate in activities.

Studies (Holaday & Turner-Henson, 1991; Weitzman et al, 1986) have demonstrated that the child with a chronic illness is likely to have a large number of absences from school because of acute illness, ongoing issues related to or exacerbations of the chronic condition, doctor's appointments, or repeated hospitalizations. These differences may become the primary identification of the child, an observation that is immediately made by peers. Often, differences in the chronically ill child stimulate fear or discomfort in other children, who may then avoid or ostracize the ill child. During this period, when friends are a crucial part of social development, such responses can be particularly devastating. With the passage and implementation of legislation mandating inclusion of children with disabilities into regular school programs, larger numbers of children may be subjected to rejection (of varying form, intensity, or source).

Children frequently respond to the pain of being different by developing feelings that their bodies are separate and unintegrated parts of their psychologic selves (Geist, 1979; Rodgers et al, 1981). This thinking is reinforced by health care professionals who refer to children as disease entities rather than as "real" people.

The time at which a child enters school often brings renewed or additional sadness to the parents of the chronically ill child. At this time, parents are made acutely aware of the physical and functional differences between their child and other children. Parents often attempt to minimize their child's differences by encouraging them not to tell peers and teachers of their illness, medications, or treatment. Additionally, this reticence in discussing their child's diagnosis with school representatives may result from frustrating past attempts to review their child's health condition or needs, during which they perceived little acknowledgment or concern for their child's academic potential or well-being (Harkins, 1991; Holaday & Turner-Hansen, 1991).

One of the most difficult problems for families at this stage is relinquishing at least part of their child's care either to the child or to another responsible adult. Children need to become more responsible for themselves and to develop self-care skills in order to begin to feel a sense of control and self-esteem in the parents' absence (Fig. 19–1). For children to become involved in school and its associated activities, the parents need to entrust part of the child's care to teachers, other parents, or caregivers. This "letting go" process may be more difficult for some families than others, so some may benefit from the support of families who have made similar adjustments. Additional support from parent groups and health team members may be particularly helpful during this time of adjustment.

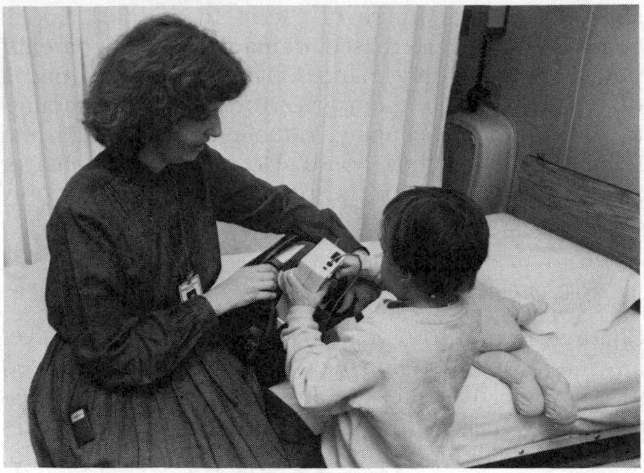

FIGURE 19 - 1. Nurses can foster independence in school-age children by letting them be responsible for their own care as they are able. Here a 10-year-old child is packing up her dialysis equipment on discharge from the hospital, as she does daily when she gets ready for school.

Adolescent

Many developmental challenges characterize the period between 13 and 18 years of age. The struggle for independence is frequently named as the major mission of adolescence. This is a broad concept that encompasses a number of aspects of what may be the most obvious struggle in this transitional phase from childhood to being an adult. Adolescents are also in the process of taking on new social roles, expectations for emotional behaviors, and responsibilities. Sexual development is also occurring, with its attendant uncertainties and anxieties. Throughout this internal struggle, as well as that for independence and loosening ties with family, the adolescent is constantly searching for peer approval. Efforts to "conform to the norm" are directly related to building an acceptable body image and individual self-esteem.

Cognitively, the adolescent phase of development coincides with Piaget's (1969) stage of formal operations, when thinking becomes less concrete and more abstract. Questioning theories, generating hypotheses, and developing an awareness of values and beliefs all are part of this new intellectual mode. When adolescents have a chronic illness, many of their developmental struggles may be intensified. Because of the illness, they may feel that their opportunity for independence and autonomy is inhibited or restricted. The evolving ability to consider intellectually the potential effects of long-term altered health status can also contribute to the decreased self-concept and self-esteem in this time of attempting to stabilize identity. The adolescent and the family may be faced with limitations that a lifelong illness or disability might place on sexual, personal, vocational, educational, and social opportunities.

During this developmental period, when "being different" is less than desirable, adolescents with chronic illness may view themselves as different, imperfect, and unacceptable. All of these physical, psychologic, and intellectual changes create an atmosphere of tension and change, which requires further adaptation. It is not unusual for adolescents to respond to these stresses in actively rebellious ways, including risk-taking behaviors. These may encompass noncompliance with or even active sabotage of the medical regimen prescribed for their disease.

In contrast, the health condition or disability may keep the adolescent physically, emotionally, and financially bound to the family. These limiting factors may contribute to the adolescent's passivity, overdependence, and even depression. Parental support and encouragement, education, and understanding by peers can promote the ability to cope with the internal and external pressures associated with the typical efforts to achieve independence, which may be compromised by a chronic health condition.

Many parents tend to encourage dependence and assume more of the adolescent's care than necessary to maintain individual and family integrity. Although not likely a conscious motivation, "smothering" is not uncommon as parents try to protect their child. Nevertheless, the adolescent needs to be allowed the freedom and responsibility of learning to manage the illness or disability. Although this process may be painful for the parents, it is a vital transition period; the adolescent builds confidence and self-esteem while assuming more responsibility for care. Appropriate, progressively decreasing parental control and direction, frequent encouragement, and support are vital. In most cases, an equilibrium is achieved between the responsibilities of illness management and the transition to further education, job-training, and independence.

Impact of Chronic Illness on Roles and Relationships

Chronic illness in a child affects each family member and the fabric of family life. Childhood chronic illness has been shown to increase stress, disrupt relationships, and interfere with family developmental tasks. Chronic illness in one member may be an underlying cause of a variety of symptoms in other family members. Chronic illness may disrupt communication patterns, impose financial hardships, and bring about changes in housing, careers, and sleep and recreation patterns. Disruptions in roles, resentment among siblings, and feelings of parental guilt, anxiety, helplessness, and despair can all be manifestations of a chronic illness in a family. These effects can be seen, to varying degrees, across the continuum that also includes families who thrive and become more cohesive (Austin & McDermott, 1981; Harkins, 1990, 1991; McCubbin & Huang, 1989). Nursing and psychosocial literature have largely considered the effect of a chronically ill child on individual family roles. Therefore, although one must consider the effect of chronic illness on family unit function and integrity, its specific effects on maternal and paternal roles, parents' marital relationship, and other family members are individually presented here.

Maternal Role

Much research on the effect of chronic illness on families has focused on the mother and the relationship she has established with her child (Anderson & Elfert, 1989; Burr, 1985; Farber, 1959, 1960; Hayes & Knox, 1984; Holaday, 1984, 1987; Holaday & Turner-Hensen, 1991; Madiros, 1982, 1985; Morrow et al, 1984; Sawyer, 1992). Reasons for this maternal focus include the fact that the mother is often the person most involved with the day-to-day care and responsibility for taking her child to the physician's office, clinic, or hospital. Thus, mothers have been most visible to health care professionals as the primary caretakers and those most available to participate in research studies. Generally, the literature reports wide variations in mothers' responses to their children's illness.

The mother may feel particularly responsible, because she gives birth to the child and tends to be most active in the child's care. Mothers experience all stages of grieving—shock, disbelief, anger, resentment, and sadness—and may become stalled at a particular stage or engage in self-blame. Mothers must be given the opportunity to mourn for the "wished-for perfect child" and accept the real child. Thoughts and feelings related to the chronically ill child may inappropriately enter relationships with other people, which is cause for concern. Most mothers are plagued with thoughts about what they did wrong and what they did not do to prevent the illness.

Many researchers have described an increased prevalence of depression in mothers of chronically ill children (Barbarin et al, 1985; Daniels et al, 1987; Gayton et al, 1977; McCrae et al, 1973; Pless & Satterwhite, 1973; Schlomann, 1988). Mercer (1974) investigated mothers' responses to infants with physical impairments for a 3-month period following birth of the child. Findings in this study indicated that evaluation of social behaviors (particularly the mothers' evaluation of how others responded to their children) was the most frequent of all behaviors engaged in by the mothers. In a later study, Mercer (1977) determined that visible impairments, particularly facial, were less socially acceptable and had the greatest influence on the parents' reactions to their children. Cohen and Martinson (1988) described the uncertainty associated with living with a child's diagnosis of cancer. In this study, mothers indicated a lack of confidence in their ability to differentiate between normal developmental changes and potentially life-threatening events.

Given the prevalence of career-oriented mothers, mothers of children with chronic illnesses are also likely to work. As mentioned, this may be not only by choice but by necessity because of the ongoing costs of health care for their child. When mothers attempt to contribute to financial stability through employment outside the home; maintain stability of the home; promote and support the developmental interest and needs of self, spouse, and siblings; and monitor the condition and care of a chronically ill child, it is obvious why they may report high levels of stress (Barbarin et al, 1985; Desmond, 1980; Harkins, 1991; Holaday & Turner-Hensen, 1991; McCubbin, 1988, 1989).

Variations in maternal responses may be attributed to multiple factors. These include her family history, the effectiveness of past and present coping strategies, her hopes or anticipations for the future of the child, her current family structure and relationships, and social support systems to which she has access.

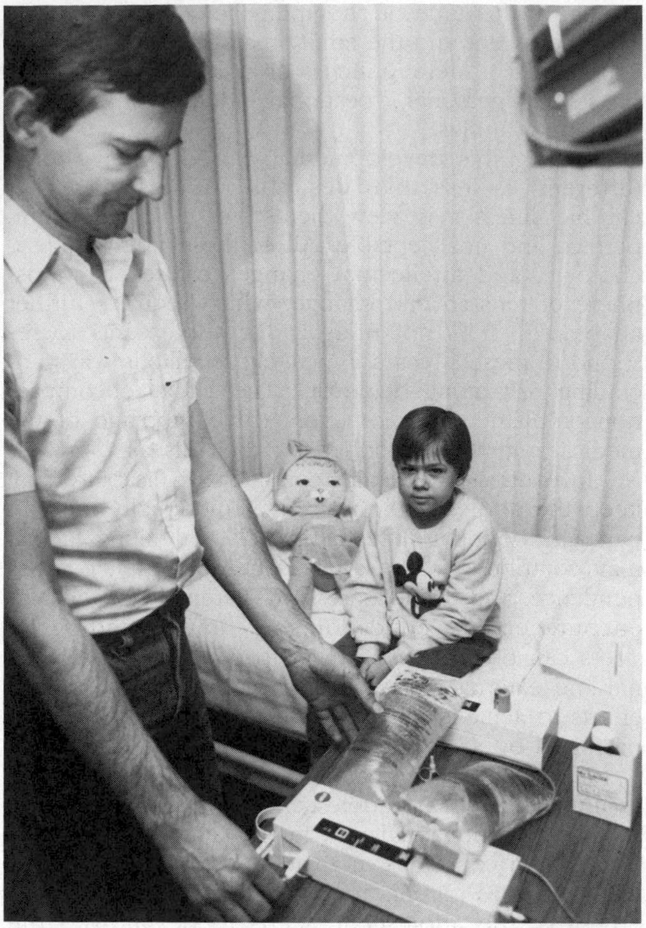

FIGURE 19-2. Many fathers share responsibility for their child's care. Although this 10-year-old can perform her own peritoneal dialysis, it is important for parents also to learn the procedure.

Paternal Role

There is considerably less information about the impact of chronic illness on fathers, largely because they have not been observed or studied to the same extent that mothers have. In North American society, the mother is often seen as the primary care provider and the father as the breadwinner. This perception is often accompanied by the belief that fathers are less involved with or emotionally affected by their child's chronic illness.

These ideas have been challenged in the literature, and the importance of the father-child relationship has been explored (McKeever, 1981; Sabbeth, 1984). Some reports are that fathers did not consider themselves as secondary to mothers in the family functioning but rather as having equal responsibility for childrearing and the daily care of their ill children. Other studies suggest that differences appear to exist between fathers of children with various illnesses in relation to the time and extent fathers participated in their child's care. For example, in an early study by Barsch (1968), 89 per cent of fathers of children with Down syndrome (compared with 38 per cent of fathers of children with organic brain disease) participated in a regular, high-quality manner in child care tasks. Some fathers may share the responsibility for the child's care with their wives, whereas others find ways to absent themselves from the situation (Fig. 19-2).

More recent nursing research (Anderson & Elfert, 1989; Harkins, 1991; Holaday & Turner-Hensen, 1991; Madiros, 1985) has shown that fathers are generally less likely to be involved with the care and management of regimens and routines for the chronically ill child. Harkins (1991) found that fathers often perceive few or no changes in their family functioning and routine after childhood chronic illness is diagnosed.

Regardless of the time that fathers actually spend on care of their children, most researchers agree that children with long-term illnesses have a significant effect on fathers (Burton, 1975). A study by Sabbeth (1984) indicated that fathers were, for the most part, psychologically very involved with their ill children. Fathers felt helpless and ineffectual when they were not able to participate in child care or because of their lack of ability to provide potentially helpful medical interventions for their children. McKeever (1981) found that fathers experienced acute grief reactions at the time of diagnosis of their child's illness. However, despite their feelings, they felt the need to demonstrate strength in order to support their wives during this crisis. Fathers also reported that their career mobility and social activities outside the family were curtailed because of having to consider first the needs of the ill child and then those of the rest of the family. Although fathers of chronically ill children may experience these reactions and have to make adjustments in their lives, they frequently receive less information or support from health professionals than do mothers. This is largely due to work schedules that often include commuting and/or long absences from home.

Marital Relationship

Family dynamics, particularly as related to marital stability or instability, is one of the variables frequently considered in the study of chronic illness in children. In an early study, Farber (1959) found marital conflict to be common in families that included boys 9 years or older with mental retardation. Other studies reporting decreased marital satisfaction include those of Gabel and associates (1983), Featherstone (1980), Tew and Laurence (1973), Morrow and colleagues (1984), and Velasco de Parra and colleagues (1983).

Another body of literature suggests that correlations of negative impact on marital satisfaction with childhood chronic illness have been exaggerated or erroneously reported (Gayton et al, 1977; Kazak & Marvin, 1984; Phillips et al, 1985; Schlomann, 1988; Sabbeth & Leventhal, 1984). In 1984, Sabbeth reviewed 34 research papers and found that marital demise occurs no more frequently than in the general population.

Attempts to equate childhood chronic illness in the family with marital dissatisfaction of the parents are, at best, equivocal, as empirical data do not unquestionably support that premise. The growing number of single parents in society in general suggests that studies reporting marital dissatisfaction may describe already existing (and perhaps unacknowledged) interpersonal conflict. In addition, one must differentiate between stress on marriage and stress on parenting. In their research, Kazak and Marvin (1984) found that the stress on parenting was more often indicated than that on the marital stability.

As health care providers and researchers (Jessop & Stein, 1989; Seligman & Darling, 1989; Cohen, 1989; Cohen & Martinson, 1988) consistently acknowledge, parents of chronically ill children experience great stress related to care and management, as well as uncertainty, associated with the diagnosis. Chronic fatigue, logistic demands of caregiving, financial effects, vigilance, and a constant state of readiness all contribute to this stress and affect the amount and quality of shared time, including time for maintaining adequate communication and social and sexual relationships.

Siblings

Healthy brothers and sisters of chronically ill children are also major contributors to family dynamics. However, they have not been a systematic focus of study until the last 2 decades. Some research reflects a sibling population that is psychologically disturbed and behaviorally disagreeable or offensive (Desmond, 1980; Farber, 1959; Phillips et al, 1985). In contrast, there is strong support for the premise that no significant differences exist between siblings of children with chronic illness and those in families without a chronically ill child (Breslau et al, 1981; Cohen & Martinson, 1988; Tritt & Esses, 1988). For example, Tritt and Esses (1988) found no significant differences in self-concept between chronically ill children's siblings and a healthy matched control group. Similar findings were reported by Dyson and colleagues (1989) in a study on adjustment of siblings of children with disabilities. Thus, research findings relative to siblings certainly are not conclusive; in fact, they are frequently contradictory.

The sources of information in studies about siblings are often parents (particularly mothers), teachers, and, infrequently, the siblings themselves. Parents often express more worry about the effect on siblings than do siblings themselves. This may be related to concerns (and guilt) about the amount of time, energy, and financial resources that are necessarily focused on the child with the chronic condition.

The intent of much of the research has been to demonstrate untoward effects on siblings; therefore, findings frequently reflect this perspective as espoused by sources other than the siblings themselves. In addition, research findings of significant differences in siblings of chronically ill children may be subsequently integrated into plans of care without the benefit of a comparison group of siblings who have no chronic illness in their families. Application of findings from these types of research may be risky and inappropriate.

This is not to say that siblings do not experience stress or act out frustrations, anger, fear, jealousy, or resentments. These emotional and behavioral reactions may be expected when one is confronted with such an intense experience. However, siblings' responses must be placed in context of stage of development of the sibling, family communication and support patterns, and individual personality.

Siblings often feel torn between loyalty to their brother or sister who is being teased or rejected and their own need for friends and acceptance. Being stigmatized is not restricted to the chronically ill child; siblings are often the victims of stigma. Healthy children struggle with loyalty to their family and ill sibling and the desire to be rid of the whole situation in the hopes of returning to "normalcy." Children in two-child families may feel an acute sense of loss when their sole sibling is ill and there are no other similar relationships to nurture. Feelings of confusion and ambivalence may be present, related not only to the ill sibling but to the entire family.

Many studies have reported siblings' responses vary according to birth order (Breslau et al, 1981; Farber, 1959; Harkins, 1991; Schlomann, 1988; Tritt & Esses, 1988) and gender. Breslau and associates (1981) found that in siblings younger than the ill child, brothers experienced more behavioral and psychologic problems (e.g., self-destructive behaviors, mentation problems, conflict with parents, regressive anxiety, fighting, isolation) than sisters. Similarly, Schlomann (1988) found that older siblings have lower negative psychosocial effects. Harkins (1991) found that older siblings indicated an initial optimistic attitude about change and the integration of changes in family functioning that accompanied the new diagnosis of a sibling; however, 3 to 6 months after initial diagnosis, there was a concomitant decrease in optimism related to ongoing change and family functioning. In contrast, younger siblings tended consistently to report optimism about change and the challenges associated with a chronically ill sibling; notwithstanding that optimism, younger siblings reported progressively more negative perceptions of inclusion in family functioning and daily routines. These studies lend credence to the importance of considering both developmental stage of siblings and their positions in the family.

Open communication among family members, especially between parents and well siblings, is often broadly advocated. Nevertheless, such communication is often uncomfortable for both parent and child. This may result from children's reluctance to ask questions or parents' uncertainty about what or how much to tell their children. The result is often a large gap in siblings' information about the illness or disability, its probable course over time, or its outcome.

Levels of information exchange are also directly related to developmental levels of well siblings. For example, younger children are more interested in concrete information about what their affected sibling can or cannot do. Older children's discussions may reflect concerns about the future. While assimilating those aspects of information, adolescents are likely to also be interested in the potential for having a child of their own with a similar disability or illness.

Family units and family members need resources and support in learning to live with the impact of childhood chronic illness in their family. Parents need to continue to experience the ability to support the accomplishments of their healthy children. Siblings need to benefit from continued parent participation and support in activities. Parent and sibling support groups are generally available for learning from and sharing with parents who have experienced similar illness in their family constellation. Sibling support groups are also becoming more prevalent, particularly in areas around medical centers that manage the care of childhood chronic illnesses. In 1989, a new support organization was established for siblings (Sibling Information Network); its newsletter is a source of information and includes a section in which siblings talk about their personal experiences of having an ill or disabled brother or sister.

Nurses can make significant direct and indirect contributions to well siblings. They can help parents anticipate the course of the illness in order to help them prepare the siblings for impending events. They can also find ways to interact directly with siblings and facilitate answering their questions. Health care professionals can encourage parents to involve others who play a significant role (e.g., grandparents and other extended family members, babysitters) in the children's lives to be aware of the siblings' needs. During family conferences, nurses can encourage inclusion of siblings in the conferences and facilitate their participation in discussions. They can assist parents in interpreting coping strategies to siblings and in finding realistic ways to participate in care. Nurses can also act as advocates for sibling hospital visitation, telephone calls, traditional recognition of special events and holidays, and interactions that will promote a supportive relationship between the children. As siblings grow older, they need to be included in discussions about future caregiving arrangements for their sibling. These nursing actions encourage the awareness that the illness is not solely the child's problem but that of everyone in the family.

Grandparents

Grandparents in some families live close enough to be emotionally and physically involved with care of the chronically ill child and the family. These older relatives may have retired from active careers and have both the time and the inclination to be involved in the lives of their grandchildren. Grandparents often view grandchildren as the rewards of their life's work. The joy that grandparents experience is reflected in their continuous stories about their grandchildren and the numerous pictures adorning their walls and mantels.

When a grandchild is diagnosed with a chronic illness, grandparents may feel intense dismay and sorrow. They may even feel guilt if the illness is hereditary. They often go through the grieving process, as do the parents. However, their grief is difficult because they are not the parents, and they are not as intimately involved in the child's life. Their grief is for their own children's sorrow as well as for themselves, and for other children in the family as well as for the ill child. Initially they may not be able to offer compassion because the child's illness forces them to face their own mortality. The grandparents' reaction may be either to overindulge or to avoid the ill grandchild. Their interaction with the grandchild may be limited because of decreased energy and a distancing exerted by the child's parents as a protective device for both the sake of the ill child and that of the grandparents. Thus, the grandparents may not feel included in the immediate family circle and may subsequently feel a sense of anguish and helplessness. Parents need to be encouraged to include willing and able grandparents in the lives of the chronically ill child and the siblings, as they often have much to offer. They often serve as a sounding board for the sick child's distraught parents. Grandparents may be able to assist with practical needs, such as providing transportation or accompanying the child and parent during outpatient care or hospitalization. Help with nonschool routines is usually greatly appreciated. They may babysit or give special attention to the siblings to help fill the void when their parents are occupied with the ill child. Grandparents often model the strength, patience, and faith that the family needs to learn as they adjust to living with chronic illness (Fig. 19–3).

Coping with Chronic Illness

Children with chronic illness experience the normative demands of age-related development. In addition, they may have to integrate numerous non-normative demands associated with the chronic illness into their life experiences. These may be episodic, recurring, or perhaps continuous. They may include numerous treatments and procedures, threats of exacerbations, lifestyle restrictions, lasting impairments, and, depending on the nature of the condition, a shortened life expectancy. These are examples of situations or events that require adaptive transactions between the person and the environment (LaMontagne, 1987a). That is, they elicit efforts to restore equilibrium as it is perceived by the child and/or family. The efforts will be a function of developmental level, personality, appraisal of the event, previous experience with the present or similar situation, history of success or failure in dealing with such experiences, and the resources available.

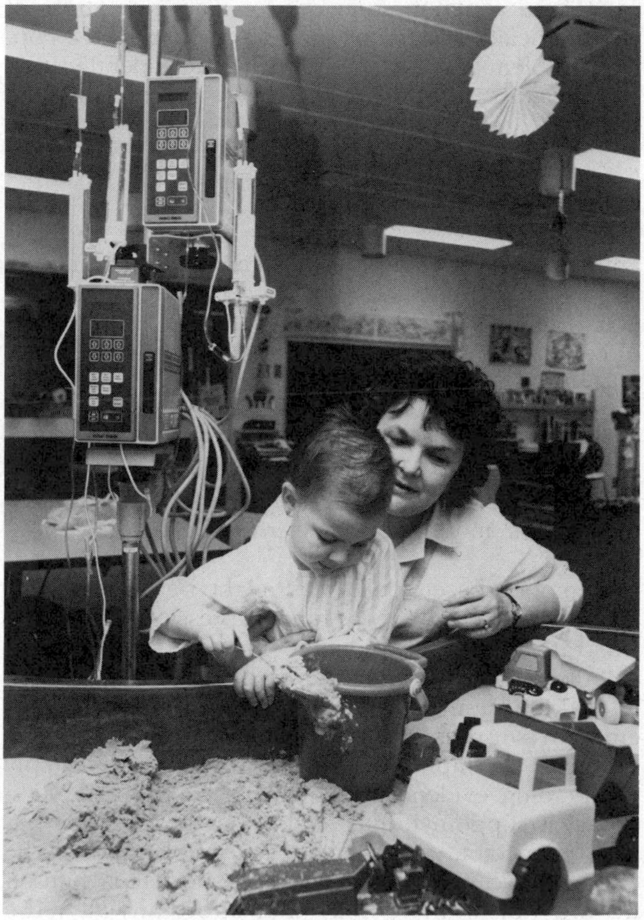

FIGURE 19 - 3. Grandparents can be a stabilizing force to the child and family and help make the hospital seem more "like home."

This is often referred to as a *coping style* and described as either cognitive or behavioral in quality (Lazarus & Folkman, 1984). Lazarus and Folkman (1984), LaMontagne (1987a, 1987b), and Ryan-Wenger (1992) submit that the concept of coping styles implies a static attribute or approach to responding to or interacting with the environment. Instead, they propose that coping is a fluid response to the environment and is therefore a *process*. Furthermore, many (LaMontagne, 1991; Ryan-Wenger, 1992; Wertlieb et al, 1987) have presented compelling arguments that this response is positively correlated with age. "Children, adolescents, and adults would vary in their views of a situation simply because their conceptualizations differ according to their cognitive developmental levels" (LaMontagne, 1987a, p 68). These views would also vary as a result of re-evaluation of a situation as information from (or about) that situation changes and as resources for handling change (LaMontagne, 1987b).

These are complementary viewpoints. While acknowledging contributing factors that alter appraisal and response as process, it is also heuristic to consider coping patterns or *strategies* as individual descriptive variables. These have been described as personal factors of perceived control. These theoretical concepts were developed to describe (and perhaps explain) adult appraisal and response to stress. For several reasons, Ryan-Wenger (1992) cautions against general application of them to children, given some obvious differences between child and adult situation and response. Specifically, children's stressors are not the same as adults' stressors; children's stressful situations are often outside their control, with less possibility for change by them; and progressive cognitive development and life experience alter the perceptions of a situation as stressful as well as the resources for responding to any associated stress.

Notwithstanding these concerns, existing theoretical views have formed much of the basis of research and discussion about children and stress responses. The strategies utilized have been described by different characteristics such as "internal" or "external" (LaMontagne, 1991), "active" or "avoidant" (LaMontagne, 1987), and "high coping" or "low coping" (Blount et al, 1991). LaMontagne (1987a, 1987b) and LaMontagne and Hepworth's (1991) research have also described the parallel between the internal-external and active-avoidant characteristics. They report that, in general, if one's perception of the situation includes the belief that one is somehow responsible for the situation and/or there is confidence in one's ability to alter the situation, more effort is likely to be expended to control events and outcome. However, if one believes that persons or things in the environment are responsible for the situation and that one has no control, that person may be passive, lack *apparent* actions, or avoid the situation.

The concept of vulnerability is closely related to appraisal and coping in chronic illness (Lazarus & Folkman, 1984). Children's interactions with people and objects in their environment may exaggerate vulnerabilities, which will affect their ability to cope with the daily challenges of being a child. Coping theorists generally agree that securing adequate information about a situation, maintaining autonomy, and using available intrapsychic (cognitive) processes are essential to the coping-adaptive process. However, in chronic illness, high levels of vulnerability have the potential to interfere with the child's ability to engage in these processes.

As children interact with an ever-enlarging environment, they become more aware of the different ways of reacting to or mastering that environment. These efforts involve behaviors or cognitive processes that promote establishing (or re-establishing) the "balance of power between a person and situational factors in any stressful encounter. Whether the person approaches or avoids the stress, the focus of the coping effort is aimed at trying to meet the demands of the situation and to manage internal conflicts engendered by the situation" (LaMontagne, 1987a).

The child and family may utilize some similar approaches or methods of coping. However, it is not unusual for family members (adults *and* children) to employ widely different patterns in attempting to manage the conflicts of childhood chronic illness. Each may have both positive and negative aspects, discussed further on.

Methods of Childhood Coping

Bullard and Dohnal (1984) suggest that children do not work through a problem, as they do a particular symptom; nor do they get over it, as they do a developmental crisis. Rather, methods of psychosocial adjustment evolve that can be invoked as they develop and meet other crises. This adjustment process involves learning, reality testing, problem solving, or perhaps withdrawal. When a child encounters a new situation, the processes of learning, testing, and coping are initiated. While learning effective coping behaviors, children may experience anger, frustration, discovery, challenge, and finally, gratification.

As previously suggested, children's coping strategies vary with age and cognitive development. For example, the infant uses coping behaviors that center primarily on motor activity. Some of these infant coping behaviors include hand-mouth activity, restlessness (i.e., fussing), crying, body rocking, clinging to familiar people, and becoming attached to transitional objects (e.g., the thumb, a favorite blanket, a special toy). Toddlers, with their increasing communication and locomotor skills, often cope in stressful situations by regressing to earlier, more familiar infant coping strategies. Toddlers use protest (temper tantrums), withdrawal, fantasy, controlling behaviors and ritualization as coping behaviors. Temporary demonstration of any of these behaviors in a stressful situation suggests effective and age-appropriate coping methods. Once children reach the age of 6 or 7 years, their cognitive function has developed (including memory, speech, language, and reality testing) to the point at which they may have an early understanding of their illness and an interest in its management. The school-age child and adolescent cope successfully by finding satisfaction in a variety of compensatory activities (physical and intellectual) and by identifying with other young patients with similar problems. The appropriate expression of anxious, sad, impatient, and angry feelings is a necessary and healthy aspect of coping.

Children with a chronic illness learn to cope with the difficult realities that they may face daily. Children free of debilitating psychologic symptoms use adaptive measures, some of which can be fostered to bring about effective coping skills. See Table 18–8 for a review of coping behaviors that all children may use. Some common strategies for managing stress of chronic health conditions include emotion-based coping, problem solving, intellectualization, identification with health care professionals, stress inoculation, ritualization, and denial and hope.

Emotion-Based Coping

Emotion-based coping is a palliative approach that attempts to alleviate the subjective (i.e., feeling, emotional) influence of the stressful situation. This method of coping is more common in younger children and is related to the child's cognitive development and problem solving skills as well as behavioral patterns. However, older children and adolescents may demonstrate some (or perhaps many) of these behaviors as alternatives to more characteristic stress management methods, if more age-characteristic behaviors are ineffective.

Emotion-based behaviors might be conspicuous indicators, such as crying and expressing anger and frustration; or they may be more obscure, as in emotion suppression. However, caution is warranted in making assumptions about the intent or use of emotion suppression. One should not assume that the child is simply being stoic or brave or is simply withholding evidence of emotions. Assessment is essential if supportive interventions are to be appropriate and accurately articulated. For example, if the child who cannot play a desired sport tells himself he did not want to play that sport anyway, the health care professional needs to distinguish between the statement as a reflection of true desire versus an indication of fatalistic withdrawal from the playing field.

Problem Solving

Problem solving is a less subjective method of responding to stress. The function of this approach is to change the situation by changing either one's own behavior or action or the problematic situation or environment. These include delayed gratification and allow for redefinition or reappraisal of the situation. For example, the child may attempt to develop or improve the skills necessary to play with the team of her chosen sport. Similarly, the child may find indoor activities to enjoy, rather than be exposed to allergens outside during school recess. This approach involves physically or cognitively altering the environment, or events, and the associated perceived stress. Children who employ this response to the stress of chronic illness effectively construct acceptable alternatives for immediate daily living and likely for the long term.

Intellectualization

Acquiring and using factual information, particularly related to anatomy, physiology, pathophysiology, medication and treatment, or even outcome potential are ways in which children employ intellectualization to deal with the stress of chronic illness. The following situation illustrates one child's use of this approach:

> I've had Crohn disease for about a year. I'm a bit young to have it, because the most common age of diagnosis is in the teen years. I know that Crohn disease is an inflammatory bowel disorder that affects part of my GI system. If I'm not careful, I may get a bowel obstruction. They have treated me with a high-protein diet, antibiotic drugs, and some steroids too. But this time I need TPN because I've lost too much weight, and my doctor doesn't want me to starve to death.

This example demonstrates Jenny's fairly broad knowledge about her disease and how she handled anxiety about her illness by providing factual information, rather than discussing her feelings about having a chronic health condition and being hospitalized. Other children who cope in this manner may also know death rates, surgical corrective procedures, hospital routines and rituals specific to their diagnosis, and equipment. They acquire this information from their own reading, by questioning people (e.g., health care providers) who know the answers, and from their own experiences.

Younger children who use this technique often know the medical jargon but may not understand it. For older children, intellectualization is a way of gaining control over something they feel is uncontrollable. It allows them to step outside their feelings and look at the chronic condition from a more objective vantage point. Facilitating this method of coping requires providing disease-specific, honest, and age-appropriate information.

Identification with Health Care Professionals

Strong identification with health care staff may accompany the intellectualization process or the child's preoccupation with the illness and its management. One explanation for identification may be a desire (whether conscious or unconscious) to acquire the same scientific aloofness or curative powers that the child believes the doctor or nurse possesses. Identification with health care staff is more likely to be utilized by children who can or want to care for themselves, rather than by those who do not have the ability or desire to influence their own physical care.

Stress Inoculation

Both of the previous two strategies may be included in this stress management method, which is based on the assumption that mitigation of stress can be accomplished by exposure to stressful situations. Exposure to precisely the same situation or event that one wishes to "immunize" against is not necessarily required. The goal is to assist the child in developing effective methods of response (coping skills) to stressful situations so that the child can generalize these other situations. Harkins (1991) reports using this technique in what was called "bravery training" for young children experiencing hospitalization, painful or frightening procedures, or therapies. Acquiring factual information about one aspect of their chronic health condition and/or assuming the "professional identification" is one aspect of illness management that may "immunize" the child against similar stresses.

Ritualization

Children with chronic illness often develop a set of ritualistic behaviors that may provide or facilitate comfort in situations over which they feel little or no control. One youngster, during his chemotherapy, insisted that a paper bag with a picture of Dracula be placed over the red intravenous fluid, because it reminded him of blood. Another child with an amputated foot demanded a particular organization of all the equipment used in his dressing change and that certain music be played during the procedure. Similarly, a 4-year-old child with aplastic anemia demanded a blue finger puppet each time her blood was drawn. Each of these rituals was the child's way of exerting control over that situation. Even though ritualistic behaviors may appear strange or even bizarre, they should be accommodated, unless they are destructive to the patient. In fact, rituals are often mutually developed between patients and caregivers and become a bond between them.

Erikson (1966) considered ritualistic behavior a means of responding to the reciprocal needs of two individuals. It heightens a sense of both belongingness and personal distinctiveness in a playful yet formalized way. For example, when the 4-year-old with aplastic anemia was readmitted to the hospital, her primary nurse sought her favorite toys—blankets and the bag of treasured blue finger puppets—hours before her arrival. When the child arrived in her room and saw her favorite things, a broad smile crept across the faces of both the child and her nurse. The adherence to the rituals served to unite the child and nurse in their attempts to cope with the difficult situation.

Denial and Hope

Chronically ill children often alternate between recognizing the realities of their illness and denying its existence. For example, a child refuses to get out of bed because he is "sick," yet yearns to be up in the playroom because he feels relatively well or not sick at all. The conflicting feelings often help to eliminate temporarily the painful reality of the illness and its threat to a child's well-being while allowing the courage and hope to endure any physical or emotional pain or suffering. Denial in the service of hope needs to be differentiated from irrational denial that interferes with the patient's ability to manage the illness on a day-to-day basis and to plan realistically for the future. This adaptive form of denial allows the child to rest from the burden of the illness and be "like every other kid." Adaptive defenses allow the child to vent frustration and anxiety and to gain some control over the illness and its treatment. Fostering a positive attitude (i.e., appropriate levels of denial *and* hope) can promote achievement of normal developmental tasks. Adult intervention is indicated only if excessive reliance or abuse of these suggests that they may be detrimental to physical health or interfere with further development. Wishful thinking and noncompliance with regimens of care cannot, in the long run, result in overall physical or psychologic well-being.

All children with chronic illnesses employ some form of coping behaviors in an attempt to manage the illness. Research indicates that the nature of the illness appears to be less influential in this adjustment process than the child's developmental level, available coping methods, and the quality of the parent-child-sibling relationships along with the family's acceptance of the disabled member (Siemon, 1987). Children who have more effective coping abilities relative to their chronic illness are more likely to achieve personal satisfaction from functioning satisfactorily at home, in school, and with their peers. Limitations imposed should be only those of the illness, not those of individuals in the child's environment. Children with chronic illnesses who evidence effective coping behaviors generally demonstrate age-appropriate dependence on their parents. Similarly, they are not likely to use their illness to elicit attention or sympathy.

However, not all children are able to use adaptive behaviors effectively to cope with their chronic condition. Exclusion from activities, learned inferiority or helplessness, and nonacceptance take their toll on emotional well-being. Table 19–3 reviews some of the common patterns of maladjustment that may be manifested in the child and family with a chronic illness. No single pattern is debilitating to the child and family. However, the cumulative effect of these approaches, perceptual distortions, and behavioral responses can contribute to detrimental attitudes and diminished motivation (Bullard & Dohnal, 1984). Accordingly, nursing interventions that can promote adjustment are also presented in Table 19–3.

Family Coping Strategies

The extent to which there are mutual effects among a chronically ill child, members of the family, and collective family functioning has been explored by nursing, social science, psychology, and medical researchers. At best, the findings have been uncertain, and often contradictory. However, they do agree on one thing: the family is a group of individuals who are *interactive* not only between members of the immediate unit but also with the larger social environment.

In writing on families and chronic illness, Wright and Leahey (1987) have identified nine assumptions for consideration when assessing and designing interventions:

- There are predictable points of family stress when a chronic illness exists.
- Families vary in their level of tolerance for the patient's [child's] physical condition.
- Families under stress tend to hold onto previously proved patterns of behavior, regardless of whether they are effective.
- Families usually go through a grief-loss process following the diagnosis of a [child with chronic illness].
- Families play a significant role in encouraging or discouraging the family member with chronic illness to participate in particular therapies.
- Families react to particular illness behavior.
- Many families have difficulty adjusting to a chronic physical illness because they have either incorrect or inadequate disease-related information.
- When there is a chronic illness, family members must adjust to changes in expectations of one another.
- A family's perception of the illness event has the most influence on its ability to cope.

TABLE 19-3
Patterns of Maladjustment in Chronic Illness and Nursing Interventions to Promote Adjustment

Child Characteristics	Family Characteristics	Nursing Interventions
Fear		
Frightened of everything Exaggerated normal fears Few friends Gives up easily on tasks	Make unrealistic demands Do not praise successes; resentful of child's limitations	Teach parents skills to enhance the child's confidence and independence
Pseudoadult		
Dependent on adults Companionship with adults instead of children Manipulative to attain the attention of adults Controlling and demanding behavior Deprived of normal peer relationships	Parents often narcissistic with little time to nurture child Resentful of care Wanting to spend less and less time with child	Encourage more normal peer relationships for child Teach parents skills to manage controlling, manipulative, and demanding behavior
Invisibility		
Unobtrusive in all social situations Wants to achieve obscurity and not draw attention to self Indifferent and withdrawn Speaks in a soft and quiet voice All child's attention goes into self-defense	Family often impulsive Allow other siblings to take control Family baby child and do not allow to be a productive member	Assist family to become less threatening to the child Establish structure and limits to create an atmosphere that enhances security and encourages the child's development
Fantasy		
Creates an imaginary world Escapes from unattractive and undesirable thoughts Real needs neglected in favor of unrealistic and unattainable daydreams Helpless and dependent deterioration Misses out on social interactions with peers	Denial by family of the child's fears and anger Allow child to be more dependent Failure to set realistic and attainable goals Feelings of helplessness	Assist child and family to face reality Develop improved problem solving skills
Overinvolvement in Medical Care		
Rigidly independent Aloof Adept at medical jargon regarding own illness and treatment Verbally assertive but makes no demands Always follows medical regimes, not upset by changes in plans Strives to please and make others feel better	Mistake child for coping maturely with illness Ignore underlying problems of child Often nonassertive, letting child take control of the situation Compliant with child's wishes	Assist family to identify child's underlying struggle Assist child in expressing anger and depression
Humor (Unrealistic/Exaggerated)		
Keeps everyone laughing Appears happy constantly Keeps a distance from others and does not form close relationships Fears others may not like him or her Frustrated with trying to prove self Insecure and has heightened dependency Often immature for age	Enjoy the child's humor Fail to identify child's underlying anger and sadness Allow child to be dependent	Assist child to express anger and sadness Encourage parents to see beyond humor and develop ways for child to express self

(continued)

TABLE 19-3
Patterns of Maladjustment in Chronic Illness and Nursing Interventions to Promote Adjustment *(Continued)*

Child Characteristics	Family Characteristics	Nursing Interventions
Encouraging Favoritism		
Liked by family and peers Considered "special" because of disability Talked to and treated as if much younger Aims to please and strives not to hurt others Very frustrated and wants to be liked for self Feels inferior and has low self-esteem	Pitied by family members Categorized as special so there is no need to relate at appropriate level Often feel guilty and embarrassed about own feelings toward child	Encourage child to recognize worth Encourage parents to treat more appropriately to promote normal development Teach child to be more assertive
"The China Doll"		
Dressed and groomed perfectly Isolated from other children Inappropriate play skills Often disruptive behavior	Parents unable to face and accept disabilities Do not meet child's internal needs Avoid situations where they have to confront the realities of their child's illness Display child but keep away from real world	Assist parents to confront own guilt and fears Encourage less perfection on the exterior and more expression of inner thoughts
Explosive Anger		
Frequent temper tantrums and rages Clings to others Unreasonable anger and physical attacks against others Blames others for misfortune and is jealous of others Feels life is unfair Does not take responsibility for actions and projects blame on others	Unresolved mourning by all family members Permit dependence Often fearful of the child's behavior and in a dilemma as to appropriate management	Assist child to recognize underlying causes of rage and take responsibility for it Encourage parents to set reasonable expectations and guidelines and stick to them
Giving Up		
No incentive or motivation to grow, care for self, or succeed Infantile helplessness Ostracized by peers Blames others for personal inadequacies Expects to be waited on	Excuse all of child's behavior Anticipate all child's needs and rescue from all problems Dependence is reinforced by doing everything for child No appropriate discipline or behavioral restrictions	Encourage parents to stop pitying, realize child's potential, and be encouraged to set realistic goals Help child to recognize helpless behavior and learn new appropriate ways of gaining attention
Overdependence		
Extreme awareness of limitations Thinks of self as unable to accomplish anything Afraid to try Fear of failing	Feel threatened by the child's chronic condition and have become very overprotective Believe in and reinforce helplessness and inability	Encourage parents to reinforce ability and give praise for trying Encourage independence and a sense of self in the child

Adapted from Siemon, M. (1987). Patterns of impairment: Cognitive/emotional. In M. Rose & R. Thomas (Eds.), *Children with chronic conditions: Nursing in a family and community context.* Orlando, FL: Grune & Stratton.

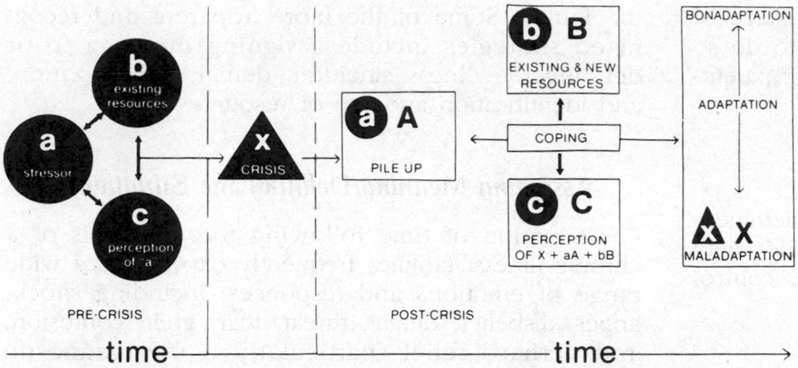

FIGURE 19-4. The double ABCX model. (From McCubbin, H., & Patterson, J. [1983]. The family stress process: The double ABCX model of adjustment and adaptation. In H. McCubbin, M. Sussman, & J. Patterson [Eds.], *Social stress and the family*. New York: Haworth Press.)

Studies, clinical observations, and empiric understanding have contributed to the development of these assumptions. They do acknowledge that families have a stability that "persists through requirements for change and adaptation to stressful situations such as illness" (Rankin & Weekes, 1989). That stability is supported within family units that provide support, promote accomplishment/fulfillment of individual and family aims, and provide reinforcement, acknowledgment, and self-esteem in those achievements. As "ideal" contributions and endeavors of family units, they are challenged and tested to greater or lesser extents over the course of normative (expected) developmental processes that have been affected by this non-normative event.

A useful theoretical model for understanding family response to stressful events has been developed by Hill (1949). The model considers the interaction of three variables (*A*, an event; *B*, resources for coping with the event; *C*, family definition of the event) to explain *X*, the crisis-proneness of the family. McCubbin and Patterson (1983) expanded Hill's model to include the basic elements, their interactions, and a recognition that other developmental and situational stresses for individual family members and for the family unit have occurred or are occurring simultaneously (Fig. 19-4). The model, called the Double ABCX Model, also recognizes the contribution of existing and new resources available to the family for responding to a stressful situation. These events contribute to both the patterns of response to stress and the ability to respond to another crisis or stressful event.

Knafl and Deatrick (1990) have advanced another conceptual model (Fig. 19-5), recognizing that "families who have an ill child do not respond in a singular fashion" (p 2) and that nursing care must integrate how families manage illness, rather than just measure or predict outcomes in terms of impact on the family. According to this model, within the given sociocultural context, each family member (the child with chronic illness, mother, father, and sibling) contributes a "definition of the situation." The combined definitions are intricately interwoven into management behaviors that blend individual accommodations and, over time, formulate the family management style (Deatrick & Knafl, 1990).

Regardless of whether they use the language of stressful events and coping behaviors or of management behaviors and management style, family members and family units demonstrate certain patterns of response and integration. Some reflect effective strategies of coping with the child's chronic health condition, whereas others are ineffective and can be detrimental to individual development and family functioning. The types and effects of both effective and ineffective coping patterns are included in the following discussion.

Once the diagnosis is confirmed, the family members may feel a profound loss. Any disability in a child is a loss for both the child and the family. A chronic illness represents loss of the "perfect" child and possible loss of bodily function, abilities, and perhaps potential for achievement of parents' aspirations for the child. Before successful adaptation can occur, it is normal for parents and children to mourn the loss of what was comfortable and familiar and the associated anticipations. Some children and parents move through this mourning period relatively quickly, whereas others may never accept the situation. A cru-

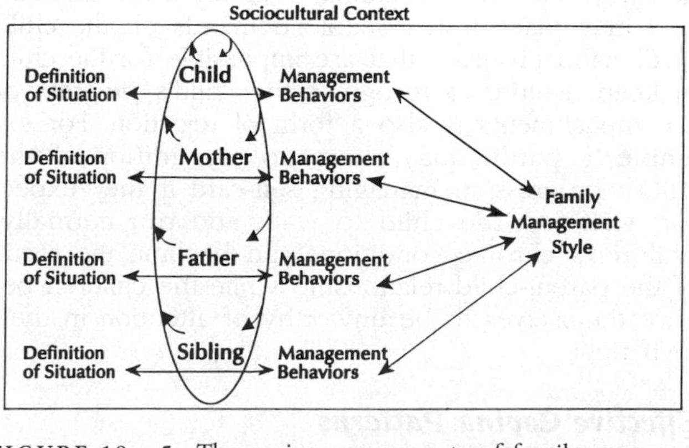

FIGURE 19-5. The major components of family management style. (From Knafl, K., & Deatrick, J. [1990]. Family management style: Concept analysis and development. *Journal of Pediatric Nursing, 5*[1], 4–14.)

cial hurdle for parents is resolution of the stage of self-blame, guilt, and inadequacy. Inability to do so may result in altered, and potentially harmful, parenting practices.

Ineffective Coping Patterns

Two ineffective coping patterns that can be detrimental are overprotection and rejection. Families may need guidance and assistance to avoid or control these tendencies.

Overprotection

As parents face the reality of their child's chronic condition, they are likely to struggle with their own feelings of guilt. The effect may be similar when parents' confidence in their assessment abilities is severely diminished (Cohen, 1988). In an attempt to relieve this guilt or lack of self-confidence, they may attempt to make their child's life as easy and pain-free as possible. This may contribute to a pattern of overindulgence or overprotection that greatly restricts the child's developmental potential. Overprotective parents attempt to shield the child from all failure, anticipate every need, and pay excessive attention to the disability. The child who is sheltered from all stress fails to develop problem solving skills necessary for successful adaptation. Despite parents' best intentions, overprotectiveness is only functional within the family system. Peers, teachers, and even extended family members are likely to find excessive demands in the interest of the "sick" child unacceptable or intolerable. The result may be further isolation and/or rejection.

Rejection

Rejection, similar to overprotection, may represent the parents' attempts to assuage their own guilt or frustration for their inability to relieve the child's discomfort or alter the event of a chronic health condition. Rejection may be overt, or it may take less obvious forms. For example, rejection may appear as either denial of love or conditional love for the child. Parents may place unreasonable demands on the child or demand promises that are impossible for the child to keep. Failure to recognize the child's progress or accomplishments is also a form of rejection. For example, a parent may show no recognition of the child's progress in managing self-care if they expect (or wish for) the child to walk and run normally. Children's chronic conditions can become the focus of the parent-child relationship while the children believe themselves to be unworthy of attention in their own right.

Effective Coping Patterns for Positive Adjustment

There are several effective coping strategies for managing and integrating childhood chronic illness within the family. Some of the more apparent and recognized strategies include assigning meaning to or defining the illness situation, denial, normalization, and identification and use of resources.

Assigning Meaning/Defining the Situation

For a period of time following the diagnosis of a chronic illness, families frequently experience a wide range of emotions and responses, including shock, anger, disbelief, denial, threat, fear, guilt, confusion, and perhaps relief (particularly if the diagnostic process has been long and difficult). They may feel overwhelmed with information, expectations, and care demands. At this time, it is not unusual for families to seek a second opinion to confirm or negate the diagnosis, especially if the condition is life-threatening.

Many parents, like their children, use intellectual processes to mitigate their pain and sorrow. This may involve an extended "career" of fact finding and knowledge building. Also like their children, whether they understand all the material they "know," many parents gather as much information as they can from all possible sources. From this bank of information, parents can also choose what they do *not want* to know. In gathering information, parents try to decrease their anxiety by becoming familiar with what lies ahead. As Holaday (1984) has indicated, "information reduces the ambiguity of the situation by assigning a meaning to the events that lead to the establishment of feelings of mastery and self-sufficiency by family members" (p 364). All family members assign meaning to, or define, the situation. Each contributes individually to the collective meaning. These meanings are not static but are modified over time as new stresses come into play, as resources and relationships vary, and as life experiences occur (Harkins, 1991).

Despite the significant disruptions that attend the diagnosis, parents have been found to be capable of realistically estimating the amount of change to expect in their lives (Goldberg & Simmons, 1988). This reflects the level of knowledge as well as the perception and interpretation of the information they have amassed. The particular meaning attached to the illness also depends on the educational and sociocultural context of the family. For example, religious, cultural, or scientific explanations may be offered for both the illness and the family's management behaviors.

Denial

At some points, conscious or unconscious disavowing or misperceptions related to the illness may be an acceptable avenue for relief from the strain of the child's illness and provide a time for re-establishing personal and family equilibrium. "This temporary disavowal of reality helps the parents master the devastating early period of loss and threat, and sets the stage for later acknowledgment of the illness and mobilization of more effective coping strategies" (Holaday, 1984, p 364).

Denial behavior may occur during crises (e.g., when diagnostic testing is being done to determine if the child with leukemia has relapses) and allows the parents the calmness and composure to tolerate subjecting their child to a painful procedure and the uncertainty and anxiety that accompany the "waiting time." When the crisis subsides, parents and children alike may experience a rebound phenomenon that is exhibited as depression or irritability, or both. This functions as a release after enormous efforts to maintain control, retain a positive attitude and confidence, and provide support for the child and others.

Rationalization

Closely related to denial is the process of rationalization. This is a process with which individuals protect themselves from painful emotions by providing explanations for any occurrence related to the child's illness. These explanations may or may not be valid. For example, the mother of a child with multiple learning disabilities explains:

> Mark's teacher has called me several times to complain about his disruptive behavior in school. She complains that he won't sit still, can't concentrate on anything, and disrupts his classmates while they are trying to work. I know it takes Mark longer to learn and his concentration is poor, but he's also 6 years old and has to burn off all his energy somehow. I think that teacher is making too much of this situation.

Instead of addressing the child's problem, the mother is attempting to explain the child's behavior by emphasizing its appropriateness for the child's developmental level and by refocusing blame on the teacher's "unreasonable expectations."

Normalization

Normalization is the most frequently mentioned strategy for adapting to and living with childhood chronic illness in families. Promoting normalcy "deconstructs" the disease label, and categorizes it in such a way that it is perceived as a small problem or no problem, so that the family can continue to function with minimal disruption. This allows parents to treat the child with the chronic illness diagnosis in minimally different ways (Anderson, 1981; Bossert et al, 1990; Cohen, 1989; Holaday, 1984; Holaday & Turner-Henson, 1991; Knafl & Deatrick, 1986, 1990; Krulik, 1980) while promoting strategies for normalizing the lives of siblings and the family unit.

When these families use normalization as a coping strategy, they are acknowledging that an impairment exists and engaging in behaviors that demonstrate that family life is relatively normal. (In contrast, families who insist that the impairment does not exist are engaged in denial rather than normalization.) Families who use normalization as a strategy for adaptation may define the social consequences of their situation as minimal, yet engage in lifestyle adjustments in an attempt to reorganize the family around the ill child. This reorganization may include changing the family's diet to that of the ill child or moving close to the treatment center, so that the child can receive outpatient treatments. Although the intent of these adjustments is to promote "normalcy," one or more family members may remain at home for career purposes and to maintain economic equilibrium. Similarly, in order to create a "normal family life," parents often plan family-centered activities or participation in special events (Deatrick et al, 1988).

Effective Use of Resources

Parents who cope effectively tend to use personal and extrapersonal resources competently. Often they use interpersonal resources in the form of increased family cohesiveness and social support systems. In addition to their own resourcefulness, families may need assistance to meet the practical demands of the child's illness, to sustain their self-esteem, and to promote and support the morale of other family members over time (Venters, 1981). Successful management of the family of a chronically ill child includes setting concrete goals and expectations for all family members. This promotes individual and collective achievement and a sense of control, which contributes to individual and family integrity (Craig & Edwards, 1983).

Role of the Nurse in Chronic Illness

When disease of a long-term or lifelong nature compounds the normal growth and development crises of childhood, the results can be potentially destructive for both the child and the family. The nurse is usually involved to some degree in the initial diagnosis of the child's chronic illness and, therefore, has the opportunity to interact and be involved with the ill child and the family from the beginning. Skill in utilizing the various steps of the nursing process—assessment, planning, intervention, and evaluation—can ensure specific and holistic nursing care both at the time of the child's diagnosis and throughout the course of the illness.

Essential nursing goals in chronic illness focus on the following:

- Assisting the child and family in the psychosocial adaptation to the child's chronic illness.
- Promoting optimal potential for the child's and family's growth and development.
- Encouraging families to make appropriate use of resources within the health care system.

Promoting Psychosocial Adaptation and Well-Being

When a child is diagnosed with a chronic, long-term, or life-threatening illness, the nurse may experience feelings of helplessness, discomfort, frustration, powerlessness, and, occasionally, incompetence. In order to deal effectively with these emotions, the nurse must recognize them and consciously redirect the focus of caring on the developmental needs of the child and family as well as on the illness and its sequelae.

Children will develop either effective or ineffective patterns of response to their chronic illness, depending on the conditions that persist in relationships with parents, peers, and society in general. Regardless of the combination of coping strategies used, underlying anxiety and stress may remain. Common nursing interventions that promote psychosocial adaptation of a child include the following:

- Assist child and parents to develop realistic goals.
- Facilitate mourning.
- Promote self-worth.
- Encourage progress along the normal developmental trajectory toward independence.
- Develop open channels of communication among parents, child, and health care system.

See Table 19–4 for a summary of how to promote psychosocial adaptation by using these interventions.

Adaptive families have confidence in their ability to handle whatever situations may arise. They have a sense of control yet allow each family member to maintain patterns of development and function that meet their needs in a variety of roles. They are tolerant and patient and can accept their own ambivalence at times. They have the capacity to handle failure and hurt as well as success. Most important, their closeness and cohesiveness allows them to laugh at themselves and start each day with a clean slate.

Parents who cope with their child's condition do not unrealistically consider their child to be limited or incapacitated; rather, they attempt to set realistic goals and challenge their child to achieve them. They attempt to be hopeful in order to allow the child to meet the challenges of normal developmental experiences while assisting the child to acquire the tools for managing the stress of living with a chronic health condition.

Promoting Optimal Potential for Growth and Development

A second goal for the nurse caring for children with chronic illnesses and their families is promotion of optimal development for each family member. The role of the nurse varies considerably and therefore is addressed separately for each developmental stage.

Infant

Parents of chronically ill infants are often devastated at the diagnosis and suffer from lowered self-esteem. A nurse who is experienced in working with families during the grieving process will be a major part of the health care team in this situation. The nurse in conjunction with other members of the health care team should meet with the parents (and, if possible, the infant) to discuss the child's illness or disability. Parents need brief, clear, concise information. Because of the complexity of the information and parents' anxiety, the explanation may need to be repeated more than once. The information should not be confusing or confounding. This means that information provided by all team members needs to be consistent. Both verbal and nonverbal (i.e., behavioral) communication should be supportive to the parents and infant.

Behaviors or comments may reflect the care provider's own grief, frustration, and sense of helplessness. Nurses need to recognize their feelings and find outlets for their emotions away from the child's family. In this way, rather than engage in meaningless or intrusive conversation with families, they can be sensitive to the parents' needs for support. Support and sensitivity can be shown by sharing silences or by engaging in frequent and empathetic visits to the parent's room.

The infant's functioning should be assessed, so that areas of normal function can be reiterated. In this way, parents can begin to balance both the positive and negative aspects of having "a less than perfect" baby.

Nurses working with infants should familiarize themselves with the most valid and reliable instruments for assessing infant functioning. Examples of instruments that assess the infant's functioning include the Bayley Scales of Infant Development (Bayley, 1969) and the Brazelton Neonatal Behavioral Assessment Scale (Brazelton, 1973). The Bayley Scales have been developed to assess the developmental status of infants from 2 to 30 months of age in the areas of mental, motor, and behavioral competency. These scales are well-standardized infant tests. The Brazelton Neonatal Behavioral Assessment Scale is an interactive examination measuring various aspects of infant behavior. This scale measures individual progress at an earlier stage than the Bayley Scales, but its administration requires more expertise on the part of the examiner. Other tools such as the Neonatal Perception Inventory (Broussard, 1978) and the Maternal Attachment Assessment Strategy (Avant, 1980), which focus on maternal perceptions of the newborn and maternal attachment strategies, may also be useful to the nurse in the initial assessment of the infant and the maternal-child relationship.

Besides assessing the maternal-child relationship, the nurse can also promote parent-infant bonding by acting as a positive role model. She can call the baby

TABLE 19-4
Nurses' Role in Promoting Psychosocial Adaptation of the Family

Developing Realistic Goals

Assist parents to gain an understanding of how their child is similar to and different from other children

Encourage parents to help their children develop realistic goals, maximizing their similarities and minimizing their differences

Encourage parents to be honest with their children about their condition by representing a realistic picture—being hopeful but not offering false promises of cures and miracles

Teach parents and children to set short-term rather than long-term goals in cases of uncertain medical courses

Facilitate evaluation of goals by the child and family on a regular basis—encourage families to let go of unrealistic goals to prevent frustration and disappointment

Facilitating Mourning

Encourage children and their families to express and share feelings of guilt, sadness, loss, anticipated physical deterioration, and fear of death

Facilitate discussion to allow families to ask questions about the chronic illness related to causation: "Why me?" "What have I done?" "How will we ever manage?"

Teach parents how to recognize and deal with their child's self-blame and personal guilt for the illness

Encourage parents to communicate about the present and future, not solely about the past

Encourage parents to re-engage in own roles within family

Allow a reasonable, but not indefinite, time for mourning, so that parents can acknowledge present limitations and future potentials

Promotion of the Child's Self-Worth

Encourage child and family to stress individual and family abilities rather than disabilities

Remind parents that how children feel about themselves is influenced by what they hear their parents say about them

Teach parents the importance of letting their children take on their normal roles within the family, enhancing their self-concept

Encourage parents to allow their child to have some say in what others know about them

Assist parents in gaining empathy with their child's situation from the child's perspective

Encourage parents not to be too overprotective, as children require exposure to real-life situations with peers in order to learn to handle cruelty, adversity, and misunderstanding

Assist parents in understanding the need to set the same rules, have similar responsibilities, and receive the same discipline with all children in the family to avoid developing feelings of partiality or favoritism for the child with the illness

Teach parents to be able to recognize the child's need to be similar to peers in hairstyles and clothes; teach parents how to make compromises to accommodate disabilities

Encourage the child and family to put their "best foot forward"

Encourage parents to promote initiative and realistic areas of accomplishment

Discuss with parents the need for children to try new activities in order to develop creativity and problem solving

Nurses and parents can support the efforts and provide role models

Developing an Appropriate Level of Independence

Assist parents in developing realistic, age-appropriate goals for independence

Encourage families to allow children to function at home, school, and play with as few limits as possible

Give children an appropriate amount of information about their condition to allow them to adapt to the necessary limits and take responsibility for their own care

Encourage family discussions to allow children and their parents to vent concerns about dependence and independence

Encourage parents to reward independence, attempts at self-care, and appropriate social interaction

Open Communication Within the Family Unit

Teach parents the importance of frequent family discussions

Encourage parents to let children speak for themselves and present their own ideas

Teach parents to recognize and communicate with their children in nonverbal ways

Assist parents to be advocates for their chidlren by insisting that others ask the children for their input and participation in discussion

by name, cuddle the child, make good eye contact with the baby, and emphasize the child's normal characteristics. Family involvement can be fostered and positive reinforcement given for parents' efforts to engage in the baby's care. Because the baby may not be able to respond to the parents' advances, the nurse can encourage parents not to become discouraged and to continue to try, since each child eventually responds in a unique way. Once parents become attached to their child, they may experience the grieving process all over again as the realities of the illness become clarified and they are reminded of the known and potential losses.

Toddler

Parents of the toddler struggle with the child's need to develop a sense of autonomy. Nursing intervention to facilitate autonomy may take many forms. First, the nurse should assess the child's developmental level by using one of a number of standardized screening tools, such as the Denver Developmental Screening Test (DDST) (see Appendix 4 and Chapter 13, Assessing Child Health). Parents should be made aware of the results of the assessment and encouraged to add stimulation in areas of developmental lag and, more important, to emphasize the child's normal development and progress.

The family needs to be assisted to understand the need for independence. This can be done by allowing the toddler to participate and make small decisions in daily care, such as taking medicine from a cup or a spoon. Note that the choice is not *whether* to take the medicine, but *how*. Power struggles should be avoided, if possible. Yet, one must emphasize to parents that in spite of the chronic illness, the toddler needs consistency, appropriate limits, and a stable routine to provide a sense of order.

Parents may need to learn how to provide activities and toys that will stimulate toddlers who have chronic illnesses. Play items such as drums, punching bags, and beanbags provide children with an outlet for their frustrations. If energy needs to be conserved, parents can be encouraged to give appropriate assistance and limit play times. Body contact, a soothing voice, and distraction (e.g., a walk) may soothe the frustrations of children of this age.

Toddlers normally experience intense anxiety when separated from their parents. Children with chronic illness are often separated from their parents during hospitalization and diagnostic and treatment procedures. Nurses can be instrumental in decreasing the amount of separation or in minimizing its impact. This is accomplished by encouraging parents to "room in" or to be present as much as possible during stressful procedures.

Primary care nursing is another effective means of assisting the child to cope with separation. This mode of care provides one or a minimal number of caretakers to interact with the child; this establishes consistency and a close relationship with a substitute caretaker. The impact of separation can also be minimized by maintaining, as closely as possible, the child's home routine. This intervention gives the child a sense of security and facilitates the child's return home on discharge. See Chapter 21 for a discussion of the hospitalized toddler and separation.

Limitations imposed by the illness may inhibit social, intellectual, and cognitive development. Parents need to be encouraged to maximize the child's competencies while acknowledging and working with limitations. Home visits by the nurse can assist parents in realizing where safety limits should be imposed and how to modify the home environment.

The diagnosis of chronic illness during the toddler years has an enormous effect on the family. Parents may find little energy and time to devote to themselves. Families need information on available community resources and how to gain access to them. This includes suitable child care arrangements that allow respite for parents.

Parents need to be encouraged to share their feelings of anger and frustration. Parent or family support groups can provide a comfortable, and comforting, forum for sharing these emotions and receiving information from parents with similar experiences. If parents know what to expect of their ill child, they can prepare for future care and begin to understand the needs of other family members.

Preschooler

During the preschool years, children develop increasing abilities to provide self-care. Preschoolers with chronic illnesses may experience limitations in the development of these self-care skills and wonder why they are different from their peers. They may blame themselves or their parents for their limitations. The parents of preschoolers need assistance to foster the developmental potential and independence of their child and to maintain family equilibrium.

To help family members maintain or achieve a balance between their own needs and the needs of their disabled preschooler, the nurse can begin to help parents identify the needs unique to their own situation. Preschoolers need to develop social skills and increase their ability to separate from the family. Therefore, support for the child and family can be provided through assistance by instituting measures such as substitute caretaking, remedial education, or visiting friends or relatives for a day or two. This brief interlude fosters the preschooler's independence and gives parents the opportunity to pursue their own needs. When parents temporarily transfer their child's care to another person, they should be aware that their concern and anxiety are normal. However, with adequate preparation, appropriate and competent care providers can be found.

As with previous stages, parents need to be aware of tasks of normal growth and development and of how their child is progressing. Preschoolers are moving from dependency to becoming more independent school-age children. For parents with a disabled child, this process is complicated by the child's additional dependency needs. Parents may gain support from other families in similar circumstances and often benefit from becoming involved in the child's remedial education program. In this setting, they gain insight into approaches that facilitate maximum development of potential while gaining reassurance that their own style of parenting for their child is appropriate.

School-Age Child

During the school-age years, peers and their influence become increasingly dominant in child development. Children need to develop a sense of industry and accomplishment, rather than feel inferior and ashamed. School often brings conflict for children with chronic illnesses. By virtue of periodic interruptions for treatments or hospitalization, peers begin to label the child as "different." School nurses or community health nurses usually provide much of the necessary medical intervention when the child is able to attend school. They also keep the teacher and others involved in supervising the child's academic activities aware of the disease status. The nurse is also an educator, providing school personnel with information and instruction about the disease and its management. This contact is necessary when the illness affects the child's school functioning or when treatment or medication must be administered during school hours.

A positive approach avoids needless restrictions, keeps the child's activity as normal as possible, and provides substitute activities when limitations are necessary. The child should be kept involved with healthy peers and included in their activities. Since there is a greater incidence of "school phobia" in children with chronic disease, the nurse should be alert to early signs of this behavior. Characteristic examples include frequent, unjustifiable complaints to the school nurse or frequent, unexplained absences, or absences with questionable explanations. The nurse, teacher, and parent should encourage and, if necessary, insist on daily school attendance. Parents may require substantial encouragement and support from the nurse while they convince their child to attend school. The school nurse is also responsible for seeing that a homebound teacher is arranged when needed.

To protect the child from additional disease or complications, school nurses may need to remind all parents to keep all childhood immunizations up to date. This will also help prevent the spread of infectious diseases. Parents of a chronically ill child should be notified of any infectious outbreaks for which their child may be at special risk. A cooperative endeavor between home and school can help eliminate or minimize the conflicts a child with chronic illness would otherwise experience at school.

School-age children should be gaining progressively more independence in their activities of daily living and in personal decision making. School-age children with chronic illnesses may experience limitations that hinder independent development in one or more areas of living. These may not necessarily be limitations resulting from the chronic conditions but may be externally imposed by parents, teachers, peers, or other segments of society that disallow progressive independence in functioning or thinking. The nurse should regularly assess the child's social environment for evidence of unnecessary restrictions. Additional education or professional counseling may help the child or the restricting individuals to see the limitations in a more realistic manner.

The health team supervising the child's long-term care should be especially alert to conflict related to school entry and school continuation. Extra support and contact should be provided by the health care team as preventive measures during this time of potential crisis. By working with teachers to plan activities that lead to increased acceptance of the child, the child's school years can be as happy and productive as they are for healthy children and those without disabilities.

Adolescent

Adolescents with a chronic illness are forced to consider the limitations that the illness places on vocational, educational, and sexual choices and decisions. Teen-agers need to be treated as developing young adults with increasing responsibility for their own care as they adapt to their illness. A major emphasis for nursing of this age group is patient education that assists with and promotes maturation.

Teen-agers need accurate, detailed information about their illness—what causes it, what to expect from it, what it means in terms of educational or vocational interests, how it will affect their appearance and sexual function, and how independent it will permit them to be. The "can do's" rather than the "can't do's" should be emphasized. To provide a model, a peer counselor could be engaged to share similar experiences.

Nurses have successfully used groups to provide patient or family support. For example, adolescent support groups or informal teen activity groups have been established for hospitalized patients. A "teen room" where groups can meet formally and informally can facilitate these support group activities. Community support groups or advocacy groups have been founded in many communities and provide physical and psychologic support as well as current information about treatment and research. Nurses can help adolescents identify acceptable, appealing activities that will allow peer contact without exceeding limitations. For example, if strenuous physical activity is limited, the student could still be a part of many team sports by acting as a student manager. Within an institutional setting, it is especially important to structure acceptable ways for an adolescent to experience social group activities and a degree of independence.

Teen-agers should be encouraged to participate in clubs, activities, and other social interaction with peers who have similar interests, not just with peers who have a similar disability. A regular school setting with modified activities is best for adjustment; however, teachers need honest information about the child's disease and capabilities. With this kind of exposure, teen-agers learn to live openly with their disabilities and to answer questions gracefully. They learn that they are special and capable.

Utilization of Resources

All families with chronically ill children, although requiring the services of health professionals from time to time, struggle to regain their family equilibrium and independence. The nurse can have a valuable role in promoting an environment that stimulates self-care activities and patient/family confidence, in both hospital and community settings.

In the hospital setting, such environmental structuring includes the following:

- Unconditional acceptance of the patient and the family by the hospital staff.
- Presenting the child's condition in a realistic manner so that the child and family can work through the grieving process appropriately.
- Providing competent and continuous patient care with increasing involvement by the child and family as they are ready, both in the hospital setting and at home.
- Providing opportunities for the child and family to feel valued in the hospital unit, thus, later at home and in the community.
- Promotion of a familiar environment and assurance that procedures and treatments will be explained.
- Promotion of privacy for the child alone and with the family.

With thoughtful structuring of the hospital setting, patients and their families can ideally feel more comfortable and supported. However, the hospital model has historically dealt primarily with acute care and only reluctantly become involved in chronicity (Haggerty, 1975). Nurses who are used to functioning in well-equipped units with the support of medical technology and the availability of emergency teams have difficulty preparing the patient and the family for community care. The issue of control over "the patient" is one that can be resolved through open communication, broad participation in goal setting, and strategy implementation. Parenting and nursing roles become blurred, with parents taking on decision making roles and attempting to adhere to the medical management of the patient while at the same time striving to integrate the child as a functioning family member.

In the community, nurses have the potential to use their knowledge and expertise in the roles of resource person, evaluator, educator, and organizer. As such, they can function as a liaison connecting the child and family, community, and broader health care community.

As resource persons, nurses can share their knowledge of various illnesses, growth and development of children and families, and common coping strategies used by children and families. This can be done by means of a formal approach, such as in a parent support group in which the nurse can take either an active educator role or a facilitative role to encourage parent leadership and directiveness. The nurse may also want to interact individually with children in the school setting and their parents in the community. In this way, the nurse can monitor the child's disease process, growth and developmental achievements; can support parents; and can be a resource person informing families about community facilities and services.

As an evaluator, the nurse in the community can monitor the child's physical and psychosocial adaptation to illness and the family's adaptation to the child's illness. Several tools for child assessment have previously been mentioned. The nurse should also evaluate the stressors that families with chronically ill children experience. These stressors may include strain on the marital relationship, decreased attention and time for siblings, and difficulty in managing caregiving tasks. Although extended families may provide assistance, they also struggle with uncertainty of the child's medical requirements and fear of interfering with the family's functioning.

Although trained personnel are usually available to assist families in metropolitan areas, resources are not always available in rural areas. Even if resources are available in these areas, there may be no adequately trained staff to respond to the needs of the child and family. Out of frustration, parents are beginning to form advocacy groups to draw attention to the needs of children with special concerns. The nurse needs to carefully evaluate both the needs of the child and the competency of available health care personnel in the community. If community adaptation to chronically ill children and their families is to be successful, careful planning is necessary, in anticipation of hospital discharge and integration into the family, school, and community.

As an educator, the nurse in the community can follow up on the activities instituted by the hospital nurse to promote self-care. In the home, the community nurse can assess the impact that particular cultures have on the child's care. The nurse can also attempt to evaluate how the family is adapting. Although some instruments have been developed to measure family adjustment to chronic illness (Pless & Satterwhite, 1973; Spitzer et al, 1971), the measurement remains limited to the field of child health. Qualitative approaches and open-ended interviewing (Satterwhite, 1976; Black et al, 1978) have been employed in some studies, but to date, few comprehensive measures that can quantify the impact of a child's illness on the family have been developed.

Stein and Riessman's (1980) Impact-on-Family Scale is an exception, but this instrument is in its early developmental stages and requires further refinements and reliability and validity testings. Hymovich (1983) has also developed the Chronicity Impact and Coping Instrument: Parent Questionnaire to measure parental perceptions of stressors, problematic situations, or resources. The instrument also provides a protocol for assessing the needs of chronically ill children. Although some initial validity and reliability have been established, more rigorous study is required before measurement properties are fully understood. Finally, Roberts and Feetham (1982) have developed the Feetham Family Functioning Survey to measure parents' perceptions of relationships among family members and their functioning in the outside world. This instrument needs to be used more widely and tested to determine if it is capable of detecting changes over time. Even with the lack of specific instruments, nurses can utilize their knowledge of chronic illness in children and families, growth and development, and coping strategies to evaluate generally the child's and family's current functional state.

The role of the case manager is one that the nurse in the community could assume. Unfortunately, there are often two case managers—one in the hospital and one in the community—contributing to duplication of efforts, increased costs, and confusion for the child and family.

As a case manager, the community nurse can assist the family in the organization and coordination of their child's health care. It is not uncommon for children with a chronic illness to see a multiplicity of health professionals regarding their illness and its sequelae, growth and developmental needs, educational needs, adjustment needs, and an array of other services in relation to financial, social, and psychological stresses. Often, many of these health professionals have no idea of the demands placed on the family by other caretakers. The family is literally "run ragged" going from one appointment to the other. The nurse can carefully collect information related to all the health care agencies with which the family is involved in an attempt to assist them in managing the many conflicting demands.

Ness and Huchala (1987) have suggested the need for a community care plan. This plan is based on the many factors that may be assessed to ensure successful community entry. Before discharge from the hospital, the issues of the availability of trained personnel, funds, equipment, and supplies need to be addressed. If nurses must be trained, this should happen in collaboration with nursing specialists within the hospital system and before the child's discharge.

The family also needs to be aggressively involved in developing the community care plan. Family members need to express a willingness to care for the child at home. They also need to know if community supports are available, if their home can accommodate equipment, and if there will be assistance for other family members during the transition. Finally, several community issues need to be addressed. Are the community medical and nursing professionals ready to accept responsibility for the child's care? Are electrical and telephone services adequate? Are transportation, emergency, and educational resources adequate? A community care plan would assist in addressing some of these issues of the hospital, family, and community. In addition, common standards of care could be developed for all health professionals practicing in both institutional and community settings.

In planning for discharge, nurses should be aware of federal and state sources of support for chronically ill children and their families. These include such programs as (1) Social Security Act, Title V, which provides monies to states for "programs for children with special needs"; (2) P.L. 94–142, a federal law mandating education for all children with disabilities; (3) P.L. 99–457 and subsequent amendments that mandate early intervention services for infants and toddlers at risk for and with disabilities; (4) maternal-child-health office resources; and (5) Supplemental Security Income (SSI).

In summary, the nurse who is assessing, providing care, role modeling, and advocating for children and families with chronic illness or disabilities must adopt and encourage a realistic and reasonable positive approach to care. The adage "What is looked for is what is obtained" was clearly demonstrated in a review of literature by Deatrick and Knafl (1987). They assert that the method and results of studying a child family member with a chronic health condition may have much to do with the perspective of the investigator. This may also be true of the care provider assessing, planning, and implementing care and support. Children and families deserve to share great expectations for one another. Most of these are children with normal development needs who also happen to have a long-term health condition.

KEY CONCEPTS

Concepts Related to Basic Information

- Currently there is no national data bank that supplies statistics or precise figures on how many children are affected by health conditions which require long-term monitoring, care, or ongoing treatment.
- When a child is diagnosed with a chronic illness, subsequent behavioral changes are due in part to characteristics of illness, in part to the family and others' reactions to the illness, and in part to the maturity and coping ability of the child and family.
- Chronic illness influences the child's physical, cognitive, social, and emotional development.
- Chronic illness during infancy can potentially disrupt the parent/child attachment and adaptation and the smooth transition into parenthood and family life.

- The presence of chronic illness in the school age group may interfere with the transition from parental to peer approval.
- Chronic fatigue, logistical demands of caretaking, financial impacts, vigilance and a constant state of readiness contribute to the stress parents of chronically ill children experience.
- Children use a variety of coping strategies to deal with the stresses of chronic illness which include emotion-based coping, problem-solving coping, identification with health care professionals, stress inoculation, ritualization, denial and hope.
- Effective coping patterns used by parents for positive adjustment include assigning meaning, denial, rationalization, normalization, and effective use of resources.
- The major nursing goals in chronic illness are facilitating psychosocial adaptation and well-being, promoting optimal child and family growth and development, and encouraging families to make appropriate use of resources.

Concepts Related to Nursing Assessment

- To assess accurately the effect of a child's illness on the family system, data on how the family functioned before and after the diagnosis are needed.
- The developmental stage for each family member, the family unit, and the affected child are important factors in considering the impact of the illness on the family's behavioral, cognitive, and emotional well-being and developmental tasks.
- In assessing sibling reactions, it is necessary to consider both their developmental stages and their positions within the family.
- Assessment of the child's coping behaviors is essential if supportive interventions are to be appropriate and accurately articulated.
- The child's level of development needs to be assessed in order to intervene effectively with the child.

Concepts Related to Nursing Intervention

- Nurses can modify both risk and vulnerability factors of the chronically child in order to improve the state of health or to prevent deterioration of illness.
- Nurses must be cautious to have neither uniform expectations nor common or universal interventions when dealing with families with a chronically ill child.
- Nurses can help parents anticipate the course of the illness in order to help them prepare the sibling for impending events, facilitate answering their questions, and involve others such as grandparents in playing a significant role.
- Nursing strategies that promote psychosocial adaptation and the well-being of the child include assisting the child and parents to develop realistic goals, facilitating mourning, promoting self-worth, encouraging progress along the normal developmental trajectory toward independence, and developing open channels of communication.
- Nursing interventions for the child with chronic illness, in order to be effective, must consider their developmental level and limitations imposed by the disease.

REFERENCES

Adams, J., & Weaver, J. (1986). Self esteem and perceived stress in young adolescents with chronic diseases: Unexpected findings. *Journal of Adolescent Health Care, 7*(3), 173–177.

Anderson, J. (1981). The social construction of illness experience: Families with a chronically ill child. *Journal of Advanced Nursing, 6,* 427–434.

Anderson, J., & Elfert, H. (1989). Managing chronic illness in the family: Women as caretakers. *Journal of Advanced Nursing, 13,* 735–743.

Anthony, E. (1974). The syndrome of the psychologically invulnerable child. In E. Anthony, C. Koupernik, & C. Chiland (Eds.), *The child in his family: Children at psychiatric risk.* New York: John Wiley & Sons.

Austin, J., & McDermott, N. (1981). Parental attitudes and coping behaviors in families of children with epilepsy. *Journal of Neuroscience Nursing, 20*(3), 174–179.

Avant, P. (1980). Maternal attachment and anxiety: An exploratory study (Doctoral dissertation, Texas Women's University, 1978). *Dissertation Abstracts International, 40,* 165B.

Barbarin, O., Hughes, D., & Chesler, M. (1985). Stress, coping and marital functioning among parents of children with cancer. *Journal of Marriage and the Family, 47,* 473–480.

Barsch, R. (1968). *The parent of a handicapped child: Study of child rearing practices.* Springfield, IL: Charles C Thomas.

Bayley, N. (1969). *Bayley scales of infant development.* New York: The Psychological Corporation.

Bibace, R., & Walsh, M. (1980). Development of children's concepts of illness. *Pediatrics, 66,* 912–917.

Black, L., Hersher, L., & Stenschneider, A. (1978). Impact of the apnea monitor on family life. *Pediatrics, 62,* 681.

Blackburn, S. (1982). The neonatal ICU: A high risk environment. *American Journal of Nursing, 82,* 1708–1712.

Blount, R. L., Landolf-Fritsche, B., Powers, S. W., & Sturges, J. W. (1991). Differences between high and low coping children and between parent and staff behaviors during painful medical procedures. *Journal of Pediatric Psychology, 16*(6), 795–809.

Bossert, E., Holaday, B., Harkins, A., Turner-Hensen, A. (1990). Strategies of normalization used by parents of chronically ill school age children. *Journal of Child and Adolescent Psychiatric and Mental Health Nursing, 3*(2), 57–61.

Bowlby, J. (1973). *Neonatal behavioral assessment scale.* Philadelphia: JB Lippincott.

Brazelton, T. B. (1973). *Neonatal behavioral assessment scale.* Philadelphia: JB Lippincott.

Breslau, N., Weitzman, M., & Messenger, K. (1981). Psychological functioning of siblings of disabled children. *Pediatrics, 67*(3), 344–353.

Brewster, A. (1982). Chronically ill hospitalized children's concepts of their illness. *Pediatrics, 62,* 355–362.

Broussard, E. R. (1978, February). Psychosocial disorders in children: Early assessment of infants at risk. *Cont Educ Fam Phys, 44,* 47–48, 55–57.

Brown, M., & Gordon, W. (1987). Impact of impairment on activity patterns of children. *Archives of Physical Medicine and Rehabilitation, 68,* 829–832.

Bullard, I., & Dohnal, J. (1984). The community deals with the child who has a handicap. *Nursing Clinics of North America, 19*(2), 309–318.

Burr, C. (1985). Impact on the family of a chronically ill child. In N. Hobbs & J. Perrin (Eds.), *Issues in the care of children with chronic illness*. San Francisco: Jossey-Bass.

Burr, B., Guyer, B., Todres, I., Abraham, B., & Chiodo, T. (1983). Home care for children on respirators. *New England Journal of Medicine, 309,* 1319–1323.

Burton, L. (1975). *The family life of sick children: A study of families coping with chronic childhood disease*. London: Routledge & Kegan Paul.

Cassel, J. (1976). The contribution of the social environment to the host resistance. *American Journal of Epidemiology, 104,* 107–123.

Cobb, S. (1976). Social support as a moderator of life stress. *Psychosomatic Medicine, 38,* 300–314.

Cohen, M. (1988). *Living under conditions of sustained uncertainty.* Doctoral dissertation, University of California, San Francisco.

Cohen, M., & Martinson, I. (1988). Chronic uncertainty: Its effects on parental appraisal of a child's health. *Journal of Pediatric Nursing, 3*(2), 89–96.

Craig, H., & Edwards, J. (1983). Adaptation in chronic illness: An eclectic model for nurses. *Journal of Advanced Nursing, 8,* 397–404.

Damrosch, S. P., & Perry, L. A. (1989). Self-report adjustment, chronic sorrow, and coping of parents of children with Down syndrome. *Nursing Research, 38*(1), 25–30.

Daniels, C., Moos, R., Billings, A., & Miller, J. (1987). Psychosocial risk and resistance factors among children with chronic illness, healthy siblings and healthy controls. *Journal of Abnormal Child Psychology, 15*(2), 295–308.

Deatrick, J., Knafl, K. (1987). Conceptualizing family response to a child's chronic illness or disability. *Family Relations, 36*(3), 300–304.

Deatrick, J., Knafl, K., & Walsh, M. (1988). The process of parenting a child with a disability: Normalization through accommodation. *Journal of Advanced Nursing, 13,* 15–21.

Deatrick, J., & Knafl, K. (1990). Management behaviors: Day to day adjustments to childhood chronic conditions. *Journal of Pediatric Nursing, 5*(1), 15–22.

Desmond, H. (1980). Two families: An observational study. In J. Kellerman (Ed.), *Psychological aspects of childhood cancer.* Springfield, IL: Charles C Thomas.

Diamond, M., & Jones, S. (1983). *Chronic illness across the life span.* Norwalk, CT: Appleton-Century-Crofts.

Dowd, E., et al. (1977, November/December). Releasing the hospitalized child from restraints. *MCN: American Journal of Maternal Child Nursing,* p. 370.

Dyson, L., Edgar, E., Crnic, K. (1989). Psychological predictors of adjustment by siblings of developmentally disabled children. *American Journal of Mental Retardation, 94*(3), 292–302.

Erikson, E. (1964). *Childhood and society* (2nd ed.). New York: WW Norton.

Erikson, E. (1966). Ontogeny of ritualization. In R. Lowerstein et al. (Eds.), *Psychoanalysis—A general psychology: Essays in honour of Heinz Hartman*. New York: International Universities Press.

Farber, B. (1959). Effects of a severely mentally retarded child on family integration. *Monographs of the Society for Research in Child Development, 71.*

Farber, B. (1960). Perceptions of crisis and related variables in the impact of a retarded child on the mother. *Journal of Health and Human Behavior, 1,* 108–118.

Featherstone, H. (1980). *A difference in the family: Life with a disabled child*. New York: Basic Books.

Feetham, S., & Roberts, C. (1982). Assessing for family functioning across three areas of relationship. *Nursing Research, 31,* 231–235.

Figley, C., & McCubbin, H. (Eds.) (1983). *Stress and the family: Vol II. Coping with catastrophe*. New York: Brunner and Mazel.

Fraser, B. (1980). The meaning of handicap in children. *Child Care, Health and Development, 6,* 83–91.

Gabel, H., McDowell, J., & Cerreto, M. (1983). Family adaptation to the handicapped infants. In S. Garwood & R. Fewell (Eds.), *Educating handicapped infants*. Rockville, MD: Aspen.

Gayton, W., Friedman, S., Tavormina, J., & Tucker, F. (1977). Children with cystic fibrosis: I. Psychological test findings of patients, siblings and parents. *Pediatrics, 59*(6), 888–894.

Geist, R. A. (1979). Onset of chronic illness in children and adolescents: Psychotherapeutic and consultative intervention. *American Journal of Orthopsychiatry, 49*(1), 4–23.

Giger, J. N., & Davidhizar, R. E. (1991). *Transculture nursing: Assessment and intervention*. St. Louis: CV Mosby.

Gliedman, J., & Roth, W. (1980). *The unexpected minority: Handicapped children in America*. New York: Harcourt Brace Jovanovich.

Goldberg, S., & Simmons, R. (1988). Chronic illness and early development. *Pediatrician, 15,* 13–20.

Haggerty, R. (1975). *Child health and the community.* New York: John Wiley & Sons.

Harkins, E. (1990). *Childhood chronic illness and development from a life-span developmental perspective.* Unpublished paper.

Harkins, E. (1991). *Childhood chronic illness and family hardiness: Integrating a new diagnosis*. Unpublished doctoral dissertation, University of California, San Francisco.

Hayes, V. E., & Knox, J. E. (1984). The experience of stress in parents of children with long-term disability. *Journal of Advanced Nursing, 9,* 333–341.

Hill, R. (1949). *Families under stress*. New York: Harper & Row.

Hobbs, N., et al. (1983). *Public policies affecting chronically ill children and their families.* Preliminary report of project: Chronically ill children in America. Nashville: Vanderbilt Institute for Public Policy Studies.

Hobbs, N., & Perrin, J. (Eds.) (1985). *Issues in the care of children with chronic illness: A sourcebook on problems, services and policies*. San Francisco: Jossey-Bass.

Holaday, B. (1984). Challenges of rearing a chronically ill child: Caring and coping. *Nursing Clinics of North America, 19*(2), 361–368.

Holaday, B. (1987). Patterns of interactions between mothers and their chronically ill infants. *Maternal-Child Nursing Journal, 16,* 29–45.

Holaday, B. (1989). The family with a chronically ill child: An interactional perspective. In C. Gilliss, B. Highley, B. Roberts, & I. Martinson (Eds.), *Toward a science of family nursing*. Reading, MA: Addison-Wesley.

Holaday, B., & Turner-Henson, A. (1991). *Final report: Growing up and going out: A survey of chronically ill schoolage children's use of time*. Rockville, MD: The Maternal and Child Research Program.

Hymovich, D. (1983). The chronicity impact and coping instrument: Parent questionnaire. *Nursing Research, 32,* 275–281.

Ireys, H. (1981). Health care for chronically disabled children and their families. In L. Shorr (Ed.), *Better health for our children: A national strategy. Vol 4: Report of the Select Panel for Promotion of Child Health* (DHHS [PHS] Publication No. 70–55071). Washington, DC: US Government Printing Office.

Isaacs, J., & McElroy, R. (1980, August). Psychosocial aspects of chronic illness in children. *Journal of School Health,* pp. 318–321.

Jessop, D., & Stein, R. (1989). Meeting the needs of individuals and families. In R. Stein (Ed.), *Caring for children with chronic illness: Issues and strategies*. New York: Springer.

Kaplan, B., Cassel, J., & Gore, S. (1977). Social support and health. *Medical Care, 15*(5, Suppl.), 47–57.

Kazak, A., & Marvin, R. (1984). Differences, difficulties, and adaptation: Stress and social networks in families with a handicapped child. *Family Relations, 33,* 66–77.

Ketterick, R. (1982). The Pennsylvania program: Case example: The ventilator dependent child (DHHS Publication No. PHS–83–50194, Report of the Surgeon General's Workshop on Children with Handicaps and Their Families). Washington, DC: US Government Printing Office.

Knafl, K., & Deatrick, J. (1986). How families manage chronic conditions: Analysis of the concept of normalization. *Research in Nursing and Health, 9,* 215–222.

Knafl, K., & Deatrick, J. (1990). Family management style: Concept analysis and development. *Journal of Pediatric Nursing, 5*(1), 4–14.

Krulik, T. (1980). Successful "normalizing" tactics of parents of chronically ill children. *Journal of Advanced Nursing, 9,* 215–222.

LaMontagne, F. (1987a). Adopting a process approach to assess children's coping. *Journal of Pediatric Nursing, 3*(3), 159–163.

LaMontagne, L. (1987b). Children's preoperative coping: Replication and extension. *Nursing Research, 36*(3), 163–167.

LaMontagne, F. (1991). Issues in the measurement of children's locus of control. *Western Journal of Nursing Research, 13*(1), 67–83.

LaMontagne, L. L., & Hepworth, J. T. (1991). Issues in the measurement of children's locus of control. *Western Journal of Nursing Research, 13*(1), 67–83.

Lazarus, R., & Folkman, S. (1984). *Stress, appraisal and coping.* New York: Springer.

Lewis, C., & Lewis, M. (1974). The impact of television commercials on health-related belief and behavior of children. *Pediatrics, 53,* 431.

Madiros, M. (1982). Mothers of disabled children: A study of parental stress. *Nursing Papers, 14*(2), 47–56.

Madiros, M. (1985). Role alterations of female parents having children with disabilities. *Canada's Mental Health, 33*(4), 24–26.

Mattsson, A. (1972). Long-term illness in childhood: A challenge to psychosocial adaptation. *Pediatrics, 50,* 801–805.

McCrae, W., Cull, A., & Burton, L. (1973). Cystic fibrosis: Parents' responses to the genetic basis of the disease. *Lancet, 2,* 11–143.

McCubbin, H., & Patterson, J. (1983). The family stress process: The double ABCX model of adjustment and adaptation. In H. McCubbin, M. Sussman, & J. Patterson (Eds.), *Social stress and the family.* New York: Haworth Press.

McCubbin, M. (1986). Family stress, resources, and family types: Chronic illness in children. *Family Relations, 37*(2), 203–210.

McCubbin, M. (1989). Family stress and family strengths: A comparison of single- and two-parent families with handicapped children. *Research in Nursing and Health, 12,* 101–110.

McCubbin, M., & Huang, S. (1989). Family strengths in the care of handicapped children: Targets for intervention. *Family Relations, 38*(4), 436–443.

McKeever, P. (1981). Fathering the chronically ill child. *Maternal-Child Nursing Journal, 6*(2), 124–128.

Mechanic, D. (1962). The concept of illness behavior. *Journal of Chronic Diseases, 15,* 189–194.

Mercer, R. (1974). Mothers' responses to their infants with defects. *Nursing Research, 23,* 133–137.

Mercer, R. (1977). When the infant has a defect. In *Nursing care for parents at risk* (pp. 41–75). Thorofare, NJ: Slack.

Morrow, D., Carpenter, P., & Hoagland, A. (1984). The role of social support in parental adjustment to pediatric cancer. *Journal of Pediatric Psychology, 9*(3), 317–329.

Murphy, L. B., & Moriarty, A. E. (1976). *Vulnerability, coping, and growth.* New Haven, CT: Yale University Press.

Neill, K. (1979). Behavioral aspects of chronic physical disease. *Nursing Clinics of North America, 14,* 443–456.

Ness, P., & Huchala, B. (1987). Adaptation of the community to children with chronic conditions and their families. In M. Rose & R. Thomas (Eds.), *Children with chronic conditions: Nursing in a family and community context.* Orlando, FL: Grune & Stratton.

Newacheck, P., Budetti, R., & Halfon, N. (1986). Prevalence of activity limiting chronic conditions among children based on household interviews. *Journal of Chronic Diseases, 39*(2), 63–71.

Olshansky, S. (1962). Chronic sorrow: A response to having a mentally defective child. *Journal of Pediatrics, 43,* 190–193.

Parson, R. (1951). *The social system.* New York: Free Press.

Perrin, E., & Gerrity, P. (1981). There's a demon in your belly: Children's understanding of illness. *Pediatrics, 67,* 841–849.

Perrin, J. M. (1985). Introduction. In N. Hobbs & J. M. Perrin (Eds.), *Issues in the care of children with chronic illness.* San Francisco: Springer.

Phillips, S., et al. (1985). Parent interview findings regarding the impact of cystic fibrosis on families. *Journal of Developmental and Behavioral Pediatrics, 6,* 122–127.

Piaget, J. (1969). *The Early Growth of Logic in the Child.* New York: WW Norton.

Pless, I. B., & Pinkerton, P. (1975). *Chronic childhood disorders: Promoting patterns of adjustment.* Chicago: Year Book Medical.

Pless, I., & Satterwhite, B. (1973). A measure of family functioning and its application. *Social Science and Medicine, 7,* 613–621.

Potter, P., & Roberts, M. (1984). Children's perceptions of chronic illness: The roles of disease symptoms, cognitive development and information. *Journal of Pediatric Psychology, 9*(1), 13–27.

Rankin, S., & Weeks, D. (1989). Life-span development: A review of theory and practice for families with chronically ill members. *Scholarly Inquiry for Nursing Practice, 3*(1), 3–27.

Ray, B. (1985). Measuring the social position of the mainstreamed handicapped child. *Exceptional Children, 52*(1), 57–62.

Richards, N. (1986). Interaction between mothers and infants with Down syndrome: Infant characteristics. *Topics in Early Special Education, 6*(3), 54–71.

Roberts, C., & Feetham, S. (1982). Assessing family functioning across three areas of relationships. *Nursing Research, 31,* 231–235.

Rodgers, B., et al. (1981). Depression in the chronically ill or handicapped school-age child. *MCN: American Journal of Maternal Child Nursing, 6,* 266–273.

Rose, M., & Killien, M. (1983). Risk and vulnerability: A case for differentiation. *Advances in Nursing Science, 5*(3), 60–73.

Ryan-Wenger, N. (1992). A taxonomy of children's coping strategies: A step toward theory development. *American Journal of Orthopsychiatry, 62*(2), 256–263.

Sabbeth, B. (1984). Understanding the impact of chronic childhood illness on families. *Pediatric Clinics of North America, 73*(6), 47–57.

Sabbeth, B., & Leventhal, J. (1984). Marital adjustment to chronic childhood illness: A critique of the literature. *Pediatrics, 73*(6), 762–768.

Sargent, J., & Liebman, R. (1985). Childhood chronic illness: Issues for psychotherapists. *Community Mental Health Journal, 21*(4), 294–311.

Satterwhite, B. (1976). *Impact of chronic illness on child and family: An overview based on five surveys with implications for management.* Paper presented at the Ambulatory Pediatric Association Annual Meeting, St. Louis.

Sawyer, E. (1992). Family functioning when children have cystic fibrosis. *Journal of Pediatric Nursing, 7*(5), 304–311.

Schlomann, P. (1988). Developmental gaps of children with a chronic condition and their impact on the family. *Journal of Pediatric Nursing, 3*(3), 180–187.

Seligman, M., & Darling, R. (1989). *Ordinary families, special children: A systems approach to childhood disability.* New York: Guilford Press.

Sibinga, M., & Friedman, D. (1971). Restraint and speech. *Pediatrics, 61,* 116.

Siemon, M. (1987). Patterns of impairment: Cognitive/emotional. In M. Rose & R. Thomas (Eds.), *Children with chronic conditions: Nursing in a family and community context.* Orlando, FL: Grune & Stratton.

Spitzer, R., Gibbon, M., Endicott, J. (1971). Family evaluation form. New York State Department of Mental Hygiene, Biometrics Research.

Stein, R. E. K. (1989). *Caring for children with chronic illness: Issues and strategies.* New York: Springer.

Stein, R., & Reissman, C. (1980). The development of an impact-on family scale: Preliminary findings. *Medical Care, 18*(4), 465–472.

Tew, B., & Laurence, K. (1973). Mothers, brothers and sisters of patients with spina bifida. *Developmental Medicine and Child Neurology, 15,* 69–76.

Thomas, R. (1983). Family response to the birth of a child with a chronic condition. Unpublished manuscript, University of Washington School of Sociology, Seattle.

Thomas, R. (1987). Introduction and conceptual framework. In M.

Rose & R. Thomas (Eds.), *Children with chronic conditions: Nursing in a family and community context*. Orlando, FL: Grune & Stratton.

Tritt, S. G., & Esses, L. M. (1988). Psychological adaptation of siblings of children with chronic medical illnesses. *American Journal of Orthopsychiatry, 58*(2), 211–220.

Velasco de Parra, M., Davila de Cortazar, S., & Covarrubias-Espinoza, G. (1983). The adaptive pattern of families with a leukemic child. *Family Systems Medicine, 1*(4), 30–35.

Venters, M. (1981). Familial coping with chronic and severe childhood illness: The case of cystic fibrosis. *Social Science Medicine,* 289–297.

Warda, M. (1992). The family and chronic sorrow: Role theory approach. *Journal of Pediatric Nursing, 7*(3), 205–210.

Weitzman, M., Walker, D., & Gortmaker, S. (1986). School absence rates of chronically ill and healthy children. *Clinical Pediatrics, 25,* 137–140.

Wertlieb, D., Weigel, C., & Feldstein, M. (1987). Measuring children's coping. *American Journal of Orthopsychiatry, 57*(4), 548–560.

Wikler, L., Wasow, M., & Hatfield, E. (1981). Chronic sorrow revisited: Parent vs. professional depiction of the adjustment of parents of mentally retarded children. *American Journal of Orthopsychiatry, 51*(1), 63–70.

Wilkinson, S. (1988). *The child's world of illness: The development of health and illness behavior*. Cambridge: Cambridge University Press.

Wright, L., & Leahey, M. (1984). *Nurses and families: A guide to family assessment and intervention*. Philadelphia: FA Davis.

Wright, L., & Leahey, M. (1987). *Families and chronic illness*. Springhouse, PA: Springhouse.

BIBLIOGRAPHY

Bank, S. (1981). *Sibling bond*. New York: Basic Books.

Bernando, M. (1982). A conceptual model of children's cognitive adaptation to physical disability. *Journal of Advanced Nursing, 7,* 595–601.

Betz, C. (1993). Pediatric community needs. *Journal of Pediatric Nursing, 8*(3), 141.

Combs, V., & Marino, B. (1993). A comparison of growth patterns in breast- and bottle-fed infants with congenital heart disease. *Pediatric Nursing, 19*(2), 175–179.

Darling, R., & Darling, J. (1982). *Children who are different: Meeting the challenges of birth defects in society*. St. Louis: CV Mosby.

Duvall, E. (1971). *Family development*. Philadelphia: JB Lippincott.

Dynesen, A., & Flensborg, E. (1978). Progosen for cystik fibrose 1 Danmark 1945–1974. *Videnskah Praksis,* 463–470.

Ferrari, M. (1986). Perceptions of social support by parents of chronically ill versus healthy children. *Children's Health Care, 15*(1), 26–31.

Freud, A. (1966). *The ego and the mechanisms of defense*. New York: International Universities Press.

Furman, R. (1973). A child's capacity for mourning. In E. Anthony & C. Koupernik (Eds.), *The child in his family: The impact of disease and death*. New York: John Wiley & Sons.

Gath, A. (1974). Sibling reactions to mental handicap: A comparison of the brothers and sisters of mongol children. *Journal of Child Psychology and Psychiatry, 15,* 187–198.

Giardino, P., Ryan, M., MacQueen, M., & Hilgartner, M. (1993). Behavioral contracting to improve adherence in patients with thalassemia. *Journal of Pediatric Nursing, 8*(2), 106–111.

Haase, J. (1987). Components of courage in chronically ill adolescents: A phenomenological study. *Advances in Nursing Science, 9*(2), 64–80.

Haber, M., & Smith, R. (1971). Disability and deviance: normative adaptations of role behavior. *American Sociological Review, 36,* 87–97.

Herdo, J., & Perry, D. (1993). Third-party payor billing and reimbursement for nursing services: Infant apnea management. *Journal of Pediatric Nursing, 8*(2), 100–105.

Holaday, B. (1981). Maternal response to their chronically ill infant's attachment behavior of crying. *Nursing Research, 30,* 383–348.

Horner, M., et al. (1987). How parents of children with chronic conditions perceive their own needs. *MCN: American Journal of Maternal Child Nursing, 12*(1), 40–43.

Klein, S. (1972). Brother to sister, sister to brother: Interview with siblings of disabled children, Parts I and II. *Exceptional Parent, 2,* 10–15, 24–27.

Kramer, R. (1984). Living with childhood cancer: Impact on the healthy sibling. *Oncology Nursing Forum, 11,* 44–51.

Krier, J. (1993). Involvment of educational staff in the health care of medically fragile children. *Pediatric Nursing, 19*(3), 251–259.

Leonard, B., Brust, J., & Paeth, S. (1993). Parental Distress: Caring for medically fragile children at home. *Journal of Pediatric Nursing, 8*(1), 22–30.

Loutzenhiser, J., & Clark, R. (1993). Physical activity and exercise in children with cystic fibrosis. *Journal of Pediatric Nursing, 8*(2), 112–119.

Mattsson, A. (1972). Long-term physical illness in childhood: A challenge to psychosocial adaptation. *Pediatrics, 50,* 801–811.

Mattsson, A., & Weisberg, I. (1970). Behavioral reactions to minor illness in preschool children. *Pediatrics, 46,* 604.

Miller, J. (1983). *Coping with chronic illness: Overcoming powerlessness*. Philadelphia: FA Davis.

Moos, R., & Tsu, V. (1977). The crisis of physical illness: An overview. In R. Moos (Ed.), *Coping with physical illness*. New York: Plenum.

Murphy, L. (1974). Coping, vulnerability and resilience in childhood. In G. Coelho et al. (Eds.), *Coping and adaptation*. New York: Basic Books.

Muscari, M. (1987). Adolescent suicide attempts by acetaminophen ingestion. *MCN: American Journal of Maternal Child Nursing, 12*(1), 32–35.

Nelms, B. (1988). More similar than different: Children with chronic illness. *Journal of Pediatric Health Care, 14*(4), 218–223.

Oremland, E. (1986). Communicating over chronic illness: Dilemmas of affected school-aged children. *Children's Health Care, 14*(4), 218–223.

Perkins, M. (1993). Parent-nurse collaboration: Using caregiver identity emergence phases to assist parents of hospitalized children with disabilities. *Journal of Pediatric Nursing, 8*(1), 2–9.

Potter, P., & Roberts, M. (1984). Children's perceptions of chronic illness: The roles of disease symptoms, cognitive development, and information. *Journal of Pediatric Psychology, 9,* 13–27.

Power, P., & Dell Orto, A. (Eds.) (1980). *Role of the family in the rehabilitation of the physically disabled*. Baltimore: University Park Press.

Rose, M. (1984). The concepts of coping and vulnerability as applied to children with chronic conditions. *Issues in Comprehensive Pediatric Nursing, 7,* 177–186.

Roskies, E. (1972). *Abnormality and normality: The mothering of thalidomide children*. Ithaca, NY: Cornell University Press.

Scannell, S., Gillies, D., Biordi, D., & Child, D. (1993). Negotiating nurse-patient authority in pediatric home health care. *Journal of Pediatric Nursing, 8*(2), 70–78.

Siemon, M. (1987). Patterns of impairment: Cognitive/emotional. In M. H. Rose & R. B. Thomas (eds.), *Children with chronic conditions: Nursing in a family and community context.* Orlando, FL: Grune & Stratton.

Siemon, M. (1984). Siblings of the chronically ill or disabled child: Meeting their needs. *Nursing Clinics of North America, 19*(2), 295–307.

Simeonsson, R., Buckley, Z., & Monson, L. (1979). Conceptions of illness causability in hospitalized children. *Journal of Pediatric Psychology, 4,* 77–84.

Sourkes, B. (1980). Siblings of the pediatric cancer patient. In J. Kellerman (Ed.), *Psychological aspects of childhood cancer*. Springfield, IL: Charles C Thomas.

Spinetta, J. (1980). Disease-related communication: How to tell. In J. Kellerman (Ed.), *Psychological aspects of childhood cancer*. Springfield, IL: Charles C Thomas.

Standiford, D., Ahlrichs, J., Carmicle, C., & Wells, P. (1993). Extended day program: Bringing preschool to the hospital. *Pediatric Nursing, 19*(3), 238–241.

Strauss, A., et al. (1984). *Chronic illness and the quality of life* (2nd ed.). St. Louis: CV Mosby.

Susser, M., & Watson, W. (1971). *Sociology in medicine* (2nd ed.). London: Oxford University Press.

Trahd, G. (1986). Siblings of chronically ill children: Helping them cope. *Pediatric Nursing, 12*(3), 191–193.

Vance, J., et al. (1980). Effects of nephrotic syndrome on the family: A controlled study. *Pediatrics, 65,* 948–956.

Vipperman, J., & Rager, P. (1980, March/April). Childhood coping: How nurses can help. *Pediatric Nursing,* pp. 11–18.

Walker, D., & Gortmaker, S. (1983). *Final report: Community child health studies* (Grant MC–R–25043). Springfield, VA: National Technical Information Service.

Weisman, A., & Worden, J. (1976). The existential plight in cancer: Significance of the first 100 days. *International Journal of Psychiatric Medicine, 7,* 1–5.

Zelter, L., & LeBaron, S. (1986). Fantasy in children and adolescents with chronic illness. *Developmental and Behavioral Pediatrics,* 7(3), 195–198.

CHAPTER • 20

Death and Dying

Darlene McCown

RELATED TOPICS
Communicating with Children and Families, Chapter 11
Stress, Crisis, and Coping, Chapter 18
Nursing Care During Hospitalization, Chapter 21
Community and Home Care, Chapter 22
Nursing Management of Pain in Children, Chapter 25

LEARNING OBJECTIVES

- **Explain the concepts of grief, mourning, and bereavement.**
- **Identify the major theoretical approaches used to describe the response to loss.**
- **Describe the development of death concepts.**
- **Recognize family responses to life-threatening illness and death of children.**
- **Identify nursing interventions to assist the family in coping with a child's terminal illness and death.**
- **Analyze the impact of caring for terminally ill children on the health care provider.**

Death touches each of us—even children. Death is usually associated with old age and is a subject people may try to avoid until they are faced with their own death or the death of their loved one. When the loved one is their child, the emotional upheaval created by the threat of loss or actual loss is immense.

Nurses assist family members in coping as they are faced with terminal illness, death, and the experience of grief. It is important for the nurse to understand the meaning of life-threatening illness and death to the child and parents, and how the family is affected by the loss of the child. This chapter presents an overview of the grieving process, children's concepts of death, the child and family's response to illness and loss, and the nurse's role in helping children and families cope with death and dying.

Definitions of Loss and Grief

The death of a loved one is followed by grief, bereavement, and mourning. "Bereavement" (from "bereave," meaning "to deprive of, to leave desolate") is the process of responding to the loss of a loved one. It has two primary aspects — grief and mourning (Averill, 1968). "Grief" reflects the intense emotional and physical feelings aroused by a loss. It is characterized by suffering, distress, sorrow, and regret and includes feelings of despair and bewilderment. Grief is an individualized process, and for this reason there is little agreement on a concept of "normal grief" (Rodgers & Cowles, 1991). Even the assumption that grief is time-limited is questioned by some (Horacek, 1991).

"Mourning" is the behavioral aspect of grieving, including expressions of sadness and weeping. Social and cultural practices associated with death are expressions of mourning. These societal rituals are believed to facilitate the mourning process.

Theoretical Approaches: The Grieving Process

Various theoretical approaches have been used to explain the process of grief. Whether the loss is an actual death of a loved one or the losses are associated with the process of dying, the grieving process is usually described by identifying stages, phases, styles, or tasks. Each of the following individuals has contributed to the present understanding of human response to loss.

Kübler-Ross' Stages of Dying

Elizabeth Kübler-Ross pioneered the study of individuals' responses to terminal illness (Kübler-Ross, 1969). Her classic work focused on dying adults, but the five coping strategies she identified have been observed in parents and family members facing a life-threatening illness in their child.

Denial and Isolation

The first stage, *denial and isolation,* begins with the initial diagnosis of a potentially fatal disease and is reflected in the response, "No, not me." Denial lessens the impact and allows time to adjust to the dreadful news of a life-threatening illness. It is temporary and gives way to a gradual awareness of reality. Facts and information given to the family during this phase often are not heard.

If possible, the nurse should be present when the family learns the medical diagnosis. The nurse helps the family during this period of anticipatory grieving by demonstrating an attitude of genuine concern and caring, by answering their questions, and by restating, interpreting, and clarifying the information given to them. The nurse's role at this time is to be supportive and ensure that the parents have adequate understanding of the situation in order to make decisions about treatment. Families in this phase may find it helpful to seek another opinion to confirm the medical diagnosis. The nurse's acceptance of the family's need to use denial (a typical characteristic of anticipatory grieving) without reinforcing it helps bring the child and family to a general awareness and psychologic adaptation to reality.

Anger

Anger occurs when denial can no longer be maintained. The parent demands, "Why my child?" This stage is associated with feelings of sadness, depression, guilt, and anger, and with somatic complaints. Guilt and anger are probably the most universal or typical reactions of parents when their child is dying. Parents need to be assured and reassured by the nurse that the child's illness is not their fault. Feelings of guilt may lead to many reactions that can cause problems for their dying child, one of which is the tendency for parents to become overly permissive or overly protective.

Anger is displaced in all directions. It is often directed at health professionals and healthy children. The family may refuse certain caregivers or particular aspects of treatment. The parents may feel they have lost control of their ability to provide the care needed by their child. The nurse helps them maintain control of as much of their child's care as possible, such as managing intravenous lines, tube feedings, and dressing changes. Participation increases parental competence and fosters feelings of closeness between the parents and their child. The demands of giving physical care also provides an outlet for emotional energy. Allowing for this kind of parental participation can alleviate some of the feelings of guilt, anger, and sorrow associated with anticipatory grieving.

In addition to the parents, the dying child and others observing the terminal illness may express anger and guilt in various ways. This anger may be expressed through open verbal hostilities or by withdrawal, rejection, or a variety of complaints. The nurse intervenes by allowing expression of angry feelings without compounding guilt.

Bargaining

Gradually, the dying child and family enter a period called *bargaining*. The person engages in an agreement that is an attempt to postpone death. The parents often set a specific time extension related to a particular event, such as starting school, a birthday, or a special day, like Christmas. Bargaining sets a deadline and includes a promise that one will not ask for more after the one favor. Bargains may be with God, the health team, or significant others. Dying children may bargain for a chance to go home. The nurse can help families make arrangements for specific activities or events.

Depression

As the process of dying demands more and more of the child and family, there comes a deep sense of loss and *depression*. Depression has two phases: reactive depression (thinking of past losses) and preparatory depression (thinking of impending losses). In "reactive depression," the concern is for loss of the happiness and joy experienced before illness (physical activity, body image, future development, and general sense of well-being). The "preparatory depression" phase is characterized by the knowledge of impending loss and separation from loved ones.

During the phase of depression, those experiencing death become quiet and sorrowful. Attempts to cheer and brighten their day are inappropriate — it is a time to be present and quiet so that their sorrow can be felt.

Acceptance

With *acceptance,* there is little interest in present or future activities. Children wish only for their parents to be present, and parents want each other or a significant other. The child and family are not happy, but not terribly sad. This is a time for tender, loving care, when touch, quietness, attention to comfort, and gentle handling become the avenues for communication. Take care not to abandon the family, but remain attentive to the needs for privacy, comfort, and meticulous physical care of the ill child.

Freud's Psychoanalytic View

The psychoanalytic view of grief emphasizes the human instinct toward life. The struggle of the neonate to breathe and to balance physiologic processes is an example of the drive for life. Psychoanalysts believe that individuals fear death and, consequently, develop grief as a symptom in response to the fear of death. Freud identified four major characteristics of mourning: dejection, lack of interest in the world, loss of capacity to love, and inhibition of activity (Freud, 1957). Freud saw grief as a departure from normal psychologic functioning and labeled it a pathologic condition.

Lindemann's Concept of Acute Grief

The concept of "acute grief" is based on Lindemann's (1944) work with 101 bereaved persons. In this population, a pattern of grief symptoms and responses became apparent. Common responses include the following:

- Sensations of somatic distress.
- Preoccupation with the image of the deceased.
- Feelings of guilt.
- Hostile reactions.
- Loss of usual patterns of conduct.
- Assuming behaviors of the deceased.

According to Lindemann (1944), grief is a normal response to the cessation of a social interaction. "Grief work" entails emancipation from emotional bondage to the deceased, readjustment to life without the deceased, and formation of new relationships. The nurse can help the family members accomplish grief work by encouraging them to face the pain and allow emotional expression of it.

Engel's Phases of Grief

Engel (1964) described four distinct phases of the grief process following a death.

Shock and Disbelief

The initial reaction is *shock and disbelief,* accompanied by a sense of numbness and immobility. As the reality of death and the meaning of associated loss penetrate one's consciousness, acute periods of anguish and pain are experienced.

Awareness

Awareness of the loss is often coupled with physical pain, emptiness, and anger. Crying typifies this period and appears to help the bereaved acknowledge the loss and the need for help by allowing a temporary dependent state. The inability to cry, according to Engel, interferes with the normal grief process.

Restitution

The third stage of grief is *restitution*. Cultural rituals, funerals, and visits with friends and family clarify the reality of the loss as well as provide comfort, activity, and support.

Resolution

As the reality of the death is accepted, *resolution* of the loss occurs. This phase takes place in stages. The bereaved feel a variety of emotions: a painful emptiness, a lessening of self-esteem, and difficulty in forming new relationships. Physical ailments similar to those experienced by the deceased may develop as a means of suffering and maintaining a bond with the deceased. Preoccupation with thoughts of the deceased range from a focus on the emotional loss experience to the physical aspects of the deceased. Gradually, a positive mental image of the deceased person develops. When the mourner's interest in new relationships and life returns, the grief process is completed. Evidence of successful healing is the ability to remember, comfortably and realistically, both the pleasures and the disappointments of the lost relationship. This stage is demonstrated by parents who return to the hospital for a visit several months or a year after the death of their child. A few moments spent with the family at these return visits, calling them by name, talking about their child, and acknowledging their specialness, contributes to their resolution.

Types of Grief

Grieving is a process that is not similarly experienced by all family members. Its character changes throughout according to the circumstances surrounding the loss. The closeness of a relationship, the duration of an illness and degree of suffering associated with it, and the suddenness of the event have an impact on the grieving process. Specific types of grief that may be associated with a loss are "anticipatory grief" and "resolving grief."

Anticipatory Grief

Anticipatory grief occurs prior to the actual loss, when the probability of the loss is realized. Unlike conventional grief, anticipatory grief has a definite ending point—the time of actual death. Conventional grief eases with time, whereas anticipatory grief increases to the point of death (Aldrich, 1974). Anticipation of the loss gives family members time to prepare and may actually give the bereaved more energy to cope at the time of death.

A study of children with cancer showed that both fathers and mothers experienced anticipatory grief (Koocher & O'Malley, 1981). The difference between mothers and fathers appears in the intensity and duration of feelings expressed. Mothers experienced stronger responses that extended over a longer period.

Anticipatory grieving, related to knowledge of the potential loss of a loved one, is a common human response. It would be considered a life process. As previously noted, the nurse can support the parents and other family members in the process of anticipatory grieving.

The nurse may care for dying children whose parents have grieved in anticipation and have begun to detach emotionally from the child prior to death. In such situations, the usually supportive family members are providing insufficient, ineffective, or compromised support, comfort, assistance, or encouragement to the dying child and to each other. The ability of the family to cope with the impending death in a supportive way is compromised. In these circumstances, family members may need assistance to understand their feelings and reactions. As parents express their feelings, nurses support the parents by explaining the normalcy of their feelings. Anticipatory grief is therapeutic since it allows time to say goodbye, express love, and fulfill the secret wishes exchanged in meaningful moments.

The nurse must remember that the death of a child is always unexpected and out of sequence with the expectations parents have for their children. Helping parents to find specific ways of parenting their child to the end is an important nursing intervention. Physical presence and holding and talking to the child will maintain a bond, relieve the parents' guilt, and provide comfort for the ill child.

Resolving Grief

Time is a great healer, but time alone is not enough to heal grief. Support in the days and months following a loss is needed to facilitate resolution of the loss and recovery. Social support systems can be both informal and formal. Friends, neighbors, and family surround the bereaved with *informal support* in the form of companionship, material assistance, such as food, and aid in decision making. Their empathetic understanding allows them to support the bereaved. The

TABLE 20-1
Community Support Groups

Candlelighters
Childhood Cancer Foundation
Suite 200
1312 18th Street NW
Washington, DC 20036 (202) 659-5136
Families of children with cancer

Compassionate Friends
P.O. Box 1347
Oak Brook, IL 60421 (312) 323-5010
Parents who have lost children of all ages

SIDS Support Groups
American SIDS Institute
275 Carpenter Drive
Atlanta, GA 30328 (800) 232-SIDS [(800) 232-7437]
Families following SIDS loss of an infant

SHARE
St. Elizabeth's Hospital
211 S. 3rd Street
Belville, IL 62222 (618) 234-2120
Perinatal loss in families

concepts of empathy and sympathy differ. *Sympathy* focuses on one's own feelings and projects those feelings to others. *Empathy* focuses on the feelings and experiences of the bereaved person; there is a loss of self with a concern and appreciation for the experience of the other. An empathetic person learns to vicariously experience and understand the feelings of another person. *Formal support* comes from organized groups, which preserve the societal responses to death and thereby facilitate and encourage the mourning process. Examples of self-help and death-related support groups that aid families in the grief process are presented in Table 20-1. The religious community is another source of comfort to the bereaved. It can offer answers to the questions of the ultimate meaning of life and thereby provide comfort and hope for the bereaved.

Grief resolution is a uniquely personal and often painful process. It requires emotional energy to let go of the familial relationship with a loved one and refocus on daily living. Facing loss *can* be a maturing experience, but if loss is denied or avoided, the individual may lose the opportunity to grow and may actually regress and experience dysfunctional grieving. In a recent study, 89 of 93 bereaved adolescents (96 per cent) identified at least one positive outcome following a death. The most common outcome was having a deeper appreciation for life, followed by greater caring for loved ones (Oltjenbruns, 1991).

If grief is not resolved before replacement of the loss, it may interfere with emotional investment in new relationships. Signs of complicated grief reactions have been categorized into four areas: (1) absent grief, in which no apparent feelings are observed, (2) distorted grief, in which anger and guilt are frequently displayed, (3) converted grief, in which the person shows symptoms of personal distress, and (4) chronic grief, in which a persistent pattern of intense grief continues (Wolfelt, 1991). The course of grief depends on the ability of the bereaved to do the work needed to separate from the lost object and invest in new interests. Recovery from grief begins at the point when the bereaved returns to normal activities with full capacity for pleasure and life.

The assumption that grieving must come to an end and that full detachment from the deceased is necessary for grief resolution has been challenged (Horacek, 1991). After reviewing the literature and clinical experiences, the Committee for the Study of Health Consequences of the Stress of Bereavement concluded that there is no clear fixed end point for the grieving process (Osterweiss et al, 1984). Furthermore, it was recognized that for many, the process continues for a lifetime and that adjustment can take place without a complete detachment from the deceased.

Development of Death Concepts

Children learn about death through the regular courses of life events and begin early to formulate a concept of death. Their understanding of death changes with developmental level, which generally corresponds to age. There is uncertainty about when a person develops the capacity to mourn the loss of a relationship. Some theorists speak of the "absence of grief" in children (Deutsch, 1937). Others advance the notion that mourning can be experienced early in childhood (Furman, 1964). According to Furman, preconditions for mourning include a concept of death and object constancy, both of which are developmental characteristics present by age 4 years. On the other hand, Wolfenstein (1966) presents the view that mourning cannot occur until after the adolescent experience of separation from the parents. In other words, not until the young person has been forced to give up the parental love object and childhood is past can true mourning occur.

Infants and Toddlers (Birth to 36 Months)

A child under 2 years of age is often described as unaware of death. However, Maurer (1966) suggests that awareness of death begins at birth, with the first physiologic struggles to obtain oxygen. Maurer contended that infant sleep/wake patterns and "peek-a-boo" games reflect infant awareness of states of existence and nonexistence.

For the young, dying infant, the experience can be one of solitude if his or her developmental requirement for a consistently available, loving person (intensified by the dying state) is not met. An infant under 4 months of age experiences a life-threatening health state primarily through overwhelming physical sensations. As the infant develops (4 to 12 months), she or he progressively experiences dying as a fear of separation and a recognizable, hurtful sensation. During the toddler years (12 to 36 months), children continue to lack understanding of death; as a child approaches 3 years of age, magical thinking makes a child think that death can be avoided or reversed.

During the process of dying, infants need a loving, consistent caregiver. Intervention, whether by the nurse or (ideally) by the parents, should provide safety, trust, and comfort. Development should be kept as normal as possible through tactile, auditory, and visual stimulation without overstimulation.

To prevent sensory-perceptual alterations, touch and sound provide valuable stimulation to the dying infant. The ill infant needs comfort from caring persons through gentle feeding, holding, rocking, and cuddling. Speaking softly before, during, and after procedures provides a sense of security.

Tapes of parents' voices can have an especially calming effect during their absence or when the infant appears anxious or restless. Singing softly or playing a music box is appropriate. The usual visual stimulation given any other child of this age should also be available to the dying infant. Placing the infant in the en face position when holding reinforces relationships with caregivers and reduces the sense of being alone to die.

All these caring tasks may best be performed by the parents, who know and love the baby, or who may need to learn to know and love the infant, before the death. These nurturing activities assist the parents to appropriately separate after the death.

The nurse caring for the dying infant does not necessarily give direct care to the infant but, rather, helps the parents provide care. The nurse reinforces their actions and decisions by teaching, counseling, and supporting them with verbal and nonverbal affirmation. Often, parents are supported solely by the nurse's presence.

Toddlers also need the closeness and loving care from those who are familiar to them. They can think of events only from their own point of view because of their egocentricity, and therefore cannot comprehend the finality of death. Although they may not express emotions about their impending death, they feel the threat of separation, intrusive procedures, and altered routine. They also are sensitive to the reactions of loved ones and can sense the seriousness of their illness through expressions of anxiety, fear, and sadness around them. When a loved one dies, they expect the person to return and may continue to talk about the deceased as though nothing happened. Open and honest communication, reinforcing the fact that the loved one will not return, helps the child to eventually adapt.

Preschoolers (3 to 5 Years)

Children between 3 and 5 years of age have a wide variety of ideas about death. They believe it is temporary and reversible (Nagy, 1948; Lonetto, 1980) and view it as departure or sleep.

Preschoolers are egocentric, believing the world revolves around them. Because of this, they are unable to differentiate self from the world or distinguish living from nonliving. Children at this age think the dead live on under new circumstances. They give life processes and thoughts to the dead. Death is generally associated with a lack of movement and with old age. Drawings of children aged 3 to 5 years show that they view death as male in gender (Lonetto, 1980). Preschoolers talk openly about death, indicating a lack of realization about its finality. They speak in fantasy about going to heaven on a cloud.

The course of a life-threatening illness is incongruent with all the landmarks young children are striving to achieve—autonomy, self-control, and initiative. As the illness progresses toward death, the 3- to 5-year old exhibits discomfort, anxiety over separation, regression, and fear because of loss of control due to irregular routines and repeated traumatic experiences. The greatest need of dying preschoolers is to be free from pain and fear of separation from their parents. It is the nurse's responsibility to relieve pain and to assure the presence of the child's parents, if at all possible, or to provide for consistency in care through primary nursing, if the parents are unavailable.

School-Age

6 to 9 Years

Children's thoughts about death at this age are based on their concrete perceptions. School-age children develop and reorganize their concept of death as they gain exposure to death and examine dead things. The dead fly on the windowsill, the dead plant, the squashed bug, the dog that was hit by a car on the road, the dead bird, the goldfish floating on its side in the fish tank, all stimulate questions about death. They move gradually from understanding death as a reversible, temporary phenomenon to one of irreversibility and permanence. School-agers develop generalizations based on observable events. They attribute specific characteristics to death and give it traits such as scary, dangerous, and mean. Death is associated with sadness and the old and sick. It comes in the night and snatches one away. Death is often identified with the dead object, not as a process (Fig. 20–1).

Children this age correctly relate biologic aspects of heart and lung activity with death and may find

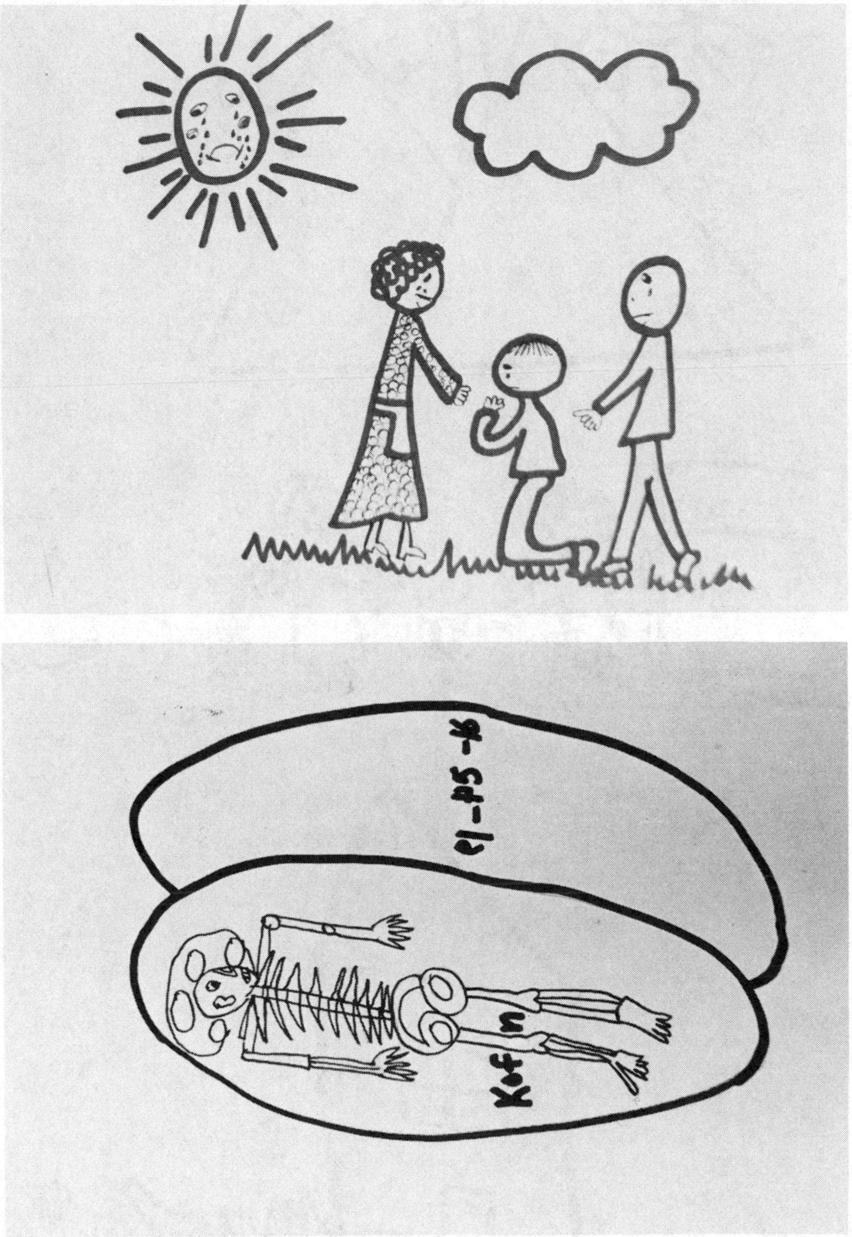

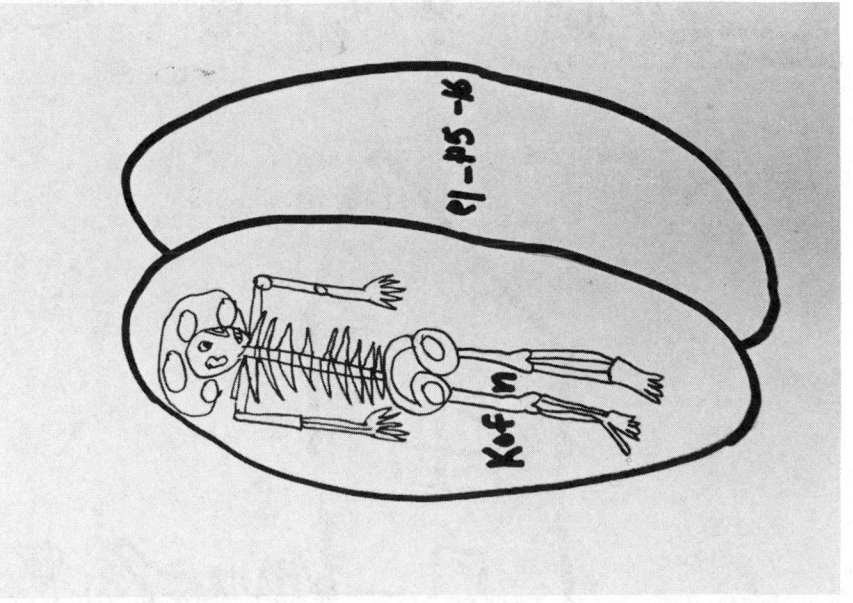

A

B

FIGURE 20-1. *A*, "A little boy dying on his front lawn—his mother and father are watching over him. They are sad. The sun is sad, too." *B*, "This is somebody dead." The school-age child is intrigued with the process of dying and with death. The two pictures illustrate a school-age child's concept of death. *(Figure continues.)*

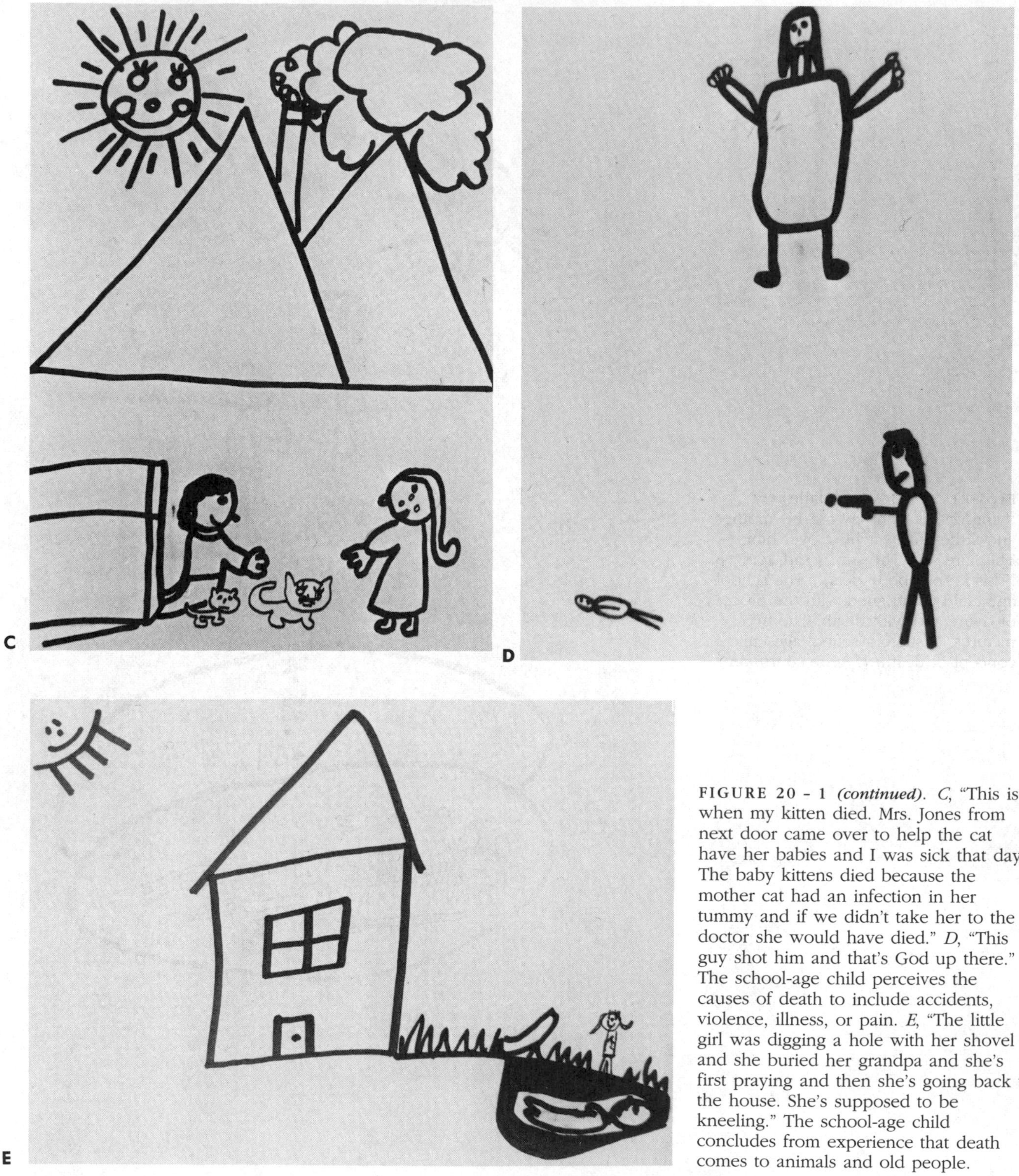

FIGURE 20 - 1 *(continued)*. *C*, "This is when my kitten died. Mrs. Jones from next door came over to help the cat have her babies and I was sick that day. The baby kittens died because the mother cat had an infection in her tummy and if we didn't take her to the doctor she would have died." *D*, "This guy shot him and that's God up there." The school-age child perceives the causes of death to include accidents, violence, illness, or pain. *E*, "The little girl was digging a hole with her shovel and she buried her grandpa and she's first praying and then she's going back to the house. She's supposed to be kneeling." The school-age child concludes from experience that death comes to animals and old people.

diseases involving these organs particularly frightening. They also focus on concrete aspects of burial and graveyards. Death is frequently linked to external forces and violence. Comfort comes from physical closeness with familiar people and things and with obeying the rules.

The nurse working with children this age may be faced with questions from the child about death—his or her own or that of others. Knowledge deficit regarding death and dying is frequently assessed as the etiology for the following nursing diagnoses: *fear, anxiety, impaired verbal communication regarding impending death, impaired social interaction and social isolation, altered family processes; ineffective individual and family coping, powerlessness, and hopelessness*. General questions about death can be answered truthfully and directly. The nurse must recognize that, unless the well-being of the child is in serious jeopardy, the *parents* must make the decision to discuss death with a child who has a life-threatening illness. They are the most effective providers of support to the child. The child can be reached and helped through the parents. Often, the decision clearly becomes one of *what* and *when* to tell rather than *whether* to tell. It is quite clear, though, that "who should tell" is the parents. The nurse can assist the parents to know what and how to explain a terminal illness and death to their child. Many resources for explaining death to children are available, some of which may be kept on a pediatric unit or in a clinic for parents to access. See Table 20–2 for a list of recommended books to use when explaining death to children.

The choice that most often proves harmful to the relationships, and that can result in a nursing diagnosis of altered family processes within the family, is maintaining a conspiracy of silence. This occurs if the family does not talk with the child about the reason for hospitalizations, treatments, or tests. During this process, the seriously ill child easily misinterprets what is happening and why it is happening, without an opportunity to validate perceptions or clarify the reasons for what is happening to her or his body. However, if the family relationship prior to the diagnosis of a terminal illness was fraught with difficulties and stress, it is unlikely that during this highly stressful time, the family will begin to communicate clearly. In fact, the added stresses may provide the stimulus for family disintegration.

10 to 12 Years

By 10 years of age, the child views death as inevitable and universal (Anthony, 1940; Nagy, 1948). It is a lawful process that happens to all living things. And, it is final. Children at this age reflect feelings of sadness, loneliness, and fear related to death (Maurer, 1966). Death becomes associated with pain as well as disease. Drawings by children at this age demonstrate progression of thought by the use of symbols, colors (black and purple), and details.

Adolescence

The response of adolescents to loss is particularly affected by their cognitive level of development. A model of adolescent grief developed by Fleming and Adolph (1986) relates loss to the tasks and conflicts of normal adolescent development. The three phases of development are (1) 11 to 14 years of age—emotional separation versus reunion; (2) 14 to 17 years of age—independence versus dependence; and (3) 17 to 21 years of age—closeness versus distance. The bereaved adolescent deals with issues that are common across the phases, but are reflective of the particular developmental level. The five core issues around which bereaved teen-agers attempt to gain resolution of personal conflicts characteristic of the age group are predictability of events, self-image, belonging, fairness/justice, and mastery/control (Fleming & Adolph, 1986). A full discussion of how each of these core issues are resolved is beyond the scope of this text. Following is a discussion of how selected core issues are resolved at the three phases of development.

Phase I: Conflict—Separation Versus Reunion

On the cognitive level, the adolescent aged 11 to 14 years recognizes that "I am different." Bereaved young teens may view the world as unsafe and feel vulnerable and recognize the unpredictability of events in life. They may be overly cautious or display risk-taking behaviors. With respect to their sense of belonging, they may believe that only peers understand them and seek peer support. Fairness and justice are issues in their search for an answer to "Why did my loved one die?" Protective or self-destructive

TABLE 20–2
Helpful Literature for Parents of Dying Children

Buscaglia, L. (1982). *Love*. Thorofare, NJ: Slack.

Colgrove, M., et al. (1977). *How to survive the loss of a love*. New York: Bantam Books.

Easson, W. (1981). *The dying child: The management of the child or adolescent who is dying*. Springfield, IL: Charles C Thomas.

Grollman, E. (1990). *Talking about death: A dialogue between parent and child* (3rd ed.). Boston: Beacon Press.

Knowles, D., & Reeves, N. (1991). *But won't Granny need her socks?* Dubuque, IA: Kendall/Hunt.

Kübler-Ross, E. (1985). *On children and death*. New York: Macmillan.

Kübler-Ross, E. (1974). *Questions and answers on death and dying*. New York: Macmillan.

Kushner, H. (1983). *When bad things happen to good people*. New York: Avon.

behaviors may be noted as evidence of the conflict about separation. Finally, as an attempt to master the event, the dead person is idealized, or perhaps characteristics very different from those of the survivor are attributed to the deceased.

Phase II: Conflict—Independence Versus Dependence

The middle adolescent sees the world from the perspective of "I can do anything," yet the conflict of independence versus dependence is evident in their bereavement behaviors. Teens between ages 14 and 17 years know that the world is unsafe and that they are vulnerable. They will face the situation with a response of independent action and risk-taking behaviors. They feel that they can handle the event, but fear loss of competence in the situation. These young people perceive that *belonging* to a group enhances their self-confidence so they seek peer recognition and approval. Many times teens have a sense of not belonging and feelings of being misunderstood. A feeling of mastery over the death is sought by believing that the teen-ager can do anything. This is indicated by intense academic and social pursuits. These children may assume additional responsibilities in an effort to show that they are capable of self-protection.

Phase III: Conflict—Closeness Versus Distance

The older adolescent, aged 17 to 21 years, operates from the cognitive principle "I can trust." This idea is disrupted with the realization that the world is unpredictable and that they cannot protect their loved ones from death. They attempt to overcome this by investing in another person in order to gain affection and safety. The *self-image* of adolescents may be threatened, and they may feel alone and isolated. They may experience a profound need for belonging in another's life. Their sense of justice may force an answer to the question, "Why?" Older adolescents may feel that they cannot risk or trust because of the threat of losing the other to death.

The adolescent at all phases of development experiences marked physical and emotional changes; these periods of rapid change are often times of vulnerability to fears and loss. Fears of death are especially acute for teens. Adolescents live in the present and future, which contributes to the impact of death as a forthcoming event. They go to extremes to challenge their fears by feats of bravado and daring. Like adults, teens understand death as a final, universal, and personal experience.

Dying adolescents fully understand what is happening to them. They struggle to find ways to accept the process. The experience of dying for teen-agers is completely incongruent with all they find important; physical appearance and prowess are replaced by dysfunction and weakness. Adolescents may react to a terminal illness with extreme anger, which drives away those they need most.

The nurse needs to recognize that overt behaviors often are not a true expression of the adolescent's needs. The nurse can encourage family and friends to maintain a supportive relationship with the teen. Peer relationships among hospitalized youth can be facilitated for mutual support and understanding. The nurse needs to allow time to just sit quietly and respond to the teen-ager. The dying, young person needs time and a trusting atmosphere that will allow facing the fact that death is happening.

The dying adolescent needs to be treated as autonomously as possible, since she or he is usually struggling to remain as independent as possible during this period of high stress. Noncompliance may be interpreted as an attempt to control self-care or as an attempt to deny the seriousness of the condition. Patience and support must be provided during this time. Parents may also be feeling a great deal of ambiguity as they try to support the independence of the adolescent and also do "what is best." They may feel extreme frustration, leading to a nursing diagnosis of *decisional conflict,* in trying to reach both these goals. Information about the disease process, treatment plans and rationale, and prognosis is essential to the adolescent at this time. The realities of the situation must be made explicit so that informed decisions about care and self-care may be made. Some parents take on the role of decision maker at this time. They become overprotective and actually set *limits to the behavior that they consider unacceptable.* Many adolescents need the security that these parameters provide, whereas others need to be able to make their own decisions regarding the quality and length of their lives.

Adolescents may find that they sometimes need to become dependent on their parents again, and they may be very angry, even enraged, at the injustice, asking, "Why me?" and declaring, "It isn't fair." The nurse can assist the adolescent and family to accept the somewhat unpredictable expressions of anger that are usually projected toward the staff and parents. By identifying the normality of the behavior under the circumstances, the nurse provides support to the family unit. The nurse can also provide opportunities for the adolescent to make decisions about self-care. The nurse can deliberately ask for the youth's opinions, suggestions, preferences, or choices. Whenever possible, these choices and preferences should be honored, thereby assisting the dying adolescent in the quest for independence and self-respect. If the death occurs in the hospital, it is helpful to discuss with the other adolescents their feelings and to explain what happened.

Explaining Death to Children

Numerous resources are available to assist parents in the task of discussing death with their dying child.

The nurse has an obligation to help parents become aware of the aids that do exist. Parents should be encouraged to begin by evaluating their own feelings about death. This introspection helps them know and understand their own feelings and fears before dealing with their child's ideas and emotions. Personal beliefs, religious orientation, cultural background, and level of comfort with the topic will influence the parents' responses to the dying child and to questions. The ultimate decision of what to tell the child must be left up to the parents. Recent research reveals parents disclose less information to children under 9 years of age with cancer than to older children, but that both groups of children report similar levels of distress (Claflin & Barbarin, 1991). Because adults tend to protect and shelter children from knowledge of or experiences with death, the decision to discuss the diagnosis of a life-threatening disease with a child is an overwhelming task for many parents. The nurse should also be aware that communication patterns of families are affected by cultural factors, making some families less inclined to disclose information about life-threatening illnesses (Munet-Vilaro & Vessey, 1990).

During the toddler and preschool years, parents can use the opportunity to explore death through natural events such as the death of a grandparent as well as the death of a pet or even a bug. Such discussions help the child to verbalize questions. Reading aloud books that discuss death or include death experiences may be another alternative for children this age. This provides information to the child and also encourages discussion between parent and child. Helping parents recognize the importance of openness and honesty with this age group is an important nursing intervention. Young children are adept at sensing inconsistencies between verbal and nonverbal messages. Fabricating stories or attempting to conceal real feelings arouses considerable anxiety in toddlers and preschoolers, and threatens the child's sense of security. Parents should also be helped to realize that children of all ages need to mourn and express their feelings in ways similar to those of adults.

How to tell the school-age child about the diagnosis of a life-threatening disease partly depends on the child's cognitive skills and previous experience. The nurse assesses the child's ability to understand those concepts necessary to comprehend death and assists parents as they provide information to the child. The nurse or parents may use questions to elicit the child's understanding of various components of the concept of death. During the discussion with the child, clarification can be provided and family values/beliefs reinforced.

At times, children's perceptions about a previous experience with death may differ from those of parents. Often parents assume that the child was too young to remember when a friend, family member, or pet died. Some questions to determine previous experience with death, such as "Did you ever have a pet that died?" and "Did you ever know a person who died?" are appropriate. Some children assume that someone is dead who has not been seen or heard from. One young school-age child, for example, was asked in a Denver Developmental Screening Test (DDST) to complete the analogy "Mother is a woman, Dad is a ________." After a few moments of thought, the child answered "soul." The mother was very shocked since the father was not dead, but the parents had been separated for a year and a half. The perception could then be clarified. Questions to help determine the child's knowledge of death include: "What happens after something dies?" "What does 'die' mean?" "Does it hurt to die?" "What do people do after they die?" Misconceptions about death can then be corrected depending on the child's responses. Books to help parents explain death to children are listed in Table 20–3.

Death Education

Parents and close family members exert a major influence on children's understanding of and reaction to death. Preparation for understanding death begins in the first years of life with the early experiences of separation from loved objects and people. Awareness of death grows as the child experiences the deaths of plants and pets. Responses to these losses and emotional recovery should not be avoided, but encouraged. Children often imitate funeral rituals of burial and graveside when a pet dies. These activities provide a chance to practice grief behaviors and say goodbye to the cherished pet. Enactment of such behaviors releases energy for emotional growth and the formation of new relationships.

Loving and caring for a pet may be a step toward deeper love, care, and assuming responsibility for another. Animals are nonjudgmental companions. They can become a sounding board for thoughts and feelings unable to be expressed to human ears. Humans often develop close, affectionate relations with companion animals. The relatively short life span of animals increases the opportunity for experiences of death and loss of the pet. Children are particularly vulnerable to being emotionally affected by the loss of a pet because it may be their first experience with death of a loved object. Immediate attempts to replace lost animals should be avoided because these tend to devalue the sanctity of life and the uniqueness of each relationship. After resolution of grief, the child will be able to welcome a new animal and a new relationship.

Family Response to Impending Death of a Child

Parental Response

If the final diagnosis forecasts a poor prognosis and a threat to life, the parents may respond with shock

TABLE 20-3
Books for Children about Death

Preschool to Age 7 Years

Brown, M. W. (1965). *The dead bird.* Reading, MA: Addison-Wesley.

A group of children find a bird and feel that its heart is not beating. They have a funeral for it before returning to their play. Each day they return to the bird's grave. They continue this ritual of mourning "until they forget."

Fassler, J. (1983). *My grandpa died today.* New York: Human Sciences Press.

A description of Grandpa slipping away to a peaceful death in his rocking chair is presented. Knowing his Grandpa was not afraid to die, David is able to cope with his grief and get on with his life.

Powell, S. (1990). *Geranium mornings.* Minneapolis: Carolrhoda Books.

The book gives information about feelings when a parent dies.

Rogers, F. (1988). *When a pet dies.* New York: Putnam's Sons.

Thomas, J. (1988). *Saying goodbye to grandma.* Boston: Clarion.

Viorst, J. (1971). *The tenth good thing about Barney.* New York: Atheneum.

The rituals of burial and mourning are observed for Barney, a pet cat. The child is led to understand that dying is as usual as living. Death is a part of life.

Zolotow, C. (1974). *My grandson Lew.* New York: Harper & Row.

Remembrances are shared between Lewis and his mother, making them a little less sad.

Ages 8 to 11 Years

Lee, V. (1972). *The magic moth.* New York: Seabury.

A very supportive family bravely copes with 10-year-old Maryanne's illness and death from a heart defect. The story tells the problems that had to be overcome for the family to work together. A moth bursting from its cocoon as Maryanne dies and seed sprouting just after her funeral symbolize that "life never ends—it just changes."

Miles, M. (1971). *Annie and the old one.* Boston: Little, Brown.

Excellent book for children.

Rofes, E. (1985). *The kids' book about death and dying.* Boston; Little, Brown.

This book is written by kids for kids. It answers questions children ask.

Smith, D. B. (1973). *A taste of blackberries.* New York: Harper & Row.

A little boy's best friend, Jamie, dies of a bee sting. The boy is confronted with grief because of the loss and comes to terms with a guilty feeling that somehow he might have saved Jamie. After a period of grief, the boy comes to accept Jamie's death.

White, E. B. (1952). *Charlotte's web.* New York: Harper & Row.

This is a story about a pig and a rat and their friendship with Charlotte, a spider. Charlotte's death and the birth of her child depict the life cycle. A classic.

Age 12 and Over

Buscaglia, L. (1982). *The fall of Freddie the leaf.* Thorofare, NJ: Slack.

Good book for all ages—both children and parents.

Gunther, J. (1971). *Death be not proud* (Memorial edition). New York: Harper & Row.

The author writes of the courage of his 17-year-old son while facing death. It is more difficult for his parents than for Johnnie to accept his death.

Hunter, M. (1972). *A sound of chariots.* New York: Harper & Row.

Bridie McShane's happy childhood during World War I in Scotland is interrupted by the death of her beloved father. As she matures, her life is marred by her sorrow, leading her to morbid reflections on time and death, which she finally learns to deal with through her desire to write poetry.

LeShun, E. (1986). *When a parent is very sick.* Boston: Little, Brown.

Zindel, B., & Zindel, P. (1980). *A star for the latecomer.* New York: Harper & Row.

A story about a teen-ager whose mother has advanced bone cancer. The daughter tries to become a star in a theatrical career before her mother dies.

and denial in the first stages of anticipatory grieving. The nurse helps them by providing a private place to recover from the impact of the terrible news and stays with them and participates as the health care team together answers their questions about the diagnosis and plan of care. Attitudes of warmth and concern and competence in providing the necessary care are important in helping families cope with the situation. Parents may also need assistance to seek out supportive friends and family who can be with them during this difficult time.

Some expression of anger, hostility, and guilt may be expected. Such feelings may be directed at the nurse, but should not be taken personally. Parents may need the help of nurses and other professionals to verbalize these feelings. As parents and older children become interested in the illness, they seek information and details about it. Parents will feel saddened as the information obtained indicates a poor prognosis and the likelihood of death. The nurse needs to recognize that the strong emotions of *anger, hostility, fear, guilt, and anxiety* experienced by the parents may cause a change in the parenting style with both their ill and their well children. Parents can be helped to understand their own behavior and be supported in their attempt to maintain their usual patterns of child care.

Guilt

Guilt is a common feeling experienced by parents of dying children. One study reported that one third of their families experienced guilt feelings (Stehbens & Lasacari, 1974). Parents often try to recall minor symptoms of the child that they overlooked and blame themselves for not seeking care sooner. They reflect on earlier events, even pregnancy, searching for reasons for their child's illness. Guilt may result in blaming one's spouse or overindulging the ill child. Parents may experience guilt after the child is dead for several reasons: (1) an ambivalent relationship while the child was alive, marked by hostility, (2) a previous desire for the child's death, (3) feelings of anger at the deceased for dying, and (4) a wish that more had been given of oneself while the child was living (Goldberg, 1973).

Relinquishing Authoritarian Role

When a child is diagnosed to have a life-threatening condition, health care personnel are granted authority in the life of the child because of their knowledge and expertise. Even the ill child transfers authority to the medical staff. Parents may feel they are losing control of their child and their parental role. Relinquishment of their parental role may explain parenting behaviors frequently observed, such as lack of discipline, permissiveness, and even neglect.

Changing Behavior Patterns

Parents may cater to or overindulge the ill child to maintain a role in the child's life and relieve their own guilt and sadness. Fear of separation surfaces, and the parents may actually cling to their child. When a child is dying, the mother's perceptions of the child's needs may be altered. In a study of 21 children and their mothers, dying children's self-perceived needs for affection, control, and inclusion were examined (Natterson & Knudson, 1960). Children with life-threatening illnesses wanted additional affection, but were unable to express this desire directly, and mothers of dying children tended not to perceive their child's needs accurately. At a time when children need understanding to help overcome the great losses they are experiencing, mothers may be unable to perceive the needs accurately. Nurses should be aware of the possible existence of the nursing diagnoses *altered parenting* and *potential altered parenting* during these times. Assessment for the defining characteristics and risk factors of these diagnoses will allow the nurse to assist the parent to create an environment that promotes the child's optimal growth and development. Nurses can point out clues that the child gives and suggest ways to meet the child's needs, such as holding, gentle touching, rubbing, and talking softly to the child.

Gender-Based Response

Fathers and mothers do not react to their child's illness and death in the same way. Parents may experience the process of mourning differently and sense a lack of support and understanding from each other. This has been labeled the "isolated wife" syndrome. It is also indicative of altered family processes. The child's mother often feels she carries the whole burden of the illness. Such feelings place a stress on the marital relationship, and the parents need to make a special effort to spend time together and each alone with the ill child to maintain relationships. The nurse can offer to stay with the child while the parents have a reprieve and can be together. Hospital policies, which allow open visiting and play activities for siblings, decrease separation of family members.

Role Adjustments

Caring for a terminally ill child demands tremendous energy and results in parental fatigue, which further compromises their relationship. They need assistance from supportive friends and relatives and are encouraged to plan time away from the demands of the situation. The stress placed on families requires altered patterns of living and a shift in expectations. The illness causes many changes, ranging from financial problems to changes in social status because of increased social isolation. Problems with siblings may arise because *of the time required* of parents to care for the ill child. The well sibling's perception of the mother as having limited time leads to feelings of hostility and rejection, especially when there is poor understanding of the child's illness. Further breakdown of relationships can occur because children may "protect" their parents from sadness by not talking about the dying child. All of the factors discussed constitute risk factors for the nursing diagnosis *altered role performance*. Often the nurse can assist family members by demonstrating the use of techniques to manage or alleviate role strains.

Grandparents' Response

During severe stress, parents may need the help and emotional support of the grandparents. In a 2-year study of 46 parents of children with cancer, grandparents tended to be less accepting of the diagnosis than the parents (Friedman et al, 1963). Reasons for grandparent difficulty with the dying child may include a fear of their own impending death; they may also feel guilty that it is not they who are facing death, but the child; they may be blaming their daughter or son, or daughter-in-law or son-in-law, for the child's ill health. All these emotions can interfere with their ability to support and help the adult children cope while their child is dying.

Following a child's death, the grief of grandparents is experienced at three levels: for their grandchild, for their adult child and family, and for themselves. A study of grandparent grief (Ponzetti & Johnson, 1991) indicates that grandparents experienced the classic grief symptoms mentioned earlier. Most grandparents expressed a need to talk about the grandchild following the death. The nurse can help grandparents grieve in a functional manner by encouraging discussion of the child's death and by listening to the grandparents. It is also important to remind the child's parents to acknowledge the importance of the death for grandparents.

Dying Child's Response

The dying child's reaction to the illness is influenced by the developmental stage of the child. Children's major concerns vary with age. The child, prior to 5 years of age, fears separation from the parent. A child 5 to 10 years old fears traumatic procedures, whereas children over 10 years of age fear death itself.

Illness and physical degeneration are a paradox for the growing, developing child. A limited awareness of life itself makes a child vulnerable to anger and resentment toward parents for allowing the hurt and suffering associated with illness and death. These feelings have been reflected in a play situation in which dying children placed distance between themselves and their families (Bluebond-Langer, 1978). The child's anger toward the parent and others or withdrawal from or clinging to the parent contribute to difficult parent-child relationships. The loss of physical function, increased dependency, and regression of the dying child further compromise the relationship because of the tendency of parents to overprotect and indulge their child at this stage.

Research using projective techniques (Waechter, 1971) and interviews (Bluebond-Langer, 1978) has demonstrated that dying children are aware of their fatal illnesses. Indications of the child's awareness of the terminal illness include a lack of interest in the future, fears of being at home and a desire to be in the hospital, decreased conversations about medications, and comments about others who have died (Bluebond-Langer, 1978). Parents need help to recognize these behaviors and need support from the nurse to establish open communication with their child to allow for exchange of love and concern and expression of fears and anxieties. Some parents are not amenable to open discussions of death. The nurse may be aided by the use of assessment tools such as the Childhood Death Awareness Inventory (Table 20–4) to introduce the topic in a neutral and nonthreatening manner. Parents' wishes need to be respected and taken into consideration.

Sibling Response

Siblings of dying children may exhibit behavior problems such as crying, school problems, somatic complaints, nightmares, death fears, enuresis, depression, excessive talking, and antisocial behavior. Research using standardized measures of behavior problems indicates that about one fourth of the siblings of deceased children have "disturbed" behavior following the death; boys and girls seem to be equally affected (McCown, 1987).

Qualitative research by Kramer (1987) of 11 healthy siblings of children dying of cancer revealed both negative and positive responses. The negative impact on the siblings resulted from three primary sources of stress: emotional realignment within the family, separation from family members, and disruptions caused by the ill child's therapeutic regimen. Emotional deprivation, decreased parental tolerance, and increased parental expectations directed at siblings contributed to emotional realignment. Lack of information, decreased family involvement, and insufficient social support resulted in feelings of separation. Watching the ill child's physical and personality changes, seeing the anxiety and pain, and adjusting to changes in family routine contributed to the negative impact of the therapeutic regimen. Positive aspects for surviving siblings included increased sensitivity and empathy for the ill child, personal maturation, and an increase in family cohesion.

Nurse's Role in Assisting the Family to Cope with Terminal Illness

Facilitating Effective Family Coping with the Length of the Illness

The parents' grief reaction and pattern of adaptation will depend a great deal on the course of illness. The progression of events leading up to the death has an impact on the parents' ability to cope. Unexpected death and anticipated death are each associated with a different set of stresses for parents.

Sudden or Unexpected Death

If the death of their child is sudden and unexpected, a variety of shock responses can be anticipated, ranging from immobilization or hysteria to complete control of the situation. Although their reactions vary, it is clear that family members do not fully comprehend

RESEARCH ISSUES
Siblings of Dying Children

Results. The effects of sibling death on surviving children has been studied from a variety of perspectives. The sample sizes of the studies vary from 12 to 65. Methods include both quantitative and qualitative measures. All but Birenbaum and co-workers (1989–1990) were retrospective studies focused on description of the effect of sibling death on the well child.

The cumulative findings support the conclusion that children who experience the death of a sibling have a higher incidence of problems. These problems are generally those associated with adult grief responses—loneliness, confusion, sleeping and eating problems, poor school performance. Approximately one fourth to one third of bereaved siblings demonstrate behavior problems above the norm on standardized tests. Furthermore, the grief behaviors extend well beyond the conventional first year after the death. Martinson (1991) reports that the negative effects of sibling death continue as long as 7 to 9 years after the event in one of six adolescent survivors.

Implications. It is clear that siblings of dying children are in need of preventive nursing interventions designed to provide emotional support and encourage expression of feelings and concerns. Research attention needs to be directed toward the identification and development of interventions that address the needs of surviving siblings.

REFERENCES

Birenbaum, L., Robinson, M., Phillips, D., Stewart, B., & McCown, D. (1989–1990). The responses of children to the death and dying of a sibling. *Omega, 20,* 213–228.

Davies, B. (1991). Long-term outcomes of adolescent sibling bereavement. *Journal of Adolescent Research, 6,* 83–96.

Lauer, M., Mulhern, R., Bohne, J., & Camitta, B. (1985). Children's perceptions of differential adjustment. *Cancer Nursing, 8,* 21–27.

Martinson, I., & Campos, R. (1991). Adolescent bereavement: Long-term responses to a sibling's death from cancer. *Journal of Adolescent Research, 6,* 54–59.

McCown, D., & Pratt, C. (1985). Impact of sibling death on children's behavior. *Death Studies, 9,* 923–935.

what is communicated during this shock stage. Once the shock begins to diminish, they have a strong need to communicate their feelings regarding what has happened. The nurse may be the only person available to help the grievers work through their feelings and thoughts about what has occurred. Because they have not had time to prepare for the death, they are deprived of the advantages of anticipatory grief. They also may feel great remorse or guilt for not having done things differently for their child. The nurse may be able to comfort them physically and psychologically through touch, active listening, or providing a comfortable, private place for the family to grieve.

Ways to help families cope vary according to family needs. Interventions available to nurses working with families following sudden loss of a child include providing information and emotional support (Murphy, 1990). Providing *information* about cognitive deficits, loss of relationships, role changes, and emotions associated with loss was found to be useful. Also, bringing people with similar losses together to share their experiences provided *emotional support.*

Anticipated Death

If the death is not immediate, but the child lingers days or weeks, family members may begin their anticipatory grief work, if they have accepted the diagnosis and are encouraged to mourn. On the other hand, a long-term life-threatening illness brings additional stresses, such as relapses and repeated hospitalizations. These events subject parents to severe emotional stress. They not only have to live with the uncertainty of the future but also must provide care for the child while they are actively mourning the expected death.

Several strategies are effective with these parents to direct their anticipatory grief into constructive actions. One is to encourage parents whose children have the same medical problems or prognosis to meet in groups. Within the group, reactions, fears, and feelings are shared with others who have experienced or are experiencing them. Support groups are helpful for some families, but not for others. Information about the groups can be made available to parents so they can decide whether they wish to participate.

Participation in the care and planning of their child's treatment is another effective strategy. Mothers may be more willing than fathers to enter into these activities, but the most benefit accrues when both parents are involved in the care. When parents are a part of the plan, their anxiety, guilt, or anger subsides; they usually become more cooperative, outgoing, and accepting of the treatment. Parents' wishes and desires regarding the care of their child should be respected; they should be allowed to take part in determining whether certain treatments should be continued if there is little hope for improvement. Parents need to be given the option to take the child home to die if they feel no cure is possible. If they choose to take their child home, parents are informed about possible problems (pain, incontinence) or com-

TABLE 20-4
Childhood Death Awareness Inventory

Family Name ______________________ Date ______________

Address ______________________

Child's Name ______________________

Age __________

Name of Deceased ______________________

Age __________

Relationship to Child ______________________

Date of Death ______________________

I. *Child's Experience with Death*

What experiences has the child had with death?

a. Pet(s) __________ Date of death __________

Child's reaction and comments:

____

____

b. Distant relative __________ Date of death __________

Name ______________________

Relationship ______________________

Child's reaction and comments:

____

____

c. Close relative __________ Date of death __________

Name ______________________

Relationship ______________________

Child's reaction and comments:

____

____

d. Friends __________ Date of death __________

Name ______________________

Relationship ______________________

Child's reaction and comments:

____

____

e. Community (teacher, pastor, schoolmates)

Name __________ Date of death __________

Relationship ______________________

Child's reaction and comments:

____

____

II. *Rituals of Death*

a. Has the child seen a dead person? Yes ___ No ___

b. Has the child seen a dead animal? Yes ___ No ___

c. Has the child attended a funeral or memorial service? Yes ___ No ___

d. Has the child visited a cemetary? Yes ___ No ___

TABLE 20-4
Childhood Death Awareness Inventory (Continued)

III. *Beliefs about Death*

a. What beliefs about death are held by the child?

b. What beliefs about death are held by the family?

c. Is the child familiar with the church (synagogue) buildings? Yes ___ No ___

IV. *Explanation of Death*

a. What has the child been told about the (possible) death?

b. What has the child been told about the disposal of the body?

c. What has the child been told about the final services (funeral, memorial service)?

V. *Expected Reaction*

a. How do you expect (child) to respond to the loss?

b. What adjustments will be difficult for the child?

VI. *Supportive Measures*

a. What actions will comfort your child?

b. Who are the people who can help your child? Have you notified them of the possible death/death?

c. What literature have you read about death and grief?

d. What questions do you have about your child and death?

From McCown, D. (1988). Helping children face death in the family. *Journal of Pediatric Health Care, 2,* 14–19.

plications they may experience at home, but are assured that someone will be available if help is needed.

Helping Siblings Cope with Life-Threatening Illness

The nurse working with dying children assesses and discusses with parents their responsibilities to their other children. It is important to promote healthy relationships for all family members to return to after the child has died. The Death Awareness Inventory (Table 20–4) may help parents focus on and recognize their well children's level of understanding about death and possible responses to it. Using the information gathered on the inventory, the nurse can discuss with the parents methods for explaining the situation to the well children. Also, stressing that quality of time spent with their children is more significant than quantity may alleviate the guilt parents experience in trying to divide their attention and time equally among the children. Parents are encouraged to be honest and open with their children and to reassure them of their love. Siblings may be fearful of having wished the child ill or dead or of becoming sick like their sibling. Expression of these fears should be encouraged through open communication with the parents.

After the death, siblings may also need help with the ongoing hostility they feel toward the dead child who took so much time from their parents. To dissipate this hostility, siblings may need to talk to parents, the nurse, or counselors about it. They need to be reassured that this hostility and these feelings are normal and that they are not bad for feeling them.

The deceased child's toys, books, and clothing may be shared with surviving siblings. Young children (those with the concept of the reversibility of death) may be afraid that the deceased child will return to reclaim the toys. Parents may need help understanding that the sibling's concern is characteristic of a young child's way of thinking about death.

Siblings may need time to think about what has happened with the family. They may need reassurance that they will not also die of the disease that has claimed brother or sister, unless, of course, they also have a genetically caused disease. If this is the case, special follow-up help will be needed as the children prepare for their own life and death.

The interactions of parents with siblings may change after the death of one child. They may become overprotective of the surviving children. The sadness that they feel is of a different nature than the sadness of the siblings. Parents may mourn well beyond the time that siblings are actively mourning, and unconscious anger may develop toward the siblings.

Decision to Discontinue Treatment

At some point, the health care team caring for a child with a life-threatening illness may suggest discontinuation of treatment because of the lack of response to medical therapy. This decision is made in conjunction with the family. There may also come a time when the family reaches this decision before the health care team mentions it. The family may request no further treatment so as to avoid further pain, frustration, or stress for their child. This decision is actually a statement that the family is giving up hope for survival, an acceptance of death as an inevitable end. It is also based on the realization that the child is not responding to treatment.

This is always a difficult decision for the family and for the health team. The nurse may help to coordinate a meeting including clergy, ethicists, teachers, family, and medical team members to provide multiple perspectives on the decision to terminate treatment. Respect for the quality of the child's remaining life must be the basis of the decision. Ultimately, the choice must be the family's. The nurse can be supportive to the family during this difficult decision making time by helping them clarify their own thoughts so that they can feel comfortable in their decision.

Decision for Home Care

The option of receiving supportive care and symptom management care, in a hospital or in the home, should be discussed with the family. Some communities have community-based programs or hospice groups to provide home care for dying children and adults. The hospice concept is that when the goal of curing cannot be realized, appropriate places other than the traditional hospitals can provide vital care during this critical time. Some cities provide hospice care to families of dying children by providing space within their hospitals; others set special places aside, such as an extended care facility. Some hospice programs are essentially home care programs. Nurses in the community are currently providing support to parents who are caring for their dying children in their own homes. Allowing a child to die in the home permits the family to design and control the environment and enables them to make themselves available to the dying child without removing themselves from their other children.

Criteria developed by Martinson and colleagues (1980) offers guidance to parents considering the option of home care. An assessment is made to determine whether the following conditions have been met:

- Cure-oriented treatment has been discontinued.
- Child wants to be at home.
- Parents desire to have the child at home.
- Parents recognize their own ability to care for their ill child; the fact that they can care for the child until death is frequently not recognized until later.
- Nurse is willing to be available 24 hours a day to facilitate care.

- Child's physician is willing to be an on-call consultant.

Making the decision to care for the dying child at home is extremely difficult. During the dying process, the parents may sometimes feel inept at providing the best care possible; they may wonder about their decision and may feel guilty that their child is not in the hospital. Inability to relieve pain is often a major reason why parents feel they cannot care for their child in the home, but, with proper instruction and support, pain management can be achieved. Medications for the relief of pain, in either oral, rectal, or parenteral form, are available to the family.

Helping Families Cope During the Final Stages of Illness

At this time, some families may begin to redirect their energies away from the child, whereas others will continue to hold on to the child until the final breath. In either case, their fears of death and pain are overwhelming. Often the greatest fear is that their child is experiencing pain. Although the child may appear comfortable, it is important to understand that the parents' anxiety may also reflect their sense of inevitable loss. Providing the child maximal comfort and relief of pain during this period is critical. Pain management in children is discussed in Chapter 25: following is a discussion of common problems associated with dying.

Common Physical Problems

Maintaining adequate nutrition leads to increased energy levels and improved physical appearance, which contribute to a sense of well-being in the ill child and family. Ill children who are dying should be allowed to eat whatever they desire. Special attention to diet may be needed to ensure comfort in regard to intake.

Nausea and Vomiting

Nausea, vomiting, and fullness are frequently associated with the terminal process and the treatment, especially if the child receives chemotherapy and radiation. Nausea and vomiting may result from obstruction of the digestive tract from physical defects or tumor or from imbalances in body fluids and electrolytes. The combination of nausea and vomiting is a common side effect of the drugs used to control many diseases.

Nausea and vomiting can be treated in part by diet. Dry foods, such as crackers, plain cookies, or toast, decrease nausea, especially in the morning. Other approaches to reduce nausea and vomiting are avoiding fried or greasy foods and offering cold, clear liquids that are easier to retain, and frequent, small quantities of food. Large amounts of food in the stomach at one time should be prevented by reducing liquids at mealtime and offering them an hour before or after meals. Have the child lie down or sit quietly after meals to aid the digestive process.

In addition to diet, medications are available to relieve nausea and vomiting. Antiemetics, such as one of the phenothiazines, can be useful and can be given rectally as well as orally.

Anorexia

Anorexia is loss of the desire for eating, often experienced by seriously ill persons. Decreased appetite may be caused by alterations in smell and taste mechanisms. Food may become associated with the unpleasantness of nausea and vomiting resulting from drugs and disease. Lack of appetite may occur from decreased activity levels and general depression of mood or an alteration in taste sensation.

Some people with life-threatening illnesses find protein foods bitter to the taste, but its ingestion should be encouraged for nutritional requirements. A metallic taste may be experienced by those on medications or chemotherapy. The taste of foods can be enhanced by adding seasonings like lemon, salt, sugar, spices, and herbs. Protein intake may be encouraged by serving the food cold or at room temperature. Cheese, pizza, luncheon meats, eggs, and puddings are easily served cold and are palatable to children. Marinating meats in fruit juices may also help. Providing small meals frequently, varying the type of food, serving it in "fun" ways, such as clown faces and animal shapes—all may increase nutritional intake for children.

High-calorie, high-protein nutritional supplements are available to increase the child's daily intake. Fruit flavors and chocolate are preferred by children. Supplements, such as Instant Breakfast, Sustocal, or Ensure, are easy to prepare but tend to be filling. These preparations taste better cold and can be enhanced by the addition of eggs or yogurt. Recipes for using supplements are available from the manufacturers of the products.

Vitamins may be added to the child's diet. If the child is on methotrexate, vitamins (without folic acid*) should be used. The ethical implications of possibly prolonging a dying child's suffering by adding supplements to the diet need to be explored with the family and health care team.

Constipation

Constipation is inability to evacuate the bowel or difficulty in passing stool. Ill children are at high risk for constipation due to disease processes, muscle weakness, decreased activity levels, medications, and diets low in fluids and fiber. Normal bowel patterns vary widely and range from three stools per day to three stools per week.

Management of constipation in the seriously ill child is best achieved by preventive interventions. Maintaining a diet sufficient in fluids and fibers and

*Methotrexate is a folic acid antagonist.

encouraging activity and regular toilet patterns assist in passing stool. This is especially difficult in anorexic young children. Oral stool-softening agents such as dioctyl sodium sulfosuccinate may be useful to keep the consistency of the stool soft enough for defecation. Glycerin suppositories may also aid stool passage by mechanical action. Chemical laxatives and enemas should be judiciously used, in consultation with the health care team.

Anemia

Anemia is a frequent problem for dying children, especially those with cancer. It may be caused by loss of blood, destruction of red blood cells by medications, and decreased production of red blood cells by the disease or treatment processes.

A diet high in iron and proteins is one measure that can be instituted at home. Often, however, blood transfusions are needed to increase the child's hemoglobin and hematocrit to normal levels. A child who is anemic will experience fatigue, decreased energy, lethargy, and irritability.

Terminal Phase

The parents of a dying child need information about the events leading to death so they can be prepared for the final moments. Many times, exhausted parents, not realizing the immediacy of the death, have gone home to rest or out to eat when the event occurs. It is difficult for nurses and doctors to predict the exact time of death, but certain signs usually precede it (Birenbaum et al, 1986). One sign of death in children is a change in normal respirations to a Cheyne-Stokes pattern (breathing with apneic periods of 10 to 60 seconds followed by gradually increasing respirations). Dying children often become less alert, and periods of wakefulness decrease. They may be difficult to arouse; their eyes are glazed and may roll back. The child's skin color becomes poor, often mottled, and cool to touch. Muscle tone decreases, and the child may become incontinent. Hearing is one of the last senses to fade, so the child may be comforted by hearing the parents' voices. Semi-comatose, dying children have been observed orienting to the mother's or father's voice in the final hours of life. If possible, parents should be encouraged to stay and comfort their child during this period, until the death occurs.

Organ and Tissue Procurement

Recent years have brought dramatic improvements in the success of organ transplantation. As these changes take place, the nurse's responsibility with the family of a dying child also changes. It is important for nurses to keep abreast of the federal and state laws that affect practice. Appropriate educational opportunities need to be made available to prepare nurses for these new responsibilities.

As the technology for organ transplantation advances, there is an urgent need for organs; the organs needed far outnumber those made available. Government has responded to the pressing need for transplantable organs by establishing laws dealing with procurement of organs. Hospitals have developed protocols that deal with organ transplantation and tissue procurement, although regulations vary. Many states require that a request be made for organ donation from family members of all patients pronounced "brain dead," whereas others require that hospitals notify local organ procurement agencies of any potential organ donors.

Enactment of laws concerning organ and tissue procurement has created ethical dilemmas and imposes a difficult responsibility on nurses. As these laws go into effect, nurses will be increasingly involved in dealing with families regarding the sensitive issue of organ and tissue donation. Nurses are often the best-known team member to families because they have spent the most time with them during their child's illness and hospitalization. Although it is a difficult task to approach a family about organ donation, it is known that parents who agree to donate their child's organ may have their own grief lessened by helping another child (Frauman & Miles, 1987).

As organ donation becomes more widespread, the need for organs will continue to increase. Areas in which the nurse needs educational opportunities include brain death criteria (Drake et al, 1986; Volpe, 1987; AAP, 1987), the specific responsibilities of the nurse (Hazinski, 1987), statutes that regulate organ donation, and a forum in which to discuss ethical issues related to organ procurement and donation (Bouressa & O'Mara, 1987). In the United States, a publication that reviews state-by-state legislation is updated annually,* and government information can be obtained from the Office of Organ Transplantation†. See Chapter 40 for discussion of brain death criteria.

After Death

After death, the body should be cleaned, carefully positioned, and covered with a blanket for viewing and goodbyes. The parents may assist in these preparations if they wish. It is a difficult time for both the parents and the nurse. It is appropriate for the nurse to express emotion and share feelings of sorrow with the family. However, total loss of control by the nurse would add a burden on the grieving family and is inappropriate. The final goodbyes may take time, and the nurse may face the dilemma of needing to remove the body and get the room ready for the next

*South-Eastern Organ Procurement Foundation (SEOPF), 3001 Hungary Spring Road, P.O. Box 28060, Richmond, VA 23228.

†Federal Register Department of Health and Human Services, Office of Organ Transplantation, Washington, DC—(301) 443–7577.

patient. The family should not be hurried when spending time with the body. Their behavior should be accepted without judgment, as part of the grief response.

An autopsy on the child will reveal answers to questions about the cause of death. It also aids physicians in obtaining exact knowledge about the disease process. By giving permission for an autopsy, parents may feel that they are contributing to medical science, which may give meaning and value to their child's death.

Helping Surviving Children

Telling about the Death

Children deserve a factual and accurate account of the death. This will help them develop a clear, real picture of the cycles of life. It will help give them an appreciation for life. The unpleasant details of death can be minimized, but not avoided. The parent may explain how the child died, what happened to the body, and discuss the plans for a funeral or memorial service. The parents can share their philosophic beliefs as well as feelings of loss and grief. Words like "went to sleep" and "God took" should be avoided, since the child may come to fear sleep as well as fear and distrust a God who destroys loved ones.

Expressing Feeling

Grief is new to children, and they may need help in expressing their feelings. Four tasks that grieving children face are as follows: (1) to make sense out of what has happened, (2) to express emotional response to loss, (3) to commemorate the loss through some type of remembrance, and (4) to learn how to go on with life (Corr, 1991). The parent should be encouraged to express sorrow and shed tears in a controlled manner when talking about the death to siblings. (Hysterical crying decreases the child's sense of security.) Many children do not cry; they should be allowed to, but not forced. They should be encouraged to ask questions if they desire. Opportunity for indirect expression of feelings through physical exercise and creative play should be provided and encouraged. Doll house items and paper, crayons, or painting materials, as well as music, poetry, and stories, allow emotional expression. It may be comforting for surviving siblings to give a gift to the deceased and place it in the casket. The surviving children and parents need private time alone with each other following a death. This allows grieving parents the chance to assure the surviving children that they too are loved and cherished equally as much as the one that is mourned.

Funerals

Should surviving children attend the funeral? Some experts say "yes" because the funeral allows children to see first-hand the reality of the death, and they may receive comfort and support from friends. A sense of closure may be helpful (Salladay & Royal, 1981; Scholwalter, 1976). Children's fantasies regarding the funeral event may be much worse than the reality. On the other hand, some studies of children and funerals show that behavior problems may develop that are related to funeral attendance (McCown, 1984). Children under 7 years of age and girls are particularly sensitive to funeral activities. This does not mean that children should not attend funerals, but it does indicate that they should be given a choice, and, if they attend, they need preparation. They should be told what they will see and what is expected. A close, friendly adult should stay with the child during the funeral service and provide encouragement and an explanation of the ritual. The adult must feel comfortable in answering difficult questions from the child, such as "Can I touch him?" and "Why is she cold?" Children and adults need to know it is OK to laugh and play at funerals. After the funeral, children need an opportunity to discuss the events. If a child chooses not to attend the funeral, he or she may go to the funeral home or church to say a private goodbye to the loved one.

Guidelines

Several clear guidelines for helping surviving children with death can be summarized:

- The child should be encouraged to discuss, ask questions, and express feelings about death.
- A specific pattern of grief behavior should not be imposed on the child.
- Adults in the child's world should feel free to cry and to share their feelings of sadness with the child in a controlled manner.
- Time with the child and loved adults should be set aside in the days immediately following the death to assure the child of her or his value and importance.
- The caretaking needs of the child should continue to be met by a warm, loving person.
- The child should be given a choice regarding funeral attendance; other important people (e.g., teacher, doctor, coach) in the child's life should be told of the death.
- The child should be allowed and encouraged to resume normal activities directly following the death.
- At each new cognitive developmental level, the child will need to review and reinterpret the death in light of a new understanding of death.

Nurse's Response to Dying Children and Death

The severe stress placed on the entire family continues to have a profound impact after the death of a child. It is critical that hospital staff continue their involvement and support during the period after death, if possible. Parents often complain that, after their child has died, they are forgotten by the staff. This period is characterized by intense grief and mourning, during which the family may also renew socialization, reorganize, and make decisions. Nurses may or may not be associated with the family during this period. They may wish to share in the funeral services or public memorial services. Phone calls, letters, or visits to the family may be appropriate and therapeutic. Whether nurses stay connected with a family after a death depends on the relationship prior to death. Yearly memorial services by the hospital or hospice or home care facility help staff to adjust to the losses experienced in their personal and professional life.

Recognizing Their Own Needs

The greatest disservice that nurses can do to themselves and a dying child and family is to disregard their own personal needs. A recent survey of 100 hospice nurses identified both losses and rewards experienced by hospice caregivers (Adams et al, 1991). Among the losses were loss of co-workers and loss of concepts and ideals key to hospice philosophy. The identified rewards of hospice care occurred when the nurse was able to be part of a peaceful death and establish a trusting relationship with the family. Appreciation and support of co-workers and families was also noted as rewarding. Certain factors were found to alleviate the stresses of working with dying patients. Self-awareness and introspection were most frequently identified as helpful techniques. These techniques included activities such as retreats, church involvement, journaling, painting, crafts, gardening, and being with children and animals. Another important helpful feature was to "celebrate and appreciate life."

Feelings of Nurses

Nurses experience a myriad of feelings in caring for a dying child. A particular child may remind nurses of their own child or a relative or close friend's child. The illness causing the suffering may remind nurses of an experience within their own family. Thus, the dynamics of each parent-child-nurse relationship are unique, and when death is imminent, the feelings that emerge are intense and stressful.

Nurses cope with stress in a manner similar to that of the child and family. Denial is used for protection from the reality of impending death. Real feelings are suppressed and a facade of "all is well" pervades in dealings with the child, family, and health team members.

Anger and guilt are commonly felt by nurses who care for a dying child. In our culture, these are results of the sentiment that it is a tremendous injustice when a child suffers or dies. Nurses may direct anger toward God, or they may blame parents for not seeking treatment earlier. When nurses are struggling to accept the death of a child, they may become intolerant of the many questions and demands from parents. Anger may also be directed toward the physician or toward themselves for not being able to cure the child. Nurses may feel guilty because painful procedures need to be done, the child is hurting, and yet there is no hope. These feelings of anger and guilt emerge out of sensitive, caring nurses who are groping to right the wrong.

Nurses' Expressions of Grief

People express grief according to their own styles of coping. Grief expression by nurses also varies according to the degree of involvement with a particular child and family, a variation that must be respected from one nurse to another. Grief needs an outlet such as the health care team, in which support is ready-made, if "stuffy professionalism" does not thwart the process of grieving. The pretense of successful coping can seriously hamper the grieving process among professionals.

Nurses need to become increasingly aware of the toll of accumulated loss. An entire staff can become depressed and lose sight of their goals if grief remains unresolved. Opportunities must be provided for nurses to share their feelings and anxieties about working with special families in stress. Support systems cannot be left to each individual's personal contacts, such as family and friends. These contacts are usually not prepared to hear out the feelings and expressions regarding a child who is dying. Professional support groups must be deliberately planned—institutional grief cannot be left to resolve itself. These periods of professional sharing should be ongoing, so that feelings during the process of death as well as after the death can be shared.

If nurses can ventilate their feelings in an atmosphere of openness, the child and family will gain. The sensitive exchange of feelings may bring to light that a nurse needs a period away from a particular child and family. The nurse who cares enough about the child and family is willing to take the professional risk of reaching out for help to face a new day; it may mean a temporary change of assignment to a work environment away from dying children.

Nurses must take an active role in planning group sessions. Group members can be asked to privately respond to a group of statements and then provide an opportunity for the sharing of feelings. A suggested list of statements for nurses to respond to is listed in Table 20–5. Statements with reference to a

TABLE 20-5
A Nurse's Feeling about Caring for a Dying Child: Statements for Nurses to Respond to in a Group Session

1. I expect to feel uncomfortable when I have to talk to a dying child and to the family
2. I feel at a loss to know what to say, especially when the child and family are aware that death is imminent
3. I cannot imagine that anyone is ever free of the fear of dying
4. I think I can help a child and family cope with the reality of death
5. I am frightened at the thought of caring for a dying child
6. I am afraid the child will ask me whether she or he is dying
7. I feel terrible about causing tiny discomforts during a treatment when I know a child is dying anyway
8. I feel I have to hide my own feelings of sadness so as not to make the child and family feel upset
9. If I cry with a child or family member it disturbs me for the rest of the day
10. I don't really have anyone to tell how I feel about (child's name) suffering

particular situation could easily be developed by the primary nurse to facilitate sharing of personal needs and feelings about experiences with other families.

Sharing of feelings and personal difficulties in regard to care of the dying brings human experiences into focus. Nurses who respect their own humaneness recognize that they are vulnerable to the same feelings of denial, anger, fear, depression, and grief that the family experiences. If nurses can support each other during this process, the pain for caring for a dying child and the family can be experienced rather than repressed (Fig. 20-2). When nurses feel the pain of loss, they can provide what the child and family need—the presence of a human being.

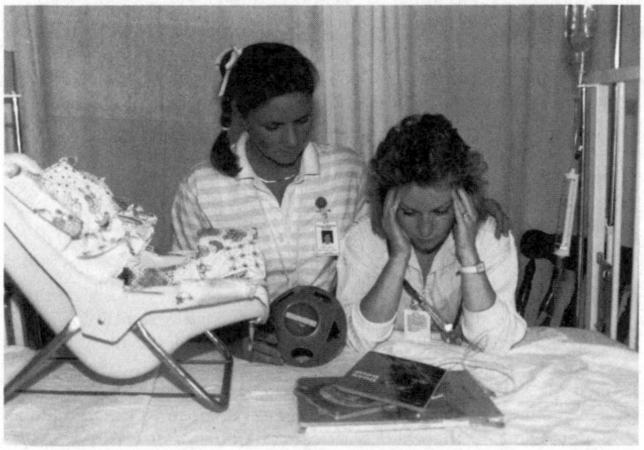

FIGURE 20-2. There is a strong sentiment in our culture that it is a tremendous injustice when a child suffers or dies. When given the needed support from another nurse, this nurse can acknowledge her own struggle in dealing with the death of an infant.

KEY CONCEPTS

Concepts Related to Basic Information

- Grieving, mourning, and bereavement are interrelated concepts with overlap in meaning. Their slightly different meanings have been described as follows: *grief* is the emotional and physical feeling aroused by a loss; *mourning* is the behavioral aspect or the expressions (e.g., societal rituals) of grief; and *bereavement* represents the process of responding to the loss of a loved one.
- Children prior to the age of 5 years cannot understand the irreversibility of death. Therefore, they think that the deceased is living under new circumstances.
- The child prior to 5 years of age fears separation from the parent; a child 5 to 10 years old fears traumatic procedures; and children over 10 years of age fear death itself.

Concepts Related to Nursing Assessment

- There is no clear fixed end point for the grieving process, and adjustment can take place without a complete detachment.
- The nurse must assess the child's perception of death and the personal meaning of the child in the family to provide support during life-threatening illness and death.
- Personal beliefs, religious orientation, cultural background, and level of comfort with the topic of death are important variables to assess when working with parents of dying children.

Concepts Related to Nursing Intervention

- The decision of discussing death with a dying child belongs to the parents; nurses help parents to know what and how to explain terminal illness and death to their child.
- When parents can be included in the plan of care, their anxiety, guilt, or anger subsides; parents need to be given the option to take the child home to die.
- Siblings need special attention to dissipate feelings of guilt or hostility; they may be fearful of having wished the child ill or dead.
- Physical problems associated with dying require special attention in trying to achieve comfort; pain, nausea and vomiting, anorexia, constipation, and anemia are common problems.

- Organ and tissue procurement are governed by regulations; each nurse who cares for dying children should be aware of these regulations as they affect his or her work setting.

REFERENCES

Adams, J., Hershatter, M., & Moritz, D. (1991, May/June). Accumulated loss phenomenon among hospice caregivers. *American Journal of Hospice and Palliative Care,* 29–37.

Aldrich, C. (1974). Some dynamics of anticipatory grief. In B. Schoenberg, et al (Eds.), *Anticipatory grief.* New York: Columbia University Press.

American Academy of Pediatrics, Task Force on Brain Death in Children. (1987, August). Guidelines for the determination of brain death in children. *Pediatrics, 80,* 298–300.

Anthony, S. (1940). *The child's discovery of death.* New York: Harcourt Press.

Averill, J. (1968). Grief: Its nature and significance. *Psychological Bulletin, 70,* 721.

Birenbaum, L., McCown, D., & Nunneley, C. (1986). *Nurses manual for family childhood cancer study.* Portland: Oregon Health Sciences University.

Bluebond-Langer, M. (1978). *The private worlds of dying children.* Princeton, NJ: Princeton University Press.

Bouressa, G., & O'Mara, M. (1987). Ethical dilemmas in organ procurement and donation. *Critical Care Nursing Quarterly, 10,* 37–47.

Claflin, C., & Barbarin, O. (1991). Does "telling" less protect more? Relationships among age, information disclosure, and what children with cancer see and feel. *Journal of Pediatric Psychology, 16,* 169–191.

Corr, C. (1991, July/August). Support for grieving children: The Dougy Center and hospice philosophy. *American Journal of Hospice and Palliative Care,* 23–27.

Deutsch, H. (1937). Absence of grief. *Psychoanalytic Quarterly, 6,* 12–22.

Drake, B., et al. (1986, July). Determination of cerebral death in the pediatric intensive care unit. *Pediatrics, 78,* 107–112.

Engel, G. (1964). Grief and grieving. *American Journal of Nursing, 64,* 93.

Fleming, S. J., & Adolph, R. (1986). Helping bereaved adolescents: Needs and responses (pp 97–118). In C. A. Corr & J. N. McNeil (Eds.), *Adolescence and death.* New York: Springer.

Frauman, A., & Miles, M. (1987, December). Parental willingness to donate organs. *ANNA Journal, Dec.*

Freud, S. (1957). Mourning and melancholia (pp 243–258). In J. Strachey (Ed. and Trans.), *The standard edition of the complete psychological works of Sigmund Freud. (vol. 14).* London: Hogarth Press.

Friedman, S., Chodoff, P., & Mason, G., et al. (1963). Behavioral observations of parents anticipating the death of a child. *Pediatrics, 32,* 610–625.

Furman, R. (1964). Death and the young child. *Psychoanalytic Study of Children, 19,* 321–333.

Goldberg, S. (1973). Family tasks and reactions in the crisis of death. *Social Work, 5497,* 398–405.

Hazinski, M. F. (1987, September/October). Pediatric organ donation: Responsibilities of the critical care nurse. *Pediatric Nursing, 13,* 354–357.

Horacek, B. J. (1991). Toward a more viable model of grieving and consequences for older persons. *Death Studies, 15,* 459–472.

Koocher, G., & O'Malley, J. (1981). *The damocles syndrome.* New York: McGraw-Hill.

Kramer, R. F. (1987). Living with childhood cancer: Impact on the healthy siblings. In J. Krulik, B. Holaday, & I. M. Martinson (Eds.), *The child and family facing life-threatening illness.* Philadelphia: JB Lippincott.

Kübler-Ross, E. (1969). *On death and dying.* New York: Macmillan.

Lindemann, E. (1944, September). Symptomatology and the management of acute grief. *American Journal of Psychiatry, 101,* 141–148.

Lonetto, R. (1980). *Children's conception of death.* New York: Springer-Verlag.

Martinson, I., et al. (1980). *Home care for the child with cancer—Final report.* National Cancer Institute Grant CA1 9490. Minneapolis: University of Minnesota.

Maurer, A. (1966). Maturation of concepts of death. *British Journal of Medical Psychology, 39,* 35–41.

McCown, D. (1984). Children cremation and funerals. *Journal of Death Education, 8,* 349–363.

McCown, D. (1987). Factors related to bereaved children's behavioral adjustment. In C. Barnes (Ed.), *Recent advances in nursing series: Caring for sick children.* London: Churchill-Livingstone.

McCown, D. (1988). Helping children face death in the family. *Journal of Pediatric Health Care, 2,* 14–19.

Munet-Vilaro, F., & Vessey, J. (1990). Children's explanation of leukemia: A hispanic perspective. *Journal of Pediatric Nursing, 5,* 274–282.

Murphy, S. (1990). Preventive intervention following accidental death of a child. *Image: Journal of Nursing Scholarship, 22,* 174–179.

Nagy, M. (1948). The child's theories concerning death. *Journal of Genetic Psychology, 73,* 3–27.

Natterson, J. H., & Knudson, A. (1960). Observations concerning fear of death in fatally ill children and their mothers. *Psychosomatic Medicine, 22,* 456–465.

Oltjenbruns, K. (1991). Positive outcomes of adolescents' experience with grief. *Journal of Adolescent Research, 6,* 43–53.

Osterweis, M., Solomon, F., & Green, M. (Eds.). (1984). *Bereavement: Reactions, consequences, and care.* Washington, DC: National Academy Press.

Ponzetti, J., & Johnson, M. (1991). The forgotten grievers: Grandparents: Reactions to the death of grandchildren. *Death Studies, 15,* 157–167.

Rodgers, B. L., & Cowles, K. V. (1991). The concept of grief: An analysis of classical and contemporary thought. *Death Studies, 15,* 443–458.

Salladay, S., & Royal, M. (1981). Children and death: Guidelines for grief work. *Child Psychiatry and Human Development, 11,* 203–212.

Scholwalter, J. (1976). How do children and funerals mix? *Journal of Pediatrics, 89,* 139–142.

Stehbens, J., & Lasacari, A. (1974). Psychological follow-ups of families with childhood leukemia. *Journal of Clinical Psychology, 30,* 394–397.

Volpe, J. J. (1987, August). Brain death determination in the newborn. *Pediatrics, 80,* 293–297.

Waechter, E. (1971, June). Children's awareness of fatal illness. *American Journal of Nursing, 71,* 1168–1172.

Wolfelt, A. (1991, March/April). Toward an understanding of complicated grief: A comprehensive overview. *American Journal of Hospice and Palliative Care,* 28–30.

Wolfenstein, M. (1966). How is mourning possible? *Psychoanalytic Study of the Child,* 21, 93–123.

BIBLIOGRAPHY

Balk, D. (1991). Death and adolescent bereavement: Current research and future directions. *Journal of Adolescent Research, 6,* 7–27.

Blechar Gibbons, M. (1992). A child dies, a child survives: The impact of sibling loss. *Journal of Pediatric Health Care, 6,* 65–72.

Bossert, E., & Martinson, J. (1990). Kinetic family drawings—Revised: A method of determining the impact of cancer on the family as perceived by the child with cancer. *Journal of Pediatric Nursing, 5,* 204–213.

Burns, C. (1992). A new assessment model and tool for pediatric nurse practitioners. *Journal of Pediatric Health Care, 6,* 73–81.

Corr, C., & McNeil, J. (1986). *Adolescence and death* (pp 97–118). New York: Springer-Verlag.

Gardner, S. L., & Merenstein, G. B. (1986). Helping families deal with perinatal loss. *Neonatal Network, 5,* 17–33.
Garland, K. R. (1986). Grief: The transitional process. *Neonatal Network, 5,* 7–10.
Garland, K. R. (1986). Unresolved grief. *Neonatal Network, 5,* 29–37.
Grogan, L. B. (1990). Grief of an adolescent when a sibling dies. *American Journal of Maternal Child Nursing, 15,* 21–24.
Hoekstra-Weebers, J. E. H. M., Littlewood, J. L., Boon, C. M. J., Postma, A., & Humphrey, G. B. (1991). A comparison of parental coping styles following the death of adolescent and preadolescent children. *Death Studies, 15,* 565–575.
Krulik, T., Holaday, B., & Martinson, I. M. (1987). *The child and family facing life-threatening illness.* Philadelphia: JB Lippincott.
Kuntz, B. (1991, January/February). Grief has no color. *American Journal of Hospice and Palliative Care, 8,* 35–37.
Leahey, M., & Wright, L. M. (1987). *Families and life-threatening illness.* Springhouse, PA: Springhouse Corporation.
Martinson, I. M., et al. (1987). The long-term effects of sibling death on self-concept. *Journal of Pediatric Nursing, 2,* 227–235.
Miles, M. (1985). Emotional symptoms and physical health in bereaved parents. *Nursing Research, 34,* 76–81.
Moody, R. A., & Moody, C. P. (1991). A family perspective: Helping children acknowledge and express grief following the death of a priest. *Death Studies, 15,* 587–602.
Morgan, J. D. (Ed.). (1991). *Young people and death.* Philadelphia: Charles Press.
Noppe, L., & Noppe, C. (1991). Dialectical themes in adolescent conceptions of death. *Journal of Adolescent Research, 6,* 43–53.
Papadatou, D., & Papadatos, C. (Eds.). (1991). *Children and death.* New York: Hemisphere Publishing.
Parry, J. K., & Thornwall, J. (1992). Death of a father. *Death Studies, 16,* 173–181.
Petix, M. (1987). Explaining death to school-age children. *Pediatric Nursing, 13,* 394–396.
Rapheal, B. (1983). *The anatomy of bereavement.* New York: Basic Books.
Report of the Task Force on Organ Transplantation. (1986, April). *Organ transplantation: Issues and recommendations.* Washington, DC: Department of Health and Human Services, Office of Organ Transplantation.
Rondo, T. (1986). *Loss and anticipatory grief.* Lexington, MA: Lexington Books.
Schowalter, J. E. (1986). Twenty years of pediatric thanatology. *Child Health Care, 14,* 157–162.
Schwab, R. (1990). Paternal and maternal coping with the death of a child. *Death Studies, 14,* 407–422.
Schwab, R. (1992). Effects of a child's death on the marital relationship: A preliminary study. *Death Studies, 16,* 141–154.
Small, M., Engler, A. J., & Rushton, C. H. (1991). Saying goodbye in the intensive care unit. *Pediatric Nursing, 17,* 103–105.
Smith, I. (1991). Preschool children "play" out their grief. *Death Studies, 15,* 169–176.
Stroebe, M., & Stroebe, W. (1991). Does "grief work" work? *Journal of Consulting and Clinical Psychology, 59,* 479–482.
Swoiskin-Schwartz, S., et al. (1988). Parents' views about having a child after a SIDS death. *Journal of Pediatric Nursing, 3,* 24–28.
Tung, T. (1990, September/October). Death, dying and hospice: An Asian-American view. *American Journal of Hospice and Palliative Care,* 23–25.
Wass, H., & Corr, C. (Eds.). (1984). *Children and death.* New York: Hemisphere Publishing.

UNIT • FIVE

Managing Illness

CHAPTER • 21

Nursing Care During Hospitalization

Astrid Hellier Wilson

NURSING PROCESS PLAN
Nursing Process Plan: The Hospitalized Child, Table 21–5

RELATED TOPICS
Therapeutic play, Chapter 17
Stress, crisis, and coping, Chapter 18
Impact of chronic illness, Chapter 19
Principles of patient education, Chapter 23
Administering medications, Chapter 24

LEARNING OBJECTIVES

- **Describe the major stressors affecting children at different ages while being hospitalized.**
- **Discuss coping mechanisms used by children at different ages to adapt to the stress of hospitalization.**
- **Discuss the balancing factors and their influence on hospitalized children at different ages.**
- **Compare and contrast different methods of preparing children for the hospital experience.**
- **Discuss how the social environment, physical environment, and admission procedures can facilitate a child's adaptation to being hospitalized.**
- **Identify key concepts in preparing children at different ages for intrusive procedures.**
- **Discuss the nurse's role in assessing hospitalized children at different ages using baseline data, ongoing assessments, and nursing diagnoses.**
- **Describe nursing planning and interventions for selected nursing diagnoses related to hospitalized children and their parents.**
- **Describe the nurse's role in teaching clients/family members to prepare for discharge from the hospital.**

Hospitalization can be a stressful experience for anyone; however, the stress easily can be compounded for children because of their lack of understanding of what is happening to them. New caretakers, different routines, fears, and separation from familiar people and places are factors that can interfere with a young child's development. Older children and adolescents may find hospitalization intimidating because of separation from peers, threats of the unknown, and vulnerabilities pertaining to their body image.

The experience of hospitalization can have numerous effects on children and their family members such as emotional and developmental damage, interference with school and work responsibilities, and the need to shift priorities. Nurses can reduce stress and promote development among families by properly managing a child's hospitalization.

Scope of the Problem

Nurses who care for children can attest to the diverse responses exhibited by both children and their parents when a child becomes hospitalized. Families respond very differently to what seem to be similar circumstances. Of utmost importance in caring for hospitalized children and their families is recognizing that each child and family unit entering the hospital brings a unique set of experiences and relationships that results in a wide range of responses.

The impact of hospitalization on children and their families has been studied for over 50 years and crosses several disciplines. A consistent problem that researchers encounter is the number of variables that affect the experience of hospitalization and the difficulty in defining and measuring the outcome of interest. Variables that can be hard to differentiate and measure are psychologic upset/anxiety (Beyer & Frick-Helms, 1992; Byrne & Cadman, 1987) and fear/anxiety (Broome et al, 1988; Gottlieb, 1990). A general belief prevails that hospitalization causes anxiety and distress in children and their families, even though further research is warranted, especially because of the dramatic changes in technology and acuity level of sick children (Kodadek et al, 1989). Some children have the resilience to actually benefit from being hospitalized and may show maturation in their coping skills. The concern for the well-being of children in hospitals is apparent in the numerous clinical approaches instituted to prevent adverse effects of hospitalization (Brazelton, 1992).

An appreciation for the evolution of child care in hospitals can be gained by reading the numerous reviews that appear in the literature (Bates & Broome, 1986; Thompson, 1985). Part of the evolution of care rendered to hospitalized children is a response to research findings. Some important variables thought to affect a child's response to hospitalization are:

- Child's age.
- Type and amount of preparation.
- Length of hospitalization.
- Frequency of hospitalization.
- Previous relevant experience.
- Child's temperament.
- Coping abilities of the child and parents.
- Parent-child relationship.
- Reason for hospitalization.
- Hospital environment (e.g., visiting policies, child care approaches, play programs).

In response to knowing the variables that influence children's reactions to hospitalization, preventive strategies have been developed by health care professionals. Five main preventive strategies instituted are: (1) preparation for hospitalization; (2) an increase in the child's contact with parents during hospitalization (Fig. 21–1); (3) pain management and procedural preparation during hospitalization; (4) child life programs; and (5) a reduction in the amount of time children spend in the hospital.

Many changes in child care in hospitals have been instituted during the last quarter of a century. Despite a rapidly expanding research base, there is still resistance to alter policies and traditional practice, which results in a gap between how we care for children and what we know reduces their stress. The basis of understanding the problem of hospitalization for a child is recognizing the stressors that affect the child and family, and the balancing factors that can be instituted to reduce stress.

Stressors of Hospitalization

Each child and family come to the hospital with their own strengths and vulnerabilities. The greatest error is

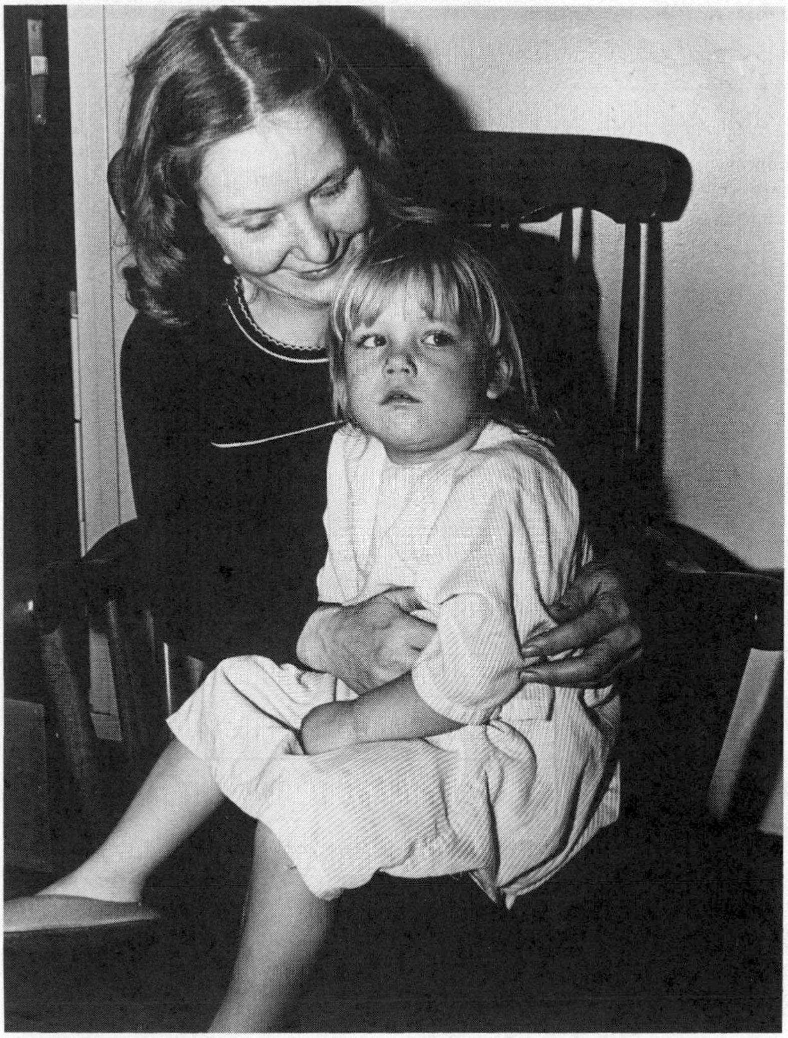

FIGURE 21 - 1. A child's stress is diminished by the presence of a parent whose anxiety has been reduced. A rocking chair is a soothing addition to a child's hospital room, for both the child and the parent.

to expect a child and family with a certain problem to adapt well because someone in a seemingly similar circumstance "adjusted so well." Although stressors to which a child and family are exposed are similar, responses to the event can be very dissimilar. Understanding the stressors associated with hospitalization provides an important knowledge base from which to make individualized assessments and plans of care.

Although the stressors of hospitalization differ according to the many variables affecting individual circumstance, there are some stressors common to many hospitalized children. They are (1) separation from parents, peers, and trusted adults; (2) harm and injury (discomfort, pain, mutilation, and death); (3) loss of control, mobility, and competence or decision making roles; (4) unknown and unfamiliar events and environment; and (5) unclear limits regarding expectations. Recognition of these stressors helps the nurse to understand potential feelings and behaviors of children related to hospitalization.

Separation from Parents and Significant Others

Separation affects children at all ages. Children's and adolescents' responses to separation vary and are influenced by their age; quality of existing parent-child and peer relationships; previous experiences with separation and hospitalization; and their temperament, which, in turn, have an impact on coping ability during hospitalization. Separation from parents is the most important stressor associated with hospitalization for children between the ages of 6 months and 4 years. Young children not only lack understanding of why there is a separation, they also lack adequate coping mechanisms to withstand the separation because of their developmental level. Thus, a child at this stage is more vulnerable to psychologic upset as a result of hospitalization than at any other age.

A major contribution in understanding children's responses to being hospitalized is identifying the

TABLE 21-1
Robertson's Stages of "Settling in"

Protest Stage

- Young children cry desperately in an effort to summon the parent's usual response; they violently protest the departure of the parents by screaming and clinging as the parents try to place them in the crib
- Parents experience ambivalence about visiting when they see their child pleading for them to stay
- Protesting behavior by a child can be seen even in a short-term hospitalization

Despair Stage

- The child experiences a continuing conscious need of a parent
- Despair, or an increasing hopelessness, results when the act of protest fails to bring the parents back
- The despair can be recognized by withdrawal from events and people in the environment
- The child rarely resists anything that is done and seldom cries during this stage; apathy and depression exist, but the complaint behavior is easily mistaken as a sign of adaptation to the hospital experience
- During this phase, the nurse must guard against misinterpreting the child's behavior when parents visit; a child is likely to cry intensely or have a temper tantrum when parents visit, as if to scold the parent for having left
- The nurse who does not understand the nature of the child's anxiety concludes that she or he is "better" when the parents do not visit

Denial (Detachment) Stage

- This can result when a young child must stay for an extended period in the hospital and is cared for by a variety of nurses
- The child has a return of interest in the environment with an appearance of having adapted; in actuality, the external appearance is the result of repression of feelings for mother
- The child no longer seems upset when parents come and go and forms superficial relationships with many staff members, but avoids closeness with any one person
- These children may become the ward favorite because they seem to be happy and respond to everyone but what they desperately need is a trusting relationship with one individual

stages of "settling in" that an institutionalized child demonstrates when separated from the mother (Robertson, 1970). These stages are protest, despair, and denial (detachment). They are not as likely to be noted in children who are separated from parents for short periods. See Table 21–1 for a description of the behaviors identified in each stage.

Older children and teen-agers tend to adapt more easily to separation from parents; their main fear is the possibility of bodily injury or deformity. These children have a better understanding of death, but they may fear being permanently separated from peers and family.

Harm, Injury, and Pain

Illness and hospitalization expose children to unfamiliar and uncomfortable sensations that adults label "pain." These sensations are frightening and produce anxiety because children usually have had little experience with pain and do not understand how one becomes ill or how recovery occurs (see Chapter 25 for discussion of pain assessment). Young children are developing an awareness about their bodies and are concerned about even the slightest injury. During the preschool and early school years, children perceive an injection as a severe threat. They fear that a large hole will be left and that blood may run out. For this reason, bandages (e.g., Band-Aids) are lifesavers to children of this age. Some school-age children also identified the use of Band-Aids as a remedy to make pain go away and to stop bleeding (Ely, 1992).

Concerns of body intactness and body integrity prevail through the preschool years. By school age, the concern encompasses fear of disability and death. By adolescence, differentiation from peers is the primary concern; therefore, the degree of change in external appearance resulting from injury is of prime importance.

Unknown and Unfamiliar Events

Admission to the hospital not only introduces a child to a threatening environment but also to anxiety-producing unfamiliarity. Young children depend on routine and familiarity for security. The strangeness of the sights, sounds, and smells in particular makes young children feel insecure. People in the environment are also a source of stress because of their unfamiliarity and different way of relating to the child.

Unclear Limits and Expectations

Illness and hospitalization often subject the child or adolescent to limits, including restricted movement, isolation, or altered dietary regimen. When a set of new rules is unclear, one's security is threatened. The number of people that become involved in a child's care introduces the potential for inconsistencies and communication of unclear expectations from one individual to another. When it is unclear to children and parents what is expected of them, they feel confused and threatened.

Loss of Control

As children grow, they become more capable of accomplishing tasks and doing things for themselves. The sense of mastery that accompanies actions of self-care fosters development of self-esteem. Hospitalization potentially endangers children's developing self-esteem unless they are permitted to participate in some way in their own care. Intrusive procedures are particularly threatening to a child's sense of control because few choices are possible and physical restraint is frequently required. The daily activities of self-care in which the child can make many personal choices are often hampered by hospital policies and rules. A child feels a sense of frustration and loss when daily self-care skills normally accomplished are not identified and encouraged. Changes in ability to participate in care occur during recovery; therefore, ongoing assessment of the child's ability to participate in care is necessary to foster a sense of control.

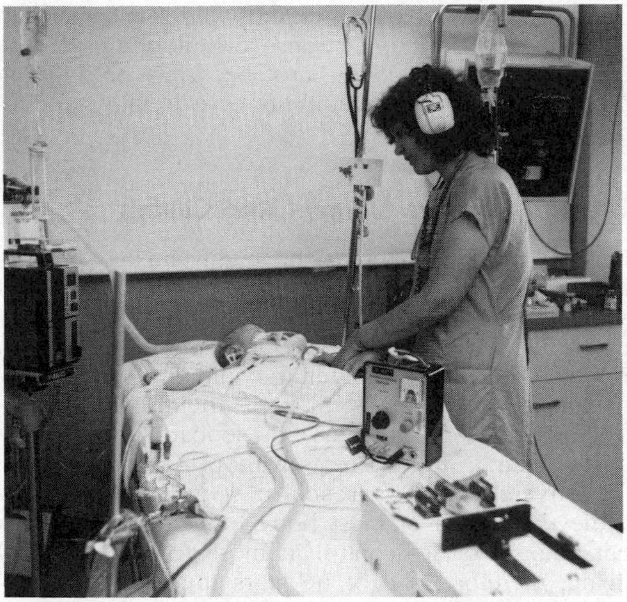

FIGURE 21-2. A strange environment with threatening sounds and equipment is disruptive to an infant.

Impact of Stressors

The impact of the stressors of hospitalization vary with the developmental age and the coping abilities of the child. Understanding development and coping at different ages provides a strong knowledge base for the nurse to plan age-specific care to hospitalized children and their parents.

Infant: Development and Coping

Disruption of routine is the major effect of hospitalization on infants under 8 months of age (Fig. 21–2). A young infant may become subdued and be less likely to exhibit outward signs of stress, such as crying and clinging to parents than an infant over 8 months of age. An infant as young as 10 days may display a response to a change in caregivers; however, in general, young infants are less affected by separation from a parent because selective attachment begins around 6 to 8 months of age.

The type of illness may influence the infant's reaction to hospitalization. The infant who is not allowed to eat or suck (e.g., because of oral surgery) may react by persistent crying or thrashing about from frustration or unmet needs.

Mobility is another important aspect in infant development. An angry or frustrated infant frequently resorts to flailing of arms and legs. Occasionally, for safety, the infant must be restrained during procedures such as intravenous therapy and nasogastric intubation, or following oral surgery. The restraint inhibits usual coping, which leads to increased tension. Infants with orthopedic anomalies often must undergo long periods of immobility and their need for stimulation is acute.

The nurse also should be alert to notice the "apparently" well-adjusted infant. It is possible for the nurse to overlook important cues from the infant because of his or her behavior, e.g., the quiet, subdued infant in Bryant traction may not attract the attention of the caregiver as readily as the crying, clinging infant.

Toddler: Development and Coping

The response of a toddler to a stressful situation does not have to be one of severe anxiety and long-term adverse effects. A toddler's security is threatened particularly by (1) separation from the parents or other significant persons; (2) an unfamiliar environment where routines and rituals are disrupted; and (3) a loss of control and autonomy because of procedures that are painful and necessitate restraints. Keeping parents with children, appropriately managing pain, and doing things consistently in the same environment enhances a toddler's security.

Hospitalization disrupts a child's familiar life of people, places, and things, making a toddler feel threatened, insecure, and even punished. As a toddler feels less secure, the spirit of "me do it" wanes. Furthermore, hospitals are run on schedules that do not allow for extra time for toddlers to do their own zippers, take off their own socks and shoes, or brush their teeth at their own pace. Toddlers dawdle to increase their sense of control, wanting to do things in their own time in their own way. Development is not interrupted when health care providers give the needed time to toddlers.

Fear of painful procedures causes considerable stress to toddlers. Their limited cognitive ability makes them likely to arrive at strange conclusions regarding painful procedures. Painful procedures may be viewed as hostile attacks and even punishment. In addition, the developing sense of autonomy may be hampered when toddlers must be firmly held during procedures or by the restraints of extremities for intravenous fluids.

Preschooler: Development and Coping

Hospitalization is likely to be highly anxiety-producing for the preschooler, even when preparation and support have occurred during their confinement (Caty et al, 1989; Galligan, 1979; Oremland et al, 1973). Hospitalization may hinder the initiative-seeking behaviors of preschoolers; threaten their sense of control over their intact body; and jeopardize their ability to separate from parents without conflict.

Physically, the preschooler has successfully achieved control of most body functions, allowing a fair amount of self-control in most activities of daily living; therefore, she or he fears the loss of control over these daily routines. Some degree of regression is seen as the hospitalized preschooler attempts to cope. This regression is frustrating and confusing to preschoolers who have just mastered self-care and who find it threatening to relinquish it. They need help to regain self-control so they do not experience shame and further regression. Preschoolers let nurses and parents know when they are not receiving adequate assistance either by becoming inactive, uncooperative, and withdrawn or by becoming hyperactive or overaggressive. The withdrawal or aggression may be expressed toward those activities in which they feel a loss of control (eating, elimination, sleeping).

Perhaps the greatest difficulty hospitalization creates for preschoolers is creating feelings of guilt and shame from the egocentric belief that being in the hospital is a punishment for something they did or thought (Brandt et al, 1972; Oremland et al, 1973; Azarnoff & Woody, 1981). A recent case study of a 5-year-old hospitalized child linked punishment and fear with being hospitalized (Abbott, 1990). Children's thinking is intuitive and magical, out of which grows a rich fantasy life. The distortion of perception that arises out of their egocentric and magical thoughts works against them during hospitalization. They tend to construct unfathomable fantasies and fears stemming from the strange hospital "Land of Oz." Even though they have usually mastered basic language skills at this age, they still may have difficulty verbalizing needs and feelings during stress. Preschoolers can be helped to avoid or master unrealistic fears during hospitalization and can progress in their ability to communicate their needs effectively even under stress.

Hospitalization can interfere with preschoolers' initiative to gain control over the environment and increase their independence, leaving them with a feeling of loss of the control they had been gaining over their environment. They may lose the initiative to try to satisfy their curiosities if they are immobilized or isolated. Nursing personnel can enhance a preschooler's sense of security and control by trying to maintain the routines and rituals used in their home.

Preschoolers still resist separation from family members during illness and other periods of stress; they tend to perceive the separation as punishment and fear abandonment. In addition, they fear body mutilation, pain, and invasion of body orifices resulting from the Oedipal crisis; this is possibly the preschoolers' greatest fear during hospitalization (Oremland et al, 1973; Petrillo & Sanger, 1980). Thus, the major tasks for the preschooler are to cope with the treatment procedures, unfamiliar individuals, and equipment required to manage the illness.

School-Age Child: Development and Coping

School-age children should have fewer adjustment problems during hospitalization because of the intellectual and emotional progress made during the preschool years. They are now better able to tolerate parental separation. Although not totally free of separation anxiety, they are more reality-oriented. Unreasonable fantasies and fears are fewer in number and severity, and children are eager to form relationships and have experiences outside the family and home. It has been suggested that hospitalization may even be a positive experience in which a child can grow in self-esteem and maturity (Brazelton, 1992).

Regressive behavior is less frequent. If regression does occur, a child typically will display fears characteristic of preschoolers (mutilation, monsters, and separation). The most feared items of medical events of school-age children include bodily injury (getting a shot, having an operation), being separated from family, and death (Broome, 1991; Broome & Hellier, 1987).

School-age children may be embarrassed by crying or screaming; therefore, alternative outlets for pain or fear may be used. Squeezing a parent's or nurse's hand, counting, engaging in diversion conversation, or clenching the teeth are common responses. School-age children appreciate the option of having or not having a parent present during procedures, even if only to passively seek contact with their eyes or through facial expressions. School-age children are able to hold still for a procedure and usually invest most of their energy in retaining self-control. Praising a child for holding still, cooperating, or participating may encourage the likelihood of future cooperation from the child.

Physically, school-age children have complete control of body functions and the physical self-care required in daily living. This independence reinforces a healthy image and builds self-confidence. They are intent on developing fine motor skills, which should continue during hospitalization, to keep up with their peers. Their industrious drive makes them eager candidates to participate actively in the treatment regi-

RESEARCH ISSUES

Instruments to Measure and Assess Children's Fears of Medical Events

Results. Children's fears of medical experiences and stresses of hospitalization have been studied (Astin, 1971; Broome et al, 1988; Broome & Hellier, 1987; Elkins & Roberts, 1984; Roberts et al, 1981; Scherer & Nakamura, 1968). This research describes the Child Medical Fear Scale (CMFS), which was developed and revised to measure children's fears of medical experiences. The items used in this instrument were generated empirically by eliciting children's perceptions of their own fears. Initial psychometric testing included measures of internal consistency and stability, and criterion validity. The empirically generated items and the initial and ongoing psychometric testing are strengths of the CMFS. The CMFS has been used in research studies measuring children's fears (Bossert, 1991; Broome et al, 1990, 1992; Broome & Hellier, 1987; Wallom, 1987, Wilson & Yorker, 1993).

Implications. The CMFS could be used by practicing nurses in the clinical setting. Nurses could identify those children who are more fearful of medical experiences and, thus, focus individual preparation for specific procedures. The CMFS is a 17-item scale that allows the child to rate his or her fear (see selected items from the CMFS below). A pictorial CMFS was developed for children 3 to 5 years of age. The preschool child is asked to view a procedure or event and then choose which of three fear pictures best describes his or her feeling.

The scale scores range from 17 to 51, with low scorers reflecting children who report fewer fears of medical experiences. The complete instruments and scoring information can be obtained by contacting Marion E. Broome, RN, PhD, Associate Professor and Assistant Chairperson, College of Nursing, Maternal-Child Nursing, Rush-Presbyterian-St. Luke's Medical Center, Chicago, IL.

Selected Items from the Child Medical Fear Scale

Not at all	A little	A lot
(1)	(2)	(3)

I am afraid of getting a shot. ____________________

I am afraid of seeing blood come out of me. ________

I am afraid of going to the hospital. ______________

I am afraid of having my finger stuck. ____________

I am afraid to throw up. _______________________

I am afraid of being away from my family if I go to the hospital. _____________________________________

REFERENCES

Astin, E. W. (1971). Self-reported fears of hospitalized and non-hospitalized children aged ten to twelve. *Maternal Child Nursing Journal, 6,* 17–24.

Bossert, E. (1991). Factors affecting stress and coping process of hospitalized school-age children. *Communicating Nursing Research,* 24, Boulder, CO: Western Institute of Nursing.

Broome, M. E., Bates, T. A., Lillis, P. P., & McGahee, T. W. (1990). Children's medical fears, coping behaviors, and pain perceptions during a lumbar puncture. *Oncology Nursing Society, 17*(3), 361–367.

Broome, M. E., & Hellier, A. (1987). School-age children's fears of medical experiences. *Issues in Comprehensive Pediatric Nursing, 10,* 77–86.

Broome, M., Hellier, A., Wilson, T., Dale, S., & Glanville, C. (1988). Development and testing of an instrument to measure children's fears of medical experiences. In C. Waltz, & O. Strickland. *Measurement of nursing outcomes.* New York: Springer.

Broome, M. E., Lillis, P., McGahee, T., & Bates, T. (1992). Use of distraction and imagery with children during painful procedures. *Oncology Nursing Forum, 19*(3), 499–502.

Elkins, P. D., & Roberts, M. X. (1984). A preliminary evaluation of hospital preparation for non-patient children: Primary prevention in a "Let's Pretend Hospital." *Children's Health Care, 12*(1), 31–35.

Roberts, M. C., Nurtele, S. R., Boone, R. R., Gentber, L. J., & Elkins, P. D. (1981). Reductions of medical fears by use of modeling: A prevention application in a general population of children. *Journal of Pediatric Psychology, 6*(3), 293–300.

Scherer, M. W., & Nakamura, C. Y. (1968). A fear survey schedule for children (FSS-FC): A factor analytic comparison with manifest anxiety (CMAF). *Behavior Research and Therapy, 6,* 173–182.

Wallom, L. (1987). The effect of hospital preparation on anxiety and fear levels of school-age children. Unpublished Master's Thesis. Medical College of Georgia.

Wilson, A. H., & Yorker, B. (1993). Use of the child medical fear scale (CMFS) among school-age children with emotional disorders. Research proposal funded by the College of Health Sciences, Georgia State University, Atlanta.

men. They still find security in a routine and willingly help structure the routine. Their understanding of time makes them capable of "helping" the nurse stay with the planned routine. Although they will require supervision, they can perform a variety of treatments after adequate instruction and practice. The opportunity to participate in planning and performing care bolsters school-age children's self-concept; provides opportunity for refinement of motor skills; and stimulates them intellectually. In addition, school-age children can be instrumental in helping teach or motivate self-care in their hospitalized peers.

Intellectually, school-age children are in the stage of concrete operations. They base perceptions on reality progressively more often than on fantasy. Most of the fears they retain involve situations that threaten to cause loss of control or bodily injury. They accept the fact that there are other points of view beyond their own. The ability to reason cause-and-effect relationships makes the school-age child intrigued with the scientific process and interested in scientific explanations about their disease. They also want explanations about the sensations they can expect during hospitalization and the rationale underlying treatments. The concepts of conservation and classification are mastered during the school-age years. They are then able to solve concrete problems that they can manipulate or visualize mentally. They can also understand the relationship between the parts and the whole. A group of school-age children having a cerebral computed tomography scan procedure were able to understand that the machine both moved and took pictures of their head at the same time, whereas younger children could not make the connection (Hellier et al, 1986).

Rules help school-age children think rationally. If rules are not provided, they will construct their own rules, which are often more rigid than those an adult would supply. Early school-age children still perceive that injuries and misfortunes that put them in the hospital are punishment for their own misdeeds; they need the same reassurances of blamelessness that preschoolers require. As they lose their egocentric focus, school-age children rely more on past memories and reason to make decisions; magical thinking disappears by middle school-age (8 to 10 years).

Language has been mastered and school-age children are now learning to use that language to express needs and feelings during stress rather than using regressive or defiant behavior to communicate. The nurse elicits the child's nonverbalized reactions, encourages communication about feelings, and teaches parents how to cope with their child's feelings and behaviors at home. Without the opportunity for verbal expression during hospitalization, school-age children may revert to the behavioral expressions characteristic of their earlier development.

Emotionally and socially, school-age children begin undertaking tasks that will lead them into healthy, productive adult relationships once the tasks are refined in adolescence. One challenge of this period (latency) is the channeling of emotional, physical, and sexual drives into socially acceptable behaviors. This period is one of general disinterest toward opposite-sex peers; same-sex peers develop gangs or clubs and engage in intimate "best friend" relationships. From these relationships comes the learning of sex roles and the "give-and-take" prerequisite to healthy heterosexual relationships that come later in life. These factors should be considered when making room assignments and structuring activities on the hospital unit.

Hospitalized school-age children worry about whether they will retain their peer group memberships and what the group is saying and thinking about them in their absence. To the extent that they are invested in nonfamily relationships, school-age children are able to bear parental and sibling separation (Erickson, 1967). At this age, assurance that they are loved and limits provided to help them maintain self-control are needed from parents. This affection and limit setting are increasingly important during crisis periods such as hospitalization.

School-age children thrive on doing things and seeing how things work. Their industrious natures are tempered by a fear of failure. They tend to depend almost entirely on external evidence of their worth and are continually self-critical. At this most crucial stage in their "concept of self" development, school-age children need much praise, frequent built-in successes, and assistance to maintain self-control (Erickson, 1967). Although they compare themselves regularly with peers and siblings, they cannot tolerate when such comparisons are made by parents or others.

Adolescent: Development and Coping

The knowledge of major issues or developmental tasks of adolescence is critical in understanding the impact of illness or hospitalization on this age group. Adolescence has been described as a period of transition, a period in which society has authorized a delay of adulthood. Time is granted for the person to integrate all the changes required to move from childhood to adulthood. Illness and hospitalization are threats to the accomplishment of the transition.

An age definition of adolescence is arbitrary because adolescence can begin and end at different ages for different people. The adolescent period is characterized by profound biologic and psychosocial changes. The biologic changes of rapid skeletal growth and reproductive development begin sometime during the preteen years. Around the age of 12 or 13 years, the young person looks to peers and explores different adult roles in defining the personality. These movements away from home signal the beginning of psychosocial changes. Adolescence culminates at 18 to 23 years with the emergence of an independent adult; to assume the adult role, adolescents must become emancipated from parents, define their role, and answer the question "Who am I?"

The age at which illness or hospitalization occurs is significant because of the wide variances in development between 12 and 23 years of age. Young adolescents are less overwhelmed by enforced dependency and allow parents to act on their behalf. The main concerns of this age group are physical appearance, function, and mobility. Illness or hospitalization is tolerated least by the adolescent in the middle years (ages 14 to 18). The dependency and decreased control imposed by hospitalization conflict with the drive for independence. Late adolescents usually use the family for support and can tolerate some dependency. A threat to the older teen-ager is a potential blocking of career goals and lifestyle through illness.

The degree to which an adolescent's development is halted by hospitalization also depends on the nature of an illness. The adolescent has the mental capability to make distinctions between short-term illnesses and permanent body changes. A long-term or chronic illness, especially if disabling, may create limitations in the amount of independence achieved.

A sudden or acute illness can be devastating to the adolescent because even a short-term illness or hospitalization causes restriction and forced dependency and can interrupt mastery and control. A group of adolescents, 12 to 17 years of age, reported four areas of stress associated with surgery: (1) anticipated and associated risks of surgery, (2) pain, (3) visible and handicapping consequences of surgery, and (4) interruption of usual lifestyles (Stevens, 1986). The more time the adolescent has for preparing for and planning the absence from school and friends, the greater the degree of acceptance of the restrictions of being hospitalized. Often the season's final football game or the class prom is more important than an operation. Consequently, a planned surgical procedure is often easier to accept than injuries sustained in an accident. Automobile accidents and trauma from other accidents are frequent causes of hospitalization for the adolescent, and the disfigurement, immobility, and guilt, especially if a friend has died in the accident, may lead to feelings of helplessness and despair.

Whatever the nature of the illness, the experience of being hospitalized produces anxiety for adolescents. Some of this anxiety can be attributed to internal factors, such as thoughts about the effect of illness on the body, but most comes from external factors. Adolescents have been removed from family and friends and now are faced with a new environment in which they have little control. Usual patterns of recreation, nutrition, sleep, and socialization are altered, and strange procedures and examinations invade their body and privacy. Health professionals tell them what needs to be done; often they are not allowed to make independent decisions. Consequently, the hospital environment may accentuate feelings of powerlessness and dependency.

Balancing Factors

Children's responses to the stress of hospitalization vary at different ages because of differing developmental needs. Factors that influence these individual responses in the direction of crisis or adaptation are called "balancing factors." Three factors determining whether a hazard will cause a crisis for an individual are: (1) perceptions of the event, a factor that is related to the child's age; (2) availability of social supports; and (3) the individual's coping skills (Zurlinden, 1985). The nurse's role is to assess the child and family to determine how these balancing factors can be adapted to reduce the stress of hospitalization.

Child's Perceptions of the Event

Children's perceptions are based on their own observations, on what is told to them, and on fantasy. A description of children's concepts of illness according to cognitive development is presented in Chapter 18. Children's ability to adapt to a stressful event depends on how they perceive the event. A child's limited cognitive ability to understand the event may result in bewilderment and misinterpretations. Nursing interventions are implemented at each developmental stage to prevent the child's perception of the event from interfering with adaptation.

Impact of Social Support

"Social support" has been described as a buffer or modifier of the potential deleterious effects resulting from stress (Cassel, 1976; Cobb, 1976; Kaplan et al, 1977). Social support refers to interpersonal transactions that make up one or more of the following: affect, affirmation, and aid (Kahn & Antonucci, 1980). "Affect" includes expressions of liking, respect, and love; "affirmation" refers to experiences of agreement or acknowledgment with respect to the appropriateness of verbal statements or actions; and "aid" includes actions of direct help (time, money, advice). Hospitalized children's and adolescents' usual sources of social support may be cut off at a time when support is crucial to cope with the stressors of hospitalization. Parents, professionals, siblings, friends, or relatives can provide the needed social support in an informal way or through organized groups. Nurses must provide individual assessment of social support and determine age-appropriate interventions aimed at alleviating various stressors.

Coping Skills

"Coping" is generally defined as the ability to make a judgment about a situation (cognitive appraisal) and then acting to solve the problem. Children's and parents' coping styles and actions differ when confronted with hospitalization. The success with which a child adapts to hospitalization is influenced by the age of the child (this affects the child's perception of the threat); the supports available to the child; and the coping skills of the child and family. When the threat of hospitalization overcomes the usual repertoire of behavioral responses, then coping strategies must be used to re-establish equilibrium.

Four modes of coping have been described: information seeking, direct action, inhibition of action, and intrapsychic processes (Lazarus & Launier, 1978). A child responds to stress using any one of these modes. Information seeking by children may include asking questions or simply watching and exploring. Active coping deals with the threat at hand and involves use of controlling, cooperative, and resistive behaviors. Avoidance, ignoring, negation, and physical or verbal attack are also forms of active coping (Rose, 1972, Stevens, 1989). Inactive coping describes children who are not involved, are silent, and display apathy. Intrapsychic processes are defense mechanisms such as regression, denial, repression, projection, sublimation, reaction formation, rationalization, and intellectualization.

Toddlers use regression predominantly; denial is the major mechanism used by school-age children (Caty, 1984). Mastery and controlling behaviors are frequent in preschool and school-age children; controlling behaviors are used by school-age children to cope more frequently than at any other age (Caty, 1984; Savedra & Tesler, 1981). Young children tend to cope by emotional expressions and by motor activity, whereas school-age children and adolescents cope through greater use of their cognitive and verbal abilities.

Six coping strategies were identified in adolescents who were hospitalized for surgery (Stevens, 1989). They include emotion-focused coping (distancing, inaction, self-control, and seeking social support) and problem-focused coping (active coping and situational control). The research was a beginning attempt to develop a taxonomy of coping for hospitalized adolescents. Adolescents in the study used distracting thoughts to replace more distressing thoughts aroused by a stressful event; inaction such as sleeping to withdraw from the situation; self-control to control their own feelings or withhold disclosure of feelings to save face in a situation; and social support (mothers, friends, nurses) to feel loved or nurtured. The nurse's recognition of age-appropriate coping behaviors and interpretation of their meaning to parents provides the basis for assessment and planning. (See Chapter 18 for further discussion of stress and coping with illness and Chapter 19 for coping with chronic illness.)

The less ambiguous the situation, the more effective is a child's coping. The child who makes attribution (assigns causation) adapts most readily. The nurse's assessment, therefore, focuses on determining what kind of information is appropriate to facilitate a child's understanding of the situation. When considering causation, it is important to know some children equate illness with punishment possibly from God; therefore, a spiritual assessment is appropriate. Belief in a benevolent and kind God could be helpful to children coping with the stress of hospitalization (Ebmeier et al, 1991). In addition, children need to know they are loved, to be given a positive image about what lies beyond death, and to know that they will be remembered (Sommer, 1989).

Preparation for Hospitalization

Communities and institutions prepare children and parents for hospitalization in a variety of ways, ranging from informal to well-organized programs. An understanding of the general purposes and methods of preparation helps the nurse make accurate assessments of an individual child's response to the experience of hospitalization.

Hospital Tours for Children in the General Population

Taking groups of young children on tours of hospitals is common practice in many communities. Guidelines for conducting hospital tours for early school-age children have been suggested (Huth, 1983). Although these guidelines are not documented by research findings, rationale is provided based on the cognitive and psychosocial development of the child (Table 21–2).

Preparation of well children using a hospital tour usually takes the following form:

1. Restricted to children over 4 years of age.
2. Group size ranges from 10 to 30 children with one to three group leaders.
3. Activities include all or some of the following: welcome speech, a stop on a pediatric unit or unused patient room, a film or slides, and a play experience with selected medical equipment.
4. Children are invited to ask questions.
5. Each child receives a coloring book about the hospital.

Robertson (1983) contends it is a fallacy to think hospital tours and discussions at school actually prepare nonpatients for hospitalization. Because some children have difficulty differentiating between "if" and "when," they actually may be troubled with thoughts of illness, pain, and separation because they think they are really going to the hospital. Unnecessary fears and anxiety can potentially be introduced by exposing very young children to random sights and sounds. An alternative to bringing healthy children into the hospital is for nurses to visit schools to discuss hospitalization; however, even this approach is discouraged by some and must be further studied. Teaching about hospitalization is thought by some to be best done by parents as the occasion arises through normal life events, e.g., when a friend, relative, or neighbor is hospitalized (Robertson, 1983; Harvey, 1983). In these circumstances, the child should be prepared before visiting the hospital. An opportunity for further questions and discussion after the visit helps the child learn about hospitals. Should the grandparent or neighbor die in the hospital, time should be spent dispelling the child's potential belief that all people who go to the hospital die there.

Preparation of healthy children for hospitalization was studied increasingly during the 1980s (Roberts et al, 1981; Azarnoff, 1983; Mather, 1983). Questions generated for further study that have not been answered in the present decade are:

> Would a small group tour be effective if such children were prepared for the tour in a nonmedical setting through play with medical equipment and related discussion?
>
> Would inclusion of prepared parents on a small group tour be an effective strategy?

TABLE 21-2
Guidelines for Conducting Hospital Tours: Early School-Age Children

Guidelines	Rationale
Keeps groups small (10 children per group)	Can assess child's reaction and promote verbal responses
Limit time length (20 to 30 min is usually long enough)	Young children have a short attention span
Encourage participation of parents	Parents can provide security and support when potentially fearful information is received; parental anxiety also may be reduced in the event of future hospitalization of their child
Incorporate use of an indirect method (puppets, films, slides) into tour; permit a period of play with dolls and hospital equipment	Child can express feelings through the medium of a "third person" to handle fears and anxieties; play provides an opportunity to satisfy curiosity and express feelings toward those objects that present real or imagined threats to body integrity
Provide information in a nonthreatening environment. In the hospital, include the playroom but avoid threatening sounds and sights; equipment, slides, and puppets also can be taken to the child's school or home	Frightening scenes such as emergency rooms or intensive care can increase a child's anxiety; if a child will be in an intensive care unit after surgery, films or pictures may be less threatening than exposure to the actual room
Present information in concrete terms; incorporate diagrams, models, or pictures; avoid extensive discussions about threatening procedures	Child is not able to comprehend invisible concepts such as pain, illness, and internal body parts; early school-age children have a multitude of fantasies and fears concerning their bodies, therefore they require factual information to help them understand but it should be brief and to the point
Allow a period for questions; questions should be phrased to encourage the child to reveal her or his perception of the information; areas of confusion should be dealt with thoroughly	A child's concrete thinking makes it necessary for answers to encompass an individual child's past experience so that misunderstandings are clarified

Adapted from Huth, M. M. (1983). Guidelines for conducting hospital tours with early school-age children. *Pediatric Nursing, 9,* 414–415, 431. Reprinted with permission of Anthony J. Jannetti, Inc., publisher.

Would children prepared in a school setting respond differently with respect to stress level and information recall than a group of hospital-prepared children?

In addition, there is a paucity of research relating to cost-effectiveness of child preparation programs.

When Hospitalization Is Imminent

Hospitals in many communities offer organized programs and tours for children prior to admission. These programs help orient children to the hospital environment and sometimes they can meet one of the nurses who will be caring for them. During the tour, children may be provided with child-sized articles of nurse's or doctor's clothing and equipment for use in dramatic play. Seeing procedures (application and removal of a cast to a doll) and handling equipment (IV tubing or an oxygen mask) may allow the child the opportunity to begin to work through some fears regarding illness and hospitalization. The experiences in organized programs allow children to become familiar with the setting when they are not under the stress of being admitted (see Chapter 17 for discussion of therapeutic play).

Books can be used by health care professionals and parents when teaching about and preparing a child for hospitalization. Lists of age-appropriate books are available through the hospital's play/library resource person or through the local children's library (a recommended list is included at the end of this chapter). These books can be read at home before admission, during hospitalization, and again when the child and family return home. When children are old enough to read the books alone, an adult should be available to discuss the child's reactions to the content, offer additional information, and correct any misconception. Well-prepared film strips and videos about the hospital experience may be available from local libraries, the hospital, or the Association for the Care of Children's Health (ACCH).*

Age-Related Preparation

Preparation of toddlers and preschoolers presents a special challenge. Most of the techniques used to prepare school-age children for hospitalization are not effective for younger children. They lack understanding of the concepts of time and causality; therefore, explanations of events that will happen in the future are not relevant to them. They also may not understand the cause of their illness or the reason for their hospitalization. Incorporating parents in the preparation of toddlers and preschoolers is essential to reduce both the anxiety in parents and the stress in the young child. To prepare the parents, the nurse helps them understand the child's illness and the reason for hospitalization; explains the events of hospital admission; and gives guidelines to prepare their child and siblings for the hospital experience.

A common approach used by parents when young children must be hospitalized is to protect them from the trauma of being told that they must go to the hospital. Parents are tempted to tell children they are going to the library, to the store, to the park, or some other pleasant place. The nurse should intervene by assisting the parents to become comfortable with telling the truth. Toddlers can be told about the hospitalization the morning of admission. The explanation should be simple and truthful, with descriptions of a few of the nonthreatening events that will occur. For example, they can be told about the environment, the nurses, doctors, and other children they will meet. It is appropriate to tell some toddlers 2 or 3 days before admission, but the explanation should not include descriptions of threatening procedures. Toddlers also can benefit from parents reading to them about hospitalization and from playing with a nurse or doctor kit a few days before admission. Preschoolers can be prepared a few days to a week in advance, whereas school-age children often know about the admission further in advance because they are more involved in their own care. Discussions that can be heard by the child concerning the imminent hospitalization should include the child.

Siblings should be prepared for the hospitalization of a brother or sister, including explanations of who will be at home to care for them, who will be spending time at the hospital, and how much time will be spent there. If a parent will be rooming-in, this should be explained. Even though a child and family members have been prepared, the nurse should recognize that hospital admission still is potentially stressful.

*ACCH has headquarters at 3615 Wisconsin Avenue, Washington, DC 20016.

The Experience of Being Admitted to the Hospital

Many factors influence the decision to admit a child to the hospital; some allow for preparation of the child and parents and others do not. An element of fear and anxiety exists for those involved despite the situation and type of preparation. There are three aspects of the admissions process that affect a child and parents: (1) the social environment, (2) the physical environment, and (3) the nature of the admitting procedures to which the child and parents are subjected.

The Social Environment

The social environment is determined by the attitudes of health professionals, hospital policies, and the hospital programs such as play, school, and social events. Introduction to other children in the room and to professionals who will be caring for the child and parents make the family feel welcome.

The Physical Environment

The physical environment of the hospital is another factor that may be stressful for the child and/or family members because of the many unfamiliar sights, sounds, and smells. In addition, children are admitted to a strange room, either alone or with children they do not know, and to an unfamiliar bed. Parents should be welcome to stay with their child, especially when young children are involved. Overnight accommodation should be explained.

An environment that allows children to decorate their own space with photos, posters, or other personal items makes children feel they are being recognized for their own individuality. Special rooms for play, socialization, and school help make the environment seem less like an institution. Whenever possible, wall hangings should be hung low for viewing at the level of children.

In some instances, additional stress occurs when a child must be isolated. Isolation is necessary either to protect a child with an impaired immune system from contracting disease or to prevent a child with an infectious disease from spreading pathogenic organisms to other children. For the young child, faces behind masks, long gowns, and strange caps are unusual and often frightening (see Chapter 23 for discussion of caring for a child in isolation).

Admission Procedures

Admission procedures can add stress to the admission process, especially if the child lacks needed preparation. Examples of admission procedures that may be unpleasant or frightening are:

TABLE 21-3
Admitting Procedure

Prior to Arrival of Child

Assess immediate needs of child based on history by telephone including:

- Developmental age of child
- Physical condition of child
- Communicability of illness
- Emotional status of child
- Available support system

Select and prepare a room, taking into consideration the above factors

Tell roommates that a child will be coming to their room; information about the child's condition is not shared with other children or their parents

Prepare the room with equipment required for the admission

Prepare any emergency equipment that might be required

Take toys into the room as appropriate for age

Orientation to Room and Unit

Greet the child and family as soon as they arrive

Introduce child and family to key members on the health team if they are available at the time of admission

Escort child and family to room and introduce to roommate(s) and family if present

Provide an orientation to the various areas of the children's unit, especially those that will be used by the child and family (i.e., playroom, school room, lounges, kitchen, bathrooms, linen areas)

Orient the child to the room and equipment; call bell, crib/bed workings, telephone, television, supplies in bedside stand or elsewhere, special equipment such as oxygen, monitors, suction

Explain hospital policies and routines (visiting hours, mealtime, bedtime, rooming-in services)

Explain how parents may participate in the care of their child

Give child/parents a booklet about the hospital if one is available

Admission Process

Check identification band that name and number correctly match admitting sheet

Apply identification band if not done in admission department

Carry out any STAT orders

Perform a nursing history

Explain routine procedures to be done and use doll-play to demonstrate, then proceed with physical assessment, including temperature, pulse, respiration, blood pressure, height, weight, and head circumference (under 2 years of age or according to hospital policy)

Obtain urine specimen

Obtain other specimens specific to diagnosis

Complete admission assessment form

Give special instructions as required to child and family concerning the diagnostic and treatment plan

Make arrangements for rooming-in as desired

Write admitting nursing diagnosis and care plan

1. Performing radiographs.
2. Drawing blood samples.
3. Collecting urine specimens.
4. Removing the child's clothing.
5. Taking blood pressure and temperature (especially rectally).

Whenever possible, admission diagnostic procedures should be done the day before admission at an outpatient clinic or physician's office. If that is not possible, ideally the procedures should be postponed until the child has had some time to adjust to the new environment. If it is not possible for a parent to be with the child during the procedure, a nurse or other professional to whom the child has already been introduced should offer comfort during the procedure and after it is completed. In many hospitals, child life workers* are used to contribute to the support and comfort of children during procedures. Table 21–3 is a summary of admitting procedures.

* Child life workers are individuals who are specifically educated to support children through a variety of approaches during hospitalization.

Preparation of Children and Parents for Intrusive Procedures

Preparation techniques vary according to a child's developmental capabilities. A description of approaches appropriate at different age levels follows. See Table 21–4 for a summary of interventions to help children cope with stressful procedures.

Infants and Young Children

Infants and young children do not understand explanations about hospital events but the nurturing caretaker can communicate in a nonverbal manner to provide a sense of security and protection to the child. The child can sense the feeling of caring and

TABLE 21-4
Interventions to Help Children Cope with Procedures

Information Through Verbal Explanations

Verbal description of the procedure explaining the steps and when and where it will take place and who will be involved is called "procedural information." Additionally, "sensory information" should be provided, including explanation of the sensations that will be felt (Johnson et al, 1975).

Stress-Point Nursing

This is the use of a combination of strategies immediately prior to stressful events (i.e., before a blood test, an injection, or just before leaving for a procedure or the OR). The intervention includes giving procedural and sensory information, identification of the child's role in the event, and rehearsal of behaviors coupled with continued supportive care (contact with the same caregiver) (Wolfer & Visintainer, 1975).

Modeling

This is the exposure of a child to another peer model in a film in a similar situation. The individual in the film demonstrates coping by first exhibiting fearful behavior but is shown to gradually overcome such fear (coping model). Another model is one who demonstrates an ideal set of behaviors from the outset, not showing fear (mastery model). The coping model has been found to be more effective than the mastery model. Melamed and Siegel (1975) indicate that a modeling film may initially increase arousal (on the Palmer Sweat Index) but that it is instrumental in reducing stress later preoperatively and postoperatively.

Presence of Parents

If parents are sufficiently supported, it is generally believed that they can in turn provide emotional support to their child. Although research to demonstrate the effectiveness of parental presence during procedures is lacking, nursing practice in many centers includes parents as a support for their child during stressful events. It should be recognized, however, that not all parents choose to accompany their child during such events and that for some procedures it may be less beneficial than others.

Motor Activities

A preverbal child lacking the cognitive coping abilities of an older child needs other means to achieve coping. Motor activities that do not interfere with the actual procedure can be encouraged; i.e., allow child to (1) squeeze Nerf ball or other object with hands or between knees; (2) squeeze hands of nurse or parent; (3) pound on a pillow (if procedure is on lower extremities); and (4) kick against a pillow (if procedure is on upper portion of body). Movement of "procedure area" can be restricted without restricting *all* movement of the child.

Play

The use of play to prepare children for procedures, hospitalization, and surgery is prevalent in many hospitals and clinics today. There is considerable anecdotal literature but only a few controlled studies to support the effectiveness of play. (See Chapter 17 for discussion of therapeutic play.)

Emotional Support

Emotional support is the provision of an environment within which the parent and child feel comfortable to express feelings and ask questions. Emotional support in combination with information provision has been demonstrated as a beneficial approach (Fassler, 1980; Wolfer & Visintainer, 1975). In some instances, emotional support is described as providing contact with the same nurse over a certain series of events (Wolfer & Visintainer, 1975).

Progressive Muscle Relaxation

This is a technique in which a child learns to relax his or her own body in a nonstressful situation. The technique must be practiced repeatedly until mastery is achieved and incorporated into their coping repertoire; otherwise, under stress children revert to their "usual" pattern of coping. If practiced, at a later time when the child is faced with a stressful situation, the previously learned relaxation techniques can be used. The technique involves learning to tense and relax certain muscle groups and performing breathing exercises. Imagery (having the child imagine a relaxing scene) is used in conjunction with the relaxation exercises. The child can gain a sense of control or mastery by using this technique during a painful procedure and it serves to refocus the child's attention from the procedure to the technique of relaxation. Progressive muscle relaxation exercises for children have been developed by Cautela and Groden (1978).

Desensitization

This technique requires considerable professional input as it is accomplished over a period of time. A threatening event is reduced to a list of events (stimuli) that lead up to the final threatening procedure. The hierarchy of events (from the least to the most frightening) is introduced one event at a time, enabling the child to cope with each event. As the child is desensitized to each stimulus, he or she moves up to the next most frightening one, until the original feared stimulus no longer elicits a fearful response.

Self-Talk

Self-talk has been used as part of a coping skills package (Siegel Peterson, 1980) in which children were taught to use relaxation, deep breathing, imagery, and calming self-talk. For example, statements such as "I will be alright soon" or "It will soon be over," are made repeatedly by the child during the procedure.

Distraction

Various methods of distraction are used during painful events. For example, relaxation, imagery, and self-talk are forms of distraction. Other suggestions are counting, squeezing someone's hand, holding a favorite toy or blanket, talking to a favorite toy animal, or actually participating in the procedure (i.e., by opening packages of 4 × 4s or preparing tape).

protection from eye contact, tone of voice, facial gestures, and physical contact.

Most educational efforts for children of this age are directed at the parents. Keeping parents informed about their child's condition and plan-of-care are useful educational strategies. Parents use problem-focused coping, such as seeking information, asking questions, talking with other parents, and being vigilant about the child's care (Miles & Carter, 1985).

Preschoolers

Preschoolers need information about their disease in simple terms, including elementary anatomy and physiology, and about the procedures and treatments used to diagnose or correct it. They are very interested in what their bodies look like and the names for various parts. They are able to comprehend simple anatomy and physiology if visual aids such as body outlines, pictures, or organ models are used. Medical equipment, dolls, and puppets for play should accompany explanations (Fig. 21–3). Body outlines are appealing to preschoolers because they are familiar with the concept of the flat body from storybooks and their own crude "people" drawings.

Before starting a session, the nurse should find out the child's perception, knowledge, and understanding about the topic to be discussed. Requests such as "Tell me how you knew you had to come to the hospital" or "Tell me what your parents told you about (topic)" reveal the child's knowledge base, fantasies that may need correcting, the areas for reassurance, and information to be emphasized. Denial of knowledge should not be taken at face value in preschoolers. They may think the disease will go away or the procedure will not take place if they deny its existence or knowledge about it.

A story approach might be useful with the denying child to elicit contributions and questions. The nurse might relate a story about a boy in the hospital who knows he is sick or needs a procedure but is afraid to ask questions because he wishes it would go away or would not happen, and then how much better he feels when he finally asks questions.

The timing of and use of words in the instruction is important. Children should have adequate time to work through the explanations but not enough time to let their imaginations get carried away with fantasies. Their attention span is limited to 10 to 15 minutes; thus, material should be presented in short sessions to avoid overwhelming them and to maintain their interest. Neutral words should be used in explanations to avoid stimulating the child's imagination or producing mutilation fears. For example, in describing an operation, the nurse should say "make an opening" instead of "cut" and "the bandage may look pinkish and wet" rather than "there may be blood on the bandage."

Preschoolers' questions should be answered honestly and briefly; repetition of information may be necessary before they fully understand explanations. Their lack of understanding may be communicated through questions and nonverbally through uncooperativeness and defiance.

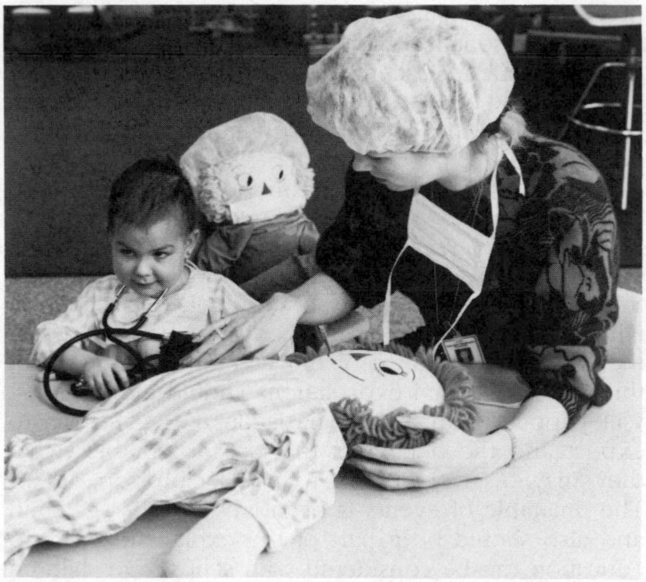

FIGURE 21-3. When toys or puppets accompany explanations of hospital events, preschoolers can better comprehend the event. (Courtesy of Child Life Department, Children's Hospital, Chedoke-McMaster University, Hamilton, Ontario.)

School-Age Children

School-age children want explanations about the disease process and treatment plan. They need to be provided with a rationale for each procedure before it is done. This knowledge helps them to maintain control and cooperate during the procedure. The teaching plan is similar to that of the preschoolers just discussed but school-age children are more enthusiastic and are able to reason, so content can be more complex. Their attention span is longer, allowing them to pay attention for 30 minutes if they are actively involved in some way; they can handle slightly more content per session than the preschooler. Questions, concerns, and feelings should be encouraged and explored. Body outlines, models, games, stuffed body-outline dolls, and puppets can be used to help them visualize verbal explanations and to solicit their active involvement (Gaynard et al, 1991; Green, 1975; Norbeta, 1976; Petrillo & Sanger, 1980). Older school-age children may not respond positively to the use of a "doll" when taught; therefore, the nurse may choose to refer to the doll as a "dummy" or "model" or use "grown up" dolls (e.g., Barbie dolls). Stuffed body-outline dolls made of muslin and devoid of any features or detail can have multiple uses with children and adolescents such as establishing rapport, assessing needs, or facilitating preparation and coping processes. The child is given the opportunity to create and personalize a doll with nontoxic, permanent markers while interacting with a child life specialist or a nurse. The doll can remain with the child during hospitalization and later can be taken home (Gaynard et al, 1991).

Procedural instruction can be provided 1 or 2 days in advance, with a quick review just before the procedure, unless knowing would upset the child, in which case instruction should immediately precede the procedure. The nurse should be honest and specific about what parts of the body will be involved in the procedure because of the fear of bodily harm at this age. Procedural explanations should include what will happen, with an emphasis on the sensations to expect and the behaviors that are acceptable (what they may or may not do to help) (Johnson, 1976). The timetable of events is of interest to this age child and also should be a part of the explanation. Group education can be considered with school-age children because they respond positively and often are supportive of each other (Shaefer, 1977).

Adolescents

Adolescents think about death; therefore, it is essential to tell them the nature of their illness. The physician should give an explanation in terms the young person can understand, including prognosis for recovery and the treatment plan. The nurse's role is to determine the adolescent's response by reviewing, supporting, and providing additional education. Adolescents will use fantasy thoughts to figure out what is happening to them if health professionals do not provide honest explanations. Recurrent questions raised spontaneously by 40 hospitalized adolescents with an acute, chronic, or terminal illness included (Craft, 1981):

1. Illness-related: What is the cause, how serious is it, and how long will I have the illness? What symptoms are likely to occur and which should I report?
2. Procedure-related: What tests and examinations will I have and why? How will I feel during them? What are my test and examination findings?
3. Lifestyle changes: How long can I expect to be in the hospital? What foods may I eat or not eat? What are the changes in exercise and athletic activities? What medications do I need and what effect do they have?
4. Future plans: Can I expect to make changes in school and future job plans, in friendships, or dating, and in future planning for marriage and children?

Adolescents have been found to show preferences for certain information providers, depending on the nature of the information. Older adolescents are more likely to prefer general information from a health professional than from a parent (Craft, 1981). However, when important topics such as cause, seriousness, symptoms, and duration of illness are discussed, adolescents seem to want the emotional support provided by the presence of their parents. The implication for the nurse is to assess each adolescent to determine their individual preference. More recent research among adolescents partially supports earlier findings that adolescents have questions and want explanations (Stevens, 1989).

Application of the Nursing Process: The Hospitalized Child

Recognition of the stressors of hospitalization as they are manifested across the developmental stages is fundamental to helping children and family members adapt. In addition, balancing factors must be carefully used throughout the nursing process to reduce the stress of hospitalization and facilitate successful adaptation.

Assessment

Nursing assessment of a hospitalized child demands a high level of skill because of the increased acuity of patients. The usual steps in the assessment process are:

1. Collecting data.
2. Validating data.
3. Organizing data.
4. Identifying patterns.
5. Communicating/recording data.

See Chapter 13 for a discussion of nursing assessment.

In a hospital situation, many factors impinge on a nurse's ability to make a comprehensive assessment. The nature of the child's illness, the impact of hospitalization, the child's age and coping abilities, and the environment or setting present a unique combination of cues that make the assessment process complex. Assessment of the child and family in this setting requires speed, sensitivity, and alertness to cues. While intervening to make the child comfortable and reduce the child's immediate fears, a thorough baseline assessment must also be made.

Baseline assessment and ongoing assessments equally require of the nurse data gathering skills, background knowledge, and data analysis skills. Assessment data can be clustered and organized according to the nurse's preferred theoretical framework or that which is practiced within the setting of employment. Assessment data, regardless of framework, encompass the physical, emotional-social, and intellectual-perceptual status of the child, as well as the adaptation of the parents and siblings.

Baseline Data

On receiving the child for admission, an immediate assessment is made to determine whether the child needs emergency care, e.g., air, breathing, and circulation (ABC), according to emergency care standards. See Chapter 46 for emergency care protocol. Additionally, a child is made comfortable by attending to the need for warmth or cooling, holding or positioning, and relief of pain. After attending to an emergency situation and the initial comfort of the child, a more thorough assessment is made using principles of interviewing, history taking, and physical assessment as presented in Chapter 13.

Regardless of the child's age or type of problem, all body systems are assessed and the findings are recorded and used as a basis for making nursing diagnoses. During this assessment, the entire body is inspected for the presence of rashes, scars, or injuries. Such markings must be documented at the time of admission. Special attention is given to assessing the body system that is involved in the presenting problem identified by the parent and child.

It is common practice to fill out an admission form to record pertinent information when a child is admitted (see Fig. 21–4 for an example of an admission form). These forms should serve only as a guide. The nurse needs to focus attention to the individual needs of the child and family. Subjective and objective assessment data for each of the categories—physical, emotional-social, and intellectual-perceptual—are presented in the Nursing Process Plan (Table 21–5).

Ongoing Assessments

Ongoing assessments are made by watching for changes in baseline data and searching for new cues that might contribute to making and revising nursing diagnoses and nursing care plans. Behavioral changes of the patient reported by a parent, change of shift reports, results of tests, or collaboration with other health care providers could provide the impetus for ongoing assessments.

Nursing Diagnostic Statements

The child's responses to specific health problems will determine the nursing diagnoses. Nursing diagnoses associated with specific illnesses are discussed in Unit Seven. This chapter deals with those diagnoses associated with hospitalization that are applicable to most illnesses. Planning and interventions for each of the following nursing diagnoses are presented in the text that follows and summarized in the Nursing Process Plan in Table 21–5.

Sleep Pattern Disturbance related to unfamiliar environment, separation from parents/family, discomfort of illness, or medications.

Altered Nutrition: Less than body requirements related to anxiety associated with unfamiliar surroundings, variation in feeding techniques among caregivers, dislike of food served associated with variations in preparation and cultural food preferences, behavioral regression in eating patterns associated with anxiety of hospitalization, anorexia, or discomfort associated with disease process.

Altered Elimination: Incontinence of urine and/or stool related to regressive behavior associated with anxiety related to hospitalization.

Diversional Activity Deficit: Altered play behavior related to separation from usual playmates/friends, lack of interesting toys/diversional materials, isolation associated with communicable disease or immobility or discomfort associated with disease process or its treatment.

Self-Care Deficit related to unfamiliar environment, regressive behavior, or illness and treatment.

Altered Growth and Development: Physical, intellectual, or emotional-social related to hospitalization.

Body Image Disturbance related to physical appearance, physical mobility/agility, intellectual function, feelings of self-worth, or feelings of competence/mastery over the environment.

Parental Role Conflict related to hospitalization of a child with an acute or chronic illness, invasive or restrictive treatment modalities, or interruptions of family life owing to treatment regimen.

Ineffective Individual Coping related to crisis of hospitalization associated with multiple stressors.

Altered Family Processes: Parents and siblings related to the crisis of hospitalization of the ill child.

- Associated with multiple stressors for the parents of unfamiliar hospital environment; loss of control over child's care; impact of the diagnosis; concern about the prognosis; potential susceptibility of other family members; guilt related to the etiology or the fact that medical help was not sought earlier; concern for the child's pain/discomfort; loss of sleep of family members; family and social role disruptions, including financial concerns, or concern about being able to manage recuperative or long-term care at home.
- Associated with multiple stressors for siblings or guilt about the illness or injury; fear of having the same illness or injury; separation from parents who are with the ill child; or loss of attention.

GENERAL INFORMATION

Health Care Provider

Grade Level Adm Date/Time

Language Spoken Interpreter

Reason for Adm

Brief Hx

Medication—Prescription/Non-Prescription

Name	Dose	Freq.	Last Dose	Comment

Way Child Takes Meds

Exposure to Contagious Illness (which, when)

Description & Time of Last Fluids & Food

Substance Use/Abuse (caffeine, alcohol, smoking, drugs)

Corrective Devices/Prosthesis/Handicaps

ALLERGIES

VITAL SIGNS/MEASUREMENTS

T	P	R	BP	Ht	Wt	OFC

ACTIVITIES OF DAILY LIVING

Breast Bottle Formula

Usual Amt

Freq

Solids (type, amt., freq.)

Cup Snacks

Feeding Skill Level/Special Utensils

Food Likes

Food Dislikes

Problems/Special Diet

Diapers Potty Chr. Toilet Toilet Trained

Date Last Stool BM Freq.

BM Character

Terms Child uses for Elim.

Problems/Devices

Bath/Hair Dental Care Dressing

Menses Hx/Care

Concerns/Problems

Naps/Rituals/Comfort Meas./Special Needs/Habits

Concerns/Problems

Adm. R.N.

A

FIGURE 21-4. Example of a nursing admission form used at The Children's Hospital, Denver, Colorado.

Planning and Implementation

The goal of nursing is to assist the child and family to adapt positively to the hospital experience by helping them draw on their strengths and support systems. Assisting families to convert limitations into strengths helps them adapt to the situations posed by hospitalization. The threat of hospitalization can be reduced by modifying the stress of hospitalization and strengthening the balancing factors. Development of positive coping mechanisms throughout the hospitalization can result in a growth experience for the child and family. Nursing interventions commonly employed to facilitate the child's and family's adjustment to hospitalization are presented here and summarized in the Nursing Process Plan in Table 21–5.

Prevent Disruption of Sleep Time

Hospitalization for any child has the potential to disrupt sleep. The comforts of bedtime routines and the security of being in one's own bed are threatened. Children's cognitive limitations amid frightening sounds and experiences lead to misinterpretation of their environment and harboring of a myriad of scary thoughts, which can interfere with the ability to sleep. The child's physical sense of well-being also is diminished with a reduction in the amount of physical activity. The physical tiredness experienced by children from a fun-filled day of activity is replaced with emotional distress; feelings of discomfort associated with the illness; and the hurts associated with diagnostic procedures or treatments. Nursing goals are:

DEVELOPMENTAL INFORMATION	PSYCHOSOCIAL BACKGROUND
Comment as appropriate on Language, Socialization, Activities/Play, Motor Levels, Sexual Behavior/Birth Control. ______	Health Care Experiences ______
	Child's Reaction to Illness/What Child Told re: Illness/Hosp. ______

	Age	Name	Usual Health Status/Comments	At Home
Mother				
Father				
Guardian				
Siblings				

UNIT ORIENTATION

Bed ___ TV ___ Phone ___ BR ___ Side Rail ___ Restraints ___
Call Light ___ Play Rm ___ Teen Lounge ___ Sib Play Ctr. ___
Smok Pol. ___ Booklets ___ Parent Facil. ___ Isol Lev. ___
Valub. ___ Prim. Nsg. ___ ID Bracelet ___ Wait for M.D. ___
Breast Pump ___ Security ___ Valet ___ Visit Rules ___
Room In ___ Visiting Plans ______
Parent Participation in Care ______
Resident/Attending notified ______

Significant Others/Pets
Dad Working (ph#, hrs)
Mom Working (ph#, hrs)
Child Care Arrangements
Transportation Arrangements
Recent Changes in Family/Situation

DISCHARGE PLANNING	AGENCIES INVOLVED WITH FAMILY		PATIENT CARE PROVIDERS
	Name/Agency	Ph. Number	Primary R.N.
			Assoc. R.N.
			Adm. R.N.

B

FIGURE 21 - 4 *Continued.*

(1) to determine usual sleep patterns and routines; (2) to provide for continuity of care; (3) to establish a record of sleep; (4) to establish naptimes; (5) to decrease the child's anxiety; (6) to effectively use medications and pain management techniques; and (7) to promote physical activity and relaxation. Nursing interventions to promote rest and sleep focus on normalizing the child's situation as much as possible within the limits of hospitalization.

Determine Usual Sleep Patterns and Routines. On admission, the usual sleep patterns are determined by appropriate questions in the admission history. The child's naptime, bedtime routines, and rituals are identified. The parents are asked to suggest methods that will assist the nurses to help their child achieve adequate rest and sleep. In the hospital, sometimes a child's routines interfere with another child's sleep, e.g., one child may read and listen to music at home, whereas these activities may keep a roommate awake. Adaptations can be made, such as encouraging the child to read earlier and to use earphones to listen to music. If parents and children understand the limitations within the hospital, they can be resourceful in adapting the routine to foster security. Younger children require their usual blanket or toy and bedtime routine; therefore, parents are encouraged to bring important security objects from home.

Provide Continuity of Care. If parents can room-in with their child, many of the bedtime fears are dispelled. To have a parent read a story and provide the usual routines is the best alternative. When parents are not available, it is not usually possible for a nurse to read a bedtime story to each child, but a short story can be read to a group of children.

Establish a Record of Sleep. Children who are frequently interrupted for procedures and require frequent nursing care may suffer sleep deprivation. To

Text continued on page 760

TABLE 9-19

Nursing Process Plan: The Hospitalized Child

Analysis: Nursing Diagnostic Statement 1

Response and Related or Risk Factors: Sleep pattern disturbance (child), *related to anxiety associated with*

- Unfamiliar environment
- Separation from parents/family
- Discomfort of illness
- Interruptions for medication administration

Projected Outcome: The child will experience no disruption in sleep time.

Defining Characteristics

Subjective:

- Verbal complaints of difficulty falling asleep, not feeling well rested
- Awakening earlier or later than desired
- Interrupted sleep
- Changes in behavior and performance (increasing irritability, restlessness, disorientation, lethargy, listlessness)

Objective:

- Mild fleeting nystagmus
- Slight hand tremor
- Ptosis of eyelid
- Expressionless face
- Dark circles under eyes
- Frequent yawning
- Changes in posture
- Thick speech with mispronunciation and incorrect words

Nursing Interventions

Sleep Enhancement

Decrease the childs anxiety related to hospitalization. (See Diagnoses 8 and 10 of this NPP)

Determine usual sleep patterns, including naptime and bedtime routines and rituals (the younger the child, the more important these familiar activities are to promote sleep)

Provide for continuity of care. When parents cannot be present to prepare the child for sleep, the primary nurse can assume this responsibility while talking to the child about the parents so he or she will know the nurse supports his or her need for parents

Establish a record of sleep.

- If the hospital uses a flow sheet, label one column for sleep; cumulatively total hours of sleep over the 24-hr period
- Compare the child's usual sleep patterns with this guide from Chapters 4–9 and determine appropriate adjustments to meet the body's increased need for sleep and rest during illness

Neonate	20–22 hrs/24 hrs
6 wks	14–16 hrs/24 hrs
6 mo–1 yr	12–16 hrs/24 hrs
1–3 yrs	10–14 hrs/24 hrs
3–5 yrs	12–14 hrs/24 hrs
6–9 yrs	11–12 hrs/24 hrs
10–12 yrs	9–10 hrs/24 hrs
Adolescent	8–10 hrs/24 hrs

Evaluation Criteria

Child or parent verbalizes ease of child in falling asleep, sleeping as long as desired without interruption, and feeling of being well rested. Absence of irritability, restlessness, disorientation, lethargy, listlessness, nystagmus, slight hand tremor, ptosis of eyelid, dark circles under eyes, yawning. Assumes usual facial expression/posture; speech is clear

TABLE 21-5 (continued)

Defining Characteristics	Nursing Interventions	Evaluation Criteria
	Enforce naptimes by posting a sign such as, "Jeremy is asleep; please come back at 3:30." Usually other health care professionals will observe the request. **Plan the administration of analgesic medications so that discomfort does not interfere with sleep.** (For example, if usual naptime is known, try to administer analgesic medications 30 min to 1 hr before naptime.) **Assess whether sleeplessness may be a side effect of medications,** e.g., theophylline. Alert the physician as appropriate.	

Analysis: Nursing Diagnostic Statement 2

Response and Related or Risk Factors: **Altered nutrition: less than body requirements,** *related to*

- Anxiety associated with unfamiliar surroundings
- Variation in feeding techniques among caregivers
- Dislike of food served associated with variations in preparation and cultural food selections
- Behavioral regression in eating patterns associated with anxiety of hospitalization
- Anorexia and/or discomfort associated with the disease process

Projected Outcome: The child's nutrient intake will be appropriate for metabolic needs.

Defining Characteristics	Nursing Interventions	Evaluation Criteria
Subjective: • Crying and irritability in response to food being offered. "I'm not hungry." "I don't want it." "Take it away." • Expressing desire to drink from a bottle or to be fed at breast after weaning to cup *Objective:* • Physically trying to move away from food or to push food away • Refusing nipple • Spitting out food put in mouth • Refusing to use eating utensils, to drink from a cup, to hold finger foods, or to chew food	*Nutrition Management* **Decrease anxiety** associated with hospitalization (see ND Statements 8, 9, and 10) **Plan for caloric requirements per 24-hr period that equal or exceed the following recommendations for the healthy child** (unless contraindicated by treatment plan): 0–6 mos: kg × 108 kcal 6–12 mos: kg × 98 kcal 1–3 yrs: 1300 kcal 4–6 yrs: 1800 kcal 7–10 yrs: 2000 kcal 11–14 yrs males: 2500 kcal 11–14 yrs females: 2200 kcal	**The child will meet caloric requirements, as evidenced by:** • Nutrient intake appropriate to age, body weight, and treatment plan • Maintenance of body weight during hospitalization • The **chronically ill** child will maintain or exceed nutrients consumed at home (unless contrary to the treatment plan) • The **terminally ill** child will receive the nutritional intake desired (unless medically contraindicated), as evidenced by saying food tastes good and voicing no complaints of increased discomfort after eating

(continued)

TABLE 21-5 (continued)

Defining Characteristics	Nursing Interventions	Evaluation Criteria
• Intake less than caloric requirements • Weight loss	15–18 yrs males 3000 kcal 15–18 yrs females 2200 kcal **Adopt age-appropriate feeding** interventions: **Infant** • Have parent feed whenever possible • Note parent's feeding technique so that it can be copied by nurse caregivers. (This will ensure as much consistency as possible and reinforce parents' self-esteem and sense of control. Of course, teaching is indicated if inappropriate techniques are observed) • Use bottle and nipple identical to that used at home and note whether parent warms formula • Determine whether solids or liquids are usually given first in the feeding and follow this pattern • If the infant is not used to commercial baby food, ask the parent to bring food from home **Toddler** • Encourage parents or siblings to be present at mealtime whenever possible • Alert parents to avoid a power struggle over food. The child should be allowed to choose the desired foods from those offered. (Given the opportunity, toddlers often use refusal of food to assert some control in a situation when they are otherwise powerless. Offered a selection of nutritious foods, usually they will choose those the body needs) • If the toddler must eat without family, allow to eat with other youngsters whenever possible to provide a semblance of normal mealtime activity. The distraction of other children temporarily may override anxiety related to the strange environment	

TABLE 21-5 *(continued)*

Defining Characteristics	Nursing Interventions	Evaluation Criteria
	• Provide highchair or booster chair as close as possible to that used at home and observe usual routines, including ritualistic food preferences • Make mealtime as pleasant as possible, avoiding administration of medication or unpleasant procedures • Plan analgesic medication administration to decrease discomfort at mealtime • Allow as much self-feeding as possible. (The toddler who feels partly in control will be more cooperative) **Preschooler** • Allow child as much control over food served as possible: assist in selecting foods from printed menu, allow to help "make" toast, milkshake, etc., and to show the nurse "how Mommy makes it." (Child will feel more in control and will be less likely to demonstrate regressive behavior if newly developed language and motor skills are acknowledged) • Encourage meals with family or other patient whenever possible • The preschooler may like to "role model" good eating behaviors for a toddler patient. (This is in keeping with the tasks of initiative and socialization) **School-Age Child** • Explain to the child which kinds of nutrients are needed for return to health, e.g., protein and vitamin C for wound healing. Allow the child to build a menu plan around favorite foods containing these nutrients. Encourage parents to supply foods from home to satisfy the choices. (Self-regulation and industry will increase the child's self-esteem	

(continued)

TABLE 21-5 *(continued)*

Defining Characteristics	Nursing Interventions	Evaluation Criteria
	and decrease anxiety; therefore, nutrient intake may also increase) • Allow the child to record the food intake on the flow chart. (This "concrete" record makes it easier for the child to keep track of progress toward a goal) • Allow the school-age child to "role model" eating and to entertain and help younger patients at mealtime (to increase a sense of self-worth) **Adolescent** • Identify with the adolescent the need for proper nutrition to regain health. (Reasons for treatment are especially important to the young person striving to make independent decisions) • Allow self-regulation in selecting food in eating, and in recording of intake • Offer the adolescent a consultation with the dietitian; this may be welcomed when weight loss or muscle building is desired after hospitalization. (Information from authorities outside the family is more likely to be valued) **Encourage family to provide food from home to meet cultural tastes.** See individual illnesses in Unit Seven of this text for treatment of anorexia, nausea, and vomiting **Acknowledge the expertise of the parents.** (In most cases they have already established the most efficient methods of care for their child and "reinventing the wheel" by planning care without them will only lead to frustration for the parents and increased anxiety for the child) • Encourage the parents (or child) to model feeding techniques used at home and duplicate these in nursing care whenever	

TABLE 21-5 *(continued)*

Defining Characteristics	Nursing Interventions	Evaluation Criteria
	appropriate. (Parents and nurses can effectively share ideas for venting a gastrostomy tube, inserting a nasogastric tube, feeding the child with tongue thrust, etc) • Recognize that while the parents (and older child) are expert in some areas, they may have questions about others. Encourage this communication. (By recognizing their expertise, the nurse thwarts defensive behavior that might otherwise impede communication) **Encourage the parents and child to identify any problems with nutrition that have arisen during home care and assist them with problem solving** **Collaborate with the home care nurse.** (His or her expertise with this child can greatly facilitate delivery of care in the hospital setting) **Determine what foods the child finds most palatable** and, with the help of the family, keep a supply in the hospital. (Something that "sounds good" to the child tonight may be refused if he or she must wait for it until tomorrow) **Identify the specific impediments to eating for this child** (e.g., stomatitis, nausea) and use all available palliative therapies. (See Chapter 42 for discussion of child on chemotherapy) **Allow the child as much self-regulation as possible** (since the goal of care is to increase quality of life)	

Analysis: Nursing Diagnostic Statement 3

Response and Related or Risk Factors: ***Altered elimination: Incontinence of urine and/or stool,*** *related to regressive behavior associated with the anxiety of hospitalization*

Projected Outcome: The child will experience no incontinence of urine and/or stool, related to regressive behavior, as a result of the anxiety or environment of hospitalization.

(continued)

TABLE 21-5 (continued)

Defining Characteristics	Nursing Interventions	Evaluation Criteria
Subjective: • Failure to express need to urinate or defecate *Objective:* • Incontinence of urine/stool after bladder/bowel training	*Bowel Incontinence Care and Urinary Incontinence Care* **Assess the source of anxiety and implement measures to alleviate it** (See Nursing Diagnostic Statements 9, 10, and 11) **Implement strategies to increase self-care.** Allowing the child as much control as possible may help lessen frustration and anxiety. (See Nursing Diagnostic Statement 5) **Avoid scolding or shaming the child for incontinence.** (If the incontinence is anxiety-related, scolding will only compound the problem) • If usual time of elimination is known, offer potty or toilet close to that time	The child who is toilet trained will return to use of toilet

Analysis: Nursing Diagnostic Statement 4

Response and Related or Risk Factors: ***Diversional activity deficit: Altered play behavior,*** *related to*

- Separation from usual playmates/friends
- Lack of interesting toys/diversional materials
- Isolation associated with communicable disease
- Immobility or discomfort associated with disease process or its treatment
- Anxiety

Projected Outcome: The child will experience no decreased stimulation from or interest or engagement in recreational or leisure activities.

Defining Characteristics	Nursing Interventions	Evaluation Criteria
Subjective: • Crying, whining, irritability • Verbal refusal to play or to participate • Statements of boredom *Objective:* • Lethargic appearance • Flat facial expression • Lies quietly, staring • Ignores available toys and diversions • Frequent dozing	**Integrate specific play times and activities into the plan of care** **Enlist the help of parents and older siblings** by explaining that therapeutic play will help the child cope with the crisis of hospitalization. See Chapter 17 for a complete discussion of play for the hospitalized child. (Laypersons may not place a high priority on play activity without this explanation) **Implement other measures to reduce the child's anxiety.** See also Nursing Diagnostic Statements	The child will participate in age-appropriate play or diversional activities The **terminally ill** child will use play to explore feelings about dying

TABLE 21-5 *(continued)*

Defining Characteristics	Nursing Interventions	Evaluation Criteria
• Watches others play but physically resists participation	9, 10, and 11. The severely anxious child will feel too threatened to engage in play activities **Provide age-appropriate toys and diversional materials** (see Chapter 17). Have a variety of toys/diversions available at the bedside; include hospital/medical toys, creative play materials, and "aggression toys." (Children often engage in anxiety-reducing play when alone with their feelings) **Infant (sensorimotor play)** • Play experienced through the senses; it elicits a motor reaction. Provide a variety of textures, colors, sounds, and movements. Human interactions are important **Toddler (parallel play)** • Active play predominant. Allow gross motor activities. Exploration of environment still important. Fine motor activities most interesting if they involve manipulation. Allow for creative, imaginative play **Preschooler (cooperative play)** • Enjoys quiet, as well as active, play. Imitation of grown-ups at its peak. Interested in activities that provide for refinement of motor skills **School-Age Child (group play)** • Play more formalized, task-oriented. Likes organized group play, games with rules, activities that refine motor and cognitive skills **Adolescent (recreational play)** • "Play" activities determined by peer acceptance. Still enjoys ways to refine motor and cognitive skills toward adult levels. Needs opportunity for motor activity as well as more quiet diversions **Offer creative materials.** (Children are often able to express their	

(continued)

TABLE 21-5 (continued)

Defining Characteristics	Nursing Interventions	Evaluation Criteria
	perceptions of death through drawings, paintings, or clay sculptures) • Use the play projects to engage the child and family in a conversation about fears and feelings associated with death • Dolls or puppets can be used to portray a family dealing with grief. (This can also help work through guilt about making others unhappy)	

Analysis: Nursing Diagnostic Statement 5

Response and Related or Risk Factors: ***Self-care deficit,*** *related to*

- Unfamiliar environment
- Regressive behavior
- Illness and treatment

Projected Outcome: The child will experience no impaired ability to perform self-care appropriate to age-related functions.

Defining Characteristics	Nursing Interventions	Evaluation Criteria
Subjective: • Verbal refusal to perform usual self-care activities (e.g., dressing, brushing teeth) • Increased irritability when self-care is suggested *Objective*: • Physical refusal to perform usual self-care • Inability to perform self-care because of illness, injury, or treatment	*Self-Care Assistance* **Assess usual self-care activities. Assess what self-care is usually performed at home rather than expecting behavior appropriate to chronologic age.** (Self-care may be delayed because of repeated exacerbations of the illness, limitations in mobility, or other factors) **Provide opportunities for, and encourage, self-care whenever possible.** (This facilitates coping by increasing self-concept and by increasing the child's sense of control.) Self-care can be enhanced by: • Carefully orienting the child to the hospital environment: bed controls, release of side rails, bathroom light, use of urinal and bedpan, etc • Allowing own pajamas with familiar closures to be worn, instead of hospital gowns and hos-	The child will perform usual self-care activities as allowed by physical condition The **chronically ill** child will maintain or exceed usual self-care, as evidenced by: • Performing self-care usually accomplished at home • Performing previously learned self-care that is specific to the illness • Learning a new self-care practice The **terminally ill** child will achieve self-care as desired

TABLE 21-5 *(continued)*

Defining Characteristics	Nursing Interventions	Evaluation Criteria
	pital pants that require tying a knot or bow • Encouraging parents to bring to the hospital the utensils used at home for eating, bathing, brushing teeth, etc • Providing a good mirror for bedfast clients so they can comb/curl their hair, apply makeup, etc • Arranging often used items near enough to be easily reached • Maintaining the attitude that the extra time (and perhaps extra mess) involved with self-care is well worth its benefit to the child **Teach the child modifications of care related to illness and treatment,** e.g., sitting on side of bed long enough to avoid orthostatic hypotension, using trapeze to move toward head of bed **Encourage self-care** • Allow the child to perform in the hospital those treatments and procedures performed at home, e.g., inserting own nasogastric tube or self-catheterization. (This enhances coping efforts and provides an excellent opportunity to evaluate the child's technique) • Use this hospital experience to teach the child new self-care behaviors and more about the illness and the treatment plan **Allow flexibility in modes of care:** the child should be supported in self-care when feeling well enough to try it but also supported with direct nursing care during periods of increased fatigue or discomfort **Encourage the child and parents to communicate about the child's self-care needs** (to avoid unnecessary feelings of guilt on either side)	

(continued)

TABLE 21-5 *(continued)*

Analysis: Nursing Diagnostic Statement 6

Response and Related or Risk Factors: Altered growth and development:

Physical, *related to*

- Prolonged immobility associated with illness, injury or treatment

Intellectual, *related to*

- Decreased environmental stimulation associated with decreased mobility and decreased energy for exploration

Emotional/social, *related to*

- Alterations in bonding associated with parental adjustments to the diagnosis and treatment, parent-child separations due to hospitalization
- Separation anxiety that reaches the state of denial

Projected Outcome: The child will demonstrate no deviations from normal from his or her age group.

Defining Characteristics	Nursing Interventions	Evaluation Criteria
Subjective: • Verbalizes inability to keep up with peers in motor and cognitive skills • Verbalizes mistrust, shame/doubt, guilt, inferiority, role diffusion • Professes to "be a loner," "not to need anyone" *Objective*: • Inability to perform gross and fine motor tasks appropriate to age • Intellectually immature for age (see Developmental Theories of Intellectual Competency, Chapter 3) • Inability to perform age-appropriate social tasks • Failure of infant and parent to display social-affective play activity	**Using a screening tool approved by the health care team** (e.g., DDST, Chapter 13), **begin development assessment upon admission and complete it during the hospital stay.** (An ill child can rarely be assessed all at one time. The nurse may have to rely upon parental reports for some behaviors. Motor behavior is especially affected by the fatigue associated with illness and should be reassessed as the condition improves) **Allow physical mobility within the limits of safety** • Remove restraints every 2 hrs under close supervision, to permit increased perfusion and movement • Allow supervised play out of the crib/bed in the room and playroom • Plan for motor play appropriate to age • Encourage exercises for bedfast clients to maintain musculoskeletal function **Provide a variety of sensory stimuli** appropriate to the child's age and condition, e.g., crib mobiles; music boxes; toys of various textures; music from a tape cassette; video movies; rides around	Any developmental delays will be identified, as evidenced by: • A charted assessment of screening for physical, intellectual, and emotional/social development • A referral for any abnormalities detected in screening that were previously undiagnosed The child will not experience developmental delays related to prolonged hospitalization, as evidenced by: • Developmental assessment at discharge showing abilities equal to or increased since admission The **chronically ill** child will continue a prescribed therapy program to promote developmental progress

TABLE 21-5 *(continued)*

Defining Characteristics	Nursing Interventions	Evaluation Criteria
	the unit in a wagon; moving crib/bed out into the hall, into the playroom, or outdoors onto a sunporch **Implement measures to reduce anxiety** (see Nursing Diagnostic Statements 9, 10, and 11) **Assess parent's knowledge of developmental tasks.** With parent, identify tasks specific to the child. Enlist parent's help, and the help of older siblings, in planning and implementing strategies to maintain or promote development during prolonged hospitalization **Collaborate with other team members** (e.g., physical therapist) **to blend care strategies to the child's advantage** **Identify** (through interviews with the child, parents, home care nurse, and therapists) **the protocol followed at home to promote development** **Enlist the aid of these experts to plan modifications to the protocol** appropriate to the illness situation **Implement the modified exercises** as tolerated, being as consistent as possible with home therapy **Evaluate frequently for developmental regression** that would signal the need to further adapt the plan of care	

Analysis: Nursing Diagnostic Statement 7

Response and Related or Risk Factors: ***Body image disturbance and/or self-esteem disturbance,*** *related to perceptions of child and family regarding effects of illness and treatment upon*

- Physical appearance
- Physical mobility/agility
- Intellectual function
- Feelings of self-worth
- Feelings of competence/mastery over the environment
- Perceived sexuality

Projected Outcome: The child will have a healthy and realistic perception of his or her body image and will have positive feelings about self or self-capabilities.

(continued)

TABLE 21-5 *(continued)*

Defining Characteristics	Nursing Interventions	Evaluation Criteria
Self-Esteem Disturbance *Subjective*: • Verbalizes feelings of inferiority, negativity, pessimism • Boasts about achievements • Declines opportunities for social activities, new experiences *Objective*: • In group situations, tends to watch rather than participate • Acting-out behavior • Poor impulse control • Poor sportsmanship • Takes little pride in appearance *Body Image Disturbance* *Subjective*: • Verbal or nonverbal response to change in appearance or function • Actual change in structure or function of the body • Not looking at or not touching affected body part • Hiding or overexposing affected body part	*Self-Esteem Enhancement and Body-Image Enhancement* **Assess self-esteem** (see Chapter 14 for specific techniques) **Facilitate the child's sense of security** • Keep hospital routines for mealtime, bedtime, etc., as close as possible to home schedule • Encourage a parent or family member to stay with the young child • Limit the number of nursing personnel giving care, to enhance trusting relationships **Facilitate the child's sense of identity** • Encourage communication of caring through verbal and physical interactions with family • Comment to the child about his or her personal strengths • Encourage the child to perform self-assessment and to think of ways the child is "special" **Facilitate the child's sense of belonging** • Encourage visits from siblings, extended family, and parents • Encourage visits, phone calls, and letters from friends and classmates **Facilitate the child's sense of purpose** • Assist the child to set realistic goals, e.g., **not** "Next time I won't cry at all," **but** "Next time I will hold my leg still, even if I cry some" **Facilitate the child's sense of personal competence** • Allow the child to make choices from those generated through discussion. (Choosing for the child thwarts autonomy, which is basic to a positive self-concept) • Encourage self-care (see Nursing Diagnostic Statement 5)	The child will display an improvement in self-esteem and body image, as evidenced by displaying one or more of the following characteristics: • Expressing feelings of being likable, worthwhile, important • Seeking activities, new experiences • Displaying pride in achievements • Being expressive, happy, optimistic • Enjoying interpersonal interactions

TABLE 21-5 *(continued)*

Analysis: Nursing Diagnostic Statement 8

Response and Related or Risk Factors: ***Altered parenting:*** *Overprotection, related to real or perceived*

- Vulnerability of child
- Environmental risks

Projected Outcome: Parents will be able to create an environment that promotes optimum growth and development of their child.

Defining Characteristics	*Nursing Interventions*	*Evaluation Criteria*
Subjective: • Child's complaints of not being allowed to do activities of peers and siblings. Parental statements, such as "Johnny has always been so sickly, he just can't do what the other children do." "No, Cindy, you can't go, you know you'll get sick if you don't have your nap" *Objective*: • Child delayed in self-care and in self-regulation of the behavior • Parent repeatedly does things for the child that child should be doing for self	**Help the parents identify major fears pertaining to the child's illness** (see Nursing Diagnostic Statement 10) **and explore any feelings of guilt they may have and use *guilt work facilitation.*** (Anxiety and guilt often lead to overprotection; this may be especially pronounced if the child is chronically or terminally ill) *Role Enhancement* **Assist the parents to clarify their role as parent of an ill child.** Allow them opportunities to supplement previous role behaviors with role behaviors that will facilitate the parents' allowance of more independence in the child • Using the child's behavior as an opportunity for discussion, comment that independence often makes the child feel better about her- or himself • Act as role model for behaviors that allow the child independence • Suggest ways for the child to attempt an age-appropriate self-care task • Evaluate with the child and parent how the child feels about the accomplishment • Written materials on parenting can be helpful adjuncts and may be less personally threatening to parents. (Issues of parenting are delicate areas to approach with parents who are already stressed and who may hold cultural and	The parents will encourage at least one new self-care activity appropriate to age

(continued)

TABLE 21-5 (continued)

Defining Characteristics	Nursing Interventions	Evaluation Criteria
	social values about parenting that differ from the nurse's. Tact and sensitivity are imperative to therapeutic interactions) • Use an appropriate opportunity to discuss the crucial parenting roles at each stage of childhood. See Chapter 12	

Analysis: Nursing Diagnostic Statement 9

Response and Related or Risk Factors: ***Ineffective individual coping*** *with the crisis of hospitalization related to anxiety from multiple stressors:*

- Separation from parents and significant others
- Unfamiliar environment
- Harm, injury, and pain
- Unclear limits and expectations
- Loss of control

Analysis: Nursing Diagnostic Statement 10

Response and Related or Risk Factors: ***Ineffective family coping: Compromised; parents and siblings,*** *related to anxiety associated with the crisis of hospitalization of the ill child associated with multiple stressors for the parents:*

- Unfamiliar hospital environment
- Loss of control over child's care
- Impact of the diagnosis
- Concern about the prognosis
- Potential susceptibility of other family members
- Guilt related to the etiology or the fact medical help was not sought earlier
- Concern for the child's pain/discomfort
- Loss of sleep
- Family and social role disruptions, including financial concerns
- Concern about being able to manage recuperative or long-term care at home

associated with multiple stressors for siblings:

- Guilt about the illness or injury
- Fear of having the same illness or injury
- Separation from parents who are with ill child
- Loss of attention

Projected Outcome: Parents and siblings will be able to provide sufficient, effective, and/or uncompromised support, comfort, assistance, or encouragement, which may be needed by the child to manage or master adaptive tasks related to his or her health challenge.

Defining Characteristics	Nursing Interventions	Evaluation Criteria
Subjective *(Patient)* • Crying • Irritability • Verbalizing specific fears	*Support System Enhancement and Family Support* **Orient child and parents to the social environment** • Communicate an attitude of caring and respect	The child/parents will experience ability to cope following the admission procedure, as evidenced by: • Decreased irritability • Increased eye contact

TABLE 21-5 *(continued)*

Defining Characteristics	Nursing Interventions	Evaluation Criteria
• Report of nightmares • Verbalizing helplessness, hopelessness, guilt, inability to "think straight" • Insomnia • Fatigue • Anorexia or nervous overeating • Diffuse somatic pains *(Parents)* • Verbalizing hopelessness, helplessness, guilt, frustration, "nowhere to turn," inability to "think straight" • Low self-esteem • Insomnia • Fatigue • Anorexia or nervous overeating • Diffuse somatic pains *(Siblings)* • Verbalizing feelings of guilt • Fear of "being punished for bad thoughts" • Fear of getting the hospitalized child's illness • Whining and crying in presence of parents and when parents leave • Complaints of diffuse somatic pains • Preoccupation with thoughts of the ill child when she or he was well • Irritability • Impatience *Objective* *(Patient)* • Physical refusal to be held and comforted • Wide-eyed expression • Frequent visual "scanning" of environment • Increased pulse and respirations • Regressive and/or acting-out behavior	• Tell the parents, "Since you know your child best, we will rely on you to help us plan the nontechnical aspects of care in the hospital." (This immediately establishes for the parents that they are in a social climate where they are respected and are being given some control. The child's anxiety will decrease if the parents are more at ease) • The primary nurse should admit the client (since this is an important step in the relating process) • Introduce the child and parents to roommates and their families • Provide both oral and written instructions for rules pertinent to unit and child's condition, e.g., isolation **Orient the child and parents to the physical environment** • Allow the child to wear own pajamas (if possible) and to have a security object. (This will decrease the threat of separation from familiar things) • Encourage one parent to stay with the child between 6 mos and 5 yrs of age. Explain rooming-in policies • Orient the family to the facilities and items needed for self-care and parental care, e.g., bathroom, urinal, bathing facilities • Leave in the room a scrapbook of pictures of hospital utensils with simple explanations. (This allows clarification at a time of reduced stress and helps the child work through fears) • If a child's condition permits, provide a tour of the unit (playroom, etc) • Encourage questions throughout the orientation and encourage the child to touch and manipulate unfamiliar articles	• More relaxed facial expression • Occasional smile • Decreased skeletal muscle tension • Increased attention span • Verbalizing feeling "more at ease" The child/parents will successfully adapt to the crisis of hospitalization, as evidenced by: • Identifying the sources of anxiety • Discussing previously used coping strategies/solution • Identifying external sources of support • Generating possible solutions to problems • Verbalizing "feeling in control again" • Verbalizing a decrease in symptoms of anxiety • Displaying fewer signs of anxiety The child will display the effective coping with the major stressors of hospitalization, as evidenced by: • Maintenance of a bond with parents and significant others • Ability to cope with unpleasant diagnostic and treatment procedures without loss of self-esteem • Demonstration of understanding of most rules and expectations, with occasional questions asked about others • Maintenance of control over some appropriate choices The **chronically ill** or **terminally ill** child will display effective coping with the relapse of illness that prompted this hospitalization, as evidenced by: • Identifying and discussing unresolved fears from previous admissions • Trying at least one new method of coping with old fears

(continued)

TABLE 21-5 *(continued)*

Defining Characteristics	Nursing Interventions	Evaluation Criteria
• Sleeplessness • Skeletal muscle tension • Shortened attention span • Clinging behavior *(Parents)* • Skeletal muscle tension • Pacing or other restless behavior • Worried facial expression • Tearfulness • Shortened attention span *(Siblings)* • Social withdrawal • Overactivity • Restlessness • Lack of initiative • Regressive behavior • Escalation of normal misbehavior • Clinging to parents • Attention-getting behaviors	**Establish the basis for a trusting relationship** • Convey an attitude of acceptance and respect • Be honest, don't be afraid to say "I don't know"; the family needs a source of **reliable** information, not just an answer for every question • Demonstrate caring and empathy • Let the child and family know when you will be available to talk to them next, then keep the appointment **Provide *crisis intervention* as needed.** (See also Chapter 18) **Facilitate identification of problems** as seen by the child/parents • Ask questions such as, "What is the most frightening/hardest/most frustrating thing for you about being in (or having your child in) the hospital?" "How do you feel about being here?" "How does this change your role as brother/sister/son/daughter/friend/sibling/student/mother/father/secretary/carpenter/etc?" • Anticipate the stressors identified for Nursing Diagnostic Statements 9 and 10; ask specific questions about these areas as indicated • Accept the answers given and reinforce the right to feelings and perceptions. (The nurse's validation can facilitate the individual's acceptance; identification and acceptance of problems precedes problem solving) • Expect identification of problems to take a period of hours to days, depending upon the meaning of the crisis to the individual **Facilitate identification of coping resources, both internal and external** • Determine personal coping strengths and patterns. Ask,	• Identifying and discussing the personal meaning of this change in health status The parents of the **chronically ill** or **terminally ill** child will display adaptive coping with this hospitalization, as evidenced by: • Exploring the personal meaning of this relapse in the child's condition • Identifying and discussing unresolved frustration and fear associated with previous admissions • Demonstrating effective problem solving The **terminally ill** child and the parents will display adaptive coping with the prognosis, as evidenced by: • Discussing their feelings about death with each other • Displaying the ability to derive pleasure from loving interactions The parents of the **terminally ill** child will cope effectively with a decision to discontinue life support, as evidenced by: • Verbalizing acceptance of death as inevitable • Displaying relief that the decision has been made • Verbalizing rationale for the decision The siblings will display adaptive behavior in response to the ill client's hospitalization, as evidenced by maintaining usual behavior patterns: • Absence of regressive behavior • No significant increase in attention-seeking behavior • No unusual withdrawal or moodiness • Maintaining usual bond with ill sibling Siblings of the **chronically ill** or **terminally ill** child will display

TABLE 21-5 *(continued)*

Defining Characteristics	Nursing Interventions	Evaluation Criteria
	"Have you ever felt this way before?" "What did you do then?" "Did it help?" "Which of the things you did helped most?" • Determine external sources of support. Ask, "Do you have family here?" "Are there friends and neighbors who can help?" "Does your church or synagogue offer help for families of hospitalized children?" • Suggest support services of which you are aware. Refer to Social Services for others **Assist with immediate needs as appropriate.** For example, Social Services may be able to provide a meal ticket or babysitting on a one-time basis. A teddy bear from the playroom may work as a replacement security object. (Beyond this initial help, allow as much self-help as possible to enhance self-esteem) **Encourage the child and/or parent to discuss possible solutions to the identified problem(s)** • Actually listing alternatives may be helpful (this "distancing" technique can help with objectivity) • Suggest solutions detailed in this chapter, e.g., one parent staying with a young child while the other cares for siblings at home • Make it clear that the choice of action is theirs but that nursing support is available **Facilitate evaluation of the outcome** • Ask questions such as, "How do you feel about it now?" "Are you still afraid Jennifer won't be your best friend after you leave the hospital?" "How is the baby sitter working out?" • If the action was not successful, support the child/parent in retracing the problem-solving steps	adaptive behavior to the hospitalization, as evidenced by: • Discussing new fears prompted by this change in health status

(continued)

TABLE 21-5 *(continued)*

Defining Characteristics	Nursing Interventions	Evaluation Criteria
	Promote relationships with family and significant others • Encourage a parent to remain with the child between 6 mos and 5 yrs of age (who is at most risk for separation anxiety) • Encourage frequent family visits for the child whose parent cannot remain at the bedside • Use pictures of family and friends, audio tapes of their voices, phone calls, and letters to help maintain the child's significant social bonds during prolonged hospitalization **Prepare for procedures according to developmental age;** see Table 23–1 **Preserve the bed/crib as a safe place.** Remove child from the room (or if in isolation, at least from the bed or crib) to perform unpleasant procedures **Reinforce adaptive coping** by focusing upon it and using it as an example of a coping strength, e.g., "You're holding your arm so still. It is OK to cry, but you're holding your arm so still, and that's wonderful!" **Provide age-appropriate explanations and rationale for rules and policies** • Parents can also be given these in written form. (If parents understand the rules, they can help the child interpret them) • Provide alternative for some of the **"Nos"** and **"can'ts,"** e.g., "You may not take the tricycle to the lobby, but you may ride it to the playroom" **Offer actual choices as often as possible,** e.g., "Do you want your medicine in the cup or syringe?" **Do not offer choices that do not exist,** e.g., whether to take a prescribed medicine	

TABLE 21-5 *(continued)*

Defining Characteristics	Nursing Interventions	Evaluation Criteria
	See also Tables 21–9 through 21–13 for strategies appropriate to needs at each developmental level **Recognize that rehospitalization may be more traumatic than the first experience** • Encourage the child to talk about previous hospitalizations. Ask, "What was the scariest part about being here before?" "What was the best part?" • Introduce the child to some new coping strategies. Let child choose one to practice and to try during a stressful situation. Help the child evaluate the effectiveness of this strategy and make modifications as necessary. • Encourage the child to explore feelings about the relapse of the long-term illness. Ask, "Why are you in the hospital this time?" "Are you sick in the same way you were before?" "What is the scariest part about being sick?" **Recognize that each relapse/readmission may represent a greater crisis than the last** because it may signal a downward spiral in the disease process. Coping may be further impaired by physical, mental, and spiritual exhaustion from the strain of home management of the illness • Encourage the parent to take time to consult with friends and clergy who can provide emotional and spiritual support • Implement the steps of crisis intervention as needed • Collaborate with the physician, home care nurse, and other involved members of the health care team to provide optimal information and support through a unified effort • Provide frequent opportunities for the parents to express their	

(continued)

TABLE 21-5 (continued)

Defining Characteristics	Nursing Interventions	Evaluation Criteria
	feelings/concerns. One way to initiate the conversation is to state an observation, such as, "You look so sad/upset/tired" • Involve the parents in the child's care and in decision making as often as possible. (This will help thwart a sense of powerlessness) • Reinforce effective coping and personal strengths by reminding parent of these qualities **Facilitate parent/child discussions about death** • If there is initial parental reluctance to "burden" the child with the prognosis, tell parents that even small children usually know instinctively that they are going to die and may be afraid to "burden" the parent • Discuss the benefits of open communication and mutual support to the quality of the child's and parents' lives **Encourage loving interactions** • Allow the child to be held and cuddled by the parent as much as is desired. (Treatment protocol is secondary to quality of life at this point) • Explain about tubes and machines to demystify them and to prevent them from forming a barrier between parent and child • Provide privacy • Reinforce the mutual support gained from these interactions by commenting to parents and child about how much each is helping the other **Encourage parents to "talk through" their feelings** during the decision process • Clarify misconceptions, offer information, listen, acknowledge their pain, but do not offer advice. (No one else can make the decision for them. The nurse can	

TABLE 21-5 *(continued)*

Defining Characteristics	Nursing Interventions	Evaluation Criteria
	be invaluable, however, in helping them to clarify their thoughts) • Support their decision by comments like "I know this was very difficult for you." "You considered all the alternatives very carefully." "I know you love your child very much" **Alert parents to common behavioral responses of siblings** Take care to do so in a manner nonthreatening to parenting abilities. (Anxiety increases sensitivity to guilt feelings) **Suggest strategies to support siblings at home and maintain their bond with the ill child.** Parents can • Plan time each day to spend with each child at home (if only a few minutes) where there is no competition for the parent's attention • Acknowledge the normal egocentricity of childhood and adolescence and not expect the siblings to be as consumed by thoughts of the ill child as the parents are • Encourage, but not force, hospital visitation, phone calls, letters, and exchange of snapshots to maintain client/sibling bonds • Suggest the ill child make a picture or other simple "gift" for each sibling at home (to keep the communication of love flowing in both directions) • Accept offers for child care and other help from extended family and friends (to reduce usual role stress and allow more time for family activities) **Alert parents to fears of siblings commonly triggered by another hospitalization:** fear of their sibling's impending death, of having the same thing happen to them, of	

(continued)

TABLE 21-5 *(continued)*

Defining Characteristics	Nursing Interventions	Evaluation Criteria
	loss of security because of parents' anxiety; of further changes in family life and structure **Discuss with parents age-appropriate ways to support siblings.** (A reminder of developmental crises and tasks can help them understand their children's behavior.) Parents can • Encourage siblings to express their fears • Discuss the child's illness and prognosis openly and honestly • Give only the information asked for (which can help each sibling adjust at his or her own pace) • Acknowledge that it is normal for siblings to feel angry at the ill child sometimes • Encourage each sibling to develop his or her own identity/potential • Keep family life and sibling responsibilities as normal as possible	

Analysis: Nursing Diagnostic Statement 11

Response and Related or Risk Factors: **High risk for knowledge deficit: Child and parents,** *about lifetime management of treatment regimen; risk factor management of the illness at home.*

Projected Outcome: The family will display a pattern of regulating and integrating into daily living a program for treatment of illness or disability that is satisfactory for meeting specific health goals.

Defining Characteristics	Nursing Interventions	Evaluation Criteria
Subjective: • Acceleration of illness symptoms *Objective:* • Verbalized desire to manage the treatment of illness and prevention of sequelae • Verbalized difficulty with regulation/integration of one or more prescribed regimens for treatment	**Begin discharge preparation on the day of admission.** (Home management is too complicated to be taught entirely on the day of discharge) • Assess teaching needs early and list on a teaching flow sheet • Allow the child and family to select the order for teaching from the list	The child and/or parents will display the knowledge and skills needed for home management of the illness, as evidenced by: • Demonstrating effective physical care (e.g., dressing change) • Demonstrating effective operation of equipment and having it installed in the home prior to discharge

TABLE 21-5 *(continued)*

Defining Characteristics	***Nursing Interventions***	***Evaluation Criteria***
of illness and its effects or prevention of complications • Verbalized that did not take action to include treatment regimens in daily routines • Verbalized that did not take action to reduce risk factors for progression of illness and sequelae	• Have the child and family check off the items as they are completed. (A sense of control and responsibility will facilitate learning) • Begin self-management and/or family management as soon as initial anxiety has decreased enough to allow it. (Repeated practice with new techniques will increase self-confidence and self-esteem and reduce anxiety.) See Table 23–1 for age-appropriate education strategies • Whenever possible, listen to the physician's final instructions to the family (so that questions can be clarified before discharge) **Allow time for questions and clarification on the day of the discharge** • Tell the family when you can spend time with them to answer any final questions. (They can then prepare for this session) • Provide written reminders of instructions whenever possible • Alert parents to the possibility of behavioral reactions to hospitalization, making it clear the child may experience no behavioral change. Encourage them to give the child extra attention for a few days after discharge **Collaborate with other members of the health care team** as appropriate to update them on the child's status after this hospitalization. Inform the parents you have called the school nurse, home care nurse, etc	• Identifying prescribed changes in diet, activity • Demonstrating safe medication administration and identifying major side effects • Identifying arrangements for child care as needed • Identifying signs and symptoms of relapse • Possessing written appointment notice and emergency numbers • Discussing strategies to use should the child display behavioral regression or excessive attention-seeking after discharge The child will show no acceleration of illness symptoms

TABLE 21-6
Normal Sleep Requirements

Neonate	20–22 hrs/24 hrs
6 wks	14–16 hrs/24 hrs
6 mos–1 yr	12–16 hrs/24 hrs
1–3 yrs	10–14 hrs/24 hrs
3–5 yrs	12–14 hrs/24 hrs
6–9 yrs	11–12 hrs/24 hrs
10–12 yrs	9–10 hrs/24 hrs
Adolescent	8–10 hrs/24 hrs

avoid sleep deprivation, a systematic recording of sleep can be used to compare against normal sleep requirements (Table 21–6). If the hospital uses a flow sheet, label one column for sleep; cumulatively total hours of sleep over the 24-hour period.

Establish Naptime. Hospital routines and schedules frequently do not take into account the child's need for sleep. During an illness, the child's sleep is frequently disrupted by procedures, medications, or monitoring of vital signs. The nurse is responsible for assessing the overall needs of the child and identifying ways to coordinate care. When primary nursing is practiced, the nursing care can more easily be planned to avoid frequent disruptions. However, the collaboration of all team members is required to reduce the number of sequential interruptions by different professionals. Some ways to help establish uninterrupted periods of sleep include:

- Discuss the child's need for sleep in team conferences.
- Specify naptimes in care plan.
- Post sign at bedside "Jeremy is asleep—Please come back at 3:30."
- Schedule treatments and medications to allow for periods of rest throughout the 24-hour period.

Decrease the Child's Anxiety Related to Hospitalization. A child's anxiety during hospitalization interferes with the ability to achieve adequate rest and sleep. Major deterrents to such anxiety are the presence of supportive parents; an opportunity to play; clear expectations about procedures; and a supportive health care team. Concern for the individual's sleep requirements is communicated by providing a comfortable environment, a story, a drink of water, a back rub, or other special measures of comfort. A few moments of the nurse's time can contribute greatly to the child's ability to fall asleep. Whenever possible, procedures that can be seen and heard by other children on the unit should be performed in the treatment room to diminish the onlooker's potential fearful thoughts that interfere with falling asleep.

Effectively Use Medications and Pain Management Techniques. If a child is experiencing discomfort, the administration of an analgesic can often be timed so it is given at bedtime to help the child relax. Sleeplessness also may result as a side effect of another medication (e.g., theophylline), in which case collaboration is needed with the physician to adjust the dosage. Nonpharmacologic methods to relieve pain should also be used to induce sleep (see Chapter 25 on management of pain).

Promote Physical Activity and Relaxation. An assessment of a child's physical activity and relaxation is necessary to promote adequate sleep and rest. If a child is physically able, movement, activity, and time spent in the playroom or recreation lounge are encouraged. Physical activity does not need to be strenuous to provide relaxation. Even a walk to a gift shop, a snack bar, or up and down the hall should be encouraged to provide physical exercise, which, in turn, promotes rest and sleep. Additionally, long periods of sleep should be avoided during the day except for naptime for younger children.

Maintain a Sufficient Intake of Nutrients to Meet Metabolic Demands

During an illness and hospitalization, a child's appetite is often dulled. Some behavioral regression in eating patterns may be noted in association with the anxiety of hospitalization. Food preparation and type of food served are often unfamiliar to the child. Cultural preferences are not as easily accommodated in an institution, and feeding techniques vary from those used at home. The reason for hospitalization may be another source of loss of appetite. As well, the physiologic process of the illness or side effects of medications may cause discomfort and anorexia. Planning for the maintenance of required caloric intakes involves careful selection of food and use of approaches that are developmentally appropriate. Nutritional intake goals are based on recommended caloric requirements (Table 21–7) unless contraindicated by treatment plan. Information about eating is obtained from the parents, and any special equipment required for feeding should be brought from home.

Feeding Infants. Infants are accustomed to the smell, touch, and voice of their caretakers. Feeding is associated with the development of a sense of trust and comfort provided by the caretaker. A comfortable place for the parents to sit to hold their infant should be provided. The following may facilitate parent/infant comfort while hospitalized:

- Have parent feed whenever possible.
- Note parents' feeding technique so it can be copied by nurse caregivers. (This will help ensure as much consistency as possible and reinforce parents' self-esteem and sense of control. Of

TABLE 21-7
Recommended Caloric Requirements

0–6 mos	kg × 108 kcal
6–12 mos	kg × 98 kcal
1–3 yrs	1300 kcal
4–6 yrs	1800 kcal
7–10 yrs	2000 kcal
females, 11–14 yrs	2200 kcal
males, 11–14 yrs	2500 kcal
females, 15–18 yrs	2200 kcal
males, 15–18 yrs	3000 kcal

Data from Food and Nutrition Board: *Recommended dietary allowances,* (10th ed.). Washington, DC: National Research Council—National Academy Press, 1989.

course, teaching is indicated if inappropriate techniques are observed).

- Use bottle and nipple similar to those used at home and inquire whether parents warm formula.
- Determine which is given first in the feeding—solids or liquids—and then follow pattern.
- If the infant does not take commercial baby food, ask the parent to bring food from home.

When possible, the comforts an infant usually enjoys at home should be implemented when fed in the hospital. If an infant's feeding time is too long (over 30 to 40 minutes), the infant tires and expends too much energy; however, the feeding should not be rushed. Infants should be held for their feedings; under no circumstances should bottles be propped. Also, the practice of leaving an infant in bed with a bottle is not condoned because it encourages dental caries. Infants are also held when being fed solids until they are able to sit alone, and then they are more comfortable and secure in a highchair. To ensure safety, a restraint should be fastened at the waist and between the legs whenever an infant is placed in a highchair in the hospital. Independence should be encouraged by providing a plastic bottle when an infant wishes to hold the bottle; finger foods can be held by the older infant. Infants and toddlers should not be left unattended in highchairs or with food.

Hospitalization of an infant can disrupt a mother's ability to breastfeed her infant; however, support and encouragement from members of the health care team can foster the mother's success at breastfeeding in the hospital. Breastfeeding mothers may feel more comfortable in a private area. A mother can pump her breasts and the milk can be used at a future feeding if an infant is having treatments or procedures or has to remain on a nothing-by-mouth (NPO) routine. Very small infants can be breastfed even though they may be dependent on monitors and machines.

Burping an infant, whether breastfed or bottlefed, can be done by holding the infant upright against the nurse's shoulder or by holding the infant in a sitting position on the nurse's lap. One hand is placed on the right side to facilitate any remaining air to rise from the stomach. Infant seats are not used if the infant has a tendency for reflux (Orenstein, 1983). (See Chapter 35 for discussion of positioning of infants with gastroesophageal reflux.)

Feeding Older Children and Adolescents. Many of the strategies used to promote an adequate intake by older hospitalized children are relevant to all ages. These include provision of:

1. An opportunity for choice and self-regulation.
2. Education about special diets and general nutrition.
3. Companionship while eating.
4. Food that is appealing in appearance.

Opportunity for Choices, Independence, and Self-Regulation. Attainment of skills in self-feeding is an important developmental landmark. Toddlers and preschoolers should be encouraged to maintain their formerly achieved level of self-feeding during hospitalization. The nurse should be alert to notice a child too tired to eat who is capable of self-feeding and offer help appropriately. Children are allowed to choose desired foods from a menu with the assistance of an adult. Special diets can be explained to school-age children and adolescents.

Teaching about Special Diets and General Nutrition. As children mature, they can understand the reasons for the need of special diets and become more cooperative when an effort is made to explain the purpose of dietary treatment plans. A pediatric nutritionist skilled in the care of children can be consulted for children having difficulty adapting to new diets.

Companionship During Meals. Young children are most comfortable if they can eat in the presence of their family members. When this is not feasible, group eating is an alternative. Small tables and chairs are often available. Older children can help younger children as needed and can be role models for proper table manners. The atmosphere of group eating encourages socialization and promotes a sense of well-being associated with eating.

Appropriate Presentation of Food. Children react to the appearance of food. Color combinations, food consistency, and the size of portions are important to consider when presenting the food tray to a child. The arrangement of food adds to its attractiveness, e.g., cutting a sandwich on the diagonal to make four small triangular sandwiches and setting them upright can be an encouragement to eat. A small cup or specially folded napkin with a happy face can change the mood of a child. Adding preferred foods, such as peanut butter, from the dietary supplies kept on the unit may be all that is needed to interest a child in food.

TABLE 21-8
Age-Appropriate Feeding Interventions for Children

Toddler

- Encourage parents and/or siblings to be present at mealtime whenever possible
- Alert parents to avoid a power struggle over food; the child should be allowed to choose the desired foods from those offered. (Given the opportunity, toddlers often use refusal of food to assert some control in a situation when they are otherwise powerless; offered a selection of nutritious foods, usually they will choose those the body needs)
- If toddlers must eat without family, allow them to eat with other youngsters whenever possible to provide a semblance of normal mealtime activity; the distraction of other children temporarily may override anxiety related to the strange environment
- Provide highchair or booster chair similar to what is used at home and observe usual routines, including ritualistic food preferences
- Make mealtime as pleasant as possible, avoiding administration of medication or unpleasant procedures
- Plan analgesic medication administration to decrease discomfort at mealtime
- Allow as much self-feeding as possible. (The toddler who feels partly in control will be more cooperative)

Preschooler

- Allow child as much control over food served as possible; assist in selecting foods from printed menu, allow to help "make" toast, milkshake, etc, and to show the nurse "how Mommy makes it." (Child will feel more in control and will be less likely to demonstrate regressive behavior if newly developed language and motor skills are acknowledged)
- Encourage meals with family or other patients whenever possible
- The preschooler may like to "role model" good eating behaviors for a toddler patient. (This is in keeping with the tasks of initiative and socialization)

School-Age Child

- Explain to the child which kinds of nutrients are needed for return to health, i.e., protein and vitamin C for wound healing; allow the child to build a menu plan around favorite foods containing these nutrients; encourage parents to supply foods from home to satisfy the choices. (Self-regulation and industry will increase the child's self-esteem and decrease anxiety; therefore, nutrient intake may also increase)
- Allow the child to record the food intake on the flow chart. (This "concrete" record makes it easier for the child to keep track of progress toward a goal)
- Allow the school-age child to "role model" eating, to entertain, and help younger patients at mealtime (to increase a sense of self-worth)

Adolescent

- Identify the need for proper nutrition to regain health with the adolescent. (Reasons for treatment are especially important to the young person striving to make independent decisions)
- Allow self-regulation in food selection, in eating, and in recording of intake
- Offer the adolescent a consultation with the dietitian as this may be welcomed when weight loss or muscle building is desired after hospitalization. (Information from authorities outside the family is more likely to be valued)

Children who are not hungry can be totally discouraged when approached with what they view as large mounds of food; therefore, large portions should be cut and some removed before serving. If a child's appetite is diminished, only a small amount of liquid should be provided with the meal. A child's small stomach can soon feel a sense of fullness if a large glass of liquid starts the meal. Additional liquids can be served between meals to meet the daily requirements. Removal of dessert from the tray initially is sometimes necessary for a child to eat adequate portions of the main course. The way desserts are managed at home influences how a child responds in the hospital. If children have learned that they must eat a balanced meal before eating their dessert, they most likely will adhere to the same rule in the hospital. Children should be encouraged to eat but food should not become a control issue between the child and the caretakers.

Children should not be forced or bribed to eat when they are not hungry. Promising to play a game if a child eats a certain amount of food is an unfair dilemma for a sick child. See Table 21–8 for specific age-appropriate interventions for children.

Promote Normal Urine and Fecal Patterns to Prevent Fluid and Electrolyte Imbalance

The stress of hospitalization and the illness can alter the child's elimination pattern. Also, changes in activity level, food, and some medications can affect elimination. Nursing goals are: (1) to alleviate anxiety; (2) to increase self-care; and (3) to avoid scolding or shaming.

Alleviate Anxiety Related to Hospitalization. Approaches to alleviate anxiety in general are presented in Table 21–5, Nursing Diagnostic Statements 9 and 10. More specifically, the nurse can alleviate anxiety by keeping parents and children (if age-appropriate) informed of the expected changes in the character of urine or stool. Young children need to be shown the location of the potty and how to call for the nurse.

Older children may tend to put off urination and defecation because of the embarrassment they sense about elimination. School-age children and older are shy and reluctant to talk about toileting, and privacy is sometimes difficult to achieve in the hospital. Hospital gowns generally are not conducive to privacy;

therefore, a second gown to be worn as a robe is offered to the older child, or parents can bring a robe from home.

Increasing Self-Care Associated with Toileting. Children and adolescents are especially embarrassed about using urinals and bedpans. They may not know how to use them or are afraid of spillage. If parents are available, they can help their child with the task of toileting until more comfort is achieved with the nurse. Any assistance that the child can give should be encouraged, so a gradual return to self-care is accomplished.

Avoid Scolding or Shaming the Child for Incontinence. A common problem resulting from the stress of hospitalization is regressive toileting behaviors. A toddler who has achieved bowel and bladder control just prior to being hospitalized frequently becomes incontinent of urine and stool. The nurse should be supportive and not reprimand the child. Parents need reassurance that temporary loss of control while in the hospital is common. Although putting diapers on a toilet-trained child consumes less of the nurse's time, it is not recommended because it does not assist the child to maintain control. On the other hand, if a toilet-trained toddler regresses to soiling, diapers should be provided without criticism. The child recovering from the illness may again take an interest in using the potty but several weeks may pass before the toddler again achieves bowel and bladder control. Thus, parents should be cautioned against expecting immediate mastery of the previously achieved task and need to be patient with their child.

Promote Play Activities That Maintain the Child's Interest and Provide Appropriate Stimulation

Play is the major activity of the waking hours of a young child. It is a natural avenue for self-expression, the medium through which children master some developmental tasks, and the major resource for learning about their world. However, intense stress at times can render a healthy child "playless." Many children tend not to play spontaneously in the hospital because of the overwhelming stress and the threat of its associated hazards (Bolig, 1984). The separation from usual playmates, lack of available toys, isolation, and immobility or discomfort associated with the disease process or its treatment can contribute to an alteration in the hospitalized child's play behavior. In addition, the acuity and complexity of pediatric patients should cause health care professionals to view play in the 1990s differently. For example, further research is needed to determine the play needs of children who are drug- and/or technology-dependent (Bolig, 1990). The goal of nursing care is: (1) to integrate play into the plan of care; (2) to explain the purpose and use of play to parents; and (3) to provide age-appropriate play and activities.

Integrate Play into the Plan of Care. Nursing care is planned incorporating play and related activities to reduce the stress of hospitalization. Although scientific validation demonstrating the effectiveness of play is limited (Bolig, 1984), it is believed that play is a primary coping mechanism used by children. Play not only promotes development but also provides an important outlet for aggressive or hostile feelings. Play allows the child to work through fears and fantasies that may be multiplied during hospital experiences. Nurses take a dominant role in normalizing the hospital experience for children and encouraging them in play. In hospitals that employ child life specialists, both professional groups take responsibility for play to be integrated into daily caregiving. Using volunteers to supplement the nurse's role is also a common approach. In any setting, the nurse must understand clearly that play for the hospitalized child is central to meeting the holistic needs of the child and not just a "nice addition."

Explain the Purpose and Stage of Play to Family Members. Parents and older siblings can assist children to engage in play in a way that is familiar and helps the child cope with the stress of hospitalization. Therefore, both parents and siblings need to understand how play is being incorporated into care.

Types of play programs vary, with some consisting of little more than a play cupboard with toys, and little focus of play being used to alleviate the stress of hospitalization. Others are based on a particular philosophy with specific goals to promote expression of feelings and mastery. It is important for the nurse to understand the various types of play and to use play effectively in nursing interventions as a balancing factor. The use of play for assessment, diversion, recreation, and reduction of anxiety common across various settings including hospitals is discussed in Chapter 17.

Provide Age-Appropriate Play and Diversional Activities. In the hospital, a child's normal growth and developmental needs cannot always be met effectively through play because of limited space, impaired mobility, reduced energy, and limited toys. Also, the opportunity for socialization is thwarted because of separation from the child's family and peers. The nurse's familiarity with developmental play at different ages is an important component of nursing care. The nurse's responsibility is to provide for the child's need to play whether or not the unit has an organized play program.

Infants. To assist in preventing regression in development and a delay in the attainment of developmental milestones, an organized play period or infant stimulation program is desirable (Fig. 21–5). Play is intellectually stimulating for an infant and provides opportunities for continued development of motor and social skills. It is most important that human interactions are maintained through play.

When feeding, dressing, or diapering, the nurse should establish eye contact and speak to the infant.

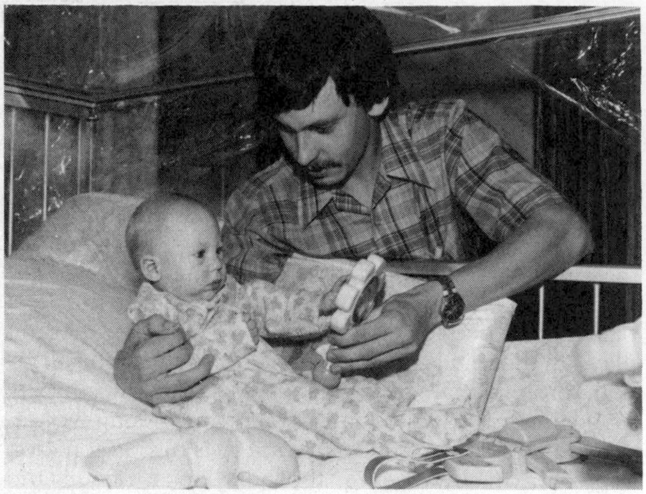

FIGURE 21 - 5. Hospitalized infants need the stimulation of play and toys to maintain their development.

Until infants are able to sit, they can be propped or placed in an infant seat at intervals, if their condition permits, so they can observe the activities around them. Mobiles, mirrors, baby gyms, and music boxes provide additional auditory and visual stimulation. Every infant should have toys within reach in the crib. Some hospital auxiliaries provide small soft toys for patients if none have been brought from home.

Activities can be planned away from the crib as well. Many units have strollers, swings, and rockers. If these are not available, a mat or bath blanket can be placed on the floor to provide the older infant opportunities for crawling, rolling, and reaching.

Toddlers and Preschoolers. As the child approaches the toddler years, play becomes more active and may be severely hampered by illness and hospitalization. Toddlers and preschoolers prefer large muscle activity, but, if such play is prohibited, toys can be brought to the child's bed or placed on a small table in the child's room. In some hospitals, enclosed outdoor play areas permit activities to exercise large muscles. If confined to bed, it is especially important to provide for the child's need to explore, to be independent, and to make discoveries through manipulation.

Coloring, painting, and manipulating toys that stack or come apart are appropriate for young children. Large puzzles, books with cardboard pages that the child can turn, and large beads to put on a heavy string are enjoyed by young children. Toys that allow the child to dissipate energy, such as a pounding board with hammer and thick crayons that can be used to scribble vigorously, can relieve a child of some of the frustration of limited physical exercise. Creative and imaginative play activities are particularly beneficial and enjoyable.

School-Age Children. Although the school-age child preserves some of the fantasy and drama from preschool days in play, play has changed in several recognizable ways. Added are rules, ritualistic behaviors, language chants ("Step on a crack, break your mother's back"), and team activities. The person who organizes structured play activities on the school-age unit should keep these facts in mind. School-age children tend to prefer games, both active and sedentary, to unstructured group play. The school-age child also enjoys the reprieve of quiet and solitary activity (playing board games, reading books, writing stories, or drawing pictures). School-age children still enjoy being read to occasionally. Therapeutic play equipment like puppets, dolls, and medical-related toys should remain available but should not be forced on them (Fig. 21–6).

Adolescents. The use of play to facilitate adjustment to hospitalization for an adolescent usually takes on the form of socialization. Group activities involving several adolescents and a place for them to gather are major recreational needs of a hospitalized adolescent. An adolescent's ability to understand explanations about procedures and events accompanying hospitalization obviates the need for use of therapeutic play as with a younger child. However, an important element in an adolescent's adjustment is participation in recreation, games, and diversionary activities. Computer games at the bedside or in a specified adolescent lounge area on the unit provide both individual and peer participation.

Promote Participation in Self-Care Activities Appropriate for Child's Age and Health State

The experience of illness and hospitalization has the potential to interfere with a child's progress toward independence in self-care. Nursing care is planned to support children in the achievement of self-care to the degree possible. The nursing goals are to: (1) assess usual self-care activities; (2) provide opportunities for self-care (Fig. 21–7); and (3) teach child self-care related to illness.

Assess Usual Self-Care Activities. Children achieve levels of self-care at varying ages and times. Each child's performance level is assessed, understanding that the child's environment and type of illness will influence their ability to maintain their normal self-care activities.

Provide Opportunities for Self-Care. Maintaining the child's usual level of self-care facilitates coping by increasing a child's self-concept and sense of control. A child can be helped to feel independent by carefully explaining the hospital environment (call bell, bed controls, bathroom light, use of urinal and bedpan). Necessary items should be arranged within reach for the child. Personal pajamas with familiar closures should be worn rather than hospital gowns requiring tying, when possible. Parents can bring personal items, such as a comb, toothbrush, or special eating utensils required to avoid spilling, from home

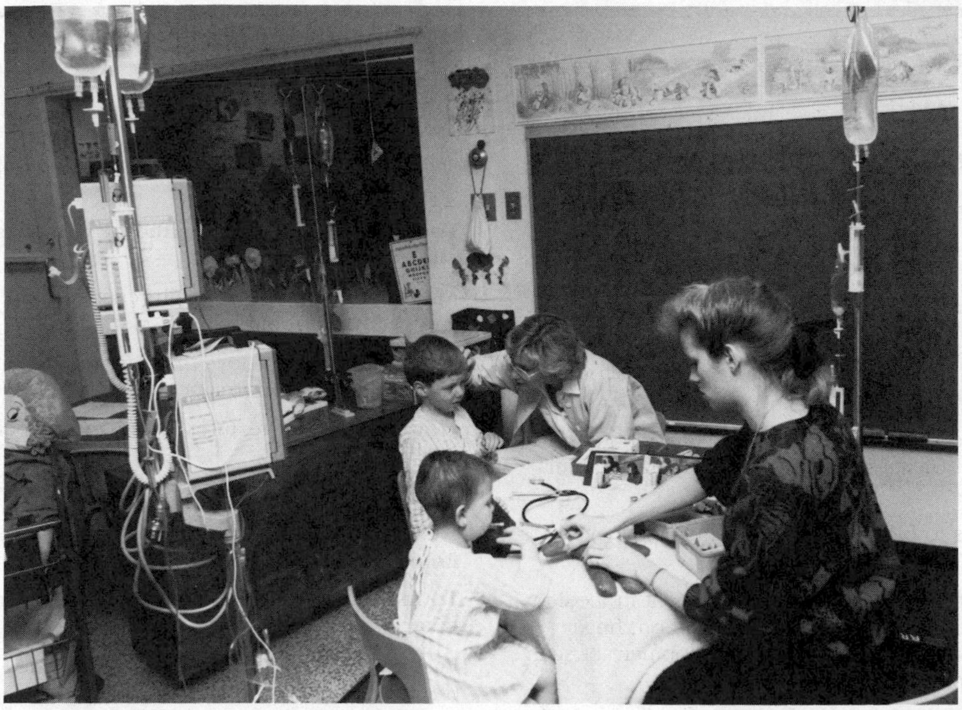

FIGURE 21 - 6. An opportunity to play with medical toys is an important strategy used in hospitals to reduce a child's anxiety. At Chedoke-McMaster Hospital, Hamilton, Ontario, a fully developed play program is provided by the Child Life Team.

for the child. Extra time (and perhaps extra mess) is needed to help promote self-care in a hospitalized child; therefore, the caregiver's support and patience are essential.

Teach the Child Self-Care Related to Illness. Modifications of care related to the child's illness and treatment are taught to the child and parents. Two examples are sitting on the side of the bed long enough to avoid orthostatic hypotension or using an over-the-bed trapeze to move toward the head of the bed. Other examples specific to various diseases can be found in Chapters 32 through 47, where specific diseases are presented.

Provide Opportunity for Activities That Promote Normal Growth and Development

Nursing care is planned to foster normal growth and development and to facilitate coping skills appropriate for the age of the child. Nursing goals are to meet normal developmental needs such as physical mobility and sensory experience. A child's developmental level is assessed, recognizing that illness affects the child's responses. Motor behavior especially is affected by the fatigue associated with illness and should be reassessed as the condition improves. The help of parents and older siblings is enlisted to plan and implement strategies to maintain or promote development during hospitalization.

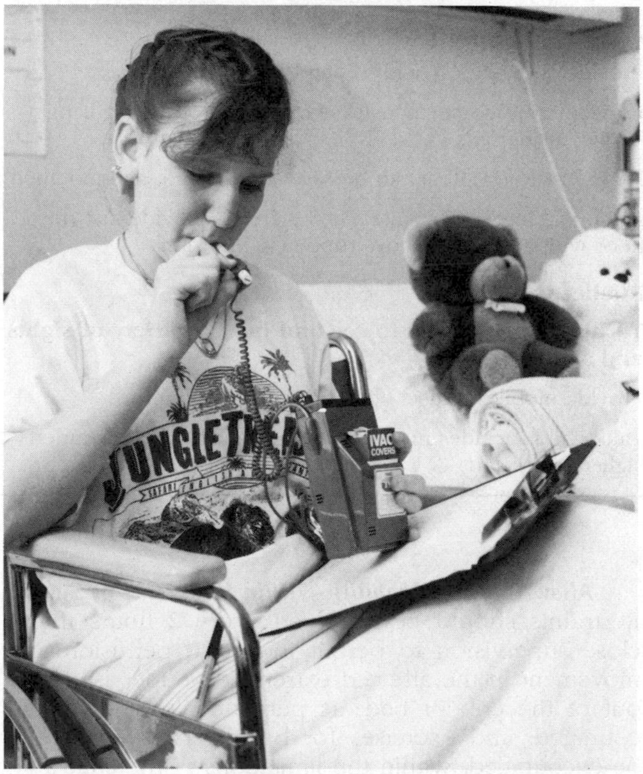

FIGURE 21 - 7. Independence and responsibility can be fostered in school-age children and adolescents by encouraging their involvement in monitoring their own vital signs.

TABLE 21-9
Developmental Needs and Nursing Interventions: Infants

Physical Needs

To be warm and dry

Check infant frequently and provide clean diapers and sheets as needed

To have hunger needs met in a consistent manner

Maintain the home feeding schedule whenever possible

Encourage the breastfeeding mother to continue; make a breast pump available if feeding must be curtailed for a period of time

On admission, check with parent for type, amount, and frequency of formula (if not breastfed), and whether formula is warmed

Encourage parents to be present for feedings whenever possible

Ask parents about the child's usual involvement in feeding (i.e., drinking from cup, self-feeding from spoon, finger foods, holding own bottle) and foster development of such skills (do not prop bottle)

Ask parents about usual position for feeding (held, highchair, infant seat, and so on)

Schedule intrusive treatments at a time other than immediately after a feeding to avoid vomiting

To have opportunity to roll and pull self up; to reach, grasp, and mouth objects in a safe environment

Ensure that side rails are locked securely

Provide "bubble-top" crib if child crawls up rails

Provide crib bumper pads to avoid injury or getting caught between side rails

Provide safe toys that can be held, transferred, and mouthed

As condition permits, take to play area—provide mat on floor with appropriate toys (under supervision)

Intellectual Needs

To have opportunity to see and hear a variety of sights and sounds

Provide mobiles, music boxes, busy boxes in crib

Take child for rides in a wagon or stroller to permit varied sights and sounds

To hear language

Speak to the infant when awake; use appropriate language (avoid baby talk)

To learn through sensorimotor experience in a safe environment

Allow infant to learn through repetition of acts, i.e., drop and pick up toy

Provide a variety of toys that can be manipulated so that infant can repeat performances

Provide variety of textures to enhance experience with the environment

Provide clean toys that can be mouthed. (Wash well after toys fall on the floor)

Emotional-Social Needs

To maintain relationship with parent or primary caretaker

Encourage parent to provide or participate in daily care (feed, bathe, hold) whenever possible

Explain to parents whether child can be held and help parent to do so

Suggest ways parent can participate in play and stimulation for their infant

If parent cannot room-in, assign the same nurse whenever possible

To develop sense of security

Handle infant gently during all care and procedures

Cuddle infant frequently, especially after procedures

Talk to infant during care and procedures

Respond to infant cues by observing when infant is tired, wants to be held, or just wants to lie in crib and play

Allow Physical Mobility Within the Limits of Safety. Restraints should be removed every 2 hours under close supervision to permit increased perfusion and movement in the affected extremities. Supervised play out of the crib or bed, as permitted, should be encouraged; and exercises for bedfast children should be encouraged, within the limitations of the child's illness, to maintain musculoskeletal function.

Provide Sensory Stimuli Appropriate to the Child's Age. For information relating to providing a variety of sensory stimuli at different ages, see Table 21–5, Nursing Diagnostic Statement 6, and Tables 21–9 to 21–13.

Foster Normal Growth and Development. Developmental needs and nursing interventions to foster normal growth and development appropriate for infants, toddlers, preschooler, school-age children, and adolescents are presented in Tables 21–9, 21–10, 21–11, 21–12, and 21–13, respectively. Another consideration is the school milieu, which contributes immensely to the growth and development of children. Hospitalization interferes with the normal benefits of

TABLE 21-10
Developmental Needs and Nursing Interventions: Toddlers

Physical Needs

To explore and develop muscle skill within a safe environment

Assess prehospitalization exploratory activities

Provide small manipulative toys (boxes with lids; stack toys; nesting toys; large beads; large puzzles; equipment to color, paint, and scribble)

Provide a crib with an enclosed see-through top when a child attempts to explore by reaching for dangerous objects or crawling out of the crib

Permit supervised activities in a playroom to explore new toys and the unfamiliar environment

Allow exploration in child's room under supervision

To have opportunity to engage in large muscle activity within safe limits

Assess degree of mobility attained

Provide for supervised out-of-bed activities consistent with patterns at home as the child's condition permits

Keep floors free of small objects

Enforce rules about wearing shoes or nonskid slippers when child is out of bed

Provide toys for the large muscles (rocking horse, soft ball, indoor slide, push-and-pull toys)

To maintain physiologic function through development of self-care skills

Assess level of self-care attained (eating, elimination, dressing, hygiene, bedtime care)

Provide opportunities for participation in self-care activities:

- Eating: Provide highchair or small table and chair, bib, and usual types of food; allow child to feed self in usual manner
- Elimination: Provide a potty chair or diapers according to usual elimination patterns; reinforce routine as established prehospitalization
- Dressing: Permit child to assist with those activities he or she is capable of doing
- Hygiene: Allow child to participate in handwashing, brushing teeth, manipulating own wash cloth in tub

Intellectual Needs

To have opportunity to learn via sensorimotor experience and express self through imitation and pretending

To engage in conversation with adults and children to enhance language development; to hear proper language and be encouraged to express self through language

Provide toys that encourage exploration and manipulation

For older toddler, provide toys and equipment that can be used to reenact hospital experience

Assess extent of child's vocabulary, especially key phrases and words pertaining to daily activities

Allow child to complete sentences; avoid speaking for the child

Reinforce words child has mastered and introduce new words

Encourage group activities (play and eating) to encourage use of language among children

To receive explanations about procedures (toddlers can understand more than they can say)

Avoid speaking about children without explanations to them as well

Explain procedures before doing them

Emotional-Social Needs

To develop sense of autonomy

Allow child to do things alone pertaining to own care

Allow child to participate in the bedtime story, and preparation for bed according to home routines

Give child control over some of own life: allow choices, restrain as little as possible, and praise for completed tasks

To learn to separate from parents

Encourage care by parents

Assist family in coping with behaviors in response to hospitalization and separation

Encourage parents to visit often even though child resists their leaving

Provide primary nurse when parents cannot be present

Keep image of parent in child's mind with a picture, personal belongings, or a tape recording

To learn to adapt socially

Reinforce those socially acceptable behaviors mastered by the child before hospitalization (eating, elimination, play)

Provide play opportunities with other children

To maintain usual routines and rituals for sense of security

Assess important rituals and routines, especially regarding bedtime (provide security objects and maintain routine; reading story, hugging, use of night light and other rituals)

Ask parents and child about preferences in foods, toys, routines regarding daily hygiene, elimination, and dressing

Maintain as many home routines as possible

TABLE 21-11
Developmental Needs and Nursing Interventions: Preschoolers

Physical Needs

To maintain control of body functions

Assess prehospitalization level of control and patterns for eating, elimination, and sleep; assess words used to describe functions

Allow normal patterns as much as possible

Reassure when accidents in elimination occur; do not reprimand or punish

Praise successes in self-control

Provide age-appropriate motor stimulation

To maintain physiologic function through increased development of self-care skills

Assess prehospitalization self-care tasks

Allow continued self-care when possible; provide some opportunities for decisions on care, especially in aspects of care in which condition or treatment prohibits self-care

Allow usual eating practices: provide foods child is used to, finger foods, favorite foods, and eating utensils from home; allow family members to eat with child if isolated or to feed if child must be fed; if not isolated, allow eating at child-sized table with hospitalized peers; follow child's usual rituals, such as prayer before eating

Allow usual elimination practices: provide potty chair (from home if preferred) or regular toilet as child is accustomed to; if mobility is restricted, offer to assist child to toilet or bedpan at usual eliminating times; keep call bell near so child may get prompt assistance at other times. (Preschoolers still have difficulty "holding off" elimination processes); stay with child or provide privacy as child is accustomed

Allow usual rest and sleep practices; allow night light if child is used to one or requests one; provide quiet, uninterrupted period during child's usual nap or rest time if nap still taken; allow usual sleep time attire to be worn; if not contraindicated, allow usual sleep position and amount of cover and pillows used at home; bring any special sleep items (blanket, pacifier, toy) from home

Permit child to dress at least partially in own clothing during daytime

Intellectual Needs

To be protected from sense of guilt, which can occur as a result of egocentric thinking

Reassure repeatedly that no one is to blame for the condition or hospitalization

Reassure that only necessary treatments will be done, and they will not be done without telling the child first

Provide activities (play, arts and crafts, stories) that stimulate intellectual development

To be protected from fears created by preoperational thinking (intuitive, magical thoughts)

Explain all procedures, especially describing what child can expect to experience through the senses, before doing them

Provide for dramatic and therapeutic play; make available safe procedural equipment and dolls during education sessions, in playroom, at bedside

Do not talk about the child unless child is included in the conversation

To have opportunity to use expressive language

Encourage questions and ask questions to learn fears, fantasies, and misperceptions (correct these when possible); give opportunity for verbal expressions during stress

Encourage child to tell stories about drawings or to tell you a "story" about hospital procedures or experiences

Teach new words related to simple anatomy and physiology, the disease or treatment, and hospital equipment and personnel

Emotional-Social Needs

To master control of the environment and develop independence

Encourage self-care in hygiene and participation in medical care and treatments. (The preschooler can cooperate if given adequate instruction and permission to participate)

Observe safety precautions

Promptly remove offensive smells and preserve orderliness; as a result of having mastered toilet functions, the preschooler is keenly aware of smells and disorder and is upset by them

Permit and encourage child's own decision making regarding care and treatments when choices exist

Praise evidence of competence in all areas of development (self-care, learning new words, helping with a treatment, cooperation during stressful procedures)

Solicit and respect child's suggestions regarding care, room environment changes, toys in room, etc

To experience limits within environment to feel security

Enforce safety rules; give simple explanations for rules (child must be in crib or bed with rails up even if used to big bed without rails at home)

Define limits on activity due to illness (isolation from other children while disease is communicable). Since time concept is undeveloped, give idea of how long the limitation will be by associating it with concrete things ("You can go to the playroom Saturday. That is the day that cartoons are on TV all morning" or "You can drink water and other drinks again when Nurse Smith comes to care for you this afternoon")

Learn during admission interview if parents want any home rules continued during hospitalization (only certain TV shows may be watched or TV is allowed only so many hours a day, teeth are to be brushed after each meal, limited beverages are allowed after suppertime) and enforce those not in conflict with treatment regimen

Explain to parents reasons any cannot be enforced

TABLE 21-11
Developmental Needs and Nursing Interventions: Preschoolers *(Continued)*

To engage in rituals to feel secure

Assess usual routines and rituals during interview; integrate rituals into care plan as possible

Encourage parents or other family members acquainted with the rituals to be present and help child carry out mealtime, bedtime, other significant rituals

Ask parents to bring from home those objects related to child's rituals and other security items

To learn to separate without conflict

Provide for a primary nurse for each shift

Permit and encourage unlimited parental visits and participation in planning and giving care

Allow parents to remain and comfort child, if desired during treatments or procedures parents cannot or do not wish to do; primary nurse is present as parent surrogate to stay with and comfort child

Let parents do as many of the "caretaking" tasks as possible

Ask parents to bring in familiar toys, family photos, personal belongings that can be left with child as reminders of them during their absence

During care, make up pleasant stories about home activities, including names of family members in the stories, or encourage child to tell stories about home and family activities

Provide opportunities for child to become acquainted with other children and parents who may "fill in" as sources of comfort during parental and sibling separations

Help parents identify ways to keep child in contact with siblings or peers who cannot visit (phone call, tape recordings, notes, pictures)

To achieve sexual identity and comfort with sexual sensations and feelings

Give thorough explanations and continued reassurance about what will happen to the child's body as a result of a treatment or procedure; it is especially important to reassure of continued presence and intactness of genitals when these body parts are involved

Handle genitalia as little as possible and use gentleness when handling is necessary; some children respond better if their hand is used with the nurse's in handling the genitalia

Avoid use of intrusive procedures or treatments whenever possible (preschoolers cope with axillary or oral thermometers better than rectal)

attending school, interacting with peers, and stimulating cognitive and social development, and may even contribute to the inability to remain in the proper grade for age. Innovative implementation of measures enabling school-age children to continue their progress is essential (Fig. 21-8). Creative programs allowing hospitalized children to keep up with their classmates can be accomplished with computers. If patients are not well enough to come to the hospital classroom, then a computer can be brought to their bedside to complete school assignments. After school hours, the computers can be used for recreation and games (Sparkman, 1991).

Promote Positive Personal Body Image

Nursing care is planned considering the child's vulnerability to personal body image. An assessment of the child's body image can be made by directing questions to assess the physical self, the personal self, and self-ideal (see Table 14-4 in Chapter 14 for examples).

Facilitate the Child's Sense of Security. Nursing care should be focused at keeping change to a minimum in a child's hospital routine. Routines such as mealtime, bedtime, and play are kept as similar as possible to the home schedule. When possible, parents are encouraged to stay with young children, and the number of nursing personnel interacting with the child is limited to allow the child to develop trusting relationships, which, in turn, enhances a sense of security for the child.

Facilitate the Child's Sense of Identity. Verbal and physical interactions with the child and family are encouraged to facilitate communication and caring. The child's personal strengths are identified and verbalized to help the child identify his or her "special" characteristics.

Facilitate the Child's Sense of Belonging. The most common way to achieve this goal is to encourage visits from siblings (Fig. 21-9), extended family, and peers (as appropriate), in addition to parents. If peers cannot visit, then contact via the phone and letters is encouraged.

Facilitate the Child's Sense of Purpose. The child is assisted to set realistic coping goals related to the illness. For example, "Next time I will hold my leg still even if I have to cry" rather than "Next time I won't cry."

Facilitate the Child's Sense of Personal Competence. Basic to a positive self-concept is achievement of autonomy. Children can be given some autonomy even though they are in the hospital, where rules and policies are enforced. Children are allowed to make choices after explanations have been given. Self-care

TABLE 21-12
Developmental Needs and Nursing Interventions: School-Age Children

Physical Needs

To complete control of body functions and self-care

Assess and maintain usual routines related to body function and self-care

Allow independent self-care to extent feasible by treatment restrictions and child's tolerance

Praise whatever self-care child does perform

To develop fine motor skills

Provide materials for fine motor activities (pencils and crayons, scissors, Lego, computer games, hospital equipment safe for play that requires finger manipulation)

Encourage drawing pictures of body and body parts during discussions of disease and treatment; this gives nurse feedback on the accuracy of the child's interpretation of information

Encourage child to "take notes" during patient education sessions—gives practice in fine motor dexterity for printing or writing

Teach child to participate in treatments that give practice in fine motor skills

Intellectual Needs

To develop rational thinking, reality orientation

Provide scientific descriptions of the child's disease and body responses during educational sessions or in reply to questions

Offer a rationale for each procedure before doing it to help the child to maintain self-control during procedures and to participate when feasible

Provide children with rules about what they may and may not do during hospitalization, because of the disease or during a treatment; suggest writing out a list or rules to post at bedside

Assess whether child perceives hospitalization as a punishment; intervene as for preschool child if so

Provide opportunities for child to make decisions about routine, treatments, and daily care whenever choices actually exist; encourage middle school-age child to help devise a care plan

To master concepts of conservation, constancy, and reversibility and to develop skills in classification and categorization

Allow child to participate in care by helping keep track on intake and output, writing down vital signs, counting the seconds or adding up the minutes it takes to complete a procedure

Encourage the child who can tell time to inform the nurse when it is time for a procedure or when it is time to stop the procedure (when to take out thermometer, when to take off soaks, etc.)

Encourage scrapbook making, collection, diary keeping (according to child's interests) during hospital stay

Use these concepts in teaching sessions

Provide games that require use of these concepts (card games, board games)

Provide hospital school or tutor schoolwork

To vocalize feelings during stress

Encourage verbalization of feelings associated with hospitalization, disease, procedures by asking questions. ("How does it make you feel to have to miss school and be away from your friends?" or "Tell me what it is like to have to lie still for 30 minutes while those compresses are on")

Schedule time to talk with child, time not associated with any specific care or procedure; let child know this is a time she or he can talk about anything or ask any questions; encourage parents to do the same

Emotional-Social Needs

To have the opportunity to channel drives into socially acceptable behaviors

Do not place girls and boys in the same room

Provide opportunities to interact with other hospitalized school-age children

Assess for preschool residual concerns re genitalia; manage as for preschool child

Help maintain peer group contact via phone calls, letter writing, tape recordings, peer visitation, photo exchanges. (Teachers and parents are usually willing to help arrange these things)

Arrange group education sessions for children with similar problems; include discussions of how problems are similar and how they differ; involve children in teaching each other about anatomy and physiology, disease process, treatment, under nurse supervision

Treat any separation anxiety as for preschool child

Encourage parents to express affection toward their hospitalized school-age child and to continue setting limits as before hospitalization

To achieve industry and associated developing self-concept

Praise cooperation efforts, self-care accomplishments, participation in treatments, and any other achievements; praise honestly and often

Provide opportunities for built-in successes several times daily. (Assign tasks the child is known to be able to accomplish)

Provide opportunities for peer cooperation (solicit roommate's help in entertaining an immobilized child)

Actively involve child in care and treatments

Balance quiet and solitary activity with action and peer interaction as tolerated

TABLE 21-13
Developmental Needs and Nursing Interventions: Adolescents

Physical Needs

Support of rapid skeletal growth

Provide nutritional information on diet, snacks, and weight control

Refer to dietitian for special dietary needs

Encourage consumption of nutritional snacks, rather than "empty calories"

To perform self-care skills associated with onset of puberty

Provide information on hygiene measures; means of independent bathing

Answer questions and provide counseling on reproductive system and function

Provide anticipatory guidance on preventive health maintenance, breast examinations, birth control

Physical exercise and mobility

Assist to move out of bed and around the unit

Recreation activities suitable to age

Acknowledge need for physical expression of frustration and provide innovative means

Encourage physical and occupational therapy to increase independence, muscle strength, and mobility

Intellectual Needs

To receive scientific explanations

Thorough explanation and preparation for procedures and instructions

Use scientific terminology to explain illness

To participate in health care management decisions

Include client in planning guide

Give all instructions to client as well as parent; orient to environment, routines, and expectations

To achieve in academics and strive toward career goals

Provide opportunity to complete schoolwork while hospitalized

Involve school teachers in health care planning

Reinforce realistic career goals

Emotional-Social Needs

To develop healthy attitudes about body image and sexuality

Encourage verbalization of fears and concerns

Provide privacy

Let youth have own belongings and wear own clothes

Assist with grooming needs (e.g., hair washing, nails)

To achieve independence

Compliment the adolescent's strengths

Encourage self-care

Provide flexible limits

Provide opportunities to participate in setting goals, planning care, and choosing options

Provide opportunities for appropriate decisions and control

To have peer contact and approval

Provide opportunities for friends to visit and call

Suggest recreation activities that stimulate adolescents to gather

Arrange for unit meeting for adolescents

Suggest passes to go home or to school or social functions

Provide opportunities for appropriate calls to friends

To receive family support

Encourage parents to visit and stay when adolescent needs or wants them

Provide opportunities for meetings where parents can discuss issues and get support

Encourage sibling visits

Give support to maintain the family unit

Encourage chaplain visits

Encourage use of appropriate community resources

Provide community agency referrals

by children is encouraged to contribute to feelings of competence (see Planning and Interventions in Nursing Diagnostic Statements 5 and 7 in Table 21–5).

Promote Positive Parental Competence During Hospitalization

During a child's hospitalization, parents can easily feel confused about their parenting competency. Nursing care is planned to support parents in the strange environment of procedures, policies, routines, and schedules, which produce a sense of loss and conflict. The role of parents of hospitalized children has changed since the 1960s. Parents have become increasingly involved with the care of their children in the hospital setting. Callery and Smith (1991) suggest that role negotiation is an important aspect of current care and nurses must be sensitive to parents' needs and not view themselves as more powerful

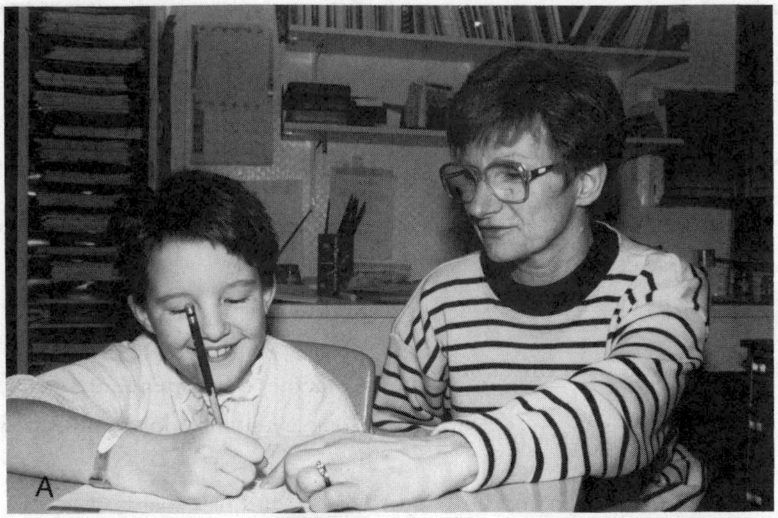

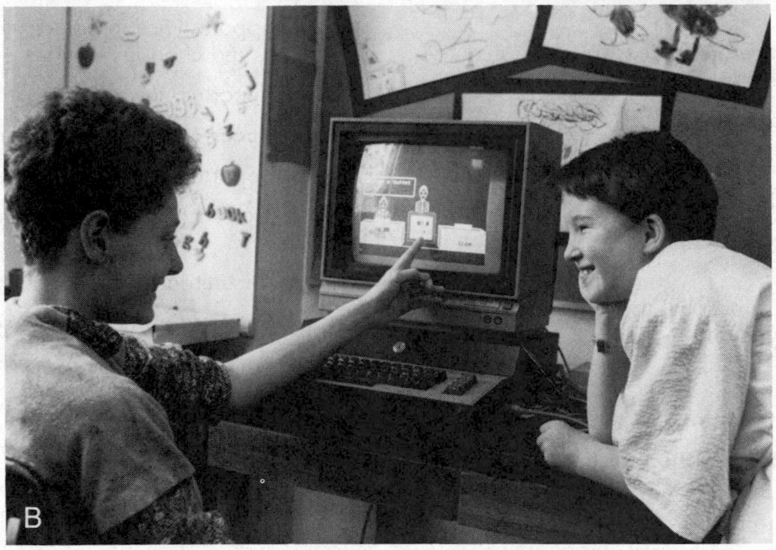

FIGURE 21 - 8. Individualized school programs are now provided to hospitalized children in some centers. Larger institutions have certified teachers and a separate classroom where equipment and supplies are available for an educational program.

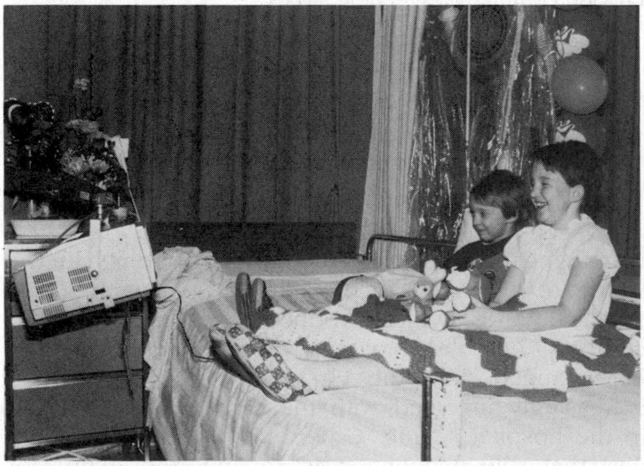

FIGURE 21 - 9. A visit from a younger brother can help to normalize a hospital environment.

than parents so appropriate negotiation for the benefit of the child, the parent, and the nurse can occur. The nursing goal is to assist parents to adapt to their parental role in the hospital, so they can accommodate the needs of their child while maintaining their own physical and mental health.

Help Parents Adapt Parenting Behaviors. It is important for the parents to continue in a parenting role during hospitalization. Nurses can assist them by encouraging them to set usual limits and to engage in behaviors such as teaching and hugging despite tubes, tents, or other equipment. Nurses should keep parents informed about their child's specialized care so they can carry out their appropriate parent role for the situation. Knowledge about tests and procedures is necessary so parents can have the understanding essential to help their child cope with stress and discomfort experienced in the hospital.

Facilitate Parents Receiving Information. Continual open communication between the nurse and the parents is an important component of supporting parents in their role. Information is made available by offering explanations, interpreting terminology, and helping them understand their child's illness. When parents cannot be with their child, information sharing is continued through telephone calls.

Support Parental Decision-Making Role. Parents should be given an opportunity to participate in formulating a plan of care. They are the experts in their child's care and have information about their child's usual responses and preferences. Parents have the expertise to make practical suggestions (e.g., how to get a child to eat, how to move a casted child in bed); these suggestions should be integrated in the child's plan of care.

Allow Parents to Participate in Child's Care. Parents should be encouraged to participate in as much of their child's care as they desire. Parents are approached to determine which tasks they wish to assume, which they want to learn, and which they want to share. Parental involvement in care changes over time; therefore, ongoing assessments are made of how parents wish to be involved. Their other responsibilities are taken into consideration and reassessed so parents do not become frustrated and made to feel guilty.

Support Parents in Normalizing the Hospital Environment. Parents are oriented to the hospital environment so they feel self-sufficient in finding the supplies they need for themselves and their child. Activities within the hospital are organized in a way that promotes a homelike atmosphere. Clothing, toys, and food may be brought from home and parents can participate in their child's activities in the playroom, teen room, or school room to normalize their child's experience.

Help Parents Verbalize Feelings about Child and Own Parenting Role Adaptation. Parents must be given an opportunity to express their feelings about their child's hospitalization and their own adaptation of their parenting role. A supportive climate encourages them to talk about any conflicts or role changes they are experiencing. Staff members who have established a therapeutic relationship with the parents are in the best position to assist and they also can facilitate the process of adjustment to the diagnoses/prognosis and planning for future care.

Provide for Parents' Physical and Emotional Needs. A major nursing role is to provide for the physical and emotional needs of the parents so they have the energy to continue their parenting role. Ongoing assessments of the parents' own needs (rest, nutrition, activity, privacy) are made and their involvement in caregiving is adjusted accordingly. Support systems are identified and family strengths are acknowledged. Additional stressors in the family are identified and referrals made to chaplains, social service, community agencies, or self-help groups, as indicated.

Research has shown that parental anxiety can influence parents' behavior by subconsciously causing parents to withdraw from their child, and parental anxiety in parents who do not room-in can increase the longer the child is hospitalized, especially if there are children at home (Alexander et al, 1986). Thus, the nurse's recognition of anxiety in parents and intervention to support parents in expressing their fears and concerns are important nursing strategies to increase the parents' comfort at the bedside. Many institutions still have limited parental visiting policies despite literature that supports the positive effects of the presence of parents. If an institution lacks a 24-hour visitation-by-parents policy, then nurses can provide leadership in establishing such a policy that provides optimal care for children.

Support groups composed of parents of children with the same or different problems can be extremely helpful in reducing stress. These groups may be planned and supervised by professionals or develop spontaneously as parents with similar needs begin to share concerns and mutually experience a relief of tension. They discuss their feelings about a treatment or test and hear how another person has coped successfully. Some of these groups continue to meet to provide information and support even after the child is discharged from the hospital.

Facilities for parents should include a lounge separate from, but close to, their child's room, where they can relax. Health care booklets, magazines, or light reading material, television, or games provide a diversion for parents. A kitchen in which parents can make coffee, toast, or soup also may help them feel welcome. Some hospitals are able to provide a shower and a dressing area for parents. In addition, some hospitals provide sleeper-lounge chairs or cots for parents, as space permits. Although comfortable facilities for parents are particularly helpful in reducing their stress, most parents respond favorably to even small attempts and gestures to make them comfortable while they stay close to their child. Referrals to appropriate resources, such as the hospital's social service department, also can help parents work through the day-to-day problems of transportation, lodging, finances, and home management. General nursing goals and interventions related to family coping are presented in Table 21–5, Nursing Diagnostic Statement 10. Following is a discussion of age-appropriate care planning and interventions.

Support of Parents with a Hospitalized Infant. The parent-infant relationship is threatened when an infant is hospitalized. Parents may see the activities of the nurse, in particular, as a threat to their own parenting abilities. Their prior responsibilities of feeding, administering medications, and the like may now be taken over by persons unknown to them. From a sense of helplessness, they may resort to criticism of their child's care. The nurse must avoid taking the criticism personally and understand this manner of coping on the part of parents to facilitate effective communication.

Every opportunity possible should be provided for parental care of the infant. Encouraging parents to touch, hold, and feed their infant is the key to fostering the ongoing development of positive interactions between infant and parents. The parents are encouraged to elicit social responses from their infant, provide play opportunities, and in all ways normalize their daily activities.

The individuality of the parenting role is an important difference for nurses to respect. First-time parents of a young infant may not feel secure in their role. The hospital setting can easily compound insecure feelings. Therefore, the nurse strives to strengthen the confidence of parents in their role by verbally pointing out the infant's responses to them and identifying the normal developmental landmarks that are being achieved.

Support of Parents with a Hospitalized Toddler. The role of parents with ill toddlers is to provide the continuity of the home situation in the hospital. Toddlers desperately need their parents to feel secure. Parents are encouraged to let the toddlers do those tasks they achieved prior to admission to maintain a sense of autonomy in a threatening environment. When a toddler is hospitalized, parents feel overwhelmed and wish to take away the hurt and anxiety they see in their child.

Parents may have difficulty setting limits in their usual way because they cannot bear to oppose their ill child's wishes. The nurse should provide an opportunity for parents to express the conflict they are experiencing and assure them that the security that the setting of limits affords toddlers is particularly important now that they are in a threatening environment. The nurse can also point out that if parents can continue to provide the limit setting in their usual manner, there will be fewer problems of readjustment for their toddler back at home.

Another area of conflict is the normal resistive behaviors of toddlers. When they feel threatened with losing control over what happens to them, they may become even more resistive, resulting in parents becoming exhausted and frustrated. Regressive behaviors like thumbsucking and soiling (by a previously potty-trained toddler) or the whining, baby cry of a toddler may be disturbing and embarrassing to parents. Parents might even feel that they are the cause of such behaviors and begin to isolate themselves emotionally from their child, even though physically present. The nurse's responsibility then is not only to encourage parents to be there but also to help them cope effectively with their child's reactions to hospitalization.

Support of Parents with a Hospitalized Preschooler. The biggest problem of the parents of hospitalized preschooler is their tendency to forget how independent their preschoolers have become. Through anticipatory guidance about the behaviors and needs of hospitalized preschoolers and through role modeling, the nurse can help parents preserve their children's independence. Involving parents in planning care communicates that they are important to their child and that they know their child best (Freiberg, 1972). They can be helped to feel capable and useful by supervising their child's self-care and helping in or doing those tasks the child is unable to handle. Probably the most valuable contribution parents make to their preschoolers' hospital adjustment is their participation in the child's preparation for procedures. To these children, parents are still essential interpreters and translators of the language of the outside world. Therefore, their involvement in their child's education is just as important as their presence and their ability to provide comfort during hospitalization encounters.

Support of Parents with a Hospitalized School-Age Child. Even though school-age children are moving away from the family toward peer influence, parents and siblings remain a major influence in their lives. They need parents now who relate as adults, not pals —someone they can turn to during stress and count on to set limits and control them when they cannot. This development becomes evident when school-age children are hospitalized. Although the continual presence of parents is not necessary, school-age children need frequent assurances that parents love them and are thinking of them (Fig. 21–10). They will want them present during painful procedures and when they are feeling acutely ill.

Parents may need help in respecting and permitting the child's contributions to the treatment regimen. The nurse can reassure them that the child's participation is welcomed by the staff and can encourage the parents' participation in the teaching process and in supervising their child in self-care.

Although the school-age child's family experiences the same needs, feelings, and concerns of other families when any of their children are hospitalized, they usually adapt better to the fact of hospitalization than do those with younger children. This is because the school-age child is more independent and can express feelings and needs; therefore, parents feel less pressured to be there continuously to interpret their child's needs to hospital staff.

Support of Parents with a Hospitalized Adolescent. In working with parents of the adolescent, the nurse

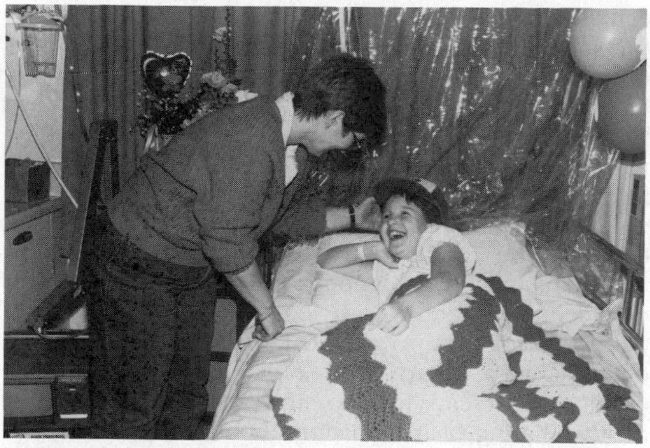

FIGURE 21-10. Although the continuous presence of parents is not necessary, school-age children need frequent assurances that parents love them.

can serve as a model, showing them how to help their child during dependency states and to allow freedom and control when dependency is not desirable. Parents are often intimidated by their adolescent's anger and anxiety. The nurse can explain the relationship between developmental issues and hospitalization. Parents usually do not volunteer information about problems with the family, such as their own feelings of guilt and frustration and sibling jealousy. Parents need to talk to the nurse and be given the opportunity to receive support instead of always being expected to be strong.

Just as hospitalization is a crisis for the adolescent, it is a crisis for the parents. They have a natural concern for their son or daughter, but their ability to be supportive is influenced by their own past experiences and fears related to hospitals and illness. Parents may interpret the illness as their punishment for neglect of the adolescent and, thus, may feel guilty. They may see themselves as failures for not preventing the illness. Parents may enjoy the nurturing role that is required when their adolescent is dependent and then may find it difficult to return to the conflicts of independence that are inevitable when the adolescent is well.

The adolescent may respond better to the staff nurse's requests than to those of the parents; this may cause the parents to resent the nurse's role as the primary caregiver. The parents and siblings may resent the time and the changes made in routines that are required to provide support to the hospitalized adolescent. The amount of support available from and contact with their parents influences the amount of anxiety experienced by adolescents. Parents are often expected to be in control and supportive without any nursing intervention or assistance. The nurse should understand the role of parents, and provide support for them when their adolescent requires hospitalization.

Promote Adaptive Behaviors and Problem-Solving

An understanding of how stressors affect children at various ages provides the basis for planning and nursing interventions. (See previous section, Impact of Stressors.) Strategies for facilitating individual coping are summarized in Tables 21-9 to 21-13 and included with interventions for the Nursing Diagnostic Statement that follows.

Promote Adaptive Family Functioning of Parents and Siblings

Care of the family begins immediately on the child's admission. Whether the parents room-in or visit sporadically, the nurse's main goals are to involve them in their child's care and to maximize the quality of the parent-child relationship. The more effective the nurse is at putting the parents at ease, the greater the child's security. Parents often have useful suggestions about special approaches that may work well with their child.

Some hospitals are establishing care-by-parent units. Nurses are available if needed, but the parents provide most of the care. These units can be especially helpful when the child does not require complex care or when a chronic problem requires complex care that the parents have learned to provide.

When parents are able to room-in with their hospitalized child, the nurse does not leave the scene because "there is nothing to do." The nurse continues to be responsible for the child by assisting with daily care and providing the specialized care pertaining to the child's illness. The more complex responsibility of the nurse, however, is that of assessing the coping level of the family and planning how to maximize the comfort of each person. At times, parents feel exhausted or frustrated by the demands of caring for their sick child. Parents experience stress when their child is hospitalized and their roles as primary caregivers are assumed by the hospital staff. Yet, they feel inadequate or too frightened to care for their child physically, especially if the condition is serious.

In these circumstances, it may be advisable to allow the parents to observe the nurse caring for the child. The nurse can use the observation time to explain the purposes of various procedures and demonstrate how they are done. As parents feel more comfortable, they may wish to increase their participation. When the parent begins to participate more actively, the nurse should assist and offer encouragement. Parents also need the opportunity to ask questions and clarify information.

The nurse should be particularly sensitive to those parents who try to take on too much responsibility. Parents need the opportunity to leave the unit for periods of time, and they need to have contact with a nurse who makes them feel at ease to express the frustrations they are experiencing. Even infants are able to sense changes in their parents, such as anxiety or fear. A child may respond with expressions of abandonment if the parent is feeling overwhelmed and unable to meet nurturing needs. The nurse needs considerable interaction with the child and the parents to assess whether the stress of caring for their sick child is overwhelming. When it is, the nurse can help the family identify how they can be assisted to cope with the stress of the hospital experience.

When parents can visit for only short periods and such visits are infrequent, the nurse must make a special effort to reduce the stress this produces. Parents who are unable to visit when a young child is hospitalized often feel extremely guilty and need the acceptance and understanding of a sensitive nurse. It is especially important that the nurse does not compound their guilt by thoughtless, judgmental remarks. When parent-child separation is inevitable because of family circumstances, the nurse must try to work out a plan with parents that will be most beneficial to the family as a unit. Some families may need assistance to re-evaluate their circumstances and search for alternatives that will increase their availability to their child.

Support of Single-Parent Families During Hospitalization of a Child. To provide the emotional support of the hospitalized child and to simultaneously maintain the family's usual level of functioning at home is often beyond what one individual can provide. The nurse's sensitivity to the special needs of single parents is an important link in effective adaptation by the child and family. Exploring alternatives with the parent and facilitating parental relief strategies can alleviate the stress experienced by both child and family.

Each family situation has its own needs and difficulties. Some alternatives to explore with a single parent are use of extended family (if available); temporary use of an adolescent in the home to take on added responsibilities; neighborhood or church group participation; or community organizations that can provide support service.

The nurse also may help by responding to the psychologic needs of a single parent. It is important for the nurse to know whether there has been a separation, divorce, or death and whether it has occurred recently. Today, an increasing number of single parents raise either biologic or adopted children; therefore, it is important to clarify the circumstances early. If a recent separation, divorce, or death has occurred, or if a family is in the process of a divorce, the nurse should know, as these determinants could result in maladaptive response to hospitalization.

Often divorced or separated parents are present at the child's bed at the same time. The hospitalized child's condition may evoke empathic, caring responses in the parents, both for the child and for each other. To the child, it may mean that the illness could be a key to the parents' reconciliation, whereas, for stepparents, this response between ex-spouses may arouse anger. On the other hand, angry divorcing couples may use the child's hospital room as a battleground. The nurse becomes directly involved when either parent tries to control the release of information, visiting privileges, or the right to give consent for procedures. In specific cases, legal consultation may be required to resolve the problems. In most circumstances, when parents are separated or divorced, the parent with legal custody has the authority to consent to medical treatment without the other parent's approval. If joint custody exists, then either parent can legally sign a consent independently. Sharing of information about the child with either parent is usually appropriate (Holder, 1977).

The nurse's role in caring for a child whose parents are separated or divorced is to support the child's psychologic and emotional well-being. The nurse, therefore, cannot risk becoming involved in the parental battles. The best choice is to permit the child or either parent to express feelings but to avoid becoming involved in focusing on the "bad" qualities of either parent.

If a parent has died, the problems of loneliness, lack of support, time, and energy exists, as it does for a divorced parent. The mourning family is vulnerable at the time of hospitalization, but the dead spouse generally remains as a "good" memory and the separation is complete and permanent. The nurse's role in this case is to support the family in the grieving process. If the dead parent was hospitalized before dying, the child's fears and anxieties about hospitalization and its relation to death must certainly be explored (Burns, 1984).

When assessing the functioning of single-parent families, it is important that the nurse does not stereotype the family and conclude that any maladaption of parent or child is caused by single parenthood. Rather, an assessment must include environmental factors, support systems, and quality of the family relationships to best provide care to single-parent families (Friedemann & Andrews, 1990).

Support of Siblings. Traditionally, hospitals caring for children have excluded children from visiting because of the belief that children are more likely than adults to be carriers of infectious diseases. As early as 1971, the American Academy of Pediatrics (AAP) stated, "Experience now indicates that visiting by children and siblings is as safe as visiting by adults if those with obvious infection or known exposure to contagion are excluded" (AAP, 1971).

Proponents of sibling visits suggest that sibling rivalry can be alleviated by increasing the sibling's active involvement in the care of the hospitalized child and that a distorted perception of the ill child's situation can be corrected (Craft, 1981). A review of the literature revealed that professionals generally believe that sibling visits are helpful to both the healthy sibling and the hospitalized child; however, there is a lack of evidence supporting the actual emotional benefits of this strategy (Shuler & Reich, 1982).

A general acceptance of the importance of maintaining the tie between the hospitalized child and the family is shown by the prevalence of sibling visitation. Visitation policies generally specify that the sibling should be screened for infectious disease, indicate where visiting is to take place (e.g., child's room, lounge), limit the length of the visit, and require preparation of the siblings; some include an age restriction—all without scientific data. The support that is believed to derive from these visits has led many institutions to allow unrestricted visiting. Research in the area of restricting visiting children in any way can be deemed unethical and hampers experimental research using a control group (Shuler & Reich, 1982).

Nurses can have considerable influence in supporting sibling visits and should promote the strategy of providing the necessary social support of a hospitalized child. In addition, nurse researchers have a responsibility to use other methods of inquiry, such as qualitative research or the case method, to provide research data for supporting sibling visitation policies.

Facilitating Home Management

The nurse's goal is to discharge the child or adolescent, along with family members, in optimal health. With appropriate interventions during hospitalization, the transition from hospital to home is facilitated.

Preparation for discharge begins when the child is admitted to the hospital. Effective discharge planning is based on nursing knowledge of the unique meaning of *this* illness for *this* child and for *this* family and specific modifications in lifestyle that will be required for home management during the recuperative process. Discharge planning is initiated with the first explanation of the disease process and the plans for treatment.

An important component of the nurse's role in preparing a child for discharge is to encourage participation of the child in self-care. The child who is forced to comply with treatment and hospitalization without any involvement in self-care suffers a loss of control and lowered self-esteem that thwarts development and reinforces regressive behaviors. Children should be encouraged to participate in their own care according to their physical and developmental abilities. They require explanations before procedures, and their ideas should be sought when plans that concern them are developed.

Active involvement and self-care help maintain and improve coordination, muscle tone, and circulation, and foster positive self-esteem and self-control. The child may have a residual chronic health problem that will require continued treatment at home. Active participation in hospital care gives the child a sense of adequacy to cope positively after hospitalization.

During the discharge phase, the nurse should be available to clarify any misconceptions the child or parent has about the hospital experience. The child should be encouraged to talk (a puppet is often helpful in initiating conversation) about her or his experiences in the hospital so that memory distortions can be identified. Photographs taken during the hospitalization will provide the child with reminders of the experience, thereby helping realistic recall and distinguishing between what was imagined and what really happened. Also, children should be allowed to take safe, disposable equipment home with them so they can continue to work through their feelings in therapeutic play (Azarnoff, 1974).

The nurse should encourage parents to keep the hospitalization experience open to discussion so that their child has opportunities to reaffirm what really happened. Also, parents should be informed that children may need continued reassurances for weeks or months that they were not responsible for the illness or hospitalization. The child and family can be invited to return for visits to the unit after discharge. Such visits can help correct memory distortions and decrease anxiety if the child needs future hospitalization.

At home, parents should be informed of the possibility of their child demonstrating reactive behaviors, such as showing regression in developmental tasks (frequently the most recently achieved task is lost first), clinging, whining, sleep disturbances, and eating disturbances. These reactions are highly individualized and relate to the child's age. Parents should be counseled to give children with reactions additional emotional support by allowing them to be more dependent for a time and gradually weaning them back to their usual, more independent behaviors. Also, parents need to be reminded that older siblings may resent the loss of parental attention because of the younger child's special needs and display attention-getting behaviors for a time.

It is equally important to realize that all young children may not regress and become more dependent at home because of a hospital experience. With careful interventions to reduce stress and to enhance normal growth and development, a child can mature and benefit from a hospital experience. The nurse and parents must make every effort to capitalize on the unique resiliency of children.

The nurse has a major role in the following list of the components of discharging a child and the parents from the hospital:

- Explanations of physical care.
- Procurement of necessary equipment to care for child's special needs.
- Instructions in activities of daily living (nutrition, school attendance, physical activity).
- Behavioral counseling (e.g., posthospitalization effects).

- Counseling to prevent further illness.
- Instructions concerning medications.
- Assessment of capabilities of family to care for their child's additional needs.
- Assessment of degree of physical and psychologic strain that care of the child imposes on family functioning.
- Assessment of appropriateness of physical environment for care of child's special needs.
- Assessment of need for referrals in conjunction with an interdisciplinary team and referrals as appropriate.
- Coordination and consultation with community or home health nurses.
- Instructions regarding date, time, place, and purpose of return appointments.

The perceptions and feelings of parents of children with medically complex needs have been studied (Diehl et al, 1991). Caring for their children was hindered by: deterioration of family structure; lack of specific information; wrong equipment recommendations; lack of financial assistance and lack of knowledge where to get information about financial assistance; concentration only on the medical problems; and the inability to keep up with normal growth and development. Careful planning at the time of discharge can facilitate a positive transition from the hospital to the home and perhaps avoid unnecessary readmission.

Evaluation

Evaluation criteria for each of the nursing diagnostic statements are listed in Table 21–5.

KEY CONCEPTS

Concepts Related to Basic Information

- Hospitalization is stressful to children and their parents; each child and family respond differently because of their unique set of experiences and relationships.
- Some variables affecting a child's response to hospitalization are age, preparation, temperament, coping abilities, parent-child relationship, hospital environment, and length, frequency, and reason for hospitalization.
- Stressors that are common for many hospitalized children are: separation from parents and peers; discomfort and pain; loss of control, mobility, and competence; unknown events and environment; and unclear limits and expectations.
- Balancing factors influence responses to crisis, and three balancing factors for hospitalized children are perceptions of the event, availability of social supports, and individual coping skills.
- Hospitals frequently offer organized programs to prepare children for hospitalization. The preparation may be individual or in small groups and usually includes a tour of the children's unit, a film or slides, a play experience, some material to take home, and an opportunity to ask questions.

Concepts Related to Nursing Assessment

- Nursing assessment of a hospitalized child demands a high level of skill because of the increased acuity of patients.
- Collecting data, validating data, organizing data, identifying patterns, and communicating/recording data are the steps of the assessment process.
- The child's and parents' responses to specific health problems will determine the nursing diagnoses from which plans, interventions, and evaluation will guide the care rendered.

Concepts Related to Nursing Intervention

- All preparation of children should be age-appropriate and should include the parents. The timing and length of the session is important and should include a simple age-appropriate explanation, some visual aids, and medical equipment that can be used in play.
- Three aspects of the admitting process that affect a child and parents are the social environment, the physical environment, and the nature of the admitting procedures.
- Discharge plans begin when a child is hospitalized to assess specific family needs. On the day of discharge, the parents should receive written instructions including: activities of daily living, medications, health-promoting information, and date, time, place, and purpose of return appointment.

REFERENCES

Abbott, K. (1990). Therapeutic use of play in the psychological preparation of preschool children undergoing cardiac surgery. *Issues in Comprehensive Pediatric Nursing, 13,* 265–277.

Alexander, D., et al. (1986, Summer). Anxiety of non-rooming-in parents of hospitalized children. *Children's Health Care, 15*(1), 14–20.

American Academy of Pediatrics. (1971). *Care of children in hospitals* (2nd ed.), Evanston, IL.

Azarnoff, A. (1974, July/August). Mediating the trauma of serious illness and hospitalization in childhood. *Children Today,* 12.

Azarnoff, P. (Ed). (1983). *Preparation of young, healthy children for possible hospitalization: The issues.* Santa Monica, CA: Pediatric Projects. (Available from Pediatric Projects, Inc., Box 1880, Santa Monica, CA 90406.)

Azarnoff, P., & Woody, P. D. (1981). Preparation for hospitalization in acute care hospitals in the United States. *Pediatrics, 68,* 361.

Bates, T. A., & Broome, M. (1986, August). Preparation of children for hospitalization and surgery: A review of the literature. *Journal of Pediatric Nursing, 1*(4), 230–239.

Beyer, J. E., & Frick-Helms, S. (1992). Guest editorial. *Children's Health Care, 21*(3), 133–135.

Bolig, P. (1984). Play in hospital settings. In T. D. Yawkey, & A. D. Pellegrini (Eds.). *Child's play; developmental and applied.* Hillsdale, NJ: Lawrence Erlbaum.

Bolig, R. (1990). Play in health care settings: A challenge for the 1990s. *Children's Health Care, 19*(4), 229–233.

Brandt, P., et al. (1972, August). Injections in children. *American Journal of Nursing,* 1402.

Brazelton, T. B. (1992). *Touchpoints: Your child's emotional and behavioral development.* Reading, MA: Addison-Wesley.

Broome, M. E. (1991). Medical fears of acutely ill hospitalized children. Unpublished paper. Chicago: Rush University.

Broome, M. E., & Hellier, A. (1987). School-age children's fears of medical experiences. *Issues in Comprehensive Pediatric Nursing, 10,* 77–86.

Broome, M., Hellier, A., Wilson, T., Dale, S., & Glanville, C. (1988). Development and testing of an instrument to measure children's fears of medical experiences. In C. Waltz, & O. Strickland (Eds.). *Measurement of nursing outcomes.* New York: Springer.

Burns, C. (1984, June). The hospitalization experience and single-parent families. *Nursing Clinics of North America, 19*(2), 285–293.

Byrne, C. M., & Cadman, D. (1987, November). Prevention of the adverse effects of hospitalization in children. *Preventive Psychiatry, 3*(2), 167–190.

Callery, P., & Smith, L. (1991). A study of role negotiation between nurses and the parents of hospitalized children. *Journal of Advanced Nursing, 16*(7), 772–781.

Cassel, J. (1976). The contribution of the social environment to host resistance. *American Journal of Epidemiology, 104,* 107–123.

Caty, S., et al. (1984). Coping in hospitalized children: An analysis of published case studies. *Nursing Research, 33,* 277–287.

Caty, S., Richie, J. A., & Ellerton, M. (1989). Helping hospitalized preschoolers manage stressful situations: The mother's role. *Children's Health Care, 18*(4), 202–209.

Cautela, J. R., & Groden, J. (1978). *Relaxation: A comprehensive manual for adults, children, and children with specific needs.* Champaign, IL, Research Press.

Cobb, S. (1976). Social support as a moderator of life stress. *Psychosomatic Medicine, 38,* 300–314.

Craft, M. (1981). Preferences of hospitalized adolescents for information providers. *Nursing Research, 30,* 205–211.

Diehl, S. F., Moffitt, K. A., & Wade, S. M. (1991). Focus group interview with parents of children with medically complex needs: An intimate look at their perceptions and feelings. *Children's Health Care, 20*(3), 170–178.

Ebmeier, C., Lough, M. A., Huth, M. M., & Autio, L. (1991). Hospitalized school-age children express ideas, feelings, and behaviors toward God. *Journal of Pediatric Nursing, 6,* 337–348.

Ely, E. (1992). The experience of pain for school-age children: Blood, band-aids, and feelings. *Children's Health Care, 21*(3), 168–176.

Erickson, F. (1967, December). Helping the sick child maintain behavioral control. *Nursing Clinics of North America,* 695.

Fassler, D. (1980). Reducing preoperative anxiety in children: Information versus emotional support. *Patient Counselling and Health Education, 2*(1), 130–134.

Freiberg, K. (1972, July). How parents react when their child is hospitalized. *American Journal of Nursing,* 1270.

Friedemann, M., & Andrews, M. (1990). Family support and child adjustment in single-parent families. *Issues in Comprehensive Pediatric Nursing, 13,* 289–301.

Galligan, A. (1979, January/February). Using Roy's concept of adaptation to care for young children. *American Journal of Nursing,* 24.

Gaynard, L., Goldberger, J., & Laidley, L. N. (1991). The use of stuffed, body-outline dolls with hospitalized children and adolescents. *Children's Health Care, 20*(4), 216–224.

Gottlieb, S. E. (1990). Documenting the efficacy of psychosocial care in the hospital setting. *Journal of Development and Behavioral Pediatrics, 11*(6), 328–329.

Green, C. (1975). Larry thought puppet-play "childish" but it helped him face his fears. *Nursing 75,* 301.

Harvey, S. (1983). Parents are the best preparers of young children. In P. Azarnoff (Ed.). *Preparation of young healthy children for possible hospitalization: The issues.* Santa Monica, CA: Pediatric Projects.

Hellier, A., Ptak, H., & Cerreto, M. (1986). CATS inside my brain: Children's understanding of the cerebral computed tomography scan procedure. *Children's Health Care, 14*(4), 211–217.

Holder, A. (1977). *Legal issues in pediatrics and adolescent medicine.* New York, John Wiley.

Huth, M. M. (1983). Guidelines for conducting hospital tours with early school age children. *Pediatric Nursing, 9,* 414–415, 431.

Johnson, J. E., et al. (1976, July/August). Easing children's fright during health care procedures. *American Journal of Maternal Child Nursing,* 206.

Johnson, J. E., et al. (1975, November/December). Altering children's distress behavior during orthopedic cast removal. *Nursing Research, 24*(6), 405–410.

Kahn, R. L., & Antonucci, T. C. (1980). Convoys over the life course: Attachment, roles, and social support. In P. B. Bates, & O. G. Brim, Jr. (Eds.). *Life span development and behavior;* Vol 3. New York: Academic Press.

Kaplan, B. H. et al. (1977). Social support and health. *Medical Care, 15*(5)Suppl, 47–57.

Kodadek, S., Massmann, T., & Wilson, C. (1989). Nursing care of children. In C. A. Tanner, & C. A. Lindeman (Eds.). *Using nursing research.* New York: National League for Nursing, Pub. No. 15-2232.

Lazarus, R. S., & Launier, R. (1978). Stress-related transactions between person and environment. In L. A. Perwin, & M. Lewis (Eds.). *Perspectives in interactional psychology.* New York: Plenum Press.

Mather, P. L. (1983). Current preparation research and practice in one community. In P. Azarnoff (Ed.). *Preparation of young, healthy children for possible hospitalization: The issues.* Santa Monica, CA: Pediatric Projects.

Melamed, B. G., & Siegel, L. J. (1975). Reduction of anxiety in children facing hospitalization and surgery by use of filmed modeling. *Journal of Consulting and Clinical Psychology, 43,* 511–521.

Miles, M. S., & Carter, M. C. (1985, Summer). Coping strategies used by parents during their child's hospitalization in an intensive care unit. *Children's Health Care, 14*(1), 14–21.

Norbeta, M. (1976, January/February). Caring for children with the help of puppets. *American Journal of Maternal Child Nursing,* 22.

Oremland, E., et al. (1973). *The effects of hospitalization on children.* Springfield, IL: Charles C Thomas.

Orenstein, S. R., et al. (1983, September). The infant seat as treatment for gastroesophageal reflux. *New England Journal of Medicine, 309,* 760–763.

Petrillo, M., & Sanger, S. (1980). *Emotional care of hospitalized children.* Philadelphia, JB Lippincott.

Roberts, M. C., Nurtele, S. R., Boone, R. R., Gentber, L. J., Elkins, P. D. (1981). Reductions of medical fears by use of modeling: A prevention application in a general population of children. *Journal of Pediatric Psychology, 6*(3), 293–300.

Robertson, J. (1970). *Young children in hospital.* (2nd ed.). London: Tavistock Publications.

Robertson, J. (1983). *The fallacy of "preparing" young healthy children for possible hospitalization: The issues.* Santa Monica, CA: Pediatric Projects.

Rose, M. H. (1972). The effects of hospitalization on coping behaviors of children. Unpublished doctoral dissertation. University of Chicago.

Savedra, M., & Tesler, M. (1981). Coping strategies of hospitalized school-age children. *Western Journal of Nursing Research, 3*(4), 371–384.

Shaefer, S. (1977, December). Communicating with children: Teaching via the play discussion group. *American Journal of Nursing, 77,* 1960–1962.

Shuler, S., & Reich, C. (1982, Fall). Sibling visitation in pediatric hospitals: Policies, opinions and issues. *Children's Health Care, 11*(2), 54–60.

Siegel, L. J., & Peterson, L. (1980). Stress reduction in young dental patients through coping skills and sensory information. *Journal of Consulting and Clinical Psychology, 48,* 785–787.

Sommer, D. R. (1989). The spiritual needs of dying children. *Issues in Comprehensive Pediatric Nursing, 12,* 225–233.

Sparkman, L. (1991, January/February). Egleston's whiz kids: Keeping up with classmates through bedside computers. *Southern Hospitals,* 15–16.

Stevens, M. (1986, October). Adolescents' perceptions of stressful events during hospitalization. *Journal of Pediatric Nursing, 1*(5), 303–313.

Stevens, M. (1989). Coping strategies of hospitalized adolescents. *Children's Health Care, 18,* 163–169.

Thompson, R. H. (1985). *Psychosocial research on pediatric hospitalization and health care: A review of the literature.* Springfield, IL: Charles C Thomas.

Wolfer, J. A., & Visintainer, M. A. (1975). Pediatric surgical patients and parents' stress responses and adjustment as a function of psychologic preparation and stress-point nursing care. *Nursing Research, 24,* 244–255.

Zurlinden, J. K. (1985, May/June). Minimizing the impact of hospitalization for children and their families. *MCN: American Journal of Maternal Child Nursing, 10,* 178–188.

BIBLIOGRAPHY

Ack, M. (1983). Psychosocial effects of illness, hospitalization and surgery. *Children's Health Care, 11,* 132–136.

Algren, C. L. (1985, Summer). Role perception of mothers who have hospitalized children. *Children's Health Care, 14*(1), 6–9.

Anderson, C. L. (1990). The adolescent ex-cultist: A nursing staff challenge. *Issues in Comprehensive Pediatric Nursing, 13,* 231–237.

Austin, J. K., Patterson, J. M., & Huberty, T. J. (1991). Development of the coping health inventory for children. *Journal of Pediatric Nursing, 6*(3), 166–174.

Beck, C. T. (1990). Qualitative research: Methodologies and use in pediatric nursing. *Issues in Comprehensive Pediatric Nursing, 13,* 231–237.

Blos, P. (1972). The child analyst looks at the young adolescent. In *Twelve to sixteen: Early adolescence.* New York: WW Norton.

Broome, M. E. (1990). Preparation of children for painful procedures. *Pediatric Nursing, 16*(6), 537–541, 556–557.

Broome, M. E., et al. (1992). The use of distraction and imagery with children during painful procedures. *Oncology Nursing Forum, 19*(3), 499–502.

Brown, J., & Ritchie, J. A. (1990). Nurses' perceptions of parent and nurse roles in caring for hospitalized children. *Children's Health Care, 19*(1), 28–36.

Charkins-Drazin, H., & Drazin, D. M. (1992). A parent's perspective: Psychosocial clinical skills. *Children's Health Care, 21*(2), 116–117.

Clatworthy, S. (1981, Spring.). Therapeutic play: effects on hospitalized children. *Children's Health Care, 9*(4), 108–113.

Cohen, D. A. (1988). Surviving your child's hospitalization. *Exceptional Parent, 18*(3), 26–29.

Coucouvanis, J. A., & Solomons, H. C. (1983, March/April). Handling complicated visitation problems of hospitalized children. *American Journal of Maternal Child Nursing, 8,* 131–134.

Davis, B. D. (1990). Loneliness in children and adolescents. *Issues in Comprehensive Pediatric Nursing, 13*(1), 59–69.

Davis, C. B. (1989). The use of art therapy and group process with grieving children. *Issues in Comprehensive Pediatric Nursing, 12,* 269–280.

Denholm, C. (1989). Reactions of adolescents following hospitalization for acute conditions. *Children's Health Care, 18*(4), 210–217.

Denholm, C. J. (1985, Winter). Hospitalization and the adolescent patient: A review and some critical questions. *Children's Health Care, 13*(3), 109–116.

Dufour, D. F. (1989). Home or hospital care for the child with end-stage cancer: Effects on the family. *Issues in Comprehensive Pediatric Nursing, 12,* 371–383.

Durst, L. M. (1990). Preoperative teaching videotape: The effect on children's behavior. *AORN Journal, 52*(3), 576–599, 581–582, 584.

Erickson, F. (1958). Play interviews of four year old hospitalized children. *Monographs of the Society for Research in Child Development, 33,* 7.

Faust, J., et al. (1991). Same-day surgery preparation: Reduction of pediatric patient arousal and distress through participant modeling. *Journal of Consulting and Clinical Psychology, 59*(3), 475–478.

Freeman, M. (1991). Therapeutic use of storytelling for older children who are critically ill. *Children's Health Care, 20*(4), 208–215.

Graves, J. K., & Ware, M. E. (1990). Parents' and health professionals' per-ceptions concerning parental stress during a child's hospitaliza-tion. *Children's Health Care, 19*(1), 37–42.

Gray, E. (1989). The emotional and play needs of the dying child. *Issues in Comprehensive Pediatric Nursing, 12,* 207–224.

Hardgrove, C. G., & Dawson, R. B. (1972). *Parents and children in the hospital: The family's role in pediatrics.* Boston: Little, Brown.

Heiney, S. P. (1991). Helping children through painful procedures. *Center for Cancer and Blood Disorders,* Columbia, SC: Richland Memorial Childrens Hospital.

Henkens-Matzke, A., & Abbott, D. A. (1990). Game playing: A method for reducing young children's fear of medical procedures. *Early Childhood Research Quarterly, 5*(1), 19–26.

Holt, L., & Maxwell, B. (1991). Pediatric orientation programs: Hospital tours allay children's fears. *AORN Journal, 54*(3), 530–532, 534, 536.

Honig, R. G. (1982). Group meetings on an adolescent medical ward. *Adolescence, 17,* 99–106.

Jansen, M. T., et al. (1989). Meeting psychosocial and developmental needs of children during prolonged intensive care unit hospitalization. *Children's Health Care, 18*(2), 91–95.

Jay, S. M. (1990). A stress inoculation program for parents whose children are undergoing painful medical procedures. *Journal of Consulting and Clinical Psychology, 58*(6), 799–804.

Jessee, P. O. (1991). Making hospitals less traumatic: Child life specialists. *Dimensions, 20,* 23–24, 37.

Klinzing, D. & Klinzing, D. (1985). *Communication for allied health professionals.* Dubuque, IA: William C. Brown Publishers.

Knafl, K. A., et al. (1988). *Pediatric hospitalization: Family and nurse perspectives.* Glenview, IL: Scott, Foresman and Company.

Knafl, K., et al. (1992). Parents' views of health care providers: An exploration of the components of a positive working relationship. *Children's Health Care, 21*(2), 90–95.

Krietemeyer, B. C., & Heiney, S. P. (1992). Storytelling as a therapeutic technique in a group for school-aged oncology patients. *Children's Health Care, 21*(1), 14–20.

Kruger, S. (1992). Parents in crisis: Helping them cope with a seriously ill child. *Journal of Pediatric Nursing, 7*(2), 133–140.

Liakopoulou, M., et al. (1983, September). Developmental interventions in infancy during lengthy hospitalizations. *Developmental Behavioral Pediatrics, 4*(3), 213–217.

Mabe, P. A., Treiber, F. A., & Riley, W. T. (1991). Examining emotional distress during pediatric hospitalization for school-aged children. *Children's Health Care, 20*(3), 162–169.

May, B. K., & Sparks, M. (1983, Winter). School-age children: Are their needs recognized and met in the hospital setting? *Children's Health Care, 11*(3), 118–121.

McCain, C. (1983, January/February). Television viewing and the hospitalized child. *Children's Health Care,* 33–35.

Melamed, B. G., et al. (1983, December). Necessary considerations for surgery preparation: Age and previous experience. *Psychosomatic Medicine, 45*(6), 517–525.

Miles, M. S., & Mathes, M. (1991). Preparation of parents for the ICU experience: What are we missing? *Children's Health Care, 20*(3), 132–137.

Ogilvie, L. (1990). Hospitalization of children for surgery: The parents' view. *Children's Health Care, 19*(1), 49–56.

Pass, M. D., & Pass, C. M. (1987). Anticipatory guidance for parents of hospitalized children. *Journal of Pediatric Nursing, II*(4), 250–258.

Penticuff, J. H. (1990). Ethics in pediatric nursing: Advocacy and the child's "determing self." *Issues in Comprehensive Pediatric Nursing, 13,* 221–229.

Porter, C. P., & Villarruel, A. M. (1991). Socialization and caring for hospitalized African and Mexican-American children. *Issues in Comprehensive Pediatric Nursing, 14*(1), 1–16.

Poster, E. C. (1983). Stress immunization: Techniques to help children cope with hospitalization. *American Journal of Maternal Child Nursing, 12,* 119–134.

Prugh, D. G. (1983). *The psychosocial aspects of pediatrics.* Philadelphia: Lea and Febiger.

Rae, W. A. (1981, Winter). Hospitalized latency-age children: Implications for psychosocial care. *Children's Health Care, 9*(3), 59–63.

Rae, W. A. (1991). Analyzing drawings of children who are physically ill and hospitalized, using the Ipsative method. *Children's Health Care, 20*(4), 198–207.

Research commentary: A research agenda for the 1990s. *Children's Health Care, 21*(2), 120–122.

Ritchie, J. A., et al. (1984). Concerns of acutely ill, chronically ill, and healthy preschool children. *Research in Nursing and Health, 7,* 265–274.

Rubin, S. (1992). What's in a name? Child life and the play lady legacy. *Children's Health Care, 21*(1), 4–13.

Rudy-Wallace, M. (1987). Temperament: Assessing individual differences in hospitalized children. *Journal of Pediatric Nursing, II*(1), 30–36.

Schepp, K. G. (1991). Factors influencing the coping effort of mothers of hospitalized children. *Nursing Research, 40*(1), 42–46.

Smitherman, C. (1979, August). Parents of hospitalized children have needs too. *American Journal of Nursing,* 1423.

Terry, G. (1979, Spring). A 5 year old boy's aggressive and compensatory behavior in response to immobilization. *Maternal Child Nursing,* 29.

Teyber, E. C., & Littlehales, D. E. (1981). Coping with feelings: Seriously ill children, their families and hospital staff. *Child Health Care, 10,* 58–62.

Thies, E. (1992). A child's perspective: The stages of having a cast and crutches in the school-age child. *Children's Health Care, 21*(2), 118–119.

Thompson, M. L. (1990). Social support, coping, and preoperative emotional adaptation among school-age children anticipating elective tonsillectomy. Syracuse University: Unpublished dissertation.

Tiedman, M. E., & Clatworthy, S. (1990). Anxiety responses of 5–11 year old children during and after hospitalization. *Journal of Pediatric Nursing, 5*(5), 334–343.

Vernon, D. T. A., et al. (1965). *The psychological response of children to hospitalization.* Springfield, IL: Charles C Thomas.

Vessey, J. A., & Mahon, M. M. (1990). Therapeutic play and the hospitalized child. *Journal of Pediatric Nursing, 5*(5), 328–333.

Vipperman, J. F., & Rager, P. M. (1980, March/April). Childhood coping: How nurses can help. *Pediatric Nursing,* 11–18.

Voepel-Lewis, T., & Andrea, C. M. (1992). Patient perception of pediatric ambulatory surgery: Using family feedback for program evaluation. *Journal of Post Anesthesia Nursing, 7*(3), 221.

Wilson, C. J. (1991). Use of children's artwork to evaluate the effectiveness of a hospital preparation program. *Children's Health Care, 20*(2), 120–121.

Wilson, C. J., & Mason, M. (1990). Preparation for routine physical examination. *Children's Health Care, 19,* 178–182.

Wolfer, J. A., & Visintainer, M. S. (1979). Prehospital psychological preparation for tonsillectomy patients: Effects on children's and parents' adjustment. *Pediatrics, 64,* 646–655.

Zeltzer, L., et al. (1980, July). Psychologic effects of illness in adolescence II. Impact of illness in adolescents—crucial issues and coping styles. *Journal of Pediatrics, 97*(1), 132–138.

Children's Books to Prepare for Hospitalization

Baznick, D. (1981). *Becky's story.* Washington, DC: Association for the Care of Children's Health.

Bemelmans, L. (1939). *Madeline.* New York: Viking Press; and (1977). *Madeline.* New York: Penguin Books (ages 3 to 9).

Berenstain, S., & Berenstain, J. (1981). *The Berenstain Bears go to the doctor.* New York: Random House.

Berenstain, S., & Berenstain, J. (1981). *The Berenstain Bears visit the dentist.* New York: Random House.

Carter, S. (1987). *Coping with a hospital stay.* New York: Rosen Publishing Group.

Clark, B. (1970). *Pop-up going to the hospital.* New York: Random House, (grades K to 3).

Collier, J. L. (1970). *Danny goes to the hospital.* New York, WW Norton, (ages 5 to 8).

Hautzig, D. (1985). *A visit to the Sesame Street hospital.* New York: Random House.

Hogan, P. Z., & Hogan, K. (1980). *The hospital scares me.* Milwaukee: Raintree Childrens Books.

Howe, J. (1970). *The hospital book.* New York: Crown Publishers.

Jessel, C. (1983). *Paul in hospital.* (2nd ed.). New York: Methuen Children's Books.

Marsoli, L. A. (1985). *Things to know about going to the doctor.* Lexington, MA: Silver Burdett, (ages 8 to 12).

Marsoli, L. A. (1985). *Things to know before you go to the hospital.* Lexington, MA: Silver Burdett, (ages 8 to 12).

Packard, M. (1981). *A visit to the dentist.* New York: Simon and Schuster.

Rey, M., & Rey, H. A. (1966). *Curious George goes to the hospital.* New York: Houghton Mifflin, (ages 3 to 8).

Rogers, F. (1988). *Going to the hospital.* New York: GP Putnam's Sons.

Stein, S. (1974). *A hospital stay: An open family book for parents and children together.* New York: Workman Publishing Company, (ages 3 to 10).

Tickle, P. (1975). *It's no fun to be sick.* Memphis: St. Luke's Press.

Watts, M. A. (1977). *Crocodile medicine.* New York: Frederick Warne, (ages 3 to 6).

Weber, A. (1970). *Elizabeth gets well.* New York: Thomas Y. Crowell, (ages 5 to 9).

Ziegler, S. (1976). *At the hospital: A surprise for Krissy.* Mankato, MN: The Child's World, Affiliate of Creative Educational Society, Inc., (ages 3 to 7).

CHAPTER • 22

Community and Home Care

Linda Waite Maurano

NURSING PROCESS PLAN:
NPP: Home Care, Table 22–1

RELATED TOPICS
Communicating with Children and Families, Chapter 11
Promoting Healthy Parenting, Chapter 12
Concepts of illness: Stress, crisis, and coping, Chapter 18
Impact of chronic illness, Chapter 19
Impact of death and dying, Chapter 20

LEARNING OBJECTIVES

- Define home care and the types of home care that are available to families.
- Trace the development of pediatric home health services.
- Identify the adaptations in nursing role and function that are necessary for delivering home care within the framework of the nursing process.
- Describe the benefits and constraints of caring for ill children at home.

Home care has expanded since the early 1980s to include the care of very ill children in the home. This change in the location and delivery of health care services to children and families has had a profound effect on pediatric health care practices, an effect that is projected to grow rapidly in the coming years. This chapter discusses the evolution of home health care, the nursing process as it relates to home care, and the future of pediatric home care. It focuses on the family in relation to nursing roles in home care. Home care specific for the ill child for all the major illnesses is presented in this text within the individual chapters devoted to illness.

Pediatric Home Care: Definitions of Services

Pediatric home care is the provision of skilled care and support services to a child in his or her place of residence. Home care for children is not characterized by any single new type of technology. It involves a fundamental change in both the site and the focus of care. Home care is a form of service that returns care and responsibility, as much as possible within the dictates of safe medical practice, to the family and community. It is a mechanism of implementing a package of services in which family values and participation can play central roles ordinarily assumed in raising healthy children.

The package of services should be designed to care for all children on the wellness-illness continuum of care. These services would fall into three major areas:

1. *Physician-directed, intermittent, skilled care delivered to homebound patients that is reasonable and necessary to their diagnosis.* These services are delivered by a federally certified Home Health Agency and usually emphasize the services of a multidisciplinary team. This highly skilled team includes a skilled nurse, physical therapist, occupational therapist, speech therapist, home health aide, and medical social services representative. Types of care that are delivered under this category include, but are not limited to, rehabilitation and skilled nursing care to trauma victims, phototherapy to newborn infants with elevated bilirubin, apnea monitoring for high-risk infants, dressing changes, and total parenteral nutrition.
2. *Physician-directed, hourly skilled services requiring the use of high technology in the home.* This is commonly called "private duty home care" and is not delivered through a federally certified home care agency because it does not meet the criteria as mentioned in number 1 for "intermittent" skilled care. Therefore, depending on the licensure laws of the state in which the services are rendered, the home care agency may or may not be licensed by the state. The services are provided by highly skilled registered nurses, licensed practical nurses, and home health aides in the patient's home on an hourly (shift) basis. Types of care that are delivered under this category include, but are not limited to, care of ventilator-dependent patients, infusion therapy, and multitherapy care requiring skilled intervention at least hourly.
3. *Hourly support services in the home designed to assist with the respite care needs of families with chronically ill children or for short-term care of a mildly ill child who cannot participate in the regular school or child care program.* This is serviced either through a private duty agency or a registry. Care is delivered by a paraprofessional, usually a home health aide. Types of care delivered under this category include, but are not limited to, respite care for children with cystic fibrosis, muscular dystrophy, or cerebral palsy; and care for ill children with mild illnesses such as chickenpox and flu.

Evolution of Home Health Care

Historical Considerations

The concept of caring for sick children at home is not new. Until the advent of modern medical technology, families were the primary caregivers and traditionally cared for ill members in the home. Before the 18th century, the family was the source not only of health care but also of work, education, religious worship, recreation, and political attitudes (Farrell & Schmitt, 1979). Family functioning and family authority were reinforced by an agrarian society. At the turn of the century, charitable dispensaries such as the Boston Dispensary were founded to provide domiciliary treatment for the indigent. These charitable dispensaries provided medical visiting for the next 150 years to those unable to meet the cost of sickness care. Physicians were often found to remark on the amazing strength of families to nurse a sick child and provide a safe environment out of their poor situations (Bergman et al, 1965). Physicians, through this experience, gained a new respect for families and their abilities. As late as 1850, the great majority of American families lived in rural areas, with health care provided by family folk remedies and by a "country doctor" who would travel among homes to tend the sick. As the industrial revolution and the lure of jobs prompted people to move to the cities, adjustments were made in family functioning. In the urban setting, family members became more dependent on persons and agencies outside the family, and the family unit began to lose some of its autonomy.

In the early 1900s, the Visiting Nurse Association and, later, the Public Health Departments made maternal and child postpartum home visits to all first-born infants, at-risk infants, and children at well child clinics. Therapeutic intervention was provided to children with diagnosed problems. As health care and medical technology became more sophisticated, care of the sick began to move out of the arms of the family and into clinics and hospitals. Provision was made within these facilities for patients only, and families were provided with schedules of "visiting hours." The message was clear: although care in the home was acceptable for some chronically ill elderly persons, acute illness care was primarily the domain of health care professionals within institutions.

This was true in the United States, but not true in England. In 1954, a pilot experiment in pediatric home care was started at St. Mary's Hospital in London to prevent hospitalization of children or to create a situation for early discharge. The study's results supported the following three theories:

1. There are few sick children who, once stabilized, cannot be treated at home.
2. It is not the gravity of the illness or the complicated care that is the main limiting factor for home care—it is usually social factors that determine the success of pediatric home care (e.g., whether a family member is willing and able and has support).
3. The use of the nurse to *support* mothering rather than take it over has appeared to have positive results in families. This support in the form of training and education succeeded in boosting the mother's confidence in her own capacity and gratification at playing a major role in assisting her child back to health (Bergman et al, 1965).

This finding is still relevant today. In November 1986, an article appeared in *Caring Magazine* written by a mother whose name was kept anonymous. Her biggest concern in caring for her ill child was not being able to care for all of her child's needs herself as she would if the child were not ill. It was important to her that her home care nurses recognized her need to be a competent caregiver. The focus of the care plan, therefore, should revolve around educating the mother to be able to meet the nursing care needs of her child rather than to take over her role. This is an important concept that nurses sometimes have trouble understanding. They feel that they must "do" for the patient and do not always understand that their teaching skills have more far-reaching effects on the long-term stability of the family unit.

In the 1950s and 1960s, while pediatric home care was dormant in the United States, hospitals in England and France accepted the challenge of caring for ventilator-dependent polio survivors at home. It became known as the Responaut Program (Goldberg, 1985). This was an interesting term coined by the polio victims themselves at the time when astronauts first embarked on the space exploration program. These persons felt that, like astronauts, they were going to venture out into the unknown—the community.

In the United States, although the caseloads of community health nurses included some stable children with chronic illnesses, home care for children requiring more sophisticated management was given little consideration until the 1970s. At that time, Ida Martinson, a professor at the University of Minnesota School of Nursing, piloted a home care program for terminally ill children. Citing enhancement of quality of life for the child and family as the rationale for the program, Martinson and her associates worked as liaisons to ensure professional support for the parents, who became the primary caregivers. In a report of their first home care program for dying children, the nurses cited a father's words of thanks (Martinson et al, 1977, p 1815):

> Seth died as we had often hoped he could—cuddled in our arms before a blazing fire, in utter quiet and peace. We have such good feelings about the peace of that moment that it has been immeasurably easier to deal with this reality. We can hardly thank you enough for permitting us the peace and dignity of that moment.

With the success of the Martinson model for home care came the question, "Why should the comfort of family support be reserved only for dying children?" Slowly, health care professionals began to experiment with parental management of other illness conditions in children. Home apnea monitoring became more common, and children were sent home with central venous catheters and on continuous ambulatory peritoneal dialysis. Today, home care extends even to children who are ventilator-dependent.

Although, in 1985, children accounted for only 5 to 10 per cent of the home health care market (Punch, 1985), continued growth is expected. There are three reasons:

1. Increased survivorship of very low birthweight children as a result of advances in medical technology.
2. Greater longevity for children with terminal illness.
3. Greater awareness and detection of chronic health problems by parents, educators, and physicians.

Now that technology in its nondiscriminating manner has saved these children and prolonged their lives, the community and the health care professionals must assist the families in caring for them in the least restrictive environment so they may achieve quality of life and, when appropriate, attain a productive life style.

Social Considerations

Although the Martinson home care model influenced social attitudes about the care of ill children, it is important to note that Martinson's work was the result of social trends. Societal influences have made an impact on home care since its inception in the United States in 1893, when Lillian Wald established The Visiting Nurse Service of New York City in response to public health concerns for the elderly. Home care for children has come about in response to several identifiable social factors. In particular, pediatric home care has been shaped by the need for cost containment, by increasing consumer demands for quality services, and by technologic developments.

Cost Containment

The issue of cost containment has become a reality for everyone in the health care industry. Costs for health care services have risen dramatically in recent years, and insurance coverage is strained by reimbursements for costly tests and procedures and by the increasing life span of persons with chronic illnesses. National estimates show that a child who is ventilator-dependent may generate hospital bills of $300,000 in 1 year. Since the majority of children who are candidates for home care will continue to live for a long time, the impact of the way their care is structured will affect the entire society for at least a whole generation. It is clear that costs must be "contained"; the challenge is to cut costs without decreasing the quality of care.

Home care has been approached as one solution to cost containment. The same technology that saved these children's lives and once was only available in the hospital now is being miniaturized for portability, enabling it to be used in the home. Fragile children can be cared for at home at tremendous cost savings when compared with the cost of an average hospital stay. Rogatz (1985) cautioned, however, that home care must be evaluated in the light of what we are trying to achieve. If we are committed to comprehensive and effective health services as well as to cost savings, then home care must be not only cheaper than hospital care but more cost-effective as well. Cost-effectiveness entails the provision of high-quality services to the most people at the most reasonable price.

With the legislation of diagnosis-related groups (DRGs), hospitals have been given an incentive to provide care that facilitates the patient's recovery in the shortest time. Although that might not appear to be an innovation, consider that, previously, hospitals could make the most money by keeping their beds full of persons whose insurance and/or Medicare plans would pay for the ongoing cost of services. DRGs dictate that, for a Medicare patient, hospitals will be paid a lump sum (or prospective fee) to treat a particular disease. That means that if the hospital can treat the illness as effectively by an alternate method of care (such as home care), a profit can be shown for that transaction.

Although DRGs at present deal only with Medicare patients, facilities that provide pediatric care are anticipating that they will be faced with similar forms of payment in the future. For this reason, and because of early reports of savings in health dollars, pediatric institutions and private pediatricians are becoming involved in home care. Home care is cost-effective if it ensures follow-up to decrease recurrent exacerbations and hospitalizations, if it minimizes the psychosocial impact of illness by maintaining a more normal environment, and if it reduces the number of salaried professionals who interact with the client.

Although home care often results in substantial savings to health care institutions, it may not be cheaper for the family. Traditionally, insurance reimbursements have been more generous for hospital-based services than for those provided in the home, and families may actually be responsible for a greater percentage of the expenses if the child is cared for in the home. Another consideration is whether one parent must relinquish gainful employment to stay at home and care for the child. Even if one parent is available to provide home care, the added physical and emotional burdens of continuous care for an ill child may necessitate extra expenses to relieve that parent of some of the usual household duties.

Insurance companies in the 1990s are realizing that they need to work together with parents, hospitals, and home care agencies to maximize the benefits they administer. These children are flourishing at home, and, therefore, their life expectancy is getting longer. To stretch the dollars and wisely spend the patient's lifetime maximum, the insurance companies are employing nurses in the role of case managers. *Case management* is a systematic approach to identifying high-cost patients, assessing opportunities to coordinate their care, developing treatment plans that improve quality by selecting alternatives best for the patient, and managing patients' total care to ensure optimal outcomes (Delaney & Aquilina, 1992). This approach includes a collaborative effort that takes place among the physician, family, home care providers, and case managers, building on the nursing process in order to assess, plan, implement, coordinate, monitor, and evaluate options and services specifically designed to meet the child's and his or her family's health needs through communication and available resources to promote quality, cost-effective outcomes.

Quality of Care

An effective quality assurance program should be designed to objectively and systematically monitor and evaluate the quality of patient care, pursue opportunities to improve patient care, and resolve identified problems (Joint Commission Accreditation for Hospital and Related Organizations, 1993). This involves monitoring and evaluating the quality of patient care and the performance of home care staff through an ongoing, planned, and systematic process. The specific activities for monitoring and evaluating patient care or services should include the identification of the important aspects of care. These aspects of care should fall into one of the following three categories:

1. *High volume:* An aspect of care or service that occurs frequently or affects large numbers of patients. *Example: apnea monitor*—parents' ability to perform cardiopulmonary resuscitation (CPR); parents' ability to be in compliance with protocols; parents' increase in knowledge from hospital teaching into and including the first days in home care. *Example: failure to thrive*—measurement of weight gain.
2. *High risk:* Patients who are at risk of serious consequences or are deprived of benefit if the care is not provided correctly. *Examples:* peripheral line site infection; ventilator management.
3. *Problem-prone:* The care has tended in the past to produce problems for staff or patients. *Examples:* medication management of a medically fragile child; coordination of services when several agencies are involved (e.g., home care, Home Medical Equipment (HME), IV company).

The common sources of data to be collected are the retrospective chart review, observation on home visits, written or verbal evaluation of care by the patient/family or caregiver, infection control reports, and incident reports. These data should be of appropriate sample size, based on total population of patients in the category and frequency of collection, to document trends in care. The quality assurance plan would clearly identify the aspects of care, method of collection, responsible person(s), and reporting path for the outcomes.

Once the data are collected, analyzed, and reported, follow-up action needs to be researched, planned, and implemented, and the results need to be monitored in order to evaluate whether the plan of action was effective in changing the outcomes. Often, this latter step is complex and could cross institution and agency lines. For example, a pediatric agency was monitoring the care of a patient who experienced a high-risk infection in a central line, causing unplanned readmission to the hospital. Normally, the agency experiences one patient with this complication every quarter; however, the incidence increased to six. The quality assurance team, through their investigation, could not find any change in home care practice that caused this outcome. Further investigation revealed that this patient's hospital stay had been shortened by 2 days because of reduced insurance coverage. The quality assurance team met with the staff at the hospital and discovered that the normal protocol for such patients was sterile dressing changes to the site for 7 days. However, the last 2 days of care did not occur because of discharge. The protocol had been that the family was taught, once the child went home, to use clean, not sterile technique. The home care staff was not informed of the change in the hospital care and continued to reinforce clean technique. The outcome of the investigation was that the home care staff would provide the care for 2 days following discharge using sterile technique, followed by a shift in care to the parents using clean technique. On further monitoring of the new plan, the incidence returned to normal.

Therefore, it is imperative that pediatric home care programs have well-established quality assurance indicators that monitor and change practice patterns. Because of the increase in technology and fast-paced changes in care, important aspects of care or services need to be identified and incorporated into the plan on an ongoing basis.

The issue of quality of life is particularly pertinent to home care of children. With the increasing emphasis in the professional and lay literature on the psychosocial and developmental aspects of childhood has come the realization that it is often detrimental to separate an ill child from family support. Normalization of the child's environment through home care can be effective in promoting recovery and in preventing hospital-induced psychologic trauma. Psychosocial, cultural, and economic factors that are easily overlooked in an acute care setting become much more apparent when the client is seen in the home. Solutions to illness-related problems (and resulting enhancement of the quality of life) are more likely to be effective when all aspects of the child's life are taken into consideration (Fig. 22–1).

Technology

The third social factor affecting pediatric home care is the technology of modern science. Recent technologic advances have resulted in the prolongation of life for infants and children who would not previously have survived. Many of these children, however, are left with chronic conditions (such as bronchopulmonary dysplasia) and need constant skilled care. Home care management, with careful teaching and follow-up by health care professionals, is often the chosen alternative for families with chronically ill children.

Another aspect of technologic advances is the equipment that has made possible home therapies that were previously only conducted in the hospital. Not only has the equipment itself become more sophisticated and reliable but, over time, health care professionals have also become more comfortable with it and therefore are more willing to teach aspects of its use and maintenance to their clients. The outcome is delivery of care in the home today that was, in some cases, considered experimental in hospitals in the early 1980s.

Support services for home care equipment have also improved. Agencies that deal in home care supplies are becoming increasingly aware of the need to provide a broad range of professional services. The competition among "provider" agencies means that it is no longer enough to employ someone to deliver large green bottles of oxygen; to be competitive, the agency may need to employ skilled respiratory therapists who can assist home care nurses in monitoring treatments and obtaining assessment data through pulse oximetry and transcutaneous monitoring.

Nursing Process in Home Health Care

The component parts of the nursing process, as it relates to home care, become a shared responsibility between the nurses (and other health care professionals) in the hospital and the nurse who will be responsible for coordination of care once the child is at home. Hospital-based nurses, in cooperation with the family and with other health care professionals, initiate the nursing process for home care by assessing whether a child and family are candidates for home care. If home care is determined to be a viable option, planning continues. Care must be taken to clarify the perceptions of the family at each step, because the family needs to have an understanding and acceptance of what it will mean to them to bring a medically fragile child home. The home care plan of treatment will not go well unless the family members

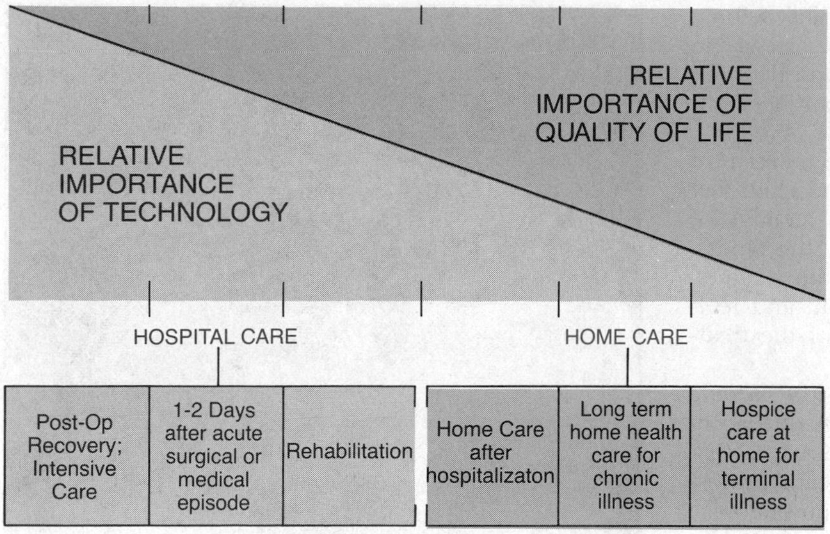

FIGURE 22-1. The relationship of acute and long-term illness to the importance of technology and quality of life. (From Rogatz, P. [1985]. Home health care: Some social and economic considerations. *Home Healthcare Nurse, 3*[1], 41.)

understand that they have an integral role to play in the care at home. They will need to be taught the treatments, how to manage the machines, when to call the physician, and what company to call depending on what the problem is. It is a role that parents need explained in detail. Their lives will change. The stress of having strangers in the home caring for their child and the need to be an advocate and master coordinator of care are difficult for even the most cohesive family to cope with. There should be no misunderstandings of the roles of home care professionals or the family. The nursing diagnoses and clinical problems are identified and goals for treatment are set. Ideally, the home health care nurse who will be responsible for implementation and evaluation of the plan is also involved in the planning process.

Assessment

The assessment process begins in the hospital with the determination of the patient's and family's needs, strengths, and limitations in relation to home-based health care management. It results in the determination of whether a child and family are candidates for home health care. Hymovich (1976) has suggested that in order to cope with chronic illness in their child parents need (1) trust, (2) information, (3) resources, and (4) guidance and support. These criteria also apply to the child with a short-term illness and form a suitable framework for assessing family readiness for home health care.

Trust

Parents* need to trust themselves, their child, the health care professionals involved, and the treatment plan. First, they must believe in their own physical and emotional ability to manage the child's care at home. Whether that care involves monitoring of equipment (such as an oxygen tank or a home apnea monitor), maintenance of indwelling tubes (such as a gastrostomy tube or central venous catheter), delivery of treatments (such as chest physical therapy or range-of-motion exercises), or administration of medications, parents need to feel confident in their ability to perform the tasks safely and effectively. This need for self-confidence also applies to children who are old enough to participate in self-care.

Before the child or the parents can trust themselves to deal with the treatment plan for illness, however, they must face the illness itself. Until the reality of the illness is accepted, there will be an emotional obstacle to the delivery of technical care. If they cannot come to accept the necessary dependency on the medical regimen, omission of parts of the treatment plan may result; the delivery of prescribed care will only serve as a painful reminder of the illness they might otherwise be able to deny. To accept the illness, parents must alter the mental and emotional image of their whole and perfect child to include the reality that their child is, temporarily or permanently, dependent on a machine or tube or on certain treatments and medications. Children, in turn, must alter their self-image to incorporate the reality of the illness.

Parents and children also need to trust the ability of the treatment plan to accomplish the desired goals, which goes hand in hand with their need to trust the health care professionals involved. *The family is unlikely to comply with the treatment plan unless it addresses the problems that they have identified in a manner that is in keeping with their values.*

Certain objective assessments contribute to an understanding of trust. Competency of return demonstrations of technical tasks by the child and parents, willingness of the child and parents to participate in

*Although it is acknowledged that the primary caregiver in the home may not be a parent, the term "parent(s)" is used in this chapter to mean "adult caregiver(s)."

the technical aspects of care in the hospital setting, observable indications of parental anxiety or ease in the presence of the child, and frequency and duration of parental hospital visits are among the pertinent observable behaviors.

Trust is also indicated subjectively. The nurse must be alert for statements from the parents and child that would reveal feelings of self-confidence, feelings of acceptance of the changes necessitated by the illness, feelings of hope that the desired goals can be met, feelings of some control over the situation, and feelings of being vital and valued members of the treatment team.

A family that is involved in the decision making process is much more likely to display signs of trust in themselves and others. A prerequisite for trust is that both parties (the family and the health care professionals) accept and value each other's contributions.

If health care professionals determine that they are unable to consider the parents (and child, when appropriate) as equal participants in the treatment, they must question whether their lack of confidence is based on legitimate concerns (such as lack of mental capacity or lack of necessary manual dexterity) or whether those concerns stem only from differences in values and lifestyle. In the former case, it may be appropriate to conclude that this family is not a candidate for home care or that professional help will be needed in the home. In the latter case, an unbiased re-examination of both facts and attitudes will be necessary.

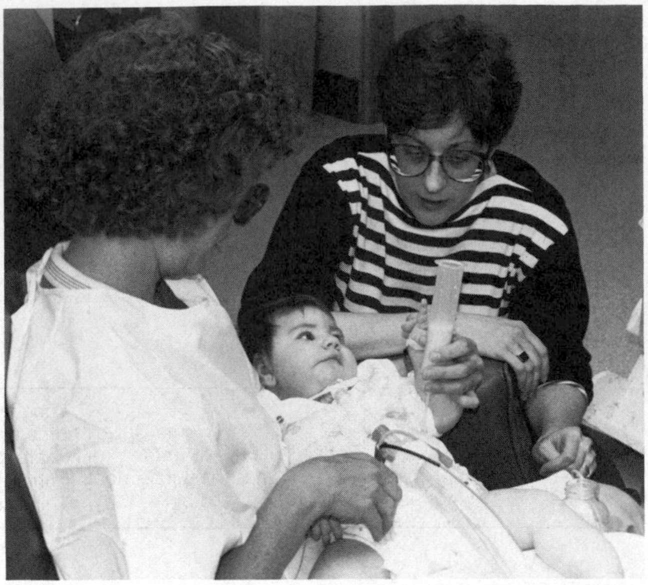

FIGURE 22-2. The home care nurse (seated) and the mother are both learning to care for the child in the hospital before discharge. Coordination with the child's primary nurse in the hospital ensures continuity of care. (Courtesy of Children's Home Care of the Children's Hospital, Denver.)

Information

Assessment of information involves the determination of what discharge teaching the family and child have received, and whether they understand and agree with the information. If the assessment reveals a lack of understanding or agreement on the part of the child and family, the method of teaching must be evaluated.

Discharge teaching is most effective when all members of the health care team understand specifically what teaching is needed, what teaching has been done, what information needs to be covered again, and when there is agreement on the way in which this information should be presented. Lacking such coordination, the process may be undermined by the family's receiving conflicting instructions, resulting in their confusion not only about the information given but also about whom to believe (Fig. 22–2).

Coordination of discharge teaching begins with a list of facts and skills to be taught.* If this list is kept at the bedside and a check list system used for items that have been addressed, potential "teachers" among the health care professionals can easily be updated on the progress made. The form should include a column for the child and family to indicate whether, after reflecting on the information or demonstration, they have achieved a level of comfort or whether they desire further teaching. It can be effective to allow the child and family to choose the order in which they want to cover the items on the discharge teaching list (Davis & Eyer, 1984). This provides them some control over one aspect of the hospital environment and enhances the chance for a receptive audience.

It is important to remember that anxiety decreases comprehension, making it necessary to discuss the same set of facts or to demonstrate the same procedure more than once. The parents and child can be "given permission" to need this additional help by statements such as, "Many children (or parents) tell me they have to do this several times before they really understand it. Would you like to do it once more?"

The issue of conflicting instructions is more likely to develop when a large number of people are interacting with and teaching the family. Control may be best achieved by designating certain "teachers" among those professionals involved and/or by frequent coordination meetings of the team responsible for discharge teaching for home care.

Assessment of whether the child and family comprehend the material and skills taught is integral to the teaching process. It is helpful, when appropriate, to listen as the child or parent explains the illness and treatment plan to other family members or friends. In

*In the illness-related chapters of this text, discharge teaching needs are itemized for many diseases under the nursing diagnosis *knowledge deficit* or *high risk for altered home health maintenance*.

fact, it can be useful to teach a procedure purposely to only one family member or to the child, and then to watch as that person teaches another of the persons who will be responsible for that part of the treatment in the home. Not only does this facilitate the nurse's evaluation of information and technical skills but it also helps to reinforce that person's confidence by attributing to him or her the status and responsibility of "teacher."

There are three possible outcomes of the assessment of the scope and depth of the family's information regarding necessary aspects of the home treatment plan: (1) they may have the necessary understanding and psychomotor skills to perform the care; (2) they may show command of part of the information but require further assessment and teaching before a final determination is made regarding readiness for home care; or (3) limitations may be identified in cognitive or psychomotor abilities. These limitations may be the result of conflicts of value or other psychosocial factors that have interfered with the family's motivation to learn the needed skills. If further teaching will correct the problem, arrangements can often be made with the home care nurse for additional technical support and teaching in the first days that the child is at home. If it does not appear that further assessment and teaching will be effective, the family will not be recommended for home care.

Resources

Assessment of the family's resources includes physical, emotional, and financial considerations. *Physical resources* include individual physical characteristics, the physical environment of the home, and sources of physical support. Parents must possess the necessary physical strength and agility to perform treatments and maintain equipment, and they must be able to do so consistently. When a primary caregiver has a chronic illness, such as asthma, modifications may be required in the plan of care. The physical strain of round-the-clock responsibility for an ill child is considerable, and even the healthiest principal caregiver will need to make provisions for respite care.

The physical environment of the home must be such that the child's safety and the effectiveness of treatments are ensured. A visit to the home prior to the child's discharge is advisable when possible. During this visit, the nurse or social worker can talk with the parents about such things as where the ill child will sleep and where equipment will be placed. At this time, assessment can be made of the ability to heat and cool the home, of the adequacy of electrical outlets or equipment and refrigeration to store food and medications, and of other potential safety and health hazards.

Sources of physical support include friends, extended family, and community support groups who are willing to provide assistance such as grocery shopping; help with laundry, cleaning, and meals; and baby-sitting for siblings of the ill child.

Emotional support resources consist of those persons within the family or community who are willing to listen to the family's problems and to assist them in the problem-solving process. Families often experience numerous offers of physical and emotional support from friends and extended family at the onset of an illness. As the illness and home care situation linger on, however, few of the support persons are able to manage the weight of the family's problems in addition to their own, and the support is withdrawn. When this occurs, the family begins to rely more and more on health care professionals to meet both physical and emotional needs.

Assessment of the family's *financial ability* to meet home care costs must include the cost to implement the medical treatment plan in the home (e.g., equipment and medications); consideration of insurance coverage for prescribed treatments, home visits, and home nursing care; and the alteration of family patterns of work outside and inside the home. Will home care necessitate one parent quitting a job outside the home? Will significant expenses be incurred (e.g., purchasing additional ready-to-eat foods, sending shirts out to be laundered, buying ready-made clothing) because the primary caregiver does not have time to perform the usual activities within the home?

Home care of the ill child need not always be abandoned if the family's resources are inadequate to sustain this type of program. A knowledgeable social worker can often help the family find sources of support for financial, emotional, and certain physical needs. It is essential, however, that the assessment process results in identification of these needs and that proper referral is made.

Guidance and Support

Guidance and support of the family by health care professionals are integral to the concept of home care. Assessment of these criteria concerns the availability of help for the family 24 hours a day, and the family's ability to reach that help. Does the family have a telephone? Can a nurse always be reached if questions arise about treatment procedures or about new signs and symptoms? If an interpreter is necessary, is there always one available? Does the family have transportation to take the child to the clinic for follow-up care? Is there ambulance service available in that area in case of an emergency? What provisions have been made, or can be made, for needed electrical equipment in case of a power outage? Is there a fire station or police station nearby that can provide oxygen and CPR in case of an emergency?

The needs of the child and family and the type of agency providing the home care will dictate the composition of the support team. If the home care is directed from a hospital or community health agency, it is likely that more disciplines will be involved in the care because of ease of access. If the home care is provided by a nursing registry, the nurses involved often draw on their knowledge and personal resources to provide many of the additional services themselves. In any case, the home care support team will include at least one nurse and one physician, with the involvement of educators, physical therapists, nutritionists, speech therapists, respiratory therapists, social workers, clergy, and psychologists as necessary.

Limitations in the availability of guidance and support for the family can often be remedied by careful coordination of health care professionals and allied health care personnel. When this is not possible, it is usually because the family's insurance will not cover the costs of the necessary support services. Although insurance carriers have been slow to provide reimbursement for pediatric home care, that trend is beginning to change as the cost-effectiveness of home care becomes more evident (Kahn, 1984; Punch, 1985). According to Kaufman and Hardy-Ribakow (1988), the majority of funding for pediatric home care is provided by private insurance companies, Supplemental Security Income (Title XVI), and state crippled children's programs. They predict that more of these costs will begin to be assumed by the Title XIX Medicaid Model Waivers, designed to help individuals who currently receive or qualify for Medicaid benefits in an institutional setting.

After all of the assessment data have been gathered, the discharge planning team will determine whether the needs of the child and family can best be met by home care, by continued hospitalization, or by another care alternative such as an extended care facility. The child and family can be identified as appropriate candidates for home care if it is determined that they demonstrate adequate trust, comprehension of information, and adequate resources, and if the necessary guidance and support are available. There is one additional element, however, that must not be overlooked. Now that the family has a good understanding of the scope of their responsibilities in home care of the child, do they still consider this to be the best option? *Have they been asked that question?* The health care professionals responsible for the hospital-based assessment and planning for home care would do well to heed Elkins' (1986) caveat to home care nurses: "When working with home care patients and their families, the home health nurse must realize that she is stepping into their environment and that when she leaves they will remain in the same environment with the responsibility of care" (p 181). Nurses and other health care professionals responsible for determining the family's readiness for home care are, at least figuratively, stepping into the lives of those persons, but they are not the ones who will carry the day-to-day burden. Care must be taken not to impose one's own values for health care on the family who will ultimately assume the responsibility for it. For home care to be successful, it is essential that the family and the professional support team have similar perceptions of the readiness for discharge and for home care.

Nursing Diagnosis

When the decision for home care has been made, nursing diagnoses form the basis for planning care. The needs of the child and family that arise from the assessment data are stated in the form of nursing diagnoses. Family involvement in identifying nursing diagnoses is not only advisable but also essential. If the family is to assume the primary responsibility for care, they must be actively involved in and informed about the basis of that care. The parents (and child, as development allows) should help establish each section of each nursing diagnosis (response, etiology, and defining characteristics) and should fully participate in assigning priorities to all the problems and needs identified. *The success of the home treatment plan will depend on the family's investment in it.*

Desired Outcomes/Evaluation Criteria

The next step in the nursing process is to set realistic goals, or outcomes, that will provide direction for the treatment plan and form a basis for evaluation. The desired outcomes of home care will reflect the individualized nursing diagnoses. In some patients (e.g., children with bronchopulmonary dysplasia or cystic fibrosis), the goals may lead to the family's independence in the care of their child. In other patients (e.g., children who have terminal cancer), the desired outcomes may reflect an increased quality of life for the child, increased opportunities for caring interactions between the child and the family, and the preservation of more normal family functioning. In the case of terminally ill children, the involvement of the professional support team usually increases as the child's condition deteriorates.

The mutual agreement on the purpose of home care (e.g., the desired outcomes or what is to be accomplished) is perhaps the pivot point for the rest of the home care experience. If the family is operating on one agenda and the health care professionals on another, neither party will be satisfied with the efforts of the other. The goals must be those of the child and family as well as of the health care professionals.

Agreement on the desired outcomes will be enhanced by (1) the family's involvement in determining needs and assigning priorities, (2) the family's participation in and understanding of the evaluation criteria, (3) evaluation criteria that are specific, realistic, and assigned appropriate time lines, and (4) frequent evaluation and restructuring of the desired outcomes and the methods of treatment.

Figure 22–3 illustrates part of a home care plan for 5-year-old Becky S., who has been diagnosed with cystic fibrosis and has been referred for home care. This care plan (which, in its entirety, includes nursing diagnoses, goals, and strategies for the scope of the child's illness) will be used by the parents as well as by the health care professionals who see Becky in her home. Becky's parents were involved in

Ineffective airway clearance, related to production of thick mucus in the bronchial tree

Recurrent wheezing, rales, and rhonchi; two episodes of *Staphylococcus aureus* pneumonia in the last 4 months; frequent cough productive of moderate-to-large amounts of thick, purulent secretions with occasional traces of bright red blood.

1. Becky will increase the clearance of mucus from her airways within 2 weeks, as evidenced by:	
a. rarely having episodes of coughing to ''get up'' mucous plugs, except when associated with respiratory treatments	Perform the respiratory therapy regimen learned in the hospital four times a day, before meals and at bedtime. (Using these times will reduce Becky's chances of vomiting. • Put the premixed solution of Alupent in the nebulizer and encourage Becky to breathe it in deeply until there are no droplets left in the nebulizer chamber. (This medicine will open Becky's airways and make it easier for the mucus to drain out.) • Clap firmly on Becky's chest for 2 minutes in each of the nine positions you were taught. Use the pictures attached to this care plan until you are more comfortable with the routine. (Percussion loosens the thick mucus in Becky's lungs and the postural drainage puts her in the best position for all of the parts of her lungs to drain.) • Encourage Becky to cough during the respiratory treatment. (Coughing is nature's way of removing mucus from the lungs.) If Becky coughs particularly hard she may still have some streaks of blood in the mucus. (This happens when small blood vessels break from the force of her coughing.) You need not be concerned about the streaks of blood unless there is considerably more bleeding than she had when she was in the hospital. If she begins coughing up a lot of blood call the home care nurse or the clinic immediately.
b. less ''noise'' and wheezing audible in her chest when parents listen to her breathe and when nurse auscultates with a stethoscope	Listen to Becky's breathing before and after the treatments. Afterwards, you should hear less wheezing and crackles and she should feel that it is easier to breathe in and out. (When the nurse visits she will take Becky's vital signs before and after a treatment, listen to her lungs, and talk with you about the effect of the treatments.)
c. *absence* of fever; chest pain; rapid, shallow breathing; a grunting sound to her breathing; and extreme tiredness	If any of these signs and symptoms of pneumonia occur, call the home care nurse or take Becky to the clinic. (If Becky develops another case of pneumonia it is important that she start on the antibiotic as soon as possible to prevent lasting effects on her lungs.)

FIGURE 22-3. An excerpt from a home care plan. The client is Becky S., age 5 years. Medical diagnosis is cystic fibrosis.

formulation of the care plan and agreed that Becky's lung involvement was the first priority of the treatment plan.

In the excerpt of the care plan shown in the figure, the nursing diagnostic response of *ineffective airway clearance* is identified. This clarifies for the parents, as well as for the health care professionals, the particular lung problem and the defining characteristics on which the nursing diagnosis is based. The goals and interventions reflect the responses to the problem. They are written in language that Becky's parents can understand and contain specific evaluation criteria that they can use to judge their daughter's progress. The interventions (implementation) list specific instructions that reflect and reinforce the teaching the family received before Becky was discharged from the hospital. Rationale for the actions is included as a reminder of their purpose.

Although it is time-consuming to construct a detailed home care plan with the family, it is cost-effective. To the extent that the care plan enhances the family's sense of comfort and competence, and their trust in the treatment plan, it will increase compliance and decrease exacerbations and future hospitalizations. To the extent that it provides the parents with a basis for making decisions about minor changes in the plan and about the need for medical or nursing consultation, it reduces the number of hours of follow-up required by health care professionals. To the extent that it provides peace of mind for the family, the care plan is of immeasurable benefit in normalizing the home environment and in enhancing loving relationships among family members.

Nursing Care/Nursing Orders

Nursing orders, or implementation of the plan of care, takes place in the home and involves the home care nurse. Before further discussion of implementation procedures, it is pertinent to explore the special qualities and preparation of the home care nurse.

Preparation of Home Care Nurses

The home care nurse's preparation should include prior hospital experience with the type of patients to be seen in home care settings. It is essential that the nurse possess competence and confidence in acute care skills such as physical assessment, venipuncture, and management of indwelling tubes and equipment. In Cherryholmes' words, "The home health nurse is a higher-leveled generalist who has to be able to recognize problems and trust her own judgment and clinical skills" (1986, p 158). She noted that knowledge of norms is necessary because there is no one in the home with whom to collaborate.

Characteristics of Home Care Nurses

Successful home care nurses tend to share certain qualities. They tend to be holistic in approach and to value flexibility and autonomy in their work settings (Mundinger, 1983; Stuart-Siddall, 1984). The home health care nurse enjoys teaching and is able to adapt teaching strategies to the full spectrum of physical and emotional climates that might be encountered. The effective nurse in the home care setting is able to communicate acceptance of a variety of lifestyles and to make judgments according to the identified outcomes for the treatment plan rather than on the basis of differences or similarities in values. In some communities, it can be very helpful to be bilingual; the family will appreciate the attempt to communicate with them in their first language. Home care nurses also tend to enjoy problem solving and have the ability to help the client identify the need for change and work through the change process (Cherryholmes, 1986).

Implementation of the home care treatment plan is, in most cases, the responsibility of the family, with the support of the home care nurse, the physician, and other professionals as needed. If the home care nurse was not involved in the creation of the care plan, time must be spent with the family clarifying the problems, outcomes, strategies, and evaluation criteria. A nursing process plan is presented in Table 22–1. This plan focuses on *family* adaptation to home care. Nursing assessments, diagnoses, client goals, strategies, and evaluation criteria can be added to address the child's illness, or the child's illness can be dealt with separately in a plan meant to be used by the family as a guideline for care (see Fig. 22–3).

Framework for Home Care Management

The home care nurse needs an organizational approach or personal conceptual framework for home care management (Hillman, 1986). Lenihan (1985) proposed adoption of the Wright and Leahy (1984) model for family interviewing as a conceptual framework for interactions in home care. This model offers a simple, commonsense approach to the intervention process. The steps of the model are engagement, assessment, intervention, and termination.

Engagement

Engagement is the introduction and trust-building stage of the nurse-family relationship. It is essential that this part of the process not be overlooked. Hillman (1986, p 164) cautioned, ". . . if the home health care nurse is insensitive to the importance of the establishment of an open, ongoing relationship, she may not be able to effect a therapeutic change, regardless of the accuracy of her assessment and problem identification." The primary tool for the engagement process is an accepting attitude that communicates to the family members that the nurse values their worth as human beings and their potential contributions to the treatment plan. Each family member should be acknowledged regardless of her or his involvement with the child's care (Elkins, 1986). The client in home care is the family; each member influences the environment and needs to be recognized for her or his role within the family.

Often engagement begins with a telephone call in which the nurse relates some personal qualifications and describes the services of the agency and the fees for service. At this time, an appointment is made for the nurse to visit the home. The initial "engagement" visit should establish the pattern for future visits (Lenihan, 1985). The family needs to know what they can expect from the nurse and what the nurse will expect from them, such as keeping appointments and providing space for physical assessment of the child.

The nurse's communication skills, both verbal and nonverbal, will never be more challenged than during this engagement stage. A successful encounter will greatly facilitate the mutually established goals,

TABLE 22-1

Nursing Process Plan: Home Care

Analysis: Nursing Diagnostic Statement 1

Response and Related or Risk Factors: *High risk for altered family processes;* risk factors related to incomplete adjustment to the physical, intellectual, emotional, and spiritual stress of home care for an ill child

Projected Outcome: The family will regain the ability to meet the physical, emotional, and spiritual needs of its members

Defining Characteristics
(Actual Responses)

Subjective:

- Verbalization of ineffective communication among family members
- Concerns about interactions with health care professionals, equipment vendors, community agencies, insurance companies
- Verbalized feelings of being overwhelmed, fatigued, having no time for self, feeling unable to cope with "all the details" of the ill child's care in addition to other family responsibilities
- Feelings of guilt and inadequacy
- Difficulty in finding meaning and purpose in life
- "Not sure we made the right decision in bringing (child) home"

Objective:

- Family members displaying poor eye contact with each other
- Tension evident in verbal exchanges
- Poor organizational skills
- Inadequate equipment, food, clean clothing for ill child
- Altered decision making skills
- Siblings demanding of parental attention

Nursing Interventions

Family Process Maintenance and Caregiver Support

Determine: (1) whether disruption in family processes likely to resolve with additional time, (2) whether family resources are adequate to meet demands of adjustment period, (3) whether additional support services needed, (4) whether to recommend continuation or discontinuation of home care.

- Assess caregivers' physical, emotional ability to implement the therapeutic regimen. Evaluate whether care being performed as prescribed
- Assess caregivers' perception of home care. Ask: "What is it like to care for (child) at home?" "What aspects of home care concern you most?" "What gives you the most satisfaction?" "Who can help you with that?" "Do you want to continue home care?" If no, "What do you see as alternatives?"
- Assess ill child's perception of home care. Ask: "What do you like best about being at home?" "Are there things about the hospital that you miss?" "What do you wish for most?"

Support adaptive behavior

- Recognize and praise adaptive behavior as appropriate: "(Child's) lungs sound so clear; you must be doing well with the

Evaluation Criteria

The family will regain the ability to meet the physical, emotional, and spiritual needs of its members as evidenced by:

- Lessening tension in interactions between/among family members
- Effective communication with health care professionals and support services
- Healthy problem solving
- Caretakers receiving adequate rest
- Adequate supplies on hand for ill child's care
- Verbalization of increased confidence, decreased stress
- Adequate organizational skills
- Behavior of siblings returning to precrisis status
- Verbalization of finding meaning and satisfaction in caring for ill child at home
- Increasing ability to coordinate ill child's care

(continued)

TABLE 22-1 (continued)

Defining Characteristics (Actual Response)	Nursing Interventions	Evaluation Criteria
	chest physical therapy." "This medication schedule is nice, I would like to tell other families about the form you've devised." "(Child) seems so content being here with the family." "How do you manage all these tasks and still find time to read bedtime stories to the other children?" "I'm glad you took some time for yourself yesterday." "Yes, that was the right person to call. It sounds as if you have resolved the problem" *Coping Enhancement* • With the caregivers, identify specific problems and goals related to care of the ill child • Modify the child's plan of care as the goals, strategies, and evaluation criteria change. See Figure 22–3 for an example • Suggest time-saving ways to organize the child's care • With the caregivers, identify problems and goals related to family processes • Reach agreement on goals to improve family processes and discuss resources and strategies to meet the goals • Encourage family consultation with members of the clergy or others who can help members regain peace of mind and a sense of purpose • Make referrals to other community agencies when family resources are inadequate. Draw on the family's resources whenever possible (Ordinarily, the overall goal is to help the family become self-reliant) • With the family's permission, contact the school nurse to obtain support for the school-age ill child and for school-age siblings	

TABLE 22-1 *(continued)*

Defining Characteristics *(Actual Response)*	Nursing Interventions	Evaluation Criteria
	• Discuss with caregivers the need for sources of respite care **Encourage the family to normalize family processes as much as possible** • Assess the family's perception of "normal" family lifestyle. Discuss with them the aspects that are most valued and encourage them to continue those activities/relationships to the extent possible • Discuss acceptable ways to modify the ill child's care to accommodate the usual family lifestyle • Reinforce the importance of planning time for self, spouse, and the other children (Without this encouragement, family members may feel guilty about planning time away from the ill child) • Suggest that siblings be allowed to help in age-appropriate ways as family responsibilities are shifted to accommodate home care (Helping can give siblings a feeling of worth and a sense of importance at a time when they might otherwise feel insecure) • Acknowledge siblings' "helper" roles when visiting the ill child (to promote their sense of self-worth and accomplishment)	

Analysis: Nursing Diagnostic Statement 2

Response and Related or Risk Factors: *High risk for knowledge deficit regarding condition and its management,* related to

- Procedures, medications
- Signs and symptoms that warrant calling the nurse or physician
- Ways to promote normal growth and development
- Well child care
- Community resources

Projected Outcome: The child/family will display the knowledge and skills needed to perform the prescribed treatment at home

(continued)

TABLE 22-1 (continued)

Defining Characteristics (Actual Responses)	Nursing Interventions	Evaluation Criteria
Subjective: • Verbalizing the need for further information/instruction *Objective*: • Unable to perform certain aspects of care related to illness management. Concentration on illness care to the exclusion of well child care	*Teaching Procedure/Treatment* **Assess the quality of physical care** • Observe therapeutic procedures instead of performing them • Ask to see the record of medication given and any other treatment or status records kept by the family • Determine caregivers' perception of progress toward the goals of therapy (to assess understanding of evaluation criteria) **Provide instructions as needed.** • Correct misconceptions and potentially harmful breaks in technique. Remain open, however, to innovations in strategies that make care easier for family members and that still accomplish the goal (e.g., evaluate whether the technique must be done exactly as taught in the hospital) • Ensure that instruction is given tactfully and that caregivers are not admonished for being novices. Use phrases like, "This takes a great deal of practice," and "You may find it easier if you . . . ." (If caregivers perceive that they are being scolded for breaks in techniques, they will be less likely to ask for help. Open communication is vital to a therapeutic relationship) • Encourage questions and discussion of care **Ensure that family is prepared for an emergency** • Ask where family keeps list of emergency numbers and when it was last updated • Ensure that the following agencies have been notified of the family's potential need for emergency service: telephone company, electric company, fire de-	**The child/family will display the knowledge and skills needed to perform the prescribed treatment at home, as evidenced by:** • Effective implementation of prescribed therapy • Proper operation and cleaning of equipment • Expected progress in child's health status • Identifying signs and symptoms that warrant medical intervention • Discussing appropriate emergency procedures • Demonstrating ability to perform cardiopulmonary resuscitation (CPR) **The child wil receive appropriate well child care, as evidenced by:** • Keeping well child appointments • Immunizations up to date • Expected progress in height and weight • Expected progress on developmental tasks

TABLE 22-1 *(continued)*

Defining Characteristics *(Actual Response)*	***Nursing Interventions***	***Evaluation Criteria***
	partment, emergency medical services, police department • Periodically assist family members to update CPR skills **Record teaching and other nursing interventions in detailed form to document the need for professional nursing care** (Proper charting is essential to document eligibility for home care and to facilitate payment for services rendered) **Emphasize well child needs** • Weigh and measure the child regularly. Discuss the child's progress on growth charts • Remind caregivers of the need to make and keep well child appointments (The child may be seeing a specialist for illness care and may need to have a separate appointment for routine well child care) • Regularly assess child's progress on developmental tasks. Alert family to pertinent tasks and discuss with them ways to help the child accomplish tasks in light of acute or chronic illness condition	

whereas a less successful beginning can haunt the remainder of the relationship.

Engagement with the child must occur concurrently with the establishment of the family's trust. The young child will take cues on trust and behavior toward the nurse from the parents, and engaging their support is certainly important. The parents' acceptance of the nurse does not ensure acceptance by the child, however. Home care nurses who care for children are usually quite experienced in introducing themselves to infants and children, but it should be emphasized that the child will feel less obliged to respond politely when on home turf than when in a health care facility. Children may resent the nurse's "invasion" of the security of their home, particularly if nurses are linked with memories of painful procedures during a recent hospitalization. It is helpful to plan extra time to spend with the child on the engagement visit. The nurse should anticipate fears based on the child's developmental stage and plan ways to reassure the child about the purpose of the home visits. As always, honesty is essential. If the home visits will occasionally involve a venipuncture or other unpleasant procedure, the child needs to know this in order to best marshal coping defenses. It is best if such procedures can be avoided on the initial visit.

Assessment

Assessment begins with the first visit and continues throughout the nurse's involvement with the family. Unlike assessment in the hospital, which focuses primarily on the child's response to disease, assessment in the home is equally concerned with the *environ-*

ment in which this response takes place. The first task in assessment within the home is to clarify the perceptions of the nurse and family regarding home care.

Clarification of perceptions can be accomplished by using the same criteria that were used by the hospital-based nurse in the initial step of the nursing process: trust, information, resources, and guidance and support. As the nurse gathers data on the feelings of the child and family, these criteria will ensure discussion of the meaning of the illness, the degree of confidence in the ability to implement the plan of treatment, the degree of confidence in involved health care professionals, the adequacy of resources, and the access to guidance and support. Assessment continues throughout the home care process to document changes in these baseline criteria as changes occur in the child's condition.

The perceptions of the child must not be equated with those of the family. Soliciting the child's impressions of the illness and of life within the family and community provides an opportunity for the nurse to correct unfounded fears and identify the child's high-priority problems. For example, Becky's mother may be most concerned about obtaining an inexpensive replacement for the broken nebulizer, whereas Becky's concern about her newly diagnosed cystic fibrosis is that the children in her class won't play with her at recess, because they think they will catch her disease. Because of their own anxiety and concerns, Becky's parents may not always realize Becky's perceptions. The nurse can facilitate family functioning by enhancing family communication.

Ongoing physical assessment of the child is the counterpart to the assessment of environmental factors. The home care nurse must be highly skilled in physical assessment in order to make judgments about the need for medical consultation or changes in the treatment plan. The nurse must be alert for untoward effects of medications, for signs and symptoms of acute secondary illnesses, and for altered growth and development. A great deal of judgment is required to distinguish between a condition that "just bears watching" and one that requires immediate referral.

Intervention

The phase of intervention combines the nurse's delivery of direct care and the supervision of the care given by the family. In both planning and implementation, it is important to realize that the nurse's role in the home is different from the nurse's role in an acute care facility. The major differences are as follows:

1. In the home care setting, the family, not the nurse, is in charge.
2. The nurse functions more often in a consultant role than in a delivery-of-care role in the home care setting.
3. The home care setting changes the focus of care from illness-oriented care to wellness-oriented care.
4. The "client" in home care is the entire family.
5. The nurse's skills of collaboration and coordination are utilized extensively.

Changes in Family Processes

Just as home care marks differences in the role of the nurse, it dictates changes in family roles and family function. Ideally, the home is a place of refuge from larger social pressures, a place where love and support are assured, a place for privacy and for being oneself. Whether the home fulfills such ideal functions, home care can be quite disruptive. The family living room or dining room may become the ill child's bedroom so that constant supervision is made easier. Equipment normally found only in hospitals may buzz and hiss during the day, and the family may be awakened by monitor alarms at night. Mealtimes may be disrupted by the ill child's treatment schedule. Privacy is threatened by the equipment vendor who walks through the house pushing a new oxygen tank on a dolly, and by the visits from the tutor, the physical therapist, the nutritionist, and the nurse. When exhaustion of one or both parents necessitates respite care or a "night nurse," the family boundaries collapse still further. Siblings, who may at first find the changes a novelty, soon wish for their former share of the parents' attention, and behavior problems are common. It is a scenario in which the family may feel an increasing loss of control. For this reason, it is important to remember that the home is the family's domain and that the family must be allowed to remain in charge. The parents must be involved in all decisions, whether those decisions involve changing the schedule for medications or whether they involve only moving the bed across the room. Only the family can determine the emotional price they are willing to pay to keep the ill child at home.

Planning Teaching Sessions

In the role of consultant, the nurse will be evaluating the adequacy of the care given and teaching modifications of care as necessary. It is important to determine *when* the child and parents are ready to learn about additional aspects of the illness or of the treatment plan. At a time when the family is reacting to the stress of a serious or prolonged illness, their coping patterns are likely to involve both emotion-focused and problem-focused behavior (Lazarus & Folkman, 1984). Emotion-focused coping is directed at the feelings evoked by the illness, the recent hospitalization, the physical and emotional discomfort, and the frustration of an altered lifestyle. Emotion-focused coping marks a time at which the distress is felt acutely by the individual and is dealt with by such actions as blaming self and others, by emotional outbursts, by talking about the situation, and by attempts to diminish the emotional effect through distraction or activity. When the individual is in this coping mode, factual information is of limited use.

Problem-focused coping is directed at managing the problem, and since information is necessary for problem-solving, teaching will be best accepted at this time. Problem-focused coping may be distinguished from emotion-focused coping by behaviors that indicate that the person is intent on the problem itself rather than on the feelings it produces. Signs of this focus in the parents and child include a less anxious demeanor, an indicated interest in learning more about the situation, close observation of the nurse's care activities, and client-initiated discussion of possible solutions to a particular aspect of the overall problem.

Treatment methods will need to be adapted to the individual home care setting, to the abilities of the caregivers, and to the family composition (e.g., small children in the home who might play with equipment settings or who might pose an increased infection risk to the ill child). Considerations specific to posthospital care of various illnesses are addressed throughout Unit 7 of this text. (Consult the index for each illness.)

Facilitating Normal Family Function

Whereas the hospital setting is illness-oriented, the home setting focuses on normalization. Meeting the needs of the child and of the family will mean facilitating normal family function. This sounds very wholesome, but nurses occasionally have trouble adjusting to the change in focus. For example, normalization of family activities and inclusion of the ill child may mean hugs from a sister with dirty hands who sneezes in the ill child's face. Although the parent may have little problem with this, it will elicit a reflex shudder in many nurses. The goals of treatment, if carefully assessed, often allow such "normalization," but the key will be the ability of the nurse to be flexible and open-minded and to consider the ill child's mental and spiritual health as well as physical health.

The fact that the client in the home care setting is the entire family makes this one of the most demanding roles in nursing. It is one thing to give lip service to family involvement in a more traditional setting and quite another to feel responsible for facilitating the holistic health of a family in their home during a health care crisis of one of the family members. Family assessment is essential to determine in what areas functioning is adaptive and where help is needed (see Chapter 2 for a discussion of family assessment and intervention).

Coordinating Care

Because of the complexity of services involved in the home care setting, someone must fill the role of care coordinator. The outcome criteria established before hospital discharge will help to determine whether the nurse is best suited for this role or whether the parents wish to assume partial or full responsibility. The nurse's collaborative skills will be important even if the parents act as care coordinators. As needs for services become apparent, the nurse is in the best position to suggest involvement of other personnel and to facilitate their smooth entry into the home care support team. If it becomes necessary for the child to be hospitalized again, the home care nurse can facilitate the hospital plan of care by sharing effective home care techniques, such as allowing the child to drink medications from a favorite red cup. *Cooperative action between home care nurses and nurses in the hospital can decrease the stress of hospitalization for the entire family.* It can also help to ensure that developmental exercises that were begun in the home are continued throughout the hospital stay so that the child does not regress unnecessarily.

Termination

Termination is that difficult, but necessary, part of the nurse-family relationship in which home visits and telephone contacts are gradually discontinued. Termination occurs when the child's condition no longer warrants professional involvement in the home, either because of death or improvement in health status or because the family is ready to assume full responsibility for the treatment plan.

The child and family should be prepared for termination at the outset of the relationship (Lenihan, 1985). During the engagement stage, the boundaries for home care involvement should be discussed in relation to the goals of treatment. This early preparation will help prevent feelings of abandonment when the support of the home care team must be terminated.

Ironically, the more successful the relationship has been, the more difficult it will be to end it. If home visits have occurred for a period of months, the termination phase may find the family at a stage in which community support resources are less available. As extended family and friends become less attentive to the family's needs, reliance on the home care nurse increases. It is important, therefore, that assessment be ongoing to help the family increase and diversify its sources of support, avoiding total dependence on the home care nurse.

The child and family should be encouraged to express their feelings about the termination of services. Feelings of sadness should be acknowledged as normal and appropriate. Family members should know that their feelings of insecurity are a common reaction to termination and should be reminded of their growth in skills and of their bonds with ongoing sources of care in the physician's office or clinic. If the relationship was therapeutic, the sadness that may occur with termination is offset by the growth that has been experienced by both the family and the nurse as a result of the interactions.

Evaluation

This final component is actually integral to each of the other components of the nursing process. Evaluation is made during assessment and analysis, is provided when desired outcomes are determined, and is an essential part of intervention techniques. The danger is that certain aspects of evaluation become so natural to many nurses that other parts of evaluation can be forgotten. For effective evaluation, the progress toward desired outcomes (client goals) must be determined. If the evaluation criteria have not been met, one must ask why. Was the initial outcome, or any part of it, unrealistic or based on inaccurate assessment data? Were the strategies used to meet the goal ineffective? If the evaluation criteria were partially met, then what, if anything, needs to be done to ensure continued progress toward the desired goal? If the criteria have been fully met, which goal replaces this one in priority?

The need for effective and timely evaluation must not be underestimated. A care plan that is appropriate this week may be ineffective next week because of changes in the child's status or in the environment. The parents and nurse should discuss the adequacy of the current plan of care at each home visit, and changes should be made accordingly. For example, a child with an inoperable tumor may be discharged to home care with the understanding that pain will be controlled by oral medications and that ambulation is permitted as tolerated. A few weeks later, this same child may be experiencing pain despite increased dosages of pain medications and may now be bedridden because of weakness and vertigo. The family, at this point, could be experiencing reduced assistance from family and community support systems, might be noticing maladaptive behavior from siblings, and might be physically and emotionally unable to manage the child's care in light of the present symptoms. If the plan of care has not been revised to accommodate the changes in the child's condition, the family's position may be, "we tried it and it didn't work." The resulting frustration will undermine the family's personal sense of competence and adequacy and will complicate their future relationships with health care professionals.

Types of Home Care

The nursing process in home care will be greatly influenced by the reason for home care. The types of home care for children can be grouped into three categories: acute, chronic, and terminal.

Acute Conditions

Care that is needed only on a short-term basis can be labeled *acute home care*. This type of care might be appropriate for a neonate undergoing home phototherapy for hyperbilirubinemia or for a child requiring one or two follow-up visits after outpatient surgery.

One type of acute home care that is becoming more prevalent is perinatal home care. The perinatal home care specialist visits mothers and their neonates who have been discharged as early as 6 hours after an uncomplicated delivery. Follow-up visits occur in the home for an average of 3 days following dismissal. The mother's postpartum status is assessed and the baby is weighed and receives a physical examination. The nurse takes care to reinforce parent-infant bonding and effective parenting practices. There is an opportunity to discuss the family's adjustment to the newcomer, including infant sleep patterns and the parents' ability to get needed rest. The parents are often asked to keep a log of the infant's sleep times, feedings, and diapers. This chart is then reviewed by the nurse and discussed with the parents so that their concerns may be addressed.

Perinatal home care can be a very rewarding nursing practice. The nurse has the opportunity to affect the remainder of the parent-child relationship positively by helping the family to get off to a good start. The home setting can be optimal for teaching, and parents of newborn infants are usually anxious to learn how to best care for their baby. Learning is facilitated in this setting because parents are less anxious in their own home, and because they have had the opportunity to anticipate the visit and to prepare questions. Learning is also enhanced by the immediate "need to know." In the hospital, when there are nurses readily available to assist with the infant's care, the full weight of parental responsibility may not be as apparent. After the family members are home with their baby, they are usually very receptive to suggestions that will facilitate the necessary adjustments.

The perinatal home care specialist may also be involved in home visits to help parents work through the grief process when an infant dies at birth. Professional intervention at this time can greatly facilitate the necessary outpouring of emotion and can provide the information needed for problem solving and grief resolution.

Chronic Conditions

This category is most accurately divided into short-term and long-term care. *Short-term care* is used to meet acute care needs in families with chronically ill children. Short-term care may also be thought of as care during the interim adjustment period between hospital-based professional management of the condition and home-based family management. A common example is the infant who is discharged from an intensive care nursery with oxygen-dependent bronchopulmonary dysplasia. Short-term home care may be instituted to ensure the family's adjustment to the baby's oxygen dependency and will be terminated as soon as the family can manage the condition with occasional clinic visits.

Long-term care for a chronically ill child occurs when the family will need continuing support to maintain home care. Children who are multiply handicapped or who are ventilator-dependent usually require home care on a long-term basis, including some in-home direct care by a home health aide or registered nurse. The cost-effectiveness of long-term care is reflected in a report from the Children's Home Health Network of Illinois. It showed that even with home care provided by a registered nurse, the cost to manage the care of a ventilator-dependent child at home was 77 per cent less than for hospital management (Kahn, 1984).

Long-term home care for chronically ill children is often the family's only alternative to long-term institutionalization. There are obvious advantages to the child in being able to accept a role within the family and to have the opportunity for development within an optimal environment. The family itself will realize both advantages and disadvantages of long-term care. The disruption of family life and the intense physical and emotional demands experienced have been previously discussed. For many families these problems are offset by the opportunity to complete the family circle and to participate fully in the child's life.

Terminal Conditions

The goal in home care for terminally ill children is to enhance the quality of life for the child and to give the family an opportunity to share their love and grief with the child in the privacy and comfort of the home setting. The Martinson (1977) model continues to provide a prototype for this kind of home care. The parents are supported in their efforts to provide pain control and physical comfort for the child, and open communication between the child and other family members is encouraged. Sometimes, the parents will need to maintain a central venous catheter or peripheral IV site, but, often, care at this stage is devoid of the trappings of modern science. The focus instead is on the psychosocial adjustment to impending death and grief.

Termination of home care for terminally ill children occurs not at the child's death, but after the involved home care professionals have attended the funeral and provided follow-up visits to ensure that family members either are attaining a healthy adjustment or are referred for further professional support.

The role of the home care nurse in terminal care or hospice care is extremely demanding. Watters (1986) observed that "hospice is an area of work in which good will, compassion, common sense, and honesty are highly valued" (p 222). The reward of this type of nursing is knowing that the therapeutic relationship has met some very special needs—that it has provided a loving atmosphere for the child during the last days of life and precious memories for the family.

Types of Agencies Delivering Service

The acute, chronic, and terminal care of the child are delivered through a variety of different types of agencies, as referred to at the beginning of this chapter. The nurse needs to have an understanding of what each encompasses in order for appropriate discharge planning to occur.

The term "certified home health agency" refers to an agency that meets the minimal standards for home care agencies as developed and enforced by the federal government. The standards are set forth in the form of conditions of participation. Annually, the agency undergoes a surprise survey conducted by the federal government to assure compliance with these guidelines. If an agency is certified, it gives them the privilege of accepting Medicare and Medicaid patients. Other insurance companies have now adopted the certified agency conditions of participation as their minimal criteria as well, which allows the agency to serve all patients. The deciding factor as to what patients are served by these agencies is found in the condition of participation that outlines the admission criteria. The criteria state that the care delivered must be intermittent skilled care that is physician-directed to homebound patients and that is reasonable and necessary to treatment of the diagnosed condition. Therefore, children who can be served by the home care staff coming in and performing skilled care on a visit basis (a visit being up to 2 hours) can qualify for service. Care can be delivered by a registered nurse, physical therapist, occupational therapist, speech therapist, home health aide, or a medical social worker.

The benefit of services being provided through this type of agency is an assurance to the parents that the minimal criteria established for a quality agency have been met. Some of these include, but are not limited to, employees who have been screened, who have been checked for references, who are free of communicable disease, who have a verified license, and who are oriented and supervised on a regular basis by in-services designed to keep their skills updated. Patient/family rights are described, as well as their recourse if they are unhappy with the care. If the normal channels cannot resolve such concerns, then the family can appeal to the state and federal agencies that certify the agency. The family is assured that the agency is established and is involved in the continuity and coordination of care between disciplines. The physician is involved, updated on any changes in the child's condition, and communicated with as to how he or she would like to change the plan of care to cope with the changes.

Agencies that deliver care outside of the admission criteria for the certified home health agency are considered private-duty home care agencies. These agencies are not certified by the federal government. However, states that have a licensure law do survey these agencies annually for adherence to their state minimal criteria for appropriate home care. The admission criteria for these patients usually revolve around hourly care as opposed to care delivered on a visit basis. Therefore, the family could receive care by a registered nurse, licensed practical nurse, or home health aide on a shift basis. This type of agency provides the same benefits to parents as consumers as does the certified agency discussed earlier.

The third type of agency to deliver home care services is the registry. This is often likened to an employment agency, and, in the states that have laws covering employment agencies, one will find registries listed. This type of service is not licensed under home health; therefore, it is rare to find any of the previously discussed minimal criteria met. The agency usually keeps a listing of registered nurses, licensed practical nurses, and home health aides and provides interviews for the family to select payment of either the agency or the professional directly for the services rendered. Some agencies conduct routine hiring practices, but others maintain a list to choose from. These employees are not usually supervised, nor are they asked to attend regular in-service training to keep their skills current. The one benefit, however, to parents is that registry services are less expensive because the type of business is not regulated. Therefore, if the parents have reached their maximum on their insurance or do not have coverage and must pay "out of pocket," a registry may be the best alternative.

Future of Home Health Care for Children

Home care for all segments of the population is expected to grow in response to the social demands for cost-effective, quality care (Coleman & Smith, 1984; Hansen, 1986). Continued growth is expected, as well, in the market for pediatric home care (Punch, 1985). The home care explosion implies an expanded role for nursing and for many allied health professionals. Hansen (1986) has predicted that, as home health care becomes recognized as a specialty, salaries will be adjusted upward. Nursing education will soon respond with increased emphasis in undergraduate areas on adaptation of technical skills to home care settings, and master's and doctoral degrees in home health care will begin to be offered. Computerization, which is currently being piloted in many community health agencies, will simplify documentation and record keeping. Technology will spawn not only increasingly sophisticated equipment for home use but also more support services for its maintenance.

The challenge to home care agencies will be their ability to temper the business aspect of home care with the noble profession of caring for people. Pediatric home care today is looked on by agencies that predominantly service adults as a means of diversifying into an aspect of the business that is less dependent on government funding. The caution, however, is not to assume that pediatric home care is the same as adult home care. Yes, the foundation and framework are the same; however, there are four key areas of difference that, if not given their due attention, will cause an agency to fail. These differences are as follows:

1. *The Focus of Care.* In adult care the focus of the intervention is on administering the procedure to the patient and teaching the patient herself or himself so as to increase her or his own level of independent functioning. In pediatric home care, the staff administers procedures to the patient as well, but the focus of the teaching is on the caregiver to deliver the appropriate care to the child. Identifying this caregiver and teaching and supporting this person, at times, is the greatest challenge.

2. *Increased Need and Use of Medical Social Services.* The child's medical condition places a tremendous amount of stress on the family unit. Most families need help in integrating their child's special health requirements with the regular functioning of the family unit, the care of their other children, or other obligations. Families also experience a period of mourning the loss of their dreams and expectations for the normal child they do not have. They must be allowed this time and assisted through their adjustment period. Approximately 90 per cent of the families served through a pediatric home health agency require social service intervention. This figure is much higher than for agencies that service adult populations.

3. *Increased Need of Support Services.* There is an increased need for specially trained home health aides and volunteers who not only deal with the child's personal care needs but should also maximize psychologic and social development. Many children with chronic health problems will be well enough to become productive members of society. Without normalization of their experiences during their formative years, children who have long-term handicaps may develop social and even cognitive deficits that may impair their functioning in later life.

4. *Medical Liability.* The final feature that distinguishes the home care needs of children from their adult counterparts is their medical liability. Children get sick very quickly, and there is less margin for error in their care compared with that of adults. They are also less able to communicate complaints to their caregivers. Situations of medical liability related to failure to recognize changes in condition or consequences of treatment errors are more likely to occur.

The impact of these differences on the process and outcome for agencies delivering services to children is significant. Staff members caring for these children must have pediatric experience. To ask a nurse whose caseload is 95 per cent elderly to occasionally care for a medically fragile child is very difficult. The diagnoses, care needs, medications, and doses are very different. The chance of error can increase significantly if the professional is not used to caring for children. Orientation and in-services must be geared toward the staff's differing role. Staff members are not caring or teaching an adult to take on the responsibility to care for themselves but are caring for the children and teaching their caregivers to deliver the service. They are not there to take on the role of the parents, but to enhance and augment the parents' ability to care for a medically fragile child who is dependent on them to make difficult choices about their welfare and management. This may be a difficult role for staff members who have been taught to "do" and who may feel they are the only ones who can do it well.

Therefore, it is imperative that the home care program that has chosen to take on medically fragile children has a dedicated pediatric staff to care for them. To provide quality pediatric home care within a full-service agency is costly. The challenge to do it well is being made at a time of cost-containment in health care and depleting professional resources. However, it also comes at a time when the pediatric home care field is characterized by burgeoning enthusiasm among parents, professionals, payers, and vendors. The future question is how best to approach the goal of designing and implementing programs to accommodate individual situations, meet community needs, and maintain or improve the quality of care and life. The future of pediatric home care revolves around three concerns:

1. *Concern over the professional role of nurses as teachers, not just caregivers.* At no time should we as nurses make parents dependent on the system to prolong our role as caregivers to our own economic advantage. Compounded by the short supply of pediatric home care nurses, we should be redefining the emphasis of our care. The family is a ready-made support system to carry out much of their child's personal care and can assume much more through the guidance and training of the professional. Parents have been verbal in their need to assume more responsibility because they perceive that this training and guidance give them a means of controlling their lives and the parade of people and machines that invade it. There will be times when this teaching will make the difference between a child staying at home and being readmitted to the hospital.

2. *Research and quality assurance.* We have very few data about the real intangible but important aspects of home care—its effect on outcomes and on the growth and development of families coping with sick children at home. Pediatric home care needs standards of care and appropriate outcome criteria to measure the quality of service provided.

3. *The nurse's role as advocate for parents, child, and professionals.* Home care must not become a one-way street. It is not appropriate for all. It may be appropriate at one time in a child's life and not at another. Home care loses its meaning when it loses the utmost respect for the sometimes fragile home environment and for the family members' constant negotiation and re-evaluation of what is best for them. Eagerness to search for good solutions within the circumstances of daily life in each family without making parents feel guilty must stand at the center of home care programs (Maurano, 1989).

Home care staff must take the lead in facilitating and permitting families and children this negotiating power. Once decisions are made, they must assist and support families in relating their decisions to physicians and third party payers.

There is one part of the future of home health care that will remain the same—the basic needs of the children and families involved. Whatever the technologic advances that the future may hold, the effectiveness of home care will still depend on the nurse who understands the effect of illness on children and families, and who is prepared to support them in their adjustment.

KEY CONCEPTS

Concepts Related to Basic Information

- Pediatric home care is in a period of rapid change because of (1) increasing numbers of children with chronic health problems and (2) changing social and political demands on the health care system, particularly those relating to cost containment.

Concepts Related to Nursing Assessment

- Assessment of children and families begins in the hospital as their readiness for home care is evaluated.
- Assessment in the home includes careful assessment of the environment.

Concepts Related to Nursing Intervention

- Many of the intervention functions of the nurse may be delegated to families. The nurses' role then becomes one of educating and monitoring parental implementation.
- Case management and coordination of care become increasingly important functions when the child is cared for at home.

REFERENCES

Bergman, A. B., Shrand, M. B., & Oppe, T. E. (1984). A pediatric home care program in London—Ten years' experience. *Pediatrics, 73*(6), 314–320.

Cherryholmes, L. G. (1986). The qualities of a home health care nurse. In S. Stuart-Siddall (Ed.). *Home health care nursing* (pp 155–162). Rockville, MD: Aspen Systems.

Coleman, J. R., & Smith, D. S. (1984). DRGs and growth of home health care. *Nursing Economics, 2,* 391–395.

Davis, J. H., & Eyer, J. (1984). Sorting out new mothers' learning priorities on home visits. *Home Healthcare Nurse, 2,* 38–42.

Delaney, B., & Aquilina, D. (1992). Case management. *Employee Benefits Journal, 12*(1), 2–8.

Elkins, J. L. (1986). Nursing the patient and family in their own environment. In S. Stuart-Siddall (Ed.). *Home health care nursing* (pp 179–188). Rockville, MD: Aspen Systems.

Farrell, M. P., & Schmitt, M. H. (1979). The American family: An historical perspective. In D. P. Hymovich & M. U. Barnard (Eds.). *Family Health Care* (Vol 1, pp 57–74). New York: McGraw-Hill.

Goldberg, A. (1985). Home care for the ventilator-dependent person in England and France. *Caring Magazine, 5,* 34–36.

Hansen, J. W. (1986). Future trends in home health care. In S. Stuart-Siddall (Ed.). *Home health care nursing* (pp 255–270). Rockville, MD: Aspen Systems.

Hillman, S. M. (1986). Assessing the patient in the home environment. In S. Stuart-Siddall (Ed.). *Home health care nursing* (pp 163–177). Rockville, MD: Aspen Systems.

Hymovich, D. P. (1976). Parents of sick children: Their needs and tasks. *Pediatric Nursing, 2,* 9–13.

Janz, K. C., & Burgess, B. (1985). Home health care. *Stanford Nurse, 7,* 9.

Joint Commission Accreditation for Hospital and Related Organizations (1993). *Accreditation manual for home care.* New York: Author.

Kahn, L. (1984). Ventilator-dependent children heading home. *Hospitals, 58,* 54–55.

Kaufman, J., & Hardy-Ribakow, D. (1988, August). Home care: A model of a comprehensive approach for technology-assisted chronically ill children. *Journal of Pediatric Nursing, 2,* 244–249.

Lazarus, R. S., & Folkman, S. (1984). *Stress, appraisal, and coping.* New York: Springer.

Lenihan, S. (1985). The young child and the home health care nurse: Problems, challenges, and intervention strategies. *Home Healthcare Nurse, 3,* 6–9.

Martinson, I. M., et al. (1977). Home care for the child. *American Journal of Nursing, 77,* 1815–1817.

Maurano, L. (1989). Pediatric home care: Past, present, and future. *Journal of Home Health Care Practice, 2*(1), 7–14.

Mundinger, M. O. (1983). *Home care controversy.* Rockville, MD: Aspen Systems.

Pierce, P. M., & Friedman, S. A. (1983). The REACH project: An innovative health delivery model for medically dependent children. *Children's Health Care, 12,* 86–89.

Punch, L. (1985). Pediatric home care expands as new technology is developed. *Modern Healthcare, 15,* 152, 154.

Rogatz, P. Home health care: Some social and economic considerations. *Home Healthcare Nurse, 3,* 38–43.

Stuart-Siddall, S. (1984). What is a home health care nurse? *Home Healthcare Nurse, 2,* 1.

Watters, P. S. (1986). Hospice nursing. In S. Stuart-Siddall (Ed.). *Home health care nursing* (pp 215–223). Rockville, MD: Aspen Systems.

Wright, L. W., & Leahy, M. (1984). *Nurses and families: A guide to family assessment and intervention.* Philadelphia: FA Davis.

BIBLIOGRAPHY

Betz, C. L. (1985). The pediatric patient: Strategies for improving interactions. *Home Healthcare Nurse, 3,* 11–17.

Edwardson, S. R. (1984). Using research in practice: Factors associated with the adoption of a nursing innovation. *Western Journal of Nursing, 6,* 141–143.

Fergusson, J., & Hobbie, W. (1985). Home visits for the child with cancer. *Nursing Clinics of North America, 20,* 109–115.

Home care for children with serious handicapping conditions (1984, May). Proceedings of a conference sponsored by the Association for the Care of Children's Health and the Division of Maternal and Child Health, Public Health Service, US Department of Health and Human Services, Houston, Texas.

Kaufman, J. (1991). An overview of public sector financing for pediatric home care: Part 1. *Pediatric Nursing, 17*(3), 280–281.

Kaufman, J. (1991). An overview of public sector financing for pediatric home care: Part 2. *Pediatric Nursing, 17*(4), 380–381.

Klug, R. M. (1992). Selecting a home care agency. *Pediatric Nursing, 18,* 504–506.

Ness, P. L., & Huchala, B. (1987). Adaptation of the community to children with chronic illnesses and their families. In M. H. Rose & R. B. Thomas (Eds.). *Children with chronic conditions: Nursing in a family and community context.* Orlando, FL: Grune & Stratton.

No huge profit potential seen in home care. (1984). *Hospitals, 58,* 70.

Norris-Berkemeyer, S., & Hutchins, K. H. (1986, July/August). Home apnea monitoring. *Pediatric Nursing, 12,* 259–262.

Reif, L. (1984). Making dollars and sense of home health policy. *Nursing Economics, 2,* 382–389.

Rossen, S. (1984). Adapting discharge planning to prospective pricing. *Hospitals, 58,* 71–79.

Shamansky, S. L., Boase, J. C., & Horn, B. M. (1984). Discharge planning: Yesterday, today, and tomorrow. *Home Healthcare Nurse, 2,* 14–20.

Smith, J. B. (1987, March). Home care is more than Medicare regs. *American Journal of Nursing,* 305–306.

Stein, R. (1985). Home care: A challenging opportunity. *Children's Health Care, 14*(2), 90–95.

Stein, R., & Jessop, D. J. (1984). Does pediatric home care make a difference for children with chronic illness? Findings from a pediatric ambulatory treatment study. *Pediatrics, 73*(6), 845–853.

Wildblood, R. A., & Strezo, P. L. (1987, January/February). The how-to's of home IV therapy. *Pediatric Nursing, 13,* 42–46, 68.

CHAPTER • 23

Principles and Skills Adapted to the Care of Children

Mabel Hunsberger

NURSING PROCESS PLAN

NPP: Perioperative Nursing Care, Table 23–7

RELATED TOPICS

Communication, Chapter 11
Physical assessment and history taking techniques, Chapter 13
Promoting Safety, Chapter 15
Use of play, Chapter 17
Nursing Care During Hospitalization, Chapter 21
Nursing Management of Pain in Children, Chapter 25
Fluid and electrolyte balance, Chapter 26

LEARNING OBJECTIVES

- **Discuss the nurse's responsibilities for ensuring the legal and ethical rights of children in circumstances requiring informed consent and assent for research.**
- **Identify assessment criteria for evaluation of patient education needs that facilitate parental and child participation in the learning process.**
- **Write nursing diagnostic statements and describe age-related strategies for teaching children and families.**
- **Identify potential safety hazards for children in health care settings and describe the nurse's role in protecting children from environmental injury.**
- **Describe age-related hygienic care for children and discuss strategies to promote child and family participation.**
- **Identify age-appropriate nursing strategies for accurate assessment of vital signs and specimen collection from children.**
- **Describe commonly used restraint procedures for children and discuss strategies to prevent associated problems.**
- **Discuss nursing care of children who require isolation.**
- **Describe universal precautions.**

- Describe the pathophysiology and management of fever in children.
- Develop an age-appropriate nursing process plan for the child undergoing a surgical procedure.
- Discuss the anesthetic management of children.

Children's needs differ from those of adults under most circumstances but especially during health care encounters. Everything a nurse does in health care is adapted according to the unique physical, intellectual, emotional, and social developmental levels of each child to ease the child's and family's experience and to promote their well-being.

An individualized approach fosters trust and cooperation from a child who does not understand the goals of care and from parents who need to be understood. The purpose of this chapter is to discuss adaptation of nursing care in specific circumstances, including

- Informed consent/assent.
- Performance of selected procedures.
- Care of children during illness.
  - When a child needs restraints.
  - When a child is placed in isolation.
  - When a child has a fever.
  - When a child requires surgery.

Informed Consent

Informed consent implies that a person has freely agreed to a specific intervention with full knowledge of (1) potential risks and benefits of the intervention, (2) consequences of intervention or nonintervention, and (3) alternative interventions. Children may not comprehend explanations of what is to be done to them or why, leaving them both *uninformed* and *unable to consent*. However, children's participation does not need to be total; it may involve selected aspects and should increase as competencies develop (Deatrick et al, 1990). For children age 7 years or older who are developmentally capable, *assent* should be obtained. Assent means that children are informed about an intervention and that they agree with the decisions made by parents or guardians. Adolescents around the age of 15 years usually have the competence to voluntarily consent to treatment (Greydanus & Patel, 1991).

Procedures and situations requiring informed consent vary according to institutional policies. Any procedure with an element of risk and all major and minor operations generally require the signing of a special form that documents informed consent. Common examples of diagnostic procedures are bronchoscopy, lumbar puncture, bone marrow aspiration, and needle biopsy. Examples of therapies are investigational drug use, blood transfusion, and radiation therapy. In some institutions, consents are also required to place a child into restraints. Other events requiring consent on the behalf of children include taking photographs, conducting research, releasing patient information, and performing postmortem examinations. Although the value of having minors participate in health care decisions is acknowledged by many health care professionals, existing hospital policies do not encourage their participation except for the purpose of research studies (Deatrick et al, 1990).

Although it is the physician's responsibility to inform the child and parents or guardians, the nurse may be responsible for requesting and witnessing the signature. Any query about the procedure to be performed should be directed to the physician responsible for the procedure. A nurse's signature on a consent form acknowledges the witnessing of a signature only, and does not represent accountability for the content of the explanation given by the physician.

Consent for Treatment

Parents or legal guardians are entrusted with the authority to give informed consent for their children who are minors. As long as the parents or legal guardians are available and the decision to be made does not involve legal and ethical dilemmas, informed consent is easily obtained. Clarification of informed consent in exceptional circumstances follows.

Mature and Emancipated Minors

States and provinces vary in their designated age of majority and definitions of emancipation. Generally, a boy or girl is considered an adult on reaching the 18th birthday, but laws vary and change over time. In many jurisdictions, provision exists for a minor to obtain treatment without parental consent under certain circumstances; such a child is classified not as an emancipated minor but rather as a "mature minor." The age is designated by the state or province and is usually set at 15 or 16 years; a policy that recognizes the rights of mature minors is a recommended undertaking for institutions (Hogue, 1989). Treatment as a mature minor may include emergency care and areas involving private and personal issues, such as contraception, drug and alcohol abuse, sexually transmitted diseases, sexual abuse, and care during pregnancy. Treatment with respect to abortion is affected by abortion laws.

An "emancipated minor" is an individual who is below the age of majority but whose life circumstances are recognized by law to set her or him free from the restrictions of childhood. Life circumstances that may qualify a minor to become emancipated include pregnancy, marriage, graduation from high school, independent living arrangements, and military service.

State or provincial laws designating mature minors and emancipated minors should be familiar to the nurse in pediatric practice.

Emergency Care When Parents (or Legal Guardian) Are Unavailable

Emergency care of minors in the absence of parents or legal guardian is handled in a variety of ways. Every attempt is made to reach the parents or legal guardian to obtain consent in person or by telephone. A second nurse can listen in on another telephone to verify such verbal consent. When all efforts to reach the parents or legal guardian fail, a search is made for grandparents or other relatives to give permission for treatment. School officials, baby sitters, and social workers cannot give permission for treatment without written authority from a parent or legal guardian to do so.

If the caretaker has no written permission, parents cannot be reached, and no relatives can be located, the health care team then has the legal right to proceed with treatment in the event of a life-threatening situation. When situations are not life-threatening, the search is continued for the parents or legal guardian, grandparents, or other relative to authorize treatment.

Consent from Divorced Parents

In situations of divorce, problems may arise concerning who has the right to give consent. The consent of both parents is generally not required, and either the custodial or the noncustodial parent can give consent.

Consent and Nontreatment

Parents have the right and responsibility to grant informed consent for medical procedures. This does not mean that they have freedom to withhold consent for procedures necessary for the survival of a child, even if the quality of life for the child is doubtful. Since the early 1970s, advancement in scientific knowledge, surgical procedures, and mechanical equipment has enabled children with severe physical problems to survive. The issue of treatment or nontreatment of children is a complex decision making process and involves the child, a team of professionals, and the parents or guardians as well as ethics committees, state or provincial agencies, and, if necessary, the courts.

Consent and Assent for Research

The ethical and legal issues surrounding the rights of children in the research process continue to evolve but, according to one review, remain unresolved (Thurber et al, 1992). A child's parents or guardians have legal authority to give informed consent for research that involves their child. A parent's or guardian's consent does not, however, fulfill a researcher's full obligation to the child.

Official regulations governing research with children issued by the US Department of Health and Human Services (DHHS) state that, in addition to parental permission, children 7 years of age and older must also give their assent to participate in research (US DHHS, 1983). *A child's assent is an expression of willingness to participate in the research after an explanation of the procedures and general purpose of the research has been provided.*

The US DHHS stipulates that children must be given an explanation, in language developmentally appropriate, that describes the study and what they would be expected to do or undergo, before they are asked to consent to the research. Assent is an affirmative agreement as opposed to simply not disagreeing (Lynn, 1986).

Children over the developmental age of 7 years are believed able to understand the basic purpose of the research and what is expected of them and to express a preference about their involvement. However, some researchers are seeking assent from children as young as 4 years of age.

Patient Education

A primary role of the nurse in health care encounters is to prepare and teach children and parents. Patient education is an interactive process that communicates an interest and concern for the client's welfare. In pediatric settings, the form and content of patient education are adapted to involve parents and to facilitate participation of the child at the appropriate developmental level. Both formal and informal teaching should occur. Specific times may be scheduled during which a formal teaching session is held (e.g., teaching cardiopulmonary resuscitation or gavage feeding). In addition, teaching is an informal process whereby the child and family are kept informed about the child's care and are involved in making decisions about care. The informal process is a *continuous and ongoing* interaction that is incorporated into all aspects of care. It is, however, not an incidental, haphazard approach but rather a systematic, goal-directed plan that involves communication and documentation of the process by all those involved in a child's care.

Assessment of Child and Family

The initial step in any teaching situation is to assess the factors that will affect outcomes of the educational process, including learning needs, child and family personal resources, anxiety level of the child and parent, family relationships, lifestyle and cultural patterns, coping styles, and the developmental level of the child.

Learning Needs

A simple but often overlooked task is to find out what the child and family initially know about the topic, to avoid the reteaching of previously learned information. This provides an opportunity to give praise and reinforce the client's correct information. Parents and children are encouraged to identify what they do not understand.

It is particularly useful to ask a child to tell you in his or her own words about an event. If the child uses technical terms, it is important to ask for clarification; some children repeat professional language because they hear it while they have only a vague understanding of its meaning. For example, a child who states "they have to take my blood" may have no concept of how that will be done or how it will feel. Many children fantasize that the procedure involves a much more extensive intrusion than actually occurs, if no true explanation is provided. A child may think "taking blood" involves going for an operation and having an IV line inserted.

In many instances, it is important to speak to the parent or to the child alone. Parents often have fears that they do not wish to discuss with the child present, yet they may not seek such clarification unless a private session is offered. It is most important that such conversations are held without the child's knowledge, so she or he does not fear that something more serious is happening. Similarly, preadolescents and adolescents appreciate being given the chance to speak to the health professional in private.

The nurse can also recognize learning needs by assessing behavior. Watching the child's and parents' facial expressions as they explain what they know can also reveal underlying fears and uncertainties. Recognizing an incongruity between what a person says and what she or he appears to be feeling is an important clue. Children cannot necessarily express their fears but demonstrate their need instead by *not* playing, *not* talking, or *not* eating.

Child and Family Personal Resources

When assessing the client's resources, three categories of human learning are taken into consideration: (1) cognitive; (2) psychomotor; and (3) affective (attitude) (Bloom, 1956). All are relevant to patient education. The three questions to be asked are

- Does the parent or child have the intellectual capacity to learn the relevant information?
- Does the parent or child have the physical capabilities to perform the task or procedure? (It is possible to understand how to perform an activity yet be unable to perform it.)
- Is the parent or child ready and motivated to perform the task? Is the parent or child responsible and accountable?

Assessment of these capabilities is an ongoing process. If outcomes are not being achieved, the nurse reassesses the client's resources and determines whether increased confidence-building is required or whether alternative approaches are needed.

Anxiety Level of Child and Parent

The nurse's perception of the severity of an illness may be a poor indicator of the degree of parental anxiety. Individuals respond differently to similar situations. A painful procedure, even though a momentary event, may produce an enormous amount of upset for some children and parents.

It should also be recognized that the parents of an injured, sick, or upset child usually feel distressed. Extremely anxious parents and children do not hear what is explained. Readiness and motivation to learn are blocked if fears and concerns distract an individual from listening. For example, parents being taught to insert a gavage tube may be distracted by the fear that the procedure is causing pain to their child; a child who is being taught how to inject insulin may be anxious about too much blood running out of the body. These concerns must be addressed before learning can take place.

Anxiety may be expressed through avoidance, forgetting, and not paying attention. Parents and children should be given the opportunity to express verbally how they feel about the learning situation. Children may not be able to describe their anxious feelings but can be encouraged to tell a story, draw a picture, or engage in a sentence-completion activity. Also, more specific tools have been developed to measure anxiety. Because fear, anxiety, and pain are interrelated feelings, assessment tools actually measure a variety of emotions. See Chapter 18 for an in-depth discussion of stress and coping and Chapter 25 for pain assessment. Some resolution of stress and pain is often necessary before education is begun.

Family Relationships

A healthy relationship between the parent and the child is an asset to learning. Children who feel supported by their parents have the freedom to express feelings of concern and will seek explanations. Parents who can encourage their children to participate in their own care are an asset to the children's adaptation.

A trusting relationship among family members also facilitates the learning process. Children need to know what will happen, and they need to have confidence that they are being told the truth. These established patterns of communication between child and parent are assessed when parental involvement in the care of the children is planned. For example, it may be necessary first to support the parents and help them cope with telling their child unpleasant information, rather than simply asking parents to tell a child unpleasant news. The nurse can role-play how to teach a child and can engage the parent in the teaching process.

Lifestyle and Cultural Patterns

The lifestyle of individuals sets the parameters within which new behaviors and responsibilities can be performed. In assessing parents and children with respect to teaching, it becomes particularly important to consider the amount of time available, the economic resources, and the feasibility of the new behavior. For example, in teaching parents how to provide a balanced meal with dietary restrictions (such as for children with diabetes), fast foods may have to be included if both parents work; guidance concerning childrearing and the discipline of children must take into account cultural beliefs and customs. It is ineffective to impart knowledge and instruct clients to adapt behaviors that are inconsistent with their lifestyle and beliefs. Breastfeeding, weaning, and toilet training are examples of issues that have cultural components.

Coping Styles

Individual differences in response to health care procedures must be taken into account when teaching strategies are planned. Some children as well as adults may benefit from detailed information that assists them to actively cope by *approaching* a situation. Others choose to cope by using an *avoidance* tactic and may feel overwhelmed and anxious in response to specific information. It is important to assess these differences to determine the most beneficial approach for teaching a particular child and family. Assessment of coping styles of families is presented in Chapter 12 and of children in Chapter 18.

Developmental Level of Child

The child's level of development in the three categories of human learning (cognitive, psychomotor, and affective) determines the content, timing, and method of education used with children. The cognitive abilities that particularly affect the child's understanding include extent of language development, concept of time, understanding of cause-and-effect relationships, and reasoning and abstracting ability. Psychomotor abilities that affect the child learner in particular are gross and fine motor development, eye-hand coordination, and organizational skills. Finally, the child's feeling state (affective) largely contributes to how much can be learned. Developmental characteristics of children are summarized in Table 23-1.

Nursing Diagnostic Statements

The nurse makes individual diagnostic statements appropriate for each child and family encountered. The nurse's effectiveness as a teacher is influenced by an understanding of the child's knowledge deficit, the child's coping skills, and the impact of the illness on the family. Nursing diagnostic statements relevant to the teaching situation include:

Ineffective individual coping, *related to*

- *Separation from family and home associated with hospitalization.*
- *Limited coping skills associated with egocentric thinking, magical thinking, and inability to abstract.*
- *Knowledge deficit.*

Altered family processes, *related to*

- *Disruption in family routines associated with care of ill child.*
- *Change in family roles associated with health care needs of ill child.*
- *Child's discomfort associated with child's illness.*
- *Knowledge deficit.*

Because knowledge deficit is not a human response, it is used here as the *related factor* in the nursing diagnostic statement rather than as the *response*. The ultimate objective of the nurse, when patient/parent teaching is used as an intervention, is to resolve a problematic response that is *caused by* or

TABLE 23-1
Educational Strategies According to Age of Child

Developmental Characteristics of Child	Educational Strategies
Infant (0–12 Mos)	
Unable to understand explanations but is sensitive to gentleness of voice, touch, and movement; infant can anticipate what will occur by physical signs (e.g., preparation of equipment, certain sounds associated with an activity)	Main focus is to teach parents and caregiver
	Tone of voice and gentle handling communicate support to infant; prepare equipment and proceed with the activity as quickly as possible to reduce the amount of anticipated distress
	Talk to and touch infant before beginning a procedure
Familiarity is a source of comfort	Provide infant with favorite toy as soon as preparation begins
Stranger anxiety occurs at 6–8 mos of age	Spend time with child before beginning a procedure or new activity; involve parent in activity
Toddler (1–3 Yrs)	
Separation from parents is primary threat	Encourage presence of parents for stressful events
Egocentric thinking	Careful explanations of reasons for events should be provided
View of world is that events are related to self	Machines and equipment should be described according to what they do and the sounds they make
Has developed limited coping skills, and ability to express emotions and feelings is limited	Use play as a method of expression; tell child it is OK to cry
Fantasizes about what will happen and why things are as they are	Use simple words child can understand; encourage expression of thoughts through doll and puppet play and verbal expression (e.g., "How does your puppet feel about. . . . ?")
Attention span short but can be increased with inclusion of sensory experiences	Teaching sessions must be short (5–10 mins) and should include equipment to touch and explore or a visual aid such as a book
Language skills limited	May interpret words literally; therefore, careful choice of simple words and short sentences is necessary
Concept of time is limited	Explanations should be given just before a procedure of short duration, such as an injection; if the procedure or event is more involved, the child should be told 2–3 hrs before it occurs
Preschooler (3–6 Yrs)	
Egocentric thinking continues	Explain why things are as they are; repeat such explanations to reduce potential for child feeling she or he has *caused* the situation
Magical thinking continues	Children should be asked to "repeat back" their perception and understanding of what has been told to them
	Reduce misconceptions by avoiding threatening words, such as "cut"; instead, say "make an opening"
Coping behaviors continue to be limited	Encourage presence of parents for stressful events
Fears of body mutilation peak at this age	Give clear explanations about which body parts will and will not be affected (be clear about *how* it will be affected); feelings can be expressed through doll play, with demonstration of the procedure (i.e., where is the tube, the bandage, or the opening)
Ability to understand how body works increases	Use visual aids of body models or picture outlines to enhance teaching; use correct anatomic terms
Attention span is increasing	Continue to provide information in short sessions (10–15 mins)
	Involve child in the teaching sessions by doing something (e.g., handling equipment, drawing, or demonstrating on a doll)
Has increased verbal skills and questions "why" (questioning is child's way to learn about the events and people in the environment)	Provide opportunity for child to phrase questions; take the time to encourage further expression of questions, then provide information in a simple, clear response; questions at this age do not require long, complicated answers

TABLE 23-1
Educational Strategies According to Age of Child ***(Continued)***

Developmental Characteristics of Child	Educational Strategies
Understands concrete explanations—only what he or she sees and touches	Actual equipment or miniature forms of equipment give child an understanding of environment
Intreprets words literally	Some words used in health care are confusing (e.g., "take your vital signs" and "take your pulse"); it is better to explain *what* you will do (e.g., "listen to your heart")
Inability to conceptualize effect of event	Explain about the sensations that will be experienced
School-Age Child (6–12 Yrs)	
Mastery becomes important at this age; is eager to learn and accomplish new skills and increase understanding of environment; has also acquired more skills, such as reading and verbal expression of ideas	Can use more books that teach the information through drawings, coloring books, and a variety of pencil and paper activities Encourage child to use language ability now to verbalize fears
Is beginning to have better understanding of causation but still cannot apply logic to abstract problems	Teaching should continue to focus on concrete aspects of the event; clarify misconceptions about causation
Concept of time has improved	Procedural information can be provided a day or two in advance
Attention span	Can pay attention for 30–45 mins if actively involved
Peers are important support	Can hold educational sessions with groups of children who have similar problems
Increased neuromuscular development	Child can now perform skills that involve manipulation of equipment
Now more interested in self-management	Parents are still required for support but child can be given more responsibility and in many instances can be given information separate from parents; children at this age may express some fears more freely to the health professional than to parents
Continues to view hospitalization as punishment	Continue to reassure and give explanations that reduce child's feelings of being the cause for the situation
Competitive behavior	Devise games that contain content to be learned
Adolescent	
Struggling with identity versus role confusion; trying to answer the question "Who am I?"	Include a clear explanation about how the body is affected by an illness or treatment
Concerned about body image	Anticipate feelings of anger and grief in response to change in body image Assist patient to identify ways to adapt to experienced changes
Peers extremely important	Invite peers with a similar experience to teach an adolescent Education sessions with a group of peers
Independence versus dependence Is struggling with autonomy Wants to be autonomous but still needs some dependence	Give adolescent some control over when teaching sessions will be held, methods of learning that are preferred; encourage collaborative decision making
Able to think abstractly and understand complex language; can verbalize fears	Scientific names (with explanations) can be used to describe illnesses, procedures, and techniques; use diagrams, literature, and pamphlets; encourage verbal expression of fears; explain what symptoms are expected in an illness and when it is necessary to seek further advice
Need for privacy	Explore with adolescent whether he or she wants parents involved in educational sessions; teach parents separately if adolescent prefers
Coping behaviors now well established	Involving the adolescent in planning can facilitate coping; assess adolescent's coping resources and provide opportunity for expression of anxieties; provide information honestly; recognize that regression is common during stress and therefore adapt teaching accordingly; increase amount of teaching according to adolescent's readiness

related to a knowledge deficit. Whenever knowledge deficit is used as a related factor, the area in which knowledge is deficient should be specified. Knowledge deficit can occur for a number of factors. The nursing intervention would be directed to the associated factor. Some of these associated factors include:

- *Cognitive limitations associated with child's developmental level.*
- *Low readiness for reception of information associated with anxiety level (parent and child), short attention span, and limited language skills.*
- *Denial of health care needs associated with threat to the personal self.*

Nursing Care

Children and parents can be motivated to participate in self-care through effective nursing approaches for the age of the child. Interest in health and in learning about one's health problem varies from child to child; but, with individualized approaches, a nurse can be a motivating force for behavior change. Strategies for teaching children at various ages are summarized in Table 23–1.

Patient Safety

Potential dangers to children in the various environments of daily living are addressed in Chapter 15. When a child enters the health care system, she or he is exposed to additional potential dangers because of special equipment and environmental variations. Needles, oxygen, medications, and various types of machinery basic to any medical environment are common dangers. Children's safety may also be jeopardized by their playful spirit. They do not realize the consequences of pretending about their identity. One child may be in another child's bed or may even try to fool the nurse by answering to the wrong name.

Assessment

Each child and family unit is individually assessed to determine how threatening an environment is to this child. One can quickly determine how active and inquisitive a child is by watching him or her explore the environment. A child who is permitted to indiscriminately explore expensive equipment and play with it as if it were a toy or who is allowed to wander away from a parent down a hall in a busy clinic can quickly become injured.

Many situations also need to be assessed for potential dangers. Placing children on carts, chairs, and wagons may put them at risk of falling if they are not appropriately restrained. Although restraints protect children, they also can cause harm if not properly applied. An ongoing discriminating approach concerning the dangers imposed by the health care setting is an important component of a nursing assessment.

Nursing Diagnostic Statements

The specific nursing diagnostic statements vary according to the age of the child, the family circumstances, and the setting. The following apply to most circumstances and health care settings:

High risk for injury; *risk factor: environmental hazards associated with*

- *Inadequate footwear to prevent falls and punctures.*
- *Improper use and placement of sockets and cords.*
- *Inadequate supervision around stairs, elevators, and doors.*
- *Use of unsafe toys and recreational equipment.*
- *Inappropriate supervision during use of faucets and bathtubs.*
- *Inappropriate supervision during meal time.*
- *Inappropriate use of supplies, equipment, and furniture.*

High risk for injury; *risk factors:*

- *Inappropriate choice of vehicle for transport.*
- *Inappropriate or lack of use of safety belt.*
- *Inadequate preparation of child about where he or she is going and what will happen.*

Nursing Care

To ensure a child's safety, the nurse identifies potential hazards in each child's immediate environment. This often involves intervening when other health professionals or parents do not adhere to safety standards. Ensuring a child's safety requires the full cooperation of all individuals involved in the child's care. The nurse also provides important input into decision making groups who set hospital or clinic safety policies.

Environmental Safety

The environment of any health care setting is unfamiliar to the child and family, compared with their home setting; thus, it is more difficult for them to predict what might happen and where dangers lie. The most fundamental environmental safety issue is that a child is correctly identified with a label on the child's bed and an identification band on the child's wrist or ankle. This is done immediately on admission and must be checked routinely thereafter before each nursing and medical activity. In addition, special attention must be given to (1) floors, sockets, and cords; (2) stairs, elevators, and doors; (3) toys and recreational supplies; (4) faucets and bathtubs; (5) eating arrangements and utensils; and (6) furniture, especially cribs. Precautions in these areas affect

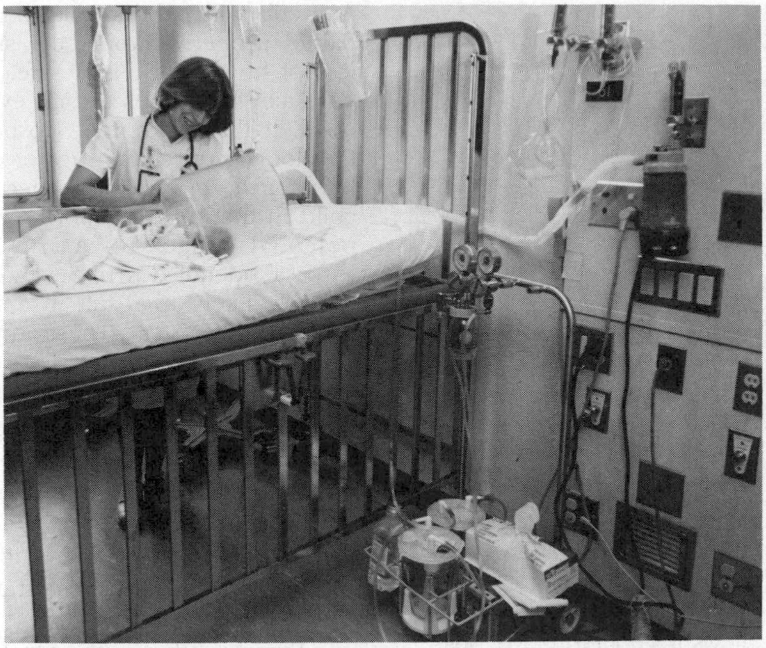

FIGURE 23-1. The wheels of cribs must be locked and the crib placed a sufficient distance from electrical outlets to prevent young children from poking objects into sockets. (Note: The crib side is in the down position for the photograph *only*.)

safety regarding the child's mobility, play and recreational activities, and activities of daily living.

The mobility of children in hospitals is to be encouraged and should not introduce unnecessary dangers. Floors should be free of clutter; they should be clean and not slippery. A highly polished, waxed floor is inappropriate for a children's unit. Children should not be allowed to walk around in bare feet or socks. Properly fitting disposable slippers or skid-free shoes from home should be worn. Slick-soled shoes can be made safe by placing a wide strip of tape along the sole. Children should be instructed to walk, not run, in corridors, and they should never be allowed to be mobile with objects on a stick (e.g., lollipops and popsicles) in their mouths.

Numerous electrical cords and sockets are necessary in most health care settings. Cribs need to be placed so that children cannot reach sockets and appliances (Fig. 23–1). Young children out of bed must be supervised to protect them from falling over cords.

In most hospitals, children may leave the unit for short periods to go to the gift shop or snack bar, if they are attended by a family member or hospital personnel; in many institutions, a sign-out board is used. On the unit, children must be protected from wandering into dangerous areas, such as treatment rooms, stairwells, and elevators. A lock placed at the upper corner of a door permits adults to enter but keeps children safe.

Safe toys and recreational equipment are basic to the care of all children. Toys and equipment must be maintained and properly cleaned and safe activities chosen for the age of the child (see Chapter 17 for discussion of age-appropriate toys and activities). Common sources of danger are removable parts that can be swallowed (especially the metal insert on squeak toys), rough and sharp edges, movable parts that readily pinch fingers, and toys and equipment that are too advanced for the child's age. Balloons are a particular threat to children because of the potential for aspiration of small fragments; many hospitals have policies that do not allow balloons to be left at the bedside unattended.

Daily care needs of the child in the hospital are the same as at home, but the unfamiliar environment may introduce additional dangers. A young child who knows which faucet is hot and which is cold at home may inadvertently turn on the hot water in the hospital. Older children who are relatively independent at home may need more supervision in the hospital because of differences in the height and contour of the tub and the placement of faucets.

Mealtime requires supervision to protect children from unfamiliar dangers. For example, some hospital kitchens use metal covers that are hot and must be removed before the meal is served. Also, a child may not be accustomed to the size of the fork or cup that is used in the hospital or may inadvertently be served food that is not age-appropriate, causing her or him to choke.

One of the greatest dangers to a child anywhere involves use of hazardous supplies, equipment, or furniture. Special precautions must be taken to avoid leaving any small objects in a child's bed. Offenses that are easy to commit are leaving plastic needle caps or small caps that cover IV tubing in a child's

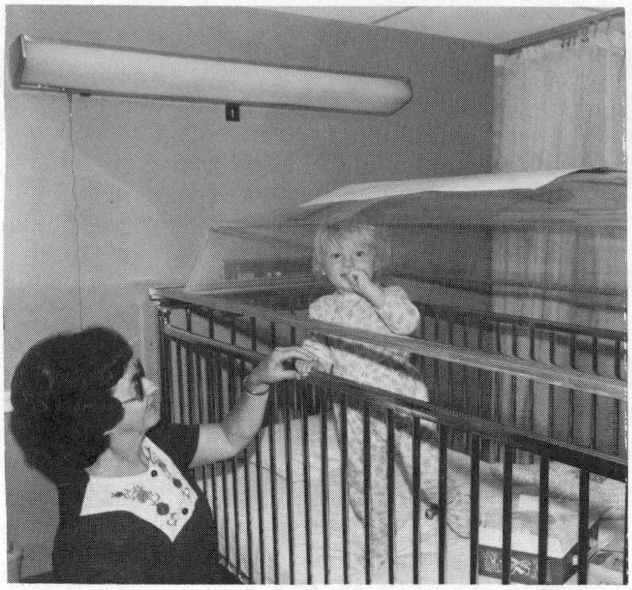

FIGURE 23 - 2. An enclosed, see-through crib keeps the toddler safe from falls but allows freedom to move. Note the large poster lying across the top of the crib to provide an interesting view for the toddler lying in the crib.

bed. A child's bed must be examined often to ensure that no dangerous pieces of equipment have inadvertently been left. Cribs must be in good repair and should be used appropriately. For example, depending on the age and size of a child, an enclosed crib (Fig. 23–2), with or without pads around its edges, may be necessary to prevent falls and injuries. These decisions are made by the nurse and require immediate attention on admission of a child to the unit. Any crib with a broken latch must immediately be repaired properly; taping the siderail in place, regardless of how firmly, is unsafe.

Falls from cribs are an even greater threat in the hospital than at home. Hospital cribs are high, and the floors rarely have rugs or carpeting to cushion the fall. Furthermore, many people who attend to the child in the crib may not be particularly familiar with potential dangers of a crib and may inadvertently leave a siderail down. Several situations that are particularly likely to result in a fall require special caution and reminders. These include:

- Infants who unexpectedly roll over.
- When a mist tent is on the bed, giving the illusion that the child cannot roll out.
- Small infants strapped into infant chairs that could tip over.
- Children who are restrained but manage to free themselves from the restraint.

Except while giving care, the nurse must insist that at all times siderails must remain up all the way.

A basic principle that must be adhered to with *all* individuals who care for children in isolettes and cribs is to keep one hand *always* securely on the child. If one's back is turned to reach for something, one hand must be firmly gripping the child to avoid a fall (Fig. 23–3). Falls from cribs are disastrous, and the nurse must rigidly adhere to these basic safety rules and ensure that parents do the same.

Another aspect of care that requires strict safety adherence is the use of highchairs. A child in a highchair should be restrained, the wheels on a chair should be locked, and the child should not be able

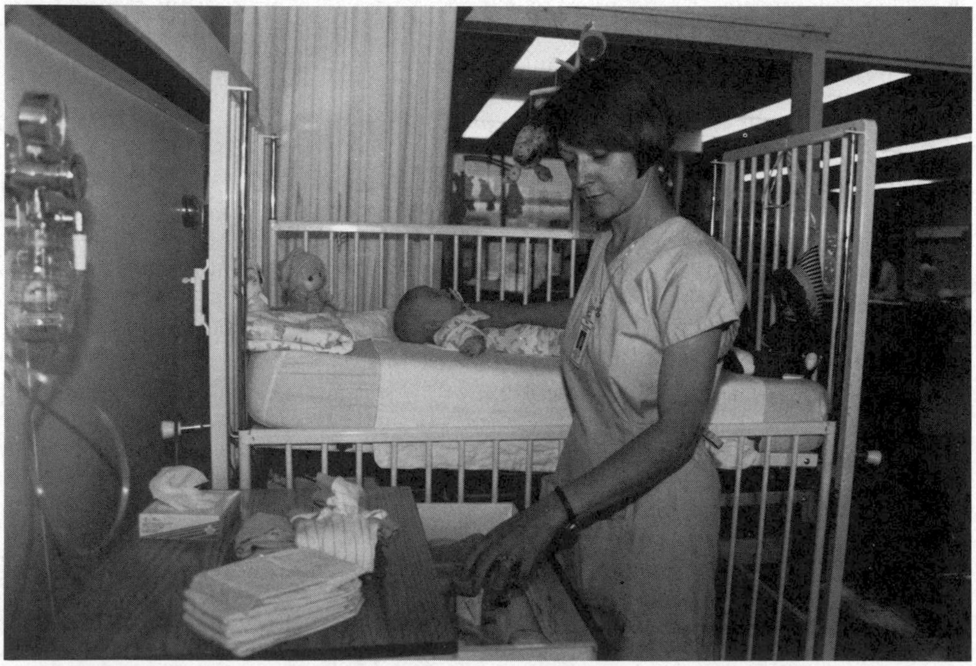

FIGURE 23 - 3. Accidents happen quickly. *Always keep one hand firmly on the child.*

to reach the wall or furniture. If these precautions are not adhered to, a child can pull on or push off from a sturdy object until the chair tips and falls. Active children can even rock themselves from side to side in a chair until it tips; restraints, regardless of how secure, are not foolproof.

Children in highchairs should be attended at all times, even if they are restrained. Even though chairs are constructed not to tip, and restraints are placed securely, it is too great a risk to leave the child unattended.

Furniture should be sturdy, and child-sized tables and chairs should be available for playing and eating. Dangerous supplies, such as electrical equipment, medications, soaps and shampoos, needles, razors, and scissors, must be appropriately stored. Rooms and cupboards where such articles are stored should be locked.

Transportation of Children

The hospitalized child frequently must be transported to another unit of the hospital for diagnostic or therapeutic procedures. An infant should not be carried to another part of the hospital by hospital personnel or by parents because of the potential to slip and fall. Appropriate ways to transport infants are by crib, baby carriage, or stroller. Older children can be transported in their bed or by stretchers, wheelchairs, wagons, or specially made carts that allow a semi-Fowler position. In any transport, the child must be securely belted for safety and be accompanied. Children on monitors and those who have been sedated for a procedure should be accompanied by a nurse, or someone of equal competence, during transport.

The same safety precautions used in transporting adults apply to children. Of particular importance is ensuring that the child is adequately identified, that the IV chamber will not run dry while the child is away from the unit, and that the child will be attended while waiting in another department. *Children may even manipulate the IV flow-rate regulator out of curiosity and seriously endanger themselves.* Careful monitoring of the IV line is always important, but especially during transport because of the additional hazards.

Children will be less resistive to procedures if they are prepared for the event. Thus, an indirect way to maintain the child's physical safety is to prepare him or her psychologically before the actual move. The type of preparation varies with the age of the child and coping styles of the child and family, as summarized in Table 23–1.

Bathing and Hygiene

During bath time, the nurse should observe the child's physical and developmental status, encourage appropriate self-care, and teach safety and daily health habits. The child's bath, grooming, and hygiene needs provide opportunities for parents to participate. It is an excellent time to assist parents with concerns about their child's health. For the older child, it is a time to exercise some control over her or his own body; for the younger child, bath time can be an enjoyable and sensual playtime.

Assessment

Decisions about how to bathe an infant or a child and whether a bath is needed are approached with various goals in mind. The child's safety, with respect to age and physical condition, largely determines whether a tub bath, shower, or bed bath is given. The nurse also assesses how to involve the parents in a way that benefits both child and family.

Nursing Diagnostic Statements

Nursing diagnostic statements related to the bathing and hygiene care of infants and children include:

***Self-care deficit: bathing and hygiene**, related to*
- *Child's physical level of development.*
- *Parents' unfamiliarity with hospital routine.*
- *Child's knowledge deficit regarding procedure.*
- *Child's fears in unfamiliar environment.*

***High risk for suffocation**; risk factors:*
- *Lack of safety precautions by caregiver during bathing of an infant/child.*
- *Leaving infant/child unattended in bath tub.*

***High risk for injury; trauma**, risk factor: excessive temperature of bath water associated with*
- *Caregiver's knowledge deficit regarding how to test water temperature.*
- *Lack of supervision by an adult during infant's/child's bath.*

***High risk for impaired skin integrity**; risk factor: child's physical condition associated with*
- *Restraint.*
- *Hyperthermia.*
- *Immobility.*
- *Excretions and secretions.*
- *Humidity.*
- *Fragility of skin.*
- *Immunologic immaturity.*

Nursing Care

The child's hospital bath routine should be as similar as possible to the home bath routine. Adhering as closely as possible to the home rituals of bathing and other routines may help minimize the trauma of hospitalization. Unless contraindicated by a child's physical condition, tubs and showers are used in the hospital. For infants, an infant tub is commonly used at the bedside.

Parents should be allowed to provide as much of the child's care as they choose to do. Because parents frequently are unsure of their role in the hospital or are reluctant to participate because of the child's physical condition, they need assistance from the nurse to understand any bathing restrictions. Parents must be given a choice about their involvement. It is important to recognize that parents need a break—hospitalization and the care of a sick child may be stressful to parents. When parents take on the responsibility of bathing and hygiene, the nurse is still responsible for the safety of these activities and must ensure that appropriate measures are taken to avoid slipping, scalding, falling, or drowning of the child in the tub. This sometimes means that if parents do not observe the necessary safety measures, the nurse must intervene to ensure the child's safety.

As with all procedures, the initial task is to gather all the necessary equipment before beginning, both for efficiency and to ensure that the child is not left unattended. The bath temperature should be about 37.8° to 40.6° C (100° to 105° F), although checking the water with a thermometer is usually not necessary. The water can be tested for comfort against the wrist or inner aspect of forearm, or older children can check the water themselves before getting into the tub.

Infants are usually bathed in a small infant tub at the bedside. *Soapy, wet infants are very slippery;* therefore, the bottom of the tub can be lined with a towel to avoid injury. For those infants unable to sit, the nurse should keep a secure grip on the baby throughout the bath. One hand grasps the infant's arm while the wrist and lower arm support the infant's head. The other hand is then free to bathe the infant (Fig. 23–4).

The eyes should be wiped with a clean washcloth, or cotton ball, without soap, working from the inner canthus outward. The auricle and external canal of the ears are washed with soapy water and a washcloth. Do not use cotton swabs (i.e., sticks with cotton tips) because this may impact the cerumen and could possibly damage the tympanic membrane or canal. To clean the female genitalia, separate the labia and gently wipe from front to back. For washing the genitalia of an uncircumcised boy, current practice is not to retract the foreskin. Retraction of the foreskin can cause tearing, with eventual scarring and phimosis. This is especially true for infants and toddlers, when retraction is impossible without damage.

The amount of supervision required for an older child varies. Many preschool- and school-age children are baffled by taking a bath in bed and usually require some instruction and explanation. To them, it is a strange request to wash themselves in bed, and, if left to their own devices, they may do a minimal job.

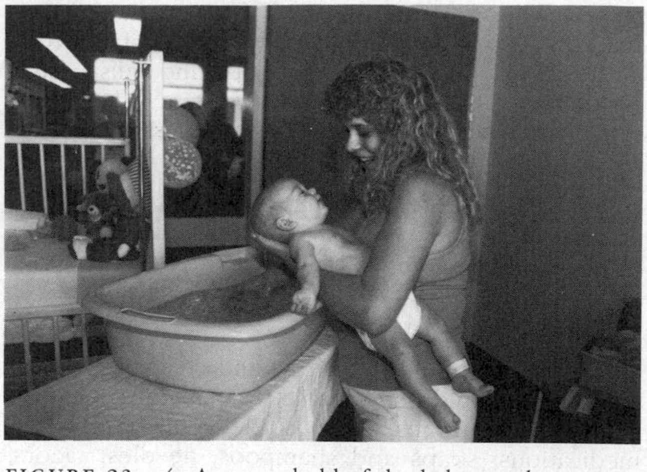

FIGURE 23-4. A secure hold of the baby can be accomplished by supporting the head and shoulders with one hand and firmly holding the baby against the caregiver's hip (football hold). The other hand is then free to wash the baby's hair.

Parents can often help supervise when the child's embarrassment makes it awkward for the nurse to check on the child's performance in bathing and hygiene.

Bubble bath products and other additives are frequently requested by children. These are contraindicated for use by children with frequent urinary tract or vaginal infections. At the first sign of skin irritation, the use of these products should be discontinued. There is routinely no need for creams or powders after a bath. A lotion is occasionally applied to dry skin, or a medicated lotion is ordered for specific dermatologic conditions.

Care of the teeth is an area of health care that is frequently neglected while children are in the hospital. If a toothbrush is not provided by the hospital, the nurse should ask the parents to bring one to the hospital for their child. Toothbrushing is an activity that some children do without reminding, but it too is an activity that requires the nurse's supervision and monitoring. It provides an excellent opportunity for nurses to teach preventive care in an important area of health.

Mouth care for children involves primarily toothbrushing, unless mouth ulcers develop. A soft sponge toothbrush is available in most hospitals and can be used if no toothbrush is available or when toothbrushing is contraindicated by the child's physical condition (e.g., low platelet count or mouth ulcers). Mouthwashes can be used in school-age children, but the child must be clearly told not to swallow the solution. Lemon glycerin swabs are composed of an alcohol, which dries the mouth, and lemon, which may be painful if the mucosa is already irritated. Neutropenic children should have their oral mucosa checked daily because of their proneness for developing mouth ulcers.

Hair care is an important comfort measure to include. An infant's head is washed as part of the daily bath. Older children may resist a hair wash; however, for any child who is hospitalized or confined to bed longer than 2 or 3 days, hair care is important. As much as possible, the technique used to wash and care for the child's hair should be similar to the one used at home. If a hair wash is impossible, then dry shampooing should be considered.

Children who have thick, coarse, or very curly hair need particular attention because this hair type mats and tangles easily, which may cause breakage. Before matted hair is shampooed, the tangles should be removed as much as possible. To do this, use a wide-toothed comb and work on a small section at a time. Beginning at the ends of the hair, gently fluff and lift the hair. Repeat this step each time, inserting the comb farther into the hair. Pulling on the scalp is painful; *be gentle*. Application of a lubricant (Dermassage, mineral oil, or commercial hair preparations) to the hair may help disentangle it and help prevent breakage if the hair is dry. This process may have to be done in several sittings, because it is uncomfortable and difficult for a child to remain still long enough for the entire head of hair to be finished. Braiding the child's hair may prevent further tangles, but care must be taken not to braid too tightly. *When special care is required, parents should be consulted and their assistance encouraged.*

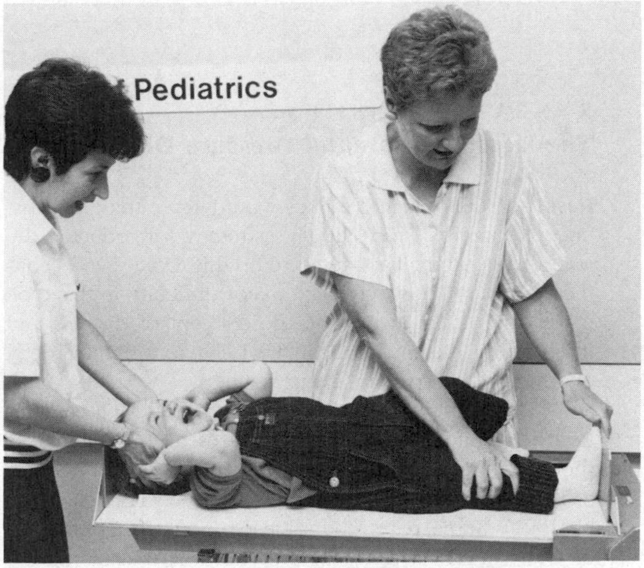

FIGURE 23-5. Such a seemingly simple procedure as measuring a toddler's length is resisted vigorously in spite of a prior explanation.

Care of Children During Specific Procedures

Nurses consider many procedures they do to be common, routine, nonthreatening events. However, for a child, having blood pressure or temperature checked may evoke anxiety and upset if the child is not prepared and supported. Procedures often involve removal of clothing, restriction of movement, and pain or discomfort. These intrusions are particularly feared by young children, who misinterpret the extent of what might occur. Thus, a child should be prepared for the event before a procedure is begun, regardless of how common and nonthreatening it may seem to the nurse (Fig. 23–5).

Proper positioning and effective restraint avoid injury to the child and shorten the procedure. One cannot generally assume that a child will hold still without some assistance. The nurse's grip must be firm but not painful to the child. The torso and arms of the nurse can be used to block the child's movement. However, care must be taken to avoid pressure from fingertips, injury to internal organs from leaning on the child, and respiratory embarrassment from occluding the airway. The goal of nursing intervention is to attain the maximal therapeutic benefit with the least amount of disruption to the child and the family.

Procedures should be done in the treatment room rather than at the child's bedside; thus, trauma is not observed by other children, and needles and equipment are not inadvertently left at a child's bedside. In the child's mind, the bed should be a place that is safe and comfortable. Parents are often invited to stay with children for traumatic procedures, but practice on this issue varies considerably.

The unique developmental needs of children dictate precautions that must be taken and serve as a guide for determining how to approach and teach the child. Many procedures need to be altered in terms of size of equipment and approach to the patient. Numerous procedures are specific to the care of children (such as the attaching of a urinary collection bag and applying a mummy restraint).

The child's illness and therapeutic regimen largely determine the procedures the child will undergo. Specific procedures are described in the chapter in which a particular illness is discussed (Chapters 32 to 47). Procedures required by most children regardless of illness include the assessment of vital signs, collection of specimens, and administration of medications and IV therapy. Medication administration and IV therapy are discussed in Chapters 24 and 26, respectively. The stress caused by procedures is a component of the stress of hospitalization and is presented in Chapter 21. Following is a discussion of the nurse's responsibility in assessment of vital signs and collection of specimens.

Assessment of Vital Signs

Children are fascinated by medical equipment; cooperation can often be gained by letting a child touch and briefly use equipment on a doll or stuffed animal. It is especially important to take the time to fa-

RESEARCH ISSUES
The Impact of Parental Presence During Procedures

Results: Most pediatric nurses would agree that the presence of parents is an effective strategy for reducing the stress of children. The literature on this topic reveals conflicting results, however. The major difficulty in this type of research is in measuring the concept of distress and interpreting the meaning of the behaviors exhibited by children when parents are present.

Those in support of this practice believe that separation of a child from parents at a stressful time increases the child's distress; others believe that parents might be too anxious and increase the child's stress (Bauchner, et al, 1991). Some researchers have reported that children of more anxious mothers are more distressed during painful procedures (Jay et al, 1983) and during anesthesia induction (Bevan, 1990). On the other hand, the presence of parents has also been reported to relieve the anxiety of children (Gauderer et al, 1989).

Relationships between the parents' and child's behavior have been studied by Broome and Endsley (1989). They found that parental behavior ranging from negative to positive was not related to the degree of the child's distress. The meaning of how a child responds to parental presence or absence is difficult to interpret. In response to brief medical procedures (injection and venipuncture), children displayed substantially more negative, distressed behaviors, that is, more crying, when parents were present than when they were absent (Gonzalez et al, 1989; Shaw & Routh, 1982). It has been hypothesized that the display of more distress by children when parents are present may indicate that the child is trying to elicit the comfort of a parent by exhibiting distress or that the parent's presence "disinhibits the expressions of the child's emotional arousal" (Gonzalez et al, 1989). One cannot, therefore, make the conclusion that a child who cries and resists more is necessarily feeling more upset; such a child may actually feel more secure, whereas a quiet child may feel more frightened. Of interest in this regard is that, when children are asked whether they want their parents to be with them, the majority indicate that they do (Gonzalez et al, 1989; Weekes & Savedra, 1988).

The relationship of the parents' behaviors to the child's distress has also been studied. In a study of 70 children ages 3 to 10 years undergoing outpatient venipuncture, it was discovered that the timing of the parents' explanations has an impact on the degree of distress experienced by children. Children who were distressed at the outset of the procedure were receptive to their parents' explanations. There was, however, also an inflammatory effect. It was hypothesized that (1) some children may respond negatively to procedure-related explanations, regardless of when they are offered, because of the child's particular coping style or that (2) an explanation offered to a nondistressed child at the beginning of a procedure may disrupt the child's successful coping efforts (Jacobson et al, 1990).

Implications: The request from children, when asked, for parents to stay with them during procedures is strong evidence in support of continuing the practice of parents being present during procedures. Furthermore, the meaning of a child's distress behavior is not understood; it may indicate psychologic comfort rather than discomfort. An important aspect to consider in determining the benefits of having a parent present is the anxiety level of the parent. If a parent is anxious about staying with a child, then additional support needs to be given to the parent. It may be that some children and parents do better if the parent is not present; the nurse should listen to the child's and parents' preferences and give them the needed support to feel successful. In some instances, this may mean that the nurse supports a parent in the decision not to stay with a child and provides extra support for the child.

REFERENCES

Bauchner, H., Waring, C., & Vinci, R. (1991). Parental presence during procedures in an emergency room: Results from 50 observations. *Pediatrics, 87,* 544–548.

Bevan, J. C., Johnston, C., Haig, M. J., et al. (1990). Preoperative parental anxiety predicts behavioural and emotional responses to induction of anaesthesia in children. *Canadian Journal of Anaesthesiology, 37,* 177–182.

Broome, M., & Endsley, R. (1989). Maternal presence, childrearing practices, and children's response to an injection. *Research in Nursing and Health, 12,* 229–235.

Gauderer, M. W. L., Lorig, J. L., & Eastwood, D. W. (1989). Is there a place for parents in the operating room? *Journal of Pediatric Surgery, 24,* 705–707.

Gonzalez, J. C., Routh, D. K., & Saab, P. G. (1989). Effects of parent presence on children's reactions to injections: Behavioral, physiological, and subjective aspects. *Journal of Pediatric Psychology, 14,* 449–462.

Jacobson, P. B., Manne, S. L., Gorfinkle, K., & Schorr, O. (1990). Analysis of child and parent behavior during painful medical procedures. *Health Psychology, 9,* 559–576.

Jay, S. M., Ozolins, M., Elliott, C. H., & Caldwell, S. (1983). Assessment of children's distress during painful medical pro cedures. *Health Psychology, 2,* 133–147.

Shaw, E. G., & Routh, D. K. (1982). Effect of mother presence on children's reaction to aversive procedures. *Journal of Pediatric Psychology, 7,* 33–42.

Weekes, D. P., & Savedra, M. C. (1988). Adolescent cancer; coping with treatment-related pain. *Journal of Pediatric Nursing, 3,* 318–328.

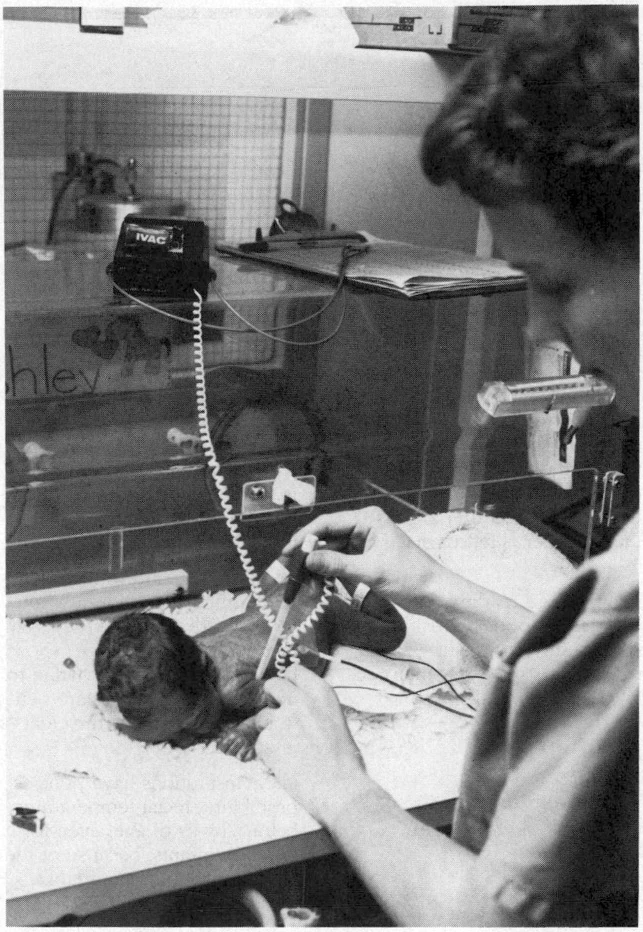

FIGURE 23-6. Use of an electronic thermometer to obtain an axillary temperature eliminates the risk of rectal perforation in the premature infant.

miliarize children with equipment when they first encounter these procedures.

Temperature. Temperature assessment in children has been made much easier, more accurate, and safer with new devices (Fig. 23–6). A summary of the various types of thermometers that are available is presented in Table 23–2. The most common type used in health care settings is the electronic thermometer; however, the glass thermometer may be used because of the cost of newer devices. The major documented disadvantage of the electronic thermometer is its inaccuracy in the measurement of axillary temperatures beyond the neonatal period (Ogren, 1990; Davis, 1993). There is considerable variation in opinion about advantages and disadvantages of thermometers. Descriptions of the glass and electronic thermometers and explanations of their uses by the oral, axillary, and rectal methods are summarized in Table 23–3.

Pulse. In assessing a child's pulse, the rate is considered as well as the rhythm and quality. The pulse should be assessed when the child is quiet; activity or crying increases the rate. For this reason, it is best to check it before beginning any procedures to be done at the same time. Common descriptive terms for quality of the pulse are "thready," "bounding," or "faint."

The apical rather than the peripheral pulse is usually assessed in young children. To do this, palpate the apical pulse (also called point of maximal impulse) and place the diaphragm of the stethoscope on this point (palpation of apical pulse is discussed in Chapter 13). Listen closely, noting the rate, rhythm, and quality of the pulsation. If, on the initial assessment, the pulse is of regular rhythm and appropriate

TABLE 23-2
Description of Thermometers*

Type and Description	Use and Accuracy
Infrared Tympanic Thermometer	
Uses infrared energy radiating from tympanic membrane; the tympanic membrane receives its blood supply from the same vessels that perfuse the hypothalamus, the temperature-regulating center of the brain	The covered probe tip is placed at the external opening of auditory canal; a reading is given in 1 sec; the desirability of this thermometer is still being studied, with some evidence that it is accurate (Newbold, 1991) but not in infants under 3 mos of age (Chamberlain et al, 1991; Muma et al, 1991; Davis, 1993)
Plastic Strip	
A plastic strip that is placed on child's forehead until a color change occurs	Used at home because it is economical and easy to use; not thought to be accurate enough for use professionally; readings tend to be higher than actual temperature (Martyn et al, 1988)
Digital	
A probe connects to a chip that translates reading to a digital display; it can be used for the oral, axillary, and rectal routes	This thermometer is easy to use and accurate; it is more expensive than a glass thermometer, but it is often preferred because of the ease of reading it

* Use of glass (mercury) and electronic thermometers is presented in Table 23–3.

TABLE 23-3
Glass and Electronic Thermometers

	Oral	Axillary	Rectal
Glass Thermometer			
A mercury thermometer that has been used traditionally but is limited in its use with children (see limitations under oral and rectal columns)	Place under the tongue slightly to right or left of midline into sublingual pocket; this site indicates changes in core body temperature; it is left in place 3–7 min with the mouth closed Factors affecting temperature: hot and cold beverages, smoking, open mouth breathing; oxygen by mask may lower temperature, but not significantly An oral temperature cannot be taken with a glass thermometer in infants and young children who cannot hold the thermometer in place or who might bite the thermometer, resulting in injury from broken glass or release of mercury into a child's mouth Some institutions have a specific age restriction (5 or 6 yrs of age) under which an oral temperature by glass thermometer is not permitted; a disoriented or mentally retarded child must also be protected from this danger	Opinion varies as to the accuracy of axillary temperatures; axillary temperatures are less intrusive than rectal temperatures and safer than oral temperatures for young children Disadvantage is length of time it takes to get an accurate reading; thermometer is placed in the axilla against the skin; care must be taken to ensure that the thermometer remains in contact with the skin during the entire procedure; a glass thermometer is left in place for 3–10 mins Temperature reading may be reduced by poor perfusion or increased by a radiant warmer; reading = 0.49°C less than rectal (Haddock et al, 1988)	To take a rectal temperature, the child is positioned on the side, prone or supine with the hips flexed; the supine position is preferred because it allows the caretaker to talk to the child and maintain eye contact, but the most important consideration is that the child is held securely to prevent squirming The thermometer is lubricated with a water-soluble jelly and is then inserted about ½ to 1 inch into the rectum and held in place for 3 to 4 mins Rectal temperatures are contraindicated for children who have severe diarrhea (they may increase stooling), those who have had rectal surgery (due to trauma), children who are neutropenic, and low birthweight infants Many institutions have policies prohibiting rectal temperatures before 6 wks of age, even for full-term infants, because of the danger of puncturing friable rectal mucosa
Electronic Thermometer			
This is a hand-held rechargeable unit that is taken to the bedside to be used; the unit has two probes (rectal has a red end, and oral has a blue end) with disposable covers Patient positioning is similar to that for the use of a glass thermometer Temperature registers within 60 sec, indicated by an audible signal After use, it is necessary to return the device to the storage unit, where it is recharged	Child's mouth can remain open; held in place until beep is heard and reading has stabilized	Accuracy of axillary route has been questioned by some (Muma et al, 1991; Ogren, 1990); held in place until beep is heard and reading has stabilized	Same position as glass thermometer; held in place until beep is heard and reading has stabilized

rate, it is acceptable to listen for 30 seconds and multiply by 2 to determine the beats per minute. An exception to this procedure is when the child has a cardiac problem, in which case auscultation for a full minute is recommended. A digital read-out of pulse is given when electronic devices that employ oscillometry are used (e.g., Dinamap, as for blood pressure measurement).

Respiration. Respiratory rate is assessed by noting the number of inspirations per minute. This is done by counting the respiratory rate through the stethoscope, by placing a hand on the abdomen (palpating), or by observing the abdomen for diaphragmatic breathing. Activity or excitement may cause an increase in the respiratory rate, so this assessment should be done when the child is quiet. In addition to rate, it is important to observe for increased respiratory effort. Indicators of this are retractions (e.g., substernal, intercostal, and supraclavicular), nasal flaring, and use of abdominal muscles to breathe. Respiratory difficulty may cause grunting or wheezing and apprehension. These signs should be noted as signals of distress that may indicate that the child needs prompt attention.

An infant's respirations are frequently irregular and must be counted for a full minute. After infancy, the respiratory rate of a child is obtained by observing chest movement for 30 seconds and multiplying by 2 unless the child has respiratory illness; in this case, auscultation for a full minute is recommended.

Blood Pressure. Blood pressure measurement is done on all children on admission to a hospital. Apprehension can cause the blood pressure reading to be higher than is normal for the child; therefore, every effort should be made to help the child relax. The procedure should be explained and equipment be made available for the child to handle before the procedure is begun.

The most important factor in taking an accurate blood pressure reading is the *size* of the cuff. Cuff size refers to the internal inflatable balloon of the apparatus. The width of the cuff should cover approximately two thirds of the upper arm. When it is wrapped around the child's arm, the internal bladder should be one fifth longer than the circumference of the child's arm. A cuff that is too narrow or too short may result in a falsely high reading, and a too-large cuff may cause a falsely low reading. The right arm is used whenever possible; this is the arm used in the development of standardized charts. The procedure of cuff application and taking of the blood pressure is the same as that for adults.

Blood pressure can be measured directly by inserting a catheter attached to a manometer into an artery. This type of measurement is used in intensive care settings. Blood pressure is more commonly measured by the indirect method using a blood pressure cuff (sphygmomanometer), which has a pressure manometer that operates by displacing air (aneroid) or a mercury column.

Electronic equipment has simplified blood pressure measurement in children. Oscillometry and Doppler techniques are now widely used in hospital settings. In oscillometry, pressure changes are detected and displayed as a digital read-out. A cuff is applied to the limb, and the cuff is pumped up by machine. Digital read-outs are displayed for systolic, diastolic, and mean arterial pressures and pulse. Equipment used to obtain these readings is known as a Dinamap or IVAC. The Doppler is an ultrasound technique that responds to blood movement within the artery to measure systolic blood pressure; it is not reliable for diastolic measurement.

Occasionally, blood pressure cannot be auscultated and electronic equipment is not available. Blood pressure measurement by palpation is an alternative method. The steps in this method are

1. Place the proper size of cuff on the arm.
2. Palpate the brachial pulse and keep fingertips over pulse site with sufficient pressure to feel the pulse but not obliterate it.
3. Inflate the cuff until the pulse is no longer felt.
4. Deflate the cuff until the pulse is again felt.

The point at which the pulse is again felt is the systolic pressure and is recorded as "98/P," indicating the palpation method has been used.

When the upper arm is not accessible, a blood pressure reading can be obtained by placing a cuff on the thigh, calf, or forearm. Sites for measurement and corresponding points for palpation are as follows:

Upper arm	Brachial artery
Lower arm	Radial artery
Thigh	Popliteal artery
Calf	Posterior tibial artery or dorsalis pedis artery.

The procedure is the same as that used to obtain a reading with the upper arm. In infants under 1 year old, the reading is normally the same in the lower and upper extremities. After age 1 year, the systolic reading is normally higher in the lower extremities than in the upper.

Collection of Specimens

Children are frequently unable to cooperate to produce the needed specimen. Young children do not have the cognitive ability to understand instructions and, in many instances, lack the physiologic capability to produce the specimen, such as for sputum collection. Special adaptations are necessary to collect specimens from children in a way that is technically accurate yet produces minimal disruption and frustration in the child. (See Fig. 23–7, which illustrates various collection devices.) Attention must also be given to self-protection, which is achieved through use of gloves and handwashing according to Universal Precautions, discussed later in this chapter.

Specimens, once collected, must be clearly labeled and immediately processed. The nurse should be sure that the correct laboratory slip accompanies the specimen when it is sent to the laboratory.

Collection of Urine Specimens. Urine specimens are collected in various ways, depending on the age of the child and the purpose of the specimen. The major difficulty is the collection of specimens from children who are not toilet trained. Routine urine specimens are collected using a clean plastic urine bag that is applied to the perineum or over the penis (Fig. 23–7*D*); Twenty-four–hour urine specimens require a special collecting bag with tubing. Specimens for culture are collected by using a sterile urine bag. In some instances, either catheterization or suprapubic needle aspiration of urine from the bladder is indicated to collect a specimen for culture.

If contamination by skin does not alter the results of the required tests (e.g., specific gravity), urine can

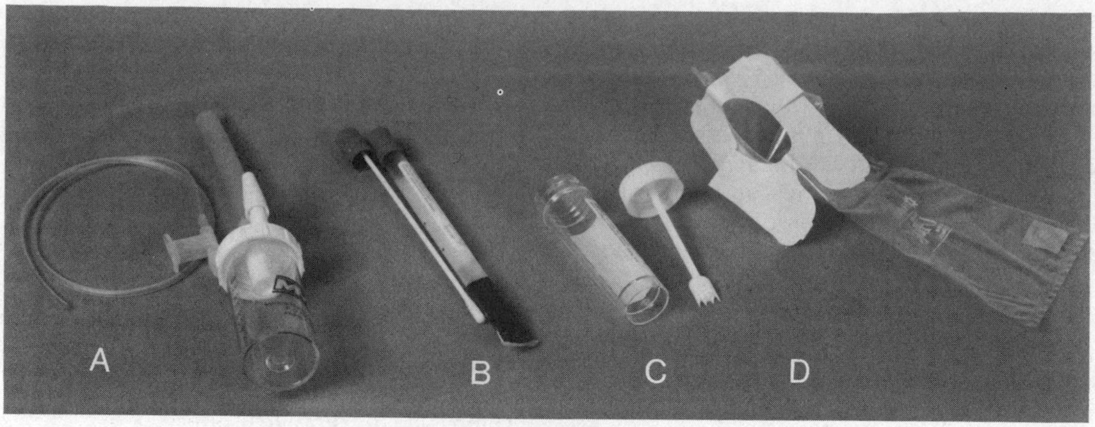

FIGURE 23 - 7. Specimen collection devices. *A*, Collecting device for sputum (also called sputum trap). Has two external openings: 1) is connected to a suction catheter (lying beside mucus trap) and 2) is connected to a wall suction that produces a vacuum in the bottle and draws the specimen into the bottle. *B*, A sterile culture swab. The tip of the swab must be kept sterile and is inserted into dark transport media after culture is taken. *C*, Stool specimen container. A specimen can be lifted with small scoop on tip of swab and inserted into tube. *D*, Urine specimen bag. Application of bag is described in text under "Collection of Urine Specimens."

be squeezed from a diaper or drawn out of a diaper with a syringe from which the needle has been removed (Reams & Deane, 1988), provided the diaper is not exposed to air, heat, or light (Lybrand et al, 1990; Stebor, 1989). The loss of moisture would affect the accuracy of specific gravity measurement. If a disposable diaper is not saturated enough, some of the wettest cotton batting can be extracted (using disposable gloves) from the diaper and squeezed to obtain the urine, or the cotton batting can be placed into the barrel of a 3-ml syringe (without a needle) and the plunger inserted to push out urine from the cotton batting. One drop of urine squeezed from a diaper is sufficient to test specific gravity with a fractometer.

Routine Urine Specimen. A specimen for routine urinalysis is collected from an infant or young child using the following guidelines.

1. Wash hands well, then cleanse the perineum or penis with soap and water; rinse and dry. This should be done before collection of any urine specimen from a child who is not toilet trained.
2. The bag can be applied by use of various techniques. If it is applied from side to side, the paper backing from one side is peeled off and that side of the bag is attached to the skin starting at the bottom and moving upward, followed by the other side. If the bag is applied from bottom to top, the paper backing from the lower half of the bag is removed and the lower portion is secured first, followed by the upper portion. In either method, the single most important factor is that the bag securely adheres to the skin, especially along the lower edge where leakage and contamination are most likely to occur. For girls, the perineum is pulled slightly taut during application of the lower portion of the bag. In young male infants, placing the penis and scrotum inside the bag facilitates a better seal at the lower edge. For older male infants and toddlers, the bag can be applied on top of the scrotum with only the penis inside.
3. Secure a diaper over the bag to prevent loosening of the bag by pulling or kicking.
4. Place the infant or child into a semi-Fowler position to facilitate flow of urine by gravity into the urine bag.
5. Give the usual amount of fluids. Overhydration may produce inaccurate results.
6. Check urine bag frequently (every 20 to 30 minutes) because the weight of the urine in the bag may cause it to loosen. Also, for the most accurate laboratory analysis, urine should be collected as soon as possible after the child has voided.
7. After the child voids, remove the bag gently to avoid skin irritation; then cleanse the area and rediaper the child.
8. When the specimen has been obtained, transfer it to a clean specimen container. Either refrigerate it or deliver it to the laboratory promptly. If a urine specimen cannot be delivered to the laboratory within 1 to 2 hours, it should be refrigerated. A urine specimen that is stored in the refrigerator preferably should not be stored longer than overnight.

Clean-Catch Specimen for Culture. With older children, the collection of a clean-catch or midstream urine specimen is done in a manner similar to that with adults. The major differences are that more supervision is required and that the required supervision may embarrass the child. Although midstream collection has not been shown to significantly reduce contamination rates, compared with nonmidstream techniques (Lohr et al, 1989; Saez-Llorens et al, 1989), it continues to be a common practice.

The nurse should explain the purpose and technique of specimen collection and forewarn the child about the coldness of the cleansing solution. Parents should be invited to accompany the child to collect the specimen if the child so desires; however, preferably the nurse should take responsibility for supervision to ensure that the urine is collected properly.

The perineum is cleansed with an antiseptic solution or soap and water by wiping from front to back along each side of the meatus and directly across the meatus with use of a clean sponge for each wipe. The perineum is then rinsed with sterile water or saline solution and patted dry with a sterile gauze sponge. The area is dried well to remove any remaining antiseptic, which has the potential to slow bacterial growth, giving a false-negative report. After the stream is started, a midstream sample of urine is collected in a sterile container.

Boys are asked to stand in the usual position to void. The meatus and glans penis are cleaned with antiseptic solution or soap and water. If the boy is uncircumcised, the foreskin is retracted slightly to cleanse the meatus and glans penis. The area is then rinsed and patted dry and a midstream urine sample collected. For an uncircumcised boy, care is taken to slide the foreskin to its original position to prevent constriction of the penis.

During specimen collection for urine culture, the open edge of the container used to collect the voided specimen is not to touch the child's skin. The container is immediately closed with a sterile lid, keeping the open edge and inside of the container clean. The specimen should be delivered to the laboratory as soon as possible and must be tested promptly because of the rapidity of bacterial growth. At room temperature, bacteria double every 20 to 30 minutes.

For infants and young children, urine for culture is collected using a sterile urine bag. The perineum or penis is cleansed in the same way as just described for a clean-catch urine specimen, with use of antiseptic solution or soap and water. After the area is thoroughly dry, a sterile urine bag is applied in the same manner as for a routine urine specimen. A sterile urine bag has a small hole on the lower edge to one side of the bag that is covered with a blue tab (Fig. 23–8). To empty the bag, it is held in such a way that the area with the tab is free of urine. After the tab is pulled off, the bag is then tipped into a position that permits drainage of the urine through the small hole that was under the tab. A urine culture requires at least 1 to 2 ml of urine.

Collection of a 24-Hour Urinary Output. For infants and children who do not have bladder control, a special collecting device is used to collect urinary output for a 24-hour period. The plastic urine bag is similar to those used for routine urine collection except that a long drainage tube is connected to one corner of the lower edge of the bag. As the child voids, the urine can be drained via this tube without removing the bag.

The urine bag is applied by the same technique as for routine urine collection, except for the use of

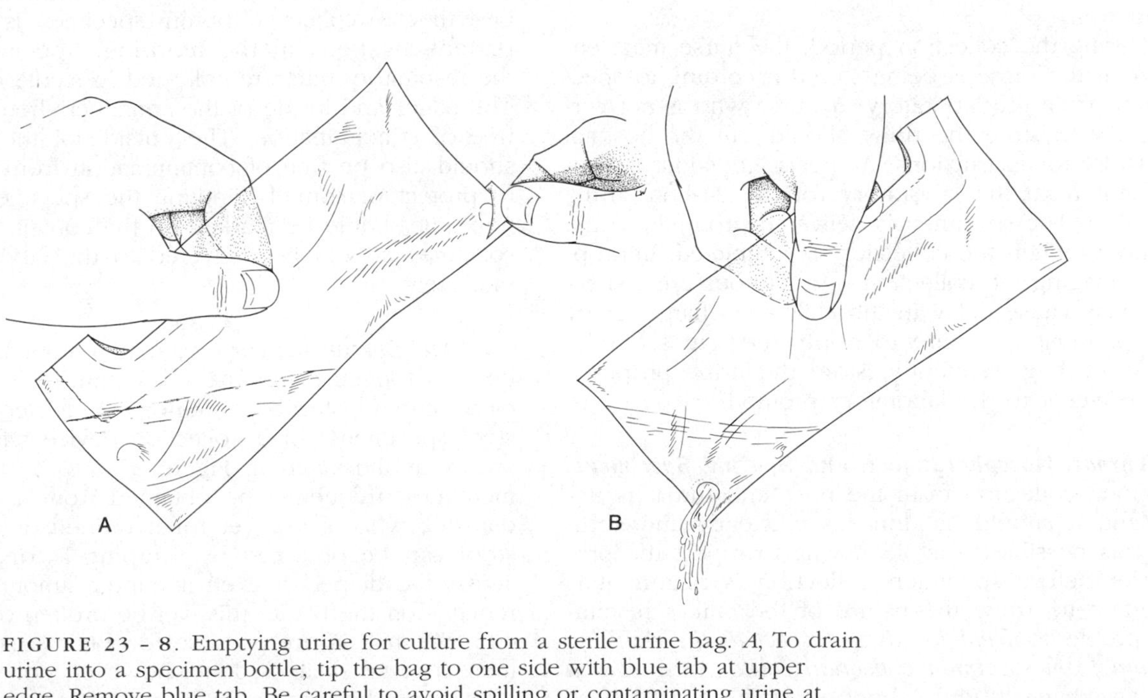

FIGURE 23-8. Emptying urine for culture from a sterile urine bag. *A*, To drain urine into a specimen bottle, tip the bag to one side with blue tab at upper edge. Remove blue tab. Be careful to avoid spilling or contaminating urine at large opening of bag. *B*, Turn bag with exposed small hole at lower edge and pour into sterile container. Apply lid, label, and send to laboratory.

an adhesive skin preparation to form a sticky surface before the bag is applied. The skin preparation is painted with a cotton-tipped applicator onto the area that will come in contact with the sealing edge of the urine bag; the area becomes sticky within a few minutes, providing an adhesive surface for attachment of the urine bag.

It is of prime importance that the bag be securely attached to prevent leakage, contamination, or loss of the entire voiding because loss of specimens interferes with the accuracy of the test. Contamination by stool is one of the most frequently occurring problems and necessitates restarting the 24-hour urine collection.

Achieving collection of a 24-hour urine specimen requires the nurse's attention to careful management of the system. The tube may be connected to a collection device or coiled within the diaper. The tube has a removable cap that is opened periodically to drain the urine from the bag. The bag must be checked and emptied frequently to reduce the likelihood of the bag coming off or of the urine becoming contaminated by stool. Parents can help the nurse decide how frequently the urine bag must be checked because they are generally aware of how frequently their child's diaper needs to be changed.

The nurse is responsible for managing the collection of a 24-hour urine specimen. It is started just after the child has voided. Urine from this first voiding is discarded, but the time of the voiding is recorded as the starting time. For infants, it is more difficult to know the exact time of voiding. A dry diaper is checked frequently until the infant voids. The bag is applied immediately after the wet diaper is noted, and the starting time is recorded when the diaper is found wet.

During the collection period, the nurse must ensure that the urine is being stored according to specification from the laboratory. A nurse who is not certain how to store the urine should call the hospital laboratory for instructions. A special container is usually sent from the laboratory for the 24-hour urine collection. The specimen is delivered promptly to the laboratory when the collection is completed. Improperly managing the collection of a 24-hour urine specimen may cause delay in the child's discharge; every attempt must be made to apply the bag securely, check the bag frequently, store the urine properly, and deliver it to the laboratory promptly.

Throat, Nasopharyngeal, and Sputum Specimens. Specimen collection from the nose and throat is unpleasant. It should be done as efficiently and accurately as possible to avoid having to repeat the procedure. Before specimen collection is begun, it is important to know the nature of the child's respiratory problem; *if epiglottitis is suspected, the resulting trauma from specimen collection could cause edema and airway occlusion.* A brief explanation just before performing a procedure is appropriate for children of all ages.

For obtaining a throat culture, a sterile swab is used. The swab should touch the most inflamed and purulent area, and it should be passed with a rolling motion deep into the throat and across the tonsils without touching the tongue on entry or exit of the mouth. This procedure should stimulate the gag reflex if done properly. If the child cannot cooperate by opening the mouth wide, a tongue depressor should be used to hold the tongue while entering the throat with the swab. The swab is returned to the holder and pushed into the lower chamber, which holds the transport medium (see Fig. 23–7*B*). Transport medium prevents specimens from drying before reaching the laboratory. Equipment varies across institutions but is similar in principle.

For collecting a sputum specimen from children who are too young to cooperate in coughing and expectorating, a device called a "mucus trap" can be used (see Fig. 23–7*A*). The catheter is inserted into the nasopharynx, stimulating a cough reflex. Suction is applied to the other tube by connecting it to a source of suction. A sputum specimen is drawn through the catheter into the mucus chamber (it is not drawn up the tube to which suction is applied). The specimen can be cleared from the catheter into the collection chamber by suctioning an appropriate liquid through the catheter. Normal saline solution can be used to clear the catheter in collecting a specimen for bacterial culture; virology medium is used for virology culture.

When a child can cough up a specimen, the nurse should monitor the activity to avoid getting a specimen that has merely been cleared from the back of the throat. Located within the bronchi and lungs, sputum can be removed only by a deep cough. The best time to collect a sputum specimen is when the patient awakens in the morning. Specimens from the respiratory tract are collected in sterile containers. The edges and inside of the container should be kept free of contamination. The outside of the container should also be free of contamination from secretions to protect personnel handling the specimen. Collection time should be marked on the container, and the specimen should be delivered to the laboratory immediately.

Stool Specimens. For obtaining a stool sample, the tip of a tongue blade is used to transfer stool into a clean cup (a sterile container is not necessary for stool specimens) or a collection device with a small scoop, as illustrated in Figure 23–7*C*. A stool specimen must frequently be obtained from a child with diarrhea who is not yet toilet trained; a sample of stool can be obtained by scraping a tongue blade across the diaper. If even a minute amount of stool remains on the blade, this can be broken off into the cup. When it is not possible to obtain a stool specimen, a rectal swab is done; however, only in shigellosis, gonorrhea, and a few other infections do the organisms live on the rectal walls rather than exclusively in the feces. A rectal swab is done by gently inserting a swab into the rectum and slightly twisting it as it is removed. The swab is inserted approximately as far as when a rectal temperature is taken. Stool specimens and rectal swabs should be sent to the laboratory immediately. Specimens for ova and parasites are placed into a fixating solution.

Blood Specimens. Collection of blood specimens is one of the most commonly performed procedures, but to a child it can be terrifying. Although most blood specimens are obtained by laboratory personnel, nurses should take an active role in supporting the child and reducing the child's fears and suffering. The appearance of the equipment and the thought of having a "hole where blood can come out" can set a child off into a state of extreme panic. Children often begin crying fretfully at the sight of the person in white who draws blood.

Anticipation of having blood drawn causes anxiety when a child in the same room is having blood drawn. Children should be protected from seeing and hearing other children go through the experience of having blood drawn. Young children, in particular, compared with older children, have been reported to be distressed by venipunctures. The use of a topical anesthetic can also reduce the suffering for a child who requires venipuncture. A topical cream, EMLA, has been available in Canada since March 1991 and is placed at the site of the venipuncture 1 to 1½ hours before the puncture. See Chapter 24 for a discussion of the use of EMLA.

Those children who do require a blood test should receive an explanation when approached. For them, the fear that is evoked can be lessened but usually not eliminated. The nurse tells the child it must be done, explains what the child can do to help, and consoles the child before and after the procedure. Giving the child a finger puppet to play with after the procedure can also help to relieve the distress. The nurse should be present, whenever possible, to assist laboratory personnel in restraining the child and to provide explanations and support to the child and parents.

Proper care of the venipuncture site after the procedure includes application of pressure to stop the bleeding and appropriate covering of the puncture site. A small Band-Aid is usually sufficient and welcomed by most children, especially if someone takes the time to draw a happy face or animal face with whiskers on the Band-Aid. Cotton balls applied with a piece of tape should be avoided because a young child may remove the cotton ball and aspirate a piece of cotton fluff.

The three sources of blood used for diagnostic purposes are venous, arterial, and capillary. Samples are obtained in a variety of ways, including arterial and venous access devices.

RESEARCH ISSUES

Saline Versus Heparin Flush Solutions for Maintaining Patency of Peripheral Venous Catheters

Results: For a number of years, study has been proceeding on whether noninfusing intravenous lines require heparin solutions for maintaining their patency. The generally accepted result is that in adults, normal saline solutions are as effective as heparin solutions. Adult-size intravenous catheters generally range from gauge 18 to gauge 22. There have been fewer studies comparing heparin with saline in children, and these are more recent. Of particular concern is the ability of saline alone to maintain patency of the 24-gauge catheters often used in infants and children. Danek and Noris (1992) found no significant difference in the length of time a 22-gauge catheter was functional when saline and heparin were compared as flushing agents, but they did find a significant difference in the 24-gauge catheters. In a study of 142 pediatric patients, McMullen and co-workers (1993) reported no significant difference in length of patency when normal saline and heparin solutions were compared as flushing agents. However, they do not report separately on 24-gauge catheters, which precludes conclusions about this small catheter size.

Implications: Use of normal saline as a flush solution for maintaining the patency of nonflowing intravenous lines has the potential of achieving considerable cost savings for health care institutions and patients. Current evidence indicates that normal saline solutions work just as effectively as heparin solutions in most catheter sizes. More evidence is needed for conclusions to be drawn about 24-gauge catheters, the smallest commonly used intravenous catheters in children.

REFERENCES

Danek, G. D., & Noris, E. M. (1992). Pediatric IV catheters: Efficacy of saline flush. *Pediatric Nursing, 18,* 111–113.

Dunn, D. L., & Lenihan, S. F. (1987). The case for the saline flush. *American Journal of Nursing, 87,* 798–799.

Epperson, E. (1984). Efficacy of 0.9% sodium chloride injection with and without heparin for maintaining indwelling intermittent injection sites. *Clinical Pharmacy, 3,* 626–629.

Geritz, M. A. (1992). Saline versus heparin in intermittent infuser patency management. *Western Journal of Nursing Research, 14,* 131–141.

Harrigan, C. A. (1985). Intermittent IV therapy without heparin: A study. *NITA: Journal of the National Intravenous Therapy Association, 8,* 519–520.

McMullen, A., Fioravanti, I. D., Pollack, V., Rideout, K., & Sciera, M. (1993). Heparinized saline or normal saline as a flush solution in intermittent intravenous lines in infants and children. *MCN: American Journal of Maternal Child Nursing, 18,* 78–85.

Venous blood samples are obtained by venipuncture or by direct aspiration from an access device placed peripherally or centrally. A sample may be taken peripherally from a saline (or heparin) lock or from an IV infusion site. However, peripheral veins used for a saline lock may be so small that drawing blood through them may make it necessary to replace the saline lock sooner than if it is not used for blood samples. The use of an IV site is not always appropriate because the type of solution being infused may affect the blood test for the sample being collected.

Veins of the antecubital fossa are usually the site of choice for venipuncture in children older than 2 years. Every attempt is made to gain the child's cooperation without restraint. If the child must be restrained, an attempt should be made to explain how the child can help. With the child in a supine position, the nurse can extend the child's arm, slightly hyperextending the elbow. The other hand is used to grasp the child's shoulder by placing it around the back of the child's neck (Fig. 23–9). The child's unused arm is secured behind the nurse's back. The nurse's torso can lean across the child but the weight is on the nurse's elbow, not on the child. This position is effective in restraining the child for the venipuncture and also allows talking and maintaining eye contact because the nurse's face will be in direct alignment with the child's face (Fig. 23–9).

In infants less than 1 year of age, the external jugular vein may be used if withdrawal from other sites has been unsuccessful. The infant is placed in a supine position with the infant's head and neck supported in the nurse's hands. The infant's head is held off the edge of the table with the shoulders resting on the table. The infant's head is turned approximately 45 to 60 degrees to one side of the midline. Key elements that enhance the success of this procedure are sufficient rotation of the head to cause stretching of the vein, stimulating the infant to cry, and ensuring that the infant's head does not move after the needle has been inserted into the vein. Stimulating the infant to cry during the procedure promotes filling of the vessel, which facilitates blood withdrawal. Immediately after withdrawal of the needle, the infant should be brought to an upright position and pressure applied to the site to reduce bleeding from the site.

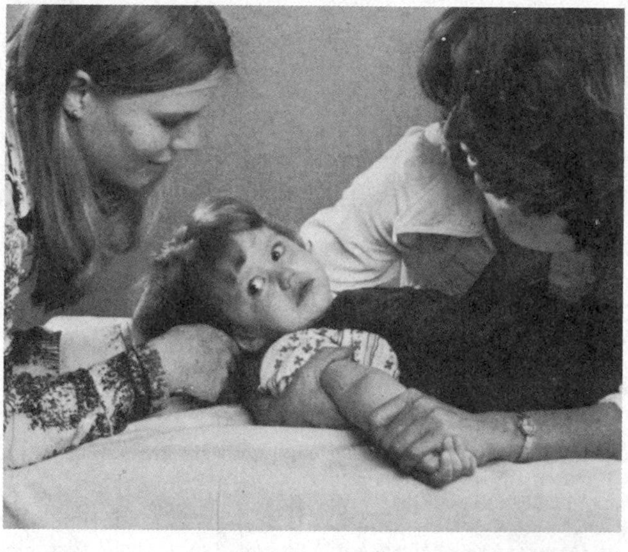

FIGURE 23-9. Venipuncture. If the child is properly restrained, both the child and the nurse can be comfortable while the arm is securely held to permit a safe venipuncture. In this photo, the child's mother assumes a comforting role while a nurse supports the child's arm for blood to be drawn by a laboratory technician.

In infants less than 1 year old, it is also possible to obtain a blood specimen from a superficial vein of the scalp. This method is reserved for times when other methods are unsuccessful (because the baby's hair must be shaved to select the vein). A rubber band placed around the head is often used as a tourniquet. For this procedure to be successful, traction is applied to the skin around the vein to stabilize it, and the needle is inserted against the direction of blood flow.

Arterial blood samples may be required for blood gas analysis, blood cultures, and selected blood chemistry. The most common reason to draw arterial blood samples has traditionally been for blood gas analysis. Noninvasive techniques, such as transcutaneous monitoring and pulse oximetry, are now the preferred methods for blood gas measurement. See Chapter 32 for a discussion of blood gas analysis. If an arterial sample is required, it may be obtained by arteriopuncture of the radial, brachial, or femoral arteries or from an indwelling arterial device. Special preparation is required to perform arterial sampling if it is required.

Capillary blood samples can be drawn from the heel for infants under age 2 years or from the finger, great toe, or ear lobe in older children. Capillary blood sampling is also less common since noninvasive devices have become available for arterial blood gas analysis.

Care of Children Who Require Restraints

Restraints are necessarily applied to children but should not be used without careful evaluation of alternatives. They are used to immobilize children for diagnostic and therapeutic procedures of varying types and duration. The nurse usually determines whether a restraint is needed and which type of restraint is most appropriate. Parents should be involved in the decision making: in many institutions, parental consent is required to use restraints.

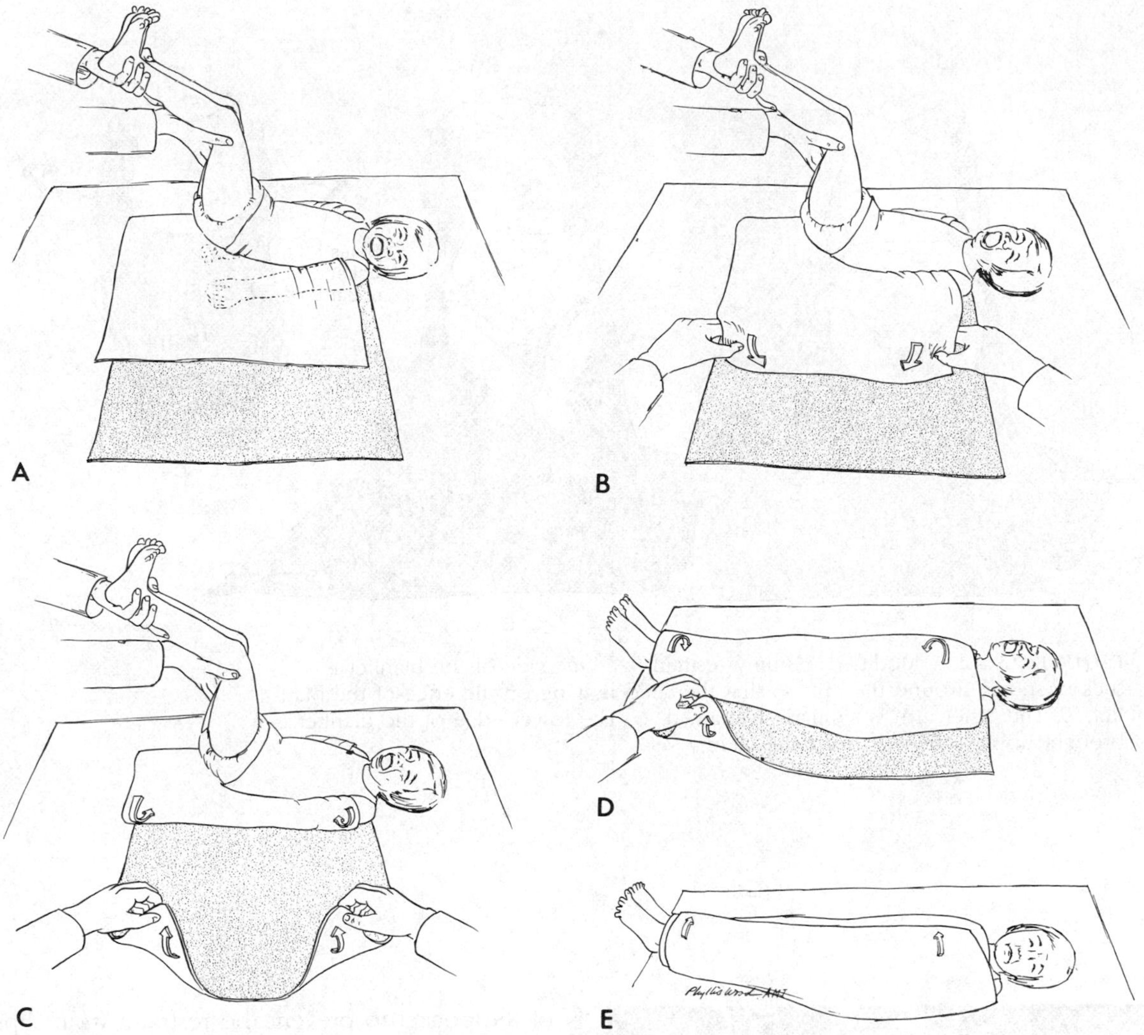

FIGURE 23 - 10. Mummy restraint. *A*, The restraining sheet is placed under the child and folded back, pinning the arms down. *B*, Next, the sheet is tucked back under the child's left arm. *C–E*, The sheet is then wrapped around the child's entire body and fastened with a safety pin.

Type of Restraint

Commonly used restraints in the care of children are (1) mummy restraints, (2) elbow restraints, (3) jacket restraints, and (4) arm and leg restraints.

A *mummy restraint* is used to immobilize an infant or small child for a short time as required for examination or treatment of the head, neck, or chest. The purpose of this technique is to secure the arms and legs within a blanket in a way that prevents the child from wriggling free. The nurse is thus free to hold the child securely to prevent movement of her or his entire body without attending to flailing arms and legs. This technique is particularly useful for jugular punctures, insertion of nasogastric tubes, scalp vein needle insertion, and detailed examination of the eye, ear, nose, and throat (Fig. 23–10).

The *modified mummy restraint* is used for procedures that require an exposed chest. Figure 23–11 details steps in securing the infant in a modified mummy restraint.

The purpose of an *elbow restraint* is to keep the child from reaching his or her face or head by preventing flexion of the elbow. This type of restraint may be needed to preserve plastic surgery of the face, a scalp vein needle, or eye patches or to prevent scratching of the face in various skin disorders. The restraint usually covers most of the arm, but it should not push into the child's axilla nor rub the wrist. A cloth restraint with pockets for tongue depressors is commonly used (Fig. 23–12). A large blade made especially for these restraints or two tongue blades taped together should be placed into *each pocket*. Each blade *must* extend the entire length

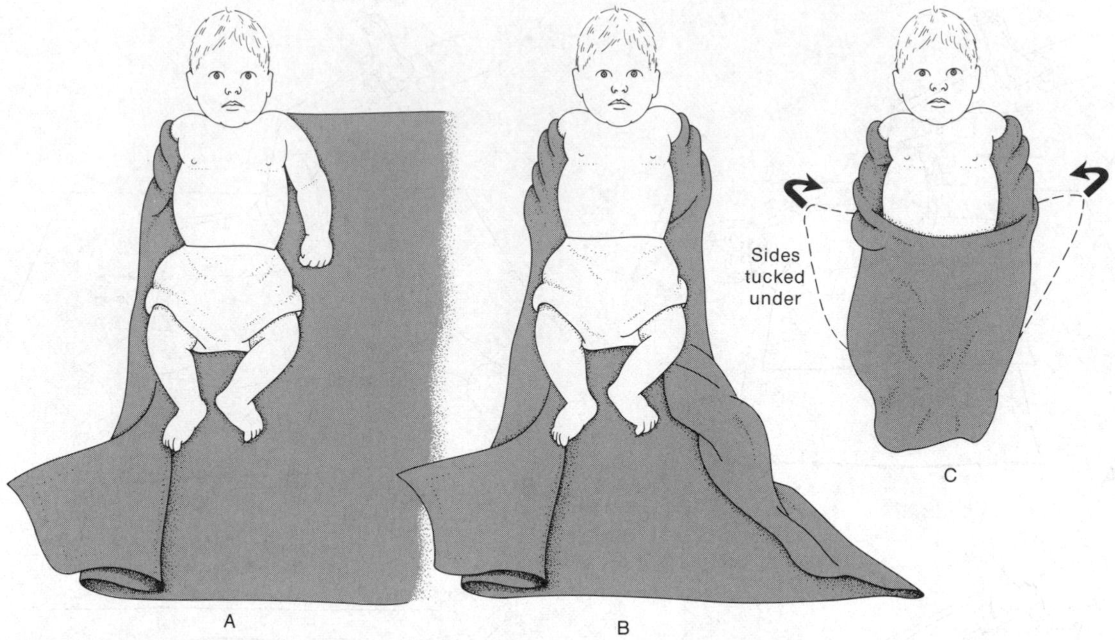

FIGURE 23 - 11. Modified mummy restraint. *A*, One side of the blanket is tucked snugly around the arm so that the child is lying on the edge of the blanket. *B*, The other arm is similarly restrained. *C*, The lower edge of the blanket is brought up and tucked *under* the child.

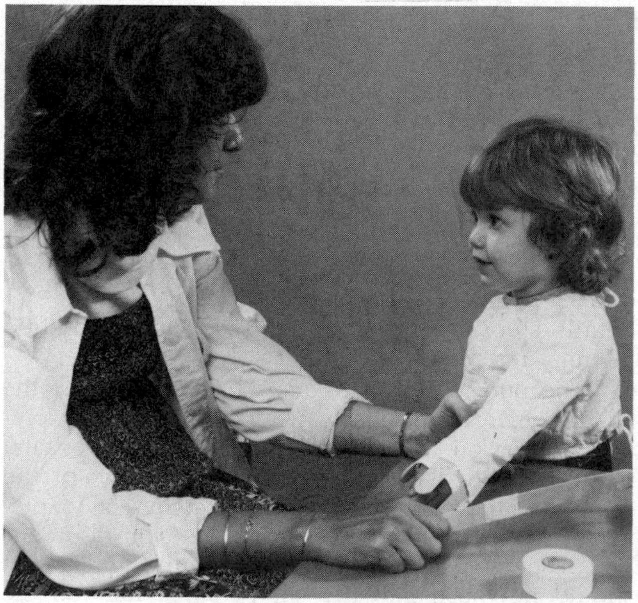

FIGURE 23 - 12. Applying an elbow restraint. Note the individual pockets in the sleeve for each tongue blade. This child requires two tongue blades taped together for sufficient length to be provided to keep her from bending her arm.

of the pocket to prevent the restraint from slipping to a position above or below the child's elbow. Care must also be taken to avoid using a tongue blade that is too long, which would result in pressure in the axilla. Restraints are commercially available, but similar types of restraints can be improvised. A padded cylinder can be made out of a cardboard or plastic container. Such a restraint must be placed over the child's shirt and secured with pins, ties, or tape to keep it from slipping off. Figure 23–13 illustrates alternative elbow restraints.

A *jacket restraint* is used to keep the child flat in bed or safe in a highchair or wheelchair. A jacket restraint should not be used to keep a child from climbing out of a crib. An enclosed crib (e.g., bubble-top as shown in Fig. 23–2) is used for that purpose. If a jacket restraint is used, it is tied at the back to keep the child from untying it, and the long tapes on the sides of the jacket should be tied to the crib frames and not to the siderails. No restraint of any kind is to be secured to the crib railing for important reasons:

1. When the siderail is inadvertently put down, the child can be seriously injured because of the abrupt pull on the limb being restrained.

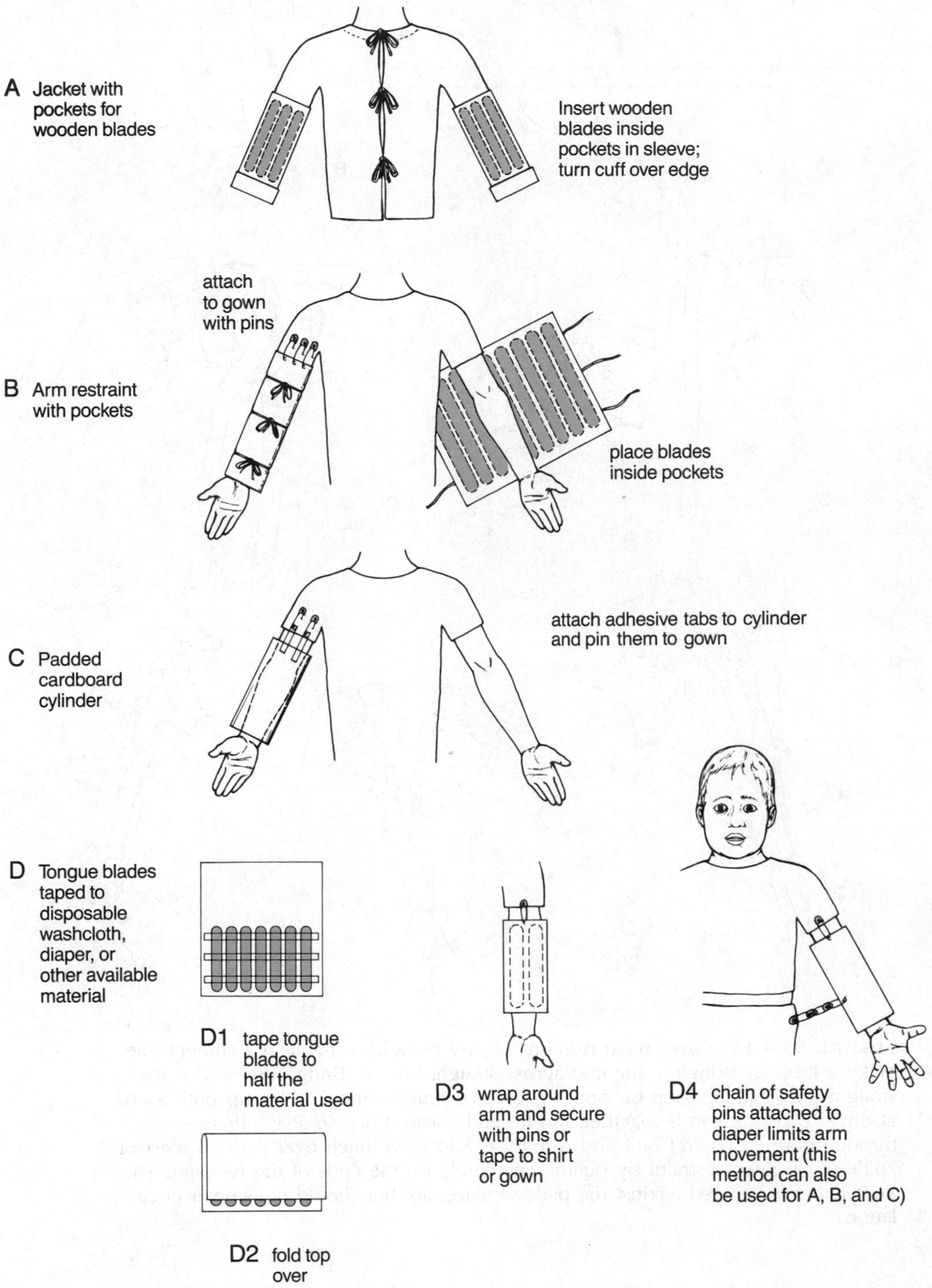
A Jacket with pockets for wooden blades
Insert wooden blades inside pockets in sleeve; turn cuff over edge
attach to gown with pins
B Arm restraint with pockets
place blades inside pockets
C Padded cardboard cylinder
attach adhesive tabs to cylinder and pin them to gown
D Tongue blades taped to disposable washcloth, diaper, or other available material
D1 tape tongue blades to half the material used
D2 fold top over
D3 wrap around arm and secure with pins or tape to shirt or gown
D4 chain of safety pins attached to diaper limits arm movement (this method can also be used for A, B, and C)

FIGURE 23 - 13. Alternative methods to restrain elbows.

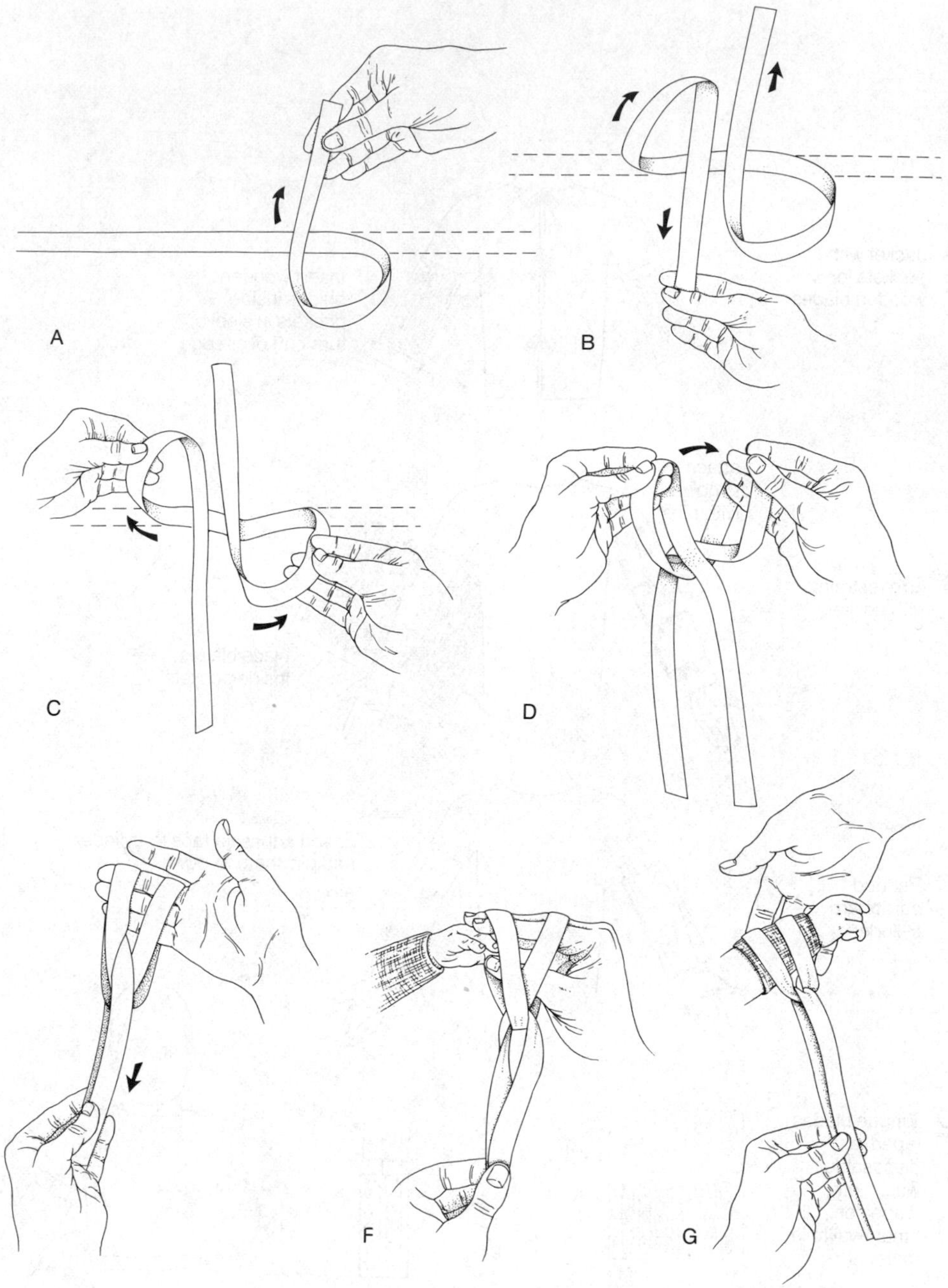

FIGURE 23 - 14. Clove hitch restraint. *A*, Lay or hold restraint in a straight line. Make a loop by bringing one end across straight line. *B*, Bring other end across straight line, making loop on opposite side of straight line. *C*, Pick up both loops at once. *D*, Bring hands together and let ends drop down. *E*, Place fingers through both loops and pull ends firmly. *F*, Slip clove hitch over padded wrist or ankle. *G*, Tighten restraint by pulling alternately on the ends of the restraint. The knot is firmly secured against the padded extremity but should not impair circulation.

2. With this method of attachment, a siderail cannot be quickly lowered in an emergency.
3. If the restraint is secured only on a vertical bar of the rail, the restraint can slide upward so that the child is not actually restrained.
4. The child could reach the place where the restraint is attached to the rail and loosen it more easily.

A jacket restraint may be used for cleft lip surgery, to keep the child from rolling onto the face, or whenever the supine position is necessary. With the prevalent use of various types of catheters for infusion rather than butterfly needles, this type of restraint is no longer used for IV therapy.

Arm and leg restraints are used to immobilize one or more extremities. The restraint can be a muslin strip, roller gauze, Kerlix, or similar material. First, the wrist or ankle is padded with gauze (one or two 4 × 4s opened and folded lengthwise), a cut abdominal pad, or small washcloth. The restraint is applied using a clove hitch technique (Fig. 23–14). The clove hitch is not a slip knot and if applied correctly does not tighten. The ends of the restraint are tied to the crib frame. The need for this type of limb restraint should be carefully evaluated and used with discretion. It is frustrating to a child to be "tied down."

Nursing Diagnostic Statements

Relevant nursing diagnostic statements applicable to most children in the various types of restraints described earlier include:

High risk for impairment of skin integrity; *risk factors:*
- *Pressure and shearing forces from restraint application.*
- *Physical immobility.*

Powerlessness, *related to*
- *Restricted movement caused by restraint.*
- *Lack of explanation accompanying the application of the restraint.*
- *Lack of opportunity for therapeutic play.*
- *Prescribed dependence on caregivers for self-care activities.*
- *Interference with usual motor coping strategies.*

High risk for injury contractures; *risk factor:*
- *Immobility.*

Diversional activity deficit, *related to*
- *Physical immobility.*
- *Lack of appropriate play materials.*
- *Ineffective use of available resources.*

Nursing Care

The child in restraints must be continually re-evaluated to see whether restraint is still needed. The minimal amount of restraint necessary to meet the therapeutic goal should be used. The basic principle is to *allow maximal mobility while meeting the need for restraint.*

The nurse should work with the family to help them understand the need for restraints. Depending on the reason for the restraint, parents can be permitted to release the child from restraints for varying lengths of time. If restraints are being used to prevent trauma to an operative site, one restraint is removed at a time.

Preventing Skin Breakdown

If restraints are applied properly, the potential for complications is minimized. If the child is not restless, each extremity should be checked at least every hour; but, for a restless child, these should be checked more frequently. The nurse should also periodically remove restraints to exercise the involved extremity and give the child freedom of movement. The nurse has a responsibility to ensure that children are released for short periods, that parents are taught how to release restraints and protect their child while unrestrained, and that children are not restrained to an unnecessary degree or for excessive duration. Meticulous bathing and drying of the skin is important for all children but especially when they are immobilized by restraints.

Increasing Child's Sense of Power and Control

Nursing interventions for a child in restraints should reduce the sense of powerlessness associated with immobility. Development of physical, intellectual, and emotional social competencies is affected by the child's inability to be mobile. When restrained, a child's major form of expression and means of coping are lost. Restrained children cannot defend themselves by running away or by physically striking out; often, they cannot even suck their thumb for comfort. They feel helpless, frustrated, and anxious.

Although children may not fully understand the explanations, the powerlessness a child experiences can be reduced by preparing the child through explanations and playing out a similar scenario using a doll.

Maintaining Joint Mobility, Muscular Strength, and Circulation

If a child requires a form of restraint over a period of several weeks, or even longer, specific interventions can promote the normal functioning of normal body processes. Children should be instructed to cough and deep breathe and perform isometric exercises by contracting and relaxing muscles. If the child is too young to follow instruction, play activities can be chosen to exercise the limb or limbs that are not restrained. Range-of-motion exercises are incorporated with bath time and play activities as well as performed at regular intervals. Parents are a great help with these activities and can often assist the nurse in getting the child's cooperation.

Providing Diversional Activities to Reduce Discomfort

Special attention is given to the child's need to engage in a form of play activity. Appropriate use of mobiles, music, and stories on records and tapes can help maintain a level of activity that engages the child's mind and attention. Although a child is restrained, she or he can be moved to the playroom with other children and be drawn into activities, if someone assists in the manipulation of materials. Caregivers must take more time with a restrained child to try to prevent the child's boredom and depression.

Care of Children Who Need to Be Isolated

Confinement of a child to a separate room within the hospital is necessary in a variety of circumstances. Short-term isolation for infectious disease is a familiar precaution in pediatric settings. Also, children who receive chemotherapy for cancer in a germ-free protected environment (laminar air flow) present a special challenge to the health care team. The most extreme example of isolation is children who are placed into a plastic "bubble" because of an immunodeficiency disease.

Children may have distorted perceptions of illness and hospitalization. One predominant perception is that hospitalization and illness are forms of punishment, mutilation, or rejection. Children may also suffer from fears of abandonment and death. Creation of physical barriers, such as masks, gloves, gowns, and closed doors, can add to the confusion of a child who is feeling threatened, fearful, and alone in a hospital.

Children and their parents often must be prepared for the need to be isolated in the midst of the crises of admission to the hospital or at the time of a new diagnosis. Too frequently, the focus of preparation is limited to giving instructions about how to gown and mask, where and when to wash hands, and clarification of rules about visitors. Some explanation about the purpose of isolation is given by the physician or nurse, or both. Besides explaining to parents, it is also important to give understandable explanations to the child according to age.

Children's perceptions of isolation have been examined by only a few researchers (Pidgeon, 1967; Broeder, 1985). Children's understanding of isolation attire has been identified as an area of misconception. The purpose of isolation attire is seen by children to be primarily associated with procedures. A child's expression about the nurse in isolation attire summarizes this misconception well: "She needs to do something to you. You don't know what, you just wait and see" (Broeder, 1985).

The child's level of language development limits comprehension about isolation. For example, the word "germ" is reported to be not well understood by young school-age children (6 to 7 years); by 9 years of age, children are more logical in explaining the concept of germs (Broeder, 1985).

The length of time and strictness of isolation are important variables affecting a child's experience. Children's responses change over time. During the first few weeks, children continue their usual patterns of talking, playing, and crying. Passivity gradually becomes a predominant characteristic, and, when children are removed from isolation, they again become more vocal (Hallenbeck et al, 1980). In a study of six children aged 6 to 9 years, feelings of deprivation were expressed in wishes for food, people, and playtime.

Nursing Diagnostic Statements

Children are isolated for a wide variety of reasons and under many circumstances. The following nursing diagnostic statements are relevant to most situations for which children require isolation.

Fear or anxiety, related to knowledge deficit, *associated with*

- *Cognitive misconceptions about purpose of isolation.*
- *Misinterpretation of purpose of gowns and masks.*

Sensory-perceptual alteration: input deficit, *related to*

- *Physical separation from other children, family, and caregivers.*
- *Social isolation due to terminal or infectious disease.*
- *Ineffective use of resources to provide stimulation.*

High risk for infection; *risk factors:*

- *Immature immune system.*
- *Invasion of a pathogenic agent.*
- *Medications that suppress immunologic function.*
- *Surgical intervention.*

Nursing Care

Children require special care during isolation because of their cognitive, social, and biologic needs. With appropriate interventions, the negative psychologic impact of isolation can be diminished and the effectiveness of the control of organisms enhanced.

Correcting Misconceptions about Isolation

Focus on helping the child understand the purpose of isolation. Misconceptions about wrongdoing and the purpose of isolation attire should be corrected. Procedures have been identified as the most stressful experience for children hospitalized and in isolation, and children tend to think that nurses are gowned for the purpose of performing a procedure. Sitting, talking, and playing games with children in isolation facilitates differentiation between isolation and procedures (Broeder, 1985).

Providing Sensory Stimulation and Psychologic Support

The feelings of aloneness, agony, and deprivation can be lessened by spending time with children in isolation and by encouraging parents to stay with their child when possible. Also, because children cannot see a person's face when it is masked, they should be allowed to see who is visiting them *before* masking to increase the sense of relationship and thereby reduce feelings of aloneness and alienation.

Feelings about being in isolation can also be expressed through drawings and therapeutic play. Favorite blankets or toys should be allowed in the room to enhance the child's sense of security. Many toys can be autoclaved, washed with disinfectants, or exposed to the sun, so play can be normal.

The decision to isolate a child should take into consideration the child's psychologic comfort. Once it has been determined that isolation is required, the procedure should be followed consistently by all professionals and visitors.

The health care team should assess regularly the child's psychologic response and physiologic status. Isolation should end at the earliest possible time the physiologic status permits.

Reducing Potential for Transmission of Organisms

Hospitalized children need to be protected from nosocomial (hospital-associated) infections, and health care personnel need protection from infectious agents transmitted by children.

Proper handwashing should be stressed at all times for all conditions and with all individuals entering and leaving the room.

Handwashing is the most important precaution to take when caring for children in isolation, especially because they do not necessarily adhere to some of the basic hygienic principles, such as covering the mouth when coughing and sneezing. Also, they may not routinely wash their hands yet tend to touch everything in the room; thus, articles tend to be more easily contaminated.

The two major isolation precaution systems outlined in the Centers for Disease Control Guidelines for Isolation are the disease-specific isolation system and the category-specific isolation system.

1. **Disease-specific isolation:** Precautions are outlined for *each* infectious disease or condition whereby transmission of a specific organism is interrupted.
2. **Category-specific isolation:** This system has been in use for some time. Similar infectious diseases are grouped into a category and precautions prescribed for each category.

Of the two systems, category-specific isolation is most commonly adopted by institutions. A disadvantage of both systems is that a diagnosis must be known before a decision concerning isolation can be made. Clinically, it is important to take precautions *before* the diagnosis is known, especially because of the inability to reliably identify patients infected with the hepatitis B virus (HBV) and the human immunodeficiency virus (HIV). For protection against the transmission of HIV and other blood-borne pathogens, the Centers for Disease Control developed the Universal Blood and Body Fluid Precautions, now referred to as "Universal Precautions." This approach stresses that all patients should be assumed to be infectious for HIV and other blood-borne pathogens. Body fluids and procedures considered potentially infectious are listed in Table 23–4; indications are given for when gloves are recommended and when only handwashing is required.

Body substance isolation is a type of isolation procedure that considers blood, feces, urine, vomitus, wound drainage, and oral secretions potentially harmful. In working with children, the likelihood of contact with these secretions cannot be readily predicted; therefore, universal precautions are more commonly used than is body substance isolation.

Regardless of type of isolation procedure, disposal and use of needles require rigid control. Needles are not recapped and must be disposed of in a designated rigid plastic container that is placed in easy access for adults but out of reach for children.

A needle is discarded in a designated box without being recapped or broken.

Care of a Child with a Fever

Fever is an obvious indicator to parents that their child is sick. Almost every child will at some time have a fever in the range of 37.8° to 40° C (100° to 104° F).

Pathophysiology of Fever

Parents become upset and worried when their child has a fever. To help parents during these crises, the nurse must have a good understanding of the phenomenon of fever. A fever is an abnormal elevation of the central body temperature caused by (1) a high thermostatic set-point, (2) metabolic heat production or excessive environmental heat that exceeds heat loss capacities, or (3) impairment of the body's heat loss capabilities (Table 23–5 gives examples of conditions).

Body temperature is regulated by the anterior hypothalamus, which contains sensitive neurons. The temperature of blood entering the brain is assessed by a hypothalamic "thermostat," which is normally set at 98.6° F (37° C); this is called the "set-point." If the

TABLE 23-4
Infection Control Recommendations for Blood, Body Fluids, and Procedures (Universal Precautions)

Handwashing is necessary after physical contact with all patients

Purpose of universal precautions: Reduce risk of HIV and other blood-borne pathogens

Body substances and procedures for which gloves are recommended (if splattering is likely, then barrier eye protection should also be used)

Body Fluids	Procedures
Blood	Intubation
Blood-contaminated fluids	Endoscopy
Amniotic fluid	Dental procedures
Pericardial fluid	Wound irrigation
Peritoneal fluid	Phlebotomy
Pleural fluid	Finger and heel sticks
Synovial fluid	Arterial puncture
Cerebrospinal fluid	Vascular catheter placement
Semen	Tracheostomy suctioning
Vaginal secretions	Rinsing of used instruments
Any other body fluid visibly contaminated with blood	Lumbar puncture
	Puncture of other cavities (e.g., pleural, peritoneal)

Body fluids and procedures for which only handwashing is recommended (if these fluids contain blood, then gloves are warranted)

Body Fluids	Procedures
Urine	Diaper change
Stool	
Vomitus	
Tears	
Sweat	
Nasal secretions	
Oral secretions	

Data from American Academy of Pediatrics Committee on Infectious Diseases (1991). *Redbook* (22nd ed., p. 83). Evanston, IL: Author.

set-point is raised, or if the thermoregulatory mechanisms do not respond adequately, then body temperature rises. Alteration in the set-point results in a *fever,* whereas ineffective regulatory mechanisms produce *hyperthermia,* a state in which the body temperature is elevated but the set-point is normal.

The way the set-point is raised in fever is as follows:

1. An endogenous pyrogen is produced in response to a foreign substance (bacterium or virus).
2. The pyrogen circulates to the anterior hypothalamus, where it stimulates the production of prostaglandins.
3. Set-point is raised (prostaglandins are suspected of being responsible for raising the hypothalamic set-point).

When the set-point has been raised, the body senses coldness and triggers compensatory mechanisms to raise body temperature until it reaches the new set-point (similar to a furnace responding to a thermostat). The mechanism of thermoregulation when the set-point has been raised (fever) is a three-phase process (Holtzclaw, 1990):

1. During the first phase, the *chill phase,* vasoconstriction and shivering occur to warm the body because the normal body temperature is sensed as cooler than the new set-point; shivering, the involuntary contraction of skeletal muscles, produces heat for the new set-point to be reached.
2. When the core temperature reaches the higher set-point, a *plateau* is reached, and shivering stops.
3. The core temperature typically exceeds the set-point, which results in a third phase called *defervescence;* vasodilatation, diaphoresis, and increased respiration dissipate heat as the body attempts to return core temperature to the set-point.

Infants typically do not have a febrile response because of the immaturity of their hypothalamus and thermoregulatory mechanisms. Also, during the first year of life, infants do not shiver but rather metabolize "brown fat" to produce heat.

TABLE 23-5
Fever: Mechanism, Causes, and Interventions

Mechanism of Temperature Elevation	Types of Condition that Cause the Mechanism	Interventions
Set-point is raised	Infection, malignancy, allergy, central nervous system lesion, radiation	Antipyretics to lower set-point; supply sufficient clothing to avoid shivering
Excessive heat production; set-point is normal	Hyperthyroidism, aspirin overdose, malignant hyperthermia	Undressing, sponging; antipyretic administration not effective
Heat loss mechanism defective; set-point is normal	Ectodermal dysplasia, burns, heat stroke	Undressing; cool environment; antipyretic administration not effective

Parents usually have greater fears and concerns about the hazards of fever than most temperature elevations warrant. Fever does not generally rise to harmful levels unless there is interference with the body's mechanism of dissipating heat. Fever by itself does not cause brain damage unless it reaches 41.7° C (107° F) (Schmitt, 1984). Fever from infection rarely poses a threat; however, heat exhaustion, thermal burns, or malignant hyperthermia are usually more serious causes of fever. In addition, fever can be harmful to children with congestive heart failure, respiratory failure, acute neurologic disease, or endotoxic shock.

Although normal children are usually not harmed by fever, parents fear their child will have a seizure. Only about 4 per cent of children who experience a fever are likely to have a convulsion. Some have even questioned whether fever per se causes a seizure or whether another mechanism associated with the illness is the cause. Many children have seizures at relatively low temperatures (e.g., 38.4° C or 101° F) at the onset of illness and during the illness, yet when the child's fever spikes, a seizure does not occur (Fruthaler, 1985).

The potential benefits of fever have been recognized. It has been hypothesized that fever may produce an environment in which endogenous pyrogen production is curtailed. Fever has also been noted to potentiate the action of antibodies and enhance defense mechanisms, such as the inflammatory response (Reeves-Swift, 1990).

Assessment

There is a normal diurnal variation of body temperature, with the lowest temperature occurring between 2 and 4 A.M. and the highest between 6 and 10 P.M. A similar diurnal pattern is demonstrated in most febrile illnesses.

In children, an oral temperature in excess of 38° C (100.4° F) or a rectal temperature in excess of 38.8° C (101.8° F) is considered by most to be a fever (Kleinman, 1984). In neonates, however, a rectal temperature of 37.5° C (99.5° F) can represent serious illness; the neonate can also have an infection without a fever and more commonly has hypothermia with sepsis.

Age is an important variable to consider in assessing fever. It is generally accepted that fever in any child under 6 months of age is more likely to be caused by serious illness than when the same degree of elevation occurs in an older child. It is also agreed by most experts that a febrile neonate should be seen promptly by a physician. Furthermore, fever in a compromised child (e.g., one who has sickle cell disease) can often indicate a more serious bacterial infection. Also, children who do *not* have associated clinical signs of infection (e.g., sore throat, runny nose) are more likely to have serious underlying disease (Younger & Brown, 1985). Fevers that persist longer than a week require diagnostic and laboratory evaluation.

The level and pattern of fever can provide important information but should be supplemented with a careful individual clinical assessment of the child. A child's spontaneous activity, play, appetite, and general behavior and disposition are significant. The child's visual movement and ability to move limbs, sit, stand, and walk should be noted. A history should consist of the fever pattern and an assessment of the child, including age, presence of a chronic condition, length of illness, presence of associated physical signs, and a general behavioral assessment. Additional data, such as complete blood count, urinalysis, urine culture, chest radiograph, and blood culture, may also be obtained. The presence of serious illness, however, cannot be predicted with accuracy. Suggested parameters (Teele et al, 1979) on which to base a prediction of bacteremia when the source of infection is not identifiable are

- Age less than 2 years.
- Fever in excess of 38.8° C (101.8° F).
- White blood cell count in excess of 20 × 1000 cell/mm^3 (μl) or 20 × 10^9 cells/L (SI units)

Therapeutic Management

Because fever is part of the body's defense mechanism, it could be argued that fever reduction is undesirable. A child with a fever, however, often has a headache or arthralgia and may suffer from malaise. It is therefore reasonable that antipyretic medication orders are prescribed not necessarily for a specific temperature level but for discomfort.

Fever management is controversial. Fluid administration is recommended to reduce fever under most circumstances. Antipyretics, removal of clothing, and sponging are other common methods, but there is some variation in how these interventions are used.

Antipyretics are to be used with caution. Aspirin should not be used for children because of its association with subsequent development of Reye syndrome. Acetaminophen is the drug most often used. A nonsteroidal anti-inflammatory drug, ibuprofen, is approved for fever reduction in children as young as 6 months of age; however, it should not be used long-term without supervision from a health professional.

There is a general overuse of antipyretics, a practice that is continually being challenged (Younger & Brown, 1985). Because antipyretics lower the setpoint, their use is appropriate in infections, malignancy, central nervous system lesions, and allergy but not when heat production is excessive (as in malignant hyperthermia) or when the mechanism for heat loss is defective (as in burns and heat stroke). In these conditions, removal of clothing and sponging are more appropriate.

The use of tepid water to moisten the child's skin

systematically is called "sponging." It can be performed while the child is lying in bed or in the bathtub. Some evidence in the literature indicates that sponging does *not* have an antipyretic effect (Newman, 1985); but because it continues to be a technique that is used, it is important for health professionals to ensure that it is performed properly to avoid disastrous results. The evaporation of water from the skin surface has a cooling effect. In the past, sponge baths to reduce a fever included the use of alcohol in water. This was believed to speed cooling by more rapid evaporation. This technique is dangerous and should not be practiced because of the absorption of alcohol and too-rapid heat loss. It is important to use tepid, not cold, water (29.4° to 32.2° C), because cold water may cause shivering. If sponging is used when the set-point is raised, antipyretic drugs must be given 30 minutes before sponging. If sponging is done *before* the antipyretic drug is given, the hypothalamus attempts to offset the lowered body temperature. The child will therefore shiver (muscle contraction to produce heat), and, as soon as sponging is discontinued, temperature will return to the previous level. However, under some circumstances, such as the presence of delirium, a seizure from fever, or a fever greater than 41.1° C (106° F), immediate sponging and use of cooler water is recommended (Schmitt, 1984).

Sponging is noted to work more quickly than immersion. A child should be placed into a bathtub with approximately 2 inches of water, while the skin is being wet continuously. Shivering is a natural mechanism that occurs with rapid cooling and causes the body temperature to increase. Thus, if a child begins to shiver, the water temperature should be raised; and if shivering continues, the cooling treatment should be discontinued (Schmitt, 1984).

Hospitalized children with persistent high fevers are frequently placed on hypothermia mattresses. These are pads with internal coils to circulate cool water. The pads should be covered with a bath blanket for comfort. It is important to watch for shivering and to discontinue the treatment if this occurs.

Parents who are treating their child's fever at home should be instructed in antipyretic therapy and told to offer fluids and not be concerned about a child's refusal to eat solids. Available antipyretic preparations and their use are summarized in Table 23–6. The nurse should review the signs of dehydration with parents and encourage them to call if the fever is not controlled.

TABLE 23-6
Acetaminophen (Tylenol and Other Brand Names) Preparations and Dosages

How Supplied

Drops	80 mg/0.8 ml
Syrup/elixir	Available in numerous preparations (e.g., 80 mg/5 ml; 120 mg/5 ml; 160 mg/5 ml; 320 mg/5 ml)
Chewable	80 mg/tab or 160 mg/tab

Dosage According to Weight

10–20 mg/kg/dose every 4–6 hrs, not to exceed 5 doses in 24 hrs

Dosage According to Age

Age	Dose
3 mos or younger	40 mg/dose q 4–6 hrs
4–11 mos	80 mg/dose q 4–6 hrs
12–23 mos	120 mg/dose q 4–6 hrs
2–4 yrs	160 mg/dose q 4–6 hrs
4–6 yrs	240 mg/dose q 4–6 hrs
6–9 yrs	320 mg/dose q 4–6 hrs
9–11 yrs	400 mg/dose q 4–6 hrs
11–12 yrs	480 mg/dose q 4–6 hrs
12 yrs and older	640 mg/dose q 4–6 hrs

Perioperative Nursing Care*

Parents expect the nurse to answer their questions and assist in the effective management of their child's perioperative experience. To meet these expectations satisfactorily, the nurse must be skilled in handling the unique responses of a child and family, allowing for the child's age and the particular family circumstances. The nurse must also be knowledgeable in caring for a child undergoing anesthesia and provide the specialized care required for the specific surgical procedure performed.

Specific age-related approaches to children requiring hospitalization and surgery are discussed in Chapter 21. Specialized nursing care for the various surgical problems is discussed throughout this text as applicable. The following is a general discussion on perioperative nursing care of a child undergoing surgery. See Table 23–7 for a Nursing Process Plan: Perioperative Nursing Care.

Preoperative Nursing Care

Pediatric patients are given anesthetics in conjunction with all surgical procedures. Anesthetics may also be administered to pediatric patients to facilitate nonsurgical procedures requiring patient immobility or pa-

* We appreciate the authorship of this section on perioperative preparation and anesthetic management of children by Mary Jean Yablonky, CRNA, MA, Staff Nurse Anesthetist, Oakwood Hospital, Dearborn; Clinical Instructor, University of Detroit–Mercy/St. Joseph Mercy Hospital Program in Nurse Anesthesiology, Pontiac, Michigan.

TABLE 23-7

Nursing Process Plan: Perioperative Nursing Care

Analysis: Nursing Diagnostic Statement 1

Response and Related or Risk Factors: ***High risk for injury: physiologic;*** *risk factor: the trauma of surgery superimposed on a concurrent febrile illness or systemic function*

Projected Outcome: The child will be free of infection.

Defining Characteristics *(Actual Response)*	**Nursing Interventions**	**Evaluation Criteria**
Subjective: • Report of aching discomfort (e.g., sore throat, stomach pain, headache) • Parental report of unusual irritability Objective: • Fever, enlarged lymph nodes, tugging at ear, vomiting, diarrhea, or other signs of infection • Increased white blood cell count, decreased hemoglobin and hematocrit, >5–10 polymorphonuclear leukocytes per high-power field in a cleanly voided urine specimen	Infection Protection **Assess for evidence of infection.** • Measure temperature every 4 hours preoperatively; report fever to physician • Perform a thorough physical assessment on admission, alerting the physician or anesthesiologist to any evidence of infection or any report from mother or child of suspicious symptoms (it is not uncommon for evidence of an infection [particularly viral] to develop quickly between the time of the doctor's preoperative examination and the time of surgery) • Alert the physician or anesthesiologist about increased white blood cell count, decreased hemoglobin and hematocrit, prolonged bleeding time, increased leukocytes in urine (laboratory results often are not available until just before surgery, and the nurse may be the first to see them; if results indicate the possibility of infection, most surgeons will appreciate being alerted before the child is prepared for surgery)	**The child will be free of detectable evidence of systemic infection at the time of surgery, as evidenced by** • Being afebrile • Showing no evidence of infection • Results of complete blood count and urinalysis within normal limits

Analysis: Nursing Diagnostic Statement 2

Response and Related or Risk Factors: ***High risk for injury: falls;*** *risk factor: the sedative effects of preoperative medications*

Projected Outcome: Environmental conditions will protect the child from injury during preoperative sedation.

(continued)

TABLE 23-7 *(continued)*

Defining Characteristics *(Actual Response)*	Nursing Interventions	Evaluation Criteria
Subjective: • Preoperative sedation administered Objective: • Sedation level that interferes with child's level of orientation and psychomotor function	Environmental Management: Safety; Fall Prevention **Institute safety precautions.** • Have the child bathe and void before administering the preoperative medication • Explain to the child and family the expected effects of the medication; caution them about the importance of the child's remaining in bed from this point on • Keep the siderails up; place the call bell, telephone, and urinal (or bedpan) within easy reach (to decrease the need to leave the bed) • Encourage family to stay with the child during this time; check back frequently	**The child will not experience a fall in association with preoperative sedation.**

Analysis: Nursing Diagnostic Statement 3

Response and Related or Risk Factors: ***High risk for aspiration;*** *risk factors:*

- Dislodging of a loose tooth during placement of an oral airway or endotracheal tube
- Vomiting during surgery
- Reduced level of consciousness
- Depressed cough and gag reflexes

Projected Outcome: The child will not aspirate secretions, vomitus, or any solids or fluids into the tracheobronchial passages.

Defining Characteristics *(Actual Response)*	Nursing Interventions	Evaluation Criteria
Subjective and Objective: • Vomiting during the surgical procedure • Signs of choking, gagging, wheezing, sternal retraction, and cough (secondary to event)	Aspiration Precautions **Implement measures to avoid aspiration.** • Assess for loose teeth; alert the anesthesiologist if any are reported or detected • Record the findings of teeth assessment on the preoperative check list • Prominently post NPO signs on the door to the child's room and on the bed • Enlist the help of family members by explaining the importance of this precaution • Remove water and all food from bedside table	**The child will not experience foreign body aspiration, as evidenced by the absence of** • Choking, gagging, wheezing, or a cough (immediate) • Stridor, wheezing, sternal retraction, and cough (secondary to event)

TABLE 23-7 (continued)

Defining Characteristics *(Actual Response)*	**Nursing Interventions**	**Evaluation Criteria**
	• Withhold fluids postoperatively until gag reflex has been re-established • Suction secretions from oropharyngeal airway until consciousness and swallowing are re-established	

Analysis: Nursing Diagnostic Statement 4

Response and Related or Risk Factors: ***Ineffective airway clearance,*** *related to poor cough effort, associated with*

- Sedative effects of anesthesia and analgesics
- Incisional pain
- Inability to cooperate because of developmental level
- Inadequate preoperative explanations and opportunity to practice cough

Projected Outcome: The child will be able to clear secretions or obstructions from the respiratory tract to keep airway patent.

Defining Characteristics	**Nursing Interventions**	**Evaluation Criteria**
Subjective and Objective: • Adventitious lung sounds • Tachypnea • Dyspnea • Tachycardia • Pallor of skin and mucous membranes	*Airway Management: Cough Enhancement; Chest Physiotherapy* **Monitor for evidence of ineffective airway clearance** every 2–4 hours, depending on postoperative status. **Institute strategies to promote airway clearance.** • Preoperatively, teach techniques for splinting incision, deep breathing, coughing, and use of incentive spirometer or blow bottles • Allow the infant or toddler to cry for a few seconds before comforting (this will ensure deep breathing in a child too young to cooperate; if secretions are present, coughing will follow the deep breaths as a reflex action) • Plan deep breathing and coughing efforts to correspond with peak effects of pain medication *Alert the physician* if evidence develops of impaired gas exchange (change in mental status, restlessness, cyanosis, dyspnea, increasing tachycardia, decrease in oxygen saturation [as monitored by pulse oximetry]).	**The child will experience effective airway clearance, as evidenced by** • Clear lung sounds • Pulse and respirations within normal limits • Mucous membranes pink, skin color normal for race

(continued)

TABLE 23-7 *(continued)*

Analysis: Nursing Diagnostic Statement 5

Response and Related or Risk Factors: ***High risk for altered tissue perfusion: systemic;*** *risk factors:*

- Hypovolemia associated with postoperative hemorrhage
- Pooling of blood in lower extremities associated with immobility

Projected Outcome: The child will maintain adequate nutrition and oxygenation of the cells to maintain capillary blood supply.

Defining Characteristics *(Actual Response)*	Nursing Interventions	Evaluation Criteria
Subjective: • Restlessness Objective: • Increased pulse and respirations • Decreased blood pressure • Decreased peripheral pulses • Capillary refill >3 seconds • Decrease in urine output • Skin cool and pale • Possible external evidence of bleeding	Surveillance; Intravenous (IV) Therapy ***Monitor for adequacy of perfusion*** every 15 minutes initially, then at least every 4 hours during the postoperative period. Check under dressings as well as on top (blood that fails to be "wicked" into dressing will run under child). ***Initiate strategies to improve tissue perfusion.*** • Maintain IV replacement of fluids (to ensure adequate vascular volume) • Ensure frequent position changes; infants and small children usually move spontaneously if pain is relieved effectively; older children and adolescents can be encouraged to change position at least every hour and taught to alternately dorsiflex and extend the feet (to facilitate venous return) • Discourage prolonged sitting positions, raising the knee gatch in the bed, or pillows under the knees (these positions compromise vascular flow) • *Alert the physician* to any sudden or significant symptoms of a perfusion deficit	***The child will maintain adequate tissue perfusion, as evidenced by*** • Usual mental status • Normal vital signs • Palpable peripheral pulses • Capillary refill <3 seconds • Urine output ≥1 ml/kg/hr or 30–50 ml/hr for a child ≥30 kg (2 ml/kg/hr for an infant) • Skin warm and of normal color for race • Dressings dry

TABLE 23-7 *(continued)*

Analysis: Nursing Diagnostic Statement 6

Response and Related or Risk Factors: ***High risk for fluid volume excess;*** *risk factor: presence of IV fluid infusion in the immediate postoperative period, when increased antidiuretic hormone and aldosterone are being produced as part of the physiologic response to stress*

Projected Outcome: The child will not experience increased fluid retention and edema.

Defining Characteristics *(Actual Response)*	Nursing Interventions	Evaluation Criteria
Subjective: • Restlessness • Anxiety Objective: • Periorbital edema • Tachycardia • Dyspnea with grunting respirations and adventitious lung sounds	Fluid Monitoring ***Monitor for fluid volume excess*** hourly in the infant and small child (whose cardiovascular systems are least well equipped to handle a sudden bolus of IV fluid) and at least every 2 hours in the older child. (Periorbital edema is often present before alterations in vital signs. Note especially the dependent eye if the child is lying on a side. If noted early, the IV rate can be decreased before cardiovascular function is compromised.) Fluid Management; Intravenous (IV) Therapy ***Institute strategies to prevent fluid volume excess.*** • Use a graduated fluid chamber for IV administration • Use an infusion pump whenever possible • Monitor and record intake and output hourly on the graphic record (because of increased antidiuretic hormone and aldosterone, intake will exceed output during the first 24 postoperative hours; output <1 ml/kg/hr, however, may signal inadequate kidney perfusion associated with heart failure) • If the infusion pump does not have childproof controls, ensure safety by putting wide adhesive tape over the controls and keeping the pump out of the child's reach *Alert the physician* immediately to evidence of fluid volume excess.	***The child will not experience hypervolemia, as evidenced by*** • Absence of periorbital edema • Pulse and respirations within normal limits • Clear lung sounds • Hourly IV intake of no more than prescribed amount of fluid

(continued)

TABLE 23-7 *(continued)*

Analysis: Collaborative Problem 1

Response and Related or Risk Factors: ***Pain,*** *related to*

- Stimulation of sensitive nerve endings in the incisional area
- Abdominal distention associated with anesthetic and narcotic analgesics, immobility, and manipulation of bowels during surgery
- Fear and anxiety associated with surgical experience

Projected Outcome: The child (or parents) do not report the presence of severe discomfort or an uncomfortable sensation.

Defining Characteristics	*Nursing Interventions*	*Evaluation Criteria*
Subjective: • Irritability • Crying • Reports of pain *Objective*: • Changes in usual behavior • Obvious "guarding" • Increased pulse, respirations • Unusual lack of movement (see Table 25–2 for other potential pain behaviors by developmental age)	*Pain Management* **Monitor for pain.** • Expect the child to experience pain similar to that of an adult in a similar situation • Enlist the help of parents in detecting pain (although the parents' objectivity in this situation is as yet unproved) • Use the pain assessment tools and techniques detailed in Chapter 25 • Assess abdominal distention and bowel function every 4 hours **Institute pain-relieving strategies.** • If abdominal distention develops, encourage ambulation rather than medicating (narcotic analgesics decrease bowel motility; ambulation increases it) *Alert the physician* if the analgesic ordered fails to relieve the pain or if abdominal distention develops that is unrelieved by ambulation.	**The child will be free of prolonged periods of intense pain, as evidenced by** • Comfort indicated by child pain assessment tools • Physical activities that approach normal • Vital signs within normal limits • Abdomen soft • Bowel sounds present in all four quadrants within 48–72 hours (or as expected by condition)

Analysis: Nursing Diagnostic Statement 7

Response and Related or Risk Factors: ***High risk for infection;*** *risk factors:*

- Original illness or trauma
- Transmission of pathogenic organisms from the hands of client, visitors, or health care professionals
- Ineffective airway clearance
- Decreased immune response associated with the physiologic stress response
- Insufficient knowledge to avoid exposure to pathogens

Projected Outcome: Decrease the child's risk for being invaded by pathogenic organisms.

TABLE 23-7 (continued)

Defining Characteristics *(Actual Response)*	Nursing Interventions	Evaluation Criteria
Subjective and Objective: • The potential for infection exists if the original illness or trauma involved infectious organisms (e.g., an inflamed or ruptured appendix may lead to peritonitis; a deep puncture wound may lead to osteomyelitis) • The potential for nosocomial infection and respiratory infection always exists postoperatively • Inadequate primary defenses (broken skin, traumatized tissue, a decrease in ciliary action, altered peristalsis) and inadequate secondary defenses (decreased hemoglobin, leukopenia, suppressed inflammatory responses) • Invasive procedures, tissue destruction, and increased environmental exposure are risk factors that increase the potential for postoperative infection	*Infection Protection; Teaching: Individual/Family* **Monitor for signs of infection** at least every 4 hours (fever, lymphadenopathy, localized inflammation) **Institute and teach the client and family strategies to prevent infection.** • The importance of meticulous handwashing cannot be overemphasized; the hands of infants and toddlers should be washed for them by parents and nurses • Encourage compliance with respiratory therapy protocol, including frequent position change • Use sterile technique for dressing changes • Encourage optimal rest, nutrients, and fluids (to enhance the body's immunologic defenses)	**The child will remain free of infection in the postoperative period, as evidenced by** • Remaining afebrile • Incision free of purulent drainage, marked redness, or induration • Clear lung sounds • Negative cultures of wound aspirate and sputum

Analysis: Nursing Diagnostic Statement 8

Response and Related or Risk Factors: ***High risk for urinary retention;*** *risk factors:*

- Effects of anesthesia on the bladder muscle
- Manipulation of the bladder during surgery
- Abnormal voiding position

Projected Outcome: The child will be able to void within 8 hours after surgery and empty bladder completely.

Defining Characteristics *(Actual Response)*	Nursing Interventions	Evaluation Criteria
Subjective: • Sensation of bladder fullness *Objective:* • Inability to void within 6–8 hours after surgery • Bladder palpable above the pubis • Dribbling, residual urine	*Urinary Retention Care* **Monitor urinary status.** • Frequently ask whether the child feels the need to void; enlist the help of the family members (especially with the child who is developing modesty) • Palpate for bladder distention • Note fluid intake since preoperative void	**The child will not experience urinary retention postoperatively, as evidenced by** • The ability to void within 8 hours after surgery • The ability to maintain a urinary output of 1–2 ml/kg/hr (infant, 2 ml/kg/hr) • The absence of • Bladder distention on palpation

(continued)

TABLE 23-7 *(continued)*

Defining Characteristics *(Actual Response)*	**Nursing Interventions**	**Evaluation Criteria**
	Facilitate normal voiding. • If possible, place toilet-trained children in the normal voiding position; often they can be carried to the bathroom or allowed to use a potty chair at bedside • If positioning alone is insufficient, try running warm water over the pubic area, letting the child hear water run into a sink, or applying moderate pressure with the hand over the bladder area; or (if not contraindicated by condition), place your hand on the child's abdomen, tell the child to take a big breath and hold it and then to push away your hand by pushing out her or his abdomen (this will apply pressure from abdominal muscles to the area of the bladder) *Alert the physician* if the child has a distended bladder and is unable to void after 8 hrs	• Sensation of bladder fullness • Dribbling/frequent voids • Dysuria

tient cooperation for an extended time, such as radiation therapy, radiographic procedures, cast applications, and certain types of examinations.

Although evidence of postoperative psychologic disturbances has not been uniformly substantiated (Davenport & Werry, 1970), the induction of general anesthesia produces a stress reaction in most children. For the potentially adverse effects of the anesthesia/surgery experience to be minimized as much as possible, children must be prepared adequately. Because parents often represent the child's primary source of information, parental comprehension of anesthesia and surgery must be ensured (Kennedy & Riddle, 1989). Some institutions provide opportunities for a prehospitalization visit for the child and parents to be familiarized with the people and facilities. Parents are encouraged to stay with their child during this preparation period; their presence is comforting to the child and provides an opportunity for the nurse and family to become acquainted.

A history and nursing assessment are completed on admission, just as for any other hospitalization (see Chapters 17 and 21). On admission for surgery, special attention is given to gathering information about the child's and the family's understanding of the operation. In many institutions, parents may visit on a 24-hour basis and may spend the entire preoperative night in the hospital. When this is not the policy, parents are told what time the surgery will take place and are encouraged to arrive at least an hour before that time to allow time to visit with their child.

Preparation to Minimize Stress

Approaches to minimize stress for surgery and anesthesia are similar to those described for procedural preparation (see earlier) and for admission to the hospital (see Chapters 17 and 21).

Specific stresses associated with surgery identified by Wolfer and Visintainer (1975) include:

1. Admission time.
2. Withdrawal of blood for blood test.
3. The afternoon of the day before surgery.

4. Preoperative medication injection.
5. Before and during transportation to the operating room.
6. Return from the recovery room.

Developmental Considerations

Specific interventions, based on the child's developmental level, are used to support the child at these particular times and throughout the surgical experience.

Infants and Young Children

The impact of hospitalization on children is discussed in Chapter 21. Because infants and young children do not comprehend the meaning of an anesthetic, the stress they experience related to surgery is primarily related to the usual stresses of hospitalization. To a young infant, the most distressing aspect of hospitalization is separation from primary caregivers. Limited cognitive development in infancy precludes adequate psychologic preparation, so reducing the length of separation from the parents and familiar surroundings is most beneficial. Outpatient surgery has had a significant impact on reducing the length of child-parent separation.

As with infants, separation from parents poses a significant threat to preschool children because they are young enough to be dependent on their parents yet old enough to be aware of their separation from them. Another reason children in this age group are vulnerable to psychologic stress is that their defense mechanisms, which would help them cope with the stress, are limited, as is their comprehension of the need for their surgery. To allay some of the fears of separation, preschoolers should be encouraged to bring a favorite toy or blanket with them to the operating room. Parents should be encouraged to stay with their child in the immediate preanesthetic period and to be there as soon as possible after the child awakens. In some institutions, parents are encouraged to accompany their child for anesthesia induction as well as to stay during recovery. (See Research Issues: The Impact of Parental Presence During Procedures, in the section "Care of Children During Specific Procedures.")

The preschool child between 2 and 5 years of age is prone to numerous fears, most notably of mutilation and physical injury. Unable to understand the rationale for specific treatments and procedures and to distinguish between reality and fantasy, preschoolers need to be reassured that their operation will "fix" their tonsils, eyes, hernia, leg, or other body part. Preschoolers should be told that they will awaken after surgery in the recovery room and that different nurses and doctors will be caring for them. They should also be told which part of their body will hurt and where a bandage will be placed.

School-Age Children

School-age children seem to worry about the actual anesthetic. They are curious as to how they will go to sleep and fearful that they may awaken during the operation. "What if I'm not tired?" and "What if I wake up before the surgery is finished?" are common questions. Explaining that "anesthesia sleep" is a special kind of sleep caused by "medicines" that work even when the child is not tired and that the "anesthesia medicines" will not be turned off until the surgery is finished may help to dispel some of these fears. School-age children may welcome the opportunity to select the method of anesthesia induction, if a choice is suitable to the child's medical condition.

The concept of sleep itself may be anxiety-provoking to some children. Children who have been told that a dead person is "sleeping" or that a pet has been "put to sleep" may equate sleep with death. These children might view anesthesia sleep as permanent. Reassure them that anesthesia is a special type of sleep from which they will awaken at the completion of their surgical procedure. Comments from parents and the nurse about seeing the child after the operation are most reassuring.

Adolescents

Adolescents suffer intense anxiety over their self-image and identity. They are often concerned about what will happen to them while under the influence of anesthetics and may feel unsure of their ability to cope appropriately. It is important to assess their level of anxiety preoperatively.

Adolescents should be given information about their proposed anesthesia and surgery to reduce psychologic stress and enlist more cooperation. If their medical condition permits a choice, they should be allowed to select the manner in which anesthesia will be induced. They should be informed that monitoring is a routine aspect of anesthesia care and told which monitors will be applied before anesthesia induction. The nurse should describe the specific sensations the adolescent can anticipate as a result of the pharmacologic agents given. The adolescent should be informed that an airway tube will be inserted after the loss of consciousness to allow oxygen and additional anesthetics to be given, ensuring unconsciousness throughout the operation. Because only the surgical site will be exposed and the anesthetic will render them immobile as well as unconscious, adolescents can be assured that they need not fear doing or saying anything in the operating room that could cause them embarrassment.

Supportive Approaches

All patients scheduled to receive an anesthetic should be assessed, ideally by the person who will be administering their anesthetic. The purpose of the visit is twofold: (1) to gather pertinent medical data critical to safe anesthetic management and (2) to establish a rapport with the patient and parents as well as to communicate with the nurses caring for the patient. Because parental anxiety is often transmitted to the child, every effort is made to gain parental confidence by explaining the anesthetic procedure and the sequence of events to them as well as to the child. Patients scheduled for same-day surgery are not always afforded the benefit of a hospital visit before their scheduled procedure. These patients are often screened through a telephone call to their parents. Preanesthetic assessment of same-day surgery patients generally occurs just before the scheduled procedure. Children prepared the morning of surgery do not seem to suffer additional anxiety or posthospital behavioral upset, compared with those prepared the day before (Kennedy & Riddle, 1989).

Parents should be informed of the need to withhold oral intake from their child for a specified time before the anesthetic is received. Parents should be told that the purpose of the fast is to reduce the risk of gastric aspiration by eliminating particulate matter from the stomach and reducing the volume of gastric fluids. The precise time after which all oral intake should cease should be told to the parents at the preanesthetic assessment or, in the case of same-day surgery patients, during a preoperative telephone call or in written instructions. Parental support is critical for ensuring an appropriately fasted child.

The technique and agent used for induction of anesthesia should also be explained to the parents. At many institutions, the child and parents can also arrange for a tour of the recovery room to familiarize themselves with the room, to meet the nurses who will be caring for them, and to have recovery-related questions answered.

Honesty is mandatory in preparing children of all ages. The anesthetic procedure should be explained in language the patient can understand to dispel some of their fears and misconceptions. The nurse should be present whenever possible for at least part of the anesthetist's visit to be able to reinforce the explanations accurately.

A guideline for teaching is presented in Table 23–8. This can be adapted to the specific needs of a particular situation and institution.

Physical Preparation

Physical preparation of the child is also the nurse's responsibility. The child must have an appropriate identification bracelet on the wrist or ankle, and the bed is clearly marked. The nurse should check that all laboratory tests that were ordered have been done. Any abnormal laboratory results or unusual clinical findings (especially an elevated temperature) should be reported to the surgeon before surgery as soon as the results are obtained as well as be documented in the patient's record.

All children who are to receive an anesthetic must undergo a period of fasting before surgery to reduce the risk of pulmonary aspiration of gastric residue during anesthesia. The length of the period between oral ingestion and induction of anesthesia is based on the patient's age and should be specified in the preoperative orders. Studies (Nicholson et al, 1992; Sandhar et al, 1989; Schreiner et al, 1990) have resulted in liberalization of preoperative feeding orders to permit clear liquids ad libitum until 2 to 3 hours before induction of anesthesia. Solid foods (including milk and formula) are generally not recommended on the day of surgery except for infants. Infants 0 to 3 months of age are generally allowed formula up to 4 hours before induction. Not all anesthesia departments have adopted these more liberal nothing-by-mouth (NPO) guidelines for pediatric patients (Table 23–9).

The nurse should explain to the child and parents the reason for the fast and should make sure the child takes nothing by mouth, as ordered. On the morning of surgery, the child is given mouth care and again reminded that she or he is not allowed to have anything to eat or drink. Children have the usual NPO signs at the bedside, but they frequently wander around the unit and into the playroom.

Placing a broad piece of tape across the front of the child's gown with "I may not eat or drink" printed on it usually ensures that an uninformed adult will not break the preoperative fast.

It is helpful if, during breakfast, the parent or a nurse can engage the child in an activity in an area away from where other children are eating. If oral intake inadvertently occurs during the specified time the child is to be fasted, the nurse should notify the anesthesia staff immediately because this may necessitate the cancellation or postponement of the child's surgery.

Children should be properly prepared for the operating room before the premedicant is administered, if one is ordered. The child is bathed either at bedtime or early in the morning. Any special surgical preparations, such as washes and scrubs, are completed. The nurse then sees that the child is properly attired and, when applicable, that jewelry, makeup, nailpolish, and any prosthetic devices have been removed.

There is considerable variation in the use of preoperative medication; the decision is usually made by the nurse anesthetist/anesthesiologist. The appropriate use of premedication minimizes the emotional trauma inherent in having anesthesia and surgery (Bogetz, 1989). Because the oral route of administration has been shown to be safe and effective for preanesthesia sedation (Feld et al, 1990; Gutstein et al, 1992; Weldon et al, 1992) and because oral premedication is clearly more acceptable to children than intramuscular medication (Schofield & White, 1989), nurses

TABLE 23-8
Pediatric Psychologic Check List For Surgery

PATIENT'S NAME:

UNIT #:

ROOM #:

SERVICE:

DIRECTIONS:

- The following items will be covered before surgery or procedures
- All explanations will include parents or some other responsible person
- All explanations will consider the child's developmental level

1. Explain operation or procedure; have patient verbalize understanding
2. Explain and get return demonstration of coughing, deep breathing, and using spirometer or blow bottles; emphasize importance and rationale
3. Explain dietary limitations, if any
4. Explain preoperative and postoperative use of equipment, bandages, tubes, restraints; use pictures if necessary; provide opportunity for therapeutic play (see Chapter 17)
5. Explain about the "stretcher person," who wears green and will take the child to the operating room on a stretcher; explain that OR personnel also wear green suits and that someone will be with the child at all times; allow the child to play with OR hats, masks, gloves, and so on
6. Ensure child has security object to take to OR
7. Let child know that parent will wait close by for child's return
8. Explain about the method of inducing anesthesia. Emphasize that the doctor will wake the child up only when the operation is over; for those 7 years old and younger, anesthesia is administered via face mask; let child play with demonstration mask; for those at least 8 years old, IV medication is used
9. Explain about the recovery room and how the child will stay there until awake; emphasize that child will be cared for by special nurses wearing green
10. Explain postoperative care and events:
    - An IV will be running on return from OR
    - Nurse will monitor vital signs
    - Medication for pain is available as needed
    - Child will be requested to cough and deep breathe
11. Inform child of preoperative injections; be honest: it will hurt; tell child, if it is known, that he or she will *not* receive an injection (discussion about an injection should be introduced at the end of other teaching so that child's anxiety level about the injection does not interfere with other learning)
12. Allow child to select gift from the toy chest
13. Answer questions

COMMENTS:

should advocate for children by working with other team members to eliminate the use of intramuscular injections (see Chapter 25). If premedication is used, the decision may be based on one of the following:

1. To prevent excessive airway secretions.
2. To allay anxiety.
3. To reduce the trauma associated with separation from their parents.
4. To facilitate induction.

TABLE 23-9
Number of Hours Child Is Kept NPO Before an Elective Surgical Procedure

Age	Solid Foods and Milk	Clear Liquids
0–3 mos	4 hrs	3 hrs
Over 3 mos	6 hrs*	3 hrs

* Solid food is best avoided on the day of surgery.

If premedication is ordered, the nurse should instruct the older child to void before administering the medication. This is necessary to eliminate the risk of having a sedated child attempt to get out of bed to go to the bathroom and possibly fall and get hurt. Voiding at this time also decreases the risk of bladder distention during anesthesia.

After the child has been prepared, the medication is brought to the room. If the premedication is an oral medication, it is usually diluted in grape juice, apple juice, or cola syrup to camouflage the taste. The child should be told she or he is drinking medicine and instructed to drink the entire contents of the cup. If it is an injection, the child is told that it will hurt for a short time and then it will make her or him sleepy. Strategies to help the child cope with the injection are used as described earlier in this chapter. After the preoperative medication is given, the child is kept in bed with the siderails up or is quietly held in the parent's arms, whichever is most soothing to the child, to derive maximal benefit from the sedative effects of the medication.

Just before the child is taken to the operating room, the nurse should check again to be sure that the names on the chart, on the child, and on the bed coincide. The nurse must also see that the young child has a source of comfort to take along, such as a special blanket, teddy bear, or other security object.

A preoperative check list is usually placed on the front of the child's chart to ensure completion of all the nurse's responsibilities (Table 23–10). These lists vary according to hospital routines. As each item on the list is completed, it may be initialed or checked off.

If the child is asleep from the premedication, the parents should be discouraged from awakening the child to give a kiss or say goodbye. Medicated children may be disoriented, and arousing them will only add to their anxiety.

Anesthetic Management of Children

Although the nurses on the unit are not required to participate in the anesthetic management of their patients, an understanding of the anesthetic period provides nurses with information to answer both patient and parental questions and to provide safe postoperative nursing care. On arrival in the operating suite, the child is quickly examined by the anesthetist to determine whether any changes have developed since the preanesthetic interview (e.g., temperature elevation or change in sensorium). The chart is reviewed, and laboratory data not available at the time of the interview are checked. If a premedicant was ordered, the time it was administered and the effect of the drug are noted. Before the child is taken into the operating room, consent forms for surgery and anesthesia are checked to determine that they are properly signed.

In the operating room, anesthesia induction should proceed as quickly as possible. Unnecessary conversation and the opening of instruments should cease. Everyone's attention should focus on the child, and every effort should be made to eliminate stress before and during the induction of anesthesia.

If parents accompany their child for the induction of anesthesia, attention is given to the preparation and support of the parent. Parents must be prepared for the appearance of the child during induction and be given step-by-step explanations about the procedure before entering the operating room. Children

TABLE 23-10
Preoperative Care Check List

1. Vital signs are taken and recorded on the chart, preferably also on the preoperative check list. Temperature, pulse, and respirations are always recorded; blood pressure is usually taken on any child over 3 yrs, varying with child's condition and institution's policy. Any abnormal findings are reported to the surgeon, and a note is attached to the front of the chart drawing attention to such findings. The nurse should also record in the chart that the surgeon has been notified, including the time.
2. The child's height and weight are recorded on the chart and check list.
3. All preopertive laboratory tests are completed (including blood type and crossmatch, if ordered). Any abnormalities have been reported to the surgeon and the chart marked accordingly.
4. The child is assessed for allergies, and these are clearly marked on the chart.
5. All external objects are removed, such as ribbons, barrettes, glasses, contact lenses, and jewelry. Long hair is kept in place by a rubber band. Nail polish is removed.
6. The mouth is checked for braces and loose teeth. Braces are removed and given to parents. Loose teeth are brought to the attention of the anesthetist.
7. The ID band is correct and secure, and the crib or bed is marked correctly.
8. Child and parents should receive appropriate information and psychologic preparation (see Table 23–8).
9. The consent form (anesthetic and operative) is placed on the chart and correctly signed and witnessed.
10. All surgical preparation procedures are completed (e.g., skin preparation, enema, NPO maintained, nasogastric tube insertion).
11. The child has voided.
12. The child is bathed and has clean gown and underpants or diaper.

can become more upset by having anxious parents present during the induction (Bevan et al, 1990); therefore, every attempt is made to prepare the parents before the experience and to support them during the event. When parents were counseled as to their role of giving silent reassurance to their child while keeping calm during induction, successful outcomes were more likely (Turner, 1989).

Induction of Anesthesia

Many methods exist for the induction of anesthesia in infants and children. No one method is effective in all situations. In general, anesthetists employ the technique they are most familiar with and one that will provide a safe and rapid onset of unconsciousness. The methods frequently used include rectally administered drugs, IV induction, and mask induction.

Inducing sleep with rectally administered drugs is beneficial to frightened children (Schreuder, 1992) for it enables them to fall asleep in the arms of their parents. This procedure is done in a room just outside the operating room, thus eliminating separation anxiety. In addition to eliminating separation anxiety, the method avoids the use of needles or placement of a mask on a frightened child's face. The major disadvantage is that occasionally the child may have a bowel movement after the drug is administered. When the child is asleep, he or she is transported to the operating room by the anesthetist. Anesthesia induction continues with one of the volatile agents.

IV induction is common for adults and older children but less common in infants and small children because the anesthetist may not be able to find a suitable vein without causing significant pain. In some instances (e.g., a hemodynamically unstable child or a child with a full stomach), IV induction is the method of choice. EMLA cream, a topical mixture of lidocaine and prilocaine, can be applied to the hand before venipuncture to attenuate pain; however, pain-free venous cannulation depends on the elimination of both the anticipatory discomfort and the actual pain of skin puncture (Ehrlich et al, 1992).

A needle is inserted into a vein, usually on the dorsum of the hand, and anesthesia is induced with a barbiturate, ketamine, or propofol. Most anesthetists use plastic cannulas rather than metal needles to start IV lines because they are less likely to infiltrate. The child's attention should be diverted during the actual IV insertion and the extremity restrained gently but firmly. The most common IV induction agents are barbiturates and propofol. The onset of unconsciousness is rapid, usually 30 to 60 seconds, and the cardiovascular effects are minimal in an otherwise healthy patient. After the child loses consciousness, a mask is placed on the face; anesthesia proceeds with a volatile agent, narcotic, and muscle relaxant or a combination of agents and IV drugs to achieve the desired result.

The most common method of inducing anesthesia in the pediatric patient population is by placing a mask over the nose and mouth and having the child breathe a potent anesthetic. This technique is generally well tolerated by children and avoids injection. The most common agent is halothane. (See Table 23–11 for a summary of inhalation anesthetic agents.)

After the induction is completed, anesthesia is maintained throughout the operative procedure. This is accomplished with a variety of agents and drugs, depending on the child's condition, the type of surgical procedure, and the anesthetist's choice. The child's physiologic response to the anesthetic is assessed throughout the procedure; adjustments are made in technique and agents are administered on the basis of response. In addition, IV fluids and, when indicated, blood products are administered.

Emergence from Anesthesia

At the conclusion of the operative procedure, the anesthetic agents are discontinued. The patient's cardiac and respiratory status are assessed. The patient is extubated if blood pressure and heart rate and rhythm are within normal limits and if respiratory rate and tidal volume are adequate. The child should be positioned on the side on the transport stretcher to ensure a patent airway and reduce the likelihood of secretion aspiration. Cardiorespiratory stability should be determined before transporting to the recovery room. Supplemental oxygen during transport to the postanesthesia recovery unit is recommended to avoid potential hypoxia (Kataria et al, 1988).

Recovering from Anesthesia

The recovery room nurse's responsibility is to see that the child emerges safely from the anesthetic. All children should receive oxygen in the immediate postanesthetic period to prevent postoperative hypoxemia. Vital signs are monitored frequently. The nurse should alert the child's physician to any signs and symptoms of shock (decreasing blood pressure; increasing heart rate; weak, thready pulse; cool, clammy skin). Because children are prone to laryngeal and tracheal edema, especially after endoscopic procedures and endotracheal intubation, they must be carefully observed for signs of postintubation croup. Children with stridor should be evaluated by the anesthetist.

The operative site should be checked for bleeding, and any increased or continual bleeding is reported to the child's physician. Some children may become delirious during emergence from anesthesia. These children need to be restrained to protect them from harm. If a muscle relaxant or narcotic was used as part of the anesthetic, the child should be observed for signs and symptoms of respiratory depression, which may be caused by narcotics or the inadequate reversal of muscle relaxants.

TABLE 23-11
Inhalation Anesthetic Agents

Nitrous Oxide (N_2O)

A weak anesthetic agent, because minimal alveolar concentration requirements cannot be achieved at atmospheric pressure

It is used frequently in pediatric anesthesia for its analgesic properties, reducing the dose requirements of the more potent inhalation anesthetics

Induction and recovery are rapid

Myocardial and respiratory depression is minimal

It is contraindicated in patients with closed air-containing spaces (i.e., pneumothorax), because the solubility difference between nitrous oxide and nitrogen would result in expansion of the space

Halothane

Introduced in 1956, this remains the most popular of the potent inhalation agents in pediatric anesthesia because of wide patient acceptance, ease of administration, and rapid onset of action and emergence

Circulatory depression occurs because of direct myocardial depression and suppression of normal baroreceptor-mediated tachycardia, an effect that can be minimized by administering atropine; it depresses airway reflexes and is a potent bronchodilator, which makes it particularly useful in asthmatic patients

A relatively poor analgesic agent; administration is often combined with nitrous oxide or narcotics

It sensitizes the myocardium to exogenous catecholamines; it decreases cerebral metabolic requirements for oxygen but increases cerebral blood flow, resulting in elevation of intracranial pressure

Enflurane

Introduced in 1973, induction times are generally longer with enflurane than with halothane because breath holding is more likely to occur, causing a prolonged period of excitement

Enflurane produces a dose-dependent, reversible depression of myocardial contractility, although bradycardia does not usually occur as with halothane; peripheral vasodilation is greater then with halothane; arrhythmias are less common because it is less sensitizing to the myocardium in the presence of exogenous catecholamines

It is a most potent respiratory depressant; it also decreases airway resistance

Because central nervous system seizure activity has been noted with higher concentrations and/or hypocarbia, it is generally avoided in patients with a seizure history

Skeletal muscle relaxation is greater, compared with halothane, and may reduce the requirement of muscle relaxants

There is evidence in adults that prolonged administration produces inorganic fluoride ion, which may cause a defect in urine-concentrating ability; this possible action may preclude its use in patients with compromised renal function

Isoflurane

Introduced in 1981, its use in pediatrics is limited by its pungent aroma and irritant effect on the airway, resulting in increased secretions, coughing, and laryngospasm during inhalation induction

Cardiac output is generally maintained because the decrease in systemic vascular resistance is offset by an increase in heart rate; it does not sensitize the heart to catecholamines

It is similar to enflurane in producing skeletal muscle relaxation

A significant advantage is its use in neurosurgical patients

It produces smaller increases in cerebral blood flow, compared with halothane or enflurane, that are more readily reversed by passive hyperventilation

It undergoes limited metabolism, and hepatic and renal toxic effects have not been reported to date

Desflurane

The first new volatile anesthetic in 20 years

Its use as an induction agent in pediatrics is doubtful, given its pungency and high incidence of airway irritability, including coughing, excessive secretions and laryngospasm

It produces hemodynamic effects similar to isoflurane (i.e., increases heart rate and decreases both mean arterial pressure and systemic vascular resistance while maintaining cardiac output)

It produces a dose-related decrease in tidal volume and depresses neuromuscular contractility

One of its heralded advantages is a rapid emergence; halothane induction followed by desflurane maintenance may become popular in pediatric patients

Sevoflurane

An anesthetic that is used in some countries. Widespread use and FDA approval are not anticipated in the U.S. at the time of this writing

A potent anesthetic with a nonirritating odor, making it useful for inhalation induction

Less hemodynamic effects, compared with halothane, in spontaneously ventilating animals (Crawford, 1992)

Has an effect similar to isoflurane on blood pressure but less of an effect on heart rate

Undergoes significant biotransformation

More rapid emergence, compared with halothane, resulting in an early need for analgesics in postanesthesia recovery unit (Eger, 1987)

Associated with a low incidence of vomiting

As children awaken from the anesthetic, their perception of pain increases. The need for postoperative analgesia should be assessed by the recovery room nurse. Adequate medication to control pain should be ordered and administered as needed. (See Chapter 25 for pain management.)

Postanesthesia Recovery

In the postanesthesia recovery unit, the anesthetist transfers the care of the child to a nurse experienced in caring for children recovering from anesthesia. The nurse is given a report on the surgical procedure that was performed, the child's physical and psychologic preoperative status, the type of anesthetic that was administered, and the response to the anesthetic agent. The recovery room nurse is always informed of all fluids and blood or blood products that were administered intraoperatively and any additional medication that was given (e.g., antibiotics) as well as the dose and time of administration. If the parents have been with their child during induction or recovery, a report should also be given on the parents' response to the experience.

If parents stay with their child during recovery, they should be given some assistance in how to be supportive of their child. An explanation is given to the parents of what is to be expected in their child's responses. Parents need to be assured that the behaviors are normal for the postanesthesia state.

Discharge from the recovery unit occurs when the child's condition is stable and predetermined discharge criteria are met. With use of a scoring system, such as shown in Table 23–12, children are discharged from the recovery unit to an inpatient general care unit when they have attained a score between 8 and 10. Children with scores less than 7 are discharged from the recovery unit if they are to be admitted to an intensive care or moderate care unit. Children whose preoperative status precludes attainment of a postanesthesia recovery score of 8 to 10 may be discharged when they have returned to their normal preanesthetic state. If a child is fully awakened from the anesthetic but the medical condition warrants additional monitoring, arrangements should be made to have the parents visit with the child in the recovery room to alleviate both parental and child anxiety caused by separation.

For every patient, the anesthetist should perform a postanesthesia assessment and document it on the patient's chart within 24 hours of discharge from the recovery unit. Any untoward developments related to the anesthetic should be noted and appropriate interventions initiated. If the recovery from anesthesia was uneventful and the patient's condition is stable, no further follow-up by the anesthetist is warranted.

TABLE 23-12
Postanesthesia Recovery Score System

	Criteria	Score
Color	Pink	2
	Pale/dusky/mottled	1
	Cyanotic	0
Airway	Clear	2
	Airway in place	1
	Obstruction/requires attention	0
Ventilation	Exchanging well	2
	Diminished	1
	Unresponsive	0
Level of consciousness	Fully awake	2
	Arousable	1
	Unresponsive	0
Movement of extremities	Purposeful/appropriate for age	2
	Involuntary	1
	No movement	0
	TOTAL	

Courtesy of C. S. Mott Children's Hospital Postanesthesia Recovery Unit, Ann Arbor, Michigan.

Postoperative Nursing Care

The nurse's responsibility in caring for a child postoperatively is multifaceted. The nurse needs to know about the effects of anesthesia, the type of surgery performed, and the effect of the experience on the child and family. The nurse also must be skilled in the various nursing procedures that must be performed and in watching for postoperative complications.

Before a child returns to the room, the nurse should have received a thorough report on his or her status. This report should contain information regarding

1. Type of operation performed and anesthesia and medication received.
2. Amount of blood loss.
3. Stability of vital signs.
4. Presence of drains, dressings, or appliances.
5. Whether the child has voided.
6. The presence, rate, and site of the IV line.
7. Presence of cough and gag reflex.
8. Level of consciousness.
9. Any difficulties encountered during surgery.
10. Any concerns expressed by the child or parents just before or since the operation.
11. What the family has been told by the surgeon regarding the success of the operation.
12. Need for any special equipment, such as mist tent, oxygen tent, cardiac monitor, or suction machine.

When the child returns to the unit, the nurse should attend to the patient immediately. The person transporting the child cannot leave until the nurse is in attendance. An immediate general assessment is done, observing the IV site, the child's color and respirations, the level of consciousness, the pain status, dressings, any tubes or drains, and the tightness of any restraints. Preferably, the nurse has immediate access to the postoperative orders and can review them at the bedside before beginning a more detailed assessment. Vital signs are then taken, and the nurse should check that the proper IV solution is being delivered at the proper rate. The patient is assessed every 15 minutes for vital signs, level of consciousness, condition and intactness of dressing, and functioning of any other tubes or appliances. The frequency of checking vital signs varies according to the surgeon's order or the policy established within the institution. A general guideline is every 15 minutes for 1 hour, or until stable, then every 4 hours during the first postoperative night.

The nurse's assessment of the child's general status is just as important as checking vital signs. For example, it is expected that in the event of hemorrhage, a change in the saturation of a patient's dressing will be noted before a change in the patient's vital signs.

Although specific postoperative care varies according to the child's age and type of operation, many aspects of care are similar regardless of these factors. Accurate monitoring of fluid and electrolyte balance is a primary nursing responsibility. Potassium should not be added to the IV solution until the child has voided (see Chapter 26). Accurate intake and output records should be kept during IV infusion, even if there is no specific order to do so.

Assessment and management of pain in children is another important aspect of postoperative care. That children require proportionately less pain medication than adults is a myth; the difference may be that the child is less able to communicate the pain. Irritability and a lowered frustration tolerance are common in children who have pain. Facial grimacing, crying, muscle rigidity, clenching of fists, and twisting and turning away from the painful stimulus are all indicators of pain. A physiologic response of elevated vital signs or pallor can also occur. In some cases, pain may cause enough fatigue so that the child finally goes to sleep. The nurse should observe for such signs of pain in addition to asking a child who can communicate about the sensation of pain. (See Chapter 25 for an in-depth discussion of pain management.)

Painful procedures and activities can be done in conjunction with the administration of pain medication. Coughing and deep breathing, change of position, and early ambulation are common postoperative activities that may cause pain. Giving medication 10 to 15 minutes before carrying out these procedures may increase the child's ability to cooperate. Pain medication is not necessarily given every time a procedure is performed, but nursing care should be adapted whenever possible to allow procedures to be done at the time pain medication has become most effective.

As soon as the nurse has read the postoperative orders, he or she should explain the required care to the parents and child. Parents can help watch the child and assist in the assessment of the child's pain level. They can also assist with coughing and deep breathing, introduction of fluids, positioning, and ambulation. Care by parents is a great asset to the child; therefore, parents should be given adequate explanations immediately postoperatively to make them feel comfortable in assisting with care.

Regardless of the type of operation, the nurse plays an important role in coordination of postoperative care. Parents frequently ask questions that must be answered by the surgeon. The nurse can reduce their anxiety by telling them how to contact the surgeon or making the telephone call for them. Questions that can be answered by the nurse should be answered promptly. Involvement of the parents throughout the postoperative course prepares them for an easier transition when it is time to take the child home.

The nurse should always clarify when the child should return to the physician's office or clinic, how to give medications and their major side effects, how to perform any procedures to be done at home, and what restrictions in activity or diet, if any, should be followed. The nurse assesses the type of care and support that is needed at home and makes a referral to agencies that may assist the family as necessary.

Same-Day Surgery

Same-day surgery reduces the stress caused by separation and staying in an unfamiliar environment. Children enter the hospital in the morning, have surgery, and return home on the same day. The introduction of this practice increases the need for excellent communication between the family's physician and the same-day surgery unit in the hospital. It is important for the nurse to be familiar with the patient's instructional needs after each type of operation because of the short time available in which to teach the family. Careful preoperative teaching is essential to ensure the patient is prepared for self-care at discharge. In these circumstances, written information given to the patient preoperatively is particularly appropriate. Nurses in the community also need to be prepared to provide the necessary follow-up care with special skills in postoperative assessment and management.

KEY CONCEPTS

Concepts Related to Basic Information

- In addition to parental permission, children 7 years of age and older must give their assent for participation in research.

- The hospital is a strange environment to the child and parent, with unfamiliar and potentially dangerous supplies and equipment (needles, needle caps, slippery floors, wall outlets, IV poles and machines, toys, bedrails, bathtubs).
- A procedure that seems routine to a nurse may be perceived as an intrusion by a child who is uninformed and fearful.
- A throat swab is not done if epiglottitis is suspected, because the trauma could cause edema and airway occlusion.
- Universal Precautions is an approach that assumes all patients to be infectious for HIV and other blood-borne pathogens.
- If parents stay with their child during the induction of anesthesia and during recovery, they require special preparation before the experience and support during the events.
- A prehospitalization visit provides an opportunity for the child and parents to become familiar with the environment and people.
- Same-day surgery is now a common practice that reduces the fears associated with being left in an unfamiliar environment.

Concepts Related to Nursing Assessment

- Factors to assess that affect teaching outcomes include learning needs, child and family personal resources, anxiety level of the child and parents, family relationships, lifestyle and cultural patterns, coping styles, and developmental level of the child.
- An important factor in taking an accurate blood pressure is the size of the cuff: too narrow a cuff results in a falsely high reading, and too large a cuff causes a falsely low reading.
- Assessment of whether a child requires restraints is a nursing role and should involve the parents.
- A temperature above 38° C (100.4° F) orally or above 38.8° C (101.8° F) rectally is a fever.
- Assessment of fever should include level of temperature, pattern of fever, behavioral changes, and appetite as well as laboratory data.
- Thorough assessment of the child's physical and psychologic condition preoperatively is the nurse's responsibility and is generally ensured by the use of check lists on the front of the chart.

Concepts Related to Nursing Intervention

- Teaching is adapted to a particular child's and family's coping style, which is to *approach* a situation actively or to use an *avoidance* tactic.
- Every child must be clearly identified by an identification band and a label on the child's bed.
- When parents participate in the care of their children in the hospital, it remains the nurse's responsibility to ensure that children are kept safe and receive the proper care.
- Parents need to be given some choice in the amount of care they wish to take on while their child is hospitalized; the care of a sick child may be stressful to a parent who may need a reprieve.
- Procedures should be done in the treatment room so that other children do not observe the trauma and so that the child's bed is seen as a safe place in the child's mind.
- If a child requires restraints, interventions should be directed at (1) increasing the child's sense of power and control, (2) providing diversional activities, and (3) maintaining joint mobility, muscular strength, and circulation.
- Proper handwashing is the most important precaution to take for all conditions and for all persons entering and leaving a patient's room.
- Needles are not recapped or broken to avoid accidental puncturing of oneself.
- Nurses should advocate for children not to receive intramuscular injections.

REFERENCES

American Academy of Pediatrics, Committee on Infectious Diseases (1991). *Red book* (22nd ed.). Evanston, IL: Author.

Bevan, J. C., Johnston, C., Haig, M. J., et al. (1990). Preoperative parental anxiety predicts behavioural and emotional responses to induction of anaesthesia in children. *Canadian Journal of Anaesthesiology, 37,* 177–182.

Bloom, B. S. (1956). *Taxonomy of educational objectives: The classification of educational goals, Handbook I: Cognitive domain.* New York: David McKay.

Bogetz, M. S. (1989). Anesthesia for pediatric outpatient surgery. *Pediatrician, 16,* 45–55.

Broeder, J. (1985). School-age children's perceptions of isolation after hospital discharge. *Maternal-Child Nursing Journal, 14*(3), 153–174.

Chamberlain, J. M., Grandner, J., Rubinoff, J. L., Klein, B. L., Waisman, Y., & Huey, M. (1991). Comparison of a tympanic thermometer to rectal and oral thermometers in a pediatric emergency department. *Clinical Pediatrics, 30*(Suppl. 4), 24–29.

Crawford, M. W., Lerman, J., Saldivia, V., & Carmichael, F. J. (1992). Hemodynamic and organ blood flow responses to halothane and sevoflurane anesthesia during spontaneous ventilation. *Anesthesia and Analgesia, 75,* 1000–1006.

Davenport, H. T., & Werry, J. S. (1970). The effect of general anesthesia, surgery, and hospitalization on the behavior of children. *American Journal of Orthopsychiatry, 40,* 806–824.

Davis, K. (1993). The accuracy of tympanic temperature measurement in children. *Pediatric Nursing, 19*(3), 267–272.

Deatrick, J. A., Woodring, B. C., & Tollefson, T. L. (1990). Children should be seen and heard: Chronically ill children should have a voice in treatment decisions. *Health Progress, 71*(3), 76–79.

Eger, E. I. II, & Johnson, B. H. (1987). Rates of awakening from anesthesia with I-653, halothane, isoflurane, and sevoflurane: A test of the effect of anesthetic concentration and duration in rats. *Anesthesia and Analgesia, 66,* 977–982.

Ehrlich, I. K., Lerman, J., Sikich, N., & Macpherson, B. (1992). Efficacy of EMLA (Eutectic Mixture of Local Anesthetic) cream for venipuncture in children. *Anesthesia and Analgesia, 74,* S82.

Feld, L. H., Negus, J. B., & White, P. F. (1990). Oral midazolam preanesthetic medication in pediatric patients. *Anesthesiology, 73,* 831–834.

Fruthaler, G. J. (1985). Fever in children: Phobia vs facts. *Hospital Practice,* 20(11A), 49–53.

Greydanus, D. E., & Patel, D. R. (1991). Consent and confidentiality in adolescent health care. *Pediatric Annals, 20*(2), 80–84.

Gutstein, H. B., Johnson, K. L., Heard, M. B., & Gregory, G. A. (1992). Oral ketamine preanesthetic medication in children. *Anesthesiology, 76,* 28–33.

Haddock, B. J., Merrow, D. L., & Vincent, P. A. (1988). Comparisons of axillary and rectal temperatures in the preterm infant. *Neonatal Network, 6*(5), 67–71.

Hallenbeck, A. R., et al. (1980). Children with serious illness: Behavioral correlates of separation and isolation. *Child Psychiatry and Human Development, 11*(1), 3–11.

Hogue, E. E. (1989). Consent for minors. *Pediatric Nursing, 15*(4), 404.

Holtzclaw, B. J. (1990). Shivering: A clinical nursing problem. *Nursing Clinics of North America, 25*(4), 977–986.

Kataria, B. K., Harnik, E. V., Mitchard, R., Kim, Y., & Admed, S. (1988). Postoperative arterial oxygen saturation in the pediatric population during transportation. *Anesthesia and Analgesia, 67,* 280–282.

Kennedy, C. M., & Riddle, I. I. (1989). The influence of the timing of preparation on the anxiety of preschool children experiencing surgery. *Maternal-Child Nursing Journal, 18,* 117–132.

Kleinman, M. B. (1984) Fever. In M. Green & R. J. Haggert (Eds.), *Ambulatory Pediatrics: Vol. 3* (pp. 106–111). Philadelphia: WB Saunders.

Lohr, J., Donowitz, L., & Dudley, S. (1989). Bacterial contamination rates in voided urine collections in girls. *Journal of Pediatrics, 114*(1), 91–93.

Lybrand, M., Bedoff-Cooper, B., & Hazard-Munro, B. (1990). Periodic comparisons of specific gravity using urine from a diaper and collecting bag. *MCN: American Journal of Maternal Child Nursing, 15,* 238–239.

Lynn, M. R. (1986). Children have rights, too. *Journal of Pediatric Nursing, 1*(5), 345–348.

Martyn, K. K., Urbano, M. T., Hayes, J. S., von Windeguth, B., & Sherrin, T. (1988). Comparison of axillary, rectal and skin-based temperature assessment in preschoolers. *Nurse Practitioner, 13*(4), 31–32, 34–36.

Muma, B. K., Treloar, D. J., Wurmlinger, K., Peterson, E., & Vitae, A. (1991). Comparison of rectal, axillary, and tympanic membrane temperatures in infants and young children. *Annals of Emergency Medicine, 20*(1), 64–67.

Newbold, J. (1991). Evaluation of a new infrared tympanic thermometer: A comparison of three brands. *Journal of Pediatric Nursing, 6*(4), 281–283.

Newman, J. (1985). Evaluation of sponging to reduce body temperature in febrile children. *Canadian Medical Association Journal, 132,* 641–642.

Nicholson, S. C., Dorsey, A. T., & Schreiner, M. S. (1992). Shortened preanesthetic fasting interval in pediatric cardiac surgical patients. *Anesthesia and Analgesia, 74,* 694–697.

Ogren, J. M. (1990). The inaccuracy of axillary temperatures measured with an electronic thermometer. *American Journal of Diseases of Children, 144*(1), 109–111.

Pidgeon, V. A. (1967). *Concepts of the rationale of isolation technique.* ANA Clinical Sessions (pp 21–27). Norwalk, CT: Appleton-Century-Crofts.

Reams, P. K., & Deane, D. M. (1988). Bagged versus diaper urine specimens and laboratory values. *Neonatal Network, 6,* 17–20.

Reeves-Swift, R. (1990). Rational management of a child's acute fever. *Maternal-Child Nursing Journal, 15*(2), 82–85.

Saez-Llorens, X., et al. (1989). Bacterial contamination rates for non–clean catch and clean catch midstream urine collections in uncircumcised boys. *Journal of Pediatrics, 114*(1), 93–95.

Sandhar, B. K., Goresky, G. V., Maltby, J. R., & Shaffer, E. A. (1989). The effect of oral liquids and ranitidine on gastric fluid volume and pH in children undergoing outpatient surgery. *Anesthesiology, 71,* 327–330.

Schmitt, B. D. (1984). Fever in childhood: 2. *Pediatrics, 74*(5), 929–936.

Schofield, N. M., & White, J. B. (1989). Interrelations among children, parents, premedication, and anaesthetists in paediatric day stay surgery. *British Medical Journal, 299*(6712), 1371–1375.

Schreiner, M. S., Triebwasser, A., & Keon, T. P. (1990). Ingestion of liquids compared with preoperative fasting in pediatric outpatients. *Anesthesiology, 72,* 593–597.

Schreuder, M. (1992). Anaesthesia without tears. *South African Medical Journal, 81,* 317–318.

Stebor, A. (1989). Post-urination time and specific gravity in infant's diapers. *Nursing Research, 38*(4), 244–245.

Teele, D. W., et al. (1979). Unsuspected bacteremia in young children. *Pediatric Clinics of North America,* 20, 773.

Thurber, F. W., Deatrick, J. A., & Grey, M. (1992). Children's participation in research: Their right to consent. *Journal of Pediatric Nursing, 7*(3), 165–170.

Tinker, J. H. (1992). First new volatile anesthetic in almost 20 years. *Anesthesia and Analgesia, 75,* 51–52.

Treloar, D. (1978). Ready, set—no: Something is missing from pediatric pre-op operation. *MCN: American Journal of Maternal Child Nursing, 3,* 50–51.

Turner, L. M. (1989). *Nursing Times, 85,* 34–35.

US Department of Health and Human Services (1983). *Protection of human subjects: Code of federal regulations* (45 CFR, 46 Sub part D, pp. 15–17). Washington, DC: US Government Printing Office.

Weldon, B. C., Watcha, M., & White, P. F. (1992). Oral midazolam in children: Effect of time and adjunctive therapy. *Anesthesia and Analgesia, 75,* 51–55.

Wolfer, J. A., & Visintainer, M. A. (1975). Pediatric surgical patients' and parents' stress responses and adjustment as a function of psychological preparation and stress-point nursing care. *Nursing Research, 24,* 244–255.

Younger, J. B., & Brown, B. S. (1985). Fever management: Rationale or ritual? *Pediatric Nursing, 11*(1), 26–29.

BIBLIOGRAPHY

Abrams, L., Buchholz, C., McKenzie, N. S., & Merenstein, G. B. (1989). Effect of peripheral I.V. infusion on neonatal axillary temperature measurement. *Pediatric Nursing, 15*(6), 630–632.

Aho, A. C., & Erickson, M. T. (1985). Effects of grade, gender, and hospitalization on children's medical fears. *Journal of Developmental and Behavioural Pediatrics, 6*(3), 146–153.

Alexander, D., & Kelly, B. (1991). Responses of children, parents, and nurses to tympanic thermometry in the pediatric office. *Clinical Pediatrics, 30*(Suppl. 4), 53–56.

American Academy of Pediatrics (1989). *Report of the committee on infectious diseases.* Elk Grove Village, IL: Author.

Banco, L., & Jayashekaramurthy, S. (1990). The ability of mothers to read a thermometer. *Clinical Pediatrics, 29*(6), 343–345.

Barber, N., & Kilmon, C. A. (1989). Reactions to tympanic temperature measurement in an ambulatory setting. *Pediatric Nursing, 15*(5), 477–481.

Berg, A. T. et al. (1990). Predictors of recurrent febrile seizures: A meta-analytic review. *Journal of Pediatrics, 116*(3), 329–337.

Bliss-Holtz, J. (1989). Comparison of rectal, axillary, and inguinal temperatures in full-term newborn infants. *Nursing Research, 38*(2), 85–87.

Broome, M. E. (1986). The relationship between children's fears and behavior during a painful event. *Children's Health Care, 14*(3), 142–145.

Broome, M. E., & Endsley, R. (1989). Maternal presence, childrearing practices, and children's response to an injection. *Research in Nursing and Health, 12,* 229–235.

Broome, M. E., Lillis, P., & Smith, M. (1989). Pain interventions in children: A meta-analysis of the research. *Nursing Research, 38*(3), 154–158.

Burnstein, S., & Meichenbaum, D. (1979). The work of worrying in children undergoing surgery. *Journal of Abnormal Child Psychology, 7,* 121–132.

Centers for Disease Control (1988). Update: Universal precautions for prevention of transmission of human immunodeficiency virus, hepatitis B virus and other bloodborne pathogens in health care settings. *Morbidity and Mortality Weekly Report, 37*(24), 377–387.

Centers for Disease Control (1989). Guidelines for prevention of transmission of human immunodeficiency virus and hepatitis B virus to health-care and public safety workers. *Morbidity and Mortality Weekly Report, 38*(S), 9–10.

Ehrhardt, B. S., & Graham, M. (1990, March). Pulse oximetry: An easy way to check oxygen saturation. *Nursing 90,* pp. 50–54.

Fradet, C., et al. (1990). A prospective survey of reactions to blood tests by children and adolescents. *Pain, 49*(1), 53–60.

Freed, G. L., & Fraley, J. K. (1991). Twenty-five percent "error rate" in ear temperature sensing device. *Pediatrics, 87*(3), 414–416.

Friedman, A. G., & Barton, L. L. (1990). Efficacy of sponging vs acetaminophen for reduction of fever. Sponging study group. *Pediatric Emergency Care, 6*(1), 6–7.

Garner, J. S., & Simmon, B. P. (1983). Guidelines for isolation precautions in hospitals. *Infection Control, 4*(Suppl.), 245.

Gillum, R. F. (1991). Resting pulse rate of children aged 1–5 years. *Journal of the National Medical Association, 83*(2), 153–158.

Iyriboz, Y. (1990). Oscillometric finger blood pressure versus brachial auscultative blood pressure recording. *Journal of Family Practice, 31*(4), 376–380.

Johnson, J. E., et al. (1975). Altering children's distress behavior during orthopedic cast removal. *Nursing Research, 24*(6), 405–410.

Joyner, M. (1988). Hair care in the black patient. *Journal of Pediatric Health Care, 2*(6), 281–287.

Katz, E. R., et al. (1981). Behavioral distress in children with cancer undergoing medical procedures: Developmental considerations. *Journal of Consulting and Clinical Psychology, 48*(3), 356–365.

Kilmon, C. A. (1987). Home management of children's fevers. *Journal of Pediatric Nursing, 2*(6), 400–404.

Lynn, M. R. (1986). Children have rights too. *Journal of Pediatric Nursing, 1*(5), 345–348.

Merritt, K., Sargent, J., & Osborn, L. (1990). Attitudes regarding parental presence during medical procedures. *American Journal of Diseases of Children, 144*(3), 270–271.

Newman, J. (1985). Evaluation of sponging to reduce body temperature in febrile children. *Canadian Medical Association Journal, 132,* 641–642.

Nix, K. S. (1991). Obtaining informed consent. In D. P. Smith, et al. (Eds.), *Comprehensive child and family nursing skills.* St. Louis: Mosby–Year Book.

Norman, E., Gadaleta, D., & Griffin, C. C. (1991). An evaluation of three blood pressure methods in a stabilized acute trauma population. *Nursing Research, 40*(2), 86–89.

Patterson, K. L., & Ware, L. L. (1988). Coping skills for children undergoing painful medical procedures. *Issues in Comprehensive Pediatric Nursing, 11,* 113–143.

Pidgeon, V. (1989). Compliance with chronic illness regimens: School-aged children and adolescents. *Journal of Pediatric Nursing, 4*(1), 36–47.

Reeves-Swift, R. (1990). Rational management of a child's acute fever. *Maternal-Child Nursing Journal, 15*(2), 82–85.

Rhodes, A. (1990). A minor's refusal of treatment. *MCN: American Journal of Maternal Child Nursing, 15*(4), 261.

Rozovsky, L. E., & Rozovsky, F. A. (1990). Consent to treatment: Four legal myths. *Canadian Critical Care Nursing Journal, 7*(1), 15–16.

Schlager, T. A., et al. (1990). Bacterial contamination rate of urine collected in a urine bag from healthy non–toilet-trained male infants. *Journal of Pediatrics, 116*(5), 738–739.

Shenep, J. L., Adair, J. R., Hughes, W. T., Roberson, P. K., Flynn, P. M., Brodkey, T. O., Fullen, G. H., Kennedy, W. T., Oakes, L. L., & Marina, N. M. (1991). Infrared, thermistor, and glass-mercury thermometry for measurement of body temperature in children with cancer. *Clinical Pediatrics, 30*(Suppl. 4), 36–41.

Snodgrass, W. R., & Dodge, W. F. (1989). Lytic "DPT" cocktail: Time for rational and safe alternatives. *Pediatric Clinics of North America, 36*(5), 1285–1291.

Suri, S. (1988). Simplifying urine collection from infants and children without losing accuracy. *Maternal-Child Nursing Journal, 13*(12), 438–441.

Talo, H., Macknin, M. L., & Medendorp, S. V. (1991). Tympanic membrane temperatures compared to rectal and oral temperatures. *Clinical Pediatrics, 30*(Suppl. 4), 30–33.

Vessey, J., Caserza, L., & Bogetz, M. (1990). In my opinion . . . Another Pandora's box? Parental participation in anesthetic induction. *Children's Health Care, 19*(2), 116–118.

Visintainer, M. A., & Wolfer, J. A. (1975). Psychological preparation for surgery pediatric patients: The effects on children's and parents' stress responses and adjustment. *Pediatrics, 56,* 187–202.

CHAPTER • 24

Pharmacologic Principles Applied to the Care of Children

Nancy Carter
John T. Wiernikowski
Mabel Hunsberger

RELATED TOPICS
Procedural preparations, Chapter 23
Mummy restraint, Chapter 23
Pain management, Chapter 25
Fluid and electrolyte maintenance, Chapter 26

LEARNING OBJECTIVES

- Describe the mechanisms of drug action in the body.
- Discuss the concepts of bioavailability, binding, and receptors.
- Describe the clinical effects that result when drugs interact with the same receptor, identical receptors located in different tissues, and different types of receptors.
- Discuss age-related differences in the absorption, distribution, metabolism, and elimination of drugs.
- Outline assessment criteria and nursing diagnostic statements pertinent to the administration of drugs to children.
- Identify nursing interventions that reduce fear, prevent injury, maintain tissue integrity, prevent discomfort, and maintain tissue perfusion when medication is given to children.
- Discuss age-appropriate techniques for administration of medication to children via the oral, nasal, inhalational, eye, ear, and rectal routes.
- Discuss nursing interventions that enhance family coping and growth.
- Outline special nursing responsibilities associated with intramuscular and intravenous administration of medication.

Getting better, in most children's minds, is associated with taking medicine. Children are introduced to medications like acetaminophen and certain antibiotics at a very young age. By 2 months of age, most children receive their first immunization, an event that many parents dread. When a more serious illness befalls a child, invasive techniques and drugs with a wide range of side effects may be required. What is most dreaded by the child is "getting a shot," and parents feel equally helpless when their child is overwhelmed with fear.

Today, injections for children are avoided whenever possible, but when an injection *must* be given, supportive techniques and a eutectic mixture of local anesthetics (EMLA) cream have greatly reduced the level of discomfort experienced by a child having an intravenous line started (Hopkins, 1988). Simultaneously, parents are given information about the drug and are involved in supporting their child during the experience.

Nurses play a key role in supporting the child and family and in decision making regarding the pharmacologic aspect of the plan of care. Although physicians *write* the order for drugs, the nurse is the one to *administer* them; therefore, the nurse has a legal responsibility to know that the drug is reasonable in kind, dose, and route for the condition and age of the child.

This chapter presents an overview of how drugs work in the body, the principles of safe administration of drugs, and practical suggestions about how to gain the cooperation of the child.

A child is completely dependent on the nurse to ensure that the right *medicine* is given in the right *dose,* to the right *patient* at the right *time* in the right way *(route).* The goal of all nurses is to meet these criteria each time a medication is administered while paying attention to the child's physiologic characteristics and psychologic needs.

Physiologic Factors

There has been a significant increase in knowledge about pediatric clinical pharmacology since the early 1970s. Much of the increase is related to pediatric pharmacokinetics, which is the study of drug absorption, distribution, metabolism, and elimination—in short, what the *body does to the drug.* Less information has been generated to bridge pharmacokinetics with pharmacodynamics, which is the study of the beneficial (or harmful) effect of a drug at a given blood concentration level—what the *drug does to the body.* In general, the disposition (i.e., pharmacokinetics) of a drug undergoes changes from the neonatal period, through infancy and into childhood, and finally to adulthood. Many of these changes can be related to changes in body composition, protein binding, maturation of metabolic pathways in the liver, and kidney function. To understand fully how the child's growth affects the disposition and actions of drugs, a review of some basic pharmacologic principles is necessary.

Principles of Drug Action

All drugs act at a cellular level to either promote (agonist drug) or disrupt (antagonist drug) some cellular activity. The choice of an agonist versus an antagonist depends on the pathophysiologic changes caused directly or indirectly by some disease process (e.g., insulin for diabetes, anti-inflammatory drugs for asthma or inflammatory bowel disease). It is generally accepted that all drugs initiate their effect by combining with a certain type of *receptor.* Many types of drug receptors have been identified and can be classified as regulatory proteins, enzymes, transport proteins (e.g., Na-K ATPase), or structural proteins. As such, drug receptors are found in every cell in the body, and the types of receptors found in any particular cell vary according to the type and/or function of the cell.

The binding of a drug to a particular receptor is only the first step in the action of the drug. The binding of a drug to a receptor forms a *drug-receptor complex.* The drug-receptor complex then initiates a series of complex biochemical steps (poorly understood for many drugs). These biochemical steps use putative "second messengers," such as cyclic adenosine 3',5'-cyclic monophosphate (a nucleotide), (cyclic AMP; cAMP), calcium, and magnesium, to ultimately bring about the clinically observed action of the drug. The relationships between drugs and various receptors can be quite complex; however, the following principles hold true for most drug-receptor interactions.

A receptor's affinity to bind a particular drug determines how much drug (i.e., concentration) is required to bind and form enough drug-receptor complexes to initiate a pharmacologic effect. Usually, increasing the drug concentration (e.g., by increasing the dose) at the receptor site (site of action) increases the magnitude of the pharmacologic effect. A maximal effect is seen at 100 per cent receptor occupancy. However, sometimes a maximum effect is seen at much less than 100 per cent, a concept often referred to as the "spare receptor phenomenon." Receptors are responsible for the selectivity of drug action. The molecular size, charge, and shape of a particular drug determine which type of receptor(s) it will bind with and the avidity of the binding. Thousands of different types of receptors are available to bind drugs in the human body. Any one drug will selectively bind to a few types of receptors more strongly than to others. As a result, any particular drug will produce both beneficial (therapeutic) effects and undesirable effects (side effects or toxicity).

The ratio of beneficial to undesirable effects of a drug is usually referred to as its "therapeutic index" and largely determines the clinical usefulness of the drug. For many drugs, the therapeutic index is favorable, yet for others (aminoglycoside antibiotics, anticonvulsants, anticoagulants, theophylline) the therapeutic index is low. For the latter drugs there is a narrow range of blood or serum concentrations within which the drug produces beneficial or desired effects. At concentrations below or above this beneficial range, the drug may produce, respectively, no therapeutic benefit or serious toxicities. Such drugs require routine measurement of blood-serum concentrations of the drug to maintain therapeutic benefits and avoid toxicity.

With these basics in mind, one can now examine some of the key factors that can influence the clinical effects of a particular drug in a child.

Route of Administration (Bioavailability)

As a rule, the intravenous (IV) route is the only route of administration that guarantees 100 per cent bioavailability. In general, bioavailability of a drug refers to the fraction of the administered dose that reaches the systemic circulation. More precisely defined, it also involves the time it takes for the drug to reach the systemic circulation. Other routes of administration (oral, buccal, rectal, subcutaneous [SC], intramuscular [IM], inhalational, topical) can have profound effects on the bioavailability of the drug and hence on the dose necessary to achieve a comparable clinical effect. Of course, properties of the drug can dictate the route of administration. Many antibiotics (aminoglycosides) are not absorbed when given orally and must be given by injection (IV or IM), whereas some drugs cannot be given by injection (acetaminophen) and must be given orally or rectally.

Protein and Other Nonspecific Binding

Once the drug reaches the blood stream, it may be "bound," to varying degrees, to plasma proteins such as albumin or nonspecifically to certain tissues (e.g., digoxin to skeletal muscle). The amount of drug bound at any one time is in equilibrium with the "free" drug, but only the free drug can interact with its relevant receptor.

Therefore, depending on the drug and the clinical circumstance, it may be necessary to measure a free drug concentration as opposed to the total (bound plus free) drug concentration that most laboratories provide.

Receptor Density, Location, and Drug Selectivity

As mentioned, virtually all drugs interact with more than one type of receptor, and the clinical effects can be classified into three broad categories.

Beneficial and Harmful Effects Mediated by Same Receptor

Beneficial or harmful effects mediated by the same receptor occur because of a direct pharmacologic extension of the therapeutic actions of a drug; for example, overanticoagulation with a drug such as heparin or warfarin results in bleeding (toxicity). Such events can be avoided by judicious alterations in dose and close monitoring of therapeutic effects via appropriate blood tests such as partial thromboplastin time (PTT) for heparin and prothrombin time (PT or INR*) for warfarin.

Beneficial and Harmful Effects Mediated by Identical Receptors Located in Different Tissues

The best example here is the use of glucocorticoid drugs such as hydrocortisone, prednisone, and methylprednisolone in clinical circumstances such as treatment for asthma, inflammatory bowel disease, and prevention of graft rejection in organ transplant patients. Glucocorticoid receptors are found on the

* International normalized ratio (INR) is being used increasingly to replace PT.

surface of a wide variety of cell types in the body, albeit in differing densities. Thus, administering one of these drugs with an anti-inflammatory or immune-suppressive intent produces the desired therapeutic effects by decreasing lymphocyte counts, neutrophil migration, and macrophage activity. Unfortunately, the glucocorticoid drugs interact with their receptor throughout the body and produce increased gluconeogenesis in the liver and increased lipogenesis in adipose tissue with net fat deposition. Catabolic effects in muscle and skin result in net protein wasting, increased mobilization of calcium from bones, and decreased absorption of calcium in the gut. These drugs also result in decreased growth in children (that is not responsive to growth hormone) and increased secretion of pepsin and acid by the stomach that may lead to ulceration.

Long-term use of drugs such as the glucocorticoids can be associated with significant adverse effects, all mediated by an identical receptor. Strategies to circumvent these adverse effects are to use such drugs in the smallest effective dose and for short periods of time. In the case of treatment for asthma, the use of inhaled steroids can provide high local concentrations of drug in the lung and achieve a good anti-inflammatory effect with minimal systemic absorption and attendant side effects.

Beneficial and Harmful Effects Mediated by Different Types of Receptors

As mentioned, many receptors can occur in more than one subtype: alpha$_1$, alpha$_2$, beta$_1$, beta$_2$ adrenoreceptors, histamine H_1 and H_2 receptors, serotonin S_1 through S_5 receptors, to name just a few. Often agonist or antagonist drugs for some of these receptors are not selective enough; for example, propranolol is a nonselective antagonist of beta receptors (i.e., beta-blocker). As mentioned, beta receptors occur in two subtypes: beta$_1$ receptors are found in high density in cardiac tissue, and beta$_2$ receptors are found in high density in the lungs.

Beta-blockers such as propranolol are useful for a patient post myocardial infarction in that antagonism of the beta$_1$ receptor by the drug results in a decrease in heart rate with a concomitant decrease in myocardial oxygen consumption (beneficial effects). If the same patient also has a history of lung disease (e.g., asthma, chronic obstructive pulmonary disease [COPD]), the beta-blocking drug also blocks beta$_2$ receptors in the lungs, resulting in bronchoconstriction and worsening of lung disease.

Drug Interactions

Drug interactions may alter the pharmacokinetics and/or pharmacodynamics of one (or more) interacting drug. Such interactions may result in changes in drug metabolism and elimination or drug absorption and distribution (e.g., changes in protein binding). Regardless of the nature of the change, ultimately there will be a change (increase or decrease) in the concentration of the drug at its receptor site and possibly a change in the pharmacologic effect observed. This necessitates a modification in drug dose and/or frequency of administration; however, in certain cases, stopping the drug or substituting another drug may be required (Bourne & Roberts, 1992).

Age-Related Differences

The goal of drug therapy is to produce the desired therapeutic effect in each child and to avoid toxicity. Variation in drug pharmacokinetics depends on age-related differences in body composition and the maturity of certain biochemical pathways in various tissues; an infant or child cannot be treated with drugs as a miniature adult. In the neonate, especially the premature infant, the physiologic immaturity results in a reduced *rate* of drug disposition (metabolism/elimination). By the age of 6 to 10 years, children utilize certain drugs twice as fast as adults do, but from this time until death the rate of drug disposition again gradually decreases (Pippenger, 1980).

It is not fully understood at what age a child's drug disposition patterns approximate those of an adult. However, drug utilization in children changes rapidly over a period of a few months at the initial onset of puberty. It has been suggested that increasing concentrations of sex hormones at this time result in a competition between sex steroids and drugs for metabolic sites in the hepatic microsomal enzymes (Pippenger, 1980).

Effect of Age on Absorption

Absorption is the process by which a drug passes into the body fluids, primarily the blood stream, which then carry it to its receptor site (site of action). The sites at which drugs can be administered are either intravascular (IV or intra-arterial) or extravascular (oral, sublingual, buccal, IM, SC, or rectal). In order for extravascularly administered drugs to reach the receptor sites, they must be absorbed. The absorption of most drugs is by passive diffusion across a concentration gradient, and is affected by the properties of the drug, the properties of the membrane it is crossing, the pH of the environment, and local blood flow (Roberts, 1984).

For a drug to be absorbed, it must generally pass through the lipid bilayer of the cell membrane, and this is best achieved if the drug remains in an unionized state. Because most drugs are either weak acids or weak bases, their ionization state can be changed by relatively minor changes in pH of the local environment. The oral route of administration is the most commonly used extravascular route of administration for most drugs, because it is convenient and the vast surface area of the gastrointestinal tract facilitates absorption of many drugs. Nevertheless, absorption of orally administered drugs is often delayed in neonates and young infants. This is primarily due to differences in the pH of their gastrointestinal tract and their reduced gastric motility.

Ionization of acidic drugs occurs in alkaline environments, and ionization of basic drugs occurs in acidic environments. Acidic drugs remain un-ionized in an acidic environment and therefore are better absorbed. Immediately after birth, gastric pH is high. By 4 months of age, gastric pH values have reached 50 per cent of the adult value, which is 1 to 3.5, and by 3 years of age, they are thought to reach adult levels (Yeh, 1985). Thus, the pH of gastric contents remains less acidic during infancy and early childhood. Acidic drugs, such as nalidixic acid, phenobarbital, and phenytoin, are therefore less well absorbed, because they are best absorbed from an acid environment. In contrast, the absorption of acid-labile drugs such as the penicillins may be enhanced (Morselli et al, 1980).

Reduced gastric motility in the neonate and young infant also affects absorption, because most of the absorption of orally administered drugs occurs in the small intestine and not in the stomach. Gastric emptying time in the neonate is 6 to 8 hours; by 6 to 8 months of age, it reaches the adult time of 2 hours (Howry et al, 1981). Prolonged exposure of certain drugs to the gastric contents can increase the risk of destroying unstable drugs. The reduced gastric motility and irregular peristalsis of the neonate and young infant can also be affected by the presence or absence of food (Milla & Fenton, 1983) and thus delay drug absorption and attainment of peak serum concentrations (recall the definition of "bioavailability").

Certain drugs (although absorbed by passive diffusion) have specific transport mechanisms that facilitate their absorption; the immaturity of intestinal transport mechanisms that carry medications to the blood stream can delay absorption of some drugs. Such drugs must be given less frequently in the neonate. For example, it has been shown that the older infant and adult can absorb riboflavin within 3 to 4 hours, whereas the neonate requires 16 hours for absorption, because riboflavin is absorbed by passive diffusion. Because the total amount of drug is eventually absorbed, overdose can occur when passively absorbed drugs are given for extended periods of time. Examples of drugs that are orally administered and absorbed slowly by the premature infant include chloramphenicol and erythromycin (Kagan, 1983). The osmolarity of the vehicle conveying the drug is also important to consider. For example, the high osmolarity of elixirs may cause diarrhea and thereby reduce drug absorption.

Rectal administration of a drug is an alternative that is used for the pediatric patient. Although information concerning the bioavailability of rectally administered drugs is limited, a few drugs are known to be effectively absorbed. Sodium valproate serum concentrations after oral and rectal administrations are comparable; a rectally administered solution of sodium diazepam is more rapidly absorbed than is an intramuscularly administered dose (Magnussen, 1979).

Absorption after IM or SC administration depends primarily on tissue perfusion in the area of administration. Absorption from IM or SC injection sites in the neonate is often reduced because of immaturity of blood flow to the various muscles and tissues and because of reduced muscle tissue and subcutaneous fat tissue (Yeh, 1985). Drug administration to the sick neonate is predominantly by the IV method to circumvent these absorption uncertainties.

Effect of Age on Distribution

After a drug is absorbed, it is carried by the blood to various organs and tissues of the body. Factors that influence distribution are composition of the body, that is, the size of the body water and fat compartments, and the quantity and binding capacity of plasma proteins to which drugs can bind.

The amount of water available in the body is an important variable determining the ultimate drug concentration achieved. In the preterm infant, total body water (TBW) constitutes 80 to 85 per cent of body weight; 75 per cent in the full-term infant; and 60 per cent (same as the adult) by the end of the second year of life. Thus, when a drug that distributes largely in total body water is administered to an infant in the same dosage (according to weight) as for an adult, lower plasma concentrations of the drug result because it is diluted by the larger proportion of body water. Consequently, the loading doses required to attain the desired plasma concentration of the drug are frequently proportionately higher in infants (Holbrook & Schaible, 1983).

Drug distribution also depends on plasma protein binding. Plasma albumin is the primary binding site for drugs. Neonatal albumin has a lower binding capacity for certain drugs (phenytoin, penicillin) compared with its binding capacity for bilirubin, although this has not been extensively studied (Udkow, 1987). (Neonatal albumin binds more bilirubin than does adult albumin.) In contrast, some drugs have an affinity for albumin (e.g., sulfonamide, warfarin, vitamin K) and compete with bilirubin for available binding sites. The competitive drug binding in the neonate increases the potential for the infant to suffer ill effects of increased concentrations of unbound, unconjugated bilirubin (Sheridan et al, 1982).

The type and amount of albumin affect binding capacity and drug disposition. The reduced capacity for neonatal albumin to bind certain drugs results in proportionately more free or unbound drug; however, the free concentration of the drug, which is a function of metabolic and elimination pathways, is probably affected very little. Thus, the clinical significance of the decreased binding capacity of neonatal albumin remains unclear. In addition, neonates—especially premature infants—may have low albumin concentrations (Udkow, 1987). This physiologic difference is compensated for by administering albumin to neonates when indicated. The variability in albumin drug-binding capacity in infants requires further research.

Effect of Age on Metabolism (Biotransformation)

Metabolism and excretion together make up the body's mechanism of eliminating drugs. Many drugs undergo metabolism to convert them into compounds that are more water-soluble for excretion via the biliary tract or by the kidney. In many instances, these compounds (metabolites) retain some pharmacologic (albeit weaker) activity. Still other drugs are inactive in their parent form and must be metabolized to an active form (e.g., prednisone, cyclophosphamide). A few drugs (penicillins, cephalosporins) are excreted largely unchanged.

Most biotransformation takes place within the liver, but it can also occur in other organs such as the lungs, kidneys, intestines, and skin. The liver metabolizes drugs through a series of reactions termed phase I (oxidation, reduction, hydrolysis) and phase II (conjugation reactions). Phase I reactions develop rapidly in the term infant and reach or exceed adult values by 6 to 12 months of age. Phase II reactions take slightly longer to mature, usually reach adult values by 1 year of age, and then continue to mature.

Children aged 2 to 6 years generally have a much greater hepatic drug-metabolizing capacity for certain drugs. After age 6 this capacity gradually declines to adult values by about puberty (Gladke, 1979). Thus, the immaturity of the liver in premature infants and neonates generally reduces the biotransformation of drugs, although this varies depending on the specific drug. Immaturity of the liver can result in prolonged excessive serum concentration of drugs and lead to drug toxicity in this patient population. Microsomal enzymes that metabolize chloramphenicol are particularly immature during the first 2 weeks. Chloramphenicol toxicity (known as the gray baby syndrome) is known to occur when the drug is administered to premature infants in a dosage based on body weight.

As mentioned, the rate of metabolism through early childhood may exceed adult values. For example, clearance rates for theophylline are low in infancy but increase fivefold by 4 years of age and then slowly decline over the years (Weinberger et al, 1981). Theophylline has also been shown to be metabolized to caffeine in the neonate. Both drugs (theophylline and caffeine) are methylxanthines with a similar pharmacologic action and, therefore, can produce toxicity through their additive effects, whereas adults rapidly metabolize theophylline to inactive metabolites (Yeh, 1985).

Another factor affecting drug metabolism is the relative change in hepatic size. A fetal liver is 4 per cent of total body weight, whereas the adult liver is 2 per cent of body weight. This helps explain why children eliminate many drugs more rapidly and have proportionately higher dosage requirements.

Effect of Age on Elimination

Urinary excretion is the major route of elimination for drugs and their metabolites; however, drugs also can be excreted in bile and feces. Although the kidney of the neonate has almost as many cells as the adult kidney, it does not function as a mature kidney. Glomerular filtration rates (GFR) and renal blood flow in the neonate are only 30 to 40 per cent of those in adults. Within the first 2 weeks of life, the GFR doubles in both preterm and full-term infants and reaches adult values at between 1 and 5 months of age.

Most drugs and their metabolites are filtered by the glomerulus in the kidney and pass into the urine. However, some drugs (i.e., penicillins) are actively secreted by the renal tubules into the urine. The tubular secretion mechanism is highly inefficient in infancy, and so in the infant, the penicillins excreted by both glomerular filtration and tubular secretion may have a half-life* 300 per cent longer than that of the adult (Howry et al, 1981). Tubule secreting abilities mature over the first few months of life and reach adult values at around 7 months of age (Giacoia & Gorodisher, 1975). Excretion of drugs is also affected by tubular reabsorption (absorption from tubule lumens back into the blood stream). The pH of the urine in the newborn infant is lower (more acidic) than that in the adult, which promotes reabsorption and prolongs the half-life of weakly acidic drugs. This occurs because acidic urine promotes non-ionization of acidic drugs, leading to greater reabsorption (Howry et al, 1981). The net effect of these immaturities is the potential for a drug to accumulate in the body, necessitating modifications in dose and frequency of administration of many drugs used in infancy.

Assessment

A large component of a child's fears in the hospital is associated with receiving medications, especially when a needle is involved. Much fear can be relieved by a nurse who approaches the child appropriately and gives medications properly. An important step is the careful assessment of the child's and family's needs for support and information about the drug. A child often needs to be assessed quickly to determine the best approach and technique. Parents can offer important information. Pertinent issues to address with parents before attempting to give any kind of medication include the following:

---

* The half-life of a drug is the length of time it takes for the concentration of the drug to decline by 50 per cent.

- What medications are taken at home? Does the child receive anything for sleep? Is the baby given gripe water? (Often parents do not consider home remedies to be medications; assessment of their use of these remedies provides a good opportunity for health teaching and home management of health problems.)
- Does the child have any allergies?
- How does the child usually respond to taking medication?
- How are medications administered at home, or how have they been given by other nurses (i.e., equipment used, child's position, drug being mixed with something)?
- What information has the parent given to the child about medication administration (should assess whether children have been told the truth, such as that needles may hurt, medications may taste bad, suppositories may be uncomfortable)?
- Has the child had any previous health care–related experiences with medications that might increase the child's fears?
- Will a parent be available to be with the child? (Leave the option open for parents not to stay, if that is their wish.)
- Is the child or parent familiar with the action, purpose, and potential side effects of the drug?
- Is there anything else the nurse should know about the child that is relevant to giving medications?

Simultaneously, the nurse makes a quick assessment of the appropriate technique to use for the situation and developmental level of the child: whether the child can swallow a capsule or requires liquid medication, and how and when to prepare the child for the medication. Some medications also require special assessments, such as checking a pulse before giving digoxin or assessing output before giving potassium chloride.

Nurses administer medications frequently and under a variety of circumstances: some are emergencies; others are routine. Sometimes the situation is administering a child's first injection; sometimes it is giving a medication with which both child and parent are familiar. In all circumstances, the nurse should prepare the child and family, involve the parents in the administration of the drug as appropriate, and respond to the individual needs of children and parents. The potential dangers involved in drug administration and the side effects of the various drugs are information fundamental to safe administration.

Nursing Diagnostic Statements

Nursing diagnostic statements applicable to most situations involving drug administration to children include the following:

Fear, related to

- *Previous negative experience associated with receiving medication.*
- *Separation from parents when receiving medication.*
- *Lack of relevant preparation for experience.*
- *Unfamiliarity of person giving medication.*
- *Too long a waiting period until injection is given, once told about it (i.e., if an injection is required because no other route is appropriate).*

High risk for injury; risk factor: inappropriate administration of medication, associated with

- *Inaccurate identification of patient.*
- *Inaccurate drug dose, time, or route.*
- *Excessive or inadequate restraint of child.*
- *Unsafe technique of administration.*
- *Inappropriate medication for child's condition.*
- *Failure to rotate sites.*

High risk for impaired tissue integrity; risk factor: damage by a chemical irritant (medication), associated with

- *Use of too short a needle for IM injection.*
- *Injection of too large a volume of medication at one site.*
- *Injection of too concentrated a medication into tissue.*
- *Injection of medication into an inappropriate site for age of child (i.e., gluteus maximus under age 6 years).*
- *Toxicity of drug.*

Altered tissue perfusion (cardiopulmonary), related to

- *Decreased cellular exchange associated with acute allergic reaction.*

Anxiety (child/family), related to knowledge deficit regarding

- *Mode of drug administration.*
- *Side effects of drugs.*
- *Purpose of drug.*
- *Pain, associated with.*
  - *Physical trauma by needle.*
  - *Tissue response to drug.*
  - *Anxiety associated with an unknown experience.*

Powerlessness, related to

- *Excessive restraint during medication administration.*
- *Lack of choice in procedure of medication administration.*
- *Lack of opportunity to be involved in decision making concerning medication regimen.*

Ineffective individual coping, related to

- *Inadequate support for developmental needs.*
- *Knowledge deficit regarding the procedure.*
- *Inability to understand explanations, associated with immaturity.*

Family coping: potential for growth, related to

- *Participation in decision making concerning child's drug regimen.*
- *Participation in preparing child for painful experience.*
- *Ability to give emotional support to child during painful experience.*
- *Involvement in providing child with diversional activity during a painful experience.*
- *Knowledge acquisition of side effects associated with child's medications.*

Planning and Implementation

Administration of medications requires skill and sensitivity from the nurse. The goal is achieving the task with the least amount of hurt to the child while obtaining the desired benefit.

Reducing Fear: Preparation and Support of Child

As is true for all procedures, parents and children (as appropriate for age) require information about the procedure and the medication. An explanation of why the drug is given, what is expected of the child, and how the parent can participate and support the child is given (see discussion on procedural preparation in Chapter 23).

The child's developmental level guides how to approach and support the child. Infants need the support of a parent and the comfort of being held and rocked after receiving a medication. Resistive toddlers and preschoolers do not necessarily understand even a simple explanation, but when one makes the effort to prepare them, a degree of trust is generated. Doll play with medical toys in this age group is a common approach to defusing a child's fears. School-age children require more specific information about the medication and specific instructions on how they can help. Participation, when appropriate, enhances cooperation and becomes a form of distraction from the potential hurt. Adolescents respond well to a full explanation and an opportunity to ask questions about the medication. They may wish to see the syringe or medication and want to be informed about the plan of therapy, including how often and how long the medication will be required.

Regardless of the child's age and the circumstances surrounding the administration of medications, certain approaches should always be used. Nurses, as well as parents, should resist the urge to bend the truth in an effort to comfort a child. Children should not be told that needles are painless or that medications will taste good. These approaches, intended to make the child more cooperative, actually have the potential to break down any trust that has developed in the relationship or to prevent the development of trust. The truth must be told, but it is supplemented with supportive statements for both the child and parents, including that the medication will help the child to get better. The task of giving medications to children can also be facilitated when nurses share information about techniques that work. If a nurse discovers a certain method that helps a particular child, it should be passed on to colleagues by leaving instructions on the care plan and in the medication profile.

Preventing Injury: Safe Technique of Administration

Until the late school-age years, children have great difficulty understanding the meaning of the events that accompany illness. To accomplish accurate and safe administration of medications with the least amount of hurt and discomfort, the nurse needs skill in the technique of administration and knowledge about a child's physiologic and developmental vulnerabilities. A child's lack of understanding results in severe physical resistance. In spite of preparation through explanations and doll play, resistive behaviors such as kicking, flailing, and hitting are often encountered. Parents may be able to suggest a method of administration for their child or give the medication themselves when appropriate.

Avoidance of physical injury to the child during the process is essential. Restraining a child too forcefully or leaning on a child can cause physical and psychologic harm. Furthermore, a struggling child can be jabbed, poked, or scratched with a syringe, cup, or needle. The way a child is positioned can guard against injury. The position depends on the type of medication being given, but in all cases one must firmly stabilize the part of the body involved, in order to avoid injury.

Preventing Injury: Appropriate Child, Drug, Dose, Time, and Route

Giving the right *drug,* in the right *dose,* at the right *time,* by the right *route,* to the right *patient,* has been called the "five rights." For parenteral medications, this list can be expanded to include the right *dilution* and the right *volume in one site* if an IM injection is given, and the right *rate* and the right *dilution* for IV administration.

Adherence to these principles protects the child from disastrous medication errors. Children do not generally speak up if they are offered a medication that is being incorrectly administered, and they may even pretend they are someone else, not understanding the potential outcomes of their play. It is essential that a nameband be on each child and that this identification be checked before a medication is given. Errors can also be prevented by having a rigorous system of checking orders against the medication profile and by repeatedly checking the profile when giving a medication: (1) when beginning to prepare it, (2) while preparing it, and (3) just before giving it to the child.

Preventing Injury: Administration of Safe Dose

A child is not a small adult; therefore, drugs are not calculated according to formulas based on adult dosages. When preparing to administer a drug, the therapeutic dosage is checked by calculating according to the weight or surface area of the child.

For example, the recommended dose of a drug is 100 to 200 mg/kg daily in three to four divided doses. You have an order for 500 mg of the drug to be given every 6 hours to a child who weighs 12 kg. Calculations to check the appropriateness of the drug dose are as follows:

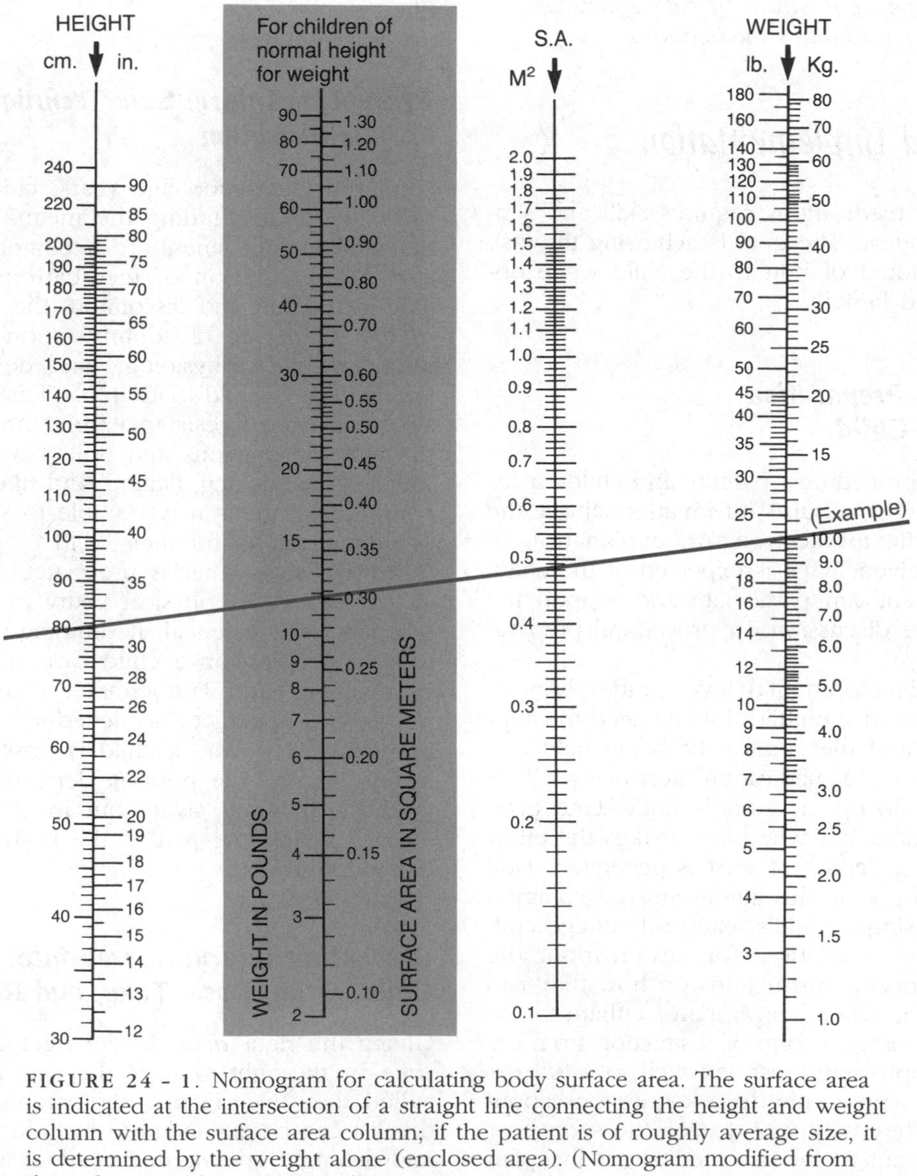

FIGURE 24-1. Nomogram for calculating body surface area. The surface area is indicated at the intersection of a straight line connecting the height and weight column with the surface area column; if the patient is of roughly average size, it is determined by the weight alone (enclosed area). (Nomogram modified from data of E. Boyd by C. D. West.)

A. Amount of drug appropriate for patient in 24 hrs:
12 kg × 200 mg (maximal dose) = 2400 mg
Amount of drug permitted per dose:
2400 mg ÷ 4 doses = 600 mg
Ordered dose of 500 mg is less than permitted dose and therefore can be administered safely

Drug dosage can also be calculated according to body surface area. The surface area is computed as a relationship between height and weight by using a nomogram (Fig. 24–1). The surface area is the point at which a straight line drawn from height to weight intersects the surface area column. The calculation to find the safe range of a drug dose is as follows:

B. Surface area of child (m^2) × dose/m^2/24 hrs = dose to be administered in a 24-hour period

To use this formula, the recommended dose/m^2/24 hrs of a specific drug is found in a reference source. That number is then multiplied by the surface area of the child (as determined from the nomogram) to calculate the recommended dose for a 24-hour period. After the dose for a 24-hour period is known, calculations as in *A* are required to determine the appropriate amount to be administered per dose.

Calculations based on body weight and surface area must include the child's age. For example, a dose based on body weight that is appropriate for a normal newborn infant may be inappropriate for a premature infant and likewise may not be suitable for an older infant or child. When one checks sources for proper dosages, one should look for any differences in recommendations across the age groups (Byington, 1991).

When one calculates the amount of medication to be given, one must not exceed the maximal recommended dose. Calculations should always be checked twice, and for certain drugs, the calculation should be checked by another nurse. If an ordered dose is not within the recommended therapeutic range (too low or too high), it is the nurse's responsibility to notify the physician of the discrepancy and have it corrected before administering it.

Becoming familiar with calculation of small doses requires supervised practice. Tables 24–1, 24–2, and 24–3 summarize key facts and principles for calculating pediatric doses.

TABLE 24-1
Most Frequently Used Equivalents in Calculation of Pediatric Doses

Volume	Weight
1 cc = 1 ml	1000 μg = 1 mg
1 tsp = 5 cc or 5 ml	1000 mg = 1 g
1 oz = 30 cc or 30 ml	1000 g = 1 kg
1 tbsp = 15 cc or 15 ml	1 kg = 2.2 lb

TABLE 24-2
Weights and Volumes

Drug calculations involve *weights* and *volumes*

The dose of the drug is *ordered* in milligrams (mg), which is the *weight* of the drug

The *volume* of the drug is what you need to know to pour it or draw it up (ml or cc)

Drug preparations are labeled to tell you how much by weight (mg) is in a designated volume (ml) (e.g., Demerol, 50 mg/ml)

When determining whether the *dose* is safe for a particular patient, you calculate milligrams

When determining how much to give, you must know how much in *volume* to pour or draw up (i.e., cc or ml)

TABLE 24-3
How to Overcome the Fear of Giving a Wrong Dose: Answer the Question, "Does It Make Sense?"

1. *Know* the recommended 24-hr dose allowed according to the weight of the child, i.e., number of mg/kg/24 hrs
2. *Check* whether the dose ordered exceeds the maximum allowed in 24 hrs
3. After validating that the ordered dose is reasonable, find the correct drug in the correct preparation
4. Look at the container to determine how many milligrams (mg) contained in each milliliter (ml)
5. Using whatever formula or system is familiar to you, calculate what is *desired (D)* from what you *have (H)*. For example, acetaminophen is prepared in 160 mg/5 ml; if the desired dose is 120 mg, the calculation may be as follows:

$$\frac{D}{H} = \frac{X}{5} \quad \text{(amount in ml to be given)}$$

$$\frac{120}{160} = \frac{X}{5}$$

$$\frac{12\not{0}}{16\not{0}} = \frac{X}{5}$$

$$16X = 60$$

$$X = \frac{60}{16}$$

$$X = 3.75 \text{ ml}$$

6. The final step is to determine mentally whether your answer *makes sense;* the mental process goes something like this:
   I had 160 mg in 5 ml
   The amount I am asked to give is 120 mg, which is more than half of 160 mg, but is less than 160 mg
   The amount I will give (in ml), therefore, will be more than half of 5 ml, but less than 5 ml
   The answer is 3.75 ml, which *makes sense*

   This process provides a check to catch any decimal point errors that might have been made in the calculation

Maintaining Tissue Integrity

It is now known that immaturity of the body systems of premature infants, neonates, and young infants can affect the disposition of a drug that is administered (see previous discussion under "Physiologic Factors"). The immature enzyme system in the liver, the reduced protein binding of drugs, and the immature renal system are factors associated with toxicity of drugs. Careful monitoring of urinary output and side effects of the drug are nursing strategies to prevent drug toxicity. In addition it is important to know whether drug levels have been ordered by the physician, and these should be checked by the nurse before the next scheduled dose is administered.

Fluid and electrolyte regulation bears extremely close monitoring during certain drug therapy. Administration of diuretics results in depletion of sodium and potassium more readily in children than in adults (Kagan, 1983). The neonate has limited ability to concentrate urine, so one must ensure adequate fluid intake for secretion of drugs and their metabolites. Intake and output should be closely monitored during drug therapy in infants, as states of dehydration can increase the potential for drug toxicity.

The immature development of the blood-brain barrier is also associated with drug toxicity. Immature myelinization of the central nervous system enhances permeability of the blood-brain barrier, making it possible for drugs and bilirubin to enter the central nervous system. For example, drugs such as morphine and phenobarbital, given for their central nervous system effect, have an intensified central nervous system response in infants compared with that in older children. Similarly, the central nervous system response to drugs given for effects on other body systems may also be exaggerated (Wink, 1991). Myelinization to create this barrier is not mature until 2 years of age (Howry et al, 1981). The nurse is particularly careful to observe for side effects of drugs in illnesses like meningitis, brain tumors, and cranial trauma in which drugs enter the central nervous system because of increased permeability of the blood-brain barrier (Russell, 1980).

The rate of absorption through a child's skin is a major consideration in topical medications. Infants and young children have a thin dermis and epidermis and a scanty stratum corneum, resulting in greater permeability than in adults (Howry et al, 1981). Also, the child's greater surface area in relation to total

RESEARCH ISSUES
Clinical Application of EMLA* Cream

Results. A new topical anesthetic ointment named EMLA* is being used in selected situations in pediatric settings in Canada. This cream provides dermal analgesia and allows for painless injections. It has been evaluated and found to be an effective topical skin anesthetic in various ages and circumstances.

Implications. The cream is applied to the skin under an occlusive dressing, and local analgesia is achieved after 60 min. The duration of analgesia is at least 2 hrs, and there is no benefit after 5 hrs. The success of the cream depends on careful planning and timing to allow the appropriate lapse of time after its application. It is recommended that a liberal amount of cream, 3–5 mm, be applied.

In children, EMLA is used for venipuncture, arterial stab, finger prick, injections, drug reservoir access, lumbar puncture, bone marrow aspirate, suture removal, removal of foreign bodies in the skin, and superficial surgical procedures, such as skin grafting and circumcision. EMLA cream must be applied 1 hour prior to a procedure, which is reasonable for in-hospital procedures, but precludes its use in emergency settings. The re-use of EMLA becomes impractical in the event of unsuccessful IV cannulations at a prepared site. Some specific limitations apply to this drug. It is not recommended for infants under 3 mos of age or for children who are hypersensitive to local anesthetics. Adverse effects include local reactions, edema, redness, or paleness. EMLA is less effective with African-American patients because of the increased density of the stratum corneum.

*Eutectic mixture of local anesthetics— 1 25 mg lidocaine/25 mg prilocaine.

REFERENCES

Broadman, L. M., Soliman, I. E., Hannallah, R. S., & McGill, W. A. (1988). Evaluation of EMLA (eutectic mixture of local anesthetics) for topical analgesia in children. *Anesthesia and Analgesia, 67,* S21.

Halperin, D. L., Koren, G., Attias, D., Pellegrine, E., Greenberg, M. L., & Wyss, M. (1989). Topical skin anesthesia for venous, subcutaneous drug reservoir, and lumbar punctures in children. *Pediatrics, 84*(2), 281–284.

Hopkins, C. S., Buckley, C. J., & Bush, G. H. (1988). Pain-free injection in infants. *Anaesthesia, 43,* 198–201.

Kapelushnik, J., Koren, G., Solh, H., Greenberg, M., & DeVeber, L. (1990). Evaluating the efficacy of EMLA in alleviating pain associated with lumbar puncture; comparison of open and double blinded protocols in children. *Pain, 42,* 31–34.

Soliman, I. E., Broadman, L. M., Hannallah, R. S., & McGill, W. A. (1988). Comparison of the analgesic effects of EMLA to intradermal lidocaine infiltration prior to venous cannulation in unpremedicated children. *Anaesthesiology, 68*(5), 804–806.

Robieux, I., Kumar, R., Radhakrishnan, S., & Koren, G. (1991). Assessing pain and analgesia with a lidocaine-prilocaine emulsion in infants and toddlers during venipuncture. *Journal of Pediatrics, 118*(6), 971–973.

body is an important factor when medications are applied to large areas of affected skin. Absorption of topical drugs through the skin can be avoided by applying a very thin layer of drug to just the affected area. Repeated topical application of steroids is avoided because of potential systemic absorption and resultant suppression of adrenal steroid production (Howry et al, 1981).

The nurse also monitors children for drug sensitivity. Sensitivity to a drug depends on the age of the child and on the developmental stage of the particular system affected by the drug. For example, inhibition of skeletal growth results when long-term therapy with adrenocortical steroids is required. Conversely, androgens such as testosterone stimulate the rate of growth but also speed up epiphyseal closure, resulting in reduced height (Kagan, 1983). The nurse's awareness of these potential side effects is an important aspect of drug administration.

Maintaining Tissue Perfusion (Cardiopulmonary)

Every effort is made to prevent acute allergic reactions to medications by taking a careful history to determine whether any allergies exist. The child's chart and medication profile are flagged, a sign is placed at the head or on the foot of the child's bed. When a new drug is ordered, the parent or child should again be asked whether the child has ever had an allergic reaction to the ordered drug.

Even though all the precautions are taken to identify drug sensitivities, an acute allergic reaction, known as "anaphylaxis," can occur; this is a serious condition. It is most commonly a response to penicillin, bee stings, contrast media, and some food and drugs. Immediate treatment is critical to prevent anaphylactic shock and death.

Anaphylaxis occurs as a result of the release of chemical mediators after antigen-antibody interaction. This interaction causes formation and/or release of chemical mediators: histamine, the kinins, and a substance called "slow-reactive substance of anaphylaxis." These mediators have three major effects: vasodilatation, smooth-muscle spasm, and increased vascular permeability with edema formation (Vanselow, 1988).

One general rule is that the sooner the signs and symptoms occur after you have administered the drug, the more severe the reaction will be. The symptoms start with pruritus, sweating, confusion, and headache. Respiratory difficulties begin with simple asthma and wheezing due to spasm of bronchial smooth muscle followed by upper-airway edema. Gastrointestinal involvement includes abdominal cramps, vomiting, and diarrhea. Cardiovascular manifestations consist of vasodilatation, hypotension, and cardiac arrhythmias (Vanselow, 1988).

If you suspect an anaphylactic reaction, first eliminate exposure to the antigen (e.g., stop the drug infusion). Put patient in a supine position, maintain an open airway, and give oxygen. IV fluids should be started, and the patient put on a cardiac monitor. Treatment may include administration of epinephrine and insertion of an endotracheal tube in severe cases (O'Neal, 1990).

Preventing Uncomfortable Sensations

Receiving medications and the associated sensations can make children feel uncomfortable and experience pain. The taste, the texture, and the side effects of medications are all factors that introduce discomfort to children. Some options can be offered to camouflage the medications, and having a child's favorite drink ready to take immediately after the medication can reduce the distastefulness of medicines. If the medication is inhaled, the coldness, irritation, and restrictiveness of a mask may produce discomfort. Giving children some control by allowing them to stabilize the mask and staying with children during inhalation to reduce their anxiety can help keep them comfortable.

When medication is required that involves a needle the use of EMLA can greatly reduce discomfort. Reducing the child's fears through appropriate preparation and support (see discussion further on) is also known to reduce the child's sensation of pain and discomfort. The person injecting a needle *must* be skilled and gentle. Proper dilution and rate of IV administration as well as careful monitoring of the site are of particular importance in maintaining comfort (see discussion under "Maintaining Tissue Integrity").

Enhancing Family Coping and Growth

The task of getting children to take medications can often be facilitated if the parents can help. Parents feel more involved if the various pharmacologic treatment strategies are explained to them, so that they feel capable of participating in decision making. For example, decisions about giving medications such as analgesics, cough syrups, or sedatives can be facilitated by including the judgment of parents. Parents also understand their child's fears and responses and can assist in the child's preparation as well as provide diversional approaches.

When children take medications, the worry about side effects is a concern to parents. One must explain to parents the purpose and action of drugs and teach them how to observe the child for side effects. If parents can be involved at this level, they feel more integral to the recovery of their child and are prepared to take this responsibility at home. If parents participate in the medication regimen of their child, the child's condition is more easily treated and family functioning is enhanced, as they experience a sense of self-management and control.

Meeting Developmental Needs of the Individual Child

Medications are administered to children at all ages through different routes. The following discussion of the nurse's approach to giving children medication by various routes of administration integrates strategies for handling children's fears, and powerlessness, preventing injury, and enhancing coping throughout the various stages of development. Table 24–4 provides guidelines for oral administration for infants, toddlers, preschoolers, school-agers, and adolescents.

Oral Medication

Infant

For security and comfort, the infant should be held on the nurse's or parent's lap when oral medications are being given. If this is not possible, the infant's head usually can be lifted off the bed and cradled in the nurse's hand. Using the thumb to press down gently on the infant's chin can help to get the infant's mouth open. Extreme caution must be taken not to lay the infant back down on the bed until the medication has been swallowed; an oral medication should never be administered while the infant is in a supine or prone position. Crying in an infant can lead to aspiration if medication is given too rapidly. As a general rule, tablets are crushed and mixed with a small amount of fluid, unless they are chewable. Depending on the medication and individual patient restrictions, suggested fluids include water, flavored syrups, juices, or flattened soda.

Various medication devices are illustrated in Figure 24–2. Oral medications are now frequently prepared in syringes under unit dose medication systems (Fig. 24–2*C*). Medication in a syringe can be administered directly into an infant's mouth. Since the sucking reflex causes the infant to push out anything placed in the front of the mouth, the tip of the syringe should be placed to one side and toward the back of the mouth; the medication should be given in small amounts. Medication by plastic dropper can be administered in the same manner. Small plastic medication cups bent slightly to form a spout or a calibrated spoon device can also be used (Fig. 24–2*A* and *B*). Since the medication is delivered at the front of the mouth, it is easily pushed out and the administration process often must be repeated for a resisting child. Putting the medication into a nipple is another alternative; this approach utilizes the infant's natural sucking responses. The nipple method is not recommended, however, in infants with sucking problems or when medication has an extremely bitter taste. Because parents often give medications with a spoon, this may be the most successful method for the nurse as well. If parents are present, they are often more effective than professionals in gaining the child's cooperation to take the medication (Fig. 24–3).

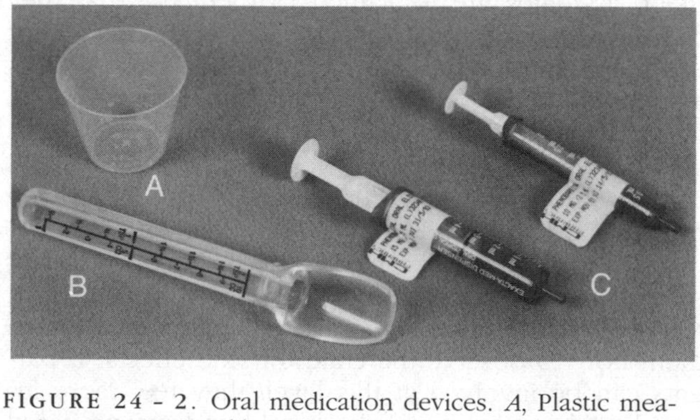

FIGURE 24 - 2. Oral medication devices. *A*, Plastic measuring cup. *B*, A calibrated spoon device. Medication is measured by holding the spoon upright; it is then tipped so the child can take the medication from the spoon. *C*, Syringes in two sizes. These syringes are prepared and labeled by the pharmacy in unit-dose systems.

Toddler

A teaspoon or calibrated spoon device, a medicine cup, or a medication syringe is used to give oral liquid medication to a toddler. The usual hospital procedure is to use a medicine cup or a syringe; however, the nurse should determine whether a spoon would be more effective. When a medicine cup is used, the toddler frequently wants to hold the cup or prefers that a parent hold it. The nurse should remain with the toddler until all the medication is swallowed.

When using a syringe, one should avoid squirting the entire contents of the syringe into the toddler's mouth at one time. The syringe should be placed to one side and toward the back of the mouth. The plunger is then pushed, injecting the portion of the medicine that the toddler is capable of swallowing at one time. (A 5-ml syringe of medication would require approximately three squirts.)

Oral medications can also be given in tablet form. Chewable tablets can usually be given to a 2-year-old. The nurse should stay with the child until the medication is chewed and swallowed. Tablets that need to be crushed can be mixed as for an infant. If the taste is extremely bitter it may be disguised in a nonessential food such as a small amount of fruit jelly. Under no circumstances, even if the medication has a pleasant taste, should it be referred to as "candy" or "a treat." Regardless of how medications are given, the nurse must approach the child with recognition of the developmental tasks and behaviors that will affect oral administration of medications.

Preschooler

Resistive behaviors to oral medications may continue to be demonstrated during the preschool years. The taste of medications cannot be as easily disguised, but resistance can more easily be counteracted with reasoning than in the younger child. Use of therapeutic play is particularly effective with this age group.

TABLE 24-4
Guidelines for Administration of Oral Medication

Nursing Actions	Rationale Based on Developmental Characteristics
1–3 Mos	
Support head well during administration	Head control is not yet developed; therefore head bobs
Keep infant's arms and palms away from face	Infant randomly moves arms and has a strong palmar grasp: may spill medication
Alternate methods of administration can be used:	
1. Medication can be put into a nipple. As a baby sucks and empties the nipple, more medication is added slowly	Infant has strong sucking reflex, which increases up to around 3 mos of age; choking or drooling, with loss of correct dosage, can occur if infant sucks medication too rapidly
2. A syringe or dropper is used by placing it to one side of the mouth along the gums toward the back of the mouth	Medication placed on front of the tongue is easily lost because of tongue thrust normally present at this stage
3. Medication can be given *slowly* from a small spoon or spouted cup in small amounts	If baby drools, medication can be caught off the face with the spoon and re-fed to baby
Hold the infant momentarily and lay on stomach or on the side after medication is given	Aspiration occurs more readily in the supine position
Medication is given slowly, regardless of method	Strong taste of medication may cause baby to choke if given too rapidly
Let parent give the medication as appropriate	Familiarity of infant with parents increases cooperation
Cradle infant in arms during medication administration, whenever possible	A comfortable, relaxed holding position makes infant feel secure and provides a situation similar to feeding, which encourages cooperation
3–12 Mos	
Comfortably hold infant during medication administration	Comfort of being held makes infant feel secure and encourages cooperation
Older infants may require gentle restraint of arms (i.e., one arm held behind nurse's back and one held by nurse's hand, or use of mummy restraint, if necessary)	Infant's increasing muscle strength may be used to refuse medication more forcefully
Take special precaution to keep medication out of reach of infant who is developing rapidly	Infant is rapidly developing gross and fine motor muscle control; therefore can reach, grasp, and open containers
Alternative methods of medication administration can be used as appropriate developmentally (syringe, spoon, cup)	By 4 mos of age, an infant can take medication from a spoon more easily. As an infant approaches 12 mos, the task of drinking from a cup is achieved; therefore, a small medicine cup is often used for medication. Medication that is spit out can be retrieved by using a spoon or medicine cup
Let parents give the medication as the nurse stands by	Around 7–8 mos, infants develop a fear of strangers; a sense of fear makes an infant resist what strangers do
Immediately after medicine is placed into infant's mouth, encourage swallowing by gently pulling up infant's chin with thumb; also can stroke infant's neck	Infant can forcefully spit out medicine
Respond to individual needs if expressed	As infant approaches 12 mos, specific wishes can be made, known by single words or gestures, i.e., the wish to be held versus sitting in a chair
Comfort infant after medication is given by holding, stroking, and rocking	Infant is responsive to tactile stimuli and facial expressions
12–18 Mos	
Keep medicine cabinets locked, and keep medicine away from child's bedside	Child advances from standing to independent walking and can crawl to reach most things in sight
Explain what the child is to do before beginning; involve the child in some choices regarding medication	Child can indicate wants by gestures; by 18 mos uses 6–20 recognizable words and understands many more; has developed independence and resists being forced to do something
Use cup, syringe, or spoon according to the needs of the child	Child may have a preference because of home routines
May need to disguise crushed tablets in small amounts of nonessential solids or liquids (e.g., pudding or soda)	Bitter-tasting medications are resisted; such medication should not be mixed into essential foods such as milk because of potential for child refusing milk thereafter

(continued)

TABLE 24-4
Guidelines for Administration of Oral Medication *(Continued)*

Nursing Actions	Rationale Based on Developmental Characteristics
18–36 Mos	
Keep medication cabinets locked, and keep medication away from child's bedside	Children wander to restricted areas and explore the environment
Prepare child by doll playing and demonstration	Cooperation is important, because at this age the mouth can be clamped tightly in resistance; imaginary play is prevalent
Be honest about the taste of medication	Resistance may be transferred to all requests, if nurse is dishonest
Alternative methods of medication administration can be used (syringe, spoon, cup, or chewable tablet) by about 2 yrs of age. Crushed tablets not of the chewable type may need to be disguised as aforementioned	Child is able to swallow well and chew a chewable tablet if instructions are given; second molars erupt at about 20 mos of age
Use a firm, consistent approach	Reactive behavior is prominent; limit setting makes a child feel more secure and cooperative
Let child make some choices and be as independent as able; e.g., choose between cup and syringe and holding the cup or syringe	Child does not experience a sense of loss of control if able to participate
Give simple directions, such as "pick up the cup, take a drink, and now swallow"	Child can follow two or three directions given at one time
Give immediate, positive tactile and verbal response for the child's participation and cooperation in taking medicine; resistive behavior is ignored	Positive feedback encourages child to participate next time to receive again the acceptance and praise
3–6 Yrs	
Continue to keep all medications under lock and key	Although beginning to comprehend the danger of medications, child will ingest dangerous amounts if unsupervised
Explain the options of medication available (i.e., chewable tablets, or capsule); let child make some choices about how the medication is administered, whenever possible	Child is able to comprehend explanations and has likely had some experience to know which option is preferred; capsules may be swallowed by some children at 5 or 6 yrs of age, depending on size and texture
Explain the purpose of the medication in simple terms	Although explanation may not be completely understandable, child attaches importance to taking medication correctly if explanation is given
Avoid prolonged reasoning and arguing; rather, firmly set limits about the need to take medication	Child may need assistance to achieve control and will feel better if such control is achieved and the task is accomplished
Parent or nurse can give medication; whoever can gain the child's cooperation should do so	Child may be more cooperative for the nurse than the parents, because the child views the nurse as an authority figure and is learning to adhere to society rules (similar to what is required of the child in school)
Use therapeutic play, letting child pretend to give medicine by syringe or cup to a doll or stuffed animal to encourage cooperation	Child achieves a sense of control and acts out feelings during such activities
Praise child immediately after giving medication	Future cooperation is encouraged if immediate feedback is given
6–12 Yrs	
Explain to child the purpose of the medication	As child approaches the age of 12 yrs, the purpose of a medication can be understood if explained simply; cooperation can be encouraged through explanation
Give medication in the form most suitable for each particular child; offer chewable tablets or liquids as required	Some 6–8-year-olds have had no experience swallowing capsules and may find it difficult to swallow them, especially large ones
Be firm and consistent in asking child to swallow medication in presence of nurse	Generally, school-age children are cooperative, but if medicine is excessively bitter, a young school-age child may willfully discard medicine, not recognizing its importance

Principles Adhered to at All Ages

1. Medications are not compared with candy
2. Medications are to be swallowed in the presence of the nurse
3. Truths are always told, e.g., regarding taste

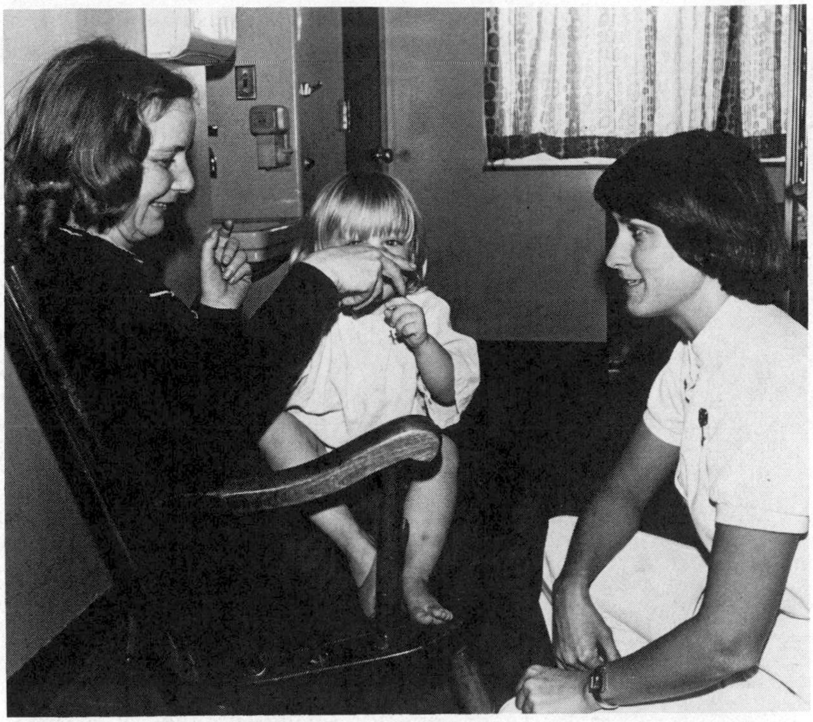

FIGURE 24-3. Oral medication administration. Children frequently cooperate in taking medications in a supportive environment. (Note that the nurse gets down to the toddler's eye level.)

School-Age Child and Adolescent

Swallowing of capsules or pills is usually achieved by most children by early school age. Physical resistance is not usually a problem during these years; rather, questions are raised about the purpose of the drug. During late school age and adolescence, decision making about therapy can often be made in discussion with the patient. Generally, drug administration should continue to be supervised by an adult during the school years, but more self-responsibility can be expected of the adolescent.

Eye Medication

Administration of eye medication is particularly resisted by older infants and young children. Children often resist when anyone comes near their face by flailing arms, kicking, screaming, and squeezing their eyes closed. It is therefore important to describe what will be done and to show the child the small amount of medication that will be used. Greatest success is achieved by moving quickly once the child has been told what will happen. Before administration, good handwashing technique by the nurse is essential. The medicine should be at room temperature, and the eyes should be gently wiped with a moist warm cloth to remove any crusted discharge.

Administration of an eye medication may often require a second individual to restrain a resisting child. If no other person is available to assist, a mummy restraint can be used (see Chapter 23).

With the child lying supine, the shoulders and neck are raised slightly with a pillow. To administer drops, the principles to adhere to are (1) stabilize the child's head and (2) avoid dropping the medication onto the eyeball. An older child should be instructed to look up when eye drops or ointments are being administered. The drops are placed into the conjunctival sac near the outer canthus of the eye, and the child is asked to close the eye(s) and blink. Contamination of the medication must be avoided by ensuring that the dropper does not touch the conjunctiva (Fig. 24–4).

To administer eye ointment, the index finger is placed on the upper eyelid, and the thumb of the same hand on the child's cheekbone. The thumb and index finger are then spread apart to open the eye. The ointment is applied by placing a thin streak along the child's lower conjunctival sac from the inner to outer canthus. When the child subsequently blinks the medication will spread across the eye. The excess is then gently wiped outward with a cotton ball or tissue; if both eyes are being medicated, the second eye should not be wiped with the same cotton ball or tissue.

If a child vigorously resists the procedure, it is extremely difficult for one person to give eye medication safely. It is advisable to stop the procedure and summon assistance from another person to ensure safe administration.

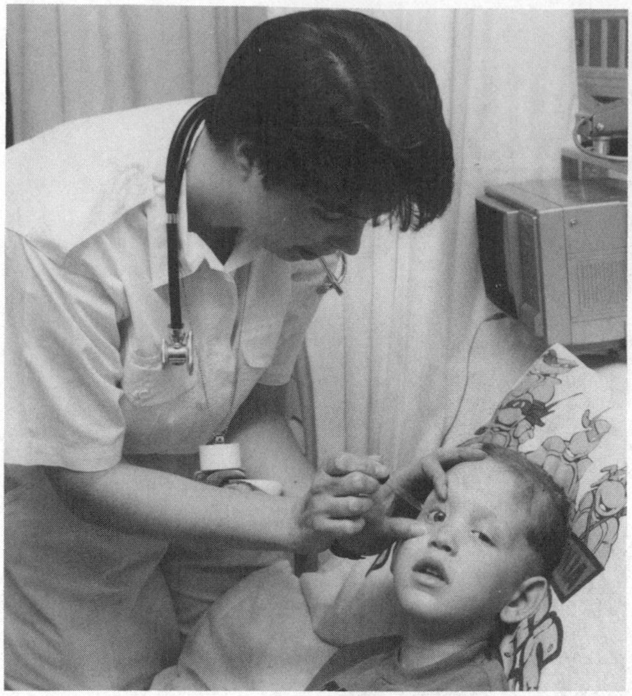

FIGURE 24 - 4. Administering eye drops. The child's head is stabilized and the lower conjunctival sac is gently pulled downward.

Nose Drops

Nose drops should be at room temperature. Preparation of the child includes an explanation of the position to be assumed, the number of drops to be administered, and a warning that the drops may be tasted momentarily after administration. If drops are being given for nasal congestion, administer them 15 to 30 minutes prior to mealtime, so that feeding will be easier; bottlefeeding is difficult for infants because they cannot breathe through the nose while sucking.

An infant can be held supine on the parent's or nurse's lap, with the head tilted back. An older child should also be supine with a pillow under the shoulders to facilitate tilting the head back. The drops are instilled into each nostril without touching the nostrils or any other part of the child's face. The nostrils can be opened farther by applying gentle upward pressure to the tip of the nose. The head must be kept in its lowered position for 1 to 2 minutes after administration to allow the drops to penetrate the swollen nasal passages by gravity flow. Vigorous sniffing should be discouraged as this may suck medication into the sinuses. Watch for signs of aspiration such as coughing; the child should sit up if coughing occurs.

Eardrops

Eardrops should be warmed to room temperature before administration to avoid pain and discomfort. The procedure is begun after an explanation has been given and questions have been answered. The external ear should be cleansed with a moistened cotton ball before drug administration.

Eardrops are most readily administered if an infant or young child is held on the nurse's or parent's lap. A young child often resists lying flat but can be held in a side-lying position while the nurse pulls down and back (in children under 3 years of age) or up and back (in children over 3 years of age) on the pinna. The ear is pulled downward and backward in a child under 3 years of age because the external auditory canal curves upward in infants, and, in children over 3 years, the ear is pulled upward and backward because the canal curves downward and forward; the direction of pull helps straighten the canal to direct the medication into the ear. An older child should lie flat in bed with the head turned to one side to make the affected ear accessible. The medication is dropped onto the wall of the external ear canal; therefore the pinna should be held in position until the medication has progressed down the canal to the eardrum. Pressing the tragus (the area directly in front of the ear) two or three times assists the drops in moving down the canal. A side-lying position should be maintained for several minutes after drops have been instilled. Placing cotton balls in the ears after administration has some disadvantages in infants and young children. A child may remove the cotton and put it into the mouth or push it into the ears farther than is recommended. If cotton is used, it should be placed gently and loosely so that, in the event of ear discharge, secretions are not trapped in the ear.

Inhalation

Medications are also administered via inhalation to facilitate a direct therapeutic effect in the respiratory tract. Inhalation medicants are often given in conjunction with percussion and postural drainage; they should not be given immediately after a meal, therefore, because of the potential for vomiting and aspiration.

Administration of a medication via inhalation is a form of aerosol therapy, usually delivered in normal saline. The prescribed medication is mixed with the prescribed amount of normal saline and placed into the nebulizer. Either compressed air or an oxygen flow forms the particles that will reach the respiratory tract. The speed of administration is controlled by the gas flow. An aerosol with medication is usually administered for 10 to 15 minutes.

A mask is placed over the mouth and nose, and the chamber containing the medication is attached below the mask (Fig. 24–5). Production of a mist indicates that the equipment is functioning properly. The mist may also be delivered via a tube on the mist chamber. The tube can be held near the nose and mouth of an infant or small child; an older child can inhale the mist through a mouthpiece on the tube.

Children often resist having a mask against their

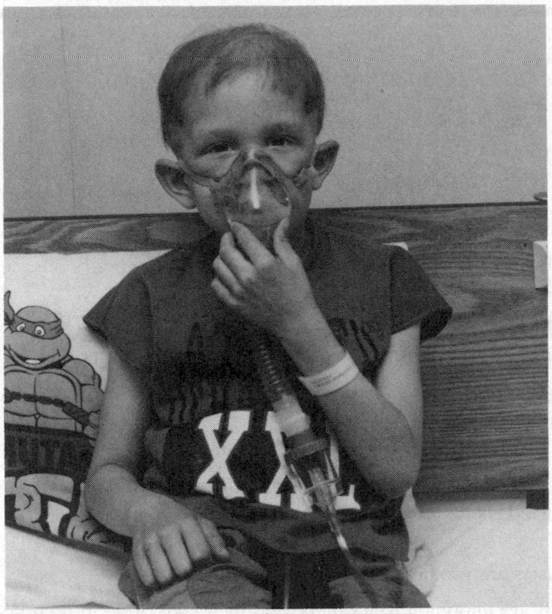

FIGURE 24 - 5. Medication administration by mask. Medication is administered through a chamber below the flexed hose and forms a mist through the mask.

face or having the mist directed toward them and may struggle and cry. Therefore, efforts are made to provide a calm environment. Parents often hold the child during the procedure but should be given a thorough explanation so that they feel comfortable. Because a parent's anxiety can readily be communicated to the child, the nurse should monitor the procedure and assist the parent if anxiety escalates. Monitoring is also required for side effects. Inhalation therapy can also be administered while a child is asleep. The medicated mist can be blown through a crib into the child's mouth and nostrils without disturbing the child's sleep. (See Chapter 32 for further discussion of respiratory therapy.)

Rectal Administration

Children's responses to insertion of a rectal suppository vary with their experience. A young child who is not accustomed to having a temperature checked rectally may find the experience anxiety-producing and threatening. Experience with toilet training also may affect how much cooperation can be achieved. A toddler who is just becoming aware of body sensations related to defecation may try to expel the suppository. Older children may perceive the procedure as an invasion of privacy and may react with embarrassment, resistance, or anger. Spending time to explain the procedure and reassure the child that it will not hurt can reduce the child's anxiety. At any age, privacy should be provided by drawing curtains or closing the door.

The suppository is inserted by using the index finger in older children and the little finger in infants and young children. A finger cot or glove covers the nurse's finger. If the suppository has become too soft for easy insertion, it can be placed under cold running water for a few seconds before the paper is removed.

Position the child on the left side with the right leg drawn up. The anus can easily be exposed by placing an infant or young child on the back with knees flexed. It is not necessary to lubricate the suppository, but if a lubricant is used, only a small amount should be applied to avoid interaction with the medication. Moistening it with water is sufficient to permit easy insertion. The suppository must be inserted past the rectal sphincter, usually as far as the first knuckle of the insertion finger. The buttocks are gently pressed together for several minutes. The suppository is not likely to dissolve for 5 to 10 minutes, but a young child generally does not tolerate having pressure applied to the buttocks for that length of time. Keeping a child quiet and briefly holding the suppository in place is usually sufficient to promote absorption. If the parents are present, they are instructed to keep their child from getting up and going to the bathroom. Holding the child and walking about to distract her or him can also be effective in preventing expulsion of the suppository. The nurse can ask the parent to check the diaper carefully the next time it is changed to be sure the suppository has not been expelled.

Intramuscular Injection

The administration of IM injections is rare in many pediatric settings because of increased awareness of the effect needles have on children. The development and success of alternative routes of drug administration have shown that the practice of routine injections is unnecessary, cruel, and preventable. The use of needles contradicts the current philosophy of children's pain management, making the practice of giving injections for pain obsolete. Most antibiotics can also be given orally or intravenously.

As a patient advocate, it is up to the nurse to question the need for any child to have an IM injection. Does the child have an IV line? If a drug is to be given routinely, would an IV line or saline lock device be suitable to prevent routine "poking"? Can the medication be given orally or rectally? Prevention of pain and anxiety is a responsibility not only of the nurse but of the whole health care team, and a team effort may be needed in your pediatric setting to make it a "no needles" zone.

In the event that an IM injection is unavoidable, there are resources to make it more bearable for the child. The development of new local anesthetic creams has made attainable the goal of making injections less painful. These creams cause a loss of feeling or "freezing" of the skin surface and are suitable for injections, IV insertions, and blood sampling. These creams have been shown to be effective in re-

TABLE 24-5
Guidelines for Administering an Injection

Nursing Action	Rationale
Birth to 12 Mos	
Spend time with the infant prior to giving an injection	This supports the development of a sense of trust
For the older infant, state what you are going to do and proceed with the injection	Child cannot understand explanations, but should not be injected without warning
Provide something to look at or a toy to hold during the injection	The infant is often distractible
Provide physical comfort after the injection	Physical comforting is more effective than verbal comforting
1–3 Yrs	
State what you are going to do and proceed with the injection; use simple words and short phrases; for example, say, "This will take only a minute and then you can play." Provide something for the child to look at, hold, or play with during the injection	At this age the child obeys simple commands and develops a sense of time beginning at about 18 mos of age; the toddler often can be distracted
Give a simple, honest reason for the injection	Fantasies are prominent at this age
Use a firm, consistent approach; reward the toddler's positive behaviors, and ignore negative ones; let the child take some part in the procedure, for example, hold the Band-Aid	Rituals are important to toddlers, and they take pride in their accomplishments
Provide a Band-Aid for covering the injection site	Toddler has an incomplete sense of body boundaries and fears body contents may leak out
3–6 Yrs	
Tell child what he or she will feel and what to do to help; for example, lying still	Child remains egocentric and is a concrete thinker but can also understand simple explanations and follow directions
Let child see and handle equipment under supervision before the injection is given	Seeing and handling equipment helps child learn and promotes coping
Tell child that injections are never used as punishment, and give a simple honest explanation	Preschoolers are developing a conscience and may view an injection as punishment for their actions, but they can understand a simple explanation
Allow youngster a choice, when possible; for example, ask in which leg to put the injection; foster development of coping mechanisms	A child this age seeks to master situations and takes pride in accomplishments
Let child play at giving injections, including handling a needle under supervision	Therapeutic play is an effective means of dealing with fantasies and fears, especially those associated with painful and/or intrusive procedures
6–12 Yrs	
Give a simple explanation of why specific injection is needed	Child has the ability to think in a logical manner and comprehend relationships
Let child help select injection site, if possible, and praise child for cooperation	Taking part in the procedure supports the child's developmental need to master situations; this age group thrives on praise
Provide time to sit and talk with child	Talking about their fears replaces play as a method of dealing with anxiety
12–16 Yrs	
Provide as much information as the adolescent requests about medication, but also tell how injections feel	Adolescent is capable of logical, abstract thinking but may also demonstrate egocentrism, especially when under stress
Provide privacy and permit choice of injection site, whenever possible.	Adolescent experiences concern over body image and likes to feel in control of a situation

From Evans, M. L., & Hansen, B. D. (1981). Administering injections to different-aged children. Reprinted from *MCN: American Journal of Maternal Child Nursing,* May/June, 1981, *6,* 194–199.

search and should be a routine part of pediatric practice (see Research Issues).

When giving IM injections, the nurse must consider the possible complications beforehand. The most frequent complications seen in pediatrics are fibrosis or contracture of a muscle because of repeated injections, abscesses at the injection site, gangrene, and nerve injury (Beecroft & Redick, 1989). Pediatric nurses must be meticulous in locating landmarks and determining boundaries for each injection. Needle length, volume of the injection fluid, rotation of sites, and adequate restraint of a child all are extremely important considerations. The nurse's assessment must include the child's size, muscle and skin condition, age, and medical diagnosis (Beecroft & Redick, 1990). Although giving medications by IM injections is now an outdated mode of therapy, a complete discussion is retained in this text. Attention to this subject underscores our belief that serious damage can be done to children physically and psychologically, and for this reason, careful description of important principles of practice are presented here, in the event that a child *must* receive an injection. Principles of practice according to the age of the child are discussed next and are listed in Table 24–5, and general guidelines for IM injection are summarized in Table 24–6.

Infants

The procedure is explained to the parents, who are asked whether they wish to stay with their child. If they wish to stay, the nurse explains how they can help. It is advisable to have an additional individual, other than a parent, to assist in immobilizing the child during the procedure. It is also preferable for the nurse to spend a brief period of time with the infant before the injection is given to establish a degree of trust.

The only acceptable site is the vastus lateralis muscle. It is the largest muscle mass in an infant and has few major blood vessels and nerves. To locate the injection site, draw an imaginary line between the trochanter to just above the knee on the outer aspect of the thigh. The middle third of the thigh should be located by visually marking off the area from the knee to the groin into thirds; the middle third is used for the injection (Fig. 24–6).

During the procedure, the infant can be talked to or given a toy for distraction. Ensuring that the infant has a favorite toy or blanket for security is also essential. The injection is usually given with a 1-inch needle, 22- or 23-gauge, to ensure that the muscle is injected. See Table 24–6 for a summary of the amounts of solution to be safely injected. Wipe the area with an antiseptic (wait for it to dry, particularly if alcohol is used). Pinch up the muscle tissue, and insert the needle into it at a 90-degree angle. Aspirate, inject, then withdraw the needle, keeping slight pressure over the area to avoid the tissue from pulling upward as the needle is withdrawn. As with any painful procedure, infants should be held and comforted, so that they do not come to associate the injection and pain with feelings of rejection.

TABLE 24–6
Guidelines for Intramuscular Injection

The nurse ensures that measures have been taken to provide the least discomfort and the greatest therapeutic effect possible. At all ages, IM injections require special precautions. As with all medications, the five rights must be ensured along with the following principles:

1. Proper hand washing and sterile technique when handling syringes, needles, and medications
2. Privacy for each patient during administration
3. Proper refrigeration of medications
4. Accurate labeling of medications in vials for future use
5. Safe and proper disposal of needles
6. Rotation of sites to reduce pain and fibrosis
7. Careful assessment of patients for the evidence of side effects
8. Avoidance of excess amount of medication in one site

Guidelines:

Deltoid muscle	6–15 yrs, 0.5 ml
	15 yrs–adulthood, 1 ml
Ventrogluteal area	3–6 yrs, 1.5 ml
	6–15 yrs, 1.5–2.0 ml
	15 yrs–adulthood, 2.0–2.5 ml
Dorsogluteal area	6–15 yrs, 1.5–2.0 ml
	15 yrs–adulthood, 2.0–2.5 ml
Vastus lateralis	Birth–1.5 yrs, 0.5 ml
	1.5–3 yrs, 1 ml
	3–6 yrs, 1.5 ml
	6–15 yrs, 1.5–2.0 ml
	(not a site preferred by older children and adults)

9. Complete and accurate documentation of drug administration
10. Evaluation of effectiveness of drug

Toddler and Preschooler

The approach to a toddler and family when giving an IM injection must take into account previous experience with injections, the parent-child relationship, and the child's developmental level. The parents should be told about the medication before the nurse enters the room. This explanation should be given when the child is not present, because it is likely to instill unnecessary fears. Injections are a source of fear because of the anticipated pain and intrusion of the body.

Toddlers and preschoolers can be prepared for injections by means of needle play during the course of hospitalization and by a brief description of what will

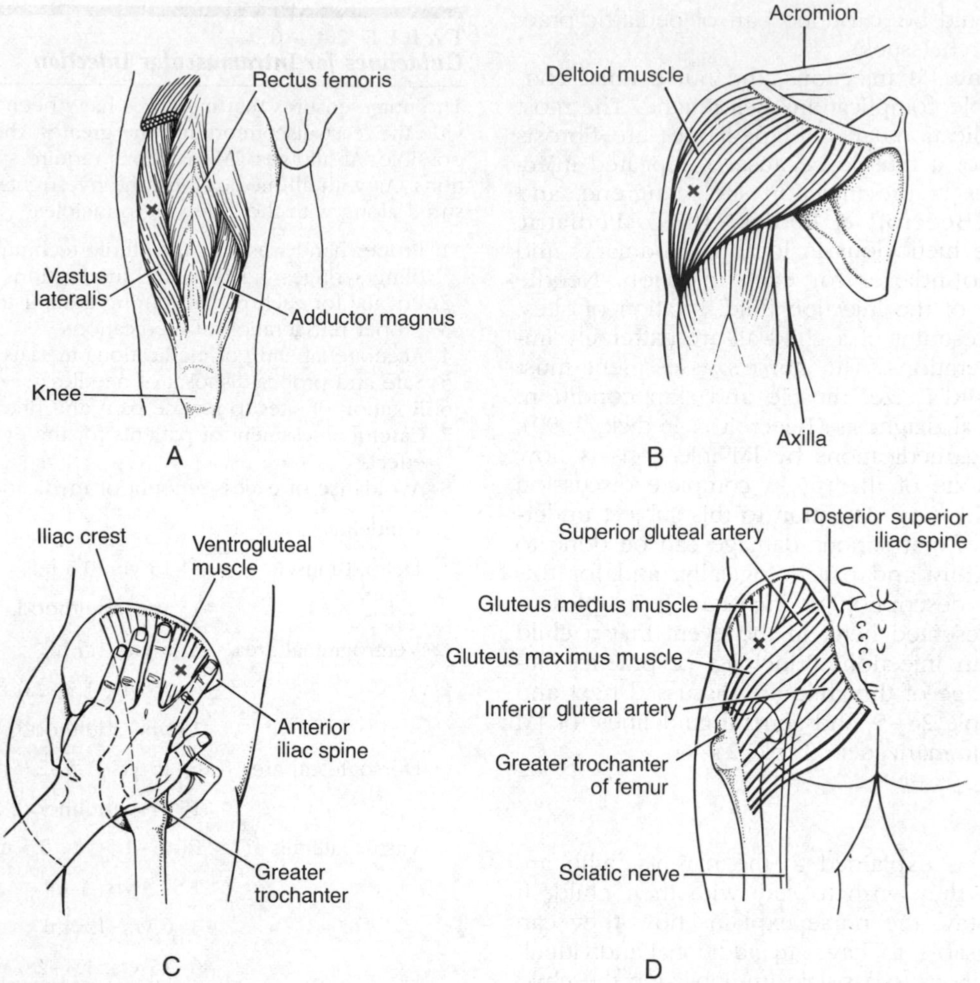

FIGURE 24-6. Injection sites. *A, Vastus lateralis site,* in the lateral middle third of the thigh. It is found by dividing the thigh into thirds from the greater trochanter to just above the knee. The area of insertion within the middle third of the thigh is found midway between imaginary lines mid-anteriorly and mid-laterally (it is the area of the leg that lies between the front crease and the side seam of a pair of pants). The needle is directed into the muscle at a right angle (90 degrees). *B, Deltoid site,* in the lower part of the upper third of the deltoid and the axilla on the lateral surface of the arm. The needle is directed into the muscle at a right angle (90 degrees) but pointed slightly toward the acromium process. *C, Ventrogluteal site:* Place the palm on the greater trochanter and the index finger on the anterior iliac spine (this may be facilitated by the flexion of the thigh at the hip). The middle finger is extended along the iliac crest as far as possible, forming a triangle between the middle and the second fingers. The injection is given in the center of the triangle, or V, formed by the hand, with the needle directed slightly upward toward the iliac crest. *D, Dorsogluteal site:* Injection is given into the gluteus medius. The site is found by locating the greater trochanter and posterior iliac spine. An imaginary line is drawn between these two points, and the injection is made above the line into the gluteus medius. The needle is directed perpendicular to the surface on which the child is lying.

occur and how it will feel immediately prior to the injection (Fig. 24–7). The needle and syringe should not be flaunted or referred to in front of the toddler or preschooler; nor should it be hidden when the nurse comes to give the injection.

Once children know they are to receive an injection, it should be given promptly. Toddlers and preschoolers are usually more receptive when the injection is given by a nurse with whom they are familiar and who has spent time with them when procedures were not involved. Children of this age should also be touched, talked to, or distracted with a toy. A toddler can best be restrained if the nurse gently leans across the torso so that arms are free to move but

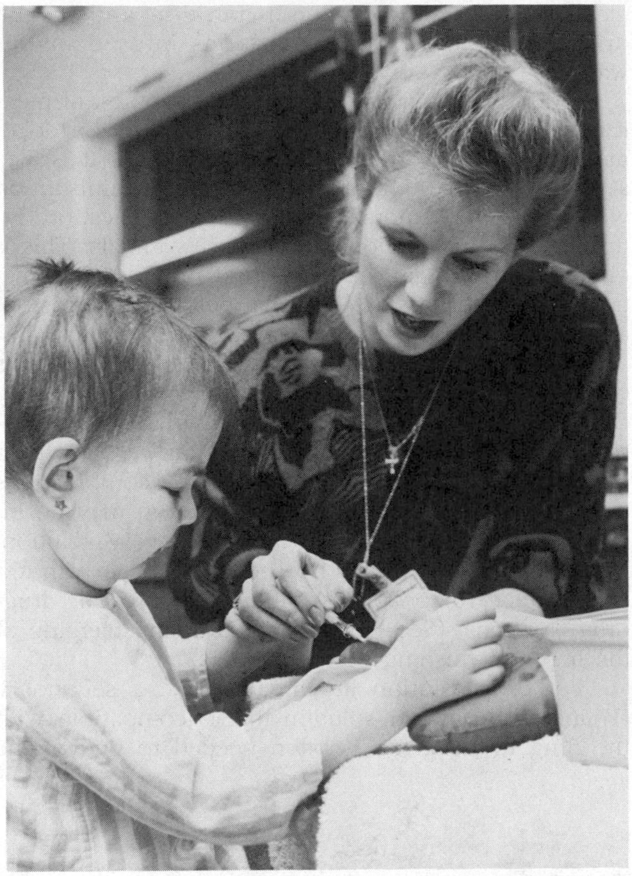

FIGURE 24 - 7. Toddlers and preschoolers eagerly participate in needle play, an activity that helps them gain a sense of mastery over their experience of receiving injections. (Courtesy of Child Life Department, Children's Hospital, Chedoke-McMaster University Medical Center, Hamilton, Ontario.)

blocked from the injection area. For many toddlers it is essential to have another nurse assist with the injection. The legs can then be restrained by one person, and the other person can give the injection. To stabilize a limb safely and firmly, it is held at the joint, that is, at the knee for restraining the upper leg and at the elbow for the upper arm. Preschoolers can often cooperate by lying still during the injection if their fears have been given time to escalate. For some children, it may be safer to have a second adult nearby to help restrain the child if necessary. While holding the child's arms in a restraining position, if needed, the second adult can preserve the child's sense of self-control by simply saying, "Let me help you hold still."

Injections are more stressful to the preschooler (because of mutilation fears, concern about body intactness, punishment perception) than to children in any other age group.

The injection technique is the same as that described for the infant. The vastus lateralis remains the only recommended site until the age of 3 years when the ventrogluteal site can be used. The ventrogluteal site is also relatively free of major nerves and vessels. The deltoid muscle is only rarely used in children under 6 years of age and then only for very small amounts of medication. The dorsogluteal site is not utilized for any child who has not walked for at least 1 year, and it is strongly recommended that children under 6 years of age do not receive injections in this site. The objection is that the muscle is very small, is poorly developed, and is located close to the sciatic nerve, which is comparatively large and takes up more space in young children than it does in older children.

After the injection is administered, a Band-Aid placed over the site gives comfort and helps reassure the child that his or her body is still intact (now all the blood cannot get out). The child is cuddled and praised for cooperation, even if he or she had difficulty holding still.

School-Age Child

A school-age child still has some fears about receiving injections, but extraordinary fears are most likely to be associated with negative previous experience. Preparation of the child, therefore, includes a brief discussion about any preconceived ideas, and misinformation is corrected. At this age, talking about their fears usually replaces play experiences, although the early school-age child may benefit from a play experience. A child of this age can understand the purpose and importance of the medication and therefore can often be more cooperative than a younger child.

The recommended injection site for school-age children is the ventrogluteal muscle. This site is easily located because of the readily palpable bony landmarks; it contains no major nerves or blood vessels and is a large muscle mass with minimal subcutaneous tissue. Use of the vastus lateralis site is frequently opposed by the school-age child, but it should be used along with the ventrogluteal and dorsogluteal sites when frequent injections or long-term IM therapy is required. The deltoid can be used for small amounts of medication (0.5 ml), but it is not a preferred site unless rapid absorption of a drug is required. Provision of privacy during IM injections is necessary for children of this age. Also, school-age children thrive on praise for "holding still"; therefore, verbal praise from the nurse is important.

Adolescent

The adolescent requires a clear explanation of the purpose of the medication. The adolescent who understands the reason for the medication is more likely to participate while in the hospital and to follow through at home. If choices and decisions are possible, the nurse should allow the adolescent some control. The preferred sites of administration are similar to those for an adult because the adolescent has adequate muscle tissue. However, caution must be taken to assess the amount of tissue, especially in emaciated or small adolescents. Generally, the dorsogluteal, deltoid, and ventrogluteal muscles are all appropriate sites. Adolescents usually prefer the arm site, which should be used if it is not contraindicated. Solutions in the deltoid should be limited to 1 ml, whereas, in other sites, 2 to 2.5 ml is permissible. When frequent injections are required, the deltoid should not be used. Injections into the thigh are resisted because they seem painful, and use of the dorsogluteus is often embarrassing. The final choice can be made in collaboration with the adolescent.

Subcutaneous Injections

The SC route is used to administer certain medications, including narcotics, insulin, heparin, and some vaccines. The procedure is similar to that for IM injections, but it requires a shorter needle length (no more than ½ inch). Aspiration is not required before an SC injection if insulin or heparin is given.

Intravenous Medications

IV medications are now used frequently in pediatric settings. The advantage of the IV route is that it provides for total absorption of medications. It also allows a noninvasive path for the child who has an existing IV line. Once a line is established and maintained, administration of medications does not depend on a child's cooperation.

IV administration of medication tends to be particularly problematic for the inexperienced nurse because of the many details that must be considered. An invaluable tool for every nurse is the hospital formulary, which should outline the institution's guidelines for IV drug administration. It usually contains material on the most appropriate way to administer IV drugs, information on solutions for dilution, maximum rate and concentrations of drugs, and common precautions. The hospital formulary also indicates which drugs nurses may administer unsupervised or supervised by a physician. Some drugs can be administered only by a physician. Co-signature by two nurses is needed with some medications; institutional policies vary, and nurses should be aware of the practice of the hospitals in which they are employed.

Medications can be delivered through an IV line in different ways. Most commonly, medication is mixed in approximately 30 to 100 ml of IV fluid and administered above the drip chamber over 15 to 60 minutes, in the Soluset or Buretrol. Minibags of 50 to 100 ml of solution can also be used if the IV does not have a Soluset. Antibiotics are frequently administered in this fashion. Some medications are given IV push, or injected into the IV tubing below the drip chamber, usually over 60 seconds; however, this procedure usually requires specialized preparation and certification. The IV push method is used when rapid administration of drugs is required and when infants who are fluid-restricted require medications. Bag or bottle administration refers to infusion of a drug, usually in at least 250 ml of IV fluid, in a plastic bag or glass bottle. Total parenteral nutrition and insulin drips are examples of medications infused in this way.

Independent of the administration route, all medications infused through the IV line should be documented properly on the medication record. It is also advisable to mark the IV line during administration with the name, amount, and time of medication administration, in addition to the nurse's initials. This is often called "flagging" the line and provides information to other nurses and hospital personnel in case of an allergic reaction or other emergency.

Before mixing medications, their compatibility is checked by referring to a compatibility chart or by calling the pharmacist. Mixing drugs that are incompatible can cause a chemical reaction and result in clouding and sediment formation. These combinations may also render drugs ineffective. A drug may be incompatible with another drug or with an IV solution. Proper flushing of the IV line between drugs with approximately 10 to 20 ml of fluid can prevent drug-drug reactions. (See Fig. 24–8, illustrating flagging of the line and flushing between drugs.)

For drug-solution incompatibilities, a secondary IV line with another solution that is compatible with the drug to be given is often needed to deliver the

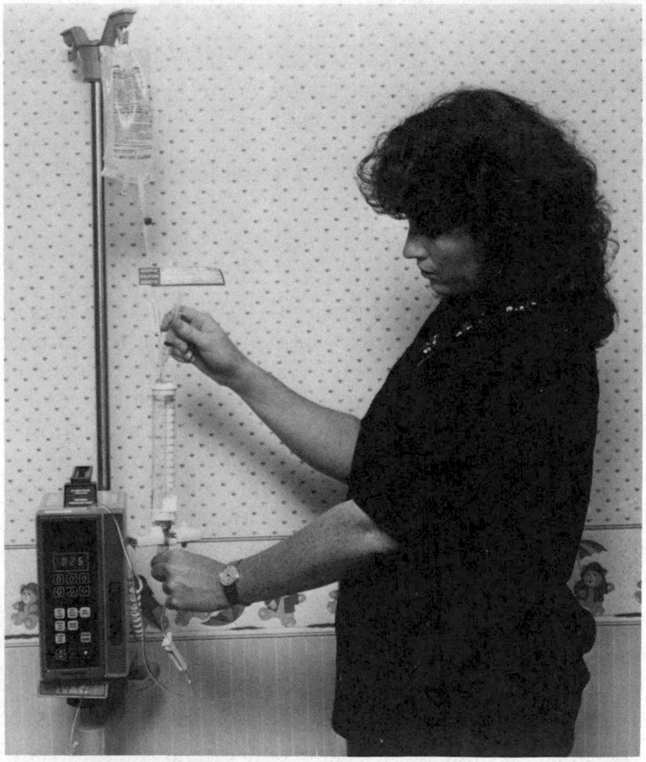

FIGURE 24-8. Administering IV medications. When IV medications are administered, the IV is "flagged" during administration to indicate which drug is infusing. Following administration of the medication, approximately 15 ml of fluid is dropped into the chamber from the bag to flush the line.

drug. For example, if the main line contains potassium and the drug to be administered is incompatible with potassium, then a secondary line without potassium is necessary. Detailed compatibility information should be available in an institution's pharmacy department.

Consideration of maximum administration time and infusion rate of a drug is important. Some drugs in solution become unstable after a certain amount of time, and must be administered within a certain time limit after mixed. The rate of infusion is significant, because some drugs are irritating. See Table 24–7 for a list of commonly used drugs that are irritating. Slower administration can offset these irritating effects.

Nursing responsibilities surrounding IV drug administration include assessment of the IV site for redness or swelling. The nurse should also be aware of the signs and symptoms of allergic reactions and anaphylactic shock. Safety is increased by teaching the child and/or parents to notify the nurse if any of these symptoms are experienced. Nursing care associated with starting and maintaining an IV is presented in Chapter 26.

Evaluation

The need to take medications may be relatively short-lived, may extend to months or years, or may be permanent. When children require medication, regardless of the length of time, the child's response to taking medications and the desired therapeutic effect are monitored.

Evaluation of interventions to resolve problematic responses associated with medication administration focuses on whether the defining characteristics of the response have disappeared or decreased. If the child shows an increasingly negative attitude, then the approach must be re-evaluated. The parents need to be consulted for their interpretation of the child's experience and about how to reduce their child's fears.

The therapeutic effect of medication is evaluated by assessing the child for a reduction in the signs and symptoms of the problem for which the drug is administered. Additionally, the child is monitored for any indication of side effects. Maintaining a balance between the therapeutic effect and side effects of the drug requires ongoing evaluation by the entire health care team; this ensures that the appropriate drug is given in the most effective dose.

TABLE 24-7
Commonly Used Irritating Intravenous Drugs

The following drugs are known to be irritating and may cause phlebitis and pain when administered intravenously:

Ampicillin	Erythromycin
Cefotaxime	Metronidazole (Flagyl)
Cefotetan	Piperacillin
Cefuroxime	Ranitidine
Cephalothin	Sodium bicarbonate
Chlorpromazine	Tobramycin
Clindamycin	Vancomycin
Cloxacillin	

Adverse effects are frequently associated with rate of infusion; therefore, slowing or temporarily stopping the infusion may ameliorate the reaction

KEY CONCEPTS

Concepts Related to Basic Information

- Pharmacokinetics is the study of drug absorption, distribution, metabolism, and elimination (what the body does to the drug).
- Pharmacodynamics is the study of the beneficial or harmful effects of a drug (what the drug does in the body).
- Drug action takes place at a cellular level and is initiated by combining with drug receptors, which are found in every cell in the body.
- A drug selectively binds to several types of receptors; to some receptors it binds more strongly than others, and this difference in binding is what causes both therapeutic effects and toxicity or side effects.
- The therapeutic index of a drug is the ratio of its beneficial to undesirable effects.
- Bioavailability of a drug refers to the fraction of the administered dose that reaches the systemic circulation (only the IV route guarantees 100 per cent bioavailability).
- Only "free" drug (that which is not bound) can interact with a receptor.
- Total drug concentration as measured by most laboratories is a measure of the total (bound and free) amount of a drug.
- Beneficial and harmful effects of drugs can occur as a result of same-receptor actions, identical receptors located in different tissues, and actions by different types of receptors.
- Drug interactions may lead to changes in the concentration of the drug at its receptor site, resulting in a change in the pharmacologic effect observed.
- Absorption of drugs is affected by the route administered, pH levels of the gastrointestinal tract, and gastric motility.
- Biologic differences across the ages of children affect drug absorption, distribution, and metabolism.

Concepts Related to Nursing Assessment

- Assessment begins with a history of the child's experience with medications, current medication regimen, knowledge about medications, past allergies, and parental involvement in the child's medication regimen.
- Before medication is given, an assessment must be made of the child's developmental capability with respect to swallowing an oral medication.
- The child must be clearly identified before medication is administered.
- When a medication is administered, regardless of the route by which it is given, the order is checked against the medication profile at least three times.
- Careful assessments are made to determine whether a child has any allergies and to identify the first signs of a drug reaction.
- The harmful effects of giving a drug intramuscularly should be heavily weighed before this route of administration is chosen.

Concepts Related to Nursing Intervention

- Involvement of parents can facilitate the cooperation of a child in all types of medication administration.
- A child's fears about medication can be reduced with appropriate preparation before the administration and by providing support during the experience.
- Forceful restraint can physically and psychologically harm a child.
- Children should be told the truth when they ask how medications taste and whether they will be painful.
- For selected drugs, blood levels are measured to check the level of the drug's concentration, and these should be checked by the nurse before the next scheduled dose is given.
- Infants must be protected against aspiration of medications by ensuring that the medication has been swallowed before the child is placed back into the crib.
- Medications should not be referred to as "candy" or "a treat" when one is trying to get a child to take the medication.
- If a child *must* receive an IM injection, preparation for and support during the procedure are essential strategies.
- The vastus lateralis is the only recommended site in the child under the age of 3 years.
- All medications are accurately documented.
- Drug-drug reactions can be prevented by proper flushing of the IV line between drug administrations.

REFERENCES

Beecroft, P. C., & Redick, S. A. (1990). Intramuscular injection practices of pediatric nurses: Site selection. *Nurse Educator, 15*(4), 23–28.

Beecroft, P. C., & Redick, S. A. (1989). Possible complications of intramuscular injections on the pediatric unit. *Pediatric Nursing, 15*(4), 333–336.

Bourne, H. R., & Roberts, J. M. (1992). Drug receptors and pharmacodynamics. In B. G. Katzung (Ed.), *Basic and clinical pharmacology*. Norwalk, CT: Appleton & Lange.

Byington, K. C. (1991). Your guide to pediatric drug administration. *Nursing 1991, 21*(8), 82.

Evans, M. L., & Hansen, B. D. (1981). Administering injections to different-aged children. *MCN: American Journal of Maternal Child Nursing, 6,* 194–199.

Giacoia, G., & Gorodisher, R. (1975). Pharmacologic principles in neonatal drug therapy. *Clinics in Perinatology, 2*(1), 125–137.

Gladke, E. (1979). The importance of pharmacokinetics for pediatrics. *European Journal of Pediatrics, 13,* 85.

Holbrook, P. R., Schaible, D. H. (1983). Pediatric pharmacotherapy. In B. Chernow (Ed.), *The pharmacological approach to the critically ill patient.* Baltimore: Williams & Wilkins.

Hopkins, C. S., Buckley, C. J., & Bush, G. H. (1988). Pain-free injection in infants; use of lidocaine-prilocaine cream to prevent pain at intravenous induction of general anaesthesia in 1–5 year old children. *Anaesthesia, 43,* 198–201.

Howry, L. B., et al. (1981). *Pediatric medications.* Philadelphia: JB Lippincott.

Kagan, B. M. (1983). Pediatric pharmacology. In J. A. Bevan & J. H. Thompson (Eds.). *Essentials of pharmacology* (3rd ed.). New York: Harper & Row.

Kearns, G. L., Reed, M. D. (1989). Clinical pharmacokinetics in infants and children, a reappraisal. *Clinical Pharmacokinetics, 17*(Suppl. 1), 29.

Magnussen, I., et al. (1979). Absorption of diazepam in man following rectal and parenteral administration. *Acta Pharmacology and Toxicology, 45,* 87–90.

Milla, P. J., & Fenton, J. R. (1983). Small intestinal motility patterns in the perinatal period. *Journal of Pediatric Gastroenterology and Nutrition, 2*(Suppl. 1): S141.

Morselli, P. L., et al. (1980). Clinical pharmacokinetics in newborns and infants: Age related differences and therapeutic implications. *Clinical Pharmacokinetics, 5,* 484–527.

O'Neill, S. P. (1990). Anaphylactic shock. *American Journal of Nursing, 90*(12), 40.

Ormerod, E., & Caulfield, C. (1976). A practical guide to giving oral medication to young children. *MCN: American Journal of Maternal Child Nursing, 2,* 320–325.

Pippenger, C. E. (1980). Rationale and clinical application of therapeutic drug monitoring. *Pediatric Clinics of North America, 27*(4), 896–925.

Roberts, R. J. (1984). *Drug therapy in infants: Pharmacologic principles and clinical experience.* Philadelphia: WB Saunders.

Russell, H. (1980). *Pediatric drugs and nursing interventions.* New York: McGraw-Hill.

Sheridan, E., et al. (1982). *Falconer's the drug, the nurse, the patient* (7th ed.). Philadelphia: WB Saunders.

Udkow, G. P. (1987). Clinical pharmacology. In R. A. Hoekelman, et al. (Eds.), *Primary pediatric care.* St. Louis: CV Mosby.

Vanselow, N. A. (1988). Minutes to counter anaphylaxis. *Emergency Medicine, 20*(15), 121–123.

Weinberger, M., et al. (1981). Clinical pharmacology of drugs used in asthma. *Pediatric Clinics of North America, 28,* 47.

Wink, D. M. (1991). Giving infants and children drugs: Precision and caution equals safety. *MCN: American Journal of Maternal Child Nursing, 16,* 317–321.

Yeh, T. F. (1985). *Drug therapy in the neonate and small infant.* Chicago: Year Book.

BIBLIOGRAPHY

Bordun, L. A., & Butt, W. (1992). Drug errors in intensive care. *Journal of Pediatric Child Health, 28*(4), 309–311.

Ferris, E. W. (1990). A neonatal home intravenous antibiotic therapy program. *Journal of Intravenous Nursing, 13*(6), 383–387.
Guyan, G. (1989). Pharmacokinetic considerations in neonatal drug therapy. *Neonatal Network, 7*(5), 9–12.
Losek, J. D., & Gyuro, J. (1992). Pediatric intramuscular injections: Do you know the procedure and complications? *Pediatric Emergency Care, 8*(2), 79–81.
Raju, T. N., Kecskes, S., Thornton, J. P., Perry, M., & Feldman, S. (1989, August 12). Medication errors in neonatal and paediatric intensive-care units. *Lancet, 2*(8659), 374–376.
Rimar, J. M. (1987). Guidelines for the intravenous administration of medications used in pediatrics. *MCN: American Journal of Maternal Child Nursing, 12*(5), 322–340.
Trang, J. M., Kluza, R. B., & Kearns, G. L. (1984). Pharmacokinetics for pediatric nurses. *Pediatric Nursing, 10*(4), 267–274.
Weatherly, K. S., Young, S., & Andresky, J. (1991). Needle stick injury in pediatric hospitals. *Pediatric Nursing, 17*(1), 95–99.
Wiggins, M. S., & Sesin, P. (1990). Guidelines for administering I.V. drugs. *Nursing, 20*(4), 145–152.

CHAPTER • 25

Nursing Management of Pain in Children

Roxie Foster
Bonnie Stevens

RELATED TOPICS
Stress, Crisis, and Coping, Chapter 18
Principles and Skills Adapted to the Care of Children, Chapter 23
Nursing Care During Hospitalization, Chapter 21
Pharmacologic principles, Chapter 24

LEARNING OBJECTIVES

- Outline the definitions and properties used to describe the concept of pain.
- Describe the Gate Control Theory.
- Identify misconceptions about pain in infants and children and discuss research findings that refute the myths.
- Summarize the research related to the pain experience in infants and children.
- Outline the components of a comprehensive nursing assessment of pain and discuss instruments used to measure pain in infants and children.
- Outline age-related pain behaviors, expressions, and fears and describe potential sources of comfort.
- Identify nursing interventions to prevent and to relieve pain and discuss developmental interventions to reduce fear, anxiety, and powerlessness.
- Discuss pharmacologic management of pain in infants and children and give examples of commonly used drugs and related nursing considerations.
- Illustrate various nonpharmacologic approaches used to relieve pain in infants and children.
- Describe methods used to evaluate the effectiveness of pain management.

Pain — a concept so familiar, yet so elusive that it has been termed the most complex of human stressors (Chapman & Bonica, 1983). Pain — a common companion to illness, a common concern for nurses who seek to comfort, and, yet, a phenomenon that is unique to the experiencing individual. By what signs and symptoms can one recognize its existence? By what measure can one determine its intensity? By what strategies can one relieve it? These and related questions have been the subject of a burgeoning body of literature associated with pain in recent years. Although fewer data exist about the experience of pain in children than in adults, progress is being made toward building a research base for pain assessment and pain relief in pediatric nursing. Despite advances in science and technology, children are not treated adequately for their pain. Resolution of undertreatment requires knowledge of the scientific base for decision making and an openness to understanding pain from the point of view of the child who is experiencing it.

Defining Pain and Pain Properties

The complexity of pain has made it difficult to define the concept in terms that are representative across individuals. As noted by Melzack (1973, p 45):

> Pain is not a single quality of experience. . . . The word "pain" represents a category of experiences, signifying a multitude of different, unique events having different causes, and characterized by different qualities varying along a number of sensory and affective dimensions.

Because of this complexity, "pain" continues to be defined in different ways by different disciplines. A neurophysiologist may think of pain in terms of patterns of action potentials in neural centers, whereas a psychologist may view pain in terms of behavioral or emotional responses. In an attempt to develop a definition of pain that could be useful to scientists and practitioners across disciplines, the International Association for the Study of Pain (IASP) proposed that pain is "an unpleasant sensory and emotional experience associated with actual or potential tissue damage, or described in terms of such damage" (Bonica, 1979, p 250). The limitation of this definition is that, although the emotional component is identified, the emphasis is on physiologic aspects of pain.

McCaffery (1972) proposed a definition of pain from the nursing perspective: "Pain is what the patient says it is and exists when he says it does." The strength of this definition is its emphasis on the uniqueness of the pain experience and the fact that most of the information about pain must come from *subjective* data. This definition has been widely accepted and used by nurses in recent years. As with all definitions, however, it has its limitations. How does one assess the preverbal child or the child who refuses to cooperate with pain assessment? It is also important to remember that *the child who chooses to tolerate pain rather than report it still suffers* (Kushner, 1985). It seems that a truly universal definition of pain, particularly one that is applicable to children, is still to be found.

It is somewhat easier to define certain properties of pain than it is to define the concept of pain itself. Pain "threshold" is the point at which an individual first perceives that an unpleasant stimulus or sensation exists. Pain "tolerance" refers to the point at which the individual can no longer endure the unpleasant sensation at that magnitude or intensity. Pain threshold is most often associated with physiologic variables, whereas pain tolerance is primarily related to psychologic factors. Pain tolerance varies from person to person and from time to time within the individual. That pain tolerance is moderated by psychologic factors can be illustrated by the boy who chooses to endure moderate pain in the presence of peers rather than appear to be a "sissy," but later asks for medication for less severe pain.

Pain "duration" is the length of time since pain onset. Duration is expressed in units of time, such as minutes, hours, days, or months. For descriptive purposes, duration is usually combined with some measure of intensity; the chart may read, "Melissa has been complaining of severe pain in her leg for the past ½ hour." Pain duration may modify pain tolerance in that pain of long duration may fatigue the child and make the pain less bearable.

Acute Versus Chronic Pain

Pain can also be classified as acute or chronic. Acute pain is often characterized by its sudden onset and limited duration. Acute pain may originate as an emotional reaction to some unpleasant or noxious stimulus and functions as an adaptive biologic warning signal (e.g., the pain of appendicitis) or a protective mechanism against injury (limiting further tissue damage by discouraging motion) (Chapman & Bonica, 1983). As noted by Ross and Ross (1988), however, the warning function is undermined by the fact that the severity of pain does not necessarily relate to the seriousness of the injury.

"Acute pain" is often modified by the suddenness with which it occurs. Fear and anxiety of the precipitating event may heighten the perception of pain. This is frequently a consideration for children undergoing diagnostic or therapeutic interventions. Fear may stem either from previous experience (e.g., an injection) or from unfamiliarity with equipment that looks "scary" but inflicts no pain (e.g., an x-ray machine). Katz and associates (1981) suggest that anxiety is the basic affective state that modulates pain perception.

"Chronic pain" is often considered to be pain lasting longer than 6 months (Escobar, 1985). Some researchers consider the psychosocial impact of pain (interference with activities of daily living) as well as its duration in defining chronicity (McGrath & Unruh, 1987). Crue (1985) described four types of long-term pain:

- "Recurrent acute," or pain from underlying continued nociceptive input (e.g., the pain from systemic juvenile rheumatoid arthritis).
- "Ongoing acute," as the pain from malignant disease and its metastasis.
- "Chronic benign pain," or the ongoing pain that has no known nociceptive cause but permits adequate coping.
- "Chronic benign intractable pain," which is chronic, long-term pain with which the patient is not able to cope adequately.

Clearly, there is some overlap in the symptoms of chronic versus acute pain. However, in acute pain, the unpleasant sensation usually disappears after the pathology or noxious stimulus is resolved, whereas, in chronic pain, the pain may persist for much longer, even after the pathology (or other cause) has been resolved.

Understanding Pain Management as a Health Care Frontier

Children often suffer needless pain. Undertreatment of pain in children was first exemplified by two studies. Swafford and Allan (1968) studied 180 children admitted to an intensive care unit over a 4-month period. Only 26 received narcotic analgesics. Of 60 children undergoing general surgery on another unit, only 2 received medications for pain. Reflecting attitudes of that time, Swafford and Allen suggested children received all the medication they "required."

In 1974, Eland compared the analgesics received by 18 adults and 18 children matched for diagnosis. Adults and children were patients on the same hospital unit and were cared for by the same nurses. The 18 adults received a total of 372 doses of narcotic analgesics and 299 doses of nonnarcotic analgesia during their hospital stay. Six of the 18 children with identical diagnoses received no medication for pain; the remaining 12 were administered a *total* of 24 doses of analgesics (Eland & Anderson, 1977).

The consciousness-raising effect of these studies launched worldwide research on pain in children in the 1970s and 1980s. Further studies comparing pain medications given to adults and children confirmed the problem of undertreatment. Some research concentrated on developing and testing better ways for children to communicate about their pain. Still other studies addressed factors thought to influence pain assessment and management. Disturbingly, the plethora of studies and subsequent publications in the professional literature had little effect on the care health professionals provided to children in pain.

Repeated descriptions of needless suffering and concern for the delay in implementing research-based practice spurred the United States Congress to commission a panel of health care experts to develop clinical practice guidelines for pain management across the life span. These guidelines, published in 1992, provide a concise outline for effective management of acute pain.*

Pain management remains a health care frontier. Knowledge has only recently reached proportions sufficient to sustain research-based judgments. For example, the chapter on pain management in the last edition of this textbook marked the first time either a medical or a nursing textbook had devoted an entire chapter to pain.

Education about pain management is critical for achieving changes in practice. The goal of effective relief of pain in children will become a reality when the barriers to pain management are exposed and addressed. Through education, the fears, myths, and half-truths that once guided decisions about the assessment and management of pain in children will be replaced by a scientific base for judgments.

---

*The "Quick Reference Guide for Clinicians—Acute Pain Management in Infants, Children, and Adolescents: Operative and Medical Procedures" (1992) (a 22-page pamphlet, AHCPR Pub. No. 92–0020) is available by calling 1–800–358–9295 or by writing to the Center for Research Dissemination and Liaison, AHCPR Publications Clearinghouse, P.O. Box 8547, Silver Spring, MD 20907.

Guidelines for management of cancer pain are also available from the Department of Health and Human Services, Public Health Service, Agency for Health Care Policy and Research, Executive Office Center, 2101 East Jefferson Street, Suite 401, Rockville, MD 20852.

The Scientific Base for Judgments about Pain in Children

Many decades of research have formed the scientific base for clinical judgments about pain. Among the important studies are those that led to the Gate Control Theory of pain (Melzack & Wall, 1965). Gate Control Theory encompasses earlier ideas of pain transmission and builds on the work of many scientists. This section provides an overview of the Gate Control Theory and its application to management of pain in children.

The Gate Control Theory

The Gate Control Theory reflects the most current understanding of how pain impulses travel between the site of injury and the brain (Bonica, 1990; Fields, 1992; Jeans & Melzack, 1992). Central to the theory is the distinction between the pain-producing impulse (nociception) and the perception of the impulse as pain.

"Nociception" or "nociceptive processing" refers to the detection of a noxious stimulus and the transduction and transmission of information about the presence and the quality of that stimulus from the site of stimulation to the brain. . . . Pain is a psychological experience, the human perception; nociception is the activity in the nervous system that may lead to pain. [McGrath, 1990, p 94]

When tissue damage occurs, distinct types of nerve receptors called "nociceptors" are activated. Nociceptive impulses travel along nerve fibers from the site of tissue damage to the dorsal horn of the spinal cord, where they synapse with T (transmission)–cells. The T-cells then transmit the impulses to action systems in the brain.

On reaching the dorsal horn, pain impulses are *modulated* (modified) before being projected to areas of the brain responsible for pain perception and response. When impulses are modified in accordance with other factors, the initial impulse may be increased or decreased (excitatory or inhibitory modulation). To the limits of current science, the modulating ("gating") mechanisms of the Gate Control Theory explain why the *same* stimulus may result in very *different* pain experiences across individuals or within the same individual at different times. As depicted in Figure 25–1, *factors within the individual (internal environment) and factors existing in the external environment sometimes play larger roles in the pain experience than the physical (somatosensory) trauma!*

Excitation and inhibition of pain impulses result from physiologic and psychologic mechanisms. "Physiologic modulation" depends on the diameter of the fiber transmitting the impulse. Small-diameter fibers have an excitatory effect on T-cells (open the gate),

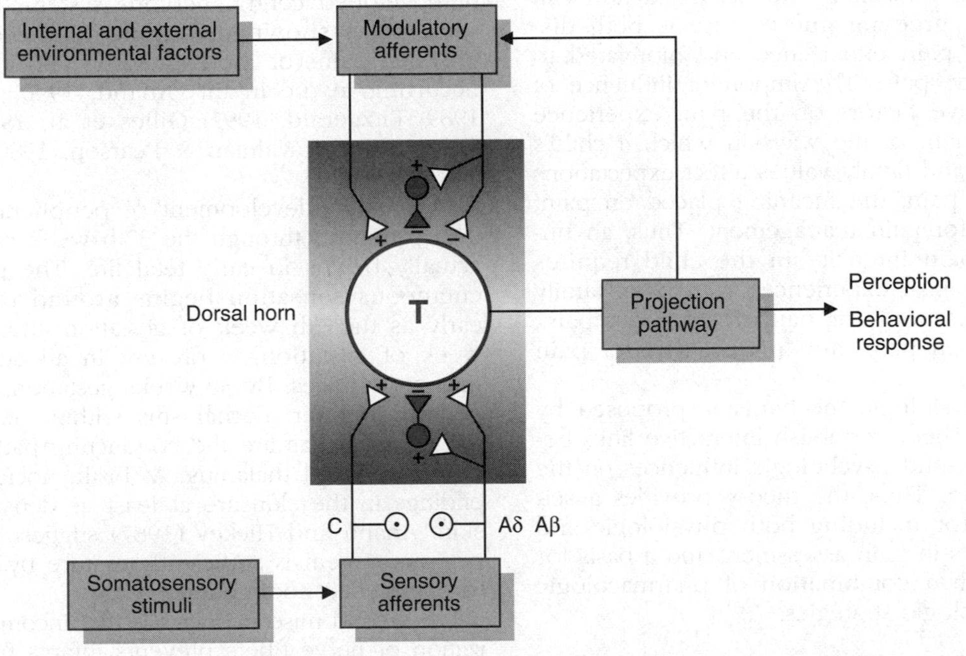

FIGURE 25 - 1. Modulatory and sensory afferents influence dorsal horn pain-transmission neurons. Although modulatory systems are clearly influenced by somatosensory stimuli, the relationship is highly variable and other environmental factors often play a greater role. (From Fields, H. L. Is there a facilitating component to central pain modulation? *American Pain Society Journal, 1*[2], 82, © 1992, Churchill Livingstone, New York.)

whereas large-diameter fibers inhibit pain impulses (close the gate). For example, if you apply firm pressure to your head after bumping it, you stimulate large-diameter fibers. The large-diameter fibers block transmission of the pain signal, and you feel the pressure of your hand instead of the pain from the bump. When the pressure is released, the intense pain returns.

"Psychologic processes" also influence the individual's pain. Melzack wrote, "We do not learn to *feel* qualities of experience: our brains are built to *produce* them" (1991, p 18). "Production" of pain is a complex process. It includes input from sensory-discriminative, motivational-affective, and cognitive-evaluative areas of the brain.

Sensory-discriminative areas of the brain provide information about the location, intensity, and duration of the noxious stimulus. An intensity monitor in the brain discriminates between levels of impulses transmitted by T-cells. Up to a critical level of intensity, impulses are thought to activate motivational-affective areas that trigger positive affect and approach tendencies (e.g., the pleasurable experience of light massage). However, when T-cell output reaches a critical intensity (as in a pinch) negative emotions are provoked and the individual tries to avoid the stimulus.

Cognitive-evaluative (cognitive control) processes provide the scientific base for the effect of attention, anxiety, cultural values, and past experiences on pain. These processes can either intensify or reduce the pain impulses. For example, fear of pain is thought to intensify the pain intensity, whereas distraction can reduce it. When greeting guests, one is both distracted from the pain experience and motivated to appear free of the pain. The important influence of cognitive-evaluative factors on the pain experience mandates assessment of the ways in which a child's past experiences and family values affect expectations for pain, fear of pain, the meaning placed on pain, and preferences for pain management. Thus, an understanding of pain intensity in the child requires knowledge about past experiences with pain, family values and expectations for pain, fears about pain, meaning placed on pain, and preferences for pain treatment.

The neurophysiologic mechanisms proposed by the Gate Control Theory establish interactive links between physiologic and psychologic influences on the perception of pain. Thus, the theory provides a scientific rationale for including both physiologic and psychologic factors in pain assessment and a basis for treating pain with a combination of pharmacologic and nonpharmacologic strategies.

Application of the Gate Control Theory to Pain in Children

Assessment of pain in infants and young children is limited by the child's verbal and comprehension abilities and the adult's ability to recognize subtle (and often different) behavioral responses. Unfortunately, the young child's inability to *express* pain in the adult sense has been generalized as an inability to *perceive* pain. Application of the Gate Control Theory to pain in children requires an understanding of those factors that modulate the child's ability to perceive and to express the pain experienced. The most important of these factors is the child's stage of development.

Developmental Aspects of Pain Perception

Perception of pain is dependent on anatomic/physiologic and cognitive/behavioral factors. These factors are influenced by the child's developmental stage. Knowledge of developmental changes in anatomy/physiology and cognitive/behavioral components of pain perception is important to pain assessment and evaluation of interventions designed to reduce or eliminate pain.

Developmental Changes in Anatomy and Physiology. Evidence firmly supports the infant's capacity for response to a painful stimulus and pain perception. Yet, many myths and misconceptions hamper pain assessment and management in this age group. The most prevalent myth is that infants do not experience pain. This myth derives from certain anatomic properties of the infant's neurologic system that include: (1) underdeveloped peripheral nerve endings, (2) incomplete myelinization of nerve fibers, and (3) an underdeveloped central nervous system. However, research has shown that none of these limitations prevents pain (or more precisely, nociception) from occurring in the infant (Anand, 1990; Anand et al, 1989; Fitzgerald, 1991; Gilles et al, 1983; Gleiss & Stuttgen, 1970; Valman & Pearson, 1980; Rizvi et al, 1987).

Although development of peripheral nerve endings continues through the 37th week of gestation, it actually begins in early fetal life. The perception of cutaneous sensation begins around the mouth as early as the 7th week of gestation and, by the 20th week of gestation, is present in all cutaneous and mucous surfaces. By 30 weeks gestation, synaptic and neurotransmitter mechanisms within the dorsal horn are complete, as are the conducting pathways to the brain stem and thalamus. At birth, nociceptive nerve endings in the skin are at least as dense as in adult skin. Anand and Hickey (1987) suggest that the fetal nervous system is sufficiently mature by midgestation to experience nociception.

A second misconception is that incomplete myelinization of nerve fibers prevents infants from fully experiencing pain. However, in adults, pain impulses are carried by both the faster myelinated and the slower nonmyelinated nerve fibers. Therefore, *the lack of a myelin sheath does not mean a lack of function in the peripheral nerves but rather a slower conduction speed.* Considering the shorter distances over which pain impulses are transmitted between the infant's periphery and the central nervous system, the speed of transmission is probably similar for infants and adults.

The third misconception is that the infant is unable to experience pain owing to the immaturity of the central nervous system. However, we now know that neurotransmitters appear as early as 8 to 10 weeks gestation and spinal cord synapses begin to develop before 14 weeks gestation. By 20 weeks, the fetal cerebral cortex has a full complement of neurons. Maturation of the pathways leading from the spinal cord to the thalamus is complete by 30 weeks gestation and from the thalamus to the cerebral cortex by 37 weeks. Thus, *mechanisms are intact to enable infants to receive and conduct pain impulses from the periphery to the sensory cortex at birth, even if born prematurely* (Fitzgerald & Anand, 1993).

During infancy and early childhood, there is continued development in nerve pathways and in the mechanisms that mediate pain. Continued refinement has two important implications for pain in preterm and term infants. *First,* research suggests that mechanisms to inhibit pain (e.g., endogenous opiates) are less well developed in early infancy than are the mechanisms to transmit pain and to excite the transmission of impulses (Fields, 1987; Fitzgerald, 1991). This means that young infants may be particularly sensitive to painful stimuli because their bodies cannot effectively inhibit pain impulses.

Second, early infancy is associated with a high degree of plasticity in the nervous system. "Plasticity" is the ability of the nociceptive system to respond differently to equal amounts of tissue damage (McGrath, 1993; Price, 1988; Wall, 1988). Different responses imply that some modification to nociceptive processing has occurred. Recent research suggests plasticity may initiate permanent structural changes in pain pathways when infants are subjected to repeated painful events without pain relief (Fitzgerald, 1991). Although this research is in the early stages, the implications are sobering.

Unrelieved pain has been linked with postoperative morbidity and mortality in neonates (Anand et al, 1992). Preterm infants have shown the ability to mount a marked stress response to surgery, as demonstrated by increased catecholamines, corticosteroids, growth hormone, and glucagon. Furthermore, the neonatal stress response has been shown to vary proportionately with the degree of surgical trauma. Although Kehlet (1991) showed that this hormonal response may be triggered by other factors such as tissue damage, fluid loss, and infection, studies by Anand and colleagues (1992) linking inhibition of stress hormones with the intraoperative administration of an analgesic argue convincingly that the stress response is at least partially related to pain.

Additionally, the actions of opioids (narcotic analgesics) are affected by physiologic development (Koren & Butt, 1985; Lynn & Slattery, 1987; Olkkola et al, 1988; Reed & Besunder, 1989). Studies have shown that, in infants younger than 6 months of age, morphine is cleared from the body more slowly than in older children and adults. Reduced activity of drug-oxidizing enzymes in the liver and reduced glomerular filtration rate in the young infant contribute to the differences in opioid metabolism.

Developmental Changes in Cognition and Behavior. Cognitive/behavioral influences on pain perception include the meaning associated with the pain, past pain experiences, emotional responses to pain, coping patterns, and social influences related to family and culture. Cognitive/behavioral influences are linked, in part, to language ability.

Research has found that age influences children's definition of pain and the meaning they associate with pain (Gaffney & Dunne, 1987; Jeans & Gordon, 1981; McGrath, 1990, 1993). Preschool children tend to define pain in terms of its location and to connect events without understanding the relationships between them. For example, a young child may think pain is the result of wrongdoing. School-age children are able to understand the cause of their pain and to describe the pain they are feeling, but their descriptions reflect the concrete thinking of that developmental stage. Adolescents can view their pain more abstractly, linking pain with physiologic processes that have been described to them but that they cannot see or completely understand.

Children's pain language depends not only on their developmental level but also on their frame of reference. For example, children evaluate pain in relation to past experiences. "Children evaluate the strength and unpleasantness of any new pain in reference to an ever-changing background of their previous pain" (McGrath, 1990, p 30). Research has shown that children with little pain experience tend to rate pictures of common pain situations as more painful than children with extensive pain experiences. Thus, *to understand the pain experience from the child's point of view, it is necessary to consider her or his basis for comparison.* For example, a child who has experienced little previous pain may rate removal of an intravenous needle as "the worst pain possible."

When talking with children about their pain, keep in mind that the child's repertoire of pain experiences is less extensive than yours. For example, the discomfort of a nasogastric tube might be considered inconsequential in relation to other pain nurses have witnessed or have experienced themselves. For the child, however, this may be the worst pain ever encountered. *Effective pain management considers the child's perspective.*

Emotions such as fear, anxiety, and sadness intensify pain. Fear is an issue for children at all ages, but the younger the child the more likely that fear is magnified by lack of understanding. Emotions affect not only psychologic responses to pain but also transmission of nociceptive impulses (Chapman & Turner,

1990). Norepinephrine released in response to emotional arousal makes nociceptors more sensitive to pain impulses. Therefore, reduction of fear and other aversive emotions is critical to pain management.

Coping patterns also influence the pain experience (Chapman & Turner, 1990; Melzack & Wall, 1988). When coping is effective, it *inhibits pain impulses* through gating mechanisms in the spinal cord. School-age children who were interviewed about their pain talked about the importance of coping. A 9-year-old girl said, "You can make it awful or you can make it OK" (Ross & Ross, 1988, p 55). Another child commented, "It just hurts and you get frustrated . . . and you've got to be real strong and not let it get to you" (Ross & Ross, 1988, p 63).

Coping strategies increase in number and sophistication as the child matures. Therefore, young children with few coping strategies are in the greatest jeopardy. Consider the plight of a 2-year-old child restrained for a painful procedure. Gross motor movement is an important coping strategy for toddlers. When movement is restricted, it is important to provide other means of comfort such as the presence of a parent and distraction techniques. Children and adolescents interviewed about their pain experiences indicated the importance of analgesic medication, attention-distraction techniques, and the support of others, especially their mothers, in coping with pain (Abu-Saad, 1984c; Branson et al, 1990; Hester, 1989; Ross & Ross, 1988).

Emotional responses and coping strategies are often associated with social learning within the family and culture. From a theoretical perspective, children learn what they see. "If the child observes significant people in his or her life showing frequent displays of verbal or nonverbal expressions of pain, overreacting to minimal pain or having difficulty obtaining pain relief . . . then the child is more vulnerable to learning noncoping pain behavior" (McGrath & Unruh, 1987, p 64). The association of family transactions and children's symptoms is also illustrated by research and clinical accounts wherein parental anxiety escalated child anxiety.

Research suggests that parental expectations of children in pain vary according to the child's age, gender, and birth order (McGrath, 1990, 1993; McGrath & Unruh, 1987). However, little substantive evidence exists to explain the influences of family and culture on the pain experience. The tendency to group individuals by ethnicity without concern for other factors can be misrepresentative. Often family values or experiences have as much influence as ethnicity. For example, parent expectations may change as children get older. In one study, interviews with Vietnamese refugees revealed the majority used traditional Vietnamese healing aids, such as coin rubbing, as the preferred treatment for pain. Children older than 8 years were expected to react stoically to pain and to refrain from physical displays of affection (Fritz et al, 1991). Results such as these must be interpreted with caution. Whereas the influence of family and culture cannot be ignored, stereotyping individuals by ethnic group ignores variables that may be more important in determining pain response.

Another approach to understanding cultural influences on the pain experience is to examine the origin of cultural values. A recent study of pain in Aztec and Mayan civilizations illuminated themes that may undergird beliefs of modern Mexican-Americans. Prominent among the themes were a stoic response to pain and alleviation of pain through restoration of balance between the person and the environment (Villarruel & Ortiz de Montellano, 1992). Additional studies like this one are needed to establish a context for understanding pain without suggesting that everyone in a particular ethnic group experiences pain in the same way.

Knowledge that emotional responses and coping skills affect the pain experience carries implications for health care professionals. "The essential ingredient is providing the patient with skills to cope with the pain and anxiety—at the very least, to provide the patient with a sense of control" (Melzack & Wall, 1988, p 25). Research with adult patients has shown that perceived control over pain reduces reported pain intensity (Toomey et al, 1991). Citing anecdotes from clinical practice with children, McGrath asserted that "understanding, predictability, and control are the most important situational factors that can minimize acute pain evoked by repeated invasive procedures" (1990, p 244). *The younger the child, the less opportunity for control over their environment* (Johnston, 1993). Yet, children as young as 3 years old can undergo painful procedures, such as finger sticks, when they can control who, when, and how the procedure is to be done. Without the option for control, learned helplessness may result, a state in which the child gives up in despair at the inability to affect or modify the situation.

Knowledge of the pain-producing stimulus, especially when combined with strategies for controlling the stimulus, can be helpful in reducing fear and anxiety (Jeans & Melzack, 1992). Information about a pain stimulus can desensitize the child by eliminating unfounded fears and increasing predictability (Chapman & Turner, 1990). This principle underlies prehospitalization preparation for children and families.

Although the efficacy of attention-distraction techniques is widely accepted, many accounts of children's success are anecdotal. The research literature is limited by small sample sizes and lack of replication. However, positive effects have been attributed to film modeling, breathing exercises, positive incentives, emotive imagery, progressive relaxation (Siegel, 1991), and other attention-distraction techniques (Engel & Rapoff, 1990; Fowler-Kerry & Ramsay-Lander, 1990; Ryan, 1989).

Developmental Aspects of Pain Expression

Developmental Changes in Physiology. Research results about physiologic and hormonal responses to pain in infants are summarized in Table 25–1. In

TABLE 25-1
Physiologic and Hormonal Responses to Pain in Infants

Response	Research Study	Results
Physiologic		
Heart rate	Berg et al (1971)	Increase
	Booth et al (1989)	Increase
	Field & Goldson (1984)	Increase
	Owens & Todt (1984)	Increase
	Johnston & Strada (1986)	Brief decrease, followed by increase
Vagal tone	Porter et al (1988)	Initial increase followed by decrease
Respiratory rate	Booth et al (1989)	Increase
	Brown (1987)	Increase
	Field & Goldson (1984)	Increase
Palmar sweating	Harpin & Rutter (1982)	Increase
	Gedally-Duff (1989)	Increase
Oxygen saturation	High & Gorski (1985)	Decrease
	Rawlings et al (1980)	Decrease
Intracranial pressure	Stevens & Johnston (1991)	Rapid Fluctuations
Hormonal		
Cortisol	Anders et al (1971)	Increase
	Gunnar et al (1987)	Increase
	Gunnar et al (1985)	Increase
Insulin	Anand & Hickey (1987)	Decrease
Catecholamines, glucagon, aldosterone, corticosteroids	Anand & Hickey (1987)	Increase

these studies, physiologic responses to noxious stimulus included increases in heart rate, respiratory rate, intracranial pressure, and palmar sweating and decreases in vagal tone and oxygen saturation. Although popular because they are relatively easy to quantify, biologic and physiologic measures of pain must be interpreted with caution. In the clinical setting, it is difficult to determine whether the response was caused by pain or by another stimulus. For example, changes in vital signs that might be attributed to pain could as easily be the result of fear of being left alone in the hospital room. Similarly, transcutaneous oxygen has been shown to decrease following painful procedures, but it also decreases in response to agitation, handling, and other stimuli.

Physiologic signs are limited, as well, by developmental differences in stability and in normal values. Further, research has failed to address the relationship of vital signs to the types of pain that can be expected for hospitalized children. For example, the endocrine response to acute pain (flight or fight response) dissipates as pain lingers. Therefore, pain that continues for days or weeks is unlikely to invoke the changes in vital signs that are associated with pain of shorter duration.

Developmental Changes in Cognition and Behavior. Vocal, verbal, and motor abilities for expressing pain vary with developmental sophistication. For example, the preterm infant may exhibit brief and subtle responses to even the most noxious stimuli, whereas the preschooler may need restraint for removal of adhesive tape. Developmental differences and the array of individual reactions to noxious stimuli make assessment of pain and evaluation of pain relief treatments problematic.

Vocalizations are an important vehicle for children who are too young to verbalize about pain (preverbal) or for those who lack language skills because of developmental delay, intubation, or injury to the vocal cords (nonverbal). Although research about pain vocalizations in nonverbal children is lacking, infant cries have been studied as an expression of pain for over a quarter of a century (Wasz-Hockert et al, 1985).

Crying is a major mode of communication in infants. As early as 300 B.C., Hippocrates suggested that the cries of infants included useful information that could augment medical diagnosis. However, infants cry for many reasons other than pain. Although nurses and parents may feel they can distinguish among the cries of pain, hunger, and irritability, methods for reliably identifying a pain cry remain under investigation.

Characteristics of the infant cry fall into three major domains: time, frequency, and intensity. Whereas some of these characteristics are easily identifiable, others require sophisticated spectrographic analysis. Cries in response to noxious stimuli have been described as high-pitched, tense, harsh, intense, and a cry that adult listeners perceive as urgent (Fuller et al, 1991; Fuller & Horii, 1988; Johnston, 1989; Johnston & O'Shaughnessy, 1988; Porter et al, 1986; Stevens et al, 1993; Zeskind et al, 1985). Research continues in the attempt to identify a specific cry pattern that is detectable by the human ear, and, thus, one that could be taught to nurses as a means of assessing pain in infants.

Language is an important skill used to express pain. As language develops, children can increasingly use words to express their pain perceptions. From the toddler's first tearful announcement of a "boo-boo," *verbal description of pain* continues to develop in concert with cognitive development. Preschool children may use words other than pain to describe their hurt (Hester et al, 1978). Therefore, when a young child is asked, "Do you have any pain?" a negative response may be given because the question is not understood. Thus, pain assessment depends on establishing a form of communication about pain that is mutually understood by the child and the caregiver.

Language difficulties have been the major impetus for developing alternate ways that children can use to communicate about pain. For example, children as young as 4 years old can communicate pain by marking on body outlines (Eland & Anderson, 1977; Savedra & Tesler, 1989). In one study of children ages 4 through 10 years, 168 of the 172 children placed an X on a body outline in a location that corresponded with their pathology, surgical procedure, or a painful event related to their hospitalization. The researchers commented, "An important lesson may be that a child can communicate by graphic means information he cannot communicate verbally, especially when the interrogator is the one hundred forty-first person that day to ask, 'How are you feeling?'" (Eland & Anderson, 1977, p 461).

As language abilities develop, children become quite proficient at describing their pain. Research has shown that school-age children from a number of cultures can discuss pain and describe strategies they use to cope with pain (Abu-Saad, 1984a, 1984b, 1984c, 1990).

Although documentation of children's ability to describe pain increases caregivers' confidence in the validity of symptoms reported by children, it does not eliminate the concern about whether children actually mean what they say. Regardless of their ability to interpret painful sensations, children (like adults) sometimes choose to deny pain. In the following example, the child was attempting to avoid pain medication (Ross & Ross, 1988, p 74):

> So even though it was killing me, like daggers right through me one after the other, I tried to act *real* surprised. And I said it didn't hurt *at all* and she [nurse] just went away. (Boy, age 8, after appendectomy).

Similarly, other researchers have reported instances in which children provided conflicting information to the nurse and the researcher during pain assessments (Hester et al, 1989). In most of these instances, the children indicated pain to the researcher but denied pain when questioned by the nurse. Thus, children's agenda for admitting pain might differ depending on the consequences of pain (e.g., an injection) and on the way in which children are asked about the presence of pain.

Behavior is another way in which children express pain. Developmental changes in *motor abilities* affect the type of pain response a child is capable of expressing. For example, reaction to a blood lance varies greatly according to the child's developmental stage.

Studies examining responses of premature infants confirm the capacity for responding behaviorally to pain (Craig et al, 1993; Davis & Calhoon, 1989; Field & Goldson, 1984; Johnston et al, 1993; Stevens et al, 1993). Behavioral responses of premature infants to a painful stimulus are similar to those seen in full-term neonates and older infants but are less vigorous and sustained and more variable. Therefore, careful observation and knowledge of how the infant responds to nonpainful stimuli is extremely important.

Infants exhibit gross body and limb movements as indicators of many stimuli, including pain. In 1941, McGraw described general diffuse movements of neonates in response to a pinprick, noting that the movements intensified during the first month of age. By 6 months, infants were exhibiting purposeful withdrawal of the affected body part, and, by 1 year, the infants also touched or rubbed the pricked area.

Since McGraw's early work, other researchers have expanded the description of body movements following acute noxious procedures (Craig et al, 1993). Although movements in response to pain from a heel lance or immunization provide some information about infants' behavioral reactions, no one movement or set of movements has been identified as specific for pain.

Several researchers have assessed facial expression as a response to tissue-damaging stimuli in infants (Dale, 1986, 1989; Grunau & Craig, 1987; Grunau et al, 1990; Izard, 1979; Johnston & Strada, 1986; Johnston & Stevens, 1991; Stevens & Johnston, 1991). Results from these studies indicate that facial expression is the most consistent response to pain across infants and may be the most promising measure of pain in infants. Facial expression (or, more precisely, the proportion of facial activity) has also been shown to vary with behavioral state or the sleep/wake patterns of the infant (Grunau & Craig, 1987). This finding is consistent with Gate Control Theory, which suggests that the infant's behavioral response is modulated by the internal factor, behavioral state. Continued research on facial expression and the factors that influence it will assist in refining this important clinical assessment parameter.

Behavioral indicators of pain have also been developed for use with older children. Unfortunately, clinical applicability of many of the scales is limited because (1) they were developed for procedural pain (rather than for pain of longer duration) and (2) the scales fail to distinguish between anxiety and pain. One of the more promising behavioral scales is the Children's Hospital of Eastern Ontario Pain Scale (CHEOPS), described later in this chapter (McGrath et al, 1985b).

A major concern about behavioral indicators stems from the difficulty in distinguishing pain behaviors from coping strategies. The following vignette illustrates the problem (LeBaron & Zeltzer, 1984, pp 736–737):

> One boy cheerfully climbed up on the treatment table and asked the nurses to hold him tightly; he then became rigid, stared at the ceiling, and proceeded to scream during the entire sterile wash and completion of the bone marrow aspiration [BMA]. In contrast to the observer's high ratings, the patient rated both his pain and anxiety as moderately low. He explained that his rigidity and screaming provided a distraction upon which he focused almost all of his attention and that, as a result, the BMA bothered him very little.

Most researchers agree that pain behaviors are, to some extent, a learned response. "Pain behavior is recognized as developing because it is adaptive, with its success in attracting the attention and help of others as one reason for its usefulness" (Craig, 1992, p 107). Therefore, infants and young children often display atypical pain behaviors. More recognizable pain behaviors develop as children learn to reproduce actions that result in pain relief and in the desired response from caregivers.

Caregivers often underestimate the adaptability of infants and young children to a painful event. For example, some pain scales suggest severe pain is accompanied by loud crying and thrashing behavior. Whereas this may be a typical response to short-term procedural pain, it rarely applies to pain of longer duration. Even young infants learn to lie quietly when crying and their movements exacerbate pain (Mills, 1989a, 1989b; Taylor, 1983). Therefore, a more appropriate guide for assessment would be to note the ways in which responses deviate from well behaviors. Using this parameter, an exaggerated lack of movement following surgery would be suspect of pain rather than assessed as "resting quietly." Although much additional research is needed to validate pain behaviors, guidelines for age-appropriate assessment are listed in Table 25–2. These guidelines reflect the available research and are augmented by the authors' clinical experiences.

Tools for Pain Assessment

Pain assessment tools are methods available to help children communicate their pain. Valid and reliable tools have undergone extensive research to determine that they actually measure pain (validity) and do so consistently (reliability) across repeated measurements. Although many pain assessment tools exist, few have undergone the research necessary to determine validity and reliability. The importance of these properties can not be overstated. *Reliability and validity signify the degree of confidence one can place in the results of the pain measure.*

Research in which Hester and colleagues (1989) tested a little-known self-report tool provides an example of the ambiguous ratings that can occur with an untested tool. The Pain Ladder consists of a picture of a nine-rung ladder; the rungs at the bottom and the top represent the extremes of pain (Hay, 1984). Although the idea of pain increasing from the bottom of the ladder to the top was understood by adults in the study, children tended to mark their pain only around the lower rungs or the top rung. Children's ratings were quite different from simultaneous ratings by parents and nurses. The researchers speculated that the children may have been overwhelmed by the number of choices for marking pain on the ladder and, thereby, shortened the scale. This speculation implies that a child who marked his or her pain on the fourth rung might have had pain of much greater intensity.

Except as noted, the assessment tools discussed in this chapter have undergone many tests of reliability and validity for use with children. The tools are compiled in Appendix 12. Additional tools are listed in Table 25–3.

Pain assessment tools can be categorized as (1) those that elicit the child's self-report of pain and (2) those that provide a format for nurses' observations of the child's behavior. Examples of self-report tools for use with children of preschool-age or older include the Color Tool, the Poker Chip Tool, and the Oucher. The verbal 0 to 10 scale and the Adolescent Pediatric Pain Tool are designed for use with children 8 years of age and older. The CHEOPS is discussed as an example of a behavioral observation tool. An additional tool, the Pain Experience History, helps to provide a context for understanding the child's pain experience and is useful in interpreting scores from other assessment measures.

Eland Color Tool. The Color Tool consists of front and back body outlines on which children indicate the location of their pain with crayons (Eland, 1975). By matching specific colored crayons to their previous pain experiences, children can also indicate the intensity of pain they are currently experiencing. Although young children may reverse left and right in their drawings, clarification with the child renders this tool valid for location of pain (Eland & Anderson, 1977). The nurse must also clarify with the child the

TABLE 25-2
Guidelines for Age-Appropriate Assessment and Management of Pain

Common Indicators of Pain/Distress*	Predominant Fears	Potential Sources of Comfort
Infant (0–12 Mos)		
Procedural Pain† Moves entire body in response to pain stimulus Withdraws limb Cries vigorously Facial expression reveals brow bulge Acute Pain‡ Restless, irritable, difficult to comfort Sleeps fitfully Reluctant to move or be moved if movement increases pain Cries quietly or whimpers if vigorous crying increases pain Must be coaxed to smile/interact Feedings altered in frequency, duration, and/or amount	Separation from parents Strangers	Analgesic as indicated Consider sedative/amnesic as appropriate for anxiety or repeated painful procedures Presence of primary caregiver or consistent nurses Bundling, holding Sucking (pacifier or feeding) Rocking or other gentle motion Comforting sounds, e.g., tape of womb sounds, lullabies, comforting voices (especially familiar voices) Security object(s) Peaceful environment§
Toddler (1–3 Yrs)		
Procedural Pain† Cries, screams Struggles against restraint (difficult to distinguish fear of restraint from actual pain) Acute Pain‡ Usually cannot localize pain unless source is visible, e.g., cut, scrape May verbalize general "hurt" or "owee" Restless, irritable, difficult to comfort Cries frequently if crying does not increase pain Cries quietly or just whimpers if vigorous crying increases pain Decreased tolerance for frustration Established sleep patterns disturbed May regress behaviorally (e.g., loss of bowel and bladder control) Reluctant to move or be moved if movement increases pain Must be coaxed to smile/interact	Separation from primary caregivers Immobility and restraint	Analgesic as indicated Consider sedative/amnesic as appropriate for anxiety or repeated painful procedures Presence of primary caregiver or consistent nurses Staying near, holding, touching Rocking or other gentle motion Comforting sounds, e.g., lullabies, familiar voices Truthful, age-appropriate explanations and frequent reassurance Security object(s) Distraction with short (3- to 5-min) activities Encouraging participation in care activities to increase sense of control Allowing movement and ambulation as possible Peaceful environment§

TABLE 25-2
Guidelines for Age-Appropriate Assessment and Management of Pain *(Continued)*

Common Indicators of Pain/Distress*	Predominant Fears	Potential Sources of Comfort
Preschooler (3–5 Yrs)		
Procedural Pain† Cries, screams Struggles against restraint (difficult to distinguish fear of pain from actual pain) Verbal barrage of questions about procedure and pleas to stop it **Acute Pain‡** By age 4, can usually localize pain verbally or with markings on body outline Restless, irritable, difficult to comfort Cries frequently if crying does not increase pain Cries quietly or just whimpers if vigorous crying increases pain Decreased tolerance for frustration Voice quality may change; e.g., child becoming very soft-spoken or whiny May regress behaviorally (e.g., clinging to parent, reverting to baby talk) Established sleep patterns disturbed Reluctant to move or be moved if movement increases pain Decreased interest in environment and usual activities	Separation from parents, siblings, home environment Pain as punishment Mutilation	Analgesic as indicated Consider sedative/amnesic as appropriate for anxiety or repeated painful procedures Presence of primary caregiver or consistent nurses; telephone contact with family Being near, holding, rocking Truthful, age-appropriate explanations and frequent reassurance Security object(s) Distraction (10- to 15-min activities) Therapeutic play Encouraging participation in care activities to increase sense of control Peaceful environment§
School-Age (6–12 Yrs)		
Procedural Pain† May cry, scream, and protest verbally and with motor behaviors or may cooperate with procedure with only facial grimacing and muscular rigidity Readily verbalizes questions, complaints, protests, instructions May grunt, groan, or sigh, but cries and screams less frequently than younger child **Acute Pain‡** Localizes pain verbally or on body outline Describes pain intensity and quality and helps to evaluate pain management interventions Restless, has difficulty finding position of comfort May cry if crying does not increase pain, but cries much less frequently than younger children Decreased tolerance for frustration; may be irritable and demanding, especially with family members Voice quality may change; e.g., child becoming very soft-spoken or whiny May regress behaviorally (e.g., increased dependence on parent) Sleep disturbances; e.g., sleeping more or less than usual, awaking frequently Reluctant or refuses to move or be moved if movement increases pain Decreased interest in environment and usual activities	Inferiority Separation from peers Loss of peer relationships Mutilation Loss of control	Analgesic (including patient-controlled analgesia [PCA]) as indicated Consider sedative/amnesic as appropriate for anxiety or repeated painful procedures Transcutaneous electrical nerve stimulation (TENS) as indicated Presence of primary caregiver or consistent nurses Telephone contact with family and friends Truthful, age-appropriate explanations and frequent reassurance Security object(s) Distraction Relaxation strategies Therapeutic play Participation in care activities to increase sense of control Peaceful environment§

(Continued)

TABLE 25-2
Guidelines for Age-Appropriate Assessment and Management of Pain *(Continued)*

Common Indicators of Pain/Distress*	Predominant Fears	Potential Sources of Comfort
Adolescent (13+ Yrs)		
Procedural Pain† Usually cooperates with procedure Often displays facial grimacing, muscular rigidity Readily verbalizes questions, complaints, protests, instructions May grunt, groan, or sigh, but rarely cries or screams **Acute Pain‡** Localizes pain verbally or on body outline Describes pain intensity and quality Adept at evaluating pain management interventions Restless, has difficulty finding position of comfort May cry if crying does not increase pain, but cries much less frequently than younger children Decreased tolerance for frustration; may be irritable and demanding, especially with family members Voice quality may change; e.g., child becoming very soft-spoken or whiny May regress behaviorally (e.g., increased dependence on parent) Sleep disturbances; e.g., sleeping more or less than usual, awaking frequently Reluctant or refuses to move or be moved if movement increases pain Decreased interest in environment and usual activities	Loss of control Loss of independence Changes in self-concept and body image Loss of peer relationships Complications in future relationships, sexual competency, ability to provide for self	As for school-age, with increased emphasis on opportunities and responsibilities for participating in pain assessment and management

*Because pain and the distress it causes are often difficult to distinguish from one another, the behaviors listed in this column may reflect either pain or distress, or some combination of pain and distress.

†Procedural pain is caused by a diagnostic technique (e.g., blood draw) or therapeutic intervention (dressing change) and typically diminishes over minutes or hours.

‡Acute pain can be caused by a natural developmental process (e.g., teething), a disease process (e.g., otitis media), or a therapeutic intervention (e.g., surgery). The pain usually diminishes over days or weeks.

§A peaceful environment is one that is (1) safe (all painful procedures should be done in the treatment room, not the child's room) and (2) devoid of stimuli annoying to the ears, nose, eyes, smell, and touch.

meaning of the colors chosen. Whereas older children often illustrate their pain meticulously, younger children may lose sight of the objective and simply color the picture.

Poker Chip Tool. The Poker Chip Tool employs four red plastic "poker" chips to measure pain intensity (Hester, 1979). The child is told that the horizontally arranged chips are pieces of hurt. The nurse explains that the first chip is a little hurt and the fourth chip is the most hurt you could ever have. Children are then asked how many pieces of hurt they have. In this way, the chips form a concrete visual aid to help children 4 years of age or older quantify their hurt. Instructions are also available in Spanish (Jordan-Marsh et al, 1990). Although the tool is effective with older children and adolescents, it is especially useful for children too young to abstractly conceptualize pain. Studies have supported the validity and reliability of this tool (Hagedorn, 1990; Hester et al, 1989, 1990).

Other studies have demonstrated that a five-chip version of the tool may be used with confidence (Aradine et al, 1988; Beyer & Aradine, 1987, 1988; Datz, 1989; Hester & Foster, 1992; Molsberry, 1979). The five-chip version adds a white chip to signify "no hurt."

Because the Poker Chip Tool conveys only the intensity of the pain, the nurse will want to question the child further. Examples of questions to clarify the response and further describe the pain are: You have a little bit of hurt? Where is the hurt? Does it hurt all the time? What makes it feel better?

Oucher. The Oucher uses pictures of children and a numeric scale to assess pain intensity (Beyer, 1984,

TABLE 25-3
Instruments Measuring Pain in Children

Approach	Instrument	Dimension Measured	Appropriate Age
Self-report	Beyer: "Oucher" (1984) (photographic scale)	Pain intensity	3–12 yrs
	Eland: "Color Tool" (1981)	Pain	4–10 yrs
	Hester: "Poker Chip Tool" (1979)	Pain intensity	4–13 yrs
	Savedra et al: Adolescent Pediatric Pain Tool (APPT) (1989a)	Location, intensity, quality	8–17 yrs
	Scott: "Projective Test" (1978)	Pain perception	4–10 yrs
	Unruh et al: "Children's Drawings" (1983)	Pain perception (categories)	5–18 yrs
	Beyer: "Oucher" (1984) (numeric scale)	Pain intensity	3–12 yrs
	Molsberry: "Hurt Thermometer" (1979)	Pain intensity	4–8 yrs
	Hawley: "Pain Communication Tool" (1984)	Frequency, duration, type of pain	3–10 yrs
	Jeans & Gordon: Drawings and interview (1981)	Quality-quantity of pain	5–13 yrs
	Jerrett: Drawings and interview (1985)	Quality-quantity of pain	5–9 yrs
	McGrath et al: "Multidimensional Pain Assessment in Children" (1985a)	Pain intensity and pain affect	Over 5 yrs
Behavioral observation	Katz et al: "Procedure Behavioral Rating Scale" (1980)	Behavioral distress Pain/anxiety	8 mos–17 yrs
	Jay et al: "Observation Scale of Behavioral Distress" (1983)	Behavioral distress Pain/anxiety	2–20 yrs
	Lollar et al: "Pediatric Pain Inventory" (1982)	Pain perception, intensity, and duration	4–19 yrs
	McGrath et al: "The Children's Hospital of Eastern Ontario Pain Scale (CHEOPS)" (1985b)	Pain expression	1–5 yrs
	Dale (1986)	Pain intensity and duration	Infants, 2–4½ mos

Adapted from Stevens, B. J., Hunsberger, M., & Browne, G. (1987, May/June). Pain in children: Theoretical, research and practice dilemmas. *Journal of Pediatric Nursing 3,* 154–166.

1988). Children who can count to 100 by ones indicate the amount of pain on the numeric scale, which ranges from 0 to 100 in increments of 10. Younger children are asked to choose one of six photographs of a white child's face. The photographs are arranged vertically and represent intensity from "no hurt" at the bottom to "worst hurt" at the top. The Oucher has been used successfully with children as young as 3 years (Beyer & Aradine, 1986). Many studies have addressed the tool's reliability and validity (Aradine et al, 1988; Belter et al, 1988; Beyer, 1984; Beyer & Aradine, 1986, 1987, 1988; Datz, 1989). African-American and Hispanic versions of this tool have been developed and are shown in Appendix 12 (Beyer et al, 1992; Neuman et al, 1990; Villarruel & Denyes, 1989).

Adolescent Pediatric Pain Tool. The Adolescent Pediatric Pain Tool (APPT) can be used with children ages 8 through adolescence (Savedra et al, 1989a). The child draws on front and back body outlines to locate the pain, indicates pain intensity on a word graphic rating scale, and circles words that describe the quality of the pain. The tool has been rigorously tested with large multiethnic samples of well and hospitalized children (Savedra et al, 1982, 1988, 1989b, 1990; Savedra & Tesler, 1989; Wilkie et al, 1990). Clinically, this multidimensional tool is especially helpful in diagnosing pain syndromes and in documenting changes in pain parameters across time.

Verbal 0 to 10 Scale. Children who can think of their pain in more abstract terms can respond to the question, "How much pain do you have on a 0 to 10 scale where 0 is no pain and 10 is the worst possible pain?" One study found this scale valid and reliable for children 8 years of age and older (Tesler, 1991). If in doubt about a child's ability to understand this verbal scale, compare responses to the verbal scale and a more concrete measure such as the rating scale on the APPT.

CHEOPS. The Children's Hospital of Eastern Ontario Pain Scale (CHEOPS) is a behavioral assessment tool scored by health care providers rather than by the child. The scale was developed by McGrath and colleagues (1985b) with input from experienced pediatric nurses. It provides for behavioral observation of the child's cry, facial expression, verbal communication, torso motion, touch, and leg motion. A scoring system transforms numeric ratings to categories of pain intensity.

The CHEOPS is limited in applicability to clinical practice because it was developed with children recovering from anesthesia. Although children may display easily observable behaviors during recovery from anesthesia, they quickly learn that pain is associated with movement and begin to limit motor activities. When children limit their behavioral responses to pain, scores on the CHEOPS may not be an accurate measure of pain (Beyer et al, 1991).

Pain Experience History. The Pain Experience History was developed in response to interviews with children about their pain experiences (Hester & Barcus, 1986). It is designed to provide a context for the current pain experience in relation to other pain experiences, usual pain behaviors, and previously effective therapies. Parents can record short answers to the questions while other admission procedures are taking place with the child. Subsequently, the parent or the nurse can obtain responses to similar questions from the verbal child. Although validity and reliability have not been substantiated, the tool appears especially useful for obtaining parental input about the preverbal or nonverbal child and is included in Appendix 12.

Making Clinical Judgments about Children in Pain

To be effective, clinical judgments about children in pain must be based on scientific knowledge of how children in various stages of development perceive and express pain. However, the scientific base provides only the raw material for decisions. The art of practice is realized as individual nurses apply the scientific base to individual children. Therefore, a discussion of clinical judgments about children in pain would be incomplete without addressing characteristics of nurses, children, and health care settings that influence those judgments.

Factors That Influence Nursing Judgments about Pain

Clinical judgment related to pain has received limited attention by researchers. The discussion in this chapter integrates previous findings with the results of recent studies.

Factors That Influence Assessment and Evaluation

Assessment of the pain experience and evaluation of the child's response to interventions are influenced by (1) the nurse's initiative in accessing information and (2) the amount of information available. Developmental limitations in children's expression of pain means that *"the burden of vigilance for pain rests with the health care provider"* (italics added) (Acute Pain Management Guideline Panel, 1992, p 54). When alert for the presence of pain, the nurse will notice clinical signs that might otherwise be overlooked among the plethora of vocal, verbal, behavioral, and physiologic cues.

Clinical judgment is enhanced by obtaining all available information. Information about pain is available through (1) direct encounters with the child, (2) conversations with other persons who have information about the child, and (3) written records.

For the nurse who is alert to the potential for pain, every encounter with the child provides information that contributes to judgments about pain. Whereas formal pain assessment may occur only a few times in a given shift, cues about pain obtained during other encounters with the child contribute significantly to clinical judgments. Information about pain is also obtained by proxy: in shift reports and in conversations with parents and other health care professionals. Finally, information is available through written records. Unfortunately, pain is often poorly documented, thus limiting the opportunity to view patterns of pain intensity and response to treatment across time.

Factors That Influence Nursing Diagnosis

Characteristics specific to each nurse influence how nurses interpret information and arrive at a nursing diagnosis. Nurse-specific characteristics include: (1) knowledge of the child's baseline, (2) expectations about pain, and (3) personal experiences with pain (Foster, 1990; Hester & Foster, 1993).

Information about the child's *baseline* establishes a point of reference for noting change and for interpreting the relative significance of various signs and symptoms. Baseline information includes pain-related behavior (1) when well or not hospitalized, (2) during previous hospitalizations, (3) during the current hospitalization, and (4) during the current shift. The Pain Experience History is helpful in establishing the child's previous experience with and responses to pain. (See Appendix 12.)

An example may help to clarify this concept. Consider a situation in which an 8-year-old child reports pain at the intravenous (IV) site in the absence of physical signs of extravasation or phlebitis. Baseline knowledge that this child had experienced IV treatment on previous hospitalizations, had no fear of the IV, and had not previously complained of pain would be important in arriving at a judgment. Research suggests *expectations* about pain and the response to treatment also influence decision making (Burokas, 1985; Bradshaw & Zeanah, 1986; Gadish et al, 1988; Hester & Foster, 1993). Awareness of the role of expectations in clinical judgment may alert individuals to instances in which their expectations are scientifically based and others in which they are not. Of particular concern are expectations associated with surgical and medical diagnoses (Foster, 1990).

Nurses tend to expect pain for children after surgery, whereas pain may be overlooked for children with medical diagnoses. A pediatric nurse in one study commented (Foster, 1990, p 177):

> Nothing's quite as obvious with medical diagnoses. I think pain assessment is much more subjective with medical patients. Because there isn't an incision. There haven't been cuts.

The nurse's comment substantiates conclusions drawn from a study of adult care nurses, "Assessments of patient suffering . . . depend largely upon the patient's presenting positive evidence of physical pathology" (Taylor et al, 1984, p 7).

Personal experiences with pain also affect judgments (Davitz & Davitz, 1981; Hester & Foster, 1993; Holm et al, 1989). In general, nurses who have experienced significant pain themselves, or have children who have been in pain, tend to infer greater pain in their patients. The implication is that nurses who have experienced severe pain wish to spare the suffering of others.

Factors That Influence Nursing Interventions

Research has shown that identification of pain does not necessarily result in an intervention for pain (Foster & Hester, 1989). Many factors influence nursing actions in response to a diagnosis of pain. These factors include personal characteristics of nurses and characteristics of the health care setting (Foster, 1990).

Personal Characteristics of Nurses. Among the important personal characteristics that influence nursing judgments is confidence in one's assessment of pain. Confidence increases with an understanding of the type of pain expected from a particular surgical intervention or disease process. When a child's pain is consistent with the pain expected, nurses are more likely to administer analgesics. Conversely, when nurses lack knowledge of pathophysiology and lack experience with children in similar circumstances, they are less likely to intervene for pain (Foster, 1990; Hester & Foster, 1993). A nurse in Foster's study captured the essence of the problem, "If I really have an understanding of the pain, then I'm willing to act on it. But if I don't understand it, then suppose they ask me why I did this" (1990, p 216).

Knowledge of pharmacology, experience in giving analgesics, and experience in evaluating therapeutic effects and adverse effects also influence whether nurses administer analgesics for pain. Where knowledge and experience are lacking, fears, myths, and half-truths often fill the void.

Personal values and beliefs are additional influences on nurses' interventions for pain (Hester & Foster, 1993). Only recently has scientific information about pain been sufficient to support clinical judgments. Most health care professionals learned little about pain in their formal education. In the absence of scientific knowledge, judgments about pain are often based on personal values and beliefs. Each professional is responsible for examining personal values and beliefs in light of the scientific knowledge about pain to clarify instances in which decisions are based more on personal opinion than on fact.

Characteristics of the Health Care Setting. The context of nursing care is currently receiving a great deal of interest in relation to the outcomes of care. Although the influence of the health care setting on nurses' judgments and actions may seem obvious, this relationship constitutes a new focus for nursing research. Characteristics of health care settings that influence nurses' administration of analgesics include unwritten standards of care, administrative factors, and resources (Foster, 1990).

Unwritten standards of care comprise *expectations* for nursing practice that arise from the values of key unit staff, such as administrators and senior staff. These standards convey the nursing actions expected under particular circumstances; the standards are sustained by peer pressure. As a nurse in one study explained, "These are the guidelines that are written nowhere, but you follow these guidelines, and everybody knows" (Foster, 1990, p 197).

Problems arise when unwritten standards guide clinical practice (Foster, 1991). Written standards are usually researched, formalized by committee action, and subject to periodic review. As such, they represent standards of excellence. In contrast, unwritten standards often reflect the minimal level of performance. Not being subject to critical review, unwritten standards are also slow to incorporate advances in knowledge. As Vladeck noted, "Given the widespread human tendency to get by, to do just enough, to satisfy rather than maximize, standards set too low or too broad may promote mediocrity" (1988, p 103).

Administrative factors and available resources also influence responses to children's pain. Nurse-patient ratios dictate the time a nurse can spend assessing and intervening with a given child. Unit practices that define parent participation in care influence the opportunity for parents to be involved in pain management. Professional relationships among nurses, physicians, pharmacists, physical therapists, and other health care professionals can limit or enhance the expertise brought to bear on pain assessment and management. Recent interest in pain management and new Joint Commission on Accreditation of Hospitals and Organizations (JCAHO) guidelines that include pain have fostered the development of pain management services in many large institutions, thus providing additional resources for staff education and for consultation about children with unrelieved pain.

Application of the Nursing Process: Children in Pain

Assessment

The goals of pain assessment are to (1) identify pain whenever it exists and (2) to obtain the best possible understanding of the location, intensity, and quality of the pain. To meet the first goal, one must *expect* pain in every ill child. The expectation for pain will ensure that pain assessment is integral to each assessment, whether the child is hospitalized or is seen in an ambulatory care setting. The second goal requires a comprehensive baseline and scheduled reassessments.

An initial baseline is established at the first office visit in ambulatory care or on hospital admission. Baseline assessments provide a point of reference for interpreting subsequent assessments.

To establish a baseline:

- Ask the parent and/or child to complete the Pain Experience History. This will help to establish words the child uses for pain, past pain experiences, and desired treatments.
- Obtain a self-report of pain from the verbal child, using a valid, reliable, age-appropriate assessment tool. (See Table 25–3.) Determine pain location, intensity, and quality. The parent or primary caregiver may be able to provide this information for the nonverbal or preverbal child.
- Ask the child/parent to describe the onset of pain and factors that exacerbate or relieve the pain.
- Determine the extent to which fear and anxiety are exacerbating the pain experience.
- Observe the child's behaviors and compare with behaviors appropriate for the child's age/developmental stage.
- Obtain the child's heart rate, respiratory rate, and blood pressure. Note the oxygen saturation as measured by pulse oximetry.

Once baseline data is available, a protocol for reassessment can be established. Reassessments determine whether the pain is resolving or intensifying. Several factors influence the frequency of reassessment. Reassess pain every 1 to 2 hours when the child is (1) an infant or toddler, (2) unattended by a parent, (3) in an unstable medical condition, or (4) experiencing unresolved pain. If pain is well controlled and pain scores vary little from one assessment to the next, reassessment at 3- to 4-hour intervals may be sufficient.

Nursing Diagnosis

Interpreting assessment data leads to a nursing diagnosis about the level of comfort. When assessment cues are consistent and congruous, the nursing diagnosis can be made with confidence. Difficulty arises when cues conflict. A common example is when children say they have moderate to severe pain but fail to display behaviors consistent with pain of that intensity.

Although the literature contends that verbal report is the gold standard of assessment parameters, pain behavior may be more important to clinicians (Craig, 1992). In our experience, when children say one thing about their pain and display behaviors that are not consistent with what they have said, nurses are often confused about what to do. Afraid to take the wrong action, nurses may take no action at all. Therefore, inconsistent cues about pain can delay interventions for pain relief.

When unsure about the presence, intensity, or quality of pain, consider that pain-relieving interventions can be diagnostic as well as therapeutic. Administer the prescribed analgesic and note the child's response.

To resolve the dilemma of inconsistent cues, consider that *pain-relieving interventions can be diagnostic as well as therapeutic*. Gordin's decision tree for distinguishing between pain and irritability in the neonate is just as appropriate for the older child

TABLE 25-4
Decision Tree for Assessing and Managing Pain/Agitation

In the presence of behavior indicative of pain/agitation:

I. Rule out respiratory cause

- Determine patency of the airway
- Check O_2 setting and integrity of oxygen tubings
- Note the pulse oximeter reading
- Take measures to correct problems discovered

If calming occurs, hypoxia was the probable cause. If the behavior persists:

II. Rule out pain

- Administer an analgesic

If calming occurs, pain was the probable cause. If the behavior persists:

III. Rule out an environmental cause

- Assess for disturbing environmental stimuli, e.g., bright lights, loud or frequent noises, noxious odors
- Reduce environmental stimuli where possible

If calming occurs, environmental stimuli were the probable cause. If the behavior persists:

IV. Rule out anxiety/agitation

- Administer a sedative

If calming occurs, anxiety/agitation was the probable cause. If the behavior persists, consider a combination of all of these therapies.

Based on Gordin, P. C. (1990). Assessing and managing agitation in a critically ill infant. Copyright 1990 The American Journal of Nursing Company. Adapted from *MCN: American Journal of Maternal Child Nursing*, January/February, 1990, *15*, 26–32. Used with permission. All rights reserved.

(Table 25–4). The decision tree proceeds from the life-threatening etiology of hypoxia, to pain, irritating environmental factors, and, finally, anxiety. Success of an intervention confirms the diagnosis.

Planning

After establishing a nursing diagnosis, collaborate with other members of the health care team to formulate a plan for pain relief. Collaboration ensures that all of the complex components of the pain experience are considered in the plan. Consult initially with the child and parent(s) and with the physician(s). Table 25–5 outlines ways in which parents can participate in the management of their child's pain. Other professionals who can make important contributions include pharmacists, psychologists, social workers, physical therapists, and child life workers.

Consider the questions in Table 25–6 when developing a plan for pain relief. The questions can help to form a logical plan that integrates assessment data.

The etiology of pain is a major consideration for planning interventions. Etiology determines pain intensity, quality, location, and duration. These qualities, in turn, determine initial intervention strategies. The following principles guide the plan for intervention:

- Mild pain can often be treated with nonsteroidal anti-inflammatory drugs (NSAIDs).
- Moderate to severe pain requires opioid (narcotic) analgesics.
- Used in combination with opioid analgesics, NSAIDs greatly potentiate pain relief. Combination therapy is especially beneficial when the opioid dose ordered fails to control the pain and when the dose of opioid cannot be increased without incurring side effects.

TABLE 25-5
Family-Centered Teaching: Participating in Management of Pain

Pain management is optimized when children and parents participate with doctors and nurses in the identification and treatment of pain

- Ask the doctor and nurse how much pain is expected with this illness or surgery and what the plan is for pain relief
- Tell hospital caregivers what words your child uses for pain
- Discuss your child's usual reaction to pain, including treatments that have been effective in the past
- Encourage your child to talk to you or others about pain and the fear of pain
- Encourage your child to use a simple device (such as a verbal 0 to 10 scale) to communicate pain to you and hospital caregivers
- Ask when the pain medication is scheduled to be given. Medicine for pain is usually not given on a set schedule. Instead, it is ordered "as needed" and will not be given until pain is identified
- Ask doctors and nurses to discuss appropriate options for pain treatment, including medicine and other comfort measures
- Assist doctors and nurses in creating a plan for pain relief that is specific for your child's needs

Data from Hester, N. O., & Foster, R. L. (1992). Children in pain: Research combats undertreatment. *Denver Medical Journal, 1*(2), 20–21.

TABLE 25-6
Planning for Pain Relief

Questions to Consider in Forming a Pain Relief Plan

What is the location, intensity, and quality of the pain?

Is the pain continuous or intermittent?

What is the child's goal for pain relief?

What has worked in the past?

What do the child and parent request for pain relief?

What is a safe dose of analgesic for this child?

How will I evaluate pain relief?

Because narcotic and non-narcotic analgesics relieve pain through different mechanisms, combinations of these drugs maximize pain relief without increasing side effects.

- Continuous pain requires a constant blood level of analgesic achieved through around-the-clock (ATC) administration or through continuous infusion.
- As-necessary (PRN) dosing is effective only for intermittent pain and for pain that occasionally "breaks through" ATC or continuous infusion administrations.
- Emotional-social and physiologic stimuli comprise the pain experience. Estimate the relative role of fear, prior pain experiences, familial expectations, and environmental factors.

Treatment of continuous pain deserves additional discussion. Analgesics are most frequently administered on a PRN basis, regardless of whether the pain is continuous or intermittent. Figure 25–2*A* illustrates why PRN administration is illogical for relief of continuous pain. Intermittent administration leads to peaks and troughs in serum levels of analgesics, initiating a cycle that often requires "overshooting" the therapeutic level to obtain the most benefit from each dose. *Somewhat like the force necessary to overcome inertia, more analgesic is required to reach the minimal effective analgesic concentration (MEAC) than to sustain it.* Therefore, ATC administration can often produce pain relief with lower doses of analgesics. Lower doses reduce the potential for side effects and adverse effects of the analgesic. An ideal therapeutic level is presented in Figure 25–2*B*. Whereas ATC administration is effective in controlling constant baseline pain, additional strategies are often indicated for situational pain that "breaks through" baseline analgesia (Fig. 25–2*C*). For example, common situations

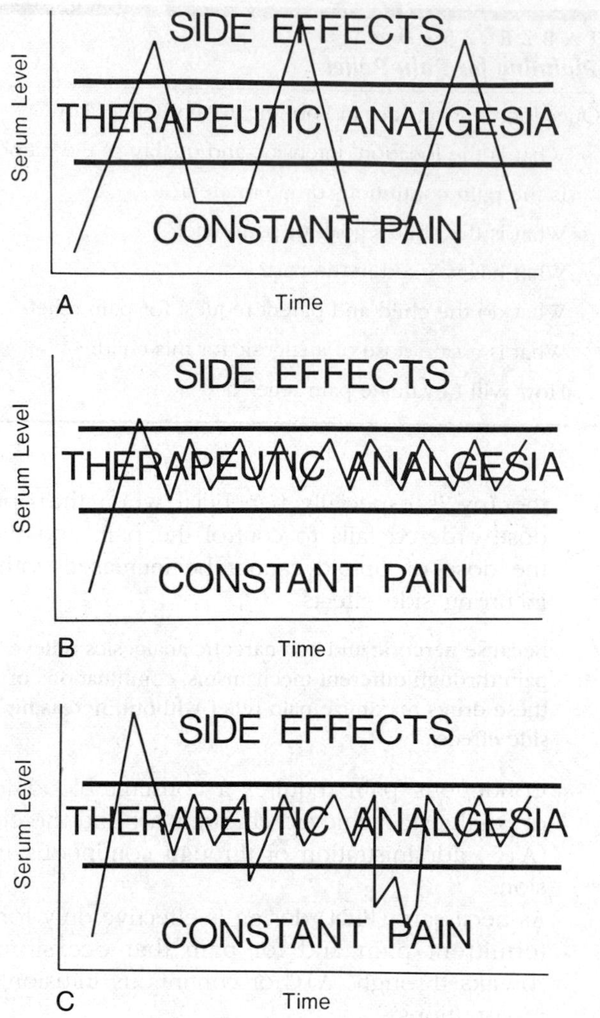

FIGURE 25-2. *A,* As-necessary (PRN) administration (big ups and downs). Graphic illustration of the effects of PRN administration of analgesics. *B,* Around-the-clock (ATC) administration (an ideal representation of therapeutic level). Graphic illustration of the effect of ATC or continuous infusion of analgesics. *C,* Clinical reality of effects of loading and breakthrough. Graphic illustration of the clinical reality of pain, showing the effects of a loading dose and the need to provide rescue doses for pain that breaks through continuous analgesia. (*A–C,* From Hester, N., & Foster, R. [in press]. Integrating pediatric postoperative pain management into clinical practice. *Journal of Pharmaceutical Care in Pain and Symptom Control.*)

that cause increased pain postoperatively include coughing, ambulating, and changes of dressings. The intensity and duration of breakthrough pain will dictate whether it can be relieved with nonpharmacologic strategies or whether additional medication is required. When painful situations can be anticipated, prophylactic administration of analgesics is usually most effective.

Intervention

Pharmacologic and nonpharmacologic interventions form the repertoire of strategies for pain relief.

Pharmacologic Strategies

Table 25–7 lists the rationale for use of NSAIDs, opioids, and local anesthetic agents.

NSAIDs *and* Acetaminophen. With the exception of ketorolac, NSAIDs are manufactured primarily as oral preparations. They share several important properties (Kuhar & Pasternak, 1984; Ready & Edwards, 1992; Wiener & Pepper, 1985):

- Analgesia is limited by a ceiling effect (i.e., medication in excess of the recommended dose fails to produce additional pain relief).
- The drugs do not produce tolerance, physical dependence, or psychologic dependence.
- All have antipyretic properties.
- With the exception of acetaminophen, all inhibit platelet function.
- The analgesic effect is attributed to inhibition of prostaglandins in the periphery. Acetaminophen is the exception; its analgesic actions are not well understood.

The key to understanding the therapeutic effects and side effects of NSAIDs lies with their action as prostaglandin inhibitors. Prostaglandins are a group of biologically active lipids produced in many organs and having broad regulatory activity in the body. Prostaglandins also function as chemical mediators in the inflammatory process that results from tissue injury. Therapeutically, NSAIDs reduce pain by inhibiting prostaglandin production and, thereby, reducing inflammation.

Side effects result when NSAIDs inhibit the necessary regulatory effects of prostaglandins as well as their role in tissue injury. Prostaglandins protect the gastrointestinal mucosa, regulate renal blood flow, and control platelet function. Thus, side effects of NSAIDs include the potential for gastrointestinal irritation, altered renal function, and increased bleeding time. However, unlike acetylsalicylic acid (ASA), which permanently alters platelet membranes, the effects of NSAIDs on platelet membranes are reversible within 24 hours of discontinuing the drug.

Table 25–8 lists acetaminophen and the NSAIDs approved for use in children. The drugs are listed in the order of their relative potency. However, *the key criterion for evaluating efficacy is the individual child's response to the drug.*

Opioids. Opioid analgesics are the mainstay of pharmacologic management for moderate to severe pain (Table 25–9). Opioids produce their potent

TABLE 25-7
Pharmacologic Interventions

Intervention	Comments
NSAIDs	
Oral (alone)	Effective for mild to moderate pain; begin preoperatively; relatively contraindicated in patients with renal disease and risk of or actual coagulopathy; may mask fever
Oral (adjunct to opioid)	Potentiating effect resulting in opioid sparing; begin preoperatively; cautions as for oral NSAIDs (alone)
Parenteral (ketorolac)	Effective for moderate to severe pain; expensive; useful where opioids contraindicated, especially to avoid respiratory depression and sedation; advance to opioid
Opioids	
Oral	As effective as parenteral in appropriate doses; use as soon as oral medication tolerated; route of choice
Intramuscular	Has been the standard parenteral route, but injections painful and absorption unreliable; hence, avoid this route when possible
Subcutaneous	Preferable to intramuscular when a low-volume continuous infusion is needed and intravenous access is difficult to maintain; injections painful and absorption unreliable; avoid this route for long-term repetitive dosing
Intravenous	Parenteral route of choice following major surgery; suitable for titrated bolus or continuous administration (including PCA), but requires monitoring; significant risk of respiratory depression with inappropriate dosing
PCA (systemic)	Intravenous or subcutaneous routes recommended; good steady level of analgesia; popular with patients but requires special infusion pumps and staff education; see cautions about opioids
Epidural and intrathecal	When suitable, provides good analgesia; significant risk of respiratory depression, sometimes delayed in onset; requires careful monitoring; use of infusion pumps requires additional equipment and staff education; expensive if infusion pumps are employed
Local Anesthetics	
Epidural and intrathecal	Limited indications; effective regional analgesia; opioid-sparing; addition of opioid to local anesthetic may improve analgesia; risks of hypotension, weakness, numbness; requires careful monitoring; use of infusion pump requires additional equipment and staff education
Peripheral nerve block	Limited indications and duration of action; effective regional analgesia; opioid-sparing

Adapted from Acute Pain Management Guideline Panel. (1992). *Acute pain management: Operative or medical procedures and trauma. Clinical practice guideline.* (AHCPR Pub. No. 92–0022). Rockville, MD: Agency for Health Care Policy and Research, Public Health Service, US Department of Health and Human Services.

Key: NSAIDs = nonsteroidal anti-inflammatory drugs; PCA = patient-controlled analgesia.

analgesic effects by binding to receptor sites both within and outside the central nervous system. These drugs share several characteristics:

- Technically, opioids have no ceiling effect; i.e., increased doses produce increased analgesia. However, a clinical ceiling effect exists in that doses are limited by side effects of the drugs.
- In comparable doses, oral opioids are as effective as those given parenterally.
- All share common adverse effects, and these side effects may occur with oral, intravenous, or epidural dosing:
  - Respiratory depression.
  - Nausea and vomiting.
  - Reduced bowel motility.
  - Urinary retention.
  - Pruritus.

Monitoring for Respiratory Depression. Because it is life-threatening, respiratory depression is the side effect of most concern. Although the incidence of respiratory depression following the administration of opioid analgesics to adults is very low, the incidence in children remains poorly documented. Some research suggests that infants of 1 month or older are no more prone to respiratory depression from opioid analgesics than are older children and adults (Hertzka et al, 1989).

In one study, researchers reported that only one incident of respiratory depression occurred out of 1678 doses of oral and intravenous opioids administered to 247 infants and children (Kotzer & Foster, 1992). Respiratory depression in one critically ill neonate was thought to be related to a weight-appropriate dose of IV morphine.

In general, neonates are more prone to respiratory depression than older infants. Research has

TABLE 25-8
Relative Doses for Acetaminophen and Nonsteroidal Anti-Inflammatory Analgesics

	Usual Dose	Comments
Parenteral		
Ketorolac (Toradol)	**IM:** 1 mg/kg q6h prn **IV:** 1 mg/kg slow IV push (IVP) (5–15 min) loading; then 0.5 mg/kg slow IVP q6h	Only IM dose approved for children at this time, but IV dosing being used under controlled conditions in some large treatment centers
Oral		
Naproxen (Naprosyn)	5 mg/kg q12h	Longer half-life than other oral NSAIDs
Ibuprofen (e.g., Motrin)	10 mg/kg q6–8h	Available as several brand names and as generic; also available as oral suspension
Aspirin	10–15 mg/kg q4h	Contraindicated in presence of fever or other evidence of viral illness; the standard against which other NSAIDs are compared; inhibits platelet aggregation; may cause postoperative bleeding
Acetaminophen (Tylenol)	10–15 mg/kg q4h	Lacks the peripheral anti-inflammatory activity of other NSAIDs; does not inhibit platelet function
Choline magnesium trisalicylate (Trilisate)	25 mg/kg bid	May have minimal antiplatelet activity; also available as oral liquid

Adapted from Acute Pain Management Guideline Panel. (1992). *Acute pain management: Operative or medical procedures and trauma. Clinical practice guideline.* (AHCPR Pub. No. 92–0032). Rockville, MD: Agency for Health Care Policy and Research, Public Health Service, U.S Department of Health and Human Services.

TABLE 25-9
Relative Dosages for Opioid Analgesics

	Recommended Starting Dose	
Drug	**Oral**	**Parenteral**
Fentanyl	Not available	**IV bolus:** 0.5–1.5 μg*/kg q½h **IV infusion:** 1–2 μg/h
Morphine	0.2–0.4 mg/kg q4–6h SR†: 0.3–0.6 mg/kg q12h	**IV bolus:** 0.02–0.1 mg/kg q2h **IM:** 0.1–0.15 mg/kg q3–4h **IV infusion:** *neonate:* 0.01–0.02 mg/kg/h *child:* 0.01–0.06 mg/kg/h
Methadone	0.1–0.2 mg/kg q6–12h	**IV bolus:** 0.05 mg/kg q4–6h
Meperidine (Demerol)	Not recommended	**IM:** 1–5 mg/kg q3–5h **IV bolus:** 0.2–1 mg/kg q2h **IV infusion:** *neonate:* 0.2 mg/kg/h *child:* 0.2–0.6 mg/kg/h
Hydromorphone (Dilaudid)	0.06 mg/kg q3–4h	**IM:** 0.02–0.1 mg/kg q3–4h **IV:** 0.015 mg/kg q3–4h
Oxycodone (e.g., Percocet, Percodan, Tylox)	0.2 mg/kg q3–4h	Not available
Hydrocodone (e.g., Lortab, Lorcet, Vicodin)	0.2 mg/kg q3–4h	Not available
Codeine	1 mg/kg q3–4h	Not recommended

*Note that fentanyl is given in micrograms (mcg), not milligrams!
†SR = sustained release.
Adapted from Acute Pain Management Guideline Panel. (1992). *Acute pain management: Operative or medical procedures and trauma. Clinical practice guideline.* (AHCPR Pub. No. 92–0032). Rockville, MD: Agency for Health Care Policy and Research, Public Health Service, US Department of Health and Human Services; and Ready, L. B., & Edwards, W. T. (1992). *Management of acute pain: A practical guide.* Seattle: IASP Publications.

shown that elimination of opioids is decreased in neonates, resulting in a longer serum half-life of the drug and in increased incidence of respiratory depression. Concern for respiratory depression in neonates makes treatment with opioid analgesics controversial. Whereas some researchers recommend opioids only for ventilated infants, others suggest that the drugs are safe in low dosages. It is safe to say that neonates receiving opioid analgesics must be monitored closely. As with older infants and children, the following principles apply:

- Maximize surveillance for respiratory depression following:
  - The first dose.
  - An increase in the dose.
  - Administration of an adjunct medication that also may depress respirations (e.g., diazepam [Valium], droperidol [Inapsine]).
  - Deterioration in medical condition.
- Use a cardiorespiratory monitor (and a pulse oximeter, as indicated) during intravenous and epidural administration of opioids.
- Assess level of consciousness as a parameter of sedation.
- Obtain a physician's order (including dose) for naloxone (Narcan) if an opioid is ordered. Maintain the naloxone syringe in a place where it can be readily accessed if needed.

Administering Naloxone (Narcan). Naloxone is used most frequently to reverse opioid-related oversedation and respiratory depression. As a narcotic antagonist, naloxone replaces the opiate at the receptor site. Although naloxone is very effective in reversing untoward effects, it also reverses the analgesic effect for a period of 15 minutes to 4 hours, depending on the dose! Therefore, naloxone should be given slowly, checking after each small increment for the desired response. Onset following IV administration occurs within a few seconds to 2 minutes.

Addressing Fears about Addiction. Some health care professionals and many families are concerned about the potential for addiction when administering opioid analgesics. In adults, the risk of addiction from opioid analgesics is very small. Although no studies exist to document the risk in children, "no known aspect of childhood development or physiology increases the risk of physiologic or psychologic vulnerability to chemical dependence" (Acute Pain Management Guideline Panel, 1992, p 50). Table 25–10 distinguishes among tolerance, physical dependence, and addiction (psychologic dependence).

The nurse should expect the child and parents to have some concern about addiction. Offer facts about addiction at the onset of opioid therapy. Facts dispel unnecessary concerns and, thus, can help optimize the use of analgesics for pain relief.

TABLE 25-10
Addiction: Fact Versus Fiction

Tolerance: A decreased response to the desired effect of the drug, largely due to compensatory physiologic responses that mitigate the drug's pharmacodynamic action. *Tolerance is not addiction!*

Physical Dependence: A state in which withdrawal of the drug produces undesirable signs and symptoms. *Physical dependence is not addiction!*

Psychologic Dependence/Addiction: Compulsive drug-seeking behavior in which the individual uses the drug repetitively not for approved medical reasons, such as pain, but for personal satisfaction. *Psychologic dependence is synonymous with addiction!*

Data from Katzung, B. G. (1989). *Basic and clinical pharmacology* (4th ed.). Norwalk, CT: Appleton & Lange; and McCaffery, M., & Beebe, A. (1989). *Pain. Clinical manual for nursing practice.* St. Louis: CV Mosby.

Administering Analgesics by Various Routes. Analgesics may be ordered for administration by a variety of routes: rectal, oral, intramuscular, intravenous (including patient-controlled analgesia), and epidural. See Table 25–7 and Chapter 23 for additional discussion of the more traditional routes.

Patient-Controlled Analgesia. Patient-controlled analgesia (PCA) is often used for IV administration of opioid analgesics. A special infusion pump is programmed to provide the drug by one of three methods: basal mode (continuous infusion) only, basal mode plus PCA mode (patient-administered boluses via a push-button device), or PCA mode only. The PCA mode is used infrequently with children younger than 7 years. Children using the PCA mode must understand that, when they push the button, additional medication is administered through the IV line. Despite the tendency to limit the PCA mode to school-age children, it is thought to be quite safe. PCA infusion pumps include a lock-out period that limits the number of times the drug can be administered in a 1-hour period, regardless of the number of times the child pushes the button. Additionally, children who become sedated from pushing the button tend to fall asleep and receive no additional boluses until they awaken.

When an IV analgesic is administered by PCA, the blood level of opioid will drop significantly at night when the child is asleep and not using the PCA device. Ask the physician to order a continuous infusion of the opioid at night so that the child does not awaken in severe pain.

A combination of the basal and PCA modes is optimum for continuous pain with occasional breakthrough pain. The basal mode delivers continuous low-dose opioid, and the PCA mode allows the child instant control over breakthrough pain. Be alert, however, for instances in which the child must continually push the button to achieve effective pain relief.

In these cases, the basal dose may need to be increased.

Epidural Analgesia. The use of epidural analgesia in noncritical care hospital units is relatively new and confined primarily to large treatment centers. However, the growing popularity of this route warrants a brief discussion. An anesthesiologist initiates the epidural by placing a tiny catheter in the epidural space or along the spine. An infusion is then administered to relieve pain in the thorax, abdomen, or lower extremities. The infusion may contain a local anesthetic (such as bupivacaine), an opioid analgesic, or a combination of anesthetic and analgesic. Because the analgesic and anesthetic agents are introduced directly to pain receptors along the spinal cord, epidural infusions can produce very effective pain relief with very small quantities of medication. Despite the small quantities of opioid delivered, concern for immediate or delayed respiratory depression necessitates careful nursing assessment and monitoring via pulse oximetry and cardiorespiratory monitors.

Titrating the Dose. Table 25–9 lists the opioid drugs in order of their relative potency, along with recommended starting doses. However, *analgesia does not come in one-size-fits-all!* The starting dose may elicit untoward effects in one child and be grossly inadequate in another child. Analgesics must be titrated to achieve maximal pain relief with minimal side effects.

Determining the Relative Dose. Often analgesic medications are ordered with a range of possible dosages, e.g., "morphine sulfate, 2 to 3 mg IV q 1 to 2 hours." Determination of the dosage to administer from this range is an important nursing responsibility. Decisions should be based on an accurate understanding of the range ordered in comparison to the recommended therapeutic range for that drug.

Administering analgesics to children is different from administering pain medications to adults because it is more difficult to determine the *relative dose* of medication being given. Whereas adult doses of narcotics and other analgesics usually vary only moderately among patients, doses for children are based individually on body weight and vary with each kilogram of difference in weight. *The only way to know the relative dose of medication being given in relation to the maximal dose recommended is to calculate the dosage.* See Table 25–11 for calculations.

The nurse who administers 2 mg of morphine (as in the foregoing order) should be aware that, for this child, 2 mg is only 35 per cent of the recommended therapeutic maximum. Perhaps this is exactly the dose the nurse desires; for example, it may be known that higher doses oversedate this particular child. However, if 2 mg is repeatedly administered for severe pain even though it fails to relieve the pain, the dosage decision is in error. The point is that 2 mg is not an appropriate dose simply because it falls within the range ordered. An appropriate dose relieves pain without undue side effects of the medication. *Dosage determination requires professional decision making and collaboration between the nurse and physician.*

TABLE 25-11
Calculation of Medication Ordered in Relation to Recommended Therapeutic Dose

1. Determine the maximal recommended therapeutic dose for the drug
2. Determine the child's weight in kilograms (usually available on the nursing admission history)
3. Calculate the maximal therapeutic dose of the drug for this child
   Example:
   Drug: Codeine elixir
   Maximal recommended therapeutic dose: 1.0 mg/kg q3–4h (Acute Pain Management Guideline Panel, 1992b)
   Child's weight: 30 kg
   Maximal dose for this child:
   1.0 mg × 30 kg = 30 mg q3–4h
4. Determine the dosage ordered
5. Divide the dosage ordered by the maximal recommended dosage to determine the relationship between the dose ordered and the maximal safe dose
   Example:
   Drug order: Codeine elixir, 20–30 mg q3–4h
   Maximal dose: 30 mg
   20 mg ordered/30 mg maximum = 66% of therapeutic maximum
   30 mg ordered/30 mg maximum = 100% of therapeutic maximum

This calculation tells the nurse that the dosage options are between 66 and 100 percent of the maximal safe dose.

Nonpharmacologic Interventions

Two nonpharmacologic interventions are essential to the care of all infants and children, regardless of the type of pain or the health care setting. Reducing fear and anxiety and enhancing control help children to cope more effectively with painful experiences.

Reducing Fear and Anxiety. Reducing fear and anxiety can alter the child's perception of pain and, therefore, enhance the child's ability to cope with the experience. Often, the first step in reducing the child's fear is reducing the parent's anxiety. Table 21–5 presents strategies to reduce the child's and family's anxiety associated with hospitalization. Many of these strategies can be adapted to other health care and home care settings. Preparation for painful procedures and for surgery can alter the cognitive perception of pain. Age-appropriate educational strategies are presented in Table 23–1.

The environment can have a significant influence on the child's pain experience. If children are isolated from their families, peers, and other patients, they are likely to be anxious and depressed. Children can also feel isolated when information is kept from them. Children can benefit from several types of information, including what will be done to them, how long it will take, and how it feels. For example, if children who are facing a cast application can first apply a cast to a toy animal or doll in the playroom, they have the opportunity to ask questions about the procedure as well as express their feelings through play. The importance of play as an intervention in managing a child's distress is discussed in more detail in Chapter 17.

Children's pain experiences can also be influenced by their observation of pain expressed by another child or parent. This observation may result in emotional sensitization, anxiety, and negative social modeling that leads children to act much like the person in pain that they have witnessed (Chapman & Turner, 1986). Conversely, if children can view another child coping well with a potentially painful situation, this can reduce pain expression and acting out behaviors. Melamed and Siegel (1975) have used this principle in the employment of social modeling. For example, slide tape shows and videotapes have been used successfully to prepare patients for a painful event. As well, handling of equipment and interactions with others who have undergone a similar procedure may also desensitize patients to painful episodes.

All these factors place emotional stress on the child in pain. As nurses, a major goal in providing optimal care is to either provide emotional support for the child or foster it within the child's existing support system. Nurses and parents alike need to be aware of the antecedent factors that cause emotional stress and the consequent reactions of the child. Children require the patience and understanding that only those who are significant in their lives can give. Nurses and others who are caring for the child also play a significant role in providing sensitive, caring support. Consultation and collaboration among the child, family, and health care professionals are essential.

To provide optimal emotional support for the child in pain, nurses may find the following guidelines useful:

1. Try to inform the children and parents what will be happening, how long it will take, and how they will feel. For younger children, it is also important for them to know that a painful experience is over. This can be accomplished by taking them from the area, picking them up and cuddling them, and telling them that the hurt is finished.
2. Use social modeling advantageously by providing examples of patients who have tolerated potentially painful situations well.
3. Incorporate appropriate pharmacologic and nonpharmacologic pain-relieving interventions throughout the child's care.
4. Encourage a parent or someone who is known to relate well with the child to stay with him or her as much as possible.
5. Try to avoid exposing the child to other children who are experiencing extreme discomfort or emotional distress.

Reducing the Sense of Powerlessness/Enhancing Control. Another method of helping children manage their pain experience is to instill in them a sense of personal control. To accomplish this, children must feel certain that they are being listened to and believed when they report their pain and that they have some role in decision making about pain-relieving strategies and their effectiveness. To help children cope with their pain is an exhausting, demanding, and often frustrating task. The coping skills that are available for children to use are influenced by their levels of cognitive development, previous experiences, and modeling provided by parents and significant others. In a study by Jerrett (1985) 5- to 9-year-olds provided a wide range of responses to the question, "When you hurt or have pain, what do you do to help yourself feel better?" Their responses indicated the use of the following coping behaviors:

1. Direct-action physical activities, such as holding or rubbing, treating with something special, or applying a bandage.
2. Avoidance activities, such as those behaviors involved in detachment or distraction, including resting, reading, or thinking of other things.
3. Help-seeking activities, such as interacting with another individual (such as a parent) and including being held or taking medications.

Although these children reported direct-action physical activities and avoidance behaviors most often, they identified behaviors that were related to the presence of a parent as the most beneficial in helping them to cope with their pain. Other studies and anecdotal clinical experience would also support that parents and significant others play a major role in the child's pain experience. Hester (1989) asked children how they comforted themselves when they were in pain and what others could do to comfort them. Excerpts from the interviews are presented in Table 25–12.

Additional Nonpharmacologic Interventions. Many other nonpharmacologic interventions exist. Table 25–13 groups interventions from the simple to more complex. Interventions used for infants include positioning and swaddling, holding and rocking, tactile stimulation, music, vocalization, diaper changes, nourishment, pacifiers (including a sucrose nipple), and environmental stimulation. Interventions for children include distraction, interaction with a parent, muscle relaxation, guided imagery, massage, coping skills

TABLE 25-12
Comfort Strategies: The Child's Perspective

The comfort strategies described by the children and adolescents who participated in this study are illustrated through interview-excerpts of Mandy, David, Cindy, Jeffrey, and Alice.

Mandy

Mandy, 5 years old (the youngest child interviewed for this study), was hospitalized for the insertion of a new stomach tube. She had had extensive experience with pain, by virtue of 35 previous hospitalizations. Mandy tried to alleviate her pain by taking medicine, telling her Mom "I'm hurting," being with her "Mom and Dad," and by holding her teddy bear or her doll. Two of these strategies were under Mandy's control: she could tell someone she hurt and she could hold her toys. However, she could not take medicine by herself nor could she determine when her parents were present. Hence, two implicit caring behaviors for Mandy were to give her medicine when she was experiencing pain and to get her parents for her or to have someone stay with her. When asked what others could do for her, Mandy replied "Hold my hand" and "Tell me to do something." *Hold my hand* was a frequent response of children of all ages in this study. *Tell me to do something* is a distraction technique. Mandy described this technique as something others could use to comfort her; older children in the study initiated various forms of distraction to alleviate the pain themselves.

David

Hospitalizations were not new to David. By 7 years of age, David had had 12 operations and approximately 30 hospitalizations. At the time of the interview, David had been surgically treated for a bowel obstruction. David, an expert on pain, cried when he hurt; he also would "Call for Mom." Although he said he would tell the nurses that he hurt, he couldn't tell the doctors. The following interview-excerpt illustrates the reason:

> Interviewer: Do you tell your doctor?
> David: My doctor? I don't have a doctor.
> Interviewer: Oh.
> David: He never comes by.
> Interviewer: Huh?
> David: He never really comes by.

David said that when he hurt he would throw his stuffed toys or blanket. But he quickly added "Well, I can hold my blanket." This blanket was a special one from home.

In response to what nurses could do for him, David said:

> "They give me some medicine."
> "They give me a shot through my IV."

For David, nurses were the dispensers of medicine for his pain. It is interesting that David, like many of the informants, stressed receiving a shot through the intravenous line. A shot was acceptable only if it went through the IV line; children viewed intramuscular shots negatively and with fear. An older girl specifically described an IM shot as totally unacceptable and would consider it only if she were in really bad pain.

Like Mandy, David wanted someone to hold his hand. He did not, however, want anyone to poke him. Other children also mentioned touching or poking places that hurt as a noncaring behavior of others. Unfortunately, assessment techniques for determining the status of the child often include touching or poking painful areas.

Being involved in decisions about his situation was important to David:

> David: I just want them to let me have my choice.
> Interviewer: Your choice? Your choice about what?
> David: Because, like they have things to make choices and (they) decide things I don't like.
> Interviewer: So you want to be a part of that decision?
> David: Uh-huh.

Most of the children emphasized, explicitly or implicitly, participation in the decision. Following this interview, the doctor told the interviewers that David would have surgery the next day. David had yet to be informed.

Cindy

Cindy, 10 years old, had broken her leg while skiing. This was her first hospitalization. Other than minor acute illnesses, knee scrapes, and cuts, Cindy had little experience with pain. She described her reaction to pain:

> Well, sometimes I can control myself and not cry too much. But if it's really bad, I do cry and I hold really tight to somebody's hand or a bar or something and squeeze real hard and pull it and everything.

Later, she stressed the importance of holding Mom's hand.

Cindy would tell the nurse when she had pain:

> Well, normally I would press the (call) button if the pain was really bad, like if I needed a pain pill or I would press the button . . . like if it's not too bad . . . but I just would tell them my toes hurt and they come in and check.

Caring behaviors for Cindy included staying with her, bringing her presents, making her feel good, talking with her, and checking her. Cindy did not want others to make a "big fuss about it."

> I don't mind . . . if they check it and ask me if I need something to drink or eat. I don't like it when they stay and fuss . . . and say "Do you want more blankets and all that? Do you want this and that closer to you? Do you want the TV on?" I don't like it when people fuss about me like that. . . .

But Cindy did not want to be ignored either:

> I don't like it when people ignore me when I'm in pain, like if I buzz the nurse and she says "Can I help you?" and I ask for a pain pill and (she) says "Well, I don't think we should give you one because you're a child."

Cindy felt ignored and she expressed her anger toward the nurse who was uninformed.

> But I've had them all the time . . . I can take them. It makes me mad because (she) should have been informed that I am able to take up to two pain pills at one time and I can take them up to three times a day.

In this situation, a nurse thwarted Cindy's efforts to be in charge of pain. The nurse rejected Cindy's need for pain medication simply on the basis of Cindy's being a child.

TABLE 25-12
Comfort Strategies: The Child's Perspective *(Continued)*

Cindy was a very take-charge individual. Her family situation provides some insight as to why.

Cindy: When I have pain it's difficult on my Mom because my Dad has MS. She has to take care of him. . . . So when I get hurt, I sort of feel guilty sometimes because that puts more pressure on my Mom and she has to work a lot harder to take care of both of us.

Interviewer: Do you ever talk to your Mom about feeling guilty?

Cindy: Yeah, I told her that I'll be all right. I can take care of myself, just take care of my Dad and just check on me once in a while and I'll be fine.

Cindy not only took care of herself; she also tried to protect her mother from being overburdened both physically and emotionally.

Jeffrey

Thirteen-year-old Jeffrey was hospitalized for an infected hip. Medically, Jeffrey had had little previous experience with pain; however, Jeffrey convincingly described extensive experience with pain as a football player. Unlike the other children in the study, Jeffrey concentrated on the noncaring behaviors of others. Jeffrey expressed a lot of anger in regard to his pain experiences and how poorly he had been treated.

Interviewer: How do you feel when you hurt?

Jeffrey: Like screaming. I get mad, I mean, I have a bad temper anyway and when I hurt, I want to get revenge . . . I want to grab my doctor's neck.

Jeffrey was particularly angry about how the health care professionals had treated him:

They gave me Valium and Demerol to calm me down . . . but they gave me that too late.

He described a lack of sensitivity and understanding on the part of his doctor:

A doctor has no way of knowing what it's going to feel like.

Later, he commented that the "doctor liked to inflict pain."

According to Jeffrey, others did not treat him in a very caring way. They ignored his requests for medication and they lacked sensitivity and understanding regarding his pain experiences. When asked what nurses did for him, he described:

It depends on how nice of a nurse. They bring painkillers and stuff. Most of them try and understand but it's hard for somebody else to understand that you're in pain . . .

Alice

Alice, a 15-year-old high school student and the oldest individual to participate in the study, was hospitalized for pancreatitis for 45 days about a year prior to the interview. The lengthy hospital stay was related to surgical complications. Although Alice described things she did to comfort herself during pain experiences, during much of her hospital stay she was very dependent on others to comfort her. As did the younger children, Alice told others when she had pain. When she was on the respirator, she wrote notes to the nurses regarding her pain. Holding a stuffed toy comforted Alice:

I got a pink bear . . . (he) was there for me the whole time . . . he was my best friend . . . I slept on him . . . (he) was like a security blanket . . . they let me take him into the operating room until they put me under . . . and when I woke he was there again and that was so nice. So I think a security blanket is just something that you have all the time . . .

Alice wanted lots of love and comfort from others. Her mother was the primary person she wanted with her:

Once in a while I would ask my Mom "Can I have a shot? Will you stay here while I go to sleep? Please stay here and don't leave until I've fallen asleep." I want that secure feeling that someone's there for me just in case I can't sleep or I need somebody to talk to for a while.

The interview-excerpts from these five children vividly illustrate children's perceptions of how they can comfort themselves, what others should and shouldn't do to comfort them, and environmental factors that prevent their comfort. This information could be useful to the nurse in comforting the child in pain.

Success in comforting the child in pain will depend on a co-partnership among the nurses, the child, and the child's family. The nurses and the child's family must acknowledge the presence of pain and be willing to comfort the child. Often, children in pain are lonely, bewildered, and frightened. They have told us how to comfort them, and this knowledge places a demand on nurses to do so.

From Hester, N. O. (1989). Comforting the child in pain. In S. G. Funk, et al (Ed.). *Key aspects of comfort: Management of pain, fatigue and nausea* (pp 290–298). Springer Publishing Company, Inc., New York 10012. Used by permission.

training, hypnosis, and transcutaneous electrical nerve stimulation (TENS). These approaches can often be used independently to relieve mild pain, but they must be used in combination with pharmacologic measures to relieve moderate to severe pain.

Distraction. Distraction is the state in which the child's attention is focused on something other than the pain or hurt. It is often used intuitively and effectively by parents or those closely associated with a particular child. Nurses can sometimes gain insight into pain relief for an individual child by closely observing the techniques used by parents. For infants, distraction may be accomplished by singing or watching a mobile. For toddlers and preschoolers, activities such as looking at a book, listening to a story, and playing with puppets or a toy may be utilized. For

TABLE 25-13
Nonpharmacologic Interventions

Intervention	Comments
Simple relaxation (begin preoperatively)	Effective in reducing mild to moderate pain and as an adjunct to analgesic drugs for severe pain; use when patients express an interest in relaxation; requires 3–5 mins of staff time for instructions
	Both patient-preferred and "easy listening" music are effective in reducing mild to moderate pain
Complex relaxation (begin preoperatively)	Effective in reducing mild to moderate pain and operative site muscle tension; requires skilled personnel and special equipment
	Effective for reduction of mild to moderate pain; requires skilled personnel
Education/instruction (begin preoperatively)	Effective for reduction of pain; should include sensory and procedural information and instruction aimed at reducing activity related pain; requires 5–15 mins of staff time
Transcutaneous electrical nerve stimulation	Effective in reducing pain and improving physical function; requires skilled personnel and special equipment; may be useful as an adjunct to drug therapy

Adapted from Acute Pain Management Guideline Panel. (1992). *Acute pain management: Operative or medical procedures and trauma. Clinical practice guideline.* (AHCPR Pub. No. 92-0032). Rockville, MD: Agency for Health Care Policy and Research, Public Health Service, US Department of Health and Human Services.

school-age children and adolescents, more complex strategies may be required. Often, these strategies need to be self-generated to be effective. Distraction in this older group could take the form of a discussion with a nurse, family, or friend, reading, watching television, or engaging in a quiet game. Music therapy has also been shown to be beneficial in treating pain patients (Bailey, 1986). Music, ideally, is selected by the patient. Music therapy can promote relaxation, provoke an alteration in mood, and be a vehicle for self-expression. For children, music and other forms of distraction can alleviate fear and anxiety while at the same time focus their attention on more pleasant sensations.

There is always the danger that effective use of distraction will be misinterpreted to mean that the severity of the child's pain has decreased. Some nurses may question the existence of pain if the child is seen playing a few minutes before requesting analgesia. Remember that *distraction can interrupt the perception of pain during the distracting activity, but has no action beyond that period.* When the activity ends, pain returns.

Interactions. Interaction with parents or a significant other (e.g., babysitter, nanny, grandparent, or sibling) is another naturally occurring event for children in pain. An examination of the interaction of children and their parents during a painful event provided information about the nature of parental support (Hunsberger et al, 1987). Child and parent behaviors were identified and categorized into an interaction scoring grid. Although generalizability of the findings is limited by a small sample size, the study suggests that parents are able to increase their efforts at comforting children and helping them cope as the pain increases. Specific behaviors that parents used included:

- Tactile: involving direct contact, as in touching, holding, rubbing, caressing, or rocking (as well as basic care needs, such as feeding and changing infants).
- Gestural: involving all forms of nonverbal communication (e.g., smiling and staying near the child).
- Verbal: communication about the pain experience (e.g., "I know it hurts") or about other, nonrelated topics.

Parents were also able to use distraction techniques or promote self-initiated distraction on the part of the child. The mere presence of the parent or significant other cannot be underrated. In a study by Jerrett (1985), children rated the presence of a parent as "the most beneficial activity and the most helpful for coping with the pain."

Relaxation. Relaxation is a widely used nonpharmacologic approach to help ease pain. It is a popular approach because it can alter the activities of the autonomic nervous system, thus affecting the pain response. Relaxation can be promoted in young children by encouraging them to cuddle a favorite toy, holding or rocking them, singing or talking in a soothing voice, or allowing them to listen to soothing music. Deep breathing and muscle relaxation are techniques that can be used with older children. Cautela and Groden (1978) have developed relaxation techniques that are specifically tailored to children.

Rhythmic breathing is a combination of distraction and relaxation. In this approach, patients are asked to stare at a pleasing object, inhale slowly and deeply, and then exhale slowly. Patients can also be asked to concentrate on how the air feels as it goes in and out of their lungs. If children are able to incorporate a more complex approach, they can be encouraged to count, do arm or leg motions, or massage the painful area (e.g., as in effleurage during preparation for childbirth).

Progressive muscle relaxation involves systematic tensing and relaxing of muscle groups. Although this may sound too complex for children, it can be utilized effectively if approached as a game. An example of a game that can be used to promote muscle contraction and relaxation is given in Table 25–14. There are also commercially produced audio tapes and videotapes that outline the steps in progressive relaxation, but similar effects can be achieved if these guidelines are followed.

1. Provide a quiet environment.
2. Children should lie on their backs, close their eyes, and totally relax. They should concentrate on how it "feels" to be relaxed.
3. Have children focus on a specific muscle group (e.g., facial muscles) and tense the muscles for 5 seconds. Have them concentrate on how it feels when the muscles are tense. Have them relax the muscles again.
4. Focus on the differences between the relaxed and the tense states.
5. Move on to another muscle group and continue this exercise in some systematic way until all muscle groups in the body have been incorporated.

Guided Imagery. If the child finds muscle relaxation exercises too difficult or too boring, guided imagery can be introduced in combination with some form of relaxation therapy or by itself. Guided imagery is similar to distraction, but it requires patients to utilize their imaginations to create pleasant images. This technique can rarely be used in children who are not capable of at least some degree of abstract thinking. If children are reluctant to try this technique it can be explained and compared with something they are familiar with—such as fantasy or daydreaming. The only difference is that imagery is selective. Children will need some assistance in choosing an image that is right for them, but they should be encouraged to pursue something that they enjoy experiencing. For example, if they enjoy swimming at the beach, this might be a useful place to start in developing a composite image. If they can be convinced to incorporate several senses, such as how the water feels, how the air smells, how the splashing sounds, and even how they look with their hair soaking wet, the exercise will be more effective in giving them mastery over their pain. Most importantly, children need to be reminded of how much fun they would be having and how good they would be feeling in the imagined scenario. Relaxation exercises may help to prepare a child for guided imagery. Questions from either the nurse or a parent may help in children's descriptions of the various sensations. Parents may also benefit from guided imagery exercises, and their participation may provide an incentive and serve as a model for the child to follow.

Massage. Another nonpharmacologic intervention is massage. As discussed earlier in relation to the Gate Control Theory, touch or rubbing the affected part is an automatic and instinctive response to pain. Examples of this behavior include young children who rub their ear when they have an ear infection or massage their gums by gnawing on a "soother" when teething. Massage is particularly useful for treating children with chronic pain, because it relaxes their muscles as well as provides comfort and sedation. Massage can be either superficial or deep, although the latter is rarely used for children.

Coping Skills Training. An approach that is often used with children suffering from recurrent pain (e.g., headaches, stomachaches) is coping skills training. This approach combines a number of nonpharmacologic interventions (such as muscle relaxation, rhythmic breathing, and guided imagery) with the major aim of helping children to manage their stress. First of all, children need to recognize what stress is and what produces it. Then they are taught how to decrease that stress using relaxation, imagery, and breathing. They also learn to engage in "invisible talking to themselves" and thought stopping. The optimal outcome is for children to obtain both pain relief and a sense of pain control (McGrath, 1983).

Hypnosis. Hypnosis is a nonpharmacologic method of pain relief that has been researched most thoroughly in children diagnosed as having cancer. Hypnosis has been shown to reduce pain during painful procedures (Hilgard & LeBaron, 1982; Kellerman et al, 1983; McGrath & DeVeber, in press). Zeltzer and

TABLE 25-14
A Game to Promote Muscle Contraction and Relaxation

The Biggest Balloon on Earth Game

1. Have children lie on the floor "in a heap" with all muscles relaxed, like a deflated balloon
2. Ask them to contract various muscle groups as they "inflate themselves, like a balloon full of air." As they are doing this, they should slowly stand up and stretch their arms up as high as they can
3. Encourage children to float around the room, with arms outstretched, muscles tense, pretending they, the biggest balloon on earth, are floating around the world
4. Tell them the balloon has sprung a leak and the air is slowly escaping. Ask them to relax various muscle groups and slowly float to the ground
5. Children end up "in a heap—a deflated balloon once more"

LeBaron (1982) compared hypnosis with a combination of deep breathing, distraction, and preparation techniques. Results of this study indicated that hypnosis reduced pain from bone marrow aspiration by a large extent and that the other methods reduced pain by a smaller, but also significant, extent. Although hypnosis has been shown to be a promising intervention for reducing pain during procedures in patients with cancer, the availability of trained personnel to perform it is limited. Self-hypnosis requires extensive training before it can be used effectively.

***Transcutaneous Electrical Nerve Stimulation* (TENS).** Transcutaneous electrical nerve stimulation (TENS) has been used in the United States with adult patients since the 1950s. This technique employs a small unit attached to electrodes that deliver varying degrees of electrical stimulation to cutaneous nerves, depending on the settings for amplitude, rate, and pulse width. Patients can operate the unit themselves to control pain. TENS has been studied more extensively in adults than in children, but Dr. Joann Eland, a nurse researcher, is currently studying the use of TENS for pain in childhood.

Eland (1988) reported successful pain relief in clinical trials of TENS units for children 4 years of age and older. TENS units were tested on children with varying types of pain, including subcutaneous chemotherapy, burning paresthesia from spinal cord compression, metastasis of cancer to the ribs, phantom limb pain, herpes zoster, and infusion of amphotericin. She concluded that TENS is a promising intervention for pain in children.

Other nonpharmacologic interventions for pain relief include biofeedback and acupuncture. Although these interventions are being used with some success in adults, they have been tested less extensively in children.

Evaluation

Evaluating the result of pain relief strategies brings us full circle in the nursing process. Evaluation might be termed "focused reassessment." To reassess, use the strategies that were effective in describing the pain initially. Interpret assessment results by comparing them against the baseline.

- Is the child expressing less pain through vocal, verbal, behavioral, and/or physiologic parameters?
- Has the child's goal for pain relief been met?
- What is the parent's estimation of pain relief?
- What side effects are present?

To access symptoms, ask the child, "Besides taking away your hurt, how does the medicine make you feel?"

Documenting Pain and Pain Relief

The importance of documentation cannot be overemphasized. Pain remains one of the most poorly documented of the critical parameters nurses assess. Documentation establishes a *pattern* of pain and of the interventions that are effective in relieving pain. Failure to document pain and pain relief is no less serious than failure to document vital signs. Imagine the confusion if the only knowledge of previous vital signs was what the last nurse had thought to pass along verbally.

An effective method of documenting the child's pain is through the use of a pain flow sheet (Stevens & Johnston, 1991). A flow sheet provides a summary of the child's pain and pain management over time. The intensity of the pain can be graphed in a manner similar to that used for vital sign charts. In addition, the location of the pain, factors that aggravate and alleviate the pain, the effect of pain on activities of daily living, and the interventions employed (medications and their effectiveness) can be recorded. Pain flow sheets can become a concise summary of the child's pain experience that can be kept either at the bedside or as part of the medical record. *Precise documentation provides the impetus for ongoing reassessment and management of the child in pain.*

KEY CONCEPTS

Concepts Related to Basic Information

- Each pain experience is the result of a unique combination of physiologic, psychologic, and social factors.
- Cognitive/emotional factors and social/contextual factors may actually be more predictive of the pain than physical trauma.
- In young infants, mechanisms to inhibit pain are less well developed than in older children and adults. Thus, infants are at increased risk for physiologic and psychologic trauma from painful stimuli.

Concepts Related to Nursing Assessment

- Pain must be identified before it can be treated. The burden for identifying pain rests with the health care provider.
- Pain assessment requires vigorous investigation. For example, when crying and movement increase pain, the infant or child soon learns to lie quietly and may even appear to be asleep.
- When educated about their roles in identifying and reporting pain, children and parents become partners in pain assessment.
- When pain assessment tools have well-established reliability and validity, the results will be a true measure of pain and will be consistent every time the tool is used, regardless of which nurse obtains the pain rating.
- Baseline assessments (including a pain history)

provide a point of reference for interpreting all subsequent pain assessments.

- Careful documentation of pain assessments establishes a pattern of pain and the response to treatment. Knowledge of this pattern is critical to effective pain management.

Concepts Related to Nursing Intervention

- Narcotic analgesics are the drug of choice for moderate to severe pain. However, combinations of narcotic analgesics with non-narcotic medications and nonpharmacologic nursing interventions can significantly increase the effectiveness of the opioid.
- Continuous pain requires a constant blood level of analgesic achieved through around-the-clock administration or continuous infusion. As-necessary (PRN) administration is effective only for break-through pain.
- Analgesia does not come in one-size-fits-all. The analgesic dose that works for one child may be either overly sedating or completely ineffective for another child.
- Every pain management program should include measures to reduce fear and anxiety and measures to enhance the child's sense of control.
- Nonpharmacologic interventions (e.g., relaxation, distraction) can be effective for the pain of short procedures and are important adjuncts to anagesics in relieving moderate to severe pain.

REFERENCES

Abu-Saad, H. (1984a). Assessing children's responses to pain. *Pain, 19,* 163–171.

Abu-Saad, H. (1984b). Cultural components of pain: The Asian-American child. *Children's Health Care, 13*(1), 11–14.

Abu-Saad, H. (1984c). Cultural group indicators of pain in children. *Maternal-Child Nursing Journal, 13,* 187–197.

Abu-Saad, H. (1990). Toward the development of an instrument to assess pain in children: Dutch study. In D. C. Tyler & E. E. J. Krane (Eds.), *Advances in Pain Research and Therapy* (Vol. 15, pp 101–106). New York: Raven Press.

Abu-Saad, H., & Holzemer, W. (1981). Measuring children's self-assessment of their pain. *Issues in Comprehensive Pediatric Nursing, 5,* 337–349.

Acute Pain Management Guideline Panel. (1992a). *Acute pain management: Operative or medical procedures and trauma. Clinical practice guideline.* (AHCPR Pub. No. 92–0032). Rockville, MD: Agency for Health Care Policy and Research, Public Health Service, US Department of Health and Human Services.

Acute Pain Management Guideline Panel (1992b). *Acute pain management in infants, children, and adolescents: Operative and medical procedures.* Quick reference guide for clinicians (AHCPR Pub. No. 92-0020). Rockville, MD: Agency for Health Care Policy and Research, Public Health Service, US Department of Health and Human Services.

Anand, K. J. S. (1990). The biology of pain perception in newborn infants. In D. C. Tyler & E. J. Krane (Eds.), *Advances in Pain Research and Therapy* (Vol. 15, pp 113–122). New York: Raven Press.

Anand, K. J. S., & Hickey, P. R. (1987). Pain and its effects in the human neonate and fetus. *New England Journal of Medicine, 317,* 1321–1329.

Anand, K. J. S., & Carr, D. B. (1989). The neuroanatomy, neurophysiology, and neurochemistry of pain, stress, and analgesia in newborns and children. *Pediatric Clinics of North America, 3*(4), 795–822.

Anand, K. J. S., & Hickey, P. R. (1992). Halothane morphine compared with high-dose sufentanil for anesthesia and postoperative analgesia in neonatal cardiac surgery. *New England Journal of Medicine, 326*(1), 1–9.

Aradine, C., Beyer, J., & Tompkins, J. (1988). Children's pain perception before and after analgesia: A study of instrument construct validity. *Journal of Pediatric Nursing, 3,* 11–23.

Bailey, I. M. (1986). Music therapy in pain management. *Journal of Pain and Symptom Management, 1*(1), 25–28.

Belter, R., McIntosh, J., Finch, A., & Saylor, C. (1988). Measurement of pain in preschool children: Three self-report methods. *Clinical Journal of Child Psychology, 17,* 327–335.

Berg, K. M., Berg, W. K., & Graham, F. K. (1971). Infant heart rate response as a function of stimulus and state. *Psychophysiology, 8,* 30–44.

Beyer, J. (1988). The Oucher: A pain intensity scale for children. In S. G. Funk, E. M. Tornquist, M. T. Champagne, L. A. Copp, & R. A. Wiese (Eds). *Key aspects of comfort: Management of pain, fatigue, and nausea* (pp 65–71). New York: Springer.

Beyer, J. (1984). *The Oucher: A User's Manual and Technical Report.* Evanston, IL: The Hospital Play Equipment Company.

Beyer, J., & Aradine, C. (1986). Content validity of an instrument to measure young children's perceptions of the intensity of their pain. *Journal of Pediatric Nursing, 1*(6), 386–395.

Beyer, J. & Aradine, C. (1988). Convergent and discriminant validity of a self-report measure of pain intensity for children. *Children's Health Care, 16*(4), 274–282.

Beyer, J. & Aradine, C. (1987). Patterns of pediatric pain intensity: A methodological investigation of a self-report scale. *Clinical Journal of Pain, 3,* 130–141.

Beyer, J. E., Denyes, M. J., & Villarruel, A. M. (1992). The creation, validation, and continuing development of the oucher: A measure of pain intensity in children. *Journal of Pediatric Nursing, 7*(5), 335–346.

Beyer, J. E., McGrath, P. J., & Berde, C. B. (1990). Discordance between self-report and behavioral measures in 3–7 year old children following surgery. *Journal of Pain and Symptom Management, 5*(6), 350–356.

Bonica, J. J. (1990). Anatomic and physiologic basis of nociception and pain. In J. J. Bonica (Ed.). *The management of pain* (Vol. 1, pp 28–94). Philadelphia: Lea & Febiger.

Bonica, J. J. (1979). The need for a taxonomy. *Pain, 6,* 247–252.

Booth, J. C., McGrath, P. A., Brigham, M. C., Frewen, T. C., & Whittall, S. (1989, June). Pain in infants: Distress responses to repeated noxious stimuli. Paper presented at the First European Conference in Pain in Children, Maastricht, the Netherlands.

Bradshaw, C., & Zeanah, P. D. (1986). Pediatric nurses' assessments of pain in children. *Journal of Pediatric Nursing, 1*(5), 314–322.

Branson, S. M., McGrath, P. J., Craig, K. D., Rubin, S. Z., & Vair, C. (1990). Spontaneous strategies for coping with pain and their origins in adolescents who undergo surgery. In D. C. Tyler & E. J. Krane (Eds.), *Advances in pain research therapy* (Vol. 15, pp 237–245). New York: Raven Press.

Brown, L. (1987). Physiologic responses to cutaneous pain in neonates. *Neonatal Network, 5,* 18.

Burokas, L. (1985). Factors affecting nurses' decisions to medicate pediatric patients after surgery. *Heart & Lung, 14*(4), 373–379.

Cautela, J. R., & Groden, J. (1978). Relaxation: *A comprehensive manual for adults, children, and children with special needs.* Champaign, IL: Research Press.

Chapman, C. R., & Bonica, J. J. (1983). *Acute pain.* Kalamazoo, MI: Upjohn.

Chapman, C. R., & Turner, J. A. (1990). Psychologic and psychosocial aspects of acute pain. In J. J. Bonica (Ed.), *The management of pain* (2nd ed., Vol. 1, pp 122–132). Philadelphia: Lea & Febiger.

Chapman, C. R., & Turner, J. A. (1986). Psychological control of acute pain medical settings. *Journal of Pain and Symptom Management, 1*(1), 9–20.

Craig, K. D. (1992). Echoes of pain. *APS Journal 1992, 1*(2), 105–108.

Craig, K. D., Whitfield, M. F., Grunau, R. V. E., Linton, J., & Hadjistavropoulos, H. (1993). Pain in the preterm neonate: Behavioural and physiological indices. *Pain, 52*(3), 287–299.

Crook, J. (1985). Concepts of pain and their relationship to measurement issues. In L. A. Copp (Ed.), *Perspective on pain*. Edinburgh: Churchill Livingstone.

Crue, B. L. (1985). Foreword. In G. M. Aronoff (Ed.). *Evaluation and treatment of chronic pain*. Baltimore: Urban & Schwarzenberg.

Dale, J. C. (1986). A multidimensional study of infants' responses to painful stimuli. *Pediatric Nursing, 12*(1), 27–31.

Dale, J. C. (1989). A multidimensional study of infants' behaviors associated with assumed painful stimuli: Phase II. *Journal of Pediatric Health Care, 3*(1), 34–38.

Datz, L. (1989). *Comparison of mother's and children's rating of children's tonsillectomy pain intensity*. Unpublished master's thesis, University of California at Los Angeles.

Davis, D. H., & Calhoon, M. (1989). Do preterm infants show behavioral responses to painful procedures? In S. G. Funk, E. M. Tornquist, M. T. Champagne, L. A. Copp, & R. A. Wiese (Eds.). *Key aspects of comfort: Management of pain, fatigue, and nausea* (pp 35–45). New York: Springer.

Davitz, J. R., & Davitz, L. L. (1981). *Inferences of patients; Pain and psychological distress. Studies of nursing behaviors*. New York: Springer.

Eland, J. M. (1974). Children's communication of pain. Unpublished master's thesis. Iowa City: University of Iowa.

Eland, J. M. (1975). *Assessment and management of pain in children*. Paper presented at The Children's Hospital, Denver.

Eland, J. M. (1981). Minimizing pain associated with prekindergarten intramuscular injections. *Issues in Comprehensive Pediatric Nursing*, 361–372

Eland, J. M. (1988, March). The use of transcutaneous electrical nerve stimulation with children in pain. Paper presented at a national conference, Key Aspects of Comfort: Management of Pain Fatigue, and Nausea, Chapel Hill, North Carolina.

Eland, J. M., & Anderson, J. E. (1977). The experience of pain in children. In A. Jacox, (Ed.). *Pain: A Sourcebook for Nurses and Other Health Professionals*. Boston: Little, Brown.

Engel, J. M., & Rapoff, M. A. (1990). A component analysis of relaxation training for children with vascular, muscle contraction, and mixed-headache disorders. In D. C. Tyler & E. J. Krane (Eds.). *Advances in Pain Research and Therapy* (Vol. 15, pp 273–290). New York: Raven Press.

Escobar, P. L. (1985, January). Management of chronic pain. *Nurse Practitioner*, 24–32.

Field, T., & Goldson, E. (1984). Pacifying effects of nonnutritive sucking on term and preterm neonates during heel stick procedures. *Pediatrics, 74*(6), 1012–1015.

Fields, H. L. (1992). Is there a facilitating component to central pain modulation? *APS Journal, 1*(2), 82–84.

Fields, H. L. (1987). *Pain*. San Francisco: McGraw-Hill.

Fitzgerald, M. (1991). The developmental neurobiology of pain. In M. R. Bond, J. E. Charlton, & C. J. Woolf (Eds.). *Pain research and clinical management: Proceedings of the VIth world congress on pain. 4* (pp 253–261). Amsterdam: Elsevier.

Fitzgerald, M., & Anand, K. J. S. (1993). Developmental neuroanatomy and neurophysiology of pain. In N. L. Schechter, C. B. Berde, & M. Yaster (Eds.). *Pain in infants, children, and adolescents* (pp 11–31). Baltimore: Williams & Wilkins.

Foster, R. L. (1990). *A multi-method approach to the description of factors influencing nurses' pharmacologic management of children's pain*. Unpublished doctoral dissertation, University of Colorado Health Sciences Center, Denver, CO.

Foster, R. L. (1991). The effect of unit culture on nurses' management of children's pain. *Journal of Pain and Symptom Management, 6*(3), 202.

Foster, R. L., & Hester, N. (1989). The relationship between assessment and pharmacologic intervention for pain in children. In S. G. Funk, E. M. Tornquist, M. T. Champagne, L. A. Copp, & R. A. Wiese (Eds.), *Key aspects of comfort: Management of pain, fatigue, and nausea* (pp 72–79). New York: Springer Publishing Co.

Fowler-Kerry, S., & Ramsay-Lander, J. (1990). Utilizing cognitive strategies to relieve pain in young children. In D. C. Tyler & E. J. Krane (Eds.). *Advances in Pain Research and Therapy* (Vol. 15, pp 247–253). New York: Raven Press.

Fritz, K. I., Schechter, N., & Bernstein, B. (1991). Cultural components of pain behavior in Vietnamese refugee children. *Journal of Pain and Symptom Management, 6*(3), 205.

Fuller, B. F., Conner, D., & Horii, Y. (1991). Potential acoustic measures of infant pain and arousal. In D. C. Tyler & E. J. Krane (Eds.). *Advances in Pain Research and Therapy* (Vol. 15, pp 137–145). New York: Raven Press.

Fuller, B. F., & Horii, Y. (1988). Spectral energy distribution in four types of infant vocalizations. *Journal of Communication Disorders, 21*, 251–261.

Gadish, H. S., Gonzalez, J. L., & Hayes, J. S. (1988). Factors affecting nurses' decisions to administer pediatric pain medication postoperatively. *Journal of Pediatric Nursing, 3*(6), 383–390.

Gaffney, A., & Dunne, E. A. (1987). Children's understanding of the causality of pain. *Pain, 29*, 91–104.

Gedaly-Duff, V. (1989). Palmar sweat index use with children in pain research. *Journal of Pediatric Nursing, 14*(1), 3–8.

Gilles, F. H., Shankle, W., & Dooling, E. C. (1983). Myelinated tracts: Growth patterns. In F. H. Gilles, A. Leviton, & E. C. Dooling (Eds.). *The developing human brain* (pp 117–183). Boston: Wright & Co.

Gleiss, J. & Stuttgen, G. (1970). Morphologic and functional development of the skin. In U. Stave (Ed.). *Physiology of the Perinatal period* (Vol. 2, pp 889–906). New York: Appleton-CenturyCrofts.

Grunau, R. V. E., & Craig, K. D. (1987). Pain expression in neonates: Facial action and cry. *Pain, 28*, 395–410.

Grunau, R. V. E., Johnston, C. C., & Craig, K. D. (1990). Neonatal facial and cry responses to invasive and non-invasive procedures. *Pain, 42*, 295–305.

Gunnar, M. R., Isensee, J., & Fust, L. S. (1987). Adrenocortical activity and the Brazelton Neonatal Assessment Scale. Moderating effects of the newborn's biobehavioral status. *Child Development, 58*, 1448–1458.

Gunnar, M. R., Malone, S., Vance, G., & Fisch, R. O. (1985). Coping with active stimulation in the neonatal period: Quiet sleep and levels of plasma cortisol during recovery from circumcision in newborns. *Child Development, 56*, 824–834.

Hagedorn, M. (1990). *Does a topical skin cooling agent alter a child's pain perception during a D.P.T. injection?* Unpublished master's thesis, University of Colorado Health Sciences Center, Denver, CO.

Harpin, V. A., & Rutter, N. (1982). Development of emotional sweating in the newborn infant. *Archives of Diseases in Childhood, 57*, 691–695.

Hawley, D. D. (1984). Postoperative pain in children: Misconceptions, descriptions and interventions. *Pediatric Nursing, 10*, 20–23.

Hay, H. (1984). *The measurement of pain intensity in children and adults—A methodological approach*. Unpublished master's research report, McGill University, Montreal, Canada.

Hertzka, R. E., Gauntlett, I. S., Fisher, D. M., & Spellman, M. J. (1989). Fentanyl-induced ventilatory depression: Effects of age. *Anesthesiology, 70*, 213–218.

Hester, N. O. (1979). The preoperational child's reaction to immunizations. *Nursing Research, 28*, 250–254.

Hester, N. O. (1989). Comforting the child in pain. In S. G. Frank, E. M. Tornquist, M. T. Champagne, L. A. Copp, & R. A. Wiese (Eds.). *Key aspects of comfort: Management of pain, fatigue, and nausea* (pp 290–298). New York: Springer.

Hester, N. O., & Barcus, C. S. (1986). Assessment and management of pain in children. *Pediatrics: Nursing update, 1*(14), 1–8.

Hester, N. O., Davis, R. C., Hanson, S. H., & Hassanein, R. S. (1978). The hospitalized child's subjective rating of painful experiences. Unpublished manuscript, University of Kansas Medical Center, Kansas City.

Hester, N. O., & Foster, R. L. (1993). *Nurse clinical decision-making: Pain in children: Final report*. Research funded by NIH, Na-

tional Center for Nursing Research under grant number R01NR01964.
Hester, N. O., & Foster, R. L. (1992). Scrutiny of the protocol for administration of the poker chip tool: Research study partially funded by RR03503, National Institutes of Health.
Hester, N. O., Foster, R. L., & Kristensen, K. (1990). Measurement of pain in children: Generalizability and validity of the pain ladder and the poker chip tool. In D. C. Tyler & E. J. Krane (Eds). *Advances in pain research and therapy* (Vol. 15, pp 79–84). New York: Raven Press.
Hester, N. O., Foster, R. L., Kristensen, K., & Bergstrom, L. (1989). *Measurement of children's pain by children, parents, and nurses: Psychometric and clinical issues related to the poker chip tool and pain ladder. Generalizability of procedures assessing pain in children: Final Report.* Research funded by NIH, National Center for Nursing Research, under grant number R23NRO1382.
High, P. C., & Gorski, P. A. (1985). Recording environmental influences on infant development in the intensive care nursery: Womb for improvement. In A. W. Gottfried, & J. L. Gaiter (Eds.). *Infant stress under intensive care: Environmental neonatology* (pp 129–136). Baltimore, University Park Press.
Hilgard, J. R., & LeBaron, S. (1982). Relief of anxiety and pain in children and adolescents with cancer: Quantitative measures and clinical observations. *International Journal of Clinical and Experimental Hypnosis, 30,* 417–442.
Holm, K., Cohen, F., Dudas, S., Medema, P., & Allen, B. (1989). Effect of personal pain experience on pain assessment. *Image, 21*(2), 72–75.
Hunsberger, M., Stevens, B., & Browne, G. (1987, March). *Children's pain: A stimulus for parent-child interaction.* Paper presented at the 2nd International Nursing Research Symposium on Clinical Care of the Child and Family, Montreal.
Izard, C. E. (1979). *The maximally discriminative facial movement coding system (MAX).* Newark, NJ: University of Delaware Istructional Resources Center.
Jay, S. M., Ozolins, M., Elliott, C., et al. (1983). Assessment of children's distress during painful medical procedures. *Health Psychology, 2,* 133–147.
Jeans, M. E., & Gordon, D. J. (1981). An investigation of the developmental characteristics of the concept of pain. *Pain* (Suppl. 1), S11.
Jeans, M. E., & Melzack, R. (1992). Conceptual basis of nursing practice: Theoretical foundations of pain. In J. H. Watt-Watson & M. I. Donovan (Eds.). *Pain management, Nursing perspective* (pp 11–35). St. Louis: CV Mosby.
Jerrett, M. D. (1985). Children and their pain experience. *Children's Health Care, 14*(2), 83–89.
Johnston, C. C. (1993). Development of psychological responses to pain in infants and toddlers. In N. L. Schechter, C. B. Berde, & M. Yaster (Eds.). *Pain in infants, children, and adolescents* (pp 65–74). Baltimore: Williams & Wilkins.
Johnston, C. C. (1989). Pain assessment and management in infants. *Pediatrician, 16,* 16–23.
Johnston, C. C., & O'Shaughnessy, D. (1988). Acoustical attributes of infant pain cries: Discriminating features. In R. Dubner, G. F. Gebhart, & M. R. Bond (Eds.). *Proceedings of the VIth world congress on pain: Pain research and clinical management* (Vol. 3, pp 336–340). New York: Elsevier.
Johnston, C. C., & Stevens, B. (1991). Pain assessment in newborns. *Journal of Perinatal and Neonatal Nursing, 4*(1), 41–52.
Johnston, C. C., Stevens, B., Craig, K., & Grunau, R. V. E. (1993). Developmental changes in pain expression in premature, full-term, two and four month-old infants. *Pain, 52*(2), 201–208.
Johnston, C. C., & Strada, M. E. (1986). Acute pain response in infants: A multidimensional description. *Pain, 24,* 373–382.
Jordan-Marsh, M., Hall, D., Yoder, L., Watson, R., McFarlane-Sosa, G., & Garcia, M. (1990). *The Harbor–UCLA medical center humor project for children.* Los Angeles: Harbor–UCLA Medical Center.
Katz, E. R., Kellerman, J., & Siegel, S. E. (1981). Anxiety as an affective focus in the clinical study of acute behavioral distress: A reply to Shachman and Daut. *Journal of Consulting and Clinical Psychology, 49*(3), 470–471.
Katz, E. R., Kellerman, J., & Siegel, S. E. (1980). Behavioral distress in children undergoing medical procedures: Developmental considerations. *Journal of Consulting and Clinical Psychology, 48*(3), 356–365.
Kehlet, H. (1991). Neurohumoral response to surgery and pain in man. In M. R. Bond, J. E. Charlton, & C. J. Woolf (Eds.). *Proceedings of the VIth world congress on pain* (pp 35–40). New York: Elsevier.
Kellerman, J., Zeltzer, L., Ellenberg, L., et al. (1983). Adolescents with cancer: Hypnosis for the reduction of the acute pain and anxiety associated with medical procedures. *Journal of Adolescent Health Care, 4,* 85–90.
Koren, G., & Butt, W. (1985). Postoperative morphine infusion in newborn infants: Assessment of disposition characteristics and safety. *Journal of Pediatrics, 107,* 963–967.
Kotzer, A. M., & Foster, R. L. (1992). Opioids: How risky are they for children? In Western Institute of Nursing, *Silver threads: 25 years of nursing excellence* (p 329). Boulder, CO: Western Institute of Nursing.
Kuhar, M. J., & Pasternak, G. W. (Eds.). (1984). *Analgesics: Neurochemical, behavioral, and clinical perspectives.* New York: Raven Press.
Kushner, H. S. (1985). When children and adults suffer. *Children's Health Care, 14*(2), 68–75.
LeBaron, S., & Zeltzer, L. (1984). Assessment of acute pain and anxiety in children and adolescents by self-reports, observer reports, and a behavior checklist. *Journal of Consulting and Clinical Psychology, 52*(5), 729–738.
Lollar, D. J., Smits, S. J., & Patterson, D. L. (1982). Assessment of pediatric pain: An empirical perspective. *Journal of Pediatric Psychology, 7,* 267–277.
Lynn, A. M., & Slattery, J. T. (1987). Morphine pharmacokinetics in early infancy. *Anesthesiology, 66,* 136–139.
McCaffery, M. (1972). *Nursing management of the patient with pain.* Philadelphia: JB Lippincott.
McGrath, P. A. (1990). *Pain in children: Nature, assessment, and treatment.* New York: Guilford.
McGrath, P. A. (1993). Psychological aspects of pain perception. In N. L. Schechter, C. B. Berde, & M. Yaster (Eds.). *Pain in infants, children, and adolescents* (pp 39–64). Baltimore: Williams & Wilkins.
McGrath, P. (1983). Psychological aspects of recurrent abdominal pain. *Canadian Family Physician, 29,* 1655–1659.
McGrath, P., & Unruh, A. (1987). *Pain in children and adolescents.* New York: Elsevier.
McGrath, P. A., DeVeber, L. L. (1986). The management of acute pain evoked by medical procedures in children with cancer. *Journal of Pain and Symptom Management, 1*(3), 145–150.
McGrath, P. A., DeVeber, L. L., & Hearn, M. T. (1985a). Multidimensional pain assessment in children. In H. L. Fields, R. Dubner, F. Cervera (Eds.). *Advances in pain research and therapy* (Vol. 9). New York: Raven Press.
McGrath, P. J., Johnson, G., Goodman, J. T., Schillinger, J., Dunn, J., & Chapman, J. A. (1985b). The CHEOPS: A behavioral scale to measure postoperative pain in children. In H. L. Fields, R. Dubner, & F. Cervero (Eds.). *Advances in pain research and therapy* (pp 395–402). New York: Raven Press.
McGraw, M. B. (1941). Neural maturation as exemplified in the changing reaction of the infant to pinprick. *Child Development, 12,* 31–42.
Melamed, B. G., & Siegel, L. J. (1975). Reduction of anxiety in children facing surgery by modeling. *Journal of Consulting and Clinical Psychology, 43,* 511–521.
Melzack, R. (1991). The gate control theory 25 years later: New perspectives on phantom limb pain. In M. R. Bond, J. E. Charlton, & C. J. Woolf (Eds.). *Proceedings of the VIth world congress on pain.* New York: Elsevier.
Melzack, R. (1973). *The puzzle of pain.* New York: Basic Books.
Melzack, R., & Wall, P. D. (1988). *The challenge of pain.* London: Penquin Books.
Melzack, R., & Wall, P. D. (1965). Pain mechanisms: A new theory. *Science, 150,* 971–979.
Mills, N. (1989a). Acute pain behavior in infants and toddlers. In S. G. Funk, E. M. Tornquist, M. T. Champagne, L. A. Copp, &

R. A. Wiese (Eds.). *Key aspects of comfort. Management of pain, fatigue, and nausea* (pp 52–59). New York: Springer.

Mills, N. (1989b). Pain behaviors in infants and toddlers. *Journal of Pain and Symptom Management, 4*(4), 184–190.

Molsberry, D. (1979). *Young children's subjective quantification of pain following surgery*. Unpublished master's thesis, University of Iowa, Iowa City.

Neuman, B. M., Denyes, M. J., Stettner, L., & Villarruel, A. M. (1990). Facial expression as an emotional response to pain: A study of instrument content validity. *Pain* (Suppl 5), S25.

Oikkola, K. T., Maunukscla, E. L., Lorpela, R., & Rosenberg, P. H. (1988). Kinetics and dynamics of postoperative intravenous morphine in children. *Clinical Pharmacology Therapy, 44,* 128–136.

Owens, M. E., & Todt, E. H. (1984). Pain in infancy: Neonatal reaction to a heel lance. *Pain, 20,* 77–84.

Porter, F. L., Miller, R. H., & Marshall, R. E. (1986). Neonatal pain cries: Effect of circumcision on acoustic features and perceived urgency. *Child Development, 57,* 790–802.

Porter, F. L., Porges, S. W., & Marshall, R. E. (1988). Newborn cries and vagal tone: Parallel changes in response to circumcision. *Child Development, 59,* 495–505.

Price, D. D. (1988). *Psychological and neural mechanisms of pain*. New York: Raven Press.

Rawlings, D. J., Miller, P. A., & Engel, R. R. (1980). The effect of circumcision on transcutaneous Po_2 in term infants. *American Journal of Diseases of Children, 134,* 676–678.

Ready, L. B., & Edwards, W. T. (Eds.). (1992). *Management of acute pain: A practical guide*. Seattle: IASP Publications.

Reed, M. D., & Besunder, J. B. Developmental pharmacology: Ontogenic basis of drug disposition. *Clinical Pharmacology, 36*(5), 1053–1074.

Rizvi, T., Wadhwa, S., & Biljani, V. (1987). Development of spinal substrate for nociception. *Pain* (Suppl), *4,* 195.

Ross, D. M., & Ross, S. A. (1988). *Childhood pain. Current issues, research, and management*. Baltimore: Urban & Schwarzenberg.

Ryan, E. A. (1989). The effect of musical distraction on pain in hospitalized school-aged children. In S. G. Funk, E. M. Tornquist, M. T. Champagne, L. A. Copp, & R. A. Wicse (Eds.). *Key aspects of comfort. Management of pain, fatigue, and nausea* (pp 101–104). New York: Springer.

Savedra, M. C., Gibbons, P., Tesler, M., Ward, J., & Wegner, C. (1982). How do children describe pain? A tentative assessment. *Pain, 14,* 95–104.

Savedra, M. C., & Tesler, M. D. (1989). Assessing children's and adolescents' pain. *Pediatrician, 16,* 24–29.

Savedra, M. C., Tesler, M. D., Holzemer, W. I., & Ward, J. A. (1989a). *Adolescent pediatric pain tool (APPT): Preliminary user's manual*. San Francisco: University of California.

Savedra, M. C., Tesler, M. D., Holzemer, W. L., Wilkie, D. J., & Ward, J. A. (1989b). Pain location: Validity and reliability of body outline markings by hospitalized children and adolescents. *Research in Nursing and Health, 12,* 307–314.

Savedra, M. C., Tesler, M. D., Holzemer, W. L., Wilkie, D. J., & Ward, J. A. (1990). Testing a tool to assess postoperative pediatric and adolescent pain. In D. C. Tyler & E. J. Krane (Eds.). *Advances in pain research and therapy* (Vol. 15, pp 85–93). New York: Raven Press.

Savedra, M. C., Tesler, M. D., Ward, J. A., & Wegner, C. (1988). How do adolescents describe pain? *Journal of Adolescent Health Care, 9,* 315–320.

Scott, R. (1978). It hurts red: A preliminary study of children's perceptions of pain. *Perceptual and Motor Skills 47,* 787–791.

Siegel, L. J. (1991). Increasing pain tolerance through self-efficacy training. *Journal of Pain and Symptom Management, 6*(3), 144.

Stevens, B., & Johnston, C. C. (1991). Premature infants' response to painful stimuli. *Journal of Pain and Symptom Management, 6,* 195.

Stevens, B., Johnston, C. C., & Horton, L. (1993). Multidimensional pain assessment in premature infants of 32–34 weeks gestational age. A pilot study. *Journal of Obstetric, Gynecologic, and Neonatal Nursing, 22*(6), 531–541.

Swafford, L. I., & Allan, D. (1968). Pain relief in the pediatric patient. *Medical Clinics of North America, 52*(1), 131–135.

Taylor, A. G., Skelton, J. A., & Butcher, J. (1984). Duration of pain condition and physical pathology as determinants of nurses' assessments of patients in pain. *Nursing Research, 33*(1), 4–8.

Taylor, P. (1983). Post-operative pain in toddler and pre-school age children. *Maternal Child Nursing Journal, 12,* 35–50.

Tesler, M. D., Savedra, M. C., Holzemer, W. L., Wilkie, D. J., Ward, J. A., & Paul, S. M. (1991). The word-graphic rating scale as a measure of children's and adolescents' pain intensity. *Research in Nursing & Health, 14,* 361–371.

Toomey, T. C., Mann, J. D., Abashian, S., & Thompson-Pope, S. (1991). Relationship between perceived self-control of pain, pain description and functioning. *Pain, 45,* 129–133.

Unruh, A., McGrath, P., Cunningham, S. I., et al. (1983). Children's drawings of their pain. *Pain, 17,* 385–392.

Valman, H. B., & Pearson, J. G. (1980). What the fetus feels. *British Medical Journal, 280,* 233–234.

Villarruel, A., & Denyes, M. (1989, May). *Cultural considerations in the assessment of pain in children*. Paper presented at the 24th Annual Conference of the Association for the Care of Children's Health, Anaheim, California.

Villarruel, A. M., & Ortiz de Montellano, B. (1992). Culture and pain: A Mesoamerican perspective. *Advances in Nursing Science, 15*(1), 21–32.

Vladek, B. C. (1988). Quality assurance through external controls. *Inquiry, 25,* 100–107.

Wall, P. D. (1988). Stability and instability of central pain mechanisms. In R. Dubner, G. F. Gebhart, & M. R. Bond (Eds.). *Proceedings of the Vth World Congress on Pain* (p 13). Amsterdam: Elsevier.

Wasz-Hochert, O., Michelsson, K., & Lind, J. (1985). Twenty-five years of Scandinavian cry research. In B. M. Lester & C. F. Boukydis (Eds.). *Infants crying: Theoretical and research perspectives* (pp 83–101). New York: Plenum Press.

Wiener, M. B., & Pepper, G. A. (1985). *Clinical pharmacology and therapeutics in nursing* (2nd ed.). New York: McGraw-Hill.

Wilkie, D. J., Holzemer, W. L., Tesler, M. D., Ward, J. A., Paul, S. M., & Savedra, M. C. (1990). Measuring pain quality: Validity and reliability of children's and adolescents' pain language. *Pain, 41,* 151–159.

Zeltzer, L., & LeBaron, S. (1982). Hypnotic and non-hypnotic techniques for the reduction of pain and anxiety during painful procedures in children and adolescents with cancer. *Journal of Pediatrics, 101,* 1032–1035.

Zeskind, P., Sale, S., Maio, J., Huntington, L., & Weiseman, J. (1985). Adult perceptions of pain and hunger cries: A synchrony of arousal. *Child Development, 56,* 549–554.

BIBLIOGRAPHY

Franck, L. S. (1991). *Pain control in critical care nursing*. Rockville, MD: Aspen.

Johnson, M. (1977). Assessment of clinical pain. In A. Jacox (Ed.), *Pain: A source book for nurses and other health professionals*. Boston: Little, Brown.

Porter, F. (1989). Pain in the newborn. *Clinics in Perinatology, 16,* 549–564.

Schechter, N. L. (1989). The undertreatment of pain in children: An overview. *Pediatric Clinics of North America, 36,* 781–794.

Stevens, B., & Johnston, C. C. (1993). Pain in the infant: Theoretical and conceptual issues. *Maternal-Child Nursing Journal, 21*(1), 3–14.

Wall, P. D., & Melzack, R. (1989). *Textbook of pain* (2nd ed). New York: Churchill Livingstone.

CHAPTER • 26

Principles of Fluid and Electrolyte Maintenance

Mabel Hunsberger

RELATED TOPICS
Stress reduction during procedures, Chapter 21
Principles and skills, Chapter 23
Pharmacologic principles, Chapter 24
Altered digestive function, Chapter 35
Development of kidney, Chapter 36

LEARNING OBJECTIVES

- Describe the regulatory mechanisms that maintain fluid and electrolyte balance in the body.
- Explain the differences in body fluid and electrolyte composition and regulation in infants and children compared with those of adults that make them especially vulnerable to imbalances.
- Describe the disturbances in regulation that contribute to the development of edema.
- Compare and contrast the types and causes of dehydration associated with sodium imbalances.
- Describe the clinical manifestations of potassium and calcium imbalances.
- Define "acid-base balance" and describe the regulation of hydrogen ion concentration in the body.

- Discuss the causes, clinical manifestations, and compensatory mechanisms associated with the four major types of acid-base disturbance.
- Outline nursing assessment criteria for evaluation of fluid and electrolyte and acid-base balance in children.
- Identify nursing diagnostic statements that describe fluid volume excesses and deficits.
- Identify the steps to calculate maintenance fluid and electrolyte therapy dosages.
- Describe nursing interventions to prevent fluid and electrolyte imbalances.
- Identify age-appropriate site selection, preparation, and evaluation of the child receiving intravenous therapy.
- Explain nursing procedures for starting, calculating, and maintaining pediatric intravenous infusions.
- Compare the advantages and disadvantages of central venous catheters and implanted devices used in the care of children.

Although alterations of function elicit predictable physiologic responses to compensate for deficits and excesses, in children developmental differences can alter the efficiency and magnitude of the body's compensatory mechanisms.

Included here is a discussion of fluid and electrolyte balance and intravenous therapy as it applies to infants and children. Those processes that have particular significance in children and the unique characteristics of children that affect fluid and electrolyte balance are addressed. Fluid and electrolyte balance and acid-base balance, interrelated mechanisms, are also addressed in this chapter. Relevant terms for understanding these concepts are reviewed in Table 26-1.

Specific illnesses that commonly result in fluid and electrolyte or acid-base imbalances are discussed in Chapters 32 to 47. For in-depth discussions of fluid and electrolytes, refer to basic science texts of biology, chemistry, and physiology.

Almost all illnesses in some way alter the intake, elimination, or need for water and electrolytes. The importance of this topic in children is that the status of infants and young children can change rapidly and insidiously when fluid and electrolyte imbalances occur.

Children, in contrast to adults, are more vulnerable to such changes because:

- Their bodies have a higher proportionate water content (therefore more can be lost rapidly).
- Greater proportion of fluid is in the extracellular space (from which it is more easily lost).
- They have a higher metabolic turnover of water (if not replaced equally rapidly, imbalance occurs).
- Their homeostatic regulation is immature (renal function, buffering capacity, calcium-phosphorus regulation).

Body Water Compartments and Internal Distribution

The greater proportionate fluid volume and its internal distribution make an infant vulnerable to fluid and electrolyte imbalances. Infants, especially premature infants, have a proportionately higher body fluid content than at any other time. Total body water (TBW) makes up 75 to 80 per cent of body weight in the full-term neonate and 90 per cent in the premature

TABLE 26-1
Fluid and Electrolyte Balance Definitions

Electrolytes

Anion: An ion with a negative charge of electricity. *Example:* Chloride (Cl^-), bicarbonate (HCO_3^-)

Cation: An ion with a positive charge of electricity. *Example:* Hydrogen (H^+), sodium (Na^+), potassium (K^+), calcium (Ca^{2+}), and magnesium (Mg^{2+})

Electrolyte: A substance that, when placed into water, dissociates into separately charged ions and conducts an electric current

Ion: A particle carrying an electric charge, consisting of an atom or group of atoms with a positive (cation) or negative (anion) charge for each electron lost or gained, respectively

Pressure and Osmolality

Hydrostatic pressure: Pressure exerted by a fluid within a closed system (e.g., pressure of the blood within the capillaries)

Oncotic pressure: The osmotic pressure exerted by colloids in solution (e.g., proteins)

Osmolality: The osmotic pressure of a solution expressed in osmols or milliosmols of the dissolved substance per kilogram of solvent (water)

Osmolarity: The osmotic pressure of a solution expressed in osmols or milliosmols of the dissolved substance per liter of the solution

Osmosis: The movement of a solvent through a semipermeable membrane to equalize the concentration of solvent on both sides

Osmotic pressure: The pressure required to prevent the movement of solvent across a semipermeable membrane that separates two solutions of different concentrations (pressure exerted by the solutes that holds or draws back water that has escaped)

Solute: The dissolved, suspended, or solid component of a solution

infant. This difference exists because of the body fat: body mass ratio. Newborn infants, and especially premature infants, have a reduced proportion of fat compared with later in life. There is an inverse relationship between TBW and total body fat.

Water is contained in two major compartments: within the cell (intracellular) and outside of the cell (extracellular). These two compartments are separated by the cell membrane, across which body fluid is freely exchanged. The extracellular fluid (ECF) includes the plasma, interstitial and lymphatic fluid, and connective tissue water. In infants, distribution of water is also different than later in life. They have a proportionately greater volume of extracellular fluid (primarily interstitial). For example, in the newborn infant, 40 per cent of body water is in the extracellular compartment, compared with 20 per cent in the adult. ECF is lost first when loss occurs (e.g., through illness, trauma, or stressful environmental conditions), increasing the vulnerability of infants. The ECF compartment also contains relatively more sodium and chloride during the period of infancy, accounting for the vulnerability of infants to electrolyte imbalances.

During the first few days of life, the normal neonate loses about 5 to 10 per cent of body weight from water loss. The infant's rapid weight gain during the first year is primarily due to an increase in adipose tissue; therefore, this is accompanied by a proportionate reduction in fluid volume. By approximately 2 years of age, both the percentage of total body water and its internal distribution approximate that of the adult. Table 26–2 compares fluid volume and its distribution at birth, at 1 year of age, and after 2 years of age.

Regulation of Fluids and Electrolytes

Despite wide variations in the dietary intake, volume and composition of body fluids are maintained in an extremely narrow range as excretion is adjusted to match intake (Rose, 1984). The regulatory mechanisms of the child, however, sometimes differ from those of the adult. Infants and young children are more vulnerable to rapid fluid and electrolyte imbalances than are adults, for various reasons including (1) their proportionately greater surface area in relation to body mass, (2) a higher basal metabolic rate, and (3) immature kidney function.

The infant's *relative greater surface area to body mass* results in a relatively higher volume of insensible perspiration through the skin and lungs (the gastrointestinal tract is considered to be an extension of surface area). The relationship of surface area to body mass is found to be five times as great in premature infants and two to three times as great in a neonate

TABLE 26-2
Approximate Total Body Water and Internal Water Distribution at Birth, 1 Year, and after 2 Years of Age

	Percentage of Total Body Weight		
	At Birth	Age 1 Yr	After 2 Yrs
Extracellular (plasma and interstitial)*	40–45	30	20–25
Intracellular†	30–35	35	35
Total body water	75–80	65	55–60

From *The body fluids in pediatrics.* Winters, R. W. (Ed.). Boston: Little, Brown, 1973. Published by Little, Brown and Company.

*The plasma portion of extracellular fluid remains relatively constant. The major difference in the newborn infant is in interstitial fluid.

†Shows relatively small variation after birth and is essentially constant after 1 yr of age.

compared with an older child or an adult (Metheney, 1992). In infancy, evaporative loss of water through the skin and lungs consumes around 50 per cent of the water requirement (Chambers, 1987).

The *increased metabolic rate* is related to (1) their greater proportionate surface area through which heat is lost, (2) increased growth needs, and (3) a child's relatively larger viscera and brain. Since metabolic processes require water for the dissipation of heat and these processes proceed twice as quickly in children as they do in adults, the rate of water turnover in children is rapid. Relative to body weight, fluid intake and output are greater in infancy than in older children and adults, resulting in a greater turnover. In an infant, half of the ECF may be exchanged compared with an adult exchange of one sixth of the ECF in a similar time period.

A relatively greater total body water content does not protect infants against fluid volume deficit at a time of loss; on the contrary, it increases their vulnerability.

Without water intake, a baby would lose the water contained in the extracellular compartments in 5 days; it would take about 10 days for that to happen in an adult. Because the homeostatic mechanisms of the body are less mature in infants and small children, they are more prone to imbalances.

The immature function of the kidney affects fluid and electrolyte regulation and acid-base balance. Glomerular filtration rate is low at birth in infants, but increases rapidly in the first few weeks of life and reaches adult values by 2 years of age. Urine concentrating capacity is also limited at birth, with considerable maturation by 2 months of age, but not reaching adult ability until 1 to 2 years of age. In contrast, diluting capacity is well developed in neonates, yet is not capable of excreting a large water load because of the slower glomerular filtration rate, which limits the available water in the diluting segments of the nephrons (Avner et al, 1990). See Chapter 36 for further discussion of the immaturity of the kidney.

Gains and Losses

Any conditions that preclude normal oral intake of fluid or food (e.g., vomiting) are particularly harmful because they deplete the body's stores of water, electrolytes, acid, and base much more rapidly in infants and children than in adults. Losses accompanying fever and diarrhea also quickly deplete the child's reserves. The body surface area through which these losses occur—the skin, the lungs, and the gastrointestinal tract—is proportionately greater in children than in adults. In most situations, though, efficient regulation of other body systems, primarily the renal system, minimizes alterations in fluid and electrolyte homeostasis in children. Infants are particularly prone to imbalance because of the limited concentrating ability of their immature kidney. More water is therefore required to excrete a given amount of solute.

Skin and Lung Regulation

Water is continually lost by evaporation through the interstices of the skin and by exhalation of water vapor through the lungs. The primary function of this loss is regulation of body temperature. Loss of body water by this route is called "insensible water loss" because the individual does not sense its occurrence. Insensible water loss consists of pure water—there are no electrolytes. Abnormal conditions, such as those that cause hyperventilation (e.g., salicylate poisoning, pneumonia), may triple water loss from the lungs. "Sensible" water loss may also occur via the skin in the form of sweat. Sweating also helps maintain temperature, but this is an intermittent rather than a continuous process. Sweat contains sodium, chloride, and potassium in addition to water.

Gastrointestinal Regulation

The gastrointestinal tract is of particular significance in maintaining homeostasis in children. Under normal conditions, there is a larger exchange of fluid in a child's gastrointestinal tract than in an adult's: water and sodium (Na^+) are reabsorbed and potassium (K^+) is excreted. Therefore, any illness that affects intestinal absorption may seriously endanger the life of a child because of large, rapid gastrointestinal losses resulting in water depletion and fluid and electrolyte imbalance.

Renal Regulation

Although the infant's kidneys are less mature than the adult's kidneys and cannot regulate fluids and electrolytes quite as effectively, they can meet the infant's homeostatic requirements under most circumstances. The capacity of the infant's kidney to dilute urine is qualitatively the same as the adult's, and the ability to adapt to changes in sodium intake is considerable. Excessive intake of water and Na^+, however, is not tolerated as well as their deprivation, since the cortical area of the kidney is less developed than the medullary region. This predisposes the infant to problems associated with fluid overload and hypernatremia. The kidney of the premature infant cannot retain sodium efficiently and is prone to *hyponatremia*.

Renal regulation of fluid and electrolytes is also affected by hormones that respond to changes in plasma volume and Na^+ content. The primary regulating hormone is the antidiuretic hormone (ADH), which is manufactured in the hypothalamus but stored in and released from the posterior pituitary gland. An extreme example of alteration in vascular volume that results in increased ADH secretion is the patient who is losing large amounts of blood. In this case, volume-sensitive receptors in the body sense the decrease in vascular volume and stimulate secretion of ADH. Water is then reabsorbed by the kidney and intravascular volume increases.

Electrolyte imbalances also affect ADH secretion. When the plasma Na^+ level is high, as in hypertonic dehydration, ADH is secreted in response to a stimulus from the hypothalamus, and the kidney conserves water to help restore electrolyte balance. On the other hand, when the plasma Na^+ levels are low, as can occur when patients are given large amounts of electrolyte-free intravenous (IV) solutions, the system is reversed: ADH secretion is inhibited and the result is diuresis. Thus, ADH decreases urine volume (conserves water), and lack of ADH increases urine volume (promotes water loss). Pain and anxiety can also increase ADH secretion, as do some drugs (morphine, barbiturates, many anesthetic agents).

Additional renal regulation is accomplished through the renin-angiotensin system and aldosterone. Reduced blood flow to the kidney stimulates a specialized area in the glomerulus to secrete renin. Renin in turn generates angiotensin (angiotensin is produced from the plasma globulin angiotensinogen) within the blood vessels. Angiotensin constricts vessels and restores blood pressure and blood flow. The release of the adrenal hormone aldosterone is also stimulated by angiotensin. Aldosterone promotes increased blood pressure by enhancing Na^+ and water reabsorption from the renal tubules, thereby increasing vascular volume.

Cardiovascular Regulation

Proper functioning of the cardiovascular system depends on adequate cardiac activity, intact vasculature, and sufficient volume, composition, and fluidity of blood. Alterations in any of these affect the entire organism, and, if they are diffuse and severe, the organism dies. An intact circulatory system facilitates maintenance of water and Na^+ balance, but it requires reasonably normal levels of water and Na^+ to function adequately. A primary problem with either the system or the fluid and electrolyte balance can adversely affect the other, which in turn can make the primary problem worse. Fortunately, the reverse is also true—improvement in one usually leads to improvement in the other.

Internal Transport of Fluids and Electrolytes

Water and electrolytes are continually exchanged between the different fluid compartments of the body. This is accomplished by active and passive mechanisms. Passive movement of fluid and particles develops spontaneously and does not require a supply of metabolic energy. Active transport, on the other hand, depends on energy derived from metabolic processes. All movement of water in the body is passive, whereas solute movement occurs by both active and passive mechanisms.

Movement of Water: Hydrostatic and Osmotic/Oncotic Pressure

The movement of water between different fluid compartments is determined by hydrostatic pressure and osmotic pressure. The highest hydrostatic pressures in the body are in the vascular space, most importantly in the capillaries, and are generated by the contraction of the heart. Capillary hydrostatic pressure is a function of arterial pressure, resistance at the precapillary sphincter, and venous pressure. This mechanical force, if unopposed, pushes plasma fluid from the capillaries (the area of higher pressure) into the interstitium (the area of lower pressure). Plasma volume, however, is preserved by the opposing osmotic forces generated by plasma proteins.

"Osmosis" is the movement of a solvent through a membrane to equalize the concentration of solvent on both sides. A shift of water occurs from a region of low solute concentration to a region of high solute concentration. Osmotic pressure is generated in cellular and extracellular fluid by exchangeable solutes, notably Na^+ and K^+, and is proportional to the number of particles per unit volume of solvent. Each unit of osmotic pressure is an osmol. "Osmolality"* (particle concentration per kilogram of water) is measured in milliosmols (mOsm). When osmolality in one fluid compartment is altered, the resultant concentration gradient causes water to shift; water diffuses passively from an area of lesser concentration of solutes to an area of greater concentration of solutes. Hypernatremia (increased serum Na^+), for example, results in water shift from the intracellular to the extracellular space, whereas hyponatremia (decreased serum Na^+) results in the opposite movement.

Osmolality, or tonicity, is an important characteristic of IV fluids. When IV fluid is added to blood and causes no change in the size of red blood cells (because it has approximately the same osmolality as the cell), the fluid is said to be "isotonic." "Hypertonic" solution has a higher osmolality than the red blood cells and causes fluid to leave the cell and the cell to shrink. "Hypotonic" fluid causes cells to swell because water enters them. A normal (isotonic) saline solution is 0.9 per cent sodium chloride. Solutions of lesser concentration are hypotonic and those of greater concentration are hypertonic.

"Plasma oncotic pressure," a type of osmotic pressure, is created by plasma proteins and effectively balances capillary hydrostatic pressure. Under normal conditions, hydrostatic and osmotic pressures are balanced. When capillary hydrostatic pressure increases

* "Osmolality" refers to the number of osmoles per kilogram of water. The total volume would be 1 L plus the volume occupied by the solute. "Osmolarity" refers to the number of osmoles per liter of solution. The total volume would be 1 L; the water volume being less than 1 L because of the volume occupied by the solute (Metheney, 1992). In clinical practice, these terms are used interchangeably; they are approximately equal in value because of the very low solute concentration in body fluids.

or plasma oncotic pressure decreases, however, the result is an accumulation of fluid in the interstitial space (edema). In allergic conditions or burns, plasma oncotic pressure is decreased because capillary membrane integrity is altered and fluid follows leaking protein into the interstitial space.

Movement of Electrolytes

Electrolytes, such as Na^+, are transported across cell membranes by a variety of mechanisms. When these solutes move in the presence of a favorable concentration and/or electrical gradient (e.g., when they simply move from an area of greater solute concentration to an area of lesser solute concentration—"downhill movement"), passive mechanisms suffice. If solutes must move *against* gradients ("uphill movement"), active mechanisms are employed—energy is required.

Passive transport of solute across a membrane occurs in three ways (Rose, 1984):

- Diffusion
  - Simple diffusion: Solutes freely move across a membrane until their concentration is equal on either side and until electroneutrality across the membrane is attained.
  - Facilitated diffusion: Solute-specific carriers exist on some cell membranes, and, when present, they facilitate more rapid diffusion of the solute than occurs during simple diffusion.
- Coupled transport: A carrier recognizes two solutes and promotes the transport of both across the membrane.
- Solvent drag: When water moves across a membrane because of an osmotic pressure gradient, frictional forces between the water and the solutes it contains result in membrane-permeable solutes being carried along with the water.

Active transport of solutes also occurs in three ways (Rose, 1984):

- Primary active transport: Mechanisms, such as the Na^+-K^+-ATPase pump* (or "sodium pump"), release energy to facilitate or prevent movement of solutes in one direction or the other.
- Secondary active transport: Energy provided by some reactions (e.g., hydrolysis of ATP to ADP) may allow the co-transport of another solute against its concentration gradient, without the usual direct energy requirement.
- Endocytosis: A portion of a cell membrane can invaginate around a particle that is too large (e.g., insulin in the proximal tubule of the kidney) to cross the membrane directly and incorporate it into the cell; the energy for endocytosis is supplied by the hydrolysis of ATP.

Fluid and Electrolyte Imbalances

Numerous childhood illnesses cause fluid and electrolyte imbalances. However, the great majority of disturbances in hydration and electrolyte balance occur secondary to vomiting and diarrhea.

Fluid and electrolyte imbalances occur when there is a total body deficit or excess of fluids and electrolytes or when the normal relationship between fluids and electrolytes has been altered. In many instances, a disturbance exists in both the total body volume and the fluid and electrolyte proportions. Edema and dehydration are two common fluid imbalances that occur in children and are often associated with electrolyte abnormalities.

Edema

"Edema" is the accumulation of excess fluid. It involves an alteration in the exchange between the capillaries and interstitial fluid. The net capillary flow of fluid outward into the interstitial space exceeds that removed by the lymphatic system (Hellerstein, 1993a). The development of edema occurs with:

- *Increased capillary hydrostatic pressure*. When hydrostatic pressure in the capillary exceeds the opposing forces in the extravascular space, fluid shifts from the vessel to the interstitial space. (Edema related to increased capillary hydrostatic pressure is seen in heart failure, renal failure, and acute pulmonary edema and with the administration of many antihypertensive and nonsteroidal anti-inflammatory drugs.)
- *Decreased plasma oncotic pressure*. Excessive loss of protein, particularly albumin, results in a decrease in the oncotic pressure of plasma while the capillary hydrostatic pressure (that is normally balanced by the oncotic pressure) remains the same; the net effect of this alteration in the balance of oncotic and hydrostatic pressure is a shift of fluid to the interstitium.
  (Protein loss is associated with nephrotic syndrome and protein-losing enteropathy; reduced albumin synthesis occurs in liver disease and malnutrition.)
- *Increased capillary permeability*. Edema develops in the presence of increased capillary permeability, because (1) fluid can simply leak into the tis-

* A system for active transport of sodium and potassium across cell membranes that is regulated by the enzyme sodium-potassium–activated adenosine triphosphate. The enzyme catalyzes hydrolysis of the high-energy compound ATP into the lower-energy compound adenosine diphosphate (ADP). The energy released by this reaction is used to transport the Na^+ and K^+ (Kaehny & Gabow, 1980).

TABLE 26-3
Clinical Signs and Symptoms Associated with Severity of Isotonic Dehydration

Signs/Symptoms	Mild Dehydration	Moderate Dehydration	Severe Dehydration
Loss of body weight	<5%	5–10%	>10%
Skin: Color	Pale	Dusky	Mottled
Turgor	Decreased	Moderately decreased	Markedly decreased
Urine output	Decreased	Oliguria	Marked oliguria and azotemia
Thirst	Slight	Moderate	Intense
Tears	Present	Decreased	Absent
Mucous membranes	Dry	Very dry	Parched
Blood pressure	Normal	Normal or slightly above or below normal	Low
Pulse	Normal or tachycardia	Tachycardia	Increased tachycardia and thready pulse
Anterior fontanelles	Level or flat	Slight sunken	Sunken

sue when the integrity of the membrane has been altered and (2) albumin also can move to the interstitium and pull fluid with it.
(Burns, trauma, inflammation, allergic reactions, and adult respiratory distress syndrome disrupt the capillary membrane and increase capillary permeability.)

- *Increased interstitial oncotic pressure.* Small amounts of protein are usually filtered across the capillary and then returned to the circulation via the lymphatics. Under certain circumstances, however, proteins enter the interstitial space more quickly than they leave. Accumulation of proteins causes increased interstitial oncotic pressure. This promotes migration of fluid into tissue.
(Lymphatic obstruction from tumors, hypothyroidism, and increased capillary permeability results in increased interstitial oncotic pressure.)

Dehydration and Sodium Imbalance

Dehydration occurs when body fluids are lost in excess of fluid gained. Common alterations that result in dehydration are due to disturbances in:

- Gastrointestinal tract (vomiting, diarrhea, malabsorption, pyloric stenosis).
- The skin (burns).
- Metabolism (fever, diabetes mellitus).
- The lungs (tachypnea, as in broncholitis).

Dehydration is often associated with Na^+ imbalance. An exception is isotonic dehydration, in which the Na^+ concentration remains within normal range. Hypotonic and hypertonic dehydration are both associated with Na^+ imbalances.

Isotonic Dehydration

This condition occurs when fluids and electrolytes are lost in approximately the same proportion as they exist in the body. In this type of dehydration, there is no fluid shift because body fluid osmolality is not affected. There simply is a deficit of total body water. The serum level of sodium accompanying isotonic dehydration remains within 130 to 150 mEq/L. This is the most common type of dehydration in children and is most typically caused by gastrointestinal losses through vomiting and diarrhea (Awazu et al, 1990b). Clinical manifestations associated with isotonic dehydration include:

- Increased heart rate.
- Sunken eyes.
- Dry mucosa.
- Cool and mottled extremities.
- Loss of elasticity of skin.
- Lack of tears.
- Weak cry.
- Decreased urine output.
- In infants, sunken fontanelle and loss of body weight.

See Table 26–3 for variations in clinical features according to degree of isotonic dehydration.

Hypertonic/Hypernatremic Dehydration

This type of dehydration is the result of a net loss of hypotonic fluid (a greater proportionate loss of water than sodium), resulting in a serum level of sodium greater than 150 mEq/L. When there is decreased intake of water, increased intake of Na^+, or a proportionately greater loss of water than Na^+, this serious condition results. It can be produced when insensible water loss from the skin and respiratory tract is high or by any clinical condition that depletes the body of water. The proportional excess of Na^+ increases the osmotic pressure of the blood, and so fluid shifts from the intracellular to the extracellular spaces. The normal defenses against this occurrence are the stimulation of thirst (i.e., intake of water) and the release of ADH (i.e., conservation of water by the kidneys). Infants, however, who likely have intact thirst mechanisms, cannot take advantage of this particular defense because they are unable to ask for water.

Conditions that may contribute to hypernatremia include the administration of hypertonic Na^+ IV fluids (Na^+ concentration > 0.9 per cent), tube feedings with high Na^+ concentrations or high-solute formulas. Diabetes insipidus, which is characterized by complete or partial failure of ADH or of renal response to ADH, also results in hypernatremia if urine output is not quickly replaced. Conditions in which there may be significant insensible loss of water, such as occurs in burns, fever, and respiratory infections, may raise serum Na^+ levels. Circulatory disturbances are usually absent in hypertonic dehydration because of the relative increase in vascular volume. Clinical manifestations that are characteristic of this type of dehydration are "doughy" skin and neurologic signs, including irritability, high-pitched cry, and seizures. These signs are related to an intracellular volume reduction of brain cells. Hyperglycemia and hypocalcemia may also be evident: hyperglycemia may be due to stress or decreased uptake of glucose by the cell; the cause of hypocalcemia is unknown (Awazu et al, 1990b).

If improper fluid therapy is initiated in patients with hypernatremia, seizures may occur because rapid rehydration may cause significant fluid shift and brain cells to swell. Mortality can be high. Early neurologic symptoms (marked lethargy and irritability on stimulation) may herald this serious complication.

Hypotonic/Hyponatremic Dehydration

This type of dehydration occurs when there is a net loss of hypertonic fluid resulting in a serum level of sodium less than 130 mEq/L (Awazu et al, 1990b). This can occur through water retention or loss of sodium.

Water retention resulting in hyponatremia occurs almost exclusively when there is a defect in renal water excretion. Excretion is impaired in:

- Circulating volume depletion (vomiting, diarrhea, tube drainage, bleeding, and intestinal obstruction).
- Renal failure.
- Diuretic therapy (thiazides, furosemide, and ethacrynic acid).
- Presence of ADH (syndrome of inappropriate antidiuretic hormone secretion).

Hyponatremia occurs commonly in those who receive disproportionately large amounts of electrolyte-free solutions (often plain water). The improper fluid can be given orally (too much plain water to a sick child or a postoperative patient), parenterally (IV fluid without sodium in it to the patient who is taking nothing by mouth [NPO]), or rectally (use of tap water rather than isotonic saline for enemas).

On the other hand, children with cystic fibrosis may have normal water content in the body, but they excrete abnormally high amounts of Na^+ in their sweat. Regardless of the cause, the lack of sufficient Na^+ to keep water from entering the cells results in water shifting from the extracellular spaces to the intracellular spaces, where Na^+ concentration is higher. If a child is dehydrated as well as hyponatremic (i.e., hypotonic dehydration), blood pressure may be reduced and the child may border on circulatory collapse. Another important cause of hyponatremia in the pediatric population is the syndrome of inappropriate antidiuretic hormone (SIADH). See Chapter 43 for further discussion of this syndrome.

Sodium is the chief extracellular ion; when a sodium deficit exists, these clinical manifestations are noted: gray pallor; cold, clammy skin; poor skin turgor; only slightly moist mucous membranes; sunken eyes; increased pulse and lowered blood pressure; and lethargy that may progress to a coma.

Potassium Imbalance

Potassium has two major physiologic functions: (1) it plays an important role in cell metabolism, participating in regulating protein and glycogen synthesis, and (2) the ratio of K^+ concentrations in the cell and the extracellular fluid is the major determinant of the resting potential across the cell membrane. The latter function helps produce normal neural and muscular function. When the plasma K^+ level is either excessive (hyperkalemia) or deficient (hypokalemia), a serious imbalance exists. The normal plasma K^+ level ranges from 4.0 to 5.6 mEq/L.

Absorption of dietary K^+ occurs readily from the small intestine. Ninety-five per cent of the body's potassium is found in intracellular fluid. The distribution of K^+ is maintained by movement of K^+ into the cells and urinary excretion of the net dietary intake. These processes are mediated by a variety of factors, including the Na^+-K^+-ATPase pump, catecholamines, insulin, and the plasma K^+ concentration. The plasma K^+ concentration is also influenced by pH. In acidemic states, some of the excess H^+ moves into the cell to be buffered, so K^+ moves out to maintain electroneutrality (i.e., equal electrical charges on both sides of the cell membrane). The result is an increased plasma K^+ concentration. This change is of most concern in some forms of metabolic acidosis due to an increase of mineral acid, as in renal failure or diarrhea, because plasma K^+ can increase 0.2 to 1.7

mEq/L for each 0.1 unit fall in blood pH in such situations. This shift is reversed in alkalemia but the change in the plasma K^+ level is less prominent. Immediate attention and constant surveillance are warranted whenever K^+ imbalance is suspected in infants and children.

Hyperkalemia

This excess of K^+ in the blood is due to increased intake of K^+; inadequate excretion of K^+, as in renal insufficiency or reduced glomerular filtration; shift of K^+ from within the cells to the extracellular compartments; congenital adrenal hyperplasia; or a primary defect in K^+ transport. An increased intake most commonly occurs in children as a result of too-rapid administration of IV potassium chloride. Inadequate excretion of K^+ occurs in the event of renal failure, adrenal insufficiency, metabolic acidosis, and the use of K^+-sparing diuretics. A shift of K^+ from within the cells to extracellular fluid occurs with (Rose, 1984):

- Tissue damage (burns, destruction of tumor tissue, and massive crushing injuries in which K^+ is released from the injured cells).
- Hemolysis (due to sudden excessive water intake).
- Digitalis overdose (results in relative inability of K^+ to enter the cells because of partial inhibition of the Na^+-K^+-ATPase pump by the drug).
- Hyperosmolality (increased plasma osmolality pulls water out of the cells, with K^+ following because of solvent drag).
- Administration of succinylcholine (the drug reduces the magnitude of the resting membrane potential, thus favoring the movement of K^+ out of the cells) or arginine (presumably due to the movement of K^+ out of the cells as the cation arginine enters the cells).

Hyperkalemia is the most dangerous of the electrolyte disorders because it can cause sudden death. It depresses sinoatrial node activity and may lead to ventricular arrhythmias and cardiac standstill (Hellerstein, 1993b).

Hypokalemia

Hypokalemia occurs when there is inadequate intake of K^+, excessive loss of K^+ (gastrointestinal and renal), or a shift of extracellular K^+ to the intracellular space. Poor food intake over an extended period or administration of IV fluids without added K^+ may result in hypokalemia. Excessive losses occur with vomiting, diarrhea, nasogastric suctioning, and when K^+-losing diuretics, notably furosemide (Lasix), or corticosteroids are administered. A shift of K^+ from extracellular compartments to within the cells occurs with alkalosis and insulin administration. With alkalosis, H^+ ions are released from the cellular buffers and move into extracellular fluid to minimize the change in pH; to preserve electroneutrality, extracellular K^+ (and Na^+) moves into the cells. Insulin promotes entry of K^+ into skeletal muscle and hepatic cells.

Calcium Imbalance

Calcium is essential not only in the process of skeletal mineralization but also in many intracellular and extracellular processes. Calcium is required for activation of numerous enzymes and for proper cardiac, neural, and muscular function. Calcium (Ca^{2+}) imbalance occurs when the Ca^{2+} level is either excessive (hypercalcemia) or deficient (hypocalcemia). The most common measure of serum calcium is the total calcium level. Normal total serum Ca^{2+} ranges from 8.8 to 10.8 mg/dl (2.25 to 2.74 mmol/L) in children and 7.0 to 12.0 mg/dl (1.80 to 3.00 mmol/L) in infants (Carpenter & Key, 1990; Schefler, 1992). Many laboratories also have the capability to measure ionized calcium (see Appendix 8 for ionized calcium values).

Calcium regulation is primarily under the control of the parathyroid hormone calcitonin and a metabolite of vitamin D calcitriol. Deposition and resorption (loss) of bone serves as an exchange mechanism for maintaining serum Ca^{2+} levels in the appropriate range. Serum Ca^{2+} measurements are influenced by the serum protein concentration; for every increment or decrement of 1.0 g/dl in albumin (or total protein), there is a corresponding change of 0.8 mg/dl in the serum Ca^{2+} level. (Metheney, 1992).

Hypercalcemia

This may result from excessive administration of vitamins A and D and some drugs, hyperparathyroidism, malignancy, and, most importantly in children, prolonged immobilization. The lack of postural changes to the skeleton disturbs the balance between bone formation and resorption, resulting in loss of bone mass and its minerals. Because children are developmentally in a state of rapid bone turnover, the kidney may be unable to excrete Ca^{2+} quickly enough to maintain normal plasma levels. Hypercalcemia may also occur in the presence of acidosis because Ca^{2+} leaves the bone and enters the plasma to allow H^+ to be buffered by the bone.

Hypocalcemia

This may occur in infants and children for many reasons. Conditions such as hypoparathyroidism, vitamin D deficiency, respiratory alkalosis, hypermagnesemia and hypomagnesemia, burns, infection, diarrhea, and renal failure, as well as a multitude of drugs, all predispose children to hypocalcemia. A disorder called "tetany of the neonate" is seen early in infancy when

TABLE 26-4
Clinical Manifestations of Imbalance of Sodium, Potassium, and Calcium

Electrolyte Imbalance	Clinical Manifestations
Sodium	
Hypernatremia: resulting from • Sodium retention • Water loss (in excess of sodium loss) Serum sodium >150 mEq/L	Dry, sticky mucous membranes Flushed skin Excessive thirst (older child) Nuchal and muscular rigidity Lethargy, weakness, irritability with stimulation Tremors, convulsions Peripheral and/or pulmonary edema Urine specific gravity (SG) >1.030
Hyponatremia: resulting from • Loss of sodium • Retention of water Serum sodium <130 mEq/L	Nausea → malaise → headache → lethargy → obtundation Twitching → convulsions Cool, clammy skin → hypotension → shock Urine SG <1.010
Potassium	
Hyperkalemia: resulting from • Increased potassium intake • Inadequate potassium excretion • Potassium shift (from intracellular to extracellular compartment) Serum potassium >5.6 mEq/L	Nausea, malaise Shallow breathing Muscle weakness → flaccid paralysis Hyper-reflexia Intestinal colic, diarrhea Oliguria → anuria Abnormal cardiac conduction: peaked, narrow T waves and shortened Q-T interval → widened QRS complex and decreased amplitude: widening and eventual loss of P wave → sine wave pattern (widened QRS merges with T wave) → ventricular fibrillation → asystole
Hypokalemia: resulting from • Inadequate potassium intake • Excessive potassium loss • Potassium shift (from extracellular to intracellular compartment) Serum potassium <4.0 mEq/L	Apathy, drowsiness Muscle weakness/cramps → flaccid paralysis Hyporeflexia Abdominal distention and ileus Shallow breathing Impaired urinary concentration, polyuria, polydipsia Mild hyperglycemia Rhabdomyolysis (disintegration of muscle) and associated myoglobinuria Arrhythmias (premature atrial and ventricular beats, sinus bradycardia, paroxysmal atrial and junctional tachycardia, atrioventricular block, ventricular tachycardia, ventricular fibrillation) Abnormal cardiac conduction: ST segment depression, decreased amplitude or inversion of T wave, increased height of U wave, increased amplitude of P wave, prolonged PR interval, widened QRS complex

TABLE 26-4
Clinical Manifestations of Imbalance of Sodium, Potassium, and Calcium *(Continued)*

Electrolyte Imbalance	Clinical Manifestations
Calcium	
Hypercalcemia: resulting from • Excessive administration of vitamin D or calcium • Hyperparathyroidism • Malignancy • Prolonged immobilization Serum calcium >10.8 mg/dl (2.70 mmol/L) in older children/adults and >12 mg/dl (3.0 mmol/L) in infants	Nausea, vomiting Abdominal/flank pain Dryness of mouth Muscle hypotonicity Stupor → coma Cardiac arrest
Hypocalcemia: resulting from • Ingestion of cow's milk with high phosphorus/calcium ratio • Hyperparathyroidism • Vitamin D deficiency • Hyper- and hypomagnesemia • Burns • Infection • Diarrhea • Renal failure • Drugs • Side effect of correction of acidosis (calcium returns to bone) Serum calcium <8.8 mg/dl (2.2 mmol/L) in older children /adults and <8.4 mg/dl (2.1 mmol/L) in infants	Tingling, numbness Muscle cramps → tetany Seizures Laryngospasm

cow's milk formulas with a high concentration of phosphate are given. This tetany associated with hypocalcemia can occur because of the reciprocal relationship of Ca^{2+} and phosphorus; when the phosphorus level in the plasma is high, the Ca^{2+} level is low. Hypocalcemia may also occur when acidosis is corrected. Some of the Ca^{2+} that moves out of the bone matrix during acidosis is lost in the urine. As the acidosis corrects, Ca^{2+} reenters the bones, resulting in a hypocalcemia. (Table 26–4 lists the clinical manifestations of electrolyte imbalances.)

Serum Electrolyte Values

During illness, disruption of regulatory mechanisms can result in *actual* depletion or excess of electrolytes in the body. Serum levels truly reflect electrolyte status at these times. Sometimes, though, disruption only *alters the distribution* of electrolytes—not the total body content. When this occurs, serum electrolyte values can be misleading. For example, a low serum K^+ is not common in patients with diabetic ketoacidosis (DKA), yet total body depletion of K^+ is common. In fact, the serum K^+ may be elevated. This apparent discrepancy occurs because K^+ moves from the intracellular to the extracellular compartment with DKA, but a rise in serum K^+ may be masked by concurrent urinary losses of the electrolyte. If treatment of DKA were to proceed based on the "normal" K^+ level, very serious complications would quickly arise as the body's K^+ stores dwindled. Knowledge of electrolyte behavior in specific childhood illnesses, therefore, is essential for the pediatric nurse.

Acid-Base Balance

Homeostasis in body fluids is a function of acid-base balance, as well as of fluid and electrolyte balance. The acidity of body fluids is determined by hydrogen ion (H^+) concentration. Hydrogen ions are the products of cell metabolism and the metabolism of dietary proteins. Sources of additional hydrogen ions include strenuous exercise (lactic acid) and diabetic ketosis (acetoacetic and beta-hydroxybutyric acid). Because free hydrogen ions are present in the body fluids in extremely small concentrations (40 nanoequivalents, or approximately one millionth of the milliequivalent per liter concentration of Na^+), the term "pH" is used to provide a means of expressing the value simply. The pH value is determined by taking the *negative* logarithm of the H^+ concentration; therefore, the *more* hydrogen ions there are, the *lower* the pH. A relatively narrow range of pH is compatible with life, from 6.80 to 7.80, because minute changes in H^+ concentration significantly affect enzymatic and physiologic processes in the body (Rose, 1984).

The terms "acidosis" and "alkalosis" refer to processes that cause acids and alkali to accumulate, and the pH tends to move in an abnormal direction when these processes occur. An abnormally low pH (an excess of acid) in the arterial blood is called "acidemia," also called "acidosis"; an abnormally high pH (too much base or too little acid) in the blood is called "alkalemia," also called "alkalosis."*

Three important points characterize the relationship of pH and H^+ concentration:

- Normal arterial blood pH is 7.40 (range: 7.35 to 7.45), or an H^+ concentration of 40 nanoequivalents.
- H^+ and pH concentration are inversely related; as the H^+ concentration rises, the pH falls, and vice versa.
- When serum pH falls below 7.35 as H^+ concentration rises, the patient is said to be acidotic; conversely, when the pH rises above 7.45 as the H^+ concentration falls, the patient is said to be alkalotic.

Regulation of H^+ *Concentration*

H^+ concentration is maintained within its narrow limits by the kidneys, the lungs, a variety of chemical buffers, and some metabolic processes.

A "buffered solution" is one that contains a weak acid and its conjugate base. Such a solution can moderate pH changes when either acid or base is added, by donating or absorbing H^+ as necessary and thereby minimizing their effect on total H^+ concentration. Body buffers that can absorb or donate H^+ in response to changes in acidity of extracellular fluids provide a defense against disastrous swings in pH. Hemoglobin, plasma proteins, and bone are effective buffers, but the most important extracellular buffer system is the bicarbonate–carbonic acid system. Buffering by this system proceeds rapidly via the following chemical reaction:

$$\text{(A)}\quad \underset{\text{(base)}}{\overset{\text{bicarbonate}}{H^+ + HCO_3^-}} \rightleftharpoons \underset{\text{(weak acid)}}{\overset{\text{carbonic acid}}{H_2CO_3}} \rightleftharpoons \overset{\text{carbon dioxide}}{CO_2} + \overset{\text{water}}{H_2O}$$

Whether carbonic acid dissociates (into hydrogen and bicarbonate or into carbon dioxide and water) or whether it is formed (from hydrogen and bicarbonate or from carbon dioxide and water) depends on which reaction(s) will restore the following important relationships:

1. The 20:1 ratio between bicarbonate and carbonic acid that is the normal ratio of base to acid in the blood (i.e., as long as the ratio is maintained, acid-base balance will exist, even if the absolute amounts of acid or base change).
2. The equilibrium of the carbonic acid and dissolved carbon dioxide levels that is normally maintained in blood.

For example, when a strong acid is added to the blood, the hydrogen ions that it releases are buffered by bicarbonate, and carbonic acid is quickly formed. The carbonic acid then dissociates into carbon dioxide and water and the carbon dioxide is quickly excreted by the lungs:

$$\text{(B)}\quad H^+ + HCO_3^- \longrightarrow H_2CO_3 \longrightarrow CO_2 + H_2O$$

The formation of carbon dioxide and water from carbonic acid occurs so that the normal balance of bicarbonate and carbonic acid (20:1) is maintained. The subsequent excretion of the carbon dioxide by the lungs then restores the carbonic acid–carbon dioxide equilibrium. This system works so well because blood carbon dioxide can be increased or decreased within minutes by changes in breathing patterns. Variations in ventilation (that is, faster, slower, deeper, or shallower breaths) can adjust carbon dioxide concentration and therefore carbonic acid and H^+/bicarbonate concentrations within minutes. If ventilation increases when pH is normal, carbon dioxide excretion is augmented (reaction *B*), resulting in

1. A drop in the partial pressure of carbon dioxide (Pco_2*).
2. A drop in carbonic acid, to match the drop in carbon dioxide and maintain their equilibrium.
3. A drop in H^+ concentration (alkalemia) as it combines with bicarbonate (to restore the 20:1 ratio) in the blood.

A decrease in ventilation causes a rise in Pco_2 and the opposite reaction, with consequent accumulation of H^+ and a drop in pH (acidemia):

$$\text{(C)}\quad CO_2 + H_2O \longrightarrow H_2CO_3 \longrightarrow H^+ + HCO_3^-$$

Although carbon dioxide is not an acid or a base, it can indirectly increase or decrease the acidity of the blood. The lungs, therefore, through regulation of the Pco_2, can *compensate* for changes in pH related to *metabolic* processes. DKA, for example, is a metabolic process. In DKA, when hydrogen ions (from the ketoacids) accumulate in the blood, they are first buffered by bicarbonate and form carbonic acid, which, in effect, holds the hydrogen ions and prevents the pH from decreasing significantly (reaction *B*). Then, the carbonic acid dissociates into water and carbon dioxide, and the carbon dioxide is excreted by the lungs with deep breathing (Kussmaul respirations). On the other hand, when H^+ concentration is low (as can occur with vomiting or nasogastric suctioning of stomach secretions, which contain high concentrations of H^+), the Pco_2 rises as ventilation re-

* The suffix "emia" refers to the plasma pH value, whereas "osis" refers to a mechanism in which acid-base homeostasis has been altered. In this chapter, "acidosis" and "alkalosis" are used because these terms are more commonly used in clinical settings.

* Since carbonic acid is in equilibrium with dissolved carbon dioxide, the measurement of partial pressure of carbon dioxide (Pco_2) can be used as a clinical estimate of carbonic acid concentration.

sponsively decreases, and the carbonic acid releases H^+, preventing a rise in the pH (reaction *C*). The net effect of reactions in the bicarbonate–carbonic acid system is maintenance of a 20:1 ratio between bicarbonate and carbonic acid.

Whereas the lungs *compensate* for pH changes caused by metabolic disorders by controlling the carbon dioxide level in the blood, the kidneys react to pH variations resulting from *respiratory* abnormalities by regulating the other end of the reaction equation—the H^+ and bicarbonate concentrations. Renal excretion or reabsorption of H^+ or bicarbonate, as compensation for changes in pH, depends on the plasma bicarbonate level and on the rate of H^+ secretion by the renal tubular cells. Bicarbonate is reabsorbed in exchange for hydrogen ions. The rate of H^+ excretion, and therefore the rate of bicarbonate reabsorption, is proportionate to the arterial Pco_2. With a respiratory disturbance, such as *hyper*ventilation, the Pco_2 drops, carbonic acid dissociates into H^+ and bicarbonate, and the bicarbonate is slowly excreted to prevent the blood pH from increasing significantly. Compensation for *hypo*ventilation, during which the carbon dioxide level rises, also occurs in the kidney. In this case, however, hydrogen ions are excreted instead of bicarbonate to minimize the drop in pH.

The interdependence of pH, bicarbonate, and carbonic acid is summarized by the Henderson-Hasselbalch equation (a mathematical formulation of the earlier equation), where pK represents the dissociation constant of the acid:

$$\text{(D)} \qquad pH = pK + \frac{\log(HCO_3^-)}{(H_2CO_3)} \quad (p = -\log)$$

The equation demonstrates that H^+ concentration (pH) of a solution is the function of the ionization constant (K)* and concentration ratio of the buffer pair (bicarbonate/carbonic acid). The key clinical message conveyed is that acidity of blood is determined by the relative availability of acid and alkali, and that plasma concentrations of bicarbonate and carbonic acid (Pco_2) reflect that availability. The H^+ concentration, and, therefore, the pH, is defined by the ratio of the Pco_2 to bicarbonate and not by the absolute value of either one alone. The components of the Henderson-Hasselbalch equation can be further described as follows (Kaehny & Gabow, 1980):

- Bicarbonate (HCO_3^-): *Metabolic component.*
  - Primarily altered in metabolic disorders.
  - Altered by buffering.
  - Altered by renal compensation for respiratory disorders.
- Carbonic acid (H_2CO_3 [or Pco_2]): *Respiratory component.*
  - Primarily altered in respiratory disorders.
  - Altered by respiratory compensation for metabolic disorders.
- pH: The result of interplay between metabolic and respiratory components.

In summary, the lungs control the Pco_2 and, in effect, the carbonic acid concentration in the body. Carbon dioxide is eliminated by the lungs and is regulated by the rate of alveolar ventilation. Hyperventilation enhances carbon dioxide excretion; carbon dioxide is "blown off," thus lowering the Pco_2 and increasing the pH (alkalosis). The plasma bicarbonate concentration is regulated by the changes in the rate of H^+ secretion from the kidney. Renal response to acid-base imbalance, however, is much slower than that of the lungs. Days, not minutes and hours, are required to restore balance.

Acid-Base Imbalance

Acid-base disturbances fall into four major categories: metabolic acidosis, metabolic alkalosis, respiratory acidosis, and respiratory alkalosis. Since the Pco_2 is regulated by respiration, primary abnormalities in the Pco_2 are called "respiratory acidosis"/(high Pco_2) and "respiratory alkalosis" (low Pco_2). On the other hand, primary changes in the plasma bicarbonate concentration are referred to as "metabolic acidosis" (low bicarbonate) and "metabolic alkalosis" (high bicarbonate). When these acid-base disturbances occur, compensatory renal or respiratory responses minimize the alteration in the Pco_2/bicarbonate ratio. Arterial blood gas analysis can provide direct measurement of pH and Pco_2 and an approximation of bicarbonate concentration. If two of these three parameters are known, the other can be calculated. Direct measurement of serum bicarbonate can also be done.

Metabolic Acidosis

The most common cause of metabolic acidosis in children is diarrhea. This is the result of

- Loss of HCO_3^- in the stool.
- Increased ketone body* production from the metabolism of fat for energy.
- Increased anaerobic metabolism secondary to dehydration and resulting in release of acids (lactic, pyruvic, and acetoacetic), free hydrogen ions, and carbon dioxide.
- Reduced blood volume causing the kidneys to

* The "ionization constant" is the term used to define an acid's strength. The pK is inversely proportional to the strength of the acid.

* Ketone bodies include acetoacetic acid, beta-hydroxybutyric acid, and acetone.

function less effectively with a reduced excretion of hydrogen ions.

Additional causes of metabolic acidosis include renal failure, ketoacidosis, and lactic acidosis. The lactic acidosis is often secondary to cellular hypoxia due to inadequate tissue perfusion. Hypoxia, in turn, causes impairment of oxidation and subsequent increased conversion of pyruvate to lactate during glucose and amino acid metabolism.

Signs and symptoms associated with metabolic acidosis are noted in the pulmonary, cardiovascular, neurologic, and skeletal systems: increased depth of respirations, tachycardia, peripheral vasoconstriction, arrhythmias (potentially fatal), lethargy through coma, and impaired growth (rickets). Anorexia, nausea, weight loss, muscle weakness, and listlessness may also be noted.

Metabolic Alkalosis

Metabolic alkalosis is the result of *H^+ loss* or *bicarbonate retention.*

Hydrogen loss may result from:

1. *Gastrointestinal tract losses:* H^+-rich gastric juices are lost with vomiting and nasogastric suctioning: The hydrogen ions from gastric juices are derived from the intracellular dissociation of carbonic acid (reaction *C* above); so, with H^+ loss, there is bicarbonate generation.

2. *Renal system regulation: Mineralocorticoid excess:* The mineralocorticoid aldosterone enhances Na^+ reabsorption; excessive Na^+ reabsorption results in concomitant H^+ excretion; again, with H^+ loss, there is bicarbonate generation; *Diuretics:* Diuretics (e.g., furosemide) that cause Na^+ and water loss decrease extracellular fluid volume but leave the bicarbonate level essentially unchanged; as a result, the plasma bicarbonate level rises (note: this is referred to as a "contraction alkalosis," and is *not* seen with K^+-sparing diuretics).

3. *Movement of hydrogen ions into the cells in the presence of hypokalemia:* As plasma K^+ falls, K^+ moves out of the cells into the extracellular fluid; to maintain electroneutrality, H^+ move into the cells, causing a rise in pH.

Bicarbonate retention may result from (Rose, 1984):

1. *Massive blood transfusion:* Most bank blood is anticoagulated with acid-citrate-dextran; citrate is rapidly metabolized and produces bicarbonate.

2. *Administration of sodium bicarbonate:* Excessive administration of sodium bicarbonate may lead to metabolic alkalosis.

3. *Milk-alkali syndrome:* The chronic ingestion of milk and antacids containing calcium carbonate (which generates bicarbonate).

Infants and children with a metabolic alkalosis may be asymptomatic or demonstrate signs of volume depletion (weakness, muscle cramps, postural dizziness) or hypokalemia.

Respiratory Acidosis

Acute respiratory acidosis in children is associated with events that depress *respiration* or interfere with *ventilation* (the movement of air in and out of the lungs). Respiration may be depressed because of head trauma or from the effect of opiates, anesthetics, sedatives, or alcohol on the respiratory center in the brain. Ingestion or administration of these substances results in too few or too shallow respirations, or both, and a subsequent rise in P_{CO_2} and a drop in pH. Aspiration of a foreign body or vomitus, severe asthma, or pneumonia directly interferes with ventilation. This also results in retention of carbon dioxide and the development of respiratory acidosis.

Neurologic abnormalities, such as headache, blurred vision, restlessness, anxiety, tremors, delirium, and somnolence (called CO_2 narcosis), may be exhibited with respiratory acidosis.

Respiratory Alkalosis

Respiratory alkalosis is often the result of hyperventilation from anxiety; fast, deep breaths cause excretion of carbon dioxide and eventual depletion of free hydrogen ions. It can, however, occur with hypoxia, pulmonary disease, and ingestion of drugs such as nicotine and salicylates. In hypoxia, a fall of Pa_{O_2} below 60 mmHg stimulates ventilation by way of peripheral chemoreceptors; in pulmonary disease, receptors within the lung parenchyma send signals via the vagus nerve to stimulate ventilation; and drugs such as salicylates and nicotine stimulate respiration by central and peripheral neural pathways (Ichikawa et al, 1990).

Manifestations associated with respiratory alkalosis are related to increased irritability of the central and peripheral nervous systems. They include lightheadedness, altered consciousness, paresthesias of the extremities and circumoral area, cramps, and syncope. Arrhythmias may also occur. (Acid-base disturbances are summarized in Table 26–5 and arterial blood gas values in uncompensated acid-base disturbance in Table 26–6.)

Assessment of Fluid and Electrolyte and Acid-Base Balance

Specific clinical and laboratory data are necessary when fluid or electrolyte imbalance is suspected. The nurse must interview the parents regarding the child's current problem and any other condition or event that may affect identification or management of the current problem. Thereafter, clinical assessment is performed as warranted by the child's condition. Lab-

TABLE 26-5
Acid-Base Imbalances: Clinical Causes, Compensatory Mechanisms, and Clinical Manifestations

Classification	Clinical Causes	Compensatory Mechanism	Clinical Manifestations and Blood Gases
Respiratory acidosis: Impaired respiratory function with CO_2 retention	Disturbance of respiratory center (drugs, head trauma); disease affecting respiratory muscles; airway obstruction; pulmonary disease; cardiac failure; right-to-left cardiac shunts	Renal compensation: Increased urinary excretion of hydrogen ion; makes and reabsorbs more bicarbonate	Respiratory distress, including tachypnea and use of accessory muscles Hypoxemia often present due to underlying cause Hypoxemia can lead to metabolic lactic acidosis* • Arterial pH low • P_{CO_2} elevated • Plasma bicarbonate moderately elevated
Respiratory alkalosis: Alveolar hyperventilation results in blowing off CO_2 in excess of its production	Acute anxiety states; hyperactivity of respiratory center in association with infection (encephalitis, meningitis); salicylate ingestion (early stages); improper use of mechanical respirators; increased sensitivity of the respiratory center to P_{CO_2}	Renal compensation: Less hydrogen ion is excreted so that less bicarbonate is produced (each time a hydrogen ion is excreted by the kidney a bicarbonate ion is produced and reabsorbed); decreased conservation of filtered bicarbonate	Tetany due to decreased ionized calcium in the presence of alkalemia • Arterial pH high • P_{CO_2} low • Plasma bicarbonate low
Metabolic acidosis • Increased production of hydrogen ions • Excessive loss of bicarbonate ions (hyperchloremia due to resulting elevated chloride level) • Decreased hydrogen ion excreted and decreased formation of new bicarbonate	Ketone acids (starvation, diabetes); lactic acids (usually secondary to tissue hypoxia); salicylate poisoning Via GI tract† (diarrhea, vomiting, suction, fistula drainage); via kidney (renal tubular acidosis) Occurs due to low glomerular filtration rate secondary to acute dehydration; reduced tubular mass (chronic renal insufficiency) limits amount of ammonia kidney can produce; excretion of hydrogen ion with ammonia is thus decreased	Respiratory compensation: Increased respirations to blow off CO_2 Renal compensation • Acidosis also stimulates kidney to produce ammonia so that hydrogen ion can be excreted with it • As hydrogen ion is excreted new bicarbonate is generated	Deep, rapid respirations (Küssmaul breathing); severe acidosis can reduce peripheral vascular resistance and cause decreased function of the ventricles of the heart; hypotension, pulmonary edema, and tissue hypoxia may result • Arterial pH low • P_{CO_2} low • Plasma bicarbonate low
Metabolic alkalosis • Loss of hydrogen ion resulting in the presence of comparatively too much base • Gain of bicarbonate • Reduced extracellular fluid volume with a greater NaCl loss than bicarbonate loss	• Loss of hydrogen ion (gastric aspiration, persistent vomiting, e.g., pyloric stenosis) • Loading with bicarbonate as: • Increased renal reabsorption of bicarbonate as in a potassium cellular deficit (reasons not clear) • When chlorides are lost, as in vomiting, the body releases more bicarbonate to keep the total number of anions equal • Administration of a diuretic	Respiratory compensation: Compensation is not effective; therefore, the problem must be eliminated	Depressed respiration: Hypertonic muscles due to decreased ionized calcium in the presence of alkalemia‡ • Arterial pH high • P_{CO_2} elevated • Plasma bicarbonate elevated

*Hypoxemia can result in metabolic acidosis due to accumulation of lactic acid in presence of reduced oxygen supply to tissues. Exercise, trauma, and infection are common causes of tissue hypoxia that can result in metabolic lactic acidosis.
†Large amounts of bicarbonate are present in gastrointestinal tract from a point distal of pylorus to anal sphincter.
‡In acidosis, there is a high ionization of calcium, and, in alkalosis, a decreased ionization.

TABLE 26-6
Arterial Blood Gas Values in Uncompensated Acid-Base Disturbances*†

Abnormality	pH	P_{CO_2}	Calculated Bicarbonate	Base Excess
Respiratory Acidosis ↓ Elimination by the lungs of CO_2 gas	↓	↑	N	N
Respiratory Alkalosis ↑ Elimination by the lungs of CO_2 gas	↑	↓	N	N
Metabolic Acidosis a. Acid is added (uses up HCO_3^-) *or* b. HCO_3^- is lost	↓	N	↓	↓
Metabolic Alkalosis a. Acid is lost, *or* b. HCO_3^- is gained	↑	N	↑	↑

*This table presents arterial blood gas values as they exist before correction or compensation by the primarily unaffected system (i.e., respiratory or renal).

†Arrows = elevated or depressed values; N = normal.

oratory evaluation of renal (urine and serum electrolytes and specific gravity) and cardiopulmonary (arterial blood gases and electrocardiogram) function is pertinent to the care of the child with potential fluid and electrolyte imbalance. The nurse should review the data during care of such a child.

Nursing History

Questions in the nursing history that are pertinent when fluid or electrolyte imbalance is suspected include:

- Has the child had any vomiting or diarrhea? If so, describe the circumstances.
- What are the type, frequency, and amount of food and fluid given at home during the illness?
- Has the child been urinating as usual? Is there an increase or decrease?
- Is the child drinking more than usual (polydipsia), especially water?
- Has the child had any appreciable weight loss or gain recently?
- Has the child had any recent change in behavior or activity level?
- If the child had a fever, what was its level and duration?
- Has the child had any recent evidence of infection?
- Is the child receiving any medication now, or has she or he received any recently?

In addition, parents should be given the opportunity to describe any change that they have noted in their child. After the interview and throughout the child's illness, the nurse evaluates vital signs, body weight, intake and output, neurologic status, and the condition of the skin, mucous membranes, fontanelles, and eyes.

Monitoring Vital Signs

A change in normal vital signs or a lack of change in abnormal vital signs must be noted and reported by the nurse to facilitate modification of the treatment plan.

Temperature

Elevation of body temperature can disrupt fluid balance in a child. Fever increases the metabolic rate. Since a heightened metabolic rate increases the amount of metabolic wastes, additional fluids are required for excretion of these wastes by the kidneys. Failure to provide the extra fluid can cause dehydration or worsen existing dehydration. Water and electrolytes are also lost in sweat, and additional fluid is lost through tachypnea, both of which can accompany fever. In hypernatremia, temperature elevation may occur owing to excessive water loss (i.e., insufficient fluid is available for sweating). A subnormal body temperature may occur in isotonic fluid volume deficit. This is likely related to a decreased basal metabolic rate (Metheney, 1992).

Pulse

Pulse is evaluated for rate, quality, and rhythm. When extravascular fluid volume is reduced, the pulse is rapid (tachycardia), weak, and thready. This can occur either in total body fluid deficit (dehydration) or when plasma shifts from intravascular to interstitial spaces (edema). A bounding pulse is a sign of increased plasma fluid volume and occurs in hypertonic dehydration or when there is an excess of total body fluid volume. Cardiac arrhythmias first may be detected when an irregular pulse is noted. The arrhythmias can be the result of a variety of problems, including a K^+ level that is either too high or too low.

Respirations

The rate and quality of respirations provide information about the body's fluid and electrolyte status. Respirations may be:

- Fast with a normal depth (tachypnea).
- Slow with a normal depth (bradypnea).
- Deep with a normal rate (hyperpnea).
- Irregular with a decreased rate (hypoventilation).
- Deep with an increased rate (hyperventilation).
- Absent (apnea).
- Normal (eupnea).

They are affected by fluid volume alterations, electrolyte imbalances, and acid-base imbalances. Metabolic acidosis, which accompanies many illnesses in children, including dehydration, is compensated for by an increased respiratory rate. Hypokalemia and hyperkalemia result in shallow breathing caused by weakness or paralysis of the respiratory muscles. (See Table 26–5 for respiratory responses in acid-base imbalance.)

Blood Pressure

Blood pressure is an important parameter to monitor. With the availability of electronic equipment, it is easier to obtain an accurate reading in children of all ages, including infants. (See Chapter 23 for a discussion of techniques used to measure blood pressure.) Increased blood pressure occurs in fluid volume excess or in the early phase of interstitial fluid-to-plasma shift. Blood pressure is decreased in a fluid volume deficit or when there is a plasma-to-interstitial fluid shift. This is more likely to occur when a condition has become advanced such as in greater than 15 per cent dehydration.

Weight

A child's weight provides important data about the state of hydration. The severity of dehydration and the degree of recovery from it are often reflected in a child's weight. To maximize the accuracy of this measurement, children should be weighed on the same scale, at the same time of day, with the same clothing, and, whenever possible, by the same nurse. Changes in weight related to changes in IV lines, dressings, or other items should be identified by documenting "with IV."

Weight gain during illness may indicate fluid retention and the presence of pulmonary edema or generalized edema. When a child gains weight suddenly, the nurse should not only recheck the weight but also look for signs of fluid retention, such as periorbital edema and pulmonary crackles.

Skin Assessment

The skin should be assessed for color, temperature, texture, moisture, and turgor* (tautness). It provides many clues to a child's state of hydration. Different types of dehydration, for example, result in characteristic skin conditions. In isotonic dehydration, the most common type of dehydration in children, the skin is pale and dry and its elasticity is poor. The peripheral blood flow may be decreased, making the extremities cool with poor capillary refill. The skin is often pale. In hypertonic dehydration, the skin may be flushed and its turgor and elasticity may be normal because the extracellular fluid compartment is relatively better preserved than in isotonic dehydration. The appearance of the child with hypotonic dehydration is the most dramatic; the skin is cool and clammy to the touch, and elasticity and turgor may be very poor. Color is generally pale and may become gray and mottled as circulatory failure progresses.

When there is increased formation or decreased removal of interstitial fluid, edema develops. This occurs with a variety of conditions and may or may not result in a net weight change.

Anterior Fontanelle and Eyes

The anterior fontanelle and the eyes should be assessed when a child has a potential or actual fluid imbalance. The anterior fontanelle, which remains open until approximately 16 to 18 months of age, should feel flat and firm. A tense and bulging fontanelle indicates increased intracranial pressure or volume, and a sunken or depressed one is evidence of dehydration. Suture lines in the skull may also become prominent when the circulating volume is decreased. The eyes appear sunken with dark circles, and the child may be unable to close eyes in severe dehydration.

Intake and Output and Urine Specific Gravity

A nurse's accurate assessment and recording of intake and output are of prime importance in caring for children with fluid and electrolyte imbalances. The nurse who deems it necessary should keep an intake and output record even if one has not been ordered by a physician. Also, the nurse should routinely check the urine specific gravity of children who are receiving all

* Skin turgor is assessed by pinching the skin and allowing it to fall back to its original position. When the skin remains slightly raised, or "tented," for a few seconds, this is called "poor skin turgor."

their intake intravenously or who have been identified to have potential fluid and/or electrolyte imbalances. However, it should be recognized that glucose, large amounts of protein, and radiographic dyes elevate the specific gravity, interfering with this parameter's ability to reflect hydration status accurately.

Infants are unable to concentrate urine as well as older children and adults, so their urine is normally dilute and will show a low specific gravity. In the immediate neonatal period, it ranges from 1.001 to 1.020 and thereafter from 1.001 to 1.030. A fluid excess in the body is reflected in a low specific gravity (1.010 or less) as the kidneys rid the body of water. A total body fluid deficit is reflected in a high specific gravity as the kidneys conserve fluid. After a period of fluid restriction, specific gravity is commonly greater than 1.025.

Oral fluid intake approximates urinary output daily. Fluid generated from metabolism roughly equals that which is lost through the skin, lungs, and stool. The normal range for 24-hour urinary output varies with age. It is common to assess a child's output according to weight; 1 ml/kg of body weight per hour is considered a normal urinary output. A markedly higher output of urine than fluid intake may be due to a shift of fluid from interstitial fluid to plasma, a high fluid intake, lack of secretion of ADH (e.g., diabetes insipidus), or renal tubular damage. Common pediatric conditions that may moderately increase urine production are fever and infection. This occurs because the higher metabolic rate results in increased wastes for the kidney to excrete; additional water is required to clear such wastes from the body.

Neurologic Status

The central nervous system displays signs and symptoms of dysfunction with many fluid and electrolyte imbalances. In dehydration, a child may become irritable and then lethargic, or simply lethargic with irritability on stimulation. Also, the child's cry may be high-pitched and weak. Marked hypokalemia and hyperkalemia cause muscle weakness, tetany, and muscle paralysis, whereas hypocalcemia may be the reason for a child's twitching, irritability, and eventual convulsions. Acute hyponatremia causes headache, confusion, muscle twitching, eventual delirium, and finally, convulsions. Severe hypernatremia may cause intracerebral bleeding, brain damage, and subsequent mental retardation, convulsions, and death (O'Brien, 1980).

Laboratory Assessment

Arterial blood gases are obtained from children with known or suspected acid-base imbalance to determine the presence of the imbalance and to provide a means of assessing the metabolic and respiratory components of the condition. Urine specific gravity and its significance in evaluating hydration have been discussed. Imbalances in various serum electrolytes have also been reviewed. Urine electrolytes are often obtained from children with both fluid and electrolyte imbalances and are interpreted in light of the corresponding serum values. When both urine and serum samples are desired for comparison, it is best to wait to draw the blood until the urine is obtained. In this way, they represent the body's status at the same point in time.

The electrocardiogram (ECG) may provide the first clues to electrolyte imbalances in children, and the abnormal findings may precede the development of life-threatening arrhythmias. Potassium and Ca^{2+} abnormalities, in particular, cause ECG changes. In hypokalemia, the T-wave is flattened and a U-wave may appear, whereas in hyperkalemia, the P-wave is flattened, the QRS is widened, and the T-wave is peaked. Hypocalcemia results in a prolonged QT interval, and hypercalcemia causes a shortened one (Catchpole, 1982). These ECG changes reflect abnormalities in the electrical activity of the heart secondary to the chemical abnormalities of the body's fluids.

It is important for the nurse to strive to gain an increased understanding of laboratory reports. The laboratory findings, however, must always be evaluated in conjunction with clinical findings. (Blood gas values in acid-base imbalance are summarized in Table 26–6.)

Nursing Diagnostic Statements and Collaborative Problems

Fluid volume excesses and deficits occur in a broad range of illnesses. Nursing diagnostic statements and collaborative problems appropriate to the situation are formulated, recognizing that imbalances can occur in vascular, cellular, or intracellular compartments of the body.

When *total* body volume loss or excess of fluid occurs, it is a *volume* deficit resulting in dehydration (isotonic) or a total volume excess resulting in edema. These imbalances occur with equal gains and losses of water and sodium. Fluid and electrolyte imbalance can also occur when there is an imbalance in the *proportion* of water and solute load, that is, hyperosmolarity or hypo-osmolarity. These imbalances can result in fluid shifts so that a certain body compartment may have an excess of fluid or solute, as discussed in the section on hypotonic and hypertonic dehydration. Nursing diagnostic statements and collaborative problems that represent volume deficit/excess and hyperosmolar or hypo-osmolar imbalances are included as possible diagnoses to use in fluid and electrolyte imbalance. As noted in Chapter 1, nursing diagnoses are formulated when the identification and treatment of the actual or potential problematic response are in nursing's independent domain. Collaborative problems are formulated when responsibilities are carried out conjointly with another discipline.

Fluid volume deficits are conditions in which vascular, cellular, or intercellular dehydration occurs. A fluid volume deficit can be related to failure of regulatory mechanisms or active loss. Fluids are lost in association with illness or therapy. Appropriate nursing diagnostic statements and collaborative problems follow. Collaborative problems include:

Fluid volume deficit *related to active fluid volume loss associated with illness or failure of regulatory mechanisms:*

- *Shock, hemorrhage.*
- *Heat prostration.*
- *Diarrhea, vomiting, diaphoresis.*
- *Burns, draining wounds, fistulas.*
- *Fever.*
- *Hyperventilation.*

Fluid volume deficit *related to active fluid loss associated with therapy:*

- *Overuse of diuretics.*
- *In-dwelling tubes.*
- *High-solute feeding.*
- *Frequent tap water enemas.*
- *Frequent irrigations with hypotonic solution.*

Alteration in cardiac output: decreased, *due to inadequate blood volume.*

A nursing diagnostic statement that may be seen is:

High risk for altered urinary elimination; *risk factor decreased plasma volume resulting in decreased renal blood flow.*

Fluid volume excess is the abnormal retention of fluids and edema. It is always secondary to an increase in total body sodium content, which in turn leads to an increase in total body water (Metheney, 1992). A collaborative problem associated with fluid volume excess is:

Fluid volume excess *related to:*

- *Excessive sodium intake.*
- *Excessive fluid intake.*
- *Compromised regulatory mechanisms associated with renal and liver disease, hormonal disturbance, nephrotic syndrome, lymphatic obstruction, congenital heart failure, and steroid excess.*

Additional nursing diagnostic statements that may be seen in children with fluid volume excess include:

High risk for impairments in skin integrity, risk factor edema.

Activity intolerance, related to ineffective breathing pattern associated with circulatory overload.

Anxiety related to feeling of inability to breathe due to development of pulmonary edema.

Hyperosmolar and hypo-osmolar states occur when there is an imbalance in the proportion of water and sodium. Additional nursing diagnostic statements that may be used in the care of children with hyperosmolar imbalances include:

High risk for altered thought process; risk factor decreased level of consciousness associated with shrinking of cells in the central nervous system.

High risk for impairment of skin integrity, risk factor dehydration.

Nursing diagnostic statements that may be used in the care of children with hypo-osmolar imbalances include:

High risk for injury; risk factors mental confusion, disorientation, and convulsions, associated with cellular edema of the brain.

Alteration in thought process, risk factor cerebral edema and dysfunction.

Therapeutic Management of Imbalances in Fluids, Electrolytes, and Acid-Base

Administration of IV fluids and electrolytes to children is a highly specialized technique. The nurse who participates in such therapy requires knowledge and a high level of clinical competence to meet this responsibility effectively. Nurses involved in the administration of IV fluids and electrolytes, as well as oral rehydration, should strive to increase their theoretical knowledge base as well as their technical skill. The care of these children and families traverses all aspects of pediatric nursing. The chemical and physiologic processes are complex and the psychologic effects on the child and parents are far-reaching. Starting and maintaining IV lines requires special skill and practice, and the mathematical calculations necessary to administer the prescribed fluid and electrolyte medication require precision. Unsupervised novice practitioners should not have sole responsibility for such potentially life-threatening procedures. Student nurses and newly practicing graduate nurses deserve the security, and the children have the right, to have another, more experienced nurse check all calculations when electrolytes are added to IV solutions.

TABLE 26-7
Maintenance Requirements of Fluids Based on Caloric Expenditure

Body Weight (Kg)	Caloric Expenditure	Fluid Requirements*
3–10	100 cal/kg/day	100 ml/kg/day
10–20	1000 cal + 50 cal/kg for each kg of body weight above 10 kg	1000 ml + 50 ml/kg for each kg of body weight above 10 kg
Over 20	1500 cal + 20 cal/kg for each kg of body weight above 20 kg	1500 ml + 20 ml/kg for each kg of body weight above 20 kg

Data from Holliday, M. A., & Segar, W. E. (1957). The maintenance need for water in parenteral fluid therapy. Reproduced by permission of *Pediatrics, 19,* 823. Copyright 1957.

*Water of oxidation provides a small daily source of fluid to the body. Water losses that must be replaced (insensible water loss and renal water loss) can be provided by 100 ml/100 cal/day; thus "cal" can be replaced by "ml" as shown in the last column.

Fluid and electrolyte therapy is employed under a variety of circumstances. The goal of therapy is to compensate for normal and abnormal losses and to replace preexisting deficits. The type of solution and the rate of administration vary according to the condition being corrected and the metabolic rate of the child.

Although nurses are not responsible for prescribing the required amount of fluids and electrolytes, they should have the knowledge to check the prescription by their own calculations and to decide whether it reflects a reasonable and safe dose for the particular child and condition being treated.

Calculation of Maintenance Fluid and Electrolyte Dose

The body is in a dynamic state. Fluids and electrolytes are normally gained and lost. "Maintenance requirements" are the fluids and electrolytes that are necessary to maintain homeostasis. Therapy must provide for:

- Insensible or evaporative losses (through skin and lungs).
- Urinary losses.
- Caloric needs.

Maintenance fluid requirements may be calculated on the basis of the patient's body weight, body surface area, or caloric expenditure. Calculation of maintenance fluid requirements gives the nurse an objective criterion for evaluation of nursing strategies for treatment of problematic human responses associated with fluid volume excesses and deficits. The method most widely used now, because of its accuracy and ease of calculation, is based on caloric expenditure. Holliday and Segar's formula (1957) (Table 26–7) can be committed to memory for easy use in the clinical area.

When the child is ill, ongoing abnormal losses (e.g., gastric secretions) must also be included in calculations. This is referred to as "replacement therapy." (Table 26–8 lists water losses under normal conditions.)

TABLE 26-8
Water Loss Metabolized under Normal Conditions*

Route	Water Lost (ml/100 Cal)
Insensible water loss	45
Sweat	0–25
Urine	50–75
Stool	5–10

Data from *The body fluids in pediatrics.* Winters, R. W. (Ed.). Boston: Little, Brown, 1973. Published by Little, Brown and Company.

*Usual loss in absence of sweating is 100 ml/100 cal metabolized.

Electrolytes must also be maintained on a daily basis to keep the body in balance. Maintenance requirements of electrolytes are (Awazu et al, 1990a):

1. Sodium: 2 to 3 mEq/100 cal.
2. Chloride: 5.0 mEq/100 cal.
3. Potassium: 2 to 3 mEq/100 cal.

In addition to electrolytes, glucose must be provided at 5 g/100 cal metabolized. A solution of 5 per cent glucose* in 0.2 per cent sodium chloride† (may be written as D5/0.2NS or D5/¼NS) with potassium chloride (KCl) provides adequate maintenance therapy for short periods of time under normal conditions.

Potassium chloride administration must be done with extreme caution. Incorrect placement of a decimal point can result in 10 times the prescribed dose being administered; this error, for a child, is lethal.

*This solution contains 50 g of glucose per L.

†Full-strength normal saline solution has 0.9 per cent sodium chloride; therefore, half-strength has 0.45, and quarter-strength has 0.22 or 0.2 per cent sodium chloride.

Some general guidelines to use for the administration of KCl:

- Always check the appropriateness of the dose.
- Give no more than 40 mEq/L.
- Never give by IV push.
- Give no more than 4 mEq/kg/day to correct hypokalemia.
- Do not administer KCl in the presence of oliguria or anuria.

Principles of Deficit Therapy

Total blood volume is 85 ml/kg of body weight in newborn infants and approximately 75 ml/kg in children over the age of 1 month (Barakat & Ichikawa, 1990). Deficit therapy is designed to evaluate and repair the losses of fluids and electrolytes that have already occurred. This can be accomplished by oral rehydration (as discussed in Chapter 35) or by IV therapy. There are three essential components of administering IV therapy (Siegel & Lattanzi, 1985):

1. Estimate the degree or severity of dehydration.
2. Determine the types of deficits that have occurred (i.e., isotonic, hypertonic, or hypotonic).
3. Plan an approach for the repair of the deficit.

IV orders are calculated and ordered by physicians, but nurses should understand the principles on which decisions are made in order to evaluate whether the IV therapy is within a reasonable range for the size and condition of the child.

IV therapy is most frequently described in three phases: *a rapid or initial phase,* in which the goal is to restore extracellular fluid—especially plasma volume—and improve renal function; *a repletion phase,* during which intracellular and extracellular deficits of water and electrolytes are replaced, but at a slower rate; and a final phase during which *re-equilibrium and stabilization occurs,* usually beginning when oral fluids are begun (Robson, 1987).

Rapid or Initial Phase

This phase of therapy is designed to restore circulation and stabilize vital signs by expanding the extracellular fluid volume. If the child is in shock, 10 to 12 ml/kg of 5 per cent human albumin or plasma should be administered within the first 30 minutes; this can be used for all types of dehydration (isotonic, hypotonic, and hypertonic). For a child with hyponatremic or isonatremic dehydration that is *not* in shock, 20 to 30 ml/kg of normal saline or Ringer's lactate solution is given over the initial 1 to 2 hours. With this therapy, adequate circulation should be re-established and the child should void (Awazu et al, 1990a). In the event of co-existence of acidosis, sodium bicarbonate may need to be added to the solution to correct the pH.

Repletion Therapy

The aim of this phase is to correct previous losses as well as to provide therapy for normal and abnormal ongoing losses. With hypotonic and isotonic dehydration, this is usually accomplished in 6 to 8 hours, but in hypertonic dehydration, correction of the deficit takes up to 48 hours. Proceeding at this slower pace allows for slow reduction of serum Na^+ to prevent swelling of the brain cells.

Another aspect of therapy in this phase is replacement of potassium. After kidney function has been established, KCl is added to the IV fluid. Replacement of other electrolytes is guided by serum electrolytes and varies according to the underlying problem.

Stabilization

Maintenance and ongoing losses, and any remaining deficit, are taken care of during this final phase. Oral intake may be resumed. Reintroduction of oral feedings usually begins with small amounts of clear liquids. Milk and solids are then gradually introduced while careful observation is being made for the body's tolerance of oral feedings.

Throughout deficit therapy, nurses have a very important role. They monitor the child's vital signs, state of consciousness, intake and output, specific gravity, and general appearance. Since these parameters reflect the success or failure of treatment, it is encumbent on nurses to make accurate observations and report abnormalities quickly.

Fluid Therapy Related to Surgery

The principles of fluid therapy already discussed also apply to the child undergoing a surgical procedure. When careful attention is paid to them, parental therapy proceeds smoothly. Errors, nonetheless, do occur, and the most common error in perioperative administration of IV fluid is overadministration, particularly of dextrose in water.

Preoperative IV therapy is rarely required unless the child has a pre-existing deficit. Fluid administration during surgery varies according to the types of losses that occur during the procedure. Postoperative fluids are provided by the parenteral route until the child has completely recovered from anesthesia and is free of nausea and vomiting. After most minor operations, fluids can be resumed gradually within the first 24 hours. IV fluids, however, are continued when the surgical intervention prohibits oral intake.

Common postoperative solutions used in pediatrics are D5/0.2NS and D5/0.45NS. Since surgery frequently causes an excess of tissue loss of K^+ secondary to trauma and an increased level of ADH related to stress, K^+ is not administered in the immediate postoperative period. Neither is it administered to the oliguric child because the primary site for secretion of potassium is the kidney, resulting in hyperkalemia in the event of kidney damage.

KCl can be safely added to IV fluids only *after* urinary output has been established.

Nursing Care: Maintaining Fluid and Electrolyte Balance

The nurse has an important role in the prevention of fluid and electrolyte imbalance, in the safe administration of IV therapy, and in the management of oral intake during recovery.

Preventing Imbalances

One of the nurse's responsibilities is to teach parents how to prevent imbalances and how to detect early symptoms. In times of minor illness, a few basic principles about fluid intake and output may help parents prevent their child from developing more serious problems.

Noting increases in air and body temperature and adjusting fluid intake and clothing accordingly may prevent development of serious imbalances. Overdressing for the environmental temperature causes increased perspiration, resulting in both fluid and electrolyte losses. Additional fluids should be offered to young children in hot weather, and time in the sun must be limited; the number of diapers used and their saturation can guide the need for additional fluids in infants. When a child becomes ill, parents also should be taught to check the child's temperature early in the illness. In the event of a fever, additional fluids should be offered, and clothing should only be sufficient to prevent shivering.

Parents should be taught to reduce solids and milk intake and to give clear fluids primarily when vomiting or diarrhea occurs. It is important, however, for parents to understand that giving plain water alone and in large amounts can be extremely dangerous and may result in seizures, coma, or death. Glucose-electrolyte solutions or a balanced combination of liquids must be used when fluid constitutes the child's only intake for a prolonged period of time. Undiluted skim milk should not be used because of its high solute content; large quantities of water are required for excretion of solutes, further depleting the body of water. How to gradually increase the child's food intake during and after illness in order to avoid starvation is also important information for parents to have (see Chapter 35 for discussion of diet for diarrhea and vomiting).

Treatment of conditions that predispose children to fluid and electrolyte imbalances can start promptly if parents have been taught to identify the early signs. Signs and symptoms they can identify:

1. *General appearance:* Sunken or bulging fontanelle and sunken eyes with dark circles, no tears with crying.
2. *Neurologic status:* Irritability, high-pitched cry, difficult to awaken.
3. *Renal status:* Fewer wet diapers.
4. *Integumentary status:* Abnormal skin color, temperature, or moistness.
5. *Respiratory status:* Increased respiratory rate or difficulty in breathing.
6. *Gastrointestinal status:* Vomiting or many loose stools.

Frequently, the nurse can help parents prevent development of more serious problems by taking the time to discuss these few early parameters and encouraging them to seek professional assistance when their child is ill. Families with infants under 6 months of age, in particular, should be cautioned to seek assistance early, because the younger child may deteriorate more rapidly than the older child when imbalances occur.

Meeting the Child's Developmental Needs

After a parenteral solution has been ordered by the physician, the nurse assumes the major responsibility for its proper, safe administration. After ascertaining that the dose prescribed (amount and rate of administration) is within safe limits, the nurse starts the IV infusion or assists another individual in doing so. The nurse:

- Prepares the child and family before bringing equipment into the room (whenever possible).
- Is aware of preferred sites and equipment options (needles or catheters and pumps or controllers).
- Evaluates whether the child needs to be restrained, and, if so, how it can be accomplished most easily.

Each of these interventions depends on the developmental characteristics of the child, which are summarized in Table 26–9.

Promoting Safety and Comfort

Choice of site varies according to the age and condition of the child and the condition of veins. The site selected should involve minimal risk and maximal efficiency, safety, and comfort. IV lines may be placed in the veins of the scalp, hand, foot, or antecubital fossa. Scalp veins are often used in infants because they are prominent and because of the difficulty in finding peripheral veins. The veins of the scalp communicate with the dural sinuses; therefore, careful cleansing of the head insertion sites is necessary. Cleansing with povidone-iodine or a similar solution is more effective than using alcohol. Positioning a needle or catheter in a vein in the front center of the head rather than toward the back and side reduces the amount of hair that must be shaved and allows the baby to lie on either side and on the back (Fig. 26–1).

Peripheral veins of the hands and feet, especially those on the dorsum of the hand, are often used in children and are gaining acceptance as choice sites for IV therapy in infants. They allow more mobility and are less disfiguring than venipunctures of the scalp (especially if infiltration occurs). Also, the sight of an IV line in the hand (and, to a lesser degree, the foot) will be less likely to cause parents distress than one in the child's head. The use of EMLA (eutectic mixture of local anesthetics), an anesthetic cream, prior to starting an elective IV line has helped to reduce the trauma associated with IV starts. (See Chapter 24 for further discussion of EMLA. This product is not recommended for infants under three months of age.)

IV lines should not be placed in the antecubital fossa unless other sites have been exhausted. The antecubital veins overlie fleshy parts of the muscle and are difficult to enter; the brachial artery lies close to the skin in this area, making it easy to puncture. Also, IV lines inserted over any joint are likely to infiltrate most rapidly. Generally, the most distal part of the vein should always be used first because the proximal continuation of the vessel may be used for future IV therapy.

Warming the limb with a warm, damp cloth helps to distend the small vessels, making access easier.

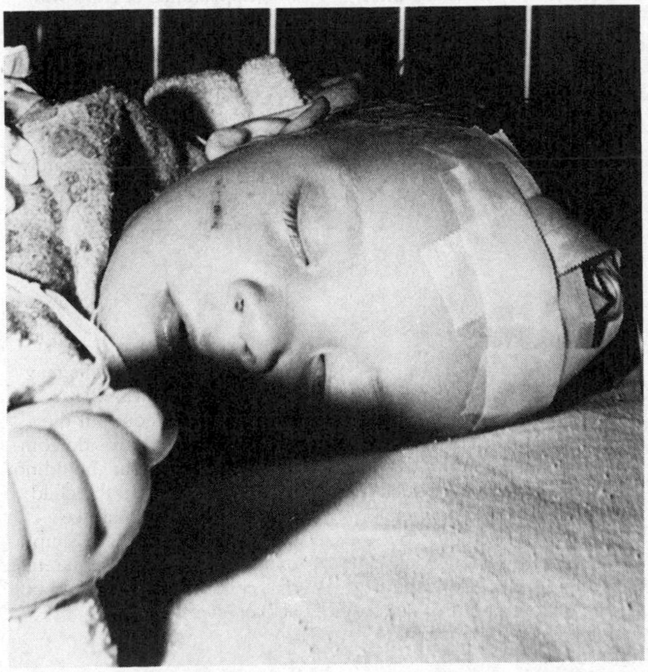

FIGURE 26-1. A scalp vein catheter inserted in a central position permits the child to be turned to either side.

Other questions to consider: Which is the infant's or child's dominant hand? How much will the child's mobility be affected (e.g., can crutches still be used)? Was an infiltrated IV line recently removed from that area (if yes, use another site)?

Plastic catheters are now used for the majority of IVs in most centers. They bend with movement of the vein and are less likely to become dislodged.

The size of the cathether used varies according to the size of the vein. In children, 20- to 27-gauge catheters are most commonly used. The higher the number, the smaller the diameter of the lumen. The smaller the lumen, the less traumatic the catheter is to the vein.

Regardless of the site or equipment used, the position of the catheter and the manner of securing it largely determine the duration of the IV therapy. The catheter must be inserted well into the vein, and a clear plastic dressing is placed over it to stabilize it.

With a scalp vein IV line, a young infant may only need positioning with a rolled blanket. Placing the tube away from the infant's body helps maintain the IV line because of random arm movements typical during this stage of development.

Starting an IV Line

Before beginning an IV, the ordered type of solution and rate of IV infusion must be checked. To prepare IV fluids and begin administration, the following steps are suggested:

1. Prepare the IV fluid by connecting the fluid chamber to the main reservoir (small bottles or bags of 250 or 500 ml are recommended to avoid unnecessary wasting of IV solutions).
2. Put enough fluid into the fluid chamber to fill the IV tubing (approximately 15 to 20 ml plus fluid for 1 to 2 hours).
3. "Prime" the system (i.e., run fluid through it).
4. Insert the catheter.
5. Connect the tubing to the catheter and check whether the IV runs by gravity.
6. Thread the tubing through the pump, set the desired rate, and start the pump.

Three basic methods are available for regulation of the flow of IV fluids:

- IV controllers regulate fluid administration at preselected rates, but they depend on gravity for proper operation.
- IV pumps automatically deliver fluid by exerting positive pressure on IV tubing (peristaltic pumps) or by pushing the fluid through a cylinder (piston and cylinder pumps) at set flow rates.
- Traditional roller clamp systems depend on gravity and are regulated by hand.

TABLE 26-9
Nursing Guidelines for Pediatric IVs at Various Stages of Child's Development

Principles common across all ages:

1. Check IV site and amount of IV flow hourly
2. Reposition restrained child and loosen restraint hourly
3. Check delivery pump for stable connections
4. Check pump settings for accuracy (IV rate, pressures)
5. Avoid restraining child whenever possible (use of catheters rather than needles has reduced the necessity for use of restraints)
6. Wear gloves for IV insertion and removal
7. Use topical anesthetic, such as EMLA cream, for all ages after 6 mos to reduce discomfort on insertion

Developmental Characteristics *Note:* Each stage builds on the earlier ones, and, during hospitalization, many children regress to behaviors appropriate to earlier levels of development	**IV Placement (Ideal Sites)**	**Preparation of Child**	**Family Involvement**
Infant (First Yr)			
Dependent on others for all needs. Needs to feel physically safe, through close relationship with one caretaking person (usually the mother). Trust develops through needs being met consistently. Mistrust and anxiety develop when needs are met inconsistently. "Stranger anxiety" begins at approximately 6 mos	Scalp vein for very small infant; foot, hand, forearm	Best not to feed infant immediately before IV insertion (vomiting and aspiration possible)	Prepare family as to need for IV therapy, insertion procedure, appearance of infant with IV, and fluid needs. Encourage family to continue providing baby with tactile and verbal stimulation and TLC. Demonstrate safe ways to hold an infant with an IV. Encourage questions and clarify misconceptions
Toddler (1–3 Yrs)			
Discovers and explores self and world. Enjoys new mobility skills. Develops egocentric thinking, and need for parallel play. Tolerates short separations from mother. Transitional objects (security blanket, special toy) provide some comfort. Oppositional syndrome ("no" stage). Separation anxiety an important problem in hospitalized toddlers separated from mother, ages 8–24 mos	Hand or arm, foot is used as a last resort because children want to stand. *Important:* From this age group on, the less dominant extremity should be used for the IV whenever possible. Determine handedness prior to IV insertion	Prepare child immediately before procedure (child has limited attention span and is likely to become more anxious if prepared sooner). Give very simple explanation in concrete terms. Show equipment to be used. See preparation for preschool age (below) and assess ability of each child to understand	Prepare family as to need for IV therapy insertion procedure, and appearance of child with IV. Whether parents remain with the child during the procedure varies. If they stay with the child, their role is to provide comfort rather than to assist with restraining. Demonstrate to parents how to safely handle child with IV
Preschool Age (4–6 Yrs)			
Magical thinking, based on what the child would like to believe. Cannot always distinguish fantasy from reality. Fears intrusive procedures. Develops conscience (guilt), while asserting independence and mastering new skills. Learning to share	Hand, forearm, upper arm (less dominant)	Prepare child just prior to procedure. Using small bottle, tubing, and doll or stuffed animal, explain in literal terms the need for IV, and insertion procedure. Allow child to see and touch equipment. Explain how child can help with procedure by cleaning site, opening packages, taping, etc. Allow some degree of control in the situation. Say you will help child hold still, and that it's OK to cry	As with toddlers, parents may or may not stay with the child during the procedure. If they stay, they should provide comfort and support but should not be asked to restrain the child for IV insertion. Reinforce child's need for honest, simple explanations. Reassure parents that child can still play and be active, even with IV

Related Nursing Actions	Protection of IV Site	Mobility Considerations *Note:* No child should be restricted to bed simply because of an IV!	Safety Needs
Infant (First Yr)			
Comfort and cuddle during and after insertion. Observe carefully during insertion for problems of vomiting, aspiration, etc. Use of pacifier diminishes stress, especially for NPO infants. Check insertion site hourly	IV may be secured with tape and is wrapped. Restraint of affected limb may or may not be necessary. A small arm board may be used	Keep restraint as loose as possible to allow for motion. Mitten hands with cotton and stockinette to prohibit infant's grasping IV. Restraining all extremities is avoided. Remember infant's need for sensory stimulation	Maintain strict I & O. Secure IV tubing out of range of kicking legs and flailing arms. Check restraint frequently for effectiveness and presence of adequate circulation
Toddler (1–3 Yrs)			
IV usually requires more than one person. Reassure child through verbal and tactile stimulation during procedure. Provide toys such as pegs to hammer for therapeutic expression of anger, after procedure and throughout hospitalization	See above (infant). A securely anchored IV is essential for the normally active toddler. Even the best site protection will not remain effective unless it is coupled with close nursing supervision, and with distracting activities for the child	Toddlers cope with the world and learn about it through action. Therefore, minimal restraint should be used. Parental presence during waking hours permits the child to be constantly supervised, and makes restraints unnecessary in many cases. However, be careful to avoid setting up a situation in which the child associates parent's departure with "punishment" of restraint	Child is unaware of danger at this age and will not know that dislodging an IV causes pain. Constant supervision needed when out of bed. Remind frequently not to touch IV tubing. Distracting activities will accomplish more than reprimand for pulling on the IV. Tape connections on tubing if child continues to handle tubing. Keep tubing clamps out of reach. Turn control panel away from child
Preschool Age (4–6 Yrs)			
Tell child this IV is *not* punishment. *Never* bribe or threaten with IVs (e.g., "Drink, or you'll get another IV"). Praise cooperation, or any efforts in that direction. Maintain patient privacy. Don't start an IV in view of other patients, visitors, or staff. Child needs support to cope with intrusiveness of this procedure. Show understanding	See above (infant). As with toddlers, securely anchored IVs are essential but inadequate unless coupled with close supervision and age-appropriate activities	Preschoolers need maximal mobility to master surroundings. Provide a range of out-of-bed activities whenever possible	Child will be curious about IV. Is capable of understanding instructions to not touch it, but needs frequent reminders. IV clamps should be out of reach or taped over. Constant supervision needed when out of bed. Child is liable to "take off" down the hall, heedless of pole, bottle, etc. Short attention span limits duration of cooperation with instructions. Turn control panel away from child

(continued)

TABLE 26-9
Nursing Guidelines for Pediatric IVs at Various Stages of Child's Development *(Continued)*

Developmental Characteristics *Note:* Each stage builds on the earlier ones, and, during hospitalization, many children regress to behaviors appropriate to earlier levels of development	**IV Placement (Ideal Sites)**	**Preparation of Child**	**Family Involvement**
School Age (7–11 Yrs)			
Struggles between mastering new skills and failure. Enjoys school, learning skills, games with rules. Needs to succeed. Fears body mutilation. May feel need to be "brave." Can understand hospital rules. World now expanding beyond family. Peer group becomes important. Competitiveness	Hand, forearm, upper arm (less dominant)	Prepare child ahead of time, but same day of insertion. Carefully explain and demonstrate equipment and reasons for IV therapy, letting patient watch you or help set up equipment. Ask child for questions about need for IV and procedure. Give child choices and let help in procedure whenever possible. Tell child crying is OK because needles hurt, and you will help him or her hold still	Whenever possible, family and child should be prepared together, so that family can reinforce what the child has been told. Stress to family the child's need for some independence in ADL, even with an IV. Parental presence or participation in IV insertion may be appropriate, but child's preference should be considered primary
Adolescent (12–18 Yrs)			
Vacillates between needs for independence and dependence. Adult cognitive abilities, deductive reasoning. Coping mechanisms: rationalization, intellectualization. Peer acceptance very important. Egocentric, rebellious at times, especially against parents and authority figures. Very concerned with body image, body changes, sexuality, and role. Searching for "who I am"	Hand, forearm, upper arm (less dominant)	Prepare child several hours to a day before procedure, if possible. Needs time between preparation and insertion to absorb explanations and ask questions. For most adolescents, approach discussions on an adult level. Explain need for IV therapy and expected duration, and show equipment. May need much support for acceptance of therapy	Explain therapy needs and duration as per patient. Decision regarding parental presence during procedure should be patient's, not parents'. Stress to family the patient's need for independence and participation in decisions affecting care

Adapted from Guhlow, L. J., & Kolb, J. (1979). Pediatric IVs: Special measures you must take. *Registered Nurse, 42,* 40–51. Published in *RN.* Copyright © 1979 Medical Economics Publishing, Montvale, NJ. Reprinted by permission.

When starting or monitoring an IV line, the nurse should carefully check the physician's orders for the type of solution and rate of infusion. An assessment is then made whether the type and rate are reasonable for the child's illness state and size. The minimal fluid requirement (Table 26-7) is used as a guide to make this clinical judgment.

The primary difference between controller and pump systems is that a controller cannot add pressure to overcome resistance to flow, whereas a pump can. A pump exerts only enough pressure to overcome the resistance but will not exceed preset limits. When the maximal preset pressure is reached, the machine's alarm sounds.

Compared with roller clamp systems, controllers or pumps help prevent fluid overload and drug overdosage. They must be used during administration of parenteral nutrition and continuous medication infusions and when fluid restriction is necessary in small children. The IV tubing is threaded through these machines, then the dial is set for the desired rate of flow (Fig. 26-2). IV pumps and controllers differ in their safety mechanisms; many have alarms that sound when the machine is not functioning properly. However, pumps often continue to infuse fluid at preset rates for a while after infiltration has occurred before alarms sound. A special control fluid chamber that holds a limited amount of solution and provides for accurate measurement is recommended for use in children. The pediatric minidrip set delivers 60 drops (gtts)

Related Nursing Actions	Protection of IV Site	Mobility Considerations *Note:* No child should be restricted to bed simply because of an IV!	Safety Needs
School Age (7–11 Yrs)			
Approach child expecting cooperation (this age group likes to please adults), but expect that child will need help holding still. Allow the child to clean the site with alcohol swab, and to cut tape, prior to insertion. Praise cooperative efforts. Give child step-by-step explanation of procedure as it progresses. Child may like to take some responsibility in keeping I & O	Will need less protection than younger children owing to interest in making IV "work" correctly. May naturally protect extremity with IV. Some children will appreciate a warning sign, "Hands Off," on a piece of tape over the IV as a reminder. Utilize the child's natural curiosity and interest in learning. Tell the "rules" of safe IV handling	Show patient and family how to safely manipulate IV for out-of-bed activities (walking in hall with pole, keeping tubing out of wheelchair wheels, etc.)	Remind patient periodically about necessary caution with IV. Show patient the clamps, and caution against handling them. Teach patient signs of IV problems. Enlist child's help in the interest of good compliance, but do not entirely depend on it. Tape tubing connections. Child may forget about IV. Emphasize need for caution in some activities, especially if play includes other children
Adolescent (12–18 Yrs)			
Be aware of IV adding to patient's dependency status, and the need for some control. Encourage patient to keep own I & O, to help in counting drip rate, etc. Privacy during insertion is very important	See above (School Age). If patient is very active, will need well-protected, well-anchored IV, as movements may be more forceful and strength greater than younger patients'	See above (School Age). Encourage mobility as much as possible as a means of independence for the adolescent	Be aware of possibility of adolescent rebellion showing itself in lack of cooperation with therapy. These patients may rebel if feeling threatened and may be very manipulative in "testing" behaviors. Consistent limits, clearly communicated to patient, parents, and staff, are needed. Instruct patient about signs of infiltration, phlebitis, etc.

per minute (Fig. 26–3). When roller clamp systems are used alone, adjust the flow rate when the child is quiet. If the rate is regulated when the child is crying, the rate may be too rapid when the crying stops.

All types of IV infusion sets require regular monitoring during use. Electronic equipment can malfunction; therefore, monitoring of the child's condition and the IV site remains an important nursing responsibility.

Calculation of IV Rates

Calculation of the proper drip rate of fluid administered to children is simplified by the use of a system that delivers 60 gtts per minute (gtts/min). Typical fluid orders are either in number of milliliters per hour (ml/hr) or in number of milliliters per 24 hours (ml/24 hrs). The simple calculations in Table 26–10 will convert such orders into gtts/min.

Maintaining the IV Infusion

Maintaining an IV infusion entails administering fluid accurately and safely to the child. The machinery available to monitor IV therapy cannot replace nurses, but it can assist them. Pump and controller systems do not reduce work, but, if used properly, they increase the safety of parenteral fluid administration.

At the beginning of each shift, the nurse respon-

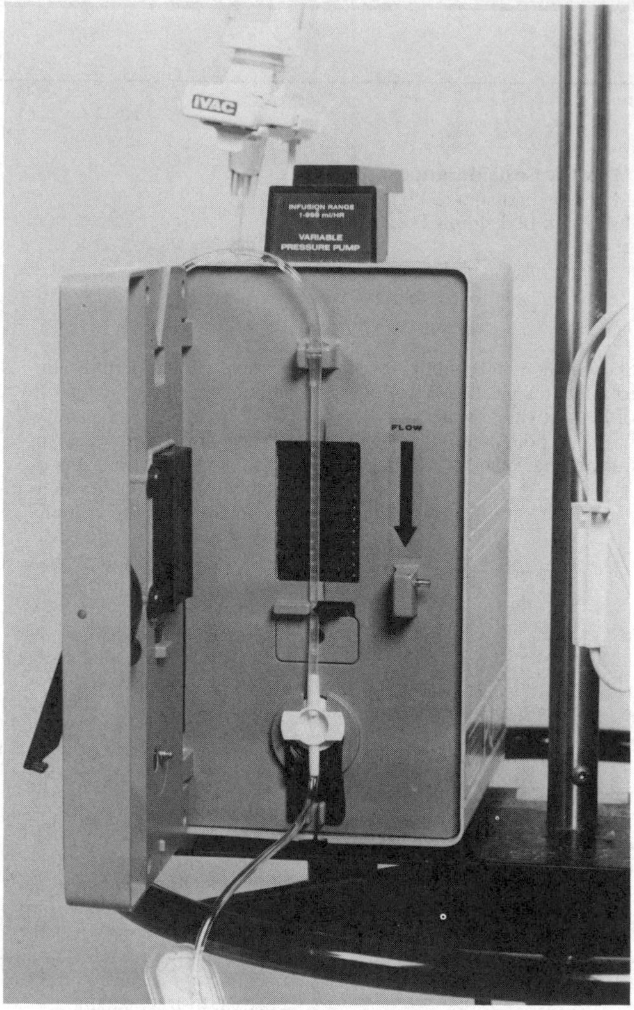

FIGURE 26 - 2. IV tubing is threaded through the pump, following the direction of the arrow on the pump. The door of the pump is then closed and the pump is started.

sible for a particular child with an IV line must make a complete check, including:

1. The type of solution and electrolyte dose.
2. The date and time the bottle and tubing were hung (usually changed every 72 hours; every 24 hours for total parenteral nutrition).
3. The machine—check the setting on the machine and count the actual gtts/min; check the pressures.
4. The tubing—check for kinks, flattening, blood, or air; check the entire length of the tubing to the insertion site.
5. The tubing for proper threading into the machine.
6. The IV site for redness, puffiness, and security of dressing over site.
7. The security and appropriateness of restraint (if used); check all involved extremities for warmth, color, and general appearance.
8. Any medication that is running; verify that the amount is absorbed on schedule as prescribed.
9. The general status of the child.
10. Vital signs and urinary output.

IV checks should be made using a flashlight if lights are out. A dim light from the hallway is not adequate. If there is any question regarding the site, overhead lights must be turned on, even though the child or other children may awaken. Hourly checks should include checking:

1. The settings on the machine and a counting of the actual drops.
2. The entire length of tubing.
3. The site and restrained extremities (if any).
4. The general status of the child.
5. The amount of fluid absorbed; enter it on an IV record sheet.

IV record sheets are used to monitor fluid administration. The types of forms used vary among institutions. Columns should be provided for the type of fluid being administered, the rate, the amount of fluid actually

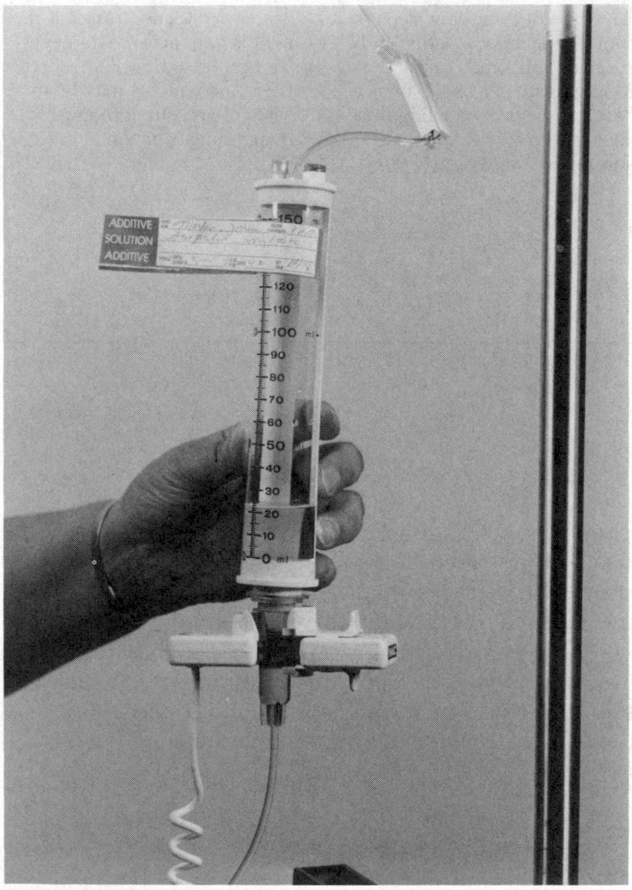

FIGURE 26 - 3. A special control chamber holds a limited amount of fluid and provides for accurate measurement of fluid administration.

TABLE 26-10
Calculations for Converting Typical Fluid Orders into Gtts/Min

When the system delivers 60 gtts/ml:
A. If the order is for ml/hr:
(*Example:* 40 ml/hr = 40 gtts/min*)
B. If the order is for ml/24 hrs:
(*Example:* 960 ml/24 hrs):
1. Change to ml/hr:

960 ÷ 24 hrs = 40 ml/hr

2. 40 ml/hr = 40 gtts/min*

The reason that ml/hr = gtts/min is explained by the following:

Step 1:

Number of ml/hr ordered	×	number of gtts/ml delivered by system	=	number of gtts/hr
40		60		2400

Step 2:

Number of gtts/hr	÷	number of min/hr	=	number of gtts/min
2400		60		40

Because the number of minutes in an hour, and the number of drops per ml are both 60, the calculations are simplified (multiplying by 60 and dividing by 60). Thus, whenever the IV set is designed to deliver 60 gtts/ml, the order of 40 ml/hr can be converted immediately to 40 gtts/min without any calculations.

*Ml/hr can be equated to gtts/min only if the system delivers 60 gtts/ml.

absorbed hourly, and a running total of fluid absorbed per shift. A column should be provided for the nurse to write her or his comments, and each hourly check should be documented with the nurse's initials.

The nurse is also responsible for making ongoing assessments of the child's fluid, electrolyte, and acid-base balance whenever parenteral therapy is being administered. The previous discussion on assessment of vital signs, weight, skin, anterior fontanelle and eyes, intake and output and urine specific gravity, and laboratory reports describes pertinent observations that must be made during IV therapy.

Some environmental and clinical situations affect fluid and electrolyte balance during fluid therapy. If a child is in a hot environment, has a fever, or is tachypneic, water loss is increased. For every degree of fever above 37.8° C, 12 per cent of fluid maintenance is added. (For each degree of fever above 100° F, 8 per cent of fluid maintenance is added.) Crying may double insensible water loss in a baby. Also, a newborn infant placed under a radiant heat warmer or receiving phototherapy has increased fluid loss through evaporation. Decreases in water loss may occur in cool environments or if humidity is high (e.g., in a mist tent). If these conditions exist when a child has renal disease or has a high concentration of ADH, water intake may need to be decreased.

Preventing Complications of IV Therapy

A major responsibility of the nurse is to prevent complications of IV therapy. Complications may include:

- Clotting.
- Infiltration.
- Phlebitis.
- Infection.
- Air embolism.

These complications are associated with the nursing diagnoses potential for injury and potential for infection.

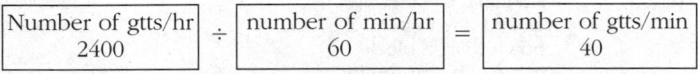

Clotting of IV lines occurs when the continuous flow of fluid is interrupted (e.g., the fluid chamber runs dry, the IV tubing kinks, or the IV pump is not turned on). It can occur very quickly, so measures

TABLE 26-11
Common Complications of Intravenous Therapy*†

Complication	Definition	Signs and Symptoms	Cause	Prevention	Nursing Action‡
Phlebitis	Inflammation in vein	Red streak, edema, tenderness, heat	Trauma to endothelial lining of vein due to: contaminated equipment or site; a difficult insertion; a catheter left in too long; a chemical irritation from some drugs or solutions	Filter irritating solutions; maintain consistent flow; routine 12-hr IV restarts unless contraindicated; monitor the site hourly; use a large vein for infusing additives that are potentially irritating; sufficiently dilute additives that are potentially irritating and run at prescribed rate; make sure all additives and solutions are compatible	Remove device, apply moist heat
Thrombosis	Injury to vessel wall, platelets adhere → clot forms	↓ Flow rate, edema below clot, tenderness			Do not apply moist heat; elevate
Thrombophlebitis	Injury to vein + presence of clot	Tenderness, edema, heat palpable cord			Do not apply moist heat; elevate extremity
Occlusion	Nonpatent system; crystallized solution or blood in IV tubing	Reduced patency of vein, ↓ IV rate, ↑ pump pressure, stopped IV drip	Mechanical, due to system malfunctioning, tubing kinks, positioning, catheter tip clotted due to bent elbow or wrist; blocking may be caused by too slow a rate, incompatible additives, or in a gravity system by backed up blood	Close observation; use of splints	Gently aspirate catheter and then flush if no resistance; if unable to flush, remove catheter
Infiltration and extravasation	Solution in subcutaneous tissue	Edema, blanching of skin, leaking fluid from insertion site; high pressure on the pump; coolness of the skin around the IV site; slowing of IV rate if run by gravity	Catheter punctures vein wall: solutions run too quickly through a small vein that cannot deal with the volume; client is very active with limb IV in; fragile veins; IV site at joints	Adequately secure and stabilize site; use of splints; frequent observation	Remove catheter, elevate extremities; notify physician if irritating or vesicant solutions go interstitial or if the limb is grossly swollen
Air embolism	Air from venous circulation goes into pulmonary artery via right side of heart	Cyanosis, hypotension, tachycardia, respiratory distress, weak pulse	Damaged IV tubing causing a leak; disconnected or loose IV tubing; tubing not properly primed	Proper securing of IV connections, use of Luer-Loks, limit number of external sets; carefully purge a new line of all air	Place patient on left side, head down; may need oxygen; clamp IV site to prevent further air entry or remove it; call the physician, may order oxygen and anticoagulants; in child with ventricle or atrial septal defect, even a small amount of air can be very dangerous
Cellulitis	Infection of fascia	Edema, pain, erythema	Poor aseptic technique	Use good aseptic technique	Remove device, apply warm compresses, usually requires antibiotics
Septicemia	Severe febrile illness due to bacteria in the blood	Chills, fever, headache, shock → death	Poor aseptic technique, contaminated equipment	Sterile solution and equipment, use a filter, aseptic technique for all IV procedures	Remove device and change IV pump, culture site, notify physician to obtain order for antibiotics
Pulmonary embolism	Free-floating air bubble goes through heart into lungs	Chest pain, cough (productive), tachycardia, ↑ shallow respiration	Dislodging of blood clot	Use filter, avoid use of veins in lower extremities, never force, flush occluded IV site	Notify physician to obtain order for anticoagulants and oxygen

TABLE 26-11
Common Complications of Intravenous Therapy*† *(Continued)*

Complication	Definition	Signs and Symptoms	Cause	Prevention	Nursing Action‡
Vein pain	Pain in vein being used for therapy	Reddened skin and/or blanching around vein	Solution with high or low pH or high or low osmolarity; some medications cause vasospasm	Good insertion technique	Dilution of medications; warm compresses to vein; an even IV rate, i.e., use of IV pumps; notify physician
Nerve damage	Damaged nerve around vein	Extreme pain; numbness of body part where IV was inserted	Improper or accidental insertion of needle into nerve; improper splinting of extremities	Good insertion technique	Remove device; notify physician

Courtesy of Kris Paton, RN, and Adrienne Austin, RN, pediatric IV and central venous line nurses at Chedoke-McMaster Hospitals, McMaster Division, Hamilton, Ontario, Canada.

*Whenever site of insertion has a discharge, swab site and send the catheter tip to microbiology.

†Because catheters are most commonly used, this table refers to catheters only, but the same principles apply to use of IV needles.

‡In all circumstances, documentation of observations and nursing actions is essential.

must be taken by the nurse to prevent these problems. IV alarms should be attended to immediately.

The infiltration of IV infusions can best be prevented by use of proper insertion and securing of the dressing. When this common complication occurs, however, early recognition will minimize the sequelae. Signs and symptoms that the nurse must watch for include local pain, swelling, tenderness, cool skin, and blanching. IV therapy must be checked by looking at the insertion site and the surrounding area, because infiltrated fluid often collects in dependent areas. Also, if the dressing appears to be becoming tighter, infiltration should be suspected. When a scalp vein site infiltrates, a generalized fullness can be noted and slight asymmetry of the head may be apparent. Lack of blood return is not always proof of infiltration in children because small-gauge catheters are often used and because a young child's venous pressure may not be high enough to cause backflow. Especially after an IV has been in place longer than 24 hours, venous flow may adjust to accommodate the catheter, resulting in no blood return.

Infiltration of IV infusions, especially when medications are in the infusate, can cause enough tissue damage to require skin grafting, so prevention is of paramount important. To guard against infiltration, take a "mental picture" of the site when the first IV check is made and carefully check its appearance hourly to compare it with its original appearance. A close monitoring of the pressure on the machine is another way to identify a problem and potential infiltration.

Complications occur for many reasons: contaminated equipment or site, length of time the catheter is in place, difficult insertion, and chemical irritation from some drugs and solutions. Phlebitis is characterized by red, hot skin, local pain, swelling, and a palpable, hardened vein. Phlebitis can be prevented by adhering to aseptic principles when inserting catheters and handling IV solutions; changing equipment (e.g., change IV tubing and solutions according to institutional policy); and using membrane filters on all IV lines through which antibiotics or other irritating drugs are administered.

Changing of IV sites varies with the type of catheter. Some catheters are recommended to be changed every 72 hours, whereas others can be left in place longer. Table 26-11 summarizes common complications of IV therapy.

It is clear from this discussion that the nurse's expertise in managing IV therapy is a skill that greatly contributes to the recovery and well-being of a child.

Supporting the Child and Family During IV Therapy

Nurses are most often responsible for the preparation of the child and the family for IV therapy. They must also guide their participation in the process. To nurses, IV therapy is a common pediatric procedure. To the child and family, however, it has a variety of meanings and is the subject of numerous fears. For example, a family may interpret their child's need for IV therapy as a sign of a deteriorating condition. Nurses, therefore, must approach IV therapy with the recognition that fears and questions need to be addressed. Responding to individual needs for reassurance and comfort is very important.

A gentle, positive approach will help gain the child's cooperation. Whether the parents should stay or leave when an IV line is started is a decision that should be made with the child, the parent, and the nurse. There is no prescribed rule. Some parents wish to stay and are able to support the child. This is appropriate if the nurse's skill is not adversely affected by their presence, and it will likely be beneficial for the child to have the parents nearby. However, if the parents' fears are easily communicated to the child or if the nurse cannot work effectively with parents present, it is usually in everyone's best interest if they wait in a lounge away from the treatment room. (See Research Issues: "The Impact of Parental Presence During Procedures" [Chapter 23]).

Children with IV lines should not be immobilized unnecessarily. Young children may require restraints when unsupervised, but parents and nurses can hold them and take them for a ride or to a playroom. Older children can be up in wheelchairs, can be allowed to walk in the halls, and can go to the play area (Fig. 26–4).

Age-appropriate independence to the degree the IV line permits should be fostered. Parents can be taught how to care for the child or assist the child in self-care. Too often parents fear dislodging the IV line and defer to the nurse when care is required. The physical isolation that is imposed by an IV line makes it particularly important that the nurse make every effort to assist parents to become involved to the degree that they can and want to be. Saline (or heparin) locks should be considered whenever possible to give the child more freedom. (Guidelines for family involvement during parenteral therapy are offered in Table 26–9.)

Venous Access Devices for Continuous or Repeated Therapy

It is becoming increasingly more common for children to require long-term IV treatment. To avoid repeated invasive IV starts, a variety of methods have been devised to make it easier for children to cope with such circumstances. The methods used to supplement the standard peripheral IV line include: (1) heparin or saline locks, (2) central venous catheters with an external exit, such as a Hickman, Broviac, or Groshong; and (3) implanted venous access devices (e.g., port-A-Cath). The type of access chosen varies according to the child's particular requirements as well as the preferences of the health care team.

A *heparin or saline lock* is used in circumstances when an IV line can be interrupted for long periods, but it still needs to be kept open for periodic access. For example, when IV medications are required by a child who can take fluids and food orally, it is unnecessary to keep the child attached continuously to an IV setup. A heparin or saline lock is like a regular IV line, except that the needle hub has a removable stopper. When a medication is required, it can be hooked up to an IV pump, and, when the treatment is completed, the line is flushed with saline (or heparin) and again capped off with a stopper.

A *central venous catheter with an external exit* is placed into the superior vena cava. These catheters are made of silicon Silastic material. They are surgically placed through the cephalic, internal, or external jugular vein with the tip lying near the junction of the superior vena cava and the right atrium. The remainder of the catheter is tunneled subcutaneously and exits the skin medial to the nipple, but at about the nipple line. A Dacron cuff at the proximal end of the catheter becomes embedded into the tissue and serves as an infection barrier and stabilizer. In the neonate and infant, this exit site is usually on the scalp; in the young child, the site may be in the neck or chest wall. Further information is given in Chapter 42.

An *implanted venous access device* is made up of two parts—a reservoir and a catheter—both of which are implanted under the skin. The catheter tip is also placed into the superior vena cava proximal to the right atrium. The port usually lies on the third or fourth rib subcutaneously. Externally, it is visible only as a small bump under the skin. No dressing or frequent flushing is required. The "port" is accessed with special bent needles (that will lie flat on the skin exterior) that puncture the skin and the chamber's septum.

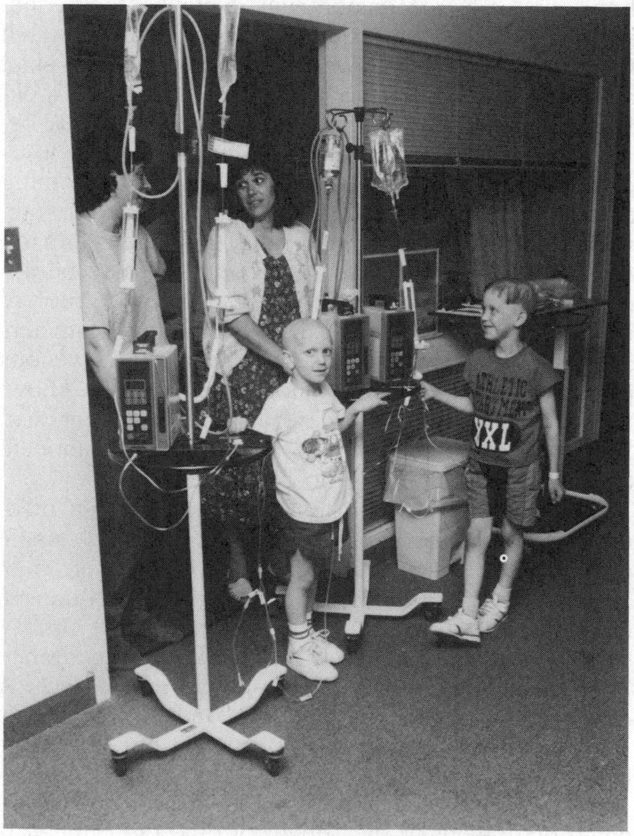

FIGURE 26-4. These children are very self-sufficient in being able to push their IV pumps to the playroom.

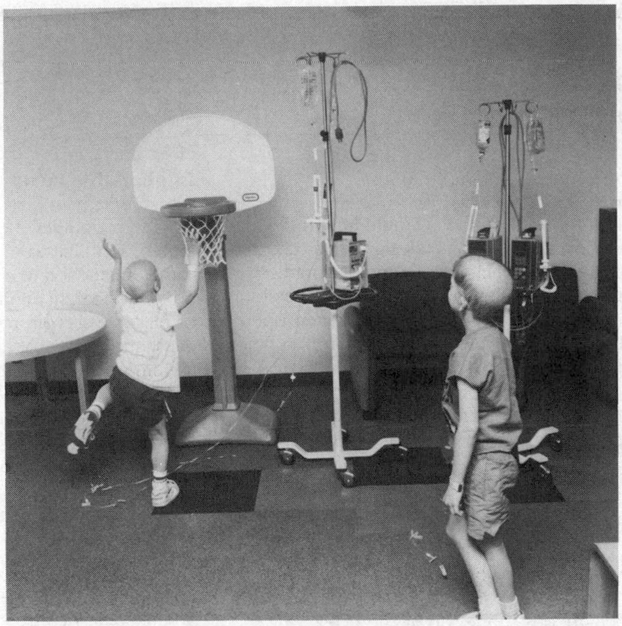

FIGURE 26-5. Children with central lines are free to be active. These children, each with a pump attached, have sufficiently long tubing, which gives them freedom to throw a basketball.

Central Venous Catheter Insertion and Care

Central venous access devices, whether fully implanted or with an external exit, are put into place while the patient is under local or general anesthesia. The position of the central venous catheter and implanted ports are confirmed by fluoroscopy or, more recently, by ECG (Hoffman et al, 1988), a method that reduces a child's exposure to radiation and is a much quicker technique. Protocols for catheter care are developed by individual institutions. Nurses receive special teaching to care for central lines, and, often, this is done by nurses on an IV team. Children with central lines are free to be mobile and push their pumps with them to participate in the many activities available on a children's unit (Fig. 26–5). General principles of catheter care are presented in Table 26–11, but many specific aspects of care may vary.

Generally, some form of daily or regular cleansing of the exit site is required with a sterile or clean dressing. In addition, most lines must be flushed daily with saline or a diluted heparin solution in order to ensure patency.

The dressing is taped occlusively with hypoallergic tape, dated, and signed. Part of the extension tubing should be looped and taped on top of the secured dressing to prevent direct tension on the catheter. There are numerous advantages and disadvantages of the implantable and nonimplantable devices. A comparison of central venous catheters and implantable venous access devices is presented in Table 26–12.

KEY CONCEPTS

Concepts Related to Basic Information

- The greater proportionate fluid volume and its internal distribution make an infant vulnerable to fluid and electrolyte imbalances.
- Infants have a proportionately greater volume of extracellular fluid (ECF) compared with older children and adults; ECF is lost first when losses occur, and ECF contains relatively more sodium and chloride during infancy compared with later in life.
- An infant's relative greater surface area to body mass results in a relatively higher volume of insensible water loss.
- Edema occurs with (1) increased capillary hydrostatic pressure; (2) decreased plasma oncotic pressure; (3) increased capillary permeability; and (4) increased interstitial oncotic pressure.
- *Isotonic dehydration* is a condition in which fluids and electrolytes are lost in approximately the same proportion; *hypertonic dehydration* is the result of a greater proportionate loss of water than sodium; and *hypotonic dehydration* is the result of water retention or loss of sodium.
- Ninety-five per cent of the body's potassium is found in intracellular fluid, and sodium is the chief extracellular ion.
- The acidity of body fluids is determined by hydrogen ion (H^+) concentration.
- The lungs, by regulating the P_{CO_2}, can compensate for changes in pH related to metabolic processes.
- The kidneys react to pH variations by regulating H^+ and bicarbonate concentrations.

Concepts Related to Nursing Assessment

- Fluid and electrolyte and acid-base balance are assessed by taking a relevant history, and by assessing vital signs, weight, skin, anterior fontanelles and eyes, intake and output, urine specific gravity, neurologic status, and reviewing relevant laboratory values, including arterial blood gases.
- The nurse assesses whether a child needs to be restrained for IV therapy (with the trend toward using IV catheters, children require fewer restraints).
- A total body fluid deficit is reflected in a high specific gravity of urine as the kidneys conserve fluid.

TABLE 26-12
Central Venous Access Devices*

		Tunneled Devices			
Device	**Percutaneous Devices**	**Hickman and Broviac**	**Groshong**	**Roko**	**Implantable Ports**
Description	Single-, double-, or triple-lumen devices; ratiopaque; stiff catheter; open ends; sutures at exit site anchor the catheter in place; each lumen is a separate identity	Single-, double-, or triple-lumen devices; radiopaque; soft Silastic catheter; open ends; two cuffs placed subcutaneously anchor the catheter and act as a bacterial barrier; each lumen is a separate identity	Single- or double-lumen devices; radiopaque; soft Silastic, clear catheter; closed end with 3-way slit valve; two cuffs placed subcutaneously anchor the catheter and act as a bacterial barrier; each lumen is a separate identity	Single-lumen device designed for use in infants; nonradiopaque; soft, flexible, clear catheter; open end; sutured in place at the venotomy site with grommets; local catheter used at Hospital for Sick Children, Toronto, and Chedoke-McMaster Hospitals	Single- or double-lumen; soft Silastic catheter attached to a stainless steel, titanium, or plastic reservoir; radiopaque; plastic or titanium reservoir is the only one that can be used with the MRI machine; septum is self-sealing; reservoir is sutured in place; needs special noncoring needles for accessing
Placement	The catheter is introduced via the jugular or subclavian vein, with the tip ending at the superior vena cava proximal to the right atrium (antecubital veins through cutdown or by venipuncture); the femoral vein may also be used as a site to introduce the catheter	The catheter is introduced via the jugular or subclavian veins, with the tip ending in the superior vena cava proximal to the right atrium; the catheter exits through a subcutaneous tunnel on to the chest			The catheter is introduced via the jugular or subclavian veins, with the tip ending in the superior vena cava proximal to the right atrium; the reservoir is placed and anchored in a subcutaneous pocket; this device is completely internal
Care of the devices					
Clamping	Side clamps on all catheters; to preserve the catheter, add a small extension with a clamp on it; use the clamps on the extension tubing; this tubing stays on for the life of the catheter, when possible	Roll clamps are on the catheter; the clamps are to be used only on the reinforced area; the clamps may need to be taped closed to keep them from opening	Clamps are not needed because of 3-way valve; increased patient safety because of minimal potential for old backflow or air embolism	There are no clamps on this catheter; a small extension stays on for the life of the catheter; the clamp on the extension is used; a bulldog clamp may be used on the catheter in emergencies	No clamps needed when not accessed; if accessed, the clamp on the small extension tubing attached to the needle is used
Dressing	Occlusive dressing, either transparent or gauze	Coil the line once under the dressing for the Hickman and Groshong		Occlusive dressing, either transparent or gauze; coil the line under the dressing	No dressing needed when the port is not accessed; when the port is accessed and the noncoring needle is left in place, an occlusive transparent or gauze dressing is used
Flushing	10 ml bacteriostatic saline daily per lumen or 5 ml heparin (10 U/ml) per lumen (p.r.n. or daily)	10 ml bacteriostatic saline p.r.n. or 5 ml heparin (10 U/ml) per lumen (p.r.n. or daily).		1–3 ml heparin (10 U/ml) daily or p.r.n.	3–5 ml heparin (100 U/ml) q 4–6 wks and p.r.n.

(continued)

TABLE 26-12
Central Venous Access Devices* *(Continued)*

Device	Percutaneous Devices	Tunneled Devices: Hickman and Broviac	Tunneled Devices: Groshong	Tunneled Devices: Roko	Implantable Ports
Advantages and disadvantages	Can be inserted at the bedside; for long-term in-hospital use; easily infected; breaks easily	Needs to be inserted in the operating room; may be used at home and in hospital; used in patients needing long-term IV treatments and will need frequent hospitalizations; not recommended to swim with these lines; causes a change in body image because the line is external; patients or family need to learn to do the dressing because they will be responsible for the dressing at home		Usually inserted in the operating room but may be inserted on the ward; rarely used at home; used in neonates who will need long-term IV infusions; breaks easily; no safe way to clamp the catheter long-term; nonradiopaque	No care needed at home when not accessed; needs to be inserted in the operating room; may be used at home and in hospital; used in patients needing long-term IV treatments and will need frequent hospitalizations; can swim with this line; does not change patient's body image because it is a totally internal line; good for 2000 needle pokes

Courtesy of Kris Paton, RN, and Adrienne Austin, RN, pediatric IV and central venous line nurses at Chedoke-McMaster Hospitals, McMaster Division, Hamilton, Ontario, Canada.

*All connections on central lines must be lumen "Luer-Loked."

- A normal urinary output is 1 ml/kg of body weight per hour.
- A major complication to prevent in peripheral IV administration is infiltration; assess for pain, swelling, tenderness, cool skin, and blanching and monitor pressures on the delivery machine.

Concepts Related to Nursing Intervention

- An important nursing responsibility is to teach parents to prevent fluid and electrolyte imbalances by avoiding overdressing, limiting time in the sun, and offering extra fluids during hot weather.
- Potassium can be safely added to IV fluids *only* after urinary flow has been established, because the primary site for secretion of potassium is the kidney.
- Administration of plain water in large amounts when a child is ill with vomiting and diarrhea can cause an electrolyte imbalance.
- The child and parents need to be prepared for the event of an IV start; the type of preparation varies with the age of the child.

REFERENCES

Avner, E. D., Ellis, P., Ichikawa, I., & Yared, A. (1990). Normal neonates and the maturational development of homeostatic mechanisms. In I. Ichikawa (Ed.). *Pediatric textbook of fluids and electrolytes* (pp 107–120). Baltimore: Williams & Wilkins.

Awazu, M., Devarajan, P., Stewart, C. L., Kaskel, F., & Ichikawa, I. (1990a). "Maintenance" therapy and treatment of dehydration and overhydration. In I. Ichikawa (Ed.). *Pediatric textbook of fluids and electrolytes* (pp 417–428). Baltimore: Williams & Wilkins.

Awazu, M., Kon, V., & Barakat, A. Y. (1990b). Volume disorders. In I. Ichikawa (Ed.). *Pediatric textbook of fluids and electrolytes* (pp 121–129). Baltimore: Williams & Wilkins.

Barakat, A. Y., & Ichikawa, I. (1990). Laboratory data. In I. Ichikawa (Ed.). *Pediatric textbook of fluids and electrolytes* (pp 478–500). Baltimore: Williams & Wilkins.

Carpenter, T. O., & Key, L. L., Jr. (1990). Disorders of the metabolism of calcium, phosphorus, and other divalent ions. In I. Ichikawa (Ed.). *Pediatric textbook of fluids and electrolytes* (pp 237–268). Baltimore: Williams & Wilkins.

Catchpole, M. (1982). Electrolytes, their physiological action and interaction: A review. *Association of Nursing Anesthetics, 50,* 476–481.

Chambers, T. L. (1987). Fluid therapy. In *Childhood*. Boston: Blackwell Scientific Publications.

Guhlow, L. J., & Kolb, J. (1979). Pediatric IVs: Special measures you must take. *RN, 42,* 40–51.

Hellerstein, S. (1993a). Fluid and electrolytes: Physiology. *Pediatrics in Review, 14*(2), 70–79.

Hellerstein, S. (1993b). Fluid and electrolytes: Clinical aspects. *Pediatrics in Review, 14*(3), 103–115.

Hoffman, M. A., Langer, J. C., Pearl, R. A., Wesson, D. E., Ein, S. H., Shandling, B., & Filler, R. M. (1988). Central venous catheters—No x-rays needed: A prospective study in 50 consecutive infants and children. *Journal of Pediatric Surgery, 23*(12), 1201–1203.

Holliday, M. A., & Segar, W. E. (1957). The maintenance need for water in parenteral fluid therapy. *Pediatrics, 19,* 823.

Ichikawa, I., Narins, R. G., & Harris, H. W., Jr. (1990). Acid-base disorders. In I. Ichikawa (Ed.). *Pediatric textbook of fluids and electrolytes* (pp 187–217). Baltimore: Williams & Wilkins.

Kaehny, W. D., & Gabow, P. A. (1980). Pathogenesis and management of metabolic acidosis and alkalosis. In R. W. Schrier (Ed.). *Renal and electrolyte disorders*. Boston: Little, Brown.

Metheney, N. M. (1992). *Fluid and electrolyte balance* (2nd ed.). Philadelphia: JB Lippincott.

O'Brien, D. (1980). Fluid and electrolyte therapy. In C. H. Kempe, H. K. Silver, & D. O'Brien (Eds.). *Current pediatric diagnosis and treatment*. Palo Alto, CA: Lange Medical Publications.

Robson, A. M. (1987). Parenteral fluid therapy. In R. E. Behrman, & V. C. Vaughan, III (Eds.). *Nelson textbook of pediatrics* (13th ed.). Philadelphia: WB Saunders.

Rose, B. D. (1984). *Clinical physiology of acid-base and electrolyte disorders*. New York: McGraw-Hill.

Schefler, A. G. (Ed.). (1992). *The HSC handbook of pediatrics* (8th ed.). St. Louis: Mosby Year Book.

Siegel, N. J., & Lattanzi, W. E. (1985). Fluid and electrolyte therapy in children. In A. I. Arieff & I. I. DeFronzo (Eds.). *Fluid electrolyte and acid-base disorders*, New York: Churchill Livingstone.

Winters, R. W. (Ed.) (1973). *The body fluids in pediatrics*. Boston: Little, Brown.

BIBLIOGRAPHY

Baker, D. L. (1990). Measuring outcome criteria: The intravenous nursing care plan. *Journal of Intravenous Nursing, 13*(4), 253–258.

Barkin, R. M. (1990). Treatment of the dehydrated child. *Pediatric Annals, 19*(10), 597–603.

Biggert, R. A., Watkins, J. L., & Crook, S. E. (1992). Home infusion service delivery system model: A conceptual framework for family-centered care in pediatric home care delivery. *Journal of Intravenous Nursing, 15*(4), 210–218.

Blatz, S., & Paes, B. A. (1990). Intravenous infusion by superficial vein in the neonate. *Journal of Intravenous Nursing, 13*(2), 122–128.

Brenner, M., & Welliver, J. (1990). Pulmonary and acid-base assessment. *Nursing Clinics of North America, 25*(4), 761–770.

Campbell, K. (1990). Pediatric home IV therapy. *Journal of Home Health Care Practice, 2*(4), 29–34.

Costarino, A., & Baumgart, S. (1986). Modern fluid and electrolyte management of the critically ill premature infant. *Pediatric Clinics of North America, 33*(1), 153–178.

Dunbar, S. B., Jarvis, A. H., & Breyer, M. (1991). The transition from nonoral to oral feeding in children. *American Journal of Occupational Therapy, 45*(5), 402–408.

Farrington, E. (1991). Treatment of hyperkalemia. *Pediatric Nursing, 17*(2), 190–192.

Halperin, D. L., Koren, G., Attias, D., Pellegrini, E., Greenberg, M. L., & Wyss, M. (1989). Topical skin anaesthesia for venous, subcutaneous drug reservoir and lumbar punctures in children. *Pediatrics, 84*(2), 281–284.

Hartsell, M. B. (1991). Home infusion pumps. *Journal of Pediatric Nursing, 6*(2), 134–136.

Holder, C., & Alexander, J. (1990). A new and improved guide to IV therapy. *American Journal of Nursing, 90*, 43–47.

Janusek, L. W. (1990). Metabolic pathophysiology, signs, and symptoms. *Nursing 90, 20*(7), 52–53.

Kandt, K. A. (1991). An implantable venous access device for children. *MCN: American Journal of Maternal Child Nursing, 16*, 88–91.

LaPook, J., & Fedorak, R. N. (1989). Oral rehydration therapy: WHO at 40, ORT at 30. *Canadian Journal of Gastroenterology, 3*(1), 7–14.

Lenox, A. C. (1990). IV therapy: Reducing the risk of infection. *Nursing 90, 20*(3), 60–61.

Lynam, L. E. (1990). Acid-base basics. *Neonatal Network, 9*(1), 67–68.

Marcoux, C., Fisher, S., & Wong, D. (1990). Central venous access devices in children. *Pediatric Nursing, 16*(2), 123–133.

McKee, J. (1991). Future dimensions in vascular access: Peripheral implantable ports. *Journal of Intravenous Nursing, 14*(6), 387–392.

Millam, D. A. (1990). Controlling the flow: Electronic infusion devices. *Nursing 90, 20*(8), 65–68.

Moss, J. R., & Craft, M. J. (1990). Accurate assessment of infant emesis volume. *Pediatric Nursing, 16*(5), 455–457.

Oellrich, R. G., Murphy, M. R., Goldberg, L. A., & Aggarwal, R. (1991). The percutaneous central venous catheter for small or ill infants. *MCN: American Journal of Maternal Child Nursing, 16*(2), 92–96.

Saavedra, J. M., Harris, G. D., Li, S., & Finberg, L. (1991). Capillary refilling (skin turgor) in the assessment of dehydration. *American Journal of Diseases of Children, 145*, 296–298.

Schaeffer, A. V., & Ditchek, S. (1991). Current social practices leading to water intoxication in infants. *American Journal of Diseases of Children, 145*, 27–28.

Taylor, J., Shannon, R., & Kilbride, H. W. (1989). Heparin lock intravenous line: Use in newborn infants. A controlled trial. *Clinical Pediatrics, 28*(5), 237–240.

Tietjen, S. D. (1990). Starting an infant's IV. *American Journal of Nursing, 90*, 44–47.

Weinstein, S. M. (1990). Math calculations for intravenous nurses. *Journal of Intravenous Nursing, 13*(4), 231–236.

Whitney, R. G. (1991). Comparing long-term central venous catheters. *Nursing 91, 21*(4), 70–71.

Zimmerman, E. (1991). The landry vein light: Increasing venipuncture success rates. *Journal of Pediatric Nursing, 6*(1), 64–66.

UNIT • SIX

Developmental-Behavioral Health Concerns

CHAPTER • 27

Understanding Altered Development

NURSING PROCESS PLAN
NPP, Long-Term Care of the Infant at Risk, Table 27–5

RELATED TOPICS
Impact of chronic illness, Chapter 19
Conduct disorders, Chapter 29
Genetic assessment, Chapter 31
Patterns of inheritance in trisomy 21, Chapter 31

LEARNING OBJECTIVES

- Compare and contrast the unique features of the diagnostic term "developmental disability" with other medical conditions.
- Explain the use of interdisciplinary assessments in the identification and care of the child with developmental disabilities.
- Describe the federal legislation and service system designed to promote the civil rights of individuals with developmental disabilities.
- Identify the purpose and function of early intervention programs.
- Describe the common nursing diagnostic statements and collaborative problems the nurse might consider in the care of the child with mental retardation.
- Apply nursing care interventions discussed to clinical practice situations involving children with mental retardation.
- Recognize the long-term impact of having a child with a developmental disability on the functioning of the family, both collectively and individually.

Nurses may work with children with developmental disabilities and their families in a variety of settings, including hospitals, clinics, physicians' offices, schools, community agencies, and the family's home. By using the nursing process, nurses play an important role in each of these settings. Although nursing interventions will vary depending on the nature of the child's disability, there are some commonalities in assessment and intervention with these children and their families. This chapter includes a discussion of some of these commonalities as well as of some of the specific interventions for selected disabilities.

Developmental Alterations

The Developmental Disabilities Act of 1978 (and Developmental Disabilities Assistance and Bill of Rights Amendment of 1987) defined a "developmental disability" as a severe chronic state that is present before the individual is 22 years of age and is likely to continue indefinitely. The disability may be caused by either a physical or a mental impairment, or a combination of the two. The person with a developmental disability has substantial limitations in at least three of the following major life activities: self-care, receptive and expressive language, learning, mobility, self-direction, capacity for independent living, and economic self-sufficiency. The person requires individually planned and coordinated interdisciplinary care, treatment, or other services for an extended period of time or throughout his or her life.

This definition of developmental disability is a unique entity. First and foremost, unlike the diagnostic labels given to illness disorders and conditions by medical, allied, and health sciences, this condition has been *legislatively* described by the United States Congress. Second, it is an umbrella term used to categorize many different types of disabilities. Erroneously, a developmental disability may be equated with mental retardation. A person may be considered to have a developmental disability and not be cognitively impaired. A child with cerebral palsy is such an example. Lastly, the state definition of a developmental disability may not be as broadly defined as the federal definition, resulting in fewer numbers of individuals considered eligible for services. For example, in California, over 108,000 individuals meet the state definition; many more could be considered eligible for services if the federal definition were used. Table 27–1 contains a selected listing of conditions that would meet the federal definition of being a developmental disability.

TABLE 27-1
Conditions Considered Developmental Disabilities

Autism
Cerebral palsy
Epilepsy
Learning disabilities
Mental retardation
Multiple handicapping conditions
Speech impaired
Emotionally disturbed
Orthopedically impaired
Visually handicapped
Deaf-blind
Hard of hearing or deaf
Chronic medical diseases
Spinal cord injuries
Stroke
Genetic disorders:
Autosomal dominant (tuberous sclerosis)
Autosomal recessive (phenylketonuria, galactosemia, Tay-Sachs disease)
X-linked recessive (Fragile X)
Multifactorial (meningomyelocele)
Chromosome disorders
(Prader-Willi syndrome, Down syndrome)
Environmental
(fetal alcohol effects, fetal rubella effects)
Sporadic syndromes—etiology unknown
(Noonan syndrome, Williams syndrome)

A developmental alteration is a variation from what is classified as "normal development" for an individual. No child is 100 per cent normal; in fact, no person is 100 per cent normal. As children grow and develop, they establish and refine a set of strengths and weaknesses that is uniquely their own. Many different patterns of strengths, weaknesses, and behaviors can be classified as "normal." The term "normal" is in itself difficult to define because it is to some extent developmentally, culturally, and socially determined. This chapter includes information about children who have experienced the following developmental alterations: developmental delays, cerebral palsy, learning disabilities, and mental retardation.

Scientists and theorists have attempted to account for the development of the human being using many different approaches. Some theorists are proponents of a strong genetic explanation, whereas others have an environmental bias. Most theorists, however, generally agree that development is a combination of both genetic and environmental influences. We have learned that a person may be genetically programmed to achieve all that is deemed normal, but be subjected to social environments that can produce pathologic problems. The right social environments, on the other hand, can produce normal or near-normal outcomes for those individuals with developmental disabilities. This principle of normal development applies to individuals both with and without disabilities (Anastasiow, 1986). Although the development of children with disabilities may be slower than those without disabilities, they *will* develop. Children with such problems may need only therapies, training, or prostheses to enhance their development. The environment needed by children without disabilities to reach their fullest potential is also beneficial to children with disabilities.

On July 26, 1990, the Americans with Disabilities Act (PL101–336) was signed into law. The Americans with Disabilities Act (ADA) extends to individuals with disabilities the civil rights afforded to all citizens regardless of race, sex, national origin, or religion.

TABLE 27-2
Key Provisions of the Americans with Disabilities Act (PL 101–336)

Prohibits discrimination against workers and job applicants with disabilities in businesses employing 15 or more individuals
Prohibits discrimination against customers by businesses open to the public such as stores, parks, schools, and stadiums
Interstate and intrastate telecommunications relay services must be made available by telephone companies for persons with disabilities
Accessible systems of publicly and privately funded transportation must be available for individuals with disabilities

The provisions of the ADA prohibit discrimination based on disability in public and private sector employment, public accommodations, and transportation services. The key provisions of the ADA are summarized in Table 27–2.

History and Physical Examination

A complete physical examination is needed to uncover any physical problems associated with the child's developmental alteration. Initially an infant or child suspected of having a developmental disability or who is at risk for developing a developmental disability is referred for more comprehensive assessment procedures. Screening procedures determine whether a developmental alteration exists. A comprehensive assessment would include the collection of data related to the genetic and health history of the child and family members and information about the environmental, behavioral, and social factors affecting the child and family.

Of particular importance on physical examination is evidence of deviation of normal growth patterns, physical stigmata, and congenital defects. The examination will cover respiratory, cardiac, renal, neurologic, perceptual, and motor problems. In infants under 6 months of age, it is especially important to observe for asymmetric movements and the expected disappearance of primitive reflexes. Also important to note are abnormalities of gait, symmetry of muscle tone, and deep tendon reflexes as well as the presence of intact cerebellar and sensory functions (Blackman, 1990).

Children with developmental alterations may have physical problems related to genetics, such as diabetes, sickle cell anemia, or cystic fibrosis. Other problems may be the result of congenital malformations, such as cardiac, neurologic, and musculoskeletal conditions. Developmental alterations may also be the result of environmental problems, such as lead poisoning, and infections, such as rubella or tuberculosis. More recently, developmental alterations have been associated with children who have AIDS.

Children with alterations in development are usually followed by a pediatrician or a physician in family practice. The physician will then establish a plan of treatment that may include referral to an agency or another professional, such as a neurologist or cardiologist.

Diagnostic Assessment

Throughout the assessment process, the nurse's role is to establish baseline measurements, gather data, give support to the child and parents, and help the family receive the appropriate services in the community. The nurse's role includes observation of the child, administration of screening tests, recording and reporting observations and results of screening, and making appropriate referrals.

Assessment of the Child in the Hospital

Nurses in hospital settings will be working with children of all ages with developmental alterations. Assessments are essential in order to detect infants who are at risk for developmental alterations. Such alterations would also constitute nursing diagnostic responses of *altered or ineffective growth and development*. A series of head measurements provides one important indicator of future problems in mental and physical development. Feeding behaviors and social-behavioral parameters are also good indicators of potential risk. If possible, auditory and visual screening should be done before the infant is discharged from the nursery.

Caesar and Eggermont (1985) summarize the "alarm signs" that should alert the nurse and other professionals to infants who are at risk for neonatal neurologic problems. These signs include infants who have difficulty feeding, continuously fuss, or persistently display abnormal eye or head positions or asymmetry in posture or movements. Other risk factors are: (1) immobility, (2) apathy, (3) floppiness, (4) hyperexcitability, (5) convulsions, (6) abnormal cry sounds, and (7) abnormal head measurements. When an infant is noted to have any of these problems, all neural functions that are testable should be evaluated, using tests that are appropriate for that infant's gestational age. Although nurses may do some of the baseline neurologic screening, the neurologist/developmentalist will do further testing.

The child's physical characteristics, treatments, x-rays, and laboratory test results should all be recorded. The results of neurologic and other testing should be noted and any changes that occur should be explained carefully. These records will be invaluable to the team who will follow the child after discharge.

Although the neonatal period is a critical time for central nervous system damage, perinatal hazards are responsible for only 15 to 20 per cent of severe de-

TABLE 27-3
Diagnostic Assessment: Developmental Function

Tool	Description
Early Screening Inventory (ESI)	Screening tool used to identify children ages 3–6 yrs for further evaluation; a Spanish version is available
Gesell Developmental Schedules (1940)	Assesses development in children from 1 mo to 6 yrs in following areas: adaptive, fine motor, gross motor, personal-social, and language
Smith-John Non-Verbal Performance Scale (1984)	Observational tool used to observe tasks performed by preschoolers ages 2–4 yrs; nonverbal test
Bayley Scales of Infant Development (1969)	Widely used scale to measure infant development; mental scales measure shape discrimination, sustained attention, imitation, etc; motor scales measure gross and fine motor abilities
Kaufman Assessment Battery for Children (KABC) (1983)	Measures mental processing composite (MPC) and achievement; used to assess children ages 2.6 to 12.6 yrs; norms are provided for culturally diverse children
McCarthy Scales of Children's Abilities (1972)	Assesses general level of intellectual functioning; measures verbal ability, nonverbal ability, number aptitude, short-term memory, and motor coordination
Peabody Picture Vocabulary Test (PPVT-R) (1981)	Assesses changes in receptive vocabulary; administered for ages 2.6 yrs to adult
Test of Early Language Development (TELD) (1981)	Assesses receptive and expressive syntax and morphology; used for ages 3–8 yrs
Sequenced Inventory of Communication Development (SICD)	Measures communication development in children ages 4 to 48 mos
Child Behavior Checklist (Achenbach) (1986)	Records behavior problems and competencies in children ages 2 yrs and above
Joseph Pre-School and Primary Self-Concept Screening Test (1979)	Assesses self-concept in preschoolers with disabilities ages 3.6 to 9 yrs
Vineland Adaptive Behavior Scales (1984)	Measures adaptive behavior needed for self sufficiency; areas assessed are (1) communication, (2) daily living, (3) socialization, and (4) nondevelopment; used from birth to 18 yrs, 11 mos
Scales of Independent Behavior (SIB) (1984)	Measures adaptive behavior in 4 areas: motor skills, personal living skills, community living skills, and social and communication skills. Age ranges from birth on
Adaptive Performance Instrument (API) (1980)	Measures functional abilities in severely disabled infants and children from birth to 9 yrs; assesses self-care, fine and gross motor abilities, reflexes and reactions, social behavior, communication, and physical interactions
Home Observation Measurement of the Environment (HOME) (1984)	Measures environmental support the child receives in the home; assesses parental discipline and involvement with the child; two inventory forms exist: infants and toddlers and preschoolers (3–6)
Stanford-Binet (4th ed.) (1985)	Measures IQ of children from age 2 yrs to adulthood; involves manipulation of objects and eye-hand coordination, vocabulary, sentence completion, and analogies
Wechsler Intelligence Scale for Children Revised (WISC-R) Wechsler Preschool and Primary Scale of Intelligence (WPPSI)	WISC-R (ages 5 to 15 yrs) and WPPSI (ages 4 to 7) measure intelligence; they cover verbal and performance subtest areas of information, comprehension, arithmetic, similarities, digit span, and vocabulary

(continued)

TABLE 27-3
Diagnostic Assessment: Developmental Function *(Continued)*

Tool	Description
Brazelton Neonatal Behavioral Assessment Scale	Includes some aspects of a neurologic test but is not a neurologic examination; it is best used as a tool to assess infant interactive behavior; useful in working with high-risk infants; requires special training for use
Denver Developmental Screening Test (DDST)	Used to identify developmental lags in children from 2 wks to 6 yrs; areas observed are personal-social, fine motor-adaptive, gross motor, and fine motor skills; reliability and validity have been demonstrated; a Spanish DDST is available
Fathering Behavior	Designed to guide nurses in observing fathers' adaptive and maladaptive behaviors; useful in observations of high-risk situations (e.g., divorce with the father in custody of the child, child abuse situations, or parent drug abuse situations)
Portage Guide to Early Development	A check list used to measure behaviors and skills of children from birth to 6 yrs; cognitive development and motor skills
School/Home Observation and Referral System (SHORS)	A general check list to observe a child for unusual behaviors in comparison to peers; for children from preschool through third grade; areas to be checked are health, motor, vision, hearing, speech, language, behavior, and learning

velopmental disabilities. Because environmental, genetic, and socioeconomic factors are responsible for 80 to 85 per cent of the damage, the child is at risk for central nervous system insults up to 2 years of age while growth of the brain is still occurring (Caesar & Eggermont, 1985). Usually, major neurologic defects are identified within the first year of life. In some rural areas, where there is no ready access to medical care, children's disabilities may not be identified until after this time period. Some disorders, such as hydrocephalus, are usually diagnosed before the third month of life, whereas others, such as cerebral palsy, may not be diagnosed until toward the end of the first year (Amiel-Tison, 1985). Some neuromotor abnormalities are transient in nature, and those persons assessing the child need to be aware of this possibility, especially in the case of very low birthweight infants.

Assessment of the Child in the Community

Usually, it is a parent or relative who first notes the presence of a problem or a difference in the child. Sometimes, a routine screening by a teacher, nurse, or member of the child's health team will reveal the first indication of a problem. All young children should be screened on a yearly basis. This screening should cover general health; auditory, visual, speech, and motor development; self-help skills; behavior; and learning or thinking. Screening may be carried out by interdisciplinary professionals in conjunction with day care providers. The medical screening may be performed by a nurse practitioner or physician. Auditory screening may be done by a nurse, audiologist, speech pathologist, or health aide (provided the aide has had special training to use an audiometer). Speech screening is usually done by a speech pathologist or therapist. Various types of screening tools can be used, such as observation check lists and commercially prepared screening instruments (Copeland & Kimmel, 1989).

Screening Tools and Observation Checklists

Nurses need to be familiar with some of the commercially prepared screening tools. Nurses may be involved in administering these tools and helping parents understand the results of the screening. These tools are used to indicate whether more definitive testing is required. *Screening is not done to measure the child's intelligence or to make a diagnosis; it is used to define a potential problem and to indicate a child's areas of strengths and weaknesses.* Some of the more common tools are listed in Table 27–3. Selection of screening tools depends on many factors, such as whether behavior or intelligence is being tested, the age of the child, cultural limitations, and the amount of training required for proficiency in its administration.

It is often difficult to use the more common intelligence tests for children with disabilities. Some tests specifically devised for these children are the Nebraska Test of Learning Aptitude for the hearing impaired, the Perkins-Binet Intelligence Scale for the visually impaired, and the Columbia Mental Maturity Scale for those with motor and language impairments. The Merrill-Palmer Scale of Mental Tests has been adapted for children who are both speaking and hearing impaired.

Check lists can be useful tools in identifying potential problems at an early age. If the nurse asks the caregiver (e.g., mother, teacher) to observe behaviors and activities, the caregiver is provided with a check list and instructions for its use. Research indicates that mothers and professionals show consistent results in their assessments of a child's development if the parent has been instructed in the same strategies used by the professional (Beckman, 1984). There are commercially prepared observation checklists, such as the Home Observation Measurement of the Environment (HOME). This tool, developed by Caldwell and Bradley, measures the environmental support the child receives in the home. It is a check list of responsibilities related to the primary caregiver and other items, such as the environment, discipline, and involvement with the child. Reliability and validity have been demonstrated. (See Appendix 5.)

The following guidelines should be followed by the caregiver when using an observational screening tool:

1. Keep an accurate description of what the child says or does during the observational period.
2. Observe the child on several different occasions to be absolutely sure the behavior you describe is a typical one.
3. Date each observation.
4. Write down exactly what is seen and heard, rather than making statements based on opinion. Objectiveness in reporting is essential.
5. In making referrals, be specific and clear about concerns and tell why the referral is being made.

Most of the observation or screening tools can be completed by teachers, health professionals, specially trained aides, or, in some cases, parents. A more definitive assessment must be done only by qualified professionals. When a child is referred to the appropriate professionals, a thorough assessment is done in an attempt to locate the problem area and to make a diagnosis. The diagnosis is made not on the basis of one test, but usually after a battery of tests is completed. This is done to ensure against labeling a child with a wrong diagnosis and condemning her or him to a lifetime of stigma and inappropriate interventions. The tests used to further assess the child will be in the areas of intellectual, emotional, behavioral, social, physical, and language skills.

Behavioral Assessment

It is important to assess children for changes in behavior and self-care activities such as toileting and eating behaviors. The child with developmental alterations may experience an improvement or deterioration in an existing problem. Skills of daily living can also be included in a form. Analysis of these data will assist the nurse and other health professionals in taking appropriate actions for correct interventions in the child's health care.

Family Assessment

After the findings of the comprehensive evaluation are analyzed, an assessment of the child's environment is made to determine its adequacy for meeting the child's safety and special needs. The parents' perceptions of the child's condition, their expectations from treatment, and their beliefs about the child's prognosis need to be determined. Assessment of

TABLE 27-4
Levels of Assessment Activities

	Purpose	Personnel	Activities
Child Find	To create awareness of typical and atypical child development among the general public	State personnel, public health professionals, volunteers, community members, early childhood personnel, parents, caregivers	Census taking, posters, brochures, media publicity
Developmental and Health Screening	To identify children who may need further diagnostic assessment	Professionals, parents, lay professionals	Administration of screening instruments, medical examinations, hearing & vision testing, parent questionnaires, and review of records
Diagnostic Assessment	To determine existence of delay or disability, to identify child and family strengths and needs, and to propose possible strategies for interventions	Multidisciplinary team of educators, psychologists, parents, clinicians, physicians, social workers, therapists, nurses	Formal testing, parent interview, home observation, team meetings
Individual Program Planning	To determine individual educational family services plan, program placement, and remedial activities	Parents, teachers, assessment team personnel, other professionals	Home and/or program observation, informal assessment, development of remedial objectives

Adapted from Meisels, S., & Provence, S. (1989). *Screening and assessment. Guidelines for identifying young disabled and developmentally vulnerable children and families.* Washington, DC: National Center for Clinical Infant Programs.

parental coping and ability to provide for the child's special needs is made. Involvement and support of all family members are ascertained. Availability of resources within the family's kinship network and in the community is determined as well (Seligman, 1991). This becomes an ongoing process throughout assessment and intervention. The nurse, along with other health care providers, will be involved in obtaining this information and helping the family deal with the problems they are facing (Failla et al, 1991).

The parent who has been dashing about with a child from one appointment to another must have a thorough explanation of all the findings and recommendations for intervention. The possible negative outcomes of the planned intervention should be discussed, along with the anticipated positive outcomes.

Therapeutic Management

Intake Procedures

A thorough assessment of the child and family is essential before an intervention program can be instituted. The assessment by use of screening tools, discussed previously, should lead to identification of children who are likely or at risk to be developmentally delayed. Some experts refer to this process as "child find" (Meisels & Provence, 1989) in early intervention programs (Table 27–4). The next step is a comprehensive evaluation by diagnosticians, such as physicians; audiologists; physical, speech, and occupational therapists; psychologists; community health and pediatric nurses; nutritionists; social workers; and special education specialists. This evaluation should include a complete physical examination with a system review, visual and auditory screening, educational assessment, laboratory and genetic testing, assessment of nutritional status and practices, anthropometric measurements, family history and pedigree, neurodevelopmental evaluations, normal 24-hour biorhythmic routine, and a dental assessment. (See Fig. 27–1 for an example of service delivery.)

Once the child's health status has been stabilized, a primary health care provider or case manager should be selected. This primary health care provider or case manager is responsible for ensuring that the child receives preventive care according to the standards of the American Academy of Pediatrics (AAP). This care includes early identification of acute and chronic problems and ongoing health interventions. Referrals that are developmentally appropriate should be made as soon as possible. A common element in all treatment is the need for an interdisciplinary approach to provide all aspects of the diverse treatment required and an ongoing evaluation.

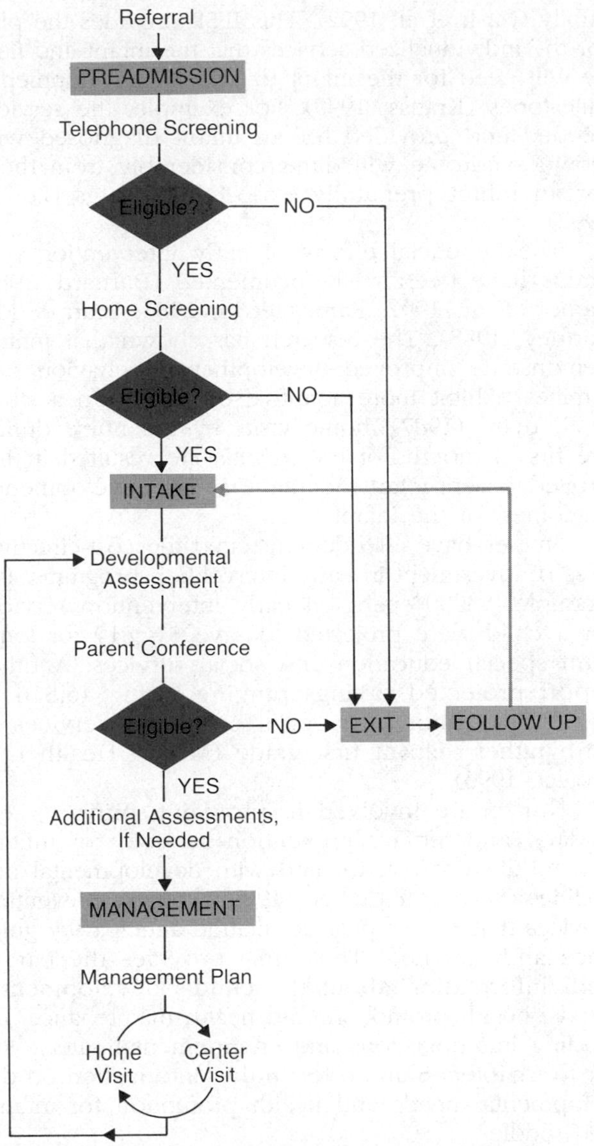

FIGURE 27-1. Flow chart of service delivery. (Reprinted with permission of D. Sue Schafer, Director, *Child success through parent training: A final report 1980–1983*. Denton, TX: Texas Woman's University School of Physical Therapy, p 15.)

Early Intervention Programs

Early intervention refers "to educational and therapeutic services provided for infants and toddlers between birth and 3 years of age who have been identified as biologically or environmentally at risk for developmental delay" (Savage & Culbert, 1989, p 339).

Early intervention services are provided by an interdisciplinary team of specialists. These specialists include language and speech therapists, occupational and physical therapists, psychologists, special education teachers, social workers, and nurses. Each of these team members conducts his or her own discipline-specific evaluation and assessment of the infant and family. Once the assessment data have been collected, the team meets and collaboratively develops an individualized family service plan (IFSP) with the family (Nash et al, 1992). This IFSP provides the plan for the individualized services that the infant and family will need for the infant to achieve developmental milestones (Krauss, 1990). For example, the services needed and provided for an infant diagnosed with Down syndrome will differ considerably from those for an infant prenatally exposed to drugs (Lewis, 1992).

The beneficial effects of early intervention programs have been well documented (Barnard, 1987; Ramey et al, 1992; Ramey et al, 1985; Scarr & McCartney, 1988). The research has shown that infants demonstrate improved developmental behaviors and families exhibit more adaptive behaviors. In a study by Barnard (1987), home visits by the nurse during the first 3 months of the infant's life resulted in improved parent-infant adaptation and developmental outcomes for the infant.

Studies have also demonstrated the cost-effectiveness of investment in early intervention programs. For example, $3000 spent on early intervention services for a child were projected to save $14,819 for long-term special education and social services. Another report projected savings ranging from $46,816 to $53,340 by initiating special education services at birth rather than at first grade (Mental Health Law Project, 1990).

Nurses are involved in providing primary, secondary, and tertiary prevention services for infants and toddlers at risk for and with developmental disabilities (Savage & Culbert, 1989). Primary prevention services that nurses provide include anticipatory guidance and teaching. The nurse provides the parent with information about the child's developmental needs, health promotion, and health maintenance, including immunizations and environmental safety. Refer to Chapters 5 and 6 for further information on developmental needs and health promotion for infants and toddlers.

Secondary prevention activities involving the nurse center on the identification and monitoring of families with a child at risk for a developmental disability. A public health nurse, school nurse, or pediatric nurse working in a community setting may identify an infant or toddler, through screening procedures, who warrants further assessment. Early identification and treatment of problems and risk factors will serve to minimize or alleviate the potential or actual problems (Lewis, 1992).

Nursing interventions make up the tertiary level of prevention. The nurse is in the ideal position to continuously assess children and parents participating in early intervention programs for health problems. The nurse can intervene when appropriate to promote child and family long-term adaptation and adjustment. The Nursing Process Plan "Long-Term Care of the Infant at Risk" (Table 27–5) discusses the nursing care issues associated in the care of the infant at risk.

The primary goal of early intervention programs is to reduce or minimize the incidence of developmental disabilities. This aim is achieved by providing structured learning experiences that foster the infant's and toddler's attainment of developmental milestones. Particular attention is directed to the needs of the family, whose participation in early intervention services are essential. Support and instruction are provided to families regarding parent-child interactions, growth and development, and parenting skills (Lewis, 1992).

Several types of early intervention programs exist: center-based, home-based, and combinations of both. In center-based programs, individual and group therapies are provided to the child and parent within the facility. In home-based programs, the early intervention therapist provides services within the home environment. Programs with combinations of home- and center-based services are adjusted to meet the needs of the child and family.

Early intervention programs have a variety of philosophic and theoretical bases. Programs that are the most effective seem to have several common components: (1) intervention beginning at a very early age, (2) the inclusion of parents as full participants in their child's program, and (3) involvement of a number of disciplines in diagnosing and planning for each child. These three elements seem to be the key to providing a program that has long-range and lasting effects (AAP, 1992).

Full Inclusion

"Full Inclusion" (an expansion of the "mainstreaming" policy) means helping people who have disabilities to learn to work in settings in which they will have the greatest opportunity to become as independent and productive as possible. In the school system, full inclusion refers to the grouping of all children with or without disabilities at the same grade level and in the same classrooms. The main purpose of fully inclusive student scheduling is to eliminate the dichotomy between special education classes and regular educational programs.

The passage of the Education for All Handicapped Children, Public Law 94–142, of 1975 ushered into existence sweeping reforms in the field of special education. Among the reforms mandated were guidelines for the rights of children with disabilities and their families. These protections included nondiscrimination testing, individualized education programs (IEP), and the concept of the "least restrictive environment," referring to the process of including students with disabilities in nondisabled settings whenever possible instead of limiting them to segregated sites. Although mainstreaming is an established practice in special education, the outcomes are still being evaluated (Hecht & Forness, 1988; Forness & Kavale, 1989). Recently, the US Circuit Court of Appeals ruled that provisions of PL 99–142 extended rights to all children no matter how severely disabled (Commu-

TABLE 27-5

Nursing Process Plan: Long-Term Care of the Infant at Risk

Analysis: Nursing Diagnostic Statement 1

Response and Related or Risk Factors: *High risk for altered growth and development: physical, intellectual, emotional/social; risk factors:*

- Physical, intellectual, and emotional/social risk factors (see Table 27–11, Risk Factors for Developmental Delay)
- Decreased environmental stimulation associated with decreased mobility and decreased energy for exploration
- Increased environmental stimulation related to overstimulation associated with hospitalization and intrusive painful treatment
- Alterations in bonding associated with parental adjustments to the diagnoses and treatment; parent-infant separations due to hospitalization
- Parental feelings of powerlessness, being overwhelmed
- Parental overprotection associated with real or perceived vulnerability of the child and possible environmental risks

Projected Outcome: The infant will achieve developmentally appropriate milestones as evidenced by progress noted on standardized methods to measure development

Defining Characteristics *(Actual Response)*	Nursing Interventions	Evaluation Criteria
Subjective: • Parent(s) reports infant is behind in developmental milestones, asks whether infant will catch up	**Assess infant from the interdisciplinary perspective in domains of physical, intellectual, and emotional/social development utilizing standardized instruments.** The infant is monitored for acquisition and achievement of developmental milestones	Any developmental delays will be identified as evidenced by a charted assessment of screening for physical, intellectual, and emotional/social development
Objective: • Delay or difficulty in performing skills (motor, social, or expressive) typical of age group • Inability to perform gross and fine motor tasks appropriate to age • Altered physical growth	**Refer to early intervention program for development stimulation interventions.** A treatment program is designed to meet the individual needs of the infant as it relates to sensorimotor, cognitive, and communicative skills	The infant will not experience developmental delays as evidenced by acquisition of developmental milestones as indicated by assessment tools The infant will continue with the prescribed therapy program to promote developmental progress
	Implement and reinforce intervention protocol. Members of the interdisciplinary intervention team will devise a protocol individualized to meet the developmental needs of the infant	
	Parent Education: Childrearing Family **Assess parental knowledge of developmental tasks.** Identify with parents and accountable family members infant's capabilities,	

(continued)

TABLE 27-5 *(continued)*

Defining Characteristics *(Actual Response)*	Nursing Interventions	Evaluation Criteria
	competencies, and anticipated outcomes of intervention strategies. Collaborate with family members in planning and implementing strategies to maintain and promote development **Collaborate with other team members to plan and implement intervention protocol. Facilitate implementation of intervention protocol at home to promote development.** Instruct parents and accountable family members on intervention techniques to be done at home; evaluate learning and reinforce teaching as indicated **Evaluate continually infant's developmental progress.** Provide emotional support to parents as means of alleviating anxiety **Help the parent(s) identify major fears pertaining to the infant's condition and explore any feelings of guilt they may have.** (Anxiety and guilt often lead to overprotection) • Written material on parenting can be a helpful adjunct and may be less personally threatening to parents. (Issues of parenting are delicate areas to approach with parents who are already stressed and who may hold cultural and social values about parenting that differ from the nurse's) • Use an appropriate opportunity to discuss the crucial parenting roles at each stage of childhood. See Chapter 12 • Allow parent(s) ample opportunity to explore how they can provide maximum freedom for their child to develop to her or his fullest potential while still keeping her or him safe • Demonstrate safe ways to assist their child in motor skill attainment	

TABLE 27-5 (continued)

Analysis: Nursing Diagnostic Statement 2

Response and Related or Risk Factors: *Ineffective family coping: temporary impairment of problem-solving abilities, related to:*

- Parent's negative perception of the diagnosis of an actual or potential developmental disability
- Lack of available coping techniques
- Lack of appropriate support systems

Projected Outcome: Parents will provide sufficient, effective, and uncompromised support, comfort, assistance, and encouragement so that the infant will have optimal resources to master adaptive tasks as he or she grows and develops

Defining Characteristics	Nursing Interventions	Evaluation Criteria
Subjective: • Parents describe preoccupation with personal reaction (e.g., fear, anticipatory grief, guilt, anxiety) to child's illness • Parents describe or confirm an inadequate understanding or knowledge base that interferes with effective assistive or supportive behaviors *Objective*: • Parents attempt assistive or supportive behaviors with less than satisfactory results • Parents display protective behavior disproportionate (too little or too much) to the child's abilities or need for autonomy	*Family Support* **Encourage ventilation of feelings about the diagnoses.** • Employ active listening techniques (see Chapter 11) • Validate expression of feelings as valid • Avoid interjecting personal bias • Recognize the pervasive emotional impact of the diagnosis upon the parents **Recognize denial as a common defense mechanism in the first weeks after diagnosis** • Repeat information in simple terms as often as necessary • Provide written information whenever possible. (Materials that can be read at home can help persons incorporate the reality of the diagnosis and generate questions) *Grief Work Facilitation* **Recognize grief as a common reaction to diagnosis.** The parents must deal with loss of the expected healthy infant and must incorporate, instead, the reality of the actual or potential diagnosis of developmental disability **Acknowledge that delays or failure in achieving developmental milestones will reactivate feelings of parental grief.** (The infant's inability to attain milestones	Family members will demonstrate ability to cope with infant's actual or potential diagnosis by • Identification and expression of feelings • Communicating with relatives and friends about the diagnosis • Provision of assistive and supportive care to the child effectively

(continued)

TABLE 27-5 *(continued)*

Defining Characteristics	Nursing Interventions	Evaluation Criteria
	within developmentally appropriate periods of time will remind parents of loss of "idealized" child) *Coping Enhancement* **Facilitate efforts toward problem-focused coping** • Ask if the client has considered how to tell relatives and friends about the diagnosis. Discuss ways to disseminate accurate information • Discuss with the parents age-appropriate ways to tell sibling(s) about the diagnosis. Caution parents that siblings may perceive themselves responsible if they had mixed emotions about the new infant *Supportive System Enhancement* • Help the client to identify family strengths and known resources for emotional, physical, and financial support • Refer parents/siblings to community-based self-help groups. (Self-help groups provide opportunities for family members to provide and elicit support from others with similar experiences. Parents gather relevant information about intervention protocols, community resources, and strategies to enhance coping and dealing with challenges of the infant's condition) **Assess the need for referral for individual counseling or marital counseling.** (Some individuals will need more in-depth help to cope with the impact of diagnosis and its implications for future life changes. Spouses may react differently and experience discordant coping and disrupted communication patterns as a potential threat to the marital relationship)	

TABLE 27-5 *(continued)*

Analysis: Nursing Diagnostic Statement 3

Response and Related or Risk Factors: *Spiritual distress (child and family), related to:*

- Worry associated with the prognosis and potential reactions to therapy
- A search for the meaning of life
- Feelings of guilt associated with the etiology or delay between onset of the condition and diagnosis
- Powerlessness associated with the uncertainty of the prognosis

Projected Outcomes: Family demonstrates continued belief in the life principle, which pervades each member's being and which integrates and transcends the biologic and psychologic nature of the family

Defining Characteristics

Subjective:

- Verbalization of concern with the meaning of life/death and/or belief systems
- Verbalization of inner conflict about beliefs
- Verbalization of concern about relationship with deity
- Verbalization of anger and resentment toward deity
- Questions meaning of child's suffering

Objective:

- Unable to participate in usual religious practices
- Seeks spiritual assistance
- "Gallows humor"
- Displacement of anger toward religious representatives
- Description of nightmares/sleep disturbances
- Increased nervousness
- Alteration in behavior/mood evidenced by anger, crying, withdrawal, preoccupation, anxiety, hostility, and apathy

Nursing Interventions

Spiritual Support

Encourage verbalization and listen with empathy and a nonjudgmental attitude. Encourage family to seek out persons (e.g., clergy) who have helped them find meaning in other situations. Refer to parents who have coped effectively with situation and who have relied on faith beliefs for assistance

Encourage participation in sectarian activities that provide source of comfort (i.e., praying).

Hope Instillation

Assist the client to correct misconceptions. (Expression of feelings with an empathetic listener will help the client gain perspective needed for problem solving)

Explore with the client the activities that are usually the most enjoyable and that produce a feeling of happiness and lightheartedness. Facilitate and encourage these activities, as permitted. (Activities that have produced this effect in the past carry a great potential for facilitating the emotional self-healing)

Refer to community-based support groups. Families with similar circumstances are credible sources of support for other families. Validation or suggestions for coping can facilitate resumption of normal affect and activities

Evaluation Criteria

The family will demonstrate received faith and confidence as evidenced by

- Verbalization of having more "peace of mind"
- Expression of a philosophic purpose for the disease
- Verbalization that life has meaning
- Verbalization of feeling at peace with the deity
- Participation in religious practices

(continued)

TABLE 27-5 *(continued)*

Analysis: Nursing Diagnostic Statement 4

Response and Related or Risk Factors: *High risk for altered health maintenance; risk factors—anxiety and knowledge deficit, regarding:*

- Administration of intervention protocol
- Diagnosis of development delay or disability
- Confusion about information presented

Projected Outcome: Family demonstrates ability to identify, manage, and/or seek out help in relation to their child's treatment regime at home

Defining Characteristics *(Actual Responses)*	Nursing Interventions	Evaluation Criteria
Subjective: • Parent(s) states unfamiliarity with treatment protocol • Stated lack of understanding regarding information presented • Reported or observed inability of parents to take responsibility for meeting health maintenance needs • Shared feelings of being overwhelmed in managing home care • History of lack of health-seeking behavior • Expressed interest in caring for child *Objective*: • Reported or observed lack of equipment or financial or other resources • Reported or observed impairment of personal support systems	*Teaching: Procedure/Treatment* **Assess the level of knowledge and reason for the knowledge deficit.** (Determine whether it is due to insufficient information, confusion about the information presented, or anxiety that prevents integration of the information) **Intervene to address the underlying problem** • Clarify what information was presented (to determine if the client failed to receive the information or failed to comprehend it). Refer back to interdisciplinary team member for reinforcement of information • Discuss the information that was presented to clarify terminology and other aspects about which the client may have questions • Incorporate return demonstration and post testing into presentation of information/client teaching **Evaluate the adequacy of the information to meet the infant's needs for problem solving** by encouraging the family members to discuss the alternatives presented in the counseling sessions *Active Listening* **Encourage verbalization** and listen with empathy *Support System Enhancement* **Encourage to seek out assistance/information** from resource person, care provider. Refer to other parents familiar with regime/case manager. Refer to home health services and organized support groups	Family members will • Verbalize increased understanding of the diagnosis and treatment protocol • Demonstrate ability to follow treatment procedures, as evidenced by correct demonstration • Verbalize motivation to adhere to intervention protocol • Know how to obtain necessary equipment, financial, and other support

nity Alliance for Special Education, 1989). A recent survey indicated that nearly 68 per cent of students with developmental disabilities were attending classes in regular school sites.

Experts are advocating the philosophy of full inclusion rather than mainstreaming of children with developmental disabilities into educational settings. Full inclusion expands on and goes beyond the concept of mainstreaming by promoting and advocating the full participation of the child with developmental disabilities in regular school programs. A child with developmental disabilities fully included in the school setting would attend classes with students without disabilities. Classroom aides, school nurses, or health aides and adaptive equipment would be available to the student to facilitate her or his full participation in academic, athletic, and social programs, rather than being segregated in special education classes even for limited periods.

In 1984, Public Law 99–457, Education of the Handicapped Amendments of 1984, was passed by Congress. PL 99–457 and subsequent amendments, PL 101–476 and PL 102–119, in the Individuals with Disabilities Education Act (IDEA), extend educational services to infants and toddlers who experience developmental delay(s) or who are at risk for developmental delay(s) or who have a diagnosed physical or mental condition that has a high probability of resulting in a developmental delay or disability. The law further requires that services be provided in a family-centered context using an IFSP. Early intervention services for infants and toddlers were discussed previously (Hansen et al, 1990; Magyary et al, 1993).

There are innovative educational programs across the nation to assist children who must be absent from school frequently because of chronic health problems. These methods include the use of closed circuit television programs, flexible scheduling that allows adjustment for children with low energy levels or those on dialysis, and contracts with schools that spell out all responsibilities when children attend school with special equipment, such as ventilators. These services, by necessity, are complex and require the services of many professionals with a wide range of specialized training.

Supportive/Independent Living

During the 1960s, a grassroots movement was championed by parents of children with developmental disabilities to create publicly funded alternatives to institutional care. As a result of the far-sighted efforts of these families, a system of care was initiated to provide community-based services. The effort to deinstitutionalize care has resulted in the creation of many types of agencies and services for individuals with developmental disabilities. Out-of-home placement options for adults with developmental disabilities include community care facilities, group homes, and independent supportive living arrangements. These are not preferred placement options for children. If an out-of-home placement is needed for a child, the optimal choice is foster care.

Generally, most children with developmental disabilities live at home with their families, receiving publicly financed support services, supplies, and equipment (Bradley et al, 1990). Although family support programs vary according to the state, the type of services available to families include respite care, medical and dental care, transportation, child care, attendant care/nursing, and counseling and therapy. Other services available are parent training and education and homemaker services. In addition, families may need assistance with vehicle modifications, architectural modifications, and procuring specialized equipment and supplies in order to manage their child at home. The range of services that a family needs depends on the nature and severity of the child's disability.

Service System

As provided by the Developmental Disabilities Assistance and Bill of Rights Act, a network of federal agencies exists to promote and develop appropriate services and supports to individuals with developmental disabilities and their families. This network of agencies across the country exists in nearly every state and is composed of three separate yet interrelated purposes to respond to the ever-changing needs of the population of persons with developmental disabilities. Within each state exists a *State Council for Developmental Disabilities.* The state council has the responsibility to plan and coordinate resources in order to protect the legal, civil, and services rights of individuals with developmental disabilities within a state. The activities of the state council focus on long-range planning for services for persons with developmental disabilities. Under contract of the state council, the boards are responsible for regional planning and program development within the state.

Protection and Advocacy (PAI) agencies exist in each state to protect the rights and liberties of individuals with developmental disabilities. These agencies provide advocacy services and legal representation for individuals with developmental disabilities. They handle discrimination suits, denial-of-service claims, and conservator issues. These agencies may file lawsuits on behalf of their clients in order to fight discriminatory practices or ensure reception of entitled services.

University Affiliated Programs (UAPs) are federally funded programs that provide services to professionals, paraprofessionals, parents, and clients in the field of developmental disabilities. The mission of UAPs since their inception has been fourfold: (1) provide interdisciplinary training of professionals in the field of developmental disabilities, (2) create and replicate exemplary services, (3) provide technical service to community-based agencies, and (4) conduct research in the field of developmental disabilities. The UAPs serve as liaisons between educational institutions and the service delivery systems. There are over 50 UAPs in the United States, representing 43 states.

State Services

The services provided to children with developmental disabilities and their families vary according to each state. Programs and their funding support depend on existing legislation. For example, some states have *entitlement programs* mandating provision of services if the child and family meet the program qualifications. That is, by law, the state must provide services because the state has legislated that these children and families are entitled to services by virtue of their developmental disability or risk for disability/delay.

Evaluation

Ongoing evaluations for preventive, maintenance, restorative, and curative activities should be carried out regularly by the health care provider to promote functional status and prevent secondary problems. Other team members should conduct regular evaluations of the child's psychosocial, motor, cognitive, and communicative development to identify actual or potential problems. Family adaptation to the child's condition should also be monitored on a regular basis, because families will vary in their ability to cope depending on their own needs and stage of development and that of the child.

Prevention Issues

Prevention is an area of great concern to children with or at risk for developmental disabilities, their parents, and the professionals providing services. The issues of prevention relate to health care issues across the life span. As discussed previously, "child find" programs and early intervention programs are designed to identify those infants and toddlers who may be at risk for developmental delay/disability and to provide services that will minimize the child's risk for developing them. Ongoing assessment and intervention by members of the interdisciplinary team of the child and of family members throughout childhood and into adulthood is essential to prevent the emergence of secondary problems or loss of functional status due to inadequate health care.

Prevention issues for the child with a developmental disability and for his or her family are concerned with the psychosocial ramifications as well. For the child and family, living with a developmental disability means facing not only the personal challenges but also the stigma, prejudice, and discrimination in society that can create obstacles to fully participating in the community. The nurse and mental health specialists in the hospital and community can assist the child and family to develop coping strategies to deal with the challenges they encounter. Additional discussion is provided throughout the chapter to address these psychosocial issues.

Referrals for future family planning and genetic counseling can be suggested to parents whose child was born with a developmental disability. For more in-depth discussion of genetics and genetic counseling, refer to Chapter 31.

Nursing Care

Nurse's Role

In many cases, clinical education for pediatric nursing is conducted in the hospital. When nursing instructors and students work with children with developmental disabilities and developmental alterations, it is usually in the context of sick children or children who are having some surgical procedure. The nurse who sees these children only in that light develops a perception of them that is somewhat biased. Nurses, however, are not unlike the general public in this respect. Many people today still believe that children with disabilities belong in a special classroom, at home, or in an institution or that they should not have been allowed to be born in the first place. All nurses need to take a good look at their own beliefs and values, and modify them, if necessary, to effectively help these children and their families.

Nurses have many hats to wear when working with children or adults who have disabilities or problems that prevent them from achieving their full potential. The nurse's role consists of any of the following activities: case finding, direct care giving, teaching, providing guidance and support, consulting, coordinating, collaborating with other professionals, and being a child and family advocate (Magyary et al, 1993). These roles may take place in a variety of settings, including the home, hospital, school, and clinic.

Assessing Actual or High-Risk Problems

An important role for nurses in any setting is that of epidemiologist. Nurses are in an excellent position to detect children with possible developmental alterations or those who are at risk for such alterations. Knowledge of the risk factors is essential for any nurse who may come in contact with children and pregnant women.

Any developmental alteration affecting a child will influence all family members. It is, therefore, essential for the nurse to be able to work with all family members to help identify their strengths and manage the problems related to their child's disability (Failla et al, 1991). The nurse's role is to identify, prevent, and reduce the problems associated with the disabling condition. The nurse has a responsibility for recognizing infants and children who are at risk for alterations in development. Nurses are also responsible for helping parents and their children gain access to appropriate resources in the community. Nurses use and develop tools for assessing children and families who are at risk for developmental alterations. Nurses who are caring for these children and their families will be working with different members of the health team; therefore, they need the skills required to function as effective team members. Nurses are uniquely qualified for many of the interventions needed by families of children with developmental alterations and are often the appropriate people to coordinate the family's care (Magyary et al, 1993).

Supporting the Family

The nurse has a unique opportunity to provide support to the family of a child with a developmental alteration. The response that parents exhibit when they first learn of the diagnosis is well documented. Their first reaction is often one of being overwhelmed with the knowledge that their child has a disability. Parents often feel guilty and begin to look for some cause of their child's disability. If they cannot find something or someone else to blame, they may turn their guilt inward. Mourning takes place for the loss of the child they had visualized in their dreams. It is quite common for parents to withdraw from friends and associates. Although such withdrawal is normal, there is a danger it may become pathologic. Parents may experience, at one time or another, feelings of rejecting their child. These feelings may lead to underexpectations for their child or to the setting of unrealistic goals (overexpectations). Trying to escape from the situation is another outcome of unresolved feelings of rejection. The feelings that have been described may ultimately lead to a diagnosis of *altered family processes*. All of these feelings are normal, but parents often need someone to help them deal with such emotions in order to resolve them, and thereby prevent the occurrence of altered family processes.

Nurses can be a source of support for the whole family as they deal with their feelings. The screening nurse can make referrals to others, such as community health nurses, school nurses, or home health nurses. The nurses can continue to assess for actual or potential family problems and, if necessary, make additional referrals to other sources of service that will meet other needs of the family. Nurses can help parents anticipate the way in which their child's disability is likely to affect the family. The impact of developmental alterations on families is similar to the impact of chronic illness as discussed in Chapter 19.

Goldfarb and colleagues (1986) state that there are roadblocks for families in developing formal support. They describe the first block as a *bureaucratic maze,* in which parents run from one agency to another seeking the services they need. As their child grows, the services they need become more complex, just as they do for nondisabled children. Families struggle to continue to be able to maintain their child's health. Nurses, concerned about the high risk for altered health maintenance, can direct the family to groups, such as the American Association for Retarded Citizens or the United Cerebral Palsy Association, where many services are centralized. Nurses should keep a ready resource notebook with referral sources on hand to assist parents (Table 27–6).

Another roadblock for families is *cost*. The services that are available to parents in and out of the hospital are the subject of much discussion at the present time. Parents of children with disabilities need to know how to finance the many treatments and medications their child may need. They need to know such things as how to find information about Social Security Disability Income and Social Security Income.

There are many other roadblocks to the families' ability to maintain their child's health, such as the *attitude of professionals* working with the family; *professional jargon* that is not explained to the family; the *stigma* that society places on the family and the person who is disabled; *time and energy* required to obtain all of the services and therapies the child requires; and, finally, *lack of support* (Goldfarb et al, 1986).

Communication Skills Needed by the Nurse

Communication skills can never be taken for granted. Although they may be competent in their various fields, professionals are not necessarily adept at meeting the many needs of parents who may be in a crisis situation. Understanding the problems faced by the parent requires certain nursing skills. Listening, gathering data, and observing the family relationships will provide the information needed to deal with the family problems brought about by the diagnosis of mental retardation or developmental delay. (See also Chapter 11 on communication strategies.)

Advocating for the Child and Family

A relatively common etiology for altered health maintenance in families of children with developmental disabilities is inability to solve problems by their own efforts. Nursing interventions that are directed to the etiology of a problem are the most effective. Perhaps the most difficult role of the nurse is the one of advocacy. Advocacy has been defined as defending and promoting the needs of a client (Monea, 1981). Collins (1983) states that advocacy is an appropriate nursing role and is used when the clients feel "alienated and unable to solve problems by their own effort."

The role of an advocate is to help the client remain independent, not to foster dependency. According to Biklen (1976), an advocate (1) helps a client remain independent and free of charity, (2) understands persons with developmental disabilities as equals and realizes that they want to be treated normally, (3) expresses not pity, but, rather, anger for the dehumanizing conditions that exist, (4) is moti-

TABLE 27-6
Resource Organizations for Children with Developmental Disabilities

National Center for Youth with Disabilities
Box 721 UMHC
University of Minnesota
Minneapolis, MN 55455

Center on Human Policy
200 Huntington Hall
Syracuse, NY 13244–2340
(315) 443–3851

Human Services Research Institute
2336 Massachusetts Avenue
Cambridge, MA 02140
(617) 876–0426

Special Olympics, Inc.
1350 New York Ave., NW
Suite 500
Washington, DC 20005

Very Special Arts
1331 F St., NW
Suite 800
Washington, DC 20004

Special Recreational, Inc.
International Center on Special Recreation
362 Koser Ave.
Iowa City, IA 52246–3038
(319) 337–7578

Young Adult Institute
460 West 34th Street
New York, NY 10001
(212) 563–7474

Association for Retarded Citizens (ARC)
2501 Avenue J
Arlington, TX 76006

Autism Society of America
1234 Massachusetts Avenue, NW
Suite 1017
Washington, DC 20005
(202) 783–0125

Epilepsy Foundation of America
4351 Garden City Dr.
Landover, MD 20785
(301) 459–3700
(800) 332–1000

National Down Syndrome Congress
1800 Dempster
Park Ridge, IL 60068

Spina Bifida Association of America (SBAA)
1700 Rockville Pike, Suite 540
Rockville, MD 20852
(301) 770–7222
(800) 621–3141

United Cerebral Palsy Association
Governmental Affairs Office
1522 K Street, NW, Suite 1112
Washington, DC 20005
(202) 842–1266

The Beach Center on Families and Disability
University of Kansas
c/o Bureau of Child Research
3111 Haworth Hall
Lawrence, KS 60645
(913) 864–7600

National Parent Network on Disabilities
1600 Prince Street, Suite 115
Alexandria, VA 22314
(703) 684–6763

National Organization for Rare Disorders (NORD)
P.O. Box 8923
New Fairfield, CT 06812
(203) 746–6518
(800) 999–NORD

TASH: The Association for Persons with Severe Handicaps
7010 Roosevelt Way, NE
Seattle, WA 98115
(206) 523–8446

National Head Injury Foundation
333 Turnpike Road
Southboro, MA 01772
(508) 485–9950
(800) 444–6443

National Health Information Center
P.O. Box 1133
Washington, DC 20013–1133
(301) 565–4167
(800) 336–4797

ICD—International Center for the Disabled
340 East 24th Street
New York, NY 10010
(212) 679–0010
(212) 889–0372

National Rehabilitation Information Center (NARIC)
8455 Colesville Road, Suite 935
Silver Spring, MD 20910
(301) 588–9284
(800) 346–2742

Social Security Administration
US Department of Health and Human Services
Local Telephone Directory, Blue Pages
US Government Section

Sibling Information Network
991 Main Street, Suite 3A
East Hartford, CT 06108

Technical Assistance for Parents Program (TAPP)
Federation for Children With Special Needs
312 Stuart St.
Boston, MA 02116
(617) 482–2915

World Institute on Disability
1720 Oregon Street, Suite 4
Berkeley, CA 94703

National Easter Seal Society
70 E. Lake Street
Chicago, IL 60601
(312) 726–2600
(312) 726–4258

National Organization on Disability (NOD)
910 16th Street, NW, Suite 600
Washington, DC 20006
(202) 293–5960
(202) 293–5968

vated to create change, and (5) must be willing to accept criticism from agencies and individuals who are challenged. Ways in which a person can perform the task of advocacy include writing, investigative forums, symbolic acts, boycotts, educating, negotiating, lobbying, and becoming a role model (Biklen, 1976).

Advocacy, however, is not without cost. Advocates may be subjected to public criticism, political pressure, and even some subtle and not so subtle discrimination from agency officials who may feel threatened. Advocates can operate within formal systems, such as the court system, or informally by promoting the respect of client rights among the general public (Johnson, 1986).

Facilitating School Adjustment

Since the passage of Public Law 94–142, the Education of All Handicapped Children, the role of those responsible for the care and education of children with developmental disabilities has been changing. The law states that all children with developmental disabilities must be afforded their right to a free and appropriate education. They must be educated with nondisabled students to the extent appropriate, and they are entitled to attend school at the expense of the district through the school year in which they become 21 years old or earn a high school diploma. The law also requires that all educational agencies must locate those children who are underserved. It mandates service for those who are mentally retarded, hearing impaired, deaf, orthopedically impaired, deaf-blind, multidisabled, speech impaired, and visually impaired and those with specific learning disabilities. In addition, the children are to receive the following related services if they need them: transportation, speech, audiology, counseling, physical and occupational therapy, recreation, psychologic services, and medical services for evaluation and diagnostic purposes (Community Alliance for Special Education, 1989).

Youngsters with developmental disabilities are entitled to a thorough evaluation, and safeguards must be clearly established to ensure that they receive it. The evaluation of the child is to be free and must be done with the consent of the parents. Children are tested using the established guidelines and standardized tests previously discussed.

Following the evaluation, an Individualized Education Plan (IEP) is written in the public school system or an Individual Personal Plan (IPP) in the day care center or home. The IEP focuses on the child's educational needs and guides special education intervention. The IPP focuses on the child's developmental needs, therapies, and related services.

The team that works with the child in developing an IEP is made up of the school administrator, a chairperson, the parent, the child (if possible), the referring teacher, the child evaluation coordinator, the child's liaison, an implementation liaison, consulting specialists, and a recorder. Goals and services and means of implementing thc child's educational plan are determined and then carried out by the appropriate school personnel. The child is placed in the least restrictive environment possible for that youngster. The least restrictive environment for a child could range from a regular classroom with no assistance needed to a special class, hospital, or residential placement with a special teacher. The least restrictive environment is determined by the needs of the child that are identified at the time of evaluation and are re-evaluated on a regular basis (Hecht & Forness, 1988). As discussed previously, advocates are promoting full inclusion of children with developmental disabilities within regular classrooms regardless of the type and severity of the disability.

Except for the requirements of Title XIX of the Social Security Act (Medicaid), the interdisciplinary team of PL 94–142 does not directly call for the inclusion of a nurse (Bureau of Community Service, 1979). However, since all children with developmental delays or disabilities have specific health problems, nurses should be included routinely on this team. The health plan should be an integral part of the total plan for each child. Unfortunately, many school and agency nurses do not see the IEP process as a function of their jobs and do not ask to be included on this team, although they could be members under the consultant classification.

Children with developmental disabilities will always be with us, and with the increasing technologic advances and the trend toward depopulating institutions, their numbers in public life will increase. Therefore, it is essential that nurses become knowledgeable and skilled in working with these children and their families.

Conditions Affecting Altered Development

Mental Retardation

The term "mental retardation" (MR) describes a constellation of symptoms consisting of impaired intellectual functioning associated with impaired social adaptation. This impaired adaptive behavior must have occurred during the time of developmental behavior (from conception through 18 years of age). According to the American Association on Mental Retardation (AAMR), mental retardation is classified as an intelligence quotient (IQ) that falls significantly below the mean for average intelligence. Average IQ is 100 on the normal curve. The 1992 AAMR report defines mental retardation as substantial limitations in present functioning characterized by the following:

- Significantly subaverage intellectual functioning.
- Limitations in two or more of these adaptive skills areas:

- communication, self-care, home living, socialization, community use, self-direction, health and safety, functional academics, leisure, and work.
- Manifests before age 18 years.

The definition of mental retardation is specifically developmental in its approach and can be differentiated from impairment that follows damage in adulthood.

Etiology/Incidence

Over 250 causes of mental retardation have been identified (President's Committee, 1975). Most causes fall into four groups of etiologic factors, but some are difficult to differentiate. These etiologic classifications involve genetic, neonatal and perinatal, infancy and childhood, and social-cultural-familial factors (Table 27–7).

There are over 6.5 million persons in the United States with a diagnosis of mental retardation. Approximately 3 per cent of the population is in the moderately to profoundly retarded range. Mild mental retardation appears to be more prevalent among the socially disadvantaged. According to the President's Committee on Mental Retardation (1975), approximately 85 to 90 per cent of cases of mild retardation that do not show identifiable organic or physical cause are associated with conditions arising from the environment.

TABLE 27–7
Factors Involved in Mental Retardation

Genetic Factors*

- Phenylketonuria
- Cerebral lipoidosis
- Galactosemia
- Hypoparathyroidism
- Hypoglycemia
- Gargoylism
- Fragile X

Neonatal and Perinatal Factors

- Inadequate prenatal care
- Premature birth
- Use of alcohol or drugs during pregnancy
- Anoxia during or after delivery
- Birth injury
- Kernicterus (Rh factor)
- Dehydration
- Maternal factors
  - Rubella in first trimester
  - Malnutrition
  - Toxemia

Factors Operative in Infancy and Childhood

- Infectious diseases
- Accidents
- Ingestion of intoxicants
- Asphyxia

Social-Cultural-Familial Factors

- Emotional rejection
- Nutritional deficiency

*Owing to an alteration of the normal genetic information stored in the DNA molecules.

Pathophysiology

Causes of mental retardation can be separated into (1) true developmental malformations of the brain and (2) those occurring from acquired destructive lesions (Kepes, 1982). True developmental malformations may be those related to normal developmental steps that have not taken place or developmental steps that have occurred in an abnormal way. Acquired destructive lesions, on the other hand, cause damage to brain tissue that has already developed in a normal way. There are many areas of overlap between these two categories.

Development of the central nervous system takes place by three separate, but interrelated, means: gross organogenesis, histogenesis, and cytogenesis. "Gross organogenesis" means development of the organs. The first sign of the neural system is development of the neural plate, neural groove, and neural tube. Failure of these areas to develop normally would lead to conditions such as spina bifida. The degree of defect can be as mild as a dimple in the lumbar region of the spinal column or as severe as a meningomyelocele or meningoencephalocele. Hydrocephalus is often a secondary result of spina bifida and a further complication. Anencephaly is a closely associated problem in which the brain is not developed. When the telencephalon does not divide into two hemispheres, a condition described as telencephalon impar can occur. In a severe form of this developmental failure facial deformities may also complicate matters. (See Chapter 40 for nursing care of children with spina bifida and hydrocephalus.)

During the third through fifth fetal months, the corpus callosum is also developing. Developmental problems at this time could cause mental retardation and seizures. There are many developmental errors that can occur which affect the brain, and those mentioned are but a few of the possibilities.)

Failure of cranial osseous development will expose the brain and cause severe damage. Premature closure of the sutures is responsible for preventing growth and expansion of the brain. Today, surgeons have perfected procedures to open prematurely closed sutures and correct facial deformities. These surgeries allow the brain to continue its growth and in some cases prevent mental retardation. Facial surgery will not prevent mental retardation, but it may aid the individual socially and psychologically by improving appearance. (See Chapter 40 for nursing care of children with premature closure of cranial sutures, termed "craniosynostosis.")

"Histogenesis" is the formation of tissues that are groupings of specialized cells that make up organs. As the brain is developing, migrating cells eventually settle in certain areas of the brain. Neuroblasts travel to the area of the basal ganglia and others to the site of the cerebral cortex (Kepes, 1982). Much of the migration activity occurs as early as the twelfth week of gestation. Genetic and environmental problems can cause the arrest of this activity. These cells then begin to develop, abnormally, in the area of the brain where they have located at the time of insult. As they develop in wrong areas this is believed to lead to epilepsy. One severe form of mental retardation occurs as a result of agyria, in which the fissures and sulci of the brain are undeveloped (Kepes, 1982).

"Cytogenesis" is the maturation of primitive neuroblasts once they have migrated to appropriate places in the brain. Depending on the role of that particular neuron, it will then enlarge and fulfill its function. Failure of development of dendrites and synapses will interfere with the progression of some neurologic impulses. This failure may result in some forms of mental retardation (Kepes, 1982).

Myelinization is not complete at birth and takes place over several years following birth. If adequate myelin is not produced to complete the process, then neurologic problems arise. Some metabolic conditions may cause this lack of production of myelin, such as maple syrup urine disease, homocystinuria, and other amino acid metabolism problems.

Genetic disorders may interfere with normal development. In some genetic conditions there is an abnormal number of chromosomes with either too few or too many chromosomes in the fertilized zygote. This results from a mishap in cell division known as "nondisjunction." Down syndrome is an example of nondisjunction of the number 21 chromosome (Cooley & Graham, 1990). Some other genetic aberrations that cause mental retardation as a result of nondisjunction of autosomes are trisomy 13 and 18. There are many others. Nondisjunction of the sex chromosomes can lead to such conditions as Turner syndrome and Klinefelter syndrome, which cause varying degrees of mental retardation.

Clinical Manifestations

Children with mental retardation are classified according to the developmental tasks that are appropriate for their ages. Mental retardation should not be confused with mental illness or emotional disturbance. Four levels of mental retardation are usually identified (Tables 27–8 and 27–9).

1. *Mild retardation.* Persons with mild retardation may be hard to identify and are often physically normal. In school, children are able to learn academic skills up to approximately a sixth grade level, and, as adults, they often acquire vocational and social skills necessary for independent living. The majority of mentally retarded individuals are mildly retarded.

TABLE 27–8
Levels of Mental Retardation (MR) and IQ Tests

Levels of MR	Stanford-Binet	Wechsler
Mild	68–52	69–55
Moderate	51–36	54–40
Severe	35–20	39–25
Profound	19 and below	24 and below

2. *Moderate retardation.* In persons with moderate retardation, intellectual functioning is of a degree that academic achievement is significantly impaired, but they can learn self-care, social, and some vocational skills.

3. *Severe retardation.* Persons with severe retardation, with special training, may be capable of a significant degree of self-care but will need supervision throughout life.

4. *Profound retardation.* Persons with profound retardation may be incapable of any self-care skills.

Diagnostic Assessment

Diagnosis of mental retardation requires a team approach. The causes of mental retardation are many, and it may be possible to make a diagnosis immediately after birth if it accompanies gross developmental lags or deformities. On the other hand, the retardation may be mild and not picked up until the child is in school and begins to fall behind peers in academic work. A variety of tests may be used to assess the child's intellectual and adaptive functioning. These tests are listed in Table 27–3.

Several other tests are useful to use with children who have language, sensory, or motor problems. Included are the Peabody Picture Vocabulary Test (PPVT), the Columbia Mental Maturity Scale (CMMS), and the Leiter International Performance Scale. The PPVT is probably the most widely used, but the most satisfactory of the three is the CMMS. The CMMS requires the child to pick out drawings on the cards. It requires perceptual discrimination of color, shape, symbols, function, missing parts, and numbers. The PPVT will produce a score slightly higher than the Wechsler and the Stanford-Binet Scales (Latham & Yando, 1982). Another test frequently used is the Vineland Social Maturity Test, which measures adaptive behavior related to specific areas of social development rather than intelligence. The tests are given under carefully controlled environmental conditions. Some measure intellectual development; some test for specific attitudes or abilities; and others test for personality related to values, problem-solving styles, interests, and attitudes.

If the child is diagnosed at a young age, the child and family may need genetic screening, medical and counseling services, and infant stimulation services.

TABLE 27-9
Significance of Clinical Manifestations of Mental Retardation

Clinical Manifestations and Explanation	Significance to the Nurse
Personal-Social Development	
Immature social behavior:	Social skills will help a child develop self-esteem and gain acceptance from others
Prefers to play with younger children	Encourage social activities
Shows defective judgment by communication that does not fit situation with other children	
Acts out to get attention	
Often shows withdrawal behavior	
Poor self-image:	Look for child who does not seem interested in new activities
Afraid to try new tasks, withdraws from any challenge	Child cries, becomes frustrated, and is anxious
Cognitive Area	
Poor problem solving:	Encourage use of games to learn colors, numbers, matching like objects
Not able to accomplish developmentally appropriate problem solving	Teach new words
Concrete thinking:	Children learn best when task is concrete or functional. Learn by feeling and touching
Cannot think abstractly	
Inability to transfer learning:	Cannot learn by observing ideas going on around them. Need to participate
Not able to apply information just learned to a new situation	Present learning in short segments
Poor informal learning	Repeat lessons to reinforce words and ideas
Short attention span	Problems learning new words and ideas
Short memory	Use Show and Tell sessions, role play, story telling, and dramatic play to help these children learn
Difficulty with concept formation	
Language and Speech Development	
Language delayed	
Speech problems owing to motor control and physical problems of speech area	The child with Down syndrome has small oral cavity and protruding tongue
Problems in following directions	Cannot remember the sequence of more directions than one at a time. Example: "Get your umbrella in the closet and bring it to me"
Motor Development	
Lacking in body control	As a general rule, motor control is not well developed, especially fine motor
Distractibility	Benefits from a learning center that cuts down on distraction from surroundings
Inability to follow directions	Needs simple directions given for one task at a time
Perseveration	Child may repeat some motor movement over and over again
Underactive	Tends to not become involved and to sit quietly for longer periods of time
Self-stimulating behaviors	May engage in rocking back and forth, head banging, manipulating fingers in front of their eyes, ruminating, or other distracting and disturbing activities
	Activities that will help children develop gross motor skills include rolling, jumping, hopping, crawling, tunneling, climbing, balancing, kicking, and kneeling. Reacting to music is also beneficial
	Fine motor skills are developed by cutting, tracing, coloring, stacking, and pasting

(continued)

TABLE 27-9
Significance of Clinical Manifestations of Mental Retardation *(Continued)*

Clinical Manifestations and Explanation	Significance to the Nurse
Perceptual Motor Development	
Visual and auditory	Children often do not hear and see things as they really are
	Children can learn by using textured materials, such as cloth, feathers, grains, sand, foam
Problem in seeing differences	Child may have problems with a moving object. Child may be unable to see difference between two objects (pictures of apple and orange and tennis ball)
Inability to distinguish between two sounds	Child is sometimes unable to tell where sound is coming from

Older children will also need an educational IEP team plus a neurologist or pediatrician, or both.

Therapeutic Management

The therapeutic management of the child with mental retardation requires an interdisciplinary approach. The nurse or, in selected cases, the social worker will serve as the child's case manager/service coordinator to ensure that the child is receiving comprehensive services and that the members of the interdisciplinary team are collaborating with one another. The members of the team—language and speech specialist, special educator, physical and occupational therapists, dentist, psychologist, physician, audiologist, nutritionist—will monitor the child's plan of care as identified by the ongoing interdisciplinary assessments to promote the child's highest developmental achievements, prevent regression in level of functional status, and prevent emergence of secondary problems and complications.

Application of the Nursing Process: Mental Retardation

Assessment

In almost every area of nursing, nurses will be involved in making referrals and working with children who are mentally retarded. Nurses are important members of the diagnostic team. Their observational skills in noting gross and fine motor movements, visual and auditory acuity, and emotional responses are important in diagnosis. Although psychologic testing is required in the evaluation of the child's mental status, the final evaluation should be made by a team of professionals, with special attention given to adaptive behavior in the child's family environment. Intelligence testing, without considering adaptive behavior, often labels a child and limits expectations. The child's cognitive lag may be due to lack of external stimuli. In this case, with exposure to positive experiences, some degree of maturation and learning will take place.

The nurse may be asked to observe a child who appears to be having difficulties or who is not keeping up. Observation should involve the child's language, social, and personal skills. Determine if the child is learning slowly or having trouble keeping up with amounts of work produced by other children. This is an important observation. The nurse should also watch the child participating in various learning areas and in different activities. An important observation is to decide whether the child is lagging in many areas or whether the child is functioning adequately but has problems in only a certain area (Hansen et al, 1990).

Nursing Diagnostic Statements and Collaborative Problems

Nurses who work with children who are diagnosed as mentally retarded will need to assess the child and family thoroughly. Nursing diagnostic statements that result from this assessment follow.

Anticipatory grieving, *related to negative parental reaction to diagnosis, as evidenced by:*
- *Anticipatory loss of idealized child.*
- *Parental guilt over having child with developmental disability.*

Uncompensated self-care deficit — dressing and grooming, toileting, feeding, *related to:*
- *Cognitive and motor impairment.*
- *Parental overprotection associated with need to "do for" child.*

Impaired social interactions, *related to:*
- *Uncompensated cognitive impairment.*
- *Prejudice and erroneous perceptions of child by peers.*
- *Difficulty in learning appropriate social skills.*
- *Engaging in "at risk" behaviors that adversely affect personal safety.*

Altered sexuality patterns, *related to:*
- *Limited level of comprehension regarding sexuality.*

- *Family members hesitant to discuss matters of sexuality with child.*

***Social isolation**, related to:*
- *Limited or impaired social skills.*
- *Segregation from mainstream of society.*
- *Self-consciousness of both child and family about child's differentness.*

***Ineffective family coping**, related to:*
- *Family feeling overwhelmed by diagnosis and treatment of condition.*
- *Shift in family responsibilities to meet demands of child's condition associated with insufficient resources to support family in coping with child's condition.*
- *Failure to meet sibling needs because of the demands of child's home management.*

***High risk for altered health maintenance, risk factor: knowledge deficit**, regarding child's condition and the long-term and home management of this condition.*

***Health-seeking behaviors**, regarding special needs for hygiene and health and dental care related to lack of accessible services.*

A collaborative problem that may result from the assessment is:

***Impaired verbal communication**, related to:*
- *Impaired cognitive skills.*
- *Speech pathology.*
- *Lack of access to speech and language services.*
- *Impatience of family members in attempting to teach child language skills.*

Planning and Implementation

Because mental retardation can accompany many other physical problems, such as cerebral palsy, hydrocephaly, spina bifida, Turner syndrome, Klinefelter syndrome, Cornelia de Lange syndrome, Down syndrome, and hundreds of other inherited or acquired disorders, the nursing care will vary. Children with mental retardation may be immobile, sensory deprived, or hearing or speech impaired. The needs of those children would be far different from those of the child who is ambulatory, aware of the environment, and able to effectively receive and express feelings and communications. Nurses are uniquely equipped to work with persons who have disabilities as a result of working with patients with other types of disease processes, such as stroke. Many of these skills can be used in working with those who have the same deficits resulting from developmental disabilities. For example, the health hazards of immobility are the same for everyone. The difference is applying this knowledge to a child.

Counseling the Family. Although it is the psychologist who will give the tests, it is imperative that nurses understand the implications of the findings. The nurse is frequently the professional sought by parents to explain the test findings to them again after they have been presented with a diagnosis. Understanding information related to the child is, therefore, of great importance for the nurse in order to assist the family (Dashiff, 1991).

Parental reactions, including guilt, require the nurse to be skilled in providing interventions to help the family explore their feelings. This is done by assisting the family members to identify their feelings and giving them feedback about the appropriateness of those feelings. It is easy to imagine feelings of guilt that could occur if a child with mental retardation is born to a mother who took drugs, either over the counter preparations or illegal drugs, or alcohol during pregnancy; to a mother involved in an accident or illness; to one who has had a positive family history of genetic problems or who knowingly did anything that would prove harmful to the developing fetus. Think of the guilt a father would feel because of poverty, abuse, or even just not being supportive enough when his wife was pregnant. A sibling might suffer guilt if he or she had not wanted another brother or sister when the mother was pregnant. Refer to Table 27–5 for long-term care of the infant at risk for additional information to assist families in coping with the long-term care issues.

Many of the family's problems will be better solved when its members can talk to each other and help each other. We know that grieving is a normal process, but the obstructions to resolution of grief are varied. When a family member becomes stuck in a phase of grieving, it can lead to depressive states. Normally, this does not mean the family member develops a psychiatric problem. It does mean that skilled intervention is needed, though, to work through the grief process.

The family members at high risk for dysfunctional grieving are the following:

- Those family members who have had problems relating to the family member who is mentally retarded.
- The family member who has shown overly cheerful, brave, or stoic behavior.
- Those who have little in the way of support systems or who perceive those systems as unsupportive.
- Those who have shown maladaptive coping mechanisms with past losses (McFarland & Wasli, 1986).

Developing Self-Feeding Skills. If the child is severely retarded, developing self-feeding skills may be problematic, but in most cases the following suggestions that the nurse can make to the parent will be helpful. Have the child sit in a comfortable position with feet on a firm surface. With your hand over the child's dominant hand, provide assistance in bringing the spoon from the dish to his or her lips. There are various wrist movements involved in getting food from a dish to a spoon and then to the mouth. This procedure will need to be repeated for many sessions and may take months. Gradually move your hand from the child's hand to the wrist, and eventually you will be assisting by only a guiding touch on the elbow. Do not be concerned about spillage but encourage neatness. The same procedure can be applied to holding a cup of milk. Begin with food the child enjoys, such as applesauce. Gradually add new textures and flavors, but reward the child with a favorite food. Encourage finger foods. Be sure that food is placed in the back of the child's mouth, not just on the tip of the tongue. Peanut butter on the upper or lower gums or between the gums and cheeks encourages tongue manipulation and mandibular movement that is necessary for both speech and chewing.

Developing Dressing/Grooming Skills. Children who are mentally retarded need to be able to believe in their own abilities. In order to do this, they must have ample opportunity to try things out and to practice. It will take them longer to master skills and learn from the environment.

Caregivers should be careful not to take over a project, but let the children have a *sense of accomplishment.* When the children are finally successful they should be rewarded. Frequently in the past we have rewarded these children with sugary treats. Dental problems and weight problems are often a result, so the rewards are best if they are of a social nature. Programs such as the Special Olympics are designed to give these children a sense of accomplishment.*

Emphasis should be placed on the child's capabilities. Children should be encouraged to use all of their abilities. Parents should be asked to tell what the child does well rather than what he or she cannot do. The adage "Build on the weakness of his strength" is frequently cited. In this process, the strengths of the child are reinforced, and gradually the unwholesome behavior is diminished. If the child has learned to tie shoelaces, this process might be enhanced by learning to tie other ribbons, thus developing improved finger dexterity.

Helpful hints for teaching dressing skills include:

1. If the child is learning to tie shoelaces, allow practice on an adult shoe. The child can slip her or his foot into the shoe and can play "pretend adult" games while learning.
2. Sew large buttons and enlarge the buttonholes on an adult blouse or shirt. The child can then lift the apparel and watch what he or she is doing.
3. Name tags on the neck bands of coats, slip-on sweaters, and tops teach the child her or his name and identify the front and back of garments.
4. For children who have trouble getting a coat on, put the coat on the table, with the lining side up and the collar toward them. The children face the coat, put an arm in each sleeve and then raise their arms over their heads. This procedure is also used for slipover sweaters and tee shirts. The neck label will identify the front and back.
5. To teach a child to put on socks, put the sock in position over the toes and let the child pull it over the heel and ankle.

Developing Toileting Skills. Toilet training for a child with mental retardation cannot be hurried. It is important that it be done at a point at which both child and mother are relaxed and ready. A routine must be established and carried out in a calm, comfortable way, with the mother explaining all actions to the child. As she takes the child to the bathroom, she says, "Here we go to the bathroom" and "Down go Jenny's pants" as she puts her hand over the child's hands and "Up goes Jenny" as the child is placed on a comfortable stool with foot support. An adult should stay with the child so that someone is there to give immediate reward when the child performs appropriately. To be effective, the reward must be something the child particularly enjoys. If there is no result in 5 minutes, wipe the child and calmly remove him or her. Again, put your hands over the child's hands as both of you pull the pants back into position.

Establish a pattern for bowel movements by noting on a calendar the time of elimination over a two-week span. Take the child to the bathroom a few minutes before the average time and repeat the procedure. Watch the child's face and listen for particular sounds. Dress the child in clothes that are simple to remove. If the child cries, discontinue and try a few weeks later when she or he may be more ready.

Promoting Development of Social Skills. These children need to learn *social skills,* which is often a very difficult project (Cole & Meyer, 1991). Other children must be taught that children with disabilities are worthwhile individuals. This is one of the problems we face in full inclusion. Built-in prejudice and wrong perceptions of the child with a developmental disability are hard to overcome. The child frequently has no peers in the neighborhood who are similar to him or her in looks and ability. The child who is mentally retarded does have some characteristics that are like those of all other children. When we teach others to look for our similarities they will find there are more instances of likenesses than differences. It all lies in what we dwell on, and this is one of the reasons the medical model fell into disfavor among those who are child advocates.

Adolescents have critical needs for learning in order to live independently and productively in the community (Siperstein & Bak, 1989). Those needs are for

- Work training.
- Group home living or supported living arrangements.

---

*Some advocacy groups are critical of Special Olympics as it serves to separate children and adults with developmental disabilities from full inclusion in recreational and social activities with nondisabled peers.

ETHICAL ISSUES

Reproductive Decisions with Adolescents Who Are Mentally Retarded

by Margaret M. Mahon, MSN, RN

Sharon is 15 years old and is mildly mentally retarded. She is independent in activities of daily living. She lives in a residential facility with five other adolescents who are mentally retarded. Sharon attends school, and it is expected that she will have a job after she completes her schooling. Sharon has regular contact with her family. During a recent medical check-up, Sharon's mother questioned, "Should we have her sterilized now, so nothing will happen?"

In the early part of the 20th century, routine and forced sterilization of people who were mentally retarded was the norm. This was the result of many factors, including eugenic philosophies, beliefs that being mentally retarded increased the likelihood of criminal or sexual behavior, or just because "it was one less thing to worry about" (e.g., neither hygiene issues related to menstruation nor pregnancy would have to be considered). Since that time, there has been a marked increase in the recognition of rights and autonomy of people who are mentally retarded. Most adolescents who are mentally retarded are likely to experience feelings of emerging sexuality, as are adolescents who are not mentally retarded. Unfortunately, the former group is much less likely to receive sex education, in large part because of an assumption that "they'll never need it." This attitude seems to come from several levels, including a lack of understanding of the sexuality of people who are mentally retarded, an unawareness that they could be sexually desirable to others, and an unawareness of their ability to choose to be sexually active and even to parent.

Laws were written to protect people who are mentally retarded from being sexually exploited, but these same laws have been used to limit legitimate sexual expression. The most important information necessary is an understanding of differences in sexuality between people who are mentally retarded and people who are not. Is it acceptable to place restrictions on the sexual expressions of people who are mentally retarded and are *different from* people who are not mentally retarded solely because of their IQ? What other factors should influence this decision?

Rarely is the developmental transition called adolescence an easy one. All adolescents have to deal with changes in their bodies; sometimes appreciated, sometimes loathed. Most adolescents deal with the ambivalence of establishing separation and the insecurities of going out alone. Life decisions are made for job as well as lifestyle. In addition, people who are mentally retarded are likely to have to deal increasingly with the fact that they are different from their peers. They may feel ostracized, and come to realize that they will never "be like everyone else." But these feelings are usually superimposed on, rather than a replacement of, feelings of all adolescents. This indicates that without information to the contrary, information about sexuality should not be withheld because of IQ.

The issue is also, who makes these decisions? Barring contravening information, IQ is not a valid reason to provide different information or opportunities. The sexual behavior of people who are mentally retarded is likely to be a function of their environment. Given appropriate information and example, there is no indication that mental retardation causes, for example, inappropriate masturbation or increased sexual drive. With the high risk of HIV, and knowing that some people will specifically try to take advantage of people who are mentally retarded, it is important that education about prevention and protection be provided.

It is important to know what information Sharon has been given about sexuality, both by her family and by those at her group home. It is essential to assess Sharon's understanding of sexuality, as well as her current level of sexual activity. Her ability to learn and integrate other information is an appropriate standard to use when estimating her ability to understand information about sexuality, as well as the accuracy of her reporting of her activities. What rules are there about sexual expression at the group home? Whose responsibility is it to establish and enforce these rules? What if an 18-year-old resident wanted contraceptive information? How is this decision different from the same decision for Sharon? Are there, or should there be, provisions in the group home for sexual intimacy?

Provision of contraceptive information must consider the ability of the person using it to be compliant, as well as how it fits with her lifestyle. Many males who are mentally retarded have demonstrated the ability to use condoms. However, some medications decrease the efficacy of oral contraceptives, such as certain anti-seizure medications.

People who are mentally retarded are often capable of parenting. Most people go through no screening prior to becoming parents. Should this be different for people who are mentally retarded? How does the "best interest of the child" standard apply here? Some people who are mentally retarded have a lower rate of fertility than people who are not retarded. In many types of mental retardation, is there an increased likelihood that a mentally retarded parent will give birth to a mentally retarded child? Is this a valid reason to limit reproductive opportunity?

The issue seems to center around the ability of the person to make an informed decision about lifestyle and options. Certainly there are cases in which one's level of disability associated with being mentally retarded precludes the ability not only to make an informed decision about sexual activity, but even to understand and manage menstruation. The options for one who is severely retarded are different because of the different abilities. Most people who are mentally retarded are mildly retarded, can often live independent lives, are capable of having sexual feelings, and can express themselves sexually. As is so often the case, before making any decisions, one must assemble accurate information.

BIBLIOGRAPHY

Abramson, P. R., Parker, T., & Weisberg, S. R. (1988). Sexual expression of mentally retarded people: Educational and legal implications. *American Journal on Mental Retardation, 3,* 328–334.

Pincus, S. (1988). Sexuality in the mentally retarded patient. *American Family Physician, 37,* 319–323.

Tasch, V. (1988). Parenting the mentally retarded adolescent: A framework for helping families. *Journal of Community Health Nursing, 5,* 97–108.

Williams, D. N. (1978). Becoming a woman: The girl who is mentally retarded. *Pediatric Nursing, 13,* 89–93.

- Sex education.
- Safety for self and others.

They now need to learn how to use the telephone, how to prepare simple meals, how to work the washing machine and dryer, and how to prevent accidents. They will also need to know how to count money and budget their funds and to tell time. They should also learn how to use transportation, such as buses and taxis.

Personal safety is a lesson that is very difficult to instill in young people regardless of mental ability. Emotions are hard to separate from reason. Pregnancy and social disease are common to people of all walks of life. There are problems with people bent on taking advantage of others, both in our general environment and within the sheltered walls of supportive environments. Adolescents must learn who they can safely ask for help and who not to ask for help. It would also be important for them to have learned what people in the community can help them, such as firefighters, police, and medical personnel.

Promoting Healthy Sexuality. One of the frustrations of the family is frequently found in the need for guidance in sexual matters. The nurse should be prepared to assist the family to establish some guidelines. The child has undoubtedly already absorbed the verbal and nonverbal cues of the family's attitude about each member's sexuality. The child's questions about sex should be answered honestly, factually, and simply. If the child has the awareness and curiosity to ask, she or he should be given an appropriate answer. Parents may need to initiate a discussion if the child does not ask. The level of comprehension (and explanation) depends on the degree of mental impairment, but the basic approach to sex education is the same.

The school-age child is faced with physical changes, and the boy may be frightened if nocturnal emissions and penile erections are not explained. A girl should certainly have received anticipatory guidance about menstruation. Children need to know that, just as it is not socially acceptable to urinate in public, so is masturbation done in private, but parents should not make the child feel guilty. The child's sexuality is part of him or her, and an open acceptance of it frees the child to develop a better self-image. The manner in which sexual matters are discussed may be more meaningful than the verbal message.

Early on, children need to be taught what are and are not appropriate areas for physical touching. These concepts can be taught in simple terms by indicating what areas of the body can be touched and by whom. The child is instructed on how to behave with strangers and what to say or do if inappropriate advances are made. Children are also instructed as to appropriate and inappropriate locations to be with others. For example, the parent would instruct the child never to allow anyone in their bed unless the parent approved such a behavior (e.g., co-sleeping with a family member).

The adolescent and young adult, like their nondisabled peers, will have need for information on sex education. Typically, adolescents with developmental disabilities receive limited information on the subject and primarily from parents who may be embarrassed or inhibited about discussing these matters openly with their children (Zetlin & Turner, 1985). Parents may dismiss their adolescent's need for information as their child is "too young" or "not interested" in the topic of sexuality and sexual activities. If the adolescent lives outside the home, the responsible caretaker may actively discourage personal relationships for fear of litigation. Failure to adequately inform the adolescent about issues pertaining to sexuality and responsible sexual behavior could result in unfortunate outcomes, such as unwanted pregnancy, sexually-transmitted diseases (including HIV infection), and sexual abuse. The nurse can provide parents and other caretakers with information and suggestions for discussing sexual matters in terms understandable and meaningful to the adolescent. Issues pertaining to fostering appropriate sexual behavior and psychosocial development can be addressed as well.

Promoting Full Inclusion. As children with mental retardation progress and have adequate preparation, they should be integrated into regular classes with their peers, or "included" (previously described in a more limited sense as "mainstreamed"). This allows for normal social activities and new experiences with peers. Segregating groups of people from the mainstream of society is seen as dehumanizing. Full inclusion gives all children an equal opportunity to participate in community and school activities. However, the teacher needs special orientation to the child and must keep open communication with the family. There is grave danger that with full inclusion, the child will no longer receive individualized help and may regress academically. Nurses can help school personnel understand the specific needs of the children with mental retardation they are working with.

The process of "normalization," first developed in Sweden, makes available to every person with mental retardation opportunities and conditions of everyday life as close as possible to the norm and patterns of other people. It implies as normal a routine of life as possible. This means that children with impairments will be integrated into as many normal experiences as they are capable of participating given their condition.

Within the past few decades, great strides have been made in creating community awareness of the needs of children who are mentally retarded. Consequently, they are more readily accepted. There will undoubtedly always be children with mental retardation, but if today's medical and nursing personnel will focus on preventive measures, a greater percentage of children previously labeled "retarded" will be able to enjoy a richer and healthier physical and emotional environment.

Promoting Family Coping. Also refer to the earlier section in this chapter on the role of the nurse as a family support for guidelines for working with families.

Mental retardation can never be an isolated diagnosis—it affects every family member. Parents and siblings need special help in understanding the pathology and their relationship with the involved child. Parents need to be especially concerned that they do not neglect other family members because of the time a child with mental retardation demands (Deatrick et al, 1988).

Professionals should encourage parents to develop interests outside the home so that no one person is responsible for providing constant care. Guilt feelings can cause overprotection. Siblings should not be expected to forfeit their social activities and relationships for the child. Although qualified babysitters are difficult to find, the family needs time away from the child with mental retardation when internal pressures become too intense. Many communities have facilities for respite care that provide families a brief reprieve. Families can be encouraged to seek support and assistance from their extended family and social support network (Seligman, 1991). Camps for children with disabilities benefit the child and the family.

Introducing one family to another that has a child of similar ability can help both find support. Many families of children with mental retardation become involved in local groups that provide the community with an understanding of children with disabilities. The National Association of Retarded Citizens (NARC) was started by a parent group. Membership in Youth NARC is open to all interested young people between the ages of 13 and 25. There are more than 600 local Youth Association for the Retarded units throughout the country.

Siblings play an important part in the child's development. When there is a healthy acceptance of the diagnosis, the child will be involved in family activities and will not be excluded from the sibling's circle of friends (Faux, 1992). The child will feel acceptance and love and will enjoy the richness of a full life. Siblings, however, need to be prepared for the onslaughts of a cruel, uninformed world that continues to tease and deride those with disabilities. Siblings have a unique role in altering public attitudes by example and education.

Nurses must remain sensitive to the daily hurts of the family and not become callous in their attitudes. They must be aware that each family situation and child is unique, and, although the family must develop its own way of adapting to changes in many life patterns, the professional team stands by, supporting, caring, and guiding.

The family sets the tone of acceptance for the community. If the family demonstrates care and concern for the child, the community will more likely respond with the same acceptance.

Teaching for Health Maintenance. *Hospitalized* children with mental retardation should be treated for the conditions for which they are admitted, but their special needs must be recognized. Their care is adapted to their specific needs, with a comprehensive and individualized plan that is geared to their developmental levels. This plan should allow for the child's self-expression, independence, and progress at a slow rate.

A significant person should be permitted to stay with the hospitalized child to provide reassurance that there will be continuity of care. The care plan should have family input on the child's specific likes and dislikes, fears, favorite activities, and any other information on the child and the rituals of daily living that will make hospitalization easier. If the child does not communicate verbally, the nurse should be aware of expressions or symbols that are important.

The child with both severe mental retardation and physical disabilities presents complex problems that require a team of experts familiar with the conditions. The child with severe brain damage may have vision and hearing deficits that may not have been discovered because the child has no way of knowing that vision or hearing is impaired. The alert nurse will observe for any signs of sensory deficit.

Children with mental retardation are incapable of abstract thinking. Most can comprehend simple explanations, but concrete examples must be given. For example, instead of nurses saying that they will return after a while, they should show the children where the hand on the clock will be when they will return.

Most children with mental retardation enjoy music. A record player and some of the child's favorite records will help ease hospital anxiety. Children should have their favorite toys with them. Toys or games that give immediate reward ("busy boxes," in which something happens when you pull a string or open a drawer) will stimulate motor activity and develop observational skills.

If the child is to have surgery, a family member, school nurse, or familiar person should stay with him or her. Procedures should be explained in simple terms. If the child is to have a tonsillectomy, a simple, "The doctor is going to fix your throat so it won't hurt as much later," might be adequate. The nurse must always be honest.

Role playing and looking at pictures of doctors in their surgical attire is therapeutic. The child could be given a mask or surgical cap to play with before surgery. If the child has a fracture, a similar cast could be applied to a doll. This can be taken off to show that the cast is not permanent (Vessey, 1988).

The physical needs of the child with mental retardation are basically no different from the physical needs of all people. Their body systems, for the most part, function normally, but mental and motor responses are restricted. Because all body systems are interdependent, any system might be directly or indirectly affected. It is the nurse's responsibility to observe verbal and nonverbal clues and know how to interpret them (Steele, 1990).

Medical information should be interpreted by the nurse to the family. Nurses will need to be comfortable in the role of consultant and confidante. They will frequently be asked questions produced by deep hurt and despair. Listening and observing are more important than pious words.

Because nurses are in leadership positions and have many opportunities for changing attitudes, they need to examine their own emotions of fear, discomfort, anger, or desire for escape when they are exposed to people with impairments. The child will quickly sense the attitude behind the all-important interactions with the nurse. There can be no therapeutic relationship if the child does not feel acceptance. Children are quick to recognize the emptiness of care given in a sense of duty. The nurse giving care will see a person of potential within an imprisoning shell.

Promoting Health-Seeking Behaviors. Body changes are occurring in the adolescent and bring special needs for understanding, hygiene, and health. Dental care, nutrition counseling, and changes in prosthetics owing to growth spurts are important areas for nurses to become involved in helping the client manage. One important activity that will prove frustrating to family, client, and nurse is finding health professionals in the private sector who can and will provide health care to those persons with cognitive limitations and disabilities (Betz, 1993).

Some health professionals have not been educated to work with clients who have disability. Owing to tight office scheduling or lack of accessibility of their facilities, these professionals are reluctant to treat individuals with special needs (Betz, 1993a, 1993b).

The nurse can facilitate the visits to health professionals by attention to such details as providing the office nurse with information about the client. Some of this information includes the following:

- The client's communication skills.
- The client's physical disabilities and use of wheelchairs and other equipment. How much lifting is required?
- Financial arrangements.
- Behaviors that might be a problem and some helpful hints to deal with these behaviors.

The nurse will note that some of the causative factors of mental retardation can be avoided. Teaching aspects of prevention cannot be overemphasized, because prevention is the most important tool in combating mental retardation. Nurses should stress the need for immunization against rubella, encourage health care during pregnancy, and recommend giving human immunoglobulin to prevent Rh hemolytic disease. They should be sure that all infants are appropriately screened for phenylketonuria. Parents should be cautioned about the danger of fetal alcohol syndrome as a result of maternal drinking. The dangers of other drugs in terms of their effects on the fetus should also be part of a prevention program. The nurse must know the community resources available and follow through on referrals from the diagnostic team. If the causative factor warrants it, nurses should encourage all siblings of children with intellectual impairments to have genetic counseling (Pueschel & Mulick, 1990).

Promoting Communication Skills. Parents are frequently concerned with communication skills they can develop with their child who has a disability. Many children with impairments have speech pathologies and should be receiving speech therapy. The following suggestions will be helpful for reinforcement at home. Parents should be reminded that facial expression and voice tone are more important than words spoken. The method of communication depends upon the degree of mental impairment.

1. Let children do their own talking. Let them try to express themselves verbally as well as they can. Take time to listen.
2. Let them be an active part of family conversation, even if they are only able to contribute an occasional "yes" or "no."
3. If the child is nonverbal, teach cues for yes and no responses, such as looking down for no and smiling for yes. Ask questions that require only a yes or no answer.
4. Plan a scheduled 15 minutes each day for speech correction if necessary. This should be the only time the child's speech is corrected. Don't nag. Give praise when the child speaks properly.

5. Speak frequently to the child, using vivid explanations (the noisy, green truck; the red book; the soft, white blanket).

6. Do not accept gestures or pointing. Name the object and encourage the child to repeat the name. If the child has the ability to speak, insist that the word be said before the object is given. For example, insist that the child say the word "milk," and do not accept pointings or gruntings. If the child makes a reasonable effort, give the milk but continue to work on quality.

7. Provide many auditory experiences by reading simple stories or playing suitable records. Allow the child to sing along or respond to rhythm.

8. Praise successful speech. Whenever the child makes an effort toward a new word, reward him or her immediately with a verbal response.

9. Use short, simple sentences, and repeat words frequently.

10. Never refrain from talking to a child with mental retardation because you do not know what to say. Speak as you would to any other child, pick cues from the child's response, and include him or her in group conversation.

Before children can learn to speak, they must know how to chew, suck, blow, and swallow. Speech can be reinforced at home by correlating the child's self-feeding skills with the speech program. Teaching self-care skills to a child with mental retardation requires much time, patience, and repetition, but the results are gratifying in terms of the family's satisfaction and the child's self-esteem. The child usually wants to become independent, and patterns must be established early before dependency habits become established. As children learn one skill, they develop more confidence in conquering the next (Downing, 1987).

Evaluation. The following outcomes will be expected as a result of the nursing and collaborative interventions.

- The family will express feelings of guilt, anger, and sadness over the diagnosis of their child, enabling the family to cope adaptively with their child's long-term needs.
- The child will learn to feed self and maintain nutritional intake necessary for growth.
- The child will learn self-care skills of dressing and grooming so as to live as independently and productively as possible.
- The child will learn self-care skills in toileting so as to function as independently and productively as possible.
- The child will socialize with peers and others in an integrated environment.
- The child/young adult will engage in developmentally appropriate and safe sexual behaviors.
- The child will communicate as effectively as possible with others as a means of living a productive and independent life.
- The child will function as independently and productively as possible in an integrated society.
- The family will demonstrate ability to manage the child's care on a long-term basis.

Down Syndrome

There is a striking similarity of the physical features of children with Down syndrome regardless of the manner of chromosomal aberration. Down syndrome is found in every race, culture, and creed.

Etiology/Incidence (Pathophysiology)

Down syndrome affects both sexes equally. It occurs approximately once in each 1000 live births. The "trisomy 21" type occurs more often in children of women over the age of 35 years. As maternal age increases, the incidence of Down syndrome increases.

Normally, cells from the male and female undergo a process known as meiosis or reduction division. During the cell division, spindle fibers within the nucleus of the cell pull the paired chromosomes apart and to opposite poles of the cell. A full complement of chromosomes is 46 prior to meiosis. During meiosis, chromosome pairs separate and 23 go to one ovum and 23 chromosomes go to the second ovum. When nondisjunction of the number 21 chromosome occurs, one ovum receives two of this chromosome and increases that cell's chromosome content to 24 instead of the normal 23. The second ovum receives no number 21 chromosome and the resulting loss of genetic material is not compatible with life. If the ovum with the 24 chromosomes is then fertilized by a sperm, which has the normal complement of 23 chromosomes, the zygote will have 47 chromosomes instead of the normal 46. The odd number of chromosomes is a result of the zygote's having three number 21 chromosomes (two from the abnormal ovum and one from the sperm), or trisomy 21 (Drapo, 1986).

The developing fetus with this abnormal chromosome count will have Down syndrome. Down syndrome also may occur as a result of other aberrations of the chromosomes. A second type of chromosomal disorder, known as "translocation," occurs when a piece of a number 21 chromosome breaks off and attaches itself to another chromosome, such as the number 15 or 14 chromosome. If, during oogenesis, the chromosome with the translocated piece of number 21 and a normal 21 chromosome are grouped in the same cell and fertilized, the result is a cell with two normal 21 chromosomes (one from the father and one from the mother) and a piece of the number

21 chromosome attached to the number 15 (or 14) chromosome. This causes the same physical problems seen in trisomy 21 and accounts for 4 per cent of cases of Down syndrome.

A third condition causing Down syndrome is "mosaicism." In this situation, some of the cells of the developing fetus are trisomy cells and some are normal cells. This occurs during early cell division following fertilization of the zygote (mitosis). Parental mosaicism accounts for about 1 per cent of Down syndrome patients (Stine, 1989).

According to Steele (1982), persons with mosaicism tend to exhibit milder manifestations of mental retardation than do children with nonmosaic forms.

Diagnostic Assessment

The characteristics of children with Down syndrome are as follows:

Head: Flat occiput, brachycephalic.

Eyes: Upslanted.
Iris speckled (Brushfield spots).
Epicanthal folds.

Nose: Short with depressed nasal bridge (owing to underdevelopment of nasal bone).

Mouth: Protruding tongue owing to small oral cavity; the mouth is usually open, tongue is furrowed, palate is short and narrow; dental abnormalities are common.

Ears: Dysplastic.

Neck: Short and broad.

Chest: Congenital heart disease is a frequent finding; lung infections are frequent.

Limbs: Short.

Hands: Hands are broad and square, and the fingers are short; clinodactyly of the fifth finger may be present; aplasia or hypoplasia of the middle phalanx also may occur.

Joints: Laxity of movement.

Stature: Short and stocky; hypotonic musculature.

Dermatoglyphics: Fingertips have marked increase of ulnar loops (with opening of loop on the ulnar side), usually on all 10 fingertips, associated with a decrease in whorls, arches, and radial loops.

Palms: Marked increase in simian creases.

Feet: Increase of fibular dermatoglyphic loops (opening of loop toward the fibular side) on the toes and a decrease of tibial loops on the great toe; in the area just under the great toe (the hallucal area), tibial arches are prominent; there is an increased space between the first and second toes.

Dermatoglyphics in children with Down syndrome are so similar to each other and so different from the population as a whole that it is possible to classify these persons on the basis of dermatoglyphics alone. Without looking at other features an observer can use certain index scores for dermatoglyphic patterns and score prints very accurately. In spite of such accuracy, this analysis can only be used as a supplement to a more precise means of diagnosis—the karyotype. (See Chapter 31 for further information on karyotypes.)

Therapeutic Management

Care for the child with Down syndrome is similar to care of the child with mental retardation. Children with Down syndrome are at higher risk for a variety of health problems. For example, approximately 40 to 50 per cent of persons with Down syndrome have congenital heart disease. They also have increased susceptibility to respiratory tract infections, acute and chronic airway obstructions, sleep apnea, and cor pulmonale. Approximately 12 per cent of infants with Down syndrome have anomalies of the gastrointestinal tract. The incidence of leukemia in these children is 10 to 30 times greater than for the general population. Five to 10 per cent of persons with Down syndrome develop seizures, with the myoclonic type being the most common. Children with Down syndrome are also at increased risk for diabetes, hypothyroidism, and spinal cord compression. Therefore, it is essential that access to specialized medical services be initiated early (Cooley & Graham, 1990). Refer to the previous section on mental retardation for further information.

Nursing Care

Down syndrome is readily diagnosed at birth because of some of the obvious signs. There are undoubtedly few other diagnoses that cause as much grief, confusion, and loneliness in parents as this one, ending their happy anticipation of a "normal," healthy baby. How the diagnosis is presented to the family is crucial, an event the family will always remember. This is a highly sensitive and emotional time; parents' acceptance of the child and the diagnosis cannot be rushed, for time is the only healer of the hurt. Parents have anticipated a child they do not have; they are mourning this normal child, and they feel guilty about their confused emotions. They should be assured that these are typical reactions and that no one is to blame for their child's anomaly (Steele, 1990). The nurse may be the most supportive person to stand by, listen, and help them formulate the questions they must ask (Damrosch & Perry, 1989; Perkins, 1993).

Acceptance of the child varies with the value orientation of the family. Parents who value academic excellence may have a great deal of difficulty accepting a child with limited intellectual potential. There is a wide range of intellectual ability among children with Down syndrome. Although some are seriously affected mentally, others function at a relatively high level. Children with Down syndrome cannot be classified in one category, although similar signs and symptoms may be present. Most children, however, continue to function at half their chronologic age up to the age of 12. They never seem to catch up with peers (Steele, 1990).

Because of recent governmental assistance in special education, it is now mandatory that education be provided for all children with disabilities. Most communities have access to special educational resources and personnel. The infant with Down syndrome is in some ways more fortunate than one with a hidden disability, because therapy can soon be initiated. Infant stimulation increases awareness and alertness. Many children who have had early intervention then participate in regular elementary classrooms with continued special assistance.

Children with Down syndrome of school age usually have delayed psychomotor development. Speech is commonly delayed; the child may need speech therapy. In the classroom, psychomotor activities are incorporated into the school day; children can learn much through play activity. Some children learn to read on a low level, but they cannot do abstract thinking. Although few achieve an IQ above 75, society has yet to learn what can be accomplished if the child is treated as a worthwhile member and given unlimited opportunities and exposures.

Siblings of children with Down syndrome are frequently embarrassed because of this child; older siblings have questions about heredity and wonder whether they too will produce a child with Down syndrome. They fear social ostracism because of the affected family member. Karyotyping should be done on siblings of persons with mental retardation for genetic counseling. Fetal cells obtained by amniocentesis as early as the eighth week of pregnancy may be cultured in vitro and the information made available.

The child with Down syndrome is a social person and enjoys contact with people. As the nurse helps the family members toward acceptance, they will become aware of the contribution the child can make to the family and the community. Children with Down syndrome should be among peers, as they learn much through imitation. They should be exposed to as many normal experiences as possible and should not be deprived of opportunities to learn and grow.

These individuals are commonly happy, frank, and honest people and have many lessons in values to teach us. As society learns to accept people for what they are, and not for competitive or intellectual performance, the person with mental retardation can be valued and accepted. When children with Down syndrome are hospitalized with any medical problem, discipline and structure should be enforced, and no concessions made "because they have mental retardation." Children soon learn whom they can manipulate. They should be treated respectfully.

Because of modern science, these children are expected to live a normal life span. Previously they usually died of respiratory illness or cardiac pathology while fairly young. Many communities now have group homes for persons with mental retardation and supported living arrangements fostering independent living.

Further information on the nursing care planning, implementation, and evaluation is given in the section on care of the child with mental retardation.

Fetal Alcohol Syndrome

Fetal alcohol syndrome (FAS) is the result of alcohol ingestion during pregnancy. Although the exact pathophysiology is not known, alcohol is thought to impair protein synthesis in the fetus (Behrman, 1992). Fetal exposure to alcohol may also increase the likelihood of cancer, especially neuroblastoma (Cohen, 1984). FAS occurs in an estimated 1 to 2 infants per 1000 live births (Kliegman & Behrman, 1992).

As reported by Cohen (1984), the Fetal Alcohol Study Group of the Research Society on Alcoholism has recommended that FAS be diagnosed only when the infant has signs in each of the following three categories: (1) growth retardation (prenatal or postnatal) with weight, length, or head circumference below the 10th percentile for gestational age, (2) central nervous system involvement, and (3) deformities of the head and face (e.g., microcephaly, small eyes, flattened maxilla, thin upper lip). If the syndrome is not diagnosed on appearance at birth, it may be identified later when the infant displays hirsutism (excess growth of body hair), a weak suck, irritability, and failure to thrive. Mental retardation is common, along with various behavioral problems.

There is no specific treatment for this disorder, and the prognosis for severely affected infants is poor. Intervention is best directed at teaching to prevent occurrence. Pregnant women should avoid alcohol consumption from the time of conception.

Nursing care of the child with mental retardation is discussed in the earlier section on mental retardation.

Cerebral Palsy

The term "cerebral palsy" is used to describe several nonprogressive disorders resulting from dysfunction of the motor centers and pathways of the brain. The severity of impairment ranges from mild to severe.

Etiology/Incidence (Pathophysiology)

Cerebral palsy is the major cause of pediatric disability in the United States and has a variety of causes. The central event is damage to the motor centers of the brain so that nerve impulses are not correctly sent

TABLE 27-10
Causes of Cerebral Palsy

Intrauterine Factors	
Rh or ABO incompatibility	
Rubella in first trimester	
Maternal toxoplasmosis infection	
Maternal diabetes	
Complications at Birth	
Prematurity	
Precipitate delivery	
Anoxia	
Toxemia	
Asphyxia from cord around neck	
Trauma during delivery	
Postnatal Period	
Infections (meningitis, encephalitis)	
Trauma	
Poisonings	
Cerebral vascular accidents	

or received. The alterations in the central nervous system reflect the type and degree of motor dysfunction. The injury may occur during gestation, during delivery, or after birth. Table 27–10 summarizes the causes of cerebral palsy. The initial neurologic deficit is nonprogressive; however, physical deformities and functional impairments may progress because of abnormal tone or postural reflexes.

Clinical Manifestations

The primary clinical manifestation of cerebral palsy is motor dysfunction. The three pure types of motor dysfunction are spastic, athetoid, and ataxic. Children with cerebral palsy may show characteristics of all types.

Spastic motor dysfunction results from a lesion in the cerebral cortex, which permits reception of excessive impulses from lower motor neurons. The result is abnormally strong tonus of muscle groups. Spasticity is found in at least 50 per cent of patients with cerebral palsy (Franco & Andrews, 1977) and a high as 90 per cent of patients (Doleysh, 1991). A child with spastic cerebral palsy shows increased deep tendon reflexes and generally holds the affected limb in flexion. Severe contractures are a common complication. Fingers are often flexed with the thumb adducted across the palm. Bilateral contractures of the hips results in scissoring of the legs. The muscles in the affected limbs are underdeveloped.

Athetoid motor dysfunction results from a subcortical lesion in the basal ganglia and extrapyramidal tract. The result is involuntary, uncontrolled movements. Athetoid motor dysfunction affects 5 to 10 per cent of patients with cerebral palsy (Doleysh, 1991). The clinical manifestations include purposeless and involuntary movements, such as writhing of the fingers and hands. The purposeless movements are exaggerated by excitement and attempts at purposeful movement.

Ataxic motor dysfunction results from a lesion in the cerebellum or its pathways, causing a disturbance in balance. Ataxic motor dysfunction occurs in 5 to 10 per cent of patients (Doleysh, 1991). The patient with ataxic motor dysfunction has no muscular control or coordination. The gait is high-stepping, stumbling, or lurching. Nystagmus is common.

Patients with cerebral palsy may have other clinical problems, which are related to hypoxic brain injury. Twenty-five per cent have seizures. Other sensory deficits, such as speech problems, visual disturbances, and hearing difficulties, may also be present. Mental retardation may be associated with cerebral palsy, although the patient may have normal intelligence and difficulty communicating because of a global motor dysfunction. Neuromuscular scoliosis may develop as a result of abnormal and unequal muscle forces.

Children with cerebral palsy often have nutritional deficits due to high energy expenditure and inadequate caloric intake due to feeding difficulties. Gastroesophageal reflux may also be a significant problem, requiring surgery.

Diagnostic Assessment

Cerebral palsy may be described by extremity involvement. *Diplegia* is the involvement of all four extremities, with the lower extremities more severely affected than the upper extremities. All the developmental milestones of the child with diplegia are delayed, although most will walk by age 4. *Hemiplegia* is the involvement of the upper and lower extremities on the same side of the body. Generally, hemiplegia is not noticed in the first year of life: the child walks at the normal times. Seizures and perceptual difficulties become apparent as development progresses. *Quadriplegia* is the involvement of all four extremities. Cranial nerves are also affected, so that vision, communication, and swallowing are abnormal. All developmental milestones are delayed. Some children will start walking by age 7, but seldom after. The non-ambulator is at risk for hip dislocation and scoliosis.

Diagnosis of cerebral palsy is made by history and physical examination. No single abnormal sign is indicative of cerebral palsy. The physical signs, with a high-risk history, will confirm the diagnosis. Significant factors include an abnormal birth history and delayed developmental milestones. Gross neurologic signs include increased deep tendon reflexes and persistent brain stem reflexes.

The brain stem reflexes included in the examination are the startle, tonic neck, labyrinthine, and parachute reflexes. All of these reflexes are present in neonates but usually disappear as the cortex matures. These primitive reflexes are abnormal in children with cerebral palsy, either persisting throughout life or being absent. With a positive labyrinthine reflex, the arms and legs extend when muscle tone is increased. When tone is reduced, the arms and legs flex. The results are that the body relaxes when the child leans forward, and muscle tone increases and the hips extend when the child leans backward. In a normal parachute reflex, a child will put both hands out protectively when the child is held with the head pointing downward. This protective reflex usually persists throughout life. In a child with cerebral palsy, spasticity will inhibit the parachute reflex.

The child will demonstrate an abnormal gait; it is important to observe the arm swing, stride length, scissoring, and stride base. A spastic gait may be the first sign of cerebral palsy. Examination in a gait lab can provide useful information as to which muscles are causing difficulty and for monitoring the effectiveness of treatment.

Beginning with the preschool years, the neurologic assessment is expanded to include assessment of fine and gross motor abilities and developmental functioning. The McCarthy Scales of Children's Ability (McCarthy, 1972), Stanford-Binet Intelligence Test (Terman & Merrill, 1973), and Vineland Adaptive Behavior Scale are examples of tools to measure developmental functioning and the extent to which problems associated with cerebral palsy interfere with it. (See Table 27–3 for listing of diagnostic assessments.)

Depending on the extent and severity of the child's condition, referral to specialized evaluation and treatment services may be indicated. Referrals for ophthalmic examinations are indicated to detect common visual problems such as strabismus, visual field defects, and amblyopia. Audiologic testing is conducted to detect sensorineural hearing loss, which occurs in approximately 5 to 15 per cent of clients with cerebral palsy. Speech and language evaluations are conducted to determine oromotor function and central processing. Referral to an educational specialist may be indicated in the presence of learning difficulties. A referral for psychologic evaluation and treatment is made when behavioral problems and difficulties in adjustment and adaptation are observed.

Early diagnosis and detection of problems can be significant factors in minimizing or ameliorating problems.

Therapeutic Management

Early intervention is crucial because of the great adaptability and elasticity of the infantile brain. The goal is not cure but treatment of symptoms and prevention of complications.

Children with cerebral palsy benefit most from an interdisciplinary approach to their physical and social needs. The needs of these children overlap many areas, including physical and occupational therapy, nutrition, medicine, nursing, orthotics, speech, and social work. An interdisciplinary visit that allows the family to talk with all the involved specialists and allows the specialists to interact as a team is the most efficient and effective.

Physical Therapy. Joint movement is limited by short muscles. Since the stimulus for growth is stretch, physical therapy may have a role in preventing the muscle shortening and resultant contractures. The therapy program is designed to promote normal tone and movement. A physical therapist will teach skills for independence in activities of daily living as well as select appropriate mobility aids. The therapist will also evaluate the child's need for special wheelchairs or adaptive equipment to help the child sit in an upright position. An upright sitting position is important for developing some motor skills, such as eating. Special inserts for a seat or wheelchair can provide support as well as help control undesired muscle movement.

Casting. Casting may be used to treat mild forms of heelcord contractures by providing a continuous, progressive stretch.

Braces and Splints. Braces and splints are used with exercise to maintain range of motion, prevent contractures, and control involuntary movements that impair functioning.

Surgery. A *selective posterior rhizotomy* will reduce tone and facilitate normal movement. The procedure can eliminate spasticity by severing the posterior spinal rootlets that cause increased electromyograph (EMG) activity. The procedure will leave contractures and lack of voluntary control unchanged. *Musculoskeletal procedures* aim to prevent serious structural changes and decreased function in adult life. Procedures include soft tissue lengthenings to correct flexion deformities and contractures, tendon transfers to restore muscle balance, and osteotomies to correct fixed bony deformities. Spinal fusion may be necessary to correct and stabilize spinal curvatures.

Application of the Nursing Process

Assessment

Nursing care needs to be highly individualized for the age of the child and the degree of pathologic involvement. Children who have CP are usually treated at home unless surgery is required. When hospitalized for orthopedic procedures, the care of their orthopedic problem is no different from that of any other child having orthopedic surgery. It may be the attendance to activities of daily living that will challenge the nurse.

Assessment of the child and family for potential and actual diagnoses is a continuous process because of the chronic nature of the condition. Given the uncertainty in predicting the course of the child's condition and changes associated with the child's progression through developmental stages, the child's condition is continually reassessed and re-evaluated.

Nursing Diagnostic Statements and Collaborative Problems

Collaborative problems that are often diagnosed in children with cerebral palsy are:

High risk for aspiration; risk factor: Impaired swallowing, *associated with dysfunction of the mouth, tongue, and pharyngeal muscles.*

Possible altered thought processes: mental retardation, *related to the brain lesion associated with cerebral palsy.*

Nursing diagnostic statements that may be diagnosed in children with cerebral palsy include:

Uncompensated impaired communication, verbal and nonverbal, *related to lack of awareness of techniques to optimize child's communication abilities.*

Alteration in nutrition, less than body requirements, *related to impaired swallowing and increased caloric demands.*

High risk for disuse syndrome, *risk factor: long-term immobility.*

Altered growth and development, *related to physical inability to participate in and accomplish age-appropriate skills.*

High risk for altered growth and development: physical, intellectual, emotional/social; *risk factors:*

- *Limitations in environmental stimulation related to motor deficits.*
- *Lack of coordination for learning motor skills.*
- *Inability to flex the muscles needed to perform such tasks as rolling and sitting.*
- *Limited social play opportunities associated with speech and motor deficits.*

High risk for body image disturbance, low self-esteem, altered role performance, and personal identity disturbance; *risk factors:*

- *Physical deformities associated with spasticity.*
- *Spastic or athetoid movements.*
- *Tendency for the public to generalize the physical deformity to include intellectual and emotional/social functioning.*
- *Personal frustration with difficulty in motor and speech behaviors.*

High risk for altered parenting: impaired attachment behavior; *risk factors:*

- *Inability of the infant to "mold" to the caregiver when held.*
- *Feelings of the parents associated with the strong social stigma of a disorder that often involves intellectual as well as physical dysfunction.*

High risk for altered health maintenance; *risk factors: knowledge deficit regarding:*

- *Cause of the disorder and the child's prognosis.*
- *Fact that not all children with cerebral palsy have mental retardation.*
- *How to perform therapeutic exercises to maintain joint mobility and muscle integrity.*
- *Administration of and side effects of anticonvulsant medications.*
- *Feeding techniques to counteract dysphagia and poor suck reflex.*
- *Ways to assist the child to meet developmental tasks despite the disabilities.*
- *Need for and availability of resources such as physical therapist, speech therapist, and special education center.*
- *United Cerebral Palsy Association and the support it offers.*

Planning and Implementation

The frequent and sustained muscle contractions of a child with cerebral palsy result in high caloric needs. Nutrition may also be complicated by impaired swallowing. It is difficult to provide adequate nutrition. Offer the child frequent, small meals to maximize caloric intake. Choose foods that are high in calories and nutrition. Consider need for a high-calorie supplement. Additional calories are also necessary during periods of stress, when muscle contractions may increase. If adequate calories cannot be provided by mouth, consult nutrition experts for evaluation of the need for nasogastric or gastrostomy tube feedings. The child should be weighed at least weekly to monitor growth so that alternative nutrition methods can be implemented if necessary.

Use and Teach Parents Safe Feeding Techniques to Avoid Aspiration and Provide for Adequate Nutrition. Children with dysfunction of the muscles of the mouth and pharynx are at increased risk for aspiration. The factors involved include persistence of infantile reflexes (tongue thrust), weak or absent ability to suck, muscular spasms during swallowing, difficulty controlling tongue and lips, and hyperactive bite and gag reflex. A Teflon-coated spoon should be used to minimize trauma due to bite reflex. Lightweight disposable plastic utensils should not be used because the child may bite down, break the plastic, and injure himself or herself.

The child should be positioned properly while eating, so that the head is upright, not tilted back. The child should be seated in a specially adapted chair, not held in the lap. The child should sit upright, not semi-reclining, with head, back, and arms well supported. The feet should be supported, not dangling.

For the child who has poor jaw control, the three-finger method helps the child close his mouth, chew, and swallow food. The technique is shown in Figure 27–2:

1. The nurse's middle finger is placed firmly under the chin and is used to help close the jaw.
2. The index finger is placed just below the cheek bone, to help control the amount the jaw moves from side to side.
3. The thumb is positioned on the chin just below the lower lip, and is used to help open the mouth and begin the motion of chewing.

The nurse allows the child's mouth to open only half way and places the spoon on top of the tongue. Firm downward pressure is applied to the tongue until the lips begin to close and the spoon is withdrawn, as the child removes food from the spoon with his lips. (Don't use the upper teeth to scrape the spoon clean.) Offer only small amounts in each bite, and check the mouth to see that the food has been swallowed before offering more. At the end of the meal check the mouth to be sure that no food is retained.

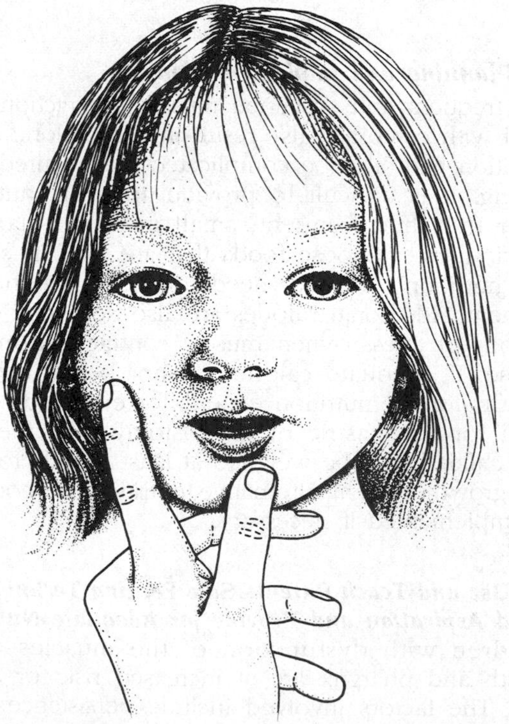

FIGURE 27-2. Feeding management: three-finger jaw control.

Promoting Cognitive Abilities/Thought Processes. If children with cerebral palsy have had only minimal exposure to learning or are limited in their abilities to respond, their IQs need to be compared with their adaptive abilities. The child should be exposed to new experiences and given opportunities for learning. Through PL 94–142 and PL 99–457 and subsequent amendments, PL 101–476 and PL 102–119 in the Individuals with Disabilities Education Act (IDEA), educational opportunities, including transportation to classes, are now the right of children with disabilities. Children with cerebral palsy should attend a regular class with peers. If needed, speech therapy or physical therapy should be provided as part of their school experiences. The children should not be singled out as being "different."

Additional information on mental retardation and associated nursing strategies can be found in this chapter. Chapter 45 details care of the child with alterations in vision, hearing, and communication.

Promote Verbal and Nonverbal Communication, Building on the Child's and Family's Strengths. Health professionals must learn the child's communication system by observing the child and by asking the family. Everyone who participates in the child's care should be made aware of the communication system. If the child uses a picture board, allow time to select letters or pictures. If the child is verbal or uses a computerized communication system, allow adequate time for response. When talking with the child, use language appropriate for the child's developmental stage. Phrase questions so that the child can use short simple phrases or "yes" or "no" to answer. Pronounce words slowly and distinctly. If the child does not have a communication system, consult speech therapy for assistance.

Promote Activity to Prevent Effects of Disuse. Although children with cerebral palsy often have uncontrollable muscle movements, they often have difficulty with intentional movement also. They may spend long periods in a wheelchair and be unable to shift position. The nurse and caregivers should assist with position changes every 2 hours to avoid prolonged pressure on body parts and compression of blood vessels. Caregivers must inspect the skin for areas of redness and institute preventive or treatment measures as necessary. Pressure-equalizing or -reducing equipment on wheelchairs or beds may be necessary to prevent skin breakdown. Children with cerebral palsy are at high risk for alteration in elimination due to abnormal muscular function. It is important to establish a baseline to monitor elimination patterns and habits. Encourage adequate fluid intake to prevent urinary stasis and constipation. The nurse should evaluate and implement home maintenance measures as appropriate.

Promote Optimal Developmental Activities. It is important for a child with cerebral palsy to maximize his or her independence and ability to participate in the activities of daily living. These activities may need to be adjusted to accommodate the child's limitations in movement. Caregivers should provide opportunities for the child to participate in self-care activities when possible. Physical and occupational therapy can assist with mobility and activities of daily living. Prolonged periods of immobility, such as after surgery, may cause a deterioration in physical skills. Aggressive physical therapy is often necessary to regain motor skills and to develop new skills.

Consistent follow-up to assess progress and any need for further interventions is essential to maximize function and mobility. A child with cerebral palsy needs to be followed so that the treatment plan can change as the child's needs change. The nurse is the primary source of accurate information on programs available in the community and technologic advances. The family will need information on services that are available to maximize the child's abilities and independence.

Promoting Optimal Development and a Healthy Self-Concept. The strategies for enhancing body image, self-esteem, role performance, and personal identity in the child with muscular dystrophy apply to the child with CP as well. Remember that the family is the most important influence on the young child's self-concept. Supporting the family and suggesting ways they can promote the child's self-concept is the best way to support the child. Refer to the chapters on growth and developmentally appropriate nursing interventions related to promoting self-concept and dealing with the stigma of a disability in the child with a sensory impairment. Many of those interventions are equally applicable to the child with cerebral palsy.

Full inclusion school experiences help these children to minimize their developmental differences from other children. Summer camps for children with special needs or Special Olympics can help these children see that they are not alone in their particular disability and they can gain strength from healthy relationships. However, it is essential that children with disabilities participate as fully as possible in age-appropriate activities with nondisabled peers (Meeropol, 1992). Segregating children with disabilities enforces their perceptions of inferiority and low self-esteem and creates feelings of discrimination in their nondisabled peers. Parents can be encouraged to enroll their children in groups such as Boy Scouts, Girl Scouts, and 4H clubs. Parents and siblings may have community support systems available to them as well. The United Cerebral Palsy Association is a source of information, guidance, and treatment in many communities.

Promoting Healthy Parenting. The nurse must be sensitive to the impact of CP on the family. Chapter 19 details strategies for helping the child and family deal with the diagnosis and with the often overwhelming care responsibilities of a chronic condition. The parenting role will be enhanced as the parent receives the support needed for personal coping (Hirose & Ueda, 1990).

Teaching to Support Care of the Child at Home. Depending on the type and severity of cerebral palsy, exercises may be prescribed to preserve muscle tone and joint function. Often these will be taught by the physical therapist, but the nurse as well should be aware of the proper technique so that he or she can answer questions and evaluate the child's progress. The nurse can determine whether home care exercises are being performed to prevent further loss of function by assessing muscular strength and joint range of motion, comparing it with the recorded baseline.

The nurse in outpatient or community settings will continually assess the child's progress on developmental tasks. Long-term care will include instructing the parents and siblings on ways to facilitate mastery of the next developmentally appropriate tasks. As the child's progress will be slow, the family will need continued reassurance and encouragement to help the child develop to potential.

Other areas of assessment will include monitoring weight gain and providing nutritional counseling as needed. The nurse will monitor for signs of respiratory infection, as a tendency for aspiration exists, and for commonly related impairments affecting the child with CP: seizure activity, vision impairments, and hearing impairments.

Anticonvulsants are frequently prescribed. Parents should receive a written list of potential side effects so that they will know when to alert the physician. Anticonvulsants and strategies for care of the child experiencing seizures is discussed further in Chapter 40.

One of the most important aspects of quality nursing care is the emotional support given to the child and family. The interdisciplinary team aids the family through periods of grief and adjustment and helps them accept the child and put the disease in perspective. The nurse can recommend available sources of support as appropriate.

Evaluation. As in all nursing care plans, evaluation of the success of the nursing and collaborative interventions described will be based on the disappearance or decrease in severity of defining characteristics of actual problematic responses.

Developmental Delay

Delays in development can occur at any time during a child's developmental period from birth through 18 years of age. Therefore, it is important that the nurse be able to recognize the risk factors that may lead to developmental delay or disabling conditions in infants and children. Table 27–11 contains a list of these risk factors. It is important to keep records of any risk factor noted in a child throughout the developmental period. Physicians and other health care workers may find clues to the probable cause of a child's disability by reading records that are well documented. For example, there is evidence to suggest that infants whose neurologic examinations show abnormalities or transient abnormalities are at risk for later difficulties, such as lesser cognitive function, hyperactivity, motor dysfunction, and learning disabilities (Ellison et al, 1985).

Genetic problems and congenital malformations can be responsible for delayed development. There are several thousand genetic disorders currently listed in the literature. Some are easy to discern at birth because of the obvious developmental problems they present. Others are metabolic in nature and are detected via blood tests (e.g., phenylketonuria [PKU], cretinism). There are some genetic problems that are not as easily assessed at birth and may not be recognized until the child is older and begins to show evidence of delayed development.

It is important for the nurse to recognize minor abnormalities that may be indicators of more serious problems, such as mental retardation, cerebral palsy, and heart or kidney disorders. Jones (1988) states that one minor anomaly may be found in 14 per cent of all newborn children without an appreciable increase in the incidence of major defects. In about 0.8 per cent of newborns, two minor anomalies are seen, in which case the incidence of a major defect is five times higher than those in the normal group. In 0.5 per cent of all newborn infants, there are three or more minor anomalies; in these infants, the incidence of major defects rises to 90 per cent. The findings of several minor defects is unusual, and the infant should be referred to a genetic screening and counseling center. Minor anomalies usually have no adverse medical or cosmetic consequences (Jones, 1988). Major anomalies, on the other hand, have an adverse effect on either the function or the social acceptance of the individual.

Examples of some major anomalies are hydrocephalus, anencephaly, severe microcephaly, hypertonicity, meningocele, severe micrognathia, severe hypertelorism, imperforate anus, cleft lip, or cleft palate. Minor anomalies are things such as bilateral epicanthal folds, upward or downward slanting of palpebral fissures, sparse eyebrows or thick eyebrows that grow together, a simian crease in the hand, clinodactyly, rudimentary polydactyly of the fingers or toes, and external ear anomalies, such as lack of the usual folds of the helix. All such deviations should be noted during the child's assessment. Following analysis of the findings, a decision should be made about an appropriate referral.

Learning Disabilities

The concept of learning disabilities as a specific and identifiable entity apart from mental retardation, neurologic impairment, or emotional disturbance has only come about since the early 1970s. Although learning disabilities share some common characteristics with attention deficit hyperactivity disorder (ADHD; as discussed in Chapter 29), they differ in definition and function. When Congress passed PL 94–142, The Education for All Handicapped Children Act, in 1975, it recognized learning disabilities as a disabling condition. The Act defines a learning disability as "a disorder in one or more of the basic psychological processes involved in understanding or in using language, spoken or written, which may manifest itself as imperfect ability to listen, speak, read, write, spell, or do mathematical calculations." The definition excludes children who have learning problems attributable to mental retardation, emotional disturbance, environmental disadvantage, or visual, hearing, or motor disabilities.

Etiology/Incidence (Pathophysiology)

Estimates of the number of children who have learning disabilities vary widely and may range from 1 to 30 per cent of the school-age population (Cowell, 1990). As with ADHD, more boys than girls are affected, in a ratio of about 4:1. There is a higher incidence of learning disabilities among the lower socioeconomic groups. Reading problems are the most common disability (Botshaw & Perret, 1981).

There are over 100 varieties of learning disabilities. Children with learning disabilities manifest problems in language, motor skills, and behavior long before they have difficulties in school. Early identification during the preschool years is important so they can be provided with appropriate educational intervention and counseling. Usually, these children are not identified until they reach the second grade. It is hoped that with the development of early childhood screening and intervention programs, children will be identified earlier.

Diagnostic Assessment

Early warning signs of learning disabilities are a child who is easily distracted, has a short attention span, needs to be told the same thing many times, and has trouble following a sequence of verbal instructions. Other early indications include delays in speech and language development, inability to repeat a sequence

TABLE 27-11
Risk Factors for Developmental Delay

I. Socioeconomic Factors
- Poverty
- Poor housing
- Social relationships
  - Divorce
  - Marital discord
  - Single parent
  - Teenage parent
- Nutritional deprivation

II. Maternal Factors
- A. Physical characteristics
  - Maternal age under 16 or over 35 yrs
  - Short stature (under 152 cm)
  - Weight (20 per cent below or above normal)
  - Family history of genetic problems
- B. Problems during past pregnancies
  - Abortions
  - Infertility
  - Multiple or closely spaced pregnancies
  - Premature or prolonged labor
  - Ectopic pregnancy
  - Cesarean delivery
  - Difficult delivery (midcavity forceps)
  - Previous infant with low birthweight
  - Previous infant weighing 4 kg or more
  - Stillborn delivery
  - Previous infant with disability
- C. Medical problems
  - No prenatal care
  - History of disease process or blood disorders
  - Drug addiction (including alcohol)

III. Risk Factors for the Fetus
- Rh sensitization (also other conditions, e.g., ABO incompatibility)
- Drugs taken during fetal developmental period of major organs
- Viral infections during the first trimester
- Radiation exposure (ionizing)
- Fetal size below or above norm
- Placental problems
- Polyhydramnios
- Ruptured membranes (premature or over 24 hours)

IV. Factors Associated with Labor
- Premature or post-term
- Prolonged labor
  - Primigravida: over 24 hrs
  - Multigravida: over 12 hrs (second stage over 2 hrs)
- Malposition
- Prolapsed cord
- Cesarean or breech delivery
- Meconium-stained amniotic fluid

V. Risk Factors in the Newborn
- Low birthweight: 2.5 kg and below
- Birth weight over 4 kg
- Apgar score 5 or below at 1 minute of life
- Fetal distress
- Resuscitation needed at birth
- Respiratory distress
- Drug-related depression
- Depression related to other causes
- Infection
- Birth injury
- Developmental malformation
- Kernicterus
- Intraventricular hemorrhage

of numbers, frequent reversing of words in sentences, taking a long time to answer questions, and frequently asking to have instructions repeated (Easter Seal Society, 1982).

These children do not learn readily from past experience and may, therefore, be difficult to discipline. They also have difficulty understanding or following instructions. For example, children with visual perceptual difficulties may not understand what they see. They may be unable to trace or draw a circle or square or copy these from a blackboard. Children with auditory perceptual disabilities may not understand a series of instructions, such as the child who may not be able to carry out three consecutive directions such as "Go to your room, turn on the light, and hang up your clothes."

Although children are not hospitalized because of their learning disabilities, the symptoms can be recognized by an alert nurse. Early referral is of prime importance in assisting the child. Parents frequently recognize symptoms but may have been told their child would outgrow the condition. Many children with learning disabilities are receiving help earlier today because teachers in day care and preschool programs recognize the symptoms and initiate referrals for therapy. Parents are usually relieved to know that someone else has also recognized the problem and that help is available.

Assessment of a child who is suspected of having a learning disability may involve an interdisciplinary approach that often includes educators, psychologists, speech pathologists, and health care personnel. It should begin with a careful history of the child's scholastic achievement and behavioral, social, and emotional adjustment. Physical and neurologic examinations are important, and generally the results are quite normal. School behavior ratings are made by teachers using checklists such as the Conners Teacher Questionnaire, Devereux Elementary School Behavior Rating Scale, and Pupil Rating Scale: Screening for Learning Disabilities. According to Cowell (1990), learning disabilities are diagnosed by excluding mental retardation, developmental disabilities, sensory deficits, and primary psychosocial problems.

Therapeutic Management

Intervention for any of the specific learning disabilities must be provided by a team. Team members should include the family, a physician, a psychologist, a teacher, a nurse, and a specialist in the discipline in which the child needs help. Various screenings must be done for auditory and visual acuity. Along with the developmental history, serologic studies, including those for lead intoxication, should be done.

Regardless of the specific diagnostic conditions, there are some general guidelines to be observed. The nurse or social worker can assist the family in implementing them:

- There must be consistency. Parents need to agree in the approach to child care. A definite time schedule for eating, sleeping, school work, and play should be planned by the family and followed consistently. Siblings and parents must evaluate their feelings, for children readily become aware of any tensions they are causing.
- Keep frustrations at a minimum. The frustration level can be increased as the child learns to function more maturely.
- Reward the child for work well done. Verbal praise is reward enough. Minimize defeats and build on strengths. Encourage positive self-concept.
- Assign simple tasks with simple directions. Show what is to be done, rather than rely on verbal commands. Give only one direction at a time.
- Special school therapy should be continued at home. Simple motor skills can be learned through play and repetition.

Some children need to attend special classes for learning disabilities until they are able to adapt to a more complex and confusing environment. Children, however, should be included in regular classes to the degree that they can tolerate. It is very important that they not be singled out from their peers as being different. Peers should be given a simple explanation of a learning disability so they can more readily accept the child.

The earlier an insult to the brain area is discovered, the greater the possibility of correction through remedial education. Earlier discovery in the preschool years will diminish problems in school. Many children's symptoms decrease after they reach puberty.

Nursing Care

One of the nurse's greatest contributions is to assist the family in using community resources. The Association for Children with Learning Disabilities (ACLD) is a parent group in which strength and support is found through exchange of concerns and ideas.

Children with learning disabilities require special attention, but this should not be given at the expense of siblings. Children with specific problems must be helped to learn to cope in their environments despite their disability and should not be allowed to use this disability as a reason for requesting special favors. Nor should they be excused from certain experiences because of lower competencies in academic skills. Nurses can encourage parents to involve the child's siblings by explaining honestly that the child has a special problem and that everyone will be required to help. This may help minimize sibling competitiveness and aid in family cooperation (Walker et al, 1989).

Children younger than the child with a learning disability may develop at a faster rate, and the child may be threatened and embarrassed by a normal younger sibling. All children should be praised for their accomplishments and allowed to grow at their own rate. Children should not be compared with their siblings, nor should there be a sense of competition. Nurses should be supportive to parents and help them in giving each child the individual attention he or she needs. Every family member is involved in building a wholesome, nonthreatening, noncompetitive, affirmative relationship.

Dyslexia

Dyslexia is the most common learning disability and is a major cause of school failure. The term "dyslexia" is loosely used to describe a condition affecting children who are two or more grades below their peers in reading level.

Etiology/Incidence (Pathophysiology)

About 15 per cent of children beginning school each year have dysfunctions in reading skills (Lubs et al, 1988). Of the children diagnosed with dyslexia, approximately 2 to 3 per cent have either primary or developmental dyslexia (DeVivo, 1991). Children with this pathologic condition should be differentiated from those with reading difficulties primarily due to lack of exposure to learning opportunities. Developmental dyslexia is more frequently found in boys than in girls. There is no known single cause of the condition.

It appears that "primary dyslexia" is usually familial. It may be due to weakness of one or several learning processes or immaturity of a certain part of the brain. "Developmental dyslexia" results from cerebral dysfunction and is evidenced in specific learning disorders of reading, spelling, and writing. The child can hear and understand statements but cannot read them. There seems to be a blockage or misconnection in the transmission of the written word from the eye to the higher brain centers in which the messages are integrated and relayed to the appropriate sensory area.

Diagnostic Assessment

The child with dyslexia may be unable to distinguish between similar-appearing letters, such as b and d. Letters may appear upside down or reversed. The children may read "on" for "no" or "was" for "saw." Letters are frequently seen in mirror image. Figure 27–3 helps illustrate the type of perceptual problems encountered by children with dyslexia.

The diagnosis of dyslexia is made through a battery of tests, including appropriate psychologic evaluations. The child is usually of average or above-average intelligence. As this is not a condition that warrants hospitalization, the nurse in that setting may have limited exposure to children with dyslexia. However, as a community health person, the nurse must be aware of the symptoms and further preventive intervention. Early recognition is the key to diminishing this problem. The child needs the assistance of a reading specialist. Individualized program planning in a structured setting with limited stimuli should be provided. If therapy is initiated early, children with dyslexia can attain the same reading level as their peers within a few years. If the problem is not recognized until the child is in the third or fourth grade, the response will be less favorable.

The nurse who does vision screening using a Snellen or an E chart can aid in the detection of visual perception problems. If a problem is suspected, the family should be informed and a referral made for a differential diagnosis by an ophthalmologist.

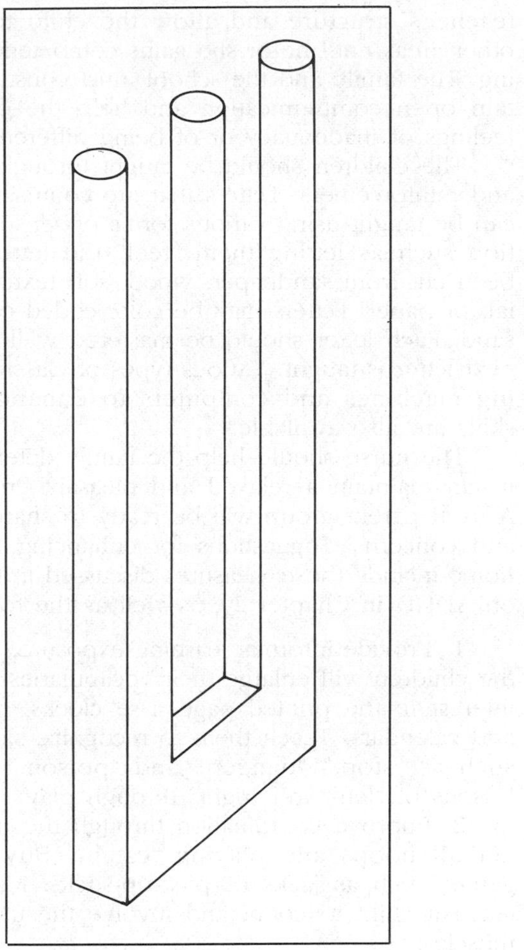

FIGURE 27-3. This drawing causes a perceptual dysfunction similar to that encountered in everyday activity by the child with dyslexia.

Arriving at a definite diagnosis will relieve family tension, as family members will have been aware of a problem and may have suspected cognitive impairment or emotional disturbance. Because children with dyslexia are usually of average intelligence, they frequently act out their frustrations by adopting an "I don't care" attitude or by using physical strength to show competencies lacking in other areas. Very sensitive children may develop feelings of inferiority and may regress in other areas. Early detection and treatment can help prevent secondary emotional scarring.

Nursing Care

Children should receive special help in remedial reading but should participate equally with their peers in other activities. There should be no discrimination because of lack of skill in one specific area. If their peers understand these children's specific needs, they can more readily accept the children as part of the group. The family should be encouraged not to emphasize reading excellence but to reinforce the teacher's structure and allow the child to excel in other areas until he or she gains competence in reading. The family and the school must constantly maintain open communication and help the child avoid feelings of inadequacy or of being different.

The children should be taught through repetition and reinforcement. Letters that are confusing to them can be taught using various forms of sensory stimulation such as letting them "feel" the letter that has been cut from sandpaper, wood, soft textured material, or paper. Letters may be color-coded or traced in sand. Each letter should be mastered well before the next letter is taught. Various types of classroom learning machines and computers to enhance reading skills are also available.

The nurse should help the family determine how it can maintain a relaxed and pleasant environment. A local parent group will be ready to share strengths and concerns. Suggestions for enhancing learning at home include those measures discussed in the section on ADHD in Chapter 29, as well as the following:

1. Provide informal learning exposure. Reading to the children will enlarge their vocabularies and create interest in the printed page. Use clocks, road maps, and calendars. Teach them to recognize safety words such as "stop," "danger," and "poison." Reinforce lessons of "left" and "right" through play.
2. Improve coordination through the use of basketball hoops and playing "catch." Buy hand-eye games such as jacks or pick-up-sticks. Many games teach a child to count and involve the use of small muscles.
3. Break down complicated tasks into small steps. Be sure the children are comfortable with each step before they attempt the next. Reward with praise. Do not scold or show impatience if they do not grasp the concept right away.
4. Assure the children that they are loved and are important family members.

KEY CONCEPTS

Concepts Related to Basic Information

- Early intervention refers to educational and therapeutic services provided for infants and toddlers between birth and 3 years of age who have been identified as biologically or environmentally at risk for developmental delay.
- Roadblocks that families face are attitudes of professionals, professional jargon, stigma attributed to having a child with a disability, time and energy to obtain services, and lack of support.
- Individualized Education Plan (IEP) written in the public school system focuses on the child's educational needs and guides special education intervention.
- Mental retardation (MR) refers to a constellation of symptoms consisting of impaired intellectual functioning associated with impaired social adaptation.
- The definition of developmental disability is a unique entity: unlike diagnostic labels given to illness disorders and conditions by medical, allied, and health sciences, this condition has been *legislatively mandated* by Congress.
- The Americans with Disabilities Act of 1990 extends to individuals with disabilities civil rights prohibiting discrimination based on disability in public and private sector employment, public accommodation, and transportation services.
- Although the neonatal period is a critical time for central nervous system damage, perinatal hazards are responsible for only 15 to 20 per cent of severe developmental disabilities. Environmental, genetic, and socioeconomic factors are responsible for 80 to 85 per cent of the damage. The child is at risk for central nervous system insults up to 2 years of age while growth of the brain is still occurring.
- "Full Inclusion" (an expansion of the "mainstreaming" policy) refers to assisting persons who have disabilities to work in settings and be educated in the same classroom where they will have the greatest opportunity to become as independent and productive as possible.
- The passage of Public Law 99–457 and subsequent amendments, PL 101–476 and PL 102–119 in the Individuals with Disabilities Education Act (IDEA), extend educational services to infants and toddlers who experience developmental delay(s) or are at risk for developmental delay(s) or with a diagnosed physical or mental condition that has a high probability of resulting in a developmental delay or disability.
- A network of federal agencies exists to promote and develop appropriate services and supports to individuals and their families; this network consists of *State Councils on Developmental Disabilities, Protection, and Advocacy* and *University Affiliated Programs*.
- Down syndrome, with its distinct physical features, affects both sexes equally, occurs in approximately 1 of every 1000 live births, and occurs with higher incidence as maternal age increases.
- Fetal alcohol syndrome (FAS) is the result of high levels of alcohol ingestion during pregnancy.
- Cerebral palsy is a neurologic problem with musculoskeletal consequences; the primary disorder involves a lack of motor control of voluntary muscles owning to a lesion in the brain that has occurred prenatally, at birth, or shortly thereafter.
- Delays in development can occur at any time during a child's developmental period, from birth through 18 years of age.

- Public Law 94–142 defines learning disability as "a disorder in one or more of the basic psychological processes involved in understanding or in using language, spoken or written, which may manifest itself as imperfect ability to listen, speak, read, write, spell, or do mathematical calculations."
- Dyslexia refers to children who are two or more grades below their peers in reading level; it is the most common learning disability and is a major cause of school failure.

Concepts Related to Nursing Assessment

- An infant or child suspected of having a developmental disability or who is "at risk" for developing a developmental disability is referred for more comprehensive interdisciplinary assessment to identify areas of delay in development.
- Diagnostic assessments are conducted throughout the life span of the child with a developmental disability as the needs of the child change.
- Throughout the assessment process the nurse's role is to establish baseline measurements, give support to child and parents, and assist the family to receive appropriate services in the community.
- Screening is not done to measure the child's intelligence or to make a diagnosis; it is used to define a potential problem and to indicate a child's areas of strength and weakness.
- Most screening tools can be completed by teachers, health professionals, and parents; more definitive assessment must be done by qualified professionals.
- Assessments are essential in order to detect infants who are at risk for developmental alterations; these alterations would also constitute nursing diagnostic responses of *altered or ineffective growth and development*.
- Ongoing assessment is done to assess parental coping and ability to provide for the child's special needs, involvement and support of all family members, and availability of resources with the family's kinship network and in the community to determine the family's ability to deal with the problems they are facing.
- A relatively common etiology for *altered health maintenance* in families of children with developmental disabilities is the inability to solve problems through their own efforts.
- Diagnosis of mental retardation requires a team approach; nurses are important members of the diagnostic team. Their observational skills in noting gross and fine motor movements, visual and auditory acuity, and emotional responses are important in diagnosis.
- Common nursing diagnostic responses and collaborative problems that result from assessment of the child with mental retardation are: *anticipatory grieving, uncompensated self-care deficit, impaired social interaction, altered sexuality patterns, impaired communication, social isolation, in-effective family coping, high risk for altered health maintenance, and health-seeking behaviors.*
- Assessment of the child with cerebral palsy and his or her family for potential and actual diagnoses is a continuous process because of the chronic nature of the child's condition.
- Assessment of a child who is suspected of having a learning disability may involve an interdisciplinary approach that often includes educators, psychologists, speech pathologists, and health care personnel.

Concepts Related to Nursing Interventions

- The case manager is responsible for ensuring that the child receives primary, secondary, and tertiary levels of preventive care; coordinates specialized services needed; and promotes child and family acquisition of goals.
- In almost every area of nursing, nurses will be involved in making referrals and working with children who are mentally retarded, whether in the hospital, clinic, community, or school settings.
- The nursing care will vary considerably for the child with mental retardation depending on the presence of other physical problems, the degree of mobility, any sensory alterations, and speech and hearing impairment.
- The primary goals of nursing care for the child with cerebral palsy include promoting physical mobility, promoting cognitive abilities, and monitoring and treating sensory perceptual alterations.
- The *individualized family service plan (IFSP)* provides the plan for the individualized services that the infant or toddler and family will need for the infant or toddler to achieve developmental milestones.
- The primary goal of early intervention programs is to reduce or minimize the incidence of developmental disabilities, which is achieved by providing structured learning experiences that foster the infant's or toddler's attainment of developmental milestones.
- Experts are advocating the philosophy of full inclusion rather than the mainstreaming of children with developmental disabilities into educational settings, as full inclusion expands on and goes beyond the concept of mainstreaming by promoting and advocating the full participation of the child with developmental disabilities in regular school programs.

- Nursing interventions are most effective that are directed to the etiology of the family's inability to solve problems through their own efforts of the nursing diagnosis, *altered health maintenance.*
- Because mental retardation can accompany many other physical problems, such as cerebral palsy, spina bifida, Turner syndrome, and hundreds of other inherited or acquired disorders, the nursing care will vary.
- The nurse in outpatient or community settings will continually assess the progress of the child with cerebral palsy with developmental tasks and determine if home care exercises are being performed to prevent further loss of function by assessing muscular strength and joint range of motion, comparing it with the recorded baseline.
- One of the nurse's greatest contributions in the long-term care of the child with a learning disability is to assist the family in using community resources.

REFERENCES

Alexander, M., & Bauer, R. (1988). Cerebral palsy. In V. Van Hasselt, P. Strain, & M. Hersen (Eds.), *Handbook of developmental and physical disabilities* (pp 215–226). New York: Pergamon Press.

American Academy of Pediatrics, Committee on Children with Disabilities (1992). Pediatrician's role in the development and implementation of an individual education plan (IEP) and/or an individual family service plan (IFSP). *Pediatrics, 89,* 340–342.

American Association on Mental Retardation (1992). *Mental retardation: Definition, classification, and system of supports.* Washington, DC: Author.

Amiel-Tison, C. (1985). Neurological assessment from birth to seven years of age. In S. Harel & N. Anastasiow (Eds.), *The at-risk infant: Psycho-social-medical aspects* (pp 239–251). Baltimore: Paul H. Brookes.

Anatasiow, N. (1986). *Development and disability: A psychological analysis for special educators.* Baltimore: Paul H. Brookes.

Barnard, K. (1987). *Interim report to National Institute of Mental Health.* Unpublished. NIMH Grant MH36894. Rockville, MD: National Institute of Mental Health.

Bayley, N. (1969). *Bayley scales of infant development.* New York: Psychological Corp.

Beckman, P. (1984). Perceptions of young children with handicaps: A comparison of mothers and program staff. *Mental Retardation, 22,* 176–181.

Behrman, R. (1992). *Nelson textbook of pediatrics* (14th ed.). Philadelphia: WB Saunders.

Betz, C. (1993a). *Opportunities for advanced clinical practice: Extending your nursing expertise.* Presentation given at Society for Pediatric Nurses, San Francisco, April 22, 1993.

Betz, C. (1993b). Pediatric community needs. *Journal of Pediatric Nursing, 8*(3), 141.

Biklen, D. (1976). Advocacy comes of age. *Exceptional Children, 2,* 309.

Blackman, J. (1990). *Medical aspects of developmental disabilities in children birth to three* (2nd ed.). Aspen, CO: Aspen Publishers.

Botshaw, M., & Perret, Y. (1981). *Children with handicaps: A medical primer* (pp 253–269). Baltimore: Paul H. Brookes.

Bradley, V., et al (1990). *Family support services in the United States: An end-of-decade status report.* Cambridge, MA: Human Services Research Institute.

Bureau of Community Health Service. (1979). *Individual service plans in the supplemental security income disabled children's program.* Rockville, MD: Office of Maternal-Child Care.

Caesar, P., & Eggermont, E. (1985). Neonatal clinical neurological assessment. In S. Harel & E. Eggermont (Eds.), *The at-risk infant* (pp 197–220). Baltimore: Paul H. Brookes.

Chin, P., Drew, C. J., & Logan, D. R. (1979). *Mental retardation: A life cycle approach.* St. Louis: CV Mosby.

Cohen, F. (1984). *Clinical genetics in nursing practice.* Philadelphia: JB Lippincott.

Cole, D., & Meyer, L. (1991). Social integration and severe disabilities: A longitudinal analysis of child outcomes. *Journal of Special Education, 25,* 340–351.

Collins, M. (1983). *Communication in health care* (2nd ed.) St. Louis: CV Mosby.

Community Alliance for Special Education (CASE) (1989). *Special education: Rights and responsibilities.* (2nd ed.) Sacramento, CA: Author.

Cooley, W., & Graham, J. (1990). Down syndrome—An update and review for the primary pediatrician. *Clinical Pediatrics, 30*(4), 233–253.

Copeland, M., & Kimmel, J. (1989). *Evaluation and management of infants and young children with developmental disabilities.* Baltimore: Paul H. Brookes.

Cowell, J. (1990). Dilemmas in assessing the health status of children with learning disabilities. *Journal of Pediatric Health Care, 4,* 24–31.

Damrosch, S., & Perry, L. (1989). Self reported adjustment, chronic sorrow and coping of parents of children with Down syndrome. *Nursing Research, 38,* 25–30.

Dashiff, C. (1991). Marital strife, social support, and the development of mentally retarded toddlers. *Journal of Child and Adolescent Psychiatric and Mental Nursing, 4*(3), 90–95.

Deatrick, J., Knafl, K., & Walsch, M. (1988). The process of parenting a child with a disability: Normalization through accommodation. *Journal of Advanced Nursing, 13,* 15–21.

DeVivo, D. (1991). Developmental dyslexia. In A. Rudolph (Ed.), *Rudolph's pediatrics* (pp 1730–1731). Norwalk, CT: Appleton & Lange.

Doleysh, N. (Chapter Ed.). (1991). Neuromuscular disorders. In S. W. Salmond, N. E. Mooney, & L. A. Verdisco (Eds.), *National association of orthopaedic nursing care curriculum for orthopaedic nursing.* Pitman, NJ: Anthony J. Jannetti.

Downing, J. (1987). Conversational skill training: Teaching adolescents with mental retardation to be verbally assertive. *Mental Retardation, 25,* 147–155.

Drapo, P. (1986). Mental retardation. In B. Johnson (Ed.), *Psychiatric-mental health nursing* (pp 433–456). Philadelphia: JB Lippincott.

Drennan, J. C. (1990). Neuromuscular disorders. In R. T. Morrissy (Ed.), *Lovell and Winter's pediatric orthopaedics* (3rd ed., pp 381–463). Philadelphia: JB Lippincott.

Easter Seal Society. (1982). *Early warning signs: Learning disabilities—A hidden handicap.* New York: Author.

Edwards-Beckett, J. (1991). Caregiver attributions of success or failure of their mentally retarded dependent. *Journal of Pediatric Nursing, 6*(2), 121–126.

Ellison, P., Prasse, D., Siewert, J., et al. (1985). The outcome of neurological abnormality in infancy. In S. Harel & N. Anastasiow (Eds.), *The at-risk infant* (pp 253–260). Baltimore: Paul H. Brookes.

Failla, S., et al. (1991). Families of children with developmental disabilities: An examination of family hardiness. *Research in Nursing and Health, 14,* 41–50.

Faux, S. (1992). Sibling relationships in families with congenitally impaired children. *Journal of Pediatric Nursing, 6*(3), 175–184.

Ferguson, A. B. (1981). *Orthopedic surgery in infancy and childhood.* Baltimore: Williams & Wilkins.

Forness, S., & Kavale, K. (1989). Identification and diagnostic issues in special education: A status report for child psychiatrists. *Child Psychiatry and Human Development, 19,* 279–301.

Franco, S., & Andrews, B. (1977). Reduction of cerebral palsy by neonatal intensive care. *Pediatric Clinics of North America, 24,* 639–649.

Frankenberger, W. (1984). A survey of state guidelines for identification of mental retardation. *Mental Retardation, 22,* 17–20.

Goldfarb, G., Brotherson, M. J., Summers, J. A., et al. (1986). *Meet-*

ing the challenge of disability or chronic illness: A family guide. Baltimore: Paul H. Brookes.

Hansen, S., Holaday, B., & Miles, M. (1990). The role of pediatric nurses in a federal program for infants and young children with handicaps. *Journal of Pediatric Nursing, 5,* 246–251.

Hecht, B., & Forness, S. (1988). Special education for handicapped and disabled children: Classification, programs, and trends. *Journal of Pediatric Nursing, 3*(2), 75–88.

Hirose, T., & Ueda, R. (1990). Long-term follow-up study of cerebral palsy children and coping behavior of parents. *Journal of Advanced Nursing, 15,* 762–770.

Johnson, B. S. (1986). The emotionally disturbed child. In Johnson, B. (Ed.), *Psychiatric-mental health nursing* (pp 370–396). Philadelphia: WB Saunders.

Jones, K. (1988). *Smith's recognizable patterns of human malformation.* Philadelphia: WB Saunders.

Kepes, J. (1982). Mental retardation: Some pathological considerations. In I. Jakab (Ed.), *Mental retardation.* New York: Karger.

Kliegman, R. M., & Behrman, R. E. (1992). Metabolic disturbances. In R. E. Behrman (Ed.), *Nelson textbook of pediatrics* (14th ed., pp 489–492). Philadelphia, WB Saunders.

Krauss, M. (1990). New precedent in family policy: Individualized family service plan. *Exceptional Children, 56,* 388–395.

Latham, C., & Yando, R. (1982). Psychological assessments of the retarded. In I. Jakab (Ed.), *Mental retardation* (pp 120–141). New York: Karger.

Lewis, K. S. (1992). Pathophysiology of prenatal drug exposure: In utero, in the newborn, in childhood, and in agencies. *Journal of Pediatric Nursing, 6*(3), 185–190.

Lubs, H., Smith, S., Kimberling, W., et al. (1988). Dyslexia subtypes: Genetics, behavior and brain imaging. *Research in Nervous and Mental Diseases, 66,* 139.

Magyary, D., Brandt, P., Fleming, J., Kieckhefer, G., & Padgett, D. (1993). Nursing specialty practice guidelines: The implications for clinical scholarship and early intervention practice. *Journal of Pediatric Nursing, 8*(4), 253–260.

McCarthy, M. (1972). *McCarthy scales of children's abilities.* New York: Psychological Corp.

McFarland, G., & Wasli, E. (1986). *Nursing diagnosis and process in psychiatric-mental health nursing.* Philadelphia: JB Lippincott.

Meisels, S., & Provence, S. (1989). *Screening and assessment: Guidelines for identifying young disabled and developmentally vulnerable children and families.* Washington, DC: National Center for Clinical Infant Programs.

Meeropol, E. (1992). One of the gang: Sexual development of adolescents with physical disabilities. *Journal of Pediatric Nursing, 6*(4), 243–250.

Mental Health Law Project (1990). Lost effectiveness. *Early Intervention Advocacy Network, 2,* 5.

Monea, H. (1981). The geropsychiatric public health nurse: A model for comprehensive mental health care. In P. Hess (Ed.), *Toward healthy aging* (pp 610–621). St. Louis: CV Mosby.

Nash, J., Rounds, K., & Bowen, G. (1992). Level of parental involvement on early childhood intervention teams. *Families in Society: The Journal of Contemporary Human Services, 73,* 93–99.

Perkins, M. (1993). Parent-nurse collaboration: Using the caregiver identity emergence phases to assist parents of hospitalized children with disabilities. *Journal of Pediatric Nursing, 8*(1), 2–9.

President's Committee on Mental Retardation. (1975). *White House Conference on Handicapped Individuals.* Vol. 5. Washington, DC: US Government Printing Office.

Pueschel, S., & Mulick, J. (1990). *Prevention of developmental disabilities.* Baltimore: Paul H. Brookes.

Ramey, C., Bryant, D., Wasik, B., Sparling, Fendt, K., & LaVange, L. (1992). Infant health and development program for low birth weight, premature infants: Program elements, family participation, and child intelligence. *Pediatrics, 3,* March, 454–465.

Ramey, C., Bryant, D., Sparling, J., & Wasik, B. (1985). Project CARE: A comparison of two early intervention strategies. *Topics in Early Childhood Special Education, 5,* 12–25.

Savage, T., & Culbert, C. (1989). Early intervention: The unique role of nursing. *Journal of Pediatric Nursing, 4*(5), 339–345.

Scarr, S., & McCartney, K. (1988). Far from home: An experimental evaluation of the mother-child home program. *Child Development, 59,* 532–543.

Schafer, S. D. (1984). *Child success through parent training: A final report.* Denton, TX: Texas Woman's University. (Available from Sue Schaffer, Texas Woman's University School of Physical Therapy, P.O. Box 22487, Denton, TX, 76204.)

Schaumann, B., & Alter, M. (1976). *Dermatoglyphics in medical disorders.* New York: Springer-Verlag.

Seligman, M. (1991). Grandparents of disabled grandchildren: Hopes, fears, and adaptation. *Families in Society: The Journal of Contemporary Human Services, 72*(3), 147–152.

Siperstein, G., & Bak, J. (1989). Social relationships of adolescents with moderate mental retardation. *Mental Retardation, 27,* 5–10.

Steele, M. (1982). Genetics of mental retardation. In I. Jakab (Ed.), *Mental retardation* (pp 27–37). New York: Karger.

Steele, S. (1990). Down syndrome: Nursing interventions newborn through preschool age years. *Issues in Comprehensive Pediatric Nursing, 13,* 111–126.

Stine, G. J. (1989). *The new human genetics.* Dubuque, IA: William C Brown.

Terman, L., & Merrill, M. (1973). *Stanford-Binet intelligence scale.* Boston: Houghton Mifflin.

Vessey, J. (1988). Care of the hospitalized child with a cognitive development delay. *Holistic Nursing Practice, 2,* 48–54.

Walker, O., et al. (1989). Mainstreaming children with handicaps: Implications for pediatricians. *Journal of Developmental and Behavioral Pediatrics, 10,* 151–156.

Zetlin, A., & Turner, J. (1985). Transition from adolescence to adulthood: Perspectives of mentally retarded individuals and their families. *American Journal of Mental Deficiency, 89*(6), 570–579.

BIBLIOGRAPHY

Early Intervention

Barnard, K., & Kelly, J. (1980). Infant intervention: Parental considerations. In *Guidelines for early intervention programs.* Salt Lake City: University of Utah, College of Nursing, pp 34–55. (Available from Office for Maternal-Child Health, Room 7–39, Parklawn Bldg., 5600 Fishers Lane, Rockville, MD 20857.)

Chasnoff, I. (1987, May). Perinatal effects of cocaine. *Contemporary Ob-Gyn,* 163–179.

Copeland, M., & Kimmel, J. (1989). Evaluation and management of infants and young children with developmental disabilities. Baltimore: Paul H. Brookes.

Dixon, S. D. (1989). Effects of transplacental exposure to cocaine and methamphetamine on the neonate. *The Western Journal of Medicine, 150,* 436–442.

Fulroth, R., et al. (1989). Perinatal outcome of infants exposed to cocaine and/or heroin in utero. *American Journal of Diseases of Children, 143,* 905.

Gawin, F. H., & Ellingwood, E. H. (1988). Cocaine and other stimulants, actions, abuse and treatment. *The New England Journal of Medicine, 318,* 1173–1182.

Gordon, B. (1988). A conceptual model for tracking high risk infants and making early service decisions. *Journal of Developmental and Behavioral Pediatrics, 9,* 279–286.

Hadeed, A. J., & Siegel, S. R. (1989). Maternal cocaine use during pregnancy: Effect on the newborn infant. *Pediatrics, 84,* 205–209.

Harms, D., & Giordano, J. (1990). Ethical issues in high-risk infant care. *Issues in Comprehensive Pediatric Nursing, 13,* 1–14.

Howard, J., et al. (1989). The development of young children of substance abusing parents: Insight from seven years of intervention. *Zero to Three, Bulletin of National Center for Clinical Infant Programs, 9.*

Jones, K. (1988). *Smith's recognizable patterns of human malformation.* Philadelphia: WB Saunders.

Katz, I., et al. (1989). *Chronically ill and at risk infants.* Palo Alto, CA: VORT.

Krehbiel, R., et al. (1991). NICU infants born at developmental risk and the individualized family service plan/process (IFSP). *Children Health Care, 20,* 26–33.
Lewis, K. DeS., Bennett, B., & Schmeder, N. (1989). The care of infants menaced by cocaine abuse. *Maternal-Child Nursing, 14,* 324–329.
Little, B., et al. (1989). Cocaine abuse during pregnancy: Maternal and neonatal correlates. *Journal of Pediatrics, 73,* 157–160.
Lott, J. W. (1989). Developmental care of the preterm infant. *Neonatal Network, 7,* 21–28.
Murphy, K. (1990). Interactional styles of parents following the birth of a high-risk infant. *Journal of Pediatric Nursing, 5*(1), 33–41.
Patterson, D. M., & Barnard, K. E. (1990). Parenting of low birth weight infants: A review of issues and interventions. *Infant Mental Health Journal, 11,* 37–56.
Plomin, R. (1990). *Nature and nuture: An introduction to human behavioral genetics.* Pacific Grove, CA: Brooks/Cole Publishing Co.
Pueschel, S., & Mulick, J. (1990). Prevention of developmental disabilities. Baltimore: Paul H. Brookes.
Ramey, C., Bryant, D., & Svarez, T. (1990). Early intervention: Why, for whom, how, and at what cost? *Clinics in Perinatology, 17,* 47–55.
Schneider, J., et al. (1989). Infants exposed to cocaine in utero: Implications for developmental assessment and intervention. *Infants and Young Children, 2,* 25–36.
Sharav, T., & Shlomo, L. (1986). Stimulation of infants with Down syndrome: Long-term effects. *Mental Retardation, 24,* 81–86.
Sparrow, S., Balla, D., & Cicchette, D. (1984). Vineland adaptive behavior scale—Interview edition. In *Survey Form Manual.* Pines, MN: American Guidance Service.
Strobel, S., & Keller, C. (1993). Metabolic screening in the NICU population: A proposal for change. *Pediatric Nursing, 19*(2), 113–121.
Turnbull, J., Turnbull, A., Bronicki, G., Summers, J., & Roeder-Gordon, C. (1989). *Disability and the family.* Baltimore: Paul H. Brookes.
Weider, S., et al. (1989). A developmental/relationship in-service training model for public health nurses serving multirisk infants and families. *Zero to Three, 10,* 16–20.
Weston, D., et al. (1989). Drug exposed babies: Research and clinical issues. *Zero to Three, Bulletin of the National Center for Clinical Infant Programs, 9.*

Technology-Assisted Children

Butler, C. (1988). High tech tots: Technology for mobility, manipulation, communication, and learning in early childhood. *Infants and Young Children, 1,* 66–73.
Cavalier, A. (1989). *Ethical issues related to technology.* Paper presented at the pre-conference for the Association for Retarded Citizens/ARK 1989 Annual Conference, Little Rock, AK.
Hazlett, D. (1989). A study of pediatric home ventilator management: Medical, psychosocial and financial management. *Journal of Pediatric Nursing, 4,* 284–294.
Joint Task Force for the Management of Children with Special Health Needs. (1990). *Guidelines for the delineation of roles and responsibilities for the safe delivery of specialized health care in the educational setting.* Reston, VA: Council for Exceptional Children.
Leonard, B., Brust, J., & Nelson, R. (1993). Parental distress: Caring for medically fragile children at home. *Journal of Pediatric Nursing, 8*(1), 22–30.
Morris, M. (1990). *State systems for the funding of assistive technology services: A workbook approach.* Paper presented at the RESNA Funding Assistive Technology for Individuals with Disabilities: A blueprint for change workshop, Washington, DC.
Odom, S. A., & Chandler, L. (1990). Transition to parenthood for parents of technology-assisted infants. *Topics in Early Childhood Special Education, 9,* 43–54.
Parette, H., & Parette, P. (1992). Young children with disabilities and assistive technology: The nurse's role on multidisciplinary technology teams. *Journal of Pediatric Nursing, 7*(4), 237–245.
RESNA. (1989). *Technology related assistance for individuals with disabilities. Summaries of 1989 successful grant applications awarded under P.L. 100–407.* Washington, DC: RESNA Press.
Scannell, S., Gillies, D., Biordi, D., & Child, D. (1993). Negotiating nurse-patient authority in pediatric home health care. *Journal of Pediatric Nursing, 8*(2), 70–78.
Steele, N., & Morgan, J. (1989). Emergency planning for technology-assisted children. *Journal of Pediatric Nursing, 4,* 81–87.

Mental Retardation

American Psychiatric Association. (1987). *Diagnostic and statistical manual of mental disorders* (3rd ed.). Washington, DC: Author.
Blackman, J. (1990). *Medical aspects of developmental disabilities in children birth to three* (2nd ed.). Aspen, CO: Aspen Publishers.
Brody, G., et al. (1991). Observations of the role relations and behavior between older children with mental retardation and their younger siblings. *American Journal of Mental Retardation, 95,* 527–536.
Cole, D., et al. (1991). Dyadic interactions between children with and without mental retardation: Effects of age discrepancy. *American Journal of Mental Deficiency, 92,* 194–202.
Cole, D. A. (1988). Difficulties in relationships between non-handicapped and severely mentally retarded children: The effect of physical impairments. *Research in Developmental Disabilities, 9,* 55–72.
Damrosch, S., & Perry, L. (1989). Self reported adjustment, chronic sorrow and coping of parents of children with Down syndrome. *Nursing Research, 38,* 25–30.
Edwards-Beckett, J. (1991). Caregiver attributions of success of their mentally-retarded dependent. *Journal of Pediatric Nursing, 6,* 121–126.
Failla, S., et al. (1991). Families of children with developmental disabilities: An examination of family hardiness. *Research in Nursing and Health, 14,* 41–50.
Flynt, S., & Wood, T. (1989). Stress and coping of mothers of children with moderate mental retardation. *American Journal of Mental Retardation, 94,* 278–283.
Foster-Gaitskell, D., & Pratt, C. (1989). Comparison of parent and teacher ratings of adaptive behavior of children with mental retardation. *American Journal on Mental Retardation, 94,* 177–181.
Frankenberger, W., & Harper, J. (1988). States' definitions and procedures for identifying children with mental retardation: Comparison of 1981–1982 and 1985–1986 guidelines. *Mental Retardation, 26,* 133–136.
Hanzrik, J. (1990). Interactions between mothers and their infants with developmental disabilities: Analysis and review. *Physical and Occupational Therapy in Pediatrics, 9,* 33–47.
Honk, V., & Thacker, S. (1989). The Centers for Disease Control program to prevent primary and secondary disabilities in the United States. *Public Health Reports, 104,* 226–231.
Kastner, T., et al. (1989). Child life services and persons with mental retardation. *Journal of Developmental and Behavioral Pediatrics, 10,* 198–200.
Kiikkala, I., & Peitsi, T. (1991). The care of children with minimal brain dysfunction: A Roy adaptation analysis. *Journal of Pediatric Nursing, 6,* 290–292.
Lombardo, E., & Lombardo, V. (1987). Attitudes of elementary, middle and high school teachers toward mainstreaming: Implications for job satisfaction. *International Journal of Rehabilitation Research, 10,* 405–410.
McCormick, P., et al. (1990). Instruction on Piagetian concepts for children with mental retardation. *Mental Retardation, 28,* 359–366.
Meeropol, E. (1991). One of the gang: Sexual development of adolescents with physical disabilities. *Journal of Pediatric Nursing, 6,* 243–251.
Nadler, A., et al. (1991). Acceptance of mental retardation and help-seeking by mothers and fathers of children with mental retardation. *Mental Retardation, 29,* 17–23.
Nelson, R. (1989). Community services for children with mental retardation. *Pediatric Annals, 18,* 615–621.
Orelove, F., & Sobsey, D. (1991). *Educating children with multiple disabilities.* Baltimore: Paul H. Brookes.

Orr, R., et al. (1991). Coping with stress in families with children who have mental retardation: An evaluation of the double ABCX model. *American Journal of Mental Retardation, 95,* 444–450.

Phillips, M., & Brostoff, M. (1989). Working collaboratively with parents of disabled children. *Pediatric Nursing, 15,* 180–185.

Rauh, J., et al. (1989). Sterilization for the mentally retarded adolescent. *Journal of Adolescent Health Care, 10,* 467–472.

Rynders, J. E., & Horrobin, J. M. (1990). Always trainable? Updating education expectations concerning children with Down syndrome. *American Journal on Mental Retardation, 95,* 77–83.

Seyfarth, J., et al. (1987). Factors influencing parents vocational aspirations for their children with mental retardation. *Mental Retardation 25,* 357–362.

Stainback, S., et al. (Eds.). (1989). *Educating all students in the mainstream of regular education.* Baltimore: Paul H. Brookes.

Steele, S., et al. (1989). Home Management of URI in Children with Down syndrome. *Journal of Pediatric Nursing, 15,* 484–488.

Stoneman, Z., et al. (1989). Role relations between children who are mentally retarded and their older siblings: Observation in three in-home contexts. *Research in Developmental Disabilities, 10,* 61–76.

Stoneman, Z., et al. (1988). Childcare responsibilities, peer relations, and sibling conflict: Older siblings of mentally retarded children. *American Journal of Mental Retardation, 93,* 174–183.

Stoneman, Z., et al. (1991). Ascribed role relations between children with mental retardation and their younger siblings. *American Journal of Mental Retardation, 95,* 537–550.

Tharinger, D., et al. (1990). Sexual abuse and exploitation of children and adults with mental retardation and other handicaps. *Child Abuse and Neglect, 14,* 301–312.

Turnbull, J., et al., (1989). *Disability and the Family.* Baltimore: Paul H. Brookes.

Turner, K., & Szymanski, E. (1990). Work adjustment of people with congenital disabilities: A longitudinal perspective from birth to adulthood. *Journal of Rehabilitation, 56,* 19–24.

Tymchuk, A., & Andron, L. (1990). Mothers with mental retardation who do or do not abuse or neglect their children. *Child Abuse and Neglect, 14,* 313–323.

Walker, O., et al. (1989). Mainstreaming children with handicaps: Implications for pediatricians. *Journal of Developmental and Behavioral Pediatrics, 10,* 151–156.

Learning Disabilities

Bender, W., & Smith, J. (1990). Classroom behavior of children and adolescents with learning disabilities: A meta-analysis. *Journal of Learning Disabilities, 23,* 298–305.

Cowell, J. (1990). Dilemmas in assessing the health status of children with learning disabilities. *Journal of Pediatric Health Care, 4,* 24–31.

Grolnick, W., & Ryan, R. (1990). Self perceptions, motivation, and adjustment in children with learning disabilities: A multiple group comparison study. *Journal of Learning Disabilities, 23,* 177–184.

Kershner, J. (1990). Self-concept and IQ as predictors of remedial success in children with learning disabilities. *Journal of Learning Disabilities, 23,* 363–374.

Meyer, S. (1989). Developmental psychology casebook. Developmental follow-up of children with multiple risks for learning disabilities. *Journal of Perinatology, 9,* 212–214.

Myles, B., & Simpson, R. (1990). Mainstreaming modification preferences of parents of elementary-age children with learning disabilities. *Journal of Learning Disabilities, 23,* 234–239.

Norhonen, T. (1991). Neuropsychological stability and prognosis of subgroups of children with learning disabilities. *Journal of Learning Disabilities, 24,* 48–57.

Priel, B., & Leshem, T. (1990). Self-perceptions of first-and second-grade children with learning disabilities. *Journal of Learning Disabilities, 23,* 637–642.

Telzrow, C. (1991). Role of the school in serving children with learning disabilities. *Seminars in Neurology, 11,* 50–56.

Torgesen, J. (1988). The cognitive and behavioral characteristics of children with learning disabilities: An overview. *Journal of Learning Disabilities, 21,* 587–589.

Toro, P., et al. (1990). A comparison of children with and without learning disabilities and social problem-solving skill: School behavior and family background. *Journal of Learning Disabilities, 23,* 115–120.

Waggoner, K., & Wilgosh, L. (1990). Concerns of families of children with learning disabilities. *Journal of Learning Disabilities, 23,* 97–98, 113.

Wansart, W. (1990). Learning to solve a problem: A microanalysis of the solution strategies of children with learning disabilities. *Journal of Learning Disabilities, 23,* 164–170, 184.

Developmental Delay

Alexander, M., & Bauer, R. (1988). *Handbook of developmental and physical disabilities.* New York: Pergamon Press.

Barnard, K., & Erikson, M. (1976). *Teaching children with developmental problems: A family care approach* (2nd ed.). St. Louis: CV Mosby.

Baron-Cohen, S. (1989). The autistic child's theory of mind: A case of specific developmental delay. *Journal of Child Psychology and Psychiatry and Allied Disciplines, 30,* 285–297.

Blackman, J. (1990). *Medical aspects of developmental disabilities in children birth to three* (2nd ed.). Aspen: Aspen Publishers.

Davis, H., & Rusthon, R. (1991). Counselling and supporting parents of children with developmental delay: A research evaluation. *Journal of Mental Deficiency Research, 35,* 89–112.

Dowdney, L., et al. (1987). Growth retardation and developmental delay amongst inner-city children. *Journal of Child Psychology and Psychiatry and Allied Disciplines, 28,* 529–541.

Fox, S., et al. (1990). Psychotherapy and developmental delay in homeless children: A pilot study. *Journal of the American Academy of Child and Adolescent Psychiatry, 29,* 732–735.

Hansen, S., Holaday, B., & Miles, M. (1990). The role of pediatric nurses in a federal program for infants and young children with handicaps. *Journal of Pediatric Nursing, 5,* 246–251.

Silva, P., et al. (1987). A longitudinal study of children with developmental language delay at age three: Later intelligence, reading and behavior problems. *Developmental Medicine and Child Neurology, 29,* 630–640.

Stainback, S., Stainback, W., & Forest, M. (Eds.). (1989). *Educating all students in the mainstream of regular education.* Baltimore: Paul H. Brookes.

Steele, S. (1991). Preschool children with developmental delay: Nursing intervention. *Journal of Pediatric Health Care, 2,* 245–252.

Vessey, J. (1988). Care of the hospitalized child with a cognitive developmental delay. *Holistic Nursing Practice, 2,* 48–54.

Whitman, T., et al. (1987). Predicting and understanding developmental delay of children of adolescent mothers: A multidimensional approach. *American Journal of Mental Deficiency, 92,* 40–56.

Cerebral Palsy

Ainojosa, J. (1990). How mothers of preschool children with cerebral palsy perceive occupational and physical therapists and their influence on family life. *Occupational Therapy Journal of Research, 10,* 144–162.

Alexander, M., & Bauer, R. (1988). Cerebral palsy. In V. Van Hasselt, P. Strain, & M. Hersen (Eds.), *Handbook of developmental and physical disabilities.* New York: Pergamon Press.

Bleck, E. (1982). Cerebral palsy. In E. Bleck (Ed.), *Physically handicapped children.* New York: Grune & Stratton.

Brucker, J. H. (1991). Selective dorsal rhizotomy. *Journal of Pediatric Nursing, 5,* 105–114.

Craft, M., et al. (1990). Siblings as change agents for promoting the functional status of children with cerebral palsy. *Developmental Medicine and Child Neurology, 32,* 1049–1057.

Ford, G., et al. (1990). Changing diagnosis of cerebral palsy in very low birthweight children. *American Journal of Perinatology, 7,* 178–181.

Giulani, C. (1991). Dorsal rhizotomy for children with cerebral palsy: Support for concepts of motor control. *Physical Therapy, 71,* 248–259.

Growth and nutrition in children with cerebral palsy. (1990). *Lancet, 335,* 1253–1254.

Hinojosa, J., & Anderson, J. (1991). Mothers' perceptions of home treatment programs for their preschool children with cerebral palsy. *American Journal of Occupational Therapy, 45,* 273–279.

Hirose, T., & Ueda, R. (1990). Long-term follow-up study of cerebral palsy children and coping behavior of parents. *Journal of Advanced Nursing, 15,* 762–770.

Issues in the management of children with spastic cerebral palsy. (1990). *Pediatrician, 17,* 230–236.

Law, M., et al. (1991). Neurodevelopmental therapy and upper-extremity inhibitive casting for children with cerebral palsy. *Developmental Medicine and Child Neurology, 33,* 379–387.

McPherson, J., et al. (1991). Analysis of upper extremity movement in four sitting positions: A comparison of persons with and without cerebral palsy. *American Journal of Occupational Therapy, 45,* 123–129.

Parette, H. (1990). Frequency and duration of therapeutic intervention with young children with cerebral palsy. *Psychology Reports, 67,* 697–698.

Peacock, W., & Staudt, L. (1991). Functional outcomes following selective posterior rhizotomy in children with cerebral palsy. *Journal of Neurosurgery, 74,* 300–305.

Philichi, L., et al. (1990). Rhizotomy surgery to relieve spasticity in young children. *MCN: American Journal of Maternal Child Nursing, 15,* 367–370.

Phillips, W., & Audet, M. (1990). Use of serial casting in the management of knee joint contractures in an adolescent with cerebral palsy. *Physical Therapy, 20,* 521–523.

Rosenbraum, P., Russell, D., Cadman, D., Gowland, C., Jarvis, S., & Hardy, S. (1990). Issues in measuring change in motor function in children with cerebral palsy: A special communication. *Physical Therapy, 70,* 125–131.

Rubin, I., & Crocker, A. (1989). Cerebral palsy in developmental disabilities: Delivery of medical care for children and adults. Philadelphia: Lea & Febiger.

Wiklund, et al. (1991). Computed tomography as an adjunct in etiological analysis of hemiplegic cerebral palsy. I: Children born preterm. *Neuropediatrics, 22,* 50–56.

Yokochi, K., et al. (1990). Gross motor patterns in children with cerebral palsy and spastic diplegie. *Pediatric Neurology, 6,* 245–250.

Other Disabilities

Alexander, M., & Steg, N. (1989). Myelomeningocele: Comprehensive treatment. *Archives of Physical Medicine and Rehabilitation, 70,* 637–641.

Green, N. (1987). The orthopaedic care of children with muscular dystrophy. *Instructional Course Lectures, 36,* 267–274.

Leger, R., & Meeropol, E. (1992). Children at risk: Latex allergy and spina bifida. *Journal of Pediatric Nursing,* 7(6), 371–377.

Monsen, R. (1992). Autonomy, coping, and self-care agency in healthy adolescents and in adolescents with spina bifida. *Journal of Pediatric Nursing,* 7(1), 9–13.

Smith, K. (1991). Bowel and bladder management of the child with myelomeningocele in the school setting. *Journal of Enterostomal Therapy, 18,* 6–10.

Steele, S. (1989). Phenylketonuria: Counseling and teaching functions of the nurse on an interdisciplinary team. *Issues in Comprehensive Pediatric Nursing, 12,* 395–409.

Van Cleve, L. (1989). Parental coping in response to their child's spina bifida. *Journal of Pediatric Nursing, 4,* 172–176.

Wharton, R., & Bresnan, M. (1989). Neonatal respiratory depression and delay in diagnosis in Prader Willi syndrome. *Developmental Medicine and Child Neurology, 3,* 231–236.

Whelan, T. (1987). Neuropsychological performance of children with Duchenne muscular dystrophy and spinal muscle atrophy. *Developmental Medicine and Child Neurology. 29,* 212–220.

CHAPTER • 28

Child Abuse and Maltreatment

B. Helen Thomas

RELATED TOPICS
Assessing and promoting family health, Chapter 2
Maternal-infant attachment, Chapter 4
Promoting Healthy Parenting, Chapter 12
Fostering Self-Esteem, Chapter 14
Understanding altered behavior, Chapter 29

LEARNING OBJECTIVES

- **Define abuse and maltreatment.**
- **Describe the extent of the problem of child abuse and maltreatment.**
- **Describe provider's legal responsibility to report child abuse and maltreatment.**
- **Relate your knowledge about the theoretical perspectives of child abuse and maltreatment.**
- **Understand and cite the nursing skills necessary to intervene with abused and maltreated children and their families at all stages (e.g., prevention, assessment, identification, and treatment).**

Child abuse and maltreatment are complex problems with serious immediate and long-term ramifications for children and adolescents, their families, and society. The problems transcend the health, social, and legal structures in society. Nurses may be involved in prevention, identification, and short-term and long-term treatment of abused and maltreated children and their families, regardless of the setting of their employment.

The purpose of this chapter is to instill in nurses a basic understanding of these problems. This chapter defines child abuse and maltreatment, describes the extent of the problem, and presents several theoretical frameworks with which to view the problem. In addition, it also discusses potential nursing roles in the prevention, identification, and treatment of child abuse and maltreatment and the knowledge and skills required to implement the nursing roles effectively.

Definition of Child Abuse and Maltreatment

One of the difficulties encountered by practitioners and researchers in the area of child abuse and maltreatment is that of definition. This difficulty exists because of deep-rooted personal values and beliefs and because of the numbers of professional disciplines and perspectives represented in the ranks of people involved in the problem. Furthermore, definitions are developed for different purposes, such as social policy, legal regulations, research, and case management (Hutchison, 1990).

On a philosophic level, very few would disagree with Gil's (1975) definition of child abuse and maltreatment:

> Any act of commission or omission by which individuals, institutions, or society as a whole deprive children of equal rights and liberties and/or interfere with their optimal development constitutes, by definition, abuse or neglectful acts or conditions . . . Child abuse, neglect, and deprivation are recognized most commonly when the parent or caretaker commits an act of omission or commission which inhibits the child's development. This may be a single incident, an occasional event, or a regular pattern.

Ultimately, the actual definition of child abuse, neglect, or maltreatment is determined by the judicial system. All states in the United States and all provinces in Canada have laws defining child abuse and specifying the actions that can be taken to protect the child and punish the perpetrator. When a child's safety and health are clearly threatened, child protection agencies are empowered to separate the child from the family.

Although child abuse and maltreatment may be perpetrated by other than family members (e.g., day care center employees, baby sitters, extended family relatives, other adults in positions of power), the primary focus in this chapter is on the nursing role with children and their abusive or maltreating families. Those wishing to explore the issue of abuse by nonrelated caregivers are referred to an article by Margolin (1991). Jonker and Jonker-Bakker (1991) provide discussions about ritual abuse. Gale and associates (1988) give an overview of the characteristics of sexual abuse.

However, strong traditions in North American culture work against a simple definition of child abuse and recognition of when such abuse is occurring. Children, in the past, have been considered the property of their parents. There has been a tradition that "parents know best" and that discipline is a parent's right.

The first child abuse case ever prosecuted in the United States occurred in 1874, when Henry Beigh, the founder of the American Society for the Prevention of Cruelty to Animals, managed to bring a case to court by arguing that a young abused girl (Mary Ellen Wilson) deserved as much protection as animals. Up to that time, no child protection statutes were in force. Over the past century, other protective laws and agencies have been created. There has been ongoing reluctance on the part of police, lawyers, physicians, and the public to interfere with the privacy of the family and the rights of parents. In the United States, the Federal Child Abuse Prevention and Treatment Act of 1974 established guidelines for all states defining what constitutes abuse, neglect, and maltreatment. This act made reporting mandatory for some groups of professionals (e.g., teachers, health care workers, police, and recreation leaders).

Table 28–1 spells out in detail a representative legal definition of child abuse and maltreatment and lists professionals who are required to report suspected abuse.

Incidence of Child Abuse and Maltreatment

Establishing the true incidence of child abuse and maltreatment is difficult for a number of reasons. Available statistics are based on reported cases. The types of cases that are reported may be different from state to state because of the differences in the laws defining abuse and governing reporting. Because the reported cases tend to be the most severe ones, the reported incidence of child abuse and maltreatment underestimates the actual incidence. Many cases are not reported because professionals fail to recognize them, or, when abuse is identified, they hesitate to report it because of ignorance of the law, fear of pos-

TABLE 28-1
A Legal Definition of Child Abuse and Maltreatment

A child suffers "abuse" in any of the following circumstances:

(a) The child has suffered physical harm, either inflicted by the person having charge of the child or caused by that person's failure to adequately: (i) care and provide for that child, or (ii) supervise the child, or (iii) protect the child;
(b) The child has been sexually molested or sexually exploited by the person having charge of the child, or by another person where the person having charge of the child: (i) knows or should know of the possibility of sexual molestation or sexual exploitation, and (ii) fails to protect the child;
(c) The child requires medical treatment to cure, prevent, or alleviate physical harm or suffering and the child's parent or the person having charge of the child: (i) does not provide the treatment, or (ii) refuses to provide the treatment, or (iii) is unavailable to consent to treatment, or (iv) is unable to consent to treatment;
(d) The child has suffered emotional harm, demonstrated by: (i) severe anxiety, or (ii) severe depression, or (iii) severe withdrawal, or (iv) severe self-destructive or aggressive behavior, and the child's parent or the person having charge of the child: (1) does not provide services or treatment to remedy or alleviate the harm, (2) refuses to provide such services or treatment, (3) is unavailable to consent to such services or treatment, or (4) is unable to consent to such services or treatment;
(e) The child suffers from a mental, emotional, or developmental condition that, if not remedied, could seriously impair the child's development, and the child's parent or the person having charge of the child either (i) does not provide treatment to remedy or alleviate the condition, (ii) refuses to do so, (iii) is unavailable to consent to treatment, or (iv) is unable to consent to treatment.

Mandatory Reporters of Child Abuse and Maltreatment

A professional or official who, in the course of his/her duties with respect to a child, has reasonable grounds to suspect that a child: (a) is abused, or (b) may be abused, or (c) may have suffered abuse, shall report forthwith his/her suspicion and the information upon which it is based to a Children's Aid Society for investigation. The professional duty to report affects the following persons: (a) a health care professional, including a physician, nurse, dentist, pharmacist, and psychologist; (b) a teacher, or school principal; (c) a social worker or family counselor; (d) a priest, rabbi, or other member of the clergy; (e) an operator or employee of a day nursery; (f) youth and recreation workers (not a volunteer); (g) a peace officer and a coroner; (h) a solicitor; (i) a service provider and an employee of a service provider, and (j) any other person who performs professional or official duties with respect to a child.

From Child and Family Services Act of Ontario, Canada: Government of Ontario.

sible court involvement, or a critical attitude toward child protective agency intervention.

Sociologic studies suggest that at least one in three children suffers some type of abuse during childhood. Although figures differ depending on the source, there is consensus that the problem is common. The rate of reported child abuse and maltreatment in the United States in 1989 to 1990 was 39 per 1000 children (Daro & McCurdy, 1992). Based on the 1989 census data, it is expected to rise to 42 per 1000 in 1990 to 1991 (Daro & McCurdy, 1992). The proportion of these cases accounted for by the various types of abuse is displayed in Table 28–2. Since 1985, the rate of fatalities from abuse and neglect has also been increasing. In 1990 it was 1.95 children per 1000, and it was expected to reach 2.15 children per 1000 in 1991 (Daro & McCurdy, 1992).

Child abuse and maltreatment are serious common problems in our society, and nurses who care for children and their families must be able to identify them and intervene appropriately.

TABLE 28-2
Child Abuse and Neglect in the United States: 1991

Type of Abuse/Neglect	Proportion of Substantiated Cases (%)*
Physical abuse	21
Sexual abuse	13
Neglect	53
Emotional maltreatment	8
Other†	7

Data from Daro, D., & McCurdy, K. (1992). Current trends in child abuse reporting and fatalities: The results of the 1991 Annual Fifty State Survey. Chicago: National Committee for Prevention of Child Abuse.
* Totals may be greater than 100 because of rounding.
† Includes abandonment and dependency.

Understanding Child Abuse and Maltreatment

Although the law dictates professional practice concerning the reporting of child abuse and maltreatment, broader definitions are useful for understanding the phenomenon and working with affected children and their families. One way to conceptualize abuse (of any type) is on a continuum of child and family health. This continuum is pictured in Figure 28–1. Although the health of families and children is dynamic and ever-changing, some families could be placed close to the "health" point (1 to 2) of the continuum. High-risk groups fall between point 3 (the midpoint) and point 4. Abusive families fall between point 4

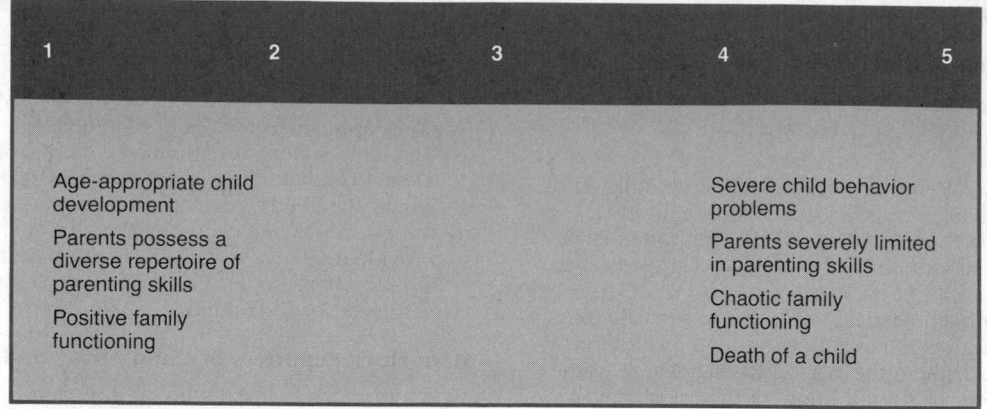

FIGURE 28 - 1. Continuum of family health related to child abuse and maltreatment.

and point 5. It is evident that the law is concerned only with the unhealthy end of the continuum, at which continuation of the abuse could lead to severe child behavior disorder, serious physical injury or illness, or even death of a child. In contrast, health care professionals can contribute to preventing families from reaching high-risk status. Chapters 12 and 14 on parenting and fostering self-esteem and Chapter 2 on family assessment present nursing interventions for promoting healthy families.

Another approach professionals frequently use to understand child abuse and maltreatment is to identify subcategories of the problem. This is particularly useful in clinical practice, because there is evidence that etiology, prevention, and treatment differ, depending on the type of abuse. Abuse is commonly subcategorized as *physical abuse, physical neglect, psychologic maltreatment,* and *sexual abuse.* The perpetrators of these types of abuse, although somewhat similar, have different specific characteristics. The children who have suffered different forms of abuse demonstrate different behavior following the abuse. The long-term sequelae of various types of abuse appear to be different. Finally, the strategies for effective treatment differ, based on the type of abuse. The subcategories of abuse and maltreatment are discussed later in this chapter.

Although using categories and labels clarifies many issues for professionals, there is much overlap among the categories of abused children. It is hard to imagine that a child who has been physically abused, physically neglected, or sexually abused has not also suffered psychologic maltreatment.

Parental drug use/abuse is frequently found in abusive and maltreating parents. Famularo and colleagues (1992) found that abuse of different drugs is associated with different forms of abuse: alcohol and physical abuse, and cocaine and sexual abuse.

Long-Term Sequelae

Regardless of how one defines child abuse and maltreatment, it is a serious problem not only because it places children at immediate risk but also because of the long-term sequelae that result if the child is not effectively treated. The long-term problems resulting from physical abuse include functional deficits from the actual injuries as well as psychologic problems that are expressed through a variety of problem behaviors. Although the scientific evidence in this field has several consistent methodologic flaws, in reviews of the literature, Lamphear (1985) and Houck and King (1989) identified a number of psychosocial problems of abused or neglected children. Children with a history of physical abuse are more physically and verbally aggressive toward parents, teachers, and peers than either those who have been neglected or those without a history of abuse. Physically abused children have attachment problems, demonstrated by their decreased likelihood of approaching caregivers for help or nurturing. Both teachers and parents report that they are more disobedient than other children. Although most of these children are of normal intelligence, they do poorly at school. Their repertoire of problem solving skills is limited. Their decreased social skills make them unpopular with peers and adults.

In a longitudinal study of children suffering various kinds of abuse, Erickson and colleagues (1989) report that physically abused children are angry, hyperactive, and noncompliant and demonstrate poor self-control and low self-esteem. Aber and associates (1989) summarized the empirical evidence of the effects of maltreatment on development during early childhood. Vondra and colleagues (1990) also found more unrealistic self-concept and less motivation and competence among maltreated children, compared with children who had not been abused or neglected. Retrospective studies of convicts indicate that a high percentage have childhood histories of physical or sexual abuse, or both.

Children who have been *physically neglected* or *psychologically maltreated,* or both, also function poorly. They are frequently emotionally withdrawn; often their physical, social, and intellectual development is delayed (Lamphear, 1985). Egeland and Erickson (1987) describe children for whom parents have been *psychologically unavailable* as very unhappy, with the least positive and most negative affect of all abused children. Their decline in intellectual functioning, attachment disturbances, and lack of social-emotional competence are enormous barriers to their subsequent development.

Sexual abuse rarely causes physical injury. McNeill and Brassard (1984) found that school-age incest victims achieve below expectations, have difficulties with peer relations, and present acting-out, hyperactive, depressive, and aggressive behaviors at home and at school. Adolescent incest victims also suffer learning difficulties. Sexual promiscuity, running away, drug abuse, somatic complaints, and increased risk for revictimization (Beitchman et al, 1991) are common behaviors shown by adolescent incest victims.

A number of studies have revealed trends of depressive anxiety, guilt, confusion over sexual identity, and fears of sexuality among these adolescents. Adult female survivors of childhood sexual exploitation or abuse can exhibit affective, somatic, social, and behavioral symptoms. These include low self-esteem, depression and suicide attempts, anxiety, eating disorders, sleeping disorders, restlessness, difficulty making friends, withdrawal from social events, difficulty relating to men, alcohol and drug abuse, sexual dysfunctions, and revictimization experiences (Rew, 1989). The impact of child sexual abuse (CSA) on the female adult's functioning depends on age of victimization, deviation of the abuse, and the relationship of the perpetrator to the victim. CSA is more traumatic if it occurs postpubertally versus prepubertally, if it goes on for a long time, and if the perpetrator is a father or stepfather (Beitchman et al, 1991). Although relatively little is known about the long-term sequelae of CSA for male adults, it appears they frequently show disturbances in sexual functioning.

Reporting Child Abuse and Maltreatment

Many state laws identify two types of reporters of child abuse. *Mandatory reporters* are those required by the law to report suspected cases of child abuse; nurses should consider themselves members of this group. *Permissive reporters* are those who may, but are not required to, report suspected child abuse (Rhodes, 1987). Mandatory reporters *must* report suspected abuse; failure to do so can result in a fine or other punishment, according to individual statutes.

Two important issues related to the reporting of child abuse and maltreatment are also addressed in most statutes. First, persons reporting suspected abuse are protected from civil action unless they acted maliciously or without reasonable grounds. Second, professionals must comply with the reporting laws, even if the information is deemed to be privileged or confidential. The only privileged information not subject to the reporting law is that between the solicitor and the client.

Professionals are *independently* responsible for their own actions. Hospitals and agencies usually have written protocols that outline procedures to be followed when child abuse or maltreatment is suspected. These protocols should be followed. After the protocol or procedure has been carried out, a professional who suspects possible abuse and is not satisfied with the outcome can make an individual report. A person can be legally liable for not reporting suspicions, even if other people in the agency or hospital do not think abuse has occurred.

Theoretical Perspectives on Child Abuse and Maltreatment

An understanding of the theoretical perspectives from which child abuse and maltreatment can be viewed is essential to effective intervention. Because abuse is a complex, multifaceted problem, theoretical frameworks provide a systematic approach. Nurses need to be familiar with these frameworks to clarify their role in the plan of care, either as individuals or as part of a multidisciplinary team in the identification, treatment, and prevention of child abuse and maltreatment. Child abuse may be just one facet in a pattern of family violence (Campbell & Humphreys, 1984). Brief descriptions of six theoretical models of abusing families are given below.

Mental Illness Model

This explanation for child abuse states that parents who abuse their children are mentally ill (Spinetta & Rigler, 1972). The goal is to cure the parent, who will then stop the abuse. This model has several limitations. First, research has shown that parental psychosis accounts for very few cases of abuse: as few as 5 per cent (Justice & Justice, 1976). Second, it implies that the illness of the parent is the sole cause of the abuse and does not consider the role of the family, child, community, or society as a whole. Third, because of its narrow focus, treatment strategies from this perspective are necessarily very limited and involve only the identified perpetrator of the abuse. This model was developed very early in the identification and treatment of abuse. Subsequent models with a broader perspective are more useful.

Environmental Stress Model

In this model, two factors interact to precipitate abuse: a violent environment and stress. The violent environment can be found either in society or the family. Sociologists and others agree that violence is tolerated to a greater degree in North American society compared with other societies, as evidenced by its frequent occurrence in entertainment media. Abusive parents ideologically belong to that segment of society that approves of physical violence against children in certain circumstances (Straus et al, 1980). This belief, coupled with the presence of increased acute or chronic stress, precipitates parental abuse of children to relieve the stress. According to this theory, the violence has to be a result of child behavior: abuse for no reason is unacceptable. Use of corporal punishment within schools is an example of abuse based on the environmental stress model. Although regulations govern this practice, the underlying theory is that when a child's behavior raises the teacher's stress level beyond acceptable limits (i.e., the student breaks the rule), corporal punishment is an acceptable way to relieve the stress. Although the numbers are decreasing, many families still subscribe to this approach. By 1990, over half of American schools had banned corporal punishment (Cohn Donnelly, 1991).

The limitations of this model are that it fails to consider the role of family functioning or individual or family stress tolerance. For instance, according to this model, it would be reasonable to expect that most poor families would be abusive because they suffer more stress than many other identifiable groups in society. Although evidence exists that the rate of abuse is higher among those of low socioeconomic status (Pelton, 1978), *abuse is not confined to this group, and many poor people do not abuse their children*. This model is used to explain intergenerational abuse: those abused as children were exposed to an environment that tolerated and even sanctioned child abuse as a method of problem solving (e.g., reducing stress).

A review of studies of parents abused as children concludes that *only about one third* of those who had been physically or sexually abused or psychologically maltreated perpetuated the behavior with their own children (Kaufman & Zigler, 1987). Since the rate of abuse and family stress appears to be increasing, this model does not appear sufficient to explain the behavior. Zeanah and Zeanah (1989) have suggested that it is not abuse per se that is intergenerational; rather, family relationship patterns contain certain themes that seem to be intergenerational. Themes identified to date include parental rejection, role reversal for parent and child, and fear of parental behavior. Not all families exhibiting these themes become abusive, but abuse and maltreatment are seen in many families in which these themes are present.

Social Learning Model

This model to explain how humans learn behavior was developed by Bandura (1973). It states that many human behaviors are learned through observation as well as through behavioral reinforcement, as proposed by Skinner. Aggression, a human behavior, can be learned in this way. Therefore, to become an aggressive or violent person, it is not necessary to experience aggression or violence but merely to observe it. Because most forms of child abuse are acts of aggression or violence, abuse can be learned by watching models. Three models that are widely available in American society are the family, the subculture, and symbolic models, especially television. This model of abuse is useful because it includes cultural and family influences.

Social-Psychologic Model

This model was proposed by Kempe and Helfer (1972), two pioneers in the field of child abuse and maltreatment research. For abuse to occur, three variables must be present: *a special parent, a special child,* and *stress.* The parent can be "special" in a number of ways, including being immature, having unrealistic expectations of the child, having poor impulse control, and failing to recognize and respect the child as a unique individual. The child can also be special or perceived by the parents to be so in several ways: "wrong" sex, physically or mentally disabled, "different" from the other children in the family, or temperamentally difficult. The stress may be acute or chronic. Helfer and Kempe state clearly that the event is perceived by the parent, not the professional, as stressful. This is important because of the frequent difference of perception of stress between the two groups and the professional's limited understanding of the parents' lifestyle and resources. This explanation of abuse is widely quoted and explains many abuse situations. Its major limitation is that it does not consider influences on abuse and maltreatment beyond the family.

Human Ecologic Model

This model to explain child abuse was developed by Garbarino (1977). It postulates that abuse is a result of interactions of the culture, the family, the parent, the child, and stress. A number of historical values in American culture lead to a predisposition to violence and to child abuse. The theoretical roots of violence in general, exploitation of children for child labor, and the belief that within families the adults are in the power position are historical cultural values. Although presently there is a sentimental belief in the great value of children to society, a comparison of the financial resources committed by government to their care and protection versus the commitment to defense or road maintenance (recognized traditional responsibilities of government) shows that children are not a public priority.

The focus on the family as opposed to the parent or the parent-abused child dyad is valuable. It identifies the family as the dysfunctional system, with abuse being a symptom. This suggests that parents, the abused child, and other children in the family interact in such a way that abuse occurs during periods of stress. Belsky (1980) explains that because the spousal relationship is the basis of the family, dysfunction within this relationship influences parent-child dynamics. This is particularly relevant in the case of intrafamilial sexual abuse of children.

The multifactorial aspect of this model makes it useful. Much previous research supports it. Its only limitation appears to be its delineation of two types of abuse: that committed by psychotic parents and that resulting from parental role dysfunction. It seems an odd separation in view of the fact that psychosis results in role dysfunction in many areas, including parenting. In spite of this limitation, this model appears promising in providing a comprehensive approach to assessment and treatment of abusive families.

Parke (1982) has developed a social interaction model similar to the human ecologic model. A nurse researcher (Millor, 1981) has described a nursing framework for research in child abuse and neglect. This is a complicated model with components similar to those outlined in the human ecologic model. Testing of this model has not yet been reported in the literature.

Belsky and Vondra (1989) have presented a model of parenting that represents multiple pathways by which individual (parent and child), historical, social, and circumstantial factors combine to shape parental functioning, which includes child abuse and maltreatment.

Psychologic-Sociologic Model for Sexual Abuse

Although all the preceding models can be used to explain child sexual abuse as well as other forms of abuse and maltreatment, Finkelhor (1984) has presented a model specifically related to sexual abuse. It has four components, developed from an individual and a sociocultural level. First, the perpetrator must be *motivated* to abuse a child sexually. This desire is fueled by the fact that sexual contact with a child will meet an important emotional need, that the contact will be sexually gratifying, and that other sources of sexual gratification are unavailable or less satisfying. The second component necessary for sexual abuse to occur is the *overcoming of internal inhibitors*. For most people, child sexual abuse bears a strong cultural taboo. Alcohol or a history of being sexually abused may reduce internal inhibitors (because of the exposure and familiarity with the practice). Third, *external inhibitors must be overcome*. Such inhibitors include the mother's ability to protect her children, and assurance that the perpetrator and the victim are never alone. In other words, external inhibitors are any variables external to the perpetrator and victim that make the abuse impossible. Finally, the *resistance of the child must be overcome*. Although they are never to blame, children can play a role in whether they are sexually abused. Children who have a history of emotional insecurity or deprivation who lack knowledge about sexual abuse, who are in a situation of unusual trust with the perpetrator (e.g., child and father), or who find themselves in a coercive situation are most likely to be sexually abused. If the perpetrator uses force, the child's vulnerability may be irrelevant. This model incorporates variables of society, family, perpetrator, and child and is supported by much research to date.

Nursing Care of Abused and Maltreated Children and Their Families

The identification and treatment of any form of child abuse or maltreatment requires the knowledge and skills of many health, social service, and legal professionals. Nurses who work with these families must be able to identify their own role and to facilitate the smooth functioning of the team of professionals.

Attitudinal Issues for Nurses

Before nurses can learn and appropriately apply the knowledge and skills necessary to work in this field, each must clarify personal values and attitudes related to this emotionally charged issue. As well as being nurses, we are all products of our own families of origin and of the broader cultural milieu within which we were raised. As a result, we have developed attitudes toward many human behaviors, including parenting and child abuse and maltreatment. For most of us the very idea of abuse raises strong negative emotions. The reality of being faced with an abused or maltreated child causes many of us to feel anger and hostility at the abusing parents or caregiver. Another common reaction is outrage at the limitations of the health and social systems that have failed to alleviate the problem. Some feel anger or disdain toward the child for being a victim: in fact, some are tempted to blame the victim. For others, an abused child revives painful childhood memories and a whole range of strong emotions toward one's own abusive or neglectful families. Those who can empathize with abusive parents may view abused and maltreated children and their families with fear: fear of their own vulnerability to the same violent behavior.

Abused children evoke a whole range of feelings among professionals who encounter them. These feelings are neither good nor bad, they just "are." The first step in clarifying one's own attitude is to recognize these feelings. As human beings, we are all entitled to personal values, beliefs, and attitudes. As professionals who wish to establish a therapeutic working relationship with such families, nurses must go beyond admitting these feelings and be able to deal with them, so that they are not inflicted on the clients with whom they work. Often, a greater understanding of the problem is helpful. Personal and professional support systems can often expand the scope of ways to view abusing families. It is necessary for the nurse to view the behavior, not the perpetrator, as unacceptable.

It is important to approach families with the belief that most people care about their children. The way families demonstrate concern for their children varies from one family to another and according to life experiences of the parents. Some questions and comments that nurses who work with abusive and maltreating families may find helpful in clarifying their attitudes are listed in Table 28–3.

Although hostility toward these parents is common, it impedes the therapeutic process in two significant ways. First, parents are usually sensitive to such negative feelings. They expend a lot of energy defending their behavior or being noncompliant with treatment, rather than becoming involved with constructive plans to improve the situation for themselves and their children. Second, nurses who view families with hostility have their *rescue fantasies** reinforced. Rescue fantasies cause the nurse to respond to the child on the basis of his or her own need to rescue, rather than on what is in the best interest of the child and family (Scharer, 1978). This can have negative consequences for everyone.

Viewing the child as "very unfortunate" promotes the nurse's feelings of having to "rescue" the child from the unworthy parents. In an effort to show unconditional caring for the child, the nurse sets no parameters on the child's behavior. This leads to reinforcement of his or her socially unacceptable, sometimes provocative behavior. Opportunities for the nurse to establish a therapeutic relationship with the family are diminished, because the nurse's verbal and nonverbal behavior indicate both disdain and hostility toward the parents. Therefore, the parents do not benefit from learning about parenting skills and may be judged or assessed unfairly. In the end, both the parents and the child may exclude the nurse. Consequently, the nurse has not successfully achieved his or her goals and the family may be discharged with no additional support, skills, or information, which can lead to another episode of child maltreatment. Awareness of personal attitudes and how they affect our professional behavior is crucial. Hostile attitudes toward parents need to be resolved before a therapeutic relationship can be established.

General Knowledge and Skills for Nurses

Although the nurse is one of many professionals who may be involved in the identification and treatment of child abuse and maltreatment, and although the precise nursing role varies according to the setting, certain knowledge and skills are required for nurses working with these children and their families, regardless of the practice setting. These are summarized in Table 28–4.

* A fantasy that the child needs rescuing from a cruel family; the nurse then reaches out to the child in a way that will negate the child's bond with the family. The nurse then becomes the sole support and thereby rescues the child.

TABLE 28–3
Exploring Personal Attitudes: Some Questions

These parents are so angry I'm afraid to get involved with them. What do I know about dealing with anger?

Anyone who could treat a child like this does not have the right to have children. How can I possibly help? How can anyone help?

Why should I help Mrs. X learn how to solve her problems —all she is interested in is herself?

This is a unit for acutely ill patients—why are abused children admitted here?

Mr. Y's relationship with Susie seems very overindulgent, but she is very uncomfortable. Will they stop coming to the clinic if I ask more questions?

None of my colleagues think this case is reportable, but Mrs. M told me she is out of control and afraid she will seriously hurt Johnny. What will I do?

Mrs. A reminds me of the people in my neighborhood. She couldn't be neglecting her youngest child, could she?

How can I help the B family? I don't know anything about parenting.

I'm here to look after sick children. Teaching parents about child development and how to care for their children isn't my job.

Child Assessment

To assess a child adequately, one must have a sound knowledge base about normal physical, social, emotional, and cognitive development of children, from neonates to adolescents. The development of children

TABLE 28–4
General Knowledge and Skills Required to Deal with Abused and Maltreated Children and Their Families

Knowledge	Skills
Normal growth and development of children from infancy to adolescence	Assessment of physical, social, and emotional development of the identified patient/client
Normal family development	Family assessment, including structural, developmental, and functional assessment
Reactions of parents	Interviewing skills: nonjudgmental, sensitive, supportive
Nursing documentation	Objective assessment summary Concise problem identification Clear interventions Ongoing evaluation
Community resources	Communication skills: clarify options and summarize plan of action

through adolescence is presented in Chapters 4 to 9 of this text. Sivan (1991) has outlined the issues of normal preschool child development and the implications for investigation of child abuse allegations. A thorough history, physical examination, and developmental assessment are outlined in Chapter 2.

Family History and Assessment

A crucial aspect of assessment of children who are suspected of being abused or maltreated is a thorough family history and family assessment.

A number of models for family assessment are available and are reviewed in Chapter 2. The Calgary Family Assessment Model (Wright & Leahey, 1984) is particularly valuable in this field, because it assesses family structure, development, and function. It includes not only present family history but also the history of parental families of origin and the cultural milieu of current family living. Many aspects of the family development and the family function assessment sections have been adapted from the McMaster Model of Family Functioning (Epstein et al, 1981). A brief questionnaire has been demonstrated to assess reliably these dimensions of family functioning (Byles et al, 1988); it could be used for an initial assessment of family functioning.

Parental Reactions

To relate to parents who may have abused their children, the nurse should be aware of the variety of reactions parents display when confronted with the possibility of having abused or maltreated their child. Of course, the reaction depends largely on the interviewing skills of the nurse. Nurses who recognize and are sensitive to the fact that parents in this situation have a number of emotions can minimize the parents' denial and hostility. At this time, parents can feel any or all of the following emotions: guilt, remorse, failure as a parent, inadequacy as a human being, fear that they will lose their child, and relief at the identification of the problem.

Interviews with the families should take place in private. Open-ended, clear, supportive questions facilitate parents' sharing appropriate data and allow them to state their perceptions of what happened or what has been going on. Parents are sensitive to any signs of punitiveness from the nurse/interviewer and invariably react with defensiveness and hostility to such negative messages. Any inconsistencies or vague explanations given by parents should be identified. Parents can then be given the opportunity to clarify them.

Reactions of parents vary according to their understanding of children and their attitudes toward them. The following comments can be useful in eliciting parental knowledge and attitudes about children.

- "All parents I've ever met get angry at their kids. How do you feel when you get angry at Mary? What do you do?"
- "Being a parent is really hard work. Some of the time parents feel like they aren't doing a very good job. What do you do when you feel that way? Do you think it works?"
- "The fact that you have brought Mike here tells me you care about him. What do you think I can do to help you and him?"
- "Two-year-olds who keep saying 'no' and having temper tantrums when they don't get what they want can be very trying. Why do you think Timmy does that? What have you done to stop the annoying behavior?"
- "How were you disciplined as a child? Do you think it was useful?"

Nursing Documentation

For the nurse, the purposes of documentation are the same when dealing with abused children as with any other child. However, more and more abuse and maltreatment cases are being handled in the courts; if litigation ensues, the chart may be part of the evidence, and the nurse may be called to explain the documentation. The time gap between charting and court appearance can vary and is often lengthy. This makes concise, clear documentation crucial both to aid recall and to facilitate explanations.

Initial assessment should include any physical injuries or abnormalities (e.g., bruises, scrapes, burns, unidentifiable marks). Drawings to illustrate the locations are helpful. Behavioral and developmental symptoms exhibited by the child should be recorded. These should be objectively stated (e.g., "does not make eye contact") and exclude personal interpretations of the behavior. Observations of parent-child interactions should also be objectively recorded. Actual quotes from parents should be included.

Accurate documentation of the history of the injury/complaint is essential. The initial family assessment should include data as outlined previously in this chapter. Ongoing documentation should fill in any gaps in the family history. On the basis of the initial assessment, short- and long-term treatment goals that are mutually negotiated with other health professionals and the family should be clearly stated. These provide direction for the development of individual patient care plans.

Ongoing nursing documentation during hospitalization includes assessment in the following areas:

- History and status of physical injuries, if any.
- Changes in the child's behavior.
- Parent-child contact—this should explain the frequency of contact, length of time the parent spends with the child, and observations of the parent-child interaction during the visit.
- Telephone inquiries by parents about their child.
- Emotional status of the parents.

Community Resources

To be able to keep children and their families informed, nurses must be knowledgeable about the community resources to which these families are likely to be referred. In situations that are by law reportable to Child Protection Services (CPS), parents should be informed about the report. This can be done in a supportive way; it is seen by many professionals as crucial in establishing a trusting, therapeutic relationship with children and families. It is necessary for parents to understand not only that the behavior must stop, but also that the professionals with whom the family will come in contact are primarily interested in assisting the family to function more effectively, so that abuse and maltreatment will not recur.

Because the long-term treatment of these children and their families is complex and requires the assistance of a variety of health and other agencies, multidisciplinary community treatment teams have been developed in many areas. Representatives of agencies frequently involved with the treatment of child abuse and maltreatment form the basic core of these teams. Team participation by specific professionals is determined by the needs of each child and family. The team formulates the overall plan of management, identifies specific individual roles in implementing the plan, and, as a group, regularly evaluates and updates the plan. Professionals frequently involved in these teams include the following:

- CPS workers who monitor the situation if the child remains in the home and determine whether removal is necessary for the child's protection.
- Community health nurses, who provide regular one-to-one sessions with families about parenting, child development, and child safety or who may facilitate the development of parenting skills by leading parent group discussions.
- Social workers, who may provide instrumental assistance (e.g., finding better housing) or therapeutic counseling, as well as assist the child who is removed from the home.
- Coordinators and providers of infant stimulation programs.
- Early childhood educators from day care centers.
- Mental health professionals.

Knowledge and Skills to Deal with Specific Types of Child Abuse and Maltreatment

The specific knowledge and skills required by nurses to care for abused or maltreated children and their families depend on the type of maltreatment and the setting in which the nurse encounters them. Each major category of child abuse is discussed here by using the human ecologic model as a framework for assessment and treatment. The nurse may encounter child abuse and maltreatment in a variety of settings. As stated earlier, the ability to carry out a comprehensive assessment of the child and family is very important. A checklist for assessing for child abuse and maltreatment has been developed by Burgess and associates (1990). TRIADS is an acronym representing the following assessment areas: *t*ype of abuse, *r*elationship of the victim to the offender; *i*ntensity of the abuse; *a*utonomic response of the child; *d*uration of the abuse; and *s*tyle of the offender.

Once abuse is strongly suspected or identified, the situation must be reported to the child protection agency. From then on, the nursing role becomes one of advocacy and support. Further investigation will be done by the CPS and/or the police.

The nursing role in relation to the type of abuse or maltreatment focuses on the inpatient pediatric setting. Because the treatment of child abuse and maltreatment usually takes place in both inpatient and community settings, the role of the community health nurse is generally addressed where appropriate. Nurses frequently deal with parents at high risk for abuse in maternity and neonatal units. The nurse's role in these settings is discussed in a later section, "Prevention of Child Abuse and Maltreatment."

Families at high risk for abuse, potential physical abuse, physical neglect, psychologic maltreatment, and sexual abuse are outlined in Tables 28–5, 28–6, and 28–8 to 28–11. The indicators are not all-inclusive, and the presence of one or two of them does not necessarily ensure that abuse or maltreatment has taken place. They are meant to be used in combination with a thorough child and family history and assessment and other diagnostic tools. The presence of several of the indicators may mean that although abuse has not occurred, preventive strategies related to improving parenting skills or reducing family stress may be needed by the family.

Nurses may encounter families at high risk for child abuse and maltreatment in a number of different settings (e.g., at prenatal examinations or classes; during labor, delivery, and the postpartum period; in emergency rooms; in pediatric inpatient units; and in the community). Indicators of high-risk families are outlined in Table 28–6. The presence of several of these indicators should alert the nurse to do a more in-depth assessment to determine the major factors causing the high-risk situation. Families can then be referred to the appropriate service to solve or minimize the problems. These are described in more detail under the various types of abuse and maltreatment later in this chapter.

Physical Abuse

Physical abuse is any nonaccidental injury to a child caused by the child's caregiver. It is most often perpetrated by parents. *These actions are rarely intentional;* rather, they result from inappropriate parental efforts to change a child's behavior. Parents with poor

TABLE 28-5
Indicators of Potential Physical Abuse

Physical Indicators	
Child	**Comments**
Unexplained bruises:	
Bruises, welts, lacerations, or abrasions	Although children sustain many injuries, normally central facial ones are unusual because children protect this area
Location:	
Face, lips, gums, mouth, eyes	
Torso, back, buttocks, back of legs	Accidental injuries to the central trunk of the body are unusual
External genitalia	
Shape:	
Clustered, forming regular patterns, teeth marks, handprint	
Same as article used to inflict injury (e.g., cord, belt buckle)	
Unexplained burns:	
Small circular burns, particularly on soles of feet, palms of hands, back of buttocks	Often result from cigar or cigarette burns
Immersion burns—clear line of demarcation is evident	Often results from holding a child in bathwater that is too hot
Rope burns on arms, legs, neck, or torso	Result from a child straining against bonds
Patterned burns indicating a hot object (e.g., stove element) on buttocks	Result from placing the child on the hot object
Unexplained fractures/dislocations:	
To skull, facial bones	Often result from hitting or throwing
Spiral fractures	Often result from pulling or twisting an arm or leg
Dislocations, particularly of shoulders or hips	
Multiple fractures in various stages of healing	On roentgenograph for the presenting complaint; other fractures in various stages of healing may be identified
Note: In children, particularly 2 yrs of age and under, fractures and dislocations usually result from blows, throws, or other inflicted force	
Other forms:	
Ingestions	Result from carelessness at best, to neglect/ignorance or forced ingestion at worst
Bald patches on the scalp	Result from pulling hair out or leaving an infant in one position for extended period of time
Subdural hematomas in children under age 2 yrs	Result from severe shaking
Retinal hemorrhages	Result from severe shaking

Behavioral Indicators	
Parent	**Child**
Explanation does not fit the injury, is inconsistent, or is absent	Is very wary of adults
May blame the child because he/she is bad, overactive, defiant, and so on	Speaks in monosyllables
Does not support the child physically or verbally (e.g., no eye contact, touching)	Has vacant stare or frozen watchfulness
Lets much time pass between occurrence of the injury and seeking medical attention	Withstands examination and painful procedures with little movement or crying or both
Reaction to the injury is inappropriate (e.g., very upset over a relatively minor injury or unconcerned over a serious one)	Does not turn to parent for support
Unaware of normal developmental stages of children	States the parent did it, but that self is to blame because he or she was bad
Views the child as capable of meeting his/her needs	Constantly tries to please the parents and to assess parental reaction to statements
	Role-reversal: child tries to take care of the parent

(continued)

TABLE 28-5
Indicators of Potential Physical Abuse *(Continued)*

Behavioral Indicators

Parent	Child
Describes own childhood as unhappy or abusive	Behavior extremes: aggressiveness or withdrawal
Routinely uses harsh unreasonable discipline	Is afraid to go home
Expresses feelings of isolation, both as an individual and as a parent; has no identifiable support system	Does not participate in gym, with no apparent reason
Demonstrates poor impulse control when questioned about how he/she handles anger	Is inappropriately dressed (e.g., long pants and long-sleeved shirts in summer) to hide bruises
	Indiscriminately seeks affection
	Shows inappropriate or precocious maturity

From Thomas, H. (1983). *Child abuse, neglect and deprivation: A handbook for Ontario nurses.* Toronto: Registered Nurses' Association of Ontario.

impulse control may vent their anger by physically lashing out at their children. Inadequate knowledge of child development or lack of parenting skills may lead to harsh, sometimes bizarre physical discipline and resulting injury to the child. Although most frequently serious among infants, physical abuse occurs in all age groups, from young children through school-age children and adolescents.

Clinical Manifestations and Diagnostic Assessment. Because children, particularly preschoolers, sustain all sorts of injuries in their normal activities, deciding which injuries are nonaccidental can sometimes be difficult. Accidental and nonaccidental sites for injury are depicted in Figure 28–2. Parental and child indicators of potential abuse are outlined in Table 28–5. The possible types of nonaccidental injuries are limited only by parental desperation or imagination. Injuries that are not age-appropriate (e.g., fractured femur in an infant) are suspect immediately. Another major warning signal is an injury that is inconsistent with the history of the incident.

As the awareness of physical abuse has increased, so have the false allegations of child abuse and accompanying tragedies for families (Wong, 1987). The cause of this increase is unknown, but it may be related to professionals' erring on the side of caution and reporting all suspicious situations to avoid possible subsequent legal proceedings. This high rate of false allegations has led to an overburdening of CPS agencies, sometimes resulting in less-than-adequate investigations (Besharov, 1985).

Unnecessary false allegations can be minimized by an awareness of signs that may be mistakenly la-

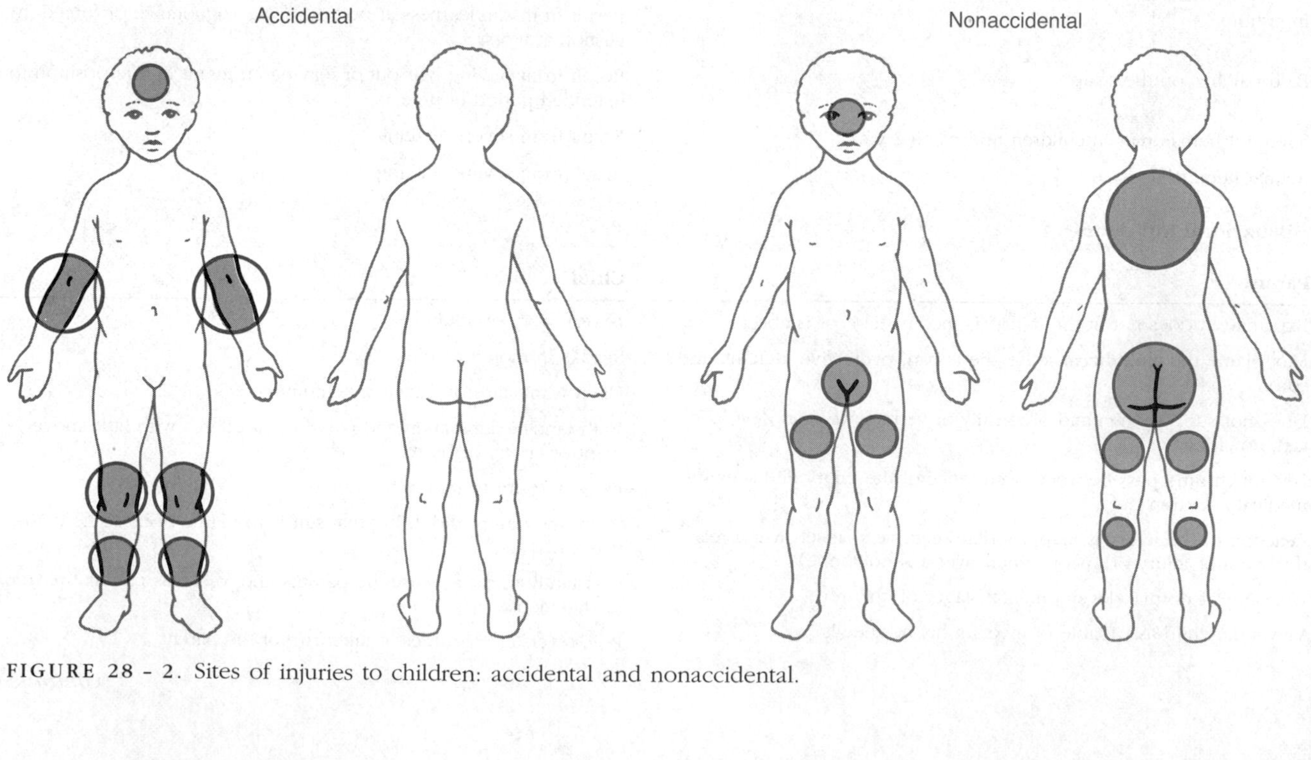

FIGURE 28-2. Sites of injuries to children: accidental and nonaccidental.

TABLE 28-6
Indicators of High-Risk Families

Prenatal Indicators

Unplanned pregnancy

Children spaced less than 1½ yrs apart

Depression related to pregnancy

One or other parent wanted either an abortion or to relinquish the child, but they did not

Denial of pregnancy

Mothers who are extremely upset about body changes during pregnancy

Young (under 20 yrs of age) mothers

Single mothers

Women who do not seek prenatal care when it is available or who ignore prenatal instructions

Parents who are overly concerned with the baby's sex

Parents who have unreal expectations of the infant

Parents who voice a lot of concern about how they will cope with an infant

Parents who make no/few preparations for the infant

Parents who have few supports and are isolated (physically or emotionally) from friends and family (e.g., no telephone)

Perinatal and Postnatal Indicators

Difficult delivery

Immediate separation of mother and infant for health reasons of either patient

Parents who avoid touching or looking at the infant after delivery

Parents who voice disappointment over sex or appearance of the infant

Parents who do not support one another

Infant with recognizable physical or mental handicaps that will require long-term treatment

Parents who do not visit the neonatal unit or inquire about the condition of the baby

Parents who do not talk to the baby

Parents who are very irritated by the infant's crying, or make little or no attempt to comfort the baby

Parents who have no understanding of infant care and appear unwilling to try, in spite of support by hospital staff

Neonatal Indicators

Premature infant

Infant with a congenital abnormality

Mentally retarded infant

Parents who express unreal expectations of the infant

Parents who feel the baby is too demanding (e.g., messy eating, changing diapers)

Parents who become unduly tense and irritable when the infant cries or who may not respond to crying

Colicky infants

Parents who express a lot of anxiety about minor or seemingly nonexistent problems (e.g., frequent calls in the middle of the night or trips to the emergency ward). As a result, they are often labeled "anxious mothers"

Fathers jealous of the time mother spends with the infant

Parents who change health care facility frequently for vague reasons. This sometimes means *their* needs are not being met, although the infant may be treated appropriately

In interview, parents who constantly refocus on themselves vs. the infant

Parents who cannot identify any support system for themselves in times of stress

Times of Crisis

Lifestyle changes such as marital separation or moving to a new setting, resulting in loss of support systems

Sudden unemployment or other situation leading to financial difficulties for the family

Death of a spouse

Diagnosis of serious illness in one of the family members

Very ill infant or child

Birth of another child—spacing

Abuse of alcohol or drugs by either parent

From Thomas, H. (1983). *Child abuse, neglect and deprivation: A handbook for Ontario nurses*. Toronto: Registered Nurses' Association of Ontario.

beled physical abuse. Hurwoltz and Castells (1987) report two cases of osteogenesis imperfecta that were misdiagnosed as physical abuse because of an absence of a family history. Certain folk medical practices common among ethnic groups have also been mistaken for physical abuse (Levin & Levin, 1982). Although such practices may lead to physical injury and are not tolerated in our society, the treatment is different from that for reportable physical abuse. Clinical signs of an underlying illness also may be misdiagnosed as child abuse. For example, bruises in various stages of healing are often a sign of physical abuse,

ETHICAL ISSUES
Medicine or Child Abuse?

by Margaret M. Mahon, PhD, RNC

Lisa and her family came to the United States from Cambodia 6 years ago. Lisa is an 8-year-old who has come to her pediatric nurse practitioner (PNP) because she has been ill since yesterday with vomiting and diarrhea. In the course of the examination, the PNP notices bruises over Lisa's abdomen, which she suspects are the result of abuse. The PNP completes the examination and then asks Lisa to wait outside the examination room. Lisa's mother is not fluent in English but is able to convey that the marks are the result of rubbing Lisa with a coin in an attempt to alleviate her stomach pain.

Health care interventions in many countries are derived from more than a physical assessment of the patient's status. Although many health care professionals attempt to integrate physical and psychologic considerations in their interactions with children and families, the extension beyond the physical realm is more systematized and more a part of daily life in non-Western health care. Only within the last 10 years have non-Western components of health care been given any validity, and although inroads have been made, they are far from being widely accepted. Furthermore, the body of evidence supporting the validity of various non-Western health care methods varies. Treatments such as acupuncture and acupressure are a routine option for some health care professionals, although for most this is not the case. Some Native American practices are more accepted in certain parts of the United States, but again, they remain separate from mainstream health care.

As in many cultures, in Cambodia and other Asian countries it is common to try "home remedies" before seeking outside help for health problems. Traditional interventions are likely to be founded on Buddhist or Taoist philosophical beliefs, which recognize the complementary nature of heat and cold in health and illness and in interventions to restore health. Coining *(kos khyal)* involves rubbing a coin along the affected area to cause "bad wind." If a red-purple discoloration results, the treatment is believed successful (Rosenberg, 1986). Besides coining, other treatments include the use of oils, cupping, pinching, and heat and cold in various forms. Situations like that described here are not uncommon and are representative of the cultural clash that can occur when a misunderstanding about treatment exists. The underlying question is "Was Lisa a victim of child abuse?"

Clearly the intent of the action was not to injure but to cure. Is that different from an adult who hits a child to demonstrate that a situation is dangerous or that a behavior is "bad" or inappropriate? Many health care interventions are painful, but are done with the intent to cure or to provide information that will help plan a cure—for example, immunizations, lumbar puncture, surgery, or chemotherapy. The intent of these procedures may be prevention, information gathering, or curative. For some, the ability to cure does not exist, but the painful procedures are undertaken with the intent to prolong life.

The unwillingness to accept coining is born largely of a lack of information about its intent. Is there any evidence to support its ability to cure? The answer to this depends on the treatment involved. Before deciding that a procedure is abuse, one must return to the first step of ethical analysis and gather appropriate information. If the procedure itself is not harmful, is it acceptable, or is it child abuse? There have been cases in which those who practiced culturally different health care were prosecuted for child abuse. The chance of this happening partly depends on the child abuse laws, which vary from state to state. In some states, child abuse is legally defined as a situation or encounter that results in severe injury to the child. In other states, the legal definition refers to the *potential* for severe injury. The question of what is severe can be subjective. If Lisa's bruises had been caused by a belt, that would most often be considered abuse. If the same degree of bruising had been caused by a fall resulting from parental negligence but no overt act, that may or may not be considered abuse, although it might be considered neglect. In deciding whether abuse is present, does one focus on the intent or the effect? The intent of the act was to cure, but the objective data reveal bruises sustained as a result of forceful contact. In Cambodia, coining is not considered abuse. How does one decide what to do in Lisa's case?

BIBLIOGRAPHY

Lawson, L. V. (1990). Culturally sensitive support for grieving parents. *MCN: American Journal of Maternal Child Nursing, 15,* 76–79.

Rosenberg, J. A. (1986). Health care for Cambodian children: Integrating treatment plans. *Pediatric Nursing, 12,* 118–120, 125.

but they also may occur as a result of undiagnosed bleeding disorders (O'Hare & Eden, 1984). The importance of thorough assessment is underlined by these examples of misdiagnosis.

When physical abuse is suspected, on the basis of parent and child indicators, assessment of the level of family functioning and stress may be accomplished quickly and systematically by using the Family Stress Check List (Orkow, 1985). This check list includes a number of variables that have been empirically demonstrated to be strongly related to the presence of abuse.

The variables include the following:

- Parental history of being abused or deprived.
- Parental history of being abusive or of using harsh punishment.
- Level of chronic and acute family stress.
- Low self-esteem, social isolation, or depression of parents.
- Poor parental impulse control.
- Rigid, unrealistic expectations of child's behavior.
- Child difficult or provocative, or perceived to be so by parents.

The presence of several of these variables strengthens the likelihood of a nonaccidental cause of injury.

Often children for whom the diagnosis of physical abuse is suspected are admitted to hospital even when treatment of the actual injury does not require inpatient care, for two reasons. First, parents are frequently emotionally overwhelmed after such an incident; hospital admission places the child in a protected environment, ensuring that immediate further abuse will not occur. It allows a cooling-off period for parents during which they are relieved of child care responsibilities. Second, having the child in the hospital allows for a thorough physical, social, and emotional assessment of the child and family, for accurate diagnosis, and for initiation of treatment of the family.

An unusual form of physical abuse, termed Munchausen syndrome by proxy, has been identified (Turk et al, 1990). In all cases reported to date, the perpetrator is a mother who is knowledgeable about illness (e.g., a nurse). The child may be seen with actual physical symptoms of an illness. However, these symptoms have been artificially induced by the mother. An example is the addition of the mother's menstrual blood to the child's urine to simulate hematuria. In some cases, the child has a history of an illness that is fictitious (e.g., seizures) and does not respond to appropriate treatment. The reported cases are dramatic—the children have been subjected to extensive diagnostic testing, multiple operations, and lengthy periods of hospitalization. The mothers of these children rarely leave them alone during hospitalization. A warning sign of this aberration is that the symptoms disappear when the mother is absent. Another sign that Munchausen syndrome by proxy may be the underlying diagnosis is that the signs and symptoms do not make clinical sense. Clinicians may be confused by this and feel that they have never seen anything like it. If nurses and other members of the health care team are aware of the possibility of this type of physical abuse, it may be detected earlier and so minimize the trauma for children and families.

Nursing Care of Physically Abused Children and Their Families. Although hospitalization may be of short duration, the nurse has an important role. In cases of serious physical injury, appropriate nursing care of the actual injury is necessary. Other nursing interventions specific to the assessment and planning phase are summarized in Table 28–7. Generally, the nursing role is to act as a parent and child advocate. Children may be frightened and confused. The nurse should explain the reason for admission and plans for care in an age-appropriate way. Involvement of child protection services means that children and parents may be separated for an indefinite period of time. Depending on the situation, the court may rule that the child be discharged to the family with supervision or to a foster home, or may permanently terminate parental rights. The disposition, of course, is based on the perceived risk of recurrence of physical abuse.

Although children may have been severely abused, being separated from their parents is a severe loss. Many children also feel guilty because they perceive that their "bad" behavior, which led to the abuse, has resulted in the family disruption. For children who can understand, the action needs to be explained, and then they need to be given an opportunity to express their feelings. A consistent nurse is likely to be most effective in this situation, because these children often have difficulty trusting others and need time to establish a relationship in which they feel safe enough to expose their true feelings.

The nursing role of parent advocate can be difficult, because parents may be hostile, frightened, and confused. The nurse who can reassure the parents that bringing the child for treatment, although frightening, was a responsible act that indicates their concern for the child will often diminish parental hostility and fear. This allows parents to ask pertinent questions, to which the nurse can provide straightforward, clear answers. Through this process, parental confusion and resulting defensiveness are often reduced. Although hospitalization of physically abused children is generally of short duration, successful nursing intervention will assist in preparing parents and children to engage constructively in long-term treatment. In some cases, hospitalization is extended because there is no satisfactory placement available for the child. A legal order may be in effect keeping the child from being returned home with the parent, but no foster home or care agency may be available. Chronic shortages of quality foster care exist in some cities.

TABLE 28-7
Assessment and Planning for the Physically Abused Child and Family

Nursing Role	Interventions
Child and family assessment	Use age-appropriate methods to assess development; preverbal and young children respond to play therapy with dolls that represent family members
	Provide age-appropriate support for the child during radiologic and other diagnostic tests
	Document physical injuries
	Document observations of child behavior that indicate psychologic and emotional status
	With other health care team members, complete the family assessment (see Chapter 2 for family assessment)
Planning and initiating care	Assess level of knowledge and skill of parent regarding child care and development
	Identify one nurse as the child's primary caregiver
	Develop a clearly defined plan of care to be followed by all nurses
	Involve older children in developing the plan for their own care
	Plan patient care to include parental participation
Interdisciplinary participation in care	Provide positive reinforcement for family/parent strengths
	Model healthy communication and parenting behaviors
	Inform parents that child protection services are being notified, without judging or accusing parents
	Explain that the objective of involvement is to strengthen family functioning and prevent future harm to children
	Support parents during initial interviews with child protection workers
	Assist parents in identifying strategies necessary to prevent future abuse (e.g., identify other professionals as supports)

Long-term treatment of the family is to prevent recurrences of abuse. Interventions with the parents are directed toward increasing their impulse control, providing alternatives for physical abuse when they are angry, increasing their knowledge of child development, and developing age-appropriate expectations of children. Many abusive parents have such low self-esteem and so few social skills that they require one-to-one treatment until they are willing to risk entering a parent group. A number of parent group programs have reported success in changing parental attitudes and behavior. Community health nurses may provide one-to-one treatment for families, and they may also lead parent groups. Self-help groups such as Parents Anonymous* provide effective support and direction for many abusive parents.

Some researchers believe that abuse results from a lack of parental empathy for the child. To empathize, parents have to recognize the emotion being demonstrated by the child and then react appropriately. Empirical evidence suggests that, compared with nonabusive mothers, abusive mothers are *unable to identify child emotions correctly,* which may explain why they respond with abuse (Kropp & Haynes, 1987). Although no programs to address this problem have been reported, the idea is an interesting one. As members of interdisciplinary child abuse teams, nurses can facilitate development and evaluation of such programs.

Programs for physically abused children have been developed to help them improve their social skills, decrease their aggression, and improve their ability to relate positively to others. These programs are often implemented within day care settings for preschool children. Interest groups for older children facilitate learning of these behaviors.

Family or marital counseling, or both, is required by some families to improve family functioning and help families learn more constructive ways to manage stress. Family stress sometimes can be reduced by instrumental assistance, such as budget counseling or providing parents a break from preschool children through part-time enrollment of children in nursery school or day care settings. Families and professionals may identify numerous other strategies to reduce stress in the home.

By being aware of the family dynamics and changes within the family, the community health nurse can be a valuable advocate for abused children and their families.

Physical Neglect

Physical neglect encompasses the failure of caregivers to provide the basic necessities of life: food, shelter, medical attention, clothing, safety, sleep, adequate supervision, and, in the case of the school-age child,

* Refer to Yellow Pages under "Crisis Intervention" or White Pages under "Parents Anonymous."

education. It tends to be chronic in nature. One must distinguish between neglect and poverty. Although children suffering from physical neglect require intervention, regardless of the cause, the interventions are different for physical neglect and for poverty resulting in inadequate physical care. Sometimes all children in the family are affected by neglect, but often one child is significantly more neglected than the others.

Clinical Manifestations and Diagnostic Assessment. The child's physical and behavioral indicators of physical neglect, as well as parental behavioral indicators, are contained in Table 28–8. A key diagnostic feature of physical neglect is the parents' inability to influence the environment. As a result, family life is chaotic, the child's needs are not recognized or met, and a sense of helplessness pervades the family. In more severe situations, a particular child in the family has been neglected because of being different or being perceived by the parents to be "different," "inferior," or "bad." These children are usually admitted to hospital because, in their neglected state, they have developed an acute illness (e.g., gastroenteritis in infants). Because of their limited resources, parents are unable to care for them at home. Accidents resulting from inadequate supervision also may result in hospitalization. For these children, physical neglect rarely occurs without being accompanied by psychologic maltreatment.

Nursing Care of Physically Neglected Children and Their Families. In the hospital, children must be treated for their acute conditions. This treatment is no different from that for any other infant or child with a similar problem. However, relatively straightforward nursing goals, such as maintaining adequate nutritional intake, become difficult because these infants and children have no established eating patterns. Furthermore, they often have not learned to eat age-appropriate or nutritious food; feeding them requires much time, patience, and creativity.

Although these families may be followed by community health nurses and other professionals for years, during the child's hospitalization the nurse can make a valuable contribution to the ongoing care. This is an opportunity to observe parenting skills and provide much-needed modeling and reinforcement of appropriate skills. Basic adequate hygiene for infants can be reinforced by observing parents as they bathe and care for their children. As with physically abused children, a consistently assigned nurse is valuable for monitoring changes in parental attitude and behavior toward the child and also for minimizing confusion for the parents. By discharge, a thorough assessment of family strengths and ongoing needs related to child care, for use by community professionals, can be documented by this consistent nurse.

Assessment of the level of parental ability or motivation to use information and people resources to effect a positive change is essential. If CPS is in-

TABLE 28–8
Indicators of Potential Physical Neglect

Physical Indicators

Child	Comments
Underweight, poor growth pattern, constant hunger, wasting of subcutaneous tissue	All result from malnutrition, if other diagnoses have been ruled out; most common cause of malnutrition is lack of food Confirmed as neglect when the child quickly gains weight when fed properly
Poor physical hygiene—severe diaper rash, skin rashes, dirty hair, dirty hands and face, persistent body odor	May result from ignorance, poverty, or neglect
Unattended physical problems or medical needs (e.g., glasses, dental work, untreated injuries)	Sometimes recognized when parents have been informed of the need and have done nothing about it
Consistent lack of supervision or abandonment	
Fatigue, listlessness, lethargy	Results from inadequate rest, sometimes a result of caring for siblings, other household tasks, or lack of suitable sleeping accommodation

Behavioral Indicators

Parent	Child
Externalizes blame for the situation	Infants may be dull and inactive
Describes a chaotic home life	Shows delay in gross motor and speech development
Lacks understanding of needs of children (e.g., food, supervision)	May be pale, listless, thin, unkempt
Lives in unsafe, dirty and/or crowded conditions	May beg for or steal food
May be mentally retarded or have a low IQ	Frequently absent from school, or arrives at school very early and leaves very late
Has little motivation or skill to effect changes in her/his life	Wears inappropriate clothing for the weather; clothing may be dirty
Is often passive, socially isolated individual who has not experienced success	Constantly squints at the board
Is unable to forego immediate gratification for long-term organization	Complains of aching teeth
Describes inappropriate parenting in his/her childhood	States there is no one to look after him or her
Reports employment instability	Assumes adult responsibilities
Lacks emotional bond to child/children	Engages in delinquent acts and/or abuse of alcohol or street drugs

From Thomas, H. (1983). *Child abuse, neglect and deprivation: A handbook for Ontario nurses.* Toronto: Registered Nurses' Association of Ontario.

volved, such assessment and evaluation often determine whether a court order for foster care or permanent termination of parental rights is sought. One factor that influences parental motivation is the teaching/learning strategies used by the nurse. Doak and associates (1985) have identified a number of issues that are useful to keep in mind when working with parents with low literacy skills. These include the following:

- A patient's perspective tends to be limited to direct personal experience.
- A patient may be insensitive to the need to give information to health care providers unless specifically asked.
- A patient does not think in terms of classes of information or of categories.
- A patient gives information in bits and pieces without an identifiable pattern.

These attributes are common among neglecting parents.

To intervene effectively, the nurse uses simple, concrete, clear questions to collect data and gives simple, concrete, step-by-step directions for care. To assess whether a child is obtaining enough sleep, the nurse does not ask, "How much sleep does Johnny get?" but rather leads the parent through Johnny's activities on a particular day and then deduces the amount of sleep he gets. In suggesting alterations in the daily pattern, the nurse must have information about the usual family activities, current sleeping arrangements, and other factors that impinge on Johnny's sleep. To obtain this information, a series of concrete, precise questions must be asked. Developing these communication techniques is essential for both inpatient and community nurses who wish to intervene effectively with physically neglecting families.

Because these families require long-term follow-up, liaison between inpatient and community nurses is essential for continuity of care. In the community, neglecting families often require assistance to build in some predictable daily routines for children. For many, developing adequate problem solving skills about child care (or anything else) can be a lifelong task that requires continuous reinforcement by others. Lay home visitors seeing these families for several hours a day, two or three times weekly, can help overcome ignorance and chaos and develop improved parenting skills.

Because recent evidence links cognitive and emotional deficits of mentally retarded parents with neglect and since empirically tested programs (Fantuzzo et al, 1986) demonstrate that mildly retarded mothers can learn to improve their parenting skills, community nurses can be instrumental in the development of such programs.

Psychologic Maltreatment

Psychologic maltreatment is defined as "acts of omission and commission which are judged on a combination of community standards and professional expertise to be psychologically damaging. Such acts are committed by individuals, singly or collectively, who by their characteristics are in a position of differential power that renders a child vulnerable" (Hart et al, 1983, p 2). Acts toward a child such as rejecting, degrading, terrorizing, isolating, corrupting, exploiting, and denying emotional responsiveness constitute psychologic maltreatment (Brassard et al, 1987).

Although few data are available, experts generally agree that this form of abuse almost always accompanies other forms of abuse, is more prevalent than other forms of abuse, and is often more destructive in its short- and long-term impact on the lives of children (Garbarino et al, 1986). It can occur at any age.

Clinical Manifestations and Diagnostic Assessment. The parental and child behavioral indicators of potential psychologic maltreatment are summarized in Table 28–9.

Parental acts of omission (e.g., ignoring the child, no involvement in the child's daily activities, disinterest in the child, lack of physical intimacy with the child) or commission (e.g., yelling, criticizing, degrading, belittling) result in a lonely child with low self-esteem and decreased ability to reach out emotionally and physically to others. Although one child may be the target of psychologic maltreatment, assessment usually reveals a family in which members have difficulty sharing their feelings and emotional support for one another is minimal. These styles of relating may have evolved over a long period of time or may have been precipitated by a family crisis or stressful event.

Nurses encounter children who have been psychologically maltreated as they care for children who have been hospitalized for other reasons. Because this type of child abuse is difficult to identify, careful nursing documentation of parent-child interactions can be helpful in the process. Parents who, when asked, are unable to identify a single positive attribute of the child, should alert the nurse to the possibility of psychologic maltreatment. Parents who without reason do not visit children or communicate with them by telephone are displaying signs of being uninvolved in their child's care. Now that open visiting hours for parents are encouraged in most inpatient settings and health care professionals recognize the value of parental participation in the care of hospitalized children, nurses must exercise caution in prematurely reaching conclusions about psychologic maltreatment as the reason for parental lack of involvement in child care. Many parents face a number of obstacles to spending regular periods of time with a hospitalized child, including lack of baby sitting services for other children; personal jobs outside the home; financial restrictions to public transportation; length of time to travel from home to hospital, to list a few. These obstacles may be compounded by feelings of discomfort or inadequacy about caring for the child with nursing supervision or by a belief that it is better if parents do not visit because the child gets upset when they leave. Nurses who encourage par-

TABLE 28-9
Indicators of Potential Psychologic Maltreatment

Parents	Child
Denies the problem or blames the child for it	Infant
Appears unconcerned about the child's welfare	Displays frozen watchfulness
Shows discrepancy between verbal and nonverbal communication to the child	Is slow developing speech
States that he/she is not involved with child in activities	Has apparent cognitive or emotional developmental lag
States child is inadequate compared with others in the family	Avoids eye contact
Uses predominantly negative comments to the child and about the child	Does not physically reach out to caregiver for comfort or attention
Refuses all offers of help	Older Child and Adolescent
	Displays hyperactive/disruptive behaviors
	Displays behavior extremes (e.g., withdrawn, aggressive, and demanding)
	Shows overly adaptive behavior (e.g., too well mannered, too clean and neat, does not cry during painful procedures)
	Displays inhibition of play
	In play, demonstrates emotional unattachment to dolls or children
	Is unusually fearful of consequences of actions, which often leads to lying
	Has sleep disorders
	States no one cares about self, that he or she is no good and cannot succeed
	Presents psychosomatic complaints (e.g., headache, nausea, abdominal pain)
	Has threatened or attempted suicide

ents to visit but appreciate the difficulties involved for some families and who are able to be flexible reinforce the parent's self-esteem and decrease guilt for "abandoning" the child.

Nursing Care of Psychologically Maltreated Children and Their Families. Psychologically maltreated infants and children present several nursing care challenges. The lack of responsiveness demonstrated by many of these infants can be frustrating for nurses. As with other abused and maltreated children, consistent care by one nurse is the model that is most likely to lead to a therapeutic relationship.

Nurses need to be prepared to expend a lot of time and energy in relating to these children and, initially, to accept meager rewards. Once a thorough assessment of current development has been completed, nursing interactions with the infant or child focus on helping the family provide an accepting, warm, nurturing atmosphere in which subsequent developmental tasks can be achieved. Play therapy can stimulate development and a sense of individual control in infants and children.

As with others who have been abused, psychologically maltreated children require clear plans of care, which include strategies to manage unacceptable behavior. Consistent adherence to these plans is crucial, so that children who are already confused about expectations and adult reactions can learn to trust this new environment.

To communicate effectively with these parents, the nurse must be supportive and empathetic to their needs. Many such parents have never known warm, supportive relationships and can initially be very suspicious. Focusing on their strengths in parent-child interactions gives parents an increased sense of self-esteem and provides positive reinforcement for the behavior.

Some parents have never learned how to enjoy their children. Through modeling games and other activities, the nurse can encourage the parent to begin to participate. Emphasizing the unique status of the parents in the child's life helps reassure parents that the nurse is not trying to assume this role. It also can contribute to making parents feel worthwhile.

When these children have been discharged from hospital, ongoing support is required to assist in the continuing improvement of family functioning. Psychologically maltreated older children can benefit from participation in adult-led activities (e.g., sports, clubs) in which adults other than parents can provide positive reinforcement and the emotional support that leads to increased self-esteem. Community health nurses and others may be involved in strategies to continue to change the behavior of family members and in psychotherapy for the family and/or particular members.

Sexual Abuse

Sexual abuse and sexual misuse are similarly defined. Brant and Tisza's (1977) definition of sexual misuse also defines sexual abuse: "exposure of the child to sexual stimulation inappropriate for the child's age, level of psychosexual development, and role in the family."

Activities that constitute sexual abuse include permitting or exposing a child to sexual acts, such as prostitution or pornography, as well as molestation, which includes exposure, fondling, masturbation, vaginal or rectal penetration, or sexual intercourse (Sgroi, 1984). About 5 to 6 per cent of all children will be victims of child sexual abuse (Finkelhor & Hotaling, 1984). Although both extrafamilial and intrafamilial sexual abuse occur, incest appears to be the most damaging to children and usually indicates severe family problems. Intrafamilial sexual abuse can involve any dyad within the family, but the most common type involves the father-daughter or the stepfather-daughter relationships. Evidence indicates that male victims are more common than previously acknowledged (Finkelhor, 1984; Vander Mey, 1988).

Child pornography and child prostitution represent big business in the United States and also inflict sexual abuse on increasing numbers of children. The plight of these children and the large number of runaways involved have been presented recently in the academic and popular press (Stiffman, 1989).

Although the media frequently report cases of false allegations of sexual abuse in custody and visitation disputes, a recent national survey indicates that slightly less than 2 per cent of these cases involve allegations of sexual abuse (Thoennes & Tjaden, 1990).

Child sexual abuse has been identified in infants as young as 6 months. Incest usually begins at about age 4 years with caressing and fondling and proceeds over time to sexual intercourse. It may continue on a regular or intermittent basis for years, until the child refuses to comply, leaves home, or discloses the behavior. The perpetrator of child sexual abuse is most frequently male, and in the cases of extrafamilial abuse is usually an individual the child knows. He may be a family member, friend, acquaintance, baby sitter, or, on rare occasion, a stranger.

Children who have been sexually abused are rarely admitted to the hospital for the problem. They are more frequently seen in emergency rooms, outpatient clinics, schools, and private offices of physicians or nurse practitioners. Along with other health professionals, nurses in these settings may be involved in the initial interview of the child, in reporting the situation to the CPS, and in the immediate aftercare of the child (Elvik et al, 1986).

Although initial disclosures may be made to a nurse, nurses do not usually conduct investigative interviews; rather they are a support for the child before and after the interview. When a disclosure occurs, the first task of the nurse, after age-appropriately reassuring the child or adolescent that to share the information was wise and that steps will be taken to stop the abuse, is to report the incident to CPS. Parents are not notified of the disclosure. They will be informed by the CPS worker and/or the police who will investigate the allegation. There are two reasons for not notifying the parents: to ensure the safety of the child; and to prevent jeopardizing the admissibility to court of evidence collected by the CPS worker and/or police. In addition, some nurses lead groups for children who have been victims of sexual abuse. Community nurses may be involved in long-term follow-up of families.

Although nurses may care for clients who have been sexually abused by any of the aforementioned perpetrators, they most frequently encounter children who are victims of repeated intrafamilial sexual abuse. Many of the manifestations of child sexual abuse and the nursing strategies for intervention outlined in this section can be applied to all types of sexual abuse, but they are particularly relevant to incest.

Clinical Manifestations and Diagnostic Assessment. Table 28–10 summarizes the child indicators of sexual abuse. The child behavior indicators are some-

TABLE 28–10
Indicators of Potential Sexual Abuse (Child)

Physical Indicators

Difficulty in walking or sitting

Pain, swelling, or itching in the genital area

Bruises, bleeding, or lacerations of the external genitalia, vaginal, or anal areas

Pregnancy, especially in early teen-age years

Poor sphincter tone

Dilatation of the vaginal opening

Torn, stained, or bloody clothing

Pain on urination

Recurrent urinary tract infections

Abdominal pain with no definitive cause

Vaginal/penile discharge

Sexually transmitted disease, especially in preadolescents

Recurrent vaginal infections in a child under 12 yrs of age

Recurrent sore throat of unknown origin

Behavioral Indicators

Reactions similar to those precipitated by any other severe stress, including the following:

- Regressive behavior in younger children (e.g., bed wetting, thumb sucking)
- Sudden onset of fears or phobias (e.g., of the dark, men, or particular settings or situations)
- Running away from home
- Abuse of drugs and alcohol
- Noticeable personality changes (e.g., depression, anger, hostility, aggression)
- Change in school performance
- Suicidal thoughts or attempts
- Somatic complaints (e.g., headaches, abdominal pain, eating disorders)

Reactions directly related to sexual abuse, including the following:

- Provocative drawings of a sexual nature
- Age-inappropriate sexual play/activity
- Excessive masturbation
- Bizarre, sophisticated, or unusual sexual behavior or knowledge
- Overtly seductive behavior toward peers
- Promiscuity among adolescents
- Prostitution among adolescents
- Withdrawal from peers
- Statement that he or she is being sexually assaulted
- Females may state relationship with mother is poor; may be very angry because mother does not protect her
- May feel it is his or her fault

From Thomas, H. (1983). *Child abuse, neglect and deprivation: A handbook for Ontario nurses*. Toronto: Registered Nurses' Association of Ontario.

what age-dependent. For example, running away from home, drug and alcohol abusc, and promiscuity or prostitution are most commonly seen in adolescent females. Among female teens, sexual abuse is the most common reason for running away. Often the sexual abuse has been accompanied by physical abuse (Felice & Friedman, 1982). Regressive behavior and age-inappropriate knowledge (advanced) about sexual activity indicate the possibility of sexual abuse in preadolescent school-age girls. Precocious sexual interest and drawings with sexual themes can reflect sexual abuse of preschool children.

Seductive behavior of children and adolescents does not cause intrafamilial sexual abuse. Normal preschool females experiment with "seducing" their father or father figure. Most fathers do not use this behavior as a rationalization for beginning sexual abuse, but rather place it within the context of the father-daughter relationship. In experimenting with female roles to use outside the home, many adolescents display provocative sexual behavior at home. Again, most fathers react to this by helping the teen to evaluate it realistically. Adults who see provocative sexual behavior of children as an opportunity to engage in incest are misinterpreting the behavior and responding inappropriately. Table 28–11 outlines behavioral indicators frequently observed in parents of girls suffering intrafamilial sexual abuse by the father or stepfather.

Because intrafamilial sexual abuse has usually gone on over a period of time, and since less than 20 per cent of the victims suffer physical trauma, identification of the problem is usually through disclosure. Disclosure can be accidental or purposeful. Accidental disclosure occurs in several ways: a third person observes the activity and reports it; during assessment of a child for an identified physical or behavioral symptom, the clinician becomes suspicious and asks the child; precocious child sexual activity arouses the suspicion of another adult who asks the child about it. Purposeful disclosure occurs when a child or adolescent reports the experience voluntarily to a teacher, health professional, or other trusted adult with whom there is contact (Sgroi, 1984). Regardless of how the disclosure occurs, it is imperative that the victim be supported in the statement. False allegations do occur, but until an initial investigative assessment has taken place, children should be believed. In the past, many professionals regarded reports of sexual abuse as a product of childish fantasy. Recent evidence indicates that most victims, particularly preadolescent children, could not describe such incidents without personal experience.

Investigative assessment of child sexual abuse includes obtaining the history from the child during an interview (or a series of interviews), physically assessing the child, and interviewing the alleged perpetrator. A number of researchers describe interviewing strategies for use with sexually abused children of various ages. The most salient aspects are presented here. Nurses wishing to expand their knowledge and skill in this area are encouraged to consult the original works (Sgroi, 1984; Kelley, 1985; Miller, 1985).

The initial investigative interview of the child or adolescent following disclosure of sexual abuse has several objectives:

- Initial engagement of the client in a therapeutic session.
- Identity of the perpetrator(s).
- History of the sexual activity (e.g., actual sexual activity, frequency, length of time from initial sexual activity to disclosure, where the activity occurred).
- Methods used to enhance victim compliance and to keep the activity a secret (e.g., bribes, physical force, rewards, threats).
- Assessment of the child's need for immediate protection.

TABLE 28-11
Indicators of Potential Sexual Abuse (Parents)

Father/Stepfather

Rigid in his perception of his role within the family

Needs to dominate the family

Sees himself as a good parent

When confronted with his behaviors, often rationalizes it as being educational and pleasurable for the child

May admit guilt and be remorseful, but is unable to change

Describes an unsatisfactory sexual and emotional relationship with wife; may be divorced, or his wife may be dead or disabled

Lacks social and emotional contacts outside the family

Pays special attention to the child victim, usually increasing sibling rivalry

Protective and jealous of the child victim, limiting child's contacts outside the family

Mother

Often aware of the incestuous relationship

Sometimes sees it as a relief for herself, and organizes time for the two to be alone

Usually states that her relationship with her husband is poor and may have terminated sexual relations with him

Usually is a passive person who is emotionally and financially dependent on her husband

May not see herself as an integral part of the family

May want the behavior to stop but will not risk exposing it

May blame the child for the relationship

Frequently was involved in an incestuous relationship in her family of origin

Frequently was poorly parented as a child and never learned how to protect herself and her children

From Thomas, H. (1983). *Child abuse, neglect and deprivation: A handbook for Ontario nurses*. Toronto: Registered Nurses' Association of Ontario.

- Assessment of the extent of the child's or adolescent's emotional trauma, to provide appropriate crisis intervention and begin planning for follow-up counseling services.

Because child sexual abuse is a health, social, and legal problem, information about the situation will be needed by several professionals. It is unnecessary and traumatic for the victim to have to recount the story several times. A tape recording of the initial session can minimize repeated questioning, since it reproduces the facts presented. In some states and provinces, these recorded interviews are accepted in court. This means that if charges are laid, the victim does not have to recount the events when the case is heard in court. An alternative is to have the participating professionals present with an identified primary interviewer. This can be intimidating for the child, but if handled effectively, it is less traumatic than having to repeat the explanation. A room with a two-way mirror for professionals other than the primary interviewer can solve this problem. Parents should not be present at the interview for two reasons. First, one of them may be the perpetrator, and second, their presence may inhibit the child who feels guilty and afraid of parental disapproval or punishment.

The purpose of the interview must be clarified, in age-appropriate terms, with the child at the outset. For victims to feel comfortable enough to describe their experience, they need to be reassured that disclosure was a good thing to do and that although what the perpetrator did was wrong, they have done nothing wrong. It is comforting for many children to know that the interviewer has talked to other children with the same problem. Because of the secrecy surrounding sexual abuse, many victims believe they are unique.

The strategies used to collect the data depend on the age of the victim. Adolescents can usually articulate answers to straightforward, clear questions. Preadolescent and younger children may have difficulty answering questions because they do not understand what is being asked or because they are too embarrassed. A number of age-appropriate aids are available to assist these children. Anatomically correct dolls have been widely used to determine exactly what has happened. Although their value is controversial and has not been empirically proved, some evidence suggests that they can be effective aids for sexually abused children between the ages of 3 and 6 years (Cohn, 1991).

Two types of art work can facilitate the explanations of children (Kelley, 1984). Anatomic drawings of males and females at the different developmental stages (preschool, school-age, adolescent, adult) can be used by children to state their names for different body parts. Then the interviewer can ask questions by using words with which the child is familiar, to help minimize confusion. Picture drawing is another useful aid for sexually abused children between 3 and 12 years of age. The children are asked to draw a picture of themselves, the perpetrator, and what happened. While they are engaged in this activity, they should be encouraged to talk about what they are drawing and how they feel about it.

Physical assessment of the child follows the investigative interview, unless the disclosure occurred during the physical examination. Physical examination of the child includes assessment for physical evidence (see Table 28–10) of sexual abuse and a pediatric or adult gynecologic examination (Pascoe & Duterte, 1981).

Because child sexual abuse is a criminal offense, the initial interview with the alleged perpetrator should be conducted by the police. They are familiar with the rules of evidence for admission of information to court proceedings. The interviewing styles of most health and social service professionals can lead to the evidence gathered being judged inadmissible in court and thus severely weaken the prosecutor's case.

Reactions of other family members to the disclosure of intrafamilial or extrafamilial sexual abuse vary. Because intrafamilial sexual abuse has many more ramifications for the family, reactions to it are strongest. The initial reactions of the father-perpetrator to the alleged sexual abuse of his daughter include denial, anger, hostility, guilt, and remorse. Initial maternal reactions are often quite hysterical. Subsequently, mothers may express many responses, such as fear, anger, denial, hostility, and apathy. Many mothers are torn between self-blame for failing to protect their daughter and the need to protect their husband. DeJong (1988) identifies three maternal responses to the sexual abuse of their children: nonsupportive; supportive with emotional changes (e.g., sleep disturbances, mood changes, crying, somatic complaints); and supportive without emotional changes. Of these three groups, the supportive mothers with emotional changes were most likely to support legal charges against the perpetrator and to seek counseling for themselves and their children. Siblings have varied reactions as well. Those who have also been sexually abused by the perpetrator may be relieved or angry at the victim for the family disruption the disclosure has caused. Sgroi (1984) points out that all family members' reactions will be based on "How will this affect me?" Often, in view of the reactions of family members, victims become less motivated to maintain their position. Pressure by parents and siblings to retract the claim of sexual abuse can result in children and adolescents changing or denying their stories. This is an excellent reason for careful assessment of the victim's emotional state and demonstrates the necessity for continued support (from others outside the family) during the investigative process.

Nursing Care of Sexually Abused Children and Their Families. As members of the multidisciplinary assessment and treatment team, nurses have an important role in the care of sexually abused children and their families. Being aware of the indicators of potential sexual abuse and maintaining a high level of suspicion will alert the nurse to the possibility of child sexual abuse, regardless of the practice setting. This can result in earlier identification of the problem and facilitate treatment for the child and family. As with any other type of abuse, the nurse who suspects child sexual abuse must report it to the CPS, following the institution or agency protocol. The idea of intrafamilial sexual abuse is so horrendous for some professionals that, even in the face of overwhelming evidence, they refuse to accept it. Knowledgeable nurses can assist these professionals in dealing with their feelings and in recognizing sexual abuse when it is apparent.

An adolescent may disclose a history of sexual abuse in an emergency setting, a clinic, the physician's office, or the school. Nurses working in these settings must be aware of the presenting symptoms that frequently mask sexual abuse (e.g., abdominal pain, somatic complaints with no identifiable cause). They must also be able to support a patient/client after disclosure. It is tempting to begin to collect further data immediately. The nurse who understands the investigative assessment procedure will be able to judge whether it is in the best interests of the client to proceed at this time or whether to wait until the other professionals have been assembled. Regardless of the role in the assessment interview, the nurse should be present to support the child or adolescent. Nurses' suggestions about age-appropriate ways to gather data can be valuable to the interviewer.

Documentation must be accurate and clear. It includes statements made by the client, physical and emotional assessment of the client, a report of procedures that have been implemented, a summary of the investigative interview, any art work done by the child, and any interaction with the parents.

In rare situations, children or adolescents who have been admitted to hospital with another problem may have been sexually abused as well. In these cases, the role of the nurse is to provide support to the patient and family and to record accurately child behavior and child-parent interactions.

As with other forms of abuse, the immediate treatment of the sexually abused child focuses on stopping the abuse. In intrafamilial sexual abuse, the initial reactions of the parents are assessed to determine whether the child can safely return home. If there appears to be a risk of further abuse, the child and perpetrator must be separated. Ideally, the perpetrator should leave the family. This is sometimes difficult to arrange and difficult to ensure. In these situations, the child is removed temporarily from the family.

A number of treatment models have been developed (Giarretto, 1982; Sgroi, 1984) that provide therapy individually or in groups for the sexually abused child, the perpetrator, the marital dyad, and the family. The details are beyond the scope of this chapter. The treatment of child sexual abuse is complex and multifaceted and to be successful usually requires a substantial investment of family time and energy. Nurses working in specialty clinics or the community may be involved in the long-term treatment process. Nurses may also refer families to self-help groups for sexually abused families. Parents United and Daughters and Sons United are examples of national self-help groups with local chapters in many cities.

The objectives of treatment are

- To aid in normal psychosexual development of the child/adolescent.
- To strengthen the marital bond.
- To reintegrate the family.

In many situations, the marital relationship is beyond repair, or adolescents do not wish to remain living with either parent. In these cases, assistance in working through the trauma and stress of separation is usually necessary. A favorable prognosis for sexually abused children and families is most likely when the father can admit his guilt and remorse to his daughter, when the mother believes and does not blame her daughter, and when the victim does not feel guilty and can forgive her father.

Because child sexual abuse is also a criminal matter, perpetrators are charged and a court appearance and case disposition takes place. The abuse of the investigation and treatment of intrafamilial child sexual abuse can be as devastating as the sexual abuse itself. Incarceration for the perpetrator results in the loss of the family unit and lifestyle, including loss of family income, family need for public assistance, change of family residence, and marital separation (Tyler & Brassard, 1984). More recently, courts have been ordering perpetrators into treatment, rather than jailing them. This has at least two positive outcomes: the perpetrators are treated, and the family is not so disrupted.

Nursing Roles in Prevention of Child Abuse and Maltreatment

A policy statement by the American Public Health Association (1987) underlines the importance of child abuse and maltreatment prevention as a national public health goal. This policy statement outlines five objectives and actions to achieve them. All have implications for nurses in practice and as concerned members of society. The nursing role in prevention of child abuse and maltreatment is addressed here by using the five objectives as a framework.

I. *Increase Public Awareness of the Nature and Extent of Efforts to Prevent Child Abuse*

As educators, nurses can assist in achieving this goal by initiating, participating in, or expanding current community education programs. Many programs* for school-age children and adolescents have been developed to heighten their awareness of child sexual abuse and what to do if they are involved in such incidents. In evaluating these programs, it is helpful to know that important topics to be included are factual information about sexual abuse, appropriate and inappropriate touch, respective role responsibilities of parents and children, and recognition of the individual's right to choose to engage in sexual behavior and the choice of partners. Nurses can be effective participants in school and community programs for children and adolescents, either by actually implementing programs or by assisting teachers or group leaders in planning age-appropriate activities.

Nurses can participate as speakers or leaders in community programs for parents related to the prevention of sexual abuse. Parents can learn to listen to the verbal and nonverbal messages children send about their interactions with other adults and possibly prevent sexual abuse. This is also an opportunity to dispel myths about child sexual abuse and to highlight specific positive communication techniques for families that enable children to discuss sexual advances of adults, if they occur.

For years, nurses have played a major role in planning and teaching prenatal classes. These classes provide an ideal setting in which to introduce the topic of parenting styles and potential problems. Providing parents with local support resources before they need them is another major goal that can be accomplished in these classes. Nurses can be influential in initiating parenting programs for new families in general, or for particular high-risk groups of parents (e.g., adolescent parents and single, poor mothers). The introduction of "family life" courses that move from prenatal to postnatal periods and through the ages and stages of child and family development is an idea that has received a lot of support but has not yet been implemented. Interested nurses could be involved in developing, carrying out, and evaluating such programs.

II. *Increase Knowledge of Health Professionals*

In the past, child abuse and maltreatment have not been emphasized in the educational curricula of health professionals. In view of their incidence, the long-term sequelae for children, and the high financial and social cost for society, they cannot be downplayed any longer. Health professionals must accept and be responsible for their role in this area of child and family care. Nurses involved in both practice and education involving the care of children and families need to provide continuing education that addresses the identification, treatment, and prevention of child abuse and maltreatment. To ensure that a multidisciplinary approach is evident, consultation with other professionals involved in this field must take place.

Nursing participation in multidisciplinary community or agency child abuse prevention and treatment programs results in a more comprehensive approach to the problem. Such participation provides nurses with the opportunity to negotiate their roles based on their identified knowledge and skills; to increase their understanding of the issues involved in the prevention, identification, and treatment of child abuse and maltreatment; and to develop respect for the roles of other involved professionals.

III. *Coordinate and Improve the Availability, Accessibility, and Quality of Health Services to Families*

There are two nursing roles related to this objective: advocacy for adequate health and social services, for all families requiring them; and early identification and treatment of families at high risk, so that child abuse and maltreatment can be prevented.

Advocacy for Expanded Health and Social Services for Children and Families. Nurses are in a position to know and understand the importance of meeting the health and social services needs of families in decreasing family stress and, thereby, diminishing the likelihood of child abuse and maltreatment. Nurses can participate in political lobbying at the community, state, or national level for stable funding for necessary health care for all children and families (including the working poor who are currently frequently uninsured and lack the financial resources for ongoing health care). Provision of quality day care and afterschool care for children is another urgent need. Neglect is often a result of family situations in which both parents (or the sole parent) work long hours to make financial ends meet and cannot afford to pay for supervision of their children. Older children are expected to supervise younger ones, and the results are often devastating for everyone.

Nurses can help focus public concerns on issues that influence the quality of family life. These include high-density living, adequate park space for inner city children, and the development of community centers where families can learn together, enjoy themselves, and meet other people. Mother-child drop-in centers are popular and decrease the social isolation of many mothers. Unfortunately, these centers do not usually have a stable funding base and are often forced to close.

Identification and Treatment of Families at High Risk for Child Abuse and Maltreatment. Families can become high risk for child abuse and maltreatment at any time. Some of the nursing diagnostic statements

* Child sexual abuse prevention resources are available from the National Committee for the Prevention of Child Abuse, Publishing Department, 332 S. Michigan Avenue, Suite 950, Chicago, IL 60604–4357; telephone: (312) 663–3520.

that should be considered include *high risk for injury, suffocation, poisoning, trauma,* and *aspiration; actual and high risk for altered parenting; altered family processes; caregiver role strain; parental role conflict; ineffective individual and family coping; low self-esteem; high risk for violence, post-trauma response; rape-trauma syndrome; anxiety;* and *fear.* The indicators for high-risk families are outlined in Table 28–6. In an attempt to provide primary prevention programs for child abuse and maltreatment, a great deal of work has been done to identify high-risk families prenatally or during the perinatal and postnatal periods. Nurses in a clinic, physician's office, or maternity setting are in an ideal position to assess these families, because they see them over time and can develop a therapeutic trusting relationship with them. This facilitates a comprehensive family history and assessment.

Several screening instruments have been developed to assist in the identification of families at high risk:

- Child Abuse Potential Inventory (Milner & Wimberley, 1979).
- Adolescent/Adult Parenting Inventory.
- Family Stress Check List (Murphy et al, 1985).
- Parenting Profile Assessment (Anderson, 1987).
- Potential Screening Scale (Avison et al, 1986).

These instruments provide a standardized, relatively quick method of assessing the level of parental risk. However, one must recognize that they have limitations. Not all have been adequately tested for reliability and validity. The Child Abuse Potential Inventory (Milner & Wimberley, 1979) is probably the best developed at this time. It has known psychometric properties, is designed for a grade 3 reading level, and asks parents to agree or disagree with 150 one-line statements. An updated version contains about 70 items, requiring less time to complete (Milner, 1988).

Selection of an instrument should be based on its purpose. For example, the Potential Screening Scale (Turner & Avison, 1985) was developed from the theory that social support is the crucial variable that differentiates abusers from nonabusers. The literature on this topic is controversial (Turner & Avison, 1985; Seagull, 1987). However, if one has a prevention program available that emphasizes the development of social support systems in preventing stress, this tool would be appropriate. Other instruments are more general and based on a multifaceted approach.

Correct identification of high-risk families is the first step in prevention. The second step, engaging these families in programs to enhance their parenting and problem solving skills, continues to be a challenge for all, including nurses. There is some evidence that providing concrete assistance (e.g., loan services for car seats, toys, or cribs; respite child care; assistance with locating and moving into new homes) can enhance early participation and continued involvement (Barth et al, 1986).

Results from a Special Families Care Project indicate that intensive health care services (2 to 4 hours per week of contact for a minimum of 18 months) for high-risk parents can reduce the incidence of reported child abuse, neglect, and out-of-home placement when compared with traditional services provided at 2- or 4-week intervals (Velasquez et al, 1984). This interdisciplinary program (nurses and social workers) provided support to high-risk parents, as well as individualized plans of care based on maternal needs (e.g., developing problem solving skills about child care, increasing knowledge about normal infant growth and development, identifying personal support systems). A unique aspect of this program was that it helped hard-to-serve clients who do not avail themselves of group programs. Because of frustration or a sense of futility, nurses often have difficulty working with these parents. This experience could be valuable to nurses working with similar clients. It underlines the necessity for ingenuity, creativity, and professional support in working with hard-to-serve clients.

IV. Develop Data Systems to Monitor the Incidence and Prevalence of All Forms of Child Abuse

As noted, the inconsistencies of data collection systems across the country make accurate assessment of the incidence or prevalence of all forms of child abuse impossible. For nurses and others interested in planning prevention or intervention programs for these children and families, up-to-date statistics would assist in determining geographic areas where the need is greatest. Most programs are situated where they are because the people who initiated them live there. This is not the most effective deployment of resources, and in these times of financial restraint for health and social services, it is an insufficient criterion on which to establish programs.

Although nurses are not directly involved in this aspect of prevention, it is hoped that their appreciation of the value of a standardized method of data collection and the resulting accurate data set will inspire some to publicly advocate for such a system.

V. Research

A number of issues in the field of child abuse and maltreatment need to be adequately addressed by empirical research:

- Prospective long-term longitudinal studies to document, in a systematic way, the nature, causes, consequences, long-term effects, and responses related to all forms of child abuse and maltreatment.
- Cross-cultural research in the areas of prevention and treatment program evaluation.

- Further clarification of high-risk families and effective prevention interventions.
- Further understanding of the critical differences between nonabusive and abusive families.

Nurses with the interest, knowledge, and skills may become investigators in multidisciplinary research projects designed to address any of these issues. Other nurses can become involved in ongoing projects in which their knowledge about and skill in identification and treatment of child abuse and maltreatment will be valued and used. All nurses need to develop an appreciation of the necessity for scientifically based nursing practice in this and other fields.

In summary, the nursing roles in the prevention of child abuse and maltreatment are several:

- Educator.
- Child and family advocate.
- Participant in identifying parents at high risk.
- Practitioner in programs designed to treat high-risk abusive families.
- Researcher or practitioner in prevention research.

KEY CONCEPTS

Concepts Related to Basic Information

- Definitions of child abuse, neglect, and maltreatment are developed for different purposes, such as social policy, legal regulations, research, and case management. Ultimately, the actual definition is determined by the judicial system.
- The actual incidence of child abuse and maltreatment is difficult to determine, because criteria for reporting differ from state to state and because of professionals' failure to recognize child abuse and hesitancy to report it.
- Child abuse is commonly subcategorized as physical abuse, physical neglect, psychologic maltreatment, and sexual abuse.
- State law identifies two types of reporters of child abuse: *mandatory reporters* who are required to report suspected abuse, such as nurses, and *permissive reporters* who may, but are not required to, report child abuse.
- Several models have been proposed to explain the complex multifaceted phenomenon of child abuse. These models are *mental illness, environmental stress, social learning, social-psychologic, human ecologic,* and *psychologic-sociologic*.

Concepts Related to Nursing Assessment

- A crucial aspect of assessment of children who are suspected of being abused or maltreated is a thorough family history and family assessment.
- Because more and more abuse and maltreatment cases are being dealt with in the courts, if litigation ensues, the chart may become part of the evidence and the nurse may be called to explain the documentation.
- Initial assessment of the child should include any physical injuries or abnormalities and an objective documentation of behavioral or developmental symptoms and observations of parent-child interactions.
- Ongoing nursing documentation during hospitalization includes assessment of history and status of physical injuries, changes in the child's behavior, parent-child interactions, telephone inquiries made by parents, and parental emotional states.

Concepts Related to Nursing Intervention

- Before the nurse can work effectively in the field of child abuse, personal values and attitudes related to child abuse must be clarified.
- Long-term treatment of abused children and their families is complex and requires the services of multiple service agencies and multidisciplinary community teams.
- Once suspected child abuse has been reported to the child protection agency, the nursing role becomes one of advocacy and support.
- Long-term interventions with parents include increasing parental impulse control, providing alternatives to physical abuse, increasing knowledge of child development, and developing age-appropriate expectations.
- The nurse's role in prevention of child abuse includes participating in public and professional education, advocating for social services and public policy changes, identifying high-risk families, and conducting research.

REFERENCES

Aber, J., Allen, J., Carlson, V., & Cicchetti, D. (1989). The effects of maltreatment on development during early childhood: Recent studies and their theoretical, clinical, and policy implication. In D. Cicchetti & V. Carlson (Eds.), *Child maltreatment: Theory and research on the causes and consequences of child abuse and neglect*. Cambridge: Cambridge University Press.

American Public Health Association (1987). Prevention of child abuse. *American Journal of Public Health, 77*(1), 111–113.

Anderson, C. (1987). Assessing parenting potential for child abuse risk. *Pediatric Nursing, 13*(5), 323–327.

Avison, W., et al. (1986). Screening for problem parenting: Preliminary evidence on a promising instrument. *Child Abuse and Neglect, 10*, 157–170.

Bandura, A. (1973). *Aggression: A social learning analysis*. Englewood Cliffs, NJ: Prentice-Hall.

Barth, R., et al. (1986). Identifying, screening, and engaging high-risk clients in private, non-profit child abuse prevention programs. *Child Abuse and Neglect, 10*(1), 99–110.

Beitchman, J., Zucker, K., Hood, J. DaCosta, G., & Akman, D. (1991). A review of the short-term effects of child sexual abuse. *Child Abuse and Neglect, 15*, 537–556.

Belsky, J. (1980). Child maltreatment: An ecological integration. *American Psychologist, 35*(4), 320–335.

Belsky, J., & Vondra, J. (1989). Lessons from child abuse: The determinants of parenting. In D. Cicchetti & V. Carlson (Eds.), *Child maltreatment: Theory and research on the causes and consequences of child abuse and neglect* (pp. 153–202). Cambridge: Cambridge University Press.

Besharov, D. (1985). Doing something about child abuse: The need to narrow the grounds for state intervention. *Harvard Journal of Law and Public Policy, 8*(3), 539–589.

Brant, R., & Tisza, V. (1977). The sexually misused child. *American Journal of Orthopsychiatry, 4*(1), 80–90.

Brassard, M., et al. (1987). *Psychological maltreatment of children and youth*. New York: Pergamon Press.

Burgess, A., Hartman, C., & Kelley, S. (1990). Assessing child abuse: The TRIADS checklist. *Journal of Psychosocial Nursing, 28*(4), 7–14.

Byles, J., et al. (1988). Ontario Child Health Study: Reliability and validity of the general functioning subscale of the McMaster Family Assessment Device. *Family Process, 27,* 97–104.

Campbell, J., & Humphreys, J. (1984). *Nursing care of victims of family violence*. Reston, VA: Reston Publishing Company.

Cohn, S. (1991). Anatomical doll play of preschoolers referred for sexual abuse and those not referred. *Child Abuse and Neglect, 15,* 455–466.

Cohn Donnelly, A. (1991). What we have learned about prevention: What we should do about it. *Child Abuse and Neglect, 15*(Suppl. 1), 99–106.

Daro, D., & McCurdy, K. (1992). *Current trends in child abuse reporting and fatalities: The results of the 1991 Annual Fifty State Survey*. Chicago: National Committee for Prevention of Child Abuse.

DeJong, A. (1988). Maternal responses of the sexual abuse of their children. *Pediatrics, 81*(1), 14–21.

Doak, C., et al. (1985). *Teaching patients with low literacy skills*. Philadelphia: JB Lippincott.

Egeland, B., & Erickson, M. (1987). Psychologically unavailable caregiving. In M. Brassard et al. (Eds.), *Psychological maltreatment of children and youth*. New York: Pergamon Press.

Elvik, S., et al. (1986). Child sexual abuse: The role of the N.P. *Nurse Practitioner, 11*(1), 15–22.

Epstein, N., et al. (1981). The McMaster model of family functioning: A view of the normal family. In F. Walsh (Ed.), *Normal family processes*. New York: Guilford Press.

Erickson, M., Egeland, B., & Pianta, R. (1989). The effects of maltreatment on the development of young children. In D. Cicchetti & V. Carlson (Eds.), *Child maltreatment: Theory and research on the causes and consequences of child abuse and neglect* (pp. 647–684). Cambridge: Cambridge University Press.

Famularo, R., Kinscherff, R., & Fenton, T. (1992). Parental substance abuse and the nature of child maltreatment. *Child Abuse and Neglect, 16,* 475–483.

Fantuzzo, J. W., et al. (1986). Parent and social-skills training for mentally retarded mothers identified as child-maltreaters. *American Journal of Mental Deficiency, 91*(2), 135–140.

Felice, M., & Friedman, S. (1982). Behavioral considerations in the health care of adolescents. *Pediatric Clinics of North America, 29,* 399–413.

Finkelhor, D. (1984). *Child sexual abuse: New research and theory*. New York: The Free Press.

Finkelhor, D., & Hotaling, G. (1984). Sexual abuse in the National Incidence Study of Child Abuse and Neglect. *Child Abuse and Neglect, 8,* 23–28.

Gale, J., et al. (1988). Sexual abuse in young children: Its clinical presentation and characteristic patterns. *Child Abuse and Neglect, 12,* 163.

Garbarino, J. (1977). The human ecology of child maltreatment. *Journal of Marriage and Family, 39,* 721–736.

Garbarino, J., et al. (1986). *The psychologically battered child: Strategies for identification, assessment and intervention*. San Francisco: Jossey-Bass.

Giarretto, H. (1982). *Integrated treatment of child sexual abuse: A treatment and training manual*. San Francisco: Science and Behavioral Books.

Gil, D. (1975). Unravelling child abuse. *American Journal of Orthopsychiatry, 45*(4), 346–356.

Hart, S., et al. (1983). *Proceedings summary of the international conference on psychological abuse of children and youth*. Indianapolis: Indiana University, Office for the Study of the Psychological Rights of the Child.

Houck, G., & King, M. (1989). Child maltreatment: Family characteristics and developmental consequences. *Issues in Mental Health Nursing, 10,* 193–208.

Hurwoltz, A., & Castells, S. (1987). Misdiagnosed child abuse and metabolic disease. *Pediatric Nursing, 13*(1), 33–36.

Hutchison, E. (1990, March). Child maltreatment: Can it be defined? *Social Service Review*, pp. 61–78.

Jonker, F., & Jonker-Bakker, P. (1991). Experiences with ritualist child sexual abuse: A case study from the Netherlands. *Child Abuse and Neglect, 15,* 191–196.

Justice, B., & Justice, R. (1976). *The abusing family*. New York: Human Science Press.

Kaufman, J., & Zigler, E. (1987). Do abused children become abusive parents? *American Journal of Orthopsychiatry, 57*(2), 186–192.

Kelley, S. (1984). The use of art therapy with sexually abused children. *Journal of Psychosocial Nursing and Mental Health Services, 22,* 12–18.

Kelley, S. (1985). Interviewing the sexually abused child: Principles and techniques. *Journal of Emergency Nursing, 11*(5), 234–241.

Kempe, C., & Helfer, R. (1972). *Helping the battered child and his family*. Philadelphia: JB Lippincott.

Kropp, J., & Haynes, O. (1987). Abusive and nonabusive mothers' ability to identify general and specific emotion signals of infants. *Child Development, 58,* 187–190.

Lamphear, U. (1985). The impact of maltreatment of children's psychosocial adjustment: A review of the research. *Child Abuse and Neglect, 9,* 251–263.

Levin, N., & Levin, D. (1982). A folk medicine practice mimicking child abuse. *Hospital Practice, 17,* 17–20.

Margolin, L. (1991). Child sexual abuse by non-related caregivers. *Child Abuse and Neglect, 15,* 213–221.

McNeill, L., & Brassard, M. (1984). *The behavioral correlates of father-daughter incest with elementary school-aged girls*. Paper presented at the Fifth International Congress on Child Abuse and Neglect, Montreal.

Miller, E. (1985). Interviewing the sexually abused child. *MCN: American Journal of Maternal Child Nursing, 10,* 103–105.

Millor, G. (1981). A theoretical framework for nursing research in child abuse and neglect. *Nursing Research, 30*(2), 78–83.

Milner, J. S. (1988). Personal communication.

Milner, J., & Wimberley, R. (1979). An inventory for the identification of child abusers. *Journal of Clinical Psychology, 35,* 95–100.

Murphy, S., et al. (1985). Prenatal prediction of child abuse and neglect: A prospective study. *Child Abuse and Neglect, 9,* 225–235.

O'Hare, A., & Eden, O. (1984). Bleeding disorders and non-accidental injury. *Archives of Diseases in Children, 59,* 860–864.

Orkow, B. (1985). Implementation of a family stress checklist. *Child Abuse and Neglect, 9,* 405–410.

Parke, R. (1982). Theoretical models of child abuse: Their implications for prediction, prevention and modification In R. Starr (Ed.), *Child abuse prediction*. Cambridge, MA: Ballinger.

Pascoe, D., & Duterte, B. (1981). The medical diagnosis of sexual abuse in the premenarchal child. *Pediatric Annals, 10*(5), 187–190.

Pelton, L. (1978). Child abuse and neglect: The myth of classlessness. *American Journal of Orthopsychiatry, 48*(4), 608–617.

Rew, L. (1989). Long-term effects of childhood sexual exploitation. *Issues in Mental Health Nursing, 10,* 229–244.

Rhodes, A. (1987). The nurse's legal obligations for reporting child abuse. *MCN: American Journal of Maternal Child Nursing, 12,* 313.

Scharer, K. (1978). Rescue fantasies: Professional impediments in working with abused families. *American Journal of Nursing, 78,* 1483–1484.

Seagull, E. (1987). Social support and child maltreatment: A review of the evidence. *Child Abuse and Neglect, 11,* 41–52.

Sgroi, S. (1984). *Handbook of clinical intervention in child sexual abuse.* Toronto: Lexington Books.

Sivan, A. (1991). Preschool child development: Implications for investigation of child abuse allegations. *Child Abuse and Neglect, 15,* 485–493.

Spinetta, S., & Rigler, D. (1972). The child abusing parent: A psychological review. *Psychological Bulletin, 77,* 296–304.

Stiffman, A. R. (1989). Physical and sexual abuse in runaway youths. *Child Abuse and Neglect, 13,* 417–426.

Straus, M., et al. (1980). *Behind closed doors: Violence in the American family.* New York: Anchor Press.

Thoennes, N., & Tjaden, P. (1990). The extent, nature and validity of sexual abuse allegations in custody/visitation disputes. *Child Abuse and Neglect, 15,* 151–163.

Thomas, H. (1983). *Child abuse, neglect and deprivation: A handbook for Ontario nurses.* Toronto: Registered Nurses' Association of Ontario.

Turk, L., Hanrahan, K., & Weber, E. (1990). Munchausen syndrome by proxy: A nursing overview. *Issues in Comprehensive Pediatric Nursing, 13,* 279–288.

Turner, R., & Avison, W. (1985, November). Assessing risk factors for problem parenting: The significance of social support. *Journal of Marriage and Family,* pp. 881–892.

Tyler, A., & Brassard, M. (1984). Abuse in the investigation and treatment of intra-familial child sexual abuse. *Child Abuse and Neglect, 8,* 47–53.

Vander Mey, B. (1988). The sexual victimization of male children: A review of previous research. *Child Abuse and Neglect, 12*(1), 61–72.

Velasquez, J., et al. (1984). Intensive services help prevent child abuse. *MCN: American Journal of Maternal Child Nursing, 9,* 113–117.

Vondra, J., Barnett, D., & Cicchetti, D. (1990). Self-concept, motivation, and competence among preschoolers from maltreating and comparison families. *Child Abuse and Neglect, 14,* 525–540.

Wong, D. (1987). False allegations of child abuse: The other side of the tragedy. *Pediatric Nursing, 13*(4), 329–333.

Wright, L., & Leahey, M. (1984). *Nurses and families: A guide to family assessment and intervention.* Philadelphia: FA Davis.

Zeanah, C., & Zeanah, P. (1989). Intergenerational transmission of maltreatment: Insights from attachment theory and research. *Psychiatry, 52,* 177–196.

BIBLIOGRAPHY

Beitchman, J., Zucker, K., Hood, J., DaCosta, G., Akman, D., & Cassavia, E. (1992). A review of the long-term effects of child sexual abuse. *Child Abuse and Neglect, 16,* 101–118.

Berowitz, C., et al. (1987). Characteristics of mother-infant interactions in non-organic failure to thrive. *Journal of Family Practice, 25*(4), 377–381.

Brown, A., & Finkelhor, D. (1986). Impact of child sexual abuse: A review of the literature. *Psychological Bulletin, 99,* 66–77.

Cavanagh, J. (1988). Child perpetrators—children who molest other children: Preliminary findings. *Child Abuse and Neglect, 12,* 219–229.

Cicchetti, D., & Carlson, V. (Eds.) (1989). *Child maltreatment: Theory and research on the causes and consequences of child abuse and neglect.* Cambridge, MA: Cambridge University Press.

Dale, P., et al. (1986). *Dangerous families: Assessment and treatment of child abuse.* London: Tavistock.

Hlady, L., & Gunter, E. (1990). Alleged child abuse in custody access disputes. *Child Abuse and Neglect, 14,* 591–593.

Kufeldt, K., Durieus, M., Nimmo, M., & McDonald, M. (1992). Providing shelter for street youth: Are we reaching those in need? *Child Abuse and Neglect, 16,* 187–199.

McCormack, A., et al. (1986). Runaway youths and sexual victimization: Gender differences in an adolescent runaway population. *Child Abuse and Neglect, 10*(3), 387–396.

Miller, A. (1983). *For your own good: Hidden cruelty in child rearing and the roots of violence.* New York: Farrar, Straus, and Giroux.

Newberger, E., & Bourne, R. (Eds.) (1985). *Unhappy families: Clinical and research perspectives on family violence.* Littleton, MA: PSG.

Powers, J., & Echenrode, J. (1988). The maltreatment of adolescents. *Child Abuse and Neglect, 12*(2), 189–200.

Strauss, S. (1986). Non-organic failure to thrive: A pediatric social illness. *Issues in Comprehensive Pediatric Nursing, 9,* 47–58.

Young, W., Sachs, R., Braun, B., & Watkins, R. (1991). Patients reporting ritual abuse in childhood: A clinical syndrome: Report of 37 cases. *Child Abuse and Neglect, 15,* 181–189.

CHAPTER • 29

Alterations in Behavior, Emotion, and Thought

RELATED TOPICS
Family health appraisals and identification of high-risk families, Chapter 2
Development of children; inborn differences in temperament, Chapter 3
Promoting Healthy Parenting, Chapter 12
Fostering Self-Esteem, Chapter 14
Stress, Crisis, and Coping, Chapter 18

LEARNING OBJECTIVES

- Identify the variables affecting psychosocial functioning.
- Describe the methods used to assess a child's mental health.
- Describe the impact the child psychiatric nurse and health providers can have in the prevention of behavioral disturbances.
- Explain the various treatment options available for the child or adolescent with alterations in behavior, thought, and emotion.
- Identify the nursing diagnostic statements frequently encountered in the care of the child or adolescent with alterations in behavior, thought, and emotion.
- Apply nursing care and treatment modalities discussed in the chapter to the care of the child or adolescent with alterations in behavior, thought, and emotion.

Many of us have heard a parent say "each of my children is so different." Individuality and uniqueness are advocated and commended in children. When individual expression of children remains within the confines of what society accepts as "normal behavior," it is met with an element of fascination and joy by family and professionals alike. However, not all children's behavior is characterized by explosions of creativity and adventure. When a child's behavior becomes maladaptive and dysfunctional, families, communities, and societies are burdened and perplexed. The complexities of how a child or adolescent becomes troubled and dysfunctional in society have created an extensive body of research and literature. This chapter discusses specific alterations that a nurse may encounter in any hospital setting, at school, or in the home. Although nurses may not be required to make independent decisions regarding the management of children with these problems, it is important to have an understanding of these alterations for appropriate assessments and referrals to be made and for working *collaboratively* with other disciplines in their therapy programs.

The genetic makeup and the experiences of each child shape the process of becoming a person. The interplay of biologic tendencies and the environmental milieu produces an individual score of vulnerability that is largely unmeasurable and unpredictable. Some difficulties that children encounter may be relatively short-lived and may cause minimal stress to the family, whereas others are enduring and cause lifelong worry, misery, or sadness to the child and to the family. The alterations included in this chapter span a wide range of problems. They have one commonality, that the child's behavior varies from that deemed adaptive by individuals and society.

Structure and Function: Alteration in Psychosocial Functioning

Alteration in a child's psychosocial functioning is generally first recognized as a behavioral alteration. These problem behaviors range on a continuum from exaggerations or deficiencies in behavior common to all children to behavior that seriously threatens the child and others. Criteria for behavior requiring intervention are presented in Table 29–1.

The problems discussed in this chapter have multiple causes. In assessing children's mental health, it is important to remember that a child's behavior is measured against the usual developmental responses characteristic of a certain age and a child's unique temperament and personality.

Variables Affecting Psychosocial Functioning

A number of variables have an impact on the child's ability to adapt successfully to society's demands. Table 29–2 summarizes these, and each is discussed in more detail.

Age and Development

An understanding of normal patterns of growth and development is needed if the health professional is to identify accurately behavioral, emotional, or thought alterations in a child (Puskar & D'Antonio, 1993). Certain behaviors that bother adults commonly occur at particular developmental stages and ages, eventually to be outgrown. Although common and appropriate at one age, the behaviors may suggest behavioral disorders at another age. For example, temper tantrums are a normal demonstration of toddlers' struggles for individuality and autonomy, but a pattern of temper tantrums in a 9-year-old is not in keeping with developmental age. Likewise, behaviors such as stuttering, phobias, and nightmares, although perplexing to parents, usually arise at certain ages and gradually disappear without any consequences. The health professional who is asked for help by parents concerned about a child's behavior must know these developmental milestones to reassure parents about a normal behavior or to initiate further assessment. (Refer to Chapters 3 through 9 for a review of developmental stage characteristics.)

Temperament

Temperament describes the way in which individuals behave or respond to their environment. (The easy, difficult, and slow-to-warm or combined temperament patterns are discussed in detail in the development chapters.) An individual's temperament is relatively consistent over time and significantly influences the spontaneity with which one adapts to new situations, the intensity with which one reacts to one's environment, and the characteristic nature of one's mood tendencies. People tend to be cheerful, positive, and optimistic or to be irritable, negative, and pessimistic in response to life situations. Children with difficult temperaments are more vulnerable to behavioral problems in early and middle childhood, with 70 per cent

TABLE 29–1
Criteria for Behavior Requiring Intervention

The behavior is to be condemned and is unacceptable regardless of how rarely it occurs (incest, intentional damage to person or property)
The behavior is not inappropriate in and of itself but is inappropriate because of its frequency, because it is exaggerated, or because of when or where it occurs
The behavior is absent or deficient in that the person rarely or never displays a behavior society deems necessary and normal (never smiles, never or rarely talks, seldom pays attention)
The behavior is a regular source of tension to the child or family members or both
The behavior is inappropriate for the person's age and stage of development, intelligence, or social situation
The behavior is compulsively enacted, appearing to "come out of the blue" without any precipitating circumstances (obscure or bizarre motivation); the child seems unable to avoid or stop the behavior even though she or he knows it is futile or that it will inevitably bring disapproval or punishment
The behavior is one of several others that together affect several areas of the child's life
The behavior brings suffering to the child and others and interferes with socialization and development

Compiled from Herbert, M. (1975). *Problems of childhood.* New York: Pan Books; Hersoo, L. (1977, June 9). Emotional disorders in childhood. *Nursing Times,* p 864; LeBow, M. (1979). *Behavior modification: A significant method in nursing practice.* Englewood Cliffs, NJ: Prentice-Hall; Levine, M., et al. (1992). *Developmental-behavioral pediatrics.* Philadelphia: WB Saunders.

demonstrating at least mild reactive behavioral alteration by age 10 years (Chess & Thomas, 1983). Carey's studies (1972) revealed that children with difficult temperaments who have disabilities or mental retardation are at even greater risk, and the difficult-temperament child with a mentally ill parent is at greatest risk for behavioral alteration. However, we emphasize that any child, regardless of temperament, is vulnerable to behavioral problems if the demands for change and adaptation are beyond his or her capabilities.

Assessing Temperament. Various methods can be used by the health professional to determine a child's temperament pattern. Questionnaires are available for the professional whose time permits. Temperament also can be determined through observation of and interaction with the child, through questions included in the health history (Ruddy-Wallace, 1987), or by questioning the child's caretakers. This assessment is pertinent from several perspectives. The assessment process is an opportunity to discuss the child's temperament with parents and to educate them regarding temperament implications in parenting approach, health management, and child care methods. Parents of the difficult or slow-to-warm child can receive reassurance that their child's behavior is characteristic for his or her temperament and not necessarily a response to their parenting style; their child is not an antisocial misfit. This discussion also affords an opportunity for preventive counseling that might alleviate future behavioral problems stemming from parent-child conflicts because the parents did not understand their child's temperament. Table 29–3 lists situations when a child's temperament should be considered by the health professional.

The demands of socialization are particularly stressful for children with difficult and, to a lesser degree, slow-to-warm temperaments because of their slow adaptability and intense negative withdrawal reactions to new situations, places, and people. The children (and later as adults) may have difficulty sleeping through the night, may have wide swings in appetite and frequent gastrointestinal complaints, and

TABLE 29–2
Variables Predisposing to Healthy Versus Altered Behavior

Variables Predisposing to Healthy Behavior	Variables Predisposing to Altered Behavior
Biologic Factors	
Easy temperament	Slow-to-warm or difficult temperament
Parents with healthy mental state	Genetically transferable mental illness in one or both parents
Physical health intact	Health erratic; or chronic illness, trauma
Normal brain function	Brain damage
Average or better intelligence	Extremely high or low intelligence
Environmental Factors	
Goodness of fit	Poorness of fit
Healthy bonding, attachment	Emotional/maternal deprivation
Parents provide role models for healthy social behavior	Parental deviance modeled
Marital/family harmony	Marital/family discord
Stable home	Unstable, broken home
Personal autonomy and self-care supported	Overprotection, dependency fostered
School success	School difficulties
Positive reinforcement predominates	Negative reinforcement predominates
Self-Concept Factors	
Intact self-concept	Vulnerable self-concept
"Good child" cognition	"Bad child" cognition

TABLE 29-3
Issues and Situations in Which Temperament May Be Significant for the Clinician

Reassurance of parents that child's deviation from culturally desirable norm does not mean pathologic change in child or bad parenting; especially true with difficult or slow-to-warm-up child
Child care advice specified in terms of child's temperament, such as approach to weaning, toilet training, and the like
Evaluation of severity of acute physical illness by estimating deviation of child's behavior from usual temperament; also, temperament may affect reaction to illness
Evaluation and management of specific symptoms such as colic, nightwaking, or "hyperactivity" as partially influenced by temperament
Child's adaptation to beginning nursery school or day care center as influenced by reactions to new situation and speed of adaptation
Ease or difficulty of child's establishment of peer relations
School functioning—optimal style of classwork and homework schedule in relation to degree of persistence and distractability
In behavior disorders, identification of influence of temperament and the specific pattern of "poorness of fit"
Special influences of temperament in the physically disabled and the mentally retarded

From Levine, M., et al. (1992). *Developmental-behavioral pediatrics*. Philadelphia: WB Saunders.

often have diarrhea or constipation. Their delay in adapting may make them less acceptable as family members and with peers, further interfering with socialization. The nurse who comes in contact with these children should keep in mind the possibility of impaired social interaction and social isolation as commonly occurring responses or related factors when formulating nursing diagnostic statements.

Goodness of Fit

How a child's attributes "fit" with those of parents, teachers, and other caretakers influences the degree of conflict and stress the child experiences in the socialization process. The phenomenon of the "problem fit" needs to be considered by the health professional (Chess et al, 1970; Chess & Thomas, 1983; Thomas & Chess, 1977, 1980). Depending on the temperaments of the parents and the child, the child develops into one described as "just like me" with goodness of fit or becomes a "problem child" with poorness of fit. It is difficult to differentiate between the child whose behavior represents a maladaptive attempt to cope with life experiences and the child whose temperament confounds the tolerance of the caretakers. A temperamentally hard-to-please child born to temperamentally hard-to-please parents portends conflict and interactional problems, whereas a temperamentally hard-to-please child born to easy-going parents may represent a joyful challenge.

A *goodness of fit* exists when the properties of a child's environment and expectations (e.g., parental demands, lifestyle, values) are in harmony with the child's own capacities, motivations, and behavioral style. Stress or conflict is not absent, but it is not excessive or continuous. *Poorness of fit* exists when discrepancies and dissonances exist between the child's characteristics and the environmental experiences. Ineffective parenting may then result. Distortions in development and maladaptive behaviors are then more likely. Some experts suggest that altered behaviors in children are the products of self-fulfilling prophecies that emerge from the parent-child conflicts resulting from poorness of fit.

Some stress and conflict foster constructive growth when in keeping with a child's developmental stage, capacity, and character. The issue in behavioral disturbances is rather one of *excessive stress* created by the poorness of fit.

Excessive Demands and Stress

Research and observation of people and animals have demonstrated that the most effective coping strategy is to engage the stressor directly. If the result is a partially or completely successful outcome or resolution, self-esteem and confidence increase, preparing one for confrontation with more stressful situations. This is the story of development and healthy living.

However, problems arise when the stressor (expectation or demand) is excessive, unrelenting, or beyond the individual's capabilities to overcome. (Overprotecting the child from normal stress can be equally detrimental.) Defensive strategies are likely to ensue, such as behavioral responses of regression, denial, or avoidance, which are attempts to cope with stressors that the individual cannot or will not confront directly (Melamud, 1992). (See Chapter 18 for a full discussion of stress and coping strategies.) These defensive strategies vary in frequency and their effect on development. Sometimes they may be employed temporarily as a stall in a healthy way to allow time to organize one's strengths and capacities for eventual positive resolution of the stressor. This behavior is common in children with slow-to-warm temperaments.

It is difficult to decide exactly when a child's behavior becomes *excessive*. Some experts suggest that any behavior lasting 3 months or more be considered long-term or excessive. It has been suggested that the behavior has reached a serious level when a consistent pattern of several deliberate behavioral alterations is seen for at least a year.

Self-Concept

Behavior is a reflection of self-concept. Self-concept is very much influenced by relationships with others. Even a well-adjusted child sometimes becomes mystified by the complexities of interrelationships. This mystification magnifies in the child whose self-concept is vulnerable. (See Chapter 14 for a discussion of self-concept development.) For example, a child who purposely breaks a toy because a sibling has just received praise from a parent is experiencing jealousy or rivalry, an angry reaction that is likely to elicit a response from the parent. Even a negative parental response is a reward, for the child is getting something (attention, consideration) in return for the behavior. The child with a vulnerable self-concept learns to use problem behavior to gain notice from others. Social interactions become highly distressful, producing intense anxiety, which results in distortion of the child's judgment of appropriate versus inappropriate behaviors. A child will "shop around" to find those behaviors that get the most responses from those whose attention is sought. The child will also use problem behavior as a strategy to dominate or manipulate people and situations over which the child otherwise feels powerless. The problem behavior, and the response it earns, reinforces the "bad me" perception of the child. A self-fulfilling prophecy is seen: "I think I'm bad—I act bad—I'm told I am bad—I must be bad." Because of this, self-esteem disturbance or chronic self-esteem disturbance is frequently seen as a response or related factor in a nursing diagnostic statement. Reinforced by this self-concept, the child becomes more and more socially ill at ease. The end result is often a lonely and estranged individual.

Interactive Model

An interplay of biologic factors and environmental forces affects the child's mental functions. Alterations of behavior, emotion, and thought may occur when these variables are influenced by precipitating events and perpetuating circumstances. Herbert (1975) has used the "loaded gun" concept to illustrate the vulnerable child: The child perceives a crisis (precipitating event). The trigger (precipitating event) only fires the already loaded (predisposing factors) gun, releasing the bullet (manifested altered behavior). Predisposing factors may exist long before their effects are seen, but they set the stage for the trigger to snap when a crisis or stressor comes along. When the crisis occurs, the behavior promptly follows. If circumstances exist to perpetuate the behavior, it will be repeated again as a coping behavior, regardless of its effectiveness or consequence. Figure 29–1 diagrams the relationship of these elements.

The health professional must recognize this interplay of variables in the assessment and identification of altered behavior, emotion, and thought. However, keep in mind that a child's developmental progress may reinforce, modify, or change specific behavior patterns. Early life experiences, although important to development, are not indicative of later behavior, nor are early behavior patterns reliable predictors of later behavior. The health professional acknowledges that there is no single cause of altered behavior patterns. An interactional approach to assessment and, later, to intervention is necessary.

Community and Family Responses

Communities, representing society at large, have handled children with altered behavior in various ways. Sometimes, the individual with behavioral problems has been socially ostracized. At other times, communities have chosen to deny the problem by segregating or isolating these persons so their existence does not have to be dealt with by the mainstream populace. More recently, communities have demonstrated empathy, acting to reform the social and legal conscience of society to provide resources and support for these persons. The greatest movement in this regard for children has been in the area of education. High as the costs for these resources may be, they are still less costly than the outcomes of neglecting the situation are likely to be.

The child can be bewildered by the reactions and responses received. Out of synchrony with peers, this child is often robbed of positive feedback and support. The unusual child's self-image may take tremendous abuse at the hands of a world he or she never made.

Differentness has its toll on the parents and family members of behaviorally altered children. The degree of impact on family members depends largely on how maladaptive they perceive the behavior to be, how much the behavior disrupts family living, and how the child is received by society (school, friends, legal institutions) (Jensen, 1991).

Other factors, unique to a particular family, may also have an impact on the family's reactions to a child's pattern of behavior. The size of the family, the health status of individual family members, the availability of support systems, and parenting style (permissive, controlling) contribute to the family's tolerance of a child's behavior (Rowe, 1992).

Diagnostic Assessment

For assessing a child's mental health, an understanding of children's behavior and how children cope is required. (See Chapter 18 for a review of childhood coping.) Whether a specific tool is used for assessment is determined by the purpose of the assessment. Assessment of the child's mental health is listed in Table 29–4. Ideally, assessment includes interviews with child and family members, observations of the child in interactions with others (particularly family members), data gathering from questionnaires or behavior check lists, and parental recordings of the child's behavior (Cromier, 1992; Scahill & Sipple, 1990).

Because a child's behavior may vary in different settings, the health professional obtains information from as many sources as possible (home, day care center, school, playground, peers' or grandparents' homes) to comprehend fully the dimensions of the

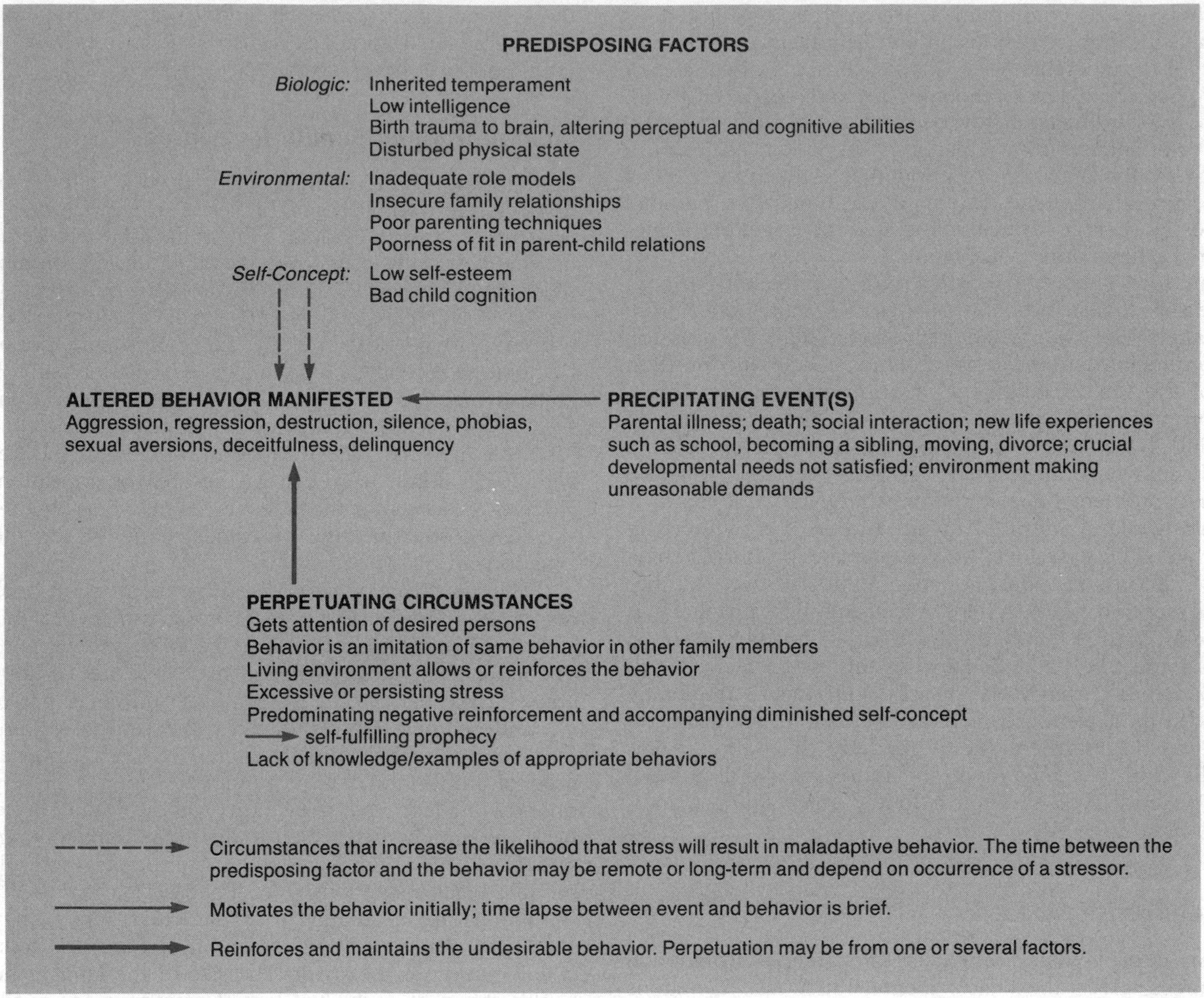
PREDISPOSING FACTORS
Biologic: Inherited temperament
Low intelligence
Birth trauma to brain, altering perceptual and cognitive abilities
Disturbed physical state
Environmental: Inadequate role models
Insecure family relationships
Poor parenting techniques
Poorness of fit in parent-child relations
Self-Concept: Low self-esteem
Bad child cognition
ALTERED BEHAVIOR MANIFESTED
Aggression, regression, destruction, silence, phobias, sexual aversions, deceitfulness, delinquency
PRECIPITATING EVENT(S)
Parental illness; death; social interaction; new life experiences such as school, becoming a sibling, moving, divorce; crucial developmental needs not satisfied; environment making unreasonable demands
PERPETUATING CIRCUMSTANCES
Gets attention of desired persons
Behavior is an imitation of same behavior in other family members
Living environment allows or reinforces the behavior
Excessive or persisting stress
Predominating negative reinforcement and accompanying diminished self-concept
self-fulfilling prophecy
Lack of knowledge/examples of appropriate behaviors
Circumstances that increase the likelihood that stress will result in maladaptive behavior. The time between the predisposing factor and the behavior may be remote or long-term and depend on occurrence of a stressor.
Motivates the behavior initially; time lapse between event and behavior is brief.
Reinforces and maintains the undesirable behavior. Perpetuation may be from one or several factors.

FIGURE 29 - 1. An interactional perspective of altered behavior causation. (Adapted from Herbert, M. [1975]. *Problems of childhood*. New York: Pan Books, Ltd.; Levine, M., et al. [1992]. *Developmental-behavioral pediatrics* [2nd ed.]. Philadelphia: WB Saunders.)

child's problem. The nurse cannot directly observe the child's behavior in all these settings; therefore, assessment relies on informant data from parents, teachers, adult significant others, siblings, peers, and other professionals who have contact with the child. When personal interviews are not possible, the telephone may be used. Also, these sources could complete a questionnaire or a behavior check list that, mailed back, could be followed by a telephone call for any clarification. At the very least, parents and, if old enough, the child should be interviewed.

During the interviews, the health professional identifies families at high risk for interactional problems. Such families may be using one child as a scapegoat to avoid facing the real issues in a situation. High-risk families usually have little or no social support, have financial difficulties, and are afflicted singly or multiply with marital instability, illness, parental depression or mental illness, or members with drug or alcohol dependencies (Hauenstein, 1992).

Just how a family contends with a behaviorally disordered child depends on the functional status of the family system itself. At the very least, the family is facing a serious threat to its equilibrium. A basically healthy family may become more closely unified because managing their "problem child" fosters improved communication and better understanding of each member's developmental needs. These are families that are not afraid to change ineffective patterns of communicating and relating. However, in many families, the effect of a "problem child" is the further disruption of family functioning (altered family processes) or even disbanding of the family unit. With assistance, these families can learn healthier coping patterns and develop constructive and supportive relationships with each other. The problem

TABLE 29-4
Components of a Mental Health Assessment

Biologic Factors

Birth History

Normal pregnancy

Complications in pregnancy or delivery

Developmental History

Milestone achievements

Feeding difficulty, sleep irregularity

Toilet training age and any difficulties

Any unusual early childhood experiences

Medical History (See Chapter 13)

Any early childhood illness, trauma, high temperatures

Any seizures or convulsions

Any severe blows to head

Any chronic illness of medical nature

Any medication taken

Temperamental History

Disposition as baby; any changes with growth

Response to new situations

Activity level of child

Environmental Factors

Early Bonding/Attachment Experiences

Primary caregiver first year of life

Involvement of each parent in infant/child care

Is child a lot "like parent" or a lot "different from parent"?

Parental attitude about this

Is child adopted; when; does child know?

Educational History

Schools attended

Was child in any special education classes?

Were any problems experienced during first year of school?

Present grade

Any grades skipped

Average grades earned

Has child ever dropped out or been expelled from school?

Any school problems

Subjects child likes, dislikes

Discipline/Parenting History

What behaviors warrant discipline?

What discipline measures are used?

Who usually administers discipline?

Child's reaction to discipline

Are siblings disciplined in same way for same thing?

In parents' families, who did the disciplining?

How were parents disciplined?

Family History

Has either parent received treatment for an emotional problem?

Has either parent a chronic illness; any siblings with chronic illness?

Any significant change in child's environment, living situation, household members

Child's response to changes in environment

Family members in home; outside home

Child living with both natural parents; if not, how long has one parent been out of the home; has that parent remarried; does child see/visit that parent?

In parents' families, were both parents present?

Where were child's parents born?

Home address; how long?

Parents' occupations

What activities are enjoyed as a family; how often?

Social History

Any change in how child spends leisure time or with whom

Does child have own room?

What behaviors prompted seeking assistance?

Does child spend more time alone or with peers?

Self-Concept Factors

Peer Relationships

Does child have friends?

What activities does child participate in with friends?

Does child prefer single play or play with peers?

Describe child's relationship with peers

Emotional Development

Has child had any losses: deaths, separation or divorce, moving?

How does child handle losses?

How does the child get attention?

Any phobias, fears, recurring nightmares; what age?

Does child experience restless sleep, nightwaking, bed wetting?

Any significant behavior change recently?

Self-Esteem Development

How does child feel about self?

What are child's strengths?

What are child's interests, hobbies?

Describe child's relationship with parents, siblings, teachers, other adults, authority figures

Compiled from Barnard, K. (1985). Studying patterns of behavior. *MCN: American Journal of Maternal Child Nursing, 54,* 358; Eyberg, S. (1985). Behavioral assessment: Methodology in pediatric psychology. *Journal of Pediatric Psychology, 2,* 123–139; Kline, K. (1986). Systematic data collection: Key to behavioral assessment in patients with behavior problems. *Perspectives, 2,* 4–6; Levine, M., et al. (1992). *Developmental-behavioral pediatrics.* Philadelphia: WB Saunders.

child may then be able to overcome or adapt to the predisposing factors that led to the maladaptive behavior (Jensen, 1991).

Therapeutic Management

Table 29–5 outlines some problem behavior patterns for which parents and teachers frequently seek help; management guidelines are included. Therapeutic management strategies employed in the care of the child and family can include any one or a combination of these treatment plans: pharmacologic methods, behavioral and operant methods, nontraditional treatments such as self-help groups, and inpatient hospitalization (Melamud, 1992). Behavioral methods include systematic desensitization, imaging procedures, relaxation training, modeling, and cognitive self-strategies (also known as stress immunization). Operant methods include techniques to extinguish the behavior or emotional response, such as continued exposure to a stimulus that evokes anxiety or fear until it disappears. In only the most serious of circumstances, as in the case of a suicidal youth, is the child or adolescent hospitalized. The usual plan of treatment for each disorder is discussed in the therapeutic management sections.

Prevention Issues

As community members and health care providers, nurses can have a significant impact on the prevention of behavioral disturbances. Many of the interventions that nurses can carry out may prevent the occurrence of the responses ineffective parenting and altered family processes. Nurses can initiate prenatal and parenting classes for parents in obstetric and pediatric clinics, in hospitals and physicians' offices, and in adult education departments of public schools. In these classes, they can discuss not only the physical effects but also the psychologic and social effects an infant may have on family life. They can help prospective parents begin to think of their unborn child as a unique individual who will have needs, feelings, and personality quirks just like they do (Hauenstein, 1992).

Nurses can intervene with parents in situations of high-risk pregnancy, in premature birth and cesarean section, and in instances of other early parent-child stress, such as the birth of a child with a physical disability. Postnatally, nurses can help parents learn and interpret their child's cues and gain positive self-esteem from their interactions. Nurses can praise parents when they observe healthy parent-child interactions. Well child examinations provide an excellent opportunity for the nurse to model and teach positive parenting techniques.

Nursing Care

Nurses often have more contact with children and their families than do other health care providers. They are therefore in key positions to identify problem behavior. The nurse is also the team member who has the greatest opportunity to intervene directly with the child and the family. Intervention is optimally aimed at two levels. The first is to assist family members, especially parents, how to change their responses to the child. The second is to help the child learn healthier coping behaviors—in particular, helping her or him unlearn self-limiting assumptions about self and the world and then to relearn what was previously misunderstood. Intervention is *individualized* to each child and family and generally requires coordination via a *multidisciplinary team*. Table 29–6 presents options for developing a characteristic multidisciplinary management program.

Perhaps the most valuable and successful approach to emphasize in working with children with behavior problems is *consistency*. A predictable, congruous approach to the child's problem behavior decreases the child's anxiety; as a consequence, the frequency and intensity of maladaptive behavior simultaneously decelerates. Consistency, coupled with praise and positive reinforcement, is critical to achieving and maintaining appropriate behavior. Neutral emotional responses from significant others when behavior is out of line are equally significant. A neutral response is calm, matter-of-fact, and confident, removing any need in the child to be defensive or offensive in response. The most challenging aspect of intervention is always to respond primarily to the child and secondarily to the behavior.

Because of parents' sense of failure and humility, one of the most difficult tasks of nurses and other team members is motivating the family to accept outside intervention. Acknowledging how difficult their situation must be, offering a no-fault suggestion that the family deserves help, and presenting tangible intervention options is often the most effective approach. Intervention is best presented in terms of possibly resolving family suffering and should capitalize on identified strengths of the child, the family members, and the family as a unit.

Specific Disorders of Behavior, Emotion, and Thought

Childhood Phobias

Fears are common to every child's experience. Children are afraid of different things at the various developmental stages, including the dark, imaginary creatures, certain animals, and natural events (storms, tornadoes) (Apter & Conoley, 1984). Most of these

TABLE 29-5

***Family-Centered Teaching:* Frequent Patterns of Disturbing Behavior and Management Guidelines**

Behavior Pattern and Characteristics	Parental Reaction/Interaction
Infantile Behavior Pattern	
Child functions below actual age; "babylike" Prone to temper tantrums, soiling, whining, crying beyond when these are age-appropriate Poor peer relations because child always wants own way, tattles on others, runs to grown ups to solve problems	Practice firm, consistent limit setting Avoid bribing or arguing with child (these are negative reinforcers that perpetuate the behavior) Ignore infantile behaviors and praise age-appropriate behaviors displayed Be supportive and kind but communicate clearly what are age-appropriate behaviors and expectations Spend positive time each day with child when he or she is not displaying infantile behavior
Excessively Shy Behavior Pattern	
Tends to stay outside a group; a "watcher" of activity Does not ask to be included in activities and avoids participation; may participate if specifically encouraged to do so Fears competition; often excels at individualized activities that are done alone Any peer friendships established are likely also to be with shy children	Approach gently Encourage initial involvement in noncompetitive group activity and, after successes, gradually introduce more competitive activities Never force group participation Praise group activity attempts Spend positive time with child daily using the time to reinforce his or her abilities
Hostile-Aggressive Behavior Pattern	
Becomes easily agitated and irritated Displays negative attitude toward almost everything May physically or mentally abuse others May be destructive to property	Requires absolute consistency in discipline and limit setting Role model appropriate management of frustration and anger Absolutely do not react with anger to child's behavior (to do so mirrors child's behavior and is a reinforcer that perpetuates the behavior) When possible, remove child from the situation before child becomes volatile Observe/supervise closely Praise attempts to handle frustrating situations and anger appropriately; spend positive time with child daily when *not* displaying the undesirable behavior
Manipulative Behavior Pattern	
Plays one person against another Often described as a "spoiled" child Capitalizes on guilt feelings and fairness values of others	Maintain absolute consistency in limit setting Remain decisive and unmoving when child attempts to persuade or change your mind about something Avoid power struggles (these are reinforcers that perpetuate the behavior) Show a caring and concerned attitude toward child without "giving in" Praise child for appropriate behavior during interaction Spend positive time with child during a time each day when child is not being manipulative
Demanding Behavior Pattern	
Wants immediate satisfaction of desires "Bossy" and insensitive to others' needs Pouts and protests vehemently when demands are not given prompt attention	Ignore demands that compete with the needs of others Praise attempts of child to wait and to consider others' needs Be patient but firm in teaching the child to wait for gratification of needs Maintain a firm position when saying no to a demand Ask if the child needs something during those times when *not* exhibiting demanding behavior; likewise, spend time with child when he or she is not making demands

TABLE 29-6
Intervention Options in a Multidisciplinary Management Program

Management Options*	Purpose
For the Child	
Psychotherapy • Based on premise that behavioral symptoms reflect unconscious conflicts and serve to reduce anxiety • Requires development of an emotional attachment by child with therapist *Health professional:* Psychiatrist, psychologist, social worker	Helps child understand psychologic conflicts and the symbolic meaning of the resulting behavior through use of symbolic play with children and dream and fantasy analysis with adolescents; deals with unconscious processes and memory, not just behavior
Behavioral Counseling *Health professional:* Psychologist, social worker, nurse with specialized psychiatric or mental health training	Provides child and family members with individual guidance and support to achieve positive changes in behavioral responses to life experiences, that is, acquiring desirable behaviors and changing undesirable behaviors
Group Therapy • Counseling sessions that involve groups of children with common behavioral symptoms, or other similar problems *Health professional:* Same as for behavioral counseling	Adds peer perspective to support for change in behavior; helps child see the effect on peers when displaying maladaptive and adaptive behaviors within a structured setting where feedback and support can be provided immediately
Behavior Management • Also called behavior modification, point system, incentive system • Applies the experience derived from principles of learning and conditioning to behavior problems • See Chapter 12 for a discussion of positive and negative reinforcement methods to achieve socialization *Health professional:* Social worker, nurse, parents, teacher	Teaches child responsibility for own behavior and effective interacting through the use of verbal and tangible incentives; focus is on correction of behavioral deficiencies, behavioral excesses, or behavioral inappropriateness
Videotherapy • May be used alone or in conjunction with group or family therapy *Health professional:* Social worker, psychologist, nurse with mental health preparation	Provides immediate feedback to child to increase self-understanding and how one affects others
Therapeutic Recreation • May be used alone or in conjunction with individual, group, or family therapy *Health professional:* Nurse, physical therapist, social worker, special education teacher, occupational therapist, recreational therapist	Develops cooperative and individual play skills relative to the child's developmental needs; meets special educational/learning needs; develops acceptable daily living skills, builds self-concept, expands problem solving skills
Relaxation Training or Desensitization • Usually used in conjunction with behavioral management *Health professional:* Nurse trained in relaxation/desensitization techniques, social worker	Inhibits undesirable responses by relaxation methods (refer to books and training guides on this subject)
Assertiveness Training *Health professional:* Nurse trained in assertiveness training techniques, social worker	Improves interpersonal relationships and related behaviors when child is a scapegoat or when child fails to stand up for own rights or cannot express feelings or thoughts in ways that respect others' rights
Self-Help Groups • Groups may use an approach similar to the 12-step concept of Alcoholics Anonymous • Tough Love is a national organization that provides assistance for the troubled child and the parents *Health professional:* Experienced parent, social workers, nurse with mental health background	Increases child's awareness of personal responsibility for behavior choices and builds external support systems for aid during periods of stress
Pediatric Psychopharmacology • Used in conjunction with other therapies sparingly and for as brief a time as possible • Psychostimulants reduce hyperactivity; hypnotics and sedatives reduce agitation; tranquilizers reduce agitation and impulsiveness *Health professional:* Physician, psychiatrist, nurse	Alleviates specific symptoms (high anxiety level, marked hyperactivity, marked apathy or withdrawal, when symptoms are so extreme that the child is unable to focus on behavior control)

TABLE 29-6
Intervention Options in a Multidisciplinary Management Program *(Continued)*

Management Options*	Purpose
For the Family—To Reinstate Child into a Healthier Family System	
Family Therapy • May be used alone or in conjunction with individual therapy *Health professional:* Psychologist, social worker, nurse with specialized mental health training	Facilitates family problem solving and reintegration of child into home that supports his or her needs in a healthy fashion; medium for reality-based interactions between child and family with professional mediation as needed
Parental Counseling • Other forms of counseling may also be indicated for individual members or the marital pair *Health professional:* Nurse, psychologist	Increases parents' role and understanding of their child's needs and behavioral management program; increases parenting skills; helps parents change their focus from organic to emotional issues
Parents and Siblings Groups *Health professional:* Experienced parents or siblings with professional resources, usually nurse or social worker	Provide support and a forum for sharing opinions, common feelings, and problems; looking at possible solutions; and increasing members' awareness and understanding of behavior disorders and their management

*The treatment plan is individualized, uses a multidisciplinary care plan that identifies methods and outcome criteria, and incorporates the child's and family's strengths.

developmental fears are transient and do not interfere with the child's daily functioning. Phobias, such as school phobia, can be debilitating. A phobia is a fear to an exaggerated degree of objects or events that in reality are not dangerous and to most people do not evoke such excessive fear (Kavanaugh & Mattson, 1987). When the fear-producing stimulus is presented, a phobic child reacts with a degree of fear that is out of proportion to the stimulus (e.g., spider, thunder, elevators). When the stimulus is not present, the child's behavior is normal.

The mechanism of how a phobia develops has been explained by various theories. The traditional psychodynamic theory proposes that an internal mental conflict (most often related to sexual and aggressive feelings) is present. Negative feelings associated with the conflict are displaced onto a specific object or event. By avoiding the specified object or event, the child's anxiety can be reduced. From the viewpoint of behaviorism, phobias develop because an originally fearful situation is repeatedly avoided. The longer the situation is avoided, the more exaggerated the fear becomes (Melamud, 1992).

Therapeutic techniques used to correct phobias vary, depending on whether the fear is based on classical conditioning or cognition (Wolpe, 1990). As Wolpe states, "Cognitively based anxiety depends on the belief that something actually harmless is dangerous, treatment depends on unlearning that belief" (1990, p 41). Classically conditioned anxiety (phobias) requires unlearning a previously learned habit of response, which can be a complex and persistent phenomenon. Confronting the patient with the phobic situation until tolerance is developed is rarely used in children (Kavanaugh & Mattson, 1987). Various forms of therapy are used: counterconditioning (use of positive images or stimuli), modeling, and cognitive behavior therapy (includes coping self-statements). Children with severe specific phobias are often referred to an appropriate therapist, such as social workers, nurse practitioners, and psychologists, for such therapies.

School Phobia

The term "school phobia" applies to a variable set of symptoms that represents an underlying anxiety in the child whose absences from school are excessive. Children suffering from severe school phobia are so immobilized that they cannot attend school, which thus results in abnormal peer relations, interrupted learning, and tremendous family stress. Hysterical, frantic behavior is manifested when any attempt is made to urge such a child to go to school. Different from the truant who does not want to go to school, the child with school phobia truly wishes to attend school but simply cannot force himself or herself to go when the hour arrives. The child who is truant does not stay at home when absent from school, whereas the child with school phobia does (Bernstein & Garfinkel, 1986).

Etiology/Incidence (Pathophysiology)

The prevalence of school phobia is difficult to estimate because many cases are handled by the school system or the child's primary health care provider, but it has been estimated to be 1.7 per cent per year (Dworkin, 1985). As teacher awareness of the problem increases, so do the number of referrals to mental health clinics. There are three peaks of frequency.

The first is at the beginning of school life when the child is between 5 and 7 years old. The second peak is between 11 and 12 years, when the child is transferred to high school; and the third peak is around 14 years (Koplewicz & Gallagher, 1992).

There are two theories about the etiology of school phobia. However, when working with school phobic children, the nurse should realize that the etiologic factors for each child may be a combination of both or part of these theories; seldom does the phobia have a single cause.

One theory held by some psychiatrists is that school phobia is basically a form of *separation anxiety* (Mansdorf & Lukens, 1987). The child is extremely fearful of leaving the home environment. In most studies, the mother is the parent the child feels closer to and is more fearful of leaving. The father has characteristically withdrawn from the situation, thus offering no or minimal support to the mother.

The parent (usually the mother) fosters a feeling of dependency in the child. The mother realizes intellectually that her child must attend school; however, her dependency on this child is so great that actually having the child separate from her is extremely difficult. Phrases like "I don't know what I'll do when you're gone" subtly reinforce the child's dependent state. It is believed that the mother has hidden hostilities toward herself of having to depend on a child and toward the child for being so dependent. In attempting to repress these unacceptable hostilities, the mother becomes overprotective of this child so that the child will not recognize these "nonmotherly" feelings. As the mother's overprotection increases, the child becomes more dependent on her and more reluctant to leave her to participate in normal activities like school.

Another theory explains why a child with normal patterns of school attendance suddenly refuses to go. Some experts believe that children with school phobia have an unrealistic view of their abilities. They overvalue themselves—think themselves capable of feats beyond their talents. For instance, they see themselves as popular, well-liked, and competent. When their peers and teachers in school do not support this view, they feel threatened and humiliated. Their self-image is damaged, perhaps to the point at which they will refuse to attend school. For these children, school becomes a difficult task because they feel constantly threatened. At home, they receive family input that reinforces their too-high opinion of themselves; at school, they feel insecure and uncomfortable. This theory would explain why a child with good school attendance later begins to find excuses to miss school and finally refuses to attend at all.

In both these theories, an unidentifiable precipitating event motivates the child's ultimate reaction to school. Such events as the birth of a sibling or unhappy experiences at school threaten the child so severely that school attendance becomes irregular, or the child may cease to attend school completely.

In considering causes for a child's refusal of school, one must remember that it could be an acquired fear, as of an object, person, or situation, such as the school setting. A child might be bullying this child, or a particular class may be too difficult. In some cases, the object of fear might not be apparent to the child or family, which may make it difficult to definitively diagnose the child as school phobic.

The theory of multicausality acknowledges that multiple factors may be involved in any given child's situation (Dworkin, 1985). A child with an unrealistically high self-image may have an overprotecting, dependent mother and additionally suffer from a particular fear.

Diagnostic Assessment

School phobia presents in the form of somatic complaints. Symptoms are varied and reflect the severity of the phobia. Abdominal pain, headaches, and general malaise are the most common symptoms; others are nausea and vomiting, anorexia, muscle aches, and occasionally a low-grade fever. The child most commonly does not complain of fear of school. Because the symptoms are so varied and nonspecific in this phobia, the primary care provider is challenged to determine the underlying issue. If a mother brings the child to the physician or nurse with the complaint of "frequent abdominal pain," an in-depth history is essential in recognizing that the primary issue is that the child does not want to go to school.

Diagnosis of the child's school phobia begins with a careful, thorough history. Clarification of statements and open-ended questions are of inestimable value. A specific area on which to concentrate is the past medical history. How much illness has the child had? How frequently did illness keep the child out of school? On careful questioning, it is often evident that the school attendance of this child has been sporadic and that somatic complaints have often been the reason. Not until the parents and child start adding up these absences do they realize their frequency.

Another phenomenon that may be apparent in assessing the child's past medical history is a pattern in the timing of symptoms. Symptoms displayed by children with school phobia are rarely seen during holidays, summer vacation, or weekends. The symptoms are most prominent Sunday evenings or on a school morning and virtually disappear by afternoon. When obtaining a history from a school-age child, the school or child psychiatric nurse always should ask the child directly about school, being alert for the attitude displayed. Information from the child regarding friends and activities at school should be obtained.

Because theories support a precipitating event in the life a child with school phobia, the nurse should pay special attention to recent life events. Such occurrences as birth of a new sibling or recent death or absence of a parent or other family member could precipitate an acute episode of school phobia. Dealing with these situations may gradually eliminate the problem of school attendance.

During the initial interview and history, the nurse should pay particular attention to the nonverbal communication taking place. How do the mother and child react to one another? Because school phobia is so intimately related to family dynamics, it is important, in obtaining the history, to have as many family members contributing as possible. In planning interventions for treatment, including all family members from the start helps ensure their commitment to participation in the management.

Because children generally present with a minor physical complaint, such as a recurrent headache or stomachache, it is important for the practitioner to perform a complete physical examination, with particular attention given to the systems involved in the "chief complaint." The physical examination is done to reassure the child and the parents that the child is physically well and to rule out an organic basis for the complaint. Simple tests, such as throat cultures or urinalysis, are sometimes performed, depending on the reason for seeking health care. Hearing and vision screening are especially important for this child because school problems are often manifestations of difficulties in hearing and vision. The nurse also evaluates parents' anxieties related to the child's blatant unhappiness, their desire to eliminate the dread of school, and their concern over how the absences will affect school work and their legal responsibility to ensure school attendance.

Therapeutic Management

These families tend to have multiple issues facing them, and long-term therapy is often the only way of managing the problems. The literature regarding school phobia generally recommends referral to a child or adolescent psychotherapist, such as psychiatrist or child nurse psychotherapist. The major goal of management is to get the child back in school as rapidly as possible. Staying home from school deprives the child of the experiences needed to mature normally. The longer the child is allowed to stay out of school, the more difficult eventual return will be.

Planning for return to school must be made cooperatively with the school, the individual child, and the family. If the plan does not include all these people, the chances of success are diminished. The plan for the child's return to school might involve a gradual return to the classroom (desensitization technique) or an immediate return to the classroom, depending on the child's ability to manage the situation (Blagg & Yule, 1989).

Nursing Care

Two fundamental considerations must be taken into account by the nurse in facilitating the plan: (1) mandatory attendance in school by law and (2) the child's capability for resuming a place in the community of peers.

As is the case in so many issues that arise in childhood, the best approach to school phobia is prevention. The nurse can assess the separation patterns that are present. As the nurse works with young families, parenting skills and communication patterns can be assessed. Anticipatory guidance and support to parents who have difficulty separating from their infant can prevent major separation problems from occurring later in the child's life. During the preschool examination, time should be spent with the family discussing feelings the parents and child have about the child's imminent school attendance.

Follow-up for guidance and support is important as the family attempts to alter long-standing patterns of behavior. The nurse is often in a position to be supportive and to help the family deal with issues that arise in school or in the family.

Enuresis

Enuresis is defined as the involuntary passage of urine by a child over the age of 3 years. It can occur during the day *(diurnal enuresis),* during the night *(nocturnal enuresis),* or at both times. A child who has never been totally continent is said to have *primary enuresis*. A child with *secondary enuresis* has experienced a period of dryness of at least 3 to 6 months after toilet training was completed (Warady et al, 1991).

Etiology/Incidence (Pathophysiology)

The prevalence of enuresis is approximately 20 per cent of 5-year-olds, 10 per cent of 6-year-olds, 7 per cent of 8-year-olds, and 3 per cent of 12-year-olds (Schmitt, 1990a). It is more prevalent in children with neurologic disorders, such as myelomeningocele (Parker & Whitehead, 1982). Enuresis occurs more frequently in boys, in children of lower socioeconomic classes, and in children of large families. Data have been reported supporting a familial tendency toward enuresis: 77 per cent of the children with two enuretic parents were enuretic, 15 per cent when neither was enuretic (Friman, 1986).

There are several theories regarding the etiology of enuresis. All or part of each one might be operating in a given child. The nurse must be aware of the possible causes of enuresis for optimal management of the problem to be offered.

The first cause that must be considered is an organic defect. There may be a physical problem or disease process present in the child. Dribbling urine may be a manifestation of an infection, diabetes, or epilepsy. There may be an anatomic abnormality of the urinary tract. In performing the physical examination, it is important to rule out all of these possible organic causes. Some investigators have reported nocturnal enuresis in children related to diet or history of food allergies, but this explanation is questionable (Granger, 1991).

There may be a psychologic cause for a child's enuresis. Some practitioners believe that the child is using enuresis to "get back" at the parents for some "unfairness." It may be a reaction to too-strict control or to the parents' unrealistically high expectations for the child's behavior and performance. Parental response to the enuresis may perpetuate this problem. Use of shaming or punishment techniques gives the child further reason for "getting even." In children with secondary enuresis having a psychologic component, a threatening event or anxiety-producing situation, such as the birth of a sibling or threatened school failure, usually precipitates the bed wetting.

There is good support for the theory that enuresis is caused by a developmental or maturational delay in the child. Some studies have shown that the child with enuresis has a smaller functional bladder capacity than that of a nonenuretic child (Schmitt, 1990b). This means some children are not physically ready for full control of urinary function at the time considered "average." Other research indicates enuresis is independent of sleep stage (Norgaard et al, 1985). They do not have adequate bladder size or sphincter control to last an entire night without voiding. Support for this theory is seen in the fact that enuresis spontaneously disappears in many children as they get older; many now believe that bladder capacity increases as the child gets older.

Diagnostic Assessment

In many instances, the enuresis has been present for months or years; therefore, it is important to know why the family has sought assistance *at this particular time*. It may be that the enuresis had not been viewed as a problem by the parents until friends or relatives began saying that the child is "not normal." Perhaps the enuresis has become a social problem for the child. "Sleeping over" at a friend's house, a popular activity, may cause the child to fear humiliation at wetting the friend's bed. Many practitioners think that enuresis should not be treated until it limits the normal activities of the child. It is believed that because so many children spontaneously stop enuresis, putting them through the regimen required to manage the problem might be more traumatic than wetting the bed.

The family history contributes to the management of enuresis. Determining that one or both parents were enuretic can help allay some of the child's concerns about the future, particularly in the area of marriage. Knowing that a parent had the same problem and was able to overcome it helps the child deal with this problem. A family history of urinary tract problems may give direction for defining the cause of this child's enuresis, suggesting that enuresis might be a symptom of an organic problem.

The past medical history of the child should be reviewed. A history of urinary tract infections may contribute to the cause of this child's enuresis. The prenatal history should be reviewed for any possible neurologic complications in the child prenatally or during birth that might contribute to incontinence. The allergic history of the child and family helps rule out allergies as the cause of enuresis. Developmental milestones should be discussed for assessing the child's progress.

Methods used by parent and child for handling enuresis are significant. Enuresis is a highly charged issue, and the nurse needs to know the attitudes and feelings of all involved. Knowledge of past attempts to deal with the problem gives important insight into management issues. *Shaming and punishing the child the next morning are of no value; in fact, these approaches are harmful.* They compound the child's existing feelings of inadequacy and "differentness" and can result in *chronic low self-esteem*. All attempts made at controlling the enuresis should be discussed, including the child's response to each attempt and the degree of success achieved with each effort.

The history should include the number of bed wetting episodes per week, the approximate amount of urine passed (at night and during the day), and the frequency with which the child urinates during the day. These facts can provide a clue as to whether the child's functional bladder capacity is small. Some practitioners feel that the enuretic child sleeps more deeply than the normal child does; depth of sleep can be assessed by inquiring about the difficulty with which the child is aroused from sleep. It is important to know whether the enuretic episodes are becoming more or less frequent and whether they can be related to any stressful event in the child's life. It should be determined whether the child has ever been continent and, if so, for how long.

Data collection should include a general physical examination with special attention to the genitourinary function. Color, stream, and odor of the urine should be assessed. Frequency, dribbling, dysuria, or hesitancy in beginning urination should be noted for ruling out organic causes. The neurologic system should be reviewed with parents and child for any abnormal behavior or activity. The child's height, weight, and weight loss should be noted; blood pressure should be checked as well as history of polydipsia or polyuria for evidence of renal disease. The abdomen should be palpated for masses or tenderness. External genitalia should be examined for any gross abnormalities. Whether the child has a history of constipation or encopresis is also important because of its association. It is difficult to achieve good bladder control without good bowel control because of the interference with bladder emptying.

Laboratory testing of urine should include a check of specific gravity and evaluation for glucose, protein, and blood. If a urinary tract infection is suspected, a urine culture should be done.

Therapeutic Management

In planning a management program, it is important to have the cooperation of the child and the parents;

otherwise, success is unlikely. The child can assume a large role in effecting cure, but parental support and reinforcement are essential. If the parents seem eager to work on the problem and the child is indifferent, positive results will not occur. This must be a joint venture. Contemporary therapies include waiting for the child to outgrow the condition, retention-control training, drug therapy, conditioning treatment, and behavior modification.

Waiting for the Child to Outgrow Bed Wetting. Many health care providers will not start a program with children of age 5 or 6 years owing to the high incidence of spontaneous resolution of enuresis in a child of this age. If the child is between 3 and 4 years of age, the health care provider should try to reduce the family's anxiety by informing them that there is no underlying kidney disorder and it is a self-limited problem. However, this period of waiting should be accompanied by the assessment and support of health care professionals for prevention of physical, social, and emotional problems that may result from the waiting approach. The potential for victimization of the child cannot be overlooked.

Retention-Control Therapy. If a small functional bladder capacity is diagnosed, efforts to enlarge the bladder may be attempted. These include having the child drink a large amount of fluids during the day and waiting to urinate until discomfort is felt at least once each day. Restriction of fluids after dinner (or after 6 P.M.) may or may not yield positive results. The child should void just before bedtime. There is some controversy as to the effectiveness of having parents wake the child to urinate when they retire. Some think this is beneficial because nocturnal urine production is highest in the early hours of sleep. Others believe that it contributes to enuresis because the child does not really wake up at this time and that it teaches the child to urinate in his or her sleep. Bladder stretching exercises have been reported to be effective in reducing enuresis by 30 per cent (Schmitt, 1990a). The procedure for these exercises is as follows: (1) have the child drink fluids and then hold the urine as long as possible, (2) measure the amount when the child voids, and (3) mark the amount on a calendar to keep track of progress.

Drug Therapy. Some physicians prescribe medication for children with enuresis. Imipramine is the drug of choice. The exact mechanism of this drug is not agreed on by practitioners. It does produce improvement in many children, but the long-term result with its use is not significantly better than in those cases that spontaneously resolve (Warady et al, 1991). In addition, the use of imipramine is not without danger to the child; neurologic side effects and overdoses are potential problems. Use of imipramine is considered inappropriate before other treatments have been employed. The two medications that are most often prescribed and that have been found most successful are imipramine hydrochloride (Tofranil) and desmopressin (DDAVP) (Warady et al, 1991).

Imipramine hydrochloride has been used for many years, and most patients will become dry if a large enough dose is given. However, side effects are relatively frequent and often lead to discontinuation of the medication. In those who become dry, the effect often wears off, and an increased dose of this drug is required (Steele, 1993). An immediate return to bed wetting is usually seen when the drug is discontinued.

Desmopressin, an intranasally administered medication, is an analogue of the antidiuretic hormone vasopressin. It is thought to work by reducing the nighttime production of urine. A decrease in both antidiuretic hormone production and nighttime volumes has been demonstrated in some enuretic children (Norgaard et al, 1991), although some children with normal nocturnal vasopressin levels have also responded to this medication. Long-term use of intranasally administered desmopressin has demonstrated persistent resolution of nocturnal enuresis in as many as 70 per cent of children. These children have been continuously maintained on the drug with minimal side effects and absence of drug tolerance (Miller et al, 1989). The cost of desmopressin can be substantial (more than $100 per month), compared with the much lower cost of imipramine hydrochloride or an alarm device. However, in many cases, the dose of desmopressin can be tapered over time or can be administered intermittently but used particularly for special occasions such as sleepovers and vacations.

Conditioning Treatment. Another method of treating children with enuresis involves use of a signal alarm device attached to the child's pajamas. An alarm goes off if the child begins to wet the bed, thus waking the child so he or she can finish urination in the toilet. In principle, this should condition the child to wake up when urination begins. When the alarm device is used for 3 to 4 months by the child with ongoing familial and professional support, the success rate reaches as high as 70 per cent (Warady et al, 1991).

Although the relapse rate may approach 25 per cent, these children usually respond to a second trial with the alarm device. Proper use of the device must be taught to the child and family. It is important that the child hear the alarm (this may take the assistance of a parent in the beginning to ensure the child awakens). Once awakened by the alarm, the child should get up, go to the bathroom, finish voiding, return to a dry bed, reset the alarm, and attach the sensor to dry pajamas. Because success with the alarm device depends on the motivation of the child, these devices are not usually recommended for children younger than 8 years of age.

Behavior Modification. Behavior modification techniques, including the principles of positive reinforcement and shaping, are also used in the treatment of enuresis. These approaches, either with or without the signal alarm devices, have been found to be more effective than use of the alarm alone (Schmitt, 1990a).

Whichever plan of treatment is chosen, the method of reinforcement is critical. None of the plans will work if the child does not receive positive reinforcement from the parents for dry nights. Special activities can be used as positive reinforcers. The reward must be meaningful to the child and must be consistently given.

Another factor to be considered is the provision of a warm, convenient place for the child to urinate. A child who must go down a long, dark hallway to the bathroom will not be likely to get up in the middle of the night to void. A warm bathroom with a night light is much more conducive to nighttime use.

Nursing Care

The management of a child with enuresis begins with a careful history. It not only serves as the principal tool with which to collect data but also offers the opportunity for the nurse to establish a caring relationship with the child and parents. This history should be obtained in a comfortable environment, with the information being given by the parents and the child. The nurse should maintain a calm, nonjudgmental attitude, supporting the strengths of the family. Many times, parents simply need to vent their feelings regarding the enuresis and to sort out the approaches they have attempted and the respective results. The nurse should emphasize the fact that the family has sought help as a positive step toward eliminating the enuresis. The history taking session itself can be an important intervention in the management of enuresis.

Both the child and parents will need ongoing support to overcome enuresis. Parents should be encouraged to share frustrations of failed or only partially successful therapies with the nurse. In this way, the nurse can help put the treatment in perspective and suggest modifications. Parents who can share frustrations with health care professionals may be less likely to vent their feelings on the child. They must be reminded that punishment is ineffective and potentially harmful to the child's developing self-concept. They should also be reminded that children with enuresis do eventually outgrow the condition, although there are groups of children that will require treatment for enuresis to be resolved.

Encopresis

The most widely accepted definition of encopresis is "persistent fecal soiling of the clothing in a child older than 4 years of age" (Ellert, 1990). In most cases, this is associated with chronic stool retention. A few children have incontinence without clear evidence of withholding. Encopresis is further differentiated into *primary encopresis,* in which bowel control has never been achieved, and *secondary encopresis,* in which the child has been continent of stool for a period of months. Fecal soiling may occur during the day as well as at night. It frequently accompanies a time of stress in the child's life (Stadtler, 1989).

Etiology/Incidence (Pathophysiology)

The incidence of encopresis is reported to be 1.5 to 3 per cent in 7- to 8-year-old children (Levine, 1975). Encopresis is seen more frequently in boys than in girls; the incidence is three to four times higher in boys than in girls (Johns, 1985). It is seen in children from disrupted families more frequently than in children with intact families.

This condition is like so many others in childhood—causes are many, and components of each theory may be involved for any given child. The role of the nurse is to identify the causal factors in each child's situation for more effectively planning a management program. For this reason, the nurse needs to be acquainted with the various etiologic theories.

Encopresis may have a *psychologic* basis arising from a variety of possible factors. For some reason, the child learns, at a very early age in some cases, to withhold stool. It could be in response to improper toilet training. Toilet training might have been started too early, or coercive tactics might have been used. Having a bowel movement may be uncomfortable to the child because of a fear of the toilet or of being left alone in the bathroom. Some deep-seated emotional problem is usually present with encopresis. Two characteristics of the young child's temperament may predispose the child to constipation: intensity and irregularity (Stadtler, 1989).

Some data indicate that there may be a *genetic cause of or predisposition to* encopresis. It is believed that children with encopresis absorb more water from the fecal mass as it passes through the colon; thus, the mass is more difficult to expel. This theory might explain why constipation is present in these children from infancy.

Encopresis may have an *organic* basis. A neurologic problem or anatomic abnormality might cause fecal soiling and constipation. The child may have internal or external anal lesions that cause pain during the passage of stool.

Diagnostic Assessment

When a child has reached school age, bowel patterns are no longer obvious to the parents. Therefore, parents may not be aware that the child is constipated; but parents are aware when fecal soiling occurs. The initial obvious conclusion of the parent is that the child has diarrhea. This complaint of diarrhea is sometimes the reason that health care is sought by a family. Other symptoms that may or may not be present are abdominal cramping, nausea, vomiting, malaise, poor appetite, and large, painful stools (Molitor, 1985).

Constipation is associated with increased incidence of urinary tract infections or vesicoureteral reflux. Many parents approach the health professional not because of diarrhea or constipation concerns but because of the frustration and embarrassment the soiling causes and the ambivalent feelings it is creating in them and the child's peers toward the child.

A physical examination is conducted, with special attention paid to neurologic aspects. By eliciting a normal anal "wink" (response to a pinprick to the anus), one can assess the neurologic status of the anus. The abdomen may be mildly distended as flatus is passed normally (Ellert, 1990). On palpation, fecal material distending the colon is noted, especially over the descending and sigmoid colon. Bowel sounds may be normal or slightly diminished. Fecal material can usually be seen around the anus. Digital examination of the rectum reveals stool (large amount) just inside the internal sphincter (Ellert, 1990).

Therapeutic Management

Once the diagnosis of encopresis has been confirmed by history and physical examination, a management program is set up. Simple and specific explanation of the problem is the first step. Various diagrams can be drawn for explaining the problem to the child and family.

The first goal of the program is to clear the impaction if it exists. The child usually has a large amount of stool distending the lower colon. Hypertonic phosphate enemas (3 ml/kg) are given on varying schedules until the impaction is removed. In most cases, this can be done over a 10-day to 2-week period (Levine, 1987). It may be done at home or in the hospital, depending on the family and the protocol being used. After the initial catharsis, a maintenance program is instituted.

Next, an oral laxative is started, and 2 tablespoons of mineral oil a day are given (refrigerated and mixed in fruit juice). Mineral oil is given between meals to minimize effects on absorption of fat-soluble vitamins. The child is gradually weaned from mineral oil for up to 6 months beyond the last painful stools and until the child has lost the fear of stooling (Fitzgerald, 1987). A program of regular elimination patterns is also established. The child is expected to sit on the toilet for a specific amount of time at regular times during the day (usually twice a day for 10 minutes each time). There should be proper foot support for the child—the feet should be at an angle whereby pushing can be comfortably done. A diet high in residue and low in milk is started; fluids are encouraged. Exercise is promoted to increase peristalsis, which also promotes elimination of stool.

If the child is doing well by 6 weeks, the oral laxative can be tapered off, but the mineral oil is continued. The child and parents are forewarned that small amounts of colorless to orange-colored mineral oil may leak into the underpants. Leakage of brown-colored mineral oil suggests another impaction requiring an enema. In most programs, a normal bowel pattern is established by 6 months. Failures in management of encopresis are most often due to failure or inability of families to follow the treatment plan. Giving an aura of hope to these children and involving families in the management are ways in which the nurse can motivate compliance. Follow-up every 6 weeks for the next 6 months is usually required (Levine, 1987).

Nursing Care

The diagnosis of encopresis and constipation begins with a careful, thorough history. This history should assess the child's daily habits and the psychosocial milieu of the family. Information about family dynamics is necessary to identify causative factors and to plan successful interventions. Parenting methods are assessed. The primary person responsible for the care of the child is identified—the mother or father, a sibling, or a baby sitter—because of the important role the primary caregiver has in the management of this condition. While obtaining the history, the nurse observes the child's interactions with the parents to assess the health of the parent-child relationship.

The history of toilet training is obtained. The child's age at which bowel continence was achieved (if ever) and the approach used are important to assess. Inconsistent or coercive means of inducing bowel control as well as beginning at too young an age have been shown to contribute to the development of encopresis.

Amount and frequency of stools should be noted, with clear descriptions. The terms "diarrhea" and "constipation" should be clearly defined, ensuring that the nurse's and parent's use of the terms are clear to both parties. If constipation has been present, the nurse will want to determine how this constipation has been treated and with what results. The issue of fecal soiling is discussed, with attention given to how it has been treated at home and with what results. Some practitioners believe that parents who actively intervene when their child soils are reinforcing the encopretic activity because the child finds satisfaction in the attention.

The goal of the program is to provide a medication, diet, and toileting ritual that encourages the child to develop normal defecation habits (Ellert, 1990). The parents and other family members will be affected by this treatment program. It may mean a diet change if they ordinarily do not eat a high-fiber diet and an exercise program for the whole family. The nurse can play a key role in ensuring the success of the program by continually instructing and reinforcing the toileting program. Shame and ridicule from family members will threaten a successful outcome.

All family members (including siblings) should be

involved in the management of encopresis. Family therapy may be warranted in some cases. Knowing the family dynamics and community resources can aid the nurse in deciding whether to refer the family for counseling.

Prevention is the key to encopresis. The nurse working with families with young children should always carefully review elimination patterns with parents. Anticipatory guidance should be given regarding toilet training (see discussion of toilet training in Chapter 6).

Attention Deficit Hyperactivity Disorder

In the past, a wide variety of terms have been used to describe attention deficit hyperactivity disorder (ADHD), including minimal brain dysfunction, hyperactive child syndrome, minimal brain damage, and minor cerebral dysfunction. Since 1980, the American Psychiatric Association has indicated that ADHD is a more appropriate term because attentional difficulties are prominent and almost always present. The onset of ADHD is before the age of 7 years. Estimates of the presence of ADHD range from 1.2 to 20 per cent of all school-age children. The syndrome occurs more often in boys than in girls and is more frequent in upper middle class families (Shaywitz & Shaywitz, 1988). ADHD was previously thought to disappear during puberty; however, more recent data suggest that ADHD persists in approximately 30 per cent of young adults diagnosed before adolescence (Gittleman, 1985). Although the hyperactivity component usually improves during adolescence, signs and symptoms of ADHD seen in adolescents are academic failure, poor peer relationships, low self-esteem, and acting-out behavior (Cromier et al, 1992). The disorder has not been identified in developing countries.

Etiology/Incidence (Pathophysiology)

The exact cause of the syndrome is unknown. In many cases, a family history reveals a possible genetic component. Often, one of the parents may have experienced some learning difficulties or hyperactivity as a child. When there is no evidence of a genetic component, the health history may reveal possible brain damage during an early developmental period. Children who were born prematurely or who suffered apnea at birth have an increased risk for ADHD (Shaywitz & Shaywitz, 1988).

Little is understood about the functions of the brain with this syndrome. Studies of the brain have identified an area called the "reticular activating system" that helps control attention (Guyton, 1991). This reticular system allows people to block out other stimuli, such as conversations, and to pay attention. A deficit of the neurochemicals active in this system can result in malfunctioning of the reticular system. Amphetamines increase the neurochemicals that are thought to be lacking in the brain of children with ADHD. This response serves as the rationale for medication therapy for these youngsters.

Clinical Manifestations

In school, the child with ADHD does not stay at tasks, has difficulty organizing and completing work, is sloppy and impulsive, and often gives the impression of not having heard or not listening when someone speaks. Group situations are especially difficult when sustained attention is required. At home, the parents note that their child does not follow through on requests and instructions and is unable to stick to activities, including play, for periods of time appropriate to age. Associated features vary with age and include obstinacy, stubbornness, negativism, bossiness, bullying, increased mood lability, low frustration tolerance, temper outbursts, low self-esteem, and lack of response to discipline. Hyperactivity in the young child is evidenced by gross motor activity, such as excessive running or climbing and being constantly on the go. The older child and adolescent may be extremely restless and fidgety. The child's behavior tends to be haphazard, poorly organized, and not goal-directed. Symptoms typically vary with the situation. For example, the child may be well organized and act appropriately on a one-to-one basis but not in a group situation or in the classroom; or adjustment may be satisfactory at home but poor at school. It is rare for the child to display signs of disorder in all settings at all times.

In some children, nonlocalized "soft" neurologic signs, motor-perceptual dysfunction (e.g., poor eye-hand coordination), and electroencephalographic abnormalities may be present. Soft signs are subtle; for example, the child may have difficulty distinguishing between the left and the right hand or may have trouble standing on one foot without falling. The children are often regarded as "clumsy" by their parents. Only about 5 per cent of the children with ADHD have an associated diagnosable neurologic disorder. Although the onset of ADHD is typically before 3 years of age, it is often not brought to the attention of a professional until the child enters school. The peak age range for referral is 8 to 10 years.

Diagnostic Assessment

The essential features of ADHD are signs of inattention, impulsivity, and hyperactivity that are developmentally inappropriate (Shaywitz & Shaywitz, 1988). For adolescents with ADHD residual deficit, excess motor activity frequently diminishes; however, attention difficulties remain. Diagnostic criteria for ADHD are listed in Table 29–7 (American Psychiatric Association, 1987).

Therapeutic Management

Early diagnosis of ADHD is important for avoiding some of the long-lasting psychologic effects this dis-

TABLE 29-7
Diagnostic Criteria for Attention Deficit Hyperactivity Disorder

When using this tool, consider a criterion met only if the behavior is considerably more frequent than that of most people of the same mental age.

A disturbance of at least 6 months, during which at least 8 of the following are present:

- Often fidgets with hands or feet or squirms in seat (in adolescents, may be limited to subjective feelings of restlessness)
- Has difficulty remaining seated when required to do so
- Is easily distracted by extraneous stimuli
- Has difficulty awaiting turn in games or group situations
- Often blurts out answers to questions before they have been completed
- Has difficulty following through on instructions from others (not due to oppositional behavior or failure of comprehension); e.g., fails to finish chores
- Has difficulty sustaining attention in tasks or play activities
- Often shifts from one uncompleted activity to another
- Has difficulty playing quietly
- Often talks excessively
- Often interrupts or intrudes on others; e.g., butts into other children's games
- Often does not seem to listen to what is being said to him or her
- Often loses things necessary for tasks or activities at school or at home (toys, pencils, books, assignments)
- Often engages in physically dangerous activities without considering possible consequences (not for the purpose of thrill-seeking); e.g., runs into street without looking

Note: The above items are listed in descending order of discriminating power based on data from a national field trial of the DSM-III-R criteria for disruptive behavior disorders.

- Onset before the age of 7 years
- Does not meet the criteria for a pervasive developmental disorder

Criteria for Severity of Attention Deficit Hyperactivity Disorder

Mild: Few, if any, symptoms in excess of those required to make the diagnosis **and** only minimal or no impairment in school and social functioning

Moderate: Symptoms or functional impairment intermediate between mild and severe

Severe: Many symptoms in excess of those required to make the diagnosis **and** significant and pervasive impairment in functioning at home and school and with peers

From American Psychiatric Association: *Diagnostic and statistical manual of mental disorders, third edition, revised.* Washington, DC: American Psychiatric Association, 1987.

order may have on a child. Treatment of the syndrome requires a team approach. A combination of medication, behavior modification, and a special education program is usually needed to treat these children. Alterations in diet have received popular support but little support from the scientific community.

Medication Therapy. Stimulant medications are still the treatment of choice for children with ADHD. They are used to help the child respond appropriately in everyday academic and social settings. The commonly used drugs are methlyphenidate (Ritalin), dextroamphetamine sulfate (Dexedrine), and amphetamine sulfate (Benzedrine). Although these drugs are often referred to on the street as "speed" or "uppers" and may be taken for their euphoric effect, they do not affect the child with ADHD in the same way. They are used to enable children with ADHD to control their impulses and to improve their attention spans.

It is estimated that medication-related improvement occurs in approximately 75 per cent of children with stimulation therapy (Woolack et al, 1991). Studies using teacher ratings have shown an improvement in behavior and attention span of children who are taking medication. These children also performed better on visual-motor tasks, such as penmanship. Some studies have noted that as the dose increased, the children became quieter; however, their academic performance also declined. The child should be monitored by a physician so that the smallest effective dose can be used (Stevenson & Wolraich, 1989).

Behavior Modification. Treatment strategies that combine medication with nondrug interventions are recommended. It is believed the most promising treatment is a combination of various forms of behavior modification and cognitive-behavioral approaches. Approaches that include contingent rewards, especially as components of token economy, or behavioral contracting programs run by highly trained parents or teachers have proved effective. Also effective are cognitive programs that teach children self-instructional and self-reinforcement skills that they can use to guide their own behavior and systematically monitor their own progress. Some programs include metacognitive training that is designed to teach children how to analyze the components and demands of a given task, to generate appropriate problem solving strategies, and to assess and modify their performance as necessary. Cognitive-behavioral approaches encourage children to become active agents in their own treatment programs; they teach "portable" coping strategies that the child can take from situation to situation without having to rely on external agents (parents, teachers, or pills). The initial results have been dramatic, but the field is still relatively new, and little is known about which techniques are best for which situations.

Nursing Diagnostic Statements and Collaborative Problems for the Child with Attention Deficit Hyperactivity Disorder

Three problem responses, which also affect the child's family, are frequently seen in the child with ADHD. Because the related factors (or etiologies) of the first problematic response cannot be *independently* changed by the nurse, this is considered a collaborative problem.

- ***Ineffective individual coping,*** *related to the child's impulsivity, lack of attention, or hyperactivity.*

- ***High risk for altered family processes;*** *risk factor: the stresses of the child's behavior on the family.*
- ***High risk for self-esteem problems;*** *risk factor: the child's inability to meet expectations at home and in school.*

Nursing Care

Improving Coping by Relieving Impulsivity/Hyperactivity. Children on medication therapy should be monitored for side effects. This task frequently becomes the responsibility of the school nurse. The nurse should be aware of possible side effects of loss of appetite and insomnia that are common if the medication is taken before meals or within 3 hours of bedtime. Stimulant medication is often prescribed to be taken in the morning or early afternoon because of the potential interference with sleep. Some children may experience stomach cramps, restlessness, or irritability. Other problems with these drugs include the risk of long-term side effects, such as suppressed growth rate or altered effects on psychosocial functioning and self-perceptions because they can undermine self-concept. Sometimes children look on their medication as "magic pills." It is important that this attitude not be tolerated and that children learn to take responsibility for their behavior.

Improving Family Functioning by Relieving Stress. Parents of these children often harbor feelings of guilt, anger, and frustration. They will need help dealing with these normal feelings. The nurse working with the family may be able to provide the support and counseling the family needs or may need to refer the family to other health professionals for these services. Referral should be made to self-help groups, such as the Association for Children with Learning Disabilities.

Preventing Self-Esteem Problems by Assisting the Child to Meet Expectations. Consistent management and a structured environment are vital for the child. The home and school environment should be adjusted to provide minimal external stimuli. Regular routines should be established for eating, sleeping, and doing school work. Situations that cause excitement, overstimulation, and fatigue should be avoided. In giving instructions or assigning tasks at school or at home, directions should be given one at a time, and the work should be divided into small parts.

Conduct Disorders

Conduct disorder is classified by the American Psychiatric Association (1987) as a subtype of attention disorder. Children may have an attention deficit disorder with or without a conduct disorder.

"Conduct disorder" is described as disturbance of conduct lasting at least 6 months, during which at least three of the following behaviors have been present.

1. Has stolen without confrontation of a victim on more than one occasion (including forgery).
2. Has run away from home overnight at least twice while living in parental or parental surrogate home (or once without returning).
3. Often lies (other than to avoid physical or sexual abuse).
4. Has deliberately engaged in setting fires.
5. Is often truant from school (for older person, absent from work).
6. Has broken into someone else's house, building, or car.
7. Has deliberately destroyed others' property (other than by fire setting).
8. Has been physically cruel to animals.
9. Has forced someone into sexual activity with him or her.
10. Has used a weapon in more than one fight.
11. Often initiates physical fights.
12. Has stolen with confrontation of a victim (e.g., mugging, purse snatching, extortion, armed robbery).
13. Has been physically cruel to people.

Contrary to the adage that a child will "outgrow" behavioral problems, studies indicate that conduct disorder at 6 years of age is a strong predictor for such a disorder at 13 or 14 years of age. Furthermore, antisocial personality in adults is strongly associated with conduct disorders in childhood (Forehand & Wells, 1987). Common manifestations of conduct disorders are lying, stealing, cheating, and aggressive behaviors.

Etiology/Incidence (Pathophysiology)

Conduct disorders are more prevalent in boys than in girls in a ratio of 3 : 1, and patients with these conditions comprise the largest group of psychiatrically disturbed children, with estimates varying from 47 to 67 per cent (Forehand & Wells, 1987). Conduct disorders in boys more than double in adolescence (Jensen, 1991). In the general population, conduct disorders have been reported to be as high as 4 per cent.

The etiology of conduct disorders is unclear. It is believed that a constitutional or organic basis exists for the behavior of these children (Wells & Forehand, 1985). Certain environmental processes are also thought to be contributing factors. Experts have suggested a "coercion hypothesis" to account for the family dynamics that contribute to conduct disorders in children. The coercive control strategies of the child, such as crying, tantrums, and screaming, are reinforced by the parent, and the parent, in turn, uses coercive tactics to control the child. Repeated coercive exchanges eventually result in disruption of all family members, with parents and child feeling depressed and anxious and lacking self-esteem.

Diagnostic Assessment

The 13 diagnostic criteria of the American Psychiatric Association for conduct disorder are presented earlier in this preceding section. The child must have at least 3 of these behaviors for at least 6 months to be classified as having a conduct disorder. However, these behaviors are often seen on a continuum, and the alert nurse will assist in their early identification (Harnett, 1989). This early identification is crucial for helping the family manage child behaviors effectively before coercive behavior patterns within the family become habitual. A discussion of these behaviors follows.

Lying. "Lying" is defined as a deliberate attempt to deceive others. Lying occurs at all ages. When parents, teachers, or others bring such a concern to a health professional, an attempt is made to discover whether such behavior constitutes a problem serious enough for professional intervention to be required.

Parents sometimes report that their young child tells lies, failing to understand that, at this developmental age, it is difficult for the child to separate reality from fantasy. Most older children tell occasional lies, especially to escape punishment. If the child lies frequently or deliberately lies about serious matters, an attempt is made to determine the motivation for such behavior.

Stealing. A certain amount of stealing is normal in children. Young children are curious about everything around them. They love to collect things and are particularly attracted to and may "borrow" brightly colored, interesting objects. School-age children are developing a superego. Although they are learning right from wrong and "mine" from "theirs," these concepts are not fully internalized. Therefore, temptations are not always resisted; if a child sees something desirable, she or he sometimes takes it.

In the adolescent, stealing is a more serious concern. Some adolescents are challenged to swipe candy bars or other items of small value from stores, school lunchrooms, and so on as a method of proving daring or of conforming to peer norms. When stealing occurs in older children, becomes frequent, or involves items of value, it indicates asocial behavior and is of concern. Stealing is a particularly disturbing problem to parents.

Cheating. Cheating is commonly seen in the early school-age years. At age 5 or 6 years, the child may not have a clear understanding of the rules of a game or activity. The child may have an extremely competitive spirit, to the extent that cheating at a particular game is more tolerable than losing. The developing superego, coupled with an inability to fully understand rules, often results in cheating behavior. It is usually of a benign, innocent nature and will disappear as the child matures. If cheating should persist and influence school or social performance, the parent or school authorities may seek help for the child. Cheating also occurs when children feel they cannot perform adequately on their own and attempt to please parents, teachers, or peers.

Aggression. "Aggression" is defined as a pattern of intentional behavior designed to produce harm to others. As a personality trait, aggressiveness is not necessarily undesirable. If channeled into socially acceptable outlets, it may serve as a positive force helping an individual become an assertive, competitive member of society. In the American culture, high value is placed on "rugged individualism." However, when aggression becomes disruptive to the community, the family, or the individual's lifestyle, aggressiveness may be seen as a behavior problem.

Child development research has identified a number of factors in aggressive behavior. A child's aggressive behavior is thought to have many causes, including genetically assigned instinctual survival responses, biologic factors such as hormone levels, and acquired response patterns to environmental stimuli (Sims & Galvin, 1990). Aggressive behavior problems are much more common in boys than in girls. Five times as many male as female adolescents are arrested for violent crimes. Expression of aggression varies with the developmental age of the child. Physical aggression, for example, may be inhibited in favor of a verbal expression of rage in older children with a higher level of cognitive functioning.

The overly aggressive child can be disruptive to family or school, causing parents anxiety as they try to cope with outbursts of anger. The behavior may cause discord with adult caregivers and peers, eventually causing the child to become isolated from friends or involved in acts outside the legal limits of the community. Parents have several options: they may permit certain behaviors, attempt to change the aggressive behavior, tolerate certain behaviors for the time being but not actually accept them, or use anticipatory planning to avoid situations that elicit the child's aggressive behavior.

Nursing Care

Lying. Several factors need to be considered in making an evaluation: the developmental stage and age of the child, the duration and frequency of the behavior, and whether there is actual intent to distort the truth. When the reason for a child's lies has been determined, proper therapy can be initiated. Depending on the clinical expertise of the nurse, the child and parents may be referred to a mental health worker. Excessive lying is often symptomatic of a deeper pathologic family process and is appropriately referred by the nurse, who will want to follow the child's progress by communicating with the mental health counselor.

If the nurse has the clinical expertise to manage this issue, a problem solving session with parents and the child might facilitate resolution. Helping the family look at communication among its members, motivation behind the child's lies, and some possible interventions may be the best approach for overcoming the problem. Parents will frequently identify behaviors that might have caused the child to lie. For example, discipline measures that are too strict may force a child into lying. Supporting the parents as they begin intervening to eliminate the child's lying may be the nurse's primary role.

Prevention of a child's lying is the first defense. Parenting that promotes open communication and realistic expectations of children is encouraged by the nurse during well child visits. (See Chapter 12 for a discussion of healthy parenting.)

Stealing. To intervene effectively with children who steal, the nurse must determine the reasons for the stealing. The reason is not likely to be discovered until a mutually trusting relationship is established between the nurse, the child, and the parents. Family dynamics may have to be explored and the cause identified. This complex issue may be resolved optimally by referring the child and family to a mental health clinic. Depending on the severity and the outcome of the stealing episodes, legal authorities may be included in the management of this problem.

The nurse with clinical expertise may work with this family regarding the issue of stealing. Suggestions from the parents about how comfortable they are in handling this problem and the intervention options that are acceptable to them should be considered first. To prevent further episodes of stealing, the parents are encouraged to handle the situation. By clearly demonstrating to the child that stealing is wrong and unacceptable behavior and will not be tolerated, further stealing may be prevented.

Parents can also help their child stop stealing by removing tempting items. Loose change should be out of sight. Pens and pencils should be in drawers, except for the items that belong to the child. By removing "stealable" items, the parents can reduce the internal conflict experienced by a child who steals.

Aggression. The nurse may become involved with families experiencing difficulties in handling aggressive acting-out behaviors. It is important for the nurse to assess the child's behavior fully in the context in which it occurs. Observation of actual parent-child interactions can give clues to incongruent communication of parental expectations. If possible, parents can keep a diary of prosocial and antisocial child behaviors to examine precipitating factors as well as to describe the aggressive act. Specific strategies for modifying aggressive behavior naturally vary with the age of the child and the degree of aggression.

Nurses can counsel parents in child management techniques, such as the need to set consistent limits, to show affection, to reward with expressions of approval for social acts, and to assist in verbalization of frustration and anger. In discussing discipline practices, the nurse can explore use of "time-outs" instead of physical punishment, use of advance warning about consequences when parental tolerance limits are about to be breeched, and immediate discussion of both the child's and the parents' perception of what happened and what precipitated an incident. A parenting style characterized by high control and coercive actions is discouraged.

Alterations Associated with Nutritional Conflicts

Nutritional conflicts can lead to a number of disorders, including obesity, anorexia nervosa, and bulimia. Prevention of obesity in infancy is discussed in Chapter 16. This section discusses the assessment and treatment of children and adolescents with obesity, anorexia nervosa, and bulimia and strategies for prevention at various stages of development. Obesity may occur at any stage of development; anorexia nervosa and bulimia usually begin in adolescence, occur predominantly in girls, and are accompanied by mood shifts and altered thought processes.

Obesity in Children and Adolescents

"Obesity" is defined as an excess of fat in ratio to lean body mass (Behrman, 1992). The diagnosis is made when weight for height is greater than the 95th percentile, skinfold thickness is greater than the 95th percentile, and the individual appears obese. "Overweight" is the term generally used to describe weight that is above average for height and age (Hammer, 1990).

Etiology/Incidence (Pathophysiology)

Obesity is a complex disorder affecting health and body image. The etiology is controversial, but current research and epidemiology suggest that both physical and environmental factors are contributory. The rate of prevalence for obesity has increased to greater than 20 per cent for boys and girls between 6 and 17 years of age (Dietz & Gortmaker, 1985). The risk of obesity is higher for children who have obese parents than for those whose parents are lean. If one parent is obese, a child has a 40 per cent chance of becoming obese; if two parents are obese, the risk rises to 80 per cent (Wilson, 1987).

A number of demographic variables have been associated with increasing the risk of obesity in children. These variables include socioeconomic status, sex of the child, birth order, birthweight, type of feeding (breast or bottle), body mass of mother, marital status of mother, presence of man in household, and person responsible for child's diet (Sherman & Alexander, 1990). Research findings suggest an increased incidence of obesity in children from lower socioeconomic strata (Golden et al, 1983; Woolston, 1987). Mothers of obese children were found to have significantly greater body mass index than that of mothers of nonobese children. A trend toward obesity was found in children who had more than one caretaker responsible for food intake (Blank & Alexander, 1988). Obese children are at risk for remaining obese throughout their lives (Sherman & Alexander, 1990).

Many theories exist about the cause of obesity, yet there are no certain answers. Bottlefeeding and early introduction of solid foods have been implicated as causes of obesity (Castiglia, 1987; Wishon & Kinnick, 1986). More recently that correlation has been challenged. See Chapter 16 for further discussion of infant obesity and infant feeding practices.

One theory is that there is a sensitive period for replication of fat cells and that obese children have an increased number and size of adipose cells (Knittle et al, 1979), which is then set for life (Brook, 1972). This theory has been challenged, and there is still much to learn about its significance in the cause and persistence of obesity. Studies of metabolic rate and regulation of energy storage do not provide irrefutable answers either. Physiologic variables may play a role in predisposition to obesity rather than causing it (Dietz, 1983).

Inactivity has been cited as a causal factor in obesity, with a cyclic pattern of inactivity, obesity, tiredness during activity, avoidance of activity, poor physical condition, and weight gain (Hammer, 1990). When activity was converted into actual energy expenditure, researchers found that obese boys did not expend less energy than lean control subjects did. It is pertinent in this study that obese boys ate much more and faster than did nonobese control subjects and that mothers served more food to their obese sons than to lean sons of close age (Waxman & Stunkard, 1980).

Many variables must be considered, most notably family variables. Obesity tends to run in families, and the risk of obesity increases as the number of obese members in the family increases (Castiglia, 1987; Woolston, 1987). This seems to indicate a genetic cause, but the tendency also exists for families with adopted children and for spouses (Kinston et al, 1987). Family correlates are strong but not explained by genetics. The epidemiology implies that conditions within the family system influence the development of obesity (Blank & Alexander, 1988).

The set-point (or *appestat*) theory proposes that there is a control system in each individual that keeps body weight at a relatively stable level. The level, or set-point, is maintained through metabolism; that is, when excess calories are taken in, the metabolic rate increases to burn the excess, and, when calories are restricted, metabolism decreases. This theory explains why it is difficult for a thin person to gain weight and an obese person to lose weight. A contributing factor worth mentioning is television, which perpetuates inactivity and the consumption of empty calories (Dietz & Gortmaker, 1985). With present knowledge, it cannot be determined why some children take in more energy or expend less than others. It is prudent to consider both physiologic and environmental variables in childhood obesity.

Diagnostic Assessment

The child's weight for height is greater than the 95th percentile, skinfold thickness is greater than the 95th percentile, and the individual appears obese. Obesity is the primary cause of hypertension, diabetes, and cardiovascular disease; orthopedic and respiratory conditions may be consequences of or aggravated by obesity (Hammer, 1990). Children's physical fitness is compromised because of obesity, and it often leads to feelings of inferiority and negative self images (Sherman & Alexander, 1990). During adolescence, there is a susceptibility to poor body image and feelings of being different from peers. The stress of normal changes can be compounded by obesity, especially puberty-onset obesity (Shestowsky, 1983). Whether poor self-concept is a precursor or a consequence of obesity remains unanswered.

A nutritional history should be performed (see Chapter 16), with particular attention being given to a child and family interactions associated with food, including:

- How is food used in the home?
- Are there rules associated with mealtime and amount of food intake?
- What attempts have been made to correct obesity?
- Are there family conflicts associated with food intake?
- Are the child and the family motivated to correct the problem of obesity?
- Does the child eat while watching television?

Other information included in the nutritional history is:

- The child's weight history.
- How did the child gain the weight? Did the child gain weight by eating more at meals? By eating higher-calorie foods? By decreasing activity level?
- How is the child maintaining weight? Is the child continuing to overeat? Is the child decreasing the activity level?

Direct observation of the child at meals provides clinical insight. Behaviors that indicate disrupted or poor eating patterns are:

- Child is eating at a rapid rate of speed.
- Child limits fluid intake at meals, possibly not drinking at all or not drinking until after eating.
- Child consistently chooses higher-calorie entrees.
- Child eats higher-calorie food first.

The major reasons for nutritional assessment are (1) to identify dietary practices of the family, (2) to obtain baseline data of calorie and nutrient intake and anthropometric measurements, (3) to promote healthful dietary practices through counseling and teaching, and (4) to provide parents with the opportunity to express concerns and ask questions about nutrition and feeding behaviors. (See Chapter 16 for discussion of performing a nutritional assessment.)

When obesity is a problem, the assessment focuses on factors that might contribute to the problem. Consideration must be given to the possibility of an underlying disease. Obesity may be part of a central nervous system disorder (trauma, tumor), an endocrine disorder (hypothyroidism, Cushing syndrome), a chromosomal abnormality (Klinefelter or Turner syndrome), or a congenital disorder such as Prader-Willi syndrome (Wilson, 1987). These factors need to be ruled out first.

Therapeutic Management

Obesity is managed according to the child's developmental stage. A growing infant or child has nutritional needs different from those of an adolescent. The problems faced at the various ages are also different because of the issue of control. Who controls what the child eats becomes an important question to consider in management.

Infant and Child. Infant obesity is managed primarily through preventive strategies and is discussed in Chapter 16. Encouragement of breastfeeding and teaching appropriate bottlefeeding and the adding of solid foods are the major areas of intervention.

For the *child* who is obese, family involvement is also essential. When obesity is seen as a family problem, it is less likely for any one person to feel ultimately responsible for the obesity and its treatment. The child will not have the burden of guilt; thus, further harm to self-esteem is prevented. Areas that the nurse would explore include:

- What are the parental boundaries related to the developmental emotional stage of the child?
- What role does the child have within the family?
- Is the child viewed as the "identified problem" or the "sick person" in the family?
- What would change within the family structure if the identified family member becomes well?

Family involvement decreases the likelihood that the child will be used as a scapegoat for other family disturbances. Thus, promotion of family involvement is an important intervention when *high risk for altered parenting* and *high risk for altered family processes* are diagnosed. Counseling regarding discipline is necessary if the related factor (etiology) is that the parents have difficulty setting limits. Implementing treatment plans will be difficult if a child is in control of the family. Unless the family and youngster are motivated to lose weight, weight loss is not likely to occur. Nurses need to motivate them to accomplish the loss.

Management of dietary intake is the main mode of treatment. The goal in calorie reduction is a slowing of the rate of weight gain while linear growth continues. A very low calorie diet is contraindicated because it can result in loss of lean body mass and nutritional deficits.

For severely obese children (over 170 per cent ideal body weight) or those with complications such as hypertension, dietary restrictions will need to be more extreme (Hammer, 1990).

For mild-to-moderate obesity, reducing intake of fat and high-carbohydrate snacks will often result in slowing weight gain. The diet must be nutritionally adequate and individualized for a child's age, activity level, and preferences (see Table 16–1 for Recommended Dietary Allowance). Family culture and socioeconomic class need to be considered. Exchange lists, like those used for diabetic diets, are helpful in teaching and in providing variety. There is no need for separate meals or expensive dietetic foods for the child. The obese child should eat at the table with the family, not alone or in front of the television. High-calorie snacks must be removed from the house and replaced with low-calorie nutritious snacks, but an occasional treat should be allowed. The child and family should be assisted not to view foods as good or bad, because foods then take on the connotation of being a reward or a punishment.

Exercise is important in improving fitness and expending energy. Toddlers and preschoolers need ample opportunity to play, jump, run, and dance. This can be encouraged if families exercise or walk together. School-age children are encouraged to participate in school, scouting, or community center activities; however, an obese child may resist these activities initially because of poor self-concept. Organized activities are especially important in the summer when a child may feel bored or lonely. Unless the child is particularly eager, competitive sports are best delayed until self-confidence is improved. Biking, walking, swimming, and dancing are noncompetitive activities families can do together. It is important for all exercises to begin slowly, with gradual expending of effort and time.

Behavioral treatments have been shown to be highly effective in weight control. On the basis of learning theory principles, children are given positive reinforcement for desirable behaviors. Children then continue to behave in ways that are rewarded (Hammer, 1990). For toddlers, praise and affection, not cookies, should be given when they remember to sit on the toilet. Preschoolers should get praise for riding a tricycle, not for emptying their plate and asking for more. A school-age child can cooperate with the family on a project of changing eating behaviors. The nurse can assist the family to agree on behaviors to be rewarded, realistic long- and short-term goals, and appropriate rewards (food should not be used for rewards).

Other behavioral methods used in obesity programs are contingency contracting, self-monitoring, stimulus control, and cognitive restructuring (Hammer, 1990). These methods are often combined into one program. Enduring behavioral changes requires persistence. If the family is highly disorganized or inconsistent in dealing with the obese child, behavioral treatments may not be effective (Bryant & Kopeski, 1986). The nurse should determine whether a family can provide the consistency needed before helping the family implement a behavior modification program.

Adolescent. Prevention counseling is implemented as a youth gains excess weight during puberty and is also recommended for adolescents who have obese parents. Balanced diet, not the need to lose weight, is stressed.

For the adolescent who is obese, family involvement in treatment from the beginning is important but with a definite structure so that the boundaries between parent and child are clearly defined and maintained. The best approach is to consider the adolescent's need for some degree of independence and desire to have free discussion with peers. A parents' support and education group allows parents to receive education about the disorder (such as diet, exercise, and programs to alter eating behaviors) and also to interact with other parents of children. With adolescents starting to deal with separation issues, parents need to provide support and nurturance but also support independence. All of these measures are important to the prevention of *personal identity disturbance* in the adolescent.

Liquid protein diets are considered controversial because of concerns about their safety and long-term efficacy. Liquid diets also create the erroneous perception that weight problems can be approached with a "quick fix." The use of drugs and surgical procedures (e.g., bypassing a portion of the intestine or occluding a large segment of the stomach) are not generally recommended for adolescents. Teens need to be warned of the hazards of overzealous dieting and encouraged to seek safe, enduring methods. The nutritionist can provide accurate information and assistance about methods of dieting and selection of foods.

Adolescents are present-oriented and want fast results. They may give up a healthy diet when fast results are not attained. They should be told that it will take time before they see the results of their efforts. They and their families will need considerable encouragement to accomplish the goal.

It is essential to work with adolescents to achieve a slow, consistent weight loss of 1 to 2 pounds per week. Exercise needs to be a part of the treatment program. An activity therapist can work with adolescents in designing an individual program that meets their needs as related to lifestyle, health needs, and personal preferences. The exercise component is started while still in thc hospital. The treatment program looks beyond the focus of weight or food and deals with the issues of body image, assertiveness, self esteem, personal identity, societal pressures, and sexuality because obesity is a symptom of a more serious personal problem (Bryant & Kopeski, 1986).

Cases of morbid obesity may require severe calorie restriction in the form of a protein-modified fast. These teens will need careful medical, nursing, and nutrition management. Because adolescents are peer oriented, the group approach is suitable. The best types of weight control programs for teens incorporate group support sessions, diet, exercise, behavior modification, and family involvement. These programs can be school-based or clinic-based. Both have been shown to be effective.

Nursing Care

A major role of nurses working with obese teens is to ensure that the total person is the focus of care. These objectives place emphasis on the adolescent and not on the fat and are more likely to assist the adolescent to establish a positive sense of identity. Evaluation is ongoing during the treatment approach. Growth variables are monitored and diet is assessed to ensure adequate nutrition. Goals and plans should be revised as appropriate to meet the final goal of designated weight loss.

Anorexia Nervosa

"Anorexia nervosa" means an abnormal or nervous lack of appetite. The term is a misnomer for a disorder that is marked by the individual's preoccupation with eating and food. The appetite may, in fact, be insatiable, but the victim engages in self-starvation. Symptoms of anxiety and fear are present but are usually consciously denied. With the onset of symptoms in puberty, issues of sexuality and independence are not resolved, and the behaviors may represent a regression to earlier stages of development. As the victim denies the need for food, she or he expresses an exaggerated need to control self and others.

Etiology/Incidence (Pathophysiology)

The individual who exhibits symptoms of anorexia nervosa is characteristically described by family members as an exceptional student, neat, compliant, overly sensitive, quiet, and perfectionist. Anorexia occurs primarily in girls (95 per cent) (American Psychiatric Association, 1987). Typically, family and teachers describe the individual as a child who "never gave us any trouble." There is some indication that anorexia nervosa is a symptom of certain family characteristics. Minuchin and colleagues (1978) identified rigidity, overprotection, enmeshment, and lack of conflict resolution as characteristics of families with an anorectic member. Selvini-Palazzoli (1985) also found denial of conflict to be a characteristic interactive pattern between the marital couple. Several explanations have been offered as etiologic factors, including sociocultural, developmental, and genetic as well as interaction of factors.

Clinical Manifestations

Identification in the early stage of anorexia may be difficult because, initially, there are no overt signs. Complaints may be vague, such as fatigue and irritability (Crawshaw, 1985), or may include gastrointestinal disturbance, a menstrual disorder, or an athletic injury due to compulsive exercise (Muscare, 1987). Food rituals may be detected early in the course of the problem, including bizarre eating habits like eating without the lips touching the utensil, weighing each bite of food, cutting food into minute pieces and pushing it around the plate, or silent chanting during the eating ritual. Other behaviors include excessive exercising and compulsive weighing of oneself; self-induced vomiting; taking diuretics, laxatives, and appetite-suppressants; and intense interest in the eating behaviors of others. Symptoms may vary as the condition becomes chronic. Initially, there is weight loss, which may be reinforced by positive comments from others, until it progresses to a significant and noticeable degree. As weight drops, the individual may experience amenorrhea, growth of lanugo, fatigue, constipation, hypotension, dependent edema, and bradycardia (Williamson, 1990). Clinical signs indicative of nutritional deficiencies are listed in Table 29–8. There is a continuum of symptoms manifested by the adolescent ranging from mild to severe. Adolescents with severe manifestations are more likely to evidence thought disorder.

TABLE 29–8
Clinical Signs of Nutritional Deficiencies

General appearance	Lethargy, excessive or inadequate body fat, muscle wasting
Skin	Dryness, flakiness, scaling, roughness (follicular hyperkeratosis), pallor
Mouth	Angular fissures, redness at corners of mouth (cheilosis); redness, swelling or atrophic papillae on tongue; red, swollen or bleeding gums
Teeth	Severe caries
Eyes	Pale conjunctivae
Nails	Spoon-shaped, brittle, or ridged
Hair	Dull, easily plucked

Diagnostic Assessment

Specific criteria for the diagnosis of anorexia nervosa, provided by the American Psychiatric Association (1987), are as follows:

- Refusal to maintain body weight over a minimal normal weight for age and height (e.g., weight loss leading to maintenance of body weight 15 per cent below that expected), or failure to make expected weight gain during period of growth, leading to body weight 15 per cent below that expected.
- Intense fear of gaining weight or becoming fat, even though underweight.
- Disturbance in the way in which one's body weight, size, or shape is experienced (e.g., the person claims to "feel fat" even when emaciated, believes that one area of the body is "too fat" even when obviously underweight).
- In women, absence of at least three consecutive menstrual cycles when they are otherwise expected to occur (primary or secondary amenorrhea). (A woman is considered to have amenorrhea if her periods occur only after hormone [e.g., estrogen] administration.)

On admission to the hospital, a variety of laboratory and diagnostic tests are done, which include electrocardiogram, electrolyte, analysis SMA-12, complete blood count with differential, liver function studies, and thyroid studies. An adolescent may eliminate all fats from the diet, which would present with abnormal values of aspartate aminotransferase, alanine aminotransferase, blood urea nitrogen, and creatinine. If the client has been refed with hyperalimentation, it is important to monitor for hypophosphatemia. Signs and symptoms of hypophosphatemia include ataxia, motor weakness, paresthesias, and eventual loss of reflexes including the gag reflex. Bone density studies may be helpful in diagnosing early osteoporosis, which may be seen in clients who are amenorrheic for a prolonged period of 3 years or more. Bone demineralization will occur in women who are amenorrheic even if they are on calcium supplements.

A thorough evaluation needs to be done at the beginning of treatment. The members of the interdisciplinary team who participate in the evaluation are physicians (internal medicine), psychiatrists, nurses, social workers, physical therapists, nutritionists, and psychologists. Psychologic screening includes the use of tools that measure depression and eating disorder behaviors, personality inventory, and clinical interviews. The adolescent is screened for medical problems that are due to eating disorders (bulimia, anorexia, or obesity).

Therapeutic Management

Without treatment, or when treatment is unsuccessful, the course of the disorder may be unremitting. Debilitation may then lead to death by starvation. Of those who do recover, many are left with phobias and compulsions that continue to dominate their lives. The treatment of the individual with anorexia nervosa depends on a number of variables, including age, length or chronicity of illness, physical and emotional symptoms of decompensation, family dynamics, and physical complications.

Three types of psychologic treatment have been used with some success and represent different theories of etiology and treatment. The psychodynamic approach of Hilde Bruch (1973) consists of intensive psychotherapy over long periods. In contrast to traditional psychotherapy, the hallmark of this therapeutic approach is to help the individual accept dependence and feel safe when receiving nurturing rather than giving it. Cognitive-behavioral approaches are often used to treat the anoretic individual. The treatment goal of this therapeutic modality is to assist the individual in addressing issues of control and autonomy in conjuction with eating patterns. Family systems therapy has been advocated by several researchers and may be used in conjunction with other psychotherapies. Behavior modification and hospitalization may also be used to supplement family systems therapy. In the paradigm, the interaction of family members is stressed; the anorectic individual is supported in communicating personal needs and anxieties within the family circle.

Behavior modification has been used extensively for those hospitalized with the disorder. With this approach, a system of rewards or privileges is established to reinforce desirable behaviors conducive to weight gain and maintenance. Short- and long-term effectiveness of this method used alone is not promising. This method can promote the client's need to meet goals, even artificially or dishonestly. Other therapeutic strategies include group therapy and individual therapy continuing after discharge. The therapy team, including the patient, primary nurse, social worker, activity therapist, attending psychiatrist, and nutritionist, works together toward common goals to

- Correct the youth's misperceptions about her or his environment and body.
- Facilitate identification of feelings.
- Develop within the patient a sense of self-worth and self-control.
- Develop a sense of competence and ease in relationships.

Hospitalization is often required when the individual has chronic symptoms. Psychoactive drugs may be needed to alter mood (particularly depression or anxiety or both), and parenteral nutrition is needed to restore electrolyte balance and nutritional deficiencies.

Nursing Diagnostic Statements for the Adolescent with Anorexia Nervosa

- ***Altered nutrition: less than body requirements,*** *related to inadequate food intake or purging (anorexia symptoms and bulimia).*
- ***Altered nutrition: more than body requirements,*** *related to intake of nutrients exceeding metabolic needs.*
- ***High risk for fluid volume deficit;*** *risk factor: decreased fluid intake.*
- ***High risk for fluid volume excess;*** *risk factors: excessive fluid intake and edema from malnutrition and hyponatremia.*
- ***High risk for ineffective individual coping;*** *risk factors: feelings of powerlessness and personal identity disturbance.*
- ***High risk for self-directed violence;*** *risk factor: feeling of powerlessness.*
- ***High risk for ineffective management of therapeutic regimen;*** *risk factors:*
  - *Anxiety.*
  - *Decisional conflicts.*
  - *Conflict between adolescent and caregivers or caregiving environment.*

Nursing Care

Nurses encounter adolescents with anorexia nervosa in a variety of professional settings. Nurses are often the first to assess behaviors, emotions, and attitudes expressed by patients or their family members that may lead to diagnosis of the disorder. Thus, it is imperative that the nurse be alert to the many symptoms that may indicate a problem. More specifically, the nurse who cares for the hospitalized adolescent with anorexia must be careful to monitor intake and output and observe eating patterns, levels of exercise, family interactions, and compulsive behaviors.

Promoting Nutrition by Promoting Intake. Because anorectic and bulimic clients fear the loss of their identity through weight gain, these adolescents may go to extreme lengths to simulate false weight gain. For monitoring this, specific structures in the program are important:

1. The adolescent is weighed every morning after the first morning void, which is monitored so that the client does not hold onto urine for extra weight. The adolescent is weighed in the hospital gown and underwear only to decrease the chance of contraband items that artificially increase weight. For example, the client may fill up pockets with coins to increase weight.
2. Bathroom use is monitored before weighing to decrease the chance of the adolescent's drinking excessive amounts of water to artificially increase weight.
3. Calorie counts will help determine if the weight gain is real or artificial.
4. The adolescent is observed for other unusual behaviors, such as keeping the room frigid and hoarding laxatives.

As the adolescent is able to participate in the treatment plan and establish a therapeutic alliance with the staff, controls can be given back to the adolescent, such as tapering the need for monitoring.

Preventing Fluid Volume Deficit by Monitoring for Dehydration. Orthostatic blood pressure and pulse are monitored at least once daily; these measures are good indicators of dehydration and poor nutrition. These orthostatic effects may be attributed to the use of antidepressants or other medications. It is essential to use proper equipment in monitoring blood pressure. Adolescents and adults will most likely need a pediatric blood pressure cuff for accurate readings to be obtained. Education is important for both the adolescent and family related to hypotension and its symptoms and how to deal with these symptoms.

Preventing Fluid Volume Excess by Monitoring for Excessive Fluid Intake. Intake and output are monitored because excessive fluid intake or output can be a signal of fluid overloading to increase weight artificially. Electrolytes are monitored because decreased serum sodium (hyponatremia) can be an indicator that the adolescent is overloading with water to increase weight. The specific gravity of urine is noted because a depressed specific gravity is a likely indicator of fluid overloading.

Promoting Coping by Empowerment and Facilitating the Development of a Positive Sense of Identity. The eating-disordered adolescent may get into a struggle and focus anger on and act out at the goals of the treatment plan (see "Therapeutic Management") and the limits used to structure them in meeting those goals of increasing food intake and weight gain. One of the nurse's challenges in providing care is to constantly reframe what the struggle really is and the adolescent's role and responsibility in wanting to be in treatment and meet that goal. The nurse reinforces the adolescent's right to be entitled to feelings of anger, loss, and sadness in meeting treatment goals. The adolescent is reinforced to take responsibility for those feelings. The nurse provides the adolescent with the support and tools/strategies to assist with this process.

Preventing Injury by Empowerment. The nurse is likely to encounter adolescents with eating disorders who are self-destructive. The adolescents' self-destructive behaviors include cutting themselves, burning themselves, and banging their heads. If the adolescent becomes self-destructive, the nurse can use written treatment contracts to set limits and provide clear, concrete expectations but in a nonpunitive manner. The adolescent is an integral part of negotiating and implementing the contract; it helps to maintain a sense of having some control and allows the staff to continue reinforcing the adolescent's ability to take responsibility for his or her behavior.

TABLE 29-9
National Organizations

National Association for Anorexia Nervosa and Related Disorders, Box 7, Highland Park, IL 60035
National Anorexic Aid Society, The Bridge Foundation, 445 East Granville Rd., Urbanton, OH 43085
Anorexia Nervosa and Bulimia Resource Center, 255 Alhambra Circle, Suite 321, Coral Gables, FL 33134

Promoting Effective Management of Therapeutic Regimen by Referral for Counseling for Feelings of Anxiety and Conflict. Inpatient treatment is often necessary after periods of improved nutritional status. The child psychiatric nurse will be involved in several types of treatment modalities for the care of the anorectic adolescent, including family and group therapy and other components of milieu treatment. The adolescent may be referred to a day treatment program after discharge.

Because individuals with the disorder have such a strong need to control all variables in their lives, the nurse must be cautious not to enter into a power struggle with them. Firm limits applied with kindness are more helpful than sympathetic permissiveness.

It can be frustrating to work with victims of anorexia nervosa because of the consistent enforcement of rules that is required. Patients require the services of a competent team in which professionals can support one another. Nurses *usually* are the professionals who monitor the individual's behavior on a daily basis during hospitalization; they particularly need the support of team members. Organizations that provide assistance and information for anorectic patients are listed in Table 29-9.

Bulimia

Bulimia is an eating disorder characterized by episodes of binge eating alternating with purge behavior. The individual is aware that the behaviors of overeating and then ridding the body of food are erratic. Patients often express fear that it is impossible to control these activities voluntarily.

Etiology/Incidence (Pathophysiology)

The precise incidence of bulimia in the United States is not known. Because of the secrecy surrounding the disorder, it is grossly underreported, thereby making estimate of incidence difficult (Laraia & Stuart, 1990). However, the pattern of binge eating, anxiety over weight gain, and subsequent purging is on the increase. It is estimated that the prevalence of bulimia in college-age women is between 4 and 13 per cent (Pyle et al, 1983). Onset of the condition is usually in adolescence, and it occurs more frequently in girls than in boys. Compulsive exercise as a method of purging has been seen in increasing numbers of boys.

Symptoms of bulimia may not be readily apparent, as most bulimic patients are of normal weight. Onset may be gradual; the condition becomes chronic with alternating periods of normal eating, fasting, binging, and purging. Binging consists of rapid intake of large amounts of food, usually with high-calorie content and sweet taste, within a short period (usually less than 2 hours). Purging may consist of self-induced vomiting, excessive use of laxatives, or a combination. Bulimia may coexist with anorexia.

Vomiting and Laxative Abuse. Adolescents with bulimia do not purge *only* after a binge. Many patients will purge after eating normal or small amounts of food, sometimes even after drinking water. Patients need education to recognize symptoms of hypokalemia.

Exercise. Adolescents will "purge" with excessive hours of exercise every day. These patients may present with sports-related injuries caused by compulsive exercise, such as skin splints and stress fractures.

Syrup of Ipecac. The use of this emetic is dangerous; it could lead to the possibility of cardiac arrhythmias and cardiac arrest. This product is easily accessible over-the-counter in any pharmacy. Adolescents need education because they do not realize the danger of using this product.

Diuretic Abuse. In addition to vomiting, exercise, and laxatives, the use of diuretics can lead to further dehydration.

Insulin. Although less commonly reported, bulimia exists within the diabetic population. Diabetics with bulimia will intentionally give themselves lower than needed insulin amounts to purposefully induce glycosuria and spill ketones, resulting in the spilling of calories. The resultant chronic binging and purging and underdosing of insulin causes widely fluctuating blood glucose levels, which may result in diabetic ketoacidosis.

Most individuals are within the normal weight range for height and age. They express undue concern about their weight and conflicts about eating and dieting. They engage in self-destructive thoughts and frequently exhibit depressed affect.

In addition to these symptoms, many individuals with the disorder experience distorted body image similar to that found in people with anorexia nervosa. They may engage in experimentation with or abuse of amphetamines, barbiturates, and alcohol. Studies have also shown that depression is common among bulimics (Walsh et al, 1985). Physical complications may include potassium depletion with subsequent cardiac arrest, spastic colitis, tetany, tooth discoloration and decay, hypertension, and esophageal or gastric perforation.

Diagnostic Assessment

Specific diagnostic criteria are provided by the American Psychiatric Association (1987) as follows:

- Recurrent episodes of binge eating (rapid consumption of a large amount of food in a discrete period of time).
- A feeling of lack of control over eating behavior during the eating binges.
- The person regularly engages in either self-induced vomiting, use of laxatives or diuretics, strict dieting or fasting, or vigorous exercise to prevent weight gain.
- A minimal average of two binge eating episodes a week for at least 3 months.
- Persistent overconcern with body shape and weight.

Therapeutic Management

The treatment of individuals with bulimia consists of physiologic regulation and cognitive and behavioral therapies in addition to psychotherapy and family counseling. Physiologic regulation of electrolyte imbalance and digestive irregularities must be provided. Antidepressive drugs may be used in conjunction with withdrawal from other abused substances.

Cognitive approaches address the self-destructive thoughts of the person. Self-affirmations and assertiveness training are used to provide cues for constructive thought processes. Behavior modification is also used to provide external rewards for appropriate eating behaviors and adaptive coping behaviors.

Psychodynamic nurturant-authoritarian, group, and family therapies are used in treating the psychologic component. Results of these approaches are highly variable, and new approaches are continuously being sought (Kelly & Liter, 1984).

Nursing Care

The nursing process is used in assessing behaviors, thoughts, and affect of the individual. As with eating disorders, the nurse is often the first person to assess the adolescent with bulimia. After diagnosis, nurses may provide inpatient physical care or counseling sessions with individuals, groups, or families. It is imperative that the nurse give attention to the physical, emotional, and social variables that interact within the patient. Resistance to treatment is common, and nurses must attend to their own feelings of frustration and self-doubt when working closely with these individuals.

Treatment modalities aimed at physical symptoms, cognitive processes, emotional coping, and interpersonal processes are provided and evaluated. Having the adolescent attend support groups with peers who are also bulimic is an invaluable adjunct to treatment. Assistance and information about eating disorders can be obtained from various organizations (see list in Table 29–9).

Substance Use and Abuse

"Substance use" refers to the use of drugs (including alcohol) or volatile inhalants for the purpose of altering mood or state of consciousness or improving performance. "Substance abuse" is the pathologic use of any substance to the extent that it interferes with an individual's relationships, school, work, or physical or emotional health or is harmful to others (Williams, 1980).

Substance use is not a new phenomenon; it has existed throughout history. Peculiar to this decade are the specific agents used and the prevalence of substance use by adolescents. The prevalence, effects on physical and psychosocial development, and possible harmful consequences of psychoactive substances give impetus for nursing involvement. Substance use by students has been identified as the most serious problem facing the school system (Palmer & Ringwalt, 1988).

Mood-altering substances have a substantial impact on the welfare of children and adolescents. The trend currently indicates an earlier age for first-time drug use. Twelve years of age is the current mean age for first-time drug use, age 11 for alcohol use (Forney et al, 1988; MacDonald, 1987). Drug and alcohol abuse are associated with each of the three leading causes of death among adolescents: accidents, homicides, and suicides (Petechers et al, 1988). Some chemical substances, such as caffeine, nicotine, tranquilizers, and alcohol (if used moderately), are sanctioned by society; however, these, too, can lead to physical and psychologic dependence.

Etiology/Incidence (Pathophysiology)

The drug scene is constantly changing. Cocaine has gained increasing popularity in various forms; users rose from 1.6 million in 1977 to 6 million in 1985. Use had leveled off until around 1984 when "crack" appeared on the scene, at which time the number of users again increased (Kleber, 1988). Cocaine is reported to have a dependence potential comparable to that of heroin, even when the route of administration is primarily intranasal (smoking or injecting is a more potent route) (Hasin, 1988).

Alcohol continues to be the most widely used illicit substance among children and adolescents in the 12- to 17-year-old age group. Since the late 1970s, the reported use of alcohol, cigarettes, marijuana, and cocaine has decreased (National Institute on Drug Abuse, 1990). Sixty-nine per cent of youths ages 12 to 17 years reported the illicit use of alcohol, cigarettes, and marijuana during the previous month (National Institute on Drug Abuse, 1990).

The principal psychoactive chemical in marijuana is tetrahydrocannabinol (THC). The THC concentration is much higher in marijuana sold today than it was in the 1960s. Therefore, marijuana may not be as harmless as its original users purported it to be (Silber et al, 1988). Furthermore, an increasingly serious problem related to substance abuse is the rapidly increasing occurrence of multiple substance abuse. Table 29–10 lists the main substances used by children and adolescents.

Developmental, familial, and societal factors contribute to substance use and abuse, and the patterns of use range from experimental to dependent. All adolescents are at risk for experimental and recreational use, but those who are at risk for chronic habits are those who are unconventional in values and behavior and who come from unstable families.

Developmental Factors. Substance use is occurring with greater frequency in school-age children. One study reported that 12.4 per cent of seventh and eighth graders had tried marijuana (Palmer & Ringwalt, 1988). If the school-age child engages in substance use, it usually denotes significant problems in the child, the family, or both, and the child and family should receive professional counseling (Myers & Anderson, 1991).

Substance use is primarily a problem of adolescents, and several etiologic factors are related to adolescent psychosocial development. Incentives for experimental and recreational drug use are often the same incentives as for other adolescent behavior. Developmental motives include rebelling against parental authority or the need to be independent and different from parents. Adolescents may see psychoactive substances, notably hallucinogens, as a means for self-discovery. Another motivation for substance use is the desire to be accepted into a peer group. Adolescents also learn behavior by modeling and may model substance use habits of adults whom they admire for being sophisticated, mature, or glamorous. Substance use becomes a symbol of a more mature status. Adolescents are often simply curious and like excitement, especially when they can share something novel with friends.

Familial Factors. Families commonly play a role in substance use, especially when the pattern is an abusive one, not merely for experimental or recreational purposes. Adolescent substance abusers frequently come from dysfunctional families (Felner et al, 1991) and may feel the need for temporary escape from prolonged family conflicts. If the youth has become the scapegoat for family problems, substance abuse can perpetuate the problems and the scapegoating and become a sequence in a cycle that is difficult to interrupt. Drug abuse may be a conscious or uncon-

TABLE 29-10
Main Addictive Substances Used by Children and Adolescents

Agents	Signs and Effects	Complications
Opiates		
Heroin ("H," "junk," "smack," "horse") *Route:* Inhaling ("snorting"), subcutaneous (SQ) ("skin-popping"), intravenous (IV) ("mainlining")	Drowsiness, euphoria, pain relief, nausea and vomiting, miosis, needle track scars from IV use, erythema of nasal mucosa from inhaling	Constipation, menstrual disturbances, duodenal ulcer, physical and psychologic dependence, skin abscesses from IV or SQ use; from IV use: acute hepatitis, septic emboli, endocarditis, HIV infection, and AIDS *Overdose:* stupor, coma, miosis, respiratory depression, cyanosis, pulmonary edema, death *Withdrawal:* usually within 8 hours of abstinence; first yawning, then tearing, rhinorrhea, mydriasis, insomnia, "gooseflesh," cramping of voluntary muscles, vomiting, diarrhea, tachycardia, and systolic hypertension
Hallucinogens		
D-Lysergic acid diethylamide (LSD, "acid"); mescaline ("acid"); psilocybin mushrooms ("mushrooms") *Route:* by mouth (PO)	Perceptual distortions, hallucinations, mydriasis, flushing, tremors, elevations in blood pressure	Paranoia, loss of control, anxiety (bad trip), accidents, spontaneous recurrence of LSD experience (flashback), psychologic dependence *Overdose:* panic
Phencyclidine (PCP, "angel dust," "peace pills," "sheets") *Route:* PO, inhaling	Euphoria, hallucinations, perceptual distortions, emotional lability, ataxia	Accidents, anxiety, paranoia, 5–15 mg—toxic psychosis: disorientation, aggression *>15 mg—overdose:* delirium, coma with alternating periods of wakefulness, arrhythmias, seizures, hypotension, dystonic posturing, muscular rigidity or myoclonic jerking, death
Marijuana—dried leaves and flower tops of *Cannabis sativa* plant; hashish—extracted resin of plant ("grass," "joint," "reefer," "hash") *Route:* inhaled (usual), PO	Elation, relaxation, intensification of mood, acute sensory perceptions, hunger, dry oral mucosa, coughing, antiemesis, injected conjunctiva, decreased intraocular pressure	Lack of coordination, accidents, decreased concentration, short-term memory loss; girls: changes in ovulation patterns; boys: decreased testosterone levels *Large dose:* hallucinations *Chronic use:* inflammatory changes in respiratory tract, apathy, psychologic dependence *Sudden withdrawal or abstinence in chronic users:* irritability, insomnia, electroencephalographic changes
Depressants		
Alcohol (beer, wine, wine coolers, whiskey) *Route:* PO	Decreased inhibitions, relaxation, diuresis, slurred speech	Impaired short-term memory, lack of coordination, impaired judgment, accidents, gastrointestinal irritation, nausea and vomiting, interactions with several other drugs *Chronic abuse:* fetal alcohol syndrome in offspring of female abuser, fatty necrosis and fibrosis of liver, nutritional deficiencies; physical and psychologic dependence (alcoholism) *Large dose:* acute gastritis, pancreatitis *Overdose:* disorientation, coma, respiratory depression, death *Withdrawal:* usually within 8 hours of abstinence; anxiety, tremors, insomnia; in adolescents who have been chronic drinkers for 1 or more years, severe with delirium tremens and seizures

(continued)

TABLE 29-10
Main Addictive Substances Used by Children and Adolescents *(Continued)*

Agents	Signs and Effects	Complications
Barbiturates; usually shorter-acting: amobarbital, pentobarbital, secobarbital ("downs," "blues," "reds," "yellow jackets") *Route:* PO (usual), IV, SQ	Decreased inhibitions, sedation, slurred speech, miosis	Lack of coordination, use of amphetamines to counteract sedation, sleep deprivation due to lack of REM sleep, increased effect when used with alcohol, depression, physical and psychologic dependence, IV or SQ complications, HIV infection, and AIDS *Overdose:* respiratory depression, coma, death *Withdrawal:* within 24 hours of abstinence, anxiety, headache, tremors, nausea and vomiting, cramps, tachycardia, hypotension, seizures, hallucinations
Nonbarbiturate sedatives; methaqualone (Quaalude) ("ludes") *Route:* PO	As above	Lack of coordination, use of amphetamines to counteract sedation, depression, psychologic dependence *Overdose:* respiratory depression, coma, death
Stimulants		
Amphetamines (amphetamine sulfate, methamphetamine, dextroamphetamine) ("speed," "uppers," "bennies," "dexies," "black beauties") *Route:* PO, IV, SQ	Euphoria, arousal, anorexia, alertness, elevated blood pressure, mydriasis	Insomnia, use of depressants to counteract wakefulness, tachycardia, nutritional deficits, weight loss, IV and SQ complications, psychologic dependence, HIV infection, and AIDS *Large dose:* anxiety, headache, tremors, impulsiveness, aggression, manic behavior, hallucinations, accidents, psychosis *Overdose:* hypertension, seizures, death *Abstinence after chronic use:* fatigue, depression
Amphetamine look-alikes (contain caffeine, ephedrine, phenylpropanolamine, and mixtures of other substances); sold to look like amphetamines and advertised with the "amine" or "caine" ending *Route:* PO	Alertness, anorexia	Restlessness, weight loss, insomnia, agitation, manic behavior, hallucinations, hypertension, death
Cocaine ("coke," "crack," "snow") *Route:* Inhaled, IV, SQ	Euphoria, increased motor activity, local anesthesia; if inhaled: injected nasal mucosa, rhinorrhea	Tachycardia, hypertension, hyperthermia, psychologic dependence, complications of IV and SQ use, HIV infection, and AIDS *Chronic use:* hallucinations, paranoid ideation, perforated nasal septum
Volatile Substances		
Substances contain toluene, hydrocarbons, or fluorocarbons: glue, gasoline, cleaning solvents, lighter fluid, typing correction fluid, thinners, lacquers, aerosol sprays *Route:* Inhaled	Giddiness, confusion, decreased inhibition, injected conjunctiva, lacrimation, rhinorrhea	Decreased coordination, hallucinations, accidents, abdominal pain, nausea and vomiting, aspiration or asphyxia from inhaling substance in plastic bag, psychologic dependence; lead poisoning from leaded gasoline, gas encephalopathy from gasoline

TABLE 29-10
Main Addictive Substances Used by Children and Adolescents (Continued)

Agents	Signs and Effects	Complications
Miscellaneous		
Agents used in sports; anabolic steroids *Route:* PO	No proven increase in muscle development and strength; larger appearance sometimes due to water and sodium retention	Sodium and water retention, hypertension; alterations in liver functions, premature closure of epiphyses, short stature; boys: decreased testosterone production, testicular atrophy, decreased libido, gynecomastia if contains female hormones; girls: hirsutism, permanent deepening of voice, acne
Diuretics, stimulants *Route:* PO	Diuresis and weight loss	Dehydration, fluid and electrolyte disturbances
Tobacco *Route:* Inhaled, chewed	Perceived maturity and sophistication	Cough, staining of teeth and nails, heart disease, emphysema, lung cancer, bronchitis, smaller infants born to female smokers, physical and psychologic dependence *Withdrawal:* nervousness, fatigue, headache, tachycardia

Data from Caddell, A. (1983). Under the influence. *Nursing Times, 79*(25), 9–10; Cohen, M. I. (1983). Marijuana—What is really known? In I. F. Litt (Ed.), *Adolescent substance abuse, report of the 14th Ross Roundtable on critical approaches to common pediatric problems* (pp 10–16). Columbus, OH: Ross Laboratories; Dietz, A. J. (1981). Amphetamine-like reactions to phenylpropanolamine. *Journal of the American Medical Association, 245,* 601–602; Hill, J. A., et al. (1983). The athletic polydrug abuse phenomenon. A case report. *American Journal of Sports Medicine, 11,* 269–271; Horowitz, J. D., et al. (1980). Hypertensive responses induced by phenylpropanolamine in anorectic and decongestant preparations. *Lancet, 1,* 60–61; Iveson, J. I. (1982, August). Barbiturates: A history of abuse. Forum 8, Drug Abuse. *Nursing Mirror,* p 155; McKerlie, L., et al. (1983, December). Solvent abuse. Community Forum 10. *Nursing Mirror* (Suppl.); Percy, E. C. (1983). Drugs and athletics. In N. J. Smith (Ed.), *Sports medicine: Health care for young athletes* (pp 176–183). American Academy of Pediatrics, Committee on Sports Medicine; Tashkin, D. P., & Cohen, S. (1981). *Marijuana smoking and its effects on the lungs.* Rockville, MD: American Council for Drug Education; Williams, D. (1980). Substance use and abuse. In J. Howe (Ed.), *Nursing care of adolescents* (pp 161–195). New York: McGraw-Hill.

scious way of redirecting attention from family difficulties. If an intolerable situation like physical abuse exists, an adolescent may desire chemical escape. It is important not to conclude that all families of substance abusers have caused the problem. Sometimes family conflicts are consequences, rather than precursors, of an adolescent's habits.

Unstable family situations increase the risk for substance abuse. Children of alcoholics, for example, are known to be at risk for alcoholism. It has not been determined whether this fact is explained by genetics, personality factors, or a combination thereof (US Department of Health and Human Services, 1987).

Societal Factors. Societal factors contribute to substance abuse. Enticements from the media make smoking and drinking appear glamorous. Antihistamine- and caffeine-containing diet and energy pills are openly advertised. Western culture is a drug-taking culture in which people expect quick pharmaceutical cures for all ailments. Psychoactive substances are readily available to adolescents (Myers & Andersen, 1991). In cities, dealers come to schools and parks to sell drugs. The availability of cocaine in a cheaper form (crack) has signaled a dramatic increase in its use. Drugs such as phencyclidine (PCP) are easily synthesized in school laboratories.

A lack of hope may engender substance use. Major defining characteristics of the problem human response *hopelessness* include "passivity, decreased verbalization; decreased affect; verbal cues with despondent content such as, 'I can't,' sighing." One frequent related factor (etiology) is "lost belief in transcendent values" (NANDA, 1992). If youths cannot feel optimistic about the future, they are likely to live for pleasures of the moment. Distraction and oblivion are appealing, particularly for adolescents who have never learned to feel competent or to feel as if anyone or anything will respond to their efforts.

Clinical Manifestations (Patterns of Substance Use)

Experimental. The experimental use of substances is inspired by curiosity and desire to experience something new. The initial experience is usually with an older friend or sibling. It is nonpatterned and does not interfere with daily activities. The risks of experimental use are further use and accidents.

Recreational. Recreational use mainly refers to using alcohol and marijuana at parties. It is usually controlled and nonprogressive, but the risks of more intensive use and accidents exist.

Circumstantial. Circumstantial use of substances occurs when the teen feels the need for help in coping with a problem or situation. For example, alcohol may be used to help numb the aftermath of a family argument, or amphetamines may be used to stay awake and study. Parents commonly notice changes in behavior, friends, and appearance. This pattern of ineffective individual coping becomes more frequent; and circumstantial use is often the dividing line between use and abuse. The dangers are interference with relationships, school, or work and, again, further use and accidents.

Intensive. Intensive use involves daily substance abuse. The teen feels a need for the drug in order to keep performing and often uses it alone and before school. Alcohol and marijuana may be the primary drugs used; the teen may have progressed to harder drugs, such as heroin; or there may be polydrug use (use of a number of drugs). There is typically school failure and truancy. Drugs are expensive, and the adolescent may steal from parents or shops or may sell drugs to others to get the money. Family problems surface, and intensify, and the substance abuse heightens in response to the family problems.

Dependent. "Substance dependence" refers to the "pathologic use and impaired social or occupational functioning for at least one month . . . plus either tolerance to the drug, which is indicated by needing increased amounts to obtain the same effect or by withdrawal (shakes, tremors, anxiety, etc.) when the drug is not used or when the amount of the drug is reduced" (Myers & Anderson, 1991, p 86).

Diagnostic Assessment

Specific diagnostic criteria for substance abuse according to the American Psychiatric Association (1987) are listed in Table 29–11. Diagnostic criteria for substance dependence according to the American Psychiatric Association (1987) are listed in Table 29–12.

The pattern of substance use is determined through the assessment. As discussed earlier, experimental or recreational use necessitates preventive measures. Circumstantial use requires counseling regarding the circumstances that are causing the substance use. Other ways of coping with stress should be addressed. Teens who are lonely, depressed, or having school or family problems require more intensive individual or family therapy.

A complete physical assessment will need to be performed. Physical signs of substance use are not usually found unless the adolescent is intoxicated at the time or the pattern of use is intensive or dependent (see Table 29–10 for physical effects of specific drugs).

Therapeutic Management

Patterns of abuse that are intensive or dependent clearly necessitate family or individual therapy or both. A physically dependent adolescent will need detoxification. Simply, "detoxification" refers to the physiologic process of reducing the toxic effects of the substance. Whether an adolescent is hospitalized or placed in a detoxification unit depends on the specific agent abused and on the teen's mental and physical condition. For example, adolescents dependent on alcohol and barbiturates will need medical supervision during withdrawal. The nurse's role during withdrawal is to calm the patient and monitor vital signs, blood pressure, fluid therapy, and intake and output. Depending on the individual situation, sedatives or seizure medicines may be ordered by the physician, and the nurse is responsible for administering the proper dose and observing the adolescent for effects of the medicine.

After detoxification, the choices for rehabilitation are either admission to residential or outpatient treatment centers or private individual, group, or family therapy. Rehabilitation is individualized and should be based on the needs of the adolescent and recommendations of the primary health care provider and specialist in adolescent drug abuse. Nurses are often employed in drug abuse rehabilitation centers and are involved in counseling the individual and family, leading group activities, and monitoring the patient's progress.

Whether the adolescent receives residential or outpatient treatment, family involvement is essential. This may be in the form of a support group for parents or conjoint family therapy. Family communication is stressed, and the focus is on the health of the family rather than the pathologic process.

TABLE 29-11
Specific Diagnostic Criteria for Substance Abuse

A maladaptive pattern of psychoactive substance use indicated by at least one of the following:

- Continued use despite knowledge of having a persistent or recurrent social, occupational, psychologic, or physical problem that is caused or exacerbated by use of the psychoactive substance
- Recurrent use in situations in which use is physically hazardous (e.g., driving while intoxicated)

Some symptoms of the disturbance have persisted for at least 1 month or have occurred repeatedly over a longer period of time

Never met the criteria for psychoactive substance dependence for this substance

From American Psychiatric Association: *Diagnostic and statistical manual of mental disorders, third edition, revised.* Washington, DC: American Psychiatric Association, 1987.

TABLE 29-12
Diagnostic Criteria for Substance Dependence

At least three of the following:

- Substance often taken in larger amounts or over a longer period than the person intended
- Persistent desire or one or more unsuccessful efforts to cut down or control substance use
- A great deal of time spent in activities necessary to get the substance (e.g., theft), taking the substance (e.g., chain smoking), or recovering from its effects
- Frequent intoxication or withdrawal symptoms when expected to fulfill major role obligations at work, school, or home (e.g., does not go to work because hung over, goes to school or work "high," intoxicated while taking care of his or her children) or when substance use is physically hazardous (e.g., drives when intoxicated)
- Important social, occupational, or recreational activities given up or reduced because of substance use
- Continued substance use despite knowledge of having a persistent or recurrent social, psychologic, or physical problem that is caused or exacerbated by the use of the substance (e.g., keeps using heroin despite family arguments about it; cocaine-induced depression; an ulcer made worse by drinking)
- Marked tolerance: need for markedly increased amounts of the substance (i.e., at least 50% increase to achieve intoxication or desired effect) or markedly diminished effect with continued use of the same amount

Note: The following items may apply to cannabis, hallucinogens, or phencyclidine (PCP):

- Characteristic withdrawal symptoms (see specific withdrawal syndromes under psychoactive substance-induced organic mental disorders)
- Substance often taken to relieve or avoid withdrawal symptoms

Some symptoms of the disturbance have persisted for at least 1 month or have occurred repeatedly over a longer period of time

The pattern of substance use will be determined through the assessment; as discussed in the text, experimental or recreational use necessitates preventive measures; circumstantial use requires counseling regarding the circumstances that are causing the substance use; other ways of dealing with stress should be addressed; teens who are lonely, depressed, or having school or family problems require more intensive individual or family therapy.

A complete physical assessment will need to be performed; physical signs of substance use are not usually found unless the adolescent is intoxicated at the time or the pattern of use is intensive or dependent (see Table 29-10 for physical effects of specific drugs)

From American Psychiatric Association: *Diagnostic and statistical manual of mental disorders, third edition, revised.* Washington, DC: American Psychiatric Association, 1987.

Nursing Diagnostic Statements for the Substance-Abusing Child or Adolescent

- ***High risk for injury and/or violence;*** *risk factors: pathologic and prolonged ingestion of illicit substances, as evidenced by*
  - *Impaired social/occupational/recreational/academic functioning.*
  - *Physiologic tolerance to illicit substance.*
  - *Heightened family problems.*
- ***Ineffective individual coping,*** *related to psychologic/physiologic dependence on illicit/abused substances.*
- ***Ineffective management of therapeutic regimen,*** *related to difficulty in making life changes to adapt to a drug-free lifestyle.*

Nursing Care

Preventing Injury and Violence. Adolescents who are using substances, or who are suspected of doing so, should be interviewed alone, by a health care professional skilled in such interviews, with the assurance of confidentiality. The teen should be told that parents will not be informed of any information given in confidence unless he or she is in danger or is hurting others.

If the youth, rather than parent or teacher, has initiated the visit, the chief complaint is rarely drug abuse but instead vague complaints of abdominal pain, headache, or fatigue (MacDonald, 1987). These physical discomforts must be evaluated first because they may be legitimate. Automatically asking "Are you doing drugs?" will close the interview fast.

After a routine history is taken, the subject of substance use may be approached. The use of drugs and alcohol among friends and classmates should be discussed in a general way first. If the interviewer is nonjudgmental and conveys a caring attitude, teens will usually continue on to discuss their own substance use. They are often relieved to have a professional who can listen and help.

It is important to ascertain the specific agents used; when, where, and how often they are used; and whether the teen is alone when using them. School, grades, and work should be discussed. In addition, vital questions to ask are, Do you feel lonely or depressed? How are you getting along with friends, boyfriends or girlfriends, and family? Do you believe that your substance use is interfering with school or home? Does your family see it as a problem? Have you ever done anything reckless while intoxicated?

Nurses may not be able to prevent experimental and recreational substance use, but they must help in the prevention of intoxicant-related accidents and in the prevention of more intense drug habits. Nurses can be active in preventive strategies at the public policy level by encouraging raising of the drinking age and by supporting initiatives to institute strict penalties for drinking and driving.

Another role of the nurse in prevention is to participate in school-based prevention programs. Panel discussions and fear tactics have not been found to be effective approaches. Today, programs are incorporating education, peer teaching, and parental involvement. Teachers are using tactics to help teens make knowledgeable and value-based choices. Programs also include teaching problem solving skills, ways for resisting social pressure, methods of improving communication with parents, and other ways of feeling good about oneself, such as creative writing or athletics. Teaching strategies can include small group discussions and role playing.

Programs should be presented in elementary school, in junior high school, and again in high school. Pediatric nurses can help plan programs and can review teaching material to see that it is age appropriate. Nurses can also educate teachers in how to identify pupils at risk for drug abuse and how to manage drug emergencies at school.

Summer is an especially drug-prone time for youths who are unemployed, bored, and frustrated. Nurses can encourage community leaders and businesses to support teens for camps or for special instruction or training.

When risk factors for substance abuse are identified, counseling is indicated. If the teen has a primary health care provider, he or she should be notified first. The family nurse practitioner or physician will usually know the family best and should be involved in the referral process if intensive therapy is needed. Otherwise, school nurses and counselors are excellent resources for counseling and screening for serious problems.

Promoting Effective Coping. The nurse's role is to identify adolescent substance users and those at risk for substance abuse, to work in the prevention of intoxicant-related accidents and prevention of substance abuse, and to provide nursing care and counseling in the treatment and rehabilitation of adolescent substance abusers.

Nurses on drug rehabilitation units should understand adolescent development and principles of communicating with adolescents. In working with troubled adolescents, it is important to treat them as individuals, not as typical adolescents. Adolescents believe that their problems are unique and resent inferences of "typical adolescent behavior." The nurse should be friendly and warm but should not behave like a peer. Teens need to feel that they are in competent hands. They need professional guidance and adult role models. Nurses who try to act like peers are often manipulated by adolescents.

Other ways nurses help in drug rehabilitation programs are by leading peer group discussions, going on group outings, and assisting with physical or creative activities. Activities are important because teens have often become so preoccupied with the substance that they forget how good other activities can feel. There are other "high" activities that can replace the chemical highs, such as drama, dancing, music, art realization techniques, meditation, and creative writing.

Promoting Effective Management of Therapeutic Regimen. Evaluation must be a part of intervention. Throughout the treatment, the nurse will evaluate the teen's response. For example, is the teen drug-free? Is the teen developing new skills to deal with problems? Is the family supportive but firm in their expectations? Are the adolescent and family communicating with one another? Is the adolescent making plans for school or work or doing things with friends? Treatment may need to be revised on the basis of evaluation of the response to the present treatment. For example, if the family can only *argue* when they are together, it might be better to have individual counseling sessions. Prognosis depends on the extent of the problems preceding substance use, the intensity of use, and the residual physical or mental effects of the substance.

Depression

Depression is generally defined as overall feelings of sadness or hopelessness. Depression as an illness is a syndrome of abnormal dejection that persists for an extended period of time and interferes with daily living (American Psychiatric Association, 1987). Depression was traditionally thought to occur only after about the age of 15 years; however, health professionals are increasingly recognizing the existence of depression in younger children.

Etiology/Incidence (Pathology)

Estimates of occurrence vary considerably because of the diverse diagnostic criteria used. A few investigations of normal children suggest a prevalence as high as 2 per cent (Kazdin, 1987). Girls are more likely than boys to suffer from depression, and it is more prevalent in adolescents than in children. There is an increase in the frequency of childhood depression presenting as ingestions or accidents. Children as young as 4 years have been seen with symptoms of depression.

Risk factors for depression can be genetic or environmental. Depression is known to occur within families, but it is difficult to separate the relative influence of genetics from environment. If one parent has a depressive disorder, the risk of depression for the offspring is 27 per cent; with two affected parents, the risk increases to 74 per cent (Aylward, 1985). There is also evidence that children who come from families with a history of alcoholism are at greater risk for depression.

Psychosocial factors also play a part in putting a child at risk for depression. Early trauma, self-blame, rigid family dynamics, a disturbance in mother-child relationships, or an unresolved loss experience have been reported to be precursors of depression (Valente, 1983). Any loss, such as the death of a loved one, rejection by a parent, a family move, divorce, abuse and maltreatment, or long-term hospitalization, puts a child at risk. Rigid parenting styles and the presence of a parental psychopathologic disorder have been cited as risk factors as well. Another contributing or related factor may be loss of self-esteem. Learning disabilities, chronic illness, or physical deformity may affect a child's self-esteem (Aylward, 1985).

A predominant risk factor for adolescent depression is female gender. Studies have shown that depression occurs twice as often in girls than in adolescent boys (Reinherz et al, 1991). The study of biologic correlates in adults has been extended to children. These studies involve investigation of growth hormone secretion, cortisol hypersecretion, and level of norepinephrine secretion.

Diagnostic Assessment

Clinical manifestations that vary with developmental level have not been clearly established during the early years. Depression can go unrecognized because it presents differently at each developmental stage. See Table 29–13 for these developmental distinctions of behavioral manifestations of depression. Depression can go unrecognized because children and adolescents have difficulties expressing their feelings and identifying their sources of distress. There are multiple sources of behaviors in youth that can mask an underlying depression. It is critical for nurses to assess for these behaviors.

According to the American Psychiatric Association (1987), the criteria for diagnosis of depression in children and adolescents may be associated with one of these psychiatric diagnoses: major depressive syndrome, adjustment disorder with depressed mood, and dysthymia. Generally, the greater the number of symptoms and the longer the duration, the more serious the depression. The criteria for diagnosis of a major depressive syndrome in children are the same as for adults and are as follows:

- At least five of the following symptoms have been present during the same 2-week period and represent a change from previous functioning; at least one of the symptoms is either (1) depressed mood or (2) loss of interest or pleasure. (Do not include symptoms that are clearly due to a physical condition, mood-incongruent delusions or hallucinations, incoherence, or marked loosening of associations.)
  - Depressed mood (or can be irritable mood in children and adolescents) most of the day, nearly every day, as indicated either by subjective account or observation by others.
  - Markedly diminished interest or pleasure in all, or almost all, activities most of the day, nearly every day (as indicated either by subjective ac count or observation by others of apathy most of the time).
  - Significant weight loss or weight gain when not dieting (e.g., more than 5 per cent of body weight in a month), or decrease or increase in appetite nearly every day (in children, consider failure to make expected weight gains).
  - Insomnia or hypersomnia nearly every day.
  - Psychomotor agitation or retardation nearly every day (observable by others, not merely subjective feelings of restlessness or being slowed down).
  - Fatigue or loss of energy nearly every day.
  - Feelings of worthlessness or excessive or inappropriate guilt (which may be delusional) nearly every day (not merely self-reproach or guilt about being sick).
  - Diminished ability to think or concentrate, or indecisiveness nearly every day (either by subjective account or as observed by others).
  - Recurrent thoughts of death (not just fear of dying), recurrent suicidal ideation without a specific plan, or a suicide attempt or a specific plan for committing suicide.

The criteria for diagnosis of an adjustment disorder with depressed mood include:

- The reaction occurs within 3 months of a stressor (change in school, parents separated, illness in family).
- The mood disturbance stems from acute stress. It is a situational depression with a clear precipitant.
- The maladaptive reaction has not persisted longer than 6 months.

The criteria for diagnosis of dysthymic disorder include:

- Quality of mood disturbance is chronic in nature.
- Depressed or irritable mood for 1 year.
- Requires the presence of at least two of the following symptoms:
  - Poor appetite or overeating.
  - Insomnia or hypersomnia.
  - Low energy/fatigue.
  - Low self-esteem.
  - Poor concentration/difficulty making decisions.
  - Sense of hopelessness.

TABLE 29-13
Developmental Distinctions in Behavioral Manifestations of Depression

Infancy	
(Biologic and deprivation syndromes)	Excessive irritability or lethargy
Feeding problems and sleep difficulty	Failure to thrive or rumination
Affective disturbances (blank stare, apathy)	Listlessness
Early Childhood (3–4 Yrs)	
(Abnormal motor activity)	Separation anxiety
High levels of activity	Social withdrawal
Physical aggressiveness, protecting behavior, and demonstrations of anger	Sleeping and eating problems
Enuresis, encopresis	Sad or irritable, emotionally labile and clinging behavior
Middle Childhood (5–8 Yrs)	
(More observable episodes of sadness; child still not reflective)	Academic underachievement
Somatization disorders	Self-esteem problems (self-blame, guilt)
Social withdrawal	Perceived rejection by parents
Lying, stealing	Excessive daydreaming
Accident proneness	School refusal
Physical aggression and oppositional behavior	Fear of death
Late Childhood (9–12 Yrs)	
(Involves low self-esteem and disappointment with self)	Unable to concentrate
Social isolation, especially from peers	School problems
Obvious sadness	Self-endangering behavior
Apathy	Suicidal ideation and suicide attempts
Sense of helplessness	Physical aggression
Irritability	Fear of death
Somatization disorders	Sleep disturbance
Anhedonia (no pleasure in usual activities)	School refusal
Psychogenic pain	Self-deprecating remarks, such as "I'm no good"
Adolescence	
Self-esteem problems	Social withdrawal
Hopelessness and fear of the future	Verbalization of suicidal thoughts and suicidal attempts
Looks at options in an inflexible all-or-none manner	Aggression toward others
Feels things will never change	Sleep disturbances
Somatization disorders	Changes in school performance
Psychogenic pain	Self-deprecating remarks, such as "I'm no good"
Anorexia nervosa	Sexual promiscuity
Substance abuse	Risk-taking behaviors
Antisocial behavior	

Therapeutic Management

The treatment plan ideally is designed in consultation with a mental health professional. Treatment methods vary and may range from short-term counseling regarding the development of coping strategies to individual or group psychotherapy, play therapy, or family therapy. Many experts believe it is essential for the family to be involved in the treatment plan to assist in identifying factors within the family that contribute to the child's problem.

Nursing Care

The nurse needs to differentiate between normal periods of depressed moods, which are brief and fade away, and profound depression, which persists and tends to get progressively worse. A youth with profound depression behaves noticeably in an irritable, tense manner and gives indications of self-esteem disturbance. In identifying depression, the nurse will note that depression takes different forms. In some situations, the depression will resemble adult depression. These youths may appear withdrawn; they may talk freely about feeling sad and lonely, rejected, and depressed; or, overwhelmed by feeling of despair and hopelessness, they may express suicidal thoughts. However, more often depression may take the form of somatic complaints, such as changes in eating patterns ranging from anorexia to overeating; digestive complaints, such as constipation; changes in sleeping habits ranging from insomnia to persistent fatigue; or changes in productivity, such as slow speech, slow thought processes, or even school failure.

Behavioral changes may present in the form of destructive, disruptive, or aggressive acting-out behavior. The youth may become defiant, truant, or delinquent or may repeatedly run away from home. In attempts to deny depression, adolescents may resort to drugs, alcohol, or sexual promiscuity. These behaviors may mask an underlying depression.

It is critical for the nurse to begin to recognize symptoms of depression and to assess the severity of depression. Data should be gathered through observation and use of interviewing skills via a social-mental health history. Losses, current stresses, and events having an impact on the child and family, as well as the child's and family's response to these events, should be assessed for directly. Nurses should assess for the loss of some significant relationship because loss is recognized as a primary etiologic agent in triggering the onset of depression.

The nurse may find that there has been a death or divorce in the family, an alteration in some significant relationship with a friend, or loss of a loved pet. Sometimes the depression may stem from shifting adolescent boyfriend-girlfriend relationships or from more serious problems, such as abortion or diagnosis of illness.

Depressive symptoms that persist for longer than 6 months, that are perceived to occur much more often in the patient than in peers, or that involve the child's serious consideration of suicide are of grave concern and require immediate further evaluation by a qualified professional. The nurse should assess for the presence and duration of depressive symptoms in any child. It can be useful to ask children what kinds of things they worry about.

An assessment of mental health status is often overlooked in dealing with pediatric clients. Incorporating a brief mental health assessment in the nursing data base obtained for each child may result in increased recognition and treatment of depression. Specific teaching about strategies for coping with stress may help prevent serious outcomes of depression, such as suicide. Once the presence and severity of the depression are recognized, the nurse's role involves seeking appropriate referrals for the child so that a therapeutic treatment plan can be established. Referral may include a child psychiatrist/psychologist or a master's prepared nurse or social worker trained in treating children and families.

In addition to making referrals, the role of the pediatric nurse is to establish a trusting relationship with the depressed youth in which the nurse is seen as a caring professional. Early nursing interventions may include acknowledging how "down" the youth seems to be and aiding in the verbal expression of his or her feelings. When a pediatric nurse observes depressive behaviors in any child or adolescent, it is important to use those behaviors to get more information via exploratory interviewing, such as "I notice you have trouble concentrating when I explain things. What are you thinking about?" Exploratory interviewing skills can be useful in providing support and data collection. Younger children may have difficulties articulating how they feel. Other ways to ascertain depression in younger children include questions such as "Do you ever feel down in the dumps?" or "Do you ever have bad feelings or an empty feeling inside?"

Listening to children is most important because it conveys respect and seriousness about their concerns. Incorporation of referral information into the current plan of care is necessary. Other interventions for the depressed child in the acute care setting may include developing schedules and routines with the child's input, providing information and teaching, and observing the child's interactions with peers.

The pediatric nurse assesses the family's response to the child's depression and begins to obtain information in regard to what the family defines as stressors and how well the family copes with them. This approach begins to place the child's symptoms in a broader context. The depressed child's family may need support, especially during the period of diagnosis and early treatment. Assessment of resources available to the family is critical at this time. It is important for both the pediatric nurse and the psychiatric clinician to maintain contact with the family, using open, honest communication. Many of the youth's behaviors reflect a long-standing maladaptive behavior pattern. The nurse needs to assess the family's expectations about treatment and to help them realize that treatment may take time to succeed. Inclusion of these interventions by the nurse may assist in prevention of ineffective family coping.

Nursing interventions that help adults develop their parenting skills will foster healthy parent-child relationships. Promoting open communication between parent and child is a goal of nursing. Other treatment modalities include cognitive therapy, social skills learning, stress management, and family therapy.

Suicide

Statistics from the National Center for Health (1990) place suicide as the second leading cause of death (preceded by accidents) in the 15- to 19-year-old age category. Suicide is the tenth leading cause of death in younger children; accidents are the leading cause. The suicide rate for adolescents and young adults between 15 and 24 years has increased more than 300 per cent over the past three decades (Blumenthal, 1990).

There is speculation that the actual numbers of deaths by suicide may be higher than reported figures. It is thought in young children and adolescents that accidents may mask actual suicide attempts. Because suicide produces tremendous guilt feelings in the survivors, death in which suicide is not clearly evident may be attributed to natural causes or labeled accidental. An example is the single-vehicle automobile accident in which a direct cause cannot be determined. Statistics may also be underestimated because suicidal gestures may not be taken seriously; thereby suicide is underreported, in addition to being underreported because of social stigma.

Furthermore, the research suggests that suicide completions represent only a small proportion of the range of suicidal behaviors. Estimates vary from 50 to 300 attempts for each suicide completion (Garfinkel, 1987). The spectrum of suicidal behavior ranges from the overt behaviors of suicide attempts to the covert behaviors of *suicidal ideation*. "Suicidal ideation" refers to the cognitive component of suicidal behavior. "Suicidal ideation" has been defined as "the domain of thoughts and ideas about: death, suicide and serious self-injurious behaviors including thoughts related to the planning, conduct and outcome (e.g., response of others) to one's suicidal behavior" (Reynolds, 1991, p 66).

Adolescents in general are most successful at suicide with the first attempt because they tend to use drastic methods with no rescue. A difference exists between adolescent boys and girls regarding successful suicidal efforts. Although girls are more likely to attempt suicide, which should be interpreted as a cry for help, boys have a much higher suicide rate, up to four times that of girls. Another fact of importance is that with each succeeding attempt at suicide, success becomes more likely.

Suicidal methods also vary between the sexes. In successful suicides, both sexes use firearms most frequently. Firearms are the leading method with boys, followed by hanging (Shaffer et al, 1988). Drug overdoses are the most common method for both sexes for attempted suicide. Girls more frequently use jumping than boys do; younger children also use jumping.

In younger children, death is not always seen as final and may be perceived to be reversible. Suicide may be sought as an escape from painful aspects of life (e.g., to join a dead loved one). Adolescents generally have a better sense of death's permanence. Younger children use more irrational thought processes in thinking about suicide (e.g., to make an important person love them or punish those who hurt them, believing they will see the effects of their action on others). Adolescents are more rational in explaining suicidal behavior (e.g., "I just can't take it anymore"). Both age groups are suggestible to suicide in different ways. The process of suicide in teens is more peer-driven and vulnerable to external factors (e.g., drugs, peers, job loss). Adolescence is also a developmental stage involving more risk taking. The process of suicide in younger children is less peer-driven and more embedded in family dynamics. Generally speaking, adolescents are more likely to attempt suicide as a result of impulsive behavior (Pfeffer, 1986, 1989).

Etiology/Incidence (Pathophysiology)

The suicide rate below age 14 years is 1.5 deaths per 100,000 per year; it rises to 9 deaths per 100,000 per year in adolescents from 15 to 19 years of age (National Center for Health Statistics, 1990). Suicide attempts seem to have a direct relationship with the amount of stress experienced by the adolescent. Statistics reveal higher suicide rates among high school dropouts than among students in high school; college students have higher suicide rates than do adolescents of the same age who are not in college. Other differences are noted in geographic locations. The Northern states show a higher suicide rate among African-American youths, whereas, in the South, the rate is higher among whites. A study of international statistics indicates that suicide is a relatively unimportant cause of death in developing countries (Barraclough, 1988).

Causative factors related to adolescent suicide or attempted suicide are difficult to isolate. Suicide most likely results from the compounding of several factors. Retrospective research studies indicate that depression is a common preceding factor in many adolescent suicides. Loss of an important relationship in the child's life is an important risk factor for suicides, as it is for depression. Another commonly cited preceding factor is social isolation. Peck (1981) reports that a substantial number of suicides occur in boys with isolated lifestyles and "loner" relationships. Adolescence seems to be a developmental period of increasing vulnerability for factors that have been associated with attempted and successful suicides. The task of gaining a sense of identity can lead to feelings of self-doubt and self-esteem disturbance, particularly when adolescents compare themselves with their peers. Feelings of social isolation result when adolescents perceive that their peers have greater independence, as interpreted from the social behaviors of the group. Modes of dress, interactions with the opposite sex, and independence in transportation and finance are but a few examples of social behaviors that have exaggerated importance in adolescence. Other factors that may indicate greater risk include (1) real or perceived public humiliation, (2) breakup of an adolescent love relationship, and (3) recent fight with parents or significant others.

Diagnostic Assessment

Most victims of adolescent suicide have had a history of chronic childhood and family problems (Matteson, 1987). Severe depression and suicide rarely occur spontaneously but are preceded by emotional conflicts associated with the onset of adolescence. Risk indicators for suicide are listed in Table 29–14. Many suicidal adolescents have experienced the warning signs for at least a month before the suicide or the attempt.

Days or weeks of loneliness precede the suicide attempt. This is often due to the loss of the few remaining relationships, such as a close relative or friend. Valente and Saunders (1987) cite the existence of a "ripple effect": bereavement and feelings of loss in response to the suicide of a friend influence other adolescents to attempt suicide (i.e., cluster suicides).

Warning signals include any threats of suicide or talk of personal death, such as questions about how many pills it would take to kill oneself or statements showing a belief that the family would be better off without the individual. Another danger signal may be a sudden upswing in mood in a previously depressed child or the sudden giving away of highly valued personal possessions. These behaviors can indicate that the adolescent has now actually made the decision to commit suicide.

Psychologic autopsies (retrospective interviews of significant others after suicide completion) have identified the following variables present at or before the time of a successful suicide: 55 per cent had history of suicidal threats; 40 per cent had history of suicide attempts; 70 per cent exhibited antisocial behavior; and 65 per cent exhibited withdrawn behavior. Any adolescent thought to be considering suicide should be asked about suicidal ideation. A referral to a mental health professional is required to evaluate the extent of the problem.

TABLE 29-14
Risk Indicators: Suicide

Depression
Expressed feelings of hopelessness
Lack of close friends
Feelings of isolation
Loss of a valued relationship through divorce, death, or separation
Feelings of sexual inadequacy
Substance abuse
Disrupted family structure or communication (divorce/separation)
School failure
School expulsion or suspension
Dramatic change in personality or behavior (e.g., marked change in sleep or eating patterns, disregard for personal appearance)
"Getting affairs in order"/"Saying goodbye" type of behavior, such as giving away valued personal possessions
Discussion of death thoughts
Threats of suicide
Talking about the future in terms demonstrating they do not expect to be a part of it
Pattern of recurrent accidental injuries
Previous suicide attempts
Family history of suicide
Perfectionist individuals
Member of an alienated group: gay/lesbian youths
Initial 3–24 hrs in jail
Incest, child abuse, runaway
Serious psychiatric problems
Low levels of 5-hydroxyindoleacetic acid

Therapeutic Management

The American Association of Suicidology has been established to coordinate national suicide prevention centers and is a source of information and educational materials. The magnitude of the adolescent suicide problem has stimulated establishment of crisis intervention centers. Suicidal behavior is the most frequently occurring psychiatric emergency in adolescents (Reynolds, 1991). One service offered through these agencies is a telephone hotline manned by professionals and trained volunteers. Callers are encouraged to talk through their concerns while the volunteer evaluates the immediate need of the caller. Crisis intervention techniques, along with referrals to appropriate agencies, constitute a large portion of services given by the telephone counselors.

Telephone interventions have been successful in helping some, but major emphasis is still needed on education for prevention. Several experts report on the development of high school–based prevention programs (Reynolds, 1991; Valente & Saunders, 1987). Although their effectiveness is questioned by some researchers, their establishment reflects society's concern about suicide among adolescents. Adolescents need to be exposed to a comprehensive education program. They should know the scope of the suicide problem in their age group and the progressive stages of deterioration leading to suicide. Adolescent participation in prevention needs to be increased; that is, adolescents need to be granted permission through education to report the indications of potential suicide in their peers. Adolescents or adults who recognize signs or suspect a suicidal intention should never dismiss the idea but should seek professional assistance immediately. It is critical that the subject of suicide be addressed directly.

When an adolescent has attempted suicide, the safest course of action is hospitalization (American Academy of Pediatrics, 1988, 1990). Inquiry is made into the events that preceded the suicide attempt. Family members are also interviewed to determine the recent stresses and current problems of the adolescent. Intervention is individualized; some require brief, crisis-oriented intervention, whereas others show evidence of depression and psychiatric illness requiring long-term care. The issue of suicide is usually not the only significant issue in therapy except during the suicide crisis itself (Valente, 1989). Adolescents who attempt suicide require carefully planned follow-up care.

Nursing Care

Because pediatric nurses, especially school nurses, have daily contact with large numbers of adolescents, they have the opportunity to contribute to the prevention of suicide. Each individual needs to be assessed in terms of his or her mental health status. Assessment of mental health should be seen as an integral part of the nursing data base. Children and adolescents can be amazingly open in communicating death thoughts to a nurse in a confidential professional setting. Nurses need to be aware that many well-adjusted adolescents report thinking of death. However, affirmative answers to the specific question "Have you ever thought about death or about killing yourself?" need to be explored in depth, with specific questions about when such thoughts occurred and about the frequency and duration of these types of thought.

Questions pertaining to the lethality of the child's or adolescent's potential for committing suicide must be assessed. The child or adolescent who indicates having a specific plan for suicide within the next 24 to 72 hours that includes the lethal method, available means, and no rescue plan must be considered at high risk for suicide. Children and adolescents are at moderate risk for suicide attempt with a less immediate plan of action and methods. Suicide attempts allowing rescue, such as wrist cutting and drug overdose, would be of this risk group. Individuals in the low-risk category would be those whose plans are vague and ambiguous with rescue plans (Valente, 1989). For additional information on suicide assessment, see Table 29–15.

TABLE 29-15
Components of Suicide Assessment

Intent

Assessment of intent directly addresses the child's desire to die; the greater the specificity with intent, the greater is the risk

Assessment includes statements such as

1. "Sometimes its not unusual for kids to have thoughts of wanting to die."
2. "Have you ever had thoughts like 'I want to die'?"

Specificity

If child/adolescent indicates intent, it is critical to ask

1. "When did you last have these thoughts?"
2. "What were you thinking of doing?" "When were you thinking of carrying it out?"
3. "What do you think would happen?"
4. "Have you ever tried to hurt yourself?"

The more specific the plan, the greater the risk

Means

Ask questions about the methods that were planned for use; the more specific and available the method, the greater the risk

1. "What method were you planning to use?"

Supports

Ask questions about what supports are available, such as

1. "Who would you like to talk to?" "Is there someone you want to call?"

All threats of suicide need to be taken seriously by parents and nurses. Immediate referral to mental health professionals should be made *whenever* there is any question about the adolescent's intent. Professionals who work with suicidal youths believe that suicide is not a sudden decision but the final result of repeated warnings given by the victims. Parents may fail to recognize behavioral changes signifying an altered emotional state. Parents may cope with such changes by denial. Nurses and teachers should be aware of the multiplicity of factors that influence adolescent behavior; they may be the first to detect significant deterioration in an adolescent's behaviors and outlook. Valente and Saunders (1987) state that school and pediatric nurses "understand that many adolescents use physical complaints as a good reason to visit the school nurse to talk about their depressions, discouragements, disappointments and feelings that life may not be worth living."

In the acute care setting, safety of the patient is the highest priority. Protocols need to be developed for the management of children with the potential for suicide. While evaluation by mental health professionals is awaited, several interventions can be made with the goal of establishing a supportive relationship, providing for safety, and further assessing the child and family. When a child is assessed as suicidal, one-to-one staffing should be implemented until further psychiatric evaluation occurs and decisions about level of observation are made. Nurses can act to secure a safe environment by removing objects that a child may use for self-harm. The child's family should be made aware and included in the process.

In addition to assessing overall mental health status, pediatric nurses need to assess and teach personalized coping strategies. Coping techniques appropriate for children and adolescents include actively seeking out friends, using daily exercise and deep breathing as tension relievers, recognizing sources of stress and of one's own limitations, and attempting to change stressful situations over which the youth has control or to change his or her own reactions to stressful situations over which the youth has no control. With guidance, children can learn to focus on the positive aspects of stressful situations and to maximize their own coping abilities.

Autism

Autism is a developmental disorder that involves alterations in developmental rates, sensory input and output, communication, and social relationships. The disorder is usually diagnosed before the age of 36 months. Autistic children have (1) problems in verbal and nonverbal communications, (2) problems in reciprocal social interactions, and (3) a restricted repertoire of activities and interests (Dalton & Howell, 1989). These children have impaired relationships with people and may exhibit other asocial behaviors.

Etiology/Incidence (Pathophysiology)

Most recent data suggest that the prevalence of autistic disorder is 4 to 5 per 10,000 children. The disorder is more common in boys (American Psychiatric Association, 1987).

Little is known about possible causative factors or conditions preceding or accompanying autism. Conditions found to be associated with autism in some children include epilepsy (Tuchman et al, 1991), mental retardation (Dalton & Howell, 1989), biochemical imbalance (Panksepp & Sahlet, 1987), and inadequate development or functioning of the left hemisphere due to early trauma with the right hemisphere assuming a compensatory role (Dawson, 1987). It is considered by some to be a neurologic abnormality (Connell, 1985). It appears to be biogenic rather than psychogenic in origin and is recognized as a behavioral outcome or underlying abnormality in brain functioning (Dalton & Howell, 1989).

There is some evidence that many different perinatal factors and autism are associated (Tsai, 1987). Numerous investigations have searched for biochemical correlates, such as hormones, amino acids, trace elements, and various metabolites. No biochemical marker has been identified (Volkmar & Cohen, 1986), although elevated serotonin concentrations, elevated levels of homovanillic acid, and elevated opioids (a newly discovered group of brain neuroregulators) have been found in individuals with autism (Elliot & Ciaranello, 1987; Yuwiler & Freedman, 1987). Although it is apparent that an abnormality in central nervous system function exists, the site or mechanism of dysfunction is not understood (Volkmar & Cohen, 1986). Researchers continue to explore different theories in understanding the cause of autism, and knowledge is expanding rapidly.

Diagnostic Assessment

The DSM-III-R places autistic disorder under the broader classification of pervasive developmental disorders. Previous diagnostic labels included symbiotic psychosis and atypical ego development. Refer to Table 29–16 for the DSM-III-R criteria.

Autism has two distinct types of clinical onset. In some children, developmental delays are observable during the first few months of life, which has been referred to as *infantile autism*. These children appear detached and demonstrate no anticipatory social responses. They exhibit an inability to form social relationships. They resist physical contact, are either unusually quiet or fussy, and do not vocalize. They fail to develop sleeping and eating cycles or interactive behavior. As toddlers, they do not imitate speech or gestures.

The second group of children display normal development until age 12 to 18 months of age. Then, they begin to regress, lose speech, withdraw from social contact, and begin to demonstrate repetitive motor behaviors. Regardless of age at onset, the preschool autistic child often demonstrates ritualistic and compulsive behavior.

The ability to communicate is severely impaired, and changes in routines or surroundings may provoke tantrumlike rages. Detached, withdrawn, and unresponsive, the child appears to have disturbance of perception, speech, language, and sometimes mobility as well as an inability to relate to people. This child does not react to either verbal commands or sounds; no response may be evinced to very loud, sudden noises. The child shows no reaction to new persons or objects in the environment and may walk into objects as if they are not seen. There is lack of response to tactile or painful stimuli. Eye contact may be less frequent or inappropriate. Speech and language may be delayed, and echolalia (repetition of sounds) is common. The child frequently flicks, twirls, or spins toy objects rather than playing with them appropriately. There is little peer interaction and infrequent or delayed social smile. The child is disinterested in people and surroundings but has an unusual interest in

TABLE 29-16
The DSM III-R Criteria for Autistic Disorder

At least 8 of the following 16 items are present, these to include at least 2 items from A, 1 from B, and 1 from C. Consider a criterion to be met only if the behavior is abnormal for the person's developmental level.

A. Qualitative impairment in reciprocal social interaction as manifested by the following:
(The examples within parentheses are arranged so that those first mentioned are more likely to apply to younger or more handicapped, and the later ones to older or less handicapped, persons with this disorder.)

- Marked lack of awareness of the existence or feelings of others (e.g., treats a person as if he or she were a piece of furniture; does not notice another person's distress; apparently has no concept of the need of others for privacy)
- No or abnormal seeking of comfort at times of distress (e.g., does not come for comfort even when ill, hurt, or tired; seeks comfort in a stereotyped way, e.g., says "cheese, cheese, cheese" whenever hurt)
- No or impaired imitation (e.g., does not wave bye-bye; does not copy mother's domestic activities; mechanical imitation of others' actions out of context)
- No or abnormal social play (e.g., does not actively participate in simple games; prefers solitary play activities; involves other children in play only as "mechanical aids")
- Gross impairment in ability to make peer friendships (e.g., no interest in making peer friendships; despite interest in making friends, demonstrates lack of understanding of conventions of social interaction, e.g., reads phone book to uninterested peer)

B. Qualitative impairment in verbal and nonverbal communication, and in imaginative activity, as manifested by the following:
(The items are arranged so that those first listed are more likely to apply to younger or more handicapped, and the later ones to older or less handicapped, persons with this disorder.)

- No mode of communication, such as communicative babbling, facial expression, gesture, mime, or spoken language
- Markedly abnormal nonverbal communication, as in the use of eye-to-eye gaze, facial expression, body posture, or gestures to initiate or modulate social interaction (e.g., does not anticipate being held, stiffens when held, does not look at the person or smile when making a social approach, does not greet parents or visitors, has a fixed stare in social situations)
- Absence of imaginative activity, such as playacting of adult roles, fantasy characters, or animals; lack of interest in stories about imaginary events
- Marked abnormalities in the production of speech, including volume, pitch, stress, rate, rhythm, and intonation (e.g., monotonous tone, questionlike melody, or high pitch)
- Marked abnormalities in the form or content of speech, including stereotyped and repetitive use of speech (e.g., immediate echolalia or mechanical repetition of television commercial); use of "you" when "I" is meant (e.g., using "You want cookie?" to mean "I want a cookie"); idiosyncratic use of words or phrases (e.g., "Go on green riding" to mean "I want to go on the swing"); or frequent irrelevant remarks (e.g., starts talking about train schedules during a conversation about sports)
- Marked impairment in the ability to initiate or sustain a conversation with others, despite adequate speech (e.g., indulging in lengthy monologues on one subject regardless of interjections from others)

C. Markedly restricted repertoire of activities and interests, as manifested by the following:

- Stereotyped body movements, e.g., hand flicking or twisting, spinning, head banging, complex whole-body movements
- Persistent preoccupation with parts of objects (e.g., sniffing or smelling objects, repetitive feeling of texture of materials, spinning wheels of toy cars) or attachment to unusual objects (e.g., insists on carrying around a piece of string)
- Marked distress over changes in trivial aspects of environment (e.g., when a vase is moved from usual position)
- Unreasonable insistence on following routines in precise detail (e.g., insisting that exactly the same route always be followed when shopping)
- Markedly restricted range of interests and a preoccupation with one narrow interest (e.g., interested only in lining up objects, in amassing facts about meteorology, or in pretending to be a fantasy character)

D. Onset during infancy or childhood

- Specify if childhood onset (after 36 mos of age)

From American Psychiatric Association: *Diagnostic and statistical manual of mental disorders, third edition, revised.* Washington, DC: American Psychiatric Association, 1987.

inanimate objects. He or she is unable to perform two tasks simultaneously. Vision appears to be more peripheral than central. The head is held to the side, and the child walks on the ball of the foot, frequently and habitually flapping the hands. Attempts to comfort the child are often ineffective, and behavior is mechanical and disconnected. They generally do not develop peer relationships. About three fourths of autistic children demonstrate some degree of mental disability. These children may engage in self-mutilative behaviors.

Therapeutic Management

Children with autism may be admitted to the hospital for diagnostic evaluation. Previously, these children were institutionalized and did not have access to a stimulating environment or a warm, symbiotic relationship with a caring person.

The trend in management is to treat these children in community-based programs. The most effective management is a structured education program in the environment of a special classroom (Haber et al, 1987). This should be begun as soon as the symptoms are recognized. Behavior modification is used in an attempt to change the child's autistic symptoms.

Positive reinforcement in the form of food, affection, or activity (feeding the gerbil, water play) should be given immediately when the child responds appropriately. Accurate and detailed recording is necessary to note change in behavior. In a group setting, aversive conditioning, such as a sharp "NO Timmy!" may eventually be effective. Any momentary awareness must immediately be rewarded to help draw the child from the world of fantasy and introversion into the world of reality.

With the assistance of a warm, caring teacher, the child will receive guidance in impulse control, gross and fine motor coordination, and language development as well as any physical contributing factors. Deafness and developmental aphasia must be ruled out.

Consistent and structured care from a limited number of receptive people can allow the child to develop at her or his own speed in an individualized academic setting. Despite the intensive, individualized treatment that many children are receiving, approximately two thirds of children with autism need supervision and support for a lifetime (Volkmar & Cohen, 1986).

The National Society for Autistic Children* is dedicated to the education, welfare, and treatment of all children with severe disorders of communication and behavior. This is an active organization with annual national meetings and continued lobbying for the rights of autistic people. Parents may benefit from the suggestions and support of other parents who have children with similar problems.

Nursing Care

Nurses may encounter children with autism in a variety of settings and have an important role in the care of these children. The nurse uses interviewing skills to gather information in regard to developmental history and precipitants to current hospitalization to formulate assessment of the child and family. Assessment criteria include:

- Unusual lags or discrepancies in areas of development, particularly in communication or social interactions.
- Observations of parent-child interactions.
- Observation of child's interaction with environment.
- Observation of child's interaction with others.
- Use of medications.
- Physical examination.
- Presence of psychosocial stresses.
- Presence/absence of self-mutilative behaviors.
- Precipitants/triggers to problem behavior.
- Management of activities of daily living.
- Presence of supports to family.
- Family response to disorder.

Regardless of where children with autism are treated, they are a challenge to care for. Whereas efforts have been made to use medication in the treatment of autism, none has altered the course of the condition. Several medications (haloperidol, fenfluramine, naltrexone), however, may be used to manage and improve the behavioral symptoms, including hyperactivity, concentration problems, sleep disturbances, withdrawal, and self-mutilation (Dalton & Howell, 1989). Nursing actions include (1) establishment of an accurate behavioral data base, which allows the nurse to monitor the effect of medications on behavioral patterns, and (2) ongoing assessment of potential side effects.

In the acute care setting, a consistent group of caregivers can be useful in decreasing the child's need to adjust to a variety of people. The environment can be made more familiar by providing the child with her or his own toys and objects. To the extent possible, familiar routines and approaches to behavior management should occur while the child is in the acute care setting.

The nurse, as part of the treatment team, can begin to increase contact by sitting near the child for brief periods. Repatterning may be used to change rocking behaviors, masturbation, and others and invokes removing the stimulus and providing an alternative acceptable behavior. Interventions for self-mutilative behaviors include (1) identification of triggering event, (2) repattern behaviors, and (3) patient safety via protective devices (e.g., helmet, pads).

Nurses can assist the family in their attempts to cope with their feelings regarding the diagnosis of autism and the lifelong alterations the diagnosis entails. The family may feel overwhelmed and require support from nursing staff. Parents may feel guilt or blame, manifested by withdrawal from the child and staff during hospitalization. It is important to be consistent in our efforts to support the family. Parental involvement in developing the care plan is encouraged to empower the family.

Schizophrenia

The term "schizophrenia" describes the type of psychotic disorder characterized by a loss of contact with reality. The term "childhood schizophrenia" generally refers to psychotic disorders that appear after the first 5 years of life. In adolescents, this disease process is noted by a gradual disintegration in several areas of mental functioning. The lack of integration in thought processes is manifested most often by disturbed behavior, emotions, and speech patterns (Haber et al, 1987).

Disruptions in cognitive processes occur and may be manifested by autistic thinking, primitive thinking, loose associations, and delusions. Hallucinations are a common symptom and reflect a disturbance in perceptual abilities. In addition, the patient's affect and emotions may be inappropriate, blunted, or ambivalent. Withdrawal and isolation from others is common.

Etiology/Incidence (Pathophysiology)

The prevalence of all forms of schizophrenia in the general population is approximately 1 per cent. Both men and women are equally affected (American Psy-

*7910 Woodmont Ave., Bethesda, MD 20814 (301) 657–0881.

chiatric Association, 1987). However, the onset of schizophrenia is usually during late adolescent or early adult years. Thus, childhood-onset schizophrenia is rare (Asarnow et al, 1989).

No one factor has been identified as the cause of schizophrenia. Theories for explaining schizophrenia fall into biologic and psychosocial categories. Current findings strongly suggest a biologic cause. Schizophrenia has been linked to deficiencies in metabolic or neural functioning, and genetic factors seem to play an important role. Current research on schizophrenia focuses on genetics, brain biochemistry, brain structure, and function. All investigators have found a higher prevalence of the disorder among family members, and especially between identical twins. However, environmental stressors and unique temperamental styles seem to interact with biologic factors.

Various psychosocial theories exist for explaining the development of schizophrenia and focus on disturbed patterns of interaction in the family. Communication theory describes the double-bind pattern of interaction in which messages are conveyed in inconsistent and contradictory ways. Often these parents fail to acknowledge the validity of their children's feelings. Family systems theory views the schizophrenic family member as reflecting larger family dysfunction. Psychoanalytic theory views pose ego functioning as critical to the development of schizophrenia. Other psychosocial stressors, such as impaired parental communication, may affect biologic predispositions.

Diagnostic Assessment

Although schizophrenia usually appears in late adolescence, children who develop schizophrenia often display alterations in normal behavior, emotion, and thought. They are more socially withdrawn, have poorer peer relationships, and have fewer interests than normal children do. They may demonstrate extreme mood lability, inappropriate clinging, unexplained rage reactions, and hyperactivity. After age 5 years, symptoms of formal thought disorder and flat or inappropriate mood first appear.

Schizophrenia may be obvious from early childhood, or it may be triggered by a developmental crisis. For example, adolescent developmental tasks early or late can overwhelm a youth with a shaky ego and heighten already existing fears, resulting in a loss of sense of self. Feelings of ambivalence in the quest for independence or hostility due to unmet dependency needs is feared. These conflicting feelings and a biologic predisposition may lead to overt schizophrenic behavior characterized by delusions, hallucinations, and inappropriate emotional reactions.

It becomes more and more difficult for the adolescent to distinguish between fantasy and reality. The earliest symptoms may be noted as behavioral changes or alterations in habits. For example, the neat child becomes sloppy, or the casual child begins to rigidly adhere to routine. In the early stages of this disorder, the child may begin to exhibit overt signs of the struggle to maintain contact with reality by displaying rituals or phobias, followed by paranoid delusions or hallucinations. Depersonalization and motor and speech disturbance become apparent.

The DSM-III-R criteria for the diagnosis of schizophrenia are listed in Table 29–17.

Therapeutic Management

The care of a child or adolescent with schizophrenia is a specialized area of practice; therefore, the reader is referred to texts in the field of psychiatry and psychiatric nursing. Inpatient evaluations, medication management, and behavioral programs are the standard of care.

Nursing Care

Nurses first encounter children and adolescents with symptoms of schizophrenia in office, school, or hospital settings. Information from parents is collected about the history and progress of the illness. Observations of parent-youth interactions and the effectiveness of the child's interactions with the environment are documented. Other needed information may include the extent of impulsivity, regression, or bizarre behavior; whether there is any self-mutilating or aggressive behavior; whether the child can distinguish between reality and fantasy; and current stresses affecting the family. The child's mental status examination is done.

Occasionally, a nurse in a pediatric setting will need to provide care for the schizophrenic child or adolescent. Such care makes unusual demands on the nursing staff. The bizarre behavior may disrupt a unit designed primarily to serve medical needs. The nurse who reacts emotionally to the disturbed behavior cannot function therapeutically. Repeated episodes of disruptive behavior can make members of the nursing staff feel they are losing control. Repeated attempts to help a schizophrenic young person may be rebuffed as she or he attempts to avoid any close interpersonal encounter. Such rejection of "helping" overtures can leave a nurse feeling helpless or inadequate. Nurses must recognize that the behavior is symptomatic of the illness. Group conferences with all health team members is essential for planning therapeutic interventions and assisting staff to understand their emotional responses to the patient. These children are often anxious and frightened, and their anxiety increases in the hospital environment.

Nursing interventions with the schizophrenic child focus on decreasing anxiety. The nurse should facilitate consistency in the schizophrenic child's environment as much as possible. Consistent caregivers can be assigned to decrease the number of staff the patient has to relate to and provide opportunities to build trust. Consistent routines can be established to provide structure, and the environment should be

TABLE 29-17
The DSM III-R Criteria for the Diagnosis of Schizophrenia

A. Presence of characteristic psychotic symptoms in the active phase: either (1), (2), or (3) for at least 1 wk (unless the symptoms are successfully treated)
   1. Two of the following:
      a. Delusions
      b. Prominent hallucinations (throughout the day for several days or several times a week for several weeks, each hallucinatory experience not being limited to a few brief moments)
      c. Incoherence of marked loosening of associations
      d. Catatonic behavior
      e. Flat or grossly inappropriate affect
   2. Bizarre delusions (e.g., involving a phenomenon that the person's culture would regard as totally implausible, e.g., thought broadcasting, being controlled by a dead person)
   3. Prominent hallucinations, as defined in 1b above, of a voice with content having no apparent relation to depression or elation, or a voice keeping up a running commentary on the person's behavior or thoughts, or two or more voices conversing with each other

B. During the course of the disturbance, functioning in such areas as work, social relations, and self-care is markedly below the highest level achieved before onset of the disturbance (or, when the onset is in childhood or adolescence, failure to achieve expected level of social development)

C. Schizoaffective disorder and mood disorder with psychotic features have been ruled out; e.g., if a major depressive or manic syndrome has ever been present during an active phase of the disturbance, the total duration of all episodes of a mood syndrome has been brief relative to the total duration of the active and residual phases of the disturbance

D. Continuous signs of the disturbance for at least 6 mos; the 6-mo period must include an active phase (at least 1 wk, or less if symptoms have been successfully treated) during which there were psychotic symptoms characteristic of schizophrenia (symptoms in A), with or without a prodromal or residual phase, as defined in the following:

   Prodromal phase: A clear deterioration in functioning before the active phase of the disturbance that is not due to a disturbance in mood or to a psychoactive substance use disorder and that involves at least two of the symptoms listed below

   Residual phase: After the active phase of the disturbance, persistence of at least two of the symptoms noted below, these not being due to a disturbance in mood or to a psychoactive substance use disorder

   Prodromal or Residual Symptoms:
   1. Marked social isolation or withdrawal
   2. Marked impairment in role functioning as wage earner, student, or homemaker
   3. Markedly peculiar behavior (e.g., collecting garbage, talking to self in public, hoarding food)
   4. Marked impairment in personal hygiene and grooming
   5. Blunted or inappropriate affect
   6. Digressive, vague, overelaborate, or circumstantial speech, or poverty of speech, or poverty of content of speech
   7. Odd beliefs or magical thinking, influencing behavior and inconsistent with cultural norms (e.g., superstitiousness, belief in clairvoyance, telepathy, "sixth sense," "others can feel my feelings," overvalued ideas, ideas of reference)
   8. Unusual perceptual experiences (e.g., recurrent illusions, sensing the presence of a force or person not actually present)
   9. Marked lack of initiative, interests, or energy

   Examples: Six months of prodromal symptoms with 1 wk of symptoms from A; no prodromal symptoms with 6 mos of symptoms from A; no prodromal symptoms with 1 wk of symptoms from A and 6 mos of residual symptoms

E. It cannot be established that an organic factor initiated and maintained the disturbance

F. If there is a history of autistic disorder, the additional diagnosis of schizophrenia is made only if prominent delusions or hallucinations are also present

From American Psychiatric Association: *Diagnostic and statistical manual of mental disorders, third edition, revised.* Washington, DC: American Psychiatric Association, 1987.

made as calm as possible to decrease anxiety. Communication and directions are kept simple, clear, and succinct. Frequent, brief, and regular contacts are made with the patient to provide contact with reality and to build trust.

Psychotropic medications may be used to lessen anxiety and other symptoms such as delusions, hallucinations, and agitation. The nurse has a critical role in monitoring the impact of medications on baseline symptoms as well as for side effects. Although it is challenging to care for these children, it can be rewarding as well.

KEY CONCEPTS

Concepts Related to Basic Information

- A child's ability to cope is influenced by a number of variables, which include age, development, temperament, "goodness of fit," stress, and self-concept.
- A phobia is a fear to an exaggerated degree of objects or events that in reality are not dangerous and to most people do not evoke such excessive fear.
- The term "school phobia" applies to a variable set of symptoms that represent an underlying anxiety in the child whose absences from school are excessive.
- The prevalence of school phobia is difficult to estimate because many cases are handled by the school system or the child's primary health care provider.
- Enuresis is defined as the involuntary passage of urine by a child over the age of 3 years; it can occur during the day (diurnal enuresis), during the night (nocturnal enuresis), or at both times.
- Encopresis refers to persistent fecal soiling in a child older than 4 years of age; the incidence of encopresis is reported to be between 1.5 and 3 per cent in 7- to 8-year-old children.

- The essential features of ADHD are signs of inattention, impulsivity, and hyperactivity that are inappropriate.
- Conduct disorders are more prevalent in boys than in girls in a ratio of 3:1 and comprise the largest group of psychiatrically disturbed children, with estimates varying from 47 to 67 per cent.
- Nutritional conflicts can lead to a number of disorders including obesity, anorexia nervosa, and bulimia.
- Bulimia is an eating disorder characterized by episodes of binge eating alternating with purge behavior.
- Alcohol is the most widely abused substance in the age group 12 to 17 years.
- Suicide is the second leading cause of death in the 15- to 19-year-old age category.
- Depression as an illness is a syndrome of abnormal dejection that persists for an extended period of time and interferes with daily living.
- Autism is a developmental disorder that involves alterations in developmental rates, sensory input and output, communication, and social relationships.
- The term "schizophrenia" describes the type of psychotic disorder characterized by a loss of contact with reality.

Concepts Related to Nursing Assessment

- Understanding the child's behavior and how the child copes is essential for assessing the child's mental health.
- Assessment ideally includes interviews with child and family members, observations of the child in interactions with others, data gathering from questionnaires or behavior check lists, and parental recordings of the child's behavior.
- Because the symptoms are so varied and nonspecific with school phobia, the primary care provider is challenged to determine the underlying issue.
- In many instances, the enuresis has been present for months or years; therefore, it is important to know why the family has sought assistance at this particular time.
- The diagnosis of encopresis begins with a thorough history that assesses the child's daily habits and psychosocial milieu of the family, history of toilet training, and amount and frequency of stools.
- Early diagnosis of ADHD is important for avoiding some of the long-lasting psychologic effects this disorder may have on a child.
- Several factors need to be considered in making an evaluation of the child's lying: developmental stage and age of the child, duration and frequency of the behavior, and whether there is actual intent to distort the truth.
- The major reasons for nutritional assessment of the child or adolescent who is obese are to identify dietary practices of the family, obtain a baseline of calorie and nutrient intake and anthropometric measurements, promote healthful dietary practices, and provide parents with the opportunity to express concerns and ask questions.
- Identification of anorexia may be difficult because initially there may be no overt signs.
- The nurse needs to differentiate between normal periods of depressed moods, which are brief and fade away, and profound depression.
- Causative factors related to adolescent suicide or attempted suicide are difficult to isolate; suicide most likely results from the compounding of several factors.

Concepts Related to Nursing Intervention

- Interventions are individualized for each child and family, requiring coordination via a multidisciplinary team.
- Perhaps the most valuable and successful intervention to emphasize in working with behaviorally disordered children is *consistency*.
- Two fundamental considerations that the nurse takes into account in working with the youth with school phobia are mandatory school attendance and the child's capability for resuming a place in the community of peers.
- In planning a management program for children with enuresis or encopresis, it is important to have the cooperation of the child and the parents; otherwise, success is unlikely.
- The goal of the management program for encopresis is to provide medication, diet, and toileting ritual that encourages the child to develop normal defecation habits.
- The major goals for the child with ADHD are to relieve impulsivity/hyperactivity, to relieve stress, and to meet expectations of the home and school environment.
- To intervene effectively with children who steal, the nurse must determine the reasons for stealing.
- Nurses can counsel parents whose child has problems with aggression about child management techniques, such as setting consistent limits, showing affection, and assisting with expressions of frustration and anger.
- The nurse who cares for the hospitalized adolescent with anorexia must be careful to monitor intake and output and observe eating patterns, levels of exercise, family interactions, and compulsive behaviors.
- Patterns of abuse that are intensive or dependent

clearly necessitate family or individual therapy or both.

- All threats of suicide need to be taken seriously by parents and nurses.

REFERENCES

American Academy of Pediatrics, Committee on Adolescence. (1988). Suicide and suicide attempts in adolescents and young adults. *Pediatrics, 81*(2), 322–324.

American Academy of Pediatrics, Committee on School Health (1990). The potentially suicidal student in the school setting. *Pediatrics, 89*(3), 481–483.

American Psychiatric Association (1987). *Diagnostic and statistical manual of mental disorders* (3rd ed., rev.). Washington, DC: Author.

Apter, S., & Conoley, J. (1984). *Childhood behavior disorders and emotional disturbance.* Englewood Cliffs, NJ: Prentice-Hall.

Asarnow, R., Asarnow, J., & Strandburg, R. (1989). Schizophrenia: A developmental perspective. In D. Cicchatti (Ed.), *The emergence of a discipline: Rochester symposium on developmental psychopathology.* Hillsdale, NJ: Erlbaum.

Aylward, G. (1985). Understanding and treatment of childhood depression. *Journal of Pediatrics, 107*(1), 1–9.

Barnard, K. (1985). Studying patterns of behavior. *MCN: American Journal of Maternal Child Nursing, 5,* 358.

Barraclough, B. (1988). International variation in the suicide rate of 15–24 year olds. *Social Psychiatry and Psychiatric Epidemiology, 23,* 75–84.

Behrman, R. (1992). *Textbook of pediatrics.* Philadelphia: WB Saunders.

Bernstein, G., & Garfinkel, B. (1986). School phobia: The overlap of affective and anxiety disorders. *Journal of the American Academy of Child Psychiatry, 25,* 235.

Blagg, N., & Yule, W. (1989). The behavioral treatment of school refusal—a comparative study. *Behavioral Research and Therapy, 22,* 119.

Blank, J., & Alexander, M. (1988). Factors associated with obesity in Mexican-American preschool children—a cardiovascular risk. *Progress in Cardiovascular Nursing, 3*(1), 27–31.

Blumenthal, S. (1990). Youth suicide: Risk factors, assessment, and treatment of adolescent and young adult suicidal patients. *Psychiatric Clinics of North America, 13,* 511–556.

Brook, C. (1972). Evidence for a sensitive period in adipose cell replication in man. *Lancet, 2,* 624–627.

Bruch, H. (1973). *Eating disorders: Obesity, anorexia nervosa, and the person within.* New York: Basic Books.

Bryant, S., & Kopeski, L. (1986, April). Psychiatric nursing assessment of the eating disorder client. *Topics in Clinical Nursing, 8*(1), 57–66.

Caddell, A. (1983, June). Under the influence. *Nursing Times, 79*(25), 9–10.

Carey, W. (1972). Clinical applications of infant temperament measurements. *Pediatrics, 81,* 823.

Castiglia, P. (1987). Obesity in infants and toddlers. *Journal of Pediatric Health Care, 4,* 218–220.

Chess, S., & Thomas, A. (1983). Individuality: Dynamics of individual behavioral development. In M. Levine, et al. (Eds.), *Developmental-behavioral pediatrics.* Philadelphia: WB Saunders.

Chess, S., Thomas, A., & Birch, H. (1970, August). The origin of personality. *Scientific American,* 102–108.

Cohen, M. I. (1983). Marijuana—What is really known? In I. F. Litt (Ed.), *Adolescent substance abuse, report of the 14th Ross Roundtable on critical approaches to common pediatric problems* (pp 10–16). Columbus, OH: Ross Laboratories.

Connell, H. (1985). *Essentials of child psychiatry (2nd ed.).* London: Blackwell Scientific Publications.

Crawshaw, J. (1985). Anorexia and bulimia: The earlier cues. *Patient Care, 19,* 80–95.

Cromier, B., et al (1992). Psychosocial screening. *Journal of Adolescent Health, 13,* 52S–57S.

Dalton, S., & Howell, C. (1989). Autism: Psychobiological perspectives. *Journal of Child and Adolescent Psychiatric and Mental Health Nursing, 2*(3), 92–96.

Dawson, G. (1987). The role of abnormal hemispheric specialization in autism. In E. Schopler & G. Mesibov (Eds.), *Neurobiological issues in autism* (pp 213–227). New York: Plenum Press.

Dietz, A. J. (1981). Amphetamine-like reactions to phenylpropanolamine. *Journal of the American Medical Association, 245,* 601–602.

Dietz, W. (1983). Childhood obesity: Susceptibility, cause and management. *Journal of Pediatrics, 103,* 676–686.

Dietz, W., & Gortmaker, S. (1985). Do we fatten out children at the television set? Obesity and television viewing in children and adolescents. *Pediatrics, 75,* 807.

Dworkin, P. (1985). *Learning and behavior problems of school children.* Philadelphia: WB Saunders.

Ellert, M. (1990). Constipation/encopresis: A nursing perspective. *Journal of Pediatric Health Care, 4,* 141–146.

Elliot, G., & Ciaranello, R. (1987). Neurochemical hypotheses of childhood psychoses. In E. Schopler & G. Mesibov (Eds.), *Neurobiological issues in autism* (pp 245–261). New York: Plenum Press.

Eyberg, S. (1985). Behavioral assessment: Methodology in pediatric psychology. *Journal of Pediatric Psychology, 2,* 123–139.

Felner, R., Silverman, M., & Adix, R. (1991). Prevention of substance abuse and related disorders in childhood and adolescence: A developmentally based, comprehensive ecological approach. *Family & Community Health, 14*(3), 12–22.

Fitzgerald, F. (1987). Constipation in children. *Pediatrics in Review, 8,* 299–302.

Forehand, R., & Wells, K. (1987). Conduct disorders. In R. Hoekelman, et al. (Eds.), *Primary pediatric care.* St. Louis: CV Mosby.

Forney, P., Forney, M., & Ripley, W. (1988). Profile of an adolescent problem drinker. *The Journal of Family Practice, 27,* 65–70.

Garfinkel, B. (1987). *Adolescent suicide.* Workshop presentation at Mendota Mental Health Institute, Madison, WI.

Gittleman, R., Mannuzza, S., Shenker, R., et al. (1985). Hyperactive boys almost grown up: I. Psychiatric status. *Archives of General Psychiatry, 42,* 937–947.

Golden, M., Saltzer, E., Depaul-Snyder, L., & Reiff, M. (1983). Obesity and socioeconomic class in children and their mothers. *Developmental and Behavioral Pediatrics, 4*(2), 113–118.

Granger, R. (1991). Bladder and bowel control disorders. In A. Rudolph (Ed.), *Rudolph's pediatrics (19th ed.).* Norwalk, CT: Appleton and Lange.

Guyton, A. (1991). *Textbook of medical physiology* (8th ed.). Philadelphia: WB Saunders.

Haber, J., et al (1987). *Comprehensive psychiatric nursing.* New York: McGraw-Hill.

Hammer, L. (1990). Obesity. In M. Green, & R. Haggerty (Eds.), *Ambulatory Pediatrics IV.* Philadelphia: WB Saunders.

Harnett, N. (1989). Conduct disorder in childhood and adolescence: An update. *Journal of Child and Adolescent Psychiatric and Mental Health Nursing, 2*(2), 74–78.

Hasin, D., et al. (1988). Cocaine and heroin dependence compared in poly-drug abusers. *American Journal of Public Health, 78*(5), 567–569.

Hauenstein, E. (1992). Shifting the paradigm: Toward integrative research on mothers and children. *Journal of Child and Adolescent Psychiatric and Mental Health Nursing, 5*(4), 18–28.

Herbert, M. (1975). *Problems of childhood.* New York: Pan Books.

Hersoo, L. (1977, June 9). Emotional disorders in childhood. *Nursing Times,* p. 864.

Hill, J. A., et al. (1983). The athletic polydrug abuse phenomenon. A case report. *American Journal of Sports Medicine, 11,* 269–271.

Horowitz, J. D., et al. (1980). Hypertensive responses induced by phenylpropanolamine in anorectic and decongestant preparations. *Lancet, 1,* 60–61.

Iveson, J. I. (1982, August). Barbiturates: A history of abuse. Forum 8, Drug Abuse. *Nursing Mirror,* p. 155.

Jensen, P. (1991). Mental health and disorder in children and adolescents: Current status and research needs. *Family & Community Health, 14*(3), 1–11.

Johns, C. (1985). Encopresis. *American Journal of Nursing, 85,* 153–156.

Kavanaugh, J., & Mattson, A. (1987). Phobias. In R. Hoekelman, et al. (Eds.), *Primary pediatric care*. St. Louis: CV Mosby.

Kazdin, A. (1987). Depression. In R. Hoekelman, et al. (Eds.), *Primary pediatric care*. St. Louis: CV Mosby.

Kelly, S., & Liter, S. (1984). *Interpersonal process group: A psychodynamic/existential approach to the treatment of bulimia*. Paper presented to the American Association for Counseling and Development. Houston, TX.

Kinston, W., Loaker, P., & Miller, L. (1987). Emotional health of families and their members where a child is obese. *Journal of Psychosomatic Research, 31*(5), 583–599.

Kleber, H. (1988). Cocaine abuse: Historical, epidemiological and psychological perspective. *Journal of Clinical Psychiatry, 49*(2), 3–6.

Kline, K. (1986). Systematic data collection: Key to behavioral assessment in patients with behavior problems. *Perspectives, 2*, 4–6.

Knittle, J., et al. (1979). The growth of adipose tissue in children and adolescents. Cross-sectional studies of adipose cell numbers and size. *Journal of Clinical Investigation, 63*, 238–246.

Koplewicz, H., & Gallagher, R. (1992). School-related anxiety and related conditions. In E. McAnarney, R. Kreipe, D. Orr, & G. Comerci (Eds.), *Textbook of adolescent medicine* (pp 994–1002). Philadelphia: WB Saunders.

Laraia, M., & Stuart, G. (1990). Bulimia. *Journal of Child and Adolescent Psychiatric and Mental Health Nursing, 3*(3), 91–97.

LeBow, M. (1979). *Behavior modification: A significant method in nursing practice*. Englewood Cliffs, NJ: Prentice-Hall.

Levine, M. (1987). Encopresis. In R. Hoekelman (Ed.), *Primary pediatric care*. St. Louis: CV Mosby.

Levine, M., et al. (1992). *Developmental-behavioral pediatrics*. Philadelphia: WB Saunders.

MacDonald, D. (1987). Patterns of alcohol and drug use among adolescents. *Pediatric Clinics of North America, 34*, 275–288.

Mansdorf, I., & Lukens, E. (1987). Cognitive-behavioral psychotherapy for separation anxious children exhibiting school phobia. *Journal of the American Academy of Child and Adolescent Psychiatry, 26*(2), 222–225.

Matteson, A. (1987). Adolescent depression and suicide. In R. Hoekelman, et al. (Eds.), *Primary pediatric care*. St. Louis: CV Mosby.

McKerlie, L., et al. (1983, December). Solvent abuse. Community Forum 10. *Nursing Mirror* (Suppl.).

Melamud, B. (1992). Fears and phobias. In E. McAnarney, R. Kreipe, D. Orr, & G. Comerci (Eds.), *Textbook of adolescent medicine* (pp 987–993). Philadelphia: WB Saunders.

Miller, K., Goldberg, S., & Atkin, B. (1989). Nocturnal enuresis: Experience with long-term use of intranasally administered desmopressin. *Journal of Pediatrics, 114*, 723–726.

Minuchin, S., et al. (1978). *Psychosomatic families: Anorexia nervosa in context*. Cambridge, MA: Harvard University Press.

Molitor, P. (1985). Constipation. *Nursing Mirror, 160*, 18–20.

Muscare, M. (1987). Identification and management of the early anorectic child. *Journal of Pediatric Health Care, 1*(4), 196–203.

Myers, D., & Anderson, A. (1991). Adolescent addiction: Assessment and identification. *Journal of Pediatric Health Care, 5*, 86–93.

National Center for Health Statistics (1990). *Advance report of final natality statistics. 1987* (Monthly vital statistics report 39 (Suppl. 3) DHHS Pub. No. PHS 90–1120). Hyattsville, MD: Public Health Service.

National Institute on Drug Abuse. *National Household Survey on Drug Abuse: Main Findings, 1990*. National Institutes of Health. Public Health Service. Unpublished data.

Norgaard, J., Hansen, J., Nielsen, J., et al. (1985). Simultaneous registration of sleep stages and bladder activity in enuresis. *Urology, 26*, 316–319.

North American Nursing Diagnosis Association. (1992). *NANDA nursing diagnoses: Definitions and classification 1992*. St. Louis: Author.

Palmer, L., & Ringwalt, C. (1988). Prevalence of alcohol and drug use among N. Carolina public school students. *Journal of School Health, 58*, 288–291.

Panksepp, J., & Sahely, T. (1987). Possible brain opioid involvement in disrupted social intent and language development of autism. In E. Schopler & G. Mesibov (Eds.), *Neurobiological issues in autism* (pp 357–372). New York: Plenum Press.

Parker, L., & Whitehead, W. (1982). Treatment of urinary and fecal incontinence in children. In D. Russo & J. Varni (Eds.), *Behavioral pediatrics: Research and practice* (pp 143–174). New York: Plenum Press.

Peck, M. (1981). The loner: An exploration of suicidal subtype in adolescence. *Adolescent Psychiatry, 9*, 461–466.

Percy, E. C. (1983). Drugs and athletics. In N. J. Smith (Ed.), *Sports medicine: Health care for young athletes* (pp 176–183). American Academy of Pediatrics, Committee on Sports Medicine.

Petechers, M., et al. (1988). Revalidation and expansion of an adolescent substance abuse screening measure. *Pediatrics, 9*(1), 25–29.

Pfeffer, C. (1986). *The suicidal child*. New York: Guilford Press.

Pfeffer, C. (1989). *Suicide among youth: Perspectives on risk and prevention*. Washington, DC: American Psychiatric Press.

Puskar, K. & D'Antonio, I. (1993). Tots and teens: Similarities in behavior and interventions for pediatric and psychiatric nurses. *Journal of Child and Adolescent Psychiatric and Mental Health Nursing, 6*(2), 18–28.

Pyle, R., Mitchell, J., Eckert, E., Halvorson, P., Newman, P., & Goff, G. (1983). The incidence of bulimia in freshmen college students. *International Journal of Eating Disorders, 2*, 75–85.

Reinherz, H., Frost, A., & Pakiz, B. (1991). Changing faces: Correlates of depressive symptoms in late adolescence. *Family & Community Health, 14*(3), 52–63.

Reynolds, W. (1991). A school-based procedure for the identification of adolescents at risk for suicidal behaviors. *Family & Community Health, 14*(3), 64–75.

Rowe, J. (1992). In support of sibling inclusion: A literature review. *Journal of Child and Adolescent Psychiatric and Mental Health Nursing, 5*(3), 27–33.

Ruddy-Wallace, M. (1987). Temperament: Assessing individual differences in hospitalized children. *Journal of Pediatric Nursing, 2*(1), 30–36.

Scahill, L., & Sipple, B. (1990). Developmental history collection on a child psychiatric inpatient service. *Journal of Child and Adolescent Psychiatric and Mental Health Nursing, 3*(2), 52–56.

Schmitt, B. (1990a). Nocturnal enuresis: Finding the treatment that fits the child. *Contemporary Pediatrics, 114*, 697–704.

Schmitt, B. (1990b). Nocturnal enuresis. In M. Green & R. Haggerty (Eds.), *Ambulatory pediatrics IV*. Philadelphia: WB Saunders.

Selvini-Palazzoli, M. (1985). Anorexia nervosa: A syndrome of an affluent society. *Transcultural Psychiatry Research Review, 22*, 3.

Shaffer, D., Garland, A., Gould, M., Fisher, P., & Troutman, P. (1988). Preventing teenage suicide. *Journal of the American Academy of Child and Adolescent Psychiatry, 27*, 675–687.

Shaywitz, S., & Shaywitz, B. (1988). Attention deficit disorder: Current perspectives. In J. Kavanagh & T. Truss (Eds.), *Learning Disabilities: Proceedings of the National Conference* (p 369). Parkton, Md: York Press.

Sherman, J., & Alexander, M. (1990, June). Obesity in children: A research update. *Journal of Pediatric Nursing, 5*(3), 161–167.

Shestowsky, B. (1983). Ego identity development and obesity in adolescent girls. *Adolescence, 18*, 551–559.

Silber, T., et al. (1988). Prevalence of PCP use among adolescent marijuana users. Clinical and laboratory observations. *Journal of Pediatrics, 112*(5), 827–829.

Sims, J., & Galvin, M. (1990). Pediatric psychopharmacologic uses of propranolol. *Journal of Child and Adolescent Psychiatric and Mental Health Nursing, 3*(1), 18–25.

Stadtler, A. (1989). Preventing encopresis. *Pediatric Nursing, 15*(3), 282–284.

Steele, B. T. (1993). Infant and neonatal peritoneal dialysis. In A. R. Nissenson & R. N. Fine (Eds.), *Pediatric dialysis in dialysis therapy* (2nd ed.). Philadelphia: Mosby–Year Book, Hanley & Belfus.

Stevenson, R., & Wolraich, M. (1989). Stimulant medication therapy in the treatment of children with attention deficit hyperactivity disorder. *Pediatric Clinics of North America, 36*, 1183.

Tashkin, D. P., & Cohen, S. (1981). *Marijuana smoking and its effects on the lungs*. Rockville, MD: American Council for Drug Education.

Thomas, A., & Chess, S. (1977). *Temperament and development*. New York: Brunner/Mazel.
Thomas, A., & Chess, S. (1980). *Dynamics of psychological development*. New York: Brunner/Mazel.
Tsai, L. (1987). Pre-, peri-, and neonatal factors in autism. In E. Schopler & G. Mesibov (Eds.), *Neurobiological issues in autism* (pp. 180–189). New York: Plenum Press.
Tuchman, R., Rapin, I., & Shinnar, S. (1991). Autistic and dysphasic children: I. Clinical characteristics. *Pediatrics, 88*(6), 1211–1218.
US Department of Health and Human Services, Public Health Service, Alcohol, Drug Abuse, and Mental Health Administration, National Institute on Alcohol Abuse and Alcoholism. (1987). *Sixth special report to the US congress on alcohol and health* (Publication ADM 87–1519). Rockville, MD: Author.
Valente, S. (1989). Adolescent suicide: Assessment and intervention. *Journal of Child and Adolescent Psychiatric and Mental Health Nursing, 1*(2), 34–39.
Valente, S. (1983). Suicide in school-aged children: Theory and assessment. *Pediatric Nursing, 9*(1), 25–29.
Valente, S., & Saunders, J. (1987). High school suicide prevention programs. *Pediatric Nursing, 13*(2), 108.
Volkmar, F., & Cohen, D. (1986). Current concepts: Infantile autism and the pervasive developmental disorders. *Journal of Developmental and Behavioral Pediatrics, 7*(5), 324–329.
Walsh, B., et al. (1985). Bulimia and depression. *Psychosomatic Medicine, 47*, 123–131.
Warady, B. A., Alon, U., & Hellerstein, S. (1991). Primary nocturnal enuresis: Current concepts about an old problem. *Pediatric Annals, 20*(5), 246–255.
Waxman, M., & Stunkard, A. (1980). Caloric intake and expenditure of obese boys. *Journal of Pediatrics, 96*, 187–193.
Wells, K., & Forehand, R. (1985). Conduct and oppositional disorders. In P. Bornstein & A. Kazadin (Eds.), *Handbook of clinical behavior therapy with children*. Homewood, IL: Dorcey Press.
Williams, D. (1980). Substance use and abuse. In J. Howe (Ed.), *Nursing care of adolescents* (pp 161–195). New York: McGraw-Hill.
Williamson, D. (1990). *Assessment of eating disorders: Obesity, anorexia and bulimia nervosa*. Elmsford, NY: Pergamon Press.
Wilson, M. (1987). Obesity. In R. Hoekelman, et al. (Eds.), *Primary pediatric care*. St. Louis: CV Mosby.
Wishon, P., & Kinnick, V. (1986). Helping infants overcome the problem of obesity. *Maternal and Child Nursing, 11*, 118–121.
Wollack, J., Low, N., & Carter, S. (1991). Static encephalopathies. In A. Rudolph (Ed.), *Rudolph's pediatric* (19th ed.). Norwalk, CT: Appleton & Lange.
Wolpe, J. (1990). *Practice of behavior therapy* (4th ed., p. 41). New York: Pergamon Press.
Woolston, J. (1987). Obesity in infancy and early childhood. *Journal of the American Academy of Child and Adolescent Psychiatry, 6*(2), 123–126.
Yuwiler, A., & Freedman, D. (1987). Neurotransmitter research in autism. In E. Schopler & G. Mesibov (Eds.), *Neurobiological issues in autism* (pp 263–284). New York: Plenum Press.

BIBLIOGRAPHY

Angold, A., Weissman, M., John, K., Wickramaratne, P., & Prusoff, B. (1991). The effects of age and sex on depression ratings in children and adolescents. *Journal of the American Academy of Child and Adolescent Psychiatry, 30*(1), 67–74.
Berlin, I. (1990). The role of the community mental health center in prevention of infant, child and adolescent disorders. *Journal of Child and Adolescent Psychiatric and Mental Health Nursing, 3*(2), 18–25.
Brady, M., Nelms, B., Albright, A., & Murphy, C. (1984). Childhood depression: Development of a screening tool. *Pediatric Nursing, 10*(4), 222–225, 227.
Busen, N. (1991). Development of an adolescent risk-taking instrument. *Journal of Child and Adolescent Psychiatric and Mental Health Nursing, 4*(1), 143–149.
Bush, C. (1992). Child and adolescent mental health: Building a base for research and practice. *Journal of Child and Adolescent Psychiatric and Mental Health Nursing, 5*(4), 5–6
Carbray, J., & Pitula, C. (1991). Trends in adolescent psychiatric hospitalization. *Journal of Child and Adolescent Psychiatric and Mental Health Nursing, 4*(2), 68–71.
Cash, R., & Pruzinsky, T. (1990). *Body images, development, deviance and change*. New York: Guilford Press.
Castiglia, P. (1990). Suicide in adolescents. *Journal of Pediatric Health Care, 4*(3), 149–151.
Coler, M. (1989). Diagnoses for child and adolescent psychiatric nursing combining NANDA and the DSM-III-R. *Journal of Child and Adolescent Psychiatric and Mental Health Nursing, 2*(3), pp .
Collins, A. (1991). Perceived stress and stress projected in spontaneous storytelling of two groups of fourth grade children. *Journal of Child and Adolescent Psychiatric and Mental Health Nursing, 4*(3), 83–89.
Committee on Substance Abuse. (1990). "Smokeless cigarettes" and other nicotine delivery devices. *Pediatrics, 87*(3), 481–483.
Dardis, P., & Hofland, S. (1990). Anorexia nervosa. *Journal of Child and Adolescent Psychiatric and Mental Health Nursing, 3*(3), 85–90.
Finney, J., Riley, A., & Cataldo, M. (1991). Psychology in primary health care: Effects of brief targeted therapy on children's medical care utilization. *Journal of Pediatric Psychology, 16*(4), 447–461.
Francell, C. (1993). Advocating for seriously emotionally disturbed children and their families: An overview. *Journal of Child and Adolescent Psychiatric and Mental Health Nursing, 6*(1), 33–37.
Freeman, B., & Ritvo, E. (1989). The syndrome of autism: Establishing the diagnosis and principles of management. *Pediatric Annals, 13*, 4.
Fremouw, W., de Perczel, M., & Ellis, T. (1990). *Suicide risk: Assessment and response guidelines*. New York, Pergamon Press.
Freitas, L., & Pieranunzi, V. (1990). Ethical issues in the behavioral treatment of children and adolescents. *Journal of Child and Adolescent Psychiatric and Mental Health Nursing, 3*(1), 3–8.
Garvey, C., Gross, D., & Freeman, L. (1991). Assessing psychotropic medication side effects among children. *Journal of Child and Adolescent Psychiatric and Mental Health Nursing, 4*(4), 127–131.
Goren, S. (1992). Practicing in partnership with families in the inpatient setting. *Journal of Child and Adolescent Psychiatric and Mental Health Nursing, 5*(3), 43–46.
Haber, J., et al. (1987). *Comprehensive psychiatric nursing*. New York: McGraw-Hill.
Hornyak, L., & Baker, E. (1989). *Experimental therapies for eating disorders*. New York: Guilford Press.
Houck G., & King, M. (1993). Cognitive functioning and behavioral and emotional adjustment in maltreated children post intervention. *Journal of Child and Adolescent Psychiatric and Mental Health Nursing, 6*(2), 5–17.
Hubbard, G. (1991). Group play therapy. *Journal of Child and Adolescent Psychiatric and Mental Health Nursing, 4*(4), 150–153.
Irwin, C., & Ryan, R. (1989). Problem behavior in adolescents. *Journal of Child and Adolescent Psychiatric and Mental Health Nursing, 3*(1), 14–17.
Jacobson, J. (1991). The relationship between social support and depression in adolescents. *Journal of Child and Adolescent Psychiatric and Mental Health Nursing, 4*(1), 20–24.
Johnson, J., & Goldman, J. (Eds.) (1990). *Development assessment in clinical child psychiatry*. Boston: Allyn & Bacon.
Kelley, S. (1992). Child maltreatment, stressful life events, and behavior problems in school-aged children in residential treatment. *Journal of Child and Adolescent Psychiatric and Mental Health Nursing, 5*(2), 5–13.
Kendall, J. (1989). Child psychiatric nursing and the family. *Journal of Child and Adolescent Psychiatric and Mental Health Nursing, 2*(4), 145–153.
Kileen, M. (1990). Challenges and choices in child and adolescent mental health–psychiatric nursing. *Journal of Child and Adolescent Psychiatric and Mental Health Nursing, 3*(4), 113–119.
Knight, M., Wigder, K., Fortsch, M., & Polcare, A. (1990). Medication education for children. *Journal of Child and Adolescent Psychiatric and Mental Health Nursing, 3*(1), 25–28.

Kuntz, B. (1991). Exploring the grief of adolescents after the death of a parent. *Journal of Child and Adolescent Psychiatric and Mental Health Nursing, 4*(3), 105–109.

Lamb, J., & Pusker, K. (1991). School-based adolescent mental health project survey of depression, suicidal ideation and anger. *Journal of Child and Adolescent Psychiatric and Mental Health Nursing, 4*(1), 101–104.

Matson, J. (1989). *Treating depression in children and adolescents.* New York: Pergamon Press.

McClowry, S. (1991). Behavioral disturbances among medically hospitalized school-age children. *Journal of Child and Adolescent Psychiatric and Mental Health Nursing, 4*(2), 62–67.

McFarland, G., & Wasle, E. (1986). *Nursing diagnoses and process in psychiatric mental health nursing*. Philadelphia: JB Lippincott.

Moreau, D. (1990). Major depression in childhood and adolescence. *Psychiatric Clinics of North America, 13*(2), 355–368.

Morris, P., & Bihan, S. (1991). The prevalence of children with a history of sexual abuse hospitalized in the psychiatric setting. *Journal of Child and Adolescent Psychiatric and Mental Health Nursing, 4*(2), 49–54.

Muse, N. (1990). *Depression and suicide in children and adolescents.* Austin, Texas: Pro-ed.

Nixon, M. (1992). Mental health rights of adolescents: What mental health nurses need to know. *Journal of Child and Adolescent Psychiatric and Mental Health Nursing, 5*(2), 14–19.

Norgaard, J., Rittig, S., Djurhuus, J. (1989). Nocturnal enuresis: An approach to treatment based on pathogenesis. *Journal of Pediatrics, 114,* 705–710.

Opie, N., & Slater, P. (1988). Mental health needs of children in school. *Journal of Child and Adolescent Psychiatric and Mental Health Nursing, 1*(1), 31–35.

Palmer, T. (1990). Anorexia nervosa, bulimia nervosa: Causal theories and treatment. *Nurse Practitioner, 15*(4), 12–18, 21.

Plehn, K. (1990). Anorexia nervosa and bulimia: Incidence and diagnosis. *Nurse Practitioner, 15*(4), 22, 25, 28.

Pierannunzi, V., & Freitas, L. (1992). Informed consent with children and adolescents. *Journal of Child and Adolescent Psychiatric and Mental Health Nursing, 5*(2), 21–27.

Provisional Committee on Substance Abuse (1990). Selection of substance abuse treatment. *Pediatrics, 86*(1), 139–140.

Puskar, K., Lamb, J., & Martsolf, D. (1990). The role of the psychiatric/mental health nurse clinical specialist in an adolescent coping skills group. *Journal of Child and Adolescent Psychiatric and Mental Health Nursing, 3*(2), 47–51.

Puskar, K., & Wargoe, K. (1992). Difficulties with teens: Can nursing consultation help? *Journal of Child and Adolescent Psychiatric and Mental Health Nursing, 5*(3) 34–41.

Reighley, J. (1988). *Nursing care planning guides for mental health.* Baltimore: Williams & Wilkins.

Rowe, J. (1988). Attachment theory and the milieu treatment of children. *Journal of Child and Adolescent Psychiatric and Mental Health Nursing, 1*(2), 66–71.

Rutter, M., & Hensov, L. (1985). *Child and adolescent psychiatry: Modern approaches*. London: Blackwell Scientific Publications.

Scahill, F. (1990). A method of screening for communication disorders in child psychiatric inpatients. *Journal of Child and Adolescent Psychiatric and Mental Health Nursing, 3*(3), 98–102.

Sullivan, D., & Everstine, L. (1989). *Sexual trauma in children and adolescents, dynamics in treatment*. New York: Brunner/Mazel.

Tuchman, R., Rapin, I., & Shinnar, S. (1991). Autistic and dysphasic children: II. Epilepsy. *Pediatrics, 88*(6), 1219–1225.

Wagner, J., Melragon, B., & Menke, E. (1993). Homeless children: Interdisciplinary drug prevention intervention. *Journal of Child and Adolescent Psychiatric and Mental Health Nursing, 6*(1), 22–30.

Williamson, D. (1990). *Assessment of eating disorders: Obesity, anorexia and bulimia nervosa*. Elmsford, NY: Pergamon Press.

Yates, A. (1991). *Compulsive exercise and the eating disorders: Towards an integrated theory of activity.* New York: Brunner/Mazel.

CHAPTER • 30

The High-Risk Infant

Janet Pinelli

NURSING PROCESS PLAN
NPP: The Premature Infant, Table 30–3

RELATED TOPICS
Family theories and assessment, Chapter 2
Attachment, families with neonates, Chapter 4
Promoting Healthy Parenting, Chapter 12
Altered Respiratory Function, Chapter 32
Altered Cardiovascular Function, Chapter 33
Altered Digestive Function, Chapter 35

LEARNING OBJECTIVES

- **Outline the age-related differences in the premature infant with respect to physical assessment and nursing diagnostic statements.**
- **Identify the age-related differences in the postmature infant with respect to physical assessment and nursing diagnostic statements.**
- **Identify the differences in the small-for-gestational-age infant with respect to nursing diagnostic statements.**
- **Identify the differences in the large-for-gestational-age infant with respect to nursing diagnostic statements.**
- **Identify the differences in multiple gestation infants with respect to nursing diagnostic statements.**
- **Outline the medical disorders commonly associated with dysmaturity.**
- **Outline the issues related to the discharge and follow-up of dysmature or ill neonates.**

Variations in the gestational age and age-appropriate size of newborns often necessitate the specialized care provided by health professionals.

The infants and their families have special problems and care needs that are different from the norm. The following section describes the differences of dysmature or ill neonates related to physical assessment, nursing diagnostic statements, and commonly associated medical disorders. Issues related to discharge home, posthospitalization follow-up, and impact on the family are also presented.

This section focuses on neonates who differ from the norm at birth because of an alteration in gestational age (the length of time from conception to birth). The general term used to describe such neonates is "dysmature."

A "term" infant is born between 38 and 42 weeks. Those infants who vary from the norm owing to gestation are called "preterm" (babies born at less than 38 weeks gestation) or "post-term" (babies born at more than 42 weeks gestation). A newborn infant of average weight for age is called "appropriate for gestational age" (AGA). An infant whose weight is not appropriate for age is called "small for gestational age" (SGA) or "large for gestational age" (LGA). Dysmature neonates are at high risk for morbidity and mortality; therefore, early identification and initiation of medical and nursing management are important. Nurses who have a good understanding of the characteristics and assessment of the normal neonate can appreciate how deviations from the norm affect the neonate's ability to survive and thrive. Most of the complications due to dysmaturity result from chemical disturbances or the inadequate functioning of organs and systems. Most disorders are described in depth in Unit 7, which covers the body systems. When mentioned here, they are cross-referenced to those chapters.

The special needs of babies who are other than healthy term infants frequently require a period of hospitalization. Sometimes this requires transfer from a community hospital to a specialized neonatal intensive care unit (NICU) away from home. Frequently, the infant and family are separated within the first minutes, hours, or days of life. Therefore, families as well as the infants need nursing intervention and support. There may also be long-term implications for these infants and families with respect to growth and development.

Prematurity

Infants are considered premature if they are born at less than 38 weeks gestation. They may also be assessed as low birthweight (less than 2500 g) or very low birthweight (less than 1500 g). Preterm infants who weigh less than 1500 g and are SGA are at the highest risk for morbidity and mortality.

The clinical status of preterm infants varies widely, but all of them must be assessed with the recognition that they were born too soon. Preterm infants differ from term infants in a number of ways. It is important to remember that preterm infants also differ markedly from one another. The physical characteristics, the behavior, and the needs of infants of 27 weeks (who weigh 1000 g or less) are obviously different from those of infants of 32 weeks (who average 1500 g) or of 36 weeks (whose weight is usually between 2000 and 2500 g).

Etiology/Incidence

In the majority of cases, the specific cause for the birth of a preterm infant is unknown. Multiple factors that have been associated with the incidence of premature and low birthweight infants are listed in Table 30–1.

With rapidly advancing technologic assistance, smaller and sicker babies are surviving. The incidence of premature births in the United States is about 9.8 per cent (US Department of Health and Human Services, 1990) and about 9 per cent in Canada (Statistics Canada, 1991). This represents no significant change in incidence since the early 1980s.

Pathophysiology/Clinical Manifestations and Related Assessment

General Appearance of Preterm Compared with Term Infants

Differences in the general appearance of term and preterm infants are evaluated through the use of the Dubowitz assessment. The external criteria used in the assessment describe some of the most obvious physical differences. Because of the cephalocaudal progression of development, the younger the gestational age of the baby, the larger its head will be in proportion to its body. Because testes do not descend until the 8th month of gestation, genitalia will be less well developed in preterm infant boys. In girls, the labia majora do not cover the labia minora until their age approaches that of a term baby.

Lanugo is abundant on the body of an immature

ETHICAL ISSUES
Infants with Disabilities

by Margaret M. Mahon, MSN, RN

Tom and Marcia Pearson had a 2-year-old daughter, and were expecting their second child. Ms. Pearson went into labor at 37 weeks gestation, and delivered a 5-lb, 4-oz boy. The infant was in moderate respiratory distress, was vomiting, and had a distended abdomen. It was suspected that the child had an intestinal obstruction. Further examination revealed that the child had duodenal atresia. In addition, the child's facies suggested trisomy 21, later confirmed by genetic examination. The parents were devastated by the diagnoses. Ms. Pearson explained: "When I was in college I did some volunteer work at a home for retarded children. They couldn't do anything! They couldn't go to the bathroom by themselves, they couldn't feed themselves! I don't want my child to live like that!" The pediatric surgeon came to Ms. Pearson's room to discuss repair of the duodenal atresia. The Pearsons refused to consent to the surgery. They said they understood the surgery was necessary for the child to survive, but that they believed "if he did survive he wouldn't have any quality of life."

The Pearsons' experience is many parents' worst nightmare. Though expectant parents often consider what they would do if their child had a disability, when it occurs the reality can be overwhelming. The first reaction is usually shock, but this is often accompanied rapidly by sadness, depression, desperation, resentment, and anger. The anger is multifocused, but is often directed, albeit rarely expressed, at the child. Some parents have said they could never love this child. Parents are often embarrassed and even horrified by their own reactions. Such reactions are valid, appropriate for the shock of the situation, and common. Knowing this can allow the nurse to intervene appropriately, and alleviate parental discomfort with her or his own reaction.

There are two patients in this situation: the mother/family and the child. When analyzing this case the perspectives must be recognized as distinct. This is different from most patient care in which the focus of treatment is the child in the context of the family. Ideally, the parent is the decision maker for the child. In this case, there is a conflict between what is medically indicated for the child and what the parents want. Most often, education and communication clarify differences, and the parent then consents. Sometimes this does not happen.

Legal considerations also influence this case and health care interventions. A helpful means of analysis is to separate the decision making based on the two conditions influencing the parents' decision making. The baby has both trisomy 21 and duodenal atresia. Surgery for duodenal atresia is common, and highly successful. Were this child born with duodenal atresia and without trisomy 21, the surgery would be expected; it is necessary to survive. To withhold surgery could be considered medical neglect.

Were the child born with trisomy 21 but without duodenal atresia, the primary consideration for the parents would remain the same: children with trisomy 21 are virtually always mentally retarded. The presence of the duodenal atresia is related to trisomy 21, but repairing the atresia will not affect the mental retardation. Without the surgery, the child is unable to eat. Although the child could be maintained on intravenous fluids, this is not a permanent option. Historically, the withholding of surgery has been with the intent of the infant's death. Not feeding or hydrating a child with trisomy 21 but without duodenal atresia would be child abuse—neglect.

So what is the difference in analysis of the case when both conditions are present? What of the question of quality of life? Most children with trisomy 21 are moderately mentally retarded, can be educated, and are likely to be employed as adults. Most children with trisomy 21 are very outgoing and loving children. People's negative reactions to a child with trisomy 21 are often based on misinformation, and sometimes perpetuated by the health care community. Many parents of newborns with trisomy 21 report being given information such as "your child will always be a vegetable," clearly at odds with the facts of the condition. The panoply of emotions erupting with the diagnosis is likely to affect parental ability to integrate new information. This has ramifications for teaching families: information should be repeated, and if feasible, provided in writing. Many parents have found it helpful to talk with a parent who has been through a similar situation. This may be difficult when a decision has to be made quickly. The goal is provision of accurate information that can facilitate decision making, within the best interest of the child standard.

Several cases like that described above have resulted in federal interventions, based on existing laws designed to protect infants, including provision of medical treatment. The US Department of Health and Human Services (DHHS) provided the following guidelines, applicable in cases in which treatment options conflict: "In cases where it is uncertain whether medical treatment will be beneficial, a person's disability must be the basis for a decision to withhold treatment." The responsibility of the nurse is to act as an advocate for the child, considering the best interest of the child standard. This has put some nurses in the difficult position of feeling pulled between parent and child, or sometimes by different members of the health care team. This exemplifies the need to be sure not only of the medical facts, but also of the legal considerations that influence one's responsibilities. If one is unsure of this information, appropriate supervisor input should be obtained whenever possible. Hospital legal counsel can also provide appropriate information. Hospital ethics committees can be a good forum for discussion and analysis of difficult cases. Ideally there is someone specifically trained in ethics on such a committee. Ethics committees

ETHICAL ISSUES
Infants with Disabilities *(continued)*

are underutilized if hospital personnel view them as decision-making and intrusive rather than supportive and objective. The Supreme Court decided in June, 1986 that the appropriate legal guidelines to be used in evaluating potential cases are the Child Abuse Amendments of 1984, a bill that prohibited the actions of health care institutions that attempted to "deprive a handicapped infant of nutrition which is necessary to sustain life, or deprive a handicapped infant of medical treatment which is necessary to remedy or ameliorate a life-threatening medical condition, if . . . any such deprivation is carried out for the purpose of causing or allowing the death of such infant; and . . . such nutrition or medical treatment generally is provided to similarly situated infants and handicapped infants."

None of the legal or ethical guidelines indicate that treatment is required in all cases. The President's Commission for the Study of Ethical Problems in Medicine and Biomedical and Behavioral Research (1983) indicates that when there is no beneficial therapy, or when therapy prolongs life but not by a substantial amount, or if the pain resulting from the therapy is too great, treatment is not ethically or legally required. There are some cases in which parents desire that a specific treatment be implemented though the health care team believes the treatment is futile. The President's Commission recommended that, if the pain resulting from the treatment is not too great, it is acceptable to initiate the therapy.

There are also cases in which it is unclear whether treatment will be beneficial. This is often the case with the birth of a premature infant. The technology exists to intervene to save or prolong the lives of infants who 20 years ago would have certainly died. The nature of premature births is often that decisions to intervene must be made rapidly—for example, artificial ventilation must be started immediately to minimize additional complications from anoxia. Additional technologies such as extracorporeal membrane oxygenation (ECMO) and surgery for hypoplastic left heart syndrome may only be available in a few places, outcomes are often unclear, and the process may be painful. Even within the need for intervention arising from technologic capabilities there is a continuum of difficulty. The ability to provide mechanical ventilation is now fairly common. Its use and continuation is usually evaluated in the context of accompanying disorders or complications such as intraventricular hemorrhage (IVH). Options about ECMO are very location-dependent.

An additional fact about health care decision making has arisen as a result of the use of machines. It often seems that the decision to use or withhold technology is made before a therapy is begun. After that there is often an attitude that once started, a technology can never be withdrawn. If a premature newborn is put on a ventilator, has the final ethical decision been made, or is it yet acceptable to withdraw treatment? Ethicists are now calling for a reexamination of this standard.

In the case described above, there may arise animosity between the family and the health care team, or within the health care team. In most of these cases, all involved believe they are acting in the best interest of the child. Use of this standard demands that one considers the child's perspective. Regardless, an understanding of the good intent of all involved is a common ground that can be used to focus communication.

BIBLIOGRAPHY

Mahon, M. (1988). Nursing involvement in treatment decision regarding newborns with congenital anomalies. *Holistic Nursing Practice, 2,* 55–67.
Mahon, M. (1990). The nurse's role in decision making for the child with disabilities. *Issues in Law & Medicine, 6,* 247–268.
H. R. 6492, 97th Congress, 2nd Session, Sec. 3, Part 202. (1982.).
Nondiscrimination on the Basis of Handicap. 45 CFR sec 84.55 (1984). Washington, DC: Congressional Federal Record.
President's Commission for the Study of Ethical Problems in Medicine and Biomedical and Behavioral Research. (1983). *Deciding to forego life-sustaining treatment.* Washington, DC: GPO.
US Commission on Civil Rights. (1989). *Medical Discrimination Against Children with Disabilities.* Washington, DC: US Government Printing Office.
Wolraich, M. L., Siperstein, G. N., & Reed, D. (1991). Doctors' decisions and prognostications for infants with Down Syndrome. *Developmental Medicine and Child Neurology, 33,* 336–342.

infant (Fig. 30–1), except in extreme prematurity, in which case it is absent. The preterm infant's head hair is in fine, woolly bunches, whereas the term baby's hair is silky and flat, with individual strands.

Skin Assessment

The skin should be assessed frequently for abrasions and lesions because of the increased risk of skin damage. This is due to the diminished cohesion between the dermis and the epidermis and to the immaturity of the stratum corneum.

The skin of a preterm infant is thin, with numerous veins and tributaries visible. Even infants as old as 34 weeks gestational age have relatively little subcutaneous fat; that layer is deposited chiefly in the 4 weeks prior to term.

Assessment of Head and Neck

The assessment of the head and neck in the preterm infant is the same as for the term infant. Particular attention should be paid to the presence of bruising because of its influence on hyperbilirubinemia.

TABLE 30-1
Factors Associated with the Incidence of Premature and Low Birthweight Infants

Maternal (Physiologic)

• Previous premature labor	• Poor maternal nutrition
• Hyperemesis	• Less than 152 cm height
• Previous abortion, stillbirth, or low birthweight infant	• Toxemia
• Maternal age under 20 or over 35 yrs	• Nonimmune status for selected infections
• Placenta abruptio or previa	• DES exposure or other toxic exposure
• Hydramnios	• Fibroids
• Antepartum hemorrhage	• Premature rupture of membranes
• Spontaneous onset of labor	• Intrauterine infection
• Incompetent cervix	• Concurrent maternal disease such as renal or heart disease
• Isoimmunization	• Genitourinary anomalies or surgery
• Anemia or abnormal hemaglobin	• Weight loss of 2.3 kg (during pregnancy)
• Hypotension	• Less than 1 yr since last birth
• Poor weight gain	
• Parity (0 or >4 children)	
• Prepregnancy weight of less than 45.5 kg (100 lbs)	

Fetal

• Multiple birth	• Head engaged at 32 wks
• Fetal anomalies	• Fetal distress

Maternal (Psychosocial)

• Single mother	• Substance abuse
• Low socioeconomic status	• High altitude
• Minority status	• Heavy work
• Low educational level	• Smoking
• Long/tiring commute	

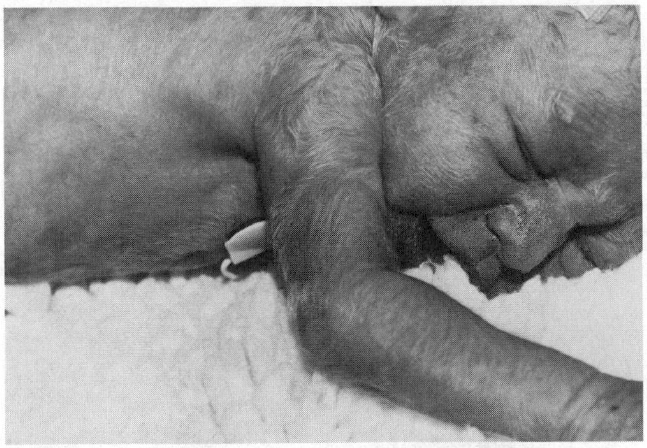

FIGURE 30-1. Lanugo, a downy distribution of fine hair over the body. It is most evident on the shoulders, back, extremities, forehead, and temples. It begins to appear on the fetus by about the 16th week of gestation and begins to disappear after the 32nd week. This infant is 24 hours old and was born at 28 weeks gestation; lanugo is therefore abundant.

Neurologic Development and Function

The nervous system of both preterm and term neonates is quite immature structurally. It is also functionally different from that of adults. In particular, neurons are immature in function, and there is limited myelination of the conduction pathways. In the premature neonate, neurologic function is largely directed by the brain stem and spinal cord rather than the cortex.

There are some distinct differences in the neurologic function of infants at various gestational ages. Some functions are present in neonates at 28 weeks and at term, but they vary in the consistency and quality of neurologic response to stimuli. These functions include vision, pupillary response, hearing, pain response, level of alertness, and limb movement. Other responses, such as primitive reflexes, are not present until a specific gestational age.

The appearance of these reflexes, or a change in their quality, forms the basis of the neurologic criteria used in the Dubowitz assessment. Generally, the development and suppression of primitive reflexes follows a specific sequence that can be used to determine gestational age. Increasing flexor responses reflect this development as the infant reaches 40 weeks gestation (Fig. 30-2). This is followed by decreasing flexion and increasing extensor responses as the infant reaches 2 to 3 months post-term. The overall posture of the baby also reflects increasing flexion. The posture of a preterm baby is one of general extension, whereas, in the term baby, the posture is one of general flexion. (Fig. 30-3). Despite these differences, it is still important to assess and document the infant's responsiveness, tone, strength, and spontaneous and elicited muscle movements.

The majority of acute neurologic problems in premature infants occur secondary to circulatory, metabolic, infectious, environmental, or physical conditions that impair function temporarily or permanently.

Skeletal Assessment

The skeletal assessment is closely related to the neurologic assessment of the infant because of the relationship between the muscles and the nervous system. The muscoleskeletal and neurologic assessments, therefore, are often carried out together. The spinal integrity can be assessed by palpating the spine from the neck to the coccyx to note whether the spinal processes are intact and whether there are dimples or hairy patches at the base of the spine. The length and symmetry of the limbs should be assessed as well as the presence of digits in the hands and feet. It is important to manipulate the hips using the Ortolani maneuver and the Barlow test (see Chapter 41 for a description of these tests). Lastly, all joints and limbs should be manipulated using a gentle range of motion technique to determine the presence or absence of contractures, the presence of pain with movement, and the extent of joint movement that is present.

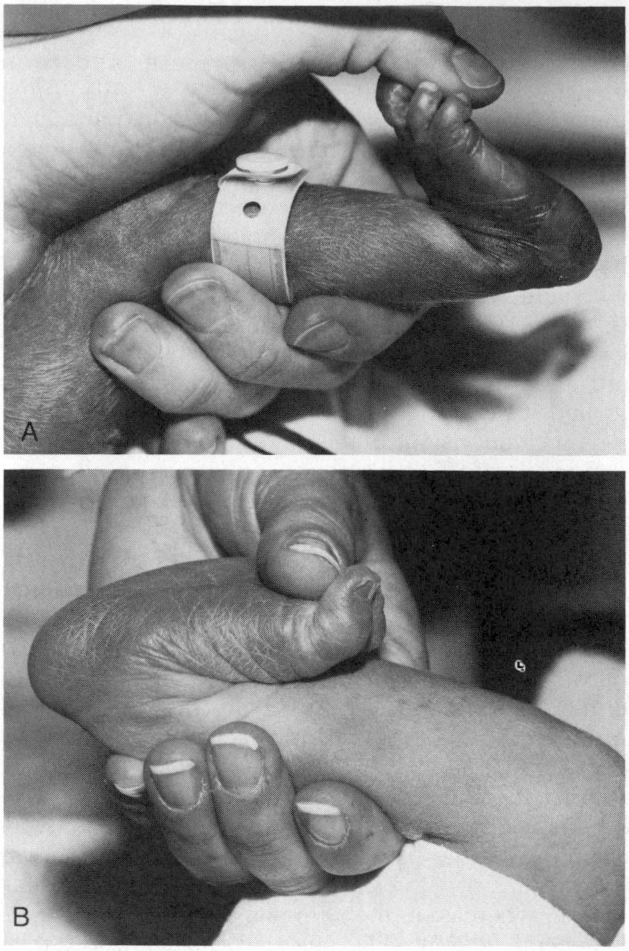

FIGURE 30-2. Ankle dorsiflexion. Increasing flexor responses reflect maturation. A decreasing angle between the dorsum of the foot and the anterior aspect of the leg occurs with maturation. *A*, Premature infant at 28 weeks gestation. *B*, Full-term infant.

Respiratory Development and Function

Of all the differences between preterm and term infants, none is more significant than the development of the respiratory tract. *Respiratory development is the crucial difference between viability and nonviability.* Before 26 to 28 weeks gestational age, there is limited development of the alveoli (the tiny air sacs at the terminal end of the respiratory system through which oxygen and carbon dioxide are exchanged) and of the alveolar capillaries. There are two types of cells within the alveoli: Type I cells give structure to the alveolus, and Type II cells produce several compounds collectively termed "surfactant." The most abundant of the surfactant compounds is lecithin, accounting for 50 to 70 per cent of surfactant. The function of lecithin and other surfactant compounds is to prevent the collapse of the alveoli on expiration. Surfactant production may be inadequate because of the immaturity, impairment, or death of the surfactant-producing cells that line the alveoli. Neonatal stress diminishes the production of surfactant, whereas stress to the fetus in utero increases production. When surfactant production is inadequate, respiratory distress syndrome (RDS or hyaline membrane disease) results.

Preterm infants also differ from term infants in the characteristics of their breathing: respirations are more irregular, with periodic apnea. Both the relative weakness of respiratory muscles and the decreased rigidity of the thoracic cage lead to hypoventilation, which in turn results in the retention of carbon dioxide and subsequent acidosis. Respiratory complications may occur because of the weak cough and gag reflexes of preterm babies, which increase the possibility of aspiration.

It is essential, therefore, that a careful and thorough assessment of respiratory function be conducted

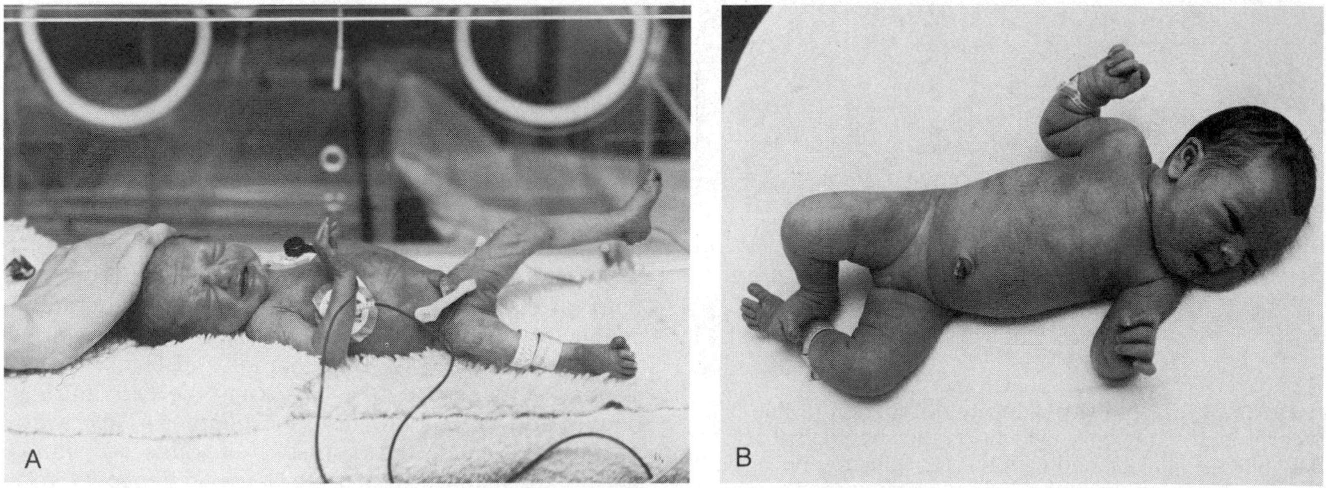

FIGURE 30-3. Muscle tone and degree of flexion increase with maturity. *A*, The posture of a premature infant is one of general extension. *B*, The posture of a term baby is one of general flexion.

on a frequent basis during the first few days of life. Dramatic changes in respiratory status can occur from one hour to the next.

Cardiovascular Function

The transition from fetal circulation to neonatal circulation is, in part, a response to the increased level of oxygen in the baby's circulatory system following initial respiration. When levels of oxygen are low, fetal circulation may persist. (Fetal circulation is shown in detail in Chapter 33). Particularly frequent in the small preterm infant is the persistence of a patent (open) ductus arteriosus (PDA) or an intermittent PDA (Chapter 33). A distinctive murmur, caused by the rush of blood through the PDA, can be heard on auscultation and should be reported and closely monitored.

In addition to detecting murmurs or other abnormal heart sounds, the assessment should include skin color and temperature, capillary refill time, peripheral pulse strength and equality, and blood pressure.

Gastrointestinal Development and Function

The gastrointestinal tract in preterm infants differs from that in the term infant in several ways. Gastrointestinal motility is decreased; stools may be infrequent, with abdominal distention.

Before 34 weeks gestation, the sucking and swallowing reflexes of the preterm baby may not be sufficiently coordinated to allow direct feeding from breast or bottle, so that alternative feeding methods may be necessary (gavage, intravenous feedings).

The immature digestive system of the preterm baby makes certain dietary adjustments necessary. Not only must the type of carbohydrate, fat, and protein be adapted to the special needs of the preterm baby but factors such as renal solute load must also be considered.

Lactose is the carbohydrate of human and cow's milk and of many commercially prepared formulas. The enzyme lactase is necessary for lactose digestion. Since lactase enzymes do not attain maximal activity until 9 months gestation, preterm infants may have impaired lactose tolerance.

Fats, even those digested rather easily by term infants, are not believed to be well assimilated by preterm babies. Triglycerides, however, are readily absorbed into the blood.

Preterm infants with respiratory distress syndrome have higher caloric needs because of an increased respiratory rate and thus an increased metabolic rate. When glucose alone is supplied to meet caloric needs, negative nitrogen balance results. Thus, protein breakdown is very high at a time when the body needs protein for brain development.

Provision of minerals is also a major problem. Lack of calcium can lead to undermineralization of the skeleton; however, it is not clear whether calcium supplementation is of any value. Since iron is stored by the fetus during the last trimester of pregnancy, preterm infants have minimal iron stores. Examination of the abdomen should include auscultation for bowel sounds and observation for changes in shape and color; the stool pattern and type should be followed as well.

Liver Function

The liver of a preterm infant is less mature than that of a term infant. A less mature liver increases the likelihood of hyperbilirubinemia and toxicity from drugs that must be excreted through the liver.

Bilirubin is a product of red blood cell destruction. Indirect bilirubin is fat-soluble and cannot be excreted in the bile or via the kidneys. Through the glucuronyl transferase enzyme system in the liver, conjugation of indirect bilirubin occurs. This converted or direct bilirubin is water-soluble and thus can be excreted in the bile or via the kidneys. It is the unconjugated, or indirect, bilirubin that may cause kernicterus, a form of serious and nonreversible brain damage in neonates.

When the liver is immature, the ability to conjugate bilirubin (convert indirect bilirubin to direct bilirubin) is decreased; this is one of the factors causing hyperbilirubinemia of preterm infants. Another factor that may be as significant, or even more important, is the decreased number of Y and Z carrier proteins in the liver cells to which bilirubin must bind in the conjugation process. There is a danger of kernicterus (1) if the level of protein is low, as when blood volume is decreased, or (2) if other substances are competing for binding sites, as when the baby is acidotic or receiving certain drugs.

Renal Function

Because of a reduced glomerular filtration rate, preterm infants are more likely to retain fluid and to excrete drugs poorly. Moreover, when blood pressure is low, kidney perfusion and, therefore, urinary output will be diminished. When body water is diminished, however, the kidneys are not able to concentrate urine in order to conserve water; consequently, the baby may become easily dehydrated.

Within the renal tubules, both reduced tubular absorption and reduced tubular secretion may occur. Reduced absorption of glucose and amino acids may result in glucose and protein being spilled into the urine at lower serum levels than in more mature infants or older children. Metabolic acidosis is more likely because of the decreased ability to retain bicarbonate. Reduced secretion in the tubules, like the reduced glomerular filtration rate, limits drug clearance. The doses of medication given to preterm infants are very small but nevertheless they may accumulate in the body and produce toxicity.

Immunologic Competence

"Immunologic competence" refers to the ability of an organism to resist infection. Immunologic competence involves cellular and humoral immune factors such as white blood cells, factors that enhance the ability of white blood cells to destroy bacteria, and immunoglobulins such as IgG, IgM, and IgA. For a variety of reasons, white blood cells are less effective in their action in these babies. The immunoglobulin IgG crosses the placenta and provides the neonate with immunity to certain infections to which the infant's mother is immune (e.g., diphtheria, measles, tetanus). The preterm infant has a deficit of IgG because transplacental passage of IgG occurs primarily in the third trimester. IgA, the primary immunoglobulin of colostrum, is not available to the baby who does not receive breast milk.

Assessment of the Preterm Infant

Descriptions of the term infant and the detailed physical examination are provided in Chapter 4. A similar approach is used to examine the dysmature infant; the initial appraisal begins at the moment of birth, with particular attention paid to the initiation of breathing and neonatal circulatory changes. After respiration is established, a brief examination of the newborn is completed in the delivery room. This examination is important to rule out the presence of major abnormalities and to determine whether birth injuries and minor anomalies exist.

Once the dysmature infant is situated in the special care nursery or intensive care unit, a more thorough assessment can be completed. As with the normal neonate, the initial physical assessment should begin with an examination of the maternal chart. Factors that are known to place infants at risk should be noted from the perinatal history. These factors can provide clues to possible abnormal findings in the physical examination and to potential clinical problems.

Premature or ill infants have less tolerance to handling than well, term infants and are more prone to temperature instability. The physical examination, therefore, may have to be conducted in several parts with rest periods in between, depending on the severity of illness and on the extent of the prematurity. The astute clinician will be able to determine the priorities with respect to the examination, until the infant can tolerate a complete and thorough assessment.

Nursing Diagnostic Statements and Collaborative Problems

Though the basic needs of preterm infants are similar to those of any neonate, nursing care necessarily becomes highly specialized in view of these infants' unique characteristics. The main nursing considerations and typical nursing diagnostic statements are as follows:

High risk for altered tissue perfusion: cardiopulmonary, renal, cerebral, peripheral, and gastrointestinal; risk factor: exchange problems.

High risk for potential fluid volume deficit; risk factors: prematurity or low birthweight.

High risk for infection; risk factors: inadequate acquired immunity, immunosuppression, tissue destruction, and increased environmental exposure.

High risk for impaired skin integrity; risk factor: inability of immature skin to tolerate mechanical and chemical aids used in care.

Fatigue related to excessive environmental stimuli and altered sensory reception, transmission, and/or integration.

Anticipatory parental grieving related to knowledge of potential loss of infant.

Typical collaborative problems are as follows:

Ineffective thermoregulation related to immaturity.

Impaired gas exchange related to ventilation-perfusion imbalance.

Altered nutrition: less than body requirements related to inability to ingest or digest food or absorb nutrients due to prematurity and/or biologic factors.

Planning and Implementation

Following are the nursing goal, nursing interventions, and evaluation for each of the identified nursing diagnoses.

Promote Nutrition and Oxygenation of the Cells by Maintaining an Adequate Capillary Blood Supply

Because alterations in tissue perfusion are related to gas exchange, the nursing care for ND3 is similar to the care for ND2. The assessment for adequate tissue perfusion of systems other than cardiopulmonary includes monitoring urine output for renal perfusion; neurologic vital signs for cerebral perfusion; capillary refill time for peripheral perfusion; and bowel sounds, movements, and abdominal shape and color for gastrointestinal perfusion. Nursing care that enhances oxygenation and ventilation will improve the tissue perfusion of all systems.

Promote Adequate Vascular, Cellular, and Intracellular Hydration

Premature infants have increased insensible water loss due to the immaturity of their skin, increased permeability of the skin epidermis to water, increased skin blood flow relative to the metabolic rate, a larger body surface in proportion to weight, and a lack of subcutaneous fat.

Fluid disturbances in neonates can be caused by a variety of disease states, but may also be caused by phototherapy, radiant warmers, increased ambient heat, increased loss by conduction or convection, increased insensible water loss (by mechanical ventilation, increased motor activity, crying, suctioning), and blood loss.

Electrolyte disturbances occur primarily as a result of fluid imbalance, malfunction of regulatory organs (e.g., kidneys, skin, respiratory tract, gastrointestinal tract), or increased demands by the body. These disturbances are usually imbalances in glucose, calcium, sodium chloride, and phosphates or acid-base imbalances.

Premature infants require frequent adjustment of their fluid and electrolyte intakes, based on careful monitoring of their status. This monitoring includes daily calculation of intake of fluids and electrolytes, measuring urine output, daily or twice-daily body weight checks, and identifying excessive loss of fluid through gastrointestinal or respiratory tracts. Assessment for physical signs of dehydration or overhydration should be included in the clinical examination.

Protect Infant Against Invasion by Pathogenic Organisms

Premature infants experience decreased transplacental transfer of immunoglobulins from the mother. Immunoglobulins provide the infant with passive immunity to a myriad of infectious agents. Not receiving such immunity, the premature infant is at risk for infection (sepsis). In addition, the premature infant's immature immunologic system is capable of only a minimal anti-inflammatory response when exposure to infectious agents occurs.

In view of the premature infant's minimal ability to resist infection, health professionals must assume major responsibility for prevention of infection. Several simple measures can be taken to diminish the likelihood of exposure to infectious agents. The most important measure, and yet the one most frequently ignored, is thorough handwashing with a bactericidal solution. Hands must be washed both before and after contact with each infant and his or her equipment. Gowning practices vary from institution to institution. Generally, gowns are worn when in direct contact with an infant and are changed between patients.

No one who is ill should be in contact with patients in a neonatal intensive care unit (NICU). As well, strict procedures for the routine cleaning of all equipment should be followed. For infants with specific infections, further isolation precautions may be initiated. Certain treatment modalities have been associated with an increased risk of infection, such as umbilical catheters, indwelling peripheral or central venous catheters, peripheral arterial catheters, and respiratory therapy equipment. Scrupulous aseptic technique must be followed by all personnel involved in these procedures. See discussion later in this chapter in neonatal sepsis.

Protect Skin from Internal and External Factors That Harm the Skin

The preterm infant is at greater risk than older infants for skin damage from the removal of tapes, electrodes, or collection bags. This is due to the diminished cohesion between the dermis and the epidermis and to the immaturity of the stratum corneum.

Part of the protective function of the skin results from the acid mantle that it produces. This acidic quality provides a barrier to the growth of normal flora on the skin. Frequent bathing with alkaline soaps and moisturizers can raise the skin pH. This may, in turn, cause bacteria to increase in number.

The nursing actions for maintaining skin integrity are as follows:

- Avoid use of caustic solutions to clean the skin.
- Minimize use of tapes.
- Minimize friction to skin.
- Avoid the use of alkaline-based soaps.
- Use mild solvent to remove adhesive tape.

Maintain an Appropriate Amount and Type of Stimuli

The premature infant's general homeostatic mechanisms are fragile and may easily be overwhelmed by almost any extra stimuli. The central nervous system of the preterm infant is sensitive to sensory information and is not very organized. The infant has difficulty in selectively processing various stimuli and becomes easily overwhelmed because of the inability to shut out the environment.

Infants born prematurely must cope with performing all the vital functions that were previously assumed by their mothers. Premature infants are also deprived of the regulatory influences of their mothers' biorhythms and of the entirety of the intrauterine sensory experience. Finally, they are exposed to the highly technologic environment of an intensive care unit that includes excessive painful and intrusive stimuli.

Several studies have documented the stressors in the NICU environment to which the premature infant is exposed. These include medical and nursing interventions, light, noise, and care patterns (Cartlett & Holditch-Davis, 1990; Becker et al, 1991; McCain, 1992). The overall goal of nursing care with respect to the infant's sensory environment is to provide a protective and nurturing setting that will conserve the infant's energy and enhance physiologic stability. Efforts should be made to incorporate routine measures that modify the infant's environment in such a way as to minimize or eliminate stressful or noxious stimuli.

Nursing care should be organized so as to disturb the premature infant as little as possible, especially during the night. It is important to observe carefully and document the infant's positive and negative responses to various stimuli. Consistency in caregivers should be promoted. Observations of the infant's responses in various situations should be shared with the parents. Any unnecessary equipment noise in the NICU should be eliminated or minimized. An example of this is keeping respiratory tubing free of excess water, which creates additional noise. The preterm infant should be handled and moved in a smooth, slow manner. Sufficient support to the spine, head, and extremities is required to avoid rapid extension and startling. The manner in which the preterm neonate is handled may influence progress in growth and development and overall health.

Promote Resolution of Parental Anticipatory Grieving to the Potential Loss of Infant

The families of infants who require intensive care at birth are confronted with many stressors. Parents are separated from their neonates because the infant is transferred either to a special unit within the hospital of birth or to a referral center some distance away. They often face the uncertainty of the initial diagnosis as well as the long-term outcome. Mothers of high-risk newborns may be ill themselves and, therefore, have additional physical stressors. These mothers also experience the normal physiologic changes that occur following all deliveries. Families may lack financial, social, and internal supports, all of which will exacerbate the stress caused by the birth of their baby (Bass, 1991).

When a baby needs specialized care because of prematurity or illness, the reactions and needs of the family are similar to those of families of an infant born with a congenital defect (see discussion in Chapter 19). Parents must grieve for the lost baby of their dreams so that they can then accept their baby as she or he really is. When the infant is critically ill, this grief may be compounded by an anticipatory grief through which parents try to prepare themselves for their infant's death. Sadness, denial, guilt, diminished self-esteem, and anger are some of the emotions parents express before reaching a stage at which adaptation to the reality of their situation begins.

Just as parents of babies with anomalies look within themselves for possible reasons for the defect, parents of preterm infants and infants who are ill at birth search for reasons. The diabetic mother of a LGA infant may feel particularly guilty if her infant has more than transient problems because she sees a direct link between her own condition and the baby's problems.

As with all parents and new babies, it is essential that a relationship of love and caring be established in the early stages of development. When the attachment process does not occur, child abuse or long-term psychologic difficulties for the child and family may result. An important goal of nursing care, therefore, is to facilitate the attachment process. This goal is applicable to all parents of high-risk newborns, even when the infant may not survive.

It is just as important to individualize care for the parents and families of ill or premature neonates as for the infants themselves. The meaning of this crisis event and its impact may be very different for the mother than for the father; it may vary considerably from family to family. Each person may have a unique way of coping with the situation (Affleck et al, 1990; Perehudoff, 1990).

To plan appropriate interventions, therefore, an assessment should be made of each parent and of the family unit as a whole. This assessment should include the parent's perception of the event, what things the parent finds stressful or helpful, how she or he is coping with the situation, and what resources are available and useful to the individual or family. With this information, an initial plan of care can then be devised and discussed with the parents. It is imperative that the plan of care be revised regularly, since parents' perceptions often change over time. A critically ill or very premature infant may remain in the hospital for many weeks, during which time the health status will change frequently. This "roller coaster" situation necessitates ongoing assessment of parental responses. In some units, the primary nurse is responsible for the family plan of care. In other units, the care of the family may be coordinated by a clinical nurse specialist or social worker.

Providing around-the-clock opportunities for visiting and telephoning, careful explanation of day-to-day changes in the baby's condition and treatments, and opportunities for participation by parents in care contribute to parental adaptation (Fig. 30–4) (Perlman et al, 1991). The opportunity for parents to discuss their feelings, particularly their negative feelings, is significant as well. Many intensive care nurseries sponsor group discussions in which parents can share feelings with one another as well as with staff members. Before their first visit to the NICU, parents should be prepared for their infant's appearance, the equipment involved in treatment, how treatment is contributing to the recovery, and what they may expect to do to help with the baby's care. The nurse should be nearby during the parents' visits but should allow them some degree of privacy. Most parents require some direction regarding the level of interaction appropriate for their baby's age and state of health. The nurse can take each opportunity available to point out the infant's positive features and progress. As the parents indicate readiness and the infant's condition warrants, they may be taught how to perform their infant's basic care. This may include changing the baby's diaper, holding the syringe during a gavage feeding, stimulating the baby orally during feed-

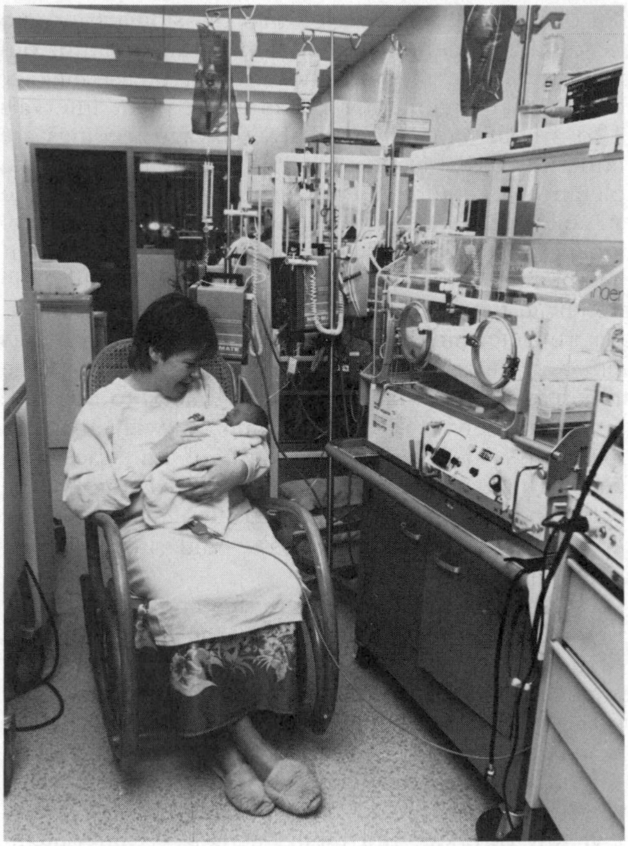

FIGURE 30 - 4. If given the support and opportunity, parents of critically ill infants can develop a relationship of love and caring even though their baby is in the midst of an overwhelming technical environment.

ing, talking to or stroking the baby, and bringing in personal items for the baby. Another important and unique contribution to the baby's care can be made by the mother: namely, the provision of breast milk for her infant. Mothers who wish to take on this task require additional support, encouragement, and teaching.

Nursing care for typical collaborative problems follows:

Assuring Protection by Maintaining Core Temperature Within Normal Range

The basic need of all neonates for warmth has been described earlier in this chapter. Thermoregulation for a preterm infant, especially an infant weighing less than 1500 g, requires special consideration. Premature and low birthweight infants are at risk for the effects of ineffective thermoregulation because of their lack of brown fat and their inability to increase their temperature through shivering. Heat loss occurs immediately following delivery so that steps must be taken to ensure that the infant is dried quickly and kept warm by an external heat source.

Infants of less than 1800 g, or infants who cannot maintain a temperature of 36.4°C (97.6°F) in room air, should be cared for in an Isolette or radiant warmer. The baby's temperature is maintained at a constant level by a heat-sensitive probe that is taped to the abdomen or back. The unit heater is activated automatically when the baby's temperature falls below the desired level of thermoneutrality. The baby's axillary temperature should also be monitored at frequent intervals as a check of the accuracy of the probe. Other important nursing interventions that will facilitate thermoregulation in the premature infant include judicious bathing, minimizing drafts into and around the Isolette/warmer, prewarming all surfaces that will contact the baby, using a radiant heat source for procedures that necessitate removal of the infant from the Isolette, use of a heat shield for very low birthweight infants, use of knitted caps and booties, and positioning to promote flexure of limbs.

Careful monitoring of ambient and infant temperature, humidity, heart rate, respiratory rate, oxygen consumption, and glucose status are also important nursing aspects.

Maintain an Adequate Passage of Oxygen and/or Carbon Dioxide Between Alveoli of Lungs and the Vascular System

Although various respiratory disorders may result in impaired gas exchange, much of the nursing care is similar and is directed toward facilitating adequate ventilation and oxygenation of the preterm infant. In general, nursing care should maximize the infant's response to the treatment modalities. Care also involves frequent monitoring of the infant's response to these treatments.

Nursing care activities should be organized so that the infant is disturbed infrequently. Excessive handling will agitate the infant and increase metabolism and energy expenditure. This will increase the need for oxygen and further compromise gas exchange. Positioning the infant on the abdomen or side will also improve oxygenation. Frequent assessment of cardiopulmonary status will indicate changes in response to treatments as well as the early development of respiratory complications (see section on medical disorders). Attention must be paid to the patency of the airway through assessment of breath sounds, suctioning, and physiotherapy.

Most of these infants will receive supplemental oxygen, and many will require assisted mechanical ventilation. Because of the risks involved in the use of too much or too little oxygen in premature infants, as discussed in the next section, continuous monitoring of the oxygen levels in the blood is a crucial part of care. This monitoring includes frequent measure of the ambient oxygen concentration and of the level of oxygen in the blood. The latter is accomplished directly by blood sampling or indirectly through the use of transcutaneous oxygen monitors and oxygen saturation monitors (refer to Chapter 32 for discussion of monitoring of oxygen levels).

Promote Sufficient Nutritional Intake to Meet Metabolic Needs

Meeting metabolic needs involves both the biochemical aspects of nutritional management and the practical aspects of delivering the nutrients themselves. The "gold standard" for growth of premature infants is controversial; a growth assessment can be performed using intrauterine or extrauterine standards, or a combination of the two standards. Frequent measurements are taken of the premature infant and include weight, length, and head circumference.

A number of studies have attempted to determine the amount of specific nutrients that are required to achieve the desired rate of growth. These studies have resulted in recommendations for the intake of protein, fat, carbohydrate, vitamins, and minerals. Generally, the recommended daily intake of protein is 3 g/kg/day; of fat is 3 g/kg/day; and of carbohydrate is 6 to 8 g/kg/day. Preterm infants also usually receive a multivitamin/mineral preparation. However, practices vary with respect to the specific nutrients given and will continue to change only as significant research data become available. (See Chapter 16 for further discussion of vitamin and mineral supplementation.)

In addition to the controversies involved in the type and amount of nutrients required for preterm infants, each method for the ideal delivery of nutrients has its proponent. Nutrients can be delivered by an enteral method (e.g., through a gastrointestinal route) or by a parenteral method (e.g., through an intravenous route).

For infants who have not yet developed the ability to suck and swallow in a coordinated fashion, or whose ability is impaired by disease, tube feedings are the method of choice. The three methods commonly used are: *gavage* (intermittent gastric), *continuous transpyloric,* and *continuous gastric feedings.* An oral or nasal tube is inserted into the stomach or into the distal duodenum or jejunum (transpyloric), depending on the method chosen, and breast milk or formula is delivered by bolus at frequent intervals (1 to 4 hours) or continuously. (Gavage feedings are further discussed in Chapter 35.) Determination of the tolerance to enteral feeding is made by noting the amount and frequency of vomiting/regurgitation, abdominal distention, and stools. In the case of intermittent feeds, the amount of residual (formula still present in the stomach just prior to the next feeding) can be determined by aspirating stomach contents with a syringe attached to the feeding tube. A large amount of residual may indicate the need to decrease the amount given at each feeding or, with an older premature, to extend the length of time between feedings (usually from 2 to 3 per hour). Intolerance to feeding also may be an indication of developing sepsis or other disease processes and should be reported and investigated.

Although intermittent gastric feeding is used most commonly, there may be indications for continuous feeding: short bowel syndrome, severe gastroesophageal reflux, delayed gastric emptying time, and so on. More clinical studies are needed to determine the effectiveness of the various feeding techniques.

Nutrients are delivered via the parenteral route when the premature or term infant is unable to receive any or enough of them enterally, as in congenital gastrointestinal anomalies, necrotizing enterocolitis, severe respiratory distress syndrome, and other conditions. Total parenteral nutrition (TPN) may be administered by either central or peripheral veins. Complete nutrient requirements can be met by TPN through a combination of specific components: protein is supplied in the form of amino acids, dextrose is the primary energy source, fats are supplied as liquid emulsions, and vitamins and minerals are added.

TABLE 30-2
Problems and Interventions in Maintaining the Preterm Infant's Nutrition

Problems	Interventions
Small energy stores	Early provision of adequate calories
Relatively higher energy needs	
Glucose intolerance	Careful monitoring of blood glucose and glucose intake
Hypoglycemia	
Hyperglycemia	
Immature gastrointestinal system	Feedings adjusted to the special needs of the preterm baby
Impaired lactose tolerance	
Relative inability to digest fats	
Increased nitrogen catabolism with respiratory distress syndrome	
Immature sucking and swallowing reflexes	Alternate routes of feeding, including gavage, intravenous feedings
Treatment for respiratory distress may interfere with oral or gavage feeding	Intravenous feeding

RESEARCH ISSUES: Breastfeeding Premature Infants

Results. The three research studies conducted by Meier and colleagues are important contributions to nursing knowledge in the area of breastfeeding premature infants. The earlier study described breastfeeding behavior in small preterm infants from initial oral feeding through discharge. The infants weighed less than 1500 g at initial oral feedings. The mother-infant pairs were videotaped while breastfeeding and bottlefeeding. Although only three pairs were studied, they were taped twice weekly for a total of 18 hours for all three pairs. These data provide important information regarding the unique breastfeeding behavior of premature infants, and demonstrated that these small infants were capable of effective breastfeeding.

In a later study, the responses of small preterm infants were compared while breastfeeding and bottlefeeding using an alternating treatment design with the infants serving as their own controls. Five infants were studied during 71 feeding sessions. The variables used to compare the two feeding methods were feeding behavior, transcutaneous Po_2, skin temperature, and duration of feeding. The results showed that infants demonstrate different sucking mechanisms for the two feeding methods and had better coordination during breastfeeding than during bottlefeeding. Infants also showed less disruption in transcutaneous Po_2 patterns with breastfeeding. The infants' mean skin temperature rose significantly more during breastfeeding, and the mean duration of feeding was greater with breastfeeding.

Implications. Although the sample sizes in these two studies were small, the results are significant with respect to challenging previously held assumptions about the limitations of preterm infants, which were not based on scientific evidence. These results have major implications for nursing in view of the fact that nurses are mainly responsible for the decision about when to put a preterm infant to breast. Nurses, then, can have the greatest impact in this area of clinical practice.

REFERENCES

Meier, P. (1988). Bottle- and breast-feeding: Effects on transcutaneous oxygen pressure and temperature in preterm infants. *Nursing Research, 37,* 36–41.

Meier, P., & Anderson, G. C. (1987). Responses of small preterm infants to bottle- and breast-feeding. *MCN: American Journal of Maternal Child Nursing, 12,* 97–105.

Meier, P., & Pugh, E. J. (1985). Breast-feeding behavior of small preterm infants. *MCN: American Journal of Maternal Child Nursing, 10,* 396–401.

Feeding implications are vitally important to nurses. Safe and effective delivery of feeding by tube includes skill in tube insertion and removal, proper positioning of the infant, instillation of milk at a controlled rate, and careful observation for signs of intolerance or distress during or following feeds.

The key aspects of nursing care during TPN are maintenance of the venous line through aseptic techniques and judicious handling and restraint of the infant so that the line does not become dislodged (see Chapter 16 for further discussion of TPN). Table 30–2 summarizes the problems and interventions related to the preterm infant's nutrition.

When the infant is able to coordinate sucking, swallowing, and breathing, it is appropriate to start the infant nursing directly from the mother's breast. It is suggested that this development occurs at about 33 to 34 weeks. The literature suggests that breastfeeding is as well tolerated as bottlefeeding, so that premature infants need not be established on bottle feeding prior to the initiation of breastfeeding (Meier, 1988; Meier & Anderson, 1987). It may also be beneficial to provide opportunities for premature infants and their mothers to begin "breastfeeding" earlier than 33 weeks. Although mainly non-nutritive in nature, these early efforts may increase the mother's milk supply and may lead to full breastfeeding being established in a shorter time. More systematic investigations of the effects of these interventions are needed before they become accepted clinical practice.

Evaluation

Each of the interventions requires specific and ongoing evaluation to determine the effectiveness of nursing approaches. See the Nursing Process Plan in Table 30–3 for evaluation of diagnoses.

Postmaturity

Infants are considered postmature if they are born at more than 42 weeks gestation. They may also be assessed as small or large for gestational age. The mortality rate is increased compared with full-term infants, especially in those born to primiparous women and women over 35 years of age.

Etiology/Incidence/Clinical Manifestations

Up to 12 per cent of neonates have a gestational age of more than 42 weeks gestation. The cause of postmaturity is unknown. With postmature infants, there is also an increased incidence of cephalopelvic disproportion, cesarean section, and birth injuries owing to their increased size.

Some of these infants have a characteristic appearance that includes absence of vernix caseosa; dry,

TABLE 30-3

Nursing Process Plan: The Premature Infant

***Analysis*:** Collaborative Problem 1

***Response and Related or Risk Factors*:** *Ineffective thermoregulation related to immaturity*

***Projected Outcome*:** Infant's core temperature will remain within normal range

Defining Characteristics	***Nursing Interventions***	***Evaluation Criteria***
Subjective: None *Objective*: • Temperature fluctuation above or below the normal range • Apnea and bradycardia episodes	*Temperature Regulation* Use appropriate sources of heat (Isolette, radiant warmer, heat shield) to maintain temperature within normal range Conserve heat during bathing and procedures Use knitted caps, booties, and flexed position Monitor *ambient* and infant temperature Monitor vital signs and metabolic state	Criteria to evaluate effective thermoregulation in premature infants include: • Warm extremities • Pink skin with no mottling • Core temperature maintained between 35.5° C and 37.5° C (96 and 99.5° F) or abdominal skin temperature between 36° C and 36.5° C (96.8 and 97.7° F)

***Analysis*:** Collaborative Problem 2

***Response and Related or Risk Factors*:** *Impaired gas exchange related to ventilation perfusion imbalance*

***Projected Outcome*:** Infant adequately passes oxygen and/or carbon dioxide between alveoli of lungs and the vascular system

Defining Characteristics	***Nursing Interventions***	***Evaluation Criteria***
Subjective: • Restlessness • Irritability • Somnolence *Objective*: • Cyanosis • Respiratory distress (e.g., tachypnea, substernal, tracheal or intercostal retractions, nasal flaring) • Abnormal blood gas values • Decreased breath sounds, rhonchi or crepitations on auscultation • Inability to move excessive secretions	*Respiratory Monitoring* Monitor infant's response to treatments Minimal disturbance for care Maintain patent airway Monitor for changes in cardiopulmonary status Monitor oxygen levels in ventilated infants **Collaborate with physician regarding the impaired gas exchange**	Criteria to evaluate effective gas exchange include: • Pink color • Equal air entry on auscultation of lung fields with no adventitia • Acceptable blood gas values, oxygen monitor parameters • Vital signs within normal limits

Analysis: Collaborative Problem 3

Response and Related or Risk Factors: *Altered tissue perfusion: cardiopulmonary, renal, cerebral, peripheral, and gastrointestinal; related to impaired gas exchange*

Projected Outcome: Infant's nutrition and level of cell oxygenation is maintained by an adequate capillary blood supply

Defining Characteristics	Nursing Interventions	Evaluation Criteria
Subjective: • Somnolence *Objective:* • Cold extremities • Dependent parts bluish to purplish • Extremities pale on elevation, color does not return on lowering • Diminished arterial pulsations • Skin shiny • Blood pressure changes • Decreased urine output • Distended abdomen	*Nutritional Monitoring and Oxygen Therapy* See Collaborative Problem 1—Nursing Interventions Monitor all body systems for adequate function **Collaborate with physician regarding the altered tissue perfusion**	Criteria for adequate effective tissue perfusion include: • Urine output between 2 and 5 ml/kg/hr • Infant responsive to stimuli, with normal neurologic vital signs • Warm extremities, capillary refill time less than 3 secs • Soft, nondistended abdomen with bowel sounds and normal stools

Analysis: Nursing Diagnostic Statement 1

Response and Related or Risk Factors: *High risk for fluid volume deficit; risk factors prematurity or low birthweight*

Proposed Outcome: Infant's hydration status is adequate (vascular, cellular, and intracellular)

Defining Characteristics *(Actual Response)*	Nursing Interventions	Evaluation Criteria
Subjective: None *Objective:* • Sunken fontanelle • Increased pulse rate (from baseline) • Decreased or excessive urine output • Weight loss in excess of expected postnatal loses • Dry skin/mucous membrane • Increased serum sodium • Excessively concentrated urine • Decreased skin turgor • Decreased venous filling • Edema	*Fluid/Electrolyte Management* Assess for signs of dehydration or overhydration Monitor fluid and electrolyte intake Accurate calculations of urine output, body weight, other fluid losses	Criteria for effective fluid and electrolyte balance in preterm infants include: • Flat fontanelle • Normal vital signs • Moist mucous membranes • Normal skin turgor • Urine output between 2 and 5 ml/kg/hr • Weight loss not greater than 15% of birthweight or gain not greater than 30 g per day • Absence of edema • Warm extremities, capillary refill time less than 3 secs • Normal serum and urine electrolytes and concentration

(continued)

TABLE 30-3 *(continued)*

Analysis: Collaborative Problem 4

Response and Related or Risk Factors: *Altered nutrition: less than body requirements related to inability to ingest or digest food or absorb nutrients due to prematurity and/or biologic factors*

Projected Outcome: Infant's nutritional intake will be sufficient to meet metabolic needs

Defining Characteristics	Nursing Interventions	Evaluation Criteria
Subjective: None *Objective*: • Signs of inadequate digestion (e.g., emesis, residuals with gavage feeding) • Pale conjunctival and mucous membranes	*Nutrition Management* Assess growth (weight, length, and head circumference) Provide 3 g/kg/day of protein; 3 g/kg/day of fat; and 6–8 g/kg/day of carbohydrate Give multivitamins/minerals Give nutrients by tube to infants where sucking and swallowing ability not developed Assess tolerance to enteral feeds Give nutrients via parenteral route, total parenteral nutrition when enteral route is not tolerated After sucking, swallowing, and breathing are coordinated, can start infant on breastfeeding or bottle feedings **Collaborate with physician in relation to maintaining nutritional intake**	Criteria to determine the effectiveness of nutritional management relate to the type of nutrients given and to the method of delivery. The major responsibility for the determination of the type of nutrients that the infant is to receive is usually not part of the nurse's role. The effectiveness of the method of delivery is determined primarily by the nurse, however, because of her role in feeding the infant Successful gavage tube feeding in preterm infants includes: • Minimal or no signs of distress during feeding • Minimal or no emesis after feeding

Analysis: Nursing Diagnostic Statement 2

Response and Related or Risk Factors: *High risk for infection; risk factors inadequate acquired immunity, immunosuppression, tissue destruction, and increased environmental exposure*

Projected Outcomes: Infant remains free from invasion of pathogenic organisms

Defining Characteristics *(Actual Response)*	Nursing Interventions	Evaluation Criteria
Subjective: None *Objective*: • Skin breakdown • Decreased hemoglobin • Leukopenia • Frequent exposure to invasive procedures	*Infection Protection* Thorough handwashing with a bactericidal solution. Prevent anyone who is ill from coming into contact with infant. Scrupulous aseptic technique during performance of procedures. Maintain caloric and protein intake Monitor for sepsis and report subtle changes Instruct family how to protect infant from infection Administer appropriate immunizations (collaborative intervention—see Chapter 10)	The successful prevention of infection in preterm infants would best be determined by the number of nosocomial or acquired infections that were identified. However, this number would also be affected by factors other than nursing care. Handwashing, maintenance of aseptic technique during procedures, and maintaining a clean environment are most likely to affect the outcome with respect to infection control. Specific criteria used to determine whether an infant has been prevented from becoming infected include:

TABLE 30-3 *(continued)*

Defining Characteristics *(Actual Response)*	Nursing Interventions	Evaluation Criteria
		• Absence of signs of sepsis • No episodes of infection • Family and hospital personnel demonstrate meticulous hand-washing • Family demonstrates knowledge of risk factors for infection

Analysis: Nursing Diagnostic Statement 3

Response and Related or Risk Factors: *High risk for impaired skin integrity; risk factors external (environmental)*

- Extremes in temperature
- Mechanical factors (pressure, restraint)
- Radiation
- Physical immobilization
- Excretion/secretions
- Humidity

Projected Outcome: Infant's skin is not harmed by internal and external factors

Defining Characteristics *(Actual Response)*	Nursing Interventions	Evaluation Criteria
Subjective: None **Objective**: None	***Skin Surveillance*** Prevent skin breakdown by: • Change position when disturbing infant for routine care • Change location of restraints when changing position • Keep skin clean, dry, and free of secretions/excretions • Avoid use of caustic solutions to clean skin • Avoid the use of alkaline-based soaps • Minimize use of tapes • Minimize friction to skin • Use mild solvent to remove adhesive tape • Maintain core temperature within normal range (see Collaborative Problem 1)	Absence of skin breakdown

Analysis: Nursing Diagnostic Statement 4

Response and Related or Risk Factors: *Sensory alterations: visual, auditory, kinesthetic, tactile, related to altered environmental stimuli and altered sensory reception, transmission, and/or integration*

Projected Outcome: Infant will experience an appropriate amount and patterning of stimuli

(continued)

TABLE 30-3 (continued)

Defining Characteristics	Nursing Interventions	Evaluation Criteria
Subjective: None ***Objective***: Avoidance behaviors: • Gaze aversion • Arching of the trunk • Finger splaying • Crying and yawning More severe responses: • Mottled or cyanotic skin • Apnea • Bradycardia • Blood pressure instability • Hypoxemia	*Sensory Management* Organize care to reduce disturbance of infant Assure consistent caregivers Minimize equipment noise Avoid bright lights as much as possible Observe infant's responses to stimuli and cues of overload Handle smoothly and slowly Support spine, head, and extremities while handling	Part of the evaluation of the nursing care that is provided to preterm infants should include the infant's response to the interventions. The recognition of distress in a preterm infant should result in the modification of the action in which the nurse is engaged. Evaluation criteria include absence or decrease of avoidance behaviors associated with overstimulation and more severe physiologic responses that are associated with overstimulation

Analysis: Nursing Diagnostic Statement 5

Response and Related or Risk Factors: *Ineffective family coping: compromised, related to parental anticipatory grieving, inadequate resources, extreme stress or anxiety, ineffective communication*

Projected Outcome: Parent(s) will be able to adapt to the stresses associated with their infant's illness or hospitalization

Defining Characteristics	Nursing Interventions	Evaluation Criteria
Subjective: • Verbal expression of being overwhelmed and unable to deal with or face the situation • Verbal expressions of continued lack of understanding reports of infant's condition • Altered sleep patterns • Inadequate nutritional intake • Verbal expression of extreme feelings of guilt, anger, depression, anxiety ***Objective***: • Prolonged denial • Avoidance behavior • Aggressive behavior toward staff, family members • Inability to leave the hospital to attend to own needs or other family members • Inability to distinguish changes in infant's status	*Coping Enhancement and Grief Work Facilitation* Assess each parent's perception of the event and coping style and teach additional coping methods if indicated Assess availability of resources and make referrals as indicated Ongoing assessment of individual parental responses Allow round-the-clock visiting and telephoning privileges Explain day-to-day changes in baby to parent(s) Explain treatments and procedures Prepare parent(s) for infant's appearance on first visit Encourage parent(s) to share concerns Assist parent(s) to provide normal infant care Support parent(s) in their grief and stress reactions	Beginning resolution of anticipatory grief and adjustment to stressors will depend on the particular situation. As the infant's outcome becomes more definitive, parents may begin to show signs of adjustment to the situation. These signs may include: • Regular visiting or phone calling • The ability to discuss with staff their concerns and their perception of the situation • Increasing interaction with the infant as the illness or prematurity permits • Ability to attend to their own needs and the needs of other family members Parents of infants who remain seriously ill, who die, or who demonstrate symptoms of long-lasting problems, may not show any further signs of adjustment, demonstrating continued feelings of sadness, denial, guilt, depression, and anger

cracking skin; long nails; decreased subcutaneous fat; oligohydramnios; meconium staining of the skin and nails; and a long, thin body.

Therapeutic Management

The therapeutic management of post term infants will depend on the clinical problems they manifest. Otherwise, the management is the same as for the healthy, term infant. Specific complications have been associated with postmaturity. These include fetal distress with subsequent hypoxic-ischemic insult and/or meconium aspiration, inadequate nutrition, thermal instability, SGA, hypoglycemia, and polycythemia-hyperviscosity syndrome.

Nursing Care

The nursing diagnostic statements and collaborative problems that are applicable to postmature infants are similar to those previously described for the premature infant. Nursing diagnostic statements are as follows:

- *High risk for altered tissue perfusion: cardiopulmonary, renal, cerebral, peripheral, and gastrointestinal; risk factors: exchange problems.*
- *Anticipatory parental grieving related to knowledge of potential loss of infant.*

Collaborative problems are as follows:

- *Ineffective thermoregulation related to postmaturity.*
- *Altered nutrition: less than body requirements related to inability to ingest or digest food or absorb nutrients due to postmaturity and/or biologic factors.*

The nursing care related to these diagnoses, which was described in the previous section, is generally the same and is not repeated here.

Small for Gestational Age

At any gestational age, an infant's weight may fall below the 10th percentile, according to standard growth charts. This infant will be termed "small for gestational age" (SGA).

Etiology/Incidence/Clinical Manifestations

Approximately one third of all babies weighing less than 2500 g at birth are SGA rather than preterm. These infants may also be said to have intrauterine growth retardation (IUGR). The clinical picture of retarded intrauterine growth is related to the duration, severity, and time of initial onset.

One type of IUGR is asymmetric or hypotrophic growth retardation, in which the neonate's length and head circumference fall within normal limits on the growth curves. Only the weight is abnormal. At birth, these infants appear thin and wasted. There is little subcutaneous tissue, so the skin appears loose; it is often peeling and meconium-stained. This type of growth failure occurs late in pregnancy; its causes include toxemia, hypertension, class C diabetes, and cardiac and renal disease. These infants are often distressed at birth and rapidly become hypoxemic and acidotic; therefore, they require resuscitation. They may also have aspirated meconium, thereby exacerbating the distress. Following birth, infants with asymmetric growth retardation do not lose weight, but rather soon experience a period of rapid weight gain. In the absence of severe hypoxic-ischemic insult or other problems, these infants usually do well.

The second type of IUGR is symmetric or hypoplastic. In this type, all the aforementioned growth parameters are below normal. The infant does not appear wasted since growth in body weight stopped weeks before birth, prior to the development of adipose tissue. This chronic growth failure occurs as a result of intrauterine infections (such as congenital rubella and cytomegalovirus), congenital and chromosomal abnormalities (such as dwarfism, cri-du-chat syndrome), and maternal malnutrition. These infants are also distressed at birth, but their distress is often due to hyaline membrane disease.

Other factors are associated with SGA infants. Multiple births may be a problem, especially with twin-to-twin transfusion. Twin-to-twin transfusion refers to an artery-to-vein anastomosis in the placenta. Blood is chronically shunted away from one twin, resulting in growth retardation. Maternal factors include high altitudes, smoking, low socioeconomic status, drug abuse, anticonvulsant therapy, antimetabolite therapy, and chronic alcoholism. There is also a 23 per cent incidence of mental deficiency in fetal alcohol syndrome. These infants commonly have dysmorphic features and cardiocirculatory abnormalities (see Chapter 27 for further discussion of fetal alcohol syndrome).

Diagnostic Assessment

Because the incidence of congenital malformation is increased in these infants, especially meticulous physical assessment is indicated.

If congenital infection is suspected, blood from both mother and baby is examined for the presence of antibodies to the TORCH group of infections (*t*oxoplasmosis, *o*thers [e.g., syphilis and infectious hepatitis], *r*ubella, *c*ytomegalovirus, and *h*erpes simplex).

Therapeutic Management

Because SGA infants have small reserves of both glycogen and fat, hypoglycemia can be a significant problem. If glucose is not supplied from the time of birth, central nervous system damage can result. Calcium is also given to SGA infants early in their treatment because of low body stores.

Polycythemia (an excess of red blood cells) is frequent and is probably an intrauterine response to chronic fetal hypoxia. When the hematocrit is greater than 65 per cent, the blood becomes sufficiently viscous to reduce its flow. This results in a high incidence of hyperbilirubinemia and treatment with phototherapy.

Nursing Care

The nursing diagnostic statements that are applicable to SGA infants are as follows:

- *High risk for fluid volume deficit; risk factor, low birthweight.*
- *High risk for infection; risk factors, inadequate acquired immunity, immunosuppression, tissue destruction, and increased environmental exposure.*
- *High risk for impaired skin integrity; risk factors, mechanical factors.*
- *Anticipatory parental grieving related to knowledge of potential loss of infant.*

Collaborative problems are as follows:

- *Ineffective thermoregulation related to low birthweight.*
- *Altered nutrition: less than body requirements related to inability to ingest or digest or absorb nutrients due to low birthweight and/or biologic factors.*

The nursing care related to these diagnoses, which was previously described, is generally the same and is not repeated in this section.

Large for Gestational Age

When an infant's birthweight exceeds the 90th percentile for gestational age, that infant is considered "large for gestational age" (LGA).

Etiology/Incidence/Clinical Manifestations

A birthweight of over 4000 g often reflects a genetic predisposition; infants of diabetic mothers are the exception. LGA babies weigh more and have proportionally larger heads and length. Infants of diabetic mothers are disproportionately heavier. This excessive weight is related to the deposition of fat from elevated maternal blood sugars. This occurs because the infant is not capable of excreting sufficient insulin to handle the elevated blood sugar.

Hypoglycemia is a major concern in infants of diabetic mothers because of the following sequence: increased maternal blood glucose results in a higher level of glucose crossing the placenta; fetal insulin production increases to metabolize the glucose that is stored as glycogen; at birth, maternal glucose is no longer available, but insulin production remains increased, leading rapidly to hypoglycemia. Respiratory distress, hypocalcemia, and hyperbilirubinemia are also common in infants of diabetic mothers.

Typical clinical complications associated with LGA infants include: hypoxic-ischemic insult, spontaneous air leaks, transposition of the great vessels, and birth trauma, all of which increase the mortality rate for LGA babies.

Diagnostic Assessment

Following initial determination of the infant's size, as LGA, tests to rule out maternal diabetes may be completed, unless this factor is already known from the history.

Therapeutic Management

The therapeutic management of LGA infants will depend on the underlying cause and on the clinical problems that they manifest. With infants of diabetic mothers, careful monitoring of serum glucose and calcium levels is required.

Nursing Care

Other than issues related to electrolyte balance, the care of these infants is not different from that of other term infants.

Multiple Gestations

Approximately 2.2 per cent of births are twin deliveries. Triplet deliveries are far less frequent, occurring in about 0.06 per cent of births (US Department of Health and Human Services, 1990).

Etiology/Incidence

Twins may be monozygotic or dizygotic. Monozygotic twins develop from a single fertilized ovum that divides to form two embryos within the first 14 days of fertilization; this occurs approximately once in every 200 pregnancies. Dizygotic, or fraternal, twins result from double ovulation. Rates of dizygotic twins are influenced by race (higher in African-American and lower in Asian-American women), by maternal age (increased incidence as maternal age increases), and by family history of dizygotic twins.

Placentas in two pregnancies may be monochorionic (i.e., with one chorion and either one or two amnions) or dichorionic (with two chorions and two amnions). When the placenta is monochorionic, a vascular connection usually exists between the twins; when this connection is artery-to-vein, there is a fetal-to-fetal transfusion (fetal transfusion syndrome). Such transfusion occurs in approximately 15 per cent of twins with monochorionic placentas.

Intrauterine development of twins is much like that of a single fetus during the first 29 to 32 weeks or to the time when the combined weight of the fetuses is approximately 3000 g. After that time, the placenta may no longer be able to meet rapidly increasing growth needs, and IUGR can occur. Intervention that enhances uterine blood flow, such as having the mother rest in the left lateral position, may enhance fetal growth.

Diagnostic Assessment

Because of the widespread use of fetal ultrasonography, most multiple pregnancies are diagnosed prior to delivery. When a multiple birth is expected, adequate nursing and medical personnel must be present at the delivery to assure that each infant receives sufficient care immediately following delivery. Twin births are considered "high risk" and include a higher risk of prematurity and being SGA.

The possibility of fetal transfusion syndrome may be suspected when maternal hydramnios occurs in a twin pregnancy. Ultrasound may reveal a major disparity in twin size; birthweights may differ by as much as 1000 g (2.2 pounds).

Therapeutic Management

In fetal transfusion syndrome, each twin will have specific problems that require immediate attention. The twin at the arterial side of the transfusion will be small, malnourished, pale, anemic, and hypovolemic. Frequently, the baby is in shock. Immediate care, as in any anemic, hypovolemic neonate, involves careful assessment of infant status and transfusion to replace volume and red blood cells. The baby is critically ill and requires all the support and intensive nursing care of a very sick neonate.

The recipient twin, in contrast, is well nourished, plethoric, polycythemic, and hypervolemic. The heart is enlarged, and the baby may have heart failure. Secondary to polycythemia, jaundice or thrombosis may occur. If the central hematocrit is greater than 65 to 70 per cent, a partial exchange transfusion may be in order to replace the more viscous blood with normal blood. At slightly lower levels, intravenous fluids may alleviate hyperviscosity if there are no symptoms of problems.

Nursing Care

The nursing diagnoses applicable to multiple gestations will depend on the gestational age of the infants (i.e., preterm or term). The unique aspects of the nursing care involved are described in the following paragraphs.

The first sight of their newborn infant and the moments of "togetherness" that follow are among the important steps in the attachment process. In multiple births, of course, the arrival of the first baby may result in a very different physical sensation for the mother; she may feel the other fetus or fetuses moving inside her. Between the delivery of the first baby and subsequent babies, both parents' attention is necessarily divided between the activities of the second stage of labor and the baby already born.

When twins are premature or ill, the period immediately following birth will be like that of any other neonate with similar problems, and nursing actions to support attachment will be similar. If the babies are term and healthy, both (all) may be with the mother during the fourth stage of labor, and breastfeeding, if desired, may be initiated.

During the first days after birth, both during hospitalization and at home, parents need extra help to integrate the babies into their lives. Not surprisingly, parents may also require additional guidance in relation to organization of time and energy. With twice the workload, fatigue is a major source of stress for parents of twins. Finances also may be a problem owing to the increased need for clothing and equipment.

Mothers-of-Twins Club, a national organization, provides emotional support and very practical advice for new parents. Ideally, contact will be made with a local group prior to the time of birth. If not, nurses who care for the mother following delivery should provide her with information. A local La Leche group may have a member experienced in the care of twins who may be particularly helpful to the breastfeeding mother. In smaller communities where no formal support structure may be available, nurses can help parents identify sources of support among their own family and friends and in the community.

Twins can be fed, just as any other infant, in a manner appropriate to gestational age, any special needs of the baby, and the desires of the mother. Though some mothers overlook the possibility of breastfeeding when multiple neonates are expected, breastfeeding offers several advantages. Because more bottles and formula will be required, breastfeeding is economical of both money and preparation time. Mother will need a well-balanced diet high in calories and protein, a high fluid intake, and opportunity for rest at intervals during the day as well as at night. If these conditions are met, milk supply is usually adequate, because the stimulus of two nursing babies enhances milk supply.

Mothers of twins may want to feed each twin individually at first, but work toward nursing both babies at the same time, allowing more time for rest and other activities between feeding time. Several positions for joint feeding are possible. The babies may be held longitudinally facing the mother (not comfortable in the first days following cesarean delivery), or in a "football" hold with feet toward the mother's sides. Other alternatives are positioning the babies in parallel, both facing the same way, or holding one baby in each arm with their bodies crossed. At first, mothers of twins, like all mothers, will need help in experimenting with positions that are most comfortable for them and their babies.

When twins are bottlefed or alternately breastfed and bottlefed, the mother may have help at feeding time, from father or others. Parents need factual information about costs and time for various feeding methods.

Alterations Commonly Associated with Dysmaturity

Respiratory Distress Syndrome

Respiratory distress syndrome (RDS), also known as hyaline membrane disease (HMD), is an acute respiratory disorder that occurs primarily in premature infants.

Etiology/Incidence

Recent reductions in the incidence of severity of RDS have occurred chiefly as a result of prenatal therapies that inhibit premature labor (e.g., bed rest, tocolytic drugs, and the use of steroids given to the mother prior to delivery to stimulate lung maturation in the fetus). The use of surfactant replacement therapy will likely also reduce the severity of RDS and the rate of occurrence (Coulter, 1992; Boeckling, 1992). The occurrence of this disease increases as birthweight decreases.

In effect, RDS occurs in infants born before completion of their lung maturation. Because of surfactant deficiency and structural immaturity, these infants are unable to establish effective respirations and, therefore, are unable to maintain adequate gas exchange. The presence of adequate surfactant allows alveoli to remain stable and not collapse following each breath. In the absence of surfactant, progressive collapse of the alveolar sacs occurs (atelectasis), leading to pulmonary hypoperfusion. These factors impair gas exchange and produce hypoxia and hypercapnia. Prolonged hypoxia results in metabolic acidosis; retention of carbon dioxide causes respiratory acidosis.

Clinical Manifestations/Diagnostic Assessment

Typical clinical symptoms include nasal flaring, expiratory grunting, use of accessory chest wall muscles in breathing (sternal and intercostal retractions), tachypnea, diminished air entry by auscultation, cyanosis, and apnea. The classic chest radiograph shows congested lung fields with a ground-glass appearance.

Therapeutic Management

Treatment in the acute phase of the disease (i.e., the first 3 to 5 days) includes the use of supplemental oxygen; providing a neutral thermal environment; intravenous therapy; and frequent monitoring of color, activity, respiratory rate and effort, heart rate, body temperature, blood pH, arterial oxygen tension (Pao_2), arterial carbon dioxide tension ($Paco_2$), and bicarbonate (HCO_3). Approximately 10 to 30 per cent of infants with RDS also require assisted mechanical ventilation to maintain adequate gas exchange and tissue perfusion (Klaus & Fanaroff, 1986). The two major modes of mechanical ventilation are continuous positive airway pressure (CPAP), alone or alternately, in conjunction with intermittent mandatory ventilation (IMV). CPAP provides positive pressure at end-expiration for infants who can breathe spontaneously, but who are experiencing alveolar collapse. IMV delivers a combination of end-expiratory pressure and inspiratory pressure at a specific respiratory rate and pattern. Both of these forms of assisted ventilation involve the use of an endotracheal or nasopharyngeal tube and, frequently, supplemental oxygen. High-frequency jet ventilation and high-frequency oscillation are two new modes of mechanical ventilation under research. It is hoped that they may decrease the long-term effects of the trauma to the lungs from current modes. (See Chapter 32 for further discussion of respiratory therapy.)

Nursing Care

Because of the risks involved in the use of too much or too little oxygen in premature infants, as discussed later in this section, continuous monitoring of the oxygen levels in the blood is a crucial part of care. This monitoring includes frequent measurement of the ambient oxygen concentration and of the level of oxygen in the blood. The latter is accomplished directly by blood sampling, or indirectly through the use of transcutaneous oxygen monitors and oxygen saturation monitors (refer to Chapter 32 for discussion of monitoring of oxygen levels).

Patent Ductus Arteriosus

Patent ductus arteriosus (PDA) closure is often delayed in premature infants and in those with RDS. The ductus arteriosus remains patent in about 20 per cent of preterm infants weighing less than 1750 g, but increases to 75 to 80 per cent of infants of less than 30 weeks gestation with HMD. It also occurs in full-term infants, and is discussed in Chapter 33.

Persistent Pulmonary Hypertension of the Neonate

Persistent pulmonary hypertension of the neonate (PPHN) has also been termed "persistence of fetal circulation" (PFC) and is associated with pulmonary hypertension, right-to-left shunting in the heart, and normal cardiac anatomy.

Etiology/Incidence

This abnormality results from pulmonary arteriolar constriction, which may be brought about by a number of causes. Basically, pulmonary vasoconstriction causes pulmonary artery pressure to rise above aortic pressure and results in a right-to-left shunt across the ductus arteriosus. Pressure in the right atrium of the heart may be greater than that in the left atrium, causing further shunting through the foramen ovale. Vasoconstriction also results in pulmonary hypoperfusion and decreased blood return to the left atrium, which causes severe hypoxemia. PPHN can occur with HMD, pneumonia (especially group B streptococcal), meconium aspiration, diaphragmatic hernia, cold stress, rapid changes in inspired oxygen concentration, and perinatal asphyxia.

Clinical Manifestations/Diagnostic Assessment

Clinically these infants present with tachypnea and cyanosis and are often critically ill. Confirmation of PPHN may be made with echocardiography. It also produces a differential in the readings from two transcutaneous Po_2 electrodes placed over the right upper chest and abdomen.

Therapeutic Management

The treatment of this disorder is difficult and complex, and includes oxygen therapy, assisted mechanical ventilation, vasodilators and vasopressors, and treatment of metabolic imbalances.

Nursing Care

It is of vital importance that infants with PPHN not be stressed unnecessarily. Any increased demands on these infants will result in a worsening of their condition. They are extremely labile and must be handled as little as possible. Careful monitoring of vital signs and oxygenation is especially important in these infants because of the rapid changes in physiologic status that can occur with PPHN.

Meconium Aspiration

Distress of the fetus in utero can result in release of meconium into the amniotic fluid, which may then be aspirated at the time of delivery.

Etiology/Incidence

Release of meconium in utero occurs predominantly in postmature infants but is also common with SGA infants. It almost never occurs in infants of less than 34 weeks gestation, and, when it does, is associated with listerial infection. The etiology of this syndrome is not well known but appears to be associated with some period of asphyxia prior to delivery. The ensuing cardiorespiratory problems result from a combination of airway obstruction and chemical inflammation. The initial fetal distress, if prolonged, can result in acidosis and hypoxemia, pulmonary vasoconstriction, and, finally, PPHN.

In addition to the effects from the intrauterine hypoxemic insult, the airway obstruction can lead to various air leak disorders of the lungs, which are discussed later in this section.

Diagnostic Assessment

The presence of meconium is detected following rupture of the membranes during labor. The infant's status is then carefully monitored in order to detect increasing fetal distress, which may necessitate a forceps-assisted delivery or an emergency cesarean section. Meconium aspiration syndrome is diagnosed following delivery by radiography. Clinically, the infant is often in significant respiratory distress and the chest appears hyperinflated or "barrel-chested."

Therapeutic Management

The most important treatment for this disorder is to minimize the aspiration of meconium at the time of delivery. This includes suctioning of the nasopharynx following delivery of the head, prior to delivery of the shoulders, and before the infant takes the first breath. In the presence of significant meconium in an infant who has not cried, a laryngoscopy should be performed to allow direct suctioning of the trachea. The need for mechanical ventilation, supplemental oxygen, and further respiratory support can then be assessed.

Nursing Care

The care of infants with meconium aspiration syndrome focuses on their respiratory status and is much the same as with any other respiratory disease. These infants are at risk for development of PPHN if they become hypoxic and should be carefully monitored for that disorder as well.

Transient Tachypnea of the Neonate

Like meconium aspiration, this disorder affects infants at, or close to, term.

Etiology/Incidence

There is no underlying lung pathology in this syndrome, and it appears to result from slow absorption of fetal lung fluid. This syndrome is frequently referred to as "wet lung." Respiratory symptoms are similar to, but usually less severe than, those of HMD.

Diagnostic Assessment

Chest radiography usually can distinguish this condition from HMD and meconium aspiration, but it may be indistinguishable from group B streptococcal pneumonia.

Therapeutic Management

These infants require frequent monitoring and may need supplemental oxygen. They rarely require mechanical ventilation or drug therapy.

Nursing Care

Because this condition is one of the respiratory disorders commonly found in neonates, nursing care of these infants will be the same as with the other respiratory diseases. The infant with transient tachypnea will be given nothing by mouth and will be monitored for changes in clinical status or in oxygen requirements.

Apnea

"Apnea is the most common respiratory event occurring in the high-risk neonate" (Marchal et al, 1987).

Etiology/Incidence/Diagnostic Assessment

Two major clinical circumstances involve apnea: (1) apnea in full-term or preterm neonates as part of respiratory distress, cardiovascular compromise, sepsis, and intrauterine hypoxic insult, and (2) apnea and bradycardia in premature neonates without other symptoms.

Severe or recurrent apneic episodes result in inadequate gas exchange, causing hypoxemia and bradycardia. This can lead to decreased cardiac output, decreased blood pressure, and decreased cerebral blood flow.

Apnea also may result from hyperthermia or hypothermia, metabolic imbalances, abdominal distention, vagal stimulation, and certain drugs. Apnea not related to any other cause is thought to occur in premature infants, from weak upper airway musculature, from decreased brain stem respiratory control, and as a response to hypoxemia by hypoventilating.

Therapeutic Management

Immediate treatment includes cutaneous stimulation; if no response is obtained, then bag and mask ventilation is applied. Recurrent apneas may be treated with low CPAP, supplemental oxygen, a pulsating waterbed, and methylxanthine or doxapram drug therapy.

Nursing Care

Nursing care includes a prompt response to stimulate the apneic infant, a neutral thermal environment, proper suctioning technique, efficient gavage tube insertion, feeding infant on the right side or in a prone position with neutral neck flexion, and monitoring for toxic drug symptoms.

Complications of Respiratory Management

The treatment for most of the preceding respiratory disorders includes supplemental oxygen therapy or assisted mechanical ventilation, or both. Note that these treatments are not without complications. Three major complications have been associated with one or both of these common therapies: air leak syndromes, chronic lung changes, and retinopathy of prematurity.

Air leak syndromes are the most frequent life-threatening complications of assisted mechanical ventilation. They can also occur spontaneously or in association with obstructive disorders, such as meconium aspiration. Pulmonary interstitial emphysema, pneumothorax, and pneumomediastinum are the most common types of air leak syndromes.

Pulmonary interstitial emphysema is characterized by air leaks that travel along the outside of the blood vessels in the lung tissue. This air causes pressure on the vessels, which compresses them, resulting in circulatory impairment. Air may also travel along the vessels toward the hilum of the lungs and invade the mediastinum (pneumomediastinum). Air bubbles can accumulate at the hilum to such an extent that the area ruptures, releasing air into the pleural space (pneumothorax). This final type of air leak may require immediate medical intervention. Pulmonary interstitial emphysema can be diagnosed only by radiologic examination and will resolve only when mechanical ventilation is discontinued as the underlying lung disease resolves. Pneumothorax and pneumomediastinum vary in the extent of their clinical manifestations. No outward clinical symptoms may be evident, and radiologic examination may be required for a diagnosis. Symptoms vary with the extent and severity of the air leak but can include tachypnea, muffled heart sounds, diminished breath sounds, and cyanosis.

Chronic lung changes can occur following oxygen therapy or mechanical ventilation. These changes, which include thickening and necrosis of alveolar walls, atelectasis, and fibrosis, have been identified as bronchopulmonary dysplasia (BPD). The majority of these infants will survive and develop normal cardiorespiratory function by 5 to 6 years of age. The disease is characterized by long-term supplemental oxygen dependency, poor weight gain, recurrent acute infections, and cardiac changes. Nursing care implications include the need to ensure adequate oxygen to avoid hypoxemia, the need to monitor the infant for signs of respiratory distress and cardiac failure, protecting from infection, and minimizing unnecessary oxygen consumption for feeding and handling. Bronchopulmonary dysplasia is covered further in Chapter 38.

Retinopathy of prematurity (ROP) is also known as retrolental fibroplasia. Etiology is discussed in Chapter 45. The incidence of ROP appears to be greatest in infants of very low birthweight. Time spent in oxygen has also been identified as an associated factor. ROP is a progressive disease of the retinal vasculature. It is characterized by the development of abnormal blood vessels on the retinal surface, following capillary constricture.

The progression of the disease involves leakage of fluid or hemorrhage from these abnormal vessels into the vitreous body. Scar tissue, which may then form, may result in detachment of the retina. ROP has a wide spectrum of severity, ranging from minimal vascular changes with no visual impairment to severe fibrovascular proliferation and retinal detachment leading to blindness. A classification system has been developed to define the extent of the disease (Shapiro, 1986). Nursing implications include cautious and judicious use of supplemental oxygen, and continuous assessment and monitoring of respiratory status, cardiac status, and activity. As the infant improves, oxygen requirements will decrease; the nurse is in a key position to recommend a decrease in therapy promptly.

Hypoxic-Ischemic Insult

Neurologic insult can occur as a result of inadequate oxygenation of brain tissue, from either decreased perfusion or decreased oxygen in the blood, or both.

Etiology/Incidence

This hypoxic-ischemic insult can be chronic and can occur prenatally from a variety of maternal conditions: toxemia, placental insufficiency, diabetes, drugs. It can also be acute, occurring at the time of birth. Common causes of hypoxic ischemia during labor and delivery include abruptio placentae, cord compression, meconium aspiration, placenta previa, and subdural and subarachnoid hemorrhage.

Diagnostic Assessment

Clinical manifestations of hypoxic-ischemic insult at the time of birth vary from severe to subtle signs and may include hypotonia or hypertonia, respiratory and cardiac depression, and decreased perfusion. Seizures are not usually visible before 6 hours of age.

Brain damage related to inadequate oxygenation can be temporary or permanent, with a wide gradation of functional impact. Cell damage and functional impairment of varying degree can also occur in organs other than the brain. These complications can be summarized by organ systems, as seen in Table 30–4.

The long-term sequelae of hypoxic-ischemic encephalopathy can include seizures, hydrocephalus, motor deficits, and mental retardation. In general, the more prolonged and extensive the hypoxic-ischemic insult, the higher the risk for severe long-term effects.

TABLE 30-4
Complications in Main Organ Systems Caused by Perinatal Hypoxic-Ischemic Insult

Respiratory
Respiratory distress
Pneumonia
Pulmonary hemorrhage
Hypercapnia
Cardiovascular
Dysrhythmias
Cardiogenic shock
Persistent pulmonary hypertension of the neonate
Disseminated intravascular coagulation
Hypotension
Gastrointestinal
Necrotizing enterocolitis
Release of meconium into amniotic fluid
Urinary
Acute tubular necrosis
Renal failure
Neurologic
Cerebral edema
Cerebral necrosis
Intraventricular-periventricular hemorrhage
Intracerebral/cerebellar hemorrhage
Subdural/subarachnoid hemorrhage
Seizures
Hypoxic-ischemic encephalopathy
Periventricular leukomalacia
Endocrine/Metabolic
Syndrome of inappropriate antidiuretic hormone secretion (SIADH)
Hypoglycemia
Acidosis

The significant damage resulting from hypoxia and decreased tissue perfusion has been discussed in relation to prenatal and intrapartum events. Note, however, that similar complications can occur in the postnatal stage. *Infants are at risk for neurologic damage whenever their systems are deprived of oxygen or adequate perfusion.* This may occur during apneic/bradycardic episodes, during cardiac arrests, from respiratory equipment malfunction, from cold stress, or from seizures.

Therapeutic Management

The overall guidelines for management include correcting the hypoxia and alleviating tissue ischemia. Although the medical management is controversial, treatment modalities are directed toward supporting the infant until there is organ recovery. These infants require close monitoring of their clinical and biochemical status, as well as ongoing assessment of organ function. Treatment of symptoms, such as seizures, oliguria, and electrolyte imbalance, and fluid restriction are the main focus in hypoxic-ischemic insults.

Nursing Care

Ongoing assessment of the neurologic status is crucial to the care of infants with hypoxic-ischemic insults. Close monitoring of the function of the affected organs (i.e., brain, heart, kidneys, bowels, and liver) is also important to the therapeutic management.

Periventricular-Intraventricular Hemorrhage

Periventricular and intraventricular hemorrhages refer to any bleeding into or around the ventricles in the brain. These types of hemorrhages are of particular significance to preterm infants because they occur in about 35 to 40 per cent of infants weighing less than 1000 g at birth (Horbar, 1992).

Etiology/Incidence

Preterm infants are susceptible to this particular type of intracerebral hemorrhage because of several factors related to their developmental immaturity. The site of hemorrhage is usually found in the subependymal germinal matrix at the head of the caudate nucleus. This matrix is composed of highly proliferative cells that are the precursors of neuronal or glial cells. The matrix is perfused by abundant but very fragile capillaries that are weakly supported by gelatinous tissue. Preterm infants also have an immature vascular autoregulatory system and increased fibrinolytic activity in the periventricular region.

The situation in which the preterm infant often finds itself contributes to these factors and can result in a hemorrhage of varying degree. Abrupt increases in arterial blood pressure, such as those secondary to resuscitation efforts or infusion of hyperosmolar solutions, can rupture the sensitive capillaries in the germinal matrix. The increased fibrinolytic activity may then allow the hemorrhage to spread throughout the subependyma or into the ventricles themselves. Abrupt changes in cerebral blood flow, such as those caused by hypoxia and rapid reperfusion, can also rupture blood vessels. Lastly, increased venous pressure, resulting from mechanical ventilation or pneumothorax, which impedes venous return, may contribute to capillary rupture.

Many hemorrhages of this type will occur on the first day of life. The smaller and younger the infant, the higher the risk of hemorrhage. The clinical features may be rapid, severe deterioration or can be much more subtle in nature.

Diagnostic Assessment

Since many intraventricular hemorrhages may be missed, most NICUs do routine real-time ultrasonography on all infants at risk, those under 1500 to 1800 g, or those with a history of trauma or hypoxia, during the first few days of life.

Therapeutic Management

It is very difficult to give parents a definite prognosis when a periventricular-intraventricular hemorrhage has occurred. There is still much that is not known about the process, and many of these infants have had other insults that complicate the prognosis. Follow-up studies will continue to provide data in this area.

Generally speaking, the more severe the hemorrhage, the poorer the outcome. The severity of the hemorrhage is determined by the extent of the bleeding and the structures involved. Hemorrhages confined to the subependymal region are more likely to have a better outcome than those that extend into the ventricles or into the cerebral parenchyma. Many of the moderate and most of the severe hemorrhages will result in the development of some degree of hydrocephalus. This is the reason that all hemorrhages initially detected by ultrasonography are then monitored by serial testing and computed tomography (Faerber, 1986).

Nursing Care

Infants who are at risk for intracranial hemorrhage should be monitored on an ongoing basis for any changes in neurologic or cardiovascular status. It is important that these infants have their head circumferences measured on a daily basis in order to detect any abnormal growth that might be indicative of hydrocephalus.

Ventricular dilatation usually begins within 2 weeks of the onset of the hemorrhage. Hydrocephalus may occur days or weeks following the dilatation. There may be no dilatation, however, and the hemorrhage will resolve over time. (Hydrocephalus is discussed in Chapter 40.)

Hyperbilirubinemia

"Hyperbilirubinemia" refers to the presence of elevated levels of conjugated and unconjugated bilirubin in the blood. Jaundice (yellowish color of the skin and sclera) is a result of the breakdown and incomplete excretion of fetal red blood cells. The normal breakdown of hemoglobin in red blood cells produces bilirubin, which must be conjugated by the liver before it can bind with albumin for excretion from the body. There are a number of causes of hyperbilirubinemia, and neurotoxicity can result if this condition is severe.

Etiology/Incidence

Because of the immaturity of a premature infant's liver, the potential for kernicterus to develop is increased compared with that for a full-term newborn. Because of the higher level of unconjugated bilirubin free to enter brain cells in a premature infant, this danger of kernicterus exists even when total bilirubin levels may not be excessively high. An increased susceptibility to bruising in preterm infants leads to increased red blood cell destruction, increasing the risk of hyperbilirubinemia. Delayed feeding, which may allow reabsorption of bilirubin from the bowel, also increases the likelihood that hyperbilirubinemia will develop. For all these reasons, serum bilirubin is monitored very closely in preterm infants.

Diagnostic Assessment

Prior to initiation of treatment, the underlying cause of the hyperbilirubinemia must be determined. This is usually done through various laboratory examinations that assess for the following:

- Hemolytic diseases.
- Infections.
- Excessive breakdown of blood products from polycythemia, bruising, cephalhematoma.
- Metabolic disorders.
- Increased enterohepatic circulation from bowel obstruction, pyloric stenosis.
- Poor fluid/caloric intake.

Therapeutic Management

The two major treatments for moderate-to-severe hyperbilirubinemia are phototherapy and exchange transfusion. Guidelines for the initiation of phototherapy vary somewhat from institution to institution. Generally, the indications depend on the infant's gestational age, birthweight, related illnesses, and rate of rise of serum bilirubin concentration. When the bilirubin in the skin surface is exposed to the special phototherapy lights, it is transformed or isomerized into water-soluble molecules. These molecules can then be excreted in the bile. The ideal light source appears to be special blue fluorescent bulbs with wavelengths ranging from 400 to 500 nm. These blue lights are used in conjunction with white lights so as not to obscure signs of cyanosis. An acrylic plastic shield is also required to block out infrared and ultraviolet light. Knowledge of the following complications should be incorporated into the nursing care of all infants receiving phototherapy:

- Phototherapy lights can increase the infant's temperature, so that special attention is given to thermoregulation.
- Insensible water loss increases because of the increased temperature, so the infant should be monitored for signs of dehydration.
- Diarrhea and lactose intolerance have been found to be complications of the gastrointestinal tract.
- Retinal damage in animals has been caused by phototherapy, so the use of opaque eye patches is an essential part of care.
- Rashes and burns have been known to occur as a result of phototherapy; therefore, careful attention is given to skin care.

The goal of exchange transfusions is to prevent the toxic effects of the bilirubin by removing it from the circulation. Specific guidelines for the use of this treatment also have not been well established. It is indicated when the bilirubin levels rise to dangerous levels too quickly. The use of phototherapy has decreased the need for exchange transfusions.

Nursing Care

The nursing care of infants receiving phototherapy for hyperbilirubinemia is vital to the success of this treatment. The nurse should ensure that the intensity of the lights is adequate and that the infant's skin is exposed to as much of the light as possible. It is also important to keep the infant's eyes covered to prevent retinal damage from the phototherapy lights. During an exchange transfusion, the nurse is usually responsible for monitoring the clinical status of the infant, including temperature, as well as for recording the amounts of blood removed and administered during the procedure.

Seizures

Because neonatal seizures are the most common neurologic problem leading to investigation, it is crucial that nurses become skilled at detecting them. Seizures of any type and of any etiology require prompt medical attention. Increasing evidence indicates that seizures may cause severe damage.

Etiology/Incidence/Diagnostic Assessment

A neonatal seizure is often not readily observable and may be initially mistaken for normal, random activity. A seizure in a preterm infant is even more difficult to detect. In neonates, jitteriness is often confused with seizure activity. Jitteriness must be distinguished from seizures. Seizures are not stimulus-dependent and will not cease, as will jitteriness, when the limb is gently restrained. Seizures are caused by a wide variety of disorders. The main causes include hypoxia, intracranial hemorrhage, infection, hypoglycemia, hypocalcemia, hyperbilirubinemia, and maternal drug use.

Behaviors associated with subtle seizures may include blinking or fluttering eyelids, sucking or mouthing movements, tonic posturing of a single limb, bicycling movements of the legs, rowing movements of the arms, and apnea. These may or may not be associated with any change in color, respiratory rate, or cardiac rate.

Therapeutic Management

Although there is little controversy over the use of anticonvulsants in the treatment of overt seizures in neonates, the actual drug of choice and length of treatment varies. The two most commonly used drugs are phenobarbital and phenytoin (Dilantin). Diazepam (Valium) and paraldehyde are also used for short-term treatment situations.

Nursing Care

Nursing care of an infant with seizures is discussed in Chapter 40.

Neonatal Sepsis

Neonatal sepsis, as the name suggests, is an infection of the blood occurring in infants during the first month of life.

Etiology/Incidence/Pathophysiology

The incidence of confirmed sepsis is 1 to 5 per 1000 live births (Gladstone et al, 1990; Ferrieri, 1990). The incidence increases in premature infants to as high as 1:230 (Ferrieri, 1990). Neonatal meningitis occurs in about 2 to 4 per 100,000 live births in North America (King, 1990).

Although neonatal sepsis may be caused by a variety of organisms, group B beta-hemolytic streptococcus and *Escherichia coli* are the most prevalent (Ferrieri, 1990). Infection may occur in utero by transplacental contamination from an infected mother, at the time of delivery (especially with aspiration of infected amniotic fluid or vaginal secretions), or after birth through contaminated articles or poor handwashing in the nursery or the home. The immature immune system of neonates makes them more prone to infection and less able to fight the organism once it has taken hold.

Clinical Manifestations

Although clinical manifestations vary somewhat, depending on the causative organism, the major signs and symptoms usually relate to thermoregulation and respiratory and gastrointestinal disturbances. Fever is less common than hypothermia, but either may result. Tachypnea and tachycardia are common, along with grunting respirations, cyanosis, intercostal and substernal retractions, and apnea. Gastrointestinal disturbances appear often as poor feeding, vomiting, abdominal distention, and diarrhea.

Meningitis may result from bacterial spread to the meninges. This is especially common with group B beta-hemolytic streptococcus infection. Clinical symptoms of meningitis vary, depending on age, length of illness, and the response to sepsis (King, 1990).

Diagnostic Assessment

Suspicion of sepsis in the neonate will usually lead to a series of diagnostic tests to attempt to identify an organism in blood, urine, cerebrospinal fluid, and possibly other body secretions. Diagnosis is confirmed when an organism is isolated. Typically a "septic work-up" includes a complete blood count with differential (preferably from a peripheral vein), a blood culture, urinalysis and urine culture, and culture of any purulent drainage, as from the eye, umbilicus, or a surgical wound. The work-up may also involve a lumbar puncture and a radiographic examination of the chest and abdomen. Since hypoglycemia may also result from sepsis in the neonate, a blood sugar test is also frequently ordered.

Therapeutic Management

Immediately after cultures are obtained, the neonate will be started on intravenous antibiotic therapy. The antibiotics ordered will vary with physician's preference, but therapy often involves both ampicillin and an aminoglycoside. With meningitis, a third-generation cephalosporin may replace the aminoglycoside (Gotoff, 1992). Once an organism has been identified, an antibiotic that is sensitive to it may replace the original antibiotics. Antibiotic therapy will be continued for 10 to 14 days or for at least 5 to 7 days after the signs and symptoms have resolved.

Neonatal meningitis should be treated for 2 to 3 weeks (King, 1990). Often, oxygen therapy is employed to ease the respiratory effort. The mortality rates for neonatal sepsis range from 10 to 60 per cent, depending on a number of factors, such as pathogen, gestational age, and time and site of occurrence (Ferrieri, 1990).

Nursing Care

The major goals for nursing care are to maintain optimal blood levels of the antibiotic ordered, to conserve the neonate's energy so the little body can use all available resources to fight the infection, and to counsel and console the family.

Maintaining Optimal Blood Levels of Antibiotic

Maintenance of the intravenous line in a neonate requires a great deal of vigilance and ingenuity. The tiny vessels are fragile, and infiltration is a common problem. See Chapter 26 for strategies related to protection of the intravenous site to prevent accidental dislodging of the needle or cannula. Inspect for infiltration and phlebitis before, during, and after each dose of antibiotic.

Conserving Energy

Attention must be given to thermoregulation, with the goal of keeping the temperature within normal limits. This includes not only intervening for fever but also preventing unnecessary heat loss during baths and other procedures when the infant is uncovered.

Infants typically expend the most energy during crying and feeding. The infant may be too ill to cry as much as healthy neonates do, but comfort measures are certainly an important consideration. Cuddling and rocking are often comforting, but the amount of time these infants are held must be based on whether they rest better in the parent's (or nurse's) arms or in the crib (or Isolette).

If the infant has been breastfeeding, more frequent feeds of shorter duration may help to expend less energy. If formula is given, a softer or "premie" nipple delivers milk with less sucking effort. Infants who are very ill with sepsis may be given intravenous nutrition and nothing by mouth or may be fed by nasogastric tube.

If the infant is receiving oxygen, it is helpful to use an oxygen monitor (e.g., transcutaneous or ear oximetry, as detailed in Chapter 32). The monitor is an indirect measure of energy expenditure because oxygen saturation will diminish with increased effort in the infant with respiratory involvement. The nurse can then gauge such things as effort expended in feeding by the infant's ability to keep the blood saturated with oxygen. A decreasing saturation is an indication to allow the infant to rest.

Counseling and Consoling the Family

The family is likely to be distraught at the sudden, severe illness of the newborn infant. See Table 30–3 regarding crisis management with families of hospitalized children.

Discharge and Follow-Up

Discharge planning from the NICU has assumed increasingly greater emphasis as smaller babies are being sent home. Planning is especially important for the 8 to 19 per cent of low birthweight infants (< 1500 g) who may have significant sequelae in the months following their discharge (Damato, 1991). Low birthweight infants are more likely to have serious congenital anomalies and are at increased risk for developing complications from respiratory tract infections.

Research indicates that earlier discharge from the NICU is not only safe but also beneficial to the infant and family (Brooten et al, 1989). The main focus for most premature infants who are discharged home is to grow and develop in the family environment, as it is for healthy infants born at term. However, for some infants, discharge planning and home care involve complex therapies.

The care discussed in the following paragraphs is appropriate for the nursing diagnostic response *high risk for altered health maintenance*. The nurse participates with the treatment team in assuring that the family is able to identify, manage, and/or seek out help to maintain the health of the infant after birth.

Planning for transfer or discharge begins at birth, with activities that enhance the developing relationship between parents and infants, and continues throughout hospitalization. Parents frequently approach the day of transfer or discharge with mixed feelings of anxiety and joy. Their anxiety results from concern regarding their own ability or the ability of the receiving unit to care for a baby who is still small or who requires highly specialized care. A smooth transition will occur only if there has been adequate planning, preparation, and support of the family and communication with the receiving unit.

Ongoing assessment is required for effective planning. A multidisciplinary approach is used in most units. Team members may include staff nurses, physicians, a community health nurse, a follow-up or home care coordinator, physical or occupational therapists, a social worker, and a clinical nurse specialist. The needs of the family and of the child dictate the type of referrals and follow-up that will be required.

Criteria for transfer or discharge may include the following: resolution of acute illnesses or stability of chronic illnesses, adequate weight gain, adequate enteral fluid and caloric intake, apnea controlled or resolved, medication levels at therapeutic range with documented side effects, and a specific plan for any special needs. Medications commonly required by infants being discharged include methylxanthines, anticonvulsants, digoxin, diuretics, and vitamin and mineral supplements (Colangelo et al, 1987).

Parents will need certain knowledge and skills to provide care for their infants at home. They must be comfortable with basic infant care tasks, such as safety, feeding, diapering, and bathing. Second, parents need to fully understand the special health needs of their infant, which may include infection and environmental control, signs and symptoms of recurrent illness, administration and side effects of medications, home monitoring, ventriculoperitoneal shunts, ostomy care, low-flow oxygen, and cardiopulmonary resuscitation.

Parents also should understand the changing aspects of the infant's development and the need for rest and stimulation. Discussion of how parents will meet their own needs and the needs of other family members should be explored throughout hospitalization. Finally, parents need to know how to obtain help when necessary and what the plans are for ongoing health care follow-up.

The nursing care of families does not end with the baby's discharge from the hospital. When the infant returns home, communication between hospital and community health agency nurses should facilitate continuity of care. If referrals are made before discharge, the community health nurse can begin to establish a relationship with and provide support to the family before discharge.

Follow-up visits for premature infants vary across the United States and Canada with respect to frequency and focus for the visit, as well as the type of infant who is referred at the time of hospital discharge. Most sources recommend that all infants with birthweights of 1500 g or less, and those who have had a neurologic insult, be referred for follow-up, with an examination at months 1, 2, 4, 6, 9, 12, 15, 18, 24, and then at 3 and 4 years corrected age. These dates are based on the infant's corrected age; that is, the age is based on weeks from 40 weeks postmenstrual age (Saigal et al, 1989). Primary care for these infants should include: body measurements (height, weight, head circumference); vision and hearing screening; development and behavior assessment; complete physical examination, including a thorough neurologic assessment; and, where appropriate, laboratory tests, immunization, and dental referral.

Another crucial component of follow-up care is providing anticipatory guidance and support for parents. In addition to the adjustments that all parents must make with a new baby at home, parents of premature infants must cope with the additional stresses of resolving their experiences from the NICU; being able to recognize the differences, and similarities, of their infant's needs from those of other infants; and learning about any special care requirements for their baby.

Health professionals who are involved in the follow-up of a premature infant should be aware of the neonatal medical course and be knowledgable of the long-term problems that are commonly associated with prematurity. This knowledge will help to focus the physical assessment of the infant as well as help with the anticipatory guidance of the parents. The following areas should be given particular attention.

Because of the premature infant's increased risk for infection, parents need to be aware of the early, subtle signs of both site-specific infections, such as otitis media, and respiratory infections. This increased risk arises from the compromised respiratory status and relative state of immunosuppression of premature infants. Generally, it is recommended that during their first year, NICU graduates be kept away from places with dense groups of people and from persons with a known infectious disease.

The neurodevelopmental assessment is one of the major areas of concern for parents. Uncertainty related to the physical and intellectual outcomes of their premature infant are heightened each time their child is examined. Neurodevelopmental examinations consist of assessment of posture, tone, reflexes, and motor performance. Findings at 40 weeks corrected age have shown a marked correlation to neuromotor outcomes at 1 year of age or older. Infants with abnormal results on the 1-year examination had significantly higher incidences of both cerebral palsy and minor neuromotor dysfunction. Abnormal findings should alert clinicians to the potential for poor outcomes and so indicate the need for careful monitoring (Allen & Capute, 1989). Infants with a history of intraventricular hemorrhage with parenchymal involvement or of meningitis are at risk for development of noncommunicating hydrocephalus. Measurement of the head circumference is done at every visit, with cranial ultrasonography included as indicated by abnormal head growth (e.g., > 1 cm per week).

Nutrition is another important concern for parents. Most premature infants grow well on their mother's milk. Special high-calorie formulas or human milk fortifiers may be needed for adequate growth in chronically ill preterm infants, SGA infants, and very low birthweight infants (< 1000 g). Preterm infants are also at risk for certain vitamin and mineral deficiencies and, therefore, require supplementation. Premature infants do not have the body stores that term infants have developed in utero and may be unable to consume adequate volumes of milk. Generally, the following supplements are recommended: vitamins A, D, C, and B for the first year; and iron beginning at about 6 to 8 weeks of age. As with term infants, cow's milk is not recommended for use until 9 to 12 months of age. If cow's milk is used, however, it should be homogeneized milk and not low-fat milk. The fat content is important for adequate neural development.

Solid foods can be introduced at 4 to 6 months of age, if the infant is ready developmentally. This is usually when the infant can sit with support and can coordinate muscular control for chewing rather than sucking.

The American Academy of Pediatrics recommends that routine immunization of premature infants begin at 2 months of age from birth, regardless of gestation. The recommendation is the same in Canada. These infants should receive the full dose and should follow the same time schedule as for term infants.

The incidence of significant inguinal hernias is higher in low birthweight infants than in term babies. The reason for this is most likely related to the immature musculature of the preterm infant. Because low birthweight infants are also at risk for complications from anesthesia and surgery, the inguinal hernia repair should be done at a medical center familiar with the problems of premature infants. These complications generally result from the preterm infant's compromised respiratory status and relative state of immunosuppression, as previously stated.

Home monitoring for apnea of prematurity is not recommended for infants who have been free of episodes for at least 1 week prior to discharge and who are not receiving methylzanthines. Normally, infants will outgrow their primary apnea by 37 weeks gestation or by term. Research has failed to demonstrate any benefit from home monitoring with respect to decreasing mortality from apparent life-threatening events (formally called sudden infant death syndrome) (Fetus and Newborn Committee, Canadian Pediatric Society, 1992). In fact, home monitoring resulted in increased parental stress due to the high number of false alarms (Phipps et al, 1989).

Infants with bronchopulmonary dysplasia or chronic lung disease may require home management on oxygen therapy for weeks or even many months. In the first year of life, half of these infants will be readmitted to the hospital for respiratory symptoms. The home care of these infants places great demands on parents' skill and patience. Careful discharge planning, which includes teaching regarding equipment management and cardiopulmonary resuscitation, and home follow-up are required for all of these patients.

The transition to home for parents of a premature infant is a stressful period. Their child's care has likely been provided for a considerable length of time by skilled health professionals. Many parents question their ability to assume full responsibility for their baby's care at the time of discharge. Adequate planning, teaching, and communication between parents and professionals will help to alleviate some of this stress. Parents may view their infant as highly vulnerable and feel the need to overprotect and overcompensate for the prematurity. This response is especially true of parents of infants with residual medical problems, who have difficulty separating normal infant needs from special needs. An important focus of the health professional's care is to help parents to interpret and resolve the early NICU experience and to try to normalize their lives.

Parents may need help in distinguishing the normal variations of infants from those issues related to the prematurity. They should be encouraged to focus on the normal aspects of their infant's behavior. Parents should be prepared for the possibility that the infant may experience transient adjustment difficulties. Often, this adjustment relates to disrupted sleep patterns. Infants who are used to constant noise and light in their environment may initially be unable to regulate their sleeping patterns in a quiet, darkened room. Appropriate air temperature in the home and taking the infant outdoors are other issues frequently raised by parents.

Parents should be encouraged to mobilize all their supports in order to assist in routine tasks and to provide care relief for them. Parents may experience guilt about taking time for themselves and about being away from the baby for whom they had waited for so long.

As the premature infant catches up developmentally to his or her peers, all of these issues are likely to be completely resolved. For those families in which the infants' outcomes are compromised and life-long problems remain, their needs will be the same as for all families with a chronically ill or special need child.

KEY CONCEPTS

Concepts Related to Basic Information

- There are multiple factors associated with the incidence of dysmature infants.
- There are a number of medical disorders that are commonly found in the preterm neonate, including patent ductus arteriosus, apnea, respiratory distress syndrome, retinopathy of prematurity, periventricular hemorrhage, bronchopulmonary dysplasia, and air leak syndromes.
- There are a number of medical disorders that are commonly found in the posterm or term neonate, including persistent pulmonary hypertension of the newborn, meconium aspiration, transient tachypnea of the newborn, air leak syndromes, and hypoxic ischemic insult.

Concepts Related to Nursing Assessment

- Dysmature neonates are at high risk for morbidity and mortality and, therefore, require a comprehensive and ongoing assessment at the time of birth.
- The physical characteristics and organ function of dysmature infants may differ significantly from those of term infants.
- Ongoing assessment of preterm and other high-risk neonates occurs at least throughout the first 2 years of life.

Concepts Related to Nursing Intervention

- Though the basic needs of preterm infants are similar to those of term infants, the nursing care of preterm infants is highly specialized in many respects.
- The care of the parents is as important as the care of the neonate in the NICU.
- Discharge planning is an integral part of the over all nursing care and has assumed greater emphasis as smaller infants are being sent home with more complex therapies.

REFERENCES

Affleck, G., Tennen, H., & Rowe, J. (1990). Mothers, fathers, and the crisis of newborn intensive care. *Infant Mental Health Journal, 11,* 12–25.

Allen, M., & Capute, A. (1989). Neonatal neurodevelopmental examination as a predictor of neuromotor outcome in premature infants. *Pediatrics, 83,* 498–506.

Bass, L. (1991). What do parents need when their infant is a patient in the NICU? *Neonatal Network, 10,* 25–33.

Becker, P., Grunwald, P., Moorman, J., & Stuhr, S. (1991). Outcomes of developmentally supportive nursing care for very low birth weight infants. *Nursing Research, 40,* 150–155.

Boeckling, A. (1992). Exogenous surfactant therapy for premature infants. *Journal of Perinatal and Neonatal Nursing, 6,* 59–66.

Brooten, D., Gennaro, S., Knapp, H., Brown, L., & York, R. (1989). Clinical specialist pre- and postdischarge teaching of parents of very low birth weight infants. *Journal of Obstetric, Gynecologic and Neonatal Nursing, 18,* 316–322.

Cartlett, A. T., & Holditch-Davis, D. (1990). Environmental stimulation of the acutely ill premature infant: Physiological effects and nursing implications. *Neonatal Network, 8,* 19–26.

Colangelo, A., Vento, T., & Taeusch, H. W. (1987). Discharge planning. In H. W. Taeusch & M. Yogman (Eds.), *Follow-up management of the high-risk infant.* Toronto and Boston: Little, Brown.

Coulter, D. (1992). The current status of replacement therapy with exogenous pulmonary surfactant for hyaline membrane disease. *Neonatal Pharmacology Quarterly, 1,* 5–18.

Damato, E. (1991). Discharge planning from the neonatal intensive care unit. *Journal of Perinatal-Neonatal Nursing, 5,* 43–53.

Faerber, E. (1986). *Cranial computed tomography in infants and children.* Oxford: Blackwell Scientific Publications.

Ferrieri, P. (1990). Neonatal susceptibility and immunity to major bacterial pathogens. *Review of Infectious Diseases, 12*(Suppl. 4), 5394–5400.

Fetus and Newborn Committee, Canadian Pediatric Society (1992). The infant home monitoring dilemma. *Canadian Medical Association Journal, 147*(11), 1661–1669.

Gladstone, I. M., EhrenKranz, R. A., Edberg, S. C., & Baltimore, R. S. (1990). A ten-year review of neonatal sepsis and comparison with the previous fifty-year experience. *Pediatric Infectious Diseases Journal, 9,* 819–825.

Gotoff, S. P. (1992). Infections of the newborn. In R. E. Behrman & V. C. Vaughan (Eds.), *Nelson textbook of pediatrics* (14th ed.). Philadelphia: WB Saunders, pp 495–524.

Horbar, J. (1992). Prevention of periventricular-intraventricular hemorrhage. In J. Sinclair & M. Bracken (Eds.), *Effective care of the newborn infant.* Oxford: Oxford University Press.

King, S. (1990). Meningitis in childhood. *Medicine North America, 9,* 1110–1118.

Klaus, M., & Fanaroff, A. (1986). *Care of the high-risk neonate* (3rd ed.). Philadelphia: WB Saunders, p 184.

Marchal, F., Bairam, A., & Vert, P. (1987). Neonatal apnea and apneic syndromes. *Clinics in Perinatology, 14,* 509–523.

McCain, G. (1992). Facilitating inactive awake states in preterm infants: A study of three interventions. *Nursing Research, 41,* 157–160.

Meier, P., & Anderson, G. C. (1987). Responses of small preterm infants to bottle and breast-feeding. *MCN: American Journal of Maternal Child Nursing, 12,* 97–105.

Meier, P. (1988). Bottle- and breast-feeding: Effects on trancutaneous oxygen pressure and temperature in preterm infants. *Nursing Research, 37,* 36–41.

Perehudoff, B. (1990). Parent's perceptions of environmental stressors in the special care nursery. *Neonatal Network, 9,* 39–44.

Perlman, N., Freedman, J., Abramovitch, R., Whyte, H., Kirpalani, H., & Perlman, M. (1991). Informational needs of parents of sick newborns. *Pediatrics, 88,* 512–518.

Phipps, S., Drotar, D., Joseph, C., Geiss, C., & Doershuck, C. (1989). Psychological impact of home apnea monitoring: Temporal effects, family resources, and maternal coping style. *Journal of Developmental and Behavioral Pediatrics, 10,* 7–12.

Saigal, S., Rosenbaum, P., Hattersley, B., & Milner, R. (1989). Decreased disability rate among 3-year-old survivors weighing 501 to 1000 grams at birth and born to residents of a geographically defined region from 1981 to 1984 compared with 1977 to 1980. *Journal of Pediatrics, 114,* 839–846.

Shapiro, C. (1986). Retrolental fibroplasia: What we know and what we don't know. *Neonatal Network, 4,* 33–44.

Statistics Canada: Canadian Centre for Health Information. (1991). *Health Reports—Births for 1989.* Suppl. 14, 3(1).

US Department of Health and Human Services. (1990). *Vital statistics of the United States*—1(Natality). (DHHS Publication No. [PHS] 90–100.) Rockville, MD: Author.

BIBLIOGRAPHY

Affonso, D., Bosque, E., Wahlberg, V., & Brady, J. P. (1993). Reconciliation and healing for mothers through skin-to-skin contact: Provided in an American tertiary-level intensive care nursery. *Neonatal Network, 12,* 25–32.

Brown, P., Rustia, J., & Schappert, P. (1991). A comparison of fathers of high-risk newborns and fathers of healthy newborns. *Journal of Pediatric Nursing, 6,* 269–273.

DeMonterice, D., Meier, P. P., Engstrom, J. L., Crichton, C. L., & Mangurten, H. H. (1992). Concurrent validity of a new instrument for measuring nutritive sucking in preterm infants. *Nursing Research, 41,* 342–346.

Farel, A. M., Freeman, V. A., Keenan, N. L., & Huber, C. J. (1991). Interaction between high-risk infants and their mothers. The NCAST as an assessment tool. *Research in Nursing and Health, 14,* 109–118.

Gross, S. J., Slagle, T. A., D'Eugenio, D. B., & Mettelman, B. B. (1992). Impact of a matched term control group on interpretation of development performance in preterm infants. *Pediatrics, 90,* 681–687.

Heird, W. (1992). Parenteral feeding. In J. Sinclair & M. Bracken (Eds.), *Effective care of the newborn infant.* Oxford: Oxford University Press.

Kurdahi Zahr, L. (1991). The relationship between maternal confidence and mother-infant behaviors in premature infants. *Research in Nursing and Health, 14,* 279–286.

Kurdahi Zahr, L., & Montijo, J. (1993). The benefits of home care for sick premature infants. *Neonatal Network, 12,* 33–27.

Leonard, B. J., Scott, S. A., & Erpestad, N. (1992). Maternal perception of first-born infants: A controlled comparative study of mothers of premature and full-term infants. *Journal of Pediatric Nursing, 7,* 90–96.

Mayes, L. C., Granger, R. H., Frank, M. A., Schottenfeld, R., & Bornstein, M. H. (1993). Neurobehavioral profiles of neonates exposed to cocaine prenatally. *Pediatrics, 91,* 778–783.

McCain, G. C. (1992). Facilitating inactive awake states in preterm infants: A study of three interventions. *Nursing Research, 41,* 157–160.

Medoff-Cooper, B., Verklan, T., & Carlson, S. (1993). The development of sucking patterns and physiologic correlates in very-low-birth-weight infants. *Nursing Research, 42,* 100–105.

Miller, D. B., & Holditch-Davis. (1992). Interactions of parents and nurses with high-risk preterm infants. *Research in Nursing and Health, 15,* 187–197.

Oehler, J. M., Goldstein, R. F., Catlett, A., Boshkoff, M., & Brazy, J. E. (1993). How to target infants at highest risk for developmental delay. *MCN: American Journal of Maternal Child Nursing, 18,* 20–23.

Schlomann, P. (1992). Ethical considerations of aggressive care of very low birth weight infants. *Neonatal Network, 11,* 31–36.

Shellabarger, S. G., & Thompson, T. L. (1993). The critical times: Meeting parental communication needs throughout the NICU experience. *Neonatal Network, 12,* 39–45.

Specker, B., DeMarini, S., & Tsang, R. (1992). Vitamin and mineral supplementation. In J. Sinclair & M. Bracken (Eds.), *Effective care of the newborn infant.* Oxford: Oxford University Press.

Steer, P., Lucas, A., & Sinclair, J. (1992). Feeding the low birthweight infant. In J. Sinclair & M. Bracken (Eds.), *Effective care of the newborn infant.* Oxford: Oxford University Press.

Strobel, S. E., & Keller, C. S. (1993). Metabolic screening in the NICU population: A proposal for change. *Pediatric Nursing, 19,* 113–117.

Vermont-Oxford Trials Network Database Project (Investigators). (1993). The Vermont-Oxford trials network: Very low birth weight outcomes for 1990. *Pediatrics, 91,* 540–545.

CHAPTER • 31

Genetic Principles and Disorders

Lynette Wright

NURSING PROCESS PLAN
NPP: The Family with a Genetic Risk, Table 31–17

RELATED TOPICS
Neonatal screening, Chapter 4
Health assessment, Chapter 13
Stress, Crisis, and Coping, Chapter 18
Alterations in development, Chapter 27

LEARNING OBJECTIVES

- Describe normal cell division and variations that may produce genetic alterations.
- List the types of genetic disorders.
- Define common terms used in describing and explaining genetic alterations.
- Name factors that place a family at risk for a genetic disorder.
- Construct a pedigree as part of a family history.
- Identify the functions of the nurse in recognizing, screening, and supporting families with genetic disorders.

Nurses who care for children have a unique responsibility to developing families. During the childbearing years, a family is most in need of counseling concerning the likelihood that their offspring will be affected by inherited tendencies or genetic alterations. Regardless of the practice setting, all nurses should recognize problems in growth or developmental delay and dysmorphic features in any client or family unit. Many of these problems have a specific genetic cause, and this is especially true in children. Genes control the development of every body structure and the regulatory processes that account for normal growth and development. The purposes of this chapter are to describe the underlying principles of human genetics, to discuss their relevance to clinical situations, and to describe applications to pediatric nursing practice. Specific genetic disorders are discussed throughout the text in relation to the involved body systems. This chapter contains symptom check lists for the common chromosomal and single gene disorders. Both a broad overview of the known single gene disorders and a glossary of terms specific to the study of genetic disorders are provided.

History

The study of human genetics is the product of the latter half of this century but has its roots in the latter half of the 19th century, particularly in relation to the concepts of unit inheritance, segregation, and independent assortment during meiosis that were demonstrated by Gregor Mendel in 1865. Mendel's work was largely ignored for almost half a century. Early in the 20th century, Beadle and Tatum espoused the one-gene, one-enzyme theory (Thompson et al, 1991), but it was not until the mid-1950s that modern genetics really emerged. In 1956, the correct number of chromosomes was identified, and by the late 1950s, Down syndrome was shown to be caused by an extra chromosome. During the 1960s, biochemical techniques had advanced to the point that a few recessive disorders could be identified and treated, and by the end of that decade, population-based neonatal screening for phenylketonuria (PKU) was beginning. The early 1970s ushered in amniocentesis as a prenatal diagnostic technique, which became a major strategy in identifying serious genetic disorders. Newborn screening expanded to include a variety of disorders, and carrier screening for Tay Sachs disease and sickle cell anemia was instituted across the country. In the 1980s, prenatal diagnosis expanded to include sophisticated ultrasonography, early amniocentesis at 12 to 14 weeks, and chorionic villus sampling. Screening for spina bifida and Down syndrome from a maternal blood sample became widespread. In the 1990s, molecular techniques have been developed that analyze genetic problems at the DNA level. As we move toward the 21st century, there is the possibility of developing strategies for therapy or even a cure for previously untreatable genetic disorders (Thompson et al, 1991).

Scope and Impact of Genetics on Pediatric Nursing Practice

In the past, many nurses have thought of genetics as a collection of a few exotic disorders that were fascinating and challenging but not part of their daily practice. In this decade and into the 21st century, genetics must become more than a disease model. Each person's individual genetic pattern forms the outside framework on which all aspects of health and illness interact. It determines our ability to adapt to specific environmental alterations, including how long we will live and whether we will develop infections or malignancies. Our genetic self reaches far beyond prenatal and neonatal variations. Techniques are being developed as part of the ongoing worldwide Human Genome Project that will include strategies to identify, during childhood, most of the predisposing genes for adult-onset disorders as well as the genetic problems of childhood (Cook-Deegan, 1991). In this generation, delivery of health services will be adapted to account for individual genetic variation and predisposition. Such advances will prevent death and disability, foster the development of new therapeutic techniques, and make actual cures for lethal genetic disorders possible (Cook-Deegan, 1991). However, the same developments raise many nursing challenges and concerns. Who will have access to these new techniques? What if they are misused? How will disabilities be viewed? What will the nurse need to know to be prepared?

Even with diagnostic techniques currently in use, recognizable genetic problems are not rare. Genetic problems account for more than 60 per cent of all pregnancy losses, with 50 per cent occurring as a result of identifiable chromosomal errors. Fifteen to 16 per cent of live-born children have genetic problems that can be identified by 1 year of age. Birth defects are the leading cause of infant mortality and the fourth leading cause of diminished life span. Genetic disorders account for 30 to 50 per cent of pediatric hospital admissions in developed countries (Centers for Disease Control, 1989). Except for those with Down syndrome, however, few patients with known genetic disorders receive genetic counseling while hospitalized.

Therefore, nurses in all areas of practice must be well grounded in genetic principles and basic counseling techniques if they are to recognize genetic problems, provide support, make appropriate referrals, provide case management, and prepare patients for testing and counseling. Appropriately trained nurse counselors may provide in-depth genetic counseling in a variety of areas, or counseling may be provided by medical geneticists (MDs), clinical geneticists (PhDs), or other master's level genetic counselors.

General Concepts

Human genetics is a science and an art. There are basic biologic principles that must be understood as amazing scientific discoveries are revealing the mechanisms by which health-producing and disease-producing genes work. Human genetics is not entirely predictable. There is considerable interaction within the genome itself and between the genes and the environment. Our understanding of less traditional concepts is just beginning (Table 31–1); however, several major concepts must be reviewed if we are to understand the "new genetics" and apply it to nursing practice.

Cell Cycle and Cell Division Review

Understanding heredity begins with a review of the individual cell and cell cycle. Within the nucleus of each human cell is the entire genetic code. Recall that

TABLE 31-1
Glossary of Genetic Terms

Allele

One of two or more alternative forms of a gene at the same site in a chromosome, which determines alternative characters in inheritance

Autosome

Somatic chromosomes; any chromosomes other than the X and Y sex chromosomes

Carrier

A person who has, and therefore can transmit, a particular gene or chromosomal abnormality but who does not show the trait

Chromosomes

Microscopic units located within the nucleus of every cell, which contain the basic hereditary factors in the form of genes. There are 46 chromosomes in every cell except the reproductive cells (egg and sperm cells), which each contain 23

Congenital

Relating to a characteristic present at or dating from birth, either of genetic or environmental origin

Consanguinity

The state of being "related by blood," that is, of being descended from at least one common ancestor

Dizygosity

Nonidentical, or fraternal, twins resulting from the fertilization of two eggs by two sperm cells. They can be of the same or opposite sex

DNA

Deoxyribonucleic acid; the nucleic acid of the chromosomes, which carries the genetic code

Dominant

A gene that produces the same characteristic when it is present in a single dose, along with a specified allele (heterozygous), as it does in a double dose (homozygous)

Familial

A condition present more often in two or more members of a family group than would be expected in the population as a whole

Gamete

The haploid cell that is the product of meiosis and that, by combination with a gamete from the opposite sex, produces a zygote

Gene

A segment of a DNA molecule

Genetic Counseling

Provision of information bearing on the problems related to the occurrence, or risk of occurrence, of a genetic disorder in a family. The process is concerned with the risk and burden of the disorder and the options available for dealing with them

Genetic Screening

Testing on a population basis to identify people at risk of having a specific genetic disorder or of having a child with a specific genetic disorder

Genotype

The genetic makeup of the individual

Haploid

Having half the number of chromosomes characteristically found in the somatic (diploid) cells

Heterozygote

A person who has two different alleles, one of which is the normal allele, at a given locus on a pair of homologous chromosomes (e.g., notation: Aa)

Homologous Chromosomes

A "matched pair" of chromosomes, one from each parent, having the same gene loci in the same order

Homozygote

A person possessing a pair of identical alleles at a given locus on a pair of homologous chromosomes (e.g., notation: aa)

Inborn Error

A genetically determined biochemical disorder in which a specific enzyme is missing or is present in insufficient quantities

Karyotype

The chromosomal constitution of the cell nucleus; by extension, the photomicrograph of chromosomes arranged in numeric order

Locus

The position of a gene on a chromosome

Meiosis

The special type of cell division occurring in the germ cells by which gametes containing the haploid chromosome number are produced from diploid cells. Two meiotic divisions occur: the first and the second (meiosis I and meiosis II). Reduction in number takes place during meiosis I. To be distinguished from mitosis

Mitosis

The ordinary process of cell division that results in the formation of two daughter cells and by which the body replaces dead cells. The two daughter cells receive identical diploid complements of chromosomes (46) that are characteristic of somatic cells

Monozygotic Twins

Twins derived from a single fertilized ovum. Identical twins

(continued)

TABLE 31-1
Glossary of Genetic Terms (Continued)

Mosaic

An individual or tissue with at least two cell lines differing in genotype or karyotype; derived from a single zygote

Multifactorial

Arising as the result of the interaction of several genes or of genetic and nongenetic factors, each with only a minor effect by itself (synonym: polygenic)

Mutation

A permanent heritable change in the genetic material

Nondisjunction

The failure of two members of the same pair of chromosomes to separate into the newly formed daughter cells, resulting in one cell with one chromosome less than the normal amount and one cell with an extra chromosome

Pedigree

A diagrammatic representation of a family history, indicating the affected people and their relationship to the person who is the basis for the genetic study

Phenotype

The entire physical, biochemical, and physiologic nature of a person, as determined by the genotype and the environment in which the person develops

Polydactyly

Extra fingers and/or toes

Polygenic

Determined by many genes at different loci

Recessive

A gene that produces its character only when present in homozygous combination (i.e., must be present in both parents)

Sex Linkage

Location of a gene on a sex chromosome: X linkage on the X chromosome and Y linkage on the Y chromosome

Teratogen

Any substance that is potentially harmful to a person or to an unborn fetus

Translocation

The transfer of a segment of one chromosome to a nonhomologous chromosome

Trisomy

The state of having three of a given chromosome instead of the usual pair, as in trisomy 21 (Down syndrome)

X Chromosome

A sex chromosome found paired in the normal female and singly in the male

Y Chromosome

The sex chromosome that occurs singly in the normal male and is absent in the normal female

Zygote

A fertilized egg

when the cell is performing biologic functions, it is not dividing. During this part of the cell cycle, the nucleus is in "interphase" and the chromatin material is less tightly coiled. When the cell prepares to divide, the chromatin condenses into discrete bodies called "chromosomes," which contain precise sequences of tightly coiled "DNA." In a human, 46 chromosomes (23 pairs) house more than 6 billion base pairs of DNA. Being tightly coiled during cell division is essential to ensure that the precise amount of DNA information on each chromosome is transmitted to the new cell. This type of somatic cell division, which ensures that daughter cells receive the appropriate set of genetic information, is called "mitosis." It is during the metaphase stage of mitosis that the chromosomes become compact enough to be individually identified under an ordinary microscope (Fig. 31–1).

"Meiosis" is the special process of cell division by which gametes (eggs and sperm) are formed. It requires a two-step process. "Meiosis I," or "reduction division," is a complex series of steps in which the 46 chromosomes are paired in homologous groups and then divided so that the egg or sperm will have one of each chromosome pair in its reduced number. Genetic information is also exchanged between chromatids during this pairing. "Meiosis II" divides the chromatids of the 23 chromosomes without further DNA replication, producing four gametes with 23 chromosomes each. Many errors can occur in both types of meiotic cell division, but certain stages of meiosis I are prone to cell division irregularities that can lead to chromosomal abnormalities in offspring (Figs. 31–2 and 31–3).

Micropackaging Information

A major concept in understanding human genetics is "micropackaging." The most sophisticated computer does not begin to store the amount of information found in the human cell (Fig. 31–4). Recall that each nucleated cell in the body contains all the genetic information for a whole person. The genomic informa-

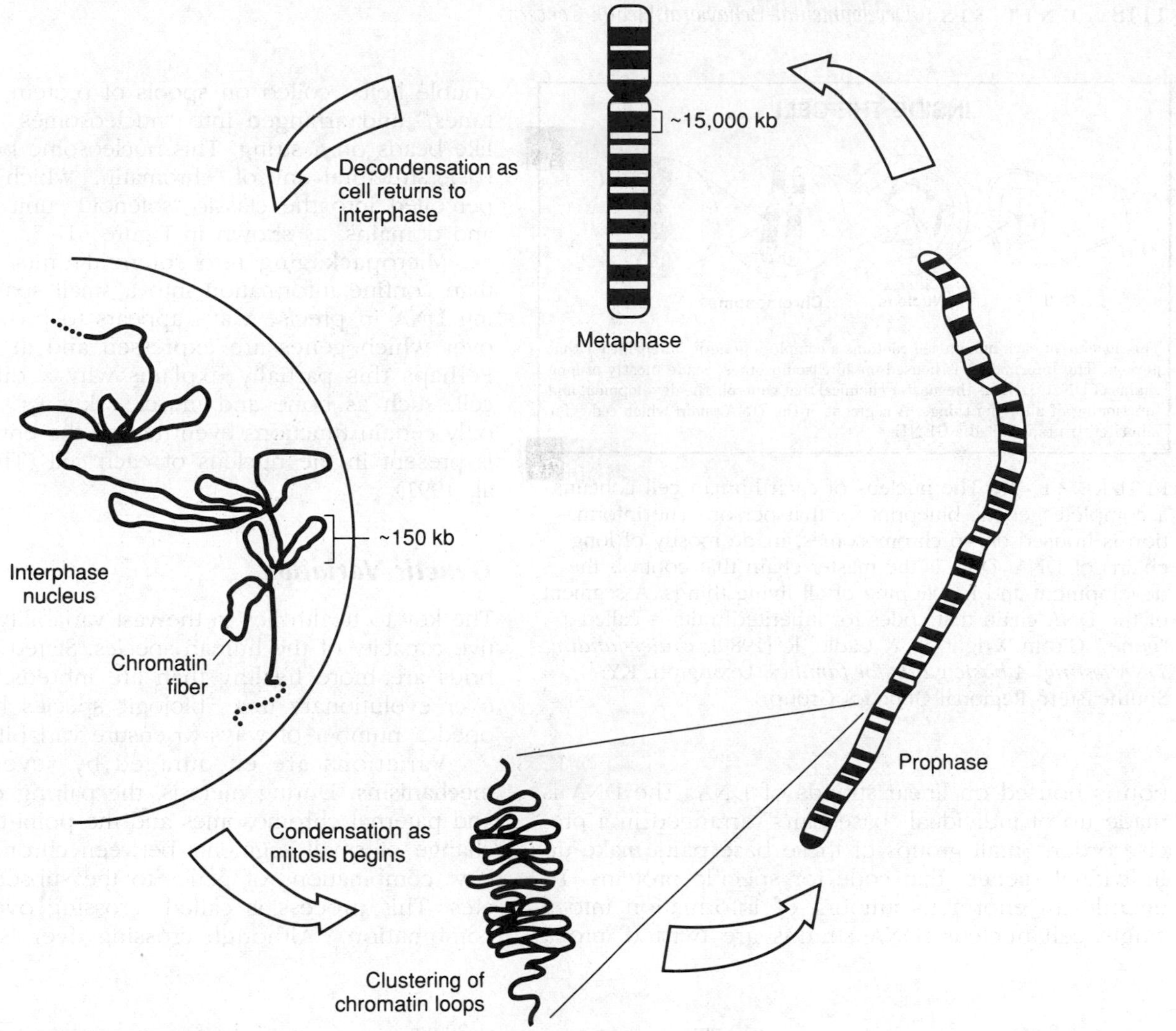

FIGURE 31 - 1. Cycle of condensation and decondensation as a chromosome proceeds through the cell cycle. (From Thompson, M. W., McInnes, R. R., & Huntington, W. F. [1991]. *Genetics in medicine* [5th ed.]. Philadelphia: WB Saunders, p 36.)

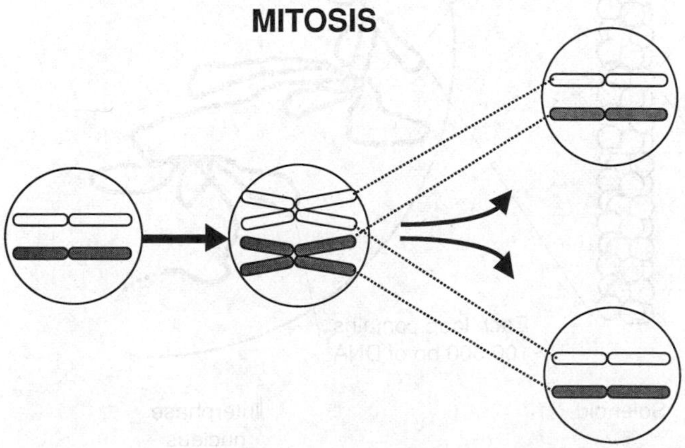

FIGURE 31 - 2. Mitosis. (Courtesy of Genetics/Screening and Counseling Service, Texas Department of Mental Health and Mental Retardation.)

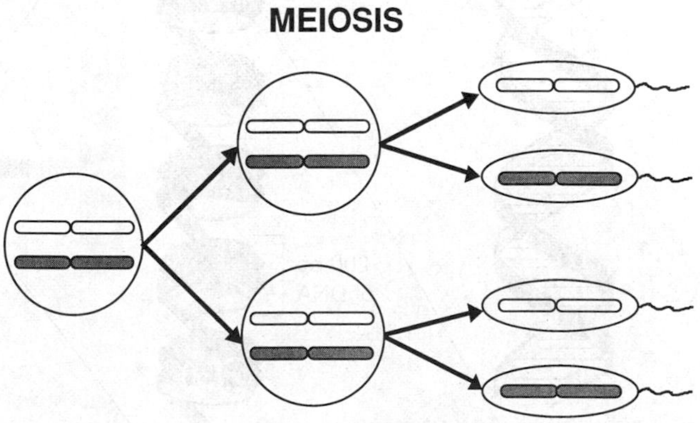

FIGURE 31 - 3. A simplified illustration of meiosis, showing the end product (sperm) with half the number of chromosomes the original had. In oogenesis, the original cell develops into three cells with half the number of chromosomes: an ovum and two polar bodies. (Courtesy of Genetics/Screening and Counseling Service, Texas Department of Mental Health and Mental Retardation.)

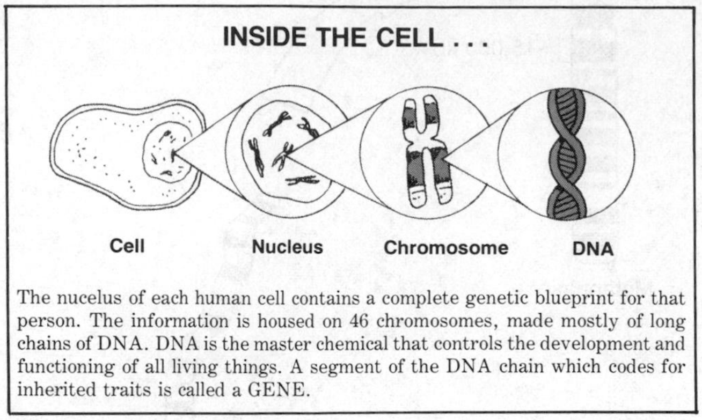

INSIDE THE CELL . . .
Cell
Nucleus
Chromosome
DNA
The nucelus of each human cell contains a complete genetic blueprint for that person. The information is housed on 46 chromosomes, made mostly of long chains of DNA. DNA is the master chemical that controls the development and functioning of all living things. A segment of the DNA chain which codes for inherited traits is called a GENE.

FIGURE 31 - 4. The nucleus of each human cell contains a complete genetic blueprint for that person. The information is housed on 46 chromosomes, made mostly of long chains of DNA. DNA is the master chain that controls the development and functioning of all living things. A segment of the DNA chain that codes for inherited traits is called a "gene." (From Wright, L., & Cadle, R. [1989]. *Understanding DNA testing: A basic guide for families.* Lexington, KY: Southeastern Regional Genetics Group.)

tion is housed on linear strands of DNA. The DNA is made up of individual "base pairs" arranged in a precise order. Small groups of these base pairs make up individual "genes" that code for specific proteins. To encode an enormous amount of information into a single cell nucleus, DNA strands are twisted into a double helix, coiled on spools of protein called "histones," and arranged into "nucleosomes," which are like beads on a string. This nucleosome becomes the basic structural unit of "chromatin," which is then supercoiled into the classic "solenoid" unit with loops and domains, as shown in Figure 31–5.

Micropackaging into solenoid units does more than confine information into a small space. Packaging DNA in precise ways appears to provide control over which genes are expressed and at what time. Perhaps this partially explains why a differentiated cell, such as bone and muscle, "knows" to perform only certain functions even though the entire genome is present in the nucleus of each cell (Thompson et al, 1991).

Genetic Variation

The key to health lies in the vast variability and adaptive capacity of the human species. Stated simply, hybrids are more healthy than are inbreds. Therefore, over evolutionary time, biologic species have developed a number of ways to ensure variability.

Variations are encouraged by several natural mechanisms. During meiosis, the pairing of maternal and paternal chromosomes and the point-to-point exchange of small segments between chromatids bring new combinations of genes to the subsequent gametes. This process is called "crossing over," or "recombination." Although crossing over is a healthy

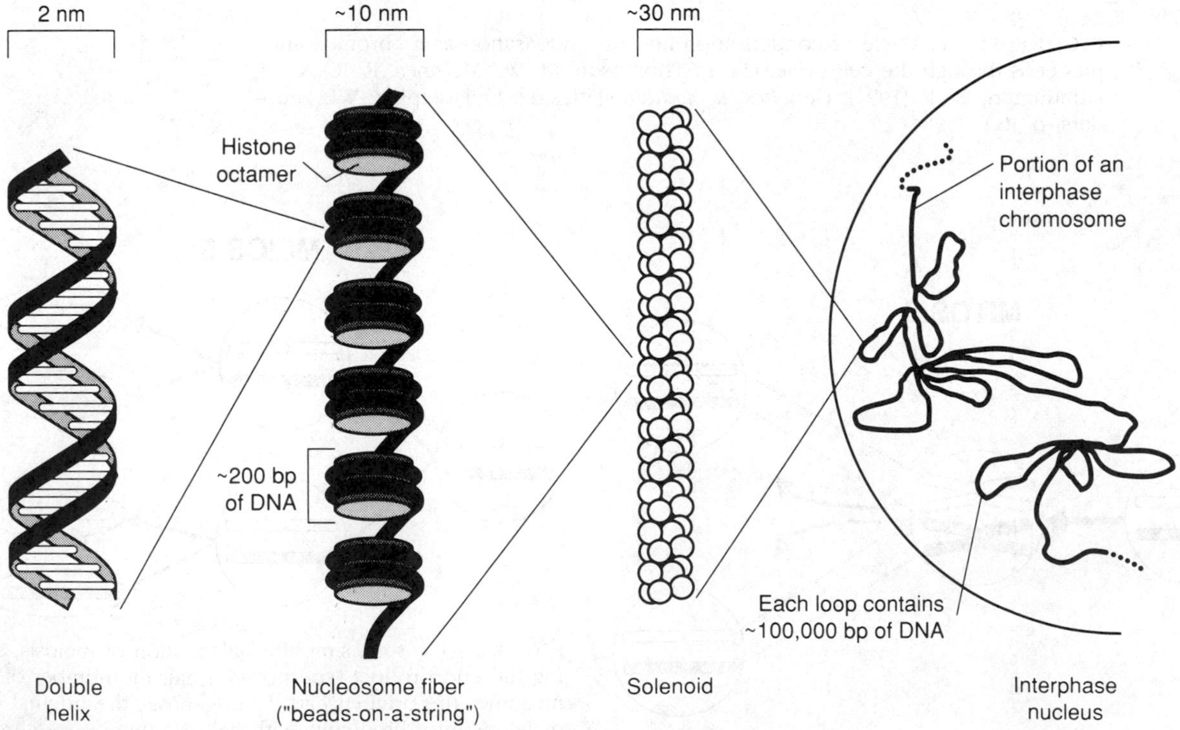

2 nm
~10 nm
~30 nm
Histone octamer
~200 bp of DNA
Portion of an interphase chromosome
Each loop contains ~100,000 bp of DNA
Double helix
Nucleosome fiber ("beads-on-a-string")
Solenoid
Interphase nucleus

FIGURE 31 - 5. Hierarchical levels of chromatin packaging in the human chromosome. (From Thompson, M. W., McInnes, R. R., & Huntington, W. F. [1991]. *Genetics in medicine* [5th ed.]. Philadelphia: WB Saunders, p 35.)

event, the presence of a recombination event can be a source of confusion when one is attempting to track a particular gene within a family unit.

Another mechanism that ensures variability is "assortment." This is the random distribution of different combinations of maternal and paternal chromosomes when gametes are formed. This was one of the major principles described by Mendel in 1865. A third way that variation is introduced into the human species is "mutation." A mutation is defined as any permanent change in the DNA, and, at a practical level, this is a change in the message or code that tells us what type of protein to produce. Once a mutation occurs, it is transmitted as part of the DNA code to subsequent generations.

Not all mutations are harmful. In fact, many proteins have several genetically different healthy forms. Alternative forms of genetic information at a particular gene location are called "alleles." Some genes have only one healthy version, but other genes have many forms. When there are at least two common normal alleles plus other rarer variations, the term "polymorphism" is used. One of the oldest and best examples of allelic variations is those types found in human blood. Various blood groups, such as the ABO and Rh systems, are examples of healthy genetic variations.

Polymorphic changes are common. Perhaps such mutations were healthy adaptations to some change in the primitive environment or simple accidental changes that persisted because the change did not affect the function of the protein. However they occurred, polymorphisms are essential tools to distinguish different inherited forms of a gene within family groups. As we begin to discuss the detection of genetic disease in families, it is important to understand polymorphisms as clues in genetic detection. Because genes are inherited in groups, nearby polymorphisms become genetic "markers" that allow us to track the presence or absence of a particular gene within family groups. Polymorphisms are useful in all of the following ways within the health care system (Thompson et al, 1991):

1. Carrier detection.
2. Presymptomatic diagnosis.
3. Prenatal diagnosis.
4. Paternity and forensic identity testing.
5. Donor-recipient matching.
6. Evaluation for predisposition to late-onset disease, such as cancer, stroke, and diabetes.
7. Gene mapping.

Recall, however, that genes—small segments of DNA arranged in a very precise order, or "sequence," on chromosomes—code for specific proteins that dictate our structural characteristics and control our regulatory functions. Even a minute variation in the sequence of base pairs or a loss of a small fraction of a chromosomal material may have profound biologic consequences. From our brief review of cell division, micropackaging, and mechanisms of genetic variation, it is easy to see that faulty transmission of genetic information may result in a variety of genetic disorders.

Classification of Genetic Disorders

Traditionally, geneticists and other health care providers have classified genetic disorders into the following major groups:

- Chromosomal disorders.
  - Variations in chromosomal number.
  - Deletions of chromosomal material.
  - Chromosomal rearrangements.
- Single gene disorders.
  - Autosomal dominant.
  - Autosomal recessive.
  - X-linked.
- Multifactorial disorders.
  - Malformations.
  - Diseases.

Recent discoveries have added the following group:

- Nontraditional inheritance.
  - Mitochondrial inheritance.
  - Genetic imprinting.
  - Uniparental disomy.

These four categories account for most malformations, variations, and childhood illnesses, including allergies and response to infection. Only childhood accidents or prenatal teratogenic exposure may be exempt from some level of genetic causation or interaction. This point further underscores the need to include a genetic assessment as a part of any evaluation of a child or family unit.

Chromosomal Disorders

Definition

A "chromosomal disorder" is any clinical presentation in which there is identifiable extra or missing chromosomal material. This may involve either a whole chromosome or a small segment of a particular chromosome. Extra or missing chromosomal material can be identified in metaphase chromosomes. Therefore, cells must be cultured, cell division suspended, metaphases identified, and nuclei visually inspected microscopically. Chromosomes are then counted in each metaphase, photographed, and paired for analysis in a karyotype format, as illustrated in Figures 31–6 and 31–7.

Causes of Chromosomal Syndromes

Chromosomal disorders often result as an alteration in chromosomal number. The mechanism by which most variations in chromosomal number occur is called "nondisjunction" because one or more chromo-

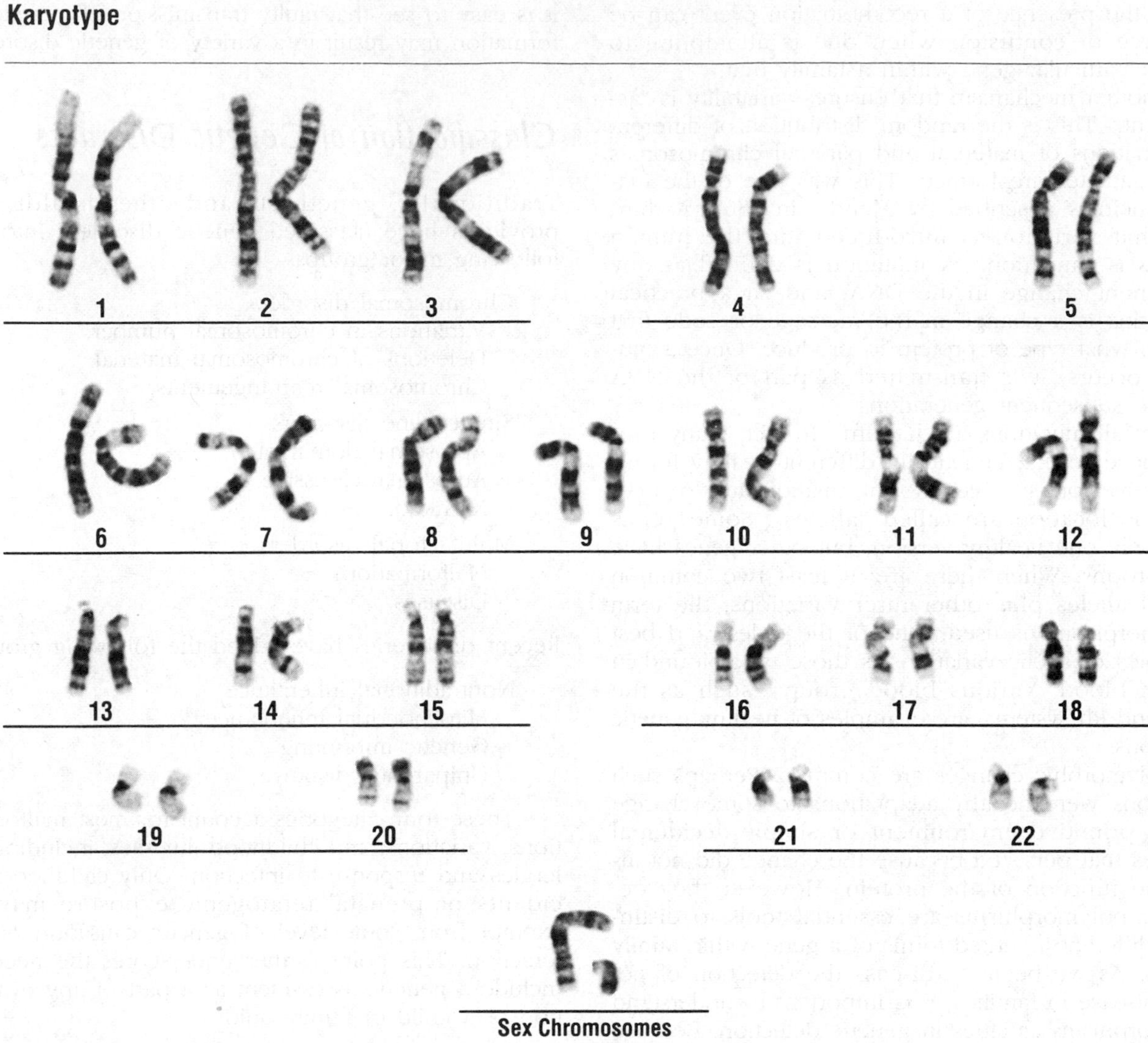

FIGURE 31-6. Normal male chromosome karyotype. (Courtesy of Integrated Genetics, West Paterson, NJ.)

somes fail to "disjoin," or separate (Fig. 31–8). The most common resulting gametes have one extra chromosome ("trisomy"), whereas others may have a missing chromosome ("monosomy"). It is possible for the entire chromosomal set to fail to disjoin during meiosis, leaving a gamete with 46 chromosomes. When paired with the other gamete at fertilization, a zygote is formed that has 69 chromosomes. These become "triploid" fetuses and are not viable; however, they are a frequent finding in abortus studies and may be noted in a family history of someone with a previous pregnancy loss. The other mechanism producing triploidy is simultaneous fertilization of an ova with two sperm.

If the gametes have the appropriate chromosomal number and fertilization proceeds normally, a chromosome problem can still be introduced by a nondisjunction error in subsequent cell division. This is called "mosaicism" and results when an error of mitosis in early embryonic development causes some cells to have an extra chromosome, some cells to have a missing chromosome, and some cells to be normal, all within the same person. Most of the time, the monosomy (missing chromosome) cell line will not survive, but the trisomy cells may persist with the normal cells, producing a clinically observable condition. Mosaic children are usually more mildly affected than are children with full trisomy conditions, but this varies, depending on the proportion of normal and abnormal cells.

Chromosomal rearrangements are called "translocations" because, in either meiosis or mitosis, chromosomes can be broken and reattached (translocated) to other chromosomes (Fig. 31–9). Translocations are permanent attachments and can be passed on to subsequent generations. A person who has a chromosomal rearrangement without extra or missing chromosomal material is called a "balanced translocation

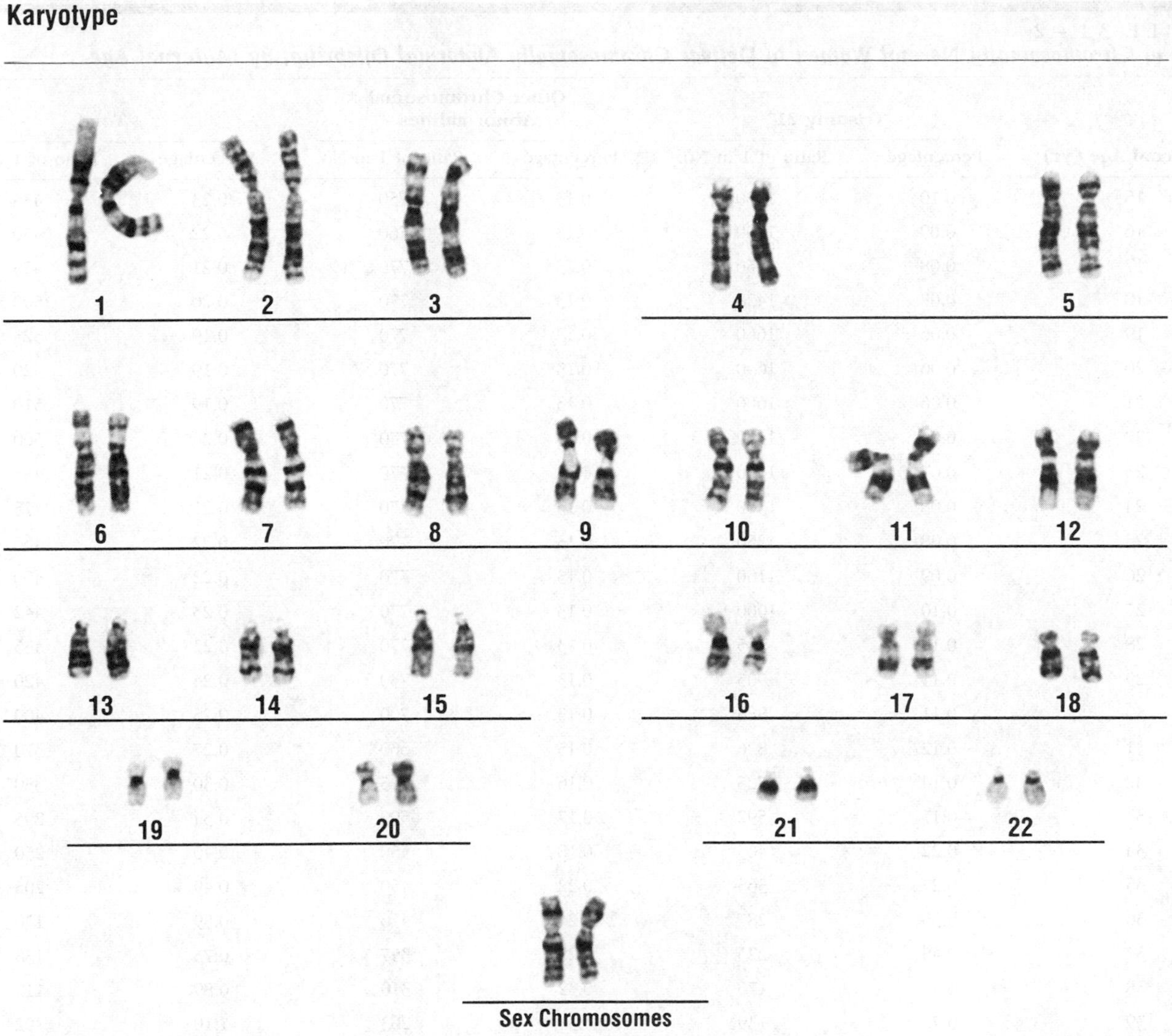

FIGURE 31 - 7. Normal female chromosome karyotype. (Courtesy of Integrated Genetics, West Paterson, NJ.)

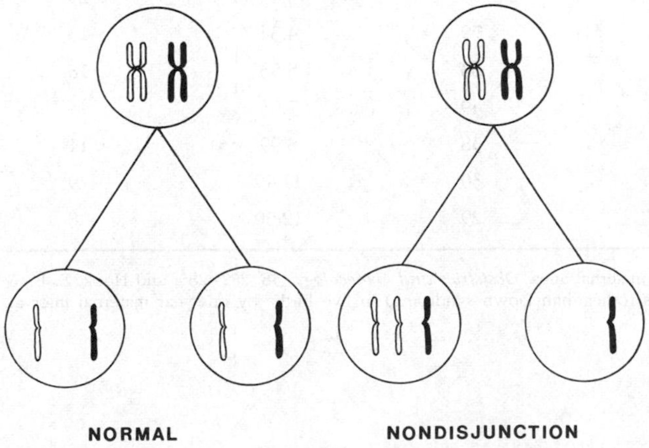

FIGURE 31 - 8. Nondisjunction. (Courtesy of Genetic Screening and Counseling Service, Texas Department of Mental Health and Mental Retardation.)

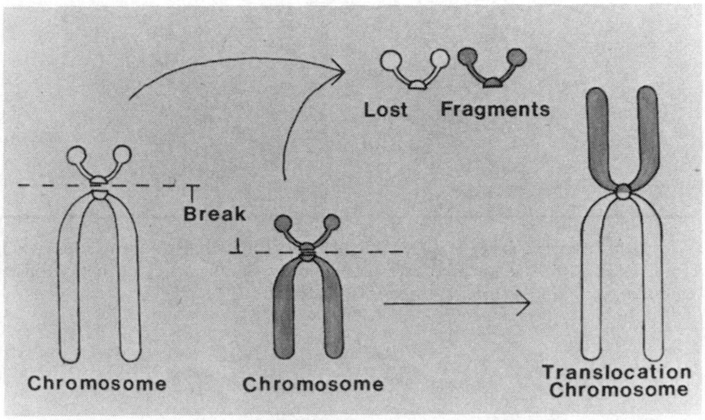

FIGURE 31 - 9. Translocation. (Courtesy of Genetics Screening and Counseling Service, Texas Department of Mental Health and Mental Retardation.)

TABLE 31-2
Risk of Chromosomally Normal Women to Deliver Chromosomally Abnormal Offspring, by Maternal Age

	Trisomy 21		Other Chromosomal Abnormalities		Total	
Maternal Age (yr)	Percentage	Ratio of 1 in No.	Percentage	Ratio of 1 in No.	Percentage	Ratio of 1 in No.
15	0.10	1000	0.13	750	0.23	435
16	0.09	1100	0.13	760	0.22	450
17	0.08	1250	0.13	770	0.21	475
18	0.07	1428	0.13	770	0.20	500
19	0.06	1660	0.13	770	0.19	525
20	0.06	1640	0.13	770	0.19	520
21	0.06	1600	0.13	770	0.19	510
22	0.06	1550	0.13	770	0.20	500
23	0.07	1400	0.13	770	0.21	485
24	0.08	1300	0.13	770	0.21	475
25	0.08	1250	0.13	770	0.22	460
26	0.09	1100	0.13	770	0.22	450
27	0.10	1000	0.13	770	0.23	442
28	0.10	965	0.13	770	0.23	435
29	0.11	905	0.13	730	0.24	420
30	0.11	885	0.13	700	0.25	400
31	0.12	826	0.15	660	0.27	370
32	0.14	725	0.16	625	0.30	330
33	0.17	592	0.17	590	0.34	295
34	0.22	465	0.18	550	0.40	250
35	0.27	365	0.22	450	0.49	205
36	0.35	287	0.24	416	0.59	170
37	0.45	225	0.28	357	0.73	138
38	0.57	176	0.32	310	0.89	112
39	0.72	139	0.38	263	1.10	92
40	0.92	110	0.45	222	1.37	73
41	1.17	85	0.54	185	1.71	58
42	1.49	67	0.66	151	2.15	47
43	1.90	53	0.81	123	2.71	37
44	2.42	41	1.01	99	3.43	29
45	3.08	32	1.26	79	4.34	23
46	3.93	25	1.60	63	5.53	18
47	5.00	20	2.03	49	7.03	14
48	6.38	16	2.61	38	8.99	11
49	8.12	12	3.37	30	11.49	9
50	9.00	11	3.45	29	12.50	8

Data from Hook, E. B. (1981). Rates of chromosome abnormalities at different maternal ages. *Obstetrics and Gynecology, 58,* 282–285; and Hook, E. B., & Cross, P. K. (1979). Estimated rates of clinically significant cytogenetic abnormalities (other than Down syndrome) in live births by one-year maternal interval. *American Journal of Human Genetics, 31,* 137A.

carrier" and is physically and mentally normal. However, when translocation carriers produce gametes, it is possible to transmit chromosomal combinations with extra or missing chromosomal material. Some of these combinations are always lethal, whereas others produce children with recognizable chromosomal syndromes. Other combinations are balanced like that of the parent or are entirely normal. Parents who are balanced translocation carriers have a significant risk of producing chromosomally abnormal offspring. Therefore, any child with a chromosomal abnormality should have a chromosomal analysis to determine if the cause was a trisomy or a translocation. If a translocation is noted, both parents should be studied to determine whether either parent is a balanced carrier or whether the original translocation occurred in the child ("de novo translocation"). Expert genetic counseling should be offered whenever a translocation is suspected.

Structural changes can also be "duplications" or "deletions." Causes can include errors during mitosis and meiosis or exposure to radiation or chemical mutagens. Large deletions have been associated with known syndromes, such as cri du chat syndrome (chromosome 5) with mental retardation, growth retardation, dysmorphic facial features, and an abnormal cry. Recently, however, molecular techniques have uncovered microdeletions and molecular duplications that account for numerous syndromes with previously unknown causes.

"Nondisjunction" is usually an accident of cell division and *not* an inherited characteristic. Therefore, chromosomal problems resulting from nondisjunctional events are less likely to recur in subsequent pregnancies than are chromosome problems caused by translocations or mosaicism. However, evidence suggests that some families are predisposed to nondisjunction. In these cases, one may find a variety of chromosomal problems scattered throughout the family history. Therefore, careful genetic evaluation is essential for any couple with a child who has a chromosomal problem, and prenatal diagnosis is available to provide reassurance for all these couples.

Maternal Age

Another important factor contributing to the presence of chromosomal disorders is "maternal age." Each month during ovulation, the individual ovum must complete meiosis as it proceeds down the fallopian tube. A woman has only one set of ova, which were established during her fetal life, and these eggs are subject to the effects of aging, the influences of illness, background radiation, or whatever else has occurred to her. These factors increase the chance for nondisjunction to occur in the ova or during meiosis in an older woman, particularly after 30 years of age. (See Table 31–2 for specific age-related risks) (Hook, 1981; Hook & Cross, 1979).

Since the early 1970s, age 35 has been the recommended age to consider prenatal diagnosis for chromosomal disorders. This is because at age 35, the risk of a chromosomal disorder is greater than the risk of the amniocentesis procedure. The age-related risk is the same whether in a first or a subsequent pregnancy. Males are not at an increased risk for nondisjunction until much later in life, because a new supply of sperm that has completed meiosis is made every 64 days.

Clinical examples of chromosomal problems include conditions such as Down syndrome, trisomy 18, trisomy 13, 4p syndrome, 5p syndrome, Prader-Willi syndrome, Turner syndrome, Klinefelter syndrome, whose clinical features are listed in the check lists found in Tables 31–3 to 31–9, and triple-X syndrome and cri du chat syndrome. These check lists can be used to document the need for a referral in a newborn nursery or pediatric setting. Because of its frequency, Down syndrome is described in greater detail in the following section.

Down Syndrome

A chromosomal cause of Down syndrome was identified in 1959, although the first clinical description was published by John Langdon Down in 1866. Down syndrome occurs commonly worldwide in all races and both sexes, with a frequency of about 1 in 1000 live births. It is also frequently identified in studies of spontaneous abortions (Stine, 1989). Down syndrome should be identifiable at birth because of the characteristic dysmorphic facial features, hand and feet findings, and hypotonia (poor muscle tone), which are almost always present in infants with Down syndrome. However, the combination of initial edema, cranial molding, and early hospital discharge may cause some of these infants to be missed in the newborn nursery. Significant cardiac findings may not be present in the first few days of life. Children with Down syndrome are more likely to have ventricular septal defects, transposition of great vessels, tetrology of Fallot, hypoplastic left heart, and other severe structural cardiac lesions than are children who are chromosomally normal. Approximately 40 per cent of these children have significant cardiac lesions (Jones, 1988).

Down syndrome should be considered following any neonatal or childhood assessment in which there is developmental delay; short stature; facies with a flat occiput, flattened profile appearance, upslanting eyes, flat nasal bridge, small nose and mouth, and protruding tongue; white specks in the irides (Brushfield spots); and low-set ears with overfolded helices. Hypotonia is a significant finding in almost all infants with Down syndrome. The hands and feet should also be examined for transverse palmar creases, incurving fifth fingers, a gap between the great toe and the other toes, and unusual fingerprints. Documenta-

TABLE 31-3
Check List for Down Syndrome

Craniofacial

____ Large or accessory fontanel (infancy)
____ Open fontanel (after ½ yr)
____ Flat occiput
____ Microcephaly (mild)
____ Flat facial profile
____ Flat nasal bridge

Eyes

____ Upslanting palpebral fissures
____ Inner epicanthal folds
____ Speckling of iris (Brushfield spots)
____ Fine lens opacities
____ Strabismus

Ears

____ Small
____ Overfold of superior helix
____ Small or absent lobes

Mouth

____ Protruding tongue
____ High-arched palate
____ Dysplastic teeth
____ Low, hoarse voice

Neck

____ Redundant or loose skin
____ Appears short

Cardiovascular System

____ Congenital heart disease
TYPE ______________________________

Gastrointestinal System

____ Umbilical hernia
____ Diastasis recti
____ Other gastrointestinal abnormality

Musculoskeletal System

____ Relatively short stature
____ Hyperflexibility of joints

Hands

____ Short
____ Clinodactyly of 5th fingers
____ Single flexion crease
____ Single horizontal palmar creases

Feet

____ Increased gap between toes 1 and 2
____ Plantar furrow

Dermatologic System

____ Cutis marmorata
____ Straight pubic hair
____ Fine, sparse hair

Genitalia

____ Underdeveloped male genitalia
____ Cryptorchidism
____ Delayed puberty
____ Menstrual irregularities

Neurologic System

____ Developmental delay
____ Mental retardation
____ Hypotonia

Other

____ Frequent infections
____ Thyroid dysfunction
____ Leukemia (1%)

Special Studies: X-rays

____ Hypoplastic iliac wings
____ Shallow acetabular angle
____ Double ossification centers in manubrium sterni
____ Vertebral body or rib abnormality

Dermatoglyphics

____ Distal palmar axial triradii
____ Ulnar loops on digits (especially 1–3)
____ True patterns in palmar 3rd interdigital
____ Arched tibia or narrow loop in plantar hallucal areas

tion of height, weight, head circumference (which should be small), and heart sounds is an essential part of the initial evaluation. Because no one symptom is diagnostic of Down syndrome, the nurse should complete a check list, including minor anomalies, and consider the constellation of findings found in these infants (see Table 31–3). Any neonate with a significant pattern of findings should be immediately referred for a complete genetic evaluation and chromosomal analysis (Jones, 1988).

With infant stimulation programs and the proper support systems, children with Down syndrome may progress well during infancy and early childhood. They learn at a slower pace but develop in the same sequence as chromosomally normal children. Short stature, speech problems, and mental retardation (IQ

TABLE 31-4
Check List for Trisomy 18

Head
____ Prominent occiput
____ Large fontanel
____ Small

Eyes
____ Epicanthal folds
____ Ptosis of lids
____ Small palpebral fissures
____ Corneal opacity

Ears
____ Low set
____ Malformed

Nose
____ Flat nasal bridge
____ Cleft lip
____ Posterior choanal atresia

Mouth
____ Small, receding mandible
____ Cleft palate
____ Bifid uvula
____ Small mouth

Neck
____ Loose skin folds

Chest
____ Shield chest and wide nipples
____ Small circumference
____ Flared
____ Short sternum
____ Cardiac abnormality

Abdomen
____ Hernias
____ Small pelvis
____ Muscular defect of diaphragm (eventration)
____ Renal abnormality
____ Malrotation of colon
____ Accessory spleen

Genitalia
____ Small or absent labia (female)
____ Cryptorchidism (male)

Trunk
____ Small birth weight
____ Failure to thrive
____ Scoliosis

Hands
____ Flexed fingers
____ Syndactyly
____ Deep transverse palmar crease
____ Long 5th finger
____ Small hypothenar muscles

Feet
____ Equinovarus
____ Rocker bottom
____ Hypoplastic dorsiflexed big toes
____ Syndactyly

Central Nervous System
____ Hypertonic
____ Mental retardation
____ Weak

General
____ Retarded bone age
____ Feeble cry
____ Decreased muscle mass
____ Hypermobility of shoulders

Special Tests
____ Extra 18 chromosomal material

Dermatoglyphics
____ Simple arches on fingers

scores usually between 25 and 50) are universal findings. Children with Down syndrome have variations in their immune system, making upper respiratory problems and other infections more frequent, and they are at increased risk for leukemia in childhood, diabetes, and hypothyroidism. There are variations in the pelvis and other bony structures. The shape of the foramen magnum and vertebral changes may place some children with Down syndrome at risk of spinal cord compromise. These children should be evaluated before gymnastics or other athletics are initiated.

Girls with Down syndrome are fertile, and there are more than 50 cases of Down syndrome females delivering live-born children documented. The theoretical risk of chromosomally abnormal offspring is 50 per cent, but the actual number of abnormal births has been about 20 per cent. Spontaneous abortion of

TABLE 31-5
Check List for Trisomy 13

Head

- ____ Sloping forehead

Eyes

- ____ Colobomas
- ____ Anophthalmia
- ____ Microphthalmia

Ears

- ____ Low set
- ____ Deformed
- ____ Deafness

Nose

- ____ Cleft lip
- ____ Absent olfactory tracts, single nares

Mouth

- ____ Cleft palate

Chest

- ____ Cardiac defects

Abdomen

- ____ Accessory spleen
- ____ Large gallbladder
- ____ Umbilical hernia
- ____ Renal anomalies
- ____ Malrotation of colon

Genitalia

- ____ Bicornuate uterus (female)
- ____ Abnormal scrotum (male)
- ____ Cryptorchidism (male)

General

- ____ Hemangiomas
- ____ Low birthweight
- ____ Failure to thrive

Hands

- ____ Deep transverse palmar lines
- ____ Hyperconvex narrow fingernails
- ____ Retroflexible thumbs
- ____ Flexion of fingers and hands
- ____ Polydactyly

Feet

- ____ Posterior prominence of heels
- ____ Polydactyly

Central Nervous System

- ____ Mental retardation
- ____ Breath holding (apneic spells)
- ____ Seizures
- ____ Hypertonic

Special Tests

- ____ Persistence of fetal hemoglobin
- ____ Extra D chromosome material

Dermatoglyphics

- ____ Distal palmar axial triradii
- ____ Plantar hallucal arch fibular pattern

TABLE 31-6
Check List for 4P− and 5P− Syndromes*

Head

____ Small (4p−, 5p−)
____ *Midline scalp defect* (4p−)

Eyes

____ Strabismus (4p−, 5p−)
____ Antimongoloid slant (4p−, 5p−)
____ Epicanthal folds (4p−, 5p−)
____ Hypertelorism (4p−, 5p−)
____ *Colobomas* (4p−)
____ *Ptosis of lids* (4p−)

Ears

____ Low set (4p−, 5p−)
____ *Simple* (4p−)
____ *Preauricular dimple or sinus* (4p−)
____ Narrow ear canals (4p−, 5p−)

Nose

____ Broad base (4P−, 5P−)
____ *Beaky* (4P−)

Mouth

____ Micrognathia (4P−, 5P−)
____ *Cleft palate* (4p−)
____ High palate (4p−, 5p−)
____ Carplike shape (4p−)

Chest

____ Congenital heart disease (4p−, 5p−)

Abdomen

____ Inguinal hernia (4p−, 5p−)

Genitalia

____ Cryptorchidism
____ *Hypospadias* (4P−)

Trunk

____ *Low birthweight*
____ Sacral dimple or sinus (4p−)

Hands

____ Deep transverse palmar lines (4p−, 5p−)
____ Short metacarpals (4p−, 5p−)
____ *Oblique nail striations* (4p−)

Feet

____ Short metatarsals (4p−, 5p−)
____ Deformities (4p−, 5p−)

Central Nervous System

____ *Psychomotor retardation, severe* (greater in 4p−)
____ Hypotonia (4p−, 5p−)
____ *Seizures* (4p−)

General

____ *Cry like a cat (cri du chat)* (5p−)
____ *Delayed bone maturation* (4p−)

Special Test

____ B chromosome, deleted short arms

Dermatoglyphics

____ *Underdeveloped dermal ridges*
____ *Low digital ridge count* (4p−)

* Distinguishing features are italicized.

TABLE 31-7
Check List for Prader-Willi Syndrome

History

____ Low birthweight
____ 3000 g (6 lb, 10 oz)
____ Slow weight gain
____ Hypotonicity in early infancy
____ Decreased prenatal fetal activity
____ Hyperphagia
____ Obesity—onset about age 2 yr

Head

____ Upsweep of frontal scalp
____ Microcephaly

Eyes

____ Almond-shaped palpebral fissures
____ Upslant to eyes
____ Strabismus

Face

____ Narrow bifrontal

Mouth

____ Down-turned mouth

Teeth

____ Thick saliva
____ Severe dental caries

Feet

____ Small for total body size (usually not evident until mid-childhood)

Hands

____ Small for total body size (quantitative measurement)
____ Clindactyly

Skin

____ Thick, insensitive erythema around hair follicles

Short Stature

____ Short stature apparent after 10 yrs of age

Mental Status

____ Delayed development
____ Mental retardation

Mild ____
Moderate ____
Severe ____

Males

____ Hypogonadism

Testicular volume (ml) ____
Penile length (cm) ____

Females

____ Scant pubic hair
____ Irregular or absent menses

TABLE 31-8
Check List for Turner Syndrome

Head

____ Abnormal sella

Eyes

____ *Strabismus

____ *Ptosis

____ *Refractive error

____ *Epicanthal folds

____ *Blue sclera

Ears

____ Anomalous

____ Low set

____ *Deafness

Nose

____ Unusual facies

Mouth

____ Narrow (high) palate

____ Small mandible

Neck

____ Low posterior hairline

____ Short

____ Webbed

Chest

____ *Idiopathic hypertension

____ Cardiac anomalies

____ Broad chest (shield)

a. Internipple distance ________

b. Chest circumference ________

c. Ratio a:b = ________ %
(ratio > 0.25 = widely spaced nipples)

____ Hypoplastic nipples

____ Pectus excavatum

Abdomen

____ Renal anomalies

____ Intestinal telangiectases

Genitalia

____ Delayed puberty

____ Delayed age of menstrual onset

____ Abnormal secondary sex development

Trunk

____ Short stature

____ *Spine defects

____ Overweight

Hands

____ Short 4th metacarpal

____ *Short 5th finger

____ *Single deep transverse palmar line

____ Nails—narrow, hyperconvex

____ Increased carrying angle (elbow >15 degrees)

____ Clinodactyly

Feet (Legs)

____ Lymphedema (by history)

____ Medial tibial exostosis

Central Nervous System

____ *Mental retardation

____ Defective space-form perception

General

____ Excessive pigmented nevi

____ *Cutis laxa

____ *Keloid formation

____ *Lax joints

Special Tests

____ Metaphyseal dysplasia or osteoporosis (x-ray)

____ Delayed bone age (x-ray)

____ Gonadal dysgenesis (biopsy)

____ Abnormal sex chromatin

____ Abnormal sex chromosomes

____ *Increased urinary gonadotropin level

____ Decreased estrogen production

Dermatoglyphics

____ Distal palmar axial triradii

____ Digital ridge count changes

*Fewer than 50% of cases.

TABLE 31-9
Check List for Klinefelter Syndrome

Head

____ * Hyperostosis of frontal bone

Face

____ Little facial hair after puberty

Eyes

____ * Refractive error

____ * Strabismus

Ears

____ * Congenital deafness

Chest

____ Gynecomastia

____ * Chronic pulmonary disease

Genitalia

____ Small testes

____ Firm testes

____ * Undescended testes

____ * Small penis

____ Sterility

Trunk

____ Tall

____ † Decreased upper/lower segment ratio

____ Obesity

____ Feminine habitus

____ Scanty body hair

____ * Scoliosis, lordosis, kyphosis

____ * Sacralization of lumbar vertebrae

Extremities

____ Long arms and legs

____ * Pes planus

____ * Abnormality of elbow

General

____ * Multiple angiomata

____ * Less regular features

____ † Upper body segment—crown to pubis ________ cm

____ † Lower body segment—pubis to sole ________ cm

Central Nervous System

____ Behavioral or mental disturbance

____ * Mental retardation

Special Tests

____ Abnormal sex chromatin

____ Abnormal sex chromosomes

____ Aspermatogenesis

____ Tubular hyalinization (testicular biopsy)

____ Interstitial cell hyperplasia (testicular biopsy)

____ Increased pituitary gonadotropin level

Dermatoglyphics

____ Decreased digital ridge count

* Fewer than 50% of cases.
† These measurements should be approximately equal in a normal person; in Klinefelter syndrome, the ratio of upper body segment to lower body segment is less than 0.93 (Nyhan & Sakati, 1987).

abnormal fetuses may account for this discrepancy (Stine, 1989). Males with Down syndrome are usually infertile. Adolescents with Down syndrome are sexually aware and should be instructed about appropriate behavior and birth control and protected from any unwanted advances. Nurses should be aware that parents may have difficulty dealing with sexuality issues in relation to adolescents with Down syndrome.

People with Down syndrome age rapidly, and they are subject to premature senility. Families should be assisted during the childhood years to make appropriate plans for as much independent living as possible in young adulthood and for supportive care as their child ages. It is essential that these plans be made during the early years, because many children with Down syndrome outlive their parents, and adult resources are limited and there are often long waiting lists.

Approximately 95 per cent of Down syndrome cases are due to trisomy 21 (Fig. 31-10). In these cases, nondisjunction occurred in the egg or sperm or at fertilization, resulting in a zygote with an extra number 21 chromosome. All other chromosomal pairs are normal. Parents of children with trisomy 21 have about a 1 per cent chance of recurrence of this problem in subsequent pregnancies. Translocations result in Down syndrome in about 4 per cent of cases; however, translocation carrier parents have a significant recurrence risk, ranging from 5 to 15 per cent, depending on the transmitting parent and the type of chromosomal rearrangement. Parental mosaicism for Down syndrome accounts for only about 1 per cent of Down syndrome cases (Stine, 1989). Parents who are mildly affected may be undiagnosed for this condition and may be reasonably functional. If the gametes have a significant percentage of trisomy 21 cells, however, there is a greatly increased chance of recurrence of Down syndrome.

All forms of Down syndrome look clinically identical. Therefore, all infants with Down syndrome

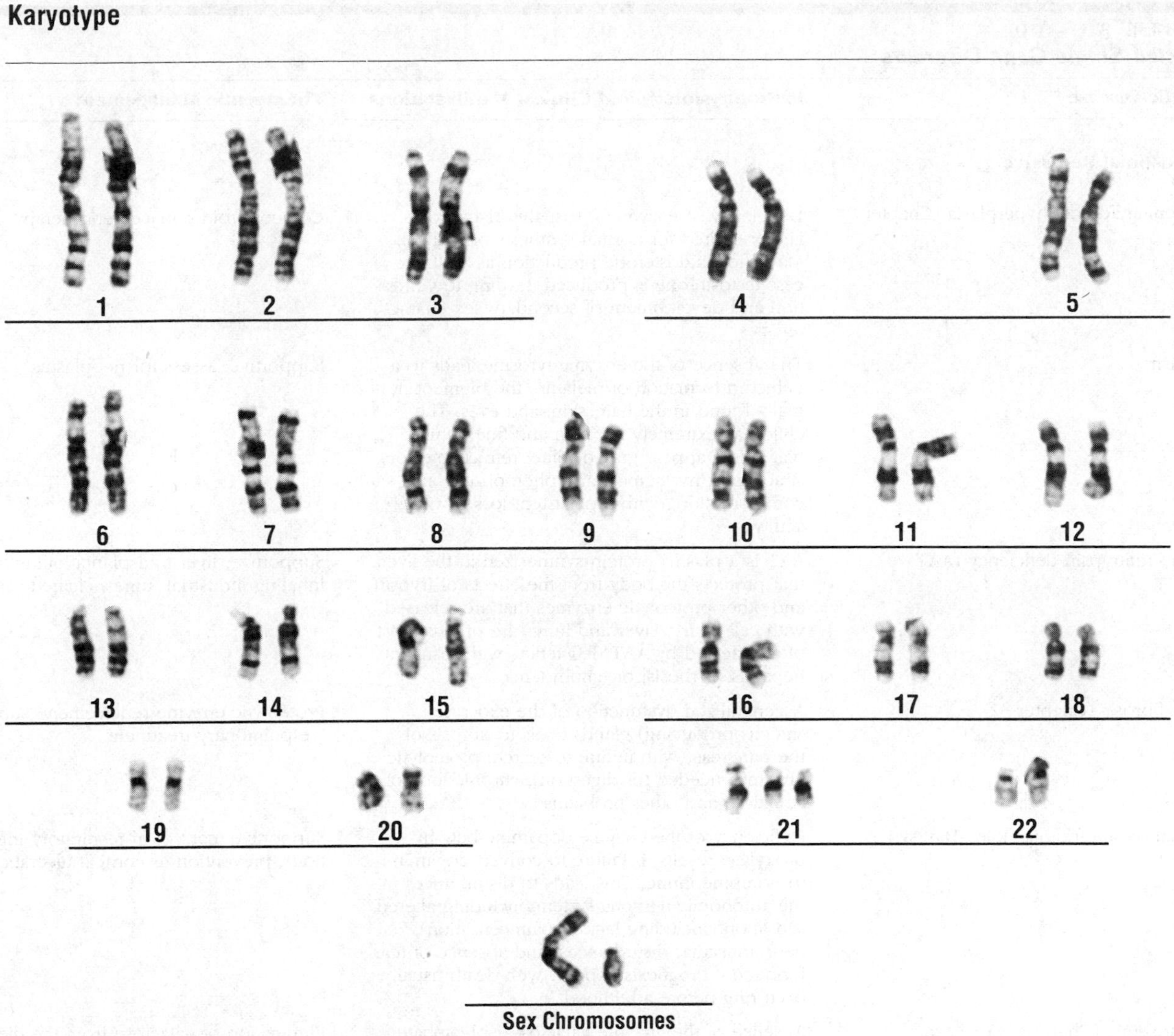

FIGURE 31-10. Trisomy 21 chromosome karyotype. (Courtesy of Integrated Genetics, West Paterson, NJ.)

should have immediate chromosomal analysis, and a family history should be obtained. If either parent has unexplained short stature or a history of developmental delay, school problems, or mild dysmorphic features, a parental Down syndrome check list should be obtained and referral for chromosomal analysis considered. See Chapter 27, Understanding Altered Development, for discussion of the nursing care of children with Down syndrome.

Single Gene Disorders

Definition

A "single gene disorder" (Table 31–10) is any condition that is caused by a variant allele or a pair of variant alleles at a particular location along a chromosome. Single gene variations sufficiently alter proteins so that a clinical effect is produced without an interaction with other genes or environmental influences.

Principles of Single Gene (Mendelian) Inheritance

One important concept in Mendelian inheritance is distinguishing the mode of transmission of single gene traits. Identifying the pattern of inheritance allows the nurse or other health care providers to predict the chance that a disorder will occur in an offspring or other relatives. Because chromosomes come in pairs, our genes, which are on the chromosomes, also come in pairs. A person should inherit one gene from the mother and one from the father. The type of trait will determine whether activity from one or both genes is necessary to produce a specified effect. If a person inherits the same allele for both of the pairs, he or she is said to be "homozygous" for that trait; if the alleles are different, the person is said to be "heterozygous." Recall that it is possible to have many alleles for a given trait in the world's population. For example, there are more than 400 different

TABLE 31-10
Selected Single Gene Disorders

Genetic Disease	Pathophysiology and Clinical Manifestations	Therapeutic Management
Autosomal Recessive		
Congenital adrenal hyperplasia (Chapter 43)	Deficiency of enzyme(s) (usually 21-hydroxylase) required for normal synthesis of cortisol. May affect aldosterone production as well. Excess testosterone is produced, leading to virilization and development of secondary sex characteristics	Corticosteroid replacement therapy
Albinism	The absence of the enzyme tyrosine leads to a defect in formation of melanin, the pigment normally found in the hair, skin, and eyes. The child has extremely fair skin and fine, white hair. Irises appear gray or blue; refractive errors, strabismus, nystagmus, and photophobia are common, along with a persistent loss of visual acuity	Supportive; assess for neoplasms
$Alpha_1$-antitrypsin deficiency (AAT)	AAT is a plasma protein synthesized in the liver that protects the body from the effects of trypsin and other proteolytic enzymes that are released with cell injury. Liver and lungs are organs most often affected by AAT deficiency, with resultant hepatitis, cirrhosis, or emphysema	Supportive; liver transplantation; avoid inhaling industrial fumes, cigarette smoke
Cystic fibrosis (Chapter 32)	A generalized dysfunction of the exocrine (mucus-producing) glands leads to fibrosis of the pancreas (with failure to secrete proteolytic enzymes needed for digestion), chronic lung obstruction, and other problems	Proteolytic enzyme replacement; supportive pulmonary treatment
Familial dysautonomia (Riley-Day syndrome)	Deficiency of the enzyme dopamine-beta-hydroxylase results in failure to convert dopamine to norepinephrine. This leads to disturbances in the autonomic nervous system, including altered sensation (including lack of pain sensation), neuromuscular disturbances, and absence of tear formation. Prognosis is poor, with death usually occurring before adulthood	Supportive: control of respiratory infections, prevention of corneal ulceration
Galactosemia (Chapter 44)	Absence of the enzyme galactose-1-phosphate uridyltransferase results in inability to convert galactose to glucose. Cellular accumulation of galactose and its abnormal metabolites leads to cirrhosis and mental retardation if diagnosis is not made at birth	Elimination of galactose from the diet
Homocystinuria (homocystinemia)	Deficiency of cystathionine synthetase results in accumulation of homocysteine, which is produced in the degradation of methionine (an essential amino acid). Progressive mental retardation and eye problems are common as well as skeletal abnormalities	High doses of vitamin B and dietary restriction of methionine
Hurler syndrome (Chapter 44)	Deficiency of the enzyme $alpha_1$-iduronidase leads to accumulation of unmetabolized mucopolysaccharides resulting in mental retardation, coarse facies, skeletal and joint deformities, deafness, dwarfism, and corneal clouding. This progressive disease usually leads to death by age 10 years	Supportive
Maple syrup urine disease (Chapter 44)	Absence of the enzymes needed for normal metabolism of leucine, isoleucine, and valine (essential amino acids) results in disrupted protein synthesis for neurologic development. Even with early, vigorous treatment, few children achieve normal physical and mental development	Dietary control of leucine, isoleucine, and valine
Metachromatic leukodystrophy	Deficiency of arylsulfatase A leads to demyelinization of the white matter of the brain with resultant loss of neuromuscular function. Children typically live only a few years after diagnosis	Supportive

TABLE 31-10
Selected Single Gene Disorders *(Continued)*

Genetic Disease	Pathophysiology and Clinical Manifestations	Therapeutic Management
Autosomal Recessive *(Continued)*		
Phenylketonuria (Chapter 44)	Absence or deficiency of the enzymes phenylethylamine and dihydropteridine reductase results in failure to convert excess phenylalanine (an essential amino acid) to tyrosine. Increased serum levels of phenylalanine and its abnormal metabolites lead to mental retardation	Dietary regulation of phenylalanine
Sanfilippo syndrome	Deficiency of heparan *N*-sulfatase leads to tissue accumulation of heparan sulfate with resulting damage to neurons and profound mental retardation. Gait disturbances and hyperactivity are characteristic. Death usually occurs during adolescence	Supportive
Sickle cell disease (Chapter 34)	Sickle hemoglobin is produced instead of normal hemoglobin, resulting in hematologic crises triggered by infection, dehydration, hypoxia, fever, high environmental temperature, high altitude, vigorous exercise, or emotional stress	Supportive: avoidance of predisposing conditions
Tay-Sachs disease	Deficiency of hexosaminidase leads to ineffective degradation of lipids found in cell membranes of the nervous system. The resulting accumulation results in neuromuscular deterioration, head enlargement, mental retardation, and blindness, with death typically occurring before age 4 years. Occurs primarily in Ashkenazi Jews	Supportive
Thalassemia major (Cooley anemia) (Chapter 34)	A defect in hemoglobin synthesis results in severe, progressive hemolytic anemia	Blood transfusion
Vitamin D–dependent rickets	Defective production of calcitriol or ineffectiveness of vitamin D at the receptor level leads to poor calcium absorption. This leads to bowing of the legs and resultant short stature.	Large daily doses of vitamin D
Werdnig-Hoffman disease (infantile spinal muscular atrophy)	Atrophy of anterior horn cells in the spinal cord and of motor nuclei in the brain results in weakness and lax muscle tone, with a characteristic frog-leg position in infants. Intelligence is normal. Death usually occurs before adulthood and is often related to respiratory failure	Supportive
Wilson disease	A defect in the synthesis of ceruloplasmin, a protein needed for copper transport, results in copper accumulation in the liver, brain, and cornea leading to cirrhosis, neurologic abnormalities, and Kayser-Fleischer rings of the cornea. Renal damage may also occur	Chelating agents to remove serum copper
Autosomal Dominant		
Achondroplasia	Abnormal skeletal growth results in short stature, short limbs, and a large head. This disease is associated with increased paternal age. The life span is usually normal	Supportive for psychosocial effects of short stature
Epidermolysis bullosa (EB)	EB is the general term for a group of diseases, some inherited through autosomal dominant genes, others as an autosomal recessive trait. The diseases are characterized by blisters brought on by mechanical trauma and high environmental temperature. They vary in severity from mild (epidermolytic EB) to life threatening (junctional EB)	Supportive; nonirritating clothes, no hot baths or tape on skin; drainage of large blisters

(continued)

TABLE 31-10
Selected Single Gene Disorders *(Continued)*

Genetic Disease	Pathophysiology and Clinical Manifestations	Therapeutic Management
Autosomal Dominant *(Continued)*		
Familial hypercholesterolemia	Lipoprotein metabolism is altered such that there is a marked increase in low density lipoproteins (LDL) from birth. Premature atherosclerosis, the most important manifestation, usually does not develop until middle age. Affected children usually have total cholesterol level >250 mg/dl	Diet low in cholesterol and oral cholestyramine
Huntington disease	Progressive degeneration of basal ganglia leads to dementia, choreiform movements, and an irregular, dancing gait. Onset is more common in middle age than in childhood	Supportive
Marfan syndrome (Chapter 31)	A disease of connective tissue, Marfan syndrome results in a tall, thin stature; long, slender fingers and hands; refractive errors in vision; and cardiac defects	Ongoing evaluation for heart disease
Neurofibromatosis (von Recklinghausen disease) (Chapter 40)	May be related to defective nerve growth factor, a neurohormone needed to differentiate neurologic cells. The classic signs include >6 café-au-lait spots and multiple cutaneous and subcutaneous neurofibromas (tumors of peripheral nerves). The tumors may become malignant, and this disease has the potential for becoming a prototype for the association between cancer and certain dominant genes. Symptoms worsen with puberty and pregnancy	Excision of tumors that cause pain or impair function; ongoing evaluation for malignancy
Noonan syndrome	Probably associated with autosomal dominant inheritance, this syndrome characterizes children who have certain anomalies in common with females with Turner syndrome. Common abnormalities include short stature, webbed neck, chest malformation, congenital heart disease, eye and ear abnormalities, and micrognathia (small chin)	Supportive
Osteogenesis imperfecta (OI)	The name for a group of hereditary diseases, some of which are transmitted by autosomal dominant traits and some by autosomal recessive inheritance. OI is characterized by bone fragility, blue sclera, presenile deafness, and a fragile appearance of skin. Cataracts are common, and teeth may be deformed	Prevention and treatment of fractures and deformity
Progeria (Hutchinson-Gilford syndrome)	Noted for the characteristic appearance of premature aging, this syndrome may be associated with autosomal dominant inheritance. Advanced paternal age seems to be an inheritance factor. Although motor and mental development are normal, profound growth failure occurs in the first year. Other common signs are characteristic facies, alopecia, loss of subcutaneous fat, abnormal posture, stiffness of joints, atherosclerosis, and "aging" skin. The median life span is about 13 years, with death from cardiac or cerebral vascular disease	Supportive
Retinoblastoma (Chapter 42)	A malignant tumor of the retina characterized by the cat's eye reflex (white reflex of the pupil instead of the normal red reflex), loss of vision, redness of the eye, and pain. Glaucoma may be present. Heterochromia (eyes of different colors or different colors within one iris) is sometimes associated	Radiation therapy, cobalt plaque applicators, cryotherapy, photocoagulation, enucleation
Treacher Collins syndrome	Characterized by deformities of facial bones, pinnas, and palate and by malocclusion of the teeth. Deafness is common	Supportive

TABLE 31-10
Selected Single Gene Disorders ***(Continued)***

Genetic Disease	Pathophysiology and Clinical Manifestations	Therapeutic Management
Autosomal Dominant *(Continued)*		
Tuberous sclerosis (Bourneville disease) (Chapter 40)	Sclerotic cerebral lesions (tubers) occur throughout the cortical gray matter. The lesions, present at birth, gradually enlarge and calcify and cause mental retardation and intractable seizures. Benign tumors develop in organs such as the kidneys, heart, liver, spleen, and lungs. Prognosis varies with the degree of involvement	Treatment of seizures, excision of large tumors
von Willebrand disease (Chapter 34)	Deficiency or absence of factor VIII (necessary for platelet aggregation) leads to prolonged bleeding time, bleeding from mucous membranes, heavy and prolonged menses	Infusion of desmopressin acetate
Waardenburg syndrome	Characterized by congenital deafness, abnormal pigmentation of the hair and eyes (a white forelock of hair and eyes that are either different colors or very pale in color). Skin also may be very light in color	Supportive for deafness
X Linked		
Color blindness	Carrier females pass this trait to their male children. It results in the inability to distinguish among certain colors: (a) red, blue, and green; (b) yellow and blue; (c) green and purple	None
Duchenne muscular dystrophy (pseudohypertrophic MD) (Chapter 41)	Primarily affecting males, this type of MD results in progressive muscular weakness, atrophy, and contractures. Death usually results from involvement of respiratory muscles	Supportive; keep active and ambulatory as long as possible
Glucose-6-phosphate dehydrogenase (G6PD) deficiency	Deficiency of this enzyme leads to episodes of hemolytic anemia associated with infections or certain drugs and to a chronic type of hemolytic anemia. Most common in males of Greek, southern Italian, Sephardic Jew, Filipino, southern Chinese, black, or Thai descent	Males of ethnic risk should be tested for G6PD before oxidant drugs are administered
Hemophilia A (factor VIII deficiency, classic hemophilia) (Chapter 34)	Deficiency of factor VIII leads to a coagulation disorder in which hemarthrosis (bleeding into a joint) is common as is bleeding into tissues following minor trauma. Severity depends on the amount of functioning factor VIII	Intravenous factor VIII replacement
Hemophilia B (factor IX deficiency, Christmas disease) (Chapter 34)	Deficiency of blood factor IX leads to a coagulation disorder as in hemophilia A	Intravenous factor IX replacement
Hunter syndrome	This mucopolysaccharide disease is similar to, but milder than, Hurler syndrome. Unmetabolized mucopolysaccharides are stored in tissues, leading to coarse facial features, short stature, joint stiffness, mental retardation, hepatosplenomegaly, and hernias	Supportive
Menkes disease	The inability to absorb copper from the gastrointestinal tract leads to failure to thrive, hypothermia, kinky hair, and progressive neurologic deterioration. Much of the damage occurs in fetal life and is irreversible, leading to death, often within the first year of life	Parenteral administration of copper
Retinitis pigmentosa	A progressive degeneration of the retina leads to vision loss, with impairment of night vision as an early symptom. This disorder may also be passed by autosomal dominant or recessive traits	Supportive
Wiskott-Aldrich syndrome	Characterized by thrombocytopenia, decreased immune competence, draining ears, and eczema	Splenectomy, bone marrow transplantation

alleles coding for hemoglobin, even though the normal hemoglobin A is the most frequent (Bowman & Murray, 1990). Although many different combinations are possible, in a given person most traits are coded for by a pair of alleles. In a few cases, multiple pairs of alleles are needed to code for a particular trait.

It is also important to distinguish between the "genotype," the genetic constitution of a person, and the "phenotype," the observed expression of the genes that involves the entire physiologic and biochemical makeup of the person. As dominant and recessive traits are discussed, realize that there are no dominant or recessive genes. For inheritance patterns, it is the observable dominant or recessive phenotype that is being described.

Genes code for the production of proteins. If an error is present within the gene that alters the protein's structure or function, an abnormality or disease may result. An easy way to remember how genes work is to think about this simple saying:

> DNA makes RNA
> RNA goes to the ribosome
> Ribosomes make proteins
> Proteins make us what we are or tell us how to function
>
> *Kathy Minor, PhD, 1979*

DNA is held within the nucleus of all cells. Therefore, it takes a single-stranded messenger RNA to leave the nucleus and travel to the cytoplasm and gather amino acid in a precise order. It is the order, or "sequence," of these amino acids that determines what type of protein is assembled in the ribosome. Once assembly is complete, the protein may be modified by several processes to produce a final product (Fig. 31–11).

Four broad categories of proteins are produced, as follows:

Structural—such as collagen, which forms the connective tissue of bone, muscle, and other parts.

Circulatory—such as hemoglobin and leukocytes.

Enzymatic—such as lactase and phenylalanine hydroxylase, which are necessary to break down

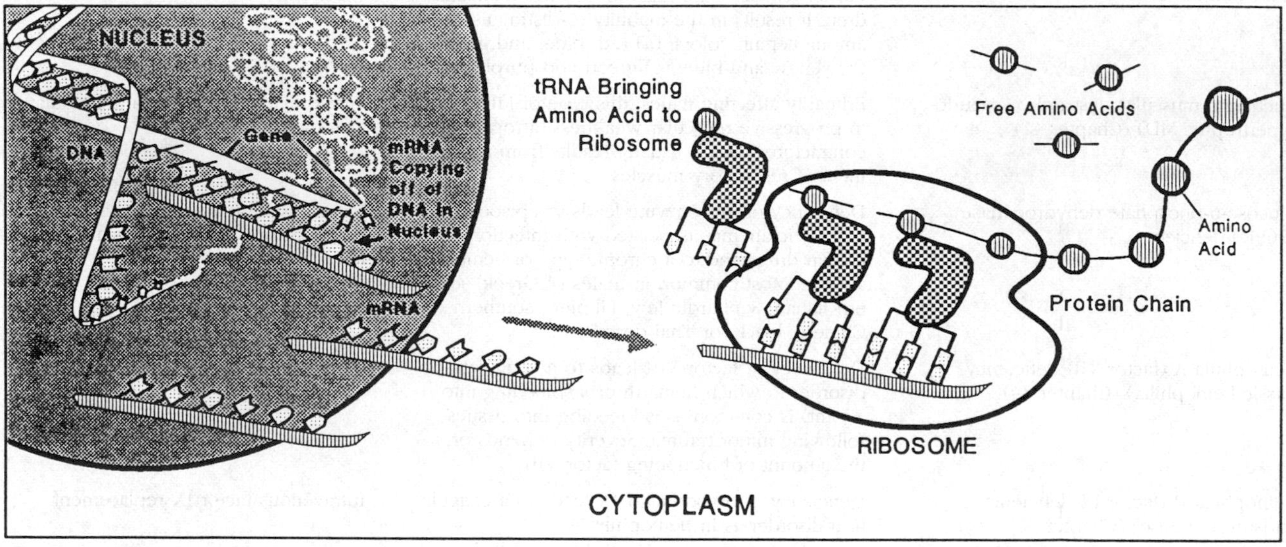

FIGURE 31-11. In the first step of gene expression, messenger RNA (mRNA) is synthesized, or transcribed, from genes by a process somewhat similar to DNA replication. In higher organisms, this process takes place in the nucleus of a cell. In response to certain signals, genes control the synthesis of mRNA. Protein synthesis, or translation, is the second major step in gene expression. Messenger RNA molecules are known as such because they carry messages specific to each of the 20 different amino acids that make up proteins. Once synthesized, mRNAs leave the nucleus of the cell and go to another cellular compartment, the cytoplasm, where their messages are translated into the chains of amino acids that make up proteins. A single amino acid is coded by a sequence of three nucleotides in the mRNA, called a "codon." The main component of the translation machinery is the ribosome—a structure composed of proteins and another class of RNAs, ribosomal RNAs. The ribosome reads the genetic code of the mRNA, and a third kind of RNA molecule, transfer RNA (tRNA), mediates protein synthesis by bringing amino acids to the ribosome for attachment to the growing amino acid chain. Transfer RNAs have three nucleotides that are complementary to the codons in the mRNA. (From US Congress, Office of Technology Assessment. [1992, August]. *Cystic fibrosis and DNA tests: Implications of carrier screening* [OTA–BA–532]. Washington, DC: US Government Printing Office, p. 89.)

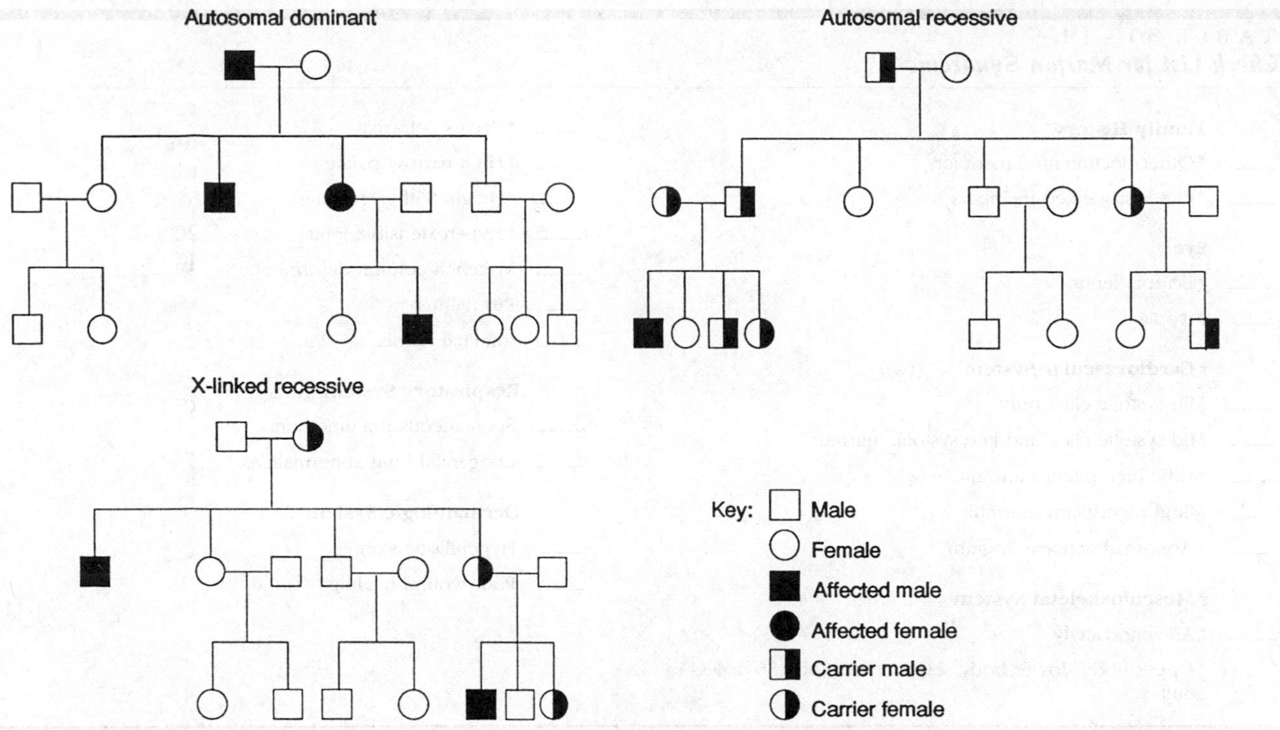

FIGURE 31-12. Autosomal dominant inheritance; autosomal recessive inheritance; and X-linked recessive inheritance. (From US Congress, Office of Technology Assessment. [1992, August]. *Cystic fibrosis and DNA tests: Implications of carrier screening* [OTA–BA–532]. Washington, DC: US Government Printing Office, p. 89.)

complex substances to simple products used by the body.

Transport—proteins, such as the cystic fibrosis transport regulator (CFTR) which help move substances across cell membranes.

Autosomal Dominant Inheritance

A trait is "dominant" if it is determined by a gene from only one of the two parents. It is expressed whenever a single copy of the gene is transmitted (Fig. 31–12). Characteristics of autosomal dominant inheritance include the following:

1. If a person is' heterozygous for one mutant allele (one normal and one variant form within the gene pair), the disorder is expressed.
2. If a person receives a "double dose," or two mutant alleles, for the same dominant trait, the result is profound, usually lethal.
3. The degree of clinical symptoms varies widely, even when the same family unit has an identical mutation; that is, some family members are mildly affected and others may be severely affected. Mildly affected persons can have severely affected offspring, and severely affected persons can have mildly affected offspring.
4. Most commonly, autosomal dominant disorders affect structural proteins.
5. In each pregnancy, there is a 50 per cent chance that an affected person will pass on the mutant gene and an equally likely chance that the normal allele will be transmitted.

Examples of common dominant inheritance that may affect the nursing care of children include most orthopedic variations such as extra digits (polydactyly), craniofacial syndromes, achondroplastic dwarfism, and osteogenesis imperfecta. Other dominant mutations include many forms of deafness, tuberous sclerosis, and neurofibromatosis (Table 31–10).

Clinical Model: Marfan Syndrome. Marfan syndrome can serve as a model for understanding structural changes that result from autosomal dominant mutations. The variant Marfan gene affects the crosslinking fibers in a certain protein, collagen. The result is a weak protein that stretches and can rupture. Such collagen changes particularly affect the vasculature, bones, and ligaments.

Children with Marfan syndrome tend to be tall (usually above the 95th percentile in height) with lanky extremities, bony knees, long fingers and toes, flat feet, scoliosis, loose joints, and dilatation of the aorta before they reach 10 years of age. They are usually nearsighted and may have dislocated lenses. Marfan syndrome does not affect mental abilities. The phenotype is like that of Abraham Lincoln, and some

TABLE 31-11
Check List for Marfan Syndrome

Family History

- ____ *Other documented members
- ____ *Other suspected members

Eye

- ____ *Ectopia lentis
- ____ Myopia

† Cardiovascular System

- ____ Mid-systolic click only
- ____ Mid-systolic click and late systolic murmur
- ____ Aortic regurgitant murmur
- ____ Mitral regurgitant murmur
- ____ † Abnormal echocardiogram

† Musculoskeletal System

- ____ *Arachnodactyly
- ____ *Upper body–lower body segment ratio of 0.85 or less in adults‡
- ____ *Pectus deformity
- ____ *High narrow palate
- ____ *Height 95th percentile
- ____ *Hyperextensible joints
- ____ Vertebral column deformity
- ____ Pes planus
- ____ Inguinal hernia

Respiratory System

- ____ Spontaneous pneumothorax
- ____ Congenital lung abnormalities

Dermatologic System

- ____ Hyperelastic skin
- ____ Poor wound healing

To meet the diagnostic criteria for classic Marfan syndrome, at least two, preferably three, of the following categories must include characteristic changes: family history, eye, cardiovascular system, and musculoskeletal system.
*Present in 50% of patients with classic Marfan syndrome.
†Present in 90% of patients with classic Marfan syndrome.
‡The usual upper body–lower body segment ratio is 0.93 in white adults (Nyhan & Sakati, 1987).

people theorize that he may have actually had Marfan syndrome (see the check list in Table 31–11).

If there is a known family history, young children should be monitored from an early age. Because Marfan syndrome is a life-threatening disorder, all school-age children should be routinely screened for Marfan syndrome using basic body measurements, such as arm span, which should be equal to height, and upper and lower segment ratios, which should be equal. The fingers of one hand should reach around the wrist and touch but not overlap. Persons with Marfan syndrome often have fingers that overlap the entire first joint. If positive signs are noted, the child should be referred for a careful evaluation, including an echocardiogram. A precise family history of heights, body types, and any sudden deaths should also be obtained.

Screening for Marfan syndrome should be completed before the child participates in school athletics. Failure to do so has resulted in several documented deaths of undiagnosed high school and college athletes. The most common cause of death is rupture of an aortic aneurysm. Central nervous system aneurysms are also common. Cardiac medication, such as beta-blockers, can reduce the life-threatening aspect of this disease.

Autosomal Recessive Inheritance

An "autosomal recessive trait" or condition is dependent on the genotype of both parents. An allele is recessive if it is expressed only when the person receives two copies (a double dose) of the variant allele (Fig. 31–12).

The characteristics of autosomal recessive inheritance are as follows:

1. The trait is expressed only when a person is homozygous for the recessive allele.
2. A person with a normal allele and a recessive variant allele will be a carrier for that trait but should be clinically healthy.
3. Most commonly, autosomal recessive disorders are due to variations in enzymatic or circulatory proteins. Thus, most recessive disorders reflect biochemical rather than structural changes.
4. If both parents are carriers of a given trait, in each pregnancy the child has a 25 per cent chance of manifesting the disorder, a 50 per cent chance of being a healthy carrier, and a 25 per cent chance of being genotypically normal for this particular allele.

Autosomal recessive disorders tend to be biochemical problems, particularly those of missing or deficient enzymes that affect the completion of a metabolic pathway. There are more than 1500 identified autosomal recessive disorders (McKusick, 1992). Examples of common recessive disorders that may be seen in pediatric practice include cystic fibrosis, sickle cell anemia, Tay-Sachs disease, PKU, galactosemia, and congenital adrenal hyperplasia.

Clinical Model: Cystic Fibrosis. Cystic fibrosis provides a model illustrating how the "new genetics" will

TABLE 31-12
Presenting Signs and Symptoms of Cystic Fibrosis in Various Age Groups

Neonatal Period
- Meconium ileus
- Meconium plug syndrome
- Intestinal atresia
- "Salty" taste

Infancy
- Failure to thrive
- "Salty" taste
- Rectal prolapse
- Heat prostration, dehydration
- Frequent, bulky stools
- Rapid finger wrinkling in water
- Steatorrhea
- Hypoproteinemia, anemia, edema
- Hypoprothrombinemia, hemorrhage
- Abdominal distention

Childhood
- Frequent, bulky, offensive stools
- Chronic secretory otitis media
- Intussusception
- Biliary cirrhosis, jaundice
- Rectal prolapse
- Heat prostration, dehydration
- Inguinal hernia
- Insulin-dependent diabetes mellitus

Adolescence/Young Adulthood
- Aspermia (male)
- Infertility
- Chronic cervicitis (female)
- Thick cervical mucus (female)
- Cervical polyps (female)
- Delayed secondary sexual development
- Poor growth/small for age
- Acute pancreatitis
- Chronic cough
- Bronchiectasis
- Glucose intolerance
- Insulin-dependent diabetes mellitus
- Intestinal obstruction
- Reactive airway disease, asthma

All Ages
- Chronic cough
- Nasal polyps (especially younger than 16 years of age)
- Cor pulmonale
- Presence of hard fecal masses in right lower quadrant of abdomen
- Recurrent pneumonia, bronchitis
- Sputum culture showing *Staphylococcus aureus* or *Pseudomonas aeruginosa*
- Elevated sweat electrolyte levels
- Absence of vas deferens (male)
- Pancreatic insufficiency and malabsorption
- Sinusitis
- Clubbed fingers
- Bronchiectasis
- Family history of similar symptoms, infant deaths
- Diarrhea

affect clinical management and nursing care in the future. Table 31-12 lists the major symptoms of cystic fibrosis in various age groups, and Figure 31-13 illustrates the major body systems affected. Chapter 32 discusses the aspects of clinical management, supportive care, and follow-up that have extended the lives of patients with cystic fibrosis from less than 2 years to young adulthood. More than one third of current cystic fibrosis patients are older than 21 years of age. However, care is still symptomatic, and cystic fibrosis remains an ultimately lethal disorder. A major breakthrough occurred in 1989 that is changing the course of cystic fibrosis management. In 1989, discovery was made of the delta F508 gene for cystic fibrosis, which accounts for about 70 per cent of cystic fibrosis cases in the United States and Canada. Before this time, the genetic basis and type of protein dysfunction were unknown. Once the gene was located, characterization began, and we now know the basis for several cystic fibrosis disease processes.

The cystic fibrosis gene is a very large gene, with more than 2500 base pairs (Fig. 31-14). Delta F508 is the location along the gene in which a three-base pair deletion has altered the function of the protein that it produces. We now know that this gene is a transport regulator gene that controls the movement of chlorides in and out of cells. In addition to the original delta F508 gene, more than 250 other mutations have been identified that alter the function of this important protein, partially explaining the extraordinary variability observed among some cystic fibrosis patients (US Congress, 1992).

Cystic fibrosis research is not yet complete, but what has developed since 1989 has changed how we approach screening, management, and research in this disorder. Screening was once limited to a "sweat

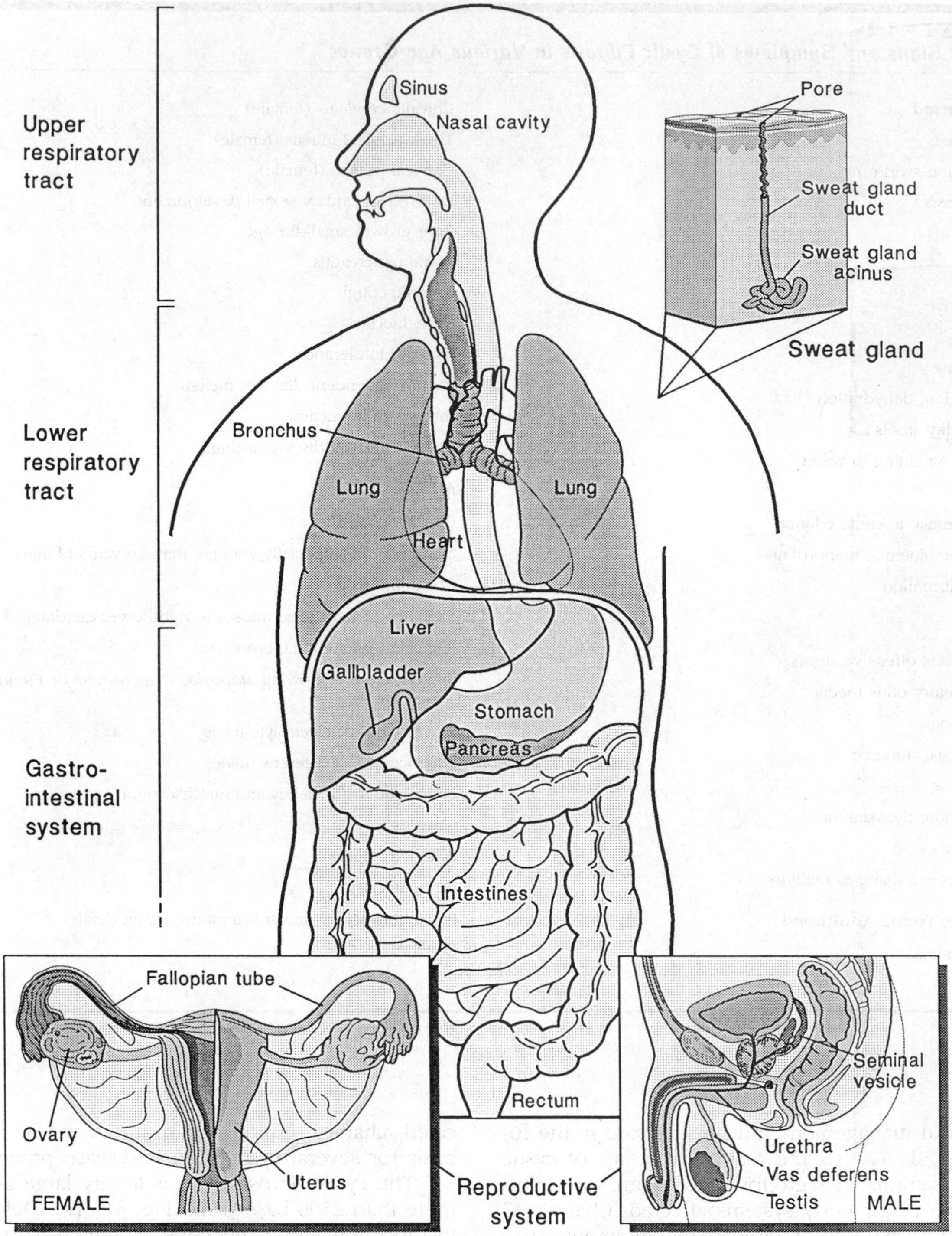

FIGURE 31-13. Organ systems affected in cystic fibrosis (CF). (From US Congress, Office of Technology Assessment. [1992, August]. *Cystic fibrosis and DNA tests: Implications of carrier screening* [OTA–BA–532]. Washington, DC: US Government Printing Office, p. 70.)

test," which measures elevations in sodium and chloride levels. DNA studies are now available that precisely identify 12 to 20 of the most frequent cystic fibrosis mutations. Efforts are being made to determine the most appropriate way to introduce neonatal screening for cystic fibrosis. A cheek brush method is available that provides DNA analysis for cystic fibrosis without the need to obtain a blood sample. The final stages of research on at least two genetically engineered therapeutic products are near completion, and clinical trials have begun. These products are designed to stop the progression of lung disease and

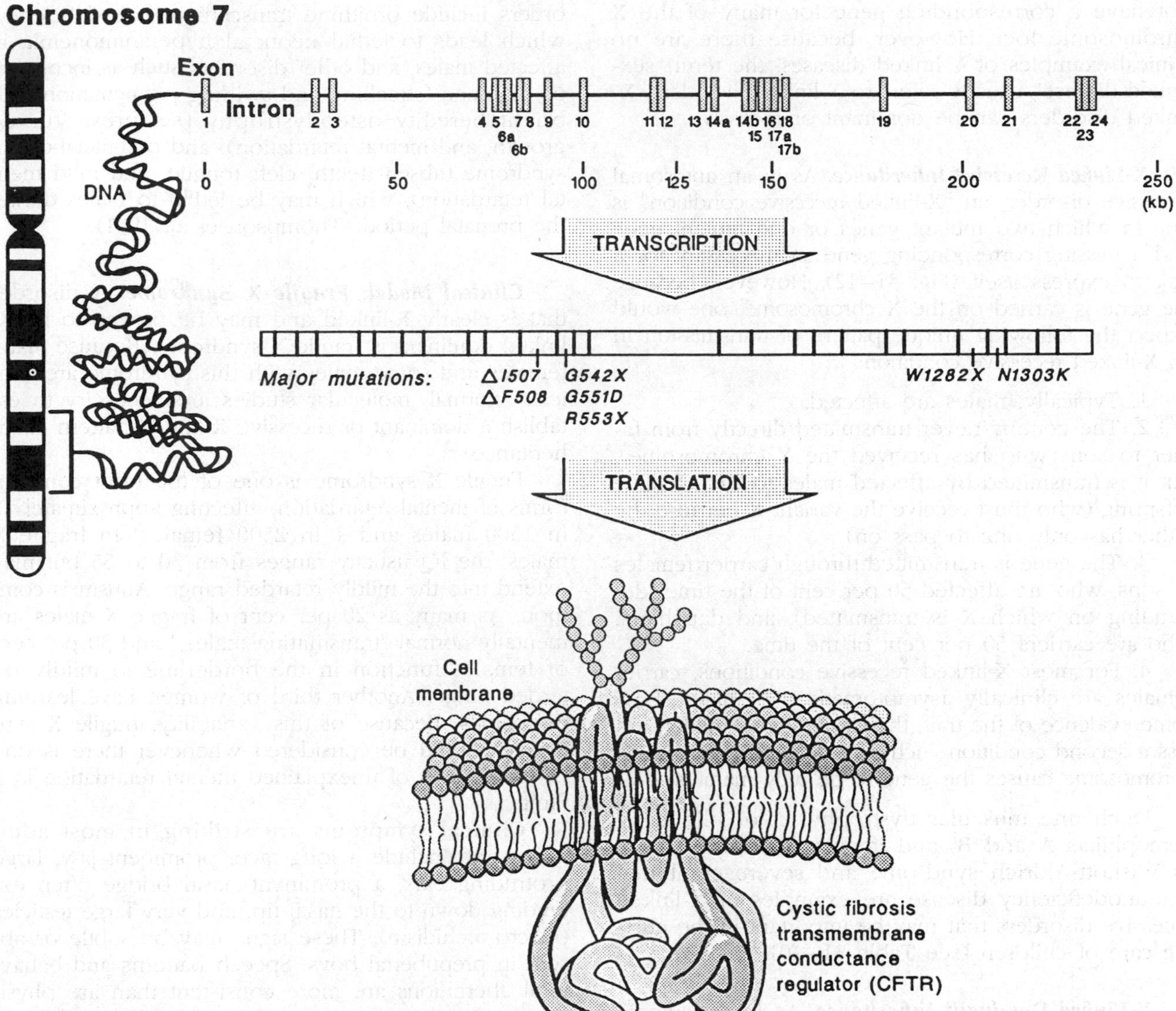

FIGURE 31-14. The CF gene is located on the long arm of chromosome 7, where it is spread over 250,000 base pairs (250 kb) of DNA. Coding regions of the DNA, or exons, are separated by noncoding regions, or introns. After the DNA is transcribed into messenger RNA (mRNA) composed of all 27 exons of the gene, the mRNA is exported from the cell nucleus. Finally, instructions in the mRNA are translated, using special structures in the cell to assemble 1480 amino acids into the final protein product. (From US Congress, Office of Technology Assessment. [1992, August]. *Cystic fibrosis and DNA tests: Implications of carrier screening* [OTA-BA-532]. Washington, DC: US Government Printing Office; based on Iannuzzi, M. C., & Collins, F. S. [1990]. Reverse genetics and cystic fibrosis. *American Journal of Respiratory Cell and Molecular Biology, 2,* 309–316.)

other clinical symptoms seen in cystic fibrosis. One genetically engineered treatment has received FDA approval and may be commercially available by the end of 1993. Basic research is ongoing to determine whether insertion of a "corrected gene" will provide a permanent cure. All these advances have been possible because researchers were able to study cystic fibrosis from a molecular rather than a symptomatic perspective.

Sex-Linked Inheritance

"Sex-linked inheritance" refers to any trait that is carried on the X or Y chromosome rather than one of the 22 autosomal pairs. The Y chromosome contains relatively few genes, primarily those associated with maleness. On the other hand, the X chromosome carries many genes related to traits other than sex. Thus, a male is "hemizygous," which means that he does not have a corresponding gene for many of the X chromosome loci. However, because there are no clinical examples of Y-linked diseases, the term "sex-linked disease" usually refers to X-linked disorders. X-linked disorders can be dominant or recessive.

X-Linked Recessive Inheritance. As in an autosomal recessive disorder, an "X-linked recessive condition" is one in which two mutant genes or one mutant gene and a missing corresponding gene are necessary for a trait to express itself (Fig. 31–12). However, because the gene is carried on the X chromosome, one would expect the following unique pattern of transmission in an X-linked recessive condition:

1. Typically, males are affected.
2. The gene is never transmitted directly from father to son (who has received the Y chromosome), but it is transmitted by affected males to each female offspring (who must receive the variant X because the father has only one to pass on).
3. The gene is transmitted through carrier females to sons, who are affected 50 per cent of the time (depending on which X is transmitted), and daughters, who are carriers 50 per cent of the time.
4. For most X-linked recessive conditions, carrier females are clinically asymptomatic. If females show some evidence of the trait, the expression is milder, unless a second condition such as a deleted or missing X chromosome causes the gene to be fully manifested.

Duchenne muscular dystrophy, color blindness, hemophilias A and B, and immunodeficiencies such as Wiskott-Aldrich syndrome and severe combined immunodeficiency disease are examples of X-linked recessive disorders that may be important in the nursing care of children (see Table 31–10).

X-Linked Dominant Inheritance. As in an autosomal dominant disorder, an X-linked dominant disorder requires only one mutant gene for the trait to be manifested. This changes the pattern of inheritance in the following ways:

1. Affected females transmit to both male and female offspring. A child of either sex has a 50 per cent chance of inheriting the mutant gene from an affected female.
2. Affected males, who have only one X chromosome, transmit the mutant X gene to all of their daughters and none of their sons.
3. On average, there are twice as many affected females as males.
4. Expression is variable but tends to be milder in affected females.
5. Some conditions may be lethal to males; therefore, X-linked dominance should be considered when all affected persons are female.

An important X-linked dominant disorder is familial hypophosphatemic rickets. Rare X-linked dominant disorders are fully penetrant, usually lethal, and severely expressed in males. X-linked dominant disorders include ornithine transcarbamylase deficiency, which leads to lethal neonatal hyperammonemia in affected males, and other disorders such as incognentia pigmenti (streaking and swirling pigmentation), Albright heredity osteodystrophy (seizures, stunted growth, and mental retardation), and oral-facial-digital syndrome (absent teeth, cleft tongue, and mild mental retardation), which may be lethal to males during the prenatal period (Thompson et al, 1991).

Clinical Model: Fragile X Syndrome. A disorder that is clearly X-linked and may be proved to be X-linked dominant is fragile X syndrome. Because many females and some males with this syndrome are clinically normal, molecular studies are necessary to establish a dominant or recessive X-linked pattern of inheritance.

Fragile X syndrome is one of the most common forms of mental retardation, affecting approximately 1 in 1500 males and 1 in 2500 females. In fragile X males, the IQ usually ranges from 30 to 55 but may extend into the mildly retarded range. Autism is common. As many as 20 per cent of fragile X males are mentally normal "transmitting males," and 30 per cent of females function in the borderline to mildly retarded range. Another third of women have learning disabilities. Because of this variability, fragile X syndrome should be considered whenever there is one or more cases of unexplained mental retardation in a family.

Clinical symptoms are striking in most adult males and include a long face, prominent jaw, large protruding ears, a prominent nasal bridge often extending down to the nasal tip, and very large testicles (macro-orchidism). These signs may be subtle or absent in prepubertal boys. Speech patterns and behavioral aberrations are more consistent than are physical signs and are more helpful in identifying children with fragile X syndrome. Hyperactivity, short attention span, poor eye contact, delayed speech and language development, and bizarre speech patterns are noted (Tables 31–13 and 31–14). Emotional instability, hand flapping, and hand biting are often seen in boys with fragile X syndrome, as are other autistic features.

Approximately 8 per cent of autistic boys have fragile X syndrome. Fragile X syndrome was named for the unraveled "fragile site" on the long arm of the X chromosome that was found in affected males and some females in family studies. Because of this fragile site, fragile X syndrome was first classified as a chromosomal disorder, but the X-linked pattern of transmission soon became apparent. Researchers have now identified the underlying gene, called "MFR-1," which follows the X-linked pattern of transmission. The underlying gene has an unstable "premutation" stretch of DNA. Clinical expression is correlated to the length of this unstable region, as is the appearance of a fragile site microscopically. Because of this variability, diagnosis should be established using the most recent DNA techniques as well as specific cytogenetic studies. Used alone, a negative fragile site on

TABLE 31-13
Check List for Fragile X Syndrome

Growth	**Integument**
____ Slightly increased birthweight	____ Increased frequency of radial loops, whorls, and arches on 3rd digits
Head circumference	____ Abnormal palmar creases (Sydney lines)
____ (>75th percentile in children)	____ Fine velvety skin
____ (>95th percentile in adults)	**Genitalia**
Facies	____ * Macro-orchidism (>23 ml volume in adults; occasionally found in children)
____ * Coarsened facial appearance	**Central Nervous System**
____ Long face	____ * Mild to profound mental retardation
____ * Prominent large ears	**Behavior**
____ Prominent high forehead	____ * Autistic features
____ High-arched palate	____ Hyperactivity
____ Thick lips	____ Violent outbursts
____ Prognathism	____ Stereotypical mannerisms
____ Epicanthal folds	____ Hand flapping
____ Dental crowding	____ Hand biting
____ Hypertelorism	**Speech**
____ Strabismus	____ Echolalia
____ Blue sclera	____ Jocular
____ Pale blue irides	____ Cluttering
Musculoskeletal System	____ Stuttering
____ Hypotonia	____ Perseveration
____ Hyperflexibility of joints	**Family History**
____ Pes planus	____ * Positive for X-linked mental retardation
____ Occasional scoliosis	
____ Large hands	
Cardiovascular System	
____ Mitral valve prolapse	

* Mental retardation *must* be present for fragile X studies to be indicated. A score of 6 or higher from the following should also be present:

Head circumference (>95th percentile)	2
Coarsened face	1
Large ears	2
Macro-orchidism	2
Positive family history for X-linked mental retardation	3
Autistic features	2
TOTAL	—

chromosomal analysis does not rule out the presence of the fragile X gene. Table 31-13 lists those people or families for whom fragile X testing should be considered (Jones, 1988; Nowak, 1992; Rousseau et al, 1991).

Multifactorial Inheritance

Most differences among humans are due to complex interactions between genes and the environment. These types of traits are referred to as "multifactorial" because they are determined by the additive effects of many genetic and environmental factors. There is a spectrum of expression of any given multifactorial trait that reflects a continuous variation. Height and IQ are examples of traits that are influenced by a combination of genetic and environmental factors. We see a continuous variation from short to tall or less to more verbal, mathematics, or performance skills, with most people somewhere in the middle range. The

TABLE 31-14
Language in Fragile X Syndrome

General language delay is noted, so specific unusual language patterns may not be detected until 7 or 8 years of age. The Denver screening tool* is not specific enough for most language problems. Use the ELM† in addition to the Denver. Remember that autism is more common in persons with fragile X.

If there is sufficient language development for speech patterns to be noted, be alert for the following unusual patterns.

Speech and Language Atypical Characteristics Check List

1. Referential gestures
2. Facial and head signals
3. Stereotyped vocalizations
4. Jargon
5. Unusual voice effects
6. Short, rapid bursts of speech
7. Dysrhythmia
8. Sound repetitions, prolongations, and interjections
9. Perseveration
10. Revision behavior
11. Echolalia
12. Affirmation by repetition
13. Conditioned statements
14. Inappropriate, tangential
15. Talks to self, objects
16. Pronominal reversal

* Denver Developmental Screening Test.
† Early language milestone scale.

same principles apply to malformations or diseases that are multifactorial: the clinical expression ranges from mild to severe along a continuum.

Important clinical examples include malformations such as cleft lip or cleft lip and palate, congenital dislocated hips, club feet, almost all isolated congenital heart malformations, and neural tube defects such as spina bifida and anencephaly. Multifactorial diseases important in pediatric practice include insulin-dependent juvenile diabetes, allergies, and immunodeficiency disorders. Most adult-onset cancer, stroke, heart disease, and psychiatric disorders fall into a multifactorial classification with significant genetic input.

The most important concept for multifactorial expression is the "threshold effect." This is the point at which the additive effects of genetic and environmental influences exceed the ability of the body to adapt and malformations or diseases become expressed. Close to the threshold, one may see minor anomalies that may be clinically insignificant but indicate a need for careful evaluation and counseling regarding risk for future offspring. Once the threshold is exceeded, one would expect to see a spectrum of clinical expression.

Because it is assumed that more than one gene locus contributes to the genetic variation (i.e., "polygenic") and that environment also plays a prominent role, multifactorial inheritance is more difficult to predict than the single gene modes of inheritance. Multifactorial traits tend to cluster in families, but there is no clear pattern of inheritance between families. However, by analyzing many families with multifactorial disorders, certain principles of recurrence within families have emerged. These principles are significantly different from those governing single gene inheritance and are listed in Table 31–15.

Nontraditional Inheritance

Recent advances in molecular genetics have helped identify other mechanisms that produce genetic disease. These mechanisms explain a variety of pediatric disorders that "looked genetic" but had no clear cause or pattern of inheritance.

- Mitochondrial inheritance—Disorders associated with genes from DNA found in the mitochondria (cytoplasmic organelles) of the ovum. Because sperm lack cytoplasm and mitochondria, this type of inheritance is always transmitted maternally. Diseases that have been associated with mitochondrial inheritance include several disorders that cause blindness, such as Leber hereditary optic neuropathy, as well as neuromuscular and epileptic syndromes.
- Imprinting—The differential expression of a chromosome or of a particular gene, depending on whether it is inherited from the male or the female parent. The classic example is that of Prader-Willi syndrome (gross obesity, mental retardation, small hands and feet, and hypogonadism) versus Angleman syndrome (ataxia, severe mental retardation, and "happy puppet" facies). If there is deletion of a particular part of chromosome 15, the child will have Prader-Willi syndrome if that chromosome was inherited from the father but Angleman syndrome if the affected chromosome was inherited from the mother. Another example is myotonic dystrophy, in which the onset is much earlier and more severe if the mother transmits the gene and milder with later onset if the father transmits the gene.
- Uniparental disomy—Two chromosomes of the same pair being inherited from the same parent

TABLE 31-15
Principles of Multifactorial Inheritance

- The incidence varies with each race
- The more severe the defect, the greater the risk of recurrence
- There is an altered sex ratio, i.e., the disorder occurs more frequently in one sex. The less likely sex has an increased risk of having an affected child
- The risk increases as the number of affected relatives increases
- The recurrence risk is usually in the range of 3–5% after one affected child, if no other relatives have expressed the disorder

with no representative chromosome from the other parent. Examples found in the literature include a child with cystic fibrosis who received two copies of chromosome 7 from her mother and a boy with hemophilia who inherited both his X and his Y chromosomes from his hemophiliac father and no X chromosome from his mother. Some cases of Prader-Willi syndrome are due to this mechanism.

We do not know if the nontraditional patterns will prove to be rare or common, but as we begin to understand humans at a molecular level, it is important that the nurse recognize these possibilities when a child presents with unusual clinical findings or an unexplainable pattern of inheritance (Hall, 1990).

The Role of the Nurse in the Recognition and Management of Genetic Variations

Family History

The most universal nursing role, regardless of clinical setting, is to obtain and analyze a family history. The advantages of taking a good history include the following:

- It can assist in establishing the diagnosis.
- It can define the natural history of the disorder.
- It provides insight into the medical and social burdens.
- It establishes the reliability of the parents, caregiver, or child.

Important characteristics of a well-conducted genetic family history include the following:

- The history centers on an identified client ("index case").
- At least first-degree and second-degree relatives are included.
- Ethnicity is identified.
- Past events that may indicate potential risks are identified, such as recurrent spontaneous abortions (miscarriages), stillbirths, children born with malformations, children who have died, conditions occurring more than once in a family, and any known genetic disorder.

Although a narrative family history may be adequate, only a pedigree can illustrate the relationships between relatives that allow the nurse or the genetic specialist to calculate risks of specific disorders. The protocol for developing a pedigree is shown in Figure 31–15.

History taking and pedigree analysis can show how genetic information relates to a comprehensive family health assessment. The pedigree includes medical, health, social, and ethnic background information about the patient and the family. All first-degree relatives (parents, siblings, and children), who are one step away from the identified patient, and second-degree relatives (grandparents, aunts, uncles, nieces, nephews, and grandchildren), who are two steps away, should be included. The family may have an informal historian who can supplement information provided by the parent and child. When combined with the objective data from the child's physical assessment, the family genetic history and the resulting pedigree chart provide the basis for decisions regarding the family's need for a comprehensive genetic evaluation.

Physical Assessment

Nurses should be prepared to assess any child for dysmorphic features, developmental delay, and problems in growth and development. If any of these factors are present, a genetic cause is likely. In addition to genetic causes, one must consider the possibility of prenatal environmental exposures that have had a teratogenic effect.

Not all genetic disorders are apparent at birth, so the nurse should include aspects of a genetic evaluation whenever a physical assessment is provided. The nurse should attempt to distinguish variations in overall appearance and development and document minor as well as major anomalies. When carefully evaluated, more than 11 per cent of infants will be found to have two or more minor anomalies (Holmes, 1974). Minor structural or developmental variations may be a clue to more serious underlying changes and require careful evaluation. Table 31–16 reviews the protocol for a genetic physical assessment of a child. If genetic alterations are noted, a referral should be made.

Clinical Examples

Assessment of the Neonate. In the neonatal nursery or well baby clinic, the nurse examines infants for obvious or suspected birth defects and for neurologic status. There may be obvious variations, such as cleft lip and polydactyly. Newborn evaluations identify serious chromosomal problems, such as Down syndrome, trisomy 18, and trisomy 13, and inherited disorders, such as dominant polydactyly and some cases of cystic fibrosis if meconium ileus is present. More often, however, subtle signs, such as poor muscle tone, ineffective sucking, wide-spaced eyes, an ear tag, and a hairy patch at the base of the spine, lead the nurse to request further genetic evaluation. Because early detection and intervention may prevent complications and reduce the severity of some disorders, the nurse should consider a genetic referral whenever any major abnormality or two or more minor anomalies are detected.

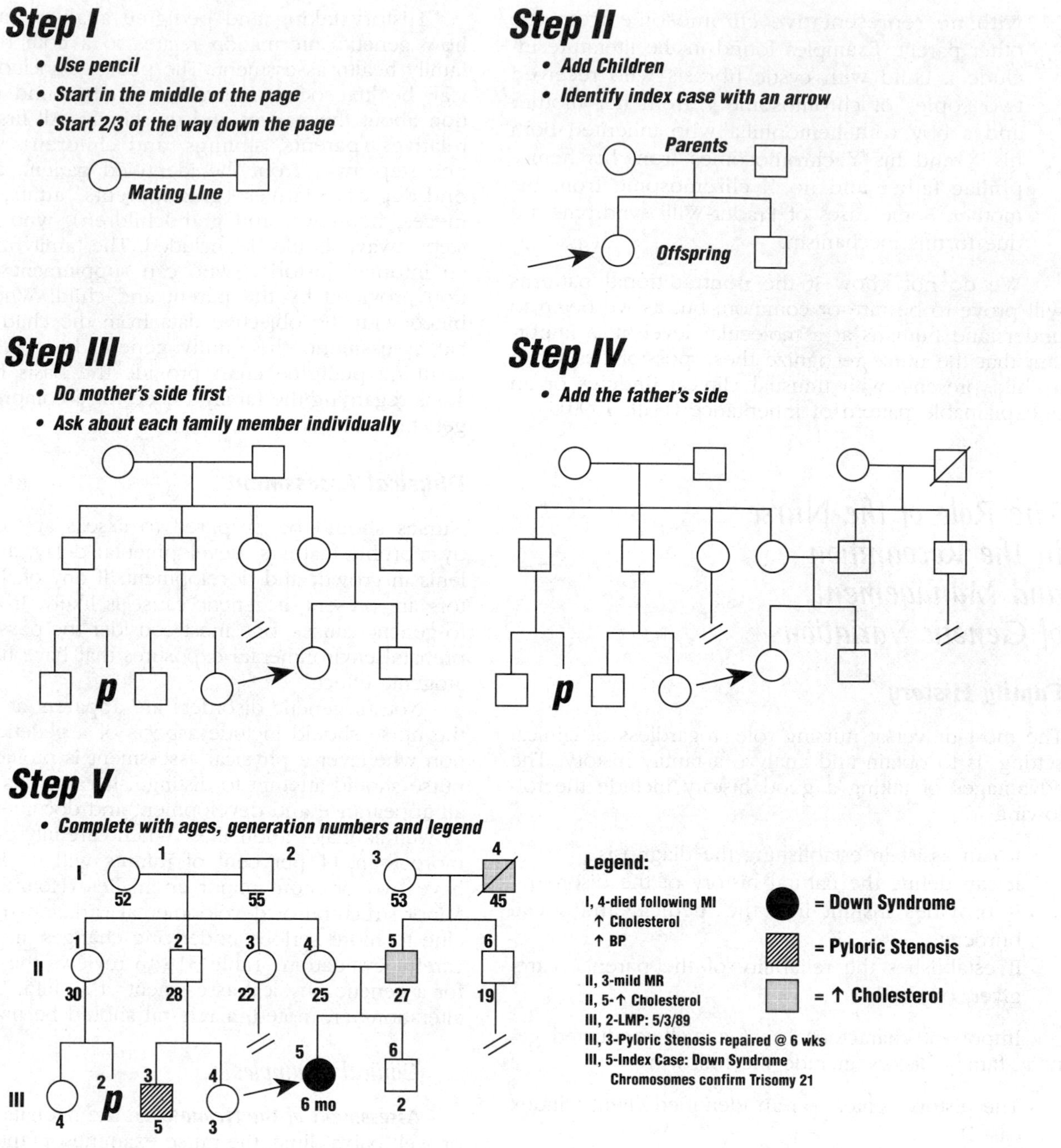

FIGURE 31 - 15. Developing a pedigree.

Genetic assessment of the neonate also includes a battery of newborn screening tests designed to identify treatable disorders that can cause death or mental retardation in the first few weeks of life (see Chapter 4). Neonatal screening tests are regulated by public health statutes and vary from state to state. The nurse should be familiar with state regulations and the types of tests provided and should be able to teach families about the reasons for neonatal testing, the difference between screening and diagnostic tests, and ways to learn about the results. By 1 month of age, most infants with autosomal chromosome disorders will have been identified, but most sex chromosome disorders will not have been diagnosed. Multifactorial conditions, such as pyloric stenosis, congenital dislocated hips, and club feet, should have been identified. Because of early hospital discharge, many forms of congenital heart disorders are identified during early well baby clinic visits.

By 1 or 2 years of age, 2 to 3 per cent of children will have an identifiable single gene disorder, and symptoms of conditions such as sickle cell anemia and cystic fibrosis can be identified. Children with chronic illness do not grow well and should be identified at this age. The nurse should also be alert for a variety of genetic causes of failure-to-thrive,

TABLE 31-16
Protocol for Genetic Assessment: Physical Examination of the Child

General Assessment

Begin the physical assessment by noting the child's general appearance and any distinctive or unusual odor. If there is anything unusual about the child's general appearance, it is helpful to take body measurements for comparison with established standards. Observe the parent(s) for the same unusual feature or minor anomaly noticed in the child. Although the appearance of the same anomaly in the parent may lessen concerns, it can also be a clue of a dominant inherited trait.

Head

The *size* of the head is extremely important because the first 2 years of the child's life are vital for brain growth. The normal size of a child's head is 34.5 cm at birth to 49 cm by 2 years of age for boys and 34 cm at birth to 48 cm at 2 years of age for girls. A series of measurements is the most useful. Measurements should be taken at the widest circumference of the head.

Among abnormal findings is *microcephaly,* which is the result of limited brain size causing the head to be 2 or more standard deviations below normal parameters. This may be caused by infection, brain trauma, or genetic abnormalities. Brain tissue may be abnormal in some cases. *Macrocephaly* is an increased head size. *Hydrocephaly* is an increase in the amount of cerebrospinal fluid. Macrocephaly with or without hydrocephaly is seen in some genetic syndromes along with other anomalies.

The *shape* of the child's head should be *normocephalic* (Fig. 31–16). Normal closure of fontanels is usually completed between 9

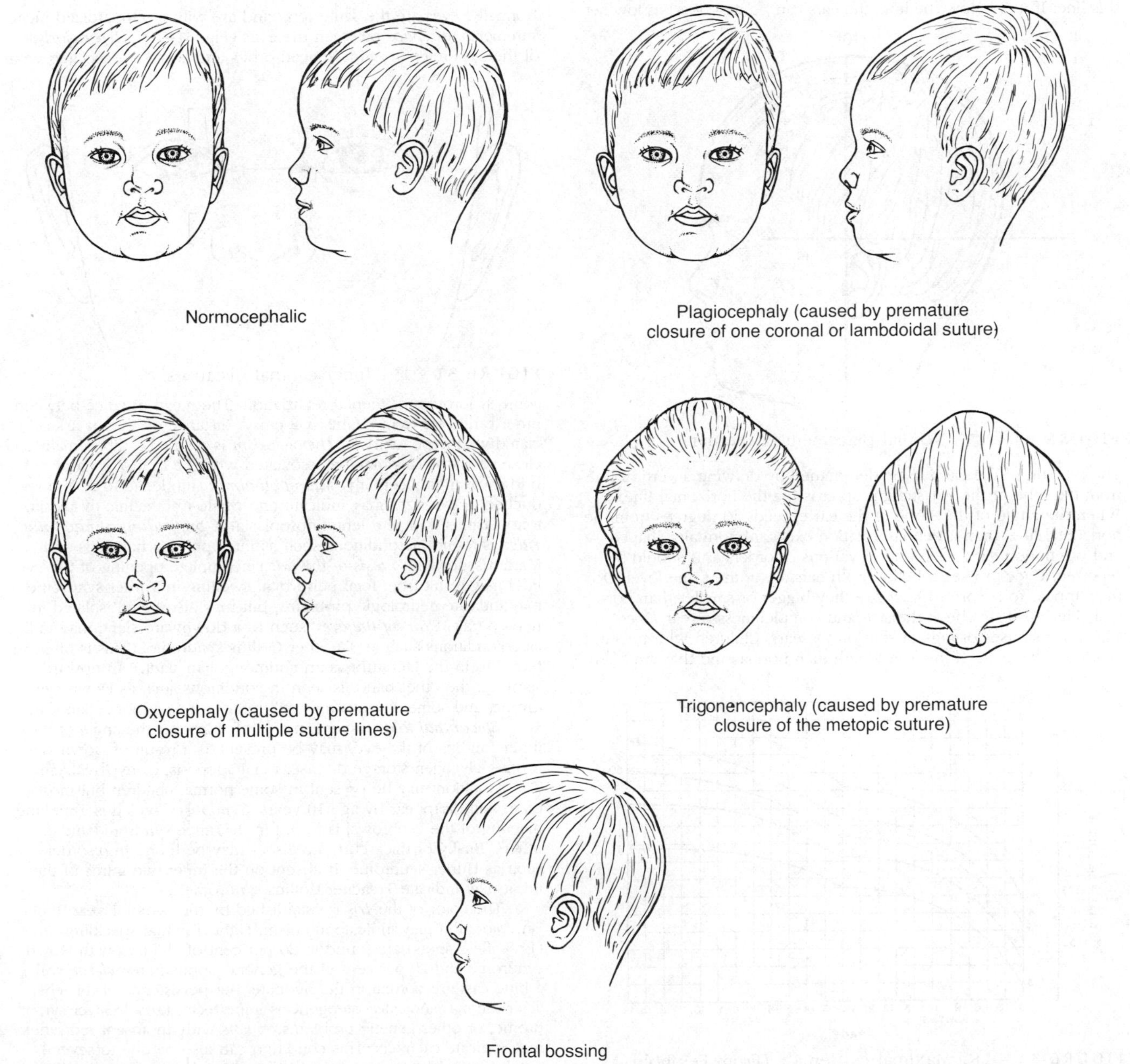

FIGURE 31-16. Head shapes.

(continued)

TABLE 31-16
Protocol for Genetic Assessment: Physical Examination of the Child *(Continued)*

and 19 months. Late closure could indicate Down syndrome, rickets, osteogenesis imperfecta, hydrocephalus, or syphilis. An anterior fontanel diameter that measures either two standard deviations above or below 2.1 cm (0.6 and 3.6 cm, respectively) is important. Posterior fontanels rarely exceed measurements of 0.5 cm. A large posterior fontanel may indicate hypothyroidism. *Premature closing of suture lines* is termed "craniosynostosis"; this disorder is detailed in Chapter 40. A prominent forehead, or *bossing* (see Fig. 31-16), is found in several genetic conditions such as Hurler syndrome and fragile X syndrome.

Ears

By drawing an imaginary line from the outside corner of the eye straight back, one can determine whether the ears are set in a normal *position* (Fig. 31-17). The upper part of the *pinna* should meet this line. If it is below the line, the ears can be described as low set.

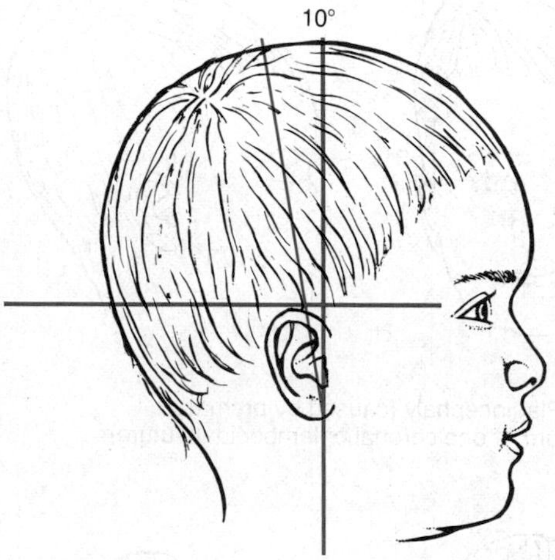

FIGURE 31-17. Normal placement of the ear.

The rotation of the ear can be determined by drawing a vertical line from the lobe of the ear straight up crossing the horizontal line. When the angle of the slope of the ear exceeds 10 degrees from the horizontal line, then a definite rotation exists. Abnormally shaped and positioned ears are found in various disorders and should be reported. Check to see whether both ears are at the same level. Do they appear to be protruding? Are they bigger or smaller than normal (Fig. 31-18)? Check the size and completeness of ear *lobes*. Check for sinuses or tags of skin on the ears. Children with fragile X syndrome have ears longer in length than normal and that are often

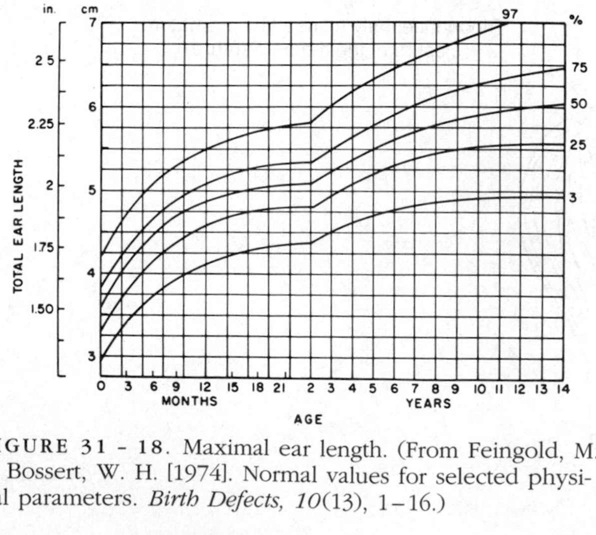

FIGURE 31-18. Maximal ear length. (From Feingold, M., & Bossert, W. H. [1974]. Normal values for selected physical parameters. *Birth Defects, 10*(13), 1-16.)

posteriorly rotated. Hypoplasia of *cartilage* causes ears to be soft and flexible. Practice looking at ears of your colleagues closely so that you can recognize minor anomalies of structure and placement.

Face

Observe for *spacing* of features, *symmetry,* and signs of *weakness* or *paralysis.* The normal *width* of a newborn infant's face is approximately 8 cm. Children with Marfan syndrome may have long, thin, narrow facies and children with trisomy 18 may have a small midface. Many genetic syndromes are associated with asymmetry of the face. Some are due to structure, as in hemifacial microsomia, and some are due to unbalanced movements of musculature, as in Moebius syndrome (maldevelopment of cranial nerves).

Eyes

Normally, eyes are the same *level* and are within standardized measurements for *space* between the eyes (Fig. 31-19). *Hypertelorism* of the eyes refers to wide-spaced orbits and is often associated with

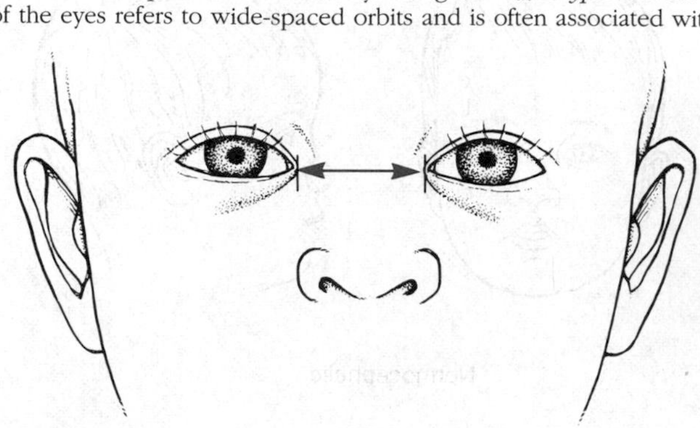

FIGURE 31-19. Inner canthal distances.

some syndromes of mental retardation. The mean distance between inner canthi for term infants is 2 cm. A distance of 3 cm is associated with hypertelorism. *Hypotelorism* is defined as abnormally close-set eyes. This may be associated with the lack of a nasal bridge, or trigonocephaly. *Microphthalmia* (moderate to severe reduction in eye size) may indicate encephalo-ophthalmic dysplasia, toxoplasmosis, or retrolental fibroplasia. A *protruding supraorbital ridge* is found in conditions such as mucopolysaccharidosis and Marfan syndrome. *Ptosis of the lids* (incomplete opening of the eyelids) may result from fetal periorbital swelling in Turner syndrome, may indicate neurologic problems, but may also be an isolated inherited trait. *Slant of the eyes,* such as a downward slant, may indicate conditions such as Treacher Collins syndrome. (This is often referred to in the literature as an antimongolian slant.) An upward slant, on the other hand, is seen in conditions such as Down syndrome, and some writings may still refer to it as a mongolian slant.

Epicanthal folds (a vertical fold of skin over the angle of the inner canthus of the eye) may be present as a result of Down syndrome, glycogen storage disease, renal agenesis, or hypercalcemia. The condition may be present in some normal children but most often will disappear by age 10 years. *Synophrys,* which is a midline meeting of the eyebrows, is found in de Lange syndrome and others. Bushy or thick curly *eyelashes* may be found in disorders such as Hurler syndrome. If absent on the inner two thirds of the lid, it may indicate Treacher Collins syndrome.

The color of the *iris* is established by the age of 1 year. Pinkish coloration may indicate albinism. Light or white speckling (Brushfield spots) are found in 80 per cent of children with Down syndrome and 20 per cent of the general population. *Sclerae* with a blue cast are normal in the neonate, but persistence of this characteristic may indicate osteogenesis imperfecta, Russell-Silver syndrome, or other genetic problems. A *lens* with an absent red reflex may indicate cataracts. This condition can also be due to several conditions leading to mental retardation, such as toxoplasmosis. A dislocated lens may be the result of Marfan syndrome or homocystinuria.

TABLE 31-16
Protocol for Genetic Assessment: Physical Examination of the Child (Continued)

Nose

A normally placed nose is found in the middle and upper portion of the face. The *shape* of the nose is important because in many syndromes one sees a great deal of variation. Notice whether the nose is broad and flat, small and up-turned, or sharply pointed. Note whether the nose is straight and whether the *nares* are symmetric. Palpate to examine the *bone* and *cartilage*. Check the *septum* with a penlight to determine whether a perforation exists by shining the light into one naris and observing to see whether the light escapes into the other naris. Occasionally the tip of the nose will have a tiny vertical indentation. Nose shape is usually unremarkable by itself, but an asymmetric nose or a nose not symmetrically placed may be important in combination with other abnormalities.

Mouth

The mouth should be symmetric. Note the *lips* to see whether they are turned down, sag to one side, or are the same size on both sides. Look for tiny dimples or pits. Are there clefts in the lip or *palate?* Drooling starts at about 3 months of age and continues until the child learns to swallow saliva at about 9 to 12 months. Examine the palate for a gentle slope. Report a high arched palate or one that is notched at the junction of the soft and hard palates. Note *micrognathia* (an excessively small lower jaw) or *macrognathia* (a large jaw), which may indicate genetic problems that should be further evaluated. For instance, a prominent jaw is found in many children with fragile X syndrome. *Teeth* that have a delayed eruption past 1 year of age may result from cretinism. *Gums* that are discolored with a dark line along the margin may indicate a high concentration of lead in the child's system. (Do not confuse this with the normal dark pigmentation seen on the gums of African-American children.)

Note the size of the *tongue*. A tongue that appears large for the mouth is found in conditions such as Down syndrome, hypothyroidism, or Hurler syndrome. Tongue protrusion is a common finding in children who are mentally retarded. Note the normal milestones in feeding patterns. It is important to note *reflexes,* such as the rooting, sucking-swallowing, gag, chewing, and bite reflexes. Rooting disappears by 2 months; the sucking-swallowing reflex disappears at approximately 6 months; the gag reflex diminishes after the chewing reflex begins at approximately 7 months; and the bite reflex ceases at about 5 months. *Lip closure* begins at about 6 to 8 months. Facial features are described as coarse if they are broad and fleshy. Always check previous pictures of the person to see if the features are becoming more coarse, a common sign of metabolic diseases.

Hair

Some syndromes are noted by hair *distribution* far down on the neck (Fig. 31–20) (Noonan or Turner syndrome) or low down on

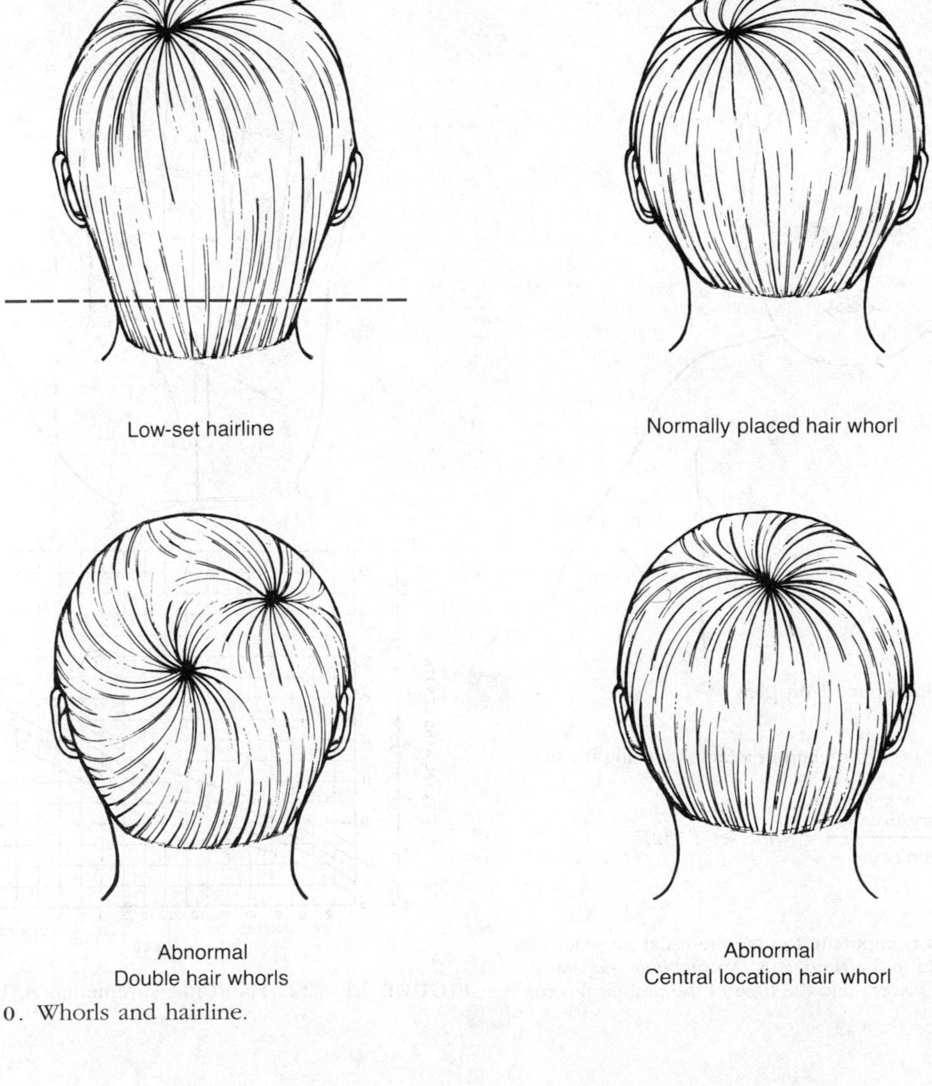

FIGURE 31-20. Whorls and hairline.

(continued)

TABLE 31-16
Protocol for Genetic Assessment: Physical Examination of the Child *(Continued)*

the forehead (Hurler syndrome). Hair on other parts of the body, such as patches low on the spine, should be reported. *Color* is important because white hair in young people may indicate albinism; a white patch may indicate Waardenburg syndrome. Diets deficient in protein cause reddish or gray color changes in hair. The majority of hair *whorls* are normally located on the left side of the crown in a clockwise rotation (see Fig. 31–20). The location of the whorl should be noted, especially if there are more than one. Note the distance between them. *Unruly* hair can be a part of a syndrome or of microcephaly. Observe the *texture* and *thickness;* some syndromes are characterized by unusually brittle and/or sparse hair.

Neck

A neck that is thick or *webbed* in appearance is abnormal. Conditions such as Noonan syndrome or Turner syndrome are indicated with such a finding. Any *primitive reflex* that persists past infancy, such as the tonic neck reflex and the startle reflex, should be noted. Primitive reflexes that do not disappear at the usual time will cause problems in the child's acquisition of other skills such as feeding.

Chest

The *shape* of the chest should be noted for any irregularities. A protruding or a funnel-shaped *sternum* is often seen in Marfan syndrome or Marquio disease. An indentation of the chest is termed "pectus excavatum" and a protrusion is "pectus carinatum." Does the chest seem to "match" the body in proportion? Look at the *nipples* and record whether they are wide set (Fig. 31–21) or hypo-

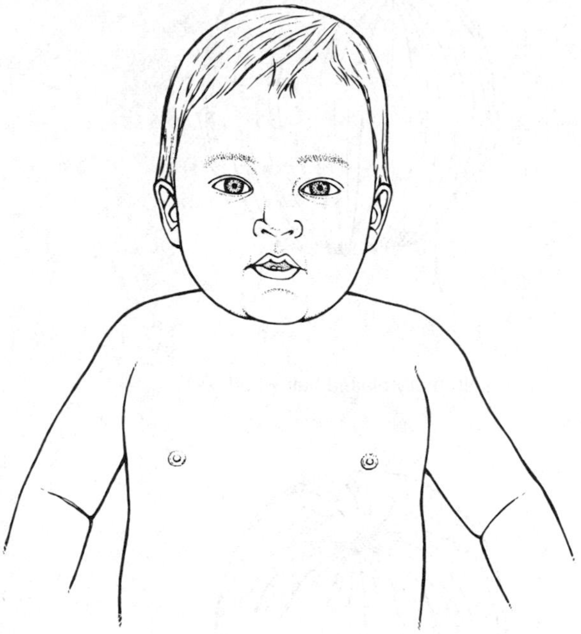

FIGURE 31 - 21. Wide-spaced nipples.

plastic. Wide-set nipples are determined in infants by using the formula:

$$\frac{\text{Intermamillary distance}}{\text{Circumference}} = \text{Wide set if } >0.25$$

Abdomen and Back

In the newborn infant, it is important to note the usual presence of two arteries and one vein in the *umbilicus*. An *omphalocele* is a herniation of abdominal viscera into the base of the umbilical cord. It is important to remember that as many as one half of children with omphalocele have other defects. Many of these associated defects are related to genetic and developmental factors. Palpate for a large liver and spleen, which may indicate a metabolic disease. A dimpling in the *spine* can be associated with *spina bifida*. The spinal column and *hips* should be evaluated radiologically for defects if dimpling is found.

Heart

Listen for adventitious heart *sounds* or sounds that are irregular, slow, or excessively fast. Many syndromes are accompanied by heart anomalies.

Arms, Legs, Hands, and Feet

Children with genetic problems often are found to have defects of the extremities. For instance, in fragile X syndrome the *hand length* (Fig. 31–22) is often found to be 2 standard deviations longer than normal, and hands are soft, fleshy, and hyperextensible. In Prader-Willi syndrome, a finding of small hands and feet is significant. Specific assessment parameters are numbers of fingers and toes, *nail growth,* and *finger or toe length*. Note any *syndactyly* (webbing) of fingers or toes and short or missing phalanges. *Enlarged* toes and fingers, such as large thumbs or an extralarge first toe, are significant. A thumb with the appearance of a finger should be reported. A large space between the first and second toe is significant in some cases. *Clinodactyly,* or an in-curving of the fingers or toes, should

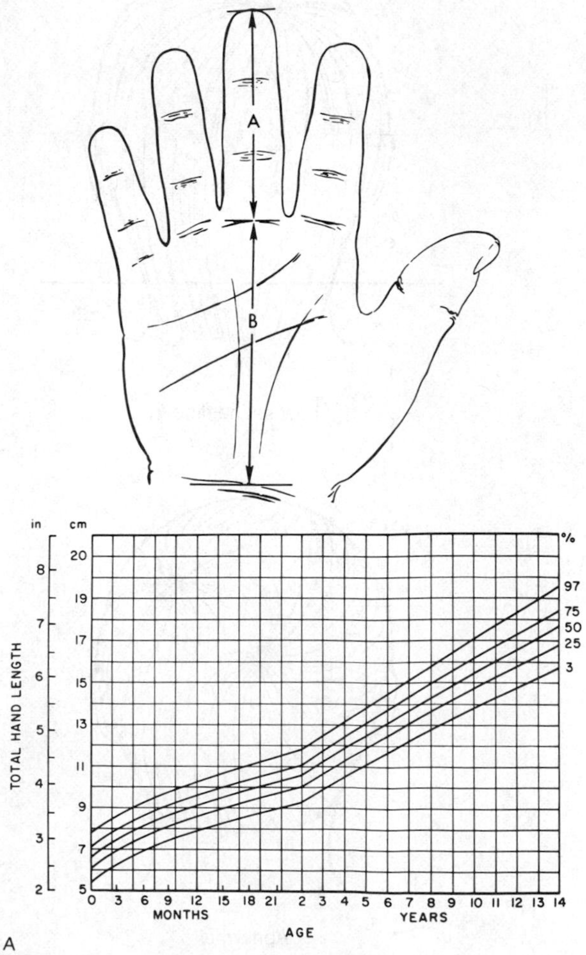

A

FIGURE 31 - 22. Hand measurements. *A*, Hand length.

TABLE 31-16
Protocol for Genetic Assessment: Physical Examination of the Child *(Continued)*

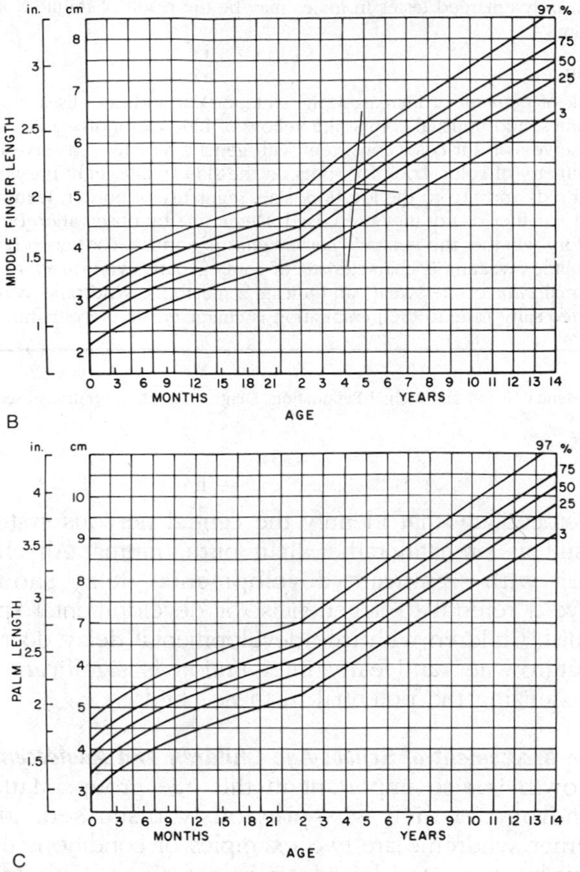

FIGURE 31-22 *(Continued) B,* Middle finger length. *C,* Palm length. (From Feingold, M., & Bossert, W. H. [1974]. Normal values for selected physical parameters. *Birth Defects, 10*(13), 1–16.)

be reported. Any *overriding* of the fingers should be noted because this is sometimes seen in children with conditions like trisomy 18. *Foot shape* is important. Look for prominent heels or the lack of an arch, which gives the foot an appearance of the bottom of a rocking chair and is called "rocker-bottom foot" (Fig. 31–23). Configurations of the lines in the palms, fingertips, and soles are known as *dermatoglyphics* (Fig. 31–24), and these sometimes vary in children with disease syndromes. Most people have a combination of loops, arches, and whorls on their fingertips. The palms normally have two horizontal and one vertical crease. Persons with Down syndrome, in particular, have different pattern configurations than the normal population. An increased *carrying angle* of the *elbows* (Fig. 31–25) should alert the nurse to the possibility of conditions such as Klinefelter syndrome in males or Turner syndrome in females.

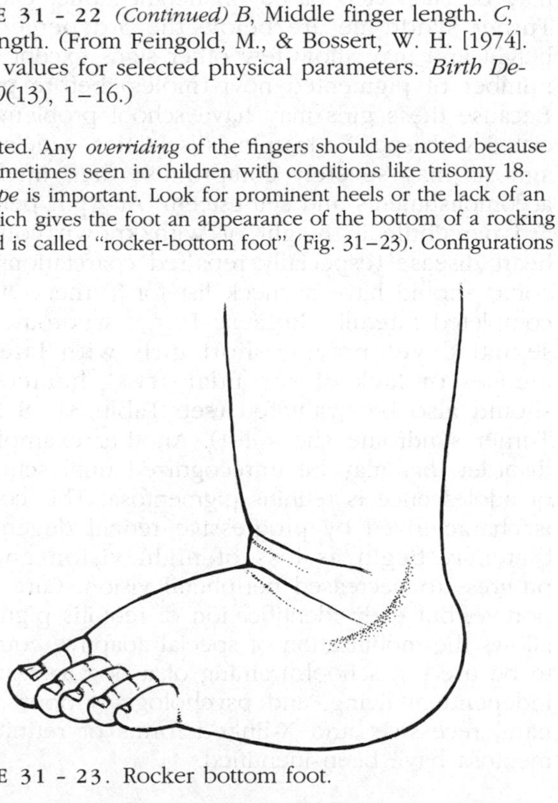

FIGURE 31-23. Rocker bottom foot.

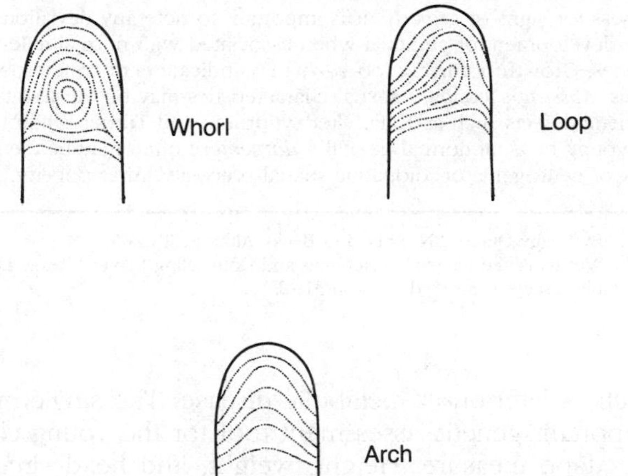

FIGURE 31-24. Fingertip dermatoglyphics.

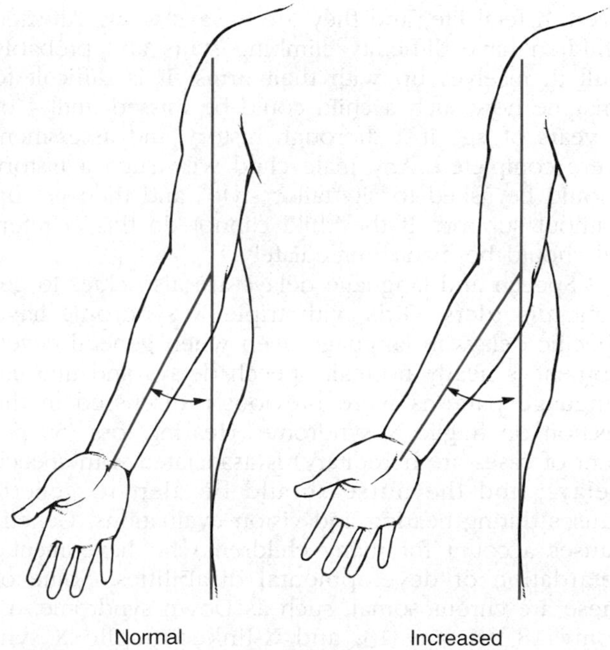

FIGURE 31-25. Carrying angle of the elbows.

Genitalia

Observe for *hypospadias* (an abnormal placement of the urethral opening), *position,* and *size* of the *penis.* A small penis is a minor

(continued)

TABLE 31-16
Protocol for Genetic Assessment: Physical Examination of the Child *(Continued)*

anomaly seen in many syndromes. Check to see whether the *testes* are descended and that the *scrotum* is placed normally and is of normal size. (Several companies sell models that can help estimate testicular volume.)

In girls, observe for hypoplastic *labia* or an enlarged *clitoris*. In some syndromes, the genitalia are ambiguous, and it is necessary to perform an emergency chromosome study to determine gender. Assess for signs of *puberty*. It is important to note any deviations in the development of genitalia when associated with normal milestones. Growth occurring too *early* may indicate endocrine problems. *Missing* secondary sexual characteristics may be the result of genetic defects such as Klinefelter syndrome and Turner syndrome. In young boys, abnormal genital *enlargement* often may be the result of neurogenic or idiopathic sexual precocity. After puberty, significantly enlarged testes in males may be the result of fragile X syndrome.

Skin

Lack of *pigment* or increased pigmentation can indicate disease syndromes, and unusual colors like yellow or blue can indicate illness. Observe skin for color consistent with genetic heritage. Observe for symmetry of color. Look for spots on the skin (white, light brown, and red) and record the location, size, regularity of border, texture, and whether or not they are raised. Determine by observation or history whether the person's *perspiration* is normal. Too much or too little sweating is characteristic of some genetic syndromes. Abnormal *odor* of the sweat can indicate a metabolic syndrome. A reported salty *taste* to the perspiration is characteristic of cystic fibrosis.

By Peggy Drapo, RN, PhD, and Becky Althaus, RN, MS.

We thank the Genetics Screening and Counseling Service, Texas Department of Mental Health and Mental Retardation, Denton, for all illustrations used in this table, except Figures 31-18 and 31-22.

such as later-onset metabolic disease. The single most important genetic assessment tool for the young child is a tape measure. Height, weight, and head circumference measurements are critical at this age, and their determination should not be delegated to less qualified personnel. General development may be a clue to genetic disorders. For example, the most consistent feature in boys with undiagnosed Duchenne muscular dystrophy is delayed walking, usually later than 18 months. These boys may "toe walk," and most are never able to run. The muscles are affected even in fetal life, and they are always weak. Affected children have difficulty climbing stairs and probably pull themselves up with their arms. It is difficult to imagine how such a child could be missed until 4 or 5 years of age if a thorough history and assessment were completed. Any male child with such a history should be asked to sit "tailor style" and then get up without support. If the child cannot do this, a referral should be made immediately.

Speech and language delays are also clues to genetic disorders. Girls with triple X syndrome have specific delays in language even when general development is nearly normal. Speech delays and unusual language patterns were previously discussed in the section on fragile X syndrome. Hearing loss (50 per cent of cases are hereditary) is associated with speech delays, and the nurse should be alert to genetic causes during hearing and vision evaluations. Genetic causes account for many children who have mental retardation or developmental disabilities. Some of these are chromosomal, such as Down syndrome, trisomy 18, trisomy 13, and X-linked fragile X syndrome, which have been described previously. Others are later-onset untreatable disorders, such as Tay-Sachs disease and adrenoleukodystrophy, which are associated with a progressive downhill course. Any child with developmental delay should be assessed for physical features such as multiple hair whorls and microcephaly that identify the central nervous system insult as prenatal rather than birth trauma. All children with significant developmental delay should have a referral to a geneticist or developmental specialist. Children with true developmental delay do not "outgrow it," and early intervention is significant in maximizing the potential in these children.

Assessment of School-Age Children and Adolescents. Growth is also important in this age group. Marfan syndrome, which was previously discussed, and Turner syndrome are two examples of conditions that may be suspected based on height alone. Girls with Turner syndrome are below the 3rd percentile in height and may show few other signs except a large number of pigmented nevi (moles) before puberty. Because these girls may have school problems associated with specific learning disabilities, a delayed diagnosis may severely compromise their intellectual accomplishments and self-esteem. Any girl below the 3rd percentile in height or with known congenital heart disease (especially repaired coarctation of the aorta) should have a check list for Turner syndrome completed carefully. Because Turner syndrome affects sexual development, short girls with late-onset menses or lack of secondary sex characteristics should also be evaluated (see Table 31-8 for the Turner syndrome check list). Another example of a disorder that may be unrecognized until school age or adolescence is retinitis pigmentosa. This condition is characterized by progressive retinal degeneration that may begin as loss of night vision and then progress to decreased peripheral vision. Care is supportive, but early identification of retinitis pigmentosa allows the mobilization of special adaptive equipment to be used in school, training of a dog to assist with independent living, and psychologic support. Dominant, recessive, and X-linked forms of retinitis pigmentosa have been identified.

Genetic Screening

Nurses in many settings are involved in screening programs to prevent disease or provide early detection. Genetic screening is based on similar principles. Genetic screening attempts to identify persons with genotypes that are associated with disease, predispose one to disease, or are capable of producing genetic disorders in subsequent offspring. The first genetic screening program in the United States began in the 1960s with the development of mass screening technology to detect PKU. This launched a nationwide neonatal screening program to detect metabolic disorders that cause mental retardation (see Chapter 44). Since then, a variety of genetic screening programs have become available. Currently, most genetic screening programs fall into one of the four groups discussed in the following sections.

Neonatal Testing

Neonatal screening focuses on identifying at-risk infants before the onset of symptoms so that therapy can begin early. This prevents infant mortality and significant infant morbidity (including mental retardation) and optimizes health in children at risk who would not be detected by conventional means until the onset of irreversible damage. State-sponsored mass neonatal screening programs for PKU and sickle cell anemia have proved the value of presymptomatic testing in reducing infant morbidity and mortality. Most of the disorders currently included in neonatal screening programs are autosomal recessive. The children are affected because they have received a double dose (two copies) of the mutant gene, one copy from each of their healthy carrier parents. Testing programs may also detect infants who are heterozygotes (carriers). It is important for the nurse to know that carriers are healthy people and to communicate that concept to families and professional staff. Pediatric nurses should be aware of the particular tests being performed in their state and ascertain the method of obtaining screening results.

Carrier Identification

Carrier identification also focuses on recessive disorders. Mass screening programs have been developed to detect recessive diseases in ethnic groups at special risk. For example, Tay-Sachs disease occurs predominantly in Ashkenazi (Eastern European) Jews. Because Tay-Sachs disease is a lethal, untreatable disorder, many Jewish synagogues and community groups have sponsored adult testing to detect carriers. Carrier couples can then be offered genetic counseling and reproductive options before conception. Other examples are people of Mediterranean origin who are at special risk for thalassemia and of African, Mediterranean, Indian, or Middle Eastern origin who are at increased risk of sickle cell anemia. Recall that being a carrier is primarily a reproductive issue. If two carriers for the same recessive trait mate, there is a 1 in 4 chance of producing an affected child.

Another type of carrier identification is within family groups. Once an affected child is identified within a family, siblings, cousins, and other family members become concerned about their reproductive risks. For example, cystic fibrosis occurs primarily in white families from Northern Europe, but no effective mass screening carrier test is available. However, since the discovery of the first cystic fibrosis gene in 1989, screening tests within families have become available. Neonatal screening has been tried in a few states, but cystic fibrosis is quite variable, and more than 250 different genes that produce the symptoms associated with CF have now been discovered. Once we identify the variant genes seen in an affected relative, however, more precise family studies are possible. Tests for cystic fibrosis genes use DNA technology that can identify the most frequent genes for anyone in the general population and can provide precise carrier identification within at-risk family groups. Research is ongoing to develop DNA-based therapy for cystic fibrosis as well as cost-effective neonatal or adult carrier mass screening methods. Another example of DNA carrier testing within families is the detection of asymptomatic female carriers for X-linked disorders such as Duchenne muscular dystrophy and fragile X syndrome.

Prenatal Screening

Prenatal genetic screening identifies fetuses at risk for specific genetic disorders. Types of prenatal screening include ultrasonography to detect structural birth defects or to identify fetal changes that increase the risk of the fetus having a genetic syndrome and maternal serum alpha-fetoprotein studies to screen for neural tube defects. More precise diagnostic sampling methods include chorionic villus sampling, early and traditional amniocentesis to detect chromosomal and other genetic disorders, and techniques to obtain a blood sample directly from the fetus. These samples may be sent for chromosomal, biochemical, or DNA analysis. Families may decide to undergo prenatal screening and diagnosis to be reassured, to optimally manage an abnormal pregnancy, to plan for the birth of a child with special needs, or to safely end a pregnancy with an abnormal fetus. The pediatric nurse should be aware that many children with special problems will be identified prenatally and will, therefore, be anticipated at delivery. For example, children with osteogenesis imperfecta ("brittle bone disease") will be identified based on ultrasonography because of multiple fractures seen during the examination. Some of these children may die, whereas others require special braces or casts after delivery. Careful parent teaching to prevent further injury to the child is essential. Anticipating these children allows for parental support, planning, and coordination.

Presymptomatic Screening

Presymptomatic screening enables a family at risk for a later-onset disorder to seek testing and, perhaps, prevention before the onset of symptoms. Such testing is possible because of the emergence of DNA technology that tests for the gene itself rather than recognizing symptomatic changes or the identification of an abnormal gene product. People being tested are usually clinically normal themselves but have relatives with the disorder. Examples of disorders for which presymptomatic testing is available include Huntington disease and myotonic dystrophy.

Within families, some people may want to know whether they carry a particular gene, whereas others may not wish to undergo testing. Some people seek testing to help them make decisions about their own childbearing as well as other life plans. Research is in progress to identify genes for diabetes, breast cancer, hypertension, hypercholesterolemia, and other common adult-onset disorders. It is likely that when persons with these genes can be identified, environmental alterations or specific treatment of the disorder will begin during childhood. In the future, nurses dealing with children should be prepared to offer nondirective support for families who seek presymptomatic testing during childhood.

Provision of Information

Families facing diagnosis of a genetic disorder need information in a variety of ways. All families who have children with birth defects or illnesses ultimately ask the question, "Why did this happen?" followed by "What is my chance this will happen again?" Genetic studies provide answers to many of these questions, and the nurse should be knowledgeable enough to supply them or find a resource person who can provide immediate, appropriate information. A nurse providing family-centered nursing care should be able to offer the following:

- Clarification of information given by genetic specialists or other health care providers.
- Explanation of procedures or tests, including the limitations of such studies.
- Clarification of genetic concepts or terminology.
- Education regarding management techniques.
- Explanations of causation and modes of inheritance.
- Specific disease information.

Genetic Counseling

A second level of information is genetic counseling. This may be provided by nurse specialists, physicians, doctoral-prepared geneticists, or master's level genetic counselors who have expertise in genetics and counseling techniques. In 1976, the American Society of Human Genetics provided a national definition of genetic counseling, as follows (Learned Management Designs, 1988, p 285):

> Genetic counseling is a communication process which deals with the human problems associated with the occurrence or risk of occurrence of a genetic disorder in a family. This process involves an attempt by one or more appropriately trained persons to help the individual or family:
>
> - Comprehend the medical facts, including the probable diagnosis, the cause of the disorder and the available management.
> - Appreciate the way heredity contributes to the disorder and the risk of recurrence in specified relatives.
> - Understand the options for dealing with the risk of recurrence.
> - Choose the course of action which seems appropriate to them, in view of their risk and the family goals, and act in accordance with that decision.
> - Make the best possible adjustment to the disorder in an affected family member and/or to the risk of recurrence of that disorder.

It is easy to recognize many appropriate nursing roles within the definition, but it is also essential that the nurse recognize when a referral is needed and not attempt to provide genetic counseling without proper training and back-up.

Any genetic counseling begins with an accurate diagnosis and, if possible, information about the prognosis. Estimates of the chance of recurrence of the problem are given. Follow-up contact is essential because anxiety often precludes "hearing," and information given in a previous visit may need to be repeated. An important nursing role is to obtain accurate information from the counseling center so that medical facts and counseling issues can be restated and clarified.

The nurse or the genetic counselor should explore the clients' perceptions of risk, because this perception will influence any decision made by the client or the family. Perhaps even more important is the family's perception of the burden of the disorder. People and families may vary widely in their perception of the seriousness of a given situation. Another influencing factor is the presence or absence of an outside support system. Misinterpretation of previous information or an earlier traumatic experience may be a negative influence. The nurse can be invaluable in providing information about the family to the counselor as well as providing support and direct help to the family itself.

Types of Counseling. In the past, most counseling was "retrospective" and attempted to determine why a particular disorder occurred in a family and to assist families in coping with a crisis situation. For example, an infant's failure-to-thrive may raise questions about the presence of a metabolic condition. A laboratory analysis may determine the cause, revealing an inherited autosomal recessive condition. In such cases, laboratory tests are often requested on an emergency basis, and counseling occurs with the family when the child is very ill. The family with no his-

TABLE 31-17

Nursing Process Plan: The Family with a Genetic Risk

Analysis: Nursing Diagnostic Statement 1

Response and Related or Risk Factors: *Decisional conflict (parental) related to knowledge deficit about the risk of occurrence or recurrence of a genetic abnormality when there is*

- A family history of a genetic disorder
- Ethnic predisposition for a genetic disorder
- Evidence of anomalies of structure or function
- Unexplained delays in growth
- Unexplained delays in physical, intellectual, and/or sexual development
- Evidence of significant environmental hazards

Projected Outcome: The family will understand and be informed about genetic risk and associated diagnoses to the extent that they will feel more certain about the course of action to be taken in their particular situations

Defining Characteristics

Subjective:

- Verbalization of uncertainty about choices
- Verbalization of undesired consequences of alternative actions being considered
- Vacillation between alternative choices
- Delay in decision making
- Verbalization of feeling of distress while attempting a decision
- Self-focusing
- Questioning of personal values and beliefs while attempting a decision

Objective:

- Physical signs of distress or tension, such as increased heart rate, increased muscle tension, and restlessness

Nursing Interventions

Genetic Counseling

Complete or *review* a three-generation *family history,* including any anomalies, infant deaths, surgical procedures, pregnancy losses, and exposures. Identify significant family member if the client cannot provide family history information

Document anomalies noted, previous studies completed or in progress. Confer with family members to determine what they understand about risk or diagnosis

Clarify general medical information. Ask if family understands genetic terms; clarify the same or notify appropriate staff for help. If diagnosis has been made, clarify and restate diagnosis, management plans, and priorities

Refer for *genetic counseling* if possible. *Note:* The actual time for referral depends on the client's emotional adjustment to the actual or potential diagnosis of a heritable disorder. Often, there is a delay of weeks or months between diagnosis and counseling

Discuss the purpose and goals* and process *of genetic counseling (to clarify the benefits to the

Evaluation Criteria

The parents will be able to

- Verbalize comfort with choice
- Make their decisions in an appropriate time period

The parents will not show any physical signs of distress

(continued)

TABLE 31-17 (continued)

Defining Characteristics	Nursing Interventions	Evaluation Criteria

	family and to reduce anxiety about the process)
	• Explain that the purpose of genetic counseling is to
	  • Define the nature of the disorder
	  • Discuss what is known and the implications of various interventions
	  • Review genetic tests that are in progress or completed
	  • Provide information about the risk of occurrence or recurrence of a genetic abnormality
	  • Discuss all available options and resources
	• Stress that the counselor provides information that can help the family make their *own* decisions about future pregnancies. (People may be fearful of being told not to have children or not to have more children)
	• Identify genetic counseling resources. Determine payment and transportation options available for genetic counseling, including insurance eligibility. Discuss options with the family
	Encourage questions and verbalization of understanding of the purpose, process, and availability of genetic counseling	

Analysis: Nursing Diagnostic Statement 2

Response and Related or Risk Factors: *Ineffective individual coping: Temporary impairment of problem-solving abilities related to the emotional impact of the diagnosis of an actual or potential genetic disorder, including grief reactions*

Projected Outcome: The parents and affected child (if not diagnosed in infancy) will regain or learn adaptive behaviors and problem-solving abilities to meet the demands of the situation and of their roles in the situation

TABLE 31-17 *(continued)*

Defining Characteristics	*Nursing Interventions*	*Evaluation Criteria*
Subjective: • Comments such as, "I can't think of anything else," "I don't know how to cope with this," or "I don't know how to ask for help with this" • Reports of inability to meet parental role expectations • Inability to problem solve • Depression • Excessive smoking, use of alcohol or prescription drugs • Chronic fatigue • Excessive sleeping • Forgetfulness • Gastrointestinal upsets *Objective*: • Alteration in societal participation • Lack of vitality in voice, movements, and general appearance • "Mechanical" aspect to behavoir • Inappropriate use of defense mechanisms • Change in usual communication patterns • Shortened attention span • Easily distracted • Weight loss • Tired, haggard appearance	*Coping Enhancement* **Encourage expression of feelings about the diagnosis** • Plan some uninterrupted periods for discussion • Practice reflective listening • Avoid interjecting personal biases **Acknowledge each person's right to the feelings expressed** • Recognize that a diagnosis that seems minor to the nurse (e.g., club foot) may carry quite a different meaning for the family • Refrain from telling the family that they are "lucky"; (the conditions of other children are not pertinent to this situation) **Recognize denial as a common defense mechanism in the first weeks after diagnosis** • Repeat information in simple terms as often as necessary • Provide written information whenever possible. (Materials that can be read at home can help people incorporate the reality of the diagnosis and generate questions) ***Grief Work Facilitation* Recognize grief as a common reaction to diagnosis.** (The parents must deal with the loss of the expected healthy infant or of the presumed healthy child and must incorporate, instead, the reality of the permanent anomaly or genetic disorder. The affected child, as well, must deal with the loss of formerly perceived health status) **Facilitate efforts toward problem-focused coping*** • Help the client identify family strengths and known resources	**The parents and affected child (if not diagnosed in infancy) will become better able to cope with the diagnosis of the anomaly or genetic disorder as evidenced by** • Verbalization of feelings of ability to cope with diagnosis and when and how to ask for help • Seeking information to help with problem solving • Identifying resources • Verbalizing planned use of resources • Reports of feeling of well-being • Reports avoidance of substances (e.g., alcohol and drugs) • Seeks out societal participation

*"Problem-focused coping" is the term used by Lazarus and Folkman (1984) to describe strategies directed at "altering environmental pressures, barriers, resources, procedures . . ." and those directed at internal "motivational or cognitive changes such as shifting the level of aspiration, reducing ego involvement, finding alternative channels of gratification, developing new standards of behavior, or learning new skills and procedures" (p. 152).

(continued)

TABLE 31-17 (continued)

Defining Characteristics	Nursing Interventions	Evaluation Criteria
	for emotional, physical, and financial support • Ask if the client has considered how to tell relatives and friends about the diagnosis. Discuss ways to disseminate accurate information • Discuss with the parents age-appropriate ways to tell siblings about the diagnosis. Caution parents that siblings may perceive themselves responsible if they had mixed emotions about the new infant or if normal feelings of sibling rivalry were present between siblings and the affected child **Assess the need for referral for individual counseling or marital counseling.** (Some people need more in-depth help to cope with the impact of the diagnosis and its implications for future life changes. Spouses may react differently and experience discordant coping, disrupted communication patterns, and a potential threat to the marital relationship)	

Analysis: Nursing Diagnostic Statement 3

Response and Related or Risk Factors: *Spiritual distress related to*

- The attempt to find meaning in the situation
- Conflict between religious or spiritual beliefs and the alternatives to giving birth to children with a heritable disorder
- Perceived guilt (parental) in having transmitted a heritable trait

Projected Outcome: The parents and affected child (if not diagnosed in infancy) will have a renewed sense of the life principle that integrates and transcends their biological and psychological nature

Defining Characteristics	Nursing Interventions	Evaluation Criteria
Subjective: • Expression of concern with the meaning of life and death and belief systems • Questions such as, "Why did this happen to me?" • Verbalization of anger at God	*Spiritual Support* **Acknowledge that the loss of "peace of mind" is a normal feeling in this situation** **Help the client identify appropriate sources of support.** Ask, "Is there a member of the clergy or a special friend who can help you	**The parent(s)/affected child will experience a renewed sense of inner peace as evidenced by** • Verbalizing feeling less anxious and more at peace • Finding strength in former religious faith

TABLE 31-17 *(continued)*

Defining Characteristics	Nursing Interventions	Evaluation Criteria
• Questions meaning of suffering • Verbalization of inner conflict about beliefs • Verbalization of concern about relationship with deity • Questions meaning of own existence • Questions moral and ethical implications of therapeutic regimen • Display of gallows humor • Displacement of anger toward religious representatives • Description of nightmares and sleep disturbances *Objective*: • Alteration in behavior and mood evidenced by anger • Crying • Withdrawal • Preoccupation, anxiety, hostility, and apathy • Significant changes in usual religious practices • Somatic signs of distress	work through the meaning of this in your life?" (Already established, trusting relationships can provide ready support) **Supplement the support of identified resources, as needed, to help the client come to terms with personal values and beliefs** • Assess the meaning of the diagnosis for this client. (Some families see the birth of a child with a congenital anomaly or genetic disorder as a special blessing from God, whereas others may feel they are being punished for real or imagined misdeeds) • Encourage expression of feelings, guiding persons to discover their own truths. Avoid interjecting personal values • Validate the normality of expressed feelings by statements such as, "Many parents (or children) tell me they feel that way" • Recognize that the affected child, siblings, and parents may repeat this search for meaning from time to time in the future, especially during the transition between developmental stages	• Verbalizing a rationale for decision making • Appearing less anxious and stressful

Analysis: Nursing Diagnostic Statement 4

Response and Related or Risk Factors: *High risk for caregiver role strain; risk factors related to*

- Overwhelming amounts of information in a time of crisis, as evidenced by confusion and difficulty in verbalizing questions
- Confusion about information presented, as presented by verbalization of misinformation
- Inability to integrate the information associated because of unsettled emotional state, as evidenced by verbalization that genetic counseling did not help with decision making and ongoing feeling of inability to cope with decision making

Projected Outcome: The caregiver will feel comfortable in performing the family caregiver role and be able to utilize information presented in genetic counseling

Defining Characteristics	Nursing Interventions	Evaluation Criteria
Subjective: • Worry about such things as the child's emotional state, having to place the child in an institution,	*Teaching: Disease Process* **Assess the reason for the knowledge deficit.** (Determine whether due to insufficient infor-	**The caregiver will receive help to utilize information presented in genetic counseling to facilitate caregiving, as evidenced by**

(continued)

TABLE 31-17 *(continued)*

Defining Characteristics	Nursing Interventions	Evaluation Criteria
and who will care for the child if something should happen to the caregiver • Feelings that caregiving interferes with other important roles in their lives • Report of finding it hard to do specific caregiving activities	mation, confusion about the information presented, or unsettling emotions that prevent integration of the information **Intervene to address the underlying problem** • Contact genetic resources to determine major counseling issues • Have family restate their understanding of the genetic problem • Clarify what information was presented (to determine if the client failed to receive the information or to comprehend it). Ask the family if they will share with you the written summary of the meeting(s), if one was prepared. Clarify terminology and other aspects about which the client may have questions • Refer, as appropriate, for further genetic or psychological counseling for on-going emotional disturbances **Evaluate the adequacy of the information to meet the client's needs for problem solving by encouraging the client to discuss the alternatives presented by the counseling team** *Caregiver Support* **Accept expressions of negative emotion** **Explore** with caregiver his or her strengths and weaknesses **Acknowledge** dependency of patient on caregiver as appropriate **Encourage** the acceptance of interdependency among family members **Provide for follow-up** health and caregiver assistance through phone calls and community nursing care **Teach** caregiver stress management techniques **Educate** caregiver about the grieving process and provide caregiver with support	• Verbalizing increased understanding of the care receiver's emotional state and interventions that may be required in the future • Demonstrating ability to do specific caregiving activities • Able to discuss a plan whereby other roles in life can be met, at least partially

TABLE 31-17 *(continued)*

Defining Characteristics	*Nursing Interventions*	*Evaluation Criteria*
	Identify sources of respite care **Teach** caregiver strategies to access and maximize health care and community resources. ***Act for caregiver if overburdening becomes apparent*** (Interventions for ***Caregiver Support*** are found in McCloskey, J. C., & Bulecheck, G. M. (1992). *Nursing interventions classification (NIC)* (p 161). St. Louis: CV Mosby.)	

tory of genetic disorders must cope with a rare diagnosis that was caused by genes that they transmitted to their child.

Prenatal diagnoses are also retrospective in that the evaluation attempts to determine whether the existing fetus is affected with a chromosomal or other severe disorder. Parents who seek prenatal counseling have wanted pregnancies and are anxious because they know they are at increased risk. The tests themselves take several days to weeks to complete, which adds to the emotional upheaval. In prenatal cases, the couple must have the test results in a timely manner to make choices. Parents either will be reassured that a particular disorder is not present or will learn that the fetus is affected. Most couples receive normal prenatal results. If the fetus is affected, however, parents must then decide whether to carry an affected fetus and plan for the birth of a child with special needs or to end this pregnancy and seek counseling about future reproduction. This is an agonizing decision for couples, and the nurse should be sensitive and supportive during this time.

In recent years, more families are considering "prospective" counseling, which attempts to identify couples at risk and provide counseling prior to conception. Such counseling may be requested by couples who are aware of a family history that includes problems such as a previous child who died or a cousin with cystic fibrosis.

Prospective counseling requires laboratory information or a diagnosis from a previously tested relative. Prospective counseling can also result from an awareness of ethnic risk learned through public information campaigns, such as Tay Sachs disease screening and education programs. In these cases, counseling requests are not emergencies. However, families may be quite anxious and fear being "less than normal" if they learn that they carry an abnormal gene. It is important for the nurse to recognize these fears. Currently, we can test preconceptionally for only a few disorders. This may cause persons concerned with those particular disorders to feel stigmatized. We know, however, that at a molecular level, 100 per cent of the population are carriers for several lethal or deleterious genes. As the Human Genome Project progresses and we identify most human genes (Cook-Deegan, 1991), the nurse should be prepared to reassure families who are seeking prospective counseling.

Supportive Care

Families experiencing any health-related crisis such as a genetic diagnosis in a child need more than information. They need help in interpreting that information and in dealing with the feelings evoked by the diagnosis. Genetic diagnoses are unique among medical evaluations in that they simultaneously influence a family's self-image—how they think about the past and how they plan for the future—and direct the management of a disorder. A genetic diagnosis may produce guilt in older family members as well as parents who "passed on" a deleterious gene or may alter the reproductive options of many family members for several generations. Families with genetic disorders need ongoing nursing support but have special needs during the phases of initial diagnosis and reproductive decision making and regarding follow-up care for affected children.

Grief

Whenever a child is diagnosed with a genetic disorder, there is grief. The parents must deal with the loss of the perceived "normal" child. The family needs support to deal with denial, anger, guilt, and bargaining responses that are part of the grieving process. This is especially true when a family realizes that this problem may be lethal or produce lifelong alterations. Parents may become depressed, overprotective of the affected child, and unresponsive to other family needs, including those of siblings.

In addition to the normal grief reaction, barriers to effective genetic intervention include the following:

- Inadequate comprehension of medical facts.
- Limited time for explanations by physicians, specialists, and geneticists—often a single visit.
- Differences in cultural and psychosocial attitudes.
- Lack of established interpersonal relationships.
- Financial and other social considerations.

Because nurses are likely to have a longer-term relationship involving the whole family unit, they are ideally suited to help families overcome these barriers.

Caring Communication

The first level of support is staff response, and nonverbal communication is the most powerful. Families are instantly aware of the nurse who is accepting of the neonate with a disfiguring birth defect or one who is dying. The nurse who honors the personhood of this individual human by touching the child, holding the child, and calling the child by name communicates support that will always be remembered. The converse is also true. Families who have been made to feel isolated and estranged will remember the lack of compassion decades later.

Families also need contact with nurses who will listen in a nonjudgmental manner. There may be no positive solutions to some genetic problems. Families often have to choose between unacceptable options, such as not treating a child who will then die versus authorizing heroic treatment in which the surviving child will have lifelong disabilities. The nurse is not expected to solve all the client's problems, but she or he needs to be a caring, active listener. Active listening (Gordon, 1970) requires that the nurse interpret what is being communicated (verbally and nonverbally) and then reflect that interpretation back to the client for clarification. In this process, the family is encouraged to explore their feelings, work through their emotional reactions to the situation, and consider the options. "The goal of the provider in active listening is to always keep the door open" (Bauer & Hill, 1986, p 99).

Active listening works equally well with children (both the affected child and the unaffected siblings) to help them clarify feelings and begin adaptive problem solving. In many cases, the genetic diagnosis is made early in life, and all the information and support are given to the parents. Adults often fail to communicate directly with children because they believe that children may not be capable of or should not be communicating about these issues. Children, however, have a great adaptive capacity and are quite capable of accepting and coping with serious and even life-threatening diagnoses. Listening and asking the child open-ended questions should precede any "telling." Explanations should then be direct and should take into account the developmental stage of the child. The nurse should discuss the use of listening and reflective techniques with parents and staff.

Siblings are affected in many ways by their brothers and sisters with a genetic disorder. They may feel slighted because of the amount of time the parents spend in caring for the affected child. They may have to assume extra family responsibilities. They may feel shame if the affected child looks "different" or is mentally retarded. They may resent the strain on family outings or other activities. They may fear death or have "survivor's guilt." Nurses who listen and who develop interventions that facilitate family communication about these issues can help resolve the siblings' trauma. Nurses can support both adult and child family members by encouraging expression of feelings, correcting misinformation, and reinforcing adaptive problem solving.

Direct Help

When a child is diagnosed with a genetic disorder, the first nursing role may be crisis intervention. Throughout the child's life, the nurse will be called to provide direct nursing care, such as hygiene, medications, fluid and nutrition management, pain relief, prevention of injury, specialized equipment, and comfort measures. In addition to the intrinsic value of these services, nursing interventions provide an opportunity to listen, educate, and continue to assess the dynamics of the family and the child's genetic condition. It is during this time that families are most open to assistance and education. Ongoing education about the child's condition should be given to parents, children, other family members, and caregivers such as baby sitters and day care facility staff. Because many health care providers are unfamiliar with most genetic diseases, the nurse should seek help in obtaining written materials and establishing a link with knowledgeable genetic specialists. Information gained can be passed on to the nurses, physicians, and other health care providers who may be caring for this family. Direct help may also be in the form of periodic examinations, which allow the nurse to promote optimal growth and development, control the effects of the genetic disorder, and assess adaptive family coping. The nurse who is providing periodic evaluations should be aware of the following developmental crisis points for families:

- Age for walking (12 to 15 months).
- Age for talking (24 to 30 months).
- Younger siblings surpassing the affected child.
- Entry into preschool, kindergarten, or school versus alternative placement.
- Onset of puberty.
- Age of driver's license eligibility (or other "rite of passage").
- Adulthood recognized (18th or 21st birthday).

If the child fails to attain these milestones, additional support may be needed.

Medical crises for the child, such as the need for surgery and development of seizures, are also, potentially, times for emotional upheaval. Because nurses are usually "on the scene," they are in the best position to intervene or refer the child and family to the most appropriate system for medical care and support. Medical problems in parents also raise critical questions: "What will happen if I die?" "Will my child ever be self-sufficient?" "Who will care for my child after I am gone?" Nurses should explore feelings with parents and evaluate the need for outside assistance. Social services, legal help, or clergy may be needed to explore spiritual needs or guardianship.

Coordination of Care

Genetic disorders are complex and require a team approach. Many different specialists and agencies may be needed to provide optimal care for the child and the family. This chapter has emphasized the need for the nurse to be part of a team approach. The nurse should be able to evaluate situations and seek help or refer rather than attempting to intervene in areas in which he or she lacks expertise. However, families can become overwhelmed by the number of persons seen, appointments to be kept, and even conflicting opinions. Even new laws designed to benefit children with special needs can create coordination problems for families.

Nurses should take a leadership role in coordinating medical and social services, educational planning, integration of physical and occupational therapy or nutrition services, and identification of peer support groups (Table 31–17: Nursing Process Plan: The Family with a Genetic Risk). Nurses who are not going to provide ongoing care should ensure that this responsibility is directly passed on to a specific person for follow-up—general notification to an agency is not sufficient.

Coordination of care in genetics includes several critical follow-up responsibilities:

1. Genetics is fast-moving, and the nurse caring for children with genetic disorders should be alert to new developments, new tests, new treatments, and new technologies.
2. Recurrence risk issues will be altered when there is a new birth, new marriage, or the appearance of other affected persons in the family.
3. The genetic situation may be altered if new medical problems develop. The family may need to be referred again for additional genetic evaluation. They may need more support or additional education about management or prognosis.

Advocacy Groups

Nurses cannot be all things to all people; therefore, they must learn how to connect families with genetic disorders into appropriate support and advocacy groups. These will vary locally, and the nurse can find resource lists through the local genetics center or state genetics coordinator. Important support services for families include the following:

- Parent support groups (e.g., parent-to-parent and Down syndrome parent groups).
- Area education agencies (local and state).
- Disease-specific organizations.
- Advocacy groups.

Most of the support organizations have regular support meetings, provide phone or direct crisis support, and offer practical day-to-day hints for managing a child with a genetic disorder. Most support groups and agencies provide a strong voice for better access to services and lobby for legislative action on behalf of the child with special needs. These groups have been effective in promoting passage of the Individuals with Disabilities Act of 1974 and the Americans with Disabilities Act of 1990, which secured the right of children with disabilities to have access to an appropriate education.

KEY CONCEPTS

Concepts Related to Basic Information

- Individual genetic patterns are the framework or basis for patterns of health and illness.
- Identification of genetic links to disease is a rapidly expanding body of knowledge.
- Genetic problems are common, accounting for 30 to 50 per cent of pediatric admissions in developed countries.
- There are four classifications of genetic disorders: chromosomal, single gene, multifactorial, and nontraditional.

Concepts Related to Nursing Assessment

- Looking for signs of genetic disorders should be part of the assessment of every child.
- Signs of genetic disorders could include major or minor anomalies, variations in appearance, or problems with growth or developmental delay.
- Minor anomalies may be a clue to more serious underlying problems.

Concepts Related to Nursing Intervention

- Genetic screening includes neonatal testing, carrier identification, prenatal screening, and presymptomatic screening.
- Explanation of procedures and tests, clarification of concepts, explanations of causation and mode of inheritance, and information about specific genetic diseases and their care are part of the nursing care of families with genetic disorders.
- Families with genetic problems will be in need of

supportive care not only at the time of diagnosis but also at various developmental points in the life of the child and family.

- Coordination of services for families and appropriate referral are vital parts of the nursing role.

REFERENCES

Bauer, B. B., & Hill, S. S. (1986). *Essentials of mental health care: Planning and interventions.* Philadelphia: WB Saunders.

Bowman, J. E., & Murray, R. F. (1990). *Genetic variations and disorders in peoples of African origin.* Baltimore: The Johns Hopkins University Press.

Centers for Disease Control. (1989). Contributions of birth defects to infant mortality—United States, 1986. *Morbidity and Mortality Weekly Report, 38,* 633–646.

Cook-Deegan, R. M. (1991). The human genome project: The formation of federal policies in the United States, 1986–1990. In K. E. Hanna (Ed.), *Biomedical politics.* Washington, DC: National Academy Press.

Feingold, M., & Bossert, W. H. (1974). Normal values for selected physical parameters. *Birth Defects, 10*(13), 1–16.

Gordon, T. (1970). *PET: Parent effectiveness training.* New York: Peter H. Wyden.

Hall, J. G. (1990). Nontraditional inheritance. *Growth: Genetics and Hormones, 7*(4), 1–3.

Holmes, L. B. (1974). Inborn errors of morphogenesis. *New England Journal of Medicine, 291,* 763–773.

Hook, E. B. (1981). Rates of chromosome abnormalities at different maternal ages. *Obstetrics and Gynecology, 58,* 282–285.

Hook, E. B., & Cross, P. K. (1979). Estimated rates of clinically significant cytogenetic abnormalities (other than Down's syndrome) in live births by one-year maternal interval. *American Journal of Human Genetics, 31,* 137A.

Jones, K. W. (1988). *Smith's recognizable patterns of human malformation* (4th ed.). Philadelphia: WB Saunders.

Lazarus, R. S., & Folkman, S. (1984). *Stress, Appraisal, and Coping:* New York: Springer Publishing Co.

Learned Managed Designs. (1988). Genetic applications: A health perspective. University of Colorado Health Sciences Center, School of Nursing/School of Medicine, Genetics Unit. Lawrence, KS: Author.

McKusick, V. (1992). *Mendelian inheritance in man: Catalogs of autosomal dominant, autosomal recessive, and X-linked phenotypes* (10th ed.). Baltimore: The Johns Hopkins University Press.

Nowak, M. E. (1992, October 12). Fragile X testing protocol (written communication). Santa Fe, NM: Vivigen Corporation.

Nyhan, W. L., & Sakati, N. O. (1987). *Diagnostic recognition of genetic disease.* Philadelphia, Lea & Febiger.

Rousseau, R., Heitz, D., Biancaiana, V., et al. (1991). Direct diagnosis by DNA analysis of the fragile X syndrome of mental retardation. *New England Journal of Medicine, 325,* 1673–1681.

Stine, G. J. (1989). *The new human genetics.* Dubuque, IA: Wm. C. Brown.

Thompson, M. W., McInnes, R. R., & Huntington, W. F. (1991). *Genetics in medicine* (5th ed.). Philadelphia: WB Saunders.

US Congress, Office of Technology Assessment. (1992, August). *Cystic fibrosis and DNA tests: Implications of carrier screening (OTA–BA–532).* Washington, DC: US Government Printing Office.

Wright, L., & Cadle, R. (1989). Understanding DNA testing: A basic guide for families. Lexington, KY: Southeastern Regional Genetics Group (SERGG).

BIBLIOGRAPHY

Bergsma, D. (1975). *Malformation syndromes.* Baltimore: The Johns Hopkins Press.

Clark, M. H., Frankel, M., & Trowbridge, D. (1989). A pedigree primer. *Journal of Pediatric Nursing, 4*(2), 112–118.

Cohen, F. L. (1984). *Clinical genetics in nursing practice.* Philadelphia: JB Lippincott.

Concise book of genetics. (1982). Scarborough, Canada: Prentice-Hall.

Emery, A., & Pullen, I. (Eds.). (1984). *Psychological aspects of genetic counseling.* London: Academic Press.

Feingold, M., & Pashayan, H. (1983). *Genetics and birth defects in clinical practice.* Boston: Little, Brown.

Fuhrmann, W., & Vogel, F. (1983). *Genetic counseling.* New York: Springer Verlag.

Hall, J. G. (Ed.). (1992). Medical genetics: I. *Pediatric Clinics of North America, 39*(1).

Hall, J. G. (Ed.). (1992). Medical genetics: II. *Pediatric Clinics of North America, 39*(2).

Kenner, C., & Berling, B. (1990). Nursing in genetics: Current and emerging issues for practice and education. *Journal of Pediatric Nursing, 5*(6), 370–374.

Nora, J. J. (1989). *Medical genetics.* Philadelphia: Lea & Febiger.

Osband, B. A. (1989). Multifactorial inheritance: Implications for perinatal and neonatal nurses. *Journal of Perinatal and Neonatal Nursing, 2*(4), 43–52.

Prows, C. A. (1992). Utilization of genetic knowledge in pediatric nursing practice. *Journal of Pediatric Nursing, 7*(1), 58–62.

Smith, D. (1982). *Recognizable patterns of human malformation.* Philadelphia: WB Saunders.

Strategies in genetic counseling. (1984). *Birth Defects, 20*(6).

Tinley, S. T. (1987). Nurses' and geneticists' role expectations for the nurse clinician. *Journal of Pediatric Nursing, 2*(4), 259–264.

Wright, L., Brown, A., & Davidson-Mundt, A. (1992). Newborn screening: The miracle and the challenge. *Journal of Pediatric Nursing, 7*(1), 26–42.

UNIT • SEVEN

Nursing Interventions in Physiologic Alterations

CHAPTER • 32
Altered Respiratory Function

Mabel Hunsberger
Lynn Feenan

NURSING PROCESS PLANS
NPP: The Child with Oxygenation Problems, Table 32–9
NPP: The Child Hospitalized with an Acute Attack of Asthma, Table 32–26

RELATED TOPICS
Principles of home care, Chapter 22
Pertussis, tuberculosis, influenza, Chapter 39
Cardiopulmonary resuscitation, Chapter 46
Airway obstruction, Chapter 46
Foreign body aspiration, foreign body in the ear, Chapter 46
Inhalation injury associated with burns or poisons, Chapter 47

LEARNING OBJECTIVES

- Identify the differences in structure and function of the respiratory system in the child.
- Identify the basic therapeutic techniques of respiratory therapy.
- Identify the priority of nursing care for the child with croup and epiglottitis.
- Identify the nursing care needs of the child with malformations of the respiratory tract.
- Identify the process of nursing care applied to the child with asthma.
- Discuss the home care management needs of the infant with bronchopulmonary dysplasia.
- Identify the nursing diagnostic statements and interventions for the care of the child with cystic fibrosis.

A continuous supply of oxygen is essential to carry out the vital processes of the human organism. One cannot "do without oxygen" for a little while as one can without food or water. The main function of respiration is to supply the body with oxygen and dispose of carbon dioxide. If the system fails, the cells die from oxygen starvation and accumulation of carbon dioxide. Alterations in the ability to consume oxygen and rid the body of carbon dioxide constitute a major segment of health problems in children. The problems discussed in this chapter cause varied degrees of distress to the family, depending on the suddenness, severity, duration, and outcome of the problem. The age of the child at the time of illness is a major variant in how a family copes and how the child is affected. Furthermore, many respiratory problems begin suddenly and frighten the child and family because of the difficulty in breathing.

Nurses need expert clinical skills to assess accurately the clinical status of children and the family's responses. Nurses also have a central role in the planning and administration of the therapeutic regimens, take responsibility for teaching children and families about their illness and how to prevent it, and provide emotional support during the illness.

This chapter presents the theoretical concepts of respiratory function applied to children, with a discussion of the most common health problems of infants and children. Nurses' roles in assessment and nursing strategies for each alteration are presented.

Many of the common respiratory alterations in children, particularly young infants, are life-threatening. For the nurse to respond effectively to the challenge of caring for children with respiratory problems, a basic understanding of respiratory function and the mechanisms of the various alterations is required.

The following is a review of the principles of altered respiratory physiology as they pertain to children and a discussion of diagnostic and therapeutic procedures that are common to respiratory problems in children. The most common alterations in children and adolescents are then discussed.

Structure and Function

To some degree, anatomic and physiologic differences related to the age of the child determine the type of problem that occurs and the degree of threat it presents.

Incidence and Etiology of Respiratory Dysfunction

Respiratory illness in children, both acute and chronic forms, is caused by intrinsic or extrinsic factors, or a combination of both. Intrinsic factors include congenital malformations of the airway, problems secondary to other organ defects (e.g., cardiac anomalies), and congenital, metabolic, or immunologic deficiencies. Extrinsic factors include infection, environment, pollution (including passive smoking), and aspirated foreign material (Randolph, 1991). Hyaline membrane disease and lung injuries during infancy and childhood are insults that have varied sequelae on long-term development.

Acute illness of the respiratory tract accounts for approximately 50 per cent of all illness in children under 5 years of age and 30 per cent in children between 5 and 12 years of age. Diseases of the respiratory system were the major cause of hospitalization for children of ages 1 through 9 (National Center for Health Statistics, 1990). The primary cause of acute respiratory illnesses is viral infections; young children contract four or five per year. Viral infections result in a broad range of illnesses, from mild to life-threatening. Many deaths still occur from bacterial infection of the respiratory tract, although early use of antibiotic treatment has reduced the morbidity and mortality rates.

Chronic respiratory disease accounts for almost half of all childhood chronic diseases. One of every ten children is affected by asthma, cystic fibrosis, bronchopulmonary dysplasia, bronchiectasis, emphysema, or congenital bronchopulmonary disorders. Children with chronic lung disease are severely affected by air pollution and cigarette smoking, including passive smoking or secondhand smoke.

Passive smoking is defined as the inhalation of mainstream smoke exhaled by the smoker and sidestream smoke that goes directly into the air from the end of a burning cigarette, pipe, or cigar (Levengood, 1988). An association between parental smoking and respiratory problems in children has been identified (Burchfiel et al, 1986), especially in relation to bronchitis and pneumonia, with the greatest impact on the first 3 years of life (Burchfiel et al, 1986).

Parental smoking also has been reported to be associated with frequent coughs in school-age children (Charlton, 1984) and to be a risk factor for recurrent otitis media, recurrent tonsillopharyngitis, and the need for tonsillectomy and adenoidectomy. Decreased pulmonary function is also reported in children of parents who smoke (Vedal et al, 1984; Ware et al, 1984), and the annual rate of lung growth in children with parents who smoke is less than expected.

Anatomy and Physiology of the Respiratory System

The process of respiration involves the same events in children as it does in adults. A basic physiology text should be reviewed to gain an understanding of the components of oxygenation, which include

- Pulmonary *ventilation* (exchange of gases between the external environment and the lung alveoli).
- *Diffusion* (exchange of oxygen and carbon dioxide between alveolar air and blood cells within the lung capillaries).
- *Transportation* of oxygen and carbon dioxide by the blood to the systemic tissue cells.
- *Exchange* of oxygen and carbon dioxide between the blood and tissue cells throughout the body as blood flows through tissue capillaries.

These physiologic processes are similar in adults and children, but some developmental differences have an impact on the effectiveness and the vulnerabilities of the respiratory system in children. Important developmental differences in respiration that the nurse should understand are as follows:

1. The predominance of diaphragmatic-abdominal breathing, normally present in the neonate, continues until around 5 years of age.
2. The chest wall is supple and very compliant, especially in infants. Because of this characteristic, when respiratory disease occurs and greater efforts at breathing are made, the chest wall is easily sucked in both substernally and intercostally (retractions).
3. Because of the small size of the airway, the infant is more susceptible to airway obstruction or collapse (smaller radius of airway creates four times the air resistance found in adults).
4. The respiratory rate of infants and children is higher than in adults, awake or asleep.
5. During the newborn and early infancy stage, the normal pattern of breathing is irregular.

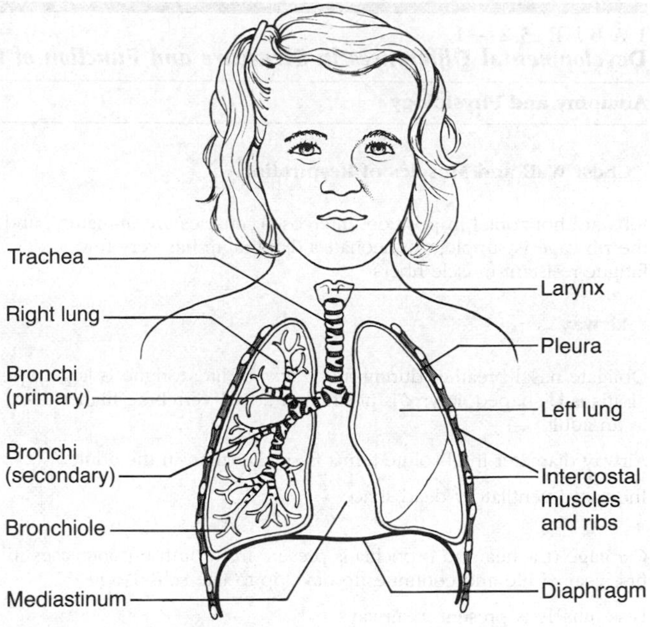

FIGURE 32-1. The respiratory unit.

6. Oxygen consumption is high in proportion to body size. The higher surface area in proportion to body weight results in increased heat loss, requiring an increased metabolic rate.

The structure and function of an infant's or child's lungs that contribute to these differences are reviewed in the next section. Table 32–1 summarizes the differences. An illustration of the respiratory system is found in Figure 32–1.

Chest Wall and Respiratory Muscles

Chest expansion in the adult is accomplished by contraction of the diaphragm (which causes the diaphragm to descend) and contraction of the external intercostal muscles (which elevates the rib cage). A major difference in the infant's chest wall affecting expansion is the *position of the ribs*. In the adult, the downward, lateral angle of the ribs permits their elevation (in a bucket handle action), which results in chest expansion. The ribs of an infant articulate with the vertebrae and sternum *horizontally,* allowing little leverage to increase the anteroposterior diameter of the chest. The infant's breathing is thus primarily diaphragmatic-abdominal. Normally the infant's chest and abdomen are raised together (synchronized). In respiratory distress, the chest falls on inspiration and rises on expiration—a symptom called paradoxical breathing. Furthermore, the abdomen moves in the direction opposite from that of the chest (falls on expiration and rises on inspiration), giving rise to the term "seesaw respirations." This phenomenon is a result of the nonrigid (compliant) chest wall. The disappearance of the seesaw characteristic of breathing

TABLE 32-1
Developmental Differences in Structure and Function of the Respiratory System

Anatomy and Physiology	Significance for Nursing Care
Chest Wall and Muscles of Respiration	
Ribs are horizontal in position; intercostal muscles are immature, and the rib cage is supple; the neonate's diaphragm has very few fatigue-resistant muscle fibers	Diaphragmatic-abdominal breathing is normal in infants; retractions occur more readily in the event of large negative intrapleural pressures
Airway	
Obligate nasal breather during first 3 wks of life; tongue is large, epiglottis is U-shaped; larynx is positioned 2 to 3 vertebrae higher than in an adult	Oxygenation compromised if nasal obstruction occurs
Airway diameter in absolute terms is smaller than in the adult	The potential for obstruction is increased
Increased ventilatory dead space	A larger increase in respiratory rate is required to increase alveolar ventilation
Cartilage (trachea and bronchi) is present from birth but increases in first year of life and continues to develop to late school age	Airway of young infant is more susceptible to collapse during expiration
Less muscle is present in airways	May be a decreased potential for bronchospasm in the very young child
Mucous membranes of airways are highly vascular	Susceptible to trauma, edema, and spasm
Diameter of airway in infants and children is proportionately larger than in adults; angle of right bronchus is reduced	Increases potential for aspiration of foreign body (right side is most common)
Alveoli and Parenchyma	
Alveoli present at birth are fewer in number and smaller in size	Although the number and size of alveoli are reduced, surface area is constant throughout life when expressed relative to body surface area
Fewer intra-alveolar pores of Kohn and bronchoalveolar canals of Lambert	Less able to achieve ventilation beyond obstructed units
Surfactant is lacking in prematurity	Absence of surfactant is the principal cause of respiratory distress syndrome
Peripheral airways contribute a larger percentage of airway resistance than in the adult	Respiration is severely compromised by illnesses that affect the peripheral airways
Related Physiologic Factors	
Infants and young children have immature thermostatic control and proportionately large surface area, compared with adults	Ability to adjust to temperature changes is decreased; respiratory rate increases appreciably to meet metabolic demands
Lymph tissue is particularly active until child is 6 yrs of age; it gradually becomes less active and atrophies after child is 12 yrs of age	Infection and edema readily result in occlusion of the upper airway in a young child
Development of accessory muscles is poor (head bobbing occurs in infants)	Reach point of respiratory insufficiency more quickly than adults

during respiratory distress is a result of the hardening of ribs/cartilage so that the framework is more stable.

The degree of stability of the chest wall affects the process of respiration. During inspiration, the diaphragm contracts and descends, thus making the pleural pressure more negative (subatmospheric). The fall in pleural pressure is transmitted through the lung and causes a slightly negative intra-alveolar pressure. Airflow from the atmosphere to the alveoli occurs because of this pressure difference between the atmosphere and the alveoli. The amount of negative pressure in the intrapleural space (between visceral and parietal pleura) that is normally seen is −4 mmHg (Guyton, 1991). The relatively rigid rib cage of an adult can be expanded and its shape maintained during this process. An infant, especially the premature infant, has a soft sternum and a less rigid rib cage. Consequently, inspiration may cause an inward movement of the rib cage because of the intrapleural subatmospheric pressure. This results in observable *retractions* (in-drawing). Such retractions can occur in a mild form during normal breathing in the neonate, but in the older infant and child they indicate that the negative intrapleural pressure required to distend the lungs is markedly below atmospheric pressure and is a sign of respiratory distress. The more marked the retractions, the greater is the negative intrapleural pressure being required to move the air from the mouth to the alveoli. This results from airflow obstruction or excessively stiff lungs. Retractions typically are intercostal, sternal, and paratracheal (tracheal tug). Retractions progressing from intercostal to sternal to paratracheal signify increasing respiratory distress and more negative pleural pressure.

Airways

The structure and components of the airway affect the ease with which air can move through the respiratory passageways. Infants are obligatory nose breathers. Therefore, intake of air is easily compromised in the event of a nasal obstruction, such as a congenital anomaly or during therapeutic procedures (suctioning, tube feeding) when nares are obstructed. Most infants do not open their mouths to maintain an airway until approximately 3 weeks of age; however, air is taken in during crying.

The potential for edema and obstruction of the airway is enhanced in infants owing to various anatomic differences, compared with adults. The tongue is larger in proportion to the mouth; therefore, occlusion of the airway is more likely. The larynx (epiglottis and glottis) of an infant or child has ciliated columnar epithelium below the glottis (vocal cord) that is loosely bound with areolar tissue, and there is greater vascularity of the mucous membrane. This area is highly susceptible to trauma, edema, and spasm. The infant epiglottis is large and U-shaped (the adult's is V-shaped), contributing to ease of obstruction. The cricoid cartilage is the narrowest part of the trachea, producing a funnel shape; a 1-mm increase in wall thickness from edema can compromise the airway 75 per cent (Behrman & Vaughan, 1987).

The airway diameter of an infant or child is in absolute terms smaller than that of an adult, increasing the potential for obstruction at all times. Proportionately, however, the diameter of the conducting airways is larger in the infant and child than in the adult. The proportionately larger diameter increases the ratio of dead space (air that fills respiratory passages with each breath) to tidal volume (volume of air inspired or expired with each breath). This anatomic difference necessitates that proportionately more air be moved in and out of the lungs each minute (minute volume) to obtain a comparable amount of alveolar ventilation where gas exchange actually takes place. This possibly is one of the reasons infants breathe at a faster resting respiratory rate.

The airways change in structure and function throughout postnatal growth. During the first few months of extrauterine life, the diameter and length of the trachea and bronchi increase rapidly (Lough et al, 1986). At birth, cartilage, mucous glands, and goblet cells are all present. Cartilage in the trachea and bronchi increases during the first year of life, providing the rigidity required to keep the airways from collapsing. The epithelium of an infant's or child's airway contains almost twice the number of submucosal glands per unit surface as does that of the adult's airway (Rudolph, 1991). Muscle in the airway wall is present at birth in the same proportion as in adults, but it is located more predominantly in central than in peripheral airways (Rudolph, 1991). The presence of smooth muscle throughout the lung from birth makes it possible for even a young infant to experience bronchospasms.

Growth of the airways in relationship to the vertebral column results in anatomic differences in the child. At birth, the bifurcation of the trachea is at the level of the third thoracic vertebra, and, by 12 years, it is at the adult position, the sixth thoracic vertebra. The left main-stem bronchus is larger in diameter than the right, and the normal angulation is sharper than that of the right. In the child, the proportionately larger diameter of the airway, the proximity of the angulation, and the reduced angle of the right bronchus make the right bronchus the most prevalent site for foreign-body aspiration.

Alveoli and Parenchyma

The developmental changes that occur in the alveoli and parenchyma during postnatal growth contribute to a gradual decrease in a child's vulnerability to obstruction and atelectasis. The newborn infant has only 20 million alveoli, compared with 300 to 600 million in the adult. Furthermore, alveoli are smaller in size, and the terminal bronchioles have not completed their branching. The number of alveolar ducts and alveoli increase dramatically in the first few months and years of life. Growth by increase in the number of alveoli is thought to continue until about 8 years of age, after which it is primarily the result of an increase in size of units (Rudolph, 1991). The growth of the lung increases surface area for exchange of gases. The primary respiratory lobule is illustrated in Figure 32–2.

The development of pulmonary surfactant within the lung is a principal factor in respiratory function at

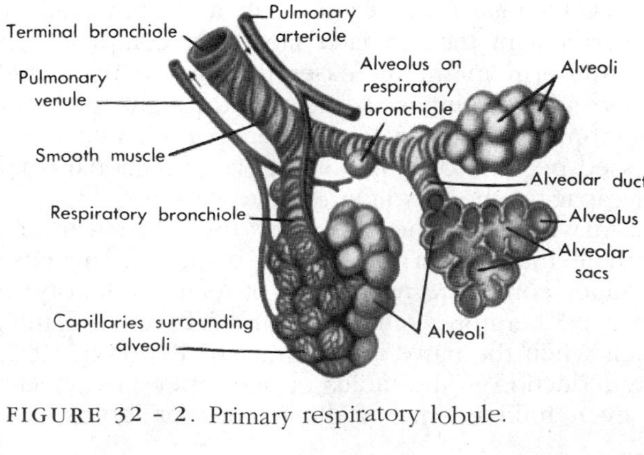

FIGURE 32-2. Primary respiratory lobule.

birth. Type II cells within the alveoli appear around 16 to 20 weeks' gestation, but secretion of surfactant does not occur until about 10 weeks later. Surfactant is a phospholipid-protein complex that lines the alveoli and has the ability to lower surface tension during expiration. Surface tension is a phenomenon in which liquid tries to minimize its surface area; for example, if water is dropped, it forms a sphere rather than a flat surface. Because the alveoli are really flat surfaces, the tendency of surface tension to form a sphere would result in collapse. A detergent-like substance such as surfactant causes the alveoli to remain open, resulting in less effort for the next inspiration. Surfactant enables the lung to remain air-filled at end-expiration; without surfactant, progressive diffuse atelectasis occurs shortly after birth, because the alveoli collapse—that is, surface tension is high and pulls the surfaces together. Absence of surfactant in the neonate is the principal cause of respiratory distress syndrome (discussed in Chapter 30). See bronchopulmonary dysplasia in this chapter for a discussion of surfactant replacement therapy.

Collateral ventilation is another mechanism that can prevent atelectasis. In the adult, alveolar air can move from one acinus to another through holes in the alveoli (pores of Kohn) and through communications in terminal bronchioles (canals of Lambert). This mechanism prevents air from being completely absorbed (leading to atelectasis) in areas distal to an airway obstruction. The absence of collateral circulation in the infant and young child is a factor that contributes to the common phenomenon of patchy atelectasis in this age group.

Work of Breathing

During normal quiet respiration, respiratory muscles contract only during inspiration, whereas expiration is a passive process. The elastic recoil of the lung and chest wall completes the ventilatory cycle, but it does not contribute to the "work of breathing." During inspiration, *compliance work* and *airway resistance work* take place.

Compliance work is required to expand the lungs and thorax against their elastic forces. We noted earlier that the neonate's rib cage is infinitely compliant. Neonatal lungs, however, are stiff and comparatively less compliant than in later life. Lung compliance in the full-term infant increases during the first week of life and continues to increase through adulthood (Guyton, 1991). However, when compliance is expressed per unit of lung volume (i.e., functional residual capacity) there is little change with age.

Airway resistance is many times greater in a neonate than in an older child or adult. The nasal passages contribute nearly half of total respiratory resistance; therefore, retractions and labored breathing result when the nares are obstructed (Rudolph, 1991). Any reduction in the radius of the upper airway, such as even mild edema of the trachea or larynx, also poses a serious threat to the neonate because of the resultant increase in airway resistance.

The resistance to airflow produced by peripheral airways (bronchioles) is proportionately higher in children than in adults. Up to age 5 years, peripheral airways may contribute up to 50 per cent of the total airway resistance, compared with only 20 per cent after age 5 years. The infant and young child's respiratory status, therefore, is severely compromised by illnesses that affect peripheral airways (e.g., bronchiolitis), whereas after this period involvement of small airways may have minimal effect on overall airway resistance.

Related Physiologic Factors

The respiratory rate and pattern of infants and children under normal circumstances are observably different from those of adults. The respiratory rate is highest at birth and gradually decreases to the adult rate during early adolescence. Most of the decrease in respiratory rate takes place during the first few years of life. Awake and sleeping respiratory rates differ considerably during early infancy (up to 3 months of age). Normally, the respiratory rate of an awake infant may be as high as 70 breaths per minute, yet the normal sleeping respiratory rate is less than 40 breaths per minute. The resting oxygen consumption and carbon dioxide output of an infant are approximately twice those of an adult (based on kilograms of body weight). In the event of increased metabolic demands, as in elevated temperature or compromised respiratory function, oxygen supply depletes more rapidly.

A young child's immature thermostatic control and the proportionately large body surface area of infants cause difficulty in maintaining body temperature. These factors can result in increased oxygen consumption, putting stress on the respiratory system.

The young child's cardiac status and function affect the child's respiratory system. The child has a lower cardiac stroke volume; therefore, the cardiac rate is higher than in the adult, to meet high metabolic demands. Consequently, when a child is in respiratory difficulty or has a fever, the pulse rate increases along with the respiratory rate in an effort to meet the metabolic demands.

History and Physical Examination

This chapter expands the health history concerning respiratory function and reviews common clinical manifestations of respiratory difficulty. Assessment of the child focuses on the following:

- The child's physical, psychologic, and social environment pertaining to respiratory status to collect data for improvement of health status (health promotion) and prevention of respiratory illnesses.
- Early identification of an existing unrecognized respiratory problem to facilitate early treatment.

TABLE 32-2
Assessment Guide: Historical Factors to Consider in Respiratory Assessment

History of Present Illness (if the illness presents with symptoms)

Past Health History

Allergies

Feeding history

Medications

Previous illnesses, injuries, or operations

Frequency of colds

Date of last chest examination

Socioeconomic and Family Factors

Stability of marriage and stress level in the home

Income level and ability to provide for food, clothing, shelter, and health care

Physical Environment

Presence of pets in the home

Exposure to cigarette smoking (parents, siblings, caretakers); does client smoke?

Family dwelling location (proximity to industry, dump, or known source of air pollution)

Conditions of crowding

Cleanliness of home

Exposure level: day care, nursery school, elementary school, high school

Health Practices

Routine immunizations

Hand washing—taught to children?

Health practices when family members have colds (covering of mouth when coughing or sneezing, disposal of tissues, avoidance of common eating and drinking utensils, and proper hand washing)

Protection from the elements (appropriate clothing)

Adequacy of diet, sleep, and exercise

Review of System (see Chapter 13)

Family Profile

A family health history is taken to determine presence of familial or hereditary disease

- Assessment and evaluation of an existing respiratory condition to determine appropriate care.

All children, whether well or ill, should be assessed at the first two levels. Even though a child is first seen with a respiratory problem, the focus of assessment and care should include health promotion and prevention of illness and early detection components as well as resolution of the immediate problem. Table 32-2 summarizes pertinent historical data to gather.

The nurse's understanding of the clinical presentation of a respiratory problem provides the base for independent decision making. Objective data noted with respiratory alterations and their significance are summarized in Table 32-3.

Accurate assessment of respiratory status helps the nurse make appropriate explanations to the child and parent. A respiratory alteration frequently is a frightening experience; the nurse can assist in the reduction of anxiety only by having accurate information.

Diagnostic Assessment

The nurse prepares the child and family for the various required diagnostic tests and procedures. Because parental anxiety can be caused by lack of knowledge, the nurse must understand how the procedure is done and the purpose of the test. In addition, an understanding of the developmental level of the child is required to give explanations appropriate for the child's age (see Chapter 23 for a discussion of the preparation of children for procedures).

Diagnostic procedures a nurse may encounter are summarized in Table 32-4. Radioisotope scanning, bronchoscopy, blood gas analysis, and pulmonary function testing are described next.

Radioisotope Lung Scanning

The preparation required for radioisotope lung scanning depends on the type of scan to be done. Usually premedication is not necessary. When a ventilatory lung scan is done, a very young or uncooperative child may require sedation. A sedated child is given nothing by mouth (NPO) for 4 hours preceding the procedure to prevent vomiting and aspiration of gastric secretions.

Perfusion Scan. The only discomfort is the intravenous injection of the radiopharmaceutical agent. A perfusion scan usually takes approximately 20 minutes when multiple views of the lungs are taken with a gamma camera.

Ventilatory Scan. The child is requested to breathe a radioactive gas or aerosol through a mouthpiece

TABLE 32-3
Clinical Manifestations of Respiratory Alterations

Objective Data and Explanation	Clinical Significance
Restlessness, irritability, and an axious expression Older children: Restlessness and mental confusion Infants: Irritability, poor activity, and seizures *Inability to breathe gives a sensation of strangulation and results in anxiety. A decrease in oxygen (hypoxemia) and an increase in carbon dioxide (hypercapnia) in arterial blood contribute to anxiety and restlessness*	A fatigued infant with labored breathing may suddenly become more active. This may indicate a general worsening of condition (i.e., respiratory failure). A $PaCO_2 > 45$ or a $PaO_2 < 60$ mmHg in 50% oxygen signifies failure
Cyanosis: Assess distribution, degree, duration, and response to oxygen *Cyanosis results from reduced alveolar ventilation, uneven distribution of oxygen relative to lung blood flow. An intrapulmonary shunt is the flow of blood past nonventilating alveoli, resulting in return of unoxygenated blood to the left side of the heart, and abnormality in diffusion. Cyanosis is seen when an excess of reduced hemoglobin (Hgb) is present (i.e., 5 or more grams of reduced Hgb/dl of blood)*	Cyanosis is difficult to assess if vasoconstriction has occurred (as in shock and acidosis). If a child is anemic, significant hypoxemia may be present without cyanosis because hemoglobin is insufficient to result in a reduced Hgb of 5 g/dl of blood. On the contrary, in polycythemia cyanosis may be present when hypoxia is minimal. When oxygen is delivered to correct cyanosis and no improvement is seen, a right-to-left cardiac shunt is highly likely
Cough: Assess onset and duration; type (dry, hacking, moist); pattern (time of day, length of time, number of times a day); associated symptoms; and productivity *A cough is a normal protective mechanism to clear the tracheobronchial tree of irritants. Mechanical factors that induce coughing are cool or dry environment, irritation or inflammation, a foreign body, and accumulation of secretions*	The high intrathoracic pressures created during coughing can cause the child's airway to collapse. Children under 8 yrs of age cannot cough on demand; therefore, a cough may need to be stimulated
Dyspnea: Observe rate and depth of respirations *Respiratory rate increases because of fever; drugs (central stimulation); stiff chest wall and/or lung; airway obstruction; stimulation of pulmonary receptors (i.e., in pulmonary edema); and weak muscles resulting in small tidal volume and faster rates*	Increased rates are associated with pneumonia, pleural effusion, and pulmonary edema. Respiratory rate can also be increased by other conditions associated with respiratory problems: fever, anxiety, acid-base imbalance
Tachycardia *Heart rate increases in response to reduced oxygen supply, or generalized increased sympathetic nervous system activity*	
Grunting *Signifies closure of the glottis, creating a positive expiratory pressure in order to stabilize alveoli and small airways. A compensatory mechanism: increases positive pressure in airway to prevent collapse of bronchioles and alveoli and prolong exchange of oxygen and carbon dioxide in the alveoli*	It is frequently associated with pneumonia. In the neonate it is associated with respiratory distress syndrome
Retractions: (nonrigid part of chest is drawn in during inspiration) Types include supraclavicular, intercostal, sternal, and paratracheal *Occurs whenever the respiratory muscles are working harder and creating a more negative pleural pressure to overcome the stiffness of the chest wall or lungs or airway obstruction. Air normally moves into lung when chest cavity is expanded; if airway entry resists, then accessory muscles are used. Retractions are common in infants and children owing to their pliable rib cage. Airway resistance causes a greater-than-normal pressure difference between the atmosphere and the intrapleural space (i.e., greater-than-normal negative pressure). Because of the flexibility of the rib cage, the greater-than-normal negative pressure draws soft tissues inward*	Slight intercostal depressions can be normal in the infant. Subcostal retractions seen at the lower anterior costal margin indicate a flattened diaphragm. This is seen in diffuse lower airway obstruction and in severe obstructive pulmonary disease
Intercostal bulging *A movement outward of the intercostal space is seen during expiration when effort is required to force air out of the lungs. When the lung is distended with trapped air and the intercostal muscles are active, bulging in the intercostal spaces occurs*	Occurs in asthma, bronchiolitis, or cystic fibrosis. Retracting and bulging can occur together: retracting on inspiration and bulging on expiration
Stridor: (a harsh sound owing to increased rate and turbulence of airflow in the larynx or trachea) *Obstruction to breathing in the larynx or trachea causes narrowing. There is an increased turbulence of airflow and an increased velocity. A greater negative intratracheal and intrathoracic pressure must be generated to overcome the obstruction. With upper airway ob-*	In younger children, the larynx and trachea are soft and pliable. They can easily be compressed by the increased negative pressure

TABLE 32-3
Clinical Manifestations of Respiratory Alterations *(Continued)*

Objective Data and Explanation	Clinical Significance
struction, the child has stridor and has more trouble getting air in. In lower airway obstruction, the child wheezes and has more difficulty getting air out. In severe cases, both sites may produce noises on inspiration and expiration, but the phase with the most trouble remains identifiable	
Head bobbing: Head bobs forward in synchrony with each respiration	Is a sign of severe respiratory effort
Accessory muscles of inspiration (scalene and sternocleidomastoid) are contracted, resulting in flexion of the neck	
Flaring of the nares	Unilateral flaring indicates facial paralysis. The presence of bilateral nasal flaring indicates respiratory difficulty
Due to contraction of muscles in the nares (controlled by the facial nerve). These accessory muscles are used because of the increased work of breathing	
Clubbing (proliferation of tissue in terminal digits of fingers, causing lifting of the nail base) (see Fig. 35–5)	Clubbing must be further investigated to search for problems other than respiratory (e.g., cardiac)
Occurs in response to prolonged hypoxemia or lung disease. The cause is unknown	
Chest pain	Pain may be a complaint of older children but may also be present in the nonverbal child. Sneezing and coughing aggravate pleural pain
Pain occurs in the chest wall, parietal pleura, bronchi, and trachea	
Breath sounds (see Chapter 13 for physical assessment of lungs and specific alterations in this chapter for explanation of breath sounds heard in various illnesses)	

with nose clips in place, or through a mask. Practice sessions of breathing with nostrils pinched should be performed before a ventilatory scan is done. The child should be told that the gas does not cause drowsiness or any unusual feelings. As the child breathes in the gas, or following inhalation if aerosol is used, scanning is begun. About 10 minutes are needed to complete a ventilatory scan with a gamma camera.

Postprocedural Care. Usually no special procedures are necessary after a perfusion or ventilatory scan, except that sputum from a productive cough should be disposed of in a closed container (Tilkian et al, 1987).

Bronchoscopy

The preparation required depends on the type of procedure and whether a general anesthetic is used. The type of scope varies in practice. The advantage of the rigid bronchoscope is that the child breathes *through* the hollow open tube. It is used when bleeding is present or for removal of a foreign body. The flexible fiberoptic bronchoscope is solid; therefore, the child must breathe *around* the tube. Fiberoptic bronchoscope tubes are now available with an external diameter of 3.5 mm or less that can be used in younger children.

An infant is usually kept NPO for at least 4 hours before the procedure; an older child is kept NPO from the midnight prior to the procedure. A preoperative sedative and atropine are given before the examination is done. A sedative increases relaxation and helps alleviate coughing and gagging. Atropine decreases bronchial secretions, relaxes the bronchial smooth muscle, and reduces the risk of laryngospasm. Laboratory work performed preprocedurally usually includes platelet count, prothrombin time, partial thromboplastin time, and bleeding time, especially if a biopsy is to be done.

General Anesthesia. One should prepare the child by explaining the following:

1. Preprocedural medication may be given intramuscularly.
2. Child will be asleep during the procedure.
3. Child will awaken with an intravenous (IV) line in the recovery room.
4. Child will return to room when awake, and the IV line will be removed when fluids are being tolerated.
5. Suctioning and postural drainage may be necessary.

Local Anesthesia. When local anesthesia is used for bronchoscopy, the nurse will want to keep these facts in mind:

1. Local anesthetic is sprayed into the mouth (cough and gag reflex are stimulated by this spraying).

TABLE 32-4
Diagnostic Assessment: Respiratory Function

Type of Procedure	Purpose	Nursing Implications
Radiology		
Posteroanterior (PA) and lateral chest radiographs	Visualize airways, lungs, heart, and great vessels	With maximal inspiration, the chest radiograph shows nine to ten ribs above the diaphragm; the trachea should be straight. Since infants cannot cooperate to take a maximal inspiration, visualization of 10 ribs indicates hyperinflation and air trapping. Movement can cause blurring of the cardiothoracic structures that can resemble pulmonary infiltrates
Lateral neck radiograph	Evaluate stridor. A swollen epiglottis is visible in epiglottitis; subglottic edema is evident in croup	
Fluoroscopy: An imaging method that records radiographic images rapidly. Images can be viewed on a television monitor	Assess regional ventilation and diaphragmatic excursion; also used during an esophagram	
Bronchography: An invasive procedure in which a radiopaque material is instilled into the trachea and bronchi	The entire tracheobronchial tree can be visualized by x-ray film; especially useful to visualize bronchi distal to area that cannot be visualized by bronchoscope	A small catheter is placed into the trachea, and contrast media is instilled to provide a fine coating of the tracheobronchial tree; performed under general anesthesia. These studies are rarely indicated
Computed tomography (CT scan): A sequence of x-rays that produces a cross-sectional view of the thorax; can also discriminate between changes in tissue density	Define lesions located anywhere within the chest wall, pleural space, mediastinum, or lung parenchyma; often used to evaluate undiagnosed masses or to assess response of known lesion to therapy	Sedation or immobilization is usually necessary, but general anesthesia is not recommended. Feedings are withheld 3–4 hrs prior to the examination because IV contrast media is often given to opacify cardiac chambers and the great vessels
Endoscopy		
Laryngoscopy: Direct inspection by inserting scope through mouth, or through nose if the newer type of small flexible fiberoptic bronchoscope is used	Evaluate stridor and local abnormalities	Indirect (mirror) laryngoscopy can be used for older children, but direct laryngoscopy is usually necessary in infants and small children. General anesthesia is usually required. Topical anesthesia and mild sedation are used with the fiberoptic bronchoscope technique
Bronchoscopy: Visualization of the tracheobronchial tree directly through a scope	For examination, for biopsy of mass lesions, to obtain specimens and to remove foreign body or mucous plugs	Types of scopes: 1. Rigid bronchoscope: a laryngoscope is first passed, then the bronchoscope is passed through it. Child can breathe through the tube 2. Flexible fiberoptic bronchoscope: used in older children whose airway permits child to breathe around the tube (inserted through nose or through a special endotracheal tube) 3. Rigid scope with fiberoptic lens: newer scopes are rigid with fiberoptic illumination and an improved telescopic lens system
Nuclear Medicine		
Radioisotope scanning: Radioactive isotopes (radionuclides) are injected IV (perfusion scan) or inhaled (ventilation scan)	Identify defects in pulmonary arterial distribution and abnormal regional ventilation (e.g., asthma, foreign-body aspiration)	Foreign-body aspiration not noted within first 24 hrs (see text for discussion of preparation of the child)
Specimen Collection		
Lung biopsy: An open thoracotomy is performed and pulmonary tissue is removed. (A closed procedure is not common in children)	Ensure an adequate specimen for histology and culture of microorganisms, and the lung can be inspected to choose the site of the biopsy	Done under general anesthesia; requires chest tube postoperatively
Lung puncture (percutaneous lung tap): A quick needle stab through a locally anesthetized intercostal space	Culture of microorganism Used when obscure interstitial pneumonia is present	Usually used only for critical cases when there is failure in response to therapy; no physical preparation for test. Complication of test is pneumothorax

2. After the spraying the tongue and throat begin to feel swollen, and there is a sensation of being unable to swallow (secretions are suctioned during the procedure).

3. Child should be reassured that he or she will be able to breathe while tube is in place.

4. Prepare the child by explaining that the room is dark and eyes will be covered to protect them.

5. Fluids will be given after normal swallowing reflexes return (usually approximately 2 hours after procedure).

6. Child will feel sleepy for about 2 hours because of the sedative.

7. Child may be placed in a mist tent to reduce laryngeal edema (child should have experience in the tent preprocedurally).

8. Child may need postural drainage.

Postprocedural Care. Following the procedure (general or local anesthesia), oral intake is withheld until the gag reflex has returned. This is an appropriate intervention for the nursing diagnosis *high risk for aspiration*. Fluids help decrease throat soreness and liquefy secretions; therefore, they should be given in small amounts after the gag reflex returns. The child should be assessed for the need to be suctioned and whether postural drainage is required. The child should be observed for complications, including hemorrhage and signs of respiratory distress (dyspnea, retractions, behavior change, change in vital signs, cyanosis). Also, the sputum should be observed for blood; slightly streaked sputum is normal following a biopsy. Following bronchoscopy, the upper airway may be irritated, which may result in increased mucous production.

Arterial Blood Gas Analysis

A frequently performed diagnostic procedure to assess respiratory function is an analysis of arterial blood gases. Arterial blood gases most commonly include values for Pao_2, $Paco_2$, pH, and HCO_3. Pao_2 and $Paco_2$ measurements are reported in millimeters of mercury (mmHg). The "P" represents the partial pressure of the gas being measured. (Partial pressure of a gas is the force it exerts in a mixture.) The "a" refers to the mixture in which the gas is being measured (i.e., arterial). For example, Pao_2 is the pressure exerted by the small amount of oxygen that is dissolved in arterial blood. This oxygen is less than 2 per cent of the total oxygen content of the arterial blood. The remainder is bound to hemoglobin. Thus, the oxygen *content* of blood depends on hemoglobin and its degree of saturation. Hemoglobin O_2 saturation (a number given in a percentage) represents the total oxygen-binding sites on the hemoglobin that are bound with oxygen. The percentage of hemoglobin saturated with oxygen depends on the Pao_2 (pressure being exerted by oxygen dissolved in the blood). In arterial blood, the relationship between Pao_2 and O_2 saturations is not a linear one and is represented by the oxygen-hemoglobin dissociation curve. The relationship depends on temperature and acidity of the blood (see Chapter 26 for further discussion of the oxygen-hemoglobin dissociation curve).

The value for $Paco_2$ is an index of the amount of carbon dioxide in arterial blood. It is a measure of the degree of alveolar ventilation. Alveolar ventilation is the amount of "fresh" air* that reaches the alveoli and with appropriate blood flow exchanges oxygen and carbon dioxide across the alveolar-capillary membrane. The pH indicates the hydrogen ion concentration (lower-than-normal pH indicates the presence of *more* hydrogen ions and acidic blood). HCO_3 is the nonrespiratory component of the acid-to-base ratio and is altered when metabolic processes are disturbed. See Table 32–5 for normal values of blood gases. Acid-base balance and the interpretation of arterial blood gases are further discussed in Chapter 26.

Arterial blood sampling is the most reliable method of blood gas determination. "Capillary" blood gases underestimate Pao_2 but usually give reliable estimates of $Paco_2$ and pH. New noninvasive techniques are being used increasingly: oximetry (ear and pulse) and transcutaneous monitoring of Po_2 and Pco_2.

Noninvasive Blood Gas Monitoring. Noninvasive electronic equipment that reflects reasonably accurate measures of oxygenation is commonly used in intensive care areas where continuous monitoring of blood gases is required. Noninvasive techniques are generally used in conjunction with direct arterial sampling. Continuous monitoring has the advantage of providing moment-to-moment information, whereas direct sampling of blood gives single readings at selected times.

Noninvasive monitoring is done by transcutaneous tension (Po_2) monitors and pulse oximetry. The transcutaneous monitor consists of a heated sensor (electrode) that is placed on the thorax or abdomen. (Extremities are generally not used in infants and young children, because reliability depends on cutaneous perfusion.) Oxygen diffuses through the skin, so the diffused oxygen is measured by the electrochemical sensor. Heating the skin causes an increased amount of oxygen to diffuse through the skin, which compensates for the normal gradient between arterial (Pao_2) and transcutaneous oxygen (Po_2). The actual measurement, therefore, correlates well with Pao_2 (Carnevale, 1986).

Transcutaneous monitoring has some limitations. Frequent calibration periods are necessary, the heated electrode may cause burns, and some wide fluctuations that cannot be detected by intermittent arterial sampling have been noted (Jennis & Peabody, 1987).

A noninvasive method is the *pulse oximeter*. It measures the oxygen saturation (Sao_2) of arterial hemoglobin. Its accuracy in adults and children has

* "Fresh" air is newly inspired air on ventilation and is differentiated from "stale" air, which is the alveolar gas left in the conducting passages at the end of expiration.

TABLE 32-5
Normal Values for Blood Gases*

		Normal Range	Normal Range in International Units
PaO_2	First day	54–95 mmHg	7.2–12.6 kPa
	Thereafter	83–108 mmHg	11.0–14.4 kPa
$PaCO_2$	Infant	27–41 mmHg	3.6–5.5 kPa
	Thereafter (M)	35–48 mmHg	4.7–6.4 kPa
	(F)	32–45 mmHg	4.3–6.0 kPa
pH	First day	7.29–7.45 mmHg	35–51 mmol/L
	Thereafter	7.35–7.45 mmHg	35–44 mmol/L
	(Must be corrected for body temperature)		
Bicarbonate (HCO_3^-)		21–28 mmol/L	21–28 mmol/L
Base excess			
	Newborn infant	(−7)–(−1) mmol/L	(−7)–(−1) mmol/L
	Child	(−4)–(+2) mmol/L	(−4)–(+2) mmol/L
	Thereafter	(−3)–(+3) mmol/L	(−3)–(+3) mmol/L

From Behrman, R., & Vaughan, V. (Eds.) (1987). *Nelson textbook of pediatrics* (13th ed.). Philadelphia: WB Saunders.

* These values are normal at sea level. Normal values for high elevations may fall outside these ranges.

been reported (Fanconi et al, 1985), as has its use in newborn infants who have no greater than 50 per cent fetal hemoglobin (Jennis & Peabody, 1987). The oximeter must be correlated with an arterial wave form to be considered accurate. It is highly susceptible to motion artifact. The oximeter may be somewhat less accurate when used on dark-skinned or jaundiced patients, because it measures Sao_2 on the basis of light absorption through the skin (Openbrier et al, 1988). The sensor is usually attached to a finger in children or to a toe or foot in neonates. Pulse oximeters display a continuous arterial oxygen saturation reading; however, periodic measurement of arterial blood gases is done as with transcutaneous monitoring.

Pulmonary Function Tests

Pulmonary function tests evaluate adequacy of pulmonary function, but they do not generally provide a diagnosis or an etiology. The primary uses of pulmonary function tests are to (1) assess the degree of pulmonary disease, (2) assess response to therapy, and (3) help distinguish between restrictive and obstructive disease. They are also valuable in detecting a respiratory limitation preoperatively and in establishing a baseline of pulmonary function. The standard terminology is diagrammed and explained in Figure 32–3.

Pulmonary function tests include two categories of testing. The first evaluates the functions contributing to movement of air in and out of the respiratory tract and the distribution of air to the alveoli. These tests are called *ventilatory function tests* (tests of lung volumes, ventilation, and pulmonary mechanics). The second category measures the transfer of gas across the blood-gas barrier (diffusion) and the effectiveness of the vascular perfusion.

The most frequently used method of pulmonary function testing is spirometry. The simplest measurement obtained by a spirometer is a single forced expiration called forced expiration volume (FEV). This test can be done in the physician's office or clinic. After an inspiration of maximal volume (to total lung capacity), the child is instructed to exhale as hard and as completely as possible. The spirometer stylus marks a curve on graph paper that can be compared with a normal curve. A good expiratory curve starts with a steep slope that levels off near end-expiration. The volume exhaled in the first second is the forced expiratory volume within 1 second (FEV_1), and the volume exhaled within the first 3 seconds is FEV_3. The total volume exhaled is the vital capacity (VC). Figure 32–3 shows that the vital capacity can be reduced by either a decrease in the total lung capacity (due to restriction of the chest wall or lung) or an increase in the residual volume (due to airway obstruction and air trapping). The ratio of FEV_1 to VC (FEV_1/VC) is used to help differentiate between obstructive and restrictive airway disease. The ratio answers the question, "Of the total amount of air that can be expelled from the lungs (VC), how much can I get out in the first second (FEV_1)?" The normal FEV_1-to-VC ratio is 0.8 (Levin & Morriss, 1990) and varies slightly with age. In obstructive airway disease, the ratio decreases (less than 0.8), whereas it is normal or increased in restrictive disease.

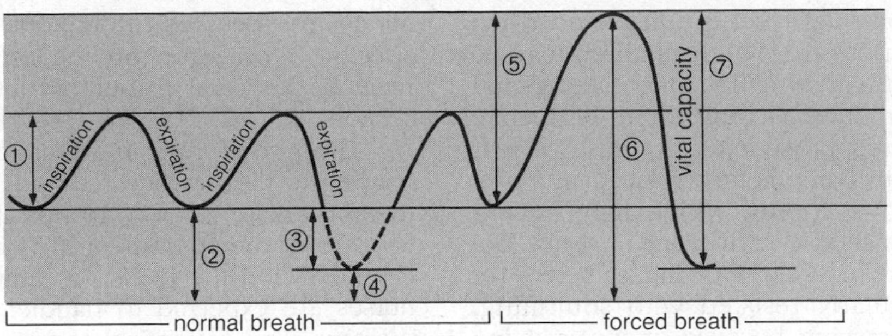

1. Normal breath—Tidal Volume
2. Air left in lungs—Functional Residual Capacity (FRC)
3. Air expelled *after* normal expiration—Expiratory Reserve Volume (ERV)
4. Air left after forced expiration—Residual Volume (RV)
5. Maximal inspiration—Inspiratory Capacity (IC)
6. Air in lungs at end of maximal inspiration—Total Lung Capacity (TLC)
7. Forced expiration after maximal inspiration—Vital Capacity (VC)

The graph depicts a normal breath and a forced breath to illustrate lung volumes and capacities. In a normal breath, the volume of gas inspired or expired during each normal respiratory cycle is called the *tidal volume*①. After a normal expiration, air remains in the lungs; this is the *functional residual capacity*②. If additional effort is exerted at the end of a normal expiration, more air can be expelled; this is the *expiratory reserve volume*③. Even after a forced expiration some air remains in the lungs; this is the *residual volume*④. If at the end of a normal expiration no additional air is forced out but rather a maximal inspiration is taken, the total amount taken in from the level of normal expiration is called the *inspiratory capacity*⑤ (this includes the tidal volume). The amount of air in the lungs at the end of maximal inspiration is called the *total lung capacity*⑥. If air is expired after maximal inspiration, forcing it beyond the normal expiration point so that maximal expiration is performed, the total amount of air expelled is called the *vital capacity*⑦.

FIGURE 32 - 3. Lung volumes and lung capacities: explanation of terminology.

Of the two categories of pulmonary involvement (obstructive and restrictive), the obstructive pattern is seen most commonly in children—namely, bronchopulmonary dysplasia, bronchiolitis, bronchial asthma, and cystic fibrosis. The restrictive problems arise from deformities of the spine (e.g., scoliosis) or neuromuscular conditions that affect the muscles and structures involved in respiration.

Preparation of the Child for Pulmonary Function Testing. Pulmonary function tests are noninvasive but still can be frightening to children if they are unprepared. Such fear can lead to ineffective individual coping in children under the age of 5 years. These younger children may have difficulty accomplishing the tasks of blowing, pushing, and stopping respirations on command and require considerable practice. At ages 5 and 6 years, children can be tested without excessive difficulty, but they also require preparation.

During spirometry and other pulmonary testing, a mouthpiece is used into which the child is asked to blow according to the technician's instructions. The nares are obstructed by a nose clip, which is not painful but may be resisted by a fearful child. A child of any age should be permitted to practice the technique and receive information about the sounds and sensations associated with this procedure. Before the procedure, terms such as "take a deep breath," "hold your breath," "blow all the way out," "pant," and "breathe naturally" should be discussed and demonstrated. These interventions are designed to assist the child to cope. Although a firm and somewhat demanding approach is required to get the child's best effort, kindness and encouragement are essential to gain a child's cooperation. *No child should be forced to complete a test that is not being performed effectively but rather should be asked to return at a later time.*

Therapeutic Management

Maintaining adequate pulmonary function in some children requires constant vigilance and specialized nursing skills. The goal is to provide maximal benefits with the least possible energy depletion and trauma to the child. The various procedures should be planned with respect to the child's total nursing plan, trying not to interfere unnecessarily with feeding or nap schedules.

A child's developmental level is considered when one formulates a plan of care. Young children may be unable to verbalize their difficulty in breathing and may be unable to produce a cough or to cooperate during these specialized procedures. A sense of fear when approached with equipment or placed in a tent can lead to ineffective coping which may be expressed through inconsolable crying and resistive behavior. Respiratory procedures involving catheters for aspiration are particularly resisted with squirming, kicking, and body thrashing because of the irritating and choking sensations they produce. The more efficient and skilled the nurse is, the more effective is the treatment with less likelihood of trauma to the child.

Many of the procedures used to care for children are similar to those for adults. Procedures discussed in this section are the most commonly performed or require special adaptation when performed on children. For step-by-step instructions on how to perform various procedures, see texts on basic skills (fundamentals) of nursing.

Medications commonly used for respiratory alterations are discussed throughout the chapter. For more specific information on the pharmacologic management of particular respiratory alterations, refer to that section.

The nurse's role in respiratory therapy varies according to the practice setting. Even when respiratory therapists take primary responsibility for therapy and for care of the equipment, it is imperative for a nurse to understand the goals of therapy. In many settings, nurses are expected to handle aspects of respiratory therapy. The following techniques are common in most pediatric settings.

Oxygen Therapy

Oxygen is indicated when Pa_{O_2} levels are significantly reduced (a decreased partial pressure of oxygen in arterial blood). Oxygen is frequently used in pediatrics because hypoxia develops early in most pediatric pulmonary problems. Its use is widespread in the treatment of most acute pediatric pulmonary problems (pneumonia, bronchiolitis, and asthma). Its use in

TABLE 32-6
Methods of Oxygen Delivery

Type of Device	Developmental Considerations	Nursing Considerations
Isolette (incubator)	Used during the neonatal period. Contact with infant is limited. Objects for visual stimuli can be placed on outside of clear Plexiglas	FiO_2* within incubator usually at 0.4 (40% oxygen concentration) or less. High flow rates can achieve between 40 and 85% oxygen concentration if only O_2 (without room air) is allowed to enter Isolette. O_2 concentration can be analyzed inside the Isolette. An Oxy-Hood (see next entry) can be placed inside an incubator. Portholes must be kept closed and opened only briefly as necessary to prevent escape of O_2 from Isolette. Humidity and temperature controls are provided by an incubator
Oxygen hood (Oxy-Hood). A clear Plexiglas dome placed over the infant's head. Gas is warmed and humidified; it should not blow directly on child's head (cold gas applied to a neonate's face may induce apnea)	The dome restricts movement and vision. Objects can be placed inside or outside the dome for visual stimulation. An infant's head is large in proportion to body; therefore, gas must be warmed to reduce heat loss and resultant oxygen consumption	Oxygen entering the hood must be sufficient to prevent the accumulation of carbon dioxide (approximately 4–8 L/min). Oxygen is analyzed within the hood with an analyzer. Edges of hood must be carefully placed and frequently checked to prevent rubbing of the neck, chin, or shoulder. Vapor collecting on the inside of the dome should be wiped away to ensure unrestricted observation. Nursing care is difficult because of limited access to child's head. For an infant who cannot tolerate being out of oxygen for feeding, the child is held and oxygen delivered via cannula for that period of time
Nasal cannula (nasal prongs)	Usually not tolerated by infants but sometimes useful for older children. Movement is not appreciably restricted; however, in very active and restless children, dislodging of the cannula is probable	Provides low-to-moderate oxygen concentration (up to 40%). Flow rates should not exceed 6 L/min, since gastric distention and regurgitation can occur as a result of high flow rates. Also, high rates by this method can cause sinus headaches
"Blow-by" nasal cannula (without nasal prongs). A catheter placed below the nose and above the mouth, so that the holes in the catheter are matched with the nares (see Figs. 32–4, 32–5, and 32–6)	Infants and children of all ages tolerate this reasonably well. Sensitivity of skin to tape must be taken into consideration and catheter changed accordingly (usually once a week if stoma adhesive is used)	Oxygen levels up to 30% can be maintained; however, one cannot measure precise concentration

chronic pulmonary disease is more complex. A lowered Pao_2 may be a significant stimulus for respiration; consequently, the response to oxygen therapy may be a decrease in ventilation, resulting in a further rise in $Paco_2$. However, significant increases in $Paco_2$ in response to oxygen administration are unusual in adults and extremely rare in children. Although oxygen administration in chronic lung disease should be monitored by assessing the response of arterial $Paco_2$, oxygen should never be withheld when needed. Only the amount of oxygen needed to maintain arterial oxygen tension at 60 mmHg (greater than 90 per cent saturated) should be given (Behrman, 1991).

Oxygen has potentially serious side effects and should be administered for the least amount of time and in the least amount of dosage that will effectively treat the condition. Although retinopathy of prematurity (retrolental fibroplasia) is now believed to be a multifactorial disorder, hyperoxia remains as one of the risk factors (Shapiro, 1986). Retinopathy of prematurity or any retinal changes are an extremely low risk for the chronic lung disease client. The benefits of low flow oxygen therapy greatly outweigh the risks. Retinopathy of prematurity and the effects of oxygen are discussed in Chapter 30.

Oxygen in elevated concentrations is thought to be associated with bronchopulmonary dysplasia, (BPD), but correlation between the degree (concentration and duration) of oxygen exposure and the severity of the disease is poor. Furthermore, infants who have received oxygen but have not needed mechanical ventilators have not developed BPD. The triggering events of BPD are thought to be oxygen-related injury and barotrauma (injury due to pressure from mechanical ventilation) in a susceptible infant with surfactant deficiency and respiratory distress syndrome (Sinkin & Phelps, 1987).

When oxygen is indicated, one must use the type of equipment that is most appropriate for the age of the child and that will deliver the percentage of oxygen needed without unnecessarily subjecting a child to excessive levels of oxygen. Oxygen blenders (a combination of oxygen and compressed air) facilitate selection and delivery of precise desired FiO_2. (See Table 32–6 for methods of oxygen delivery.)

TABLE 32-6
Methods of Oxygen Delivery *(Continued)*

Type of Device	Developmental Considerations	Nursing Considerations
Nasal catheter. A tube inserted into the nares and taped into place	Gives child mobility and unrestricted interaction with caretaker. Has been recommended when sending oxygen-dependent children home (Glassanos, 1980) but is increasingly being replaced by a nasal cannula placed across and under the nose (Voyles, 1981)	Cannot measure precise concentration of inhaled O_2 because end of catheter is inside nares. Tube must be changed every 8 hrs, alternating between nares, to prevent nasal infection and necrosis. Provides an extremely variable FiO_2 (0.22 to 0.50). Flow rates should not exceed 6 L/min to prevent tissue irritation and gastric distention
Simple oxygen mask†	Not well tolerated for continuous therapy. Older children may tolerate a mask for a short period, but young children pull them off	O_2 concentration is 35–55% with 6–10 L/min of pure oxygen as room air is inhaled through side parts of mask. Used for short-term therapy but should not be used for comatose children because of danger of aspiration
Venturi mask (diluter mask).† Placed over child's mouth and nose	Young children may resist even short-term therapy; therefore, they have to be held in place during aerosol therapy	Delivers between 24 and 50% oxygen. Designed to deliver a specific oxygen concentration. Air entrainment ports (openings that permit room air to enter) vary in size and determine oxygen concentration. Not well tolerated for continuous therapy. Can be used for intermittent administration of O_2 with aerosol therapy
Tents. A canopy placed over a metal frame and placed on the bed *Types: Croup tent,* cooled by ice and cold water. *Ohio tent,* cooled by refrigeration system. No ice is required	For most children beyond infancy, tents are the preferred method for continuous delivery of O_2. Child can play in tent (toys inside). Safety precautions are necessary (plastic, sparks). Child resists separation from parents (see text for further discussion of developmental considerations)	Delivers oxygen and mist simultaneously and has a cooling mechanism. Approximate FiO_2 (0.4–0.5) can be provided by 6–10 L/min. Monitor temperature of infant (avoid overcooling). Check O_2 concentration. Keep edges of plastic tucked in well. Keep moisture off inside of tent for easy visibility. Parent teaching about the tent needed. Assess ongoing need for tent. Feeding can be done in the tent (see text for further discussion)

From Burgess, W. R., & Chernick, V. (1982). *Respiratory therapy in newborn infants and children.* New York: Thieme-Stratton; Glassamos, M. R. (1980, January/February). Infants who are oxygen-dependent—sending them home. *MCN: American Journal of Maternal Child Nursing,* pp 42–45; Voyles, J. B. (1981). Bronchopulmonary dysplasia. *American Journal of Nursing, 81*(3), 510–514.

* FiO_2 reading of 0.4 is the same as 40 per cent oxygen concentration; FiO_2 means "fraction of inspired oxygen."

† Flow rates to any mask must be sufficient to eliminate CO_2 accumulation (3–6 L/min depending on type of mask) (Burgess & Chernick, 1982).

Regardless of the equipment used to administer oxygen, some basic principles and nursing care considerations are common to all methods. Hospital oxygen is derived from compressed tank sources and is desiccated. If used directly, it would have a drying effect on the mucous membranes; therefore, it is humidified. In addition, dry oxygen induces bronchoconstriction and must be avoided. Home oxygen at a flow of less than 1 L/min is generally not humidified. Whenever possible, oxygen is analyzed with an analyzer to determine the actual percentage of oxygen inspired. The number of liters at which the flow meter is set is adjusted to maintain the desired oxygen concentration for inhalation. When oxygen concentration is analyzed, the measurement should be done close to the child's mouth and nose (that is, the air the child is actually inhaling).

Care of the Child in a Tent. A popular method of delivering a low-to-moderate concentration of oxygen is via a mist tent, known in pediatrics as a "croup tent." A tent is designed to provide an enclosed space in which a child can rest comfortably and breathe in air with a higher oxygen concentration than room air. A tent may be used to deliver oxygen *and* humidity or *only* humidity.

Humidity refers to the amount of water vapor present in a gas. Devices that add water vapor (humidity) to a gas are humidifiers. The amount of humidity that can be contained in a gas is proportional to the temperature of the gas. (As temperature increases, the water content of air increases.) A common way to provide humidity in the home is to use a room vaporizer or to run a hot shower in the bathroom.

In the hospital, mist tent therapy is used for the treatment of various respiratory problems. Humidity is thought to prevent water loss and mobilize secretions. The droplets produced by mist therapy vary according to the type of equipment used.

If only humidity is required, then the tent is connected to an air outlet rather than to oxygen. When oxygen is required, the level of concentration that can be maintained is directly related to the number and length of times that a tent is opened. An environment of up to 50 per cent oxygen concentration can be maintained if leaks are minimized. Careful tucking-in of the canopy under the mattress on both sides and at the upper end of the crib is necessary to achieve a high concentration. Nursing care must be organized effectively to avoid repeated opening of the tent. Using the side zippers rather than lifting the tent is one way to prevent repeated escape of large amounts of oxygen. Excessive amounts of oxygen can accumulate; therefore, the oxygen concentration should be routinely measured with an oxygen analyzer.

Numerous safety hazards accompany the use of oxygen tents. If a high-humidity environment is also desired, mist and droplets on the inside of the tent may interfere with the nurse's observation of the child's condition. If the mist cannot be reduced, it may be necessary to wipe the inside of the tent periodically. A tent is usually cooled by means of ice or a refrigeration unit, the goal being to maintain an environment cooler than room air. A small infant could easily be overcooled; therefore, the child's temperature must be carefully monitored because of the *high risk for altered body temperature,* including hypothermia. If the baby's temperature drops, oxygen and mist can be continued, but the refrigeration unit must be turned down; if a croupette with ice is being used, water is kept in the ice chamber, but no ice is added. Because of the blowing effect of the oxygen and the dampness resulting from humidity, a child should be dressed when in a tent. Linens and clothing must be changed frequently to prevent overcooling.

The usual safety precautions must be observed when oxygen is in use. No smoking is allowed in the room, and electrical devices like hair dryers and shavers should not be used inside the tent. Additionally, toys that produce sparks or "rev-up" toy trucks and cars should not be allowed inside the tent. The plastic canopy can be a hazard to young children, especially if they are agitated and try to get out of the tent. Keeping the tent tucked tightly under the mattress and tucking a folded sheet across the bottom of the tent help keep the plastic away from the child's face. The potential exists for nurses, physicians, and parents to walk away from a crib without putting up side rails, because the tent gives one the false impression that the child is enclosed, even though the rail is down. Side rails must be put all the way up as for any other child. The nurse should monitor parents and other professionals closely to ensure that they do not leave a side rail down. All of these precautions are interventions for the nursing diagnosis *high risk for injury.*

The willingness of a child to get into a tent varies according to the child's age and previous experiences, and the parents' reactions. The greatest source of discomfort that a tent creates is separation from parents. Additionally, an anxious parent contributes to the fear and distress and consequent inability to cope that a child experiences when enclosed inside the plastic walls of a tent. Various techniques can be tried to get the child to stay in the tent. First, it is important to elicit the parents' cooperation. A brief explanation about the need for oxygen and mist should be given to the parents. The toddler and preschooler may be fearful about the noise the tent makes and need assurance that no part of the machine is hurtful. While the child is being placed into the tent, the parent is encouraged to remain at the bedside within the child's field of vision. Furthermore, the nurse and the parents reassure the child that the parent will stay, if this is possible. Permitting the child to take a favorite toy or blanket inside the tent can also provide some security. If a young child is screaming excessively after being put into the tent, the parent is encouraged to reach through the side of the tent and stroke the child's head or back. One must not keep taking the child out each time he or she cries. By doing so, one is inadvertently rewarding the child for crying and conditioning the child to expect removal from the tent by crying long and hard. The nurse's collaboration with the parents is a major element in gaining the cooperation of the child. Parental suggestions of techniques to keep the child in the tent are elicited and used as appropriate.

In the early stages of illness, it may be necessary to feed the child in the tent. The child can be assisted by an adult reaching into the tent or lifting the canopy up and leaning into the tent. The decision to begin feeding the child outside the tent is frequently made by the nurse in collaboration with the physician. It should be recognized that sucking requires energy and increases the demand for oxygen *(high risk for impaired gas exchange);* therefore, infants must be evaluated and monitored closely when taken out of the tent for feeding. As soon as the infant can tolerate being out of the tent, parents should be encouraged to hold and feed their child to re-establish the patterns of care that provide comfort and security to the infant. The child may require oxygen per nasal cannula when out of the tent for feeding.

Low Flow Oxygen Therapy. Low flow oxygen therapy is a method of oxygen delivery for infants and children who are oxygen-dependent for prolonged periods and do not require high oxygen concentration. Low flow oxygen is delivered by hood, by nasal cannula (a feeding tube inserted 1 to 2 cm into one or two nostrils), or by a catheter placed on the philtrum without entering the nares (catheter with two holes in a horizontal position below the child's nostrils) (Fig. 32–4). This is sometimes called a moustache catheter because of its position. Taping the catheter on the side of a baby's face may be problematic because of skin excoriation. Stoma adhesive, which needs to be changed only once a week, has been recommended as an effective alternative (Fig. 32–5), and, for older children, a child's cap can be used to stabilize the cannula (Fig. 32–6).

Low flow oxygen is used when oxygen requirements are less than 55 per cent and when the infant weighs more than 1500 g. The difficulty in its use is that the exact amount of inspired oxygen is not known. When oxygen is delivered by hood or Isolette, oxygen concentration can be measured by using an oxygen analyzer. In the case of the nasal or moustache catheter, 100 per cent oxygen is delivered via a flow meter, and oxygen tubing is attached to the nasal catheter. The infant is breathing predominantly room air, and the actual inspired oxygen concentration is unknown.

The danger of this technique is that the inspired oxygen concentration (FiO_2) may be unnecessarily high or too low in the infant whose oxygen requirements are greater than the inspired concentration. The

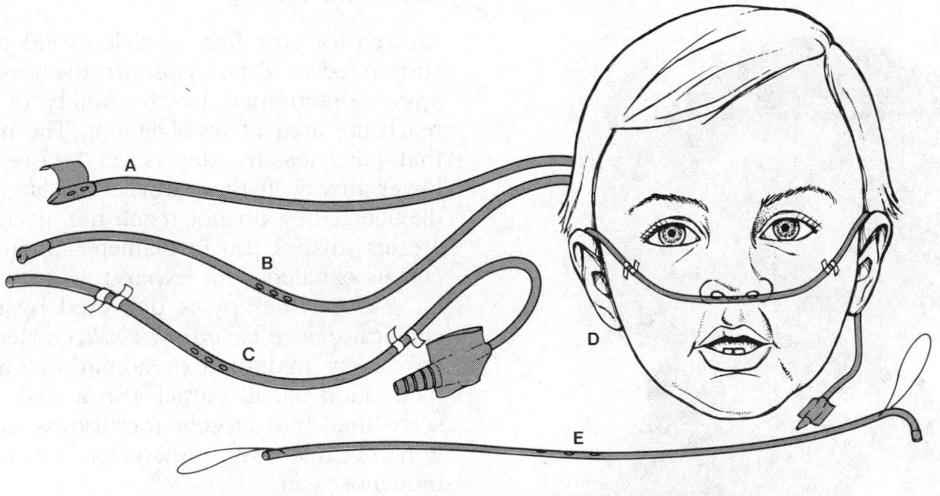

A. Occlude all the holes on a small feeding or suction catheter with tape.

B. Cut three to four small holes in catheter. Judge placement of holes by measuring from front of baby's ear to nares.

C. Place tape on cannula so that it can be attached to the baby's face. Make sure the holes point upward toward nares.

D. Paint area under tape with tincture of benzoin to protect the skin. Tape on one side of face, pull cannula tight, and secure on other side to prevent cannula from rolling over.

E. Attach umbilical or twill tape to the ends of the cannula and fit around the ears for an older child who is receiving long-term oxygen therapy.

FIGURE 32-4. How to devise your own nasal cannula.

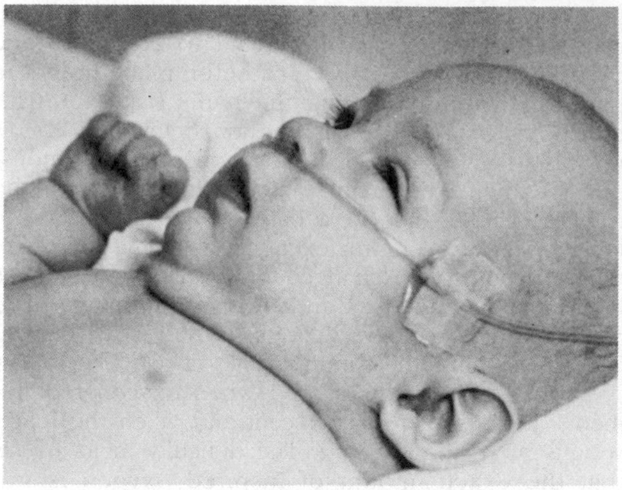

FIGURE 32-5. Five-month-old boy with bronchopulmonary dysplasia, illustrating the use of stoma adhesive to secure the cannula for continuous low flow oxygen therapy. The cannula is positioned on the philtrum without entering the nares. (From Koops, B. L., et al. [1984, February]. Outpatient management and follow-up of bronchopulmonary dysplasia. *Clinics in Perinatology,* pp 101–122.)

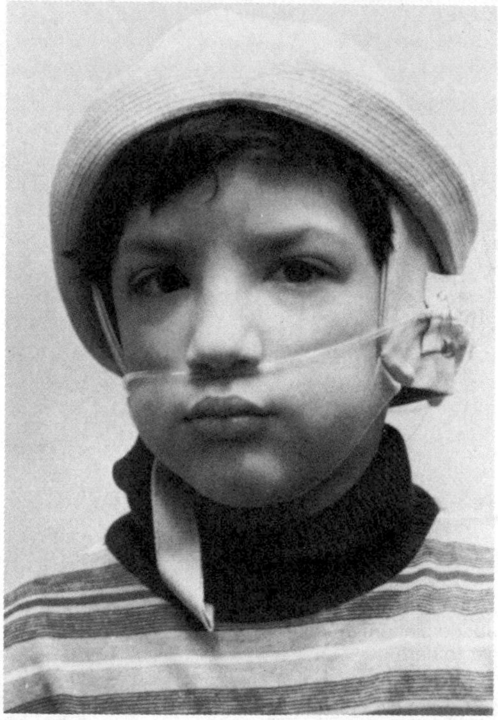

FIGURE 32-6. Four-year-old boy with bronchopulmonary dysplasia, illustrating the use of a cap to secure the cannula for continuous low flow oxygen therapy. The cannula is positioned on the philtrum without entering the nares. (From Koops, B. L., et al. [1984, February]. Outpatient management and follow-up of bronchopulmonary dysplasia. *Clinics in Perinatology,* pp 101–122.)

recommended range of low flow oxygen is from 0.05 to 0.5 L/min if a nasal catheter is used. (These low flow rates require special flow meters, as the usual hospital flow meter is inaccurate in these ranges.) When labial or moustache catheters are used, higher flow rates (1 to 3 L/min) are required and can be administered by the usual hospital flow meter. When hoods are used, the flow rate is also higher, with the flow meter being graduated from 3 to 10 L/min (Monin & Vert, 1987).

Home Use of Low Flow Oxygen. Home care on low flow oxygen is widespread in current practice. Recommended criteria for discharge on low flow oxygen vary and include postconceptual age greater than 41 weeks, a weight above 2000 g and an otherwise medically stable condition, absence of any change in FiO_2 or medications (diuretics) during the few days prior to discharge, absence of high pulmonary arterial blood pressure, acceptance by parents, a community support system (physician and community health nurse), a satisfactory home assessment by a health care professional, and the presence of more than one adult in the home (Monin & Vert, 1987). Intensive predischarge teaching and follow-up care are essential for home management of infants on low-flow oxygen. Most of the time parents are taught to assess clinical symptoms and adjust FiO_2 accordingly, within certain parameters.

Aerosol Therapy

An aerosol is a fine particle (solid or liquid) that is suspended in a gas. The effectiveness of aerosol therapy is determined by the ability of the particles to reach the area of involvement. The major difficulty is that particles are deposited before they reach the lower airway. If the particles are larger than 3 μm* in diameter, they do not reach the alveolar level; if they are less than 1 μm in diameter, approximately 90 per cent is exhaled with expired air.

Aerosol therapy is delivered by means of a mechanical device called a *nebulizer.* Nebulizers are used for airway hydration or administration of aerosolized medication (small particles in a gas). One should observe the child closely for distress during aerosolization, because any aerosolized substance may cause bronchospasm.

Aerosol therapy may be administered *continuously* or *intermittently.* Continuous aerosolization can be provided by a nebulizer device in a tent. Intermittent therapy can be administered via the aerosol mask. Such a device consists of a nebulizer attached to a mask. The aerosolization is produced by either a flow meter or a compressor. Hand-held devices, called *metered-dose inhalers,* also can be used (see following section, "Home Use of the Nebulizer") (Fig. 32–7).

* 0.001 mm = 1 micrometer (μm).

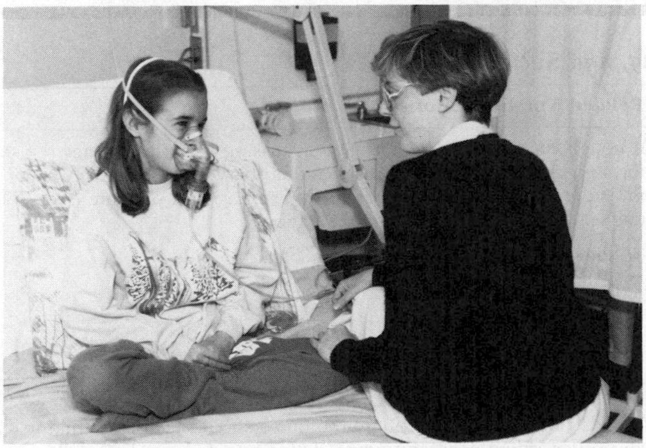

FIGURE 32-7. Intermittent aerosol therapy by mask is common for children hospitalized for respiratory conditions. This 11-year-old girl has cystic fibrosis and is highly accustomed to this therapy.

An *ultrasonic nebulizer* is an electrically powered device that produces a vibration by means of a transducer, resulting in a particle that averages approximately 3 μm in diameter. It has been used in the treatment of illnesses like cystic fibrosis, in which secretions are thick and tenacious. Although this device is highly efficient, absorption of water and fluid overload are hazards in small infants and children. Mobilization of secretions via ultrasonic nebulization should be accompanied by attempts to evacuate the secretions in order to prevent their accumulation and resultant ineffective airway clearance. This form of therapy can be delivered by tent (usually only at night to prevent overhydration) or by intermittent ultrasonic nebulization treatments every 4 to 6 hours. Administration by tent requires a canopy that drapes over the crib, but it does not require tight tucking of plastic under the mattress. Therefore, physical contact with the infant is easy (Fig. 32–8).

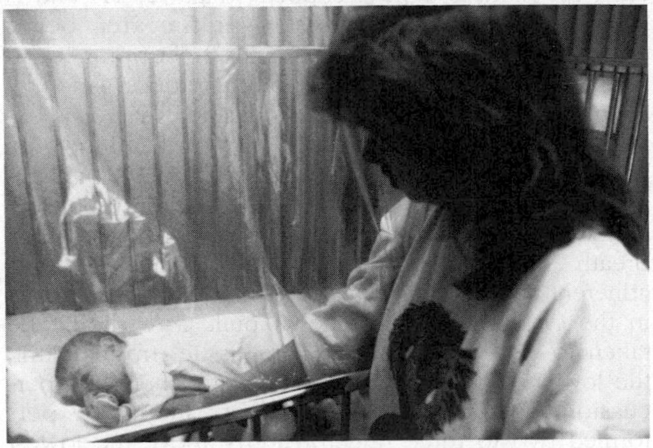

FIGURE 32-8. If time is taken to explain the purpose of therapy, parents become very effective in calming their infant who is in a tent.

Aerosol therapy is used in the treatment of upper and lower respiratory tract problems. The type of medication depends on the effect desired. Bronchodilators are the most common type. Others are mucolytic agents (propylene glycol, acetylcysteine [Mucomyst]), antibiotics, and expectorants.

The nurse collaborates with the respiratory therapist to ensure the safe and proper functioning of all equipment. A careful procedure for cleaning the equipment is important to decrease the potential for bacterial growth and transmission of pathogens.

Home Use of the Nebulizer. Older children can use the hand nebulizer, a device with a rubber bulb. When the bulb is compressed, the aerosolized medication is released and the child breathes in at the proper time. After inhaling the aerosol, the child is instructed to hold the breath 5 seconds and then repeat the procedure. Various portable inert gas nebulizers are available to deliver a premetered dose of the aerosol. They all require coordination of breathing with release of the medication. Nebulizers with a rebreathing chamber are called *aerochambers*. These are easier for children to use, because they do not require breathing in coordination with release of the medication.

Chest Physical Therapy

Chest physical therapy is a frequently used intervention in the pulmonary care of children when pulmonary secretions cannot be removed by the normal processes. It can include any or all of the following activities: deep breathing games or exercises, coughing, huffing, splinting, tracheal tickling, suctioning, postural drainage, percussion, and vibration. These techniques are used singly or in combination in an effort to assist the infant or child in clearing excess or abnormal secretions from the lungs and avoid ineffective airway clearance. The techniques in chest physical therapy often need to be modified for children because of their size and their inability to follow verbal instructions. Table 32–7 lists developmental considerations in breathing, coughing, and suctioning.

Techniques for Chest Physical Therapy

Chest physical therapy involves a combination of techniques, including (1) positioning (postural drainage), (2) mechanical stimulation of the chest (percussion and vibration), and (3) suctioning.

Postural Drainage. In postural drainage, the child is placed in a series of positions, so that gravity secretions from the periphery of the lung move centrally toward the trachea. There are 18 lung segments and 12 classic postural drainage positions. In each classic drainage position, one or more segmental bronchi are perpendicular to the floor, so that the force of gravity is optimal. Figures 32–9 and 32–10

TABLE 32-7
Nursing Interventions to Facilitate Deep Breathing, Coughing, and Suctioning

Developmental Considerations	Related Nursing Actions
Infants and young children do not understand the directions to take a deep breath or cough Even when the direction to take a deep breath and to cough is understood, child often needs to be encouraged to do so by being engaged in developmentally appropriate activities	A cough can be stimulated by slowly passing a sterile catheter through child's nose until it reaches the pharynx or trachea. A natural cough reflex can be stimulated by exerting firm pressure over trachea at sternal notch during expiration To facilitate deep breathing, the nurse can provide • Balloons • Soap bubbles • Incentive spirometry • Pinwheels • Variety of blowing games To facilitate an effective cough, the nurse should (1) place child in an upright sitting position to provide for maximal expansion of chest and mechanical advantage for abdominal muscles; (2) prepare child with appropriate pain medication and, in postoperative cases, splint the operative area with a pillow; and (3) demonstrate the desired cough and ask the child to imitate
Mucous membranes are thin and easily traumatized; special precautions must be taken in technique of suctioning	*Oral suctioning* Insert catheter at each side of the mouth and advance to the back of the mouth. Gently rotate catheter; do not poke in and out of back of mouth. Suction each area once and then reassess the child and allow rest. Repeat procedure only if secretions are abundant *Nasopharyngeal suctioning* Catheter is measured by spanning it from tip of child's nose to earlobe. The measured distance on catheter is inserted through one nostril, then the other, smoothly and gently. On withdrawal, suction is applied and catheter is rotated between the fingers. Avoid a jerky in-and-out motion. Assess respiratory status, and repeat procedure only if indicated *Nasotracheal suctioning* This potentially traumatizing procedure must be done with extreme caution (can result in laryngospasm and/or bradycardia). It is not a routine pediatric procedure but rather a specialized technique usually used for children in intensive care units

show correlation of the segment being drained and the position of the child. The recommended positions for a particular child will vary according to the lung segments most involved. Children are generally not able to tolerate more than four to six positions at one session; therefore, it may be necessary to rotate positions from one session to the next. For a young child, a comfortable position can be attained by placing him or her on a pillow while in bed or on the therapist's or parent's lap. A neonate in an Isolette can be positioned by using a rolled blanket and by raising and lowering the Isolette tray. With older children and adolescents, use of the knee gatch and pillows facilitates effective positioning for postural drainage. At home, an inverted chair, a home-made padded board, or a stack of newspapers with couch cushions over them may be used. A commercially made drainage board is available on the market.

Percussion. Percussion is performed intermittently during postural drainage to speed movement of the mucus. Percussion must always be comfortable for the child, so that deep breathing can continue throughout the postural drainage treatment. To protect the skin from irritation, the child's chest should be covered with a light cotton shirt and no rings or bracelets should be worn by the therapist or the nurse. To percuss, the hand is tightly "cupped" (Fig. 32–11) and is "clapped" against the chest over the area being drained. (Percussion is also called "cupping" and "clapping.") This procedure should produce a hollow sound (not a slapping sound), indicating that air is being compressed between the therapist's hand and the child's chest wall. The compression wave is presumably transmitted to the bronchi, stimulating turbulence in the air the child is moving in and out with each breath. The turbulent airflow catches the secretions adherent to bronchial walls and moves the secretions in the direction of gravitational pull. Care should be taken to percuss only over lung tissue. In an infant, the lower ribs cover liver and kidneys; therefore, percussion, even for the lower lobes, should be performed two to three fingerbreadths above the lowest rib. When the size of the infant's chest does not accommodate the therapist's hand, other means of percussion are used. To percuss an infant's chest, two or three fingers are tented together (Fig. 32–12), or a

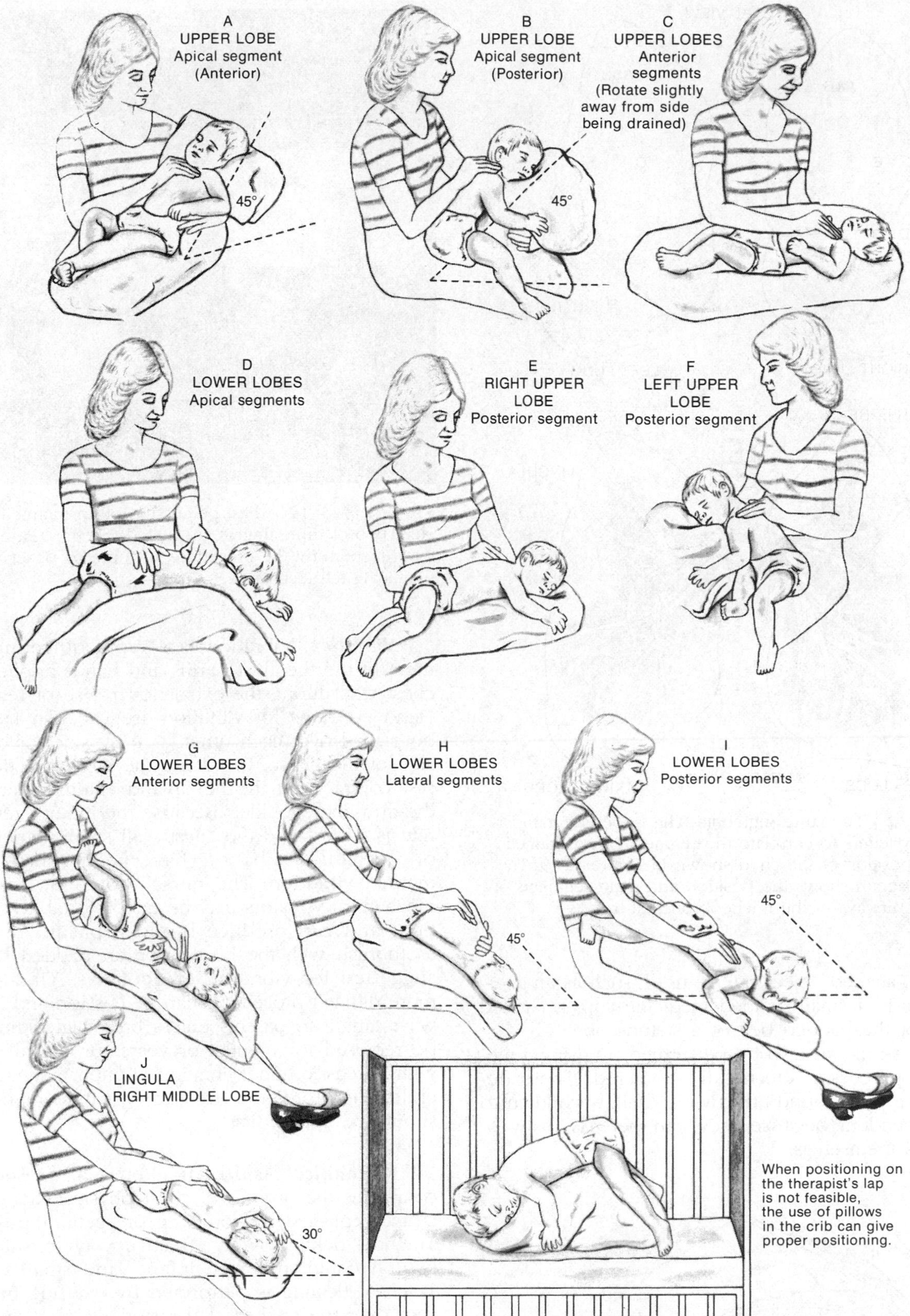

FIGURE 32-9. Postural drainage. The positions for postural drainage are correlated with the segment being drained (see Fig. 32–10). In positions *H* and *J*, the child is shown on the right side; however, the boy must also be turned to the left side to drain both lobes. (Adapted from materials used by the Chest Physical Therapy Department, Physical Therapy Division, Department of Physical Medicine and Rehabilitation, Hospital of the University of Michigan, Ann Arbor, Michigan.)

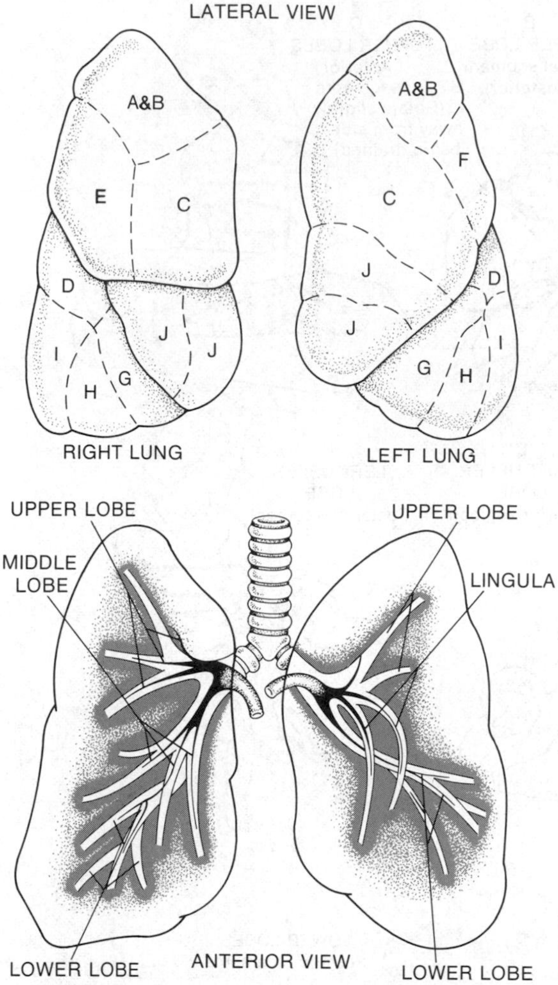

FIGURE 32-10. Lung segments. The upper diagram is labeled by letters to correlate the segment being drained with the position of the child shown in Figure 32–9. The bottom diagram shows the position and main segments of the lower airways of the tracheobronchial tree.

small cup-shaped object can be used, such as an anesthesia mask, a small padded medicine cup, a padded nipple, or the padded bell of a stethoscope.

Percussion can also be performed by using a mechanical percussor, electrically powered. These devices have been found effective and allow children to be independent because they can percuss many of the lobes themselves.

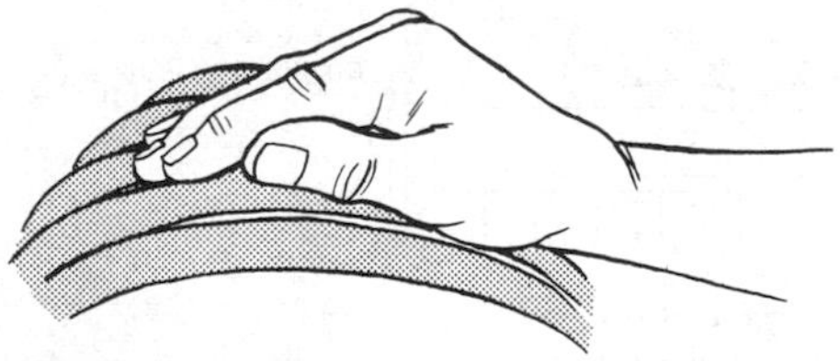

FIGURE 32-11. Position of hand cupped for percussion. The wrist movement involves a brisk relaxed flexion and extension. The examiner should be careful not to use only the fingers or only the heel of the hand.

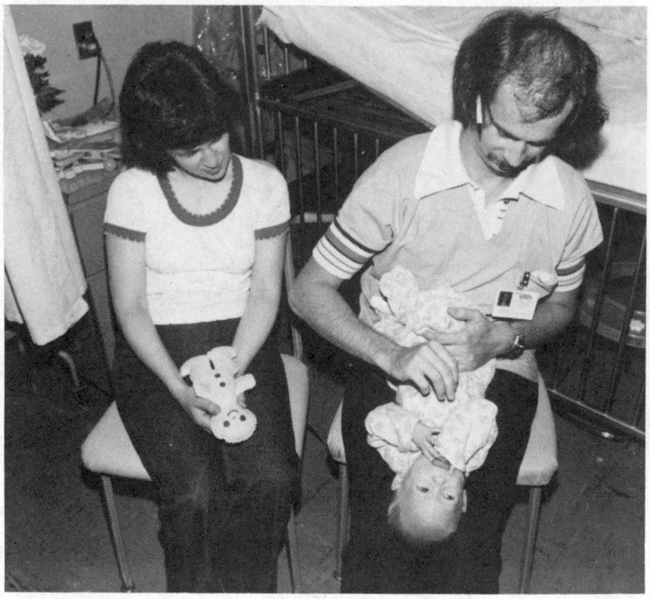

FIGURE 32-12. Chest percussion of an infant. To percuss, two or three fingers are tented together. Parents can learn to perform the procedure at home by observing and practicing the technique.

Vibration. Vibration is a rapid quivering movement of the therapist's arms and hands applied to the chest wall during the exhalation phase of respiration. Hand positions for vibration are variable; hands can be placed over each other, side by side, or on either side of the chest. To initiate the vibration, the therapist contracts all the flexor and extensor muscles of the arm and shoulder. Because the infant's respiratory rate is so fast and the chest wall small, various types of mechanical vibrators have been substituted for manual vibration. The nurse should be aware that mechanical vibrators may be uncomfortable to the patient and can produce bronchospasm. An electric toothbrush with the bristle portion padded has been suggested for vibration of neonates. Vibration is a more difficult procedure than percussion and is not always taught to parents unless bronchial drainage will be required for months or years. Bronchial drainage with percussion and vibration is often fatiguing to the child; therefore, the areas of greatest involvement should be treated first.

Mechanical Aspiration. Removal of secretions completes the process of chest physical therapy. This is accomplished by coughing or suctioning, or both. Tracheal tickling is an effective way to stimulate a natural cough reflex in infants and small children. Tracheal tickling is performed by exerting firm pressure over the trachea at the sternal notch during expiration. If secretions cannot be removed by coughing, mechanical aspiration is indicated.

Prior to suctioning, the amount of negative pressure produced by the suction apparatus must be checked. This is done by clamping off the tubing (i.e., producing suction) and noting on the dial the amount of negative pressure produced. Infants require 80 to 100 mmHg negative pressure. For older children, 100 mmHg negative pressure is usually sufficient, but up to 120 mmHg is within a safe range.

Safety precautions include (1) use of sterile technique (at home, clean technique is adequate), (2) application of suction on withdrawal only, and (3) gentle and quick suctioning to avoid hypoxia and apnea. The catheter is removed in one continuous motion as it is pill-rolled between the thumb and forefinger to avoid trauma to the mucosa. Catheters used on infants may induce a vagal response causing apnea and bradycardia; therefore, a bulb syringe may be preferred. Also, prolonged suctioning under any circumstances is to be avoided without bagging (giving oxygen via an Ambu bag) in between, or else the lungs are deflated merely by aspirating the air.

Nursing Care

The nurse participates in chest physical therapy in a variety of ways, depending on the patient's needs and the setting. Nurses may be in complete charge of carrying out the procedures; however, in many centers a respiratory therapist performs the procedures and plays a major role in teaching the family. Regardless of the type of setting, the nurse retains responsibility for the total care of the child. This means that the nurse should listen to chest sounds to identify any child who could benefit from chest physical therapy. The nurse evaluates the effectiveness of chest physical therapy and assists the physical therapist in teaching the family the necessary home program. Furthermore, the nurse checks that the chest physical therapy is being done and that it is being coordinated with other treatments the patient is receiving. For example, if a child requires a bronchodilator, it should be given prior to physical therapy. If the child requires an inhaled antibiotic, it should be administered following physical therapy. Chest physical therapy is usually done two to three times a day and should be done before meals and at bedtime. Unless contraindicated, the child is encouraged to drink fluids to help liquefy pulmonary secretions.

The treatment is documented in the medical record by the nurse or respiratory therapist. Notes should include response to treatment, amount and type of secretions, duration of the treatment, the lung segments being drained, and a statement about the participation of the patient and parents.

Parents need to understand the purpose of each of the chest physical therapy procedures and the benefit their child can derive from them. The nurse and physical therapist involve the parents in the care of their child, so that they learn to perform the chest physical therapy techniques effectively. If a home program is necessary, the parents are given written guidelines before discharge, including illustrations of the various positions. The nurse can also assist the family by demonstrating with puppets, dolls, horns, balloons, and bubbles. Parents of a critically ill child need information and support from the health care team, especially if the child is in pain or resistive to parts of the treatment program.

Incentive Spirometry

Incentive spirometry uses specially designed devices to effect maximal inspiration that results in optimal lung inflation. This technique is useful only in the treatment of older children, because it requires the child's cooperation.

The devices that have been designed provide immediate feedback to the child and provide some entertainment as well. They have a preset volume that must be reached to accomplish the goal. The goal varies with the particular model of equipment used. In one device, the child's inspiration illuminates a clown's nose; in another one, it lifts a colored ball in a plastic column. The preset volume can be adjusted from time to time to increase the inspiratory flow required. The number of times that the child is asked to perform incentive spirometry varies according to the condition of the child. Performing the activity five to six times every 2 hours is usually tolerated. If the procedure is explained and the child is not forced to the point of exhaustion, cooperation is usual. If this form of therapy is to be used postoperatively, the child should practice the maneuver before undergoing surgery.

Breathing Exercises

Breathing exercises can be taught to older children and are employed particularly in chronic lung problems (cystic fibrosis, asthma). The purpose is to promote a normal pattern of breathing through the correct use of the diaphragm and to avoid involving the accessory muscles of respiration (scalene, intercostal, sternocleidomastoid, trapezius, and pectoral). A common breathing exercise that is taught to children is diaphragmatic breathing. To teach a child diaphragmatic breathing, do the following:

- Place child in semi-Fowler position with knees flexed.
- Place one hand on upper chest and one on abdomen to feel movement of air.
- Instruct child to breathe in gently.
- Instruct child to exhale through pursed lips (this produces back pressure on the airway and holds the airway open, allowing exhalation of air trapped in alveoli). Press gently with both hands during expiration.
- Emphasize relaxation of shoulders and upper chest throughout respiration.

Once the technique is mastered in the semi-Fowler position, it is practiced in other positions, so that it can be performed while sitting or walking and especially during episodes of dyspnea.

Maintaining Airway of the Child with Tracheostomy

A tracheostomy is a surgical procedure of cutting into the trachea through the neck. It is performed for three major reasons: when an obstruction in the upper respiratory tract prevents adequate flow of oxygen through the trachea, to allow for chronic mechanical ventilation, and to allow a way for care providers to remove aspirated oral secretions by suctioning, for children with chronic aspiration. An indwelling tracheostomy tube is placed to keep the artificial tracheal opening patent. (See Figure 32–13.)

Tracheal tubes are made of soft, pliable materials that comfortably conform to the contour of the trachea. Most tubes for children today do not have an inner cannula. The inner cannula is unnecessary, because the smooth plastic surface reduces collection of secretions and crust formation.

Maintaining Skin Integrity. Generally, it is not beneficial to place a gauze pad between the skin and the tube, since secretions gather here and wetness can cause skin breakdown. If secretions are heavy, patting the area dry with gauze is preferred. The skin

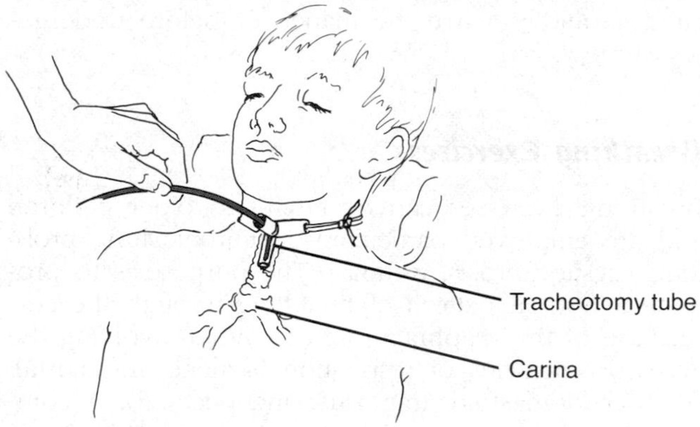

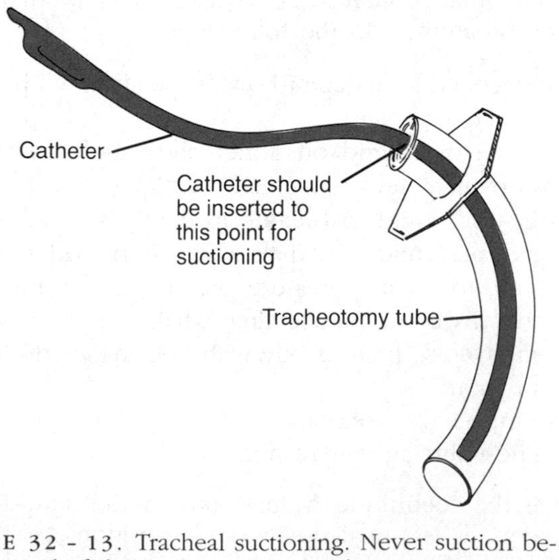

FIGURE 32 - 13. Tracheal suctioning. Never suction below the end of the tracheotomy tube, because it can cause severe damage to the tracheobronchial tree.

around the tracheostomy is kept clean and inspected for excoriation. Dip a Q-tip into a half-strength hydrogen peroxide (H_2O_2) solution, roll over the skin under the tube to remove crusted secretions, rinse by using a Q-tip dipped in clear water, and dry. Powders and lotions are not recommended, and any prescribed ointment is applied sparingly. It has been suggested that stoma adhesive is effective in protecting the skin.

Safety Issues. Infants and young children may need to be restrained (elbow restraints are preferable to wrist restraints) to prevent pulling at the tracheal tube. Special precaution is taken that children do not play with small toys or toys with removable parts that could be inserted into the tracheal tube. The tube must be protected from food spillage during mealtime with a bib that fits the contour of the neck and has short ties. For infants with particularly chubby necks, a small towel rolled to support the neck prevents occlusion of the opening by skinfolds. Aerosols are not recommended around children since they have no way of filtering the air they breath directly into the tracheostomy. Cigarette smoke is a severe airway irritant and should be kept away from these children.

A bath is permitted, but children are supervised to ensure that water does not enter the trachea. Showers are not recommended (Lichtenstein, 1986).

Humidification to Prevent Drying. The normal process of filtering, warming, and humidification of air by the upper airway is bypassed when a tracheostomy is necessary. Air can be humidified in a variety of ways, depending on the age and mobility of the child. A mist tent or a collar (special mask) is placed over the tracheostomy opening, or a mechanical ventilator may be used. Humidification prevents drying of the tissues and aids in loosening secretions. A device known as an "artificial nose" can be placed over the opening of the tracheostomy tube. The child breathes in and out through the device, and air is warmed and humidified.

Assessment for Signs of Obstruction. The nurse frequently checks a child with a tracheostomy to detect the need for suctioning. An increased pulse, restlessness, bubbling of secretions from the tracheostomy, changes in color (cyanosis or pallor), dyspnea, retractions, and noisy respirations are indications that the child's airway is being partially occluded with secretions. Infants and children require constant surveillance to identify these signs. Adults and older children have various means of summoning help. Infants or young children have only a cry to alert the caregiver to discomfort; with a tracheostomy, the cry is silent, since the vocal cords are not vibrated by air moving through them. Consequently, these children must be placed where the nurse can easily see their movements at all times. It is also recommended that infants and young children with tracheostomies be placed on an apnea monitor to signal breathing problems.

Emergency equipment—including an extra tracheostomy tube and equipment, a suction machine, suction catheters, and obturator—is kept at the bedside.

Suctioning Through a Tracheostomy. A child's vulnerability to infection is great; therefore, sterile technique must be carefully observed and trauma to the tissues must be minimized. Bagging (giving oxygen via bag and mask) is sometimes necessary between repeated suctionings, if the child becomes compromised during the suctioning procedure. Although the exact procedure may vary, the following guidelines can be used for suctioning infants and children:

1. Sterile technique is used to prevent secondary infection.
2. Normal saline solution, 0.5 to 2 ml, may be instilled into the trachea just before suctioning to loosen secretions. (If a child requires bagging, saline solution is instilled just before bagging.) This may produce coughing or gagging.
3. After saline solution is instilled, the child should be suctioned with a sterile catheter moistened by saline.
4. The suction catheter should be inserted (without applying suction) the length of the tracheostomy tube. This should be measured against a tube of the same size at the child's bedside. Suction is then applied intermittently (80 to 100 mmHg) as the catheter is withdrawn in a continuous rotating motion. Withdrawing the catheter should take approximately 5 seconds (see Fig. 32–13).
5. Between suctionings, the child should be allowed to take a few breaths and rest. If necessary, the child may need to be bagged. The care provider should listen for secretions and assess whether the child needs repeated suctioning. Auscultation to listen for air exchange and evaluation of the child's general condition should be part of the assessment.
6. The child is allowed to rest, the chest is auscultated to listen for air exchange, and the child's general condition is evaluated before the procedure is repeated.
7. It also may be necessary occasionally to suction the oropharynx to remove accumulated secretions.
8. The suction catheter should be rinsed with normal saline between passes to clear the tube of secretions.
9. The suction tube and glove are discarded after each use.

Suctioning is done only as needed. If a child has an adequate cough, she or he should be encouraged to do so to clear secretions. Most commonly, suctioning may be necessary in the morning, before meals, and at bedtime. The color, quantity, consistency, and odor of secretions are noted. Infection in the trachea or lungs results in a yellowish to green color change in the mucus and causes it to have an odor. Blood-tinged mucus can indicate that suctioning is done too frequently or with too great a negative pressure. Pressure is the same as for nasopharyngeal suctioning (80 to 100 mmHg for infants and 100 to 120 for older children). Signs of infection should be reported to the physician, as the child may need antibiotic treatment.

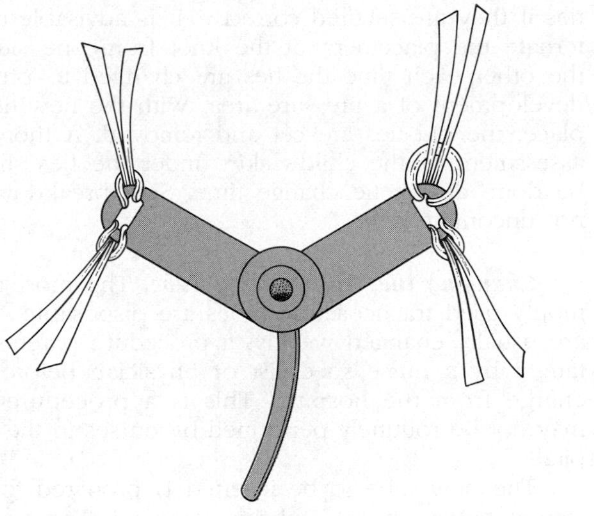

FIGURE 32-14. A lark knot.

Changing the Tracheostomy Ties. The tracheostomy tube is kept in place by securing it with ties. Twill tape is attached to the wings of the tracheostomy tube and firmly secured around the child's neck. Various methods are used to attach the twill tape to the tube wings. Some recommend securing it with a lark knot (Fig. 32–14), and others simply thread it through the tube wing holes (Fig. 32–15). In both methods, the free ends are secured with a square knot on the side of the child's neck. (Tying at the back of a child's neck may cause confusion with the ties of a gown or bib.)

Two people are required to change the ties. The child is positioned by elevating the shoulders slightly with a pad or blanket roll to expose the tracheostomy area. The old ties are slid to the upper edge of the tube wings (on both sides) so that new ties can be threaded through the wing holes by using a lark knot (Fig. 32–14). The new ties are then secured with a square knot. One finger should fit snugly under the

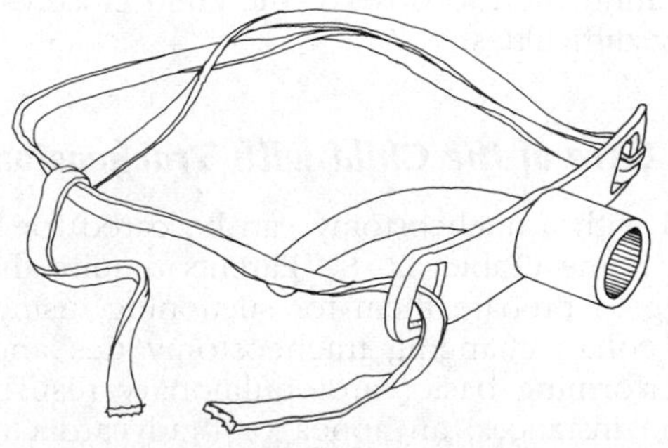

FIGURE 32-15. Placement of tie for tracheal tube. (From Hughes, W., & Buescher, E. [1980]. *Pediatric procedures* [p. 229]. Philadelphia: WB Saunders.

ties if they are secured correctly. It is advisable to alternate the placement of the knot from one side to the other each time the ties are changed to prevent development of a pressure area. With the new ties in place, the old ties are cut and removed. A thorough assessment of the child's skin under the ties should be done during tie change time. Skin breakdown is not uncommon.

Changing the Tracheostomy Tube. The most commonly used tracheostomy tubes are disposable. They are usually changed weekly, a procedure parents are taught by a nurse specialist or physician before discharge from the hospital. This is a procedure that may not be routinely performed by nurses in the hospital.

The new tube to be inserted is prepared for insertion before the old tube is removed. The ties are attached through the tracheostomy wings, an obturator is inserted into the tube, and the tube's sterility is maintained for insertion. A sterile, *water-soluble* lubricant should be spread on the bottom 2 to 3 cm of the tube to ease insertion. With the new tube ready for insertion, the old ties are cut and the tube removed. The new tube is then inserted, directed backward, then downward. The old tube is drawn out with one hand, and the new tube is in the other hand ready for immediate insertion. The old tube is inspected for any odor, mucous plugs, and any color change of mucus.

Decannulation. The tracheostomy tube is generally removed when it is no longer needed (e.g., the child is off the ventilator, the obstruction is relieved). Some children need their tracheostomies for a lifetime. There are many options for decannulation. "Downsizing" from the original size tube to a smaller tube size is one option. When the smallest size is reached, the tube may be plugged to see how the child does breathing through the upper airway. If this is well tolerated, the tube is removed and the stoma closes in a few weeks. Air leakage through the wound is not uncommon but generally ceases within 72 hours after removal of the plugged tube. Often a bronchoscopy is done prior to decannulation to evaluate the child's airway before the tube is removed. At least 24 to 48 hours of hospitalization is required after decannulation to observe the child closely for respiratory difficulties.

Home Care of the Child with Tracheostomy

A child with a tracheostomy can be cared for by parents at home (Table 32–8). Parents require thorough teaching to prepare them for suctioning, using a humidity collar, changing tracheostomy ties and tube, and performing basic cardiopulmonary resuscitation. In some instances, an apnea or bradycardia monitor is recommended, although this practice varies.

TABLE 32-8
Family-Centered Teaching: Tracheostomy Home Care—Developmental/Safety Considerations

Play
Avoid use of toys with small removable parts
Avoid use of stuffed animals and furry toys
Instruct other children not to put toys, food, or other small objects into the tracheostomy tube
Feeding
Prevent food from entering tracheostomy by using a bib (placed loosely to avoid occlusion)
Position infant on side after eating to prevent aspiration
Environment
Stay with the child during bathing or playing in a wading pool (humidity collar or an artificial nose can be used to protect the tracheostomy from water splashes)
Protect child from irritants (hair sprays, talcum powder, perfume, smoke, and ammonia products)
Avoid exposure to extremely cold air (it causes tracheal spasm) and dust particles (tracheostomy can be loosely covered on extremely cold or dusty, windy days)
Clothing
Keep clothing away from airway (light covering used to prevent extreme cold, irritants, food, or dust from entering tracheostomy)

Emergency telephone numbers should always be posted by the telephone. If the airway becomes obstructed, parents are taught to attempt to clear it by suction, but if this is not successful the tube must be changed. The child's breathing is evaluated by placing an ear over the tracheostomy and watching the chest for respiratory movements. If the child does not respond after a new tube is inserted, the child's nose and mouth are covered with one hand and four quick puffs of air are given by placing the mouth over the tracheostomy to form a seal. Cardiopulmonary resuscitation is instituted by giving one breath to five compressions.

Nursing Care

Assessment of the respiratory status of a child is one of the most frequently performed functions of a nurse. See Chapter 13 for the review of systems and how to perform a physical assessment of the chest and lungs (observation, palpation, percussion, and auscultation). Table 32–9 is designed for general care of the child with respiratory illness. It augments the discussions of specific nursing care for disease entities in this chapter.

TABLE 32-9

Nursing Process Plan: The Child with Oxygenation Problems

Oxygenation problems can occur in patients for a variety of reasons. Whether the antecedent of the problem is vascular, cardiac, or respiratory, similar conditions may result and care will be the same. In this nursing process plan, related nursing diagnostic statements and collaborative problems are treated simultaneously. Nursing diagnostic statements 1 through 6 and collaborative problem 1 are treated first.

Analysis: Nursing Diagnostic Statement 1

Response and Related or Risk Factors: *Ineffective airway clearance, related to*

- Obstructed nares
- Increased mucous production
- Inadequate expectoration of mucus
- Pooling of secretions in dependent lobes of lungs associated with immobility and pull of gravity

Projected Outcome: The child will be able to clear secretions or obstructions from the respiratory tract to maintain airway patency

Analysis: Collaborative Problem Statement 1

Response and Related or Risk Factors: *Altered tissue perfusion, related to*

- Fear/anxiety
- Impaired gas exchange
- Decreased cardiac output

Projected Outcome: The child will experience adequate nutrition and oxygenation at the cellular level. The capillary blood supply will be within normal limits

Analysis: Nursing Diagnostic Statement 2

Response and Related or Risk Factors: *High risk for suffocation; risk factors*

- Ineffective airway clearance
- Impaired gas exchange
- Ineffective breathing patterns

Projected Outcome: There will be adequate air available for inhalation

Analysis: Nursing Diagnostic Statement 3

Response and Related Risk Factors: *High risk for aspiration; risk factors*

- Hemorrhage
- Ineffective airway clearance
- Immobility

Projected Outcome: The child's tracheobronchial passages will remain patent without entry of gastrointestinal secretions, oropharyngeal secretions, solids, or fluids into them

Analysis: Nursing Diagnostic Statement 4

Response and Related or Risk Factors: *High risk for ineffective breathing pattern; risk factors*

- Impaired gas exchange
- Anxiety

(continued)

TABLE 32-9 (continued)

Projected Outcome: The child's inhalation and exhalation patterns will enable adequate pulmonary inflation or emptying

Analysis: Nursing Diagnostic Statement 5

Response and Related or Risk Factors: *Impaired physical mobility and fatigue, related to activity intolerance secondary to*

- Altered cardiac output

Projected Outcome: The child will be able to have some independent physical movement; the child will be rested enough to have capacity for age-appropriate physical and mental activity

Analysis: Nursing Diagnostic Statement 6

Response and Related or Risk Factors: *High risk for altered growth and development; risk factors*

- Inadequate tissue perfusion to promote healthy tissue growth
- Lack of energy to accomplish developmental tasks (partially secondary to nutritional deficit)

Projected Outcome: The child will grow and develop according to developmental norms

Defining Characteristics	Nursing Interventions	Evaluation Criteria
Ineffective Airway Clearance *Objective:* • Abnormal breath sounds • Changes in rate or depth of respiration • Tachypnea • Cough, effective/ineffective, with or without sputum • Cyanosis • Dyspnea ***Altered Tissue Perfusion*** *Objective:* • Cold extremities • Dependent blue or purple skin • Skin pale on elevation, and color does not return on lowering • Diminished arterial pulsation • Skin shiny • Lack of lanugo • Gangrene • Slow-growing, dry brittle nails • Claudication • Blood pressure changes in extremities	*Surveillance* **Assess air exchange** • Take vital signs and auscultate chest every 2–4 hrs as dictated for respiratory distress and fluctuations in temperature • Monitor for and immediately report to physician the signs of impending respiratory failure: increasing pallor or cyanosis; fatigue; restlessness; significant tachypnea (>60 breaths/min at rest for an infant) or an increase of ≥10 breaths/min at rest in an older child; tachycardia > 160–170 beats/min at rest for an infant) or an increase of ≥20 beats/min at rest for an older child; $Po_2 < 70$ mmHg; decreasing breath sounds **Institute measures to facilitate air exchange; balance activity and rest** (to reduce metabolic O_2 needs) • Assess child's tolerance of activity by checking pulse, respirations, and color before, during, and after activity such as crying, feeding, bathing • Allow time between activities for	**The child will achieve optimal air exchange, as evidenced by** • Pulse and respirations within normal limits for age or at normal baseline for child • Breath sounds clear and equal • Color pink (or normal for race) • Absence of retractions and nasal flaring • No abnormal increase in pulse or heart rate, nor unusual fatigue with activity that is appropriate to age • Arterial blood gases within normal limits **The child will experience no observable increase in respiratory distress related to mucus, as evidenced by** • No observable increase in mucous production or dyspnea

TABLE 32-9 *(continued)*

Defining Characteristics	Nursing Interventions	Evaluation Criteria
• Bruits • Slow healing lesions • See NANDA (1992) for additional information regarding definitions ***Ineffective Breathing Pattern*** Objective: • Dyspnea • Shortness of breath • Tachypnea • Fremitus • Abdominal arterial blood gas • Cyanosis • Cough • Nasal flaring • Respiratory depth changes • Assumption of three-point position • Pursed-lip breathing, prolonged expiratory phase • Increased anteroposterior diameter • Use of accessory muscles • Altered chest excursion • Seeming short of breath while feeding and at rest • Sweating with feeding and at rest • Having a weak cry • Poor weight gain ***Impaired Physical Mobility*** Objective: • Inability to purposefully move within the physical environment, including bed mobility, transfer, and ambulation • Reluctance to attempt movement • Limited range of motion • Decreased muscle strength, control and/or mass • Imposed restrictions of movement, including mechanical, medical protocol	vital signs to return to baseline and for child to recover from fatigue *Anxiety Reduction* • Allow parent to participate in care as much as possible • Encourage parents to hold and cuddle child • Make sure that staff assignments to care for child allow for a consistent caregiver • Always speak softly before touching child *Oxygen Therapy* **Administer O_2 and respiratory treatments as ordered, and evaluate effects** • Determine whether oxygen equipment is functioning properly, with correct setting, patent and intact tubing, and proper humidification • Determine whether O_2 equipment, i.e., tubing, humidification bottle, has been replaced within the time dictated by hospital policy (bacteria may multiply within O_2 equipment that is not routinely replaced) • By means of transcutaneous monitoring, pulse oximetry, or vital signs, assess whether oxygen setting is adequate, both at rest and during activity; notify physician if PO_2 or cardiac output drops below prescribed limits, or if vital signs rise significantly during an activity like feeding • Auscultate chest before and after chest physical therapy to determine therapeutic effects *Chest Physiotherapy* • Position child with lung segment to be drained in dependent position. Apply gentle tapping or vibration over chest wall; this is	

(continued)

TABLE 32-9 *(continued)*

Defining Characteristics	Nursing Interventions	Evaluation Criteria
• See *NANDA Nursing Diagnoses* (1990) for suggested functional level classification • Periorbital edema and edema of face, hands, and feet • Neck vein distention (in older child) • Urine output less than 1 ml/kg/hr • Failure-to-thrive: less than third percentile for height and weight on growth chart • Cardiomegaly, hepatomegaly ***Fatigue*** *Objective*: • Verbalization of child's unremitting and overwhelming lack of energy and inability to maintain usual and perceived need for additional energy to accomplish routine tasks • Parental report of infant's inability to take an adequate amount per feeding • Falling asleep at feedings and spending little time awake ***Altered Growth and Development*** • Not yet accomplishing; delay in performing skills (motor, social, expressive) typical of age group • Altered physical growth • Inability to perform self-care or self-control activities appropriate for age	sometimes done with the handle of an electric toothbrush for infants • Use ultrasonic nebulizer as ordered • Encourage coughing afterwards • When administering chest physical therapy, pay particular attention to the involved lobes • Evaluate whether the fatigue resulting from chest physical therapy outweighs the benefits of the amount of sputum expectorated *Airway Management* **Clean nares regularly** with small cotton "wicks" and suction secretions from nares with bulb syringe as needed **Anticipate the need for suction equipment** and have at the bedside a suction machine, tubings, suction catheters, and an ear bulb syringe • Suction following chest physical therapy and episodes of crying (crying more fully inflates the lungs and displaces secretions) **Change the position of a small infant or immobile child every 1–2 hrs** (to prevent pooling of fluid in the lungs) **Include position with buttocks elevated on pillow** (to allow for drainage of secretions from dependent lobes of lungs) **Place the dyspneic child in a Fowler position** and slightly hyperextend the neck (to straighten the trachea, thereby opening the airway; note that marked hyperextension will narrow the airway in a young infant with immature cartilaginous rings • An infant can be put in an infant seat; for an older child, the head of the bed or top of the crib mattress can be raised 30 de-	

TABLE 32-9 *(continued)*

Defining Characteristics	***Nursing Interventions***	***Evaluation Criteria***
	grees; place a small towel or blanket under the shoulders to straighten the airway (elevation of the head decreases upward pressure, from gravity, of abdominal organs on the diaphragm) *Medication Administration* **Administer prescribed medications and observe for therapeutic effects versus side effects** • Administer *antibiotics* and observe for therapeutic effects (decreased fever, increased respiratory function) and for side effects (phlebitis from IV administration, diarrhea, rashes); yogurt given PO may help relieve diarrhea (by replacing *Lactobacillus* organisms) • Obtain specimen for culture before the first dose of antibiotic is given (this will ensure optimal colonies of the organism for culture growth); if antibiotics have been administered, note this on the laboratory slip accompanying the specimen • If *theophylline* preparations are in use, monitor serum theophylline levels and signs of toxicity, especially agitation, vomiting, and tachycardia • Control continued elevations in temperature with *antipyretics* as ordered; only lightly clothe and cover the child; keep the room cool and well ventilated (fever increases metabolic O_2 needs and may predispose to febrile seizure) **Institute isolation measures** as ordered or as appropriate to culture results	

(continued)

TABLE 32-9 *(continued)*

Analysis: Nursing Diagnostic Statement 7

Response and Related or Risk Factors: *Sleep pattern disturbance related to*

- Obstructed nares
- Cough
- Fear/anxiety

Projected Outcome: The child will experience adequate rest and sleep that allows pursuance of usual activities without discomfort

Defining Characteristics	Nursing Interventions	Evaluation Criteria
Subjective: Self- or parental report of sleeplessness, interrupted sleep, restlessness, marked irritability, disorientation, lethargy, listlessness *Objective:* • Dark circles under eyes • Mild, fleeting nystagmus • Slight hand tremor • Ptosis of eyelid • Expressionless face • Frequent yawning • Changes in posture • Thick speech with mispronunciation and incorrect words	*Airway Management* **Cleanse nares frequently, and suction as necessary** *Anxiety Reduction* **Carry out measures as previously mentioned to decrease anxiety and fear** *Sleep Enhancement* **Determine usual sleep patterns,** including naptime and bedtime routines and rituals (the younger the child, the more important these familiar activities are to promote sleep) **Prepare for continuity of care;** when parents cannot be present to prepare the child for sleep, the primary nurse can assume this responsibility **Establish a record of sleep** • If the hospital uses a flow sheet, label one column for sleep; cumulatively total hours of sleep over the 24-hr period • Compare the child's usual sleep patterns with the following guide, and determine appropriate adjustments needed to meet the body's increased need for sleep and rest during illness. Neonate 20–22 hrs/24 hrs 6 wks 14–16 hrs/24 hrs 6 mos–1 yr 12–16 hrs/24 hrs 1–3 yrs 10–14 hrs/24 hrs 3–5 yrs 12–14 hrs/24 hrs 6–9 yrs 11–12 hrs/24 hrs 10–12 yrs 9–10 hrs/24 hrs Adolescent 8–10 hrs/24 hrs	**The child will obtain sufficient sleep to meet needs, as evidenced by** • Agreeing to sleep and rest at times client usually does so at home • Rested appearance • Increased energy for interest in play

TABLE 32-9 *(continued)*

Defining Characteristics	Nursing Interventions	Evaluation Criteria
	Enforce naptimes by posting a sign; usually other health care professionals will observe the request **Assess whether sleeplessness may be a side effect of medications,** e.g., theophylline; alert the physician, as appropriate	

Analysis: Nursing Diagnostic Statement 8

Response and Related or Risk Factors: *Altered nutrition: less than body requirements, related to*

- Elevated basal metabolic rate, which results in increased caloric expenditure associated with the work of breathing
- Anorexia associated with decreased perfusion of gastrointestinal tract and/or the side effects of medications
- Decreased energy available for sucking/chewing
- Obstructed nares

Projected Outcome: The child's intake of nutrients will be sufficient to meet metabolic needs

Analysis: Nursing Diagnostic Statement 9

Response and Related or Risk Factors: *High risk for fluid volume deficit; risk factors*

- Mucus related dyspnea associated with effect of dairy products on mucous production
- Anorexia
- Increased basal metabolic rate

Projected Outcome: The child will remain well hydrated

Defining Characteristics	Nursing Interventions	Evaluation Criteria
Subjective: • Self- or parental report of anorexia or of being "too tired to eat" • Parental report of caloric or nutrient intake that is less than body requirements, falling asleep during feeding • Pale conjunctival and mucous membranes • Poor muscle tone *Objective*: • Failure to maintain the weight percentile (and usually also the length percentile) on the growth chart established by the birth-weight and length of full-term infant	Nutrition Management **Assess the effect of formula and dairy products on mucus production, and adjust diet accordingly** • Obtain order to dilute infant feedings to ¼ to ½ strength with water, if needed, to control mucus-related dyspnea • Avoid dairy products in the older child and the infant who cannot tolerate even diluted feedings; offer *clear liquids* frequently • *Suction nares with bulb syringe prior to feeding the infant or young child* (nasal obstruction will make sucking and chewing very difficult)	**The child will maintain adequate hydration during the initial period of anorexia, as evidenced by** • Adequate urine output • Normal urine concentration • Stability of weight • Normal serum sodium levels **The child will increase caloric intake appropriate to age as initial symptoms subside, as evidenced by** • No further weight loss • Replacement of weight lost during initial phase of illness • Resumption of usual eating patterns

(continued)

TABLE 32-9 *(continued)*

Defining Characteristics	*Nursing Interventions*	*Evaluation Criteria*
• Body weight 20% or more under ideal	**Gradually increase normal caloric intake** (i.e., increase formula dilution from ¼ to ½ to full strength, as tolerated) **Monitor progress;** weigh daily **Make mealtime as pleasant as possible** • Encourage family to eat with the hospitalized child • Counsel parents not to force the child to eat (this may lead to a power struggle that will exaggerate feeding difficulties) • Assure the family that decreased caloric intake can usually be well tolerated during the first 48 to 72 hrs of the illness, provided hydration is maintained	• Self- or parental report of desire to eat and of increased intake

Analysis: Nursing Diagnostic Statement 10*

Response and Related or Risk Factors: *High risk for ineffective individual/family coping (compromised); risk factors*

- Fear/anxiety regarding child's illness and its meaning
- Pain
- Lack of available means to cope with the stress of a chronic or potentially fatal disease
- Inadequate support systems
- Knowledge deficit regarding the care of the child including home monitoring
- Knowledge deficit regarding resources available
- Feelings of inadequacy

Projected Outcome: The child and parent(s) will display adaptive behaviors and problem solving abilities to address effectively tasks essential to the health challenge

Analysis: Nursing Diagnostic Statement 11

Response and Related or Risk Factors: *Altered family processes, related to*

- Anxiety regarding possible death of child
- Parental feelings of inadequacy about health care function
- Difficulty obtaining baby sitters
- Difficulty in meeting demands of child

Projected Outcome: The family will return to its pre-illness mode of effective functioning

Analysis: Nursing Diagnostic Statement 12

Response and Related or Risk Factors: *Anticipatory grieving, related to*

- Perceptions regarding diagnosis of chronic and/or potentially fatal illness
- Perceived loss of a healthy child

* Nursing diagnostic statements 10 through 12 are presented together because the interventions are interrelated.

TABLE 32-9 *(continued)*

Projected Outcome: The parents will be able to verbalize and reach some level of acceptance of living with their child as he now is

Defining Characteristics

Ineffective Individual Coping

Subjective:

- Verbalization (child/parent) of inability to cope or ask for help
- Inability to meet role expectations (e.g., cannot hold still during procedures—kicks, bites, etc.)

Ineffective Family Coping: Compromised

Subjective:

- Parents verbalize preoccupation with own reactions (e.g., fear, anticipatory grief, guilt, anxiety)
- Parents describe or confirm an inadequate knowledge base, which interferes with their ability to give the child effective assistance and/or support

Objective:

- Parents attempt assistive or supportive behaviors with less than satisfactory results
- One or both parents withdraw from communication with the child or decrease communication at times that are most stressful for the child
- Parents display protective behavior disproportionate (too little or too much) to the child's abilities or need for autonomy

Altered Family Processes

Objective:

- Vocalizations by child or family members of inability to meet physical and/or emotional and spiritual needs of members

Nursing Interventions

Coping Enhancement, Child

- Use preparation methods, appropriate to child's age, before carrying out procedures, e.g., medical play (see Chapters 21 and 23)
- Allow the child opportunities to "play out" procedures after they have been performed
- Teach and practice with the child coping methods that assist him or her to hold still, e.g., deep breathing ("pant like a puppy")
- When restraining the child for a procedure, explain that you are helping her or him to hold still
- Tell the child it is "OK to cry when things hurt or are scary"
- Whenever possible, give the child a choice (e.g., which medicine first) to enhance sense of control
- Allow the parents to stay with the child to provide support (*never* ask the parents to assist with restraining the child)
- Use a calm, reassuring manner in carrying out procedures on the child

Coping Enhancement, Parents

- Ask questions of the parent and the older child, such as, "What frightens you most about caring for your child (or about being cared for) at home?" and "How do you visualize your child's (your) future?"

Supply information needed for problem solving

- Give clear, concrete answers to questions (anxiety decreases comprehension)

Evaluation Criteria

The family will be able to return to effective functioning

- Child will be able to hold still when necessary for a procedure
- Child will display alternative coping methods when undergoing a procedure
- Parents will show ability to attend to child's reactions
- Parents will verbalize correctly and will give their child effective assistance and support when it is needed by the child

(continued)

TABLE 32-9 *(continued)*

Defining Characteristics	Nursing Interventions	Evaluation Criteria
• Inability of family members to express/accept a wide range of feelings • Family unable to meet security needs of members • Inability of family members to accept/receive help appropriately • Family unable to adapt to change/deal with child's condition; unlikely family decision making processes • Inappropriate boundary maintenance and level and direction of energy	• Explain every nursing care activity (this will help the child and family relate to the treatment and will decrease their feelings of helplessness and hopelessness) • Encourage parents to ask questions and to discuss their feelings • Discuss the relationship between the physical problems and the child's behavior, e.g., poor sucking response, to help diminish frustration with the behavior • Clarify misconceptions (effective problem solving is based on accurate information)	
Anticipatory Grieving *Subjective*: • Potential loss of child • Expression of distress at potential loss • Denial of potential loss • Guilt • Anger • Sorrow • Choked feelings	**Decrease family role strain by assisting the child and family to set realistic goals and possible methods of attaining them** • Assist in identification of coping strategies that have been effective in the past • Refer to external sources of support and counseling as these needs are identified **Actively involve the child and family in the treatment plan** • Invite participation in the nursing plan of care and in its implementation (this will greatly help dispel feelings of powerlessness and increase self-esteem) • Take every opportunity to reinforce with the family ways in which the child benefits by their participation ("doing for" a loved one can provide a healthy outlet for grief and frustration) **Assist the family to explore ways to work together toward common goals** **Encourage child and family coping abilities through expression of feelings and emotions and identification of sources of anxiety**	

TABLE 32-9 *(continued)*

Defining Characteristics	Nursing Interventions	Evaluation Criteria
	• Determine the family's past experience with illness and diseases and their related health beliefs • Convey that anxiety is normal and expected • Encourage the parents to air guilt feelings about hereditary and perinatal factors; clarify misconceptions; refer to genetic counseling when appropriate • Use leading statements, such as "Many parents tell me they feel inadequate when their baby won't take enough milk" *Support System Enhancement* • Make the family aware of support groups available through the hospital or local heart association that can bring them together with others who have experienced similar conditions in their child	

Analysis: Nursing Diagnostic Statement 13

Response and Related or Risk Factors: *High risk for altered health maintenance; risk factor: knowledge deficit regarding importance of follow-up care in the home or clinic*

Projected Outcome: Parents will be able to identify, manage, and/or seek out help through follow-up care to maintain their child's health

Defining Characteristics	Nursing Interventions	Evaluation Criteria
Subjective: • Parents state they do not understand treatment regime • Ask nurse for information *Objective*: • Parents are not able to demonstrate ability to duplicate return demonstration	*Teaching: Individual* Inform the parents of the appropriate schedule for follow-up in the clinic or home, and provide them with information regarding what activities will take place during follow-up care	**Parents demonstrate knowledge and ability regarding how to care for their child at home**

Impact of Respiratory Alterations on the Family

When a child is ill with a respiratory problem, the entire family is affected. A respiratory problem usually represents nights of coughing, irritable behavior, and audible respiratory sounds that are distressing to parents; sometimes there is fever. The fatigue of parents after a series of almost sleepless nights is particularly pronounced when both parents work outside the home and when there are other siblings who require care for the hours during which a parent would ordinarily get some additional rest. The day-to-day planning surrounding school attendance or baby-sitting arrangements presents special problems when both parents work or when there is a single parent. The uncertainty of how sick a child is and whether he or she is infectious presents difficulty in making these arrangements.

The potential for a rapid worsening of their child's condition is a cause of worry for parents, especially if they go to work. Particularly when an *infant* is ill, parents are frequently anxious because of their own inexperience or because of the fear that the baby's condition will worsen and not be noticed by a baby sitter. Some parents may be concerned that their infant will be a victim of the sudden infant death syndrome.

The overall discomfort associated with respiratory illness can range from minor problems to a high level of anxiety related to the inability to breathe. Mouth breathing, skin excoriation, headaches, and cough are nuisances that children do not cope with particularly well. The more severe situation of severely compromised air exchange results in an element of panic and struggle for survival.

The generalized effect of struggling to breathe is externally obvious and brings about a panic response in those responsible for the child's care. Frequently there are audible symptoms associated with the exaggerated chest movements. The color changes and facial expressions that accompany these symptoms compound the stressfulness of the situation for the observer. The rapidity with which a child's appearance worsens is overwhelming to parents and can be the source of guilt feelings if immediate help was not solicited.

Respiratory problems often require some special form of therapy that can add an additional burden to the planning and organizing of family activities. The refusal to take medications and the resistance if inhalation or chest physical therapy is required are additional burdens to a stressed family. In the event of long-term respiratory problems, special equipment, such as monitors, oxygen and mist devices, and suction equipment, restricts the family's time away from home and involvement in community activities.

Nursing strategies are presented for the various respiratory illnesses discussed in this chapter. In many instances, the nurse can provide specific support through telephone counseling. The difficult decisions that parents must make can be made less stressful if they have access to counsel by telephone.

When communicating with parents, whether on the telephone or in a health care setting, one must recognize the multitude of stresses that parents endure when their child has a respiratory problem. These stresses put them at risk for ineffective family coping. Their anxiety, fatigue, and irritability require a nonjudgmental attitude and a willingness to respond sensitively to their needs. Often they require repeated explanations because they were too anxious to hear when told the first time. The plan of care must be explained to parents, because they urgently want to know what will be done for their child. The nurse permits the parents to stay near, since they may still fear losing their child. Special attention to the fatigue of a parent is given by offering a comfortable chair and by assisting them to make arrangements to care for their own needs of rest and meals.

Infections of the Respiratory Tract and Related Structures

Respiratory infections of infants and children can cause serious illness requiring hospitalization and intensive therapy. Factors that contribute to an infant's or a young child's susceptibility to infection include (1) immunologic immaturity, (2) a relatively small airway from the trachea to the end of the bronchioles, (3) accessory muscles that are not well developed, and (4) ineffectual coughing efforts. The net result is that even small amounts of secretions and edema within the lumen of the respiratory tract can cause obstruction and respiratory distress.

Prevention of respiratory illnesses by counseling families in proper nutrition, rest, and personal hygiene is an important role of the nurse. When an infant has repeated respiratory infections, the nurse takes a careful history in search of underlying problems such as cystic fibrosis, foreign-body aspiration, immunodeficiency, or allergies.

Infants and young children (birth to 3 years of age) are more susceptible to respiratory tract infection than older children and adults. Of particular concern is the neonate, especially if premature. The clinical manifestations of respiratory tract infection in infants and children can be more generalized and more severe than one expects in older children and adults (Table 32–10). A child who has any combination of these signs and symptoms can cause parents to become extremely anxious; in severe cases, parents may be in a state of panic. The onset of symptoms may be abrupt, often following a minor upper respiratory infection. This kind of situation has the potential to make parents feel guilty for not having sought treatment earlier. Although immediate lifesaving measures are frequently necessary, the nurse should encourage parents to stay with their child and hold her or him as soon as the condition permits.

TABLE 32-10
Clinical Manifestations of Respiratory Tract Infection

Clinical Manifestation	Developmental Considerations	Clinical Considerations
Fever	Neonates may have serious infections without fever Fever is associated with infection at 6 mos to 3 yrs of age	Temperatures of 39.4–40.6°C (103–105°F) can occur with mild infections Fever often precedes other signs of infection; therefore, a child with fever requires careful watching Behavior can be listless or irritable Elevated temperature occurs in both viral and bacterial infection May be accompanied by meningeal signs (headaches, pain and stiffness in neck, positive Kernig and Brudzinski signs)
Febrile Convulsions	Do not usually occur after 4 yrs of age	Convulsions result when there is a rapid change in temperature Only a small percentage of children with febrile convulsions later develop epilepsy
Anorexia	Infants and young children do not verbalize loss of appetite	May be demonstrated by refusal to suck and by lassitude May precede fever and other signs; loss of appetite may continue through most of illness
Vomiting and Diarrhea	Fluid and electrolyte imbalance can occur in small children if vomiting or diarrhea continues throughout the course of illness	Vomiting usually occurs at the onset of illness but may continue throughout entire illness and become severe; mild transient diarrhea is a common characteristic
Abdominal Pain	Children have difficulty explaining the source and character of pain	May be due to mesenteric lymphadenitis accompanying throat infection
Sore Throat	The elasticity of the tissues results in less pressure on sensitive nerve endings	Often the throat is inflamed, but the child does not complain of a sore throat

Nasopharyngitis (Common Cold)

The common cold is a self-limiting viral infection of the upper respiratory tract.

Etiology/Incidence (Pathophysiology)

Typically, three epidemic waves of the common cold occur annually. The greatest incidence seems to be during the fall with the opening of school, whereas the more severe cases with a greater tendency for complications tend to occur in midwinter. Another round of mild cases occurs in the spring. The common cold is, in fact, the most prevalent infectious disease among all ages, with older children and adults averaging two colds per year, and children under 4 years, three to eight per year. Infants and toddlers can have severe responses to upper respiratory infections and more frequently develop complications.

The common cold is caused by a wide variety of viruses; however, rhinoviruses are the cause of approximately 90 per cent; there are about 100 rhinoviruses. These viruses have an incubation period of 2 to 4 days. During the latter part of the incubation period, the virus begins to spread and may continue to spread throughout the period of acute illness. The virus invades the mucous membranes of the upper respiratory tract and causes swelling and hypersecretion of mucus. Rhinoviruses are spread mainly by direct contact with nasal secretions, whereas viruses that infect the lower respiratory tract are transmitted by air droplets resulting from coughs and sneezes.

Other agents that cause the common cold include parainfluenza virus, respiratory syncytial virus, adenovirus, coronavirus, and enterovirus.

Clinical Manifestations

Symptoms usually last 2 to 10 days and in young children begin with fever. Excessively high fever, however, does not usually accompany the common cold and should raise one's suspicions that other disease processes or complications are present. Neonates and premature infants often have no fever or may even show a reduction in temperature during infections. Older children and adults usually run a low-grade fever, under 37.8° C (100° F) on an oral thermometer. Mucous membrane irritation by the virus results in rhinorrhea (a thin, watery nasal discharge), stuffy nose, and generalized nasopharyngeal congestion. The obstruction these symptoms pose to respirations causes the child to experience restlessness, malaise, and anorexia (because difficulty in sucking consumes energy and increases oxygen needs). The irritation to membranes also causes sneezing, increased lacrimation, and a raspy sensation in the back of the throat. Hypersecretion of mucus causes coughing, especially at night when secretions pool in the nasopharyngeal cavity. Viral enteritis may be present and may account for an associated diarrhea. Bacterial superinfections of the tonsils, ears, sinuses, or lower respiratory tract are frequent, especially in infancy. Secondary dehydration and a mild degree of ketoacidosis can occur when fever is present. The crankiness and acetone breath so common in young children with minor infection are a result of this condition (Gellis & Kagan, 1990).

Diagnostic Assessment

Diagnosis is based on history and clinical manifestations. A culture of nasal discharge may be made to determine whether bacterial involvement exists. Allergic rhinitis must be differentiated from an infectious process. Allergic rhinitis is not accompanied by fever; nasal discharge generally is not purulent; and it is seen in combination with itching of the eyes and nose and nasal mucous membranes that are pale rather than inflamed. (See Chapter 37 for discussion of allergic rhinitis.)

Therapeutic Management

The common cold is self-limiting. Although it affects millions each year, its cure eludes medical science. Treatment, therefore, is symptomatic in nature, focusing on (1) general comfort measures, (2) procedures to relieve local irritation, (3) relief through use of antipyretics, and (4) prevention of the complications of dehydration, otitis media, and secondary bacterial infection. The most common complication is otitis media. No specific treatment exists for the common cold, and antibiotics are not thought to affect the course of illness or to reduce the incidence of bacterial infection.

Most of the discomfort is caused by the nasal obstruction and the effect of fever. Vasoconstrictive decongestant nose drops such as pseudoephedrine (Sudafed), phenylephrine (Neo-Synephrine), or phenylpropylmethylamine (Vonedrine) are commonly used in infants over age 3 months. They shrink congested nasal membranes, making breathing easier. In younger infants, sterile saline nose drops are used, because a sympathomimetic decongestant may cause irritability and tachycardia. The addition of corticosteroids and antibiotics has not proved to be effective (Behrman, 1992).

Decongestant nasal sprays can be used by older children, but only with supervision. No nasal medication should be continued for more than 4 to 5 days, to prevent rebound engorgement from chemical irritation. With prolonged administration of decongestants, the involved capillaries lose their tone, resulting in a permanent state of nasal congestion (O'Grady, 1987). Orally administered decongestants are also widely given to older children to shrink engorged nasal mucosa.

Antihistamines are largely ineffective for treating the common cold, although some studies report they are effective to relieve nasal congestion in children with acute nasopharyngitis (Behrman, 1992).

Acetaminophen is recommended for the first few days to reduce irritability, aching, and malaise. Aspirin is not prescribed for children with respiratory tract infections, because when given to a child with influenza viral infection, the risk of developing Reye syndrome increases (Behrman, 1992). Antitussives, if indicated, are used cautiously, because they can depress the cough reflex, leading to aspiration. An antitussive may be desirable if coughing is paroxysmal or if needed at bedtime to facilitate adequate rest. The effectiveness of vitamin C as an effective agent in treating a cold is greatly debated, but it has not been shown to have significant therapeutic or prophylactic value (Gellis & Kagan, 1990). Furthermore, vitamin C in higher doses than required nutritionally (approximately 50 mg/day) may be toxic.

Nursing Diagnostic Statements

Ineffective airway clearance, *related to obstructed nares.*

High risk for altered oral mucous membrane; *risk factors:*
- *Dehydration.*
- *Mouth breathing.*
- *Infection.*

High risk for fluid volume deficit; *risk factors: hyperthermia from*
- *Infectious process.*
- *Inadequate fluid intake.*

Sleep pattern disturbance, *related to*
- *Inability to breathe through nose.*
- *Paroxysmal cough.*

High risk for impaired home health maintenance; *risk factor: knowledge deficit regarding complications of a common cold.*

Nursing Care

Maintaining Effective Airway. Saline nose drops (1 teaspoon of salt in 1 pint of warm water) are usually satisfactory to clear secretions in young infants; in older children, decongestants may be used.

To administer nose drops, the child's head is lowered and turned to the side. Several drops are placed into the lower nostril and the position maintained for 1 minute; the procedure is repeated in the opposite nostril.

Postural drainage facilitates loosening and drainage of secretions from the upper airway. A cold steam vaporizer also liquefies and loosens secretions of the upper airway as well as soothes irritated membranes and relieves coughing. Gentle removal of excessive mucous exudate with an infant aspirator or ear bulb syringe four to five times a day (especially before feeding) increases the effectiveness of nose drops or vaporizer.

Placing the infant on the stomach facilitates drainage of nasal secretions and prevents fluid from draining via the eustachian tube to the middle ear during swallowing.

Maintaining Tissue Integrity. A vaporizer prevents drying of the mucosa. In addition, petroleum jelly or similar lubricants applied in a very thin film on chapped lips and irritated nose both soothe and prevent further excoriation. Excessive amounts are avoided, as they can be aspirated.

Maintaining fluid intake promotes tissue integrity by liquefying secretions, preventing dehydration, and helping rid the body of the virus. Anorexia is often frustrating to the parent. Urging food often leads to vomiting or diarrhea, and forcing it may cause food aversions. Parents should be reassured that a brief interval without normal intake will not create malnutrition, but every effort is made to provide appealing fluids frequently and in small amounts. Diluting or temporarily eliminating formula, providing a liquid diet, and suctioning the nose with a bulb syringe to remove excess secretions prior to feedings are helpful suggestions for maintaining adequate intake.

Reducing Fever and Promoting Comfort. Rest in bed until the fever subsides helps reduce the likelihood of secondary complications. Bed rest is hard to achieve in the older infant, but a satisfactory compromise is quiet play in a playpen. Relief from the discomforts caused by fever is achieved by dressing the child in light clothing, keeping room temperatures somewhat cool, administering antipyretics, and sponging with tepid water when temperatures reach 39.5° C (103° F) or higher. Fever management and its various controversies are discussed in Chapter 23.

Acetaminophen is recommended for the acute phase of illness and is usually administered prior to sponging. Parents are taught the correct preparation and dosage of medication. (See Chapter 23 for dosage and preparations.) Explain to parents that the use of aspirin in the presence of an influenza viral infection is associated with Reye syndrome.

Providing Information That Assists Family in Identifying Complications. When a child under age 4 years is being treated for a cold at home, telephone follow-up by the nurse is recommended. The nurse calls to assess whether the cold is resolving or complications are developing, since colds in young children often are a precursor to streptococcal infections. Parents should also be told to seek medical help if their child develops retractions, nasal flaring, or grunting; if nasal discharge becomes purulent, foul-smelling, thick, or bloody; if fever persists beyond 48 to 72 hours; or if the child has a cold without fever and fever occurs after 3 or 4 days, indicating bacterial involvement (Table 32–11).

TABLE 32–11
Family-Centered Teaching: Home Care for Nasopharyngitis

Promote fluid intake

- Clear liquids are well tolerated (broth, flavored water, Jello)

Use the following measures to reduce fever:

- Bed rest
- Administration of antipyretics
- Sponging with tepid water
- Environmental temperature control

Know the appropriate response if signs and symptoms of complications develop

Otitis Media

Otitis media is an inflammation of the middle ear that may occur with or without effusion. Middle ear effusion is the collection of a liquid in the middle ear space; the effusion may be serous (thin and watery), mucoid (thick and mucuslike), or purulent* (pus-like). Otitis media is further defined by its temporal relation, by means of the terms "acute" (rapid onset lasting approximately 3 weeks), "subacute" (a 3-week to 3-month period during which an acute phase resolves), and "chronic" (persists longer than 3 months). These terms have been used inconsistently in the literature, which has led to some confusion.

"Acute otitis media" (AOM) is the term used to describe otitis with *purulent* effusion (even though the word "effusion" is not used in its description). The collection of fluid in the middle ear is of infectious (purulent) etiology. "Otitis media with effusion" (OME) is the term that is usually used to describe a collection of fluid in the middle ear that is *not* infectious (nonpurulent), formerly called serous otitis media. (See Table 32–12 for terminology and definitions.) The distinction between purulent and nonpurulent cannot be clearly made either by otoscopic criteria or by the type of presenting symptoms (Marchant & Shurin, 1983). Table 32–13 compares OME and AOM.

Etiology/Incidence (Pathophysiology)

Otitis media is one of the most common infectious diseases of childhood. It is estimated that 50 per cent of all children will have had one episode of otitis media by 1 year of age and 76 per cent by 2 years of age (Mitchell, 1987). After age 5 years, the incidence and prevalence of otitis media decline.

Otitis media is the most common complication of upper respiratory infections. Infants and children under 3 years of age are particularly predisposed be-

* "Purulent" and "suppurative" are used interchangeably.

TABLE 32-12
Terminology and Definitions for Otitis Media and Related Disorders

Terms	Definition
Otitis media	An inflammation of the middle ear; this term does not make reference to etiology or pathogenesis
Middle ear effusion	Fluid resulting from otitis media; the fluid may be • Serous (thin, watery) • Mucoid (thick, viscid, mucus-like) • Purulent (pus-like)
Otorrhea	A discharge from the ear
Otitis media without effusion	Inflammation of the middle ear mucous membrane and tympanic membrane without evidence of middle ear effusion
Acute otitis media	A rapid or short onset of signs and symptoms of inflammation in the middle ear. Other terms used are "suppurative" or "purulent otitis media"
Otitis media with effusion	Inflammation of the middle ear in which fluid has collected in the middle ear; other terms used include "nonpurulent, nonsuppurative, serous, secretory, or glue ear"; subdivision are • Acute (less than 3 wks) • Subacute (3 wks to 2–3 mos) • Chronic (more than 2–3 mos)

cause of their shorter, more horizontal, wider, and more distensible eustachian tube, which more readily allows passage of foreign matter up the tube. (See Chapter 13, Assessing Child Health.) The infant's humoral defenses are also less developed. The usual lying down position increases susceptibility, because fluid pools in the pharyngeal cavity and hinders tube drainage. The abundance of nasopharyngeal lymphoid tissue normally present in infants and children is also thought to predispose to local infection and to eustachian tube obstruction (Paradise, 1980).

The primary factor causing recurrent otitis media is abnormal functioning of the eustachian tube. The three functions of the eustachian tube are (1) ventilation of the middle ear, (2) protection from nasopharyngeal secretions and sound pressure, and (3) drainage of secretions from the middle ear into the nasopharynx (Bluestone & Klein, 1988). Normally, the eustachian tube is closed and flat, opening only long enough to permit drainage of middle ear secretions. With blockage, drainage is impaired and a negative middle ear pressure is created. Causes of eustachian tube dysfunction are shown in Table 32–14. Normally, the eustachian tube equalizes the pressure between the atmosphere and the middle ear and replenishes oxygen that has been absorbed. With obstruction, trapped air is absorbed during circulation and a vacuum is created. If this condition persists, secretions collect within the middle ear, resulting in otitis media with effusion (serous liquid). This is sometimes referred to as a "sterile effusion."

TABLE 32-13
Comparison of Otitis Media with Effusion and Acute Otitis Media

Type	Clinical Signs	Indicative Behaviors or Complaints
Otitis Media with Effusion		
Also called "nonpurulent" or "nonsuppurative otitis media" and "serous, secretory, and glue ear" *Pathology:* Nonpurulent middle ear effusion *Etiology:* Blocked eustachian tube causes retention of middle ear secretions	May be relatively asymptomatic; light reflex obscured; varying degrees of hyperemia; redness of tympanic membrane (eardrum). Bony landmarks are visible, with handle of malleus prominent and more horizontal; umbo is stark white. Fluid level (meniscus) sometimes is visible through the eardrum. Membrane is retracted, usually in posterosuperior region. Frequent otoscopic finding is opacification of the tympanic membrane. Pneumatic otoscopy reveals a retracted or convex tympanic membrane in which mobility is impaired	May be none; may have fullness in ear; may feel some pain in early stage. Snapping sensation occurs when child swallows or yawns. Diminished hearing is expressed by listlessness and general inattentiveness to voice in infant; may be restless. Signs and symptoms of acute infection (otalgia, fever) are lacking
Acute Otitis Media		
Also called "purulent" or "suppurative otitis media" *Pathology:* Purulent accumulation of exudate in middle ear *Etiology:* Bacterial or viral invasion of middle ear secretions, often secondary to middle ear effusion (negative pressure draws infectious organisms in)	Light reflex is obscured or absent. Fluid meniscus or bubbling visible through membrane; obscuring of bony landmarks. Membrane bulging and has limited or no mobility to pneumatic otoscopy; spontaneous rupture is possible. Erythema of the eardrum is an inconsistent finding	Discomfort expressed when ear is touched, or child pulls at ear. Acute onset of ear pain and fever. May have purulent ear drainage if eardrum ruptures; inconsolable irritability and restlessness; persistent crying; anorexia, vomiting, or diarrhea. May have cervical lymph node involvement

TABLE 32-14
Causes of Eustachian Tube Dysfunction

Type	Cause
Functional	A decreased tubal stiffness related to immature development of cartilage, resulting in easy collapsibility
	An inefficient active opening mechanism
	An unrepaired cleft palate*
	Down syndrome*
Mechanical	
Intrinsic	Inflammatory mucosal edema of the tube related to allergy or infection
Extrinsic	Obstructive adenoids
	Nasopharyngeal tumors

Compiled from Bluestone, C. D., & Klein, J. O. (1988). *Otitis media in infants and children*. Philadelphia, WB Saunders; and Paradise, J. L., et al. (1987). Efficacy of adenoidectomy for recurrent otitis media: Results from parallel random and nonrandom trials. *Pediatric Research, 21,* 286A.

* The reason for the dysfunction in these conditions is not clearly understood.

When the eustachian tube is not totally obstructed, infectious organisms can enter the middle ear by aspiration, owing to negative middle ear pressure, and by insufflation during crying, nose blowing, and swallowing when the nose is obstructed. This results in acute AOM. The most common offending organisms in AOM are *Streptococcus pneumoniae* (approximately 40 per cent) and *Haemophilus influenzae* (approximately 20 per cent). Additional organisms, each accounting for 5 per cent of the cases, are group A beta-hemolytic streptococcus, *Staphylococcus aureus,* and *Branhamella catarrhalis*. In addition, gram-negative enteric bacilli are found in neonates. Sterile effusions (nonpurulent) account for approximately 25 per cent of cases.

Complications and Sequelae of Otitis Media

Hearing Loss. This is the most prevalent complication of otitis media. The presence of effusion or high-negative pressure within the middle ear during each bout of otitis media is associated with temporary hearing loss. This episodic hearing loss is usually reversible, but permanent conductive hearing loss may develop, owing to the complications of recurrent middle ear inflammation. Frequent episodes of otitis media and its related hearing loss may interfere eventually with the development of language and cognitive skills. The degree and duration of hearing loss necessary to interfere with development have not been defined.

Acute Mastoiditis. A frequent complication of suppurative otitis media in the past, acute mastoiditis is now rare because of the availability of antibiotics. It does still occur in children with untreated otitis media or in those whose antibiotic course was inadequate in dose or duration of administration. The anatomic communication between the mastoid process and middle ear invites infectious exchange.

Clinically, mastoiditis reveals pain over the mastoid process, erythema, edema, and tenderness to pressure. Diagnosis may be difficult to establish if the infection has been partially suppressed by antibiotics.

Once the condition is diagnosed, antibiotic therapy should commence immediately. Sedation may be necessary to allay restlessness until pain subsides. Pain is lessened by application of a cold compress or ice bag to the mastoid process. Fever is relieved with antipyretics. Mastoidectomy is indicated only if subperiosteal abscess occurs or if antibiotic therapy fails.

Acquired Cholesteatoma. A cholesteatoma is a saclike structure lined with squamous epithelial cells. It develops primarily in association with chronic otitis media. Impaired ventilation apparently is the primary factor leading to its development. A sustained high negative pressure in the middle ear and the loss of elasticity result in a flaccid and eventually atelectatic tympanic membrane. The most flaccid part of the tympanic membrane, the pars flaccida, is drawn inward to form a pocket. This pocket, called a *retraction pocket,* eventually adheres to the ossicles and surrounding structures. It fills with desquamated cells and forms a cholesteatoma. Shiny white pieces of debris collect that may create a foul-smelling discharge. On otoscopic examination, the flakes of debris are observed through a large perforation or in a defect of the membrane in the involved area. The cholesteatoma is surgically excised to prevent destruction of the temporal bone and intracranial involvement. If the discharge is profuse, a preoperative antibiotic is administered.

Clinical Manifestations

An upper respiratory infection with persistent fever always suggests otitis media. Although the distinction between suppurative and nonsuppurative (serous) otitis media cannot always be clearly made, some differentiating criteria can be helpful (see Table 32–13). If persistent or recurrent middle ear infection occurs, the tympanic membrane (eardrum) becomes stretched enough that retraction or bulging does not create pain. Table 32–13 also describes the typical behavior or complaints and systemic signs that suggest otitis media.

Diagnostic Assessment

The tympanic membrane (eardrum) is usually easily visible on otoscopic examination, but its appearance varies. Table 38–9 describes the usual otologic manifestations in AOM and OME. Mobility of the eardrum is tested by applying negative and positive pressure with a pneumatic otoscope. An airtight seal is achieved by putting a piece of rubber over the tip of the speculum that is placed in the external auditory canal. Pressure (negative and positive) is applied by squeezing the bulb.

Nasopharyngeal cultures are not helpful in diagnosing purulent otitis media organisms, as the infectious agent of the ear is most often not the same one that is causing nasopharyngeal symptoms (Hughes, 1984). Any purulent ear drainage should be cultured for specific organisms.

If the mobility of the tympanic membrane is greater than normal, the drum is said to be *compliant* (i.e., it moves when even slight positive or negative external canal pressure is applied). In AOM and in OME, mobility is poor when either positive or negative pressure is applied. Mobility also can be examined by placing a soft rubber cuff over the external ear canal to achieve an airtight seal, at which time air pressure registers on an attached hand-held probe.

Electroacoustic impedance measurement, including tympanometry, is useful for screening OME to prevent hearing loss (see Chapter 45, Sensory and Communication Alterations, for further explanation of technique).

Therapeutic Management

Management options for otitis media with effusion range from watchful waiting to aggressive surgical intervention. The option to wait and observe is based on the belief that, in most children, otitis media will follow a benign course and resolve (Gellis & Kagan, 1990).

Pharmacologic Therapy. AOM is treated with vigorous antibiotic therapy for 10 to 14 days. Oral ampicillin, 50 to 100 mg/kg per 24 hours in four divided doses, or amoxicillin, 40 mg/kg per 24 hours in three divided doses, is the recommended initial treatment (Bluestone & Klein, 1988). Amoxicillin is as effective as ampicillin and has fewer side effects, such as diarrhea. Trimethoprim-sulfamethoxazole or cefaclor is also chosen because of the increasing prevalence of *H. influenzae* resistance to ampicillin and amoxicillin.

Decongestants to reduce edema and improve eustachian tube function and antihistamines have not been established as efficacious in the treatment of AOM (Zenk et al, 1990). However, these medications seem to provide some comfort and continue to be used. Analgesic and antipyretic drugs may be administered to relieve earache and fever. Topical intranasal and systemic corticosteroids lack convincing evidence of their efficacy (Bluestone & Klein, 1988). Application of heat or cold to the affected ear region may relieve discomfort.

Young children should be watched closely for signs of secondary mastoiditis, meningitis (especially those under 4 months of age), or hearing loss.

Aeration of the Middle Ear. This procedure has been recommended by some and can be taught to the older child. It is done by pinching the nose and forcing air into the ear by blowing up balloons or closing the lips while chewing sugarless gum. The reason some object to this procedure is that bacteria may be blown from the nose to the middle ear. If allergy is contributing to serous otitis, its evaluation and treatment are important to prevent recurrent otitis involvement.

Myringotomy. Aspiration of fluid by surgical incision of the eardrum (myringotomy) or placement of tympanostomy tubes to facilitate drainage may be indicated if OME persists after nonsurgical methods of treatment have been tried. If myringotomy is elected and a general anesthetic is required, a tympanostomy tube is inserted at the same time. The incision allows for removal of the accumulated fluid, and tubes function as accessory eustachian tubes, allowing for air exchange between the middle and outer ear. The tubes work their way out in 2 to 9 months. A small amount of bloody drainage and slight pain are normal when the tubes work their way out.

Myringotomy with tube (M & T) insertion is not without some complications. Scarring (tympanosclerosis) and otorrhea may result, but they do not appear to have long-term sequelae (Behrman, 1992). The major issue surrounding M & T is timing in relation to prevention of hearing loss. It is felt that children can tolerate effusion for around 3 months without significant hearing loss, and 90 per cent of such effusions will resolve if kept free from recurrent disease. The role of adenoidectomy continues to be unclear, but there is increasing evidence that removal of enlarged adenoids reduces the recurrence rate of OME (Paradise et al, 1987); however, some children do not improve after the procedure, and others improve without undergoing the procedure.

Pneumococcal Vaccine. Pneumococcal vaccine continues to be experimental and is not routinely recommended for prevention of otitis media in children under 2 years of age. It may be of value, however, in children older than 2 years who suffer from recurrent episodes of AOM (Bluestone & Klein, 1988).

Nursing Diagnostic Statements and Collaborative Problems

High risk for (or actual) infection: middle ear inflammation; *risk factors: dysfunction of the eustachian tube, associated with*

- *Anatomy of eustachian tubes in children under 3 years of age.*
- *Pooling of fluid in the pharyngeal cavity.*
- *Abundant nasopharyngeal lymphoid tissue.*

High risk for fluid volume deficit; *risk factors: increase in sensible loss, fever, decreased fluid intake.*

High risk for impaired home health maintenance; risk factor: knowledge deficit, regarding care of child with tympanostomy tubes and home care management.

Nursing Care

Preventing Middle Ear Infection and Promoting Its Resolution. To prevent middle ear infection, parents are taught to feed infants in the upright position and avoid laying them in their cribs with a bottle of milk. Children are taught to blow their noses properly during respiratory infections and not to hold one nostril closed while blowing.

In an infection requiring antibiotics, symptoms usually subside in 24 to 48 hours after instituting therapy. The nurse gives adequate explanations to parents, so they understand that the full course of drug therapy is necessary to eradicate the infection, despite the child's apparent early improvement. A telephone follow-up in 2 to 5 days after therapy is initiated is appropriate to determine whether symptoms are being relieved. The child should be re-evaluated at the end of the antibiotic course to determine whether the infection has resolved. Ideally, another checkup is done in 2 to 3 months to ensure that a chronic condition does not exist.

Preventing Fluid Loss. The nurse will ensure that the child is well hydrated. This is accomplished by offering small frequent feedings of clear, preferred liquids. Oral electrolyte solutions flavored with Jello powder, weak tea, and flat soda can be offered to the child. The child is assessed for signs of dehydration. Intake and output are recorded, and urine specific gravity is measured during each shift.

A collaborative problem of pain can also be made for children with otitis media. In addition to dependent interventions involving medication administration, the nurse can relieve the severe earache that accompanies otitis media. Acetaminophen is used to reduce pain and is also effective for fever management. Either warm or cool compresses can be recommended, whichever provides the greatest comfort to the child. Care must be taken not to burn the child if a heating pad is used. A pain-relieving prescription of eardrops may be ordered by the physician, if pain cannot otherwise be managed effectively.

Preventing Dislodging of Tubes and Middle Ear Contamination. The child's activity around water when tympanostomy tubes are in place is controversial. Parents are instructed to plug the child's ears lightly with sterile cotton coated with petroleum jelly during baths or shampooing to keep water from entering the ear canal. Also, diving or swimming deeply under water is not permitted, because it leads to contamination of the middle ear. Surface swimming can be permitted if ear plugs or specially designed ear defenders are worn, although some reports suggest that surface swimming without ear protection does not increase the risk for otitis media (Lounsbury, 1985).

Facilitating Home Care Management. The nurse provides parents with other home care instructions for management of otitis media. Nurses need to emphasize that antibiotics must be continued, although the child's symptoms may have been relieved (refer to previous discussion). For younger children, the nurse can describe nonverbal symptoms of pain the child may demonstrate, such as pulling the ear, "splinting" the ear against a surface such as pillow, or irritable and fussy behavior. Scheduling for follow-up appointments to assess placement for tympanostomy tubes and conduct hearing tests is reviewed. Parents are instructed to observe for signs and symptoms of complications such as mastoiditis, which include pain over the mastoid process, erythema, edema, and tenderness to pressure as well as a foul-smelling discharge that suggests an acquired cholesteatoma, and to contact the physician without delay.

Parents are instructed to assess for signs and symptoms of complications. Parents can be taught to screen for hearing loss of low, middle, and high tones through age-appropriate methods. Symptoms of mastoiditis are discussed with parents; these include pain over the mastoid process, erythema, edema, and tenderness to pressure. If the parents detect a foul-smelling discharge, the child should be brought to the pediatrician, as it may be an acquired cholesteatoma.

Diseased Tonsils and Adenoids

In its common usage, the word "tonsils" refers to the two faucial (palatine) tonsils on either side of the opening of the oral cavity into the pharynx (see Fig. 13–22).

Etiology/Incidence (Pathophysiology)

Adenoids (pharyngeal tonsils) are located superiorly in the midline of the posterior wall of the nasopharynx. Tonsils and adenoids, along with other lymphoid tissue, trap infection from the upper respiratory tract; tonsils also have the capacity to produce antibodies and have a major function in immunity. The size of lymphoid tissue increases to that of an adult when the child is around 6 years of age, almost doubles by age 10 years, then gradually shrinks to normal adult size by age 20 years. During early childhood, lymphoid tissue (including tonsils and adenoids) responds to infection by becoming larger.

The close proximity of the palatine tonsils and the pharyngeal tonsils (adenoids) to the opening of the eustachian tubes has resulted in tonsillectomy and adenoidectomy as a treatment for recurrent otitis media. Removal of tonsils and adenoids is a subject of much controversy. Although the nurse may not play a primary role in the decision, an awareness of the nature of the controversy is helpful in discussions with the family. The nurse must have a clear understanding of the explanation that has been given to the family by the physician regarding the need for tonsillectomy and adenoidectomy (T & A).

Clinical Manifestations

The child presents with a sore throat, in many cases accompanied by a fever. The young child may complain that the throat "hurts," "is hot," or is "so sore I can't eat." The child's pharynx and tonsils are reddened and inflamed. The nurse may observe exudate on the tonsils, petechiae on the soft palate, and ulceration of the tonsils or pharynx. The cervical lymph nodes may be enlarged.

Diagnostic Assessment

The need for T & A is evaluated by weighing the potential benefits it can provide against potential risks. Some physicians still perform T & A to treat recurrent sore throats, whereas others recommend that it be done only in rare circumstances. A more conservative attitude is now prevailing. The number of procedures done yearly has been reduced by more than half since the 1960s and 1970s (Kornblut, 1987). It is generally agreed that adenoidectomy alone may be indicated in children under 4 years of age and that tonsillectomy is preferably deferred until after 5 years of age. Removal of both tonsils and adenoids in very young children may stimulate hyperplasia of other lymphoid tissue in the oropharynx (Gellis & Kagan, 1990). Some of the common indications with explanations for T & A are summarized in Table 32–15.

Therapeutic Management

Anesthesia may be given by endotracheal intubation or inhalation. Adenoidectomy by curettage is usually performed first, followed by the tonsillectomy. The tonsils are removed by surgical dissection, with the lower pole of the tonsil being severed by scissors or a snare. Tonsillectomy and adenoidectomy may also be done separately or in conjunction with myringotomy and tube insertion. Bleeding should be controlled before the child leaves the operating room. (See Table 32–15 for contraindications to T & A.)

Nursing Diagnostic Statements

***Anxiety**, related to knowledge deficit, regarding scheduled T & A*

***High risk for injury: physiologic**; risk factors: the following contraindications for surgery:*
- *Acute upper respiratory infection.*
- *Fever.*
- *History of untoward reactions to anesthesia or bleeding tendencies.*
- *Evidence of a submucous cleft palate.*
- *Hemorrhage from the surgical site.*

***High risk for aspiration**; risk factor:*
- *Loose tooth.*
- *Hemorrhage from surgical site.*
- *Impaired swallowing.*

***Impaired swallowing**, related to*
- *Throat pain.*

***High risk for altered home health maintenance management**; risk factor: knowledge deficit, regarding*
- *Lack of information about the postoperative course in the hospital.*
- *Lack of information about home care during the recovery period.*
- *Lack of understanding of reasoning for T & A.*
- *Altered health.*

TABLE 32–15
Indications and Contraindications for Tonsillectomy and Adenoidectomy

Tonsillectomy Indications

Severe recurrent tonsillitis: One method of reducing incidence of beta-hemolytic streptococcal infection; penicillin prophylaxis may be a desired or indicated alternative

Peritonsillar abscess

Cervical adenitis: Chronic (minimum of 6 mos duration) enlargement or tenderness of cervical lymph nodes, after trials of appropriate antibiotic treatment, is an indication for tonsillectomy

Neoplasm: Unilateral removal of a tonsil is supported when a neoplasm is suspected and tissue is needed to establish a diagnosis

Adenoidectomy Indications

Persisent nasal or airway obstruction: If adenoid enlargement results in obstructive sleep apnea, mouth breathing, and nasal congestion with discharge, adenoidectomy alone is indicated (provided symptoms are not due to allergy)

Tonsillectomy and Adenoidectomy Indications

Recurrent tonsillitis/pharyngitis

Peritonsillar abscess

Suspected malignancy

Lymphoid hyperplasia (in cases causing severe upper airway obstruction)

Tonsillectomy and Adenoidectomy Contraindications

Children who cannot tolerate general anesthesia

Cleft palate, short palate, submucous cleft of palate

Severe upper airway obstruction secondary to lymphoid hyperplasia

Cleft palate (tonsils help reduce air escape during speech)

Under 3 yrs of age

Acute infection (local inflammation increases risk of hemorrhage)

Blood dyscrasias (leukemia, purpura, aplastic anemia, hemophilia)

Uncontrolled systemic disease (diabetes, heart disease, seizure disorder)

Nursing Care

Relieving Anxiety Associated with Lack of Information about the Surgery. Once the decision has been made that removal of tonsils and adenoids is necessary, the nurse focuses on preparing the child and family for the surgical experience and providing optimal postoperative nursing care to prevent complications. Frequently the child is admitted to the hospital the evening before surgery, although some recommend that the child sleep at home the night before surgery and be admitted the morning of surgery. The child should be prepared for hospitalization and various procedures according to age.

Preoperatively, the child and parents should be prepared for what the child will experience before and following surgery. Many hospitals have special programs, including a film or slide-tape, a prehospitalization tour, and a play program that provides an opportunity for the child to manipulate equipment and supplies that she or he will see during the preoperative and postoperative experience.

Physical preparation of the child should also be explained to the child and family. Platelet count, prothrombin time, and partial thromboplastin time evaluations may be done in addition to routine admission laboratory tests of hemoglobin, hematocrit, complete blood count, and urinalysis. Foods and liquids are withheld for 8 hours before the operation to prevent vomiting with aspiration. Preoperative medication varies in type and method of administration.

Special attention is given to the child's understanding of the procedure. A young child may fear "being cut" and may not understand that the operation will be done through the mouth and that an incision is not made through the neck. The child and the parents should be prepared for the child's sore throat after surgery, including explanations of what will be done for it. (See Chapters 21 and 23 on hospitalization and preparations for procedures and Table 23–7.) Nursing management of pain in children is discussed in Chapter 25.

Assessing for Contraindications to Surgery and Preventing Postoperative Complications. The nurse performs a complete health assessment on admission, including a careful evaluation of the child's respiratory status. T & A should not be performed until several weeks after an upper respiratory infection has cleared. An elevated temperature should be reported to the surgeon. The child and the family are assessed to identify medication allergies, a history of bleeding tendency, an uncontrolled illness, or a family history of any reactions to anesthetics. In addition to these factors, a submucous cleft palate (soft palate with little or no muscle) is a contraindication for adenoidectomy. A submucous cleft palate may be recognized by hypernasal speech, a history of frequent cases of otitis media, a bifid uvula, and a palpable U-shaped notch in the posterior edge of the hard palate. The nurse also assesses for and reports any loose teeth, which could become dislodged and aspirated during surgery. The physician will usually extract loose teeth to prevent aspiration.

Preventing Aspiration. Postoperatively, the bed is kept in a flat position, and the child is placed in a side-lying or abdominal position with the upper knee flexed and the head tilted slightly forward. This permits the tongue and jaw to come forward and secretions and vomitus to drain from the mouth, preventing aspiration. Vital signs are checked frequently beginning immediately after the child returns from the recovery room. The nurse should watch for tachycardia, pallor, and excessive swallowing. (Swallowing indicates that blood is trickling down the child's throat.) The throat is checked with a flashlight to assess for bleeding. Almost all cases of fatal bleeding occur within the first 24 hours postoperatively (Rasmussen, 1987).

On return to the ward, the child alternates between periods of sleep and restlessness, owing to the effect of the anesthetic. When the child is fully awake and vital signs are stable, fluids are given cautiously. Small amounts of liquids should be given until the danger of vomiting has passed. Sucking through a straw produces a vacuum that could potentially stimulate bleeding; therefore drinking from a cup is recommended. A well-tolerated form of intake is a popsicle. Red liquids are avoided during the postoperative period to prevent their confusion with frank blood in secretions and vomitus.

Parents are encouraged to stay with their child. Having a parent quietly sit at the bedside is comforting to children as they periodically awaken. A suction machine should be immediately available in the event of obstruction from vomitus or secretions or if hemorrhage occurs.

Facilitating Swallowing by Relieving Throat Pain. An ice collar wrapped in a soft material and applied to fit comfortably the contour of the child's neck may provide some relief of pain, but this effect varies. Analgesics need to be administered on the basis of the nurse's judgment rather than the child's verbal expression of pain. The first postoperative dose of analgesics should be administered routinely to keep the child from experiencing excessive throat pain. Children may resist taking the medication because it hurts to swallow, but with encouragement and explanation they usually cooperate. One must explain the purpose of the medication and acknowledge the child's resistance and fears. A comfortable child is more likely to take fluids, which in turn promotes recovery and early discharge. Oral codeine and acetaminophen are the drugs frequently administered for pain as needed. Aspirin should be avoided because of the risk of hemorrhage.

Promoting Effective Home Health Management. Children can be discharged the same day or the next morning following surgery. Parents should be advised against giving their child hot, coarse, or spicy foods for

5 to 7 days; swimming is generally discouraged until the follow-up visit in 10 to 14 days; and any signs of bleeding should promptly be reported to the physician. A late hemorrhage (5 to 10 days after surgery) is associated with infection of the upper respiratory tract. Thus it is advisable during the recovery period to limit exposure to other children who are known to have colds. The hemorrhage occurs when the tissue (eschar) that normally forms over the raw surface separates prematurely during infection; parents should be aware of this. Analgesics may be necessary for the first few days after surgery for throat pain and referred pain to the ears, but pain should not persist beyond the first week. Many institutions have developed an instruction sheet for parents (see Table 32–16 for an example).

TABLE 32-16
Family-Centered Teaching: Postoperative Tonsillectomy and Adenoidectomy Home Care

Dietary Instructions

First Day

Avoid hot and highly seasoned foods

Encourage intake of several glasses of water and other fluids (e.g., bland fruit juices, gelatin, broth)

Second Day

Add soft foods as desired/tolerated (e.g., gelatin, chocolate pudding, mashed potato, pureed vegetables, cottage cheese)

Third to Fifth Days

Resume normal diet gradually, but avoid hot foods, potato chips, nuts, dry toast, and crackers until 1 to 2 wks after surgery

General Instructions

The child should be kept relatively quiet for the first 3 days

Avoid frequent coughing and clearing the throat

Fluid intake alleviates objectionable mouth odor

A gray membrane on the sides of the throat is normal and should disappear in 1–2 wks

Earache or a slight fever is expected and may be disregarded unless condition worsens

Child may return to school 1 wk after discharge

Do not use aspirin for 2 wks, because it increases the possibility of bleeding; use acetaminophen (Tylenol) for pain

Avoid drinking citrus-containing fluids (orange juice, grapefruit juice, and tomato juice) for 1 wk after the operation, as they will make the throat burn

Observe for bleeding; in 2% of patients, slight bleeding is seen after 5–6 days postoperatively

Instruct child to be quiet, lie down, and spit the blood out gently; gargle gently with ice water. If the bleeding does not stop promptly, call your doctor; if doctor is not available and bleeding continues, call the nearest emergency room

Croup (Acute Laryngotracheobronchitis)

Croup is a syndrome characterized by a brassy, barking cough, a hoarse cry, inspiratory stridor, and varying degrees of respiratory distress. These symptoms are the result of laryngeal obstruction due to edema and spasm. "Croup syndrome" refers to infections of the epiglottis, larynx, trachea, and bronchi. Epiglottitis, although a form of croup, is discussed as a separate entity because of its uniqueness in presentation and management. The croup syndromes are summarized in Table 32–17. Acute viral laryngotracheobronchitis (LTB) is the most common form of croup and is discussed here.

Etiology/Incidence (Pathophysiology)

Acute viral LTB, or croup, is most common in children between 3 months and 3 years of age. It usually follows an upper respiratory infection and is most often seen in late fall or winter, during the cold season. It tends to recur, but as the child grows, attacks tend to disappear.

LTB is most commonly caused by the parainfluenza viruses. Other organisms include the adenoviruses and respiratory syncytial, influenza, and measles viruses.

The symptoms associated with croup primarily result from inflammation and edema with subsequent narrowing of air passages. In children, the laryngeal airway is relatively smaller, and the mucous membrane is more loosely attached and more vascular, resulting in rapid compromise by edema and spasm.

As the infection extends down the respiratory tract, breathing becomes more difficult. Symptoms appear gradually, often initially in the evening, and worsen progressively. After several days of respiratory symptoms, there is a gradually increasing brassy or barking cough (like a seal's bark), a hoarse cry, and inspiratory stridor. Stridor is a harsh sound caused by increased rate and turbulence of airflow in the larynx or trachea. Stridor is predominantly inspiratory.

Clinical Manifestations

Varying degrees of respiratory distress, including labored breathing, flaring of the nares, prolonged expiratory phase, and use of accessory muscles (substernal, intercostal, suprasternal retractions) accompany the typical cough and stridor of croup. Breath sounds may be diminished. Fever is generally present but not as severely as in epiglottitis.

Signs of increasing respiratory obstruction include increasing stridor and retractions at rest, respiratory rate above 60 breaths/min, tachycardia, cyanosis (circumoral and orbital), pallor, and restlessness. Restlessness and tachycardia are signs of increasing hypoxia.

TABLE 32-17
Differentiating Croup Symptoms

Common Symptoms: hoarseness; brassy, barking cough; inspiratory stridor; respiratory distress

Differentiating Features	Acute LTB*	Spasmodic Croup	Acute Epiglottitis	Aspirated Foreign Body
Age	<3 yrs	1–4 yrs	>3 yrs	Any age
History	Gradual onset; preceded by upper respiratory infection	Child awakens in night with symptoms	Sudden onset; symptoms worsen over a few hours	Sudden onset of symptoms; child playing or eating; environmental hazards present; adult supervision absent
Etiologic agent	Viral	Unknown	Bacterial *(Haemophilus influenzae)*	Foreign body
Symptoms	Fever (<40°C); mild-to-severe respiratory distress, worse at night	Afebrile; mild-to-moderate respiratory distress	Child's chin may be thrust forward; drooling; difficulty swallowing; epiglottis cherry-red; febrile (>40°C); child appears toxic	Mild-to-severe respiratory distress; afebrile; possibly clutching at throat
Comments	Most common	Sometimes relieved by vomiting; asymptomatic in day, symptoms recur during night	No attempt should be made to visualize child's epiglottis; child should be kept calm; emergency tracheotomy may be needed; high morbidity	Heimlich maneuver may help older child but not necessarily infants; emergency tracheotomy may be needed

* LTB = laryngotracheobronchitis.

Diagnostic Assessment

Diagnosis of viral croup is made on the basis of history and clinical manifestations and the exclusion of bacterial infection. An assessment of the symptoms of croup is summarized in Table 32–17.

Therapeutic Management

Medical treatment for croup focuses on maintenance of a patent airway. Initial medical assessment determines whether the illness is so severe as to require emergency treatment. It is rare that sufficient obstruction occurs to warrant tracheotomy or nasotracheal intubation (Boat, 1992). If complete obstruction does occur, insertion of a large-bore needle into the trachea will provide a temporary airway; this procedure is to be followed immediately by tracheostomy. A 14-gauge intercatheter is ideal for this procedure, since the needle can be withdrawn and the catheter left in place.

The child who has an adequate airway but has stridor at rest is usually admitted to the hospital. Therapy during the acute phase usually involves bronchodilating medications, racemic epinephrine by aerosol, cool mist administered within a croup tent, and intravenous hydration. Oxygen may be used to alleviate hypoxia, but the child must be observed particularly closely, because cyanosis, a sign of impending obstruction, is masked. Sedatives are contraindicated because they mask restlessness, which is one of the principal clinical indications that the child's condition is worsening.

Corticosteroids are sometimes administered for their anti-inflammatory properties when croup fails to respond to conventional treatment. The most beneficial results of steroid therapy have resulted when a single dose was given early in the course of illness (Gellis & Kagan, 1990). Because croup is of viral origin, antibiotics are not ordered unless a secondary bacterial infection exists.

Nursing Diagnostic Statements*

High risk for suffocation and aspiration; *risk factor: ineffective airway clearance, due to inflammation and edema of laryngeal, tracheal, and bronchial tissues.*

High risk for fluid volume deficit; *risk factors:*

- *Fever.*
- *Increased insensible water loss associated with increased respiratory effort.*
- *Decreased fluid intake associated with respiratory distress.*

Ineffective breathing pattern, *related to fear/anxiety (child) caused by*

- *Respiratory distress.*

*To be used with Table 32–9.

- *Croup tent and other unfamiliar surroundings.*
- *Parental anxiety.*

High risk for altered health maintenance; *risk factor: knowledge deficit regarding care of child at home.*

Nursing Care

Maintaining Airway Clearance. Maintenance of an adequate airway is central to the care of a child with croup, whether hospitalized or cared for at home. The child must be carefully and frequently observed for signs of increasing obstruction (Table 32–18) and hypoxia (see Table 32–9).

Dramatic changes in the child's condition can occur quickly, and respiratory arrest from complete obstruction is always a possibility. Any progression of symptoms must be reported to the physician immediately. In the event of impending obstruction, giving humidified oxygen via positive pressure (Ambu bag and mask) may force enough oxygen through the narrowing airway to maintain respiration until the physician arrives. Equipment to perform intubations or tracheostomy should be kept at the bedside or in a place of immediate access when a child with severe croup is hospitalized.

Cool mist relieves some of the distress of croup by decreasing laryngeal edema. If the child is hospitalized, a croup tent provides the ideal environment. A child may be frightened and resist staying in the tent at first. Parents should be nearby and encourage the child by distracting with toys or a game. The child's parents may have other suggestions as to how to keep their child in the tent.

Racemic epinephrine and 40 per cent oxygen may be administered in aerosol form with or without intermittent positive pressure breathing to relieve temporarily the moderately severe symptoms of airway obstruction. Racemic epinephrine by aerosol is administered over a 10- to 15-minute period. Thirty minutes is the minimum time that should be allowed between treatments.

Epinephrine is a potent adrenergic agent that is effective in croup because of its ability to increase oxygenation through bronchodilation and to decrease edema through vasoconstriction. When given by inhalation, epinephrine produces its effects very quickly, with onset at 1 minute and a peak of action at 3 to 5 minutes (Loebl & Spratto, 1986).

Epinephrine has yet another effect, which is *not* advantageous for treatment of respiratory problems. It causes a marked increase in both heart rate and force of contraction. For this reason, it is essential that the pulse rate and quality be closely monitored during and after inhalation of racemic epinephrine. Depending on institutional policy, administration of racemic epinephrine may be limited to an intensive care unit where electronic monitoring of cardiac status is instituted.

Not all children receive relief from this therapy, and repeated attempts should not be tried. In children who do not respond to racemic epinephrine, the nurse should observe for a rebound effect. (A rebound effect is a worsening of symptoms in response to therapy.)

Maintaining Fluid Balance. Adequate hydration is necessary and is provided orally in cases of mild respiratory distress. Intravenous therapy is advisable when respiratory difficulty interferes with oral intake. As the child improves, clear fluids are gradually increased while diet is increased. Refer to Table 32–9 for specific nursing strategies related to hydration.

Facilitating Normal Breathing Pattern by Relieving Fear and Anxiety. A significant aspect of nursing management of croup is decreasing the child's and the family's anxiety. Croup is dramatic and frightening, and it usually worsens at night. Respiratory distress is aggravated by anxiety. Upsetting the child should be avoided. Unnecessary procedures or extensive examinations should be deferred until the child is in less distress. The child's perception of the situation is significantly influenced by parental behaviors; therefore, the focus should be on calming the parents. Parents can then be encouraged to remain with the child to hold and comfort him or her. Rhythmic movements, such as rocking, and gentle touches help calm the child. While in a croup tent, the child should assume a comfortable position and be able to maintain physical contact with the parents. Parents should be encouraged to reach in and touch the child to provide reassurance and prevent feelings of isolation.

Parents who understand the purpose of cool mist

TABLE 32-18
Clinical Manifestations of Acute Narrowing of Lower Airway

Symptoms	Signs
Anxiety	Prolonged expiratory phase
Dyspnea	Sitting or standing position preferred (leans forward)
Shortness of breath	Expiratory wheezing or silent "breath sounds"
Cough	Nasal flaring
Vomiting	Cyanosis
Dehydration	Use of accessory muscles, particularly sternocleidomastoid
Fever	Retractions
Infection	Pulsus paradoxus greater than 20 mmHg
	Grunting respirations in infants

therapy are more likely to cooperate with treatment. They should know that the cool mist is effective in reducing fever, in liquefying secretions for easy expectoration, and in reducing edema of the affected portions of the airway. These effects are often demonstrated within the first hours that the child is in the tent, and the results can be discussed with the parent.

When the child's condition begins to improve (i.e., when stridor and retractions have significantly decreased), attempts are made to "wean" the child from the croup tent. In some institutions, physicians make the decision for weaning; in others, it is a nurse's prerogative. Weaning from the croup tent is accomplished by allowing the child to be out of the tent for short periods that are gradually lengthened if the child tolerates room air without an increased respiratory effort. Periods spent outside the tent are first tried during the day rather than at night. After successful weaning from the croup tent, the child is usually discharged to finish recuperating at home.

Parents need to understand the course of illness and what to expect. Acute LTB lasts from several days to several weeks, sometimes with a persistent barking cough. The prognosis of acute LTB is excellent. Although it may recur during childhood, it eventually is outgrown as the child grows and airway dimensions increase.

Preparing Family to Care for Child at Home. Because croup tends to recur, once a child has an attack, the nurse should provide the necessary information to parents for preventing future attacks or to minimize their stressful effects. Although there are no definite preventive measures, environmental control of temperature and humidity may be helpful. When a child has a cold, the possibility of an attack should be anticipated. Air passages should be kept clear and the child adequately hydrated.

Symptoms of croup at home can often be relieved by special techniques. A croup tent can be improvised by placing a sheet over the top of a crib or playpen and securing it. A vaporizer (warm or cool mist) is then directed into the crib. Safety precautions must be taken, so that the child is not burned or otherwise injured by the equipment. Serious accidents can occur with warm humidifiers in the home. Plastic should not be used because of the possibility that the child might pull it down and smother. The child should frequently be observed while in a croup tent. If it is impractical to improvise a croup tent, the shower or tub water can be run in a bathroom with the door closed to provide an environment high enough in humidity to relieve the distress. The child should never be left alone under these conditions. Parents should be aware of signs of increasing obstruction and instructed to return the child to the hospital if the condition worsens. Exposure to the cold night air during transport to the hospital frequently has been reported by parents to give temporary relief.

Epiglottitis (Supraglottitis)

Epiglottitis is an acute infection of the epiglottis with a potentially fatal outcome.

Etiology/Incidence (Pathophysiology)

In epiglottitis, the epiglottis is swollen, cherry-red in appearance, and surrounded by copious secretions. The infection occurs most commonly in children between 2 and 4 years of age and is almost always caused by *H. influenzae* (type B) (Committee on Infectious Diseases, American Academy of Pediatrics, 1991). The incidence of epiglottitis and other illnesses due to *H. influenzae* is declining as a result of *H. influenzae* type B conjugate vaccine.

The epiglottis is a thin, leaf-shaped flap that covers the entrance to the larynx when a person swallows. It prevents food or liquid from entering the airway. Epiglottitis, an inflammation of this structure, generally occurs subsequent to an upper respiratory tract infection. The characteristically rapid and marked inflammatory response of the epiglottis and surrounding structures causes mechanical obstruction. The edematous epiglottis, like a ball valve, is pulled down into the larynx during inspiration. Inspiratory obstruction may occur because of the narrowing force that occurs with the negative intrathoracic pressure (Hall & Hall, 1987).

Clinical Manifestations

Symptoms of mild upper respiratory infection may or may not precede the sudden onset of the classic symptoms of epiglottitis. Over a period of several hours, the child develops high fever and severe sore throat with dysphagia and rapidly progresses to a state of severe respiratory distress with some inspiratory stridor, a prominent respiratory snore, and retractions. The general appearance of the child is suggestive of the diagnosis: leaning forward with chin thrust out and mouth open with drooling that occurs because swallowing is too painful. The condition may worsen rapidly, with complete obstruction occurring within 6 to 12 hours from the time of onset.

Diagnostic Assessment

A tentative diagnosis is based on the history and clinical presentation. Treatment is immediately instituted when there is clinical evidence that the child has epiglottitis. A throat swab should not be attempted before an airway is established. Placing the child in a recumbent position or using a tongue depressor may produce instant obstruction and is avoided until the child is moved to a facility in which skilled personnel have appropriate equipment to establish an airway. A lateral radiograph of the neck may show the swollen epiglottis. Radiographs are usually made with personnel in attendance who are capable of establishing an airway, and oxygen is administered on the way to the operating room.

Therapeutic Management

A child diagnosed to have epiglottitis is immediately treated with an artificial airway. Until the early 1960s, tracheostomy was generally the accepted method of treatment, but because of the associated morbidity, mortality, and length of hospital stay, alternative methods have been investigated. Nasotracheal intubation has now become the preferred method and is performed in hospitals that have facilities to care for intubated children.

The child with an artificial airway requires respiratory care, including direct humidification of the airway, physical therapy, tracheal suctioning, and constant observation for signs of respiratory difficulty (increased pulse and respiration, retractions, restlessness, cyanosis). Mist can be delivered through a hood or a mist tent, whichever is most comfortable for the child. An IV line is required to deliver antibiotics and maintenance fluids, although these children are usually not dehydrated because they have been well until just before the rapid onset of symptoms.

Appropriate antibiotic therapy is initiated immediately and continued for 7 to 10 days. With increasing reports of infections from ampicillin-resistant *H. influenzae,* the recommended treatment is now combined therapy using chloramphenicol (50 mg/kg per 24 hours) and ampicillin (200 mg/kg per 24 hours) IV. Cefuroxime (100 mg/kg per 24 hours) may also be effective (Boat, 1987). When results of antibiotic sensitivity testing are obtained, the specific effective antibiotic is continued and the other one discontinued. Racemic epinephrine and corticosteroids are not effective.

A nasotracheal tube is usually kept in place for a minimum of 24 to 36 hours (Fig. 32–16). After extubation, the child is observed in the intensive care unit in a mist tent for 24 hours, then transferred to a pediatric unit. One or two days later, the child is discharged on antibiotics. There is some evidence that racemic epinephrine and hydrocortisone facilitate extubation and are useful in the treatment of croup associated with extubation.

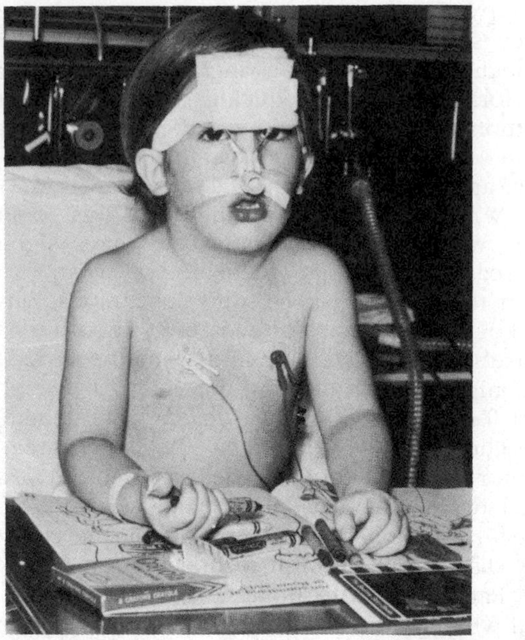

FIGURE 32 - 16. Young child with intubation treatment for supraglottitis. Nasotracheal tubes are well tolerated by most children. (From Barker, G. [1979, August]. Current management of croup and epiglottitis. *Pediatric Clinics of North America,* pp 5–6.)

Nursing Diagnostic Statements

High risk for suffocation; *risk factors: ineffective airway clearance, due to progressive airway obstruction, associated with inflammation of the epiglottis.*

High risk for injury: respiratory arrest; *risk factor: accidental extubation.*

Ineffective breathing pattern, *related to fear/anxiety, resulting from acute respiratory distress.*

High risk for ineffective individual coping: posthospital behavior changes; *risk factors: the fear and anxiety associated with epiglottitis*

Nursing Care

Promoting Adequate Oxygenation. The nurse has a major role in the early management of epiglottitis. To avoid the catastrophe of bringing on obstruction of the airway, all team members must recognize the clinical presentation of epiglottitis. The nurse's ability to remain calm can reduce the child's and parent's anxiety during the emergency phase. The child is not left unattended, even momentarily, until an artificial airway is established. The child is allowed to assume a position of comfort and is not asked to lie down. The child is left undisturbed: no procedures are done that would cause crying or excitement.

The nurse is an important member of the skilled team that intervenes immediately to establish an artificial airway. The nurse's familiarity with the equipment and the technique can facilitate an efficient, skillful procedure.

Preventing Accidental Extubation. Accidental extubation must be prevented by applying appropriate restraints when the child is unattended; elbow restraints are usually sufficient. Taping of the endotracheal tube with regular adhesive tape or umbilical tape rather than clear plastic waterproof tape helps secure the tube. Excessive tape is avoided, because secretions from the nose and mouth can seep between the layers of tape and cause the tube to slip, resulting in accidental extubation.

Positioning of an intubated child is done carefully to avoid movement of the tube. The head, neck, and shoulders must be rotated as one unit, and neck extension and flexion are prevented.

Preparing the Family for Potential Posthospital Behavior Changes. Epiglottitis seldom recurs, but the frightening experience is not easily forgotten by the child or the family. Because of the fear-producing experience that the child has been through, the nurse should prepare the parents for potential posthospital behavior changes according to the age of the child. (See Chapter 21 on Hospitalization.)

Bronchiolitis

Bronchiolitis, an inflammation of the bronchioles, is most frequently caused by respiratory syncytial virus (RSV). Other identified causative organisms include adenovirus and parainfluenza and influenza viruses.

Etiology/Incidence (Pathophysiology)

Bronchiolitis rarely occurs after 2 years of age and has a peak incidence at 6 months of age, occurring most commonly during the winter and early spring months. Boys are affected more frequently than girls. It is primarily a condition treated on an outpatient basis, with only one of five children requiring hospitalization.

Inflammation of the bronchioles results in edema of the airway passages and eventual accumulation of mucus and exudate from cellular destruction. The bronchioles consequently become occluded; some are partially obstructed, and some may become totally obstructed. The alveoli are usually normal, except those in the immediate vicinity of the inflamed bronchioles.

Under normal circumstances, expiration is an entirely passive process whereby relaxation and upward movement of the diaphragm move air out of the alveoli. Normally, the bronchial passages narrow during expiration, but when the lumen is further compromised by edema and exudate, air enters the alveoli and becomes trapped. Sufficient air is taken into the lungs, but there is difficulty in expelling the air, resulting in hyperinflation of the lungs and air trapping. When the obstruction is complete, the air is absorbed by the blood flowing in the pulmonary capillaries and the walls of the alveoli are pulled together, resulting in atelectasis. The impaired ventilation can result in hypoxemia and hypercapnia (carbon dioxide retention), leading to respiratory acidosis.

Clinical Manifestations

After a few days of serous nasal discharge and sneezing, diminished appetite, coughing, and a low-grade fever, an acute phase begins. The infant's condition worsens rapidly, with tachypnea (up to 80 breaths/minute), chest retractions, and a paroxysmal wheezy cough. The infant may be irritable, appear anxious, and have some cyanosis, flaring of the nares, and wheezing, with a prolonged expiratory phase. *When air exchange is severely compromised, a wheeze may not be heard because insufficient air is being exchanged.* Fine crackles may be heard, especially on deep inspiration. When obstruction of the bronchioles is nearly complete, breath sounds are diminished. *A sudden absence of breath sounds, cyanosis, pallor, and listlessness are signs of impending respiratory failure.*

Feeding is often a problem because of the difficulty of breathing experienced by the infant while sucking. The pulse rate is usually increased, and body temperature may range from normal to as high as 41° C (105.8° F).

Diagnostic Assessment

Chest radiographs may be normal but usually show hyperinflation and occasional areas of atelectasis. Areas of consolidation on chest radiographs are thought to be due to atelectasis or inflammation. Certainty of diagnosis requires virus isolation techniques. Immunofluorescent techniques applied to nasal aspirates are highly reliable (Committee on Infectious Diseases, American Academy of Pediatrics, 1991). Routine laboratory tests are not specific for the diagnosis of bronchiolitis. The age of the infant and the clinical manifestations in the face of an epidemic of RSV in a community are highly suggestive of bronchiolitis.

Therapeutic Management

Most infants can be treated conservatively with rest, fluids, and high humidity. Careful handwashing and protection of other children are essential, because RSV continues to be shed for an average of 9 days in children less than 1 year of age. The virus is transmitted by droplets; therefore, respiratory isolation is necessary. Mist therapy, combined with oxygen, loosens secretions and alleviates dyspnea and hypoxia. Clear fluids or hydration by IV therapy is provided, depending on the severity of illness.

A conservative approach is used in the administration of medications. Ribavirin (Virazole), an antiviral agent, is effective against RSV infection causing bronchiolitis if administered early in the illness (Boat, 1992). It is used in selected cases of severe infection or in children with underlying chronic illnesses. Concerns have been raised regarding the safety of ribavirin for health care providers. Although clinical evidence is limited, certain precautionary practices should be followed. These include use of surgical filter masks, good room ventilation, and good handwashing. Gowns and gloves are not indicated, as dermal absorption is negligible. Pregnant women should probably avoid caring for children receiving ribavirin as it has known teratogenic effects in animal studies. (Committee on Infectious Diseases, American Academy of Pediatrics, 1991).

Antibiotics generally are not indicated, and sedatives that depress respirations should be avoided. The role of bronchodilator remains controversial. Children under 18 months of age do not seem to respond to bronchodilators (Corey & Clore, 1991). However, bronchodilators are frequently used in infants with *severe* bronchiolitis or for those who have a positive family history of asthma. Although corticosteroids are not warranted in the usual cases of bronchiolitis, they may be selected for the treatment of acute wheezing in infants. Antibiotics may be chosen for small, acutely ill infants when there is uncertainty about the causative organism. Also, the fact that viral infection predisposes an infant to secondary bacterial invasion is sometimes used to justify administration of antibiotics (Corey & Clore, 1991).

Most infants improve within 3 to 4 days if given adequate supportive care, but usually 2 weeks are required to attain normal ventilation. However, in some cases, the clinical course is longer. Approximately 20 per cent of the infants develop persistent wheezing and hyperinflation of the lungs with abnormal gas exchange that may last for many months (Wohl, 1983). Abnormalities in respiratory function have been found in some children many years after an infection of the bronchioles. Also, there is a high incidence of asthma in children who have had bronchiolitis in infancy. It is unclear whether damage to the lungs from bronchiolitis predisposes these infants to asthma or whether the diagnosis of bronchiolitis was made when the first attacks of asthma were experienced.

Nursing Diagnostic Statements

Ineffective airway clearance, *related to increased mucous secretion, associated with inflammation of the bronchioles (especially with RSV etiology).*

High risk for suffocation; *risk factors: impaired gas exchange, caused by air trapping in the alveoli, associated with narrowing of bronchioles by edema and exudate.*

High risk for fluid volume deficit; *risk factors:*

- *Insensible fluid losses associated with tachypnea.*
- *Reduced fluid intake associated with feeding difficulties.*

High risk for ineffective family coping; *risk factor: anxiety associated with the child's respiratory distress.*

High risk for altered health maintenance regarding assessment and care factors at home; *risk factor: knowledge deficit.*

Nursing Care

Promoting Effective Airway Clearance and Breathing Pattern. The nurse gives careful attention to placing the infant where observation is easy and where other infants are not readily exposed. Constant surveillance is necessary to monitor respiratory status. Frequent assessment for tachypnea, retractions, flaring of the nares, cyanosis, and restlessness is necessary. Apnea monitoring is often indicated during the acute phase. A sudden increase in respiratory and cardiac rates and a dramatic increase in audible crackles are signs of cardiac failure. These findings should be reported immediately to allow rapid treatment by digitalization. Although uncommon, a small percentage (about 1 per cent) of hospitalized infants with bronchiolitis progress to respiratory failure and require intubation and ventilatory assistance.

The major consequence of inadequate ventilation is hypoxemia. Humidified oxygen is delivered via an Isolette, oxygen hood, or nasal catheter. An inspired oxygen concentration of 35 to 40 per cent is usually adequate to correct the hypoxemia (Wohl, 1983). The temperature within the device used for oxygen administration must be controlled to avoid increased oxygen consumption by the infant with hypothermia.

Mist therapy has not been proved to have a beneficial effect on the pulmonary problem. If mist tent therapy is used, a small-particle mist delivered by an ultrasonic nebulizer is desired to aid in thinning secretions. (A large-particle mist does not reach the lower respiratory tract.) These secretions can then be more readily removed by suctioning and postural drainage. Percussion and postural drainage may be ordered if moist crackles are present. Although treatments may be administered by the respiratory therapist, the nurse is also responsible for evaluating response to treatment. Frequently this procedure cannot be tolerated by the acutely ill infant.

Promoting Adequate Hydration. Some infants have dehydration and mild metabolic acidosis. Dehydration may occur as a result of insensible losses of fluid from tachypnea and because of reduced intake related to feeding difficulty. IV fluids hydrate the child, resulting in thinner secretions, which enhances their removal. If IV fluids are administered, they should be given cautiously because unresolved bronchiolitis can eventually lead to heart failure. Specific gravity of urine can be monitored with the goal to maintain a value of not greater than 1.015.

Promoting Adaptive Family Coping. Parents are often anxious and fearful throughout the course of the illness. Therapy is supportive, and they may need help to understand that antibiotics and other medications are not indicated. The anxious appearance and respiratory difficulty of their infant are distressing to parents.

Nursing care provides maximal comfort for the infant and the parents. Care should be organized to avoid unnecessary disturbance of an infant who is already experiencing an energy deficit. Although infant-parent contact is hampered to some degree by an Isolette or mist therapy, parents should be encouraged to touch, hold, and cuddle the infant, as tolerated. When these anxious infants are extremely ill, the best sedative is cuddling by parents. It is the nurse's responsibility to help the parents feel sufficiently calm to provide that comfort.

Facilitating Home Care. Before discharge, parents can be instructed on how to assess adequately for breath sounds by listening for crackles and/or wheezing. Parents are forewarned that their child will not have the same level of energy as before until completely recovered. It is not unusual for their child to need naps, because he or she will tire easily. The child may not feed as well following hospitalization because of being lethargic and perhaps having persistent nasal congestion. The nurse needs to emphasize to parents the need for regular follow-up care and the need for medical intervention if respiratory signs and symptoms recur.

Bronchitis

"Bronchitis" is a term inconsistently used to describe conditions in which the primary symptom is a cough. Chronic bronchitis is usually associated with an underlying disease and rarely exists as an isolated entity. This discussion is limited to acute bronchitis, a condition that can be transient or recurrent.

Etiology/Incidence (Pathophysiology)

Acute bronchitis is an inflammatory process involving the lower trachea and upper bronchi. The terms "tracheobronchitis" and "bronchitis" are not clearly differentiated in the literature. In this discussion, *acute bronchitis* is used, with the recognition that bronchitis is usually accompanied by some degree of tracheitis.

Attacks occur most commonly during the winter months, the peak season for respiratory viral illnesses accounting for 50 to 75 per cent of diagnosed cases (Gellis & Kagan, 1990). Acute bronchitis is usually associated with an upper respiratory tract infection of viral origin, most commonly rhinovirus. It can also be associated with pertussis, rubeola, diphtheria, influenza, scarlet fever, and pneumonia. Factors that may contribute to a child's susceptibility include allergy, environmental factors (climate, cigarette smoke, air pollution), and chronic upper respiratory infections (Behrman, 1992). In some children with frequent or recurring bronchitis for whom an underlying cause is not established, it has been suggested that susceptibility may be genetically determined.

Diagnostic Assessment

Acute bronchitis is usually preceded by a viral upper respiratory infection. After 3 to 4 days of common cold symptoms, the child is seen with a persistent, nonproductive, hacking cough that becomes loose and productive in a few days. The child is usually afebrile or may have a low-grade fever. As the illness progresses, coarse and fine crackles can be heard on auscultation. The cough usually subsides in 7 to 10 days, unless it is a symptom of an underlying problem. Malaise may extend for a week or more after the cough has subsided.

Therapeutic Management

Most children do not require therapy and recover with palliative treatment. Cough suppressants are generally avoided but may be administered in severe cases when sleep is interrupted by cough. Antihistamines cause drying of secretions and are not recommended; the efficacy of expectorants is doubtful. Antibiotics should be reserved for conditions in which a bacterial organism is identified. There is some support for a trial of theophylline for children with severe symptoms that disturb sleep and interfere with exercise and performance in school.

If the cough persists beyond 10 days, secondary bacterial infection or a complication such as pneumonia or atelectasis should be considered. A chest radiograph and sputum examination may be required for confirmation. Children with recurrent or chronic cough should be evaluated for an underlying cause (Table 32–19). Viral infections at the various levels of the respiratory tract are summarized in Table 32–20.

Nursing Care

Maintenance of adequate fluid intake to liquefy secretions, humidification of inspired air, and chest physiotherapy help remove secretions. Adequate rest and avoidance of cigarette smoke are encouraged. If the child is afebrile, moderate activity helps free the secretions from the bronchial tree. General principles of care are provided in Table 32–9.

Pneumonia

"Pneumonia" is a term that describes the presence of an acute inflammation of the lung parenchyma (tissue), including the smallest airways and alveoli.

TABLE 32-19
Causes of Chronic or Recurrent Cough According to Age

Infant (Under 1 Yr of Age)
Congenital malformations (e.g., tracheoesophageal fistula)
Infections (viral, bacterial [pertussis], chlamydial)
Aspiration (milk, gastric contents)
Asthma
Cystic fibrosis
Toddler and Preschooler
Aspirated foreign body
Infections (tonsillar and adenoid hypertrophy, bronchiectasis, pneumonia)
Asthma
Cystic fibrosis
School-Age Child to Adolescent
Cigarette smoking
Mycoplasma pneumonia
Asthma
Cystic fibrosis
Psychogenic cough
Sinusitis
Nasopharyngitis (postnasal drip)

Etiology/Incidence (Pathophysiology)

Pneumonia is most commonly caused by a virus or bacteria (Tables 32–20 and 32–21), *Mycoplasma* (Mycoplasma pneumoniae), and in more recent years *Chlamydia,* a bacteria-like organism (see Table 32–21 for further information on *Mycoplasma* and chlamydial pneumonia). Certain causative organisms are more prevalent in certain age groups than others. Also, the same organism can result in varied clinical responses, depending on the age and general health of the child. The neonate and young infant are particularly vulnerable to serious consequences of pneumonia.

Pneumonia seen in infants and children can be acquired before birth, during birth, or after birth. Pneumonia acquired during birth (perinatal) is thought to be due to aspiration of infected amniotic fluid or secretions from the birth canal. Common organisms transferred are *Escherichia coli, Klebsiella,* group B beta-hemolytic streptococcus, herpes, and *Chlamydia.* Sources of infection of pneumonia acquired after birth (postnatal) include human contact and contaminated equipment (staphylococcal infections). See Table 32–20 for a summary of viral pneumonias and Table 32–21 for the various bacterial pneumonias.

With pneumonia, the lungs are involved in varying degrees, depending on the type of organism and the severity of the infection. The various forms of pneumonia are as follows:

- Lobar—consolidation of all or part of a lobe or several lobes of the lung; exudate is chiefly within the alveoli. Bilateral involvement may occur (also called "double pneumonia").
- Disseminated lobular—a patchy distribution of infectious areas in both lung fields, surrounding and involving the bronchi.
- Interstitial—a diffuse bronchiolitis and peribronchiolitis in both lung fields; inflammation is confined to the alveolar walls and the peribronchial and interlobular tissues.

"Bronchopneumonia" is a loose term that describes a combination of disseminated lobular and interstitial pneumonia. Lobar and lobular involvement is characteristic of bacterial pneumonia, whereas viral pneumonia is characterized by an interstitial inflammation.

Clinical Manifestations

Pneumonia during the neonatal period is predominantly bacterial in origin. Perinatal and postnatal infections are usually manifested by nonspecific signs of illness. Initially, an infant has signs such as poor feeding, lethargy, and fever. Respiratory distress may develop at the onset of the illness or sometime later. When the pneumonia is acquired perinatally, illness manifests itself during the first several days of life, whereas pneumonia acquired after birth manifests itself during the first month of life.

After the neonatal period, pneumonia in infants and children is predominantly of viral origin (see Table 32–20 for a summary of viral pneumonias). Although most patients recover without sequelae, viral pneumonia cannot be viewed as a benign illness. Adenovirus can cause a particularly serious illness with potential fatality. Many infants and children can be treated at home, but severely ill patients should be hospitalized for IV fluids, oxygen, or in some cases ventilator assistance.

Bacterial pneumonia is often preceded by a viral respiratory disease. The lower respiratory tract is made more susceptible to bacterial pneumonia in the presence of a viral respiratory disease in the following ways: (1) secretions are increased; therefore, aspiration of bacteria-laden fluid is more probable; (2) there may be temporary disruption of the ciliary activity, causing less efficient clearing of bacteria from the respiratory tract; (3) phagocytosis and bactericidal activity of alveolar macrophages may be decreased; and (4) the immune response may be reduced (see Table 32–21 for a summary of various bacteria-caused pneumonias).

TABLE 32-20
Viral Infections of the Lower Respiratory Tract*

Bronchitis† and Tracheobronchitis	Bronchiolitis	Viral Pneumonia
Definition		
Infection of upper bronchi and lower trachea	Inflammation of bronchioles	Inflammation of lung parenchyma
Organism		
Usually viral agents (paramyxovirus, respiratory syncytial virus (RSV), and adenovirus)	RSV; adenovirus (rarely)	Respiratory syncytial virus, parainfluenza virus, and adenoviruses
Age		
Occurs most frequently during the first 4 yrs of life	Peak incidence at 6 mos of age; rarely occurs after 2 yrs of age	Can occur in any age group; most of the pneumonia caused by RSV occurs in the first 3 yrs of life
Onset		
Usually preceded by a viral upper respiratory infection, but it can also follow illnesses such as croup or pneumonia	Begins as a mild upper respiratory infection	Insidious or acute symptoms usually precede pulmonary illness
Clinical Manifestations		
Persistent nonproductive, hacking cough that becomes loose and productive in a few days; rhonchi and rales can be heard as illness progresses; cough subsides in 7–10 days	Tachypnea, chest retractions, and a paroxysmal wheezy cough; patient may be irritable, dyspneic, and have prolonged expirations. Rhonchi, wheezes, or rales are heard throughout lungs; breath sound diminished where obstructed. X-ray films show diffuse hyperinflation of lungs and peribronchial infiltrates suggestive of interstitial pneumonia. Scattered areas of consolidation are due to atelectasis or inflammation of alveoli	Cough, wheezing, coarse rhonchi, and frequently a high fever. Headache, malaise, and myalgia are present in older children
Treatment		
Cough suppression by medication is generally avoided (sometimes given in severe cases when sleep is interrupted by cough). Expectorants can be given. Mask inhalations of nebulized solutions and chest physiotherapy help raise secretions. Humidification of inspired air must produce small droplets to be effective. Hydration by increased oral fluids or IV fluids	Treated with rest, fluids, and humidified oxygen. Bronchodilators, sedatives, and corticosteroids not recommended. Antibiotics usually not indicated. IV fluids for hydration, electrolytes, and pH balance are often necessary. Mist therapy delivering large droplets does not affect lower airway; therefore, ultrasonic nebulization is recommended	Treatment is symptomatic; no antibiotics; treat with bed rest, analgesics, and antipyretics with adequate fluid intake and increased humidity. In severe illness, postural drainage and oxygen may be indicated. Ventilator assistance may be required.
Nursing Considerations		
Counsel family against use of over-the-counter drugs to suppress cough; a vaporizer that produces a sufficiently small droplet is recommended	Most critical phase is the first 48–72 hrs. RSV highly contagious—isolate from other infants. Infant needs to be observed closely. Parent-infant contact extremely important because of infant's anxiety. Stress of parents must be reduced by frequent explanations of status of infant	RSV highly contagious—isolate from other infants
Complications and/or Prognosis		
Complications of otitis media, sinusitis, and pneumonia may occur in children who are undernourished or in poor health	Most improve within 3–4 days and in 2 wks respiratory rate is normal, but in some instances illness is prolonged	Most recover in 7–10 days. Otitis media is common in children with RSV infections. Adenovirus can cause severe and fatal pneumonia in infants. There is some evidence that chronic lung disease in adulthood may be caused by viral pneumonia in childhood

* Also see Table 32–17 for acute laryngotracheobronchitis, which is a viral disease.
† Bronchitis is usually accompanied by some degree of tracheitis.

TABLE 32-21
Bacterial Pneumonias Most Common in Infants and Children

Streptococcal*	Streptococcal (Group A)	Staphylococcal†	Pneumococcal‡
Organism			
Group B beta-hemolytic streptococcus	Group A beta-hemolytic streptococcus	*Staphylococcus aureus*	*Streptococcus pneumoniae*
Age			
Occurs in neonates less than 5 days old (early onset) as an intrapartum infection or in infants up to 6 wks of age (late onset). In early-onset, pneumonia is more common; in late-onset, meningitis predominates	Occurs most commonly in children 5–6 yrs of age through young adulthood	Occurs in infants more frequently than in older children. 30% of patients under 3 mos of age; 70% under 1 yr	Children under 4 yrs have a higher incidence. Children under 3 yrs with sickle cell disease have an attack rate of 20%
Onset			
History of prolonged rupture of membranes and low birth weight	Onset is extremely variable; frequently associated with rubeola, varicella, or scarlet fever	History of mild upper respiratory infection (varies in duration from a few days to a week or sometimes longer)	In infants, onset is abrupt, with a temperature of 39.5–40.6°C (103–105°F) and generalized convulsions; sometimes vomiting and diarrhea
Clinical Findings			
Apnea and shock within 24 hrs of birth; hypoxia and hypercapnia. Pulmonary lesions may be patchy or extensive. It is difficult to differentiate from respiratory distress syndrome of newborn infant	May be sudden with fever, chills, and pleuritic pain or may present with mild illness (low-grade fever and cough). Leukocytosis, increased ASO titer, diffuse bronchopneumonia, and pleural effusion may be present. Pleural tap required for identification of organism	Extremely variable. Usually cough, high fever, abdominal distention, rapid grunting respirations. In more severe cases, cyanosis and shock may occur. Chest auscultation may be misleading. In infants breath sound may be heard even with serious pneumonia. Progresses from a bronchopneumonia to consolidation of an entire lobe within hours. Pneumatocele, empyema, and pyopneumothorax are common	Rapid, shallow respirations with grunting, tachycardia, and circumoral cyanosis are seen. Cough is not usual. Abdominal distention and nuchal rigidity occur. Auscultatory findings are not reliable. Patchy bronchopneumonia is most typical in infants. Lobar consolidation is more common in older children
Treatment			
Penicillin G and intensive supportive therapy	Penicillin G (100,000 U/kg/24 hrs). Initial dose is given parenterally followed by a 2–3 wk course of oral administration. Erythromycin, clindamycin, and cephalosporins are used in the event of a penicillin allergy	A penicillinase-resistant penicillin (methicillin) is used. If organism sensitive to penicillin G, then methicillin is not used because of its nephrotoxicity. (Methicillin-resistant strains have also been reported.) Chest tube drainage of fluid or pus from pleural cavity is done. Blood transfusions for anemia may be necessary. Supportive therapy is given	Penicillin G is usual. Ampicillin is used for young children, because it is effective for both pneumocococcus and *H. influenzae*. If pneumonia is complicated by otitis media, medication is prescribed for a period longer than the usual course
Specific Nursing Concerns			
Avoid inaccurate encouraging remarks about an illness with	Compliance by family in administering full course of anti-	Nephrotoxicity of methicillin. Observe infection control pro-	A pneumococcal vaccine is available that is recommended

* Since the early 1970s, the incidence of Group B beta-hemolytic streptococcus has increased as a cause of mortality and serious morbidity in neonates.
† Staphylococcal pneumonia has decreased in recent years.
‡ Beyond the neonatal period, pneumococcal and *H. influenzae* are by far the most common.

TABLE 32-21
Bacterial Pneumonias Most Common in Infants and Children *(Continued)*

Streptococcal*	Streptococcal (Group A)	Staphylococcal†	Pneumococcal‡
Specific Nursing Concerns *(Continued)*			
an extremely high mortality rate. These neonates are seriously ill; the mother is likely to be hospitalized in the obstetric department. Nurse caring for infant should facilitate communication with both parents	biotics. Early and vigorous chest physical therapy may be required to prevent complications	cedure strictly. (Hand washing, gown, and mask are required.) Long duration of hospitalization places entire family under severe stress	for persons 2 yrs of age or older who are especially vulnerable to high morbidity and mortality from pneumococcal infections
Complications and/or Prognosis			
Mortality rate is 60–90%	Bacteremia in 10%; empyema and septic foci (bones or joints)	Septic lesions outside the respiratory tract. Mortality rate is 10–30%	Meningitis, otitis media, sinusitis, and purulent conjunctivitis. Empyema and pneumatoceles may develop. Mortality rate below 1%

Haemophilus Influenzae‡	*Mycoplasma*	Chlamydial
Organism		
Haemophilus influenzae type B	*Mycoplasma pneumoniae*	*Chlamydia trachomatis*
Age		
Most frequent in children under 1 yr. Gram-negative organisms account for only a small percentage of pneumonia in infants and children (after the neonatal period), but they are becoming increasingly prevalent	Although it occurs predominantly in children 5 to 15 yrs of age, younger children are also infected but are not usually ill	It is the most common cause of ophthalmia neonatorum and is an important cause of pneumonia in infants in the first 3 mos of life
Onset		
Similar to pneumococcal but often with a more insidious onset. Most are preceded by a mild upper respiratory infection	The onset is usually gradual, with fever, headache, malaise, myalgia, cough, and sore throat	Chlamydial pneumonia is characterized by a gradual onset of upper respiratory tract signs in infants between 4 and 12 wks of age
Clinical Findings		
Cough is almost always present (can be productive or nonproductive). Rales, fever, tachypnea, retractions, and nasal flaring; dullness to percussion. Can be either lobar or disseminated (bronchopneumonia). Empyema is often present. Pneumatoceles have been seen (difficult to differentiate from pneumococcal)	The cough can increase in severity, taking on a hacking, paroxysmal nature, and is sometimes productive with blood-tinged sputum. These symptoms often indicate a very ill child, but a physical assessment may reveal only a reddened pharynx and slightly enlarged lymph nodes. Later in the illness, fine crackles are common, and chest radiography reveals interstitial pneumonia involving one or more of the lower lobes. The white blood cell count is unusually normal	Nasal obstruction, with or without discharge, a gradually worsening cough, and tachypnea (40 to 80/min) are the predominant respiratory signs. The cough can become paroxysmal and cause vomiting and cyanosis. With lack of fever and only minor complaints of poor weight gain and malaise, the condition may exist for days or weeks before pneumonia is considered the cause. On auscultation, breath sounds are heard throughout the chest, crackles may be heard, but wheezing is uncommon. Chest radiographs show hyperexpansion of the lungs with diffuse interstitial infiltrates

(continued)

TABLE 32-21
Bacterial Pneumonias Most Common in Infants and Children *(Continued)*

Haemophilus Influenzae‡	***Mycoplasma***	**Chlamydial**
Treatment		
Ampicillin and chloramphenicol. Ampicillin is required in large doses. Ampicillin-resistant strains occur; therefore, simultaneous chloramphenicol therapy is recommended	Erythromycin (50 mg/kg/24 hrs in four daily doses for 7 days) is recommended for children younger than 9 yrs of age and tetracycline (25 to 50 mg/kg/24 hrs in four doses) for children above 9 yrs of age	Erythromycin (40 mg/kg/24 hrs) or sulfisoxazole (150 mg/kg/24 hrs) for duration of 3 wks)
Specific Nursing Concerns		
Observe for chloramphenicol side effects	Compliance by family in administering full course of antibiotics	Compliance by family in administering full course of antibiotics
Complications and/or Prognosis		
Frequent complications include bacteremia, pericarditis, cellulitis, empyema, meningitis, and pyarthrosis	Children with *Mycoplasma* pneumonia recover without complications, but there have been reports of fatalities. It has been suggested that this organism could possibly have some part in the development of chronic lung disease	Improvement will be noted in 5 to 7 days, and in 2 wks the infant is usually asymptomatic and normal on physical examination

Diagnostic Assessment

Radiography. Chest films have limitations in establishing a diagnosis; they identify the location of involvement but do not verify etiology. However, certain findings are suggestive of specific organisms. For example, pleural effusion signifies a bacterial pneumonia, and the presence of empyema early in the illness is suggestive of pneumonia due to *H. influenzae* or *Staphylococcus.* Consolidation of a lobe or segment is suggestive of pneumococcal pneumonia. Consolidation is also seen in pneumonia caused by *Klebsiella,* but pneumococcal infections occur more frequently.

White Blood Count. White blood counts are variable. In viral pneumonia, the white blood cell (WBC) count is usually less than 20,000/mm^3 or 20×10^9 cells/L. Bacterial pneumonia is generally associated with more extreme WBC elevations and the presence of many immature cells. The elevated WBC count is primarily due to an increase of polymorphonuclear cells. In severe illness, leukopenia may occur. Leukopenia, a poor prognostic sign, occurs when white cells leave the circulation faster than they are being produced by the bone marrow. (See Chapters 34 and 39 for further discussion of WBC counts during infection.)

Approaches to identifying the causative organism in pneumonia include cultures and Gram stains of secretions in the posterior pharynx and of the blood, tests to detect bacterial antigen, and, when indicated, lung punctures. Results of throat cultures have been found not to correlate well with those of blood cultures and autopsy findings. Countercurrent immunoelectrophoresis and latex particle agglutination are used on serum, urine, pleural fluid, and spinal fluid to detect specific bacterial antigens. The severity of the illness is suggested by the amount of antigen present, with an increased amount present in more severe illness. These tests are particularly useful for cases in which there is no clinical response to the usual course of antibiotics. Lung punctures are recommended in some cases when immediate diagnosis is essential for prompt therapy.

In addition to radiographs, WBCs with differential, and various cultures, the physician takes into account the child's age, the clinical manifestations, and existence of an epidemic in establishing a diagnosis.

Therapeutic Management

Medical treatment for pneumonia, as for many of the respiratory diseases, focuses on improving oxygenation and preventing dehydration. For the child hospitalized with pneumonia, the physician usually orders oxygen as well as ultrasonic mist, and chest physical therapy. Antipyretics may be needed to control fever, and IV hydration is usually instituted.

If the pneumonia is of bacterial origin, IV antibiotics will be used. Antibiotic regimens (types and dosage) change rapidly as resistant strains of organisms emerge. The physician's medication order is based on the most potent available antibiotic for the identified organism, with considerations for cost per dose, number of doses needed per day, and severity of potential side effects. (See Tables 32–20 and 32–21.)

In the event of fluid accumulation in the pleural cavity, drainage is accomplished either by continuous drainage by chest tube or by numerous thoracenteses. Fluid accumulation is most common when pneumonia is caused by *Staphylococcus aureus*. Pain medications may be ordered on an as-needed basis to control the discomfort of invasive drainage procedures.

Nursing Diagnostic Statements and Collaborative Problems*

Impaired gas exchange, *related to ineffective breathing pattern and pain from inflammation of lung tissue.*

Ineffective airway clearance, *related to increased mucus production associated with the infectious process in the lungs.*

High risk for hyperthermia; *risk factor: the infectious process.*

High risk for fluid volume deficit; *risk factors:*
- *Fever.*
- *Increased insensible water loss associated with tachypnea.*
- *Decreased fluid intake associated with dyspnea.*

High risk for ineffective child and family coping; *risk factors:*
- *Anxiety associated with the child's respiratory distress.*
- *Anxiety associated with treatment measures that are perceived as stressful for the child.*
- *Disruption in usual physical interactions associated with oxygen and IV therapy.*

High risk for altered health maintenance regarding residual effects of pneumonia and home care of these effects; *risk factor: knowledge deficit.*

Nursing Care: Facilitating Effective Breathing Patterns. *Changing the child's position* every 2 hours facilitates pulmonary drainage, helps prevent skin breakdown, and provides comfort. Such measures promote gas exchange. Respirations are generally eased by placing the child in a semi-Fowler position with the neck slightly hyperextended. Raising the head of the mattress 30 degrees and placing a small folded blanket or towel under the shoulders straightens the airway and facilitates respiration. Older children assume a position of comfort. Suction should be available whenever secretions are not being handled effectively by the child's respiratory system.

Providing Optimal Comfort and Pain Relief. The nurse must be aware that inflammation of lung tissue often results in pain with the normal effort of breathing. Pain further taxes the child's ability to cope. Careful assessment is indicated to determine whether an analgesic should be administered. If pain is suspected and the physician has not ordered an analgesic, the nurse, in the advocate role, should request such an order.

An analgesic will almost always be warranted for relief of the discomfort associated with chest tubes and thoracentesis. The child in greatest comfort is more likely to obtain the rest needed for healing of infected tissues. Nonpharmacologic comfort measures can provide an effective adjunct to analgesic therapy. (See Chapter 25 for a complete discussion of pain control in children.)

Promoting Effective Airway Clearance. Clearance of secretions is accomplished through a combination of mist therapy and chest physiotherapy, which loosens and removes secretions from the respiratory tract. Ultrasonic nebulizers are capable of producing a dense mist of the small particles that are more likely to reach the lower respiratory tract than are the large particles produced by a mist tent. Percussion, vibration, and postural drainage are usually done every 4 to 6 hours; times vary with the severity of the pneumonia and tolerance of the child. Chest radiograph reports can be used by the nurse to identify the lobes that need particular emphasis when chest physiotherapy is performed.

Parents should be taught to do percussion and postural drainage when their child is hospitalized. They should be given the opportunity to participate

*To be used with Table 32–9, Nursing Process Plan: The Child with Oxygenation Problems.

in the treatment and should be able to demonstrate the entire procedure at least once before their child is discharged. (See discussion "Chest Physical Therapy" under "Therapeutic Management.")

Controlling Hyperthermia. Fever is closely monitored and treated to prevent convulsions. Antipyretics, fluids, and a cool mist environment are provided to reduce fever. A sponge bath with tepid water is recommended by some physicians for a rectal temperature of 39.4° C (103° F), although extended cooling is controversial. Cool mist moistens the airway and helps reduce fever, but chilling must be avoided. Acetaminophen (Tylenol) is prescribed to control fever and make the child more comfortable.

Promoting Adequate Hydration. The nurse also assesses for dehydration that is caused by high fever, insensible water loss from tachypnea, and poor fluid intake due to dyspnea. The nurse should monitor intake and output, check specific gravity of urine, and make ongoing assessments of hydration status. An elevated specific gravity indicates dehydration. Oral fluids are encouraged, but IV fluid therapy may be indicated when intake is poor. Infants in particular have difficulty maintaining an adequate intake because of dyspnea while sucking.

Promoting Adaptive Family Coping. The nurse should also respond to the stresses that parents experience because of the nature of the illness. The need for oxygen, mist, chest physiotherapy, IV fluids, and antibiotics is distressing to parents, especially when it interferes with their ability to hold their child. When a child can tolerate brief periods out of the oxygen tent or Isolette, the nurse can show parents how to properly handle the child to prevent IV infiltration or dislodgment. Parents should also be shown how to support and cradle an infant while feeding the child inside a tent. Providing for child-parent contact during all phases of the illness helps parents feel prepared to take their child home after discharge.

Before discharge, the nurse should discuss the use of antipyretics, antibiotic administration and side effects, percussion and postural drainage, and signs of respiratory distress. A discussion of adequate fluids, rest, and diet for age will help parents take preventive measures in maintaining the health of their child.

Facilitating Home Care. Prior to discharge, parents can be instructed on how to adequately assess for breath sounds by listening for crackles and/or wheezing, which are residual effects of pneumonia. The nurse instructs parents about the importance of taking the entire prescription of medication. The purpose and untoward effects of prescribed medications are reviewed with parents. The parents should be encouraged to give pain medication (Tylenol), should the child have chest discomfort. The nurse instructs the parents to inspect wounds from chest tubes or thoracentesis for signs of infection. Parents are forewarned that their child will not have the same level of energy as before until completely recovered. It will not be unusual for their child to require and need naps, as he or she will tire easily. The nurse needs to emphasize that parents should contact the nurse to discuss questions pertaining to resumption of normal activity and measures to prevent recurrence.

Acute Pharyngitis

Acute pharyngitis is an inflammation of the structures in the pharynx, including tonsillitis and pharyngotonsillitis.

Etiology/Incidence (Pathophysiology)

It occurs at all ages, but the peak incidence is during the late preschool and early school-age years.

The two most common causes of acute pharyngitis are viruses and group A beta-hemolytic streptococcus (referred to as strep throat). About 80 per cent of cases are caused by a virus, and 20 per cent or less are bacterial in origin. In children less than 3 years of age, the bacterium *H. influenzae* is common; streptococcal pharyngitis is rare before age 2 years. The most susceptible ages for acute pharyngitis are 5 to 15 years of age. At this time a child is more consistently exposed to infections outside the home. A natural hypertrophy of lymphoid tissue also develops at this time, shown in enlarged tonsils and adenoids.

Diagnostic Assessment

Viral and streptococcal pharyngitis cannot be reliably differentiated by clinical manifestations. Some characteristics of each are summarized in Table 32–22, but even these overlap considerably. Streptococcal pharyngitis cannot be reliably diagnosed without a throat culture.

Therapeutic Management

Viral pharyngitis is treated symptomatically, whereas streptococcal infections require antibiotics to prevent complications (especially rheumatic fever and glomerulonephritis). In viral pharyngitis, acetaminophen generally brings about a prompt reduction in fever, whereas in streptococcal infections, fever usually persists. On the other hand, antimicrobial therapy (penicillin) is so effective in streptococcal pharyngitis that fever does not usually persist longer than 24 hours after initiation of therapy.

The method of administering antibiotics varies. It is generally safe to wait for the results of the throat culture before instituting therapy (Widome, 1987). If there is concern that a patient will not return for treatment, then therapy may be initiated sooner.

TABLE 32-22
Characteristics of Bacterial and Viral Pharyngotonsillitis*

	Streptococcal Pharyngotonsillitis		Viral Pharyngotonsillitis
	<2 Yrs of Age	>2 Yrs of Age	(Any Age)
Onset	Gradual or sudden	Sudden	Gradual
Presenting signs	Nasopharyngitis	Abdominal pain, vomiting, headache	Moderate sore throat (often preceded by malaise and anorexia)
Fever	Slight to moderate (rarely, 39°C, 102° F), often irregular	Usually high (39.4–40°C, 103–104°F), but may be moderate; may continue for 1–4 days; severe cases, 2 wks	Slight to moderate, sometimes high
Tonsillar involvement	Little or none	May have any or all of following: follicular exudation, erythema of tonsils and pillars, petechial mottling of soft palate, lymphadenopathy; or mild-to-moderate tonsillar or pharyngeal inflammation	Similar to streptococcal, although petechial mottling is less common and erythema is often less; small ulcers may form on soft palate and posterior pharyngeal wall
Clinical complaints	Anorexia, runny nose, listlessness, failure to thrive, vomiting	Sore throat	Sore throat, hoarseness, cough, rhinitis, conjunctivitis. May last less than 24 hrs; does not persist beyond 5 days
Laboratory results	Leukocytosis	Leukocytosis	Leukocyte count normal to high

* In many children there is considerable overlap in symptoms of viral and streptococcal disease.

Penicillin is the drug of choice. It can be administered orally for 10 days or by one (IM) injection. The advantage of IM injection is that the patient who might not return is treated effectively, but this is a painful mode of treatment, and, unless streptococcal disease has been confirmed, it is thought to be unreasonable to subject a child to such therapy without proof of need. If compliance is a problem and streptococcal infection is confirmed, one dose of benzathine penicillin is given intramuscularly to ensure adequate penicillin levels for a 10-day period. If the child is allergic to penicillin, the drug of choice is erythromycin for 10 days.

Nursing Care

The nurse has an important role in obtaining a complete health history, giving particular attention to the history of the illness. The nurse also gathers sufficient data to recommend the mode of therapy (oral or intramuscular) that would be most appropriate for the particular family.

Promoting Compliance with Antibiotic Therapy. If the child is to receive a 10-day course of antibiotics, the nurse emphasizes the importance of continuing the medication even though the child feels well and is free of symptoms. If IM penicillin is to be administered, both the child and parents are forewarned of the pain associated with the injection. Local measures can be suggested to provide relief at home, including warm baths and a warm water bottle.

Relieving Throat Discomfort. Additional symptomatic measures for sore throat include cool, bland liquids, acetaminophen (Tylenol), warm compresses to the neck, and warm normal saline gargles (if the child is able to gargle). Parents should be counseled not to force the child to eat and to avoid liquids and foods that are irritating to the throat, especially citrus and spicy foods. The nurse also advises the family to report similar symptoms in other family members. Recurrent streptococcal pharyngitis within the family is an indication for all family members to have throat specimens cultured.

Explaining the Need for Follow-Up Care. Viral pharyngitis is usually self-limiting, requiring only symptomatic treatment. Streptococcal pharyngitis, if adequately treated, generally results in complete recovery. Both nonsuppurative complications (rheumatic fever and glomerulonephritis) and suppurative complications (peritonsillar abscess, otitis media, mastoiditis, cervical adenitis, meningitis, osteomyelitis, pneumonia) can usually be prevented with prompt treatment. Follow-up practices for streptococcal infections vary. Many practitioners believe a reculture should be done 14 days after treatment with antibiotics. If the repeat culture is positive for group A beta-hemolytic streptococci, three possibilities should be considered: (1) the child did not complete the 14-day antibiotic therapy, (2) an organism that is resistant to the antibiotic is present, and (3) a new infection has been acquired. The question of whether the child is a carrier is also of concern. Most clinicians believe that a second course of antibiotics is warranted; however, if a third throat culture remains positive, one should consider that the child is probably a carrier. (It has been estimated that 15 to 20 per cent of healthy children might be carrying group A streptococci as normal flora.)

Retropharyngeal Abscess

Etiology/Incidence (Pathophysiology)

A retropharyngeal abscess develops when lymph glands located behind the posterior pharyngeal wall become infected. This may result from pharyngitis (group A hemolytic streptococcus) in which the infection extends to the lymph nodes via the lymphatic system. Purulent infection of contiguous areas (sinuses, adenoids, nasopharynx) causes the nodes to become infected, with resultant swelling and suppuration.

Diagnostic Assessment

The illness usually follows an upper respiratory infection and produces an abrupt onset of fever, dyspnea, and difficulty swallowing. A typical response of the nurse may be to suction the nasopharynx to maintain the child's airway. This imprudent action could have disastrous results: rupture and aspiration of the contents of the abscess. If suctioning is necessary to prevent aspiration of oral secretions, it should be of the mouth only.

The diagnosis is established by a lateral radiograph of the neck and by digital palpation of a fluctuant mass on one side of the posterior pharyngeal wall. The child is placed in the Trendelenburg position for the digital examination to prevent aspiration. A suction apparatus must be immediately available in the event of rupture of the abscess during the examination.

Therapeutic Management

A fluctuant abscess is treated by incision and drainage in conjunction with preoperative and postoperative antibiotic administration. Postoperatively, it is important to observe the child for signs of respiratory distress and frequent swallowing (a sign of bleeding) and to keep the child in a prone position to facilitate drainage of secretions. Parents should be kept informed of the child's condition and be given explanations of how they can participate in the care.

Chronic Alterations Affecting Respiratory Function

Asthma (Reactive Airway Disease)

Asthma is a chronic pulmonary disease resulting from a wide variety of stimuli (pollen, dust, viruses), causing increased irritability of the tracheobronchial tree with varying degrees of airway obstruction. The condition is usually reversible either spontaneously or following therapy (Sly, 1985).

Etiology/Incidence

Approximately 8 million children (12 per cent) in the United States experience at least one attack of bronchospasm in their lifetime; 5 per cent of children in the United States suffer from chronic asthma. The prevalence appears to be increasing (Traver & Martinez, 1988).

Asthma, also termed "reactive airway disease," is most common in children, with onset usually before 3 years of age. During childhood, boys experience asthma more frequently than girls. Age is believed to affect the course of asthma. Young children (infants, toddlers, preschoolers), in comparison with adults, have anatomic and physiologic airway differences (see Table 32–1). Among these differences are smaller airways and compromised collateral ventilation. This makes young children more vulnerable to airway obstruction and makes the asthmatic attack more dangerous. Children may have severe symptoms, with acute attack symptoms progressing more rapidly and leading more often to respiratory failure. It is estimated that respiratory failure leads to death in 1 to 2 per cent of children with asthma. Pediatric deaths have occurred prior to therapy, during therapy, and as a result of treatment complications (Friedman, 1984). This emphasizes the child's fragile respiratory state during acute episodes.

Asthma is characterized by an extreme reaction of the trachea and bronchial tissues to chemicals released by the body in response to allergens, psychologic or physiologic stress, or infection. An asthmatic reaction occurs in some individuals in response to allergens, but in others, allergic factors play little if any role. For further information on the inflammatory response, refer to Chapter 37.

Even when allergy is present, it rarely is the only important factor (Pearlman & Bierman, 1988). There is often, however, a family history of allergy when a child is diagnosed with asthma. Chapter 37 describes in detail the allergic response. As identified by Pearlman and Bierman (1988), the following factors can precipitate or aggravate an asthmatic episode:

- *Allergens,* including foods, animal dander, mold spores, pollens, insects, infesting agents, and drugs.
- *Irritants,* including paint odors, hair sprays, perfumes, chemicals, air pollutants, active and passive cigarette smoke (also cigar and pipe smoke), cold air, cold water, coughing, and positive ions.
- *Weather changes* (atmospheric changes).
- *Infections,* especially viral respiratory.
- *Exercise* that is strenuous and associated with breathlessness.
- *Emotional factors;* however, there is no evidence that psychologic factors are the *basis* for asthma.

- *Gastroesophageal reflux,* which is considered to be a cause of nocturnal asthma.
- *Allergic rhinitis, sinusitis,* and *upper respiratory tract inflammation,* related to irritation of the upper respiratory tract.
- *Nonallergic hypersensitivity* to drugs and chemicals, such as aspirin and nonsteroidal anti-inflammatory drugs and tartrazine (yellow food dye number 5).
- *Endocrine factors,* including the menstrual cycle, birth control pills, and hyperthyroidism.
- *Interaction* of various of the preceding factors.

The term "extrinsic" asthma is sometimes used to denote an atopic or allergic cause. "Intrinsic" usually refers to nonallergic factors. Regardless of the cause, the result of asthmatic triggers is bronchoconstriction or narrowing of the airways, edema formation, and secretion of mucus.

Pathophysiology

The airway-narrowing characteristic of an asthma attack (Fig. 32–17) is caused by three mechanisms: (1) *the contraction of the airway's smooth muscle,* (2) *edema of the tracheobronchial mucosa,* and (3) *excessive secretion of the submucosal glands* resulting in mucous plugging (Sly, 1985). The narrowing may be partial or complete, leading to impaired ventilation and gas exchange. Frequently, the child with asthma also has sinusitis, nasal polyps, or concurrent chronic bronchitis that further compromises oxygenation. The characteristic mouth breathing caused by nasal congestion thickens secretions, which further aggravates

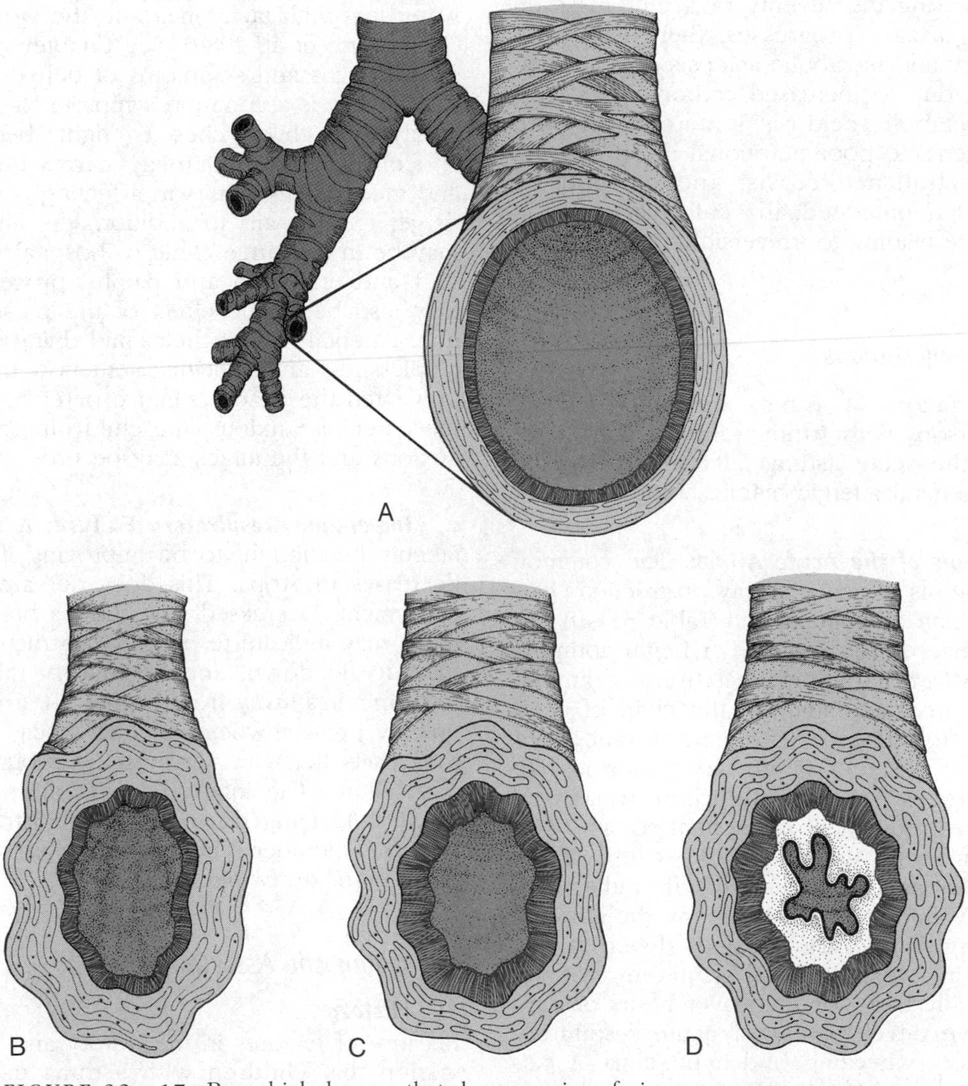

FIGURE 32-17. Bronchial changes that decrease size of air passageway occur during an asthma attack. The narrowed bronchi increase airway resistance to the flow of inspired and expired air. *A,* Cross-section of a normal bronchus, with mucous membrane shown in red. *B,* Bronchospasm: the smooth muscle surrounding the bronchus contracts, causing narrowing of the airway. *C,* Edema of the mucous membrane further narrowing the airway. *D,* Increased mucus secretion by the submucosal glands.

obstruction. If these physiologic responses are not reversed early, air becomes trapped in the alveoli, causing air hunger and resultant hyperinflation of these tissues. The blocked inspiratory air and poor oxygen–carbon dioxide exchange lead progressively to hypoxia and acidosis.

The child's major physiologic problems from the nurse's perspective are as follows:

- *Ineffective airway clearance* related to bronchospasm, mucosal edema, hypersecretion of mucus, and tenacious bronchial secretions.
- *Impaired gas exchange* related to air trapping in the alveoli.

During the early stage, the hypoxemia and metabolic acidosis may be offset by the child's increased respiratory rate. The fright and the vagal stimulation created by air hunger further aggravate the bronchospasm, increasing the severity of symptoms even further. As the disease progresses, there is a combined respiratory and metabolic acidosis. The respiratory acidosis is due to increased carbon dioxide retention; the metabolic acidosis is a result of both decreased oxygen and poor nutritional intake causing anaerobic metabolism, ketosis, and build-up of metabolites. If left untreated, the child can develop respiratory failure leading to irreversible brain damage or even death.

Clinical Manifestations

Clinical manifestations of asthma are either general, common to persons with various allergic conditions, or specific to the acute asthma attack. (Chapter 37 elaborates on general allergic manifestations.)

Manifestations of the Acute Attack. The common signs and symptoms of acute airway obstruction characteristic of asthma are outlined in Table 32–18. An asthma attack may develop slowly or begin abruptly.

Impending Attack. Early manifestations of an impending attack are complaints by the child of chest congestion or tightness, exercise intolerance evidenced by early onset of fatigue and shortness of breath, and increased sputum production, usually accompanied by a productive, paroxysmal cough. Vomiting may occur in the young child because of the tendency to swallow coughed-up mucus rather than expectorate it. Vomiting may accompany the effort of severe coughing. Wheezing often is absent at this stage. Without intervention these symptoms may resolve, but typically they continue over hours or days with progressive development of acute respiratory distress, expiratory wheezing, and hypoxemia. A pattern of apparent resolution of symptoms and their reappearance 6 to 8 hours later, often with increased severity, may be observed.

Progressive Distress. Wheezing is usually worse at night, may be sudden or gradual, and is often preceded by rhinorrhea. The child's cough, although it may be nonproductive, may sound loose because of an increase in secretions. Signs and symptoms indicating progressive or increased severity of airway obstruction are sternocleidomastoid contraction (indicating increased expiratory effort), supraclavicular retractions (indicating increased inspiratory effort), audible prolonged expiratory wheezing, and a prolonged expiratory phase, and pulsus paradoxus greater than 10 mmHg (Lockey & Bukantz, 1987; Mansmann et al, 1988). Subclavicular and intercostal retractions are common, as are nasal flaring and grunting respirations. Pallor occurs as oxygen saturation drops and the child becomes increasingly restless. At this point, the child may assume a tripod position, leaning forward and using all accessory muscles for respiration.

The child experiencing an acute attack may become dehydrated. Dehydration may occur from vomiting, decreased fluid intake, and increased insensible water loss with tachypnea and the work of breathing (Mansmann et al, 1988). See Chapter 26 for a discussion of signs and symptoms of dehydration.

Anxiety is a common symptom for both child and family. The child's chest is "tight" because of bronchoconstriction and airway narrowing from edema and mucus. This results in a feeling of not being able to get enough air. In addition, the child and family may be in a strange clinic or hospital with unfamiliar staff and unknown and painful procedures. Anxiety may also be a side effect of the prescribed medication. Parental fear of their child dying and feelings of helplessness and guilt that somehow they could have prevented the attack enhance parental anxiety. When the parent is anxious, the child often becomes more anxious and the attack may become more severe.

Impending Respiratory Failure. A child can mistakenly be thought to be improving if the wheezing decreases or stops. This does not always mean improvement. Decreased adventitious breath sounds actually may indicate respiratory obstruction, fatigue, refusal to lie down, and respiratory failure, with the child minutes away from having an arrest. Infants frequently present wheezing, tachypnea, and intercostal retractions that can very rapidly progress to respiratory failure. The infant also manifests increased distress while lying down and less distress while held over the shoulder. Therefore, frequent chest auscultation for *air exchange* is critical.

Diagnostic Assessment

History

Because of features in the history and physical examination that children with asthma usually share in common, diagnosis often is possible on the basis of these alone. The history often includes eczema (atopic dermatitis), recurrent bouts of bronchitis, pneumonia, and persistent coughing with or without colds, or perhaps merely a chronic chest rattle throughout infancy and early childhood. Symptoms during these episodes historically have abated after treatment with adrenergic drugs. Symptoms are also typically more severe at night or during early morning hours, with noticeable improvement through the daytime.

Episodes of coughing or coughing spells accompanied by expiratory wheezing are often reported. These episodes may clear spontaneously after 5 to 7 days. Up to 5 per cent of affected children may present with history of coughing without wheezing (Traver & Martinez, 1988). Observant parents or the child may even be able to identify "triggers," or factors that precipitate these episodes. The child's contribution to the history should be solicited, because children often can identify factors that parents have overlooked or misunderstood. Documentation of any known allergies or of any family history of asthma or other allergic disorders should also be made.

Physical Examination

The physical findings depend on the child's age, the severity and chronicity of the asthma, and the timing of the assessment. Physical parameters for growth retardation may reflect a decrease in both weight and height, resulting from diminished appetite, and chronic hypoxemia or obesity associated with the side effects of steroids. Physical growth increases once the asthma is successfully managed.

Blood pressure should be recorded as a baseline for comparison after drug therapy for asthma has been initiated. (Steroids and adrenergic agents may cause elevations.) Respirations should be evaluated for rate, prolonged expiration, dyspnea, retractions or nasal flaring, and use of accessory muscles (shoulders rise). Use of neck muscles to facilitate inspiration is also called "tracheal tugging" or "chin lag." Skin color and capillary return of the nailbeds should be documented. A round shoulder posture indicates alveolar hyperinflation. If hyperinflation is marked, the liver is pushed downward and is palpable. The heart, too, is displaced downward, shifting the location of the apical area for cardiac auscultation or point of maximal impulse. The lungs should be auscultated for unequal breath sounds, crackles that clear with coughing, and overt or latent wheezing produced with forced expiration. The child is asked to force expiration by taking deep breaths and breathing through the mouth during auscultation. Cardiac rate and rhythm should be carefully assessed, because asthma drug therapy can alter cardiac function. Assessment should be done for concomitant aggravating factors such as otitis media, the swollen turbinates and gray boggy nasal mucosa of sinusitis, and healed or active eczematous skin lesions.

Laboratory Tests

Table 32–23 summarizes the usual laboratory tests done for the differential diagnosis and ongoing evaluation of asthma. Blood tests indicate elevated eosinophils and serum immunoglobulin E. Sputum cytology assesses for elevated eosinophils commonly associated with asthma. Pulmonary function tests evaluate lung volumes and flow rates. The most common and the easiest test to perform with children is the peak expiratory flow rate. Most children can learn this technique by 3 years of age. The peak expiratory flow rate reflects the degree of airway obstruction in large airways, which correlates with the degree of small airway obstruction and can be readily used for routine monitoring of health status.

A peak flow meter can be used at home to monitor the child's health status continuously by measuring the peak expired flow of air. Daily use of the peak flow meter is necessary to establish proper technique and baseline measures.

Pulmonary function tests that quantify additional parameters aid in the diagnosis of asthma, provide information regarding the severity of an attack or disease, and evaluate the child's response to treatment or exercise. Sometimes a chest film is needed to assess the airway obstruction caused by atelectasis or the degree of obstruction based on lung hyperinflation. Chest x-ray films are rarely helpful in diagnosing asthma. However, during an acute episode, they may help identify a concurrent infection. Chest radiography is also used to evaluate possible cardiomegaly secondary to pulmonary hypertension from chronic obstruction. Skin testing or elimination diets may be indicated when allergic inhalants or ingestant allergens are suspected.

Therapeutic Management

Asthma management is aimed at avoidance of specific allergens (if applicable), at reducing hypersensitivity reactions by medication and immunotherapy (if indicated), and at preventing attacks via exercise and infection.

Avoidance of Allergens. According to Sly (1986), the most effective treatment for allergy is the elimination of exposure to the antigen. Common house dust is the allergen most often identified in asthma. Mold, mildew, animal dander, and air pollution (notably cigarette smoke) are other common offenders. See Table 37–33 for allergy-proofing techniques involving reduction of common allergens. The subject of allergen avoidance is further addressed under management of allergy in Chapter 37.

Asthma in children can be classified as mild, moderately severe, or severe (Rudolph, 1991). Mild asthma describes the child who has infrequent, intermittent attacks responsive to oral theophylline or adrenergics and who is symptom-free between attacks. The child with moderate-to-severe asthma may require medications around the clock (oral theophylline or oral adrenergics, or both, or aerosol), and the chronicity of the disease has a much greater impact on the family. The latter condition interferes with activity, such as school, sports, academics, play, sleep, and family relationships, although with proper management these children may be symptom-free between attacks.

TABLE 32-23
Laboratory Tests in Asthma

Test	Possible Abnormalities in Asthma	Comments
Complete blood count	Leukocytosis (occasionally)	Induced by infection, epinephrine administration, "stress" (?)
	Eosinophilia (frequently)	Varies with medication, time of day, adrenal function; not necessarily related to "allergy" (often higher in "intrinsic" than "extrinsic" asthma)
Sputum examination	Eosinophils, Charcot-Leyden crystals	In both intrinsic and extrinsic asthma
White or "clear" and small yellow plugs		
Nasal smear	Eosinophils	Suggests concomitant nasal allergy
	Lymphocytes, PMNs, macrophages	Replace eosinophils in upper respiratory infections
	PMNs with ingested bacteria	Bacterial rhinitis or sinusitis
Serum tests	IgG, IgA, IgM	Often normal; may be abnormal—various patterns seen
	IgE	Sometimes elevated in "allergic" asthma Often normal
	Aspergillus-precipitating antibody	Suggestive, not diagnostic of bronchopulmonary aspergillosis
Sweat test	Normal in asthma	Cystic fibrosis and asthma can co-exist
	Perform to rule out cystic fibrosis	
Chest radiograph	Hyperinflation, infiltrates, pneumomediastinum, pneumothorax	Indicated once in all children with asthma Indicated on hospitalization for asthma
	Rule out tuberculosis	
Pulmonary function tests	↓ FEV_1, ↓ FVC, ↓ $FEF_{25-75\%}$, ↓ PEFR; $FEV_1/FVC < 75\%$	Useful for following course of disease, response to treatment
Response to bronchodilators	>15% improvement FEV_1; PEFR	Safest diagnostic test for asthma
Exercise tests	Decreased lung function after 6 mins exercise	Useful to diagnose asthma in children
	PEFR and FEV_1 > 15% ↓	Often abnormal when resting lung function is normal
	$FEF_{25-75\%}$ > 25% ↓	
Methacholine inhalation test (Mecholyl test)	20% fall in lung function with dose tolerated by "normal" subjects	Should be performed only by specialists
Antigen inhalation tests	20% fall in lung function immediately after challenge; may cause delayed response 6–8 hrs later	Potentially dangerous; specialist only
Allergy skin tests	Identifies allergic factors that *might* be causative factors	Test only likely factors—selected by history
Serologic tests for IgE antibody (e.g., radioallergosorbent test [RAST])	Same significance as skin tests	More expensive than skin tests

Modified from Pearlman, D., & Bierman, C. (1988). Asthma (bronchial asthma, reactive airways disorder). In C. Bierman & D. Pearlman (Eds.), *Allergic diseases of infancy, children, and adolescence* (2nd ed.) (p. 559). Philadelphia: WB Saunders.
PMNs = polymorphonuclear leukocytes; FEV_1 = forced expiratory volume; volume of air expired in 1 sec; FVC = forced vital capacity; total volume of air released in one expiration; $FEF_{25-75\%}$ = forced expiratory flow; 25–75% = maximal flow at midexpiration; PEFR = peak expiratory flow rate; an assessment of airflow through all airways.

Pharmacologic Therapy. Pharmacologic management is complex and individualized; it is summarized in Table 32-24. The dosage of theophylline preparation is individualized for the infant and child, because individuals vary widely in metabolism and clearance rates. Desirable blood therapeutic levels are between 10 and 20 μg/ml. To promote adherence to medication for the child with moderate-to-severe asthma, long-acting sustained-release preparations are prescribed to decrease the child's rapid clearance rate, improve compliance, and provide clinical control. Beaded sustained-release theophylline preparations such as Theo-Dur can be sprinkled on food; however, the beads must not be chewed. Beta-adrenergic aerosol treatments

TABLE 32-24
Pharmacologic Treatment for Asthma

Drug	Drug Action	Nursing Implications
Adrenergic drugs (e.g., aerosolized albuterol)	Relaxation of bronchial smooth muscles; possible depression of the inflammatory response in the lungs	Aerosol medications provide good bronchodilating effects at a dose 10–20 times less than would be needed for oral or parenteral administration. Teach the child to use the inhaler after a normal expiration. The child should breathe in the medication slowly and hold the breath to a count of 10. Results are better if a few minutes elapse between inhalations
Theophylline	Bronchodilator; exact mechanism of action is unclear	Often administered in a sustained-release capsule, because it is excreted from the body rapidly when taken in liquid or uncoated tablet form. The family should know the child will need periodic blood tests for serum drug levels; concentrations >20 μg/ml are associated with toxicity. Classic manifestations of toxicity are irritability, marked restlessness, tachycardia, and vomiting
Cromolyn sodium	By an unidentified mechanism, cromolyn inhibits the release of chemicals that activate the inflammatory response, also reduces the hyper-reactivity of the airways	The family must understand that cromolyn is used exclusively for prevention of attacks; it will not open airways during an attack. It is an expensive medication that is inhaled. It is now available in a metered-dose inhaler. It is usually used in combination with adrenergic drugs
Glucocorticosteroids	Reduce the inflammatory and allergic responses and help dilate smooth bronchial muscles	New surface-active aerosol agents have been developed that produce bronchial steroid effects with relatively few systemic effects. The inhaler may be difficult for children under 5 yrs of age. The child must be taught to hold the canister outside the mouth rather than inside, to use the inhaler before meals, and to rinse the mouth and throat after inhalation. There is some concern that aerosolized glucocorticosteroids may damage the pharynx and airways in children

(e.g., albuterol, terbutaline) are preferred over oral preparations for children, because they are faster and more effective in decreasing pulmonary obstruction and have fewer systemic side effects.

Cromolyn sodium, a mast cell stabilizer, prevents the release of histamine. This medication can be inhaled and helps prevent cold-induced or exercise-induced asthma. Its pharmacologic action is effective only in prevention, not after an attack has started. Cromolyn is not an episode treatment but must be taken continuously to achieve optimum control. Corticosteroids enhance bronchodilator effects, decrease mucosal edema, and improve oxygenation (Rudolph, 1991). Current practice is to use corticosteroids by inhalation much more freely than previously, both to prevent an attack and to halt one.

Corticosteroids are given to prevent or treat status asthmaticus if asthma is unresponsive to bronchodilators. Corticosteroids are usually continued in daily doses for 4 to 10 days after the acute attack (Gellis & Kagan, 1990).

Immunotherapy is sometimes given in inhalant-stimulated asthma, particularly when the specific inhalants are ones that cannot be eliminated from the environment or whose elimination would require drastic lifestyle changes. Additional information about immunotherapy is located in Chapter 37.

Therapeutic Management of the Acute Attack

Management of the child's acute asthma attack begins at home. Prompt, effective treatment of early symptoms of an asthma attack significantly reduces the severity of the attack. The family and physician should formulate an individualized asthma attack plan for the use of medications and when to seek medical treatment or hospital care. When symptoms appear, the child and parent can intervene by having the child practice abdominal breathing and self-relaxation techniques along with prescribed oral bronchodilators or beta-adrenergic aerosol treatments (Rudolph, 1991).

Parents can give their child lukewarm fluids during an acute asthma attack. This will liquefy secretions and prevent dehydration.

If the child does not respond, an emergency visit to the clinic, doctor's office, or hospital emergency room is indicated.

The nurse receiving the child and family in an emergency situation needs to provide a calm, relaxed atmosphere. This type of encouragement and support can diminish the anxiety-related increase in oxygen consumption.

On arrival, the child is immediately given oxygen, because hypoxemia is a common consequence of airway obstruction. Although children may prefer nasal prongs to a mask, the prongs are effective only if the child is nose breathing and oxygen requirements are low. The child should be encouraged to assume a position of comfort. (Usually, a Fowler or semi-Fowler position is preferred, but no specific position should be forced.)

The child should be evaluated quickly for signs of hypoxemia (headache, anxiety, confusion, dizziness) or impending respiratory failure (drowsiness, diaphoresis, decreased oxygen saturation per pulse oximetry). Lung auscultation should be done to evaluate airflow. In severe bronchoconstriction, no wheezing is audible or it occurs with inspiration—a sign of impending respiratory failure. In less severe episodes, wheezing is heard on both expiration and inspiration. Wheezing that clears with change of position or coughing is due to mucus that narrows large airways. Arterial blood gas levels are obtained to assess carbon dioxide and oxygen levels. The accumulation of carbon dioxide is a major problem in an acute asthma attack.

The assessment continues with evaluation of the child's hydration status and a family interview. Interview questions are presented calmly and focus on precipitating factors, duration of attack, course of previous episodes, medications taken (especially when last dose of theophylline was taken if that drug is in use), and known allergies. These questions assist in understanding how the child usually responds during an attack, how the child is currently reacting, and what treatments may be necessary to control the child's present attack.

A bronchodilator should be given prior to postural drainage. An antibiotic should be given following postural drainage.

Pharmacologic intervention with subcutaneous injections of epinephrine, or nebulized beta-adrenergics (e.g., albuterol) over a specified time, usually control the attack. If the child is responsive and stops wheezing and the pulmonary function values return to baseline, the child is usually able to return home. If the child is not responsive, an IV line is then started for fluid and electrolyte maintenance* and for the administration of IV aminophylline and steroids. If response was poor to initial adrenergic drugs, oral or IV corticosteroid therapy may be initiated early in an acute attack to help reduce inflammation. Early corticosteroid administration is necessary because 6 or more hours are required for the drug to take effect. Corticosteroids may prevent or reverse status asthmaticus.

An IV infusion pump ensures effective titration levels of the IV drug in the blood. Aminophylline is initially given in a loading dose, then a maintenance dosage is achieved by continuous infusion. Because aminophylline is a form of theophylline, serum theophylline levels need to be therapeutic to be most effective. Theophylline blood levels should be determined before the maintenance dosage is begun; the goal is to maintain theophylline blood levels at 10 to 20 g/ml. Additional doses of inhaled adrenergic drugs may be given to control bronchospasm. Heart rate must be monitored, because these drugs can cause tachycardia.

This therapy is continued until the patient has stopped wheezing and pulmonary function is stable. If after 4 to 6 hours there is no deterioration, the child may be sent home; however, if there is deterioration or pulmonary clearing is incomplete, hospitalization for further evaluation is in order. Expectorants are occasionally prescribed to help bring up secretions but require adequate hydration to be effective. If infection exists (this may be verified by an otoscopic examination, sputum culture, or chest film), an antibiotic is prescribed.

During emergency care, questions posed to the child should be minimal and limited to those that can be answered "yes" or "no." The parents should be permitted to stay with the child to offer reassurance and comfort. Likewise, any security item the child has brought along should remain as additional emotional support. Once the attack has diminished so that the child can swallow fluids without gasping, small but frequent drinks of liquid should be offered to help liquefy and bring up secretions. Chest physical therapy may be ordered to help remove secretions after the child has become stabilized.

Therapeutic Management of Status Asthmaticus

Status asthmaticus refers to continuing respiratory distress that *does not* respond to previous prescribed therapy or to subcutaneous epinephrine or aerosol bronchodilators. This child requires continuing observation, monitoring, and interventions to prevent respiratory failure and is, therefore, hospitalized.

Table 32–25 outlines common management techniques used in the treatment of status asthmaticus. Preparation of the child and family diminishes fears and anxieties regarding unexpected procedures or medications and helps the child manage a very frightening situation. One must initiate steroids early, as they enhance the aminophylline effects, improve oxygenation, and decrease edema.

Any child requiring an isoproterenol drip or intubation requires skilled pediatric intensive care personnel to provide cardiac and respiratory monitoring, because both therapies increase the potential for serious complications.

Nursing Diagnostic Statements

Fear/anxiety, related to
- *Severe dyspnea.*
- *Perception of hospital environment as threatening.*

*Urine specific gravities help establish hydration needs. Serum electrolytes should be used to determine the need for potassium replacement.

TABLE 32-25
Management of Status Asthmaticus

Administer oxygen
Hospitalize
Be calm while continuing to monitor the child's respiratory, oxygen, mental, and hydration status
Provide opportunity for the child to rest
Prepare the child and family for laboratory diagnostic work: • Arterial blood gases (to assess decreased PaO_2 and increased $PaCO_2$, O_2 saturation, and acid-base balance) • Complete blood count (to assess for infection, hydration) • Urine specific gravity (to assess hydration) • Chest radiograph (may be needed to rule out pneumonia and assess air trapping)
Prepare child and family for IV fluids: • Need to rehydrate child • Need to provide IV medications
Administer prescribed medications to child; explain actions, side effects to child (age-appropriate) and family; medications commonly administered are • Subcutaneous epinephrine or terbutaline • IV aminophylline • IV steroids (need to be started early to be effective therapy) • Atropine is sometimes used in the management of status asthmaticus • *Never* administer sedatives (may mask the signs and symptoms of impending respiratory failure) • Expectorants have not been shown to be effective • Continue with bronchodilator aerosol treatment with O_2
If child is unresponsive to previous treatment and displaying signs of respiratory failure, an isoproterenol (Isuprel) drip may be started, *requiring pediatric intensive care monitoring*
Institute intubation and respiratory ventilator support, if not responsive to Isuprel drip

***Ineffective airway clearance**, related to*
- *Bronchospasm.*
- *Mucosal edema.*
- *Hypersecretion of mucus.*

***Impaired gas exchange**, related to air trapping in the alveoli.*

***High risk for ineffective family and individual coping**; risk factors: emotional, physical, and financial impact of asthma.*

***High risk for altered growth and development**: emotional-social development; risk factor: stigma of a chronic illness. intellectual development; risk factor: frequent school absences.*

***Altered health maintenence**, related to knowledge deficit, regarding management of asthma at home.*

Nursing Care

The nurse has a primary role in the early identification of allergenic substances, referral to an allergy specialist, and support and education of the family to promote adaptive coping and effective home management. The nurse in the acute care setting is also directly involved with symptomatic relief of the acute attack. The first two nursing diagnoses deal with the pathophysiology of asthma, which governs specific therapy during an acute attack and prompts the therapeutic regimen designed to prevent episodes of airway obstruction.

The five nursing diagnoses identified can provide the basis for a plan of care during an acute episode or during long-term home management. The nursing process plan in Table 32-26 details nursing interventions for care of the child during an acute attack of asthma. The remainder of this section considers nursing interventions for long-term management of asthma.

Improving Airway Clearance and Gas Exchange. Involving the child and family in the child's asthma management is accomplished by the following:

- Providing information about causes, signs, and treatments of asthma.
- Providing information and discussions on environmental control to decrease contact with known antigens and reduce precipitating factors.
- Teaching them to decrease the incidence of infections and administer asthma medications.
- Promoting self-management techniques in asthma-associated attacks.
- Assessing the effectiveness of therapy or evaluating complaints by reviewing recent peak expiratory flow rate.

Avoiding Allergens and Reducing Precipitating Factors. *Environmental factors* known to precipitate or aggravate asthma attacks should be eliminated or avoided when possible, but not to the extent of inhibiting experiences valuable to the child's normal growth and development or to the degree that constant family discord is created. The nurse can help the family determine how vigorously allergy proofing should be done and how to evaluate its utility.

Exercise-induced asthma in children can have crippling effects on the child's social development, affecting relationships with peers and having negative effects on self-image, if participating in certain sports or activities is perceived as critical to self-esteem. Exercise-induced asthma is commonly caused by activities that require prolonged vigorous effort, such as distance running (Blue, 1988). Sports such as tennis and swimming do not have the same debilitating effects as running and provide alternatives for peer and social involvement. Inhaled cromolyn and bronchodilators used before activity, along with a few minutes

TABLE 32-26

Nursing Process Plan: The Child Hospitalized with an Acute Attack of Asthma

Analysis: Nursing Diagnostic Statement 1

Response and Related or Risk Factors: *Fear/anxiety, related to*

- Severe dyspnea
- Perception of hospital environment as threatening

Projected Outcome: The child will not experience a vague uneasy feeling or feeling of dread

Defining Characteristics

Subjective:

- Self- or parental report of being afraid
- Pleading, telling nurse "I can't breathe"
- Crying in response to hospital personnel, equipment, therapies

Objective:

- Fearful, worried expression
- Sympathetic stimulation—cardiovascular excitation, superficial vasoconstriction, pupil dilatation, increased respiratory effort
- Appearing "wild-eyed" and clinging to parent in response to attempts at diagnostic or therapeutic interventions
- Restlessness
- Trembling
- Voice quivering
- Increased wariness
- Increased perspiration

Nursing Interventions

Airway Management: Admission Care

Quickly implement strategies to relieve hypoxemia and increase airway clearance and gas exchange (see Collaborative Problems 1 and 2)

- Restrict questions to the child as much as possible during the admission period (to reduce oxygen demands)

Security Enhancement

Implement strategies to reassure the child and parents and to reduce the threat of the unknown

- Approach the family with a *calm, quiet, caring* attitude that establishes your competence (their anxiety will be reduced by a feeling that someone knows what to do to relieve the child's distress; therefore, less anxiety will be communicated to child)
- Allow the child to assume a *position of comfort* and to sit on the parent's lap if desired; approach the child with deliberate movements, *explaining* action
- If the child resists a necessary intervention, such as the oxygen mask or prongs, encourage the parent to reassure the child. If this technique fails, perform the action *quickly* (and with the appropriate restraints to prevent self-injury by the child), despite the child's protests and without pleading or bargaining (which

Evaluation Criteria

The client will experience a reduction in fear and anxiety as evidenced by

- More relaxed posture and expression
- Verbalizing "easier breathing"
- Less physical withdrawal from health care personnel, equipment, and interventions
- Return of cardiovascular and respiratory characteristics to baseline
- Dry skin

TABLE 32-26 *(continued)*

Defining Characteristics	Nursing Interventions	Evaluation Criteria
	would delay therapy and cause prolonged protest behavior on the part of the child); explain calmly why the action is necessary (the child's anxiety will usually decrease as the parent's anxiety diminishes) • For additional measures to reduce anxiety of the child and parents, see Table 21–5, Nursing Process Plan: The Hospitalized Child	

Analysis: Collaborative Problem 1

Response and Related or Risk Factors: *Ineffective airway clearance, related to*

- Bronchospasm
- Mucosal edema
- Hypersecretion of mucus

Analysis: Collaborative Problem 2

Response and Related or Risk Factors: *Impaired gas exchange, related to*

- Air trapping in the alveoli

Projected Outcome: The child will experience ability to clear secretions from the respiratory tract and improved ventilation

Defining Characteristics	Nursing Interventions	Evaluation Criteria
(For Collaborative Problems 1 and 2) *Subjective:* • Statements such as "It's hard to breathe" and "My chest feels so tight" • Report of contact with known or suspected allergens • Report of ineffectiveness of home therapies (breathing and relaxation techniques, bronchodilators) to arrest the attack • Irritability *Objective:* • Expiratory wheezing with occasional crackles (rales) and diminished airflow • Retractions (especially intercostal) • Inability to move secretions, cough	**Assess air exchange** • Take vital signs and auscultate lungs frequently, at least every hour initially (to ensure that any changes are noted promptly) • Assess carefully for changes in airflow, alerting the physician if diminished airflow is not resolved by change of position or coughing (this could signal increasing airway obstruction and impending respiratory failure) • Assess for other signs of respiratory failure (see Table 32–3) • **Alert the physician should evidence indicate increasing airway obstruction** *Ventilation Assistance; Oxygen Therapy; Teaching: Procedure/Treatment* **Teach and implement strategies to increase airway clearance and gas exchange**	**The client will experience increased airway clearance and increased gas exchange as evidenced by** • Increased air movement on lung auscultation • Decreased retrations • Expectoration of mucus • Vital signs within normal limits for age • Absence of headache, fatigue, confusion, dizziness • Arterial blood gases within normal limits • Urine specific gravity 1.015 • Absence of abnormal breath sounds • Absence of pallor and cyanosis • Calm appearance and verbalizations of relief

(continued)

TABLE 32-26 *(continued)*

Defining Characteristics	**Nursing Interventions**	**Evaluation Criteria**

• Pallor with circumoral cyanosis
• Tachycardia, increased effort on expiration
• Hypoxemia indicated by arterial blood gases (decreased pH, decreased PaO_2) and by fatigue from respiratory effort
• Restlessness
• Increased urine specific gravity
	• Reduce hypoxemia
	  • Administer *oxygen,* as ordered, to ease the respiratory effort and resolve hypoxemia (related to the obstructive effects of mucus, bronchospasm, and edema
	• Reduce bronchospasm
	  • Administer *bronchodilators,* as ordered, e.g., SC epinephrine or SC terbutaline, IV aminophylline, nebulized beta-adrenergic agents (to relieve bronchospasm by relaxing smooth muscles)
	  • Monitor *blood* levels of *theophylline* during IV administration of and before administering the next oral dose of aminophylline (theophylline is the largest component of aminophylline; blood levels >20 μg/ml may lead to toxicity)
	  • Use a *cardiorespiratory monitor* with IV aminophylline, if use of monitor is a nursing prerogative in the institution (aminophylline increases heart rate and force of contraction; high blood levels may lead to tachycardia)
	• Teach the cooperative child to inhale deeply on the nebulizer airway, hold the breath to a count of 10 (if possible), and exhale through pursed lips (to increase the penetration and effect of the medication on the bronchial tree)
	• Reduce bronchial edema
	  • Administer *corticosteroids* as ordered for severe asthma (to reduce pulmonary inflammation and edema, and to potentiate the action of beta-adrenergic bronchodilators). Assure parents that short-term use of corticosteroids will not result in cushingoid effects or steroid dependency	

TABLE 32-26 (continued)

Defining Characteristics	Nursing Interventions	Evaluation Criteria

	• Evaluate effectiveness of medications against evaluation criteria
	• Promote expectoration of mucus
	  • Keep the child well *hydrated* (to help liquefy secretions); calculate the child's fluid needs per kilogram of body weight (see Chapter 26), and ensure that the child receives at least this much fluid (IV + PO) every 24 hrs
	  • Measure urine specific gravity every shift (if this is done with a spectrometer on the unit, it does not need a physician's order)
	  • After bronchospasm has resolved, perform chest physical therapy (CPT) as ordered, or if this is a function of the respiratory therapy department, assist the therapist to evaluate the benefits of CPT in clearing the airway	

Analysis: Nursing Diagnostic Statement 2

Response and Related or Risk Factors: *Altered health maintenance, related to knowledge deficit of child and/or parents, about management of asthma at home*

Projected Outcome: The child and family will demonstrate ability to manage care at home

Defining Characteristics	Nursing Interventions	Evaluation Criteria
Subjective and/or Objective: • Demonstrated lack of adaptive behaviors to and/or observed inability to take responsibility for meeting home care needs • Expressed interest in learning how to care for self/child at home	*Discharge Planning* **Assure adequate time for learning home management** • Begin discharge teaching on the day of admission • Plan time for questions and clarification on the day of discharge • Table 21–5 provides details of these strategies *Teaching: Disease Process* **Ensure that the child and parent are aware of factors that may precipitate another attack** • Discuss with them avoidance of allergens and irritants	**The child and/or parents will display the knowledge and skills needed for home management, as evidenced by** • Demonstrating effective physical care • Demonstrating effective operation of equipment • Demonstrating safe medication administration and identifying side effects

(continued)

TABLE 32-26 (continued)

Defining Characteristics	Nursing Interventions	Evaluation Criteria
	• As appropriate to the client, include house dust, animal dander, mold and mildew, seasonal pollens, particular foods, cigarette smoke, odors from paints and chemicals, weather and climatic changes, air pollution, exercise, infections, and/or emotional stress *Teaching: Prescribed Activity/Exercise* **Ensure that the child and parents understand physical restrictions, if any apply** • Discuss with them plans for exercise • Suggest these strategies to minimize the threat of bronchospasm: minimize intake of cold air by wrapping a muffler around the nose and mouth; precede physical exercise with a warm-up period; consider activities that do not require sudden bursts of activity, which increase airflow; consider using medications prior to exercise to increase tolerance **Request that the child and parents list signs and symptoms requiring medical attention:** increasing wheezing and difficulty breathing; cough; increasing fatigue and lethargy; a respiratory infection; decreasing effectiveness of medications; and emotional dependency on prn inhalant bronchodilators *Teaching: Procedure/Treatment* **Discuss with the family their plans for well child care; ensure that the child and parents can competently operate and clean necessary equipment, such as a nebulizer** • Institute self-treatments or parental treatments with the equipment in question as soon as initial anxiety has decreased (repeated practice will increase competence)	

TABLE 32-26 *(continued)*

Defining Characteristics	Nursing Interventions	Evaluation Criteria
	Teaching: Prescribed Medication **Provide verbal and written instructions about medication and allow self-administration or parental administration as often as possible** • Provide information about the administration of *theophyllyine* products: • Common side effects: agitation, nausea and vomiting, tachycardia • Large quantities of chocolate, coffee, tea, or colas may increase action of theophylline (by reducing clearance from body) • Smoking tobacco or marijuana, ingestion of charcoal-broiled beef, or high-protein diet may reduce action of theophylline (by increasing clearance rate) • Provide information about metered-dose inhaler for *cromolyn* administration	
	Self-Esteem Enhancement **Address the issue of adherence to therapeutic regimen associated with feelings about being stigmatized** • Encourage the child to voice feelings about taking the medications at home and at school • Help the child identify feelings that may present a problem with regular administration • Help the child plan ways to take the medications and still avoid unpleasant feelings about administration, e.g., taking the medications before and after school, going home for lunchtime therapies, taking the medications in the school nurse's office during a recess break • Help the parents realize the benefits of self-management to the child's self-esteem • Reinforce the family's efforts at the child's self-management	

of warm-up exercise, have demonstrated their ability to control the reactive airway disease associated with exercise-induced asthma.

Preventing Infections. For the child with asthma, infection is a double threat. Not only is there the usual concern about infectious illness, but that illness may trigger an asthma episode, especially if it involves the respiratory tract. Prevention involves promoting optimal general health and avoiding exposure to pathogens.

Children with asthma need to maintain their general health with balanced nutrition, adequate rest, and a relatively routine, calm home and school environment. Consultation with the child's allergist determines which immunizations may be safely given. The culture media for some vaccines are highly allergenic for some persons. Most children with asthma should have all the usual immunizations at the recommended ages.

Avoiding pathogens is, of course, impossible in the literal sense, but the nurse can support the family's own common-sense methods of keeping the child away from infectious persons. In addition, the nurse can teach the family about ways in which bacteria, viruses, and fungi are spread and can impress on them the importance of good hand washing. (The family can also consult with the allergist about the advisability of flu vaccine prior to flu season.) Yearly flu and pneumococcal vaccines are often recommended if the child is not allergic to them.

Achieving Compliance with Medication Therapy. The current long-acting theophyllines have improved medication adherence, because the medication is required less frequently, usually only twice a day. In spite of the recent pharmacologic improvements, peer pressures and the social activities of school-age children and adolescents may result in irresponsible behavior regarding medications. Lack of compliance may result from fear of peer nonacceptance or an unconscious effort to avoid feelings of dependency or vulnerability.

For children on round-the-clock medications, the schedule should be as convenient as possible.

Parents may be noncompliant in administering any bronchodilator (aminophylline), as the child may exhibit increased activity levels and insomnia.

Ideally the schedule avoids school hours; when medication is necessary at school, arrangements should be made for the child to take the medication privately, with no undue attention.

Adequate information should be provided as growth and development progress in order to enhance the child's capability for self-management of the medical and environmental therapies. The dangers of attempting to manage asthma with unprescribed over-the-counter drugs advertised to relieve allergic symptoms should be emphasized. Parents should be cautioned that even under the most careful management, occasional asthma attacks may occur, and they should be reassured that these attacks are not evidence of parental failure.

Promoting Optimal Development. The intermittent acute asthma attacks and the chronicity of a complicated, burdensome medical regimen have an emotional, physical, developmental, and financial impact on the child and family. The growing child faces many stresses associated with asthma, which make it difficult to function independently.

Recognizing and Reducing the Impact of Illness on the Child. During acute attacks, the asthmatic child may have to cope with anxiety, irritability, sadness, and fears of suffocation and dying. The long-term consequences of this chronic condition create fear and uncertainty about future attacks, emergency visits, hospitalization, separation from family and peers, and painful or misunderstood procedures. The side effects of prescribed medications, along with the disease's behavioral aspects, may result in changes in psychologic functioning affecting school attendance and achievements and the child's participation in social activities. Psychologic changes include central nervous system stimulation, inability to sleep, fatigue, decreased ability to concentrate, irritability, and anxiety.

Stress at home for the asthmatic child and parent usually involves fears of an attack that could occur when help and appropriate remedial treatment would not be immediately available. The parents may fear sending the child to a day care center, leaving the child with a baby sitter, and taking vacations very far from the local doctor or hospital. This leads to unnecessary restrictions on family activity and overprotectiveness of the child, with resulting limitations on initiative and cognitive growth.

The child and family can deal with this insecurity by having a plan for daily preventive activities to control symptoms and an attack plan to halt symptoms. The plan is mutually designed by child, family, nurse, and physician. The plan is reviewed about every 6 months to adjust for growth. After age 5 years, the child can be taught to use and carry an inhaler. With proper allergenic control, the symptoms lessen and restrictions can be minimized. The more responsibility the child takes for self-management, the greater is the feeling of control with respect to the asthmatic symptoms. A sense of control contributes to self-confidence in mastering developmental tasks and in achieving self-esteem and competence. Self-management must be linked, however, to developmental readiness. Parents must remain involved in care at least through the school-age years.

Some children with asthma have learned that wheezing behavior can manipulate others. Limit setting should start early and remain consistent. The parent must be cautioned not to make threats that cannot be enforced. The child needs frequent assurance from health personnel and from parents that there is no cause for guilt, even though everyone involved sometimes feels frustration because of the asthma. Asthma is, in fact, something beyond anyone's control. Parents may need to be cautioned against using their child's asthma as a conversation topic. (Children react to overheard conversations about themselves long before they master language.) Some parents may need counseling if they persistently use the child's asthma as a convenient excuse for misbehavior. There are numerous asthma management programs in the community that can assist parents and children together to learn about asthma management.

If conflicts and anxieties in the family perpetuate the child's asthma episodes or the child frequently uses asthma behavior to express and meet emotional needs, counseling should be sought. Parents need help in developing in their child an increasing responsibility for self-care. The goal is to raise the child as normally as possible.

Recognizing and Reducing the Impact on Parents and Siblings. Parents may have the same experiences and feelings as their asthmatic child. Parents face physical fatigue from loss of sleep, anxiety, guilt, frustration, financial hardships, and restriction of family activities. Parental guilt may be compounded by financial constraints, such as not having enough money to allergy-proof their home. Interventions such as financial aid, finding a baby sitter qualified to care for the child in an emergency, and avoiding precipitants that stimulate attacks may help diminish family stress.

Conflicts over dependency-independency needs often occur in families of children with asthma. Some parents experience difficulty both in separating from their school-age children and in encouraging independence and self-responsibility. Parental overprotection, rejection, neglect, and discipline issues may become evident. Inconsistent limit setting may become the parental style of discipline. The inconsistency and lack of structure can result from parental fears that discipline may precipitate an attack.

Parent groups led by qualified professionals help in solving day-to-day health and childrearing problems and emotional concerns. Suppressed parental anger about lifestyle changes can cause conflicts. Resolution of anger is essential to the management regimen. Parents who are in touch with their feelings about the chronic nature of asthma are better prepared to support their child in the therapeutic regimen.

Siblings may exhibit behavior demonstrating resentment toward the "sick" child, or anxiety and overconcern for well-being. Sibling jealousy over preferential treatment given the child or restrictions on freedom imposed on the entire family may lead to suppressed anger. The angry younger sibling may benefit from activities, such as modeling clay and pounding tables, that allow release of pent-up emotions. Sibling rivalry is often reduced by ensuring that all children in the family share equally in family responsibilities. Sibling involvement in the family teaching and counseling is necessary for optimal family functioning. Through counseling, parents and siblings can learn to identify and accept their feelings and to seek appropriate outlets.

The nurse can be supportive of the family by recognizing their need for intervention and by referring them to appropriate counseling and/or support groups. The nurse who has the opportunity for long-term follow-up with the family can be supportive by reinforcing effective problem solving.

Promoting Home Management. The goal of nursing strategies with the asthmatic child and family is to provide information, education, and counseling to support the child's and family's self-management of asthma (Zahr et al, 1989). The effects of self-management lessen the disease's disruptive influence within the home and foster the independence and development of both the child and the family.

Counseling regarding styles of discipline is frequently a family need. One should encourage consistency in the style of parental discipline. If parental discipline precedes an attack, the family is encouraged to continue to be consistent with limit setting and to deal with the attacks as they occur. Parental love and attention given to the child when well will help minimize the use of wheezing to gain attention.

The nurse involved in the community may identify ways to educate schoolteachers and the asthmatic child's peers. The nurse must provide information regarding

- Causes of asthma.
- Signs of asthma attack.
- Participation in physical education activities.
- Medications taken at school (including side effects) and importance of having some medications (e.g., inhalers) with the child at all times.
- Possible hearing loss from otitis media.
- What to do if the child has trouble with asthma (is doing more than just wheezing).
- Effect of animals in the classroom on the asthmatic child.
- Foods the child can eat at school parties.
- Effect that missing school for illness or doctor visits has on the child.
- Ways to promote the child's strength and normalize their school interactions.
- Avoid special treatment.

This information facilitates understanding and a supportive environment for the child with asthma.

Long-term asthma management involves both child and family. Family education commitment is critical to promote adherence to the treatment protocol, to improve outcome, and to lessen emergency room visits and hospitalization. The nurse can use therapeutic approaches to enhance family motivation and commitment.

Improper use of inhalers is a problem for many children. It is an area of family-centered teaching that requires continued monitoring for optimal outcomes.

Cystic Fibrosis

Cystic fibrosis is a multisystem disorder with the predominant characteristics of chronic pulmonary disease, pancreatic enzyme deficiency (resulting in digestive problems), and abnormally high sweat chlorides.

Etiology/Incidence

The life span of children with cystic fibrosis continues to increase. The average age at death in the 1940s was 1 year; with the advent of antibiotics and various modes of treatment, children with cystic fibrosis are now living through adolescence to early adulthood. Approximately 95 per cent live to the age of 16 years, 50 per cent live to age 28 years, and a number live into their thirties and early forties (McQuitty & Lewis, 1991). Cystic fibrosis occurs equally in males and females, but affected males generally outlive females, six to one, by 20 years of age. It is the most common life-threatening genetic disease in caucasians. It occurs less commonly in African-Americans. It is estimated to affect 1 in 2000 and 1 in 17,000 white and African-American neonates, respectively, but this varies according to ethnic composition within a population. Cystic fibrosis is less common in populations of Asian descent; it is rare in Native Americans.

The mode of transmission of cystic fibrosis is an area of continuing research, but it is transmitted by the autosomal recessive mode of inheritance.

The gene responsible for cystic fibrosis is located on chromosome 7 (Riordan, 1989). This gene codes for the membrane protein in epithelial cells that regulates the movement of chloride and sodium in these cells. Several alterations of this gene appear to cause cystic fibrosis. One of the most common alterations (70 per cent of genes, ΔF508) results in the omission of the amino acid phenylalanine from the cystic fibrosis transmembrane regulator protein. Approximately 100 other different mutations of the gene are thought to exist and to affect the protein in different ways. This variation of mutations serves to explain the varied presentations of the disease.

This discovery may enable families with a history of cystic fibrosis to determine whether they are carriers of the gene. It is estimated that 5 per cent of the white population are carriers (heterozygous) and that 1 in 400 marriages are between two individuals who are carriers of the disease (Hodson, 1983). When two individuals are carriers of the abnormal gene, there is a 1 in 4 risk with each pregnancy for their offspring to be a child with cystic fibrosis. The unaffected sibling of a child with cystic fibrosis has a 2 in 3 chance of being a carrier for cystic fibrosis. (See Chapter 31 for further discussion of patterns of inheritance.)

Pathophysiology

The exact cause of cystic fibrosis remains undetermined; however, it involves a generalized dysfunction of the exocrine (mucus-producing) glands with varying degrees of severity. The basic problem is thought to occur at the cellular level and to involve an alteration in a protein, possibly an enzyme, primarily affecting the movement of chloride and water into and out of the cell. The *primary pathophysiology* is an abnormal accumulation of viscid mucus, which leads to the obstruction and dilatation of many glands and organs. Although many organs may be affected, the pathology in the lung and the pancreas presents the greatest clinical problems. The degree of organ system involvement varies: digestive system involvement occurs in 75 to 80 per cent, whereas some degree of pulmonary involvement is eventually seen in most cases. However, a few patients have only enzyme deficiency without pulmonary disease (Gellis & Kagan, 1990).

Although the lungs are not exocrine glands, they are composed largely of epithelial cells. The lung usually appears normal at birth, but soon thereafter, obstruction of the airways with viscid mucus leads to infection and a chronic inflammatory process. At autopsy, the trachea and bronchi are generally filled with a mucopurulent material, the lungs are emphysematous with adhesions and areas of consolidation, and atelectasis is present. The mucopurulent material is thought to be a combined product of the tracheobronchial gland secretions and the infectious process (Schwachman, 1983).

Involvement of the pancreas is clinically important because of its effect on the digestive system. The exocrine glands of the pancreas, clogged with thick mucus, show dilatation of ducts and, in later stages, diffuse fibrosis associated with autodigestion from trapped proteolytic enzymes. Failure of the pancreas to secrete enzymes results in digestive disorders that are characterized by malabsorption, with excessive fat and protein in the stools.

The most consistent pathophysiologic observation is the presence of elevated chloride and sodium in sweat. It occurs in 98 to 99 per cent of affected children. This clinical finding is now thought to be related to a decreased absorption in the sweat glands associated with a decreased cellular permeability to chloride (Quinton & Bisman, 1983; Rosenstein, 1988).

A link may exist between thick mucous secretions and abnormal sweat electrolyte concentrations, or each may be the independent result of a more basic defect affecting secretory and transport mechanisms of cells (Schwartz, 1987). Other organs affected are paranasal sinuses, salivary glands, liver, intestine, the reproductive tract, and tear glands. The number of involved organs and degree of organ involvement vary considerably from one child to another.

Clinical Manifestations

Because the two main organ systems involved in the disease are the respiratory and gastrointestinal tracts, the presenting signs and symptoms generally result in complications of these systems. Approximately 10 per cent of infants with cystic fibrosis show symptoms as early as the newborn period, with meconium ileus (an impaction of meconium). In the remaining children, symptoms of the disease are variable, differing in degree of severity; in fact, many are not readily apparent until quite late in life. The most common presenting signs are recurrent respiratory infections, poor weight gain despite voracious appetite, persistent coughing with excessive mucus, and wheezing. Additional signs are salty taste of the skin, nasal polyps, and bulky, foul-smelling, numerous stools.

Respiratory Manifestations. Many affected children have a history of chronic pulmonary disease with onset as early as birth, but their condition is sometimes not diagnosed for years. Initial symptoms include a chronic cough followed by obstruction of bronchioles, resulting in secondary infection and respiratory distress.

As the thick, tenacious mucus accumulates, obstruction occurs and the flow of air is impaired, with an increase in residual volume and subsequent decrease in the vital capacity of the lungs. Auscultatory findings may be normal in the early stages, but as the disease progresses, moist crackles and harsh breath sounds are heard. As the functioning alveoli become overaerated, the chest distends, resulting in a barrel shape. If ventilation is significantly impaired, cyanosis is observed. Clubbing of the fingers and toes is observed in patients, with at least some level of chronic respiratory compromise (see elsewhere in this text for a description of clubbing). The course of these symptoms follows a pattern of remissions and exacerbations. Major pulmonary complications include hemoptysis, pneumothorax, cor pulmonale, congestive heart failure, and eventual respiratory failure.

Gastrointestinal Manifestations. Pancreatic involvement is apparent in approximately 85 per cent of children with cystic fibrosis. The earliest possible clinical manifestation is meconium ileus. Meconium ileus with intestinal obstruction is due to abnormal mucous secretion from the intestinal mucosal glands and the deficit of pancreatic enzymes. Intestinal obstruction is a sign of meconium ileus, including abdominal distention, dehydration, vomiting, and absence of stools.

As cystic fibrosis progresses, children have a markedly impaired ability to digest food, resulting in malabsorption. Causes of malabsorption include obstruction of the pancreatic ducts and absence of the enzymes necessary for conversion of food into products that can be absorbed by the intestines. Because the enzymes (protease, lipase, and amylase) capable of breaking down fats and proteins are absent, the child characteristically has large, loose, foul-smelling stools caused by fat in the stool (steatorrhea). The stool may actually appear greasy.

Although the child has a voracious appetite, the nutrient loss from the intestinal tract causes the child to lose weight and appear malnourished, with a distended abdomen and thin extremities. A common gastrointestinal complication is rectal prolapse. Because of the inability to absorb fats, variable degrees of deficiencies of the fat-soluble vitamins A, D, E, and K can occur in children with cystic fibrosis; however, only occasionally do they have vitamin deficiency symptoms (Doershuk & Boat, 1987). Vitamin K, which is provided primarily through intestinal synthesis, may be deficient, causing hypoprothrombinemia requiring vitamin K supplementation.

Problems pertaining to reproduction are also frequent. In the male, the epididymis, vas deferens, and seminal vesicles are usually poorly developed or absent, resulting in most males being sterile. Sexual function is usually not impaired. Female fertility is low, owing to plugging of the cervix with a thick mucus that is abnormal in physical and chemical properties and blocks entry of the sperm (Rudolph, 1991).

Diagnostic Assessment

Neonatal screening for cystic fibrosis remains unproven as beneficial and is still being researched. The only reliable and valid diagnostic test for cystic fibrosis is the sweat test by pilocarpine iontophoresis (quantitative pilocarpine iontophoresis test) followed by Gibson-Cooke quantification of chloride concentration. This test is difficult to perform in the first few weeks of life owing to the paucity of sweat and is ideally done between 4 and 6 weeks of age. Furthermore, it is not known whether early treatment of an asymptomatic infant affects prognosis. The fact that a false-positive result could interfere with early infant-parent relationships is a serious concern. False-negative results also raise serious medical and legal issues.

Research continues in search of an appropriate screening test, including prenatal and postnatal tests. DNA analysis techniques can detect sibling heterozygotes or fetuses with cystic fibrosis when both parents and the sibling with cystic fibrosis are available (Doershuk & Boat, 1987). Evaluation of meconium for albumin content is not widely accepted. A relatively simple test—the dried blood immunoreactive trypsinogen assay—continues to be studied. This assay measures a manifestation of the disease, deficient pancreatic enzymes, but has false-positive results and misses the 10 per cent of cystic fibrosis children with normal pancreatic function. The reliability and validity of this test have not yet been determined, and the test is not recommended for mass screening (Ad Hoc Committee Report, 1983). Positive identification of the cystic fibrosis gene in 1990 will lead, one hopes, to improved detection and/or treatment potentials.

The diagnosis of cystic fibrosis is based on a positive sweat test in combination with one or more of the following: chronic lung disease, pancreatic insufficiency, and a family history of the disease (Doershuk & Boat, 1987). The sweat test is believed to be the most reliable diagnostic test, and a diagnosis is not made without it. The sweat test involves a painless collection of sweat from the forearm of the child. To ensure an accurate test, it is strongly recommended that the test be done in a cystic fibrosis center that performs at least 100 of these tests each year. Measurements of sodium and chloride levels above 60 mEq/L are considered diagnostic: levels between 45 and 50 mEq/L are considered suggestive. The test should be repeated for children with the latter finding. The diagnosis in a family should alert the physician to have sweat tests performed on all siblings.

In addition to the sweat test, chest x-ray films confirm chronic obstructive lung disease. Pulmonary function studies reveal decreased vital capacity and tidal volume, increased airway resistance, and decreased FEV_1 and FEV_1/VC ratio. These are the result of chronic pulmonary infection, which eventually progresses to bronchiectasis.

To determine pancreatic involvement, stool samples are studied for trypsin and fat content. (The stool sample must be fresh or one that was frozen immediately.) Trypsin is either absent or markedly diminished in children with cystic fibrosis. A 3-day collection of stool with documented and measured intake is required to document steatorrhea (fatty stools). A comparison is made between dietary fat intake and stool output. Absorption of less than 95 per cent fat is considered malabsorption.

The nurse can help relieve some of the family's anxiety during the diagnostic period. Although the diagnostic tests are not traumatic, the child and the parents need to have a thorough explanation of the procedure and equipment involved. Encouraging a parent to stay with a child and even hold her or him during a procedure whenever possible is recommended. In the sweat test, a small electric current and the drug pilocarpine are placed on the forearm (thigh of infants) of the child to stimulate the sweat gland (iontophoresis). The sweat is then collected by overlying filter paper or gauze. A simple explanation of the procedure and allowing the young child to handle the apparatus are helpful in alleviating anxieties. The electrodes cause no discomfort, but the appearance of the apparatus may be frightening, and the infant or young child does not like to be held still.

Therapeutic Management

Treatment is individualized and aimed at promoting an independent life as adolescence and adulthood are approached. Promotion of good nutrition, prevention of pulmonary infection, and a healthy psychosocial adjustment to the disease by the child and family are the goals of therapy. A variety of treatments are used to deter the disease.

Digestive and nutritional therapy consists of pancreatic enzyme replacement, diet adjustment, and fat-soluble vitamin supplementation (in some instances) to promote growth, adequate nutrition, and normal bowel movements. A tablet or powdered form of animal pancreatic enzymes is taken orally whenever food is consumed, including snacks. The most frequently prescribed supplement is a capsule containing enterically coated microspheres that are designed to release the active enzyme in the duodenum. Infants under 12 months of age, however, may lack sufficient gastric acid to remove the enteric-coated microspheres (Lester & Rothberg, 1986); therefore, a powdered supplement is preferred.

The amount of extract needed varies with the child's diet, activity level, number of bowel movements per day, and type of stool. If stools become large and bulky, more enzymes are required; if constipation is a problem, fewer enzymes may be required. Whenever a protein fluid such as a milkshake is consumed, enzymes need to be taken; if a high-fat meal is anticipated, enzymes should be increased. Because the enzymes are specific and only partially replace normal pancreatic function, a moderate-fat, high-protein, high-calorie diet may be prescribed to promote weight gain and digestion of foods. Medium-chain triglyceride (MCT) oil, a dietary supplement of medium-chain triglycerides, is sometimes given to increase calories. MCTs are more readily digested and provide 8.4 cal/g. Infants may require a special, partially digested formula. When failure to thrive is severe, the insertion of a gastrostomy or jejunostomy tube may be recommended. This allows the addition of high-calorie nighttime feeds and has been successful for weight gain.

Because of the severe fat malabsorption, supplements of liposoluble vitamins in water-miscible liquid may be given to children with pancreatic involvement. When administered, vitamins A, D, and E are given in amounts of twice the usual daily dose. Vitamin K is given as necessary for infants with vitamin K deficiency and to older patients with hemoptysis and cirrhosis of the liver. The addition of vitamin B complex is usually recommended for patients receiving oral antibiotics. Iron is usually prescribed, because pancreatic enzyme supplementation causes a reduction in iron absorption.

Salt is allowed in generous amounts to prevent salt depletion through sweating. Sweating complications usually do not occur, except during excessive sweating, when loss of salt can lead to dehydration and collapse; therefore, additional salt is usually taken during hot weather.

Pulmonary therapy is designed to prevent and treat pulmonary infection. Therapy aims to clear secretions from the airways, improve aeration, and reduce the intensity of pulmonary infection. It consists of chest physical therapy, breathing exercises, inhalation therapy, and antibiotic administration.

The purpose of *chest physical therapy* is to maintain good pulmonary hygiene. The lungs are drained by placing the patient in various positions and percussing and vibrating the chest. Chest physical therapy is carried out two to four times daily prophylactically and more often during acute infections or bed rest. Other devices, such as chest vibrating vests and positive expiratory pressure (PEP) masks, are being used in conjunction with or instead of chest physical therapy as ways of aiding in secretion mobilization and clearing (Fig. 32–18).

Inhalation therapy prevents and treats infections. Intermittent aerosol therapy is usually done for 5 to 10 minutes prior to chest physical therapy to administer medications (bronchodilators) to the lower respiratory tract. If thick, tenacious secretions are difficult to mobilize, direct inhalation from an ultrasonic nebulizer may help break up the mucus. With excessive amounts of sputum, and if the child can tolerate it, postural drainage before and after aerosol therapy may be necessary. Drainage before aerosol therapy allows the droplets to reach areas previously filled with secretions. Aerosol delivery of some antibiotics is sometimes done after chest physical therapy.

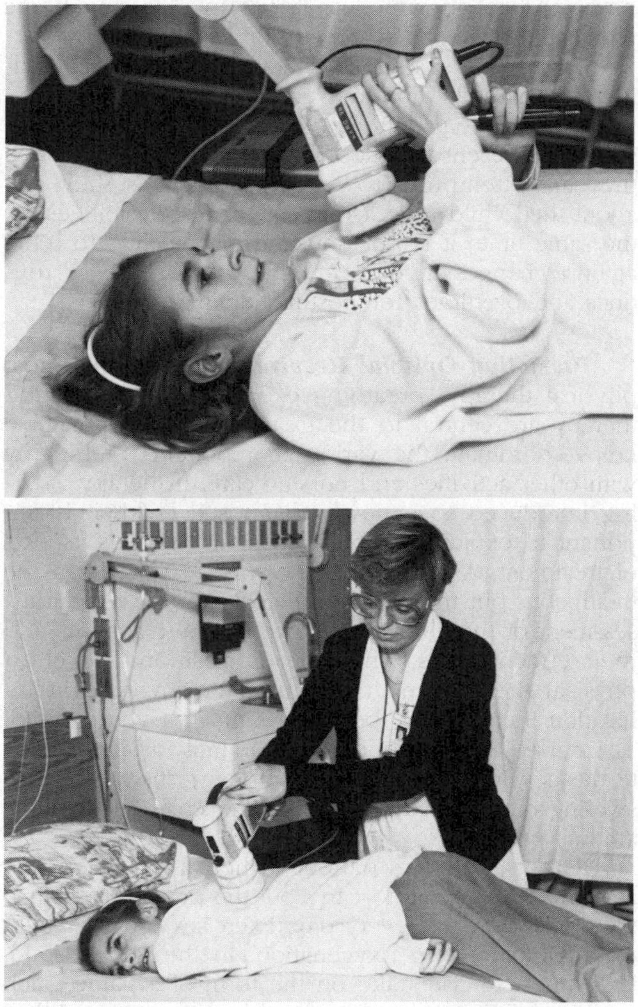

FIGURE 32 - 18. Hospitalized for cystic fibrosis, this 11-year-old girl performs parts of her own percussion. The nurse percusses the areas that the patient cannot reach. Mechanical percussion is now widely used and replaces manual percussion.

Breathing exercises help aerate the lungs to maximal capacity. These exercises are carried out daily before, after, or during postural drainage. Regular *exercise programs* are recommended for patients with cystic fibrosis as a means to improve breathing mechanics, posture, chest mobility, muscle strength, and aerobic fitness (Rose & Jay, 1986).

The use of *antibiotics* as a preventive measure is controversial. Many physicians prescribe antibiotic therapy only if there is an infection; others use it prophylactically. Prophylactically, different antibiotics are given in rotation to prevent drug resistance. The most common organisms recovered in the sputum are penicillin-resistant *S. aureus, H. influenzae,* and *Pseudomonas aeruginosa.* Two- to three-week courses of IV antibiotic therapy are given during acute exacerbations. Aerosol antibiotic therapy may be given in conjunction with systemic therapy.

Genetic counseling is a major component of care. A geneticist provides information to the family to assist them in decision making about reproductive plans. An interdisciplinary team may work together to provide the necessary guidance and support as these difficult decisions are made.

Members of the team include the nurse, nutritionist, social worker, physical therapist, and physician. Heart and lung or lung transplants have become successful treatment options for some clients with cystic fibrosis. Although the client receives an unaffected organ donation, the problems associated with cystic fibrosis persist. The client with cystic fibrosis is still not cured of the disease and assumes the experiences of transplant recipient.

Nursing Process for Cystic Fibrosis

Assessment

The child's medical history and treatment regimen are obtained to aid in the development of the nursing care plan. The nurse's observations of respiratory status and response to treatment are noted throughout hospitalization and the course of long-term management.

Nursing Diagnostic Statements and Collaborative Problems

Anticipatory grieving, related to perceptions regarding the diagnosis of an eventually fatal disease.

High risk for altered health maintenance; *risk factor: knowledge deficit about the disease process and its management.*

Ineffective airway clearance, *related to difficulty in expelling thick mucus within the airways.*

Ineffective breathing pattern, *related to impaired gas change, due to air trapping in the alveoli, associated with airways narrowed by tenacious mucus.*

High risk for infection: pulmonary; *risk factor: chronic tenacious pulmonary secretions and lack of compliance with physical therapy regimen.*

Altered nutrition: less than body requirements, *related to impaired metabolism of nutrients and vitamins, associated with insufficient pancreatic enzymes and malabsorption.*

High risk for ineffective individual and family coping; *risk factor: lack of available mechanisms to cope with the stress of a chronic and eventually fatal disease.*

Planning and Implementation

Nursing care is focused on promoting respiratory and gastrointestinal function, providing psychosocial support to the child and family, and preparing the family for effective home management.

Providing Support During the Period of Anticipatory Grief. *Emotional adjustment* to the diagnosis is often overwhelmingly difficult. The thought of an eventually fatal illness stimulates an acute anticipatory mourning reaction in family members, including feelings of denial, avoidance, shock, and disbelief, followed by information seeking. Anger is also a common manifestation of this stage. Often parents who have "known something was wrong" express ambivalent feelings about the diagnosis. They experience shock and guilt in learning the poor prognosis but are relieved finally to have a diagnosis for their child's chronic condition (Cowen, 1986).

When parents are informed of the diagnosis, the nurse should make every effort to be with them to clarify it and to provide support, because the response and understanding of parents at this early phase can have long-lasting effects on the child's perception of self and the illness. Parents need careful explanation of the disease, information regarding the therapy involved, and additional support because they have been faced with not only the fatal outcome of the disease but also the treatment for which they must assume responsibility. The ability of many parents to absorb information about the disease during this early stage is limited. Reiteration and provision of written material are beneficial.

Counseling should also be offered at the time of diagnosis (see Chapter 31 for the nursing process plan for genetic counseling). A common response of parents is to become overprotective, creating anxiety and a poor self-image in the child. Knowing that children with cystic fibrosis are now living into adulthood aids in decreasing parents' feelings of hopelessness.

Teaching to Facilitate Care in the Home. From the time of diagnosis, the goal is to involve the patient and family in self-care. Through education about the disease and the therapy required, the child and family are, from the beginning, prepared for discharge and home care. The National Cystic Fibrosis Foundation* has available many publications and educational aids for parents and for patients in their teens and twenties.

Preparation for home care includes teaching the parents and child how to carry out chest physical therapy, how to provide inhalation therapy by nebulizer, and how to give enzymes and other necessary medication at home. To teach postural drainage correctly, it is necessary to demonstrate through pictures and to have parents practice the technique (see elsewhere in this text for illustrations of postural drainage). Return demonstrations are important to assess parents technique. Areas on which to focus in assessing home management are presented in Table 32–27.

Care of the sick child at home, although demanding of a parent's time and energy, may be very satisfying. The initial stage of care following diagnosis seems to present the most problems for parents, since they are attempting to learn as much as they can about their child's disease and their responsibilities. At the same time, it is not unusual for the child to rebel against changes in diet and the interference of routines and playtimes for postural drainage.

Promoting Optimal Respiratory Function. Chest physical therapy, breathing exercises, and inhalation therapy are central to the treatment plan. The nurse helps coordinate the various components of therapy with other activities and nursing care. If therapy is being introduced to a newly diagnosed child, it is important to explain the purpose of the various aspects of treatment. A respiratory therapist may perform the treatments, but the nurse participates in the overall assessment of the child's tolerance of the treatments and their effectiveness. The various positions for chest physical therapy and the equipment involved in inhalation therapy may be frightening to a young child. The nurse supports the child and family as they adjust to the new routines and discomforts of therapy by answering questions and keeping the child as comfortable as possible.

Parents and the patient (when appropriate for age) are taught how to carry out the procedures, since they must be done every day. Exercises can be taught to children to help oxygenation. In the young child, breathing exercises take on the form of a game, such as blowing soap bubbles or blowing out candles.

---

*National Cystic Fibrosis Foundation, 6000 Executive Blvd., Suite 309, Rockville, MD 20852; Canadian Cystic Fibrosis Foundation 2221 Yonge St., Toronto, Ontario M4S 2B4; phone: (416) 485–9149.

TABLE 32-27
Nursing Focus in Assessing Home Management for the Child with Cystic Fibrosis

Plot height and weight on the growth curve and assess for steady progress
Assess vital signs, breath sounds, and energy available to perform usual activities of daily living
Determine effectiveness of expectoration with home chest physical therapy and inhalation therapy; have caregivers demonstrate technique
Ask the child and parent about gastrointestinal symptoms that would indicate malabsorption and inadequate enzyme replacement: bloating, abdominal cramping and distention, and diarrhea (Lester & Rothberg, 1986)
Have the child and parent record the dietary intake for the previous 24–48 hrs to assess nutrient and caloric adequacy
When appropriate, determine adherence to prescribed antibiotic therapy
Encourage the child and parent to discuss psychosocial and developmental concerns and to ask questions about the technical aspects of home management • Yearly chest radiograph; unless chest condition changes between visits, then more often • Pulmonary function tests done on all children over 5 yrs every 3–6 mos • Blood and urine testing as necessary • Exercise testing every 6 mos • Sputum culture every 6 mos

Older children are encouraged to place their hands over the upper and lower portion of their chest to feel movement as they inhale and exhale.

Children with a chronic chest condition frequently develop poor posture. Daily exercises that help maintain good posture include back extension, shoulder exercises, and standing erect against a wall (Orenstein, 1988). Another major part of therapy for the child with cystic fibrosis is swimming or hydrotherapy. This type of exercise helps build the muscles of respiration while encouraging good breathing habits. Children and adolescents are encouraged to participate in sports and activities that promote good breathing habits. Participation in team sports is more difficult because of small stature, low weight, and coughing.

When children with known cystic fibrosis are admitted to the hospital for care, the child and parents should be permitted to adopt a routine that is similar to the one they usually follow at home. Letting the child and parents be responsible for as much of the treatments as possible is a way to foster independence and responsibility and to avoid making them feel powerless.

Preventing Pulmonary Infection. The nurse ensures that the child and parents understand the need to take antibiotics for the prescribed course of treatment. During acute infections, antibiotics may be administered parenterally. Families are prepared to administer IV antibiotics at home, since most children undergo placement of a port-A-Cath or other type of central venous access device (i.e., Hickman or Broviac catheter). Home therapy requires thorough family and patient education, evaluation of appropriateness for the family, and anticipatory guidance before discharge.

Recurrent infections may result in frequent hospitalizations. Children may feel discouraged during bouts of pulmonary infection and need encouragement from the nurse to be cooperative in the full medical regimen. The usual treatments as done at home are continued, with an increase in the amount of percussion and postural drainage because of the decreased activity of the child.

Measures to prevent pulmonary exacerbations are an important aspect of management. Although unrestricted living style is the goal, some precautions should be taken to avoid exposure to respiratory infection. Avoiding large crowds during the flu season and avoiding contact with individuals who obviously have a respiratory infection may limit some exposure. Flu immunizations are strongly recommended on a yearly basis.

Promoting Optimal Nutrition. The underlying problem in children with cystic fibrosis is the inability of the pancreas to produce sufficient amounts of the enzymes to digest protein, fat, and carbohydrates adequately. Some cystic fibrosis centers are no longer imposing dietary restrictions. The rationale is to provide a better psychologic adjustment for the children, especially for those who are at an age during which peer relationships and independence are important. The suggested alternative is to increase enzymes to match intake. Because enzymes are prescribed by the physician, inadequate nutrition is considered a problem that is handled collaboratively by the physician and the nurse. Experience has shown that older children are able to determine for themselves what their systems can best handle and to decide what needs to be eliminated. During acute illness, the child may become anorexic and the ordered diet may be restrictive. Ensuring adequate calorie intake is essential and usually requires the assistance of a nutritionist.

Enzymes should be mixed with carbohydrate foods (applesauce is often used) and administered at the beginning of the meal or snack. Enzymes are not mixed with protein foods, because proteins would immediately be broken down and the mixture would become watery. Breakdown of skin can occur if enzymes remain on the lips or skin for an extended period of time.

MCT oil preparations are usually unpalatable to older children* but can be readily mixed into food or formula for infants.

*Recipes for using MCT oil are available from Mead Johnson and Company, Evansville, IN 47701.

Promoting Adaptive Individual and Family Coping: Recognizing Common Stressors. Major stresses are fears related to suffocation or dying while asleep, embarrassment associated with odorous flatulence and stools, altered body image due to thin body and possible short stature, frequent uncontrolled bouts of coughing, and the agony of engaging in the daily time-consuming activity of bronchial drainage (Canam, 1986). With the increasing life expectancy of these children, the family and the child will need additional

ETHICAL ISSUES
Adolescent Compliance

by Margaret M. Mahon, PhD, RN

Carmen is a 14-year-old who was diagnosed with cystic fibrosis (CF) at age 8 mos. She has two sisters, ages 11 and 7 yrs. One sister also has CF. Carmen is a freshman in high school, and is a B student. Management of her CF consists of PO enzymes, diet modification, and respiratory treatments administered at home, usually by her mother. After school and on weekends Carmen spends most of the time with her friends, frequently missing meals. When she eats away from home, she eats food that is unhealthy for her, and misses her enzymes. When it is suggested that she take her enzymes with her, she either refuses or brings the enzymes with her but does not use them. In addition, Carmen frequently misses her respiratory treatments. She has been hospitalized twice in the past year for respiratory infections. Carmen is aware that not following her recommended protocol can endanger her health, but she is unwilling to perform her treatment regimen around her friends. Carmen's mother is afraid that Carmen's next infection will be fatal.

This case exemplifies some of the issues in caring for adolescents with chronic conditions. Knowledge of child development explains many of these issues. For ill and chronically ill adolescents, there is a conflict between personal needs of affiliation and belonging, and the intricacies of ongoing management of conditions such as CF, spina bifida, diabetes, end-stage renal disease, asthma, scoliosis, and other conditions. For these conditions, a range of interventions are necessary. Factors such as visibility, time required, and physical differences affect the likelihood of adolescents' utilizing treatments. In some cases, it is not in the adolescents' best interest to manage their own health care. What would lead to this decision?

The nature of adolescence is to develop and assert independence of thought and action. If Carmen did not have CF, her behavior (missing meals, going out with her friends, spending time away from home) might go unchallenged. Indeed, these behaviors are not being questioned; the extent to which these activities have or might compromise Carmen's health is of concern. Can Carmen make an informed decision not to follow all aspects of her protocol? Is it ever acceptable to allow behavior that is potentially life-threatening? If such behavior is not acceptable, how does one intervene?

Compliance is the adherence to one's prescribed health care regimen. However, it has been recognized that a plan of care may fit the needs of health care professionals more than needs of the child and family. For example, times for administering medications that worked while a child was hospitalized may be impractical at home. Labels of noncompliance may not indicate that a patient is abrogating health care responsibilities. When a patient is labeled as noncompliant, one should determine why there is a discrepancy between what was recommended and what is being done.

Compliance partly depends on one's understanding of the disease as well as the required treatments. Many children with chronic conditions have an advanced understanding of their disease but in all other ways are typical for their age. Because she has had the condition for so long, it is likely that Carmen understands her condition and treatments.

Many adolescents engage in risk-taking behavior. If adolescents without chronic conditions are not permitted to endanger their health, neither should adolescents with chronic conditions. Is there a difference because Carmen shows no other risk-taking behavior? Because Carmen has not demonstrated competence in her own health care, is adult intervention required? As with most adolescents, changing Carmen's behavior is likely to be difficult and may in fact be sabotaged; the desire to conform, to be like one's peers, is greater than the desire to be compliant with a necessary regimen. The process may be more difficult with children who had previously assumed a more responsible role in their health care. If Carmen is making an informed decision, is this situation different from allowing adults to smoke cigarettes? Does Carmen have a responsibility to be an example to her sister with CF?

Many health care providers establish relationships with adolescents apart from their parents. An agreement for compliance may be established between the adolescent and the health care provider. If this occurs, what is the role of the parent in "enforcement"? If noncompliance does occur, what responsibility does the health care provider have to intervene with the adolescent?

BIBLIOGRAPHY

Mann, L., Harmoni, R., & Power, C. (1989). Adolescent decision-making: The development of competence. *Journal of Adolescence, 12,* 265–278.

Sigman, G. S., & O'Connor, C. (1991). Exploration for physicians of the mature minor doctrine. *Journal of Pediatrics, 119,* 520–525.

support as adolescence is approached. The older school-age child and adolescent may require reevaluation for the need for more information. A child who grows up with a disease needs additional information as cognition expands and as new problems are encountered through the various developmental stages. The effect of the disease on physical appearance, the difficulties surrounding reproduction (*not* sexuality), and the fear of diminished job opportunities become meaningful as the child matures. The shortened life expectancy and facts about the disease are reconsidered at this time. An adolescent may require individual or group therapy to cope successfully with the illness during this stage of development. Refer to the box for a discussion of the ethical issues of adolescent compliance.

The family as a unit must adapt to the hardships imposed by the disease. The severe financial strain on the family budget, interruption of family routine, intrafamily communication breakdown, social isolation, sexual difficulties, and general depression are some of the usual problems. It has been found, however, that by the end of the first year after diagnosis, life becomes less stressful for the parents of cystic fibrosis children (Cowen et al, 1986). Negative emotions subside, and a degree of reorganization in daily family activities is established.

Bronchopulmonary Dysplasia

Bronchopulmonary dysplasia (BPD) is an iatrogenic chronic lung disease that develops in premature infants following a period of intensive respiratory therapy. In the past, infants born prematurely either died or recovered fully during the first few days of life; few infants survived to develop residual lung disease. Improvement in the survival rate of very low birth-weight infants has resulted in the emergence of respiratory insufficiency in the perinatal period, followed by chronic lung disease in subsequent years (Saigal & O'Brodovich, 1987).

Lifesaving measures and intensive therapy of these infants are confined to the specialty area of neonatal intensive care; long-term care is provided by nurses in clinics, on general pediatric inpatient units, through public health agencies, in schools, and in the child's home. The survival of these infants presents a new health care challenge.

Etiology/Incidence

The wide variation in the reported incidence of BPD (5 to 68 per cent) is primarily due to the lack of consistency in defining BPD. Incidence is particularly high in premature infants treated with mechanical ventilation for respiratory distress. The more immature the infant and the more intensive the respiratory movement required, the greater is the likelihood that chronic lung changes will occur (Brown, 1987).

Overall, the incidence of BPD has increased because of the increased survival rate of very low birth-weight infants (Monin & Vert, 1987). However, it is not established that chronic lung disease is associated with hyaline membrane disease itself. The incidence of BPD in infants with respiratory distress syndrome who receive intermittent positive pressure ventilation and survive varies between 10 and 20 per cent. The incidence of infants surviving with milder forms of chronic lung damage is much higher (Bancalari & Gerhardt, 1986; McElheny, 1989). The triggering events of BPD are oxygen-related injury and barotrauma (trauma associated with the pressure required in mechanical ventilation) in an infant who is susceptible because of the surfactant-deficient state of the respiratory distress syndrome. Some evidence indicates that the presence of an endotracheal tube alone can cause mechanical damage to the tracheal epithelium (Sinkin & Phelps, 1987). Onset appears to be within minutes to hours after birth.

Other factors that place the infant at risk for BPD are meconium aspiration, persistent pulmonary hypertension, congenital pneumonia, pulmonary edema from a patent ductus arteriosus (PDA), excessive fluid administration, and any disorders that require prolonged mechanical ventilation in neonates.

The relative role of oxygen as a causative factor in BPD is debated in the literature and remains unclear (Sinkin & Phelps, 1987). Exposure of immature lungs to inhalation of high oxygen concentrations is thought to damage the protective system of the lungs. Existing alveolar Type I cells are damaged and replaced with poorly functioning type II alveolar cells. This pathologic response results in an alveolar-capillary leak.

Pathophysiology

Edema and inflammation of the capillary bed and alveolar wall interfere with lung function. Some of the alveoli collapse, whereas others are overinflated. Tissue cells in the lung are infiltrated with polymorphonuclear leukocytes that release free oxygen radicals and protease (a proteolytic enzyme). As a result of the collection of proteinaceous debris in the alveoli, any surfactant that is present is inactivated (see elsewhere in this text for discussion of the role of surfactant in the alveoli).

Edema and inflammation in the lungs make the lung tissue more susceptible to barotrauma. Barotrauma causes alveolar rupture, leading to interstitial emphysema, pneumothorax, and airway damage. The combined effect of high oxygen concentrations and barotrauma thus damages the small airways and cells of the alveolar lining. This causes an increased capillary permeability and leakage of plasma proteins and fluid into the alveoli and interstitium.

Prolonged respiratory failure can lead to right heart failure secondary to pulmonary hypertension with cardiomegaly, hepatomegaly, and fluid retention. Right ventricular hypertrophy, cardiac enlargement, edema, and venous congestion are a consequence of pulmonary vasoconstriction (pulmonary vasoconstriction is the result of hypoxemia). Cardiac involvement is also related to the presence of a PDA because of left-to-right shunting through a PDA and associated pulmonary edema.

Clinical Manifestations

Clinical manifestations of BPD vary widely, with most infants exhibiting signs of respiratory distress such as wheezes, crackles, retractions, copious secretions, and cyanosis on crying, feeding, agitation, or stress. The fussiness and irritability commonly seen in these infants is likely associated with the instability in arterial oxygen levels and transient hypoxia.

Diagnostic Assessment

The diagnosis of BPD is based on clinical and radiographic characteristics, but no *specific* clinical signs or laboratory results confirm the diagnosis. It is characterized by hypoxia, hypercapnia, and oxygen dependence with a diagnostic chest radiograph. Stages of BPD have been described progressing from stage I to stage IV with mild, moderate, severe, and advanced-chronic phases. These stages were first described by Northway and colleagues (1967). Toce and colleagues (1984) have developed a BPD clinical scoring system including measures of gas exchange, respiratory distress criteria, growth parameters, and a chest radiograph assessment to be used at 21 days of age.

A variety of criteria are used to diagnose BPD:

- Intermittent positive pressure ventilation required during the first week of life for at least 3 days.
- Clinical evidence of chronic respiratory distress persisting beyond around 30 days of age.
- Supplemental oxygen requirement for more than 28 days to maintain a Pao_2 over 50 mmHg.
- An abnormal chest radiograph showing hyperinflation, dense linear opacities, and scattered hyperlucent foci (translucent cysts).

Other tests that contribute to the diagnosis are an electrocardiogram and an echocardiogram to confirm the diagnosis of hypertrophy of a ventricle and pulmonary function tests to evaluate the degree of interference in lung function. Lung compliance and functional residual capacity are found to be low, and airway resistance is high (Scherf, 1985).

Therapeutic Management

Avoidance of the factors that contribute to BPD is the key to prevention. Precautions are taken to *prevent* respiratory distress syndrome and to *reduce* barotrauma and oxygen toxicity.

Prevention by Drug Therapy. Numerous research studies concerning prevention of BPD are under way. These include administration of dexamethasone to induce maturation of surfactant synthesis prior to premature birth (Avery, 1984), surfactant replacement therapy (Merritt et al, 1986; Cummings et al, 1989), and the administration of antioxidants to reduce oxygen toxicity (i.e., vitamin E, N-acetylcysteine, and superoxide dismutase). Surfactant replacement therapy is a successful therapeutic approach that has been shown to be beneficial in treating some infants with neonatal RDS (Notter & Shapiro, 1987). Formulation of synthetic lung surfactant that has negligible toxicity and is as effective as human lung surfactant is the goal of current research.

Monitored Ventilation and Oxygen Administration to Prevent Bronchopulmonary Dysplasia. Because barotrauma and oxygen toxicity contribute to the development of BPD, mechanical ventilation and oxygen administration are necessarily managed meticulously. The goal is to use the lowest inspired oxygen concentration and the lowest peak pressures and mean airway pressure that will maintain adequate gas exchange. Short inspiratory times (0.3 to 0.5 second) are recommended to reduce risk for BPD.

The acceptable ranges of blood gas levels maintained to prevent BPD are $Paco_2$ at 35 to 45 mmHg and Pao_2 at 50 to 70 mmHg. However, higher $Paco_2$ levels may be acceptable to prevent excessively high inspired FiO_2 concentration and mean airway pressure.

New concepts in ventilation, introduced in the early 1980s, use greater-than-normal breathing frequencies. High-frequency oscillatory ventilation (rates of 300 to 800 per minute) and high-frequency jet ventilation are used in some cases to reduce mean airway pressure and tidal volumes and thus reduce barotrauma. These high-frequency methods have not yet demonstrated a reduced incidence of BPD, despite encouraging results (see Table 32–3) (Monin & Vert, 1987).

An infant must be weaned from the ventilator gradually, with careful monitoring of fluids to avoid pulmonary interstitial fluid and pulmonary resistance. Diuretics and intermittent mandatory ventilation (IMV) are often used during the weaning process. IMV means that mechanical ventilations are at slow rates, allowing for spontaneous respirations between the ventilator-driven breaths.

Bronchodilators (theophylline) and salbutamol (albuterol) may shorten the duration of ventilator weaning by decreasing airway resistance and increasing compliance (Rotschild et al, 1989; Wilkie & Bryan, 1987). The ability of the infant to tolerate weaning is evaluated by the stability of pH, $Paco_2$, and Pao_2 during the period of progressive reduction of ventilator settings.

Fluid Therapy. Fluid restriction may be required to reduce pulmonary congestion and prevent cardiac failure. Diuretic therapy may be beneficial in chronic lung disease. Frequently used diuretics include

- Furosemide (Lasix), 1 to 2 mg/kg per day given in a single dose, IV or PO.
- Spironolactone (Aldactone), 3 to 6 mg/kg per day given in divided doses every 12 hours.
- Chlorothiazide (Diuril), 10 to 40 mg/kg per day given in divided doses every 12 hours PO.

Chronic administration of furosemide requires monitoring, as it results in urinary losses of calcium and potassium and can contribute to the development of osteopenia of prematurity (Monin & Vert, 1987) and renal calcification as a result of hypercalciuria. Chlorothiazide in combination with furosemide decreases urinary calcium excretion (Korones, 1988).

Adequate Oxygenation During Chronic Lung Disease. Adequate and stable oxygenation is required for the growth of the lung tissue and the healing process. Oxygen is administered in a variety of ways during the chronic phase, including Oxy-Hood, nasal cannula, or pharyngeal catheter (for FiO_2 above 35 per cent).

Nutrition. Very low birthweight infants have a functional limitation of the gastrointestinal tract, yet require a proportionately greater calorie intake compared with an older child. In the early phase of respiratory distress, calorie requirements are 50 to 70 cal/kg per day. These infants have a higher metabolic rate, secondary to BPD; therefore, fluid overload may become a problem.

In the convalescent phase, the calorie needs are 120 to 130 cal/kg per day (Monin & Vert, 1987). Nutritional requirements are met through total parenteral nutrition early in treatment and later on by nasogastric tube, gavage, gastrostomy, and breast or bottle feedings. A constant challenge is providing adequate calorie nutrition while maintaining strict fluid restrictions.

Prognosis

With supportive care, many of these infants seem to recover by growing new lung tissue. However, some infants with BPD continue to have poor health, with numerous hospital admissions for respiratory infections. Most studies show that infants with BPD have a higher incidence of neurodevelopmental disorders and developmental lag, compared with other very low birthweight infants (Saigal & O'Brodovich, 1987), although they tend to improve after the first 2 to 3 years of life (Sauve & Singhal, 1985). Pulmonary problems also tend to decline during the first 2 to 3 years of life; however, the long-term pulmonary function of these infants remains to be determined. Many older children with BPD have reactive airway disease requiring chronic therapy. The ultimate outcome of infants with BPD is unknown, since follow-up studies are few and none of these children has yet reached adulthood (Sinkin & Phelps, 1987).

Nursing Process for Bronchopulmonary Dysplasia

Assessment

Assessment of the infant's respiratory status is an important function of the nurse. Changes in the infant's clinical presentation are evaluated in relation to other diagnostic findings, such as chest radiographs and blood gases.

Nursing Diagnostic Statements and Collaborative Problems

High risk for suffocation, impaired gas exchange; *risk factors: caused by*

- *Alveolar-capillary membrane damage associated with oxygen toxicity and barotrauma.*
- *Atelectasis associated with surfactant deficiency.*
- *Ineffective breathing pattern, caused by decreased lung expansion (compliance) associated with fibrotic changes.*
- *Fatigue and decreased energy associated with hypoxia.*
- *Inflammatory process associated with secondary respiratory infection.*

High risk for infection; *risk factor: inadequate primary defense, associated with fibrotic lung changes of BPD.*

Altered nutrition: less than body requirements, *related to*

- *Increase of 25 per cent in metabolic rate associated with increased respiratory effort (Hodgman, 1986).*
- *Feeding difficulties associated with dyspnea and prematurity.*
- *Increased calorie expenditure associated with work of breathing.*

High risk for altered fluid volume: excess; *risk factor: increased workload of the right side of the heart, associated with increased pulmonary interstitial fluid.*

Activity intolerance, related to altered cardiac output, *due to*

- *Cardiac failure associated with presence of a left-to-right shunt (in the presence of a PDA).*
- *Cardiac failure associated with pulmonary vasoconstriction (pulmonary hypertension) due to hypoxemia.*
- *Cor pulmonale associated with pulmonary edema and right ventricular hypertrophy.*

High risk for altered growth and development; *risk factors:*

- *Reduced oxygenation associated with fibrotic lung changes.*
- *Overprotection from caretakers and significant others associated with BPD.*

- *Lack of adequate stimulation and developmentally appropriate activities.*
- *Prolonged and frequent hospitalization.*
- *Reduced energy associated with hypoxia/dyspnea.*

High risk for ineffective family coping: compromised; *risk factors:*

- *Stresses of long-term intensive management of BPD at home.*
- *Inadequate support systems.*
- *Inadequate information about the care of the infant.*

High risk for altered home health maintenance; *risk factor: knowledge deficit about the infant's condition and treatment regimen.*

Planning and Implementation

Intensive care of the infant at risk for BPD is described in neonatal intensive care literature. The focus of this discussion is management of the infant with chronic lung disease.

Maintaining Adequate Oxygenation. As airway damage progresses, a barrel chest is apparent; oxygenation becomes more difficult, and CO_2 retention increases. Careful assessment for increased signs of respiratory distress and close monitoring of blood gases are required. An increase in pulmonary vascular pressure is generally observed when arterial Pao_2 drops below 55 mmHg (Monin & Vert, 1987). Special attention is also given to maintaining the infant's body temperature, because hypothermia and hyperthermia increase oxygen consumption. During stress (feeding, crying, suctioning, and any procedures), oxygen may need to be temporarily increased. Home care issues concerning oxygenation are summarized in Table 32–28.

Preventing Infection. Children with BPD are at risk for lower respiratory tract infections. Parents are counseled to avoid close proximity with those who are known to have a respiratory infection and to seek early treatment of any signs of respiratory distress in their infant. Chest physical therapy and suctioning may be necessary for removal of secretions to prevent infections. Yearly flu vaccinations are recommended. See Table 32–28 for issues to discuss with parents regarding home care.

Maintaining Adequate Nutritional Intake. The nurse monitors the caloric intake of these infants to ensure adequate growth. A delicate balance must be maintained between caloric and fluid requirements and the child's feeding behaviors (Pridham et al, 1989). Early in the phase of treatment, intake is parenteral. Because fluid overload complicates BPD, the required caloric intake cannot be easily achieved; therefore, formula that contains 24 or 30 cal/oz may be required. Feeding difficulties and intolerances are often seen in babies with BPD. They may develop significant feeding aversions that require gastrostomy nutrition and extensive speech and occupational therapy. Home care issues to be raised with parents are summarized in Table 32–28.

Maintaining Fluid Balance. Fluid intake and output are monitored, and infants are often weighed daily because they are at risk for development of pulmonary edema. Caloric requirements must be met in the lowest volume of fluids possible. Any increase in respiratory or heart rate; retractions; cyanosis; change in chest sounds, such as the presence or increase of rales; or a decrease in breath sounds is an indication of increased respiratory difficulty and possible pulmonary edema.

Maintaining Adequate Cardiac Output. When an infant is in cardiac failure, fluid intake and output are very strictly monitored, as is the infant's weight. Episodes of stress, which would represent exercise and would be poorly tolerated by the infant, are avoided by adopting a "minimal touch" policy organizing nursing care and tests to reduce interruptions of the infant's rest.

Fostering Normal Growth and Development. Prolonged respiratory dysfunction has been found to be associated with growth retardation (McElheny, 1989; Sauve & Singhal, 1985). Infants with BPD often have severe visual impairment, poor growth, recurrent respiratory infections, and frequent hospitalizations (Saigal & O'Brodovich, 1987). Parents need to understand the effects of BPD on growth and development to avoid the worry and self-blame that might occur if they feel these delays are related to their inadequate care. Parents are aided in providing adequate nutrition that will promote growth (see section on normal nutrition in Table 32–28). Although no controlled studies demonstrate the effectiveness of programs for sensory stimulation and movement and motor patterns, such interventions are prevalent in clinical practice. In one study, individualization of behavioral and environmental care for very low birthweight infants at risk for developing BPD has been shown to reduce the length of ventilation time and oxygen requirements and to improve behavioral organization and mental development at 9 months of age (Als et al, 1986).

Regardless of whether a formal stimulation program is instituted, as soon after birth as possible nurses encourage parents to stroke, hold, and talk to their infant. Slow motor development, hypotonia or hypertonia, and asymmetry of movement frequently make it necessary for parents to perform specific exercises in the home; however, many of these children have normal development for corrected age, after some initial lag.

TABLE 32-28
Family-Centered Teaching: Home Care Management of Child with Bronchopulmonary Dysplasia

Maintaining Fluid and Nutritional Balance	Maintaining Oxygenation
Oxygen administration during feeding is usually necessary because of the work of breathing and sucking	The oxygen-dependent infant or child usually can tolerate a cannula for oxygen administration. It can be taped to a stoma-adhesive patch (see Fig. 32–5). This needs to be changed only once a week and protects the skin (Koops et al, 1984). A nasopharyngeal catheter is used for oxygen concentration of 35% or greater
Infants with cardiac involvement may require fluid restriction	Oxygen for home care is supplied by concentrates, tanks, or liquid oxygen systems. Of these, the concentrates seem to be preferred because no tank changing is necessary. However, the availability of liquid oxygen enables portability.
Sometimes the use of medium-chain triglycerides (MCT) or 24- or 30-cal/oz formulas are required to meet caloric needs for growth	Financial considerations may limit availability, as it is very costly
Occasional gavage feedings may be necessary if baby is especially tired; therefore, parents may need to learn this type of feeding	Chest physical therapy and suctioning may be required three to four times a day. Parents must have had supervised practice and demonstrate the necessary skills
Gastrostomy tube may be necessary if adequate weight gain is not accomplished with PO or gavage methods	
Preventing Infection	**Maintaining Family Coping**
The usual preventive measures appropriate for a child with a chronic respiratory problem must be stressed: avoidance of smoking near the infant, avoidance of close proximity with those known to have a respiratory infection, and early treatment of signs of respiratory illness in the infants	Lack of identified support system. Encourage the family to find a few support people to help them during this period of adjustment
Careful feeding techniques to avoid aspiration are taught to parents as a way to reduce risk of infection	The interruption of family life may sometimes lead to marital stress. A competent baby sitter should be taught how to care for the infant to allow parents to have time together and to themselves
Chest physical therapy and suctioning need to be increased for removal of secretions from the lungs to prevent lower respiratory infections	Parents should have an understanding about the illness, recognizing that respiratory infections may require readmission to the hospital, but this does not mean they have failed
Bronchodilators (by inhalation) for wheezing may be required, especially during respiratory infections. Parents must be helped to secure the equipment from a supply company and be taught proper administration	

Promoting Adaptive Family Coping. The problems associated with BPD demand the services of a dedicated interdisciplinary team (composed of nurses, physicians, nutritionist, social worker, and respiratory, speech, physical, and occupational therapists) and care by a family able and willing to commit a large proportion of time and energy to their child. Multidisciplinary care begins immediately on diagnosis, in recognition of the scope and complexity of needs represented by these children and their families. Home management of a child with BPD often involves sending an oxygen-dependent child home, which presents a challenge to the nurse. Early involvement of the parents in the care of their infant, accompanied by ongoing teaching regarding the nature of the lung problem, is essential for successful management in the home.

Parents should be prepared for the extent of care that will be required of them at home. The preparation for discharge involves all team members and a coordination of efforts to facilitate consistency of instructions. An ongoing assessment of the parent's ability to care for the child and comfort in doing so provides the necessary information to determine readiness for discharge. Even after they realize the extent of care that is required, parents must still want to care for their child at home and demonstrate a capability to do so.

Factors to be evaluated when home care is being considered include the following:

- Weight gain. A steady weight gain should be demonstrated, and the baby should weigh more than 2 kg.
- Complexity of care. Nurse should evaluate parents' ability to feed infant, frequency of feedings, number of medications, and need for chest physical therapy and suctioning.
- Percentage of supplemental oxygen required. Maintenance of oximetry at 92 per cent saturation during caregiving, feedings, and sleep is recommended. (Note: oximeters are less invasive and used more frequently now than transcutaneous O_2 monitors).

Facilitating Home Care. The infant's care following discharge from the hospital requires long-term management. It is therefore essential that parents be well informed about their infant and their care needs. Parents are expected to monitor closely their infant's growth together with the team of specialists. The infant's growth and weight is monitored on the growth grid. The infant's pattern of growth is of more concern than any particular measure. Accurate measurement must account for age correction between chronologic and gestational age on the growth chart. The infant's progress on developmental tasks is assessed. Parents are instructed to assess vital signs, skin color, and breath sounds and to observe their infant's response to feeding and playing to screen for respiratory competency and for signs of infection. Feeding difficulties or intolerances are referred to the team.

Parents are encouraged to voice concerns about growth and development, technical management, and stresses on family functioning. The family are referred to available social services and support systems, as appropriate.

Evaluation

The nurse collaborates with other health team members to evaluate the complexity of care and the realistic goals that can be set for home care. Some families are too overwhelmed to learn to care for their baby at home in the time expected by the health care team. In some cases, the family's socioeconomic status imposes significant challenges to home care. Very poor families may lack the most basic of necessities, such as electricity and running water. The most important outcome is that parents enjoy their baby and establish a loving, trusting relationship with the child (Koops et al, 1984). Consequently, a highly individualistic approach must be taken in assessing the appropriateness of home care for a child with BPD.

The first visit after discharge is recommended at 1 week and the second visit 1 to 2 weeks thereafter. Interdisciplinary care must continue to provide the necessary support and evaluation of progress. The anticipated problems encountered in children with BPD are summarized in Table 32–28.

Apnea-Related Disorders

Apnea of Prematurity

Apnea of prematurity is differentiated from periodic breathing in Table 32–29. *Periodic breathing* is characteristic of premature infants (is present in many term infants as well) and can be a normal event. When the pauses of periodic breathing are 20 or more seconds or when the pause is associated with other signs of distress (see Table 32–29), the episode is classified as *apnea of prematurity*. Apnea of prematurity usually is manifested at 1 or 2 days of age and resolves around 34 to 36 weeks gestational age. Conversely, *apnea of infancy* occurs at or near term (onset of greater than 37 weeks gestation) and is usually associated with serious causes.

Etiology/Incidence (Pathophysiology)

As many as 25 per cent of all premature infants under 1800 g (around 34 weeks gestational age) have at least one apneic episode. The incidence of apnea increases as gestational age decreases. Almost all premature infants under 30 weeks gestational age have occasional apneic spells.

Usually no single factor can be identified as the cause of apnea of prematurity. The respiratory control mechanisms and reflexes of the premature infant are immature with characteristic responses, one of which is the response to hypoxia. Immature infants respond to hypoxia with an initial increase in respiratory effort, followed by periodic breathing, with eventual respiratory depression and apnea (Marchal et al, 1987). Hypoxia is thus suspected to be a primary factor that depresses the respiratory system, leading to apnea in the premature infant. As hypoxia increases, the ventilatory response to CO_2 decreases, a phenomenon that is the reverse of that of an older infant or an adult (Avery, 1987).

Stimulation of certain reflexes in the premature infant elicits responses different from those of an adult. Stimulation of receptors in the upper airway (especially laryngeal mucosa) produces apnea. This laryngeal reflex explains the apnea observed during tube feeding, upper airway suction, and gastric content regurgitation. Overheating or excessive cooling, poor positioning, and airway obstruction with mucus are additional stimuli that produce apnea.

The relationship of apnea to sleep is not entirely clear. Apnea is believed to be more common during rapid-eye-movement (REM) sleep and less common during quiet sleep and waking. The more highly organized quiet state of sleep does not exist in the immature infant; the stimuli in an intensive care unit further disrupt a poorly organized circadian rhythm. Apnea in association with REM sleep may be due to an obstructive phenomenon associated with temporary loss of muscle tone in the upper airway structures (Rudolph, 1991).

Apnea that persists without evidence of its cause is a perplexing problem. If apneic spells occur during the first few days of life, they are more commonly associated with an underlying disorder (Avery, 1987), such as the following:

- Sepsis.
- Metabolic disorders (hypoglycemia, hypocalcemia, hyponatremia).
- Anemia.
- Patent ductus arteriosus.
- Seizures.
- Gastroesophageal reflux.
- Central nervous system depression from drugs.
- Intracranial hemorrhage.
- Pulmonary disease.
- Temperature fluctuations and instability.

TABLE 32-29
Definitions and Terminology for Apnea

Apnea

Cessation of respiratory air flow due to the following causes:

- Central or diaphragmatic
- Obstructive (usually upper airway)
- Mixed

Central apnea of ≤15 secs can be normal at all ages

Pathologic Apnea

A respiratory pause that is 20 secs or longer or is associated with the following:

- Cyanosis
- Abruptness
- Marked pallor or hypotonia
- Bradycardia

Periodic Breathing

A breathing pattern in which there are three or more respiratory pauses of greater than 3 secs' duration and that occur less than 20 secs apart. Periodic breathing can be a normal event

Apnea of Prematurity

Periodic breathing with pathologic apnea in a premature infant. Apnea of prematurity usually ceases by 37 wks gestation but can persist for several weeks past term

Apparent Life-Threatening Event (ALTE)

This event is frightening to the observer; it is characterized by some combination of the following:

- Apnea
- Color change (cyanotic, pale, or on occasion reddened)
- Marked change in muscle tone (limpness usually)
- Choking or gagging

Terminology such as "aborted crib death" or "near-miss SIDS" should not be used, because these terms make an association between the event and SIDS that could be incorrect

Apnea of Infancy

This term usually refers to infants greater than 37 wks gestation at onset

An unexplained cessation of breathing for 20 secs or longer or a respiratory pause of shorter duration but that is associated with the following:

- Bradycardia
- Cyanosis
- Pallor and/or marked hypotonia

Clinical Manifestations

The clinical manifestations of apnea of infancy are described in Table 32-29.

Diagnostic Assessment

The diagnostic tests used vary according to the disorder being investigated. During the diagnostic phase, the nurse must carefully monitor and record apneic episodes, with a clear description of the degree of cyanosis and the degree of bradycardia, if any. The nurse must also note whether oropharyngeal secretions, gavage feedings, and suctioning are causing apneic spells. See next discussion, "Apnea of Infancy," for further coverage of diagnostic assessment.

Therapeutic Management

Premature infants considered to be at risk for apnea (those less than 32 weeks' gestational age or less than 1500 g birthweight) are placed on continuous cardiorespiratory monitors in neonatal intensive care units (Avery, 1987).

Specialized nursing care is the major form of treatment for these infants, but if spells longer than 20 seconds occur more than three times a day, symptomatic therapy is instituted, including preventive stimulation, continuous positive airway pressure, and pharmacologic treatment.

Preventive stimulation can be provided in the form of cutaneous stimulation or by placing the infant on a water or rocking bed. Motion is thought to stimulate the labyrinthine passages and reduce apnea frequency (Marchal et al, 1987). *Continuous positive airway pressure* increases Pa_{O_2}, lung volume, and lung compliance and decreases the work of breathing, all of which contribute to reduced apneic episodes.

Pharmacologic therapy includes use of methylxanthines (oral theophylline or IV aminophylline). One of the ways that methylxanthines are thought to work is by increasing the ventilatory response to carbon dioxide; however, other mechanisms continue to be researched. Caffeine citrate also can be used to decrease the frequency of apneic episodes and may be less toxic (Marchal et al, 1987).

Doxapram, a respiratory stimulant, may be useful if the treatment of apnea with other drugs is ineffective (Barrington et al, 1986). Home apnea monitoring may be indicated for some infants and is covered in the next discussion, "Apnea of Infancy."

Nursing Diagnostic Statements

See nursing diagnostic statements and nursing care in the discussion that follows, "Apnea of Infancy."

Apnea of Infancy

Apnea can also occur in healthy, full-term infants. This is called *apnea of infancy*.

Etiology/Incidence (Pathophysiology)

Episodes of apnea that are frightening to the observer are called *apparent life-threatening events* (ALTEs) (see Table 32–29 for definition). Approximately 50 per cent of infants with apnea have diagnosable conditions; however, infants experiencing significant apnea without a known cause are thought to be at risk for *sudden infant death syndrome* (SIDS) (Spitzer & Fox, 1986). Apnea and SIDS have been linked because pathology findings suggest that SIDS infants have tissue changes consistent with chronic hypoxia. Infants with apnea (as diagnosed by polysomnography) do not die of SIDS at any greater rate than the normal population. However, there are many other probable causes of SIDS and, conversely, apnea can be a symptom of many other underlying determinable conditions.

Clinical Manifestations

The clinical manifestations of apnea of infancy are described in Table 32–29.

Diagnostic Assessment

The specific type of diagnostic testing is determined by the clinical indications and may include exploration of seizures, feeding problems, an infection, or other presenting clues to the etiology of apnea.

Detection of primary causes of apnea may require a period of hospitalization during which the infant is placed on a cardiorespiratory monitor. A diagnostic workup may include a complete blood count, blood chemistry, chest film, electrocardiogram, and electroencephalogram. A specific test to evaluate for apnea is the pneumocardiogram, which simultaneously records heart rate and chest wall movements. However, these are not recommended as screening tools, because their predictability has not been sufficiently documented.

Polysomnography (a sleep study) is a more elaborate study; it records brainwaves and movements of the eye and body, and measures oxygen. Polysomnography can distinguish central from obstructive apnea. These tests, however, are not definitive for apnea of infancy.

Therapeutic Management

The most commonly used therapy for infants with apnea is home cardiorespiratory monitoring. Home cardiorespiratory monitoring does *not* deter apnea; it simply alerts caregivers that apnea may be occurring, so that appropriate stimulation or treatment can be initiated. Widespread controversy prevails about the indications for home monitoring. Certain circumstances clearly indicate a need for it. These include the following:

- Infants with one or more severe ALTEs requiring mouth-to-mouth resuscitation or vigorous stimulation.
- Symptomatic preterm infants.
- Siblings of two or more SIDS victims.
- Infants with certain diseases or conditions, such as central hypoventilation.

Situations in which the evidence is not conclusive include the following:

- Any sibling of a SIDS victim.
- Infants with less severe episodes of ALTE.
- Infants with tracheostomies need a monitor as a way to signal possible obstruction or decannulation.
- Infants with opiate- or cocaine-abusing mothers.
- Infants with gastroesophageal reflux.

Before home monitoring is recommended, treatable causes of apnea are managed with appropriate therapy. In addition to home monitoring, a child with episodes of apnea or the preterm infant with apnea may require pharmacologic management (see discussion "Apnea of Prematurity" for description of pharmacologic management).

The decision to discontinue home monitoring varies according to the individual circumstances. Table 32–30 lists the criteria used.

Nursing Diagnostic Statements and Collaborative Problems

High risk for suffocation, ineffective breathing patterns; *risk factors:*

- *A paradoxical failure in the premature infant to increase respirations in response to hypoxia.*

TABLE 32-30
Criteria for Monitor Discontinuation in Apnea

Each of the following criteria are met:

- No life-threatening events requiring vigorous stimulation or resuscitation for 2–3 mos *or* no critical problems for 2 mos following the present episode
- No *real* monitor alarm for 2 mos (with apnea setting at 20 secs and heart rate at 60 beats/min)
- Infant must have had an upper respiratory tract infection, or a DPT immunization, or another illness without a recurrence of apnea
- Assessments (neurologic, developmental, and physical) must show that any initial reason for monitoring has resolved, and the child is otherwise growing and thriving normally
- No significant abnormalities on cardiorespiratory recordings

- *Recurrent cessation of breathing in the full-term infant associated with either known or unknown etiology.*

Anticipatory grieving, related to the perceived loss of a healthy infant associated with the diagnosis of apnea.

High risk for altered health maintenance, *risk factor: knowledge deficit about*

- *The technical aspects of home apnea monitoring.*
- *Cardiopulmonary resuscitation.*

Altered family processes, related to

- *Anxiety associated with the threat of infant death.*
- *Feelings of inadequacy associated with home management.*
- *Difficulty in obtaining baby sitters.*
- *Feelings of isolation and social deprivation.*
- *Difficulty in meeting the demands of other children.*

Nursing Care

Maintaining Effective Breathing Patterns. Nursing strategies to prevent and reduce the frequency of apnea during the acute phase of care are numerous. Precautions are taken in the method of handling and positioning of infants and the manner in which procedures are carried out. Hyperflexion of the neck is avoided to maintain maximal air entry. Placing infants in the prone position is associated with higher oxygen tension and shorter gastric emptying and reduces the frequency of regurgitation and aspiration.

Procedures that can produce apnea include suctioning and orogastric feedings. Pharyngeal suctioning is done gently and for the shortest time and least number of times possible. An orogastric tube must be carefully inserted; sudden gastric distention is avoided to reduce the likelihood of regurgitation (Marchal et al, 1987).

The environment should be maintained at a comfortable temperature, and extremes avoided. If oxygen is administered via a hood, it should be warmed to incubator temperature.

Supporting the Family in the Initial Period of Grief. Whenever an infant requires home monitoring, parents can be expected to go through a grieving process, because they experience the loss of their "perfect" child. The dilemma to be faced is that home apnea monitoring is potentially stress-producing for the family, yet its use is recommended, even though there are no data from which to conclude that home monitoring reduces the incidence of SIDS (Weese-Mayer et al, 1989).

Teaching to Support Home Care. In view of the limitations of our knowledge about the effectiveness of monitors to prevent SIDS, the major task confronting the health team is assisting the family to accept the ambiguities surrounding the diagnosis of being "at risk" for SIDS. The decision to place the infant on a monitor must be explained to the family. The nurse participates in the process of providing the explanation and handles ongoing doubts and questions that are raised by parents.

It is a team responsibility to prepare the family for all aspects of home monitoring. Parents are taught to use the monitor, respond to an alarm, and perform cardiopulmonary resuscitation (CPR). The nurse can serve as a liaison with the equipment vendor, as needed. Videotapes provide the opportunity for extended family members and baby sitters to learn the technique.

Promoting Effective Family Functioning. A thorough teaching approach to help parents learn how to operate the monitor, assess the infant, and perform CPR is essential. In addition to the technical aspects of preparation, responding to the psychosocial aspects of home monitoring, based on current research findings, should be considered. An *adequate support system* (family members and baby sitters) that can provide respite care, an *open communication system with a knowledgeable health care team* to discuss concerns and fears, and *contact with a parents' group* or telephone network with other parents who have monitored their infants should be incorporated.

Heightened levels of anxiety have also been reported by Lyman and coworkers (1985), whereas McElroy et al (1986) did not find a difference in the anxiety of two groups of mothers at 12 weeks or 1 year after the birth of their infant who required home apnea monitoring.

Further research is required to understand the ongoing needs of families who monitor their infants at home. *Home visiting by a community health nurse* is essential to provide the necessary assessment of the family's adjustment to home monitoring. Also needed is adequate technical support from the monitor vendor. Technical failure and malfunction (i.e., frequent false alarms) are constant problems with home monitoring. It is especially important that a health care professional intervene during the first week, when the highest level of anxiety is being experienced by the family. From the onset, a plan is developed in collaboration with parents for eventual discontinuation of monitoring. Ongoing assessments and interventions should focus on maintaining the infant's health status, restoring the mother's physical condition, establishing normal parent-infant relationships, and optimal family functioning.

Sudden Infant Death Syndrome

SIDS has been defined by the National Institutes of Health Panels (1987) as "the sudden death of an infant under 1 year of age which remains unexplained after a complete postmortem examination, including an investigation of the death scene and a review of the case history. Cases failing to meet the standards of this definition, including those without postmortem examinations, should not be diagnosed as SIDS." Although SIDS (also called "crib death" or "cot death") has only in recent years been described as a specific syndrome, its existence has been noted since biblical times. In spite of significant research advances, the cause of SIDS remains elusive.

Etiology/Incidence (Pathophysiology)

Approximately one third of all deaths occurring in infants from the ages of 1 week to 1 year are the result of SIDS. During the third and fourth months of life, the condition apparently accounts for more than one half of all infant mortality. The general risk is 2 in 1000 live births, but occurrence varies with ethnic background. Although Native Americans and African-Americans are reported to be at greater risk for SIDS, the determining factor is believed to be socioeconomic status, not race (Rudolph, 1991). The recurrence risk in siblings of SIDS is now thought to be 4 in 1000. Almost every study has shown a male preponderance.

A variety of epidemiologic factors have been investigated in relationship to the incidence of SIDS. Many theories emerge that are well publicized by the media—often prior to the completion of the scientific research. Parents of SIDS victims who are exposed to the publicity may grasp each theory as it comes along as an answer to questions regarding the death of their infant. It is essential that the nurses keep abreast of current research, so that they can provide accurate information. Nurses must learn to discriminate between sensationalized reports that are essentially opinions and sound, reproducible research findings.

No single predictive or diagnostic criterion can be employed to identify those at risk for SIDS. However, some demographic and environmental factors and characteristics of the infant and mother have been identified as probable risk factors.

Demographic and Environmental Risk Factors. SIDS can occur in any family but is more frequent in families who are poor or live in crowded housing. It is reasonable to suspect that maternal health and prenatal care are the critical factors underlying this association. The temporal distribution of SIDS shows a seasonal variation, with the peak incidence during the coldest months of the year and the fewest cases during the summer months. The SIDS event often occurs during the normal period of sleep. SIDS infants have been found in car seats or strollers, but most generally death occurs in the crib or parents' bed.

Characteristics of the Infant. SIDS babies are usually well developed and apparently normal and healthy. In some instances, there is a history of preterm birth, low Apgar scores, the need for oxygen and resuscitation at birth, or intrauterine growth retardation.

Neonatal characteristics identified retrospectively that were found to be associated with SIDS include jitteriness and irritability, feeding difficulties, growth lag, and muscle hypotonicity. These risk factors and infant characteristics are present in vast numbers of infants who do not succumb to SIDS; furthermore, not all SIDS victims have had these problems.

Characteristics of the Mother. Some of the maternal risk factors associated with SIDS are related to fetal environment. Reported maternal risk factors include severe anemia, cigarette smoking, third trimester bleeding, and maternal sedation or anesthesia. Infants of mothers who use methadone (Dolophine HCl) are at 10 times the usual risk for dying from SIDS (Herbst et al, 1988). Maternal age is a risk factor, with the highest rate of SIDS occurring when mothers are less than 20 years of age. An inverse association of SIDS and maternal age may be a significant clue to causation. Maternal nutrition during pregnancy has been suggested as a major direction for future research.

Circumstances of the Event. There is no audible outcry at the approximate time of death. Even though death apparently occurs in silence, often evidence indicates activity prior to death. Often the parents find the infant face down or with blankets pulled over the head, or wedged in a corner of the bed. Some infants are found face up with bedding clutched in their hands. These findings usually lead the caregivers to suspect suffocation and to feel guilty. The nurse must be aware of the developmental abilities of infants at various ages in order to reassure the parents and relatives of the unreasonableness of this hypothesis. The peak incidence of SIDS is 2 to 3 months of age, by which time the infant is able to reposition the head to maintain adequate ventilation. Also, evidence indicates that ordinary bedding is incapable of causing hypoxia to the point of suffocation. The suffocation hypothesis is also refuted by the fact that pathologic findings at autopsy are identical in SIDS cases, regardless of the position in which the infant was found.

Theories of Causation. The conviction is growing that SIDS has multiple causes. It is difficult to stay abreast of the extensive research that is being conducted on causation. Parents may seek information or may have read in the popular literature or newspapers about the following causes of SIDS.

Feeding History. Early studies indicating that SIDS does not occur in breastfed infants have since been refuted. Therefore, apparently no immunity to SIDS is passed to the infant from breast milk.

Infectious Disease. Because of the age distribution, the seasonal variations, the evidence of upper respiratory tract infections in SIDS victims, and the autopsy finding of mild inflammation, researchers are continuing to study this area of possible causation. Most studies exploring viral infections as a possible cause conclude that they do not *cause* SIDS but rather predispose the infant at risk (Guntheroth, 1989).

Genetic Factors. No convincing evidence exists that SIDS is a genetic disease. Even though the risk of SIDS is increased four to ten times in the subsequent siblings of SIDS victims, genetic factors have not been shown to be the cause. It is suggested that intrauterine or extrauterine environmental deficits could be the associated factors of causation (Kelly & Shannon, 1982).

Apnea Hypothesis. The apnea hypothesis continues to be only speculative. It suggests that periods of apnea during sleep eventually may result in an apneic episode that results in SIDS. The question of carbon dioxide responsiveness of infants and parents has been evaluated in an attempt to identify a predictor for SIDS. The results of these studies have varied, but the majority of parents and siblings of SIDS victims have not shown an abnormal carbon dioxide responsiveness (Guilleminault and Ariagno, 1989).

A major body of research has developed in response to the belief that SIDS is associated with hypoxia and hypoxemia, a result of repeated apneic episodes. These findings continue to be researched in an effort to understand the pathogenesis of SIDS (Glotzbach et al, 1989).

The mechanism of the relationship between apnea and SIDS is not well substantiated. It is thought that a sleeping infant can become hypoxic with positional narrowing of the airway and respiratory inflammation. Additional factors such as autonomic-neurologic instability, the control of ventilation (Brady & McCann, 1985), and chemical factors such as pH balance, hypercalcemia, and others may place the hypoxic sleeping infant on the path toward obstructive apnea. The infant's floppy pharynx, the large muscular tongue, and neck flexion all may contribute to these obstructive episodes. The infant may either revert to normalcy after recuperating from an apneic episode or may die. The difficulty with this hypothesis is that infants who die from SIDS are almost invariably a "white" ashen color, not cyanotic as would be expected if obstruction were the cause.

Gastroesophageal Reflux. Supporters of this hypothesis believe that reflux of gastric contents can cause a fatal reflex apnea. This hypothesis continues to be developed and researched. The high incidence of gastroesophageal reflux in infants, however, makes this association difficult to prove.

Prolongation of the Q-T Intervals. Disturbance in cardiac conduction (Q-T interval) has been researched by some investigators, but in a review of research findings the evidence supporting this hypothesis has been found to be inconclusive (Guntheroth et al, 1989).

Diagnostic Assessment

Development of a profile of infants at risk for SIDS is receiving extensive study. Common SIDS characteristics have been identified but cannot be used as predictive or diagnostic criteria. Based on McClain (1985) and Black et al (1986), the following characteristics represent findings drawn from retrospective epidemiologic studies (Chan, 1987).

- Boys 2 to 4 months of age.
- African-American infants.
- Multiple births and/or low birthweight infants.
- Infants born to teen-age mothers.
- Infant deaths in winter months.
- Time of death between 12 midnight and 8:00 A.M.
- Lower socioeconomic status (despite normal development and adequate nourishment).
- Maternal factors.

Signs and Symptoms Found During Autopsy

External examination of the infant reveals the typical victim to be in a normal state of nutrition and hydration. Over half exhibit frothy fluids in the mouth and nostrils, indicative of pulmonary edema. Often this fluid is tinged with blood. The diapers usually are filled with urine and stool. These findings lead one to suspect that vigorous motor activity has occurred. Vomitus may be found on the face, and the hands may be clutching fibers of blanket materials.

Internal examination reveals intrathoracic petechiae. Typically, these dot the surfaces of lungs, pericardium, and thymus, and frequently they also involve the parietal serosal surfaces of the chest. Experts propose that these petechiae may indicate intrathoracic negative pressure during the final moments of life. Typically, pulmonary congestion, edema, and inflammatory infiltrates in the upper airway and lungs are discovered. These findings, however, are not marked and do not provide an explanation of death.

Therapeutic Management

The National Foundation for Sudden Infant Death (NFSID) has advocated a management plan for SIDS. The four aspects of this program are as follows:

- Performance of autopsies on all infants dying suddenly and unexpectedly.
- Prompt notification of the results of that autopsy to the parents.
- Use of the term "sudden infant death syndrome" on the death certificate.
- Follow-up information and counseling for all families, provided by a knowledgeable health professional.

In the Home. Paramedical personnel are frequently the first persons called to the home when the nonbreathing infant is found. Therefore, it is imperative that they possess adequate information about SIDS. They must be trained to deal with the death in an empathetic and nonjudgmental manner. Local police, county coroner, and other community officials are informed by the community health care personnel about the special needs of SIDS families at the time of death.

In the Emergency Room. Emergency room personnel may have an overwhelming reaction to the SIDS event. Because they are geared toward preservation of life, dealing with the family of a SIDS victim can be extremely difficult—so difficult that at times the family is left alone in grief and confusion. Emergency room personnel need assistance in dealing with their own feelings of grief, so that they can provide the intervention families need at this critical time. Families need someone to stay with them and to reassure them that what has happened is not their fault. They need someone to listen to their pain, minister to their simple needs (get a cup of coffee for them), and help them make the important, immediate decision about an autopsy consent and perhaps organ donation. Parents also need to make funeral arrangements and handle the reactions of siblings.

At Autopsy. Autopsy serves two functions: in approximately 15 per cent of the cases a cause other than SIDS may be found, and the mysterious cause of death then may be clarified. Otherwise, families are left with doubt for the rest of their lives. It has been suggested that the health team member who conveys the results of the autopsy be the pathologist or family physician. After this information is relayed (preferably in person and within the first 24 hours after the death of the infant), a letter summarizing the cause of death should be sent.

Community Follow-Up. A community outreach program, including counseling at four critical periods, has been advocated. This program would include four steps: (1) when the baby is found dead, immediate intervention must be provided; (2) during the year following the death, counseling must follow in the form of either one-to-one intervention or group intervention and support; (3) counseling is again critical at the time of subsequent pregnancy and birth; and (4) continued support is needed until the subsequent child's age passes that of the SIDS infant.

Every effort should be made to have contact with the family within the week following the SIDS event. Often a follow-up program involving community health nurses can be developed within the community health care network. Parents also need opportunities to draw support from other parents of SIDS infants if they so desire. During the first home visit the nurse specialist assesses the family's level of understanding of the SIDS event. Information that has been misunderstood needs to be clarified at this time. Rather than commence an involved discussion of etiologic theories, the nurse needs to focus on the family members' reactions to the SIDS event. During this time, the nurse can provide continual reassurance that the parents could have done nothing to prevent, and that they did nothing to cause, the SIDS event.

During the next few months the nurse specialist needs to be available to the parents by telephone, letters, or visits. Assisting the family in their grief work is a prime function. Throughout this period, the nurse must be aware that special days within the year—the child's birthday, Thanksgiving, religious holidays, the anniversary of the infant's death—have significance to the family members. The nurse should make every effort to prepare the parents for the extra stress that often exists on these days and see that they have support systems to lean on during these times. A subsequent pregnancy initiates a period of renewed anxiety, and the nurse should be prepared to provide additional information, reassurance, and support. The issue of apnea monitoring must be faced and discussed at this time.

The support these families need is great and long-range. Support is often derived from a SIDS parents' group.* Films provided by these groups not only offer clarification of SIDS but also provide a focus for discussions about feelings and grief work. A unique relationship is shared among parents of SIDS infants. The strength of that relationship should not be underplayed by the health team.

Organizations that provide special information to health professionals and families are listed in Table 32–31.

Nursing Care

Impact of SIDS on the Family. Following the SIDS event, severe stress is experienced by all members of the family, including parents, grandparents, and siblings. Friends of the family, including the baby sitter, also are affected by the sudden unexpected death of an infant. This stress occurs without a noticeable precursor—the benefit of anticipatory grief is not experienced by the family.

The initial response to the child's confirmed death is extreme shock that produces varying degrees of confusion. This may be followed by outrage so intense that injury to self or others may occur. The absence of an explanation for the death increases the difficulty of resolving the loss. Family members commonly experience guilt, either self-blaming or projecting the blame onto another family member (often the spouse). A typical psychologic reaction of parents is that they review over and over every detail of the pregnancy, the birth, the life, and death of their child in search of a cause of the death (Swoiskin-Schwartz, 1988). These are the typical mixtures of responses experienced by all involved in the sudden death event. The nurse must be prepared to recognize these reactions.

During this critical period, the parents of the SIDS infant need tremendous support. Reality orientation helps the family cope with their confusion and guilt. The first essential step in reality orientation is the physician's confirmation of the death to the family. This should not be done by telephone. Because of the

*Information is available from the SIDS Alliance, 10500 Little Patuxent Parkway, Suite 420, Columbia, Maryland 21044; (800) 221-7437.

TABLE 32-31
SIDS Support Agencies

International Council for Infant Survival 9178 Nadine River Ct. Fountain Valley, CA 92708 Phone: (714) 968-7623 or (319) 322-4870
SIDS Alliance 10500 Little Patuxent Parkway, Suite 420 Columbia, MD 21044 Phone: (800) 638-7437 or (410) 964-8000; 24-hr answering service is (800) 221-7437
National Sudden Infant Death Resource Center 8201 Greensboro Dr., Suite 600 McLean, VA 22102 Phone: (703) 821-8955

extreme shock of sudden death, no family member should be told of the death without the presence of another family member, relative, or friend. Family members have less difficulty accepting the death and resolving their grief when they are permitted to view or even hold their dead infant. The family should always be prepared before seeing the dead infant. Stressful as it is, seeing or holding their child facilitates the family's acceptance of the death; however, no family member should ever be forced to have this experience.

The family members need an opportunity to sort their feelings and to begin to cope with their outrage. A place for the family to be alone affords them the privacy they need to regain composure and release feelings they do not wish to display publicly. An individual family member should never be left alone; nor should the family feel abandoned by the nurse. At this time the nurse serves as a therapeutic person by listening to fears and answering questions about the death.

Some families find that this event draws them closer together, whereas other families are immobilized to the extent that they are unable to support each other. Families who are drawn apart are more likely to project their guilt. Providing the family with printed information about SIDS helps allay some of the blame and guilt.

Inadequate parenting, the infant's suffocation by blankets or choking on vomitus, or the infant's inability to mouth breathe, as well as parents' failure to take the infant to the physician in time to cure a slight cold, are false explanations for the death often voiced by parents. These misunderstandings must be dispelled at the first visit with the family (in the emergency room or wherever the nurse first has contact with the family members). The crucial piece of information that parents and relatives must have is that *the death was not preventable.*

Impact of SIDS on Siblings. The inability of parents to cope with the needs of their other children during the initial period of shock and confusion can cause stress for the remaining siblings. They are often temporarily housed with relatives or friends to "protect" them from the pain of the mourning process and the funeral events. Such actions do not recognize the need of siblings to remain with their parents during this intense stress or work through their own grief. Only their parents can continue to provide the security needed by the surviving children through this stressful time.

Young children may also develop their own explanations for the baby's absence from the family. They may experience intense guilt or anxiety associated with the baby's death. Sending the children away from home at this time further increases their anxiety, confusion, and sense of guilt. Although the parents are having an extremely difficult time supporting one another, they must somehow share in their children's grief as well. The nurse intervenes to provide information about childhood grief to the parents and facilitate the family's unique grief work. Play therapy with siblings may assist younger children to express fear, guilt, and anxiety. Older siblings may need time to talk about the death with the nurse or their parents. The nurse can facilitate their grief work by providing an opportunity for it to occur.

Malformations of the Respiratory Tract

Choanal Atresia

Each nasal cavity communicates with the nasopharynx by posterior nasal openings (choanae). Choanal atresia is an obstruction of one or both of these openings due to the presence of a membranous or bony septum located between the nose and the pharynx. The atresia is approximately 2 to 3 cm anterior to the posterior margin of the hard palate. Congenital obstruction of the choanae is relatively common, with twice as many girls being affected as boys.

Etiology/Incidence (Pathophysiology)

An infant with unilateral choanal atresia may be asymptomatic and require no treatment for a prolonged period of time. With bilateral choanal atresia, prompt provision of an adequate airway is essential. Most newborn infants do not breathe through their mouths; therefore, when this anomaly is present, an infant develops varying degrees of respiratory distress, depending on the degree of obstruction and whether it is unilateral or bilateral. Unilateral choanal atresia can be overlooked, because the infant may be asymptomatic until the time of a respiratory infection. Signs of unilateral choanal atresia are nasal obstruction and nasal discharge from the involved side. Both signs may be pronounced during a respiratory infection, giving the first diagnostic sign of choanal atresia.

Clinical Manifestations

Infants with bilateral choanal atresia usually severe signs of distress after the initial cry at birth. When the infant quiets and attempts to breathe through the nose, cyanosis and severe retractions follow. Vigorous attempts to inspire air are made by a sucking-in motion of the lips. The greater the sucking effort the more tightly the tongue is drawn against the pharyngeal wall. This distress can be relieved by opening the infant's mouth. Sucking is almost impossible in the presence of bilateral atresia.

Diagnostic Assessment

Diagnosis of choanal atresia is considered if the dyspnea is increased by placing one's hand over the infant's mouth and if a firm catheter cannot be passed through the nostril. Instillation of a small amount of radiopaque dye into the affected side followed by a lateral x-ray film of the nasal region documents the presence of an atresia (Bingham, 1987).

Therapeutic Management

An oral airway is mandatory to accommodate mouth breathing pending surgery. Once an oral airway is established, the infant can be fed (see later discussion on nutrition). Carbon dioxide laser-resection technology allows for definitive surgical repair, usually within the first month of life.

Nursing Diagnostic Statements and Collaborative Problems

High risk for suffocation, ineffective airway clearance; *risk factor, congenital obstruction of one or both posterior nasal openings.*

Altered nutrition: less than body requirements, *related to sucking difficulties associated with airway obstruction.*

High risk for ineffective parenting (new parent); disrupted parent-infant bonding; *related to decreased opportunities for parent-infant contact.*

High risk for impaired home health maintenance; *risk factor: the knowledge deficit about child's needs for nutrition and attachment.*

Nursing Care

Recognizing Ineffective Airway Clearance. The clinical signs of severe respiratory distress are cause to suspect bilateral choanal atresia and should be identified by the nurse. Unilateral choanal atresia should be suspected if, during suctioning of the nares, the nurse observes respiratory difficulty and cyanosis. As the uninvolved side is being suctioned, the only open airway is being blocked by the catheter; therefore, signs of respiratory distress may be manifested.

The nurse's astute observations in the first moments of life can lead to early recognition and management of this condition.

Providing Adequate Nutrition. Gavage feedings are administered until the infant learns to eat and mouth breathe without the assisted airway. Surgical correction of the anomaly can be deferred until much later, although some surgeons advise immediate operation when the atresia is bilateral (Boat, 1992). If it is postponed until the child is 1 year of age or older, cautious bottle and spoon feeding can be introduced after the initial period of gavage feeding.

Facilitating Parent-Infant Bonding. Parents are under considerable stress during the treatment process. The nurse must recognize that the respiratory distress manifested by the infant with bilateral obstruction is frightening for parents to see. The early feelings of closeness and satisfaction that feeding brings are delayed because of the need for gavage feedings and surgical intervention. The nurse intervenes by providing opportunities for the parents to have physical contact with their baby and to participate in the daily physical care, including holding the infant for gavage feedings.

Facilitating Home Care. The nurse instructs parents about the most effective technique for feeding their child. The method of feeding is determined by the child's ability to tolerate feeding; the nurse instructs parents on signs to observe while feeding the child. Initially, the parents may be taught proper gavage feeding of their infant. Information on gavage feeding can be found in Chapter 35. Later, if the infant's condition warrants it, bottle and spoon feeding may be tolerated. Parents may feel uncomfortable and anxious about caring for their child at home, fearing they may not properly provide the care their child needs or not knowing what to do should an emergency arise. Parental anxieties can be dispelled by means of discharge teaching, which includes guided instruction and returned demonstrations of procedures to be provided at home. Printed instructions with telephone numbers of the health care team with indications for calling for advice and information are given to parents.

Parents may need encouragement and support in parenting their infant. The parents may have a tendency to view their child only in terms of the illness rather than as a child *with* an illness. The nurse can assist parents in bonding with their infant by emphasizing the child's unique personality characteristics and behaviors as well as the infant's response to the parent's nurturing and caregiving behaviors. Parents may require additional emotional and advocacy support following discharge, necessitating a referral to a social worker, parent group, or community agency such as home respite services.

Congenital Laryngeal Stridor (Laryngomalacia)

The term "laryngomalacia" describes an excessively flabby larynx, which results in stridor (noisy breathing). In stridor caused by laryngomalacia, no underlying structural anomaly is present: it is an exaggeration of the normally flaccid infant larynx.

Etiology/Incidence (Pathophysiology)

Laryngomalacia is the most common congenital laryngeal abnormality, with boys being affected twice as often as girls. It occurs in approximately 1 in 8000 births. The inheritance pattern is multifactorial, with a risk to siblings of less than 5 per cent.

The larynx is composed of three regions: supraglottis, glottis, and subglottis. It is a musculocartilaginous structure that provides for airway protection, clearance of secretions by a vigorous cough, and production of sound. The larynx is normally flaccid during infancy. When the laryngeal cartilage is especially soft and flaccid, the supraglottic structures are not well supported and collapse into the airway, causing a partial obstruction.

Clinical Manifestations

The most characteristic sign is a noisy crowing sound on *inspiration* (stridor). Noisy breathing may be accompanied by retractions and is usually compounded by a supine position. When the child is in the prone position, the supraglottic structures fall away from the airway, causing less obstruction. The infant's cry is usually normal, cyanosis is uncommon, and weight gain is within normal limits.

Stridor may bc present after the first few days of life, or it may not be noted until 2 months of age. In contrast, infectious croup (laryngotracheobronchitis) occurs late in infancy and is associated with low-grade fever.

Diagnostic Assessment

The nurse can assist in making a diagnosis by taking a thorough history: (1) duration and type of symptoms (intermittent, progressive, positional), (2) any association of symptoms with feeding, (3) worsening of symptoms with agitation, and (4) an incident of trauma or foreign-body aspiration. A diagnosis of laryngomalacia can be made on direct laryngoscopy by the physician. Although no treatment is necessary if laryngomalacia is the cause of stridor, direct laryngoscopy is done to rule out other anatomic abnormalities that may require treatment.

Therapeutic Management

Congenital stridor caused by laryngomalacia is a self-limiting condition. The condition improves over 6 to 12 months as the supporting cartilage matures, and symptoms usually subside by 1 to 2 years of age. On rare occasions, the condition is severe enough to cause airway obstruction. In these cases, a tracheostomy may be necessary until the child's cartilage matures. However, stridor without the presence of laryngomalacia during the first year of life may indicate a different and more serious condition and requires the attention of the nurse and physician for early identification.

Nursing Diagnostic Statements

High risk for suffocation, ineffective airway clearance; *risk factor: due to partial obstruction of the airway by supraglottic structures.*

High risk for injury: severe respiratory distress, *associated with increased oxygen demands associated with an upper respiratory infection.*

Ineffective family coping, related to anxiety; parental, *associated with*

- *The infant's respiratory distress.*
- *Feelings of inadequacy in dealing with the clinical manifestations.*

High risk for impaired home health maintenance; *risk factor: knowledge deficit about home care.*

Nursing Care

Promoting Optimal Airway Clearance. Stridor may be more pronounced during crying or feeding; therefore, the nurse discusses these aspects of infant care with the parents. The prone position can be suggested as a means of easing the baby's respirations. The baby should be watched when in the prone position. Feeding slowly and allowing time for the baby to breathe between sucking is recommended.

Preventing Respiratory Distress Associated with Infection. Parents are encouraged to call for assistance if they note any changes in the respiratory status of their infant, because these changes may indicate an infection or other problems requiring treatment. Although the infant may be able to compensate physiologically for the partial airway obstruction, the added burden of a respiratory infection may lead to severe respiratory distress.

An infection may increase the body's demands for oxygen through such processes as fever, further airway obstruction from mucous secretions and laryngeal edema, and decreased lung area for gas exchange. Parents can be taught general techniques for infection control, notably good hand washing, proper cleansing of articles that enter the infant's mouth, and isolation of the infant from persons with an active infection.

Relieving Parental Anxiety. The nurse is an important resource to the family when the infant is a noisy breather. Parents are apprehensive about their baby's symptoms and need reassurance that the condition will resolve as their baby develops. The nurse should be prepared to answer repeated questions about the baby's symptoms and to offer suggestions for increasing the baby's comfort and reducing the parents' anxiety.

Facilitating Home Care. Before discharge, the nurse instructs the parents to assess their infant's respiratory status, especially as related to positioning and signs and symptoms of an infectious process. Parents are instructed and given written instructions for observing and reporting respiratory changes in their infant. The nurse encourages parents to vent anxieties and concerns about their ability to care for their infant. Support, encouragement, correction of misconceptions, and provision of information facilitate their independent management of the infant's respiratory condition.

KEY CONCEPTS

Concepts Related to Basic Information

- Chronic respiratory disease accounts for almost half of all childhood chronic diseases.
- Low flow oxygen therapy is a method of oxygen delivery for infants and children who are oxygen-dependent for prolonged periods and do not require high oxygen concentration (oxygen requirements less than 55 per cent).
- Chest physical therapy is frequently used when pulmonary secretions cannot be removed by means of the normal process.
- The multiple stresses parents endure when their child has a respiratory problem put them at risk for ineffective family coping.
- Otitis media is one of the most common infectious diseases of childhood; it is the most common complication of upper respiratory infections.
- Epiglottitis is an acute infection of the epiglottis with a potentially fatal outcome.
- Approximately 8 million children in the United States experience at least one attack of bronchospasm in their lifetime.

Concepts Related to Nursing Assessment

- Signs of increasing respiratory obstruction include increasing stridor, retractions at rest, respiratory rate above 60 breaths per minute, tachycardia, circumoral and orbital cyanosis, pallor, and restlessness.
- When air exchange is severely compromised, a wheeze may not be heard because insufficient air is being exchanged.
- When assessing vital signs, the nurse checks the child for color, quality of respirations, nasal flaring, and restlessness.

Concepts Related to Nursing Intervention

- The nurse's role in respiratory therapy varies according to the setting; if the respiratory therapist has primary responsibility for respiratory treatment, the nurse needs to understand the goals of treatment.
- Maintenance of an adequate airway is central to the care of a child with croup.
- Maintenance of adequate fluid intake, humidification of inspired air, and chest physiotherapy to remove secretions are the goals of nursing care for the child with acute bronchitis.
- The nursing care of the child with cystic fibrosis is focused on promoting respiratory and gastrointestinal function, providing psychosocial support to child and family, and preparing the family for effective home management.
- Early involvement of the parents in the care of the infant with bronchopulmonary dysplasia, accompanied by ongoing teaching, is essential for successful management in the home.
- Reality orientation assists parents of the SIDS infant to cope with their initial shock and guilt; the essential first step is the physician's confirmation of the death to the family.

REFERENCES

Introduction (Principles, Respiration and Oxygenation, Malformations)

Behrman, R. (Ed.) (1992). *Nelson textbook of pediatrics* (14th ed.). Philadelphia: WB Saunders.

Burchfiel, C., et al. (1986). Passive smoking in children. *American Review of Respiratory Disease, 133,* 966–967.

Burgess, W. R., & Chernick, V. (1982). *Respiratory therapy in newborn infants and children*. New York: Thieme-Stratton.

Carnevale, F. (1986). Transcutaneous oxygen monitoring: Assessment techniques. *Dimensions in Critical Care Nursing, 5*(5), 264–269.

Charlton, A. (1984, June). Children's coughs related to parental smoking. *British Medical Journal, 288,* 1647–1649.

Committee on Environmental Hazards, American Academy of Pediatrics (1982). Involuntary smoking—A hazard to children. *Pediatrics, 77,* 755–757.

Fanconi, S., et al. (1985). Pulse oximetry in pediatric intensive care: Comparison with measured saturations and transcutaneous oxygen tension. *Journal of Pediatrics, 107,* 362–366.

Gellis, S., & Kagan, B. (1990). *Current pediatric therapy 13*. Philadelphia: WB Saunders.

Glassanos, M. R. (1980, January/February). Infants who are oxygen dependent—Sending them home. *MCN: American Journal Maternal Child Nursing,* pp. 42–45.
Guyton, A. (1991). *Textbook of medical physiology.* Philadelphia: WB Saunders.
Jennis, M. S., & Peabody, J. L. (1987). Pulse oximetry: An alternative for the assessment of oxygenation in newborn infants. *Pediatrics, 79,* 524–527.
Levengood, T. (1988). Involuntary smoking: Children in crises. *Pediatric Nursing, 14*(2), 93–95.
Levin, D., & Morriss, F. (1990). *Essentials of pediatric intensive care.* St. Louis: Quality Medical Publishing.
Lough, M., Doershuk, C., & Stern, R. (Eds.) (1986). *Pediatric respiratory therapy.* Chicago: Year Book Medical.
Lichtenstein, M. A. (1986). Pediatric home tracheostomy care: A parent's guide. *Pediatric Nursing, 12*(1), 41–48.
Monin, P., & Vert, P. (1987). The management of bronchopulmonary dysplasia. *Clinical Perinatology, 14,* 531–549.
National Center for Health Statistics. (1990). [National Health Interview Survey 1989. Public Health Service.] Unpublished data.
North American Nursing Diagnosis Association (NANDA) (1992). *NANDA nursing diagnoses: definition and classifications.* St. Louis: Author.
Openbrier, D. R., et al. (1988, February). Home oxygen therapy. Evaluation and prescription. *American Journal of Nursing,* pp. 192–197.
Randolph, A. (1991). *Randolph's pediatrics* (19th ed.). Norwalk, CT: Appleton & Lange.
Shapiro, C. (1986). Retrolental fibroplasia: What we know and what we don't know. *Neonatal Network, 4*(6), 33–44.
Sinkin, R. A., & Phelps, D. L. (1987). New strategies for the prevention of bronchopulmonary dysplasia. *Clinical Perinatology, 14*(3), 599–620.
Tilikian, S., Conover, M., & Tilikian, A. (1987). *Clinical implications of laboratory tests.* St. Louis: CV Mosby.
Vedal, S., et al. (1984). Risk factors for childhood respiratory disease. Analysis of pulmonary function. *American Review of Respiratory Diseases, 130,* 187–192.
Ware, I., et al. (1984). Passive smoking, gas cooking and respiratory health of children living in six cities. *American Review of Respiratory Diseases, 129,* 366–374.

Nasopharyngitis

Behrman, R. (Ed.) (1992). *Nelson textbook of pediatrics* (14th ed.). Philadelphia: WB Saunders.
Gellis, S., & Kagan, B. (1990). *Current pediatric therapy 13.* Philadelphia: WB Saunders.
O'Grady, M. (1987). Rhinitis: Allergic and nonallergic. *Canadian Family Physician, 33,* 1459–1463.

Otitis Media

Behrman, R. E. (Ed.) (1992). *Nelson textbook of pediatrics* (14th ed.). Philadelphia: WB Saunders.
Bluestone, C. D., & Klein, J. O. (1988). *Otitis media in infants and children.* Philadelphia: WB Saunders.
Gellis, S., & Kagan, B. (1990). *Current pediatric therapy 13.* Philadelphia: WB Saunders.
Hughes, J. (1984). *Synopsis of pediatrics.* St. Louis: CV Mosby.
Lounsbury, B. F. (1985). Swimming unprotected with long-shafted middle ear ventilation tubes. *Laryngoscope, 95,* 340–343.
Marchant, C. D., & Shurin, P. A. (1983, April). Therapy of otitis media. *Pediatric Clinics of North America,* pp. 281–296.
Mitchell, D. (1987). Otitis media in children. *Canadian Family Physician, 33,* 1497–1499.
Paradise, J. (1980, May). Otitis media in infants and children. *Pediatrics,* pp. 917–943.
Paradise, J. L., et al. (1987). Efficacy of adenoidectomy for recurrent otitis media: Results from parallel random and nonrandom trials. *Pediatric Research, 21,* 286A.
Zenk, K., & Ma, H. (1990). Pharmacologic treatment of otitis media and sinusitis in pediatrics. *Journal of Pediatric Health Care, 4*(6), 297–303.

Croup

Boat, T. (1992). Infectious croup. In R. Behrman (Ed.), *Nelson textbook of pediatrics* (14th ed.) (pp. 1065–1068). Philadelphia: WB Saunders.
Gellis, S., & Kagan, B. (1990). *Current pediatric therapy 13.* Philadelphia: WB Saunders.
Loebl, S., & Spratto, G. (1986). *The nurse's drug handbook* (4th ed.). New York: John Wiley & Sons.

Epiglottitis

Committee on Infectious Diseases, American Academy of Pediatrics (1991). *Report of the Committee on Infectious Diseases* (22nd ed.). Elk Grove Village, IL: Author.
Hall, C. B., Hall, W. J. (1987). Epiglottitis. In R. A. Hoekelman et al. (Eds.), *Primary pediatric care.* St. Louis: CV Mosby, 1591–1594.

Bronchiolitis

Boat, T. (1992). Acute bronchiolitis. In R. Behrman (Ed.), *Nelson textbook of pediatrics* (14th ed.) (pp. 1075–1076). Philadelphia: WB Saunders.
Committee on Infectious Diseases, American Academy of Pediatrics (1991). *Report of the Committee on Infectious Diseases* (22nd ed.). Elk Grove Village: IL: American Academy of Pediatrics.
Corey, M., & Clore, E. (1991). Management of the infant with respiratory syncytial virus. *Journal of Pediatric Nursing, 6*(2), 93–98.
Wohl, M. E. B. (1983). Bronchiolitis. In E. L. Kendig & V. Chernick (Eds.), *Disorders of the respiratory tract in children* (pp. 283–294). Philadelphia: WB Saunders.

Pharyngitis and Tonsillitis

Kornblut, A. B. (1987). A traditional approach to surgery of the tonsils and adenoids. *Otolaryngology Clinics of North America, 20,* 349–367.
Rasmussen, N. (1987). Complications of tonsillectomy and adenoidectomy. *Otolaryngology Clinics of North America, 20,* 383–393.
Widome, M., et al. (1987). Pharyngitis and tonsillitis. R. Hoekelman (Ed.), *Pediatric primary care.* St. Louis: CV Mosby.

Asthma

Blue, C. (1988). Exercise-induced asthma: "The silent asthma." *Journal of Pediatric Health Care, 2*(4), 167–174.
Friedman, M. (1984). Psychological factors associated with pediatric asthma death: A review. *Journal of Asthma, 21,* 97–117.
Gellis, S., & Kagan, B. (1990). *Current pediatric therapy 13.* Philadelphia: WB Saunders.
Lockey, R., & Bukantz, S. (1987). *Principles of immunology and allergy.* Philadelphia, WB Saunders.
Mansmann, H. C., et al. (1988). Treatment of acute asthma in children. In C. Bierman, & D. Pearlman (Eds.), *Allergic diseases from infancy to adulthood* (2nd ed.) (pp. 571–586). Philadelphia: WB Saunders.
Pearlman, D., & Bierman, C. (1988). Asthma (bronchial asthma, re active airways disorder). In C. Bierman, & D. Pearlman, (Eds.), *Allergic diseases from infancy to adulthood* (2nd ed.) (p. 559). Philadelphia: WB Saunders.
Rudolph, A. (1991). *Rudolph's pediatrics* (14th ed.). Norwalk, CT: Appleton & Lange.
Sly, R. M. (1985). *Pediatric allergy.* New York: Medical Examination Publishing Company.
Traver, G., & Martinez, M. (1988). Asthma update I. Mechanisms, pathophysiology, and diagnosis. *Journal of Pediatric Health Care 2,* 221–226.
Zahr, L., Connolly, M., & Pago, D. (1989). Assessment and management of the child with asthma. *Pediatric Nursing, 15*(2), 109–114.

Cystic Fibrosis

Ad Hoc Committee Task Force on Neonatal Screening. Cystic Fibrosis Foundation (1983, November). Neonatal screening for cystic fibrosis: Position paper. *Pediatrics,* pp. 741–745.

Canam, C. (1986). Talking about cystic fibrosis within the family—what parents need to know. *Issues in Comprehensive Pediatric Nursing, 9,* 167–178.

Cowen, L., et al. (1986). Psychologic adjustment of the family with a member who has cystic fibrosis. *Pediatrics, 77,* 745–753.

Boat, T. F. (1992). Cystic fibrosis. In R. E. Behrman (Ed.), *Nelson textbook of pediatrics* (14th ed.) (pp. 1106–1116). Philadelphia: WB Saunders.

Gellis, S. S., & Kagan, B. M. (1990). *Current pediatric therapy 13.* Philadelphia: WB Saunders.

Hodson, M. E. (1983, November). Cystic fibrosis in adolescents and adults. *Practitioner,* pp. 1723–1729.

Lester, L. A., & Rothberg, R. M. (1986). Cystic fibrosis. In S. S. Gellis & B. M. Kagan (Eds.). *Current pediatric therapy 12* (pp. 225–231). Philadelphia: WB Saunders.

McQuitty, J., & Lewis, N. (1991). Cystic fibrosis. In A. Rudolph, *Rudolph's pediatrics* (19th ed.) (pp. 1526–1532). Norwalk, CT: Appleton & Lange.

Orenstein, D. M. (1988). Exercise tolerance and exercise conditioning in children with chronic lung disease. *Journal of Pediatrics, 118,* 1043–1047.

Quinton, P. M., & Bisman, J. (1983). Higher bioelectric potential due to decreased absorption in the sweat glands of patients with cystic fibrosis. *New England Journal of Medicine, 308,* 1185.

Riordan, J., et al. (1989). Identification of the cystic fibrosis gene: Cloning and characterization of complementary DNA. *Science, 245,* 245.

Rose, J., & Jay, S. (1986). A comprehensive exercise program for persons with cystic fibrosis. *Journal of Pediatric Nursing, 1,* 323–334.

Rosenstein, B. J. (1987). A clearer—and somewhat brighter—picture of cystic fibrosis. *Contemporary Pediatrics, 4*(7), 71–91.

Rudolph, A. (1991). *Rudolph's pediatrics* (14th ed.). Norwalk, CT: Appleton & Lange.

Schwachman, H. (1983). Cystic fibrosis. In E. L. Kendig & V. Chernick (Eds.), *Disorders of the respiratory tract in children* (pp. 640–661). Philadelphia: WB Saunders.

Schwartz, R. H. (1987). Cystic fibrosis. In R. A. Hoekelman et al. (Eds.), *Pediatric primary care* (pp. 1203–1210). St. Louis: CV Mosby.

Bronchopulmonary Dysplasia

Als, H., et al. (1986). Individual behavioral and environmental care for the very low birth weight preterm infant at high risk for bronchopulmonary dysplasia: Neonatal intensive care unit and development outcome. *Pediatrics, 78,* 1123–1132.

Avery, M. E. (1984). The argument for prenatal doses of dexamethasone to prevent respiratory distress syndrome. *Journal of Pediatrics, 104,* 240.

Bancalari, E., & Gerhardt, T. (1986). Bronchopulmonary dysplasia. *Pediatric Clinics of North America, 33,* 1–23.

Brown, E. (1987). In H. W. Tawusch, & M. W. Yogman (Eds.), *Follow-up management of the high-risk infant.* Boston: Little, Brown.

Cummings, J., et al. (1989). A controlled trial of dexamethasone in preterm infants at high risk for bronchopulmonary dysplasia. *New England Journal of Medicine, 320*(23), 1505–1510.

Koops, B. L., et al. (1984, February). Outpatient management and follow-up of bronchopulmonary dysplasia. *Clinical Perinatology,* pp. 101–122.

Korones, S. B. (1988). Complications. In J. L. Goldsmith et al. (Eds.), *Assisted ventilation of the neonate.* Philadelphia: WB Saunders.

McElheny, J. (1989). Parental adaptation to a child with bronchopulmonary dysplasia. *Journal of Pediatric Nursing, 5*(5), 346–352.

Merritt, C. M. (1986). Prophylactic treatment of very premature infants with human surfactant. *New England Journal of Medicine, 315,* 785–790.

Monin, P., & Vert, P. (1987). The management of bronchopulmonary dysplasia. *Clinical Perinatology, 14,* 531–549.

Northway, W. H., et al. (1967). Pulmonary disease following respiratory therapy of hyaline membrane disease: BPD. *New England Journal of Medicine, 276,* 357–368.

Notter, R. H., & Shapiro, D. L. (1987). Lung surfactants for replacement therapy: Biochemical, biophysical and clinical aspects. *Clinical Perinatology, 14,* 433–479.

Pridham, K., et al. (1989). Parental issues in feeding young children with bronchopulmonary dysplasia. *Journal of Pediatric Nursing, 4*(3), 177–185.

Rotschild, A., et al. (1989). Increased compliance in response to solbutamol in premature infants with developing bronchopulmonary dysplasia. *Journal of Pediatrics, 115,* 984.

Saigal, S., & O'Brodovich, H. (1987). Long-term outcome of preterm infants with respiratory disease. *Clinics in Perinatology, 14*(3), 635–650.

Sauve, R. S., & Singhal, N. (1985). Long-term morbidity of infants with bronchopulmonary dysplasia. *Pediatrics, 76,* 725–733.

Scherf, R. F. (1985). Total patient care of the newborn infant who develops bronchopulmonary dysplasia. *Neonatal Network,* 3, 28–37.

Sinkin, R. A., & Phelps, D. L. (1987). New strategies for the prevention of bronchopulmonary dysplasia. *Clinical Perinatology, 14*(3), 599–620.

Soll, R. F., et al. (1990). Multicenter trial of single-dose modified bovine surfactant extract (Survanta) for prevention of respiratory distress syndrome. *Pediatrics, 85,* 1092.

Stevens, M. (1990). A comparison of mothers' and fathers' perceptions of caring for an infant requiring home cardio-respiratory monitoring. *Issues in Comprehensive Pediatric Nursing, 13*(2), 81–95.

Toce, S. S. et al. (1984). Clinical and roentgenographic scoring systems for assessing bronchopulmonary dysplasia. *American Journal of Diseases of Children, 138,* 581–585.

Wilkie, R., & Bryan, M. (1987). Effect of bronchodilators or airway resistance in ventilator-dependent neonates with chronic lung disease. *Journal of Pediatrics, 11,* 278.

Apnea-Related Disorders

Avery, G. (Ed.) (1987). *Neonatology* (3rd ed.). Philadelphia: JB Lippincott.

Barrington, K. J. et al. (1986). Physiologic effects of doxapram in idiopathic apnea of prematurity. *Journal of Pediatrics, 108,* 125–129.

Brady, J., & McCann, E. (1985). Control of ventilation in subsequent siblings of victims of sudden infant death syndrome. *Journal of Pediatrics, 106*(2), 212–217.

Kelly, D., & Shannon, D. C. (1982, October). Sudden infant death syndrome and near sudden infant death syndrome: A review of the literature. *Pediatric Clinics of North America,* pp. 1241–1261.

Lockey, R., & Bukantz, S. (1987). *Principles of immunology and allergy.* Philadelphia, WB Saunders.

Loebl, S., & Spratto, G. (1986). *The nurse's drug handbook* (4th ed.). New York: John Wiley & Sons.

Lyman, R. D., et al. (1985). Psychological effects on parents of home and hospital apnea monitoring. *Journal of Pediatric Psychology, 10*(4), 439–448.

Marchal, F., et al. (1987). Neonatal apnea and apneic syndrome. *Clinical Perinatology, 14*(3), 509–529.

McElroy, E., et al. (1986). Emotional and health impact of home monitoring on mothers: A controlled retrospective study. *Pediatrics, 78*(5), 780–786.

Rudolph, A. (1991). *Rudolph's pediatrics* (14th ed.). Norwalk, CT: Appleton & Lange.

Spitzer, A., & Fox, W. (1986). Infant apnea. *Pediatric Clinics in North America, 33*(3), 561–581.

Weese-Mayer, D., Brouillette, R., Morrow, A., et al. (1989). Assessing validity of infant monitor alarms with event recording. *Journal of Pediatrics, 115,* 702.

Sudden Infant Death Syndrome

Black, L., David, R. J., Brouillette, R. T., et al. (1986). Effects of birth weight and ethnicity on incidences of sudden infant death syndrome. *Journal of Pediatrics, 108*(2), 209–214.

Chan, M. M. (1987). Sudden infant death syndrome and families at risk. *Pediatric Nursing, 13*(3), 166–168.

Glotzbach, S., Baldwin, R., Lederer, N., Tansey, P., & Ariagno, R. (1989). Periodic breathing in preterm infants: Incidence and characteristics. *Pediatrics, 84,* 785.

Glotzbach, S., & Heller, H. (1989). Thermoregulation. In M. Kryger, T. Roth, & W. Dement (Eds.). *Principles and practice of sleep medicine* (pp. 300–309). Philadelphia: WB Saunders.

Glotzbach, S., Tansey, P., Baldwin, R., & Ariagno, R. (1989). Periodic breathing in preterm infants: Influence of bronchopulmonary dysplasia and theophylline. *Pediatric Pulmonology, 7,* 78.

Guilleminault, C., & Ariagno, R. (1989). Apnea during sleep in infants and children. In M. Kryger, T. Roth, & W. Dement (Eds.), *Principles and practice of sleep medicine* (pp. 655–664). Philadelphia: WB Saunders.

Guntheroth, W. (1989). Interleukin-1 as intermediary causing prolonged sleep apnea and SIDS during respiratory infections. *Medical Hypotheses, 28*(2), 121–123.

Herbst, J. J., et al. (1988). New findings shed light on SIDS. *Patient Care, 22*(9), 61–76.

McClain, M. Sudden infant death syndrome: An update. *Journal of Emergency Nursing, 11*(5): 227–233.

Rudolph, A. (1991). *Rudolph's pediatrics* (14th ed.). Norwalk, CT: Appleton & Lange.

Swoiskin, S., Schwartz, S., Deatrick, J., & Hanson, D. (1988). Parents' views about having a child after a SIDS death. *Journal of Pediatric Nursing, 3*(1), 24–28.

Congenital Anomalies

Bingham, W. T. (1987). The neonatal airway: Problems and management. *Canadian Family Physician, 33,* 1467–1470.

Boat, T. (1992). Congenital disorders of the nose. In R. Behrman (Ed.), *Nelson textbook of pediatrics*. (14th ed.) (p. 1053). Philadelphia: WB Saunders.

Rudolph, A. (1991). *Rudolph's pediatrics* (14th ed.). Norwalk, CT: Appleton & Lange.

BIBLIOGRAPHY

Introduction (Principles, Respiration and Oxygenation, Malformations)

Ballard, P. L. (1989). Hormonal regulation of pulmonary surfactant. *Endocrine Review, 10,* 165.

Blanchette, T., et al. (1991). Pulse oximetry and normoxemia in neonatal intensive care. *Respiratory Care, 36*(1), 25–32.

Chen, Y., & Yu, S. (1986). Influence of passive smoking on admissions for respiratory illness in early childhood. *British Medical Journal, 293,* 303–305.

Committee on Infectious Diseases, American Academy of Pediatrics (1991). Report of the Committee on Infectious Diseases. Elk Grove Village, IL: American Academy of Pediatrics.

Kitterman, J. (1988). Physiological factors in fetal lung growth. *Canadian Journal of Physiologic Pharmacology, 66,* 1122.

Mammel, M., & Boros, S. (1988). High frequency ventilation. In J. Goldsmith & E. Karitkin (Eds.), *Assisted ventilation of neonate.* Philadelphia: WB Saunders.

Murray, A., & Morrison, B. (1989). Passive smoking by asthmatics: Its greater effect on boys than on girls and on older than on younger children. *Pediatrics, 84,* 451–459.

Panico, G., et al. (1990). Pediatric respiratory infections of nosocomial importance. *Asepsis, 12*(3), 2–9.

Paynton, A. (1991). Synthetic surfactant: Giving premature infants a better chance for survival. *Nursing, 21*(3), 64.

Pedreira, F., et al. (1985). Involuntary smoking and incidence of respiratory illness during the first year of life. *Pediatrics, 75,* 594–597.

Ramanathan, R., Durand, M., & Larrazabal, C. (1987). Pulse oximetry in very low birth weight infants with acute and chronic lung disease. *Pediatrics, 79,* 612.

Riggato, H., et al. (1989). High frequency oscillation ventilation compared with conventional mechanical ventilation in the treatment of respiratory failure in preterm infants. *New England Journal of Medicine, 320,* 88.

Wright, J. R., & Clements, J. A. (1987). Metabolism and turnover of lung surfactant. *American Review of Respiratory Disease, 136,* 426.

Tracheostomy

Aday, L., & Wegner, D. (1988). Home care for ventilator-assisted children: Implications for the children, their families, and health policy. *Children's Health Care, 17,* 112–120.

Andrews, M., & Nielson, D. (1988). Technology dependent children in the home. *Pediatric Nursing, 14,* 111–114, 151.

Briggs, N. (1987). Selecting a pediatric home care program. *Pediatric Nursing, 13,* 191.

Campbell, J., et al. (1989). Experience with the homecare of tracheostomised paediatic patients. *Archives of Otorhinolaryngology, 246,* 345–348.

Carabott, J., et al. (1991). Teaching families tracheostomy care. *Canadian Nurse, 87*(3), 21–22.

Grundfast, K., et al. (1988). Gaining access to school for the child with a tracheostomy. *International Journal of Pediatric Otorhinolaryngology, 16,* 101–112.

Hall, S., & Weatherly, K. (1989). Using sign language with tracheostomized infants and children. *Pediatric Nursing, 15,* 362–367.

Hazinski, M. (1986). Pediatric home tracheostomy care: A parent's guide. *Pediatric Nursing, 12,* 41–48.

Hill, B., & Singer, L. (1990). Speech and language development after infant tracheostomy. *Journal of Speech and Hearing Disorders, 55,* 1–20.

Kaufman, J., & Hardy-Ribakow, D. (1988). What parents need to know about trach care. *RN, 51,* 99–104.

Kennelly, C. (1987). Tracheostomy care: Parents as learners. *MCN: American Journal of Maternal Child Nursing, 12*(4), 264–267.

Kenney, M. (1987). Hospital to home: Care of the child with a tracheostomy. *Neonatal Network, 6*(1), 21–24.

Kirkhart, K., et al. (1988). Louisiana's ventilator assisted care program: Case management services to link tertiary with community-based care. *Children's Health Care, 17,* 106–111.

Leighton, E., Davis, R., & Anderson, L. (1990). An orientation program for high-technology home care nursing. *Pediatric Nursing, 16,* 182–185.

Lucas, J., Golesi, J., Sleeper, G., & Ryan, J. (1988). *Home respiratory care.* Norwalk, CT: Appleton & Lange.

McCarthy, M. (1986). A home discharge program for ventilator-assisted children. *Pediatric Nursing, 12,* 331–335, 380.

Runton, N., & Zalzal, G. (1989). The decannulation process in children. *Journal of Pediatric Nursing, 4,* 370–373.

Schreiner, M., Donar, M., & Kettrick, R. (1987). Pediatric home mechanical ventilation. *Pediatric Clinics of North America, 34,* 47–60.

Sherman, L., & Rosen, C. (1990). Development of a preschool program for tracheostomy dependent children. *Pediatric Nursing, 16*(4), 357–361.

Singer, L., et al. (1989). Developmental sequelae of long-term infant tracheostomy. *Developmental Medicine and Child Neurology, 31,* 224–230.

Simon, B., & McGowan, J. (1989). Tracheostomy in young children: Implications for assessment and treatment of communication and feeding disorders. *Infants and Young Children, 1*(3), 1–9.

Steele, N., & Harrison, B. (1986). Technology-assisted children: Assessing discharge preparation. *Journal of Pediatric Nursing, 1*(3), 150–158.

Steele, N., & Morgan, J. (1989). Emergency planning for technology-assisted children. *Journal of Pediatric Nursing, 4,* 81–87.

Stroup, K., Wylie, P., & Bull, M. (1987). Car seats for children with mechanically assisted ventilation. *Pediatrics, 80,* 290–292.

Thilo, E., Comito, J., & McCulliss, D. (1987). Home oxygen therapy in the newborn. *American Journal of Diseases of Children, 141,* 766–768.

Waisn, C., et al. (1987). Controlled supplemental oxygenation during tracheobronchial hygiene. *Nursing Research, 36,* 211–215.

Wegerer, D., & Aday, L. (1989). Home care for ventilator-assisted children: Predicting family stress. *Pediatric Nursing, 15,* 371–376.

Wessel, G., Prumo, M., & Harrison, P. (1989). School placement and the oxygen-dependent child. *Pediatric Nursing, 6,* 435–436.

Whitford, K. (1988). Health care needs of ventilator-dependent children. *Pediatric Nursing, 14,* 216–219.

Otitis Media

Dyson, A., et al. (1987). Speech characteristics of children after otitis media. *Journal of Pediatric Health Care, 1*(5), 261.

Hendrickse, W., et al. (1988). Five vs. 10 days of therapy for acute otitis media. *Pediatric Infectious Disease Journal, 7*(1), 14.

Kaufman, D., Grothe, G., & Brasser, B. (1987, January/February). Early identification of ear infection and hearing loss in early childhood population. *School Nurse,* pp. 18–21.

Le, C. (1988). Otitis revisited: Are ear tubes the answer? *Contemporary Pediatrics, 9*(9), 24–45.

Roberts, J., et al. (1989). Otitis media in early childhood and cognitive, academic and classroom performance of the school age child. *Pediatrics, 83,* 477–485.

Weiss, J., et al. (1988). Cost effectiveness in the choice of antibiotics for the initial treatment of otitis media in children: A decision analysis approach. *Pediatric Infectious Disease Journal, 7*(1), 23.

Croup

Kairys, S., Olmstead, E., & O'Conner, G. (1989). Steroid treatment of laryngotracheitis: A meta-analysis of the evidence from randomized trials. *Pediatrics, 83,* 683.

Kuusela, A., & Vesikari, T. (1988). A randomized double-blind placebo controlled trial of dexamethasone and racemic epinephrine in the treatment of croup. *Acta Paediatrica Scandinavica, 77,* 99.

Lepow, M., & Hethington, S. (1990). Respiratory tract infections. In M. Green & R. Haggerty (Eds.), *Ambulatory pediatrics*. Philadelphia: WB Saunders.

Mauro, R., Poole, S., & Lockhart, M. (1988). Differentiation of epiglottitis from laryngotracheitis in the child with stridor. *American Journal of Diseases of Children, 142,* 408.

Skolnik, N. (1989). Treatment of croup. A critical review. *American Journal of Diseases of Children, 143,* 1045.

Stokes, D. (1990). The croup syndrome. In S. Gellis & E. Kagan (Eds.). *Current pediatric therapy 13* (pp. 111–114). Philadelphia: WB Saunders.

Stool, S. (1988). Croup syndrome: Historical perspective. *Pediatric Infectious Disease Journal, S157.*

Super, D., et al. (1989). A prospective randomized double-blind study to evaluate the effect of dexamethasone in acute laryngotracheitis. *Journal of Pediatrics, 115,* 323–329.

Epiglottitis

Butt, W., Shann, F., Walker, C., et al. (1988). Acute epiglottitis: A different approach to management. *Critical Care Medicine, 16,* 43.

Mauro, R., Poole, S., & Lockhart, M. (1988). Differentiation of epiglottitis from laryngotracheitis in the child with stridor. *American Journal of Diseases of Children, 142,* 679.

Tooley, W. (1991). Inspiratory obstruction. In A. Rudolph (Ed.), *Rudolph's pediatrics* (19th ed.). Norwalk, CT: Appleton & Lange.

Bronchiolitis

Agah, R., Cherry, J., Garakian, A., & Chapin, M. (1987). Respiratory syncytial virus (RSV) infection rate in personnel caring for children with RSV infections. *American Journal of Diseases of Children, 141,* 695–697.

Arlo, O., et al. (1990). Risk factors for recurrent acute otitis media and respiratory infection in infancy. *International Journal of Pediatric Otorhinolaryngology, 19*(2), 151–161.

Englund, J., Piedra, P., Jefferson, L., Wilson, S., Taber, L., & Gilbert, B. (1990). High-dose, short-duration ribavirin aerosol therapy in children with suspected respiratory syncytial virus infection. *Journal of Pediatrics, 117,* 313–320.

Fackler, J., Flannery, K., Zipkin, M., & McIntosh, K. (1990). Precautions in the use of ribavirin at the Children's Hospital. *New England Journal of Medicine, 322,* 634.

Fiascone, J., Grandgeorge, S., Rhodes, T., & Knapp, M. (1989). *Current Problems in Pediatrics.* Chicago: Year Book.

Gozal, D., Colin, A., Joffel, M., & Hochberg, Z. (1990). Water, electrolyte and endocrine homeostasis in infants with bronchiolitis. *Pediatric Research, 27,* 204.

Groothius, J., Salbenblatt, C., & Lauer, B. (1990). Severe respiratory syncytial virus infection in older children. *American Journal of Diseases of Children, 144,* 346.

Hall, C. (1987). Respiratory syncytial virus. In R. D. Feigin, & J. D. Cherry (Eds.), *Textbook of pediatric infectious diseases* (2nd ed.) (pp. 1653–1669). Philadelphia: WB Saunders.

Lebel, M., et al. (1989). Respiratory failure and mechanical ventilation in severe bronchiolitis. *Archives of Disease in Childhood, 64*(10), 1431–1437.

Mallory, G., Motoyama, E., et al. (1989). Bronchial reactivity in infants in acute respiratory failure with viral bronchiolitis. *Pediatric Pulmonology, 6,* 253.

Mertsola, J., et al. (1991). Recurrent wheezing bronchitis and viral respiratory infections. *Archives of Disease in Childhood, 66*(1), 124–129.

Nederharid, K., et al. (1989). Respiratory syncytial virus: A nursing perspective. *Pediatric Nursing, 15,* 342–345.

Piontek-Lentz, T. (1988). Ribavirin: Ready for RSV season. *Neonatal Network, 7*(2), 29–35.

Rimar, J. (1986). Ribavirin for treatment of RSV infection. *MCN: American Journal of Maternal Child Nursing, 11,* 413.

Rodriguez, W., Bui, R., Connor, J., Kim, H., Brandt, C., Parrott, R., Burch, B., & Mace, J. (1987). Environmental exposure of primary care personnel to ribavirin aerosol when supervising treatment of infants with respiratory syncytial virus infections. *Antimicrobial Agents and Chemotherapy, 31,* 1143–1146.

Shaw, K., et al. (1991). Outpatient assessment of infants with bronchiolitis. *American Journal of Diseases of Children, 145*(2), 151–155.

Steinhorn, R., et al. (1990). Use of extra-corporeal membrane oxygenation in the treatment of respiratory syncytial virus bronchiolitis: The national experience 1983–1988. *Journal of Pediatrics, 116*(3), 338–342.

Welliver, R., Sun, M., Rinaldo, D., & Ogra, P. (1986). Predictive value of respiratory syncytial virus-specific IgE response for recurrent wheezing following bronchiolitis. *Journal of Pediatrics, 109,* 776–780.

Pneumonia

Committee on Infectious Diseases, American Academy of Pediatrics (1991). *Report of the Committee on Infectious Diseases* (22nd ed.). Elk Grove Village, IL: American Academy of Pediatrics.

Gellis, S., & Kayan, B. (1990). *Current pediatric therapy 13.* Philadelphia: WB Saunders.

Green, M., & Haggenty, R. (1990). *Ambulatory pediatrics.* Philadelphia: WB Saunders.

Ledbetter, E. (1988). The many faces of pneumococcal pneumonia. *Contemporary Pediatrics, 5*(11), 50–72.

Moffet, H. (1989). *Pediatric infectious disease* (3rd ed.). Philadelphia: JB Lippincott.

Swischuk, L., & Hayden, C. (19867). Viral vs. bacterial pulmonary infections in children: (Is roentgenographic differentiation possible?) *Pediatric Radiology, 16,* 278.

Lodisco, T., de Benedictis, F., & Dottorins, M. (1989). Viral and *Mycoplasma pneumoniae* pneumonias in school-age children: Three year follow-up of respiratory function. *Pediatric Pulmonology, 6,* 232–236.

Sheahan, S., & Seabolt, J. (1989). *Chlamydia trachomatis* infections. A health problem of infants. *Journal of Pediatric Health Care, 3,* 144–149.

Turner, N., et al. (1987). Pneumonia in pediatric outpatients: Cause and clinical manifestations. *Journal of Pediatrics, 111,* 194–200.

Wright, A., Taussig, L., Ray, G., et al. (1989). The Tuscon children's respiratory study II. Lower respiratory infection in the first year of life. *American Journal of Epidemiology, 129,* 1232.

Pharyngitis and Tonsillitis

Committee on Infectious Diseases, American Academy of Pediatrics. (1991). *Report of the Committee on Infectious Diseases* (22nd ed.). Elk Grove Village, IL: American Academy of Pediatrics.

Denny, F. (1987). Current problems in managing streptococcal pharyngitis. *Journal of Pediatrics, 111,* 797–805.
Gellis, S., & Kagan, B. (1990). *Current pediatric therapy 13.* Philadelphia: WB Saunders.
Gerber, M. (1989). Comparison of throat cultures and rapid strep tests for diagnosis of stretococcal pharyngitis. *Pediatric Infectious Disease Journal, 8,* 820.
Gerber, M., Randolph, M., & Tilton, R. (1986). Enzyme fluorescence procedure for rapid diagnosis of streptococcal pharyngitis. *Journal of Pediatrics, 108,* 421–423.
McMillian, J. (1988). Sore throats in teens: Strep and beyond. *Contemporary Pediatrics, 5*(3), 20–30.
Moffet, H. (1989). *Pediatric infectious disease* (3rd ed.). Philadelphia: JB Lippincott.
Montgomery, J., et al. (1987). Anesthesia for tonsillectomy and adenoidectomy. *Otolaryngology Clinics of North America, 20,* 331–347.
O'Grady, M. (1987). Rhinitis: Allergic and nonallergic. *Canadian Family Physician, 33,* 1459–1463.
Pearlman, D. (1988). Chronic rhinitis in children. *Journal of Allergy and Clinical Immunology, 81,* 962–966.
Putto, A. (1987). Febrile exudative tonsillitis—viral or streptococcal? *Pediatrics,* 8–11.
Oski, F., et al. (Eds.) (1990). *Principles and practice of pediatrics.* Philadelphia: JB Lippincott.
Randolph, M., Gerber, M., De Meo, K., & Wright, C. (1985). The effect of antibiotic therapy on the clinical course of streptococcal pharyngitis. *Journal of Pediatrics, 106,* 870.
Simons, F. (1988). Allergic rhinitis: Recent advances. *Pediatric Clinics of North America, 35,* 1053–1074.

Asthma

Attaway, N. J., & Strunk, R. C. (1989). Death due to asthma in children: What the pediatrician can do. *Pediatric Annals, 18*(12), 819–823.
Brim, S. (1989). A quick guide for home use of inhalant medications. *Pediatric Nursing, 15*(1), 87–88.
Conboy, K. (1989). Self-management skills for cooperative care in asthma. *Journal of Pediatrics, 5*(2), 863–866.
Dworkin, G., & Kattan, M. (1989). Mechanical ventilation for status asthmaticus. *Journal of Pediatrics, 114*(4), 545–549.
Geelhoed, G. C., et al. (1990). Oximetry and peak expiratory flow in assessment of acute childhood asthma. *Journal of Pediatrics, 117,* 907.
Lewiston, N. (1986). Asthma self management programs and education. *Pediatric Annals, 15,* 127–136.
Littenberg, B. (1988). Aminophylline treatment in severe acute asthma. A meta-analysis. *Journal of the American Medical Association, 259,* 1678.
Litwack, K., et al. (1989). Practical points in the management of asthma. *Journal of Post Anesthesia Nursing, 4*(4), 251–253.
Mellis, C. M. (1988). Important changes in the emergency management of acute asthma in children. *Medical Journal of Australia, 148,* 215.
Murray, A., et al. (1988). Passive smoking and the seasonal difference of severity of asthma in children. *Chest, 94*(4), 701–708.
Miller, B. D., & Strunk, R. C. (1989). Circumstances surrounding the deaths of children due to asthma. *American Journal of Diseases of Children, 143,* 1294–1299.
Nurses Drug Alert. (1989). Psychological effect of theophylline in children. *Nurses Drug Alert, 13*(7), 51.
Pierson, W. (1988). Exercise-induced bronchopasm in children and adolescents. *Pediatric Clinics of North America, 35,* 1031–1040.
Rachelefsy, G., et al. (1986). Behavior abnormalities and poor school performance due to oral theophylline use. *Pediatrics, 78,* 1133–1138.
Rappaport, L., et al. (1989). Effects of theophylline on behavior and learning in children with asthma. *American Journal of Diseases of Children, 143,* 368–372.
Ramsey, A. M., & Siroky, A. S. (1998). The use of puppets to teach schoolage children with asthma. *Pediatrics Nursing, 14*(3), 187–190.
Richards, W. (1989). Hospitalization of children with status asthmaticus: A review. *Pediatrics, 84*(1), 111–118.
Robin, E. D., & Lewiston, N. (1989). Unexpected, unexplained sudden death in young asthmatic subjects. *Chest, 96*(4), 790.
Salmeron, S., et al. (1989). High doses of inhaled corticosteroids in unstable chronic asthma. *American Review of Respiratory Diseases, 140,* 164.
Sly, P. D., & Hibbut, M. E. (1989). Childhood asthma following hospitalization with acute viral bronchiolitis in infancy. *Pediatric Pulmonology, 7,* 153–158.
Stein, R., et al. (1989). Severe acute asthma in a pediatric intensive care unit: 6 years experience. *Pediatrics, 83*(6), 1023–1028.
Weinberger, M. (1989). *Managing asthma.* Baltimore: Williams & Wilkins.
Weinberger, M. (1989). Antiasthmatic therapy in children. *Pediatric Clinics of North America, 36*(5), 1251–1284.
Wynn, S. R. (1989). Alternative approaches to asthma. *Journal of Pediatrics, 115,* 846.
Zimo, D. A., et al. (1989). The efficacy and safety of home nebulizer therapy for children with asthma. *American Journal of Diseases in Children, 143,* 208–211.

Cystic Fibrosis

Brissette, S., et al. (1987). Nursing care plan for adolescents and young adults with advanced cystic fibrosis. *Issues in Comprehensive Pediatric Nursing, 10,* 87–97.
Boat, T., Welsh, M., & Beaudet, A. (1989). Cystic fibrosis. In C. Scriver, A. Beaudet, W. Sly, & D. Valle (Eds.), *The metabolic basis of inherited disease* (6th ed.). New York: McGraw-Hill, 2649–2680.
Brock, D. (1990). Population screening for cystic fibrosis. *American Journal of Human Genetics, 47,* 164–165.
Buffone, G., et al. (1988). Prenatal diagnosis of cystic fibrosis: Microvillar enzymes and DNA analysis compared. *Clinical Chemistry, 34,* 933–937.
Cassey, J., et al. (1988). Totally implantable system for venous access in children with cystic fibrosis. *Clinical Pediatric, 27,* 91–95.
Dibble, S. L., & Savedra, M. C. (1988). Cystic fibrosis in adolescence: A new challenge. *Pediatric Nursing, 14,* 299–303.
Gellis, S. S., & Kagan, B. M. (1990). *Current pediatric therapy 13.* Philadelphia: WB Saunders.
Gibson, C. (1988). Perspective in parental coping with a chronically ill child: The case of cystic fibrosis. *Issues in Comprehensive Pediatric Nursing, 11,* 33–41.
Gilbert, F. (1990). Is population screening for cystic fibrosis appropriate now? *American Journal of Human Genetics, 46,* 394–395.
Huang, N., et al. (1987). Clinical features survival rate and prognostic factors in young adults with cystic fibrosis. *American Journal of Medicine, 82,* 871.
Johnson, J. P. (1988). Genetic counseling using linked DNA probes: Cystic fibrosis as a prototype. *Journal of Pediatrics, 113,* 957–964.
Kerem, B., Commens, J., & Buchannan, J. (1989). Identification of the cystic fibrosis gene: Genetic analysis. *Science, 245,* 1073–1080.
MacLusky, I., et al. (1989). Long term effects of inhaled tobramycin in patients with cystic fibrosis colonized with *Pseudomonas aeruginosa. Pediatric Pulmonology, 7,* 42.
Myer, P. A. (1988). Parental adaptation to cystic fibrosis. *Journal of Pediatric Health Care, 2,* 20–28.
Orenstein, D. M. (1988). Exercise tolerance and exercise conditioning in children with chronic lung disease. *Journal of Pediatrics, 118,* 1043–1047.
Stullenberger, B., et al. (1987). Family adaptation to cystic fibrosis. *Pediatric Nursing, 13,* 29–31.
Strom, C., Verlinsky, Y., Milayeva, S., et al. (1990). Preconception genetic diagnosis of cystic fibrosis. *Lancet, 336,* 306–307.
Strauss, G., et al. (1987). Variable weight training in cystic fibrosis. *Chest, 92,* 273–276.

Bronchopulmonary Dysplasia

Abman, S., et al. (1989). Late unexpected deaths in hospitalized infants with bronchopulmonary dysplasia. *American Journal of Diseases of Children, 143,* 815–819.
Avery, M. E. (1986). Surfactant replacement. *New England Journal of Medicine, 315,* 825–826.

Berry, D. (1991). Neonatology in the 1990's: Surfactant replacement therapy becomes a reality. *Clinical Pediatrics, 30*(3), 167–182.
Blanchette, T., et al. (1991). Pulse oximetry and normoxemia in neonatal intensive care. *Respiratory Care, 36*(1), 25–32.
Campbell, L., et al. (1988). Neurologic aspects of bronchopulmonary dysplasia. *Clinical Pediatrics, 27*(1), 7–13.
Charon, A., et al. (1989). Factors associated with surfactant treatment response in infants with severe respiratory distress syndrome. *Pediatrics, 83,* 348.
Fiascone, J., et al. (1989). *Current problems in pediatrics.* Chicago: Year Book.
Groothius, J., et al. (1988). Respiratory syncytial virus infection in children with bronchopulmonary dysplasia. *Pediatrics, 82*(2), 199–203.
Harkavy, K., et al. (1986). Dexamethasone therapy for chronic lung disease. *Journal of Pediatrics, 115*(6), 979–983.
Harkavy, K., et al. (1989). Dexamethasone therapy for chronic lung disease in ventilator- and oxygen-dependent infants: A controlled trial. *Journal of Pediatrics, 115,* 979.
Hartley, S., et al. (1989). Maintenance sedation of agitated infants in the neonatal intensive care unit with chloral hydrate: New concerns. *Journal of Perinatology, 9*(2), 162–164.
Hazlett, D. (1989). A study of pediatric home ventilator management: Medical, psychosocial, and financial aspects. *Journal of Pediatric Nursing, 4*(4), 284–293.
Horbar, J., et al. (1989). A multicenter randomized, placebo-controlled trial of surfactant therapy for respiratory distress syndrome. *New England Journal of Medicine, 320,* 959.
Kurzner, S., et al. (1988). Growth failure in infants with bronchopulmonary dysplasia: Nutrition and elevated resting metabolic expenditure. *Pediatrics, 81*(3), 379.
Lund, C., & Collier, S. (1990). Nutrition and bronchopulmonary dysplasia. In C. Lund (Ed.), *Bronchopulmonary dysplasia: Strategies for total patient care.* Petaluma, CA: Neonatal Network Publishing.
Manisclo, W., et al. (1989). Surfactant replacement therapy: Impact on hospital changes for premature infants with respiratory distress syndrome. *Pediatrics, 83*(1), 1–6.
Panico, G., et al. (1990). Pediatric respiratory infections of nosocomial importance. *Asepsis, 12*(3), 2–9.
Paynton, A. (1991). Synthetic surfactant: Giving premature infants a better chance for survival. *Nursing, 21*(3), 64.
Scharer, K., & Dixon, M. (1989). Managing chronic illness: Parents with a ventilator dependent child. *Journal of Pediatric Nursing, 4*(4), 236–247.
Soll, R. F., et al. (1990). Multicenter trial of single-dose modified bovine surfactant extract (Survanta) for prevention of respiratory distress syndrome. *Pediatrics, 85,* 1092.
Stevens, M. (1990). A comparison of mothers' and fathers' perceptions of caring for an infant requiring home cardio-respiratory monitoring. *Issues in Comprehensive Pediatric Nursing, 13*(2), 81–95.
Tay-Uyboco, J., et al. (1989). Hypoxic airway constriction in infants of very low birth weight recovering from moderate to severe bronchopulmonary dysplasia. *Journal of Pediatrics, 115,* 456.

Apnea-Related Disorders

Andrews, M., et al. (1987). Home apnea: Monitoring in the Intermountain West. *Journal of Pediatric Health Care, 1*(5), 255–260.
Bairam, A., et al. (1987). Theophylline versus caffeine: Comparative effects in treatment of idiopathic apnea in the preterm infant. *Journal of Pediatrics, 110*(4), 636–639.
Booten, D., Keemar, S., et al. (1986). A randomized clinical trial of early hospital discharge and home follow-up of very low-weight infants. *New England Journal of Medicine, 315*(15), 934–939.
Brooks, J. (1988). Apnea and home monitoring. *Pediatrician, 15,* 212.
Consensus statement. National Institutes of Health Consensus Development Conference on Infantile Apnea and Home Monitoring (1989). *Pediatrics, 79,* 292.
Hartsell, M. (1986). Selecting home monitors. *Journal of Pediatric Nursing, 1*(1), 54–57.
Kahn, A., Rebuffat, E., Sottiaux, M., & Blum, B. (1988). Management of an infant with an apparent life-threatening event. *Pediatrician, 15,* 204.
Komelasky, A. (1990). The effect of home nursing visits on parental anxiety and CPR knowledge retention of parents of apnea-monitored infants. *Journal of Pediatric Nursing, 5*(6), 387–392.
Motoyoma, E. (1988). Respiratory physiology. In D. Cook & J. Marcy (Eds.), *Neonatal anesthesia.* Menlo Park, CA: Appleton Davies.
Muttitt, S., et al. (1988). Neonatal apnea: Diagnosis by nurse versus computer. *Pediatrics, 82*(5), 713–720.
Oren, J., Kelly, D., & Shannon, D. (1986). Identification of a high-risk group for sudden infant death syndrome among infants who were resuscitated for sleep apnea. *Pediatrics, 77,* 495.
Saylor, C., et al. (1989). Anxiety in mothers of infants on apnea monitors. *Children's Health Care, 18*(2), 117.
Spitzer, A., et al. (1989). Anxiety in mothers of infants on apnea monitors. *Children's Health Care, 18*(2), 117.
Weese-Mayer, D., Brouillette, R., Morrow, A., et al. (1989). Assessing validity of infant monitor alarms with event recording. *Journal of Pediatrics, 115,* 702.
Wright, S., Norton, C., & Kesten, K. (1989). Retention of infant CPR instruction by parents. *Pediatric Nursing, 15*(1), 37–41.

Sudden Infant Death Syndrome

Ariagno, R. L. (1988). Management of apnea in the ICN graduate. In R. A. Ballard, *Pediatric care of the ICN graduate* (pp. 264–280). Philadelphia: WB Saunders.
Bentele, K. H. P., & Albani, M. (1988). Are there tests predictive for prolonged apnea and SIDS? A review of epidemiological and functional studies. *Acta Paediatrica Scandanavica, 342* (Suppl), 3.
Brazy, J. E., Kinney, H. C., & Oakes, W. J. (1987). Central nervous system structural lesion: Causing apnea at birth. *Journal of Pediatrics, 111,* 163.
Chasnoff, I., Hunt, C., Kletter, R., & Kaplan, D. (1989). Prenatal cocaine exposure is associated with respiratory pattern abnomalities. *American Journal of Diseases of Children, 143,* 583.
Consensus Statement: National Institutes of Health Consensus Development Conference on Infantile Apnea and Home Monitoring (1987). *Pediatrics, 79,* 292.
Denmead, D., Aariagno, R., Carson, S., & Benirschke, K. (1987). Placental pathology is not predictive for sudden infant death syndrome (SIDS). *American Journal of Perinatology, 4,* 308.
Forsyth, K., Weeks, S., Koh, L., et al. (1989). Lung immunoglobulins in the sudden infant death syndrome. *British Medical Journal, 298,* 23.
Grether, J., & Schulman, J. (1989). Sudden infant death syndrome and birth weight. *Journal of Pediatrics, 114,* 561.
Grether, J., Schulman, J., & Croen, L. (1990). Sudden infant death syndrome among Asians in California. *Journal of Pediatrics, 116,* 525.
Griffin, M., Ray, W., Livengood, J., & Schaffner, W. (1988). Risk of sudden infant death syndrome after immunization with the diphtheria-tetanus-pertussis vaccine. *New England Journal of Medicine, 319,* 618.
Guntheroth, W., Lohmann, R., & Spiers, P. (1990). Risk of sudden infant death syndrome in subsequent siblings. *Journal of Pediatrics, 116,* 520.
Hunt, C., & Brouillette, R. (1987). Sudden infant death syndrome: 1987 perspective. *Pediatrics, 110,* 669.
Kerfoot, T. (1989). The perils of pertussis. *Journal of Pediatric Nursing, 4*(4), 277–283.
Krous, H. (1988). Pathological considerations of sudden infant death syndrome. *Pediatrician, 15,* 231.
Mortimer, E. (1987). DTP and SIDS: When data differ. *American Journal of Public Health, 77*(8), 945–950.
Smialek, J., & Lambros, Z. (1988). Investigation of sudden infant deaths. *Pediatrician,* 191.
Swoiskin, S., Schwartz, S., Deatrick, J., & Hanson, D. (1988). Parents' views about having a child after a SIDS death. *Journal of Pediatric Nursing, 3*(1), 24–28.
Swoiskin, S. (1986). Sudden infant death: Nursing care for the survivors. *Journal of Pediatric Nursing, 1*(1), 33–39.

Valdes-Dapena, M. (1988). Sudden infant death syndrome: Overview of recent research developments from a pediatric pathologist's perspective. *Pediatrician, 15,* 222.

Walker, A., et al. (1987). Diphtheria-tetanus-pertussis immunization and sudden infant death syndrome. *American Journal of Public Health, 77*(8), 945–950.

Weese-Mayer, D., et al. (1989). Assessing validity of infant monitor alarms with event recording. *Journal of Pediatrics, 115,* 702.

Zielke, H. R., et al. (1989). Normal fetal hemoglobin levels in the sudden infant death syndrome. *New England Journal of Medicine, 321,* 1359.

Zylke, J. W. (1989). Sudden infant death syndrome: Resurgent research offers hope. *JAMA, 262,* 1565.

Congenital Anomalies

Davenport, S., Hefner, M., & Mitchell, J. (1986). The spectrum of clinical features in CHARGE syndrome. *Clinical Genetics, 29,* 298.

MacFarlane, P., Olinsky, A., & Phelan, P. (1985). Proximal airway function 8 to 16 years after laryngomalacia: Follow-up using low volume loop studies. *Journal of Pediatrics, 107,* 216.

McCray, P., et al. (1988). Hypoxia and hypercapnea in infants with mild laryngomalacia. *American Journal of Diseases of Children, 142,* 896.

Richardson, M., & Osguthorpe, J. (1988). Surgical management of choanal atresia. *Laryngoscope, 98,* 915.

Stahl, R., & Jurkiewicz, M. (1985). Congenital posterior choanal atresia. *Pediatrics, 76,* 429.

CHAPTER • 33

Altered Cardiovascular Function

Elaine Daberkow-Carson
Patricia Smith

NURSING PROCESS PLANS
NPP: The Child with Congestive Heart Failure, Table 33–3.
NPP: Care of the Child Having Cardiac Surgery, Table 33–4.

RELATED TOPICS
Impact of chronic illness, Chapter 19
Nursing Process Plan: Perioperative Care, Table 23–7
Nursing Process Plan: The Hospitalized Child, Table 21–5
Organic failure-to-thrive, Chapter 28
Genetic counseling, Chapter 31
Kawasaki disease, Chapter 37
Rheumatic fever, Chapter 37

LEARNING OBJECTIVES

- Explain the transitional differences in structure and function of the cardiovascular system.
- Discuss the nursing implications that are specific to various types of heart defects.
- Describe the general principles of nursing care applied to the care of the child having cardiac catheterization.

- **Describe the general principles of nursing care applied to the child having cardiac surgery.**
- **Identify the nursing interventions to apply to the care of the child with congestive heart failure.**
- **Identify the nursing interventions to apply to the care of the child with cyanosis.**
- **List the health maintenance issues for the child with hypertension.**
- **List the health maintenance issues for the child with congenital/acquired heart disease.**

When an infant is born with any type of birth defect, the parents' coping abilities are challenged. Because the heart is vital to human existence and is viewed by many as the "life force" of the human body, a defect of the cardiac structure may be of heightened significance to the parents and family. The nurse caring for the child with a cardiac defect must help the parents cope with their feelings of grief and fear so that they are able to deal with the facts related to their infant's illness.

In the United States, most alterations in cardiovascular function in children are the result of defects in the heart that are present at birth, or "congenital" heart disease. "Acquired" heart disease (e.g., infective endocarditis, hypertension, cardiomyopathy, dysrhythmias) occurs less than one tenth as often as congenital disease.

An estimated 40,000 babies are born with congenital heart disease (CHD) in the United States yearly. Of these, about one third become critically ill in the first year of life, one third develop problems later in childhood or as young adults, and one third never experience serious handicaps (Nadas, 1990). Management of CHD is primarily surgical. Usually, cardiac catheterization, an invasive diagnostic procedure, precedes surgery.

Approximately 1 in 100 infants has one or more congenital cardiovascular abnormalities (Adams et al, 1989). The risk of CHD occurring in offspring of an affected parent, as well as the risk of occurrence in newborn siblings of an affected child, varies widely depending on the specific heart defect and the etiologic circumstance.

Ninety per cent of CHD is thought to be due to multifactorial inheritance, in which there is a genetic predisposition for CHD that interacts with an environmental trigger during a vulnerable period of gestation. Environmental triggers (Table 33–1) can be separated into three main categories: drugs, infections, and maternal conditions.

Development of the heart and great vessels takes place during the first 14 to 60 days of gestation. This is considered the vulnerable period of gestation for cardiac malformation. The specific type of cardiac malformation produced varies depending on the environmental trigger and its timing within the vulnerable period.

Approximately 8 per cent of CHD is associated with other abnormalities such as trisomies 21, 18, and 13, Turner syndrome, and Noonan syndrome. Approximately 2 per cent of CHD is thought to be due to environmental factors alone, not requiring a genetic predisposition. Alcohol, thalidomide, rubella, and, possibly, cytomegalovirus are environmental triggers in this category (Adams et al, 1989). Multiple environmental triggers such as coxsackie B virus, mumps virus, and influenza B virus have been identified since the early 1970s, but many more have yet to be discovered. In most cases of CHD, the specific cause cannot be identified. It is hoped that ongoing research in this area will delineate more clearly the full range of environmental influences that cause CHD. Table 33–2 outlines nursing interventions for prevention of congenital heart anomalies.

This chapter deals with nursing interventions related to recognition, diagnosis, and management of the child with congenital or acquired heart disease, cardiac surgery, and long-term care (health maintenance). The impact of heart disease on the child and family will be both acute and long-term. Because congestive heart failure (CHF) is a condition common to many cardiac disorders, nursing care for the child

TABLE 33-1
Environmental Triggers of Congenital Heart Defects

Environmental Triggers	Frequency (Per Cent)
Drugs	
Alcohol	25–30
Chemotherapy	5
Amphetamines	5–10
Hydantoin	2–3
Trimethadione	15–30
Lithium	10
Thalidomide	5–10
Sex hormones	2–4
Infections	
Rubella	35
Cytomegalovirus	?
Maternal Conditions	
Diabetes	3–5
Lupus erythematosus	?
Phenylketonuria	25–50

From Daberkow, E. D., & Washington, R. (1985). Congenital heart disease. In G. Merenstein, et al (Eds.), *Handbook of neonatal intensive care*. St. Louis: CV Mosby.

with CHF is detailed in Table 33–3. The Nursing Process Plan, "Care of the Child Having Cardiac Surgery" (Table 33–4), details the nursing care provided to the child undergoing cardiac surgery.

Structure and Function

In order to adequately assess anatomic and circulatory changes for cardiac abnormalities, the nurse must be aware of normal differences in structure and function that result from anatomic and physiologic immaturity. Table 33–5 summarizes these developmental differences. The remainder of this section describes fetal circulation and the physiologic changes that occur at birth. Knowledge of these cardiopulmonary changes provides a base for understanding congenital heart disease.

Fetal Circulation

A thorough understanding of fetal circulation and physiologic changes occurring in the neonate from birth through the first few weeks of life is important in order to understand CHD and its presentation. Fetal circulation (Fig. 33–1) differs from neonatal circulation in many significant ways. In the former, the placenta is the major route of gas exchange, excretion, and acquisition of essential fetal chemicals. The lungs are fluid-filled and extract oxygen from the blood instead of providing oxygen for it. In addition, the pulmonary blood vessels are constricted and have a thick muscle coating, which offers a high resistance to blood flow. Therefore, in fetal circulation, the right ventricle pumps against a higher resistance than the

TABLE 33-2
Congenital Heart Anomalies: Nurse's Role in Prevention

Assessing for Children and Families at Risk

- Genetic counseling for parents with one child with CHD or a parent with CHD
- Screening infants of mothers with maternal rubella, diabetes, or lupus erythematosus
- Screening of premature infants
- Screening of infants with other congenital anomalies, or with chromosomal aberrations

Implementing Preventive Measures

- Rubella vaccine by 15 mos of age
- Rubella titer on women with questionable history of rubella
- Genetic counseling of women over 35 yrs of age
- Maintaining a positive maternal environment
  1. No cigarette smoking
  2. No alcohol ingestion
  3. Adequate nutrition, rest, and exercise
  4. Prevention of illness during pregnancy
  5. No self-prescribed drugs

TABLE 33-3

Nursing Process Plan: The Child with Congestive Heart Failure

Analysis: Nursing Diagnostic Statement 1

Response and Related or Risk Factors: *Impaired physical mobility and fatigue related to activity intolerance secondary to the heart's inability to pump an adequate supply of blood to meet the body's metabolic needs*

Projected Outcome: The child will be able to have some independent physical movement. The child will be rested enough to have capacity for age-appropriate physical and mental activity

Defining Characteristics

Subjective:

- Verbalization by child and/or parents of lack of energy and inability to maintain usual routines and perceived need for additional energy to accomplish routine tasks with or without exercise
- Parental report of infant's inability to take an adequate amount per feeding, falling asleep at feedings and spending little time awake, seeming short of breath with feeding and at rest, sweating with feedings and at rest, becoming pale, having a weak cry, not yet accomplishing developmental tasks expected for age
- Poor weight gain

Objective:

- Inability to purposefully move within the physical environment, including bed mobility, transfer, and ambulation
- Reluctance to attempt movement

Increase in physical complaints

- Emotionally labile
- Impaired ability to concentrate
- Decreased performance
- Lethargic or listless

Nursing Interventions

Activity Therapy

Increase activity tolerance.

- Provide feeding, dry diapers, and tactile stimulation before infant cries (crying uses oxygen, further decreasing activity tolerance)
- Use a pacifier while preparing feedings, or during fussy times (crying increases energy expenditure)
- Feed the infant frequently and in small amounts (large feedings tire the infant)
- Allow frequent rest periods during feeding
- Use a soft nipple (to reduce the work of sucking)
- Breastfed babies may need additional rest periods (breastfeeding requires slightly more energy expenditure than bottle feeding)
- Limit feeding at breast to 8–10 mins on the first side and 10–15 mins on the second side (this will usually meet caloric needs; further sucking may burn more calories than it adds)
- Some infants may require high-calorie formulas to increase the caloric intake per energy expenditure
- Continuous nasogastric drip formula feedings may be required to further decrease the work of feeding for the infant while providing optimal calories. Notify physician if this judgment is made

Evaluation Criteria

The child will balance energy demands with the cardiac output and the heart's ability to perfuse the tissues as evidenced by:

- Ability to maintain physical exercise (crying, feeding) for longer period without fatigue
- Developmentally appropriate ability and willingness to move within the physical environment
- Continuation of muscle strength at previous level or increase
- Verbalization by child and/or parents of adequate energy and ability to maintain usual routines

(continued)

TABLE 33-3 *(continued)*

Defining Characteristics	Nursing Interventions	Evaluation Criteria
	• Ensure uninterrupted sleep/rest periods • Schedule activities, such as bathing, after rest and at other than feeding times • Maintain normal body temperature (to decrease energy demands of hyperthermia or hypothermia) by keeping the environment at a moderate temperature; preventing chilling during bathing; adjusting clothing and blanket coverings to the environmental temperature	

Analysis: Collaborative Problem 1

Response and Related or Risk Factors: *Altered tissue perfusion: systemic, related to* decreased cardiac output

Projected Outcome: The child will experience adequate nutrition and oxygenation at the cellular level

Defining Characteristics	Nursing Interventions	Evaluation Criteria
Objective: • Skin color pale and cool to touch, becoming mottled or cyanotic with increased oxygen demands (e.g., crying, feeding, playing) • Periorbital edema and edema of face, hands, and feet • Neck vein distention (in older child) • Blood pressure changes in extremities • Skin quality, shining, lack of lanugo, slow healing of lesions • Urine output <1 ml/kg/hr • Failure to thrive: 3rd percentile for height and weight on growth chart • Cardiomegaly • Hepatomegaly	*Surveillance; Cardiac Care: Rehabilitative* • Decrease the cardiac workload (see interventions to increase activity tolerance) • Administer O_2 if ordered • Monitor O_2 saturation (per pulse oximetry or ABGs) • Treat infection promptly • Attempt to reduce exposures to infectious contacts • Administer digoxin as ordered (to increase ventricular contractility and decrease heart rate). Ensure safe administration by checking the dosage with another registered nurse and by taking the apical pulse for 1 min • Check with physician if pulse is <100 for a neonate, <90 for a 1-year-old, <85 for a 2-year-old, <80 for a 4-year-old, <75 for a 6-year old, <70 for an 8-year-old, <60 for a 14-year-old • Monitor for the following therapeutic effects of digoxin: de-	**The child will show adequate tissue perfusion as evidenced by:** • Absence of edema or neck vein distention • Blood pressure within normal limits • Weight gain • Skin warm to touch; color normal, appropriate to race, mucous membrane pink • Pulse and respirations within normal range for age • Peripheral pulses palpable • Urine output ≥1 ml/kg/hr

TABLE 33-3 *(continued)*

Defining Characteristics	Nursing Interventions	Evaluation Criteria
	crease in pulse and respirations, increase in urine output (signaling better kidney perfusion), improvement in skin color and temperature (with better perfusion to the peripheral tissues) • Monitor for the classic signs of digoxin toxicity: nausea (manifests as anorexia in the infant), vomiting, lethargy, bradycardia, and dysrhythmia (noted on ECG or cardiac monitor, and in irregular apical pulse) • Monitor serum digoxin levels: >2.1 mg/ml may indicate toxicity • Blood for digoxin levels should be drawn at least 6–8 hrs after the last dose (to ensure equilibrium between serum and tissue levels) • Administer diuretics as ordered (to decrease salt and water retention related to decreased renal perfusion and the resulting rise in antidiuretic hormone and aldosterone levels) • Monitor for therapeutic effects of diuretic administration: urine output, decreased peripheral edema, decreased neck vein distention, clearing of lung sounds • Monitor diuresis by recording input/output and by daily weights. (Weight is a sensitive indicator of fluid balance.) Weigh before breakfast or the first A.M. feeding. Weigh the infant and toddler nude; weigh the preschooler or older child with only a hospital gown • Counsel the parents that the infant should wet at least 6–8 diapers per day to ensure adequate output. Have them notify you if this does not occur • Monitor for side effects: dehydration and electrolyte imbalance, especially hypokalemia (which potentiates digoxin and may lead	

(continued)

TABLE 33-3 *(continued)*

Defining Characteristics	Nursing Interventions	Evaluation Criteria
	to toxicity) (common symptoms: muscle weakness and cramping, decrease in peristalsis, dysrhythmia) and hyponatremia (common symptoms: muscle weakness, leg cramps, dry mouth, dizziness, and gastrointestinal disturbances) • Prevent respiratory infections by teaching the family good handwashing techniques and alerting them to the most common sources of pathogens (infection increases O_2 demands) • Discuss *fomite*-transmitted respiratory illnesses such as respiratory syncytial virus (RSV)	

Analysis: Nursing Diagnostic Statement 2

Response and Related or Risk Factors: *Altered nutrition: less than body requirements, related to:*

- Anorexia associated with decreased perfusion of the GI tract and/or the side effects of medications
- Decreased energy available for sucking/chewing
- Increased metabolic demands associated with the increased workload of the overloaded heart

Projected Outcome: The child will receive caloric intake to meet metabolic demands for growth and development

Defining Characteristics	Nursing Interventions	Evaluation Criteria
Subjective: • Self-report of anorexia or of "being too tired to eat" • Parental report of caloric/nutrient intake that is less than body requirements • Falling asleep during feeding *Objective*: • Failure to maintain the weight percentile (and usually also the length percentile) on the growth chart established by the birth weight and length of the full-term infant • Pale conjunctival and mucous membranes	*Nutrition Therapy* **Ensure caloric requirements per 24-hr period that equal or exceed these recommendations for the healthy child (congestive heart failure [CHF] increases metabolic needs)** **Note:** Infants in CHF require ≥150 kcal/kg/day to grow **Normal Requirements:** 0–6 mos — kg × 115 kcal 6–12 mos — kg × 105 kcal 1–3 yrs — 1300 kcal (average) 4–6 yrs — 1700 kcal (average) 7–10 yrs — 2400 kcal (average) 11–14 yrs — 2200–2700 kcal average for girls/boys	**The child will experience adequate response to metabolic demands as evidenced by:** • Gradual increase in weight • Maintenance of or increase in weight/length percentiles on the growth chart • Ingestion of enough calories to meet metabolic needs

TABLE 33-3 *(continued)*

Defining Characteristics	*Nursing Interventions*	*Evaluation Criteria*
• Poor muscle tone	15–18 yrs 2100–2800 kcal (average) • Recommended gavage feeding to physician if necessary (to ensure adequate intake and reduce caloric expenditure) • Follow measures to decrease energy expenditure (see Nursing Diagnostic Statement 1) • Administer 24 kcal/oz formula (amount usually ordered to increase caloric intake per feeding). Monitor for therapeutic benefit (steady weight gain) versus intolerance (diarrhea and/or vomiting with weight loss) **Encourage attainment of emotional, social, and cognitive tasks** • Provide visual, auditory, and tactile stimulation appropriate to the child's age and energy level • Encourage loving and playful interactions with family members • Assure parents that most of the child's emotional, social, and cognitive tasks can be met despite the CHF, and that motor tasks will develop quickly once physical health improves	

Analysis: Nursing Diagnostic Statement 3

Response and Related or Risk Factors: *High risk for altered growth and development, risk factors:*

- Inadequate tissue perfusion to promote healthy tissue growth
- Lack of energy to accomplish developmental tasks (partially secondary to nutritional deficit)

Projected Outcome: The child will maintain own growth curves; child will demonstrate no deviations in norms from his or her age group

Defining Characteristics *(Actual Response)*	*Nursing Interventions*	*Evaluation Criteria*
Subjective: Parental report of delay or difficulty in performing skills (motor, social, or expressive) typical of age group	*Energy Management; Support System Enhancement* **Assess factors contributing to altered growth and development** (evidence of infant/child/adolescent's behavior deviating from	**The child will demonstrate growth and development appropriate for age as evidenced by:** • Gradual increase in ability to perform skills

(continued)

TABLE 33-3 *(continued)*

Defining Characteristics	Nursing Interventions	Evaluation Criteria
Objective: • Observed delay in performing skills (motor, social, or expressive) typical of age group • Altered physical growth • Inability to perform self-care or self-control activities appropriate for age (these delays can be measured using a valid developmental assessment inventory) • Flat affect • Listlessness, decreased responses	age-appropriate levels will be observed and documented according to theoretical basis of growth and development; peer support, parent-child relationships; social support; knowledge of physiologic effects of disease on the child and family) **Instruct caregivers regarding acquisition of age-appropriate developmental tasks and anticipatory guidance** (refer to information on developmental norms in each chapter related to specific age groups) **Refer child/adolescent and family to appropriate community resources as needed:** • Appropriate agency for counseling for child and family treatment • Appropriate agency for supportive services (e.g., occupational therapy, physical therapy, home care services) • Community programs specific to factors affecting the child's altered growth and development (e.g., child protection services, early intervention services, Women, Infants, and Children [WIC], educational services, and social services) • Provide information on community self-help groups, parent and sibling support groups, advocacy groups (e.g., Epilepsy Foundation of America, American Heart Association, Association of Retarded Citizens) • Referrals to community resources will be made as needed	• Maintenance of or increase in weight/length percentiles on growth chart

Analysis: Nursing Diagnostic Statement 4

Response and Related or Risk Factors: *High risk for ineffective child/family coping: compromised; risk factors:* family role strain associated with financial, emotional, and time demands of the child's heart condition

- Fear, anxiety
- Knowledge deficit, child/parent regarding condition and treatment

Projected Outcome: The child and family will show adaptive behavior and problem solving abilities in adequately meeting life's demands and roles

TABLE 33-3 *(continued)*

Defining Characteristics *(Actual Response)*	Nursing Interventions	Evaluation Criteria
Subjective: • Verbalization (child/parent) of inability to cope or ask for help • Inability to meet role expectation • Parents verbalize preoccupation with own reactions (e.g., fear, anticipatory grief, guilt, anxiety) • Parents describe or confirm an inadequate knowledge base that interferes with their ability to give the child effective assistance and/or support *Objective:* • Parents attempt assistive or supportive behaviors with less than satisfactory results • One or both parents withdrawn from communication with the child or decreases communication at times that are most stressful for the child • Parents display protective behavior disproportionate (too little or too much) to the child's abilities or need for autonomy	*Coping Enhancement* **Encourage child/family coping abilities through expression of feelings and emotions and identification of sources of anxiety** • Assist the child to cope with procedures associated with his/her condition (see ***Coping Enhancement, Child*** in Table 32–9) • Determine the family's past experience with heart defects and diseases and their related health beliefs • Convey that anxiety is normal and expected • Encourage the parents to air guilt feelings about hereditary and perinatal factors; clarify misconceptions; refer to genetic counseling when appropriate • Use leading statements, such as, "Many parents tell me they feel inadequate when their baby won't take enough milk." • Ask questions of the parent and the older child, such as, "What frightens you most about caring for your child (being cared for) at home?" and "How do you visualize your child's (your) future?" • Make the family aware of support groups available through the hospital or local heart association that can bring them together with others who have experienced heart disease in their child. **Supply information needed for problem solving** • Give clear, concrete answers to questions (anxiety decreases comprehension) • Explain every nursing care activity (this will help the child and family relate to the treatment of	**The parents/child will demonstrate ability to cope with situation as evidenced by:** • Expressing feelings • Following up with referral to community resources • Identifying resources • Seeking information to assist with problem solving

(continued)

TABLE 33-3 (continued)

Defining Characteristics *(Actual Response)*	Nursing Interventions	Evaluation Criteria
	CHF and will decrease their feelings of helplessness and hopelessness) • Discuss the relationship between the physical problems and the child's behavior (e.g., poor sucking response) to help diminish frustration with the behavior • Clarify misconceptions (effective problem solving is based on accurate information) • Decrease family role strain by assisting the child and the family to set realistic goals and possible methods of attaining them • Assist in identification of coping strategies that have been effective in the past • Refer to external sources of support and counseling as these needs are identified **Actively involve the child and family in the treatment plan** • Invite participation in the nursing plan of care and in its implementation (this will greatly dispel feelings of powerlessness and increase self-esteem) • Take every opportunity to reinforce with the family ways in which the child benefits by their participation ("doing for" a loved one can provide a healthy outlet for grief and frustration) **Assist the family in exploring ways to work together toward common goals**	

Analysis: Nursing Diagnostic Statement 5

Response and Related or Risk Factors: *High risk for altered health maintenance; risk factor:* parental knowledge deficit regarding follow-up care in home or clinic

Projected Outcome: Parents will be able to identify, manage, and/or seek out help through follow-up care to maintain their child's health

TABLE 33-3 (continued)

Defining Characteristics (Actual Response)	Nursing Interventions	Evaluation Criteria
Subjective: • Parents express anxiety about managing child's care at home *Objective*: • Repeated calls to hospital, visits to hospital, worsening of child's condition • Demonstrated lack of behaviors indicating ability to care for child at home	*Discharge Planning; Teaching: Prescribed Activity/Exercise* Inform the parents of the appropriate schedule for follow-up in the clinic or home and provide them with information regarding what activities will take place Review, with parents, activities their child will be able to carry out and any limitations on the child's actions Obtain feedback from parents to ascertain if what was reviewed was learned correctly Call parents 1 wk after discharge to determine how well they are doing	Parents express confidence in their ability to care for child at home. Parents are able to correctly state activities allowed and limitations on activity of their child

left ventricle does. The left ventricle pumps against the low resistance of the placenta (Moller & Neal, 1990). The pressures in the right side of the heart are greater than the pressures in the left side in utero.

The three shunts present in fetal circulation—the ductus venosus, the foramen ovale, and the ductus arteriosus—enable the fetus to receive highly oxygenated blood from the umbilical veins and deliver it to the tissues with the highest oxygen demand, the fetal myocardium and the brain.* The *ductus venosus* shunts highly oxygenated blood from the umbilical veins to the inferior vena cava. The blood then enters the right atrium and most of it is directed through the *foramen ovale* into the left atrium. Here, it mixes with blood returning from the lungs through the pulmonary veins to the left atrium and passes into the left ventricle. It then flows from the left ventricle into the aorta, perfusing the coronary, carotid, and subclavian arteries before entering the descending aorta and returning ultimately to the placenta. Blood returning from the head and upper limbs of the fetus enters the right atrium via the superior vena cava, passes into the right ventricle, and exits through the pulmonary artery. Eight to 10 per cent of the blood flows to the left and right lungs via the left and right pulmonary arteries. The greatest percentage of blood, however, flows through the *ductus arteriosus* and into the descending aorta to return to the placenta. Blood flow through the ductus arteriosus is from pulmonary artery to aorta (right to left) because of the high resistance to flow in the lungs and the low resistance to flow in the aorta.

For normal development of the cardiac structure, including chambers, valves, and vessels, it is essential that blood flows in appropriate quantities unobstructed throughout the developing heart and great vessels. Lack of blood flow through a chamber or vessel results in hypoplasia of that chamber or vessel. For example, in tricuspid atresia with intact ventricular septum there is no forward blood flow to the right ventricle, and the right ventricle is usually very hypoplastic.

Changes in Circulation after Birth

Profound hemodynamic changes occurring immediately after birth allow the neonate to adapt to the external environment. With the first breaths, the alveoli expand and the resistance to blood flow in the lungs (pulmonary vascular resistance) decreases, allowing more blood flow to the lungs. The resistance to blood flow in the systemic circulation (systemic vascular resistance) and left ventricular pressure are greatly increased owing to clamping of the umbilical cord and removal of the placenta, which offered low resistance to blood flow (Moller & Neal, 1990). Systemic vascular resistance is now higher than pulmonary vascular resistance, and blood flow through the ductus arteriosus is therefore from left to right (from aorta to pulmonary artery).

The volume of blood returning to the left atrium is greatly increased by two factors: (1) the decrease in pulmonary vascular resistance, allowing for more

* In utero, the umbilical artery carries the desaturated or unoxygenated blood from the fetus to the maternal circulation. The umbilical veins carry the highly oxygenated blood from the maternal circulation to the fetus.

TABLE 33-4

Nursing Process Plan: Care of the Child Having Cardiac Surgery

Analysis: Nursing Diagnostic Statement 1

Response and Related or Risk Factors: *Ineffective individual and family (child and parent) coping related to* knowledge deficit about hospitalization, operative procedures, and postoperative care

Projected Outcome: The family will provide sufficient, effective, uncompromised support, comfort, assistance, or encouragement as needed by the child to manage or master adaptive tasks related to his or her hospitalization and surgery

Defining Characteristics

Subjective:

- Parents admit to being preoccupied with their own fears and concerns (e.g., parents make statements such as: "I don't know what to expect." "I feel overwhelmed with my child's upcoming surgery." "I can't cope.")
- Child makes statements such as "What are you going to do?" "What is that?" "Are you going to hurt me?"
- Parent(s) show inability to meet parental role expectations (support, comfort, assistance)
- Parent(s) show change in communication patterns with each other and with child
- Child regresses

Objective:

- Child makes repeated requests for support, comfort, etc. from parent, which are not responded to
- Parents are obsessed in attempts to provide assistive or supportive behaviors to their child with less than satisfactory results
- Parents withdraw or enter into limited personal communication with the child
- Parents display overprotective behavior toward the child

Nursing Interventions

Teaching: Preoperative

Instruct parents to begin preparing child for surgery prior to coming to hospital

Arrange for parents to have *anticipatory guidance* regarding what preparation of their child will entail

Preoperative teaching should include information regarding the operative procedure and hospital course in the following areas:

Preparatory Sensory Information:

- Describe and allow, as much as possible, the child and parents to experience the physical sensations (sight, smell, taste, temperature, kinesthetic) they will experience before and after surgery. Use *medical play* (see Chapter 17) when appropriate to the child's age
- Description and visual representation of the experience in the operating room
- Rationale for and description and visual representation of ICU environment and experience
- Postoperative procedures done and equipment used
- Home care management
- Preoperative physical preparation, which includes: a complete history, thorough physical examination, laboratory studies (complete blood count, platelet count, hemoglobin, hematocrit, determi-

Evaluation Criteria

The child will be able to ask for help (if old enough) and will use age-appropriate defense mechanisms effectively

The parents will verbalize ability to cope or ability to ask for help; be able to meet role expectations and basic needs and to problem solve; use defense mechanisms appropriately

The parents will carry out assistive and supportive behaviors for their child with satisfactory results; will communicate appropriately with their child; and will display protective behavior that is proportionate to their child's abilities and need for autonomy

TABLE 33-4 *(continued)*

Defining Characteristics	Nursing Interventions	Evaluation Criteria
	nation of clotting time, electrolyte levels, blood urea nitrogen, creatinine, calcium, type and cross-match for 2–5 units of blood and urinalysis), chest radiograph, ECG, echocardiogram, and results of a recent cardiac catheterization • Description of preoperative procedure, which includes: an endotracheal tube is placed in the throat to help with breathing (an infant cannot cry, or an older child talk, while tube is in place) • The child will be allowed nothing by mouth, or NPO, after midnight the evening before surgery; the time for fasting will be determined by the age and scheduled time for surgery; it is important to post a sign on the door to the child's room and on the crib so that nothing is given by mouth before surgery. For infants and very small children, it is important to provide nourishment around 10:00 P.M. Preoperative medications vary considerably among institutions **Information regarding procedures and equipment to expect after surgery should be included** • A nasogastric tube is placed through the nose and into the stomach to keep the stomach empty until digestive function is restored • Three or four intravenous lines may be present to replace fluids and blood and to provide a means of checking pressures within the heart • There will be a large chest incision with a dressing or metal staples • Two or more chest tubes will be present to remove air and blood that enter the chest during surgery	

(continued)

TABLE 33-4 (continued)

Defining Characteristics	Nursing Interventions	Evaluation Criteria
	• Urine will be collected by either a catheter or a plastic bag placed on the perineum • Disks with wires (cardiac leads) on the child's chest are placed to monitor the heart rate and observe the heart pattern • The nurse will be monitoring the child at least every 15 mins until his or her condition stabilizes • Child and parents may visit the ICU and meet the members of the nursing staff **After age-appropriate teaching of the foregoing, the child between 2 and 8 yrs of age should be allowed the opportunity to "play out" all procedures** **Identify significant milestones of the cardiac experience:** • Admitted to hospital 1 day prior to surgery for preoperative work-up • Child is in ICU following surgery for 1 to 3 days • Child is transferred to ward for an additional 3 to 5 days, gradually resuming normal activities	

Analysis: Nursing Diagnostic Statement 2

Response and Related or Risk Factors: *High risk for aspiration; risk factor:* reduced level of consciousness while anesthetized

Projected Outcome: The child will not experience aspiration of gastric contents.

Defining Characteristics *(Actual Response)*	Nursing Interventions	Evaluation Criteria
Subjective: • Fear or anxiety *Objective*: • Severe respiratory distress • Mechanical obstruction of airway • Pneumonitis, which may progress to pneumonia	*Aspiration Precautions* Keep NPO after midnight the evening before surgery. Post sign on door to child's room or crib so nothing is provided by mouth before surgery (aspirated contents can cause mechanical blockage, aspiration pneumonia, or chemical pneumonitis)	Child does not aspirate as evidenced by: • Normal respiratory function • No mechanical blockage of airway • No aspiration pneumonia • No chemical pneumonitis

TABLE 33-4 (continued)

Analysis: Nursing Diagnostic Statement 3

Response and Related or Risk Factors: *High risk for injury: physiologic; risk factors:*

Preoperative

- Cardiac enlargement
- Conduction abnormalities, dysrhythmia
- Valve regurgitation or prolapse
- Complications of diagnostic procedures
- Obstruction or constriction
- Pulmonary vascular disease
- Persistent hypertension
- Bacterial endocarditis

Postoperative

- Complications of cardiac surgery, including dysrhythmias
- Residual septal defects
- Pulmonary venous obstruction
- Heart block
- Bacterial endocarditis
- Stenosis of one of the great vessels

Projected Outcome: The client will be free from adverse responses related to cardiac surgery

Defining Characteristics (Actual Response)	Nursing Interventions	Evaluation Criteria
Subjective: • Self-report from child of presence of fatigue, rapid heart beat, shortness of breath • Parental report for infant or young child: feeding and sleep patterns, sweating with feeding or while sleeping, respiration patterns, exercise not well tolerated (e.g., feeding, crying) **Objective:** • Altered heart rate and respiratory rate • Presence of adventitious heart sounds • Faintness or absence of peripheral pulses • Skin color pale or cyanotic (circumoral, hands and feet) and temperature cool at rest and with activity • Diaphoresis, presence of edema, neck vein distention • Abnormal CVP readings	*Cardiac Care* • Check vital signs and apical pulse every 15 mins to 1 hr depending on status • Auscultate the apical pulse for a full minute to assess for arrhythmias • Check level of consciousness with vital signs (child may be heavily sedated) • Assess for and report to physician any signs of tachycardia, stridor, tachypnea, retractions, nasal flaring, expiratory wheezing, or grunting • Assess for skin color and temperature, and check for diaphoresis and circumoral or circumorbital cyanosis; observe the tongue and mucous membrane for central cyanosis. Monitor and maintain temperature (hypothermia used during cardiac surgery to reduce oxygen needs). Infant will usually be without clothing for maximal observations and placed on	• Heart rate, blood pressure, and respiratory rate within normal range for age • Palpable peripheral pulses • Urine output ≥1 ml/kg/hr • Absence of cardiac arrhythmias • Adequate peripheral perfusion • Pale or pink mucous membranes and lips • Central venous pressure (CVP) readings within expected parameters • Gradual reduction in chest drainage and change in color from bloody, to serous-sanguineous, then to serous

(continued)

TABLE 33-4 *(continued)*

Defining Characteristics *(Actual Response)*	**Nursing Interventions**	**Evaluation Criteria**
• Decreased urine output • Failure to gain weight • Placement on growth chart indicating inadequate physical growth • Delay in expected developmental accomplishments • Cardiomegaly, hepatomegaly	radiant heated table or ak-pad to maintain temperature Palpate right and left peripheral pulses simultaneously and assess for rate, rhythm, and strength (weak thready pulses indicate decreased cardiac output) • Assess capillary refill on all four extremities (cool extremities indicate sluggish capillary refill) • Frequently check that monitor leads are in place and that monitor alarms are properly set • Monitor and record CVP (via a right atrial catheter to measure cardiac output) with vital signs (low readings may be indicative of hypovolemia; high readings of worsening cardiac status, bleeding into the pericardial sac, or fluid overload) • Observe and record, with vital signs, mean arterial pressure (assesses circulatory blood volume) • Keep all lines free of kinks; compare intra-arterial blood pressure with reading from manual cuff on extremity • Weigh daily or twice a day on the same scale, nude • Assess fontanel, lips, and mucous membranes for hydration status • Maintain strict intake and output; maintain fluid restriction as ordered (prevent overload of cardiovascular system) • Inspect incision each shift for presence of redness, swelling, or drainage; report any new occurrence • When moving child do not pick up under arms (puts stress on suture line and causes pain)	

TABLE 33-4 *(continued)*

Analysis: Nursing Diagnostic Statement 4

Response and Related or Risk Factors: *High risk for ineffective breathing patterns; risk factors:*

- Weakness
- Pain
- Pre-existing pulmonary hypertension

Projected Outcome: The child's inhalation and exhalation pattern will enable adequate pulmonary inflation or emptying.

Defining Characteristics *(Actual Response)*	Nursing Interventions	Evaluation Criteria
Subjective:	*Respiratory Monitoring*	
• Parental report of infant's inability to take an adequate amount per feeding, falling asleep at feedings and spending little time awake, seeming short of breath with feeding and at rest, sweating with feedings and at rest, becoming pale, having a weak cry, not yet accomplishing developmental tasks expected for age, poor weight gain	• Assess for absence or presence of decreased breath sounds bilaterally, all lobes • Maintain chest drainage system below level of chest • Check that chest tubes are patent and free of kinks, and that all connections are taped and secured • Stabilize tubes so as to prevent any tension and to allow for movement	• Normal rate and depth of respiration for age • Absence of nasal flaring or retractions • Arterial blood gases within normal limits • Breath sounds present and clear all lobes • Chest radiographs show improvement; no atelectasis and no effusions
Objective: • Blood pressure changes in extremities • Skin color pale and cool to touch, becoming mottled or cyanotic with increased oxygen demands (e.g., crying, feeding, playing). Skin quality: shining lack of lanugo; slow healing of lesions • Arterial blood gases show inadequate oxygenation • Nasal flaring • Retractions • Periorbital edema and edema of face, hands, feet, and neck; vein distention (in older child) • Urine output <1 ml/kg/hr • Failure to thrive: <3rd percentile for height and weight on growth chart • Cardiomegaly, hepatomegaly	• Record character and amount of drainage hourly; significant increases in drainage should be reported to physician • When indicated, vibration of chest and suction via endotracheal tube is done. Increased peak inspiratory pressures, visible secretions, rising CO_2, and decreased PO_2 are all indications for suctioning • Nasotracheal suction, performed cautiously (when not intubated), stimulates coughing and removes secretions • Provide 100% O_2 before, during, and after suctioning by bagging or mask • Turn from side to side every 1–2 hrs (prevent pooling of secretions and promote increased depth of respirations), unless otherwise ordered	

(continued)

TABLE 33-4 (continued)

Defining Characteristics *(Actual Response)*	Nursing Interventions	Evaluation Criteria
	• Monitor arterial blood gases or pulse oximetry and report deviation from preoperative levels and expected postoperative levels • Institute as needed ***chest physiotherapy*** as ordered, 2–3 days postoperatively. Administer pain medication ½ hr prior to chest percussion (decreases incisional pain and promotes more effective healing)	

Analysis: Collaborative Problem 1

Response and Related or Risk Factors: *Impaired physical mobility and fatigue related to activity intolerance, secondary to:*

- Increased cardiac workload and excessive pulmonary blood flow
- Heart's inability to pump an adequate supply of blood to meet the body's metabolic demands
- Insufficient oxygenation resulting from obstruction of blood flow from right ventricle

Projected Outcome:

- The child will be able to have some independent physical movement
- The child will be rested enough to have capacity for age-appropriate physical and mental activity

Analysis: Collaborative Problem 2

Response and Related or Risk Factors: *High risk for altered tissue perfusion: lower extremity hypertension; risk factor:* decreased blood flow to the lower part of the body

Projected Outcome:

- The child will experience adequate nutrition and oxygenation at the cellular level
- The child's skin temperature and color will not worsen

Defining Characteristics *(Actual Response)*	Nursing Interventions	Evaluation Criteria
Subjective: • Verbalization by child and/or parents of lack of energy and inability to maintain usual routines and perceived need for additional energy to accomplish routine tasks • Parental reports of infant's inability to take adequate amount per feeding, falling asleep with feeding and spending little time awake, shortness of breath at	Cardiac Care *Independent Interventions:* **Increased activity tolerance:** • Provide feeding, dry diapers, and tactile stimulation before infant cries • Use a pacifier while preparing feedings and during fussy times (crying increases energy expenditure) • Feed the infant frequently and in	• Developmentally appropriate ability and willingness to move within the physical environment. Muscle strength remains at previous level or increases • Child and/or parents verbalize adequate energy and ability to maintain usual routines **The child's physical status will improve:** • Peripheral pulses palpable

TABLE 33-4 *(continued)*

Defining Characteristics *(Actual Response)*	Nursing Interventions	Evaluation Criteria
rest, sweating with feeding and at rest, becoming pale, having a weak cry, delay in accomplishing developmental tasks expected for age, poor weight gain *Objective*: • Inability to purposefully move within the physical environment, including bed mobility, transfer, and ambulation, reluctance to attempt movement • Decreased muscle strength (hypertonicity and unusual posturing in newborns), control, and/or mass **Increase in physical complaints** • Emotionally labile or irritable • Impaired ability to concentrate • Decreased performance • Lethargic or listless • Disinterest in surroundings (lack of cry when disturbed in infants; blood pressure changes in extremities • Skin color pale and cool to touch, becoming mottled or cyanotic with increased oxygen demands (e.g., crying, feeding, playing) • Periorbital edema and edema of face, hands, and feet • Neck vein distention (in older child) • Blood pressure changes in extremities • Skin quality: shining, lack of lanugo, slow healing of lesions • Urine output <1 ml/kg/hr • Failure to thrive: <3rd percentile for height and weight on growth chart • Cardiomegaly • Hepatomegaly	small amounts (large feedings tire the infant) • Allow frequent rest periods during feeding • Use a soft nipple (to reduce the work of sucking) • Breastfed babies may need additional rest periods (breastfeeding requires slightly more energy expenditure than bottle feeding). Breast milk can be fed via bottles or via nasogastic tubes • Prevent respiratory infections by teaching the family good handwashing techniques and alerting them to the most common sources of pathogens (infection increases O_2 demands) • Limit feeding at breast to 8–10 mins on the first side and 10–15 mins on the second side (this will usually meet caloric needs; further sucking may burn more calories than it adds) • Some infants may require high-caloric formulas to increase the caloric intake per energy expenditure • Continuous nasogastric drip formula feedings may be required to further decrease the work of feeding for the infant while providing optimal calories (dependent intervention) • Ensure uninterrupted sleep/rest periods • Schedule activities such as bathing after rest and at other than feeding times • Maintain normal body temperature (to decrease energy demands of hyperthermia or hypothermia) by keeping the environment at a moderate temperature. Prevent chilling during bathing, adjusting clothing and blanket coverings to the environmental temperature	• Skin color normal, mucous membrane pink, skin warm to touch • Urine output ≥1 ml/kg/hr • Able to maintain physical exercise (crying, feeding) for longer period without fatigue • Edema and neck vein distention decreases

(continued)

TABLE 33-4 *(continued)*

Defining Characteristics *(Actual Response)*	**Nursing Interventions**	**Evaluation Criteria**
	Collaborative interventions with associated independent interventions/responsibilities: **Decrease the cardiac load** • Administer O_2 if ordered • Monitor O_2 saturation (per pulse oximetry or ABGs) • Administer digoxin as ordered (to increase ventricular contractility and decrease heart rate) (see Table 33–10). Ensure safe administration by checking the dosage with another registered nurse and by taking the apical pulse for 1 min. Withhold the digoxin if the pulse is <100 for a neonate, <90 for a 1-year-old, <85 for a 2-year old, <80 for a 4-year-old, <75 for a 6-year old, <70 for an 8-year-old, <60 for a 14-year-old • Measure P-R interval prior to digoxin administration. If P-R interval prolonged, notify physician before administering digoxin. When digoxin is given, monitor for the therapeutic effects: decrease in pulse and respirations, increase in urine output (signaling better kidney perfusion), improvement in skin color and temperature (with better perfusion to the peripheral tissues) • Monitor for the classic signs of digoxin toxicity; nausea (manifested as anorexia in the infant), vomiting, lethargy, bradycardia, and dysrhythmia (noted on ECG or cardiac monitor, and in irregular apical pulse) • Monitor serum digoxin levels; levels 2.1 ng/ml may indicate toxicity • Blood for digoxin levels should be drawn at least 6–8 hrs after the last dose (to ensure equilibrium between serum and tissue levels) • Administer diuretics as ordered	

TABLE 33-4 *(continued)*

Defining Characteristics *(Actual Response)*	**Nursing Interventions**	**Evaluation Criteria**
	(to decrease salt and water retention related to decreased renal perfusion and the resulting rise in ADH and aldosterone levels) • Monitor for therapeutic effects of diuretics: increased urine output, decreased peripheral edema, decreased neck vein distention, clearing of lung sounds, and increased O_2/CO_2 exchange • Monitor diuresis by recording input/output and daily weights. (Weight is a sensitive indicator of fluid balance.) Weigh before breakfast or the first A.M. feeding. Weigh the infant and toddler nude; weigh the preschooler or older child with only a hospital gown • Counsel the parents that the infant should wet at least 6–8 diapers per day to ensure adequate output • Monitor for side effects: dehydration and electrolyte imbalance, especially hypokalemia (which potentiates digoxin and may lead to toxicity) and hyponatremia (common symptoms: muscle weakness, leg cramps, dry mouth, dizziness, and gastrointestinal disturbances)	

***Analysis*:** Nursing Diagnostic Statement 5

***Response and Related or Risk Factors*:** *High risk for infection; risk factors:*

- Surgical procedures
- Invasive monitoring
- Insertion of prosthetic material
- Altered nutrition
- Postcardiotomy syndrome

***Projected Outcome*:** The child will demonstrate no evidence of infection

- Postcardiotomy syndrome
- Pericarditis
- Upper respiratory infection (URI)
- Urinary tract infection (UTI)
- Endocarditis
- Wound

(continued)

TABLE 33-4 *(continued)*

Defining Characteristics *(Actual Response)*	**Nursing Interventions**	**Evaluation Criteria**
Subjective: • Child reports being fatigued or "sleepy" • Child cries, is irritable • Parent reports child "feels hot," acting "out of sorts," sleepy Objective: • Redness, inflammation of incisional site • Exudate from incision • Dyspnea • Tachypnea • Low-grade fever • Substernal pain • Friction rub • Pleural effusion • Increased WBCs • Elevated viral titers • Malaise • Lethargy • Pericardial effusion	Infection Control • Monitor vital signs, including temperatures • Assess for signs and symptoms of postcardiotomy syndrome. (This is seen 7–14 days after the operation: low-grade fever, malaise, lethargy, friction rub, pleural effusions, pericardial effusion, ↑ ESR, ↑ WBC, ↑ viral titers, substernal pain) • Maintain strict aseptic techniques • Obtain cultures as ordered • Clean catheter entrance sites and incisional sites (refer to institutional manual for procedure; nature of procedure will vary according to institutional policy) • Administer antipyretics and antibiotics as ordered; monitor child's response to medications • Observe for signs of URI and UTI • Promote nutritional intake (TPN, PO, NG)	The child will not manifest signs of infection

Analysis: Nursing Diagnostic Statement 6

Response and Related or Risk Factors: *Altered nutrition: less than body requirements, related to:*

- Anorexia associated with decreased perfusion of the GI tract and/or the side effects of medications
- Decreased energy available for sucking/chewing
- Increased metabolic demands associated with the increased workload of the overloaded heart

Projected Outcome: The child will receive caloric intake to meet metabolic demands for growth and development. (Refer to Table 33–3, Diagnostic Statement 2)

Analysis: Nursing Diagnostic Statement 7

Response and Related or Risk Factors: *Parental anticipatory grieving, related to* perception of the loss of their fantasized normal child and, after child's cardiac defect has been repaired, loss of ill child

Projected Outcome: Parents will express feelings of grief about fantasized child; and later after repair of cardiac defect loss of ill child

TABLE 33-4 *(continued)*

Defining Characteristics	Nursing Interventions	Evaluation Criteria
Subjective: • Expression of feelings of grief, "I never expected this"—denial of feelings of grief such as: refusal to listen to diagnoses, or learn about child's condition, pay little attention to medical/surgical plans of management, lack of compliance with treatment plan • Displaced anger at other parent, physician, nurse *Objective*: • Altered patterns of sleeping • Increased nervousness • Acting out behavior • Altered pattern of eating (overeating, anorexia) • Aggressive behavior • Depression	*Griefwork Facilitation* • Conduct a complete assessment for anticipatory grieving and dysfunctional grieving (many parents block feelings of loss and deny the problem. Denial is especially prevalent in parents of asymptomatic children. Refer to behavior demonstrated under subjective assessment • Refer parents to community/school nurse for continued follow-up and support • Refer to community-based support groups. Talking with parents who have been through same experiences helps • Encourage parental expression of feelings • Assist expression of feelings with calm acceptance of their anger followed by reassurance (parental anger and resentment may be expressed toward ill children by overprotective behavior leading to infantilization or by detachment from and decreased contact with the child) *Presence* • Encourage questions • Provide concrete and factual answers to parents' questions (often parents are uncomfortable asking questions of health professionals and do not want to take up their time; unanswered questions can add to parental stress)	**The parent/child will demonstrate ability to express grief feelings as evidenced by:** • Following-up with referral to community resources • Identifying resources • Seeking information to assist with problem solving

Analysis: Nursing Diagnostic Statement 8

Response and Related or Risk Factors: *High risk for altered growth and development; risk factors:*

- Inadequate tissue perfusion to promote healthy tissue growth
- Lack of energy to accomplish developmental tasks (partially secondary to nutritional deficit)

Projected Outcome: The child will demonstrate no deviations in norms from his or her age group

(continued)

TABLE 33-4 *(continued)*

Defining Characteristics *(Actual Response)*	Nursing Interventions	Evaluation Criteria
Subjective: Parental report of delay or difficulty in performing skills typical of age group *Objective:* • Observed delay in performing skills (motor, social, or expressive) typical of age group: • Altered physical growth • Inability to perform self-control activities appropriate for age (these delays can be measured using a valid developmental assessment inventory) • Flat affect • Listlessness, decreased response	*Parent Education: Childrearing Family* **Encourage parents to assist child in attainment of physical, emotional, social, and cognitive developmental tasks** • Provide visual, auditory, and tactile stimulation appropriate to the child's age and energy level (see Chapter 17 for ways to do this through play) • Encourage loving and playful interactions with family members • Assure parent that most of the child's emotional, social, and cognitive tasks can be met despite the CHF, and that motor tasks will develop quickly once physical health improves	• Gradual increase in ability to perform developmental skills • Gradual increase in physical growth

Analysis: Nursing Diagnostic Statement 9

Response and Related or Risk Factors: *High risk for altered health maintenance; risk factor:* parental knowledge deficit regarding importance of follow-up care in home or clinic

Projected Outcome: Parents will be able to identify, manage, and/or seek out help through follow-up care to maintain their child's health

Defining Characteristics *(Actual Response)*	Nursing Interventions	Evaluation Criteria
Subjective: Parents make statements such as: "I don't know how to do this procedure." "Who do I call with a problem?" "What do I do in an emergency?" *Objective:* • Repeated calls to hospitals, visits to the emergency room, postoperative complications, child's resumption of activities is delayed • Child remains isolated from friends, social activities	*Teaching: Disease Process* • Instruct parents on signs of problems specifically related to their child's cardiac defect and repair (e.g., CHF following repair of AV canal: labored or rapid breathing, feeding difficulties, perspiration, swelling around eyes, irritability) *Teaching: Procedure/Treatment* Instruct parents on wound care: • Soap and H_2O best • Avoid baths and showers until wound healed • Notify physician if any of the following develops: fever, redness or swelling around incision, separation of incision, drainage from incision	**The child remains healthy and develops at an appropriate rate**

TABLE 33-4 *(continued)*

Defining Characteristics *(Actual Response)*	**Nursing Interventions**	**Evaluation Criteria**
	• Instruct child not to scratch incision; keep fingernails short and clean *Teaching: Prescribed Medications* Instruct parents on administration of medications: • Drug actions and doses • Time schedule • Medication side effects (see Table 39–13C for digoxin administration) Instruct parents on activity restrictions Provide parents with phone number to call for assistance should problems arise Refer for community nursing services if indicated Reinforce need for return visit at cardiology clinic or private physician's office 2 wks following discharge (based on institutional policy)	

Analysis: Nursing Diagnostic Statement 10

Response and Related or Risk Factors: *High risk for spiritual distress (child and family): risk factors:*

- Worry associated with the prognosis and potential reactions to therapy
- A search for the meaning of the illness
- Feelings of guilt associated with the diagnosis
- Feelings of powerlessness associated with the child's condition

Projected Outcome: Child and family will find meaning in their situation and demonstrate a renewed reliance on the life principle by which they live

Defining Characteristics *(Actual Response)*	**Nursing Interventions**	**Evaluation Criteria**
Subjective: • Expresses concern with the meaning of life and death and/or belief systems • Questions such as, "Why did this happen to me?" • Verbalizes anger at God • Questions meaning of suffering • Verbalizes inner conflict about beliefs	*Spiritual Support* Encourage verbalization and listen with empathy and a nonjudgmental attitude • Encourage family to seek out person (e.g., clergy) who has helped them find meaning in other situations. Refer to parents who have coped effectively with situation and who have relied on faith beliefs for assistance	**The parents/affected child will experience a renewed sense of inner peace as evidenced by:** • Verbalizing feeling less anxious and more at peace • Finding strength in former religious faith • Verbalizing a rationale for decision-making

(continued)

TABLE 33-4 *(continued)*

Defining Characteristics *(Actual Response)*	Nursing Interventions	Evaluation Criteria
• Questions meaning of own existence • Questions moral/ethical implications of therapeutic regimen • Uses gallows humor • Displaces anger toward religious representatives • Describes nightmares/sleep disturbances *Objective*: • Alteration in behavior/mood evidenced by anger • Crying • Withdrawal • Preoccupation, anxiety, hostility, apathy, etc • Significant changes in usual religious practices • Somatic signs of distress	• Assist the client in correcting misconceptions (expression of feelings with an empathetic listener will help the client gain perspective needed for problem solving) • Explore with the client the activities that are usually the most enjoyable and produce a feeling of happiness and lightheartedness. Facilitate and encourage these activities, as permitted (activities that have produced this effect in the past carry a great potential for facilitating emotional self-healing) • Refer to community-based support groups (families with similar circumstances are credible sources of support for other families. Validation or suggestions for coping can facilitate resumption of normal affect and activities) • Encourage participation in sectarian activities that provide comfort (e.g., praying)	• Appearing less anxious and stressful

Analysis: Nursing Diagnostic Statement 11

Response and Related or Risk Factors: *Altered parenting: (overprotection) related to fear of real or perceived risks:*

- Vulnerability of the child
- Environmental risks

Projected Outcome: Parents will interact with child in an age-appropriate manner and create an environment that promotes optimum growth and development of their child

Defining Characteristics	Nursing Interventions	Evaluation Criteria
Subjective: Parents express concern that "My baby cannot keep up with other children of the same age"; "My baby is blue." *Objective*: Parent repeatedly does things for the infant that infant could be doing for self	*Parent Education: Childrearing Family* Help the parents identify major fears pertaining to the infant's condition (see nursing diagnostic statement) and explore any feelings of guilt they may have. (Anxiety and guilt often lead to overprotection.) Use an appropriate opportunity to discuss the crucial parenting roles at each stage of childhood (see Chapter 12)	**Parents will demonstrate fewer overprotective behaviors as evidenced by:** • Expression of feelings of guilt associated with child's diagnosis • Demonstration of developmentally appropriate parenting behaviors • Questions regarding parenting practices

TABLE 33-5
Developmental Differences in Structure and Function of the Cardiovascular System

Anatomy and Physiology	Significance
Preterm	
Prostaglandin E_1: Preterm infants may have increased prostaglandin E_1 levels (in fetal life prostaglandin E_1 and decreased PO_2 maintain patency of the ductus arteriosus)	In the presence of lung disease (e.g., respiratory distress syndrome), which causes hypoxia, increased prostaglandin E_1 results in ductus arteriosus remaining patent
Pulmonary vascular resistance and myocardial capacity: Preterm infants have a proportionately faster decline in pulmonary vascular resistance, leading to increased left-to-right shunting through anomalous connections in the heart. In addition, their heart muscles are immature and poorly equipped to handle the increased volume that results with shunting	Preterm infants with congenital heart defects are more prone to congestive heart failure than are full-term infants
Full-Term Infant	
Pulmonary and cardiac pressures: Neonate retains increased pulmonary vascular resistance due to pulmonary vessel hypertrophy; this increases pressures on the right side of the heart	Detection of L → R shunts may be delayed because increased right atrial and ventricular pressures decrease the left-to-right shunting
Stroke volume: Infants have limited ability to increase stroke volume in response to decreased cardiac output	When cardiac output decreases the child will respond with tachycardia
Infants and Young Children	
Chest wall: Chest walls are thin in infants and young children because of the relative lack of subcutaneous and muscle tissue compared with older children	"Innocent" murmurs can be auscultated in structurally normal hearts because the normal turbulence is audible through the thin chest wall

blood flow to the lungs from the right side of the heart, and (2) the shunting of blood from left to right through the ductus arteriosus to the lungs. The increased volume of blood returning to the left atrium distends the left atrium and increases left atrial pressure, which assists in closure of the foramen ovale. This takes place usually within the first few hours to days of life.

The ductus arteriosus closes functionally within the first several days after birth; however, it does not become obliterated until several months to a year later (Moller & Neal, 1990). The left-to-right shunt through the ductus arteriosus usually persists for 15 to 20 hours after birth, or it may last for several days. The increased oxygen tension (PaO_2) in the neonate's arterial blood from increased pulmonary blood flow and oxygenation in the lungs initiates constriction of the ductus arteriosus. The umbilical veins, umbilical arteries, and ductus venosus no longer carry blood so the blood in these structures clots and they atrophy (Merenstein et al, 1985).

The neonate's circulation (Fig. 33-2) now resembles that of the adult in that desaturated blood returns from the body via the superior and inferior vena cavae to the right atrium and passes through the tricuspid valve to the right ventricle. From the right ventricle, blood passes through the pulmonary valve into the main pulmonary artery, then into the left and right pulmonary arteries, and finally into the lungs, where oxygenation occurs. Oxygen-saturated blood returns via the pulmonary veins to the left atrium and passes through the mitral valve into the left ventricle. From the left ventricle, blood flows through the aortic valve into the aorta and the systemic arterial system. Neonatal circulation is unique, however, in that the newborn infant retains elevated pulmonary vascular resistance and elevated pressures in the right ventricle and pulmonary system owing to the hypertrophy of the pulmonary vessels. This hypertrophy slowly resolves, and the pulmonary vascular resistance and right heart pressures decrease to normal by 1 to 2 months of age (Adams et al, 1989). Adjustments in cardiopulmonary physiology at birth are summarized in Table 33-6.

Cardiac Function (Physiology)

The primary function of the heart is as a circulatory pump, which, in conjunction with the pulmonary system, delivers oxygen to the tissues of the body to meet its metabolic demands. "Cardiac output," the amount of blood ejected in 1 minute, is vital to accomplishing this goal. Cardiac output is a function of heart rate times the stroke volume ($HR \times SV = CO$).

The "heart rate," the number of beats per minute, is regulated by the autonomic nervous system. An increase in heart rate results in an increase in cardiac output. A decrease in heart rate results in a decrease in cardiac output, unless there is a concurrent increase in stroke volume. An increase in heart rate is the most common initial response to a decrease in cardiac output or an increase in oxygen demand, such as occurs during exercise.

"Stroke volume" is the amount of blood ejected during one contraction. Stroke volume is influenced by three factors: (1) preload, (2) afterload, and (3) contractility. These factors do not function as single, isolated variables, but as interacting components that adjust to maintain a steady state.

"Preload" is the amount of myocardial fiber stretch present before contraction. The fiber length stretch is a combination of the circulating blood volume and the compliance (distensibility) of the ven-

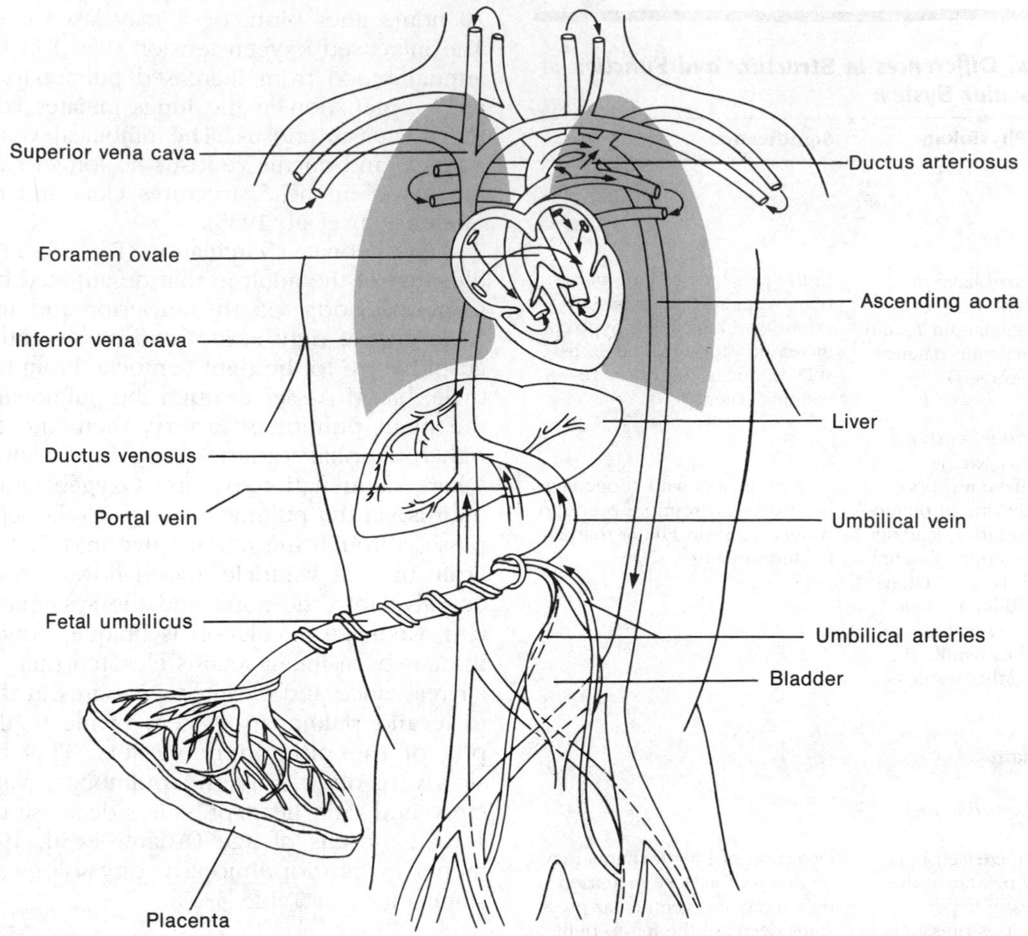

FIGURE 33-1. Fetal circulation.

tricular wall. The Frank-Starling law demonstrates that normal myocardium generates greater tension during contraction if it is stretched. This will produce an increase in ventricular work and, therefore, an increased stroke volume. Preload is most easily assessed by measuring central venous pressure (CVP).

"Afterload" is the impedance to ventricular ejection of blood. "Pulmonary vascular resistance" (PVR) and "systemic vascular resistance" (SVR) are both measures of afterload. If the afterload is increased because of an anatomic abnormality, or resistances increase as a physiologic response to cold or a low output state, this increases cardiac work. Blood pressure measurement can give a basic idea of changes in afterload.

"Contractility" is the efficiency and velocity of myocardial fiber shortening. It is the force generated by the myocardium. Contractility is usually assessed by echocardiogram. It is affected by electrolyte imbalance, hypoxia, acidosis, and anemia.

History and Physical Examination

An infant who has symptoms of cardiac disease in the first few hours to days or weeks of life most likely has a significant defect. Complex lesions such as transposition of the great arteries, tetralogy of Fallot, pulmonary atresia, hypoplastic left heart, coarctation of the aorta, and truncus arteriosus are likely to be diagnosed within the first 2 weeks of life. Clinical manifestations of alterations in cardiovascular function that the nurse may observe are summarized in Table 33–7.

CHD may not be discovered while the infant is in the hospital. Parents may bring the infant to the physician's office with a number of concerns. During the history the parents may mention that the infant is having feeding problems. These problems may be characterized by profuse sweating or fatigue during feeding, tachypnea, irritability, reflux, and the desire to feed coupled with the inability to do so. Concern may be expressed that the infant has failed to gain weight appropriately. Parents should be asked to detail the infant's feeding behavior. How often does the infant eat? How long do feedings take? How does the infant act during the feedings? How much formula is taken during one feeding? How much formula is taken during 24 hours? How does the infant respond after a feeding? Is there any vomiting?

The toddler and the older child may be described as a "picky" or "slow" eater. The parents' main concern may be that the child has had poor weight gain.

Respiratory difficulties such as rapid respirations,

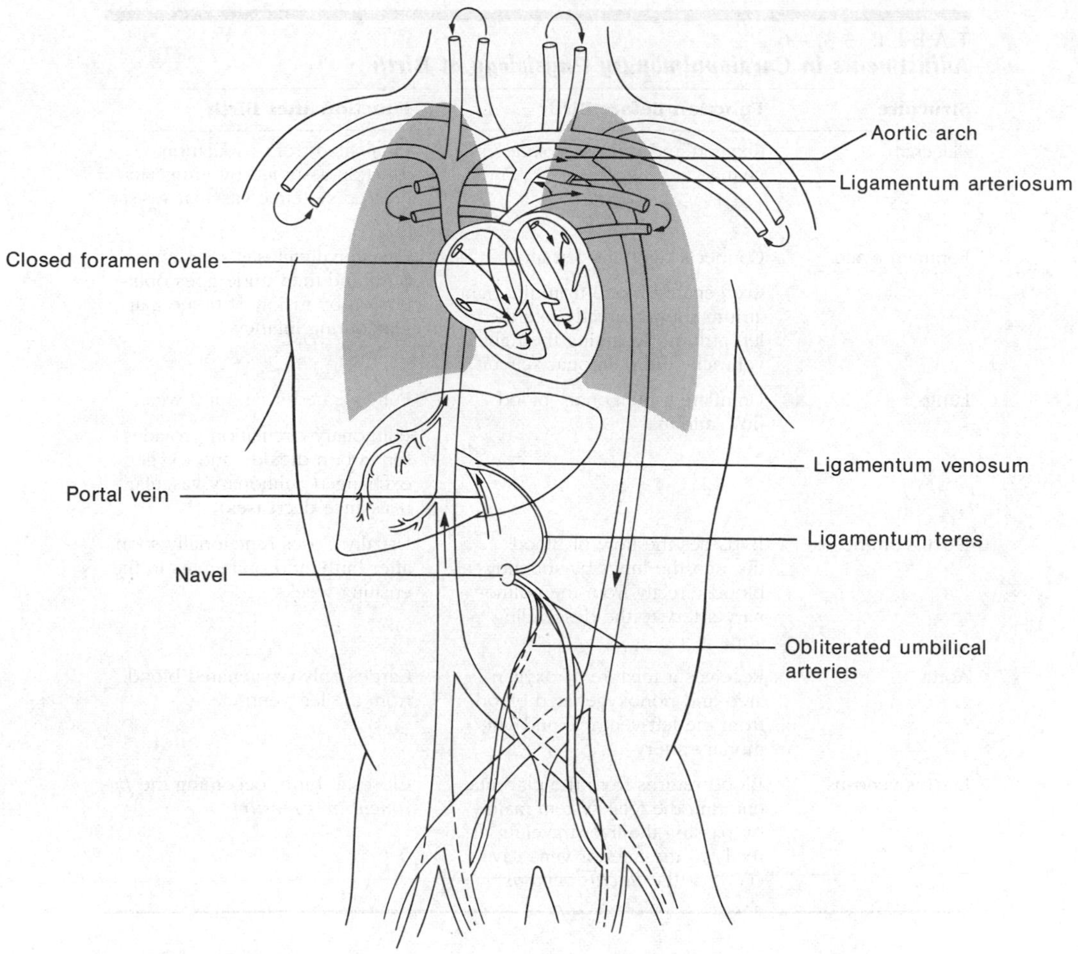

FIGURE 33-2. Neonatal circulation.

difficulty breathing (retractions, nasal flaring, grunting, stridor, deep "sighing" respirations), anoxic spells, or respiratory infections may be reported by the parents. Parents should be asked to elaborate on any respiratory problems. Does the infant or child have a chronic cough or frequent choking episodes? If respiratory infections have been reported, how frequent have they been and of what severity? If the parents have been concerned about their infant having rapid breathing, it is important to discern how rapid the respirations have been and of what duration.

Parents may report pallor and a bluish cast (termed "cyanosis") to the skin, mucous membranes, lips, nailbeds, and conjunctivae, either persistent or intermittent. Questions to ask include: Does the infant's color change when crying? when feeding? when defecating? when position is changed suddenly? Has the infant ever turned blue, and, if so, under what circumstances and room temperature? For the toddler and older child, parents should be asked if the child's color changes during exercise, crying, respiratory infections, or rest.

Activity level or activity intolerance must be investigated. Parents may complain that their infant is continuously restless, becomes tired easily during feedings, or is lethargic and sleeps all the time. Parents should be asked to describe the position the infant usually assumes when asleep or resting. Often, infants with cardiac problems sleep with the upper extremities flaccidly extended above the head or favor the knee-chest position. The parents may say that the infant is persistently "sweaty," especially during feedings, but even while at complete rest. When asked to describe their toddler or older child's activity level, many parents may feel their child has normal exercise tolerance. Further questions can help clarify what "normal" means to them: What activities does the child perform? Are there siblings or other children the child plays with, so parents can compare his or her activity level with that of other children? Does the child keep up with other children at play or require frequent rest periods? Is there a tendency toward performing sedentary tasks? Does the child ever complain of headaches, dizziness, leg cramps, chest pain, or shortness of breath with exercise? Has he or she ever "passed out" or fainted? Does the child frequently squat during play or activities? Does the child feel palpitations (possibly described as a "funny" feeling in the chest or as chest pain) or a fast heart rate?

It is important to explore any other parental concerns. In addition, the school-age and adolescent child should be included in the interview and asked

TABLE 33-6
Adjustments in Cardiopulmonary Physiology at Birth

Structure	Function Before Birth	Function after Birth
Placenta	Oxygen and carbon dioxide exchange	Eliminated from circulation: function assumed by lungs (increased systemic vascular resistance)
Foramen ovale	Connects right and left atria Oxygenated blood from the right atrium shunts directly into the left atrium, bypassing the right ventricle and pulmonary circuit	Functionally closes soon after birth and then undergoes obliteration by fusion of tissue margins during infancy
Lungs	Uninflated, pulmonary blood flow minimal	Fully aerated in about 2 wks Pulmonary circulation provides for carbon dioxide and oxygen exchange (pulmonary vascular resistance decreases)
Ductus arteriosus	Bypasses the flow of blood through the lungs by shunting blood directly from the pulmonary artery to the descending aorta	Usually closes functionally soon after birth, and obliterates in the ensuing weeks
Aorta	Receives a mixture of oxygenated and nonoxygenated blood from the left ventricle and pulmonary artery	Carries only oxygenated blood from the left ventricle
Ductus venosus	Blood returns from the placenta, entering the fetal system mainly by passing the liver traveling directly to the inferior vena cava (IVC) or the *ductus venosus*	Closes at birth, becoming the *ligamentum venosum*

about her or his symptoms and concerns. It is important for the child to feel included and an integral part of the discussions. This will enhance the child's understanding, help to allay fears, and increase the child's sense of control.

The mother's history regarding the pregnancy, birth, and neonatal period should be elicited. Special inquiry should be made as to the maternal health history during the first trimester of pregnancy, including rubella, viral infections, medications, and radiographs. Family history is obtained related to congenital heart disease as well as connective tissue disorders, diabetes, hypercalcemia, and glycogen storage disease.

In addition to the concerns expressed by parents, the nurse may recognize signs indicative of CHD as evidenced by alterations in general appearance, skin, vital signs, chest, and abdomen. The nurse who performs a physical assessment of cardiac function will want to keep in mind those differences in cardiovascular structure and function that are related to development.

General Appearance

General body position and level of activity should be noted. Is the infant or child resting comfortably or is he or she fretful or agitated? Does the child respond to stimuli appropriately or appear flaccid and lethargic? What is the nutritional status? Is the child small for his or her age? Does there seem to be inadequate subcutaneous tissue or malnourishment? Are there any obvious features or syndromes that may be associated with congenital heart defects, such as Down syndrome?

Skin

Assess the infant's color for cyanosis or pallor, or both. Central cyanosis may be the only evidence of a cardiac lesion during the first weeks of life. Mild cyanosis may appear as "high" or "ruddy" color, with unusually red cheeks, lips, and fingertips, all unrelated to the temperature of the environment.

Also, the infant or child should be kept warm and assessed both while at rest and during activity. Because activity increases the body's requirement for oxygen, cyanosis will be more pronounced during activity. In dark-skinned children, cyanosis is more difficult to assess; thus, these children should be assessed primarily by checking mucous membranes. Moistness of the skin should be observed. Diaphoresis may occur in children with left-to-right shunts. The presence of mottling on examination of the skin may be observed as well.

TABLE 33-7
Clinical Manifestations of Alterations in Cardiovascular Function

Clinical Manifestation	Possible Cause	Physical Finding	Clinical Significance
Murmur	Sound created by turbulent blood flow	"Swish" sound with the presence or absence of a thrill, graded according to loudness and presence of thrill; can increase with fever and activity; "innocent" murmur disappears with age	• Monitor vital signs • Auscultate heart sounds and note character, position • Presence/absence of thrill
Delayed/decreased/absent pulses in lower extremities	May be a sign of coarctation of the aorta	Grading system to assess peripheral pulses from absent (0) to full and bounding (+4)	• Palpate all pulses, brachial/femoral timing • Monitor warmth, color of extremities
BP difference upper/lower extremities	May be due to coarctation of aorta	A difference of 20 mmHg or greater between upper extremities and lower extremities	• Monitor vital signs, especially BP • Notify physician of difference in pressure greater than 20 mmHg
Cyanosis	Bluish discoloration; R/T reduced hemoglobin in arterial/peripheral capillary blood and in lesion causing right-to-left cardiac shunts and conditions causing vasoconstriction and decreased cardiac output	(a) Mild cyanosis: "high" or "ruddy" color, unusually red cheeks, lips, fingertips; (b) Moderate cyanosis: varying shades of bluish tint in mucous membranes, lips, tongue, and gums	• Monitor vital signs • Hgb/Hct indices • Assess activity tolerance • Oximetry
Wide pulse pressure	May be indication of aortic insufficiency or patent ductus arteriosus	Pulse pressure greater than 40–50 mmHg should be reported; may also have bounding peripheral pulses	• Monitor blood pressure
Clubbing	Capillary proliferation in fingertips and toes due to decreased peripheral tissue perfusion	Broadening of fingertips	
Diaphoresis	Caused by stimulation of sympathetic cholinergic fibers	May first be seen on forehead across nose and upper lip	• Monitor precipitating events • Allow rest periods
Edema	Excessive amount of extracellular fluid in body caused by increased capillary pressure due to causes such as heart failure, venous obstruction, fluid and electrolyte imbalances	*Infants:* Weight gain, facial (especially periorbital) edema; *toddlers and older children:* generalized edema, seen in face, hands, and feet	• Monitor I & O • Monitor administration of diuretics • Comfort measures • Protect edematous tissues from injury

Presence or absence of edema should be noted. Infants usually manifest fluid retention as weight gain; however, they may have facial, especially periorbital, edema. The toddler and older child may have generalized edema, noticeable in the face, hands, and feet.

Vital Signs

Respiratory status must be assessed. Respirations are counted for 1 full minute with the infant or child undressed and at rest. Observe for "tachypnea" (a resting respiratory rate greater than 60 respirations per minute in an infant up to 1 year of age, greater than 50 per minute in a 2-year-old, and greater than 35 per minute in a 3-year-old), expiratory grunting, stridor, nasal flaring, retractions (between and below the ribs), and dyspnea (Adams et al, 1989).

An apical pulse must be carefully assessed. A resting heart rate over 160 beats per minute in an infant, over 120 beats per minute in a 1-year-old, and over 100 beats per minute in a 3-year-old is considered "tachycardia" (Adams et al, 1989). Fever and other existing illness must be taken into account when evaluating heart rate. The apical pulse is assessed for 1 full minute, with its character, regularity, and rate noted. Peripheral pulses are assessed and any pulse deficit or other abnormalities are noted. Palpate pulses at the brachial, femoral, and pedal points. Decreased, delayed, or absent pulses in the lower extremities may be a sign of coarctation of the aorta. Bounding pulses may indicate a patent ductus arteriosus. The following grades are commonly used to assess peripheral pulses:

0 = Absent pulse.
1+ = Palpable.
2+ = Normal.
3+ = Full.
4+ = Full and bounding.

Blood pressure, another important parameter that the nurse must assess, should be measured in both upper and lower extremities. It is crucial in assessing accurate blood pressures that the appropriate-sized cuff be used. Using too small a cuff will give a falsely elevated blood pressure reading. The bladder inside the cuff should be two thirds the length of the upper arm for upper extremity pressures and two thirds the length of the thigh for lower extremity pressures. Since most infants and children have larger thighs than upper arms, a range of cuff sizes should be available to obtain accurate pressures. When blood pressure is measured in the lower extremities, the infant or child should be positioned supine and the popliteal artery auscultated in the popliteal fossa. The infant or child should be at rest and as relaxed as possible. The upper extremity pressure should be taken in the supine position. A wide difference of blood pressure readings between the two upper extremities is a significant finding.* In addition, if the lower extremities have a blood pressure reading 20 mmHg or more lower than the upper extremities, the child should be evaluated further for coarctation of the aorta (Uzark, 1983).

Chest

The chest is examined to see if there is any bulging or prominence on the chest wall, especially on the left side where the apex of the heart is most commonly situated. The "point of maximum impulse" (PMI) is ascertained (see Fig. 13–24). Sometimes the PMI is visually apparent as a pulsation in children with thin chest walls or with enlarged hearts. Palpation is done to locate the PMI and the presence of a thrill (see Chapter 13). A "thrill" (a vibration caused by turbulence of blood flow in the heart) may be felt by placing the tips of the fingers on the anterior chest wall. The vibration has been described as like a purring kitten.

Auscultation of the heart using a stethoscope is done to check the quality, rate, and rhythm of the heart sounds and to identify murmurs. Murmurs are the most common means of identifying congenital heart disease. A "murmur" is a sound created by turbulent blood flow through the heart.

When assessing a murmur, it should be described in terms of several parameters: its location (aortic, pulmonic, tricuspid, and mitral areas), its position in the cardiac cycle, and its duration, configuration, pitch, intensity, quality, and response to exercise and movement. There are two categories of murmurs: innocent and organic. "Innocent murmurs" are not associated with any underlying pathology; the heart is structurally normal. Innocent murmurs represent the turbulence of normal blood flow through the heart and are commonly heard in infants and young children because of their thin chest walls. These murmurs increase in intensity with fever and exercise owing to increased heart rate and cardiac output. Innocent murmurs usually are no longer heard as the child reaches school age and adolescence. Parents require thorough explanations and reassurances that their child with an innocent murmur has a "normal" heart. "Organic murmurs" are associated with either acquired or congenital heart disease.

Heart murmurs are classified according to their loudness and the presence or absence of a thrill. Murmurs are graded from I (softest) to VI (loudest) and are described as follows:†

- Grade I— Very faint, difficult to hear unless child is very quiet, may be heard faintly after a period of attentive listening.
- Grade II— Soft, though readily heard; louder than grade I.
- Grade III— Moderately loud; no thrill.
- Grade IV— Loud with a thrill.
- Grade V— Loud enough to be heard with a stethoscope barely on the chest wall; thrill is present.
- Grade VI—Can be heard without having the stethoscope on the chest wall; accompanied by a thrill.

Abdomen

The abdomen should be palpated for hepatomegaly, defined as enlargement of the liver greater than 3 cm below the right costal margin (see section on "Congestive Heart Failure").

Diagnostic Assessment

Vital to the diagnosis of CHD is a thorough history and physical examination. A variety of diagnostic procedures and tests may also be ordered. Diagnostic assessment is summarized in Table 33–8.

Electrocardiogram

An electrocardiogram (ECG or EKG) is a graphic tracing of the electrical activity produced by the heart muscle from different sides and from different planes of the body. The heart action that accompanies each phase of electrical activity is described in Figure 33–3. The ECG shows the sequence of electrical events in the heart, the heart rate and rhythm, damage to the heart muscle, and conduction disturbances.

* A 10 to 15 mmHg difference between the upper extremities can be found in normal individuals.

† Note: Intensity of murmur is not necessarily associated with severity of defect.

TABLE 33-8
Diagnostic Assessment: Cardiac Function

Name of Test	Description/Purpose	Nursing Implications
Thoracic radiograph	Provides four types of information about the cardiovascular system: (1) cardiac size and size of specific chambers or great vessels, (2) cardiac contour, (3) status of pulmonary blood flow, and (4) status of lungs and other noncardiac tissue (e.g., size of thymus, rib notching, scoliosis)	Inform child/parent about reason for radiograph; radiation exposure is minimal; assure chest area is clear of ECG leads, O_2 tubing, zippers, snaps, etc.
Electrocardiography	Records the electrical activity of the cardiac muscle from different sites and in different planes of the body to assess myocardial ischemia or drainage, chamber enlargement or hypertrophy, electrolyte imbalance, or irregular rhythms	Inform child/parent about reason for test; child needs to lie still during test
Echocardiography	Identifies and records, by means of reflected sound waves, intracardiac structures and their motion, whether normal or abnormal; there are several types: 2-D, M-mode, contrast, and Doppler	Explain details of the procedure including use of conductive jelly applied to different places on chest; child may be asked to inhale, exhale, or hold breath during the procedure; sedation may be used in children 3 mos to 2–3 yrs of age to obtain an accurate study
Hemoglobin and hematocrit with indices	Reflects magnitude of desaturation and cyanosis; also measures for anemia	Red blood cell count, hemoglobin, and hematocrit increase to compensate for decreased systemic arterial oxygen saturation (as in cyanosis); a high hematocrit (polycythemia) results in increased blood viscosity and may lead to cerebral thrombosis
Cardiac catheterization	Allows determination of oxygen saturation and pressure in the various cardiac chambers and vessels; cardiac output and vascular resistances can be calculated; the response of the heart to exercise and drugs can be evaluated using these data	Obstructive lesions and shunting of blood from one side of the heart to the other are identified; heavy sedation is used for the procedure; inform parent/child about purpose of test; prepare child for experience
Angiography	Injection of dye is often used in evaluating cardiac anatomy; provides visualization of cardiac chambers and vessels; radiopaque media are injected into cardiac chambers or vessels, and a record is made by means of serial x-ray films or movies; usually included as a part of catheterization procedure	Demonstrates shunts, type of obstruction, and site and abnormal location of chambers or vessels; constitutes a permanent record; explain to child/parent that ECG electrodes will be applied, intravenous injection will be given, and passage of contrast media (dye) through circulation system will be recorded by camera
Magnetic resonance imaging (MRI)	Imaging technique that uses strong magnetic field to cause movement of nuclei that results in a resonant picture	Increasingly used in this area to visualize coarctation of aorta and peripheral pulmonary arteries; children are sedated; no metal can be in use

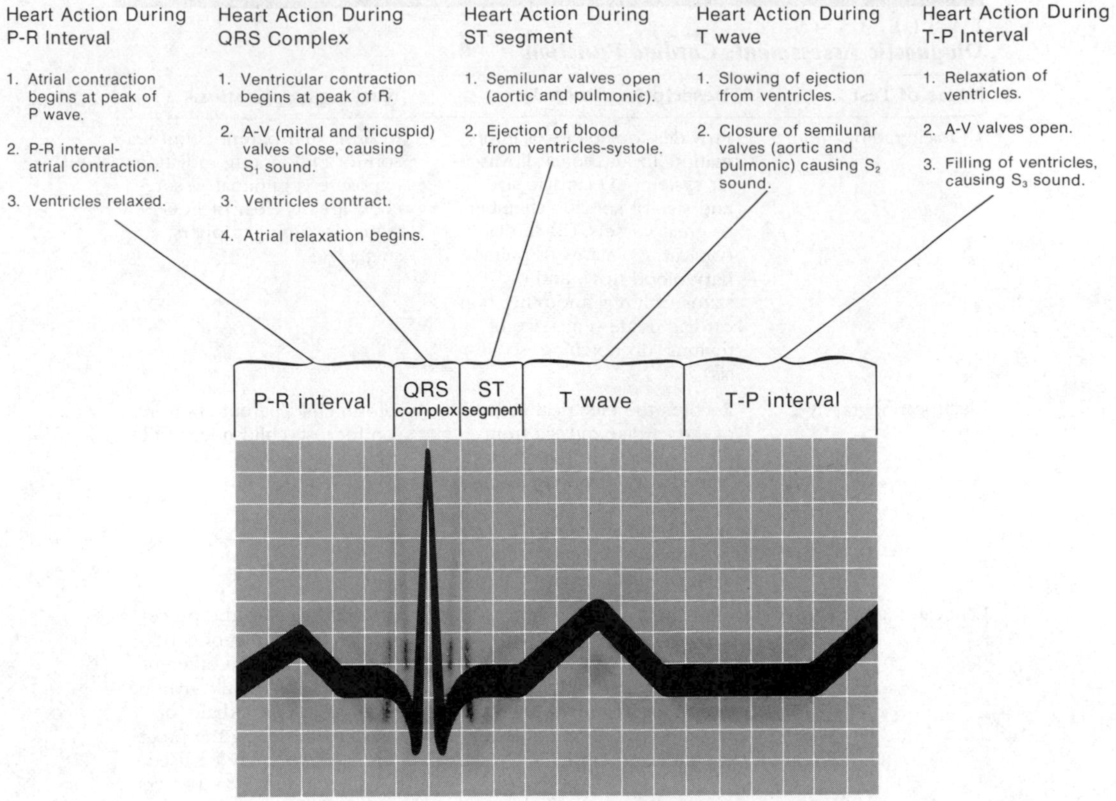

Heart Action During P-R Interval
1. Atrial contraction begins at peak of P wave.
2. P-R interval-atrial contraction.
3. Ventricles relaxed.
Heart Action During QRS Complex
1. Ventricular contraction begins at peak of R.
2. A-V (mitral and tricuspid) valves close, causing S_1 sound.
3. Ventricles contract.
4. Atrial relaxation begins.
Heart Action During ST segment
1. Semilunar valves open (aortic and pulmonic).
2. Ejection of blood from ventricles-systole.
Heart Action During T wave
1. Slowing of ejection from ventricles.
2. Closure of semilunar valves (aortic and pulmonic) causing S_2 sound.
Heart Action During T-P Interval
1. Relaxation of ventricles.
2. A-V valves open.
3. Filling of ventricles, causing S_3 sound.
P-R interval
QRS complex
ST segment
T wave
T-P interval

FIGURE 33 - 3. Electrocardiogram (ECG) with description of heart action in each phase of electrical activity.

In addition, hypertrophy or enlargement of cardiac chambers can be determined from the ECG. Leads are placed on the extremities and the chest for recording of the ECG; this is a noninvasive technique.

Echocardiography

Echocardiography is a noninvasive technique using ultrasound (high-frequency sound waves) to obtain an image of the structure of the heart. It graphically records the position and motion of the heart walls and the internal structures of the heart and neighboring tissue by the echo obtained from beams of ultrasonic waves directed through the chest wall. M-mode echocardiography provides a single-dimension view, whereas 2-D echocardiography gives a two-dimensional picture. When Doppler ultrasonography is used with 2-D echocardiography, the physician can estimate the pressure on either side of valves in the heart and determine cardiac output and blood flow patterns within the heart and great arteries (Friedman, 1988). Color flow echocardiography adds the advantage of representing blood flow abnormalities in color. Sedation is required for the young child, 3 months to 2 years, to ensure a thorough and accurate study.

Fetal echocardiography provides information about the fetal cardiovascular system and function not previously possible. The fetal heart can be examined for structure and function as early as 18 to 20 weeks.

Chest Radiograph

Chest radiographs provide information regarding the cardiac size and the size of specific chambers or great vessels, the cardiac contour, the status of pulmonary blood flow, and the status of the lungs and other noncardiac tissues (e.g., size of thymus, rib notching).

Magnetic Resonance Imaging (MRI)

Magnetic resonance imaging (MRI) has proved to be extremely useful in the diagnosis and evaluation of coarctation of the aorta and peripheral pulmonary arteries. It is a new, noninvasive imaging technique that gives high-resolution tomographic images without either contrast injection or radiation. This is accomplished by the application of low-energy radio waves in combination with a strong magnetic field. The magnet aligns hydrogen atoms while the radio waves cause the protons to resonate and generate low-frequency signals. This, in turn, is translated into tomographic images.

Because this technique is fairly new and the equipment costly, it is not available in all institutions. Sedation is required for most children because of the need for the patient to be very still throughout the study.

Transcutaneous Pulse Oximetry

Transcutaneous pulse oximetry is a noninvasive means of assessing arterial oxygen saturation. Accuracy depends on tracking of the pulse perfusion, which is influenced by movement of the child. Oximetry is less accurate secondary to skin color and light absorption through the skin. However, it is an effective, nonthreatening way of evaluating suspected cyanosis in infants and children at rest and during rapidly changing circulatory states (see Chapter 32).

Although many of these diagnostic studies are noninvasive techniques that are not painful, careful explanation of each test must be given to the parents and to the child. The strangeness of the environment and the equipment is frightening; therefore, nursing intervention is aimed at informing the parents and the child to lessen their anxiety.

Hematologic Testing

Hematologic tests are done to help in the work-up and follow-up of congenital heart disease. A complete blood count is ordered. The child with a cyanotic defect will usually show an increased hemoglobin and hematocrit. The tissue hypoxia associated with cyanosis stimulates the production of the hormone erythropoietin, which in turn stimulates the bone marrow to produce increased red blood cells (polycythemia) for additional oxygen-carrying capacity. Polycythemia may lead to problems because of increased viscosity of the blood.

Arterial blood gases may also be ordered to determine the oxygen saturation of the arterial blood. In cyanotic newborn infants, the oxygen challenge test is often ordered to evaluate the etiology of the cyanosis.

Cardiac Catheterization

A diagnostic test that requires special nursing care is cardiac catheterization.

The objectives of cardiac catheterization are as follows:

- Measure the pressures within the different chambers.
- Measure cardiac output and function.
- Measure oxygen saturation within the chambers of the heart.
- Visualize the structures of the heart to determine any anomalies.
- Evaluate the flow of blood through the heart.

This is an invasive, definitive procedure used to diagnose CHD. It involves passing a thin, flexible, radiopaque catheter (Fig. 33–4) into the chambers of the heart via a peripheral vessel, usually the femoral vein or artery. A percutaneous needle puncture is usually all that is needed to introduce the catheter into the femoral vessel. In the neonate, the umbilical vein or artery may be used. However, in very small infants or in children with vessels that are difficult to reach, a cutdown may be done. Catheterization of the right side of the heart is done by passing the catheter into the femoral vein and advancing it through the inferior vena cava and into the right atrium, the right ventricle, and the pulmonary artery. Pressure measurements are recorded and saturations obtained. If the foramen ovale is patent or an atrial septal defect is present, the catheter may be advanced into the left atrium through this opening and the left side of the heart catheterized. If there is no atrial or ventricular level communication, then the left side of the heart may be catheterized by passing the catheter into the femoral artery and into the descending aorta to the left. The catheterization is usually done in combina-

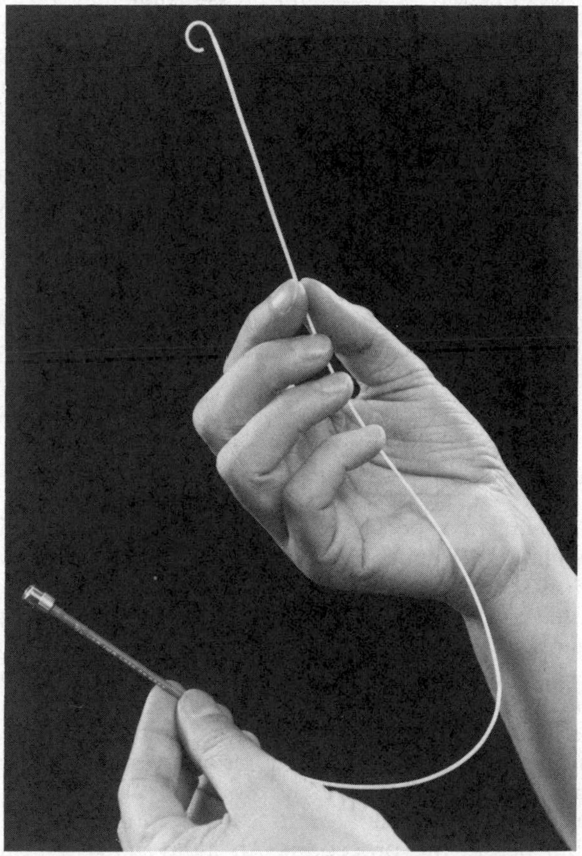

FIGURE 33-4. Catheter used for cardiac catheterization of an infant. This is called a "pigtail catheter" because of the curled end. This end has small holes out of which dye is injected into the heart chamber.

tion with angiography. In this procedure, a contrast medium is injected into a chamber or vessel (aorta, pulmonary artery) of the heart and a video recording of the x-ray films is made. This allows for later replay and detailed examination of the cardiac structure (Agamalion, 1986).

Precatheterization Nursing Care

For cardiac catheterization, the infant or child may be admitted to the hospital for 24 to 48 hours. In some situations, the catheterization may be an outpatient procedure. This is becoming a more common practice and requires some alteration in precatheterization care.

The child is admitted or seen as an outpatient the day before the procedure, during which time the physical examination, chest radiograph, electrocardiogram, echocardiogram, and hematologic studies are performed as necessary. Hematologic studies usually include a complete blood count to identify a potential infection and obtain values necessary for hemodynamic calculations in the catheterization laboratory. Because the contrast solution (dye) used in angiography is excreted by the kidneys, a blood urea nitrogen (BUN) and creatinine are obtained to rule out any renal dysfunction. A type and cross-match may be obtained to ensure availability of blood should any excessive bleeding occur during or after the catheterization, especially for certain interventional procedures and infants less than 1 year of age. Blood should not be drawn from the catheterization site. At this time, more detailed preparation of the child is carried out at an appropriate developmental level (see Chapter 21) with continued assessment of the child's tolerance for the information and anxiety levels. The preparation should include experiential information about the catheterization procedure, such as positioning on the table with the arms over the head, restraining legs with a safety belt, washing the groin areas, injecting lidocaine, and the positioning and noise of the cameras during cineangiography. Explanation of expectations following the catheterization is also important. The child should be told about returning to the room, the need to stay in bed with the extremity straight, and frequent assessment by the nurse. Preparation at this time may also include a tour of the catheterization laboratory and therapeutic play (Agamalion, 1986).

The following day, the catheterization is done, which lasts approximately 2 hours for a routine diagnostic procedure. Difficulty getting vascular access, complex intracardiac anatomy, or interventional procedures will lengthen the time of the catheterization. The child is not allowed to eat or drink for 4 to 6 hours before the procedure. An intravenous (IV) line may be placed. Preoperative medications vary among institutions, but they usually include an analgesic, such as meperidine or morphine, and a sedative, which are administered 30 to 45 minutes before the catheterization to help the child relax.

Intracatheterization Nursing Care

It is important to understand that, in addition to preparation of the child prior to the procedure, it is the responsibility of the nurse to be supportive and informative during the procedure. Although many children sleep through the catheterization, the sedative is generally mild enough that the child is rousable during local anesthetic administration and, occasionally, during the procedure itself. One of the nurse's roles, then, is reinforcement of teaching with provision of emotional support. Parents are usually very anxious during the catheterization. Providing information to them about the progress of the procedure is very helpful.

Cardiac catheterization laboratories may vary as to the number of nurses present and their responsibilities. For the most part, though, technical responsibilities include setting up for the procedure; preparing and draping the patient; monitoring vital signs, intravenous fluids, and general status; assisting the physician; preparing medication, and, generally, overseeing the functioning of the laboratory. Specialized training is important, especially in sterile technique and in detection and treatment of dysrhythmias, as well as a thorough understanding of normal cardiac anatomy and physiology and of congenital cardiac lesions.

Postcatheterization Nursing Care

From the moment the procedure is over and the child returns to the unit, the nurse begins immediate, careful, systematic observations. The child must be observed closely for any complications. When moved from the stretcher to the bed, the child's color and level of consciousness are noted. The child will have a pressure dressing over the catheterization site, which must be checked to see that it is snug and that no bleeding is present. For infants, the diaper should be unfastened to allow for complete examination of the dressing on each assessment because blood can pool under the child. These interventions are carried out for the nursing diagnosis *high risk for hemorrhage*. The pulse, color, temperature, and capillary refill of the extremity distal to the catheterization site should be checked, because arterial thrombosis and spasm of the vessels are the most frequent complications of the cardiac catheterization procedure. All of the vital signs are checked immediately on return from the procedure and monitored closely for several hours.

The child may have a transient *temperature elevation* due to physiologic dehydration from being without fluids for 4 to 6 hours (if an IV was not started) before the procedure or from the contrast media, or both. (Many children have this very mild reaction to the contrast media.) If the fever persists, it may be due to the introduction of pathogens during the procedure.

The patient must be observed closely for signs of *bradycardia, tachycardia,* and *dysrhythmias*. The introduction of catheters into the cardiac chambers can cause irritation and/or stimulation of the myocardium, resulting in dysrhythmias. Usually, any dysrhythmia, bradycardia, or tachycardia is temporary. However, occasionally it will persist and require therapeutic intervention. *Apnea, dyspnea with retractions, hypotension, and asymmetric or decreased motion of the extremities* are also signs of complications. *Stroke* can occur from catheterization owing to thrombus formation on the catheter. Cyanotic children have an increased risk of stroke occurring from catheterization.

The extremity distal to the catheterization site must remain extended until the pressure dressing is removed, usually 6 to 12 hours after the catheterization. An older child will usually respond to instructions to keep the leg straight with frequent reminders to do so. For infants, attempt to position the leg in a position that is as extended as possible. Restraint of the leg should be avoided because it may actually increase the potential for *bleeding from the catheterization site* if the child pulls against this restraint. If the infant or toddler is awake and crying, it may be more beneficial to allow the parents to hold the child on a pillow on their lap or in their arms, keeping the child supine and keeping the leg as straight as possible. In addition, attaching a urine bag for urine collection helps prevent contamination of the catheterization site. It is important to note any urination following the test because it is possible that the bladder may have been perforated by the guide wire or catheter. The contrast medium is a hypertonic solution and tends, therefore, to result in diuresis post catheterization. Newer lower osmolarity contrast solutions cause fewer complications.

Clear liquids are usually reintroduced immediately following the catheterization. If clear liquids are tolerated, the infant or child may advance to a regular diet. If nausea or vomiting, or both, should occur, the infant or child is kept on clear liquids until this ceases. The following morning, the child is usually discharged from the hospital, provided there is a good pulse in the affected extremity, vital signs are stable, and the child is tolerating a regular diet. For children undergoing cardiac catheterization on an outpatient basis, discharge will take place 6 to 8 hours after the procedure if stable. The parent instruction sheet should be given to reinforce teaching about the procedure and about postprocedural care at home. A sample parent instruction sheet is found in Table 33–9.

Congestive Heart Failure

In the majority of cases, congestive heart failure (CHF) is the result of a surgically correctable structural abnormality of the heart. CHF can also be caused by arrhythmias, anemia, myocardial disease (e.g., myocarditis), sepsis, or hypertension.

Etiology/Incidence (Pathophysiology)

CHF is a clinical syndrome that reflects the inability of the heart to meet the metabolic needs of the body. However, in the infant or young child with an anatomic abnormality, the condition described is actually one of pulmonary arterial overperfusion and pulmonary venous congestion caused by a large left-to-right shunt (Sapire, 1991). Ventricular function is usually not impaired as in the older child or adult. *The following clinical manifestations of CHF therefore reflect the decreased cardiac output or decreased perfusion of various organ systems* (Merenstein et al, 1985).

Clinical Manifestations

Cardiac Enlargement. The heart will dilate or hypertrophy, or both, in the presence of a volume overload, pressure overload, cardiomyopathy, or dysrhythmias. Cardiac enlargement can be identified on chest roentgenogram.

Tachycardia. Tachycardia is a compensatory mechanism for increasing cardiac output and providing increased oxygen delivery to the tissues. Cardiac output can be enhanced through two mechanisms—increasing heart rate or increasing stroke volume ($CO = HR \times SV$). Infants have very little ability to increase stroke volume, so they increase heart rate. The older child with a dilated heart from CHF also has limited ability to increase stroke volume and will become tachycardic.

Tachypnea. Inefficient emptying or overloading of the pulmonary system results in interstitial pulmonary congestion. Tachypnea is the first clinical manifestation of pulmonary congestion; however, as pulmonary congestion progresses, alveolar and bronchiolar edema occur, resulting in intercostal retractions, grunting, nasal flaring, dyspnea, rales, cough, and possibly cyanosis.

Gallop Rhythm. A gallop rhythm is an abnormal filling sound heard as a triple heart sound on auscultation. It is related to dilatation of the ventricles.

Decreased Urine Output and Edema. Decreased perfusion to the kidneys results in decreased glomerular filtration. This is interpreted by the body as a decrease in intravascular volume so compensatory mechanisms such as vasoconstriction and fluid and sodium retention are initiated. Infants normally manifest this as weight gain or puffy eyelids. Edema of the face, hands, and feet can occur in the older child.

Decreased Peripheral Pulses and Mottling of the Extremities. Poor cardiac output results in a compensatory redistribution of blood flow to vital tissues. The resulting decreased peripheral tissue perfusion causes mottling of the skin, a grayish or pale skin color, and decreased pulses.

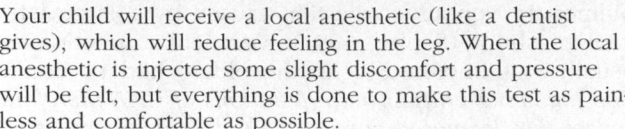

TABLE 33-9
Family-Centered Teaching: Cardiac Catheterization

Your child will receive a local anesthetic (like a dentist gives), which will reduce feeling in the leg. When the local anesthetic is injected some slight discomfort and pressure will be felt, but everything is done to make this test as painless and comfortable as possible.

During the procedure thin plastic tubes, called catheters, are inserted into a vein or artery in the leg. When the catheters are in place the cardiologist is able to learn the nature of your child's heart trouble by analyzing blood samples and by measuring blood pressures through these tubes. A special fluid that is visible on x-ray is injected into the heart chambers through the catheters. Heart malformations are identified by x-ray films as the fluid travels through the circulatory system.

The test usually takes about 2 hrs. When it is over, a bandage is placed over the area where the catheters were inserted. Sometimes, a small incision is needed to reach the vein or artery, instead of just a needle stick. The incision will be closed with several stitches, which will be removed within a week.

Following the catheterization your child will return to his or her room and will most likely be very sleepy the remainder of the afternoon. Your child will need to keep his or her leg straight (and not bend the knees) to prevent bleeding from the catheterization site. You may hold your child in your arms if this is more comfortable; however, it is important to keep your child's leg straight while you are holding him or her.

Your child may begin taking clear liquids soon after returning. If he or she can drink clear liquids without becoming nauseated or sick to the stomach, regular food can be eaten.

The nurses will be checking your child's pulses, blood pressure, temperature, and catheterization site frequently for the first hour. When the cardiologist feels your child is ready, he or she may go home.

Home Care Instructions

Diet: Your child may return to a regular diet as soon as he or she reaches home. Once in a great while the effects of the catheterization may make a child lose appetite, in which case you should start with liquids and slowly return to solid foods over the next 24 hrs. If nausea and vomiting do not stop, call your physician.

Cleanliness: It is best to keep the child out of the bathtub for 24 hrs, using sponge baths instead. If there are stitches, it is better to use sponge bathing (staying clear of the wound) until the stitches are removed by your doctor.

Keep the catheterization site clean and dry. It is usually best to leave this area open to the air (without a bandage) after the child is home. The area may be gently cleaned with a wash cloth and air dried. (Discharge instructions will depend on physician judgments and institutional policies.)

Activity: The child should be up and around the house playing quietly on the first day home. After the first day, he or she may return to previous activities. If there *are no stitches,* very active physical activities, such as gym, should be skipped for several days. (Discharge instructions will depend on physician judgments and institutional policies.)

What to Watch For:

1. Check temperature once the evening after catheterization and twice the next day. Report to your doctor any reading over 101°F.
2. Watch the catheterization site for signs of infection, such as redness, swelling, or the presence of any drainage.
3. If bleeding should occur, it can be controlled by firm pressure directly over the wound applied for 3–4 mins. If this does not stop the bleeding, bring the child to your physician, or the nearest general hospital emergency room.
4. If there is a slight bruise around the wound site, do not become alarmed, as this sometimes occurs and is not serious.
5. If there is pain at the catheterization site you may use acetaminophen (Tylenol); *please do not use aspirin.*
6. Your child may not be able to sleep for a short time after any hospitalization, particularly if an anesthetic has been given. This will go away with time and is not serious.

If your child has had an arterial as well as a venous puncture catheterization, watch the leg for pale color associated with pain or numbness. Call your doctor if paleness, pain, or numbness begins.

Sweating. Sweating represents an increased metabolic rate with CHF and probably increased activity of the autonomic nervous system. The increased metabolic rate is in response to the increased workload of the heart in failure.

Hepatomegaly. Hepatomegaly represents hepatic congestion due to elevated central venous pressure (CVP). In older children with an elevated CVP, neck vein distention can also be seen. The right ventricle in CHF is less compliant and may not adequately empty, leading to elevated pressures in the right atrium, central venous system, and hepatic system.

Failure-to-Thrive and Feeding Difficulties. Failure-to-thrive and feeding difficulties result from multiple factors. Respiratory difficulties compromise the infant's ability to feed. The basal metabolic rate increases in infants with CHF, requiring a higher caloric intake (150 cal/kg/day or more). The infant must expend more energy to consume the calories but lacks the energy reserve to do so, resulting in a malnutrition state. In addition, the decreased tissue perfusion may curtail the infant's ability to grow. All of these factors lead to failure-to-thrive.

Decreased Exercise Tolerance. Infants may sleep a majority of the time; fall asleep during feedings; and be delayed in motor activities, such as turning over, crawling, and sitting. The older child may show fatigue and inability to keep up with peers during physical activities owing to decreased perfusion to peripheral tissues and the energy required by the heart in failure. Other situations that increase metabolic demands, such as fever and heat, may not be well tolerated.

Diagnostic Assessment

Diagnosis of CHF will include pertinent findings from the history and physical examination, chest roentgenograms, an ECG, and results of arterial blood gases and electrolytes. In addition, echocardiography and radionuclide studies may be used to assess ventricular function (Gersony, 1988).

Therapeutic Management

Medical management of CHF takes into account the underlying cause. Since, in the majority of cases, the cause is a surgically treatable congenital anomaly, medical management comes into play before surgery and is often continued during the postoperative recovery period (Kaplan, 1986). The major goals of medical treatment are improvement of myocardial function (most often through the use of digitalis and diuretics) and the supply and conservation of energy (through nutritional support and prescribed rest).

Nursing Diagnostic Statements and Collaborative Problems

Impaired physical mobility and fatigue *related to activity intolerance, secondary to the heart's inability to pump an adequate supply of blood to meet the body's metabolic oxygen needs.*

Altered tissue perfusion: Systemic, *related to decreased cardiac output.*

High risk for infection: Respiratory, *risk factors:*

- *Decreased immune competence associated with the stress of inadequate cardiac function.*
- *Compromised pulmonary function related to inefficient emptying or overloading of the pulmonary vasculature.*

Altered nutrition: Less than body requirements, *related to*

- *Anorexia associated with decreased perfusion of the gastrointestinal tract, medication side effects, or both.*
- *Decreased energy available for sucking/chewing.*
- *Increased metabolic demands associated with the increased workload of the incompetent heart.*

High risk for altered growth and development, *risk factors:*

- *Inadequate tissue perfusion to promote healthy tissue growth.*
- *Lack of energy to accomplish developmental tasks.*

Fear and anxiety *in the child and family related to*

- *Inability to cope with potential for the long-term and lasting effects of CHF on growth and development.*
- *Parental perception of inability to be an adequate caregiver.*
- *Perception of inability to cope with possibility of death.*
- *Knowledge deficit, child/parent, regarding condition, diagnostic procedures, and treatment.*
- *Altered family process related to family role strain associated with financial, emotional, and time demands of child's heart condition.*
- *Parental perception of inability to maintain child's health at home.*

Nursing Care

Major goals of nursing care for the child with CHF relate to the identified nursing diagnostic responses. Interventions are geared to removing or alleviating the etiologies of actual problems and preventing the occurrence of potential problems. The infant or child must be assisted to compensate for activity intolerance and decreased cardiac output, increased nutritional demands with decreased energy for feeding, high risk for infection, and developmental delays.

Children in CHF have many specific needs requiring carefully structured nursing interventions. The Nursing Process Plan in Table 33–3 summarizes nursing diagnostic responses and interventions related to the impact of CHF on the child and family.

Compensating for Activity Intolerance and Decreased Cardiac Output

Compensation for activity intolerance and decreased cardiac output involves (1) adequate rest so that the young patient can conserve energy and (2) medications to enhance cardiac function. In both instances, the nurse has a vital role in family teaching as well as in direct care delivery during hospitalization.

Increasing Activity Tolerance

Identify the child's normal pattern for sleep, feedings, playtime, and so on. Often the best time for feeding is on awakening. Infants with CHF quickly tire and become short of breath if allowed to cry when hungry; therefore, the infant should not be allowed to cry for extended periods. This does not mean that all crying should be prevented, but only that the infant should be soothed and satisfied before crying depletes his or her energy.

Baths should be given when the child feels relaxed and playful and should be a pleasurable interaction time for parents and infant alike. If the child is especially fatigued, skip the bath for that day.

Teach parents to recognize cues that indicate the infant or young child is ready for play and stimulation. Although the young patient may not have the energy for prolonged interaction, even short intervals of cuddling, playing, and stimulation are beneficial for bonding and developmental progress.

Administering Medications to Enhance Cardiac Function

The medications for the infant or child in CHF are determined by the child's symptoms and the severity of CHF. Digoxin (Lanoxin) is a positive inotropic agent that improves myocardial contractility and slows the heart rate. As a side effect of improving cardiac function, the urine output will increase. Digoxin comes either as a lime-flavored elixir or in tablet form (Table 33–10 gives usual dosages).

Digoxin elixirs are administered via a calibrated dropper or an oral syringe. Have the parent practice drawing up the medicine. The infant's head and shoulders should be elevated (to prevent aspiration) as the digoxin is slowly dropped into the side of the mouth. The infant must be given time to swallow a few drops at a time. To ensure the infant's receiving the entire dose, never mix the medication with formula or food.

Occasionally the infant or child may have a little emesis after taking the medication. *Do not repeat* the dose. It is impossible to ascertain how much has already been absorbed. Serum levels of digoxin that are temporarily too high are more dangerous than those that are temporarily too low.

Digoxin is given at regular intervals, usually every 12 hours, to ensure uniform serum levels. The family needs to maintain the same schedule each day. If a dose is forgotten for more than 6 hours, advise the parents to skip that dose and continue with the next dose as scheduled. Should the forgotten dose be remembered in less than 6 hours, the parent can give the late dose and then adjust the following dose to be given somewhat later. After that they can return to regular times of administration.

Vomiting can often be decreased by giving the digoxin between meals, about 1 hour before feeding or 2 hours after. If the child vomits two or more consecutive doses of digoxin, the physician should be informed. The most common signs of digoxin toxicity are:

- Nausea and vomiting.
- Anorexia.
- Listlessness.
- Dysrhythmias.
- Bradycardia.

The family must notify the physician at the first suspicion of digoxin toxicity. In addition, digoxin's effect on the heart may be altered by the loss of body fluids. Therefore, the physician should be notified any time the child has vomiting, diarrhea, or an elevated temperature.

Because the dose of digoxin is determined in part by the child's weight, an increase in dosage will usually be prescribed by the physician following a weight gain. Parents need reassurance that the increased dose is not related to increasing severity of the disease.

Digoxin is potentially lethal. It must be placed out of the reach of the ill child and the siblings. Table 33–11 summarizes answers to questions frequently asked about digoxin.

Diuretics such as furosemide (Lasix), chlorthiazide (Diuril), and ethacrynic acid (Edecrin) are used to decrease total body water and to increase urine output. Diuretics can deplete the potassium stores of infants and children. A potassium supplement may be prescribed to compensate for this loss, or spironolactone (Aldactone), a diuretic that inhibits potassium excretion, may be used. Potassium supplements are usually poorly tolerated by infants and children. They have a disagreeable taste and tend to stimulate emesis. Because spironolactone has a weak diuretic effect when used alone, it is usually prescribed in conjunction with a more powerful diuretic such as Diuril or Lasix.

Occasionally, parents may experience difficulty complying with prescribed medication times. This problem is more likely to occur in a very busy household with several children or when the infant or child is receiving several drugs. These families may be helped by devising a daily check-off chart that may be placed, with an attached pencil, in a conspicuous spot.

TABLE 33-10
Usual Dosages for Digoxin

Total PO Digitalizing Dose*	PO Maintenance Dose*
Prematures:	
20 μg/kg	5 μg/kg in two divided doses
Newborn to 6 mos:	
30 μg/kg	10 μg/kg in two divided doses
Greater than 6 mos:	
50 μg/kg	10 μg/kg in two divided doses

* IV dose is 75% of PO dose.

Preventing Infection

Infants and children in CHF are much more susceptible to respiratory infections. Avoiding crowded public places during cold and flu season and asking friends and relatives not to visit when they have an active infection are sensible precautions. There is no point, however, in trying to isolate the infant or child: not only is this impossible, it is also inadvisable from the standpoint of the child's emotional development. Support the parents' efforts in caring for their ill child by advising them that it may be impossible to avoid the introduction of viral illnesses from siblings during the

TABLE 33-11
Answering Parents' Questions about Digoxin Administration

1. What if one dose is missed?
   Give the next dose on time. Do not double the dosage to make up for the missed one.
2. What if more than one dose is missed in a row or one dose is missed for several days in a row?
   Notify your physician of the number of doses missed and the times they were missed.
   It is helpful to make the administration of this medication part of your child's daily routine so that it will not be forgotten and to help with the child's acceptance of it.
3. How often is the medication given?
   Digoxin is usually given every 12 hrs. It takes about 1 hr to take effect. It reaches its peak between 1 and 2 hrs after it was given. The effects decrease over 24 to 35 hrs.
4. What is the best time to give the digoxin?
   Digoxin is best absorbed when the stomach is empty because food may interfere with its absorption. For this reason it is best to give the digoxin 1 hour before or 2 hrs after eating.
5. What if my child vomits after receiving the medication?
   The dose should not be repeated because some of the digoxin may have been absorbed. If your child continues to vomit notify your physician because this may be a sign of some other problem.
6. What shall I do if my child has the flu with vomiting, diarrhea, and fever?
   Your physician should be notified immediately. If your child becomes dehydrated through loss of fluid the effects of digoxin on the body may be altered. Continue to give the digoxin as prescribed and encourage fluids. The type of fluid will vary with the degree of illness.
7. Where should digoxin be stored?
   Digoxin, like any medication, should be stored in a secure place out of the reach of children.
8. What should be done if a child accidentally swallows digoxin?
   Follow the instructions that your doctor or nurse has given you for emergency care following accidental ingestion of digoxin. However, if you have not received instructions, do the following: If ingestion has been within the last 30 mins and the child is alert with good gag reflexes, induce vomiting with syrup of ipecac and proceed to the emergency department with the bottle of the remaining digoxin. If it has been longer than 30 mins and/or the child is NOT alert and/or DOES NOT have a good gag reflex, call 911 for emergency help. Time should not be wasted. Remember to take the digoxin bottle with you to the emergency room.

peak of flu and cold season. *Because tobacco smoke is particularly irritating for the child with CHF, smoking in the child's presence or home should be strongly discouraged.*

Increasing Appetite and Energy Available

It can be difficult and frustrating to feed infants with CHF. They may have trouble sucking, swallowing, and breathing, simultaneously. They may need to rest frequently during a feeding, thus prolonging feeding time, and then may fall asleep exhausted before adequate intake is achieved. Older children may display an increasing loss of appetite and refuse food. To achieve optimal nutrition for the child, the nurse will ensure that caloric intake is adequate, that energy is conserved, and that the parents receive support and encouragement.

Observe the infant feeding and watch parent-child interaction during the feeding. Each infant is different and any feeding plan must reflect individual needs. Include the parents in every aspect of nutritional planning and work together in developing an optimal feeding plan. Take into consideration the household schedule, presence or absence of other family members, food preferences, and ethnic background.

Anticipate the infant's hunger and provide feedings before energy is spent in crying. Smaller, more frequent feedings may help conserve energy and increase total intake. Position the infant in a semi-erect position in the parent's arms. If the infant tends to have "wet burps" or actual emesis after feeding, place her or him with head and torso semi-elevated for 30 minutes following each feeding. Burp the infant before, during, and after each feeding. Many babies with CHF have a poor suck and draw in large amounts of air with their food, which can result in colic. Burping the infant after every half ounce will help minimize this problem and will reduce the chance of emesis.

Never prop the bottle. Feeding the infant with CHF requires constant attention to feeding tolerance. Small infants do best with a soft, free-flowing (premature) nipple. This helps to ensure adequate intake in a shorter time with less energy expended in sucking. The nipple hole should be large enough to deliver the formula easily, but not so large as to increase the chance of aspiration. Infants with additional congenital disorders, such as cleft lip or cleft palate, may require special nipples and may need feeding appliances adapted to their individual needs.

Review formula preparation with the family. Most commercially prepared formulas contain 20 cal/oz. Sometimes infants with CHF are placed on a formula containing 24 cal or more per ounce. This is aimed at increasing the caloric consumption without extra energy expenditure for additional feedings. Higher-calorie formulas are not always well tolerated, however. The infant may develop diarrhea, vomiting, or both. If this occurs, the formula will be changed to a lower-calorie preparation and then gradually the more concentrated form will be reintroduced. Gradual introduction of the higher-calorie formula often increases tolerance. Low-salt formulas are rarely used for infants in CHF because these promote anorexia and may deplete normal sodium intake.

When an infant fails to grow, it is important to assess exactly how much intake he or she is receiving. Calculation of the formula consumed in 24 hours will help to determine whether the volume of formula is adequate.

Breastfeeding is slightly harder work for infants than bottlefeeding. Breast milk is, however, considered to be more easily digested than formula. In addition, breastfeeding can be a very special time for mother-infant bonding. The mother who chooses breastfeeding should be supported in her choice. The success of breastfeeding can be enhanced by following these guidelines:

- Encourage offering both breasts at each feeding, alternating the starting breast.
- If the infant fatigues easily, limit the feeding time. Ninety per cent of the milk is ingested in the first 5 minutes of vigorous sucking at breast. Allowing 8 to 10 minutes on the first breast and 10 to 15 minutes on the second should provide adequate intake and satisfy the infant's sucking needs. Some infants may need to be fed as often as every 2 hours. Other infants may not need such frequent feedings, but the infant with CHF should never go longer than 4 hours between feedings.
- If the mother's breasts become very engorged, it is difficult for the infant to grasp the nipple. Manual expression of a small amount of milk will soften the breast and decrease the sucking effort.
- Nursing mothers use 600 to 1000 cal/day for breast feeding; therefore, they need to consume adequate calories and a nutritionally balanced diet.
- The breastfed infant is receiving enough milk if there are 6 to 8 wet diapers per day, and if the infant feeds at least every 4 hours and is alert.

An important fact for families to understand is that many infants will not gain weight or will gain it very slowly, regardless of the method of feeding, owing to their cardiac defect.

For the older child, meals should be well balanced, with small, attractive, and tasty portions. Empty calories, such as carbonated beverages, cookies, candy, and potato chips, should be avoided. Asking parents to keep a 7-day record of dietary intake helps to determine quantity and quality of nutrients taken in. It can also serve as a tool for nutritional counseling. Review with the parents the amount of milk the child is drinking each day. If large volumes of milk are being consumed, needed nutrients may be missing and iron deficiency anemia may occur.

Promoting Healthy Growth and Development

Growth needs have been addressed with regard to conservation of energy, adequate nutritional intake, and enhancement of cardiac function. Developmental needs will be partially met by loving interactions between the family and the child. The family should be counseled, however, that some developmental delays are common and unavoidable because the infant's available energy will be used first for maintaining vital functions, such as breathing and feeding, leaving little energy for pursuit of developmental tasks. They should be reassured that, after the infant is stabilized by either medical or surgical treatment, she or he will catch up to her or his peers.

Facilitating Coping, Altering Problematic Perceptions, and Providing Information

The family of an infant or child in CHF needs detailed teaching and emotional support from the nurse. Explanation of the term "congestive heart failure" should be given early, as it is a frightening term for parents. The words "heart failure" often give rise to thoughts of a heart on the brink of stopping. It is important that parents understand that stating a child is in heart failure does not imply that the child's heart is ready to stop. To decrease the family's anxiety, it is helpful to explain heart failure as any situation in which the heart shows signs of being unable to pump enough blood to meet all the needs of the body.

Cyanosis

Cyanosis is a blue discoloration of the skin, nail beds, and mucous membranes caused by systemic arterial oxygen desaturation in surface blood vessels (hypoxemia). Cyanosis becomes clinically evident when there is at least 5 g of reduced (unoxygenated) hemoglobin per 100 ml of blood. The presence of cyanosis correlates with an arterial O_2 saturation of 75 to 85 per cent (Hazinski, 1992). The degree of cyanosis is related to arterial oxygen saturation, the concentration of hemoglobin, and the rate of capillary blood flow. The lower the arterial oxygen saturation, the greater the cyanosis. The child with low hemoglobin concentration (anemic) will appear less cyanotic than the child with normal or increased (polycythemic) hemoglobin concentration at the same level of arterial oxygen saturation. Slower capillary blood flow will result in greater extraction of oxygen from the hemoglobin, causing increased desaturation at the capillary level. Assessment of cyanosis is influenced by skin color, ambient lighting in examination area, and the child's clothing.

Causes of Cyanosis from Hypoxemia

Peripheral cyanosis, sometimes called "acrocyanosis," is usually seen in the hands, feet, and around the mouth. This condition is thought to be due to vasomotor instability in the newborn infant or a normal response to retain heat. The mucous membranes will remain pink. It is extremely unlikely for peripheral cyanosis alone to be an indication of CHD (Sapire, 1991).

Central cyanosis is discoloration of the mucous membranes, especially in the mouth on the buccal mucosa, the inner aspect of the lips, and the gums. It is almost always pathologic. There are various causes of central cyanosis, most of which can be classified as pulmonary or cardiac in origin. When central cyanosis is observed, it is then critical to determine the physiologic cause. Cyanosis that decreases with crying is usually pulmonary in origin; cyanosis that increases with crying is usually cardiac in origin.

A technique that may help differentiate pulmonary or cardiac causes is the hyperoxia test. An arterial blood gas sample is obtained when the child is in room air, and then after a 15- to 20-minute interval in 100 per cent oxygen. If the arterial oxygen tension increases by more than 20 torr, or rises above 200 torr while in 100 per cent oxygen, the cyanosis is probably pulmonary in origin (Hazinski, 1992). If the oxygen tension does not increase significantly, this indicates that venous (desaturated) blood is directly entering the arterial circulation as a result of an anatomic cardiac abnormality that causes decreased pulmonary blood flow and/or arteriovenous admixture. The hyperoxia test is somewhat controversial at this time with regard to its efficacy and safety, but it is still used in practice.

Physiologic Responses to Hypoxemia

Chronic hypoxemia of any etiology will produce polycythemia or an increased production of red blood cells due to stimulation of erythropoietin by the kidney. The concentration of hemoglobin is also elevated. This process increases the oxygen-carrying capacity of the blood. Monitoring of the hematocrit/hemoglobin with red blood cell (RBC) indices is an important clinical parameter in the follow-up of children with cyanotic heart disease. Stability of the hematocrit/hemoglobin is an indication of stable arterial oxygen saturation. If hematocrit/hemoglobin begin to rise, it is probably in response to a change in the child's overall cardiac status.

Dyspnea will frequently be observed, especially with exertion. Exercise increases the oxygen demands of the tissues, and, in the cyanotic (hypoxemic) child, these demands cannot be met because of the arterial desaturation. Respiratory efforts increase in an attempt to improve oxygenation.

A prominent physical finding is clubbing of the fingers and toes. Clubbing is a rounding and enlargement of the tips of the fingers (especially the thumb) and the toes, resembling a matchstick (Fig. 33–5) (Sapire, 1991). There is thickening and shininess of the terminal phalanges, with disappearance of the normal creases. The degree of clubbing is related to the amount of hypoxemia and the length of time that the condition has persisted. The exact etiology of clubbing is unclear. There appears to be an increased amount of capillaries, soft tissue fibrosis, and increased blood flow through a myriad of arteriovenous aneurysms, related to hypoxemia, and polycythemia. Clubbing will resolve over time when arterial saturation is improved with surgical intervention.

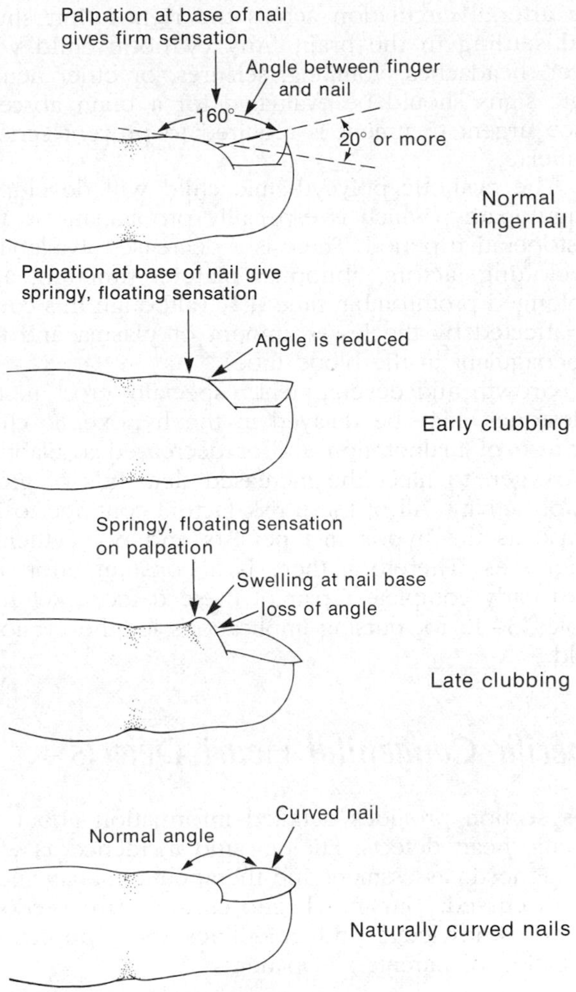

FIGURE 33-5. Clubbing in infant's fingers, caused by poor oxygenation.

Complications

The cyanotic child is at risk for cerebral vascular accidents (CVAs) or brain infarction. This may be from various causes, which are not fully understood. Because of the polycythemia and increased viscosity of the blood, there is thought to be microemboli formation that can cause strokes. Dehydration must be avoided. Iron deficiency anemia can also cause hypoxic stroke because of decreased oxygen-carrying capacity of the blood cells. Brain abscess can occur because of bacteria in the blood stream passing into the arterial circulation across the right-to-left shunt and settling in the brain. Any cyanotic child with fever, headaches, vomiting, seizures, or other neurologic signs should be evaluated for a brain abscess, since urgent treatment is required to prevent serious sequelae.

The cyanotic polycythemic child will develop a coagulopathy, which is especially problematic in the postoperative period. There is a decreased availability of clotting factors, abnormal platelet function, and prolonged prothrombin time (PT) (although this could be affected by the lesser amount of plasma and the anticoagulant in the blood tube).

Growth and development, especially gross motor milestones, may be delayed in the hypoxemic child because of malnutrition and/or decreased availability of oxygen to meet the increased demands of gross motor activity. All of these risk factors continue to increase as the hypoxemia persists and polycythemia progresses. Therefore, there is a constant effort toward early complete repair of these defects. Refer to Table 33–12 for nursing implications for the cyanotic child.

Specific Congenital Heart Defects

This section provides detailed information about 15 specific heart defects. Etiology and incidence as well as diagnostic assessment and therapeutic management are discussed. Nursing diagnoses and care sections provide knowledge and guidelines for support and education of parents and patients.

TABLE 33-12
Nursing Implications for the Cyanotic Child

Laboratory samples require more blood (less plasma available secondary to polycythemia)
Absolutely no air in IV lines (right-to-left shunt risk factor for emboli)
Puncture sites may bleed longer
Higher risk for bleeding postoperatively
Avoid dehydration
Provide increased rest periods
Time ABGs appropriately (crying reduces oxygen saturation)
Note changes in color, causes of increased cyanosis
Minor stresses can cause significant deterioration
Growth chart percentiles are important indicators of chronic changes in hemodynamics
Be alert to changes in neurologic status, especially after hypercyanotic spells
Cyanosis will be more evident with elevated hematocrit/hemoglobin (more desaturated hemoglobin present)
Keep child warm (cold increases vasoconstriction, decreases blood flow and oxygen delivery)

Guidelines for Learning about CHD

Because of the amount of detailed information in this section, guidelines for learning are provided. If one learns the path of altered blood flow from each defect and the pathophysiology that prompts each flow pattern, the associated medical, surgical, and nursing interventions will follow quite logically. It is recommended, therefore, that the illustrations accompanying the description of the heart anomaly be used to locate the structural defect(s) and to trace the resulting alteration in blood flow. The following questions can help structure learning. (The answers that appear here for illustrative purposes apply to ventricular septal defect.)

- What is (are) the structural defect(s)?
  There is a hole between the ventricles.
- How does (do) the defect(s) change normal blood flow?
  Some oxygenated blood now flows from the left ventricle to the right ventricle.
- Why does blood flow in this direction (or in this manner)?
  Pressure is greater in the left ventricle than in the right (after the neonatal period).
- Does the altered flow result in increased work for any of the heart chambers? What are the associated complications?
  Both ventricles must deal with extra blood volume. Over time, this can lead to congestive heart failure.
- Will the defect(s) affect the lungs? The peripheral circulation? How?
  The lungs will receive an increased volume of blood through the pulmonary artery that arises from the right ventricle. Over time, this can damage the pulmonary vessels.
- What are the special considerations for perioperative nursing care for a child with this disorder (e.g., in addition to general perioperative care)?
  High risk for altered cardiac output: decreased; high risk for altered growth and development: failure-to-thrive; high risk for injury: physiologic, related to damage to the pulmonary vessels, conduction abnormalities (dysrhythmias), and bacterial endocarditis.

Mastery of the answers to these questions for each of the major CHDs will provide a sound basis for planning nursing care.

Hemodynamics of CHD

For a better understanding of the hemodynamics of individual cardiac defects, it is helpful to know the normal pressures and oxygen saturations within the cardiac chambers and great vessels.

In the heart and great vessels, blood will flow from an area of higher pressure to that of lower pressure (Fig. 33–6). Therefore, if abnormal communications exist between the left and the right sides of the heart, the direction of blood flow through the communication will be determined by the relative pressures on the right and left sides of the heart.

Blood flowing from one chamber, artery, or vein to another, resulting in the mixing of oxygenated and unoxygenated blood, is called a "shunt." Shunts are described in terms of the ratio of pulmonary blood flow to systemic blood flow (Qp/Qs). The amount of blood flow from the right ventricle to the lungs should be equal to the amount of blood flow from the left ventricle to the systemic circulation. The ratio should be 1:1. A left-to-right shunt of 3:1 would mean that three times as much blood would be flowing to the lungs as to the systemic circulation. This would be classified as a lesion with increased pulmonary blood flow because blood flow to the lungs is increased and no unoxygenated blood is reaching the systemic circulation. A right-to-left shunt exists when right heart pressures are greater than left, and unoxygenated blood flows from the right side of the heart to the left side and out to the systemic circulation, resulting in cyanosis. This would be classified as a lesion with decreased pulmonary blood flow.

An important consideration with shunts is their effect on the pulmonary vasculature. Three stimuli can cause constriction of the pulmonary vessels and increase pulmonary vascular resistance: (1) *increased pulmonary blood flow,* (2) *blood flow to the lungs under increased pressure,* and (3) *hypoxia.* If these stimuli persist individually or in combination, irreversible damage can occur in the pulmonary vessels. Early changes in the pulmonary vessels, such as medial hypertrophy and abnormal extension of muscle into small peripheral arteries, are usually reversible. However, progressive damage, such as occlusion of the vessels, fibrosis, and decreased number of vessels, are irreversible, resulting in permanently elevated pulmonary vascular resistance and pulmonary hypertension. *Eisenmenger syndrome* is the term used to describe the condition in which increased pulmonary blood flow secondary to left-to-right shunting has resulted in a progressive elevation in PVR and permanent damage to the pulmonary vessels. A reversal of the shunt and cyanosis result. Eisenmenger syndrome is a terminal condition.

Once pulmonary vessels are damaged irreversibly, the child becomes progressively hypoxic and dies (Adams et al, 1989). Therefore, medical management of any cardiac lesion must take into consideration the effects of the lesion on the pulmonary vasculature. Nursing care for children with different defects varies, depending on the physiologic effects of the altered blood flow. This will be reviewed individually with each cardiac lesion. Various shunts and their effects on pulmonary blood flow are summarized in Table 33–13.

Therapeutic Management

The majority of CHDs can be surgically repaired or palliated sufficiently for the child to live a normal life.

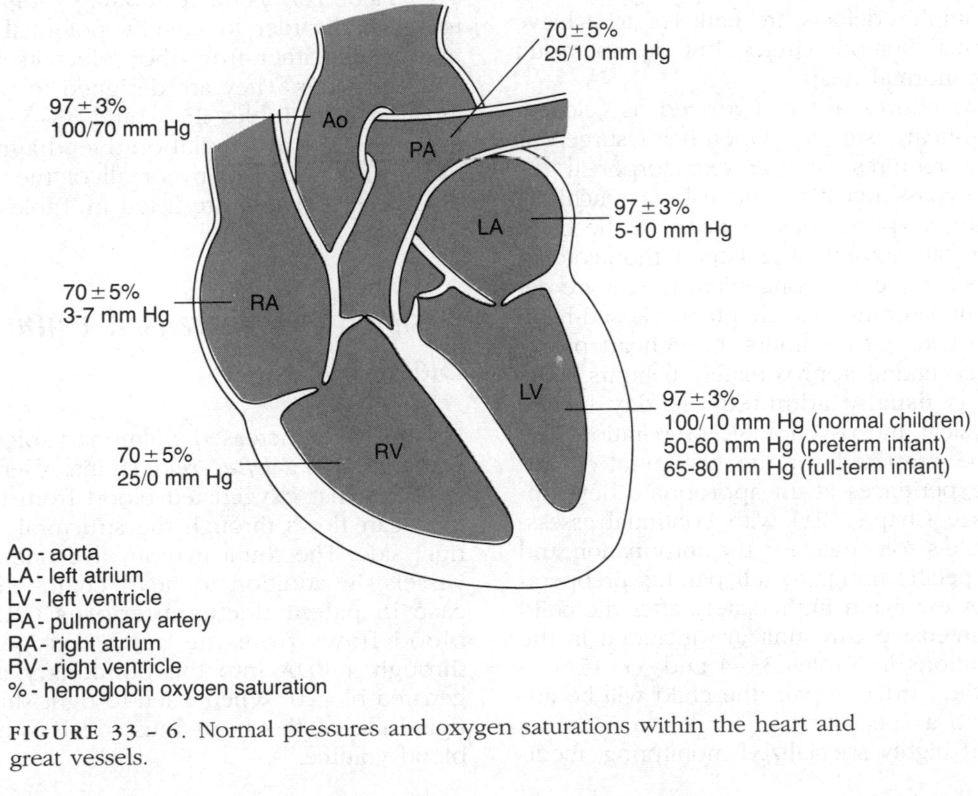

FIGURE 33 - 6. Normal pressures and oxygen saturations within the heart and great vessels.

TABLE 33-13
Cardiac Anomalies with Hemodynamic Alterations

State of Pulmonary Blood Flow	Acyanotic Left-to-Right Shunts	Cyanotic Right-to-Left Shunts
Increased	Atrial septal defect Patent ductus arteriosus Ventrical septal defect Atrioventricular canal defect	Transposition of great arteries Truncus arteriosus Total anomalous pulmonary venous connection Hypoplastic left heart syndrome
Normal	*Obstructive Lesions:* Aortic stenosis Pulmonary stenosis Coarctation of aorta	None
Decreased		Tetralogy of Fallot Ebstein anomaly Tricuspid atresia Pulmonary atresia

Symptoms such as CHF may be managed with medications until surgery can be performed safely. Medications used in the management of children with cardiac problems are presented in Table 33-14. Only the simplest defects, such as atrial septal defect or patent ductus arteriosus, can be completely repaired. Other, more complex defects are palliated to achieve reasonably normal hemodynamics, but do not result in a completely normal heart.

Surgical procedures are categorized as "closed-heart" or "open-heart" surgery. Open-heart surgery is a procedure that requires using an extracorporeal cardiopulmonary bypass machine (heart-lung machine). The most common approaches to opening the chest are the median sternotomy and lateral thoracotomy (surgical repairs for specific congenital defects are described in detail later in this chapter). Closed-heart procedures can take 3 to 4 hours; open-heart procedures are longer, taking approximately 6 hours.

The child is usually admitted the day before surgery for physical and psychologic preparation. The child should be prepared for the preoperative and postoperative experiences at an appropriate developmental level (see Chapter 21) with continual assessment of the child's tolerance for the information and anxiety level. Specific things to tell parents preoperatively and to review again immediately after the child returns to the intensive care unit are included in the nursing interventions in Tables 33-4 and 33-15.

Following the cardiac repair, the child will be admitted directly to a specialty unit for 24 to 72 hours of intensive and highly specialized monitoring, medical management, and nursing care. When the child no longer requires ventilatory support and is considered hemodynamically stable, he or she will be transferred to a general unit for 5 to 7 days of continued assessment and recuperation. The child's vital functions, circulatory status, respiratory status, level of consciousness, and fluid and electrolyte balance are monitored while normal diet and physical activity are gradually resumed. Usually, infants and toddlers resume activity on their own, whereas older children may need some encouragement. Nursing interventions to modify defining characteristics associated with the nursing diagnostic response ***high risk for altered health maintenance*** are discussed in Table 33-4.

Perioperative Care

Nurses who practice in acute care settings will most often encounter children with CHD during the perioperative period. In planning perioperative care for the child undergoing heart surgery, the nurse builds on knowledge of nursing care in any surgical procedure, as described in Table 23-7 (Nursing Process Plan: Perioperative Nursing Care) and the care of the hospitalized child (Table 21-5: Nursing Process Plan: The Hospitalized Child). Table 33-3 details the perioperative care of the child having cardiac surgery.

In addition to knowledge of *general* perioperative nursing diagnoses and nursing interventions, the nurse who cares for the child with CHD must be aware of implications for care that are *specific* to heart surgery and to the specific type of heart defect. The major *perioperative nursing diagnoses* are listed for each disorder to identify potential problems that may result either from the defect itself or following surgical repair. They are designed to be used in conjunction with Tables 23-7 and 33-3. There are several nursing and collaborative diagnoses that are likely to occur in many or all of the congenital cardiac defects. These are listed in Table 33-3.

Lesions with Increased Pulmonary Blood Flow

Lesions with increased pulmonary blood flow result when there is a *left-to-right* shunt. A left-to-right shunt indicates that oxygenated blood from the left side of the heart flows through the structural defect into the right side. The shunt may involve one or more major vessels, in addition to heart chambers. Such is the case in patent ductus arteriosus (PDA), in which blood flows from the aorta (oxygenated blood) through a PDA into the pulmonary artery (unoxygenated blood). When a left-to-right shunt occurs, the right side of the heart must deal with an increased blood volume.

TABLE 33-14
Medications for Cardiovascular Alterations

Drug	Action	Dose/Route	Side Effects/Toxicity	Nursing Implications
Antiarrhythmics				
Atropine	• Vagolytic (anticholinergic) • Increases SA node rate • Increases SA and AV node conduction velocity	0.01 mg/kg IV/SQ (0.1 mg min/0.4 mg max)	• Tachycardia, headaches, restlessness, flushed skin, blurred vision, decreased GI motility, urinary retention, hyperpyrexia • *Treat overdose with physostigmine and supportive measures*	• Monitor urine output, neurologic status • Ice chips, cool drinks for dry mouth • May cause parodoxical bradycardia in infants at dose less than 0.1 mg
Digoxin (Lanoxin)	• Cardiotonic glycoside • Increases contractility resulting in increased cardiac output • Decreases SA node rate, atrial automaticity • Increases AV node conduction time	See Table 33–10	• Arrhythmias, visual disturbances, GI upset • *Toxicity is enhanced by hypokalemia* • *Toxicity can be fatal* • *Toxicity treated by:* Withholding drug Determine serum level Supportive therapy Administer Digibind (digoxin immune FAB)	• Monitor vital signs • Monitor for arrhythmias • Monitor serum potassium level • Check with MD if arrhythmias, decreased heart rate, prolonged PR interval noted • Instruct parents re: medication administration, signs and symptoms of toxicity, potency of drug, when to call MD, what to do in case of accidental overdose
Lidocaine	• Decreases spontaneous ventricular depolarization • Used to treat ventricular ectopy	• 1 mg/kg/dose IV bolus • 10–20 μg/kg/min continuous IV infusion	• Apprehension, agitation, sedation, loss of consciousness, confusion, seizures, myocardial depression, hypotension, blurred or double vision • *Toxicity treated by discontinuing drug, supportive measures*	• Monitor ECG • Maintain infusion on rate control pump • Assess neurologic status • Monitor vital signs, emergency equipment available
Phenytoin (Dilantin)	Used to treat ventricular dysrhythmias that are unresponsive to lidocaine or procainamide or induced by digoxin	• IV: 2–4 mg/kg/dose • Give over 5 mins • Give in normal saline • Not compatible with other drugs • PO: 2–8 mg/kg/day	Bradycardia, hypotension, decreased myocardial contractility, slurred speech, confusion, dizziness, visual disturbance, gingival hyperplasia, blood dyscrasias	• Oral suspension must be thoroughly shaken before administration • Monitor baseline liver function • Observe for side effects at beginning of therapy • Good dental hygiene is important • Be aware of potential drug interactions • Monitor serum levels and avoid IM administration
Propranolol (Inderal)	Beta-adrenergic blocker; decreases heart rate, AV conduction, and ventricular contractility; used to treat arrhythmias, hypertension, and hypercyanotic spells in tetralogy of Fallot	• IV: 0.01–0.1 mg/kg • Give over 10 mins • PO: 0.2–8 mg/kg/day	Bradycardia, myocardial depression, drowsiness, wheezing	• Monitor for bradycardia, decreased myocardial function • ECG and BP monitoring when given IV
Quinidine	Decreases atrial and ventricular excitability; prolongs conduction through AV node; useful in treatment of atrial fibrillation and atrial flutter	*Gluconate* • IV: 0.5 mg/kg slowly; mix in dextrose • IM: 2–10 mg/kg q 3–6 hrs p.r.n. • PO: 10–30 mg/kg/day; give in two divided doses	Tachyarrhythmias, decreased myocardial contractility, blood dyscrasias, vertigo, headache, confusion, hypotension, increased AV block, ECG changes, abdominal pain, nausea, vomiting	• Patients are usually digitalized before starting quinidine to prevent accelerated conduction through AV node • Quinidine will increase digoxin level, so digoxin dose is decreased when quinidine starts

(continued)

TABLE 33-14
Medications for Cardiovascular Alterations *(Continued)*

		Sulfate • PO: Begin with 3–6 mg/kg q 2–3 hrs ×5 maintenance: 7–12 mg/kg/day in divided doses		• Monitor ECG and vital signs before initiation of therapy • GI side effects are signs of toxicity; check serum levels • Instruct parents to report all side effects
Diuretics				
Chlorothiazide (Diuril)	• Inhibits reabsorption of sodium in distal tubule • Inhibits reabsorption of water in the ascending limb • Peak effect 2–4 hrs	PO: 20–40 mg/kg/day	Decreased serum potassium, dehydration, postural hypotension, anorexia, nausea, blood dyscrasias, electrolyte imbalances	• Discontinue if BUN and creatinine increased • Monitor weight and serum electrolytes regularly • Instruct in diet rich in potassium • Instruction in signs and symptoms of hyperkalemia • Give with food • Give medications at times to avoid nocturia
Furosemide (Lasix)	• Inhibits sodium and chloride reabsorption in the proximal loop of Henle • Promotes excretion of sodium, water, chloride, and potassium • Peak effect 5–20 mins IV, 1–2 hrs PO	IV: 1–2 mg/kg/dose (max = 6 mg/kg/day) PO: 2 mg/kg/dose (max = 6 mg/kg/day)	Fluid and electrolyte imbalance; diarrhea may occur with liquid preparation (contains sorbitol); significantly decreases serum potassium, orthostatic hypotension, ototoxicity	• Discontinue if BUN and creatinine increase • Discontinue if dehydration occurs • Potassium supplement important • Monitor fluid and electrolyte status • Access to bathroom facilities important after dose • Don't give before bedtime • Teach parents signs and symptoms of hypokalemia, when to call MD
Hydrochlorothiazide (Hydrodiuril)	• Inhibits sodium reabsorption in cortical diluting tubule • Peak effect 2–4 hrs	2–3 kg/day PO in two divided doses (q 12 hrs)	• Decreased serum potassium, fluid and electrolyte imbalance, orthostatic hypotension, pancreatitis, blood dyscrasias • *Overdose treated with ipecac or gastric lavage, supportive measures, monitoring fluid and electrolyte balance*	• Discontinue if BUN and creatinine increased • Monitor fluid and electrolytes • Teach parents signs and symptoms of hypokalemia, when to call MD • Potassium-rich foods, access to bathroom facilities important after dosing • Do not give just before bedtime
Spironolactone (Aldactone)	• Aldosterone antagonist; inhibits exchange of sodium for potassium in the distal tubule (potassium-sparing) • Peak effect 1–4 days (prolonged effect 2–3 days after discontinuing medication)	2–3 mg/kg/day PO	• *Hyperkalemia may cause false elevations of digoxin level assay, headache, drowsiness, rash, GI upset, gynecomastia in males*	• Crush tablets and administer in food or liquid • Monitor serum electrolytes • Do not administer before bedtime • Teach parents signs and symptoms of toxicity • Administer with food • Avoid potassium-rich foods

TABLE 33-14
Medications for Cardiovascular Alterations *(Continued)*

Sympathomimetics/Inotropes				
Dobutamine (Dobutrex)	• Selective beta-adrenergic agonist • Increases cardiac contractility • May increase heart rate • Decreases systemic vascular resistance	2–20 μg/kg/min (continuous IV infusion)	Arrhythmias, pulmonary venoconstriction, nausea, vomiting, hypertension, dyspnea	• Continuous ECG and BP monitoring • Correct hypovolemia • Titrate dose to meet individual needs • Rate-controlled infusion pump must be used • Change infusion every 24 hrs
Dopamine (Intropin)	• Dopaminergic effect—increases renal glomerular filtration rate, increases urine output • Dopaminergic effect continues and beta-1 effects begin—increase in heart rate, blood pressure • Alpha-adrenergic effects—increased peripheral vascular resistance, renal vasoconstriction	1–5 μg/kg/min 2–10 μg/kg/min 8–20 μg/kg/min	Arrhythmias, nausea, vomiting, headache, local necrosis and sloughing of tissue with extravasation	• Do not infuse in peripheral IV • See Dobutamine
Epinephrine	• Alpha, beta-1, beta-2 adrenergic effects • Vasopressor, cardiac stimulant • Low dose: beta-1 dominates • High dose: alpha dominates (vasoconstriction)	0.05–0.15 mg/kg/min (continuous IV infusion) 0.2–0.3 μg/kg/min	Increased myocardial oxygen consumption, restlessness, headache, dizziness, excitability, irritability, ECG changes, dysrhythmias, hypertension, visual disturbances, GI upset	• Correct hypovolemia • Continuous ECG and BP monitoring • Strict intake and output intracardiac • Administration requires cardiac massage to disperse drug
Isoproterenol (Isuprel)	• Beta-adrenergic effect • Increases heart rate and cardiac output • May cause peripheral vasodilation, may treat bronchoconstriction	0.05–0.1 μg/kg/min (continuous IV infusion)	• Increased myocardial oxygen consumption, tachydysrhythmias, restlessness, irritability, headache, dizziness, mild tremors, GI upset, hyperglycemia • *Discontinue if ventricular arrhythmias occur*	• Continuous ECG and BP monitoring • Titrate infusion rate to achieve expected response • Correct hypovolemia • Correct hypotension before administration • Infuse on rate-control pump
Amrinone	• Nonadrenergic inotrope • Phosphodiesterase inhibition • Increased intracellular cyclic AMP • Improves myocardial contractility and vasodilates	• 0.75–5 mg/kg (loading dose, give slowly) • 5–10 μg/kg/min (continuous infusion)	Dysrhythmias, hypotension, thrombocytopenia, GI upset	• Continuous ECG and BP monitoring • Correct hypovolemia • Limited experience in children
Other Medications				
Indomethacin (Indocin)	Pharmacologic closure of patent ductus arteriosus in premature infants; exact mechanism is unknown; may inhibit prostaglandin synthesis	IV: 0.2 mg/kg; may repeat twice at 12–24 hr intervals	• GI upset and bleeding, acute renal failure, hyperkalemia, hematuria, blood dyscrasias, decreased platelet aggregation, elevated liver enzymes • *Overdose treated with supportive measures*	• Check renal function parameters before administering • Monitor for signs of decreased renal function • Do not administer second dose if renal impairment occurs • Monitor for signs and symptoms of bleeding

(continued)

TABLE 33-14
Medications for Cardiovascular Alterations (Continued)

Alprostadil (Prostin VR)	Prostaglandin E_1 (PGE_1); relaxes the smooth muscle of the ductus arteriosus to maintain patency	IV: 0.05–0.1 μg/kg/min (continuous infusion)	• Fever, apnea, lethargy, seizures, flushing, bradycardia, hypotension, GI upset, blood dyscrasias, decreased platelet aggregation, bronchospasm • *Adverse reactions are treated with supportive measures and decreasing infusion rate*	• Infuse on rate-controlled pump • Monitor ECG and BP continuously • Frequent monitoring of blood gases and pulse oximetry • Have ventilatory assistance available • Ampules should be stored in refrigerator
Captopril (Capoten)	• ACE inhibitor • Decreases systemic vascular resistance (afterload) and pulmonary capillary wedge pressure (preload) resulting in increased cardiac output • Antihypertensive	• PO: neonates 0.1–0.4 mg/kg q 6–24 hrs • *Infants:* 0.6–0.6 mg/kg/day divided q 6–12 hrs • *Children to 12 yrs:* 25 mg/day divided q 12 hrs	Dizziness, orthostatic hypotension, rash, anorexia, proteinuria, nephrotic syndrome, renal failure, hyperkalemia, fever, leukopenia, neutropenia	• Check baseline WBC with differential, BUN, and creatinine • Monitor WBC and serum potassium frequently for 3 mos, then periodically • Do not give with food • Antacids decrease effects • Advise parents to watch for dizziness and other side effects; report immediately • Instruct to change position slowly early in treatment
Enalapril (Vasotec)	See Captopril	PO: can be given once or twice daily	See Captopril	• See Captopril
Hydralazine	Antihypertensive (peripheral vasodilator) • Dominant dilating effect is arterial, decreasing peripheral vascular resistance	• PO: 0.75 mg/kg/day in four divided doses • Increase gradually for therapeutic effect • IV: 0.1–0.8 mg/kg q 3–6 hrs	Headache, dizziness, orthostatic hypotension, dysrhythmias, rash, GI upset, neutropenia, leukopenia	• Check baseline CBC • Advise against sudden changes in position • Administer with food • Monitor ECG and BP if giving IV • Instruct in signs and symptoms to report

Atrial Septal Defect (Fig. 33-7)

Atrial septal defects (ASDs) are openings in the wall separating the right and left atria. They account for about 17 per cent of all congenital cardiac defects, and occur more frequently in girls than in boys (Adams et al, 1989).

Etiology/Incidence (Pathophysiology)

There are three common forms of ASD: ostium secundum (the most common), ostium primum (also called a partial atrioventricular canal defect), and sinus venosus. Secundum ASDs are located in the midseptal wall near the foramen ovale and are frequently isolated defects. Primum ASDs, located in the septum just above the tricuspid valve, are associated with a cleft in the mitral valve and defects of the atrioventricular septum. Sinus venosus ASDs, located adjacent to the superior vena cava, are commonly associated with anomalous connection of the right pulmonary veins to the right atrium or right superior vena cava (Borow & Braunwald, 1988).

In the presence of an ASD, a portion of the oxygenated blood returning to the left atrium from the lungs crosses through the ASD to the right atrium and right ventricle and returns to the pulmonary circulation. The amount of left-to-right shunting depends on the size of the defect, its location, and the difference in pressures in the right and left atria. The pressures in the atria are determined in part by the outflow resistances of the ventricles. In the early months of life, right ventricular pressures are still elevated. As the pulmonary vascular bed matures, PVR decreases and right-side pressures decrease. Shunting across the ASD is minimal until the decrease in right ventricular pressure occurs. Most ASDs are not diagnosed until after the neonatal period and may not be detected until the school-age years. The major stimulus to the pulmonary vasculature with an ASD is increased blood flow (see section on classification of defects, "Effects on the Pulmonary Vasculature"). Changes in

TABLE 33-15
Family-Centered Teaching: Infants with a Cardiac Condition

What caused my child's heart defect? Am I responsible?

Tell parents: You are not responsible for the defect—we do not know the exact cause. (There are exceptions when the cause is known.) Heart development occurs in the first 2 mos of gestation. Part of the heart sometimes fails to develop beyond this early stage. Many factors may be related, including maternal rubella during pregnancy, prematurity, chromosomal aberrations. The condition is not related to a family history of heart attacks

Why did it take so long to diagnose the problem?

Often a murmur is not heard until 6 wks of age and it may not have been apparent at birth. Therefore, to identify problems early it is necessary to examine infants frequently in the first months of life

What causes the murmur? What is the defect?

Review flow of blood through normal heart. Using a diagram, explain the defect to parents. (This may have to be done two or three times.) Use the same terminology the physician has used (and explain it). Explain that the murmur is caused by abnormal flow of blood through the heart. Give diagram, name, and definition of defect to the parents to keep at home for reference

What will my child look like when he gets sick?

Provide parents with a list of signs they may expect to see their child display: cyanosis, difficulty breathing, difficulty feeding, edema, perspiring, easy tiring, exhaustion; and directions for responding to child's problem (e.g., call 911, call physician)

What does it mean to treat him normally?

Tell parents: Treat this child as you do your other children. Discipline and set limits for him. Physical education is okay unless physician advises against it. Infants usually limit their own activity. Reinforce information on diet, usually a normal diet, rarely a salt-restricted diet. Instruct parents how and when to feed—small frequent feedings may prevent fatigue of infants. Allow parents ample time to feed and handle baby while in the hospital. Reinforce child's normal, desirable features: for example, remark on all normal aspects of the child when doing bath demonstration for parents

What is my child's future?

Outline the long range problems so that surprises in treatment are kept to a minimum: hospitalization, cardiac catheterization, surgical repair, if appropriate. Explain medications to be given, their purpose, name, dose, time, and side effects

What should I tell my child and my other children?

Explain that the child has a heart defect. Be honest with the other children. As the child grows older, explanations can be in greater depth

Adapted from Garson, A., et al. (1978). Parental reactions to children with congenital heart disease. *Child Psychiatry and Human Development, Feb.*, 86.

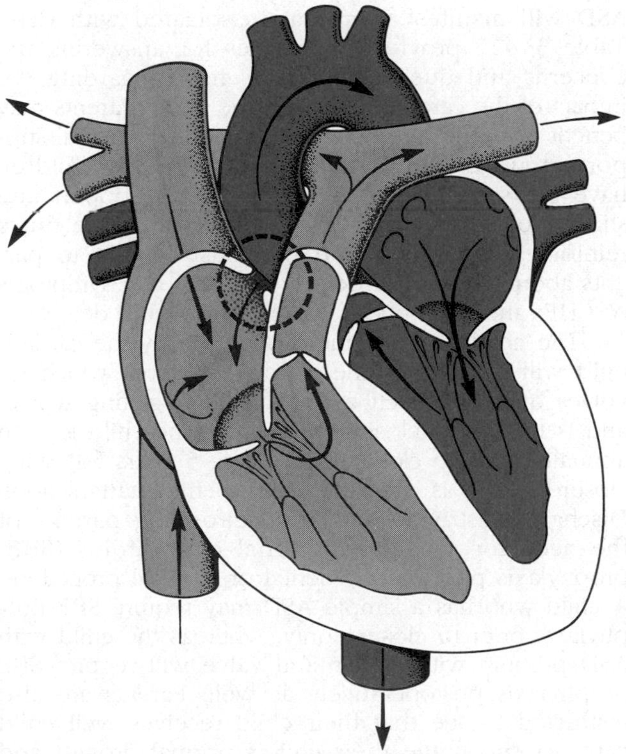

FIGURE 33-7. Atrial septal defect (ASD). The shunt is from left atrium to right atrium.

the pulmonary vessels usually occur very slowly. Pulmonary hypertension and increased PVR rarely develop during the childhood years, although they have been reported in the first and second decades of life (Adams et al, 1989).

Clinical Manifestations

Infants and children with secundum and sinus venosus ASDs are usually asymptomatic. Development of CHF is rare, and the only symptoms may be decreased exercise tolerance and dyspnea.

Diagnostic Assessment

Cardiac Examination. The increased flow of blood across the pulmonary valve produces a systolic ejection murmur heard best in the upper left sternal border. Fixed splitting of the second heart sound can usually be heard in older children. If the left-to-right shunt is large, a diastolic murmur of increased blood flow across the tricuspid valve may be heard.

Electrocardiogram. An RSR' pattern—incomplete right bundle branch block, which can be normal in this age group—and possibly atrial enlargement are usually present.

Chest Radiograph. Enlargement of the heart, a prominent pulmonary artery segment, and increased pulmonary vascular markings are usually seen.

Echocardiogram. 2-D echocardiography can usually define the location and size of the ASD as well as dilatation of the atria and size and wall thickness of the right ventricle. In addition, color flow echocardiography can identify the presence of anomalous pulmonary veins.

Therapeutic Management

Small ASDs may occasionally close spontaneously, requiring no intervention. Surgical correction for hemodynamically significant ASDs is recommended between 2 and 4 years of age (Friedman, 1988). Earlier surgical repair may be done if the child is symptomatic. The surgical repair is most often done through a median sternotomy (an incision made along the midline of the sternum) and requires cardiopulmonary bypass. Closure of secundum ASD can be accomplished by suturing the edges of the defect together, or, with large ASDs, a pericardial or dacron patch is sewn over the defect. Clinical trials with transcatheter closure devices for secundum ASDs are promising. Longer follow-up is necessary in this area.

When anomalous pulmonary venus connection to the superior vena cava is present with a sinus venosus ASD, a tunnel is surgically constructed to divert the pulmonary venous flow through the ASD to the left atrium. Operative risk is usually rare. Postoperative complications include cardiac enlargement and dysrhythmias. Mitral valve prolapse (MVP) may also be present. Associated MVP is present in more than 15 per cent of patients with secundum ASD (Merenstein et al, 1985). Cardiology follow-up is required for the patient with the repaired defect, since MVP may not occur until adolescence or adulthood.

Ostium primum ASDs or partial atrioventricular canal defects are associated with a cleft in the mitral valve and mitral valve insufficiency. These defects in infants are usually diagnosed early, owing to the prominence of cardiac murmurs. The left-to-right shunt is usually large and the infant has a pulmonary flow murmur as well as a murmur of mitral insufficiency. These infants can present with CHF due to the combination of a large left-to-right shunt and mitral insufficiency. Growth failure, dyspnea, decreased exercise tolerance, and increased respiratory infections are common signs and symptoms. Surgical correction is usually performed earlier than with secundum ASDs and involves closure of the cleft in the mitral valve and patch closure of the ASD. Seven to 10 per cent of these infants will later require replacement of the mitral valve for residual mitral insufficiency (Adams et al, 1989).

Nursing Diagnostic Statements and Collaborative Problems

Preoperative:

Altered nutrition: less than body requirements*, related to*
- *Anorexia.*
- *Decreased energy.*
- *Increased metabolic demands.*

Postoperative:

High risk for injury: physiologic*; risk factors:*
- *Cardiac enlargement and dysrhythmias.*
- *MVP.*

High risk for ineffective breathing pattern*; risk factors:*
- *Weakness.*
- *Pain.*
- *Pre-existing pulmonary hypertension.*

High risk for ineffective coping: child and parent*; risk factor: Knowledge deficit regarding operative procedure and postoperative and home care.*

Nursing Care

Very few children with ASD are symptomatic, which may make parental acceptance of their child's defect difficult to acknowledge. This denial of their child's condition may actually result in delay of surgical intervention, as their child does not appear or act ill to them. Children who have a large ASD or primum ASD will manifest symptoms associated with CHF. Table 33–15 provides guidelines for answering the concerns and questions parents have regarding the impact of the cardiac defect on the child. Parents may benefit from the referral to a community parental support group or network of parents whose children have the same diagnosis for emotional support and sharing of information. Prior to discharge, the nurse reinforces the information previously taught to parents about the cardiac defect, the signs and symptoms of CHF, and the options for closure of the defect.

The need for continued follow-up by the cardiologist will depend on the child's condition, which involves questions such as: Is the child getting worse? and Is the defect closing? Generally, the child is seen annually prior to closure and every 5 years following closure, which is done before the child starts school. Discharge instructions include informing parents of the need for subacute bacterial endocarditis (SBE) prophylaxis prior to any dental or surgical procedure. A child who has a simple ASD may require SBE prophylaxis prior to closure only, whereas the child with ASD primum with cleft mitral valve will require SBE prophylaxis postoperatively as well. Parents are also instructed to see that their child receives well child care, to encourage their child's normal growth and development, and to utilize the necessary community resources to assist in raising their child.

Patent Ductus Arteriosus (Fig. 33–8)

The ductus arteriosus is a normal pathway in the fetal circulatory system. It is a large channel (roughly the same size as the descending aorta) between the pulmonary artery and the descending aorta that allows fetal blood to pass from the pulmonary artery to the descending aorta and, ultimately, to the placenta.

Etiology/Incidence (Pathophysiology)

Functional closure of the PDA usually occurs spontaneously during the first 10 to 15 hours after birth. Permanent closure occurs within 5 to 7 days in most infants, but may take up to several weeks.

The exact mechanisms of closure of the ductus arteriosus are not fully understood. However, two major factors play an important role in ductal closure: a rise in the infant's arterial oxygen saturation (Po_2) with respirations, and the fall in circulating prostaglandins (PGE) with removal of placenta. If the neonate's O_2 saturation does not increase, closure may be delayed. If passage is needed in the presence of some CHD, the ductus arteriosus may be kept open with infusion of PGE.

Failure of closure of the ductus arteriosus or PDA accounts for about 5 to 10 per cent of congenital heart defects in term infants (Adams et al, 1989). The incidence in preterm infants is higher. Generally, the shunt is left to right (oxygenated blood from the aorta flowing into unoxygenated blood in the pulmonary artery) owing to higher pressures and resistance in the aorta than the pulmonary artery. Preterm infants have a higher incidence of PDA because of several factors. The younger the gestational age of the infant, the more the response of the ductus to oxygen is decreased. In addition, the very preterm infant may have lung disease causing hypoxia, which dilates the ductus. The preterm infant may also have high concentrations of prostaglandins, causing the ductus to remain dilated.

The stimuli to the pulmonary vasculature with a PDA are both increased flow and increased pressure owing to the higher systemic pressure shunting blood to the lungs across the ductus. Irreversible pulmonary vascular disease can develop with large PDAs that go uncorrected.

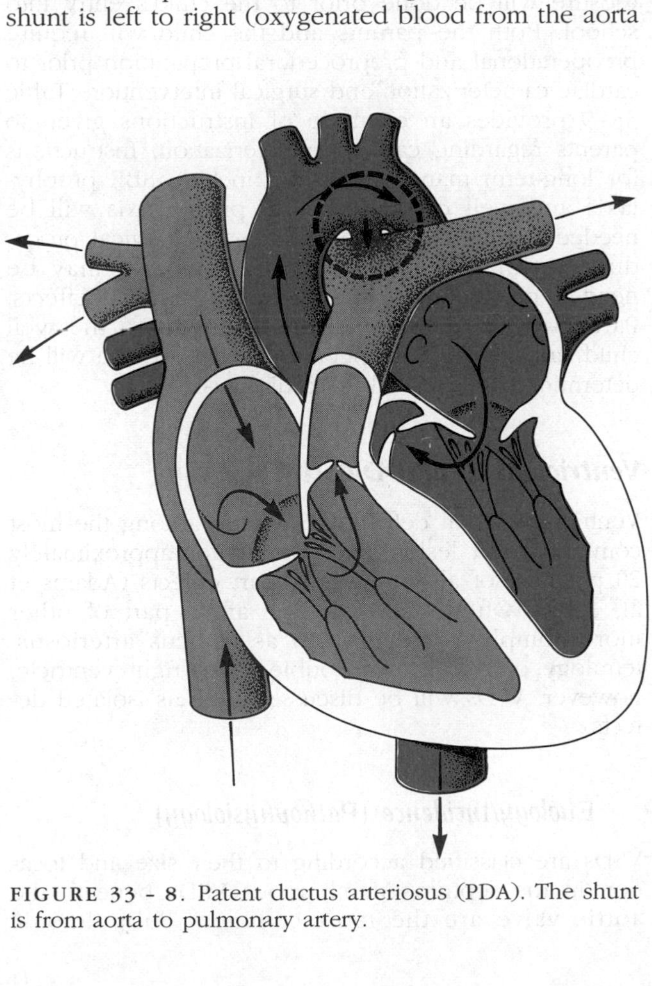

FIGURE 33 - 8. Patent ductus arteriosus (PDA). The shunt is from aorta to pulmonary artery.

Clinical Manifestations

The clinical presentation of a PDA depends on the size of the PDA, the systemic and pulmonary vascular resistance, and the ability of the myocardium (the heart muscle) to handle the extra load. Preterm infants are usually symptomatic earlier. Because their PVR falls more rapidly, allowing more left-to-right shunting, and their myocardiums are immature and less able to handle the extra load, they go into CHF more readily. The symptoms of the term infant are usually determined by the size of the ductus. Term infants with a small PDA are usually asymptomatic, whereas those with a large PDA may present in CHF. Any conditions that put extra demands on the heart for increased systemic flow will exaggerate the symptoms of cardiac failure. Such conditions include infection, fever, poor nutrition, decreased hemoglobin, increased environmental temperature, and increased activity. Older children may be identified for the first time during a routine examination. They may have slight growth retardation and easy fatigability as their only symptoms.

Diagnostic Assessment

Cardiac Examination. Preterm and term newborn infants may or may not have a murmur. When present, the murmur is usually systolic or continuous and is best heard in the second to third left intercostal space. The second heart sound is split normally and pulmonic closure is normal unless lung disease is present; then it may be accentuated. With large PDAs a diastolic rumble and a gallop may be heard. The older child may have the classic "machinery"-type murmur from blood flow across the PDA during systole and diastole. Pulses are usually described as bounding in any age group.

Electrocardiogram. The ECG is usually normal; however, it may show left ventricular hypertrophy and left atrial dilatation in the older child.

Chest Radiograph. The chest radiograph typically shows increased pulmonary vascularity with normal or increased heart size.

Echocardiogram. An M-mode echocardiogram may show increased left atrial size. With a color flow 2-D echocardiogram, the PDA can be visualized, and, with Doppler, the amount of blood flow across the PDA can be estimated. 2-D echocardiography also helps to identify the presence or absence of other cardiac defects.

Therapeutic Management

Some PDAs will close spontaneously; however, preterm infants who are symptomatic and require increasing ventilatory support require early intervention, such as surgical closure or closure with indomethacin, a prostaglandin inhibitor. By inhibiting prostaglandin, indomethacin allows the PDA to close. This agent is more effective in preterm than in term infants and should be administered before 10 days of age. It is given orally or intravenously at a dose of 0.2 mg/kg and may be repeated up to three times, 12 to 24 hours apart.

Surgical closure is indicated when indomethacin has been unsuccessful in young infants. Surgical closure is accomplished through a lateral thoracotomy. The ductus is either ligated with suture or ligated and divided completely. This is closed-heart surgery and is low risk. Clinical trials of transcatheter closure devices are promising; more data are required. The presence of a PDA in an older infant or child, even if very small, is still an indication for surgery, since operative risk is low compared with that of endocarditis in subsequent years (see the later section on endocarditis).

Nursing Diagnostic Statements and Collaborative Problems

Preoperative:

Impaired physical mobility and fatigue related to activity intolerance, *secondary to CHF secondary to increased cardiac workload and excessive pulmonary blood flow.*

High risk for altered growth and development: failure to thrive, *risk factor: metabolic demands of the myocardium:*

- *Increased basal metabolic rate.*
- *Increased tissue perfusion (bounding pulses).*

High risk for injury: physiologic, *risk factor:*

- *Bacterial endocarditis.*

Postoperative:

High risk for ineffective breathing patterns, *risk factors:*

- *Weakness.*
- *Pain.*
- *Pre-existing pulmonary hypertension.*

Nursing Care

Prior to discharge and with follow-up care, parents are likely to need reinforcement of information about their child's cardiac defect. Parental concern and anxiety may make it difficult for parents to hear information previously provided, and to hear it *accurately*. Table 33–15 offers guidelines for responding to parent's concerns and questions about their child's cardiac defect. Parents are taught to observe for the signs and symptoms of CHF (refer to section on "Congestive Heart Failure") and the indications for contacting the cardiologist. An infant with a large defect with CHF will be seen by the cardiologist every few weeks. If the infant has problems feeding, has failure-to-thrive, or signs of CHF, surgical intervention will be performed early. Open-heart surgery is not required; complications are rare.

It may be difficult for the parent to accept the child's condition if the child demonstrates no symptoms. As a result, parents may delay surgical intervention, believing the child's condition does not require it. Prior to discharge and with follow-up care, options for closure are discussed with the parents. Closure will be done prior to the child's entry into school. Both the parents and the child will require preoperational and preprocedural preparation prior to cardiac catheterization and surgical intervention. Table 33–9 provides an example of instructions given to parents regarding cardiac catheterization. Instructions for long-term management will include SBE prophylaxis and well child care. SBE prophylaxis will be needed preoperatively for dental and surgical procedures prior to closure; SBE prophylaxis may be needed postoperatively if there are residual effects. Parents need encouragement to attend to the well child care needs. Postoperative follow-up care will be determined by the child's cardiologist.

Ventricular Septal Defect (Fig. 33–9)

Ventricular septal defects (VSDs) are among the most common heart lesions, accounting for approximately 20 per cent of all congenital heart defects (Adams et al, 1989). Often, these defects are a part of other more complex defects such as truncus arteriosus, tetralogy of Fallot, and double-outlet right ventricle; however, VSDs will be discussed here as isolated defects.

Etiology/Incidence (Pathophysiology)

VSDs are classified according to their size and location in the septum. Membranous VSDs beneath the aortic valve are the most common. Subpulmonic

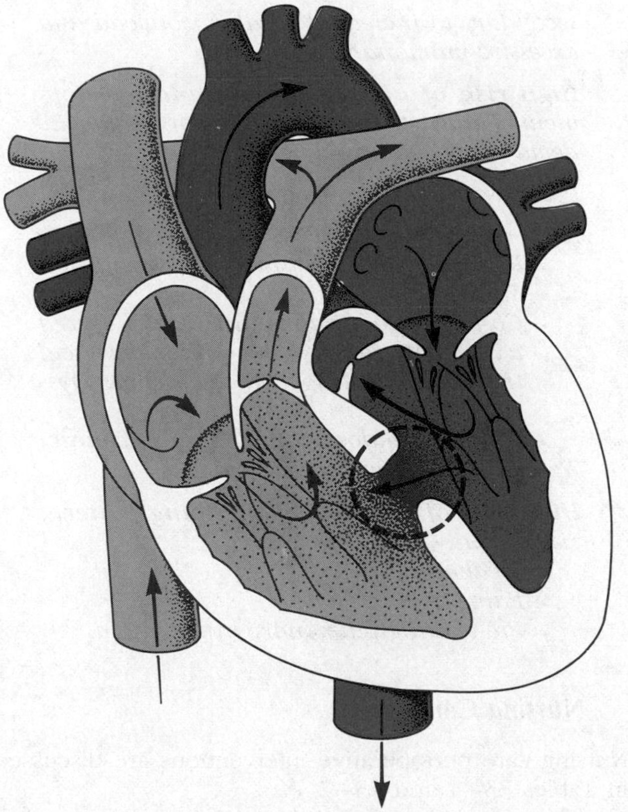

FIGURE 33 - 9. Ventricular septal defect (VSD). Shunt is from left ventricle to right ventricle.

VSDs beneath the pulmonary valve account for about 5 to 7 per cent of VSDs, atrioventricular canal–type VSDs or posterior defects approximately 8 per cent. Muscular VSDs are frequently multiple and represent 5 to 20 per cent of VSDs (Moller & Neal, 1990).

In the presence of a VSD, a portion of the oxygenated blood returning from the lungs to the left atrium and left ventricle crosses the VSD into the right ventricle and returns to the pulmonary circulation. The shunt is left to right. The magnitude of the shunt is determined by the size of the VSD and the amount of PVR present. High PVR will elevate pulmonary pressure (making it approximate left ventricular pressure) and decrease shunting across the VSD. In the newborn period, PVR is still high; therefore, little shunting may occur at this time and the child may be asymptomatic. As PVR decreases over the first 1 to 2 months of life, the child may become very symptomatic. The size of the VSD also plays an important role, with small defects having little shunting and with moderate to large defects permitting unrestricted shunting in the presence of low PVR.

With a VSD, the blood vessels in the lungs receive increased blood flow and experience increased pressure. The combination of these stimuli with the moderate to large VSD can cause changes in the pulmonary vessels even within the first year of life. Irreversible pulmonary vascular changes usually do not occur before 2 years of age, although studies have shown irreversible changes as early as age 1 year (Adams et al, 1989).

Clinical Manifestations

Symptoms depend on the size of the defect, the degree of shunting, the age of the child, and the PVR. With small VSDs, there is little shunting and the infant or child is usually asymptomatic. In addition, there are rarely any changes in the pulmonary vasculature. With moderate to large VSDs and a large left-to-right shunt, the infant or child may experience failure-to-thrive and CHF (see Chapter 16 for failure-to-thrive and the section in this chapter on "Congestive Heart Failure" for signs and symptoms). The child over age 2 may present with frequent respiratory infections and increased fatigue.

Diagnostic Assessment

Cardiac Examination. Blood flow across the VSD produces a systolic murmur that can be grade II to IV/VI,* heard best at the mid to lower left sternal border. In the presence of large left-to-right shunts (2:1 or greater), the increased blood flow returning from the lungs across the mitral valve produces a diastolic flow rumble. When increased PVR is present, the second component of the second heart sound, P_2, will be accentuated.

Electrocardiogram. In the presence of small VSDs, the ECG is usually normal. With moderate to large VSDs, left ventricular hypertrophy is usually present. Children with large VSDs may have left atrial enlargement, right ventricular hypertrophy, combined ventricular hypertrophy, or any combination of these.

Chest Radiograph. With small VSDs, the chest radiograph is usually normal. With moderate-sized VSDs, heart size and pulmonary vascular markings will be increased. With large VSDs, heart size and pulmonary vascular markings will be increased and a prominent pulmonary artery segment will be present.

Echocardiogram. Color flow 2-D echocardiography is helpful in determining the size and location of the VSD as well as the presence of more than one VSD. The degree of left-to-right shunting and the PVR can also be assessed.

Therapeutic Management

Seventy-five to eighty per cent of small VSDs and 5 to 10 per cent of large VSDs will spontaneously close, usually sometime during the first 2 years of life (Adams et al, 1989). Infants with small VSDs usually

* Murmurs are often denoted in this manner to indicate both the grade of murmur and the scale on which it is based, e.g., II/VI means a grade II murmur on a scale where VI is the highest.

require no medical or surgical therapy except antibiotics to prevent endocarditis during susceptible periods. Infants with moderate to large VSDs who are symptomatic, showing signs of CHF, and failing to grow, are usually medically managed with a combination of digoxin and diuretics. If the infant continues to fail-to-thrive or continues to show signs of CHF, or both, then early surgical repair is indicated. Other indications for early surgical repair are increasing pulmonary pressures and frequent respiratory infections.

Infants or children with large VSDs who respond to medical management but have a persistent shunt of 2:1 or greater at 1 to 2 years of age usually undergo surgical repair. An important aspect of management for infants and children with moderate to large VSDs is careful assessment of pulmonary pressures and PVR. Surgical intervention is necessary before irreversible pulmonary vascular disease develops.

Surgical repair of VSDs is an open-heart procedure; VSDs of children weighing less than 7 kg are usually repaired with the child in deep hypothermia with circulatory arrest (Merenstein et al, 1985). In larger children, cardiopulmonary bypass is used. VSDs are closed through a median sternotomy and an incision in the right atrium rather than an incision through the left or right ventricle. The VSD can be closed by directly suturing the edges of the defect together, or, with larger defects, a synthetic patch (e.g., of Dacron) is used to close the defect. The patch is not rejected because it is an inert substance and cardiac tissue completely covers the patch within 6 months after surgery. Complications of surgical repair include residual VSDs and conduction abnormalities. Most conduction abnormalities are temporary because of edema and trauma to the conduction system; however, rarely, permanent interruption of the conduction system occurs, necessitating placement of a permanent pacemaker. (See Fig. 33–23.)

Pulmonary artery banding is a palliative procedure used to decrease pulmonary blood flow until total repair can be done. It is not an open-heart procedure and is performed through a left lateral thoracotomy incision. This procedure is rarely used anymore because the combined risk of pulmonary artery banding, debanding, and total repair is greater than that of total repair alone.

The surgical risk for any infant or child undergoing VSD repair is determined by the child's age, size, and condition, as well as the size and location of the VSD. Following surgical repair, these children may require continued antibiotic prophylaxis for endocarditis for certain procedures and continued cardiology follow-up.

Nursing Diagnostic Statements and Collaborative Problems

Preoperative:

Impaired physical mobility and fatigue related to activity tolerance, *secondary to CHF secondary to increased cardiac workload and excessive pulmonary blood flow.*

High risk of altered growth and development: Failure-to-thrive; *risk factor: metabolic demands of the myocardium.*

Postoperative:

High risk for injury: Physiologic; *risk factors:*
- *Residual VSDs; Defining characteristics: Murmur.*
- *Conduction abnormalities associated with temporary edema and/or surgical trauma; Defining characteristics: Dysrhythmias, heart block.*
- *Bacterial endocarditis; Defining characteristics: Fever, bacteremia.*

High risk of ineffective breathing pattern; *risk factors:*
- *Weakness.*
- *Pain.*
- *Pre-existing pulmonary hypertension.*

Nursing Care

Nursing care perioperative interventions are discussed in Tables 33–4 and 23–7.

The parents will need continued information about their child's cardiac defect and the signs and symptoms of CHF (see section on "Congestive Heart Failure") to observe for. The signs and symptoms the child demonstrates will depend on the size of the defect and the amount of pulmonary blood flow. The child may have a very small VSD and have insignificant hemodynamic effects. Very small defects may not have to be closed. Regardless of the size of the child's defect, parents will have questions regarding the impact on the child's life, as well as on their own lives. For more detailed information, refer to Table 33–15. Instructions on long-term management will include the need for SBE prophylaxis and the need for follow-up care, which will be determined by the cardiologist. The parents and child will need to be prepared prior to surgical intervention. SBE prophylaxis will be necessary preoperatively prior to dental and surgical procedures; postoperative prophylaxis will be decided by the child's cardiologist.

Atrioventricular Canal Defect (Fig. 33–10)

Atrioventricular (AV) canal defect is also called atrioventricular septal defect and endocardial cushion defect.

Etiology/Incidence (Pathophysiology)

Complete AV canal defects account for approximately 4 per cent of all congenital heart defects and are the most common defect associated with Down syndrome (Moller & Neal, 1990). The endocardial cushions are

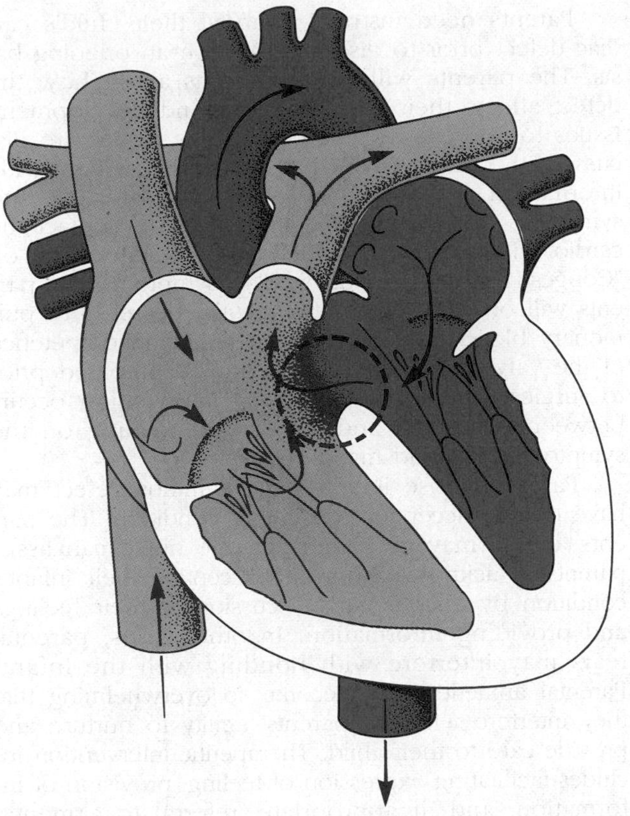

FIGURE 33-10. Great vessels are cut away to reveal the atrioventricular canal defect. The shunt is from left to right atria, left to right ventricle; mitral regurgitation occurs from the abnormal mitral valve (not depicted in this figure).

large projections of endomyocardial jelly that separate the AV canal into the atria and ventricles during fetal development. There are four cushions arising from the sides of the canal, with the posterior and anterior cushions contributing to most of the division. These two cushions also contribute to formation of the mitral and tricuspid valves. AV canal defects result from arrested or abnormal development of these cushions in utero. These defects are classified as complete or partial, each having varied clinical manifestations that depend on the size of the defect as well as the involvement of the AV valves.

The most common form of AV canal defect is partial AV canal or ostium primum septal defect, in which there is a large atrial septal defect, a cleft in the anterior mitral valve leaflet, and an intact ventricular septum. Complete AV canal defects involve a large atrial septal defect, a ventricular septal defect of varying size, and a common or single AV valve originating from both atria. Congenital heart lesions associated with AV canal defects include pulmonary stenosis and PDA.

Blood flow resulting from this defect depends on the size of the septal defect as well as the degree of involvement of the atrioventricular valves. *Essentially, there is a large central hole in the heart.* Mitral regurgitation (the backward flow of blood from the left ventricle into the left atrium through an inadequate mitral valve), tricuspid regurgitation, and shunts—either left to right or right to left—may exist. The direction of the shunt is determined by pulmonic and systemic resistance and compliance of each chamber of the heart.

The major stressors on the pulmonary vessels with an AV canal are increased pulmonary blood flow and increased pressure. If a large VSD exists, increased PVR and pulmonary hypertension may develop, causing the shunting to be bidirectional. This combination of stimuli may cause early pulmonary vascular changes and early onset of irreversible pulmonary vascular disease. In both partial and complete defects, the AV node and the bundle of His may be interrupted or displaced, creating conduction abnormalities (altered transfer of electrical impulses through the heart) (Adams et al, 1989).

Clinical Manifestations

Patients with partial AV canal defects may present with symptoms similar to those with secundum atrial septal defects, depending on the degree of mitral regurgitation present. Clinical manifestations of complete AV canal defects can be quite severe. The amount of AV valve regurgitation varies; however, most defects involve significant AV valve regurgitation. Symptoms develop in early infancy and include tachypnea, dyspnea, poor weight gain, and diaphoresis. CHF and cardiomegaly (increased heart size) develop early. Cyanosis may result from bidirectional shunting. Usually, these infants are pale and prone to recurrent respiratory infections.

Diagnostic Assessment

Cardiac Examination. Mitral regurgitation will produce a loud systolic murmur heard best at the lower left sternal border and at the apex. There may be an additional systolic murmur, heard best at the upper left sternal border, from increased blood flow across the pulmonary valve. A diastolic flow rumble may be present from increased blood flow returning from the lungs and flowing across the mitral valve. The first heart sound may be accentuated, and, if pulmonary hypertension is present, the second component of the second heart sound (P_2) will be accentuated.

Electrocardiogram. With complete AV canal, the ECG will demonstrate classic features of the counterclockwise rotation of the QRS loop, left axis deviation, and right ventricular hypertrophy. A prolonged PR interval is also frequently present.

Chest Radiograph. With complete AV canal, there is an increased heart size, a prominent pulmonary artery segment, and increased pulmonary vascular markings.

Echocardiogram. Color flow 2-D echocardiograms are extremely helpful in identifying and classifying partial versus complete AV canal and in determining the AV valve structure.

Therapeutic Management

Infants with a complete AV canal defect who are symptomatic are usually medically managed with digoxin and diuretics early on. If medical management fails and the infant persists in CHF and fails to thrive or has pulmonary hypertension, early surgical repair is indicated. If the child grows well and does not develop pulmonary hypertension, then surgical repair is performed electively before 2 years of age.

Surgical repair usually consists of total correction. Total repair is an open-heart procedure requiring deep hypothermia and circulatory arrest in infants, or cardiopulmonary bypass. It is performed through a median sternotomy. With total repair, the common AV valve is divided into separate tricuspid and mitral valves, and a patch (usually Dacron or Teflon) is sewn over the VSD and ASD. The mitral and tricuspid septal leaflets are then attached to the septal patch. The most difficult part of this repair involves the AV valves. The surgeon must reconstruct the mitral valve to make it as competent as possible. Complications of the surgery include CHF, residual septal defects, conduction abnormalities, and AV valve regurgitation. A small percentage of these children will require a mitral valve replacement later in life. All of these children require life-long prophylaxis for endocarditis and continued cardiology follow-up.

Nursing Diagnostic Statements and Collaborative Problems

Preoperative:

High risk for impaired gas exchange; *risk factors: increased volume of pulmonary blood flow and pressure.*

Impaired physical mobility and fatigue related to activity intolerance se*condary to CHF, increased cardiac workload, and excessive pulmonary blood flow.*

Postoperative:

High risk for injury: physiologic; *risk factors:*

- *Residual septal defects.*
- *Conduction abnormalities.*
- *AV valve regurgitation; Defining characteristics: Loud systolic murmurs, diastolic flow rumble.*
- *Bacterial endocarditis; Defining characteristics: Fever, bacteremia.*

Nursing Care

Nursing interventions for perioperative care are found in Table 33–4.

Parents need instruction about their child's cardiac defect prior to discharge and on an ongoing basis. The parents will have concerns about how the defect affects their child's growth and development. Issues to address with parents in this regard are discussed in Table 33–15. The nurse also will provide information to parents on assessment for signs and symptoms of CHF and the indications to contact the cardiologist or specialty nurse (see earlier section on "Congestive Heart Failure"). The symptoms the parents will observe for depend on the decrease of pulmonary blood flow and the degree of incompetence of the valve. Parents will need to be prepared prior to surgical intervention. Surgical intervention occurs between 6 months and 2 years, depending on the symptoms the child manifests.

Parents whose infants have a minor defect may have trouble accepting the child's condition. The parents' denial may be significant; the nurse can assist parents in acknowledging and accepting their infant's condition by encouraging discussion of their feelings and providing information. In other cases, parental fears may interfere with bonding with the infant. Parental anxieties may become so overwhelming that they interfere with the parents' ability to nurture and provide care to their child. Therapeutic intervention includes facilitating expression of feeling, provision of information, and, if appropriate, referral to a mental health specialist. Referral to a community-parent support group may be beneficial for support and information.

Long-term management will include SBE prophylaxis and routine well child care. SBE prophylaxis will be required preoperatively and postoperatively prior to dental and surgical procedures. Many children with Down syndrome have AV canal defect. In these circumstances, parents will need referral to appropriate community resources that provide services to children with developmental disabilities. Refer to Chapter 27 on "Developmental Alterations" for further information on developmental disabilities.

Lesions with Decreased Pulmonary Blood Flow

"Lesions with decreased pulmonary blood flow" refers to obstruction of flow to the pulmonary system with resultant shunting of the unoxygenated blood to the arterial system (right-to-left shunt) through ASD, VSD, or PDA. In this case, the blood perfusing the tissues contains less than the normal amount of oxygen (hypoxemia). In lesions with mildly decreased pulmonary blood flow, the amount of unoxygenated blood may be negligible and result in no visible cyanosis or other manifestations. In more severe conditions, however, the heart is unable to supply the tissues with the oxygen needed for such common activities as feeding and exercise.

Tetralogy of Fallot (Fig. 33–11)

Tetralogy of Fallot (TOF) accounts for 10 per cent of all congenital heart defects and is the most common heart defect with decreased pulmonary blood flow.

Etiology/Incidence (Pathophysiology)

Described by Fallot more than 100 years ago, this anomaly has four components: (a) *pulmonary stenosis,* (b) *VSD,* (c) *an overriding aorta,* and (d) *right ventricular hypertrophy.* The VSD is usually large and located high in the septum. The pulmonary stenosis involves the infundibular region and may include the pulmonary valve and/or the pulmonary arteries. The right ventricular hypertrophy results from the pulmonary stenosis.

A wide range of types and degrees of pulmonary stenosis can be present in TOF. The degree of pulmonary stenosis determines the pattern of blood flow in the heart. With mild pulmonary stenosis, right ventricular pressure is lower than left ventricular pressure, which allows oxygenated blood from the left side of the heart to pass through the VSD and out the pulmonary artery to the lungs. This is a left-to-right shunt, and these infants and children will be acyanotic. TOF with mild pulmonary stenosis is often referred to as "pink" TOF. With severe pulmonary stenosis, right ventricular pressure is equal to or greater than left ventricular pressure. Unoxygenated blood therefore passes from the right ventricle through the VSD and out the overriding aorta to the systemic circulation. These infants and children have a right-to-left shunt and are cyanotic.

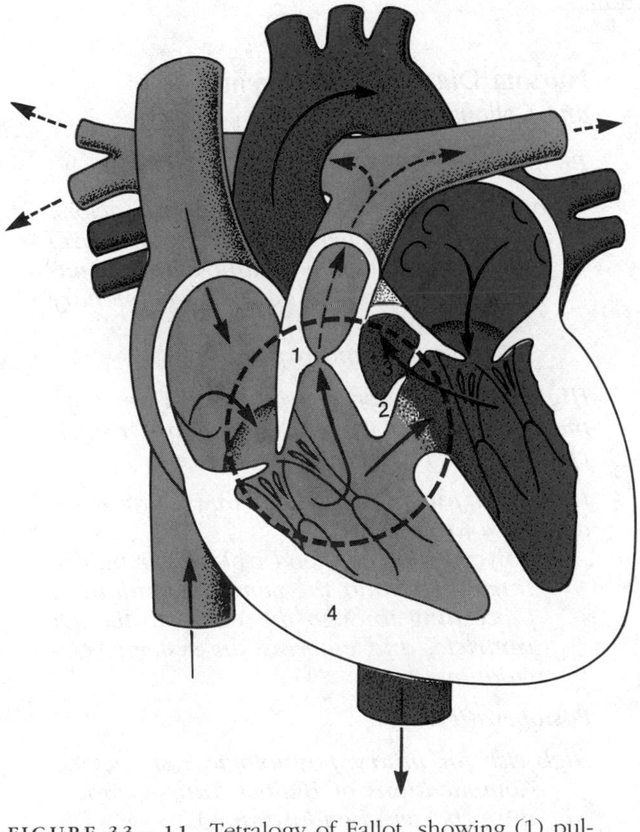

FIGURE 33-11. Tetralogy of Fallot, showing (1) pulmonary stenosis, (2) VSD, (3) overriding aorta, and (4) right ventricular hypertrophy. Flow patterns are determined by the degree of pulmonary stenosis.

The infundibular pulmonary stenosis associated with TOF usually increases in severity with time. These infants and children will become more cyanotic as pulmonary blood flow decreases. Even infants who are originally acyanotic or "pink" will eventually become cyanotic because of the progression in infundibular stenosis.

Clinical Manifestations

The most significant symptom seen in TOF is cyanosis. The degree of cyanosis depends on the severity of the pulmonary stenosis, which influences the amount of right-to-left shunting. The infant with mild stenosis may be pink at rest and only demonstrate cyanosis with crying or activity. The more severe obstructions will cause cyanosis even at rest. As the infant grows, the stenosis increases. This presents a fixed obstruction to pulmonary flow; therefore, the child cannot meet increased oxygen demands. Cyanosis increases and exercise tolerance decreases. Before the trend toward early repair, "squatting" was observed in the older child who was engaged in physical activities.

Infants who are cyanotic in the first month of life usually have severe pulmonary stenosis. These infants commonly have TET spells (see next paragraph), polycythemia, dyspnea on exertion, irritability, and poor exercise tolerance. In addition, poor growth and development are typical. If polycythemia becomes severe, CVAs and brain abscesses can occur.

"TET" (from "tetralogy") or hypercyanotic spells may occur in children with TOF. *TET spells* are characterized by acutely increased cyanosis, irritability, pallor, and tachypnea. Flaccidity and possible loss of consciousness occur as the spell progresses. They commonly occur in the morning after a night's sleep and are most frequently precipitated by crying, defecation, and feeding, all of which cause an increased oxygen need. These spells may be the result of a transient increase in the obstruction of the right ventricular outflow tract (usually increased contraction of the muscular infundibular area). Softening or elimination of murmur and narrowing on angiography are observed during catheterization (Fyler, 1992). As the obstruction increases, more unoxygenated blood is passed through the VSD to the systemic circulation, causing severe hypoxia. TET spells can progress to seizures, CVAs, and death.

Treatment of TET spells includes placing the infant or child in a knee-chest position or administering morphine or propranolol, or a combination of these agents and O_2 therapy. The knee-chest position enhances systemic venous return, which helps to dilate the right ventricle, decreasing the obstruction. The older child will squat on her or his own. Propranolol, usually administered at 1 mg/kg up to four times a day, aids in decreasing infundibular muscle spasm. Morphine, 0.1 mg/kg, aids in decreasing infundibular spasms and helps to calm and sedate the infant. These therapies are useful for halting TET spells. Propranolol is sometimes given on a routine basis to prevent further TET spells if the child is not a surgical candidate.

Diagnostic Assessment

Cardiac Examination. A harsh systolic murmur of grades II–IV/VI is heard along the left sternal border. The second heart sound is single, representing aortic valve closure. Pulmonic valve closure is usually not heard.

Electrocardiogram. Right ventricular hypertrophy is almost always present on the ECG.

Chest Radiograph. The heart size is usually normal, with a characteristic "boot-shaped" contour resulting from the small main pulmonary artery and the right ventricular hypertrophy. The pulmonary vascularity may be normal or decreased. Twenty-five per cent will have a right aortic arch.

Echocardiogram. With color flow 2-D echocardiography and continuous wave Doppler, the VSD, the overriding aorta, and the pulmonary stenosis can be visualized and evaluated or graded.

Therapeutic Management

Infants who are severely cyanotic in the first few months of life or who have TET spells require either a palliative procedure to increase blood flow to the lungs or a total repair. Total repair is not usually recommended in the neonatal period. The earliest age at which total repair is performed varies among institutions.

Palliative procedures for TOF consist of systemic to pulmonary shunts and are indicated if the infant is too young for a full repair or if the pulmonary arteries are of small size. After a shunt procedure, the pulmonary arteries hopefully will grow. The most common shunt used today is the *Blalock-Taussig shunt.* In this procedure, the right or left subclavian artery is connected to the ipsilateral (on the same side) pulmonary artery. This allows for increased blood flow to the lungs. Although the Blalock-Taussig shunt increases blood flow to the lungs, the overall volume of blood reaching the lungs is still limited. Following the shunt procedure, the child will continue to be cyanotic but to a lesser degree. The Blalock-Taussig shunt is not an open-heart procedure and is performed through a lateral thoracotomy incision. Complications of the Blalock-Taussig procedure include a diminished or absent pulse in the affected arm (BP in that arm will be inaccurate), CHF from too large a shunt, or an inadequate shunt.

When a Blalock-Taussig shunt cannot be performed, a central shunt with Gore-Tex graft between the aorta and the pulmonary artery can be performed. Central shunts, however, are at risk for too much pulmonary blood flow, leading to severe CHF and systemic hypoperfusion.

Total repair of TOF consists of a patch (usually Dacron) closure of the VSD and relief of the pulmonary stenosis. Resection of the infundibular muscle, a patch (pericardium or Dacron) widening of the infundibular region, a pulmonary valvulotomy, and, if necessary, an extension of a patch across the annulus of the pulmonary valve to widen it may all be required to relieve the pulmonary stenosis. In some instances, the pulmonary stenosis is severe and a homograft conduit is placed from the right ventricle to the pulmonary artery to bypass the obstruction. The surgical approach is through a median sternotomy and it is an open-heart surgery requiring cardiopulmonary bypass or deep hypothermia with circulatory arrest. If the child has had a previous shunt, it will be closed.

Complications of total repair include conduction abnormalities (heart block), a residual VSD, residual pulmonary stenosis, and pulmonary valve regurgitation.

Nursing Diagnostic Statements and Collaborative Problems

Preoperative:

High risk for activity intolerance; *risk factors:*

- *Altered tissue perfusion: hypoxic (TET) spells, secondary to insufficient oxygenation associated with decreased pulmonary blood flow.*
- *Polycythemia and hypoxia.*

High risk for altered growth and development: failure to thrive; *risk factor: insufficient oxygen to meet metabolic needs.*

High risk for injury: cerebrovascular accident; *risk factors:*

- *Polycythemia, a blood clot, or air bubble introduced into the venous circulation, proceeding through the VSD into the left ventricle, and entering the systemic circulation.*

Postoperative:

High risk for injury: physiologic; *risk factors:*

- *Complications of Blalock-Taussig procedure (bacterial endocarditis).*
- *Complications of total repair (dysrhythmias [heart block or ventricular ectopy]),*

residual VSD, residual pulmonary stenosis, pulmonary valve regurgitation, bacterial endocarditis.

Nursing Care

Care for these infants and children *prior to surgical repair* should include special emphasis on (1) the provision of *adequate* iron intake (with hypoxia, the need for increased oxygen-carrying capacity requires increased iron for hemoglobin) and (2) scrupulous dental hygiene to reduce the risk of endocarditis.* In addition, when these infants and children have an IV line in place, great care should be taken to avoid forceful unplugging of a clotted needle or other actions that could lead to air in the line. Because these infants or children are cyanotic with a right-to-left shunt, air or a clot may be transported directly to the systemic circulation causing a CVA. Life-long antibiotic prophylaxis for endocarditis for certain procedures is required by all children with TOF.

Parents will require ongoing information about their child's defect and observation of the signs and symptoms their child may exhibit. This information will be provided prior to discharge and on a continuing basis. The symptoms the child exhibits will depend on the obstruction to pulmonary outflow. It is important for the nurse to impress on parents how to assess for increasing cyanosis and decreased exercise tolerance and when to call the physician and the specialty nurse. Parents will need to learn how to recognize and treat a TET spell and notify the doctor. On hearing their child's diagnosis, parents will have numerous concerns and questions. Guidelines for addressing these concerns are addressed in Table 33–15. Parents will require preoperative and preprocedural preparation prior to cardiac catheterization and open-heart surgery, which occurs between 3 months and 2 years. For more in-depth information on cardiac catheterization, refer to Table 33–9 for parental instruction related to cardiac catheterization. Instruction on long-term management will include SBE prophylaxis, school issues, and well child care. The child will require ongoing follow-up after surgery; the frequency will depend on how the child is doing. The nurse must impress on parents the need for long-term follow-up and the potential of long-term sequelae. SBE prophylaxis is necessary preoperatively and postoperatively for dental and surgical procedures. School issues will need to be addressed; these are discussed in detail in the later section entitled "School Environment." Parents need to be encouraged to get well child care for their child.

* Poor dental hygiene can result in swollen, bleeding gums. Bacteria in the mouth can enter the blood stream through the gum lesions and cause endocarditis.

Ebstein Anomaly (Fig. 33–12)

Ebstein anomaly represents approximately 0.5 per cent of congenital heart defects (Adams et al, 1989).

Etiology/Incidence (Pathophysiology)

Ebstein anomaly consists of an abnormally low placement of the tricuspid valve, resulting in a portion of the right ventricle being part of the right atrium. The remaining right ventricular cavity is small. Tricuspid regurgitation is present in varying degrees. Commonly associated cardiac defects are ASD (present in greater than 50 per cent), pulmonary stenosis, pulmonary atresia, and VSD. Ebstein anomaly occurs frequently in infants of mothers who have received lithium during their pregnancy.

The physiology and clinical manifestations of Ebstein anomaly vary widely, depending on the size of the right ventricle and the degree of tricuspid regurgitation. If the tricuspid valve is only minimally displaced downward and mild regurgitation is present, then blood flow approximates normal and symptoms are absent. However, if the tricuspid valve is very displaced and moderate to severe tricuspid regurgitation is present, there is backflow of blood into the right atrium. This backflow of blood elevates right atrial

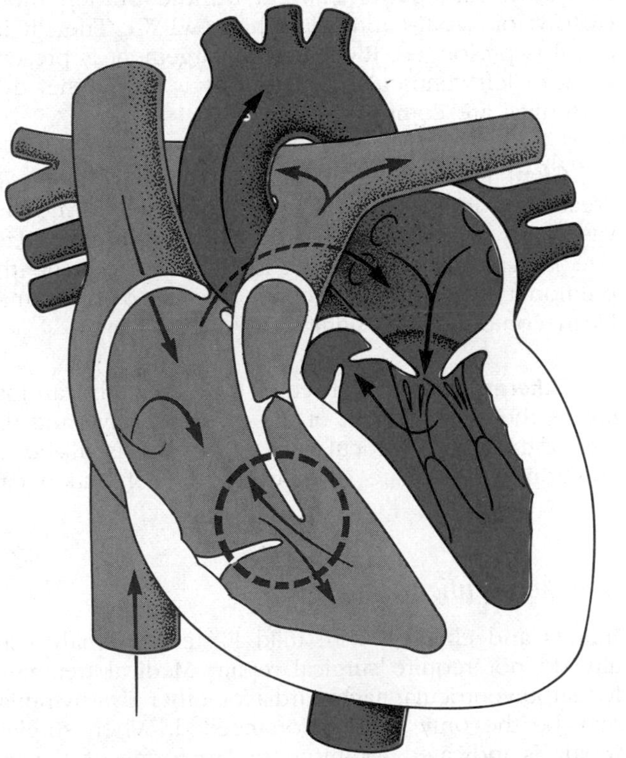

FIGURE 33-12. Ebstein anomaly with tricuspid valve significantly displaced downward in the right ventricle. Leakage occurs through the tricuspid valve back to the right atrium, and unoxygenated blood is shunted across the ASD into the left atrium.

pressure, causing unoxygenated blood to be shunted across the foramen ovale or ASD to the systemic circulation resulting in cyanosis. In addition, infants or children with Ebstein anomaly commonly have paroxysmal supraventricular tachycardia (25 per cent).

Clinical Manifestations

Symptoms vary tremendously with variation of anatomic pathology. Infants may be asymptomatic or may present with cyanosis, CHF, tachycardiac episodes, or some combination of these. The older child commonly has dyspnea on exertion, cyanosis, fatigue, and tachycardiac episodes. Symptoms of tachycardiac episodes include dizzy spells, fatigue, syncope, headaches, chest pain, and a sensation of palpitations or a "racing" heart. Thromboembolism can occur as a sequela of right atrial dilatation with stasis of blood.

Diagnostic Assessment

Cardiac Examination. There is commonly a systolic murmur of grades I–V/VI heard along the lower left sternal border, representing tricuspid regurgitation. Diastolic murmurs are also common.

Electrocardiogram. The ECG usually shows one of two abnormal patterns: right bundle branch block (RBBB) or Wolff-Parkinson-White (WPW). The PR interval is prolonged. Right atrial enlargement is present. Right or left ventricular hypertrophy is rare. Other dysrhythmias are commonly found.

Chest Radiograph. In infants, the heart size is increased (sometimes massively) and the pulmonary vascularity is decreased. In the older child, the heart size is typically normal or slightly increased and the pulmonary vascularity is either decreased or normal. Heart contour varies significantly.

Echocardiogram. With color flow 2-D echocardiography, the displacement of the tricuspid valve and the size of the right ventricular cavity can be visualized. In addition, an estimate of tricuspid valve function can be obtained.

Therapeutic Management

Infants and children with mild Ebstein anomaly usually do not require surgical repair. Medical treatment for supraventricular tachycardia or other dysrhythmias may be the only intervention needed. When surgical repair is indicated for more severe forms of Ebstein anomaly, it is usually not performed in infancy. The surgical procedure involves repositioning and repairing the tricuspid valve to improve its competency. Atrial defects are closed. Sometimes the tricuspid valve needs to be replaced. In addition, plication (stitching folds or tucks in the wall) of the atrialized right ventricle (the portion of the right ventricle that is part of the right atrium) is performed to eliminate supraventricular tachycardias. The surgical approach is through a median sternotomy. This is an open-heart surgery requiring cardiopulmonary bypass.

Antibiotic prophylaxis for certain procedures is necessary in these children to reduce the risk of endocarditis.

Nursing Diagnostic Statements and Collaborative Problems

Preoperative:

High risk for injury; *risk factors: altered tissue perfusion, cerebral, secondary to*

- *Tachycardiac episodes.*
- *CHF in infant.*

Postoperative:

High risk for injury: physiologic; *risk factors: complications, including:*

- *Residual tricuspid regurgitation.*
- *Persistent dysrhythmias.*
- *Bacterial endocarditis.*

Nursing Care

Nursing interventions for perioperative care are found in Table 33–4.

Parents will need information about their child's cardiac defect and associated signs and symptoms in order to effectively observe and manage their child at home. The child's symptoms will depend on the child's cardiac defect. Parental concerns and anxieties will need to be addressed and supported by the nurse. Table 33–15 provides guidelines for responding to these parental needs. Instruction on long-term management will address SBE prophylaxis and well child care. Parents will require instructions on when to notify the cardiologist and the specialty nurse. Parents need to be informed that the child will require SBE prophylaxis preoperatively and postoperatively.

Tricuspid Atresia (Fig. 33–13)

Tricuspid atresia accounts for approximately 2 to 3 per cent of all congenital heart defects (Moller & Neal, 1990).

Etiology/Incidence (Pathophysiology)

The tricuspid valve in this lesion fails to develop and *no communication* exists between the right atrium and the right ventricle. The right ventricle is usually hypoplastic (small) and an ASD or patent foramen ovale is present. A VSD is also commonly present. The pulmonary arteries may be small or normal in size. Additional cardiac defects are present in 30 per

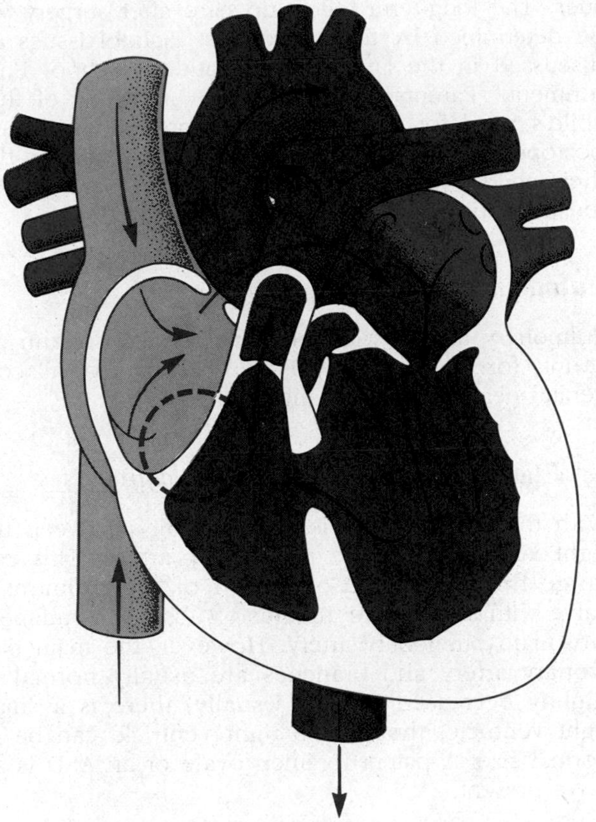

FIGURE 33 - 13. Tricuspid atresia, showing no communication between the right heart chambers. Blood is shunted through the ASD to the left atrium and through the VSD to the pulmonary artery.

cent of these patients, the most common being transposition of the great arteries, persistent left superior vena cava, coarctation of the aorta, and PDA.

In the presence of tricuspid atresia, unoxygenated blood returning to the right atrium cannot pass into the right ventricle. It must therefore pass through an ASD or patent foramen ovale into the left atrium and left ventricle. From the left ventricle, a portion of the blood flow passes through the VSD, if present, into the small right ventricle and the pulmonary circulation. The remaining blood flow goes to the systemic circulation. If no VSD is present, then blood flow to the lungs is solely through the PDA.

Clinical Manifestations

Infants with tricuspid atresia are usually cyanotic at birth. If no VSD is present, then the infant is totally dependent on the PDA for pulmonary blood flow. As the PDA closes, the infant will become profoundly cyanotic, tachypneic, and acidotic. Infants with a large VSD may have excessive pulmonary blood flow and present in CHF. This, however, is uncommon. Older infants and children with a moderate-sized VSD and decreased pulmonary blood flow may have hypoxic spells, delayed growth, and clubbing.

Diagnostic Assessment

Cardiac Examination. Murmurs of associated heart defects such as VSD and PDA are usually present.

Electrocardiogram. Right and left atrial enlargement, decreased or absent right ventricular forces, and left ventricular hypertrophy are typically found.

Chest Radiograph. The heart size can be normal or increased. The pulmonary vascularity may be decreased (most common), normal, or increased.

Echocardiogram. The absence of a tricuspid valve, the size of the right ventricle, and the presence of other cardiac defects, such as a VSD, can be identified with 2-D echocardiography.

Therapeutic Management

Infants who are dependent on the PDA for pulmonary blood flow are given continuous infusion of prostaglandin E_1 (PGE_1) to maintain patency of the ductus arteriosus until a systemic-to-pulmonary shunt such as the *Blalock-Taussig shunt* (see previous description) can be performed. PGE_1 is administered at dosages of 0.05 to 0.1 μg/kg/minute intravenously; *it must be administered with a continuous infusion pump.* Intermittent delivery of PGE_1 may allow the PDA to close. Apnea is the most common side effect of PGE_1, followed by hypotension from vasodilatation. Intubation and ventilatory support may be needed (Merenstein et al, 1985). The infant must be continually monitored for signs of hypotension. Appropriate agents to support blood pressure, if necessary, should be on hand.

Infants with a VSD and adequate pulmonary blood flow do not require a systemic-to-pulmonary shunt. If inadequate atrial communication exists (3 mmHg pressure gradient), a *balloon atrial septostomy* (see later description) may be performed in the cardiac catheterization laboratory to ensure a large interatrial communication. The right atrium has no outlet other than through the interatrial communication.

The total repair for tricuspid atresia involves creation of a communication between the right atrium and the pulmonary artery or the right ventricle by direct anastomosis or a conduit. The ASD and VSD, if present, as well as any previous systemic-to-pulmonary shunts, such as the Blalock-Taussig, are closed. This repair is typically referred to as the *Fontan procedure;* however, there are numerous variations of the procedure. Ideally, the procedure is performed at 4 to 5 years of age. Some institutions are having success with patients 2 years of age. The surgical approach is through a median sternotomy, and is an open-heart procedure requiring cardiopulmonary bypass. Complications of surgical repair include CHF, pleural effusions, renal failure, residual VSD, conduit obstruction, and dysrhythmias. Children with tricuspid atresia require life-long antibiotic prophylaxis for endocarditis for certain procedures.

Nursing Diagnostic Statements and Collaborative Problems

Preoperative:

Altered tissue perfusion: *systemic hypoxia related to decreased pulmonary blood flow.*

Impaired physical mobility and fatigue *related to activity intolerance secondary to insufficient oxygenation resulting from decreased pulmonary blood flow or shunting of unoxygenated blood into the systemic circulation.*

High risk for altered growth and development: failure to thrive; *risk factor: inadequate oxygenation of blood to meet metabolic needs.*

Postoperative:

High risk for injury: physiologic; *risk factors:*
- *Complications of Blalock-Taussig procedure (see under "Tetralogy of Fallot").*
- *Complications of Fontan procedure:*
  CHF.
  Pleural effusions. Defining characteristics: If small effusion, asymptomatic; if large accumulation, cough, dyspnea, retractions, tachypnea, cyanosis.
  Renal failure. Defining characteristics: Urine output less than 1 ml/kg/hr, rising BUN and creatinine.
  Residual VSD.
  Conduit obstruction.
  Dysrhythmias.

Nursing Care

Nursing interventions related to perioperative care are discussed in Tables 33–4 and 23–7.

Parents will need information about their child's defect and signs and symptoms of changes in their child's condition. These symptoms will include cyanosis, decreased exercise tolerance, increased irritability and fussiness, changes in neurologic status, and signs of stroke (see section on cyanosis for more detailed information). The nurse will review medical and surgical treatment plans with parents and discuss timing and indications for palliation and surgical repair. Total repair is done at approximately 2 years of age. Initially, on hearing their child's diagnosis, parents will have numerous questions and concerns. Table 33–15 provides guidelines for addressing some of these concerns with parents. The child and family will require preparation prior to surgical intervention. Instruction on long-term needs will include follow-up care, SBE prophylaxis, well child care, and school issues. The long-term follow-up care after surgery will be determined by the cardiologist. School issues are discussed in the later section entitled "School Environment." Parents will need to be informed of their child's need for SBE prophylaxis preoperatively and postoperatively. Parents will need to be reminded that their child's well child care should be managed by the pediatrician.

Pulmonary Atresia (Fig. 33–14)

Pulmonary atresia with intact ventricular septum accounts for approximately 1 to 3 per cent of all congenital heart defects (Adams et al, 1989).

Etiology/Incidence (Pathophysiology)

With this lesion, there is no continuity between the right ventricle and the pulmonary artery. This can range from complete occlusion of the pulmonary valve with small valve annulus to absent or rudimentary main pulmonary artery. However, the main pulmonary artery and branches are usually normal to slightly decreased in size. Usually, there is a small right ventricle, though the right ventricle can be of normal size. A patent foramen ovale or an ASD is always present.

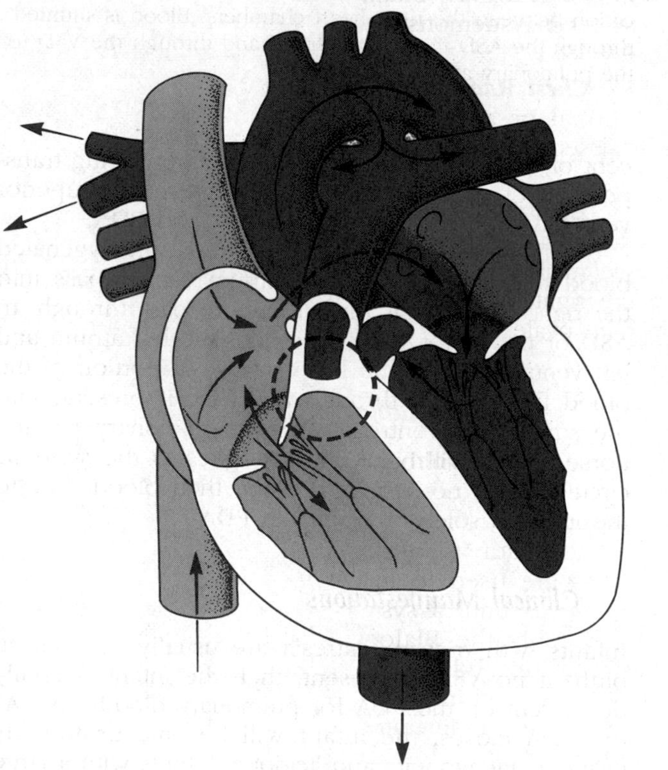

FIGURE 33-14. Pulmonary atresia with small right ventricle, ASD, and patent ductus arteriosus. Abnormal blood flow is from the right chambers through the ASD to the left side of the heart. Blood can reach the lungs only through a patent ductus arteriosus.

The blood flow in the presence of pulmonary atresia is similar to that of tricuspid atresia. Unoxygenated blood returning to the right atrium bypasses the right ventricle, flowing through the interatrial communication to the left atrium and left ventricle. Some blood may enter the right ventricle through the tricuspid valve; however, because no outlet exists to the right ventricle, the blood then flows back through the triscuspid into the right atrium. The only pathway through which blood can reach the lungs is the PDA. The PDA varies in size and determines the amount of pulmonary blood flow.

Clinical Manifestations

These infants become cyanotic and tachypneic shortly after birth. The degree of cyanosis depends on the amount of pulmonary blood flow through the PDA.

Diagnostic Assessment

Cardiac Examination. The second heart sound is single because the pulmonary valve closure component is absent. There may be systolic murmurs of either the PDA or tricuspid regurgitation.

Electrocardiogram. Right atrial enlargement is present, and, typically, left ventricular hypertrophy is found. However, infants with normal-sized right ventricles may demonstrate right ventricular hypertrophy.

Chest Radiograph. The chest radiograph may be normal or show an increased heart size and decreased pulmonary vascularity.

Echocardiogram. 2-D echocardiography can demonstrate the atretic pulmonary valve, the size of the main and branch pulmonary arteries, the size of the right ventricle, and the size of the ASD or foramen ovale.

Therapeutic Management

These infants will be cyanotic shortly after birth, and, if the PDA closes, they will become profoundly hypoxemic with severe cyanosis and acidosis progressing to death if no intervention is made. PGE_1 infusions are used to maintain patency of the ductus arteriosus until a systemic-to-pulmonary shunt (most commonly the Blalock-Taussig shunt) can be performed. In addition, a balloon atrial septostomy may be performed in the cardiac catheterization laboratory to enlarge the interatrial communication from right to left atrium, if pulmonary valvotomy is not planned.

If the right ventricle is of adequate size, some institutions perform a pulmonary valvulotomy or a pulmonary outflow patch procedure in addition to a shunt. This establishes an open pathway through the atretic valve area between the pulmonary artery and the right ventricle. Blood flow through the right ventricle and pulmonary artery will then promote growth of these areas.

Total repair of pulmonary atresia depends on the size of the right ventricle. If there has been adequate growth of the ventricle, followed by closure of any previous systemic-to-pulmonary shunts, closure of the ASD will be performed. The pulmonary outflow tract will be enlarged. A patch or a conduit will be placed, connecting the right ventricle to right atrium. The timing of total repair varies among institutions. Complications of surgery include CHF, pleural effusions, renal or liver failure, conduit obstruction, and dysrhythmias. A Fontan procedure is used in cases of pulmonary atresia and hypoplastic right ventricle.

Life-long antibiotic prophylaxis for endocarditis when undergoing certain procedures is required by these children, as well as long-term follow-up by a cardiologist.

Nursing Diagnostic Statements and Collaborative Problems

Preoperative:

Altered tissue perfusion: systemic hypoxia, *related to the inability to pump an adequate amount of blood to the lungs, associated with obstruction of the pulmonary artery.*

Impaired physical mobility and fatigue *related to activity intolerance, secondary to insufficient oxygen resulting from decreased pulmonary blood flow or shunting of unoxygenated blood into the systemic circulation.*

Postoperative:

High risk for injury: physiologic; *risk factors:*

- *Complications of Blalock-Taussig procedure (see under "Tetralogy of Fallot").*
- *Complications of Fontan procedure (see under "Tricuspid Atresia").*
- *Bacterial endocarditis (with both procedures). Defining characteristics: Fever, bacteremia.*
- *Complications of conduit placement.*

Nursing Care

Nursing interventions related to the perioperative care are discussed in Tables 33–4 and 23–7.

The nurse will need to inform and reinforce information previously provided to parents about the nature of their child's cardiac defect and about observation of symptoms that indicate changes in their child's cardiac status. Changes parents should be alerted to are increased cyanosis and decreased exercise tolerance. (These are discussed in detail in the section entitled "Cyanosis.") On hearing their child's diagnosis, parents will have questions and concerns about how this cardiac defect will affect their child's life and that of their family. Table 33–15 provides guidelines for addressing these issues with parents. The nurse will provide parents with preoperative preparation as palliative repair is done. Instruction on long-term management and the child's requirement for SBE prophylaxis will be needed preoperatively and postoperatively.

Mixed Circulation Defects

Complete D-Transposition of the Great Arteries (Fig. 33–15)

Complete d-transposition of the great arteries (TGA) is a cyanotic defect that accounts for about 9 per cent of congenital heart defects (Gersony, 1987).

Etiology/Incidence (Pathophysiology)

The aorta arises from the right ventricle and the pulmonary artery arises from the left ventricle, resulting in *two separate and parallel circulatory systems*. TGA occurs much more often in males than in females and usually in term infants (Adams et al, 1989). Cardiac defects commonly associated with TGA are PDA, ASD, VSD, and VSD with or without pulmonary stenosis.

With the great arteries transposed, the pulmonary artery, arising from the left ventricle, delivers blood to the lungs for oxygenation. This oxygenated blood returns to the left atrium and left ventricle and is recycled again through the pulmonary circulation. The aorta, arising from the right side of the heart, delivers unoxygenated blood to the systemic circulation. This blood then returns to the right atrium and ventricle and, without being oxygenated, is circulated back to the systemic circulation via the aorta with progressive hypoxemia. The major physiologic abnormalities in TGA are an oxygen deficiency in the tissues and an excessive workload on the right and left ventricles. The only mixing of oxygenated and unoxygenated blood occurs in the presence of associated lesions (patent foramen ovale, ASD, VSD, PDA, or collateral circulation). The extent of the mixing depends on the number, size, and position of the anatomic communications, and the pressure differential between the two systems. Without the presence of an associated lesion, death results.

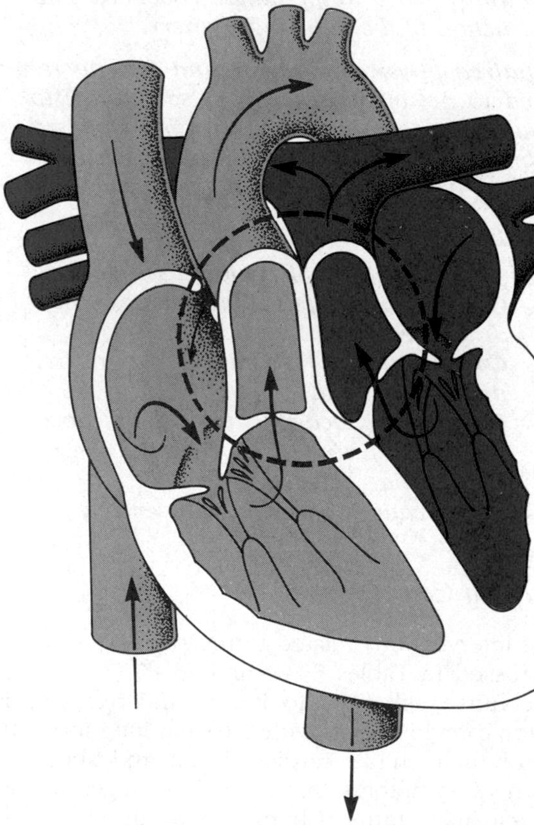

FIGURE 33-15. Complete D-transposition of the great arteries with an associated ASD. Blood flow exists as two parallel systems—one recirculating oxygenated blood, the other recirculating unoxygenated blood. Mixing occurs only through defects such as the ASD shown here.

Clinical Manifestations

TGA is diagnosed in infancy. Cyanosis is always present and the degree will depend on the amount of intercirculatory mixing present. Cyanosis may be mild if the mixing occurs through a large VSD or PDA. Cyanosis is profound if the ventricular septum is intact or the PDA is closing, or both. Hypoxic spells may be frequent, especially during crying or exertion. Infants, especially those with a large VSD, may present in CHF. Clubbing secondary to cyanosis may be seen in older children.

Diagnostic Assessment

Cardiac Examination. Murmurs, if present, are usually those of associated cardiac defects such as a PDA or a VSD. The second heart sound is single and increased in intensity because of the aorta rising from the right ventricle (the anterior ventricle).

Electrocardiogram. The ECG may be normal for a neonate or demonstrate right ventricular hypertrophy. Left ventricular hypertrophy or combined ventricular hypertrophy is uncommon.

Chest Radiograph. Heart size may be normal or moderately enlarged. The cardiac silhouette may assume the shape of an egg lying on a string and the pulmonary vascularity may be normal, increased, or decreased, depending on the extent of the defect.

Echocardiogram. The color flow 2-D echocardiogram is extremely useful in establishing the diagnosis and evaluating the presence of associated cardiac defects.

Therapeutic Management

Oxygen therapy in the profoundly cyanotic neonate with TGA may be harmful. It may enhance closure of the PDA, which may be the only source of mixing in TGA. Only a certain amount of oxygenated blood is able to reach the systemic circulation, and administration of additional oxygen does not improve this situation.* Enlargement of the interatrial communication by *atrial balloon septostomy (Rashkind procedure)* during cardiac catheterization is critical in establishing adequate mixing of oxygenated and unoxygenated blood for these infants. A Rashkind procedure is performed by passing a balloon catheter through the foramen ovale, inflating the balloon, and pulling the catheter back to tear and stretch open the foramen ovale and create an enlarged opening between the two atria. Creation of an ASD or enlargement of the foramen ovale surgically is termed a *Blalock-Hanlon procedure*. Following these palliative procedures, the infant will continue to be cyanotic, especially in times of stress (crying, feeding, or exposure to cold temperatures). However, oxygenation should be sufficient for the infant to thrive until the time for total repair.

Several surgical procedures exist for total repair of TGA; three are discussed here.

The *arterial switch operation* is the preferred surgical repair for TGA at this time. The Mustard and Senning procedures involve intra-atrial redirection of blood flow. With the *Mustard procedure*, a new atrial septum is created by using pericardium to make a baffle. This baffle alters the blood flow by redirecting unoxygenated blood from the right atrium through the mitral valve to the left ventricle and out to the lungs via the pulmonary artery; oxygenated blood from the left atrium is redirected through the tricuspid valve to the right ventricle and to the systemic circulation via the aorta. The *Senning procedure* creates the same redirection of blood flow, but without the use of a pericardial patch. The atrial septum and a portion of the atrial wall are used to reroute the blood flow. Both the Mustard and the Senning procedures have been very successful, with a low mortality rate. Timing of repair varies among institutions; however, most commonly, repair is recommended in the first year of life. Surgical repair should be performed before pulmonary vascular changes develop.

Complications of the Mustard and Senning procedures include: (1) superior vena cava or inferior vena cava obstruction, (2) dysrhythmias, (3) tricuspid regurgitation, and (4) obstruction of the pulmonary veins (a severe complication requiring immediate correction).

The third type of total repair is the arterial anatomic correction or the *arterial switch procedure*. In this procedure, the pulmonary artery and the aorta are transected above the respective valves and "switched" back to the appropriate ventricles. The pulmonary artery then arises from the right ventricle and the aorta from the left ventricle. The coronary arteries are resected with a button of surrounding tissue and reanastomosed to the supravalvar area of the new ascending aorta. In performing this procedure, it is essential that the left ventricular pressure be near systemic. In infants with a VSD, the pressure tends to be equal in both ventricles, in which case this procedure may be postponed for several days or even months. However, infants with intact ventricular septa require surgery within the first month of life before left ventricular pressures begin to decrease. Once left ventricle pressure has decreased, the left ventricle is no longer prepared to pump to the systemic circulation. This procedure has been performed successfully and has been the procedure of choice in many institutions since 1975. Complications include (1) coronary artery stenosis, (2) myocardial ischemia and infarction, and (3) dysrhythmias. The Le Compte procedure is done to prevent pulmonary stenosis (Adams et al, 1989).

The three total repair procedures described are all performed through a median sternotomy and are open-heart procedures requiring cardiopulmonary bypass or deep hypothermia. Children with TGA require antibiotic prophylaxis for endocarditis for certain procedures and close cardiology follow-up. Without treatment, 90 per cent of infants with TGA will die within the first year of life.

*Prostaglandins may be used to keep the ductus open until a palliative procedure or surgery is performed.

Nursing Diagnostic Statements and Collaborative Problems

Preoperative:

High risk for altered protection; *risk factor: altered tissue perfusion, systemic hypoxia, secondary to oxygenated blood being recirculated through the lungs and unoxygenated blood being recirculated through the body. Defining characteristics: Cyanosis, activity intolerance.*

Postoperative:

High risk for injury: physiologic; *risk factors:*

- *Complications of Mustard or Senning procedures, such as obstruction of the vena cavae, dysrhythmias, tricuspid regurgitation, obstruction of the pulmonary veins.*
- *Complications of the arterial switch procedure, such as coronary artery stenosis, dysrhythmias, pulmonary stenosis, aortic insufficiency.*

Nursing Care

Nursing interventions for perioperative care are found in Table 33–4.

Prior to discharge and on an ongoing basis, parents will require information and reinforcement of information about their child's cardiac defect as well as about signs and symptoms the child may demonstrate that would indicate a worsening of the child's condition. Parents will have many questions and concerns about their child's diagnosis and the impact it will have on their child. Table 33–15 provides guidelines for addressing these concerns. Parents will need preoperative preparation prior to the arterial switch, which is done within the first few weeks of the infant's life. Discharge instructions will include the child's need to be on medications including digoxin, furosemide, or potassium-sparing diuretic and potassium supplements. The parents will need information about the reasons for the medication, methods of administration, and untoward effects to observe for. Instructions also will include indications for contacting the cardiologist. Parents will need to know that SBE prophylaxis will be required preoperatively and postoperatively with any dental or surgical procedure. Parents will need to follow up on their child's well child care, since the child has other medical needs common to all children.

Total Anomalous Pulmonary Venous Connection (Fig. 33–16)

Total anomalous pulmonary venous connection (TAPVC) accounts for approximately 2 per cent of all congenital heart defects (Moller & Neal, 1990).

Etiology/Incidence (Pathophysiology)

In TAPVC, the pulmonary veins do not connect with the left atrium; rather, they connect directly to the right atrium or one of the systemic veins. The four main types of TAPVC are (1) supracardiac (most common), in which the pulmonary veins drain into the superior vena cava through the innominate vein; (2) cardiac, in which the pulmonary veins drain into the coronary sinus or directly into the right atrium; (3) infracardiac, in which the four veins join behind the heart and travel through the diaphragm connecting to the portal venous system; and (4) mixed, in which the pulmonary veins enter the systemic venous system at more than one site (Merenstein et al, 1985). Each of these types of anomalous connections can occur with or without

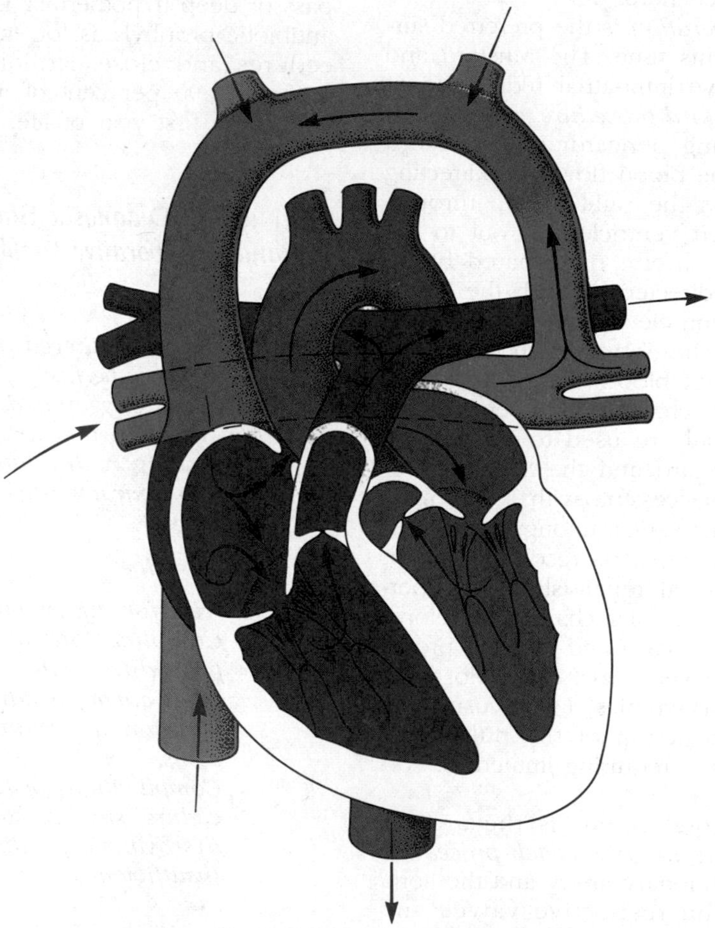

FIGURE 33-16. Total anomalous pulmonary venous connection (supracardiac, showing pulmonary veins connected to left innominate vein). The presence of an ASD is necessary to allow blood to reach the left side of the heart.

obstruction of the pulmonary veins. Approximately 33 per cent of patients with TAPVC have other associated cardiac defects or a congenitally absent spleen.

In the presence of TAPVC, blood flow depends on where the pulmonary veins connect and the presence or absence of pulmonary venous obstruction. In all varieties of TAPVC, both systemic (unoxygenated) and pulmonary venous (oxygenated) blood is returning ultimately to the right atrium. The only pathway for blood to reach the left atrium, left ventricle, and the body is through an ASD or patent foramen ovale. If there is no pulmonary venous obstruction, then blood flow to the lungs is excessive and only mild cyanosis is present. These infants often present with heart failure. If pulmonary venous obstruction is present, then blood flow to the lungs is limited and cyanosis is severe. In addition, pulmonary edema usually occurs owing to increased pulmonary venous pressure.

Clinical Manifestations

Infants with TAPVC without pulmonary venous obstruction may not exhibit symptoms until several weeks to months of life when PVR drops. These infants are usually only mildly cyanotic and present with tachypnea, feeding difficulties, failure-to-thrive, increased respiratory infections, and heart failure. Infants with pulmonary venous obstruction are symptomatic very early, usually at birth. Cyanosis, tachypnea, dyspnea, feeding difficulties, and heart failure are present within the first few days of life.

Diagnostic Assessment

Cardiac Examination. In patients without pulmonary venous obstruction, the cardiac examination may be similar to that of a child with an ASD including a systolic murmur; wide, fixed splitting of the second heart sound; and a tricuspid diastolic flow murmur. In patients with pulmonary venous obstruction, there are usually no murmurs and the pulmonary component of the second heart sound is accentuated.

Electrocardiogram. The ECG may show right ventricular hypertrophy and right atrial enlargement.

Chest Radiograph. With pulmonary venous obstruction, the heart size is usually normal; however, a pattern of pulmonary edema may be seen. Without pulmonary venous obstruction, heart size and pulmonary vascularity are both increased.

Echocardiogram. A color flow 2-D echocardiogram is helpful in determining the presence and type of TAPVC; however, it is difficult to visualize this cardiac defect on echocardiogram. A single large pulmonary vein can sometimes be seen draining into the superior vena cava or an extra cavity visualized behind the left atrium. Doppler can document the presence of obstruction.

Therapeutic Management

Infants with obstructed pulmonary veins require surgical repair urgently. Infants with unobstructed pulmonary veins may be treated medically for heart failure, if necessary, before undergoing surgical repair. The surgical repair will depend on the type of TAPVC present. Surgery is performed through a median sternotomy and is an open-heart procedure requiring cardiopulmonary bypass or deep hypothermia with circulatory arrest. Supracardiac and infracardiac TAPVC require reimplantation of the pulmonary veins into the left atrium and closure of the ASD. Intracardiac TAPVC is repaired by realigning the atrial septum during closure of the ASD and directing the anomalous veins to the left atrial side.

Complications of surgical repair for all types of TAPVC are pulmonary venous obstruction and dysrhythmias.

Nursing Diagnostic Statements and Collaborative Problems

Preoperative:

High risk for activity intolerance; *risk factors: CHF secondary to increased cardiac workload and excessive pulmonary blood flow.*

High risk for injury: physiologic; *risk factors:*
- *Pulmonary venous obstruction.*
- *Dysrhythmias.*
- *Altered tissue perfusion: systemic secondary to lack of oxygenated blood reaching left ventricle.*

High risk for altered growth and development: failure to thrive; *risk factors:*
- *Feeding difficulties associated with respiratory distress and fatigue.*
- *Increased basal metabolic rate.*
- *Increased tissue perfusion (bounding pulses). Defining characteristics: Height and weight less than the 3rd percentile; developmental delays.*

Postoperative:

High risk for injury: physiologic; *risk factor: bacterial endocarditis.*

Impaired physical mobility and fatigue related to activity intolerance *secondary to heart's inability to pump an adequate supply of blood to meet the body's metabolic needs.*

High risk for ineffective breathing patterns; *risk factors:*
- *Weakness.*
- *Pain.*
- *Pre-existing pulmonary hypertension.*

Nursing Care

Nursing diagnostic responses and nursing interventions for postoperative care are found in Tables 33–4 and 23–7.

Prior to discharge and on an ongoing basis, information on the child's defect and the surgical interventions the child will undergo to correct the defect need to be discussed with the parents. Parents will need to be instructed on the recognition of changes in the child's cardiac status related to cyanosis and CHF prior to having the repair done (see sections on "Cyanosis" and "Congestive Heart Failure" for more detailed discussion). Parents will have many questions and concerns on hearing their child's diagnosis. Table 33–15 addresses these parental concerns. Prior to total correction the child will undergo a cardiac catheterization. Parents will require preparation prior to the catheterization and surgical preparation. Refer to Table 33–9 for parental instruction about cardiac catheterization. Prior to correction, parents will need instruction regarding medication administration, monitoring for untoward reactions, and preparation for cardiac catheterization. Following correction, parents will be instructed by the nurse to observe for signs and symptoms of CHF since it is the first sign observed that indicates that the correction is being obstructed (see section on "Congestive Heart Failure" for detailed discussion). Instructions on long-term management will include the child's need for lifelong follow-up on an annual basis, and the requirement for SBE prophylaxis preoperatively and postoperatively with any dental or surgical procedure. Lastly, parents will need to be reminded of the child's need for well child care to attend to the health care needs common to all children.

Truncus Arteriosus (Fig. 33–17)

Truncus arteriosus accounts for approximately 1 to 4 per cent of congenital heart defects (Adams et al, 1989).

Etiology/Incidence (Pathophysiology)

Truncus arteriosus results from the incomplete septation and division of the common truncal vessel. It is characterized by one great artery arising from the left and right ventricles overriding a large VSD. This common artery has one valve, usually with two to four cusps, and gives rise to the pulmonary, coronary, and systemic arteries. Truncus arteriosus is classified into three types, depending on the origin of the pulmonary arteries.

Type I—A short, main pulmonary artery arises from the common trunk and divides into the right and left pulmonary arteries.

Type II—The right and left pulmonary arteries arise directly from the posterior surface of the common trunk.

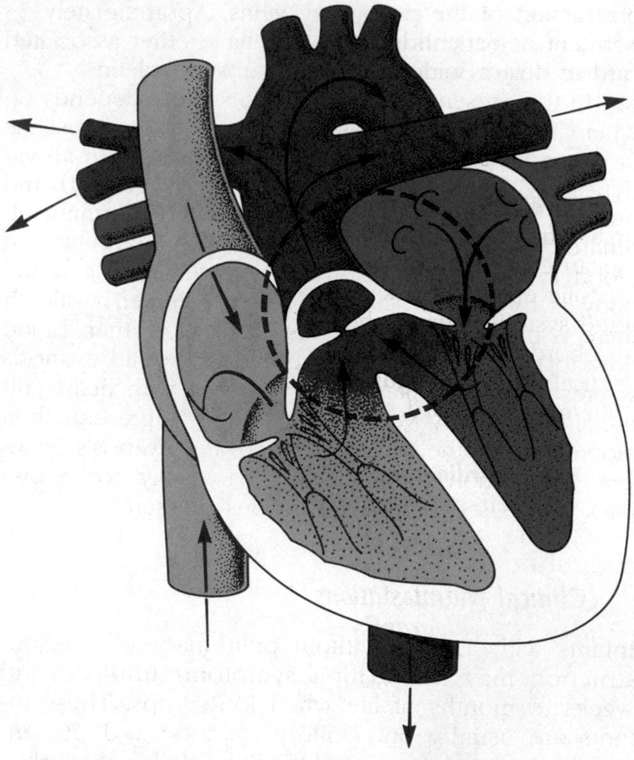

FIGURE 33-17. Type II truncus arteriosus. Blood flow is from both ventricles into a common great artery that overrides a VSD.

Type III—The right and left pulmonary arteries arise directly from the lateral walls of the common trunk (Merenstein et al, 1985).

Commonly associated cardiac anomalies include a right aortic arch (30 to 35 per cent), an interrupted aortic arch, absent ductus arteriosus, PDA, ASD, unilateral absence of a pulmonary artery, and truncal valve regurgitation.

In the presence of truncus arteriosus, the common trunk receives a mixture of unoxygenated blood from the right ventricle and oxygenated blood from the left ventricle. Blood flow to the lungs varies with the type of truncus and the PVR but is usually increased and at systemic level pressure. When pulmonary blood flow is adequate or increased, minimal cyanosis is present. These infants with increased pulmonary blood flow (at systemic level pressure) are at high risk for developing early pulmonary vascular disease.

Clinical Manifestations

Infants may present in CHF and/or cyanosis shortly after birth or between 2 and 3 weeks of age. The presence of CHF will depend on the amount of pulmonary blood flow. The persistent high PVR in the first few weeks of life (see section on "Changes in Circulation after Birth") will decrease pulmonary blood flow and CHF may not be present. However, if the truncal valve is regurgitant, then CHF will be present shortly after birth. If pulmonary blood flow is increased, the child may have bounding peripheral pulses and a widened pulse pressure.

Diagnostic Assessment

Cardiac Examination. The first heart sound is normal. The second heart sound will be single and loud because of the single valve of the common trunk. A systolic ejection click may be heard. There may be a loud systolic murmur heard best at the lower left sternal border and radiating throughout the chest. If the truncal valve is regurgitant, a blowing diastolic murmur may be heard.

Electrocardiogram. Combined ventricular hypertrophy and left atrial enlargement are most often seen. Right ventricular hypertrophy alone may be seen with normal or decreased pulmonary blood flow.

Chest Radiograph. Increased heart size and increased pulmonary vascularity as well as an absent pulmonary artery segment are typically found.

Echocardiogram. With a color flow 2-D echocardiogram and continuous wave Doppler the truncus arteriosus defect can be visualized and most often the type can be identified as well as the presence of truncal valve stenosis or regurgitation, or both.

Therapeutic Management

Infants with truncus arteriosus are treated medically, if possible, during the first few months of life. They generally require treatment for CHF and/or preventing complications of hypoxemia. Surgical repair can be either palliative or total. Palliative surgery consists of placing a band around the pulmonary artery or arteries to decrease pulmonary blood flow until full surgical repair can be performed. This procedure is thought to prevent pulmonary vascular damage until the child is older and can undergo a full repair. Pulmonary artery banding, however, is not always successful in preventing pulmonary vascular disease and can distort the pulmonary arteries. Therefore, the trend is to perform a total repair as soon as is safely possible. Complete surgical repair consists of separating the pulmonary artery or arteries from the common trunk, closing the VSD with a patch (ensuring that the common trunk now arises from the left ventricle), and inserting a right ventricular-to-pulmonary artery valved conduit. The conduit may be of prosthetic material with a porcine valve or may be a homograft conduit. The surgical approach is through a median sternotomy and is an open-heart procedure requiring cardiopulmonary bypass or deep hypothermia with circulatory arrest.

Complications and residual effects include residual VSDs, truncal valve regurgitation, conduit obstruction, and pulmonary vascular disease. These children require antibiotic prophylaxis for endocarditis for certain procedures, and continued follow-up with a cardiologist. Repeat operations are required to replace the conduit as the child grows.

Nursing Diagnostic Statements and Collaborative Problems

Preoperative:

High risk for activity intolerance; *risk factor: CHF secondary to increased cardiac workload and excessive pulmonary blood flow.*

High risk for impaired gas exchange; *risk factors:*

- *Lungs receiving more blood at higher pressure.*
- *Mixing of oxygenated and unoxygenated blood.*

Postoperative:

High risk for injury: physiologic; *risk factors:*

- *Residual VSDs.*
- *Truncal valve regurgitation/obstruction.*
- *Conduit obstruction.*
- *Pulmonary vascular disease.*
- *Conduction disturbance (from VSD closure).*

Nursing Care

Nursing interventions for perioperative care are found in Tables 33–4 and 27–3.

Prior to discharge and on an ongoing basis, parents will need information about their child's cardiac defect and about observing the signs and symptoms of CHF and cyanosis (refer to sections on "Congestive Heart Failure" and "Cyanosis"). On receiving the child's diagnosis of truncus arteriosus, parents will have many questions, concerns, and anxieties about the impact of the cardiac defect on their child. Table 33–15 provides guidelines for addressing these parental concerns and questions. The parents will require instruction about administration of medications, since the infant will likely be on digoxin, furosemide, or a potassium-sparing diuretic and potassium supplement. Parents, and later the child, will need preparation prior to this surgery, as well as other operations, since the child usually undergoes surgical intervention during the first few months. The child will require multiple operations to replace the conduits as he or she grows. Instruction on long-term management will include follow-up care, SBE prophylaxis, school issues, and well child care. Parents will need to know that the cardiologist will see their child every few months prior to surgery and postoperatively, semiannually and annually, on a lifelong basis. The child will require SBE prophylaxis preoperatively and postoperatively. School issues will be of particular concern to parents and child. These school issues are discussed in the later section entitled "School Environment." Parents will need to be encouraged to continue well child and adolescent care for their child to address the other health needs of the child.

Hypoplastic Left Heart Syndrome

Hypoplastic left heart syndrome (HLHS) accounts for approximately 3 per cent of all congenital heart defects (Hoffman, 1990).

Etiology/Incidence (Pathophysiology)

HLHS is characterized by a range of left-sided heart defects including hypoplasia of the aorta, severe aortic valve stenosis or atresia, and severe mitral valve stenosis or atresia. The left ventricle and ascending aorta are usually small or hypoplastic. Blood flow to the coronary arteries is usually retrograde (having a backward flow) through the hypoplastic ascending aorta.

Typically, the small left ventricle is unable to sustain adequate cardiac output to the systemic circulation. In the presence of aortic or mitral atresia, or both, the only blood flow to the systemic circulation is through the PDA.

Clinical Manifestations

These infants may be cyanotic or have severe pallor and grayish skin as the ductus arteriosus begins to close. They may present in a state of vascular collapse with tachypnea, dyspnea, decreased blood pressures in all extremities, grunting, nasal flaring, and hypothermia. Heart failure is almost always present.

Diagnostic Assessment

Cardiac Examination. The second heart sound is single, owing to the absence of the aortic valve closure component. A soft systolic ejection murmur is heard in most infants.

Electrocardiogram. Right atrial enlargement and right ventricular hypertrophy are usually present.

Chest Radiograph. The heart size is increased, and increased pulmonary vascularity as well as pulmonary edema are seen.

Echocardiogram. With 2-D echocardiography the size of the left ventricle, presence or absence of the aortic and mitral valves, and sizes of the ascending aorta, right ventricle, right atrium, and pulmonary artery can be visualized.

Therapeutic Management

Without surgical intervention, approximately 95 per cent of these infants will die within the first month of life (Adams et al, 1989). PGE is necessary for survival until treatment decisions can be made. However, the surgical repair currently available is a palliative procedure that has had limited but increasing success over time and is often dependent on the institution doing the procedure. The *Norwood procedure* is a surgical palliation of two to three stages approved to treat infants with HLHS. Stage I creates continuity from the single right ventricle to the aorta to ensure adequate systemic perfusion, places an aorta-to-pulmonary shunt to establish near-normal pulmonary blood flow and pressures, and provides interatrial communication, which decreases pulmonary obstruction. Stages II and III of the repair are modifications of the Fontan procedure. The mortality rates of infants who have undergone first-stage palliation operations vary from 53 to 91 per cent. Overall outcomes are uncertain because of the small numbers and lack of long-term follow-up. Recently, cardiac transplantation has been performed in some infants with HLHS (Bailey & Gundry, 1990). Cardiac transplantation in infants, however, is considered a controversial procedure. Ethical considerations require that all three options should be presented to parents—that is, do nothing, the Norwood procedure, and cardiac transplantation. Parents will require support from members of the team for whatever decision they make.

The families of these infants require maximal support if they take their infants home to die. Public health nurses and community hospice programs can provide the family with daily support (if necessary) and long-term counseling. The infant may survive at home as long as several months. The family attempting to cope with this situation will be under enormous stress. Not all families are able to deal with the stress of having their infant at home. The family should always be given the option of hospitalization, placing the infant in an alternative treatment facility, or surgical palliation at any time. Regardless of whether the infant is in the home or at a treatment facility, the family will require ongoing support and help with the grieving process. After the death of the infant, it is particularly important that the support be continued for as long as the family needs it.

Nursing Diagnostic Statements and Collaborative Problems

Preoperative:

Impaired physical mobility and fatigue related to activity intolerance *secondary to ineffective left ventricle.*

Impaired physical mobility and fatigue related to activity intolerance *secondary to insufficient oxygenation resulting from obstruction of blood flow from right ventricle.*

High risk for injury: physiologic; risk factors:
- *Profound ductal constriction, resulting in myocardial ischemia.*
- *Ineffective muscular structure of septal wall.*

Nursing Care

Initially, parents will require supportive care while in the hospital as they decide what course to pursue—to do nothing and let their child die, or to consent to surgical intervention such as heart transplantation or the Norwood procedure. If parents choose to let their child die, they will require physical and emotional support while the infant is extubated. If the infant survives long enough to be taken home, then home care support is needed to assist parents to cope with their child's death and dying. Parents will need to understand the reasons for the death, and they need to be forewarned that they may find their infant dead in bed. (See Chapter 20, "Death and Dying," for nursing care for parents anticipating their child's death.)

If the child undergoes the Norwood procedure, parents will need instruction on what to anticipate when their infant is in pediatric intensive care. Parents will require information about the Norwood procedure, and postoperatively how to assess for signs and symptoms of CHF, changes in cyanosis, and changes in neurologic status (see sections on "Congestive Heart Failure" and "Cyanosis" for more detailed information). Other postoperative instruction will include information on the administration of medications and the observation of side effects. If parents decide to choose transplantation, then the nurse reinforces information given about transplantation and the ongoing issues associated with it. Following the cardiac transplant, parents will require information regarding the administration of medications, issues related to transplantation, and psychosocial and developmental concerns.

Obstructive Lesions

Pulmonary Stenosis (Fig. 33–18)

Isolated pulmonary stenosis, which exists in 5 to 10 per cent of all patients with congenital heart disease (Adams et al, 1989), is an obstructive lesion that interferes with blood flow out of the right ventricle.

Etiology/Incidence (Pathophysiology)

Obstruction may occur below the pulmonary valve in the infundibular area (subvalvar), above the valve (supravalvar), or at the valve (valvar). Pulmonary stenosis is often associated with other anomalies such as TOF, TGA, double-outlet right ventricle defects, AV canal defects, VSD, ASD, and PDA. It is the most common defect found with Noonan syndrome and may also be found with rubella syndrome and William syndrome. Isolated pulmonary stenosis with intact ventricular septum is described in this section.

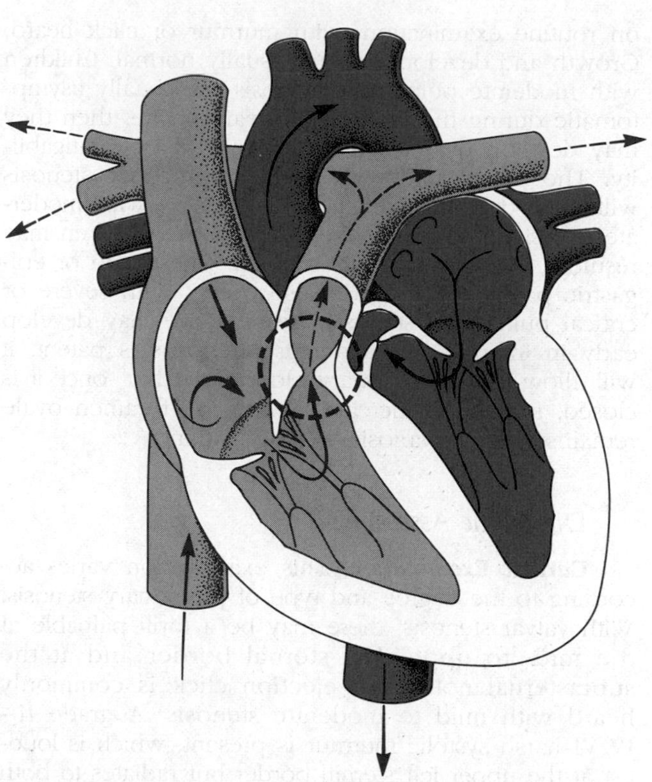

FIGURE 33-18. Pulmonary stenosis (valvar) with right ventricular hypertrophy. Blood flow patterns are normal.

Pulmonary stenosis involves malformation of the cusps of the pulmonic valve that controls the flow of blood from the right ventricle into the pulmonary artery. It can vary in degree from mild to severe or critical. As the obstruction increases, right ventricular pressure increases and thickening of the right ventricular wall (hypertrophy) develops. If right ventricular hypertrophy is severe, as in critical pulmonary stenosis, right atrial pressure can increase, resulting in right-to-left shunting through the foramen ovale. The infant or child would then be cyanotic. However, most infants and children are acyanotic with mild to moderate pulmonary stenosis. When the obstruction is at the *valvar* level, there is a "jetting" of blood through the stenotic valve, which dilates the main pulmonary artery. *Infundibular,* or subvalvar, stenosis may occur alone or in conjunction with valvar stenosis. *Supravalvar* pulmonary stenosis can be an isolated constriction involving the main pulmonary artery, the left and right pulmonary arteries, and the smaller peripheral arterial branches.

Clinical Manifestations

Symptoms vary according to the degree of obstruction. The majority of children with pulmonary stenosis are asymptomatic, and their cardiac defect is discovered on routine examination, with murmur or click heard. Growth and development are usually normal. Children with moderate pulmonary stenosis are usually asymptomatic during the first 2 to 3 years of life, then they may develop dyspnea on exertion and easy fatigability. The older child with severe pulmonary stenosis will have dyspnea and fatigability, even with moderate exercise. Strenuous exercise in these children may result in syncope or sudden death. Chest pain or epigastric pain, or both, may also occur. With severe or critical pulmonary stenosis, heart failure may develop early in infancy. If the ductus arteriosus is patent, it will allow some pulmonary blood flow, but, once it is closed, symptoms increase. When the foramen ovale remains patent, cyanosis will be evident.

Diagnostic Assessment

Cardiac Examination. This examination varies according to the degree and type of pulmonary stenosis. With valvar stenosis, there may be a thrill palpable at the mid- to upper left sternal border and at the suprasternal notch. An ejection click is commonly heard with mild to moderate stenosis. A grade II–IV/VI harsh systolic murmur is present, which is loudest at the upper left sternal border but radiates to both axillae and can be heard throughout the chest. The first heart sound is normal. The second heart sound is usually normal; however, with severe pulmonary stenosis, the murmur may be prolonged, obliterating a portion of the second heart sound. In this case, the second heart sound would be a single sound. Diastolic murmurs are not typically present. The cardiac examination with infundibular stenosis is generally the same as with valvar stenosis, except that there is usually no ejection click. As with infundibular stenosis, supravalvar stenosis does not have an associated ejection click.

Electrocardiogram. With mild to moderate pulmonary stenosis, the ECG may be normal or show right ventricular hypertrophy. In severe pulmonary stenosis, the ECG almost always shows right ventricular hypertrophy and right atrial enlargement.

Chest Radiograph. The heart size is most often normal, as is the pulmonary vascularity. With valvar pulmonary stenosis, there is a prominent main pulmonary artery segment distinguishable on the chest radiograph. With infundibular and supravalvar pulmonary stenosis, the main pulmonary artery segment is not prominent.

Echocardiogram. Color flow 2-D echocardiography can demonstrate the size of the right ventricle and its outflow tract, the pulmonary valve, main pulmonary artery, and the left and right pulmonary arteries. The level(s) of obstruction can be visualized, as can the presence of other cardiac defects. With the addition of continuous wave Doppler measurements, the actual pressure gradient across the obstruction can be estimated.

Therapeutic Management

Symptomatic infants or older children with severe pulmonary stenosis need balloon valvuloplasty (dilatation of the stenotic valve with a balloon catheter) or surgical repair. When right ventricular pressure exceeds left ventricular pressure the pulmonary stenosis is considered severe or critical. In newborn infants, PGE_1 has been used to maintain the patency of the ductus arteriosus, allowing adequate pulmonary blood flow until relief of obstruction can be achieved. Balloon dilatation is the treatment of choice in these infants, but surgical intervention can also be utilized.

If the valve annulus (the ring of tissue to which the leaflets are attached) itself is small, an incision into the annulus is made and a patch is used to enlarge the annulus. When infundibular stenosis is present, resection of the hypertrophied muscle is performed, and, if necessary, a pericardial or Dacron patch is used to widen the outflow tract. For supravalvar stenosis, the area of obstruction is incised and a patch graft inserted to widen the area. Moderate pulmonary stenosis is not surgically repaired in infancy but rather followed throughout early childhood. If the stenosis increases, right ventricular hypertrophy increases, and/or the child becomes symptomatic, the stenosis is repaired electively. Mild pulmonary stenosis does not need intervention.

As an alternative to surgery for pulmonary valvar stenosis, a technique called pulmonary balloon valvuloplasty has been utilized quite successfully in many institutions. In the procedure, a balloon catheter is placed across the stenotic pulmonary valve during cardiac catheterization. The balloon is inflated, opening the stenotic valve and relieving the obstruction. This technique can only be used for valvar stenosis when the valve annulus is of adequate size. Balloon valvuloplasty is ineffective in relieving infundibular pulmonary stenosis. Some forms of supravalvar pulmonary stenosis have been successfully relieved by balloon valvuloplasty. The benefit of balloon valvuloplasty is obvious, in that it eliminates the need for a surgical repair. The long-term results of balloon valvuloplasty (e.g., degree of residual obstruction, rate and degree of reobstruction, rate and degree of pulmonary regurgitation) need further study. Residual obstruction, reobstruction, and pulmonary regurgitation are complications seen after both surgical repair and balloon valvuloplasty. Children with pulmonary stenosis require life-long antibiotic prophylaxis for endocarditis for certain procedures.

Nursing Diagnostic Statements and Collaborative Problems

Preoperative:

High risk for activity intolerance; *risk factors: obstruction of blood flow from the right ventricle associated with pulmonary artery valve obstruction.*

Postoperative:

High risk for injury: physiologic; risk factors:

- *Residual obstruction or reobstruction or both.*
- *Pulmonary valve regurgitation; Defining characteristics: Diastolic murmur; bacterial endocarditis.*

Nursing Care

Nursing interventions for care are detailed in Tables 33–4 and 27–3.

The symptoms the child will manifest will vary according to the severity of the child's defect. The child will be asymptomatic unless the stenosis is severe. Regardless of the severity of the child's defect, the parents will have questions and concerns about the impact of the cardiac condition on their child's life. Table 33–15 provides guidelines for addressing these concerns. If the child's stenosis is mild, long-term follow-up will not be necessary, although SBE prophylaxis may be necessary. For children who have moderate to severe pulmonary stenosis, balloon dilatation will be done in the cardiac catheterization laboratory on diagnosis. Parents will need information about the procedure prior to the balloon dilatation. As with mild pulmonary stenosis, long-term follow-up will not be necessary except for SBE prophylaxis. Children with severe pulmonary stenosis will require immediate balloon dilatation in the catheterization laboratory or surgical intervention. Parents will need information and support from the nurse to cope with the urgency of their child's condition. Parents will need to know that, for children with severe pulmonary stenosis, SBE prophylaxis will be necessary prior to dental and surgical procedures on a lifelong basis.

Aortic Stenosis (Fig. 33–19)

Aortic stenosis (narrowing) constitutes about 5 per cent of all CHD (Gersony, 1987).

Etiology/Incidence (Pathophysiology)

The aortic valve controls blood flow between the left ventricle and the aorta. Aortic stenosis in infants and small children is always regarded as a congenital defect, whereas adults may develop aortic stenosis following rheumatic fever or from progressive atherosclerotic disease. The incidence of congenital aortic stenosis in males is four times greater than it is in females (Adams et al, 1989). Males are also more commonly affected by the valvar type. Other CHDs associated with aortic stenosis are PDA, coarctation of the aorta, VSD, and pulmonary stenosis.

Aortic stenosis is divided into three related types: (1) valvar, (2) subvalvar, and (3) supravalvar. Valvar aortic stenosis (stricture of the aortic valve) is the type most frequently encountered. The aortic valve may be unicuspid, bicuspid, or tricuspid. In most cases, the valve is bicuspid and thickened or the commissures are fused. Discrete subvalvar stenosis (narrowing below the valve) results from a thin membrane or thick, fibrous ring in the subvalvar region of the aortic valve. Supravalvar aortic stenosis occurs above the aortic valve. This type of stenosis is fairly uncommon and is usually associated with other defects such as mental retardation, defective dental development, abnormal facies, infantile hypercalcemia, and pulmonary stenosis. This is also referred to as Williams syndrome.

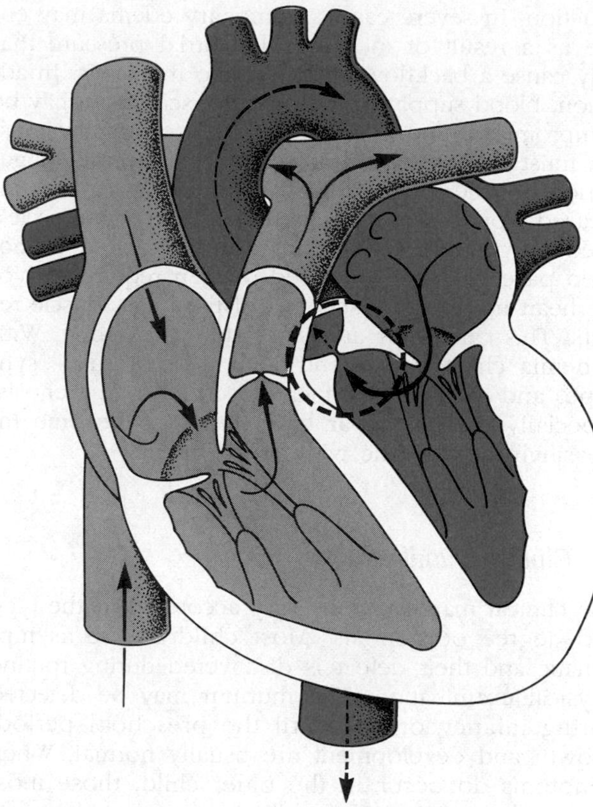

FIGURE 33-19. Aortic stenosis (valvar) with left ventricular hypertrophy. Flow patterns are normal.

In the presence of aortic stenosis, there is obstruction to blood flow from the left ventricle. This results in thickening, or hypertrophy, of the left ventricle in response to the increased workload required to eject blood. The degree of obstruction varies from mild to severe or critical. Pressure in the ventricle increases in direct correlation with the degree of obstruction.

With mild aortic stenosis, there is minimal obstruction to blood flow from the left ventricle and, consequently, minimal, if any, left ventricular hypertrophy. With moderate to severe or critical aortic stenosis, however, the left ventricle is very hypertrophied and left ventricular pressure is quite high. Heart failure can develop due to the excessive workload placed on the left ventricle pumping against the obstruction. In severe cases, pulmonary edema may ensue as a result of increased left atrial pressure that may cause a backflow of blood into the lungs. In addition, blood supply to the heart muscle itself may be compromised. The hypertrophied left ventricular muscle must contract with stronger force over a longer period of time to eject blood from the heart. This increased workload in turn increases the heart muscle's need for oxygen. The coronary arteries often cannot keep pace with the increased oxygen requirement of the heart muscle and ischemia of the heart muscle results. This can occur at rest or during exercise. With ischemia chest pain, ventricular dysrhythmias, syncope, and sudden death can occur. Aortic stenosis, especially the subvalvar type, tends to become increasingly problematic without treatment.

Clinical Manifestations

The clinical manifestations vary according to the type and degree of stenosis. Most children are asymptomatic and their defect is discovered during routine physical examination. The murmur may be detected during infancy or not until the preschool period. Growth and development are usually normal. When symptoms do occur in the older child, those most commonly seen are fatigability, exertional dyspnea, chest pain, and syncope. Infants with critical aortic stenosis may present in heart failure in the neonatal period or in the first few months of life. These infants will be irritable, pale, hypotensive, tachycardic, and tachypneic and have decreased perfusion and pulmonary congestion.

Diagnostic Assessment

Cardiac Examination. The cardiac examination will vary with the degree and type of aortic stenosis. In general there will be a harsh systolic murmur, grade II–IV/VI, heard typically at the upper right sternal border radiating to the upper left sternal border and the neck. An ejection click may be heard at the apex and lower left sternal border. A suprasternal notch thrill is palpable.

Electrocardiogram. The ECG may be normal or demonstrate left ventricular hypertrophy. There is often very poor correlation between the ECG and the degree of aortic stenosis, e.g., in the presence of severe aortic stenosis, the ECG may be normal or show only mild left ventricular hypertrophy. ST segment depression indicates myocardial ischemia and the need for immediate intervention.

Chest Radiograph. The heart size is most often normal, even when severe aortic stenosis is present. Dilatation of the ascending aorta may be seen with valvar aortic stenosis. Infants may have an increased heart size, especially if they are in heart failure.

Echocardiogram. With 2-D echocardiogram, the type of aortic stenosis, as well as the presence of other cardiac defects, can be visualized. Left ventricular wall thickness and left ventricular function can also be evaluated. With the continuous wave Doppler, an estimate of the pressure gradient across the obstruction can be made.

Cardiac Catheterization. The area of obstruction is localized, and the valve motion is demonstrated.

Therapeutic Management

Infants and children with mild to moderate aortic stenosis are usually followed clinically with no surgical intervention unless their aortic stenosis progresses. Infants with critical valvar aortic stenosis need surgical intervention or balloon dilatation in the cardiac catheterization laboratory as soon as possible. Valvar aortic stenosis is repaired through a median sternotomy. The aorta is incised and the aortic valve commissures incised, permitting the leaflets to open freely during systole. With balloon dilatation, a catheter is placed across the aortic valve, inflated to tear or separate the leaflets, then deflated and removed. With either intervention, the valve will never be normal, however; and residual obstruction is common, as is aortic insufficiency. There is no medical management for aortic insufficiency. If the aortic insufficiency becomes significant, the child may require an aortic valve replacement at some time.

Repair of discrete subvalvar aortic stenosis involves removing the obstructing membrane or fibrous ring below the aortic valve. Diffuse tunnel or muscular subvalvar aortic stenosis is a difficult lesion to repair. The traditional approach has been to remove surgically as much of the obstructing muscle as possible. However, residual obstruction is almost always present and the muscular obstruction most often progresses, necessitating further surgical repairs. Several surgical approaches have been devised to repair residual and/or recurring muscular subvalvar aortic stenosis. The Konno procedure is a surgical procedure that involves removing obstructing muscle, widening the outflow area of the left ventricle, including the aortic valve annulus, with a patch, and replacing the aortic valve with a larger valve. This procedure is relatively new but appears to be successful in relieving diffuse tunnel or muscular subvalvar aortic stenosis. Further studies are needed to evaluate the long-term effectiveness of this procedure.

If obstruction to outflow cannot be relieved with either of these procedures, a valved conduit may be placed from left ventricle to descending aorta. This procedure is somewhat controversial. Supravalvar stenosis is repaired by incising the narrowed segment of the aorta and widening the area with a patch graft.

When *replacing the aortic valve,* there is a wide variety of valve types available. Three common types of valves are (1) tissue heterograft valves (porcine valves and bovine pericardium valves), (2) prosthetic valves, and (3) homograft valves (human donor valves). Porcine valves and bovine pericardium valves are used less often on the left side of the heart in infants and children because they tend to calcify rapidly and need to be replaced often. Prosthetic valves are commonly used on the left side of the heart because they seldom calcify. However, infants and children with a prosthetic valve require continuous anticoagulation therapy to prevent clot formation on the valve. The third type of valve, the homograft, has been used relatively recently in most areas of the world. Preliminary results show minimal calcification of the valve, and these children do not require continuous anticoagulation. Further studies are needed to evaluate the long-term effectiveness of the homograft valve. Another advantage to using the homograft valve is its flexibility and pliability during surgical insertion. In addition, it is possible to use a larger size in the homograft valve than can be used with a prosthetic or porcine valve. This allows the child a longer period of growth before a second valve replacement is required, and, in some children, it is possible to place an adult-sized homograft, which would eliminate the need to replace the valve with a larger one later.

Aortic balloon valvuloplasty (see description of balloon valvuloplasty procedure under "Pulmonary Stenosis") is a relatively new technique for relieving valvar aortic stenosis in infants and older children. This procedure may carry a higher risk than pulmonary balloon valvuloplasty. Complications of aortic balloon valvuloplasty include aortic aneurysms, rupture of the aortic wall, and tearing of aortic leaflets creating severe aortic regurgitation. However, if this procedure can be implemented when early intervention is indicated, the need for surgical intervention and the placement of an artificial valve may be delayed until adolescence or adulthood. This would decrease the number of operations needed and lessen the risk of complications.

All children with aortic stenosis require antibiotic prophylaxis for endocarditis for certain procedures. These children also require close continued follow-up by a cardiologist for evaluation of progressive obstruction, development of aortic regurgitation, and other complications.

Nursing Diagnostic Statements and Collaborative Problems

Preoperative:

High risk for altered tissue perfusion: myocardium; *risk factor: inability of the left ventricle to meet metabolic demands of the myocardium.*

Postoperative:

High risk for injury: physiologic; *risk factors:*

- *Residual obstruction and aortic insufficiency.*
- *Bacterial endocarditis.*

Nursing Care

Nursing interventions for perioperative care are found in Tables 33–4 and 27–3.

Prior to the child's discharge, parents will require information about the child's defect. The child will be asymptomatic unless the defect is severe. Information regarding the long-term care needs of the child will vary according to the type of defect. Regardless of the type of defect their child has, parents will have numerous questions and concerns about its impact on the child's life. Table 33–15 provides guidelines for addressing these issues with parents. The child with a mild defect may not require follow-up. Parents whose child has a moderate to severe defect will need preparation for surgical intervention/balloon dilatation and support, since the child may be initially treated with balloon dilatation and may require subsequent surgical intervention. The child with a severe aortic stenosis requires immediate surgical intervention/balloon dilatation. Instruction on long-term management will include information on SBE prophylaxis, well child care, participation in sports activity, and school issues. SBE prophylaxis will always be necessary prior to dental and surgical procedures. As the child gets older, he or she will need to be counseled about not participating in contact sports and about upper trunk isometric exercises such as weightlifting. Parents will need to be instructed to have their child receive well child care pertaining to health care needs common to all children. As the child enters school, these issues will be of concern to the child and family. School issues are addressed in the later section entitled "School Environment."

Coarctation of the Aorta (Fig. 33–20)

Coarctation of the aorta constitutes approximately 7 per cent of all congenital heart defects (Hoffman, 1990).

Etiology/Incidence (Pathophysiology)

It is a narrowing of the aorta in the region of the ductus arteriosus and left subclavian artery, commonly referred to as "juxtaductal." The narrowing can be either discrete or involve a long segment and can vary in severity from a mild constriction to total occlusion such as in interrupted aortic arch. This impedes blood flow to the lower portion of the body, creating increased pressure proximal to the obstruction. Bicuspid aortic valve is the most frequently associated anomaly (85

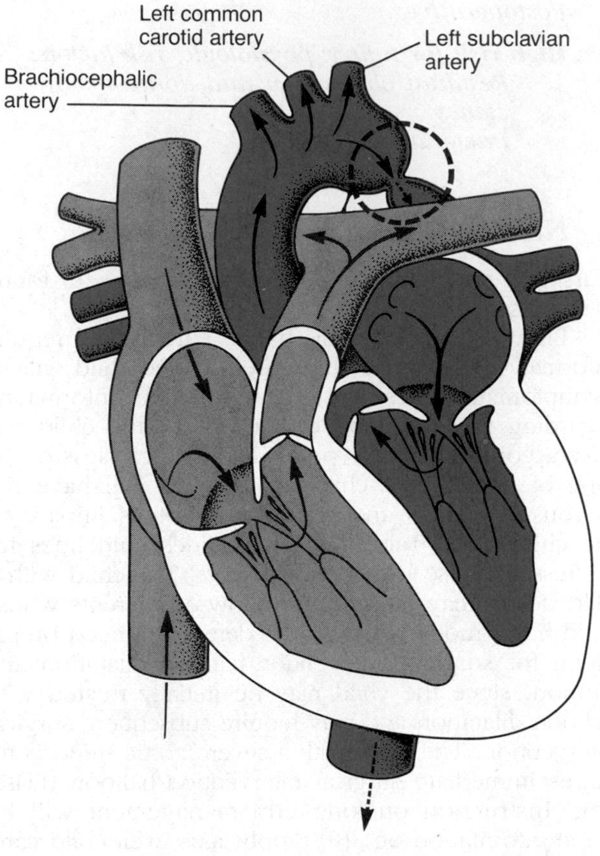

FIGURE 33 - 20. Coarctation of the aorta. Flow patterns are normal but are diminished distal to the coarctation. Blood pressure is increased in vessels leaving aorta proximal to the coarctation.

per cent). However, PDA, VSD, aortic stenosis, aortic regurgitation, mitral valve abnormalities, TGA, and double-outlet right ventricle are also associated anomalies. Coarctation is the most common congenital heart defect found with Turner syndrome (Adams et al, 1989).

Clinical Manifestations

There are two groups of patients with coarctation: (1) those who are symptomatic in infancy and (2) those who remain asymptomatic and are diagnosed during routine physical examination in later years. If symptoms do not develop during infancy, the child will most likely grow normally and remain asymptomatic until later childhood. Occasionally, these children will present with complaints of weakness or pain in their legs with exercise. However, most often they are identified through a differential in upper and lower extremity blood pressures, hypertension of the upper extremities, and absent or diminished femoral and pedal pulses. Infants usually present with CHF and failure-to-thrive. Symptoms include respiratory distress, poor weight gain, feeding problems, irritability, and tachycardia. Mottling is often evident in lower extremities. Infants with coarctation and a PDA may have adequate blood flow to the lower extremities, good pedal pulses, and no differential in blood pressure. Once the PDA closes, however, they will have absent or diminished femoral and pedal pulses and a differential in upper and lower extremity blood pressures.

Severe obstruction that depends on ductal pathway results in cardiovascular collapse when the PDA closes, a moribund presentation.

Diagnostic Assessment

Cardiac Examination. The first and second heart sounds are usually normal. There may be no murmurs present, or there may be a systolic murmur along the left mid to upper sternal border that radiates to the back. In addition, murmurs of associated cardiac defects such as a VSD may be heard. An additional systolic or continuous murmur may be present from collateral circulation. It is especially important to evaluate *both* upper extremity blood pressures and *both* lower extremity pressures with appropriate-sized cuffs. In the presence of a coarctation, upper extremity pressures will be at least 20 mmHg higher than lower extremity pressures. Femoral and pedal pulses are diminished or absent. Brachial/femoral delay is noted.

Electrocardiogram. Left or right ventricular hypertrophy is seen on ECG in the infant with coarctation. The older child may have left ventricular hypertrophy or a normal ECG.

Chest Radiograph. Increased heart size and increased pulmonary vascularity are often seen on the infant's radiograph. The older child may have a normal heart size but display such findings as rib notching and a prominent descending aorta.

Echocardiogram. The presence of a coarctation and the degree of isthmic narrowing, as well as the presence of other cardiac defects, may be determined by the echocardiogram.

MRI and cardiac catheterization are both procedures that are useful in clearly defining the area and extent of narrowing.

Therapeutic Management

Infants presenting in CHF and with failure-to-thrive are stabilized with medical therapy (see section on "Congestive Heart Failure") and are surgically corrected once stabilized. If other cardiac defects, such as a VSD, are present, the coarctation is repaired first, and, if possible, the other cardiac lesions are repaired when the infant is older. Coarctation may be surgically corrected using numerous approaches. The *end-to-end anastomosis,* where the narrowed portion of the aorta is removed and the two parts of the aorta on either side of the defect are joined, is the surgery of choice today. Narrowing may occur but can be balloon-dilated. Introduction of the use of absorbable sutures has made a significant difference in eliminating future problems of recoarctation.

The *subclavian flap aortoplasty* is a procedure in which a longitudinal incision is made in the aorta across the coarctated site and continued to the end of the distally divided left subclavian artery. The left subclavian artery is used as a patch or flap to increase the diameter of the aorta. *Patch aortoplasty* is still another technique, in which the coarcted area is excised and a patch graft placed on the aorta to widen the area. This technique is not in general use today.

If the child is asymptomatic, surgical repair is still recommended between the ages of 2 and 4. Delayed repair beyond 4 years of age may lead to prolonged or permanent hypertension, greater risk of premature death, and cardiovascular disease (Adams et al, 1989). Older children usually have an end-to-end anastomosis because there is less risk of recoarctation owing to the size of the aorta. Surgical repair of coarctation is not an open-heart procedure and, therefore, usually does not require cardiopulmonary bypass. It is performed through a lateral thoracotomy incision. Postoperative complications pertinent to nursing care include diminished or absent pulses in the left arm (with the subclavian flap aortoplasty) and persistent hypertension. Rebound hypertension immediately postoperatively is commonly present in patients, regardless of the procedure, and is treated with vigorous medical therapy. The severity of the hypertension and its duration are related to the child's age at the time of repair and the degree of preoperative hypertension.

Balloon aortoplasty, a special procedure in which a balloon catheter is introduced into the aorta during cardiac catheterization and inflated at the site of the coarctation to relieve the obstruction, has been tried in recent years with varying success. In some centers, this procedure has successfully been used in all age groups for native (unoperated) and renarrowed, previously operated coarctation. The advantages are no general anesthesia, no incision, and short hospital stay. Patients are followed closely for restenosis or aneurysm formation. However, consistent success has been reported in relieving recoarctations in older children with this procedure.

Continued antibiotic prophylaxis for certain procedures is necessary, as is cardiology follow-up at least every 1 to 2 years. Without correction, coarctation can pose life-threatening dangers. CVAs, aneurysms, and rupture of the aorta occur as a result of the increased pressure and formation of collateral circulation. If left untreated, calcification of the aorta, hypertension, and left ventricular hypertrophy develop, leading to ventricular dysfunction.

Nursing Diagnostic Statements and Collaborative Problems

Preoperative:

High risk for altered tissue perfusion: upper extremity hypertension; *risk factor: increased pressure in the left ventricle and ascending aorta associated with obstructed blood flow in the aorta.*

High risk for altered tissue perfusion: lower extremity hypotension; *risk factor: decreased blood flow to the lower part of the body.*

High risk for altered cardiac output: decreased; *risk factor: decreased blood flow through the descending aorta.*

High risk for altered growth and development: failure-to-thrive; risk factors: CHF, feeding problems.

Postoperative:

High risk for injury: physiologic; risk factors:

- *Persistent hypertension.*
- *Bacterial endocarditis;.*

Nursing Care

Nursing interventions for perioperative care are found in Tables 33–4 and 27–3.

The child with mild coarctation of the aorta may go undiagnosed for a long period. For children with more serious defects, the parents will need instruction on monitoring of blood pressure, the administration of antihypertensives, and monitoring of untoward side effects of the medications. Parents will need preparation for cardiac catheterization, possible balloon dilatation, and surgical repair. Coarctation frequently recurs if the child required intervention during the first 3 months, thereby requiring close follow-up to monitor the child's blood pressure. During follow-up visits, the child will need upper and lower blood pressure and pulse assessments by the specialty nurses. Instruction on long-term management will include SBE prophylaxis, monitoring of blood pressure, administration of medications, well child care, and school issues. The parents will be instructed to have their child given SBE prophylaxis prior to any dental and surgical procedures, to have their child's blood pressure monitored on a regular basis, and to attend to well child care. School issues will be of concern to the child and parents, and are discussed in the later section entitled "School Environment."

Impact of CHD

Emotional and Social Ramifications

The diagnosis of CHD in an infant has a tremendous impact on the family unit and those individuals involved in caring for the child in the community.

These children not only must adapt to the physical stress of hospitalization, evaluative testing, and palliative and corrective surgery but also may have to contend with an altered psychologic, social, and emotional environment.

Parents of the child with a congenital heart defect usually experience extreme stress, which may be compounded by guilt feelings and many fears. The nursing diagnosis patterns of *relating, valuing, choosing, and perceiving* should be assessed thoroughly. The family of this child requires support and practical guidance at the initial diagnosis and throughout the management of the disease to maintain and promote a healthy lifestyle for the child and the family's other members. Long-term psychologic outcomes for the child will depend on the family's response to the child. In turn, the family's response is greatly influenced by the health care team. *Effective nursing support can, therefore, directly influence the way in which heart disease affects a child and family.*

Often, congenital anomalies are corrected by surgery. Whenever possible, however, surgery is postponed until the child is beyond the neonatal period and can better tolerate the procedure. This means that, for a period of months or years, the family must manage the child's care at home. *Nursing care* during this period will occur most often in the home or clinic setting and will focus on preparing the family to administer medications to improve heart function (e.g., digitalis), provide optimal nutrition, and conserve the child's limited energy. CHF is a common complication of congenital heart disease in the period before surgical correction. Table 33–3 provides a nursing process plan for the child with CHF. Chapter 19 deals further with the impact of chronic illness on the child and family.

It has also been observed that parents may experience difficulty interacting with their infants who have congenital heart defects. This alteration in parenting may be due to parental perceptions of the infant's behavior—poor feeding, lethargy, restlessness. The parents may interpret these as reflections of poor parenting.

Parents of a child with CHD go through a grieving process; therefore, a complete assessment for anticipatory grieving and dysfunctional grieving is included in the plan of care. They must mourn the loss of their fantasized normal child before they are able to accept this child. Many parents block these feelings of loss and cope by denying the problem. Denial is especially prevalent in parents of asymptomatic children. These parents may exhibit behaviors indicative of ineffective denial, such as refusal to discuss the diagnosis or to learn about the heart disease, pay little attention to plans for medical and/or surgical management, and fail to comply with the treatment plan for medications or follow-up visits. Anger may be displaced on the other parent (e.g., arguing or placing blame), the physician (e.g., distrust, discontinuance of care), or the nurse (e.g., hostility toward the nurse, angry complaints about care, interference with care). The nurse can help the parents express their feelings. Anger and resentment are normal feelings but they must be dealt with appropriately. Parents can be helped to deal with anger by calm acceptance of their outbursts followed by reassurance and a discussion of the feelings that prompted the behavior. Parents' anger and resentment may be expressed toward ill children by overprotective behavior leading to infantilization or by detachment from and decreased contact with the child.

Parents may go through a second grieving process after the repair of the cardiac defect. During this grieving, they mourn the loss of the defective child who now may be essentially normal. This is usually apparent in the children who are quite symptomatic and who, after repair, improve remarkably.

Nursing Interventions for Long-Term Care

The majority of children with CHD will be able to lead normal lives. It is important that parents and family members see the child as a productive member of the family with individual strengths and weaknesses like every other member of the family. The nurse responsible for monitoring these children will carry out ongoing assessment for the nursing diagnostic responses in the perceiving pattern including *body image* and *personal identity disturbance, self-esteem problems,* and *hopelessness* and *powerlessness.*

If the child with CHD is seen as a severely limited, disabled child, then that is the self-image the child will have. Many families, because of their anxiety about CHD, overemphasize the cardiac condition and any limitations their child may have. They may even impose unwarranted limitations. These children may become very anxious about their cardiac condition and fearful of attempting physical activities, new experiences, and so forth. They may become very dependent and unfortunately may fail to develop to their fullest potential socially, physically, and emotionally. Parents should be encouraged to emphasize the positive. They should emphasize what the child *can* rather than cannot do.

At developmental stages throughout life, individuals need to feel a sense of accomplishment and control over their environment. Helping their child with CHD progress through developmental stages successfully offers special challenges for parents. Adolescents, for example, must complete developmental tasks such as (1) accepting one's body, (2) expanding peer relationships to include both sexes, (3) gaining emotional independence from family members, (4) achieving economic independence, (5) selecting and preparing for a vocation, and (6) becoming socially responsible. The adolescent with CHD can accomplish these tasks with family support and guidance and a healthy perspective. Adolescents who are fearful of their cardiac condition, who feel different from their peers, and who feel inadequate to complete tasks or goals will be unable to achieve these developmental tasks. Acceptance of one's body and gaining emotional independence from family members are particularly difficult for these adolescents.

To foster a positive self-image and a sense of accomplishment, parents need to identify and emphasize what is uniquely special about their child. What talents and special skills does the child possess which can be developed further? If the child with CHD must be limited in exercise (uncommon) or self-limits her or his activity, the family should emphasize another area of achievement. For many families, however, competitive sports and athletic activity are a priority. These families may have difficulty accepting and reacting in a positive manner to their child's physical limitations. These families in particular need special counseling regarding the influence they will have on their child's self-perception.

Exercise

Most children with CHD are not restricted in exercise. Rather, they are usually allowed to self-limit, stopping when they are fatigued. Nurses can assist the parents in determining their child's activity level. Parents need to recognize early if their child will have a limited ability to tolerate strenuous physical activity. They should then consult with their physician regarding the level of tolerance for exercise and sports. On the other hand, children who have no limitations to physical activity should not be restricted because of their parents' anxiety about the cardiac condition. Parents need the guidance of the cardiologist in making decisions about their child's exercise. The cardiologist should provide specific exercise parameters for the family and child. Commonly, when the child reaches school age, an exercise stress test is performed to determine the child's exercise capabilities and physiologic response (such as ECG and blood pressure response) to exercise. Exercise stress tests have been very beneficial in identifying specific safe exercise parameters for these children. In addition, both the child and the parents usually gain reassurance from the stress test and feel more comfortable regarding exercise.

School Environment

The school nurse is in a unique position to help the child with CHD in the school environment. The nurse should obtain information about the child's cardiac condition, any medications being given, and what the child's specific exercise parameters are. The nurse can then provide an optimal environment for the child by educating the teachers and others interacting with the child regarding his or her specific needs. Many teachers either "overprotect" or "overexert" these children, owing to fears or misconceptions about CHD. The nurse, as the child's advocate in the school environment, can do much to influence how the child is treated.

For example, the child who is unable to participate in normal physical education classes should not view this as a "punishment." Taking an alternative class, acting as a teacher's assistant, or performing some enjoyable task should be offered in place of the physical education class. The child needs to see it as a positive experience. Open communication among parents, the cardiologist, and the school is important in providing an optimal home and school life for the child.

Occasionally, children with CHD have additional needs that require special planning on the part of the school nurse. Two circumstances that would require additional planning would be (1) if the child had a pacemaker and (2) if the child were receiving anticoagulant therapy for a prosthetic valve.

Pacemakers

The child with a pacemaker may be totally pacemaker-dependent or may need the pacemaker only as a backup in case of dysrhythmias. The location of the pulse generator (pacemaker battery pack) may be subxyphoid (most common in young children), abdominal, or in the right or left upper thorax. The pacemaker function is generally checked once a month by the cardiologist. This is usually done over the telephone (transtelephonic) from the child's home or school. The child will have a transmitter that is placed directly over the chest or connected by electrodes to the fingers. The cardiology office or pacemaker clinic is then telephoned and the mouthpiece of the telephone is placed over the transmitter. The receiver in the cardiology office or pacemaker clinic will print out an ECG and a digital readout of pacemaker parameters. In this way, the cardiologist can monitor pacemaker function and determine when reprogramming is necessary and when battery life is depleted. Because the pacemaker is a risk factor for the nursing diagnostic response, *high risk for injury,* the school nurse may be called on to perform these pacemaker checks. *Precautions* for the child with a pacemaker in school include avoidance of hard blows to the chest, participation in contact sports such as football, and jumping on trampolines or from heights (such as from trees or fences).

All of these activities or circumstances may cause damage to the pacemaker lead wires. Electrical current, strong magnets, and strong radio waves may actually change the pacemaker program and function. Microwave ovens may affect pacemaker function, but this is uncommon with the new and better-insulated microwave ovens. Usually, the child simply needs to move away from the area. Vigorous physical activity is not contraindicated; it is the *type* of activity that is important. Swimming, running, bicycle riding, and baseball are all generally permitted because they do not involve extensive hard body contact or vigorous up-and-down jarring motion. More specific exercise parameters can be obtained from the cardiologist.

Signs and symptoms of pacemaker malfunction include dizziness, fatigue, pallor, syncope, and a pulse rate below the pacemaker's minimal heart rate setting. If pacemaker malfunction is suspected, the child's pulse should be taken immediately and the physician notified.

Anticoagulant Therapy

It is sometimes necessary to replace natural valves with prosthetic ones. Children with prosthetic valves will be maintained on anticoagulants, which constitute risk factors for the nursing diagnostic response *altered protection: hemorrhage*. Therefore, they require special precautions in the school and home environments to prevent serious injury, such as a blow to the head. A list of instructions, signs and symptoms of bleeding, and emergency treatments should be provided the school and the family.

Blood clotting or prothrombin time may be affected by major changes in the child's diet or activity level. Wide swings in anticoagulation levels occur, producing overcoagulation or undercoagulation if the child lacks a consistent, well-balanced dietary intake and consistent levels of activity. Vomiting, diarrhea, febrile illnesses, and medications also significantly affect anticoagulation levels.

Children receiving anticoagulants should refrain from taking any other medications (including aspirin, cold remedies, vitamins) without first checking with their cardiologist. In addition, loss of appetite, decreased exercise, and illnesses should be reported immediately, so that appropriate adjustments in anticoagulation therapy can be made.

Children receiving anticoagulant therapy should not bleed excessively from minor cuts and scrapes. Parents should be taught to hold pressure over the cut or scrape until the bleeding has stopped. The child may bleed longer than normal but the blood should clot. Frequent nosebleeds, blood in the urine or stool, excessive bruising, bleeding from an injury, or significant trauma such as hard blows to the chest or abdomen should be reported to the physician. Each child should wear a medical identification bracelet stating that she or he is on anticoagulants (blood thinners). If the child is in a car accident or suffers other physical trauma, an examination for internal bleeding by a physician is necessary. Signs of external bleeding may be absent, even when there are significant internal injuries. Safe, effective management of these children, which allows them the maximum of independence and activity, requires close cooperation and communication among parents, school personnel, and physician.

Acquired Heart Disease

Infective Endocarditis

Other common terms used for infective endocarditis are "subacute" (SBE) and "acute bacterial endocarditis" (BE).

Etiology/Incidence (Pathophysiology)

Infective endocarditis is an inflammatory process resulting from infection of the valves, the endocardium, or the endothelium of the heart. The infectious agent may be bacterial (such as staphylococcus and streptococcus) or fungal (such as *Candida albicans*).

Congenital heart defects increase susceptibility to infections within the heart or blood vessels because of turbulent blood flow. Abnormal communications (VSD), stenotic valves, and so forth will produce turbulent blood flow that results in areas of tissue damage in the heart. Bacteria or fungi circulating in the blood stream become entrapped at these sites and form vegetations. These vegetations can grow, interfere with cardiac function, and deteriorate valves (Fig. 33–21). In addition, vegetations can break off and become emboli causing CVAs and other infarcts. Infectious agents may be introduced into the systemic circulation during dental procedures such as teeth cleaning, cavity filling, tooth extraction, or any oral surgery. Other procedures at risk for introducing bacteria or fungi into the circulation are upper respiratory tract, gastrointestinal tract, and genitourinary tract operations (American Heart Association [AHA], 1990). Postoperative intracardiac lines are also a potential source of bacterial contamination. To decrease the risk of infection, antibiotic prophylaxis is given before and after these procedures.

Diagnostic Assessment

SBE or BE may be suspected in the presence of low-grade fever, anorexia, malaise, joint pain, and weight loss. Other signs include petechiae of skin and mucous membranes or Janeway spots, hemorrhagic areas on the palms of the hands and soles of the feet. There may be a new murmur or a change in a mur-

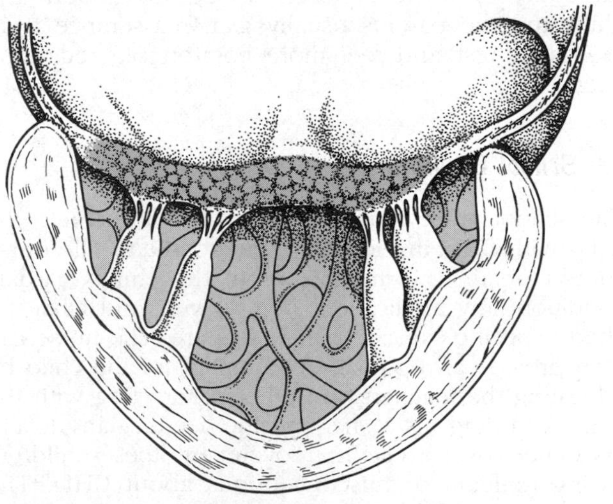

FIGURE 33-21. Endocarditis is characterized by the presence of vegetations (called "Aschoff bodies") on the surface of the endocardium, most commonly the mitral valve.

mur. Diagnosis is confirmed with positive blood cultures and the visualization of vegetations with echocardiogram.

Therapeutic Management

Infective endocarditis is a serious complication and must be treated vigorously. After culture identification of the infectious agent is made, IV antibiotics are administered for up to 6 weeks or more. If the valves are extensively involved or significant emboli have occurred, surgery is usually needed. Infants or children who have had a previous valve replacement and who have a tissue or prosthetic valve in place may require replacement of that valve.

Nursing Care

Care of the child with infective endocarditis requires hospitalization for the administration of prescribed medications, monitoring for fever and emboli, and providing information and emotional support for the child and family.

Administering Medication. Treatment of infective endocarditis will involve administration of IV antibiotics. In some situations, if the child is stable, IV antibiotics can be administered at home with the support of home nursing services.

Monitoring for Fever. Temperature readings are recorded every 4 hours, and more often if the child has a fever. If the child remains febrile on antibiotics or becomes febrile after having been on antibiotics for several days or weeks, further cultures will be required to ascertain whether other organisms are involved that will require different antibiotics.

Monitoring for Emboli. Because emboli are a potential complication of infective endocarditis, the nurse's recording must reflect assessment for clinical manifestations. These include seizures, slurred speech, neurologic impairment, and asymmetric movement of the extremities. The kidney, spleen, and bowel can also be damaged.

Providing Information and Support for the Child and Family. Teaching needs will include explanation of diagnostic procedures (such as blood tests and echocardiograms) and an explanation of the disease process, potential complications, and the treatment plan. Use of diagrams and a heart model can enhance teaching effectiveness.

Because of the serious nature of infective endocarditis and the prolonged hospital stay, the child and family will have a particular need for nursing support. The child's diversional needs may involve in-depth planning with the recreational therapist and the family. Children of school age and older may benefit from having a large calendar in their room so that they can mark off the days of antibiotic therapy or the number of days until discharge. This can help to make the date of discharge seem more attainable.

Parents and the child require extensive teaching before discharge to prevent recurrence of infective endocarditis. Prevention consists of antibiotic prophylaxis for at-risk procedures. Typically, an oral dose of amoxicillin is given 1 hour before the procedure and a second dose 6 hours after the initial dose. Children who are allergic to amoxicillin may receive erythromycin or clindamycin (AHA, 1990).

Hypertension

Etiology/Incidence (Pathophysiology)

Primary hypertension in adults is one of the greatest health risks facing our nation. Research indicates that hypertension may have its inception during childhood. Hypertension in children may be secondary to other conditions such as coarctation of the aorta, renal artery stenosis, renal disease, oral contraception, steroids, obesity, and adrenal disorders (Cushing disease, adrenogenital syndrome, primary aldosteronism). When a child is identified as being hypertensive, a secondary cause such as those just listed should be ruled out. If a secondary cause is indeed present, then treatment of the secondary cause will be initiated.

Some children will have primary hypertension with no apparent etiology. The exact incidence of this in the pediatric population is still being researched through long-term longitudinal studies on large populations of children. Geographic, ethnic, and racial differences in blood pressure readings in children are being investigated.

Diagnostic Assessment

The child who is identified as having primary hypertension is usually followed closely with regular blood pressure checks and evaluation of serum lipids, serum cholesterol, and serum triglyceride levels. A careful family history is obtained to determine the presence of hypertension and coronary artery disease in other family members. The severity of the hypertension will dictate treatment. The definition of mild, moderate, and severe hypertension remains variable among institutions and in different areas of the world.

Therapeutic Management

Mild hypertension is usually just monitored on a regular basis. Appropriate cuff size and measurement of blood pressure in children is discussed in the section on "Coarctation of the Aorta." Treatment for moderate hypertension is usually close monitoring as well; however, some physicians institute medical therapy including sodium-restricted diets (no added salt) and occasionally the use of antihypertensive medications. Severe hypertension requires antihypertensive drug therapy and possibly dietary alterations. It is not yet known whether control of hypertension in childhood will have an effect on development of arteriosclerotic disease and hypertension in adulthood.

Nursing Care

The role of the nurse in caring for a child with hypertension includes extensive teaching of the child and family. Lifelong health habits such as diet, exercise, weight control, and attitudes toward smoking are established during childhood. The family as a whole must model a healthy lifestyle in order for the child to develop healthy patterns of living.

When teaching the child about exercise and healthy dietary practices, the information should be presented as a positive approach to life with enjoyable benefits such as feeling better with exercise, becoming more fit, being able to participate in more activities, and feeling a sense of accomplishment. Dietary restrictions and institution of an exercise routine should never be seen by the child as punishment for the hypertension. Family participation in lifestyle changes is particularly important so that the child will not feel singled out or punished. In addition, when the whole family participates, lifestyle changes tend to be more consistent and long-lasting. The nurse has an important role as a health advocate in teaching healthy lifestyles for the prevention of disease and the promotion of health.

Cardiomyopathy

Etiology/Incidence (Pathophysiology)

Cardiomyopathy is defined as all entities in which myocardial pathology is the dominant feature (Fyler, 1992). Primary cardiomyopathy is not associated with any other cardiovascular or systemic diseases. Secondary cardiomyopathy is thought to be related to an associated disease. Three general categories of cardiomyopathy are usually identified: (1) hypertrophic, (2) dilated, and (3) restrictive. Although cardiomyopathies can be caused by genetic, infectious, metabolic, or pharmacologic factors, in most cases the exact etiology is unknown.

Diagnostic Assessment

Hypertrophic cardiomyopathy is characterized by asymmetric thickening of the left ventricle. This causes the left ventricle to be stiff; systolic function may not be impaired, and may even be hyperkinetic (progressive diastolic dysfunction). Left ventricular outflow tract obstruction (LVOTO) can be present, but is not as common as once thought (Adams et al, 1989).

Clinical presentation can include a soft murmur or murmur of LVOTO or mitral insufficiency, failure-to-thrive, signs and symptoms of CHF (which usually occur late), cardiomegaly on chest radiograph, no particular ECG pattern (can be "bizarre"), and asymmetric left ventricle wall thickening on echocardiogram.

Clinical course is variable, and generalized prognosis is difficult. Most children will be stable for many years; however, the occurrence of important symptoms in childhood is a poor prognostic sign that indicates early progression of the disease. Sudden death is rare in infants, but more common in individuals between 12 and 35 years. Sudden death is most likely due to ventricular arrhythmias.

Dilated cardiomyopathy is characterized by a dilated, poorly contractile left ventricle and sometimes left and right ventricles. The left atrium is dilated, and valve regurgitation is often present. Dysrhythmias may also occur. Thrombi often form in the atrial appendage or the left ventricular apex.

Clinical presentation almost always includes signs and symptoms of CHF. There will be no murmur unless there is valve regurgitation. Chest radiograph shows cardiomegaly. ECG shows ST segment and T-wave abnormalities.

The clinical course and prognosis are difficult to predict. The prognosis is worse when the disease presents in childhood and adolescence with CHF. According to Moss (1989), two thirds of patients survive 1 year, one third survive 5 years, and a minority improve function with long-term survival.

Restrictive cardiomyopathy is characterized by endocardial or myocardial disease that restricts ventricular diastolic expansion, thereby reducing ventricular filling. This form of cardiomyopathy is rarely seen in children.

Therapeutic Management

Treatment is directed toward reversing cardiac dysfunction or correcting the underlying cause, when known. Treatment must be individualized with careful monitoring of response. Digoxin and other inotropic agents can be helpful in dilated cardiomyopathies. If LVOTO is present in hypertrophic cardiomyopathy, digoxin can increase the obstruction and is not recommended. Digoxin can cause arrhythmias in an acutely inflamed myocardium in the presence of myocarditis. Beta blockers can help relieve LVOTO in hypertrophic cardiomyopathy, but can also cause myocardial depression. Afterload-reducing agents (vasodilators) and diuretic therapy can decrease cardiac workload. Antiarrhythmics are used as needed. Anticoagulation reduces the risk of dangerous emboli.

In more severe episodes of CHF, IV inotropic, diuretic, and vasodilator therapy may be necessary, along with mechanical ventilation. There is some evidence that IV dobutamine therapy has beneficial effects that last for a time after discontinuation of treatment. If maximal medical management fails, cardiac transplantation may be considered.

Heart Transplantation

Each year about 40,000 children are born with CHD. Of this number, about 5 to 10 per cent are not suitable candidates for conventional cardiac surgical procedures. The option for this group of children is heart transplantation. Table 33–16 identifies the major conditions for heart transplantation. Eighty per cent of children transplanted had cardiomyopathy. Congenital heart defects account for 16 to 20 per cent of transplants performed. The first pediatric heart transplant was performed in 1967, only days after the first adult heart transplant in Capetown, South Africa. That first transplant was performed on a 2-week-old neonate with severe heart failure due to Ebstein anomaly; the neonate survived only a few hours.

Initially, the survival of heart transplant recipients was poor; less than 10 per cent survived. The life expectancy of heart transplant recipients increased significantly with the introduction of cyclosporine for immunosuppression. From 1984 to 1988, more than 200 transplants were performed in children less than 10 years of age, and 60 were performed in infants less than 1 year of age (Heck et al, 1989).

A comprehensive medical and psychosocial evaluation is conducted to determine the eligibility of the recipient and family. Careful selection of an appropriate recipient is the most important determinant of a favorable outcome. Diagnostic assessment includes evaluation of major organ functioning. The diagnostic and laboratory tests used to evaluate recipient eligibility are listed in Table 33–17.

Donors for transplant are evaluated for suitability according to criteria specified by the uniform Anatomical Gift Act. Donor hearts are distributed according to guidelines developed by the United Network for Organ Sharing. The donor should be within 20 per cent of the recipient's body weight. Furthermore, the donor's harvested organ should be able to reach the patient within 4 hours so as to circumvent the problem of organ ischemia. Unfortunately, the availability of donor organs is a major problem with heart transplantation. Some experts have suggested the use of anencephalic donors; however, this option is controversial and lacks legislative guidelines. It is unlikely that anencephalic infants would be used as donors.

The recipient is placed on cardiopulmonary bypass through a median sternotomy. Depending on the age and condition of the recipient, one of several surgical techniques is used. An *orthotopic* heart transplantation involves the removal of the recipient's heart and replacement with the donor's. A *heterotopic* transplantation uses the recipient's atria as cuffs for anastomosis for the donor heart. This type of transplant is rarely done in children.

Follow-up care includes weekly outpatient examinations for 2 months, followed by monthly visits for 4 months. The child is seen every 3 to 6 months thereafter. The child is on immunosuppressants for life. Long-term problems to monitor are listed in Table 33–18. The survival rate at 1 year post transplantation is 74 per cent, and at 5 years 70 per cent. Research studies indicate that the majority of recipients have attained high-level functioning and psychosocial adaptation (Trento et al, 1989; Fricker et al, 1987).

TABLE 33-16
Indicators for Heart Transplantation

Primary myocardial heart disease
End-stage acquired cardiac myopathy
End-stage ischemic heart disease
End-stage congenital heart disease
Intractable life-threatening dysrhythmias
Primary cardiac tumor
Failed cardiac transplant growth

Adapted from Ring, W. S., Mahony, L. (1990). Heart and heart-lung transplantation. In D. L. Levin & F. C. Morris (Eds.), *Essentials of pediatric intensive care*. St Louis: Quality Medical; and Adams, F., Emmanouilides, G., & Riemenschneider, T. (1989). *Moss' heart disease in infants, children, and adolescents* (4th ed.). Baltimore: Williams & Wilkins.

Nursing Care

The nurse may be best able to offer parental/patient support and education concerning diagnosis, prognosis, activity restrictions, medications, and diagnostic studies. Involvement will be intense and long-term if transplantation is considered and carried out.

Perioperative care of the child with a heart transplant is similar to the care of the child undergoing open-heart procedures. For further information on perioperative nursing diagnoses and interventions, refer to the section on perioperative care, Tables 23–7, and 33–4. Some early complications can occur more commonly in children with heart transplants. These are listed in Table 33–18. An uncomplicated postoperative course is approximately 3 weeks.

Dysrhythmias

Etiology/Incidence (Pathophysiology)

Normal Conduction System

Electrical conduction stimulates the muscular contraction of the heart. Disease processes and surgery may disrupt this system, producing a variety of results. In the normal heart, the impulse originates in the right atrium from the sinoatrial (SA) node, located at the junction of the superior vena cava and the right atrium (Fig. 33–22). Cardiac cells are of either the pacemaker or the nonpacemaker type. Pacemaker cells have the ability to depolarize spontaneously (automaticity); nonpacemaker cells require an unusual

TABLE 33-17
Diagnostic and Laboratory Assessment for Cardiac Transplantation

Cardiac
Cardiac catheterization
Rest and exercise; multiple gated acquisition (MUGA) scan
Thallium stress examination
Metabolic stress testing
Myocardial enzymes

Hepatic
Hepatitis screen
Coagulation profile
Liver function test

Renal
BUN
Creatinine
Creatinine clearance

Pulmonary
Chest radiograph
Pulmonary function tests

Neurologic
Cranial CT or MRI
EEG

Musculoskeletal
Skeletal survey
Bone age
Densitometry

Endocrine/Metabolic
Serum glucose
Serum calcium
Serum magnesium
Thyroid function

Immunologic
ABO typing
Transfusion and pregnancy history typing
Antileukocyte antibody screen
Serologic testing for viruses (HIV, CMV, Epstein-Barr virus, herpes simplex virus, varicella-zoster virus)
Serologic testing for toxoplasmosis
Tuberculin skin test

Dental
Dental examination
Dental radiograph

Psychosocial
Adequacy and availability of support systems
History of medical noncompliance
History of substance abuse
Financial resources

Data from Levin, D., & Morris, F. (1990). *Essentials of pediatric intensive care.* St. Louis: Quality Medical.

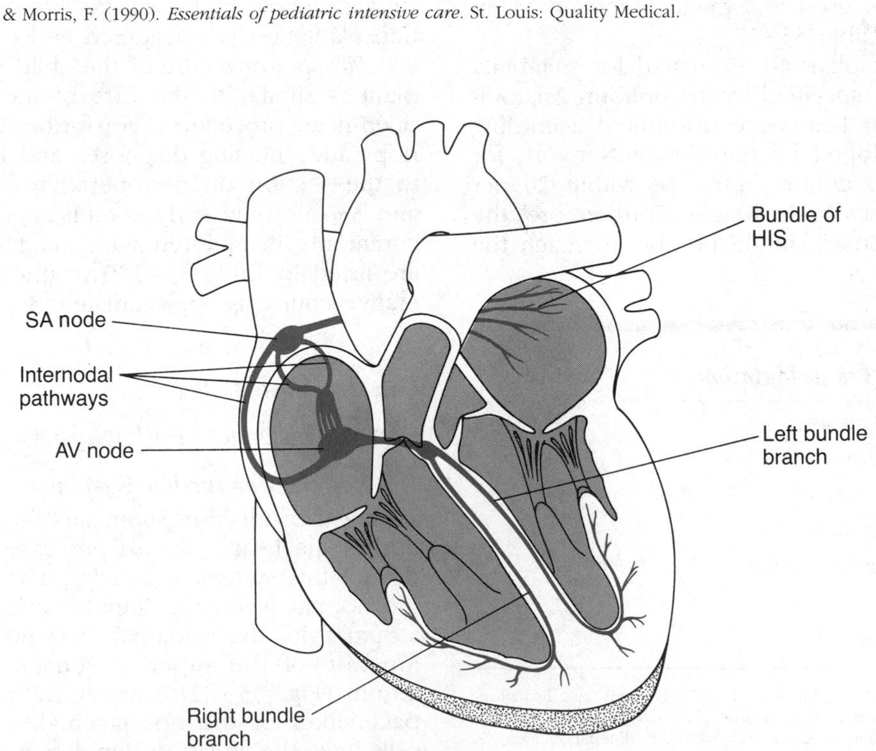

FIGURE 33-22. Internodal pathways.

TABLE 33-18
Complications of Heart Transplantation

Early Complications
- Cardiac dysfunction
  - Right ventricle more than left ventricle
- Dysrhythmias
- Sinus node dysfunction
- Reversible renal insufficiency
- Neurologic dysfunction
  - Seizures
  - Stroke
- Infection
- Side effects of immunosuppression
  - Nephrotoxicity
  - Neurotoxicity
  - Hypomagnesemia
  - Hypertension
  - Hirsutism

Later Complications
- Infection (accounts for 38% of deaths following transplantation)
- Rejection (accounts for 28% of deaths following transplantation)
  - Acute rejection
  - Maintenance rejection
- Side effects of immunosuppressive drugs
- Malignancy
- Psychiatric complications
- Medical noncompliance

Adapted from Chartrand, C., Dumont, L., & Stanley, P. (1989). Cardiac transplantation. *Transplant Proceedings, 21,* 3349–3350; © 1989. Reprinted by permission of Appleton & Lange, Inc.; Fricker, F., et al. (1987). Experience with heart transplantation in children. Reproduced by permission of *Pediatrics, 79,* 138–146, copyright 1987; and Levin, D., & Morris, F. (1990). *Essentials of pediatric intensive care.* St. Louis. Quality Medical.

stimulus (such as severe hypoxia) to depolarize spontaneously. Pacemaker cells with the highest rate of automaticity occur in the SA node. Therefore, the SA node functions as the pacemaker of the heart. Nerve centers in the brain control the release of impulses from the SA node by sympathetic fiber stimulation, which increases the heart rate, and by vagus (parasympathetic) nerve fiber stimulation, which decreases it.

Impulses originating in the SA node travel through the right and left atria via three internodal pathways to the AV node, located at the lower atrial septum, where there is a slight delay of the impulses. Impulses then continue from the AV node through the bundle of His and bifurcate into the right and left bundle branches located in the ventricular septum. The impulses then continue through the Purkinje fibers in the myocardium and stimulate ventricular contraction (Fig. 33–23).

An ECG tracing shows the electrical stimulation and contraction of the atria (the P wave) and the ventricles (the QRS complex), as well as the recovery phase of the ventricles (the T wave). The PR interval represents the time for the original impulse to reach the ventricles and stimulate contraction. The ST segment represents the period between the completion of contraction and the recovery of the ventricular muscle. Table 33–19 provides a detailed outline of fetal and neonatal dysrhythmias. This detailed information is provided primarily for reference purposes.

Abnormal Rhythms

Cardiac dysrhythmias are abnormalities in the rate, rhythm, or conduction of the electrical impulse (Table 33–19). They can be further categorized as *bradycardias*—slower than normal for the child's age; *tachycardias*—faster than normal for the child's age; *heart block*—interference with conduction resulting in an irregular or slow heart beat; and *ectopic beats*—beats originating from a focus other than the underlying rhythm. Dysrhythmias can occur in otherwise healthy children, in conjunction with a congenital heart defect, or as a result of surgical repair of complex congenital heart defects.

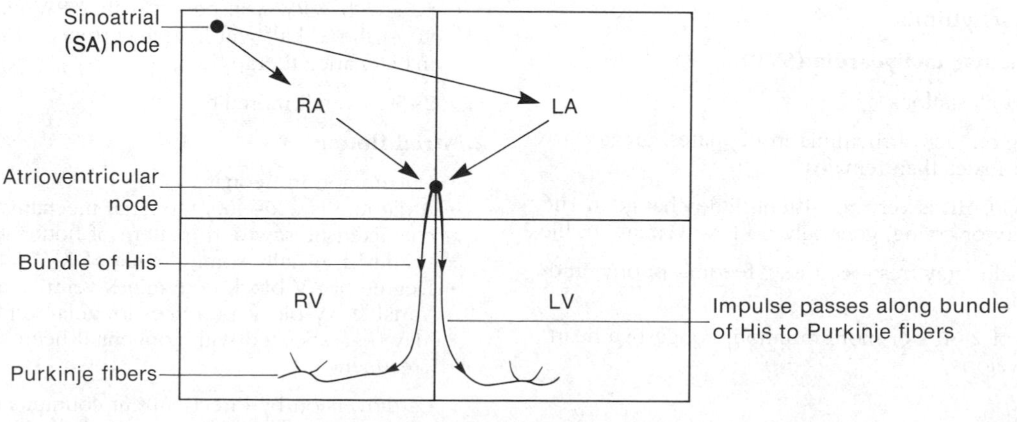

FIGURE 33-23. The conduction system of the heart.

TABLE 33-19
Fetal and Neonatal Dysrhythmias

Fetal Dysrhythmias

Fetal heart (HR) range is ~120–160

Estimated 1–2% incidence of dysrhythmias

Most dysrhythmias are supraventricular premature beats which disappear after birth

Serious dysrhythmias can occur, i.e., complete heart block (CHB) and supraventricular tachycardia (SVT)

Treatment in utero is limited to infants in congestive heart failure:

CHB—delivery is induced if gestational age is appropriate, and a pacemaker is placed
SVT—Digoxin or propranolol have been used by giving the mother PO or IV doses

Neonatal Dysrhythmias

Average HR of the newborn is ~130–145 with considerable variation (90–195).

Benign dysrhythmias:

1. Sinus bradycardia

- Repeated episodes of HR <80
- Up to 35% of normal premature infants have episodes of bradycardia
- Short episodes are associated with eating, defecating, hiccuping, and nasopharyngeal suctioning
- Most likely due to functional or developmental responses of the SA node
- No intervention necessary

2. Sinus tachycardia

- Intermittent episodes of HR >195
- Associated with periods of increased activity, crying, fever, loud noise stimulation
- Can be associated with underlying problems, i.e., sepsis, congestive heart failure, hyperthyroidism
- No intervention necessary unless treating an underlying problem

3. Sinus arrhythmia

- Phasic variation in HR with normal P-R interval usually associated with respirations in the older child but not in neonates

Pathologic Dysrhythmias

1. Supraventricular tachycardia (SVT)

- Clinical manifestations

Most common tachyarrhythmia in neonates, greater incidence in males than females

HR 210–350, HR is very consistent, little change in HR with activity or crying, generally no P waves are visible

Infant is pale, gray, restless, fussy, feeding poorly, and/or vomiting

With SVT of 24 hrs or more duration, congestive heart failure develops

- Etiology

8–26% have congenital heart disease, e.g., Ebstein anomaly, corrected transposition, tricuspid atresia

Myocarditis, cardiomyopathies, and myocardial tumors

10% have Wolff-Parkinson-White (WPW) syndrome with an accessory pathway (bundle of Kent) present

There is a classic short P-R interval giving a delta wave with a wide QRS complex

- Treatment *(done by specialist)*

Vagal stimulation—gagging or carotid pressure—usually ineffective in neonates

Ice bag to the face or facial immersion in cold water; occlude nostrils and immerse face in 5°C water for <5 secs. Causes bradycardia from parasympathetic stimulation

Caution must be used to avoid aspiration or asphyxia

- Drug therapy

Digoxin

Digitalizing dose (initially, half the digitalizing dose is given, then in 6–8 hrs one fourth of the digitalizing dose and in 12–16 hrs one fourth of the digitalizing dose)

Premature	20 μg/kg PO
Newborn	30 μg/kg PO
Infant	50 μg/kg PO

Maintenance dose 5–10 μg/kg/day PO given B.I.D. (IV dose is 75% of PO dose)

Propranolol, verapamil, quinidine, and procainamide also used, although verapamil not used in neonates

- Cardioversion by direct current countershock 0.5–1.0 watt sec/kg

Used if the infant is in severe congestive heart failure or the SVT is long-term or does not respond to other management

Maintenance drug therapy, e.g., digoxin, must be used following shock conversion to prevent recurrence

- Prognosis

Digoxin or drug therapy usually maintained for 1 yr, after which SVT in most cases does not recur

50% with WPW will persist with WPW pattern after 1 yr; of these, half will have recurrence of SVT despite maintenance therapy

2–5% overall mortality

2. Atrial flutter

- Uncommon in neonates
- Atrial rate is 220–460, the atrial mechanism is regular, characteristic sawtooth pattern of flutter wave in leads II and III, usually some degree of AV block
- Degree of AV block determines ventricular rate
  Variable AV block produces irregular ventricular rate
- May be associated with congenital heart disease
- Treatment

Cardioversion by direct current countershock

Digoxin

TABLE 33-19
Fetal and Neonatal Dysrhythmias (Continued)

3. Atrial fibrillation

- Rare in neonates
- Almost always associated with some form of congenital heart disease
- ECG shows extremely rapid atrial depolarization and a rapid irregular ventricular rate, a chaotic-appearing rhythm
- Neonate may have severe congestive heart failure with symptoms similar to those of SVT
- Treatment

Cardioversion by direct current countershock

Digoxin

Quinidine

4. Ventricular tachycardia

- Rare in neonates
- Usually associated with congenital heart disease, electrolyte disturbance, myocardial tumor, or myocarditis
- Treatment

Cardioversion by direct current countershock

Infusion of lidocaine, 0.5–1 mg/kg/hr

Diphenylhydantoin (Dilantin), 3–8 mg/kg/dose

5. Heart block (AV block)

- Uncommon in newborns
- First-degree AV block

Prolonged P-R interval, >0.12 sec in neonates

One-to-one conduction ratio (every P wave is conducted through with a ventricular response)

Most common cause is digoxin effect (does not necessarily mean digoxin toxicity)

Can be caused by electrolyte abnormalities, e.g., hypokalemia or hyperkalemia

No specific intervention is necessary except to watch digoxin levels or correct electrolyte imbalance

- Second-degree AV block

Not all atrial beats are conducted to the ventricle

Type I (Wenckebach) is progressive lengthening of the P-R interval until an atrial beat fails to be conducted and a dropped beat occurs; may be due to digoxin toxicity

Type II is present when ventricular beats are dropped without preceding prolongation of the P-R interval. Type II tends to progress to complete heart block

- Third-degree (complete) AV block

The ventricular rate is totally independent of the atrial rate with the ventricular rate being slower

The higher the level of block, the higher the ventricular rate

Owing to an anatomic discontinuity within the AV node or distal conduction system

30% have associated congenital heart disease

Associated with myocardial rhabdomyoma and endocardial fibroelastosis, infection, metabolic or vascular disorders, and maternal lupus erythematosus

Clinically, the infant may be asymptomatic especially if the ventricular rate is 50–80. If the ventricular rate is <50, the infant may have CHF, dyspnea, tachypnea, peripheral cyanosis, cardiomegaly, and other arrhythmias (e.g., atrial flutter, PVCs, and bundle branch block)

Treatment

Not indicated in an asymptomatic, well infant with a ventricular rate >50; in symptomatic infants atropine or isoproterenol may be used until pacemaker insertion; indications for pacemaker include CHF, underlying congenital heart disease, HR <50 especially if associated with syncope and wide QRS complex

Prognosis

Death can occur from infection, and cardiomyopathy despite adequate pacing

Good prognosis if the infant is asymptomatic, HR >50, and has a narrow QRS

The ventricular rate tends to become slower as the infant gets older; many children require pacemakers during school age or adolescence

6. Ectopic beats

- Common in healthy newborns: 31% incidence
- Supraventricular ectopic beats are more common and are identified by an abnormal P wave (abnormal configuration or timing); these are usually considered benign and no treatment is necessary
- Ventricular ectopic beats are characterized by a wide, bizarre QRS complex, not preceded by a P wave; these can be benign but bear close monitoring if multifocal, frequent, and/or paired

Diagnostic Assessment: Monitoring Dysrhythmias

Holter Monitor

Infants and children suspected of having dysrhythmia will usually undergo a Holter monitor evaluation. This is a 24-hour recording of the child's ECG. The Holter monitor itself is a portable device approximately the size of a transistor radio. The leads are attached to the child's chest and taped securely in place, and the recorder is turned on. The monitor itself is attached to the child's belt or carried in a small pouch or backpack. The device is worn for 24 hours, during which time the child should perform all normal activities, being as active as possible. An hourly diary of the child's activity is kept by the parents, child, or nurse when the child is hospitalized. Accurate diaries are very helpful in interpreting the Holter monitor recordings and determining what activities precipitate dysrhythmias. *Caution should be used while the monitor is on to avoid immersion in water (e.g., swimming, bathing, or showering).* At the end of 24 hours, the Holter monitor is removed from the child and the tape is deciphered and interpreted.

Ambulatory Dysrhythmia Event Monitor

At times, a child's dysrhythmia occurs infrequently and does not occur while the Holter monitor is in place. For these children, a portable dysrhythmia event monitor may be used. This monitor is placed over the child's chest (anywhere on the chest) only when the child is symptomatic. A button is pushed and a 38-second ECG is recorded automatically. The ECG is stored in the device and is then transmitted over the telephone by the parents to a receiver in the cardiologist's office. This particular monitor allows more flexibility in recording symptomatic episodes and in determining whether a dysrhythmia is occurring. Other event-recording monitors can be worn continuously, and a button is pushed when symptoms occur.

An electrophysiologic study is a more extensive and invasive look at the conduction system in the presence of persistent dysrhythmias that are refractory to medical management. The study is performed via cardiac catheterization; attempts are made to identify a more specific area of stimulation or dysrhythmia. The information can be used to choose a more appropriate medical management or to ablate the problem area with radiofrequency waves. This study can take 6 to 8 hours.

Therapeutic Management

The treatment of dysrhythmias should first focus on identifying and treating the underlying cause. If the cause is not external (cold, heat, agitation, catheter) and the abnormal rhythm compromises cardiac output, medical management is necessary. Medications are chosen based on the source of the rhythm disturbance and the specific manner in which the drug works (Table 33–14). Conduction abnormalities that result in irreversible bradycardia may require the placement of a permanent pacemaker. This is an invasive, surgical procedure with lifelong follow-up.

A multitude of types of pacemakers are used today. The type of pacemaker a child will have depends on the underlying cardiac condition and reason for pacing. A ventricular demand (VVI) pacemaker was the standard pacemaker used most often in the past. With this pacemaker, one (unipolar) or two (bipolar) lead wires are attached to the ventricle and deliver an electrical impulse to stimulate a heartbeat if an intrinsic (the child's own) heartbeat is not sensed. The heart rate is "fixed," in that the rate at which the pacemaker is set will be the child's heart rate unless the child's intrinsic heart rate is higher. Heart rate will not vary with exercise unless the child can increase her or his intrinsic heart rate.

A second type of pacemaker is the physiologic or AV synchronous pacemaker. There are many varieties of this pacemaker; in general, it has atrial and ventricular lead wires that sense atrial and ventricular activity. If no atrial activity occurs, an atrial beat is stimulated, followed by stimulation of a ventricular beat if no ventricular activity is sensed. The advantage to this type of pacing is the synchrony between atrial and ventricular contractions, allowing the ventricles time to fill. This type of pacing most closely simulates normal cardiac conduction and function.

A third type of pacemaker is a rate-responsive, activity-triggered, or activity-responsive pacemaker. It paces the atrium or ventricle but at a variable, not a "fixed," rate. This pacemaker has the ability to sense large muscle activity and to increase the child's heart rate according to his or her activity. Therefore, depending on how it is programmed, the pacemaker will increase the heart rate when children are running and slow it down when they are resting. This rate-responsive pacemaker has improved exercise capacity for many children.

Nursing Care

The nurse has the ability to provide support and education to the parents and child concerning diagnoses, prognosis, medications, activity levels, surgery, and follow-up care. Tables 33–4 and 27–3 discuss interventions for cardiac surgery.

KEY CONCEPTS

Concepts Related to Basic Information

- An estimated 40,000 infants are born annually with congenital heart disease (CHD). Ninety per cent of CHD is thought to be associated with multifactorial inheritance.
- Approximately 8 per cent of CHD is associated with other abnormalities such as trisomies 21, 18, and 13, Turner syndrome, and Noonan syndrome.
- Central cyanosis may be the only evidence of a cardiac lesion during the first weeks of life.
- In the majority of cases, congestive heart failure (CHF) is the result of a surgically correctable structural abnormality of the heart. CHF can also be caused by arrhythmias, anemia, myocardial diseases, sepsis, or hypertension.
- Cyanosis is a blue discoloration of the skin, nailbeds, and mucous membranes caused by systemic arterial oxygen desaturation in surface

blood vessels. Cyanosis becomes clinically evident when there is at least 5 g of reduced hemoglobin per 100 ml of blood.

- Lesions with increased pulmonary blood flow are those which result when there is communication between the left (high-pressure) and the right (low-pressure) sides of the heart, allowing blood to shunt left to right.
- Ventricular septal defects (VSDs) are among the most common heart lesions, accounting for approximately 20 per cent of all CHDs.
- Lesions with decreased pulmonary blood flow result from obstruction of blood flow to the pulmonary artery with subsequent right-to-left shunting through an existing septal defect.
- Cardiac output equals the heart rate × stroke volume.
- Stroke volume is affected by preload, afterload, and contractility.

Concepts Related to Nursing Assessment

- An infant who has symptoms of cardiac disease in the first few hours to days or weeks of life most likely has a significant defect.
- Nursing diagnostic responses for the child with CHD in the perceiving pattern include *body image disturbance, personal identity disturbance, self-esteem problems, hopelessness, and powerlessness.*
- Nursing diagnostic responses and collaborative problems likely to occur in many or all of the CHDs are *altered nutrition, high risk for ineffective breathing pattern, high risk for ineffective coping, high risk for altered health maintenance, and altered tissue perfusion.*
- Perioperative nursing concerns for the child with CHD are *high risk for altered growth and development; failure to thrive; and high risk for injury: physiologic,* related to damage to the pulmonary vessels, conduction abnormalities, and bacterial endocarditis.
- Major preoperative nursing diagnostic responses for the child with tetralogy of Fallot are *high risk for activity intolerance; high risk for altered growth and development; high risk for injury: cerebrovascular accident; and high risk for injury: physiologic,* risk factors, complications of total repair.
- A major postoperative nursing diagnostic statement for the child with complete transposition of the great arteries is *high risk for injury: physiologic,* risk factors: complications of Mustard, Senning, or arterial procedures.
- Parents of a child with CHD go through a grieving process; therefore, a complete assessment for anticipatory grieving and dysfunctional grieving is included in the plan of care.

Concepts Related to Nursing Intervention

- Nursing care for the child having cardiac surgery includes assessing for problems of the following risk factors: dysrhythmia, pulmonary venous obstruction, stenosis of one of the great vessels, heart block, and bacterial endocarditis.
- Nursing care of the child with endocarditis involves administration of medications, monitoring for fever and emboli, and providing information and emotional support to the child and family.
- Nursing care for the child with congenital/acquired heart disease includes teaching for long-term health maintenance.
- Effective nursing support can directly influence the way in which heart disease affects a child and family.
- Prevention of rheumatic fever is a primary responsibility of the nurse in ambulatory or school settings, where screening sore throats for group A streptococcal infection is possible.

REFERENCES

Adams, F., Emmanouilides, G., & Riemenschneider, T. (1989). *Moss' heart disease in infants, children and adolescents* (4th ed.). Baltimore: Williams & Wilkins.

Agamalion, B. (1986). Pediatric cardiac catheterization. *Journal of Pediatric Nursing, 1,* 73–79.

American Heart Association Committee on Rheumatic Fever, Endocarditis and Kawasaki Disease (1990). Prevention of bacterial endocarditis. *JAMA, 264,* 2919–2922.

Bailey, L., & Gundry, S. (1990). Hypoplastic left heart syndrome. *Pediatric Clinics of North America, 37,* 137–150.

Borow, K., & Braunwald, E. (1988). Congenital heart disease in the adult. In E. Braunwald (Ed.), *Heart disease: A textbook of cardiovascular medicine* (3rd ed.). Philadelphia: WB Saunders, pp 1057–1078.

Fricker, F., et al. (1987). Experience with heart transplantation in children. *Pediatrics, 79,* 138–146.

Friedman, W. (1988). Congenital heart disease in infancy and childhood. In E. Braunwald (Ed.), *Heart disease: A textbook of cardiovascular medicine* (3rd ed.). Philadelphia: WB Saunders, pp 967–1056.

Fyler, P. (Ed.). (1992). *Nadas' pediatric cardiology.* Philadelphia: Hanely & Belfus Publishers.

Gersony, W. (1988). Congenital heart disease. In R. Behrman & V. Vaughan (Eds.), *Nelson textbook of pediatrics* (13th ed.). Philadelphia: WB Saunders, pp 962–1004.

Hazinski, M. (1992). *Care of the critically ill child* (2nd ed.). St. Louis: CV Mosby.

Heck, C., et al. (1989). The Registry of the International Society for Heart Transplantation Sixth Official Report—1989. *Journal of Heart Transplantation, 8,* 271–276.

Hoffman, J. (1990). Congenital heart disease: Incidence and inheritance. *Pediatric Clinics of North America, 37,* 31.

Kaplan, E. (1987). The startling comeback of rheumatic fever. *Contemporary Pediatrics, 4,* 20–34.

Merenstein, G., et al. (1985). *Handbook of neonatal intensive care.* St. Louis: CV Mosby.

Moller, J., & Neal, W. (1990). *Fetal, neonatal and infant cardiac disease.* Norwalk, CT: Appleton & Lange.

Nadas, A. (1990). Congenital heart disease. In S. Gellis & B. Kagan, *Current Pediatric Therapy, 13,* 133–137.
Sapire, D. (1991). *Understanding and diagnosing pediatric heart disease.* Norwalk, CT: Appleton & Lange.
Trento, A., et al. (1990). Lessons learned in pediatric heart transplantation. *Annals of Thoracic Surgery, 48,* 617–623.
Uzark, K. (1983). *Obstructive lesions: pulmonic stenosis, aortic stenosis, coarctation of the aorta. Unit 5 in Series 3: Cardiovascular disease in the young: nursing intervention.* Norwalk, CT: Appleton-Century-Crofts.

BIBLIOGRAPHY

Abelson, W., & Smith, R. (1987). *Resident's Handbook of Pediatrics* (7th ed.). Toronto: BC Decker.
American Heart Association. (1988). *If your child has a congenital heart defect: A guide for parents.* Dallas: AHA.
Arfken, C., et al. (1990). Mitral valve prolapse, associations with symptoms and anxiety. *Pediatrics, 85,* 311–315.
Bartz, B. (1988). Long-term patient outcomes after Fontan repair. *Progress in Cardiovascular Nursing, 3,* 19–26.
Bartz, C. (1988). Pharmacologic augmentation of cardiac output following cardiac arrest. *Critical Care Nursing Quarterly, 10,* 43–49.
Becker, K. L., & Stevens, G. A. (1988). Get in touch and in tune with cardiac assessment. Part 1. *Nursing 88,* Mar, 18, 51–55.
Bellet, P. (1989). *The diagnostic approach to common symptoms and signs in infants, children and adolescents.* Philadelphia: Lea & Febiger.
Benitz, W., & Tatro, D. (1988). *The pediatric drug handbook.* Chicago: Yearbook Medical Publishers.
Benson, L., & Freedom, R. (1989). Interventional cardiac catheterization. *Current Opinion Pediatrics, 1,* 106–109.
Broome, G. (1990). Differentiating between pain and agitation in premature neonates. *Journal of Perinatology Neonatal Nursing, 4,* 53–56.
Campbell, R., et al. (1987). Surgical treatment of pediatric cardiac arrhythmia. *Journal of Pediatrics, 110,* 501–508.
Carpenito, J. J. (1987). *Nursing diagnosis—Application to clinical practice.* Philadelphia: JB Lippincott.
Chernow, B. (1988). *The pharmacologic approach to the critically ill patient.* Baltimore: Williams & Wilkins.
Cleary, J. (1988). Two inotropic agents: Dopamine and dobutamine. *Pediatric Nursing, 14,* 414.
Cullen, L., & Laxson, C. (1988). Ballooning open a stenotic valve. *American Journal of Nursing,* July, *88,* 987–992.
Danaher, R. R. (1987). Complete congenital heart block: A case study. *Neonatal Network, 5,* 19–23.
Delgizzi, L. J., & Ueda, J. N. (1990). Using vasodilating agents in pediatric patients with cardiac disease. *AACN's Critical Care Nursing Clinics, 1,* 131–147.
DesRosier, M. B. (1988). Taking a baby. *American Journal of Nursing,* Jan, *88,* 67.
Driscoll, D. J. (1990). Evaluation of the cyanotic newborn. *The Pediatric Clinics of North America, 37,* 1–24.
Elixson, E. (1989). Hemodynamic monitoring modalities in pediatric cardiac surgical patients. *Critical Care Nursing Clinics of North America, 1,* 263–274.
Ferencz, C. H. D., et al. (1989). Congenital cardiovascular malformations associated with chromosome abnormalities: An epidemiologic study. *Journal of Pediatrics, 114,* 79–85.
Ferry, P. (1990). Neurologic sequelae of open-heart surgery in children. *American Journal of Diseases in Children, 144,* 369–373.
Foldy, S., & Gorman, J. (1989). Perioperative nursing care for congenital cardiac defects. *Critical Care Nursing Clinics of North America, 1,* 289–296.
Garson, A. (1987). Medicolegal problems in the management of cardiac arrhythmias in children. *Pediatrics, 79,* 84–88.
Gerraughty, A. B. (1989). Caring for patients with lesions obstructing systemic blood flow. *Critical Care Nursing Clinics of North America, 1,* 231–244.
Glasier, C., et al. (1989). Extracardiac chest ultrasonography in infants and children: Radiographic and clinical implications. *Journal of Pediatrics, 114,* 540–544.
Heart transplantation in newborns with inoperable malformations. (1989, January). *Pediatrics News, 23,* 17.
Hellenbrand, W., & Mullins, C. (1989). Catheter closure of congenital cardiac defects. *Cardiology Clinics, 7,* 351–368.
Hudgins, R. J., et al. (1988). Natural history of fetal ventriculomegaly. *Pediatrics, 82,* 692–697.
Ino, T., et al. (1988). Dilated cardiomyopathy with neutropenia, short statures and abnormal carnitine metabolism. *Journal of Pediatrics, 113,* 511–514.
Jonas, R., & Lang, P. (1988). Open repair of cardiac defects in neonates and young infants. *Clinics in Perinatology, 15,* 659–680.
Karch, A., & Boyd, E. (1989). *Handbook of drugs and the nursing process.* Philadelphia: JB Lippincott.
Kenner, C., & Hern, M. (1989). Writing a nursing diagnoses for a complex client: The infant with a congenital heart defect. *Journal of Pediatric Nursing, 3,* 256–264.
Kriett, J., & Kaye, M. (1990). The Registry of the International Society for Heart Transplantation Seventh Office Report—1990. *Journal of Heart Transplantation, 9,* 323–330.
Kulik, L. A. (1989). Caring for patients with lesions decreasing pulmonary blood flow. *Critical Care Nursing Clinics of North America, 1,* 215–230.
Levin, D., & Morriss, F. (1990). *Essentials of pediatric intensive care.* St. Louis: Quality Medical Publishing.
Maguire, P., & Maloney, P. (1988). A comparison of fentanyl and morphine use in neonates. *Neonatal Network, 7,* 27–35.
Mair, D. (1989). The Fontan procedure: The first 20 years. *Current Opinion in Pediatrics, 1,* 94–99.
Moynihan, P. J., & King, R. (1989). Caring for patients with lesions increasing pulmonary blood flow. *Critical Care Nursing Clinics of North America, 1,* 195–214.
Norton, S. (1988). After effects of morphine and fentanyl analgesia: A retrospective study. *Neonatal Network, 7,* 25–28.
Porterfield, L., & Porterfield, J. (1987). What you need to know about today's pacemakers. *Registered Nurse,* March, 44–49.
Radtke, W., & Lock, J. (1990). Balloon dilation. *Pediatric Clinics of North America, 37,* 193–214.
Rao, P. (1989). Balloon valvuloplasty and angioplasty in infants and children. *Journal of Pediatrics, 114,* 907–914.
Reidy, S., O'Hara, P., & O'Brien, P. (1989). Streptokinase use in children undergoing cardiac catheterization. *Journal of Cardiovascular Nursing, 4,* 46–56.
Rigby, M. (1989). The trend to primary repair of congenital heart defects in the first 3 months of life. *Current Opinion in Pediatrics, 1,* 82–84.
Rosen, K. R., & Rosen, D. A. (1989). Caudal epidural morphine for control of pain following open heart surgery in children. *Anesthesiology, 70,* 418–421.
Rudolph, A. (1991). *Rudolph's pediatrics* (19th ed.). Norwalk, CT: Appleton & Lange.
Runton, N. (1988). Congenital cardiac anomalies. A reference guide for nurses. *Journal of Cardiovascular Nursing, 2,* 56–70.
Sherman, F., & Sahn, D. J. (1987). Pediatric doppler echocardiography 1987: Major advances in technology. *Journal of Pediatrics, 110,* 333–342.
Smith, J. (1988). Big differences in little people. *American Journal of Nursing, 88,* 458–462.
Smith, M., et al. (1989). Symptomatic mitral valve prolapse in children and adolescents: Catecholamines, anxiety and biofeedback. *Pediatrics, 84,* 290–295.
Sondheimer, H. M. (1990). Cardiac catheterization—A new role in the 90s. *Contemporary Pediatrics, 7,* 91–106.
Swetnam, S., Yabek, S., & Alverson, D. (1987). Hemodynamic consequences of neonatal polycythemia. *Journal of Pediatrics, 110,* 443–447.

Congestive Heart Failure

American Heart Association. (1988). *Caring for an infant with congestive heart failure: A guide for parents.* San Francisco: AHA.
Artman, M., & Graham. (1987). Guidelines for vasodilator therapy of

congestive heart failure in infants and children. *American Heart Journal, 113,* 994–1005.
Dahlman, A. (1989). Captopril. *Neonatal Network, 7,* 41–43.
Lloyd, T. R., et al. (1989). Orally administered enalapril for infants with congestive heart failure: A dose-finding study. *Journal of Pediatrics, 114,* 650–654.
Montigny M. (1990). Captopril in infants for congestive heart failure secondary to a large ventricular left-to-right shunt. *American Journal of Cardiology, 63,* 631–633.
Rheuban, K. S., et al. (1990). Acute hemodynamic effects of converting enzyme inhibition in infants with congestive heart failure. *Journal of Pediatrics, 117,* 668–670.
Rose, R., Bollinger, R., & Pinsky, W. (1992). Grading the severity of congestive heart failure in infants. *Pediatric Cardiology, 13,* 72–75.
Ross, R., et al. (1987). Plasma norepinephrine levels in infants and children with congestive heart failure. *American Journal of Cardiology, 59,* 911–914.
Salmon, A., et al. (1989). Sodium balance in infants with severe congestive heart failure [letter]. *Lancet, 2,* 875.
Shaddy, R. E., et al. (1988). Short-term hemodynamic effects of captopril in infants with congestive heart failure. *American Journal of Diseases of Children, 142,* 100–105.
Stone, J., Bentur, Y., Zalstein, E., et al. (1990). Effect of endogenous digoxin-like substances on the interpretation of high concentrations of digoxin in children. *Journal of Pediatrics, 117,* 321–325.

Congenital Heart Disease

Benson, D. (1989). Changing profile of congenital heart disease. *Pediatrics, 83,* 790–791.
Brandhagen, D., et al. (1991). Long-term psychologic implications of congenital heart disease: A 25-year follow-up. *Mayo Clinic Proceedings, 66,* 474–479.
Case, C. L., Trippael, D. L., & Gillette, P. C. (1989). New antiarrhythmic agents in pediatrics. *Pediatric Clinics of North America, 36,* 1293–1320.
De Maso, D., Campis, L., Wypy, D., et al. (1991). The impact of maternal perceptions and medical severity on the adjustment of children with congenital heart disease. *Journal of Pediatric Psychology, 16,* 137–149.
Driscoll, J. (1990). Evaluation of the cyanotic newborn. *Pediatric Clinics of North America, 37,* 1–23.
Gellis, S. S., & Kagan, B. M. (1990). *Current pediatric therapy 13.* Philadelphia: WB Saunders.
Hoffman, J. (1990). Congenital heart disease: Incidence and inheritance. *Pediatric Clinics of North America, 37,* 31.
Horner, M., & Rawlins, K. (1987). How parents of children with chronic conditions perceive their own needs. *MCN: American Journal of Maternal Child Nursing, 12,* 40–43.
Kulik, L., Hickey, P., & Lawrence, P. (1991). Pharmacologic interventions for the neonate with compromised cardiac function. *Journal of Perinatology and Neonatology Nursing, 5,* 71–83.
Linday, L., et al. (1987). Digoxin inactivation by the gut flora in infancy and childhood. *Pediatrics, 79,* 544–548.
Lock, J., Keane, J., & Fellows, K. (1987). *Diagnostic and interventional catheterization in congenital heart disease.* Boston: Martinus, Nijhoff.
Monetl, Z., & Moynihan, P. (1991). Cardiovascular assessment of the neonatal heart. *Journal of Perinatology and Neonatology Nursing, 5,* 50–59.
O'Brien, P., & Boisvert, J. (1989). Discharge planning for children with heart disease. *Critical Care Nursing Clinics of North America, 1,* 297–305.
Perloff, J. (1987). *The clinical recognition of congenital heart disease* (3rd ed.). Philadelphia: WB Saunders.
Purcell, J. (1989). Cardiomyopathy. *American Journal of Nursing, 89,* 57–75.
Rotundi, P. (Issue Ed.). (1989). Cardiac disease in infants and children. *Critical Care Nursing Clinics of North America, 1,* (2).
Salzer, H., et al. (1989). Growth and nutritional intake of infants with congenital heart disease. *Pediatric Cardiology, 10,* 17–23.
Younger, J. (1991). A primary care focus on pediatric cardiology. *Nurse Practitioner Forum, 2,* Mar, 27–32.
Zalstein, E., et al. (1990). Once-daily versus twice-daily dosing of digoxin in the pediatric age group. *Journal of Pediatrics, 116,* 137–139.

Cardiac Surgery

Anella, J., McCloskey, A., & Vieweg, C. (1990). Nursing dynamics of pediatric intra-aortic balloon pumping. *Critical Care Nurse, 4,* 24–37.
Craig, J. (1991). The postoperative cardiac infant: Physiologic basis for neonatal nursing interventions. *Journal of Perinatal and Neonatal Nursing, 5,* 60–70.
Drinkwater, D., & Laks, H. (1989). Principles of pediatric heart surgery. In F. Adams, G. Emmanouilides, & Riemenschneider (Eds.), *Moss' heart disease in infants, children, and adolescents* (4th ed.). Baltimore: Williams & Wilkins.
Girlando, R. M., Belew, B., & Klarn, J. (1988). Coarctation of the aorta. *Critical Care Nurse, 8,* 38–50.
Rao, P. S., Solymar, L., Mardini, M. K., et al. (1989). Anticoagulant therapy in children with prosthetic valves. *Annals of Thoracic Surgery, 47,* 589–592.

Pulmonary Atresia

Freedom, R., et al. (1989). Tricuspid and pulmonary atresia with coarctation of the aorta: A rare combination possibly explained by persistence of the fifth aortic arch with a systemic-to-pulmonary arterial connection. *International Journal of Cardiology, 24,* 241–245.
Hawkins, J., et al. (1990). Early and late results in pulmonary atresia and intact ventricular septum. *Journal of Thoracic and Cardiovascular Surgery, 100,* 492–497.
Iyer, K., & Mee, R. (1991). Staged repair of pulmonary atresia with ventricular septal defect and major systemic to pulmonary artery collaterals. *Annals of Thoracic Surgery, 51,* 65–72.
Shimazaki, Y., et al. (1991). Pulmonary artery morphology and hemodynamics in pulmonic valve atresia with ventricular septal defect before and after repair. *American Journal of Cardiology, 67,* 744–748.
Smyllie, J., et al. (1989). The value of Doppler color flow mapping in determining pulmonary blood supply in infants with pulmonary atresia with ventricular septal defect. *Journal of the American College of Cardiology, 14,* 1759–1765.

Tricuspid Atresia

Gewillig, M., et al. (1990). Impact of Fontan operation on left ventricular size and contractility in tricuspid atresia. *Circulation, 8,* 118–127.
Imai, Y., et al. (1991). Palliative repair of aortic atresia associated with tricuspid atresia and transposition of the great arteries. *Annals of Thoracic Surgery, 51,* 646–648.
Powell, M., & Costenzo, J. (1990). Tricuspid atresia. Surgical treatment, pediatric nursing care. *AORN Journal, 52,* 567–574.
Rao, P. (1992). *Tricuspid atresia* (2nd ed.). Mt. Kisco, NY: Futura.
Sade, R. M., & Fyle, D. (1990). Tricuspid atresia: Current concepts in diagnosis and treatment. *Pediatric Clinics of North America, 37,* 151.

Transposition of the Great Arteries

Callow, L. B. (1989). A new beginning: Nursing care of the infant undergoing the arterial switch operation for transposition of the great arteries. *Heart and Lung, 18,* 248–257.
Castaneda, A. (1989). Correction of transposition: Arterial switch procedure. In H. Grello (Ed.), *Current therapy in cardiothoracic surgery.* Toronto: BC Decker.
Deanfield, J. (1989). Transposition of the great arteries: To switch or not to switch? *Current Opinion in Pediatrics, 1,* 85–89.
Kirklin, J. W., Colvin, E. V., McConnell, M. E., & Bargeron, L. M. (1990). Complete transposition of the great arteries: Treatment

in the current era. *Pediatric Clinics of North America, 37,* 171–178.

Malinowski, P., & Elixson, M. (1985). Transposition of the great arteries. *Critical Care Nurse, 5,* 35–48.

Moynihan, P., & King, R. (1989). Caring for patients with lesions increasing pulmonary blood flow. *Critical Care Nursing Clinics of North America, 1,* 195–214.

Tetralogy of Fallot

Amato, J., et al. (1990). The central shunt: Aortopulmonary Gore-Tex shunt. *Seminars in Thoracic and Cardiovascular Surgery, 2,* 34–45.

Barbero-Marcial, M., & Jatene, A. (1990). Surgical management of the anomalies of the pulmonary arteries in the tetralogy of Fallot with pulmonary atresia. *Seminars in Thoracic and Cardiovascular Surgery, 2,* 93–107.

Castaneda, A. (1990). Classical repair of tetralogy of Fallot: Timing, technique and results. *Seminars in Thoracic and Cardiovascular Surgery, 2,* 70–75.

Deanfield, J. (1991). Late ventricular arrhythmias occurring after repair of tetralogy of Fallot: Do they matter? *International Journal of Cardiology, 30,* 143–150.

Giddings, S., Bessel, M., & Liao, Y. (1990). Determinants of hemoglobin concentration in cyanotic heart disease. *Pediatric Cardiology, 11,* 121–125.

Kirklin, J., et al. (1990). Predicting the degree of relief of the pulmonary stenosis or atresia after the repair of tetralogy of Fallot. *Seminars in Thoracic Cardiovascular Surgery, 2,* 55–60.

Kulik, L. (1989). Caring for patients with lesions decreasing pulmonary blood flow. *Critical Care Nursing Clinics of North America, 1,* 215–230.

McConnell, M. (1990). Echocardiography in classical tetralogy of Fallot. *Seminars in Thoracic and Cardiovascular Surgery, 2,* 2–11.

Pacifico, A., et al. (1990). Tetralogy of Fallot: Late results and reoperations. *Seminars in Thoracic and Cardiovascular Surgery, 2,* 108–116.

Page, G. (1986). Tetralogy of Fallot. *Heart and Lung, 15,* 390–399.

Pinsky, W., & Arciniegas, E. (1990). Tetralogy of Fallot. *Pediatric Clinics of North America, 37,* 179–192.

Rosenkranz, E. (1990). Modified Blalock-Taussig shunts in the treatment of tetralogy of Fallot. *Seminars in Thoracic and Cardiovascular Surgery, 2,* 27–33.

Rosenthal, G., et al. (1991). Birth weight and cardiovascular malformations: A population-based study. The Baltimore-Washington Infant Study. *American Journal of Epidemiology, 133,* 1273–1281.

Sreeram, N., et al. (1991). Results of balloon pulmonary valvuloplasty as a palliative procedure in tetralogy of Fallot. *Journal of the American College of Cardiology, 18,* 159–165.

Ventricular Septal Defect

Gersony, W. (1989). Coarctation of the aorta and ventricular septal defect in infancy: Left ventricular volume and management issues. *Journal of the American College of Cardiology, 14,* 1553–1554.

Kimball, T. (1991). Relation of symptoms to contractility and defect size in infants with ventricular septal defect. *American Journal of Cardiology, 67,* 1097–1102.

Marino, B., et al. (1990). Ventricular septal defect in Down syndrome: Anatomic types and associated malformations. *American Journal of Diseases of Children, 144,* 544–545.

Martin, G. R. (1989). Increased prevalence of ventricular septal defect: Epidemic or improved diagnosis. *Pediatrics, 83,* 200–203.

Moynihan, P., & King, P. (1989). Caring for patients with lesions increasing blood flow. *Critical Care Nursing Clinics of North America, 1,* 215–230.

Nordenberg, D., et al. (1989). Atrial septal defect, ventricular septal defect, and coarctation of the aorta in sibs: An autosomal recessive disorder? *American Journal of Medical Genetics, 32,* 182–183.

O'Laughlin, M., & Mullins, C. (1989). Transcatheter occlusion of ventricular septal defect. *Catheterization and Cardiovascular Diagnosis, 17,* 175–179.

Pacifico, A. D. (1989). Surgical treatment of complex atrioventricular septal defects. *Cardiology Clinics, 7,* 399–410.

Perrault, H., et al. (1989). Comparison of cardiovascular adjustments to exercise in adolescents 8 to 15 years of age after correction of tetralogy of Fallot, ventricular septal defect or atrial septal defect. *American Journal of Cardiology, 64,* 213–217.

Vermilion, R., et al. (1989). Transient atrioventricular block resulting from left ventricular angiography in infants with ventricular septal defect. *American Journal of Cardiology, 64,* 128–130.

Atrial Septal Defect

Borow, K., & Karp, R. (1990). Atrial septal defect—Lessons from the past, directions for the future. *New England Journal of Medicine, 323,* 1698–1700.

Finley, J., et al. (1989). Sinus arrhythmia in children with atrial septal defect: An analysis of heart rate variability before and after surgical repair. *British Heart Journal, 61,* 280–284.

Hamilton, J., et al. (1991). Alternative technique for repair of sinus venosus atrial septal defect. *Annals of Thoracic Surgery, 51,* 144–146.

Kronzon, I., et al. (1991). Transesophageal echocardiography is superior to transthoracic echocardiography in the diagnosis of sinus venosus atrial septal defect. *Journal of the American College of Cardiology, 17,* 537–542.

Moynihan, P., & King, R. (1989). Caring for patients with lesions increasing pulmonary blood flow. *Critical Care Nursing Clinics of North America, 1,* 195–214.

Murphy, J., et al. (1990). Long-term outcome after surgical repair of isolated atrial septal defect. Follow-up at 27 to 32 years. *New England Journal of Medicine, 323,* 1645–1650.

Rao, P. (1991). Transcatheter occlusion of cardiac septal defects. *Indian Journal of Pediatrics, 58,* 605–621.

Rao, P., et al. (1992). Transcatheter closure of atrial septal defect by "buttoned" devices. *American Journal of Cardiology,* April, *69,* 1056–1061.

Vet, T., & Ottenkamp, J. (1989). Correction of atrioventricular septal defect. *American Journal of Diseases in Children, 143,* 1361–1365.

Pulmonary Stenosis

Beekman, R., Rocchini, A., & Rosenthal, A. (1989). Therapeutic cardiac catheterization for pulmonary valve and pulmonary artery stenosis. *Cardiology Clinics, 7,* 331–340.

Dubois, J., et al. (1991). Modified Blalock-Taussig shunt anastomosis in a three month old child with pulmonary stenosis: Embolization therapy. *Pediatric Radiology, 21,* 198–199.

Engelhardt, W., et al. (1990). Transient transcatheter balloon closure of patent foramen ovale following surgical repair of critical pulmonary stenosis. *Thoracic and Cardiovascular Surgeon, 38,* 377–378.

McCrindle, B., Kan, J. (1991). Long term results after balloon pulmonary valvuloplasty. *Circulation, 83,* 1915–1922.

Rheuban, K., et al. (1991). Successful balloon pulmonary valvuloplasty in a neonate with Ebstein's anomaly and critical pulmonic stenosis. *American Heart Journal, 121,* 1565–1567.

Rodriguez, R., & Riggs, T. (1990). Physiologic peripheral pulmonic stenosis in infancy. *American Journal of Cardiology, 66,* 1478–1481.

Tometzki, A., et al. (1991). Balloon valvuloplasty of critical aortic and pulmonary stenosis in the premature neonate. *International Journal of Cardiology, 30,* 248–249.

Vogel, M., Eger, R., et al. (1990). Brock transventricular pulmonary valvotomy in patients with pulmonary stenosis: Long-term results. *Pediatric Cardiology, 11,* 191–194.

Zacharisen, M., & Friedberg, D. (1991). Percutaneous balloon pulmonary valvuloplasty in children. *Wisconsin Medical Journal, 90,* 15–18.

Hypoplastic Left Heart Syndrome

Aiello, V., et al. (1990). Morphologic features of the hypoplastic left heart syndrome—A reappraisal. *Pediatric Pathology, 10,* 931–943.

Backer, C., et al. (1990). Cardiac transplantation for hypoplastic left heart syndrome: A modified technique. *Annals of Thoracic Surgery, 50,* 894–898.

Bailey, L., & Gundry, S. (1990). Hypoplastic left heart syndrome. *Pediatric Clinics of North America, 37,* 137–150.

Freedom, R. (1989). The hypoplastic left heart syndrome: Evolving trends and therapy and present concerns. *Current Opinion in Pediatrics, 1,* 90–93.

Glauser, T., et al. (1990). Congenital brain anomalies associated with the hypoplastic left heart syndrome. *Pediatrics, 85,* 984–990.

Johnson, A., & Downs, J. (1991). Treatment options for the neonate with hypoplastic left heart syndrome. *Journal of Perinatology and Neonatology Nursing, 5,* 84–92.

Hedenkamp, E. (1988). Hypoplastic left heart syndrome—options for the infant and family. *Progress in Cardiovascular Nursing, 2,* 80–85.

Meliones, J., et al. (1990). Longitudinal results after first-stage palliation for hypoplastic left heart syndrome. *Circulation, 82* (Suppl. 5), 151–156.

Morris, C., et al. (1990). Hypoplastic left heart syndrome: Natural history in a geographically defined population. *Pediatrics, 85,* 977–983.

Murdison, K., et al. (1990). Hypoplastic left heart syndrome. Outcome after initial reconstruction and before modified Fontan procedure. *Circulation, 82* (Suppl. 5), 199–207.

Noonan, D., Koster, N., & White-Traut, R. (1991). Nursing considerations for the neonate awaiting heart transplantation for the hypoplastic left heart syndrome. *Journal of Pediatric Nursing,* Oct., *6,* 322–330.

Norwood, W., & Pigott, J. (1989). Reconstructive surgery for hypoplastic left heart syndrome. In H. C. Gillo, W. G. Austen, & E. W. Wilkins (Eds.), *Current therapy in cardiothoracic surgery.* Toronto: BC Decker.

Panyard, J., & Kaneta, M. (1988). Hypoplastic left heart syndrome: Clinical manifestations and treatment. *Neonatal Network, 7,* 17–35.

Pigott, J., Murphy, J., et al. (1988). Palliative reconstructive surgery for hypoplastic left heart syndrome. *Annals of Thoracic Surgery, 45,* 122–128.

Smith, J., & Vernon-Levett, P. (1989). Hypoplastic left heart syndrome: Treatment and options. *MCN: American Journal of Maternal Child Nursing, 14,* 180–183.

Zuberbuhler, J., Fricker, F., & Griffith, B. (1989). Cardiac transplantation in children. *Cardiology Clinics, 7,* 411–418.

Ebstein Anomaly

Bennett, M., & Shiu, M. (1991). Ebstein's anomaly associated with splenomegaly and reversible hypersplenism. *British Heart Journal, 65,* 223–224.

Chan, K., et al. (1989). Surgical correction of tetralogy of Fallot in the presence of Ebstein's anomaly of the tricuspid valve. *International Journal of Cardiology, 25,* 242–243.

Choe, K., et al. (1990). Atrioventricular septal defect and Ebstein's malformation. *American Journal of Cardiology, 65,* 939–941.

Kulik, L. (1989). Caring for patients with lesions decreasing pulmonary blood flow. *Critical Care Nursing Clinics of North America, 1,* 215–230.

Plowden, J., et al. (1991). The use of extracorporeal membrane oxygenation in critically ill neonates with Ebstein's anomaly. *American Heart Journal, 121,* 619–622.

Quaeqebeur, J., et al. (1991). Surgery for Ebstein's anomaly: The clinical and echocardiographic evaluation of a new technique. *Journal of the American College of Cardiology, 17,* 722–728.

Rheuban, K., et al. (1991). Successful balloon pulmonary valvuloplasty in a neonate with Ebstein's anomaly and critical pulmonic stenosis. *American Heart Journal, 121,* 1565–1567.

Roberson, D., & Silverman, N. (1989). Ebstein's anomaly: Echocardiographic and clinical features in the fetus and neonate. *Journal of the American College of Cardiology, 14,* 1300–1307.

Siebert, J., et al. (1989). Ebstein's anomaly and extracardiac defects. *American Journal of Diseases in Children, 143,* 570–572.

Starnes, V., et al. (1991). Ebstein's anomaly appearing in the neonate. A new surgical approach. *Journal of Thoracic and Cardiovascular Surgery, 101,* 1082–1087.

Heart Transplantation

Chartrand, C., et al. (1989). Pediatric cardiac transplantation. *Transplant Proceedings, 21,* 3349–3350.

deLeval, M., et al. (1988). Total cavopulmonary connection: A logical alternative to autopulmonary connection for complex Fontan operation. *Journal of Thoracic Cardiovascular Surgery, 96,* 682–695.

Dunn, J., & Donner, R. (Eds.) (1990). *Heart transplantation in children.* Mt. Kisco, NY: Futura.

Fricker, F., et al. (1987). Experience with heart transplantation in children. *Pediatrics, 79,* 138–146.

Heck, C., et al. (1989). The Registry of the International Society for Heart Transplantation Sixth Official Report—1989. *Journal of Heart Transplantation, 8,* 271–276.

Hutchings, S., & Monett, Z. (1989). Caring for the cardiac transplant patient. *Critical Care Nursing Clinics of North America, 1,* 245–262.

Kahan, B. (1989). Pharmacokinetics and pharmacodynamics of cyclosporine. *Transplant Proceedings, 21,* 9–15.

Kahan, B. (1987). Immunosuppressive therapy with cyclosporine for cardiac transplantation. *Circulation, 75,* 40–56.

Kauffman, R. (1990). Cardiac transplantation in infants and children. *Journal of Pediatrics, 116,* 266–268.

Lawrence, K., & Fricker, F. (1987). Pediatric heart transplantation: Quality of life. *Journal of Heart Transplantation, 6,* 329–333.

Aortic Stenosis

Beekman, R., et al. (1991). Balloon valvuloplasty for critical aortic stenosis in the newborn: Influence of new catheter technology. *Journal of the American College of Cardiology, 17,* 1172–1176.

Gerraughty, A. (1989). Caring for patients with lesions obstructing systemic blood flow. *Critical Care Nursing Clinics of North America, 1,* 231–244.

Hata, T., et al. (1990). Prenatal diagnosis of valvar aortic stenosis by Doppler echocardiography and magnetic resonance imaging. *American Journal of Obstetrics and Gynecology, 162,* 1068–1070.

Hofstetter, R., et al. (1990). Echocardiographic evaluation of systolic left-ventricular function in infants with critical aortic stenosis before and after aortic valvotomy. *Thoracic and Cardiovascular Surgeon, 38,* 236–240.

Karl, T., et al. (1990). Critical aortic stenosis in the first month of life: Surgical results in 26 infants. *Annals of Thoracic Surgery, 50,* 105–109.

Leung, M., et al. (1991). Critical aortic stenosis in early infancy. Anatomic and echocardiographic substrates of successful open valvotomy. *Journal of Thoracic and Cardiovascular Surgery, 101,* 526–535.

Ludomirsky, A., et al. (1991). Left ventricular mid-cavitary obstruction after balloon dilation in isolated aortic valve stenosis in children. *Catheterization and Cardiovascular Diagnosis, 22,* 89–92.

Perry, A. B., et al. (1989). Interventional catheterization of left heart lesions, including aortic and mitral valve stenosis and coarctation of the aorta. *Cardiology Clinic, 7,* 341–349.

Tometzki, A., et al. (1991). Balloon valvoplasty of critical aortic and pulmonary stenosis in the premature neonate. *International Journal of Cardiology, 30,* 248–249.

Turley, K., et al. (1990). Neonatal aortic stenosis. *Journal of Thoracic and Cardiovascular Surgery, 99,* 679–834.

Acquired Heart Disease

Dajani, A., et al. (1990). Prevention of bacterial endocarditis: Recommendations by the American Heart Association. *JAMA, 264,* 2919–2922.

Ho, S., et al. (1989). Endocarditis in an infant causing "tricuspid atresia." *International Journal of Cardiology, 22,* 393–394.

Hohn, H., & Stanton, R. (1987). Myocarditis in children. *Pediatric Review, 9,* 83–88.

Howard, J., Bindler, R., Dimico, G., et al. (1991). Cardiovascular risk factors in children: A Bloomsday research report. *Journal of Pediatric Nursing,* Aug., *6,* 222–229.

Lux, K. (1991). New hope for children with Kawasaki disease. *Journal of Pediatric Nursing,* June, *6,* 159–165.

Muirhead, J. (1989). Heart and heart-lung transplantation. *Nursing Clinics of North America, 24,* 865–880.

Murdock, D., et al. (1987). Rejection of the transplanted heart. *Heart and Lung, 16,* 237–245.

Pahl, E., et al. (1990). Coronary arteriosclerosis in pediatric heart transplant survivors: Limitation of long-term survival. *Journal of Pediatrics, 116,* 177–183.

Radley-Smith, R. (1989). Cardiac transplantation in the management of congenital and acquired heart disease. *Current Opinion in Pediatrics, 1,* 100–102.

Schnepf, C. (1987). The pediatric heart transplant patient: Immunosuppressive drugs and organ rejection. *Journal of Pediatric Health Care, 1,* 91–97.

Scrima, D. (1987). Infective endocarditis: Nursing considerations. *Critical Care Nursing, 7,* 47–56.

Shrivastava, S., & Radhakrishnan, S. (1989). Infective endocarditis following patch closure of ventricular septal defect: A cross-sectional Doppler echocardiographic study. *International Journal of Cardiology, 25,* 27–31.

Wensley, K. T., et al. (1987). Infective endocarditis in children with congenital heart disease: Comparison of selected features in patients with surgical correction of palliation and those without. *British Medical Journal, 58,* 57–65.

Hypertension

American Academy of Pediatrics: Report of the Second Task Force on Blood Pressure Control—1987. *Pediatrics, 79,* 1–25.

Berenson, G., et al. (1989). Pathogenesis of hypertension in black and white children. *Clinical Cardiology, 12* (Suppl. 4), 3–8.

Danforth, J. (1990). Exercise as a treatment for hypertension in low-socioeconomic-status black children. *Journal of Consulting and Clinical Psychology, 58,* 237–279.

Daniels, S. (1991). The prevalence of retinal vascular abnormalities in children and adolescents with essential hypertension. *American Journal of Ophthalmology, 111,* 205–208.

DeSwiet, M., & Dillon, M. (1989). Hypertension in children. *British Medical Journal, 299,* 469–470.

Dillon, M. (1987). Investigation and management of hypertension in children. A personal perspective. *Pediatric Nephrology, 1,* 59–68.

Falkner, B. (1989). Essential hypertension in children. *Current Opinion in Pediatrics, 1,* 131–134.

Kanai, H., et al. (1990). Hypertension in obese children: Fasting serum insulin levels are closely correlated with blood pressure. *International Journal of Obesity, 14,* 1047–1056.

Liu, Z., et al. (1990). Endogenous digoxin-like substance as an important factor in the development of hypertension in children. *International Journal of Cardiology, 29,* 343–348.

Mendoza, S. (1990). Hypertension in infants and children. *Nephron, 54,* 289–295.

National Heart, Lung, and Blood Institute Task Force on Blood Pressure Control in Children. (1987). *Report of the second task force on blood pressure control in children.* Washington, DC: US Department of Health and Human Services, Public Health Service, National Institutes of Health.

Rocchini, A. P., et al. (1988). Blood pressure in obese adolescents: Effect of weight loss. *Pediatrics, 82,* 16–23.

Scharer, K. (1987). Hypertension in children and adolescents—1986. *Pediatric Nephrology, 1,* 50–58.

Sinaiko, A. R., Gomez-Marin, O., & Prineas, R. (1989). Prevalence of "significant" hypertension in junior high school-aged children: The children and adolescent blood pressure program. *Journal of Pediatrics, 114,* 664–669.

Whincup, P. H., Cook, D. V., & Shaper, A. G. (1989). Early influences on blood pressure: A study of children aged 5–7 years. *British Medical Journal, 299,* 587–591.

Psychosocial Care

Alpern, D., Uzark, K., & Dick, M. (1989). Psychosocial responses of children to cardiac pacemakers. *Journal of Pediatrics, 114,* 494–501.

Curley, M. A. Q. (1988). Effects of the nursing mutual participation model of care and parental stress in the pediatric intensive care unit. *Heart & Lung, 17,* 682–688.

DeMaso, D., Campis, L., et al. (1991). The impact of maternal perceptions and medical severity on the adjustment of children with congenital heart disease. *Journal of Pediatric Psychology, 16,* 137–149.

Johnson, P. A., Nelson, G. L., & Brunnquell, D. J. (1988). Parent and nurse perceptions of parental stressors in the pediatric intensive care unit. *Children's Health Care, 17,* 98–105.

Kasper, J. W., & Nyamathi, A. M. (1988). Parents of children in the pediatric intensive care unit: What are their needs? *Heart & Lung, 17,* 574–581.

Philichi, L. M. (1989). Family adaptation during a pediatric intensive care hospitalization. *Journal of Pediatric Nursing, 4,* 268–276.

Proctor, D. L. (1987). Relationship between visitation policy in a pediatric intensive care unit and parental anxiety. *Children's Health Care, 16,* 13–17.

Shelton, T. L., Jeppson, E. S., & Johnson, B. H. (1987). *Family-centered care for children with special health care needs.* Washington, DC: Association for the Care of Children's Health.

Vulcan, B. M., Nikulich-Barrett, M. (1988). The effect of selected information on mothers' anxiety levels during their children's hospitalizations. *Journal of Pediatric Nursing, 3,* 97–102.

Wilson, T., & Broom, M. (1989). Promoting the young child's development in the intensive care unit. *Heart and Lung, 18,* 247–281.

Youngbult, J. M., & Jay, S. S. (1991). Emergent admission to the pediatric intensive care unit: Parent concerns. *AACN Clinical Issues in Critical Care Nursing, 2,* 329–337.

CHAPTER • 34

Altered Hematologic Function

Marcia Sosnowski Leonard

NURSING CARE PLAN
NPP: The Child with Altered Tissue Perfusion: Anemia, Table 34–8

RELATED TOPICS
The impact of chronic illness, Chapter 19
Interventions for pain management, Chapter 25
Genetic counseling, Chapter 31
Patterns of inheritance, Chapter 31
NPP: The Family with a Genetic Risk, Table 31–17
AIDS, Chapter 37

LEARNING OBJECTIVES

- Describe the anatomy and physiology of blood that includes the function and production of RBC, WBC, and platelets.
- Identify the age-related differences in RBC concentration and WBC values.
- Identify the key elements in the history and physical examination of the child with anemia.
- Demonstrate an understanding of the pathologic features and the therapeutic management of childhood blood disorders.
- Identify the major nursing diagnostic statements associated with childhood blood disorders and nursing interventions used to ameliorate or modify the defining characteristics of those statements.
- Synthesize and apply information to the nursing care of children with childhood blood disorders.

Childhood blood disorders are a heterogeneous group of diseases with wide ranges of etiology, severity, treatment, and prognoses. This is due in great part to the complex structure and function of blood and to the independent functions of each of its components. Blood components affect every cell in the body. The constituents of blood are so vital to homeostasis that severe disorders or deficiencies may be incompatible with life, and even mild dysfunctions have systemic effects.

Nursing care of children with blood disorders requires a sound knowledge of normal blood anatomy and physiology as well as an understanding of the inheritance patterns of genetic disorders, nutrition, and, as in all pediatric disorders, growth and development.

Structure and Function: Anatomy and Physiology of Blood

Blood is composed of a liquid called "plasma," which contains dissolved proteins (albumin, globulin, and the clotting factors), metabolites and electrolytes, and the formed elements *erythrocytes* (red blood cells), *leukocytes* (white blood cells), and *thrombocytes* (platelets). The constant movement of blood throughout the cardiovascular system keeps the formed elements suspended in the plasma, but when a sample of blood is removed from the body and spun down in a centrifuge, it is possible to separate the solid components from the liquid plasma. The cellular components are quantified via a measurement called "hematocrit," which represents the percentage of blood volume composed of blood cells. Because most (about 97 per cent) of the cells in blood are red blood cells, the hematocrit is a reliable indicator of red cell population. However, it cannot be used to predict white cell or platelet levels (Fig. 34–1).*

Red Blood Cells

Red blood cells are the most abundant cells in the blood. Red blood cells have a biconcave disk form that easily adapts to small blood vessels. In fact, Guyton (1991) likens a red blood cell to a "bag" because it can conform to almost any shape.

Production of Red Blood Cells

Red blood cells are produced in the marrow of bones. Essentially all bones are employed in red cell production during the first 5 years of life. After that time, production in the shafts of the long bones (e.g., tibia, femur) is gradually reduced and hematopoiesis occurs only in the ribs, sternum, and vertebrae as well as the pelvis, skull, clavicles, and scapulas. "Erythropoiesis" is the term used for the process of red blood cell formation. It is illustrated in Figure 34–2.

Red blood cell production is stimulated by decreased tissue oxygenation. That is, red blood cell production depends not on the absolute numbers of red blood cells but on their ability to carry oxygen and carbon dioxide. When tissue oxygenation decreases, the hormone *erythropoietin* stimulates stem cells in the bone marrow to progress to mature red blood cells. Whereas some erythropoietin is thought to be produced in tissues such as the liver, the majority (80 to 90 per cent) is produced in the kidney, probably either in or near the glomeruli (Guyton, 1991). Therefore, kidney disease can affect the body's response to tissue hypoxia.

* White blood cells and platelets are measured in thousands per cubic millimeter and red blood cells are measured in millions per cubic millimeter.

Normal red blood cells have a life span of about 120 days. As they become older, their membranes become more fragile and may rupture when the cells squeeze through a small capillary. Many of the red cells break up in the spleen where they must squeeze through small spaces in the red pulp of that organ. When red cells burst, the hemoglobin is taken up by macrophages, to be released back into the blood for transfer to the bone marrow where it is used for production of new red blood cells. If no more iron is needed for that purpose, iron may be stored in the liver and other tissues in the form of ferritin (Guyton, 1991).

Function of Red Blood Cells

Red blood cells transport oxygen and carbon dioxide to and from the cells of the body, via a mechanism in which oxygen and carbon dioxide bind chemically to *hemoglobin* molecules, the major physiologic component of red cells.

Hemoglobin. Hemoglobin is a complex protein consisting of *heme* (iron-containing) molecules and globin molecules. Its primary function is to bind to oxygen easily and reversibly and then release it at a tissue site. Oxygenated hemoglobin is bright red in color and gives arterial blood its characteristic color. Because most of the red cell weight is made up of hemoglobin, hemoglobin and hematocrit levels vary directly with each other (Fig. 34–3). Normally the hematocrit value is three times greater than the hemoglobin value (Table 34–1).

A secondary function of hemoglobin is its role in the acid-base buffer system. Hemoglobin acts as a weak base to minimize the change in blood pH that occurs as oxygen is absorbed and carbon dioxide released in the lungs, and as oxygen is delivered and carbon dioxide taken up at the tissue level.

Red Blood Cell Indices. Red blood cell indices indicate the size of the cells and their hemoglobin content. They are useful in differentiating types of anemias and are discussed in the section on anemias.

White Blood Cells

White blood cells can be classified into three major groups: lymphocytes, monocytes, and granulocytes. The white blood cell count, or WBC (part of the complete blood count, CBC), expresses the total amount of all white cells in the blood. The white cell *differential* describes the types of white cells present (Table 34–2).

Production of White Blood Cells

Figure 34–2 illustrates the genesis of white blood cells. Pluripotential hematopoietic stem cells exist,

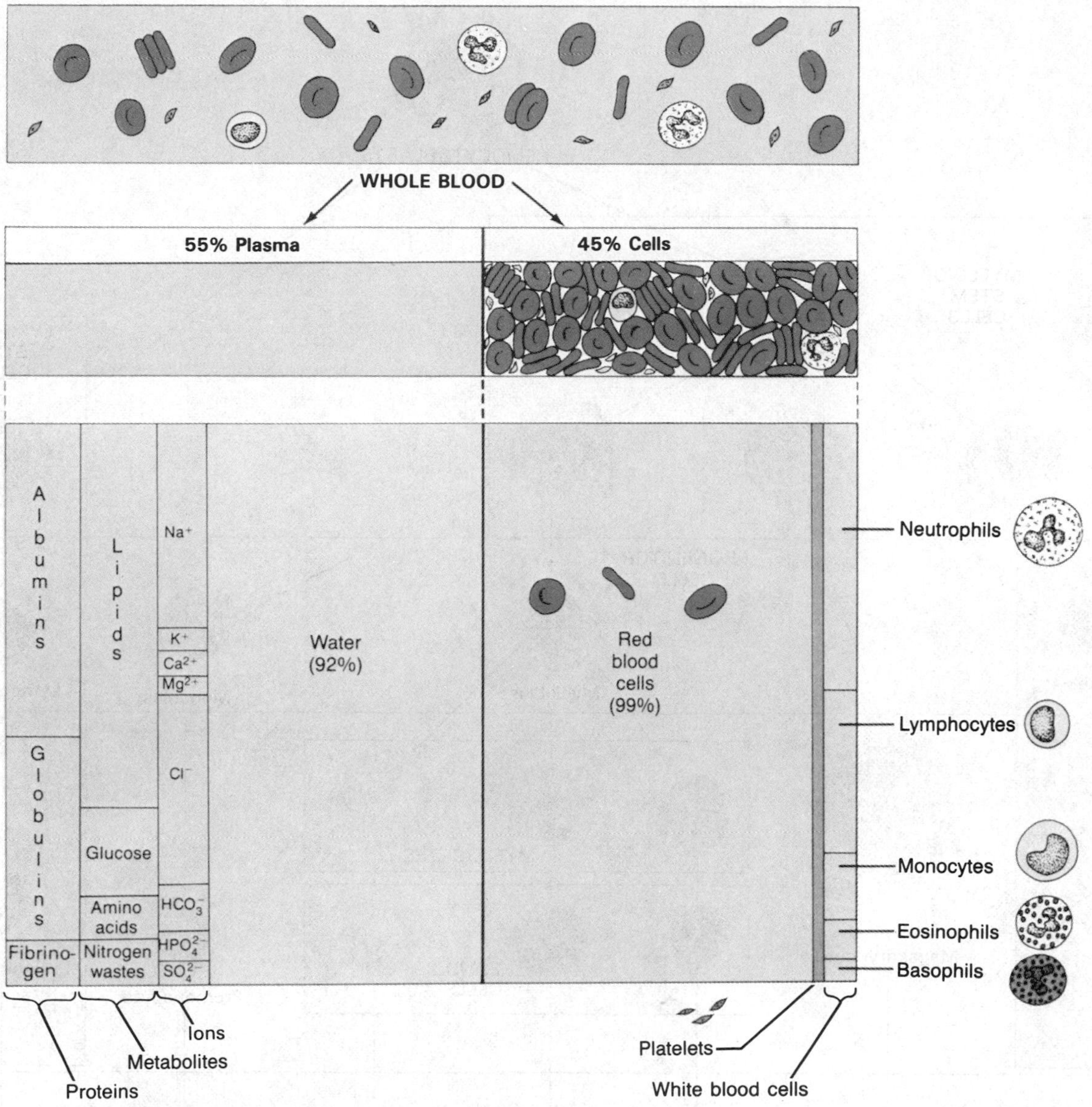

FIGURE 34-1. The composition of whole blood. (From Frederic Martini, *Fundamentals of anatomy and physiology,* 2e, © 1992, p 607. Reprinted by permission of Prentice-Hall, Englewood Cliffs, New Jersey.)

from which any type of blood cell may be formed. These cells give rise to myeloid and lymphoid stem cells. Myeloid and lymphoid stem cells are restricted in their subsequent development. They are called "committed" stem cells, because further reproduction occurs only along a particular cell line. Committed stem cells differentiate to precursors of monocytes and granulocytes as well as platelets and erythrocytes. Lymphoid stem cells form T-lymphocytes and B-lymphocytes. Chapter 37 contains additional information on the immune functions of T-cells and B-cells.

Most white blood stem cells originate in the bone marrow. Granulocytes are completely matured in the marrow; monocytes migrate into body tissue and develop into macrophages. Lymphocytes are produced in the bone marrow but are also produced in the thymus, spleen, and lymph nodes (Guyton, 1991). White blood cells formed in the bone marrow, especially the granulocytes, are stored until needed. Normally, the bone marrow has about a 6-day supply of granulocytes.

Function of White Blood Cells

White blood cells are a component of the body's immune system. Most of those produced reside in peripheral tissues; only a small fraction actually circulate in the blood. There are five types of leukocytes normally present in the blood; they are divided into two

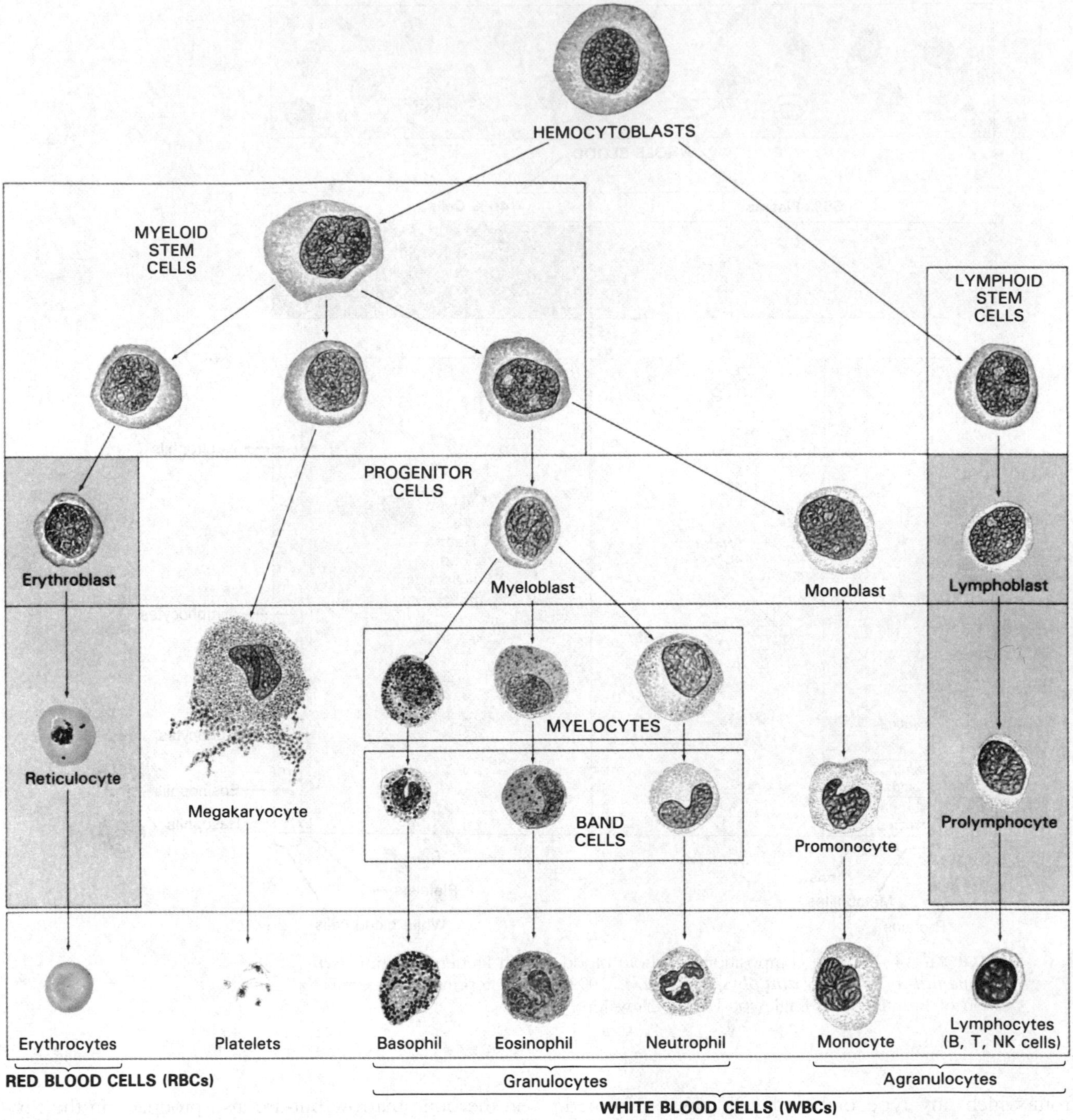

FIGURE 34 - 2. The origins and differentiation of blood cells. (From Frederic Martini, *Fundamentals of anatomy and physiology,* 2e, © 1992, p 629. Reprinted by permission of Prentice-Hall, Englewood Cliffs, New Jersey.)

main groups: the granulocytes (neutrophils, eosinophils, and basophils), and the agranulocytes (monocytes and lymphocytes). An important function of white blood cells is to attack and destroy invading bacteria, viruses, fungi, and other foreign cells.

This function falls primarily to the *neutrophils*. Neutrophils are the most numerous white blood cells throughout most of the life cycle. They are highly mobile and are the first white blood cells to arrive at the site of an injury. Their life span is very short, 10 to 12 hours, the shorter span for cells actively ingesting bacteria (a process called phagocytosis). The number of neutrophils can increase dramatically—four- to fivefold—within a few hours after inflammation begins (Guyton, 1991).

Eosinophils function mainly in response to para-

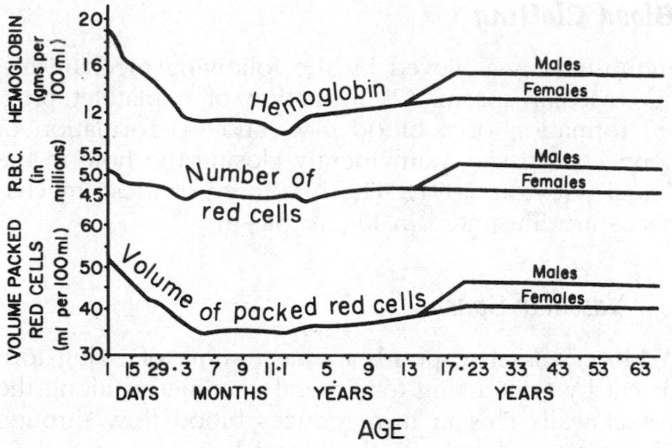

FIGURE 34-3. Relationship of age and sex to the hemoglobin content, red blood cell (R.B.C.) count, and volume of packed red cells (hematocrit) of the blood. (From Guyton, A. [1986]. *Textbook of medical physiology* [8th ed.]. Philadelphia: WB Saunders.)

TABLE 34-1
Age-Specific Parameters: Hemoglobin and Hematocrit

Age	Hemoglobin (g/dl)	Hematocrit (%)
6–23 mos	<10	<31
2–5 yrs	<11	<34
6–12 yrs	<12	<37

Data from U. S. Department of Health Education and Health Services, Centers for Disease Control (1976, June). *Nutrition.* Washington, DC: US Government Printing Office.

sites and allergens. They are mobile cells that migrate to the tissues diseased by parasites, where they attach to the invading organisms. They can kill immature forms of parasites by secreting chemicals toxic to the parasites. Eosinophils also appear in great numbers at sites of an allergic reaction (see Table 37–12). They help mediate the untoward effects of the allergic response by deactivating substances such as histamine.

Basophils secrete heparin into the blood stream to prevent blood coagulation and to facilitate the removal of fat particles from the blood after a fatty meal. Basophils are important to the inflammatory reaction and the allergic response, because they release histamine, bradykinin, serotonin, and other substances into the injured tissues. (See further on for more discussion of basophils, mast cells, and the inflammatory response.)

Lymphocytes respond to specific microorganisms, foreign proteins, and toxins. The two types of lymphocytes, T-cells and B-cells, respond very differently. T-cells enter the peripheral tissues and directly attack the offending agent. B-cells produce and secrete antibodies that can attack and kill invading pathogens.

Stimulus for Production of White Cells

Tissue damage is the stimulus for increased production of neutrophils. Tissue damage may be related to an inflammatory response to infection, malignancy, acute hemorrhage, poisoning, operative procedures, or injection of foreign protein into the body (Guyton, 1991). In response to tissue damage, both the total white blood cell count and the proportion of neutrophils increase (Pearson, 1987). In its haste to supply neutrophils to fight bacteria (or another cause of tissue damage), the body often releases immature band cells or even less mature neutrophil precursors.

TABLE 34-2
Hematologic Values During Infancy and Childhood

	Hemoglobin g/dl		Hematocrit %		Reticulocytes %	Leukocytes WBC/mm³		Differential Counts: Neutrophils %		Lymphocytes %	Eosinophils %	Monocytes %
Age	Mean	Range	Mean	Range	Mean	Mean	Range	Mean	Range	Mean*	Mean	Mean
Cord blood	16.8	13.7–20.1	55	45–65	5.0	18,000	(9–30,000)	61	(40–80)	31	2	6
2 wks	16.5	13.0–20.0	50	42–66	1.0	12,000	(5–21,000)	40		48	3	9
3 mos	12.0	9.5–14.5	36	31–41	1.0	12,000	(6–18,000)	30		63	2	5
6 mos–6 yrs	12.0	10.5–14.0	37	33–42	1.0	10,000	(6–15,000)	45		48	2	5
7–12 yrs	13.0	11.0–16.0	38	34–40	1.0	8000	(4500–13,500)	55		38	2	5
Adult												
Female	14	12.0–16.0	42	37–47	1.6	7500	(5–10,000)	55	(35–70)	35	3	7
Male	16	14.0–18.0	47	42–52								

From Behrman, R. (Ed.) (1992). *Nelson textbook of pediatrics* (14th ed.). Philadelphia: WB Saunders.
*Relatively wide range.

This phenomenon is called a "shift to the left." Presumably the name reflects the fact that neutrophils are usually reported as the first column on the *left* of a differential count and that a *shift* has taken place in which neutrophils now occupy a higher percentage of the total white blood cell population.

Whereas an increased number of neutrophils characterizes an acute infection or tissue damage, the response to a chronic infection is often an increase in monocytes rather than neutrophils. This results in an increased ratio of macrophages to neutrophils in the damaged tissue. See Table 34–2 for normal values of the white cells differential at various ages.

Platelets

Platelets are fragments of megakaryocytes (see Fig. 34–2. Megakaryocytes mature in the bone marrow, where they eventually break up, each releasing some 5000 platelets into the blood (Andreoli et al, 1986). Platelets have a circulating life span of 7 to 10 days and are an integral component in blood *hemostasis* (prevention of bleeding). Among other hemostatic functions, platelets adhere to damaged blood vessel walls and aggregate, or clump together, to form plugs at the site of tissue injury. Blood flow can usually continue through the platelet plug so that the vessel remains functional. Platelet numbers normally remain stable, ranging from 150,000 to 400,000/mm^3 throughout life.

Blood Clotting

Hemostasis is achieved by the following mechanisms: (1) vascular spasm, (2) formation of a platelet plug, (3) formation of a blood clot, and (4) formation of connective tissue, permanently closing the hole in the vessel (Guyton, 1991). The first three of these mechanisms are illustrated in Figure 34–4.

Vascular Spasm

A blood vessel responds to the trauma of being torn or cut by contracting for several centimeters along the vessel wall. This in turn reduces blood flow through the vessel and reduces the blood loss.

Formation of a Platelet Plug

Small holes in vessel walls can be repaired by platelet plugs. When platelets come in contact with damaged vessels, they swell, assume irregular forms, and adhere to the walls of the vessel at the site of the damage. Further, they activate other platelets in the area, and these cells adhere to the first. Through this succession platelets group together to "plug" the hole. The effect of decreased platelets *(thrombocytopenia)* can be seen in the multiple petechiae that occur when platelets are not available in sufficient numbers to plug the normally occurring holes in small blood vessels.

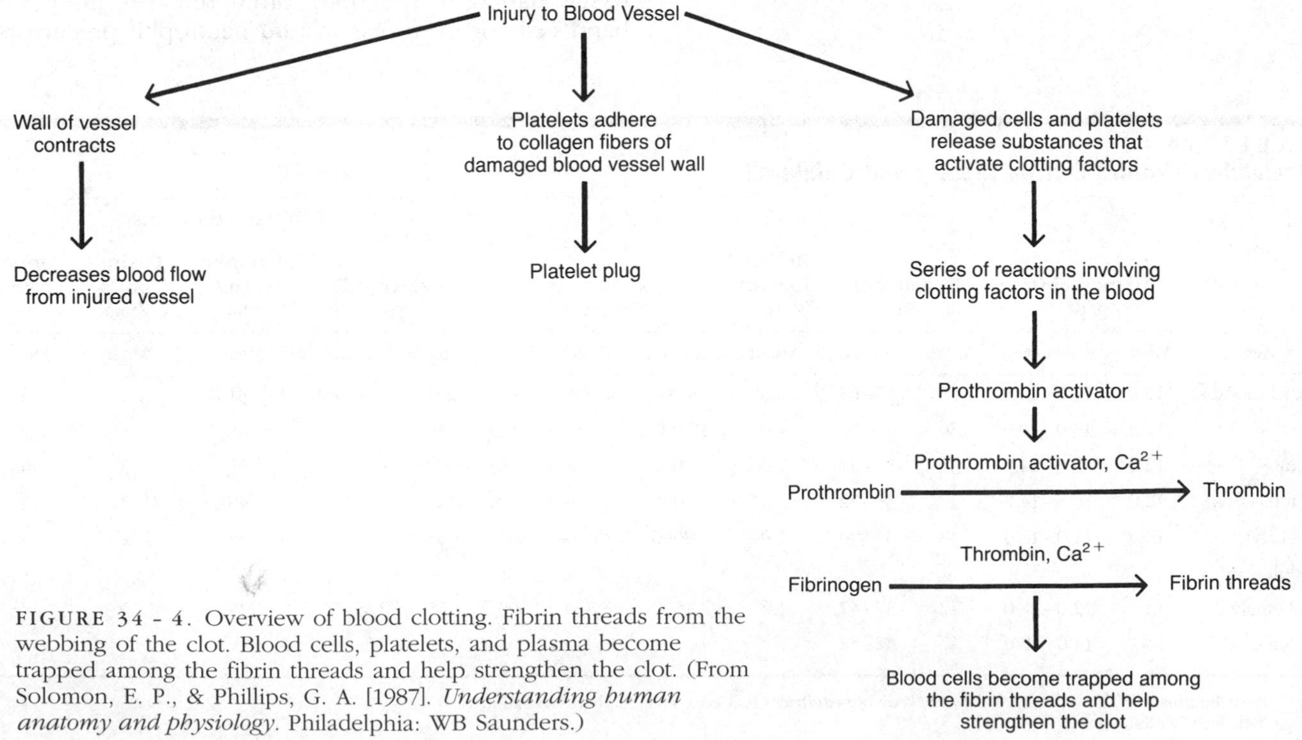

FIGURE 34-4. Overview of blood clotting. Fibrin threads from the webbing of the clot. Blood cells, platelets, and plasma become trapped among the fibrin threads and help strengthen the clot. (From Solomon, E. P., & Phillips, G. A. [1987]. *Understanding human anatomy and physiology*. Philadelphia: WB Saunders.)

Formation of a Blood Clot

Clotting is generally agreed to occur in three steps: (1) the formation of prothrombin activator, (2) the conversion of prothrombin to thrombin, and (3) the conversion of fibrinogen into fibrin threads (Fig. 34–4). The first step is the most complex because it involves a group of clotting factors (involved in the intrinsic and extrinsic pathways). Each clotting factor depends on the presence and activation of the one before it in the pathway and, in some cases, on additional clotting factors. Table 34–3 lists the clotting factors and their synonyms.

Step One: The Formation of Prothrombin Activator. The *extrinsic pathway* is set in motion by trauma to the vascular wall and surrounding tissues. It involves conversion of factor X to activated factor X with the assistance of factor VII and chemicals released into the tissues at the time of injury (tissue factor). With the help of factor V, activated factor X forms prothrombin activator. Calcium ions are important for conversions all along the pathway.

The *intrinsic pathway* is stimulated by contact of factor XII and platelets with collagen in the wall of a damaged vessel. This pathway is even more complex, forming prothrombin activator only after a series of steps (sometimes called a "cascade") in which factors XII, XI, IX, and X are each activated in sequence. Factor VIII (which results in classic hemophilia [or hemophilia A] when quantities are decreased) is also necessary for activation of factor X. Factor V also comes into play in the last phase of the process before prothrombin activator is formed.

TABLE 34-3
Blood Clotting Factors

Clotting Factor	Synonyms
Fibrinogen	Factor I
Prothrombin	Factor II
Tissue thromboplastin	Factor III; tissue factor
Calcium	Factor IV
Factor V	Proaccelerin; labile factor; Ac-globulin; Ac-G
Factor VII	Serum prothrombin conversion accelerator; proconvertin; SPCA; stable factor
Factor VIII	Antihemophilic factor (AHF); antihemophilic globulin (AHG); antihemophilic factor A
Factor IX	Plasma thromboplastin component (PTC); Christmas factor; antihemophilic factor B
Factor X	Stuart factor; Stuart-Prower factor
Factor XI	Plasma thromboplastin antecedent (PTA); antihemophilic factor C
Factor XII	Hageman factor
Factor XIII	Fibrin-stabilizing factor
Platelets	Thrombocytes

From Guyton, A. (1991). *Textbook of medical physiology* (8th ed.). Philadelphia: WB Saunders.

Step Two: The Conversion of Prothrombin to Thrombin. Once prothrombin activator is formed, it does just as its name implies and, with the assistance of calcium ions, activates available prothrombin. Prothrombin is continually formed in the healthy liver, but in the event of liver disease or lack of vitamin K (needed for prothrombin formation), clotting may be impaired.

Step Three: The Conversion of Fibrinogen into Fibrin Threads. In the presence of thrombin and calcium ions, fibrinogen (also formed in the liver) is converted to fibrin threads. These threads form a fine meshwork across the damaged section of the vessel to trap blood cells, platelets, and plasma. These cells enmeshed in the fibrin strands form the blood clot and prevent further leakage through the damaged vessel wall. Within minutes after clot formation, clot retraction begins, pulling the sides of the damaged vessel closer together as the clot retracts. Platelets are essential for bonding to fibrin threads to form the meshwork for the clot.*

Once formed, the clot either can form the base for new connective tissue or can undergo a process of lysis and dissipate. Often the clot is invaded by fibroblasts, in which case fibrous connective tissue is formed within 7 to 10 days (Guyton, 1991). If the clot is very large, however, such as a site of tissue hemorrhage, the clot itself secretes lytic enzymes (such as fibrinolysin) that digest the clot.

Age-Related Differences

Differences in Red Blood Cell Concentration

The number of red blood cells varies with age, gender, and the altitude at which a person lives. As illustrated in Figure 34–3, hemoglobin and hematocrit are higher at birth than ever again. The high levels at birth reflect the extra red blood cells and hemoglobin required in utero for oxygenation under conditions of lower oxygen tension. When the infant initiates respirations at birth, the oxygen saturation rises from 65 per cent (normal fetal level) to 95 per cent (Miller, 1990). In response to this relatively oxygen-rich environment erythropoiesis shuts down and allows the neonate to enter a 6- to 12-week period of physiologic adaptation to extrauterine life. During this adaptive period, fetal red cells are destroyed, and hemoglobin and hematocrit levels drop to a low point

* Procoagulant substances are released by entrapped platelets, creating further bonding activity. In addition, the platelets activate contractile proteins (platelet thrombosthein, actin, and myosin molecules), thereby enhancing the bonding process of platelets to the fibrin threads (Guyton, 1991).

called the "nadir." The decline is commonly referred to as "physiologic anemia of infancy," but as Pearson (1987) points out, this term is a misnomer, because hemoglobin levels rarely fall below 9 g/dl. Once hemoglobin reaches 9 to 11 g/dl, erythropoiesis resumes to maintain hemoglobin at a mean of 12 g/dl and hematocrit at a mean of 37 per cent during the first 6 years of life (Table 34–2).

At puberty, gender differences in red blood cell concentration become evident (Fig. 34–3). From that time throughout adulthood, males have higher mean values of red blood cells, hemoglobin, and hematocrit.

Persons living at very high altitudes, where the quantity of oxygen in the air is significantly reduced, produce more red blood cells (and consequently have higher hemoglobin and hematocrit levels). Nurses practicing in or near mountainous regions will be aware that clients not only have higher red blood cell levels but also require these higher levels to function in their home environments. This means that resumption of functional hemoglobin and hematocrit levels for these clients after blood loss or bone marrow suppression must be measured against their normal baseline values, not against norms calculated at sea level.

Differences in White Blood Cell Values

The ratio of neutrophils to lymphocytes changes with age (Table 34–2). Neutrophils predominate at birth but then decrease rapidly in the first weeks to reach a low point at 3 months that corresponds with the nadir of red cells. At about 5 years of age, neutrophils and lymphocytes are rather even in number. From that point, neutrophils again increase in proportion until the adult mean of 55 per cent is reached at puberty. If the clientele of the laboratory primarily consists of children, as in a children's hospital, the forms on which the blood values are reported will often "correct for" age of the child. If this is not the case, however, the nurse must keep in mind the age-related differences in white blood cell components, especially in the young infant.

In general, younger children demonstrate a more pronounced *neutrophilia* (increased neutrophil count) in response to infection than do older children and adults. Younger children also tend to display greater numbers of immature neutrophils when neutrophil production is increased. (Refer to Table 34–2.)

History and Physical Examination

The diagnostic workup for a child with a blood disorder will include a complete history and physical examination. Children with blood disorders have usually been diagnosed early in infancy or childhood. Age at onset of symptoms is a distinguishing diagnostic feature, because disorders of red cell membrane and enzymes are evident at birth. In contrast, the hemoglobinopathies such as beta-thalassemia or sickle cell are not evident before 3 months of age. A thorough family history is essential, because certain blood disorders have a hereditary basis, as do sickle cell anemia, beta-thalassemia, and congenital aplastic anemia.

In caring for adolescents and young adults, it is now important to determine whether they received any blood products before April 1985. Blood was not screened for human immunodeficiency virus (HIV) prior to this time (Seeler, 1992). Any who received blood products under these circumstances should be counseled and tested for HIV antibodies.

Symptoms in the child or adolescent are associated with underlying causes. For example, bruising in a child suggests a blood loss due to alteration in the clotting factors. Jaundice is a sign associated with a hemolytic process.

Diagnostic Assessment

The common diagnostic tests used to measure the type and number of blood cells and characteristics of blood clotting capacity are listed in Table 34–4. Normal values for these tests can be found in Table 34–2 and in Appendix 7.

Therapeutic Management

The child with a blood disorder will be treated according to the management protocol that addresses the etiology of the disorder. The treatment for a child with an erythrocyte disorder is different from that for the child with a disorder affecting the white blood cells or a disorder of hemostasis. The student is referred to the therapeutic management sections throughout the chapter that discuss the specific treatment options for a particular disorder.

Prevention Issues

The concept of prevention of blood disorders has relevance for genetic and nutritional counseling and health maintenance. Nutritional counseling is pertinent to not only the treatment but the prevention of iron deficiency anemia. An infant is at risk for iron deficiency anemia if fed with cow's milk or formula not fortified with iron, a situation that can be prevented with appropriate follow-up newborn and postpartum care. See further on in this chapter for more information on iron deficiency anemia.

Genetic counseling should be offered to parents of children born with a heritable blood disorder, such as sickle cell anemia and beta-thalassemia. Follow-up evaluation should be offered to siblings to determine their status and assist in making informed reproductive decisions in the future. The topic of future reproductive options is highly charged for family members, because it is so deeply personal. As discussed later in the chapter, prenatal diagnosis is possible and enables prompt referral and treatment.

TABLE 34-4
Diagnostic Assessment: Hematologic Function

Test	Purpose	Nursing Implications
Complete blood count	Frequently ordered for screening purposes	Explain reasons for test Do not use hand or arm that has an IV line infusion Capillary blood (finger stick) may be obtained from infants and very young children
White blood cell count (WBC)	Total number of circulating white blood cells	Leukocytosis (increase in white blood cells) results from various causes, such as infections
Differential white blood count (Diff)	Percentage of the total WBC made up of neutrophils, eosinophils, basophils, lymphocytes, monocytes, and, less frequently, other less mature white blood cells	"Shift to the left" may indicate a severe bacterial disease or acute stress on the bone marrow Medications may increase neutrophil count Medications may decrease the lymphocyte, eosinophil, and neutrophil counts Blast forms indicate possibility of leukemia
Red blood cell count (RBC)	Total number of circulating red blood cells	Used to calculate red cell indices Assists in the diagnosis of anemia
Hematocrit (Hct)	The percentage of red blood cells in a volume of whole blood	Decrease seen in significant blood loss, anemia, leukemia Increase seen in severe burns, severe dehydration, shock, surgery, polycythemia vera
Hemoglobin (Hgb)	Measures the oxygen-carrying capacity of blood	Hemoglobin levels below normal may reflect an anemic condition Hemoglobin levels usually correspond to hematocrit levels
Mean corpuscular hemoglobin (MCH)	A measure of the average weight of hemoglobin in the individual red blood cell; less accurate than the MCHC because it uses the red cell count in its calculation, and that count may be inaccurate	Calculated by dividing the hemoglobin value by the RBC Increase in macrocytosis Decrease in microcytosis
Mean corpuscular volume (MCV)	Express the volume occupied by a single red blood cell; it indicates whether the red blood cells appear • *Normocytic*—of normal size • *Microcytic*—smaller than normal • *Macrocytic*—larger than normal	Increased in acute bleeding, hemolytic anemia, malignancy, aplastic anemia, cytotoxic drugs Decreased in anemia, polycythemia
Mean corpuscular hemoglobin concentration (MCHC)	A calculated value, MCHC is an expression of the average concentration of hemoglobin in the red blood cells; i.e., the ratio of the weight of hemoglobin to the volume of red blood cells	Decreased in chronic iron deficiency anemia
Platelet count	Total number of circulating platelets	Elevation of platelet count above normal (thrombocytosis) seen in polycythemia, infections, anemia, hemorrhage, malignancies
Erythrocyte sedimentation rate	The rate at which red blood cells settle out of unclotted blood in 1 hr	Elevated in chronic inflammations, neoplasms
Hemoglobin electrophoresis	Identifies the types and percentages of hemoglobin in the blood; distinguishes between sickle cell trait and disease	
Sickledex	Identifies the presence (but not the percentage) of sickle hemoglobin	Positive for sickle cell anemia
Reticulocyte count	Numbers of immature red blood cells (reticulocytes) compared with total red blood cells	Indicates an increase in red blood cell production and/or an increase in red blood cell destruction
Partial thromboplastin time (PTT)	Time required for clotting of plasma; fibrin clot formation; assesses *phase I* of clotting mechanism; adequacy of factors XII, XI, IX, and VIII	Apply pressure following venipuncture to stop bleeding Abnormal values with defects of platelet functioning

(continued)

TABLE 34-4
Diagnostic Assessment: Hematologic Function *(Continued)*

Test	Purpose	Nursing Implications
Activated partial thromboplastin time (APTT)	Same as for PTT but more sensitive and performed more quickly	Same as PTT Store in ice if not immediately transported to laboratory
Prothrombin time (Pro time, PT)	The time it takes plasma to clot after thromboplastin and calcium are added; directly measures a defect in any of the *phase II* clotting mechanisms: prothrombin, fibrinogen, factor V, factor VII, and factor X	Same as PTT Send to laboratory as soon as possible; factor V begins to deteriorate at room temperature after 4 hours
Prothrombin consumption test (PCT)	Determination of prothrombin in serum after coagulation of whole blood; test for *phase I* factors	Same as PTT Store in ice if not transported immediately
Thromboplastin generation test	A deficiency of any of the *phase I* factors will lead to an abnormal generation of thromboplastin	Same as PTT
Thrombin time	Time required for plasma to clot after the addition of bovine thrombin; detects inadequate levels of fibrinogen; *phase III*	Same as PTT Store in ice if cannot be transported immediately to laboratory

Nursing Care

Throughout this chapter, nursing care issues related to the spectrum of blood disorders are discussed. Although profiles of presentation in the child or adolescent differ, depending on the etiology and organ systems affected, the nurse constantly monitors the child or adolescent for signs and symptoms reflecting clinical status.

Conservation of energy is a nursing priority for the child who has anemia, regardless of etiology. The subjective assessment includes a report of the youth's fatigability during activities appropriate to developmental age and a report of the child's progress on developmental tasks, especially as related to motor activity. Insights about the etiology of the child's anemia can be gathered by assessing the child's and family's eating patterns.

Objective assessments collected include pulse and respirations at rest and with activity, signs of infection (including temperature), and the child's growth pattern as indicated on the growth charts. Color of the skin and mucous membranes is noted, as is tissue perfusion. Refer to Table 34-8 for a description of the process of nursing care.

Disorders of Red Blood Cells

Anemias constitute the most common hematologic disorders in children. "Anemia" is defined as a reduction in either the total number of circulating red blood cells or a decrease in the concentration of hemoglobin, or both (see Table 34-1 for age-specific parameters defining anemia). Anemias can be classified on the basis of etiology or by the morphologic description of the red cells. Etiologic classification divides anemia into three categories:

- Blood loss, which may occur from acute or chronic hemorrhage.
- Excessive blood destruction (hemolysis), which may be due to structural defects of the red blood cells.
- Decreased or impaired production, which originates in the bone marrow and may be acquired or constitutional.

The red blood cell indices reported on the complete blood count are measurements of the erythrocyte size and hemoglobin content. Indices tell whether the red cell size is *microcytic* (small), *normocytic* (normal), or *macrocytic* (large) and whether the color is *hypochromic* (pale, indicating less than normal hemoglobin concentration) or *normochromic* (normal). The morphologically descriptive name may be used to define an anemia, for example, "normochromic, microcytic," especially if the etiology has not been determined. The red blood cell indices are as follows:

- *MCV,* the mean cell volume or size of an individual red blood cell.
- *MCHC,* the mean cell hemoglobin concentration; a measure of the hemoglobin concentration in 100 ml of red blood cells.
- *MCH,* the mean cell hemoglobin or the hemoglobin concentration of each individual red blood cell. Table 34-5 correlates the indices with the descriptive terms.

TABLE 34-5
Red Blood Cells: Morphology and Indices

	MCV (mean cell volume, femtoliters)	MCH (mean cell hemoglobin, picograms)	MCHC (mean cell hemoglobin concentration, %)
Macrocytic	>94	35–40	>30
Microcytic	<70	12–29	<30
Normocytic	80–94	26–34	>30

Modified from Klopovich, P. (1983). An overview of anemia in children. *Issues in Comprehensive Pediatric Nursing, 6*(5–6), 281.

Regardless of etiology or morphology, *tissue hypoxia* is the major consequence of anemia. The degree of hypoxia determines the severity of symptoms. Mild anemia is most often asymptomatic and may not be diagnosed, except in the presence of another unrelated illness or during routine screening. Severe anemia, however, affects virtually every organ system and if untreated, eventually results in death.

Sickle Cell Disease

Sickle cell disease represents a spectrum of clinical disorders that result from abnormalities of the globin genes of the hemoglobin molecule. The disorders are transmitted genetically in an autosomal recessive fashion and are chronic in nature. The child with sickle cell anemia produces abnormal sickle hemoglobin (hemoglobin S [Hb S]), rather than hemoglobin A (Hb A). Sickle cell anemia is now designated as Hb SS, which indicates the homozygosity of sickle hemoglobin. The child with *sickle cell trait* has inherited a sickle gene (Hb S) from one parent and a normal hemoglobin gene (Hb A) from the other parent. Sickle cell trait is designated as Hb AS. Sickle cell trait does not develop into sickle cell anemia. The child with sickle cell trait is a carrier of the disease, sickle cell anemia, and is almost always asymptomatic.

Etiology/Incidence

Sickle cell anemia results when the child inherits two abnormal recessive Hb S genes, one from each parent (see the discussion of autosomal recessive inheritance elsewhere in this text). Children with sickle cell anemia have red cells that contain up to 80 to 100 per cent Hb S, the remainder being fetal hemoglobin (Hb F) and Hb A, a minor adult hemoglobin. Sickle cell anemia is a potentially fatal disease that occurs in African-Americans and less frequently in persons of Mediterranean, Asian, Indian, and Middle-Eastern descent. Approximately 8 to 10 per cent of African-Americans have sickle cell trait (Nathan, 1987). In African-Americans, the incidence is 1 in 500 births (Kinny & Ware, 1988; Rodgers, 1991).

Pathophysiology

The child with sickle cell trait synthesizes Hb S but, because of the heterozygous state, has the ability to produce Hb A as well and usually does not experience symptoms. The red blood cells of children with sickle cell trait contain 30 to 40 per cent Hb S. There are many variants of Hb SS disease; at least 500 have been recognized to date. Most are rare. The more common variants are listed in order of frequency in Table 34–6.

Hemoglobin S, sickle hemoglobin, is much less soluble than normal hemoglobin when deoxygenated. This is a direct result of the amino acid substitution in the hemoglobin molecule that occurs in this disorder. The decreased solubility of Hb S causes it to become more viscous and to precipitate into long crystal shapes, thereby deforming the shape of the cell. "Sickling" is the term used to describe the red blood cell change from the normal roundness to a crescent, or sickle shape. Sickling occurs in the red blood cells of persons with sickle cell disease when oxygen tension or concentration is reduced as a result of acidosis or other forms of stress (Fig. 34–5). Some degree of sickling occurs continuously throughout life.

Once sickled, red blood cells are more rigid, fragile, and rapidly destroyed. They lose the ability to flow easily through tiny capillary beds. When the rate

TABLE 34-6
Variants of Sickle Cell Anemia (Hb SS)

Hemoglobin (Hb) Defect	Comments
Hb SC	Higher hemoglobin level generally less severe than Hb SS
Hb SB thalassemia	Two distinct forms:
	Hb SB thalassemia—severe
	Hb SB thalassemia—mild
Hb SD	Moderately severe
Hb SE	Most common form in Asia, usually occurs in offspring of African-American and Asian-American parents

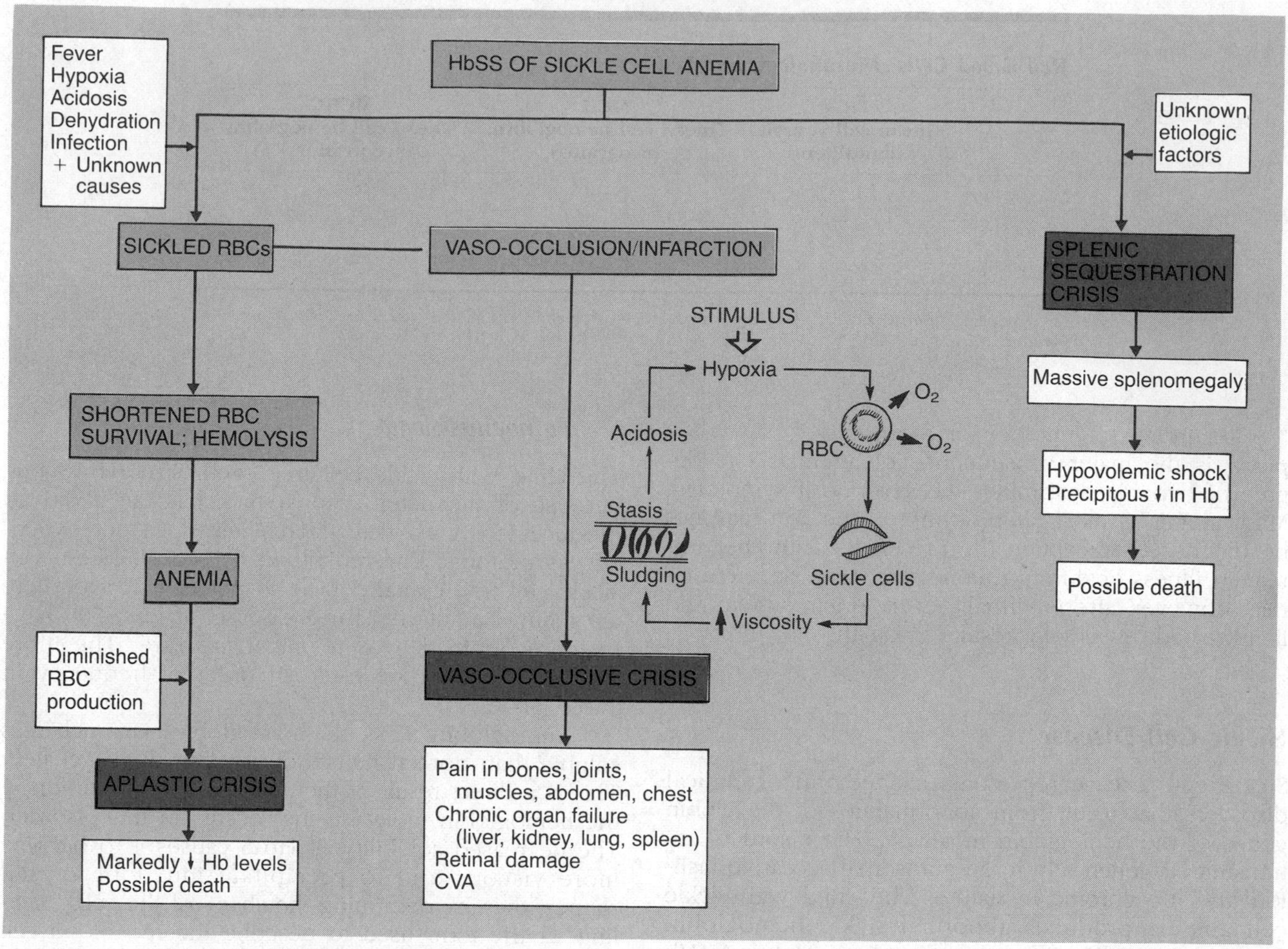

FIGURE 34-5. The pathophysiology of sickle cell anemia, including the three types of sickle cell crisis and the resulting clinical manifestations.

of sickling is increased, the sickled cells may become clumped, causing obstructions and impairment of blood flow beyond the obstruction. This results in severe tissue hypoxia and, subsequently, more sickling. As the hypoxia worsens, infarcts and necrosis may develop. The duration and size of the ischemic area determine the extent of the injury. Conditions that predispose one to sickling include infection, dehydration, cold, hypoxia, fever, high altitudes, vigorous exercise, and emotional stress.

Clinical Manifestations

Clinical symptoms of sickle cell anemia are the results of (1) the decreased life span of the red cells—that is, hemolysis and the compensatory mechanisms evoked by the subsequent anemia and (2) the formation of thrombi in the small vessels of various organs as a result of sickling. General manifestations of sickle cell anemia include pallor, weakness, easy fatigability and jaundice as a result of hemolysis, and tissue hypoxia. Children with sickle cell anemia begin to demonstrate growth abnormalities at around 7 years of age. Both height and weight are below average, and puberty is usually delayed. The heart becomes progressively enlarged as a result of increased cardiac output associated with chronic anemia. The kidneys lose the ability to concentrate urine effectively, as a result of renal medulla damage from tissue hypoxia, which results in enuresis and nocturia in 50 per cent of children with sickle cell disease. In addition, microthrombi from clumped sickled cells cause progressive damage to multiple organs, including the eye, liver, and lungs. Table 34-7 lists clinical manifestations at various stages.

Sickle Cell Crisis

A "crisis" is not a specific disease entity. Rather, it is the term used to describe an acute, painful event of various, sometimes unknown, etiologies that occurs throughout the life of the person with sickle cell anemia. The frequency of these crises may range from an almost constant occurrence to a nearly asymptomatic life. Most patients fall between these two extremes. Greenberg and associates (1990) report that in a 21-month period of close monitoring for vaso-occlusive

TABLE 34-7
Clinical Manifestations of Sickle Cell Anemia at Various Developmental Stages

6 Mos–2 Yrs	School Age	Adolescence
Normal appearance	Pallor	Impaired growth
Dactylitis	Fatigue	Delayed sexual maturity
Hepatomegaly	Scleral icterus	Frontal bossing
Splenomegaly	Splenomegaly	Retinal changes (especially Hb SC)
	Functional asplenia by age 5 yrs (Hb SS)	Gallstones
	Cardiomegaly with or without murmur	Avascular necrosis of long bones
	Enlarged nodes	Leg ulcers
	Dilute urine	Neurologic changes secondary to stroke

pain episodes, 25 per cent of patients had four or more crises that required hospitalization, and 71 per cent had two or fewer.

Crises can be classified into three main groups: (1) vaso-occlusive, (2) sequestration, and (3) aplastic.

Vaso-Occlusive Crisis. This is the most common, or classic, type of crisis. It is often referred to as a "pain crisis."

Sickled cells become massed and clogged, obstructing blood flow to more distal areas which results in tissue hypoxia and infarction (Fabry & Kaul, 1991). There is a rapid onset of deep, gnawing, throbbing pain, often without physical findings (see Fig. 34–5). The onset is acute, and often no precipitating factor can be determined. Vaso-occlusive crises rarely begin before the age of 4 or 5 months, because of the high levels of fetal hemoglobin present during the first few months of life. The back and extremities are the most commonly affected areas. Areas less frequently involved are the lungs, ("acute chest syndrome"); the abdomen; the central nervous system, where symptoms are suggestive of stroke; and the penis.

Hand-foot syndrome, or *dactylitis,* is a distinct type of vaso-occlusive crisis that occurs in infants and toddlers (Fabry & Kaul, 1991). Hand-foot syndrome is often the first clinical symptom of sickle cell anemia. This crisis causes symmetric infarction of the bones in the hands and feet, with resultant painful swelling of the soft tissues over the metacarpals or metatarsals of the hands and feet. Ten to 45 per cent of all patients experience at least one episode of hand-foot syndrome (Ohini-Frempong & Schwartz, 1990). *Acute chest syndrome* includes a constellation of symptoms including chest pain, fever, hypoxia, cough, and leukocytosis. These features are common to pneumonia as well. The diagnosis of infection versus infarction is difficult to make, and often both conditions are present simultaneously.

Sequestration Crisis. Children with sickle cell anemia eventually lose function of the spleen as a result of frequent infarction from sickling episodes. Prior to the onset of this "autosplenectomy," the infant or young child may suddenly pool enormous volumes of blood within the spleen. The organ becomes massively enlarged, and the hemoglobin level drops precipitously. This type of crisis is potentially fatal, and death may occur within hours of onset of symptoms. Parents must be instructed to bring their child to the hospital if sudden pallor, faintness, rapid breathing (signs of shock or deficient intravascular blood volume), and/or acute enlargement of the abdomen develops. Young children between the ages of 8 months and 2 years are at the highest risk.

Aplastic Crisis. The red blood cells of the child with sickle cell anemia survive only about 10 to 20 days in the circulation (Ohini-Frempong & Schwartz, 1990) (normal life span of red blood cells is approximately 120 days). Because red blood cells are destroyed so quickly, the child with sickle cell anemia is highly dependent on a strong compensatory mechanism that continually produces new red blood cells at a rate five to eight times normal. Infections, especially of viral origin, can often cause a temporary cessation of bone marrow activity, even in otherwise healthy persons. The need for new red blood cells is so profound in patients with sickle cell anemia that even a 1-day arrest of bone marrow activity during an infection can cause a drop of 10 to 15 per cent in the hematocrit and result in aplastic crisis.

Aplastic crisis is characterized by a lack of reticulocytes in the blood. Platelet and white blood cell counts usually are not depressed. Hemoglobin levels may fall as low as 1 g/dl; in this case, death from congestive heart failure often results (Ohini-Frempong & Schwartz, 1990).

Aplastic crisis is usually self-limited, lasting 5 to 10

days. More severe aplastic crises are treated with transfusions of packed red blood cells. Milder degrees of aplasia frequently require no treatment. Parents should know to seek immediate medical care if the child becomes weak and pale, especially in the midst of an ongoing or recent infection.

Daily penicillin administration has been proved to dramatically decrease mortality in children with sickle cell anemia. Penicillin prophylaxis should begin immediately after the diagnosis is made.

Diagnostic Assessment

Sickle cell anemia and sickle cell trait are easily diagnosed with a blood test called hemoglobin electrophoresis. Electrophoresis applies an electrical charge to a blood specimen and separates the various types of hemoglobin. This test also quantifies the percentages of various hemoglobins present. Less sensitive laboratory tests that indicate the presence of any Hb S are available (e.g., Sickledex). These tests cannot differentiate between heterozygosity or homozygosity for sickle hemoglobin. They merely indicate the presence or absence of Hb S. Such tests are used for large screening programs. Positive results require further testing with hemoglobin electrophoresis.

Early identification of children with sickle cell disease is desirable. Such identification allows parent education and facilitates the beginning of early treatment for sequestration and vaso-occlusive crisis and administration of prophylactic antibiotics (Earles, 1989). Hemoglobin electrophoresis should be performed at birth on all infants. In May, 1972, Congress passed the National Sickle Cell Anemia Control Act. Under this act, services for voluntary screening and diagnosis, counseling and education, medical referral, follow-up, and research are mandated. Because sickle cell screening is available on request and since sickle cell anemia and sickle cell trait are most prevalent in the African-American population, the nurse should discuss the importance and need for testing with parents of African-American infants. Genetic counseling should be offered to the parents with sickle cell anemia, as should follow-up evaluation of siblings to determine their hemoglobin type. At least 35 states have infant screening programs in place (Tsevat et al, 1991). (See Chapter 31 for a discussion of genetic counseling, and Table 31–17 for a nursing process plan for the family with genetic risk.)

Accurate prenatal diagnosis of sickle cell disease is possible by utilizing fetal blood or fetal cells obtained by means of amniocentesis or fetoscopy. Chorionic villus sampling (CVS) can be done much earlier, between 9 and 11 weeks of gestation (Pearson, 1987b; Tsevat et al, 1991). Parents should be made aware of centers that provide this testing. The nurse must present this information in a sensitive manner, realizing that the decision to obtain prenatal screening for future pregnancies is personal and involves strong emotions. Parents should not feel pressured to obtain this service; nor should they be made to feel guilty if they refuse it.

Therapeutic Management

Currently there is no cure for sickle cell anemia. Treatment is palliative at best. The child and family are counseled to avoid the known "triggers" of sickle cell crisis: infection, dehydration, hypoxia, high altitude, vigorous exercise, and stress. Management of vaso-occlusive crisis includes increased hydration, effective analgesia, and identification and treatment of any precipitating event (Vichinsky & Lubin, 1987). Anemia associated with sequestration or aplastic crises is treated with transfusion of packed red blood cells.

"Hypertransfusion" programs describe regimens that provide routine packed red blood cell transfusions to maintain hemoglobin levels greater than 12 g/dl. Hemoglobin levels greater than 12 g/dl shut down erythropoiesis, thereby preventing manufacture of Hb S and subsequent sickling. Hypertransfusion programs may be used as treatment for life-threatening complications, especially cerebrovascular accidents (CVAs).

CVA can be one of the most devastating complications in sickle cell disease (Fig. 34–6). Damage is variable, depending on the area of the infarct. Once a CVA has occurred, the incidence of recurrence within the next 3 years is 70 per cent. A subsequent CVA generally causes more severe neurologic consequences than the earlier episode. Long-term transfusion programs are generally very effective but carry the risk of possible hepatitis, HIV, alloimmunization, and eventually iron overload (described later in the discussion of thalassemia). The duration of long-term transfusion programs following CVA is currently unknown.

Application of the Nursing Process: Sickle Cell Disease

Assessment

Objective data that the nurse considers in assessing the child are pulse and respiration rates at rest and during activity, fever, and other indications of infection and tissue perfusion (especially in the central nervous system and the periphery). Height, weight, and status on the growth chart are noted. The child's developmental status is recorded, because the child with moderate to severe anemia will be delayed in achieving developmental tasks owing to fatigue. The color of the skin and mucous membranes of the anemic child is pale. In dark-skinned children, the color of the oral cavity is assessed. Laboratory tests performed during the diagnostic workup for the child with anemia are complete blood count, blood smear, reticulocyte count, serum iron and iron binding test, stool and urine for occult blood, and serum bilirubin. Refer to Table 34–8 for additional assessment parameters the

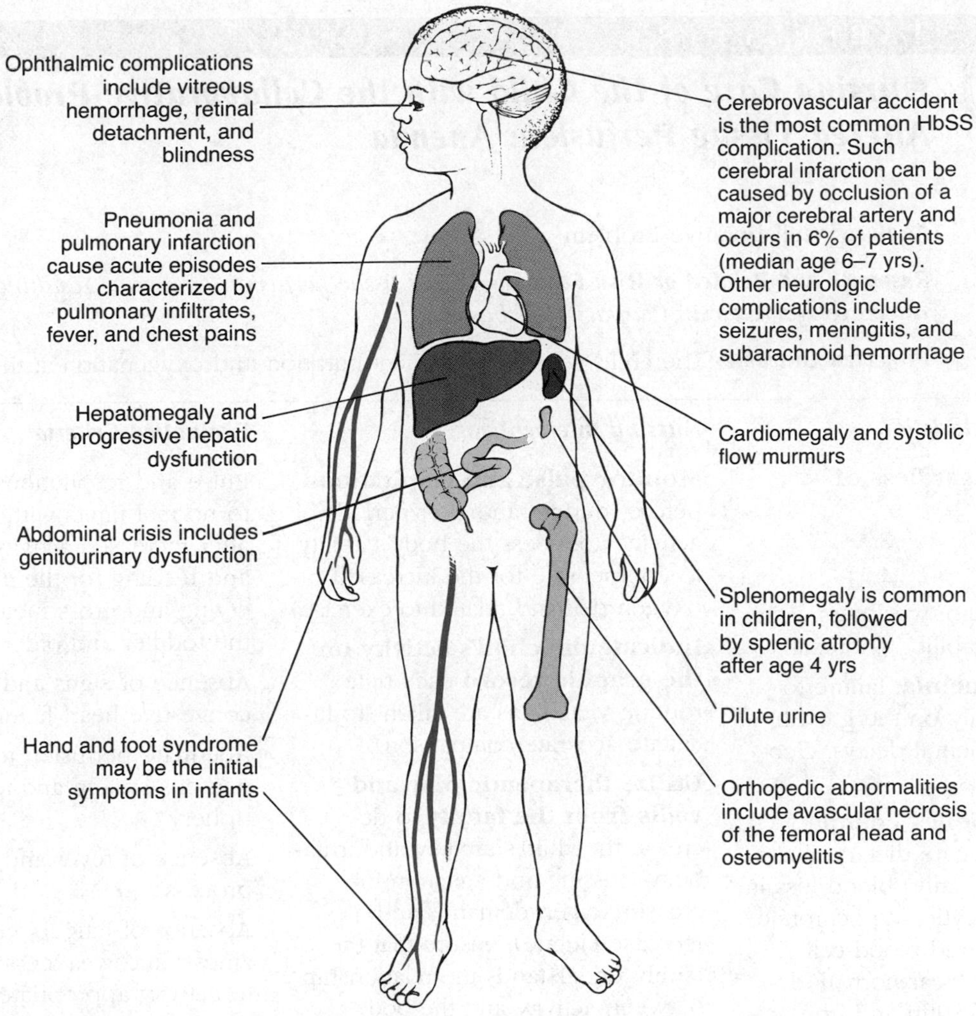
Ophthalmic complications include vitreous hemorrhage, retinal detachment, and blindness
Pneumonia and pulmonary infarction cause acute episodes characterized by pulmonary infiltrates, fever, and chest pains
Hepatomegaly and progressive hepatic dysfunction
Abdominal crisis includes genitourinary dysfunction
Hand and foot syndrome may be the initial symptoms in infants
Cerebrovascular accident is the most common HbSS complication. Such cerebral infarction can be caused by occlusion of a major cerebral artery and occurs in 6% of patients (median age 6–7 yrs). Other neurologic complications include seizures, meningitis, and subarachnoid hemorrhage
Cardiomegaly and systolic flow murmurs
Splenomegaly is common in children, followed by splenic atrophy after age 4 yrs
Dilute urine
Orthopedic abnormalities include avascular necrosis of the femoral head and osteomyelitis

FIGURE 34 - 6. Common complications of sickle cell disease.

nurse must consider when caring for a child with sickle cell anemia.

Nursing Diagnostic Statements and Collaborative Problems

Pain related to altered tissue perfusion: systemic; *associated with*

- *Occlusion of vessels by sickled cells (vaso-occlusive crisis).*
- *Pooling of blood in the spleen (splenic sequestration crisis).*
- *Temporary cessation of red blood cell production associated with effects of infectious agents on bone marrow function (aplastic crisis).*

Altered tissue perfusion; *(anemia) resulting from impaired oxygen-carrying capacity of the blood associated with hemolysis of red blood cells and subsequent anemia.*

Ineffective individual and family coping, *related to pain, secondary to tissue ischemia associated with vascular occlusion.*

High risk for infection; *risk factor: splenic dysfunction.*

High risk for low self-esteem and body image disturbance; *risk factors:*

- *Physical restrictions associated with sickle cell anemia.*
- *Delayed growth and onset of sexual maturity.*
- *Potential for transmission of the recessive trait to offspring.*

High risk for altered family process: sibling rivalry; *risk factors:*

- *Inadequate knowledge of the disease process and treatment.*
- *Parental tendency to spend more time with the ill child and less time with well siblings.*

TABLE 34-8

Nursing Care of the Child with the Collaborative Problem Altered Tissue Perfusion: Anemia

Analysis: Collaborative Problem

Response and Related or Risk Factors: *Altered tissue perfusion (anemia) resulting from reduced oxygen-carrying capacity of the blood*

Projected Outcome: The child will have sufficient nutrition and oxygenation at the cellular level

Defining Characteristics

For anemia regardless of etiology:

Subjective:

Headache, vertigo, weakness, irritability, easy fatigability, anorexia

For chronic anemia: failure to progress normally on the growth chart; developmental delays; clubbing of the digits

For iron deficiency anemia: Evidence of inadequate dietary intake of iron; (occasionally) blood loss in the stool; microcytic, hypochromic red blood cells; red blood cell count normal or near normal; decreased serum ferritin and iron, increased iron-binding capacity and free erythrocyte porphyrin

For aplastic anemia: normochromic, normocytic red blood cells in reduced numbers; leukopenia; thrombocytopenia

For anemia related to infectious processes: decreased red blood cell count; normochromic, normocytic red blood cells; leukocytosis; possible fever and other evidence of infection

Objective:

Tachycardia and dyspnea, especially with activity; pallor of skin and mucous membranes; hemoglobin < 10 g/dl and/or red blood cell count < 4 million/mm^3

For anemia associated with prematurity: nadir* at 1 to 3 mos of age with hemoglobin at 7–8 g/dl

Nursing Interventions

Monitor pulse and respirations before, during, and after periods of activity (to assess the body's ability to compensate for the increased oxygen demand related to exercise)

Indicate the child's activity on the graphic record each time routine vital signs are taken (to facilitate accurate comparison)

Utilize therapeutic play and visits from the family to decrease the child's anxiety and irritability (fussing and agitation increase oxygen demands and increase fatigue); ensure that the family understands the relationship between activity and the body's demand for oxygen (to facilitate home care)

Monitor for signs and symptoms of congestive heart failure (related to the heart's inability to compensate, through tachycardia, for decreased oxygen-carrying capacity); if found, report immediately to physician

Monitor heart and lung sounds; report adventitious sounds; if congestive heart failure is suspected, record weight daily (weight is a sensitive indicator of fluid retention)

Assess, monitor, and chart change in mental status and in color of skin and mucous membranes

Measure temperature every 4 hrs; monitor for prodromal signs and symptoms of illness, such as

Evaluation Criteria

Pulse and respirations that return to normal limits within 15 mins after increased activity (e.g., crying and feeding for the infant, loud crying and gross motor activity for the toddler and older child)

Absence of signs and symptoms of congestive heart failure

Adequate perfusion to the central nervous system and to the periphery

Absence of fever and infectious process

Absence of fatigue, headache, dizziness, and weakness in response to activity appropriate for age

Increased appetite

Increased ability to perform skills typical of age group

Increased progress on growth chart

Absence of nausea, vomiting, diarrhea, and abdominal pain

TABLE 34-8 (continued)

Defining Characteristics	Nursing Interventions	Evaluation Criteria
for infants weighing 1000–1500 g at birth; 9.5 g/dl for infants with birthweights between 2000 and 2500 g **For hemolytic anemia:** Nausea, vomiting, diarrhea, abdominal pain, jaundice, hepatosplenomegaly **For anemia related to blood loss:** normochromic, normocytic anemia; leukocytosis; reticulocytosis; possible evidence of blood in the urine and/or stool	irritability, malaise, nasal discharge, sore throat, dullness of the eyes **Protect the child from nosocomial infection** by careful hand washing (especially in aplastic anemia because of the reduced lymphocytes) **Plan and implement rest periods for the hospitalized child** that produce the desired outcomes	

*Nadir is that time in infancy when hemoglobin level is at its lowest; stores from the mother are depleted, and bone marrow activity in the infant has not yet compensated.

High risk for altered health maintenance; risk factor: knowledge deficit, regarding:

- *Management of sickle cell disease at home:*
- *Nature and course of the disease, including the signs and symptoms of crisis.*
- *Plan of treatment as it relates to infection, hydration, analgesia, and physical activity.*
- *Genetic counseling.*

Planning and Implementation

Strategies for the child with sickle cell anemia will be based on the following principles related to (1) teaching self-management of the disease, (2) nursing management of sickle cell crises, and (3) techniques for facilitating family coping. Because the diagnosis of *high risk for activity intolerance* is common to all children with anemia, interventions for this diagnosis are addressed in Table 34–8.

Promoting Tissue Perfusion and Relieving Pain. Treatment of the collaborative problem pain, resulting from vaso-occlusive crisis is aimed at relieving symptoms and providing supportive care. One must ascertain that a pain crisis alone is occurring and that there is no underlying cause or serious complication. For example, the patient admitted with abdominal pain crisis should undergo a complete workup for a possible surgical problem.

Fluids, analgesia, and general comfort measures are the mainstay of sickle crisis therapy. Maintaining an adequate level of *hydration* is a primary intervention measure for the child in crisis, because the sickling process is enhanced by dehydration. Both oral and parenteral fluids are used to improve the level of hydration (Davies & Brozovic, 1989). Fluid intake should be increased to one and a half times the normal maintenance volume, assuming cardiac function is adequate. The oral route of hydration maintenance is preferable, if possible.

The close monitoring of vital signs while the child is receiving hydration is critical (Table 34–9). There is little evidence to support application of heat to areas of infarction for pain relief. Application of cold is contraindicated, because it may enhance sickling.

Administering Transfusions to Relieve Anemia. The nurse is usually responsible for carrying out the regimen prescribed by physicians in the management of sickle cell anemia. Often this entails transfusions of packed red blood cells. Other blood components may also be indicated (Table 34–10). During aplastic crisis, the slow transfusion (2 to 3 ml/kg every 6 to 8 hours) of packed red blood cells to increase the hemoglobin by 5 g/dl is required (Miller, 1990, p 399). During splenic sequestration, vigorous replacement of blood volume with whole blood or packed red blood cells and support of the child in shock are indicated. Table 34–9 lists guidelines for blood transfusion safety and transfusion reactions.

Many physicians believe that anesthesia poses increased risk for the child with sickle cell anemia. Hypoxia, dehydration, circulatory stasis, acidosis, cold, and infections may result from the surgical procedure itself or as a result of general anesthesia. Some studies dispute these beliefs; however, most physicians give patients transfusions to achieve Hb S levels of 30 per cent or less before surgery. Controlled studies may determine that this is no longer necessary (Miller, 1990).

Preparation for surgery may require 10 days to 2 weeks. The transfusion of packed red blood cells every few days results in suppression of the production of sickle cells, causing an overall decrease in Hb S

TABLE 34-9
Blood Transfusion Safety

Nursing Considerations

Determine patient's transfusion history. Assess nature of previous adverse reactions and notify physician and blood bank if there is a positive history

Always identify patient/blood product. Check ID wrist band and blood tag—ask child to state full name if possible

The most severe and potentially fatal transfusion reaction—acute hemolytic crisis—is most often a result of patient-blood mix-up. You *must* double-check this information with another person (hospital policy dictates appropriate personnel)

Be sure that the proper filter is in place for the product being infused

Be prepared to hang product immediately after received from the blood bank—if not possible, send product back to the blood bank (once unrefrigerated for more than 30 mins, the bank will refuse unit)

All IV lines should be primed with normal saline. This helps decrease hemolysis. Packed red blood cell transfusions can be infused with the use of Y-tubing and normal saline

Never add medications to blood

Vital signs (temperature, pulse, respiration, and blood pressure) should be obtained prior to the start of the transfusion as a baseline. If abnormal, check with the child's physician before starting the infusion

Vital signs should be repeated frequently during the transfusion, usually every 15–30 mins. However, close observation and inspection of child, especially during the first 15–30 mins of the transfusion, are mandatory

Begin the transfusion slowly—the rate should not exceed 2 ml/min during the first 15 mins

Transfusion should last no longer than 4 hrs

Most transfusions in children require an infusion pump to maintain proper rate. The IV site must be checked for infiltration frequently. If the transfusion is not being monitored on an infusion device, the following measures may help restore a proper rate if rate has slowed considerably and IV site is intact: raise the IV pole, use a pressure sleeve, agitate the blood bag frequently, change the filter or tubing

Blood-warming devices may be used with rapid transfusions that are infused through central lines (the cold blood may cause cardiac arrhythmias). Blood warming is also required for exchange transfusions in infants

Transfusion Reactions

Febrile

Extremely common, probably caused by host white cell antibodies reacting with white cells in the transfused blood. Usually occur during or immediately after the transfusion. Symptoms include fever and chills

Allergic

Caused by reaction to foreign plasma protein. May occur during and immediately after transfusion. Symptoms include urticaria and hives; usually, mild antihistamines may be given to relieve symptoms

Acute Hemolytic Reactions

Transfused red blood cells react with circulating antibody in the recipient, resulting in intravascular hemolysis. Occur most frequently when group O patients mistakenly receive group A, B, or AB blood. Usually occur within the first 15 mins of the transfusion. Occur most often as a result of error in blood/recipient. Symptoms include fever, chills, pain in lumbar region, chest pain, apprehension, hemoglobinuria, tachycardia, burning along veins in which blood is being transfused

Delayed Hemolytic Reactions

Occur 4–8 days after transfusion in patients who have developed antibodies previously but in whom the level is too low to be detected at the time of pretransfusion screening. Signs include falling hematocrit and positive Coombs test. Most delayed hemolytic reactions are benign, but subsequent transfusions may cause more severe problems

If a Transfusion Reaction Occurs

Stop the infusion immediately

Keep vein open with normal saline

Call physician

Closely monitor patient and vital signs. Follow hospital policy regarding blood and urine specimens and completing blood bank forms. Do not discard blood product

Antihistamines, diphenhydramine, 1 to 2 mg/kg IM, IV, or oral (PO) medication may be ordered for allergic reactions. Aminophylline, 3 mg/kg IV over 20 minutes, may be ordered for wheezing in an allergic reaction; epinephrine, if the reaction is very severe

Antipyretics—acetaminophen will be ordered for febrile reactions; diphenhydramine (1 mg/kg) or meperidine (Demerol, 10 mg/kg) for severe shaking, chills

TABLE 34-10
Blood Component Transfusion

Blood Product	Description	Volume	Uses
Whole blood		500 ml	Rarely used to replace massive blood loss due to acute hemorrhage
Packed red blood cells (PRBCs)	The red blood cells extracted from 1 unit of whole blood Small amount of plasma and white blood cells present	300 ml–400 ml May be available in partial units (50–100 ml/unit)	Relieve symptomatic deficit of oxygen-carrying capacity
Special filter PRBCs	Blood is issued with a special filter to produce a 95–99% reduction in white blood cells	300–400 ml	History of documented significant febrile reactions to previous infusions
Washed PRBCs	Blood is washed and resuspended in saline to reduce white blood cells by 80%	200 ml	History of severe allergic reactions to plasma proteins (e.g., IgA deficiency)
Frozen deglycerolyzed PRBCs	Process reduces number of WBCs by ~90%; allows rare blood types longer storage time	200 ml	Freezing allows longer storage in blood bank
Single-donor plasma (SDP)	Plasma separated from 1 unit of whole blood Does not contain platelets or factors V and VIII	200–275 ml	Volume expander Replacement of stable coagulation factors or fibrinogen
Fresh frozen plasma	SDP frozen within 6 hrs to preserve factors V and VIII	200–275 ml	Factor V deficiency; disseminated intravascular coagulation (DIC)
Platelet concentrates (random donor)	Platelets harvested from 1 unit of fresh blood suspended in 50 ml of donor plasma	50 ml/unit (units can be pooled and concentrated to reduce volume for small children)	Relieve bleeding due to thrombocytopenia or to elevate low platelet count
Platelet concentrates (single donor)	Obtained by platelet pheresis from one donor, equivalent to 6–8 units of random donor	250–350 ml (may be concentrated)	Patients refractory to random donor platelets
Platelet concentrations (human lymphocyte antigen [HLA]-matched donor)	Obtained by platelet pheresis from one donor with identical HLA markings	250–300 ml	Patients refractory to single-donor platelets
Platelet concentrates (leukocyte-poor)	Any of the above platelet concentrates processed to remove 90–99% of white blood cells	250–300 ml	History of severe febrile reaction to platelets
Granulocyte concentrates (single donor)	1×10^{10} white blood cell obtained from donors must be ABO- and RH-compatible	250–350 ml	Absolute neutrophil count < 500 with proven bacterial sepsis unresponsive to antibiotics
Cryoprecipitate	Derived from the plasma from 1 unit of blood; each bag contains ~100 units factor VIII and 170 mg fibrinogen	10 ml/bag	Type III von Willebrand disease; DIC, hemophilia A

Infusion Time

Rates should be ordered by physician for each individual case; the following are typical rates:

Whole blood, PRBCs, Plasma	10 ml/kg typically can be transfused over 2 hrs (no more than 2 ml/kg per hr for child in heart failure) Must be infused over 4 hrs maximum
Platelets	Run in as rapidly as possible—concentrate units if volume is a problem
Cryoprecipitate	Run in as rapidly as possible—concentrate units if volume is a problem; wash bag with 10–15 ml of normal saline after empty to ensure complete usage
Granulocytes	Administer slowly over 2–4 hrs; premedication with acetaminophen, diphenhydramine, or hydrocortisone is usually mandatory; chills and fever frequently occur; stop transfusion for high temperature, dyspnea, cyanosis, hypoxia; use with caution in patients receiving amphotericin B

and a presumed lower risk of problems occurring because of the surgery or anesthesia.

Promoting Coping by Comforting the Child in Pain. Propoxyphene hydrochloride (Darvon), acetaminophen, or codeine-containing compounds may be useful for children during mildly painful episodes. Some physicians believe aspirin can increase acidosis, which enhances sickling and should therefore be avoided. Others (Vichinsky & Lubin, 1987) recommend aspirin as an adjunct to narcotic analgesics. More potent narcotics may be required for children in severe pain. The nurse is responsible for pain assessment and drug administration during the course of each crisis. Most often the nurse must interpret the child's pain because analgesic orders are commonly written as needed. Pain medication should not be denied because a child does not ask for it or because of the nurse's belief that the child's pain cannot last longer than 48 to 72 hours.

The pediatric nurse must observe nonverbal signs of pain and also realize that younger children may actually deny pain because they are afraid of the analgesics or the route required for administration (see also Chapter 25). The nurse may recommend that pain medication be ordered at regular intervals around the clock, rather than as needed, because this may reduce the child's anxiety about asking for pain relief. It may also allow a drug of lower potency to be more effective because of consistent blood levels and eliminate the dulling side effects of more potent medications. Patient-controlled analgesia (PCA) delivered via intravenous (IV) infusion with electronic pumps can be used with children as young as 5 years of age and is a highly effective means of controlling the pain of a severe vaso-occlusive crisis. Morphine sulfate is the drug of choice (Gillespie & Morton, 1992; Miller, 1990; Schechter et al, 1988).

Communication between child and nurse should be fostered, so that the child becomes a partner in pain control. Increased participation allows the child a greater sense of control and decreased anxiety. Adjuvant therapies (e.g., massage, guided imagery, and transcutaneous electrical nerve stimulation [TENS]) for relief of pain can be incorporated into the child's plan of care.

If immobilization is necessary for parenteral infusions, the nurse must provide for the child's physical, psychosocial, and safety needs. Providing an infant seat may facilitate comfort and safety. Restraints, if essential for safety, must be removed at least every 45 to 90 minutes.

All children with a painful crisis episode should be kept as free from stress as possible. The opportunity for rooming-in is an essential component of basic care to the family. The caregiver's presence affords the child more security and thereby facilitates coping. Rooming-in should be permitted and encouraged in a manner that does not place guilt on parents unable to stay because of other family obligations. The presence of another person is important to a child in pain; it gives the feeling that the pain is "shared." If the parents cannot stay with the child, it is helpful for nurses to plan time to sit with the child and offer support by their presence. Each nurse should make every effort to anticipate and provide for the needs of the sick child within the family. Parents should be provided with adequate information about the latest episode to facilitate their own problem solving and support the child.

Preventing Infection. The child with sickle cell disease is prone to serious bacterial infection because of splenic dysfunction. Young children (less than 3 to 4 years of age) are frequently infected with *Pneumococcus* and *Haemophilus influenzae* organisms, and older children have a high incidence of *Salmonella, Escherichia coli,* and *Staphylococcus aureus* infection. Infection is the most common cause of death in young children with sickle cell anemia. The risk of acquiring sepsis or meningitis is higher than 15 per cent in children younger than 5 years, and the associated mortality is 30 per cent. In young children, the risk of pneumococcal sepsis appears to be 400 times that of healthy children (Nathan, 1987).

The parents need information regarding common childhood illnesses and how to interpret the symptoms that may occur. The nurse should help parents learn the proper method of taking their child's temperature. They should be taught to recognize subtle changes in their child's behavior and to realize that picky eating or fussy behavior may be the first signs of infection. Daily penicillin prophylaxis has had a significant impact on preventing acute overwhelming bacterial infections. Gaston et al (1986) showed a dramatic 84 per cent decrease in the incidence of pneumococcal sepsis with twice-daily oral penicillin, compared with placebo. The nurse should ascertain that parents understand the importance of penicillin usage and should stress that it does not imply that medical care is not needed at times of fever or illness. The need for immediate medical attention, regardless of time of day, cannot be overemphasized when a temperature of 101°F (38.3°C) develops. In addition, all children should receive a pneumococcal vaccine and hepatitis B vaccine to reduce the incidence of infections with these organisms. *H. influenzae* type B vaccine is given to all children at 2, 4, and 6 months of age. A booster dose (fourth dose) is given at 15 months of age or as soon as possible (American Academy of Pediatrics, 1990).

Promoting Self-Esteem and Positive Body Image by Normalizing the Environment. In all dealings with the child with sickle cell disease and the family, the nurse should strive to keep the emphasis on the normalcy of life. The child's painful crises can often be circumvented through prevention and early intervention; many episodes can be controlled at home by oral pain medication, increased fluids, and rest. The family should help the child to master various coping skills, such as relaxation training and distraction, at an early age to help reduce anxiety during crisis periods. (These techniques are taught in most comprehensive sickle cell programs.) The nurse, along with the parents, should appeal to the school system to permit the child with sickle cell disease to have rest periods, analgesia, increased fluids, and frequent trips to the bathroom (secondary to hyposthenuria, which is voiding urine of low specific gravity).

Undue absenteeism may be prevented by these measures, thus allowing the child a greater chance for success in life. The availability of a homebound program should be explored when frequent crises prevent regular attendance (Hernandez, 1989). Counseling and participation with peers in sickle cell support groups can assist the preadolescent and adolescent dealing with the anguish, shame, and embarrassment associated with delayed growth and sexual maturation.

Promoting Healthy Family Functioning. Siblings should be encouraged to play an active role in caregiving for their affected brother or sister. Depending on the sibling child's developmental level, factual explanations must be given for the repeated admissions to the hospital and the other events surrounding the management of the ill child's unique needs. Siblings should have an opportunity to participate in the child's care to the degree they wish. This may include accompanying the child to the doctor's office, clinic, or the hospital. Such visits can help clarify questions and help the sibling understand the ill child's needs.

It is not uncommon for siblings to feel concern for their ill brother or sister, and factual information reduces the possibility of frightening fantasies. At the same time, siblings are likely to feel jealous and left out because their parents are forced to spend extra time with their ill sibling. They may direct their anger at the sibling or at their parents. Parents should be counseled that these feelings are normal and encouraged to spend "special time" with the healthy child to prevent him or her from feeling neglected. Special times need not be elaborate, planned events. Parents can take advantage of daily activities such as performing a household chore together, reading a bedtime story, having a bedtime chat, or accompanying the child on trips to the mailbox or to the local store. Less frequent events, such as a special afternoon or a day trip, can also provide "quality" interactions (Craft, 1993). (See Chapter 19 for further discussion of the impact of chronic illness on the family.)

Facilitating Home Health Maintenance. Parental teaching should always be specific rather than general. Telling parents to "force fluids" gives no helpful guidelines to parents. Instead, the nurse should calculate the required maintenance fluids for the child and provide the parents with the amount measured in common household terms. Lists of alternatives that provide high levels of fluids (e.g., popsicles, soups, Jello) and their equivalent liquid values should also be given. Parents need to be reminded not to withhold fluids at bedtime. This is often done in an attempt to control bed wetting, which results from the damaged kidneys' loss of concentrating ability. Parental support and bladder training programs are needed to manage the enuresis. Parents should be made aware that fluid restriction may precipitate other problems, such as vaso-occlusive crisis.

Anticipatory guidance should be offered to parents for normal developmental changes, appropriate level of activity, and symptoms particular to sickle cell anemia, such as short stature, delayed puberty, and cardiovascular limitations.

Maintaining the child's general health is necessary preventive action. Comprehensive care of the child is indicated and is most optimally delivered from a sickle cell treatment center. The special needs of the child and family with sickle cell anemia should be addressed along with routine "well child" management. Assessment of growth and development, routine immunizations, nutrition counseling, auditory and visual screening, and education should be available to families. Genetic counseling should be an integral part of family education (see Chapter 31).

The child with sickle cell disease has a better prognosis today than previously. As adults, many affected individuals must make decisions about parenting. Women with sickle cell disease have been able to conceive and deliver normal children. However, early prenatal medical and nursing management are essential to foster a healthy outcome for both mother and newborn child. Even though the prognosis has improved, there remains a high mortality rate as a result of sequestration crisis but mostly because of overwhelming infections. Screening of all infants at birth and subsequent prompt referral to a comprehensive facility that emphasizes prevention and parental education should cause these high mortality rates to begin to decline dramatically.

Evaluation

The nurse can evaluate how well the interventions met the projected outcomes by assessing for a decrease or disappearance of defining characteristics of actual problems and some risk factors of potential problems. Interventions to prevent high risk problems are successful when the high risk problems do not occur.

Beta-Thalassemia

Beta-thalassemia major (Cooley anemia) is a disorder of hemoglobin synthesis resulting in a severe hemolytic anemia.

Etiology/Incidence (Pathophysiology)

Normal hemoglobin (hemoglobin A) is composed of two polypeptide chains designated as alpha and beta. Children with Cooley anemia have severe deficiencies or total suppression of the beta-chain synthesis. As a result, the circulating red cells are small and contain markedly reduced amounts of hemoglobin. The hemoglobin is severely compromised and is unable to support life for more than a few years. The disorder occurs mainly in persons of Mediterranean origin, especially persons of Greek or Italian ancestry, but the genes are distributed in the Middle East, India, Pakistan, Southeast Asia, Africa, and China.

The disease is inherited in an autosomal recessive pattern. The child who inherits only one gene for beta-thalassemia is said to have "thalassemia trait" or thalassemia minor. Generally, the child with thalassemia trait is asymptomatic; however, a very mild degree of anemia may occur. This anemia may be misdiagnosed as iron deficiency anemia, as the red cells in both disorders are hypochromic and microcytic. Genetic counseling should be made available to parents of children with thalassemia trait and later to the children themselves. If the child later marries a person who also carries the thalassemia gene, the couple has a 1 in 4 chance of producing a child with beta-thalassemia major (Loukopoulos, 1991). (See the discussion of autosomal recessive inheritance in Chapter 31.)

Clinical Manifestations

Historically, older children with beta-thalassemia presented with similar physical changes. This constellation of signs and symptoms includes prominent forehead and cheeks, eyes slanted slightly downward, and an enlarged maxilla with poorly aligned and misshapen teeth. The facial abnormalities are a direct result of bone marrow hypertrophy subsequent to severe anemia. Growth retardation usually occurs also as a consequence of severe anemia, and there is delayed or absent development of puberty and secondary sexual characteristics. Often, cardiac enlargement occurs, as does a flow murmur. Other features include gallstones, pericarditis, and leg ulcers. Unfortunately, the compensatory activity of the marrow does not alleviate the severe anemia, because the defective gene does not allow for the production of useful hemoglobin. Without red blood cell transfusions, the child with beta-thalassemia would die as a result of severe anemia.

Diagnostic Assessment

The child with beta-thalassemia major is asymptomatic during the first 6 months of life because of the presence of hemoglobin F. Some children continue to produce high levels of hemoglobin F and may escape diagnosis until 2 to 3 years of age. Diagnostic presenting symptoms are those of anemia: pallor, listless or fussy behavior, poor appetite, and often frequent infections. Hemoglobin electrophoresis provides laboratory confirmation. As the child becomes older, without treatment the symptoms of anemia become more profound. The body attempts to overcome the anemia by increasing the production of red blood cells. This compensatory mechanism in turn causes enlargement of the liver and spleen and hypertrophy of the bone marrow, resulting in marked changes in the skeletal system. Prenatal diagnosis of beta-thalassemia can be made by amniocentesis or at an earlier gestational age by chorionic villous sampling.

Therapeutic Management

In the past, and in many parts of the world still, transfusion was delayed until clinical symptoms of anemia developed—generally at hemoglobin levels of 5 to 6 g/dl. Life expectancy of these children was only 15 to 20 years (Miller, 1990). Since 1965, hypertransfusion—the maintenance of hemoglobin levels greater than 9 g/dl—has become the accepted treatment. Hypertransfusion has had a dramatic effect on the normal progression of Cooley anemia and prevents many of the aforementioned bone marrow changes and stigmata as well as hepatosplenomegaly. The major drawback of repeated transfusions is the inevitable development of hemosiderosis, the accumulation of iron in body tissue from the breakdown of transfused red blood cells. Iron overload is a well-described phenomenon and causes endocrine dysfunction, liver failure, and cardiac abnormalities (Giardina & Hilgartner, 1992).

Agents that help mobilize (chelate) excess iron and allow for its excretion from the body have been developed. Only desferoxamine (Desferal, DF), an agent that is administered as a continuous subcutaneous or IV infusion, appears to be effective with relatively low toxicity (Miller, 1990). The use of chelating agents early and continuously throughout life prevents the side effects of hypertransfusion programs.

Hepatitis A, B, and C infection remains a serious complication of frequent blood transfusions. In addition, there is risk of infection with cytomegalovirus (Chapter 39) and HIV. (See Chapter 37 for a discussion of AIDS.)

The long-term outlook for children with beta-thalassemia who have not had optimal iron chelation is poor. Death occurs no later than the third decade, most often from congestive heart failure or other complications of iron overload. Children who begin iron chelation early, usually by age 5 or 6 years, may prevent the onset of cardiac complications. Results are encouraging, but follow-up of these children is only 10 to 15 years so far.

Nursing Diagnostic Statements and Collaborative Problems

Altered tissue perfusion (anemia), *owing to decreased oxygen-carrying ability of red blood cells.*

Body image disturbance, self-esteem problems and personal identity disturbance, *related to child's perceptions about altered appearance and self-imposed or other imposed social isolation.*

Altered home health maintenance, *related to knowledge deficit, child and parent about:*

- *The disease process and its treatment.*
- *Necessity for routine immunizations.*
- *Procedures and techniques to be carried out in home care of the child.*

Planning and Implementation

Central to any plan of care is teaching specific to the identified knowledge deficit. Care of the child with beta-thalassemia also involves management of blood transfusions to improve tissue perfusion (see "Therapeutic Management") and support of the child in relationship to altered physical appearance.

Relieving Anemia Through Transfusion. Transfusions for the child with beta-thalassemia are best managed on an outpatient basis. The primary dependent function of the nurse who cares for the child with beta-thalassemia is administration of transfusion. This approach is least disruptive to the child's schedule and may help the child remain in school and in contact with the peer group. Effective transfusion programs usually administer 1 to 3 units of blood every 3 to 5 weeks, depending on the age and size of the patient; 3 weeks is probably the norm. In later years, transfusions may be complicated by increased sensitization to minor blood group antigens and development of antibodies to substances in blood. This results in increased difficulty in finding appropriate blood to transfuse and greater incidence of blood transfusion reactions. Any cardiac involvement requires slower rates of transfusion as well.

Parents and children (when they are old enough to understand) must be taught the correct and safe use of chelating agents. The importance of consistent usage cannot be overstressed. Desferal has traditionally been infused into the subcutaneous tissue via a small needle and a portable infusion pump. The infusion is administered over 8 to 10 hours, usually during the night. Hard, painful lumps sometimes develop at the site of the infusion, rendering the site unusable for days or weeks. Long-term Desferal use is also inconvenient and expensive. Compliance can become a serious problem if the entire family is not highly motivated. Venous access devices (surgically implanted IV lines) can decrease some of the difficulties involved in iron chelation therapy. The nurse should continually encourage and praise the child and family for their efforts, if appropriate, while providing sympathetic acknowledgement of the inconvenience and frustration of the therapy.

Promoting Healthy Body Image, Self-Esteem, and Sense of Identity. Children and adolescents with beta-thalassemia may feel extremely isolated. They are unlike peers in their ability, and the adolescent may have an altered appearance. In addition, they may have substantial feelings of guilt for placing such a burden on their family. Often, they have no one with whom to share feelings of loneliness, fear, and despair. The nurse who consistently cares for the child or adolescent with beta-thalassemia should provide the opportunity for sharing these feelings. Appropriate words of praise and encouragement can also mean a great deal to the young person. Referral to a peer support group or counseling may be appropriate.

Teaching to Address the Knowledge Deficit and Facilitate Home Health Maintenance. The nurse offers comfort to parents who may be grieving at the time of diagnosis. Repeated reinforcement of the physician's explanations of the treatment of beta-thalassemia will be necessary but should be offered when the parents are emotionally ready to hear them. This may not be for several months in some families. Many parents feel overwhelming guilt at the time of diagnosis. The nurse should acknowledge this emotion but encourage parents to overcome it and focus their energies on a more positive area. Often, parents find comfort in support groups of families with chronically ill children. Information on the Cooley's Anemia Foundation should be given (address at the end of this chapter). The nurse should encourage all family members (grandparents, aunts, uncles, siblings) to be tested for the beta-thalassemia trait.

As with all chronic diseases, care of the whole child must not be overlooked. Routine immunizations as well as hepatitis B vaccine and health maintenance should be a priority.

The nurse is responsible for the use of proper products (leukocyte-poor, glycol-washed), monitoring for transfusion reactions, and pretreating with diphenhydramine and acetaminophen, if frequent reactions occur. A nursing study found that adherence was improved with the use of behavioral contracting and a reward system (Koch et al, 1993). Instruction is needed to assess the severity of signs and symptoms of anemia and any complications of hypertransfusion therapy. The complications of hypertransfusion therapy parents should look for include local inflammation at the Desferal injection sites and signs of hemosiderosis (congestive heart failure, endocrine dysfunction, and hepatomegaly). Lastly, the nurse must ensure that the family has been referred for genetic counseling (Martin & Butler, 1993).

Disseminated Intravascular Coagulation

Disseminated intravascular coagulation, most commonly referred to as *DIC,* is by itself not a disease entity. Rather, it is the potential consequence of various pathologic conditions that may occur during the course of severe illness.

Etiology/Incidence (Pathophysiology)

The pathologic conditions that may predispose an individual to DIC include hypoxia, acidosis, tissue necrosis, endotoxic shock, and endothelial damage.

Disorders or diseases that may cause these altered states are numerous but can broadly be classified into the following: (1) infections, (2) neoplasms (e.g., promyelocytic leukemia), (3) immunologic disorders (e.g., blood transfusion reactions), (4) extensive tissue damage (e.g., burns, severe trauma), and (5) other disorders, such as snake bites and giant hemangiomas. The most common causes of DIC in infants and children are fulminant bacterial septic shock, severe respiratory distress syndrome, disseminated viruses, and massive head injuries (Lusher, 1984).

The mechanism of DIC is complex and multifaceted. The DIC spectrum is triggered by the release of thromboplastic material, such as snake venom, endotoxin, or leukemic or tumor cell content, into the circulation, thereby activating the coagulation process. The continued release of coagulation-inducing substances causes abnormal levels of thrombin within the plasma. In addition to its key role in the coagulation cascade, thrombin is also essential to transforming plasminogen into plasmin. Plasmin breaks down fibrinogen and fibrin clots in the normal functioning fibrinolytic system. Fibrin degradation products (FDPs) are formed as a result of plasmin's action on a blood clot. In DIC the excess thrombin not only converts fibrinogen to fibrin at an accelerated rate; it likewise activates the fibrinolytic system. The FDPs have an affinity to bind with circulatory fibrinogen, causing emboli to form. These emboli can be deposited in the microvasculature and may ultimately cause tissue necrosis. Bleeding ensues as the components required for hemostasis, the coagulation factors and platelets, are consumed by the ongoing intravascular coagulation process and are eventually depleted.

Clinical Manifestations

Clinical manifestations of DIC are often first noted by the nurse. Oozing from previous puncture sites and significant ecchymosis or purpura in a seriously ill child are the hallmarks of the disorder. Signs of circulatory failure (hypovolemia) are manifested by pallor, tachycardia, and decreased blood pressure; hypoperfusion of fingers and toes ensues secondarily.

Diagnostic Assessment

Laboratory confirmation of DIC demonstrates a decreased or falling platelet count, prolonged bleeding time, and significantly prolonged coagulation assays: prothrombin time (PT), activated partial thromboplastin time (PTT), and thrombin clotting time (TCT). The fibrinogen, factor V, and factor VIII levels are low, and, in addition, an assay of FDPs is significantly elevated.

Therapeutic Management

Treatment of DIC is aimed primarily at resolving the underlying disease responsible for triggering DIC. Supportive measures are necessary during the acute phase. Whole blood or packed red blood cells are indicated for treatment of hypovolemia or shock. Fresh frozen plasma and/or cryoprecipitate may be used to help restore the previous homeostasis of the child's plasma, although this is often achieved by alleviating the underlying disease. Heparin therapy is controversial and is used mainly in cases of severe tissue or organ necrosis resulting from thrombi. The administration of heparin in a bleeding disorder seems paradoxical. Its use in children with DIC may be indicated, however, because "by its inactivation of thrombin and other clotting factors, heparin can interrupt the coagulation process and diminish fibrinolysis" (Flug & Karpatkin, 1985). As fibrinolysis decreases, bleeding and thrombus formation also diminish. The overall prognosis for the child with DIC depends on the outcome of the disease causing the coagulation disorder.

Nursing Diagnostic Statements and Collaborative Problems for the Child with Disseminated Intravascular Coagulation

Altered tissue perfusion: hypovolemia, *related to hemorrhage.*
Fear/anxiety: child and family, *related to perceptions regarding life-threatening nature and treatment of the disease and knowledge deficit: child and family, regarding nature and treatment of DIC.*

Nursing Care

Children who do develop the full clinical picture of DIC are severely ill and should be managed in an intensive care setting. The nurse should make every attempt to inform the child about every action he or she is experiencing. The parents are often relegated to waiting rooms for long periods. When the parents are with the child, it is helpful for the nurse to volunteer information on any changes that have taken place since their last report. The nurse should point out any obvious equipment being used on or around the child. The parents often become keenly aware of the technical aspects of treatment and may seem to focus more on this than on their child. This may be the parents' only means of maintaining some control of their child's life, and parents should not be discouraged from doing so.

The nursing diagnoses and collaborative problems identified will facilitate care planning for the nurse in the intensive care unit. Because DIC is managed in this specialized care setting, the nurse generalist is seldom involved with direct nursing management. The principal responsibility of the nonspecialist is in recognizing disease states that may lead to DIC and in astutely assessing and quickly reporting unusual signs of bleeding. Early medical intervention can often prevent the disease from becoming fulminant.

Acquired Aplastic Anemia

Aplastic anemia may be defined as bone marrow failure characterized by reduction or absence of the solid elements (red cells, white cells, platelets) of blood. The disease can be congenital (Fanconi anemia), or it can be acquired.

Etiology/Incidence (Pathophysiology)

Approximately 1000 new cases of the acquired form are diagnosed yearly, of which 30 to 50 per cent have no established etiology (Miller & O'Reilly, 1990). Known agents capable of inducing aplastic anemia include chemicals such as benzene; drugs, most notably the antibiotic chloramphenicol; radiation; and antineoplastics. It can also occur as a complication of infections such as hepatitis or mononucleosis.

Diagnostic Assessment

Patients present with the typical symptoms of depressed bone marrow function: bruises, petechiae, and epistaxis as a result of decreased platelets; anemia, pallor, and fatigue from decreased red blood cells; and often infections due to low white blood cell count. A complete blood count shows that anemia is often profound (3 to 7 g/dl) with few or no reticulocytes (red blood cell precursors) present. Thrombocytopenia and neutropenia are constant presenting features. A bone marrow biopsy shows a marked decrease in all the normally present cells.

Aplastic anemia is classified as moderate or severe. By definition, severe aplastic anemia includes two of the following three parameters at diagnosis:

1. Neutrophil count less than 500.
2. Platelet count less than 20,000.
3 Reticulocytes less than 1 per cent as well as a bone marrow with severe or moderately decreased cellularity.

Fewer than 20 per cent of patients who fit the "severe" category were alive 1 year after diagnosis (Miller & O'Reilly, 1990). Assigning severity assumes great importance in treatment decisions. Children with severe aplasia have little choice other than to undergo a bone marrow transplant, despite the risks and complications. Children with moderate disease at presentation may be candidates for immunotherapy with antilymphocyte globulin or antithymocyte globulin. Survival rates following immunotherapy are 60 per cent (Miller & O'Reilly, 1990). If a bone marrow transplant donor is deemed acceptable, blood product support in the form of transfusions should be withheld or used sparingly. No family member's blood may be given.

Therapeutic Management

Treatment aimed at a cure includes androgen and steroid therapy, bone marrow transplantation, and in some centers immunotherapy. If a compatible donor is available, bone marrow transplantation is the preferred treatment of choice. This modality has a 3-year survival rate of 80 per cent (Nathan, 1987).

Tissue typing of family members should immediately be performed at diagnosis, before any transfusions have been administered. Transfusions can seriously compromise a subsequent bone marrow transplant. Thirty per cent of patients with a history of prior transfusions reject their marrow graft (Miller & O'Reilly, 1990). If the child has no acceptable donor, or bone marrow transplant is not an option, then transfusion support is ordered.

Nursing Care

Nursing care for children with aplastic anemia is similar to that for children with leukemia. Parental education about home care of the child with low blood counts is essential. Chapter 42 contains further information on bone marrow transplantation and care of the child with low blood counts.

Table 42–5 details a nursing process plan for the child with cancer undergoing chemotherapy. Chemotherapeutic drugs cause bone marrow suppression that is similar in presentation to aplastic anemia. This nursing process plan, therefore, addresses care of the child with decreased white blood cells, red blood cells, and platelets.

Congenital Aplastic Anemia: Fanconi Anemia

Congenital aplastic anemia, or Fanconi anemia, is a rare disorder inherited in an autosomal recessive fashion. Many patients are recognized at birth because of the associated congenital anomalies, although hematologic abnormalities rarely become evident before 17 months of age and may not develop until the second decade. Congenital anomalies include café-au-lait spots and skin hyperpigmentation, especially involving the neck, axilla, abdomen, umbilicus, and genitalia. Absence of thumbs and radii is associated, and other skeletal anomalies such as short stature (as a result of short trunk) may occur. Hypoplastic thumbnails have frequently been noted. Renal abnormalities may occur; these include horseshoe kidneys, hydronephrosis, or absence of one kidney. In addition, central nervous system findings such as microcephaly, mental retardation, deafness, ptosis, nystagmus, and hyper-reflexia may occur. However, 37 per cent of persons listed in the International Fanconi Anemia Registry had no noted abnormalities (Alter, 1992). Treatment is similar to that for acquired aplastic anemia and includes supportive care, androgens, and steroids. The majority of children with Fanconi anemia may have long-term disease remission with androgens and steroids alone; however, there is little potential for cure. The remission period may be several, even as many as 20, years in duration (Alter, 1992). Bone marrow transplantation is the only cure for the aplastic anemia. This generally requires a human leukocyte antigen (HLA)-matched sibling donor (see Chapter 42 for further discussion of bone marrow transplant donors). Transplants using unrelated or mismatched donors have not produced good results (Alter, 1992).

Hemophilia

"Hemophilia" is a term that has a high index of familiarity to most people. The disease has many historic references, and images of "bleeding to death from a pin prick" are common in the public's eye. In truth, children with hemophilia may experience prolonged troublesome bleeding from such minor events as tooth loss or nosebleeds, but these events are rarely, if ever, life-threatening. Superficial cuts and scrapes do not require treatment other than cleansing and pressure. Rather, *the hallmark of hemophilia is repeated oozing of blood into soft tissue, muscles, and, most frequently, joint capsules.* Indeed, the joint bleeding and subsequent limitations of movement and eventual crippling places hemophilia well within the scope of an orthopedic disorder.

Etiology/Incidence

Hemophilia occurs in 1 in 10,000 males born in the United States. The disease is transmitted in an X-linked recessive manner. The disease primarily affects males but can rarely be present in females. (See Chapter 31, "X-Linked Recessive Inheritance," for futher discussion.)

The nurse must fully understand and help explain the genetic rules of the disease to the parents and later to the child. It is crucial that parents understand that the overall risk is the same for each pregnancy, regardless of what has occurred in prior births. Female relatives of the affected child can be tested for carrier status by a laboratory blood test with a fairly high rate of accuracy.

Pathophysiology

Hemophilia occurs as the result of a deficiency in one of the clotting factors; all other aspects of coagulation are typically normal. The most common form of hemophilia is known as hemophilia A, which is also known as classical hemophilia or simply factor VIII deficiency (Lusher & Warrier, 1991, 1992). The second most frequent type is called hemophilia B, also known as Christmas disease or factor IX deficiency. Approximately 80 per cent of those affected have classic hemophilia. Although they are two separate diseases, both forms of hemophilia have similar symptoms, genetic rules, and treatment policies. For ease of writing, "hemophilia" will be generic for both disorders, unless specifically noted otherwise.

Clinical Manifestations

Any part of the body has the potential to become the site of a bleeding incident. Young boys tend to have more oral bleeding and perhaps more bruises during the unsteady toddler period. Nosebleeds may be more frequent in young children, probably as a result of "wandering fingers" more than anything else (Helgartner & McMillan, 1984). Nosebleeds can generally be stopped with pressure alone and, although bothersome, do not present a significant health risk.

Central nervous system bleeding can occur at any age and most often follows trauma to the head but can be spontaneous in origin. Central nervous system hemorrhage accounts for more deaths in hemophilic persons than any other type of bleeding.

Oozing of blood into soft tissue can occur and may appear as a nodular mass with definitive borders. No treatment is usually required, unless the bleeding is in a critical area, such as the neck or wrist, where obstruction from the blood-filled mass could result in serious injury from pressure on major vessels and nerves.

Bleeding may occur deep within a muscle belly, normally well supplied with blood vessels. This may result from blows, sudden twists, sprains, or deep intramuscular injections. The area is very painful, and the child may refuse to use an affected limb. Abdominal and retroperitoneal muscle bleeds may be indistinguishable from other serious abdominal conditions.

Bleeding into the joint spaces, *hemarthrosis,* is the most common complication in severe hemophilia. The knee is the joint most frequently involved, followed in frequency by the elbow, ankle, hip, shoulder, and wrist. The bleeding begins with a slight tear in the synovial tissue; if no treatment is given, it continues until the joint capsule is fully expanded and no more

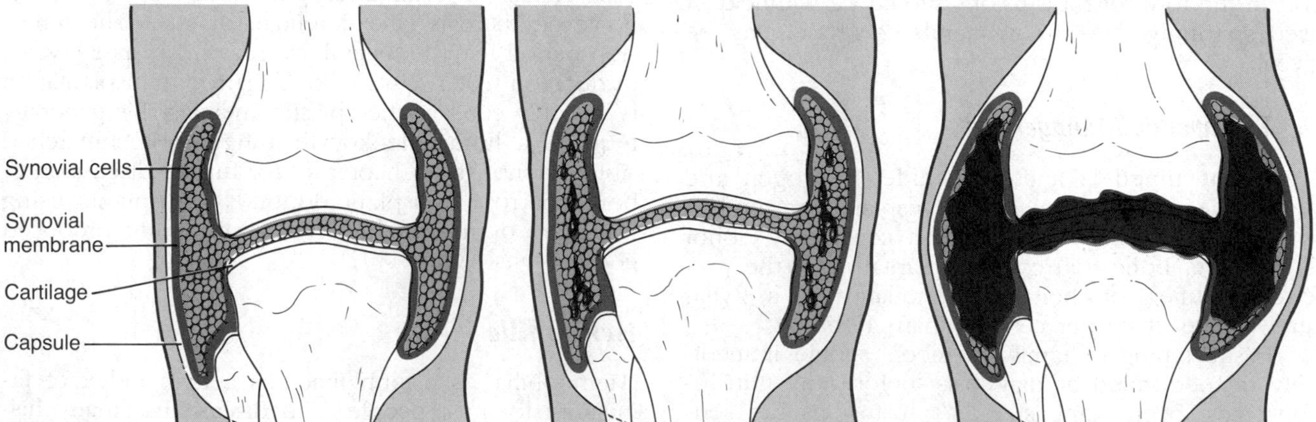

FIGURE 34-7. Hemarthrosis in hemophilia. *A*, Normal knee joint; *B*, bleeding; *C*, joint capsule swollen with blood.

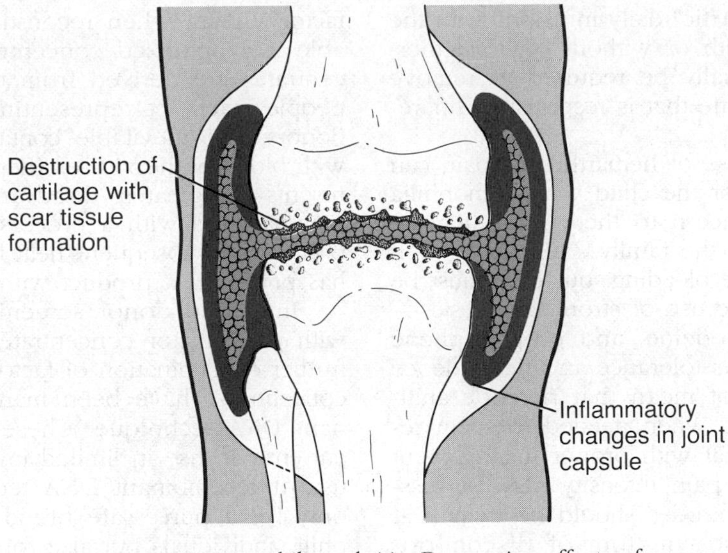

FIGURE 34-8. Hemophilic arthritis. Destructive effects of successive episodes of bleeding into the joint.

blood can leak into the capsule (Fig. 34–7). Discomfort occurs at the onset of bleeding and progresses to severe pain and refusal to use the affected joint. Once the bleeding is stopped, the blood is gradually reabsorbed; however, with repeated bleeding episodes into the capsule, progressive destruction of the joint occurs (Fig. 34–8).

Diagnostic Assessment

In hemophilia A or B, factor VIII or factor IX, respectively, is present but in a diminished capacity. The defective factor is unable to perform its function in the coagulation "cascade." The cascade sequence is halted, and no fibrin clot can be formed. (Refer to "Structure and Function: Anatomy and Physiology of Blood.")

The severity of hemophilia is dependent on the percentage of the functioning factor present. Severely affected hemophilic individuals* have less than 1 per cent factor coagulant activity. Those moderately affected have 1 to 5 per cent, and those with mild disease have 5 to 50 per cent coagulant activity. The person with mild hemophilia may be diagnosed only after surgery or major trauma. The moderately affected child may experience one or two bleeding episodes per year. The severely affected individual may have as many as two or three bleeding episodes per week, many of them "spontaneous" in origin (no known trauma).

Hemophilia can be diagnosed at birth because maternal factor VIII is not transferred to the fetus. Diagnostic evaluation is likely to be done in families with a positive family history. Prenatal diagnosis can be made from fetal blood. Laboratory confirmation of hemophilia would show a prolonged PTT, a normal PT, normal bleeding time, normal platelet count, normal factor VIII antigen (or factor IX), and low levels of factor VIII coagulant level (or factor IX in hemophilia B).

Twenty-five per cent of all new cases of hemophilia have no family history and are thought to be genetic mutations. These children are often diagnosed following prolonged bleeding after circumcision, but the majority of hemophilic boys have no substantial bleeding during the first year of life. Most begin to have difficulty when they begin to walk and undergo subsequent bumps and falls. A common first injury in toddlers is oral mucous membrane bleeding following trauma to the tongue, frenulum, buccal mucosa, or gums.

Therapeutic Management

In most cases, treatment of hemophilic bleeding consists of replacement of the deficient factor; local control measures, such as ice packs and elastic bandages; and analgesia if necessary. Immobilization is mandatory for comfort and to avoid further bleeding. Initially, the nurse should take care not to aggravate the bleeding further by moving the affected area, particularly a painful joint. Once the bleeding has been stopped—within 24 to 48 hours in most cases—the child's physician may order gentle, passive range-of-motion exercises several times a day to the affected joint. This is done to prevent stiffening and eventual contractures of the joint. It is not unusual for one particular joint to become especially troublesome for an individual child; the reasons for this are not clear. Such a situation can be extremely trying and frustrating for both the child and family. To break the cycle of frequent bleeding, the physician may order night-

* In an effort to promote better self-concept, the National Hemophilia Foundation and hemophilia consumer groups advocate the use of the terms "hemophilic individual" or "person with hemophilia," rather than "hemophiliac."

time splints and "prophylactic" daily infusions with the missing clotting factor with or without physical therapy. Surgery may eventually be required to remove the damaged synovial tissue that is responsible for repeated bleeding.

During the acute phase of hemarthrosis, pain can be severe. Pain control for the child with hemophilia must be an issue of concern to the comprehensive care team, the child, and the family. Pain medication should be used for severe bleeding, but care must be exercised to avoid chronic use of strong analgesics—meperidine (Demerol), codeine, and propoxyphene (Darvon), for example—as tolerance and dependence may occur. This does not mean that narcotic analgesics should be withheld when needed for pain relief. Rather, it indicates that with proper management of the bleeding episode, pain intensity may be lessened. Ideally, bleeding episodes should be treated at the onset of the earliest symptom of discomfort, thereby requiring only 24 hours of immobilization and acetaminophen (Tylenol) for pain relief. Aspirin is avoided in children with bleeding disorders because of its antiaggregating effects on platelet function.

To stop bleeding effectively, the child needs a circulating factor VIII (or IX) level of 20 to 100 per cent. The location and severity of the bleeding incident dictate the level of factor replacement required, thus accounting for the wide range of acceptable treatment levels. For example, significant head trauma (e.g., falling down steps, tumbling from a bicycle) requires immediate factor replacement to the 100 per cent level. However, bleeding into a joint capsule that is detected very early may be successfully treated with a 20 to 40 per cent level (Aronstram, 1980).

Factor replacement is achieved by infusion of plasma, cryoprecipitate, or factor concentrates. Fresh frozen plasma contains 1 unit of factor (VIII or IX) per milliliter. An infusion of 1 unit/kg of factor VIII (1 ml/kg plasma) raises the factor VIII blood level by 2 per cent. Factor IX (1 unit/kg) raises the blood level by 1.5 per cent. To achieve 100 per cent replacement, a 10-kg child with factor VIII deficiency would require 50 ml plasma per kilogram, or 500 ml. This large volume is impossible to give safely to a small child. Factor levels of 15 to 20 per cent are the highest levels possible in plasma treatment because of the volume required.

Cryoprecipitate is formed when fresh frozen plasma is thawed at 4°C. This substance is rich in factor VIII and fibrinogen as well as in the von Willebrand factor. One bag of "cryo," as cryoprecipitate is commonly known, contains approximately 100 units of factor VIII (range 60 to 125 units/bag). The volume of one bag is approximately 10 ml. Our theoretical 10-kg child could now achieve 100 per cent factor VIII levels with only 50 ml volume of cryoprecipitate. Cryoprecipitate does not contain factor IX and must be stored at −20°C until ready to use. Several pharmaceutical firms prepare lyophilized (freeze-dried) factor VIII concentrates. These products are conveniently packaged, have a long shelf-life, can be stored or carried at room temperature, and provide high levels of factor VIII/ml when reconstituted. Factor IX is available in lyophilized concentrate as well. Factor concentrates are derived from the plasma of numerous people, each lot representing 20,000 to 30,000 paid donors. The inevitable contamination of the product with blood-borne viruses (hepatitis B and C, HIV) represents the greatest disadvantage. Factor concentrate manufactured with a process using more clonal antibodies and subsequent heat treatment (pasteurization) has produced a product with much greater purity.

Improved donor screening and testing coupled with purer factor concentrate will hopefully eliminate further contamination of factor concentrate. Factor VIII concentrates have been manufactured with recombinant DNA technique. These factor concentrates are currently in use in limited investigational settings. The use of recombinant DNA techniques gives hope not only for a pure, safe blood replacement for hemophilic individuals but also for the possibility of a cure.

The availability of factor concentrates have dramatically improved the quality of life for hemophilic individuals over the past 20 years. Before 1980 and the AIDS epidemic (see further on), the life expectancy of hemophilic persons had improved dramatically; males with mild disease had survival rates equivalent to those of unaffected males (Jones & Ralnoff, 1991). The convenience and accessibility of the manufactured concentrate made "home care" a reasonable alternative. Home care programs allow the parent or child to treat a suspected or actual bleeding incident themselves at home as early as possible. Logically, the sooner a bleeding episode is stopped, the fewer sequelae (e.g., pain, immobility, follow-up treatments, joint damage) will be experienced. Parents and patients are instructed how to recognize early signs and symptoms of bleeding episodes and are taught the proper dosage of the factor needed for the various types of bleeding incidents. In addition, they become proficient in the technical aspects of factor usage, such as reconstitution and IV administration of factor concentrate. Home infusion also encourages the child and family to function more normally, by decreasing and often totally eliminating in-hospital treatment.

Dosages of factor concentrates are calculated in the same manner as for plasma or cryoprecipitate. The desired percentage of circulating factor must be decided by the patient's physician and the following formula used to calculate the dose (Agle et al, 1977):

$$\frac{\text{weight in pounds}}{4.4} \times \text{\% factor VIII or factor IX activity desired} = \text{number of units of factor needed}$$

Almost all patients who require frequent factor infusions are on home care programs. Ineligible patients may include young children or babies with poor venous access, patients or parents with severe emotional problems, and in some treatment centers patients who have developed inhibitors (described in the following discussion "Complications"). It is not unusual for children enrolled in home care programs to receive all care as outpatients and to require infrequent hospitalization only for surgery or for treatment of a major bleed. Home care has meant a dramatic change for the families of children with hemophilia. The benefits include prompt treatment of bleeding episodes with a subsequent decrease in serious arthropathy, decrease in hospital time, increase in school and work time, and greater sense of control by families and patients. (See Chapter 22 for a discussion of principles and interventions related to home care.)

Complications. Approximately 10 per cent of children with hemophilia develop inhibitors. Inhibitors are circulating antibodies that render the infused factor VIII (or IX) molecule useless. Inhibitors are measured in Bethesda units (BU). One BU inactivates the factor in 1 ml plasma. Hemophilic persons must have had at least one exposure to infused factor before they develop an inhibitor; however, the tendency appears to be genetically determined. There is no evidence that frequent factor infusions predispose an individual to develop inhibitors.

The treatment of patients who have developed inhibitors is controversial. Some centers do not treat bleeding episodes in children with inhibitors unless they are life-threatening. In other centers, the treatment is massive doses of factor VIII. The number of units of factor that would be bound by the inhibitor is mathematically calculated; units above this level are then administered. In still other centers, a product that contains activated factor X (Xa) (FeIBA) has been used with some success, as has therapy with high doses of prothrombin concentrates (Konyne, Proplex), which also contain appreciable levels of factor X. The high level of factor X is thought to "bypass" the need for factor VIII in the coagulation cascade. None of these methods has been highly successful, and the last three methods are very expensive. The patient with an inhibitor is likely to spend more time hospitalized and is likely to have more severe joint disease.

AIDS has come to the forefront as the most devastating complication of transfusion therapy. It is ironic that the therapy that changed the natural history of hemophilia from a crippling disease with a low life expectancy—factor concentrates—is also responsible for the current epidemic levels of HIV positivity among hemophilic patients. Factor concentrate produced between 1978 and 1985, with the years 1981 to 1983 most implicated, was frequently contaminated with HIV. Consequently, 80 to 90 per cent of hemophilia A patients and 50 per cent of hemophilia B patients are HIV-positive. AIDS has replaced hemorrhage as the most common cause of death among this population. The ultimate outcome of the current generation of hemophilic patients remains unknown. The prognosis for HIV-positive hemophilic patients is no different from that for other risk groups: 25 per cent will develop AIDS within 8 to 9 years (Rosendaal, 1991).

AIDS is discussed in detail in Chapter 37. Infants and young children born after 1986 when preventive measures were in place have been spared exposure to contaminated plasma and do not have the same levels of HIV infection.

Hepatitis, both type B and type C (the primary etiologic agent for non-A, non-B hepatitis), is a significant problem for the same group of patients at risk for HIV. Chronic hepatitis and liver disease account for more deaths than does bleeding. Recognition of this danger has prompted new methods of factor preparation. The development of tests to determine the presence of hepatitis C virus and improvements in the detection of hepatitis B, in addition to the hepatitis B vaccine, should prevent infection in the younger patients. As in the case of HIV, the fate of those currently hepatitis-positive (more than 90 per cent) is unknown.

Application of the Nursing Process: Hemophilia

Assessment

Assessment data that the nurse collects are vital signs, including pulse and respirations at rest and the color of skin and mucous membranes. Height, weight, placement on the growth chart, and developmental status are noted, because the child may have delays in these areas. As discussed in "Diagnostic Assessment," a variety of tests are conducted during the diagnostic workup. Refer to Table 34–8 for additional assessment parameters the nurse considers when caring for a child with hemophilia.

Nursing Diagnostic Statements and Collaborative Problems

High risk for injury: localized hemorrhage; *risk factor:*

- *A significant decrease in clotting factor VIII (or IX) associated with a sex-linked genetic trait.*
- *Parental knowledge deficit regarding factor replacement.*

Altered comfort: pain, *related to hemarthrosis associated with trauma to a limb.*

High risk for altered health maintenance; *risk factor: knowledge deficit, regarding home care.*

High risk for altered growth and development; *risk factors:*

- *Parental overprotection.*
- *Poor school attendance associated with treatment for bleeding episodes.*
- *Stigma associated with a chronic disease and with physical restrictions.*

High risk for altered parenting: impaired patterns of discipline; *risk factors:*

- *Guilt associated with genetic transmission of the disease.*
- *Concern for the child's physical well-being.*

Planning and Implementation

Administering and Teaching Intravenous Factor Replacement. The nurse is often responsible for preparing and administering factor replacement to the hospitalized hemophilic patient. Detailed instructions for reconstitution accompany each bottle of factor concentrate. The units of each bottle vary, and this may sometimes cause confusion. The calculated factor replacement level should be approached as closely as possible without waste of any reconstituted factor. For example, if the physician calculates the required dose to be "500 units factor VIII," any number of units *in that range* is acceptable. If the pharmacy or blood bank has only 550 unit vials available, then all the units should be given. However, if only 480 unit vials are available, it would not be necessary to obtain an additional 20 units elsewhere. The calculated factor level should be regarded as an estimate.

The nurse should encourage the child and family to assist in mixing and administering the factor if they are not enrolled in a home care program. If the family is on home care, the nurse should not feel threatened by the family's desire to mix and perform venipuncture themselves. The nurse should encourage and reinforce this desire for independence. The child should be encouraged to participate in factor administration at an early age. He may begin by mixing the factor bottles or helping to push the plunger on the syringe. His responsibilities should increase gradually, and all children should be using the self-infusion technique by their teen-age years (Fig. 34–9).

Comforting the Child in Pain. Strategies for pain management are addressed under "Therapeutic Management." Additional strategies for pain assessment and management can be found in Table 25–2.

Facilitating Home Health Maintenance. The nurse instructs family members on assessment techniques. Families are taught to assess for evidence of bleeding within the musculoskeletal and central nervous systems, and the function of joints previously involved in hemorrhage into the joint capsule. Parents are instructed to monitor HIV status, lymphocyte function, hepatitis studies, and liver function tests. The family must be given current information about the risk for AIDS infection related to transfusion of blood products. Teen-agers and young adults are given information on modes of AIDS transmission and methods of prevention.

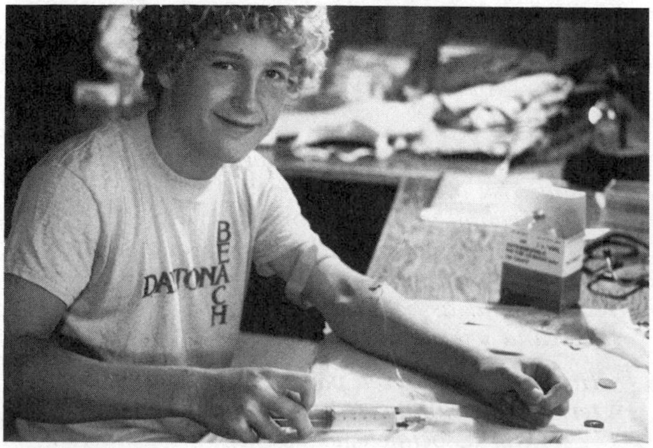

FIGURE 34-9. Self-infusion helps promote positive self-esteem and a sense of normality.

Hemophilic individuals may be ostracized and exposed to hostility because of their HIV status. Hemophilia has been recognized as one of the high-risk groups for development of AIDS within the lay press. Many people are ignorant about HIV transmission and extremely fearful of themselves or their children contracting the virus. The medical community may be of great support to the child and family and should advocate for the child with the school and community.

Updated information can be obtained from the Centers for Disease Control (telephone numbers: [800]342-AIDS or [800]342-7514). See Chapter 37 for further discussion of AIDS.

Routine Health Promotion Is Part of Home Health Maintenance. The hemophilic child should receive routine childhood immunizations. Hepatitis B vaccination should begin in infancy. These shots are not deeply injected, and firm pressure over the site or wrapping with an elastic bandage most often prevents muscle bleeding. Ice is probably of little benefit and must be used cautiously to prevent skin damage in young children. Other medications, such as antibiotics or pain medications, should be administered by oral or rectal routes if possible.

The nurse should reinforce the importance of a sound dental hygiene program. Preventive care avoids an additional source of potential bleeding problems. Children should learn the proper technique of toothbrushing early. The child should be expected to brush at least twice a day with a soft-bristled brush. Visits to a dentist who is familiar with hemophilia should start at age 2 years and should be maintained every 6 months. Dental anesthesia can be administered, but pretreatment with factor replacement is often necessary to prevent bleeding or hematoma at the injection site.

Provision of a Safe but Normal Environment Is also Part of Home Health Maintenance. Parents are instructed to provide a safe environment for their child with hemophilia but also to normalize the environment as much as possible. The nurse can assist families by reviewing the various developmental and emotional stages of early childhood with the family and providing anticipatory guidance before each new stage.

Infancy is rarely a period of stress or bleeding problems. The infant is safely bundled and usually is not exposed to significant trauma. As previously stated, toddlerhood exposes the child to new sources of trauma, and this is the time during which most cases of hemophilia are diagnosed. In general, safety measures that should be employed for all children of this age are sufficient for the child with hemophilia.

This includes installing gates or doors over stairs, locking cabinets, removing dangling cords, removing throw rugs, and placing obtrusive furniture in unobtrusive places as well as other well-described child-proofing measures. Padded clothing, padded furniture, helmets, and other similar measures are usually not recommended. These are largely ineffective in preventing hemophilic bleeding, and may cause the child to feel ostracized. In addition, parents must be cautioned not to reprimand or remind the child continually with comments such as "Be careful" and "Don't hurt yourself." It is inevitable that these children will hurt themselves and have bleeding episodes. The parents must realize early on that this in no way reflects on their parenting ability. They must also be cautioned never to tell or even insinuate to their child that factor replacement is a form of punishment for participating in a forbidden activity.

Parents may have questions about appropriate toys for their children. Once again, age-appropriate and safe toys that any child would use are suitable. A Big Wheel tricycle may help prevent a few falls and subsequent bleeding, because it is so low to the ground. A slightly longer period of training wheels on a new bike may also prevent some injuries. Working with scissors and, later, woodworking or doing similar shop-type activities should not be forbidden as long as the child has been instructed in safe use and is supervised until he or she can use the tools safely.

The parents should be taught that physical activities and sports are vital to the child's muscular development and coordination as well as emotional well-being. Certain sports that predispose to injury and trauma such as football, soccer, ice hockey, and karate must be avoided, but activities such as swimming, softball, running, hiking, and bicycling should be encouraged.

The nurse should inform all families of all new patients about the existence of the National Hemophilia Foundation (address listed at the end of this chapter). Nurses should encourage parents to obtain the literature available through this group and to become involved in local chapters. Advice and support from a parent who has been through the same experience can be invaluable.

All children with hemophilia should wear Medic-alert tags, even as infants. Young children should refrain from wearing necklaces for safety reasons and rely instead on wearing bracelets or merely pinning the tag onto clothing.

Promoting Healthy Development. With the availability of factor replacement therapy, home care programs, and strong comprehensive hemophilia medical programs, families are encouraged to allow their children to run and play with friends, to attend regular classrooms, and, most importantly, to learn to set their own limits. Families and children require frequent interventions and counseling about psychosocial issues by the medical staff. The nurse who consistently cares for the child with hemophilia can develop a trusting relationship with the family. This nurse may be the medical team member to whom the family feels most comfortable addressing their problems and concerns (Spitzer, 1992).

It is easy to understand why children with hemophilia are at high risk of developing low self-esteem. The children may be thwarted in attempts to achieve mastery of specific developmental tasks. The early wanderings and discoveries of toddlerhood may be restricted, as may normal play activities when they become older. School performance may be affected by poor attendance and by taunts or rejection by peers. Sadly, in some families most of the time that the children and parents spend together is medically related. Children can sense very early the burden they have placed on the family. The additional burden of HIV infection has placed considerable strain on these children. Once again, the reader is referred to Chapter 37 for a detailed discussion of the psychologic effects of AIDS.

Families must be alerted to the subtle signs of overprotection that they may manifest. Constant admonishments to be careful, refusing to allow participation in normal play activities, or not permitting visits away from home for extended periods leads children to believe they are helpless and encourages a passive-dependent personality.

Promoting Parenting: Healthy Patterns of Discipline. Like any child, the child with hemophilia needs lots of love and encouragement but must not have "ultraspecial" status within the family. Allowing chronically ill children to "use" their disease to avoid discipline, household tasks, or homework must not be allowed. The same form of discipline should be used consistently with all children in the family, and the same expectations for achievements should be maintained. Allowing children free reign of the home and school destroys their sense of industry and independence.

School personnel should be contacted by the medical team at the time of the child's entry into the system. Ideally, the nurse can make a school visit to facilitate the process. This can help correct misconceptions about the disease, and it helps teachers to develop a realistic approach with the child. The value of a good education cannot be overestimated for these children. This can best be achieved by early intervention with the school and open, honest communication among the school, family, and medical staff.

Von Willebrand Disease

Von Willebrand disease is a complex and not fully understood disorder of coagulation. It is usually inherited in an autosomal dominant fashion, although rarely it can be autosomal recessive (see Chapter 31 for a discussion of these inheritance patterns).

Etiology/Incidence (Pathophysiology)

The disease results in low levels of the factor VIII molecule and its component, the von Willebrand factor. Unlike the child with classic hemophilia, in which the factor VIII molecule is present but defective, the child with classic or type I von Willebrand disease has diminished levels and in very severe cases (type III), complete absence of the entire factor VIII complex. The von Willebrand component of the factor VIII molecule is thought to be necessary for platelet aggregation (sticking together) to stop bleeding. Type II von Willebrand disease has four subtypes and variable laboratory parameters (Lusher, 1984).

Clinical Manifestations

Clinical symptoms of von Willebrand disease vary greatly from person to person and may even vary within an individual's lifetime. Many children with the disorder escape diagnosis entirely, unless routine coagulation studies are done before an unrelated surgical procedure.

Children with severe disorders may present with frequent nosebleeds, bruising, gum bleeding, prolonged oozing of blood from minor wounds, and in teen-age girls, heavy and prolonged menses. Hemarthrosis, the bleeding most common in hemophilia, occurs very rarely in von Willebrand disease and only in type III in which the factor VIII deficiency is severe.

Therapeutic Management

Most bleeding episodes in the child with classic von Willebrand disease stop with conventional measures (i.e., pressure to the site of bleeding).

The bleeding defect in von Willebrand disease has responded to infusions of desmopressin acetate (DDAVP) (Lusher, 1984). DDAVP is a synthetic analogue of the natural hormone arginine vasopressin that is commonly used to treat diabetes insipidus. DDAVP causes immediate but transient release of factor VIII normally held in storage in the endothelium of blood vessels. The transient rise may be sufficient to protect a patient during minor surgery or dental work. DDAVP does not carry the risk of hepatitis or other blood product contamination and is the treatment of choice for most children with von Willebrand disease. Desmopressin commonly causes facial warming and flushing and occasionally transient headache and nausea. Rarely, hypertension and fluid and electrolyte imbalances may occur. Desmopressin cannot be used for severe type III disease. Children with severe disease have no stores of factor VIII molecule to be released. Cryoprecipitate is indicated for treatment of bleeding episodes for these children.

Menstrual periods may be a problem for young women with severe disease. Routine cryoprecipitate infusions may be necessary to control bleeding. A moderate degree of success has been achieved with hormonal modification of the menstrual cycle with anovulatory birth control pills. Pregnancy and childbirth can be safely achieved, but it is imperative that the young woman receive care from both obstetrician and hematologist. Cryoprecipitate infusions should begin before the delivery and should continue for several days post partum.

The overall prognosis for the child with von Willebrand disease is very good. Those with mildly and even moderately decreased levels of factor VIII are apt to have no problems with routine activities. Children with severe disease are likely to be homozygous (inheritance of gene from both parents), and their occurrence is uncommon (the actual incidence is unknown).

Nursing Care

The family whose child is diagnosed with von Willebrand disease requires education about the disorder. Truthful reassurance is best for the parents of moderate or mildly affected children. Medic-alert tags should be worn by the child, and physically demanding occupations should be discouraged. Children with von Willebrand disease are eligible for referral for services from the local and national levels of the Hemophilia Foundation.

Idiopathic Thrombocytopenic Purpura

Idiopathic thrombocytopenic purpura, commonly referred to as ITP, is an acquired blood disorder characterized by increased destruction of circulating platelets.

Etiology/Incidence (Pathophysiology)

ITP occurs most frequently in the age range of 2 to 5 years, although it can occur at any age. White children have a higher incidence than African-American children.

As its name suggests, the etiology of ITP is unknown. However, current theories of an autoimmune phenomenon are widely accepted (see Chapter 37 for a discussion of autoimmune mechanisms). For unknown reasons, platelets become coated with antiplatelet antibody, are recognized as foreign material, and are subsequently destroyed by the spleen.

Diagnostic Assessment

Signs and symptoms of ITP include the sudden onset of easy bruising and randomly distributed petechiae and ecchymoses all over the body. Twenty to thirty per cent of children present with epistaxis or bleeding from other mucous membranes. About 80 per cent of children with ITP have a positive history of a recent febrile illness, usually a nonspecific upper respiratory infection, although rubella and rubeola have also been implicated (Corrigan, 1990). At presentation, despite their severely bruised appearance, these children do not look "sick." Careful assessment is indicated to differentiate the bruising of ITP from that of child abuse.

Laboratory studies show a reduced platelet count, usually below 20,000 to 30,000 mm^3/dl. A bone marrow aspiration should be performed to rule out malignant infiltration of the marrow; in ITP, the aspiration is normal, except for higher than normal levels of megakaryocytes—the parent cells of platelets. Laboratory tests that measure platelet function, specifically the bleeding time and tourniquet test, are prolonged in children with ITP; all other blood studies are typically normal (see Table 34–4).

Therapeutic Management

Platelet transfusions are of little value in ITP, because the transfused platelets become coated with antibody and are destroyed as easily as autologous platelets. Transfusions may be indicated in life-threatening hemorrhage, such as an intracranial hemorrhage, but the incidence of such bleeding in ITP is less than 1 per cent (Bussel & Hilgartner, 1987). The majority of patients (80 to 90 per cent) recover spontaneously in 6 months; in fact, most of these within 8 weeks of diagnosis (Bussel & Hilgartner, 1987).

The unresponsive 10 per cent of patients with persistent thrombocytopenia beyond 6 months of diagnosis are said to have chronic ITP. This form tends to occur more often in older children and girls.

Treatment of acute ITP is not standard throughout the country. In the past, no treatment was instituted, and the vast majority of children had no major problem. There is a small (1 per cent or less) but very serious threat of intracranial hemorrhage. Because of this risk, many hematologists treat children, especially those with platelet counts of less than 20,000. Treatment options include steroids, either IV (methylprednisolone) or oral (prednisone), and/or IV immunoglobin (IVIG).

IVIG often causes an immediate rise (within 24 hours) in platelet count with few if any minor side effects. However, it is very expensive. IVIG may be given as a single dose or daily over 2 to 5 days.

Steroids, although cheap compared with IVIG, are associated with significant side effects. Most children develop cushingoid symptoms; they may have trouble sleeping and become emotionally labile. Long-term use of steroids is associated with a myriad of serious side effects.

Treatment of chronic ITP is not clearly defined. Steroids, immunosuppressive therapy (vincristine, cyclophosphamide), and high-dose gamma globulin have been used with varying success. Splenectomy may be performed after 1 year of refractory thrombocytopenia but should be reserved for children older than 5 years of age because of the potential for serious bacterial sepsis in splenectomized youngsters.

Nursing assessment of the child with ITP can be found in Table 34–8.

Nursing Diagnostic Statements and Collaborative Problems

High risk for injury, hemorrhage; risk factor: *autoimmune destruction of platelets.*

Fear/anxiety: family and individual, *related to perceptions that the child may have a life-threatening illness.*

High risk for altered health maintenance; risk factor: knowledge deficit, *regarding management of ITP at home:*

- *Nature of the disease and the encouraging prognosis.*
- *Protection from bleeding.*
- *Signs and symptoms of central nervous system hemorrhage and emergency telephone numbers.*
- *Administration of immunosuppressive medications, if ordered, and the child's increased susceptibility to infection during this therapy.*

Planning and Implementation

Preventing Unnecessary Bruising and Bleeding. Interventions will be directed toward limiting new petechiae and areas of ecchymosis and preventing prolonged bleeding. The child must be protected from either accidental or therapeutically induced trauma.

Invasive procedures, such as intramuscular injections, suctioning, catheterization, and venipuncture, must be performed by experienced, skillful clinicians. Aspirin and aspirin-containing products inhibit platelet aggregation and, therefore, should not be used. Inspect the child's entire body daily to check for new areas of petechiae and purpura.

Allaying Unnecessary Fears. Nursing care of the child with ITP must include family education. Parents are often extremely frightened to discover their child suddenly covered with bruises. Most people have never heard of ITP, and parents of these children may assume that the child has a life-threatening catastrophic disease, such as leukemia. It may be difficult for parents to accept that "no treatment" may be the acceptable treatment. Frequent reassurance is indicated, with ample time provided for questions from the child and family.

Facilitating Home Health Maintenance. Children with ITP are discharged from the hospital before the platelet count has returned to normal. Parents must be taught to help the child avoid injury. The child should avoid rough, injury-prone activities such as contact sports, climbing up trees or jungle gyms, and motorcycle riding. Parents of younger children need to be reassured that the normal toppling over and frequent falls of a toddler just beginning to walk are not dangerous. They should be advised, however, to move furniture with sharp edges into nonobtrusive places and to remove throw rugs for the duration of the illness. A soft toothbrush is often advised to minimize bleeding from the gums.

Parents must be cautioned to avoid giving their child aspirin or aspirin-containing products. They need to read labels of over-the-counter preparations to ascertain that acetylsalicylic acid is not an ingredient.

If bruising appears to be increasing or if bleeding from mucous membranes occurs, parents should notify the health center or their physician. In addition, if the child undergoes significant head trauma or if symptoms of central nervous system bleeding, such as headaches, diplopia, projectile vomiting, lethargy, or sensorium changes occur, the parents must immediately contact their doctor. Although rarely needed, the parent should be provided with a telephone number that will provide telephone assistance 24 hours a day.

The child's platelet count is normally measured every 1 to 2 weeks following discharge. Once the levels are back to normal, parents should lift all restrictions and treat the child just as before. The incidence of recurrence is small, approximately 3 per cent (Gaady-Cohen, 1983).

Age-appropriate explanations should be given to the child and the parents. Children may be more apprehensive than is typical because of their parents' fears and also because of their dramatic body changes. The sight of blood causes many people to panic, and children are no exception. Children need frequent reassurance that they probably will be better and back to normal in a short while. See the discussion of nursing care of the child with thrombocytopenia related to leukemia (Chapter 42) for a summary of special considerations for planning nursing care.

Iron Deficiency Anemia

Iron deficiency anemia is the most common nutritional deficiency during childhood. It is the most frequently encountered form of anemia in children in the United States and in the world. Nurses can play a major role in both the prevention and the treatment of this disorder.

Etiology

Infancy is the period of the greatest postnatal growth velocity in the life cycle. Infants normally triple their birthweight during the first year of life. Accompanying the weight increase is a corresponding increase in blood volume. During the first year of life, 150 to 200 mg of iron must be absorbed to provide enough iron to double the total volume of red blood cells (and therefore hemoglobin). A daily iron absorption of 0.50 to 0.75 mg is required to meet this need (Lukens, 1990).

Full-term infants are born with some iron stores. The iron is stored at numerous sites but principally in the liver, bone marrow, spleen, and skeletal muscles. Essentially, all of this iron storage occurs during the third trimester of gestation, paralleling the period of greatest fetal weight gain. The iron stores of the full-term infant normally meet the baby's needs for 4 to 6 months. Premature babies miss this period of rapidly increasing iron storage and, therefore, are born with a substantially smaller iron reserve. The premature baby's iron supply lasts significantly less time and is depleted by 2 to 3 months of age.

After complete utilization of the iron stores available at birth, the baby must rely solely on dietary sources to meet minimum daily iron requirements. Milk is the primary (and often the sole) source of nutrition for infants. Breast and cow's milk are poor sources of iron, containing only 0.5 mg to 1.5 mg iron per liter (Oski, 1987).

Not all the iron available in a food source is absorbed by the body. In fact, the "bioavailability" of iron from most food sources ranges from 1 to 20 per cent. Foods in the vegetable family rank on the lower end of the spectrum; meat sources are on the higher end. The average diet of combined food sources is generally believed to provide an iron absorption rate of 10 per cent. Infant formulas and cow's milk likewise provide only about 10 per cent iron absorption (Oski, 1987). In addition, the phosphate in milk binds with iron, removing it from the body. In other words, a food source containing 10 mg of iron per serving would have 1 mg (or 10 per cent) of iron actually absorbed by the intestine. A notable exception is breast milk, which has an iron absorption rate of about 50 per cent (Oski, 1987).

To meet the daily requirement of 0.50 to 0.75 mg absorbed iron, the non-breastfed infant requires a diet containing 5.0 to 7.5 mg of iron per day. If a diet consists of only nonfortified milk or formula, approximately 2 gallons per day are needed to meet the iron requirements! Consider that the recommended daily allowance for iron is the same for infants and men. These examples help illustrate why infants are at high risk for developing iron deficiency anemia.

Toddlers are also at risk because of their rapid growth during this period and the likelihood of inadequate iron intake. Milk is still a major food and caloric source at this age. Many high-iron-content foods are not preferred by picky toddlers. The high-bulk diet characteristic of some ethnic groups also reduces the body's utilization of iron, because the foodstuffs are moved out of the gastrointestinal tract faster, resulting in less opportunity for iron absorption.

Causes of iron deficiency anemia other than dietary deficiency in toddlers are less common. Impaired iron absorption associated with conditions such as persistent or severe diarrhea or malabsorption syndromes may lead to iron deficiency anemia. This anemia may also be secondary to pica (compulsive eating of nonfood items, such as dirt, hair, plaster, clay, or laundry starch), lead poisoning, or intestinal parasite infection—all of which have a high incidence during toddlerhood. Intestinal bleeding from cow's milk allergy may also cause anemia. Unless an iron supplement is given, children with chronic illness may have difficulty ingesting or utilizing adequate iron because of excessive need or poor absorption related to infection, the disease process, or the iron-absorption-inhibiting effects of medications used to treat the chronic illness.

Incidence

Iron deficiency anemia can occur at any age, but it occurs most frequently between the ages of 6 months and 3 years and during adolescence. The child with small iron stores at birth (i.e., preterm infants) is at particular risk. Various surveys showed prior to the onset of the WIC Program (Special Supplemental Food Program for *W*omen, *I*nfants, and *C*hildren) that between 17 and 76 per cent of infants had some degree of iron deficiency anemia (Lukens, 1990). The disorder occurs most frequently in lower socioeconomic groups in which both the knowledge of and the ability to procure iron-rich foods may be limited but, of course, can occur in any child.

The WIC program provides iron-fortified formula for the first year of life and is a wonderful example of preventive medicine at its best (Hervada and Newman, 1992). In data obtained on a yearly basis in state health departments and the Centers for Disease Control, the prevalence of anemia in children younger than 2 years fell to 3 per cent, and severe anemia was virtually eliminated (Lukens, 1990). The use of iron-fortified infant formulas and cereal and an increase in the popularity of breastfeeding are undoubtedly the causes.

The incidence of iron deficiency anemia in adolescents may range from 11 to 27 per cent (Lukens, 1990). The adolescent is experiencing a growth spurt, second in velocity only to that occurring in the first year of life. The red blood cell mass of the adolescent is rapidly expanding to accompany the increased body mass. The increase in circulating hemoglobin mass is two times greater in adolescent boys than in female counterparts. However, girls have the additional burden of blood loss during menstruation (20 mg of iron per menses) (Lukens, 1990). Both male and female adolescents are notorious for diets that are low in absorbable iron. Fast food, fad diets, and skipped meals all contribute to the development of iron deficiency anemia.

Pathophysiology

Hemoglobin synthesis is dependent on a constant supply of iron. In fact, 3.4 mg of iron is required to make 1 gm of hemoglobin (or 1 mg of iron is needed for every 1 ml of packed red cells). On the average, 0.5 mg to 1.5 mg of iron must be absorbed daily to maintain iron balance in the nonpregnant, nonbleeding adult (Lanzkowsky, 1980). In this adult population, the body's iron needs are normally met by absorption of iron from dietary sources. If an iron deficit occurs, the production of hemoglobin decreases and anemia develops, resulting in a reduced oxygen-carrying capacity of the blood.

Clinical Manifestations

Children with slowly developing anemias may show no clinical symptoms, even though their hemoglobin may be as low as 6 g/dl. If signs and symptoms are present, they are likely to be vague and nonspecific. Symptoms of irritability and anorexia and signs such as pallor of skin and mucous membranes may have occurred insidiously; the parents are frequently unaware of their presence. Children with anemia of long duration may have some degree of growth retardation. Thirty to fifty-six per cent of iron-deficient children are below the tenth percentile for weight at the time of diagnosis, but the heights of these children are normally distributed (Lukens, 1990). Exercise intolerance—impairing both performance and endurance—frequently occurs in iron-deficient states, but once again, the onset is so gradual that caregivers may accept this as the child's norm. Often, a coincidental infection is the parent's sole reason for seeking medical help.

In the past, it was assumed that iron deficiency anemia had no serious consequences other than risk of heart failure as a result of profoundly low hemoglobin levels. However, many studies have disproved this. Long-term effects on behavior, development, and cognition that persist at least 5 years after the anemia was corrected have been documented (Hervada & Newman, 1992). Iron deficiency anemia in infants and toddlers must be regarded as a potentially devastating disease that causes irreversible damage to the brain during its period of greatest growth.

Diagnostic Assessment

The diagnostic process involves obtaining (1) a careful history and physical examination, (2) blood smear and red blood cell indices, and (3) serum iron and iron-binding studies.

The history must include information on the child's diet, activity, appetite, rate of growth, recent blood loss, and birth history. Mucosal and skin pallor and deficient capillary refill along with a history of iron-deficient diet or pica are suggestive of anemia.

Blood Studies

Tissue hypoxia, produced by the decreased supply of oxygen being carried by the blood as a result of decreased hemoglobin production, stimulates the bone marrow to continue producing red blood cells. Therefore, the red blood cell count is usually normal or only slightly reduced in anemia and typically is disproportionate to the decreased hemoglobin concentration. Hemoglobin is low, because the iron required to form it is not available. Because the red cells are not fully filled with hemoglobin when they are released into the blood, they are microcytic and hypochromic. The red cell indices in iron deficiency anemia show MCV less than 80 femtoliters, MCH less than 27 pg, and MCHC less than 30 per cent (Waskerwitz, 1983).

The diagnosis of iron deficiency anemia can most often be made from a standard blood smear and the clinical history. Additional studies may be required to distinguish iron deficiency anemia from other microcytic, hypochromic anemias and to re-examine patients with anemia who do not respond to iron therapy.

The three most useful additional studies are (1) serum ferritin, (2) transferrin saturation, and (3) free erythrocyte porphyrin (FEP). FEP levels greater than

10 to 11 mg/dl are characteristic of iron deficiency anemia. See Table 34–4 and Appendix 7 for further information on laboratory testing.

Therapeutic Management

Unless permanent dietary changes are made, the child is in danger of recurrences. The American Academy of Pediatrics Committee on Nutrition makes the following recommendations for infants:

- Iron supplements from one or more sources should start no later than at 4 months of age in full-term infants and no later than at 2 months in preterm infants.
- In formula-fed infants, the most convenient and best sources of supplemental iron are iron-fortified formulas and 2 servings per day of iron-fortified cereal.
- The intake of supplemental iron should not exceed 1 mg/kg per day for a full-term infant and 2 mg/kg per day for preterm infants to a maximum intake of 15 mg/day.
- The maintenance of breastfeeding for 6 months or more should protect against the development of iron deficiency anemia in full-term infants, but preterm infants require ferrous sulfate drops after 2 months of age. Iron-fortified cereals should be given when solids are introduced.
- Commercially available infant formulas are preferable to fresh milk during the first 6 to 12 months of life. Excessive ingestion of fresh cow's milk may contribute to iron deficiency by causing increased gastrointestinal blood loss. (There is a substance in fresh cow's milk, which unless inactivated by heating, may induce protein-losing enteropathy and gastrointestinal bleeding in infants, probably on the basis of hypersensitivity or allergy [Oski, 1981].)
- If infants receive fresh cow's milk after 6 months of age, their total daily milk intake should not exceed ¾ quart (24 oz). Infants who continue to receive formula after 6 months of age should receive no more than 1 quart (32 oz) of formula per day in order to encourage the introduction of iron-rich solid foods and set the pattern for a more varied diet.

Iron deficiency anemia can be easily treated with oral iron therapy. Daily administration of an oral iron supplement is prescribed. The therapeutic dose is 6 mg/kg per day given in three divided doses. The elemental or ferrous form (ferrous sulfate) is normally used, because it is better absorbed than the ferric form and is less likely to cause gastrointestinal irritation. It should be offered between meals, when digestive acid concentration is highest, in order to facilitate absorption. The supplement may be given with a citrus fruit or juice high in ascorbic acid to enhance its solubility and absorption.

Nursing Diagnostic Statements and Collaborative Problems

Activity intolerance, *related to altered nutrition: less than body requirements; dietary sources of iron.*

High risk for impaired tissue integrity: subcutaneous; *risk factor: improper injection technique.*

High risk for poisoning: child or siblings; *risk factor: accidental ingestion of iron supplement tablets.*

High risk for ineffective management, by parents, of therapeutic regimen; *risk factor: knowledge deficit about administration and side effects of iron preparations, related to management of iron deficiency anemia.*

Planning and Implementation

Interventions pertaining to the nursing diagnosis of activity intolerance are common to any type of anemia and are addressed in Table 34–8. The following additional interventions designed to eliminate the decreased oxygen-carrying capacity of blood are specific to iron deficiency anemia.

Providing Dietary Sources of Iron. Guidelines for infant nutrition with regard to iron intake were listed previously. The nurse needs to be aware of iron sources for the older child. Children need iron-rich foods every day. Organ meats, dried legumes, shellfish, and muscle meats are the richest sources of iron and have the highest iron absorption rate. Other good iron sources include nuts, green vegetables, unsweetened chocolate, dried fruits, and whole wheat or iron-enriched flours and breads, although the iron in these foods is less well absorbed than the iron from meats and legumes. The iron in eggs is poorly absorbed, unless the eggs are eaten with a good food source of vitamin C. Substantial sources of vitamin C are provided by citrus fruits, green vegetables, and liver.

Protein intake, especially from animal sources, and vitamin C intake should also be increased, as both enhance the intestinal absorption of iron from foodstuffs. If the previous diet was high in bulk, bulk intake should be reduced. Milk intake should be limited to a *maximum* of 1 qt/day, allowing calories to be provided by other food sources to lower levels of phosphate, which inhibits iron absorption.

The nurse must provide nutrition information that is realistic for the family's economic resources, attitudes regarding food, and cultural practices. For example, if beef is not a practical source of iron and protein because of the family's finances or religious and cultural beliefs, the nurse might instead encourage increased intake of dried beans, peanut butter, or turkey, which also are iron-rich protein sources. The caregiver who plans meals and does the grocery shopping may need the nurse's assistance to learn how to plan balanced meals rich in vitamin C, protein, and iron or how to shop for low-cost foods high in these nutrients. Parents unfamiliar with high-iron foods may appreciate recipes and preparation guidelines for these foods. Positive reinforcement of the caregiver's efforts and successes in providing the child with the proper nutrition to prevent or correct an iron-deficient diet should continue until these dietary measures become habitual practices. Often, parents need simple instruction in basic nutrition before being taught special dietary measures. Instruction should always include the reasons for and intended effect of these foods on the child's health.

Safely Administering Parenteral Iron. In some instances, an anemic child cannot take an oral iron supplement for the following reasons: severe intolerance, pre-existing gastrointestinal disorders interfering with intestinal absorption, surgery with anesthesia, or concurrent, serious systemic infection and persistent noncompliance. Under these circumstances, parenteral iron therapy may be ordered. The preferred route for parenteral iron (Imferon) is by intramuscular injection. The Z-track technique (displace skin laterally before injecting) should be used to minimize skin discoloration and irritation. In addition, a fresh needle should be used to inject the medicine after drawing it from the vial, and a small amount of air should be allowed in the syringe. Both actions avoid tracking the medicine through the subcutaneous tissue.

Avoiding Accidental Ingestion of Iron Supplement. Iron poisoning has been known to cause death in children who have ingested as few as 6 iron tablets at one time (Pearson, 1987). Therefore, teaching parents to keep the medication out of the reach of children cannot be overstressed. No more than 1 month's supply of iron should be kept in the home. Additional responsibilities of the nurse in relation to high risk for poisoning are found in Chapter 15.

Teaching Parents to Administer Iron Supplements. The nurse has a major responsibility in educating parents to carry out the treatment regimen. This must be done tactfully and within the framework of the family's income, customs, and food preferences. The nurse also has a role in helping parents overcome their feeling that they are to blame for their child's anemia and rebuilding the wavering confidence they have in their parenting abilities. Positive reinforcement of even minor efforts to comply with the treatment regimen, frequent pointing out of signs of the child's improved health state, and support by means of regular telephone calls or home visits help restore feelings of parental adequacy. These feelings, in turn, yield greater cooperation for what needs to be done currently and on a long-term basis to resolve the child's anemia and prevent its recurrence.

The nurse should ensure that parents know the proper medication dose and how much to withdraw. Parents can be taught to assess for signs of therapeutic action of the iron supplement, which include a gradual increase in activity, decreasing irritability, return of appetite, increased reticulocyte count within 3 to 5 days of beginning the iron supplement, and return of hemoglobin levels to normal limits after 2 months of therapy (Lukens, 1990). They should be cautioned that liquid iron preparations may temporarily stain the child's teeth. Therefore, liquid iron should be taken through a straw or administered with a dropper to the back of the mouth. As an extra precaution, the child's teeth may be brushed after each administration. Parents should also be informed that the child's stool will turn a tarry green when adequate iron levels are reached. The nurse should assess for this occurrence periodically as an indicator of adequacy of administration or dose.

Although side effects are rare in children, oral iron does sometimes cause gastrointestinal irritation, nausea and vomiting, diarrhea or constipation, and anorexia. If gastrointestinal side effects do occur, the iron should be given with meals or right after meals. Sometimes the iron is initially prescribed with meals so the intestinal mucosa has time to build up some tolerance to the drug; after 3 or 4 days, the iron is administered between meals so that absorption is greater. Another alternative is to give lower doses of the iron initially, and gradually increase to a therapeutic dose within 3 to 5 days in an effort to avoid the adverse effects of the drug.

Hemoglobin and hematocrit levels begin improving immediately after oral iron therapy is begun. This can be observed or monitored via the reticulocyte count. Normally, 1 per cent of the circulating red blood cells are very immature forms called reticulocytes. In a child with iron deficiency anemia, 3 to 5 days of iron therapy will increase the production of red blood cells. The reticulocyte count will rise dramatically and reach maximum levels at 5 to 10 days. Lack of improvement is often attributable to inconsistent or inaccurate oral iron administration. If this is the suspected cause, a community health nurse may be assigned to administer the oral supplement or to teach, supervise, and support caregivers to comply with the prescribed regimen.

Normal hemoglobin values are usually attained 2 months after oral iron therapy begins. The iron preparation should be continued for at least 2 months longer to replenish the depleted iron stores. Children treated only until the anemia is corrected are likely to have recurrences of iron deficiency anemia.

Information Resources

Nurses and parents may contact the following agencies for additional information about blood-related disorders.

- Aplastic Anemia Foundation of America, P.O. Box 22689, Baltimore, MD 21203, (301)955-2803.
- Cooley's Anemia Foundation, 105 East 22nd Street, Suite 911, New York, NY 10010, (800)221-3071.
- Fanconi Anemia Research Fund, 66 Club Road, Suite 398, Eugene, OR 97401, (503)687-4658.

- National Hemophilia Foundation, 25 West 39th Street, New York, NY 10018, (212)869-9740.
- National Association for Sickle Cell Disease, Inc., 34601 Wilshire Blvd., Suite 1012, Los Angeles, CA 90010, (213)736-5455.

KEY CONCEPTS

Concepts Related to Basic Information

- Plasma contains dissolved proteins, metabolites, electrolytes, and formed elements that include erythrocytes, leukocytes, and thrombocytes.
- Hematocrit represents the percentage of blood volume composed of blood cells.
- "Erythropoiesis" is the term used for the process of red blood cell formation.
- Red blood cell production is stimulated by decreased tissue oxygenation.
- White blood cells can be classified into three major groups: lymphocytes, monocytes, and granulocytes.
- Hemostasis is achieved by the following mechanisms: (1) vascular spasm; (2) formation of a platelet plug; (3) formation of a blood clot; (4) formation of connective tissue.
- The number of red blood cells varies with age, gender, and the altitude at which a person lives.
- Younger children demonstrate a more pronounced neutrophilia in response to infection than do older children and adults.
- Anemias are the most common hematologic disorders in children; they are classified on the basis of etiology or morphologic description of red blood cells.
- Sickle cell disease represents a spectrum of clinical disorders that result from abnormalities of globin genes of the hemoglobin molecule; the disorders are transmitted genetically in autosomal recessive fashion and are chronic in nature.
- Beta-thalassemia major is a disorder of hemoglobin synthesis that results in severe hemolytic anemia.
- DIC is the potential consequence of various pathologic conditions that may occur during the course of severe illness.
- Aplastic anemia can be defined as bone marrow failure characterized by reduction or absence of red blood cells, white blood cells, and platelets of the blood; the disease can be congenital or acquired.
- The hallmark of hemophilia is repeated oozing of blood into soft tissue, muscles, and most frequently, joint capsules.
- Hemarthrosis refers to bleeding into the joint spaces, which are the most common site of injury in severe hemophilia.
- Idiopathic thrombocytopenic purpura is an acquired blood disorder characterized by increased destruction of circulating platelets.
- Iron deficiency anemia is the most common nutritional deficiency seen during childhood.

Concepts Related to Nursing Assessment

- Objective data that the nurse considers in assessing the child with anemia are pulse and respirations, at rest and with activity, indicators of infection and tissue perfusion, height, weight, and position on the growth chart.
- The major nursing diagnostic statements the nurse considers in providing care to the child with sickle cell are *high risk for altered tissue perfusion, high risk for activity intolerance,* and *high risk for altered health maintenance.*
- The principal responsibility of the nonspecialist is recognizing disease states that may potentially lead to DIC and astutely assessing and quickly reporting unusual signs of bleeding.
- The major collaborative problems the nurse considers in the care of the child with hemophilia are *high risk for injury: localized hemorrhage* and *altered comfort: pain;* the major nursing diagnostic statements are *high risk for altered growth and development,* and *high risk for altered parenting.*
- The nursing diagnostic statements the nurse considers in the care of the child with ITP are *high risk for injury: hemorrhage, fear/anxiety: family and individual,* and *high risk for altered health maintenance.*
- The collaborative problem altered tissue perfusion is central to the care of the child with any type of anemia.

Concepts Related to Nursing Intervention

- Nursing care for the child with sickle cell anemia is based on the following principles: (1) teaching self-management of the disease, (2) management of sickle cell crisis, and (3) techniques to facilitate family coping.
- The primary dependent function of the nurse who cares for the child with beta-thalassemia is administration of transfusion.
- Central to the plan of care for the child with beta-thalassemia is teaching specific to the identified knowledge deficit and support of the child in relationship to altered physical appearance.
- Children who develop the full clinical picture of DIC are severely ill and are managed in the intensive care setting.
- Home management instructions for the child with hemophilia and family members include assessment techniques, current information about the risk of AIDS infection, pain management and en-

couraging health promotion, providing a safe but normalizing environment, and promotion of normal growth and development.

REFERENCES

Agle, D. P., et al. (1977). *Home therapy for hemophilia, a physician's manual.* New York: National Hemophilia Foundation.
Alter, B. (1992). Fanconi's anemia. *American Journal of Pediatric Hematology/Oncology, 14*(2), 170–176.
American Academy of Pediatrics (1990).
Andreoli, T., et al. (1986). *Cecil essentials of medicine.* Philadelphia: WB Saunders.
Aronstram, A., et al. (1980, January 26). Double-blind controlled trial of three dosage regimens in treatment of hemarthrosis in hemophilia A. *Lancet, 1,* 169–171.
Behrman, R. (Ed.) (1992). *Nelson textbook of pediatrics* (14th ed.). Philadelphia: WB Saunders.
Bussel, J., & Hilgartner, M. (1987). Intravenous immunoglobin therapy of idiopathic thrombocytopenic purpura in childhood and adolescence. *Hematology/Oncology Clinics of North America, 1*(3), 465–482.
Craft, M. (1993). Siblings of hospitalized children: Assessment and intervention. *Journal of Pediatric Nursing, 8*(5), 289–297.
Corrigan (1990).
Davies, S., & Brozovic, M. (1989). The presentation, management and prophylaxis of sickle cell disease. *Blood Reviews, 3,* 29–44.
Earles, A. (1989). Nursing perspective. *Pediatrics, 83*(Suppl), 901–902.
Fabry, M, & Kaul, D. (1991). Sickle cell–vaso-occlusion. *Hematology/Oncology Clinics of North America, 5,* 375–394.
Flug, F., & Karpatkin, M. (1985). Acquired disorders of homeostasis. In S. Zimmerman & J. Gildea (Eds.), *Critical care pediatrics* (pp. 426–439). Philadelphia: WB Saunders.
Gaady-Cohen, D. (1983). Idiopathic thrombocytopenia in children. *Issues in Comprehensive Pediatric Nursing, 6*(5–6), 311.
Gaston, M., et al. (1986). Prophylaxis with oral penicillin in children with sickle cell anemia. *New England Journal of Medicine, 314*(25), 1593–1599.
Giardina, P., & Hilgartner, M. (1992). Update on thalassemia. *Pediatrics in Review, 13*(2), 55–62.
Gillespie, J., & Morton, N. (1992). Patient-controlled analgesia for children: A review. *Paedric Anaesthesia, 2,* 51–59.
Greenberg et al. (1990).
Guyton, A. (1986). *Textbook of medical physiology* (7th ed.). Philadelphia: WB Saunders.
Guyton, A. (1991). *Textbook of medical physiology* (8th ed.). Philadelphia: WB Saunders.
Hernandez, S. (1989). Social work perspective. *Pediatrics, 83*(Suppl), 903–905.
Hervada, A., & Newman, D. (1992, May/June). Weaning: Historical, practical recommendations and current controversies. *Current Problems in Pediatrics,* pp. 223–240.
Hilgartner, M., & McMillan, C. (1984). Coagulation disorders. In D. Miller et al. (Eds.), *Smith's diseases of infancy and childhood* (5th ed.). St. Louis: CV Mosby.
Jones, P., & Ratnoff, O. (1991). The changing prognosis of classic hemophilia. *Annals of Internal Medicine, 114*(8), 641–644.
Kinny, T., & Ware, D. (1988). Advances in the management of sickle cell disease. *Pediatric Consult, 7*(3), 1–7.
Klopovich, P. (1983). An overview of anemia in children. *Issues in Comprehensive Pediatric Nursing, 6*(5–6), 281.
Koch, D., Giardina, P., Ryan, M., MacQueen, M., & Hilgartner, M. (1993). Behavioral contracting to improve adherence in patients with thalassemia. *Journal of Pediatric Nursing, 8*(2), 106–111.
Lanzkowsky, P. (1980). Iron deficiency anemia. In *Pediatric hematology-oncology.* New York: McGraw-Hill.
Loukopoulos, D. (1991). Thalassemia: Genotypes and phenotypes. *Annals of Hematology, 62*(5), 145–150.
Lukens, J. (1990). Iron metabolism and iron deficiency anemia. In D. Miller et al. (Eds.), *Smith's diseases of infancy and childhood* (6th ed.). St. Louis: CV Mosby.
Lusher, J. M. (1984). Desmopressin acetate (DDAVP): Its use in disorders of hemostasis. *Thrombosis and Haemostasis, 6*(5).
Lusher, J., & Warrier, I. (1991). Hemophilia. *Pediatrics in Review, 12*(9), 275–281.
Lusher, J., & Warrier, I. (1992). Hemophilia A. *Hematology/Oncology Clinics of North America, 6*(5), 1021–1033.
Martin, M., & Butler, R. (1993). Understanding the basics of β thalassemia major. *Pediatric Nursing, 19*(2), 143–145.
Martini, F. (1990). The cardiovascular system: The blood. In F. Martini (Ed.), *Fundamentals of anatomy and physiology.* Englewood Cliffs, NJ: Prentice-Hall.
Miller, D. (1990). Normal blood values from birth through adolescence. In D. Miller et al. (Eds.), *Smith's blood diseases of infancy and childhood* (6th ed.). St. Louis: CV Mosby.
Miller, D., & O'Reilly, R. (1990). Aplastic anemia. In D. Miller et al. (Eds.), *Smith's blood diseases of infancy and childhood* (6th ed.). St. Louis: CV Mosby.
Nathan, D. (1987). Sickle cell disease. In D. Nathan & F. Oski (Eds.), *Hematology of infancy and childhood* (3rd ed.). Philadelphia: WB Saunders.
Ohini-Frempong, K., & Schwartz, E. (1990). Sickle cell disease and other disorders of abnormal hemoglobin. In D. Miller et al. (Eds.), *Smith's blood diseases of infancy and childhood* (6th ed.). St. Louis: CV Mosby.
Oski, F. (1981). Differential diagnosis of anemia. In D. Nathan & F. Oski (Eds.), *Hematology of infancy and childhood* (2nd ed.) (pp. 311–312, 328). Philadelphia: WB Saunders.
Oski, F. (1987). Differential diagnosis of anemia. In D. Nathan & F. Oski (Eds.), *Hematology of infancy and childhood* (3rd ed.). Philadelphia: WB Saunders.
Pearson, H. (1987a). Diseases of the blood. In R. Behrman & V. Vaughan (Eds.), *Nelson textbook of pediatrics* (13th ed.) (pp. 1033–1078). Philadelphia: WB Saunders.
Pearson, H. (1987b). Sickle cell diseases: Diagnosis and management in infancy and childhood. *Pediatrics in Review, 9*(4), 121–124.
Rodgers, G. (1991). Recent approaches to the treatment of sickle cell anemia. *Journal of the American Medical Association, 265,* 2097–2101.
Rosendaal, F., Smit, C., & Briet, E. (1991). Hemophilia treatment in historical perspectives: A review of medical and social developments. *Annals of Hematology, 62*(1), 5–15.
Schechter, N., Berrien, F., & Katz, S. (1988). PCA for adolescents in sickle cell crisis. *American Journal of Nursing,* May, 719–722.
Seeler, R. (1992). Developmental overview of hematology and oncology. In E. McAnorney, R. Kreipe, D. Orr, G. Comerci. *Textbook of adolescent medicine.* Philadelphia: WB Saunders.
Shapiro, B. (1989). The management of pain in sickle cell disease. *Pediatric Clinics of North America, 36*(4), 1029–1045.
Spitzer, A. (1992). Children's knowledge of illness and treatment experiences in hemophilia. *Journal of Pediatric Nursing, 7*(1), 43–51.
Tsevat, J., Wong, J., Pauker, S., & Steinberg, M. (1991). Neonatal screening for sickle cell disease: a cost effective analysis. *The Journal of Pediatrics, 118*(4), 546–554.
Vichinsky, E., & Lubin, B. (1987). Suggested guidelines for the treatment of children with sickle cell anemia. *Hematology/Oncology Clinics of North America, 1*(3), 483–501.
Waskerwitz, M. (1983, September/December). Iron deficiency anemia in children. *Issues in Comprehensive Pediatric Nursing,* pp. 287–288.

BIBLIOGRAPHY

Aach, R. (1992, May). The emergency clinical significance of hepatitis C. *Hospital Practice,* pp. 19–22.
Agle, D. P., et al. (1980). *Psychological factors in hemophilia.* New York: National Hemophilia Foundation.
American Academy of Pediatrics (1976). *Iron Supplementation for Infants* [Policy reference guide]. Elk Grove, IL: Author.
Blanchette, V., Vorstman, E., Shore, A., Wang, E., Petric, M., Jett, B., & Alter, H. (1991). Hepatitis C infection in children with hemophilia A and B. *Blood, 78*(2), 285–289.

Bowman, J., & Murray, D. (1990). *Genetic variation and disorders in people of African origin.* New Haven, CT: Johns Hopkins University Press, 191–228.

Bray, B. (1990). Recent advances in the preparation of plasma-derived and recombinant coagulation factor VIII. *Journal of Pediatrics, 117*(3), 503–507.

Bray, G. (1990). Recent advances in the preparation of plasma derived and recombinant coagulation factor VIII. *Journal of Pediatrics, 117*(3), 503–507.

Brettler, D., & Levine, P. (1989). Factor concentrates for treatment of hemophilia: Which one to choose? *Blood, 73*(8), 2067–2073.

Byssel, J. (1990). Thrombocytopenia in newborns, infants and children. *Pediatric Annals, 19*(3), 187–193.

Carrai, E., & Linney, D. (1983). *Employment issues in hemophilia: Questions and answers.* New York: National Hemophilia Foundation.

Carroll, P. (1988). Cyanosis: The sign you can't count on. *Nursing 88, 18*(3), 50.

Charache, S., Lubin, B., & Reid, C. (Eds.). (1989). *Management and therapy of sickle cell disease.* U.S. Department of Health and Human Services, Public Health Services, National Institute of Health, NIH Publication #8921117, Revised. September, 1989.

Clements, M., & Mattison, A. (1980). *Prevention of social and emotional problems in boys with hemophilia.* New York: National Hemophilia Foundation.

Cohen, A. (1987). Management of iron overload in the pediatric patient. *Hematology/Oncology Clinics of North America, 13,* 521–551.

Consensus Conference (1989). Newborn screening for sickle cell disease and other hemoglobinopathies. *JAMA, 258*(9), 1205–1209.

Eyster, M., Schaefer, J., Ragni, M., Gorenc, T., Shapiro, S., Cutter, S., Kajani, M., Abrams, J., Barron, L., Odenwelder, A., et al. (1992). Changing causes of death in Pennsylvania's hemophiliacs 1976 to 1991: Impact of liver disease and acquired immunodeficiency syndrome. *Blood, 79*(9), 2494–2495.

Fischbach, F. (1984). *A manual of laboratory diagnostic tests* (2nd ed.). Philadelphia: WB Saunders.

Freedman, M. (1990). Aplastic anemia in children: New concepts in etiology and therapy. Introduction. *American Journal of Pediatric Hematology/ Oncology, 12*(4), 383–384.

Gallo, A., Breitmayer, B., Knafl, K., & Zoeller, C. (1993). Mothers' perceptions of sibling adjustment and family life in childhood chronic illness. *Journal of Pediatric Nursing, 8*(5), 318–324.

Giver, L. (1980, August). New thinking about parenteral iron supplements. *Nursing 80.*

Gomperts, E. (1990). HIV infection in hemophiliac children: Clinical manifestations and therapy. *American Journal of Pediatric Hematology/Oncology, 12*(4), 497–504.

Gradolf, B. (1983). Sickle cell anemia in children. *Issues in Comprehensive Pediatric Nursing, 6*(5–6), 295–307.

Green, M. (1986). *Green and Richmond pediatric diagnosis* (4th ed.). Philadelphia: WB Saunders.

Hubner, C. (1986). Altered clotting. In V. Carrieri, et al. (Eds.), *Pathophysiological phenomena in nursing human responses to illness* (pp. 367–389). Philadelphia: WB Saunders.

Imbach, P. (1991). Immune thrombocytopenic purpura and intravenous immunoglobulin. *Cancer, 16*(6 Suppl.), 1422–1425.

Jones, P. (1991). HIV infection and hemophilia. *Archives of Disease in Childhood, 66*(3), 364–368.

Kogan, S., Doherty, M., & Gitschier, J. (1987). An improved method for prenatal diagnosis of genetic diseases by analysis of amplified DNA sequences: Application to hemophilia A. *New England Journal of Medicine, 317*(16), 985–990.

Landler, W., et al. (1987). How to administer blood components to children. *Maternal Child Nursing, 12*(3), 178–184.

Lanzkowsky, P. (1980). Iron deficiency anemia. In *Pediatric hematology-oncology.* New York: McGraw-Hill.

Lipton, J., & Nathan, D. (1980). Aplastic and hypoplastic anemia. *Pediatric Clinics of North America, 27,* 217–235.

Lukens, J. (1986). Anemia of iron deficiency, blood loss, renal disease, and chronic infection. In S. Gellis & B. Kagan (Eds.), *Current pediatric therapy* (Vol. 12) (pp. 243–246). Philadelphia: WB Saunders.

Martin, M., & Armstrong, M. (1987). Busting the blood gas blues. *American Journal of Nursing, 87*(10), 1354.

Masoorli, S., & Piercy, S. (1984, September). A lifesaving guide to blood products. *RN,* pp. 32–37.

Miller, J. (1990). von Willebrand disease. *Hematology/ Oncology Clinics of North America, 4*(1), 107–128.

Nagrl, A., et al. (1984, May). New insights on sickle cell anemia. *Diagnostic Medicine,* pp. 26–37.

Overall, J. (1987). Infections of the newborn. In R. Behrman & V. Vaughan (Eds.), *Nelson textbook of pediatrics* (13th ed.) (pp. 422–435). Philadelphia: WB Saunders.

Pearson, H. (1985). Sickle cell disease and its crises. In J. Dickerman & J. Lucey (Eds.), *Smith's the critically ill child: Diagnosis and medical management* (3rd ed.) (pp. 229–241). Philadelphia: WB Saunders.

Querin, J., & Stabl, L. (1983, November). Twelve simple sensible steps for successful blood transfusions. *Nursing 83,* pp. 36–42.

Quintero, C. (1993). Blood administration in pediatric Jehovah's witnesses. *Pediatric Nursing, 19*(1), 46–48.

Reynolds, M. (1989). Role of immune globulin in the treatment of idiopathic thrombocytopenia purpura. *Journal of Pediatric Health Care, 3*(2), 109–112.

Roako, Y., & Pack, B. (1983). A profile of sickle cell disease. *Nursing Clinics of North America, 18*(1), 131–191.

Rodgers, G., Dover, G., Uyesaka, N., Noguchi, C., Schecter, A., & Nienhus, A. (1993). Augmentation by erythropoietin of the fetal-hemoglobin response to hydroxyurea in sickle cell disease. *New England Journal of Medicine, 328,* 73–80.

Rooney, A., & Hoveley, C. (1985). Nursing management of disseminated intravascular coagulation. *Oncology Nursing Forum, 12*(1), 15–23.

Rose, E., & Aledort, L. (1991). Nasal spray desmopressin (DDAVP) for mild hemophilia A and von Willebrand disease. *Annals of Internal Medicine, 114*(7), 563–568.

Rozzell, M., et al. (1983). The painful episode. *Nursing Clinics of North America, 18*(1).

Sergis-Davenport, E., et al. (1983). Overview of hemophilia. *Issues in Comprehensive Pediatric Nursing, 6*(5–6), 317–329.

Solomon, E. P., & Phillips, G. A. (1987). *Understanding human anatomy and physiology.* Philadelphia: WB Saunders.

Stevens, D. (1991). Epidemiology of hypochromic anemia in young children. *Archives of Disease in Childhood, 66,* 886–889.

Vichinsky, E., et al. (1983, September). Sickle cell disease: Basic concepts. *Hospital Medicine,* pp. 128–158.

Wayne, A., Kevy, S., & Nathan, D. (1993). Transfusion management of sickle cell disease. *Blood, 81,* 1109–1123.

Weatherall, D., et al. (1983). Editorial retrospective: Iron loading in thalassemia—5 years with the pump. *New England Journal of Medicine, 308,* 456.

Webb, D., et al. (1991). Acquired aplastic anemia: Still a severe disease. *Archives of Disease in Childhood, 66,* 858–861.

Weetman, R., & Boxer, L. (1980). Childhood neutropenias. *Pediatric Clinics of North America, 27,* 361–375.

CHAPTER • 35

Altered Digestive Function

Regina M. Cusson

NURSING PROCESS PLAN
NPP: Care of the Child after Abdominal Surgery, Table 35–15

RELATED TOPICS
Dietary practices and failure-to-thrive, Chapter 16
Skills adapted to children, Chapter 23
Nursing Management of Pain in Children, Chapter 25
Fluid and electrolyte balance, Chapter 26
Genetic counseling, Chapter 31

LEARNING OBJECTIVES

- Identify developmental differences in gastrointestinal function.
- Apply specialized skill techniques in caring for a child with altered digestive function.
- Describe the impact of an alteration in gastrointestinal function on the family.
- Discuss alterations in nursing care needed for a child with a congenital gastrointestinal anomaly or obstruction.
- Describe gastrointestinal alterations associated with an inflammatory process, functional disorders, and malabsorption.
- Identify therapeutic modalities and nursing care for the child with hepatic alterations.

Digestive alterations can involve the gastrointestinal tract or its accessory organs, the liver, gallbladder, and pancreas. Such changes interfere with ingestion, transport, digestion, and absorption of nutrients. The child's growth and development may therefore be hindered, and chronic malnutritional disturbances may occur. Although some alterations cause minor disruption, others, such as diaphragmatic hernia or intestinal obstruction, can be life-threatening and require immediate treatment.

This chapter focuses on problems associated with altered digestive function. The nurse's role in assessment and management of these disorders is addressed. Major nursing diagnostic statements and nursing care are included for those disorders that are encountered more frequently and for which nursing care is most complex.

Principles of Digestive Function

The gastrointestinal system is responsible for breaking down fats, proteins, and carbohydrates into molecules that can be used by the cells as fuel. The gastrointestinal tract also defends the body against pathogens via lymphatic tissue in the small intestine (Peyer patches); intestinal and gastric secretions containing immunoglobulins; and gastric acid in the stomach, which destroys pathogens because of its acidity. An alteration in the gastrointestinal system may affect the overall health of a child and can lead to fatal illness. Refer to Figure 35–1 for an illustration of components of the gastrointestinal tract.

Developmental Differences Affecting Gastrointestinal Function

Developmental differences in absorption, immunity, membrane permeability, hepatic function, and type of gastric secretions affect gastrointestinal function of infants and children. In comparison with an adult, the newborn infant has a highly ineffective gastrointestinal system because function is still immature (see summary in Table 35–1).

By the first birthday, the major differences between the child and adult reflect the child's higher nutrient and energy needs for growth and a higher metabolic rate rather than inefficiency or immaturity of organ systems. Behavioral development also strongly influences the function of the gastrointestinal tract after the first year and may lead to problems of eating, digestion, and toileting.

Differences in Intestinal Absorption

The loose stools of the newborn infant reflect a degree of malabsorption that would be thought pathologic for an adult. Lactose is incompletely absorbed because of lower lactase levels in the intestinal mucosa during the first 3 months of life. The normal infant absorbs only 90 per cent of ingested fat because of a smaller pool of bile acid. Less is known about protein digestion. It is not clear whether this relative inefficiency serves some purpose or whether the newborn infant has insufficient resources to completely match the enormous metabolic demands that require 100 kcal/kg, compared with 30 to 40 kcal/kg characteristic of adult requirements.

However, certain relative deficiencies are compensated for by properties of human milk. Many stud-

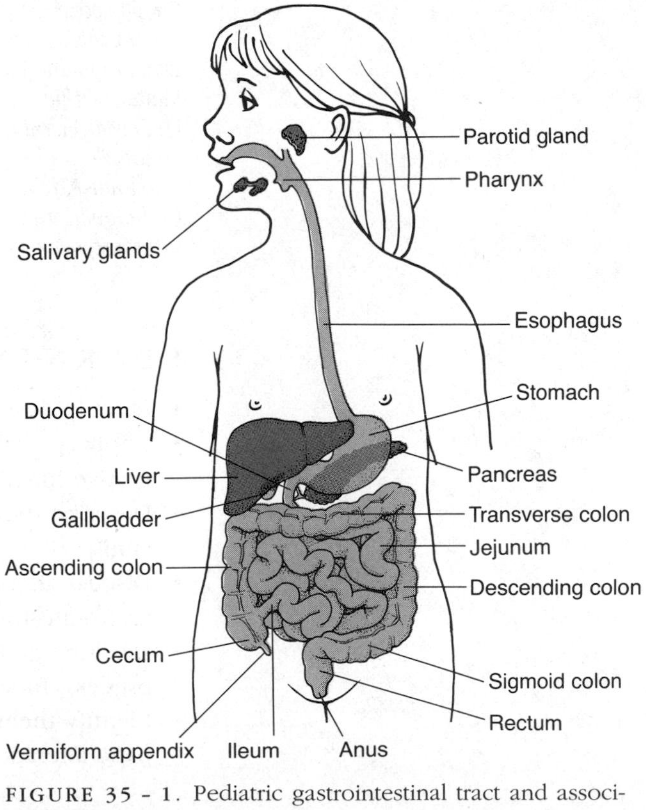

FIGURE 35 - 1. Pediatric gastrointestinal tract and associated structures.

TABLE 35-1
Developmental Differences in Structure and Function of the Gastrointestinal System

Structure and Function	Significance for Nursing Care
Increased Metabolic Rate	
Calories needed per kilogram of body weight vary with age and illness	Calories per kilogram for infants are greater than for other ages; additional calories are needed with illness; caloric needs in acute illness often exceed normal nutrition and may require tube feeding or total parenteral nutrition
Evaporative Fluid Loss	
Ratio of body surface area to volume is highest during infancy and childhood	Evaporation results in significant fluid losses, which can be exacerbated by fever, radiant warmers, or phototherapy lights
Lactose Intolerance	
Decreased lactase levels in the intestinal mucosa	Lactose is incompletely absorbed, which can cause diarrhea
Fat Absorption	
Only 90 per cent of infant's ingested fats is absorbed because of decreased pool of bile acid	Fat in human milk is better absorbed owing to lipase (in mother's milk)
Immunocompromised	
Immunoglobulin levels are generally lower; anergic to skin tests (deficit in T-cell function)*	Infants are immunocompromised; however, human milk provides immunologic protective factors; also, lactoferrin, a milk product, has an antibacterial effect
Intestinal Permeability to Whole Proteins	
An increased permeability facilitates uptake of immunoglobulin proteins	Cow's milk protein and other potential allergens also cross intestinal wall and may increase susceptibility to allergy
Immature Neonatal Liver	
Hepatic glucuronyl transferase levels not sufficient to conjugate water-insoluble bilirubin, and physiologic jaundice results	Physiologic jaundice gradually clears and hepatic efficiency improves as liver matures
Toxic substances inefficiently detoxified	
Medications inefficiently processed	Therapeutic drug dosage adjustment necessary during first few months of life
Altered Gastric Activity	
Gastrointestinal motility is decreased, gastric emptying is increased, and gastroesophageal reflux is common	Changes in gastric activity are responsible for the standard infant feeding practices
Increased Gastrin and Stomach Acid	
May represent response to stress of birth or an adaptive response to help destroy ingested bacteria before breastfeeding is established	High levels of secretion occur in the first few days of life, which then gradually lower; infants can develop stress ulcers

* See also Table 37-2.

ies suggest increased bioavailability of nutrients from human milk compared with cow's milk; for instance, fat in breast milk is absorbed more readily than the butterfat of cow's milk because of the activation of lipase present in mother's milk. Although iron levels are low in human milk, absorption is relatively complete.

Differences in Immune Competence

By most standards, the human infant is also immunocompromised. Immunoglobulin levels are generally lower, and infants are anergic (do not react) to skin tests, reflecting a relative deficit in T-cell function. It has become known that human milk provides a variety of immunologically protective factors. Lactoferrin, a milk protein, has an antibacterial effect. Breast milk provides immunoglobulins, which may be surface active and are absorbed to a certain extent, possibly playing a role in systemic defenses.

Differences in Intestinal Permeability to Protein

Increased intestinal permeability to whole proteins, which facilitates uptake of protective immunoglobulin proteins, has been demonstrated in infants. However, the infant's system also allows cow's milk protein and other potential allergens to cross from the intestine into the blood stream. This perhaps explains the young child's higher susceptibility to gastrointestinal allergic problems. The tendency toward these allergic responses decreases after 1 year of age, when the child's immunologic system becomes more like that of the adult.

Differences in Hepatic Function

Physiologic jaundice is one of the most consistent observations reflecting the unique metabolism of the newborn infant. For several days after birth, the child's hepatic glucuronyl transferase levels are incapable of conjugating all of the water-insoluble bilirubin created by the breakdown of old red blood cells. Consequently, most newborn infants have some degree of jaundice. This gradually clears as hepatic efficiency improves. For the same reasons, the liver of an infant has more difficulty metabolizing drugs. Consequently, medications must be given to infants in proportionately lower dosages or at longer intervals. (See Chapter 24 for further discussion on principles of pharmacology.)

Differences in Digestive Tract Activity and Secretions

Gastrointestinal activity is altered in the infant and young child. Gastrointestinal motility is decreased, whereas gastric emptying is increased. Gastroesophageal reflux is common during the first 4 to 6 months of life because of immaturity of the lower esophageal sphincter.

Most secretory elements of the human digestive tract are present in lower amounts in the first few months after birth, compared with later in life. However, some factors are produced in higher amounts. Serum gastrin and stomach acid, for instance, are produced in relatively high amounts in the first few days of life and then gradually decrease. This may represent a response to the stress of birth or an adaptive response to help kill ingested bacteria in the days before breastfeeding is firmly established. However, the high levels of gastric hydrochloric acid may not be entirely beneficial; although it is rare, certain infants develop stress ulcers. Such ulcers gradually resolve a few days after birth.

Assessment of Gastrointestinal Function

Health History and Physical Assessment

An assessment of the child with a gastrointestinal problem should begin with a standard history (see Chapter 13). The presenting symptom or symptoms should be assessed in depth, and relevant areas that might be associated with gastrointestinal function should be explored. (See Table 35–2 for a summary of relevant historical information.)

A prenatal history, including a child's estimated duration of gestation and birthweight, yields important baselines to use when assessing growth patterns. Information about prenatal care should be gathered to determine any deficits or trauma during prenatal development.

Data from the neonatal and early infancy period are often relevant to gastrointestinal problems, which are often subtle and unrecognized in their early stages (such as feeding disturbances). Past and current history should therefore include a broad range of gastrointestinal system–related information including defecation. (See Past and Current Health History in Table 35–2.) It is especially important to note whether a presenting symptom is associated in any way with a change in food or water intake. Information on recent travel or change of location is significant because of the potential for ingestion of contaminated food or water. Lifestyle and family factors are also explored (see Table 35–2). A family history should be obtained to seek a similar problem in other family members. Socioeconomic status and living conditions of the family should be considered because of their effect on general hygiene and health practices. The ability to provide an adequate diet and the presence of running water and indoor plumbing are often relevant factors. The number of children in the family and type of housing can affect the general health of children, especially in the case of infectious gastrointestinal problems. Finally, the stress, general happiness, and well-being within a family affect how children use food and relate to the experience of eating. Changes that have occurred in a child's life that might cause stress (e.g., starting school, new sibling, death of a pet, a recent move) are particularly influential.

Because it is often a balance of intake and output that must be addressed in assessing gastrointestinal status, an important component in analyzing digestive function is a 24-hour nutritional history (see Chapter 16).

A complete physical examination is performed (see Chapter 13), including examination of the mouth for clefts, dental problems, or infections, and a thorough abdominal and rectal assessment for the presence or absence of clinical manifestations (see Table

TABLE 35-2
Historical Factors to Consider in the Assessment of Gastrointestinal Alterations

Presenting Symptom

Prenatal and Perinatal History

Estimated gestation and birthweight

Prenatal care

Maternal nutrition

Polyhydramnios

Past and Current Health History

Prolonged jaundice at birth

History of gastrointestinal tract anomaly or surgery

Feeding history (ability to suck, episodes of aspiration or respiratory distress, frequency and amount of intake)

Regurgitation and vomiting

Defecation history (stooling pattern, frequency, consistency, relationship to feedings, presence or absence of blood or mucus in stool)

Gastric distention

General appetite

Bowel pattern (failure to pass meconium, diarrhea, constipation)

Abdominal pain

Weight gain or loss

Chronic illness (inflammatory bowel disease, necrotizing enterocolitis)

Medications (related to gastrointestinal problem or other)

Lifestyle and Family Factors

Family history of anomaly, or gastrointestinal problem

Recent travel or move

Socioeconomic status

Health practices (food preparation, handwashing, general hygiene)

Stress within the family (social contacts, degree of isolation)

Individual stress for child

35-3; see also Tables 35-4 through 35-6). The data gained from this assessment will contribute to the nurse's ability to make valid diagnoses as well as to carry out dependent and collaborative functions.

Laboratory and Diagnostic Studies

Gastrointestinal symptoms are often vague and frequently involve other body systems. Diagnostic tests are uncomfortable, may require long periods of fasting, and may be both frightening and embarrassing to a child. However, with adequate preparation aimed at the developmental level of the child, many of these problems can be avoided. In addition, patients undergoing tests of gastrointestinal function require the nurse's attention and special support. Because many of these tests interfere with one another, the nurse must be clear about the order in which certain tests should be done as well as how to prepare the patient.

In addition to physical preparation, the child and family should be given accurate explanations. Further explanations may be given during the test, and steps are taken to reduce the discomfort and anxiety that accompany these procedures. Sedation and analgesia are recommended for invasive procedures. Young children or patients at risk may require general anesthesia.

After an examination, a child is given the opportunity to express his or her feelings about the experience and is encouraged to resume usual activities (unless physical activity is restricted by the medical condition).

Laboratory tests and diagnostic procedures commonly used to assess gastrointestinal alterations are summarized in Tables 35-7 and 35-8, respectively.

Nursing Care

The overall goal of nursing care is to foster normal growth and development by maintaining a balanced nutritional state. The nurse's role is important because of the meticulous monitoring of nutritional intake and output that is needed and the clinical judgment that is required concerning feeding methods and approaches. The nurse's observations during feeding and assessment of the child's overall behavior and physiologic status provide important data on which management decisions are made. The nurse needs to understand the importance of precise monitoring, the use of a variety of nutrition and elimination procedures, principles of postoperative care, and the psychosocial impact of gastrointestinal disturbances on the child and family.

Ensuring Precision in Monitoring and Measurement

Successful management of children with gastrointestinal problems rests primarily in the hands of those who calculate and record the daily nutritional and fluid balance data. Although these activities are easy to perform, if they are not done properly and consistently, the nurse's efforts will be of little value. Inaccurate recording can actually present a danger to the patient because management decisions are then based on wrong information. A basic question to ask in any situation of measurement and calculation is, "Does this number make sense?" For example, if an infant's

TABLE 35-3
Clinical Manifestations of Gastrointestinal Problems

Clinical Manifestation	Clinical Significance
Regurgitation	
Lower esophageal sphincter is immature; muscle is atonic (relaxed); pressure on the fundus of the stomach exceeds that in the lower esophagus, resulting in spitting up	Many normal babies regurgitate one or more times a day; as long as normal weight gain progresses, there is no cause for concern, regurgitation usually disappears by 8 months of age, but if it persists and is associated with failure to thrive, further evaluation is required
Vomiting	
Vomiting results from a coordinated sequence of abdominal muscle contractions and reverse esophageal peristalsis; it is usually associated with nausea except when projectile; vomiting is classified as follows:	Vomiting is a common sign of gastrointestinal tract disturbance, but it also occurs in many other conditions; character of vomitus is assessed to determine type of problem (see Table 35–4) and recognize clinical significance (see Table 35–5)
Mechanical: secondary to an obstructive lesion.	Infants have immature cough and gag reflexes; therefore, they should be positioned on the side or abdomen to reduce aspiration
Reflexive: Due to gastrointestinal tract stimuli (e.g., infection, allergy)	
Central: (1) central nervous system involvement (e.g., neoplasm, meningitis); (2) caused by other than primary central nervous system involvement (e.g., abnormal metabolites, sepsis, psychogenic vomiting)	Note the onset, frequency, and severity (quantity, degree of forcefulness, presence of bile); find out type of formula, amount ingested and amount expelled, feeding technique, and postfeeding position
	Protracted vomiting may result in significant loss of hydrochloric acid, resulting in hypochloremic alkalosis; urine is often paradoxically acidic because of intracellular deficits; note associated symptoms such as fever, diarrhea, abdominal pain, bloody stools, and failure to thrive
Abdominal Distention	
Distention results from accumulation of fluid or gas (or both) within the gastrointestinal tract or peritoneal cavity	A young child's abdomen is normally rounded, thus making distention more difficult to evaluate; also, children normally swallow air when eating or crying, and therefore they have louder tympany; palpation is easier because the abdominal wall is less developed
	Gastrointestinal distention may be caused by congenital gastrointestinal tract malformations, constipation, hernia, gastrointestinal tract perforation, cirrhosis, or other problems, such as nephrosis, heart failure, or abdominal masses; abdominal girth is measured at the umbilicus daily and marked with a pen
Abdominal Pain	
Abdominal pain may be acute, chronic, diffuse, or localized; it arises from the abdominopelvic viscera, the parietal peritoneum, or the capsules of the liver, kidney, or spleen; it is produced as a result of stretching or tension of the gut wall, traction on the peritoneum or mesentery, intestinal contraction, inflammation, ischemia, or sensory nerve irritation	Abdominal pain may herald an emergency, and therefore immediate assessment is required; children cannot verbally describe pain as readily as adults, and thus behavioral indices should be evaluated (grimacing, pulling legs up); constant, steady pain may indicate organ perforation, ischemia, inflammation, or the presence of blood in the peritoneal cavity
Diarrhea	
Diarrhea is an increase in the frequency and fluidity of bowel movements; it may be *acute* as a result of infection, stress, a reaction to drugs, or fecal impaction, or *chronic* as a result of chronic infection, obstructive and inflammatory bowel disease, or malabsorption syndrome; diarrhea may also result from food allergy, gastrointestinal tract anomalies, or gastrointestinal surgery	Note onset, duration, frequency, pattern, severity, and character of stool; assess for associated gastrointestinal symptoms, such as vomiting, abdominal pain, and anorexia; systemic symptoms, such as fever, coryza, weight loss, and reduced general activity, are often associated with gastrointestinal disorders; assess hydration, circulatory status, and mental status
Diarrhea occurs when there is excess fluid in the small intestine; this occurs as the result of	*Mildly ill:* patient is alert, is active, appears well hydrated, and has normal urinary output
1. Stimulation of cyclic AMP by bacterial toxins or other factors, resulting in active transport of electrolytes into small intestine	*Moderately ill:* patient may be lethargic, have reduced tearing, dry skin, decreased urine output
2. Disrupted integrity of small intestinal mucosa, impairing intestinal absorption 3. Increased intestinal motility, resulting in decreased intestinal absorption	*Severely ill:* patient has altered mental status (irritability or lethargy), rapid pulse, poor skin turgor, delayed capillary refill, no tears (see Table 35–6 for causes of diarrhea and associated symptoms)

TABLE 35-4
Symptoms Associated with Common Gastrointestinal Disturbances

Appendicitis

May follow or accompany abdominal pain

Gastritis

Vomitus may contain mucus or blood and be associated with belching and pain; slowly bleeding gastric or duodenal lesion can result in coffee-ground vomitus (digested blood)

Gastroenteritis

Vomitus often contains undigested food and is associated with diarrhea, hyperactive bowel sounds, fever, and abdominal pain

Intestinal Obstruction

Obstruction below pylorus (bile-stained or greenish vomitus); intestinal obstruction or infarction (brown vomitus with fecal odor)

Pyloric Stenosis

Projectile vomiting associated with visible peristaltic waves across epigastrium

Intussusception

Vomiting associated with bloody stools

TABLE 35-5
Clinical Significance of Character of Vomitus

Undigested Food

In a newborn infant, undigested food suggests esophageal atresia; in older children, it suggests an obstruction or stricture at or above the cardia

Absence of Bile

Absence of bile suggests an obstruction proximal to the ampulla of Vater; in freshly passed vomitus, bile may not be apparent because food and gastric juice may camouflage the yellow color of bile; on exposure to air, oxidation of bile causes it to turn green

Bilious Vomiting

A sign of intestinal obstruction

Fecal Vomiting

A sign of peritonitis or an obstruction of the lower bowel or colon

Hematemesis

Bright red color indicates that the blood has not been in contact with gastric juices; therefore, acute bleeding must be occurring at or above the cardia or in the stomach

Coffee-Ground Emesis

Vomitus that appears like coffee grounds indicates that blood has been altered by gastric contents and suggests slow bleeding from the esophagus, stomach, or duodenum

TABLE 35-6
Causes of Diarrhea and Associated Symptoms

Malabsorption

Occurs after meals; diarrhea accompanied by distention, cramps, steatorrhea, anorexia, weight loss, fatigue

Infection

Extremely watery and contains mucus; associated with pain, cramps, nausea, vomiting, and fever; may lead to dehydration, weight loss, and possibly blood in the stool

Crohn Disease

Patient may have 10 to 20 stools a day; associated with crampy abdominal pain, nausea, fever, chills, weakness, anorexia, and weight loss

Ulcerative Colitis

Bloody diarrhea and abdominal pain

Intestinal Obstruction

Partial obstruction increases intestinal motility, resulting in diarrhea, pain, nausea, and sometimes distention; bloody stools may occur

Irritable Bowel Syndrome

Diarrhea alternates with constipation or normal bowel function; associated with pain, distention, dyspepsia, and nausea

Lactose Intolerance

Diarrhea occurs after milk ingestion and is accompanied by pain and flatus

weight has dropped significantly but the intake has been maintained, the nurse should search either for an explanation (e.g., such as administration of a diuretic) or for an error in recording or calculation. *Record keeping thus involves, to a great extent, the process of analyzing and interpreting the meaning of what has been calculated and recorded.* See Table 35–9 for a description of parameters frequently measured in caring for children with gastrointestinal problems.

Providing Altered Means for Nutrition and Elimination

Disruptions in digestive function frequently make it necessary to use alternative diets and feeding methods. When normal digestive processes are altered, intake is adjusted accordingly. Various types of dietary adjustments and nursing considerations are summarized in Table 35–10. Children with gastrointestinal problems require a variety of specialized procedures to re-establish and maintain digestive function. Following is a discussion on the care of children who require (1) a nasogastric tube, (2) a gastrostomy tube, (3) an enema, and (4) a colostomy or ileostomy.

TABLE 35-7
Laboratory Tests Commonly Used to Diagnose Gastrointestinal Disturbances

Laboratory Test	Purpose or Use	Interpretation of Test or Other Information
Complete blood count (CBC)	Measures the hemoglobin (Hgb), hematocrit (Hct), and red and white blood cell counts (RBC, WBC); used to assess for infection, anemia, or hemorrhage	Low Hgb and Hct indicate blood loss, poor iron intake, or absorption; Hgb and Hct are elevated in dehydration because of vascular fluid volume deficit
Erythrocyte sedimentation rate (ESR)	Measures the rate at which red blood cells settle to the bottom of a calibrated tube in the laboratory; used to assess for inflammation	Reflects inflammation in the body but does not predict exactly where the problem lies; useful as a screening test to indicate underlying disease, such as Crohn disease
Serum electrolytes (Na, K, Cl)	Serum sodium, potassium, and chloride are measured to assess electrolyte balance; balance among electrolytes is critical to normal metabolism and cellular function	Disturbed by poor intake, metabolic disturbance, excess losses, or poorly regulated intravenous fluids
Liver Enzymes	A group of enzymes reflecting important liver functions	
Alanine aminotransferase (ALT)	Elevated when damage to liver (or heart) cells has occurred	Reflects cell *integrity* rather than *function*. ALT and AST are similar; ALT is liver specific, whereas AST is derived from other organs in addition to the liver; in most cases, there are parallel rises
Aspartate aminotransferase (AST)	Similar to ALT	
Alkaline phosphatase (Alk phos)	Measures hepatic obstruction	Also raised by bone turnover, so it is always higher in the growing child (also in rickets)
Bilirubin	Increased with hemolysis or liver damage	Primary excretion product from the breakdown of red blood cells
Serum ammonia	Measures impaired hepatic detoxification of protein	Measures liver *function;* other liver enzymes reflect liver *cell integrity*
Serum amylase	An important pancreatic enzyme	One of the few measures of pancreatic function
Hepatitis antigens	Measure components of the hepatitis B virus	Different components appear at different times in hepatic infection
Hepatitis antibodies	Measure the immune response to infection	Can reflect present hepatic infection as well as past infection and immunity
Absorption Tests		
Xylose tolerance test	An indicator of intestinal mucosal function	Xylose, a passively absorbed sugar, is given by mouth after 8-hr fast; a blood level taken 1 hr later gives an index of intestinal absorption
Breath hydrogen test	Measures functioning of intestinal disaccharidase enzymes	Measured excretion of hydrogen in the breath reflects lactase, sucrase, or other sugar, depending on the sugar ingested; breath samples are taken at ½-hr intervals after ingestion of the index sugar in solution
Carbohydrate tolerance	Measures uptake of sugar into the bloodstream	Blood specimens are taken at ½-hr intervals to check serum glucose levels; less a measure of absorption than of metabolic regulation
Stool Tests		
Reducing substance	Measures certain sugars when they are not completely absorbed	Depends on which sugars are fed (lactose and glucose are reducing substances; sucrose is not)
Stool pH	Measures the acidity of the stool	Stool turns acid with the malabsorption of sugars
Stool fat	Measured as a stain on a random sample or a 72- to 96-hr timed collection correlated to fat intake	Useful measure of malabsorption because fat accounts for such a high proportion of ingested calories; the time when the test is initiated and completed should be carefully recorded; in children, concurrent food intake over the same interval is recorded so that the dietitian can determine the fat content of the food ingested

TABLE 35-7
Laboratory Tests Commonly Used to Diagnose Gastrointestinal Disturbances *(Continued)*

Laboratory Test	Purpose or Use	Interpretation of Test or Other Information
Stool trypsin	A random sample of the pancreatic enzyme	Normally found only in stools of infants; its absence may indicate cystic fibrosis
Stool culture	Pathogenic bacteria are grown in the laboratory	Selective media are used to depress growth, except of the specific problem organisms; hence, samples may be taken from the diaper, the floor, and so forth
Ova and parasites	Parasites or their eggs are sought in the stool	Specimens must be freshly examined or preserved in fixative solution
Pinworm test	Uses anal Scotch tape imprint to locate the pinworm eggs	Tape is placed on the perianal folds as parasite emerges at night to lay eggs in the anal tissues; the sticky surface of tape is then placed on a slide; a commercially prepared swab with a sticky surface is also available
Occult blood	A variety of tests are available, specifically developed to detect blood loss itself or minute traces, as in cancer	Denotes blood in the stool, indicating blood loss or inflammation

TABLE 35-8
Diagnostic Procedures Commonly Performed to Diagnose Gastrointestinal Disturbances

Diagnostic Procedure	Purpose or Use	Nursing Considerations
Upper gastrointestinal endoscopy	Direct examination of the esophagus, stomach, and duodenum using a fiberoptic endoscope	Usually accomplished by anesthetizing the throat and using sedation or general anesthetic
Colonoscopy	Direct endoscopic examination of the colon as far as the ileocecal junction	The colon must be entirely empty; study done with sedation or general anesthetic
Sigmoidoscopy	Examination of the rectum and sigmoid colon using a rigid or flexible fiberoptic tube	A more limited examination than a colonoscopy; may only take 5 mins; sedation is used in infants and children, especially if they are apprehensive
Upper gastrointestinal radiography	Radiologic examination of the esophagus, stomach, and upper small bowel by use of a contrast agent (e.g., barium)	Patient must have taken nothing by mouth; contrast medium is taken from a bottle or cup but is resisted by some children
Small bowel follow-through	Radiologic examination of the lower small bowel using contrast; barium is followed by sequential x-ray films as it progresses down the intestinal tract; most useful to detect Crohn disease or low small bowel lesions	Patient must have taken nothing by mouth; test may take up to 90 mins, depending on intestinal transit; occasionally barium is introduced by tube; sequential films are made, and it is necessary to tilt the table in various positions
Barium enema	Radiologic examination of the colon using contrast; may be used to diagnose Hirschsprung disease, causes of rectal bleeding, or polyps; hydrostatic pressure can at times reduce an intussusception	Barium is run into the bowel from an enema bag; sometimes air is introduced to give "double contrast" for greater detail; an uncomfortable test because cramps are felt when the colon is distended; children will be asked to "hold" barium as the various x-ray films are taken
Flat plate of abdomen	Radiologic examination of the abdomen without contrast; demonstrates air-fluid levels in obstruction, constipation, or stones	Can be done without bowel preparation; a simple x-ray of the abdomen

(continued)

TABLE 35-8
Diagnostic Procedures Commonly Performed to Diagnose Gastrointestinal Disturbances *(Continued)*

Diagnostic Procedure	Purpose or Use	Nursing Considerations
Three views of abdomen	Radiologic examination of the abdomen without contrast but includes a standing film and one with patient lying on the side	Moving the patient causes air to float to the top, and different features can be visualized
Duodenal-jejunal biopsy or aspirate	These techniques are used to find parasites or to diagnose celiac disease	The child is sedated; a sample of tissue and fluid is taken from the upper small bowel either through an endoscope or through a sampling tube, which is passed down the alimentary canal until it lodges in the small bowel; by use of a special capsule on the tube with a small cutting edge, the specimen is taken and removed for examination
Cholangiography: oral cholecystogram (OCG); intravenous cholangiogram (ICG); endoscopic retrograde cholangiopancreatography (ERCP); transhepatic cholangiogram	Radiologic examination of the gallbladder and biliary tree	Contrast medium is administered orally; if more concentration is required, contrast agent may be given intravenously (ICG), or pushed into the biliary tree from an endoscope in the duodenum (ERCP), or injected directly through the liver (transhepatic)
Liver biopsy	Many liver diseases can be diagnosed only by examining the liver tissue	A sample of liver tissue is obtained by putting a needle into the liver; it is done with sedation or a general anesthetic; coagulation must be normal or corrected with vitamin K or plasma
Rose bengal, tech HIDA, tech BIDA (liver scan)	Nuclear imaging is used to track a radioactive tracer through the course of the liver; an abnormal test indicates obstruction	These tracers are injected intravenously and excreted much like bilirubin in the liver; the radioactive "tag" allows them to be recognized by the scanner; involves less radiation than a chest radiograph
Ultrasonography of abdomen	Uses sound waves to examine abdomen; works best to view cysts, masses, and the gallbladder	Not an invasive test, but the patient must lie still; helpful for a parent to accompany a small child
Ultrasonography of abdomen with Doppler	Used to examine vasculature and blood flow	Same as Ultrasonography of abdomen
Computed tomography scan of abdomen	Multiple radiographs combined and interpreted by a computer; contrast medium may be used	Can visualize "invisible" pancreas, adrenals, and blood vessels
Manometry of motility	Measures the pressures in the esophagus and stomach through a tube; can measure transmission of a peristaltic wave	Child must lie quietly despite presence of a nasal tube
24-hour pH monitoring	Uses an "acid-sensitive" probe left in the esophagus and connected to a portable recorder to measure the number of times acid refluxes from stomach into esophagus; most reliable test of acid reflux	Usually done overnight as an inpatient or outpatient procedure
Meckel scan	Uses radioactive-labeled technetium, which is taken up in "ectopic" stomach tissue in the Meckel diverticulum to locate its presence	A noninvasive test but not always accurate
Rectal biopsy	A small amount of tissue is removed from the rectum by a direct incision, punch biopsy, or suction biopsy; special stains are used in processing the tissue to locate absence of nerves in Hirschsprung disease	Although the procedure does not cause pain, a child may be fearful because of the equipment and setting; also, parents often think biopsy means looking for cancer

TABLE 35-9
Nursing Assessment of Gastrointestinal Status

Description	Nursing Implications
Calorie Count	
All food is measured and recorded; the exact amount of food eaten is recorded (e.g., by teaspoons, tablespoons, or cups); the nutritionist then calculates caloric intake; calorie-containing liquids must also be recorded	Parents can be taught to measure and record the amount of food eaten Calorie count sheets should be kept at the bedside to facilitate recording after each meal and snack
Intake and Output Record	
Intake and output is recorded to assess fluid balance All fluid intake orally, intravenously, or by other means is entered in separate columns and totaled Urinary output is measured, as well as any other measureable liquid (e.g., secretions from a nasogastric decompression tube) Stool is generally not measured unless accurate intake and output is required; however, the number, character, and color of stools is recorded The number of voids for infants is generally counted unless accurate intake and output is required; then diapers are weighed	Foods such as Popsicles and gelatin can be calculated as a liquid when child is on liquid diet; ½ standard Popsicle = 50 ml
Accurate Intake and Output (Stool Collection, Diaper Weights, Emesis, Intravenous, and Nasogastric)	
All intake and output is measured, including food, liquid intake, urine output, stool, emesis, and body secretions Urinary output for infants can be measured by weighing diapers; each diaper is weighed before use and again after it is wet; the difference is calculated in grams and converted to milliliters (1 g = 1 ml) Vomitus is calculated whenever it can be measured Intravenous intake is calculated according to fluid in the chamber (not the intravenous bag); additionally, any intravenous fluid that is used to administer medications is added to intake Collection from a nasogastric tube is calculated as output, but any amount instilled to irrigate the tube must be either subtracted from the total collection or counted as input	When 72-hr stool is collected, the best method is to place a plastic bag over the anal area to keep stool and urine separate To calculate accurate output, diapers should be weighed individually to increase accuracy Diapers must be weighed on the same scale before and after use; to increase accuracy, they should be weighed as soon as possible after use because a diaper that has dried will not provide a correct measure of output
Daily Weight	
An infant is weighed with no clothes and no diaper Weights should be done at the same time daily and *before* a feeding; the same scale should be used from day to day; if there is a large discrepancy in a weight compared with the previous weight, it should be checked by two nurses for verification and charted accordingly	Struggling, kicking infants are difficult to weigh; the job can be made easier if the previous weight is known so that the actual weight can be found more quickly; even when electronic scales are used, the previous weight should be known to be able to identify a discrepancy
Urine Specific Gravity	
Specific gravity of urine can be monitored by nurses on the unit by using a fractometer or a specific gravity set from the laboratory Specific gravity range is normally as follows: 1.001–1.020 (neonate or infant) 1.001–1.030 (thereafter) 1.025 (after fluid restriction)	As specific gravity rises, the patient is becoming less hydrated A low specific gravity occurs when patient has increased secretion of urine (diuresis)

(continued)

TABLE 35-9
Nursing Assessment of Gastrointestinal Status *(Continued)*

Description	Nursing Implications
Abdominal Girth	
The circumference of the abdomen is measured by placing a tape around the abdomen at the level of the largest diameter; the tape must be level from front to back	It is useful to mark the skin at two points (both sides or front and back) to indicate point of measurement from day to day; use a tape that does not stretch (paper rather than cloth), and measure when patient is in same position from day to day
Stool Chart	
When a stool chart is kept, descriptions of the stool should be included; e.g., amount (scant, small, medium, large), color (yellow, green, brown, black, or combinations, such as yellowish-green), character (meconium, mucousy, watery, seedy, loose, solid or formed, hard pellets, greasy, bulky), odor (foul-smelling, musty, sour, or vinegar-like)	Interpretation of stool varies from one individual to another; parents help provide continuity in assessment

Caring for a Child with a Nasogastric Tube

Children require nasogastric tubes to provide a route for gavage feedings (given when a child is unable to take nourishment by mouth), for abdominal decompression, or for lavage (washing out of the stomach). The largest tube possible that will go into the nares is used for decompression; the smallest tube that will deliver the feeding is used for nourishment. Regardless of intended use, the principles for insertion are the same. Insertion of this tube is a frightening experience and should be explained to the child and the parents. The parents should also be told how they may assist. The child is helped to sit quietly by the parents or a nurse during the insertion. A choking sensation occurs as the tube stimulates the gag reflex, but this will subside as the tube passes beyond the pharynx.

Inserting a nasogastric tube in an infant is much easier because of diminished gag reflex. Ease of insertion can be enhanced by the use of a pacifier, which may also decrease distress during the procedure. An older child may complain of a sore throat, earache, or dry mouth and lips (altered oral mucous membrane) while a tube is in place. Providing frequent mouth care and lubrication for the lips will lessen the discomfort. With the permission of the physician, a child can be allowed to suck on hard candy or ice chips to soothe the sore throat. Sucking on ice may also numb the throat before tube insertion. After insertion of the nasogastric tube, correct placement needs to be assessed. There are several methods of ensuring correct placement (see Research Issues). Injecting air through the tube and auscultating in the epigastric region is commonly recommended. This should produce a loud "whooshing" sound as the air is injected. Gastric contents can be aspirated with a syringe. Presence of fluid is not a definitive sign of gastric placement; confirmation is needed with a test of pH. Gastric fluid should be acidic, with a pH in the range of 5 or less. Inability to aspirate gastric fluid is not unusual, especially with small bore feeding tubes. Excessive force in injecting or aspirating should be avoided to prevent mucosal injury.

Nasogastric Tube Feeding. Nasogastric feeding may be given by a continuous drip feeding or an intermittent feeding. Continuous feeding can be scheduled at night, and bolus (or intermittent) feedings during the day. The formula and amount are prescribed by the physician (see Chapter 16). The continuous drip formula should be infused slowly to avoid distention or discomfort. Continuous drip feeding can be administered via an enteral feeding pump. If the patient complains of nausea, the feeding should be slowed or discontinued temporarily. This intervention can prevent the occurrence of aspiration. The amount of formula that is hung should not exceed that which will be used in 8 hours because the milk-based formula is an excellent medium for bacterial growth.

When administering a formula to an infant, provide the same stimulation that would be given if the feeding were taken orally. The infant should be held and talked to during the feeding. Providing the infant with a pacifier during tube feeding has been documented to ease the transition to oral feeding. In addition, the use of pacifiers has been associated with many positive outcomes, including decreased length of stay and increased weight gain in preterm infants (Anderson, 1986).

With intermittent feeding of infants, the tube may be inserted before each feeding and taken out after the feeding is completed. In this instance, the tube is usually inserted through the mouth rather than the nose. If a tube is to stay in place between feedings, it can be cleared with several milliliters of water after the feeding is completed. To remove the tube, the procedure is explained to the child, as appropriate,

TABLE 35-10
Nutritional Interventions and Nursing Considerations

Description	Nursing Considerations
NPO (Nothing by Mouth)	
Children frequently are not permitted to ingest anything by mouth because there is an anatomic abnormality (e.g., tracheoesophageal fistula), a digestive problem (e.g., Crohn disease), a temporary infectious process (e.g., gastroenteritis), or sucking inadequacy (e.g., low birthweight infants) Children also are put on NPO in preparation for diagnostic procedures and surgery and for a period of time postoperatively until postoperative ileus resolves	Children who are not permitted to have anything by mouth should have a sign placed above their bed; it is also humane to take children from their rooms to the playroom when breakfast is served the morning of a procedure or surgery, if possible
Clear Liquid Diets	
Clear liquid diets consist of water, gelatin-water, Popsicles, gelatin, broth, glucose water, flat sodas, and clear juice (apple or cranberry juice)	Liquids with high sugar content need to be kept to a minimum in conditions such as osmotic diarrhea (the high sugar content causes an influx of water into the small bowel and prevents absorption of water and electrolytes)
Thickened Feedings	
Thickened feeds are prepared by adding cereal to milk to a thickness that permits infants to take milk from bottle; these feeds reduce tendency for regurgitation	Avoid making the nipple hole so large that an infant would obtain too much too fast, causing aspiration
Elemental Diet	
Elemental diets are used when regular food is not tolerated but the condition does not require total parenteral nutrition Elemental diets are a complete nutritional regimen containing essential and nonessential amino acids, simple sugars, minimal fat, minerals, trace elements, and vitamins These diets are nutritionally balanced, bulk- and residue-free, low in fat, and digested primarily in the upper jejunum; they are more rapidly absorbed than regular food	Elemental diets are generally unpalatable; therefore, they are given by tube feeding Bolus feeding of these diets produces nausea, cramps, and diarrhea because of the high osmolarity Feedings are started in one-fourth strength or one-half strength and increased in volume, then given in full concentration
Positioning after Feeding	
Placing an infant on the right side during and after feeding facilitates emptying of the stomach because the pyloric sphincter muscle, which opens into the duodenum, is on the right side The danger of aspiration is reduced by placing infants on either side Elevation of the head slightly relieves the pressure of a full stomach on the diaphragm	Placing infants into infant seats after feeding when there is a potential for vomiting can result in aspiration

and the tube is clamped and then gently withdrawn. Mouth care is provided, as soon as possible, after removal of the tube. (See Table 35–11 for summary of gavage feeding procedure.)

Decompression by a Nasogastric Tube. A nasogastric tube may be inserted to remove air and secretions from the stomach and intestines (decompression) preoperatively or postoperatively (or both) to prevent vomiting and bowel distention. Peristalsis is inhibited after abdominal surgery owing to handling of the abdominal organs and analgesia/anesthesia, necessitating decompression by a nasogastric tube. Drainage is achieved by intermittent suction or by gravity. Continuous suction is used frequently. The tube must have an air vent (Salem sump) and use the lowest pressure possible to remove secretions (less than 80 mmHg; usually 30 to 40 mmHg is effective).

When a child has a nasogastric tube for decompression, the amount, consistency, and color of drainage are observed and recorded. The drainage contains important electrolytes; therefore, it must be measured accurately to allow replacement. Drainage is replaced by giving an amount of intravenous fluids as ordered by the physician depending on the child's

RESEARCH ISSUES

Methods of Estimating Appropriate Length of Nasogastric Tubes and Accuracy of Placement

Results: Differences exist in recommendations for measurement of tube length of nasogastric tubes and confirming correct placement. Standard methods have been to measure the distance from the nose to the ear to the xiphoid with the addition of up to 2 cm or to measure from the nose to the ear to the umbilicus. These measurements have been found by Hanson (1979) and Stroebel and colleagues (1979) to underestimate length and result in esophageal placement of tubes, especially in premature infants. The researchers found that height correlated more closely with esophageal length than did the standard measurement techniques. Stroebel suggests an equation based on regression of esophageal length on height as a measurement estimation. Stroebel's equation was retested by Beckstrand and associates (1990) and Ellett and colleagues (1992), who found it fairly accurate for estimates of orogastric length but less accurate at estimating nasogastric length in children. Ellett suggests a new regression equation.

Methods of confirming placement have included auscultation for sounds associated with insufflation of air; observing for coughing, choking, and inability to speak (as evidence of entrance into airway); aspiration of fluid with the appearance of gastric fluid; and checking for pH of fluid aspirate. Metheny and co-workers (1990) found auscultation of insufflated air to function poorly for classifying tube placement within various portions of the gastrointestinal tract, correctly classifying placement only 34.4 per cent of the time. Fewer data on differentiation of respiratory from gastrointestinal placement are available because of infrequent occurrence of this misplacement. However, Metheny and co-workers report on two cases of respiratory placement in which air insufflations were clearly heard in the epigastric region.

Measurement of pH appears to be a more promising method for differentiating respiratory and gastrointestinal placement and identifying location within the gastrointestinal tract. Metheny and co-workers (1989, 1993) found highly significant agreement between x-ray confirmation of tube placement and pH. Use of pH is less accurate when patients receive H_2 receptor antagonists.

Clinical symptoms of choking, coughing, and inability to speak are not useful indicators in patients with reduced level of consciousness. Also, the use of very small bore feeding tubes may not produce these symptoms.

Implications: No clear answer exists on the best method for estimating gastric tube length. Estimates based on height appear more accurate than nose to ear to xiphoid measurements. Testing pH of tube aspirate currently appears to be the most reliable method of confirmation of gastric tube placement. Considerably more research is needed for clear conclusions on both of these clinical problems.

REFERENCES

Beckstrand, J., Ellett, M., Welch, J., Dye, J., Games, C., Henrie, S., & Barlow, R. S. (1990). The distance to the stomach for feeding tube placement in children predicted from regression on height. *Research in Nursing and Health, 13,* 411–420.

Ellett, M., Beckstrand, J., Welch, J., Dye, J., & Games, C. (1992). Predicting the distance for gavage tube placement in children. *Pediatric Nursing, 18*(2), 119–127.

Hanson, R. L. (1979). Predictive criteria for length of nasogastric tube insertion for tube feeding. *Journal of Parenteral and Enteral Nutrition, 3,* 160–163.

Metheny, N., McSweeney, M., Wehrle, M. A., & Wiersema, L. (1990). Effectiveness of the auscultatory method in predicting feeding tube location. *Nursing Research, 39*(5), 252–267.

Metheny, N., Williams, P., Wiersema, L., Wehrle, M. A., Eisenberg, P., & McSweeney, M. (1989). Effectiveness of pH measurements in predicting feeding tube placement. *Nursing Research, 38*(5), 280–285.

Metheny, N., et al (1993). Effectiveness of pH measurements in predicting feeding tube placement: An update. *Nursing Research, 42*(6), 324–331.

Stroebel, C. T., Byrne, W. J., Ament, M. E., & Euler, A. R. (1979). Correlation of esophageal lengths in children with height: Application to the Tuttle test without prior esophageal manometry. *Journal of Pediatrics, 94,* 81–84.

Weibley, T. T., Adamson, M., Clinkscales, N., Curran, J., & Bramson, R. (1987). Gavage tube insertion in the premature infant. *American Journal of Maternal Child Nursing, 12,* 24–27.

response, ranging from half to equal the amount of drainage. (This is in addition to the daily 24-hour intravenous fluids.)

Ensuring patency of the tube is accomplished by irrigating the tube with normal saline according to the physician's order. The usual order is for irrigation with a specified amount of normal saline every 2 hours and as necessary. The saline is gently instilled with a syringe and then gently drawn back. The same amount that is instilled is withdrawn to ensure accurate calculation of the drainage. An alternative method is to reconnect the tube to suction after instilling saline, noting that the fluid is freely drawn back by suction. The amount of saline instilled each shift or each 24 hours must then be calculated and subtracted from the total amount of drainage to calculate the actual drainage. In either method, force is never used while instilling or while drawing back because the stomach mucosa is easily damaged. The ease with which the tube irrigates and the consistency, color, and amount of the fluid returned at the time of irrigation are recorded. Bowel sounds should be checked whenever a child has a nasogastric tube for abdominal decompression.

TABLE 35-11
Gavage Feeding Procedure

1. Warm formula and measure
2. Assemble:

   Feeding tube No. 5–8 French

   Syringes One 3-ml syringe
   One 10- to 20-ml syringe (separate barrel from plunger) to hold formula

   Tape

   Stethoscope

   Blanket
3. Explain procedure to parents
4. Change diaper if needed and wash hands
5. Wrap patient in blanket and position with head elevated (may not be necessary)
6. Measure tube:
   a. From tip of nose to earlobe (or earlobe to tip of nose), then to a point between the xiphoid process and umbilicus for nasogastric insertion
   b. From mouth to earlobe (or earlobe to mouth), then to a point between xiphoid process and umbilicus for orogastric insertion

   Mark tube at measured level with tape
7. Dip tip of tube into water (this step is often omitted in nasogastric insertion and is not necessary for orogastric insertion)
8. Insert tube

   Nasogastric: Inspect nostril and begin inserting tube into nostril at a slight downward angle; nose may be pressed slightly upward; do not force

   Orogastric: Hold infant's mouth open, direct tube to back of mouth, and insert gently with a downward angle; insert to designated mark; observe for signs of distress during insertion; ask child to swallow during insertion (if age-appropriate)
9. Check for proper position with air insertion

   Instill air into tube with a syringe: premature infants receive 0.5 ml, full-term infants receive 1–2 ml; listen with stethoscope for "whoosh"
10. Secure tube with tape

    Do not tape on nose, but rather directly below nose; tube should not create pressure on the nares because this may cause necrosis, especially in compromised infants
11. Check for gastric secretions

    The withdrawal of gastric secretions further verifies proper position

    When gavage feeding infants, it is often advisable to check for residual formula (i.e., withdraw stomach contents and measure); reinsert contents into stomach through tube to avoid loss of electrolytes (if excessively mucousy, small amounts may be discarded)

    Usually the amount of residual is subtracted from the amount to be fed
12. Attach syringe barrel to tube

    Clamp tube or hold tube below level of stomach

    Pour prepared formula into syringe

    Remove clamp and elevate tube above level of stomach
13. Begin feeding

    Insert plunger into tip of barrel and give one quick push of formula to begin flow; remove plunger; hold infant to feed and give pacifier (unless size or condition does not permit)

    Raise syringe only high enough to maintain flow by gravity; keep refilling syringe and avoid letting syringe get empty until completed

    Feeding should take 15 to 20 minutes

    Note: An orogastric tube becomes dislodged easily; therefore, it should be held in place between fingers while feeding
14. Ensure that formula in tube has run in by raising syringe
15. Remove by pinching tube and pulling it all the way out

    Pinching tube is done to avoid leakage of formula as it is pulled

    Flush with sterile water if it is to be left in place; this should be done before syringe is completely empty to avoid letting air enter

    Insert 1 to 2 ml of water, close end of tube, and burp infant (especially if pacifier used during feeding) or keep tube elevated and open for 30 minutes to provide a vent for air to escape

    Check that tape is secure

Note: Sometimes an infant is bottlefed followed by a gavage feeding if the infant in unable to take the entire amount by bottle; in this case, a nasogastric tube is inserted before the bottlefeeding is begun to avoid stimulation of vomiting during the feeding; nasogastric tube may be left indwelling

Lavage by Nasogastric Tube. When a nasogastric tube is inserted as a consequence of poison ingestion, the child is positioned with his or her head to one side and slightly lowered to avoid the potential for aspiration in the event of vomiting. Suction should also be available for immediate removal of vomitus whenever stomach contents are removed by lavage. (See Chapter 46 for further discussion of lavage in the event of poisoning.)

Lavage is also used for control of gastric bleeding

associated with gastrointestinal disruptions, such as trauma, acute hepatic failure, and coagulopathy. Gastric lavage with room temperature normal saline can aid in the removal of blood and clots. It also allows the stomach to contract, which slows gastric bleeding. Iced saline lavage is contraindicated because of shivering hypothermia, which impairs systemic coagulation.

Caring for a Child with a Gastrostomy Tube

A gastrostomy tube is a catheter that enters the stomach either through a surgical incision in the abdominal wall or percutaneously through endoscopy. The tube that is inserted has either a "mushroom" or a balloon close to its tip, which remains snug against the inside wall of the stomach. The gastrostomy tube is used for temporary postoperative conditions or for long-term management of children who are unable to receive adequate nutrition through oral feedings.

The catheter is secured in place on the surface of the abdomen by using tape. The tape is wrapped around the tube and secured to the skin. The tube may also be secured by using gauze or a Holister drain tube attachment device to maintain the tube at a 90-degree angle to the skin. The tube may also be passed through a nipple with a hole cut at the tip. The nipple is moved along the tube and positioned on the gauze placed around the entrance of the tube through the skin. Securing the nipple and gauze to the skin holds the balloon of the gastrostomy tube firmly against the stomach wall.

The tube may come out regardless of the method used to secure it. If this happens with a child on tube feedings at home, the family should be instructed as follows:

1. Stomach contents may leak out; do not be alarmed.
2. Cover the opening with a diaper or other absorbent cloth.
3. Go to the emergency department of the local hospital or to the clinic of the hospital at which the tube was inserted. Do this before the next feeding time or within 2 hours.
4. Take the old tube with you; this will let the staff know the size of tube the child needs. You may have been given an extra sterile tube when the child was discharged. If you were, take this tube to the clinic or emergency department.

A family can, however, be taught to change a gastrostomy tube at home (Paarlberg & Balint, 1985).

A reddened area about the size of a quarter around the tube may be observed. There may be a small amount of drainage around the tube, but if a bad odor develops, or if the drainage changes in any way, the site should be checked for possible infection. A fever may also indicate an infection. Assessment should also be carried out for potential skin breakdown. To keep the area clean, wash around the tube with soap and water or other mild antiseptic solution. The child can be bathed as usual.

During feedings, an infant should be held and cuddled; an older child can sit in a highchair. Type and amount of formula will be prescribed by the physician. The position of the tube can be checked by gently pulling until resistance is felt. To complete the feeding:

1. Wash your hands.
2. Check the temperature of the formula. It should be room temperature.
3. Attach the end of the tube to a syringe (10 to 50 ml, varying with size of the infant) or feeding bag with or without an enteral feeding pump.
4. Clamp the tube.
5. Fill the syringe with formula.
6. Holding the tube above the height of the opening, unclamp the tube.
7. Add more formula to the syringe before it empties to prevent air from entering the stomach.
8. Follow the formula with one-half ounce of water to clear the tube.
9. Clamp the tube, fold it over, wrap it with a 4 × 4 gauze pad, and secure it with a rubber band.
10. Position the child side-lying or with head elevated after the feeding.
11. Wash the materials in hot soapy water, rinse well, and store in a clean place.
12. The feeding should take approximately as long as a feeding by mouth.
13. Infants should be allowed to suck on a pacifier to satisfy normal developmental needs.

Medication may be given through the tube. Using the same syringe, give one-half ounce of water after the medicine to ensure that the medication has not remained in the tube.

The tube can be pinned to the child's undershirt or covered with soft, stretchy tube gauze. With a gastrostomy tube, the child can resume regular play activities. Problems that might arise during the use of a gastrostomy tube are summarized in Table 35–12.

A new type of apparatus called the gastrostomy feeding button is gaining favor as an alternative to the traditional types of tubes (Huth & O'Brien, 1987). It is a small, flexible silicone device that has a mushroom-like dome on the end, which is inserted. A one-way valve inside the device prevents reflux of stomach contents. The external device (two small wings with an opening in the center covered by some type of cap) lies flat against the abdomen, thus eliminating the need for an external tube. Advantages, disadvantages, and use of this type of device have been reviewed by Huddleston and Palmer (1990). Feeding through a gastrostomy button may require a special adapter or tubing, depending on the manufacturer. The principles and procedure of feeding through the button are similar to those of a gastrostomy tube.

TABLE 35-12
Common Problems with Gastrostomy Tubes

Problem	Possible Causes	Nursing Actions
Leaking around tube (risk factor for potential skin breakdown)	1. Balloon/mushroom of catheter has slipped away from wall of stomach	1. Gently pull back on catheter or tube to ensure that balloon is snug against stomach wall
	2. Balloon/mushroom of catheter may have become somewhat deflated	2. Reinflate balloon or change catheter
	3. Tube is too small for size of stoma	3. Consult physician to evaluate further; placing larger catheter may only exacerbate the problem
Blocked tube (risk factor for aspiration)	1. Obstruction due to food or medication	1a. Gently milk tube to dislodge obstruction b. Use liquid medication when possible or well-suspended, finely ground medication c. Change tube
Erythema or drainage around tube or stoma	1. Some erythema or drainage is normal	1. Clean area frequently with mild soap and water; keep dressing dry
	2. Skin irritation may result from dampness or gastric leaking around tube	2a. Clean area more frequently b. Karaya powder sprinkled on area and covered with dressing may heal area c. Topical antibiotics are generally not indicated d. Call physician if problem persists
Vomiting or diarrhea* or both (risk factor for aspiration)	1. In an otherwise healthy child, this may indicate that the tube has migrated into the stomach or beyond the stomach a. Migration into the duodenum or jejunum may cause "dumping," resulting in liquid stool during or immediately after a feeding b. Blockage or irritation of the pylorus by the gastrostomy tube may cause vomiting	1. Measure external length of catheter; gently pull back on the tube to assess tube position; check tube position at each feeding
	2. Vomiting may result from too rapid administration of a feeding	2. Feed over a longer period of time
	3. Vomiting or diarrhea may result from too large a feeding	3. Smaller, more frequent or continuous feedings should be considered
Bleeding around tube or stoma	1. Bleeding may occur during a tube change	1a. Minimal bleeding is insignificant b. The physician should be consulted if larger amounts of bleeding occur c. Cauterization of the stoma may be necessary
	2. The stoma may become irritated from movement of the tube in the stoma	2a. Secure the tube to the child's shirt between feedings b. Same as 1a, b, c
Tissue build-up around gastrostomy tube	1. A small amount of epithelial tissue is normal and not painful	1a. If tissue build-up is excessive and interferes with care, notify the physician b. Cauterization may be necessary

Adapted from Paarlberg, J., & Balint, J. P. (1985, March/April). Gastrostomy tubes: practical guidelines for home care. *Pediatric Nursing,* pp. 99–102. © 1985 Pediatric Nursing. Adapted with permission of Jannetti Publications, Inc., Publisher.
**Note:* In each instance, consult the physician if vomiting or diarrhea persists.

Caring for a Child Who Requires an Enema

An enema is used for the same purpose in children as it is in adults: (1) to facilitate defecation when normal physiologic processes of elimination are ineffective and (2) to cleanse the bowel in preparation for surgery or diagnostic procedures. The procedure for enema administration to a child, specific differences between children and adults, and related nursing actions to consider are discussed in Table 35–13.

There are three special considerations in giving an enema. First, comparing the sensation of the catheter tip insertion to the taking of rectal temperature is useful for some children, but the child should not be led to believe that an enema is "just like having your temperature taken." Second, a potty-trained child should be encouraged to expel the enema while sitting on a potty chair. Also, potty-trained children need special reassurance that it is alright if they do not make it to the potty chair to expel the enema. Third, preschool-

TABLE 35-13
Procedure for Enema Administration to a Child*

Developmental Considerations	Nursing Actions
The child's bowel capacity and anal opening vary according to size; a young child's rectal mucosa is thin and easily traumatized	Approximate normal saline* solution amounts according to age of child: • Infant, 150–250 ml • Toddler and preschooler, 250–350 ml • School-age child, 300–500 ml • Adolescent, 500–750 ml Enema tips should be soft, well lubricated, and appropriate in size for age of child (French catheter No. 10–12 for young children); for older school-agers and adolescents, the standard enema tip can be used; the enema tip is inserted 1½ to 4 inches (3.7 to 10 cm), varying according to size of child†
Young children are particularly vulnerable to fluid and electrolyte imbalances	An isotonic (normal saline) solution (warmed) is used to prevent rapid fluid shift from bowel; plain water is hypotonic, and water intoxication and fluid overload can result with repeated enemas
A child's bowel is more easily perforated under pressure	The enema reservoir is elevated gradually until the solution begins to slowly flow by gravity; for young children, greater control of administration is achieved by using a 50-ml syringe attached to a cathether
Young children do not have the cognitive or physiologic ability to "hold" the enema	With child in supine position, head and back can be supported with pillow; the bedpan must be in position during administration because there is immediate return of the solution; after the solution has been administered, the buttocks can be gently pinched together to facilitate "holding" of the enema; a child who is old enough (school-age and adolescent) to understand the instruction to "hold the enema" is positioned on the left side with right leg flexed and asked to hold the enema for 3–5 mins

* When instructions are given to administer an enema at home, instructions should be given in cups (240 ml = 1 cup). A normal saline solution can be prepared by adding ½ teaspoon of table salt per cup of lukewarm water.

† Commercially prepared enemas are administered similarly. The tip is prelubricated. Warm the solution. The tip is inserted, then the enema container is gently squeezed; it is not usually possible to empty it completely.

ers require special explanations and understanding because they do not clearly mentally separate rectal and genital regions of the body. Administration of an enema thus has the potential to arouse fears related to the genitalia.

Caring for a Child with a Colostomy/Ileostomy

The surgical creation of an opening between the intestine and the surface of the body can be either a colostomy (large intestine; colon) or an ileostomy (small intestine; ileum). In many instances, a temporary procedure colostomy is done during infancy, with the definitive procedure being performed at a later time (often when the child reaches 1 year of age). A colostomy/ileostomy may also be necessary for various reasons later in childhood. Parents and children, including siblings, benefit from explanations and demonstrations, using a doll or special models designed for teaching about a colostomy/ileostomy and ostomy care.

After surgery, the child and parents are encouraged to become familiar with the stoma (colostomy/ileostomy opening) and gradually increase their involvement in ostomy care. This is done to ensure that health maintenance of the child will be unimpaired. For preventing impaired adjustment, extra care is taken to provide an atmosphere that encourages them to discuss their concerns, fears, and feelings about caring for a colostomy/ileostomy. Adjustment by the child and parents is affected by the reason the colostomy/ileostomy is required and whether it is to be temporary or permanent. A child's adjustment also is determined by his or her particular developmental level and by how well the parents can accept their child's need for a colostomy/ileostomy.

As much as possible, nursing care should be provided by the same individuals to help the family learn and to ease their adjustment. Table 35–14 provides specific directions for care of an ostomy.

Colostomy irrigation is performed to completely cleanse fecal material from the bowel. The equipment necessary for this procedure includes an enema bag, warmed irrigation solution, a soft and pliable catheter, a nipple, lubricant, and an intravenous pole. The irrigation solution is placed in the enema bag, and the tubing is filled with fluid. The pliable catheter is attached to the enema tubing. The catheter is inserted through the nipple. The catheter is then inserted into the stoma, followed by the nipple. The nipple is used to prevent leakage around the catheter as the enema is administered. The enema bag is placed 18 inches above the stoma, and the solution is administered gradually. This procedure should be done slowly. If the child complains of crampy abdominal pain, stop the solution for several minutes and then restart.

TABLE 35-14
Family-Centered Teaching: Care of an Ostomy

Pouch Application

1. Gather equipment and wash your hands
2. Remove the old pouch with use of adhesive remover or warm water; discard pouch into plastic bag
3. Measure the stoma by use of the measuring guide provided in each box of flanges or pouches
4. Trace the pattern on the flange or adhesive backing of the pouch and cut out the opening; remove the release paper and set aside
5. Wash peristomal skin with warm water; a tub bath may also be taken; pat the skin dry
6. If the peristomal skin is excoriated, apply karaya powder or Stomahesive powder to peristomal skin and dust off excess; apply skin sealant (Ex-Skin Prep, Bard Protective Wipe, Alkare) over same area and let dry
7. Center the pouch or flange over the stoma and apply to peristomal skin; press into place
8. Apply tail closure to the bottom of the pouch

Emptying the Pouch

1. Remove tail closure
2. Empty the drainage into a container or into the toilet
3. Using an ear syringe or Asepto syringe, place warm water into the pouch; swish around in pouch and empty into container or toilet
4. Special deodorants are available for use, if necessary
5. Dry the end of the pouch with toilet paper and apply the tail closure

Helpful Hints

1. Always carry extra pouches and skin care products with you when traveling
2. Cut out a few pouches or flanges in advance for quick changes
3. Change the pouch when the child is calm
4. For excoriated skin, apply a small amount of egg white to the peristomal skin and let dry; the albumin in the egg white promotes healing

Many one-piece and two-piece appliances are available to the pediatric client:

Hollister Pediatric Pouch

Convatec Little Ones Drainable/Urostomy Pouch

Convatec Sur-Fit Flexible Wafer with Mini Pouch

Smith/Nephew Pediatric Transfer Pouch

Nu-Hope Pediatric Pouch

Information supplied by Joan Selekof, RN, BSN, CETN.

Caring for a Child after Abdominal Surgery

Care after abdominal surgery requires close monitoring by the nurse as for any other surgery. Depending on the type of surgical procedure, specific care, such as irrigation of abdominal wounds, shortening of incisional drains, care of colostomy/ileostomy, or irrigation of a nasogastric tube, may be required. General principles of care are presented in Table 35-15, Nursing Process Plan: Care of the Child after Abdominal Surgery.

This Nursing Process Plan is applicable regardless of the reason for the operation and, for the most part, can be used after most surgical procedures.

Impact of Gastrointestinal Alterations on the Child and Family

Although many of the alterations discussed in this chapter can be surgically corrected early in life, the extent of the disruption to the individual family can be great. Some disorders are life-threatening (e.g., diaphragmatic hernia, severe gastroenteritis), whereas many are chronic and require a lifetime of adjustment (e.g., Crohn disease and ulcerative colitis). Frequent hospitalizations and a series of surgical procedures are disruptive at any age and cause stress to both child and family. The nurse should carefully assess for diagnoses in the relating, valuing, choosing, perceiving, and feeding patterns.

Positive feeding experiences, nutritional intake, and the growth of children are evidence to parents that they have a normal child and that they themselves are succeeding as parents. Disturbances that interfere with these feelings of satisfaction and achievement can lead to ineffective family coping or altered family processes. Negative feelings may arise toward the infant if food is either rejected or regurgitated. Disturbances in nutritional intake and absorption also interfere with the infant's oral gratification and available energy for mobility. *The infant's and family's general sense of well-being is affected by interruptions in the normal process of feeding and the social exchanges that normally accompany these experiences.*

Frequently, gastrointestinal problems involve the use of tubes, appliances, and cumbersome equipment. Although parents become skilled at providing food through tubes and other apparatus, extensive adaptation is required. This adaptation can be aided by encouraging the parents to become involved when they are ready, which may not necessarily be at a time the nurse thinks they should be. The parents must first adjust and cope with the child's condition and then learn new skills in the care of their child; however, involvement from the beginning is important in enhancing adjustment.

Generally, when eating habits and digestion are altered, a person's sense of well-being is disrupted. In some instances, the alterations in nutritional state and in fluid and electrolyte imbalance become so severe that the individual does not feel well, and in some conditions even the appearance is altered. Need for a nasogastric tube, an ileostomy or colostomy, and the cachectic appearance associated with illnesses such as severe Crohn disease may lower the patient's self-esteem, body image, sense of identity, and acceptance among peers.

It is difficult for children and their families to accept a problem that concerns such a personal, private aspect of life as elimination. Parents often find it hard to explain to friends and other people the nature of

TABLE 35-15

Nursing Process Plan: Care of the Child after Abdominal Surgery*

Analysis: Collaborative Problem 1

Response and Related or Risk Factors: *High risk for altered tissue perfusion: systemic;* risk factor: hypovolemia associated with postoperative hemorrhage

Projected Outcome: The child will maintain adequate nutrition and oxygenation at the cellular level

Defining Characteristics
(Actual Response)

Objective:

- Blood pressure changes in extremities
- Diminished arterial pulsations
- Skin color, dependent, blue or purple
- Skin color, pale on elevation, color does not return on lowering of leg
- Skin temperature, cold extremities
- Skin quality, shining
- Claudication
- Bruits

Nursing Interventions

Surveillance, Intravenous (IV) Therapy

Monitor for adequacy of perfusion every 15 minutes initially, then at least every 4 hours during the postoperative period.

Check under dressings as well as on top (Blood that fails to be "wicked" into dressing will run under child)

Initiate interventions to improve tissue perfusion.

- Maintain IV replacement of fluids (to ensure adequate vascular volume)
- Ensure frequent position changes; infants and small children usually move spontaneously if pain is kept under control; older children and adolescents can be encouraged to change position at least every hour and taught to alternately dorsiflex and extend the feet (to facilitate venous return)
- Discourage prolonged sitting positions, raising the knee gatch in the bed, or placing pillows under the knees (these positions compromise vascular flow)
- *Alert the physician* to any sudden or significant change in perfusion

Evaluation Criteria

The child will maintain adequate tissue perfusion, as evidenced by

- Normal blood pressure
- Palpable arterial pulsations
- Skin warm and of normal color and texture for race

* This table is designed to detail care particular to the child after abdominal surgery. For supporting information, see (1) Table 21–5. Nursing Process Plan: The Hospitalized Child and (2) the beginning of this chapter for care of the child with a nasogastric tube.

TABLE 35-15 *(continued)*

Analysis: Nursing Diagnostic Statement 1

Response and Related or Risk Factors: *High risk for ineffective airway clearance;* risk factor: poor cough effort associated with

- Sedative effects of anesthesia and analgesics
- Incisional pain
- Inability to cooperate because of developmental level

Projected Outcome: The child will maintain ability to clear secretions or obstructions from the respiratory tract to maintain airway patency.

Defining Characteristics *(Actual Response)*	Nursing Interventions	Evaluation Criteria
Objective: • Adventitious lung sounds (rales, rhonchi) • Changes in rate or depth of respiration • Tachypnea • Cough, effective/ineffective, with or without sputum • Cyanosis of skin and mucous membranes • Dyspnea	*Airway Management* **Monitor for evidence of ineffective airway clearance** every 2–4 hours, depending on postoperative status. **Institute interventions to promote airway clearance.** • Preoperatively, teach techniques for splinting incision, deep breathing, coughing, and use of incentive spirometer or blow bottles • Position to facilitate airway drainage (side-lying) or patency (semi-Fowler) • Perform chest physical therapy as appropriate • Allow the infant or toddler to cry for a few seconds before comforting (this ensures deep breathing in a child too young to cooperate; if secretions are present, coughing follows the deep breaths as a reflex action) • Plan deep-breathing and coughing efforts to correspond with peak effects of pain medication (because respiratory exercises should be carried out every 2 hours, continual analgesic administration [i.e., every 3–4 hours as ordered] should be considered in the immediate postoperative period); instruct how to cough effectively *Alert physician* if evidence develops of impaired gas exchange	**The child will maintain airway patency, as evidenced by** • Clear lung sounds • Respirations within normal limits • Mucous membranes pink, skin color normal for race

(continued)

TABLE 35-15 *(continued)*

Defining Characteristics *(Actual Response)*	**Nursing Interventions**	**Evaluation Criteria**
	(change in mental status, restlessness, cyanosis, dyspnea, increasing tachycardia, decrease in SO_2 [as monitored by pulse oximetry]).	

Analysis: Nursing Diagnostic Statement 2

Response and Related or Risk Factors: *High risk for urinary retention;* risk factors:

- Postoperative effects of anesthesia on the bladder muscle
- Manipulation of the bladder during surgery
- Abnormal voiding position

Projected Outcome: The child will void within 8 hours after surgery.

Defining Characteristics *(Actual Response)*	**Nursing Interventions**	**Evaluation Criteria**
Subjective: • Verbalization of sensation of bladder fullness *Objective:* • Inability to void within 6–8 hours after surgery • Bladder palpable above the pubis • Dribbling • Residual urine • Dysuria • Overflow incontinence	*Urinary Retention Care* **Monitor urinary status.** • Frequently ask whether the child feels the need to void; enlist the help of the family members (especially with the child who is developing modesty) • Palpate for bladder distention • Note fluid intake since preoperative void **Facilitate normal voiding.** • If possible, place toilet-trained children in the normal voiding position; they can often be carried to the bathroom or allowed to use a potty chair at bedside • If positioning alone is insufficient, try running warm water over the pubic area, letting the child hear water run into a sink, or applying moderate pressure with the hand over the bladder area; or (if not contraindicated by condition), place your hand on the child's abdomen and tell the child to take a big breath, hold it, and then push away your hand by pushing out his or her abdomen (this will apply pressure from abdominal muscles to the area of the bladder)	**The child voids within 8 hours after surgery and experiences complete emptying of the bladder.**

TABLE 35-15 (continued)

Defining Characteristics *(Actual Response)*	Nursing Interventions	Evaluation Criteria
	Alert the physician if the child has a distended bladder and is unable to void after 8 hours.	

Analysis: Collaborative Problem 2

Response and Related or Risk Factors: *Abdominal pain,* related to altered bowel elimination and decreased peristalsis, associated with

- Manipulation of the bowel during surgery
- Effects of anesthesia
- Effects of morphine sulfate or codeine, or both
- Immobility

Projected Outcome: The child will experience a pain-free state.†

Defining Characteristics *(Actual Response)*	Nursing Interventions	Evaluation Criteria
Subjective: • Complaints of crampy abdominal pain • Feeling of "fullness" • Anorexia *Objective:* • Guarding behavior • Self-focusing • Narrowed focus • Withdrawal from social contact • Impaired thought process • Distraction behaviors • Facial mask of pain • Alteration in muscle tone	Bowel Management **Assess bowel status.** • Measure abdominal girth at the umbilicus preoperatively if possible, or immediately postoperatively (to establish a baseline); then record *abdominal girth every shift* during the first 48–72 hrs, or until normal bowel function has returned • Auscultate for bowel sounds every 4 hrs, listening in all four quadrants; *record actual number* of sounds per minute (using terms such as "decreased" or "increased" is too subjective to be of much value to the next evaluator) • Palpate the abdomen every 4 hours and record whether soft or firm, flat or distended • Listen for passage of flatus and ask the parent or older child about passage of flatus • Question the child about abdominal comfort	**The child will** • Verbalize abdominal comfort • Show interest in surroundings • Be relaxed

† Realistic goals for return of peristalsis depend on the type and length of surgery, the amount of bowel manipulation, and the presence of peritonitis; return of peristalsis may vary from 24 hours to several days.

(continued)

TABLE 35-15 (continued)

Defining Characteristics *(Actual Response)*	Nursing Interventions	Evaluation Criteria

	Implement interventions to facilitate return of peristalsis and to decrease gaseous distention.
	• Assist the child with frequent position changes
	• Ambulate as soon as and as often as ordered:
	  • Set specific ambulation goals for time and distance with the child and family and reinforce (verbally, with colored stickers, etc.) the child's progress in walking
	  • Medicate the child for incisional pain *before ambulation,* planning the ambulation time during the medication's peak effect
	• Reduce air swallowing whenever possible
	  • Reduce crying in the infant through pharmacologic and nonpharmacologic comfort measures
	  • Ensure that the nipple is full of liquid (to prevent taking in air with feeding)
	  • Discourage gum chewing and sucking on hard candy (these activities increase air swallowing)
	• Maintain patency of the nasogastric tube (if present)
	  • Observe for withdrawal of fluid during intermittent suction (because the suction will usually be set at "low" intensity, fluid fluctuation in the tubing may not be dramatic, but it should gradually move toward the collection bag)
	  • Irrigate the nasogastric tube gently if it appears plugged and if orders have been written for irrigation
	• Substitute non-narcotic analgesics for morphine sulfate and acetaminophen (Tylenol) with co-	

TABLE 35-15 *(continued)*

Defining Characteristics *(Actual Response)*	**Nursing Interventions**	**Evaluation Criteria**
	deine once severe pain has subsided; this can usually be done after the first 48 hours without sacrificing the child's comfort (narcotics can decrease peristalsis) • Differentiate between gas pain and incisional pain (ambulation and a rectal tube or flush-type of enema are appropriate interventions for gas pain; narcotic analgesics will be counterproductive) • Begin oral fluids slowly, assessing frequently for abdominal distention and discomfort • As oral intake is advanced, caution the child and parents about gas-forming foods: onions, cabbage, popcorn, carbonated beverages	

Analysis: Nursing Diagnostic Statement 3

Response and Related or Risk Factors: *High risk for infection: peritonitis;* risk factors: release of intestinal contents into the abdominal cavity through

- Rupture or penetration of a part of the bowel
- Leakage through the bowel wall or suture line associated with the build-up of pressure within the bowel

Projected Outcome: The child will be free of peritonitis.

Defining Characteristics *(Actual Response)*	**Nursing Interventions**	**Evaluation Criteria**
Subjective: • Severe abdominal pain and rebound tenderness *Objective:* • Fever • Distention and "boardlike" rigidity of the abdomen • Absent or diminished bowel sounds • Tachycardia • Tachypnea • Increased white blood cell count	Surveillance, Infection Protection **Assess for evidence of peritonitis.** • Record vital signs, contour and tension of abdomen, bowel sounds, and level of comfort every 4 hours • Monitor white blood cell count; report counts that are increasing or that fail to return to normal **Implement interventions to prevent peritonitis.** • Prevent disruption of drains placed during surgery by re-	**The child will be free of peritonitis, as evidenced by** • Increasing abdominal comfort after the first postoperative day • Soft, nondistended abdomen • Returning bowel sounds • Absence of fever, tachycardia, tachypnea • White blood cell count returning to normal levels

(continued)

TABLE 35-15 *(continued)*

Defining Characteristics *(Actual Response)*	**Nursing Interventions**	**Evaluation Criteria**
	straining the infant or young child as needed • Take measures to facilitate peristalsis and reduce gaseous distention; see interventions for Collaborative Problem 1 **If evidence of peritonitis occurs:** • *Place the child in a semi-Fowler position* to localize pooling of intestinal contents. • *Alert the physician* immediately.	

Analysis: Nursing Diagnostic Statement 4

Response and Related or Risk Factors: *High risk for impaired skin integrity;* risk factors:

- Leakage of abdominal fluids onto skin
- Tape associated with dressings

Projected Outcome: The child will maintain skin integrity.

Defining Characteristics *(Actual Response)*	**Nursing Interventions**	**Evaluation Criteria**
Subjective: • Verbalization of itching, tenderness *Objective*: • Erythema • Excoriation • Maculopapular rash	*Skin Surveillance* **Implement interventions to protect skin integrity.** • Ask the child and parent if allergies to tape exist • Use Montgomery straps whenever possible (to reduce irritation from frequent tape removal) • Use *paper tape* (which is less adhesive and less irritating) when tape must be used • Consider the use of tincture of benzoin to make skin less sensitive to tape and other irritants • Cleanse skin of wound drainage (observing sterile technique) whenever dressings are changed; keep skin as clean and dry as possible	**The child will maintain skin integrity, as evidenced by** • Verbalizing comfort of skin around incision, drains • Absence of erythema, excoriation, or rash

their child's problem and therefore may need to discuss such feelings with health professionals. Particular problems that parents can anticipate, depending on the alteration, are problems in toilet training, resistance to participation in gym and in sports that involve changing clothes and sleepovers (especially if the child has a colostomy/ileostomy). In some instances, children or parents, or both, can participate in a group conducted by a health professional or organized as a self-help group.

To promote adequate health maintenance, it is important that adequate time and attention be paid to providing information and teaching the child and family how to care for themselves. The initial step for the nurse is to accept patients' unwillingness to care for themselves. Recognizing that the child or parent is experiencing a loss by having to learn new techniques of care is part of this initial phase. Even though the procedure may be a temporary one, some resistance may develop because of the "abnormalcy" that it represents. Involving the child or parent gradually and consistently on a daily basis can eventually result in sufficient acceptance and support to initiate self-care. Many of the technical procedures discussed in the previous section are learned by children and parents. Regardless of the type of problem, the *individual* responses of children and their families must be explored and recognized. The nurse cannot predict any individual's response on the basis of how previous patients with similar disorders responded. Although the disruptions are similar from a physiologic viewpoint, the coping mechanisms, the support systems, and the person's perception of the disorder all determine adaptation in each specific situation.

Anomalies and Obstructions of the Digestive Tract

Disorders included in this section require surgical intervention ranging from facial surgery for cleft lip or palate to simple repair of an inguinal hernia to complex staged repairs of the intestines. In most instances of digestive tract surgery, the infant's greatest source of gratification—eating—must be interrupted for a time. When an infant requires the withholding of oral feeding, other sources of comfort must be provided. Some parents may resist the use of a pacifier, but it is an appropriate option to suggest during this time, especially in an infant under 3 months of age, for whom the need to suck is particularly great.

Surgery on the gastrointestinal tract may affect toilet training. Because the majority of operations are done during infancy, the potential for normal bowel control remains in question for several years. These children may need extra time and support from parents to become continent.

Cleft Lip and Cleft Palate

Cleft lip, cleft palate, and combinations of these are the most common of all facial anomalies. Cleft lip with or without cleft palate is more common in boys. Cleft palate alone is more common in girls. Boys more commonly have a combined cleft lip and cleft palate, usually of more severe degree than in girls.

Etiology/Incidence

Accurate incidence data are difficult to obtain, but it is generally believed that cleft lip with or without cleft palate occurs in 1 per 1000 births and cleft palate alone in 1 per 2500 births. The incidence varies by race, with a higher incidence rate in the Japanese (twice that of the white population), and a lower incidence rate in the African-American population (less than half as many as the white population).

A strong genetic component exists for cleft lip and cleft palate, yet environmental factors are likely as well (Owens et al, 1985). Available data indicate that cleft lip with or without cleft palate is etiologically and genetically distinct from isolated cleft palate (Aylsworth, 1985; McWilliams et al, 1984). Genetic factors are believed to be of greater significance in cleft lip with or without cleft palate than in isolated cleft palate. Children with isolated cleft palate have a greater incidence of associated anomalies than is noted in children with cleft lip with or without cleft palate.

Sometimes the family history reveals no previous occurrence of cleft lip or cleft palate. It is, however, possible for a small, nondetected cleft to have been present in a family; therefore, it is important not to falsely assure parents that there is no genetic basis present.

The role of nonhereditary factors remains unclear. Environmental studies in utero have been done primarily on laboratory animals; causative environmental factors in humans have not yet been clearly identified (McWilliams et al, 1984). However, some evidence has suggested that phenytoin (Dilantin) taken during pregnancy has possible teratogenic effects, such as formation of clefts (McWilliams et al, 1984).

The most widely accepted view is that the great majority of clefts are caused by multifactorial inheritance. Probably many genes contribute to clefting. Each is of minor importance individually, but their interaction together with negative environmental conditions may cause clefting (McWilliams et al, 1984).

Pathophysiology

Even though the embryologic development of the palate and lip takes place around the same time, it occurs independently; therefore, cleft lip and cleft palate may occur together, or either defect may occur separately. The facial structures develop between 5 and 9 weeks after conception. The lips (primary palate) form at 7 weeks; the hard and soft palates (secondary palate) develop at 9 weeks. The lips are formed from three processes—a midline central nasal process and two wings of a branchial arch, which are called the maxillary processes. When fusion of the nasal process and maxillary processes does not occur, a clefting of the lip results.

Complete separation of the oral and nasal cavities normally results when the primary and secondary palates fuse to form a continuous structure. Early in development, the tongue pushes into the nasal cavity, and two structures (palatal shelves) occur in a vertical position on either side of the tongue. During the seventh and eighth weeks the tongue drops, and the palatal shelves elevate into a horizontal plane and fuse. When fusion of the palate does not occur, a cleft palate results.

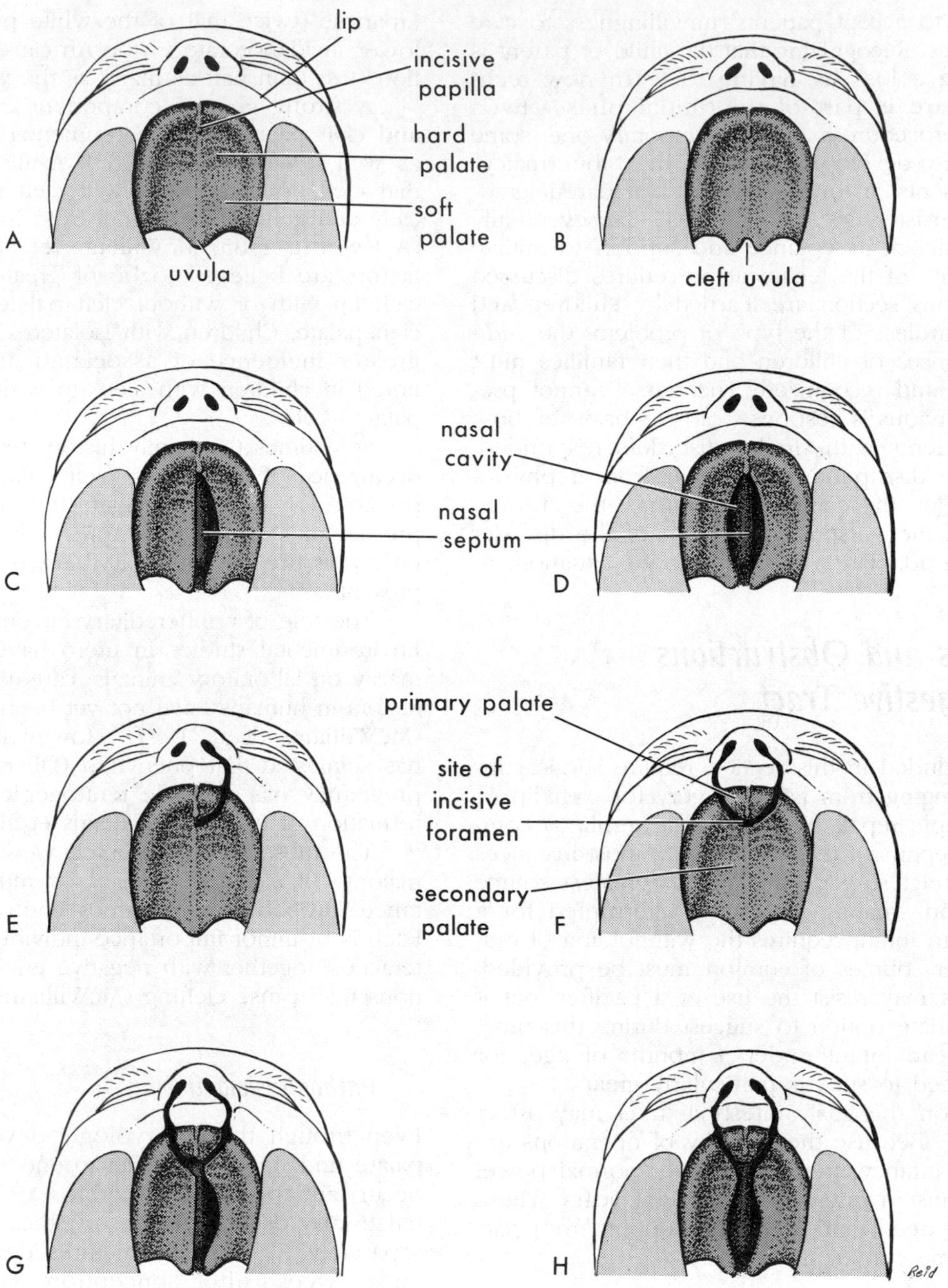

FIGURE 35 - 2. Drawings of various types of cleft lip and cleft palate. *A,* Normal lip and palate. *B,* Cleft uvula. *C,* Unilateral cleft of the posterior or secondary palate. *D,* Bilateral cleft of the posterior palate. *E,* Complete unilateral cleft of the lip and alveolar process of the maxilla with a unilateral cleft of the anterior or primary palate. *F,* Complete bilateral cleft of the lip and alveolar processes of the maxillae with bilateral cleft of the anterior palate. *G,* Complete bilateral cleft of the lip and alveolar processes of the maxillae with bilateral cleft of the anterior palate and unilateral cleft of the posterior palate. *H,* Complete bilateral cleft of the lip and alveolar processes of the maxillae with complete bilateral cleft of the anterior and posterior palates.

Clinical Manifestations

Cleft lip and cleft palate appear in various forms. In some cases, the defect is obvious, but in others it is not. The cleft lip can be unilateral or bilateral (Figs. 35–2 and 35–3). Midline cleft lips are rare. The extent of clefting can vary from a slight indentation (incomplete) to a widely opened (complete) cleft. Varying degrees of nasal distortion usually accompany the cleft lip, and the defect may also involve supernumerary, deformed, or absent teeth.

The degree of deformity of the cleft palate also varies (Fig. 35–2). Because it is less obvious than the cleft lip, it may not be detected without a thorough assessment of the mouth. It can be identified by placing the fingers directly on the palate. The defect may involve only the uvula (incomplete cleft) or may extend to both the soft palate (posterior portion) and hard palate (anterior portion) (complete cleft). The isolated cleft palate occurs in the midline and may involve the uvula or extend to the soft and hard palates. Cleft palate associated with a cleft lip may take a variety of forms. It may involve the uvula and midline of the soft palate, and if it extends into the hard palate, it may involve one or both sides (unilateral or bilateral cleft palate) (Fig. 35–2).

Diagnostic Assessment

Before surgery, the infant should be in good health and gaining weight. The infant should be robust in behavior and have good skin turgor. If the infant is not gaining weight and demonstrating delays in development, a referral is made to the cleft palate team for instruction in feeding technique (Fisher, 1991). Once the infant is evaluated as ready for the surgical repair, preoperative laboratory tests are done, such as complete blood count with bleeding time, urinalysis, serum electrolyte analysis, and chest x-ray examination. Explanations to parents regarding the rationale and description of the preoperative workup alleviate their anxiety about the unknown aspects of procedures, thereby enabling parents to provide the emotional support their infant needs during threatening and painful procedures.

Therapeutic Management

Surgical repair of the cleft lip precedes repair of the palate and is done within the first 3 months of life (usually at 1 month) if the infant is gaining weight and is free of infection. Z-plasty, the most commonly per-

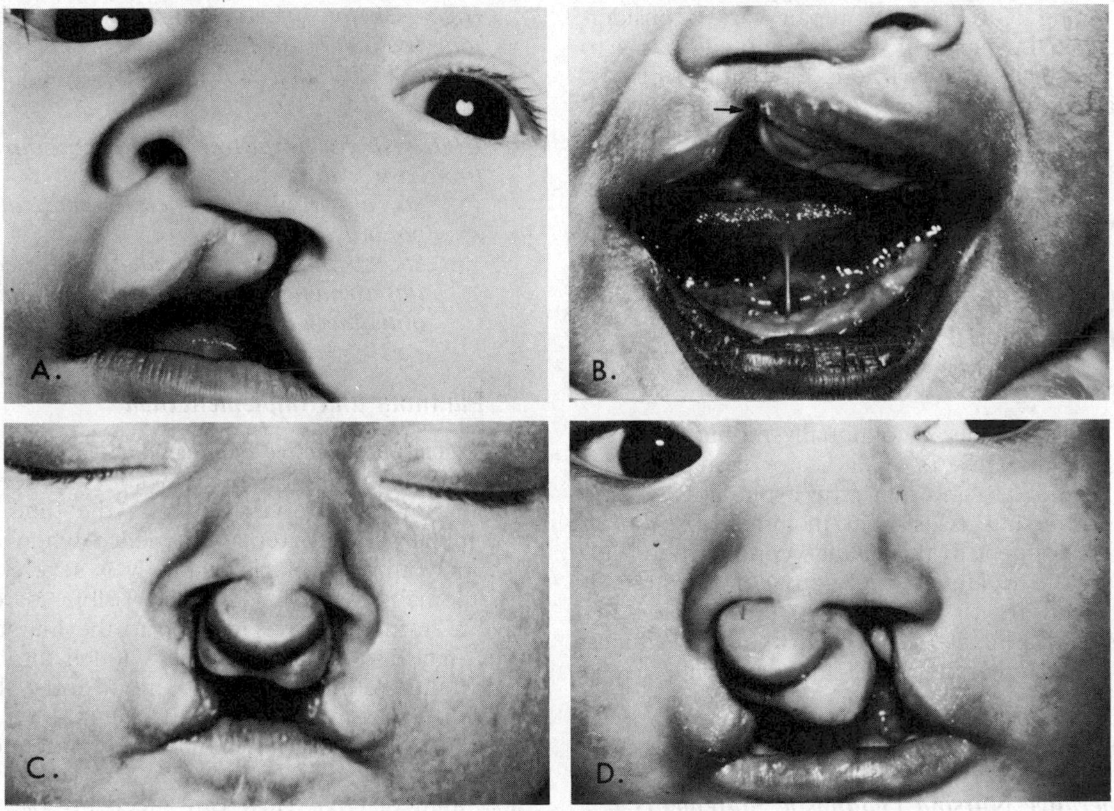

FIGURE 35 - 3. Photographs illustrating clefts of the lip. This malformation used to be referred to as harelip; this is an inappropriate term because the hare's lip is divided in the median plane. *A* and *B,* Unilateral cleft lip. The cleft in *B* is incomplete; the arrow indicates a band of tissue (Simonart band) connecting the parts of the lip. *C* and *D,* Bilateral cleft lip. (*A–D,* Courtesy of Dr. D. A. Kernahan, The Children's Memorial Hospital, Chicago.)

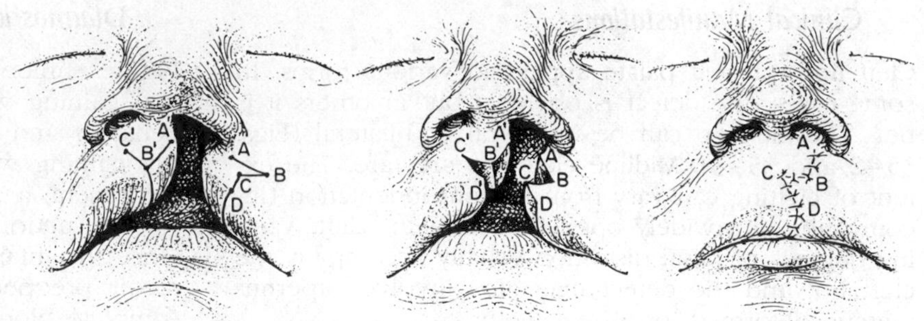

FIGURE 35-4. A procedure for cleft lip repair. The surgeon makes several incisions, then sutures the lip together. (Reprinted with permission from Fochtman, D., & Raffensperger, J. [1976]. Principles of nursing care for the pediatric surgery patient [2nd ed.]. Boston: Little, Brown and Company.)

formed surgical technique, uses a staggered Z-shaped suture line (Fig. 35–4). The goal is to approximate the vermilion border and minimize notching.

A Logan clamp (a curved metal bow taped down on both sides of the suture line over the lip) or a butterfly adhesive restraint is applied immediately after surgery to prevent tension on the suture line. The cosmetic results of the surgery will depend on the extent of the original defect and the absence of infection or trauma. Additional surgery may be needed at a later age to improve the child's appearance.

The timing of cleft palate repair varies considerably. The initial repair may be done as early as 4 to 6 months. It may be done in one operation, as in the case of a soft palate defect, or may require several stages of repair, depending on the severity of the defect. Most surgeons prefer to close the palate before the age of 2 years to prevent the development of faulty speech habits (Lindsay, 1986).

Application of the Nursing Process: Cleft Lip and Cleft Palate

Assessment

Before surgery, the nurse continually monitors weight gain and health status as an indicator that the infant is eating adequately and injury by aspiration is being prevented. Nursing assessment includes observation of family adjustment to the infant's condition and adherence to the treatment regimen. For example, it may be necessary to reinstruct parents on feeding technique if the infant fails to gain weight. Families' adherence and adjustment will be continually tested as the infant encounters the need for surgery and possibly years of corrective treatments.

Preoperative Nursing Diagnostic Statements and Collaborative Problems

High risk for ineffective family or altered family processes; *risk factors:*
- *The shock of the newborn infant's facial or palatal anomaly.*
- *Knowledge deficit regarding the defect.*

High risk for altered nutrition: less than body requirements; *risk factors:*
- *Sucking difficulties: ineffective suction on the nipple associated with the cleft.*
- *Parental anxiety and frustration associated with the infant's tendency to choke on feedings.*

High risk for aspiration; *risk factor: a direct pathway into the nasopharynx created by the cleft.*

High risk for infection: middle ear; *risk factors: inefficient drainage of the middle ear associated with altered functioning of soft palate muscles.*

High risk for impaired verbal communication; *risk factors:*
- *Speech problems associated with altered palatal arch.*
- *Speech problems associated with hearing impairment during repeated episodes of otitis media.*

Planning and Implementation

Promoting Effective Family Functioning. Supporting the parents toward unimpaired family processes is a critical nursing intervention from the time of birth. The initial shock parents experience when an infant is born with an orofacial anomaly is severe. Because the anomaly is on the face and visible, parents may have a strong negative reaction to the infant initially. They may find it hard to hold or touch the baby and may delay telling relatives and friends about the problem or letting them see the infant.

Parents will have many immediate concerns: "Why did this happen?" "What can be done?" and, most immediately, "How can I feed my baby?" Families vary in how they respond, depending on their usual coping styles, relationship between the parents, and social support network.

As discussed in Chapter 31, reaction to a defect includes a period of sorrow and grieving for the loss of the "idealized" child. The initial period of shock may be followed by a turning away from the infant in disbelief or denial. Some parents may not be ready immediately to learn about feeding the infant, whereas others find release in aggressively questioning staff about all aspects of care, seeking out literature on the anomaly, and consulting specialists in the field.

Encouraging and supporting parents in holding and touching their infant in the earliest hours and days is a nursing responsibility. Some parents may be afraid to touch the infant's face. The nurse, by handling and holding the baby in a natural manner, can lessen their anxiety. The nurse should remember that the parents may need basic education about newborn infant care (e.g., how to hold the infant, how to wrap a blanket, or how to change a diaper).

A cleft lip can be very disfiguring; therefore, it is especially important for nurses to emphasize the positive aspects of the infant's appearance and express optimism about the possibility for correction. The infant may be at home with the parents for 1 to 2 months before surgical repair of the lip is initiated. Parents usually adjust fairly well to this cosmetic defect if they have been given reasonable explanations concerning its cause, are supported by a nurse specialist who maintains phone or home visit contact during this interval, and are shown evidence of the improvement that surgery will make in their child's appearance and functioning. Parents are particularly interested in seeing before and after photographs of successful repairs. Photographs are more impressive and reassuring than is verbal assurance that improvement will be significant. An opportunity to talk with other parents who have been through the experience is the most useful intervention the health team can offer the parents. A hospital will generally have a support group service with names of other parents willing to talk to new parents.

Infants with cleft palate present a different problem. Because further growth of the secondary palate is desirable, definitive surgery may be delayed until the baby is 6 months to 18 months of age. Parents must be helped to take care of the child at home and counseled if they have difficulty in accepting the baby as part of the family.

Accurate and consistent answers to parents' questions from the first day are important. The treatment plan for an infant depends on the type and severity of the anomaly; therefore, the nurse should provide accurate information in conjunction with other professionals involved in immediate and long-term care. The timing and type of surgical repair are discussed with parents early to allow them to develop realistic goals concerning their family life. Financial concerns about surgery and long-term treatment need to be discussed with the physician, hospital, and social worker. A cleft lip may require early surgical treatment with short-term adaptations required of the family, whereas a severe cleft lip and cleft palate may necessitate a complete program of habilitation, requiring years of special care by physicians, surgeons, dentists, orthodontists, speech therapists, and social workers. It is therefore important that a team approach be established early, ensuring accurate, consistent information to the family.

Providing Adequate Nutrition and Preventing Aspiration. The difficulty of feeding an infant with a cleft lip or cleft palate varies according to the extent and type of cleft. Many infants born with a cleft of the lip only or with a very small cleft of the soft palate may have little or no difficulty sucking. An infant born with a cleft of the lip *and* palate or a complete cleft of the palate may have difficulty creating a seal to produce suction in the mouth. The usual bottle nipples frequently can be used for these infants. The nipple hole can be crosscut in four directions to enlarge it. The nurse should be aware that feeding is initially a frightening experience for the parent because frequently in cleft palate, formula returns through the nose, accompanied by episodes of gagging and choking. Holding the infant in an upright position at a 60- to 80-degree angle with the head resting in the bend of the parent's elbow decreases the likelihood of aspiration. In this position, the natural cough reflex can more readily clear the airway. The nipple should be positioned firmly in the baby's mouth in a normal position. Observation of the infant's face is important because it provides clues as to how the infant is tolerating the feeding. Before gagging or choking, the infant will elevate eyebrows and wrinkle the forehead. The nipple can then be removed.

Mothers who wish to breastfeed their infants should be encouraged to do so. In cleft lip alone, breastfeeding can usually be achieved with minor adjustments. If the baby has difficulty making a seal, the cleft in the lip can be filled with the mother's thumb or the breast can be molded to fill the gap. Breastfeeding can be made easier for the infant if the breast is massaged before nursing to bring the milk down. The local LaLeche League chapter may be able to help a new mother who would like to breastfeed her infant or express breast milk to save and feed the baby later. Assistance and support to discuss the alternatives are required from the health team during this time of adjustment.

Preventing Middle Ear Infection and Language Difficulties. Ear infections, speech difficulties, and hearing problems are common in children with cleft palate. Under normal conditions, the muscles of the soft palate aid in proper functioning of the eustachian tube. In the presence of a cleft palate, involvement of these muscles results in inefficient drainage of the middle ear, causing a greater susceptibility to ear infections. Because ear and upper respiratory tract infections are frequent, precautions against infection should be taken. The pharyngeal opening of the eustachian tube is often in an abnormal position; consequently, the infant should not be fed in a lying-down position, nor should the baby be confined to a supine position for long periods. Good mouth care is also important in reducing infections. A milk feeding should be followed with a small amount of clear water to rinse the mouth. If an infection occurs and fluid accumulates, movement of the eardrum is inhibited, and a hearing loss may occur. Thus, when a child has a cleft palate, language acquisition may be hampered by inability to hear if careful attention is not given to early treatment of middle ear infections.

In many cases, myringotomy and placement of ventilation tubes are necessary. This surgery can be performed at the time of lip repair or in early infancy but can commonly be delayed until the time of palate repair (Trier, 1985). Another approach is to use a prosthesis that occludes the cleft palate. There is no evidence, however, that such prostheses assist in feeding or lessen the amount of orthodontic work required (Trier, 1985). Before the child is sent for either of the surgical procedures, parents should be informed about postoperative care, especially the restraints that are necessary to protect the repair from self-inflicted injury.

Evaluation

As in all high-risk diagnoses, the effectiveness of intervention in meeting projected outcomes is evaluated by observing for the absence of defining characteristics of the actual problem.

Postoperative Nursing Diagnostic Statements and Collaborative Problems

High risk for impaired tissue integrity; *risk factors:*

- *Rubbing of the surgical site.*
- *Suture line tension associated with sucking or crying.*

High risk for aspiration; *risk factor: ineffective positioning of the infant postoperatively.*

High risk for infection: surgical site; *risk factors:*

- *Inadequate handwashing by persons coming in contact with the infant.*
- *Remnants of milk or formula that collect on the incision and form a culture medium for pathogens.*

Ineffective individual and family coping, *related to pain resulting from surgical repair of the cleft.*

High risk for ineffective health maintenance; *risk factors:*

- *Parental stress.*
- *Knowledge deficit.*

Planning and Implementation

Preventing Disturbance of the Surgical Site after Cleft Lip/Palate Repair. The major emphasis in nursing care after cleft lip repair is on protecting the operative site. Arm restraints should be used to prevent the child from rubbing or otherwise disturbing the suture line, such as by thumbsucking or putting objects into the mouth. Children who are old enough to roll over will also need a jacket restraint to prevent them from rolling onto the abdomen and rubbing the face on the bed. (See Figs. 23–12 and 23–13 for examples of arm restraints.) The arm restraints are removed periodically to exercise the arms and to check for skin irritation. Also, because the child is placed only on the back or side after repair, periodic positioning in an infant seat increases comfort and stimulation.

The watchfulness required to maintain the surgical repair of a cleft lip is demanding of the nurse and the parents. The parents require assistance in understanding the importance of keeping the baby's hands away from the face. Parents also need to be shown how to hold their baby safely and provide physical contact even though restraints are in place. Mobiles and toys with various sounds, colors, and textures are essential for these babies' developmental progress. Parents should be encouraged to participate in the provision of an appropriately stimulating environment.

Feeding methods postoperatively are similar to those used before surgery. Preoperatively, however, these methods were employed to reduce the threat of aspiration and to enhance sucking. Postoperative feeding methods are designed to reduce trauma to the surgical site. Some surgeons may permit the infant to breastfeed early in the postoperative period. Immediately postoperatively, a medicine dropper or Asepto syringe may be used. These should be placed in the mouth from the side to avoid the suture line, and care should be taken to prevent the infant from sucking. Because sucking would disrupt the suture line, a pacifier cannot be used until sufficient healing has taken place.

After cleft palate repair, injury to the newly closed palate must be prevented. No sharp objects, such as spoons or forks, are permitted in the child's mouth. Liquids are given by mouth, but straws are not used. Soft foods can be fed from the side of a spoon, but self-feeding by a spoon could result in damage to the operative site.

Preventing Aspiration. Positioning of the infant postoperatively is critical for preventing aspiration of secretions. The position will vary, depending on the surgical procedure. An infant who has had a cleft lip repair cannot be placed in a prone position without damaging the surgical site. Therefore, the position of choice for this infant is on either side, but well protected with sandbags or blanket rolls to prevent the child from turning onto the abdomen.

After cleft palate repair, the infant may be safely placed either on the abdomen or on the side; the palatal sutures will not be damaged by a prone position. A mist tent may occasionally be used to ensure that the secretions remain liquid.

Strategies for suctioning of secretions also differ,

depending on the type of surgical repair. Although a bulb syringe may be used safely to gently suction secretions after a cleft lip repair, suctioning of any kind is contraindicated after surgery for cleft palate because introduction of a bulb syringe tip or a suction catheter may inadvertently damage the palatal suture line.

Preventing Infection. The importance of good handwashing should be impressed on parents and other visitors who come in direct contact with the infant. Needless to say, the nurse's hands carry the greatest potential for cross-contamination because of contact with other ill children and with contaminated surfaces. The nurse's careful handwashing (basic to nursing practice) is always a key to control of iatrogenic infection.

Initial feedings will be of clear liquids as tolerated. When feeding with milk or formula resumes, the mouth should be gently rinsed with water after each feeding. This is particularly important after surgery for cleft palate because there is no other way to clean the suture line. After cleft lip repair, the suture line should be cleaned with a cotton-tipped applicator and cleansing solution. The physician will often order an antibiotic ointment as well. Protection and astute care of the suture line are essential to provide for optimal healing and cosmetic results.

Promoting Effective Coping with Pain. The infant can be expected to have pain postoperatively from the surgical manipulation and suturing of tissues. Both analgesic medication and nonpharmacologic strategies should be considered. The provision of comfort is important not only for humane reasons but also because crying will place pressure on delicate suture lines.

Acetaminophen (Tylenol) is often ordered for postoperative analgesia after such procedures. Tylenol can be effective in controlling pain if it is administered routinely (i.e., every 3 to 4 hours as ordered) during the first 24 hours or at the time when the infant can be expected to have the most pain. A single dose or widely spaced doses of a mild analgesic, such as Tylenol, will probably not accomplish the goal of providing optimal comfort.

Infants seem to derive a good deal of comfort from being held and cuddled after cleft lip or cleft palate repair. Physical closeness with their infant can promote family coping by giving parents an opportunity to express their love and concern and to assure themselves that the baby is fine. The nurse can facilitate this nonpharmacologic comfort measure by showing the parents how to prevent suture line disturbance and how to prevent aspiration of secretions while holding the infant.

Promoting Health Maintenance. Aside from surgical repairs, the complete program of rehabilitation for the child with a cleft lip or palate will require the care of other specialists, particularly with respect to dental corrections and the development of normal speech. A speech pathologist can help the child develop normal speech early in life and can assist parents in early speech training as needed.

Treatment is most effective when provided by a cleft palate team. The American Cleft Palate Association (ACPA) registers cleft palate teams and sets guidelines about team membership. A list of cleft palate teams or centers can be obtained from the ACPA National Office.* The Cleft Palate Foundation is an educational arm of the ACPA and is located at the same address. A 24-hour telephone service is available for referrals and information.

Remarkable progress in the management of children born with a cleft lip or cleft palate, or both, has made it possible for these children to look like other children, speak like other children, and essentially live a normal life. The team approach provides the supportive care and coordinated treatment that is needed by these families. The nurse has an important role in helping families cope with the stress of having a baby with a defect and assisting them to understand and participate in the treatment and management program for their child.

Evaluation

Evaluation of the effectiveness of interventions in meeting projected outcomes is accomplished by assessing for the absence of defining characteristics of actual problems.

Pyloric Stenosis

In pyloric stenosis, there is an overgrowth (hypertrophy and hyperplasia) of the circular muscle of the pylorus, which results in obstruction of the pyloric sphincter.

Etiology/Incidence/Pathophysiology

Although the cause of pyloric stenosis is unknown, there seems to be a hereditary component; a family history of the problem is present in about 15 per cent of cases. It is thought to be more common in boys (1:150) than in girls (1:750) and especially in first-born boys, although some authors believe these factors have been overemphasized (Filston & Izant, 1985).

The pylorus is the opening through which food passes from the stomach to the intestines. This opening is surrounded by a muscular ring called the pyloric sphincter. In pyloric stenosis, the sphincter is in a state of spasm that causes hypertrophy of the muscle, resulting in a narrowed opening (Fig. 35–5). The

* The national office is located at The American Cleft Palate Association, 1218 Grandview Avenue, Pittsburgh, PA 15211; (800) 24–CLEFT ([800] 242–5338).

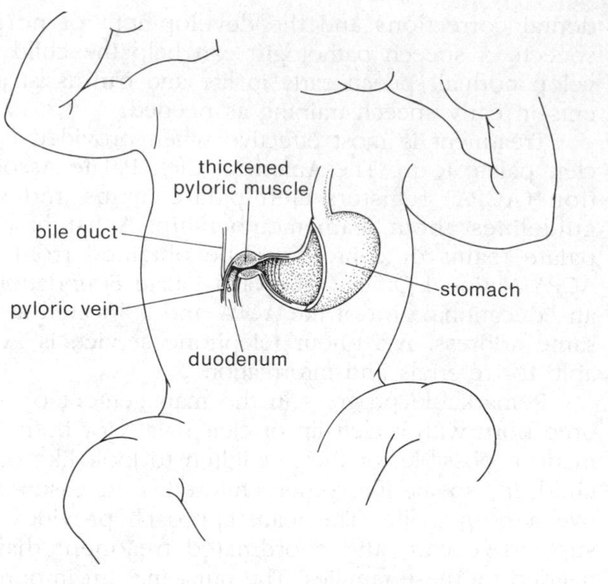

FIGURE 35 - 5. Pyloric stenosis. Hypertrophy, or thickening, of the pyloric sphincter blocks the stomach contents, causing the infant to regurgitate forcefully. Serious electrolyte imbalances ultimately occur, and surgery is necessary to correct the condition.

stomach's peristaltic movements do not effectively move contents through the obstructed pylorus; consequently, the overworked stomach musculature hypertrophies. The stomach contractions increase in frequency and force as they attempt to push stomach contents through the elongated, partially obstructed pyloric canal.

Clinical Manifestations

The history may vary; typically, at about 3 weeks of age, the infant begins to regurgitate small amounts of milk immediately after a feeding. Within a week, the pattern and type of vomiting can change dramatically, becoming projectile in character (vomitus propelled distances of several feet) and occurring with almost every feeding. The vomiting usually occurs during the feeding or shortly thereafter but, in some instances, may occur several hours later. The infant is hungry in spite of the vomiting and will usually take milk again. The vomitus contains no bile because the constriction is proximal to the ampulla of Vater, the site at which the common bile duct enters the duodenum.

Gastritis may occur owing to the irritation caused by stomach contents remaining in the stomach for prolonged periods. In gastritis, the vomitus may be blood-tinged (brownish discoloration).

The initial pattern of regurgitation after feedings may not result in any decrease in the baby's weight, nutritional state, or fluid and electrolyte balance; but with continuous, progressive vomiting, some serious alterations eventually develop. If untreated, the infant will lose weight. With eventual nutritional depletion, the child will show signs of dehydration and become alkalotic. With excessive loss of gastric juices, the electrolytes sodium, potassium, and chloride are lost. Gastric juice contains more chloride than sodium; therefore, hypochloremic alkalosis develops. As vomiting continues, a state of hypochloremia and hypokalemia results. Hydrochloric acid is lost, resulting in an increased pH and increased bicarbonate (carbon dioxide content) level. The fluid and electrolyte imbalance that results from excessive vomiting must be corrected before surgery is attempted.

Diagnostic Assessment

The nurse in a clinic or similar primary care setting may be the first to hear a parent's account of an infant who shows the beginning signs of pyloric stenosis. A careful history must be taken to differentiate this infant from the one who is vomiting owing to a poor feeding experience, such as might occur with an overly anxious caregiver or inadequate bonding. In 90 per cent of the infants with pyloric stenosis, a mass (the hypertrophied pylorus) can be palpated in the right epigastrium under the edge of the liver. The mass feels hard and is movable and shaped like an olive. Successful palpation requires a relaxed abdominal muscle and an empty stomach. A nasogastric tube may be passed and placed on continuous suction to facilitate palpation. Abdominal muscle relaxation can be achieved by holding the infant to quiet him or her, offering a pacifier with sugar or a bottle of warm sugar water, and elevating the baby's feet or flexing the knees and hips. After feeding, peristaltic waves can sometimes be noted moving from left to right toward the pylorus.

Radiographs are indicated only when the mass cannot be palpated after several examinations. If pyloric stenosis is present, barium contrast studies reveal delayed gastric emptying and an elongated, narrow pyloric canal (string sign), which may appear as a small or double streak of barium. Frequently, the pyloric mass can also be identified on ultrasonographic examination of the abdomen. If the results of diagnostic studies are normal, other conditions must be considered. However, the infant may be examined again in a week or 10 days because it can take some time for the typical diagnostic findings to develop in the presence of pyloric stenosis.

Therapeutic Management

In infants who are well hydrated and have no evidence of electrolyte and acid-base abnormalities, surgery is performed without delay. If an infant is dehydrated and has electrolyte imbalance, it is imperative that these conditions be corrected before surgery.

The stenosis is corrected by the Ramstedt-Fredet-Weber pyloromyotomy, which involves a longitudinal splitting of the hypertrophied muscle down to the mucosa so that the mucosa bulges between the split muscle. The mucosa and submucosa are left intact so that the lumen of the duodenum is not entered. The time for introduction of oral feedings varies.

Nursing Diagnostic Statements and Collaborative Problems

Ineffective family coping: disabling, *related to delay of surgery and apprehension about the surgery.*

High risk for fluid volume deficit; risk factor: *persistent preoperative vomiting.*

High risk for aspiration; *risk factor: persistent preoperative vomiting.*

Ineffective family coping, preoperative, *related to fear/anxiety: parental, regarding the infant's impending surgery.*

High risk for fluid volume deficit: postoperative; *risk factor: vomiting.*

High risk for aspiration, postoperative; *risk factor: vomiting.*

Ineffective individual/family coping, postoperative, *related to pain associated with tissue trauma.*

High risk for altered health maintenance; *risk factor: knowledge deficit regarding home care.*

Planning and Implementation

Supporting the Parents Preoperatively. If the infant is dehydrated and experiencing an electrolyte imbalance, surgery may be delayed from 24 to 36 hours while the infant receives intravenous fluids containing potassium. The baby may be irritable and crying because of not receiving any oral fluids. It is disturbing to parents to see their tiny baby distressed; they should be encouraged to discuss their feelings. Parents are taught how to protect the intravenous site while holding their infant and are encouraged to be present during this period to hold, comfort, and talk to the baby.

Parents are prepared for the surgery and the postoperative period by being told what to expect. The operation is a short procedure (15 to 30 minutes), and the infant will probably return from surgery with an intravenous line. Parents are told about the potential for vomiting in the immediate postoperative period and the need for gradual reintroduction of fluids, with clarification about when breastfeeding can be resumed.

Preventing Postoperative Fluid Volume Deficit and Aspiration. For a bottlefed infant, diluted formula is given postoperatively in small amounts, and gradually the quantity and strength of formula are increased. A basic rule to follow is not to change quantity and content of feeding at the same time (Filston & Izant, 1985). An infant who is breastfed can be allowed a gradual increase in the length of time at the breast.

Postoperative vomiting may occur for various reasons such as air swallowing with feeding and vigorous activity after feeding, and the nurse must make every effort to ensure that improper feeding technique is not the cause. These infants need to be fed using a firm nipple with a hole small enough so that milk is not taken too quickly. The nurse should emphasize that the nipple must be kept full of milk at all times to minimize swallowing of air, and the infant should be burped at any sign of discomfort. Also, these infants are often hungry and should not be allowed to suck on an empty bottle. If the infant must be disturbed after feeding, he or she should be handled with extra care to prevent vomiting related to the activity.

Helping parents to feel at ease by staying with them, helping them feed the baby correctly, and reassuring them that they are playing an important part in the recovery of their infant gives them support and courage during this sometimes difficult period.

Promoting Effective Coping with Pain. The infant can be expected to experience pain, especially in the first 24 to 48 hours after surgery. Because infants react to pain differently from older children or adults, assessment is difficult, and comfort measures often need to be instituted on the nurse's judgment that pain *must* be present. As always, both pharmacologic and nonpharmacologic strategies should be employed to ensure that the infant experiences no unnecessary distress. (See Chapter 25 for a discussion of pain assessment and management.)

Facilitating Home Health Maintenance. Care of the surgical site includes observation for signs of drainage or inflammation. The infant can usually be bathed, but care is taken to avoid immersing the surgical site in water until it is completely healed.

These infants can usually be discharged on the morning of the second postoperative day on an unrestricted diet. The incision is often sealed with collodion (a viscous liquid that is sprayed or applied with an applicator over an incision, which dries to form a strong, thin, transparent film) so that no dressing changes are required. Parents can resume their usual infant care routine and should be encouraged to plan their responsibilities in a way that will allow a relaxed, quiet feeding environment. It is important that parents feel positive about the feeding experience at discharge; otherwise, preconditioned feelings of failure may again make feeding an unpleasant and unsuccessful experience.

The mortality rate is well below 1 per cent in infants whose conditions have been identified early and who have been properly prepared for surgery. The nurse, as a member of the health team, has an important role in both of these areas.

Esophageal Atresia and Tracheoesophageal Fistula

Esophageal atresia and tracheoesophageal fistula can each occur as a single entity, but usually they occur together.

Etiology/Incidence/Pathophysiology

The reported prevalence of atresia (with or without tracheoesophageal fistula) is approximately 1 per 3000 live births. There are numerous types of esophageal atresia with or without tracheoesophageal fistula. Atresia with a distal fistula constitutes 80 to 90 per cent of all cases (Fig. 35–6*A*). In this type, the upper (proximal) esophagus ends in a blind pouch, and the lower (distal) esophagus exits from the stomach and joins the trachea instead of forming a continuous tube with the upper esophagus. The second most frequent type (Fig. 35–6*B*) is atresia without a fistula, accounting for 5 to 8 per cent of all cases. In this type, there is a proximal dilated pouch, and the distal end of the esophagus is narrowed and short. The third type, an isolated tracheoesophageal fistula without esophageal atresia, constitutes about 2 per cent of all cases. It is sometimes called the H-type because a fistula connects the trachea and esophagus in a way that resembles the letter H (Fig. 35–6*C*). Rare types occur in varying combinations of fistulas and atresia but are not discussed here.

Clinical Manifestations

Aspiration of secretions into the lungs has a major effect on prognosis. Aspiration can be prevented or diminished by early diagnosis and placement of a nasogastric sump tube in the proximal pouch to remove secretions.

Only a few clues can be relied on to identify an infant with esophageal atresia and tracheoesophageal fistula early. Prematurity and hydramnios (excess amniotic fluid) are two conditions that should alert the nurse to make further assessments. Eighty-five per cent of infants with atresia accompanied by fistula have a maternal history of hydramnios (Ashcraft & Holder, 1976). This suggests that effective swallowing

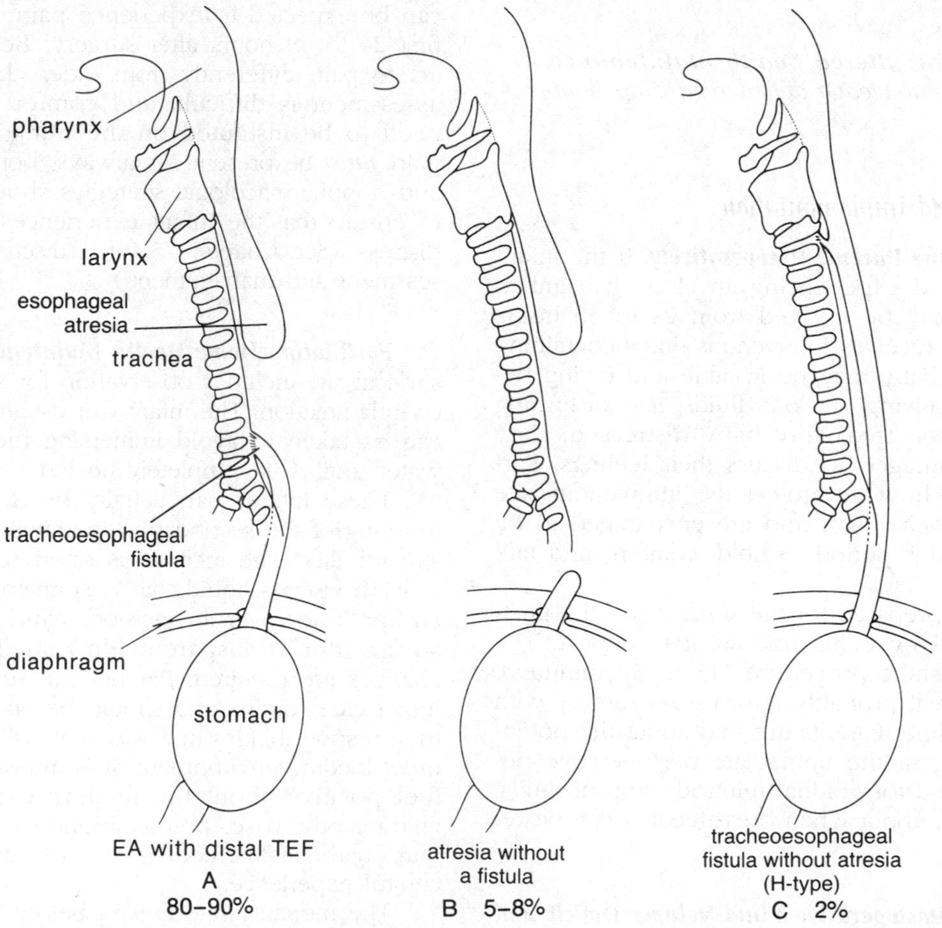

FIGURE 35 - 6. The three most common types of esophageal atresia and transesophageal fistula. *A*, Esophageal atresia with a distal fistula constitutes 80 to 90 per cent of all cases. *B*, Atresia without a fistula, 5 to 8 per cent. *C*, Isolated tracheoesophageal fistula without esophageal atresia (H-type), 2 per cent.

and absorption of amniotic fluid in utero is prevented. Approximately one third of the affected infants are premature. When prematurity, hydramnios, or both are present and the nurse suspects esophageal atresia or tracheoesophageal fistula, other signs to look for include excessive pharyngeal secretions, such as drooling or bubbling from the nostrils. Unfortunately, atresia is often first suspected when an infant coughs, chokes, regurgitates, or becomes cyanotic on feeding. In the H-type fistula, drooling does not occur (because this type does not consist of a proximal esophageal pouch), and choking and coughing on feeding are the first signs. Abdominal distention is noted with crying because air is shunted across the fistula.

When the fistula is small, the symptoms are not so obvious, but repeated pneumonia in the first few months of life should raise the suspicion of an H-type tracheoesophageal fistula. These episodes of pneumonia result from reflux of gastric secretions into the trachea.

When atresia is suspected, the presence of a blind pouch of the proximal esophagus can be confirmed by the inability to pass a radiopaque No. 8 to 10 French catheter into the stomach. Curling of the tube in the proximal esophagus is shown on radiographs. If a fistula is present, the radiographs will show air in the stomach and intestines because of the esophageal connection to the trachea. When there is no connection to the distal esophagus, neither air nor food enters the stomach. In these infants, the abdomen is flat and scaphoid in appearance.

Diagnostic Assessment

The procedure of choice for diagnosis is bronchoscopy with telescopic endoscopy. Other diagnostic methods are considered less accurate and introduce delay and the risk of aspiration (Filston & Izant, 1985).

In 30 per cent of cases of esophageal atresia, additional abnormalities are present, especially cardiac anomalies; therefore, a thorough physical examination and appropriate diagnostic studies in search of other anomalies are also done before surgery.

The parents are under a great deal of stress during the diagnostic period. If they witness the choking, coughing, and cyanosis produced by feeding, they may be particularly frightened; they need careful explanation of what the existing problem is and why their baby cannot be fed by mouth. Once the diagnosis is established, the family must be prepared for the necessary procedures and surgery that will follow.

Therapeutic Management

The goals of initial therapy are to prevent pulmonary complications and to ensure adequate nutrition (Gryboski, 1986). Preoperatively, the infant is placed in a position with head elevated (45 to 60 degrees) to reduce the likelihood of regurgitation of stomach con-

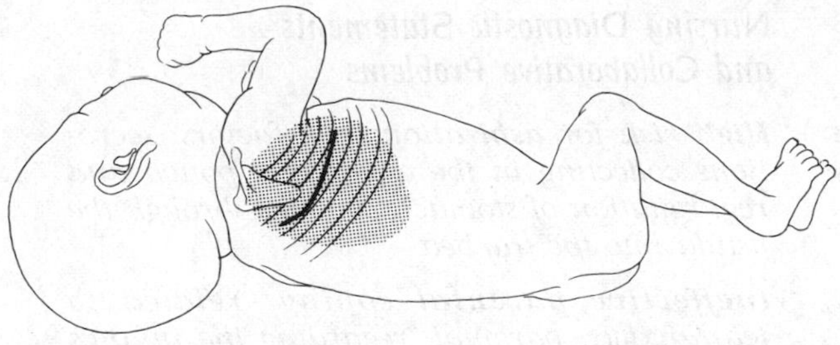

FIGURE 35-7. Incision for primary repair of tracheoesophageal fistula. (From *Surgery of the neonate,* A. Coran, Boston: Little, Brown, 1979, p 48. Published by Little, Brown and Company.)

tents into the trachea. A sump tube* (usually a Replogle) will be placed in the proximal esophageal pouch to remove pooled secretions and to decrease the chance of aspiration. The infant's respiratory status is closely monitored. A gastrostomy tube may be placed to decompress the stomach, although this varies with the type of defect. The infant is placed in an Isolette, where oxygen, humidity, and thermoregulation can be provided.

Primary repair consists of ligation of the fistula and anastomosis of the upper and lower segments of the esophagus. This is done through a right posterolateral thoracotomy (Fig. 35–7). When the anastomosis is completed, the tube in the esophageal pouch is removed. At the end of the operation, a retropleural chest tube is placed through a stab wound. Primary repair may be delayed if the infant is at risk owing to low birthweight, pneumonia, or another congenital anomaly. In these cases, a gastrostomy is performed (Randolph, 1986).

Postoperatively, fluid and electrolyte balance is maintained by an intravenous line, and prophylactic antibiotics may be ordered. Intravenous overload and pulmonary congestion are avoided by keeping intravenous fluid volumes at low maintenance levels (Canty, 1986). Respiratory management is the major concern in the immediate postoperative period. Mechanical ventilation may be required during the first few days. Oral feedings are recommended by some to begin on the second day unless there is concern about the anastomosis (Leape, 1987). Other approaches of nutritional maintenance are total parenteral nutrition or gastrostomy feedings. The anastomosis is weakest at 5 to 7 days; therefore, if there is concern about the anastomosis, oral feedings are delayed until 10 days postoperatively (Leape, 1987). In 5 to 10 per cent of patients, dilatations of the anastomosis are necessary.

* A sump tube has side holes over only the distal 1 inch of the tube. A standard nasogastric tube should not be used because it has side holes over the distal 2 to 3 inches. If a nasogastric tube is used in the pouch, too much available air would be suctioned from the pharynx.

Nursing Diagnostic Statements and Collaborative Problems

High risk for aspiration; *risk factors: secretions collecting in the esophageal pouch and regurgitation of stomach contents through the fistula into the trachea.*

Ineffective parental coping, *related to fear/anxiety: parental, regarding the infant's diagnosis and impending surgery.*

High risk for ineffective airway clearance: postoperative; *risk factors: increased mucus production and edema.*

High risk for impaired tissue integrity: surgical site; *risk factors: improper suctioning techniques and pressure against the suture line.*

High risk for altered health maintenance (home care); *risk factor: knowledge deficit, regarding infant care in the recuperative phase.*

Planning and Implementation

Preventing Aspiration. In the most common type of esophageal atresia (with fistula), the goals of preoperative care are to prevent aspiration of the secretions from the proximal esophageal pouch and prevent regurgitation of stomach contents through the fistula into the trachea. The latter condition is the more serious in that it causes chemical pneumonitis. Immediate nursing care includes allowing nothing by mouth and performing suctioning* of the nasopharynx until the pouch is drained via a sump tube. This tube requires frequent irrigation to ensure its patency.

Preoperatively, the infant is positioned with head and chest elevated 45 to 60 degrees and on abdomen. This accomplishes two goals: (1) secretions are pooled in the bottom of the esophageal pouch, facilitating withdrawal by constant suction, and (2) gravity counteracts gastric reflux into the trachea and lungs. In spite of this position, distention of the stomach during crying causes gastric regurgitation. Therefore, keeping the baby quiet by stroking and gentle handling are important measures during this period of frequent stimulation that occurs as a result of the required emergency care. Although use of a pacifier may increase salivation, once the sump tube is in the esophageal pouch, the mucus is easily removed; a pacifier will help to diminish crying and satisfy the infant's need to suck.

Promoting Parental Coping. The family of a child with esophageal atresia experiences stress because of the immediacy and intensity of the care required. The nurse supports the parents before surgery by keeping them informed of the status of their infant. The need for suctioning, intravenous therapy, placement of a sump tube, and preparation for the impending surgery are distressing to parents and seemingly disruptive to the infant. They have not yet recovered from the shock of learning that something is wrong with their baby when they need to face yet another stress, the surgery itself. The nurse can be supportive by answering their questions about the purpose of the various procedures and kinds of equipment required. The careful monitoring their baby requires may actually make parents fear that something has gone wrong. The nurse makes ongoing explanations about the routine aspects of the infant's care to alleviate such fears and encourages parents to hold their infant as the condition improves.

Maintaining a Patent Airway and Preventing Trauma to the Surgical Site. Postoperatively, two of the nurse's most important goals are to maintain a patent airway and prevent trauma to the anastomosis. To meet both of these goals, a suction catheter is marked by the surgeon to the maximum length that it can be inserted when suctioning through the nares to ensure that it is not passed farther than a point just above the anastomosis. The nurse should place this premeasured catheter in a clearly visible location with careful instructions so that each person suctioning the infant will measure the catheter used against the premeasured catheter. The nurse carefully observes the infant for early signs of airway obstruction. An anxious expression on the infant's face is often the first sign, followed by an increase in respiratory rate and, when there is serious trouble, the onset of retractions.

Suctioning technique is extremely important. It must be done gently to avoid trauma to the tissues, quickly to avoid oxygen deficiency, and frequently to maintain the airway. The nurse must use judgment regarding frequency of suctioning, realizing that it increases the edema that already exists from the operation. On occasion, endotracheal suctioning may be necessary. This is usually done by a physician under direct vision with a laryngoscope (Canty, 1986).

If ventilatory support is required because of prematurity or respiratory distress, the ventilator is kept at the lowest setting that will achieve adequate ventilation but avoid barotrauma to the lungs and the surgical areas.

Postoperatively, the infant is usually positioned with the head slightly elevated, in a warm, humidified environment. Hyperextension of the neck must be avoided to prevent pull on the sutured esophagus. In the immediate postoperative period, the upright position and placement of the gastrostomy tube (if present) on gravity drainage prevent gastric regurgitation, thereby decreasing pressure on the anastomosis. The infant's position should be changed from back to either side at least every 2 hours to prevent pneumonia and provide comfort. Percussion and postural drainage are also employed as preventive measures; for the

* Suctioning may be necessary every 10 to 15 minutes but must be done gently to avoid traumatizing the mucosa and risk of edema.

first 3 to 4 days, only vibration is performed while the suture line heals (Cassani, 1984).

Oral feedings may be started by the second day, or they may be delayed for 10 days. If the infant is NPO for 10 days, total parenteral nutrition is administered. If gastrostomy has been done, it is placed on gravity drainage for 2 to 3 days, then elevated. Gastrostomy feedings of formula or expressed breast milk are then administered, cautiously increasing volume and strength.

When oral feeding is begun, the nurse should immediately begin teaching the family effective feeding techniques. Extreme care must be taken to prevent the baby from swallowing large amounts of air that would potentiate regurgitation. If the infant is being given gastrostomy feedings while awaiting primary repair, parents are taught the feeding procedure.

Facilitating Home Health Maintenance. The amount of family involvement varies with each institution and family situation. In many cases, parents can be helped to feed their baby after the first oral feeding has been given. Parents also readily learn the technique of gastrostomy feeding and are encouraged to feed their baby as they feel comfortable. If the family has been included in the infant's care during hospitalization, discharge preparation requires little additional time by the nurse.

Parents should become familiar with signs of respiratory distress and be instructed to report any pronounced coughing, gagging, or dysphagia that may indicate anastomotic stricture. Parents should also be informed that the infant will have a raspy cough. Referral is frequently indicated for follow-up visits in the home, particularly when special procedures are necessary.

Esophageal Atresia Without Fistula

Cases of esophageal atresia without a fistula (see Fig. 35–6) require some variations in treatment and care from those described for esophageal atresia with tracheoesophageal fistula. The presenting symptoms are similar, but radiographs demonstrate absence of gastrointestinal gas. In esophageal atresia without fistula, the distance between the proximal and distal esophageal segments is often too great to allow a primary repair.

When direct anastomosis cannot be performed, cervical esophagostomy may be necessary. The proximal esophagus is brought to the exterior (opens on the neck above the left clavicle) to prevent aspiration of secretions from the blind pouch (Fig. 35–8). During this period, the infant is fed by gastrostomy tube, and sham oral feedings are offered to maintain swallowing reflexes and meet the infant's need to suck.

The infant is maintained by gastrostomy feedings until a colon interposition is performed. A segment of the colon is mobilized from the abdomen and interposed in the chest to connect the proximal and distal ends of the esophagus (Fig. 35–8). This procedure is usually done after 6 months of age and before the child reaches 24 months of age. Other surgical procedures include reverse gastric tube and jejunal interposition.

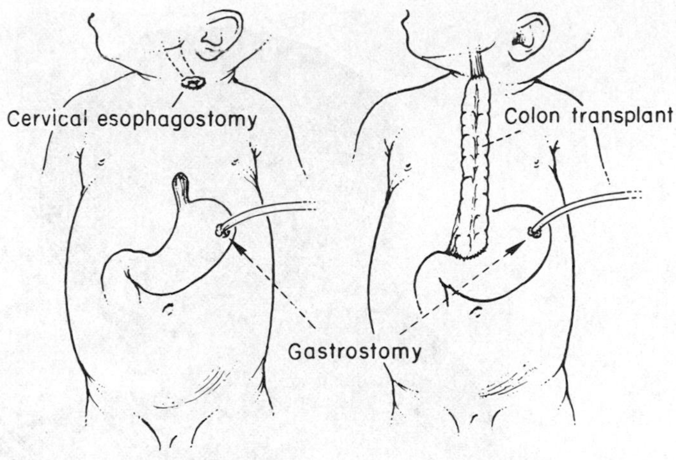

FIGURE 35-8. Stages in treatment of esophageal atresia. Cervical esophagostomy and gastrostomy, which are performed on newborns infants, and colon interposition between the esophagus in the neck and the stomach. (From *Principles of nursing care for the pediatric surgery patient* [2nd ed.], D. Fochtman & J. Raffensperger, Boston: Little, Brown, 1976, p 39. Published by Little, Brown and Company.)

Almost all full-term infants with esophageal atresia survive if no other serious anomalies are present. Pneumonia is a frequent complication in patients with tracheoesophageal fistula. Other complications are a leak at the anastomosis, recurrent fistula, and gastroesophageal reflux, but the most common late complication is stricture at the anastomosis.

Nursing Diagnostic Statements and Collaborative Problems

High risk for aspiration; *risk factor: accumulation of saliva.*

High risk for impaired skin integrity; *risk factor: cervical esophagostomy.*

High risk for altered growth and development; sense of trust; *risk factor: lack of sucking gratification.*

High risk for injury, esophageal stricture; *risk factor: esophageal suture line.*

Planning and Implementation

Preventing Aspiration, Promoting Adequate Nutrition, and Promoting Skin Integrity. Meticulous nursing care is required in the interim period with the cervical esophagostomy to avoid aspiration of saliva and to ensure adequate nutrition. Constant suction of the

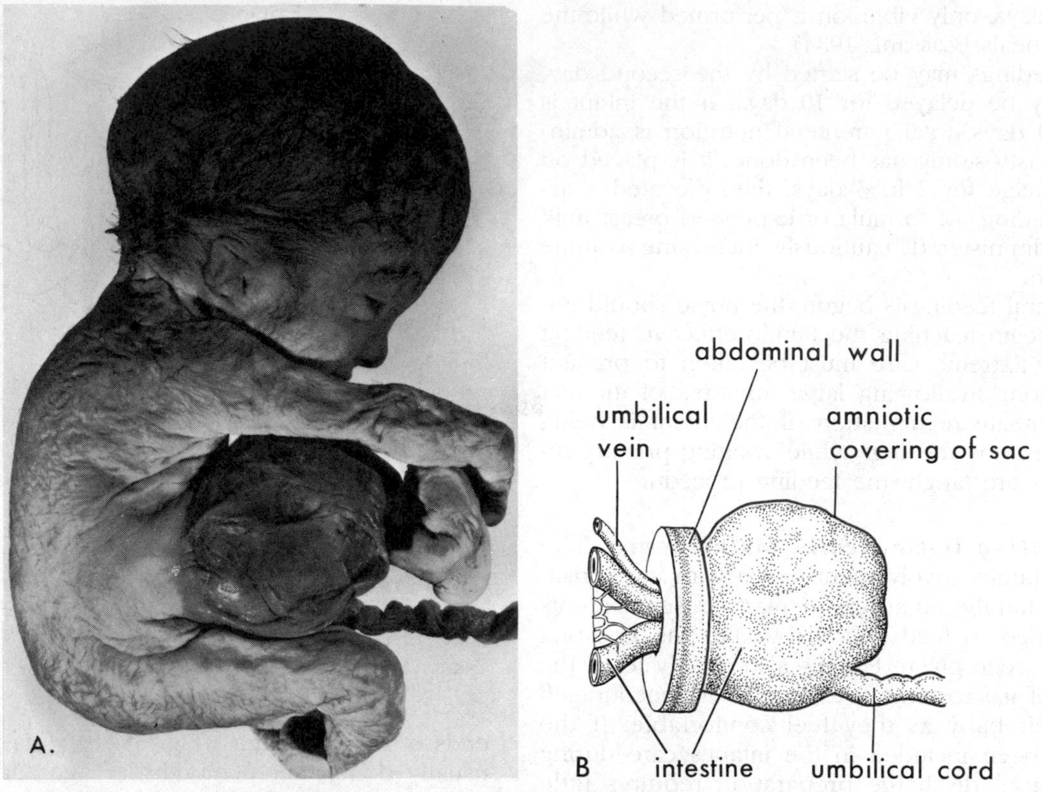

FIGURE 35-9. *A,* Large omphalocele in an immature 28-week fetus. Half actual size. *B,* Drawing illustrating the structure and contents of the hernial sac. The protruding mass of intestine is covered by a transparent, bilaminar membrane composed of peritoneum and amnion. This membrane occasionally ruptures before or during birth. In this case, the eviscerated intestine lies freely around the gaping defect in the abdominal wall.

pouch by a sump tube is used and must be maintained at all times.

Promoting Normal Development by Providing Sucking Development. Sham oral feedings* take additional time and do not provide any nutritive value, but a nurse should not overlook the importance of meeting these normal developmental needs. Parents should be encouraged to give these feedings after their purpose is explained. The skin around the esophagostomy becomes easily excoriated from saliva, which contains digestive enzymes. A protective ointment can be applied, or a pad of soft, absorbent material can be placed over the area and held in place by the infant's shirt. Tape should be avoided because it increases skin breakdown. The pad must be changed frequently and the ointment removed daily to allow thorough cleansing and drying of the skin.

Preventing Esophageal Strictures after a Colon Interposition Has Been Performed. Parents need to be informed about signs of stricture, such as inability to tolerate solid foods, increased drooling, frequent coughing and choking, and dysphagia. It has been reported that one to several dozen dilatations are required in 50 per cent of patients until the esophagus is wide enough to permit passage of food. These dilatations may be required over a period of weeks, months, or years. Therefore, the help the family needs from the professional team varies with the occurrence of complications and the type and length of follow-up treatment required.

Omphalocele

An omphalocele is a herniation of variable amounts of abdominal viscera through the open umbilical ring into the base of the umbilical cord. The size of the defect ranges from 2 to 15 cm. The herniated viscera are enclosed by a translucent membrane with the umbilical cord extending from its surface. A small sac may contain only one or two loops of bowel, but a large sac may contain the liver, spleen, and most of the bowel (Fig. 35-9). A peritoneal sac is always

* Sham feedings are any fluids given orally. These feedings drain immediately from the opening on the neck (esophagostomy) but provide a sucking experience for the infant. When such feedings are given at the time of gastrostomy feeding, the act of sucking is associated with the comfort of satiety.

present in an omphalocele but may be ruptured during or after delivery.

Etiology/Incidence/Pathophysiology

Omphalocele occurs in approximately 1 per 5000 live births and is associated with many other anomalies. Almost all affected infants have malrotation and abnormalities in bowel fixation (Frentner, 1987).

Between the 5th and the 10th weeks of development, the midgut grows rapidly and projects from the abdomen through the umbilical ring into the umbilical cord. Herniation of the midgut into the umbilical cord in this period of embryonic life is a normal developmental process. The intestines thus grow outside the abdominal wall for a portion of fetal life. As the midgut grows, it rotates counterclockwise within the cord. Re-entry of the intestines into the abdominal cavity takes place around the 11th week of fetal life. The intestines continue to rotate as re-entry takes place. If re-entry fails to occur, a persistence of herniation of the intestines (omphalocele) exists, and the abdominal cavity remains small. (It is the presence of abdominal contents within the cavity that causes the cavity to grow and develop; consequently, the larger the omphalocele, the smaller the abdominal cavity.)

Therapeutic Management

The sac must be protected to prevent rupture and infection. Exposure of the sac is also dangerous to the infant because of hypothermia, which results from radiant heat loss. A variety of approaches are used to protect the sac preoperatively. The sac can be covered with warm, sterile, moist saline gauze. A bowel bag (a large plastic bag covering the lower half of the baby's body) is also used and often is preferred because it protects the sac and helps to prevent hypothermia by interfering with radiant heat loss (Frentner, 1987).

Care of the omphalocele is done with sterile gloves and without placing undue pressure on the omphalocele. A nasogastric tube must be inserted and placed on low suction to prevent distention of the stomach and intestines. The infant is kept in an incubator and prepared for immediate surgery, including fluid therapy, administration of antibiotics, and overall stabilization.

Surgical Repair. The ideal form of treatment is primary closure. The sac is excised, the bowel and abdominal organs are examined, the abdomen is stretched, and the abdominal contents are returned to the abdominal cavity, followed by abdominal wall closure. Although this technique may cause pressure within the abdomen and compromise the diaphragm, it is now the most common approach because ventilatory support is highly advanced in neonatal care units. For those infants in whom primary closure is not feasible, a staged repair is done (Frentner, 1987).

In a staged repair, the omphalocele is encased in a Silastic mesh sac. The mesh is sutured in place all around the defect to create a tall, cylindrical silo, which is then tied with umbilical tape or other device to form a pouch over the defect (Fig. 35–10). The contact area between the skin and the mesh is sus-

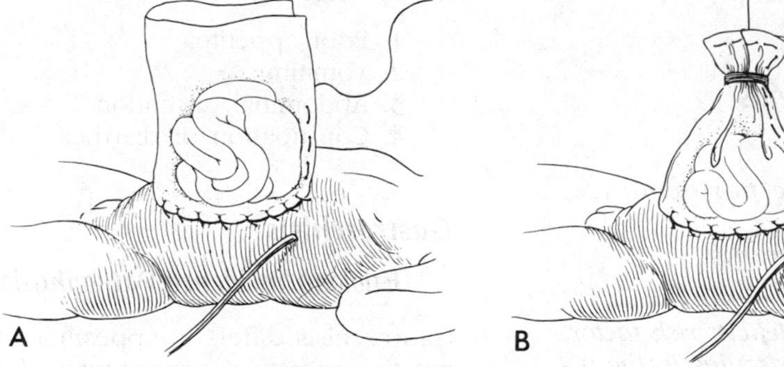

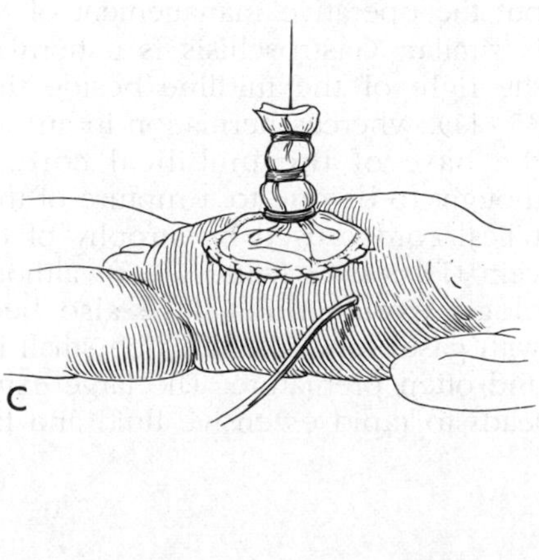

FIGURE 35 - 10. Staged repair of omphalocele. Silastic mesh is used to create a silo, and the viscera are gradually pushed into the abdominal cavity by a system of lower levels of ties. (From *Surgery of the neonate,* A. Coran, Boston: Little, Brown, 1979, p 193. Published by Little, Brown and Company.)

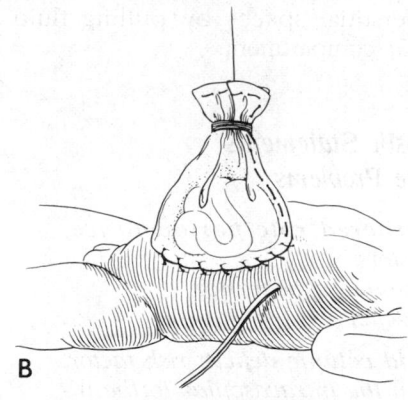

ceptible to infection and can be protected by wrapping the silo with gauze that has been saturated with half-strength Betadine solution. The top of the silo is loosely supported by attaching it to a flexible device suspended from the top of the incubator. This is done to prevent it from falling to one side.

The viscera are moved gradually into the abdominal cavity without causing undue pressure on the vena cava or diaphragm. In stages, the surgeon gently pushes more of the viscera into the abdomen and ties a new tape at the lower level (Fig. 35–10). Within 5 to 10 days, the viscera are usually reduced into the abdominal cavity.

Postoperative Care. When a primary repair is performed, the enclosed abdominal contents cause pressure on the diaphragm. These infants are commonly placed on a ventilator for 7 to 10 days. As third space fluids* cause increasing intra-abdominal pressure, ventilator settings are increased to maintain oxygenation.

If the infant has a staged repair, the bowel is reduced in stages. As the intestines are gradually pushed back into the abdominal cavity, there is increased pressure on the inferior vena cava. This can result in circulatory overload problems manifested by edema in the lower extremities, and the incision must be inspected carefully for signs of dehiscence. After reduction of the viscera is complete, the infant must be returned to surgery for closure of the abdomen.

The type of fluid and method of feeding vary with the severity of the defect. Total parenteral nutrition, gastrostomy feedings, or nasogastric feedings are approaches that are used during the postoperative period, depending on the infant's needs.

A colloid, such as albumin, is generally required to increase osmotic pressure, which will re-establish equilibrium and interstitial spaces by pulling fluid back into the vascular compartment.

Nursing Diagnostic Statements and Collaborative Problems

High risk for altered role performance, parental*; risk factors:*

- *Infant's grotesque appearance.*
- *Knowledge deficit.*

High risk for fluid volume deficit*; risk factor: loss of fluids from the intravascular to the interstitial space.*

High risk for injury, complications of surgery*; risk factor: parental knowledge deficit regarding complications after surgery.*

* Third space fluids are fluids lost from the intravascular space to the interstitial space because of capillary permeability associated with the trauma of surgery. As proteins are lost from the intravascular space, fluids also shift.

Planning and Implementation

Promoting Parental Role Performance. The family will be shocked by the appearance of their infant. When the omphalocele is large, the parents may feel repulsed by the gross abnormality. It may be difficult for them to comprehend that an anomaly of this magnitude can be corrected with excellent results when there are no associated anomalies. They may be pessimistic about the surgery and show little interest in their infant. Because of these factors, the parents may be at risk for experiencing *altered role performance,* such as denial of the parental role and change in perception of the parental role. It is the nurse's role to encourage parents to talk about their infant and help them express what they are experiencing. The nurse needs to be patient with the parents who do not seem to hear or believe that their child can be helped. In this early phase of bonding, the infant's appearance may be a drawback. Even with explanation and encouragement, parents feel overwhelmed. Once the abdomen is closed, the nurse can more easily help them make contact with their infant by touching and holding when possible.

Maintaining Fluid Balance. During the postoperative period, the nurse keeps careful intake and output records and assesses the infant for symptoms of hypovolemia, including tachycardia, decreased urinary output, increased urine specific gravity, and decreased blood pressure.

Teaching to Ensure Prompt Treatment of Complications. The potential complications after surgery include the development of intestinal obstruction or malabsorption. Parents should alert the physician if any of the following signs occur after discharge (Kenner et al, 1988):

1. Poor appetite.
2. Vomiting.
3. Abdominal distention.
4. Constipation or diarrhea.

Gastroschisis

Etiology/Incidence/Pathophysiology

Gastroschisis differs in appearance from omphalocele, but the operative management of the two anomalies is similar. Gastroschisis is a herniation of bowel to the right of the midline beside the umbilicus (Fig. 35–11), whereas herniation in an omphalocele is into the base of the umbilical cord. Gastroschisis is thought to be due to a rupture of the base of the umbilical cord caused by atrophy of the right umbilical vein (Filston & Izant, 1985), although other embryologic explanations have also been given. Infants with gastroschisis tend to be small for gestational age and often premature. The large exposed surface area leads to rapid extensive fluid and heat loss.

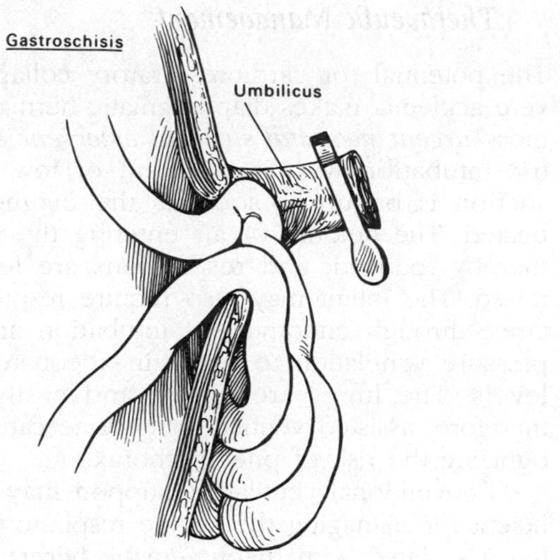

FIGURE 35 - 11. Gastroschisis: a defect in the abdominal wall that allows the intestines to protrude from the abdomen in utero. (From Schwartz, S. I., et al. [1979]. *Principles of surgery*. New York: McGraw-Hill, p 1653. Reproduced with permission of McGraw-Hill.)

Therapeutic Management and Nursing Care

In gastroschisis, the bowel is not protected by a sac, as in omphalocele. Nursing and collaborative diagnoses in these two conditions are often similar. The bowel is irritated by amniotic fluid, and there is considerable inflammation and edema, which interfere with normal bowel activity after surgical repair. The infant should be positioned on the side to permit the bowel to rest on a surface and avoid creating a pull on the bowel as it exits from the abdominal wall defect. Broad-spectrum antibiotics are initiated preoperatively, and nasogastric tube decompression is begun to avert aspiration pneumonia and to decompress the bowel to allow as much bowel as possible to be placed into the abdomen during surgery.

Treatment varies with the amount of bowel outside the abdomen. The bowel should be protected with warmed, saline-soaked sponges and a bowel bag. The intestines can be placed into the abdomen and closed (primary repair); or, for some cases of gastroschisis that are excessively large, a staged repair as for omphalocele is done.

Postoperatively, the infant is managed in a way similar to the infant with omphalocele (see previous discussion). Most of these infants survive and lead normal lives.

Diaphragmatic Hernia

A diaphragmatic hernia is an opening in the diaphragm through which abdominal contents herniate into the thoracic cavity.

Etiology/Incidence/Pathophysiology

Normally, the strong musculature of the diaphragm prevents entrance of abdominal viscera into the chest. When defective embryonic development occurs, an aperture persists in the posterior lateral segment of the diaphragm, located most often on the left side (foramen of Bochdalek) in approximately 90 per cent of the cases (Molenaar, 1991). Abdominal contents protrude through the defect and cause a group of symptoms that nurses should be able to recognize as indicative of diaphragmatic hernia. Abdominal contents in the left thorax compress the lung on the left and displace the heart to the right (dextrocardia) (Fig. 35–12). Congenital hypoplasia of the lung is usually

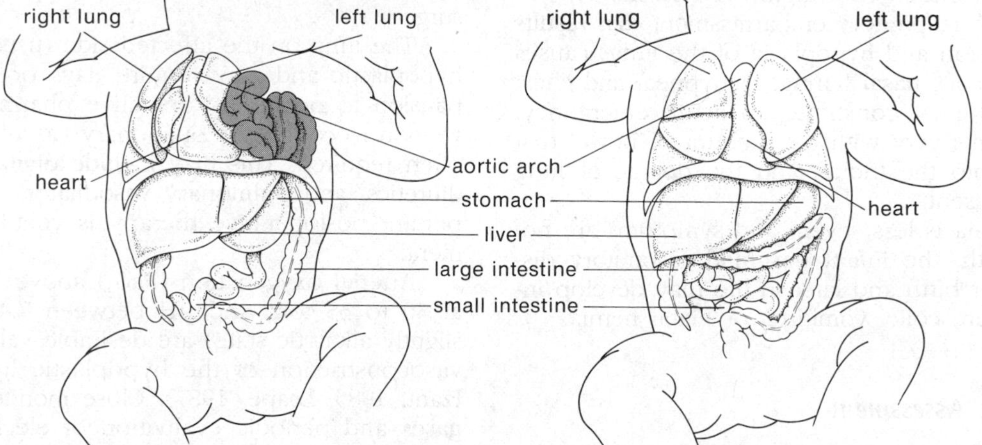

FIGURE 35 - 12. Diaphragmatic hernia; the normal relationship of the heart, lungs, and diaphragm is shown on the right. When an abnormal hole exists in the diaphragm (left), abdominal contents can crowd the lungs. Respiratory embarrassment can result, with severity of symptoms depending on the amount of bowel displaced into the thorax.

present on the affected side; it has also been observed on the opposite side. There is also an increased muscularity of small pulmonary arteries that may contribute to increased pulmonary resistance and hypertension (Behrman, 1987). Respiratory acidosis, hypoxemia, and hypercapnia occur as a result of inadequate exchange of oxygen and carbon dioxide. Metabolic acidosis rapidly develops as peripheral tissues are inadequately perfused. These infants are highly susceptible to development of persistent pulmonary hypertension (severe pulmonary hypertension with a pulmonary artery pressure that is equal to or greater than systemic pressure). Right-to-left shunting then occurs through a patent ductus arteriosus and foramen ovale. A knowledge of the physiologic alterations allows the nurse to help identify this condition and contribute to the care of these infants. Congenital diaphragmatic hernia occurs in 1 per 2500 live births (Molenaar, 1991). Mortality rate is approximately 50 per cent within 6 hours of birth in infants who present with respiratory distress syndrome secondary to diaphragmatic hernia.

Clinical Manifestations

The nurse should expect to find diminished or absent breath sounds on the affected side and listen carefully for bowel sounds that may be audible over the chest. The apical heartbeat will be heard at a point to the right of the usual position owing to dextrocardia. A barrel chest and scaphoid abdomen result, depending on the degree of visceral displacement into the thorax. Respiratory distress usually develops soon after birth. As the infant begins to breathe, the negative intrathoracic pressure causes increasingly more bowel to be drawn into the chest. Further compression of the heart occurs as the infant cries and swallows air, causing the bowel loops within the chest to become increasingly distended (Burrington & Powers, 1985).

The severe respiratory embarrassment that results from compression and hypoplasia of the lungs causes dyspnea, cyanosis, nasal flaring, tachypnea, and chest retraction that may constitute an acute emergency. These symptoms vary with the amount of bowel that is displaced into the thorax and the degree of lung hypoplasia present.

If the hernia is less severe and symptoms are not present at birth, the infant has mild respiratory distress soon after birth and later in life may develop indigestion, severe colic, vomiting, or hiatal hernia.

Diagnostic Assessment

A typical radiograph shows fluid and air-filled loops of the intestine in the chest and a shift of the mediastinum to the unaffected side. The presence of bowel sounds in the chest, a scaphoid abdomen, and a typical radiographic film are indications for surgery (Molenaar, 1991).

Therapeutic Management

The potential for cardiorespiratory collapse and severe acidemia makes diaphragmatic hernia one of the most *urgent neonatal surgical emergencies*. Nasogastric intubation with intermittent or low continuous suction is begun as soon as the diagnosis is suspected. The amount of air entering the intestines is thereby reduced, and respirations are less compromised. The infant may also require respiratory assistance through endotracheal intubation and positive-pressure ventilation to maintain adequate blood gas levels. The lungs are fragile and easily ruptured; therefore, assisted ventilation is done cautiously, recognizing the risk of pneumothorax.

Conventional ventilatory support may not be sufficient for managing the severe respiratory failure often associated with diaphragmatic hernia. New technologies, such as extracorporeal membrane oxygenation and jet ventilation, have had some success. However, the amount of viable lung tissue may be inadequate for meeting the body's needs for oxygenation and ventilation even with these advanced methods (White et al, 1990).

Metabolic acidosis is corrected by the administration of bicarbonate, and ventilatory insufficiency is corrected through positive-pressure ventilation. In patients with an increased carbon dioxide level, metabolic acidosis may be corrected with tromethamine (Williams, 1982).

The surgical procedure involves repositioning the abdominal contents into the abdomen and closing the defect. In most cases, malrotation of the intestines accompanies a diaphragmatic hernia and is also corrected. A gastrostomy tube is inserted through a separate stab wound. In some instances, the peritoneal cavity is too small to contain the abdominal contents; therefore, it is necessary to leave the fascia open and close only the skin. This results in a ventral hernia that is repaired several months after the initial surgery.

The lung on the affected side (usually the left) is hypoplastic and may require days or weeks for expansion to occur. Postoperative pharmacologic intervention to counteract pulmonary vascular resistance is often required. This may include digitalis derivatives, diuretics, and pulmonary vasodilators. The most important postoperative therapy is ventilatory management.

Arterial oxygenation (Pao_2) above 100 torr, $Paco_2$ at 30 to 35 torr, and pH between 7.45 and 7.50 (a slightly alkalotic state) are desirable values to prevent vasoconstriction of the hypoplastic lung (Filston & Izant, 1985; Leape, 1987). Close monitoring of blood gases and periodic evaluation of electrolyte, hematocrit, and blood glucose levels are required.

Survival rate is about 50 per cent for severely affected infants diagnosed within the first 24 to 72 hours (Williams, 1982). When resuscitation and surgery have been managed optimally, the prognosis still depends on three factors: (1) the size of the defect, (2) the degree of hypoplasia of the lung, and (3) the condition of the lung on the unaffected side. In general, the earlier symptoms appear, the poorer the prognosis. The final determinant of success is the total amount of pulmonary function available for gas exchange. Many infants who do not survive are found to have associated severe congenital anomalies (especially of the heart).

Nursing Diagnostic Statements and Collaborative Problems

Impaired gas exchange and ineffective breathing pattern, *related to reduced intrathoracic area available for respiratory excursions.*

High risk for ineffective family coping; *risk factor: threat of loss of child.*

High risk for altered home health maintenance; *risk factor: knowledge deficit.*

Planning and Implementation

Promoting Adequate Gas Exchange and Effective Breathing Pattern. The nurse can improve the infant's condition by instituting some immediate nursing measures: (1) placing the infant in semi-Fowler position reduces intrathoracic pressure and facilitates downward position of the abdominal viscera, and (2) placing the infant on the affected side aids in expansion of the good lung. Facilitating rapid and efficient treatment to relieve respiratory distress is an important nursing role. Infants with diaphragmatic hernia are at high risk for developing persistent pulmonary hypertension. Infants with persistent pulmonary hypertension will not tolerate handling or suctioning without severe respiratory compromise. Progressive distention of the intestines is prevented by maintaining suction and patency of the nasogastric tube. Heat loss increases oxygen demands and compounds the acidosis. Minimal handling and careful thermoregulation are essential strategies to reduce respiratory distress.

Careful monitoring of intravenous fluids and respiratory assessment are nursing responsibilities. If mechanical ventilation is necessary, precautions against pneumothorax must be taken (i.e., low ventilation pressures). Poor lung function continues to be a threat during the postoperative period.

Promoting Family Coping. The nurse must be attentive to the stress that the parents are experiencing during these emergency procedures. Although little time is available to explain the emergency treatment in any detail to parents, briefly telling them what is being done while the baby is being treated is appreciated. Before surgery, the family should be told about the procedure and the postoperative appearance of the infant.

In the postoperative period, parents will continue to feel anxious because of the constant threat of respiratory complications and fear of the equipment needed to maintain their infant. *Extreme caution is taken in the handling of these infants.* No holding, touching, or stimulation is permitted by parents because the infant is at risk for developing persistent pulmonary hypertension. Nurses can intervene by helping the parents understand the reason for this restriction. They also must be kept informed of the general status of their infant.

Facilitating Home Health Maintenance. The family should feed the infant for at least several days before discharge. After surgery, the infant may be lethargic, and coaxing him or her to eat may cause vomiting or gagging. Parents should be taught to burp the infant frequently and not to force the baby to eat when there is disinterest in feeding. Parents should report to the physician

1. An increase in respiratory rate or effort.
2. Cyanosis, whether it occurs during feeding or at rest.
3. Feeding intolerance: vomiting or refusing to eat (Kenner et al, 1988).

Hiatal Hernia

Hiatal hernia is the intermittent or constant displacement of the proximal segment of the stomach through the esophageal hiatus of the diaphragm. This protrusion causes a displacement of the esophagogastric junction and portions of the proximal part of the stomach through the esophageal hiatus into the mediastinum, resulting in the regurgitation of food and fluid. As a consequence, the child may experience recurrent emesis severe enough to result in failure to thrive, aspiration pneumonia, or septic esophagitis with anemia due to gastrointestinal bleeding. Hiatal hernias are rare in the neonatal period, but the frequency increases after the first few months of life.

A hiatal hernia is manifested by symptoms similar to the condition known as gastroesophageal reflux (chalasia). Documentation of the frequency, volume, and presence of bile or blood in the emesis and respiratory symptoms such as coughing, wheezing, or short apneic periods facilitates diagnosis. It is important to determine the adequacy of weight gain by referring to the child's placement on a growth chart.

In addition to the history, diagnosis involves a barium swallow, which will demonstrate reflux from a segment of the stomach situated above the diaphragm into the esophagus.

Management is similar to that for gastroesophageal reflux, including a period of conservative medical management followed by a Nissen-Hill fundoplication if reflux does not resolve after several months of therapy. (See discussion under "Gastrointestinal Dysfunctional Disorders.")

Umbilical Hernia, Inguinal Hernia, and Hydrocele

A hernia is the protrusion of a part of the bowel, ovary, or testis through an abnormal opening in the containing walls of the abdomen. It consists of three parts: the sac or outpouching of the peritoneum, the coverings of the sac that are derived from the abdominal wall, and the contents of the sac—bowel, ovary, or testis. The most frequent locations for hernias are the umbilical and inguinal regions. Although congenital, the hernia may not appear until the infant is several months old.

Etiology/Incidence/Pathophysiology

Umbilical Hernia. During fetal development, the intestines return to the abdominal cavity around the eleventh week of fetal life. Failure of the umbilical ring to close completely as the intestine returns to the abdominal cavity leaves a fascial defect at the base of the umbilical cord. An umbilical hernia is the protrusion of the intestines at the umbilicus through this fascial defect.

Inguinal Hernia. An inguinal hernia is the protrusion of bowel into the groin region (Fig. 35–13*B*). In the boy, the testis descends from the abdominal cavity into the scrotum. The testis carries the parietal peritoneum with it, thus forming a tube (processus vaginalis) from the abdomen to the scrotum. Normally, the processus vaginalis will close spontaneously during development; if not, the descent of the intestine into the patent processus produces an inguinal hernia.

In the girl, the round ligament extends from the uterus through the inguinal canal to its attachment in the labia majora. Weakness of the tissue around the round ligament together with increased abdominal pressure produces an inguinal hernia.

Hydrocele. A hydrocele is a collection of fluid within the processus vaginalis. Hydroceles are most

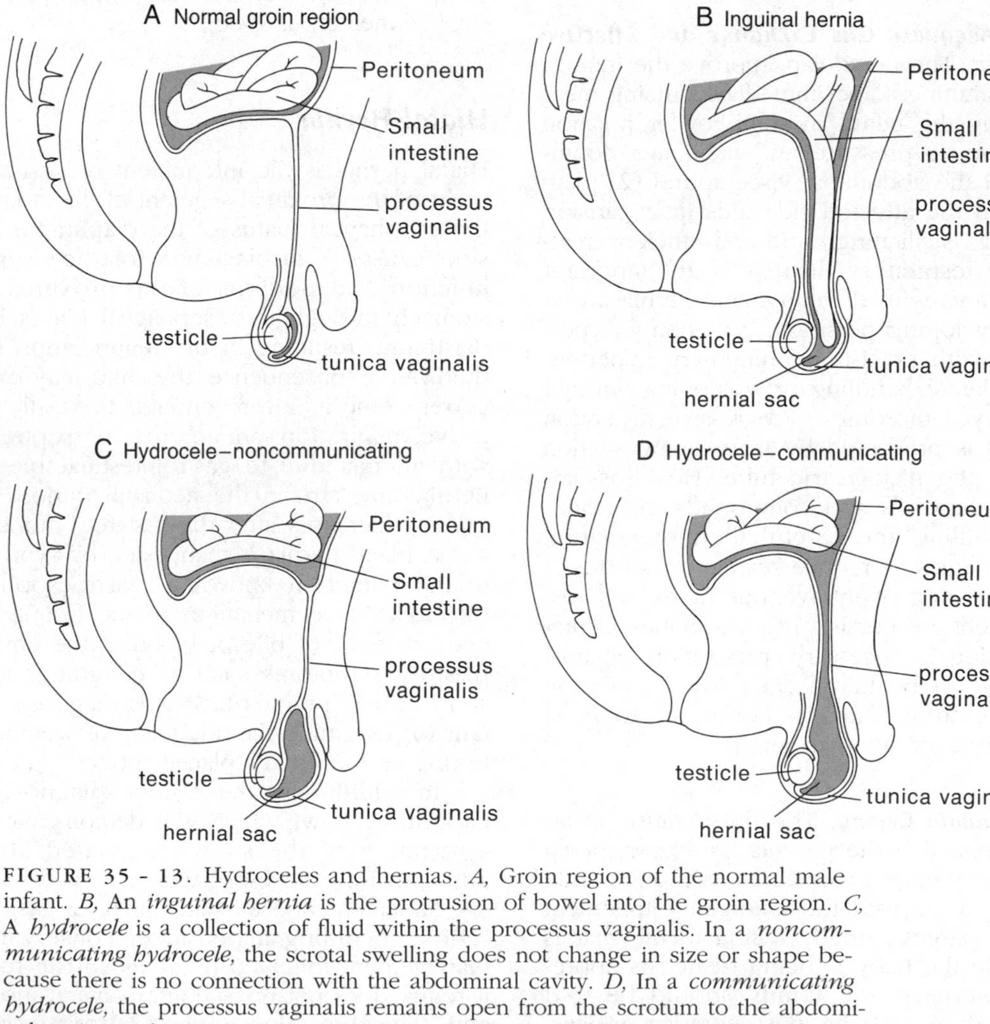

FIGURE 35 - 13. Hydroceles and hernias. *A,* Groin region of the normal male infant. *B,* An *inguinal hernia* is the protrusion of bowel into the groin region. *C,* A *hydrocele* is a collection of fluid within the processus vaginalis. In a *noncommunicating hydrocele,* the scrotal swelling does not change in size or shape because there is no connection with the abdominal cavity. *D,* In a *communicating hydrocele,* the processus vaginalis remains open from the scrotum to the abdominal cavity, and scrotal swelling may vary in size during the course of an infant's day.

commonly seen in boys. The type seen at birth presents as a soft scrotal swelling. In this type, the upper portion of the processus vaginalis is obliterated, but the portion within the scrotum (tunica vaginalis) remains open. Peritoneal fluid is trapped within the tunica vaginalis. There is no communication with the peritoneal cavity—thus, it is referred to as a *noncommunicating* hydrocele (Fig. 35–13*C*). The scrotal swelling is painless and does not change in size or shape when the baby cries or changes position. It is not reducible, but it can be easily transilluminated. The fluid is gradually absorbed, and usually this type does not require surgery.

A *communicating* hydrocele is more often associated with a hernia because the processus vaginalis remains open from the scrotum to the abdominal cavity (Fig. 35–13*D*). Scrotal swelling may not be noticed until a few weeks after birth or even later in infancy. When a hydrocele communicates with the abdominal cavity, it may vary in size from one time to another. During sleep, decreased intra-abdominal pressure and a supine position effect a decrease in scrotal swelling by morning. With an upright position and activity during the day, the scrotum again gradually enlarges. If a hydrocele is present after 3 months of age, it usually means that a hernia is present and should be repaired.

Diagnostic Assessment

Umbilical Hernia. Diagnosis is made by observation and palpation of the defect. Parents should be advised that 90 per cent of these hernias resolve on their own. It is rare for an umbilical hernia to become incarcerated. (If the hernia has not resolved by age 5 years, surgery is scheduled, usually on an outpatient basis.) Parents should be advised not to use binders, tape, or other materials to compress the hernia. It has never been documented that these remedies aid in the closure of the defect, and they can cause infection.

Inguinal Hernia or Hydrocele. Diagnosis of inguinal hernia is made by observation and palpation of a bulge in the groin area. Frequently, the diagnosis must be made on the basis of a history of a bulge in the groin that a parent has noted while the infant was crying or straining to defecate. During the examination, it is important to check that both testes are in the scrotal sac and to determine the presence or absence of a scrotal or cord hydrocele (a collection of fluid in the tunica vaginalis of the testicle or along the spermatic cord). See Chapter 13 for assessment strategies.

The hernia causes the infant little discomfort unless it becomes incarcerated. There is a high frequency of incarceration of an inguinal hernia in the first 3 months of life. Parents must be advised to watch for redness in the area of the hernia, increased swelling of the hernia, and an inability to reduce the hernia. Under any of these circumstances, they should be advised to contact their pediatrician immediately.

Therapeutic Management

Umbilical Hernia. The umbilical hernia is repaired through a transverse incision, which is made within the fold of the inferior aspect of the umbilicus. The incision is then carried through the subcutaneous fat and areolar tissue to the linea alba at the inferior rim of the umbilical ring. A plane is dissected around the ring at the level of the linea alba, and the sac is dissected away from the umbilical skin. The sac is then transected and closed along with the fibrous umbilical ring in one to two layers. The incision is coated with a protective sealant, and a compression dressing is applied for 7 days.

Inguinal Hernia or Hydrocele. Surgery to correct either inguinal hernia or hydrocele, or both, is done on an outpatient basis. It is believed that this is less stressful for the child and family. Preoperative teaching begins in the surgeon's office; the procedure, the need for blood work, and restrictions for food and fluids are explained to the parents.

All inguinal hernias should be promptly repaired to avoid incarceration. Surgical treatment is rarely indicated for a hydrocele (90 per cent resolve spontaneously). If surgery is indicated (i.e., large, symptomatic, or one that does not disappear by age 5 years), the procedure is the same as for inguinal hernia: ligation of the processus vaginalis.

Parents should be advised that the scrotum may become edematous and appear bruised. This is due to the manipulation of the testis during the operation and should resolve in 1 to 3 weeks after the operation. The incision is coated with a protective sealant, and no dressing is applied.

Nursing Diagnostic Statement

Altered health maintenance, related to parental knowledge deficit regarding home care after surgery.

Planning and Implementation

Facilitating Health Maintenance after Umbilical Hernia Repair. The child is ready for discharge from the recovery room within 2 hours. The parents are requested to sponge bathe the child and to maintain the compression dressing for a week. It is important that the parents attempt to limit the child's physical activities for several weeks, although this is not easy to accomplish. Otherwise, there are no dietary or activity restrictions. The child is seen 1 week after surgery, and the dressing is removed. The parents should be advised that edema will still be present and that this will decrease over time.

Facilitating Health Maintenance after Repair of Inguinal Hernia or Hydrocele. The major concern for home care of the child after surgery for inguinal hernia or hydrocele is protection of the incision. Parents should be advised to change diapers frequently and to gently remove feces from the skin with soap and water. Sponge baths (versus tub) should be given for 1 week. In an older child, parents should attempt to limit physical activities for several weeks. Otherwise, the child has no restrictions.

The nurse should make sure that the family receives a prescription for an analgesic before discharge. The infant or young child is likely to be uncomfortable in the first day or two after surgery. Parents who understand the principles of correct dosage and regular administration can often manage the child's discomfort effectively even with an analgesic as mild as acetaminophen.

Parents should be given a telephone number through which they can obtain nursing or medical advice at any time of the day or night during the immediate postoperative period. The nurse should anticipate the family's anxiety about caring for the infant or young child after outpatient surgery. Confident, well-planned, and unhurried explanations can be invaluable to a concerned family.

Intestinal Atresia

Etiology/Incidence/Pathophysiology

Intestinal atresia is the complete obliteration of the intestinal lumen. The most common sites of intestinal atresia are the duodenum and ileum, followed by the jejunum, then the colon. Atresia is believed to be the result of a vascular accident in utero. It occurs about once in 1500 to 3000 live births. A large number of children with duodenal atresia have other anomalies, such as Down syndrome.

Clinical Manifestations

Polyhydramnios (excess amniotic fluid) should raise the suspicion that esophageal or duodenal atresia is present. The clinical manifestations of atresia are signs of intestinal obstruction that include bilious vomiting, jaundice, abdominal distention (more pronounced in ileal atresia), and failure to pass meconium. Distention of the abdomen causes an elevation of the diaphragm, necessitating close observation for respiratory distress.

Diagnostic Assessment

Atresia is documented on an abdominal radiograph by evidence of dilated loops of bowel and air-fluid levels. Ileal atresia can be differentiated by noting dilated proximal loops of bowel and small, unused distal bowel. In duodenal atresia, an upright abdominal film will document a distended stomach with the appearance of a "double bubble." This strongly suggests that the obstruction is in the duodenum. The two distinct bubbles are formed by the air that rises to the top of the duodenum and to the top of the stomach. The rest of the abdomen is devoid of gas. An upper gastrointestinal and small bowel series is performed to distinguish between small and large bowel distention, to determine if the colon is functional or nonfunctional, and to locate the position of the cecum to rule out the presence of an abnormal rotation of the cecum and duodenum. It is important to obtain results of these tests quickly. The infant is at risk of developing volvulus (a twisting of the bowel on itself).

Therapeutic Management

Preoperatively, the infant is maintained in the incubator, and a nasogastric tube is inserted through the mouth or nose to decompress the abdomen and prevent further vomiting and gaseous distention. It is essential that this tube remain patent; this may require irrigation with air or water once every 4 to 6 hours. Baseline laboratory studies (complete blood count and electrolytes) are done, and the infant is maintained on intravenous hydration. Broad-spectrum antibiotics are administered; fluid and electrolyte deficits must be corrected before surgery.

During the surgical procedure, the entire bowel is inspected for evidence of malrotation, volvulus, and atresia. Various types of anastomosis (side-to-side, end-to-end) are performed between the proximal and distal segments of the bowel. A gastrostomy may be performed if early recovery is not anticipated. In some instances, an end-to-end anastomosis is not possible because of the size disparity of the two ends. In these circumstances, an ostomy is performed with a nearby fistula (Burrington & Powers, 1985). The two ends can be anastomosed at a later time. No ostomy will be performed if the atresia is proximal duodenum or jejunum.

Postoperatively, gastric decompression is maintained until there is evidence of gastric emptying and bowel sounds are heard. Parenteral nutrition may be required, depending on the speed of recovery. Oral or gastrostomy feedings are begun in small amounts and are increased in volume and strength gradually. It is important to document the consistency and number of stools per shift.

Ninety per cent or more of the infants operated on for duodenal atresia survive the operation; the major complication is anastomotic strictures. Malabsorption may be a problem in jejunal or ileal atresia because of an inadequate intestinal surface for absorption.

Nursing Care

Many times, the parents are able to see the infant only briefly before he or she is taken to the operating room or is transferred to another hospital. It is essential to spend time with the family, to answer their questions, and to encourage involvement in the infant's care. Postoperatively, the nurse ensures proper functioning of gastric decompression (see "Decompression by a Nasogastric Tube" under "Caring for a Child with a Nasogastric Tube" for further information). Maintenance and monitoring of intake via parenteral nutrition or gastrostomy tube is a nursing priority.

Malrotation and Volvulus

Volvulus is the twisting of the intestine on itself. Malrotation is an abnormal rotation of the cecum and duodenum (Fig. 35–14).

Etiology/Incidence/Pathophysiology

During fetal development, the abdominal cavity is not able to accommodate the rapidly developing intestine; therefore, a large portion of it herniates into the umbilical sac outside the abdomen. The position of the intestine at this time is reversed from its later normal position; the ascending colon is on the left instead of its later normal position on the right. Around the eleventh week of gestation, the intestinal loops return to the abdominal cavity. As the bowel moves into the abdomen, it rotates until the colon is in its normal position in the lower right quadrant, and the mesentery of the ascending colon fixes to the posterior abdominal wall. Three abnormalities can occur during this process: malrotation of the colon, volvulus of the midgut, and formation of adhesive bands that constrict the duodenum.

If rotation of the bowel is incomplete, the mesentery cannot attach in its usual position. The duodenum then becomes trapped behind peritoneal bands that fix the abnormally placed cecum. The inadequate fixation of the mesentery allows twisting of the small intestine (volvulus), resulting in compromise of the bowel's blood supply and sometimes leading to life-threatening necrosis.

Clinical Manifestations

The symptoms are usually evident during the first postnatal week. The nurse should watch for any signs of intestinal obstruction: bilious vomiting or increased vomiting of feedings, passage of bloody stool, and distention of the abdomen. The physician should be notified of any of these signs.

Diagnostic Assessment

A radiographic film of the abdomen will show multiple distended bowel loops and a large bowel that is devoid of gas. It is essential to obtain a barium enema study or an upper gastrointestinal radiograph as soon as the diagnosis is suspected. The barium enema will show the cecum abnormally placed. The upper gastrointestinal radiograph will reveal the position of the ligament of Treitz. Surgery is scheduled immediately to prevent the development of intestinal gangrene.

It is important to explain the anomaly to the family. This is a stressful period because the parents ini-

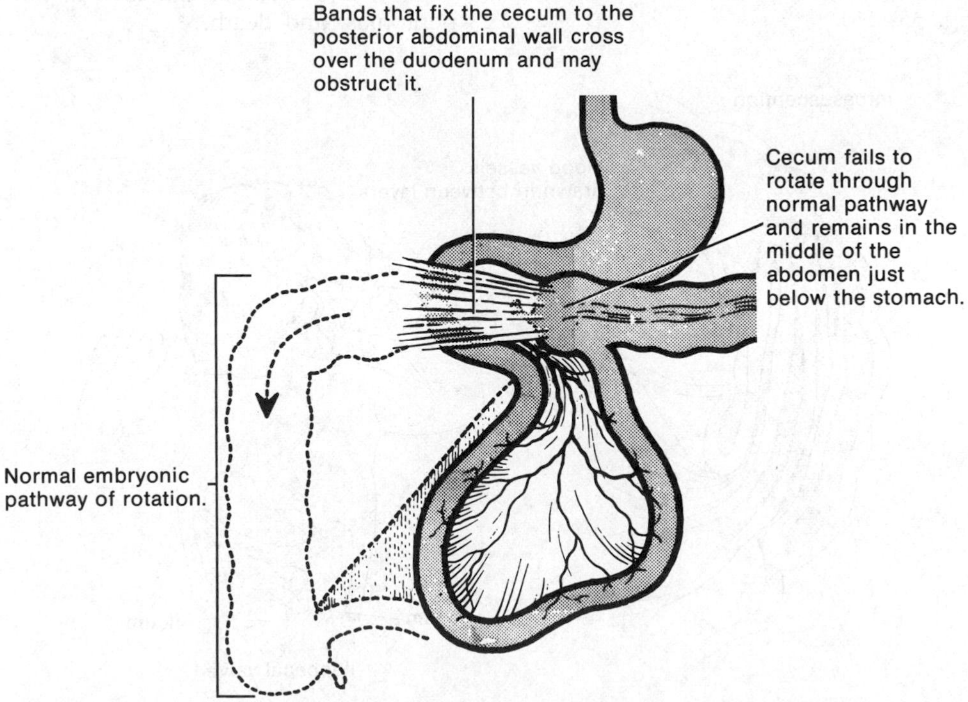
Bands that fix the cecum to the posterior abdominal wall cross over the duodenum and may obstruct it.
Cecum fails to rotate through normal pathway and remains in the middle of the abdomen just below the stomach.
Normal embryonic pathway of rotation.

FIGURE 35-14. Malrotation of the intestine. (From Nixon, H., & O'Donnell, B. [1961]. *The essentials of pediatric surgery*. Philadelphia: JB Lippincott.)

tially have perceived the infant as healthy. The parents will have questions concerning the cause of the anomaly, the operation, and postoperative care.

Therapeutic Management

The infant is given broad-spectrum antibiotics intravenously, vitamin K is administered, and a nasogastric tube is placed in the stomach as a means of decompression. During the operation, the bowel is inspected for areas of obstruction. The intestine is untwisted to relieve the vascular obstruction. The bands of tissue (Ladd bands) between the cecum and abdominal wall are divided. The duodenum is then positioned vertically on the right side of the abdomen, and the cecum is placed in the left lower quadrant. An appendectomy is also performed.

Nursing Care

The child is maintained on intravenous hydration postoperatively. If stooling does not occur by the third or fourth postoperative day, parenteral hyperalimentation should be considered. Once the infant has begun to defecate, oral feedings are initiated. The feedings are increased slowly in volume and strength. Parents are encouraged to hold, feed, and care for their infant during this period, which will help them establish a positive infant-parent relationship.

Intussusception

Intussusception is an invagination or telescoping of part of the intestine into an adjacent distal portion of the intestine (Fig. 35–15).

Etiology/Incidence/Pathophysiology

Intussusception occurs most commonly in healthy, well-nourished male infants around 6 months of age. It can occur in children of any age but is rare before 3 months and occurs with decreasing frequency after the age of 3 years.

The cause of intussusception is unknown in most cases. An etiologic factor is determined in fewer than 10 per cent of afflicted children. Some of the identifiable causes are Meckel diverticulum, an ileal polyp, lymphosarcoma, and duplication of the bowel. There is a seasonal incidence that has been linked to the prevalence of adenovirus infections in the early summer and early winter months.

During an infection, there is hypertrophy of the Peyer patches (configuration of lymph nodules, single or in groups, in the ileum near its junction with the colon). It is thought that the presence of the resultant swelling may stimulate peristalsis (Shandling, 1992). The ileum, with its greater number of Peyer patches, thus has greater potential to become the lead point for invagination into adjacent bowel.

The most common type of intussusception begins at or near the ileocecal valve, pushing into the cecum and onto the colon (referred to as ileocecocolic or ileocolic). The lumen of the bowel is compromised, and vascular flow is obstructed. The involved intestine becomes inflamed and edematous, with eventual bleeding from the mucosa. The initial incomplete obstruction progresses to a state of complete obstruction, producing distention and vomiting. Strangulation of the bowel can result, although this does not usually occur in the first 24 hours (Shandling, 1992). Intussusception, if untreated, can lead to intestinal gangrene, peritonitis, and death.

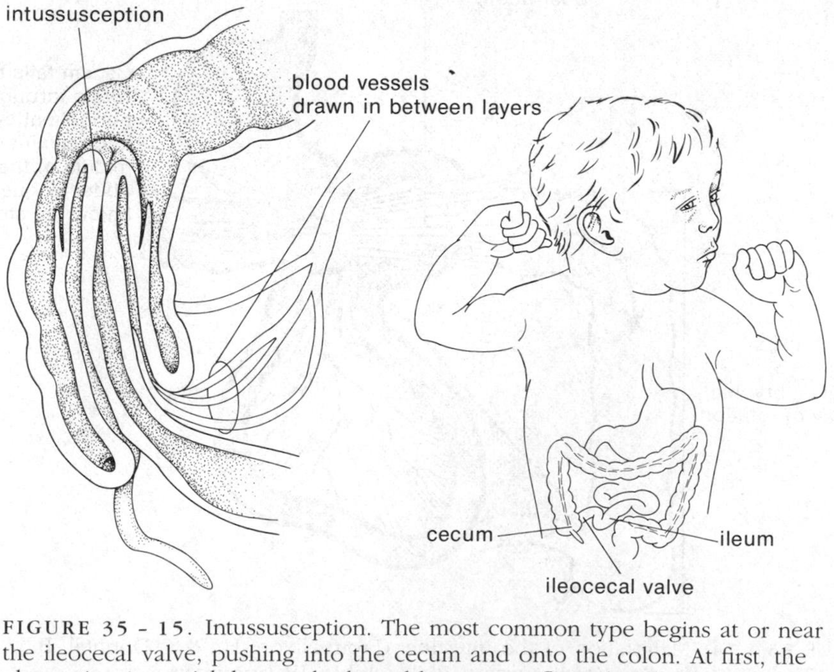

FIGURE 35-15. Intussusception. The most common type begins at or near the ileocecal valve, pushing into the cecum and onto the colon. At first, the obstruction is partial; but as the bowel becomes inflamed and edematous, complete obstruction occurs.

Clinical Manifestations

The infant with intussusception has symptoms that are frightening and disturbing to parents. A healthy infant suddenly shows symptoms of severe abdominal pain, which recurs at frequent intervals. The infant draws the legs up sharply with a piercing cry. The infant usually vomits, becomes extremely restless, and often appears diaphoretic and pale. Normal stool may be passed during the initial phase. The attack then subsides, and the infant shows no abnormal signs between the severe attacks of abdominal pain.

As the condition worsens, the infant becomes lethargic and progressively weaker. Vital signs reflect a shocklike state, vomitus may now be bile stained, and abdominal distention is apparent. There will be either no stool or a stool characteristically described as currant jelly–like in appearance owing to the presence of blood and mucus as a result of intestinal irritation. This type of stool occurs in about 50 per cent of cases (Filston & Izant, 1985). Blood usually appears in the stool within 12 hours of the onset of symptoms. Between attacks of pain, in some cases a sausage-shaped mass can be palpated in the right upper quadrant of the abdomen.

Diagnostic Assessment

A barium enema study confirms the diagnosis and in many cases can successfully treat the intussusception through hydrostatic reduction.

The nurse must be able to give accurate guidance when parents initially report symptoms. Because the infant may sleep and is comfortable between attacks, the seriousness of the symptoms can be overlooked by a nurse who is not familiar with the characteristic pattern of their onset. Nurses must advise the family to seek immediate medical attention and explain to them that even though the baby seems normal between attacks, the condition may change rapidly.

Therapeutic Management

Three types of treatment are used for intussusception: (1) reduction by the hydrostatic pressure of a barium enema, (2) reduction by surgical manipulation, and (3) surgical resection of a nonreducible involved intestine.

Reduction by Barium Enema. During the first 24 hours of symptoms, the intussusception can be reduced by hydrostatic pressure. The success rate varies, but in one review, it was found to be 70 per cent (Liu et al, 1986). Contraindications for reduction by barium enema are (1) a complete mechanical obstruction and (2) a high temperature, vomiting, and signs of peritonitis, sepsis, or shock (Welch, 1986).

The infant must be prepared for a barium enema as though surgery will follow, because if reduction by barium enema is unsuccessful, the infant undergoes an operation immediately. The family must understand the purpose of the barium enema and must realize that surgery may be necessary. Preparation for the barium enema includes giving the infant nothing by mouth, insertion of a nasogastric tube to prevent aspiration during the barium enema, and administration of intravenous fluids. Sedating the infant with morphine is helpful because it calms the infant and relaxes the bowel. Preparation for such treatment occurs rapidly and may leave parents stunned. They can be helped to calm the infant if the nurse attends to their need for a description of the problem and gives frequent explanations of what is occurring. (The nurse can use a rubber glove or tube gauze to describe telescoping of the bowel, inverting a finger of the glove or the gauze into itself to illustrate intussusception.) Barium is administered rectally from a height of 30 to 36 inches above the tube, and the pathway of the barium is observed by fluoroscopy. The pressure caused by the flow of barium frequently results in extension of the bowel to its normal position. Even when reduction is successful, however, hospitalization is recommended until feedings are tolerated, stool is passed, and the infant is asymptomatic.

When feedings are started, parents should be encouraged to feed the infant, with clear instructions about the amount to be fed. They should be forewarned that stool will contain grayish white barium and that each diaper should be checked by the nurse.

Surgical Treatment. As noted previously, surgical intervention is necessary when the barium enema is not successful in reduction and when there is clinical evidence of intestinal obstruction with abdominal distention. The intussusception is reduced surgically by milking the intestine (distal to proximal) to move the invaginated portion back to its normal position. (Attempts lasting longer than 10 minutes are not recommended.) If this is not successful, intestinal resection and anastomosis may be necessary.

Spontaneous reduction occasionally occurs. When an intussusception is reduced by barium enema, there is a recurrence rate of 5 to 10 per cent. Recurrence is also possible after surgical reduction; it is least common after intestinal resection. The length of time that elapses between onset and reduction of the intestines affects prognosis. Prognosis is excellent if the condition is treated within 12 to 24 hours and grave in the event of strangulation.

Nursing Care

Postoperatively, the nurse must help the family cope with the stress of caring for the infant, who is not allowed to eat, requires frequent position changes, and needs to be restrained to prevent dislodging of the nasogastric tube and intravenous needle or catheter. Also, the nurse must frequently assess the infant's vital signs (particularly a high fever), blood pressure, bowel sounds, sutures and dressing, level of pain, proper functioning of the nasogastric tube, and accurate infusion of intravenous fluids. (See also Table 35–15, Care of the Child after Abdominal Surgery.)

Meckel Diverticulum

Meckel diverticulum is a congenital anomaly characterized by an outpouching of the ileum. This outpouching is caused by a persistent duct that in early embryonic development connected the primitive gut to the yolk sac (omphalomesenteric duct). Failure of the duct to atrophy results in a Meckel diverticulum.

Etiology/Incidence/Pathophysiology

The condition may be asymptomatic for many years and may be found only in the course of abdominal surgery. It is the most common gastrointestinal anomaly and is present in 1 to 2 per cent of the population. It is usually asymptomatic. Meckel diverticulum may manifest itself at any age, but the majority of symptomatic cases become apparent before the child reaches 2 years of age. This anomaly is significant because it can cause intestinal obstruction, massive bleeding, perforation, and peritonitis. The diverticulum may be attached to the anterior abdominal wall directly or by a fibrous cord. Most often, it is free from the abdominal wall. The band may compress another loop of intestine and cause obstruction, or it may be the focal point of a volvulus (twisting of the intestines). The free outpouching ileum can act as a lead point for intussusception, with resulting symptoms.

Clinical Manifestations

Bleeding occurs because the tip of the outpouched ileum frequently contains ectopic gastric mucosa rather than ileal mucosa (Fig. 35–16). The gastric secretions are an irritant to the surrounding tissue. Eventually there is severe ulceration of the ileal mucosa at the base of the diverticulum or within the adjacent ileum to which it is connected. The eroded area hemorrhages, resulting in painless rectal bleeding, the most common sign in children. Rectal bleeding is dark red or bright red and is usually passed without stool. Less frequently, the diverticulum becomes inflamed and may perforate.

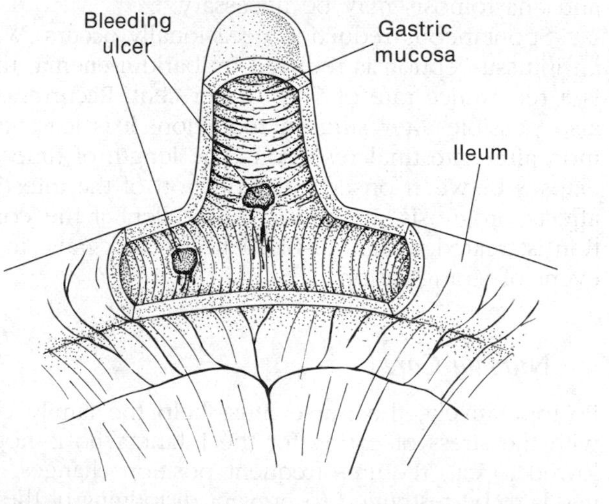

FIGURE 35 - 16. Meckel diverticulum is an outpouching of the ileum. This anomaly may remain asymptomatic for years, may become a source of intestinal bleeding, may become inflamed and lead to perforation, or may become the focal point for intussusception, obstruction, or volvulus.

Diagnostic Assessment

Meckel diverticulum is generally not demonstrated on radiographs. Diagnosis is made by the history and on clinical manifestations (i.e., massive rectal bleeding). A technetium scan shows an area of radioactivity suggestive of gastric mucosa in the diverticulum but is negative in about half of symptomatic patients.

Therapeutic Management

The immediate concern is to remove the lesion surgically to prevent hypovolemic shock from bleeding. When a peptic ulcer is present in the adjacent ileum, excision of the involved bowel is necessary. Postoperatively, the child has a nasogastric tube and requires the usual postoperative care indicated for bowel surgery.

Nursing Care

Postoperative nursing responsibilities are to maintain patency of the nasogastric tube, administer intravenous fluid, check vital signs and bowel sounds, calculate intake and output until eating is resumed, and provide for the early resumption of a normal level of activity. (See also Table 35–15.)

It is frightening to parents when their otherwise healthy child develops massive rectal bleeding and requires immediate surgery. The family needs frequent reassurance that the child is recuperating satisfactorily. The nurse can reduce the stress the child and family have experienced by keeping parents informed and ensuring that their questions are answered.

Hirschsprung Disease (Congenital Aganglionosis or Aganglionic Megacolon)

Hirschsprung disease is a congenital abnormality in which obstruction is caused by reduced motility in the colon.

Etiology/Incidence/Pathophysiology

Hirschsprung disease occurs in 1 in 5000 full-term births and predominantly affects boys. It has been associated with other anomalies, such as Down syndrome and genitourinary abnormalities. It is usually diagnosed in infancy.

Hirschsprung disease is also referred to as congenital megacolon (large colon present since birth). The anomaly is characterized by partial to complete obstruction associated with the distal alimentary tract (Fig. 35–17*A*). The absence of intramural ganglion cells (nerve cells) involves both the submucosal and intermuscular nerve plexuses. This may involve as small an area as the lower rectum (short-segment Hirschsprung disease) or as large an area as the entire colon (long-segment Hirschsprung disease). The lack of ganglion cells prevents the bowel from transmitting the coordinated peristaltic waves that normally enable fecal material to pass through the alimentary tract. The internal sphincter is unable to relax; evacuation of solids, liquids, and gases is prevented. Thus, the patient has a mechanical intestinal obstruction (Sieber, 1986).

Clinical Manifestations

The onset of symptoms is usually noted in the first 24 to 48 hours of life. The nurse should consider Hirschsprung disease as a possible diagnosis for any infant who does not pass meconium within the first 24 hours of life and alert the physician. The nurse should watch the infant closely for passage of meconium or for bile-stained vomitus and abdominal distention. In older infants, the initial symptom is constipation or overflow diarrhea or both. In addition, abdominal dis-

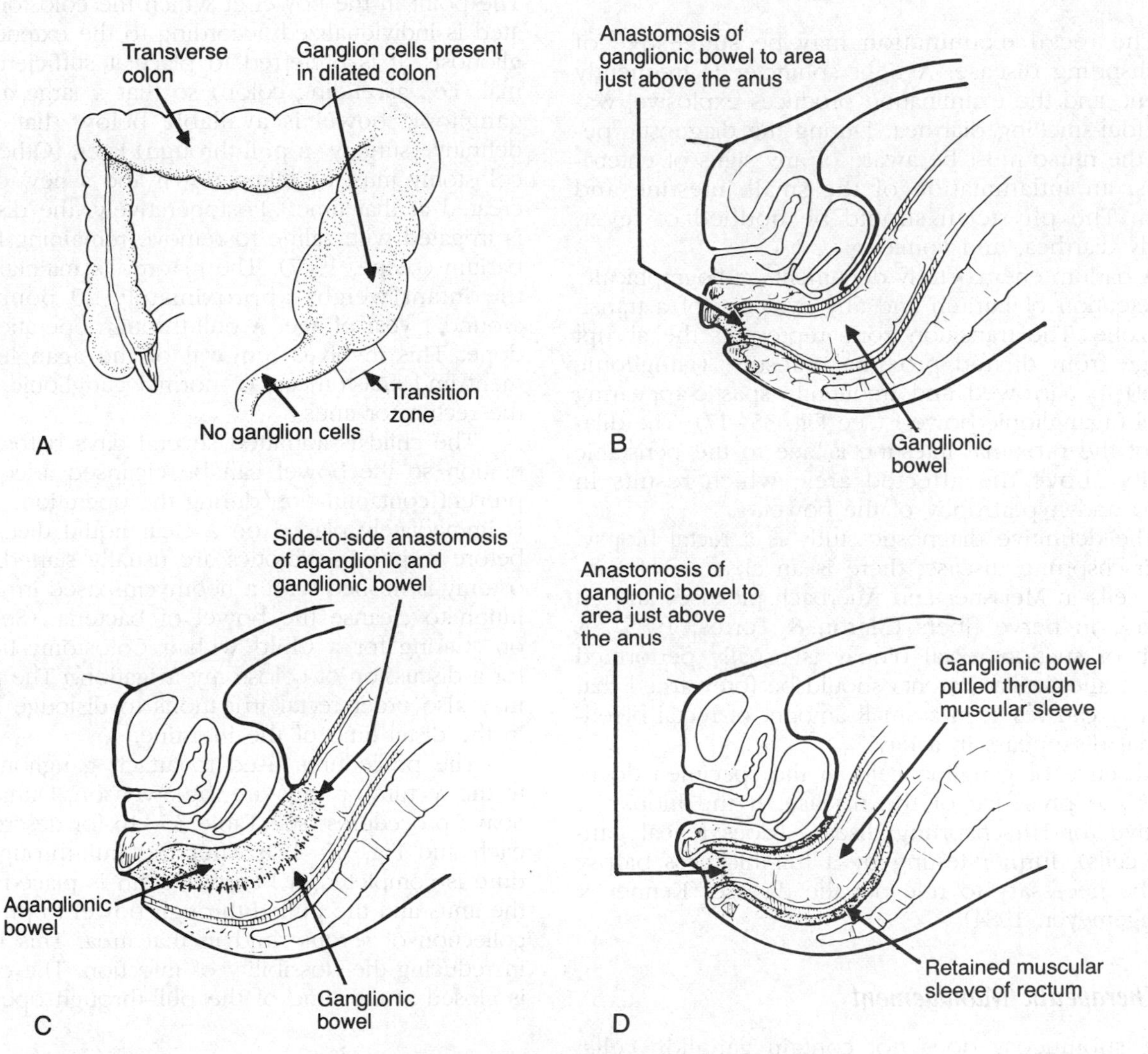

FIGURE 35-17. Hirschsprung disease and surgical procedures for repair. *A*, Lack of ganglion cells in a segment of the colon prevents the transmission of normal peristaltic waves and results in intestinal obstruction. *B*, Swenson procedure. Aganglionic bowel is completely resected, and ganglionic bowel is anastomosed to the anus (see Table 35–16 for further description). *C*, Duhamel procedure. Ganglionic bowel is anastomosed side-to-side to aganglionic bowel and to the anus. *D*, Soave procedure. Ganglionic bowel is brought through a retained muscular sleeve of the rectum and anastomosed to the rectum.

tention is present, and a large fecal mass may be palpated. Anorexia, malnutrition, muscle wasting, nausea, and lethargy are manifestations of more advanced involvement.

Diagnostic Assessment

The history obtained should include a detailed documentation of family members with stooling difficulties. A genetic factor has been associated with Hirschsprung disease in 3 to 5 per cent of all cases. There is an 18 per cent frequency for brothers of girls with long aganglionic segments to also have the disease and a 0.6 per cent frequency for sisters of boys with short aganglionic segments to likewise be affected. This is an important consideration for genetic counseling. (See Chapter 31 for a discussion of genetic counseling.)

The rectal examination may be suggestive of Hirschsprung disease. A tight sphincter is frequently evident, and the examination produces explosive, watery, foul-smelling diarrhea. During the diagnostic period, the nurse must be aware of any signs of enterocolitis, an inflammation of the small intestine and colon. The physician should be notified of fever, bloody diarrhea, and vomiting.

A barium enema study documents radiographically the retention of barium and any evidence of a transition zone. The transition zone represents the abrupt change from dilated proximal intestine (ganglionic bowel) to narrowed and frequently spastic-appearing bowel (aganglionic bowel) (see Fig. 35–17). The dilation of the proximal intestine is due to the peristaltic activity above the affected area, which results in edema and hypertrophy of the bowel.

The definitive diagnostic study is a rectal biopsy. In Hirschsprung disease, there is an absence of ganglion cells in Meissner and Auerbach plexuses and an increase in nerve fibers (Martin & Torres, 1985). A punch or suction rectal biopsy is usually performed without anesthesia. Parents should be forewarned that a biopsy can result in a small amount of rectal bleeding that disappears in a day.

Absence of ganglion cells in the specimen documents the presence of the disease. If the biopsy is negative for Hirschsprung disease (does reveal ganglion cells), further testing by a full-thickness biopsy may be necessary to rule out the disease (Kenner & Breuggemeyer, 1984).

Therapeutic Management

If the submucosa does not contain ganglion cells, surgery is scheduled. The infant is prepared for surgery by placement of a nasogastric tube to low suction for abdominal decompression, administration of broad-spectrum antibiotics and vitamin K (depending on the age of the child and whether these were already given in the newborn nursery), and initiation of intravenous fluids with electrolytes. A cleansing isotonic enema is given to empty the bowel.

Once the infant has been anesthetized, the surgeon must determine where the junction of aganglionic and ganglionic bowel lies. This is accomplished by obtaining multiple specimens for histologic evaluation. It is important to explain to the parents that this can be time-consuming, thus lengthening the time of the operation. A temporary colostomy (an opening of the colon through the abdominal wall) is created just above the determined level of ganglionic bowel.

The colostomy is created to provide the infant with the means to defecate and to allow the distended bowel to become normal in size. The bowel is incised, the distal end is closed, and the proximal end is sutured to the abdominal wall to create a colostomy. The point in the bowel at which the colostomy is created is individualized according to the extent of aganglionosis. It is preferred to place it sufficiently proximal (i.e., ascending colon) so that a large amount of ganglionic bowel is available below that point for definitive surgery (a pull-through) later. (Otherwise the colostomy must be taken down and a new colostomy created at that time.) Postoperatively, the distal colon is irrigated with saline to remove remaining feces and barium (Leape, 1987). The ostomy is maintained until the infant weighs approximately 20 pounds or is around 1 year of age. A pull-through operation is then done. This involves removal of the aganglionic segment and anastomosis of normal ganglionic bowel to the rectum or anus.

The child is admitted several days before the operation so the bowel can be cleansed adequately to prevent contamination during the operation. The child is immediately placed on a clear liquid diet. The day before surgery, antibiotics are usually started, and the ostomy is flushed with a neomycin-based irrigation solution to cleanse the bowel of bacteria. (See section on "Caring for a Child with a Colostomy/Ileostomy" for a discussion of colostomy irrigation.) The physician may also order rectal irrigations to dislodge any stool in the distal limb of the intestine.

The procedures used to attach ganglionic bowel to the rectum or anus are the Swenson, Duhamel, and Soave procedures (see Table 35–16 for descriptions of each and Fig. 35–17). After the pull-through procedure is completed, a Penrose drain is placed between the anus and the pulled-through bowel to prevent any collection of serous fluid in that area. This is helpful in reducing the possibility of infection. The colostomy is closed at the time of the pull-through operation.

Nursing Diagnostic Responses and Collaborative Problems

These diagnoses are meant to be used with those listed in Table 35–15, Nursing Process Plan: Care of the Child after Abdominal Surgery.

TABLE 35-16
Corrective Surgical Procedures for Hirschsprung Disease

Swenson Pull-Through Operation
After resection of the aganglionic segment from just above the anus, the normal bowel is brought down, and a direct end-to-end anastomosis of the proximal colon just above the rectum is performed
Duhamel Procedure
The aganglionic rectum is left in place, and the ganglion-containing colon is brought through the pelvis behind the retained rectum; a side-to-side anastomosis between the ganglion-containing colon and the aganglionic rectum is performed
Soave Procedure
The rectum is retained, but the mucosa is removed; the aganglionic colon above the rectum is resected; the outer layer of the rectum then forms a conduit through which the aganglionic bowel is pulled until it reaches the anus; the ganglionic bowel is then sutured to the anal opening; the sphincters (muscles of continence) in the rectal region are preserved

Adapted from Martin, L. W., & Torres, A. M. (1985). Hirschsprung's disease. *Surgical Clinics of North America, 65,* 1171–1180; Leape, L. L. (1987). *Patient care in pediatric surgery.* Boston: Little, Brown.

During Temporary Colostomy Phase

High risk for altered health maintenance, home care; *risk factor: knowledge deficit regarding*
- *Colostomy care.*
- *High risk for impaired skin integrity from ostomy drainage.*

High risk for altered role performances, parental; *risk factor: difficulty accepting the infant's altered appearance and bowel function.*

During Pull-Through Phase

High risk for injury site; *risk factor: mechanical trauma to rectal tissue (e.g., taking rectal temperature, rectal examination).*

Impaired skin integrity: buttocks, related to frequent acidic stools after closure of the colostomy.

High risk for altered health maintenance, home care; *risk factor: knowledge deficit.*

Planning and Implementation

Temporary Colostomy Phase

The infant remains on intravenous hydration and antibiotics for 3 to 5 days. The nasogastric tube is discontinued after defecation through the colostomy has begun, usually on the third postoperative day. It is important for the parents to hold and comfort the infant during this period so they can develop a relationship with the baby. (See Table 35–15 for detailed strategies for postoperative care.)

Facilitating Health Maintenance at Home. Initially, the parents should be advised that the stoma will decrease in size. The bowel has a good vascular supply and few nerves, so parents can be assured that they will not hurt the infant when they touch the stoma. The infant can be placed on the abdomen and can be held on the shoulder without pain.

Postoperative teaching of ostomy care is the primary responsibility of the nursing staff. Many hospitals have enterostomal therapists who can help the nurse and family in selection of the appropriate equipment for proper care of the ostomy. Parents should be given time initially to adjust to the physical appearance of the infant with an ostomy and then to become more involved in the actual care of the ostomy.

Parents must be taught to empty, cleanse, and change the ostomy bag. Skin care is essential because the stool is irritating. (See Table 35–14 for a description of ostomy care.) Parents may prefer to allow their infants to stool into the diaper. The nurse can establish a discharge teaching plan cooperatively with the parents. Because ostomy equipment is expensive, in appropriate cases parents should be referred to a social worker for financial assistance. A community health nurse referral provides continued help for the family after discharge.

Supporting Effective Parenting. When a trusting relationship has been established, the nurse can aid parents in voicing their perceptions of their infant and in working toward an acceptance of the baby and the condition. Although body image is not an issue for the infant, it is for the parents who must care for the child with an ostomy. Also, when they are provided with an atmosphere of support, participation, and understanding, the family will be prepared when the infant is medically ready for discharge.

Pull-Through Phase

Providing Effective Postoperative Care and Preventing Trauma to Rectal Tissues. Postoperatively, the child is fed intravenously, a nasogastric tube is inserted to prevent distention of the abdomen,* urinary output is measured through a Foley catheter, and a Penrose drain provides drainage of serous fluid through the rectum. The child is restrained to prevent dislodging of the various tubes. The nasogastric tube is placed to intermittent suction to decompress the stomach. It

* The stomach and upper gastrointestinal tract continuously secrete digestive juices. The nasogastric tube allows these juices to be drained, which reduces the child's feeling of nausea and prevents vomiting. It also prevents pressure of the distended abdomen on the new suture line.

should be irrigated routinely (every 4 hours) with air or saline to ensure its patency. The Penrose drain is removed by the physician within the first 48 hours postoperatively. The child should be turned every 2 hours. This can be done in conjunction with postural drainage, with cupping and clapping or nasopharyngeal suctioning. These nursing measures are important to prevent atelectasis or pneumonia. *It is essential that rectal temperature not be taken and rectal examinations not be done postoperatively.*

When the child begins to pass flatus (usually on the third postoperative day), intermittent suction of the nasogastric tube is no longer necessary, and the nasogastric tube is placed on dependent drainage (drained by gravity). Once the child has begun to pass stools, the nasogastric tube is removed. The Foley catheter is removed on the third to fifth postoperative day. A urine culture may be obtained after removal of the catheter to identify any possible source of infection. Diet is slowly advanced from clear liquids to full liquids and eventually to a regular diet. Intravenous antibiotics are given for 5 days or as indicated.

Maintaining Skin Integrity in the Diaper Area. Before discharge, the surgeon may perform a rectal examination to assess the sphincter tone and the site of anastomosis. The child is medically ready for discharge if he or she is afebrile, has a white blood cell count within normal limits, tolerates a full diet, and has a healed wound and the parents understand the care of diaper dermatitis. The child may have frequent stools, and excoriation of the skin of the buttocks is the major concern before and after discharge. The stool lacks consistency and is very acidic, causing excoriation.

The reason for the excoriation should be explained to the parents before discharge. They should be encouraged to apply an ointment as prescribed with each diaper change and to air-dry the area whenever possible. Skin excoriation can be a problem for 2 to 3 months after the operation. Parents need to be supported and their diligent care of the skin acknowledged.

Facilitating Health Maintenance at Home. After discharge, the infant is followed closely according to need. A rectal examination is done at each clinic visit. The purpose of this is to dilate and assess the patency of the anastomosis site. The segment of intestine that has been pulled through may undergo stricture, and it is essential that it remain patent and functioning. The rectal examinations are upsetting and uncomfortable for the child. There is usually a moderate amount of bloody discharge from the rectum for about 24 hours after the examination.

After the initial postoperative period, the child has rectal examinations in the clinic every 6 months. These rectal examinations are intrusive and uncomfortable for the child. This may result in the child's being fearful of health professionals and of the return visits because of the examination. Suggestions that may help alleviate some of the trauma of these procedures include allowing the parent to hold the child during as much of the examination as possible, providing the child with a rectal examination glove and lubricant and allowing the child to "act out" the procedure on a doll, providing other toys and distractions to make the visit less threatening, and not having the child wait any longer than absolutely necessary for the examination.

It is important to emphasize to the parents that the child may be slow to toilet train but that most children achieve continence after the definitive operative procedure is performed. They are encouraged not to attempt toilet training until the child is over 2 years of age. Once toilet trained, the child is observed on a yearly basis to monitor the stooling patterns.

Anorectal Malformations

Congenital anomalies of the anus and rectum occur in various forms with or without fistulas.

Etiology/Incidence/Pathophysiology

Anorectal malformations occur in approximately 1 per 3000 to 4000 live births and are more common in boys.

The various anorectal malformations occur as a result of abnormal separation of the cloaca (caudal hindgut). The cloaca normally divides into the rectum dorsally and the urogenital sinus ventrally as a result of inward migration of mesoderm from the lateral sides of the cloaca at around the seventh week of gestation. The ridges created on either side of the cloaca meet in the midline. Malformations occur when this process is impeded in any way. Whenever the passage of fecal material is obstructed by a structural anomaly of the anus and rectum, the anus is described as imperforate. There are four main types of imperforate anus: (1) anal stenosis, (2) imperforate anal membrane, (3) anal agenesis, and (4) rectal atresia (Fig. 35–18 and Table 35–17).

Anal agenesis is described as high if the blind pouch of the rectum lies above the levator sling. (The pubococcygeal and puborectalis muscles constitute the levator sling.) For rectal continence to be accomplished, the rectum must be placed within the sling. A line drawn from the tip of the coccyx to the symphysis pubis would approximate the level of the levator sling. If the blind pouch lies below this line, it has theoretically traversed the levator sling and is referred to as a low lesion. Most boys have high lesions, whereas most girls have low lesions. Fistulas occur in 80 to 90 per cent of patients with anal agenesis.

The specific variations of anal agenesis are identified in Table 35–18 and Figures 35–19 and 35–20.

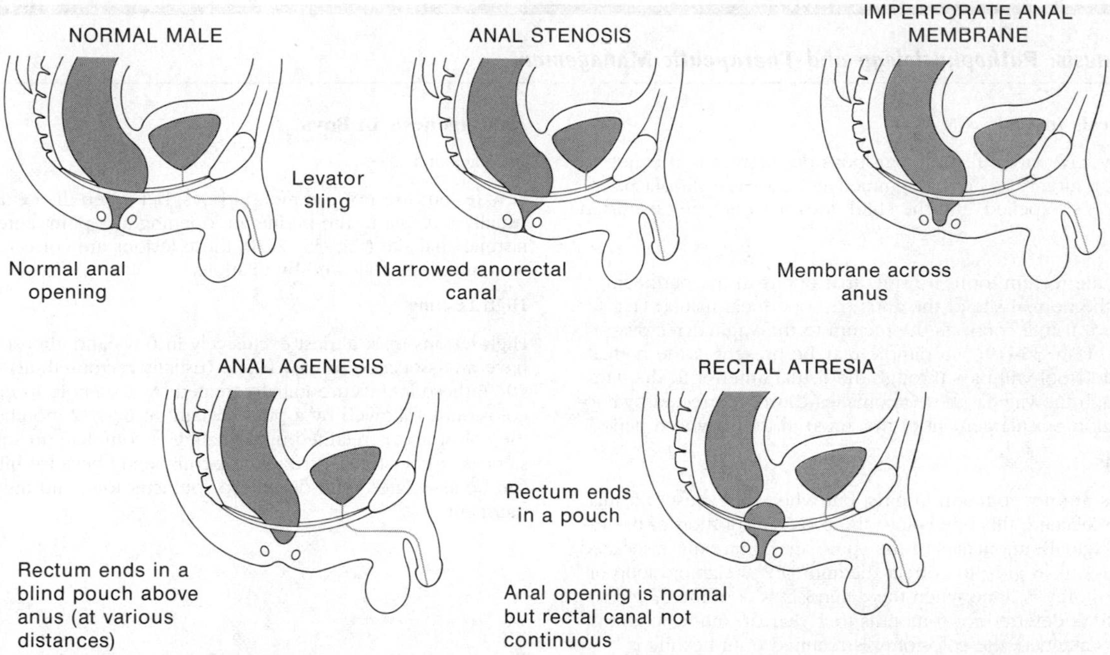

FIGURE 35 - 18. Normal anal anatomy and four main types of imperforate anus. Type I, anal stenosis. Type II, imperforate anal membrane. Type III, anal agenesis (this is the most common type, occurring in about 80 per cent of cases of imperforate anus). Type IV, rectal atresia.

TABLE 35 - 17
Types and Treatment of Imperforate Anus

Type I

Congenital anal stenosis is a narrowing of the anorectal canal that may occur at any point or extend its entire length; diagnosis can be established by digital and endoscopic examination; manual dilatations can often correct this type of malformation

Type II

In imperforate anal membrane atresia, a thin cutaneous membrane persists across the anal opening; meconium fills the rectum and can frequently be seen as a discoloration of the membrane; treatment consists of incision or excision of the membrane followed by anal dilations until bowel function is normal

Type III

In anal agenesis, the rectum ends in a blind pouch at variable distances above the anus; this type accounts for approximately 80 per cent of anorectal malformations; most of these infants have associated fistulas of various types; treatment is surgical and varies with the type of lesion and fistula

Type IV

In rectal atresia, there is a normal anus, but the rectal canal is not continuous; the lower rectal pouch can be identified by careful digital examination; usually a complete block is encountered when one examines with the little finger; this rare anomaly is corrected by anastomosis through an abdominoperineal approach.

Clinical Manifestations

When checking temperature rectally on a newborn infant, the nurse should always inspect the anus to be sure the thermometer is being inserted into the anus and not into a perineal fistula. The anal area should always be inspected for a dimple as a clue to imperforate anus. The nurse must carefully check that there is a normal anal opening and that there is no membrane present.

An understanding of the various anorectal malformations assists the nurse to make accurate observations. If meconium is not passed, the perineum, urethra, and vagina are inspected for a speck of meconium. Fistulas may not be apparent at birth, but usually during the first 24 hours of life, meconium is gradually forced through the fistula by peristalsis and is seen as a tiny speck at the opening of a fistula. Each voiding must be inspected for meconium, which may have passed via a rectourethral fistula (most common in boys). Also, abdominal distention observed by the nurse could lead to the diagnosis of an undetected anorectal anomaly.

Diagnostic Assessment

Definitive diagnosis is made by x-ray examination. The infant is placed prone in the Trendelenburg position to allow air to rise to outline the rectal pouch;

TABLE 35-18
Anal Agenesis: Pathophysiology and Therapeutic Management

Anal Agenesis in Girls

Girls usually have larger fistulas than boys do; therefore, it is not necessary for surgery to be done immediately; a larger fistula permits stool to be expelled, and the child does not become obstructed

Low Lesions

The end of the rectum forms a fistula that opens in the perineum anterior to the normal site of the anus (rectoperineal fistula) (Fig. 35–19*B*), or a fistula connects the rectum to the vagina (rectovaginal fistula) (Fig. 35–19*C*); a dimple may be present at the normal anal site, and stool will pass through the fistula anterior to the dimple or through the vagina; these anomalies can be corrected by anoplasty (creation or enlargement of the anus) in the newborn period

High Lesions

High lesions are not common in girls, but when they exist, a fistula is usually associated; this opens into the proximal portion of the vagina (rectovaginal); anomalies of the spine are commonly associated with high lesions in girls; to correct the anomaly, a sigmoid loop or divided colostomy is done when the diagnosis is confirmed, and a pull-through* is deferred for 6 months to 1 year or until a weight of 8 to 10 kg is attained; the colostomy is retained until healing is complete

Anal Agenesis in Boys

Low Lesions

Low lesions are not common in boys, but when they exist, there is usually a fistula to the perineum, opening at a point anterior to the normal anal site (Fig. 35–20*B*); these lesions are corrected by perineal anoplasty followed by dilations

High Lesions

High lesions exist almost exclusively in boys and almost always have an associated urinary fistula (usually rectourethral) (Fig. 35–20*C*); these infants are initially treated by a sigmoid loop or divided colostomy, followed by a pull-through* at 6 to 12 months of age; the colostomy is retained until healing is complete; in some instances, a colostomy is required permanently because high lesions can be associated with decreased sphincter tone and muscular impairment

*"Pull-through" is the terminology used to describe corrective surgery in which the rectum is brought through the muscles of control (i.e., puborectalis, levator ani, and external sphincter).

this indicates whether a high or low lesion exists. A retrograde urethrocystogram usually confirms the presence of a rectourethral fistula. Other anomalies are common, and the infant should be inspected for their presence. The nurse should be in communication with the physician about the various procedures to be done. It is a comfort to parents when the nurse is informed and can reinforce explanations given by the physician. Also, the fact that stool can be expelled from any body orifice other than the rectum is difficult for many parents to accept. They may believe their infant is abnormal, and they need special attention from the health team to help them understand the available treatment.

Therapeutic Management

Treatment required will vary according to type of anorectal malformation. Refer to Tables 35–17 and 35–18 for treatment modalities for imperforate anus and anal agenesis.

Nursing care of patients with anorectal malformations varies according to the type of treatment required. To prepare an infant for surgery, oral feedings are withheld and intravenous hydration is maintained; the nurse continues to observe for any signs of abdominal distention. When stool is expelled, it should be gently wiped from the opening of the fistula with cotton balls and soap and water.

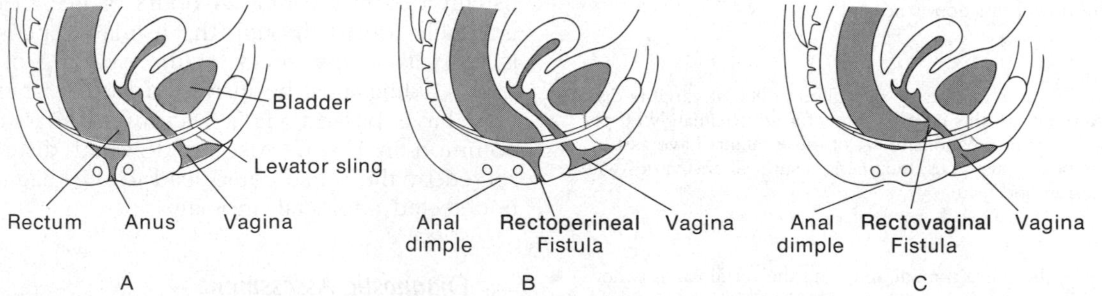

FIGURE 35-19. Anal agenesis in girls. *A,* Normal configuration. *B,* A low lesion in which the terminus of the rectum opens in the perineum in front of the normal site of the anus *(rectoperineal fistula.) C,* A low lesion in which the rectum is connected to the vagina *(rectovaginal fistula).* The openings are large enough for stool to be expelled through the fistulas.

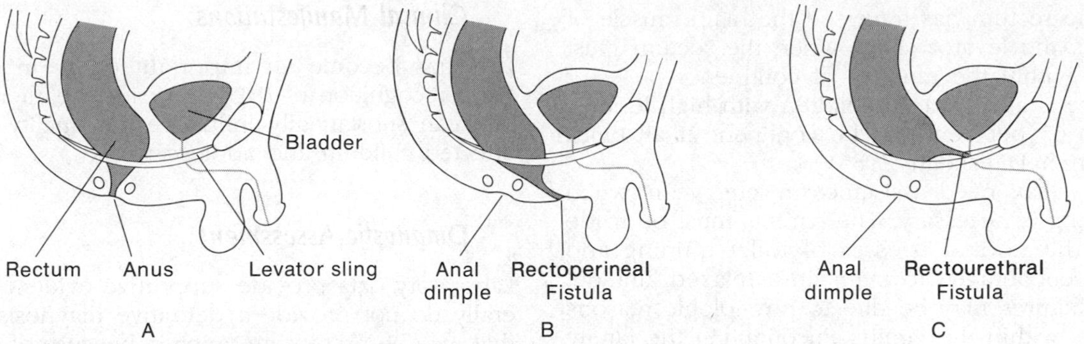

FIGURE 35 - 20. Anal agenesis in boys. *A*, Normal configuration. *B*, A fistula to the perineum, with the opening anterior to the normal anal opening. *C*, A high lesion in a male, in which there is a connection between the rectum and the urethra.

Nursing Diagnostic Statements and Collaborative Problems

High risk for ineffective family coping: compromised; risk factors:

- *Inability of parents to accept the need for surgery and/or colostomy.*
- *Perceptions regarding emergency nature of the condition.*

High risk for injury, operative site; risk factors:

- *Exposure of suture line to feces and urine.*
- *Excessive spreading of buttocks owing to improper positioning.*

Family coping: potential for growth related to desire of parents to safely care for infant after discharge.

Planning and Implementation

Promoting Effective Family Coping. The nurse must be available to parents as they begin to adjust to the fact that surgery is required. If a colostomy is to be done, they may have difficulty seeing beyond the immediate crisis. The nurse must be sensitive to their feelings and avoid discounting their concerns with the reply, "But it's only temporary." An opportunity to speak with the parents of a child who has had a similar procedure with subsequent closure of the colostomy is a great comfort to these parents.

Preventing Injury after Anoplasty. Postoperative nursing care varies according to the type of lesion corrected. When an anoplasty is done for low lesions, the diaper is left off to expose the perineum to air to promote healing. The suture line should be kept clean by removing stool from the anoplasty with a soft cloth and mild soap and water. Care must be taken to avoid disrupting the sutures; a material that will not catch on the sutures should be used for wiping. After the stool has been removed, meticulous cleaning can be done with cotton-tipped applicators and water or a solution as ordered by the physician. Urine generally does not come in contact with the surgical site (i.e., rectal area) when the infant is in a prone position. If the surgical area becomes contaminated with urine, it is cleansed in a similar way as for stool (i.e., cotton-tipped applicators). In the event of excoriation of the skin, a bland ointment may be used to promote healing. The baby is generally allowed to assume a position of comfort. Side-lying and prone positions prevent excessive spreading of the buttocks and also permit easy removal of stool. Temperatures are not to be taken rectally; the nurse must make this known, by way of written and verbal communication, to the family and all team members who care for the infant. Regular diet is resumed as soon as peristalsis returns. Dilations may be required for several months after anoplasty, and parents are taught to perform them daily.

Assisting Parents to Care for the Child after Discharge. When a colostomy is performed for high lesions, parents are taught how to care for the colostomy (see Table 35–14). The nurse should recognize that although the colostomy is temporary, it is necessary for approximately an entire year. This can be an overwhelming thought to parents; they may not adequately understand, in spite of careful explanation, about the care their infant requires. The nurse should not be judgmental of parents who have difficulty accepting the need for a colostomy, even though it is temporary.

Parents wait expectantly and with great hope for permanent closure of the colostomy. Fecal continence varies according to the type of lesion and surgical technique; therefore, specific information should be given by the surgeon and reinforced by the nurse.

Normal or near-normal bowel control is achieved in 85 to 90 per cent of the infants with low lesions because the rectum has traversed the main muscle of continence, the levator sling. When the rectum must be placed within the muscles of continence, a lesser success rate is achieved. In children with high lesions, only 50 to 65 per cent will be continent at all times (Templeton & Ditesheim, 1985).

Parents may need assistance in later years when toilet training is necessary. The parents must be made aware of the normal stresses of toilet training and should be encouraged to maintain a relaxed attitude. Repeated failures may be due to physiologic reasons or to stress within the family. Encouraging the family and the child during this stressful time is an important nursing role.

Alterations Associated with an Inflammatory Process

Disorders caused by an inflammatory process occur at any age. Some may result from a known infectious disease, whereas others are not associated with any recognized infection. The cause of the noninfectious inflammatory disorders remains obscure. Inflammatory (infectious and noninfectious) alterations discussed in this section include necrotizing enterocolitis, ulcerative colitis, Crohn disease, peptic ulcer, appendicitis, and gastroenteritis.

Inflammatory Bowel Disease (Ulcerative Colitis and Crohn Disease)

Ulcerative colitis and Crohn disease are two diseases of the bowel not caused by recognizable infection. They are viewed as distinct but related diseases whose common features are described by the term inflammatory bowel disease (IBD).

Etiology/Incidence/Pathophysiology

The causes of ulcerative colitis and Crohn disease are unknown. Many potential etiologic factors continue to be investigated, including heredity, environmental and infectious agents, and immunologic mechanisms. Psychogenic factors may exacerbate the condition. Both are diseases of young people and frequently arise in the second decade, with a peak incidence in the twenties. Younger children under 5 years of age are also diagnosed. IBD occurs more frequently in whites than in African-Americans and is particularly common among persons of Jewish descent. About 20 per cent of patients will have a first-degree relative with one or the other of these diseases. Refer to Table 35–19 for a comparison of pathophysiology and diagnosis of ulcerative colitis and Crohn disease.

Clinical Manifestations

IBD has become an important entity in pediatrics. Early recognition of IBD can lead to earlier treatment and can substantially influence the quality of life for affected children and adolescents.

Diagnostic Assessment

Laboratory data provide supportive evidence but generally do not provide a definitive diagnosis. Findings that may be present are anemia because of blood loss and malnutrition, electrolyte imbalance (especially hypokalemia), reduced serum protein levels because of losses through diarrhea and inadequate protein intake, and an elevated white blood cell count and sedimentation rate because of inflammation and blood in the stool.

Diagnostic studies include a barium enema and upper gastrointestinal series with small bowel follow-through, and sigmoidoscopy or colonoscopy. (See Table 35–19 for summary of their use and findings in each disease.)

Therapeutic Management

Pharmacologic Management. The treatment of IBD remains limited. The medications available include sulfasalazine (Salazopyrin), mesalamine (5-ASA) (a newer, more purified form of sulfasalazine), and corticosteroids. Salazopyrin and 5-ASA are most useful in the treatment of disease involving the colon, whether in Crohn disease or ulcerative colitis. Occasionally a patient with Crohn disease of the small bowel seems to respond to these drugs despite the findings of the National Collaborative Crohn's Disease Study, which suggested they would be ineffective (Summers, 1979).

Corticosteroids may be used in the form of intravenous hydrocortisone or methylprednisone, prednisone, and prednisolone. They will usually induce a remission but will not halt progression of the disease despite making the patient feel much better. Corticosteroids must be used judiciously because of the multitude of side effects that can be produced. These include weight gain, moon face, dowager's hump, acne, cataracts, muscle weakness, salt retention, hypertension, glycosuria, osteomalacia, growth failure, aseptic necrosis of the hip, increased susceptibility to infections, and euphoria. However, used in the smallest effective dose with monitoring for side effects, they can be very safe. The nurse must be sure the parents understand the side effects and dangers to be watched for. Monitoring for side effects should be part of the nursing care plan for both inpatients and outpatients. Rectal suppositories of steroids and derivatives of 5-ASA may be ordered for adolescents with involvement primarily in the distal intestine. Patients should acquire a medical alert bracelet indicating corticosteroid use and the possibility of adrenal suppression

TABLE 35-19
Comparison of Pathophysiology and Diagnosis of Ulcerative Colitis and Crohn Disease

Ulcerative Colitis	Crohn Disease
Location	
Primarily a disease of the rectum and distal colon, but in children usually involves the entire colon; the most severe disease occurs distally	The distal small intestine (terminal ileum) is most frequently involved (80% of cases), but it may involve any area of the alimentary tract
Character	
An inflammation of the colonic mucosa; vascular engorgement of the mucosa and submucosa is present with increased leukocytes; the lesion rarely extends beyond the mucosa into deeper layers; acute edema and inflammation result in thickening of the bowel	Inflammation is characterized by transmural or deep bowel wall involvement; lesion penetrates bowel wall; thickened intestinal wall, mucosal fissures, and fistulas are typical; granulomas occur in 50% of cases
Pattern	
Lesion is continuous; when a lesion develops, it spreads to adjacent areas without skipping healthy bowel	Lesion occurs as a skip lesion (i.e., diseased bowel is separated by normal bowel)
Long-Term Changes and Complications	
As the disease becomes chronic, the bowel takes on a lead-pipe appearance (i.e., shortening of colon, loss of mucosal folds, loss of haustral folds [scalloped appearance of colon], and development of fibrous tissue and linear strictures); complications include toxic megacolon, in which the colon suddenly dilates and perforates, spreading infection into the abdominal cavity and blood stream; this is a rare complication	Chronic inflammation is characterized by the presence of granulomas, scarring, and formation of fibrotic strictures; strictures can eventually cause bowel obstruction; the transmural nature of the lesion results in fistula formations, but the inflammation and engorgement on the serosal surface inhibits perforation; as a result, spillage of intestinal contents into the peritoneal cavity is rare
Presentation of Illness	
Children are usually healthy with sudden onset; the most frequent manifestations are bloody diarrhea and abdominal pain; blood loss can be profound; patients experience cramping sensations (tenesmus) with bowel movements, which frequently come on with a sense of urgency; extraintestinal manifestations (skin rash, arthritis, iritis) are rare in children but occur in adolescents and young adults; occasionally anorexia, nausea, fever of undetermined origin, anemia, and dehydration accompany the presenting symptoms; physical examination reveals a tender and distended abdomen with signs of peritoneal irritation	Onset is insidious, with failure to thrive a reason for seeking care; crampy abdominal pain is the most common initial complaint; many have diarrhea, and constitutional symptoms characteristic of the disease include fever, malaise, and anorexia; pain is most frequent in the right lower quadrant; abscess formation is common, and therefore a spiking fever and leukocytosis may be noted; extraintestinal symptoms often accompany the disease and include mouth ulcers, iritis, arthritis, arthralgia, or skin rashes
Making the Diagnosis	
A barium enema reveals the characteristic lead-pipe appearance of a previously inflamed bowel; a barium enema also identifies the extent of ulcerative colitis; direct examination of the large bowel by sigmoidoscopy or colonoscopy will reveal friability and ulceration confirmed by characteristic changes in the biopsy specimens taken during the procedure	Because the symptoms are often nonspecific and difficult to localize in the intestinal tract, the diagnosis may not be made for months to years after the onset of symptoms; a small bowel follow-through study or barium enema is initially done to allow the entire colon to be visualized; a colonoscopy may be performed to document the extent of disease; the presence of skip lesions on radiographs or colonoscopy is confirmed by finding granulomas in the biopsy specimens
Effect of Inflammatory Bowel Disease on Growth and Development	
Inflammatory bowel disease results in growth retardation; growth is retarded if a child falls below the third percentile on standard growth charts in height and fails to develop sexually at the normal rate; growth retardation is considered a common occurrence in inflammatory bowel disease; originally it was believed that growth retardation was due to low levels of growth hormone, but it is now thought to be due to chronic inadequate caloric intake (Kirschner, 1988); after puberty, the chances of recovery from growth retardation are reduced	

in the event of severe illness or accident. Alternate-day corticosteroids are used more frequently in children with Crohn disease than in adults because they stimulate appetite and promote a sense of well-being, thus encouraging normal growth and development while minimizing side effects. See also Table 37–4, Nursing Process Plan: The Child on Corticosteroid Therapy.

Immunosuppressive drugs, such as 6-mercaptopurine (6-MP), azathioprine (Imuran), and cyclosporine, are being used in patients who cannot be tapered off steroid therapy or who have chronic and severe problems with fistula formation. Steroids are administered for approximately 2 to 3 months after the institution of immunosuppressives because of their slow onset of action. Approximately half of the patients on immunosuppressives can discontinue steroid use.

Nursing responsibilities include monitoring blood counts, especially for leukopenia, every 2 to 4 weeks. Therapy may be discontinued with severe hematologic effects. The child will need to be protected from exposure to infectious contacts, whether in the hospital or at home; the nurse will instruct parents about specific measures to be taken relating to family members, friends, and peers.

Nutritional Management. Nutritional management is becoming increasingly important in IBD. Most patients with Crohn disease will go into remission on total parenteral nutrition or elemental feeding. Elemental feeding may be provided at home by nasogastric tube given overnight. Most teenagers prefer to remove the tube in the morning and reinsert it in the evening rather than go to school with a tube in the nose. Elemental diet by tube feeding or orally is used most often to correct growth failure in Crohn disease. For most patients, a relapse of the disease can be expected several months after the elemental feeding regimen is stopped. These techniques are not effective for ulcerative colitis, although total parenteral nutrition may be necessary to prepare a chronically malnourished patient for surgery or when tube feedings are not tolerated.

Surgical Management. Neither of these bowel diseases can be cured medically, although operative removal of the entire colon will cure ulcerative colitis. Colectomy and subsequent ileostomy is understandably resisted by patients and families until they have experienced the full ravages of the disease. However, the severity of the disease in young people and the increasing chance that cancer will arise in the colon after 10 years of disease means that many young patients with ulcerative colitis will eventually have the colon removed surgically. Consequently, there is great enthusiasm for the techniques that produce the "continent ileostomy" or ileoanal continuity so that the patient can go to the bathroom in the normal fashion. These newer techniques are rarely done immediately after the removal of the colon, particularly if surgery was performed because the patient had been acutely ill.

Application of the Nursing Process: Inflammatory Bowel Disease

Assessment

The presenting symptoms are explored, including a search for historical factors that might contribute to the development or exacerbation of IBD (see Table 35–19 for presenting symptoms of each disease). Extraintestinal symptoms are common and include oral sores, fever, rashes, and arthritic joints. Urinary tract complications, such as renal calculi and hematuria, may also occur. Eye disorders, such as conjunctivitis, episcleritis, and iritis, may also occur. The family history in particular is reviewed to search for other similar problems in other family members, not necessarily diagnosed as IBD. Stresses in the home, in school, or on the job (for an adolescent) are potential aggravators of the disease.

The history should rule out other causes of symptoms, such as infectious diarrhea and allergy. Details of travel, source of drinking water, and recent changes in food intake may provide important clues. If growth retardation is present, a review of height and weight since birth should be included. During the assessment phase, an environment is promoted in which the child or parent feels comfortable in describing the symptoms. Fear and embarrassment about bloody bowel movements may lead the child to conceal the problem from parents. Once the condition is diagnosed, the child or adolescent will often minimize the description of symptoms to avoid visits to the doctor or further medical tests. Appreciating the feelings that are associated with the symptoms is an important aspect of the communication process during assessment.

Nursing Diagnostic Statements and Collaborative Problems

Altered bowel elimination: diarrhea, *resulting from intestinal inflammation.*

High risk for injury: physiologic; *risk factors:*

- *Untoward effects of prescribed medications.*
- *Complications of IBD, caused by chronic inflammation and ulceration of the bowel.*

Altered comfort: pain, *related to abdominal cramping associated with intestinal inflammation and ulceration.*

Altered nutrition: less than body requirements, *resulting from poor absorption of essential nutrients associated with chronic inflammation of the bowel.*

High risk for altered growth and development: failure to thrive; *risk factors:*
- *Poor absorption of essential nutrients.*
- *Knowledge deficit regarding nutritional therapy at home.*
- *Child's fear of pain resulting from eating.*

Activity intolerance: acute phase, *related to the tendency for exercise to increase intestinal motility.*

Impaired skin integrity *related to frequent and prolonged contact of the skin with feces.*

Ineffective individual and family coping, *related to knowledge deficit regarding diagnostic process and prognosis.*

High risk for impaired adjustment; *risk factor: lack of available coping mechanism to deal with the ongoing alterations in daily living associated with chronic inflammatory bowel disease.*

High risk for altered growth and development, cognitive and emotional; *risk factor: effects of IBD on activities of daily living.*

Planning and Implementation

Controlling Diarrhea. The usual recording of stools is supplemented with a notation of any relationship of the diarrhea to types of food, emotional stress, or activity.

Antidiarrheal drugs, such as diphenoxylate (Lomotil) or loperamide (Imodium), or anticholinergics should be given as ordered and their effectiveness evaluated. These medications reduce cramping as well as diarrhea. The nurse and the family must monitor for side effects of the medications used in the management of IBD. The preceding section on pharmacologic management includes nursing strategies to address potential untoward effects of medications.

The problem of diarrhea is often embarrassing to patients and is associated with abdominal discomfort and problems of skin irritation. Maintaining an odor-free environment by promptly removing linens, supplying appropriate pain medication, using comfort measures, and carefully cleansing the perineal area are important nursing interventions. When severe skin irritation is present, application of a thin film of protective ointment may prevent further irritation.

Providing Optimal Comfort and Assessing for Complications. Pain management involves administration of pain medication, repositioning, alleviation of anxiety through supportive conversation, and quiet diversional activities.

Pain of increased intensity that is not responsive to therapy should be monitored closely because this may indicate a complication (obstruction, peritonitis, or hemorrhage). Careful documentation of the character and pattern of pain and its relationship to meals is important.

Providing Essential Nutrients and Facilitating Development. Dietary management of IBD may involve total parenteral nutrition, elemental feeding by mouth or tube, a low-residue bland diet, or, in some cases, a regular diet. Care of the patient with total parenteral nutrition is discussed in Chapter 16.

Instruction in tube placement and feeding techniques is usually done by the nurse. The timing of education is important. After the therapy has been discussed and the technique is explained, it is important to proceed with the placement of the tube. Delaying its use for days or weeks simply gives the child or adolescent time to experience increased anxiety.

Elemental diets are nutritionally balanced, bulk and residue free, and low in fat. They are digested mainly in the upper jejunum and are relatively nonstimulating, allowing the bowel to rest. *Any signs of intolerance* (abdominal distention, diarrhea, nausea, vomiting) *to the feedings should be consistently documented by the nurse.* Children who are required to receive an elemental diet by tube feeding need the support of parents and relatives. Preparation for therapy at home should include the counsel of a nutritionist. The nurse should be involved, devising the plan for home care with the goal of providing the parents and child with adequate information and supervision to carry out the procedure at home.

Dietary counseling for maintenance of nutritional status is provided. The nutritionist and also the nurse spend time with the child to identify which foods may aggravate symptoms. Sometimes children need to be persuaded to eat because they associate pain and diarrhea with eating. Foods that cannot be tolerated should be eliminated, but involvement of the child in these decisions may increase overall intake and satisfaction with the diet. Keeping an accurate record of food and fluid intake and output provides important information for management during acute phases. Management at home is more relaxed, and usually measurement of intake and output is unnecessary.

Monitoring Physical Activity. During the acute phase, physical activity may be kept to a minimum to decrease intestinal motility. Patients on parenteral nutrition can be encouraged to exercise if they are feeling strong enough and free of symptoms. Exercise, in these cases, is promoted to use the dextrose and protein supplied in parenteral nutrition to build muscle tissue (Simmons, 1984).

Preserving Skin Integrity. Skin breakdown in the form of fistulas and fissures is common in Crohn disease. Patients with ulcerative colitis and Crohn disease suffer from excoriation of the anal region owing to diarrhea. Sitz baths, meticulous skin care, and medicated wipes such as Tucks provide some relief. Care around a draining fistula site is important to prevent further breakdown. Although care varies greatly from center to center, one nursing specialist recommends that small fistulas be cared for by using a small, sterile saline packing, which is changed every 4 to 6 hours. For excessively large fistulas, a stoma adhesive around the fistula can provide a skin barrier. A pouch can be attached to the stoma adhesive and accurate drainage measured (Simmons, 1984).

In acute phases, when a patient is on bed rest, the usual measures to prevent skin breakdown must be instituted, including use of sheepskin, a foam mattress, or a waterbed; repositioning; and gradual ambulation.

Promoting Coping. Health professionals must realize that the diagnostic investigations performed for IBD are highly stressful. Patients and families will usually need assistance to develop mechanisms that they can use for coping with events associated with IBD. Parents and relatives may be even more fearful than the patient because most adults associate the use of barium enema, endoscopy, and especially biopsy with the possibility of cancer. This fear is seldom spoken and should be specifically addressed. Ulcerative colitis and Crohn disease both have a tendency to relapse and remit, and the course is highly variable from individual to individual. An acquaintance will often tell patients and families about those IBD victims who have had the most severe disease and complications. Families should be warned about this in advance. Similarly, all chronic incurable diseases sooner or later become the subject of sensational media reports of miraculous cures. Parents and grandparents should be encouraged to bring these items in to be discussed openly so that a foundation of trust is maintained. It is the nurse's responsibility to ensure that patients are informed and prepared for the various procedures that are required to arrive at a diagnosis. The tests required during the diagnostic phase are uncomfortable and may be embarrassing to some children or teenagers. The nurse's role during this phase involves a sensitive response to the child's and family's particular reactions.

Supporting Adjustment of the Child and Family to IBD. Inflammatory bowel disease considerably disrupts the patient's life. This puts the child and family at risk for being unable to modify their lifestyle and behavior in a manner consistent with the change in health status. The way the patient can participate in society and the impact on daily life must be appreciated by the nurse who cares for these individuals and their families.

Psychologic support is essential. The psychologist, social worker, or nurse on the team should be prepared to cope with behaviors of a chronically ill patient. Anger, denial, and often perfectionism are behaviors that are expressed during illness. Loss of control over bowel function, eating, and daily activities arouses feelings of frustration and anger. Having the patient identify those aspects that are providing the greatest burden may be helpful. Additional information about the treatment plan, drugs, and feedings may correct or expand the patient's understanding.

Careful attention should be given to how patients can participate and gain some control in their own care. Nonverbal messages are of particular importance during the care of an ostomy or cleaning up soiled linens and bedpans. Patients are particularly sensitive to any signs of disgust or revulsion.

The nurse should discuss with the parent and child ways to increase intake of essential nutrients without creating a power struggle between the child and family over the issue of eating (e.g., eliminate low-nutrient "junk food" from the home, allow the child to choose favorite foods from a list of nutritional foods, allow the child to help shop and plan menus for the family, and reinforce with the child that good nutrition is important for all members of the family to decrease any feelings of being a martyr on the part of the child). Encourage the child to discuss the ways in which he or she manages the symptoms of IBD. Verbally reinforce adaptive coping to enhance the child's sense of control.

Adjustment can be facilitated if expression of the patient's fears and frustrations is encouraged. Questions should be answered honestly and in collaboration with other health team members.

Assistance from specialized nurses called stomal therapists should be sought for preparation of the patient before surgery, for management of the ostomy after surgery, and for skin problems associated with ostomies or fistulas (see Table 35–14). Patients with ostomies require counseling concerning sexual issues, an area that requires specialized support. The United Ostomy Association* has pamphlets available on sex, courtship, and pregnancy for male and female ostomy patients. Information concerning fertility and sexuality can be obtained from the Crohn-Colitis Foundation of America.†

Promoting Cognitive and Emotional Development. The prognosis for both these diseases is surprisingly good considering the trouble they cause when they are active. Both are compatible with a full life, including employment, marriage, and childbearing. Young patients with ulcerative colitis often have sporadic school attendance. The combination of embarrassment and a tendency for symptoms to worsen under stress often leads to school avoidance. School attendance and well-being should be checked at every visit. Similarly, patients with Crohn disease frequently do not feel well even though objective signs and symptoms of disease are not apparent. If the child or adolescent is not active in school and participating in

---

* United Ostomy Association, 36 Executive Park, Suite 120, Irvine, CA 92714; ([800] 826–0826).

† Crohn-Colitis Foundation of America, 444 Park Ave South, New York, NY 10016; ([800] 932–2423).

sports and activities or not growing, some element in the program should be adjusted. The nurse plays a critical role in these assessments because patients frequently confide their true feelings and complaints to a sympathetic nursing professional. This sense of trust is necessary to the effective understanding and management of the young person with IBD.

Evaluation

Evaluation of nursing action carried out for intervention in collaborative problems will also be a collaborative process carried out by the nurse and physician. As always, evaluation of the effectiveness of nursing interventions designed for nursing diagnoses is accompanied by assessing for absence or decrease of the defining characteristics of the actual problems.

Acute Infectious Diarrhea

Diarrhea is a frequent symptom of illness in infants and young children. Causes of diarrhea are numerous, one of which is the presence of infectious organisms. When diarrhea is presumed or known to be due to an infection, the terms "infectious gastroenteritis" and "acute infectious diarrhea" are used. Gastroenteritis can be mild or severe and is caused by a virus, bacterium, or parasite. It is an alteration of the gastrointestinal tract resulting in increased motility and rapid emptying of the intestinal contents. This rapid excretion interferes with the absorption and causes loss of necessary nutrients, electrolytes, and water.

Etiology/Incidence/Pathophysiology

In children, infectious gastroenteritis is second only to upper respiratory tract infections as a cause of illness. Although the illness is generally benign and self-limited, it accounts for 3 to 5 per cent of pediatric hospital admissions. In developing countries, it remains the largest single cause of death because of the prevalence of malnutrition, parasites, and poor hygiene (Cusson, 1992).

The majority of acute diarrheal illnesses in infants and young children are of viral origin (LeBaron et al, 1990). *Rotavirus* is the major cause of viral diarrhea and has been consistently associated with 50 to 70 per cent of wintertime gastroenteritis in children (LeBaron et al, 1990). Rotavirus may cause a prolonged illness because of its ability to cause a secondary lactose malabsorption or monosaccharide intolerance (Davidson, 1986). The Norwalk-like viruses are thought to be the etiologic agents in about one third of the epidemics of diarrhea (Davidson, 1986).

Organisms responsible for bacterial diarrhea are many and vary according to environmental factors. *Campylobacter* and *Yersinia* have recently been isolated more frequently because of improved culture techniques. *Shigella, Salmonella, Staphylococcus aureus,* enterotoxigenic *Escherichia coli* (ETEC), and pathogenic *E. coli* are other pathogens that cause bacterial diarrhea. *Giardia lamblia* and *Dientamoeba fragilis* are the most common parasitic agents affecting children.

The pathogenic mechanism of viral infection is not well understood. The infection damages or destroys some of the epithelial cells lining the intestinal tract. Recovery entails regeneration of epithelial cells and their associated enzyme systems. Illness continues while this regeneration occurs (48 to 96 hours).

Bacteria may act on the intestinal mucosa, causing (1) enterotoxin production, (2) mucosal invasion and destruction, or (3) penetration.

Enterotoxin Production. In this mechanism, the organism does not invade the mucosal epithelium but rather multiplies in the small intestine, then adheres to the mucosa, and releases an enterotoxin. The interaction between the toxin and the epithelium activates adenyl cyclase in the cell membrane, leading to an increase in cyclic adenosine monophosphate (cyclic AMP), which causes active electrolyte and water secretion. Diarrhea resulting from this process is called *secretory diarrhea.* Action of the enterotoxin reduces the absorptive function of the surface area in the upper small bowel. The organisms that cause this reaction are *Vibrio cholerae,* enterotoxigenic *E. coli* (predominates in infants), and certain strains of *Shigella* (e.g., *S. dysenteriae* type 1). In addition, food poisoning caused by the enterotoxins of *S. aureus* or *Clostridium perfringens* is associated with this type of diarrhea. Diarrhea associated with these organisms is profuse and watery, leading to dehydration and acidosis, particularly in children under 2 years of age.

Invasion and Destruction of Epithelial Cells. In this process, enterocytes (cells in the epithelium) are invaded by organisms, which results in mucosal inflammation and destruction. On histologic examination, bacterial organisms are seen within epithelial cells, where they multiply and cause superficial mucosal ulcerations. Organisms that cause an inflammatory reaction in this way include *Shigella, Campylobacter jejuni, Salmonella,* certain strains of *E. coli* (e.g., enteroinvasive *E. coli*) and antibiotic-associated *Clostridium difficile* (Guerrant et al, 1986). The inflammatory nature of this type of infection often results in high fever and tenesmus associated with blood, mucus, and pus (leukocytes) in the stool on microscopic examination. Superficial ulcerations of the mucosa occur as a result of the inflammatory process.

Penetration and Systemic Invasion. This type of process involves penetration of the gut wall (often through Peyer patches in the ileum) followed by multiplication of organisms intracellularly. Eventually, the organism may reach the systemic circulation. Organisms causing infection in this way include *Salmonella typhi, Yersinia,* and *Campylobacter fetus.* Clinical symptoms include a febrile illness that often begins without diarrhea and is diagnosed by blood, bone marrow, or involved lymph node culture (Guerrant et al, 1986).

Transmission of Organisms. Children are particularly at risk for infections because subclinical infection in an adult may be transmitted to a child. Most organisms that cause diarrhea are spread by the fecal-oral route. When an organism can be spread by a relatively small dose or inoculum, person-to-person contact may be sufficient to transmit the disease. For example, *Shigella, Giardia,* and possibly *Campylobacter* are spread by direct contact. Transmission through contaminated food or water usually requires a larger dose or inoculum. An example is *Salmonella,* which is ingested with milk, meat, or eggs contaminated by the organisms during preparation or storage. The contamination may occur in the home or in commercial preparation. Staphylococcal gastroenteritis is caused by ingestion of *Staphylococcus*. Frequently, the foods affected are dairy products that have been stored improperly.

Clinical Manifestations

The major complication from gastroenteritis, regardless of cause, is dehydration and accompanying electrolyte imbalance. Signs of dehydration are not always apparent to parents. These signs are depressed fontanels, sunken eyes, loss of skin turgor, oliguria, or concentrated urine. Parents should be informed of these signs and should report them. A decreased urinary output, indicated by fewer than six wet diapers per 24 hours or a period of longer than 4 hours without urination, is significant in an infant. Skin turgor can be checked by pinching the skin on the abdomen. If the skin returns to normal after being released, there is no loss of skin turgor. Skin that remains elevated after being released signifies loss of subcutaneous fluid and is indicative of dehydration. Other signs for parents to watch for are the absence of tears, increasing lethargy or irritability, and dry lips and tongue.

Potassium and sodium are normally lost through stool but replaced through oral intake. During diarrheal disease, these losses are greater than can be replaced by normal oral intake. Sodium losses in turn create additional extracellular fluid loss, compounding the problem of volume deficit. Potassium losses cause muscle weakness, abdominal distention, and possible electrocardiographic changes.

Diagnostic Assessment

Diagnosis is made largely by history. Parents report a large number of watery stools. These stools are frequently green from the excretion of bile. Stools resulting from bacterial infection may contain pus and, infrequently, blood. The child often has a history of vomiting and a low-grade fever. An accurate history is important in differentiating normal stool changes, which occur with age and diet changes, from diarrhea, which reflects a pathologic process.

Routine total and differential white blood cell counts are of little value in identifying the causative organism. The total white blood cell count may be normal, increased, or decreased. Over 50 per cent of children with infectious diarrhea have an increased percentage of band forms (immature white blood cells) (Feigin & Stoller, 1992).

Laboratory studies include microscopic examination of the stool for leukocytes, examination for occult blood by the guaiac test (Hemoccult), stool culture and sensitivity, and stool virology. Stool pH of 5.5 or less and a positive Clinitest (0.5 per cent glucose or greater) suggest impaired carbohydrate utilization, which may be due to a noninfectious process or be found in children with acquired lactase deficiency that follows persistent infectious diarrhea (Feigin & Stoller, 1992). The presence of fat and neutrophils suggests steatorrhea or an inflammatory process. A stool that is positive for polymorphonuclear cells is usually sent for cultures for *Salmonella, Shigella,* and *Campylobacter.* A fresh stool specimen is required when ova and parasites are suspected (which must be delivered to the laboratory immediately), or the stool can be put into a fixating solution for transport.

Therapeutic Management

The management of infectious gastroenteritis has three components: (1) to maintain or restore fluid and electrolyte balance, (2) to restore the bowel to normal functioning, and (3) to prevent the infection of others in contact with the child. Mild cases of the disease can be treated at home by the parents. While the child is actively vomiting, little is given by mouth for 2 to 6 hours. Fluids recommended for parents to use at home are various soft drinks, clear juices, flavored gelatin water, and an oral electrolyte solution such as Pedialyte.

The parents should be informed of specific minimal fluid intake required for the individual infant. Controversy exists over how to reintroduce the oral feedings. Small, frequent feedings are most often given, yet larger quantities offered less frequently may be recommended because frequent feedings have the potential to induce peristalsis. Also, the timing of advancing from clear fluids is debated. Early reintroduction of feeding has generally replaced the concept of "resting the bowel." Feeding after 24 to 36 hours may provide a surge of diarrhea, yet the children recover more quickly.

Breastfed infants with mild diarrhea are able to remain on breast milk. The diarrhea will usually resolve when the infant takes nothing orally for several hours and then continues with breastfeeding. Other infants advance from clear fluids to a lactose hydrolyzed milk or soy substitute after 24 hours and toddlers to a bland milk-free diet. Bananas, rice, applesauce, and toast (known as BRAT) or rice, applesauce, and bananas (known as RAB) are diets that have traditionally been prescribed for children after diarrhea and continue to be used.

Infants and children with severe diarrhea, those with symptoms of dehydration, and those in whom vomiting accompanies diarrhea are usually hospitalized for observation and fluid and electrolyte therapy. Medical treatment during hospitalization is aimed at restoring normal fluid and electrolyte balance and allowing the bowel to resume normal function. This is accomplished by the use of normal saline intravenous feeding with potassium added as necessary. Before intravenous potassium is added, kidney function must be established.

It has been demonstrated that dehydration from diarrhea can also be treated effectively with use of a glucose-electrolyte oral solution (Listernick et al, 1986; Tolia & Dubois, 1985). The oral rehydrating solution provides a 2 per cent glucose solution, which enhances sodium transport in the small intestine (glucose-coupled sodium transport is the physiologic basis of oral rehydration therapy). If sufficient sodium is provided, water will follow the osmotic gradient produced by the sodium transport, thus maximizing the absorptive potential of the gut.

Oral rehydrating solutions have been evaluated in developed and developing countries. The composition of the oral rehydration solution recommended by the Diarrhea Disease Control Program of the World Health Organization contains sodium, 90 mmol/L; potassium, 20 mmol/L; chloride, 80 mmol/L; bicarbonate, 30 mmol/L; and glucose, 111 mmol/L (2 per cent) (Robson, 1987). The amount and rate of oral rehydration vary according to the patient's condition. The purpose is to meet maintenance requirements, replenish previous losses, and meet ongoing requirements. Vomiting that occurs in the first 2 hours of rehydration is not a contraindication to continuation of therapy.

Rice-based oral rehydration solutions offer significant advantages. Whereas glucose solutions are effective in restoring fluid balance, rice carbohydrate actually decreases diarrhea stool volume. In addition, rice-based solutions can be more highly concentrated, delivering up to four times the calories of a glucose solution. This increased calorie solution is especially important in developing countries where malnutrition is also a significant problem. Rice-based solutions are also cheaper and more readily available in many parts of the world (Cusson, 1992).

As with the child treated at home, the hospitalized child gradually advances to a more solid diet. The introduction of milk may cause the child's diarrhea to begin again because of possible lactase deficiency. For this reason, formula may be introduced at a lower strength, with slow advance to full strength. In some instances it may be necessary to give the infant a soy formula until the deficiency is corrected naturally. It has, however, increasingly been recognized that steadily advancing the diet hastens recovery and prevents iatrogenic malnutrition.

Nursing Assessment

The hydration status of the child is closely monitored. This includes observation and monitoring for electrolyte and hydrogen ion imbalance. Signs and symptoms of dehydration and clinical manifestations of electrolyte imbalances, such as hyponatremia, hypokalemia, and metabolic acidosis, are continually assessed. The assessment data provide the basis for decision making pertaining to treatment modalities and nursing care.

Nursing Diagnostic Statements and Collaborative Problems

High risk for injury: electrolyte and hydrogen ion imbalance; *risk factors:*

- *Loss of Na^+, K^+, and HCO_3^- in diarrheal stools.*
- *Increased production of keto acids associated with starvation and dehydration.*
- *Increase in lactic acid associated with decreased tissue perfusion.*
- *Retention of nonvolatile H^+ associated with decreased urine output.*

High risk for altered health maintenance; *risk factor: knowledge deficit regarding home care of the child with mild acute infectious diarrhea.*

Ineffective individual coping, *related to altered comfort: pain, with abdominal cramping.*

Impaired skin integrity, *related to repeated perineal contact with acidic stools.*

Planning and Implementation

Monitoring Fluid, Electrolyte, and Hydrogen Ion Status. The child with dehydration and electrolyte and hydrogen ion imbalances will usually be hospitalized for intravenous therapy. Nursing responsibilities include administration of intravenous fluids and electrolytes and, with the physician, evaluation of this therapy.

Monitoring of fluid balance necessitates accurate daily weights, recording of intake and output, and close monitoring of specific gravity. The most accurate assessment of fluid loss is through body weight. Weight is the basis for assessing the success of management during the acute phase of the disease, and weighing must be done on an accurate scale with the child completely undressed. The child is weighed on admission, and all subsequent weighings should be done on the same scale. A precise record of oral and parenteral intake and of output is important. Stool and urinary output is most easily measured by weighing the diapers dry and again after soiling. Urine specific gravity is done to measure the state of hydration. The urine specific gravity reflects the density of the urine: the higher the reading, the more concentrated the urine. A urine specific gravity of 1.025 or greater is indicative of dehydration; a reading of approximately 1.015 indicates normal hydration. As intravenous fluids are begun, the urine specific gravity will decrease. During the acute phase of hospitalization, urine specific gravity should be checked every 4 hours.

Monitoring electrolyte and hydrogen ion status entails assessment for signs of imbalance. See Tables 26–4 and 26–5 for clinical manifestations of hyponatremia, hypokalemia, and metabolic acidosis. The nurse also monitors results of serum electrolyte studies.

Facilitating Home Health Maintenance. During the course of an illness, specific instructions are needed by parents who are managing gastroenteritis at home. Detailed dietary guidelines must be given. Other important information includes handwashing technique and proper disposal of soiled articles. Families should also be familiar with the signs of dehydration and instructed to seek additional assistance if these signs are present or if the diarrhea continues beyond a few days.

When giving soft drinks to the child with diarrhea, the parents should be told to allow the drink to become "flat" by stirring until the carbonation is no longer present. Gelatin water is made by mixing 2 tablespoons of flavored gelatin powder in 8 ounces of water. It is important to inform parents that the child's stools will be the color of the gelatin water, and this is not cause for alarm. Liquids should be offered at room temperature because cold liquids may increase bowel motility.

Acute infectious diarrhea may sometimes be avoided by instituting basic hygiene measures. The nurse functioning in a variety of settings is in an excellent position to teach families and children correct methods of storage and preparation of meat and dairy products. Discussing the importance of handwashing after diapering, after using the toilet, and before food preparation and feeding is an important measure in decreasing the frequency of gastroenteritis. In addition, good handwashing and proper disposal of contaminated articles by personnel within institutions will discourage the spread of the disease.

In some hospitals, children with gastroenteritis are in enteric isolation. Proper handwashing and disposal of soiled articles will prevent the spread of the disease. Parents need to be instructed in these techniques and on the rationale for their use. (See Chapter 23 for further discussion of principles of isolation.)

Promoting Coping. During the acute phase of excessive stooling, the infant or child can be expected to experience discomfort from abdominal cramping. In addition, lack of oral intake will be frustrating to most infants and small children. These discomforts are best addressed by nonpharmacologic means.

During periods without oral feedings, the infant's need to suck is not decreased; not being able to do so is often a source of great frustration to the child. Offering a pacifier or allowing the child who normally sucks the thumb to continue to do so often relieves some of the frustration.

Normalization of activity enhances the young child's motor coping patterns and reduces frustration. Parents can be shown safe positions in which to hold an infant without disturbing the intravenous line, thus providing security and comfort.

Preventing and Treating Perineal Excoriation. The stools in diarrhea are acidic and irritating to the skin around the perineum. If the child is not cleaned promptly after defecation, the skin quickly becomes excoriated. To prevent this, the area should be gently cleaned immediately with soap and water and dried thoroughly. Excoriation frequently responds quickly to air-drying; the area can simply be cleaned and then left uncovered to the air. The area is painful, and the child will be uncomfortable during diaper changes. Applying a protective ointment to the area will keep the diaper from sticking to the skin and also prevent contact of the skin with stool.

Evaluation

As in all plans of care, evaluation of nursing interventions is accomplished by assessing for the absence or decrease of defining characteristics of actual problems.

Appendicitis

Acute appendicitis is the most common surgical emergency in children.

Etiology/Incidence/Pathophysiology

Although the mortality rate has declined steadily, appendicitis is still the cause of many preventable deaths. The disease tends to occur slightly more often in boys and is rare under 2 years of age.

The appendix is located at the end of the cecum and has no apparent function. The cause of appendicitis is an obstruction of the appendiceal lumen, usually by a fecalith (hardened feces). Appendiceal perforation occurs more easily because of the thin-walled appendix and the inability of the immature omentum to prevent peritonitis. Secondary obstruction may result from inflammatory changes of blood-borne or enteric infections or from parasites, stenosis, or kinking. The obstruction causes inflammatory changes in the mucosal wall, which becomes edematous and filled with leukocytes. This distention relays pain via stretch receptors through visceral nerve fibers so that pain is first perceived in the periumbilical region. Inflammation of the appendix leads to vomiting and fever; with increased inflammation, the pain localizes to the right lower quadrant. Distention also compromises the blood supply. Gangrene and perforation may result. Perforation of the appendix allows bacteria to escape and produces a generalized peritonitis or a localized abscess (confined by the adjoining omentum).

Clinical Manifestations

Appendicitis has a wide variation in onset and pattern of symptoms; however, symptoms usually do not come to the attention of a health professional until they are acute. It is not uncommon for the child with appendicitis to appear in the school nurse's office complaining of severe abdominal pain. Many children will not be comfortable standing upright and will attempt to lessen discomfort by bending over and guarding the abdomen with their hands. It is difficult to assess the location of pain because the child is fearful of anyone's touching the abdomen. However, the nurse can ask the child to show "where it hurts" and avoid palpation. *The presence of low-grade fever, periumbilical or right lower quadrant pain (at McBurney's point), and vomiting should alert the nurse to seek immediate medical assistance for the child.* In young children (toddlers and preschool-age children), appendicitis does not necessarily present with the classic symptoms of pain, vomiting, and fever. The first symptoms may be irritability or listlessness, followed by vomiting. Diarrhea is more common and more extensive than in the older child. Nausea and vomiting occur after the onset of pain, whereas in gastroenteritis the reverse is true. This is an important difference in differentiating appendicitis from gastroenteritis (Leape, 1987).

Diagnostic Assessment

Because appendicitis is an emergency, there is little time available to prepare the child adequately for the diagnostic workup. If at all possible, parents should be encouraged to stay with the child. Letting the parents know that the nurse is aware of their concern and will answer their questions helps them cope with their anxiety.

The abdomen is palpated to assess for rigidity and tenderness. Adequate preparation will decrease the child's tendency to tense the abdominal muscles. Sedation can be used to allay the child's anxiety and overcome voluntary guarding without masking the underlying process (Kottmeier, 1986).

The examination is started in an area opposite the suspected region of the inflamed appendix. Bowel sounds during the early acute phase of appendicitis are usually normal or occasionally may be high-pitched. Advanced inflammation and perforation result in diminished or absent bowel sounds. Tenderness at McBurney's point (right lower quadrant) is the most important finding on physical examination. With progressive inflammation, involuntary spasm is present; and with the onset of peritonitis, rebound tenderness is noted. Rebound tenderness is elicited by applying deep pressure to the abdomen followed by a quick release of pressure. Pain (localized or general) felt on release of pressure indicates peritoneal irritation. If the inflammation is located in the pelvic area, the abdominal examination may be negative. A rectal examination should be done last. School-age children are particularly modest, and it is important to explain the need for rectal examination and to provide privacy. Although the rectal examination is questioned as a diagnostic tool, it remains an essential part of the examination to rule out other causes (Kottmeier, 1986).

Diagnostic tests will include blood studies, x-ray examination, sonography, or computed tomography scans of the abdomen. A leukocyte count of 14,000 to 16,000 cells/mm^3 is a significant finding. Visualization studies may show the presence of a fecalith or a swollen and inflamed appendix. The physician must also rule out other possible causes of acute abdominal pain, including severe constipation, urinary tract infection, and acute gastroenteritis as well as pelvic inflammatory disease and discomfort associated with ovulation in postpubescent girls.

Therapeutic Management

Perforation occurs frequently in children, so when a diagnosis of appendicitis is made, an emergency appendectomy is scheduled. Contraindications to immediate surgery include the presence of a high fever, dehydration, or sepsis, all of which must be quickly controlled before the child is anesthetized.

Preoperatively, the patient may require pain medication or sedation to relieve anxiety if the child was not sedated during the physical examination. The use of prophylactic antibiotics preoperatively has been shown to lower postoperative wound infection (Winslow et al, 1983). Prophylactic antibiotics are also given for 24 hours postoperatively in nonperforated appendicitis and 10 days for perforated or gangrenous appendicitis. If perforation occurs, wound drainage and delayed wound closure may also be indicated.

Nursing Care

If perforation did not occur and there was no abscess, the child usually remains in the hospital for 3 to 4 days. Nursing care includes monitoring the intravenous fluids and vital signs; assessing the incision at dressing changes; encouraging ambulation, deep breathing, and coughing; and observing for signs of abscess formation (increased pain, restlessness, irritability, and a decrease in ambulation). Table 35–15 details an appropriate plan of care for the child after appendectomy.

The child will experience pain from the incision, and pain medication should be offered. Many children hesitate to ask for medication because they are afraid of a "shot." The nurse should obtain an order for oral medication to be given as soon as the child can tolerate liquids, usually 24 hours after surgery. Intravenous analgesia is another alternative.

The child with an abscess or perforated appendix will return from surgery with an intravenous line, a drain in the incision, and a nasogastric tube. The child will be given parenteral antibiotics for the period of hospitalization, usually 10 days. The child is acutely ill and needs intensive nursing care during the immediate postoperative period.

The child without peritonitis recovers rapidly and may return to school a week or two after surgery. Strenuous exercise should be curtailed for several weeks, however. School personnel will need to be informed of these restrictions to ensure the child's recovery.

Necrotizing Enterocolitis

Necrotizing enterocolitis (NEC) continues to be the most serious and most frequently seen gastrointestinal disorder in neonatal intensive care units (Walsh & Kliegman, 1986). In this condition, a diffuse or patchy necrosis of the mucosa or submucosa occurs in the large and small bowel. Intestinal perforation, peritonitis, and shock are potential outcomes of this disturbance.

Etiology/Incidence/Pathophysiology

Neonatal NEC is primarily a disease of low birthweight infants (usually less than 34 weeks' gestation) but can also occur in full-term infants. Reported frequency varies, ranging from 1 to 5 per cent of all admissions to the neonatal intensive care unit. In the very low birthweight infant (less than 1500 g), frequency approaches 12 per cent (Walsh & Kliegman, 1986).

No single explanation is currently accepted for the pathogenesis of NEC. Most investigators believe that NEC is a multifactorial disease. Mechanisms thought to be important in the pathogenesis of NEC are summarized in Table 35–20. The best hypothesis that can be formulated at this time is that NEC results as a response of the immature gastrointestinal system to multiple potentially injurious factors and may be caused by their producing synergistic damage (Fanaroff & Kliegman, 1993).

Clinical Manifestations

Over 90 per cent of patients develop symptoms within the first 5 days of life and the remainder usually within 2 weeks after birth. Almost all infants who develop NEC have been fed formula or breast milk. Sys-

TABLE 35-20
Probable Mechanisms in the Pathogenesis of Necrotizing Enterocolitis

Gastrointestinal and Immunologic Immaturity

There is some evidence that enteral feeding may be the critical element that initiates intestinal maturation; it is unknown whether prolonged periods without enteral feedings or the effect of timed bolus feedings by nasogastric tube contributes to the pathogenesis of necrotizing enterocolitis (NEC); a hyperosmolar substrate, such as medication or even formula, may cause mucosal injury; immunologic immaturity may also be a factor in the development of NEC; infants fed exclusively human milk (which contains many immunoactive components) have, however, not been protected against developing NEC

Hypoxic-Ischemic Insult to the Bowel

Intestinal hypoperfusion with ischemia of the bowel is thought to occur as a result of events associated with high-risk premature infants (e.g., perinatal asphyxia, respiratory distress syndrome, shock, localized vasospasm, or thromboembolic phenomena); the "diving reflex" phenomenon, in which blood is shunted away from the intestines during systemic hypoxia with selective perfusion of the brain and heart, has been proposed as an explanation for bowel ischemia; also, the mucosal cells cease secretion of mucin, and proteolytic autodigestion of the mucosa occurs; clinical factors such as umbilical arterial catheterization (because of the potential for large vessel thromboemboli) and neonatal polycythemia (because of sluggish gastrointestinal blood flow) continue to be studied as potential causes of bowel ischemia; maternal cocaine use has also been associated with NEC—it is hypothesized that cocaine crosses the placenta and causes vasoconstriction of the fetal gastrointestinal tract

Bacterial Invasion of the Bowel

Infection is thought to play a prominent role in NEC; bacteria penetrate the intestinal wall after proteolytic autodigestion occurs; NEC occurs endemically and epidemically; organisms associated with outbreaks of NEC include *Escherichia coli, Klebsiella, Enterobacter, Pseudomonas, Salmonella, Clostridium* species, coronavirus, rotavirus, and enteroviruses; intestinal mucosa is thought to allow passage of intraluminal bacteria through the wall into the blood stream

Substrate for Bacterial Replication Through Excess Feeding

Conflicting opinions exist regarding the role of enteral feeding in the development of NEC; 90 to 95 per cent of all infants who develop NEC have been fed enterally; the mechanism by which excess feeding may contribute to NEC remains obscure; it has been postulated that excess formula may be malabsorbed and pass to the colon, where it may serve as a substrate for the bacterial flora in the colon

From Walsh, M. C., & Kliegman, R. M. (1986). Necrotizing enterocolitis: treatment based on staging criteria. *Pediatric Clinics of North America, 33,* 179–201; Rushton, C. (1990). Necrotizing enterocolitis, 1: Pathogenesis and diagnosis. *MCN, 15,* 296–300.

temic manifestations that raise the nurse's suspicion include temperature instability, lethargy or irritability, apnea, or bradycardia. Signs and symptoms associated with feeding and gastrointestinal function include difficulty with feedings, increased pregavage residuals (feeding retained in the stomach or from the previous feeding), abdominal distention, inability to defecate (may indicate a developing ileus), and occult blood in emesis or stool (Holtzman & Brown, 1986). The infant may be tolerating feedings and requiring decreasing amounts of oxygen and then unexpectedly develop this disease. The changes can occur rapidly and must be dealt with immediately; however, it is essential that explanations and support for the parents be provided (Korones, 1986).

Diagnostic Assessment

The earliest radiologic sign is segmented distention of the small bowel. The cardinal sign of the disease is pneumatosis intestinalis, which is the presence of air pockets within the intestinal wall caused by invading bacteria that can result in perforation of the bowel. This most commonly affects the terminal ileum and right colon, but it can be much more extensive. Portal vein gas seen on x-ray examination is indicative of extensive disease.

Therapeutic Management

Nonoperative treatment is successful in a high percentage of infants with NEC if therapy is instituted before there is extensive bowel necrosis. The goal of therapy is complete bowel rest. A sump tube (a nasogastric tube attached to suction) can be used to decompress the abdomen. The infant is given nothing orally; hydration and nutrition are maintained via peripheral or central parenteral nutrition for approximately 2 weeks, although the timing of the reinstitution of feeding is controversial. After blood, urine, stool, and spinal fluid cultures are taken, antibiotics are administered, both intravenously and orally. The use of oral antibiotics also is controversial. If they are administered, it is to decrease the risk of septicemia and reduce intestinal colonization (Holtzman & Brown, 1986). Blood studies are carried out to monitor the infant's electrolyte and blood gas levels and to obtain complete blood count and platelet count. Intubation of the infant may be necessary if respiratory compromise develops.

Abdominal radiographs are taken every 8 to 12 hours to look for distention of bowel loops, pneumatosis intestinalis (air in the intramural wall of the intestines), pneumoperitoneum (air in the peritoneum), or air in the hepatic vein. A left lateral decubitus radiograph is needed to detect free air from an intestinal perforation. The only absolute indication for surgery is intestinal perforation. The challenge in management is to "avoid operating on the infant with NEC who does not have necrosis yet not delay operating on the infant who does" (Leape, 1987).

If surgery is performed, the entire bowel is examined for perforations and necrotic tissue. Only the *obviously* necrotic intestine is removed (Embron, 1990). Intestinal diversion is performed by creating an enterostomy (opening into the intestine and creating a stoma on the abdomen). The final stage of treatment is removal of the ostomy and reanastomosis of the two ends of the intestine 1 to 2 months later after distal bowel resting. When the majority of the intestine appears to be necrotic, massive resection leads to a short-bowel syndrome, but *not* resecting is fatal.

Postoperative management requires a qualified intensive care team. These infants may require ventilatory support, large amounts of fluids, and repeated infusions of platelets and clotting factors to correct disseminated intravascular coagulation (see Chapter 34).

Nursing Diagnostic Statements and Collaborative Problems

Altered nutrition: less than body requirements; need for parenteral feedings.

High risk for altered health maintenance; *risk factors:*

- *Increased family stress.*
- *Lack of resources to promote effective breastfeeding.*

Planning and Implementation

Providing Nutrition Postoperatively. Postoperatively, the infant is maintained on parenteral nutrition. Nasogastric low-osmotic feedings are begun gradually. Breast milk or predigested formula in small amounts and diluted strengths is used for feedings. The infant must be watched closely for residuals before feedings and for diarrhea, bloody feces, or occult blood in the stool, which would signify further irritation or necrosis of the bowel.

As the infant continues to improve, attempts are made to give feedings via the nipple. The infant is given the opportunity to take a designated amount by mouth, and the remainder is given via gavage.

Facilitating Home Management. Necrotizing enterocolitis is a debilitating disease that results in prolonged hospitalization with the potential of at least two major operative procedures for the infant. This places added stress on the family and on the bonding process between the infant and parents. The nursing staff can minimize family members' anxieties by establishing a trusting relationship with them. This is done through honestly answering their questions and being available to hear their concerns. This relationship will foster the exchange of information and support the development of plans for discharge. These families have been under a great deal of stress and usually require referral to community resources, such as a visiting nurse, to facilitate adjustment to home care of the infant.

The nurse should explore with the mother the possibility of breastfeeding her infant who is at risk for NEC. *Fresh* breast milk contains lymphocytes, macrophages, and lactoferrin, which aid the infant's natural defenses against bacterial invasion of the intestinal mucosa; however, NEC is also known to occur in breastfed infants. (Protective elements of breast milk are lost when breast milk is stored.) Many hospitals have breast pumps that can be used during the infant's long hospitalization to aid the mother in continuing to feed her baby. Resource groups, such as the Leche League, may be supportive referrals.

Peptic Ulcer

Peptic ulcer is a general term describing any erosion of the mucosal wall of the stomach (gastric ulcer) or duodenum (duodenal ulcer).

Etiology/Incidence/Pathophysiology

Peptic ulcers are more common in adults; however, now that fiberoptic technology has made endoscopy practical for infants and children, the diagnosis is increasingly encountered in pediatric patients. No firm prevalence figures exist, but peptic ulceration is encountered in 1 to 2 per cent of hospitalized pediatric patients. Boys are affected more often than girls are. Peptic ulcers are more common in late school-age children and adolescents than in younger children.

The exact cause of peptic ulcers is unknown. In most instances, the ulcers arise as a complication of the stress of other diseases. These secondary ulcers typically are multiple and superficial. They may occur equally in the stomach and duodenum. They are associated with more serious insults, such as head injury, multiple trauma, or severe burns (Curling ulcer). However, they may also accompany sepsis and respiratory, renal, or hepatic failure.

"Primary ulcers" are usually deeper and solitary and are most often found in the gastric antrum or duodenum. These ulcers occur in genetically predisposed individuals with a strong family history of peptic ulcer disease. Research has indicated two mechanisms as possible causes: (1) increased gastric acid secretion or (2) impaired mucosal defense against back-diffusion of acid. In addition, stress is thought to be an important contributing factor in the development of peptic ulcers. A spiral bacterium, *Helicobacter pylori,* has been identified as a possible etiologic factor in peptic ulcers and gastritis in both adults and children (Nord, 1988; Gryboski, 1991).

Clinical Manifestations

Bleeding is the most common presentation of peptic ulceration. This may take the form of *hematemesis*—the vomiting of blood from the stomach, which usually gives the appearance of coffee grounds because of the interaction of blood and stomach acid. Bright red blood is more likely vomited from the pharynx or the esophagus. Parents are usually more alarmed by the appearance of recognizable blood. Some reassurance can be offered that the problem is rarely as dramatic as it appears. By contrast, the vomiting of large amounts of coffee-ground material may not worry parents but should be recognized by professionals as an alarming sign.

When blood is passed in the stools, they take on a tarry black appearance known as melena. A characteristic foul metallic odor is present.

Chronic abdominal pain or even weight loss may be the only sign of chronic primary peptic ulcer disease. This is seen most often in children and adolescents with a strong family history of ulcers but may occur acutely after unusual stress. Abdominal pain may be nonspecific, particularly in younger children, but epigastric pain, especially if it penetrates to the back and is relieved temporarily by eating, points to the possibility of an ulcer. Most children with abdominal pain have no serious organic process, but complaints that are specific are more suggestive of disease. Presence of anemia or occult blood in the stool is a strong indication for further investigation for peptic ulcer disease.

Diagnostic Assessment

Differential diagnosis includes any of the causes of acute upper gastrointestinal tract bleeding. Parents should be questioned about all possible factors when a child has bleeding. Hematemesis is often the result of blood ingested from a posterior nose bleed. Individuals with a bleeding tendency may bleed more easily from this and other causes. These conditions are exacerbated by aspirin ingestion, which impairs platelet function. Forceful vomiting accompanying gastritis may tear the esophageal mucosa, a condition known as a Mallory-Weiss tear. Erosions of the esophagus, stomach, and duodenum result from the ingestion of corrosives. These may be caused by lye, the residue from automatic dishwasher soap, or medications such as aspirin. Rarely, upper gastrointestinal bleeding results from esophageal varices, a complication of chronic liver disease in both children and adults.

In adult patients, older children, and adolescents, upper gastrointestinal tract barium studies are probably as effective as endoscopy in making a diagnosis of ulcer. (See Table 35–8.) However, it is difficult for infants and young children to cooperate fully during the radiographic techniques that make reliable diagnosis possible. Accordingly, endoscopy is preferable in infants and children. This can now be performed in most children without the need for general anesthesia. However, few children with nonspecific abdominal pain will be found to have ulcers and are spared endoscopy unless there are specific signs pointing to the diagnosis. If upper gastrointestinal tract bleeding is present, endoscopy will most frequently lead to a diagnosis.

Therapeutic Management

As in most conditions, the best treatment for ulcer disease is prevention. Children at risk for the development of secondary ulcers should be treated prophylactically. The intensive care unit patient with an indwelling nasogastric tube should be given sufficient liquid antacid to keep gastric acid pH above 5 as measured at the bedside. This may require 10 to 30 ml of antacid instilled every 1 to 2 hours. Alternatively or in addition, one of the histamine H_2 receptor antagonists, such as cimetidine or ranitidine, can be effective in blocking secretion of stomach acid. Again, the effect on gastric pH is checked and the dose adjusted because metabolism of these drugs varies considerably in severely ill patients. Antacids and histamine H_2 receptor antagonists should not be given at the same time because antacids may inhibit absorption of the drug. In the presence of mucosal erosions, sucralfate is used. This is a medication that combines with fibrin to form an occlusion over the ulcer site to protect it from the effects of acid and digestive enzymes and allow healing. Antacids interfere with the action of sucralfate, so they should not be administered concurrently.

The prognosis for "secondary ulcers" depends on effective treatment at the time they occur and the course of the underlying disease. Once the acute phase is over, the ulcers are not likely to recur, and the antiulcer medications may be discontinued within days. Primary ulcers in children follow the well-described adult pattern. The tendency to ulcer formation is a chronic condition; in about one half of patients, they will recur. These may have a seasonal pattern, flaring in the spring or fall or coming on at times of stress. In adults, prophylaxis for 4 to 6 weeks with half the therapeutic dose of antiulcer medications can prevent recurrence. This has not been tested in children. However, with the availability of modern diagnostic and therapeutic approaches, few children will require surgery because of recurring ulcers. Despite this, many myths about the origin and treatment of ulcers persist. It is up to the nurse as part of the health care team to inquire about the family's attitude toward the disease and to guide them to remedies.

The nurse plays an important role in all phases of care. During diagnosis, careful use of Hematest tablets or Hemoccult paper to test for occult blood in the stool and accurate documentation facilitate early recognition. Helping to identify the child at risk for secondary peptic ulcer disease is an important nursing responsibility as well.

Nursing Diagnostic Statement

***Family coping: potential for growth** related to expressed desire to learn management of therapeutic regimen.*

Planning and Implementation

Teaching to Control Symptoms and to Promote a Healthier Lifestyle. The nurse's role in teaching includes the areas of medication, stress management, and dietary management. Medications both aid in healing and help to control the pain associated with a peptic ulcer. The child (when old enough) and family should be thoroughly familiar with the use of prescribed medications and should be given written instructions to refer to as questions arise during home management.

Stress management deals with both illness-related stressors and chronic stressors encountered as the result of individual and family lifestyles. Nursing strategies to minimize the stress of acute illness and hospitalization are detailed in Table 21–5, Nursing Process Plan: The Hospitalized Child. Chapter 18 deals with the general topics of stress, coping, and related nursing strategies.

Most parents think that peptic ulcers should be treated by diet. There are few dietary regimens that are truly necessary, however. The family is asked what they believe about the relation between diet and ulcers. It has been appreciated that milk products probably cause more harm than good in ulcer patients. Initially, milk buffers the acid and provides symptomatic relief. However, the high levels of calcium present in milk are potent stimulators of acid secretion and result in a rebound effect, which produces more stomach acid. Alcohol, caffeine, and cigarettes are potent stimulants to acid secretion and should be particularly avoided by the adolescent patient. The nurse should encourage the patient to eat a normal well-balanced diet for age, and relatives should be counseled to avoid aggravating the patient at mealtime with unnecessary suggestions about food.

Healthy dietary patterns are also encouraged. Striving to maintain a regular mealtime schedule, avoiding overeating, and eating a small snack between meals are preventive measures.

Gastrointestinal Dysfunctional Disorders

Children who have gastrointestinal dysfunctional disorders are generally healthy children with chronic digestive symptoms. Although only a few of the problems are life-threatening, they can cause considerable personal stress and interruption in family life. Accurate delineation of the problem and early prescription of an effective strategy can allay anxiety and may well prevent a brief interlude of dysfunction from developing into an entrenched maladaptive problem.

The following conditions are categorized as dysfunctional: (1) colic, (2) gastroesophageal reflux (chalasia), (3) irritable bowel syndrome, and (4) chronic constipation.

Colic

Colic is characterized by vigorous crying and drawing the legs up to the abdomen as if the baby were in severe pain.

Etiology/Incidence/Pathophysiology

Colic occurs in infants under 3 months old and rarely persists past 6 months of age, although parents cannot be guaranteed of this. It usually begins in the first 3 weeks of life and is suspected to be the result of paroxysmal abdominal cramping, although a specific cause is rarely uncovered. Crying is intermittent, occurring one or more times a day, with each episode lasting from 30 minutes to 2 hours (Schmitt, 1986). Gas may rumble in the stomach, and temporary relief seems to occur if this is passed. Some infants can be quieted with handling but will cry incessantly as soon as they are put down. Colicky babies are healthy and between crying spells are usually happy. If the crying is continuous, other causes should be suspected. Factors thought to be associated with colic include the absorptive immaturity of the gastrointestinal tract, food allergy, maternal factors, infant characteristics, and feeding practices.

Absorptive Immaturity. In comparison with the adult, the normal term infant has malabsorption of many nutrient classes. Virtually all infants have some degree of lactose malabsorption (Balistreri et al, 1983). This gradually improves until maximal efficiency is achieved by 3 to 4 months of age (Maclean & Fink, 1980). Similarly, most term infants fail to absorb as much as 15 per cent of ingested fat from formula, in contrast to the adult's normal malabsorption of 5 per cent. Part of this is due to a reduced bile acid pool (Balistreri et al, 1983).

Allergy. The extent to which food allergy contributes to colic continues to be studied and debated. It is speculated that the ability for whole protein to cross the mucosal barrier in the intestinal tract of a newborn renders the infant more susceptible to allergy. Allergy is questioned as a cause because colic occurs with equal frequency in bottlefed and breastfed infants (Iacono, 1991).

Maternal Factors. If the mother's pregnancy or delivery was particularly arduous, if perinatal complications have developed, and if the mother has been sleep deprived, her ability to tolerate a crying infant may be limited. Parental frustration and anger after the appearance of colic may aggravate symptoms or at least affect the family's tolerance. The physical demands made of the mother or the amount of support she is receiving may well contribute to the likelihood of the baby's being viewed as colicky by the mother.

Infant Characteristics. The infant's temperament also influences the degree to which colic will affect the child. The average infant cries about 2 hours daily at 2 weeks. This increases to 3 hours at 6 weeks, with some infants crying for close to a mean of 4 hours. Infants differ in temperament, and infants who are described by their parents as difficult cry more. These differences may also be indicated in utero by fetal activity levels.

Feeding Practices. Colic can occasionally be connected with improper feeding techniques or inadequate burping, but this cause is not nearly as prevalent as it was once thought to be; changes in diet or burping and feeding methods rarely eliminate colic.

Diagnostic Assessment

The vast majority of infants with symptoms of colic have a self-limiting syndrome of multifactorial causation. The distinction from diseases requiring investigation or remediation begins with a careful history.

Careful determination of the timing and volume of feeds provides helpful clues concerning overfeeding, underfeeding, or chaotic schedule, all of which may be contributing to the child's symptoms. Colic associated with improper feeding methods, although rare, is readily halted by teaching better technique. Caregivers should be asked to demonstrate the feeding process to rule out this possible source of colic. A detailed history of daily events helps establish any pattern to the colic attacks or any precipitating factors and to document caregiver reactions and efforts taken to relieve the crying.

On physical examination, comparison of height, weight, and head circumference with the norms is the single most valuable tool. If the infant's development is normal and the child is well nourished, most concerns for underlying disease can be eliminated.

Therapeutic Management

Despite the fact that colic disappears spontaneously and is frequently given only minor attention by health care professionals, it often has a strong emotional impact on the family. Any family that has lived through only a few days of the crying episodes of an infant who is unresponsive to any efforts to comfort or console feels extremely exhausted and emotionally drained. This is especially true for the main caregiver. The disruption that a crying, irritable infant causes to family relationships and routines produces a vicious cycle of fatigue, frustration, anger, and helplessness. This can be destructive to the functioning of the family unit if empathetic intervention is not begun early and maintained until the colicky period is outgrown.

In some circumstances, management includes a change of formula. The rationale for making more than a single formula change is highly questionable. The findings of studies suggesting that colic is affected by intake of milk are inconclusive. Carey (1989) observed that changing formula may create a placebo effect initially, resulting in less crying; but after a few days, previous levels of crying return. Although rarely used, a mild sedative for the infant may carry a family through the most difficult period. This may include the use of phenobarbital elixir or one of the antihistamines, such as hydroxyzine hydrochloride (Atarax) or diphenhydramine hydrochloride (Benadryl). Antispasmodics such as dicyclomine hydrochloride (Bentyl) are no longer used because of an association with infant death under 6 months of age (Pinyerd & Zipf, 1989).

The most effective tool available to the family with a colicky infant is professional support. Scheduled weekly visits or telephone calls can contribute to their growth as confident caregivers during this difficult period.

Nursing Diagnostic Statements

High risk for caregiver role strain, mother; *risk factors:*

- *Maternal guilt feelings.*
- *Maternal fear that infant's well-being is threatened.*
- *Lack of respite from care of the infant.*
- *Repeated nature of episodes of colic.*

High risk for parental role conflict; *risk factor: negative parental feelings about the infant.*

Planning and Implementation

Promoting Effective Caregiving. Emotional support involves reassurances to the caregiver that despite the crying and pain, the infant is gaining weight and developing normally. Regular emphasis should be placed on the fact that colic is not the result of poor mothering and that maternal feelings of inadequacy, anger, or periodic dislike of the baby and of mothering are universal. The caregiver should be offered regular opportunities to talk about feelings and be encouraged to do so. Some communities have parental stress hot lines (COPE, CALM), of which parents of colicky infants should be informed. They should be encouraged to keep the phone number available even if they never need to use it. Some parents find solace just in knowing there are resources in case the stress becomes too much.

The caregiver should be urged to spend time away from the colicky infant on a fairly regular basis. Some relief from constant full responsibility makes most caregivers better able to handle themselves when they are "on duty." Some parents need help to overcome guilt feelings associated with "getting away" for awhile.

TABLE 35-21
Family-Centered Teaching: Diversional Activities to Assist Care of an Infant with Colic

- Place infant in a front pouch carried close to the body
- Provide rhythmic vibration, such as a car ride in an approved car seat
- Place the infant prone across the knees and gently pat the back
- Use infant massage techniques, especially of the abdomen
- Provide rhythmic motion for the infant through walking, rocking, or placing in a swing
- Swaddle the infant in a soft blanket
- Place the infant on a warmed heating pad or covered hot water bottle, taking care not to make it too hot
- Provide soothing auditory stimuli, such as taped intrauterine sounds, white noise, and lullabies

Efforts to prevent or reduce colic episodes require experimentation; the success of a given method is highly individualistic. Some infants respond to measures that stimulate peristalsis. This may be achieved by carrying the infant close,* placing the baby prone over a warm towel or warm water bottle, or giving the infant a few ounces of warm diluted tea. Much caution should be used with a warm water bottle; burns can occur with too much heat. The infant's skin does not tolerate as much heat as that of older children or adults. The warm water bottle should be securely closed and covered with a towel before placing the baby on it. The infant's skin should be checked frequently to ensure that overheating of the skin does not occur. Another suggested approach is walking and placing the infant over the caregiver's arm, which provides gentle pressure on the abdomen (Gillies, 1987).

Other infants show improvement when their position is changed often, when they are burped by the shoulder method and with massaging rather than patting, and when smaller feedings are offered more frequently. Taking time to relax and play with the baby before beginning feeding and placing the baby in an infant seat for at least 30 minutes after feedings are sometimes effective in reducing colic episodes. Assisting the parents with the development of diversional strategies is also an important task (Table 35–21).

Some infants can be distracted successfully from their colicky episodes with brightly colored wrapping paper, pictures of varying complexity and depth, or music of varied rhythm and loudness. Some colicky

* An infant carrier allows the caregiver to keep the infant close in either a chest or back position while leaving the hands free to carry out other activities.

infants respond to the rhythm of an automatic infant swing or to being placed (with proper securement and continued presence of the caregiver) on top of a running clothes dryer. (In this case, it may be the sound, vibration, or warmth that quiets the baby.) An automobile ride may have a similar effect.

Fostering Parental Role Performance. Fostering attachment is important because frequent negative feelings can eventually disrupt development of a healthy parent-child attachment. Pointing out the infant's desirable features and signs of normal development regularly helps the parents view the child more positively, which encourages attachment feelings. Acknowledging and praising good interaction between parent and infant as well as helping the parent notice how the infant responds to parental overtures also nurture healthy bonds.

Gastroesophageal Reflux (Chalasia)

Gastroesophageal reflux occurs as a result of relaxation or incompetence of the lower esophageal sphincter, permitting reflux of gastric contents into the esophagus. This condition may exist with or without a hiatal hernia.

Etiology/Incidence/Pathophysiology

The cause of gastroesophageal reflux is not known. Although many infants have some degree of incompetence of the lower esophageal sphincter, in more severe cases the infant is threatened because of chronic esophageal inflammation or pulmonary aspiration. Failure to thrive may also result, requiring intervention.

The advent of newer diagnostic techniques has complicated the once simplistic picture of gastroesophageal reflux. A physiologic high-pressure zone of 1 to 3 cm of the distal esophagus is termed the lower esophageal sphincter. Pressures in this zone increase steadily from birth to 2 months of age in healthy infants. However, competence of the valve depends on coordinated relaxation and closure. The entrance of the esophagus into the stomach at an acute angle enhances effectiveness of closure. Delayed gastric emptying is associated with reflux (Orenstein, 1991).

Some reflux of gastric contents has been shown to occur even in healthy subjects. Total number and duration of episodes of reflux, documented by prolonged pH monitoring, seem to be important determinants in the development of esophagitis (Andze et al, 1991). This in turn may affect the functioning of the lower esophageal sphincter. Shortened esophagus is probably a consequence of chronic esophagitis from chronic reflux rather than the cause. Likewise, a demonstrable hiatus hernia is probably an associated factor rather than a causative one.

Most infants will improve spontaneously. In healthy infants, regurgitation should have stopped by the time the child begins to walk at 10 to 12 months. Neurologically impaired children have a much higher prevalence of significant reflux. In fact, some authors distinguish two groups of children, those with simple reflux and those in whom it occurs in association with other significant problems. Many of these are older children.

Clinical Manifestations

Signs of gastroesophageal reflux usually appear in the first week of life and most commonly consist of chronic vomiting or regurgitation. There are usually no signs of discomfort or gastrointestinal dysfunction, and the infant readily eats again if given the opportunity after vomiting. Vomiting may be effortless, is usually quite forceful, and does not contain bile. Because of a possible significant loss of calories, the infant may show weight loss and eventually failure to thrive. A variety of cardiorespiratory symptoms may accompany the vomiting. Reflux into the pharynx predisposes to aspiration and may cause respiratory symptoms, including apnea, bradycardia, sudden infant death syndrome, severe aspiration episodes, recurrent upper respiratory infections, and aspiration pneumonia. Repeated reflux of gastric acid can cause irritation of the esophagus leading to esophagitis and esophageal bleeding manifested as hematemesis, melena (blood in stools), or occult blood.

Diagnostic Assessment

The presence of reflux is evaluated through use of a barium esophagogram or radionuclide scan. Because reflux is an intermittent phenomenon, it may not occur at the exact time that the barium esophagogram is done. Therefore, the sensitivity of this method is in question (Johnson et al, 1981). Reflux can also be evaluated by intraesophageal pH monitoring, in which a probe is inserted (2 to 3 cm proximal to the esophageal sphincter) to measure reflux of acid from the stomach. With an indwelling electrode, reflux episodes can be evaluated during a 24-hour period. Ambulatory pH monitoring systems are available, making home monitoring an acceptable alternative (Petersen, 1986).

Therapeutic Management

Medical Management. Medical management of the infant with gastroesophageal reflux is aimed at reducing the likelihood of reflux and its consequences. This is done by use of (1) cereal-thickened formula, (2) small-volume feedings, (3) slow feedings, (4) burping during feedings (after each 1 to $1^1/_2$ ozs) and after each feeding, and (5) an upright (30-degree angle) prone position after feeding.

Elevation of the upper body is used for one to several hours after each feeding, depending on the severity of the problem. Antacids or a histamine H_2 receptor antagonist is sometimes required to treat esophagitis. Other medications used to treat gastroesophageal reflux are bethanechol chloride (parasympathomimetic) and metoclopramide (dopaminergic blocking drug) to accelerate emptying of the stomach. Symptoms and weight gain are monitored carefully during this trial period of conservative medical management.

The length of conservative treatment varies. Gastroesophageal reflux resolves in most infants by 18 months of age if treated medically with good positional therapy. However, it is recommended that children with an esophageal stricture be treated surgically.

Surgical Management. Unsuccessful medical therapy usually warrants re-evaluation and often surgical intervention (e.g., Nissen-Hill or Thal fundoplication), depending on the severity of complications. In this procedure, the distal esophagus is wrapped with the adjacent gastric fundus and secured with plicating sutures to create a new gastroesophageal junction and thereby curtail reflux. During the immediate postoperative period, gastric decompression by nasogastric tube is necessary to prevent tearing of the sutures. A gastrostomy may be performed, depending on the surgeon's preference.

Nursing Diagnostic Statement

High risk for injury: postoperative complications; risk factors:

- *Stasis of respiratory secretions.*
- *Intolerance to oral feedings.*

Planning and Implementation

Nurses participate in all phases of care. Assisting parents to promote the child's normal development and helping them understand the treatment modalities are important nursing roles. Management during conservative medical therapy requires careful monitoring and documentation of nursing observations.

Nursing Strategies Related to Prevention of Complications. A major focus of postoperative care is the preservation of good respiratory function. The surgical procedure is commonly done before the age when cooperation with requests to cough and deep breathe is possible; therefore, repositioning every 2 hours is necessary. An additional important measure is postural drainage. This should be done before feedings to prevent regurgitation.

Small amounts of oral feedings are gradually given; the child is observed for any signs of intolerance, such as distention, vomiting, or discomfort. A blenderized diet is required for approximately 2 weeks until the operative swelling has subsided.

It is essential that older children be encouraged to chew their food thoroughly when they eat. Parents should be advised that the child may complain of a bloated sensation after eating. This is due to delayed gastric emptying. Hiccupping may also be occasionally seen but gradually resolves. Parents are advised to see the surgeon for follow-up care and further evaluation.

Irritable Bowel Syndrome

Irritable bowel syndrome is characterized by intermittent episodes of large, loose stools or crampy abdominal pain. Although there is an increase in numbers of stools per day, there is no evidence of malabsorption or impaired growth. In the toddler, recurrent diarrhea is the common presentation of irritable bowel syndrome; school-age children usually have recurrent, abdominal pain.

Etiology/Incidence/Pathophysiology

Fat intake and increased fluid intake have been identified as causes of irritable bowel syndrome. It is postulated that fat delays gastric emptying time, thereby influencing transit through the small bowel. Excessive fluid intake overwhelms the child's intestinal capacity for absorption of fluid or solute. Restriction of fat and fluids to normal amounts restores most patients to an acceptable bowel pattern. Other explanations for the phenomenon include disordered motility, rapid transit, artificial sweeteners, dietary factors, emotional factors, and family dysfunction.

An excessive number of children are considered allergic and placed on progressively more restrictive diets as an ever-widening selection of food groups appear to be responsible for the essentially random nature of the loose stools. Often the child with irritable bowel syndrome has a parent with the same condition; and in some instances, children with irritable colon had colic as an infant. No sex difference is noted until adolescence, when girls outnumber boys.

Undoubtedly, some of these children's symptoms result from previous infection with subclinical damage to the small bowel. Examining intestinal mucosa by scanning electron microscopy, Poley (1983) noted evidence of excessive bacterial adherence to the mucosal surface, increased cell shedding associated with more surface mucus, and damage to the brush border. Disturbed fat absorption follows viral infection, possibly as a result of impaired bile acid uptake. However, it is possible that initial fat intolerance eventually resolves and a state of chronic diarrhea persists because of prolonged fat deprivation.

Clinical Manifestations

Clinical manifestations vary according to the age of the child, as does management. The presentation and management of irritable bowel syndrome in the toddler and school-age child are therefore presented separately.

Toddler. Recurrent diarrhea is the common presentation of irritable bowel syndrome in toddlers. The definition relies on the observation of an increased number of loose movements lasting more than 3 weeks without evidence of malabsorption or impaired growth. The usual onset occurs at 6 to 18 months. The problem starts insidiously. The parent describes three to eight stools per day, which initially are slightly formed but become progressively watery throughout the day (Jonas & Dever-Haber, 1982). The child often has an intense thirst. Toddlers generally do not become dehydrated, nor do they lose weight unless their diet is markedly restricted. Infants with diarrhea or dietary restrictions are more easily affected adversely.

School-Age Child. Irritable bowel syndrome in school-age children may present as recurrent abdominal pain. Recurrent abdominal pain is described as repeated complaints of nonspecific stomachaches occurring at least three times over a period of months. Pain is severe enough to interfere with normal functioning but does not usually awaken the child from sleep. The pain is usually periumbilical, although location is variable. It is not associated with eating or a bowel movement. The stool varies in consistency, but constipation is common. Other symptoms, such as headaches, dizziness, blurred vision, and dysuria or frequency, may also be present. Other causes of abdominal pain, including food allergy and lactose intolerance, must be ruled out.

Therapeutic Management

Toddler. The goal of management is to have the child on a diet that does not have excess fluid and contains sufficient fat. This may be accomplished easily by suggesting that the child have some form of fat with every meal with increased amounts early in the day, such as formula or homogenized milk, peanut butter, bacon, margarine, or butter. A maximum of 8 ounces per day of juice and sweetened drinks should be allowed, with the rest of the desired fluid offered as water. Intake of milk can be encouraged; fluids are limited to 24 to 30 ounces per day. Some children should no longer be given the "bottle" because this fosters habitual excessive fluid intake. The rare person with a strong family history of the irritable bowel syndrome may respond to the judicious inclusion of increased fiber in the diet. By contrast, some toddlers seem exquisitely sensitive to large morsels of chewed food, such as raisins or carrots, which may be eliminated from the diet or pureed.

School-Age Child. Management of these children calls for open supportive communication with the family. Antispasmodics may benefit some children, but many respond to increased dietary fiber.

Nursing Care

Nurses can provide supportive counseling for families who are faced with trying to alter their basic approach to a child's dietary habits. It is difficult to change a toddler's habits because of the ritualism in this phase of development. Parents can be encouraged to replace the bottle and the usual sweet juices with water from a cup and simultaneously engage the toddler in favorite activities to divert attention from the habit.

Families with school-age children can benefit from the nurse's support and encouragement as they cope with their child's variable pain. Strategies to strengthen the child's self-image and sense of security are used. (See Chapter 12 on parenting and Chapter 14 on self-esteem.) The nurse can help the child and parents identify environmental factors that might be exacerbating the symptoms. The child's school situation and relationships with friends and family may be stressful and should be discussed. Interviewing the child separately from the parents is often appropriate.

The nurse should recognize that some families may need additional professional counseling and should make an appropriate referral to community resources.

Constipation

Some infants and children have recurrent or chronic constipation; stool is passed infrequently or, if passed daily, consists of hard, small masses. The cause is often a diet that contains too much milk or insufficient amounts of fluids or bulk-forming foods.

Etiology/Incidence/Pathophysiology

Conditions that make defecation painful may promote constipation because the child withholds feces to avoid pain. The most common condition is anal fissures that have developed during the previous passage of hard stool. Inspection of the anus to identify fissures is done by placing a thumb on either side of the anus and retracting the anal tissues laterally. Until healing is complete, an anesthetic ointment and stool softener may be prescribed to relieve defecatory distress.

Mechanical obstruction may also precipitate constipation. Rectal stenosis and Hirschsprung disease are occasional etiologic factors. Rectal stenosis can be confirmed by digital examination. The little finger will be difficult to insert into the anus, and it will seem to meet with resistance in the presence of stenosis. The stenosis is corrected by frequent dilation of the anal canal with the finger until the stenosis is eliminated. Hirschsprung disease and rectal malformations are discussed earlier in this chapter.

In older infants and children, constipation may be due to a chronic misuse of laxatives by apprehensive parents or a psychologic response to faulty toilet training, producing poor bowel evacuation habits.

Regardless of the cause of constipation, measures may be taken to promote adequate defecation while the etiologic factor is being remedied. The child is placed on a high-fiber diet. If medications are used, docusate sodium (Colace) is a frequent first choice as a stool softener. Stimulant laxatives stronger than senna glycerides (Senokot) should not be employed. (There is a common tendency to use glycerin suppositories excessively in young infants.) Accordingly, suppositories should be recommended only with caution against their overuse. If impaction exists, an isotonic enema solution (1 level teaspoon of salt to a pint of water) may be administered to clear the bowel. It should be stressed, however, that most constipation in infancy is readily managed by diet alone.

Functional constipation is treated by first clearing the bowel of stool with enemas, stool softeners, or laxatives. Next, a behavioral program is instituted. The child is put on the toilet two or three times during the day. The child is reinforced with stars or stickers on a calendar or chart when stooling occurs. A predetermined reward mutually agreed on by the child and parent will be awarded once the child has reached the goal. The child is placed on a high-fiber diet and receives stool lubricant or laxatives to promote stooling and promote the return of the bowel to normal size.

Nursing Care

An important role of the nurse in the prevention of constipation is to counsel parents about elimination patterns and dietary habits during well child visits. After 6 months of age, infants can have some foods that are finely chopped rather than pureed to increase bulk. Corn syrup or molasses may be added to milk for infants who are prone to constipation. Nurses can advise parents to offer prunes or prune juice regularly to infants who have hard stools. Providing fluids in addition to milk is an important preventive measure at all ages.

Diets adequate in fiber constitute another preventive measure to encourage for older children. There can be no doubt that the greatest deficiency in the standard North American child's diet is the absence of fiber. This is probably the biggest problem of the so-called junk foods. Even the much maligned "fast foods" probably provide sufficient vitamins, minerals, and protein, but they consistently lack a significant amount of fiber. High-fiber diets have not been well studied in infants, however, and there is concern about binding of essential nutrients if high-fiber diets are given to infants (Cummings & Stephen, 1981).

Parents may also need information about the normal variations in bowel habits among children. Excessive attention and coerciveness about toilet training should be avoided (see Chapter 6 for a discussion of toilet training).

Any treatment approaches to be carried out at home should be explained (i.e., suppository, other medication, an enema). Both verbal and written instructions should be given to parents regarding treatment measures to be conducted at home. One or two demonstrations should also be given if parents seem unsure of instructions or if the nurse judges it necessary.

Malabsorptive Alterations

Intestinal malabsorption in a mild and transient form may produce only temporary indigestion. If it is severe and persistent, however, it can lead to serious consequences, such as nutritional deficits and clinical starvation. Malabsorption occurs when there is a disruption in any step of the digestive process that interferes with the absorption of water and electrolytes, vitamins, minerals, carbohydrates, proteins, and fats. Malabsorptive alterations have diverse causes, including inadequate production of digestive juices, growth of organisms, inflammation of the lining of the intestines, disturbed lymphatic or vascular flow, loss of surface area of bowel (such as in surgical resection), lactose intolerance, and mild malnutrition. Common causes of malabsorption in infancy and childhood discussed in this section include celiac disease and lactose intolerance. Infectious and inflammatory disorders are discussed earlier in this chapter. Cystic fibrosis is discussed in Chapter 32, and milk allergy in Chapter 37.

Gluten-Sensitive Enteropathy (Celiac Disease)

Gluten-sensitive enteropathy is second only to cystic fibrosis as the most common cause of malabsorption in children.

Etiology/Incidence/Pathophysiology

The exact prevalence of the disease is unknown because treatment is not sought for many asymptomatic children. Prevalence is higher in parts of Europe and in Canada than in the United States. The highest frequency of gluten-sensitive enteropathy (1:597) has been found in west Ireland (Silverman & Roy, 1983). Peak frequency is between the age of 9 and 18 months. There is some indication that the incidence of celiac disease coincides with introduction of gluten-containing foods. The mucosa of the small bowel is damaged by gluten-containing foods, resulting in nutrient malabsorption. Gluten is a form of protein contained in wheat, barley, rye, and oats. The toxicity of gluten derived from wheat and rye is more clearly established than that from barley and oats. The gluten itself consists of two protein fractions, glutenin and gliadin. Of these, gliadin appears to be the causative agent. The exact means by which gluten damages the mucosa of the small bowel remains obscure. However, two explanations currently exist. In the first, an enzymatic insufficiency (intestinal) is thought to cause an accumulation of toxic gluten peptides. However, because this deficiency appears to be reversed by dietary management, it may be a consequence of the disease rather than a cause (Silverman & Roy, 1983). It may well be that the peptidase deficiency is secondary to the epithelial damage (Gryboski & Walker, 1983). A second theory, which is now gaining increasing support, holds that the gluten toxicity results from an alteration in immunologic response. Gliadin is thought to play the role of an antigen that causes an injurious immune response. This theory is supported by the striking response to corticosteroid therapy.

The intestinal mucosa is normally lined with tall villi whose function is the absorption of nutrients. In celiac disease, sensitivity to the undigested gluten causes the villi to gradually flatten out, resulting in a reduced absorptive surface area. Digestion of fats is affected primarily, but there is also some interference with carbohydrate and vitamin absorption.

Clinical Manifestations

The resulting malabsorption, if untreated, leads to chronic diarrhea with large amounts of digested but unabsorbed fats being excreted (steatorrhea). The stools are characteristically bulky and foul smelling. As the disease progresses, absorption of proteins, carbohydrates, calcium, iron, and vitamins D, K, B_{12}, and B_6 (folic acid) is greatly impaired. Abdominal distention develops, and the child appears malnourished. Owing to the failure to use ingested calories, wasting is seen in normal areas of fat distribution, particularly the buttocks. Vitamin D malabsorption can cause bone changes, and rickets or tetany may develop. Anemia may be present owing to malabsorption of iron or vitamins B_{12} or B_6, or of all three, and bleeding disorders may result from vitamin K deficiency.

Symptoms may begin at any time after the introduction of gluten into the diet, usually at the time cereals are first given. Affected children may have a history of digestive disturbances starting at 6 to 12 months of age.

The disease is insidious, marked by poor weight gain and failure to grow, which may persist throughout childhood without notable gastrointestinal symptoms. Other persons with the disease may, however, be well during childhood and not manifest symptoms until adult life.

Certain changes in behavior often correlate with the presence of celiac disease. These changes include irritability, lack of cooperation, and eventually apathy. However, 30 per cent of children do not exhibit behavioral changes (Hamilton, 1992).

The child with celiac disease may initially appear irritable and anorexic, with chronic diarrhea, failure to thrive, a pot belly, and muscle wasting. The child may first come to medical attention in a state of celiac crisis. This is an acute episode of watery diarrhea and vomiting leading to severe electrolyte imbalance and dehydration, which may progress to metabolic acidosis. The crisis may be precipitated by infection, alteration in diet, or use of anticholinergic drugs, commonly for preoperative medication. Because celiac disease may have a genetic basis, the nurse should be aware of significant family history when gathering assessment data. This would include information on family members who may have had obscure complaints of digestive problems, intermittent diarrhea, or failure to thrive and gain weight. The child's dietary history should be reviewed to ascertain at what age new foods were introduced.

Diagnostic Assessment

In evaluating the physical status of a child who is not thriving, the nurse should observe for body distribution of fat. A protuberant abdomen in conjunction with frequent, foul-smelling, fatty stools that float in the toilet bowl lends credence to the diagnosis. Although the family and child must make adaptations to the disorder, celiac disease is usually well controlled by strict adherence to the dietary regimen; and in other respects, a normal lifestyle can be maintained.

Although a jejunal biopsy is mandatory to make the diagnosis, malabsorptive screening tests can be carried out before the biopsy is performed (Gryboski & Walker, 1983). The serum D-xylose absorption test is used as a screening test to assess upper small bowel surface area. After the ingestion of D-xylose, a serum level of 20 mg/dl or less at 1 to $1^1/_2$ hours suggests reduced small bowel surface area (Gryboski & Walker, 1983). A 72-hour stool test for fat may be done to confirm the presence of steatorrhea.

Before the intestinal biopsy, blood clotting function should be assessed. A complete blood count, platelet count, prothrombin time, and partial thromboplastin time should be obtained. The nurse should know the results of clotting function tests before biopsy and identify any abnormalities. After a 6- to 8-hour fast and appropriate sedation, the biopsy is done.

Atrophy of the villi demonstrated by biopsy coupled with a dietary history consistent with the disease supports the diagnosis. Serum protein and immunoglobulin levels may be low owing to the protein-losing enteropathy. On radiologic examination, bone age may be retarded, and osteoporosis and osteomalacia are often present. If the child responds favorably to a withdrawal of gluten from the diet and subsequently the condition is exacerbated in response to gluten challenge,* the diagnosis is confirmed.

Therapeutic Management

Nursing responsibility during the diagnostic period is diverse. Most times, diagnostic workup is done on an outpatient basis; only the very ill child is hospitalized.

* Gluten challenge means the reintroduction of gluten (usually in 10- to 30-g daily amounts) to the diet under controlled conditions. This may be continued for 2 to 3 weeks if symptoms are absent. Patients with true celiac disease develop steatorrhea and have decreased xylose absorption.

The nurse assists in collection of 72-hour stool specimens to be examined for fecal fat and coordinates collection of hematologic specimens for evaluation of anemia, protein and prothrombin levels, and electrolyte imbalance. Radiographic studies may be done to determine bone age and lower gastrointestinal tract function. While coordinating these procedures, the nurse should be aware of the importance of timing. If possible, tests should be scheduled so that they do not interfere with mealtimes. Honest, concise explanations should be given to the child, without exaggeration. These are best given immediately before the procedure to avoid increasing the young child's anxiety level. This is particularly important to ensure co-operation in the future. The comfort and safety needs of the child should be met before, during, and after each procedure.

The treatment of celiac disease centers on correct dietary management. This involves the institution and maintenance of a lifetime diet free of gluten. Corn and rice as well as soybean flour may be substituted for the grain portion of the diet. Health food stores are a good source for many appropriate foods. Care must be taken in purchasing *all* foods because grains are frequently used as fillers or thickeners. Labels must be read carefully to avoid ingestion of grains. Foods labeled "with hydrolyzed vegetable protein" or "vegetable protein added" must be avoided. Because of the suppression of disaccharidase activity, a lactose-free diet is advocated initially to help lessen the diarrhea. A nutritionist is involved from the beginning of treatment to assist the family with careful dietary management.

If the diet is followed carefully and consistently, a dramatic response is seen. Within the first few days, the child's disposition improves; he or she becomes less irritable and less apathetic. A progressive improvement in muscle tone and lessening of diarrhea and decreased abdominal distention are seen.

Those seriously ill children who are in crisis may need replacement therapy with intravenous fluids, parenteral nutrition, and vitamin administration. A dramatic improvement has been seen in crisis when corticosteroid therapy is initiated to decrease the inflammation of the bowel. A nasogastric tube may be passed to decrease abdominal distention and should be attached to intermittent suction. When the crisis is resolved, the child returns to diet therapy for maintenance.

Before the child's discharge, parents should understand what precipitates a celiac crisis and have a good knowledge of the dietary regimen. Other members of the health care team who may be required to treat the child should be made aware of the celiac disease status so that anticholinergic drugs will not be prescribed to treat the symptoms.

Within 6 months to 1 year after beginning the diet, the child with celiac disease should be within normal weight for age. Height and bone age take somewhat longer to become normal, usually 2 years. Relapses occur whenever the child eats gluten-containing foods.

The possible correlation between celiac disease and intestinal lymphoma and other forms of gastrointestinal cancer is a sufficient reason to remain on a gluten-free diet for life, and this should be brought to the parents' attention.

Nursing Diagnostic Statements

Altered nutrition: less than body requirements, *related to:*

- *Knowledge deficit, concerning components of a gluten-free diet, and*
- *Parental perception of the impact of the disease as overwhelming.*

High risk for ineffective family coping; *risk factor: perceptions of inability to care for child.*

Nursing Care

Nursing responsibility involves care during diagnosis and crisis, dietary management and instruction, facilitating the adaptation to a modified diet, and stimulation of appropriate emotional and developmental responses.

Nutritional Education. Careful explanation of the role of gluten in the disease as well as a copy of the diet and recipes to bring variety to meals should be given to the family. The family just learning of this diagnosis can contact another family with more experience in dealing with this disease, who can share methods of coping that have worked for them. This will also provide an opportunity to ask for recipe ideas. Suggestions are helpful for making special treats and favorite foods for the child, such as gluten-free cookies, birthday cakes, and pizza. Appropriate snack foods, such as fruit chunks, cheese, and carrot sticks, are suggested for between-meal snacks. The nutritionist also can provide specialized information that helps the family adjust to the restrictions of the disease.

A special diet is expensive and may place an added financial burden on a family. Means of rebudgeting or working out a more economical method of preparing the diet may need to be explored. Incorporating low- or no-gluten foods into the family diet may be beneficial; cooking special foods for one individual is more expensive and will set the child apart.

As the child's condition improves, appropriate physical, social, and intellectual activities should be initiated. Children with celiac disease learn early that their diet will always be a little different; and if they also learn at an early age to make the correct decisions, they will adapt well throughout life. The adolescent may be tempted to "cheat" with the dietary restrictions in the attempt to be like everyone else. The normality of their lives should be stressed. In essence, celiac disease is a dietary problem; with correct dietary control, other limitations on lifestyle are not major.

Enhancing the Family's Coping. The nurse responds to the family's needs throughout all diagnostic procedures. Because of the slow, insidious onset of the condition, the parents' abilities to cope with the situation may be severely altered. Parents will be extremely worried about their child and may question their own abilities to provide adequate care. Every effort should be made to give them as much information as they are able to absorb and allow time for them to express their fears and concerns.

The child with celiac disease may be irritable, anorexic, unsociable, and withdrawn during the diagnostic phase and may be difficult for the parents and the nurse to deal with. The parents may be on the verge of exhaustion and occasionally need opportunities to have time out from the stress of this situation. They should also be informed that the child's irritability will quickly disappear once the diet is initiated and the intestinal tract becomes normal.

As is true for many other situations, the parents initially have to adjust to the potential changes in their own lives as well as feelings of guilt, and they may not readily absorb large amounts of information. Parents will not necessarily adjust at the same pace. Explanations may need to be detailed, and repeated and frequent feedback sessions are helpful to determine the parents' level of understanding.

Lactose Intolerance

Lactose intolerance is the result of a lack or deficiency of the enzyme lactase, which is present within the border of the intestinal villi and is required to hydrolyze (or reduce) the disaccharide lactose into the monosaccharides glucose and galactose. The term "lactose intolerance" is used interchangeably with lactase deficiency. Milk allergy, however, is a sensitization to one of the milk proteins and should not be confused with lactose intolerance. (See Chapter 37 for a discussion of food allergy.)

Etiology/Incidence/Pathophysiology

Congenital lactose intolerance is a rare form of the disorder and is genetically determined. Normal intestinal mucosa is found on small bowel biopsy, but lactase activity is markedly diminished or absent, resulting in malabsorption. At birth, the infant appears normal; but after one or two feedings of milk, irritability and abdominal distention develop with explosive, watery, frothy stools having a sour or vinegar-like smell.

Late-onset lactose intolerance occurs after infancy. Prevalence of the disorder in Jews, Indians, Asians, and African-Americans ranges between 50 and 90 per cent (Gryboski & Walker, 1983). The frequency of this disorder increases with age; lactase activity is known to be maximal during infancy. As part of normal development, up to 70 per cent of the world's population gradually loses lactase activity beginning at age 4 years (Wald et al, 1982), at which time symptoms begin to be more prominent. Up until age 4 or 5, the only symptom may be an aversion to milk. Some children have complaints that may mimic appendicitis, including recurrent abdominal pain and flatulence. Diarrhea often does not begin until months after repeated episodes of abdominal pain.

TABLE 35-22
Disorders Associated with Secondary Lactase Deficiency

Infection	Viral gastroenteritis
	Bacterial enteritis
	Giardiasis
Inflammation	Protein-losing enteropathy
	Chronic inflammatory bowel disease
	Immunodeficiency
	Eosinophilic gastroenteritis
	Nonspecific enterocolitis
Reduced surface area	Short bowel syndrome
	Malnutrition
	Hypoxia
	Radiation enteritis

Secondary (acquired) lactose intolerance develops when the maturation of gastrointestinal epithelial villi becomes disrupted. Reductions in lactase activity are associated with disorders of infection and inflammation and with conditions that reduce the intestinal surface area (see Table 35–22 for a list of common conditions associated with secondary lactase deficiency).

The mucosal enzyme lactase splits lactose, a disaccharide, into the monosaccharides glucose and galactose for absorption. Inadequate levels of the enzyme lactase (disaccharidase) on either a congenital or an acquired basis results in the presence of unabsorbed lactose in the gut. Unabsorbed lactose remains osmotically active, drawing water into the intestinal lumen, which in turn stimulates intestinal motility and shortens transit time. When the unabsorbed lactose reaches the distal intestine and colon, the sugar is fermented to hydrogen, carbon dioxide, and organic acids (especially lactic acid). As a result, osmotic activity increases, the pH of the stool drops to below 5.5, and there is reduced absorption of water and electrolytes from the colon. Some of the sugars are not fermented and can be found in stools as reducing substances.

Clinical Manifestations

Symptoms are produced as a result of ingestion of lactose-containing foods (especially milk). In infants, lactose intolerance produces severe diarrhea, acid stools, dehydration, and failure to thrive. After infancy, symptoms are less dramatic. The gas generated from the fermentation of sugar may produce a sensation of bloating or belching and flatulence. This may be associated with abdominal pain, loose stools, and urgency.

Diagnostic Assessment

Lactose intolerance can sometimes be identified by the presence of symptoms after ingestion of lactose-containing products and the absence of symptoms after withdrawal of these foods. Laboratory tests can be used to diagnose lactose intolerance. In infants, a high level of reducing sugars in the stool (above 0.5 per cent glucose using a Clinitest tablet) and an acid pH (below 5.5) are seen in the presence of lactose intolerance. Another test, breath hydrogen testing, is performed to identify increased levels of hydrogen in expired air after lactose ingestion. Hydrogen production increases during the fermentation of the disaccharide, and therefore its presence in expired air also increases. A biopsy of a segment of the small intestine will also identify lactase deficiency. The breath hydrogen test for lactose has the advantage of being relatively inexpensive, noninvasive, and applicable throughout childhood.

Therapeutic Management

Elimination or reduction of lactose intake is the initial approach, depending on whether the deficiency is partial or complete. After 6 months of age or more, many infants can tolerate diets containing low levels of lactose, whereas some cannot tolerate even the smallest amount. For infants, a lactose-free formula such as Isomil, Soyalac, or Prosobee is prescribed; however, older children rarely find these palatable. Elimination of lactose from the diet entails exclusion of milk and milk products. Milk products are ingredients in many unexpected substances; therefore, labels must be checked carefully. When milk is excluded from an infant's diet, adequate calcium and vitamins must be provided in the form of supplementation. Several brands of commercially prepared lactase enzyme are available in liquid and capsule form. The liquid can be added to milk to predigest the lactose. In some areas, milk treated with lactase enzyme is available. Some individuals, usually those with milder forms of lactose intolerance, can tolerate limited quantities of dairy products if they are ingested in conjunction with commercial lactase liquid or capsules. A lactose-free diet is summarized in Table 35–23.

Hepatic Alterations

Biliary Atresia

Biliary atresia, a defect in which an infant is born with fibrotic or absent bile ducts, occurs in 1 per 10,000 live births. The disruption may be intrahepatic, affecting bile ducts within the liver, or extrahepatic, affecting the conduits outside the liver.

Etiology/Incidence/Pathophysiology

The cause of biliary atresia is unknown; however, a viral infection before or immediately after birth may be responsible for the disruption that develops. Research has focused on the type of viral infection, with reovirus type 3 being the most commonly cited virus believed to cause biliary atresia (Morecki et al, 1982). Rubella virus, cytomegalovirus, hepatitis A and B virus, and prenatal infection by *Listeria monocytogenes* have also been associated with biliary atresia (Oellrich & Cusmano, 1987; Oski, 1984). Prevalence is higher in girls than in boys.

Normally, the liver secretes bile, which passes through the bile ducts in the liver to the hepatic duct. The hepatic duct joins with the cystic duct from the gallbladder to form the common bile duct, which empties bile into the duodenum. Atresia may occur in any part or all of this duct system. Untreated, this condition eventually causes cirrhosis and death. Intrahepatic atresia occurs when the liver has no internal duct system. The only long-term successful therapy for these patients is a liver transplant. Extrahepatic atresia is the most common type. It involves defects of the hepatic or common bile duct and can be corrected surgically with the Kasai procedure (Kasai et al, 1968).

Diagnostic Assessment

Diagnosis is based on the history of jaundice at 3 to 4 weeks of age, the physical examination, and laboratory and diagnostic tests. Conjugated serum bilirubin, serum alkaline phosphatase, and cholesterol levels are elevated, indicating blockage of the bile ducts; however, these and other tests are not specific for biliary atresia. Biochemical studies are helpful in ruling out other disease entities, but making a diagnosis requires more specific tests, such as ultrasonography and radionuclide scan.

A liver biopsy with operative cholangiogram can identify the presence or absence of the intrahepatic biliary tree. A core of liver tissue is obtained under local anesthesia by inserting a suction biopsy needle (Menghini needle) into the liver. The tissue sample is sent for laboratory examination. *Hemorrhage* is the most frequent and serious complication of this procedure. Adequate immobilization of the infant's abdomen during the biopsy by holding the infant securely on the examining table is an important assistive nursing intervention. Moderate pressure is maintained over the biopsy site for 5 to 10 minutes after the procedure. Movement is restricted for several hours after the biopsy, and the child is positioned on the right side.

Therapeutic Management

The infant with biliary atresia has no chance for survival without surgical correction. Parents must deal initially with the news that their infant has a defect

TABLE 35-23
Lactose-Free Diet*

Foods Allowed	Foods Not Allowed
Milk: None (exception: use of LactAid additive to predigest lactose)	All milk and milk drinks—including whole, skim, low-fat, dried, evaporated, and condensed milk and human breast milk; yogurt—any type; cream—sweet or sour; infant formulas other than those permitted; ice cream sodas, milkshakes
Beverages: Powdered fruit-flavored drinks, ginger ale, tonics	Any made with milk, such as milkshakes, eggnog, hot chocolate
Eggs: As desired	Eggs prepared with milk—use specific formula; do not prepare with butter
Meats: Any baked, broiled, roasted, or boiled, except those to be avoided	Creamed or breaded meat, fish, or poultry; prepared meats that may contain dried milk solids, including bologna and cold cuts, frankfurters, salami, commerically prepared fish sticks, and some sausage
Although made from milk, cheeses vary in their lactose content; lactose is water-soluble, therefore, cheeses that are dry and hard have less lactose present (e.g., parmesan); there are some cheeses available made from lactose-reduced milk; soy cheeses are a possible substitute	All types of cheese and cheese dishes not listed as allowed
Breads: Only breads made without milk, such as French bread, Italian bread, water bagels, or "parva" breads	Breads made with any form of milk; any baked product made with milk; muffins, biscuits, waffles, pancakes, doughnuts, sweet rolls, commercial mixes
Cereal: Any made without milk, cooked or ready to eat; macaroni, spaghetti, pasta, rice—all prepared without milk or cheese	Any prepared cereal that contains dry milk solids
Vegetables and potatoes: All—cooked, canned, frozen, or fresh	Any vegetable prepared with milk, butter, milk solids, bread, or bread crumbs; no cheese or cream sauces
Fruits: All	All are allowed
Desserts: Any made without milk or milk products, such as gelatin desserts, fruit crisp, snow puddings, fruit and water sherbets, pie with fruit filling, angel cake	All commercial cake and cookie mixes, ice cream, custard puddings, junket, ice milk or sherbets that contain milk; frosting made with milk or butter, dessert sauces, cheese cakes
Soup: Any prepared without milk or milk products; homemade or canned, e.g., chicken rice	All creamed soups, chowders
Fats: Milk-free margarine or "parva" margarine; oils, nuts, peanut butter	Butter, margarine, some commercial salad dressings (check labels)
Sugar and seasonings: Sugar, honey, molasses, maple syrup, corn syrup, jelly and jam, hard candy, gumdrops, marshmallows, hard peppermints, fondant; salt, pepper, spices, herbs, condiments, vinegar, catsup, relish, pickles, olives, tomato sauce, coconut, wheat germ; artificial flavoring and extracts	Any product made from milk, butter, cream, chocolate, toffee, cream mints, caramel candy, candy with cream centers Miscellaneous: Medications that may contain lactose as filler or bulk agents; party dips; nonprescription vitamins; spice blends; Easter egg dyes; dietetic foods and foods advertised as "high-protein" sometimes contain lactose or dry milk solids *Check all labels carefully*†

* This diet is for the patient who must eliminate *all* sources of lactose from the diet. Lactose is the sugar found in milk, so all foods containing milk are to be excluded from the diet.

† *Read the label carefully.* Avoid any food containing *milk, nonfat milk solids, skim milk, butter, cream, lactose, casein, caseinate,* or *sodium caseinate.*

Adapted from Gryboski, J., & Walker, W. A. (1983). *Gastrointestinal problems in the infant* (2nd ed.). Philadelphia: WB Saunders.

that is often fatal. Surgery and transplantation hold new hope for some of these families, but these procedures have high risks and high mortality rates.

Surgical success is greatest when surgery is performed within the first few months of life and before the liver is permanently damaged by the trapped bile. Surgical correction of biliary atresia depends on the type and extent of atresia present. The best results are obtained when the atresia is distal to the liver, at the area where the biliary tree empties into the duodenum. In this case, the atresia can generally be resected and a direct anastomosis made between the healthy segments of tissue. When the atresia is of the proximal biliary tree, major reconstruction is required. Even then, however, correction is difficult because proximal atresia often involves intrahepatic atresia as well. Intrahepatic atresia is not surgically correctable, and the only treatment available is liver transplantation. When the proximal atresia does not involve intrahepatic atresia, the Kasai procedure is the most common surgical correction.

The Kasai procedure was developed by a Japanese surgeon in 1959. The purpose of this procedure is surgical correction of proximal extrahepatic biliary atresia. The operation involves the creation of an extrahepatic substitute biliary tree from the liver to the duodenum. The obstructed biliary tree is removed, and a resected segment of jejunum is anastomosed between the liver and the duodenum. If the operation is successful, the substitute biliary tree serves as a conduit for bile drainage. Other variants of the procedure involve the creation of a portoenterostomy, or stoma, that drains bile externally. Advantages of this procedure that have been identified include decreased postoperative infection and enhanced assessment of bile drainage. The stoma is usually closed after 12 to 24 months.

If surgical correction is not possible or is unsuccessful, liver transplantation is carried out for infants with biliary atresia (Kasai et al, 1989). Liver transplantation has become increasingly more successful with the wider use of immunosuppressive drugs, such as cyclosporin A (Starzl et al, 1982), azathioprine, and cytaltic agents in combination with corticosteroids (Lake & Kilkenny, 1992). New transplantation strategies include living-related donations and reduced-size liver transplants. Both of these strategies increase the availability of organs to small children (Boone et al, 1992; Treacy, 1992).

Nursing Diagnostic Statements

High risk for ineffective family coping; risk factor: stress of impending surgery.

High risk for altered health maintenance; risk factor: knowledge deficit regarding care of the child at home.

Planning and Implementation

Nursing intervention for the parents under stress during this time requires active listening and the development of a supportive relationship.

Promoting Family Coping. Preparation of the parents for the infant's surgery and appropriate support while they cope with the postoperative course are the mainstays of nursing care for the family. Preoperatively, the infant may be irritable and uncomfortable. The physical closeness of the parents will comfort the infant and will help the parents prepare for the reality of the surgery.

Facilitating Home Health Maintenance. Questions concerning the surgical procedure and the anticipated postsurgical course should be answered by the surgeon. Nurses should also be informed about the expected outcome and participate in preparing the family to care for the child at home. Signs and symptoms of infection should be reviewed, and parents should demonstrate competence in taking and interpreting the results of rectal temperatures. The reduced bile salts in the intestine may lead to poor uptake of the fat-soluble vitamins A, D, E, and K; therefore, oral supplements are necessary.

A special diet, which includes predigested fats and water-miscible vitamins, is prescribed for 6 to 12 months after surgery. Breastfeeding is encouraged; however, a formula such as Portagen, Alimentum, or Pregestimil may be used. Such a formula is a high-calorie one, but it contains fats (medium-chain fatty acid) that can be digested without the need for bile and contains water-miscible vitamins. Parents should feel comfortable with the dietary regimen before the infant returns home. Plans for the necessary long-term medical follow-up are made with the parents before they leave the hospital. (See discussion on cirrhosis of the liver in the next section.)

Cirrhosis/Liver Failure

Cirrhosis is an alteration in hepatic lobular structure and function that is the result of injury to the hepatocytes (liver tissue cells). Hepatocytes have a remarkable capacity for regeneration. Therefore, injury to cells results in a process of destruction and regeneration, which eventually leads to permanent scarring of the liver tissue.

Etiology/Incidence/Pathophysiology

Cirrhosis is the result of a variety of diseases with varying mechanisms of injury. It is believed that hepatic injury must be prolonged and repeated for cirrhosis to develop (Hughes & Griffith, 1984). Injury to hepatocytes occurs as a consequence of metabolic diseases, toxins, biliary obstructions, infections, and vascular conditions. Table 35–24 describes the three types of cirrhosis and related pathologic changes.

Some of the more common causes of cirrhosis in infancy, childhood, and adolescence are cystic fibrosis, alpha$_1$-antitrypsin deficiency, biliary atresia, and hepatitis. The adolescent population is at particular risk for cirrhosis as hepatitis B becomes more widespread among teenage illicit parenteral drug users.

When hepatocytes suffer an insult, a regeneration process is initiated by the activation of fibroblasts. Although, in some instances, regeneration can lead to repair, a continuing process of destruction and regeneration results in excessive growth of fibrotic tissue. The fibrotic process compounds cellular damage because it interferes with blood flow to the cells.

TABLE 35-24
Types of Cirrhosis

Type	Cause	Pathology
Postnecrotic cirrhosis	Previous acute viral hepatitis	Replacement of liver tissue with nodules of fibrous tissue
Biliary cirrhosis	Chronic biliary infection and obstruction	Scarring around bile ducts and the lobes of the liver
Portal or Laennec cirrhosis	Chronic alcoholism	Scarring around the portal area

Hepatic dysfunction causes major alterations in the body because of interruption in the important functions of the liver, including synthesis and storage of glycogen, deamination of amino acids and synthesis of proteins, biotransformation of bile pigments, synthesis of fibrinogen and prothrombin, destruction of bacteria, storage of vitamin B and fat-soluble vitamins, and lipid metabolism. Hepatic dysfunction leads to a group of interrelated pathophysiologic processes resulting in jaundice, portal hypertension, ascites, impairment of fat digestion, reduced clotting mechanisms, encephalopathy, and renal dysfunction.

Jaundice occurs because damaged parenchymal hepatic cells fail to conjugate and excrete bilirubin into the bile. Instead, it accumulates in the blood, resulting in yellowing of the skin, dark-colored urine, and clay-colored stools. The clay color of feces is caused by the lack of stercobilin. Bilirubin is normally excreted into the biliary tree and then into the gastrointestinal tract, where it is converted to urobilinogen and then to stercobilin. Retained components of bile salts can also cause pruritus; however, the degree of itching is not related to the degree of hyperbilirubinemia (Balistreri, 1992).

Portal hypertension occurs because the hepatic fibrotic process obstructs blood flow through the liver, causing a back pressure into the portal system. The hepatic portal vein normally carries blood *to* the liver from the abdominal portion of the gastrointestinal tract, pancreas, and spleen. In the presence of portal hypertension, collateral flow around the liver increases with the development of varices (particularly esophageal) and spider angiomas as a result of dilated abdominal wall veins. Hypersplenism can also occur, resulting in damage to the blood cells and a diminished production of platelets.

Ascites, an accumulation of serous fluid in the peritoneal cavity, commonly occurs with cirrhosis. The mechanism of its formation is poorly understood. A major contributing factor is the reduced amount of albumin that is synthesized by an injured liver. The resultant hypoalbuminemia reduces vascular osmotic pressure, thereby contributing to fluid loss from the vascular space. Portal hypertension further contributes to ascites because of increased vascular hydrostatic pressure. Another explanation is that lymph is formed in the hepatic sinusoids in excess of what can be drained by the thoracic duct; therefore, lymph accumulates in the peritoneal cavity as ascites (Balistreri, 1992).

Impairment of fat digestion occurs because there is a decrease in intestinal bile salts. Furthermore, decreased fat digestion interferes with the absorption of the fat-soluble vitamins A, D, E, and K. The vitamin K deficiency that results contributes to the bleeding tendency seen in advanced cirrhosis.

Reduced clotting mechanisms occur because of altered synthesis of the clotting factors fibrinogen and prothrombin and altered production and function of platelets in the presence of hypersplenism (Balistreri, 1992).

Encephalopathy in hepatic dysfunction is thought to occur because a primary *inhibitory* neurotransmitter is not cleared from the blood and crosses the blood-brain barrier to inhibit brain activity (Balistreri, 1992). Also, ammonia is thought to have a role in hepatic encephalopathy. Increased serum ammonia levels interfere with metabolism within the brain. Ammonia levels increase because there is a reduction in the ability of the liver to convert ammonia to urea for excretion by the kidney. Ammonia (which is formed in the intestine) is also allowed to bypass the liver and enter the general circulation because of the collateral circulation that develops in the presence of portal hypertension.

Renal dysfunction may be caused by the same systemic disease or toxins that affect the liver. Liver and renal dysfunction are closely related. Renal alterations include impaired concentrating ability, altered potassium metabolism, and alterations in sodium and water retention.

Diagnostic Assessment

A diagnosis is made by gathering historical information, doing a physical examination, and performing selected laboratory tests and diagnostic procedures. A history of loss of appetite, nausea and vomiting, and prior liver disease such as hepatitis may contribute to making a diagnosis. In the adolescent population, information that might reveal drug and alcohol abuse should be sought. A physical examination will reveal clinical manifestations as discussed earlier, although symptoms may be vague. In biliary atresia, jaundice is usually evident; in cirrhosis from other causes, an insidious onset can be expected. Findings with advanced disease also include finger clubbing, skin ecchymosis, and signs of hepatic encephalopathy. A classic early neurologic sign is asterixis, a flapping tremor elicited when arms are outstretched with dorsiflexion of the hand. Later signs include tremors, incoordination, muscle twitching, decreased level of consciousness, and coma. Laboratory tests used for diagnosis of cirrhosis are included in Table 35–8.

Definitive diagnosis is made by liver biopsy if coagulation is normal or corrected. Hepatic failure with unknown cause requires further diagnostic study, including toxicology screen, liver function studies, angiology, and blood cultures.

Therapeutic Management

Because liver failure is not treatable, therapeutic regimens are supportive, awaiting the resumption of liver function. Prevention of major complications, such as increased intracranial pressure, hemorrhage, fluid and electrolyte imbalance, and renal failure, is an important goal. However, prolonged liver failure requires additional supports.

Nutritional support is necessary with a high-calorie, low-fat, and low-protein diet. A low-protein diet is necessary to decrease ammonia production, which contributes to encephalopathy. Total parenteral nutrition and vitamin supplementation may be necessary. Deficiencies in fat-soluble vitamins A, D, E, and K are replaced orally or parenterally. Levels of water-soluble vitamin deficiencies are monitored to determine adequate supplementation.

Coagulopathies are managed through transfusion of necessary blood components. Plasmapheresis may also be used, especially if the child is awaiting liver transplant.

Gastrointestinal hemorrhage, which can be due to gastritis, peptic ulcer, or esophageal varices, is managed according to its cause. Blood transfusions, fluid and electrolyte replacement, administration of vitamin B complex and vitamin K, stomach gavage with room-temperature solutions, vasoconstrictive agents such as vasopressin, and a Sengstaken-Blakemore tube are therapeutic approaches that are used. Additionally, esophageal varices are increasingly being treated by sclerosis during endoscopy.

Ascites is controlled by restricting dietary salt to 0.5 g/day. If urinary output is adequate, it is not usually necessary to restrict fluid intake. Diuretics are administered, and serum and urinary electrolyte levels are monitored.

Pruritus is a troublesome problem in cirrhosis. Bile acid binders, such as cholestyramine (Questran), 8 to 16 g/day, are given. Cholestyramine can be administered to stimulate bile flow and inhibit reabsorption of bile salts through the normal route of enterohepatic circulation (bile salts are normally reabsorbed from the intestine to the liver via the enterohepatic circulation). Cholestyramine is given with caution because it can decrease absorption of fats and fat-soluble vitamins as well.

Nursing Care

Nursing care is directed toward reducing the potential for further damage to the liver, keeping the child comfortable, and helping the child and family cope with the child's current condition and plan for the future realistically.

The child's *activity level* is kept to the limits tolerated by the child during the acute phase to conserve energy. A child with cirrhosis is usually tired and weak and probably will not want to engage in exercise.

Adequate nutrition is difficult to maintain when a child has nausea and vomiting. The dietary restrictions of limited salt, fat, and protein can further decrease the appetite of a child who does not feel like eating. Tube feeding may become necessary, particularly if the child is being prepared for liver transplantation. Total parenteral nutrition is also used to ensure adequate nutritional intake.

Skin assessment is an important function of the nurse. Hyperbilirubinema is assessed by checking the skin for jaundice, the child's sclera for increased yellow staining, the urine for a dark color, and the stool for clay color. If pruritus is present, warm baths can be used without soap followed by application of a lotion.

Assessments for signs of bleeding are made by checking gums for bleeding (especially during toothbrushing), assessing the skin for signs of bruising, testing stool and urine for occult blood, and assessing prolonged oozing from puncture sites.

Nursing care varies according to the therapeutic regimen that is instituted and consists of accurate assessment of the child's status and effect of therapy. The family and child (as appropriate for age) are kept informed of the purpose of the various procedures being performed, and the child is kept comfortable. Parents are also encouraged to express their feelings of loss and fear surrounding the uncertainty of their child's illness.

KEY CONCEPTS

Concepts Related to Basic Information

- The gastrointestinal system is responsible for breaking down food into nutrients that can be used at the cellular level and defending the body against pathogens.
- The overall goal of nursing care of the pediatric patient with a gastrointestinal disorder is to foster normal growth and development by maintaining a balanced nutritional state.
- Many congenital anomalies appear during the neonatal period, which can result in a severe psychologic burden on the parents.
- Alterations associated with an inflammatory process may be acute and urgent (e.g., appendicitis) or chronic (e.g., inflammatory bowel disease) in nature.
- Disruptions characterized by malabsorption result from an inability to absorb nutrients and can lead to failure to thrive and malnutrition if not adequately managed.
- Hepatic alterations result in life-threatening, severe illness that requires advanced nursing and medical management.

Concepts Related to Nursing Assessment

- Developmental differences in gastrointestinal function necessitate careful assessment of the pediatric patient's nutritional status.
- Gastrointestinal functional disorders, such as colic and irritable bowel syndrome, present a challenge to parents' coping skills because they must learn to care for an infant who is in pain or uncomfortable for a significant period.

Concepts Related to Nursing Intervention

- Caring for a child with a gastrointestinal alteration may require specialized skills in feeding techniques (nasogastric tubes and gastrostomy) and support of elimination (enemas, colostomy/ileostomy care).
- The nurse must be knowledgeable about congenital anomalies and obstructions of the digestive tract to facilitate nursing interventions that restore altered digestive function.
- The nurse's role in enhancing parental acceptance of nutritional alterations and understanding alternatives for treatment is crucial.
- Nurses and parents must establish collaborative partnerships in care to facilitate meeting the nutritional needs of a child with a complex gastrointestinal disorder.

REFERENCES

Anderson, G. C. (1986). Pacifiers: The positive side. *MCN: American Journal of Maternal Child Nursing, 11*(2), 122–124.

Andze, G., et al. (1991). Diagnosis and treatment of gastroesophageal reflux in patients with esophageal atresia: The value of pH monitoring. *Journal of Pediatric Surgery, 26*(3), 295–300.

Ashcraft, K. W., & Holder, T. M. (1976). Esophageal atresia and tracheoesophageal fistula malformations. *Surgical Clinics of North America, 56,* 299.

Aylsworth, A. S. (1985). Genetic considerations in clefts of the lip and palate. *Clinics in Plastic Surgery, 12,* 533–542.

Balistreri, W. F. (1992). Liver and biliary system. In R. E. Behrman, (Ed.), *Nelson textbook of pediatrics* (pp 1001–1013). Philadelphia: WB Saunders.

Balistreri, W. F., et al. (1983). Immaturity of the enterohepatic circulation in early life: Factors predisposing to "physiologic" maldigestion and cholestasis. *Journal of Pediatric Gastroenterology and Nutrition, 2,* 346.

Barnett, B. (1983). Viral gastroenteritis. *Medical Clinics of North America, 67,* 1031–1058.

Behrman, R. E. (1987). Peritoneum and allied structures. In R. E. Behrman & V. C. Vaughan (Eds.), *Nelson textbook of pediatrics* (13th ed., pp. 850–853). Philadelphia: WB Saunders.

Boone, P., et al. (1992). Liver transplantation: Living-related donations. *Critical Care Nursing Clinics of North America, 4*(2), 243–248.

Burrington, J., & Powers, L. (1985). Pediatric surgery. In G. B. Merenstein & S. L. Gardner (Eds.), *Handbook of neonatal intensive care* (pp. 373–393). St. Louis: CV Mosby.

Canty, T. G. (1986, July-August). Esophageal atresia and tracheoesophageal fistula. Aspects of respiratory care. *Perinatology-Neonatology,* pp. 42–47.

Carey, W. (1989). Colic: Exasperating but fascinating and gratifying. *Pediatrics, 84*(3), 568–569.

Cassani, V. L. (1984). Tracheoesophageal anomalies. *Neonatal Network, 3*(2), 20–26.

Cummings, J. H., & Stephen, A. M. (1981). The role of dietary fibre in the human colon. *Canadian Medical Association Journal, 123,* 1109.

Cusson, R. M. (1992). Rice-based oral rehydration fluid in the treatment of infant diarrhea. *Journal of Pediatric Nursing, 7*(6), 1–2.

Davidson, G. F. (1986). Viral diarrhea. *Clinics in Gastroenterology, 15,* 39–53.

Embron, C. (1990). Ostomy care for the infant with necrotizing enterocolitis: Nursing considerations. *Journal of Pediatric and Neonatal Nursing, 4*(3), 56–63.

Fanaroff, A. A., & Kliegman, R. M. (1993). Necrotizing enterocolitis. In M. H. Klaus & A. A. Fanaroff (Eds.), *Care of the high-risk neonate.* Philadelphia: WB Saunders.

Feigin, R. D., & Stoller, M. L. (1992). Diarrhea. In R. E. Behrman (Ed.), *Nelson textbook of pediatrics* (pp. 662–664). Philadelphia: WB Saunders.

Filston, H. C., & Izant, R. J. (1993). *The surgical neonate* (2nd ed.). New York: Appleton-Century-Crofts.

Fisher, J. (1991). Feeding children who have cleft lip or palate. *Western Journal of Medicine, 154*(2), 207.

Frentner, S. (1987). Abdominal wall defects: Omphalocele and gastroschisis. *Neonatal Network, 6*(3), 29–40.

Gillies, C. (1987). Infant colic: Is there anything new? *Journal of Pediatric Health Care, 1*(6), 305–312.

Gryboski, J. (1991). Peptic ulcer disease in children. *Medical Clinics of North America, 75*(4), 889–902.

Gryboski, J. D. (1986). Disorders of the esophagus. In S. S. Gellis & B. M. Kagan (Eds.), *Current pediatric therapy 12* (pp. 178–181). Philadelphia: WB Saunders.

Gryboski, J., & Walker, W. A. (1983). *Gastrointestinal problems in the infant* (2nd ed.). Philadelphia: WB Saunders.

Guerrant, R. L., et al. (1986). Acute infectious diarrhea. I. Epidemiology, etiology, and pathogenesis. *Pediatric Infectious Disease, 5,* 353–359.

Hamilton, J. R. (1992). Celiac disease. In R. E. Behrman (Ed.), R. M. Kliegman, W. E. Nelson, & V. C. Vaughan III (Eds.), *Nelson textbook of pediatrics* (pp 977–979). Philadelphia: WB Saunders.

Holtzman, I. R., & Brown, D. R. (1986). Necrotizing enterocolitis: A complication of prematurity. *Seminars in Perinatology, 10*(3), 208–216.

Huddleston, K. C., & Palmer, K. L. (1990). A button for gastrostomy feedings. *MCN: American Journal of Maternal Child Nursing, 15,* 315–319.

Hughest, J. G., & Griffith, J. F. (1984). *Synopsis of pediatrics* (6th ed.). St. Louis: CV Mosby.

Huth, M. M., & O'Brien, M. E. (1987, July-August). The gastrostomy feeding button. *Pediatric Nursing, 13*(4), 241–245.

Iacono, G., et al. (1991). Severe infantile colic and food intolerance: A long term prospective study. *Journal of Gastroenterology and Nutrition, 12*(3), 332–335.

Johnson, D. G., et al. (1981). Gastroesophageal reflux in infants and children: Recognition and treatment. *Surgical Clinics of North America, 61,* 1101–1115.

Jonas, A., & Dever-Haber, A. (1982). Stool output and composition in chronic non-specific diarrhea syndrome. *Archives of Disease in Childhood, 57,* 35.

Kasai, M., et al. (1968). Surgical treatment of biliary atresia. *Journal of Pediatric Surgery, 3,* 1968–1972.

Kasai, M., et al. (1989). Surgical limitation for biliary atresia: Indication for liver transplantation. *Journal of Pediatric Surgery, 24*(9), 851–854.

Kenner, C., et al. (1988). *Neonatal surgery.* Orlando, FL, Grune & Stratton (Division of Harcourt-Brace-Jovanovich).

Kenner, C., & Breuggemeyer, A. (1984). Hirschsprung's disease: Current trends and practices. *Neonatal Network, 3*(1), 7–16.

Kirschner, B. S. (1988). Inflammatory bowel disease in children. *Pediatric Clinics of North America, 35*(1), 189–208.

Korones, S. B. (1986). *High-risk newborn infants* (4th ed., pp. 364–392). St. Louis: CV Mosby.

Kottmeier, P. K. (1986). Appendicitis. In K. J. Welch, et al. (Eds.), *Pediatric Surgery: Vol. 2* (4th ed.). Chicago: Year Book Medical Publishers.

Lake, K., & Kilkenny, J. (1992). The pharmacokinetics and pharmacodynamics of immunosuppressive agents. *Critical Care Nursing Clinics of North America, 4*(2), 205–220.

Leape, L. L. (1987). *Patient care in pediatric surgery.* Boston: Little Brown.

LeBaron, C. W., et al. (1990). Annual rotavirus patterns in North America. *Journal of the American Medical Association, 264,* 983–988.

Lindsay, W. K. (1986). Cleft lip and cleft palate. In K. J. Welch, et al. (Eds.), *Pediatric Surgery: Vol. 2* (4th ed.). Chicago: Year Book Medical Publishers.

Listernick, R., et al. (1986). Outpatient oral rehydration in the United States. *American Journal of Diseases of Children, 140,* 211–215.
Liu, K. W., et al. (1986). Intussusception—current trends in management. *Archives of Disease in Childhood, 61,* 75–77.
Maclean, W. C., & Fink, B. B. (1980). Lactose malabsorption by premature infants. Magnitude and clinical significance. *Journal of Pediatrics, 97,* 383.
Martin, L. W., & Torres, A. M. (1985). Hirschsprung's disease. *Surgical Clinics of North America, 65,* 1171–1180.
McWilliams, B. J., et al. (1984). *Cleft palate speech.* St. Louis: CV Mosby.
Molenaar, J., et al. (1991). Congenital diaphragmatic hernia, what defect? *Journal of Pediatric Surgery, 26*(3), 596–599.
Morecki, R., et al. (1982). Biliary atresia and reovirus type III infection. *New England Journal of Medicine, 307,* 481.
Nord, K. S. (1988). Peptic ulcer disease in the pediatric population. *Pediatric Clinics of North America, 35,* 117–140.
Oellrich, R. G., & Cusmano, M. M. (1987). Biliary atresia. *Neonatal Network, 5*(5), 25–35.
Orenstein, S. (1991). Gastroesophageal reflux. *Current Problems in Pediatrics, 21*(5), 193–241.
Oski, F. (1984). Obstructive jaundice due to biliary atresia and neonatal hepatitis. In M. E. Avery, & H. W. Taeusch (Eds.), *Schaffer's diseases of the newborn* (pp 637–643). Philadelphia: WB Saunders.
Owens, J., et al. (1985). Epidemiology of facial clefting. *Archives of Disease in Childhood, 60,* 521–524.
Paarlberg, J., & Balint, J. P. (1985, March-April). Gastrostomy tubes: Practical guidelines for home care. *Pediatric Nursing,* pp. 99–102.
Petersen, M. (1986). Esophageal pH monitoring. *Journal of Pediatric Nursing, 1*(5), 354–357.
Pinyerd, B., & Zipf, W. (1989). Colic: Idiopathic, excessive infant crying. *Journal of Pediatric Nursing, 4*(3), 147–161.
Poley, J. R. (1983). Chronic non-specific diarrhea, investigation of the surface morphology of small bowel mucosa utilizing the scanning electron microscope. *Journal of Pediatric Gastroenterology and Nutrition, 2,* 71.
Randolph, J. G. (1986). Esophageal atresia and congenital stenosis. In K. J. Welch, et al. (Eds.), *Pediatric surgery: Vol. I* (4th ed., pp 682–693). Chicago: Year Book Medical Publishers.
Robson, A. M. (1987). The pathophysiology of body fluids. In R. E. Behrman & V. C. Vaughan (Eds.), *Nelson textbook of pediatrics* (pp 172–207). Philadelphia: WB Saunders.
Rushton, C. (1990). Necrotizing enterocolitis: 1. Pathogenesis and diagnosis. *MCN: American Journal of Maternal Child Nursing, 15*(5), 296–300.
Schmitt, B. C. (1986). The prevention of sleep problems and colic. *Pediatric Clinics of North America, 33,* 763–774.
Shandling, B. (1992). Congenital anomalies of the gastrointestinal tract and intestinal obstruction. In R. E. Behrman (Ed.), R. M. Kliegman, W. E. Nelson, & V. C. Vaughan III (Eds.), *Nelson textbook of pediatrics* (pp. 958–959). Philadelphia: WB Saunders.
Sieber, W. K. (1986). Hirschsprung's disease. In S. S. Gellis & B. M. Kagan (Eds.), *Current pediatric therapy 12* (pp 206–207). Philadelphia: WB Saunders.
Silverman, A., & Roy, C. C. (1983). *Pediatric clinical gastroenterology* (3rd ed.). St. Louis: CV Mosby.
Simmons, M. A. (1984). Using the nursing process in treating inflammatory bowel disease. *Nursing Clinics of North America, 19,* 11–25.
Starzl, T. E., et al. (1982). Liver and kidney transplantation in children receiving cyclosporin-A and steroids. *Journal of Pediatrics, 100,* 681.
Summers, R. W., et al. (1979). National Cooperative Crohn's Disease Study: Results of drug treatment. *Gastroenterology, 77,* 847.
Templeton, J. M., & Ditesheim, J. A. (1985). High imperforate anus—quantitative results of long-term fecal continence. *Journal of Pediatric Surgery, 20*(6), 645–652.
Tolia, V. K., & Dubois, R. S. (1985). Update on oral rehydration: Its place in treatment of acute gastroenteritis. *Pediatric Annals, 14*(4), 295–303.
Treacy, S. (1992). Reduced-size liver transplantation for infants and children. *Critical Care Nursing Clinics of North America, 4*(2), 235–242.
Trier, W. C. (1985). Primary palatoplasty. *Clinics in Plastic Surgery, 12,* 659–675.
Wald, A., et al. (1982). Lactose malabsorption in recurrent abdominal pain in children. *Journal of Pediatrics 100,* 65.
Walsh, M. C., & Kliegman, R. M. (1986). Necrotizing enterocolitis: Treatment based on staging criteria. *Pediatric Clinics of North America, 33,* 179–201.
Welch, K. J. (1986). Intussusception. In R. A. Hoekelman, et al. (Eds.), *Principles of pediatrics.* New York: McGraw-Hill.
White, C., et al. (1990). High frequency ventilation and extracorporeal membrane oxygenation. *AACN Clinical Issues in Critical Care Nursing, 1,* 427–444.
Williams, R. (1982). Congenital diaphragmatic hernia: A review. *Heart and Lung, 11,* 532–538.
Winslow, R. E., et al. (1983). Acute nonperforating appendicitis. Efficacy of brief antibiotic prophylaxis. *Archives of Surgery, 118,* 651–655.

BIBLIOGRAPHY

Appendicitis

Bell, M. J., et al. (1983). Antimicrobial prophylaxis in pediatric surgical patients. *Communication AAP Committee on Infectious Disease,* pp. 1–7.
Gamal, R., & Moore, T. (1990). Appendicitis in children aged 13 years and younger. *American Journal of Surgery, 159*(6), 589–592.
Neilson, I., et al. (1990). Appendicitis in children: Current therapeutic recommendations. *Journal of Pediatric Surgery, 25*(11), 1113–1116.
O'Shea, J., et al. (1988). Diagnosing appendicitis in children with acute abdominal pain. *Pediatric Emergency Care, 4*(3), 172–176.
Putnam, T., et al. (1991). Appendicitis in children. *Surgery, Gynecology and Obstetrics, 170*(6), 527–532.
Rothrock, S., et al. (1991). Clinical features of misdiagnosed appendicitis in children. *Annals of Emergency Medicine, 20*(1), 45–50.

Biliary Atresia

Esquivel, C., et al. (1987). Indications for pediatric liver transplantation. *Journal of Pediatrics, 111*(6, Pt. 2), 1039–1045.
Falchetti, D., et al. (1991). Liver transplantation in children with biliary atresia and polysplenia syndrome. *Journal of Pediatric Surgery, 26*(5), 528–531.
Lally, K., et al. (1989). Perioperative factors affecting the outcome following repair of biliary atresia. *Pediatrics, 83*(5), 723–726.
Laurent, J., et al. (1990). Long-term outcome after surgery for biliary atresia. Study of 40 patients surviving for more than 10 years. *Gastroenterology, 99*(6), 1793–1797.
Lilly, J., et al. (1989). The surgery of biliary atresia. *Annals of Surgery, 210*(3), 289–296.
MacDonald, C. (1991). Biliary atresia. *Journal of Pediatric Nursing, 6*(6), 379–383.
Stewart, B., et al. (1988). Liver transplantation and the Kasai operation in biliary atresia. *Journal of Pediatric Surgery, 23*(7), 623–662.

Cleft Lip and Palate

Chapman, K. (1991). Vocalizations of toddlers with cleft lip and palate. *Cleft Palate Craniofacial Journal, 28*(2), 172–178.
Chapman, K., & Hardin, M. (1991). Language input of mothers interacting with their young children with cleft lip and palate. *Cleft Palate Craniofacial Journal, 28*(1), 78–85; discussion 85–86.
Curtin, G. (1990). The infant with cleft lip or palate: More than a surgical problem. *Journal of Perinatal Neonatal Nursing, 3*(3), 80–89.

Eliason, M. (1991). Cleft lip and palate: Developmental effects. *Journal of Pediatric Nursing, 6*(2), 107–113.

Eliason, M., et al. (1991). Factors that influence ratings of facial appearance for children with cleft lip and palate. *Cleft Palate Craniofacial Journal, 28*(2), 190–194.

Enemark, H., et al. (1990). Evaluation of unilateral cleft lip and palate treatment; long term results. *Cleft Palate Journal, 27*(4), 354–361.

Farnan, S. (1988). Nutrition and feeding of children with cleft lip/palate. *Nutrition News, 3,* 1–4.

Sauter, S. (1989). Cleft lip and palate: Types, repairs, nursing care. *Journal of Association of Operating Room Nurses, 50*(4), 813–815, 817–820.

Strauss, R., & Broder, H. (1991). Directions and issues in psychosocial research and methods as applied to cleft lip and palate and craniofacial anomalies. *Cleft Palate Craniofacial Journal, 28*(2), 150–156.

Wellman, C., & Coughlin, S. (1991). Preoperative and postoperative nutritional management of the infant with cleft palate. *Journal of Pediatric Nursing, 6*(3), 154–158.

Colic

Colon, A., & DiPalma, J. (1989). Colic. *American Family Physician, 40*(6), 122–124.

Hartsell, M. (1990). New products. *Journal of Pediatric Nursing, 5*(1), 59–60.

Larsen, J. (1990). Infant colic and belly massage. *Practitioner, 234*(1487), 396–397.

Larson, K., & Ayllon, T. (1990). The effects of contingent music and differential reinforcement on infantile colic. *Behaviour Research and Therapy, 28*(2), 119–125.

Sampson, H. (1989). Infantile colic and food allergy: Fact or fiction? *Journal of Pediatrics, 115*(4), 583–584.

Sloman, J., et al. (1990). Infantile colic and transient developmental lag in the first year of life. *Child Psychiatry and Human Development, 21*(1), 25–36.

Constipation

Hatch, T. (1988). Encopresis and constipation in children. *Pediatric Clinics of North America, 35*(2), 257–280.

Loening-Baucke, V. (1991). Constipation in infants and children. *Iowa Medicine, 81*(2), 59–62.

Loening-Baucke, V. (1991). Persistence of chronic constipation in children after biofeedback treatment. *Digestive Diseases and Sciences, 36*(2), 153–160.

Loening-Baucke, V. (1989). Factors determining outcome in children with chronic constipation and faecal soiling. *Gut, 30*(7), 999–1006.

Loening-Baucke, VA. (1987). Factors responsible for persistence of childhood constipation. *Journal of Pediatric Gastroenterology and Nutrition, 6*(6), 915–922.

Diarrhea

Brown, K. (1991). Dietary management of acute childhood diarrhea: Optimal timing of feeding and appropriate use of milks and mixed diets. *Journal of Pediatrics, 118*(4, Pt. 2), 92–98.

Brown, K., et al. (1988). Effect of continued oral feeding on clinical and nutritional outcomes of acute diarrhea in children. *Journal of Pediatrics, 112*(2), 191–200.

Brown, K., et al. (1991). Clinical trial of modified whole milk, lactose-hydrolyzed whole milk, or cereal-milk mixtures for the dietary management of acute childhood diarrhea. *Journal of Pediatric Gastroenterology and Nutrition, 12*(3), 340–350.

Campbell, R., et al. (1988). Effects of diaper types on diaper dermatitis associated with diarrhea and antibiotic use in children in day-care centers. *Pediatric Dermatology, 5*(2), 83–87.

Delucchi, M., et al. (1989). The use of oral hydration in the treatment of children with acute diarrhea in primary care. *Journal of Pediatric Gastroenterology and Nutrition, 9*(3), 328–334.

Kotloff, K., et al. (1989). Enteric adenovirus infection and childhood diarrhea: An epidemiologic study in three clinical settings. *Pediatrics, 84*(2), 219–225.

Leung, A., & Robson, E. (1989). Acute diarrhea in children. What to do and what not to do. *Postgraduate Medicine, 86*(8), 161–164, 167–174.

Pickering, L. (1991). Therapy for acute infectious diarrhea in children. *Journal of Pediatrics, 118*(4, Pt. 2), 5118–5128.

Smith, L. (1988). Home treatment of mild, acute diarrhea and secondary dehydration of infants and small children: An educational program for parents in a shelter for the homeless. *Journal of Professional Nursing, 4*(1), 60–63.

Staat, M., et al. (1991). Diarrhea in children newly enrolled in daycare centers in Houston. *Pediatric Infectious Disease Journal, 10*(4), 282–286.

Thomas, D. (1989). Bloody diarrhea in children. *Gastroenterology Nursing, 12*(2), 100–103.

Esophageal Atresia and Tracheoesophageal Fistula

Black, T., et al. (1991). The effect of tube gastrostomy on gastroesophageal reflux in patients with esophageal atresia. *Journal of Pediatric Surgery, 26*(2), 168–170.

Chittmittrapap, S., et al. (1990). Anastomotic stricture following repair of esophageal atresia. *Journal of Pediatric Surgery, 25*(5), 508–511.

Curci, M., & Dibbins, A. (1988). Problems associated with a Nissen fundoplication following tracheoesophageal fistula and esophageal atresia repair. *Archives of Surgery, 123*(5), 618–620.

Goh, D., et al. (1991). Esophageal atresia with obstructed tracheoesophageal fistula and gasless abdomen. *Journal of Pediatric Surgery, 26*(2), 160–162.

Holder, T., et al. (1987). Care of infants with esophageal atresia, tracheoesophageal fistula and associated anomalies. *Journal of Thoracic and Cardiovascular Surgery, 94*(6), 828–835.

McKinnon, L., & Kosloske, A. (1990). Prediction and prevention of anastomotic complications of esophageal atresia and tracheoesophageal fistula. *Journal of Pediatric Surgery, 25*(7), 778–781.

Poenaru, D., et al. (1991). A more than 25-year experience with end-to-end versus end-to-side repair for esophageal atresia. *Journal of Pediatric Surgery, 26*(4), 472–477.

Reves, H., et al. (1989). Management of esophageal atresia and tracheoesophageal fistula. *Clinics in Perinatology, 16*(1), 79–84.

Shaul, D., et al. (1989). Primary repair without routine gastrostomy is the treatment of choice for neonates with esophageal atresia and tracheoesophageal fistula. *Archives of Surgery, 124*(10), 1188–1191.

Sillen, U., et al. (1988). Management of esophageal atresia: Review of 16 years' experience. *Journal of Pediatric Surgery, 23*(9), 805–809.

Gastroesophageal Reflux

Andze, G., et al. (1991). Diagnosis and treatment of gastroesophageal reflux in 500 children with respiratory symptoms: The value of pH monitoring. *Journal of Pediatric Surgery, 26*(3), 295–300.

Black, T., et al. (1991). The effect of tube gastrostomy on gastroesophageal reflux in patients with esophageal atresia. *Journal of Pediatric Surgery, 26*(2), 168–170.

Dipalma, J., & Colon, A. (1991). Gastroesophageal reflux in infants. *American Family Physician, 43*(3), 857–864.

Dupont, C., et al. (1990). How to treat gastroesophageal reflux in children. *Clinical Reviews in Allergy, 8*(4), 471–487.

Gaynor, E. (1991). Otolaryngologic manifestations of gastroesophageal reflux. *American Journal of Gastroenterology, 86*(7), 801–808.

Lynn, M. (1986). Use of infant seats for gastroesophageal reflux. *Journal of Pediatric Nursing, 1*(2), 127–129.

Orenstein, S. (1991). Gastroesophageal reflux. *Current Problems in Pediatrics, 21*(5), 193–241.

Orenstein, S. R., et al. (1983). The infant seat as treatment for gastroesophageal reflux. *New England Journal of Medicine, 309,* 760–763.

Petersen, M. (1986). Esophageal pH monitoring. *Journal of Pediatric Nursing, 1*(6), 354–357.

Sutphan, J. (1990). Pediatric gastroesophageal reflux disease. *Gastroenterology Clinics of North America, 19*(3), 617–629.

Tovar, J., et al. (1991). Surgery for gastroesophageal reflux in children with normal pH studies. *Journal of Pediatric Surgery, 26*(5), 541–545.

Gastroschisis and Omphalocele

Caniano, D., et al. (1990). An individualized approach to the management of gastroschisis. *Journal of Pediatric Surgery, 25*(3), 297–300.

Carlan S., et al. (1990). Antenatal fetal diagnosis and maternal transport gastroschisis. A maternal-infant case report. *Clinical Pediatrics, 29*(7), 378–381.

Frentner, S. (1987). Abdominal wall defects: Omphalocele and gastroschisis (continuing education credit). *Neonatal Network, 6*(3), 29–41.

Goldbaum, G., et al. (1990). Risk factors for gastroschisis. *Teratology, 42*(4), 397–403.

Gornall, P. (1989). Management of intestinal atresia complicating gastroschisis. *Journal of Pediatric Surgery, 24*(6), 522–524.

Guzman, E. (1990). Early prenatal diagnosis of gastroschisis with transvaginal ultrasonography. *American Journal of Obstetrics and Gynecology, 162*(5), 1253–1254.

Hughes, M., et al. (1989). Fetal omphalocele: Prenatal US detection of concurrent anomalies and other predictors of outcome. *Radiology, 173*(2), 371–376.

Lloyd, D. (1991). Gastroschisis, malrotation, and chylous ascites. *Journal of Pediatric Surgery, 26*(1), 106–107.

Meller, J., et al. (1989). Gastroschisis and omphalocele. *Clinics in Perinatology, 16*(1), 113–122.

Muraji, T., et al. (1989). Gastroschisis: A 17-year experience. *Journal of Pediatric Surgery, 24*(4), 343–345.

Sauter, E., et al. (1991). Is primary repair of gastroschisis and omphalocele always the best operation? *American Surgeon, 57*(3), 142–144.

Sipes, S., et al. (1990). Gastroschisis and omphalocele; does either antenatal diagnosis or route of delivery make a difference in perinatal outcome? *Obstetrics and Gynecology, 76*(2), 195–199.

Stringer, M., et al. (1991). Controversies in the management of gastroschisis: A study of 40 patients. *Archives of Disease in Childhood, 66*(1 Spec. No.), 34–36.

Hernias and Hydrocele

Byard, R., et al. (1990). Unsuspected diaphragmatic hernia: A potential cause of sudden and unexpected death in infancy and early childhood. *Journal of Pediatric Surgery, 25*(11), 1166–1168.

Caplan, M., & MacGregor, S. (1989). Perinatal management of congenital diaphragmatic hernia and anterior abdominal wall defects. *Clinics in Perinatology, 16*(4), 917–938.

Connors, R., et al. (1990). Congenital diaphragmatic hernia repair on ECMO. *Journal of Pediatric Surgery, 25*(10), 1043–1047.

Davies, N., et al. (1990). Irreducible inguinal hernia in children below two years of age. *British Journal of Surgery, 77*(11), 1291–1292.

Given, J., & Rubin, S. (1989). Occurrence of contralateral inguinal hernia following unilateral repair in a pediatric hospital. *Journal of Pediatric Surgery, 24*(10), 963–965.

Gleeson, F., & Spitz, L. (1991). Pitfalls in the diagnosis of congenital diaphragmatic hernia. *Archives of Disease in Childhood, 66*(6), 670–671.

Grosfeld, J. (1989). Current concepts in inguinal hernia in infants and children. *World Journal of Surgery, 13*(5), 506–515.

Grosfeld, J., et al. (1991). Inguinal hernia in children: Factors affecting recurrence in 62 cases. *Journal of Pediatric Surgery, 26*(3), 283–287.

Henderson, R., et al. (1988). Review of the surgical management of recurrent hiatal hernia: 5-year follow-up. *Canadian Journal of Surgery, 31*(5), 341–345.

Molenaar, J., et al. (1991). Congenital diaphragmatic hernia, what defect? *Journal of Pediatric Surgery, 26*(3), 248–254.

Moss, R., & Hatch, E. (1991). Inguinal hernia repair in early infancy. *American Journal of Surgery, 161*(5), 596–599.

Nagaya, M., et al. (1991). Management of congenital diaphragmatic hernia by extracorporeal membrane oxygenation (ECMO). *European Journal of Pediatric Surgery, 1*(1), 10–14.

Nakayama, D., & Rowe, M. (1989). Inguinal hernia and the acute scrotum in infants and children. *Pediatrics in Review, 11*(3), 87–93.

Nyhus, L., et al. (1990). Inguinal hernia repairs. Types, patient care. *AORN Journal, 52*(2), 292–304.

Petrikovsky, B., & Shmoys, S. (1990). Fetal hydrocele: A persistent finding? *Pediatric Radiology, 20*(5), 362.

Shenbhogue, L., et al. (1990). Preoperative stabilization in congenital diaphragmatic hernia. *Archives of Disease in Childhood, 65*(10 Spec. No.), 1043–1044.

Theorell, C. (1990). Congenital diaphragmatic hernia: A physiologic approach to management. *Journal of Perinatal and Neonatal Nursing, 3*(3), 66–79.

Van Meurs, K., et al. (1990). Effect of extracorporeal membrane oxygenation on survival of infants with congenital diaphragmatic hernia. *Journal of Pediatrics, 117*(6), 954–960.

Webster, A., et al. (1991). Spinal anaesthesia for inguinal hernia repair in high-risk neonates. *Canadian Journal of Anaesthesia, 38*(3), 281–286.

Your child's umbilical hernia. (1988). *Australian Family Physician, 17*(9), 777.

Hirschsprung Disease

Adams, D. A., & Selekof, J. L. (1986). Children with ostomies: Comprehensive care planning. *Pediatric Nursing, 12*(6), 429–433.

Arliss, J., & Holgersen, L. (1990). Neonatal appendiceal perforation and Hirschsprung's disease. *Journal of Pediatric Surgery, 25*(6), 694–695.

Badner, J., et al. (1990). A genetic study of Hirschsprung disease. *American Journal of Human Genetics, 46*(3), 568–580.

Boocock, G., & Donnai, D. (1987). Anorectal malformation: Familial aspects and associated anomalies. *Archives of Disease in Childhood, 62*(6), 576–579.

Carcassone, M., et al. (1989). Management of Hirschsprung's disease: Curative surgery before 3 months of age. *Journal of Pediatric Surgery, 24*(10), 1032–1034.

Doig, C. (1991). Hirschsprung's disease—a review. *International Journal of Colorectal Disease, 6*(1), 52–62.

Foster, P., et al. (1990). Twenty-five years' experience with Hirschsprung's disease. *Journal of Pediatric Surgery, 23*(5), 531–534.

Joseph, U., & Sim, C. (1988). Problems and pitfalls in the management of Hirschsprung's disease. *Journal of Pediatric Surgery, 23*(5), 398–402.

Stannard, V., et al. (1991). Familial Hirschsprung's disease: Report of autosomal dominant and probable recessive X-linked kindreds. *Journal of Pediatric Surgery, 26*(5), 591–594.

Watanatittian, S., et al. (1991). Association of Hirschsprung's disease and anorectal malformation. *Journal of Pediatric Surgery, 26*(2), 192–195.

Intestinal Atresia

Adejuyigbe, O., & Odesanmi, W. (1990). Intrauterine intussusception causing intestinal atresia. *Journal of Pediatric Surgery, 25*(5), 562–563.

Davenport, M., & Bianchi, A. (1990). Congenital intestinal atresia. *British Journal of Hospital Medicine, 44*(3), 174, 176, 178–180.

Gornall, P. (1989). Management of intestinal atresia complicating gastroschisis. *Journal of Pediatric Surgery, 24*(6), 522–524.

Smith, G., & Glasson, M. (1989). Intestinal atresia: Factors affecting survival. *Australian and New Zealand Journal of Surgery, 59*(2), 151–156.

Intussusception

Holmes, M., et al. (1991). Intussusception in cystic fibrosis. *Archives of Disease in Childhood, 66*(6), 726–727.

Johnston, J., & Harnsberger, J. (1990). Episodic vomiting due to intermittent duodenal intussusception. *Journal of Pediatric Gastroenterology and Nutrition, 10*(3), 405–408.
Kim, Y., & Rhy, J. (1989). Intussusception in infancy and childhood. Analysis of 385 cases. *International Surgery, 74*(2), 114–118.
Krasna, I., et al. (1990). Intussusception in childhood. *New Jersey Medicine, 87*(9), 715–720.
Ong, N., & Beasley, S. (1990). Progression of intussusception. *Journal of Pediatric Surgery, 25*(6), 644–646.
Page, A., et al. (1990). Chronic intussusception. *Archives of Disease in Childhood, 65*(1), 134–135.
Palder, S., et al. (1991). Intussusception: Barium or air? *Journal of Pediatric Surgery, 26*(3), 271–275.
Reijnen, J., et al. (1990). Intussusception: Factors related to treatment. *Archives of Disease in Childhood, 65*(8), 871–873.
Skipper, R., et al. (1990). Childhood intussusception. *Surgery, Gynecology and Obstetrics, 171*(2), 151–153.
Yadav, K., et al. (1990). Transanal and intraperitoneal prolapse in intussusception. *Journal of Pediatrics and Child Health, 26*(2), 99–100.

Lactose Intolerance

American Academy of Pediatrics Committee on Nutrition: Practical significance of lactose intolerance in children. *Pediatrics, 86*(Suppl. 4), 643–644.
Barr, R. (1989). Infantile color and lactose intolerance [Letter]. *Journal of Pediatrics, 115*(3), 501–502.
Montes, R., & Perman, J. (1991). Lactose intolerance. Pinpointing the source of nonspecific gastrointestinal symptoms. *Postgraduate Medicine, 89*(8), 175–178, 181–184.
Shavedra, J., & Perman, J. (1989). Current concepts in lactose malabsorption and intolerance. *Annual Review of Nutrition, 9,* 475–502.
Murphy, M., & Walker, W. (1991). Celiac disease. *Pediatrics in Review, 12*(11), 325–330.
Vajro, P., et al. (1990). Incidence of cirrhosis in children with chronic hepatitis. *Journal of Pediatrics, 117*(3), 392–396.

Malrotation and Volvulus

Jackson, A., Bisset, R., & Dickson, A. (1989). Malrotation and midgut volvulus presenting as malabsorption. *Clinical Radiology, 40*(5), 536–537.
Mori, H., Hayashi, K., Futagawa, S., Uetani, M., Yanagi, T., & Kurosaki, N. (1987). Vascular compromise in chronic volvulus with midgut malrotation. *Pediatric Radiology, 17*(4), 277–281.

Necrotizing Enterocolitis

Amspacher, K. (1989). Necrotizing enterocolitis: The never-ending challenge. *Journal of Perinatal and Neonatal Nursing, 3*(2), 58–68.
Anderson, D., & Kliegman, R. (1991). The relationship of neonatal alimentation practices to the occurrence of endemic necrotizing enterocolitis. *American Journal of Perinatology, 8*(1), 62–67.
Ballance, W., et al. (1990). Pathology of neonatal necrotizing enterocolitis: A ten-year experience. *Journal of Pediatrics, 117*(1, Pt. 2), S6–S13.
Carrion, V., & Egan, E. (1990). Prevention of neonatal necrotizing enterocolitis. *Journal of Pediatric Gastroenterology and Nutrition, 11*(3), 317–323.
Embon, C. (1990). Ostomy care for the infant with necrotizing enterocolitis: Nursing considerations. *Journal of Perinatal and Neonatal Nursing, 4*(3), 56–63.
Kliegman, R. (1990). Neonatal necrotizing enterocolitis: Bridging the basic science with the clinical disease. *Journal of Pediatrics, 117*(5), 833–835.
Neonatal necrotizing enterocolitis: Current concepts and controversies. Proceedings of the Second International Wexner Symposium on Developmental Gastroenterology and Nutrition. September 25–27, 1989. *Journal of Pediatrics, 117*(1, Pt. 2), 51–74.
Porat, R., & Brodsky, N. (1991). Cocaine: A risk factor for necrotizing enterocolitis. *Journal of Perinatology, 11*(i), 30–32.
Roberts, P. (1991). Neonatal necrotizing enterocolitis: Etiology, treatment, prevention, and nursing care. *Critical Care Nurse, 10*(4), 38–53.
Rushton, C. (1990). Necrotizing enterocolitis: I. Pathogenesis and diagnosis. *MCN: American Journal of Maternal Child Nursing, 15*(5), 296–300.
Rushton, C. (1990). Necrotizing enterocolitis: II. Treatment and nursing care. *MCN: American Journal of Maternal Child Nursing, 15*(5), 309–313.
Smith, S., et al. (1990). The hidden mortality in surgically treated necrotizing enterocolitis: Fungal sepsis. *Journal of Pediatric Surgery, 25*(10), 1030–1033.

Peptic Ulcer

Gryboski, J. (1991). Peptic ulcer disease in children. *Medical Clinics of North America, 75*(4), 889–902.
Gryboski, J. (1990). Peptic ulcer disease in children. *Pediatrics in Review, 12*(1), 15–21.
Harnsberger, J. (1988). Peptic ulcer disease in infants and children. *Postgraduate Medicine, 83*(4), 60–63, 67–71.
Tam, P., & Saing, H. (1989). The use of H_2-receptor antagonist in the treatment of peptic ulcer disease in children. *Journal of Pediatric Gastroenterology and Nutrition, 8*(1), 41–46.
Tsang, T., et al. (1990). Peptic ulcer in children. *Journal of Pediatric Surgery, 25*(7), 744–748.

Pyloric Stenosis

Eriksen, C., & Anders, C. (1991). Audit of results of operations for infantile pyloric stenosis in a district general hospital. *Archives of Disease in Childhood, 66*(1), 130–133.
Forman, H., et al. (1990). A rational approach to the diagnosis of hypertrophic pyloric stenosis: Do the results match the claims? *Journal of Pediatric Surgery, 25*(2), 262–266.
Garcia, V., & Randolph, J. (1990). Pyloric stenosis: Diagnosis and management. *Pediatrics in Review, 11*(10), 292–296.
Habbick, B., & To, T. (1989). Incidence of infantile hypertrophic pyloric stenosis in Saskatchewan, 1970–85. *Canadian Medical Association Journal, 140*(4), 395–398.
Habbick, B., et al. (1989). Infantile hypertrophic pyloric stenosis: A study of feeding practices and other possible causes. *Canadian Medical Association Journal, 140*(4), 401–404.
Hayashi, A., et al. (1990). Balloon catheter dilatation for hypertrophic pyloric stenosis. *Journal of Pediatric Surgery, 25*(11), 1119–1121.
Latchaw, L., et al. (1989). The development of pyloric stenosis during transpyloric feedings. *Journal of Pediatric Surgery, 24*(8), 823–824.
Milne, C. (1989). Congenital pyloric stenosis. *Nursing Standard, 3*(17), 22–23.
Reilly, D., & Hershman, M. (1989). Diagnosis of infantile hypertrophic pyloric stenosis by ultrasound. *British Journal of Clinical Practice, 43*(9), 339–340.
Rollins, M., et al. (1989). Pyloric stenosis: Congenital or acquired? *Archives of Disease in Childhood, 64*(1), 138–139.
Swift, P., & Prossor, J. (1991). Modern management of pyloric stenosis—must it always be surgical? [Letter]. *Archives of Disease in Childhood, 66*(5), 667.
Tam P., & Chan, J. (1991). Increasing incidence of hypertrophic pyloric stenosis. *Archives of Disease in Childhood, 66*(4), 530–531.

Ulcerative Colitis and Crohn Disease

Belli, D., et al. (1988). Chronic intermittent elemental diet improves growth failure in children with Crohn's disease. *Gastroenterology, 94*(3), 603–610.
Ellet, M., & Schibler, K. (1988). Adolescent psychosocial adaptation to inflammatory bowel disease. *Journal of Pediatric Health Care, 2,* 57–66.
Griffiths, A., et al. (1991). Factors influencing postoperative recurrence of Crohn's disease in childhood. *Gut, 32*(5), 491–495.
Kanof, M., et al. (1988). Decreased height velocity in children and

adolescents before the diagnosis of Crohn's disease. *Gastroenterology, 95*(6), 1523–1527.

Kirschner, B. (1988). Inflammatory bowel disease in children. *Pediatric Clinics of North America, 35,* 189–208.

Lenaerts, C., et al. (1989). High incidence of upper gastrointestinal tract involvement in children with Crohn disease. *Pediatrics, 83*(5), 777–781.

Motil, K., & Grand, R. (1987). Ulcerative colitis and Crohn disease in children. *Pediatrics in Review, 9*(4), 109–120.

Schmidt-Sommerfeld, E., et al. (1990). Endoscopic and histologic findings in the upper gastrointestinal tract of children with Crohn's disease. *Journal of Pediatric Gastroenterology and Nutrition, 11*(4), 448–454.

Seidman, E., et al. (1987). Nutritional therapy of Crohn's disease in childhood. *Digestive Diseases and Sciences, 32*(Suppl. 12), 825–885.

Stapleford, P., & Long, S. (1990). Crohn's disease in children. *Nursing Standard, 4*(48), 25–27.

CHAPTER • 36
Altered Genitourinary/Renal Function

Annette Vigneux
Mabel Hunsberger

NURSING PROCESS PLAN
NPP: The Child Undergoing Dialysis Secondary to Chronic Renal Failure, Table 36–15

RELATED TOPICS
Fostering Self-Esteem, Chapter 14
Impact of chronic illness, Chapter 19
Principles of fluids and electrolytes, Chapter 26
Immune function, Chapter 37
Nursing Process Plan: Perioperative Care, Table 23–7

LEARNING OBJECTIVES

- Outline the normal anatomy and physiology of the urinary system and discuss pediatric variations.
- Identify assessment criteria and diagnostic procedures relevant to history taking and physical examination for evaluation of genitourinary function in children.
- Describe interventions for nursing care of the child with a urinary drainage device.
- Discuss the developmental impact of genitourinary disorders on the child and family.
- Describe the major genitourinary tract anomalies and discuss their therapeutic management.

- Identify the etiology and clinical manifestations of urinary tract infection in children and describe interventions to facilitate management compliance and follow-up care.
- Discuss medical management of the child with vesicourethral reflux and perioperative care.
- Compare and contrast the etiology, clinical manifestations, and nursing care of the child with nephrotic syndrome and the child with acute glomerulonephritis.
- List foods high in sodium and potassium.
- Describe acute and chronic renal failure and develop a nursing process plan for the child undergoing dialysis.

Genitourinary/renal disorders in children encompass a wide range of problems, from common ones such as enuresis or cystitis to rare ones such as exstrophy of the bladder. Congenital anomalies affect a significant percentage of children with sequelae that may be minor or life-threatening. Urinary tract infections are fairly common and constitute one of the most frequently seen bacterial diseases in children.

The role of the nurse includes the assessment, planning, intervention, and evaluation of children with disorders of the genitourinary/renal system. Because these disorders have such a wide variety of manifestations and treatment plans, the nursing role is diverse and requires a sound knowledge base. In order to better understand genitourinary disorders, a review of the anatomy and physiology of the genitourinary system is presented. Common laboratory and diagnostic studies including pertinent nursing interventions are discussed. A comprehensive description of genitourinary system disorders and anomalies, including the nursing role and current modes of therapy, is included.

Structure and Function

The discussion on structure and function of the genitourinary system is presented in two sections: (1) anatomy and physiology of the urinary system, and (2) anatomy of the genitalia. Developmental differences in structure and function of the genitourinary system are presented in Table 36–1.

Anatomy of the Urinary System

The urinary system comprises the *kidneys, ureters, urinary bladder,* and *urethra.* Urine is formed by the kidneys and transported outside the body by the remainder of the system (Fig. 36–1).

The kidneys are located retroperitoneally to the right and left of the lumbar spine. Each kidney is supported by fascia, covered by a tough capsule, and surrounded by a cushion of fat. The right kidney is displaced by the liver and lies lower than the left kidney.

The production of urine takes place in the kidney. From the kidney, the urine flows through the ureters to the urinary bladder. The ureters are a pair of mucosa-lined tubes that have no sphincters but use peristalsis to transport the urine. The ureters join the bladder at an oblique angle, which helps to prevent the occurrence of reflux (backflow) when the bladder empties.

The urinary bladder is a hollow, muscular sac that is located in the pelvis posterior to the pelvic bones. The urethral orifice is located at the inferior portion of the bladder, joining the bladder to the urethra.

The urethra is a hollow tube that leads to the urinary meatus. In males, the urethra is long (approximately 20 cm in the adult male), and, in females, it is relatively short (3 to 5 cm in the adult female). In children, the length of the urethra is proportionately shorter according to their growth and age.

TABLE 36-1
Developmental Differences in Structure and Function of the Genitourinary System

Anatomy and Physiology	Significance
Urine Concentration	
Infants do not gain the ability to concentrate urine until about 3 mos of age	• A low specific gravity for the young infant is not necessarily indicative of adequate hydration • The lack of concentrating ability makes the young infant particularly prone to dehydration
Urine Dilution	
Although the infant's capacity to dilute urine is comparable with that of an adult, the infant kidney is less well equipped to process a sudden large quantity of fluid (Drummond, 1983)	• The infant is more prone to fluid volume excess; IV fluids must be carefully monitored to prevent volume overload
External Genitalia of the Newborn Female	
Labia: The labia minora may be relatively prominent and protrude beyond the labia majora in preterm and some full-term infants. In addition, the edges of the labia minora are typically darkly pigmented at birth. Swelling of the external genitalia may be present in the first days of life. *Vaginal discharge:* In the first 2 wks of life, alterations in circulating hormones may produce a grayish or milky, thin or mucoid discharge, which may also be blood-tinged	• The nurse who recognizes normal developmental immaturity from anatomic and physiologic anomalies can reassure parents about their baby's health and can appropriately refer signs and symptoms of concern
External Genitalia of Newborn Male	
The nonerect newborn penis is typically 2–3 cm in length. Transient penile erection is common in the infant and small child. At birth, the testicles often appear large for the infant's size	• The nurse can reassure parents about the normalcy of their son's anatomy
The uncircumcised foreskin is usually difficult to retract during the first 2–3 mos, becoming more easily retractable at 4 mos, and fully retractable at 4 yrs of age	• The private physician's advice should be followed regarding whether to routinely retract the uncircumcised foreskin in early infancy; practices and opinions vary

Three general regions may be identified within the kidney: the *renal cortex,* the *renal medulla,* and the *renal pelvis* (Fig. 36–2).

The renal cortex is the outer section of the kidney. This section arches over the renal pyramids of the medulla. The sections that extend inward between the pyramids are called the *renal columns.*

The renal medulla is composed of approximately 18 to 20 triangular wedge-shaped masses called the *renal pyramids.* Each pyramid projects centrally toward the renal pelvis to form a *papilla.* The papilla has a number of openings that allow urine to flow into the cup-shaped extension *(calyx)* of the renal pelvis.

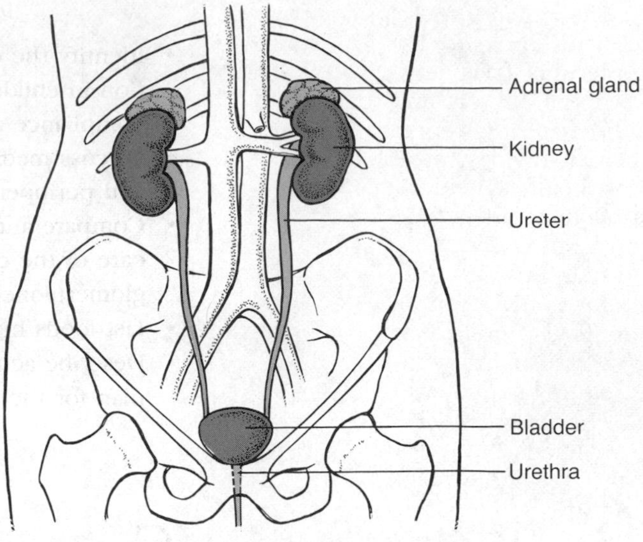

FIGURE 36-1. Components of the urinary system.

The renal pelvis is a funnel-shaped sac that receives urine from all parts of the kidney via the calyces. The renal pelvis is attached to the ureter. Urine collects in the renal calyces and pelvis and drains into the ureters, from which it is transported by active peristalsis to the bladder.

The basic functional unit of the kidney is the *nephron.* There are approximately 1 to 1.5 million nephrons in each kidney. Each nephron consists of a renal tubule and a renal corpuscle.

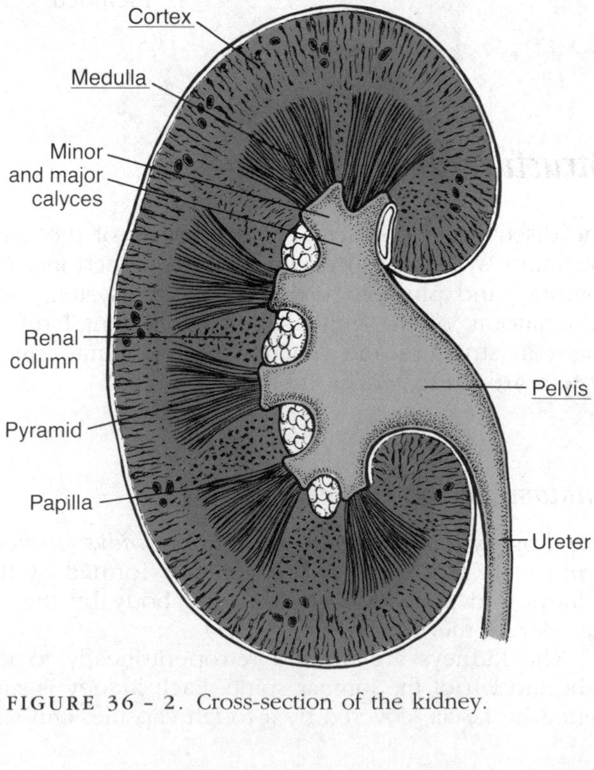

FIGURE 36-2. Cross-section of the kidney.

The renal corpuscle is made up of the *glomerulus* and encased by the *Bowman capsule*. The glomerulus is a network of capillaries that lie between the afferent and the efferent arterioles. The *afferent arteriole* transports blood to the glomerulus where it divides into up to 50 capillary loops inside the structure. These loops join to form the *efferent arteriole* that carries blood away from the glomerulus to the *peritubular capillaries*. The peritubular capillaries and hairpin loops, called the *vasa recta,* surround the tubule of the nephron (Fig. 36–3). The diameter of the afferent arteriole is twice that of the efferent arteriole; it also has a more substantial layer of smooth muscle compared with the efferent arteriole.

The Bowman capsule serves two purposes: to filter materials in and out of the glomerulus and to act as the beginning point for the renal tubule. The renal tubule begins its course at the Bowman capsule and ends at the collecting tubule. The tubule changes names as it progresses through the nephron—the *proximal convoluted tubule;* the *loop of Henle;* and the *distal convoluted tubule*. The collecting tubule passes through a renal pyramid and joins other collecting tubules or ducts to form one of the papillary ducts that opens into a calyx. Several nephrons drain into each collecting tubule.

The renal corpuscles of the nephrons lie within the renal cortex. The renal corpuscles of *cortical nephrons* are located in the outer two thirds of the cortex. These nephrons usually have small glomeruli and short loops of Henle. The nephrons that remain within the inner third of the cortex are called *juxtamedullary nephrons*. These nephrons have long loops of Henle that extend downward in variable distances to the medulla.

Physiology of the Renal System

The kidneys are major body organs that serve many functions: the detoxification of the blood and elimination of metabolic wastes such as urea, creatinine, uric acid, phosphate, sulfates, potassium, nitrates, and phenols; the regulation of volume, electrolyte concentration of body fluids, and acid-base balance; the regulation of blood pressure through the release of renin and prostaglandins; the release of erythropoietin to stimulate new red blood cell production; and the

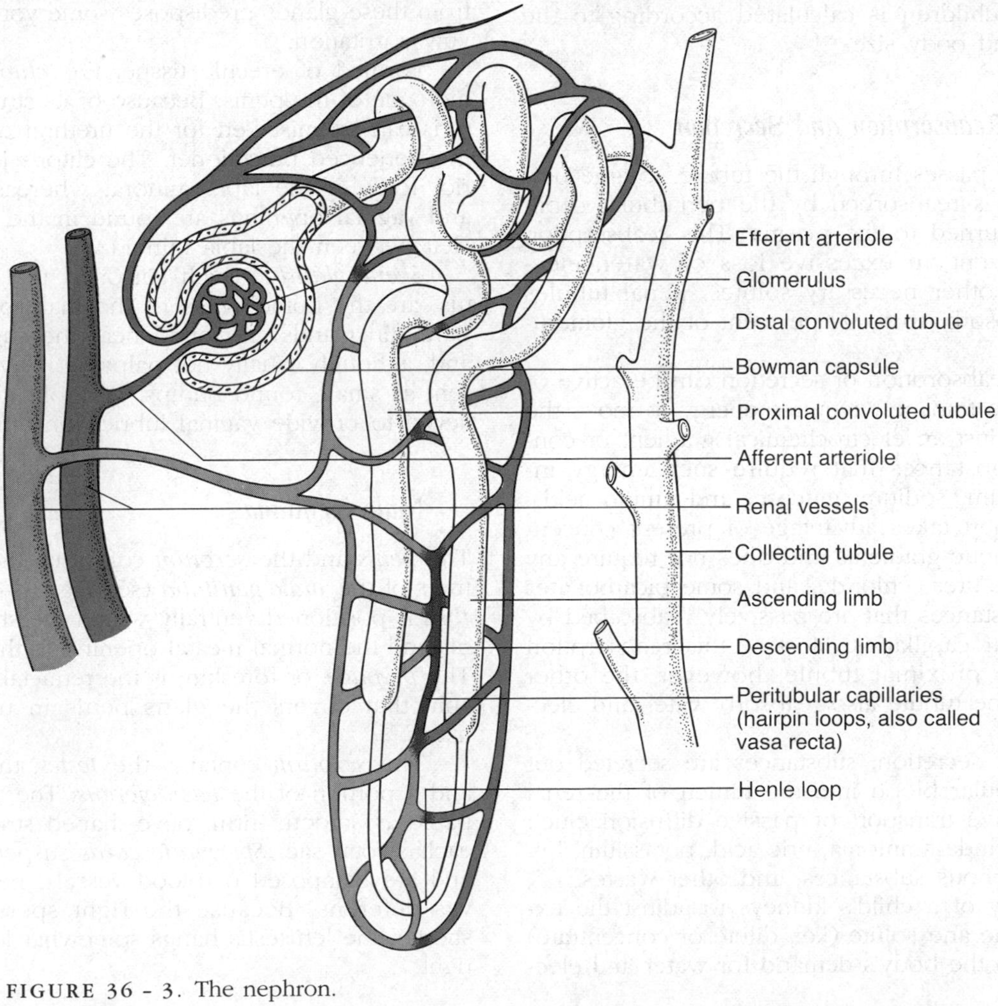

FIGURE 36 - 3. The nephron.

regulation of calcium balance through vitamin D metabolism.

The production of urine by the kidney provides the body with a mechanism to excrete waste products, to clear foreign substances, and to detoxify substances. The processes involved in urine formation are (1) glomerular filtration and (2) tubular reabsorption and secretion.

Glomerular Filtration

The blood entering the glomerulus through the afferent arteriole is at a high pressure. The force of this pressure creates a difference among the glomerular capillary pressure, the colloidal osmotic pressure, and the capsular pressure. The difference in these pressures is called *net filtration pressure.* The net filtration pressure forces substances of a small molecular weight across the glomerular membrane into the lumen of the surrounding Bowman capsule. However, large molecules such as proteins are unable to pass and are retained in the blood.

The glomerular filtration rate (GFR) is determined by the blood pressure, the effective filtration pressure, and the permeability of the capillary walls. If abnormalities in any of these exist, the GFR will be altered. The GFR in children is calculated according to the child's age and body size.

Tubular Reabsorption and Secretion

As the filtrate passes through the tubule, a large percentage of it is reabsorbed by the peritubular capillaries and returned to the plasma. This reabsorption helps to prevent an excessive loss of water, electrolytes, and other necessary solutes. Renal tubules normally reabsorb up to 99 per cent of the glomerular filtrate.

Tubular reabsorption or secretion can be active or passive. Active transport requires energy to move the substance against an electrochemical gradient or concentration. Substances that require such energy include potassium, sodium, glucose, and amino acids. Passive transport takes advantage of present concentration or osmotic gradients and does not require any energy. Water, urea, chloride, and some bicarbonates represent substances that are passively reabsorbed by the peritubular capillaries. Most of this reabsorption occurs in the proximal tubule; however, the other segments of the tubule also reabsorb water and electrolytes.

In tubular secretion, substances are secreted out of the peritubular blood into the lumen of the renal tubule by active transport or passive diffusion. Such substances include ammonia, uric acid, potassium, hydrogen, exogenous substances, and other wastes.

The ability of a child's kidneys to adjust the excretion of urine and solute (i.e., dilute or concentrate) in response to the body's demand for water and electrolyte balance is normally adequate but is less adaptable than an adult's kidneys in times of emergency. Infants gain the ability to dilute their urine on approximately the 14th day of life and the ability to concentrate urine during the 3rd month of life. Although the ability to dilute urine is comparable with that of an adult, a newborn infant cannot excrete a water load because of reduced GFR (Bergstein, 1992).

Anatomy of the Genitalia

Female Genitalia

The female genitalia involve both internal and external structures. The *internal organs* include the *ovaries, fallopian tubes, uterus,* and *vagina.* The reader is directed to a textbook of gynecologic and obstetric nursing for a description of the complex hormonal physiology of these internal structures.

The *external genitalia* include the *mons pubis, labia majora, labia minora, clitoris, vestibule,* and *Bartholin* and *Skene glands.* The labia majora and labia minora form the outer and inner lips of the female genitalia or vulva (see Fig. 13–26). The inner surfaces of the labia contain many sebaceous glands, which become active at puberty. The perspiration from these glands predisposes some young women to vulvar irritation.

Formed of erectile tissue, the *clitoris* is the homologue of the penis. Because of its structure, the clitoris can be mistaken for the urethral opening by an inexperienced practitioner. The clitoris joins the anterior folds of the labia minora, whereas the urethral and vaginal openings are found in the vestibule, the cleft between the labia minora.

Skene glands, which surround the urethral meatus, are the homologues of the male prostate gland. Bartholin glands are found near the vaginal opening and, although usually not palpable, may at times present as small, round bumps. Bartholin glands are believed to provide vaginal lubrication during coitus.

Male Genitalia

The *penis* and the *scrotum* constitute the major structures of the *male genitalia* (see Fig. 13–27). The *urethra* is positioned ventrally within the shaft of the penis and the normal meatal opening in the glans penis. The *prepuce,* or foreskin, is the retractable fold of the skin that covers the glans penis in uncircumcised males.

The *scrotum* contains the *testes,* the *epididymis,* and a portion of the *vas deferens.* The testes are palpable as smooth, firm, olive-shaped structures within each scrotal sac. *Spermatic cords* suspend each testis and are composed of blood vessels, nerves, and the vas deferens. Because the right spermatic cord is shorter, the left testis hangs somewhat lower than the right.

The vas deferens carries sperm from the testis to the *ejaculatory duct* formed by the union of the vas deferens and the vesicles. The semen is propelled from the ejaculatory duct into the urethra. The *prostate gland* is located within the abdominal cavity, and surrounds the urethra and the ejaculatory ducts. Abnormalities of the prostate gland are rare before adulthood.

History and Physical Examination

Because the kidneys play a major role in maintaining homeostasis in the body, an impairment of renal functioning has the potential to affect other body systems. Therefore, a wide range of signs and symptoms must be considered related to the potential for or presence of renal dysfunction.

The child's age and level of maturation in assessment are important. The type of disorder and the incidence of its occurrence may be more significant in a child of one age group than another. For example, the implications for an infant with a urinary tract infection (UTI) differ vastly from those for a sexually active female adolescent with the same problem.

The components of the assessment are the history and physical examination. If the child is young, the presence of the parents is helpful in obtaining the information and in gaining the child's cooperation.

Assessment of genitourinary and renal function should be included in every history. Many disorders may have only subtle manifestations in their early stages, with ensuing serious complications if not detected early. Therefore, a comprehensive history is imperative. Although a previous history or physical examination, or both, may not reflect a disorder, this should not deter the nurse from searching for a subtle abnormality. In assessing a child with a genitourinary or renal disorder, specific factors should be noted that will be pertinent to the nursing care and treatment (Table 36–2).

The goal of physical assessment is to identify abnormalities. A complete physical examination should be performed as described in Chapter 13. Common clinical manifestations of genitourinary or renal alterations are presented in Table 36–3.

Diagnostic Assessment

Children with genitourinary disorders frequently undergo numerous laboratory tests and diagnostic procedures. Procedures associated with the genitalia or with the function of urination usually produce a great deal of anxiety. Laboratory tests and diagnostic procedures required for children are frequently more difficult to do than they are in adults because of the child's anxiety and limited ability to understand and cooperate during specimen collection procedures.

TABLE 36–2
Nursing History for a Child with a Genitourinary or Renal Disorder

History of Present Illness

1. Identify complaint
2. Identify duration, location, severity, past and current treatment of the genitourinary problem

Birth History

1. Presence of polyhydramnios or oligohydramnios during the pregnancy
2. Number of umbilical vessels at birth
3. Presence of congenital anomalies
4. What were the neonatal voiding patterns?

Past Health History

1. Previous serious illnesses
2. Exposure to nephrotoxic agents
3. Exposure to potentially nephrotoxic drugs
4. Previous bladder infections or obstructions
5. Has the child ever had headaches, irritability, seizures, visual disturbances (suggestive of hypertension)?
6. Has the child ever been fatigued, anorectic, had failure-to-thrive, or stopped growing (suggestive of chronic renal failure)?

Developmental History

Has the child reached developmental milestones (e.g., toilet training)?

What words does the child use for elimination?

Habits

Diet

Alterations in feeding or changes in fluid intake

Alterations in the child's appetite

An increased thirst for water in particular

Elimination

Bowel: Identify the child's bowel patterns, consistency of stool, frequency of elimination

Bladder—child's voiding pattern: Is there any frequency, change in volume, dysuria, alterations in urinary stream, dribbling, pain in the genital area, urgency? Color and odor of urine

Presence of daytime or nocturnal enuresis

Sleep

Alteration in the sleeping pattern

Behavior

Does the child fatigue easily?

Is the child irritable?

TABLE 36-3
Clinical Manifestations of Genitourinary or Renal Alterations

Clinical Manifestation	Clinical Significance
Headaches, irritability, visual disturbances, seizures	Indicative of hypertension, acidosis, or alkalosis
Paleness of conjunctivae, skin, and mucous membranes	Indicative of anemia
Breath odor may be ammoniac or urinelike	Indicative of uremia
Heart murmur, arrhythmia, or pericardial friction rub	Cardiovascular abnormalities may result from anemia, hypertension, or fluid overload
Tachypnea, rales, rhonchi, Kussmaul respirations. Infant may have nasal flaring, retractions	Respiratory alterations may indicate fluid overload, metabolic acidosis
Abdominal masses, abdominal or flank pain, palpation of enlarged kidneys	Indicative of hydronephrotic kidneys, tumor, presence of infection
Urine color, odor, urinary stream, pain on urination, hematuria, frequency. *In younger children:* child may complain of abdominal pain, cry with urination. *In older children:* child may have enuresis, complain of dysuria	Alteration may indicate presence of infection, obstruction, or dehydration
Skin color—pale, sallow, or jaundiced	Indicative of obstruction, anemia, or uremia
Edema, weight gain	Indicative of fluid retention
Growth retardation	Indicative of chronic infection or renal failure
Poor nutritional intake, vomiting, weight loss	Indicative of renal failure
Congenital anomalies: low-set ears, widely spaced nipples, absence of abdominal musculature (prune belly syndrome), spina bifida, abnormalities of the external genitalia	These anomalies are associated with genitourinary disorders

Some of the procedures are intrusive and painful or uncomfortable. Preparation for the procedures with explanations about sensations that are likely to be experienced can help the child and family members feel more in control of themselves and their situation. Preparation of children for procedures is presented in Chapter 23.

The most commonly performed test used in the diagnostic assessment of genitourinary problems is a routine urinalysis. This test is performed routinely on hospital admission as well as in primary care settings. The definitive study for the presence of bacteria in the urine (bacteriuria) is urine culture and sensitivity. This is the test that should be used to determine the appropriate treatment for UTI. Unfortunately, abnormal results are not consistently pursued to reap the potential benefits of early diagnosis (Mitchell & Stapleton, 1990). Although it is a team responsibility to ensure that abnormal test results are followed up, nurses should take a major role in ensuring that the necessary surveillance takes place.

A summary of laboratory tests is presented in Table 36-4, and diagnostic procedures are listed in Table 36-5. Test results in children are frequently different from those in adults and are noted in these tables.

Therapeutic Management

Management of genitourinary and renal problems frequently requires the use of devices to facilitate urinary drainage. Nurses must understand the purpose of the various devices and know how to maintain their function properly and safely in order to promote recovery of the patient.

Understanding the Purpose of Catheters, Stents, and Drains

Children who have had urinary tract surgery frequently return from the operating room with multiple appliances that require expert nursing knowledge and care. These appliances fall into three main categories: catheters, stents, and drains. Open catheter drainage using a double diaper system is also used following urethral surgery (Montagnino et al, 1988). *Catheters* transport urine from any part of the urinary tract to a drainage bag and are named according to the anatomic part they drain, e.g., nephrostomy tube (kidney), ureterostomy tube (ureter). Because the bladder can be drained in several ways, bladder catheters are named according to the route of drainage: urethral catheter (through the urethra), suprapubic tube (through the bladder and abdominal walls), or perineal urethrostomy (through the middle portion of the urethra).

Stents are very thin catheters that serve also as internal splints for surgical sites within the urinary tract. They promote tissue healing and, by draining urine, prevent pressure on the surgical site from the build-up of fluid. The terms "ureteral tube" and "ureteral stent" are frequently used interchangeably. Stents usually exit the body through the urethra or through an incision in the abdominal wall.

Drains are placed outside the urinary tract to allow urine that has leaked from surgical sites to reach the outside of the body, thereby preventing infection and scarring caused by urine build-up in the tissues surrounding the urinary structure. When the child has more than one drainage tube or catheter, the nurse must carefully label the tubes according to their origin within the body. The volume of urine from each catheter or tube should be recorded separately.

Parents may become disconcerted on seeing their child return from surgery with multiple tubes and bandages and, as a result, may have difficulty supporting the child. The nurse should prepare parents

TABLE 36-4
Laboratory Assessment: Genitourinary or Renal Disorders

Name of Test/ Normal Range	Alteration/ Clinical Significance	Nursing Implications
Urine Tests (Routine)		Explore intake and output patterns and assess hydration status; assess for recent injury; assess for other signs of infection (dysuria, frequency, odor, malaise, and fever)
Appearance Clear, pale yellow to gold color	The color of normal urine is determined by a pigment that is excreted at a uniform rate: *Cloudy:* Indicates white cells from infection or precipitation of phosphate *Tea-colored:* Indicates blood loss from the filtering system—usually nephritis *Frank red:* Blood from kidney, bladder, or urethra A dark urine is a concentrated urine	
Odor	Foul, fishy, indicating infection; assess for source of infection; evaluate need for urine culture	
Specific gravity (SG) 1.002–1.030 *Neonate* 1.001–1.020	SG of a solution is a measure of its density; it is obtained by comparing the weight of urine with an equal amount of water; it provides information about hydration status and the kidney's ability to concentrate/dilute urine *Increased:* Dehydration, presence of glucose or protein, excretion of radiopaque contrast media *Decreased:* Diuresis, diabetes insipidus In chronic renal disease, the kidney loses the ability to concentrate urine first; later the ability to dilute urine is lost as well; SG is fixed at 1.010, the same as SG of plasma; this occurs when 50% of the nephron mass has been destroyed	Assess hydration status; monitor intake and output; assess for other signs of diseases associated with increased and decreased SG; one cannot re-establish SG within normal range by increasing and decreasing fluids in the presence of renal disease
pH 4.6–8.0 (depends on time of day and freshness of specimen) average = 6.0 *Neonate* 5–7	Indicates the acid-base balance; affected by medications and diet *Alkaline urine* (pH 7.5): Can develop in presence of urea-splitting bacteria (e.g., *Proteus*) *Acid urine* (pH 5.0): Results from metabolic or respiratory acidosis, nephritis First morning urine is acid; a meal lacking protein will usually result in an alkaline urine	
Glucose Negative	*Present in* 1. Hyperglycemia caused by diabetes mellitus and infusion of glucose-containing fluids, administration of hormones, central nervous system disorders, or other drugs 2. Conditions of renal tubular origin when there is decreased ability to reabsorb glucose (nephrosis, cystinosis)	Assess for signs of related disease (i.e., diabetes, renal disease)
Protein Negative-trace (trace protein may or may not be normal)	*Positive* Positive in a variety of acute and chronic renal diseases (e.g., nephrotic syndrome)	When more than a trace of protein is present, a 24-hr urine is usually done; may be positive intermittently (1+ or 2+) in many neonates and adolescents; is important to repeat test being sure to use first morning sample eliminating "postural proteinuria" (related to activity)

(continued)

TABLE 36-4
Laboratory Assessment: Genitourinary or Renal Disorders *(Continued)*

Name of Test/ Normal Range	Alteration/ Clinical Significance	Nursing Implications
Urine Tests (Routine)		
Ketones Negative	*Positive* Increased in conditions resulting in acidosis (e.g., diabetes mellitus, starvation, fever, high-fat diet)	
Red blood cells (RBCs) Not seen normally Dipstix positive for greater than 4 RBCs per high-power field (HPF)	RBCs of glomerular origin are identified by the presence of RBC casts and dysmorphic RBCs	Hematuria occurs in pathologic conditions that involve the mucosa of the collecting system; bleeding from the kidneys produces dark red urine, from the urinary tract, bright red urine; microscopic hematuria is more commonly nephrogenic and gross hematuria (evident to naked eye) is more commonly urogenic
White blood cells (WBCs) >5/HPF	More than five polymorphonuclear leukocytes/HPF Increased in urinary tract inflammatory process	Dipstix can detect white cells with leukocyte strip
Casts Occasional	Specific types of casts are frequently associated with certain renal disorders (but can vary); hyaline casts: dehydration; granular/waxy casts: chronic renal failure, renal transplant rejection; WBC casts: pyelonephritis; RBC casts: glomerulonephritis	
Bacteria	More than 100,000/ml of centrifuged specimen indicates urinary tract infection	Dipstix can detect bacteria with nitrite strip
Crystals	Seen in some types of renal calculi	Uric acid crystals may stain the diaper red—rarely signifies disease
Other Urine Tests		
Creatinine clearance	Reflects glomerular filtration rate (GFR) Decreases when GFR decreases; secondary to disease process (e.g., glomerulonephritis)	Based on 24-hr urine collection and is compared with *serum* creatinine levels
Osmolality 50–1400 Osm/kg water (usual urine : serum ratio = 4 : 1)	More accurate than SG in evaluating renal-concentrating mechanisms because does not vary with diet or changes in urine content Compared with *serum* osmolality	Increases and decreases occur in conditions as for SG (see above)
Volume (age-related) *Age (ml/24 hrs)* Neonate (30–60) 1–7 days (100–300) 10–60 days (250–450) 2–12 mos (400–500) 1–3 yrs (500–600) 3–5 yrs (600–700) 5–8 yrs (650–1000) 8–14 yrs (800–1400) Adults (600–1600)	Output less than 1 ml/kg/hr is usually pathologic Polyuria can result from ingestion of excess fluid, chronic renal failure, and diabetes mellitus and diabetes insipidus; anuria or oliguria can be caused by an obstruction or acute renal failure	Measurement of urine is done to identify polyuria, oliguria, and anuria
Blood Tests		
Creatinine *Newborn infant* (0.3–1.0 mg/dl) *Child* (0.3–0.7 mg/dl)	Increased with impaired renal function	Glomerular filtration rate must be reduced by at least 50% before a significant increase in serum creatinine occurs

TABLE 36-4
Laboratory Assessment: Genitourinary or Renal Disorders (Continued)

Name of Test/ Normal Range	Alteration/ Clinical Significance	Nursing Implications
Blood Tests		
Blood urea nitrogen (BUN) *Newborn infant* (3–12 mg/dl) *Infant/child* (5–18 mg/dl)	Increased with impaired renal function, or in any condition causing reduced renal blood flow (e.g., shock, salt and water depletion, cardiac failure); decreased with overhydration, low-protein diet, liver failure	In chronic renal disease, BUN correlates better than creatinine with symptoms of uremia
Uric acid 2.0–5.5 mg/dl	Increased in severe renal disease	

TABLE 36-5
Radiologic and Other Renal Function Tests

Name of Test	Description and Purpose	Nursing Implications
Renal ultrasonography (abdominal/renal ultrasonography) *Easiest and best*	Sound waves bounced off anatomic structures result in an electronic image (noninvasive); lubricant is applied to abdomen and/or flank and transducer is moved over the area (total time: approx. 15 mins); useful procedure in the diagnosis of congenital anomalies, hydronephrosis, renal tumors, cysts, calculi, and abscesses; also used to diagnose prenatal structural abnormalities	Preparation or sedation rarely required
Voiding cystourethrogram (VCUG)	Catheterization and filling of the bladder with contrast medium; visualizes bladder outline and urethra; shows reflux of urine into ureters or kidneys; series of radiographs before, during, and after voiding (total time: approx. 15 mins); useful in the diagnosis of vesicoureteral reflux, urethral valves, and strictures	Prepare the child for catheter insertion. Explain that the feeling is similar to having to go to the bathroom as the bladder is filling with the special liquid—contrast material; explain to the child that she or he will be a little sore the first few times going to the bathroom after the procedure, but reassure that the soreness will go away soon *Note:* radiology department may request that a pediatric physician or nurse catheterize child for procedure
Intravenous pyelogram (IVP)	Intravenous injection of radiopaque contrast medium; excretion of medium through kidneys with concentration in the collecting tubules allowing visualization of calyces, renal pelvis, ureters, and bladder; films are often taken at 1 min, 5 mins, and at 10 mins postcontrast; a postvoiding bladder film is frequently not obtained in children (total time: approx. 30 mins); useful in the diagnosis of hydronephrosis, renal scarring, cysts, tumors, and calculi; ultrasound and radionuclide scanning often more useful	*Preprocedural care* Prepare child for feelings associated with injection of contrast medium: general feeling of warmth, burning at IV site, nausea; avoid use of word "dye," as this may frighten younger children (may confuse with "die"); verify that child has had no past allergic reactions to radiopaque contrast medium; administer cathartics/enemas as indicated in adolescents; bowel preparation is not indicated in children
Radionuclide scanning	Radioactive material is injected intravenously; an imaging device detects radioactivity in each kidney, which is analyzed by computer; best visualization of excretory function, shows differences between two kidneys as well as areas of renal scarring	Preparation as for IVP (above)
Plain film or flat plate of abdomen (KUB—kidneys, ureters, bladder)	Routine radiograph of abdomen; older children may be asked to hold breath for a few seconds; useful in diagnosis of renal calculi	As for routine radiograph

(continued)

TABLE 36–5
Radiologic and Other Renal Function Tests *(Continued)*

Name of Test	Description and Purpose	Nursing Implications
Computed tomography (CT)	Oral contrast medium is administered the evening before the study to visualize bowel and avoid confusion of fluid-filled bowel with masses; x-ray with a thin beam is directed at an area at multiple angles to produce an image; this is combined with computer analysis to assign density values to specific points in the body; is useful to detect a renal mass or calculi, differentiate tumors and cysts, determine level of hydronephrosis, and evaluate renal transplants	Patient has to remain still up to 30 mins; sedation usually required
Cystoscopy	General anaesthesia required; insertion of thin tubelike cystoscope into the urethra and visualization of the urethra and the interior of the bladder; useful in the assessment of bladder wall anomalies, urethral valves, and strictures prior to possible surgery	*Preprocedural care* NPO as ordered Premedication as ordered *Postprocedural care* Reassure parents and child that urination after procedure is frequently uncomfortable; having child urinate in a tub of warm water may be helpful; encourage fluids; monitor urine volume and character for small amounts of bleeding; monitor temperature carefully; bacteremia can occur after instrumentation of the urinary tract; notify physician if temperature over 101°F (38.4°C); administer prophylactic antibiotics if ordered, prior to procedure and for several days afterward
Renal angiography	Contrast medium is injected via a catheter placed into a femoral artery and threaded into renal artery (umbilical artery used in newborn infants); is used only when other, less invasive techniques are not adequate	*Preprocedural care* Withhold food and fluid as ordered; verify that child has no past allergic reactions to contrast medium; sedation or general anesthesia required *Postprocedural care* Observe for allergic reactions to contrast medium during procedure; monitor vital signs
Renal biopsy	A large-bore needle is guided into the kidney by ultrasonography; required for a definitive diagnosis of some cases of nephrotic syndrome or nephritis	Prepare for local anesthetic while child lies prone; sedation also required; observe and save blood-stained urine after biopsy; vital signs required to recognize severe or continued bleeding

and children preoperatively for postoperative appearances and procedures, using words that can be understood by both. In preparing the child, the nurse can describe the catheter as a "tube"; surgery can be described as "fixing." Indiscriminate use of frightening words like "cut" or "bleed" should be avoided.

General principles of catheter care that apply to all categories of drainage devices are summarized in Table 36–6.

Teaching Clean Intermittent Catheterization

Clean intermittent catheterization is most frequently used in children with neurogenic bladder dysfunction. It is based on the theory that the bladder is resistant to infection as long as it is emptied frequently and does not become overdistended. Catheterization is done at least every 3 to 4 hours; the frequency depends on the type of neurogenic bladder dysfunction, bladder capacity, sphincter function, and fluid intake.

The nurse's assessment of the parent's and child's willingness and ability to perform routine frequent catheterizations is of the utmost importance. Serious UTIs can result if the bladder is not routinely emptied and becomes overdistended. Clean intermittent catheterization can be taught to parents, as outlined in Table 36–7. Under Public Law 94–142 in the United States and B.1182 in Canada, the law mandating certain educational services for handicapped children, clean intermittent catheterization is a mandated school health service. For children who cannot catheterize themselves, school personnel, ideally the

TABLE 36-6
Guidelines for Care of Catheters and Drainage Devices

1. Always wash hands before and after doing catheter care. Wear gloves (it is not necessary for gloves to be sterile)
2. Position child carefully to prevent kinking or looping of tubing. Infants and very young children may need gauze mittens or restraints to keep them from pulling at the catheter
3. Prevent movement of the catheter by taping it to the thigh/flank/abdomen and allowing some slack in the tubing
4. Keep a careful record of urine output and character (e.g., clear, cloudy, blood-tinged, clots) from each catheter. Prepare parents and child for appearance of drainage postoperatively (watery and bright red 24 hrs after surgery, progressing to reddish-brown with small clots, to clear within 4–7 days). Notify physician if significant amount of bleeding occurs at any time
5. Watch for signs of obstruction: No output for more than an hour, urine leaking around the catheter, bladder distention, large blood clots, or tissue shreds inside the catheter. If no external obstruction (e.g., kinks) can be found, gently "milk" the tubing and/or irrigate with sterile normal saline, if ordered. Notify physician immediately if not successful with preceding procedures
6. Always keep the collecting bag below the level of the child's bladder to facilitate gravity drainage of urine. Never fasten bag to bed siderails as it could inadvertently become caught when siderails are raised or lowered
7. Carefully cleanse catheter entry site at least twice a day according to institutional policy. Apply antimicrobial ointment and/or dressing if indicated
8. Maintain sterile closed drainage system. Open the system only for irrigation or collection of specimens as ordered. Always thoroughly cleanse site where system will be opened before and after opening
9. Administer comfort measures and pain medication as ordered for bladder spasms. Check for kinking or obstruction of tubing as cause for pain
10. Encourage adequate oral intake
11. After catheter removal, prepare parents and child for some discomfort over next 24 hrs. Keep careful record of intake/output; notify physician if child does not void within 6 hrs after catheter removal.

TABLE 36-7
***Family-Centered Teaching:* Clean Intermittent Catheterization**

1. Wash hands with soap and water or with a towelette, if possible. Because the avoidance of bladder overdistention is so important, catheterization should be done even if unable to wash
2. Preferably, catheterization is done with the child sitting on the toilet or standing beside it. However, any position that is comfortable, including supine, is acceptable
3. Lubricate catheter (optional for females)
4. Insert catheter
   A. *Male:* Grasp penis, holding on sides, and hold it erect, then insert catheter slowly
   B. *Female:* Separate labia and insert catheter. A mirror may be helpful while learning but child can usually learn to locate meatus by palpation

   Note: Catheter sizes range from 8 to 14 French. A clear plastic No. 8 feeding tube may be used to catheterize infants and young children
5. Insert 1–2 inches farther than point at which urine begins to flow
6. Allow urine to flow into a cup or other container until flow stops
7. Remove catheter slowly; hold catheter tip up after withdrawal to avoid spilling urine
8. Wash catheter in soap and water; rinse and dry. Store in dry clean bottle, plastic bag, or other small container
9. Replace catheter as directed. A wide range of schedules is used by parents (i.e., daily, weekly, or monthly)

school nurse, must be available to perform the procedure. The hospital or clinic nurse can work with school personnel to ensure their understanding of the child's health care needs. A private area with a sink, a place to store equipment, and a change of clothing are all necessary.

Nursing Care

This chapter addresses a broad range of surgical and medical conditions affecting the genitourinary system. A commonality across conditions is that the nature of these illnesses focuses attention on body parts and body functions that are generally personal and private. Because of the close association between the urinary tract and the reproductive system, genitourinary disorders may raise concerns, frequently unspoken, about virginity, future fertility, and sexual functioning.

The process of making a diagnosis and treating the child's condition often involves invasive, frequently painful, procedures. Although surgical correction is possible for many of the structural anomalies, loss of renal function introduces the child and family to a long period of uncertainty and stress associated with any chronic illness. These psychologic stresses are compounded when repeated treatment and long-term therapy are required. The uncertainty, for example, involved in waiting for a kidney transplant puts the entire family under severe stress.

The group of illnesses discussed in this chapter thus presents a particular challenge to the nurse. Parents and children may have many questions and concerns they have difficulty expressing. Not only do they need help to verbalize these concerns but the parents may also need someone to help them talk to their child about the condition, its treatment, and its prognosis. It may also be difficult in some cases for parents and children to explain their child's condition to relatives and neighbors. Genitourinary conditions are generally not observable to the public and may even present a degree of mystery to those outside of the family.

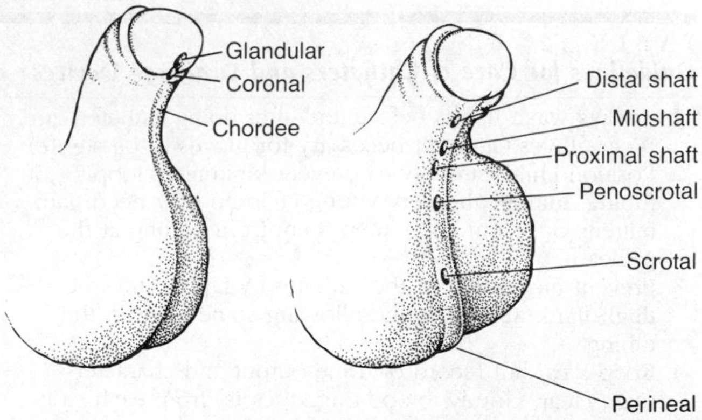

FIGURE 36 - 4. Hypospadias anomalies. In all but a few cases, hypospadias is accompanied by chordee, with the curvature proportional to the severity of hypospadias. It is best to classify hypospadias severity according to the site of the proximally displaced meatus, as shown here, rather than by imprecise quantification of "degrees of hypospadias."

Congenital Anomalies of Genitourinary Function

Genitourinary tract anomalies range from those that are visible at birth to those that are not easily detected but cause progressive damage to the urinary tract. The nurse plays an important role in facilitating the early identification of urinary tract anomalies at birth and throughout childhood and adolescence. Urinary tract anomalies may have a considerable effect on the child and family. The nursing role is vital in assessment, planning, and intervention in order to minimize the impact of the disorder.

Nursing care in the perioperative period specific to that anomaly is included with the discussion of each disorder. The interventions that are included should be considered *in addition to* the general perioperative care detailed in Table 23–7.

Hypospadias

In hypospadias, the urethral meatus opens below the glans penis or at any point along the ventral surface of the penis, or on the scrotum or perineum. Undescended testes and inguinal hernia are two commonly associated anomalies.

Etiology/Incidence

The cause of hypospadias is unknown. There are familial tendencies for the development of this disorder. Genetic factors are thought to contribute, although the mode of inheritance is not known. It is the most common anomaly of the penis, occurring in about 1 in 500 live male births.

Clinical Manifestations

This disorder results when the urethral folds fail to fuse in the midline, and the urethral meatus opens on the ventral surface of the penis. The prepuce (foreskin) is smaller ventrally and presents as a hood or flap. Hypospadias is categorized into types according to the position of the urethral opening. The types of hypospadias are glandular (urethra opens at the base of the glans penis); coronal (urethra opens at the junction of the glans and the penis); distal, mid, or proximal shaft (urethra opens on the shaft between the glans and the scrotum); penoscrotal (urethra opens at the junction of the penis and scrotum); scrotal; or perineal (urethra opens on the perineum) (Fig. 36–4).

Chordee, a ventral curvature of the penis, is present in almost all forms of hypospadias. This curvature is caused by tough, fibrous bands that extend ventrally behind the urethra to the glans. The chordee will vary in severity and is generally proportional to the degree of hypospadias.

Diagnostic Assessment

The nurse can assist in the identification of hypospadias by performing a genital examination on all neonates. Mild degrees of hypospadias may be missed on casual examination. A thorough examination is essential because if any degree of hypospadias is present circumcision should not be performed without urologic consultation. Urinary incontinence is not usually manifested, since the urethral abnormality in this condition occurs distal to the urinary sphincter.

After the neonatal period, the nurse should continue to assess for mild degrees of hypospadias in all males. Often, less severe cases of hypospadias are missed in early infancy and diagnosed later. Thus, inspection of the position of the urinary meatus and examination for penile curvature should be included in routine physical assessments.

The anomaly most commonly associated with hypospadias is undescended testes (cryptorchidism) (see discussion of cryptorchidism later in this section). If hypospadias occurs with one or both testes not palpable, the child may have ambiguous genitalia. In this situation, an extensive investigation should be done to determine the appropriate assignment of the infant's sex. Care of the child with ambiguous genitalia is presented in Chapter 43 (endocrine alterations).

Hypospadias, as either an isolated anomaly or part of a more complex syndrome, may be difficult for the family to understand and accept. The nurse, with other health team members, can help the family understand the condition, its long-term implications, and methods of management.

Therapeutic Management

Surgical repair of hypospadias is being performed at an increasingly younger age. Concerns surrounding surgery are that the penile shaft is large enough to achieve successful surgical repair and that the child suffers the least amount of psychologic trauma possible. There is some variation in the recommended age for surgery. Some recommend 3 to 9 months of age as an ideal time (Duckett, 1992), whereas others prefer 2 years of age, especially for complex repairs (Kodoma & Winslow, 1991). Surgery during the first year of life is now technically possible because of improved instrumentation. The major accomplishment through early repair is prevention of the child's suffering embarrassment because he looks different from his friends and other males in the family. However, there is some limitation on how early the repair can be done because penile development must be sufficient to make the operation technically possible.

The goal of surgical management is to normalize the appearance and function of the penis. Although the surgery performed varies according to the extent of the disorder, the aim is to reconstruct a straight penis with a meatus at the tip of the glans, to allow a urinary stream that is directed forward, and to make normal coitus a possibility. To achieve this, the fibrous bands and skin adhesions causing the ventral curvature must be completely released, and a urethral tube must be created to allow the urethra to terminate in its expected location. The prepuce is used for reconstructive surgery; therefore, circumcision is not done on infants with hypospadias.

Nursing Care

No special physical preparation is required prior to surgery for hypospadias. Psychologic preparation varies according to the age of the child. The toddler will not necessarily verbalize his fears, nor will he understand what is happening to him. He should be told that the doctor will make an opening at the tip of his penis and that he will urinate from that opening after the area is healed. The likelihood of pain and discomfort following surgery should also be explained, with the assurance that medication will be available to keep him comfortable. All of these explanations are difficult for a young child to understand; parents should be involved in the process, an element of the process that brings comfort to a young child. Telling the child that surgery will make his penis "look better" should be avoided as it suggests that he does not currently appear normal. Preoperatively, the child can be given a simple explanation about the dressing and the catheter that will be in place postoperatively. The family should be made aware of the hospitalization procedures as well as what they may reasonably expect during the preoperative and postoperative periods.

After the operation, a pressure dressing is often used to reduce bleeding and tissue swelling. This dressing is not to be removed by the nurse, and the child's hands must be kept away from his penis so that the dressing is not dislodged and the surgical area is kept free of trauma. Although this may require temporary restraint, a parent sitting at the bedside during the critical period is the most comforting and safe approach. The tip of the penis should be checked frequently to be sure that it is pink and viable. The dressing is usually left in place for several days to encourage healing of the grafted skin flap. It is then changed by the surgeon and should not be removed unless this has been ordered. Some form of urinary diversion such as a suprapubic catheter is often used to allow the urine to temporarily bypass the operative site. Early ambulation is encouraged, often the same day as surgery. The catheter and urinary bag can be fastened to the child so that he can ambulate. Care is taken not to put pressure on the catheter, not to kink it, and to keep it at or below the level of the bladder. Parents often feel overwhelmed in caring for their child because of the dressing, catheter, urinary bag, and the discomfort experienced by their child.

The child's comfort is a major concern during the postoperative period. Sedation may be necessary because of the child's irritability and inability to rest. Use of analgesics to reduce the child's pain is also necessary.

After catheter removal (usually by the 7th to 10th postoperative day), urinary infection, dysuria, hematuria, or frequency may develop. Parents should be cautioned about symptoms of infection so that they can report them early. Discomfort on initial voiding after catheter removal is common; children and parents usually manage this well if they have been prepared for the temporary discomfort.

The most common complication of hypospadias repair is a fistula in which an opening forms between the urethra and the skin of the shaft. If the fistula is small, it may close spontaneously; larger fistulas may require further surgical intervention. Persistent chordee, meatal stenosis, urethral stricture and stenosis, and urethral diverticula are other complications of hypospadias repair; all require additional surgical intervention.

Epispadias

Although hypospadias is a common congenital anomaly, epispadias is rare. It involves location of the urethral orifice along the dorsal surface of the penis.

The severity of epispadias varies from a mild anomaly, in which the meatal opening is proximal to the glans penis, to the severe epispadias that is associated with exstrophy of the bladder (see the discussion of exstrophy of the bladder later in this chapter). Epispadias can be surgically repaired. The goals of treatment and strategies for nursing care are similar to those discussed for hypospadias.

Cryptorchidism

Cryptorchidism refers to a condition in which a testis has not descended into the scrotal sac but has been arrested in descent at some point between the kidneys and the scrotal sac.

Incidence/Etiology

The incidence of cryptorchidism increases as the degree of prematurity increases. For example, in full-term male neonates, the incidence is 3 to 4 per cent; in those with birthweights between 2000 and 2500 g, it is 17 per cent; it rises to 100 per cent for those under 900 g at birth. It is thought that descent of the testes from the inguinal canal into the scrotum takes place around the 7th month of gestation; spontaneous descent does not usually occur after 1 year of age. The incidence of cryptorchidism after 1 year of age drops to 0.7 per cent, reflecting the high numbers of spontaneous descent that occur during the first year of life (Gonzales, 1992).

The etiology of cryptorchidism is unknown; however, several theories are prevalent. The first is that an undescended testis is inherently an abnormal organ, and failure of descent reflects this disordered embryologic state. The second theory points to lack of sufficient gonadotropic stimulation (particularly applicable to bilateral cryptorchidism) as the cause. The third theory cites mechanical obstruction to descent caused by fibrous bands, a short spermatic cord, or an ectopic location (commonly noted in unilateral undescended testis) (Hadziselimovic et al, 1975; Hadziselimovic and Herzog, 1976).

Pathophysiology

The classification of undescended testes is based on whether the testes are palpable or impalpable on clinical examination. Impalpable testes are totally absent from the body or located in a position where they are never palpated by a clinician. Palpable testes are divided into three categories: retractile, ectopic, or truly undescended testes within the canal.

Retractile testes are most commonly found in the groin but may be palpated at any level along the line of descent. These testes are normally descended but have been pulled back into an extrascrotal position because of a hyperactive cremasteric reflex, which retracts the testes into the upper part of the scrotum or into the inguinal canal in response to cold, pain, fear, or touch. Retractile testes may be manually drawn into the scrotum, where they will remain.

The second type of palpable cryptorchid testis is the *ectopic* type. An ectopic testis is one that has deviated from the normal path of descent after emerging from the inguinal canal. The testis may be located in the superficial inguinal pouch, the perineum, over the pubic bone, or in the femoral region.

Truly undescended testes, the third category of palpable undescended testes, are intermittently palpable to the clinician and may be palpated in the abdomen, scrotal canal, or inguinal ring. In truly undescended testes, the spermatic vessels are felt to be shorter, thus preventing the testes' normal descent into the scrotum.

Diagnostic Assessment

Accurate documentation of the position of both testes immediately after birth and during well baby examinations is an essential part of medical and nursing assessment. Before the child reaches 6 months of age, the scrotal contents are easily examined and the cremasteric reflex is absent or rudimentary. After 6 months of age, the cremasteric reflex becomes quite active and may simulate the empty scrotum of cryptorchidism in up to 50 per cent of boys (retractile testes). A reassuring attitude and thorough explanation of what the child or parent should expect will facilitate the examination. If examination of the inguinal and scrotal regions in the upright and supine positions suggests an undescended testis, it is often helpful to repeat the examination if the child is able to be seated with his knees drawn up to his chest. This will diminish the cremasteric reflex. Early documentation of a testis in its normal scrotal position (4 cm below the pubic tubercle) eliminates confusion in later years. Whenever a nurse is unable to palpate a testis in the scrotum he or she should bring it to the attention of a physician for further examination. If, on repeated examination, a testis is not palpable in its normal position by the time the child reaches 1 year of age, the diagnosis of cryptorchidism can be made and appropriate management instituted.

When cryptorchidism is suspected, the child by age 1 year should be referred to a surgeon skilled in pediatric urologic procedures.

Therapeutic Management

Treatment is instituted early to reduce the potential for the development of the various consequences of undescended testes. An undescended testis is unable to produce mature sperm, which is thought to be due to the higher temperature in the abdominal cavity or the inguinal canal (Moore, 1988). Also, true undescended testes are accompanied by indirect inguinal hernias; hernias are also common with ectopic undescended testicles. The goal of treatment is to avoid the consequences that follow if the testes remain undescended; these include infertility in adulthood, tumor development in the undescended testes, associated hernias and their complications, torsion of the undescended testes, and the psychologic effects of an abnormal-appearing scrotum because it is empty.

The treatment for undescended testes is surgical. Testes located extra-abdominally can be brought down and treated with a procedure called "orchidopexy"; this procedure is performed at around 2 years of age. In the case of a unilateral testis, ultrasonography is used to identify the location of an unpalpable testis. For bilateral undescended testes, the child must be evaluated for absent testes; this is done by measuring serum testosterone. This differential diagnosis is done by giving human chorionic gonadotropin (hCG) to stimulate the production of testosterone. If the testosterone level rises, it indicates the presence of testes; therefore, an abdominal exploration and orchidopexy follows.

Treatment with hCG to bring down the testes is generally unsuccessful to replace surgery, but some believe its use may facilitate surgery. It is generally agreed that hCG is effective only for retractile testes; its effect is that it induces an early pseudopuberty, thereby stimulating the permanent descent of the testes (Gonzalez, 1992). Retractile testes usually become permanently lodged in the scrotum during puberty.

To perform an orchidopexy, a small transverse incision is made in the lower abdominal skinfold and the testes and spermatic cord are freed from surrounding tissues. A hernial sac is present in up to 90 per cent of cases, although it is not usually detectable preoperatively and is only occasionally symptomatic. After an adequate length of spermatic cord is obtained, an incision is made through the skin of the lower portion of the scrotum, a pouch created, and the testis is pulled down into the pouch and then sutured to the inner wall of the scrotum. Subcutaneous sutures that do not require removal are used to close the skin incisions. The child may be discharged on the afternoon of surgery or the following morning and may resume normal activities as tolerated. Tub bathing is usually withheld for several days; showers, however, are permitted.

The potential for reduced fertility and the long-term risk of testicular malignancy should be discussed with the patient and his parents. Although the physician plays the primary role in this discussion, the nurse should have sufficient knowledge to participate effectively in counseling these families. It is important for the nurse to be present when the physician discusses these issues with the family so that she or he is aware of specific information that has been given by the physician. The nurse is then prepared to be supportive of family members as they deal with the effects of this information.

Specific information given to a family will vary; however, there are some facts that will assist the nurse in understanding the approach to management of cryptorchidism. Spermatogenesis may be significantly impaired in undescended testes. Although orchidopexy improves the situation, the fertility rate among these patients, even when only one testis is undescended, is reduced in comparison to that of unaffected men. Additionally, the risk of developing a malignant testicular tumor is increased 20 to 44 per cent in the 3rd or 4th decade of life. Males who remain untreated for intra-abdominal cryptorchidism or those who had corrective surgery during or after puberty are at greatest risk (Gonzalez, 1992).

Nursing Care

The nurse, working together with other members of the health care team, can play a central role in the management of these children. Early examination and documentation of the position of the testes by the nurse may obviate a false diagnosis later in life, thus eliminating needless anxiety, costly examinations, and unnecessary testing. Postoperatively, the operative site is kept free of urine and stool to prevent infection. Discussions with the patient and his family on the importance of long-term follow-up for development of tumor and for evaluation of fertility are essential. Additionally, instructing the child, when old enough, in the method and importance of self-examination of the testes to check for tumor is critical because of the length of time between surgery for undescended testes at 1 to 2 years of age, and the possible development of a tumor at about 30 to 40 years of age.

Exstrophy of the Bladder

Exstrophy of the bladder is a rare congenital malformation that occurs in 1 of 30,000 live births (Duckett & Caldamone, 1985). It affects males three times more often than females and is rarely familial.

Pathophysiology/Clinical Manifestations

Exstrophy of the bladder results from a deficiency in the development of the anterior abdominal wall, the symphysis pubis, the bladder, and the urethra during gestation. When the child is born, the bladder appears in the suprapubic region as a protruding red mass that constantly seeps urine. There is a wide separation in the symphysis pubis, and the hip sockets are rotated posterolaterally. These abnormalities cause the child to have difficulty walking, perhaps exhibiting a waddling gait. In the female, the clitoris is often bifid, the labia are widely separated, and the vaginal opening is tilted slightly anteriorly. Bilateral inguinal hernias and undescended testes in males may accompany exstrophy of the bladder. The penis is often epispadic, points upward, is short and stubby, and has an open urethral strip on the dorsum. The exposed mucosa is very sensitive to touch because the parasympathetic nerves are intact. Repair of the epispadias often involves cosmetic and functional reconstruction of the penis and urethra and is usually done after the other repairs are complete.

Therapeutic Management

Various surgical treatment modalities and philosophies are used in the management of exstrophy of the bladder. The success of the intervention depends on the severity of the defect. The major goals for treatment are to prevent and treat any infection, avoid trauma to the bladder, and promote the child's growth and development.

Current recommendations for treatment of exstrophy of the bladder are to intervene surgically within the first 48 hours of life (Gonzalez, 1992). Surgical closure of the defect and repair of the abdominal wall create a closed system. By surgically intervening during the neonatal period, the bladder has an opportunity to grow and expand safely, without trauma, during the first few years of life. Complications following this initial surgery include infection and hydronephrosis. The majority of infants have vesicoureteral reflux, and, usually, antibiotics are ordered. Also, antispasmodics for bladder spasms, analgesics and sedatives for comfort, and immobilization by use of Gallows traction or modified Bryant traction is required.

Repair of the epispadias with construction of an anterior urethra and correction of the form of the penis take place around 1 to 2 years of age.

When the child is 3 to 4 years old, a bladder neck tightening procedure is done. This involves reconstruction of the bladder neck and reimplantation of the ureters. The goal of this procedure is to help the child gain urinary control and prevent reflux from the ureters. However, it may take months or years before the child gains complete urinary control.

In some exceptional conditions, the anomaly is so extensive it cannot be repaired by reconstructive surgery at birth. In these rare circumstances, a type of temporary urinary diversion will be performed, such as a *bilateral ureterostomy,* an ileal conduit, or a ureterosigmoidostomy. A bilateral ureterostomy involves attaching the ureters directly to the abdominal wall, where urine is passed onto the abdomen. A diaper is placed around the abdomen, and urine drains into the diaper.

The creation of an *ileal conduit* involves resecting a small section of the colon or ileum and attaching one end of the resected bowel to the distal ends of the ureters and the other end of the bowel to a small opening (stoma) in the lower abdomen. This conduit provides transport for the urine from the ureters to the stoma. The child wears an ileostomy appliance over the stoma to collect the continuously flowing urine.

Ureterosigmoidostomy is now less commonly used than it was in the past but it is still used in some centers. It involves the anastomosis of the ureters to the sigmoid portion of the colon, thus permitting urinary excretion through the bowels. This form of urinary excretion occurs without the use of an abdominal stoma, enhancing the child's body image and continence. Because the urine is passed with the stool, complications may result from ascending bacteria or reflux. Common problems that are associated with a ureterosigmoidostomy include recurrent pyelonephritis, hyperchloremic acidosis due to the absorption of chloride, hypokalemia, and growth impairment.

Nursing Care

The major goals of nursing care are to promote parent-infant bonding, protect the bladder mucosa (prior to surgery), promote postoperative protection and healing of the surgical area, provide comfort, and provide parent support and teaching.

Parents of a child born with exstrophy of the bladder experience grief related to loss of the "perfect" child. The birth of a defective child may create anxiety, guilt, and much stress within the family. Because this defect is physically obvious and not well known to the general public, parents of children with exstrophic bladders have an added burden; however, in 75 per cent of cases, the anomaly can be corrected at birth with abdominal wall closure.

Prior to surgery, the bladder mucosa is protected with a Silastic shield or other appropriate dressing that will permit drainage but prevent desiccation of the bladder mucosa. Prompt transfer to a center where the bladder can be repaired is essential. Application of gauze or petrolatum or other ointments is avoided. A cord tie is used rather than a cord clamp to prevent the clamp from damaging the bladder (Bernhardt, 1993).

Following surgery, the infant is placed in Gallows or modified Bryant traction to promote healing by immobilization for 3 to 4 weeks. During this period, the infant must be given antispasmodics as ordered to prevent bladder spasms. Antibiotics are administered as ordered to prevent infection. The infant is monitored for signs of urinary tract infection (UTI). The infant must also be kept comfortable with analgesics, and excessive crying and irritability are reduced with the use of sedatives. A quiet, comfortable infant reduces the potential for disruption of the surgical closure.

Support and teaching of parents is determined by the type and results of surgical intervention. Parents can help to keep the infant comfortable following the surgical intervention. They need to be kept informed about the purpose for the various aspects of nursing interventions and to be told about the stages of treatment that may be required. They will need to know the signs and symptoms of UTI (e.g., fever, malodorous urine, and hematuria). If the child has undergone a ureterosigmoidostomy, the parents will require information about the symptoms of hypokalemia and acidosis that may result from the ostomy.

Although reconstructive surgery has improved the prognosis for children with exstrophy of the bladder, the child will still require multiple hospitalizations, tests, and frequent health care visits. The psychologic, social, and physical impact of this anomaly are felt by the child and family throughout the child's life.

Obstructive Renal Conditions

Obstructed urinary flow can be the result of congenital or acquired conditions affecting the flow of urine anywhere in the urinary tract. The obstruction may be unilateral or bilateral, complete or incomplete, and it may result in an acute or chronic condition.

The obstruction can occur anywhere in the urinary tract, as depicted in Figure 36–5. Conditions of the urinary tract that obstruct the outflow of urine are summarized in Table 36–8. Any partial or complete obstruction of the urinary tract can cause hydronephrosis. A discussion of this condition follows.

Hydronephrosis

Hydronephrosis is the accumulation of urine in the renal pelvis and calyces. If a urinary tract obstruction is not corrected, the kidney becomes distended with urine and the renal pressure rises. Cyst formation can result, and renal parenchyma destruction occurs as a result of the pressure. The extent and seriousness of the damage that occurs depend on the type of obstruction, how long it is present before correction, and whether the obstruction is unilateral or bilateral. When obstruction occurs within the pelvis or at the ureteropelvic junction, renal pelvic distention and subsequent damage can occur within hours. On the other hand, obstructions distal to the kidney, such as urethral stricture, result in bladder distention before hydronephrosis. (See Table 36–8 for further description of levels of obstruction.)

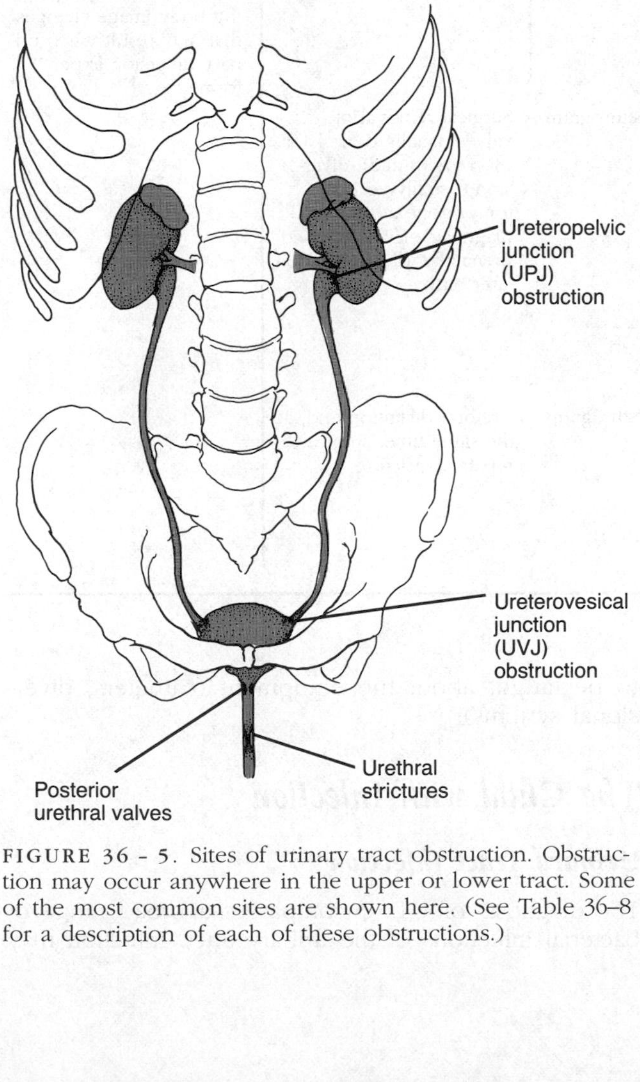

FIGURE 36 - 5. Sites of urinary tract obstruction. Obstruction may occur anywhere in the upper or lower tract. Some of the most common sites are shown here. (See Table 36–8 for a description of each of these obstructions.)

Etiology/Pathophysiology

As urine accumulates in the renal pelvis and calyces, the intrarenal pressure rises; eventually it rises to a level equal to the filtration pressure in the glomerular capillaries. Once this occurs, glomerular filtration stops. If the obstruction is uncorrected, circulation to the kidney is reduced; atrophy of the kidney follows, leading to renal insufficiency.

Clinical Manifestations

The severity and duration of obstruction, and whether one or both kidneys are affected, will determine the degree of renal function. The infant may present with signs of UTI caused by urine stasis. Flank pain and hematuria may be the first symptom in older children (>3 years). Urinary concentrating ability may also be impaired, which is characterized by increasing polydipsia and polyuria. If the condition becomes chronic, renal damage may also cause anemia because erythropoietin secretion is impaired (erythropoietin is a hormone that stimulates red blood cell production and is produced primarily in the kidney).

Diagnostic Assessment

The diagnosis of urinary tract obstruction and hydronephrosis can be made by prenatal ultrasonography as early as 15 weeks gestation. Postnatally, the structure of the kidneys and diagnosis of an obstruction can usually be made by ultrasonography. Intravenous pyelography and voiding cystourethrography may be indicated. Assessment of voiding patterns is helpful (e.g., dribbling without a full stream in boys may mean urethral obstruction).

Therapeutic Management

Early diagnosis allows for corrective surgery, urinary diversion, and perhaps early use of prophylactic antibiotics to prevent UTIs that may lead to renal scarring.

TABLE 36-8
Obstructions of the Urinary System

Name	Description and Clinical Manifestations	Diagnostic Assessment	Treatment	Nursing Care
Ureteropelvic junction (UPJ) obstruction	Most common site of obstruction in infancy and childhood; may affect one or both kidneys and may present as mild to severe obstruction; severe form may present early with failure-to-thrive and renal failure; later, colicky flank pain, hematuria	Renal ultrasonography Radionuclide scan to evaluate function of kidneys; reflux may need to be excluded with voiding cystourethrogram	Surgical correction	
Ureterovesical junction (UVJ) obstruction	May affect one or both ureters to varying degrees Hydronephrosis with enlargement of ureter	Renal ultrasonography		
Ectopic ureter	Ureter opens in a position other than usual and may occur in one or both ureters; usually associated with duplex urinary system	Renal ultrasonography, intravenous pyelogram, and cystourethrogram may be necessary	Surgical correction	Early recognition of symptoms to facilitate early diagnosis; education about tests and emotional support at time of diagnosis and treatment; avoid infection, and teach family and child early recognition of infection; give support to child and family regarding body image changes that may result when urinary diversion is performed
Ectopic ureterocele	Cystic dilatation of a ureter in which some part of it is situated at the bladder neck; occurs more commonly in girls and may be associated with a duplex urinary system		Surgical excision of the ureterocele	
Posterior urethral valves (PUVs)	Affects boys; PUVs are located in the posterior urethra, which constitutes the urethral passage extending a few centimeters below the bladder neck; the commonest form consists of membranous folds that are present at the posterior urethra and that obstruct the flow of urine from the bladder	Voiding cystourethrogram cystoscopy	Surgical removal of valves usually done later (3–5 yrs of age); diversion (usually vesicostomy) done at time of diagnosis or if diagnosed prenatally, diversion soon after birth	
Urethral strictures	Congenital stenosis along the urethra almost exclusively in boys; may present with varying degrees of symptoms (e.g., poor urinary stream, dribbling, infection)	Voiding cystourethrogram	Urethral dilatation and, at the same time, surgical repair of stricture	

Nursing Care

Early detection of urinary tract obstruction is a major nursing role. For example, a simple approach is to observe the urinary stream in infant boys for a forceful, steady stream. There are numerous tests and diagnostic procedures for which the child must be prepared; the parents need information about the purpose and nature of tests, as well. These children often require treatment at home and, therefore, need to be taught about the equipment (catheters, diversional systems).

The Child with Infection

Urinary Tract Infection

The diagnosis of UTI encompasses a broad range of bacterial infections of the urinary tract. Infection may be limited to the urethra *(urethritis)* or the bladder *(cystitis),* or may involve the kidney *(pyelonephritis).* In young children, it is often difficult to establish whether infection is present only in the lower urinary tract (the urethra and the bladder) or has spread to the upper tract (the ureters and the kidneys).

In the neonatal period, UTIs occur most frequently in males, possibly because of the higher incidence of anatomic abnormalities in male neonates. Recent evidence suggests that UTIs may also be directly linked to whether the male infant is circumcised. Uncircumcised infants seem to have significantly more UTIs than circumcised infants (Gonzalez, 1992). By 4 months of age, UTIs are 10 times more common in girls than in boys (Stull & Lipuma, 1991). This increased incidence in girls continues throughout childhood and into adulthood.

In infancy, bacteria frequently enter the urinary tract through the blood and cause infection (hematogenous). After infancy, nearly all urinary infections occur when bacteria enter the urethra and ascend into the urinary tract. Females are therefore especially at risk for infection because the female urethra is much shorter than the male urethra. The female urethra is also more subject than the male urethra to contamination because of its proximity to the anal opening.

Escherichia coli causes approximately 75 to 90 per cent of all UTIs in females. No one fully understands why and how bacteria that are normally found in the stools invade the urinary tract and cause infection. It seems, however, that the ability of some bacteria to adhere to the cells of the genitourinary tract may be linked to their ability to cause infection. However, congenital anomalies of the urinary tract, neurogenic bladder dysfunction, vaginal foreign bodies, and indwelling urethral catheters all predispose an individual to UTI. Other factors such as sexual intercourse, use of bubble bath, and constipation have also been suggested as contributing factors in the development of UTIs; however, scientific evidence that supports these factors as causal is limited.

Pathophysiology

In an acute, uncomplicated infection, inflammation is usually limited to the bladder (cystitis). Urinary urgency and frequency develop when the inflammation causes irritability and spasm of the bladder wall. Bleeding secondary to inflammation may result in the appearance of blood in the urine (hematuria).

Repeated infection of the bladder and chronic inflammation may lead to changes in the bladder wall, especially at the site where the ureters enter the bladder (the vesicoureteral valves). Damage to these valves can allow urine to reflux into the ureters, especially during voiding. The ureters may become dilated. Urine and bacteria then have easy access to the kidneys, and kidney infections (pyelonephritis) may result (see discussion of vesicoureteral reflux later in this chapter).

Pyelonephritis may interfere with the normal concentrating and filtering mechanisms of the kidney. With chronic infection, scarring and loss of renal tissue may also result. The development of scarring in association with reflux appears to occur primarily in children under 5 years of age (White, 1987). Identification of UTIs in this age group is therefore of particular concern.

Clinical Manifestations

UTIs may be the result of underlying pathology. Renal anomalies are found in 5 to 15 per cent of children with UTI (Durbin & Peter, 1984). Renal scarring occurs in as many as 20 per cent of children with UTI, especially in children with significant reflux (Smellie, 1992). The challenge is to detect the infection early. To do this, the nurse must have a high index of suspicion for a variety of signs and symptoms.

In neonates and infants, nonspecific symptoms predominate and include vomiting, diarrhea, irritability, lethargy, poor feeding, slow weight gain, and unexplained jaundice. Fever or hypothermia can be present. The prevalence of UTI in infants who have fever, failure-to-thrive, jaundice, and other nonspecific symptoms ranges from 4 to 20 per cent (Spencer & Schaeffer, 1986). Specific urinary signs such as a weak urine stream, frequency, and foul-smelling urine may be present but difficult to document. In older children, dysuria, urgency, fever, abdominal or flank pain, and enuresis prevail. Fever is less common in the younger age group and, if present, may signify renal parenchymal infection or infection in an obstructed urinary tract.

UTIs are frequently missed because the diagnosis is not considered before antibiotic therapy for undiagnosed fever is started. Urine cultures should be obtained whenever possible in ill children, especially if any of the aforementioned signs and symptoms are present.

Up to two thirds of children with urinary tract complaints may not have a documented infection. Alternative explanations for dysuria are numerous and include vaginitis, urethritis (secondary to bubble bath, irritating clothing, masturbation, sexual intercourse, pinworms, or diaper rash), or falsely negative urine culture results.

Diagnostic Assessment

Specimen Collection for Laboratory Studies

The diagnosis of UTI rests on the detection of significant amounts of bacteria in the urine. Urine for culture can be collected in one of three ways: (1) clean-voided (preferably midstream) specimen, (2) catheterization, or (3) suprapubic aspiration. The method of collection determines, in part, the interpretation of the urine culture results.

Clean-voided urine specimens can easily become contaminated with bacteria from stool and vaginal secretions, despite cleansing of the external genitalia before collection. Contaminated urine, however, usually contains fewer than 10,000 (10^4) bacterial colonies per milliliter. Frequently, two or more species of organisms will grow in culture when there has been contamination. In contrast, truly infected urine usually contains over 100,000 (10^5) colonies/ml, usually of only a single organism. When culture results are equivocal (between 10,000 and 100,000 colonies/ml), the urine culture may need to be repeated.

The above guidelines for bacterial counts apply only to urine collected as a clean-voided specimen. Urine obtained by suprapubic aspiration with more than 1000 colonies/ml indicates infection. Likewise, urine obtained by catheterization that contains more than 10,000 colonies/ml indicates infection (Sherbotie & Cornfeld, 1991).

In addition to contamination from the external genitalia, delays in getting the collected urine to the laboratory and storing the urine at a warm room temperature give false-positive results because these practices allow bacteria to proliferate. False-negative results can occur with a very dilute urine (low specific gravity), a low urine pH, the presence of antibacterial drugs (possibly for the treatment of another infection), or inappropriate culture techniques (Vickers et al, 1991). Microscopy by a clinician has been found to be as effective as urine culture in the identification of bacteria. Furthermore, it is an inexpensive and rapid investigation that can be combined with clinical urine analyses (Vickers et al, 1991).

Radiographic Studies

Once a UTI is diagnosed, decisions must be made about the need for diagnostic imaging. A renal ultrasound examination and a voiding cystourethrogram (VCUG) should be performed in (1) all boys with their first UTI, (2) all girls under the age of 3 years with their first UTI, and (3) all children with pyelonephritis (Travis & Brouhard, 1991). Renal ultrasonography in experienced hands can be used to detect obstruction, to assess renal size and contour, and to detect lower tract abnormalities and stones. It should always include careful evaluation of the kidneys, ureters, and bladder before and after voiding. Although ultrasonography may detect renal scars, other techniques such as intravenous pyelogram (IVP) or nuclear scanning using isotope may be necessary. Girls between the ages of 3 and 12 may also be candidates for radiographic studies if they have a history of an abnormal pattern of urination, poor physical development, elevated blood pressure; an abnormal flank, abdominal, or genital examination; previous UTI; or a poor response to antibiotic treatment for infection (Sherbotie & Cornfeld, 1991). The nurse should compile a careful history of the child's past health. Up to 40 per cent of UTIs may be asymptomatic or may have been mistakenly diagnosed as respiratory or gastrointestinal infections. What seems to be a first infection may actually be a recurrent infection.

Ultrasonography and VCUG are usually done 2 to 6 weeks after diagnosis because transient inflammatory changes of the urinary tract are at times difficult to distinguish from permanent abnormalities. Children may be given prophylactic antibiotics in the interim to prevent recurrent infection. Radiographic studies at the time of diagnosis are indicated if the child has any sign of urinary obstruction, abdominal masses, or poor response to antibiotic therapy.

Urologic tests and procedures and their nursing implications are presented in Tables 36–4 and 36–5. Toddlers and preschoolers may benefit from explanations using dolls. Simple drawings of the urethra, bladder, ureters, and kidneys can be used with parents and older children.

Therapeutic Management

Management of UTIs is aimed at achieving three goals: (1) cure of the infection, (2) identification and correction of any factors that predispose the child to infection, and (3) prevention of recurrent infections. Treatment approaches for three categories of infection are discussed next.

Acute, Uncomplicated Infection

A child with an acute, uncomplicated UTI typically is school-age and has no symptoms of kidney infection (fever, flank pain); lower urinary tract symptoms (dysuria, frequency, urgency) predominate. Antibiotics that are most effective against the infecting bacteria are chosen to treat the infection. Because approximately 80 per cent of all UTIs are caused by *E. coli*, a 7- to 10-day course of trimethoprim-sulfamethoxazole or amoxicillin is usually given. Cefixime only taken once each day is gaining acceptance. Sulfisoxazole and the new quinolones frequently used in adults with UTI are not safe for use in children. Shorter courses (3 to 5 days) with antibiotics are becoming more common.

Single-dose amikacin given intramuscularly has been shown to be effective in the treatment of UTI caused by *E. coli* (Wallen et al, 1985). Potential advantages of single-dose therapy are fewer side effects and less toxicity, excellent compliance, and reduced potential for the growth of resistant organisms that result in response to frequent therapeutic doses of antibiotics. At times, a urinary analgesic such as phenazopyridine hydrochloride (Pyridium) is also given to relieve the pain of dysuria. Parents and children should be warned that this medicine turns urine an orange-red color.

Recurrent Infections

A recurrent UTI is one that occurs after a previous infection has been successfully treated. Recurrent infections are frequently caused by organisms different from those that caused the previous infection. Therefore, antibiotics should be chosen based on culture and sensitivity reports. Indications for radiographic studies with recurrent UTIs were discussed earlier. Children who have normal urinary tracts but have had three or more infections frequently are given prophylactic antibiotics to prevent recurrent infection. Trimethoprim-sulfamethoxazole or nitrofurantoin given daily at bedtime in half the usual dose is the drug of choice. The nurse needs to be knowledgeable about possible side effects of long-term antibiotic therapy.

Complicated Infections

Complicated UTIs are those in which the child is febrile, less than 3 years of age, or a male of any age. They are classified as "complicated" because of the high likelihood of renal infection (pyelonephritis) or structural abnormalities of the urinary tract, or both. *Proteus, Klebsiella, Pseudomonas,* and *Enterococci* are the most common infecting organisms. These children are frequently hospitalized and treated, at least initially, with intravenous antibiotics. Ampicillin, aminoglycosides, and cefamandole are the usual drugs of choice.

Nursing Diagnostic Statements and Collaborative Problems

- ***High risk for ineffective management of therapeutic regimen;*** *risk factor: knowledge deficit regarding home care and early signs of UTI.*
- ***High risk for injury: complications of UTI, e.g., chronic renal disease;*** *risk factor: inflammatory changes associated with severe or recurrent pyelonephritis.*
- ***High risk for infection;*** *risk factor: insufficient knowledge of child and parents about ways to avoid recurrence.*

Planning and Implementation

Ensuring Effective Management of Therapeutic Regimen. The nurse needs to work with the child and family to ensure that the correct amount of the antibiotic will be given at the correct time. Medication names, dosages, and administration times, as well as follow-up instructions, should be given to the family in writing. Families frequently need to be encouraged to complete the full prescribed course of the medicine, even though the child is feeling better. If the child does not feel better within 24 to 48 hours, the parents should call their health care provider. If the child is in school, the school nurse should be contacted about the prescribed medicine, and any required forms for the administration of medication in school should be completed.

The diagnosis of a UTI necessitates a number of follow-up urine cultures. A culture may be done 2 days after the initiation of antibiotic treatment to ensure that the antibiotic is working effectively. Urine is usually sterile after 48 hours of antibiotics. Routine follow-up urine cultures are usually obtained 2 to 3 days after the cessation of treatment, but routine cultures when the child is asymptomatic have not been proved to be useful (White, 1987). The child and family should be taught the early signs of UTI and the correct technique for obtaining a urine specimen and providing prompt delivery to their local laboratory to ensure prompt treatment of recurrence.

Assessing for Signs and Symptoms of Chronic Renal Disease. When pyelonephritis is present, in addition to urine culture follow-up, other indices of renal function including urine concentration (specific gravity), blood urea nitrogen (BUN), and serum creatinine must be assessed periodically. The development of elevated blood pressure and growth failure may also indicate chronic renal problems. The nurse assists in the assessment of the child with a complicated UTI through careful monitoring of temperature, blood pressure, weight, input and output, and routine urine dipsticks to test for blood or protein in the urine.

Teaching Preventive Measures. The nurse needs to work with the child and family to prevent recurrent infection. Adequate fluid intake and regular emptying of the bladder (every 3 to 4 hours) may be beneficial. Traditionally, girls have been taught to wipe themselves from front to back after using the bathroom. To date, there is no evidence that this decreases the risk for UTI. We have only to look at the incidence of UTI in a 5-month-old infant girl (which is very low) to realize that contamination of the urethra with stool does not easily cause UTI. Other preventive measures include avoidance of tight-fitting and potentially irritating nylon underwear, bubble baths, and constipation, which may cause urethritis or poor bladder emptying and lead to UTI. Adolescent girls who seem to develop UTIs in association with sexual activity can be encouraged to urinate both before and immediately after sexual intercourse to wash away any bacteria that may have entered the urethra.

The actual effectiveness of these preventive measures is poorly documented. It is important not to mistakenly attribute an infection to a child's failure to practice these preventive measures.

When poor hygienic practices are evident, one should not assume it to be the cause of a UTI; to do so diverts attention from a possible underlying abnormality.

Vesicoureteral Reflux

Vesicoureteral reflux (VUR) is the abnormal backflow of urine from the bladder into the ureters and possibly the kidneys. Experts estimate that the prevalence of VUR in healthy children is less than 1 per cent. VUR is found, however, in 29 to 50 per cent of children following UTIs and is the most common radiographic abnormality associated with UTIs in children. Development of reflux may be, at least in part, genetically determined. Siblings of children with VUR are 10 times more likely to have reflux than other children (Levitt & Weiss, 1985). Some researchers recommend that all siblings of children with reflux, whether symptomatic or asymptomatic, undergo a screening cystourethrogram (van den Abbecle, 1987).

Pathophysiology

Normally, the ureters enter the musculature of the bladder at an oblique angle and travel through the bladder mucosa before opening into the interior of the bladder (Fig. 36–6). When bladder pressures rise, during voiding and during the accumulation of urine, the length of this submucosal segment of ureter becomes compressed and acts as a valve to prevent urine from backflowing into the ureter and the kidney. This valvular mechanism malfunctions when the submucosal ureter is either congenitally abnormally short (primary reflux) or has been damaged by chronic infection or increased pressures caused by bladder outlet obstruction (secondary reflux).

The ultimate danger of reflux is the development of renal scarring and atrophy (reflux nephropathy). Urine that has backed into the ureters during voiding returns to the bladder and remains there until the child voids again. This residual urine (urine that stays in the bladder) serves as an excellent medium for bacterial growth. Bladder infections can quickly lead to renal infections when infected urine refluxes from the bladder into the kidneys.

Diagnostic Assessment

The diagnosis of vesicoureteral reflux is made by VCUG (see Table 36–5). Classification of reflux depends on the degree of filling and dilatation of the ureter and renal pelvis as depicted in Figure 36–7. Grading is usually based on a scale of 1 through 5, with 1 representing reflux into the ureter with no dilatation and 5 representing gross reflux and dilatation of the ureter, renal pelvis, and calyces (International Reflux Study in Children, 1985).

Therapeutic Management

The ultimate goal of treatment is to protect the kidneys from scarring and allow them to grow as normally as possible. Factors predisposing children to reflux (e.g., bladder outlet obstruction, neurogenic bladder dysfunction) must be identified. Reflux can be treated either medically or surgically. There continues to be some controversy about the preferred treatment.

Medical Management

Medical management is based on the assumption that sterile reflux does not damage the kidney (White, 1989). Studies have documented spontaneous resolution in 60 to 85 per cent of VUR (Steele & DeMaria, 1992). In an attempt to prevent infection, continuous low-dose prophylactic antibiotics are administered to the child until resolution of the reflux is documented or up to 7 years of age, when renal scarring associated with VUR no longer occurs (White, 1989). Other medical management includes the encouragement of a liberal fluid intake to create a bladder washout effect and a regular (every 3 hours) voiding program, which may include double voiding at bedtime. An important but poorly recognized feature of recurrent UTIs and VUR is constipation. Thus, it is essential to increase fecal bulk and softness with a high-fiber diet,

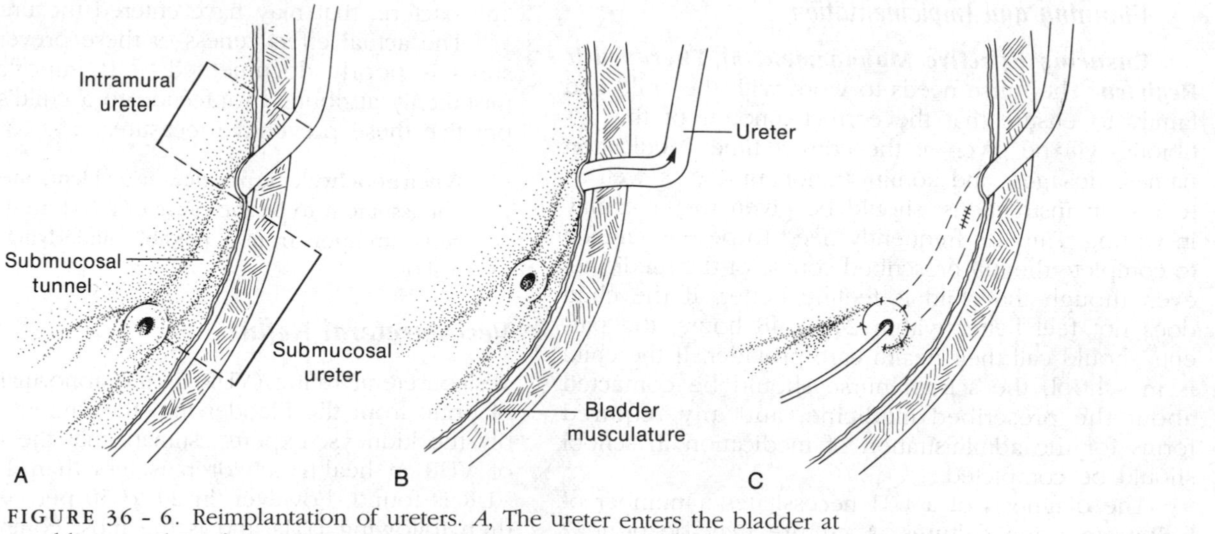

FIGURE 36 - 6. Reimplantation of ureters. *A*, The ureter enters the bladder at an oblique angle to form a normal ureterovesical junction. Normally, as pressure in the bladder rises, the angled position of the ureter causes a temporary closing off of the lumen, preventing urine backflow (reflux). *B*, In vesicoureteral reflux, the ureter enters the bladder at an acute angle and the submucosal tunnel is shortened. As pressure in the bladder rises, urine is directed up the ureter (reflux). *C*, Reimplantation of the ureter is done to correct the ureterovesical angle and lengthen the submucosal tunnel to prevent reflux.

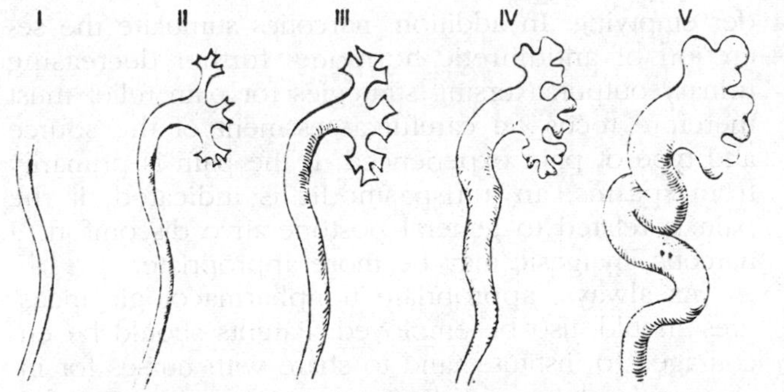

FIGURE 36-7. Grades of reflux—International Study Classifications. *I,* Ureter only. *II,* Ureter, pelvis, and calyces. No dilatation, normal calyceal fornices. *III,* Mild or moderate dilatation and/or tortuosity of ureter and mild or moderate dilatation of renal pelvis, but no or slight blunting of fornices. *IV,* Moderate dilatation and/or tortuosity of ureter and moderate dilatation of renal pelvis and calyces. Complete obliteration of sharp angle of fornices but maintenance of papillary impressions in majority of calyces. *V,* Gross dilatation and tortuosity of ureter. Gross dilatation of renal pelvis and calyces. Papillary impressions are no longer visible in the majority of calyces. (From Anderson, G. F., & Smey, P. [1985]. Current concepts in the management of common urologic problems in infants and children. *Pediatric Clinics of North America, 32,* 1145.)

which often facilitates muscular relaxation and thereby helps to reduce residual urine.

The Birmingham Reflux Study Group (1987) reported a 5-year prospective study of medical versus surgical management of severe VUR. Their results confirmed that there was no significant difference between the treatment groups in the incidence of breakthrough UTIs, renal function, renal growth, progression of existing scars, and development of new ones.

Surgical Management

Surgical management of reflux may be indicated when there is: (1) recurrent infection despite prophylactic antibiotics; (2) noncompliance with medical management; (3) ureteral obstruction in association with reflux; (4) no submucosal ureteral segments; or (5) persistent severe reflux (Levitt & Weiss, 1985). The corrective surgical procedure is called *ureteroneocystostomy,* or reimplantation of the ureter. A variety of different surgical techniques are used, but they all focus on lengthening the submucosal segment of the ureter and/or moving the site where the ureter opens into the bladder closer to the bladder neck, thereby correcting the angle at which the ureter enters the bladder (see Fig. 36-7).

Recently, a new technique, the subureteric injection of Teflon, has been shown to be successful in correcting VUR. Under cystoscopy, Teflon is injected around the distal end of the ureter to narrow the lumen. This technique is simple, but it has not yet been accepted universally because of concerns regarding the safety of Teflon.

Nursing Diagnostic Statements and Collaborative Problems

When treated by medical management:

High risk for infection: urinary tract, related to:
- *Stasis of urine and subsequent backflow to kidney.*

Ineffective management by parents of therapeutic regimen (antibiotic administration), related to:
- *Mistrust of the effect of the regimen and potential side effects of medication.*
- *Insufficient information to recognize seriousness of condition and implications of not giving antibiotics.*
- *Insufficient cues to remember the medication and note established routine.*

Constipation, related to reduced bowel tone.

When treated by surgery:

High risk for injury: surgical site, related to pressure exerted on site of reimplantation by:
- *Tension on the stent.*
- *Obstruction of urinary drainage devices.*

High risk for infection: urinary tract, related to introduction of pathogens by:
- *Surgical intervention.*
- *Contamination of urinary drainage devices.*

Altered comfort: pain, related to:
- *Bladder spasms.*
- *Inflammation and edema associated with surgical manipulation.*

Planning and Implementation

Medical Management

Preventing Infection. During the course of medical management an attempt can be made to modify the condition of reflux. Liberal fluid intake can be achieved by setting up routines whereby the child and parents will remember to offer fluids. Involvement of the child in planning the fluid intake can achieve better results. This effort should be combined with a regular (every 3 hours) voiding program.

Achieving Goals of Antibiotic Regimen. Education of the child and family is important, because they need to understand what happens in VUR and the high risk of UTI. They also need to be informed regarding the efficacy of prophylactic antibiotics and their safety with long-term use.

Preventing Constipation. Relief of constipation will lead to better bladder emptying, and, thus, less risk of UTI. There seems to be an association between constipation and poor bladder emptying. Use of extra fluid, increased bulk in diet, exercise, and, in some cases, use of laxatives correct the problems. Parents need to be encouraged to follow through with this approach without drawing excessive attention to bowel patterns.

Surgical Site

Preventing Trauma to the Surgical Site. The child will usually return from surgery with either a suprapubic or a urethral catheter. In addition, stents may be placed in the ureters to maintain patency and divert urine while healing occurs. Stents are very small, soft, supple catheters with multiple perforations along their length. They exit the body through small incisions in the lower abdomen and are attached to drainage tubing and collection bags. Stents do not occlude the ureters, and, therefore, some urine drains around them and into the bladder.

In order to prevent trauma to the site of ureteral reimplantation, it is important that the stent(s) be free of tension and that all catheters are patent. Tubing attached to stents must be taped to the child's leg and a stress loop (a loop of tubing that is taped or otherwise secured below the first taping site) should be formed in the tubing for additional protection. Securing the drainage tubing will protect against accidental trauma to the ureter that could occur with tension on the stent. Wrist restraints for unattended children may sometimes be necessary to prevent a child from pulling on the drainage tubings.

Patency of drainage devices is essential to prevent back pressure of urine upon the surgical site. Urine flow should be checked and recorded hourly for the first 24 hours, and at least every 4 hours thereafter.

Preventing Infection. Antibiotics to suppress infection will be ordered postoperatively and will usually be continued for several weeks to 3 months. Teaching in preparation for discharge must include the importance of continuous administration of the antibiotics. The family needs to be aware of signs and symptoms of side effects of long-term antibiotic therapy so that early medical intervention may be sought.

Nursing responsibility for postoperative infection control includes meticulous care of drainage devices to ensure their sterility.

Providing Pain Relief. In addition to general postoperative discomfort, painful spasms of the bladder and involved ureter(s) are common after reimplantation. Physicians' orders frequently include antispasmodics or sedatives as well as narcotic pain relievers. The informed nurse will be aware that antispasmodics may be more effective than narcotic analgesics for relief of pain associated with smooth muscle spasms. Antispasmodics are designed to relieve spasticity of smooth muscles (such as those of the bladder and ureter); narcotic analgesics may actually increase the tone and spasms of these organs and may delay bladder emptying. In addition, narcotics stimulate the secretion of antidiuretic hormone, further decreasing urinary output. Nursing strategies for pain relief must therefore focus on careful assessment of the source and type of pain experienced. If the pain is primarily from spasms, an antispasmodic is indicated; if the pain is related to general postoperative discomfort, a narcotic analgesic may be more appropriate.

As always, appropriate nonpharmacologic measures should also be employed. Parents should be encouraged to institute (and to share with nurses for inclusion in the care plan) any appropriate comfort measures that have been beneficial to the child in the past. These might include close physical contact with parents and significant others, diversionary activities, gentle massage, and music of the child's choice.

Adequate rest will increase the child's ability to cope with postoperative discomfort and will enhance rapid healing. It is the nurse's responsibility to schedule some rest periods for the child that are uninterrupted by procedures, medications, and visits by other health care professionals.

Renal Calculi

Urolithiasis (renal calculi) is an uncommon pediatric disorder among children in the United States. This condition, however, has been found to be endemic among children from low socioeconomic classes who live in Asia and is the most common pediatric urologic problem in that part of the world. Urolithiasis occurs more often in males and affects children with equal frequency between the ages of 1 and 15 years (Malek, 1985).

Etiology/Pathophysiology

The etiology of renal calculi is either *idiopathic* or *secondary* to disorders such as UTIs, hypercalciuria, or a variety of metabolic disorders.

Idiopathic calculi are composed of calcium oxalate. Children with idiopathic calculi have a genetic predisposition. The symptoms of calculi, however, usually will not occur until the child is between the ages of 10 and 15 years.

Secondary calculi may form in children with frequent UTIs as a result of urease, which is produced by bacteria. Urease converts urea to ammonia; this increases the alkalinity of the urine, favoring the formation of calculi. These calculi are mostly composed of magnesium ammonium phosphate. They usually form in the upper collecting system and may be associated with congenital structural anomalies.

Calculi resulting from hypercalciuria are created by an increased deposit of calcium in the kidneys. Hypercalciuria is a disorder that results from several conditions, including hyperparathyroidism, uncontrolled renal tubular acidosis, Cushing syndrome, neoplasms, and prolonged immobilization, such as occurs when a child is in traction.

Metabolic abnormalities may cause renal calculi and account for 10 per cent of urolithiasis in children.

Clinical Manifestations

The main symptoms of urolithiasis include colicky flank or abdominal pain, hematuria, and sepsis. Spontaneous passage of the stone may occur without previous symptoms. Less commonly, patients with renal calculi may exhibit enuresis, polydipsia, and urethral obstruction. If an underlying disease or infection exists, symptoms of this disorder may also be present.

Diagnostic Assessment

During the acute phase, assessment should include a family history; the child's medical history; an assessment of the child's growth and development; a diet history, including the use of vitamin or calcium supplements; and an assessment of exposure to medical or surgical procedures. This information will help determine whether a predisposition to renal calculi exists.

A urinalysis is done to check for the presence of infection or blood. Blood tests are done to check for increases in calcium, phosphorus, alkaline phosphatase, and uric acid. The child may undergo a plain radiograph of the abdomen, renal ultrasonography, a computed tomography (CT) scan, or an IVP to evaluate the presence and location of stones.

Therapeutic Management

Surgical intervention or lithotripsy (crushing of a calculus in the bladder or urethra) during the acute phase of urolithiasis is usually unnecessary, unless emergency conditions such as complete obstruction or hemorrhage exist. As mentioned, some renal calculi will pass spontaneously. If this does not occur, the acute phase will be managed supportively. The decision to intervene surgically in the event of renal calculi will be made on an individual basis and will be determined by the size and location of the calculi (Gearhart et al, 1991).

Nursing Care

The primary goals for nursing care are to (1) dilute the urine, (2) administer analgesics for colicky pain, (3) monitor urine output for passage of the stone, and (4) provide information and guidance to support home management. A high intake of dilute fluids is almost always recommended, to ensure a reduction in the concentration of crystalloids. The nurse will be responsible for maintaining specific gravity of the urine within the prescribed limits (usually under 1.005). In order to prevent increased specific gravity of urine during the night, it may be necessary to give large amounts of fluid at bedtime and to awaken the child in the night to give additional fluids. Parents may need support to temporarily abandon attempts to toilet train the child during this period.

Adults who have experienced renal colic will attest to the excruciating pain that may be associated with the body's attempt to pass a renal stone. The nurse is responsible for pain assessment and for providing optimal comfort through pharmacologic and other supportive means (see Chapter 25).

Urine must be strained in order to determine when the stone is passed. This can be accomplished by passing the urine through filter paper before discarding. Signs should be prominently posted in the child's hospital room and bathroom to prevent a well-meaning visitor from emptying urine that has not been strained. If a stone is found, it should be sent to the laboratory for analysis.

If the cause of the stone can be determined, treatment may include medications to reduce the particular crystals that caused the problem. Parents will need to be advised of appropriate medication techniques and of potential side effects. Prevention of recurrence will almost always involve a continued high fluid intake.

Hereditary Renal Disorders

Hereditary renal disease consists of a group of renal disorders that have a genetic basis and involve the capillary or tubular basement membranes. The incidence of these diseases is unknown, but they may account for as much as 13 to 25 per cent of renal failure in children (Brouhard, 1991). These disorders include Alport syndrome, polycystic disease, cystinosis, Bartter syndrome, and renal tubular acidosis. See Table 36–9 for a summary of these alterations.

Nephrotic Syndrome (Nephrosis)

Nephrotic syndrome is an alteration in renal function due to glomerular injury, characterized by proteinuria, hypoproteinemia, edema, and hyperlipidemia. It may be congenital, idiopathic, or secondary to another disease.

The most common of these is idiopathic, accounting for approximately 90 per cent of nephrosis in childhood. It is more common in boys than in girls (2:1) and is most common between 2 and 6 years of age, although it has occurred in infants as young as 6 to 12 months of age (Bergstein, 1992). The most common type of idiopathic nephrotic syndrome is minimal change nephrotic syndrome (MCNS). The discussion that follows addresses MCNS, and Table 36–10 summarizes the remaining, less-common types of nephrotic syndrome. The prognosis of children with MCNS is generally quite good. Although relapses are common, most children respond to treatment. For children with lesions other than those of MCNS, the

TABLE 36-9
Hereditary Renal Disorders

Name	Description and Clinical Manifestations	Diagnostic Assessment	Treatment	Nursing Care
Alport syndrome	Also known as hereditary progressive nephritis—autosomal dominant; characterized by recurrent hematuria and progressive renal failure; deafness and ocular defects occur with varying frequency; males are affected earlier and more severely than females; usually presents in early adolescence	Family history of disorder; hypertension, urinalysis shows hematuria and possibly proteinuria; audiometry, kidney biopsy	No form of treatment affects the course of the disease; antihypertensives when indicated; treatment of urinary tract infection (UTI); dialysis and transplantation; genetic counseling	Early recognition of hypertension and UTI; education of child and family about the disease and treatment; support child and family during diagnostic tests and throughout dialysis and transplantation
Polycystic disease	Bilateral renal cystic disease; infantile form is autosomal recessive and may present at birth; accompanied with liver abnormalities that can lead to portal hypertension in older children; progresses to renal failure at birth or in early childhood; adult form is autosomal dominant and may progress to hypertension and renal failure in adulthood	Family history of disorder; kidneys palpable on examination; renal ultrasonography; urinalysis—hematuria, hypertension, kidney biopsy	Prevention and management of hypertension; dialysis and transplantation may be necessary; genetic counseling	
Cystinosis	Rare metabolic disease characterized by intracellular accumulation of free cystine in many organs, including the kidney; autosomal recessive; infantile cystinosis leads to progressive tubular, glomerular impairment, and renal failure	Family history of disorder, skin biopsy, cystine crystals seen in cornea by slit-lamp examination; history of failure-to-thrive in infancy with episodes of unexplained fevers, vomiting, polydipsia, renal biopsy	Symptomatic correction of acidosis; trials ongoing with cysteamine, which may mobilize cystine and delay renal failure; dialysis and transplantation; genetic counseling	
Bartter syndrome	Sporadic or familial syndrome characterized by impaired urinary concentration ability, hyperplasia of the juxtaglomerular apparatus and normal blood pressure; may present in infancy or early childhood with failure-to-thrive, weakness, salt-craving, polyuria, and polydipsia	Delayed growth and development Urinalysis: dilute urine Blood analysis: ↓ potassium ↓ magnesium ↓ bicarbonate	Potassium replacement and magnesium; genetic counseling	Early recognition of failure-to-thrive, increased thirst, polydipsia; education of family to prevent dehydration, administration of medication; provide information about the disease and therapeutic regimen
Renal tubular acidosis (RTA)	Syndrome of impaired renal acidification manifested by chronic hypochloremic metabolic acidosis; several types of RTA identified and may be categorized according to segment of the nephron that is impaired; frequently associated with hypokalemia; proximal RTA is frequently acquired, but may be genetically transmitted according to an autosomal dominant, autosomal recessive, or sex-linked inheritance; most common in boys	Family history of RTA; failure-to-thrive: polyuria and polydipsia Urinalysis: dilute, acidic Blood analysis: hyperchloremia Metabolic acidosis: ↓ potassium	Correction of acidosis; potassium replacement; genetic counseling	

TABLE 36-10
Congenital and Secondary Nephrotic Syndromes

Name	Description	Diagnosis	Management
Congenital nephrotic syndrome	This form of nephrotic syndrome, also known as Finnish-type nephrotic syndrome, is commonly associated with toxemia or pregnancy, an enlarged placenta, and prematurity; the presence of other clinical signs such as proteinuria, distended abdomen, and atypical facies with wide-set cranial sutures, low-set ears, and a small snub nose should alert the nurse to the possibility of nephrotic syndrome; astute observation in the delivery room for identification of infants at risk is essential	Careful screening and developmental assessment throughout infancy will help in making the diagnosis of congenital nephrotic syndrome; these children may fail to gain weight as they should, despite conscientious efforts to help them feed; investigation may identify other members of the family with renal disease, since the congenital form of nephrotic syndrome is believed to be transmitted by an autosomal recessive gene (see Chapter 3 for a discussion of patterns of inheritance); the child should be observed for an edematous abdomen, which may be indicated by an arched-back position and increases in abdominal girth measurements	The congenital form of nephrotic syndrome is rare; infants born with this disorder are small for gestational age and have proteinuria and edema; they usually fail to respond to corticosteroid or cytotoxic drug therapy and develop end-stage renal disease within the first or second year of life; renal transplants have been tried in children with congenital nephrotic syndrome with limited success
Secondary nephrotic syndrome	Since the secondary causes of nephrotic syndrome are diverse, the morphologic features of each of these are also variable; the child with secondary nephrotic syndrome usually presents with the features of minimal-change nephrotic syndrome (MCNS) as well as hematuria, hypertension, a decreased C_3 concentration, and possibly azotemia	The secondary form of nephrotic syndrome develops during the course of a diverse group of diseases including systemic lupus erythematosus, Henoch-Schönlein purpura, diabetes mellitus, sickle cell disease, syphilis, and many others; it may also occur secondary to systemic infections (infected atrioventricular shunt, subacute bacterial endocarditis) or as the result of drug toxicity	These children respond poorly to glucocorticoid therapy and require renal biopsy; management varies according to the type of secondary nephrotic syndrome (see below for a discussion of four types)
Focal segmental glomerular sclerosis	Focal segmental glomerular sclerosis (FSGS) initially is difficult to distinguish from MCNS in childhood; FSGS constitutes 6–12% of all cases of nephrotic syndrome in childhood; children with FSGS are slightly older at onset (median age 6 yrs) than those with MCNS; a predominance in boys is also seen	Although some researchers believe that FSGS represents a progression from MCNS, most believe it is a separate process. The frequent detection of deposits with electron microscopy and the finding of mesangial immunofluorescence suggest a pathogenesis different from that of MCNS (Travis, 1991)	There is no proven effective therapy, although trials with cyclophosphamide and cyclosporine are suggested; less than 15% of all children with FSGS achieve a remission with normal function; approximately 25% progress to end-stage renal disease within 2–5 yrs, and the majority of the others have significant proteinuria or reduced renal function; children with FSGS who receive a transplant have a 25% likelihood of recurrence in the transplanted kidney
Membranoproliferative glomerulonephritis	Membranoproliferative glomerulonephritis (MPGN), also known as mesangiocapillary or hypocomplementemic glomerulonephritis, accounts for about 8% of children who present with nephrotic syndrome; it affects older children more frequently and is twice as common in girls; a familial occurrence has sometimes been noted; the cause of MPGN is unknown; the complement system appears to be involved, though the precise mechanisms are not completely understood; biopsy examination indicates that there are two distinct types of disease (and possibly a third), the differences involving the nature and location of deposits within the kidney	Most children present with a nephritic-nephrotic picture; that is, all the signs and symptoms of MCNS, as well as hematuria, hypertension, azotemia, and a low C_3 concentration	Many believe that intensive daily steroid use in those with MPGN can hasten deterioration and worsen the disease by accelerating hypertension; symptomatic therapy is the only uniformly accepted approach to management (Travis, 1991)

(continued)

TABLE 36-10
Congenital and Secondary Nephrotic Syndromes (Continued)

Name	Description	Diagnosis	Management
Membranous glomerulonephritis	Membranous glomerulonephritis (MGN) is characterized by generalized thickness of the basement membrane of the glomerular vessels without cell proliferation; although MGN accounts for only 1% of nephrotic syndrome in children, it is important to recognize because it may be caused by a number of potentially curable systemic diseases such as syphilis, toxoplasmosis, malaria, and hepatitis; the disease is often seen with renal vein thrombosis, but most investigators believe MGN to be the cause of the thrombosis, rather than the reverse (Travis, 1991)	These children usually present with edema, hematuria, hypertension, and azotemia	Eradicating the cause, when it can be found, is most important, and symptomatic treatment is helpful; several studies have suggested that steroid therapy can prevent progression of MGN (Remirez et al, 1982); the course in children with MGN is variable, but children who are less than 7 yrs old at onset have a better prognosis
Mesangial proliferative glomerulonephritis	Mesangial proliferative glomerulonephritis (MPN) is seen with systemic lupus erythematosus, polyarteritis, Henoch-Schönlein purpura, resolving poststreptococcal glomerulonephritis, shunt nephritis, and recurrent hematuria	With MPN, the basement membranes are normal, but there is a diffuse increase in the number of mesangial cells and moderate increase in mesangial matrix; minimal mesangial proliferation is seen in children with MCNS, but when the changes are marked, the disease is classified as MPN; approximately 2–3% of children with MCNS have MPN	The course of MPN is not yet clear, although response to steroid therapy correlates with a good prognosis

outlook is less optimistic, with possible progression to end-stage renal disease (ESRD) necessitating dialysis or transplantation.

Pathophysiology

This disorder is characterized by massive proteinuria, hypoproteinemia, oliguria, generalized edema, and hyperlipidemia (Fig. 36–8). In nephrotic syndrome, proteinuria occurs owing to a defect in the glomerular basement membrane that allows protein to pass freely into the urine. Hypoproteinemia may result if the liver is unable to synthesize enough protein to compensate for the loss of protein in the urine. Generalized edema occurs in nephrotic syndrome in two ways. First, there is a reduction of plasma colloid osmotic pressure in response to a decrease in circulating serum protein. This reduction in pressure causes fluid to leave the intravascular spaces and fill the interstitial spaces, resulting in edema. As a result of this fluid shift, there is a reduced blood volume. Second, there is an increase in the reabsorption of sodium and water in response to the decreased blood volume. This occurs in response to increased secretion of aldosterone. This reabsorption further compounds the edema because the decreased plasma oncotic pressure allows the reabsorbed sodium and water to collect in the interstitial spaces. The reduced intravascular volume also stimulates the release of antidiuretic hormone, which contributes further to reabsorption of water and eventual edema. The mechanism for the hyperlipidemia is not clearly understood but is believed to occur secondarily to the hypoproteinemia.

The initiating event that produces proteinuria is unknown. Although pathogenesis is not clearly understood, it is thought that the kidney may be impaired in nephrotic syndrome as the result of an undefined immunologic response. The glomeruli appear essentially normal under routine microscopy. However, electron microscopy reveals a change in the outer surface of the basement membrane, which allows the leak of protein into the urine. MCNS is readily responsive to corticosteroid therapy, with eventual clearing of proteinuria and reversion to normal status.

Clinical Manifestations

Children with MCNS will usually present with insidious edema that has developed over a period of several weeks. Parents may report that the child has periorbital edema on arising, which diminishes throughout the day. They may also indicate that it is difficult to find clothes and shoes that fit properly and that ankle and pedal edema seem to develop in the later hours of the day. Volume and frequency of urination are decreased, and the urine is foamy and dark in color. Hematuria is uncommon. The edema is more prevalent where subcutaneous tissues are loose,

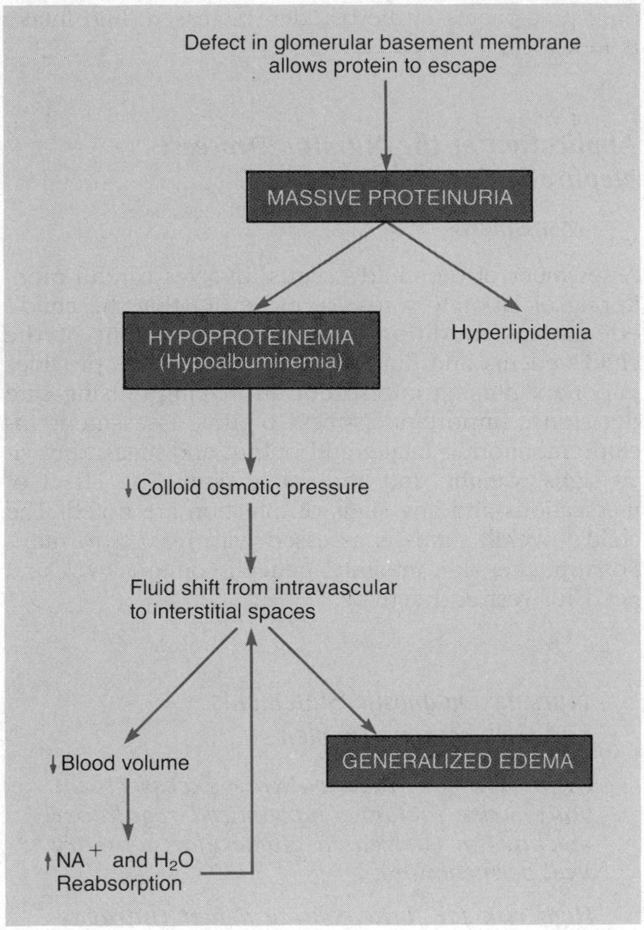

FIGURE 36-8. Pathophysiology of minimal change nephrotic syndrome.

such as around the eyes, neck, and genitalia. Ascites and pleural effusion may be present.

Respiratory difficulty may occur if ascites produces sufficient pressure on the diaphragm. With an increase in edema, the child may become anorexic, irritable, and lethargic. Changes in behavior and eating patterns may be valuable clues. The blood pressure is usually normal or slightly decreased; in only 5 to 10 per cent of cases is it elevated. See Table 36–11 for comparison of MCNS and poststreptococcal acute glomerulonephritis.

Diagnostic Assessment

The diagnosis is made on the basis of the clinical presentation combined with various laboratory tests. A urinalysis usually reveals a 3+ or 4+ proteinuria; protein excretion exceeds 2 g/24 hrs. Gross hematuria is rare, although microscopic hematuria may be present. Other findings contributing to the diagnosis are elevated serum cholesterol and triglyceride levels, low creatinine clearance due to lowered renal perfusion, reduced serum albumin level (less than 2 g/dl), and reduced total serum calcium levels because of the reduction in the albumin-bound fraction of calcium. Serum sodium concentration is low (130 to 135 mEq/L) because of the tubular reabsorption of sodium, but the total body sodium level is high. With high levels of protein in the urine, specific gravity is elevated. Hemoconcentration, due to the reduction in intravascular volume, may result in elevated hemoglobin and hematocrit levels, although they are usually normal; the platelet count is usually high (500 to $1000 \times 10^3/mm^3$).

Renal biopsy may be done to éxamine glomerular tissue. However, usually a trial test of prednisone is given first to assess response to corticosteroids. If

TABLE 36-11
Comparison of Minimal Change Nephrotic Syndrome and Poststreptococcal Acute Glomerulonephritis

	Nephrotic Syndrome	Glomerulonephritis
Etiology	Probably autoimmune responses leading to changes in glomerular membrane	Streptococcal infection leading to autoimmune response, which produces changes in glomerular membrane
Glomerular filtration rate	Normal	Decreased
Proteinuria	Massive	Usually moderate
Hematuria	Rare	Often grossly evident
Fluid volume	Hypovolemia (fluid shifts to interstitial spaces)	Hypervolemia (fluid remains in intravascular compartment)
Blood pressure	Usually normal	Hypertensive
Edema	Pronounced—systemic	Usually confined to face

the response is favorable, steroid treatment is usually continued and the biopsy is deferred. If a renal biopsy is done, the child must be prepared for a surgical procedure with appropriate play techniques and simple explanations. (See Chapter 23 for age-appropriate teaching interventions.)

Therapeutic Management

Treatment with pharmacologic agents should be initiated as soon as possible. Bed rest may be instituted to bring about a mild spontaneous diuresis, but generally ambulation is encouraged except when significant edema interferes. Children may determine their own level of activity. The male child may find comfort in a scrotal support during periods of ambulation.

Sodium restriction in the diet is usually beneficial in the edematous phase or while the child is receiving daily prednisone. This restriction may prevent further retention of sodium and subsequent increases in edema. Care must be taken not to severely restrict salt because this may make food unpalatable just at a time when an increase in nutritional intake is desired. Occasionally, diuretics are ordered. Fluids are not usually restricted unless edema progresses despite sodium restriction.

Corticosteroids will usually induce remission in children with MCNS. A daily dose of 2 mg/kg of prednisone is given in three or four divided doses. Remission usually occurs in 6 to 14 days and is indicated by an abrupt diuresis and the absence of urinary protein. Care must be taken to observe the child for side effects of the steroids. An increase in weight and appetite, an elevation of blood pressure, obesity, moon facies, and striae may occur. Serious infections may be masked, and growth may be stunted with prolonged therapy. As soon as feasible, steroids are gradually tapered and only reinstituted in cases of relapse. Approximately 92 per cent of children with MCNS respond to standard courses of steroids. The remaining 8 per cent are divided into three groups: those who rarely relapse, those who relapse infrequently, and those who relapse frequently. Children who frequently relapse will show side effects of prolonged steroid therapy related to repeated courses of daily prednisone. See Table 37–4 for care of a child on corticosteroids.

Patients who fail to respond to prednisone after 4 weeks of therapy are considered steroid-resistant and may be treated with an alkylating agent such as cyclophosphamide or chlorambucil in combination with the steroid. The severe side effect of cyclophosphamide is leukopenia, which will drastically increase the child's susceptibility to infection. Hair loss may result from cyclophosphamide and may be a distressing problem to children who are already experiencing body image concerns because of the edema. If treatment continues for more than approximately 3 months, there is a potential for it to cause sterility in males. Because chemical cystitis may occur if the drug precipitates in the bladder, increased fluid intake is indicated.

Application of the Nursing Process: Nephrotic Syndrome

Assessment

Assessment of the child's status involves careful monitoring of laboratory results and evaluating the child's edematous condition. Ongoing assessment of the child's edema and fluid and electrolyte status provides important nursing information in making nursing care decisions. Important aspects of this assessment include monitoring intake and output and measuring vital signs, weight, and abdominal girth. The effect of medications and any signs of infection are noted. The child's overall status is assessed with respect to nutritional intake, skin integrity, general comfort level, and need for rest and activity.

Nursing Diagnostic Statements and Collaborative Problems

High risk for fluid volume excess (total body); *risk factor, compromised regulatory mechanism (increased glomerular capillary wall permeability).*

High risk for fluid volume deficit (intravascular); *risk factor, failure of regulatory mechanism.*

High risk for impaired tissue integrity; *risk factor, edema.*

High risk for altered nutrition: less than body requirements; *risk factor, anorexia and lethargy.*

High risk for infection; *risk factor, altered immune response associated with corticosteroid therapy.*

Body image disturbance, *related to perception of self during period of marked edema.*

High risk for sensory-perceptual alteration: visual; *risk factor, marked periorbital edema.*

High risk for injury: falls; *risk factor, altered coordination associated with marked edema.*

High risk for ineffective management of therapeutic regimen; *risk factor, inadequate knowledge about:*

- *Signs and symptoms requiring medical attention.*
- *Importance of follow-up care.*
- *Urine testing for protein.*
- *Drug therapy dosages and side effects.*
- *Low-salt diet during edematous phase and prednisone therapy.*

Planning and Implementation

Nursing care for the child with nephrotic syndrome includes planning for the care of the child and family during the acute phase and preparing the family to assume care at home following the child's discharge from the hospital.

Reducing Edema and Hypovolemia. Careful monitoring of the child's edema is essential to effective management of this condition. Although fluid is not usually restricted unless edema progresses, it is essential that intake and output be accurately measured and recorded to determine the relative balance of fluid. An accurate daily weight, recorded at the same time each day, is essential to effective monitoring. It is important that the nurse compare the weight with that of the previous day and recheck the weight immediately if there is an unexpected difference. Abdominal girth taken at the umbilicus is another important measure that is used to assess the child's response to therapy. Other aspects of monitoring the child's progress are testing urine for specific gravity and albumin and taking and recording vital signs, including blood pressure. The child's hypovolemic state also requires close monitoring of hemoglobin and hematocrit levels. Rapid positional changes should be avoided to reduce the potential for postural hypotension.

Corticosteroids, given to treat the disease process, require that the nurse be alert for associated fluid retention (which would aggravate existing edema), hypokalemia, gastric irritation, hyperglycemia, and neurologic changes. (See Table 37–4 for further discussion of care of children requiring corticosteroid therapy.) It is important to assist the child in adhering to a low-salt diet during this phase.

The nurse's role while the child is on corticosteroid therapy is to administer the drug accurately and to participate in the monitoring of the effectiveness of the drug. In most children, diuresis does not begin in the first few days of therapy but occurs as the amount of protein excreted into the urine decreases; this usually occurs within approximately 1 week following initiation of therapy. Along with the responsibility of administering the medication and monitoring its effectiveness, it is important to explain the side effects of the drug and expectations of therapy to the parents. Cyclophosphamide has serious side effects, including leukopenia and potential sterility in males when they are treated for 2 to 3 months. If this drug is prescribed, parents should be taught to give it in the morning, followed by plenty of fluids during the day to prevent bladder irritation and hematuria.

Protecting Edematous Body Surfaces. Careful attention and meticulous cleansing of touching skin surfaces is essential; skin creases should be padded with a soft material. Supporting edematous areas with pillows may provide a measure of comfort. The child should be turned, positioned, and gently massaged frequently. A bed cradle may be helpful in lifting bed covers off the child's skin and allowing air to flow.

Encouraging Adequate Nutritional Intake. As the edema diminishes, the child's malnourished appearance may become visible. Getting the child to eat may become a challenge. The nurse should make meals as attractive as possible, and smaller portions should be offered more frequently. Although food is not salted liberally, enough salt can usually be allowed to make the food more palatable. Using a small glass with a small amount of fluid will help gain the child's cooperation to drink.

Protecting the Child from Known Sources of Infection. Because infection is the leading cause of death in nephrosis (Kim & Grupe, 1986), the nurse's role is critical in protecting the child from known sources of infection. The child's resistance to all infections is lowered and compromised by corticosteroid therapy. Whether hospitalized or at home, the child should be protected from exposure to other children with infections, especially varicella (chickenpox). A child exposed to chickenpox may require Zoster immune plasma or serum globulin. In the event a child acquires chickenpox while on high-dose steroids, intravenous antiviral agents are indicated for up to 1 week of therapy. Appropriate handwashing is an emphasis for family teaching.

Promoting a Positive Body Image. Body image is just beginning to emerge in the younger child. During the edematous phase, the child may become concerned when parts of his or her body are no longer visible. Boys need reassurance that their penis is still there, even if edema conceals it from their view. Opportunities should be provided for the child and family to express their fears and concerns about the rapid changes in body size.

Reducing Periorbital Edema. Edema about the eyes may interfere with sensory perception and comfort. The use of eye irrigations or ophthalmic creams may be indicated. Allowing the child to sleep with the head elevated on a pillow may prevent the eyes from swelling closed and eliminate the fear associated with this.

Ensuring Safety from Falls. Safety must be constantly monitored, as changes in body size may alter the child's ability to move and maintain position. Bed siderails are usually necessary and are absolutely essential for the younger child. Parents should be made particularly aware of the need for safety as they prepare to take the child home.

Ensuring Effective Home Management of Therapeutic Regimen. Effective management at home requires that the nurse prepare a family for care at home through education and emotional support. It is particularly important that the family understand the disease process and how drug therapy and a low-salt diet affect the child's progress. Parents should also be taught to assess for fever and signs and symptoms of infections that may follow nephrotic syndrome, such as pneumonia, bronchitis, peritonitis, cellulitis, UTI, and septic arthritis (Kim & Grupe, 1986). Instruction for urine testing for protein should be practiced as soon as the parents' level of readiness is deemed appropriate. The protracted course of the disease with remissions, relapses, and occasional admissions to the hospital may place severe stress on the family. Although outpatient treatment is usually practical for children with moderate edema, parents must learn the importance of complying with a regimen of regular office or clinic visits.

Parents should be encouraged to keep a diary of the child's illness events. A record of relapses, therapy, responses, and progress provides information that is useful when repetitive therapy is necessary.

Evaluation

The child's status is evaluated by assessing for signs of remission. As the child responds to drug therapy, it is expected that the permeability of the glomeruli will be decreased and that no further loss of proteins will occur. With an improved condition, it is expected that the child will have a normal amount of fluid (interstitial and intravascular), as evidenced by:

- Urine specific gravity within normal limits (1.010 to 1.025).
- Electrolyte levels within normal limits.
- Weight within normal limits and stable.
- A balance in fluid intake and output.
- Reduced edema.
- Lack of proteinuria, ascites, hypoproteinemia, and hyperlipidemia.
- Clear, pale yellow urine.
- Blood pressure within acceptable range.
- Intact skin without evidence of lesion.
- A well-balanced diet.
- No signs of infection.
- A positive body image.
- Usual response to stimuli.
- Ability to be mobile and coordinated.

Acute Renal Failure

Acute renal failure (ARF) is an abrupt deterioration or cessation of renal function. It is the sudden loss of the kidney's ability to excrete water, electrolytes, and waste products of cell metabolism in sufficient quantities to maintain homeostasis. ARF develops in response to a variety of conditions and is classified according to the mechanism that causes the disturbance in renal function: prerenal; intrinsic renal; or postrenal (Table 36–12). Common conditions that cause ARF in children include poststreptococcal glomerulonephritis, hemolytic-uremic syndrome, and others such as postcardiac surgery.

Pathophysiology

Prerenal Failure. In prerenal ARF, an impairment of renal perfusion (a marked decrease in blood flow to the kidneys) occurs, leading to decreased glomerular filtration and increased proximal tubular absorption. The urine sodium concentration remains low, while the urine osmolality, urea, and creatinine concentrations are high. Acute prerenal ARF is often readily reversible when the cause of the renal hypoperfusion is corrected.

Intrinsic Renal Failure. The second type of ARF is intrinsic renal failure. The renal cortex and medulla are the principal sites damaged in intrinsic ARF, resulting in an oliguric or anuric state.

Postrenal Failure. Postrenal ARF, a relatively rare condition in children, results from obstruction of urine flow at a point within the pelvicalyceal collecting system, in the ureters, or within the urethra. Renal calculi, a tumor, or, more commonly, a congenital malformation may cause this obstruction.

Clinical Manifestations

The clinical manifestations of ARF may be overshadowed by the precipitating disorder; therefore, the clinician must be astute to recognize the symptoms of ARF. *The principal manifestation of ARF is oliguria or anuria.* Other common symptoms include edema, drowsiness, tachypnea, and laboratory abnormalities. The urine may contain red blood cells, protein, casts, and tubular cells. The urine sodium may be low or elevated, depending on the type of ARF. Blood abnormalities that are the hallmark of ARF include an elevated BUN, creatinine, and uric acid concentration.

Diagnostic Assessment

The condition causing ARF must be determined immediately, because the treatment for prerenal, intrinsic, and postrenal failure will vary according to the precipitating problem.

To determine the cause of ARF, the following interventions are needed: a complete history; a thorough physical examination, including weight, blood pressure, and evaluation of hydration; accurate measurement of any urinary output; a urinalysis, a urine culture, osmolality, and pH; blood studies, including BUN, creatinine, uric acid concentration, sodium, potassium, chloride, phosphorus, calcium, bicarbonate, complete blood count, and platelet count; and an

TABLE 36-12
Major Causes of Renal Failure in Children

Prerenal Failure

Hypovolemia and hypotension caused by:

- Dehydration
  - Vomiting
  - Diarrhea
  - Febrile illness
  - Massive reduction in colloid oncotic pressure (protein-losing enteropathy, nephrotic syndrome)
  - Septic shock
  - Congestive heart failure
  - Hemorrhage
  - Hyponatremia

Intrinsic Renal Failure

Acute tubular necrosis

- Prolonged secondary hypotension
  - Vomiting
  - Diarrhea
  - Shock
  - Nephrotoxins
  - Organ perfusion
- Glomerulonephritis
  - Primary
  - Secondary

Interstitial nephritis

- Primary
- Secondary
  - Drugs
  - Toxins

Vascular

- Venous thrombosis
- Cortical necrosis
- Disseminated intravascular coagulation

Pigmenturia (myoglobinuria, hemoglobinuria)

Postrenal Obstruction

Urethral obstruction

- Stricture
- Posterior urethral valves
- Diverticulum

Ureterocele

Solitary renal unit with ureterovesical or ureteropelvic juncture obstruction

Extrinsic tumors compressing bladder outlet

Intrinsic urinary tract tumors

Neurogenic bladder

From Osofsky, S. G., & Lewy, J. E. (1985). Acute renal failure. In J. D. Dickerman & J. F. Lucey (Eds.). *Smith's The critically ill child: Diagnosis and medical management*. Philadelphia: WB Saunders.

ECG to evaluate any dysrhythmias. Ultrasonography may be used to assess for the presence of obstruction. Radiographs of the chest and abdomen may be indicated to determine the presence of congestive heart failure, pulmonary edema, or renal calculi.

Therapeutic Management

If prerenal failure is suspected, the immediate approach will be to infuse a bolus of normal saline solution intravenously over 1 hour. If the child responds to this intervention with an increased urinary output, then hypoperfusion of the kidney, or intrinsic ARF, is the likely diagnosis. This therapy is not attempted if the child manifests symptoms of fluid overload, such as congestive heart failure.

ARF can be reversed or may lead to chronic renal failure or death. Prompt and aggressive treatment of ARF and the underlying disorder will minimize mortality. The three major goals of treatment of ARF are to correct the cause of ARF, to manage the complications of renal failure, and to support the child until the tubular epithelial cells regenerate and normal renal function returns.

Reversible ARF progresses through three phases: oliguric; early diuretic; and late diuretic. The *oliguric phase* may last from 7 to 21 days. During this phase, BUN levels will be elevated and oliguria will be present. The child will require intensive nursing care and may require dialysis or continuous arteriovenous hemofiltration at this time. Dialysis and hemofiltration are described later in this chapter.

The second phase, the *early diuretic phase,* may last up to several weeks. During this phase, the urine volume may be high and the BUN level ceases to rise.

The *late diuretic phase* may last from several months to 1 year. During this stage, the BUN level and urine output begin to return to normal. The tubular epithelium begins to regenerate and normal renal function will return.

Nursing Diagnostic Statements and Collaborative Problems

High risk for injury: metabolic imbalance; *risk factors:*

- *Electrolyte and hydrogen ion imbalance associated with impaired excretion or intravascular dilution.*
- *Elevation of urea and creatinine associated with decreased excretion.*

High risk for altered fluid volume: excess; *risk factors:*

- *Decreased renal perfusion.*
- *Damage to renal tissue.*
- *Obstruction of urine flow.*

High risk for infection; *risk factor, altered immune responses associated with serious illness.*

Fear/anxiety: child and family, *related to the serious nature of ARF.*

High risk for altered fluid volume: deficit; *risk factor, rapid diuresis.*

Planning and Implementation

Although the initial care of the child with ARF will usually take place in a specialty unit, the nurse generalist will often be involved with care of the child before hospital discharge. The nursing diagnoses and goals of care are directed by the fact that ARF renders the kidneys unable to maintain their usual functions of excreting nitrogenous wastes and maintaining fluid, electrolyte, and acid-base balance. Both medical treatment and nursing care are focused, then, on assisting the body to maintain these functions until the kidneys recover.

Dietary potassium will usually be restricted. Restrictions in diet commonly include sodium as well, in order to prevent the sodium from drawing additional fluid into the vascular compartment. Table 36–13 lists common foods that are high in sodium and potassium and can guide the nurse in monitoring the child's diet.

Metabolic acidosis may result from decreased renal excretion of nonvolatile hydrogen ions and from catabolism of body protein. Kussmaul respirations are a common sign of this disorder. Sodium bicarbonate or sodium lactate may be given orally or intravenously to control the acidosis.

Azotemia denotes accumulation of nitrogenous wastes in the blood. It is reflected by BUN levels greater than 20 mg/dl and elevated creatinine levels. As noted in Table 36–4, glomerular filtration rate (GFR) must be decreased by at least 50 per cent before creatinine level is affected. If the child is not oliguric, fluid therapy will be ordered to optimize urinary output and thereby reduce serum accumulation of nitrogenous wastes.

Urea also rises in response to catabolism and is reflected in an increased BUN. The goal of dietary management will be to meet the child's metabolic demands for calories. Protein catabolism can be minimized if nonprotein caloric intake (glucose) is increased to as much as 50 to 60 kcal/kg/day as a mixture of essential and nonessential amino acids while restricting proteins to approximately 0.5 mg/kg/day (Bock, 1992). Protein may be restricted in ARF because it is assumed to be a temporary measure, whereas in chronic renal failure, it is not as commonly restricted because of the effect that protein restriction has on the growth of the child.

Monitoring and Reducing Metabolic Imbalances. Metabolic imbalances include electrolyte disturbances, metabolic acidosis, and azotemia. The most common electrolyte disturbances in ARF are hyperkalemia (resulting from decreased renal excretion and release of potassium by injured tissues), hyponatremia (resulting from dilution of body fluids), hyperphosphatemia (related to reduced renal excretion), and hypocalcemia (which occurs in response to hyperphosphatemia). The nurse must be alert for physical evidence of electrolyte imbalance. Serum electrolytes will be measured frequently in renal failure. Because the nurse may often be the first to see the laboratory report, it is important that she or he be able to evaluate the findings and alert the physician appropriately.

Hyperkalemia is a life-threatening imbalance because potassium levels that approach 6 mEq/L cause cardiac conduction abnormalities (Schact, 1985). The child with renal failure should have a cardiorespiratory monitor to aid in detection of cardiac dysrhythmias. Kayexalate, a cation-exchange resin, may be given orally or by enema to reduce serum potassium levels.

Monitoring and Reducing Complications of Fluid Excess. Since decreased urine output is the hallmark of ARF, knowledge of hourly urine output (and hourly fluid intake) is essential for many medical and nursing decisions. If a urinary catheter is in place, a special collection system will be attached to the catheter when hourly output is to be recorded. The catheter will drain into a small, graduated plastic chamber. After the hour's output is recorded, the contents of the chamber can be released into an attached, larger collection bag. Some systems include ports through which a sterile needle may be inserted to collect a urine specimen for analysis.

Weight may be recorded as often as every 12 hours to help determine fluid balance. Because of the critical nature of these measurements, it is essential that all extraneous variables (scales, clothing, relation to meals) be held constant so that any differences in measures reflect actual changes in fluid balance.

Complications of excess intravascular fluid include hypertension, edema, and pulmonary edema. *Hypertension* is usually the direct result of sodium and water retention. Nursing responsibilities include judg-

TABLE 36-13
Foods High in Sodium and/or Potassium

Food Source	Sodium (mg)	Potassium (mg)
Fruits		
Apricots, dried, 17 large halves	26	*979**
Banana, raw 1 medium	2	*550*
Dates, domestic, 10 medium, pitted	1	*648*
Watermelon, 1 slice 6 × 1½ in	6	*600*
Meats		
Beef, ground chuck, 3½ oz	60	*370*
Beef, dried, chipped, 3 oz	*3660*	170
Chicken, light meat, fried, 3½ oz	68	*434*
Ham, 1 slice, 2 oz	*518*	239
Hot, dog, 1 average	*542*	108
Lamb, loin chop, 3½ oz	49	*466*
Liver, calf, fried, 3½ oz	118	*453*
Pork chop, loin 1 chop, 2 oz	41	*386*
Salami, dry, 1 oz slice	*540*	102
Turkey, light meat 3½ oz	82	*411*
Vegetables		
Artichoke, raw, 1 large bud	86	*860*
Asparagus, frozen, in butter sauce, 1 cup	*747*	270
Avocado, ½	10	*574*
Beans, canned, with pork and tomato, ½ cup	*579*	263
Beans, frijoles, 1 serving	*1102*	*693*
Beans, green, canned ½ cup	*565*	227
Spinach, raw, 3½ oz	159	*795*
Potato, white, baked without skin, 3¼ in diameter	6	*755*
Potato, dehydrated flakes 3½ oz	80	*1600*
Potato chips, 3½ oz	*1130*	197
Seaweed, kelp, raw 3½ oz	*3007*	*5273*
Squash, winter, baked, ½ cup	1	*461*
Squash, acorn ½ baked squash	2	*749*
Tomato, canned, 1 cup	*1000*	*1060*
Miscellaneous		
Hershey bar	24	*456*
Meat tenderizer, 1 tsp	*1745*	Trace
Meat tenderizer, low-sodium, 1 tsp	1	*2392*
Milk, whole, 1 cup	120	*370*
Peanuts, roasted, salted, 3½ oz	*460*	*700*

* The values in italics represent the high electrolyte content for that food source.

ments related to frequency and techniques of blood pressure measurement. In order to ensure the most accurate measurement, the blood pressure should always be taken with the child in the same position (to avoid alterations related to position change), in as restful a state as possible (to avoid temporary increases in systolic pressure), and with the same equipment (to avoid alterations associated with cuff size and manometer settings). Strategies to reduce the risk of hypertension (and other complications of fluid overload) include careful regulation of intravenous fluids.

Edema may result from vascular overload. It may present as periorbital, pretibial, or pedal edema; ascites; or pleural or pericardial effusion. Nursing assessment for edema should be reflected in the chart. If edema is present, particular care will be needed to prevent skin breakdown.

Pulmonary edema, a very serious complication, results when vascular fluid backs up in the lungs because the heart is unable to deal with the increased vascular load. Pulmonary edema presents with tachypnea, tachycardia, rales (crackles), rhonchi (wheezes), and increased respiratory secretions. Expert nursing assessment is essential to aid in early diagnosis and treatment.

Reducing the Risk of Infection. As discussed in Chapter 37, significant physical and psychologic stress can alter immune processes. In addition, immune function may be impaired by the disease that caused ARF, such as glomerulonephritis. Add to this increased risk of infection, the probability for invasive diagnostic and therapeutic procedures, and *potential for infection* becomes an important nursing diagnosis.

The strategies involved with reducing the risk for infection may seem repetitious and mundane, until one considers that infection is a major cause of death in ARF. *The nurse's responsibility for reducing the risk of infection is critical to a favorable outcome for the child.* The importance of handwashing before each contact with the child cannot be overemphasized. Instruct family members about proper handwashing. Posting signs can be helpful and is often less threatening than a verbal reminder. Health care professionals who know they have an infectious condition should refrain from caring for children with ARF.

Urinary and central venous catheters are potential avenues for pathogens. These will be removed as quickly as possible, but, while in place, aseptic technique and assessment for signs of infection are imperative. Intermittent straight catheterization may sometimes be used instead of an indwelling Foley catheter. Cultures should be obtained from suspected infection sites. Insertion and care of central venous catheters is discussed in Chapter 23.

Antibiotics are rarely used prophylactically, and those prescribed for infection should be the least nephrotoxic. When administering any medication to the child with renal failure, particularly if the child is oliguric, the nurse must be aware of the drug's mechanism for elimination from the body. Pharmacologic agents and their metabolites that rely on glomerular filtration for excretion (e.g., digitalis) will be retained by the body. The physician may alter the dose or time interval between doses to offset some of these effects. The nurse, who is in constant attendance, can provide valuable assessments for evaluating the child's response to medications.

Supporting the Child and Family. The child with ARF is seriously ill and requires multiple tests and procedures. Throughout all phases of the disease, the child and family will require emotional support to deal with this crisis. Because the course of ARF covers several months, the child and family will require repeated information and reassurance about the child's progress.

Care During the Diuretic Phase. Careful management of fluid and electrolyte balance will extend through the diuretic phase of ARF. If the GFR improves faster than function of the tubules, a fluid balance deficit may result. Nursing assessment of intake and output, urine specific gravity, and evidence of dehydration are important in this phase of recovery from ARF. Medication dosages will be adjusted in accordance with increased glomerular filtration.

Poststreptococcal Acute Glomerulonephritis

Glomerulonephritis is a common cause of ARF. It is an inflammation of the glomeruli of the kidneys. The diagnosis represents a number of different disease processes, some causing glomerular inflammation as the primary disorder and others in which glomerular inflammation is only one manifestation of an overall systemic disease. Poststreptococcal acute glomerulonephritis (PSAGN) is the most common form of glomerulonephritis in children and typically follows a streptococcal infection of the throat or skin.

Acute glomerulonephritis associated with pharyngeal streptococcal infections is most common in temperate or cold climates; it occurs 8 to 14 days after the pharyngitis and has a peak incidence during the winter and spring months (Travis, 1991). Early school-age children are most frequently affected, boys twice as often as girls, for unknown reasons.

In contrast, glomerulonephritis associated with streptococcal infections of the skin (e.g., impetigo) is most common in hot, tropical climates; this form occurs 14 to 21 days after the skin infection and has a peak incidence during the late summer and early fall (Travis, 1991). Preschool children, with equal distribution to both sexes, are most often affected.

If one family member develops PSAGN, other family members are at high risk for developing the same disease. Second attacks of acute glomerulonephritis rarely occur in the same individual (Bergstein, 1992).

Etiology/Pathophysiology

The glomeruli initiate the formation of urine by filtering the blood as it passes through the kidneys. Glomerulonephritis results when immune complexes (antigen-antibody complexes) formed during the streptococcal infection become entrapped in the glomerular membrane and cause inflammation. White blood cells, specifically polymorphonuclear leukocytes, collect in the glomeruli; the cells of the membrane proliferate, become edematous, and occlude the affected glomeruli. The GFR decreases, resulting in sodium and water retention and eventual circulatory congestion and edema. Those parts of the glomerular membrane that are not occluded malfunction and allow large amounts of protein to leak into the glomerular filtrate (proteinuria). Red blood cells may also pass into the filtrate if the membrane ruptures (hematuria) (Fig. 36–9). Permanent damage to the glomeruli, although rare, can occur with severe disease.

Only certain types of group A beta-hemolytic streptococci cause PSAGN. The most common nephritogenic strains are types 12 and 49, associated with streptococcal infections of the pharynx and skin, respectively (Bergstein, 1992).

As streptococcal infection of the upper respiratory tract or the skin frequently precedes PSAGN, the nurse must elicit a careful history to determine whether such an infection in fact did occur 1 to 3 weeks prior to the present symptoms. Documented prior infections will not always occur, however; viruses, parasites, and bacteria other than streptococci have also been implicated in the development of acute glomerulonephritis.

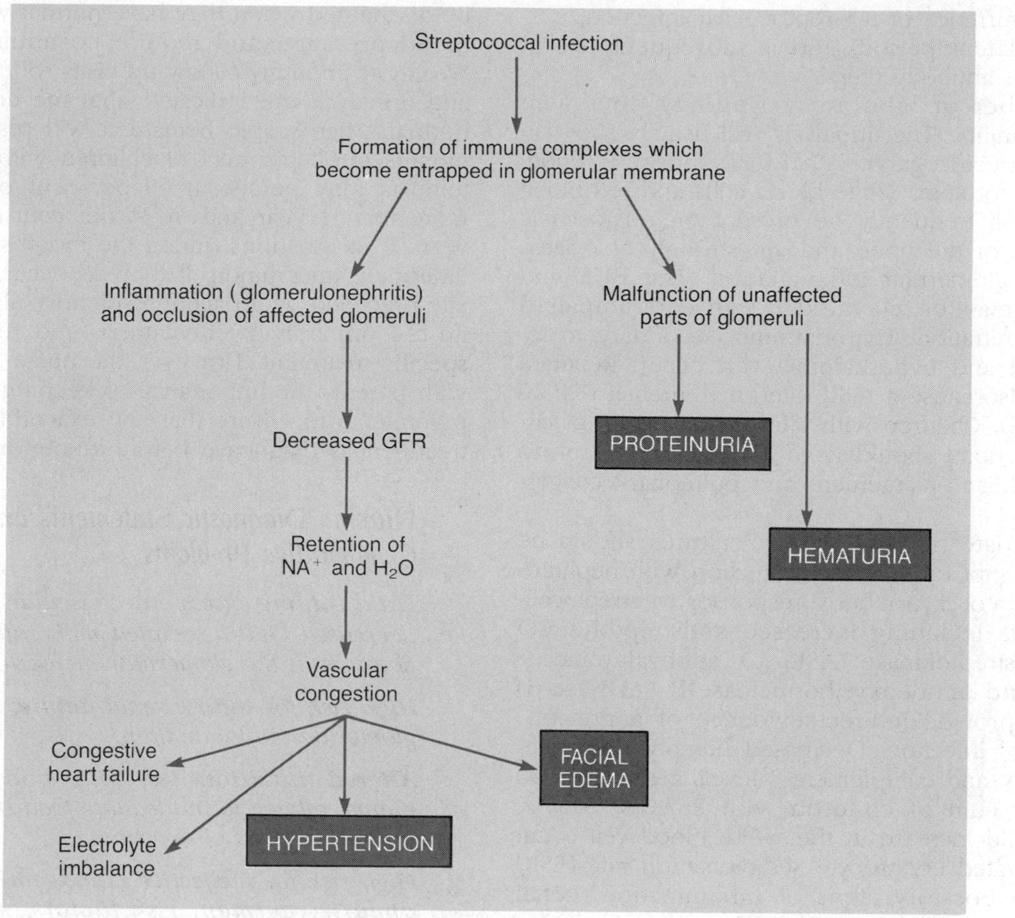

FIGURE 36-9. Pathophysiology of poststreptococcal acute glomerulonephritis.

Early diagnosis of PSAGN is especially important because prevention does not seem possible. Early antibiotic treatment of streptococcal infections as a method of preventing the subsequent development of glomerulonephritis is not well supported, although it may be somewhat effective in reducing the severity of the disease. Because there may be a familial incidence of infection with nephritogenic strains of streptococci, family members of a child with PSAGN should have throat cultures done; those with streptococcal infections should be treated with antibiotics prophylactically (Bergstein, 1992). Routine screening throat cultures of all children are not indicated, however, because healthy, asymptomatic individuals can have nonnephritogenic streptococci cultured from their throats. Appropriate treatment of insect bites, cuts, and abrasions may inhibit the development of streptococcal impetigo. If impetigo does develop, systemic antibiotics are superior to local antibiotic creams and ointments for treatment.

Clinical Manifestations

Signs and symptoms are acute in onset and range from very mild to extremely severe. A puffy face (edema) and discolored urine (hematuria) are the two most common presenting complaints. Edema frequently involves the periorbital area and is usually confined to the face, except in severe disease when it may be more generalized. Gross hematuria, often described as cola- or tea-colored, rusty or reddish-brown, occurs in 30 to 50 per cent of children hospitalized with acute glomerulonephritis (Travis, 1991). Microscopic hematuria is present in nearly all children with the disease. A decreased urine output, flank or abdominal pain, anorexia, weight gain, pallor, and low-grade fever are other common manifestations.

Hypertension is a frequent complication; it is usually mild to moderate (120–180/80–120 mmHg), asymptomatic, and found only by checking blood pressure. Occasionally, hypertension can be severe enough to cause headaches, visual disturbances, sleepiness, coma, or seizures. Other signs of circulatory overload, such as dyspnea, tachypnea, and cough, may also be present. Table 36–11 compares the etiology and clinical manifestations of glomerulonephritis and MCNS.

Diagnostic Assessment

The diagnosis of PSAGN rests on (1) evidence of injury of the glomeruli (hematuria, proteinuria, or casts); (2) identification of a nephritogenic type of group A beta-hemolytic streptococcus; and (3) the sequential occurrence of a streptococcal infection, a 1- to 3-week latent period, and a subsequent rise in streptococcal antibody titers.

A number of laboratory findings document glomerular injury. The urinalysis will usually show an increased specific gravity (>1.030), positive blood, and positive protein. White blood cells and red blood cell casts will frequently be present on microscopic examination of the urine and are strongly associated with acute glomerular inflammation. The BUN and creatinine may be elevated because of impaired glomerular filtration. Hyponatremia secondary to retained fluid and hyperkalemia can occur. Retained fluid may also cause a mild dilutional anemia (Hb 10 to 11 mg/dl). Children with clinical symptoms of circulatory overload should have a chest radiograph to rule out cardiac enlargement and pulmonary congestion.

Appropriate throat and skin cultures should be done to attempt to document infection with nephritogenic streptococci. Antibody responses to streptococcal products including increased antistreptolysin-O (ASO), antistreptokinase (ASKase), antihyaluronidase (AHase), and antideoxyribonuclease-B (ADNase-B) titers also provide indirect evidence of a previous streptococcal infection. Decreased hemolytic complement activity and complement-3 levels are seen in 90 to 100 per cent of children with PSAGN (Travis, 1991). A mild increase in the white blood cell count and an elevated erythrocyte sedimentation rate (ESR) are other laboratory signs of inflammation. Renal biopsy is rarely needed for diagnosis.

Therapeutic Management

The acute phase of glomerulonephritis usually lasts 1 to 2 weeks; however, the severity of the illness is unpredictable, and ranges from very mild to life-threatening. Children who have normal blood pressure, an adequate urine output, and very mild symptoms may be managed carefully as outpatients. Children who develop hypertension, oliguria, or acute weight gain secondary to fluid retention will need to be hospitalized. Criteria for admission will vary with the institution.

The major danger during the acute phase of glomerulonephritis is renal failure with subsequent hypertension and circulatory congestion. Intervention focuses on preserving renal function and preventing circulatory overload. Children who are sick generally restrict their activities according to how they feel; therefore, enforced bed rest is usually not needed unless severe hypertension is present.

Fluid restrictions and diets high in carbohydrates and fats and low in sodium, potassium, or both, may be implemented. Antihypertensives and diuretics may be ordered if the diastolic pressure is elevated for age. Antibiotics may be prescribed if the child still has a positive streptococcal culture.

Diuresis occurs after the initial 1- to 3-week edematous phase of the illness. Hospitalized children can be discharged when they have normal weight, normal blood pressure, and require no antihypertensives. Weekly to monthly follow-up visits for blood pressure and urinalysis are indicated until the urine returns to normal. Microscopic hematuria will resolve within 6 months in 90 per cent of children with PSAGN. Proteinuria may persist in 60 per cent of patients for more than 1 year and in 36 per cent for 2 or more years. Exacerbations during the months following the illness are uncommon. If they do occur, they are usually preceded by an acute respiratory illness, are manifested primarily by hematuria, and resolve without specific treatment. However, the nurse should discuss with parents the importance of keeping follow-up appointments to ensure that any exacerbation requiring treatment is diagnosed before kidney injury occurs.

Nursing Diagnostic Statements and Collaborative Problems

Fluid volume excess: intravascular; *caused by decreased GFR associated with inflammatory changes in the glomerular membrane.*

High risk for injury: renal failure; *risk factor, glomerular inflammation.*

Altered nutrition: less than body requirements, *related to inadequate food intake associated with loss of appetite.*

High risk for ineffective management of therapeutic regimen; *risk factors, knowledge deficit regarding:*

- *Measurements of blood pressure, weight, intake, and output.*
- *Administration of prescribed medications.*
- *Identification of evidence of congestive heart failure, electrolyte imbalance, and renal failure.*
- *Expected course of the disease.*

Planning and Implementation

The nursing diagnoses direct the nursing goals: monitoring and reducing excess intravascular fluid volume, assessing for evidence of renal failure, providing adequate nutritional intake, and providing information and guidance needed to support home care. Strategies to meet these goals are discussed subsequently.

Maintaining Fluid Balance. The child hospitalized with acute glomerulonephritis will require careful monitoring of fluid balance. An accurate intake/output record will be needed, as well as daily weights and blood pressure measurement at least every 4 hours. The physician must be alerted to increasing oliguria, weight gain, or increasing hypertension.

The oliguric state (inadequate excretion) may predispose to electrolyte imbalances—most notably, hyperkalemia. The nurse can monitor for this complication by checking laboratory reports and by assessing for muscle weakness, bradycardia, hyperreflexia, flaccid paralysis, malaise, nausea, shallow breathing, and intestinal colic and diarrhea. Intravascular congestion may also lead to congestive heart failure. Careful assessment for classic signs and symptoms of this complication is an important nursing responsibility. (See Chapter 33.)

Nursing interventions can assist in reducing intravascular volume. Antihypertensives and diuretics may be ordered if hypertension becomes severe. Correct administration, patient and family teaching, and evaluation of the drugs' therapeutic effects are among nursing responsibilities. In addition, the nurse will be the one to explain and enforce fluid and dietary restrictions. The child and family will be more cooperative if they are aware of the reasons for the restrictions and are allowed to exercise as much control as possible within the prescribed guidelines. Fluid restriction is less obvious to the child if liquids are served in a small cup.

Assessing for Evidence of Renal Failure. Because renal failure is the major threat to the child with glomerulonephritis, nursing assessment for this complication cannot be overemphasized. The section on ARF in this chapter provides a complete list of clinical manifestations.

Promoting Adequate Food Intake. The nurse can help stimulate the child's already decreased appetite by working with the parents to plan a diet that appeals to the child, serving small portions, and encouraging family members to be there to eat with the child at meal times.

Facilitating Home Management of Therapeutic Regimen. The nurse must be sensitive to what this illness means for the child and family. Facial edema and dark-colored urine can be frightening for the child. The nurse can help by listening to these and other concerns and by stressing the temporary nature of these bodily changes.

"Kidney disease" sounds frightening to parents and often is associated with the words "dialysis" and "kidney transplant." The family needs to be supported in the care of their child in the home by receiving adequate information about the nature of their child's condition and the reason for the plan of care. An explanation of the importance of monitoring blood pressure, weight, and intake and output helps to gain their cooperation in keeping follow-up appointments. Parents are also told about the importance of giving medication as prescribed and are taught about signs and symptoms to watch for that indicate exacerbation requiring treatment.

Long-Term Outcome

The expected outcome for children with PSAGN is excellent. A few children, however, will develop chronic glomerular disease. Most experts believe that the severity of the initial illness correlates with the development of chronicity. Documentation of this belief is difficult because chronic glomerulonephritis develops through a variety of different disease processes. The disease may go undetected for years; therefore, it is seen primarily in adolescents and adults. The signs and symptoms of the illness reflect progressive renal failure as the glomeruli gradually become replaced with fibrous tissue. Treatment is predominantly symptomatic, dialysis and renal transplant may ultimately be needed.

Hemolytic-Uremic Syndrome

Hemolytic-uremic syndrome (HUS) is by far the most common cause of ARF in children between 1 and 4 years of age. HUS is an acute disease characterized by renal failure, hemolytic anemia, and thrombocytopenia. The syndrome predominates in whites and affects males and females equally. In its most common form in North America, it affects children under 5 years of age following an enteric illness. This disease predominates also in certain geographic areas in the world, including the western United States, Argentina, Southern Africa, and The Netherlands.

Etiology/Pathophysiology

The frequency of gastroenteritis as a predecessor has marshaled medical research to look for enteric pathogens related to HUS. The majority of cases of typical HUS are associated with either *Escherichia coli* or *Shigella dysenteriae*. The verotoxin-producing *E. coli* 0157:H7 serotype (VTEC), usually implicated with this disease, is spread by both person-to-person contact and contaminated food (typically beef or unpasteurized milk). There are numerous other bacteria as well as viruses that have been associated with HUS.

There is also an atypical form that is rare in children under 2 years of age. This type of HUS occurs in all seasons, and no diarrheal prodrome is observed. Familial occurrence is possible. Relapses can occur, and most atypical HUS results in ESRD, although the role of genetics is unknown (Loirat et al, 1993).

In HUS, the glomeruli and arterioles are damaged. The actual process by which *E. coli* and *S. dysenteriae* produce the cell damage remains unknown. It is known, however, that this damage directly alters the endothelial barrier of the arterioles and leads to coagulation of fibrin strands in the capillary walls. As platelets and red blood cells pass through these abnormal capillary walls, they fragment and are damaged. The red blood cells become fragmented or helmet-shaped and eventually are trapped by the spleen. This reduction and damage to the red blood cells results in severe hemolytic anemia. Thrombocytopenia occurs from the platelet aggregation within the damaged vessels or from the damage occurring to the platelets as they pass through the capillary walls.

Clinical Manifestations

HUS is characterized by occurrence in the summer, sometimes in epidemics, and usually follows a gastroenteritis or viral illness within several days to 2 weeks. The onset of this disorder is acute, characterized by a prodrome of bloody diarrhea, extreme pallor, lethargy, irritability, anorexia, bruising, and a decreased urine output. The child may have associated problems with hypertension, edema, mild jaundice, splenomegaly, seizures, and symptoms of circulatory congestion. The urine may remain amber or be brownish-red in color.

Diagnostic Assessment

The history should include a diet history and information about the recent health of family members and friends. HUS associated with VTEC may be seen in outbreaks involving several family members and immediate contacts.

The diagnosis of HUS is made by identifying the presence of hemolytic anemia, renal failure, and thrombocytopenia in the child. In order to confirm the diagnosis, numerous blood and urine tests are done. A complete blood count with differential and reticulocyte count will confirm the presence of anemia and hemolysis. Often, the hemoglobin will be 5 to 7 g/dl and there will be an elevated reticulocyte count. The platelet count will initially be normal, but it decreases during the first few days of the illness. Serum electrolytes, BUN, and creatinine values are usually consistent with renal failure. Uric acid concentrates will be elevated. Urinalysis will reflect renal damage, manifested by hematuria, proteinuria, and the presence of urinary casts.

Therapeutic Management

The acute phase of HUS usually lasts for 1 to 2 weeks, with gradual improvement over 1 to 2 months. In more severe cases, the acute phase may lead to renal failure or death. Drugs such as corticosteroids, anticoagulants, or antiplatelet agents have not been found to be effective and are not used in the treatment of HUS.

During the acute phase of the illness, therapeutic measures are supportive and aimed at alleviating complications associated with the anemia, thrombocytopenia, and renal failure. Peritoneal dialysis is often necessary to alleviate problems associated with renal failure.

If the child experiences a severe anemia, transfusion with fresh-washed, packed red blood cells may be necessary. If bleeding occurs secondary to the thrombocytopenia, the child may be transfused with platelets. If the child is acutely ill, a nutritional diet may be provided through nasogastric feedings or by total parenteral nutrition.

Nursing Care

The nurse generalist will seldom be involved in the initial care of the child with HUS. Specialized care is usually necessary and is often provided in an intensive care setting. Goals of nursing care will be similar to those detailed in this chapter for ARF.

The child with bloody diarrhea should be placed in a private room if possible with strict handwashing enforced. HUS has been reported to have been transmitted to a nurse in at least one instance (Karmali et al, 1988). Throughout the course of the illness, the nurse assists with the collection of specimens, ensures the child's comfort and safety, monitors the child's vital signs, and observes for alterations in skin integrity, neurologic status, and renal and cardiovascular functioning. As each test or procedure is done, the parents and child should be informed about the purpose of the test and what is involved in carrying it out.

The nurse may be responsible for administering blood transfusions, monitoring intravenous fluids, assessing for evidence of hypertension and pulmonary edema, monitoring hourly urine output, and monitoring for signs and symptoms of electrolyte imbalance, especially hyperkalemia and uremia. Nutritional support may be unusually challenging because of associated anorexia. If oral intake is not sufficient to prevent tissue catabolism, parenteral nutrition may be ordered. Neurologic involvement may occur (Siegler, 1988) and requires careful nursing assessment and seizure precautions.

During the course of the illness, nurses should be available to talk to the family about the disease and collaborate with the physician and other health care professionals to keep the family informed. Because HUS is relatively uncommon, yet serious, the family will require ongoing explanations.

Long-Term Outcome

The expected outcome for the child with HUS is fairly good, with the majority of the patients surviving the acute phase. Approximately 15 per cent of the patients have adverse sequelae, including hypertension, proteinuria, and azotemia. Approximately 10 per cent of the children with HUS develop ESRD.

Chronic Renal Failure

In chronic renal failure (CRF), a reduction in renal function occurs over time in response to *irreversible* damage to the nephrons. This alteration in renal function decreases the GFR and causes metabolic, biochemical, and clinical disturbances. However, the onset of CRF is insidious, and the symptoms are often present only after severe damage to the kidneys has occurred.

Etiology

The etiology of CRF is closely associated with the age of the child at the time of diagnosis. Congenital urologic abnormalities and chronic glomerulonephritis are the two leading causes of CRF in children. Children up to age 5 years with congenital anomalies of the kidney or urinary tract (particularly renal hypoplasia and severe bilateral vesicoureteral reflux) make up the greatest number of children with CRF. During the school-age and adolescent years, glomerulonephritis is responsible for the majority of the cases of CRF. Other causes in this age group are HUS and various hereditary disorders.

The kidney may also become involved in a systemic disease such as lupus erythematosus or HUS. Rare causes of CRF in children include cortical necrosis from renal anoxia, nephrotoxic drugs and poisons, and inborn errors of metabolism such as cystinosis.

Pathophysiology

The actual mechanism of deterioration that causes progression to ESRD remains unclear. Some factors thought to contribute to the process include (1) inflammation and scarring resulting from deposition of immune complexes in the glomerulus, (2) hyperfiltration injury as a result of increased glomerular blood flow and hypertrophy of nephrons, (3) dietary protein and phosphorus intake through a mechanism that is unclear, (4) persistent proteinuria, and (5) systemic hypertension.

Compensatory mechanisms operate early in the course of the disease, resulting in an asymptomatic condition. As nephrons become damaged, the GFR eventually falls, impairing the body's ability to excrete nitrogenous wastes. When it reaches a level of 20 per cent below normal, a combination of metabolic and biochemical disturbances occur that result in a set of clinical manifestations that are known as a *uremic state*. See Table 36–14 for a summary of the pathophysiologic mechanism and related clinical manifestations.

Clinical Manifestations

The signs and symptoms of CRF are vague and nonspecific in the early stages and progress to affect every body system in the final stages of the disease. CRF progresses in three stages: decreased renal reserve, renal insufficiency, and ESRD. During the decreased renal reserve stage, the child is asymptomatic and BUN and serum creatinine levels are normal. In renal insufficiency, more than 75 per cent of the nephrons have been destroyed and the GFR is approximately 25 per cent of normal. The BUN and serum creatinine levels begin to rise and nocturia or polyuria may occur.

In ESRD, or uremia, 90 per cent of the nephrons are destroyed and the GFR is 10 per cent of normal or less. The serum creatinine and BUN levels rise sharply and the child becomes oliguric. The kidneys cease to function effectively and dialysis or kidney transplant must be considered.

Most children with CRF do not come to the attention of the health care personnel during the decreased renal reserve stage but are diagnosed after the damage to the kidney is quite severe. They may have a history suggestive of recurrent UTIs and vague complaints of decreased appetite, increased thirst, diminished physical activity, fatigue, a decline in school performance, polyuria, secondary enuresis, and poor growth. Often, the renal failure is detected only when the child manifests symptoms of edema, symptomatic hypertension, or gross hematuria, or develops a urinary tract infection.

During the renal insufficiency phase, the child may have nocturia, bone or joint pain, growth retardation, skin dryness or itchiness (uremic frost), muscle cramps, and signs of motor or sensory neuropathy. Physical findings include a pale or sallow complexion, growth retardation with bony deformities (osteodystrophy), diastolic and systolic hypertension, uremic breath (uremic fetor), and signs of neuropathy and retinopathy. Signs of circulatory overload may be present, manifested by tachycardia, tachypnea, cardiomegaly, and an ejection murmur.

In the later stages of the disease, the child may have vomiting, bloody diarrhea, confusion, edema, bruising, headache, seizures, and a decreasing urine output. Symptoms of cardiac failure may be present.

The electrolyte, metabolic, and chemical manifestations of CRF are quite complex and are described in Table 36–14.

Diagnostic Assessment

The diagnostic criteria used in ARF can be applied to the evaluation of a child with CRF. The presence of anemia (with the exception of HUS) is suggestive of the chronicity of the renal failure. The main cause of anemia in CRF is lack of the hormone erythropoietin, which is produced mainly in the kidneys. This hormone is essential in the production of red blood cells. A second cause of anemia is the decreased lifespan (decreased by two thirds) of red blood cells because of uremic toxins.

In addition, the physical examination of children with CRF may confirm growth failure and the presence of renal osteodystrophy (ROD). Two interrelated but distinct pathophysiologic events lead to ROD: (1) secondary hyperparathyroidism and (2) derangements in vitamin D metabolism. Vitamin D is metabolized into its active form by the healthy kidneys; this active form of vitamin D is essential in calcium absorption. The presence of hyperparathyroidism and ROD on

TABLE 36-14
Chronic Renal Failure: Pathophysiology, Clinical Manifestations, and Therapeutic Management

Pathophysiology	Clinical Manifestations	Therapeutic Management
Renal insufficiency prevents sodium excretion and leads to retention of sodium and water	Edema and hypertension	Restriction of sodium and water intake; administer diuretics; monitor weight; monitor vital signs frequently; monitor electrolyte values
Renal insufficiency causes decreased renal excretion of potassium; acidosis and catabolism also increase extracellular potassium (hyperkalemia)	Cardiac arrhythmias, high serum potassium levels	Provide adequate caloric intake; provide low-potassium diet; monitor vital signs; monitor electrolyte values; administer sodium polystyrene sulfonate (Kayexalate); monitor electrocardiogram; observe for prolonged PR intervals and peaked T-waves
Renal insufficiency causes reduced GFR, which leads to retention of nitrogenous wastes	Uremia-anorexia, nausea, vomiting, lethargy	Provide adequate caloric intake; monitor protein intake
Damaged kidney results in decreased acid excretion, decreased ammonia excretion, bicarbonate reabsorption impaired, resulting in metabolic acidosis	Deep and rapid respirations	Monitor respiratory status; administer bicarbonate
Diseased kidney produces a decreased amount of vitamin D, resulting in decreased calcium absorption; reduced GFR and excretion of inorganic phosphates cause elevated plasma phosphate, resulting in hypocalcemia and hyperphosphatemia (renal osteodystrophy)	Growth arrest or retardation, osteomalacia, valgus deformites of lower extremities	Administration of phosphate binders, vitamin D, and calcium supplements; reduction of milk and other dairy products
Plasma insulin levels are elevated, which cause an inhibition of cellular glucose uptake	Hyperglycemia, abnormal glucose tolerance test	Monitor urine and blood glucose levels
The renal diluting and concentrating mechanism is frequently absent	Dehydration or pulmonary edema	Intravenous or oral fluids; accurately monitor urine output; monitor weight
Reduction of red blood cell production from a lack of renal erythropoietin; sequestration of red blood cells by spleen may contribute to anemia	Pallor, fatigue, low hemoglobin and hematocrit	Provide diet high in iron and folic acid; administer erythropoietin; administer supplementary iron; transfuse packed red blood cells
Salt and water retention causes hypervolemia, which increases blood pressure; overproduction of renin by damaged kidney may also cause hypertension	Increased blood pressure, headaches, dizziness, flushing	Monitor vital signs, including blood pressure; provide low-sodium diet; restrict fluids; give hypertensives; monitor output; monitor weight
Hypervolemia and hypertension may cause congestive heart failure; pericardial effusion may be associated with severe uremia	Tachycardia, gallop heart rhythm, poor peripheral perfusion, dyspnea, tachypnea, hepatomegaly, edema	Restrict sodium and fluid intake; monitor vital signs and cardiac function; monitor weight; administer diuretics and digoxin
Factors affecting growth include age of onset of renal disease, etiology of primary disease, acidosis, and presence of renal osteodystrophy	Retardation of height, bone growth	Monitor child's height, weight, and growth velocity and plot on growth chart; provide child with nutritional caloric intake; supportive measures around body image

bone radiographs would contribute to a diagnosis of CRF.

Determination of renal size by ultrasonographic examination is also helpful since children with CRF may have small and scarred kidneys or other obvious congenital defects such as hypoplasia, dysplasia, and polycystic kidney disease. Children with ARF usually have normal renal ultrasonographs.

Therapeutic Management

The treatment of CRF demands an understanding of the complex physiologic disturbances that occur and an appreciation of the impact this disease process has on the child and family (Frauman & Gilman, 1990). CRF affects all aspects of a child's life and impedes the child's activity level, school participation, and peer and family relationships. The child faces dietary and activity restrictions and experiences altered elimination patterns. Children with CRF may have varying degrees of growth retardation that can affect the development of body image and self-esteem. The child's daily routine may include medications, multiple visits to the hospital or physician, invasive procedures, and often dialysis.

The family members also face multiple stressors. The financial burden of multiple tests, hospitalizations, and perhaps dialysis can be overwhelming. Knowing that the child has a life-threatening illness creates anxiety and may cause conflict among family relationships.

Many children with CRF may be treated with drug, dietetic, and supportive therapy to combat the metabolic and chemical imbalances of renal failure. Human recombinant erythropoietin is now available and is very important in treating the anemia associated with CRF (Sinai-Frieman et al, 1989). The prevention and management of bone disease necessitates prescribing vitamin D available in its active form. However, when conservative management becomes ineffective in permitting the child to function normally in her or his environment or in preventing the symptoms of uremia, then dialysis or kidney transplant, or both, should be considered. ESRD requiring dialysis or transplantation develops in 2 to 3.5 children per million population per year. See section on treatment modalities for ESRD in this chapter.

Nursing Diagnostic Statements and Collaborative Problems

High risk for injury: metabolic imbalance; *risk factors:*

- *Electrolyte and hydrogen ion imbalance associated with impaired excretion or intravascular dilution.*
- *Elevation of urea and creatinine associated with decreased excretion.*

High risk for altered fluid volume: excess; *risk factor, oliguria/anuria associated with:*

- *Decreased renal perfusion.*
- *Damage to renal tissue.*
- *Obstruction of urine flow.*

High risk for impaired gas exchange; *risk factor, anemia associated with:*

- *Decreased production of erythropoietin by the diseased kidney.*
- *Hemolysis.*
- *Blood loss from hemodialysis.*

Altered nutrition; less than body requirements, *related to:*

- *Anorexia, nausea, and vomiting.*
- *Inadequate intake due to diet restrictions.*
- *Catabolic state.*

Body image disturbance, *related to perceptions of the child regarding delayed physical growth.*

High risk for caregiver role strain; *risk factors:*

- *Excessive demands associated with care of a child with chronic illness.*
- *Dependency on medications and dialysis machine.*

Planning and Implementation

The nursing care associated with the first two diagnoses is the same as for children with ARF. Nursing care for diagnoses *high risk for injury* and *high risk for altered fluid volume: excess* are found in the section, "Acute Renal Failure." In the section that follows, nursing care associated with the remaining nursing diagnoses is presented.

Reduce Metabolic Demands for Oxygen. Hemoglobin and hematocrit values must be closely monitored in children with CRF. Anemia occurs as a complication of CRF because of decreased production of erythropoietin by the diseased kidney, due to hemolysis, and through blood loss from hemodialysis equipment. Measures to reduce anemia are use of erythropoietin and selection of hemodialysis equipment that causes the least amount of blood loss. Because erythropoietin is now available, blood transfusions are rarely required. Erythropoietin is a very painful injection when given subcutaneously, and appropriate comfort measures are essential.

Promote Sufficient Nutritional Intake to Meet Metabolic Demands. Careful management of nutritional intake can appreciably reduce the nitrogenous waste products that must be excreted. The goal in dietary management is to promote growth by providing sufficient calories but to do so without making excessive demands on the kidney. Caloric intake can be increased by giving high amounts of carbohydrate and fat. Aspects of the diet that are to be restricted and that affect the kidney are proteins and phosphorus.

Protein intake is kept at the level of 1.5 g/kg/24 hrs because of the protein required for growth. Proteins should be of high biologic value to reduce the quantity of nitrogenous wastes produced. Examples of such foods are eggs, milk, meat, fish, and fowl. However, cow's milk has a high level of phosphorus; therefore, it should be restricted or given in combination with an oral phosphate binder. Potassium is not restricted unless creatinine clearance is reduced below 30 to 35 ml/min, or in the case of oliguria or anuria.

As the child's condition worsens, more restrictions may be required and parents may need increasing help with reading labels and keeping nutritional intake at an adequate level. If intake becomes inadequate, water-soluble vitamins may be required; supplementation with fat-soluble vitamins A, E, and K is not required; these vitamins may even accumulate if given as supplements. A major component of fostering growth and development is to ensure proper nutritional intake as described previously. Additionally, the nurse gives phosphate binders, vitamin D, and calcium supplements as ordered to prevent ROD.

Promote Improvement in Child's Perceptions Toward His or Her Body. Throughout the course of the disease, the child needs to receive realistic and simple explanations about the disease process. Encouraging participation in self-care to the degree the child is able promotes feelings of competence and can increase the child's feelings of worth. It is also important to involve the child to the degree possible in decision making concerning treatment plans.

The child should be encouraged to express in words the emotions felt with respect to body changes that are occurring. Coping strategies used by the child should be identified and acknowledged to make the child feel self-sufficient. In some cases it may also be helpful to use self-picture drawing approaches to promote the child's expression and to provide a means of evaluating the child's body image perceptions.

Decrease Caregiver Role Strain. Parents of a child with CRF face daily stresses with respect to management of their child's illness. Their child's loss of appetite, the need for dietary restrictions, and the general sense of not feeling well are daily concerns. The uncertainty of outcome for their child's future is particularly stressful and can lead to tensions within the family and can interfere with open communications. The nurse can support the family by providing information about the child's progress and eventually assist in the decision making concerning the methods of therapy, including dialysis and kidney transplantation.

Modalities of Treatment for End-Stage Renal Disease

Dialysis

The decision to institute dialysis will be made by the child and family in collaboration with the health care team. All dialytic options as well as transplantation should be evaluated. Renal transplantation is considered to be the optimal therapy for a child with ESRD. Some children may need bilateral nephrectomy prior to transplantation for the treatment of severe uncontrolled hypertension or severely malformed and chronically infected urinary tract. These children will need dialysis to maintain them as they prepare for transplantation. The choice of dialysis modality must be individualized to suit each child and family. The child's age, developmental status, and underlying renal disease, as well as whether the parents are willing and able to carry out dialysis in their home, must be considered.

Indications

The decision to institute dialysis should be made prior to the need for it so that the necessary surgical procedure can be performed while the child is in an optimal clinical state. Indications for initiating chronic dialysis therapy in children are not as clear as they are in adults (Leichter & Kanwal, 1992). Residual renal function is important and measurable, but clinical observations—such as the impact of CRF on growth, bone disease, increasingly poor nutrition, neurologic development, and the general health of the child—must be considered. Additionally, hypertension, edema, and electrolyte abnormalities such as hyperkalemia and metabolic acidosis may be management problems without dialysis. Six absolute indications for initiating dialysis in a child with CRF are fluid overload, congestive heart failure, uncontrolled hyperkalemia, pericarditis, uremic encephalopathy, and uremic peripheral neuropathy (Leichter & Kanwal, 1992). The options for dialysis include hemodialysis, intermittent peritoneal dialysis, continuous ambulatory peritoneal dialysis, and continuous cycling peritoneal dialysis. These may be conducted in a treatment center or at home.

Choosing the Dialysis Modality

Short-term and acute hemodialysis in infants and young children is feasible. It is generally avoided for long-term therapy because of long-term problems with vascular access and because it requires highly specialized staff and equipment available only in tertiary care pediatric centers. Peritoneal dialysis can usually be done safely and effectively in the home with infants and children of all ages, which minimizes the number of hospital visits for the child and family. Children who have previously undergone extensive abdominal surgery may not be candidates for peritoneal dialysis because of peritoneal scarring and adhesions, which decrease the peritoneal surface area available for dialysis. Peritoneal dialysis is usually not considered in children with ventriculoperitoneal shunts or in the presence of ileostomy or ureterostomy.

Peritoneal Dialysis

Peritoneal dialysis (PD) is now considered, by many, the dialysis therapy of choice in children with ESRD (Holloway, 1993). PD uses the peritoneal cavity as the semipermeable membrane through which water and solutes move by osmosis and diffusion. Access to the peritoneum is created by the surgical placement of a catheter into the peritoneal cavity. This catheter remains permanently in place in the abdomen for as long as peritoneal dialysis is needed (Steele, 1993). Dialysis fluid is aseptically instilled in the peritoneal cavity, allowed to "dwell" for a prescribed time while dialysis takes place, then drained (a peritoneal dialysis exchange). This exchange of dialysis fluid is done by gravity and can be performed manually or with an automated cycler. Most families can be taught PD at home.

Intermittent Peritoneal Dialysis. Intermittent peritoneal dialysis (IPD) requires that the child's catheter be attached to manual dialysis tubing or an automatic cycler for 10 to 12 hours at a time (usually overnight) 3 to 4 times weekly. This form of PD is used for *acute peritoneal dialysis* and is rarely used in long-term care.

Continuous Ambulatory Peritoneal Dialysis. Continuous ambulatory peritoneal dialysis (CAPD) is being used with increasing frequency. The dialysate is instilled intraperitoneally through a bag to the catheter over a period of 5 to 10 minutes. The dialysate is supplied in collapsible bags that can be clamped, folded up, and placed in the patient's pocket until the dialysate must be drained. Four to 6 hours later, the patient unclamps the catheter and allows the bag to drain by gravity. After 10 to 15 minutes, the bag fills with the solute-laden dialysate and may be discarded. A fresh bag of dialysate is then instilled. This procedure is done three to five times daily. The connection to the dialysis bag must be done using aseptic technique and is usually done using ultraviolet or heat technology.

CAPD is often preferred in children for several reasons. It provides a more continuous control of uremia and salt and water balance. This permits the child's diet to be more liberal and gives the child "machine-free" mobility. Because of the simplicity of the procedure, the child and family are able to perform the procedure simply and safely outside the hospital. The child can participate in more activities at school and with his or her peers.

Continuous Cycling Peritoneal Dialysis. Continuous cycling peritoneal dialysis (CCPD) combines the techniques of IPD and CAPD. A cycler is used for dialysis every night and a small amount of solution is left in the abdomen during the day. This solution is then drawn off in the first cycle when the machine is reattached (Fig. 36–10) (Holloway, 1993). Nightly dialysis decreases the chances of hernia related to increased abdominal pressure over a 24-hour period as in CAPD and does not interfere with the child's appetite during the day. CCPD also frees the child from interruptions during the day, allowing the parents to work and the child a full school day.

The complications of PD include peritonitis secondary to faulty sterile technique or chronic catheter infection, obstruction of the catheter, or metabolic consequences of glucose absorption from the dialysate. Over time, the efficiency of the peritoneum to act as a dialyzer may diminish. Parental fatigue and possible burnout related to daily responsibilities with home dialysis are becoming the focus for social support programs.

Hemodialysis

Hemodialysis (HD) is an extracorporeal procedure, requiring vascular access in order to remove blood from a child, circulate it through an "artificial kidney" or dialyzer, which allows the removal of solute and water by diffusive and convective transport, and return it to the body.

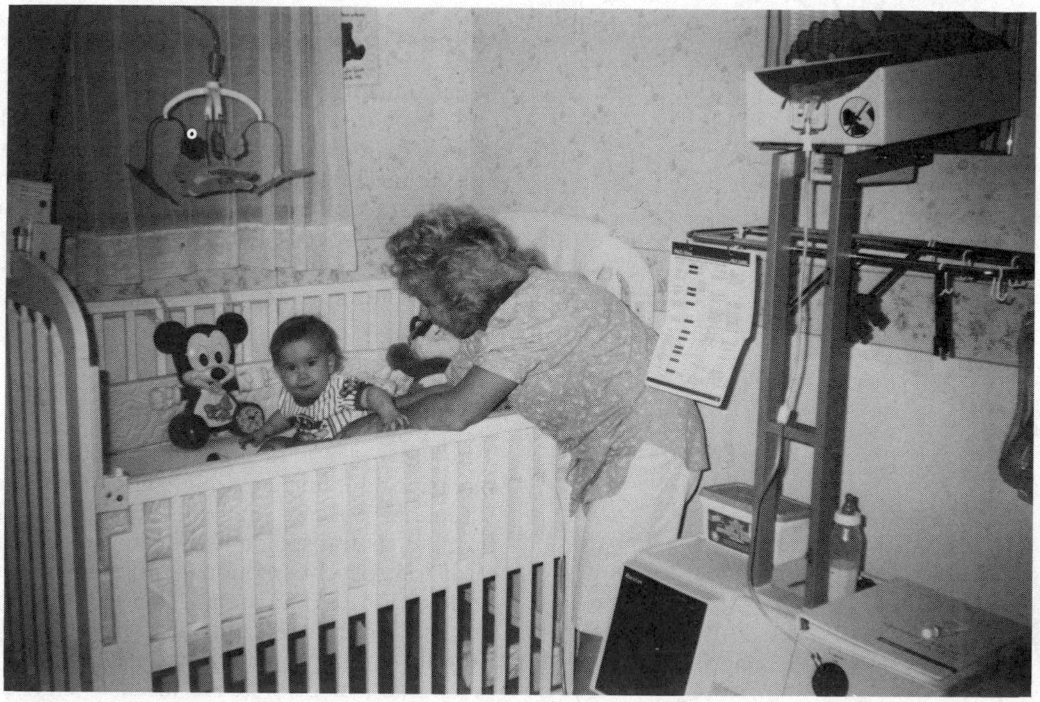

FIGURE 36 - 10. Continuous cycling peritoneal dialysis. This 1-year-old child is able to be at home because his family has taken on the responsibility to perform dialysis each night. This is the child's own bedroom in his home, with the cycler placed beside the crib where it can be attached each night to the child via a permanent dialysis catheter. This allows the child to be free all day for normal play activities. Here, the child's grandmother is providing the care required.

Vascular access for HD is frequently needed on an emergency basis. A central venous catheter (Fig. 36–11) that is specially designed for HD is usually inserted into the subclavian vein with the patient under general anesthesia. Although complications from long-term indwelling catheters are infrequent (Sherman, 1993), central venous access catheters are reserved for short-term HD.

When chronic vascular access is needed, two types are considered: (1) the arteriovenous fistula and (2) the bridging of an artery or vein with a synthetic graft (Fig. 36–12).

Once vascular access is established, the child will undergo HD approximately three times per week for 3 to 4 hours per dialysis. During this time, the child must be attached to the dialyzer and closely monitored. HD is usually performed in a hospital center with qualified people present to monitor the child during the procedure. A text on HD can supply additional information about this procedure.

Dietary restrictions must be quite severe in children receiving HD in order to prevent metabolic imbalances, hypertension, or episodes of congestive heart failure. The child should be restricted to a fluid intake of 400 ml/m^2 per day plus urinary output. The child's diet shoud be low in sodium, potassium, and phosphorus. Adherence to these restrictions will be quite difficult for the child because many "favorite" foods must be limited (e.g., soda, chocolate) (see also Table 36–13).

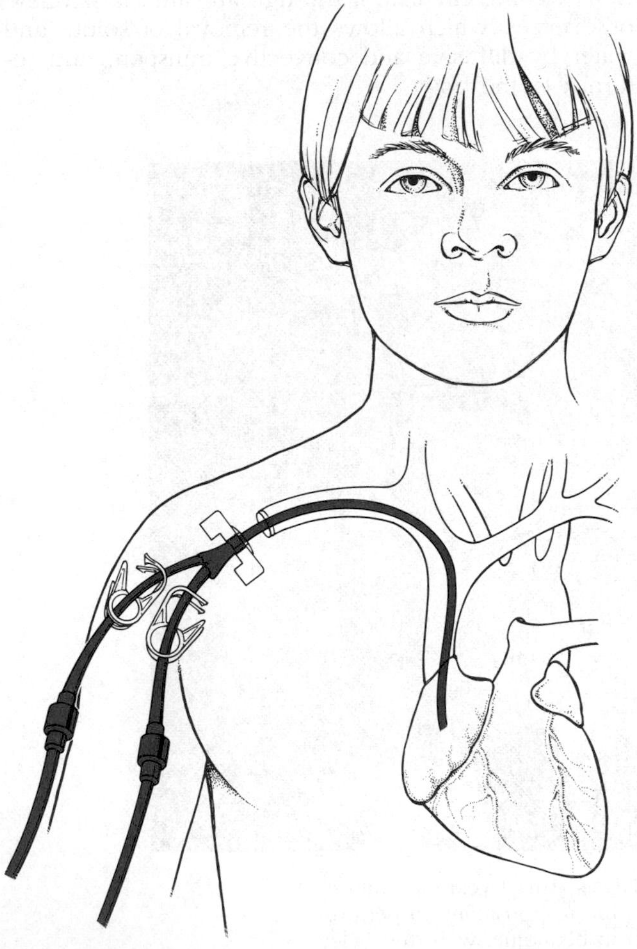

FIGURE 36 - 11. Central venous catheter for dialysis access. Usually it is inserted into the subclavian vein and the tip is advanced into the right atrium.

The child and family will require much counseling, support, and guidance concerning HD. The need for repetitive needle insertions and the strict diet may create anxiety in the child and family. The dialysis sessions are lengthy and require that the child remain somewhat immobile during the procedure. This may cause the child to be socially isolated and limit educational opportunities.

Hemofiltration

Hemofiltration or continuous arteriovenous hemofiltration (CAVH) is the slow, continuous removal of water using an artificial membrane called a "hemofilter." Like HD, it involves access to the blood stream and the use of an extracorporeal circuit and blood pump. The hemofilter removes fluid at a slow, controlled rate, preventing the rapid shifts of fluid seen with hemodialysis. CAVH is recommended for oliguria when waste products and electrolytes such as potassium are in an acceptable range. This form of water removal is used commonly in intensive care settings in children who have oliguria following cardiac surgery. The controlled removal of water (such as in normal urine excretion) allows for more efficient nourishment in the form of total parenteral nutrition.

Renal Transplantation

Renal transplantation is considered to be the optimal choice of treatment for children with ESRD, particularly with respect to restoration of the child's growth and rehabilitation. With renal transplant, the child may attain normal or near-normal renal function. The problems associated with long-term dialysis (chronic uremia, frequent invasive procedures, restricted diet) are avoided and the child is able to lead a relatively normal life.

Recipient Selection

The selected criteria used for performing renal transplants in children are quite liberal but vary with institutional policies. In general, children are excluded from renal transplant if they have severe mental retardation, psychoemotional problems, or active malignancy (Fine & Ehrlich, 1985). The presence of a lower urinary tract abnormality (e.g., obstructive uropathy), of primary renal disease (e.g., nephrotic syndrome), or of systemic disease (e.g., diabetes mellitus or systemic lupus erythematosus) does not contraindicate transplantation. Each child must be individually evaluated and the effect of the underlying disease considered.

Renal transplantation in children less than 10 kg has not been proved to be uniformly successful (Fine

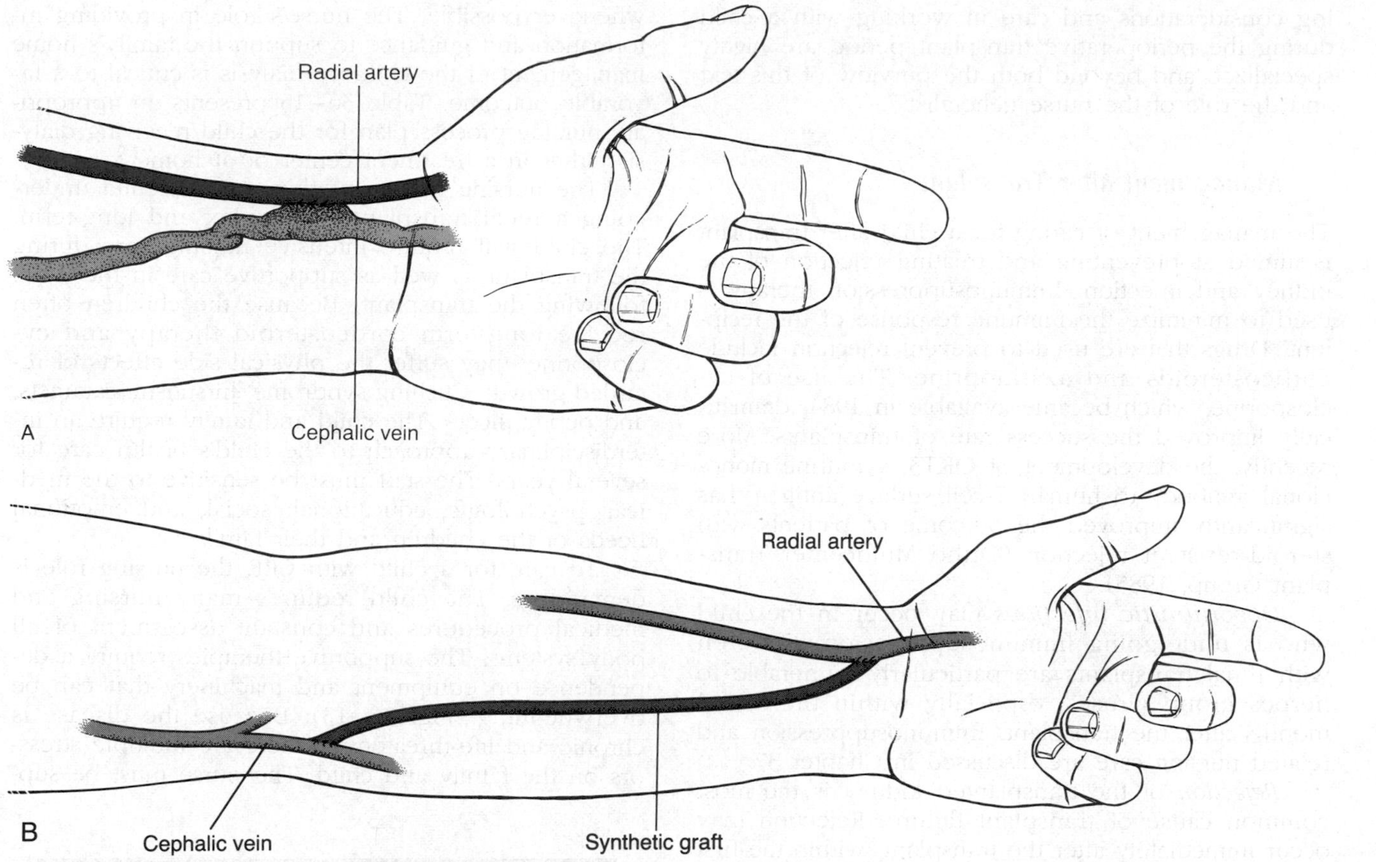

FIGURE 36 - 12. *A*, Arteriovenous fistula. Surgical creation of an anastomosis between an artery and a vein provides easy access to blood for hemodialysis. This reduces the risk of infection and makes external shunts unnecessary. *B*, Synthetic graft. An artificial conduit is created to conduct blood from an artery to a vein. This artificial conduit is the site of needle puncture for hemodialysis. Both the arteriovenous fistula and the synthetic graft must be created 2 to 6 weeks before either can be used. Although blood vessels are colored gray and red here for illustrative purposes, there is of course, significant mixing of unoxygenated blood proximal to the fistula, shunt, or graft.

& Ehrlich, 1985). These children present technical and management problems because of their small size. If possible, the transplant will be deferred until the child grows, and dialysis or supportive management meanwhile used.

Donor Selection

Children with ESRD who are eligible candidates for a renal transplant may receive the kidney from a live donor or from a cadaver (a donor who died a few hours earlier). Immunologically, the transplant has a higher survival rate if the donor is a relative to the child. Twin siblings are often the best donors because the tissue typing is almost identical. Siblings (if they are above the legal age of consent), parents, aunts, and uncles are also optimal donors.

If a relative is not available as a donor, a cadaver source may be used. The cadaver kidney is closely matched in terms of tissue type and ABO grouping to minimize rejection.

Procedure

The transplanted kidney is usually placed retroperitoneally in the anterior iliac fossa. However, in small children who weigh less than 20 kg, a transperitoneal incision is used with intraperitoneal placement. If a congenital anomaly of the lower urinary tract exists, a urinary conduit may be necessary in order to prevent reflux to the new kidney and allow for urinary drainage.

The recipient's kidneys are usually left in place. However, a bilateral nephrectomy is indicated if the kidneys are harmful to the child, as in cases of severe hypertension, persistent massive proteinuria in nephrotic syndrome, or persistent clinical pyelonephritis.

Large adult kidneys that are transplanted into children will function adequately, although they are quite large initially. Over time, the kidney will decrease in size. Conversely, cadaveric kidneys from small children that are transplanted into adolescents will hypertrophy and increase in function. The nursing considerations and care in working with a child during the perioperative transplant period are highly specialized and beyond both the purview of this text and the role of the nurse generalist.

Management after Transplant

The management of caring for a child after transplant is aimed at preventing and treating rejection of the kidney and infection. Immunosuppression therapy is used to minimize the immune response of the recipient. Drugs that are used to prevent rejection include corticosteroids and azathioprine. The use of cyclosporine, which became available in 1984, dramatically improved the success rate of transplants. More recently, the development of OKT3, a murine monoclonal antibody to human T-cell surface antigen, has significantly improved the outcome of patients with steroid-resistant rejection (Ortho Multicenter Transplant Group, 1985).

Opportunistic infections may occur in the child who is undergoing immunosuppression. Children with renal transplants are particularly vulnerable to herpes group viruses, especially within the first 3 months after the transplant. Immunosuppression and related nursing care are discussed in Chapter 37.

Rejection of the transplanted kidney is the most common cause of transplant failure. Rejection may occur immediately after the transplant, within the first few days to 1 to 2 years after the transplant, or as a chronic rejection over time.

If rejection occurs immediately after the transplant, it is related to the inability of the recipient's antibodies to accept the foreign organ. The child will manifest symptoms of fever, abdominal discomfort over the graft site, hypertension, and a decreased urine output. Serum creatinine and BUN levels will increase, reflecting the diminishing renal function. In an attempt to prevent rejection, intravenous methylprednisolone should be administered.

Chronic rejection occurs gradually and reflects diminishing renal function. The child may manifest hematuria or proteinuria, or both, and may develop symptoms of CRF. Inevitably, the loss of the transplanted kidney will occur.

The rate of growth may be enhanced in some children following transplantation, but it remains unpredictable. The cause of growth retardation has not been clearly evaluated, but most children do not attain normal adult height. Recently, recombinant growth hormone has been advocated for these children (Kher et al, 1993). Initial results from these studies appear to be promising, but long-term follow-up of patients has not yet been reported.

Nursing Care

When the child with CRF reaches ESRD, dialysis or kidney transplantation will be necessary. There is a national trend to allow home dialysis for children whenever possible. The nurse's role in providing information and guidance to support the family's home management of the child on dialysis is critical to a favorable outcome. Table 36–15 presents an appropriate nursing process plan for the child receiving dialysis either in a treatment center or at home.

The nursing role in working with a child undergoing a renal transplant is complex and long-term. The child will require intensive nursing care during the transplant as well as supportive care in the years following the transplant. Because the children often receive long-term corticosteroid therapy and cyclosporine, they suffer the physical side effects of retarded growth, Cushing syndrome, hirsutism, cataracts, and peptic ulcers. The child and family require an interdisciplinary approach to the child's health care for several years. The staff must be sensitive to the medical, psychologic, educational, social, and emotional needs of the children and their families.

To care for a child with CRF, the nursing role is demanding. The child requires many nursing and medical procedures and constant assessment of all body systems. The supportive therapies require a dependence on equipment and machinery that can be overwhelming (Fig. 36–13). Because the disease is chronic and life-threatening, there are multiple stressors on the family and child. The nurse must be sup-

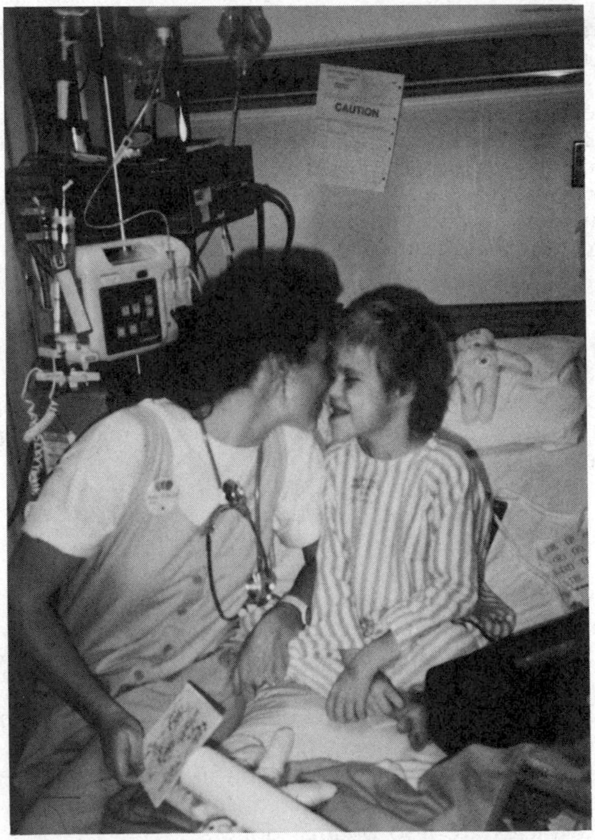

FIGURE 36-13. The nurse's focus on the specialness of the child makes the extensive equipment associated with dialysis and nutritional balance recede into the background.

TABLE 36-15

Nursing Process Plan: The Child Undergoing Dialysis Secondary to Chronic Renal Failure*

Analysis: Nursing Diagnostic Statement 1

Response and Related or Risk Factors: *High risk for injury: complications of hemodialysis:*

- *Infection,* related to repeated cannulation of the vascular access site
- *Vascular obstruction,* related to blood clots or vascular damage associated with repeated cannulation
- *Hemorrhage,* related to leakage or accidental disconnection of external shunt
- *Seizures,* related (probably) to cerebral edema associated with the response of cerebral tissue to rapid shifts in extracellular fluid osmolality

Projected Outcome: The child will undergo uncomplicated hemodialysis without the occurrence of injury (complications of hemodialysis)

Defining Characteristics

(Actual Response)

Infection:

- Redness
- Swelling
- Pain
- Warmth
- Drainage
- Fever
- Malaise
- Increased WBC

Vascular Obstruction:

- Absent or diminished bruit and thrill
- Decreased pulse below arteriovenous connection
- Decreasing redness and warmth of blood in external tubing (if an external shunt)

Hemorrhage:

- Frank bleeding from connection site

Seizures:

- Seizure activity during or after hemodialysis

Nursing Interventions

Infection Protection

Assess for evidence of infection

- Assess cannula insertion site and associated limb every 4–8 hrs
- Ask child and family to report immediately any changes in sensation, warmth, comfort, or appearance of the site
- Monitor blood values for WBC count

Initiate strategies to prevent infection

- Use and teach meticulous aseptic technique when connecting and disconnecting tubings†
- Arteriovenous fistula cannulation sites should be covered with small dressings and are well occluded
- Swimming and tub bathing are contraindicated for the child with an external shunt
- Teach child and family to assess frequently for cracks or leaks in an external shunt
- Ensure that the child, family, and other health care professionals

Evaluation Criteria

The child will be free of infection related to the site of venous access as evidenced by:

- Normal skin color
- Warm skin temperature
- Absence of swelling
- Absence of pain
- Absence of drainage
- Absence of fever
- WBC within normal limits

The child's arteriovenous connection will remain patent as evidenced by:

- Bruit heard over site
- Thrill felt over site
- Normal pulse below access site
- Warm, red blood in external shunt tubing

The child will be free of bleeding from vascular access

- The child will suffer no preventable seizure during or after dialysis
- The child will suffer no injury from preventable seizure

*This plan is appropriate for inpatient care or home care (see Chapter 22 to modify this care guide for use by the family or other lay caretakers).

†Treatment centers will vary somewhat on techniques used. Institutional policy records should be consulted.

(continued)

TABLE 36-15 *(continued)*

Defining Characteristics *(Actual Response)*	**Nursing Interventions**	**Evaluation Criteria**
	know that the limb with the access site is not to be used for IVs or for venipunctures **Assess for patency of the arteriovenous connection** • Auscultate for a bruit and feel for a thrill over the site • Check radial (or pedal) pulses bilaterally (in order to detect a decrease in arterial flow below the site) • Inspect the character of blood visible in external shunt tubing; leave part of the tubing exposed when dressing the site **Initiate strategies to reduce the incidence of obstruction** • Monitor BP carefully (a decrease in BP can cause clotting or collapse of the vein) • Alert family to the need for medical attention if child is at risk for dehydration (e.g., with vomiting and diarrhea) • Monitor closely for orthostatic hypotension if new antihypertensive is begun; teach child to change positions more slowly in the first several days after beginning drug • Ensure that child, family, and other health care professionals know that BP should *never* be measured in the limb containing the access site • Instruct child not to lie on the limb containing the access site. **Assess the integrity of the shunt tubing and connections** • Teach child and family to assess for leaks and cracks, and how to ensure connections are firmly in place after disconnecting the tubings from home hemodialysis equipment • Ensure that the child understands the consequences of accidentally disconnecting the tubing	

TABLE 36-15 (continued)

Defining Characteristics *(Actual Response)*	**Nursing Interventions**	**Evaluation Criteria**
	• Keep two bulldog clamps attached to the shunt dressing or the child's clothing for ready access in case of accidental disconnection; ensure that the child and all family members know how to use them **Assist in prescribed measures to reduce the threat of seizure** • Administer prescribed dialysate solution (to decrease rapid clearance of urea) • Administer prescribed IV mannitol during dialysis (to reduce cerebral edema) • Administer prescribed phenobarbital (to decrease risk of seizures) **Institute seizure precautions to reduce the risk of injury (see Chapter 40)**	

Analysis: Nursing Diagnostic Statement 1

Response and Related or Risk Factors: *High risk for injury: complications of peritoneal dialysis:*

- *Peritonitis,* related to repeatedly connecting and disconnecting the peritoneal catheter
- *Tunnel infection,* resulting from pathogen invasion along the insertion site of the peritoneal catheter
- *Pain,* related to peritoneal irritation associated with initial dialysis treatments, infusion of cold dialysate or hypertonic solution, and stretching and irritation of the diaphragm
- *Insufficient return of dialysate,* related to constipation
- *Protein deficiency,* related to loss of protein to the returning dialysate
- *Blood in returning solution,* related to peritoneal or intra-abdominal irritation from the catheter or to other intra-abdominal lesions

Projected Outcome: The child will undergo uncomplicated peritoneal dialysis without the occurrence of injury (complication of peritoneal dialysis)

Defining Characteristics *(Actual Response)*	**Nursing Interventions**	**Evaluation Criteria**
Peritonitis: • Fever • Rebound tenderness • General malaise • Cloudy output • CAPD effluent (dialysate return) with WBC > 100	Infection Protection **Assess for evidence of peritonitis:** • Assess and record each shift/visit: vital signs, abdominal comfort, energy level, character of effluent	**The client will be free of peritonitis as evidenced by:** • Absence of fever • Absence of nausea or rebound tenderness • Usual energy level • Clear effluent

(continued)

TABLE 36-15 *(continued)*

Defining Characteristics *(Actual Response)*	Nursing Interventions	Evaluation Criteria

• IPD or CCPD effluent with WBC > 300	• Obtain effluent specimen if peritonitis is suspected
	Initiate strategies to reduce the risk of peritonitis
	• Ensure that child, family, and other health care professionals understand that child is at risk for entry of pathogens *every* time peritoneal catheter is connected and disconnected
	• Use and teach meticulous aseptic technique in connecting and disconnecting tubings
	• Use and teach use of any of the following techniques as appropriate and as the family can afford the cost (Binkley, 1984):
	  • A Betadine block (Betadine in the distal, clamped portion of the catheter after dialysis)
	  • An in-line filter
	  • A sterile connection device to form a heat weld between dialysate bag and the catheter)
	  • An ultraviolet light (to irradiate the conduction assembly before the dialysis bag is connected)
		• WBC of CAPD effluent < 100
		• WBC of IPD or CCPD effluent < 300

Tunnel Infection: • Fever • Malaise • Warmth • Redness • Drainage at insertion site • Increased WBC • Positive wound culture	**Assess the insertion site for evidence of infection each shift/visit** • Culture any wound drainage • Obtain a blood specimen for analysis as appropriate **Institute strategies to reduce the risk of tunnel infection** • Instruct the child to shower (rather than bathe) and to avoid swimming (to reduce concentration of bacteria at insertion site) • Keep insertion site clean and dry; apply Betadine or other antiseptic according to treatment center protocol	**The client will remain free of tunnel infection as evidenced by:** • Absence of fever • Absence of warmth, redness, or drainage at insertion site • WBC within normal limits • Negative wound culture
Pain: • Report of discomfort associated with inflow or "dwell" stages of dialysis		**The client will be free of pain associated with insertion or retention of dialysate as evidenced by:** • Verbal report • Usual activity and behavior
Insufficient Return of Dialysate: • Failure after the first month of therapy to return most of the dialysate • Palpable bowel • Infrequent, hard stools that fail to achieve evacuation		**The client will remain free of constipation as evidenced by stool number and character normal for age**
Protein Deficiency: • Growth delay • Wasting of muscle tissue		**The child will not suffer a protein deficiency as evidenced by:** • Consuming the prescribed mg/kg of protein per day • Steady (although often slow) growth • Maintenance of muscle mass
Blood in Returning Solution: • Effluent positive for blood on visual inspection or upon hematest		**The client will obtain early diagnosis and treatment for significant intra-abdominal bleeding**

TABLE 36-15 *(continued)*

Defining Characteristics *(Actual Response)*	**Nursing Interventions**	**Evaluation Criteria**
	Pain Management **Assess for pain associated with dialysis; provide comfort measures** • Assure the child and family that discomfort associated with inflow on initial treatments is not uncommon and usually subsides within the first 2 wks (Binkley, 1984) • Prewarm the dialysate before instilling it • Avoid continuous use of hypertonic solution when possible • If pain exists between the shoulder blades, it may be referred from diaphragm and may be an indication to decrease amount of dialysate instilled **Assess for problems related to insufficient return of dialysate. Assess and record adequacy of bowel evacuation** • Ask child/parent about stool patterns • Palpate abdomen for evidence of full bowel **Initiate strategies to reduce the risk of constipation** • Ensure that child receives a diet adequate in natural fiber and fluids (within prescribed limits) • Encourage exercise appropriate to age and physical condition • Consult physician about use of dark syrup or mineral oil in the diet to facilitate evacuation **Assess protein intake** • Ask family to keep a food diary for a week • Weigh and measure child monthly and plot growth curve • Assess muscle mass of limbs **Assist in increasing inadequate protein intake**	

(continued)

TABLE 36-15 (continued)

Defining Characteristics (Actual Response)	Nursing Interventions	Evaluation Criteria
	• Share with family high-protein recipes and lists of protein foods that might be palatable to child • Consult with physician or nutritional clinical specialist about supplemental nutrition such as N/G tube feedings while child sleeps **Assess for blood in the returning dialysate** • Instruct the family to notify the physician of visible bloody return • Monitor hemoglobin and hematocrit levels	

Analysis: Nursing Diagnostic Statements 2 and 3

Response and Related or Risk Factors: *Body image disturbance and self-esteem disturbance, related to:*

- Negative reactions to dependency on a dialysis machine
- Possible inability to wear fashionable clothing because of peritoneal dialysis tubing
- Negative reaction to short stature associated with chronic renal disease
- Delayed appearance of secondary sexual characteristics

Projected Outcome: The child will perceive his body in a positive way. The child will express positive self-evaluation/feelings about self or self capabilities

Analysis: Nursing Diagnostic Statement 4

Response and Related or Risk Factors: *Altered role performance, related to* difficulty in achieving developmental tasks associated with the physical and social restrictions of dialysis

Projected Outcome: The child will be able to assume role behaviors necessitated by condition.

Defining Characteristics	Nursing Interventions	Evaluation Criteria
Body Image Disturbance *Subjective:* • Verbal or nonverbal response to actual or perceived change in structure (e.g., presence of cannula, short stature) and/or function of body • Verbalization of change in lifestyle as a result of body change(s) • Fear of rejection or reaction by others	Self-Esteem Enhancement **Assess the child's self-concept (see Table 14–2). Institute strategies to enhance self-concept** • Discuss with family ways they can facilitate healthy development of self-concept (see Table 14–1) • Ensure that family receives physical and emotional support for their needs so they can, in turn, meet the child's needs • Assess the family's support system	**The client will display self-valuing behaviors as evidenced by:** • Describing herself or himself (including the body) positively • Maintenance of a healthy level of social involvement with peers • Verbalizing understanding of role capabilities and making realistic plans for the future based on these capabilities

TABLE 36-15 *(continued)*

Defining Characteristics	*Nursing Interventions*	*Evaluation Criteria*
• Focus on past strength, function, or appearance • Negative feelings about body • Feelings of helplessness, hopelessness, or powerlessness • Preoccupation with change or loss • Emphasis on remaining strengths • Heightened achievement • Refusal to verify actual change *Objective*: • Not looking at body part • Not touching body part • Hiding or overexposing body part • Change in social involvement *Self-Esteem Disturbance* *Subjective*: • Self-negating verbalization (e.g., verbalizes feelings of inferiority, negativity, pessimism, shame) • Evaluates self as unable to deal with events • Rationalizes away/rejects positive feedback and exaggerates negative feedback about self *Objective*: • Change in social involvement • Acting out behavior • Poor impulse control *Altered Role Performance* *Subjective*: • Change in self-perception of role • Change in physical capacity to resume role • Change in usual patterns of responsibility	• Refer to appropriate agencies and support groups for financial, physical, and emotional support	

portive of the child and family, encouraging as normal a lifestyle as possible for the family (Frauman & Gilman, 1985). Families will require information about numerous medications, procedures, and symptoms so they can be involved in and informed about the child's care.

KEY CONCEPTS

Concepts Related to Basic Information

- Bowman capsule serves two purposes: to filter materials in and out of the glomerulus and to mark the beginning point of the renal tubule.
- Early repair of hypospadias is important, because it prevents the child from feeling embarrassed because he looks different.
- An infant with hypospadias is not circumcised because the foreskin is used in the surgical repair.
- When obstruction occurs within the pelvis or at the ureteropelvic junction, renal pelvic distention and subsequent damage can occur within hours.
- Renal scarring occurs in as many as 20 per cent of children under 5 years of age with UTI.
- Stasis of urine and subsequent backflow to the kidney places a child at high risk for infection.
- Respiratory difficulty may occur if ascites produces pressure on the diaphragm.
- Severe and continuous hydronephrosis leads to decreased GFR.
- Research shows that VUR leads to scarring at same rate, whether treatment is medical or surgical.

Concepts Related to Nursing Assessment

- Assessment of genitourinary function should be included in every history.
- Assessment of the urinary stream is a simple approach to detect urinary tract obstruction in a boy.
- Fever is less common in infants than in older children with UTI. Common signs are anorexia, vomiting, and failure-to-thrive.
- Serum creatinine does not rise until at least 50 per cent of nephrons are damaged and "stop working."
- Siblings of children with VUR should be investigated with ultrasonography since VUR is 10 times more likely to occur in siblings.
- Polydipsia and polyuria may be a sign of the kidney's inability to concentrate urine.
- Complicated UTI is suspected when child is febrile, less than 3 years of age, or a male of any age.

Concepts Related to Nursing Intervention

- Clean intermittent catheterization is based on the principle that the bladder is resistant to infection if it is emptied frequently and not overdistended.
- The postoperative dressing following hypospadias repair is removed by the surgeon.
- It is important to teach a child (when he is old enough) self-examination of testes to check for tumor following surgery for undescended testes.
- "Enteric precautions" or "careful handwashing" or "isolation" is important in children with HUS caused by VTEC (verotoxin-producing *E. coli*), since VTEC can be passed from child to nurse.
- It is important to have parents of children with nephrotic syndrome keep a permanent record of their child's course of illness, listing time of diagnoses, treatment progress, and relapses.
- Relief of constipation leads to better bladder emptying, and thus less risk of UTI.
- In nephrotic syndrome, fluids are not usually restricted unless edema progresses despite sodium restriction.
- It is preferred that HD be done in a hospital setting with children because of the rapid fluid shifts that can lead to shock and other complications.

REFERENCES

Anderson, G. F., & Smey, P. (1985). Current concepts in the management of common urologic problems in infants and children. *Pediatric Clinics of North America, 32,* 1145.

Bergstein, J. M. (1992). Nephrologic diseases. In R. E. Behrman (Ed.), *Nelson textbook of pediatrics* (14th ed., pp 1323–1358). Philadelphia: WB Saunders.

Bernhardt, J. (1993). Renal/genitourinary disorders. In P. Beachy & J. Deacon (Eds.), *Core curriculum for neonatal intensive care nursing (NAACOG)* (pp 365–393). Philadelphia: WB Saunders.

Birmingham Reflux Study (1987). Prospective trial of operative vs. non-operative treatment of severe vesicoureteric reflux: 5 year observation in 96 children. *British Medical Journal, 295,* 237-241.

Bock, G. (1992). Acute renal failure. In K. K. Kher, & S. P. Makker (Eds.), *Clinical pediatric nephrology.* New York: McGraw-Hill.

Brouhard, B. H. (1991). Hereditary renal disorders. In A. M. Rudolph, *Rudolph's pediatrics* (19th ed. pp 1273–1276). Norwalk, CT: Appleton & Lange.

Duckett, J. W. (1992). Hypospadias, epispadias, and exstrophy. In C. M. Edelmann (Jr.), J. Bernstein, S. R. Meadow, A. Spitzer, and L. B. Travis (Eds.), *Pediatric kidney disease* (2nd ed.), Vol II. Boston: Little Brown & Company, pp 2111–2120.

Duckett, J. W., & Caldamone, A. A. (1985). Bladder and urachus. In P. P. Kelalis, L. R. King, A. B. Belman (Eds.). *Clinical pediatric urology* (2nd ed.). Philadelphia: WB Saunders.

Durbin, W. A., Peter, G. (1984). Management of urinary tract infections in infants and children. *Pediatric Infectious Disease, 3,* 564–574.

Fernandes, E., Vernier, R., & Gonzalez, R. (1991). The unstable bladder in children. *Journal of Pediatrics, 118,* 831–837.

Frauman, A. C., & Gilman, C. M. (1990). Care of the family of the child with end-stage renal disease. *American Nephrology Nurse Association Journal, 17,* 383–386.

Gearhart, J. P., Herzberg, G., & Jeffs, R. D. (1991). Childhood urolithiasis: Experiences and advances. *Pediatrics, 87,* 445–450.

Gonzales, R. (1992). Urologic disorders in infants and children. In R. E. Behrman (Ed.), *Nelson textbook of pediatrics* (14th ed.). Philadelphia: WB Saunders.

Hadziselimovic, F., et al. (1975). Surgical correction of cryptorchidism at 2 years. *Journal of Pediatric Surgery, 10,* 19–26.

Hadziselimovic, F., & Herzog, B. (1976). The meaning of the Leydig cell in relation to the etiology of cryptorchidism. *Journal of Pediatric Surgery, 11,* 1–8.

Holloway, M. S. (1993). CAPD/CCPD disorders in children. In A. R. Nissenson, & R. N. Fine (Eds.), *Pediatric dialysis in dialysis therapy* (2nd ed.). Philadelphia: Hanley & Belfus.

International Reflux Study in Children. (1985). International system of radiographic grading of vesicoureteric reflux. *Pediatric Radiology, 15,* 105–109.

Karmali, M. A., Arbus, G. S., Petric, M., Patrick, M. L., Roscoe, M., Shair, J., & Lior, H. (1988). Hospital-acquired *Escherichia coli* 0157:147 associated haemolytic uraemic syndrome in a nurse. *Lancet, 1,* 526 (letter to editor).

Kher, K. K., Buzzetta, P. C., & Alarif, L. (1992). Renal transplantation. In K. K. Kher, & S. P. Makker (Eds.), *Clinical pediatric nephrology*. New York: McGraw-Hill.

Kim, M. S., & Grupe, W. E. (1986). The nephrotic syndrome. In S. S. Gellis, & B. M. Kagan (Eds.), *Current pediatric therapy 12* (pp 366–369). Philadelphia: WB Saunders.

Kodama, B. H., & Winslow, R. T. (1991). Hypospadias. In F. F. Marshall (Ed.), *Operative urology* (pp 513–527). Philadelphia: WB Saunders.

Leichter, H. E., & Kanwal, K. K. (1992). Management of end-stage renal failure—Dialysis therapy. In K. K. Kher & S. P. Makker (Eds.), *Clinical pediatric nephrology*. New York: McGraw-Hill.

Levitt, S. B., & Weiss, R. A. (1985). Vesicoureteral reflux. In P. P. Kelalis, L. R. King, & A. B. Belman (Eds.), *Clinical pediatric urology* (2nd ed.). Philadelphia: WB Saunders.

Loirat, C., Baudouin, V., Sonsino, E., Mariani-Kurdjian, P., & Elion, J. (1993). Hemolytic uremic syndrome in the child. In J. P. Grümfeld, J. F. Bach, H. Kreis, & M. Maxwell (Eds.), *Advances in nephrology*. St. Louis: Mosby Year Book.

Malek, R. S. (1985). Urolithiasis. In P. P. Kelalis, L. R. King, & A. B. Belman (Eds.), *Clinical pediatric urology* (2nd ed.). Philadelphia: WB Saunders.

Mitchell, N., & Stapleton, F. B. (1990). Routine admission urinalysis examination in pediatric patients: A poor value. *Pediatrics, 86,* 345–349.

Montagnino, B. A., Gonzales, E. T. Jr., & Roth, D. R. (1988). Open catheter drainage after urethral surgery. *Journal of Urology, 140,* 1250–1252.

Moore, K. I. (1988). The urogenital system In *The developing human* (4th ed., pp 246–285). Philadelphia: WB Saunders.

Ortho Multicenter Transplant Study Group. (1985). A randomized clinical trial of OKT3 monoclonal antibody for acute rejection of cadaveric renal transplants. *New England Journal of Medicine, 314,* 1219.

Osofsky, S. G., & Lewy, J. E. (1985). Acute renal failure. In J. D. Dickerman & J. F. Lucey (Eds.), *Smith's The critically ill child: Diagnosis and medical management* (3rd ed., p 288). Philadelphia: WB Saunders.

Ramirez, F., Brouhard, B. H., Travis, L. B., & Ellis, E. N. (1982). Ideopathic membranous nephropathy in children. *Journal of Pediatrics, 101,* 667.

Schact, R. G. (1985). Acute renal failure. In S. S. Zimmerman & J. H. Gilden (Eds.), *Critical care pediatrics* (pp 313–327). Philadelphia: WB Saunders.

Sherbotie, J. R., & Cornfeld, D. (1991). Management of urinary tract infections in children. *Medical Clinics of North America, 75,* 327–338.

Sherman, N. J. (1993). Acute and chronic vascular access in children. In A. R. Nissenson & R. N. Fine (Eds.), *Pediatric dialysis in dialysis therapy* (2nd ed.). Philadelphia: Mosby Year Book, Hanley & Belfus.

Siegler, R. L. (1988). Management of hemoloytic uremic syndrome. *Journal of Pediatrics, 112,* 1014–1020.

Sinai-Frieman, L., Salusky, I. B., & Fine, R. N. (1989). Use of subcutaneous recombinant human erythropoietin in children undergoing continuous cycling peritoneal dialysis. *Journal of Pediatrics, 114,* 550–554.

Spencer, J. R., & Schaeffer, A. J. (1986). Pediatric urinary tract infections. *Urologic Clinics of North America, 13,* 661–672.

Steele, B. T. (1993). Infant and neonatal peritoneal dialysis. In A. R. Nissenson & R. N. Fine (Eds.), *Pediatric dialysis in dialysis therapy* (2nd ed.). Philadelphia: Mosby Year Book, Hanley & Belfus.

Steele, B. T., & DeMaria, J. (1992). A new perspective on the natural history of vesicoureteric reflux. *Pediatrics, 90,* 3–32.

Stull, T. L., & Lipuma, J. J. (1991). Epidemiology and natural history of urinary tract infections in children. *Medical Clinics of North America, 75,* 287–297.

Travis, L. B., & Brouhard, B. H. (1991). Infections of the urinary tract. In M. R. Abraham (Ed.), *Rudolph's pediatrics* (19th ed.). Norwalk, CT: Appleton & Lange.

Travis, L. B. (1991). The kidneys and the urinary tract. In M. R. Abraham (Ed.), *Rudolph's pediatrics* (19th ed.). Norwalk, CT: Appleton & Lange.

van den Abbecle, A. D., et al. (1987). Vesicoureteral reflux in asymptomatic siblings of patients with known reflux: Radionuclide cystography. *Pediatrics, 79,* 147–153.

Vickers, D., Ahmad, T., Coulthard, M. G. (1991). Diagnosis of urinary tract infection in children: Fresh urine microscopy or culture? *Lancet, 338,* 767–770.

Wallen, L., Zeller, P., Goessler, M., Connor, E., & Yogev, R. (1985). Single-dose amikacin treatment of first childhood *E. coli* lower urinary tract infections. *Journal of Pediatrics, 103,* 315–319.

White, R. H. R. (1987). Management of urinary tract infection. *Archives of Disease in Childhood, 62,* 421–427.

White, R. H. R. (1989). Vesicoureteric reflux and renal scarring. *Archives of Disease in Childhood, 64,* 407–412.

BIBLIOGRAPHY

Ashcraft, K. W. (1990). *Pediatric urology*. Philadelphia: WB Saunders.

Briscoe, D. M., Kim, M. S., Lillehei, C., Eraklis, A. J., Levey, R. H., & Harmon, W. E. (1992). Outcome of renal transplantation in children less than two years of age. *Kidney International, 42,* 657–662.

Callaway, T. W., Lingardh, G., Basata, S., & Sylven, M. (1992). Percutaneous nephrolithotomy in children. *Journal of Urology, 148,* 1067–1068.

Dagan, R., Einhorn, M., Lang, R., Pomeranz, A., Wolach, B., Miron, D., Raz, R., Weintraub, A., Steinberger, J., & Isaachson, M. (1992). Once daily cefixime compared with twice daily trimethoprim/sulfamethoxazole for treatment of urinary tract infection in infants and children. *Journal of Pediatric Infectious Diseases, 11,* 198–203.

Elder, J. S., Snyder, H. M., Peters, C., Arant, B., Hawtrey, C. E., Hurwitz, R. S., Parrott, T. S., & Weiss, R. A. (1992). Variations in practice among urologists and nephrologists treating children with vesicoureteral reflux. *Journal of Urology, 148,* 714–717.

Fine, R. N., Ehrlich, R. M. (1985). Renal transplantation in children. In P. P. Kelalis, L. R. King, & A. B. Belman (Eds.). *Clinical pediatric urology* (2nd ed.). Philadelphia: WB Saunders.

Frauman, A. C., & Gilman, C. M. (1985). Normal life: A goal for the child with chronic renal failure. *American Nephrology Nurse Association Journal, 12,* 192–195.

Kelalis, P., King, L., & Belman, A. (Eds.) (1992). *Clinical pediatric urology* (3rd ed.). Philadelphia: WB Saunders.

Lopez, E. L., Devoto, S., Fayad, A., Canepa, C., Morrow, A. L., & Cleary, T. G. (1992). Association between severity of gastrointestinal prodrome and long-term prognosis in classic hemolytic-uremic syndrome. *Journal of Pediatrics, 120,* 210–215.

Miller, K., Goldberg, S., & Atkin, B. (1989). Nocturnal enuresis: Experience with long-term use of intranasally administered desmopressin. *Journal of Pediatrics, 114,* 723–726.

Moffat, M. (1989). Nocturnal enuresis: Psychologic implications of treatment and nontreatment. *Journal of Pediatrics, 114,* 697–704.

Nissenson, A. R., & Fine, R. N. (Eds.). (1993). *Dialysis therapy* (2nd ed.). St. Louis: CV Mosby.

Norgaards, J., Rittig, S., & Djurhuus, J. (1989). Nocturnal enuresis: An approach to treatment based on pathogenesis. *Journal of Pediatrics, 114,* 705–710.

Peratoner, L., Messi, G., Mascarin, M., & Marchi, A. G. (1992). Long-term effect of a protocol for the diagnosis and treatment of urinary tract infection. *Child Nephrology and Urology, 12,* 19–23.

Reinberg, V., DeCastano, I., Gonzalez, R. (1992). Influence of initial therapy on progression of renal failure and body growth in children with posterior urethral valves. *Journal of Urology, 148,* 532–533.

Scott, J. E. S., Lee, R. E. J., Hunter, E. W., Coulthard, M. G., & Matthews, J. N. S. (1991). Ultrasound screening of newborn urinary tract. *Lancet, 338,* 782–788, 1571–1573.

Smellie, J. M. (1992). Commentary: Management of children with severe vesicureteral reflux. *Journal of Urology, 148,* 1676–1678.

Southwest Pediatric Nephrology Study Group. (1985). Focal segmental glomerulosclerosis in children with idiopathic nephrotic syndrome. *Kidney International, 27,* 442.

Springate, J. E., Christensen, S. L., & Feld, L. G. (1992). Serum creatinine level and renal function in children. *American Journal of Diseases of Children, 146,* 1232–1235.

Warady, B. A., Alon, U., & Hellerstein, S. (1991). Primary nocturnal enuresis: Current concepts about an old problem. *Pediatric Annals, 20,* 246–255.

CHAPTER • 37

Altered Immune Function

Ann Harkins

NURSING PROCESS PLANS

NPP: The Child on Corticosteroid Therapy, Table 37–4

NPP: The Child with Atopic Dermatitis, Table 37–18

RELATED TOPICS

Immunizations, Chapter 10

Impact of chronic illness, Chapter 19

Impact of death and dying, Chapter 20

Techniques for administration of eye and nose drops, Chapter 23

Asthma, Chapter 32

Seborrheic dermatitis, diaper dermatitis, oral thrush, Chapter 38

Graft-versus-host disease, Chapter 42

LEARNING OBJECTIVES

- **Identify the components of the normal immune response.**
- **List the mitigating factors that affect immune response.**
- **Describe the types of altered immune disorders and the major diseases within each type.**
- **Discuss the nurse's role in educating parents about immune disorders.**
- **Plan appropriate nursing care for a child with an immune disorder.**

The immunologic system is designed to protect the body through the mechanisms of defense, homeostasis, and surveillance (Bellanti, 1985). It defends against invasion by microorganisms, promotes homeostasis by removing cellular wastes and worn-out cells, and monitors for and destroys abnormal cells (e.g., tumor cells) that may arise within the body. Considering the importance of these functions, it may seem curious that the immune system has remained relatively obscure. Whereas even elementary school children can recite the basic functions of the heart and lungs, the functions of such immune system organs as the thymus and spleen may puzzle considerably more sophisticated students. Although theories of cellular and humoral immunity were postulated in 1908, not until the 1930s were functions of specific antibodies identified; not until the 1960s did the role of the thymus become better understood; in the 1980s the role of heredity became central to the understanding of the immune response (Bellanti, 1985). Current and future research

promises to further explain individual differences in the ability of the immune system to protect the body from pathogens, to eradicate mutant cells arising within the body, and to differentiate between *self* and foreign proteins.

Although normally protective in function, the immune system is subject to physiologic alterations that can be quite harmful to the host. The immune elements that defend against invading organisms may react inappropriately, leading to *hypersensitivity* (allergy), or underreact, resulting in *hyposensitivity* (immunodeficiency disorders). The homeostatic mechanisms that catabolize cellular wastes may malfunction and selectively destroy healthy tissues, a phenomenon termed "autosensitivity" (autoimmune disease). The surveillance mechanism may fail to identify and dispose of cell mutations, the proliferation of which may lead to malignant disease. This chapter presents the normal immune response and the alterations in that response that lead to (1) certain autoimmune or chronic inflammatory diseases, (2) allergy, and (3) immunodeficiency. Malignant diseases are discussed in Chapter 42.

Structure and Function of the Immune System

The Normal Immune Response

The organs and tissues that constitute the immune system are spread diffusely throughout the body. Lockey and Bukantz (1987a) defined the nature and function of the immune system according to primary and secondary organs. Lymphocytes designated as "T-cells" and "B-cells" develop in the primary (or central) organs and then migrate to secondary (or peripheral) organs where they reside in their mature form. The primary organs and tissues of the immune system are the thymus and the bone marrow. The secondary organs and tissues are the spleen, lymph nodules and nodes (e.g., tonsils, Peyer patches), gut-associated lymphoid tissue (GALT), bronchus-associated lymphoid tissue (BALT), skin-associated lymphoid tissue (SALT), and the blood (Fig. 37–1). These organs and tissues are important to immunity because of their relationship to both nonspecific and specific immune mechanisms.

Both T-lymphocytes and B-lymphocytes originate from the same type of stem cell (Fig. 37–2), but they are prepared for their unique immune functions in different organs. T-lymphocytes further differentiate in the thymus, and B-lymphocytes mature in the bone marrow.

The spleen functions as a filter for blood and lymph. It screens out foreign particles and organisms, along with worn-out blood cells, to allow phagocytosis by the many macrophages that reside in splenic tissue. Children who sustain splenic injury resulting in splenectomy, or who have a disease that leads to splenic atrophy, are at increased risk of infection without this protective mechanism.

The lymph nodes and nodules (including the tonsils and Peyer patches of the intestine) are filters within the lymphatic drainage system that remove particulate matter and microorganisms. Lymphatic channels are found in all body tissues except the cornea and the central nervous system (CNS); the CNS is protected by the lymphocytes within its rich blood supply (Lockey & Bukantz, 1987a).

The GALT, BALT, and SALT represent conceptual "subdivisions" of the immune system that emphasize the importance of the gastrointestinal and respiratory tracts and the skin as defenses between the body and foreign antigens. All these subsystems contain macrophages. In addition, the GALT and BALT are protected by immunoglobulin A (IgA), a class of antibodies that are secreted by mucous membranes.

Because the immune system is designed to protect the body from foreign proteins, it is essential for immunologic cells to differentiate between the body's own healthy tissues and the foreign proteins that they seek to destroy. This differentiation is based on a genetic code that determines cell surface protein configurations in body cells.

Human Leukocyte Antigen

Cells of the immune system identify foreign proteins according to a "self" versus "nonself" scheme of recognition that is determined by the arrangement of genes on the short arm of the sixth chromosome. This chromosomal region is referred to as the "human leukocyte antigen" (HLA). The unique arrangement of surface proteins that results from the HLA blueprint acts as a signal for immune cells.* Cells with surface

* The configuration of cell surface proteins is also pertinent for cells other than the leukocyte. Leukocytes, however, are the cells that have been most thoroughly studied at this time, and that is why HLA configurations are frequently denoted in the genetics literature. As cell surface mapping is completed on other types of cells, scientists will begin using those designations as well.

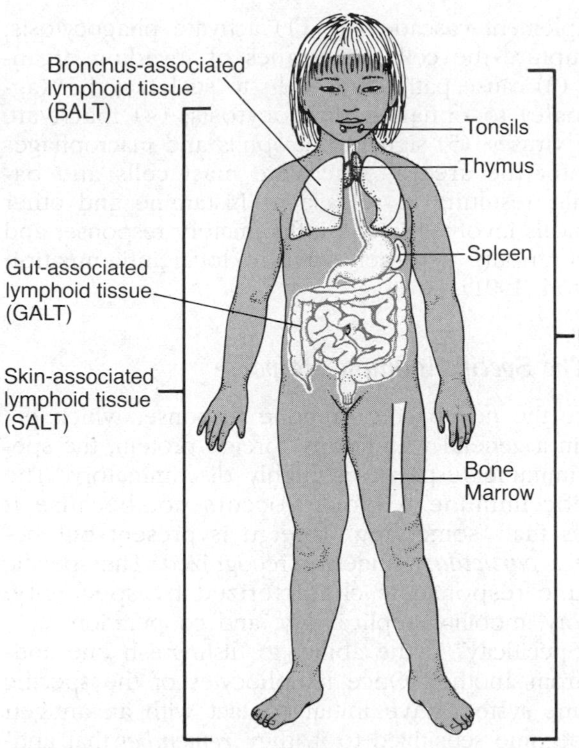

FIGURE 37-1. Organs and tissues of the immune system.

proteins in a configuration matching that individual's HLA are recognized as "self"; proteins configured in any other way are identified as "foreign." Foreign proteins are dealt with in one of the following ways:

1. A state of *tolerance* develops in which the body fails to respond to that protein (for example, as when repeated small doses of an antigen are injected to desensitize an allergic individual to that antigen).

2. A nonspecific immune reaction occurs involving phagocytosis and inflammation.

3. A specific immune response occurs with involvement of cellular and humoral mechanisms.

Tolerance is discussed further in the section on allergy. A description of the nonspecific and specific immune responses follows.

The Nonspecific Immune Response

The nonspecific immune response is the first immune reaction to a foreign protein, such as a bacterium and a virus. Phagocytosis, the inflammatory response, and the complement system constitute this primary immune response.*

Phagocytosis. The major phagocytes are *monocytes* (which become macrophages) and *neutrophils* (also known as polymorphonuclear leukocytes [PMLs]). Both monocytes and neutrophils are produced from nonlymphoid stem cells in the bone marrow. Monocytes circulate in the blood for only a brief time before they migrate to the body tissues and develop into macrophages. Tissue *macrophages* can respond quickly to infectious organisms because they are already present in the tissue. The macrophages are highly specialized to engulf and destroy certain bacteria, damaged or worn-out body cells, neoplastic cells, colloidal materials, and macromolecules such as antigen-antibody complexes (Bellanti, 1985).

Neutrophils, unlike tissue macrophages, remain in the circulating blood until they are signaled by an infectious or inflammatory process to enter the tissues. Chemicals released within injured tissues during the inflammatory process facilitate the escape of neutrophils through the vascular walls. These chemical mediators and others stimulated by encounters of microorganisms with the complement cascade (de-

* The complement system also comes into play as a result of the antigen-antibody reaction within the specific immune response.

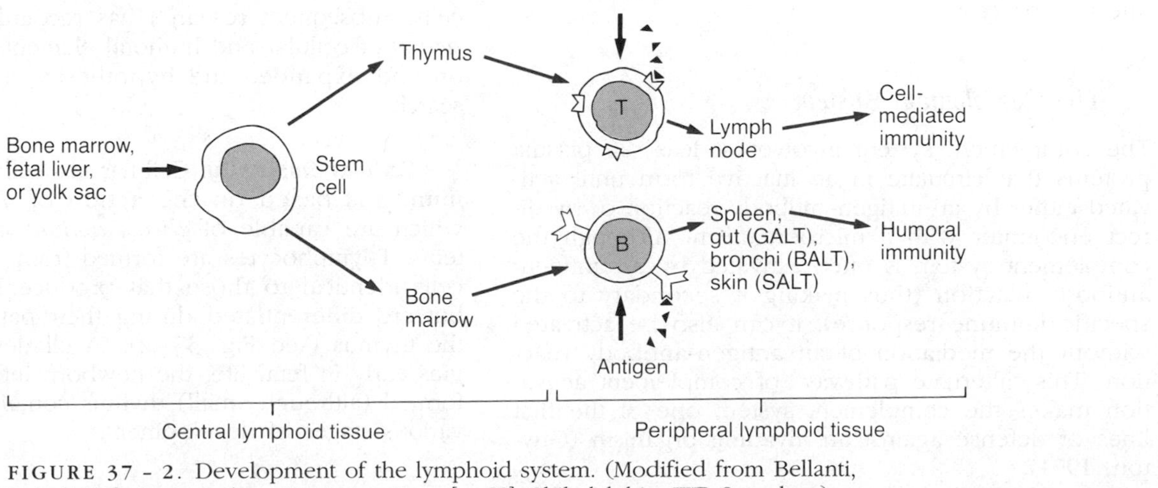

FIGURE 37-2. Development of the lymphoid system. (Modified from Bellanti, J. A. [1985]. *Immunology: Basic processes.* [p. 33]. Philadelphia: WB Saunders.)

scribed later) provide a directional signal for neutrophils to follow as they migrate to the area of tissue injury (Lockey & Bukantz, 1987a). Once at the tissue site, neutrophils engulf and digest susceptible organisms in a phagocytic manner similar to that of macrophages.

The Inflammatory Response. The inflammatory response is not unique to immune reactions. It occurs in response to tissue injury, whether that injury is caused by bacteria, trauma, chemicals, heat, or other phenomena. In the inflammatory response, damaged cells release large quantities of histamine, bradykinin, serotonin, and prostaglandins. These chemicals increase the blood flow to the localized site and increase the permeability of venous capillaries, allowing large quantities of fluid and proteins to leak into the tissues. The chemicals that cause capillary permeability facilitate the immune response by (1) allowing entry of phagocytic neutrophils into the tissues and (2) drawing the neutrophils to the site of greatest antigen concentration. This "drawing" power is termed "chemotaxis" and is essential to phagocytosis. Chemotaxis is augmented by the complement system.

The *cardinal signs of inflammation* are redness, heat, swelling, and pain. Despite these unpleasant effects of the inflammatory response, *inflammation is a protective mechanism* that facilitates phagocytosis and limits the spread and replication of at least some organisms (Fulginiti, 1992). Increased blood flow manifests as erythema and heat; the local heat and characteristic systemic fever of microbial invasion are thought to inhibit the multiplication of microbes. The inflammatory exudate that develops from the fluids that escape the blood stream provides a medium for the phagocytic process.

Pain associated with inflammation may occur for several reasons. Endogenous chemical substances such as bradykinin, serotonin, histamines, and prostaglandins are known to have an irritating effect on the tissues. The tissue tension-pressure exerted by the edema also may be a source of pain. Pain, in itself, is protective, however, by alerting the host to the infective process.

The Complement System

The complement system involves at least 20 plasma proteins that circulate in an inactive form until activated either by an antigen-antibody reaction or by direct encounter with a microorganism. Although the complement system is often activated by an antigen-antibody reaction (thus making it secondary to the specific immune response), it can also be activated without the mediation of an antigen-antibody reaction. This "alternate pathway" of complement activation makes the complement system one of the first lines of defense against an invading organism (Guyton, 1991).

Once activated, the proteins grouped within the nine complement components work sequentially (the "complement cascade") to (1) activate phagocytosis; (2) rupture the cell membranes of invading organisms; (3) cause pathogenic cells to stick together (agglutinate) to enhance phagocytosis; (4) inactivate some viruses; (5) signal neutrophils and macrophages to enter the area; (6) activate mast cells and basophils, resulting in release of histamine and other chemicals involved in the inflammatory response; and (7) contribute in other ways to local inflammation (Guyton, 1991).

The Specific Immune Response

Unlike the nonspecific immune response, which occurs in a general way to any foreign protein, the specific immune response is highly discriminatory. The specific immune response occurs not because it senses that "something" foreign is present but because a *particular* antigen is recognized. The specific immune response is characterized by specificity, memory, mobility, replicability, and cooperation.

"Specificity" is the ability to distinguish one antigen from another. Once lymphocytes of the specific immune system have initial contact with an antigen and become sensitized to it, they *remember* that antigen and, on subsequent exposure, react more swiftly and effectively to eliminate it. The elements of the specific immune system are mobile; they travel throughout the body. They also frequently reproduce, or *replicate,* when activated. The nonspecific and specific immune responses interact *cooperatively* to rid the body of potentially harmful proteins. There is constant interaction among lymphoid and nonlymphoid cells, antibodies, and secretory chemical mediators.

"Lymphocytes" are the essential element of both cellular and humoral immunity. Cellular and humoral immunity began as separate theories proposed by different immunologic researchers. The emphasis of the cellular theory was on the "biologic effects of intact cells involved in the host's response to foreignness" (Bellanti, 1985, p 4), whereas the humoral theory emphasized the study of chemical products produced by cells. Subsequent research has recognized the *interaction* of cellular and humoral elements and has built on and expanded the hypotheses of the early researchers.

Cellular Immunity. Cellular (or cell-mediated) immunity is based on the action of *T-lymphocytes,* which are capable of *direct action* on foreign proteins. T-lymphocytes are formed from lymphoid stem cells identical to those that produce B-lymphocytes but are differentiated during their pathway through the thymus (see Fig. 37–2). T-cell development begins early in fetal life; the newborn infant has a fully formed (although small) thymus containing T-cells at various stages of development.*

* The thymus reaches adult size at about 12 years of age.

T-lymphocytes are not a single cell type but a family of cells with different effector and regulatory functions. "Effector T-cells" recognize and destroy foreign proteins (antigens) without the aid of antibodies. The two types of effector T-cells are cytotoxic (Tc) cells and delayed hypersensitivity (Tdh) cells. Cytotoxic cells act directly on a virus-infected cell. In killing the virus, however, the host cell is usually killed as well. Tdh cells, as their name implies, are responsible for delayed hypersensitivity (allergic) reactions such as contact dermatitis. Tdh cells are activated directly by an antigen and secrete chemical mediator substances, lymphokines, which produce localized inflammation and enhance phagocytosis.

"Regulator T-cells" help regulate the actions of B-lymphocytes. They include T-helper cells (Th or T4 cells) and T-suppressor cells (Ts or T8 cells). T4 cells help activate B-lymphocytes. T8 cells secrete chemicals that decrease the action of B-lymphocytes, leading to "down-regulation" of immune activity (Lockey & Bukantz, 1987a).

Humoral Immunity. Contrary to early speculation, the fetus and neonate have an active, although immature, immunologic system (Lawton & Cooper, 1989). The progressive development of the immune system can be noted in normal variations of humoral components found in serum levels (Table 37–1).

Humoral immunity depends on the antibody-producing properties of B-lymphocytes. B-lymphocytes originate in the bone marrow and are activated in response to antigen. On activation, these lymphocytes

TABLE 37–1
Normal Variations in Humoral Components (unit/ml ± 2 SD) Found in Serum Levels (mg/dl ± 2 SD)

			IgM		
Age	**IgG**	**IgA**	**Male**	**Female**	**IgE**
Birth	800–1792	0–8	0–23	0–23	0–26
1 mo	513–1183	4–21	17–67	22–85	0–26
2 mos	313–827	8–55	23–89	29–114	0–44
3 mos	261–687	13–71	26–106	33–136	0–60
4 mos	224–661	15–84	28–117	36–150	0–54
5 mos	261–713	15–88	30–123	39–157	0–54
6 mos	278–766	17–95	32–128	40–164	0–57
7 mos	305–809	17–105	33–134	43–171	0–57
8 mos	322–879	19–109	35–140	44–178	0–57
9 mos	365–948	19–120	36–145	46–185	0–480
10 mos	392–1027	21–126	36–150	47–192	0–480
11 mos	426–1122	23–137	38–156	49–200	0–480
1 yr	452–1192	25–158	39–156	50–200	1–525
2 yrs	539–1401	34–168	47–184	61–236	<20–100
3 yrs	600–1575	40–235	51–201	66–257	<20–200
4 yrs	626–1653	46–288	53–201	67–257	<20–300
5 yrs	661–1749	59–328	54–201	68–257	<20–400
6 yrs	687–1879	65–368	54–201	68–257	<20–400
7 yrs	713–1905	69–393	54–201	68–257	<20–400
8 yrs	722–1940	76–420	54–202	68–257	<20–400
9 yrs	740–2001	84–445	54–203	68–258	<20–400
10 yrs	748–2001	92–473	54–206	68–260	20–500
11 yrs	748–2001	96–498	54–212	68–264	20–500
12 yrs	748–2001	97–525	54–217	68–267	20–500
13 yrs	748–2001	99–550	54–217	70–271	20–500
14 yrs	748–2001	103–578	56–223	71–278	20–500
15 yrs	748–2001	105–603	56–233	71–285	20–500
Adult	800–1801	113–563	54–222	62–250	<20–300

Adapted from Steele, R. (1983). *Immunology for the practicing physician.* Norwalk CT: Appleton-Century-Croft.

mature into plasma cells that synthesize immunoglobulins (antibodies) specific to the presenting antigen. The major classes of immunoglobulins are IgM, IgG, IgA, IgD, and IgE. These classes contain various antigen-specific antibodies. Their functions are the following (Lockey & Bukantz, 1987a, b; Miller, 1988; Young & Geha, 1985):

- IgM First line of defense; first antibody formed in response to an antigen; activates complement.
- IgG Major antibody against bacteria and viruses; neutralizes toxins and enhances phagocytosis. Activates complement. The only antibody to cross the placenta; the basis for passive immunity in the first 3 to 6 months of life.
- IgA Protects mainly secretory surfaces of mucous membranes where antigen contact is nonvascular; found in saliva, tears, bronchial mucosa, nasal mucosa, mucous secretions of the small intestine, vagina, and breast milk.
- IgD Functions remain largely unknown. May have a role in the differentiation of B-cells.
- IgE Responsible for stimulating mast cells to release chemical agents that cause allergic reactions; effective against parasitic infections and may defend against antigens penetrating the mucosa of the skin and the gastrointestinal and respiratory tracts. Appears to be involved in some viral infections such as respiratory syncytial virus (Ch. 32) and to be instrumental in potentiating the inflammatory response.

The various elements of the immune system have been discussed separately. To understand the complex protective immune functions, however, it is necessary to consider the ways in which these elements interact. The reactions that occur on initial and prolonged or subsequent antigen invasion are described in the following section.

Initial Immune Response to an Antigen

The body's response to a new antigen is nonspecific. The foreign protein (antigen) activates the immune system in one of two ways: either by activating the complement cascade (which promotes both the inflammatory response and phagocytosis) or by direct contact with tissue macrophages. Activated macrophages secrete chemicals that, in turn, stimulate activation and proliferation of both T-lymphocytes and B-lymphocytes. More specifically, activation of lymphocytes involves

- "Presentation" of the antigen to a T-cell by a macrophage.
- Activation of the T-cell by the encounter with the antigen and by the chemicals secreted by the macrophage.
- Activation of B-cells by T-helper cells.
- Production (by B-cells) of antigen-specific antibodies.

This process of lymphocyte activation requires some time, and several days pass before a rise in serum antibodies can be detected (Lockey & Bukantz, 1987a). Because of this lag time in enlisting the help of lymphocytes, phagocytosis and the cell-killing effects of complement are the major weapons in the initial immune response.

The invading protein may be contained and killed by phagocytosis that occurs within the inflammatory exudate or by the attack of late-acting proteins of the complement system on the foreign cell membrane. This initial response may, however, be unsuccessful either because of characteristics of the antigen, such as large quantities of antigenic cells and antiphagocytic properties of the cells, or because of an immature or unhealthy immune system (Fig. 37–3). When the antigen persists despite the initial nonspecific immune response, the outcome of the attack is governed by the efficiency of the specific immune response (T-lymphocytes and B-lymphocytes).

Immune Response to Prolonged or Subsequent Encounters with an Antigen

In prolonged or subsequent encounters with an antigen, the specific immune response becomes the major protective mechanism. The specific response *does not replace* the actions of the nonspecific immune elements but rather enhances phagocytosis and adds the cell-killing effects of cytotoxic T-cells. A subsequent response to the antigen results in a shorter lag period, a more rapid rise in serum antibodies (with IgG predominating), and a higher antibody affinity for the antigen (i.e., greater binding power) (Lockey & Bukantz, 1987a).

An antigen that survived the nonspecific response is now attacked additionally by cytotoxic T-cells and is covered with antibodies that enhance phagocytosis by breaking down antiphagocytic capsules and promoting the binding of the antigen with macrophages and neutrophils (and subsequent engulfment and destruction). Antigen-antibody reactions also activate the complement system.* If the specific immune response fails to contain the invader, the host may be overwhelmed by the antigen unless there is medical intervention.

Factors that Affect the Immune Response

Considering the important protective properties of the immune system, it is pertinent to consider factors that enhance or limit immune competence. Recognition of

* When complement is activated by an antigen-antibody response, the "classical pathway" for activation is said to have been used. If complement is activated by properties of the antigen itself (during the nonspecific response), the process is termed the "alternate pathway."

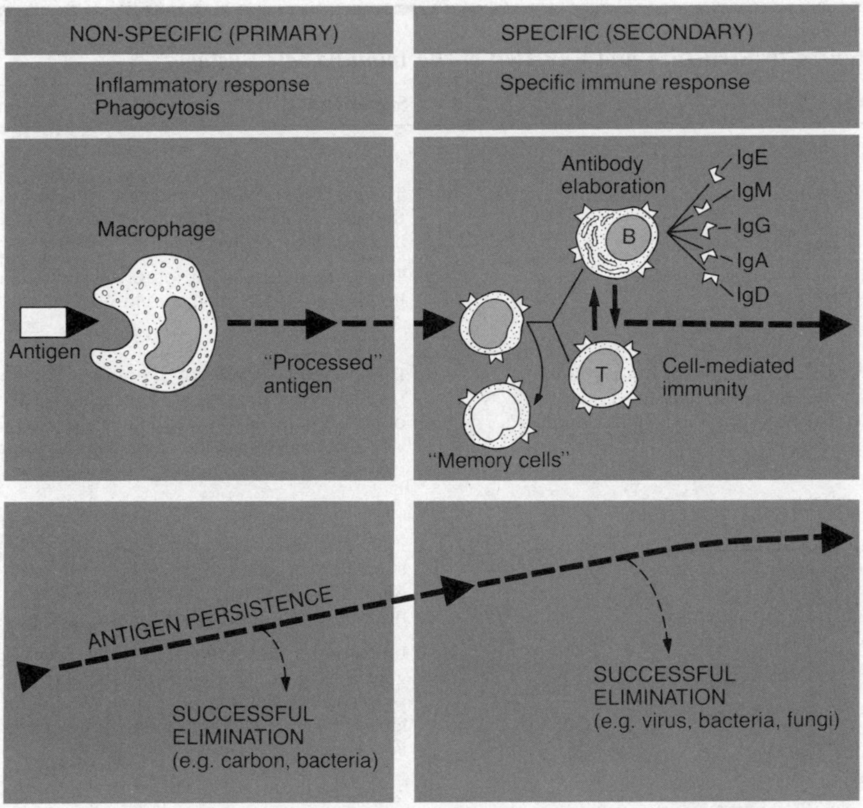

FIGURE 37-3. Schematic representation of the nonspecific and specific immune responses. (From Bellanti, J. A. [1985]. *Immunology: Basic processes.* [p. 187]. Philadelphia: WB Saunders.)

these factors increases the nurse's ability to correctly diagnose many potential nursing diagnoses and collaborative problems. Because immunology is a relatively new field, there remain more questions than answers in relation to maintaining a healthy immune system. Several areas, however, have been examined for their effect on immune competence; these include genetic, age-related, nutritional and metabolic, environmental, anatomic, microbial, physiologic, and stress factors.

Genetic Factors

The entire immune system is under genetic control (Bellanti, 1985). Genes control the body's ability to respond to antigens, as well as the level and duration of the response. Genetic defects in immune elements result in an increased susceptibility to disease. One example is the increased susceptibility to infection that is characteristic of children with Down syndrome (see Chapters 27 and 31). Although the mechanisms are poorly understood, children with this genetic disorder have deficits of both cellular and humoral immune elements (Anderson, 1987).

Alterations in HLA have been associated with increased incidence of certain inflammatory, autoimmune, and endocrine disorders. The exact mechanisms of this predisposition remain poorly defined. Recent research suggests that other genetic factors related but not linked to HLA may be partly responsible for this predisposition (Stastny, 1987).

Age-Related Factors

At birth, the immune response is compromised by the immaturity of phagocytic cells, T-lymphocytes, and complement proteins, as well as by decreased levels of immunoglobulins (antibodies). Premature infants possess considerably less immunocompetence than do full-term infants. Table 37–1 demonstrates characteristic levels of humoral immune development after birth of full-term infants, and Table 37–2 details developmental differences in structure and function of the immune system.

Nutritional and Metabolic Factors

Malnutrition has been linked with (Feigin & Garg, 1987)

- Diminished secretory IgA, which decreases the effectiveness of the mucous membrane barrier to infection.
- Depression of complement proteins.
- Depletion of T-lymphocytes (although B-lymphocytes remain at normal levels).

Breast milk supplies the infant with additional IgA that protects secretory surfaces of mucous mem-

TABLE 37-2
Developmental Differences in Structure and Function of the Immunologic System

Structure and Function	Significance
Organ Structure	
The skin of premature infants and neonates is thinner and more permeable	Thinner skin is more vulnerable to skin breakdown, thus destroying the body's first line of passive defense, which places this age group at great risk for infections
In later childhood, lymphoid tissue mass increases	The increased mass size of tonsils and adenoids is a normal physical finding in the school-age child
Nonspecific Response	
Neonate demonstrates immaturity of inflammatory response; phagocytic cells have less effective chemotactic (cell movement) activity with immature phagocytic (cell-ingesting) ability. The neonate's complement system is deficient	Diminished responses of the nonspecific immune system place the neonate at greater risk for infection and allow for more rapid spread of infection leading, potentially, to sepsis. The lessened inflammatory response masks the more common signs and symptoms of infection (e.g., fever), making clinical diagnosis more difficult
Cell-Mediated Immunity (T-Cell)	
Altered T-cell activity with neonates and stressed infants (e.g., those who are small for gestational age [SGA] and premature)	Immature and inexperienced immune cells place the neonate and stressed SGA infant at greater risk for viral and bacterial infections. Altered T-cell activity may affect neonates' responsiveness to immunizations (e.g., pneumococcal vaccine)
	Immature or inexperienced cell-mediated responses to certain antigens during first few years of life affect the reliability of delayed hypersensitivity skin reactions. The reliability is influenced by the infants' immature skin and inflammatory response. Therefore, the test is not routinely used with infants
Humoral Immunity (B-Cell)	
IgM, IgE, IgA, IgD, IgG normally at low levels at birth. IgM, IgE, IgA, IgD do not cross the placenta. The immunoglobulins reach adult levels at different ages (Miller, 1988):	Lower immunoglobulin levels place infant and young child at greater risk for bacterial infections. As child's exposure and response to specific antigens become more experienced, the child will develop higher levels and be less vulnerable. Lower IgE level may account for lack of immediate hypersensitivity type allergies in the first 2–3 mos of life (Bierman et al, 1988)
IgG crosses placenta and provides protective transmission to infant from mother	Passive placental transfer may affect infants' response to active immunization, i.e., pertussis and/or diphtheria. Because of transplacental IgG, most immunodeficiency diseases do not become apparent until 1 mo of age (Regelmann et al, 1987)
	Prematures born less than 30 wks gestation receive very little IgG from mother and are unable to produce own. This enhances the infection risks for fatal outcomes

Immunoglobulin	Age (yrs) at which serum concentration reaches ≥ 80% adult level
IgM	9–11
IgG	3–5
IgE	10–15
IgA	12–16

branes. Breastfeeding, therefore, has been associated with a decreased incidence of upper respiratory, ear, and gastrointestinal infections.

Increased susceptibility to infection is associated with hypoadrenal and hypothyroid states. Steroid administration also alters the immune response by inhibiting the secretion of interleukin-1,* and thus decreasing replication and development of "killer" (cytotoxic) T-cells (Fuller, 1985).

* Substance released into body fluids by blood leukocytes, tissue macrophages, and large granular killer lymphocytes following phagocytosis of bacteria and bacterial byproducts. Interleukin-1 then acts on the hypothalamus to produce fever (Guyton, 1991).

Environmental Factors

Environmental factors involve conditions in which exposure to pathogens is increased. These conditions include feeding contaminated formula, poor handwashing among caregivers (including health care professionals), repeated exposure to siblings or adults with frequent infections, day care facilities that allow attendance of infectious children, infrequent bathing, use of contaminated linens and clothing, mouthing of dirty toys, and others. In addition, climate, weather, air pollution, and other environmental factors are known to affect the presentation and aggravation of allergic symptoms (see the following section on allergy).

Anatomic Factors

Breaks in the skin and mucous membranes decrease the competence of these anatomic barriers to infection. This principle underlies the need for extra precautions to prevent infection in children with burns, eczema, and other tissue damage.

Microbial Factors

The normal body flora (nonpathogens) help protect the body from pathogenic organisms. To gain entry into the body, invading bacteria must first "dislodge" the normal flora at a given site; thus, when normal flora are present in sufficient numbers, it is more difficult for pathogens to gain entry (Fulginiti, 1992). Treatment with broad-spectrum antibiotics, however, is known to kill normal flora along with pathogenic organisms and thereby to depress this protective mechanism. Staphylococci and yeast organisms are particularly likely to invade while normal flora are depressed.

Physiologic Factors

Many physiologic factors provide protection against foreign antigens. Gastric juice is known to kill certain bacteria. The ciliary action of the respiratory tract and the cough reflex help remove organisms and other particles that enter through the upper respiratory tract. Normal urine flow flushes pathogens from the urinary tract. The blood contains bactericidal substances sometimes referred to as "natural antibodies" (Bellanti, 1985). In addition, normal flow of phagocytic cells from the circulation to tissues and onto endothelial surfaces provides a broad surveillance for foreign proteins (Fulginiti, 1992).

Stress Factors

In recent years, both the popular and professional literature have made numerous references to the notion that stress alters immune function and predisposes individuals to disorders such as infection, cancer, and autoimmune diseases. Reviews of relevant research by Fuller (1983) and Dorian and Garfinkel (1987) support the premise that stress alters immune function. In light of studies showing that immune responses may be either depressed or enhanced at different times in relation to a stressor, Dorian and Garfinkel (1987) concluded that stress tends to exert *dysregulatory* effects on immune function. The implication for clinical nursing is that persons under increased physiologic and psychologic stress are likely to experience periods of increased susceptibility to organisms and other immune-related conditions such as asthma, gastric ulcers, and inflammatory bowel disease.

History and Physical Examination

The focus of the history and physical examination will have different points of emphasis depending on the child's presenting complaint(s) and symptoms. More in-depth information can be found in Chapter 13 and in Tables 37–2 and 37–3 on components of the physical examination for the child with altered immune function.

Diagnostic Assessment: Immune Function

Tables 37–1 and 37–2 present laboratory data relevant to the function of the immunologic system. Specific diagnostic and laboratory tests done for each immune disorder are found in those sections under "Diagnostic Assessment."

Therapeutic Management

The management strategies used in the treatment of children with immune dysfunctions are specific to the individual disorder and described within each section discussion.

Nursing Care

To enhance immune function, assessment and analysis of factors that potentiate or interfere with immunity must be made. Immune function is compromised when genetic defects, immaturity, nutritional deficiencies, environmental hazards, anatomic and physiologic alterations, depression of normal body flora, or significant physiologic or psychologic stress is present. When the body's own protective responses malfunction or are overtaxed, the plan of care should include the diagnosis *High Risk for infection* with implementation of appropriate precautionary measures to reduce transmission of microorganisms. The Nursing Process Plan: The Child on Corticosteroid Therapy (Table 37–4) details the plan of care for children on corticosteroids, a component of the therapeutic management for children with immune disorders.

Altered Immune Response: Autoimmune and Immune-Related Inflammatory Disorders

Autoimmunity is an immune response launched by lymphocytes against the body's own healthy tissues. It represents a failure in the body's ability to recognize

TABLE 37-3
Physical Assessment for Allergic Disorders

Signs/Symptoms	Explanation for Clinical Manifestations
Skin	
Rash/hives Dryness, scaliness Itching involves cheeks, forehead, extensor or flexor surfaces Nails buffed from rubbing skin Contact dermatitis involves exposed area	Elevated IgE levels suggest allergy. Mast cells and basophils release histamine, resulting in inflammation, rash, and itching. Chronic itching causes buffed nails, skin breakdown, and dryness. Reason for anatomic location of rash unknown, with the exception of contact reaction. In these situations, exposed area in contact with allergen elicits a rash
Eyes	
Conjunctivitis Itching, burning, excessive lacrimation Puffiness of eyelids Allergic shiners (dark circles under eyes) (Fig. 37–4) Deep transverse crease, lower eyelid Dennie folds (lines progressing from the inner eye, slanting downward and ending in slight swing located in the lower orbitopalpebral grooves)	Chemical release of histamine from sensitized IgE mast cells and basophils causes swelling, itching, and excessive lacrimation (conjunctivitis). Dennie folds and allergic shiners are associated with swelling and discoloration of tissue located below the lower eyelid (orbitopalpebral groove)
Nose	
Broadened nose bridge (chronic nasal allergy) Nasal salute, with transverse nasal crease above tip of nose from nose rubbing (Fig. 37–5) Persistent nasal discharge Mucosa pale, swollen, congested External irritation from chronic discharge Paroxysmal sneezing	Chemical release of histamine by nasal mucosa mast cells causes vascular dilatation and swelling, hypersecretion, and itching. This involves frequent wiping of nasal discharge (nasal salute), with subsequent nasal crease and broadened nose bridge if allergic response is chronic. Nasal swelling is associated with nasal obstruction and inability to breathe through the nose (check obstruction by having child sniff from each nostril with other nostril closed)
Mouth	
Mouth breathing High-arched palate Geographic tongue (Fig. 37–6) Throat clearing continuous	Nasal swelling and obstruction associated with allergic rhinitis leads to mouth breathing. Mouth breathing is associated with oral dryness. Geographic tongue involves red patches with gray margins. Red patches result from desquamation of tongue epithelium. Gray area is thickening of tongue epithelium. Chronic oral breathing is believed to be associated with the development of a high-arched palate. Increased nasopharyngeal mucus leads to frequent attempts to clear the throat
Ears	
Otitis media Pain, drainage Hearing loss	Swelling and fluid accumulation is medium for infection (otitis media) and affects hearing ability. Pain is a common symptom with otitis media. Chronic ear infections may result in hearing loss
Chest/Respiration	
Accessory muscle use Increased breathing rate Prolonged inspiration or expiration, shortness of breath Wheezing Pear-shaped chest Barrel-shaped chest Increased mucus Chronic cough	Increased pulmonary mucus production, edematous airway walls, and bronchospasm result in increased respiratory work effort, air trapping, and more resistance to air movement. Increased respiratory effort results in accessory muscle use (retractions) and faster breathing rates. Obstructed airways cause the wheezing sound. The anatomic appearance of pear/barrel chest is associated with air trapping

TABLE 37-3
Physical Assessment for Allergic Disorders *(Continued)*

Signs/Symptoms	Explanation for Clinical Manifestations
Gastrointestinal System	
Diarrhea, vomiting Stomachaches, flatulence, cramps Colic Food intolerances	Antigenic substances from food can pass the intestinal mucosa despite mucous barrier and IgA, IgE-mediated reaction may occur with submucosal edema, dilated blood vessels, and smooth muscle spasm. These pathologic findings are associated with diarrhea, stomachache, cramps, and flatus
Central Nervous System	
Tension-fatigue syndrome Irritability Tiredness Depression Headaches	No definitive cause is identified for symptoms of tiredness, irritability, depression, and headache

Figures from Marks, M. (1977). *Stigmata of respiratory tract allergies.* Kalamazoo, MI, Upjohn.

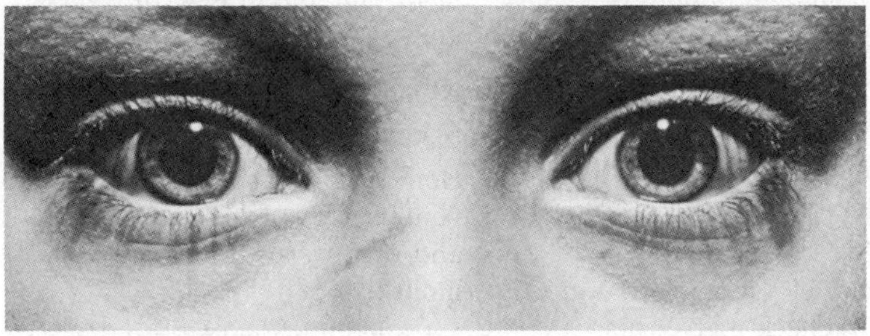

FIGURE 37-4. Allergic shiners. (From Marks, M. [1977]. *Stigmata of respiratory tract allergies.* Kalamazoo, MI: Upjohn.)

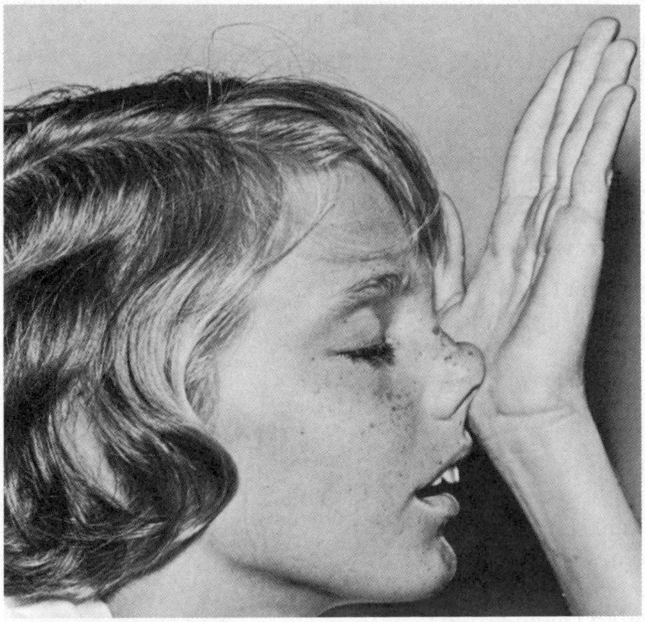

FIGURE 37-5. Allergic salute. (From Marks, M. [1977]. *Stigmata of respiratory tract allergies.* Kalamazoo, MI: Upjohn.)

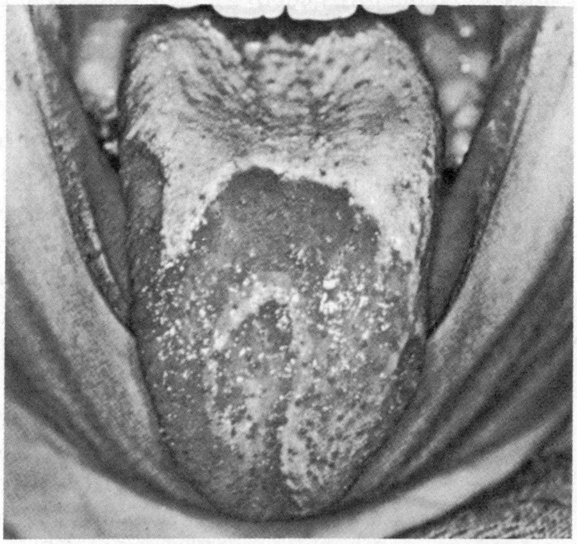

FIGURE 37-6. Geographic tongue. (From Marks, M. [1977]. *Stigmata of respiratory tract allergies.* Kalamazoo, MI: Upjohn.)

TABLE 37-4

Nursing Process Plan: The Child on Corticosteroid Therapy

***Analysis*:** Nursing Diagnostic Statement 1

***Response and Related or Risk Factors*:** *High risk for fluid volume excess; risk factors:*

- Mineralocorticoid activity associated with the prescribed corticosteroid
- Child and/or parent(s) knowledge deficit regarding interventions to control fluid retention

***Projected Outcome*:** The child will not experience increased fluid retention and edema

---

Defining Characteristics
(Actual Response)

Subjective:

- Shortness of breath
- Change in mental status
- Restlessness
- Anxiety

Objective:

- Increase in weight and blood pressure
- Palpable edema, anasarca
- Intake significantly greater than output
- Orthopnea
- S3 heart sounds
- Pulmonary congestion (x-ray, auscultation) and abnormal breath sounds, rales (crackles)
- Change in respiratory pattern
- Decreased hemoglobin and hematocrit
- Central venous pressure changes
- Jugular vein distention
- Positive hepatojugular reflex
- Oliguria, urine specific gravity changes
- Azotemia
- Altered electrolytes

Nursing Interventions

Hypovolemia Management to include

Monitor for edema

- Assess for edema of extremities and sacrum every shift and record findings
- Measure intake and output
- Weigh daily on same scale with only diaper or underwear
- Measure blood pressure every shift with child under like conditions (i.e., preferably with child at rest, not crying or protesting)
- Monitor any elevations in blood pressure; recheck in 1–2 hrs; correlate with weight, urinary output
- Report to physician elevations judged to be associated with fluid retention

Teaching: Disease Process; Prescribed Activity and/or Procedure, Prescribed Diet

Teach and implement interventions to control fluid retention

- Teach parent(s) and child how to assess for edema (to support home management)
- Implement a "no-added-salt" diet for the child prone to fluid retention
- Discuss with parent the need for regular follow-up care. Explain that if edema becomes significant, physician may change to different corticosteroid (with a weaker mineralocorticoid activity)

Evaluation Criteria

- Absent or only slight edema of the extremities
- No sudden increases in weight
- Output balanced with intake
- Vital signs within normal limits for age and weight, including heart rate, blood pressure, respiratory rate and character
- Lungs clear
- Normal breath sounds
- Hemoglobin, hematocrit, central venous pressure, electrolytes, and urinalysis within normal limits
- Negative hepatojugular reflex
- Appears calm, and mental status as at baseline

TABLE 37-4 (continued)

Analysis: Nursing Diagnostic Statement 2

Response and Related or Risk Factors: *High risk for injury: physiologic, hypokalemia; risk factors:*

- Increased excretion of potassium associated with corticosteroid therapy
- Child and/or parent(s) knowledge deficit regarding measures to avoid hypokalemia

Projected Outcome: The child will not experience hypokalemia

Defining Characteristics *(Actual Response)*	Nursing Interventions	Evaluation Criteria
Subjective: • Muscle cramps • Nausea • Paresthesias *Objective:* • Diarrhea • Vomiting • Tetany • Dysrhythmias • Potassium < 3.5 mEq/L	*Electrolyte Management: Hypokalemia* **Monitor for hypokalemia** • Question child if he or she is experiencing classic signs and symptoms • Monitor laboratory reports for serum potassium level • Monitor cardiac status carefully. Monitor apical pulse for 1 full min, being alert for dysrhythmia. Institute use of a cardiorespiratory monitor, if indicated *Teaching: Prescribed Medications; Prescribed Diet* **Teach and implement measures to avoid hypokalemia** • Avoid potassium-depleting diuretics • Increase potassium-rich foods in the diet	• Serum potassium between 3.5 and 5 mEq/L • Absence of muscle cramps, nausea and vomiting, paresthesias, diarrhea, tetany, and dysrhythmias

Analysis: Collaborative Problem 1

Response and Related or Risk Factors: *High risk for injury, physiologic, gastric irritation; risk factors:*

- Ulcerogenic effects of corticosteroids
- Child and/or parent(s) knowledge deficit about measures to prevent gastric irritation

Projected Outcome: The child will not experience physiologic injury as a result of gastric irritation

Defining Characteristics *(Actual Response)*	Nursing Interventions	Evaluation Criteria
Subjective: • Nausea • Anorexia • Epigastric pain that may or may not be relieved by eating or antacids	**Monitor for gastric irritation** • Ask the child about comfort level. Use measures designed to assess pain in children; see Chapter 25	• Denies epigastric distress • Usual or baseline appetite (or slight increase) • Absence of blood in vomitus or stool

(continued)

TABLE 37-4 *(continued)*

Defining Characteristics *(Actual Response)*	Nursing Interventions	Evaluation Criteria
Objective: • Heme-positive stools or vomitus	• Monitor appetite; if food and fluid intake is decreased, determine whether related to medication or to other factors *Bleeding Reduction: Gastrointestinal* • Routinely test vomitus and stool for blood • Alert parents to contact the physician if evidence of gastric irritation occurs *Teaching: Disease Process* **Teach and implement measures to prevent gastric irritation** • Administer corticosteroid, as ordered, with food or milk • Avoid known gastric irritants (aspirin and other nonsteroidal anti-inflammatory drugs, alcohol) • Limit intake of caffeine in chocolate, coffee, tea; (caffeine increases gastric acidity)	

Analysis: Nursing Diagnostic Statement 3

Response and Related or Risk Factors: *High risk for injury: physiologic, hyperglycemia; risk factors:*

- Promotion of gluconeogenesis
- Decreased glucose utilization effects of corticosteroids
- Child and/or parent(s) knowledge deficit regarding schedule of needed follow-up care

Projected Outcome: The child will not experience hyperglycemia

Defining Characteristics *(Actual Response)*	Nursing Interventions	Evaluation Criteria
Subjective: • Hunger • Thirst *Objective*: • Polyuria • Glycosuria • Increased blood sugar	*Hyperglycemia Management* **Monitor for signs of hyperglycemia** • Monitor for polydipsia, polyuria, polyphagia • Measure urine sugar and acetone every shift during initial therapy, periodically thereafter • Monitor laboratory reports of serum glucose *Teaching: Disease Process* • Teach child and parents symptoms of hyperglycemia and how to test blood or urine for sugar	• Absence of unusual hunger or thirst • Absence of polyuria • Absence of glycosuria • Fasting blood sugar < 120 mg/dl

TABLE 37-4 (continued)

Defining Characteristics *(Actual Response)*	Nursing Interventions	Evaluation Criteria
	• Alert the family to contact the physician if evidence of hyperglycemia occurs • Caution the child and parent to obtain regular follow-up care. More insulin may be needed while on corticosteroid therapy	

Analysis: Nursing Diagnostic Statement 4

Response and Related or Risk Factors: *High risk for altered growth and development: linear growth; risk factor*

- Protein catabolism and inhibition of growth hormone associated with corticosteroid therapy

Projected Outcome: The child will demonstrate linear growth within norms for his or her age group

Defining Characteristics *(Actual Response)*	Nursing Interventions	Evaluation Criteria
Subjective: None *Objective:* • Failure to maintain height and weight at pretherapy percentiles on standardized growth chart	**Monitor growth parameters** Measure and plot height and weight on appropriate growth charts at every follow-up visit *Nutrition Management* **Encourage a high-protein diet** (to help offset the effect of protein catabolism) **Alert the physician to the first evidence of growth failure.** (It may be possible to use an alternate-day dosage schedule that minimizes protein catabolism)	The child will maintain pretherapy percentiles or better for height and weight on standardized growth chart

Analysis: Nursing Diagnostic Statement 5

Response and Related or Risk Factors: *High risk for infection; risk factors:*

- Altered immune function, after discharge, associated with corticosteroid therapy
- Child and/or family knowledge deficit concerning ways to prevent infection

Projected Outcome: The child will remain free of avoidable infections

Defining Characteristics *(Actual Response)*	Nursing Interventions	Evaluation Criteria
Subjective: • Verbalization of signs of infection	*Teaching: Disease Process* **Teach the child and family** • How infections are acquired and transmitted	The child will remain infection free

(continued)

TABLE 37-4 *(continued)*

Defining Characteristics *(Actual Response)*	**Nursing Interventions**	**Evaluation Criteria**
Objective: • Evidence of infectious process (although not necessarily with the typical signs)	• Meticulous handwashing at appropriate times • Maintenance of general health **Alert the family to the contraindication for immunization with live virus: trivalent oral poliovirus vaccine; measles, mumps, rubella** (because of immunosuppressive effects of corticosteroids) **Explain the necessity to seek medical advice for wounds that are slow to heal, persistent inflammation, or persistent malaise** (because of immunosuppression and the potential of corticosteroids to mask other illness)	

Analysis: Collaborative Problem 2

Response and Related or Risk Factors: *Activity intolerance related to impaired physical mobility, associated with muscle weakness, associated with the protein-catabolizing effects of corticosteroids*

Projected Outcome: The child will have sufficient physiologic energy to endure or complete required and/or desired daily activities

Defining Characteristics	**Nursing Interventions**	**Evaluation Criteria**
Subjective: • Verbal report of fatigue or weakness • Exertional discomfort or dyspnea *Objective:* • Abnormal heart rate or blood pressure response to activity • Electrocardiographic changes reflecting arrhythmias or ischemia	*Exercise Therapy: Muscle Control* **In collaboration with physical therapist, determine muscle strength,** subjectively and objectively, at each follow-up visit **Collaborate with physical and occupational therapist to teach the child to promote muscle strength** through a planned program of regular exercise *Teaching: Prescribed Diet* Collaborate with the nutritionist to promote a high-protein, high-calcium diet	• Denying changes in muscle strength • Exhibiting normal and equal strength in extremities on examination

Analysis: Nursing Diagnostic Statement 6

Response and Related or Risk Factors: *High risk for injury: neurologic; risk factor* untoward reactions to corticosteroids (e.g., cerebral edema)

Projected Outcome: The child will not experience adverse neurologic effects of corticosteroids

TABLE 37-4 *(continued)*

Defining Characteristics *(Actual Response)*	**Nursing Interventions**	**Evaluation Criteria**
Subjective: • Headache **Objective:** • Papilledema • Oculomotor or abducens nerve paralysis • Visual loss	*Cerebral Edema Management* **Monitor for evidence of neurologic reactions** (e.g., changes in mental status, complaints of dizziness) • Alert the physician to evidence of neurologic effects (because this signals an untoward reaction to the corticosteroid) • Assure the child and family that the syndrome is reversible	• Absence of papilledema or vision changes • Absence of nerve paralysis • Absence of persistent headache

Analysis: Nursing Diagnostic Statement 7

Response and Related or Risk Factors: *High risk for altered health maintenance; risk factor:*

• Knowledge deficit of child and family regarding safe administration of corticosteroid

Projected Outcome: The child and/or family will be able to identify, manage, and/or seek out help to maintain the child in a healthy state

Defining Characteristics *(Actual Response)*	**Nursing Interventions**	**Evaluation Criteria**
• Subjective or objective indication of being unfamiliar with corticosteroid actions and potential side effects • Lack of adaptation of family to need to follow health maintenance procedures • Reported or observed inability to take responsibility for corticosteroid administration • History of inability to manage health maintenance procedures • Expressed interest in learning how to safely administer corticosteroids • Lack of appropriate equipment • Lack of financial or other resources	*Teaching: Prescribed Medication* **Teach and implement the following aspects of safe corticosteroid administration** • Inject intramuscular corticosteroids deeply into approved site with largest muscle mass (to avoid tissue atrophy at site)* • Avoid subcutaneous injection or reuse of injection site • Explain that morning administration, before 9 A.M., will minimize immunosuppression • Instruct the family that the child should receive NO over-the-counter drugs without consulting the physician • Consult the physician if severe infection, injury, or other significant stress occurs (that may necessitate an increased dose of corticosteroid)	• Observed ability to safely administer corticosteroids • All necessary equipment is available, and family has resources to obtain equipment as needed • Correct verbalization of administration time and precautions to follow while administering • Correct verbalization of factors to report to physician or home health nurse

*Corticosteroids are rarely ordered for children by the intramuscular route. However, when this route is chosen, careful technique is indicated

(continued)

TABLE 37-4 *(continued)*

Defining Characteristics *(Actual Response)*	**Nursing Interventions**	**Evaluation Criteria**
	• Explain that the corticosteroid should not be stopped abruptly; (withdrawal syndrome and hypoadrenalism may occur) • The child on long-term corticosteroids should wear a Medic-Alert bracelet to inform emergency personnel of the medication	

***Analysis*:** Nursing Diagnostic Statement 8

***Response and Related or Risk Factors*:** *Self-esteem disturbance related to*

- Body image disturbance associated with Cushing syndrome due to prolonged high corticosteroid dosages
- Medical necessity to curtail certain high-risk physical activities

***Projected Outcome*:** The child will verbalize and display a positive self-evaluation about self and self-capabilities

Defining Characteristics	**Nursing Interventions**	**Evaluation Criteria**
Subjective: • Self-negating verbalization • Expressions of shame and guilt • Evaluates self as unable to deal with events because of embarrassment about appearance • Rationalizes away or rejects positive feedback • Hesitant to try new things and situations and avoids social interactions • Projection of blame and responsibility for problems • Hypersensitive to slight or criticism *Objective*: • Moon facies • Hirsutism • Acne • Muscular weakness • Cervicothoracic hump • Hypertension • Osteoporosis • Amenorrhea	**Monitor for the signs of Cushing syndrome listed under objective defining characteristics** • Report concerns to physician for consideration of dose adjustment *Body Image Enhancement* **Promote adaptive behavior** • Encourage the child to express feelings about changes in appearance and facilitate problem solving • Suggest the use of depilatories for hirsutism • Counsel the child with acne about skin care; see Chapter 38 • Suggest the use of artificial nails and full or partial wigs (especially for the female adolescent) • Counsel the child about the need to prevent injury. Help the child think of suitable alternatives for activities that must be sacrificed (e.g., tennis or track versus football). Bone demineralization associated with corticosteroid therapy makes one more prone to injury	• Positive verbalizations about self and ability to deal with events • Discusses plans to manage aspects of appearance that can be enhanced • Initiates social relationships • Reports "feeling better about self" • Begins to try new activities

TABLE 37-4 *(continued)*

Defining Characteristics	Nursing Interventions	Evaluation Criteria
• Striae • Thinning of hair and nails • Ecchymosis		

Analysis: Nursing Diagnostic Statement 9

Response and Related or Risk Factors: *Fear [child and parent(s)] related to* perception that side effects of corticosteroids are permanent

Projected Outcome: The child and parent(s) will verbalize that the feeling of dread about permanence of corticosteroid side effects is decreased or eliminated

Defining Characteristics	Nursing Interventions	Evaluation Criteria
Subjective: • Verbalization of fear and ability to identify object of fear (perception regarding corticosteroids) • Restlessness • Complaints of insomnia *Objective:* • Sympathetic stimulation: cardiovascular excitation, superficial vasoconstriction, pupil dilatation • Glancing about • Poor eye contact • Trembling/hand tremors • Extraneous movement (foot shuffling, hand/arm movements) • Facial tension • Voice quivering • Increased perspiration	*Emotional Support* • Encourage verbalization of feelings • Assist child and/or family to find ways to deal with their fear • Stay with the patient while verbalization of feelings is occurring *Teaching: Disease Process; Prescribed Medication* Assure the child and family that side effects of corticosteroid therapy are reversible. Provide resources such as pamphlets to the family to reinforce the information given *Support Group* Arrange for child and parent(s) to meet with other people who have undergone corticosteroid therapy	• Verbalization that fear is no longer present • Physiologic parameters within normal limits • Able to focus • Calm appearance and voice • Absence of tremors, extraneous movements • Skin warm, dry

"self" versus "nonself." Although several hypotheses have been postulated to account for this untoward immune reaction, the mechanisms resulting in autoimmunity remain largely unexplained. The diseases presented in this section are all thought to be related to altered responses of the immune system.

The disorders in this section are also grouped together because they all involve inflammation of connective tissue. Connective tissue is a fibrous type of tissue that is spread throughout the body. It supports and connects internal organs, forms bones and the walls of blood vessels, attaches muscles to bones, and makes up the scar tissue formed after an injury. Connective tissue contains a protein called "collagen," thus disorders of connective tissue are also termed "collagen diseases."

Because connective tissue is found everywhere within the body, inflammatory diseases of connective tissue usually involve many tissues and organs and exhibit systemic symptoms. The tissue and organ involvement described in the following disorders varies, but these diseases often include arthritic involvement of joints, inflammation of blood vessels, and damage to organ tissues.

Systemic Lupus Erythematosus

Systemic lupus erythematosus (SLE) is a complex, chronic inflammatory disorder characterized by circulating autoantibodies that affect connective tissue. Because connective tissue is present in the body as fibroelastic, reticular, adipose, and elastic tissue, as well as bone, cartilage, synovial membrane, and the vascular system tissue, multiple systems of the body (including the skin, joints, pleural and pericardial membranes, kidney, and hematologic and nervous systems) may be affected (Fig. 37–7). There seem to be several different types of lupus; therefore, the disease may appear as a trivial problem in one child, whereas in another it is catastrophic (Miller et al, 1986). Typically, remissions and exacerbations occur, and death can result from cardiovascular, renal, or neurologic complications or overwhelming bacterial sepsis.

Etiology/Incidence

Affecting approximately 500,000 individuals in the United States, lupus is most commonly seen in the second and later decades of life. Twenty per cent of cases of SLE occur in childhood, however, predominantly in females (with an approximate ratio of 3 to 1) 8 years of age and older (Behrman, 1992). All races are affected, but the incidence is approximately three times greater in dark-skinned females (e.g., African-Americans, Hispanics, Asian-Americans, and some Native Americans).

The etiology of SLE is thought to be multifactorial, with involvement of immunologic, genetic, environmental, and infectious factors. SLE is considered the prototype for immune complex disease because of the significant defects in both humoral and cell-mediated immunity and in the complement system (Lockey & Bukantz, 1987b).

Support for the genetic theory of cause is found in the high rate of occurrence of SLE in both persons of a pair of monozygotic twins. Environmental causes include medications such as procainamide, hydralazine, anticonvulsants, oral contraceptives, and some antibiotics. In addition, photosensitivity, stress, immunizations, and pregnancy have been linked to the onset of SLE. Viruses also may be a factor.

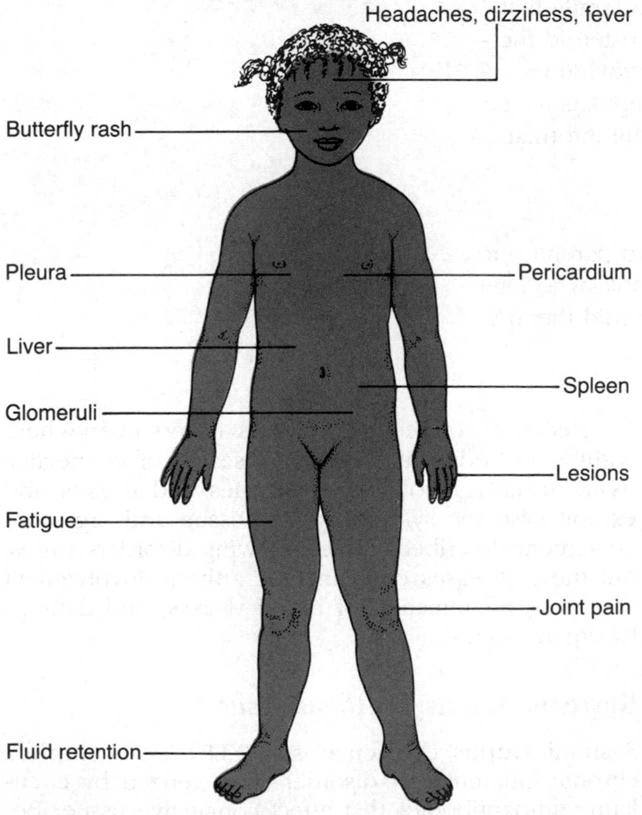

FIGURE 37-7. Symptoms and sites of pathologic changes in systemic lupus erythematosus.

Pathophysiology

The involvement of connective tissue leads to widespread inflammatory changes and vasculitis in many tissues and organs. SLE may take on many appearances, manifesting in one or many ways and in widely varying degrees of severity. As a chronic process, unpredictable exacerbations and remissions of one or more of these manifestations are common. All the pathologic changes in SLE are the result, either directly or indirectly, of antibodies formed against "self-antigens." Antibody activity may directly damage tissues (e.g., blood cells) or cause indirect damage secondary to deposition of antigen-antibody complexes in the tissues (e.g., glomerulonephritis) (Miller et al, 1986). The skin and kidney are the most frequently and severely affected organs in SLE. A progressive retinopathy also can occur, with the potential for blindness. Vasculitis in the spleen results in characteristic "onion ring" lesions around affected vessels. The CNS can be affected also, but involvement is usually mild.

Clinical Manifestations

Although symptoms vary widely, general systemic complaints are common at first. A typical presentation for a child with SLE is arthralgia or arthritis, fever, and rashes. Myalgia, malaise, fatigue, and/or weight loss may also occur. During the course of the disease, symptoms may vary in appearance, location, and intensity. A discussion of specific manifestations follows.

Joints/Musculoskeletal. Joint disease is the most common manifestation, appearing in approximately 95 per cent of patients with SLE. In fact, joint discomforts may be the first symptom of active SLE, preceding other signs or symptoms, and may be migratory or rheumatoid. The child may have complaints of pain on movement or tenderness, and these complaints may be out of proportion to physical findings. Involvement is symmetric and occurs most commonly in the proximal interphalangeal joints, knees, wrists, and metacarpophalangeal joints. Effusions also may be seen. Rheumatoid nodules may appear with disease exacerbations and disappear when disease activity is suppressed. Deformities of fingers may appear, but permanent joint changes are rare.

Myalgias (muscle pains) are seen in about 25 per cent of patients with SLE. When they occur, they are most common in proximal muscles. Muscle weakness also may be noted, but this is relatively rare.

Skin. Skin and mucous membranes are frequent targets of SLE. The lesions include rashes, erythematous macules, photosensitivity, oral ulcerations, and alopecia. Exposure to bright sunlight and other sources of ultraviolet radiation, especially if prolonged, can precipitate skin eruptions and serious vital organ involvement.

The classic butterfly rash was first described by Hebra in 1845. It is an erythematous rash distributed across the bridge of the nose and cheeks, seen in approximately 50 per cent of patients (Fig. 37–8). A similar rash may appear on the palmar surface of the hands and the soles, as well as on the chest.

Discoid lesions occur in approximately 15 per cent of patients. Beginning as a small area of erythematous plaque or a papule, the lesions spread outward and leave a hyperkeratotic area with follicular plugging and atrophy.

Vasculitic lesions with ulceration, purpuric lesions, and subcutaneous nodules also may be seen on the hands and arms. Vasculitis may be found as periungual (around the nails) erythema and spider hemorrhages. Livedo reticularis (a mottled discoloration of the skin) is common in these patients, especially when exposed to cold. Other cutaneous lesions less frequently observed include periorbital edema, bullous lesions, and ulcerations of the buccal mucosa.

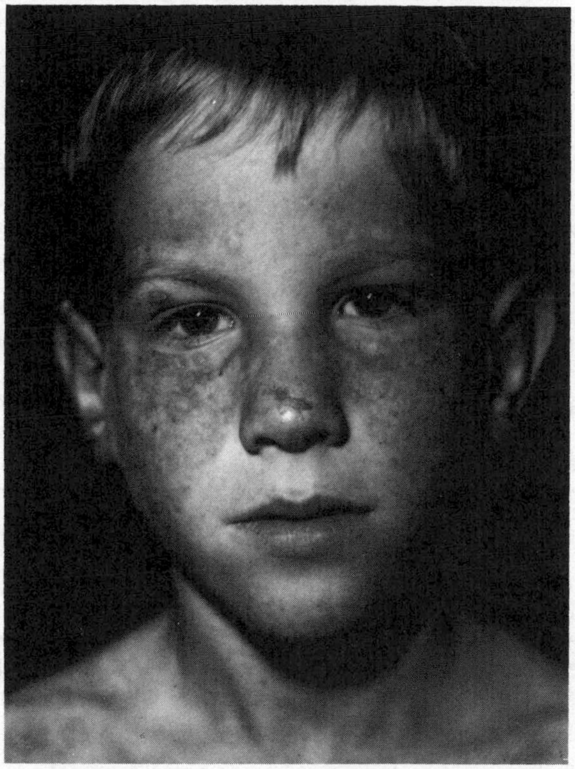

FIGURE 37 - 8. Discoid lupus erythematosus with typical butterfly distribution, atrophy, and depigmentation of skin. (Courtesy of Dr. L. Schweich. From Kornreich, H. K. [1976]. Systemic lupus erythematosus in childhood. *Clinics in Rheumatic Diseases, 2*[2], 429.)

Alopecia (loss of hair) is a common feature, occurring in about 65 per cent of patients with SLE, particularly in periods of active systemic disease. This occurs as patchy losses rather than total loss. Hair may become thin and brittle, prone to breaking.

Renal. Renal involvement is present in 50 to 70 per cent of children with SLE and is potentially the most life-threatening complication (McCurdy et al, 1992). Nephrotic syndrome and glomerulonephritis (see Chapter 36) are the forms of renal disease typically seen. Symptoms are usually noted early in the disease and include microscopic hematuria, proteinuria, and increased urinary sediment. These may vary from one urine specimen to the next and do not necessarily accurately reflect disease activity. Increased serum creatinine and decreased creatinine clearance reflect renal insufficiency. Other manifestations of renal disease include edema (secondary to sodium and water retention), weight gain, and hypertension.

Gastrointestinal. Recurrent abdominal pain is a common complaint in children with lupus; its cause is often unclear (Eberhard et al, 1991). Pancreatitis and serositis may be responsible for some of this discomfort, but it also may result from irritation caused by medications. Sepsis must be considered if these complaints occur with fever.

Pulmonary. Pleurisy and pleural effusion are the most common pulmonary manifestations of SLE. Pulmonary function tests are characteristically abnormal (Pohlgeers et al, 1990). The child may be dyspneic owing to the pain associated with breathing. Effusions are not usually large and on chest radiographs usually are seen as streaky lesions at the base of the affected lung. Because of defective immunologic function, as well as the immunosuppressive medications prescribed, pneumonia is relatively common. Symptoms include a nonproductive cough, fever, and rales.

Cardiac/Cardiovascular. Cardiovascular symptoms are seen in more than 50 per cent of lupus patients. Pericarditis, the most frequent cardiac manifestation, occurs in approximately 25 per cent. Its presence may vary from a transient friction rub to a pericardial effusion. The child may complain of substernal or precordial pain. Murmurs, persistent tachycardia, and transient dysrhythmias may be noted. Pleural and pericardial effusions may be seen repeatedly when disease activity flares. Congestive heart failure may be the presenting indication of myocarditis.

Cardiovascular manifestations may present in a number of ways. Raynaud syndrome may be seen; in this condition, vasoconstriction occurs in peripheral vessels in response to cold or emotional stress. Distal portions of fingers and toes may appear blue, whereas proximal portions appear to have more normal circulation. Gangrene may result from decreased circulation, possibly with loss of digits.

Hematologic. Nearly all children with SLE have one or more hematologic abnormalities, including anemia, leukopenia (neutropenia and most commonly lymphopenia), and thrombocytopenia. A prolonged partial thromboplastin time (PTT) may be found, as a result of antibodies to phospholipid antigens. Circulating lupus anticoagulants also cause a false-positive test for syphilis. Other hematologic findings, in varying frequency of occurrence, include positive lupus erythematosus (LE) cells, antinuclear antibodies (ANAs), and rheumatoid factor (RF).

Eye. Conjunctivitis is frequently an initial symptom. Other parts of the eye affected by inflammation include the sclera, the uveal tract, and the retina. Fundoscopic examination may reveal cytoid bodies (white fluffy patches) in the retina. These inflammatory processes are usually associated with the acute disease and do not result in visual impairment.

Central Nervous System. CNS symptoms can be divided into three groups: organic disorder secondary to CNS lupus, toxic disorder secondary to medications, and behavioral disorder as a reaction to the diagnosis.

Organic Disorder. Symptoms include irritability, depression, headache, lethargy, dizziness, seizures, hallucinations, loss of orientation to time and place, ataxia, cranial nerve palsies, chorea, and, rarely, coma.

The headache may be one of the presenting symptoms and generally subsides as disease activity remits. Like a migraine, these headaches may begin with a visual aura. In general, headaches in lupus are not cause for concern. However, it must be determined that they are not an indication of hypertension, increased intracranial pressure, or an adverse effect of medication.

Toxic Disorder. Corticosteroids are part of the primary treatment regimen for SLE. However, they lower the threshold for seizure and may also precipitate personality changes, depression, or euphoria. It is important to determine whether these occur because they are medication-induced behavior changes or CNS changes resulting from disease activity.

Behavioral Disorder. Depression may be a reaction to being told one has SLE. Denial also may be a compensatory coping mechanism. Refer to Chapter 19 on Chronic Illness for further information on the child's and family's response to chronic illness.

Lymphoid System. Hepatomegaly is common in children with SLE. This is not directly correlated with disease activity, as is the more prominent splenomegaly. Generalized lymphadenopathy may also occur.

Diagnostic Assessment

The criteria established in 1971 and revised in 1982 by the American Rheumatism Association were designed to classify or identify patients with a diagnosis of SLE more clearly. Serologic tests that reveal LE cells or ANAs provide a clear-cut diagnosis because these are relatively specific for lupus. However, SLE rarely makes a dramatic presentation with all or most symptoms present at any given time. Rather, the symptoms usually unfold episodically over time. Therefore, diagnosis is based on a group of overt symptoms and confirmed by serologic, histopathologic, and other laboratory findings. As indicated in Table 37–5, patient identification is made if any four or more of the 11 diagnostic criteria are present, serially or simultaneously, during any period of observation.

Therapeutic Management

Death is no longer a "given" expectation when a diagnosis of SLE is made. Although a significant portion of the patients have systemic involvement and do die, advances in early diagnosis, intervention, and ongoing care have made it possible to anticipate a relatively normal lifestyle, albeit with restrictions, precautions, and monitoring. The goals of the care are control of symptoms, minimizing or preventing exacerbations of systemic symptoms and complications, and promotion of as nearly normal a lifestyle as possible. With coordinated efforts of a broad interdisciplinary health care team and the cooperation and compliance of the child and family, this goal is not unrealistic.

There is no "protocol" for treating the diagnostic label of SLE. Treatment must be flexible and directed toward specific problems of a specific patient during any given time of disease activity, supporting and promoting appropriate developmental tasks. The intensity and length of therapy depend on the clinical and laboratory measures of disease. The patient with mild or no overt symptoms of active SLE may be managed with regular monitoring but no medication. At the other extreme, the child with gradually increasing or sudden onset of symptoms must be treated quickly and aggressively to minimize the potential for permanent tissue damage.

The components of drug therapy include antiinflammatory and immunosuppressive agents, cytotoxic drugs, and antimalarial medications. Prophylactic measures such as phototherapy, and general health measures, including rest and diet, are important. Patient and family education is a critical part of the management of lupus. A regimen that includes any or all of these components must be geared to control the disease to allow the child to lead as nearly normal a life as possible; to minimize or prevent scarring, which can result from extensive inflammation; and to minimize or prevent serious side effects of the medications.

TABLE 37-5
Classification Criteria (Revised) of Systemic Lupus Erythematosus*

1. Malar Rash

Fixed erythema, flat or raised, over the malar eminences, tending to spare the nasolabial folds

2. Discoid Rash

Erythematous raised patches with adherent keratotic scaling and follicular plugging; atrophic scarring may occur in older lesions

3. Photosensitivity

Skin rash as a result of unusual reaction to sunlight, by patient history, or by physician observation

4. Oral Ulcers

Oral or nasopharyngeal ulceration, usually painless, observed by a physician

5. Arthritis

Nonerosive arthritis involving two or more peripheral joints, characterized by tenderness, swelling, or effusion

6. Serositis

a. Pleuritis—convincing history of pleuritic pain or rub heard by a physician or evidence of pleural effusion

OR

b. Pericarditis—documented by electrocardiogram or rub or evidence of pericardial effusion

7. Renal Disorder

a. Persistent proteinuria >0.5 g/day or greater than 3+ if quantitation not performed

OR

b. Cellular casts—may be red blood cell, hemoglobin, granular, tubular, or mixed

8. Neurologic Disorder

a. Seizures—in the absence of offending drugs or known metabolic derangements, e.g., uremia, ketoacidosis, or electrolyte imbalance

OR

b. Psychosis—in the absence of offending drugs or known metabolic derangements, e.g., uremia, ketoacidosis, or electrolyte imbalance

9. Hematologic Disorder

a. Hemolytic anemia—with reticulocytosis

OR

b. Leukopenia—<4000/mm^3 total on two or more occasions

OR

c. Lymphopenia—<1500/mm^3 on two or more occasions

OR

d. Thrombocytopenia—<100,000/mm^3 in the absence of offending drugs

10. Immunologic Disorder

a. Positive LE cell preparation

OR

b. Anti-DNA: antibody to native DNA in abnormal titer

OR

c. Anti-Sm: presence of antibody to Sm nuclear antigen

OR

d. False-positive serologic test for syphilis known to be positive for at least 6 months and confirmed by *Treponema pallidum* immobilization or fluorescent treponemal antibody absorption test

11. Antinuclear Antibody

An abnormal titer of antinuclear antibody by immunofluorescence or an equivalent assay at any time and in the absence of drugs known to be associated with "drug-induced lupus" syndrome

From Tan, E. M., et al. (1982). The 1982 revised criteria for the classification of systemic lupus erythematosus. *Arthritis and Rheumatism, 25*(11), 1271–1274.

* For the purpose of identifying patients in clinical studies, a person shall be said to have systemic lupus erythematosus if any 4 or more of the 11 criteria are present, serially or simultaneously, during any interval of observation.

Aspirin and other nonsteroidal anti-inflammatory drugs (NSAIDs) are used to control arthritis and arthralgias, serositis, and fevers. When a fever occurs, great caution must be taken in ruling out the possibility of infection as a cause of the fever. If aspirin is ineffective in reducing or eliminating these symptoms or is poorly tolerated, other NSAIDs can be selected, such as ibuprofen and tolmetin.

If rash or other cutaneous lesions occur that are not responsive to aspirin therapy, antimalarial drugs such as hydroxychloroquine may be used. Because of its ability to diminish penetration of ultraviolet light, this is the drug of choice for the child who is photosensitive as well. Regular eye examinations every 6 to 8 months are important for the child receiving antimalarial agents because of the progressive retinopathy that may be induced by these drugs.

For patients who do not respond to aspirin, NSAIDs, or antimalarial drugs, or who have involvement of other major organ systems (e.g., hematologic, CNS, renal), steroids are necessary. These have both anti-inflammatory and immunosuppressive functions. Dosage and route may vary, from maintenance doses of prednisone every other day to high-dose steroids in divided doses several times a day, to "pulse" doses (high-dose intravenous administration) to interrupt or control severe exacerbations. When symptoms have been controlled and the child has been asymptomatic for a period, a carefully designed "tapering" schedule can begin. Attention must always be given to the possibility of infection that may be masked by steroid administration. Table 37–4 is a Nursing Process Plan for the child on corticosteroid therapy.

Cytotoxic drugs, particularly azathioprine, may be given to intervene in progressive renal disease. These drugs, especially in combination with steroids, have been shown to delay or interrupt lupus nephritis. When disease progression has been stabilized, these drugs may be tapered to minimal maintenance doses.

Application of the Nursing Process: Systemic Lupus Erythematosis

Assessment

Painful and swollen joints are one of the most frequent presenting symptoms. As therapy is begun and therapeutic serum levels of aspirin or other NSAIDs are obtained, any objective or subjective changes should be noted.

Thorough cardiovascular and pulmonary assessments are important components of routine evaluations of the child with SLE. These should include heart sounds, rate, and rhythm; breath sounds and respiratory rate; and the vascular status of the extremities. Hands and feet should be protected from the cold to facilitate circulation.

Deterioration in renal function is the most significant potential complication. Nursing assessment for adequate renal function, therefore, should include monitoring blood pressure, intake and output, daily weight, and laboratory reports, in addition to routine evaluations of urine specimens.

Nursing Diagnostic Statements and Collaborative Problems

Impaired physical mobility related to joint inflammation.

High risk for altered tissue perfusion: peripheral; *risk factor: abnormal vasoconstriction.*

High risk for altered cardiac output: decreased; *risk factor: inflammation of the pericardium.*

High risk for altered patterns of urinary elimination; *risk factor: inflammatory changes in the glomerular capillaries.*

High risk for impaired skin integrity; *risk factors:*

- *Rash.*
- *Discoid lesions.*
- *Impaired circulation.*
- *Photosensitivity.*

High risk for injury: physiologic; *risk factor: untoward reactions to medications.*

High risk for infection; *risk factors: alterations in humoral and cell-mediated immunity.*

Altered thought processes: powerlessness related to/associated with *inflammation of CNS and side effects of steroid therapy.*

Body image disturbance and/or situational low self-esteem and/or altered role performance related to social-emotional impact of the disease and changes in physical appearance.

High risk for ineffective coping: individual/family; *risk factor: negative or dysfunctional perceptions of the disease.*

High risk for altered home health maintenance; *risk factor: knowledge deficit about home care.*

Planning and Implementation

Managing Joint Inflammation. Effectiveness of medications can be monitored by changes in comfort levels with movement of fingers, elbows, ankles, and toes. Early signs of exacerbations may be noted by increases in discomfort or swelling. A physical therapist can help develop an exercise program that includes range-of-motion exercises, positioning of joints to prevent contractures, and activities to maintain strength and endurance. As the most consistent contact in the health care team, the nurse can help the child practice and reinforce these "routines," explain their rationale, and encourage the child and/or family to participate actively in this aspect of maintaining normalcy.

The nurse may also ask an occupational therapist to recommend appropriate activities to facilitate a physical therapy program. Such a program accommodates any decrease in energy level and increased need for rest while being responsive to the needs and tasks appropriate to the child's stage of growth and development.

A medication regimen should be developed to maximize the effectiveness of medications while minimizing interruptions in rest times or activities (both therapeutic and recreational). Refer to further discussion of drug therapy under "Juvenile Arthritis." In addition, warm baths may be helpful in reducing pain associated with inflamed joints.

Preventing Peripheral Tissue Ischemia and Alterations in Cardiac Output. Cardiovascular assessments should detect possible indications of carditis, which has a potential for permanent damage. Tachycardia, possible dysrhythmias, pericardial rub, complaints of chest pain, lethargy, and perhaps dyspnea all suggest a change in cardiac status. As noted earlier, changes in cardiac function can lead to congestive heart failure. Daily weight measurements may provide early indication of congestive failure. If cardiac function changes significantly, the pumping action of the heart and, subsequently, vascular sufficiency may be compromised. The problems may be further complicated if Raynaud phenomenon is present.

Maintaining Normal Urinary Elimination. Deterioration of renal function is the most significant potential complication. Early detection of renal compromise is essential to minimize or prevent permanent renal damage and, ultimately, failure. A 24-hour urine collection for creatinine clearance will indicate adequacy of or changes in renal function. Routine evaluations of urine should include tests for hematuria, proteinuria, increased urine sediment, and casts—all measures of adequate kidney function. Other symptoms of renal involvement are hypertension and weight gain.

Maintaining and/or Promoting Skin Integrity. Skin integrity may be compromised as a result of rashes (especially if pruritic, causing the child to scratch) or discoid lesions or as a result of impaired circulation to extremities. Monitor any increase of rash or lesions and decreases in vascular competence. Fingers and toes will become numb and painful if exposed to cold. Socks, gloves, and warm, layered clothing will help encourage peripheral circulation and provide warmth and protection. Tight clothing should be avoided. The nurse must be alert to early evidence of infections either in lesion sites or as the result of scratching. If erythema, induration, or pustules occur, the physician is informed and treatment begun.

Monitoring Medication Therapy. The effects of medication, both therapeutic and adverse, are also important assessments. Some are effective in a brief time, whereas others (e.g., hydroxychloroquine) require several weeks to take effect. As a mainstay of therapy, aspirin may have adverse effects, such as gastritis, tinnitus, or increased bleeding, when platelet competency may be already compromised by the disease process. Documentation of the positive effects of steroids must be made, but the nurse needs to be aware of their side effects, some of which may be difficult to distinguish from the disease manifestations. Hypertension, irritability, capillary fragility, and depression may be characteristic of both. Therefore, awareness of both the individual child's symptoms as well as any changes, especially as they relate to possible undesired responses to medications, is important.

Preventing Infection. Any child with an altered immune response has an increased potential for infection. Susceptibility for the child with SLE is related specifically to genetic, anatomic, physiologic, metabolic, and microbial factors. It is thought that at least some of the immune defects of cellular and humoral immunity are linked to genetic inheritance. Anatomically, the child is at risk during periods of skin involvement that cause a break in this barrier to infection. Physiologically, the decreased B-cell function may affect the normal antibody protection of the genitourinary system, and renal complications may alter normal urine flow that tends to flush out bacteria. Metabolic factors include steroid administration, which further alters the immune response. Microbial factors may be involved during periods of antibiotic administration for systemic infection. The nurse (and family) must be alert to signs and symptoms of overgrowth of nonsusceptible bacteria.

The child's immune competence can be bolstered by insurance of adequate calories consumed in a balanced diet. The importance of good handwashing in reducing the spread of infection cannot be overemphasized. The child and all family members should be taught proper handwashing techniques. In addition, the family will need guidance about the mode of transmission of common cold and flu viruses so that they can adequately protect the child without being unduly restrictive.

Assisting the Child and Family to Deal with CNS Alterations. CNS involvement can be a frustrating and depressing aspect of SLE for the patient. Although the causes of the headaches, anxiety, mood swings, mental confusion, disorientation, personality changes, chorea (involuntary contraction of muscles resulting in jerky movements), or seizures may be either organic or psychological, steroid therapy is usually effective management. However, if the patient is already receiving steroids, it may be difficult to distinguish between exacerbation of the illness with CNS involvement and a steroid-induced psychiatric disorder. It is important for the nurse to assess and document actions and interactions carefully, particularly as they relate to medication administration, environmental factors, or other symptoms that might signal increased disease activity (see Table 37–4).

Both the patient and family need to be helped to understand that once the systemic illness is under control, the symptoms will most likely disappear. However, these are frightening symptoms for the family and the child (especially if he or she is an adolescent). Building and encouraging an ongoing, trusting relationship between members of the health care team and the child and family is an important aspect of care.

Regular assessment of neurologic status is important. Appropriate precautions should be taken for any indication of seizures. Chorea also may occur as one of the neurologic symptoms. The child with chorea needs to be protected from injury and given physical assistance with whatever basic tasks may be difficult or impossible to perform. Both the child and family need to hear that these uncontrollable movements are not permanent nor do they impair intellectual abilities.

Enhancing Self-Esteem, Body Image, and Role Performance. Unsightly rashes, joint pain, fatigue, changes in body weight distribution, and a cushingoid appearance that may result from medications may affect self-concept (including body image and self-esteem). In addition, photophobia may inhibit outdoor activities. Some suggestions that the nurse can make to enable the child or adolescent to feel like one of the crowd and acceptable to self are the use of hypoallergenic cosmetics to cover rashes, pacing of activities to keep fatigue at bay, choosing styles of clothing that help camouflage weight gain, and structuring outdoor activities in the early morning or evening hours. Assisting the family in locating a support group of children with similar problems for their child may be beneficial. The nurse can assist parents in emphasizing the child's positive attributes and areas of accomplishment and skill that are not being affected by the treatment regimen.

Promoting Child and Family Coping. Ongoing emotional support, in sickness and in health, for the child and family will be an important aspect of nursing care. They will likely have many questions, fears, anxieties, angers, and frustrations. The nurse is a primary source for information, comfort, and care and can respond to many of the physical, emotional, and educational needs that exist and will continue to evolve for these patients and families. The nurse can also refer them to community resources and support groups. Some of these include the Arthritis Foundation, the American Lupus Society, and various published materials (videos and written) for patients and families.

Facilitating Home Health Maintenance. Patients and families need to learn about SLE, its cause(s), its course and prognosis, therapeutic aims, and general health care. Some aspects of the disease process may be frightening; some are frustrating because there are no definite answers. Therefore, it is important to assess the levels of knowledge and stress and begin teaching at a level where the child and family can hear and understand. An important first step is for the child and family to *begin* to verbalize their fears and anxieties, as well as their knowledge and self-confidence in their abilities to manage this chronic illness.

The child and family must know the side effects of medications and realize that some of these are difficult to distinguish from symptoms of the disease process. They should be instructed to inform their physician of any of these unusual occurrences rather than try to determine cause and effect themselves. They should also be reminded that if antimalarials are part of the medication regimen, regular eye examinations are important, even after the medication has been discontinued. Discussion of the administration procedure for steroids will help the patient and family understand dosage variations and the rationale for a dramatically increased dosage with subsequent slow tapering. Steroids also may be used topically for skin and scalp lesions (see Table 37–4).

When renal involvement is a component of the disease process, steroids will most likely be part of the medication regimen. Diet, then, becomes an important issue for teaching for both these factors. Fluid retention occurs in patients taking steroids. With renal compromise and fluid retention due to medications, the child and family need to be taught the need for low-sodium, low-protein foods. A dietitian may be helpful as a resource and facilitator.

If monitoring for proteinuria or hematuria is indicated, the nurse can teach the child and family to use and read one of the commercial dipsticks for urine testing. Weekly weights (or more often if there is concern) are a good indicator of renal ability to regulate body fluid. Any sudden weight gain needs to be reported.

Photophobia may appear at any point and is an issue for discussion with the patient and family. Exposure to sunlight is not necessarily totally avoided, but because of the potential for serious systemic exacerbations caused by ultraviolet rays, exposure should be limited. To minimize exposure, the patient should be fully clothed (including a hat) when outdoors in bright, intense sunlight and should use sunscreening lotions (sun protection factor of 15 or higher).

Rest is a significant component of care for the child with SLE. Unfortunately, it is frequently either forgotten or ignored. Energy levels are usually much lower when a child is ill, and this is also true of the child with SLE. *Increased fatigue, stress, and anxiety can trigger exacerbations* of the disease process; therefore, the nurse helps the child and family formulate a schedule that allows for adequate uninterrupted rest.

Some symptoms are "signals" for concern that the child and family need to know about. When the child has a fever, chills, pain in the abdomen, chest, or joints, urine changes, or undue fatigue, the physician should be notified. Doubts or concerns should be shared with either the nurse or the physician for validation.

Because female sex hormones appear to accelerate autoimmune disease (Miller et al, 1986), mechanical modes of contraception are recommended instead of oral contraceptives. Pregnancy is not absolutely contraindicated in the patient with SLE, especially if the disease is quiescent. However, pregnancy and delivery can precipitate a flare, including nephritis, which can present an unpredictable hazard for both mother and child. Therefore, the anticipation of pregnancy should be discussed in depth (including genetic counseling) and progress through it should be closely monitored by a physician who is aware of the disease process and its potential hazards.

Juvenile Arthritis

"Juvenile rheumatoid arthritis" is the term applied to inflammatory arthritis in children. Since 1977, there has been controversy about the name given this disorder. Based on studies and the accumulation of statistics reported from centers where these children are diagnosed and cared for, there is only a 5 to 6 per cent correlation (clinically and serologically) between arthritic children and adults with *rheumatoid* arthritis. We join the movement to designate this childhood inflammatory process as simply "juvenile arthritis" (JA) and will so designate this disorder within this chapter.

Arthritis is defined by the American Rheumatology Association as joint swelling or restriction of motion, with pain, tenderness, or heat. Pain and tenderness alone are not enough to diagnose JA. JA is a systemic disorder of connective tissue, joints, and viscera and includes several arthritislike manifestations that are designated into three onset types: systemic onset, pauciarticular onset, and polyarticular onset. The onset type is determined by the manifestations during the first 6 months of illness. Although symptoms resembling another type may appear later, the type that was present during the initial 6 months remains the designated type of JA for a particular patient. The course of the disease is marked by remissions and exacerbations.

Each subtype of JA has its defining characteristic and prognosis.

- Systemic-onset JA is defined by the presence of a recurrent intermittent high fever (103° F and higher). The rheumatoid rash and other organ involvement may or may not be present.
- Pauciarticular-onset JA is defined by the presence of arthritis in fewer than five joints.
- Polyarticular-onset JA is defined as the presence of arthritis in more than four joints.

Patients whose diagnosis is systemic-onset JA are excluded from the latter two types.

Although the cause of JA remains unknown and there are no criteria for accurate prediction of outcome in an individual patient, the outlook for most children with this disorder is good. For some children, the condition will be chronic. But approximately 75 per cent of children emerge 10 to 15 years after onset to lead normal lives without crippling (Brewer, 1986). In addition, studies have shown that these young adults fare as well as or better than their siblings in educational level, marriage, childbearing, and income (Miller, 1982).

Etiology/Incidence

Statistics are incomplete but, based on those available, the prevalence of JA appears to be approximately 0.5 per 1000 children. Asian-American children seem to be less affected than white children. It appears that fewer black than white children are affected.

Objective onset of JA may occur as early as 6 weeks of age; however, in general, the age of onset occurs between the ages of 2 and 16 years. Each of the onset types appears to have its own characteristic incidence, just as it has its own characteristic areas of symptoms and degree of involvement (Table 37–6). Thirty per cent of children with JA have systemic-on-

TABLE 37-6
Classification of Juvenile Arthritis (JA)

Mode of Onset	Incidence: Age (Years)	Incidence: Sex F:M	Prognosis
Systemic (30% of all JRA* cases)	10	1.5:1	All JA mortality is in this group (1–2% of all JRA patients); 40% evidence of joint destruction
Polyarticular (>4 joints) (<25% of all JRA cases)			Mortality—0; duration longer; more crippling; 25% remission
Subtype 1 (RF+)	>10	mostly female	
Subtype 2 (RF−)			Less crippling than RF+
Pauciarticular (<5 joints) (45% of all JRA cases)	<10	6:1	Continuous—25%. Arthritis rarely erosive, 5-yr remission 60%
Subtype (iritis)	<10	almost all girls	10%—functional blindness 55%—acute 45%—chronic
Subtype 2 (HLA-B27+)	>10	1:9	Possible juvenile ankylosing spondylitis later
Subtype 3 (Arthritis only)			Best outlook for recovery

Data from Brewer, E. J. (1986). Collagen vascular disease. In S. S. Gellis & B. M. Kagan (Eds.), *Current pediatric therapy 12.* (pp 353–357). Philadelphia: WB Saunders.
* JRA, juvenile rheumatoid arthritis; JA, juvenile arthritis.

set JA. It occurs often around 10 years of age; girls are affected slightly more often than boys. Approximately 25 per cent of children with JA have polyarticular-onset JA. In this group more than twice as many girls as boys are affected, and symptoms usually appear after 10 years of age. The remaining 45 per cent of children with JA have the pauciarticular-onset type and are most commonly girls under age 10 years (Page-Goertz, 1989).

Research studies continue to identify causes for juvenile arthritis, but the cause remains unclear. Several theories have been postulated, including the relationship among JA, infections, and an autoimmune response. Although their relationship to JA remains unclear, several factors, including upper respiratory infections and trauma, may precipitate this inflammatory process. Genetic factors (HLA type) are also suspected (Bellanti, 1985).

Pathophysiology

The inflammatory process of JA may begin insidiously, being almost unnoticeable, or may appear as sudden joint swelling that might cause one to suspect trauma. Swelling is caused by inflammation of the synovial membranes and the adjacent joint capsule. Inflammation of the synovial tissues causes increased secretions of joint fluids. As this fluid volume increases, it causes swollen, boggy joints and is termed "joint effusion." The joints are edematous and feel warm to the touch. The normally clear joint fluid becomes cloudy as it is infiltrated with lymphocytes and plasma cells. Pain and stiffness result from the pressure on sensory nerves in the area. In later stages of JA, stiffness and limited mobility may result from joint destruction or contractures.

Children may have long periods of synovitis before permanent joint damage occurs. "Once joint destruction has commenced, erosions of subchondral bone, narrowing of the joint spaces (loss of articular cartilage), destruction of fusion of bones, and deformity, subluxation, or ankylosis of joints may result" (Fig. 37–9) (Schaller, 1992).

Other pathologic changes that may occur as the result of the inflammatory process include serositis of the pleura, pericardium, and peritoneum. The rash

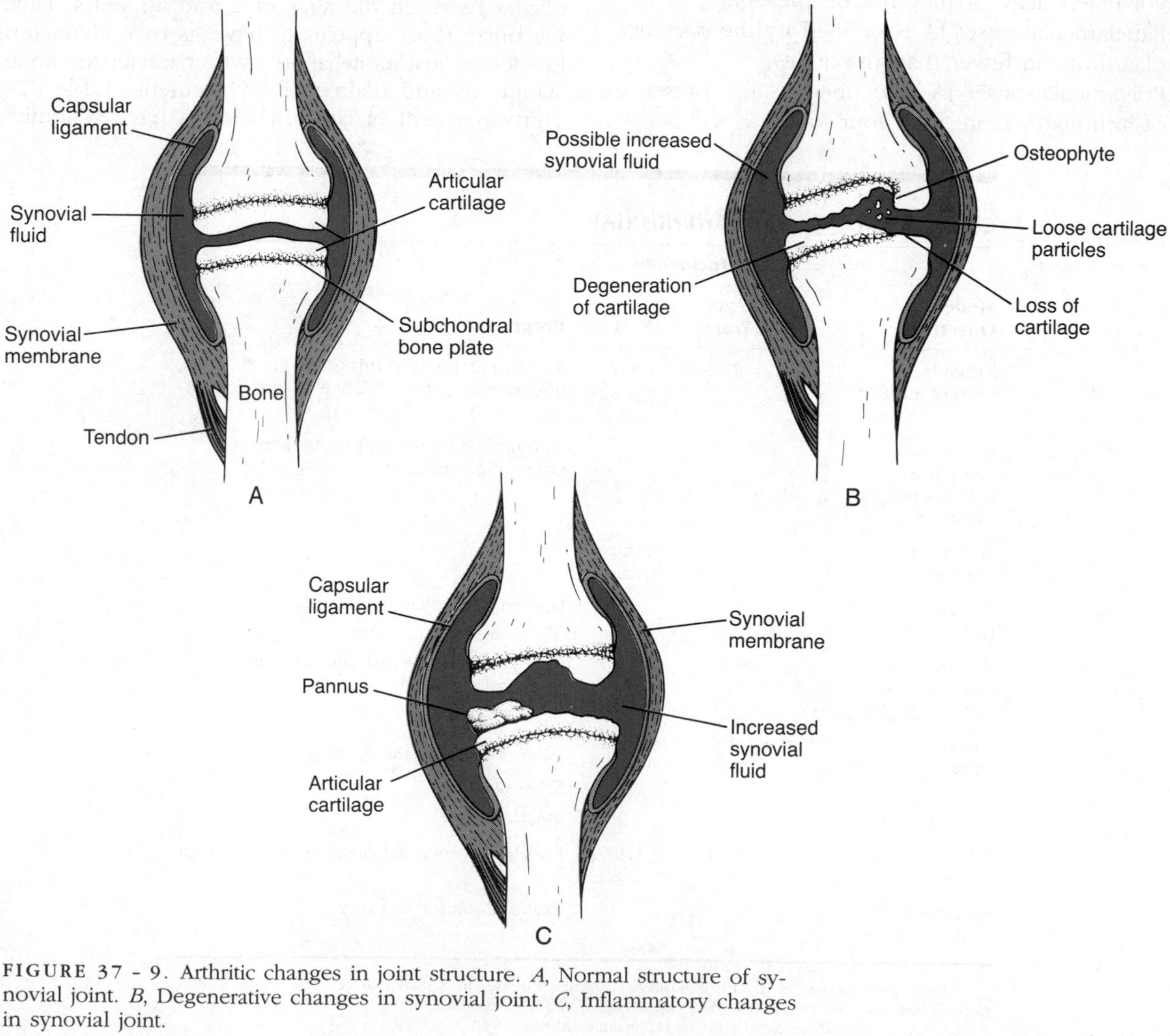

FIGURE 37-9. Arthritic changes in joint structure. *A*, Normal structure of synovial joint. *B*, Degenerative changes in synovial joint. *C*, Inflammatory changes in synovial joint.

that may be seen in systemic-onset JA occurs as the result of a mild vasculitis in the subepithelial tissues. Fever, loss of appetite, weight loss, fatigue, and generalized weakness also may be associated with systemic inflammation.

Inflammation of the iris and ciliary body of the eye, termed "anterior uveitis" or "iridocyclitis," may occur. Uveitis is a potentially serious and frequent complication in young girls with pauciarticular onset. Typically, this inflammatory process is asymptomatic, but eye pain and diminished vision have been reported. Although some cases of iridocyclitis are acute in nature and respond to topical corticosteroids or are self-limiting, about 70 per cent of children with this type of inflammation have a chronic relapsing course with resulting visual impairment (Petty, 1987).

Growth disturbances may result from generalized growth retardation associated with chronic childhood illness, including overgrowth or undergrowth around the affected joints, localized effects of inflammation on the epiphyseal growth, and growth failure of the mandible (micrognathia, Fig. 37–10).

Clinical Manifestations

Arthritis may be a manifestation of many different diseases, including SLE, rheumatic fever, and dermatomyositis. However, each of these has its own characteristic rash and diagnostic laboratory data. No specific diagnostic laboratory tests are available for JA. Tests such as rheumatoid factor, ANAs, and HLA antigens can be used to help classify the different types of JA. However, the diagnosis of JA is made only after many other diseases have been ruled out.

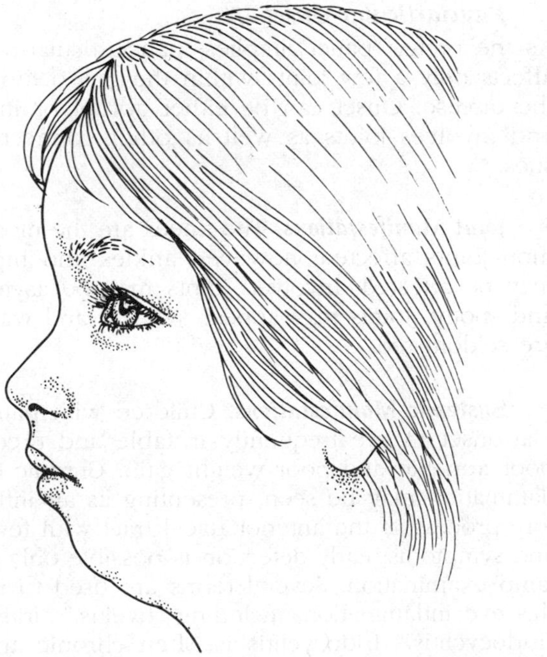

FIGURE 37-10. Micrognathia. A receding chin is the hallmark of the child with arthritis of the neck or joints of the jaw. Not shown—the angle of the jawbone is reduced or nearly absent.

JA has many signs and symptoms. Some are general and occur in all three types, whereas others are characteristic of one specific onset type. The signs and symptoms include (1) fever, (2) rash, (3) iridocyclitis, (4) cardiac involvement, (5) nodules, (6) stiffness, (7) tenosynovitis, (8) cervical spine involvement, (9) rheumatoid factor, (10) ANAs, (11) growth disturbances, (12) anemia and leukocytosis, and (13) hepatosplenomegaly and lymphadenopathy. As indicated, exacerbations and remissions of symptoms are common. Accurate diagnosis and optimal management depend on an understanding of these symptoms and their association with each type of JA.

Systemic-Onset JA (Still Disease)

Systemic-onset juvenile arthritis (previously known as "Still disease") is characterized by fever, rash, joint involvement, and other systemic manifestations. Laboratory data most often show an elevated erythrocyte sedimentation rate (ESR), leukocytosis with a significant percentage of PMLs, and anemia.

Fever. Fever occurs intermittently, usually in a diurnal pattern with spikes to at least 39.5° C (103° F). Between spikes, the child's temperature is usually normal or below (Fig. 37–11).

Rash. The rash associated with JA is most commonly seen in children with systemic-onset JA. This rash is an evanescent, pale red, nonpruritic, macular rash. The macules frequently coalesce. It will most often decrease or disappear during afebrile periods but, when present, is usually seen on the trunk and extremities (except the soles and palms). In addition to appearing during periods of fever, the rash may also appear when the skin is irritated (e.g., from scratching, heat, or trauma).

Joint Manifestations. Joint manifestations may be present at onset but go unnoticed for several months, especially if the joint problems are mild and systemic

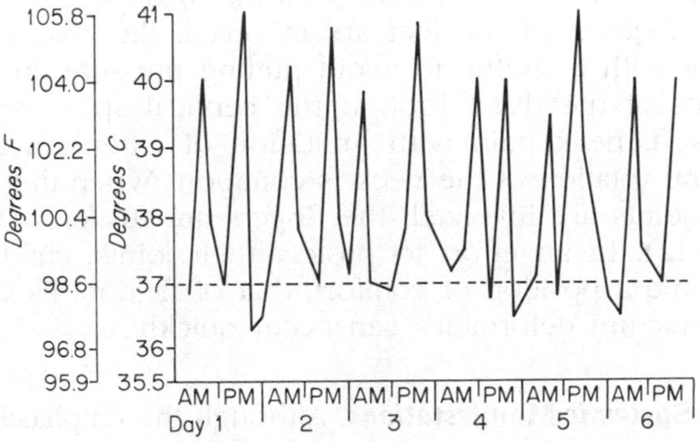

FIGURE 37-11. Fever patterns in systemic-onset juvenile arthritis. There are one or two daily temperature elevations to 39°C or greater, with rapid return of temperature to normal or subnormal levels. (From Behrman, R. E. [Ed.]. [1992]. *Nelson textbook of pediatrics* [14th ed., p. 617]. Philadelphia: WB Saunders.)

symptoms are severe and demand attention. Ultimately, these children have joint involvement that is similar to polyarticular onset, with five or more joints being affected. All joints, large and small, including the cervical spine, may be involved. During febrile periods the patients may have incapacitating myalgias and arthralgias.

Systemic Manifestations. In addition to fever and rash, other systemic manifestations are common: hepatosplenomegaly and/or lymphadenopathy, pleuritis and/or pericarditis, leukocytosis, and severe anemia. These signs and symptoms may occur over a period of months, fluctuate through periods of remission and exacerbations, and then abate, but they rarely continue into adulthood. Articular symptoms may follow a similar course, but they may also persist as chronic arthritis.

Polyarticular-Onset JA

The polyarticular-onset type of juvenile arthritis is defined as involvement of more than four joints. The type is further broken down into those patients who have positive tests for IgM rheumatoid factor (antibodies that react with gamma globulin) and those who are negative for the factor. The child with RF-negative polyarticular JA has the same characteristic signs and symptoms as one with systemic-onset JA, except that according to the American Rheumatism Association, the fever is below 39.5° C (103° F). Fever, rash, anemias, fatigue, anorexia, and failure to gain weight will be present.

Joint Manifestations. Generally speaking, children with polyarticular-onset juvenile arthritis have fewer systemic manifestations, so attention is focused on the articular manifestations. The joints most commonly affected include the wrists, knees, ankles, elbows, and feet. Affected joints are often symmetric but may also be asymmetric or even unilateral. Occasionally, polyarticular-onset JA can affect the large joints such as the cervical spine, hips, and shoulders. Regardless of location, the joints usually become swollen and tender. If joints of the feet are involved, the child may walk with a shuffle to avoid putting pressure on the joints of the distal foot. If the cervical spine is involved, neck pain with limitation of extension and lateral rotation of the neck is common. When the finger joints are involved, the fingers are fusiform (Fig. 37–12). In an effort to protect their joints, children assume a position of comfort, that of flexion. Flexion contracture deformities can occur quickly.

Systemic Manifestations. Although the emphasis in this type of JA is on joint involvement, systemic manifestations are present in most patients. Malaise, low-grade fever, organomegaly, adenopathy, anemia, and growth retardation or weight loss are commonly found (Zerin et al, 1991).

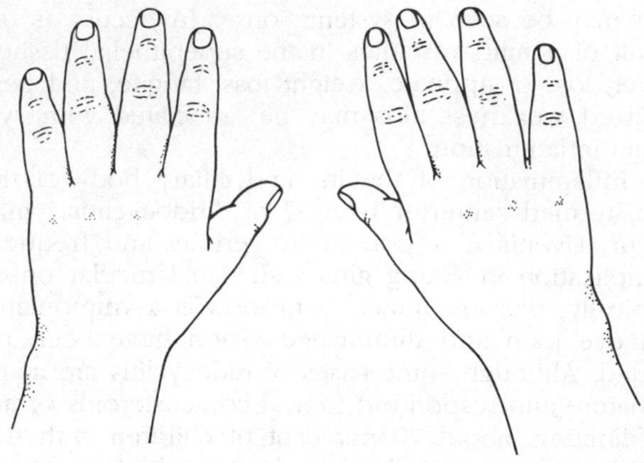

FIGURE 37-12. Arthritic involvement of the hands and wrists. The fingers of children with arthritis become fusiform, with fat central portions around the swollen near (proximal) joint and pointed toward the tips. The joint nearest the fingertip (distal) is rarely involved.

Variations in Clinical Manifestations by Subtype. In polyarticular-onset juvenile arthritis, it is important to distinguish between those children who have RF-positive and RF-negative JA because the probable manifestations as well as the prognosis of each differ significantly. RF-positive JA closely resembles adult-onset rheumatoid arthritis. Children with positive RF tests are more likely to develop severe chronic arthritis than children with negative RF. Rheumatoid nodules and rheumatoid vasculitis are likely to occur in RF-positive JA patients. There is a strong correlation between this type of JA and a genetic cause.

Pauciarticular-Onset JA

As the prefix "pauci" implies, pauciarticular-onset JA affects only a few joints within the first 6 months of the disease. Onset can be either abrupt or insidious and involves joints as well as other connective tissues.

Joint Manifestations. The knees are the most common joints affected; however, ankles and hips also may be affected. Involved joints may be asymmetric and spotty. Joints may appear swollen and warm but are seldom red.

Systemic Manifestations. Children with pauciarticular-onset JA are frequently irritable and tired, with poor appetite and poor weight gain. Chronic eye inflammation may be seen, presenting as an inflammatory process of the anterior uveal tract with few signs and symptoms; early detection is possible only by slit-lamp examination. Several terms are used to identify this eye inflammation, including "uveitis," "iritis," and "iridocyclitis." Iridocyclitis is often chronic and, because it is insidious, has great potential for damage (including cataracts and glaucoma) and vision loss or blindness.

Variations in Clinical Manifestations by Subtype. Pauciarticular JA is frequently divided into types or subsets according to age of onset, sex, presence of RF, presence of ANAs, and certain HLA-B27* characteristics. Of these, three subsets are significant: ANA-positive girls, HLA-B27–positive older boys, and RF-positive patients. The first of these subsets is primarily girls with age of onset at 5 years or younger, who have a high incidence of iridocyclitis. The second significant subset is that of boys for whom the age of onset is generally after 8 years of age and who have a greater incidence of HLA-B27 than do JA patients in general. These boys tend to develop changes typical of ankylosing spondylitis. The third subset is a small group of pauciarticular-onset patients who have a positive RF. These children tend to follow a polyarticular course and may develop erosive disease.

Diagnostic Assessment

The JA subcommittee of the American Rheumatism Association has proposed the following criteria for diagnosis of JA:

- Objective evidence of arthritis (defined as joint swelling or joint limitation of motion with heat, pain, or tenderness) in one or more joints. (Pain or tenderness alone is not sufficient for a diagnosis of arthritis.)
- Persistence of arthritis for at least 6 weeks in a given joint.
- Exclusion of other specific diseases that may cause or be associated with arthritis.

This differential diagnosis may include ruling out childhood disorders such as malignancies, other inflammatory disorders (e.g., rheumatic fever, ankylosing spondylitis, and SLE), infections of bacterial or viral origin, "growing pains," or congenital anomalies.

Laboratory Tests. No specific laboratory data are absolutely diagnostic for JA, but some tests and values are characteristically associated with JA. The ESR is usually elevated; anemia is common; the white blood cell count is frequently elevated; any or all of the serum immunoglobulins may be elevated; and ANAs are found in 25 per cent of children with RF-negative JA, 75 per cent of children with RF-positive JA, and about 60 per cent of young girls with pauciarticular arthritis. RFs (antibodies that react with gamma globulin) are not specific for rheumatoid arthritis. They are found in other rheumatic diseases such as SLE and scleroderma and in association with certain infections and malignancies.

* HLA is the major human histocompatibility complex. The letter B represents one genetic locus on the short arm of chromosome 6; the number 27 represents the allele at that site. See also the previous discussion of HLA in this chapter.

Therapeutic Management

Drug therapy and physical therapy are the bases for treatment of JA. The goals of therapy include reduction of inflammation, relief of symptoms of active disease, and maintenance or restoration of joint position, function, and strength. Accomplishment of these goals may require a concerted, well-orchestrated interdisciplinary effort; frequently, it is the nurse who can or must coordinate such an endeavor.

Drug Therapy. The drugs used are the same as those for treatment of adult rheumatoid arthritis, some of which have not been specifically approved for use in children. The first-line drug is aspirin.

Aspirin. Aspirin administration in children has come under scrutiny because of its possible relationship to Reye syndrome. In addition, dental caries have been linked to the chewing of baby aspirin (Brewer, 1986). Despite these concerns, aspirin remains the drug of choice for JA. It is more effective than any other single NSAID* and costs significantly less (Brewer, 1986).

The major effects of aspirin (and the other NSAIDs) are analgesic, antipyretic, and anti-inflammatory. A serum salicylate level of 20 to 30 mg/dl is considered therapeutic. The usual dosage is 60 to 100 mg/kg/day, administered in four daily doses spread to maintain a consistent salicylate level as nearly as possible. Because there is a wide variation in metabolism of aspirin, patients must be watched for signs of salicylate toxicity, decrease in platelet count, and bruising. It is important to monitor for evidence of gastritis or gastric ulcers (including blood in the stool). Because small children rarely complain of tinnitus, an apparent hearing loss may be an early clue of salicylate toxicity.

The anti-inflammatory effect of aspirin may not be achieved for several weeks. It is evaluated by reduction in swelling, reduced pain on movement, reduced tenderness, and increased range of motion in involved joints (Brewer, 1986).

Other NSAIDs. The development of new NSAIDs has provided a significant alternative or adjunctive drug treatment for all types of arthritis. Some of these drugs, however, have not yet been approved for use in children and are still being studied. In general, they are considerably more expensive than aspirin but have the advantages of fewer gastrointestinal side effects and less frequent administration.

Indomethacin is an older NSAID that is recognized as one of the most effective drugs for treating severe forms of systemic JA, particularly if the child is not doing well on aspirin alone. If the child is started on an NSAID because of toxicity to aspirin, the nurse must be alert for signs of toxicity to the new drug. Patients who react to one NSAID have a 50 per cent

* Despite the tendency to think of aspirin as being in a class by itself where arthritis is concerned, it is actually classified as an NSAID.

chance of developing toxicity to another drug within this classification and often show similar toxic symptoms (Brewer, 1986).

Slower-Acting Antirheumatic Drugs. Another classification of drug therapy is the slower-acting antirheumatic drugs (SAARDs). These drugs are used for their effect on the immune system but do not have anti-inflammatory properties. SAARDs include gold (Myochrysine, Solganal) and antimalarials (penicillamine, hydroxychloroquine). They are generally administered in conjunction with aspirin and other NSAIDs when these two types of drugs cannot effectively control the disease after a 4- to 6-month trial.

Of the SAARDs, gold is the treatment of choice. It is given by intramuscular injection. Prior to administering a therapeutic dose, test doses may be given to assess for allergic response. The gold preparation is usually given weekly for 20 weeks, subsequently tapering administration to every 2 to 4 weeks. A response to gold will probably not be seen for at least 2 to 6 months. The effects, if present, will be long-lasting.

Toxicities, including oral ulcerations, proteinuria, and alterations in polymorphonuclear, white blood cell or platelet counts, are not uncommon. These may be mild and reversible, or they may be severe, requiring complete cessation of the medication. Therefore, it is necessary to monitor blood counts, urine, and transaminases prior to each injection. Auranofin is an oral preparation of gold with doses beginning at 0.25 mg/kg/dose the first week, and weekly incremental 0.25 mg/kg increases. The maintenance dose is 0.75 to 1 mg/kg/dose weekly, not to exceed 25 mg/dose, to a total of 20 doses; then the dose is given every 2 to 4 weeks. Diarrhea, gastrointestinal bleeding, hematuria, and anemia may occur.

Hydroxychloroquine (Plaquenil) and penicillamine are oral agents that are also slow acting; their effects may not be seen for several weeks or months after their initiation. Side effects of hydroxychloroquine may include visual complications, bleaching and loss of hair, anorexia, abdominal discomfort, and neuromuscular weakness. Therefore, it is important for the child taking this drug to be examined by an ophthalmologist once every 6 months. Side effects of penicillamine are similar to those associated with gold, and monitoring of blood counts, urine, and platelets, as well as liver function, is important.

Steroids. The use of steroids in children with JA is usually inappropriate. Although they are the most potent anti-inflammatory drugs available and can dramatically suppress symptoms, there are few indications for their use. They neither alter the overall course of the disease nor prevent joint destruction. Furthermore, their side effects, particularly that of growth impairment, make them undesirable. However, they may be indicated in life-threatening situations, such as in myocarditis, pericarditis, and progressive iridocyclitis, or in children who are immobilized by severe debilitating disease that does not respond to other anti-inflammatory medications. In children with pauciarticular-onset JA in which only one or two inflamed joints are involved, intra-articular injection of steroids may control inflammation for 4 to 6 weeks, facilitating exercise and rehabilitation. This is a painful procedure, however, and repeated injections can result in steroidal damage to the cartilage and bone necrosis.

Immunosuppressive Drugs. Immunosuppressive drugs are being used experimentally in children with JA whose disease simply will not respond to any other medical treatment. These include cyclophosphamide (Cytoxan), chlorambucil (Leukeran), azathioprine (Imuran), and methotrexate (Ansell, 1991). Each of these has serious potential side effects, including bladder inflammation, infertility, and severe immunosuppression predisposing to malignancy. As a result, their use is controversial and is limited to extreme cases.

Physical Therapy. Drug therapy is only one aspect of care for the patient with JA. A balanced program of medication, rest, and a regular schedule of exercise that includes physical therapy is necessary in most instances. Goals often include (1) increasing or maintaining strength and range of motion, (2) promoting independence in ambulation and other activities of daily living, and (3) controlling pain (Scull et al, 1986).

Considerations for Rest and Exercise. Rest has long been acknowledged as an effective treatment for joint swelling and heat. In fact, casting has long been used to facilitate periods of rest. However, muscle atrophy quickly occurs with this type of immobilization. Therefore, for the body as a whole as well as for individual joints, rest must be balanced with exercise (see discussion under "Planning and Implementation").

Surgical Intervention. Surgery may be necessary for some patients with JA. Contractures that do not respond to splinting, exercise, or other therapies should be released before cartilage destruction makes them immovable. Joint replacements in children continue to be controversial. Hip, knee, wrist, and shoulder replacements are done but must be postponed until late adolescence or until bone growth has ceased (Witt et al, 1991). Surgical interventions present other problems, including lack of motivation by the child to participate actively in rehabilitation and anesthesia for the child who has temporomandibular or cervical spine disease.

Application of the Nursing Process: Juvenile Arthritis

Assessment

The acute care nurse may encounter the child during acute exacerbations of the disease. The child will be hospitalized (1) when the disease process "flares" and intensive occupational therapy/physical therapy

(OT/PT) are required, (2) when medications need to be re-evaluated, or (3) when surgical procedures are required (synovectomies, muscle/tendon releases for treatment of contracture, serial casting, joint replacements). The acute care nurse begins management responsibilities which, at the patient's discharge, become the domain of the home care nurse. These include facilitating and monitoring the involvement of the parent and child in the therapy regimen, assessing the psychological impact of illness on an ongoing basis, making referrals for counseling as needed for promoting positive attitudes toward school and psychosocial development, intervening with community resources (school, OT, PT), and recognizing needs for teaching. Teaching needs include aspects such as medications, physical assessment, appropriate activities, nutrition, availability of community resources, use of splints and braces, and use of community resources.

Management of the child with JA occurs primarily in the home. The child and family benefit from a disciplined daily routine that balances time for individual and collective needs for therapies, rest, relaxation, pleasure, school, adequate nutrition, and normal or routine family activities. This balance may be delicate and precarious, but it is essential for facing the challenges of JA and promoting the most positive passage through each stage of growth and development. Therefore, the role of the nurse may be extremely broad, encompassing that of caregiver, teacher, advocate, and coordinator.

Nursing Diagnostic Statements and Collaborative Problems

Impaired physical mobility and sleep pattern disturbance *related to pain from chronic joint inflammation.*

Altered nutrition: less than body requirements *related to altered metabolism.*

High risk for altered growth and development; *risk factors:*

- *Overprotective behavior of parents.*
- *Physical limitations associated with joint involvement and systemic symptoms.*
- *Irregular school attendance.*

High risk for self-esteem or body image disturbance; *risk factor: the perceptions of the child and significant others to the physical limitations.*

High risk for ineffective family coping; *risk factors:*

- *Anxiety.*
- *Sibling problems.*

High risk for altered home health maintenance; *risk factor: knowledge deficit about home care.*

Planning and Implementation

Promoting Physical Mobility and Adequate Rest. Pain control should incorporate physical care, such as application of heat, positioning, and limitation of activities. Although it is not clear how they work, cutaneous application of menthol ointments may provide temporary relief of joint pain. Techniques such as distraction and relaxation can be effective. Redirection of attention by story-telling, singing, or other areas of concentration may be helpful. Relaxation techniques may be more effective in the older child and may vary from meditation to breathing exercises to relaxing with music. The use of imagery or self-hypnosis also has been shown to be effective in pain relief for children with JA and may enhance the child's sense of mastery and control (Olness & Gardner, 1988). Benefits of the techniques listed include reducing anxiety, easing muscle tension, promoting rest (may be as effective as napping), and increasing the effectiveness of other interventions used for pain relief.

Exercise for the child occurs both in normal play and directed school activities. It is tempting to consider this "normal activity" adequate exercise for the child with JA, but a formal exercise program that takes all areas of the body through maximum active range of motion is essential to maintain function. A well-developed, integrated PT program maintains mobility by (1) providing invigorating physical activities that strengthen muscles and put joints through full range of motion, and (2) promoting a positive attitude about physical capabilities. A major challenge is the development of a program that is interesting and stimulating and will encourage compliance. A coordinated program needs to be developed with OT and PT and may also involve school nurses and teachers. It is important to select activities that maintain mobility and range of motion but do not strain inflamed joints, particularly weight bearing strain, which aggravates synovitis. Suggestions for activities include the following:

- Noncompetitive swimming, which is particularly good because it provides total body exercise and protects joints against strain while strengthening muscles and improving range of motion.
- Directed slow movements imitating birds or animals, which may be effective for younger children. Toddlers may enjoy kicking a balloon or soft beach ball.
- Riding a tricycle or bicycle, which can help reduce stiffness of knees and hips.
- Rolling clay, which exercises hands and wrists.
- For adolescents, t'ai-chi routines, which can be used as progressive resistive exercises with common sense and reasonable caution when the adolescent is free of pain. However, they are contraindicated when joints are inflamed and painful.
- ADLs (activities of daily living), which are natural, automatic sources of action and range of motion.

Dressing, bathing, and grooming activities provide natural, routine exercises that are also therapeutic. Adaptations of both function and equipment may be necessary to facilitate these activities and allow more independent self-care while protecting joints from excessive strain.

Activities that are "in harmony with" the natural or acquired interests or inclinations can be used or modified to meet individual needs. Running, jumping, and prolonged walking should be avoided, however, if active lower extremity synovitis is present. Long periods of reading or watching television weaken muscles and cause fixed joint deformities.

Early morning stiffness may make normal activities as well as exercises extremely painful and difficult. A warm shower or soaking in warm (32° to 36.5° C) water can help reduce early morning stiffness and relax muscles. Pain relief methods, as described under "Reducing Pain," can also be used.

Occupational and physical therapists can develop appropriate orthoses. When joints are inflamed and painful, splints may provide comfort and rest. The child may object to wearing the splints, but they are important in maintaining function and reducing the possibility of deformity. The most frequently used splints are night-time knee splints prescribed to prevent knee flexion (or contracture) and to improve knee extension. Splints for wrists are also commonly used to improve wrist dorsiflexion.

A home visit may be necessary to determine the need for assistive devices or the presence of factors in the home that may be a problem for the child or the family. A bathroom not wheelchair accessible, or multiple steps into or within the home, is an example of problems that make daily living difficult for the family and the child and that must be resolved for the goal of normal living. Adaptive devices for the bathroom for toileting and bathing are relatively easy to obtain and can make these intimate aspects of daily living possible on a more independent basis. The physical therapist can assess the need for these and other aids and provide information and assistance in locating these resources.

Many children with JA experience increased fatigability. The demands of school and routine ADLs may be very tiring. Excessive emotional and physical fatigue may trigger exacerbations of JA. Younger children usually respond more appropriately to feelings of fatigue, pacing physical activities and rest time. School-age children and adolescents who tend to get caught up in peer activities and possibly job responsibilities may need encouragement to allow themselves extra rest. Rest, relaxation, leisure activities, and relief from emotional distress may relieve fatigue and reduce exacerbations and therefore become an important aspect of management.

Promoting Optimal Nutrition. For the child with JA, no evidence suggests that any food or vitamin has either a causative or curative role, but there are nutritional concerns for these children. Decreased mobility may reduce metabolic needs, predisposing to weight gain. However, the inflammatory process coupled with anemia may increase metabolic needs, leading to weight loss or inadequate weight gain. Obesity is a concern for the child with JA because excessive weight places more stress on already inflamed joints and because the overweight child tends to be less active and, therefore, stiffer. Being too thin is a problem as well if caloric intake is insufficient for normal growth. Recognizing the potential for caloric intake that either exceeds or fails to meet nutritional needs and incorporating nutritional aspects into teaching can prevent unnecessary physical and emotional stress for the child.

Promoting Normal Development. The key to promoting normal development is normalization of the environment to the extent possible. This can often be accomplished by focusing on the *abilities* of the ill child rather than on the limitations. For example, assignment of appropriate household chores and responsibilities fosters a sense of normality, acceptance, and accomplishment for the child and promotes more normal family functioning. Attention to normal development also includes the enhancement of self-esteem and promotion of regular school attendance. (See Chapter 19 for additional strategies related to normal development for the child with a chronic illness.)

School is an integral part of growth and development, and regular attendance should be encouraged. Some adjustments may be necessary, however, to accommodate some of the limitations imposed by JA. Climbing stairs or walking long distances may be difficult or impossible, and access to classes may need to be arranged. Early morning stiffness may make getting to school difficult. Because of the child's increased fatigability, the school day may need to be shortened by temporary withdrawal from less essential classes. Participation in physical education programs may need to be adapted to account for the child's physical limitations.

Social interactions in the school setting are an important part of normal development, so part-time school attendance or home tutoring on a regular basis is discouraged. Tutoring, however, occasionally may be advisable to allow the child to "keep up" when mobility is further restricted by disease exacerbations or surgery.

Enhancing Self-Esteem and Body Image. The limitations imposed on the child by inflamed joints and by any permanent limitations and disfigurements can significantly alter the child's perception of both self-abilities and self-worth. Assessment of what is real or accurate in these perceptions is an important role of nurses. They should assist the child to a realistic perception and expectation while affirming the positive characteristics and abilities of the child, thereby affirming his or her worth.

Children, as well as parents, must have an accurate perception of the disease process to understand which aspects of the process can be altered by their interventions and which are beyond their control. This understanding helps assuage guilt feelings that somehow they are getting worse because of failure to comply with prescribed therapy. The child (particularly the preschooler) also needs to be absolved of guilt by understanding that the illness was not caused by thinking "forbidden" thoughts or by "naughty" behavior.

For the adolescent, JA presents concerns about vocational preparation, heterosexual interactions, and realistic expectations for marriage and family. Adolescent support groups are one way of providing a safe environment for exchange of ideas, concerns, frustrations, and feelings. For further information on the impact of a chronic illness on the child and family, refer to Chapter 19.

Supporting Adaptive Coping. Diagnosis of JA may be a long and tedious process requiring more than one physician to complete the diagnostic workup. The anxiety associated with the child's discomfort and the fear and frustration of the diagnostic process can take an incredible toll on the whole family. The fears and frustrations of the parents are further increased when the child is unable to either understand or articulate discomforts.

An additional anxiety-producing experience is the hospitalization of the child for "flares," control of fevers, acute joint inflammation, or complications such as pericarditis and myocarditis. The nurse may be the single member of the large interdisciplinary health care team most consistently present, and, as such, must function as a resource/comfort/support person throughout all these periods.

Siblings of the ill child often require special consideration by parents and health care professionals. Siblings should be allowed to vent their feelings of guilt, frustration, and anxiety during the long, tedious, physically and emotionally draining course of the illness. Support groups for these family members can provide education, encouragement, and understanding. In addition, organizations such as Crippled Children's Service and the American Juvenile Arthritis Organization, which is sponsored by the Arthritis Foundation, may provide educational materials, specialized services, and financial aid to qualified families.

Facilitating Home Health Maintenance. The goal of patient and family teaching is to assist the child and family to be active, knowledgeable, and responsible participants in disease assessment and management.

The purpose of teaching disease-specific assessment skills is to provide the family with a framework for judgments. For example, the child and family need to be aware of any pattern of fevers so that they can feel comfortable with differentiating between what may be normally associated with the disease process and what indicates other illness or possible complications and therefore should be communicated to a physician. The presence of a rash that is associated with temperature spikes needs to be differentiated from a rash that might be an allergic response or associated with some other illness.

Aspirin therapy is the most common form of treatment. Instruction must include the therapeutic dosage that has been calculated specifically for the child. Brushing the teeth after chewing baby aspirin reduces the risk for cavities associated with residual aspirin packed into indentations on chewing surfaces. Aspirin should be administered with food or milk to reduce gastric irritation. Antacids should be discouraged, except as recommended and monitored by the physician, because they interfere with medication absorption. Parents may be concerned about the side effects of aspirin and inquire about acetaminophen. It is necessary for parents to understand that acetaminophen does not have anti-inflammatory properties.

The risks of aspirin administration during flu season and during outbreaks of chickenpox cannot be ignored in light of the probable link among these infections, aspirin, and Reye syndrome. Parents should be cautioned to contact the physician for potential changes in medication at these times.

If aspirin therapy and other NSAIDs are ineffective in controlling the disease process, immunosuppressive drugs may be necessary. This presents another concern for the nurse, both when the patient is hospitalized and at home. The child will be more susceptible to infectious diseases because of the immunosuppression. The child and family should be counseled to avoid large groups or enclosed public areas during flu season to prevent unnecessary exposure to infection. The child also is at risk for septic conditions that may be masked by the steroids. This possibility must always be considered when the patient has otherwise nonspecific symptoms. When the immunosuppressed child is hospitalized, room assignment must reflect the need to protect the child from a nosocomial infection (see Table 37–4).

Parents should be reminded that aspirin and all medications should be kept out of reach of children who are too young to be responsible for their own medication administration. Overdoses of aspirin can cause gastrointestinal bleeding and severe acid-base disturbances in children. (Chapter 24 provides detailed strategies related to age-appropriate administration of medications.)

Other aspects of teaching for which the nurse may be responsible include discussion of assessments that need to be made by the child or parents, such as temperature patterns, rashes, changes in mobility or ability to function, and use of orthoses (splints or braces).

Identification of affected joints and the characteristics of their involvement is important. The status of and changes in warmth and color of joints, the presence or absence of effusions, and joint position are all significant assessments that should be made on a regular basis. Orthoses should be assessed on a regular basis for fit, changes due to normal growth, or skin irritation that may result from poor placement or unsatisfactory fit. The child and family need to know how to evaluate the therapeutic and side effects of medications. Assessments for visual changes that might indicate iridocyclitis are important to prevent permanent visual impairment. Assessments for any changes in physical and emotional stability or endurance need to be made by both the nurse and the family. Early assessments and evaluations can often prevent further complications.

Rheumatic Fever

Rheumatic fever, named for its joint involvement and increased temperature in the acute stage, is a systemic inflammatory disease of childhood that can involve the heart, joints, CNS, skin, and connective tissue.

Although the incidence of rheumatic fever has decreased in the Western world, it is still considered the most common cause of heart disease in people younger than 40 years of age. The natural history of the disease has been altered by environmental as well as medical factors. Industrialization, urbanization with improved socioeconomic conditions, the advent and increasingly widespread administration of antibiotics, as well as improved health care practices, and better criteria for identification are all factors that have contributed to this reduced incidence.

Etiology/Incidence (Pathophysiology)

Even though the incidence of rheumatic fever has decreased, the disease has not been eradicated. An estimated 100,000 cases occur each year in the United States, and studies have shown an increased incidence in New York City (Lockey & Bukantz, 1987b). It is more often found in school-age children between 6 and 15 years old, with a peak incidence at about 8 years of age. It also appears to be more commonly seen in cold, humid climates. Statistics suggest that there may be an increased familial incidence, but it is not known whether this is due to heredity, environment, or other factors. Rheumatic fever is known to recur.

Rheumatic fever is a potential sequelae of group A beta-hemolytic streptococcal infections and may occur after illnesses such as Streptococcal tonsillitis, pharyngitis, or impetigo. A direct relationship between a group A beta-streptococcal infection and the occurrence of rheumatic fever has been firmly established, but the exact pathologic mechanism responsible for development of rheumatic fever is still unknown. It has been documented, however, that when a beta-hemolytic streptococcal infection (e.g., pharyngitis, scarlet fever, or middle ear infection) occurs, antibodies are formed against the toxin released by the streptococci. The antibodies formed in this immune response react with tissue antigens and can cause damage in different tissues of the body (an autoimmune response), specifically the heart, joints, glomeruli of the kidney, CNS, and skin. Some tissues are more susceptible to damage than others, particularly the heart. The fact that only 3 per cent or fewer (Behrman, 1992) of children with streptococcal infections contract rheumatic fever suggests, however, that undefined genetic or other factors may be operating.

The acute stage of rheumatic fever is characterized by inflammation of connective tissue in the heart, joints, and skin. The acute stage usually lasts 2 to 3 weeks and is followed by a proliferation phase that involves primarily the heart. During this second phase, Aschoff bodies (large, multinucleated cells) may accumulate on heart valves weakened by inflammation. (Fig. 33–21 illustrates this phenomenon.) Cardiac valve injury, the most serious complication, occurs as the valve leaflets become scarred. The extent of resulting valvular stenosis and regurgitation depends on the degree of the initial insult and any added damage with recurrence of rheumatic fever. The mitral valve is the most commonly affected, followed by the aortic valve.

Clinical Manifestations

As indicated, rheumatic fever characteristically follows a group A beta-hemolytic streptococcal infection. The initial infection may have occurred a few days to 6 weeks earlier. The entire episode of rheumatic fever lasts from 1 to 3 months and is self-limiting. The Jones criteria for guidance in the diagnosis of rheumatic fever have identified major and minor manifestations of the disease (Table 37–7). The sequence

TABLE 37–7
Jones Criteria (Revised) for Guidance in the Diagnosis of Rheumatic Fever*

Major Manifestations	Minor Manifestations: Clinical	Minor Manifestations: Laboratory
Carditis Polyarthritis Chorea Erythema marginatum Subcutaneous nodules	Previous rheumatic fever or rheumatic heart disease Arthralgia Fever	Acute-phase reactants: erythrocyte sedimentation rate, C-reactive protein, leukocytosis Prolonged P-R interval

Supporting Evidence of Streptococcal Infection
Increased titer of antistreptococcal antibodies (antistreptolysin O), others
Positive throat culture for group A *Streptococcus*
Recent scarlet fever

From American Heart Association. (1982). Data from Committee on Rheumatic Fever and Bacterial Endocarditis. Dallas: Author.

* The presence of two major criteria, or of one major and two minor criteria, indicates a high probability of acute rheumatic fever, *if supported by evidence of preceding group A streptococcal infection.*

of signs and symptoms is fairly predictable, with inflammation of joints, heart, and erythematous rash appearing and often associated with a temperature of 38°C (100.4°F) or higher. The major manifestations identified in the revised Jones criteria are discussed next.

Arthritis. The onset of rheumatic fever may be insidious, with the child merely appearing tired and apathetic. One of the first complaints may be that of joint tenderness. The area may appear swollen, red, and warm. However, these *complaints may seem out of proportion* to evidence of arthritis. The joints most frequently affected by these arthritic changes are the large joints: knees, elbows, and wrists. Other joints that may be affected are shoulders, ankles, and finger joints. These arthritic pains, usually migratory, generally last from 1 to 4 weeks and rarely cause permanent deformities. Three fourths of children with rheumatic fever experience arthritic symptoms (Behrman, 1992).

Carditis. Carditis (cardiac inflammation) is the most severe manifestation of rheumatic fever and occurs in most children with the disease (Griffiths, 1986). It may involve the myocardium, endocardium, and pericardium as well as the heart valves, most commonly the mitral and aortic valves. The other signs and symptoms of the acute illness will disappear, but children who have had carditis may experience some degree of residual valvular damage.

The mildest cases of carditis may not exhibit signs and symptoms. Indeed, on radiography, the chest may appear normal. The first indication may be a new systolic murmur. If pericarditis is present, a pericardial friction rub may be heard. Conduction abnormalities (prolonged P-R intervals or atrial fibrillation) may be seen on electrocardiogram (ECG).

Other signs of carditis may include tachycardia (particularly a persistent increase in the sleeping pulse rate); shortness of breath with exertion; muffled heart sounds as a result of pericardial effusion; edema of the face, abdomen, or ankles as a result of increased cardiac workload or cardiac insufficiency; pericardial friction rub; and enlargement of the liver. As the inflammation resolves, scarring or fusing of the leaflets of the valves can result in valvular stenosis, which may subsequently lead to left-sided heart failure. Changes in electrical conductivity of the heart (prolonged P-R interval) may be seen in a significant number of patients, but this alone is not diagnostic or prognostic of rheumatic carditis.

Erythema Marginatum. Erythema marginatum is a rare skin manifestation found in children with rheumatic fever (Kaplan, 1992). It is characterized by an erythematous, nonpruritic, macular rash with a circular pattern on the trunk, buttocks, and proximal limbs. It blanches when pressed and is accentuated with heat. Erythema marginatum is a transitory skin manifestation and leaves no residual tissue damage. It may occur in the acute phase of illness but may come and go for several months. Erythema marginatum usually occurs in patients who also have carditis.

Subcutaneous Nodules. These are usually visible nodules that are found on the flexor surfaces of the joints and bony prominences, such as feet, hands, scapula, scalp, and vertebrae. They are small, firm, nontender swellings that occur during the febrile stage of illness and persist for relatively long periods, eventually resolving with no permanent damage. This manifestation also usually occurs in patients with carditis.

Chorea. Chorea is also known as "Sydenham chorea," "St. Vitus dance," and "encephalitis rheumatica." It is an infrequent manifestation of rheumatic fever, and its cause is unknown. It is rare in children younger than 3 years and older than 15 years of age. As the incidence of rheumatic fever declines, so does this unusual associated symptom.

Like erythema marginatum and subcutaneous nodules, chorea appears in patients with carditis; however, it may have a later occurrence than do other sequelae. Its occurrence also varies with age relative to the appearance of other major manifestations.

Chorea is characterized by involuntary movements of facial muscles as well as muscles of the limbs, particularly the upper extremities. Signs and symptoms may be insidious and nonspecific, beginning with irritability and emotional lability. The child may at first be thought to have behavioral problems, such as being fidgety and showing altered school performance. This process may progress to the point of interference with normal activities of daily living through uncontrollable jerky movements that interfere with voluntary control. Slurred speech may be present.

The CNS changes typically occur 2 or more months after the initial streptococcal infection or after the other symptoms of rheumatic fever have subsided. There may be electroencephalogram (EEG) abnormalities; however, these usually return to normal. The symptoms may persist for as briefly as a week or for as long as 1.5 to 2 years. Chorea is generally a benign and self-limited aspect of rheumatic fever, and full recovery is expected.

Less significant manifestations of rheumatic fever include abdominal pain, pleurisy, and rheumatic pneumonitis. Figure 37–13 summarizes the major and minor manifestations of rheumatic fever.

Diagnostic Assessment

The revised Jones criteria for diagnosing rheumatic fever have been significant for differentiating this disease from other illnesses with which it may be confused. Diagnosis depends on recognition of the classic symptoms and a detailed patient history. Most children with an acute pharyngitis have a viral rather than a bacterial infection. A throat culture, therefore, is im-

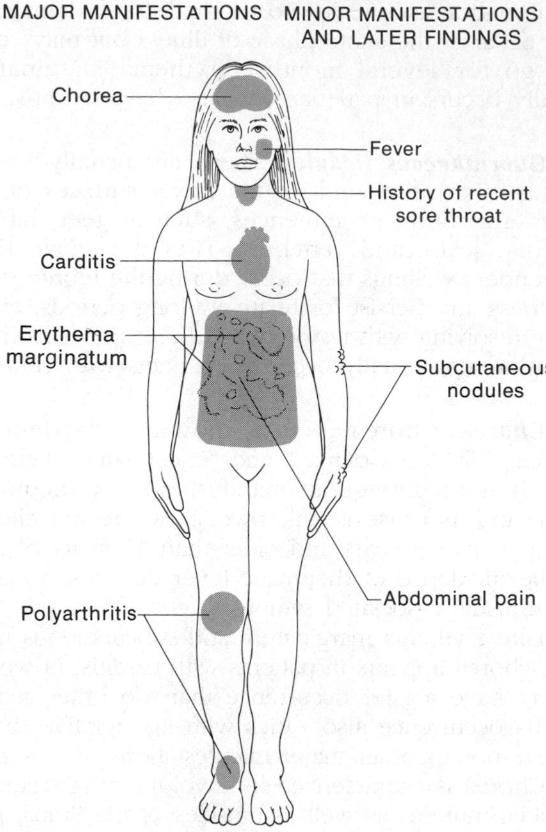

FIGURE 37 - 13. Manifestations of rheumatic fever (Jones criteria).

portant for determining the presence of group A beta-hemolytic streptococcus. Rheumatic fever may follow a streptococcal infection anywhere in the body; the risk is not limited to pharyngitis.

Although no diagnostic laboratory tests are specific for rheumatic fever, elevations in the ESR, C-reactive protein, and white blood count will usually be seen, indicating the presence of an inflammatory process. A mild anemia is also common and is due to suppressed erythropoiesis during inflammation. Cardiac enzymes may be increased if severe carditis occurs. If the pharyngitis has resolved within the previous 2 months, the presence of an increased streptococcal antibody titer will indicate the preceding infection. The test for identifying streptococcal antibodies is the antistreptolysin O (ASO) test. Streptolysin O is a streptococcal extracellular byproduct that causes lysis of red blood cells. ASO titers indicate the presence of antibodies to these products within the blood. Echocardiography and cardiac catheterization can identify and evaluate valvular damage and ventricular function.

Therapeutic Management

Prevention of rheumatic fever is the best "treatment." Effective management of beta-streptococcal infections can prevent the development of rheumatic fever. Early recognition of the symptoms of streptococcal infection and appropriate treatment can also prevent recurrence of rheumatic fever, which then reduces the chance of permanent cardiac damage.

If the child has a positive streptococcal culture from the throat, impetigo lesions, or elsewhere at the time of inflammatory symptoms, the active streptococcal infection will be treated.

The treatment of choice to eradicate beta-streptococcal infection is penicillin, usually in the form of an intramuscular injection of benzathine penicillin G. This form of penicillin is a long-acting drug, and, therefore, treatment may be limited to a single injection. Other penicillins may be administered parenterally or in a combination of parenteral and oral doses.

During the acute phase of the disease, bed rest is recommended to decrease the workload of the heart. Children with carditis are kept on bed rest until the ESR returns to normal and congestive heart failure (if present) is controlled (Kaplan, 1992).

Salicylates are often administered in the acute phase. These help control inflammation, particularly in the joints. They also provide analgesia for palliation of other symptoms. In cases involving severe carditis, steroids may be prescribed for their anti-inflammatory properties. However, there is still controversy about the long-term benefits of steroids in preventing rheumatic heart disease and their advisability in view of the significant potential side effects (Behrman, 1992). Follow-up care is important.

Residual heart disease is the most destructive long-term complication of rheumatic fever; the incidence is proportional to the degree of carditis. If valvular or other cardiac damage is present, the physician will be alert for subsequent signs of congestive heart failure. (See Chapter 33 for management of congestive heart failure.)

Cardiac valvular damage increases the susceptibility to bacterial endocarditis, particularly if procedures are carried out that could cause septicemia (e.g., dental procedures that may cause entry of mouth bacteria into gum lesions). Prophylactic antibiotics are therefore ordered, usually throughout childhood and adolescence, or for at least 5 years in the older adolescent, even in patients with no residual heart disease. If valvular heart disease is present, lifelong prophylaxis may be recommended. (See Chapter 33 for further discussion of bacterial endocarditis.)

Nursing Diagnostic Statements and Collaborative Problems

High risk for injury, physiologic (carditis); *risk factors:*

- *Noncompliance with bed rest owing to lack of alerting symptoms of damage.*
- *Knowledge deficit about reasons for activity limitations.*

Altered comfort: pain related to *joint inflammation.*

High risk for impaired skin integrity; *risk factor: bed rest.*

High risk for altered nutrition: less than body requirements; *risk factor: disease-associated anorexia.*

High risk for altered growth and development; *risk factors: social isolation, abnormal movements of chorea.*

High risk for diversional activity deficit; *risk factors:*

- *Social isolation.*
- *Bed rest.*

High risk for ineffective family coping; *risk factor: impact of the chronicity of the disease.*

High risk for altered home health maintenance; *risk factor: knowledge deficit about home care.*

Planning and Implementation

Care of the child with rheumatic fever now occurs primarily in the home rather than in the hospital. In general, interventions are manifestation-specific or symptom-specific. Referral likely will be made to a community health nurse who can both assess and anticipate the needs of the child and the family. The nurse will be instrumental in helping the family secure needed supplies.

An important responsibility of the nurse is participation in screening programs aimed at preventing rheumatic fever. Community health nurses as well as school nurses should be alert to children who exhibit signs and symptoms of group A beta-hemolytic streptococcal infections, particularly if these children live in "at risk" environments. On diagnosis of a streptococcal infection, emphasis is placed on completion of antibiotic therapy to ensure eradication of the bacteria. Compliance with this regimen will reduce the risk of rheumatic fever.

Promoting Compliance with Bed Rest and Activity Restrictions. Maintaining bed rest for the child with rheumatic fever may prove to be one of the greatest challenges for the nurse and the family. Because the child may not feel ill, bed rest may seem unreasonable or unnecessary. One way to maintain bed rest is to plan appropriate low-activity diversions, such as board games, puzzles, reading, and paper dolls. The parents and child need to understand that to feel well does not mean that the body has recovered. Explaining the reason for activity restrictions often helps the child and family cope with the frustration and inconvenience. The discussion should explain the relationship between activity and cardiac workload, thus providing a rationale for activity restrictions. The child and family will need clarification of the physician's intent for activity. The nurse can clarify what the specific expectations of "bed rest" are (i.e., does this include bathroom privileges, ADLs such as out of bed to dress, eat meals, and walk, or does this mean strict or absolute bed rest?).

Once it is clear why extra rest is needed and exactly what the activity restrictions are, the nurse can talk with the family about allowing the child some self-management responsibilities. The child who is allowed to exercise some autonomy is usually more willing to follow the prescribed treatment. During follow-up visits, the nurse can reinforce the child's sense of accomplishment for self-management by commenting on appropriate choices and evidence of good judgment. A gradual increase in activities can be anticipated as the ESR returns to normal, inflammation subsides, and any cardiac involvement stabilizes. Despite explanations and promises of being able to normalize activity after a few weeks, restrictions may cause the child to feel angry, frustrated, frightened, and anxious. The nurse can be supportive by communicating understanding and by providing a safe environment for sharing of these feelings and concerns.

Alleviating Discomfort. Discomforts occur throughout the course of rheumatic fever as a result of fever, arthritis, and arthralgias. Analgesics (aspirin and acetaminophen) are given to reduce the fever and discomfort. Equipment such as bed cradles can be used to lift linens and reduce pressure on sensitive skin and joints. Bed rails (which can be rented from a home care supply service) can aid the child in moving in bed and also prevent falls. Care should be organized to minimize handling of the child if the child is having acute arthritic pain. Massage, manipulation of joints, and heat or cold may aggravate discomforts. Proper body alignment will help reduce joint discomfort.

Preventing Skin Breakdown. Because of fever, discomfort associated with movement, joint pains, and stiffness, skin breakdown is a potential problem. Breakdown can be avoided by regular repositioning and making sure that the skin is kept clean and well lubricated, that linens are clean and wrinkle free, and that bony prominences are well lubricated and protected from irritation and pressure.

Promoting Optimal Nutrition. The child with rheumatic fever often experiences an increased metabolic rate associated with fever and inflammation. This increased metabolic rate means the child will need an increased amount of nutrients. However, immobility, boredom, and discomfort may lead to anorexia. In addition, aspirin and steroids can cause gastric irritation, further diminishing appetite. The additional need for calories, coupled with anorexia, can lead to insufficient intake.

During convalescence, the diet should have adequate protein and calories to meet the recovery needs of the body, especially when fever or infection is present. (It is also important, however, to avoid excessive weight gain.) Fluid intake should be monitored to prevent either dehydration or overhydration. This can be accomplished by calculating the child's maintenance fluid volume and using this amount as a guideline for 24-hour fluid intake. (See discussion of calculation of fluid maintenance requirements in Chapter 26.) The febrile patient needs additional fluids, but hypervolemia increases the workload of the heart. Medications should be taken with milk or food to minimize stomach upsets. Parents should be encouraged to be tolerant when the child's appetite is poor, offering small frequent meals in lieu of large meals. Intake may increase if the child is allowed some control by selecting from choices of nutritious foods for meals and snacks.

Promoting Normal Development. Emotional and social development may be temporarily interrupted because of prescribed bed rest that takes the child out of the classroom and away from normal peer activities. When the disease is complicated by the occurrence of chorea, development is further obstructed. The nurse can alert the family to age-appropriate developmental tasks and help them normalize the child's environment as much as possible. When chorea is present, the family will need reassurance of its temporary nature, and practical advice for management.

The nurse can clarify that "bed rest" need not mean "in the bedroom." The child can be kept near the family activities by lying on a cot in the kitchen or on a sofa in the living room. At times when the child is alone in a bedroom, anticipation of needs may help reduce feelings of isolation. Some means should be provided (e.g., a bell) to allow the child to indicate the need for assistance or attention. Family pets can be wonderful companions, and a telephone can provide an important link to peers and extended family.

Children with uncontrollable body movements related to chorea are usually frightened and frustrated, as are their families. The child and family will need reassurance that this is only a temporary disorder and that while it is a neurologic phenomenon, the child's intellect is not affected. It may be necessary to intervene with teachers and perhaps students to explain the child's problem and to ensure all concerned that this is not a behavioral or learning disorder. With family support, interruptions in development encountered during chorea need not result in significant delays.

Caregivers should anticipate that the child will probably need assistance with basic care such as feeding, toileting, and bathing. In addition, the child must be protected from injury related to uncontrollable movements. Persons who assist with feeding should be reminded that sudden choreic movements of the head make use of a fork or a straw dangerous. Plastic (rather than glass) is advised for plates and drinking glasses. The child's bed should have rails (or some other protection) that prevent falling out of bed. Rails or protective barriers should be padded to prevent injury. Mittens and head covering may be indicated at times. Toys and games should be assessed for sharp edges.

Choreiform movements disappear during sleep; therefore, sedatives may be prescribed. In the acute phase of chorea the child may rest better in a room where stimulation is minimized.

Promoting Diversional Activity. Boredom becomes a problem for the child confined to bed. The child can be encouraged to participate in development of a daily schedule, which should include as many of the usual activities as possible, for example, getting dressed, eating meals with the family, and attending to studies. All the activities must be geared to decrease boredom while conforming to the limits imposed by the degree of restrictions, expectations, and implications of "bed rest." Age-appropriate diversional activities can be encouraged or provided, for example, quiet games, art activities, books, video recordings, and television. Family and friends can be encouraged to write, call, or visit (after being screened for upper respiratory infections or other illnesses). When the child's condition permits, a tutor should be provided to help keep the child current with school assignments.

Supporting Family Coping. Assisting families to cope effectively is an important aspect of care. The nurse should encourage expression of anger, guilt, frustration, fears, and concerns. The nurse can act as a liaison between the family and community resources (e.g., the Crippled Children's Service and the American Heart Association), which can provide information and possibly financial assistance.

Facilitating Home Health Maintenance. Family teaching may include all or part of the following areas:

- The disease and its treatment (characteristics and progress of the illness, possible complications, expected outcome, and potential effects of noncompliance with prescribed therapy).
- Relationship of exercise to cardiac workload.
- Rationale, side effects, and expected length of administration of each medication.
- Psychological and physical preparation for procedures (purpose of the test, the procedure itself, and any follow-up).
- Importance of minimizing contact with other infections, particularly respiratory.
- Recognition of signs of recurrent strep infections and the importance of seeing the physician for prompt treatment of sore throat after the initial recovery period.

- Reassurance that, except for possible valvular damage, all other symptoms are temporary.

Managing Medications. Penicillin to eradicate streptococcal infection is often given by injection and is therefore the responsibility of the nurse rather than the family. Intramuscular injections of benzathine penicillin G must be administered with care. Gluteal injections can cause vasospasms and sciatic nerve damage if injected into the neural area. The midlateral thigh is the recommended site for injection for small children. The ventral gluteal site is appropriate when the muscle has developed more fully. The site must be carefully identified. If oral penicillin is prescribed instead of, or in addition to, the injection, the family must realize the importance of administering all of the pills.

Alertness to signs of an allergic response to medications is essential. In the initial assessment, the nurse should inquire about any previous adverse reactions to penicillin, and the child should remain in the clinic for 20 minutes following the injection in case an anaphylactic reaction occurs. Epinephrine must be available for this emergency. The child and parents should be taught the side effects of oral penicillin, including any indications of hypersensitivity, such as rash, pruritus, chills, and dyspnea. Erythromycin is the usual drug of choice if the child is allergic to penicillin.

Aspirin and steroids may be used to minimize the inflammatory process. Fever, arthritis, arthralgias, and myalgias are generally controlled well with aspirin. Children's ability to tolerate aspirin is variable. Side effects of aspirin include gastrointestinal disturbances, decreased platelet count, tinnitus, headaches, and possible mental disturbances.

Steroids, which may be prescribed if the child has an associated carditis, have significant anti-inflammatory properties but also have serious side effects. See Table 37–4 for the nursing process plan related to corticosteroid administration.

Digoxin may be added to the medication regimen. It slows conduction (and therefore the heart rate) and strengthens the contractions of the myocardium, thereby improving cardiac efficiency. If there are changes in pulse rate or quality, particularly if there is a significant decrease in rate, the digoxin dose should not be administered and the physician should be notified. Parents need to be taught to take an apical pulse. (See Chapter 33 for additional information on administration of digoxin.)

Managing Associated Carditis. The presence of carditis with its associated potential for permanent cardiac damage requires careful follow-up and management. Often the child with mild-to-moderate carditis can be treated in the home. Severe carditis usually involves congestive heart failure and requires hospitalization.

A change in the quality of the pulse may be the first indication of cardiac involvement. Nursing assessment on follow-up visits will therefore include careful respiratory and cardiac assessment. The pulse parameters and the rate and rhythm of the apical pulse will be compared with the child's baseline at the time of diagnosis. Any irregularities or significant changes must be referred to the physician for diagnosis.

The administration of oxygen may be indicated with carditis to reduce the workload of the heart. The nurse can facilitate home oxygen therapy by serving as a liaison between the family and the company supplying the equipment. The family will need a 24-hour-per-day phone number in case of questions or malfunction of the equipment.

If oxygen is required, a nasal cannula provides the most accurate method of administration. Children also consider it the least restrictive. Appropriate explanation of the rationale and benefit of oxygen is important to promote compliance with therapy and reduce anxiety for both parents and child. Instructions on the use of safety precautions with home administration of oxygen must be given.

Vital signs (particularly heart rate and blood pressure) are good indicators of progress or status of cardiac function. As the acute stage resolves, the heart rate should be more nearly normal for age, and decompensation with activities should be less significant (e.g., the heart rate returns more quickly to normal).

Kawasaki Disease

"Kawasaki disease" (KD) is the name currently given to the syndrome previously known as "mucocutaneous lymph node syndrome." It is a febrile, multisystem disorder in which vasculitis is the most potentially dangerous characteristic. Generally considered a self-limiting disease, KD can also be fatal if aneurysms or myocardial infarction occurs.

Etiology/Incidence (Pathophysiology)

KD may be seen at any age but is virtually restricted to prepubertal children. It is most common in boys younger than 2 years and in persons of Japanese ancestry (Hicks & Melish, 1986). Genetics has been suggested as a possible explanation for a higher incidence among Japanese children, but the evidence to support this is inconclusive. KD has a seasonal pattern, with a significantly greater number of cases in the winter and spring months.

It is generally agreed that Kawasaki disease is not a new pathologic entity. In the past, KD was probably misdiagnosed as other types of vasculitis before criteria were established to clearly define it from other disease processes. KD appears to be occurring more frequently, sporadically and in clusters, than at the time it was first described by Kawasaki in 1967. However, this may be the result of more accurate diagnosis or reporting.

Although the cause of KD remains unknown, several possible causes have been proposed. Environmental factors (e.g., rug shampoo) have been implicated but remain unconfirmed. When "epidemics" have occurred, the affected children have had a significantly higher-than-average occurrence of mild respiratory upset. No specific etiologic organism was identified, however, and no person-to-person infectious tendency was found. This suggests that hypersensitivity or an altered immune system may play a role in the pathogenesis of KD. Melish (1987) summarized studies that have shown a sharp rise in antibody production in the first 4 weeks of the disease (probably related to depression of T-suppressor cells) and then a subsequent fall in all the immunoglobulins. The rise in immunoglobulins supplies additional antibodies for reaction with antigens, and circulating immune (antigen-antibody) complexes are frequently detected in KD. It is thought these immune complexes may bind directly to the vascular endothelium, causing inflammation of the vessels.

The most common and potentially dangerous effect of the KD process is vasculitis, which can result in occlusive or ischemic manifestations during the acute disease process or at a later period in life. Over the course of illness, any or all parts of the vascular system can be involved, beginning with the microvessels (arterioles, capillaries, and venules) and progressing to involve small- and medium-sized vessels.

The inflammatory process begins in the perivascular tissues and moves into the other layers of vascular tissue. The combination of vascular inflammation (probably associated with binding of immune complexes to vessel walls) and the typically increased thrombocyte count may result in clot formation (thrombi). The vascular changes in the heart muscle and the coronary arteries are of most concern because they can lead to lifelong morbidity or mortality.

Clinical Manifestations

Typically, the child with acute KD has an unexplained fever of 38.9° to 41.1° C (102° to 106° F) that does not remit with administration of antipyretics. Additionally, a pruritic, polymorphic rash; a marked cervical lymphadenopathy; dry, red, cracked lips; a "strawberry" tongue; bilateral conjunctivitis; and striking erythema (perhaps with desquamation) of the palms and soles are likely. The child is also likely to be irritable and lethargic.

The clinical course of the disease occurs in three phases. Symptoms appear and resolve in a typical pattern. In the acute phase (the first 8 to 10 days), fever, strawberry tongue, cracked-fissured lips, rash, erythema and edema of the palms and soles, and lymphadenopathy are seen. In the subacute period (10 to 35 days), desquamation of the toes, feet, fingers, and palms occurs. The child will likely continue to be irritable and anorectic and have conjunctival injection. Also during this period, arthritis, thrombocytosis, and cardiac and vascular manifestations occur. The recovery phase is said to continue until the ESR becomes normal (perhaps as long as 10 weeks after onset).

Diagnostic Assessment

Criteria developed for diagnosis require that the child meet five of the following six criteria and that other diseases are ruled out: (1) abrupt onset of fever unresponsive to antibiotics; (2) bilateral conjunctivitis; (3) changes in the mouth: dry, chapped, fissured, or reddened lips; strawberry tongue; or reddened mucosa; (4) changes in the extremities: reddened palms or soles, indurative edema of hands or feet, or desquamation (peeling skin) from the fingertips or toes; (5) rash on the trunk; and (6) enlargement of cervical lymph nodes (Hicks & Melish, 1986).

Laboratory Tests. Laboratory data used for diagnosis are fairly nonspecific. Complete blood count (CBC) with differential, ESR, and platelet count are the tests most commonly used for both diagnosis and monitoring of the course of the disease. A markedly elevated ESR is common in the early stages of illness and helps distinguish this illness from viral illnesses that otherwise might be suspected. The white blood count is significantly elevated (leukocytosis), with a shift to the left (a high percentage of polymorphonuclear cells). A marked thrombocytosis (increased platelet count) occurs 10 to 12 days after onset of the fever. In the early period of illness, abnormal liver function tests may be seen in a slightly elevated level of transaminase. An echocardiogram is done for a baseline measurement.

Therapeutic Management

Therapy for KD continues to be controversial. Aspirin has been the primary means of therapy for both its anti-inflammatory and antiplatelet effects (i.e., to counteract thrombocytosis). In the acute period, dosages of up to 100 mg/kg/day of aspirin are prescribed for the anti-inflammatory effect. For unexplained reasons, therapeutic aspirin levels are difficult to achieve in the acute period. The most widely accepted explanation for this is a markedly impaired absorption of aspirin. Serum aspirin levels of 20 to 25 mg/dl appear to be adequate to achieve an anti-inflammatory effect, abolish the high fever, and reduce the incidence of further cardiac involvement. As the course of disease progresses into the subacute phase, the aspirin dose can be reduced because there is improved absorption and, therefore, higher serum levels. In addition, at this point, the indication for aspirin becomes its antiplatelet effect rather than its anti-inflammatory effect, and this effect can be gained at a much lower serum level (10 mg/dl). Accordingly, aspirin levels must be regularly monitored to ensure that appropriate therapeutic levels are achieved to accomplish the specific purpose without producing toxicity.

Low-dose aspirin is continued until the child's platelet count and ESR return to normal. This therapy may also be continued as long as coronary artery dilatation persists. If the child has difficulty taking aspirin (owing to gastritis, for example), other anti-inflammatory preparations may be prescribed.

Recent studies indicate that aspirin has not been shown to reduce the occurrence of coronary artery abnormalities. High-dose intravenous gamma globulin given in conjunction with aspirin, however, appears to be effective in rapidly reducing fever as well as having a rapid, generalized anti-inflammatory effect (Melish, 1987; Newburger, 1986). In addition, as shown on echocardiogram, the number of children with coronary artery abnormalities is greatly reduced.

Nursing Diagnostic Statements and Collaborative Problems

High risk for injury, physiologic; *risk factor: inflammation of blood vessels.*

High risk for impaired skin integrity; *risk factors:*

- *Erythema.*
- *Possible desquamation of the palms and soles.*

High risk for altered comfort, pain, and pruritis; *risk factors:*

- *Edema.*
- *Skin irritation.*

Hyperthermia.

High risk for altered nutrition, less than body requirements; *risk factor: disease-related anorexia.*

Ineffective child and family coping *related to fear and anxiety about diagnostic tests and prognosis.*

High risk for altered home health maintenance; *risk factor: knowledge deficit about disease process and home care.*

Planning and Implementation

Preventing Cardiovascular Damage. Assessment of cardiac status is critical. A cardiopulmonary monitor is indicated if there are signs and symptoms of myocarditis. Tachycardia, gallop rhythm, chest pain, and ECG changes (depressed ST segment) suggest myocarditis. Tachypnea or dyspnea, rales or other noisy respirations, costal retractions, nasal flaring, orthopnea, distended neck veins, and edema are all signs and symptoms of congestive heart failure. Unusual dysrhythmias may indicate impairment or disruption of the electric conduction system of the heart. Signs of cardiac tamponade may be similar to those of congestive heart failure. This also may present as distant heart sounds, narrowing of pulse pressure, and/or presence of pulsus paradoxus.

Careful assessment of the circulatory status of the extremities is important, particularly in the subacute phase of illness when thrombi are more likely to cause circulatory impairment that could contribute to progression of infection or necrosis of fingers or toes.

Promoting Optimal Skin Integrity. It is important to note the presence and status of any rash and edema. As the desquamation occurs, the skin condition should be assessed to note early signs of infection that may occur. Keeping the skin clean, dry, free of irritation from linens and clothing, and well lubricated helps preserve the integumentary barrier to infection and makes the child more comfortable as well. Protect edematous areas from friction and prolonged pressure. Gentle handling of the child is indicated in light of altered skin integrity but does not override the child's need for physical comfort.

Reducing Discomfort. Edematous hands and feet may be painful because of the pressure exerted on tissues by the inflammatory exudate. There is also discomfort associated with the pruritic rash. Systemic antipruritic medications may be used to reduce itching. The aspirin administered for anti-inflammatory and antiplatelet properties also provides analgesia. Nonpharmacologic comfort measures of holding, rocking, singing, reading stories, and other distraction techniques should also be included in the plan of care (McEnhill & Vitale, 1989).

Monitoring and Managing Fever. Because the fever associated with KD tends to be high and unrelieved by medication, careful monitoring is indicated. Because the etiology for the hyperthermia cannot be changed by the nurse, management is symptomatic and includes increased fluid intake and the removal of clothing and blankets. Sponging at times may be indicated, but it is a controversial intervention and must be done carefully to avoid injury. See Chapter 23 for detailed information about sponging.

Maintaining Adequate Nutrition. Adequacy of the nutritional status may be difficult to maintain, and ongoing assessment of intake and output (both fluids and solids) is important. Intravenous fluids are administered to maintain hydration during the acute stage. The discomfort of the mucous membranes may be one deterrent to adequate nutrition. Pain that results from gastritis or other organ involvement may also decrease appetite and willingness to eat and drink and requires intervention. Application of a water-soluble lubricant to the lips, cleaning of the mouth with a soft sponge saturated with dilute hydrogen peroxide, and perhaps a topical anesthetic applied at eating time can provide comfort and a sense of control and independence.

Reducing Fear and Anxiety. The vascular and potential cardiac involvement associated with KD often arouses fear regarding the child's prognosis. Some children may have coronary artery aneurysms, experience infarctions (which may occur in any organ system or part of the body), or die in the acute, subacute, or recuperative phase of the disease process, but families should be reassured that 95 to 99 per cent of patients with KD totally recover without any sequelae.

Fear and anxiety may interfere with the family's ongoing ability to cope with (or manage) the adaptive tasks related to the child's health challenge. The child and family need preparation and emotional support for several procedures. These may include frequent blood tests, possible intravenous infusions, lumbar puncture, echocardiogram, cardiac monitoring, collection of urine specimens, and perhaps angiograms. Support for anxious parents can be provided by regular updates on the child's status and information regarding the symptoms that are present. Parents can participate in the child's care to support their needs for parenting as well as the comfort needs of the child.

Facilitating Home Health Maintenance. Management of the child at home requires continued monitoring of the child's cardiovascular status. Adherence to the prescribed medical regimen is essential to full recovery. The child requires follow-up diagnostic and laboratory assessments as part of the long-term management.

Stevens-Johnson Syndrome

Stevens-Johnson syndrome (SJS), first reported in 1922, is classified as a severe form of erythema multiforme. Of diverse etiology and affecting many systems, it is characterized by distinctive skin lesions, mucosal involvement, and often severe systemic symptoms. Unless it is quickly and carefully treated, SJS can be fatal.

SJS is an uncommon disease seen most frequently in children and young adults; boys are affected more often than girls, and it is more often seen in the winter months (Strom et al, 1991).

Etiology/Incidence (Pathophysiology)

The exact etiology of SJS remains unknown, but it is generally considered to be a hypersensitive-immunologic reaction to one or more of many different stimuli, including diverse disease states and drugs. Viral, bacterial, and fungal infections, as well as collagen diseases, some vaccines, foods, and contactants, have been implicated. When drugs are suspected as an etiologic factor, symptoms may appear within hours as long as 3 weeks after administration. Barbiturates, penicillins, sulfonamides, and many others have been identified as possible causes of SJS; the penicillins appear to be more frequently associated with this syndrome than the others (Strom et al, 1991). A significant number of patients who develop SJS are noted to have chronic or recurring infectious processes, suggesting a possible immune deficiency. Exactly what the relationship or role any of these agents play is not clear, and each may, in fact, be only one of several interacting factors. In SJS, a split occurs in the dermal-epidermal junction and an inflammatory response develops in the dermis. Tissue damage occurs, and the skin actually peels off the body.

Complications are of significant concern in SJS. The most common complications are those associated with the eye. Acute lesions or conjunctival scarring can lead to permanent visual impairment. Tear duct atrophy, corneal ulceration, and adhesions also may occur. Gastrointestinal problems that may occur include esophageal strictures resulting from esophagitis. Respiratory complications are also common. Upper airway involvement and different types of pneumonia, particularly that caused by *Mycoplasma pneumoniae,* are frequently seen. As with burn patients, when skin damage is severe, complications such as fluid and electrolyte imbalances and sepsis are the significant concerns. Mortality rate can be as high as 10 per cent in the acute phase, especially if there is respiratory involvement (Schaller, 1992).

Clinical Manifestations

A description of skin lesions is difficult because they evolve and change appearance throughout the course of the disease. Typical early lesions look like an insect bite with an erythematous papule. A blister may develop, or a central area of epidermal necrosis may occur without a blister. These are known as "target" or "iris" lesions. These lesions may progress from fine maculopapular lesions to confluent areas of erythema to toxic epidermal necrosis, which is a massive denudation (peeling) of the epidermis. Skin pigmentation may also affect the appearance of the lesions. Lesions commonly appear over a 3- to 5-day period, but new eruptions may occur for as long as 2 weeks. Depending on the severity of the mucosal damage, the course of the disease process from eruption to healing may take as long as 6 weeks, not including recurrent lesions.

The distribution of lesions is commonly symmetric on the extremities, spreading to the trunk, but it is extremely variable. Mucosal involvement is frequently present; these lesions are characteristically found in the mouth and eyes but may also be accompanied by genital, pharyngeal, and upper respiratory lesions. Serious sequelae or morbidity results from damage to the mucous membranes. Itching, burning, and pain may be associated with mucosal lesions. Systemic symptoms associated with the disease process include fever, myalgias, and prostration.

Diagnostic Assessment

Diagnosis is made on the following minimum characteristics: target lesions, bullae, vesicles, involvement of two or more mucous membranes, purulent conjunctivitis, and systemic toxicity. A prodromal phase may be seen in which there is fever, sore throat, cough, and malaise. Differential diagnosis must rule out contact dermatitis, Reiter disease, chickenpox, impetigo, and herpes simplex.

Laboratory Tests. Laboratory data are not likely to be helpful in making a diagnosis. There are no specific laboratory tests for SJS, and the most common abnormal hematologic criteria—elevated ESR and leukocytosis—are too general to be of value in making a diagnosis. To complicate the picture even further, there are some contrasting reports (Ruiz-Maldonado, 1985; Westley & Wechsler, 1984) of marked reduction in leukocytes that has yet to be explained. In fact, when this occurs and does not improve within 5 to 7 days, the prognosis appears to be grave.

Therapeutic Management

Treatment should be supportive and appropriate for symptoms that occur. This includes maintenance of fluid balance, debridement of crusted lesions, and aggressive pulmonary care to limit or prevent pulmonary complications. Mouth care is important to treat stomatitis (oral mucous membrane lesions). Warm saline mouthwashes and topical anesthetics may provide relief. Any eye involvement must be closely monitored. Irrigations, warm compresses, and topical steroids may be helpful. If the eye lesions are severe, it may be necessary to instill artificial tear solution.

A method of management of severe cutaneous involvement that seems to be most effective in minimizing complications and reducing mortality has been to use a regimen similar to that followed in caring for burn patients. This appears to reduce the incidence of septicemia and fluid and electrolyte imbalances.

Despite a variety of management philosophies and methods, the outcome for the patient with SJS is unpredictable. Severe skin involvement or continuous leukopenia usually indicates poor prognosis. Although many children recuperate without residual problems, some permanent disabilities can result, including corneal and conjunctival scarring, dermal scarring secondary to infections, prolonged gastric ulceration, and esophageal strictures. Respiratory compromise resulting from an initiating factor of *Mycoplasma pneumoniae* infection may contribute further to this mortality rate. Aggressive, meticulous care and careful monitoring of status may minimize or prevent complications and death.

Nursing Diagnostic Statements and Collaborative Problems

High risk for infection; *risk factor: loss of skin defense.*

High risk for fluid volume deficit; *risk factors:*

- *Increased insensitive loss.*
- *Altered immune response.*

High risk for altered nutrition, less than body requirements; *risk factor: painful stomatitis and esophagitis.*

High risk for infection and pain; *risk factor: impaired skin integrity; skin lesions.*

Ineffective child and family coping *related to fear and anxiety about altered appearance, prognosis, and social isolation.*

High risk for altered home health maintenance; *risk factor: knowledge deficit about disease process and home care.*

Planning and Implementation

Preventing Infections. The presence of open or draining lesions presents an inviting medium for sepsis. If leukopenia occurs as a part of the disease process, immune status is compromised. Good handwashing technique, meticulous management of intravenous lines, monitoring of visitors to screen for infectious disease, and instructions for visitors regarding interactions and contact with the child are important physical concerns.*

Thorough assessments of respiratory status are critical. With the high incidence of *Mycoplasma pneumoniae* as a precipitating factor of this disease, continuous monitoring, documentation, and aggressive management are essential.

Maintaining Fluid and Electrolyte Balance. Fluid requirements increase as larger surface areas become denuded. Attention to intake and output records and to urine specific gravity aids judgments related to administration of fluids. The nurse must also monitor for urinary retention, which can be associated with inflammation of the genitalia. Intake that is significantly greater than output and a palpable bladder are signs of urinary retention.

Managing Nutritional Intake. Lesions in the mouth and mucous membranes of the gastrointestinal tract may necessitate nasogastric (NG) feeding. Adequate nutrition is essential for replacement of lost fluids and for healing of what may be a large percentage of the cutaneous and mucocutaneous surfaces. Maintaining a nasogastric tube in these children, however, presents a special challenge. If there are esophageal lesions, insertion (and replacement) may be irritating and quite painful. Maintaining correct placement of the tube can be difficult if there are le-

* In the past, "reverse" isolation or "protective" isolation practices were used with an immunocompromised child. This involved donning various combinations of gown, gloves, and mask to protect the child from the caregiver. Reverse and protective isolation procedures have been discontinued in most institutions (Kirkis & Grier, 1988) because they provided a false sense of security and led to breakdown in certain strategies (such as handwashing) that have proved effective in reducing the spread of microorganisms.

sions on the face and nose, making tape a contraindication. Nursing ingenuity is often essential in safeguarding tube placement. Careful intake and output records must be maintained to determine nutritional adequacy.

Promoting Integrity of Skin and Mucous Membranes. Frequent, thorough observations should be made, and any changes in the status of the lesions documented. This includes the appearance of new lesions and changes in eye lesions. Record the type and amount of drainage from the eyes.

Soothing soaks may be ordered, which, for the young child, can be administered like a bath in a tub that has been meticulously disinfected. Bath toys can decrease fear of this procedure. Ointments may also be ordered and are usually scheduled to follow soaks. Application of the ointment with a sterile glove can help prevent transfer of organisms from caregiver to child and increases comfort by reducing friction with the denuded skin.

Comfort measures are important when lesions are pruritic or painful. Careful administration of antihistamines and analgesics can provide relief. However, because of the high correlation between medications and SJS, nonessential drugs should be avoided. Most comfort measures are nonpharmacologic, although rocking and cuddling may cause additional discomfort to denuded areas of the skin. The nurse who collaborates with the parent and other family members concerning potential nonpharmacologic measures will be more successful in comforting the child.

Promoting Coping. Thoughtful, appropriate explanations of procedures should be made before they are done. Time should be allowed for listening to the child's concerns. Diversional activities consistent with the stage of growth and development and appropriate for the limitations imposed by the disease process can help the child cope with the stress of the illness. The child must be ensured that the skin will heal and that the itching and discomfort will then be gone.

Facilitating Home Health Maintenance During Recuperation. Because of the potential for severe complications of SJS, care during the acute phase will occur in the hospital. The recuperative phase of the illness, however, will be managed primarily on an outpatient basis and parents will need information and support for home management. Anticipating that the child will be maintained on salicylates or steroids, the nurse can begin teaching early in the hospitalization about administration techniques and side effects of the drugs.

The child's activities may also be curtailed during the recovery phase, and the nurse can use the interactions with family during the period of hospitalization to facilitate planning of appropriate, quiet activities, including a rationale for the activity restriction, and perhaps including a consultation with the play therapist. Care of skin lesions at home will follow techniques used during hospitalization, and, once again, it will be advantageous to involve the parents in this therapy early in the hospitalization. The family also will need instruction in preventing skin and systemic infections.

Altered Immune Response: Allergy (Hypersensitivity)

The term "allergy" brings to mind sneezing, wheezing, itching, general discomfort, and even life-threatening anaphylaxis. Despite this well-deserved connotation, allergy is largely a protective function. In all cases, allergic reactions occur in response to a cell that the body recognizes as foreign (i.e., an antigen). The problem is that, for genetic or other undefined reasons, the immune response in these instances occurs with such intensity (i.e., *hypersensitivity*) that host tissues are damaged in the process.

"Allergy" is a general term for a broad group of disorders. To help in classifying these disorders, Coombs and Gell (1975) proposed the four (now classic) types of allergic response (Table 37–8). The first three of these hypersensitivity reactions involve the humoral immune response (antibodies); the fourth is mediated by the cellular immune response (Tdh cells). This section begins with a general overview of assessment and management of allergy in childhood and nursing strategies to promote effective family coping with chronic allergy. Allergic disorders are then presented, which represent two of the four types of allergic reactions, Types I and IV. Categorized as Type I reactions are allergic rhinitis, conjunctivitis, atopic dermatitis, urticaria and angioedema, insect sting allergy (may also be Type IV), and food allergies. Contact dermatitis is presented as an example of the Type IV reaction. Table 37–8 lists chapters dealing with certain Type II and III disorders.

Assessment of Allergic Disorders

Assessment of the child for a suspected allergic disorder involves a careful history, physical findings, and diagnostic laboratory data. A thorough history is the first and most significant aspect in identifying an allergy (Table 37–9).

History

The history includes the child, family, and environment as essential components. Many children with atopic allergies have a family history of allergies. Assessing the family provides information of the child's genetic predisposition and assists in ruling out allergic manifestations associated with immunologic disorders. Assessment of the child's chief complaint focuses on three basic questions. They reflect the *when,*

TABLE 37–8
Classification of Allergic Reactions

Type I	**Immediate Hypersensitivity** Features antigen interaction with IgE (and possibly some IgM molecules) bound to a mast cell or basophil. The cell releases histamine and other chemical mediators to produce a local inflammatory reaction. Reactions include hay fever, allergic rhinitis, allergic asthma, many urticarias, and anaphylaxis (the most severe form of hypersensitivity)
Type II	**Antibody-Mediated Cytolysis** Involves lysis of the cell membranes of foreign-appearing blood cells. Lysis occurs as the result of antigen binding to IgM or IgG antibodies on the cells and initiating complement activation. Reactions include blood transfusion reactions (see Chapter 34); hemolytic disease of the newborn; drug-induced hemolytic anemia, leukopenia, and thrombocytopenia (see acquired aplastic anemia, Chapter 34); and hyperacute kidney transplant rejection.
Type III	**Immune Complex—Dependent Tissue Injury** Certain circulating antigen-antibody complexes (immune complexes) deposit within tissues such as the kidneys, choroid plexus, joints, skin, or lungs. Chemical mediators are released that stimulate inflammation (with phagocytosis) and activate the complement system. Phagocytosis and complement reactions cause injury to the tissues containing the immune complexes. Reactions include serum sickness, systemic lupus erythematosus, glomerulonephritis (see Chapter 36), and juvenile arthritis
Type IV	**Delayed Hypersensitivity** This response is *not* antibody related. Caused by interaction of antigen with certain T-lymphocytes (delayed hypersensitivity T-cell, Tdh), which release lymphokines, causing inflammation and tissue injury. The response is usually well localized. Reactions include contact dermatitis, organ rejection, and graft-versus-host disease. May play a part in resistance to certain tumors.

Adapted from Bierman, C. W., Pearlman, D. S., & Berman, B. A. (1988). Injection therapy for allergic diseases. In C. W. Bierman & D. S. Pearlman (Eds.), *Allergic diseases from infancy to adulthood*. (2nd ed., pp. 279–293). Philadelphia: WB Saunders; Coombs, R. R. A., & Gell, P. G. H. (1975). Classification of allergic reactions responsible for clinical hypersensitivity and disease. In P. G. H. Gell, et al. (Eds.), *Clinical aspects of immunology* (3rd ed.). London: Blackwell; and Lockey, R. F., & Bukantz, S. C. (1987). *Principles of immunology and allergy*. Philadelphia: WB Saunders.

TABLE 37–9
Assessment Data for Allergic Disorders

History of Present Complaint

Assess when, what, and where of child's symptom state and symptom-free state

When refers to time of day, week, month, and year

What refers to what child and family assess the cause is

Where refers to place or geographic location

Past Health History

Pulmonary manifestations

Nasal, ear, sinus symptoms

Dermatitis, urticaria

Gastrointestinal symptoms

Irritability, fatigue, headache (tension-fatigue syndrome)

Drug reaction(s)

Feeding history

Socioeconomic and Family Factors

Family history of allergies (family profile)

Stability of family members' relationships and stress level in home

Income level and ability to provide food, clothing, shelter, and health care

Physical Environment

Structural description of home (air/heating system, carpets, cellar, plants, etc.)

Description of child's toys, bedroom, bedding, other rooms of the house where child spends waking hours (e.g., TV room)

Presence of pets in home

Exposure to irritants and/or pollutants (cigarette smoking, proximity to industry, dump or known source of air pollution, household cleaning supplies)

Cleanliness of home

Exposure level: baby sitters, relatives, day care facility, school

Health Practices

Routine immunizations

Child's daily routine, including adequacy of eating, activities, rest, sleep

Reaction to Common Allergens

See Table 37–10

Family Profile

A family history taken to determine presence of immunologic or allergic disorder(s)

what, and *where* of the child's symptom state as well as symptom-free state (Korenblat & Wedner, 1984) (Table 37–9). Additionally, any present or past history of the following should be documented:

- Bronchial manifestations.
- Nasal and sinus symptoms.
- Skin disorders.
- Gastrointestinal symptoms.
- Recurrent periods of inactivity or lassitude.
- Colic or irritable behavior.
- Dietary history.
- Drug reaction history.
- Environmental reaction history.
- Exercise history.

A thorough history of the child's environment is obtained with a focus on the child's bedroom or sleeping area. Information is obtained on other environments in which the child spends considerable time, such as preschool or baby sitter's or grandparents' homes. It should be noted if the child is exposed to secondary smoke.

The presence or absence of symptoms in all these areas should be noted. The source of this information (often parents) is important because valid recall of times and events associated with symptomatology is critical in providing clues to the causal antigen as well as in establishing the diagnosis. Table 37–10 contains a list of common allergens.

Physical Examination

The physical examination is a systems approach that takes into consideration the child's age and understanding (see Table 37–3). Infants and toddlers may

TABLE 37-10
Common Allergens

Inhalants	**Ingestants**
Pollen	Food
Mold	Cow's milk
House dust	Eggs
Animal dander	Wheat
Fabric fiber	Chocolate
Feathers	Cola products
Dyes	Fish, pork, chicken
Chemicals	Corn, legumes
Injectants	Citrus fruits, strawberries, nuts
Vaccines	Drugs
Injected drugs	Aspirin
Animal serum	Antibiotics
Animal saliva	Barbiturates
Animal venom	Food Additives
Insect stings	**Contactants**
Bacterial Infectants	Plants
Viral Infectants	Topical drugs
	Resins
	Metals
	Cosmetics
	Dyes
	Chemicals
	Other Environmental Factors
	Sunshine
	Temperature changes
	Air pollution

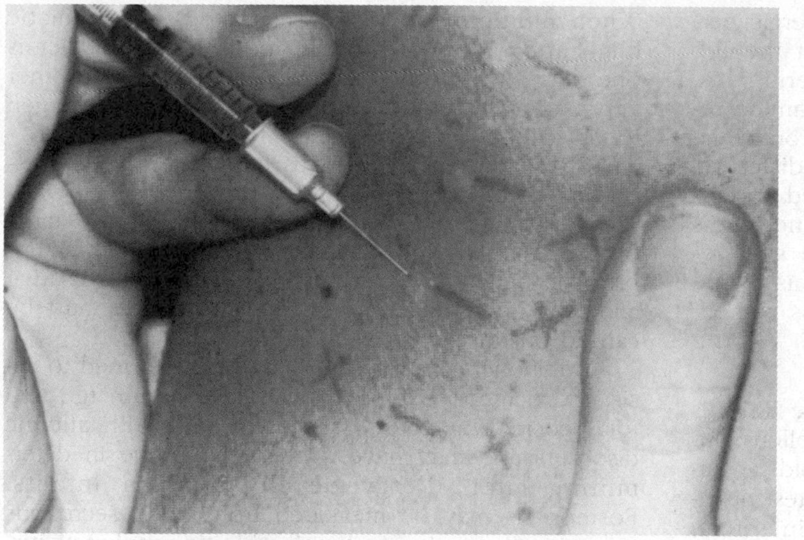

FIGURE 37 - 14. Intradermal skin testing for allergy. A 27-gauge needle is used for the intradermal injection of a small amount (0.2 ml) of allergen extract. (From Bierman, C. W., & Pearlman, D. S. [1988]. *Allergic diseases from infancy to adulthood.* [2nd ed., p. 236]. Philadelphia: WB Saunders.)

cry during the examination; therefore, it may be best to assess their lungs and respirations before they become upset. In all cases, the child's weight and length are measured and plotted on appropriate growth charts to assess for long-term effects of the allergic condition or medications (steroids) resulting in growth failure. During the physical examination, particular attention should be given to the skin, eyes, mucous membranes, and breath sounds.

Laboratory and Diagnostic Studies

Laboratory and diagnostic studies may be necessary. The need to perform these studies is based on the child's history, physical assessment, and inability to control the allergic reaction by elimination or avoidance measures. (Elimination procedures can be valuable in the improvement of symptoms and diagnosis of allergies.) Skin testing and the serum radioallergosorbent test (RAST) are useful diagnostic methods to identify specific antigen(s) or causative agent(s). There are many variations of this test (e.g., MAST, FAST, ELISA), each of which uses different carriers for antigen (Shapiro, 1988).

Skin Testing. The skin test procedure involves skin exposure through scratch, prick, or intradermal injection (Fig. 37–14) of minute quantities of suspected allergens followed by observation for the type of skin reaction. This test is useful because there is usually a high correlation between antibodies in the skin and those in the blood and respiratory tract (Shapiro, 1988). See Table 37–11 for details of allergy skin testing.

TABLE 37-11
Allergy Skin Testing

Allergy skin testing involves the use of extracts from numerous common antigens. Scratch, prick, or intradermal injection are the common techniques used. Prick testing involves dropping the extract onto the skin through which a light puncture is made. Scratch testing is very similar, except that small scratches (⅓″ long) are made. The intradermal method constitutes injecting a small amount of allergens just under the skin. Which antigen extracts are tested is determined by the child's age and size, geographic and environmental exposure, history, and physical findings. The extracts are injected in rows, in a specific pattern, and a control substance is injected for comparison. The usual test site is the back or arm. The back is commonly used for scratch or prick testing. The forearm is most desirable for intradermal testing because it is more accessible to a tourniquet should an extreme allergic response occur to one of the antigen extracts. No antihistamines should be given to a child within 96 hrs prior to testing.

Preparation of the child for skin testing is based on the child's level of cognitive development. Preparation of the child and family includes explanation of the possible itching and swelling of the tested area, the reaction appearance, length of time for testing, and methods the child and parent can use to assist the child in holding still during the procedure. Sitting on the parent's lap and distractions such as reading stories, imagery, and music may comfort and support the child.

A child is never to be left alone during the testing procedure or in the following period when reactions may occur. Reactions will occur within 10 to 30 minutes after exposure, if the child is allergic. The tests are usually read in 15–20 mins and scored according to the skin reaction. A positive reaction is evidenced by erythema and wheal formation at the site. In the prick or scratch test, once a reaction occurs, the area should be immediately wiped off to prevent further reaction. All the extracts should be removed in approximately 30 mins after the testing. Reactive manifestations may persist for 8–12 hrs. The family should be instructed to report delayed reactions (occurring 24–48 hrs later).

When allergens are introduced to an allergic person, the allergen commonly interacts with the IgE molecule attached to the mast cell, triggering histamine release (Wasserman, 1988). The histamine release causes a wheal or flare to develop around the tested area. The skin reaction may be immediate (occurring within 15 to 30 minutes) or delayed (occurring up to 48 hours after testing). Skin testing is less often performed with infants because the skin response is usually delayed or incomplete. This is due to a slower rate of IgE synthesis and a less responsive immunologic system.

***The Radioallergosorbent Test* (RAST).** The RAST is a blood test for specific IgE antibodies to pollens, animal danders, house dust, mites, foods, molds, penicillins, and stinging insect bites. This blood test quantifies the amount of specific IgE present in serum. RAST testing, instead of skin testing, is used to identify allergens in infants, pregnant women, children with dermatitis, and asthmatics in whom a severe reaction to skin testing is suspected or who are wheezing. This test is easier and safer to perform, but it is much more expensive and is believed to be less sensitive (and therefore less accurate) than skin testing for identifying the antigen (Sampson & Albergo, 1984; Shapiro, 1988). Both skin testing and the RAST are used as aids in the development of environmental control and as guides to immunotherapy with those allergens that cannot be avoided.

Other Diagnostic Tests. Patch tests are done when the child is suspected of having a contact allergy. The suspected material is taped to the skin for 1 to 2 days. The test is then read and scored.

Echograph, using the technique of ultrasonography, is a diagnostic tool to assess the presence of sinusitis in children with rhinitis. This quick and noninvasive tool causes little discomfort.

When food allergies are suspected, removal of the suspected food from the diet may provide definite diagnosis of the child's adverse reaction to the food. When multiple foods are suspected, a systematic blind approach to removing foods from the diet is one way to sort out the actual allergen(s). Another approach includes a diet beginning with low-allergen foods, with the gradual addition of other foods.

Challenge testing involves administering the suspected allergen and observing the child's response. This testing may be done for diagnosing food allergy or causes of asthma. Challenge testing, particularly bronchial challenge testing for identifying causative allergens for asthma, can be dangerous and must be carried out in a controlled setting.

Additional serum testing may be performed to assist the diagnosis of allergy. Elevated serum IgE and total eosinophil counts are associated with allergic disorders and may have a predictive value in determining later allergy development in infants. Eosinophils may be measured from body secretions to assist diagnosis of allergic rhinitis, conjunctivitis, and food allergies (Sly, 1985). See Table 37–12 for specimen collection.

Therapeutic Management

Three basic goals in the treatment of allergic children are to (1) identify and remove the allergen, (2) relieve the symptoms, and (3) control severity of future attacks. Treatment is provided while helping the child and family achieve an environment supportive of the child's growth and development.

Removing the Allergen

When proper diagnosis and identification of causative allergen(s) are possible, elimination or removal of the allergen is the most logical step to take. For example, if the antigen is from animal dander or cow's milk, removal or avoidance will relieve the allergic symptoms. Success with removal or avoidance of the allergen depends on the family's willingness to adhere to recommendations. This may be particularly difficult when the family pet is to be avoided. Keeping the

TABLE 37-12
Eosinophil Collection and Results Indicative of Allergic Disease

Test	Obtaining Specimen	Significant Results
Mucous cytology (rhinitis)	Infant: aspirate nasal secretions in bulb syringe. Older child: blow nose into wax paper	10% + eosinophils
Conjunctival cytology (conjunctivitis)	Swab (sterile) inner canthus of conjunctiva	10% + eosinophils
Bronchial secretion cytology (asthma)	Infant: aspirate bronchial secretions by suctioning; seldom done. Older child: rinse mouth several times with mouthwash, then cough sputum into sterile container	10% + eosinophils
Stool mucus (food allergy)	Stool specimen with mucus (if present)	10% + eosinophils
Complete blood count	Peripheral blood smear from finger, earlobe, or heel prick	7–25% eosinophils

pet outdoors may be more acceptable to the family than giving the pet away. Home allergy-proofing techniques and environmental controls are valuable information to the child and family (Table 37–13). This information may help the family eliminate causative agents and have some control over the effects the allergy has on their child.

Relieving the Symptoms

If avoidance or removal of causative agents cannot be achieved, symptomatic relief is indicated. Medications commonly used for relief of symptoms are antihistamines and bronchodilators. Antihistamines are the most frequently used drugs for the treatment of allergies. Antihistamines are most effective when taken before or early in an allergic reaction.

Immunotherapy. When the allergen cannot be avoided, immunotherapy or hyposensitization is also an option. Bierman and colleagues (1988) caution, however, that immunotherapy "is an adjunct to allergic management, not a substitute for it" (p 283). Patients should understand that this treatment can help control symptoms but does not cure the allergy.

Immunotherapy provides an estimated 75 per cent reduction of signs and symptoms associated with seasonal pollen (Korenblat & Wedner, 1984). Once the allergen is identified, it is given subcutaneously in the form of a dilute extract at weekly or more frequent intervals, with a gradual increase in strength over succeeding doses. The strength is increased until the child develops *tolerance* to the allergen (i.e., the immune system becomes *desensitized* to that antigen). The strength that accomplishes tolerance be-

TABLE 37-13
***Family-Centered Teaching*: Home Allergy Proofing**

For Mild Allergy

House Dust (Focusing on Child's Bedroom)

Vacuum and dust frequently

Damp mop to reduce dust

Change filters monthly on central air conditioner/furnace

Use bedroom for sleeping; close door during the day

Keep pets out of bedroom

No smoking in the house

For Severe Allergy

House Dust (Focusing on Child's Bedroom)

Bed

- Plastic mattress cover with zipper for mattress and box springs
- Washable synthetic blankets and bedspread and nonallergenic (not foam or feathers) pillows

Washable toys in bed at night

Washable curtains

No carpeting or scatter rugs

Cover heat ducts with cheesecloth to reduce dust circulation. Tape the cheesecloth to floor or ceiling. Wash and change at least every 2 wks. Do not place bed directly under, over, or beside duct

Avoid using closet as storage area. Avoid keeping extra materials on floor or shelves. Clean with rest of room

Keep organization of room simple. Avoid having open shelves and dust-gathering collections (planes, cars, stuffed toys, dolls) or books. Keep toys in storage box

Keep doors and windows closed if using an electrolytic furnace filter

Wood or linoleum floor recommended. Damp mop. If carpeting present, vacuum daily

Mold, Mildew

Eliminate plants and aquariums from child's bedroom and play area; keep to minimum throughout home

Avoid use of cellar as play or living area

Clean bathroom and tile areas with antimold agent (e.g., Lysol) regularly

Always clean water jar on vaporizers or humidifiers with vinegar solution (2 parts vinegar to 3 parts water) before filling. Have vinegar solution run through machine for 15–20 mins. Follow with a water rinse. Dry with clean cloth. Clean a minimum of three times per week

Use dehumidifier in humid or damp areas

Clean drip pans under frost-free refrigerators at least monthly

Prevent mold and mildew by airing tennis shoes and boots. Teach children not to put damp towels with other laundry

Danders, Feathers

Find new homes for pets, or limit them to outdoors

Avoid stuffed animals and upholstered furniture; including clothing stuffed or insulated with feathers (down)

Contactants

Do not buy wool clothing

Wash all new clothing and linens before using

Double-rinse infant's clothing and diapers

Wash baby articles in mild soap

Use mild soap to bathe baby, and rinse well

Avoid use of perfumed lotions, powders, oils

Avoid tobacco smoke

comes the maintenance dose. The injections are received one or two times weekly until the maintenance dose is reached. (This may take 2 months to a year or longer.) The maintenance dose is then administered on a regular basis at 2- to 4-week intervals.

The immunotherapy may be given preseasonally (before the time of year when the antigen is present in quantity) or perennially (throughout the whole year), which is the most common approach. The goal of this therapy is desensitization to the antigen. The series of regularly injected antigen stimulates development of IgG antibodies. IgG has a higher or greater affinity for the allergen than does IgE. Therefore, the allergen binds with the IgG first, preventing the antigen-antibody IgE reaction from occurring and the subsequent Type I hypersensitivity reaction that releases histamine. The allergen is subsequently destroyed by phagocytosis or complement proteins.

For the child receiving frequent injections, it will be necessary to rotate the injection site and document the dosage and injection site reactions. Prior to injection, the child should be assessed to establish absence of conditions that require other treatment or signal likelihood of an adverse reaction (e.g., significant wheeze) and so that there is a baseline for comparison if a reaction occurs. *Monitoring of the child is critical during and for at least 20 minutes after the antigen injection because anaphylaxis may occur that requires emergency intervention.* Emergency equipment and supplies (epinephrine and oxygen) must be readily available. Local reactions can be treated with cold compresses and oral antihistamines. If a dose causes a systemic response or creates local erythema or edema the size of a nickel or larger, the next dose should not be given until an allergist is consulted.

Preventing Future Attacks

The risk for the infant of developing an allergic disorder is 70 per cent if both parents have allergies and 54 per cent if one parent has allergies (Johnstone, 1988). Therefore, it is recommended that allergic parents consider breastfeeding their infant because human milk contains fewer antigens to which the infant may become sensitized. The breastfeeding mother is advised to eliminate highly allergenic foods from her diet to further reduce the infant's exposure to allergens (Buscinco & Cantani, 1984). Delaying introduction of solid foods until the second 6 months of life may be indicated.

Reduction of allergens in the home can also help protect the allergy-prone infant. Exposure should be reduced as much as possible to house dust, house dust mites, indoor mold, animal allergens, cigarette smoke, and fur-bearing pets (Johnstone, 1988).

Impact of Allergy on the Family

The chronicity and periodic crisis of the allergic child's illness impact emotionally, socially, and financially on the child and members of the family (White & Owsley, 1983).

The child with an allergic illness may experience complicated treatment, daily medication(s), lack of sleep from acute asthmatic attacks, intense itching from atopic dermatitis, decreased ability to learn in school, and diminished involvement in social activities. The demands of the chronic illness may result in anxiety, fatigue, poor self-esteem, nonadherence to the medical regimen, and feelings of guilt that somehow the child is responsible for the illness. During an acute asthmatic attack, feelings of suffocation and death have been described by children.

Parents have similar emotional and psychological reactions to their child's allergic disorder. Both parents and children experience fear, anxiety, and uncertainty about future emergency hospital admissions and frequent visits to the clinic or physician. In addition, they experience feelings of separation from home and friends, they may not fully understand medical procedures, and they live with the effects of the allergy on family activities, leisure, trips, and school attendance. Parents may experience fear, helplessness, self-blame, and guilt for their child's illness. In addition, parents may feel anger at lifestyle changes, financial costs, and time demands for routine follow-up care. These feelings can result in alterations in parenting behavior. The resulting impact may affect the child's growth and development, the quality of support for the child, and, therefore, the child's ability to cope with the allergy.

Siblings are also affected by the allergy. Feelings of resentment and anger may develop, based on their perception that their parents are always spending time with the "sick" child. Feelings of guilt and self-blame for their sibling's illness may occur, if the well siblings perceive themselves as responsible for causing the allergy. They may also be afraid of developing the same disorder. Environmental and dietary adjustments are likely to be extended to include siblings. These changes may be generally accepted by siblings, or they may add further to feelings of anger and resentment. Siblings may be included in the teaching and monitoring processes. When included in these processes, they are less likely to experience separation, guilt, and anger.

The financial impact on the family may be tremendous. The cost of medications; special allergy-proofing of the home; frequent physician, hospital, and clinic visits; time lost from work or perhaps the necessity for one parent to quit his or her job to provide special care for the child puts a tremendous financial strain on the family. The monetary and time commitment by the parents may contribute to feelings of resentment, anger, and anxiety.

Enhancing Family Coping

Nursing care of the allergic child needs to focus both on minimizing future allergic exacerbations and supporting the family's strengths so it can adapt and manage the allergic disorder. Nursing care is directed toward the child with severe allergic involvement and should be modified in keeping with the severity and frequency of symptoms.

Supporting the Family in the Health Care System. Family support involves orienting the child and family to new environments, clarifying the role of the nurse, and involving the parent and child in the care and ongoing follow-up. For example, the child receiving immunotherapy for the first time in the clinic may be anxious and uncooperative. As part of the family's preparation, the nurse can provide information to both the child and caregiver about the play area, restrooms, what they can do while waiting, who will be giving immunotherapy, and what the procedure involves. Informing the child and family of examinations, procedures, and care usually diminishes their anxiety, enhances their sense of control, and assists them in coping with the medical demands of the allergy. The parent will need instruction on symptoms of anaphylaxis and appropriate treatment with epinephrine.

Supporting the Family in the Community. Community follow-up is based on the nursing assessment of the family's functioning and resources. The school nurse can be an invaluable resource to the child and family by supporting the child's transition from home to school and meeting the child's health needs in the school system.

Collaborative planning strengthens the family unit's resources and coping. A family-centered approach to counseling and education is critical for the child to adhere to medical treatments and medications. These actions reinforce the child's and family's strengths. Collaborative problem solving with the child and parent regarding timing of medications, treatments, and social and daily activities individualizes the physical, psychological, and developmental care of the child and parent, thus promoting commitment and adherence to recommended care. An example of collaborative planning is a school-age child with asthma who required bronchodilator aerosol treatment three times a day to manage acute seasonal attacks. The nurse who interviewed the child and parent discovered that the child received only two treatments a day, which did not control his wheezing. Both parents worked outside the home, and the school nurse was not always available to provide the treatment. Through problem solving with the family, it was recognized that the child's baby sitter could be taught to provide the third treatment. In fact, the youngster participated in the teaching of his baby sitter. The listening and collaborative problem solving provided effective options for treatment.

Supporting the Family Through Teaching. Education involves information regarding causes, management, and prognosis of allergic disorders. The discussion will focus on environmental control, medications, and treatments. The goal of education is to promote parental responsibility with the infant and young child and self-care that emphasizes increasing responsibility and independence with age for the older school-age child and adolescent. The preparation of a child with an allergy is as important as the parents' understanding. When assessing the child's understanding, the child's coping style and cognitive level are considered. Written information reinforcing the teaching is provided to both parents and older children to improve understanding of home care needs and adherence to treatment (Kruger & Rawlings, 1984).

The following sections describe specific allergic disorders that fall within the Type I and Type IV classifications. (See Table 37–8 for an overview of the four types of allergic reactions.) Type II responses often result in blood dyscrasias, such as those described in Chapter 34. Type III responses include SLE and JA, discussed earlier in this chapter.

Type I Allergic Disorders

Pathophysiology of the Type I Response

Type I allergic responses result in the signs and symptoms most often associated with the word "allergy." Among those manifestations are sneezing, watery eyes, nasal congestion, hives, and anaphylaxis. The Type I allergic response is mediated primarily by IgE antibodies. IgE is known for its extremely high binding capacity with tissue mast cells and blood basophils; any open receptor sites on these cells tend to be filled by available IgE molecules. The significance of this binding action is that when the mast cell (or basophil) carrying IgE antibodies on its surface encounters an antigen, the mast cell releases a sudden burst of histamine and other chemical mediators into the tissues (or, in the case of a basophil, into the blood stream) (Fig. 37–15). These chemicals may cause a variety of allergic responses, including local or systemic anaphylaxis, asthma, allergic rhinitis, urticaria, and angioedema (Buckley, 1988).

Histamine is the chemical most commonly associated with Type I allergic reactions. It is known to

- Contract smooth muscles of the bronchial tree (with resultant wheezing as air passes through narrowed passages).
- Contract smooth muscles of the gastrointestinal tract (leading to nausea, cramping, diarrhea, and other gastrointestinal symptoms).
- Enhance vascular permeability (leading to release of inflammatory elements, neutrophils, and plasma into the tissues).
- Cause constriction of pulmonary vessels (decreasing the capacity for oxygen exchange and leading to shortness of breath).
- Stimulate nasal mucous production (Wasserman, 1988).

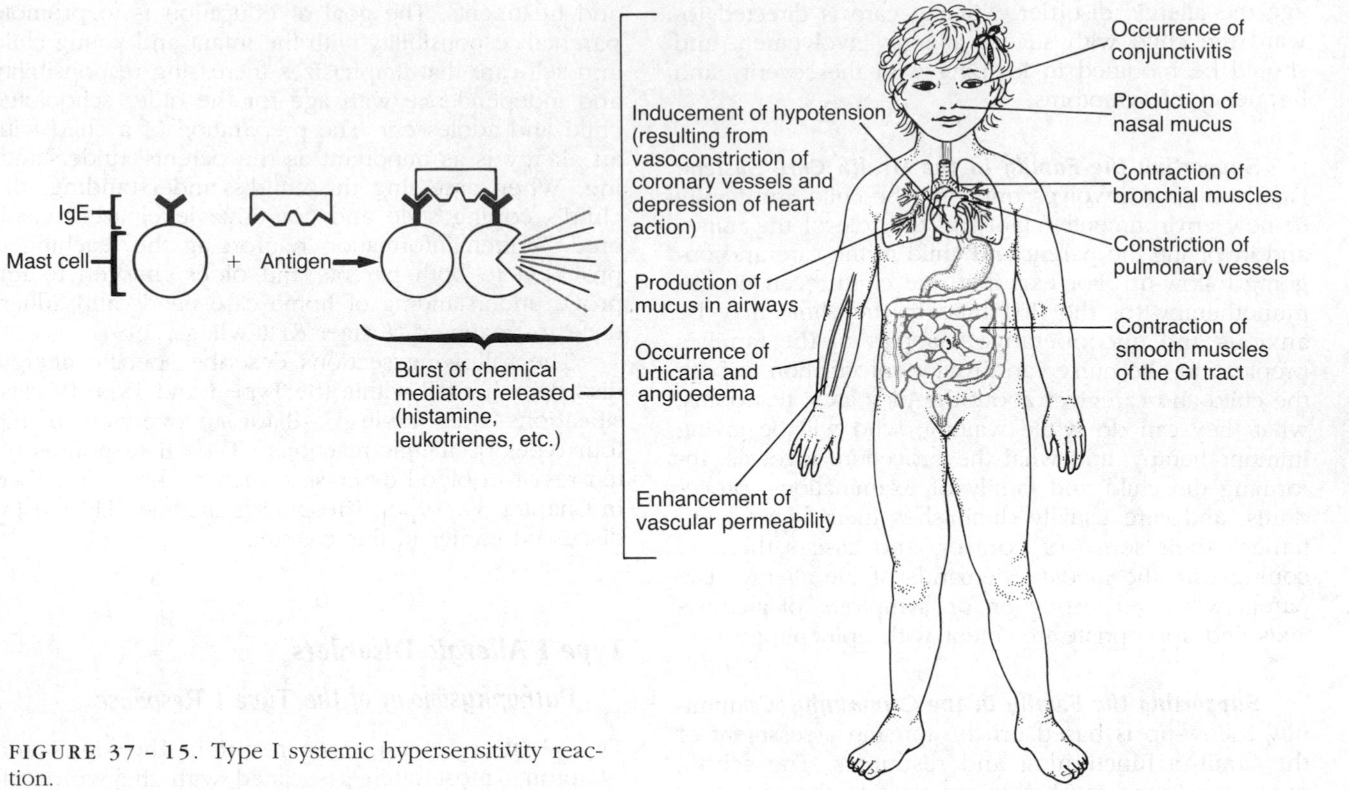

FIGURE 37-15. Type I systemic hypersensitivity reaction.

Histamine released from cutaneous mast cells can cause urticaria and angioedema (Fineman, 1987). It may also cause inflammation of the conjunctiva of the eye.

Leukotrienes (formerly called "slow-reacting substance of anaphylaxis") are among the other chemicals released by the mast cell or basophil. These substances have several actions in common with histamine. In addition, they increase mucous production in the airways (leading to reduced diameter of airways, wheezing, and coughing), induce hypotension (resulting in symptoms of faintness or light-headedness), produce localized wheal and flare responses (urticaria and angioedema) (Table 37–14), and may inhibit lymphocyte function (Wasserman, 1988).

The Type I allergic disorders discussed in this section are allergic rhinitis, allergic conjunctivitis, atopic dermatitis, urticaria and angioedema, insect sting allergy, and food allergies.

Allergic Rhinitis

Allergic rhinitis may be seasonal, commonly referred to as "hay fever," or perennial (chronic), in which symptoms are present throughout the year.

Etiology/Incidence (Pathophysiology)

Allergic rhinitis is the most common allergic disorder, occurring in 10 per cent of all children (Korenblat & Wedner, 1984). Although the condition can occur at any age, it is most common in children older than 5 years of age. Common causes of chronic rhinitis are house dust and dander. In the winter, the chronic symptoms may become worse because the child spends more time indoors. Seasonal pollens, molds, or foods can result in either seasonal or chronic symptoms.

Rhinitis is an inflammation of the nasal mucosa resulting from the chemical release of histamine by the mucosal mast cells. The histamine causes local

TABLE 37-14
Comparison of Urticaria and Angioedema

	Urticaria	Angioedema
Onset	Acute (usually occurs within minutes)	Subacute (may develop more slowly)
Location	Dermis	Deeper layers of skin, including subcutaneous tissue
Clinical Manifestations	Multiple reddened lesions that look like wheals Itching	Usually single lesion Lesions smaller in size, with less itching and redness Lesions evolve more slowly Stinging, tingling, or burning feeling Commonly involves face, extremities

vascular dilatation, edema, sneezing, and hypersecretion from stimulation of nerve fibers (Sly, 1985). This Type I hypersensitivity reaction (local anaphylaxis) is responsible for the mild-to-moderate nasal eosinophilia counts, supporting the diagnosis.

Clinical Manifestations

The symptoms of allergic rhinitis may vary in duration, severity, and pattern, based on the child's hypersensitivity to the antigen or allergen and the extent of exposure. Common symptoms are nasal congestion, clear watery discharge (a change in color may mean infection or extreme abundance of eosinophils), sneezing, and itching. Children may also complain of an itchy throat or headache. The child may become irritable and experience both lack of appetite and decreased ability to smell. Table 37–15 summarizes characteristic symptoms of the child with chronic rhinitis. Complications may result, including sinus infection, tonsil or adenoid hypertrophy, epistaxis, serous otitis, otitis media, and oral-facial abnormalities resulting in malocclusion.

TABLE 37–15
Clinical Manifestations of Chronic Allergic Rhinitis

Allergic Shiners

Dark circles noted around the eyes from chronic nasal and sinus congestion (see Fig. 37–4 in Table 37–3)

Allergic Salute

Upward brushing of the nose tip to allay pruritus and open nasal passages; a white crease across bridge of nose may be present (see Fig. 37–5 in Table 37–3)

Allergic Gaping

Open-mouth breathing, particularly during times of rest; often accompanied by a high, V-shaped palate and aseptic red throat

Transient Hearing Loss with Immobile or Scarred Tympanic Membrane

Results from chronic serous otitis media associated with persistent (allergic) rhinitis and blockage of the eustachian tubes

Abnormal Nasal Mucosa

Pale or blue and swollen, with gray, boggy, enlarged nasal turbinates

Conjunctivitis

Common finding with allergic rhinitis. Itching, excessive lacrimation, eye vessels look hardened

Hypernasal Voice

Vowels are heard to be muffled during episodes of seasonal rhinitis

Diagnostic Assessment

Diagnosis is based on previously described physical findings and history. Nasal eosinophil counts may support the diagnosis; skin testing will assist in identifying causative allergens. An echogram of the sinuses is frequently done to rule out sinusitis, a common complication.

Therapeutic Management

Treatment involves avoidance or elimination of causative allergens, immunotherapy if indicated, and pharmacologic interventions. Common drugs used in management are antihistamines and decongestants. Intranasal steroids have been found useful with severe cases. Cromolyn sodium spray is sometimes effective in preventing and managing symptoms associated with allergic rhinitis (Sly, 1985). Nasal irrigations with saline nose drops can also be helpful.

Nursing Diagnostic Statements

Ineffective airway clearance: upper respiratory system, *related to nasal congestion and discharge.*

High risk for altered health maintenance; *risk factor:* knowledge deficit about management of symptoms at home.

Planning and Implementation

Relieving Nasal Congestion. Because of chronic irritation and frequent nasal drainage, nasal passages tend to become dry, irritated, and prone to small painful cracks in the mucosa. This nasal congestion is caused by increased nasal mucus produced by antigen-triggered histamine. Humidification of the air can help maintain moist mucous membranes in a dry climate or during winter months when the home is heated. If the family does not own and cannot afford a central humidification system, a portable humidifier can be effective. Even a cool-mist vaporizer operated in the child's room during hours of sleep helps reduce nasal dryness and stuffiness.

Exercise and an upright position cause nasal vasoconstriction and thus help relieve stuffiness. Because nasal congestion is often most severe on arising in the morning, a regimen of morning exercise may increase comfort.

Facilitating Home Health Maintenance. Nursing support focuses on teaching the child and family about environmental control of the allergen, medication administration, and, if indicated, immunotherapy procedures. Side effects of commonly used antihistamines include fatigue, insomnia, anorexia, rebound congestion, and nausea or vomiting. Knowledge of side effects assists both the child and parent to deal more competently with the impact of the allergic disorder. The family should be aware that, over time, a temporary tolerance to medications develops and a particular antihistamine may become less effective in controlling symptoms. This is the time to contact the physician, who can order another medication. For most persons, tolerance is not permanent, and a medication previously used may be effective later.

The nurse can also instruct about supportive measures such as those suggested by Kaliner and Slater (1986). A stuffy nose may be relieved by saline nose drops that help reduce discomfort and promote mucus drainage. For best results, the child should remain in a position with his or her head back (neck hyperextended) for a few minutes after the drops are instilled. (See Chapter 24 for detailed techniques of nose drop administration.) Distraction techniques can help accomplish this positioning in the infant and toddler. Tell children they may feel and taste the salty drops running down the throat, and explain how the drops get from the nose to the throat. Assure the child that this feeling will be temporary and that this will not reduce the effectiveness of the saline drops.

With the realization that allergic rhinitis will probably be a lifelong condition, it is advisable for the family to begin assigning responsibility for management to the child as soon as feasible. The child who controls symptoms through self-management is likely to develop a more positive self-image and to feel less debilitated by the symptoms.

Food Allergies

Food allergies may occur at any age, although infants are at greater risk for developing them. The infant's immature digestive system and immune capability allow for an easier absorption of larger amounts of incompletely catabolized proteins that can be antigenic (Bierman & Pearlman, 1988; Buscinco & Cantani, 1984). Also, infants may develop food sensitivities from intrauterine sensitization or from antigens ingested from their mother's breast milk. Another reason why food allergy is common in infants is because this is the time when the child is introduced to many new (and potentially antigenic) foods. In addition, diarrhea or other inflammation of the intestinal lining may enhance the absorption of antigens, causing an allergic reaction to certain foods in some children.

Etiology/Incidence (Pathophysiology)

Any food can produce allergic symptoms, but some foods are considered highly allergenic. The most common food allergens in children are cow's milk, eggs (largely due to egg white), wheat, corn, chocolate, cola, citrus fruits, legumes, and shellfish. Allergy to legumes and shellfish is not outgrown as often as allergy to other foods. Occasionally, vitamins and drugs (e.g., antibiotics) with lactose fillers also cause gastrointestinal allergic responses.

Cow's milk is the most common allergic food, with a 2 to 7.5 per cent incidence in childhood. Three fourths of the children with cow's milk allergy show allergic signs and symptoms within the first few months of life, most likely owing to the infant's immature digestive and immunologic systems (Jalonen, 1991). Any infant on cow's milk with a history of colic, irritability, or repeated bouts of respiratory infection is suspect. Metabisulfites, which are preservatives used on fruits and vegetables, have demonstrated food sensitivity in asthmatic children. These preservatives have provoked signs and symptoms of bronchoconstriction, flushing, weakness, urticaria, and angioedema (Sly, 1985).

Certain physiologic and immunologic intestinal properties provide barriers to food proteins (antigens) that have the potential for causing food allergies in children (May & Block, 1978; Sly, 1985). The intestinal physiologic and immunologic properties are the low pH of secretions and the intestinal mucus, secretory IgA on the intestinal lining, and Peyer patches. These patches possess the capacity to impede the absorption or digestion of the food antigen. If this is not accomplished, the antigen may penetrate the mucosa, enter the circulation, and stimulate the allergic response in sensitive children.

Clinical Manifestations

Clinical features have been shown to involve the gastrointestinal tract, skin, respiratory system, and nervous system (Hill et al, 1984). Infants experiencing acute reactions to cow's milk within a few hours after ingestion may exhibit metabolic acidosis, gastroenteritis, or septicemia-like features. Delayed reactions in infants are manifested as failure-to-thrive, chronic cutaneous eruption, anemia, and food malabsorption.

As with allergic reactions from cow's milk, the child sensitized to other foods may experience reactions that are mild or severe. The reaction may occur immediately after ingestion, leading to anaphylaxis, or be delayed, occurring 48 to 72 hours after ingestion. The child's allergic symptoms may be diverse and multiple (Walker, 1980; White & Owsley, 1983). Clinical manifestations are presented in Table 37–16. An immediate response is usually due to the food substance itself, whereas a delayed response is usually caused by some product formed during the digestion of the food.

Diagnostic Assessment

Diagnosis of food allergies is focused primarily on the child's nutritional history, the family's history, and the child's response to dietary elimination of a suspected food. Dietary elimination is done by removing the suspected food from the diet for approximately 3 weeks, followed by reintroduction of the food (Sly, 1985). Diagnosis is confirmed after two more elimination food trials; it is made more difficult if the offending antigen is in a food that is eaten only occasionally or is antigenic only under certain conditions (e.g., causes a reaction only when eaten raw). Sometimes certain food combinations or certain quantities of a food produce the reaction, or the food may produce a reaction only when ingested during certain seasons or with exercise. In this situation, the infant or child is placed on a restricted diet eliminating the

TABLE 37-16
Clinical Manifestations of Food Allergy

Integumentary	
Eczema	
Urticaria	
Angioedema	
Geographic tongue	
Gastrointestinal	
Vomiting	
Diarrhea	
Abnormal pain or colic	
Colitis	
Malabsorption	
Iron deficiency	
Failure-to-thrive	
Respiratory	
Rhinitis	
Otitis media	
Wheezing, asthma	
Neurologic	
Fatigue	Tension-fatigue syndrome
Irritability	Tension-fatigue syndrome
Drowsiness	Tension-fatigue syndrome
Inability to concentrate	Tension-fatigue syndrome
Headache	Tension-fatigue syndrome
Systemic	
Anaphylactic shock	

more highly allergenic foods. Foods that are removed are reintroduced one at a time, with 3 days allowed between each food added back to the diet.

Food challenges are not recommended for children who have histories of severe anaphylaxis. Food challenges involve the introduction of the suspected food(s) into the child's restricted diet. One suspected food at a time is introduced to avoid confusion. When the suspected food is introduced, the amount is slowly increased while the child is closely monitored for signs of an antigen reaction. Children who experience severe anaphylaxis are extremely vulnerable to this test. In this case, skin testing or RAST provides the best alternative in diagnosing the allergen(s). Skin testing (in contrast to the RAST) is believed to be more accurate in predicting allergies to wheat and milk. As mentioned earlier, infants usually are not responsive to skin testing. Therefore, when the infant's history suggests there may be a systemic anaphylaxis, food challenge needs to be performed in a controlled environment, such as a hospital.

Therapeutic Management

Treatment involves the dietary elimination of the allergic food(s) while maintaining and supporting the child's nutritional needs for growth. Infants with cow's milk allergy may be switched to a soybean formula, only to discover an intolerance to soy (Hill et al, 1984). In this situation, the diet is changed to an alternative formula such as Pregestimil or Nutramigen or an elemental formula (Vivonex) (Table 37-17). When the breastfeeding infant develops sensitivities to foods ingested by the mother and secreted in the breast milk, an elimination diet or restricted diet may be necessary for the mother to control her infant's food sensitivities. If the maternal elimination diet is unsuccessful, the infant may need to be switched to a milk-free or elemental formula.

Symptomatic relief of gastrointestinal reactions may be initiated until the reaction subsides or the causative food is identified and eliminated. An antihistamine may be used to control intestinal spasms or abdominal pain (colic). Reducing the spasms and pains usually results in eliminating other complaints such as nausea, diarrhea, and constipation.

Nursing Diagnostic Statements

***Altered nutrition, less than body requirements** related to inability to eat certain foods.*

***High risk for altered parenting, overprotection;** risk factor: fear of anaphylaxis.*

***High risk for altered home health maintenance;** risk factor: knowledge deficit about management of food allergy at home.*

Planning and Implementation

Promoting Nutrition. In highly allergic families, prevention may start during pregnancy with the maternal elimination of highly allergenic foods. This hypoallergenic diet is maintained during breastfeeding. Infants who develop acute gastroenteritis benefit from the restriction of suspected allergens (thereby limiting the possible absorption of allergenic antigen during this vulnerable period when the intestine is inflamed).

Prevention of allergy by beginning appropriate teaching before the child is born, especially when a strong family history for allergy exists, cannot be overemphasized. Avoiding introduction of solid foods until after the infant is 6 months old also helps reduce the likelihood of food allergy. See detailed strategies for anticipatory guidance related to introduction of solid foods, Chapter 5. These actions by the nurse can aid significantly in reducing the incidence of food allergy in infancy.

The prognosis is good for children with food allergies. Children whose food allergies start during the

TABLE 37-17
Common Alternatives to Cow's Milk Formulas*†

Formula	Kilocalories per Ounce	Protein Source	Carbohydrate Source	Fat Source	Indication
Infant Formulas					
Human milk	22	Lactalbumin, casein	Lactose	Human milk	CMPA, soy allergy
Isomil (Ross)	20	Soy protein	Sucrose, corn syrup solids (lactose free)	Coconut oil, soy oil	CMPA, lactose intolerance, galactosemia
Prosobee (Mead Johnson)	20	Soy protein	Corn syrup solids (lactose free, sucrose free)	Soy oil	CMPA, lactose intolerance, galactosemia, postgastroenteritis
Nutramigen (Mead Johnson)	20	Casein hydrolysate	Modified tapioca, sucrose	Corn oil	CMPA, lactose intolerance, soy allergy, multiple food allergies, galactosemia
Portagen (Mead Johnson)	20	Sodium caseinate	Corn syrup solids, sucrose	Corn oil, MCT oil (86%)	Steatorrhea in cystic fibrosis, intestinal resections, pancreatic insufficiency, celiac disease, biliary atresia
Pregestimil (Mead Johnson)	22	Casein hydrolysate	Modified tapioca, corn syrup solids	MCT oil (40%), corn oil	CMPA, soy allergy, multiple food allergies, disaccharidase
Elemental Formulas					
Precision (Doyle Pharmaceutical)	30	Egg albumin, sodium caseinate	Glucose oligosaccharides, sucrose	Vegetable oil	Multiple food allergies, disorders of digestion and absorption
Vital (Ross)	30	Partially hydrolyzed whey, soy and meat protein, free amino acids	Glucose oligosaccharides, glucose polysaccharides	MCT oil, safflower oil	Multiple food allergies, disorders of digestion and absorption
Vivonex (Norwich Eaton)	30	Amino acids	Glucose, glucose oligosaccharides	Safflower oil	Multiple food allergies, disorders of digestion and absorption

Adapted from Grant, J. A., & Kennedy-Caldwell, C. (1988). *Nutritional support in nursing*. Philadelphia: Grune & Stratton; and Krause, M. V., & Mahan, L. K. (1984). *Food, nutrition, and diet therapy* (7th ed.). Philadelphia: WB Saunders.

* Formulations change frequently; to ensure updated information, it is best to contact the company representative.

† MCT, medium-chain triglycerides; CMPA, cow's milk protein allergy.

first 3 years of life are likely to be allergy-free within a few years.

Helping the Family Reduce Overprotective Tendencies. Home management of a food allergy requires a great deal of vigilance on the part of the parent and other caregivers (such as the baby sitter, day care center, and extended family). It is not uncommon for a child with a food allergy to react violently to a food antigen just from *touching* the food. One child who is allergic to wheat flour developed a significant reaction (with hives and marked facial edema) from holding a soda cracker someone had "kindly" given her while she was in the church nursery. Such accidental encounters with allergens, despite unusual vigilance, may cause the parent to feel that overprotection is not only justified but imperative. The nurse can be instrumental in helping the family cope with the threat of allergen contact and balance that threat with the child's developmental needs for independence. One strategy is to help the family separate actual threats from those that are only perceived and then to assist them with problem solving to protect the child. Another strategy is to discuss with them the child's developmental tasks and then help them balance the benefits of meeting tasks for independence against the threat of time away from the primary caregiver. (See the discussion on "Phenylketonuria" in Chapter 44 for further suggestions about avoiding contact with forbidden foods.)

Facilitating Home Health Maintenance of Food Allergy. Teaching methods to avoid allergens involves, first of all, clarifying exactly what the allergen is. If the allergy is reported to be to wheat flour, does that mean barley flour is all right? Is the wheat flour found in canned soup really off limits, or is it allowed because "there can't be much of it"? When this clarification has been made, the problem has been identified and a plan can be formulated. Parents must be alerted to read labels carefully to be sure the eliminated food(s) is not contained in other products. This can be as confusing as it is time consuming. The nurse or nutritionist can be helpful in providing for the parent a list of other names for the food; for example, milk products may be listed as whey or lactose. In some instances, the parent will need to prepare special foods. A list of health food stores and other suppliers of ingredients (such as rye flour) can be an invaluable resource.

One recommended approach to avoiding allergens is to be strict long enough for symptoms to be gone, approximately 3 to 6 months. If the allergen is especially difficult to eliminate or the parents really want the child to have it, then small amounts of the food can be tried. The longer parents can be strict, the greater the likelihood the child will tolerate small amounts of the allergenic foods later.

Another resource can be a family who is experiencing similar management problems. The nurse is often in a position to provide support links among families for both emotional and informational help. For example, families may be able to share special recipes and cookbooks.

Children can benefit from family support groups as well. It is helpful for them to know they are not alone in dietary restrictions. As children get older and begin assuming more self-management, their support group of peers with food allergies can help them with problem solving, such as ways to avoid "feeling different" and ways to avoid pressure from other friends to "have one just this once."

Atopic Dermatitis (Eczema)

Atopic dermatitis is a chronic, severely pruritic skin disorder. It is a relatively common allergic skin response in children between 2 months and 5 years of age, usually developing in the first year of life. Although some children outgrow this disorder, for many others it becomes a lifelong malady. At least 50 per cent of children with atopic dermatitis at age 2 years will have it into adulthood (Jacobs & Goldsobel, 1988).

Etiology/Incidence (Pathophysiology)

The term "atopic" refers to the hereditary predisposition to develop some form of allergy. Seventy per cent of children with atopic dermatitis have a family history of allergy (asthma, hay fever, or allergic conjunctivitis) (Paller, 1987a). The exact mode of genetic transmission has not been established. Although the susceptibility to atopic dermatitis is inherited, environmental factors greatly influence whether and how the tendency for dermatitis will be expressed.

When allergens do gain entry, they are thought to interact with IgE molecules to produce the Type I allergic reaction previously described. The skin of affected children, however, has been shown to release twice as much histamine as that of normal children. The inflammatory response that follows histamine release causes erythema and edema, which aggravate the pruritus.

Skin lesions resulting from frequent scratching are prone to infection. It is notable that children with atopic dermatitis have an increased susceptibility to viral, fungal, and staphylococcal skin infections (Jacobs & Goldsobel, 1988). Therefore, herpes simplex and impetigo are commonly associated with exacerbations of eczema.

Clinical Manifestations

Clinical manifestations vary with the age of the child. In infancy, a red, papular rash often appears first on the cheeks and spreads to the forehead and scalp and down the extensor surfaces of the arms and legs. Eventually, it may cover the entire body. In older children, the rash is more commonly seen on the flexor surface of the elbows and knees, the neck, sides of the face, eyelids, and dorsum of the hands and feet (Nicol, 1987). The pruritus is intense, and the child scratches the lesions, causing excoriation of the skin. Jacobs and Goldsobel (1988) quote the old axiom, *"Atopic dermatitis is not a rash that itches but an itch that rashes."* The trauma of scratching plays a major role in the occurrence and progression of the dermatitis. The child with atopic dermatitis has a higher-than-normal colonization of *Staphylococcus aureus* on the skin, and secondary infection is common. Infection leads to the typical vesiculation, oozing, and crusting (Jacobs & Goldsobel, 1988) (Fig. 37–16). As the crusts heal, they fall off, leaving healthy new epithelium.

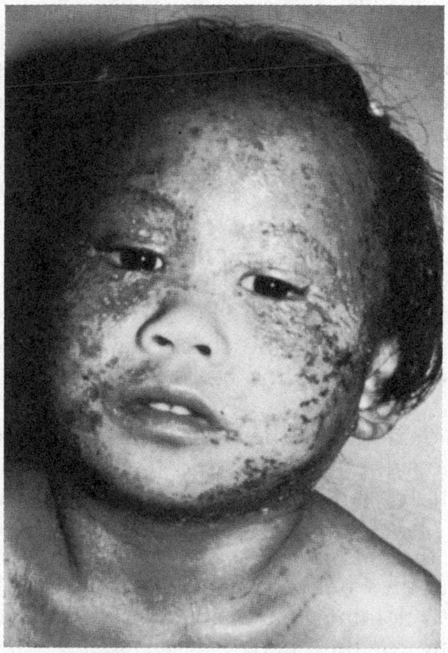

FIGURE 37 - 16. Three-year-old child with severe atopic dermatitis. (From Bierman, C. W., & Pearlman, D. S. [1988]. *Allergic diseases from infancy to adulthood.* [2nd ed., p. 393]. Philadelphia: WB Saunders.)

If atopic dermatitis develops, the parents are usually concerned about the facial rash and seek medical attention as it spreads and becomes excoriated by the child's scratching. The diagnosis is made based on the positive family history, the character and distribution of the lesions, the intense pruritus, and the pattern of exacerbation and remission of the condition. As with all types of dermatitis, a thorough history is imperative to establishing an accurate diagnosis (see Table 37–9).

Physical examination of the child with eczema often reveals an array of several types of dermatitides in varying stages of healing. The child's discomfort and fatigue are usually apparent in a forlorn, sallow appearance. The children are usually very unhappy and cry a great deal. Once symptoms have been controlled with treatment, parents may comment, "That child behaves like a new person."

Therapeutic Management

The goals of therapeutic management are hydration, control of pruritus, prevention of secondary infection, and identification and removal of allergens.

Hydration. Hydrating the skin through the use of bathing, wet wraps, and occlusive creams (e.g., Eucerin, between exacerbations) or ointments is thought to be the key in relieving the cycle of drying, cracking, itching, and scratching (Nicol, 1987). Drying soaps need to be avoided. Oatmeal soap or pH neutral moisturizing soap is used only when the skin is dirty and needs cleansing. Prolonged baths should be avoided because they act to dehydrate the skin. Nursing care related to these techniques is detailed in Table 37–18, Nursing Process Plan: The Child with Atopic Dermatitis.

Controlling Pruritus and Preventing Secondary Infection. Arm and hand restraints may be needed for the infant or small child to prevent scratching. (Restraints need to be covered with nonabrasive material.) Fingernails should be kept short and clean. The young infant's hands can be covered with long socks that are then taped or pinned to the shirt sleeves. This allows free movement of the arms while reducing scratching. Scratching can also be a learned, unconscious behavior. Some children, when old enough, are helped by behavior modification techniques to decrease scratching.

Consideration of the adverse effect of increased environmental temperature and humidity on itching is important. In particular, overheating aggravates itching. The child should be kept out of the direct sun. Dressing the infant in lightweight cotton or cotton-blend garments helps minimize this effect. The same amount of clothing that is comfortable for an adult is appropriate for the child.

Care of the skin is important in minimizing itching. In the acute exudative phase, a carefully followed topical skin regimen as described for the management of contact dermatitis can control the symptoms.

Inflammation is controlled by the application of a steroid cream or ointment following the hydrating bath or wet soaks. A fluoridated steroid cream is never used on the face because it causes unsightly acnelike eruptions and capillary dilation. One per cent hydrocortisone cream or ointment is most often used on the face. Other local steroids often used on the rest of the body include Kenalog cream 0.1 per cent, Cordran cream 0.05 per cent, Synalar cream 0.025 per cent, and Valisone cream 0.1 per cent. During the acute exudative phase, a cream or lotion base is used to avoid the occlusive effects of an ointment. Applied to large areas of damaged skin, steroids may be absorbed in quantities sufficient to depress adrenal function. Parents are taught to apply thin applications of steroid cream twice daily gently massaged into the skin. Small areas may be wrapped with a plastic film (such as Saran Wrap) or, as suggested by Nicol (1987), with wet Kerlex dressings followed by bandages to enhance the effectiveness of the medication. Because this practice increases the risk of adverse systemic effects, large body areas should not be wrapped. Another teaching point related to topical therapy is that steroids have a tendency to mask infection. The skin must be inspected carefully for subtle signs of bacterial and yeast infections. Increased inflammation, pain, or pruritus may indicate infection. Systemic antibiotics such as erythromycin are prescribed for infection. The antibiotic dosage and administration schedule should be thoroughly discussed with parents to promote compliance with treatment.

Atopic dermatitis can be controlled but not cured. By 2 years of age, 50 per cent of children may undergo permanent remission. They have little scarring, and the changes in pigmentation that occur after inflammation are temporary. Not reassuring is the fact that half of the remaining infants with atopic dermatitis develop asthma or hay fever later in life. For those in whom there is not a permanent remission, a childhood stage of atopic dermatitis usually appears during the preschool years. It is characterized by less redness and beginning lichenification (thickening of the dermal and epidermal skin layers). The third stage, the adult stage, is characterized by dermatitis on the face, neck, and flexural spaces such as the antecubital fossa and axillary areas. Popliteal lichenification is common.

Eliminating Allergens. Elimination of identified or common allergens is an approach that may be used in treating infants with atopic dermatitis. Allergy-proofing the home may be recommended (see Table 37–13). The results, however, are often disappointing. Although foods have sometimes been identified as antigens in atopic dermatitis (Paller, 1987b), many authorities now believe that unless a specific allergy to a specific food can be demonstrated, the trial elimination diet (discussed in the following section on food allergies) is of questionable value.

TABLE 37-18

Nursing Process Plan: The Child with Atopic Dermatitis

Analysis: Collaborative Problem 1

Response and Related or Risk Factors: *Impaired skin integrity: cutaneous dryness related to the inability to hold moisture in the stratum corneum*

Projected Outcome: The child's skin will return to its intact state

Analysis: Collaborative Problem 2

Response and Related or Risk Factors: *Altered comfort: pruritus, related to*

- Dry skin
- External irritants (e.g., scratching, woolen or synthetic clothing, secondary infection)
- Low threshold for itching

Projected Outcome: The child will experience and report (or give behaviors indicative of) relief from the presence of the sensation of itching

Analysis: Nursing Diagnostic Statement 1

Response and Related or Risk Factors: *Parental desire for health maintenance related to verbalized intention to learn home care of their child*

Projected Outcome: Parents will be able to identify, manage, and/or seek out help to maintain optimal health of their child

---

The following are applicable to CP 1 and 2 and ND 1.

Defining Characteristics

Impaired Skin Integrity

Subjective:

- Complaints of dry, itching, chapped skin
- Seasonal variation in symptoms

Objective:

- Skin dry, with some scaling (evidence of disruption of skin surface layers)
- Erythema and excoriation (destruction of skin layers) present from scratching
- Gooseflesh appearance of skin

Pruritus

Objective:

- Verbalization of itching
- Scratching self
- Restlessness during napping and sleeping
- Skin excoriation

Nursing Interventions

Skin Surveillance

Inspect skin regularly, and observe for signs of further skin breakdown, e.g., larger areas of dryness and scaling, extension of areas of excoriation, new areas of redness. Also observe for signs of improvement

Teaching: Prescribed Activity/Exercise

Skin Care: Topical Treatments

Institute and teach the following interventions regarding topical treatments

- Apply hypoallergenic creams or ointments as ordered by the physician *immediately* after bathing (to help seal in moisture). Avoid perfumed lubricants and bubble baths (that may trigger an allergic skin response)
- Collaborate with physician in planning to use a topical preparation like Eucerin Creme, Moisturel cream, or Aquaphor ointment. (Creams and ointments seal better than lotions)

Evaluation Criteria

The child will experience reduced dryness and skin irritation as evidenced by:

- Verbalizing increased skin comfort
- Decreased scaling
- Decreased (or absence of) redness
- Decreased excoriation from scratching
- Smooth and dry appearance of skin

The child will experience a decrease in pruritus, as evidenced by:

- Verbalizing increased comfort
- Decreased or absent scratching behaviors
- Decreased restlessness during napping and sleeping
- Decreased excoriation from scratching

(continued)

TABLE 37-18 (continued)

Defining Characteristics	Nursing Interventions	Evaluation Criteria
	Maintenance of appropriate atmospheric conditions • Avoid extremes in temperature and humidity. Use a humidifier, especially in dry climates and in winter months when heating lowers humidity indoors. If the family cannot afford a humidifier, a cool-mist vaporizer used in the child's room will help. (Provision of atmospheric humidity maintains moisture content in skin and/or prevents loss of moisture from skin) *Teaching: Prescribed Activity/Exercise* **Institute and teach, as necessary, the following interventions to promote skin hydration** (children with atopic dermatitis are usually treated at home) • Bathe at least once every day, soaking for 15–20 mins in warm, not hot, water. Bathe more often when signs and symptoms increase. (Bathing in warm water allows water to enter the pores and hydrate the skin) **Institute and teach the following interventions to reduce external irritants** • Break the scratch-itch-scratch cycle by keeping skin clean and well lubricated, keeping fingernails short, putting mitts on small infants, using elbow restraints, and administering topical steroids, antipruritics, antihistamines, or sedatives, as ordered, if needed. When creams and ointments are applied, use long, *firm* strokes, downward on the skin. (Firm application downward is less irritating.) Avoid dabbing or patting creams and ointments because this method of application can induce itching. These measures are especially important at naptime and at night (because pruritus caused by atopic dermatitis typically increases at night)	**Parents, and child as appropriate to age level, correctly verbalize all aspects of care** to promote skin hydration; reduce external skin irritants, and apply topical treatments. **Parents correctly demonstrate ability to carry out interventions required** to promote skin hydration, reduce external skin irritants, and apply topical dressings

TABLE 37-18 *(continued)*

Defining Characteristics	Nursing Interventions	Evaluation Criteria
	• Apply wet compress of Burow solution as ordered (to dry weeping lesions, rehydrate skin, and cool inflammation through evaporation) • Use material for compresses that is soft, lightweight, and loosely woven, such as a single-thickness diaper or Kerlix • Use solution at room temperature or heat just until tepid. (Extremes of temperature increase pruritus) • Wet compresses thoroughly, but avoid dripping (because solution that runs off the body is of no value) • Keep soaks wet; do not allow to dry on skin • Use *soft cotton clothing* when possible. Avoid clothing with rough, tightly woven fibers (that prevent natural evaporation from the skin) and wool (which may cause an allergic skin response) • Avoid exposure to *potential allergens*. Do not let the child crawl on a wool carpet. Stuffed animals and fuzzy toys may also be suspect. It is best to avoid exposure to dogs and cats (see Tables 37–9 and 37–10) • Wash new clothing and sheets before use (to remove formaldehyde and sizing). Avoid strong detergents and fabric softeners. Rinse clothing thoroughly • Administer *systemic antibiotics* to alleviate secondary bacterial infection. (Topical antibiotics are of no value, and their use on excoriated skin may cause the child to become allergic to the drug.) Assess for therapeutic side effects • Reduce sweating (which increases pruritus) • Avoid excessive clothing and high environmental temperatures, when possible	

(continued)

TABLE 37-18 *(continued)*

Defining Characteristics	Nursing Interventions	Evaluation Criteria
	• Alert child of preschool age and older that physical activity may increase itching **Assist parents to find appropriate and appealing play activities that do not increase itching** • Reduce anxiety (which also increases pruritus). Table 21–5 discusses anxiety reduction for the hospitalized child and the family. Parents who are aware of the relationship between anxiety and pruritus often can increase comfort measures and teach the child appropriate coping strategies	

Analysis: Nursing Diagnostic Statement 2

Response and Related or Risk Factors: *High risk for infection: secondary; risk factors:*

- Skin excoriation
- Decreased resistance to cutaneous viral, fungal, and staphylococcal organisms
- Accentuated skin folds
- Knowledge deficit of parents regarding signs of infection

Projected Outcome: The child will not experience invasion of pathogenic organisms in disrupted skin surface

Defining Characteristics *(Actual Response)*	Nursing Interventions	Evaluation Criteria
Subjective: • Pruritus • Loss of sleep • Irritability *Objective:* • Vesicles in various weeping and crusted stages	*Infection Protection* **Monitor for evidence of infection.** Teach parent(s) the signs of infection; ensure that they understand that presence of these signs indicates the need for medical intervention **Teach parent(s) the relationship between scratching and infection.** Encourage appropriate skin care techniques, as discussed earlier **If prophylactic antibiotics have been ordered, teach parent(s) proper administration** • Explain the virulence of the identified pathogen (usually *Staphylococcus*), and emphasize the importance of administering the medication according to schedule and until gone	The child will experience a reduction in infectious lesions, as evidenced by absence of erythema with vesiculation, exudation, and crusting

TABLE 37-18 (continued)

Defining Characteristics *(Actual Response)*	**Nursing Interventions**	**Evaluation Criteria**
	• Assist parent(s) in devising a schedule that will ensure dosage at the proper time • Ensure that caregivers realize the need for re-evaluation with each outbreak of pustular lesions and that they do not attempt to use "left-over" medication • If a humidifier or vaporizer is used, ensure that the family understands the necessity of cleaning before each water refill (to avoid aerosolization of mold or bacteria)	

Analysis: Nursing Diagnostic Statement 3

Response and Related or Risk Factors: *Self-esteem disturbance related to* body image disturbance associated with negative perceptions due to

- Inaccurate perceptions of others regarding the skin lesions
- Response of significant others to appearance

Projected Outcome: The child's perception of his or her body will return to baseline. The child will evaluate self in a positive way and have positive feelings about self

Defining Characteristics	**Nursing Interventions**	**Evaluation Criteria**
Body Image Disturbance *Subjective:* • Verbalizes a response to the actual change in skin integrity • Fears rejection • Focuses on past appearance • Negative feelings about body • Feelings of helplessness, hopelessness, or powerlessness • Preoccupation with change *Objective:* • Actual change in skin integrity • Change in social involvement *Self-Esteem Disturbance* *Subjective:* • Expressions of inferiority, negativity, pessimism	*Self-Esteem Enhancement and Body Image Enhancement* **Teach parent(s) that the young child's self-esteem is closely related to the responses of significant others.** Encourage parent(s) to prepare others for the child's appearance, and explain to others that eczema is not contagious unless severely infected. (It may otherwise be mistaken for impetigo or as an indication of uncleanliness) • Encourage family members to express their feelings about the child's appearance and the chronic nature of eczema (unidentified fears and concerns may hinder the relationship of parents and siblings with the child) and to discuss the changes in appearance with the child	**The child will exhibit a positive body image and a high self-esteem, as evidenced by:** • Displaying social development appropriate to age • Expressing feelings of importance, self-worth • Enjoying interpersonal interactions

(continued)

TABLE 37-18 *(continued)*

Defining Characteristics	Nursing Interventions	Evaluation Criteria
• Rationalizes away or rejects positive feedback • Reports few friends, limited social interactions • Expresses shame and guilt • Evaluates self as unable to deal with the change • Exaggerates the negative feedback about self • Denial of the presence of lesions *Objective*: • Delayed social development • Absence of expected comfort response in interactions with significant others	• Determine the parents' and significant others' perceptions regarding the child's altered body appearance. (Allow the nurse to determine if inaccurate or distorted perceptions are present) • Assure parents that it is not uncommon to experience occasional feelings of rejection toward the child because of skin lesions and the fussing and crying that tend to accompany the pruritus of an acute exacerbation. (Acknowledging and understanding these feelings can help allay guilt that might otherwise interfere with adaptive coping) • Monitor the frequency of statements by the child that indicate fear of rejection and negative feelings about self and appearance. (Knowing the frequency and intensity of the child's concerns can help the parents know how and when to address these concerns) **Assist family members to identify and carry out ways to enhance the child's self-esteem and body image** • *Reinforce* the child's sense of *identity*. Encourage the expression of caring between the child and significant others. Talk to the child about ways in which he or she excels • *Reinforce* the child's sense of *personal competence*. Encourage self-management of eczema as appropriate for age. Ensure that the child understands that controlling scratching will greatly reduce lesions. Allow the child to make age-appropriate decisions about when to use palliative measures such as wet soaks	

TABLE 37-18 *(continued)*

Analysis: Nursing Diagnostic Statement 4

Response and Related or Risk Factors: *High risk for altered health maintenance; risk factor: parental knowledge deficit regarding home care of the child*

Projected Outcome: The parent(s) will be able to identify, manage, and/or seek out help to maintain health

Defining Characteristics *(Actual Response)*	***Nursing Interventions***	***Evaluation Criteria***
Subjective: • Asking questions • Requesting demonstration of procedure(s) • Expressing interest in improving health of the child *Objective*: • Inability to demonstrate physical care behaviors or to verbalize what was previously taught • History of lack of health seeking behaviors by parents • Reported or observed lack of equipment or resources to obtain equipment • Reported or observed impairment of support systems to encourage continuation of home care as needed	**Teach the family about the allergy regimen prescribed** *Teaching: Prescribed Diet* • Ensure that they realize hypoallergenic diets and allergy-proofing do not cure eczema and may provide only limited control. (If they do not understand this, they may believe that increased eczematous symptoms are the fault of their inadequate management) • Identify the relationship between contact with certain substances and an increase in cutaneous signs and symptoms • If a hypoallergenic diet is prescribed, teach parents to read food labels carefully for alternate names of prohibited ingredients *Teaching: Procedure/Treatment* • Support the family's efforts to control allergen contact • Acknowledge the time and energy involved in controlling possible allergens • Because allergy-proofing requires drastic measures to reduce dust in the home, help the family assess the resources available to enforce this regimen. Make referrals to appropriate agencies that can assist in allergy proofing • Reinforce the family's attempts to identify possible allergens by commenting on accurate assessment of signs and symptoms • Arrange ways that parents can contact nursing staff (e.g., by telephone), or arrange for home health nursing visits	**The family will correctly identify and use appropriate measures to eliminate allergens** **The family will correctly demonstrate strategies to control dry skin, pruritus, and secondary infection**

(continued)

TABLE 37-18 *(continued)*

Defining Characteristics *(Actual Response)*	**Nursing Interventions**	**Evaluation Criteria**
	Assist the family to evaluate the outcome of their interventions and to modify home management as necessary. Take into account the perceptions, health beliefs, and cultural values identified in assessment	
	Discuss with parents and siblings ways to normalize the child's life despite the chronic nature of eczema	

Nursing Care

Teaching the family about home management of eczema involves hydration and skin care, symptomatic control of pruritus, and secondary bacterial infection, as described in "Therapeutic Management." The child and family need a great deal of support in dealing with the visible and frustrating exacerbations of the illness during childhood. Additional nursing strategies for the child with atopic dermatitis are detailed in Table 37–18.

Urticaria and Angioedema

Urticaria (hives) is easily recognized and may occur either alone or with angioedema. Both skin conditions result in interstitial edema and dilated blood vessels (Korenblat & Wedner, 1984). Reactions are acute and are believed due to Type I hypersensitivity reaction (Sly, 1985). Table 37–14 compares urticaria and angioedema.

Etiology/Incidence (Pathophysiology)

Some of the causes of angioedema and urticaria involve drugs, especially penicillin; food; blood products; insect stings or bites; inhalants; physical factors (cold, heat) and emotional factors; parasitic infections; and exercise. Special attention must be paid to allergic urticarial reactions to medications. The reintroduction of the drug may cause a more severe reaction or systemic anaphylaxis. The medication should be avoided along with similarly structured drugs. Inhalant urticaria is less common and may be seen with seasonal exacerbations of rhinitis, conjunctivitis, or asthma (Bierman & Pearlman, 1988). A complication associated with urticaria and angioedema is systemic anaphylactic shock involving upper airway obstruction. If untreated, this can lead to death. Although urticaria and angioedema can also be caused by Types II and III hypersensitivity reactions, Type I is the most common. The reaction is believed to be the result of antigen contact with IgE-bearing cutaneous mast cells.

Diagnostic Assessment

Diagnosis results from a careful history, physical assessment of lesions, and laboratory studies. The cause of urticaria often is easily recognized owing to the acute reaction. Serum eosinophils are occasionally elevated. Allergy skin testing and an elimination diet may be helpful in diagnosing possible allergens. The elimination diet involves either removing the suspected allergen or restricting the child's diet and slowly reintroducing the suspected foods. Both approaches require careful monitoring by the parents. The dietary challenge is conducted in a controlled setting if there is the potential for an anaphylactic reaction (life-threatening respiratory distress usually followed by vascular collapse and shock). Stool collection for laboratory analysis for ova and parasites is valuable if parasitic infection is suspected. In spite of these tests, the child's history and physical assessment are most helpful in establishing a diagnosis.

Therapeutic Management

Treatment for urticaria and angioedema is avoidance of the causative agents. Epinephrine injections may be necessary to prevent life-threatening angioedema or severe urticaria. Antihistamines are effective in controlling skin lesions but must be given soon after the onset of symptoms to be effective.

Urticaria and angioedema are usually transient and are usually more frightening and bothersome than they are serious.

Nursing Care

Nursing interventions include educating the family about procedures for avoiding allergens, administering medication, screening of children for drug allergies, and monitoring and organizing emergency supplies and equipment in hospitals, clinics, and physicians' offices to prevent systemic anaphylaxis. Parents need to carry and learn to use an emergency kit containing epinephrine.

Insect Sting Allergy

Honeybees, bumblebees, wasps, hornets, yellow jackets, and fire ants are responsible for most insect hypersensitivity reactions. These insects are of the Hymenoptera order (Sly, 1985). Refer to Table 46–8 in The Injured Child chapter for further information about insect bites and stings.

Etiology/Incidence (Pathophysiology)

Insect stings cause 40 to 50 deaths each year. Reactions vary from local to systemic. A normal reaction occurs even without a hypersensitivity to the venom, because pharmacologic properties in the venom do cause skin responses of pain lasting for a few minutes, followed by local erythema and a pruritic wheal that disappears within a few hours. Cellulitis has been known to develop after wasp and yellow jacket stings because these may transmit bacteria. A local reaction involves edema confined either to a small area or involving an entire extremity. The edema may persist for several days. Multiple stings may result in a toxic systemic reaction with vomiting, diarrhea, fever, headache, or convulsions.

Diagnostic Assessment

Type I hypersensitivity reaction (systemic anaphylaxis) may also occur with an onset within minutes of the sting or at any time up to 6 hours and cause death from angioedema progressing to upper airway obstruction (Sly, 1985). Delayed reactions (Type IV) may occur several days after a sting. Some findings associated with delayed reaction are bloody diarrhea, thrombocytopenic purpura, and nephrotic syndrome. Diagnosis is based on reported history from the child or parent, physical findings, and skin testing.

Therapeutic Management

Treatment is available to children with sting or bite reactions that cause large local reactions, that are increasing in severity from repeated stings, or that produce systemic reactions. Treatment of severe reactions to insect bites includes emergency management airway maintenance, administration of oxygen, and, often, administration of epinephrine. A short course of corticosteroids may be administered after anaphylactic episodes (McLean, 1987). Although some authorities recommend immunotherapy with insect venom only for adults (Yunginger, 1988), other clinics report successful results with this form of treatment in children.

People with a history of severe reaction to insect bites should be instructed in methods to avoid being stung or bitten (Table 37–19). Patients and older children should be taught emergency care, including the use of subcutaneous epinephrine, if indicated. Epinephrine (1:10,000 strength) should be available at all times.

Allergists are beginning to obtain data suggesting that immunotherapy can be stopped after several years with no increase in reaction to stings.

TABLE 37–19
Family-Centered Teaching: Avoiding Stinging Insects

Avoid loose-fitting clothes outdoors (may entrap bee)
Avoid brightly colored clothes. White is least likely to attract bees
Avoid scented cosmetics, hairsprays, deodorants, and perfume
Avoid going barefoot outdoors
Avoid areas harboring stinging insects (e.g., flower beds, orchards, garbage cans, picnic grounds)
Have a professional exterminator destroy wasp nests or beehives near the home
Keep automobile windows closed
Keep windows and doors closed unless screens are available
When away from home, take an insecticide spray

Nursing Care

Table 46–8 details nursing strategies appropriate to an insect sting in a child for whom there is no immediate danger of anaphylaxis. When the child is allergic to the venom, additional teaching is indicated. The nurse helps the family obtain a Medic-Alert bracelet, indicating the child's hypersensitivity, and acquire an emergency kit containing oral antihistamines and a prefilled epinephrine syringe. They should, of course, be taught the technique of subcutaneous injection. A medication emergency kit may be kept at several areas (at school, home, or baby sitter's place). Additional instructions on how to handle emergency situations need to be provided to other people involved in the child's care. A child experiencing systemic reactions with or without administration of medication should be seen at an emergency facility.

Allergic Conjunctivitis

Conjunctivitis is the inflammation of the delicate membrane that lines the eye and is associated with a discharge. Allergic conjunctivitis is a common finding associated with allergic rhinitis, and it is believed to result from chemically mediated release of histamine from sensitized IgE mast cells, usually in response to environmental allergens such as pollen (Sly, 1985). Common physical findings are itching, excessive lacrimation, and edema of the eyelids and periorbital tissues. These findings may affect the child's attention span, ability to read, and participation in classroom activities or sports.

Therapeutic Management

Treatment consists of topical vasoconstrictors, Opticrom (cromolyn sodium for optical use), and oral antihistamines to relieve the swelling and itching. In rare instances, topical steroids are used to decrease the inflammation and swelling. It has been documented that frequent acute reactions may result in corneal changes and abnormal tear patterns (Bierman & Pearlman, 1988). Wetting agents to help lubricate the eye may be needed. Cold water compresses may be soothing and reduce swelling.

The family may require instruction in ophthalmic medicine administration (Chapter 24) and the effect of conjunctivitis on the child's behavior. For example, the child with conjunctivitis may appear inattentive and uncooperative with learning activities. The itching, edema, and excessive tearing may make it difficult for the child to concentrate or focus on tasks demanding visual attentiveness.

Type IV Allergic Disorders

Type IV allergic disorders are characterized by the response of Tdh. The general pathophysiology of Type IV allergic disorders is summarized in Table 37–8. The pathophysiology of allergic contact dermatitis illustrates one specific example of this type of allergic response.

Allergic Contact Dermatitis

Allergic contact dermatitis is an acquired immune reaction resulting from skin contact with allergens. Common sensitizers in children include poison ivy, shoes, metals, preservatives, and topical medications. (See Chapter 46 for additional nursing care strategies for the child with poison ivy.)

Etiology/Incidence (Pathophysiology)

Boys show a greater tendency for allergic contact dermatitis than do girls. It occurs more often in infants and toddlers, usually beginning around 3 to 4 months of age. Susceptible children tend to have unusually dry skin from birth and a family history of allergy.

Allergic contact dermatitis begins with penetration of the skin by small antigenic particles (called "haptens"). Once inside the stratum corneum, they combine with other proteins in the skin to form a complete antigen. This antigen is then processed by skin macrophages (Langerhans cells) and presented to T-lymphocytes. Only a few T-cells need be present at the skin site to trigger the sensitization process. After the initial antigen–T-cell contact, lymphokines are released that cause further activation and proliferation of T-cells. The T-cells then migrate from the epidermis to area lymph nodes where they proliferate into large numbers of T-effector and T-memory cells. Clones of these effector and memory cells circulate in the blood to reach all parts of the lymphatic system. Circulation of the sensitized cells is a key component of the Type IV reaction in allergic contact dermatitis. It means that subsequent skin contact with that antigen, anywhere on the body, will result in T-cell recognition of the antigen and the activation of a cell-mediated immune response (Parker, 1988).

Allergic sensitization in this manner generally takes 7 to 10 days after the allergen is first contacted, but it is not uncommon for sensitization to occur over a period of many years. Once sensitization (allergy) develops, all future contacts with the allergen will result in an inflammatory reaction at the contact site, usually within 24 to 72 hours. Contact allergies tend to persist indefinitely (Parker, 1988).

Clinical Manifestations

The inflamed skin area may be configured to match the antigen contact with the skin. The exposed skin area is erythematous, edematous, and pruritic. Papules and vesicles form, which weep, ooze, and crust if scratched. Lichenification (hardened, leathery skin) develops if the dermatitis becomes chronic.

Diagnostic Assessment

A history of dry skin, family members with allergies, and ready skin blanching (tendency toward vasoconstriction of cutaneous vessels), coupled with localized inflammatory configuration and distribution, are evidence of contact dermatitis. Diagnostic evaluation usually includes patch testing to identify the cause. Suspected allergens are applied to the back on adhesive strips. After 48 hours, the strips are removed and the skin is observed for reactions. A positive reaction usually appears as vesicles on an edematous, red base and exactly outlines the area covered by the adhesive patch (Parker, 1988).

Therapeutic Management

Because this allergic disease is self-limiting, treatment is primarily symptomatic. In most instances, topical treatment is sufficient. Steroid creams such as Kenalog or Valisone may be used during the acute phase. Antihistamines may be necessary to control itching. The physician also usually orders cool wet dressings; these may be soaked in a soothing solution such as Burow solution. This not only cools and soothes the skin but helps clean and dry the lesions.

Because secondary bacterial infection is common, a wound culture will be obtained if purulent lesions, fever, and/or increased erythema develop. Antimicrobial drugs are ordered to combat identified organisms.

Nursing Diagnostic Statements

High risk for infection, secondary; risk factor: open skin lesions.

Altered comfort: pruritus related to effects of allergens.

Sleep pattern disturbance, related to pruritus.

Body image disturbance related to negative perception regarding skin lesions.

High risk for altered home health maintenance; risk factor: knowledge deficit about home care.

Planning and Implementation

Once the antigen is identified, its elimination, if possible, prevents further episodes of contact dermatitis. If the allergy can be traced to an allergen such as perfume, a metal, a detergent, or a type of fabric, elimination may be manageable. If, however, the allergen is something like the dichromate used in leather processing or a chemical compound found in printer's ink, the task will be more difficult. Desensitization therapy is hardly ever successful in managing this dermatitis, although it may decrease the severity of reaction if the antigen is a plant source that cannot be eliminated. In these instances, it is usually used preseasonally for a few weeks.

Promoting Sleep. Discomfort severe enough to disturb sleep should be controlled with temporary use of antihistamines or steroid ointments administered at bedtime. Antihistamines' sedative properties are often sufficient. In some instances, sedatives may be prescribed.

Preventing Further Allergic Responses. Emotional distress increases susceptibility to allergic response and intensifies reaction severity. Once the dermatitis is present, such distress increases the pruritus experienced. Therefore, a calm environment, void of as much friction and emotional pressure as possible, is of utmost importance to the child.

Promoting Home Health Management. Preparing the family for home management of allergic contact dermatitis includes preventive strategies and treatment of symptoms. Preventive management involves keeping the skin lubricated, clean, and healthy to increase its resistance and to minimize infection secondary to allergic response. Daily tepid baths without soap and lasting 15 to 20 minutes, followed by application of a bland lubricant (e.g., Eucerin Creme) while the skin is still wet, are usually sufficient to maintain general integumentary health and to promote absorption of topical agents. Use of a humidifier in the home during dry months also helps combat an infant's dry skin condition. Daily cleaning of the humidifier is recommended to prevent aerosolizing mold and bacteria that can colonize this device.

Nursing care pertaining to nursing diagnostic responses *impaired skin integrity; altered comfort: pruritus; high risk for infection: secondary;* and *body image and/or self-esteem disturbance* can be found in Table 37–18.

Altered Immune Response: Immune Deficiency

As newsworthy as immune deficiency is today, it is interesting to note that the first identified immune deficiency disease, agammaglobulinemia, was not described until the 1950s. Since that time, many other immunodeficiency disorders have been identified. These disorders can involve any part of the immune system, including T- and B-lymphocytes, phagocytes, complement proteins, or organs of the immune system (Lockey & Bukantz, 1987a, 1987b). Some immune deficiencies have been related to genetic causes (e.g., X-linked agammaglobulinemia), whereas others are acquired (e.g., acquired immunodeficiency syndrome [AIDS]). The exact cause of many of these disorders remains unknown. What is known is that immunodeficiency leaves the body without adequate protection from microorganisms, and people with these diseases experience repeated, and often life-threatening, infections.

Acquired Immunodeficiency Syndrome

Etiology/Incidence

AIDS is an irreversible, fatal disease of the immune system. The first official case of AIDS in the United States in a child was reported in November 1982, about 18 months after the first reported adult case (Rogers et al, 1987). Since that time, the incidence of AIDS, including that in children, has been steadily increasing despite public education efforts. The World Health Organization (WHO) estimates that 1 million children worldwide have been infected with HIV, and they project that 10 million will be infected by the year 2000 (Baum, 1992).

AIDS is caused by infection with HIV. The virus is carried primarily in blood and semen and is transmitted through contact with these body fluids from an infected person. Primary risk factors (Table 37–20) for children contracting the virus include (1) infants born to at-risk or documented HIV-positive mother or (2) transfusion of contaminated blood or blood products (e.g., factor replacement products used in children with clotting factor deficiencies) (Edmundson, 1988). Depending on the age of the child, geographic location, and other variables, such as the method of childbirth and the mother's stage of HIV infection, percentages of perinatal transmission (also called "vertical transmission") from HIV-infected mothers to their infants vary widely. Reported percentages range from as low as 13 per cent to as high as 50 per cent (Butler & Pizzo, 1992; Evans, 1992). Most evidence indicates that the virus is primarily transmitted to the infant in utero through the placenta (Butler & Pizzo,

TABLE 37-20
Children at Risk for AIDS

Mother or father an intravenous drug user
Mother having sexual relations with person(s) at risk for AIDS
Father bisexual
Parent recent immigrant from Haiti or central Africa
Infant/child exposure to contaminated blood:
1. at time of delivery
2. through transfusion of blood or blood components (e.g., children with hemophilia)

1992; Rubinstein & Bernstein, 1986). However, other routes of transmission are hypothesized, including exposure to maternal blood and body fluids during the birth process and through breast milk. However, these other factors remain speculative and in study. Explanations of why children at equal risk do not manifest the infection are still undetermined. At least one case has been reported in which one identical twin contracted the HIV virus and the other (at age 3 years) was still seronegative (Menez-Bautista et al, 1986). This example demonstrates the gaps in understanding of mechanisms that contribute to or inhibit virus transmission.

The suggested mode of postnatal transmission of breast milk has some basis for concern. HIV has been isolated from colostrum as well as breast milk, per se. However, conflicting results are reported from studies seeking to confirm the relationship of transmission risk to breastfed infants and their HIV-positive mothers. Some reports suggest that "HIV transmission through breast milk may occur only when the mother is acutely infected and before maternal antibody has been generated" (Butler & Pizzo, 1992). Given this uncertainty, in the United States and other developed countries, breastfeeding is discouraged for seropositive mothers or mothers who are considered high-risk for the virus. In underdeveloped countries, the risk of transmission by this route is considered preferable to that posed by unreliable milk supplies or substitutes and the serious potential for diarrheal syndromes that contribute to mortality among bottlefed infants in those countries.

The immature immunologic system of premature and newborn infants makes them especially susceptible to transfusions of contaminated blood (Rubinstein & Bernstein, 1986). Most children who contracted HIV through transfusions of contaminated blood did so prior to the HIV *antibody* (not virus antigen) screening that began in May 1985. Nevertheless, it should be noted that blood donated soon after exposure to HIV, before antibodies have been formed, can transmit the virus in an undetectable state, thus placing those with immature and/or compromised immune systems at significant risk.

Although one focus of HIV transmission and infection is newborn infants, another significant at-risk groups is adolescents. In this age group, in which childhood AIDS was the seventh leading cause of death in 1989, modification of high-risk sexual and drug-abusing behavioral patterns has been limited despite extensive educational efforts. A high percentage of adolescents are admittedly sexually active, yet less than one third report use of condoms (Hein, 1989). Unprotected sexual and drug-abusing practices have important implications for infection and transmission of the HIV virus. The adolescent's characteristic belief in his or her invincibility and the notably fewer resources for coping with the serious ramifications of HIV infection, together with the typically longer latency period for symptom development in this age group, make the adolescent a particularly important target for intervention, education, and support.

Pathophysiology

The HIV that causes AIDS produces abnormalities in both T-cell function (cellular immunity) and, indirectly, in B-cell function (humoral immunity). The initial attack is on the T-lymphocytes, leading to a marked depression of the T-helper cells that regulate B-cell function (Lockey & Bukantz, 1987a). Depression of T4 cells reverses the usual ratio of T4 to T8 (T-suppressor) cells. Although antibodies (IgG, IgA, and IgM) are typically increased in the serum of persons with HIV infection, the T8 effect on B-lymphocytes renders the B-cells incapable of forming antibodies to new microorganisms. Thus, the patient is somewhat protected against those microorganisms to which antibodies have been previously formed but cannot defend against newly introduced pathogens. Because children have had fewer exposures to pathogens, they have fewer circulating antibodies than do adults. In addition, phagocytic macrophages in HIV-infected patients have a decreased ability to process and kill antigens and to interact with T-cells (Ammann, 1987). This means that the child (or adult) with HIV is extremely susceptible to infection, and, once infected, has little defense against the invading organism.

The effect of the HIV virus on levels of T4 and T8 and the T4/T8 ratio levels is important for several reasons. They are laboratory values by which progression of the disease is monitored and are also important factors in the development of intervention strategies. However, absolute values in children can be misleading unless interpretation of levels has been corrected for age because children have significantly higher T4 levels than those in normal adults. Niven and associates (1990) and the Centers for Disease Control (CDC) (1991) have provided comparative data of developmental T4 (CD4+) counts in children (Table 37-21). The normal progressively decreasing absolute numbers of T4 concentrations as well as the T4/T8 ratio must be considered in evaluating the immunologic competence along with the stage of HIV

TABLE 37-21
Age-Adjusted T4 (CD4) Levels and T4/T8 (CD4/CD8) Ratios in Children (Compared with Adults)

	Child's Age (Mos)				
	1-6	7-12	13-24	25-74	Adults
Absolute T4 (CD4) Count					
Median (cells/mm³)	3211	3128	2601	1668	1027
5th to 95th percentiles	1153-5285	967-5289	739-4463	505-2831	237-1817
Percentage of T4 (CD4) Cells					
Median (%)	52	48	46	42	51
5th to 95th percentiles	36-67	33-63	31-60	32-52	35-67
T4/T8 (CD4/CD8) Ratio					
Median	2.2	2.1	2.0	1.4	1.7
5th to 95th percentiles	0.9-3.5	0.8-3.4	0.6-3.4	0.7-2.1	0.4-3

(Data from Centers for Disease Control [1991].)

infection. Defects in T4 function may precede the reduction in count and must be taken into consideration in planning intervention.

HIV *Infection and Classification (Stage) of Disease*

The CDC has created a definition and system for classifying stages of illness progression from presumed HIV infection to a diagnosis of AIDS (Table 37-22). As indicated, the P-0 classification includes infants, usually younger than 15 months, in whom infection has neither been conclusively determined nor excluded. Children in class P-1 have documented HIV infection and are asymptomatic. Classification is based on level of immunologic function. Children in class P-2 have documented infection *and* demonstrate signs and symptoms of HIV infection. As indicated, this class is further subdivided to specify some, but not all, categories of symptoms considered "AIDS indicator conditions."

TABLE 37-22
Classification of HIV Infection in Children Younger than 13 Yrs of Age

Type	Description
Class P-0	Indeterminate infection (perinatally exposed infants younger than 15 mos of age who have antibodies to HIV)
Class P-1	Asymptomatic infection
Subclass A	Normal immune function
Subclass B	Abnormal immune function
Subclass C	Immune function not tested
Class P-2	Symptomatic infection
Subclass A	Nonspecific findings
Subclass B	Progressive neurologic disease
Subclass C	Lymphoid interstitial pneumonitis
Subclass D	Secondary infectious diseases
Subclass E	Secondary cancers
Subclass F	Other diseases possibly due to HIV infections

Centers for Disease Control (1987). Classification system for human immunodeficiency virus (HIV) in children under 13 years of age. *Morbidity and Mortality Weekly Report, 36*(15), 227.

Clinical Manifestations

Symptomatic evidence of HIV infection varies, depending on the source of infection and age of the child at the time of infection. There are reports of delays in symptom expression, with an average of 0 to 36 months, during which the child may be essentially asymptomatic. Children infected in utero appear to have shorter incubation periods and more rapid progression of the disease (Borkowsky et al, 1992; Butler & Pizzo, 1992; Dowe et al, 1992). Young children such as those with hemophilia who contracted HIV infection through blood or blood products appear to be more likely to have a longer incubation period than similarly infected older children (Butler & Pizzo, 1992). Because children infected with HIV have not usually been exposed to common pathogens, and, therefore, have not developed an immune response capability to them, they often present with recurrent infections to familiar pathogens. For example, 80 per cent of HIV-infected children will have serous otitis media, acute otitis media, or chronic otitis media (Dowe et al, 1992).

In some children, manifestations of illness may be subtle and insidious. Nonspecific symptoms such as failure-to-thrive, developmental delays, organomegaly, lymphadenopathy, recurrent respiratory tract infections, recurrent diarrhea, malaise, and fevers may be the primary indicators of HIV infection. Etiologically, these are bacterial assaults to which the immature and/or compromised immune system cannot mount an effective response. Common invading organisms include *Streptococcus pneumoniae, Haemophilus influenzae, Staphylococcus aureus,* and *Meningococcus* (Butler & Pizzo, 1992).

The HIV-infected child is also subject to "opportunistic infections."* Of these, *Pneumocystis carinii* pneumonia is the most common and is the leading cause of death among these children. Because of the swiftness with which it can develop, *P. carinii* pneumonia must always be considered as a primary possible diagnosis, especially if symptoms include tachypnea and cough with a fever, even if low grade.

Almost invariably, HIV-infected children have gastrointestinal symptoms. Because of the integral relationship between nutrition and health, it is frequently difficult to discern whether the infection induces anorexia, diarrhea, and, ultimately, malnutrition or if the result of these symptoms augments the progressive nature of the infection. Abdominal pain, persistent or recurrent diarrhea, and colitis are all common symptoms in HIV-infected children (Butler & Pizzo, 1992).

Another common symptom of HIV infection in children is CNS involvement. Mounting evidence indicates that CNS damage begins early in the course of the disease and likely begins in utero in infants born to HIV-infected mothers. The incidence of neurologic abnormalities increases as the disease progresses; however, there is no characteristic pattern for the development of encephalopathy. It may appear acutely, or it may be more insidious in both its initial presentation and development. This aspect of HIV infection may contribute to a loss of previously achieved developmental milestones and a limited ability to progress toward other milestones. Attention span, ability to concentrate, and even physical coordination may be reduced so that learning, playing, or other developmentally appropriate activities may be hindered.

Because of the nature of the invading virus, no physiologic system is unaffected by HIV infection. However, the type or extent of symptom expression in the child includes some notable differences from those seen in the HIV-infected adult. Although fluid and electrolyte and acid-base balance problems are common in HIV-infected children, primary renal disease is relatively uncommon. Thyroid and adrenal dysfunction are among the endocrine abnormalities that have been described in afflicted adults but are less frequently seen in children. Kaposi sarcoma, widely described in adult patients, is extremely rare in children.

Diagnostic Assessment

Detection of antibodies to HIV is the means for establishing a differential diagnosis. HIV antibody testing is usually accomplished using a test known as the "enzyme-linked immunosorbent assay" (ELISA) for screening, followed by the Western Blot technique as the confirmatory test. Because of the potential for false-positive or false-negative results using only one of these diagnostic tools, one test is rarely used independently of the other. There are ongoing efforts to develop more reliable methods for diagnosis. These include methods to detect the virus, virus antigens, and viral deoxyribonucleic acid (DNA) (Arpadi & Caspe, 1991).

The ELISA and Western Blot techniques are relatively effective in identifying HIV antibodies in older children and adults. However, nearly all infants born to HIV-positive mothers have positive test results because of the persistence of maternal antibodies in the infant's circulation, which are not eliminated until approximately 12 to 15 months of age. Until recently, the presence of maternal antibodies has made it impossible to know if an infant is infected unless the infant shows signs of immunosuppression (Butler & Pizzo, 1992). Detection of the HIV p24 antigen in the blood of infants appears to be able to distinguish infected and noninfected infants with relative accuracy (Miles et al, 1993). Further refinement of identification techniques for exposed infants will not only relieve parental anxiety but make earlier treatment with antiretroviral agents possible.

Currently, none of the diagnostic tests can distinguish between an acute infection and a carrier state (Coulis & DiSiena, 1987) or between maternal and infant antibodies. Ultimate diagnosis depends on physical findings and is structured according to the CDC's criteria for classification of stage of the disease. The terminology "AIDS-related complex" (ARC) has been used to identify persons who do not meet the criteria for a diagnosis of AIDS. However, the term "HIV positive" is replacing "ARC" for referring to patients whose disease has not progressed to being classified as AIDS. HIV-positive adults may live symptom free for several years, but children do not usually fare as well.

During the diagnostic process and throughout the course of the disease, blood counts should be routinely followed. The white blood cell count with differential allows a gross evaluation of infectious status. Closer examination of lymphocytes to assess the total number, the percentage of T4 lymphocytes, and the T4/T8 ratio is an ongoing aspect of monitoring for progressive disease.

Therapeutic Management

Management of HIV in children parallels that for adults. It includes (1) reduction of viral replication within the T-lymphocyte with the use of antiretroviral drug therapy, (2) treatment of infections, and (3) immunopotentiation. Normal lymphocyte replication occurs through synthesis of ribonucleic acid (RNA), with DNA serving as the template. In HIV infection, the virus reverses the process of information transcription, with RNA altering the DNA genome of the host cell.

*The term "opportunistic" refers to the fact that the person with HIV may be so immunocompromised that pathogens that do not usually cause disease may result in infection.

Antiretroviral therapy attempts to inhibit virus-encoded reverse transcriptase early in the virus's life cycle, thereby interrupting the critical transfer of information from RNA to DNA (Butler & Pizzo, 1992). However, these drugs are not effective once the reverse transcription has occurred. In 1992, the only drug in this classification licensed for use in HIV infection was zidovudine (AZT). AZT is currently approved for use in HIV-infected infants and children who are older than 3 months and are symptomatic or for those who are asymptomatic but have values indicating significant immunosuppression. Because maternal antibodies do not disappear from the infant's system until 12 to 15 months of age, decisions about treatment with antiretroviral agents must be made based on an evaluation of the infant for signs of immunosuppression (changes in T4 and T8 levels or clinical symptoms) or the use of HIV p24 antigen detection tests (Miles et al, 1993). This therapy is being used more with children while the search is continued for a vaccine as well as other drugs that are effective in HIV-positive patients.

Doses of intravenous gamma globulin every 3 or 4 weeks are used to reduce or prevent infection in children who are HIV positive or who have AIDS and cannot make their own antibodies. Although this therapy does not prevent infection indefinitely in the HIV-positive child, it has been shown to reduce recurrent bacterial and viral infections and prolong life in clinical trials (Ammann, 1987; Fischer, 1988; Gupta et al, 1986; Rubinstein, 1986; Shyur & Hill, 1991).

Once diagnosis of HIV infection is made, the treatment program for infectious episodes is primarily with antibiotic, antiviral, and antifungal agents specific to the infecting organism. Prophylactic use of these agents as therapy against opportunistic infections may be initiated and continued over an extended period.

Application of the Nursing Process: Acquired Immunodeficiency Syndrome

Assessment

Nursing assessment of the child who is HIV positive involves the observation and monitoring of signs and symptoms discussed in the Clinical Manifestations section. The data collected formulate the basis for identification of nursing diagnoses and collaborative problems.

Nursing Diagnostic Statements and Collaborative Problems

High risk for infection; *risk factors:*
- *Suppression of immune system by virus.*
- *Presence of virus in body fluids.*

High risk for altered growth and development; *risk factors:*
- *Failure-to-thrive related to unknown mechanisms associated with HIV infection.*
- *Chronic infection.*
- *Poor attachment associated with a terminal prognosis.*
- *CNS involvement.*

High risk for injury, allergic reaction; *risk factor: administration of intravenous gamma globulin.*

Ineffective family coping; *related to:*
- *Parental feelings of guilt.*
- *Terminal prognosis of one or more family members.*
- *Loss of social support associated with fear of HIV transmission.*

High risk for altered home health maintenance; *risk factor: knowledge deficit about management of HIV-positive child at home.*

Planning and Implementation

Preventing Infection in the Nurse. The nursing plan of care must address the safety of the nurse as well as that of the child. The facts about AIDS transmission are that although HIV has been found in blood, semen, saliva, and tears, the disease has been known only to be transmitted sexually, perinatally, and by direct inoculation (Blattner, 1987; Lilleyman, 1986; US Public Health Service, 1988). The concern for health care professionals, then, is to prevent direct inoculation, that is, to ensure that body secretions, especially blood, from the patient do not enter the blood stream of the caregiver.

Universal Precautions. In August 1987, the CDC published a document entitled "Recommendations for Prevention of HIV Transmission in Health-Care Settings." It was recommended that blood and body fluid precautions be consistently observed for ALL patients, regardless of their diagnosis or blood-borne infection status. The extension of blood and body fluid precautions to all patients has come to be known as "universal precautions." In universal precautions, blood and certain body fluids for any patient are considered potentially infectious for HIV, hepatitis B virus (HBV), and other blood-borne pathogens (Table 37–23). *The implementation of universal precautions is intended to supplement, not replace, other category-specific or disease-specific isolation precautions.* (General isolation guidelines are discussed in Chapter 23.)

Blood and Body Fluid Precautions. Specific policies for *blood and body fluid precautions* vary somewhat among institutions. However, most institutions have adopted policies similar to the guidelines outlined by Kirkis and Grier (1988):

- Put the patient in a private room if hygiene is poor or if the environment is likely to become contaminated with blood. Two patients with the same disease can be in the same room.
- *Wash hands* thoroughly before and after patient care and after handling contaminated articles.

TABLE 37-23
Universal Precautions (Blood and Body Fluid Precautions)*

ALWAYS use blood and body fluid precautions for these substances (see Table 23–4):
Blood†
Body fluids containing visible blood†
Semen
Vaginal secretions
Tissues
Cerebrospinal fluid
Synovial fluid
Pleural fluid
Peritoneal fluid
Pericardial fluid
Amniotic fluid
Universal precautions do not apply (unless visible blood is present):
Feces
Nasal secretions
Sputum
Sweat
Tears
Urine
Vomitus
Saliva

* *Note:* The implementation of universal precautions does not eliminate the need for other disease-specific or category-specific precautions as outlined in Chapter 23.

† These are the only sources of HIV and hepatitis B virus that have been implicated in transmission of infection from patient to health care worker. Semen and vaginal secretions have been associated with sexual transmission of bloodborne organisms but not with patient-to-nurse transfer. The other fluids listed in this column are potential sources of infection and are the subject of ongoing epidemiologic studies.

Handwashing is the most cost effective, practice effective method to reduce the spread of infection.

- Always wear *gloves* when touching blood or body fluids.
- Wear a *mask* only if aerosolization of secretions is likely (e.g., during suctioning).
- Wear a *gown* only if soiling of clothes is likely.
- Discard contaminated disposable articles; bag and send reusables for reprocessing.
- Avoid needle-stick injuries. Handle needles and sharps carefully.
- Clean up blood spills promptly with a solution of bleach diluted 1:10 with water.

The CDC recommends that needles not be recapped, bent, removed, or otherwise manipulated, because this increases the risk of accidental puncture. Syringes with needles attached should be disposed of, intact, in an impervious container in the room. If an incident of contamination occurs (i.e., needle stick, breaking the skin with a contaminated sharp object, splash contamination), report it immediately to the employee health service department for that institution. Tests will be conducted to determine whether the patient carries antibodies for hepatitis or AIDS. Follow-up testing of the nurse for AIDS or provision of hepatitis B immune globulin will be carried out as indicated.

The precautions for hospital personnel exceed the precautions recommended for families in home care because of the repeated risks of exposure for these professionals.

Exemption Policies. The practice of providing exemption for the pregnant nurse from the care of persons with AIDS, cytomegalovirus (CMV), and certain other communicable diseases is becoming much less prevalent as a direct result of CDC recommendations for universal precautions. It is becoming increasingly evident that nurses and other health care professionals are at greater risk for exposure from the patient presumed free of infection (but who may in fact be infectious) than from the patient with a diagnosed communicable disease for whom appropriate precautions are observed. If blood and body fluid precautions are consistently followed for all patients, regardless of health status (universal precautions), the risk of exposure is greatly reduced for all members of the staff.

Preventing Infection and Caring for the Child with Opportunistic Infection. AIDS destroys the body's natural defenses against bacterial, viral, and fungal infections, making it imperative that precautions be taken to protect the child from pathogens. Despite precautions, however, it can be expected that some opportunistic infections will develop. The infections common in children vary somewhat from those found in adults with AIDS. The body organs most often attacked by opportunistic infections are the lungs and the skin; chronic bacterial infections are an additional concern.

P. carinii pneumonia is the most frequent opportunistic infection in children (Ammann, 1987). Less frequently, *Mycobacterium avium* or *Candida albicans* may be the cause of lung infection.

Recognizing the child's tendency toward lung infection, the nurse can meticulously assess for changes in pulmonary status and can teach and implement good pulmonary hygiene. Assessment findings of concern are fever, increased pulse and respirations, adventitious lung sounds, a cough, pallor on exertion, and retractions or other signs of increased respiratory effort.

Preventive hygienic measures include ensuring that the child's lungs are fully inflated at regular intervals and that secretions have no opportunity to pool within the lung because of immobility. Young children with AIDS who are feeling well enough to play usually meet these criteria for pulmonary hygiene on their own through running, jumping, yelling, and other activities that stimulate movement and deep breathing. The child hospitalized with a serious infection may need some innovative nursing help to accomplish this goal, however. The nurse can draw on techniques used to promote turning and deep breathing after anesthesia. Gentle oral suctioning may be warranted if the child is unable to expectorate secretions.

Another important preventive measure is to ensure that the child is not needlessly exposed to pathogens. Research has shown that the most effective way to prevent the spread of infection is through good handwashing. When the child is hospitalized, nurses and other health care professionals must remember that *the child is in more danger of contracting an infection from the nurse than the nurse is in peril of contracting AIDS from the child.* Parents, siblings, and the ill child should be taught proper handwashing techniques and counseled about avoiding exposure to crowds and to persons with active infections of any kind.

Infections of the integument in children are frequently either oral thrush (candidiasis) or chronic herpes simplex. Thrush is considered an opportunistic infection in children when it also involves the esophagus (Rubinstein, 1986). Oral antiseptic rinses such as nystatin and fluconazole are used to treat thrush.

Herpes simplex is more common in children than in adults (Rubinstein, 1986). The blisters may occur in the perianal as well as the oral region. Perianal lesions are in danger of secondary infection from fecal contamination, so gentle cleansing is needed after bowel movements. Severe infections may involve hospitalization and treatment with acyclovir.

Kaposi sarcoma, although not common among children with AIDS, may be found in adolescents with the disease. The raised purple tumors may be seen through the skin or mucous membranes. They are disfiguring because of their dark color but are usually not painful or irritating unless they involve the mucous membranes of the intestinal tract, where they often cause malabsorption and chronic diarrhea (Schietinger, 1986).

Nurses are often the persons responsible for teaching and implementing assessment and preventive measures. Parents can be taught to check the child's body daily for evidence of rashes, redness, bruises, blisters, or other unusual findings. Evidence of abrasions, such as "skinned" knees, means extra precautions using universal precaution measures (including gloves) to prevent secondary infection until a protective scab is formed. Usually such "scrapes" can safely be treated with half-strength hydrogen peroxide three to four times per day and protected with an ointment such as Neosporin. When in doubt, consult with the physician regarding a specific protocol for each child. Preventing infections of the skin and mucous membranes involves keeping the skin clean, dry, and well lubricated and reporting the first evidence of an infectious process before a full-blown infection occurs.

Bacterial infections are common among children with AIDS (Ammann, 1987). It is important to alert parents that common childhood illnesses, such as ear aches, gastroenteritis, and impetigo, can become serious illnesses in the child with AIDS because of the lack of usual body defenses. Adolescents should be advised that opiates, alcohol, and marijuana can act as immunosuppressants and therefore may increase the susceptibility to infection (Dhundale & Hubbard, 1986).

Teach families that milk or formula is an excellent medium for bacterial growth. Infants should not be put to bed with a bottle that may be only partially consumed before sleep and finished hours later because bottle caries can develop. Baby food, too, can become a culture medium. Teach parents not to feed directly from the baby food jar; bacteria from saliva can contaminate the remaining food. Fruits and vegetables should be washed and peeled or cooked before they are eaten (Berry, 1988).

If a gastrostomy tube or nasogastric tube is required for supplemental feeding, it should be rinsed with water following feedings and clamped to avoid regurgitation. Strict aseptic technique is indicated in the care of central venous catheters to reduce the risk of localized infections or sepsis. Signs of sepsis include marked changes in temperature of the skin or body, tachycardia, hypotension, weak peripheral pulses, mottling, and altered mental status (Iazzeti, 1986). Prompt assessment and treatment of infection and compliance with prophylactic antimicrobial therapy are the best protection currently available for the child with AIDS.

Safe Administration of Intravenous Gamma Globulin. As outlined by Iazzeti (1986), certain precautions should be observed when administering intravenous gamma globulin. The vial containing gamma globulin should not be shaken or rotated because bubbles may form in the solution. Gamma globulin is compatible *only* with a 5 per cent dextrose intravenous solution. No other medications or solutions should be administered through the same line.

Assessment for side effects of gamma globulin is similar to that for a transfusion reaction. Vital signs, including temperature, should be taken immediately before, and frequently during, administration. The most common side effects are skin rash, urticaria, fever, and dyspnea. If any of these signs or symptoms occur, stop the transfusion. Keep the line open with 5 per cent dextrose, record the vital signs and physical assessment, and alert the physician.

Enhancing Growth and Development. Some part of growth retardation and developmental delays seems attributable to actions of the AIDS virus, but enhancement of growth and development is still an attainable goal (Thurber & Berry, 1990). Why should one be concerned about growth and development in a child with an incurable disease? It is the position of the scientific community that AIDS *is* curable and that it is only a matter of time until those cures are found. Drug research continues. Currently, intravenous gamma globulin and AZT are proving effective in preventing infections in children and prolonging their lives. Care must be structured to ensure that those children who will benefit from chemotherapeutic and other advances in AIDS treatment will have the capacity to lead normal lives and not be scarred by early neglect of well-child practices.

Height and weight should be assessed and plotted regularly, and developmental milestones should be traced and recorded. Neurologic assessments are important as a basis for interpreting developmental progress. Significant delays in growth and development should be reported to the physician.

Growth can sometimes be enhanced through nutritional supplements. Children may be placed on enteral feedings or hyperalimentation, especially if chronic diarrhea or frequent vomiting is present. Monitoring of these therapies will include assurance that enteral feedings are being digested (i.e., little residual feeding is left in the stomach when the next feeding is due and no increase in diarrhea is evident) and that hyperalimentation is not producing glycosuria or ketonuria (i.e., Clinitest and Acetest are negative).

Older children and adolescents may be encouraged to supplement their diets with nutritious foods such as fruit, vegetables, and milk shakes. They should be cautioned to eat only peeled or cooked fruit and vegetables to avoid infectious organisms and to make sure their milk products are pasteurized (Dhundale & Hubbard, 1986).

Development will be affected by frequent infections and the child's lack of energy to achieve new tasks. Hospitalizations that involve separation from parents and siblings also may have detrimental effects. The nurse who is aware of these hazards can discuss with the family the child's current tasks and plan with them ways to help the child master them despite illness. In the severely ill child, developmental delays may have to be accepted, but continuing to work with the child at her or his own pace will usually enhance the quality of life.

Supporting Family Coping. There is no single scenario that describes families experiencing the diagnosis of HIV in a child family member. Understanding the impact of the diagnosis of HIV infection in a child requires consideration of factors that contributed to the contraction of virus, the developmental characteristics of family members, and the psychosocial state of family members and the family unit. The family whose child contracts HIV from a transfusion experiences the same fear, anxiety, social exclusion, grief, and pain as those for whom there are other contributing factors. That most HIV infections in children occur at the ends of the pediatric age range (i.e., infancy and adolescence) clearly demonstrates the implicitness of developmental issues. Given the admonition that nurses and all health care providers must avoid using a stereotypic approach to care and support for families that include an HIV-infected child, the exemplar that will be used in this discussion is that of the family of the HIV-positive infant.

When HIV has been contracted in utero, the presence of maternal HIV infection is implied. In addition, it is possible that other family members are also seropositive. HIV in women is most prevalent among intravenous drug abusers, prostitutes, and those whose partners are bisexual. There is strong evidence of a greater role for heterosexual spread of the virus in the adolescent age group, with a higher female to male ratio of HIV-positive persons than in the adult population. A correspondingly significant number of seropositive infants are born to HIV-positive adolescent women. Thus, the family environment is likely to have multiple stressors and be one in which much intervention is indicated. The nurse who recognizes the needs associated with the stress and additional disruption of individual and family functioning will involve social service agencies early and collaborate with them in providing support for the family as a whole.

Families must deal with the guilt associated with infection transmission to the child, the anxieties related to access to and cost of ongoing medical care, the uncertainties of living with a chronic and life-threatening illness (Brown & Powell-Cope, 1991; Cohen, 1988), and their anticipatory grief owing to a probable terminal prognosis. Compounding the crisis is the fact that they may lose essential support from friends and family because of the fear of "catching" the disease. In an environment of AIDS phobia, the nurse can be instrumental in separating the facts of transmission from the public panic about AIDS. Referral to support groups in the community can provide a valuable resource for family members. Hospitals, physicians' offices, public health departments, the American Red Cross, and the CDC are some sources of information.

The most important goal of the nurse supporting the families of an HIV-positive child is establishing practice based on the facts versus the emotional fears about transmission while refraining from judging the personal values and practices that led to exposure. This is essential in providing care for the family in crisis whose needs may not be acknowledged or addressed if that practice remains at the level of public hysteria.

Facilitating Home Health Maintenance. Teaching the family to manage the care of the child or adolescent with AIDS includes information about transmission of the virus, normalization of the child's lifestyle, protection of the child from infection, and protection of the adolescent's sexual partners or fellow drug-users (Thurber & Berry, 1990). Care of the child in relation to infectious processes was discussed under the section dealing with the first nursing diagnosis.

Transmission of the Virus. Consistent reinforcement of the fact that there are *no* reported cases of transmission of the virus by *casual* contact between family members will provide comfort and support to families (Berry, 1988). The one reported case of a mother contracting HIV from her child involved extensive, unprotected exposure to the child's blood (CDC,

1986). Studies such as the one conducted by Rubinstein (1986) involved not-so-casual contact. In many homes, children shared beds, toothbrushes, toys, and food and lived under crowded conditions without transmission of HIV. Although these practices are not recommended, the study gives credence to the safety of family members. In the words of the US Surgeon General, "We would know by now if AIDS were passed by casual, non-sexual contact" (Koop, 1987).

It is recommended that precautions be taken to protect family members. The nurse can counsel the family to avoid the mixing of the ill child's body secretions and excretions with their own. That means having separate linens, a separate toothbrush, a separate razor for the adolescent, and not sharing eating utensils without washing them. Linens and clothing can be washed with detergent (and for extra protection with 1 cup of bleach or Lysol per load) and dried in the dryer. Dishes are considered properly disinfected if washed with detergent in hot water or in a dishwasher.

More stringent precautions are indicated for blood and body excretions. Gloves should be worn to change dressings. Spills of blood or excretions can be disinfected with a 1:10 bleach solution (Dhundale & Hubbard, 1986; Schietinger, 1986). Trash can be kept in closed plastic containers for normal trash pickup (Berry, 1988). Feces, urine, and other body fluids or secretions can be flushed down the toilet. The nurse can help the family obtain a safe container for needles or sharps. This container should be taken to the hospital for proper disposal or picked up by the needle vendor.

Normalizing the Child's Lifestyle. Normalization necessarily begins with understanding of the disease process and of child behavior. As expressed by Schietinger (1986), "Having a life-threatening illness yet feeling healthy can be confusing" (p 1021). It can also be confusing for the family to see the child active and playing one day and hospitalized with an overwhelming infection a few days later. The fact that the child will look and act quite well between infections can lead to denial of the illness and doubt about the diagnosis. The nurse can be instrumental in helping the family understand the disease process. The family must also come to understand that "children with AIDS can be touched, hugged, and loved" (Berry, 1988, p 344).

Immunizations can be given on a normal schedule. Measles, mumps, and rubella vaccine is given in most cases; *H. influenzae* B vaccine should be administered as well as influenza vaccine. Inactivated polio immunization is given instead of live attenuated oral polio vaccine. All healthy family members should receive the inactivated vaccine if they need to be immunized so that HIV-infected family members do not contract polio from the shed virus.

The issue of school attendance for children with HIV has received national press coverage. This media attention has generated fear and anxiety among families whose children attend classes where the HIV-positive child is also in school. Mills and associates (1986) report that "AIDS poses the most profound issues of constitutional law and public health since the Supreme Court approved compulsory immunization in 1905" (p 931). Guidelines regarding school placement and attendance were released by the CDC (1985) and the American Academy of Pediatrics (1986). In 1986, the Baltimore public school system adopted a plan that incorporates these guidelines and is a model for integration of public policy for meeting the child's social and educational needs (Table 37–24). These guidelines consider the risks and benefits to both the infected child and to students and education professionals. Authorities in both the United States and Great Britain support the position that the need for public education for the child with HIV far outweighs the risk of acquiring or transmitting infection (CDC, 1985; Lilleyman, 1986).

School and community health nurses can be instrumental in helping the public sort the facts about transmission of HIV from the fears (Hughes & Bailey, 1987). As stated by the CDC, "It should be emphasized that any theoretical transmission would most likely involve exposure of open skin lesions or mucous membranes to blood and possible other body fluids of an infected person" (CDC, 1985, p 519). Education professionals (including nursery and day care facility personnel) should be taught about use of universal precautions in situations where exposure to bodily secretions may occur. The reader is referred to Chapter 19 for further discussion of the impact of a chronic condition on the child and family.

In addition to protection measures discussed previously, the child at home may be in danger of infection from household pets. Avoid contact between the ill child and young animals that may bite or scratch. Because children often have responsibility for pet care, certain precautions, as outlined by Dhundale and Hubbard (1986), should be discussed with the family.

TABLE 37-24
National Guidelines Regarding School Placement for HIV-Infected Children

- In general, infected school-age children should be allowed to attend school in an unrestricted setting. The benefits of school attendance outweigh the remote possibility of transmission occurring in school
- Some children, such as preschoolers and children with neurologic impairments, open skin lesions, or behavior problems such as biting, may need a more restricted setting
- In determining an individual educational placement, a team approach should be employed, using representatives of health and education departments as well as family members and/or the child's pediatrician
- Staff knowledge about a child's HIV status should be based on a "need to know." A child's right to privacy should be respected
- Universal hygiene precautions should be adopted by schools
- Mandatory or universal screening is not warranted
- Education about HIV/AIDS should be encouraged for parents, students, and educational staff

From Santelli, J. S., Birn, A., & Linde, J. (1992). School placement for human immunodeficiency virus–infected children: The Baltimore city experience. Reproduced by permission of *Pediatrics, 89*(5), 843–848. Copyright 1992.

If the family has a cat, neither the HIV-infected child nor any HIV-infected adult should clean the litter box. Family members should wear gloves and mask should also be worn when cleaning the bird cage to protect against psittacosis. Because of the danger of mycobacterial infection, the child should *never* clean the fish tank.

Protecting the Adolescent's Friends from AIDS. Because AIDS in adolescence is most likely to be acquired by sexual or intravenous drug practices, the adolescent must take responsibility for protecting his or her friends from the disease. The nurse's rapport with the adolescent plays a large part in whether there is compliance with the teaching.

As reported by Bennett (1986), transmission of AIDS appears to be dose-related—that is, semen is more likely to transmit HIV than is simple contact with vaginal or rectal mucosa. Rectal intercourse is particularly contraindicated because even small breaks in the mucosa provide a direct route to the blood stream. Heterosexual transmission has been reported, however, with only vaginal intercourse. The key to safe sexual practice is to avoid the mixing of body secretions. This means using a condom and diaphragm for intercourse in addition to a water-soluble lubricant with 5 per cent nonoxynol 9 (Dhundale & Hubbard, 1986). In addition, great care should be taken not to damage rectal or vaginal mucosa. The need to inform the sexual partner should also be discussed with the adolescent.

Drug users should avoid sharing needles or syringes with friends. Further, they should be taught aseptic technique so that if they are unable to stop drug use, they can at least do it with less risk of infection.

Evaluation

No other persons, family, or health care workers will contract the virus.

The child will:

- Not experience infection.
- Experience normal growth and attain normal developmental milestones for as long as possible.
- Not experience injury related to allergic reaction to gamma globulin.

The family will cope effectively, without excessive guilt, and will find sources of social support.

The family will have sufficient knowledge to care for their child at home.

KEY CONCEPTS

Concepts Related to Basic Information

- The primary organs of the immune system are the thymus and the bone marrow; the secondary organs and tissues are the spleen, lymph nodes, gut-associated lymphoid tissues, bronchus-associated lymphoid tissues, and skin-associated lymphoid tissues.
- The factors that impact on immune system function include genetic, age related, nutritional, metabolic, environmental, anatomic, microbial, physiologic, and stress related.
- Connective tissue is found everywhere within the body; inflammatory diseases of the connective tissue usually involve many tissues and organs, resulting in many systemic symptoms.
- Alterations in immune function often result in disorders that have life-long implications.

Concepts Related to Nursing Assessment

- Patients with immune disorders require assessment of many body systems.
- Many immune disorders predispose the patient to infection; children require careful assessment for infection as well as their immune problem.

Concepts Related to Nursing Intervention

- One of the nurse's primary responsibilities will be teaching parents appropriate care of the child with an immune disorder.
- Many immune disorders are poorly understood by lay persons; appropriate education by the nurse is indicated.

REFERENCES

American Academy of Pediatrics, Committee on School Health and Committee on Infectious Diseases. (1986). School attendance of children and adolescents with human T-lymphocyte virus III/lymphadenopathy-induced virus infection. *Pediatrics, 77,* 430–432.

American Heart Association. (1982). Data from Committee on Rheumatic Fever and Bacterial Endocarditis. Dallas: Author.

Ammann, A. J. (1987). Pediatric acquired immunodeficiency syndrome. In R. D. Feigin & J. D. Cherry (Eds.), *Textbook of pediatric infectious diseases* (2nd ed., pp 1044–1049). Philadelphia: WB Saunders.

Anderson, D. C. (1987). Infectious complications resulting from phagocytic cell dysfunction. In R. D. Feigin & J. D. Cherry (Eds.), *Textbook of pediatric infectious diseases* (2nd ed., pp 41–78). Philadelphia: WB Saunders.

Ansell, B. M. (1991). Still's disease. *British Journal of Clinical Practice, 45*(3), 212–215.

Arpadi, S., & Caspe, W. B. (1991). HIV testing. *Journal of Pediatrics, 119*(1), Part 2 (Suppl.), S8–S13.

Baum, R. M. (1992). Progress fitful on understanding AIDS, developing therapies. *Chemical and Engineering News, 70*(34), 26.

Behrman, R. E. (Ed.) (1992). *Nelson textbook of pediatrics* (14th ed.). Philadelphia: WB Saunders.

Bellanti, J. A. (1985). *Immunology: Basic processes* (2nd ed.). Philadelphia: WB Saunders.

Bennett, J. A. (1986). What we know about AIDS. *American Journal of Nursing, 86*(9):1016–1021.

Berry, R. K. (1988, July/August). Home care of the child with AIDS. *Pediatric Nursing, 14*(4), 341–344.

Bierman, C. W., Pearlman, D. S., & Berman, B. A. (1988). Injection therapy for allergic diseases. In C. W. Bierman & D. S. Pearlman (Eds.), *Allergic diseases from infancy to adulthood* (2nd ed., pp 279–293). Philadelphia: WB Saunders.

Blattner, W. A. (1987). Human retroviruses. In R. D. Feigin & J. D. Cherry (Eds.), *Textbook of pediatric infectious diseases* (2nd ed., pp 1795–1810). Philadelphia: WB Saunders.

Borkowsky, W., Rigaud, M., Krasinski, K., Moore, T., Lawrence, R., & Pollack, H. (1992). Cell-mediated and humoral immune responses in children infected with human immunodeficiency virus during the first four years of life. *Journal of Pediatrics, 120*(3), 371–375.

Brewer, E. J. (1986). Collagen vascular disease. In S. S. Gellis & B. M. Kagan (Eds.), *Current pediatric therapy 12* (pp 353–357). Philadelphia: WB Saunders.

Brown, M. A., & Powell-Cope, G. M. (1991). AIDS family caregiving: Transitions through uncertainty. *Nursing Research, 40*(6), 338–345.

Buckley, R. H. (1988). IgE antibody in health and disease. In C. W. Bierman & D. S. Pearlman (Eds.), *Allergic diseases from infancy to adulthood* (2nd ed., pp 75–94). Philadelphia: WB Saunders.

Buscinco, L., & Cantani, A. (1984). Prevention of atopy—current concepts and personal experience. *Clinical Reviews in Allergy, 2,* 107–123.

Butler, K. M., & Pizzo, P. A. (1992). HIV infection in children. In V. T. DeVita, S. Hellman, & S. A. Rosenberg (Eds.), *AIDS: Etiology, diagnosis, treatment, and prevention.* Philadelphia: JB Lippincott.

Centers for Disease Control (1986, February). Apparent transmission of human T-lymphotropic virus type III/lymphadenopathy-associated virus from a child to a mother providing health care. *Morbidity and Mortality Weekly Report, 35*(5), 76–77.

Centers for Disease Control (1985). Guidelines for education and foster care of children infected with human T-lymphotropic virus type III/lymphadenopathy-associated virus. *Morbidity and Mortality Weekly Report, 34,* 517–520.

Centers for Disease Control (1991). Guidelines for prophylaxis against *Pneumocystis carinii* pneumonia for children infected with human immunodeficiency virus infection/exposure. *Morbidity and Mortality Weekly Report, 40,* RR–2.

Centers for Disease Control (1987). Revision of the CDC surveillance case definition for acquired immunodeficiency syndrome. *Morbidity and Mortality Weekly Report, 36,* 225–230; 235–236.

Centers for Disease Control (1987). Recommendations for prevention of HIV transmission in health-care settings. *Morbidity & Mortality Weekly Report, 36* (Suppl. 2S), 3S–12S.

Cohen, M. (1988). Living under conditions of sustained uncertainty [Unpublished dissertations]. San Francisco: University of California, San Francisco.

Coombs, R. R. A., & Gell, P. G. H. (1975). Classification of allergic reactions responsible for clinical hypersensitivity and disease. In P. G. H. Gell, et al (Eds.), *Clinical aspects of immunology* (3rd ed). London: Blackwell.

Coulis, P. A., & DiSiena, J. J. (1987). AIDS immunodiagnosis: Questions and answers about screening tests. *AIDS Patient Care, 1*(1), 25–27.

Dhundale, K., & Hubbard, P. M. (1986). Home care for the AIDS patient: Safety first. *Nursing 86, 1*(9), 34–36.

Dorian, B., & Garfinkel, P. E. (1987). Stress, immunity and illness—A review. *Psychological Medicine, 17,* 393–407.

Dowe, D. A., Heitzman, E. R., & Larkin, J. J. (1992). Human immunodeficiency virus infection in children. *Clinical Imaging, 16*(3), 145–151.

Eberhard, A., Shore, A., Silverman, E., & Laxer, R. (1991). Bowel perforation and interstitial cystitis in childhood systemic lupus erythematosus. *Journal of Rheumatology, 18*(5), 746–747.

Edmundson, K. S. (1988, February). Acquired immune deficiency syndrome in the neonate. *Neonatal Network,* 7–12.

Evans, H. E. (1992). Human immunodeficiency virus (HIV) infection. Infectious diseases: Viral infections and those presumed to be caused by viruses. In R. E. Behrman (Ed.), *Nelson textbook of pediatrics* (14th ed., pp 835–842). Philadelphia: WB Saunders.

Feigin, R. D., & Garg, R. (1987). Interaction of infection and nutrition. In R. D. Feigin & J. D. Cherry (Eds.), *Textbook of pediatric infectious diseases* (2nd ed., pp 17–27). Philadelphia: WB Saunders.

Fineman, S. M. (1987). Urticaria and angioedema. *Immunology and Allergy Clinics of North America, 7*(2), 265–276.

Fischer, G. W. (1988, June). Therapeutic uses of intravenous gammaglobulin for pediatric infections. *Pediatric Clinics of North America, 35*(3), 517–533.

Fulginiti, V. A. (1992). Immunologic responses to infection. In R. D. Feigin & J. D. Cherry (Eds.), *Textbook of pediatric infectious diseases* (3rd ed., pp 24–30). Philadelphia: WB Saunders.

Fuller, B. F. (1985, April). Organ graft rejection: The biological process. *AORN Journal, 41*(4), 738–745.

Fuller, B. F. (1983). Using research in practice: Some beneficial effects of stress. *Western Journal of Nursing Research, 5*(1), 99–104.

Grant, J. A., & Kennedy-Caldwell, C. (1988). *Nutritional support in nursing.* Philadelphia: Grune & Stratton.

Griffiths, S. P. (1986). Acute rheumatic fever. In S. S. Gellis & B. M. Kagan (Eds.), *Current pediatric therapy 12* (pp 167–169). Philadelphia: WB Saunders.

Gupta, A., et al. (1986). Restoration of suppressor T-cell functions in children with AIDS following intravenous gamma globulin treatment. *American Journal of Diseases of Children, 140*(2), 143–146.

Guyton, A. C. (1991). *Textbook of medical physiology* (8th ed.). Philadelphia: WB Saunders.

Hein, K. (1989). Commentary on adolescent acquired immunodeficiency syndrome: The next wave of the human immunodeficiency virus epidemic. *Journal of Pediatrics, 114,* 144.

Hicks, R. V., & Melish, M. E. (1986, October). Kawasaki syndrome. *Pediatric Clinics of North America, 33*(5), 1151–1175.

Hill, D., et al. (1984). A study of 100 infants and young children with cow's milk allergy. *Clinical Reviews in Allergy, 2,* 125–142.

Hughes, R. B., & Bailey, F. K. (1987, May/June). AIDS from a school health perspective. *Pediatric Nursing, 13*(3), 155–156.

Iazzeti, L. (1986). Nursing management of the pediatric AIDS patient. *Issues in Comprehensive Pediatric Nursing, 9*(2), 119–129.

Jacobs, A. H., & Goldsobel, A. B. (1988). Atopic dermatitis. In C. W. Bierman & D. S. Pearlman (Eds.), *Allergic diseases from infancy to adulthood* (2nd ed., pp 385–404). Philadelphia: WB Saunders.

Jalonen, T. (1991). Identical intestinal permeability changes in children with different clinical manifestations of cow's milk allergy. *Journal of Allergy and Clinical Immunology, 88*(5), 737–742.

Johnstone, D. E. (1988). Prevention of allergic diseases. In C. W. Bierman & D. S. Pearlman (Eds.), *Allergic diseases from infancy to adulthood* (2nd ed., pp 294–299). Philadelphia: WB Saunders.

Kaliner, M., & Slater, J. (1986). Allergic rhinitis. In S. S. Gellis & B. M. Kagan (Eds.), *Current pediatric therapy 12* (pp 628–630). Philadelphia: WB Saunders.

Kaplan, E. L. (1992). Rheumatic fever. In R. E. Behrman (Ed.), *Nelson textbook of pediatrics* (14th ed., pp 640–645). Philadelphia: WB Saunders.

Kelley, W., et al. (1981). *Textbook of rheumatology.* Philadelphia: WB Saunders.

Kirkis, E. J., & Grier, M. (1988). *Nurse's guide to infection control practice.* Philadelphia: WB Saunders.

Koop, C. E. (1987, Fall). Surgeon general report. *Professional Nursing Quarterly, 2*(3).

Korenblat, P., & Wedner, H. (1984). *Allergy theory and practice.* Orlando, FL: Grune & Stratton.

Krause, M. V., & Mahan, L. K. (1984). *Food, nutrition and diet therapy* (7th ed.). Philadelphia: WB Saunders.

Kruger, S., & Rawlings, P. (1984, Fall). Pediatric dismissal protocol to aid the transition from hospital to home care. *Image, 16*(4), 120–125.

Lawton, A. R., & Cooper, M. D. (1989). Ontogeny of immunity. In E. R. Stiehm (Ed.), *Immunologic disorders in infants and children* (3rd ed.). Philadelphia: WB Saunders.

Lilleyman, J. S. (1986). Haemophilia, blood transfusion, and the AIDS virus. *Archives of Disease in Childhood, 61,* 105–107.

Lockey, R. F., & Bukantz, S. C. (1987a). *Fundamentals of immunology and allergy.* Philadelphia: WB Saunders.

Lockey, R. F., & Bukantz, S. C. (1987b). *Principles of immunology and allergy.* Philadelphia: WB Saunders.

Marks, M. (1977). *Stigmata of respiratory tract allergies.* Kalamazoo, MI: Upjohn.

May, C., & Block, S. (1978). A modern clinical approach to food hypersensitivity. *Allergy, 33,* 166–188.

McCurdy, D. K., Lehman, T. J., Bernstein, B., Hanson, V., King, K. K., et al. (1992). Lupus nephritis: Prognostic factors in children. *Pediatrics, 89*(2), 240–246.

McEnhill, M., & Vitale, K. (1989). Kawasaki disease: New challenges in care. *MCN: American Journal of Maternal Child Nursing, 14*(6), 406–410.

McLean, D. C. (1987). Stinging insect allergy. *Immunology and Allergy Clinics of North America, 7*(2), 277–283.

Melish, J. E. (1981). Kawasaki syndrome: A new infectious disease? *Journal of Infectious Diseases, 143*(3), 317–324.

Melish, M. E. (1987, April). Kawasaki syndrome: A 1986 perspective. *Rheumatic Disease Clinics of North America, 13*(1), 7–17.

Menez-Bautista, R., et al. (1986). Monozygotic twins discordant for the acquired immunodeficiency syndrome. *American Journal of Diseases of Children, 140*(7), 678–679.

Miles, S. A., Balden, E., Magpantay, L., Wei, L., Leiblein, A., Hofheinz, D., Toedter, G., Stiehm, E. R., Bryson, Y., & the Southern California Pediatric AIDS Consortium. (1993). Rapid serologic testing with immune-complex–dissociated HIV p24 antigen for early detection of HIV infection in neonates. *New England Journal of Medicine, 328*(5), 297–302.

Miller, J. J. (1982, March). The social function of young adults who had arthritis in childhood. *Journal of Pediatrics, 100*(3), 378–382.

Miller, M. E. (1988). The immune system. In C. W. Bierman & D. S. Pearlman (Eds.), *Allergic diseases from infancy to adulthood* (2nd ed., pp 1–19). Philadelphia: WB Saunders.

Miller, M. L., et al. (1986, October). The immunologic basis of lupus. *Pediatric Clinics of North America, 33*(5), 1191–1219.

Mills, M., et al. (1986). The acquired immunodeficiency syndrome: Infection control and public law. *New England Journal of Medicine, 314*(14), 931–936.

Newburger, J. W., et al. (1986). The treatment of Kawasaki syndrome with intravenous gamma globulin. *New England Journal of Medicine, 315*(6), 341–347.

Nicol, N. H. (1987). Atopic dermatitis: The (wet) wrap-up. *American Journal of Nursing, 87*(12), 1560–1565.

Niven, P., Skuza, C., Chadwick, E., et al. (1990). Age-related changes of lymphocyte phenotypes in healthy children. *Pediatric Research, 27,* 155.

Olness, K., & Gardner, G. G. (1988). *Hypnosis and hypnotherapy with children.* Philadelphia: Grune & Stratton.

Page-Goertz, S. S. (1989). Even children have arthritis. *Pediatric Nursing, 15*(1), 11–16, 30.

Paller, A. S. (1987a, August). Allergy and atopic dermatitis. *Immunology and Allergy Clinics of North America, 7*(2), 255–264.

Paller, A. S. (1987b, September). Allergy in atopic dermatitis. *Primary Care 14*(3), 491–501.

Parker, F. (1988). Contact dermatitis. In C. W. Bierman & D. S. Pearlman (Eds.), *Allergic diseases from infancy to adulthood* (2nd ed., pp 405–414). Philadelphia: WB Saunders.

Petty, R. E. (1987). Current knowledge of the etiology and pathogenesis of chronic uveitis accompanying juvenile rheumatoid arthritis. *Rheumatic Disease Clinics of North America, 13*(1), 19–36.

Pohlgeers, A. P., Eid, N. S., Schikler, K. N., & Shearer, L. T. (1990). Systemic lupus erythematosus: Pulmonary presentation in childhood. *Southern Medical Journal, 83*(6), 712–714.

Regelmann, W. E., et al. (1987). Immunology of the newborn. In R. D. Feigin & J. D. Cherry (Eds.), *Textbook of pediatric infectious diseases* (2nd ed., pp 921–939). Philadelphia: WB Saunders.

Rogers, M. F., et al. (1987). Acquired immunodeficiency syndrome in children: Report of the Centers for Disease Control National Surveillance, 1982 to 1985. *Pediatrics, 79*(6), 1008–1014.

Rubinstein, A. (1986). Pediatric AIDS. *Current Problems in Pediatrics, 16*(7), 367–409.

Rubinstein, A., & Bernstein, L. (1986). The epidemiology of pediatric acquired immunodeficiency syndrome. *Clinical Immunology and Immunopathology, 40,* 115–121.

Ruiz-Maldonado, R. (1985, October). Acute disseminated epidermal necrosis—Types 1, 2, and 3: Study of sixty cases. *Journal of the American Academy of Dermatology, 13*(4), 523–535.

Sampson, H., & Albergo, R. (1984). Comparison of results of skin tests, RAST, and double-blind, placebo-controlled food challenges in children with atopic dermatitis. *Journal of Allergy and Clinical Immunology, 74,* 26–33.

Santelli, J. S., Birn, A., & Linde, J. (1992). School placement for human immunodeficiency virus–infected children: The Baltimore city experience. *Pediatrics, 89*(5), 843–848.

Schaller, J. G. (1992). Juvenile rheumatoid arthritis. In R. E. Behrman (Ed.), *Nelson textbook of pediatrics* (14th ed., pp 612–621). Philadelphia: WB Saunders.

Schietinger, H. (1986). A home care plan for AIDS. *American Journal of Nursing, 86*(9), 1021–1028.

Scull, S. A., et al. (1986, October). Physical and occupational therapy for children with rheumatic diseases. *Pediatric Clinics of North America, 33*(5), 1053–1077.

Shapiro, G. G. (1988). Diagnostic methods for assessing the patient with possible allergic disease. In C. W. Bierman & D. S. Pearlman (Eds.), *Allergic diseases from infancy to adulthood* (2nd ed. pp 224–238). Philadelphia: WB Saunders.

Shyur, S., & Hill, H. R. (1991). Immunodeficiency in the 1990's. *Pediatric Infectious Disease Journal, 10*(8), 595–611.

Sly, M. (1985). *Pediatric allergy.* New York: Medical Examination.

Stastny, P. (1987, April). HLA and the role of T cells in the predisposition to disease. *Rheumatic Disease Clinics of North America, 12*(1), 1–6.

Strom, B. L., Carson, J. L., Halpern, A. C., Schinner, R., Snyder, E. S., et al. (1991). A population-based study of Stevens-Johnson syndrome: Incidence and antecedent drug exposures. *Archives of Dermatology, 127*(6), 831–838.

Tan, E. M., et al. (1982). The 1982 revised criteria for the classification of systemic lupus erythematosus. *Arthritis and Rheumatism, 25*(11), 1271–1274.

Thurber, F., & Berry, B. (1990). Children with AIDS: Issues and future directions. *Journal of Pediatric Nursing, 5*(3), 168–178.

US Public Health Service. (1988). *Understanding AIDS.* (DHHS Publication No. [CDC] HHS–88–8404). Rockville, MD: Department of Health and Human Services.

Walker, J. (1980). Childhood gastrointestinal allergy: Forbidden fruits. *Nursing Mirror, 151,* 32–36.

Wasserman, S. I. (1988). Chemical mediators of inflammation. In C. W. Bierman & D. S. Pearlman (Eds.), *Allergic diseases from infancy to adulthood* (2nd ed., pp 65–74). Philadelphia: WB Saunders.

Westley, E. D., & Wechsler, H. L. (1984, June). Toxic epidermal necrolysis. *Archives of Dermatology, 120,* 721–726.

White, J., Owsley, V. (1983, November/December). Helping families cope with milk, wheat and soy allergies. *MCN: American Journal of Maternal Child Nursing, 8*(6), 423–428.

Witt, J. D., Swann, M., & Ansell, B. M. (1991). Total hip replacement for juvenile chronic arthritis. *Journal of Bone and Joint Surgery, 73*(6), 770–773.

Young, M. C., & Geha, R. S. (1985). Ontogeny and control of human IgE synthesis. *Clinical Immunology and Allergy, 5*(2), 339–349.

Yunginger, J. W. (1988). Insect allergy (adults and children). In C. W. Bierman & D. S. Pearlman (Eds.), *Allergic diseases from infancy to adulthood* (2nd ed., pp 678–683). Philadelphia: WB Saunders.

Zerin, J. M., Rockwell, D. T., Garn, S. M., Schlesinger, A. E., & Sullivan, D. B. (1991). Carpo-metacarpal growth disturbance and the assessment of carpal narrowing in children with juvenile rheumatoid arthritis. *Investigative Radiology, 26*(8), 727–733.

BIBLIOGRAPHY

American Academy of Pediatrics Task Force on Pediatric AIDS. (1991). Education of children with human immunodeficiency virus infection. *Pediatrics, 88*(3), 645–648.

American Academy of Pediatrics Task Force on Pediatric AIDS. (1992). Perinatal human immunodeficiency virus (HIV) testing. *Pediatrics, 89*(4), 791–794.

Araujo, O. E., & Flowers, F. P. (1984). Stevens-Johnson syndrome. *Journal of Emergency Medicine, 2,* 129–135.

Bierman, C. W., & Pearlman, D. S. (1980). *Allergic diseases of infancy, childhood, and adolescence*. Philadelphia: WB Saunders.

Brewer, E. J., et al. (1982). *Juvenile rheumatoid arthritis* (2nd ed., p 120). Philadelphia: WB Saunders.

Brouwers, P., Belman, A., & Epstein, L. (1990). Central nervous system involvement: Manifestations and evaluation. *Pediatric AIDS, 1,* 318.

Centers for Disease Control. (1988, July 18). *AIDS weekly surveillance report— United States*. Atlanta: Author.

Centers for Disease Control. (1986). Recommendations for preventing transmission of infection with human T-lymphotropic virus type III/lymphadenopathy–associated virus during invasive procedures. *Morbidity and Mortality Weekly Report, 35*(4), 221–223.

Cohen, D. G. (1990). Similarities between the nursing care needs of children with cancer and the child with immunodeficiency virus infection. *Journal of Pediatric Oncology Nursing, 7*(4), 149–153.

DeVita, V. T., Hellman, S., & Rosenberg, S. A. (1992). *AIDS: Etiology, diagnosis, treatment, and prevention*. Philadelphia: JB Lippincott.

European Collaborative Study: Risk factors for mother to child transmission of HIV-1. (1992). *Lancet, 339,* 1007–1012.

Foster, W. P., Somerville, M. A., & Duckett, M. (1990). HIV/AIDS and school boards: A policy approach. *Social Science Medicine, 30*(3), 267–279.

Guyton, A. C. (1987). *Human physiology and mechanism of disease* (4th ed.). Philadelphia: WB Saunders.

King, J., & Ziegler, S. (1981, Summer). The effects of hospitalization on children's behavior: A review of the literature. *Child Health Care, 10,* 20–28.

King, K., & Hanson, V. (1986). Psychological aspects of juvenile rheumatoid arthritis. *Pediatric Clinics of North America, 33*(5), 1221–1237.

Kline, S. W., & Shearer, W. T. (1992). Impact of human immunodeficiency virus infection on women and infants. *Infectious Disease Clinics of North America, 6*(1), 1–17.

Koren, G. K., & MacLeod, S. M. (1984). Difficulty in achieving therapeutic serum concentration of salicylate in Kawasaki disease. *Journal of Pediatrics, 105*(6), 991–995.

Loebl, S., & Spratto, G. R. (1986). *The nurse's drug handbook* (4th ed.). New York: John Wiley & Sons.

Mann, J. M. (1992). AIDS—the second decade: A global perspective. *Journal of Infectious Diseases, 165*(2), 245–250.

Marion, R. W., et al. (1986). Human T-cell lymphotropic virus type III (HTLV-III) embryopathy: A new dysmorphic syndrome associated with intrauterine HTLV-III infection. *American Journal of Diseases of Children, 140*(7), 638–640.

Marvin, J. A., et al. (1984, May). Improved treatment of the Stevens-Johnson syndrome. *Archives of Surgery, 119,* 601–605.

Mischel, M., & Braden, C. (1987). Uncertainty: A mediator between support and adjustment. *Western Journal of Nursing Research, 91*(1), 43–57.

Pizzo, P. A., & Wilfert, C. M. (1991). *Pediatric AIDS: The challenge of HIV infection in infants, children, and adolescents*. Baltimore: Williams & Wilkins.

Rose, C. D., & Doughty, R. A. (1992). Pharmacologic management of juvenile rheumatoid arthritis. *Drugs, 43*(6), 849–863.

Steele, R. (1983). *Immunology for the practicing physician*. Norwalk, CT: Appleton-Century-Croft.

Stutman, O. (1985). Ontogeny on T cells. *Clinical Immunology and Allergy, 5*(2), 191–234.

Understanding AIDS and HIV Infection: Information for Hospitals and Health Professionals. (1988). Ontario, Canada: Queen's Printer for Ontario.

Urbano, M. T., & Von Windemuth, B. J. (1992). Preparing preschool programs to care for children with HIV infection. *Journal of Pediatric Health Care, 6*(2), 60–64.

Virant, F. S., et al. (1984, July). Multiple pulmonary complications in a patient with Stevens-Johnson syndrome. *Clinical Pediatrics, 23*(7), 412–414.

Voyles, J., & Menendez, R. (1983). Role of patient compliance in the management of asthma. *Journal of Asthma, 20,* 411–418.

Wiener, M. B., & Pepper, G. A. (1985). *Clinical pharmacology and therapeutics in nursing* (2nd ed.). New York: McGraw-Hill.

Ziegler, J. B., et al. (1985). Postnatal transmission of AIDS-associated retrovirus from mother to infant. *Lancet, 1,* 896–897.

CHAPTER • 38

Altered Skin Integrity

Noreen Heer Nicol
Marcia J. Hill

RELATED TOPICS
Birthmarks, Chapter 4
Immune response, Chapter 37
Contact dermatitis, Chapter 37
Atopic dermatitis, Chapter 37
Poison ivy, Chapter 46
Thrush, Chapter 39
Measles, chickenpox, Chapter 39
Fungal skin infections, Chapter 39
Parasitic infections, Chapter 39
Burns, Chapter 47
Allergic contact dermatitis, Chapter 37

LEARNING OBJECTIVES

- Describe the normal protective functions of the skin.
- Identify the developmental differences that affect skin function in children.
- Recognize the importance of the skin in the assessment of many other disorders.
- Identify the common types of skin lesions.
- List the common noninfectious and infectious skin disorders of children.
- Plan appropriate nursing care for a child with a skin condition and their families.

The skin is often underrated for its service to the body. "Skin" may bring to mind the softness of a baby's hand, the rosiness of a preschooler's cheek, or the emotional upset caused by a teen-ager's blemish. Less often are the skin and mucous membranes credited for their vital function as *the body's primary physical barrier* against the rather inhospitable environment. As Lookingbill and Marks (1993) observed, it is the integumentary system that keeps *us* within and the world without.

This chapter discusses the structure and function of the skin, including developmental differences for infants and children; factors that affect the skin's ability to protect the body; assessment and identification of primary skin lesions, principles of topical therapy, and the impact of integumentary disorders on children and families. Skin disorders covered in this chapter include certain dermatitis conditions, bacterial and viral skin infections, and acne.

The Structure and Function of the Skin

The skin is composed of three major layers, the epidermis, the dermis, and the subcutaneous fat (hypodermis). The epidermis is further divided into five distinct layers, each functionally related. Figure 38-1 shows a cross-section of the skin, revealing its stratified structure and the appendages that originate there. The skin serves several important functions (Table 38-1). The epidermis provides a barrier against physical injury, light, and infectious organisms. The dermal layer supplies a support structure for body tissues.

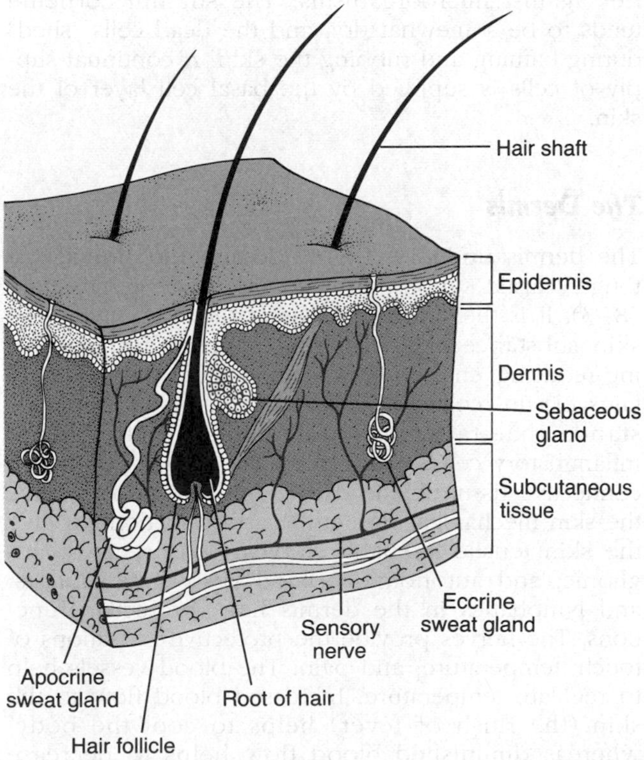

FIGURE 38-1. Structure of the skin and the subcutaneous tissue.

The skin facilitates temperature regulation, provides for touch sensation, insulates from cold and trauma, and serves as a calorie reservoir. In addition, the skin is important to one's appearance. Skin disorders in childhood and adolescence can greatly influence the development of self-concept.

The Epidermis

The epidermis is made up of five layers of highly differentiated, avascular tissue (Fig. 38-2). These layers are—from the deepest to the outermost—basal cell (stratum basale), prickle cell (stratum spinosum), granular layer (stratum granulosum), stratum lucidum (found only in palms and soles), and horny layer (stratum corneum). The epidermis can actively regenerate developing new skin cells approximately every 28 days.

TABLE 38-1
Skin Functions

Function	Responsible Structure
Barrier	Epidermis
Physical	Stratum corneum
Light	Melanocytes
Immunologic	Langerhans cells
Tough, flexible foundation	Dermis
Temperature regulation	Blood vessels
	Eccrine sweat glands
Sensation	Nerves
Grasp	Nails
Decorative	Hair
Unknown	Sebaceous glands
Insulation from cold and trauma	Subcutaneous fat
Calorie reservoir	Subcutaneous fat

From Lookingbill, D. P., & Marks, J. D., Jr. (1993). *Principles of dermatology* (2nd ed.). Philadelphia: WB Saunders.

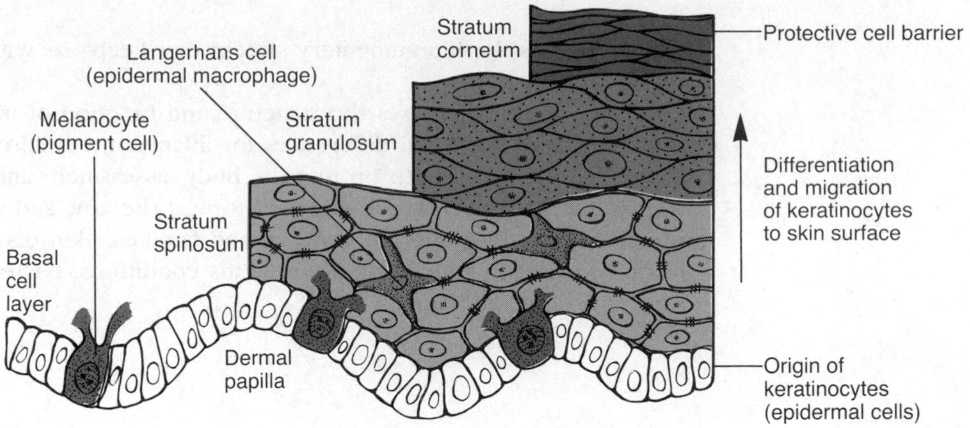

FIGURE 38-2. Structure of the epidermis.

Basal Cell Layer

The primary cell of the epidermis is the keratinocyte. Keratinocytes produce a specialized protein, keratin, that is vital to the protective barrier function of the skin. Keratinocytes originate as basal cells and go through three phases in their development: germative, differentiation, and protective. In the germative phase, the keratinocyte divides leaving one cell in the basal layer while the other progresses up through the various layers of the epidermis. During the progression through the different layers, the keratinocyte flattens, or differentiates (differentiation phase), until it reaches the horny layer as an anucleated cell of low water content. Keratin is produced by these keratinocytes, giving the skin its protective quality (protective phase). Keratinocytes make up 95 per cent of the epidermis, with the other 5 per cent consisting of dendritic melanocytes. Melanocytes are found within the basal cell layer and function to give color to skin, eyes, and hair and to afford some protection from ultraviolet rays.

Prickle Cell Layer (Stratum Spinosum)

By the time the basal cells reach the stratum spinosum, they have differentiated into keratinocytes, cells that produce the fibrous keratin that is a major component of the stratum corneum. Within the stratum spinosum are the *Langerhans* cells, skin macrophages that mount a phagocytic response to microorganisms that manage to penetrate the stratum corneum. (Langerhans cells are found in all layers of the epidermis except the stratum corneum.) The importance of these macrophages and the normal skin flora (nonpathogenic microorganisms that discourage pathogenic invasion) has been given increasing recognition in recent years and is now designated the skin-associated lymphoid tissue (SALT) (see Chapter 37 for further discussion).

Granular Layer (Stratum Granulosum)

Within this layer the differentiation of epidermal cells is completed. The cells are degraded by enzymes, lose their nuclei and cytoplasm, and are pushed upward to form the stratum corneum.

Horny Layer (Stratum Corneum)

The horny layer (stratum corneum) is the outermost layer of skin. It is composed of dead skin cells that are tightly joined to form an almost impenetrable barrier against microorganisms. The stratum corneum tends to be somewhat dry, and the dead cells "shed" during bathing and rubbing the skin. A continual supply of cells is supplied by the basal cell layer of the skin.

The Dermis

The dermis underlies the epidermis and provides a tough, elastic support structure for body tissues (Fig. 38–3). It is the principle mass of the skin, giving the skin substance and structural support and absorbing/reducing environmental stress and strain. It contains elastin, collagen, reticulum, and a ground substance that facilitates movement of fluids and inflammatory cells. Collagen makes up the majority of connective tissue in the dermis and functions to give the skin mechanical strength. Elastin functions to give the skin tensile strength. Nerves (sensory, postganglionic, and autonomic), blood vessels, fibroblasts, and lymphatics in the dermis have protective functions. The nerves provide the protective sensations of touch, temperature, and pain. The blood vessels help to regulate temperature. Increased blood flow to the skin (the flush of fever) helps to cool the body, whereas diminished blood flow helps to decrease heat loss (the pallor associated with being cold). The

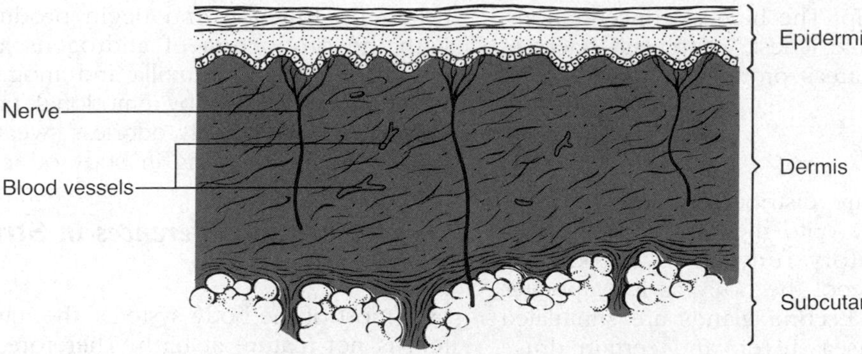

FIGURE 38 - 3. Structure of the dermis. (From Lookingbill, D. P., & Marks, J. D., Jr. [1993]. *Principles of dermatology* [2nd ed.]. Philadelphia: WB Saunders, p 7.)

blood vessels supply both the dermis tissue and the nonvascular epidermis with nutrients and oxygen. Fibroblasts are important to the repair process and, to some extent, to the synthesis of collagen and elastin fibers. The lymphatics function to remove foreign bodies, combat infections, and mediate certain reactions in the skin.

Subcutaneous Fat Layer (Hypodermis)

The layer of fat (adipose tissue/panniculus adiposus) below the dermis has achieved so much infamy for its "pinch-an-inch" characteristics that its protective functions often go unheralded. This layer helps to insulate the body from cold (as witnessed by the decreased thermoregulatory ability of the premature infant and the neonate who have not yet formed a functional layer and of the elderly person who has lost much of this layer). In addition, the subcutaneous fat provides a cushion that absorbs trauma, generates heat, and serves as a calorie reserve for the body.

Skin Appendages

Skin appendages include nails, hair, and eccrine, apocrine, and sebaceous glands. All of these appendages are composed of specialized epidermal cells; therefore, they are referred to as "epidermal appendages."

Nails, Hair, and Sebaceous Glands

Nails and hair are made of keratin. The pink color of the nail is due to the highly vascular dermis underneath. That is why depressing the nail (blanching) and awaiting return of color is an indication of peripheral circulation. Nails are composed of hardened keratin. The components of the nail are the nail plate, the root, the nail bed, the hyponychium, the eponychium, and the lunula.

Hair grows from a hair follicle in the dermis and receives its color from melanocytes in the bottom of the hair follicle (Fig. 38–4). The fine hair of the neonate is replaced by coarser and sometimes more darkly pigmented hair as the child grows. Genital hair growth is stimulated by hormones and does not develop until puberty. Hair grows in defined cycles: anagen (growth), catagen (atrophy), and telogen (rest).

Sebaceous glands are attached to hair follicles. In response to sex hormones, they secrete a complex lipid product, sebum, into the hair follicle, from which it progresses to the epidermal surface. Sebum functions to lubricate the skin, waterproof the hair and skin, and promote absorption of fat-soluble substances and may also function in vitamin D synthesis (Hill, 1990). Sebaceous glands are located everywhere except on the palms, soles, and dorsa of the feet and

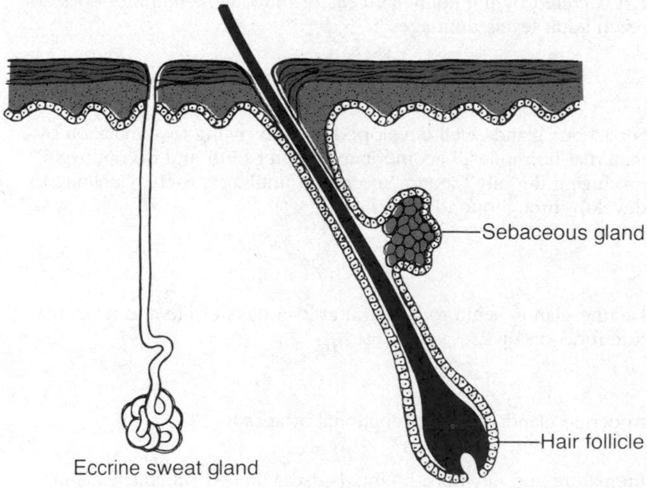

FIGURE 38 - 4. Normal hair follicle, sebaceous gland, and eccrine sweat gland. (From Lookingbill, D. P., & Marks, J. D., Jr. [1993]. *Principles of dermatology* [2nd ed.]. Philadelphia: WB Saunders, p 9.)

perhaps on the lower lip. The highest concentrations, however, are on the face, chest, scalp, and back, as evidenced by the skin areas prone to acne.

Sweat Glands

Eccrine sweat glands are distributed over the entire body and open directly onto the skin surface. They fulfill a thermoregulatory function by producing sweat, which helps to cool the body as it evaporates from the skin surface. Eccrine glands are stimulated by heat, exertion, nausea, fever, and certain drugs (e.g. alcohol, pilocarpine) (Kahn, 1988). Eccrine sweat glands are found everywhere except the lip margins, eardrums, nail beds, inner surface of the prepuce, and the glans penis (Siedel et al, 1991).

Apocrine sweat glands are found in the axillae, the periumbilical region, nipples, areolae, anogenital area, eyelids, and external ears. They appear to have no useful function and begin producing secretions with the production of androgens at puberty. The glands located in the axilla and anogenital region are stimulated primarily by emotional factors, and it is here where the initially odorless sweat is acted on by body bacteria, resulting in body odor.

Developmental Differences in Structure and Function

Like most of the body systems, the integumentary system is not mature at birth. Therefore, it is not as effective a barrier to physical elements or microorganisms at birth and in infancy as it is later in childhood (Table 38-2). These limitations in skin protection make infants and young children more prone to infection. The skin also appears smoother than that of adults because of less terminal hair and owing to the fact that it has not been subjected to long-term expo-

TABLE 38-2
Developmental Differences in Structure and Function of the Skin

Anatomy and Physiology	Significance
Thin epidermis, especially in the premature infant	Absorption through the skin is dramatically increased. Most compounds placed on the skin of premature infants can be found in the urine and saliva in a matter of minutes. No topical ointments or other skin preparations should be used without a physician's order. The thin epidermis is fragile and requires careful handling The thin epidermis blisters easily. The younger the child, the more easily the skin will blister. This characteristic makes it more difficult to assess the trauma that caused blistering
Melanocytes do not function until birth	Soon after birth, skin pigmentation changes with darkening first in the nipples, face, and genitalia. This is the reason for a light complexion in a black neonate
Skin pH more alkaline in first week of life	A more acidic skin surface discourages microorganisms. The neonate is, therefore, more susceptible to infection
IgA secreted by the epithelial cells of mucous membranes does not reach adult levels until ages 2-5	Diminished ability to produce these antibodies reduces the mucosal resistance to organisms. Objects "mouthed" by infants need to be cleaned frequently, and young children should be taught good handwashing as early as possible because their hands are often in contact with their mouths, noses, and other vulnerable surfaces
Sebaceous glands well developed at birth owing to stimulation by maternal hormones; become inactive after birth and do not begin producing the oily "sebum" secretion until ages 8-10. Continue to develop throughout adolescence	Newborn "acne" may result from androgen stimulation of sebaceous glands in utero. Evaporation of sebum helps to lower skin pH, thus increasing skin resistance to infection in later childhood. Teen-age acne is related to function of the sebaceous glands. Without lubrication by sebum, the skin is more prone to dryness and chapping, making hydration precautions important in infancy and early childhood
Eccrine glands begin to function at 2-5 days of life and reach mature function by 2-3 yrs of age	The ability to perspire freely gives the toddler and older child better thermoregulatory function than is possessed by the infant. The evaporation of eccrine sweat lowers skin pH and thus increases resistance to microorganisms
Apocrine glands become functional at ages 8-10	Because axillary sweating begins a few years before puberty, its appearance can be a sign of normal progress toward the pubertal stage
Premature and newborn infants possess limited subcutaneous fat	They are more sensitive to changes in environmental temperature because they are less well "insulated" than older infants and children. The lack of subcutaneous fat provides better conduction, however, when transcutaneous oxygen is being monitored

Based on Kahn, G. (1988). Principles of diagnosis and treatment of skin disorders. In C. W. Bierman & D. S. Pearlman (Eds.). *Allergic disorders from infancy to adulthood* (2nd ed., pp 377-384). Philadelphia: WB Saunders.

sure to environmental elements. In addition to limitations in skin protection, infants have poorly developed subcutaneous fat, predisposing them to hypothermia. The eccrine sweat glands will not begin to function until after the first month of life, which will also inhibit the infant's ability to control body temperature.

With the onset of adolescence, apocrine glands enlarge and become active. This activity leads to axillary sweating and characteristic body odor. The sebaceous glands begin to produce sebum in response to hormone activity (primarily androgens), which predisposes the individual to acne. Along with the skin glands becoming active, coarse terminal hair grows in the axillae and pubic areas of both sexes and on the faces of males.

Factors that Affect the Skin's Protective Function

Skin function is affected by genetic inheritance and hormonal factors and by cleanliness, hydration, and nutrition.

Genetic Factors

Skin cells are affected by their genetic blueprint just as other body cells are. Alterations in skin integrity that are thought to be genetically inherited include albinism (a defect in pigment production), neurofibromatosis (which results in multiple café-au-lait spots), atopic dermatitis (which predisposes the skin to persistent dryness and pruritus), and psoriasis (which manifests as scaling plaques).

Hormonal Factors

Skin is affected by both increased and decreased hormone production. The classic example of hormone-induced skin problems is acne, which may result from pubertal androgens. Increased glucocorticoids also can cause acne, along with hirsutism, atrophy, purpura, and moon facies. Decreased secretion of glucocorticoids (Addison disease) leads to hyperpigmentation of the skin. Hyperthyroidism results in a warm, moist skin, and hyposecretion of the thyroid gland causes the skin to be dry and cool. Effects of hormone secretion on the skin are further discussed in Chapter 43.

Cleanliness and Hydration

Skin that is clean and well hydrated is less prone to breaks in its integrity. Dirt and body secretions (e.g., urine and feces) not only have the potential to cause skin irritation but also may "seal" microorganisms against the skin, thus prolonging their contact and increasing the chance for penetration of the stratum corneum.

Skin must be well hydrated, however, as well as clean. Dry skin is prone to irritation and cracking. If soap is used, it should be a mild preparation such as Keri, Purpose, Neutrogena, Oilatum, or Dove. Among the harshest soaps are Ivory, Lowila, Zest, and Irish Spring (Kahn, 1988).

Baths can actually help to hydrate dry skin, if the skin pores are allowed time to absorb the water (15 to 20 minutes) and are then quickly sealed against evaporation. Skin (preferably still damp) should be sealed after the bath with an occlusive application such as petrolatum ointment or a good moisturizing cream or lotion (Nicol, 1987).

Nutritional Factors

The skin is a rapidly dividing tissue and, therefore, has a high demand for nutrients (Table 38–3). Vitamins A and C are particularly important to healthy skin. Vitamin A regulates the process of keratinization (differentiation and migration of epidermal cells toward the surface). Vitamin A deficiency leads to skin dryness and scaling. Vitamin C is necessary for normal development of connective tissue within the dermis. Vitamin C deficiency delays wound healing (scar tissue is primarily connective tissue) and leads to skin fragility and easy bleeding.

TABLE 38-3
Nutritional Factors in Skin Integrity

Deficiency	Cutaneous Manifestations
Vitamin A	Dry eyes—corneal scarring
	Generalized scaling with hyperkeratosis
Vitamin B	
Niacin (pellagra)	Dermatitis in sun-exposed areas
Biotin*	Dermatitis with desquamation
	Alopecia
Vitamin C (scurvy)	Impaired wound healing
	Perifollicular purpura
	Red, swollen, bleeding gums
Zinc*	Seborrheic dermatitis–like rash
	Alopecia
Amino acids (glucagonoma)	Glossitis
	Dermatitis with superficial epidermal necrosis
Essential fatty acids*	Scaling rash starting in flexural folds—then generalized
	Alopecia

From Lookingbill, D. P., & Marks, J. D., Jr. (1993). *Principles of dermatology* (2nd ed.). Philadelphia: WB Saunders.
*Has been associated with total parenteral nutrition.

Emotional Factors

Emotions also affect the skin. Emotions stimulate itching, flushing, and sweating, and stress can exacerbate acne, possibly through the increased glucocorticoids associated with the stress response.

Skin as a Mirror of Health

Skin is often a mirror of one's health and one's lifestyle. Skin characteristics change with circulation and oxygenation (e.g., cyanosis), with altered excretion of body wastes (e.g., jaundice), with fatigue (e.g., circles under the eyes), with nutrition (e.g., scaling), with hydration (e.g., loss of turgor, maceration), with changes in environmental temperature (e.g., flushing, pallor, goose flesh), with response to antigens (e.g., hives), with hormonal cycles (e.g., blemishes with menstruation), with emotions (e.g., blushing, sweating, itching), with caloric intake (e.g., amount of subcutaneous fat), and with the loss of collagen in aging. Since these and so many other physiologic and psychologic processes are "written" on the skin, it is little wonder that the skin is so important to diagnostic assessment.

Skin assessment is included throughout the chapters of this unit as it relates to assessment of the various body systems. In the following section, skin assessment is discussed as it relates to alteration of the integument itself.

Diagnostic Assessment of Skin Lesions

History

The nurse is often the one who first recognizes signs of skin breakdown or to whom parents and teachers bring their concerns about a child. Therefore, the nurse's assessment skills in identifying and differentiating various skin lesions and in associating them with other symptoms are important to proper management of these conditions. Recognition depends as much on a thorough history as it does on assessment of physical factors. A history should cover three areas: (1) local, systemic, or prodromal symptoms, (2) exposure to causative agents, and (3) risk factors (Table 38–4).

TABLE 38-4
Considerations in Obtaining a History of the Integumentary System

Symptomatic History
- Time of onset and changes in lesions
- Whether lesions itch or burn
- Systemic signs and symptoms
- Home treatment
- What makes condition better or worse
- Prodromal symptoms in the last 7 to 10 days

History of Exposure in the Last Month
- Environmental irritants
- Infectious organisms
- Local epidemic or pandemic disease patterns

Risk Factors
- Immunization status
- History of infectious disease
- Immunosuppressive and other drugs
- Genetic predisposition
- Family lifestyle

Symptomatic History

The nurse will want to determine (1) where the skin lesions started, (2) whether they have changed in appearance since the onset, (3) whether they "bother" the child (e.g., burn or itch), (4) whether there are systemic signs or symptoms, (5) what home remedies and over-the-counter medications have been tried, (6) what makes the condition better or worse, and (7) whether the child has had this or other skin conditions in the past. The nurse must always be alert to any cutaneous signs of child abuse, such as perianal or genital disorders that would not normally be seen in infants and children (e.g., venereal warts) or unusual lesions that do not fit neatly into some disease pattern.

Many infectious diseases of childhood have a prodromal phase of systemic symptoms that precedes the skin lesions. Of particular significance are any symptoms reported within the past 7 to 10 days. Common manifestations involve enlarged lymph nodes, respiratory complaints (e.g., sniffling, nasal stuffiness), fever, anorexia, malaise, or various neurologic complaints. Prodromal symptoms are often near resolution by the time the nurse has contact with the child, making the nurse dependent on the child's or parent's recall of the symptoms and their onset. See Chapter 39 for a further discussion of childhood infectious diseases.

Exposure History

The child and parent(s) should be questioned regarding exposure within the past month to environmental irritants or infectious organisms that might cause integumentary diseases. Inquiry should be made as to recent changes in environment, recent exposure to a crowd or large numbers of people, or recent illness of family members, playmates, or others with whom the child has regular contact. The nurse should also be familiar with any epidemic (regional outbreak) or pandemic (widespread) disease patterns in the locale, particularly within the schools.

Risk Factors

Because some of the infectious integumentary disorders are preventable with immunizations, knowledge of the child's immunization status is imperative for a thorough assessment. Ask whether the child has had any of the childhood infectious diseases involving the skin (e.g., measles, chickenpox).

Medications, including over-the-counter and home remedies, that the child is taking or has just finished should be noted. Sensitivity to antibiotics and other drugs may result in a rash. Children who are taking immunosuppressive drugs (e.g., azathioprine [Imuran], corticosteroids) are at increased risk for infection because of diminished immune response to microorganisms.

A family history is pertinent to determine genetic predisposition to skin disorders. Atopic dermatitis, for example, is more common in the child whose parents have a history of allergies or asthma. In addition, aspects of the family's lifestyle and living environment should be explored for the potential of various parasitic conditions. Questions should include whether the family has recently visited another country and whether children routinely walk barefoot outside. Chapter 39 presents further information on parasitic infections.

The ethnic and cultural background of the child can also be a factor. For example, a condition known as "traction alopecia" is commonly seen in African-American female children. This condition is a result of a cultural influence on hair styles. The practice of pulling the child's hair into tight braids for an extended length of time will result in alopecia. Other habits, such as routine cleansing habits, types of soaps, lotions, pomades, or other substances that are routinely used on the hair or skin, must be considered.

In infants, a feeding history should be elicited. Determine whether an infant is formula-fed or breast-fed and what types of foods have been introduced into the diet and when. The parent(s) should be asked about cleansing routines at diaper changes, whether rubber pants are used, what type of diapers are used (disposable versus washable), and what kind of detergent is used for washing clothes and diapers. Discuss the frequency of bathing and types of soaps, oils, or lotions are used. It is also important to find out about the amount and type of clothing that is worn, the temperature and humidity of the home environment, and whether the infant has a habit of rubbing skin surfaces on bed surfaces, furniture, rug, or crib.

In older children, in addition to these risk factors, it is important to ask about eating habits and types of food eaten. Exposure to household pets or other animals may lead to the diagnosis of a suspicious skin lesion (e.g., ringworm). Nail biting and hair twisting may lead to nail infections or loss of hair, respectively.

Physical Assessment

Examination of the integument should be done in a systematic way, beginning with the head and working down the body. Inspection and palpation are the primary assessment techniques for skin disorders. The child should be clothed in an examination gown to provide visual access to all areas of the skin. The diaper should be removed when that area of the body is examined. Be sure to respect the privacy of the child who has begun to develop modesty (some preschoolers and all school-age children). Mucous membranes, scalp, hair, and nails should be included in inspection of the integumentary system (see Chapter 13). Adequate lighting is necessary.

Lesions should be described according to characteristics, exudates, pattern of arrangement, location, and distribution. The characteristics of lesions include size, shape or configuration, color, texture, elevation or depression, and pedunculation. Figure 38–5 gives examples of common skin lesions. In describing the exudates, the nurse should note color, odor, amount, and consistency. Pattern of arrangement may be described as annular, grouped, linear, arciform, or diffuse. Location and distribution can be important clues to diagnosis. The lesions may be generalized or localized. The region of the body where lesions are found should be documented, and the pattern of distribution (dermatomal, flexor or extensor, random, relation to clothing lines or jewelry) should be noted. Whether the lesions are discrete or confluent should also be noted. The nurse will need a small, flexible ruler for measuring of skin lesions, a flashlight, and a magnifying glass for closer inspection of some lesions.

The condition of the hair and nails gives a clue about the patient's level of self-care and some sense of emotional order and social integration (particularly in children and adolescents) (Siedel et al, 1991). Hair should be examined for texture, color, distribution, and quantity. If there is a suspicion of hair loss, gently pulling on a few strands of hair to discern whether hair will come out easily will help discern whether hair loss is spontaneous or possibly from manipulation. Distribution and type of hair on the body may help the nurse to determine hormonal problems.

Nails should be inspected for color, length, configuration, symmetry, and cleanliness. The nails can exhibit numerous changes that may be due to chronic or acute states. White spots on the nail plate may be a result of trauma to a nail from nervous picking, from being injured, or from nutritional deficiencies. Eczema may produce longitudinal ridges, which may be seen in older children. Clubbing of the nails may

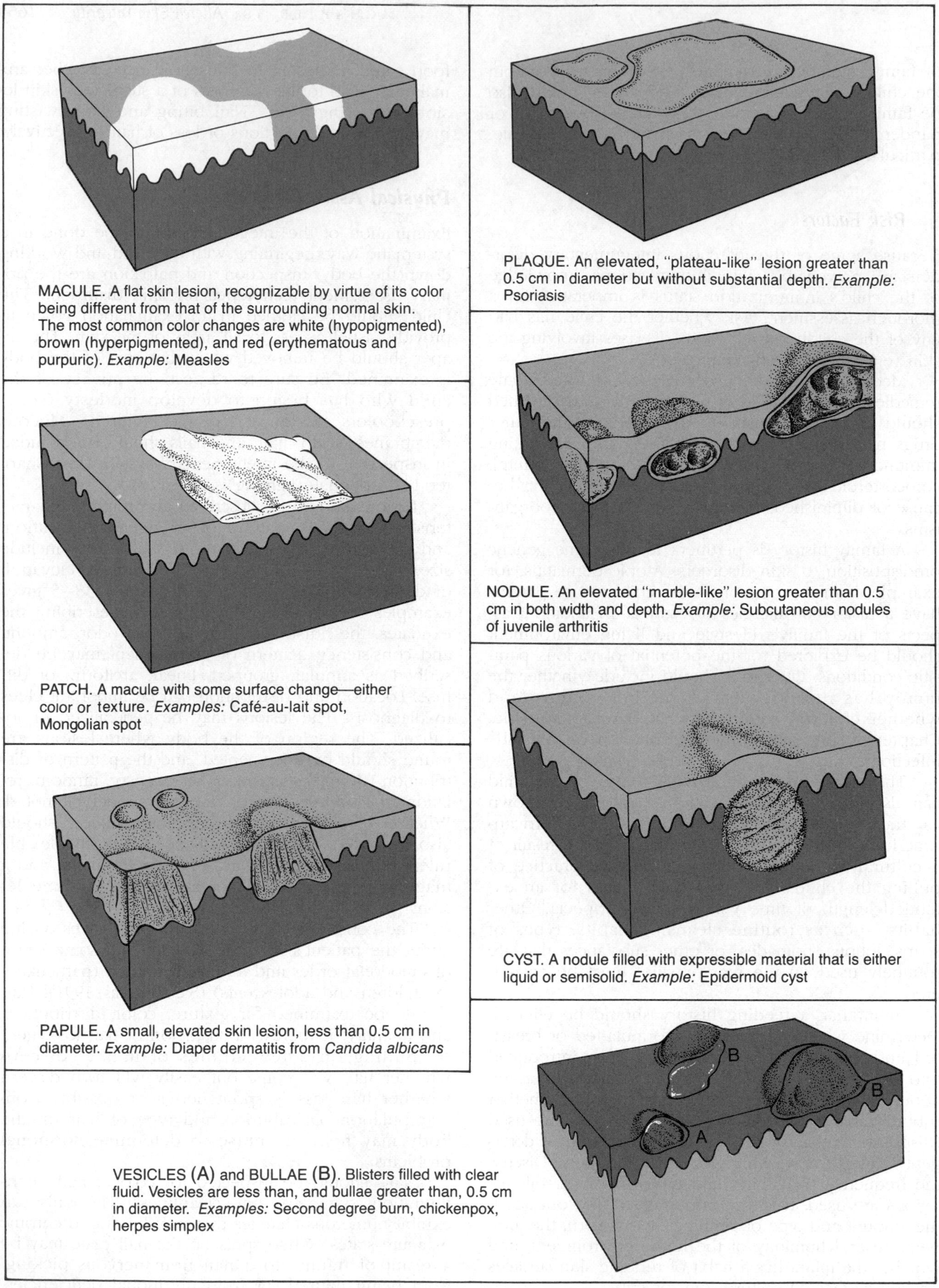

MACULE. A flat skin lesion, recognizable by virtue of its color being different from that of the surrounding normal skin. The most common color changes are white (hypopigmented), brown (hyperpigmented), and red (erythematous and purpuric). *Example:* Measles

PLAQUE. An elevated, "plateau-like" lesion greater than 0.5 cm in diameter but without substantial depth. *Example:* Psoriasis

PATCH. A macule with some surface change—either color or texture. *Examples:* Café-au-lait spot, Mongolian spot

NODULE. An elevated "marble-like" lesion greater than 0.5 cm in both width and depth. *Example:* Subcutaneous nodules of juvenile arthritis

PAPULE. A small, elevated skin lesion, less than 0.5 cm in diameter. *Example:* Diaper dermatitis from *Candida albicans*

CYST. A nodule filled with expressible material that is either liquid or semisolid. *Example:* Epidermoid cyst

VESICLES (A) and BULLAE (B). Blisters filled with clear fluid. Vesicles are less than, and bullae greater than, 0.5 cm in diameter. *Examples:* Second degree burn, chickenpox, herpes simplex

FIGURE 38 - 5.

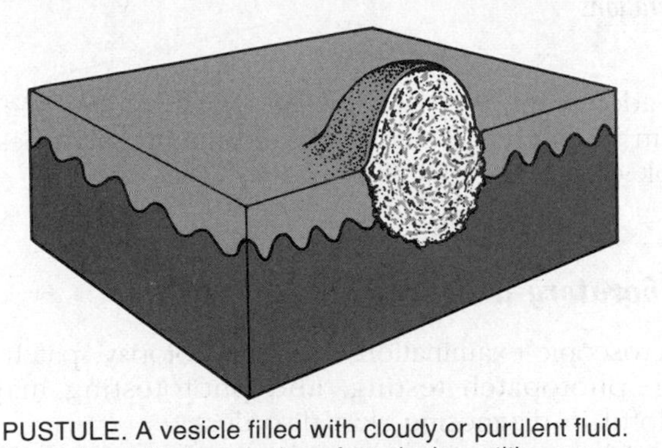

PUSTULE. A vesicle filled with cloudy or purulent fluid. *Examples:* Infectious lesion of atopic dermatitis, acne

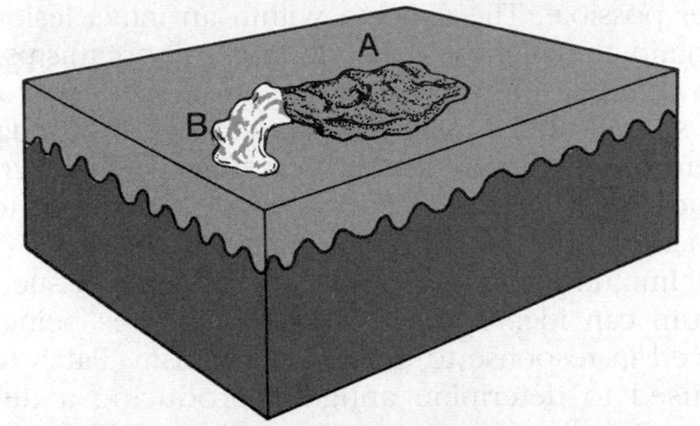

CRUST (A) and OOZING CRUST (B). Liquid debris (e.g., serum or pus) that has dried on the surface of the skin. Most frequently crusts result from breakage of vesicles, pustules, or bullae. *Example:* Impetigo

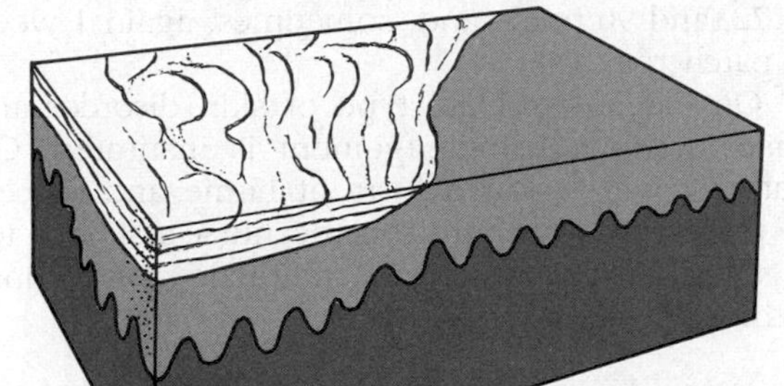

SCALE. Visibly thickened stratum corneum. Scales are dry and usually whitish in color. These features help distinguish scales from crusts, which are often moist and usually yellowish or brown. *Example:* Psoriasis

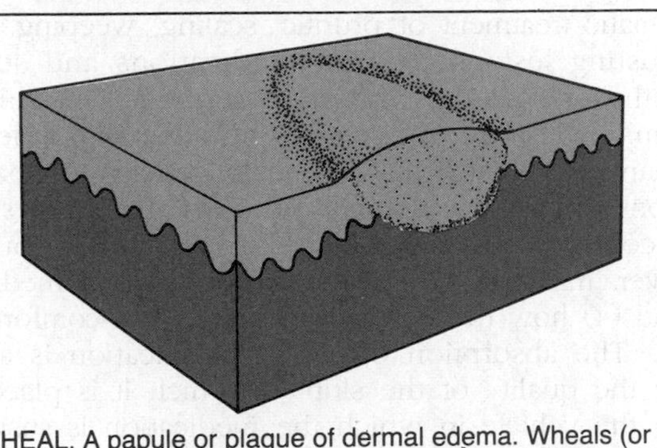

WHEAL. A papule or plaque of dermal edema. Wheals (or *hives*) often have central pallor and irregular borders. *Examples:* Type I hypersensitivity reaction, urticaria

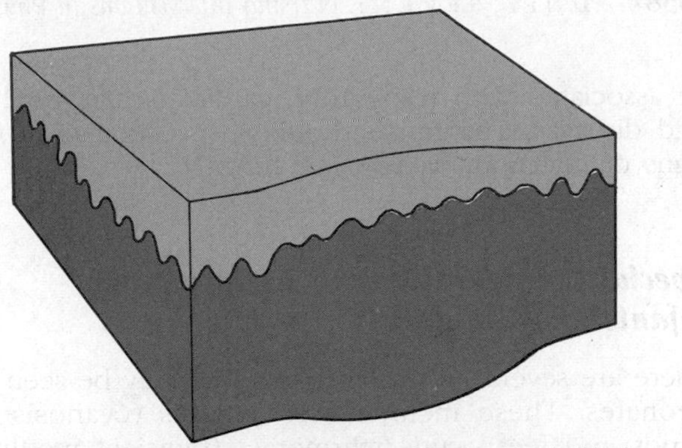

INDURATION. Dermal thickening resulting in skin that *feels* thicker and firmer than normal. *Example:* Poorly approximated edges of an inflamed wound

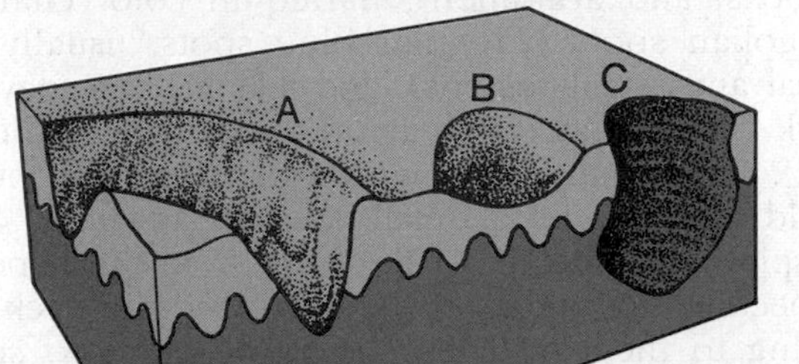

FISSURE (A), EROSION (B), and ULCER (C). A fissure is a thin linear tear in the epidermis. An erosion is wider but is limited in depth, being confined to the epidermis. An ulcer is a defect devoid of epidermis as well as part or all of the dermis. *Example:* Anal fissure

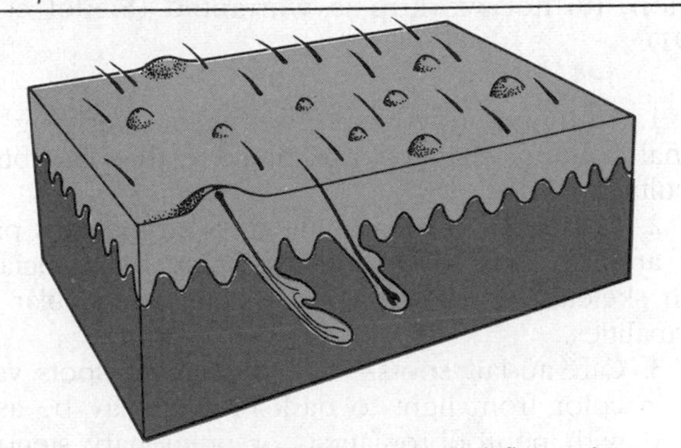

COMEDO (plural, COMEDONES). The noninflammatory lesions of acne that result from keratin impaction in the outlet of the pilosebaceous canal. *Example:* Acne

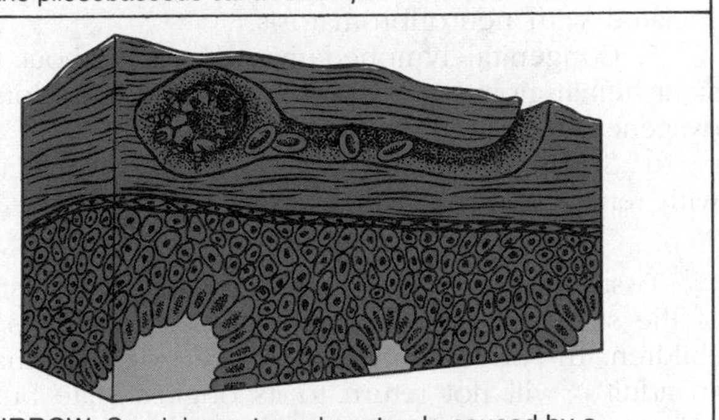

BURROW. Serpiginous tunnel or streak, caused by a burrowing organism. *Example:* Scabies

FIGURE 38 - 5. *Continued*

be associated with respiratory, cardiovascular, or thyroid diseases. The nurse should inspect the nails for signs of infection, bacterial or fungal.

Special Considerations in Assessing Infants and Children

There are several normal variants that may be seen in neonates. These include acrocyanosis (cyanosis of hands and feet), cutis marmorata (transient mottling secondary to decreased temperature), erythema toxicum (pink papular rash with vesicles on thorax, back, buttocks, and abdomen), harlequin color change, mongolian spots (irregular blue spots, usually on gluteal and sacral regions), and telangiectatic nevi or "stork bites" (flat, pink areas, usually on nape of neck). In examining the newborn infant, the nurse should be cognizant of small defects, particularly over the spine, the midline of the head from the nape of the neck to the bridge of the nose, and the neck extending to the ear. These could be clues to sinus tracts, brachial clefts, or cysts (Siedel et al, 1991). The infant's skin should be examined for texture and should be soft and smooth. Vernix caseosa may be present and is normal.

There are several cutaneous lesions that may give clues to congenital problems. If any of the following (only a partial list) are seen during an initial examination, further workup is warranted (Siedel et al, 1991):

1. Faun tail nevus—tuft of hair overlying the spinal column; may be associated with spina bifida occulta.
2. Epidermal verrucous nevi—warty lesions present at birth or early childhood; may be associated with skeletal, central nervous system, and ocular abnormalities.
3. Café-au-lait spots—flat, pigmented spots varying in color from light to dark brown; may be associated with neurofibromatosis or pulmonary stenosis, temporal lobe dysrhythmia, and tuberous sclerosis.
4. Freckling in the axillary or inguinal area—associated with neurofibromatosis.
5. Congenital lymphedema with or without transient hemangiomas—may be associated with gonadal dysgenesis.
6. Supernumerary nipples—may be associated with renal abnormalities.

Tissue turgor will very quickly give an assessment of the state of hydration and nutrition in infants and children. In serious dehydration, the skin, like that of an adult's, will not return to its original state but remain in the "tented" position caused by gentle pinching. Dennie lines (Morgan fold) may be seen in children with atopic dermatitis. This is a line, or fold, seen under the eye, caused by chronic rubbing and inflammation. It is important for the nurse to remember that, when assessing the skin of an infant, child, or adolescent, they are not just small adults. The skin is in a different level of development and does not look or act like that of an adult.

Laboratory and Diagnostic Tests

Microscopic examinations, cultures, biopsy, patch testing, photopatch testing, and phototesting may be helpful in diagnosing skin disorders.

When collecting an exudate specimen for culture, obtain material from an intact vesicle or pustule whenever possible. The exudate within an intact lesion will contain the highest concentration of organisms. The top of the lesion can be carefully removed with a sterile scalpel and a swab inserted to obtain exudate. If there are no intact lesions, carefully remove crusted exudate (by soaking and gentle débridement) to obtain the liquid material underneath.

Immunofluorescence tests of biopsied tissue or of serum can identify the type of antibodies being produced in response to the microorganism. Patch testing is used to determine antigens producing a delayed (type IV) allergic response. (See Chapter 37 for further information about the type IV response.) Antigenic test materials are placed on the upper back or forearm under occlusive patches and removed 48 hours later. The sites are then assessed for local inflammation at 48, 72, and 96 hours and, sometimes, again 1 week after patch removal.

On diagnosis of the type of skin disorder and its cause, therapeutic management is instituted. Often, treatment will be carried out at home and success of the therapy may depend on the nurse's skill in teaching the child and family the rationale and techniques of the prescribed regimen.

Therapeutic Management: Principles of Topical Therapy

Management of many skin disorders will involve symptomatic treatment of pruritic, scaling, weeping, and/or crusting lesions. Topical medications and soothing baths or soaks are often prescribed. The child and family will need to know (1) how the skin lesions will change as they heal (e.g., from vesicles to oozing lesions to crusts and finally to clear skin), (2) signs of secondary infection (increased erythema, pustules, fever, malaise), (3) how to apply topical medication, and (4) how to decrease itching and discomfort.

The absorption of topical medication is affected by the quality of the skin on which it is placed and by the vehicle in which the medication is suspended (e.g., cream, ointment). The barrier capacity of the stratum corneum is lowest in warm, moist skin, so absorption is usually best when a cream or ointment is applied after a bath. Topical medications should be applied with downward strokes. Always apply in the direction of hair growth. Rubbing in circles, or using

TABLE 38-5
Properties of Topical Preparations

Preparation	Properties	Nursing Implications
Cream (e.g., Unibase, Plastibase, Polysorb, Hydrosorb, Keri, Lubriderm)	Water-based, semisolid emulsion of *oil in water;* white, nongreasy	Not occlusive; rubs completely into skin. Can be made into a lotion by adding water. Contains several preservatives to prevent the compound from becoming rancid; may rarely cause allergic reaction. For use on oily, moist, opposing skin surfaces and on weeping eruptions
Ointment (e.g., petrolatum, Eucerin, Aquaphor, lard, Crisco)	Oil-based emulsion of *water in oil;* clear, greasy	The most occlusive vehicle for medication; does not easily rub off or wash off. Petrolatum considered by some to be the standard ointment of dermatologic therapy; inexpensive and hypoallergenic. Ointments often used on dry and lichenified skin when absorption otherwise limited
Lotion (e.g., calamine)	Suspension of powder in water	More drying than creams and ointments. Relieves itching by cooling effect as water evaporates; leaves protective powder on skin. Shake before using to suspend powder evenly in the liquid. Often effective on scalp lesions
Tincture, aerosol spray	Suspension of active ingredient in alcohol	Alcohol evaporates, cooling skin, reducing itching, and leaving active ingredient on skin. Sprays are especially useful for hairy areas
Gel	Transparent, colorless, semisolid emulsion	Nonocclusive; liquefies when applied to skin. May be used in place of cream

Based on Lookingbill, D. P., & Marks, J. D., Jr. (1993). *Principles of dermatology* (2nd ed.). Philadelphia: WB Saunders.

a back-and-forth action may cause folliculitis as medication is rubbed into hair follicles. Occlusive vehicles (e.g., petrolatum) generally deliver the highest concentration of medication because they increase local skin temperature and resist being rubbed from the skin. Table 38–5 details the properties of common topical preparations. Table 38–6 describes the use of dressings and therapeutic baths.

TABLE 38-6
Therapeutic Use of Dressings and Baths

Treatment	Nursing Implications
Nonadherent (Dry) Dressing (e.g., petroleum gauze, semipermeable plastic membrane)	Used to prevent disruption of new tissue. Should not stick to wound when removed. Preserves skin moisture, which enhances healing
Adherent (Dry) Dressing (e.g., absorbent gauze-type dressing, fine-mesh gauze)	Used to nonselectively débride moist wounds. When removed, dressing pulls off dead tissue and dried secretions, which adhere to it. Fine-mesh gauze often used to prevent cotton fibers sticking to lesions. Removal is painful; check with the physician to see whether dressings may be soaked to ease removal. Prepare the child by administering analgesia, and allow the child as much control as possible during dressing changes (to decrease feelings of anxiety, helplessness, hopelessness); (e.g., allow child to pull off old dressings, apply new tape)
Wet to Dry Dressings (e.g., gauze [usually fine mesh] soaked in saline, water, or an antiseptic solution, covered by dry gauze dressings/pads)	Used to nonselectively débride crusts, dead tissue. Allow to dry, then remove (see débridement comments under "Adherent Dressings")
Wet Dressings (e.g., gauze, cotton-filled pads, or towels soaked and kept wet with water, astringent such as Burow solution, or antimicrobial solution such as povidone-iodine)	Used to treat acute inflammation. They soothe, cool, and dry skin by evaporation. Help to remove crusts and exudate. Towels, wash cloths, or wet clothing can be just as effective as expensive gauze material. Cover with dry clothing to prevent chilling. Skin may become macerated if plastic wrapping is used to keep soaks wet. Plastic wrap also a safety hazard for young child. Tubular bandage retainer (Surgitube, American Span) can secure soaks even to the face if holes are cut for the eyes, nose, and mouth (Nicol, 1987). Soaks are often best tolerated by the young child during naptime. Child can be rocked or otherwise lulled to sleep as the soaks begin to provide comfort; child may then associate treatment with comfort rather than the frustration of immobility and "wet towels"
Therapeutic Baths Tar emulsions, colloidal oatmeal, baking soda	Used for acute eruptions that crust and weep. Soothe, clean, relax, decrease itching

Based on Lookingbill, D. P., & Marks, J. D., Jr. (1993). *Principles of dermatology* (2nd ed.). Philadelphia: WB Saunders; and Kahn, G. (1988). *Principles of diagnosis and treatment of skin disorders*. In C. W. Bierman & D. S. Pearlman (Eds.). *Allergic disorders from infancy to adulthood* (2nd ed., pp 377–384). Philadelphia: WB Saunders.

Psychosocial Aspects of Skin Disorders

Anger, frustration, and anxiety are commonly experienced by children and families with skin disease, and this often exacerbates the disorder. Individuals with underlying skin disease are more likely to respond to stress, frustration, embarrassment, or any emotionally upsetting event with itching and scratching. Excitability and arousal of the central nervous system from an emotional upset can intensify the vasomotor and sweat responses in the skin and lead to the itch-scratch cycle. In some instances, scratching is used as an expression of the child's anger, as typically it will get an immediate response from those nearby. The added dimension of family hostility, rejection, and guilt can damage the family structure.

Learning about the acute or chronic nature of the given disorder, exacerbating factors, and the management measures that can control it is important to both the child and the family members. Maintaining a healthy outlook is important. Counseling and other psychosocial intervention are often very helpful when dealing with the frustrations of skin disease. It is especially helpful to adolescents and young adults who may consider the lesions disfiguring or unattractive.

The education needs of those affected by skin disease are vast. Health care providers need to consistently provide information that includes detailed skin care plans, general disease information, and availability of client-oriented support organizations, as well as updates on hopeful research results. Most will forget or confuse the important skin care recommendations without written instructions. Clearly outlining to the client, in both a verbal and a written manner, the skin care recommendations is essential for good outcomes. Nursing plays the major role in providing this important aspect of care. Adequate time and client teaching materials are needed to provide education in an effective manner. Nurses should be resourceful in obtaining or writing educational materials and instruction sheets. Educational pamphlets are available through a variety of sources, including the many dermatologically oriented client support groups and professional dermatology agencies, such as the Dermatology Nurses' Association and American Academy of Dermatology (Table 38–7). Introducing clients and families to these professional organizations can add a notable dimension to the client's care.

Remember that each child or family requires individualized therapy. What works for one may not work for another, or the preferred outlined regimen may not be acceptable to them. Individuals need to have a choice and a role in deciding their care. Nurses have an invaluable role in helping to determine what is the most acceptable therapy. It is important to use only the medications and therapies that have been agreed on by the client and the caregiver. When compliance is high with outlined skin care recommendations, the outcomes are generally very rewarding for the children, families, and caregivers alike, even with the most difficult skin disease.

Noninfectious Skin Disorders of Childhood

Eczema

Eczema is not a specific disease. "Dermatitis" and "eczema" are terms that may be used interchangeably and describe a group of diseases that have a characteristic appearance. A few examples of eczema seen frequently in children include allergic contact dermatitis (eruptions from allergy to poison ivy, sumac, or oak or to a proven allergen like nickel), irritant contact dermatitis (eruption from direct contact with cosmetics, chemicals, dyes, or detergents), nummular eczema (appearance of coin-shaped, oozing, crusting patches), seborrheic dermatitis (yellowish-pink scaling of scalp, face, and trunk), and atopic dermatitis (characteristic distribution of ezcema in persons with a family history of allergic disease).

Eczema/dermatitis has three primary stages; different types of ezcema may manifest in any one of the three stages or the three stages may coexist in a given client.

"Acute dermatitis" is characterized by extensive erosions with serous exudate or by intensely pruritic, erythematous papules and vesicles on a background of erythema.

"Subacute dermatitis" is characterized by erythematous, excoriated, scaling papules or plaques that are either grouped or scattered over erythematous skin. Often, the scaling is so fine and diffuse that the skin acquires a silvery sheen.

"Chronic dermatitis" is characterized by thickened skin and increased skin markings secondary to rubbing and scratching (lichenification); excoriated papules, fibrotic papules, and nodules (prurigo nodularis); and postinflammatory hyperpigmentation and hypopigmentation.

"Atopic dermatitis" is a common, chronic, relapsing, pruritic type of eczema that usually occurs in individuals with a personal or family history of allergic diseases. It is discussed in Chapter 37.

Diaper Dermatitis

"Contact dermatitis" is an inflammatory skin reaction either to allergens (Chapter 37) or to external irritants. Diaper dermatitis (diaper rash) is the most common form of nonallergic, irritant contact dermatitis in infancy and early childhood. Diaper dermatitis is not a specific disease but rather a variety of inflammatory disorders affecting the lower aspect of the abdomen, genitalia, buttock, and upper portion of the thigh. It is a form of contact dermatitis that is initiated by a combination of factors, including prolonged exposure to and irritation by urine and feces and maceration by wet diapers and airtight plastic diaper covers. Frequently, diaper dermatitis is secondarily infected with *Candida albicans*.

TABLE 38-7
Agencies and Patient Support Groups for Dermatologic Disorders

American Academy of Dermatology, 930 N. Meacham Road, P.O. Box 4014, Schaumburg, IL 60168–4014

American Cancer Society, 235 Montgomery Street, Suite 320, San Francisco, CA 94104

Dermatology Nurses' Association, East Holly Avenue, Box 56, Pitman, NJ 08071–0056

Alopecia Areata, National Alopecia Areata Foundation, 710 C Street, Suite 11, P.O. Box 150760, San Rafael, CA 94915–0760

Ataxia-Telangiectasia and Other Immunodeficiency/Cancer Syndromes, National Ataxia Foundation, 15500 Wayzata Boulevard, Wayzata, MN 55391–3750

Bloom's Syndrome, Bloom's Syndrome Registry, ℅ Laboratory of Human Genetics, The New York Blood Center, 310 E. 67th Street, New York, NY 10021

Ectodermal Dysplasias, National Foundation for Ectodermal Dysplasias, 219 East Main Street, Box 114, Mascoutah, IL 62258

Eczema Association for Science & Education, 1221 S.W. Yamhill, Suite 303, Portland, OR 97205

Epidermolysis Bullosa, Dystrophic Epidermolysis Bullosa Research Association of America, Inc., 141 Fifth Avenue, New York, NY 10010

Fanconi's Anemia, Fanconi Anemia International Registry, ℅ Dr. Arleen Auerbach, Laboratory for Investigative Dermatology, The Rockefeller University, 1230 York Avenue, New York, NY 10021–6399

Gardner's Syndrome, Familial Polyposis and Gardner's Syndrome Registry, ℅ Dr. Martin Lipkin, Memorial Hospital for Cancer Research, 1275 York Avenue, New York, NY 10021

Gluten Sensitivity, Gluten Intolerance Group, Elaine Hartsock, Ph.D., P.O. Box 23053, Seattle, WA 98102

Herpes, Herpes Resource Center, American Social Health Association, Palo Alto, CA 94302

Ichthyosis Foundation of America, 710 Laurel Avenue, B–8, San Mateo, CA 94401

Lupus Erythematosus, The Lupus Foundation of America, 1717 Massachusetts Avenue N.W., Suite 203, Washington, DC 20036

National Lupus Erythematosus Foundation, 2635 North First Street, Suite 206, San Jose, CA 95134

Neurofibromatosis, The National Neurofibromatosis Foundation, Inc., 141 Fifth Avenue, Suite 7S, New York, NY 10010

Pediculosis, National Pediculosis Association, P.O. Box 149, Newton, MA 02161

Porphyria, American Porphyria Foundation, P.O. Box 11163, Montgomery, AL 36111

Port Wine Stains, The National Congenital Port Wine Stain Foundation, 125 East 63rd Street, New York, NY 10021

Psoriasis, National Psoriasis Foundation, 6443 S.W. Beaverton Highway, Suite 210, Portland, OR 97221

Scleroderma, United Scleroderma Foundation, Inc., P.O. Box 399, Watsonville, CA 95077

Skin Cancer, The Skin Cancer Foundation, 245 Fifth Avenue, Suite 2402, New York, NY 10016

Skin Phototrauma Foundation, P.O. Box 6312, Parsippany, NJ 07054

Tuberous Sclerosis, National Tuberous Sclerosis Association, Inc., 8000 Corporate Drive, Suite 120, Landover, MD 20785

Vitiligo, National Vitiligo Foundation, Inc., P.O. Box 6337, Tyler, TX 75711

Xeroderma Pigmentosa, Xeroderma Pigmentosa Registry, ℅ Department of Pathology, UMDNJ–New Jersey Medical School, 185 South Orange Avenue, Newark, NJ 07103

Clinical Manifestations and Therapeutic Management

Diaper rashes involve inflammatory response in areas normally covered by a diaper (Figs. 38–6 and 38–7). They are extremely common in infants and untrained toddlers. Intertrigo (Fig. 38–7), a dermatitis that develops in skinfolds, is also fairly common in toddler and preschool girls who forget to wipe after voiding or who do so inadequately. Table 38–8 describes the most frequent diaper eruptions, their characteristic appearance, and specific treatments. Diagnosis is readily made by inspection of the rash characteristics and the area involved.

Nursing Diagnostic Statements

Impaired skin integrity: inflammation and rash, *related to irritation of the diaper area by*

- *Urea and ammonia salts.*
- *Feces.*
- *Detergent left in cloth diapers.*

Altered health maintenance, related to knowledge deficit (caregiver), *concerning*

- *Cause of rash and prevention of recurrence.*
- *Symptomatic treatment.*

Nursing Care

Relieving Diaper Area Irritation. General treatment of any of the diaper rashes requires basic diaper and skin care. The goal is "clean and dry." Prompt, thorough cleansing of the diaper region with a mild soap and water after each defecation or voiding is imperative to rid the skin of irritant byproducts and reduce the pathogen population. The caretaker should be in-

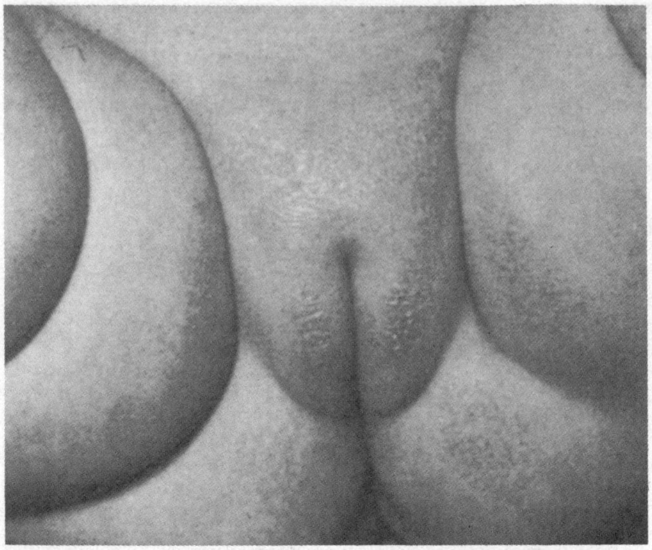

FIGURE 38-6. Primary irritant contact dermatitis (ammoniacal). Note involvement of convex surfaces but not the folds. (From Jacobs, A. H. [1975, May]. Eruptions in the diaper area. *Pediatric Clinics of North America,* p 212.)

structed to check every hour for elimination in the newborn and young infant and every 2 hours in the older infant.

Teaching to Address Knowledge Deficit. Maintenance of healthy skin is more likely when the caretaker(s) understands the reasons for the diaper rash and is given a clear explanation of how adequate skin hygiene and cleansing of diapers will help prevent or eliminate diaper rash. The region should be air-dried and exposed to the air at additional frequent intervals to promote faster healing. Because diaper rash is exacerbated by heat, moisture, and the friction and restriction of a diaper, exposing the skin surface to air helps to soothe irritation and dry any lesions present (see Table 38–8).

A topical antifungal medication is used to treat *C. albicans,* when present. Short-term use of low-potency topical steroids, alternately with antifungals at each diaper change, helps to reduce inflammation. A protective ointment such as Desitin or zinc oxide is used after inflammation is reduced, or prophylactically. An antibiotic may also be prescribed if secondary infection exists. Suggesting that the diaper and ointment be removed when the infant is resting or sleeping and that ointment and a loosely applied diaper be put on when the child is up or being held may be helpful to the caretakers.

Rubber pants and disposable diapers should be avoided either during bouts of diaper rash or continuously in very susceptible infants. Parents need explanations that the rubber and plastic prevent evaporation, thereby increasing maceration from urine breakdown. Even though disposable diapers are advertised to reduce wetness by pulling the urine toward the liner and away from baby's skin, the urea and ammonia salts that cause the breakdown are left behind as a residue on the diaper surface touching the child's skin, just as they are in cloth diapers. Parents need to know that the "wicking" action of disposable diapers does not eliminate the need to change them frequently. Use of powders, especially those containing cornstarch, should be avoided. Cornstarch promotes the growth of fungi. Powders, in general, are discouraged owing to danger of inhalation.

If diaper laundering has been inadequate or the parent has never used cloth diapers before, instruction should be given to launder them separately, using a mild soap and a *double rinsing*. Soaking rinsed, soiled diapers in a quaternary ammonium compound such as Diaparene helps to disinfect them.

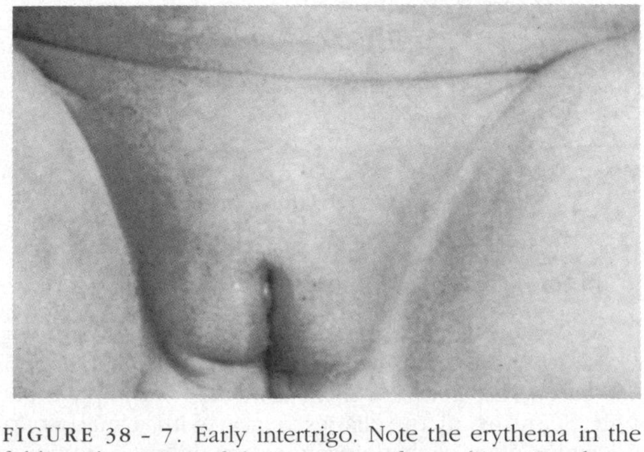

FIGURE 38-7. Early intertrigo. Note the erythema in the folds with sparing of the convex surfaces. (From Jacobs, A. H. [1975, May]. Eruptions in the diaper area. *Pediatric Clinics of North America,* p 213.)

Seborrheic Dermatitis

Etiology and Pathophysiology

Seborrheic dermatitis (cradle cap, seborrheic eczema) is an inflammatory skin disease thought to be related to a dysfunction of the sebaceous glands (Hurwitz, 1981). It usually appears shortly after birth when hormone levels are high, disappears after several weeks even without treatment, then reappears at adolescence when hormone levels again rise (Hurwitz, 1981). This dermatitis occurs most often on the scalp (cradle cap) (Fig. 38–8), although it may also involve the eyelids and eyebrows (blepharitis), the external ear canal (otitis externa), the postauricular region (behind the ears), the axillae and neck folds (Fig. 38–9), and the inguinal region (seborrheic diaper dermatitis). The lesions appear as thick, greasy crusts of a salmon color or as waxy yellow plaques with large scales. Transient alopecia may be present over the area of the crusty or scaly patches.

TABLE 38-8
Clinical Manifestations and Therapeutic Management of Diaper Rashes

Area Involved	Source	Treatment	Comments
Primary Irritant Contact Dermatitis: Parchmentlike Erythema (Similar to Scald)			
Convex area of buttocks, medial thighs, mons pubis, and scrotum, but not the folds Occurs at age 3 mos or older	Ammonia (urine) and putrefactive enzymes (feces) interact to create byproducts. In older infants, the contact dermatitis may be an allergic response to enzyme detergent or rubber	Topical corticosteroid cream (2½% hydrocortisone): add 1 cup of vinegar to last diaper rinse and let soak ½ hr before spinning (acidifies urine); basic diaper and skin care	Increasing risk of secondary infection with *Candida*
Intertrigo: Red Macerated Area of Sharp Demarcation			
Area where skin surfaces are in opposition, particularly groin folds Occurs at any age	Heat, moisture, and sweat retention combine to irritate and macerate the skin	Basic diaper and skin care. Teach appropriate wiping to child being potty-trained	Bacterial populations grow with maceration, increasing risk of secondary infections
Seborrheic Dermatitis: Characteristic Salmon-Colored Greasy Lesion with Yellowish Scale, Found Primarily in Intertriginous Areas; Nonpruritic (Differentiates It from Eczema)			
Presence of intertrigo in groin and in other skinfolds (neck or axilla) plus cradle cap indicates seborrheic dermatitis Occurs at age 3 wks–4 mos	Inborn physiologic trait	Same as for contact dermatitis	May spread to entire diaper region after initial appearance in folds; highly susceptible to secondary yeast or bacterial infection; subsides spontaneously
Miliaria: Small, Sterile, Clear Vesicopustules			
Anywhere that heat and moisture accumulate, especially diaper area Occurs at any age	Reaction to concentrated heat and humidity	Basic diaper and skin care	Also known as heat rash or prickly heat
Primary Candidiasis: Small Red Papules with Peripheral Scaling			
Sharply marginated area, usually involving the anterior thighs and abdomen, as well as the diaper area Occurs at any age, usually after age 2 wks	*Candida albicans* from gastrointestinal tract or an untreated infected caretaker	Topical antimonilial (e.g., Vioform, Nilstat, Mycostatin, Micatin). Oral Nilstat or Mycostatin is often indicated; basic diaper and skin care	Often secondary to seborrheic dermatitis; usually occurs following oral thrush. Do not use cornstarch on rash as it may be metabolized by microorganisms, promoting disease

Clinical Manifestations and Diagnostic Assessment

Cradle cap usually occurs in the first month of life. The lesion surfaces of seborrhea are a pink or yellow greasy scale. Seborrhea responds rapidly to treatment. Seborrhea is not pruritic. Diagnosis is based on the characteristic appearance of the crusts and the absence of pruritus.

Nursing Care

Preventive and symptomatic intervention are essentially the same. The most important aspect is adequate and frequent scalp hygiene measures. The scalp should be shampooed vigorously and thoroughly every other day. Parents usually have some reservations about vigorous scalp hygiene because of misconceptions about the durability of the "soft spots," or fontanels. They should be informed that these spots are as durable as the skin anywhere else on the body and will not be punctured by the pressure required for vigorous scrubbing. For some families, a demonstration shampoo may be more convincing than verbal descriptions. The "no tears" shampoos or those containing mild concentrations of salicylic acid or coal tars are most effective.

Measures may be taken to soften and remove some of the crusts prior to shampooing. Slightly warmed mineral oil or petrolatum can be massaged

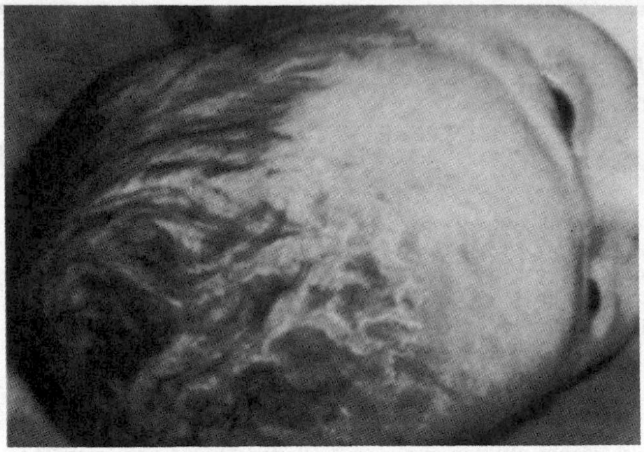

FIGURE 38 - 8. Cradle cap, a seborrheic dermatitis of the scalp, is extremely common in young infants. (From Jacobs, A. H. [1975, May]. Eruptions in the diaper area. *Pediatric Clinics of North America,* p 214.)

into the scalp 15 to 20 minutes before shampooing. A soft brush or fine-toothed comb can then be used during the shampoo to loosen and remove crusts and scales. Two to three treatments of this sort may be needed to clear the scalp but scrubbing should be limited to once a day to prevent scalp irritation.

If lesions are extensive or inflamed, low-potency topical corticosteroids applied twice daily for 1 to 2 weeks are effective in producing remission. Secondarily infected lesions, although infrequent, may require treatment with either topical or systemic antibiotic or antifungal therapy. Parents should be cautioned to avoid getting these ointments in the infant's eyes.

Although the lesions are of concern to parents and the crust-softening techniques somewhat bothersome, the child's behavior is generally unaltered by this disorder because it produces little if any discomfort. Seborrhea is a self-limiting disease in infancy and often clears by 8 to 12 months of age, even without treatment (Hurwitz, 1981). Parents can generally institute the prescribed treatment without difficulty, however, given adequate instruction. Recurrence can be prevented by regular shampooing.

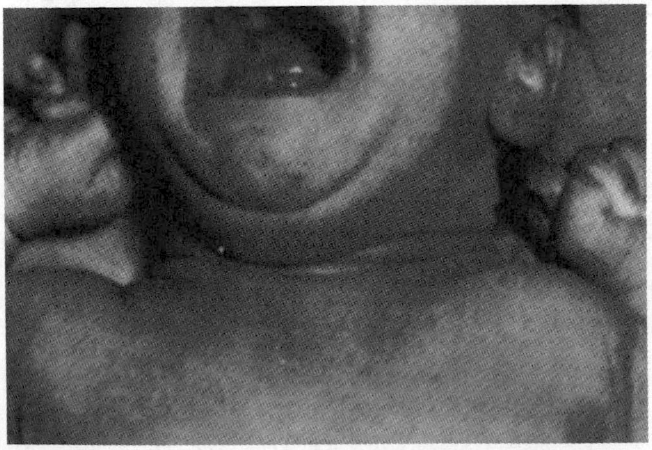

FIGURE 38 - 9. Seborrheic dermatitis may involve the axillae and neck folds. (From Jacobs, A. H. [1975, May]. Eruptions in the diaper area. *Pediatric Clinics of North America,* p 214.)

Psoriasis

Psoriasis vulgaris is a chronic, recurrent, erythematous, inflammatory disorder involving keratin synthesis. It may begin at any age, with onset before 15 years of age in 27 per cent of patients. In the childhood form, males are affected twice as often as females (Hurwitz, 1981). Although the exact etiology is unknown, there is a family history of psoriasis in 35 per cent of the cases (Lookingbill & Marks, 1993).

Pathophysiology

Psoriasis is a disease of the stratum corneum in which the usual differentiation and migration of keratinocytes through the layers of epidermal tissue is dramatically accelerated. Ordinarily it takes 28 days for a cell to travel from the basal cell layer to the stratum corneum. In psoriasis, cells make that transition in 3 to 4 days. The problem results when the outer layer of skin fails to shed the cells as quickly as they are produced. Cells of the stratum corneum then accumulate, with resulting scales and inflammation of the dermal layer (Lookingbill & Marks, 1993). The course of psoriasis is prolonged and unpredictable. Psoriatics have a greater than normal colonization of *Staphylococcus* on plaques. HIV-positive psoriatics are at high risk of infection from self-innoculation.

Clinical Manifestations

The scales of psoriasis are distinctive for their silver "micalike" color and the fact that they attach at the center rather than at the periphery. If scales are removed, they leave a small bleeding point associated with a ruptured capillary (Hurwitz, 1981). Classically, the lesions begin as tiny, red papules covered by scales. They grow together (coalesce) to form plaques that may measure several centimeters in diameter. The lesions are most common on the scalp, knees, and elbows and between the gluteal folds. The appearance of lesions at the site of a previous injury is known as "Koebner phenomenon." Koebner phenomenon is a useful diagnostic feature of psoriasis. These lesions are usually precipated by a scratch, laceration, sunburn, insect bite, or pressure. Guttate psoriasis begins on the trunk and proximal extremities as multiple erythematous macules that progress to "droplike" papules with a silver scale. Guttate psoriasis may follow a streptococcal pharyngitis. Nails may be involved with the appearance of small depressions or pits in the nail plate.

Diagnosis is often made on signs and symptoms and a family history of the disease. Cell studies can be done to confirm the diagnosis.

Therapeutic Management

Because psoriasis cannot be cured, management focuses on control of the recurrent exacerbations. Specifically, therapy seeks to decrease both the dermal inflammation and the proliferation of cells in the stratum corneum. Topical steroids, topical tar preparations, and ultraviolet (UV) light have proved effective.

Nursing Diagnostic Statements

High risk for ineffective management of therapeutic regimen, *risk factor: knowledge deficit concerning the nature and usual course of psoriasis.*

High risk for infection: secondary staphylococcal or streptococcal, *risk factors:*

- *Scratching associated with characteristic pruritus.*
- *Characteristic staphylococcal colonization of the skin in persons with psoriasis.*

High risk for disturbance in body image, *risk factor: chronic and unpredictable skin outbreaks affecting perceptions of self and others.*

Altered comfort: pruritus, *related to*

- *Dry skin.*
- *Low threshold for itching.*

Nursing Care

Assisting the Child and Family to Manage Topical Skin Care. The child and family will need some knowledge of the nature and usual course of psoriasis to manage the disease effectively at home. They should be aware that outbreaks are unpredictable and seemingly without cause; otherwise, they may become frustrated with the prescribed treatment or blame themselves unjustly. Parents and child should understand that prescribed steroid and tar preparations do more than just "soothe." They reduce the rapid cell division and decrease the dermal inflammation to help bring about remission. Tar preparations are available for baths (e.g., Polytar Bath, Zetar emulsion) and may be an acceptable alternative for young children who insist on rubbing off topical ointments.

Ultraviolet light (UVL), either alone or in combination with other treatments, remains the mainstay of therapy for moderate to severe psoriasis that is unresponsive to topical agents. Several types of phototherapy are available. The most practical form of UVL is sunlight. Children will often be happy to hear that playing outdoors is part of the "prescription" and adolescents are frequently pleased to further their suntans. Precautions are necessary to avoid overexposure. A sunburn can damage tissue enough to bring about an exacerbation of the disease. In climates and seasons where sunlight is not plentiful, UVL treatments can be administered by a dermatologist. In a controlled setting, either UVA or UVB light waves can be administered. UVB therapy can be used alone or in combinations with topical therapy like coal tar products or anthralin. UVA is given in combination with oral psoralens; this type of photochemotherapy is known as "PUVA." PUVA is reserved for children whose psoriasis has failed to respond to standard therapies. There are various side effects that must be discussed. The young person must be warned to protect the eyes with specially made goggles or with moist cotton balls to avoid damage to the corneas and to avoid overexposure. The most serious risk of UVL therapy is skin cancer (see discussion under "Sunburn").

Preventing Infection and Relieving Itching. Secondary infection in psoriasis results for the same reason as it does in many of the other inflammatory skin disorders—pruritus leads to scratching, which results in breaks in the skin barrier and penetration by bacteria. Proper use of the prescribed topical gel, cream, or ointment can reduce pruritus significantly. Young children should always have short, smooth fingernails and should be taught techniques such as applying pressure over the pruritic area rather than scratching it. Strange as it may sound, gently rubbing the opposite limb in the corresponding spot may help relieve itching (McCaffery, 1972). Infants may need to wear mits during naptime or when the caretaker cannot distract them from scratching. Children should be taught proper skin care, with attention to cleanliness, hydration, and good nutrition (see factors that affect skin function in the first part of this chapter). Skin that is generally healthy will recover more quickly from exacerbations of psoriasis and will be better able to resist infection.

Promoting a Positive Body Image. Psoriatic lesions can be a very real source of embarrassment for the child and adolescent. Their peers may express concerns of "catching" the skin lesions or may taunt and tease. In early childhood, the child may look on each new outbreak as retribution for some real or imagined wrongdoing (see Chapter 7 on cognitive development of preschoolers). The preschooler will need reassurance that the new outbreak of lesions was unpreventable.

Children who are allowed age-appropriate self-management may feel somewhat more in control and less frustrated. They may find that prompt application of the prescribed topical preparation can limit the spread of a new attack and thus feel that there is, after all, something they can do about the disorder. Support and understanding from the parent and the nurse can be invaluable in helping the youngster build a positive body image. Focusing on strengths and refusing to "generalize" the limitations of this skin disease to other aspects of the child's personality are effective strategies.

Acne Vulgaris

Acne vulgaris is the most common skin disorder affecting 85 per cent of the population between the ages of 12 and 25 years. It encompasses a wide spectrum of clinical presentations (Leyden & Shalita, 1986). Caused primarily by androgen stimulation of pilosebaceous units (hair follicle/sebaceous gland structures) in the skin, acne occurs in nearly all males and in 80 per cent of females in their teen-age years (Strauss, 1987). Genetic influences may determine the patient's susceptibility and the severity of the condition. Severe acne tends to run in families and affects males more frequently. The term "acne vulgaris" describes ordinary acne. The word "acne" is derived from a Greek word meaning "eruption on the face" and "vulgaris" comes from the Latin for "ordinary or common."

Pathophysiology

The exact cause of acne is unknown. The principal factors are abnormal keratinization of the follicular epithelium, excessive sebum production, proliferation of *Proprionibacterium acnes (P. acnes),* and inflammation secondary to the action of extracellular inflammatory products produced by *P. acnes.*

As long as sebum is secreted into an open follicle, it flows out onto the skin and evaporates. In acne vulgaris, however, follicles tend to *obstruct.* Epithelial cells, keratinocytes, accumulate within the follicle and seem to adhere to the follicular lining, thus clogging the channel through which sebum would normally be excreted. It is thought that this accumulation of cells may also be the result of androgen stimulation (Lookingbill & Marks, 1993). *P. acnes* are ordinarily harmless *bacteria* that live within the hair follicles. When follicular contents become stagnant, however, these bacteria appear to increase the inflammatory process, possibly by secreting chemicals that attract neutrophils (Lookingbill & Marks, 1993). (See Chapter 37 for the role of neutrophils in the inflammatory response.)

Clinical Manifestations

The microcomedo is the precursor of all clinical acne lesions. This lesion is not visible on the skin surface and only detectable by microscopy. It forms when a keratinous plug obstructs the follicular canal, causing a build-up of sebum and bacteria. The microcomedo may divide into a visible comedo or lead to development of an inflammatory lesion such as a pustule, papule, or nodule. Open comedones are often called

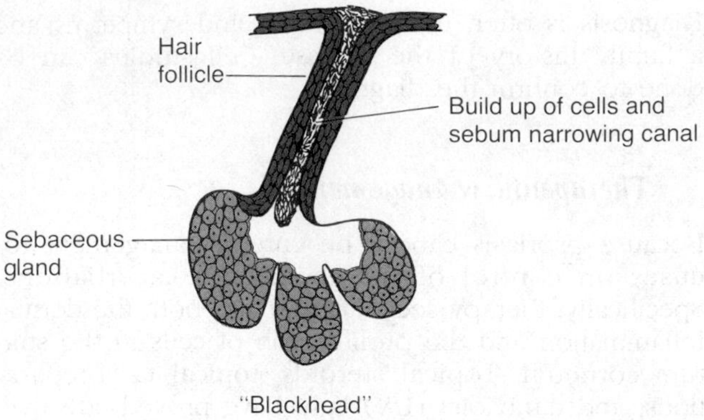

FIGURE 38-10. Open comedo with widely dilated follicle opening.

"blackheads." These result from the continuing accumulation of horny cells and sebum, which dilates the follicle (Fig. 38-10). (Blackheads, although unsightly, do not progress to inflammatory lesions unless squeezed and manipulated.)

Closed comedones are called "whiteheads," a term that is not to be confused with a white pustular lesion. These whiteheads are small, nonerythematous papules (bumps) just under the skin surface. The closed comedone is essentially that—a closed follicle that prevents sebum and other accumulations from escaping to the skin surface. As cells and sebum continue to accumulate, the lesion can become inflammatory if the follicular wall ruptures (Fig. 38-11). The lesion that results depends on the size of the ruptured follicle and on the location of the rupture within the dermis (Hurwitz, 1981). If the rupture was high in the dermis, the lesion will be a pustule, pushing out against the thin epidermis and disclosing the white inflammatory exudate underneath. If the rupture was deeper within the dermis, the lesion will present as a larger papule or firm nodule. Nodular lesions are especially bothersome because of the intense feeling of pressure from the deep inflammation. Squeezing in an attempt to "pop" the lesion and relieve the pressure is useless, however, because there is no channel through which the inflammatory contents can exit. This sort of manipulation increases tissue injury, further increasing the inflammation and predisposing to secondary infection through breaks in the epidermis.

Therapeutic Management

An individual plan of care is important. Many factors, such as type of acne, age, severity of onset, and family history, play a role in determining recommended therapy. Therapeutic management is aimed at (1) normalizing keratinization within the follicle, (2) decreasing sebum production, (3) inhibiting *P. acnes,* and (4) producing an anti-inflammatory effect. These aims are accomplished primarily through drug therapy (Strauss, 1987). Drugs that affect *keratinization* include a topi-

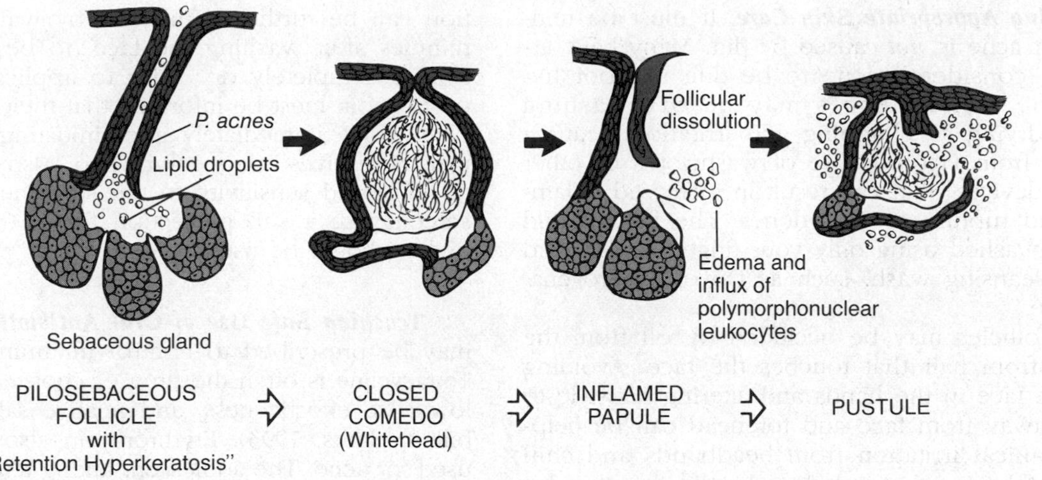

FIGURE 38 - 11. The development of an inflammatory acne lesion. (Adapted from Hurwitz, S. [1981]. *Clinical pediatric dermatology*. Philadelphia: WB Saunders, p 108.)

cally active derivative of vitamin A (tretinoin [Retin-A]); benzoyl peroxide, topical salicylic acid, and oral retinoids (isotretinoin [Accutane]). Drugs that decrease *sebum* production include oral estrogens, low-dose corticosteroids, and oral retinoids. The actions of *P. acnes* are inhibited by topical benzoyl peroxide, topical and oral antibiotics, and oral retinoids. *Anti-inflammatory* drugs include locally injected corticosteroids, oral corticosteroids, and oral retinoids. Acne surgery, including comedo extraction, intralesional steroids, and cryosurgery, is useful in selected patients.

Whereas in the early 1980s, adolescents deprived themselves of chocolate, cola drinks, refined sugars, milk, ice cream, fried foods, potato chips, shellfish, and iodides in an attempt to "clear their complexions," it is now thought that diet has little effect on acne. Most acne sufferers will benefit most from a well-rounded nutritious diet combined with adequate sleep and exercise.

It is impossible to predict how long any one individual will have acne. The natural history of acne is a remitting and exacerbating course. There is no cure for acne; however, many therapies improve the disease. The goal of therapy is to achieve optimal control. It is important that the nurse be honest but positive about likely outcomes. Explain carefully that it takes 4 to 8 weeks for noticeable improvement with any therapy.

Nursing Diagnostic Statements

High risk for ineffective management of therapeutic regimen, *risk factors: regarding*

- *Pathophysiology and etiology of acne.*
- *Proper skin care.*
- *Safe use of prescribed medications.*

High risk for body image disturbance, self-esteem disturbance, and personal identity disturbance (disturbance in self concept), *risk factor: negative perceptions about self associated with*

- *Presence of skin lesions.*
- *Scarring associated with chronic pustule or nodule formation.*

Nursing Care

Teaching to Address Knowledge Deficit. Whatever treatment regimen is tried, health professionals intervening need to begin by educating the adolescent about the pathophysiology and etiology of acne. Myths and fears need to be replaced with factual information. Youths need to understand that treatment will be lengthy and will not totally prevent or cure their acne state. They must be impressed with the importance of faithfully complying with the treatment regimen, despite a seeming lack of improvement, if successful results are eventually to occur. Understanding of these facts by parents is also important to their cooperation with and reinforcement of the plan of care.

Once treatment is prescribed, the nurse can help interpret the therapy as specific and practical actions the adolescent can understand. The patient's ability to complete the recommended program of care should be evaluated. Lack of understanding of the disease or treatment, low motivation, a treatment schedule inappropriate for day-to-day activities, or inability to pay for prescribed therapy are frequent reasons for treatment failures.

Nurses can periodically monitor teens' ability to manage the treatment regimen and help them to see the gradual improvement of their condition. (Color snapshot close-ups every 3 to 6 months provide visual evidence of the steady changes in their skin condition that go unnoticed under daily observation.)

Teaching Appropriate Skin Care. It must be reinforced that acne is *not* caused by dirt. Many have erroneously considered acne to be due to poor hygiene. The consequences may be overwashing inducing drying or chapping and irritation. Trauma can result from vigorous use of washcloths or other "cleaning devices" that can result in increased inflammation and rupture of comedones. The face should be gently washed using only your fingers and a mild soap or cleansing wash, such as Dove, Neutrogena, or Purpose.

Hair follicles may be occluded by oil from the hands or from hair that touches the face. Avoiding resting the face in the hands and altering hairstyle to pull hair away from face and forehead can be helpful. Mechanical irritation from headbands and chin straps of athletic gear can induce localized outbreaks, especially when combined with heat and humidity. Certain oil-based cosmetic agents can be comedogenic. Nurses can counsel their female patients to buy only water-based cosmetics, which they apply sparingly and remove completely each night. "Noncomedogenic" moisturizers should be utilized for dryness. Patient education needs to clarify that there is no "best" product for everyone.

One of the nurse's greatest challenges will be to convince the patient not to pick the lesions. The temptation is almost overwhelming! They should know that much of acne skin damage is self-inflicted. When one understands the cause for lesions and realizes that pushing against lesions to extract their contents causes a good deal of damage to the surrounding tissues, that temptation may be somewhat abated.

Teaching Appropriate Use of Topical Agents. Topical treatment should be the first line of therapy because it is the least invasive. Frequently used topicals in acne therapy include antibiotics, benzoyl peroxide, salicylic acid, and tretinoin. Many times, these topicals are used in combination by applying one product in the morning and another in the evening. Choice of which topicals depends on the type of acne. Topical medications may come in solution, lotion, gel, pledget, cream, or ointment vehicles. All specific instructions supplied with the medications should be followed unless other clear written instruction is given. In general, these are usually applied in the morning and/or evening after washing the face with a gentle soap. If drying occurs, be sure to instruct the patient regarding choices of approriate noncomedogenic moisturizers.

Tretinoin (Retin-A) is commonly used because it is the topical agent that most significantly inhibits comedo formation. Most patients' skin needs time to adjust to tretinoin. This can be accomplished by instructing the patient to initiate therapy with low-strength, pea-sized applications, once a night or, if necessary, every other night. To minimize skin drying, patients should be cautious if using other topicals containing alcohol, resorcinol, or salicylic acid. Irritation can be further minimized by waiting 20 to 30 minutes after washing the face, to be sure that the skin is completely dry prior to application. Patients on tretinoin must be informed that their acne may appear worse immediately after initiating therapy; this usually resolves in a week or two. Also, there may be an increased sensitivity to the sun; therefore, a sunscreen with a sun protection factor (SPF) of 15 or higher should be used daily.

Teaching Safe Use of Oral Antibiotics. Antibiotics may be prescribed to control inflammatory lesions. Tetracycline is often the drug of choice because of its low cost, effectiveness, and relative safety (Lookingbill & Marks, 1993). Erythromycin also is commonly used for acne. The adolescent taking tetracycline must be taught to take it on an empty stomach because food, particularly dairy products, interferes with absorption. Persons with asthma or other disorders who also take theophylline preparations should know that tetracycline potentiates the action of theophylline. Patients should call their physician if they experience symptoms of theophylline toxicity: nausea, a feeling of agitation, or a racing pulse. Tetracycline also may render oral contraceptives less effective and cause increased photosensitivity.

Teaching about Other Oral Agents. Isotretinoin (Accutane) has been found extremely effective in inducing remission of severe acne but should only be used when all other methods have failed. It inhibits sebaceous gland function, decreases sebum production, reduces *P. acnes* colonization indirectly and possesses anti-inflammatory and antikeratinizing effects. Although it has dramatic effects on acne, isotretinoin is reserved for use in cases of severe cystic acne because of its significant side effects. These effects include cheilitis, dry skin, pruritus, skin eruptions, drying of the mucous membranes, conjunctivitis, and nosebleeds. The most disturbing side effect of isotretinoin, however, is its ability to cause severe birth defects. Male patients are in no danger because there is no effect on sperm. All females of childbearing potential must agree and consent, in writing, through standardized forms, to: (1) using effective forms of contraception 1 month before, during, and 1 month after using the drug; (2) having a mandatory serum pregnancy test within 2 weeks before starting the drug; (3) waiting until the second or third day of their menstrual period to begin therapy; (4) having recommended pregnancy testing monthly; (5) having the drug prescribed in only 1 month quantities; (6) participating in a follow-up survey (Laudano et al, 1990). The risk of serious birth defects is so great that some physicians will not prescribe isotretinoin unless the patient signs an agreement that, should she become pregnant while on the medication, she will seek a therapeutic abortion.

Estrogen may be administered to females in the form of certain birth control pills to reduce hyperfunction of sebaceous glands. Because of the risks associated with high doses of estrogen, however, it is restricted to cases of acne resistant to other forms of therapy (except isotretinoin) (Dobson, 1984).

Addressing the Disturbance in Self-Concept. Acne should never be dismissed as an inevitable fact of growing up that must simply be tolerated and ignored to the extent possible. Such attitudes on the part of parents or health professionals lead to unnecessary physical discomfort and possibly disfigurement associated with permanent scarring. Even more destructive is the injury to self-concept as a result of the embarrassment and self-consciousness acne causes at a time when identity development is crucial. It is important to discuss the impact acne has made in the individual's life. In severe cases, referral for psychosocial intervention is appropriate.

Sunburn

Pathophysiology and Etiology

Sunburn is an acute inflammatory skin response, characterized by delayed redness and tenderness, that occurs as a reaction to excessive exposure to sunlight. Dermatopathologic changes include the production of epidermal cells that have cytoplasmic and nuclear changes. The dermis shows vasodilatation of blood capillaries, vascular permeability, and leukocyte migration. "Photodamage" is the term used to describe the broad spectrum of presumably permanent undesirable changes that result from repeated sun exposure. The spectrum of damage ranges from sunburn to skin cancer.

Clinical Manifestations

A "first-degree" sunburn produces mild, tender erythema followed by desquamation (peeling) that heals without scarring. "Second-degree" sunburn causes more extreme erythema and edema, and blistering results from damage to the epidermal cells. "Third-degree" burns involve damage to the dermis, leaving black eschar formation often associated with lack of pain secondary to nerve damage. Third-degree burns rarely occur with sunburn unless induced with artificial sources such as tanning lamps or booths. Usually, healing takes from 1 to 14 days and is without scarring if there are no complications. Severe and/or extensive sunburn may cause systemic manifestations (e.g., chills, nausea, headache, abdominal cramping). These signal dehydration and electrolyte imbalance.

Therapeutic Management and Nursing Care

Prevention is obviously the best therapy for sunburn. There is growing concern in the health care community regarding the dangers of excessive UV radiation exposure. The numbers of nonmelanoma and melanoma skin cancers are escalating at alarming rates (Nicol, 1989). Children require special consideration. Experts believe that by age 18, a child has received the majority of the lifetime dose of UV light. Regular use of a sunscreen with an SPF of 15 during those first 18 years of life would reduce a person's lifetime risk of nonmelanoma skin cancer by 78 per cent (Stern et al, 1986). One of the most effective ways to protect skin is through the proper use of sunscreens. (See Table 38–9 for tips on using sunscreens.) Creating safe sun habits in children is critical.

However, when the skin does become sunburned, treatment involves decreasing inflammation and rehydrating the damaged skin. For localized, first-degree sunburn, apply cool tap water soaks for 20 minutes or until the skin is cool. This limits skin destruction, prevents edema, and, potentially, reduces blisters. Tepid tap water baths are indicated for large sunburned areas. After a bath or soak, apply water-based emollients, preferably after refrigerating them for an additional cooling effect. Emollients should also be applied throughout the day to soothe and relieve dryness. Lotions or foams containing camphor and/or menthol (e.g., Sarna) can also be beneficial.

For second-degree sunburn, apply continuous cool, normal saline soaks or soaking baths to reduce oozing and edema. Apply sterile dressings and try to avoid unroofing blisters. Avoid débridement unless there is evidence of secondary bacterial infection. Although topical antibiotics are not usually necessary, 1 per cent silver sulfadiazine may be prescribed for its bacteriostatic effect. Systemic antibiotics may be prescribed for secondary infection after a bacterial culture is taken. Avoid use of over-the-counter remedies containing local anesthetics (benzocaine, dibucaine, or lidocaine) because they are rarely effective and have the potential of contact sensitivity.

Prostaglandin inhibitors (aspirin, indomethacin) may be used to reduce the erythema and inflammation. Because of its analgesic and anti-inflammatory properties, aspirin is recommended in adults for first- and second-degree sunburn in the first 24 to 48 hours on a routine basis every 4 to 6 hours; however, aspirin is not generally recommended for children owing to the possibility of Reye syndrome. Topical corticosteroids may be prescribed to be used sparingly in nonocclusive vehicles (i.e., cream or lotion) for their vasoconstrictive effects. Systemic corticosteroids are prescribed only for patients with very extensive, painful burns, but their use has declined in favor of prostaglandin inhibitors. The treatment of choice for sunburn is prevention.

Infectious Skin Disorders of Childhood

Infectious diseases of the skin are generally caused by bacteria, viruses, or fungi. These infections usually

TABLE 38-9
Family-Centered Teaching Guide: Protecting the Child's Skin from Sun Damage

How Sun Damages Skin

Sunburn (redness and sometimes blistering or peeling) is a sign of damage to the skin. Repeated exposure to sun over the years can cause premature aging, deep wrinkling, roughness, "age spots," freckles, and yellowing of the skin. This "photodamage" can also lead to the development of skin cancer

How to Protect Skin from Photodamage

Use a sunscreen with a minimal sun protection factor (SPF) of 15

Whenever possible, dress the child in dry, tightly woven, protective cotton clothing and a broad-brimmed hat

Avoid the sun's peak hours—between 10 A.M. and 3 P.M.

Protect the child with sunscreen, even on cloudy or hazy days. A thin cloud cover reduces ultraviolet radiation (UVR) by less than 20%

Sitting under a beach umbrella is not complete protection. Sand, concrete, and water can reflect up to 90% of the sun's rays. The beach umbrella may reduce sun exposure by only 50%

Some medications make skin more sensitive to the sun. Check with your doctor or pharmacist

How to Use Sunscreens for the Best Protection

Photoprotection of children is especially important. Estimates indicate that at least 50% of lifetime exposure to UVR occurs by age 18

Sunscreens should not be used routinely on children under 6 mos of age. Preferably, they should be kept out of the direct sunlight altogether

A broad-spectrum sunscreen is ideal, as it protects against both ultraviolet A (UVA) and ultraviolet B (UVB) wavelengths of the sun

Apply sunscreen to all sun-exposed areas, including the nose, cheeks, ears, back of the neck, backs of the hands, and arms

Sunscreens are most effective when applied liberally and absorbed completely over all exposed skin at least 30 mins before exposure

Be sure to reapply sunscreen after swimming (or splashing in a wading pool, sprinkler, or garden hose), exercising, rubbing the skin with a towel, or perspiring. Use waterproof sunscreen when needed

Sunscreen is important in the winter, too, because snow reflects up to 90% of the sun's rays; so use sunscreen for children during outdoor play

A sunscreen is an important part of sun protection, but does not shield completely from the sun's damaging rays

If irritation or an allergic reaction occurs, stop using the sunscreen and consult your health professional

Adapted from Skin Phototrauma Foundation (1992). *Sun smart guide.* The Skin Phototrauma Foundation (SPF) is a nonprofit organization whose mission is to educate the health care community about trauma to the skin induced by ultraviolet radiation (UVR). Its mission is accomplished through health care professional and patient education materials, symposia, lectures, and attendance at medical/nursing society conventions. All material and membership information are available by writing to the SPF at: P.O. Box 6312, Parsippany, NJ 07054.

develop in skin previously damaged by mechanical or thermal trauma or inflammation. Uncommonly, impaired host immunity from deficiencies in immunoglobulins, complement, or granulocytic function is the major predisposing factor. Most infections occur superficially; however, systemic signs and symptoms develop. Many of these diseases have significant nursing implications.

Diagnostic Assessment and Therapeutic Management

Diagnosis of each of the integumentary infections discussed in this section is made by visual recognition of the characteristic lesion and by culture of the lesion to establish origin and the appropriate choice of therapy. Typically, a topical and/or systemic antibiotic, antiviral, or antifungal agent is prescribed to facilitate resolution of the infectious process. Conscientious good daily skin care and good hygiene are important both in preventing the development of these skin infections and in reducing the likelihood of spread or transfer of the infectious organisms.

The effect of integumentary infections on the child and family members is related to three factors primarily: (1) the unpleasant appearance of the lesions that occur primarily on the face; (2) the potential transfer of the infection to other members; and (3) hygienic implications.

Education and teaching and reinforcing meticulous hygiene measures and good daily skin care are the most appropriate nursing interventions to facilitate physical resolution of the infection and to minimize the psychosocial effects on the child and family members. Parents, siblings, and peers should be urged to continue to communicate acceptance and to avoid making derogatory statements or teasing the child about her or his appearance. This is especially imperative for the adolescent for whom appearance is developmentally bound to self-concept.

Good daily skin care, including good hydration, adequate moisturizers, and appropriate hygienic practices, is key to maintaining optimal skin integrity.

Well-hydrated, intact skin is the best defense against the invasion of microorganisms, viruses, and fungi. Hygienic practices that emphasize cleanliness and frequent handwashing, careful cleansing of wounds and insect bites, and individual use of bath and bed linens should be taught to all children from the time they are toddlers. These practices should be reviewed and re-emphasized when skin infections do occur.

Patient education and allowing the child and family to have a role in deciding their care will greatly enhance compliance and treatment outcomes.

Impetigo

Etiology

Impetigo is a common superficial bacterial skin infection in infants and children due to *Streptococcus pyogenes* (group A streptococcus) and *Staphylococcus aureus,* alone or together. The disease is more common in middle to late summer, with a higher incidence in hot, humid climates. Impetigo is particularly infectious among those living in crowded conditions with poor sanitary facilities. It affects children in good health, but conditions such as anemia and malnutrition are predisposing factors. There are two types of impetigo: bullous and vesicular. This discussion focuses on the more common vesicular type, impetigo contagiosum.

Impetigo contagiosum is a contagious, acute, superficial, vesiculopustular form of impetigo. The organism is disseminated by direct physicial contact from another infected individual or through insect bites. The most common sites of involvement are exposed areas such as the face and extremities. Multiple lesions are often present.

Clinical Manifestations and Diagnostic Assessment

The lesions begin as small vesicles with a honey-colored serum. Yellow to white-brown crusts form (Fig. 38–12) as the vesicles rupture and extend radially. These lesions have a rapid peripheral spread, so the nurse typically will see a group of lesions forming a circle or arc. The lesions are highly contagious for as long as they exist. Diagnosis is generally possible based on the characteristics of the lesions. Regional lymph nodes may be enlarged.

Therapeutic Management

Treatment of choice for both types of impetigo is systemic antibiotics, unless it is a very localized infection when topical mupirocin (Bactroban) is the drug of choice. Antibiotic therapy should be determined by bacterial culture and sensitivity. While waiting for these laboratory results, empiric treatment with drugs such as oral erythromycin or dicloxacillin or topical mupirocin, which give good coverage against staphylocci and streptococci, should be used. If streptococci are cultured, penicillin V (Pen-Vee K) may be used. Removal of crusts and scrubbing the lesions with antibacterial soaps have not been shown to be effective (Weston & Lane, 1991). Good handwashing techniques and isolation of the infected child's washcloth, towels, drinking glass, and linen are important. The highly contagious nature of this disease should be emphasized. Poststreptococcal glomerulonephritis may follow impetigo if nephritogenic strains of streptococci are involved. The risk of nephritogenic strains of streptococci varies considerably in North America. (Acute glomerulonephritis is covered in Chapter 36.)

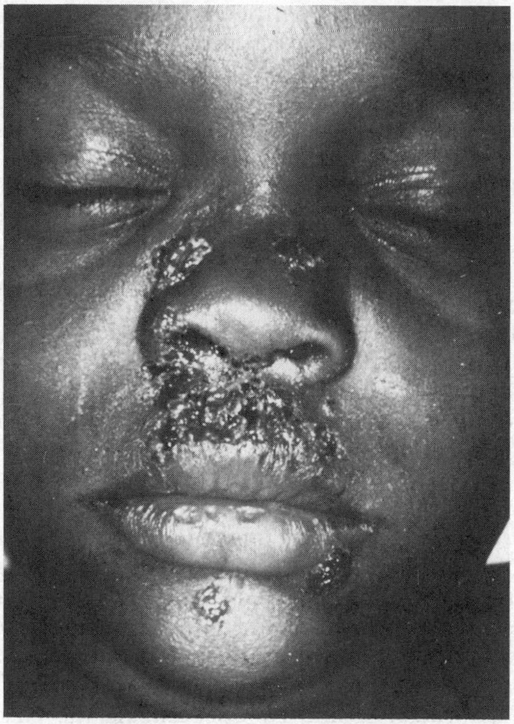

FIGURE 38 - 12. The characteristic distribution of impetigo is about the nose and chin. (From Green, M., & Haggerty, R. J. [1990]. *Ambulatory pediatrics* IV. Philadelphia: WB Saunders.)

Nursing Diagnostic Statements

High risk for ineffective management of therapeutic regimen (parents and child), *risk factor: knowledge deficit, regarding*

- *Antibiotic administration.*
- *Preventing spread of the infection to family members and playmates.*
- *Care of lesions and skin.*
- *Signs and symptoms of disease complication, acute glomerulonephritis.*

Nursing Care

Teaching Antibiotic Administration. The family must be instructed how often to give the antibiotic and impressed with the importance of giving the child all of the medication in properly spaced doses so that an antibiotic-resistant strain of streptococci will not develop. Penicillin V (Pen-Vee K) is better absorbed when taken after a meal than on an empty stomach. Question the child and parent about previous reactions to penicillin or other medications. Instruct them to call the physician should any signs of drug hypersensitivity result: rash, fever, hives, pruritus, or difficulty breathing.

Erythromycin is probably the most frequently used oral antibiotic. It is less effective in an acid medium; pills that have been crushed or chewed will be partially inactivated by stomach acid. Erythromycin should not be given with fruit juice. Generally, it is best to administer it on an empty stomach, 1 hour before meals or 3 hours after.

Preventing Spread of Impetigo. Parents should be cautioned that impetigo lesions are highly contagious. Children in school or in day care should remain at home until they have been taking antibiotics for 48 hours and/or the lesions are dry. Contamination among siblings can be limited by frequent and thorough handwashing and by encouraging the child not to touch the lesions. The infected child should not share towels and washcloths with other family members.

Teaching Care of Lesions and Skin. Good daily skin care is important while treating impetigo and to prevent it from recurring. Once- or twice-daily soaking baths followed by application of an antibiotic ointment (Bacitracin) or a simple bland emollient (Vaseline or Aquaphor Ointment) to the base of cleansed lesions is helpful to promote healing and decrease itching if present. Scratching the lesions may result in secondary infection despite the administration of antibiotics. Mits may be necessary for the infant or small child. Children are best discouraged from scratching by distraction and comfort techniques.

Routine bathing and moisturizing of the skin are the best prevention because they keep the skin barrier intact and inhibit the invasion of microorganisms. Minor breaks in the skin and insect bites should be washed with soap and water, and a topical antibiotic preparation applied to any minor wound that begins to appear inflamed.

Alerting the Family to Signs and Symptoms of Acute Poststreptococcal Glomerulonephritis. In geographic areas where impetigo often leads to acute glomerulonephritis, a urinalysis should be performed at the time of diagnosis and the child should be followed for at least 7 weeks following healing of the lesions (Hurwitz, 1981). Parents should alert the physician if the child's urine output significantly decreases (decreased wet diapers or voiding) or if the urine changes color. (Acute glomerulonephritis is covered in Chapter 36.)

Cellulitis

Cellulitis is a bacterial infection of the subcutaneous tissue and the dermis. The most common causative organisms are staphylococci, group A beta-hemolytic streptococci, and, in children under 5 years of age, *Haemophilus influenzae,* type b (Melish, 1992). The infection usually occurs at or near the site of a wound or previous trauma. Often, the initial wound is so minor it was overlooked.

Clinical Manifestations

In the classic course of cellulitis, a red, tender, warm swelling appears within a day or two of the original skin trauma. The swelling rapidly increases to produce a large, firm area of edema. A bluish hue within the lesion is seen, particularly with *H. influenzae* cellulitis in infants, but can be seen with other bacterial origins as well. The child experiences pain as a result of the intense pressure of the inflammatory exudate on skin tissues. Fever, lethargy, and regional lymphadenopathy are also common findings. Cellulitis can occur anywhere, but some of the common sites are fingertips, periorbital cheeks, and over large joints.

Therapeutic Management

Whereas mild cases of cellulitis may be treated with oral antibiotics at home, children are often admitted to the hospital for intravenous antibiotics, especially if acutely ill or with periorbital cellulitis. Prompt administration of the appropriate antibiotic is essential. Antibiotic choice is often penicillin, dicloxacillin, ampicillin (alone or in combination with chloramphenicol) or cephalosporins, depending on suspected etiology. Intravenous therapy is continued until there is a noticeable reduction in the redness and edema.

Nursing Care

The antibiotics given for cellulitis are frequently quite irritating to veins, and special attention must be given to the onset of phlebitis. The child with venous irritation will often complain of burning during administration, the site of intravenous injection will be especially tender, and the redness may begin creeping up the vein. Irritation can be lessened by reducing the rate of administration and by mixing the drug to the maximal dilution. If more than one antibiotic is being administered, the nurse must check whether the drugs can be safely administered through the same intravenous line.

The child with cellulitis will often be irritable from the discomfort of the edematous area and from fear of or discomfort from the intravenous therapy. Palpation of the edematous area is especially painful, and assessment of this nature should be held to the minimum needed to ensure that edema is not increasing. A mild analgesic such as acetaminophen

(Tylenol) can significantly decrease pain, and the child can be further comforted by rocking, being distracted with toys for quiet play, and having the presence of a parent or family member. Warm soaks may also help to relieve pain and may enhance healing by increasing blood circulation (and thereby circulation of antibiotic) to the area.

Furuncles and Carbuncles

Pathophysiology and Etiology

A "furuncle," or boil, is an acute localized perifollicular staphylococcal abscess of the skin and subcutaneous tissue that undergoes necrosis and suppuration.

Development of a furuncle results from obstruction of a sebaceous gland or ingrowth of a hair follicle. Typically, a furuncle is preceded by a superficial staphylococcal folliculitis. A small pustule enlarges around the hair follicle, becoming firm, red, and tender. The lesion becomes fluctuant and will eventually drain purulent material, allowing healing to occur in 1 to 2 weeks. Furuncles may occur at any age. In children, they are most commonly seen in staphylococcal carriers and those with chronic nutrition problems, immunodeficiency states, and other debilitating diseases (Demis et al, 1979).

"Carbuncles" represent a more severe and extensive skin infection than furuncles. The incidence of carbuncles is greater in males and is seen most often in children with diabetes, hypogammaglobulinemia, and other resistance-lowering diseases. This perifollicular abscess affects adjacent hair follicles and drains through multiple openings in the skin; thus, carbuncles are often described as multiple furuncles. The neck, back, and thighs are common sites for abscess development. The simple pustule develops slowly, enlarges to the size of an egg or an orange, and causes extensive pain. When carbuncles drain, the entire center lesion may slough off a large amount of necrotic material, leaving a large ulcerated area. The ulcer will granulate in several weeks, but a scar is usually present.

Diagnostic Assessment and Therapeutic Management

Furuncles occur most commonly in the neck, buttocks, extremities, perineum, axillae, and face. The child may initially experience itching but usually will ignore the pustule until it enlarges and causes pain. Malaise and an elevated temperature (38.3 to 38.9° C or 101 to 102° F) are other presenting symptoms. Diagnosis is made by isolation of *S. aureus* from the purulent drainage. Simple furuncles can be treated with heat alone. Referral to a physician is warranted if the child is experiencing intense pain and the lesion does not drain spontaneously. Large boils are carefully incised and drained and treated with topical antibiotics. Occasionally, a systemic antibiotic is ordered, depending on the results of culture and sensitivity tests and if extensive surrounding cellulitis or fever is present.

Children with carbuncles will usually experience general malaise, fever, and chills and complain of severe pain. The nurse will easily recognize a carbuncle from its large size, red color, and tenderness. Any child presenting with this skin condition should be referred to the physician for diagnosis and immediate treatment. Management usually includes systemic antibiotics, rest, and warm, moist compresses. Analgesics may be needed if the pain is severe.

Nursing Diagnostic Statements

Altered health maintenance (home management of condition), *related to knowledge deficit regarding*
- *Treatment.*
- *Prevention of spread of the staphylococcal organism to other breaks in skin integrity or to other persons.*
- *Hygiene practices to prevent recurrence.*
- *Measures to alleviate discomfort.*

High risk for occurrence and recurrence of furuncles and carbuncles, *risk factors:*
- *Previous exposure to staphylococcal infection(s).*
- *Chronic nutrition problems.*
- *Concurrent immunodeficiency state or other debilitating disease.*

High risk for ineffective family coping with need for excision, *risk factor: family unprepared for procedure.*

Nursing Care

Nursing care for home management of a boil includes careful instruction on good handwashing, a daily bath and shampoo, avoiding hand contact with the pustule, and disposing of drainage in a closed container. Fingernails should be kept short and clean. The child's towels, washcloths, sheets, and clothing should be separated from those used by the rest of the family and should be washed daily.

The application of warm, moist compresses may alleviate some of the child's discomfort. Children with draining lesions may attend school if bandages are used to cover the area. Clean, dry gauze is placed over the area but may need to be changed while the child is in school. The nurse can help change the bandage and evaluate whether further treatment is necessary. This is also an opportunity for the nurse to demonstrate proper handwashing and disposal of the soiled dressing. Also, assess the child's discomfort; if pain is severe, attendance at school should be evaluated. The school nurse can contact the child's teacher and arrange for make-up work to be done at home.

Children with furuncles will benefit from knowing that the skin infection is only temporary and there will be no residual scarring.

Nurses working with children identified as "at risk" should facilitate early treatment by teaching the signs and symptoms of furuncles. When teaching good skin care to children, they should include a description of furuncles, and children should be cautioned against "picking" at infected hairs. Recurring furuncles may require checking family members for staphylococcal carriers.

Recurrence of carbuncles is common, and children prone to development of this skin condition should avoid skin irritation from constrictive clothing.

Occasionally, excision of the carbuncle is necessary to promote drainage. The nurse should prepare the child and parents for the excision in these ways: (1) describe the procedure and equipment to be used, (2) describe possible pain the child may feel, and (3) discuss whether the child wants to have his or her parents present during the treatment. Adequate preparation for treatment enhances the child's coping abilities and promotes parental support. (See Chapter 17 for specific measures to use in preparing children and families for procedures.)

Hordeolum (Stye)

Clinical Manifestations

A "stye" is the result of an acute staphylococcal infection of the glands on the margin of the eyelid that produces a small abscess. There will be pain and redness, localized on the lid margin, with preauricular lymph node enlargement. The lid around the area may become tender and swollen. Superficial abscesses come to a head, rupture spontaneously, and heal completely without treatment.

Nursing Care

If the abscess does not either reabsorb or come to a head (point) on its own within 1 to 2 days, treatment consists of localizing the abscess by applying warm, wet compresses for 20 to 30 minutes four to six times a day, followed when necessary by application of a topical ophthalmic antibiotic or sulfa ointment. If the condition does not improve, a culture and sensitivity test may be necessary to find an effective medication. Children who have repeated styes should have their vision checked because, although styes have nothing to do with vision problems, children with a refractive error do a lot of rubbing, which can contribute to the development of styes. Rarely, incision and drainage of the abscess by a physician may be required.

Herpes Simplex Virus Type I

There are four types of human herpesviruses: herpes simplex virus (HSV types 1 and 2), cytomegalovirus (CMV), Epstein-Barr virus (infectious mononucleosis), and varicella-zoster virus. Other herpesvirus infections are covered in Chapter 39. With all types of herpesvirus, the immune status of the host determines whether and to what degree the virus will be manifested.

HSV type 1 is classically the "oral" type of herpes ("cold sores," "fever blisters") and type 2 has been known as the "genital" type. Clinical distinction between the two types has become less clear, however, with increasing practices of oral-genital sex, and it is now known that either type can affect any given region of the body (Kohl, 1992). This discussion is confined to the type 1 virus, which is not classically passed through sexual contact.

Incidence and Etiology

Exposure to herpesvirus is widespread. Among young children from a lower socioeconomic environment, 40 to 60 per cent are seropositive by the age of 5 years. Most of these children will, by adulthood, exhibit HSV type 1 antibodies. The incidence is somewhat less in higher socioeconomic populations, with only about 30 per cent of university students showing serologic evidence of HSV infection.

HSV is transmitted by infected body fluids, such as saliva, coming in contact with microscopic or larger breaks in the skin or mucous membranes. Newborn infants may acquire HSV in passage through an infected birth canal. Nurses and other health care workers can (and do) transmit HSV between patients when handwashing protocols are overlooked. Children especially susceptible to HSV are those with burns, infants with diaper rash or eczema, and those immunosuppressed by illnesses or drug therapy (e.g., children with leukemia or other cancers) (Kohl, 1992).

Pathophysiology

In most cases HSV type 1 infection occurs at the site of entry on the skin or mucous membranes. HSV shows particular affinity for tissues that arise from the ectoderm (epidermis, hair, nails, cutaneous and mammary glands, anterior pituitary gland, tooth enamel, inner ear, lens of the eye, and nervous tissue). The infected cells swell and degenerate, leading to local inflammation (nonspecific immune response) and subsequent formation of antibodies (specific immune response). Vesicles form, become infected by resident bacteria on the skin, form pustules, ooze, dry, and crust. Lesions on mucous membranes usually present as shallow ulcers. HSV type 1 lesions are superficial and do not leave scars, although following pronounced lesions, skin color under the lesion may be altered for a few weeks. The incubation period between contact with the virus and appearance of infection is 2 to 20 days.

Once a patient is infected with HSV, the virus remains latent, probably within nerve cells innervating that portion of the skin originally infected. HSV can be reactivated by several factors, including fever, emotional upset, exposure to sunlight, trauma, menstruation, and immunodepression.

Clinical Manifestations

The most common form of HSV type 1 in children is gingivostomatitis, herpes infection of the mouth. Vesicular lesions can be found on the lips, gums, tongue, and hard palate. The breath may have a particularly foul smell. Cervical and submental lymph nodes are usually enlarged. As the vesicles break, shallow gray ulcers are left that are extremely painful. The child usually refuses to eat or drink and dehydration becomes a concern. Resolution of the lesions occurs spontaneously within 10 days to 2 weeks. In adolescents, HSV type 1 may present as pharyngitis with painful, ulcerative lesions on markedly swollen tonsils.

Therapeutic Management

Management of oral herpes is usually symptomatic and can be handled in the home unless fear of dehydration results in hospitalization for administration of intravenous fluids. Intravenous, oral, or topical acyclovir (Zovirax) may be effective in severe cases but has had little testing in children (Kohl, 1992).

Nursing Care

Gingivostomatitis is a particularly distressing illness for both the child and the family caretaker. The child will be extremely irritable because every swallow of saliva or liquids brings intense pain from oral lesions and, perhaps, from lesions in the throat. The fetid breath is unpleasant for caretakers, and, even if one can convince the child to swish with a diluted mouthwash (e.g., quarter-strength hydrogen peroxide) or gently brush the teeth, the odor returns almost immediately. Parents become exhausted because comfort measures and other care are often necessary throughout the night. Attempting to swallow during sleep may cause the child to awaken with a cry.

The nurse who is aware of the discomfort associated with this disorder can provide the family with a good deal of support and reassurance. In addition, the nurse can advocate prescription of oral anesthetics and analgesics to reduce the pain.

Parents will need to be reassured that the child will not be harmed by a few days without solid food. They must realize the necessity of fluids, however. Minimal fluid requirements to prevent dehydration should be calculated on the basis of body weight (see Chapter 26) and translated for the parent into household measures. The nurse may suggest keeping a chart to mark down the sips of fluid taken and suggest that "success" be measured by the ability to entice the child to take one sip at a time throughout the day and night. Fluids must be bland, and parents will need an explanation of that term, e.g., no fruit juices or salty liquids. Milk-based fluids (including pudding), noncarbonated or "flattened" soft drinks, gelatin, electrolyte solutions (Gatorade), and Kool-aid preparations are often best tolerated. Parents should know that the first overt sign of dehydration will be decreased urination, with increased color and odor to the urine. The physician should be contacted at the first sign of dehydration. Guidelines for care that are as specific as possible can help to relieve unnecessary anxiety. If the nurse works in a setting that allows time to do so, a phone call to the family can support their efforts and answer questions that have arisen since diagnosis.

Molluscum Contagiosum

Etiology

"Molluscum contagiosum" is a common, highly contagious, viral infection of the skin and, occasionally, conjunctiva that frequently affects children. A poxvirus that induces epidermal cell proliferation causes this disease. The characteristic molluscum body is composed of mature, immature, and incomplete viruses and cellular debris.

Clinical Manifestations

The lesions are discrete, skin-colored or pearly white, slightly umbilicated, dome-shaped papules that appear anywhere on the skin or conjunctiva. The distribution in children is mainly on the trunk, face, and extremities. In sexually active young adults, they are commonly seen in the pubic area and genitalia. The prevalence of this viral, sexually transmitted disease has increased dramatically since the early 1970s. There is usually no inflammation surrounding the molluscum lesions unless they are manipulated. Scarring can occur with healing.

The best diagnostic procedures are (1) staining smears of expressed molluscum body, (2) examining a biopsy, or (3) inoculating a suspension into cell culture to demonstrate cytotoxic reactions. The diagnosis most often confused with molluscum is warts.

Therapeutic Management

Most lesions are self-limiting and clear in 6 to 9 months if not manipulated. However, many times it is difficult to keep from manipulating the lesions. When manipulated, they often spread. The papules can be removed by curet or destroyed with liquid nitrogen. However, if multiple lesions are present, these procedures are painful to children and not justified. Measures to prevent the spread of infection must be taken. Children must be taught not to manipulate or stratch these lesions. Recurrences are common.

Other Infectious Skin Conditions

Other skin conditions that are infectious by nature are described in Chapter 39. These conditions include fungal infections (tinea pedis, tinea capitus, tinea corporis) and parasitic conditions (scabies, pediculosis).

KEY CONCEPTS

Concepts Related to Basic Information

- The skin is the body's primary physical barrier and has a vital protective function.
- Children's skin is thinner and more easily damaged than adult's skin.
- The skin of young children is not as effective a physical barrier as mature skin.
- Infants have poorly developed subcutaneous fat, making them more prone to hypothermia.
- Skin function is influenced by genetic and hormonal factors, cleanliness, hydration, nutrition, and emotional state.

Concepts Related to Nursing Assessment

- Because the skin often reflects health or illness conditions in the body, assessment of the skin is an extremely important facet of physical assessment of any child.
- Neonates have a number of normal skin variants that the nurse must be aware of when assessing newborn infants, including acrocyanosis, mottling, harlequin color change, erythema toxicum, mongolian spots, and "stork bites."
- Skin lesions can be an important clue to congenital problems.
- Skin turgor is one of the primary methods of assessing hydration.

Concepts Related to Nursing Intervention

- Skin is the most visible part of our body and skin changes can greatly influence developing self-concept.
- Nursing care of many skin disorders involves symptomatic treatment of itching, scaling, weeping, and/or crusting lesions, including the application of topical preparations.
- Teaching protection of skin from sun damage is an important part of anticipatory guidance for parents, school-age children, and adolescents.
- A vital part of the nursing care of adolescents with acne is addressing the effect it has on self-concept.

REFERENCES

Demis, D., et al (Eds.). (1979). Furuncles and carbuncles. In *Clinical dermatology*. New York: Harper & Row.

Dobson, R. (1984, August). An interview with the president of the American Academy of Dermatologists. In *Stress tied to problems with skin. St. Louis Post-Dispatch,* p. 19.

Green, M., & Haggerty, R. J. (1990). *Ambulatory pediatrics (IV)*. Philadelphia: WB Saunders.

Hill, M. J. (1990, February). The skin: anatomy and physiology, *Dermatology Nursing, 2*(1), 13–17.

Hurwitz, S. (1981). *Clinical pediatric dermatology*. Philadelphia: WB Saunders.

Kahn, G. (1988). Principles of diagnosis and treatment of skin disorders. In C. W. Bierman & D. S. Pearlman (Eds.). *Allergic disorders from infancy to adulthood* (2nd ed., pp 377–384). Philadelphia: WB Saunders.

Kohl, S. (1992). Postnatal herpes simplex virus infection. In R. D. Feigin & J. D. Cherry (Eds.). *Textbook of pediatric infectious diseases* (3rd ed., pp 1558–1582). Philadelphia: WB Saunders.

Laudano, J. B., Leach, E. E., & Armstrong, R. B. (1990). Acne: Therapeutic perspectives with an emphasis on the role of isoretinoin. *Dermatology Nursing, 2*(6), 328–377.

Leyden, J. J., & Shalita, A. R. (1986). Rational therapy for acne vulgaris: An update on topical treatment. *Journal of the American Academy of Dermatology, 15*(4, Pt. 2), 907–915.

Lookingbill, D. P., & Marks, J. D., Jr. (1993). *Principles of dermatology* (2nd ed.). Philadelphia: WB Saunders.

McCaffery, M. (1972). *Nursing management of the patient with pain*. Philadelphia: JB Lippincott.

Melish, M. E. (1992). Bacterial skin infections. In R. D. Feigin & J. D. Cherry (Eds.). *Textbook of pediatric infectious diseases* (3rd ed., pp 820–830). Philadelphia: WB Saunders.

Nicol, N. H. (1987). Atopic dermatitis: The wet wrap. *American Journal of Nursing, 87*(12), 1560–1563.

Nicol, N. H. (1989). Early detection and prevention of skin cancer. *Dermatology Nursing, 89*(1), 11–20.

Siedel, H., Ball, J., Davis, J., & Benedict, G. (1991). Skin, hair and nails. In *Mosby guide to physical examination* (pp 91–140). St. Louis: Mosby Year Book.

Stern, R. S., Weinstein, M. C., & Baker, S. G. (1986). Risk reduction for nonmelanoma skin cancer with childhood sunscreen use. *Archives of Dermatology, 122,* 537–544.

Strauss, J. S. (1987). Update on acne. *Primary Care, 14*(1), 167–176.

Weston, W. L., & Lane, A. T. (1991). *Color textbook of pediatric dermatology*. St. Louis: Mosby Year Book.

BIBLIOGRAPHY

Books

Arndt, K. W. (1989). *Manual of dermatologic therapeutics* (4th ed.). Boston, Toronto: Little, Brown.

Bondi, E. E., Jegasothy, B. V., & Lazarus, G. S. (1991). *Dermatology diagnosis and therapy*. Norwalk, CT, San Mateo, CA: Appleton & Lange.

Fitzpatrick, T. B., et al. (1987). *Dermatology in general medicine: Textbook and Atlas* (3rd ed.). New York: McGraw-Hill.

Sams, W. M., & Lynch, P. J. (1990). *Principles and practice of dermatology*. New York: Churchill Livingstone.

Schachner, L. A., & Hansen, R. C. (1988). *Pediatric dermatology*. New York: Churchill Livingstone.

Rosen, T., Lanning, M., & Hill, M. (1983). *The nurse's atlas of dermatology*. Boston, Toronto: Little, Brown.

Weston, W. L., & Lane, A. T. (1991). *Color textbook of pediatric dermatology*. St. Louis: Mosby Year Book.

Articles

Acne

Laudano, J. B., Leach, E. E., & Armstrong, R. B. (1990). Acne: Therapeutic perspectives with an emphasis on the role of isotretinoin. *Dermatology Nursing, 2*(6), 328–337.

Nicol, N. H. (1992). All about acne: A model workshop. Pitman, NJ: Dermatology Nurses' Association.

Pochi, P. E., Shalita, A. R., & Whiting, D. A. (1989). An update on acne management. *Patient Care, 23,* 85–88, 91–92.

Shalita, A. R., Pochi, P. E., & Leyden, J. D. (1991). Symposium: Acne therapy in the 90s. *Journal of International Postgraduate Medicine, 4,* 3–16.
Stern, R. S., Rosa, F., & Baum, C. (1984). Isotretinoin and pregnancy. *Journal of the American Academy of Dermatology, 10,* 851–854.
Strauss, J. S. (1987). Sebaceous glands. In T. B. Fitzpatrick et al (Eds.). *Dermatology in general medicine: Textbook and atlas* (3rd ed.). New York: McGraw-Hill.

Atopic Dermatitis

Clark, R. A. F., Nicol, N. H., & Adinoff, A. D. (1990). Atopic dermatitis. In M. Sams & P. Lynch (Eds.). *Principles and practice of dermatology* (pp 365–380). Philadelphia: WB Saunders.
Clark, R. A. F., Nicol, N., & Adinoff, A. (1990). Current concepts in the management of the patient with atopic dermatitis. *Modern Medicine, 58*(3), 78–94.
Nicol, N. H. (1987). Atopic dermatitis: The (wet) wrap-up. *American Journal of Nursing, 87*(12), 1560–1564.
Nicol, N. H. (1990). Current considerations and management of atopic dermatitis. *Dermatology Nursing, 2,* 129–138.
Nicol, N. H., & Clark, R. A. F. (1988). Therapy of atopic dermatitis. In E. Farmer & T. Provost (Eds.). *Current therapy in dermatology—2.* Philadelphia: BC Decker.

Psoriasis

Abel, E. A., et al. (1986). Drugs in exacerbation of psoriasis. *Journal of the American Academy of Dermatology, 15,* 1007–1022.
Dunn, M. L., et al. (1988, August). Treatment options for psoriasis. *American Journal of Nursing, 88*(8), 1082–1087.
Ellis, C. N., & Voorhees, J. J. (1987). Etretinate therapy. *Journal of the American Academy of Dermatology, 1,* 267–291.
Farber, E. M., & Nall, L. (1984). An appraisal of measures to prevent and control psoriasis. *Journal of the American Academy of Dermatology, 10,* 511–517.

Pruritus

Smith, D. P., & Nicol, N. H. (1991). Controlling pruritus. In D. P. Smith (Ed.). *Comprehensive child and family nursing skills: Assessment and intervention* (pp 503–510). St. Louis: CV Mosby.

Skin Cancer Prevention

Keesling, B., & Friedman, H. S. (1987). Psychosocial factors in sunbathing and sunscreen use. *Health Psychology, 6*(5), 477–493.
Klingman, A. M. (1969). Early destructive effects of sunlight on human skin. *Journal of the American Medical Association, 210*(13), 2377–2380.
Nicol, N. H. (1989). Actinic keratosis: Preventable and treatable like other precancerous and cancerous skin lesions. *Plastic Surgical Nursing, 9,* 49–55.
Nicol, N. H. (1989). Early detection and prevention of skin cancer. *Dermatology Nursing, 89,* 11–20.
Nicol, N. H. (1989). What's new in sunscreens? Choices, choices, choices. *Pediatric Nursing, 15,* 417–418.
Pathak, M. A., Fitzpatrick, T. B., Greiter, F., & Kraus, E. W. (1987). Preventive treatment of sunburn, dermatoheliosis and skin cancer with sunprotective agents. In T. B. Fitzpatrick et al. (Eds.). *Dermatology in general medicine: Textbook and Atlas.* (pp 1507–1522). New York: McGraw-Hill.
Rumsfield, J. (1990). Sunscreens: What you and your patients should know. *Dermatology Nursing 2*(3), 139–147.
Scotto, J., & Fears, T. R. (1987). The association of solar ultraviolet and skin melanoma incidence among caucasians in the United States. *Cancer Investigation, 5*(4), 275–283.
Stern, R. S., Weinstein, M. C., & Baker, S. G. (1986). Risk reduction for nonmelanoma skin cancer with childhood sunscreen use. *Archives of Dermatology, 122,* 537–544.

CHAPTER • 39

Infectious Disease

Kathleen Lord Feroli

RELATED TOPICS
Isolation procedures, Chapter 23
Developmental delays, Chapter 27
Child abuse, Chapter 28
Other respiratory infections, Chapter 32
Infective endocarditis, Chapter 33
Pinworms, Chapter 35
Other gastrointestinal infections, Chapter 35
Other genitourinary tract infections, Chapter 36
Neurologic infections, Chapter 40
AIDS, Chapter 37

LEARNING OBJECTIVES

At the conclusion of reading the chapter, the reader will be able to:

- Discuss the normal immune responses to viruses, bacteria, parasites, and fungi.
- Describe the common communicable diseases of childhood.
- List the important preventive measures for communicable diseases that parents need to know.
- Discuss the nurse's role in providing education concerning communicable diseases.
- Identify the common sexually transmitted diseases.
- Describe educational strategies that nurses may use to combat the spread of sexually transmitted diseases.

During an individual's lifetime, a multitude of microbial contacts are experienced. Infants and children generally experience successive exposure to a variety of viruses and bacteria. Children in generally good health rarely experience devastating illness from these infections, and on recovery, the immunologic response to the microbe that has occurred often renders the child immune to further infection from that particular organism. For some of these diseases, the child can acquire immunity without experiencing the disease through specific vaccinations.

This chapter deals with viral and bacterial infections that are not covered in the body systems chapters. Additionally, diseases that are caused by parasites, fungi, rickettsiae, and protozoa are covered. Vaginal infections and the sexually transmitted diseases other than AIDS are addressed in the final section.

Specific Immune Responses

The general immune response is detailed in Chapter 37. Specific responses to viruses, bacteria, parasites, and fungi are addressed here.

Viruses

Viruses are pathogens that have the capacity to penetrate healthy cells. They possess a special coating that makes them seem benign until they are internalized. When the body cell tries to digest the virus, however, the protective coating is destroyed, releasing viral nucleic acid that takes over the function of healthy cells. Instead of serving the purpose for which the body cell was created, the diseased body cell puts most of its energy into the replication of the virus.

Immune mechanisms that protect against viruses are (1) the anatomic and physiologic barriers (intact skin and mucous membranes, intact cellular layers of the respiratory and gastrointestinal tracts); (2) phagocytes that engulf and destroy viruses; (3) interferon that renders noninfected cells resistant to the virus; and (4) the specific immune response, including macrophages, T-cells, and antibodies. The barrier effect of intact skin and mucous membranes is enhanced by immunoglobulin A (IgA) antibodies, which neutralize many viruses (Fulginiti, 1992).

Bacteria

Intact skin and mucous membranes protect against bacteria as well. Tissue macrophages that reside in the liver, spleen, bone marrow, kidney, and lung help remove bacteria before they gain hold in the body. Bacteria stimulate both T-cell and B-cell responses, and antibodies produced by B-cells (as well as complement components) destroy bacteria. One component of the immune attack against both bacteria and viruses is the inflammatory response, which manifests as fever and malaise in the infected person.

Parasites

The immune mechanisms against parasites are poorly understood. Parasite antigens are complex and elicit a host of responses, which may or may not play any role in immunity: The primary antigens of helminths appear to be secreted by the worm itself. It is known that certain of the helminthic antigens stimulate mononuclear inflammatory cells in the host (Fulginiti, 1992).

Fungi

Fungi gain hold primarily in hosts who are immunocompromised. Fungal diseases that act on the surface of the body (e.g., *Candida albicans* and tinea) produce a localized infection that results in little, if any, immune response. These surface fungi are transmitted to areas within the body by indwelling vascular catheters, endotracheal tubes, and artificial organ parts, especially when antimicrobial therapy is being administered. Antimicrobials alter the normal bacteria that protect against fungi colonization. Prevention is imperative in the immunosuppressed child because fungal invasion of body organs can be lethal.

Diseases of Viral and Bacterial Origin

Childhood Communicable Diseases

A communicable disease occurs when an infectious agent or its toxic products cause an illness or disease. The mode of transmission may be direct or indirect contact. In direct transmission, the person has actual contact with the infected person or reservoir (environment), whereas indirect contact relates to the interaction with contaminated objects (fomites).

Diagnosis of the various childhood communicable diseases is made from visualization of the characteristic lesions and their location and by history of exposure and prodromal symptoms.

The commonalities of treatment are those interventions related to comfort from fever and/or pruritus and to helping the child. Family members must adjust to the temporary isolation measures and prevent transmission of the disease.

Many of the childhood communicable diseases are not highly stress producing for either the child or family members as long as comfort measures are understood and employed. The greater concern for the nurse is to help parents take responsibility for preventing most of the childhood communicable diseases by ensuring current and complete immunization of their children (see Chapter 10 for additional information about immunizations). Table 39–1 gives specific information about each of the childhood infectious diseases and other commonly known viral and bacterial infections.

Cytomegalovirus Infection

Etiology

Cytomegalovirus (CMV) infection, cytomegalic inclusion disease (CID), cytomegaly, and salivary gland disease are synonymous. Cytomegalovirus belongs to a unique group of viruses, the herpes family, in which the primary infection is followed by a latent form that may reactivate in the body at any time. All ages may be affected by CMV, beginning even before birth. It is the most common cause of intrauterine infection. Most infections take place during the childbearing years, between ages 15 and 35.

Transmission of CMV occurs horizontally (direct person-to-person contact) as well as vertically. Salivary contamination is a major source of contact, and infected urine also plays a role in transmission. CMV is not highly contagious, yet spread has been documented in households and day care facilities.

There are three types of CMV infections: congenital, perinatal, and other acquired forms. The congenital form is caused by a primary infection in the mother. The virus crosses the placenta and infects the fetus, causing inflammation and necrosis, especially of the central nervous system (CNS), resulting in brain damage and mental deficiency. Fetuses of mothers infected during the second trimester are most at risk for developing symptoms.

Clinical Manifestations

Ninety per cent of congenitally infected infants are healthy and asymptomatic at birth. The remaining 10 per cent of these infants exhibit symptoms. A small percentage of these infants present with "classic" newborn CID. Perinatally acquired CMV is transmitted at birth through contact with maternal cervical secretions, and the infant experiences mild transient illness. Other acquired forms of the disease are generally asymptomatic, except in immunocompromised patients who may exhibit signs of pneumonia or retinitis. During the early months of life, the infection may be acquired from the mother's breast milk. Table 39–2 lists the clinical manifestations and prognosis of CMV.

Diagnosis

Both congenitally infected infants and those affected perinatally or postnatally excrete large amounts of the virus in the throat and urine, often for many months or years. Diagnosis of CMV depends on isolating the virus from the throat, body fluids, or blood. In the congenitally infected neonate, an elevated IgM (specific CMV antibody) correlates with active disease. In acquired CMV, significantly rising antibody titers are usually sufficient for diagnosis.

Other diagnostic signs that may be found on surface appraisal or in monitoring the child's health status include a petechial rash on the first day after birth, failure to thrive, or repeated respiratory infection with a high incidence of chronic interstitial pneumonia during infancy.

Therapeutic Management

No effective treatment of CMV is known; therefore, preventive measures must be stressed. Recent attempts have been made to treat affected neonates with cytosine arabinoside and adenine arabinoside (metabolic inhibitors that interfere with in vitro synthesis of CMV), and although urinary excretion of the virus was suppressed, the long-term beneficial effects need further study before such drugs can become widely available. Treatment with interferon inducers and various antiviral agents has to date produced minimal effects.

A live vaccine is under active investigation. Research suggests that it is possible to prepare a vaccine that is well tolerated and antigenic and that results in both neutralizing and complement-fixing antibodies. Further work needs to be undertaken specifically in relation to mothers and infants. The safety of widescale use of this vaccine has not been established. Whether the vaccine would increase the potential for neoplastic disease and increase susceptibility to infection and whether giving the vaccine to pregnant women will also afford immunity to the fetus are questions that remain unanswered.

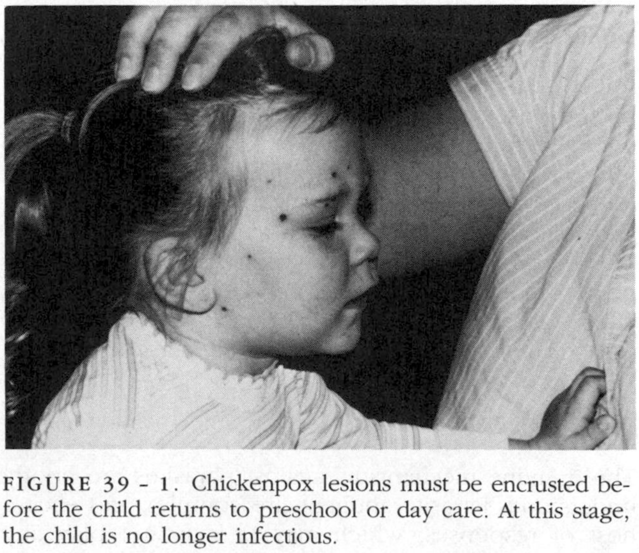

FIGURE 39-1. Chickenpox lesions must be encrusted before the child returns to preschool or day care. At this stage, the child is no longer infectious.

TABLE 39-1
Characteristics of Commonly Known Infectious Diseases

Disease (Agent)	Clinical Manifestations	Complications	Family Teaching	Prevention
Chickenpox (Herpesvirus; also called "varicella-zoster")				
Epidemiology: Highly contagious *Transmission:* Contact, air *Incubation:* 10–21 days *Infectious period:* From 1–2 days before lesions appear until all lesions are crusted (usually 5–6 days from onset) (see Fig. 39–1) *Most common:* Late winter, early spring *Immunity:* Usually lifelong after illness but second occurrences have been reported **Isolation**: Strict†	*Prodromal:* Low-grade fever, malaise, anorexia, occasionally accompanied by a scarlet uniform rash *Acute phase:* Lesions begin as red maculopapular rash, which turns almost immediately to vesicles, each on an erythematous base. Vesicles ooze and crust. New crops of vesicles continue to form for 3–5 days, spreading from the trunk to the extremities. *Pruritus* is an outstanding symptom. Mucous membranes of the mouth and genitalia may be involved, and these lesions may be quite painful. Disease course varies from mild with a few lesions to severe with hundreds of lesions and a high fever *Immunosuppressed child:* Lesions may continue to erupt with fever of up to 40.5° C (105° F) up to 7–10 days from onset. The mortality rate in progressive varicella is 20%	Secondary skin infection with *Staphylococcus* or *Streptococcus,* especially with poor hygiene and increased temperature and humidity. CNS: postinfectious encephalitis most common, also aseptic meningitis, Reye syndrome **Therapeutic Management**: Supportive: antihistamines, antipruritics, mild analgesia (acetaminophen, *not* aspirin), Calamine lotion. Acyclovir for immunosuppressed child or those susceptible to severe varicella lesions	Avoid use of aspirin or aspirin-containing products (because of association with Reye syndrome). Cut nails to decrease irritation from scratching. Cool sponge bath without soap; light, loose-fitting clothing; fluids for fever. Avoid cornstarch soaks (may increase chance for infection). Aveeno baths are particularly helpful and soothing. May use paste of baking soda and water on lesions to control itching. Alert family that premature removal of crusts by scratching may cause permanent scars. Frequent handwashing by child and caregiver. Avoid excessive contact with siblings; successive cases in the same family may be more severe because of overwhelming exposure to virus	Vaccine now available for children at high risk (e.g., children with leukemia). Used with caution in general population because of risk of latent disease and untoward effects of the herpesvirus in later life. Passive immunity with intramuscular serum globulin or zoster immune globulin within 3 days after exposure to children at high risk for complication or fatality. Isolation of high-risk children from known cases
Cholera *(Vibrio cholerae)*				
Epidemiology *Transmission:* Ingestion of contaminated water and food, particularly shellfish *Incubation:* 2–3 days; may be as long as 5 days *Infectious period:* Unknown *Immunity:* Vaccine protects for only a short period in about ½ of people vaccinated **Isolation**: Enteric precautions	Acute onset of watery, painless diarrhea—stool is colorless and contains mucus. Dehydration and electrolyte imbalance often follow. May progress to seizures and coma	Rare **Therapeutic management**: Oral tetracycline 50 mg/kg/day; given for 3–5 days to eradicate the organism. In children younger than 9 yrs, use trimethoprim-sulfamethoxazole	Rehydration is imperative using oral or parenteral fluids. Monitor specific gravity, intake and output, and skin turgor. Follow and report electrolyte results	Drink only boiled water when traveling. Cook thoroughly all shellfish. Cholera vaccine is required for travel outside of the United States to areas of Asia, Africa, and Middle East

(continued)

TABLE 39 - 1
Characteristics of Commonly Known Infectious Diseases *(Continued)*

Disease (Agent)	Clinical Manifestations	Complications	Family Teaching	Prevention
Herpes Zoster (Herpesvirus hominis; also called "shingles") A latent infection produced by same virus that causes chickenpox				
Epidemiology *Transmission:* Contact, air *Incubation:* 4–24 days; person with shingles may give chickenpox to someone who has never had the disease *Infectious period:* As for chickenpox *Immunity:* Second attacks occur in fewer than 1% **Isolation:** Same as chickenpox†	*Prodromal:* Pain and itching along ganglion lines for 1–5 days before lesions erupt. Pain is burning, stabbing, worse at night and with movement *Acute phase:* Lesions located along the ganglion of peripheral nerve roots, most commonly in the thoracic area. Always unilateral eruption that does not cross midline. Successive crops of vesicles for 1–4 (or up to 7) days. Eruptions clear in 7–14 days	Rare. Encephalitis, secondary bacterial infection. **Therapeutic Management:** As for chickenpox. May employ soaks of Burow solution to aid drying of lesions. Analgesia for pain. Acyclovir or vidarabine to retard viral activity	Avoid use of aspirin. Cut nails to decrease irritation from scratching. Frequent handwashing. Attention to comfort—both pharmacologic and nonpharmacologic; plan diversion for child whose mobility is limited by zoster lesions	Isolate from those who have not had varicella
Mumps (Paramyxovirus; also called "parotitis")				
Epidemiology: Only slightly less contagious than rubella and measles *Transmission:* Contact, air *Incubation:* 12–25 days (usually 16–18 days) *Most common:* Late winter, early spring *Immunity:* Considered lifelong from clinical or subclinical infections, although rarely a second case occurs **Isolation:** Respiratory†	*Prodromal:* Rare, but possibly fever, muscular pain, headache, malaise *Acute phase:* Unilateral or bilateral swelling of parotid glands (lymphocyte infiltration of glands with cell necrosis and blockage of openings) and/or other salivary glands; ⅔ of cases symptomatic; ⅓ subclinical. Swelling peaks by 3rd day, returns to normal by 10th day. Chewing and sour liquids or foods aggravate the earache-like pain	Meningoencephalitis; orchitis, epididymitis (especially in adolescents) with atrophy of the affected testes occurring in 30–40%, impaired fertility in 13%; pancreatitis, nephritis; thyroiditis; myocarditis; mastitis, deafness; visual complications, arthritis **Therapeutic Management:** Symptomatic	Liquid or soft bland diet as tolerated; bed rest with testicular support for orchitis. Acetaminophen for pain. Warm or cold compresses for swelling, whichever increases comfort.	Vaccine (with measles, mumps, rubella [MMR]) given at or after 15 mos of age. Second MMR given at age 11–12 yr unless given previously at school age. Permanent immunity with vaccine or disease, whether or not disease symptomatic
Rubella (Rubella virus; also called "3-day measles," "German measles")				
Epidemiology *Transmission:* Air, transplacental *Incubation:* 14–21 days *Infectious period:* From up to 7 days before rash until rash disappears *Immunity:* Permanent immunity from disease or vaccine **Isolation:** Contact†	*Prodromal:* Young children: none, except for possible lymphadenopathy Older children: lymphadenopathy, low-grade fever, anorexia, mild conjunctivitis, runny nose, sore throat *Acute phase:* Begins on face and hairline and, as it clears, moves to trunk, then extremities. Also pinpoint rose-red spots on soft palate. Rosy red, dry, maculopapular rash, diffuse configuration, lasts 3 days	Postinfectious encephalitis, arthritis, thrombocytopenia. Virus crosses placenta in pregnancy, causing birth defects, especially if mother exposed in first trimester. Congenital rubella may lead to deafness, visual anomalies, congenital heart defects, musculoskeletal defects, CNS anomalies, immunologic defects **Therapeutic Management:** Supportive	Self-limiting activity, acetaminophen for fever or headache	Vaccine (with MMR) at or after 15 mos of age. Second MMR given at age 11–12 yr unless given previously. *Isolate from pregnant females*

Measles, Rubeola (Paramyxovirus; also called "hard measles," "red measles," "regular measles")				
Epidemiology *Transmission:* Contact, air *Incubation:* 8–12 days *Infectious period:* From 7 days after exposure until 5 days after rash appears *Immunity:* Permanent from vaccine or disease **Isolation:** Respiratory†	*Prodromal:* Fever and cold-like symptoms, conjunctivitis, photophobia, nasal congestion, hacky cough. Koplik spots (white spots circumscribed in red, opposite lower molars). Fever increases to about 39.5° C (103° F) *Acute phase:* Rash begins as fever peaks; fever then subsides. Dark-red, dry, maculopapular rash begins behind ears and at hairline and spreads from head to feet. Lasts 10–15 days. Rash turns brown and scaly after 5–6 days. Young children may have associated vomiting, diarrhea, or otitis media	Otitis media, laryngotracheitis, pneumonia, encephalitis, appendicitis **Therapeutic Management:** Supportive for uncomplicated cases: acetaminophen, antitussives	Bed rest or quiet activities as tolerated during febrile period, then gradual return to normal activity. Increased fluids during fever; sponge baths for comfort; room humidification for cough; dimly lit room or sunglasses for photophobia; cleanse eyes to remove crusts, discourage rubbing of eyes; pharmacologic and nonpharmacologic comfort measures; diversionary activities	Vaccine (with rubella, mumps; MMR) at or after 15 mos of age. Second MMR given at age 11–12 yr unless given previously
Roseola Infantum (Herpesvirus 6, sixth disease, 3-day fever)				
Epidemiology *Transmission:* Unknown *Incubation:* Unknown *Infectious period:* Unknown; most cases in children 6–24 mo of age **Isolation:** None†	Sudden onset high fever—39.4–41.2° C (103–106° F), possibly with slight irritability and mild coldlike symptoms. Fever falls rapidly on the 3rd–4th day, and a macular or maculopapular rash appears on the trunk, spreading to the rest of the body. Rash fades within 24 hr	Febrile seizures, rarely: encephalitis, hemiplegia, permanent paresis, mental retardation **Therapeutic Management:** No specific treatment. Acetaminophen for fever	Often child not diagnosed until fever crisis is over and rash beginning. If seen at this time, reassure parent that the rash will fade quickly and child will soon feel well. If seen during febrile period, teach regarding temperature measurement and methods to safely lower temperature	None at present because of multiple viruses linked to cause
Erythema Infectiosum (Human parvovirus; also called "fifth disease")				
Epidemiology *Transmission:* Air *Incubation:* 7–28 days (commonly 16 days) *Infectious period:* Uncertain; probably only during prodrome; no longer infectious when rash appears; therefore, isolation not required **Isolation:** None†	*Prodromal:* headache, chills, muscle aches, malaise, then free of symptoms for about 7 days before acute phase *Acute phase:* Three rash stages. Stage 1 rash: bright-red cheeks (slapped-cheek appearance) with circumoral pallor; fades in 1–4 days. Stage 2 rash: red, symmetric, maculopapular; begins 1 day after stage 1 rash disappears. Starts on trunk, then extremities and buttocks. Lasts 2–40 days (average 11 days). Frequently pruritic; headaches common. Stage 3 rash: periodic recurrence, especially with exercise, environmental temperatures, emotional upset, or skin irritation. Fades from center in lacy appearance	Arthralgia to arthritis (less than 10% of children), transient hemolytic anemia, encephalitis **Therapeutic Management:** No specific treatment, analgesics for joint involvement	Parents may need help in explaining disease to school personnel. School attendance allowed. Saline baths or Calamine lotion for pruritus. Acetaminophen for joint aches or headache. Prepare family for prolonged nature of rash and recurrence in stage 3	No vaccine available

(continued)

TABLE 39-1
Characteristics of Commonly Known Infectious Diseases *(Continued)*

Disease (Agent)	Clinical Manifestations	Complications	Family Teaching	Prevention
Pertussis (*Bordetella pertussis;* also called "whooping cough")				
Epidemiology: Highly contagious *Transmission:* Air, direct contact with nasopharyngeal secretions, contact with contaminated fomites* *Incubation:* 6–20 days (average, 7 days) *Infectious period:* From catarrhal stage through the 4th wk *Immunity:* Vaccine provides limited immunity (wanes with age); antibody for pertussis does not cross placenta–newborn has no protection; permanent immunity with disease **Isolation:** Respiratory†	*Catarrhal stage:* Lasts 1–2 wks. Upper respiratory infection–like symptoms, headache, low-grade fever, sneezing, irritating cough, anorexia *Paroxysmal stage:* Lasts 4–6 wks. Cough worsens, developing to spasms and ends with prolonged inspiration (crowing or "whoop" sound). Cough spasm often followed by vomiting of large amounts of thick, stringy mucus; may appear to be strangling during paroxysm. Paroxysms initially occur several times per hour, decrease to 3–4 per day. Attacks triggered by yawning, sneezing, eating, drinking, exertion. *Not* all children will have whoop-type cough. Young infants in particular tend not to have whoop but often exhibit apnea *Convalescent stage:* Lasts 1–2 wks, although cough may persist for months. Any intercurrent respiratory infections may result in cough, vomiting. Cough gradually decreases, vomiting stops, appetite and strength return	Pneumonia responsible for >90% of deaths from pertussis in children <3 yr old. Otitis media, seizures, ulcer of the frenulum of the tongue, epistaxis, melena, subconjunctival hemorrhages, rupture of the diaphragm, umbilical or inguinal hernia, rectal prolapse, dehydration, CNS and nutritional disturbances **Therapeutic Management:** Erythromycin to shorten period of communicability (to 3–4 days from start of administration). Supportive care with oxygen, hospitalization in early stages	During hospitalization: *Maintain patent airway* with gentle suction during paroxysms; monitor respiratory and cardiac effort per noninvasive oxygen monitor and cardiorespiratory monitor. *Maintain hydration* via oral and intravenous fluids as ordered; monitor urine specific gravity, skin color and turgor. Small, frequent feedings; often best tolerated immediately after a vomiting episode. *Conserve energy:* cool room with good ventilation, antipyretics and decreased clothing to control fever; calm, supportive manner to comfort child during paroxysms; plan for uninterrupted naps when possible; plan care to avoid tiring infant/child *Monitor for signs of pneumonia. Support family in home care during convalescent stage* • Teach to use and clean room humidifier; keep room free of dust, smoke, temperature extremes • Encourage tepid liquids often; small, frequent feedings after vomiting • Teach to suction as necessary to relieve strangling effects of mucus expectoration during paroxysms • Teach signs of impending respiratory distress (see Chapter 32) • Teach signs of pneumonia, otitis media. Encourage follow-up care	Vaccine (with diphtheria, tetanus [DPT]). Despite risk of neurologic sequelae from vaccine, children are at *much* greater risk for neurologic damage, pneumonia, and death if they contract the disease. Siblings and others <7 yrs exposed to disease who have not completed 4 doses of DPT or who have not received DPT within 3 yrs of exposure should receive DPT vaccine; oral erythromycin may also be given to close contacts
Diphtheria *(Corynebacterium diphtheriae)*				
Epidemiology: Transmission: Air, direct contact, fomites* *Incubation:* 1–6 days *Infectious period:* 2–4 wks without therapy, 1–2 days after start of therapy; until child no longer harbors or-	Depends on site of diptheritic membrane: *Nasal:* Most common in infants. Mild coldlike symptoms, few systemic signs. Nasal discharge becomes serosanguineous, then mucopurulent, ex-	Respiratory obstruction leading to death, vocal cord paralysis, myocarditis, neurologic complications, paralysis of eye muscles or diaphragm, gastritis, hepatitis, nephritis **Therapeutic Management:** Intrave-	Initial care will be in the hospital. Maintain patent airway. Maintain hydration by oral and intravenous fluids as ordered. High-calorie liquid or soft diet. Suction excess secretions. Monitor quality of voice, gag reflex. Gavage feedings for pharyn-	Vaccine (given with pertussis and tetanus [DPT]). No permanent immunity; must be maintained through boosters (Tb) at 10-yr intervals

ganism (determined by three consecutive negative cultures) *Immunity:* Vaccine may not always give complete protection; disease gives immunity for 50% of children for 1 yr or more, but immunization needed after recovery **Isolation:** Strict†	coriates upper lip. Foul odor; white membrane on nasal septum *Tonsillar/pharyngeal:* Initially anorexia, malaise, low-grade fever, pharyngitis. White or gray adherent membrane covers tonsils, pharyngeal surfaces, possibly into larynx, trachea; bleeding results if membrane disturbed; possible cervical lymphadenopathy. In mild cases, membrane sloughs in 7–10 days followed by recovery. In severe cases cardiopulmonary collapse may occur *Cutaneous:* Ulcerative skin lesions on a membranous base	nous antitoxin to neutralize free toxins; skin or conjunctival test for sensitivity to horse serum must precede administration. Antibiotics; bed rest for 2–3 wks to reduce risk of myocarditis; tracheostomy for laryngeal obstruction	geal or palatal paralysis. Place on cardiorespiratory monitor; auscultate chest regularly. Alert parents to need for follow-up care and regular immunizations after recovery	
Tetanus *(Clostridium tetani)*				
C. tetani is a spore-forming bacillus. Spores are harmless until body conditions are right for their conversion to vegetative forms that multiply. The clinical symptoms are caused by toxins from the vegetative cells **Epidemiology** *Transmission:* Introduced into an area of injury from contaminated soil or intestinal contents *Incubation:* 1 day to several months (commonly 3–21 days) *Immunity:* Vaccine gives time-limited immunity; second attacks after disease are rare **Isolation:** None†	Classically trismus (lockjaw), spasm of the masticatory muscles with difficulty opening the jaw. Also irritability, restlessness, stiff neck, dysphagia, rigidity of the abdominal or thoracic muscles. Tonic spasms may also involve the neck, back, and abdomen, leading to opisthotonus. Generalized seizures triggered by very slight external stimuli	Lethal glottal and laryngeal spasms, hyperpyrexia, tachycardia, hypotension, cardiac arrest, death in 45–55% **Therapeutic Management**: Administration of tetanus antitoxin; surgical removal of the site of entry of the organism (to eliminate the toxin "factory"); sedatives, muscle relaxants, neuromuscular blocking agents, penicillin; close monitoring of fluid, electrolyte, and calorie balance	Because of the extremely serious nature of this disease, the child will be cared for in an intensive care unit. Nursing strategies, for the nurse generalist, pertain to prevention, particularly the proper cleaning and débriding of all wounds	Vaccine (given with diphtheria and pertussis [DPT]) as a basic series in childhood with follow-up boosters, and every 10 yrs in the adult *The importance of vaccination is underscored by the fact that the portal of entry in 80% of cases is an insignificant wound!* The environment of the tissue is optimal for tetanus to develop in the following wounds: burns, injuries induced by blank cartridges, deep punctures, furunculosis, dental extraction, embedded splinters, decubitus ulcers, hypodermic injections, compound fractures complicated by chronic active osteomyelitis
Poliomyelitis (Poliovirus)				
Epidemiology *Transmission:* Air, contact (fecal-oral) *Incubation:* 14–21 days *Infectious period:* Virus in throat for 1 wk after onset, in feces intermittently for 3–4 wk **Isolation:** Enteric precautions†	*Abortive type:* Brief febrile illness—fever seldom >39.5° C (103° F) along with one or more of the following: malaise, anorexia, nausea, vomiting, headache, sore throat, constipation, abdominal pain *Nonparalytic type:* As for abortive, but headache, nausea, becoming more intense with muscle stiffness of neck, trunk, limbs. Progresses to nuchal and spinal rigidity, changes in reflexes	Paralytic polio: intestinal erosion, hypertension, cardiac irregularities, acute pulmonary edema, pulmonary embolism, skeletal decalcification, renal calculi **Therapeutic Management** *Abortive:* Supportive treatment at home with analgesics, sedatives, bed rest until fever is normal for several days. Antibiotics and immunoglobulins not effective. Careful follow-up	*Abortive:* Teach regarding use of analgesics, nutritious diet, emphasize need for bed rest with gradual return to activity; need for follow-up care *Nonparalytic:* As for abortive, with addition of application of hot packs or warm tub baths for stiff muscles, firm bed, footboard *Paralytic:* In hospital: total care as for paralysis from other causes (see Chapter 40)	Vaccine (oral polio vaccine) given at 2 months, 4 months, 15–18 months, and prior to entry into elementary school

(continued)

TABLE 39-1
Characteristics of Commonly Known Infectious Diseases *(Continued)*

Disease (Agent)	Clinical Manifestations	Complications	Family Teaching	Prevention
	Paralytic type: As for nonparalytic, plus weakness of one or more skeletal or cranial muscle groups progressing to paralysis, including paralysis of bowel and bladder muscles and paresis of respiratory muscles. Vital signs reflect damage to medullary centers	*Nonparalytic:* As for abortive *Paralytic:* Hospitalization with attention to airway maintenance, maintenance of joint and muscle function, bowel and bladder programs		
Scarlet Fever (Group A beta-hemolytic *Streptococcus;* also called scarletina and septic sore throat)				
Epidemiology *Transmission:* Air, direct contact *Incubation:* 1–7 days (average, 3 days) *Infectious period:* Variable, until 1–2 days after start of therapy **Isolation:** Drainage precautions if pharyngitis present†	Abrupt high fever, abdominal pain, vomiting, sore throat, headache, malaise. In early days, tongue has white coat through which edematous red papillae project (white strawberry tongue); white coat sloughs, leaving prominent papillae (strawberry tongue). Rash appears within 12–48 hr of onset: red, papular sandpaper-like rash; appears first in axillae, groin, neck, but then becomes generalized; fades on pressure, almost always leads to desquamation. Flaking begins on face, spreads to entire body	Extension of *Streptococcus:* otitis media, pneumonia, peritonsillar abscess, rheumatic fever, acute glomerulonephritis **Therapeutic Management:** Penicillin is drug of choice (prevents rheumatic fever). Bed rest during febrile stage, analgesics for comfort	Ensure compliance with complete 10-day course of therapy. Monitor fever, antipyretics as needed. Maintain bed rest; provide diversion. Cool-mist humidification; liquid or soft diet for sore throat. Alert family to need for follow-up care. Instruct regarding signs and symptoms of complications	Throat cultures for suspected streptococcal infection; administration of *all* of antibiotic ordered. For repeated recurrent infections, all family members should be cultured

Influenza (Orthomyxoviruses of 3 types—A, B, C—and multiple subtypes)				
Epidemiology *Transmission:* Air, direct or indirect contact *Incubation:* 1–7 days (commonly 2–3 days) *Infectious period:* Influenza A—6 days before onset of symptoms until 1 wk after onset Influenza B—1 day before onset of symptoms to 2 wk after recovery *Immunity:* Persists *for that type of virus* for several years after natural infection in older children but is probably of shorter duration in infants and young children. Immunity from vaccine is time limited and restricted to viruses in the vaccine **Isolation:** Contact†	*Influenza A:* Sudden onset with systemic symptoms of fever (>38.9° C or 102° F) and chills, headache, anorexia, malaise, muscle aches, cervical adenopathy. Respiratory symptoms of cough, runny nose, sore throat, sputum production, hoarseness; sometimes accompanied by abdominal pain, vomiting, nausea, diarrhea *Influenzas B and C:* Similar signs and symptoms but less severe and of shorter duration	Pneumonia, otitis media, sinusitis most common. Also acute myositis, Reye syndrome, neurologic disease, pericarditis, myocarditis, glomerulonephritis, sudden death **Therapeutic Management:** Symptomatic: bed rest, adequate oral hydration, control of fever and muscle aches with acetaminophen, nasal decongestants, humidified air, cough suppressants for persistent cough during convalescence. Amantadine given orally twice a day for 2–7 days will decrease the severity of influenza A	Teach caregiver to take the child's temperature and appropriate methods for temperature control. Talk with the family about the amount of fluid that should be ingested in 24 hrs and suggest age-appropriate measures to encourage this consumption. Alert them to signs of dehydration (e.g., significant decrease in number of wet diapers). Teach signs and symptoms of impending airway obstruction so that family may seek medical assistance before an emergency arises. Teach caregiver how to suction nares with bulb syringe to relieve mucus plugging in infant and small child. Encourage follow-up care to rule out secondary infection or other complications	Vaccine for high-risk children (chronic illness or immunosuppression). Keep child away from crowds during flu season

Data from Behrman, R. E., & Vaughan, V. C. (Eds.) (1992). *Nelson textbook of pediatrics* (14th ed.). Philadelphia: WB Saunders; Feigin, R. D., & Cherry, J. D. (Eds.). *Textbook of pediatric infectious diseases* (3rd ed.). Philadelphia: WB Saunders; Farrar, W. E., & Lambert, H. E. (1984). *Infectious diseases*. Baltimore: Williams & Wilkins; and Lookingbill, D. P., & Marks, J. D. (1993). *Principles of dermatology*. 2nd. ed.). Philadelphia: WB Saunders.

*Fomites are any substances to which infectious agents adhere, e.g., articles of personal grooming, clothing, and linens.

†Isolation procedure related only to hospitalized children.

TABLE 39-2
Description of Cytomegalovirus Infections

Classification			Clinical Manifestations	Prognosis
Congenital		90% asymptomatic	Normal development	Occasional mental retardation
	10%	Symptomatic	Transient jaundice	High recovery
			Purpura	Some with brain damage and mental retardation
			Respiratory illness	
			Hepatosplenomegaly	
			Failure to thrive	
		Symptomatic Classic	Severe jaundice	High mortality
			Thrombocytopenia	Survivors have severe brain damage, mental retardation, microcephaly
			Chorioretinitis	
			Hepatosplenomegaly	
			Pneumonia	
			Encephalitis	
			Seizures	
			Microcephaly	
Acquired		Perinatal	Mild transient illness with symptoms similar to those of congenital symptomatic cytomegalovirus	CNS damage may become evident at school entry
		Neontal and early childhood	Asymptomatic	CNS damage may become evident at school entry
			Occasionally:	
			Respiratory symptoms → pneumonia	
			Hepatosplenomegaly	
			Petechial rash	
		Late childhood and adult	Mononucleosis-type symptoms	

Nursing Care

During the hospitalization of the child with CMV, isolation procedures are instituted, because infants excrete the virus in saliva for approximately 6 months and in urine for 4 months or more. The degree of thoroughness of isolation practices is controversial, varying from careful handwashing to strict isolation. Universal precautions should be instituted. Pregnant women and also children are prohibited from rooms as a preventive measure.

Because the disease seems to occur more commonly in conditions of poor sanitation and overcrowding, the nurse may help families to ensure adequate sanitation.

Complications of congenital CMV may include spastic quadriplegia, mental retardation, obstructive hydrocephalus, or acute respiratory problems. Therefore, management of the child must be individualized and long term. The nurse is especially helpful in coordinating the efforts of the health team and community services involved. Most parental concerns result from the child's failure to attain developmental milestones. Support, understanding and proper referral to agencies designed to work with children with development delays are important.

In patients who are immunosuppressed and require blood or blood products, the CMV status must be checked. If the child is CMV negative, they must be given CMV-negative blood.

The families of children with CMV may be socially isolated owing to the stigma attached to the child who will be excreting the virus over many months. Although the virus is believed to be contagious only on intimate contact, encouraging good hygiene and proper disposal of diapers is imperative in such families. Discussing the rationale for protection of pregnant women and of children may alleviate anxieties.

Infectious Mononucleosis

Infectious mononucleosis is a viral disease often attributed to the dating years. In actuality, it can occur at any age, although rarely before age 2 or after age 40, when most adults are immune. The overall incidence is 50:100,000 population per year, rising to about 1:1000 per year in adolescents and young adults (Plotkin, 1992).

Etiology

Infectious mononucleosis is caused primarily by the Epstein-Barr virus (EBV), a member of the herpesvirus group. In Western countries, 60 to 80 per cent of adolescents are seropositive for EBV, the more affluent being somewhat less likely to have been exposed. Seroconversion increases with age until in the United States nearly all adults test positive for the virus (Plotkin & Henle, 1987). Other infectious agents associated with mononucleosis include CMV, *Toxoplasma gondii,* adenoviruses, rubella, and hepatitis A virus (Brown, 1992).

Clinical Manifestations

The cardinal symptoms of infectious mononucleosis are fever, exudative pharyngitis, malaise, and fatigue, accompanied by lymphadenopathy and hepatosplenomegaly. Frequently there is a 2- to 5-day prodromal period of malaise and fatigue, with or without fever. Fever in the acute phase may be quite high but usually resolves within 2 weeks. Pain may be significant, owing to tonsillitis and pressure from enlarged lymph glands. Swallowing may be impaired, and the adolescent and family caregivers should be alerted to the possibility of pharyngeal occlusion so that they will seek care before a medical emergency arises. Splenomegaly develops in about 50 per cent of cases and hepatomegaly in about 10 per cent (Brown, 1992). Organomegaly usually resolves within 3 months. Other possible clinical signs include a rash, petechiae of the soft palate, bilateral edema of the eyelids, and jaundice. Neurologic complications and aplastic anemia are potential sequelae.

A particularly unpleasant aspect of mononucleosis may be the development of acute ulcerative gingivitis (Vincent infection). The gum margins become swollen with areas of bacterial invasion and necrosis. The breath takes on a persistently fetid odor. Treatment of this infection may be complicated by the contraindication of antibiotics during mononucleosis, especially ampicillin, which causes a rash in persons with mononucleosis.

Diagnostic Assessment and Therapeutic Management

Laboratory analysis usually reveals lymphocytosis (at least 50 per cent lymphocytes), an increase in atypical lymphocytes, a mild to moderate rise in liver enzymes, and a positive mononucleosis test (e.g., Mono-Test, Mono-Diff, and Mono-Spot).

Treatment is primarily supportive, because no effective chemotherapeutic agent has been found other than interferon, which is scarce and expensive. Adenine arabinoside has little activity against EBV, and acyclovir is typically reserved for immunosuppressed patients because it is effective only in high concentrations (Brown, 1992). Several experimental drugs are currently being tested for their clinical efficiency and safety for use against the Epstein-Barr virus.

Nursing Care

The young person may be diagnosed in the prodromal phase of the disease and leave the clinic or physician's office feeling no worse than if he or she had a common virus. The onset of the acute phase of the disease may proceed in this same mild fashion, with only moderate curtailment of activities necessary, or it may result in severe prostration. The adolescent and the family should be alerted to the latter possibility. The severely affected young person should observe bed rest during the acute phase and will often need supportive care from family members. In case of a severely sore throat, an anesthetic gargle can be prescribed to increase comfort. Acetaminophen (Tylenol) may also help for sore throat, fever, and muscle aches.

Fluid intake must be preserved despite the sore throat to offset the dehydrating effects of the fever. Bland, thin liquids or puddings may be best tolerated. Fluid intake should be nutritious as well because significant weight loss may occur from tissue catabolism in relation to the virus.

No isolation precautions are instituted in the hospitalized child with mononucleosis. Once the acute phase resolves, adolescents will need guidance about their return to normal activities. School attendance on a half-day basis is one way to ease back into activities until the student feels stronger. Vigorous athletic activities and contact sports should be avoided until organomegaly has resolved because of the danger of splenic rupture. Whereas recovery may be prompt for some people, it is not unusual for a return to full vigor to require several months. If this should be the case, adolescents may need repeated support and encouragement that they will indeed recover.

Hepatitis

Hepatitis (inflammation of the liver) is a viral disease of three major distinct types: hepatitis A, hepatitis B, and hepatitis C. Recently, hepatitis D and an enterically transmitted non-A, non-B hepatitis (hepatitis E) have been identified. In the United States, there are estimated to be 70,000 cases of hepatitis yearly (Brunell, 1992).

Hepatitis A and hepatitis B were for a long time referred to as "infectious hepatitis" and "serum hepatitis," respectively, because of a recognized oral-fecal mode of transmission in A and parenteral mode of transmission in B. However, research has shown that both types can be transmitted parenterally and nonparenterally so that the names "serum hepatitis" and

TABLE 39-3
Characteristics of Hepatitis A, Hepatitis B, and Hepatitis C

Characteristic	Hepatitis A (Short-Incubation Hepatitis)	Hepatitis B (Long-Incubation Hepatitis)	Hepatitis C (Long-Incubation Hepatitis)
Agent	Hepatitis A virus	Hepatitis B virus	Unknown; more than one agent
Mode of transmission (direct or indirect transmission possible in all three types)	Primarily fecal-oral secretions (stool, urine, semen, tears, menses) and in contaminated food (especially shellfish), breast milk, and water. Transmitted rarely, if at all, by blood transfusion. Virus will cross placental barrier in third trimester	Primarily parenteral route via serum, blood, and blood products; also detected in saliva, semen, vaginal secretions, and even breast milk. Virus will cross placental barrier in third trimester	Parenteral route (accounts for approximately 90% of post-transfusion hepatitis). Other routes suspected but not well defined. Perinatal transmission is rare
Incubation period	15–50 days	60–180 days	14–115 days
Recovery time	Average 28–30 days	Average 90 days	Average 45 days
Carrier state	No	Yes (persistence of HB_sAg† in blood for years or life)	Yes
Isolation	Enteric isolation	Blood and body fluids precautions	Enteric isolation
Seasonal variation	Greatest incidence in winter; rare in summer	None	None
Pre-exposure or postexposure prophylaxis	Ig* 80–90% effective; may cause long-lasting natural immunity	HBIg‡ or Ig effective for 3–4 mos; hepatitis B vaccine gives long-lasting immunity	Unknown; effectiveness of Ig unproved

Adapted from Aach, R. D. (1992). In R. D. Feigin & J. D. Cherry (Eds.), *Textbook of pediatric infectious diseases.* (3rd ed., pp 677–697). Philadelphia: WB Saunders; and Brunnell, P. A. (1992). Hepatitis. In R. E. Behrman & V. C. Vaughan (Eds.), *Nelson textbook of pediatrics* (14th ed., pp 818–823). Philadelphia: WB Saunders.

*Ig = immunoglobulin.
†HB_sAg = Hepatitis B surface antigen.
‡HBIg = Hepatitis B immunoglobulin.

"infectious hepatitis" are no longer meaningful. "Hepatitis A" refers to an acute clinical disease with a short incubation period (average 25 to 30 days) and hepatitis B to clinical disease with a long incubation period (average 120 days). "Hepatitis C" refers to clinical disease resembling hepatitis B, but in which tests do not confirm hepatitis A or B antigens. Table 39-3 summarizes the similarities and differences in characteristics of each of the hepatitis forms.

Pathophysiology and Clinical Manifestations

Characteristic liver changes in hepatitis are liver cell damage, spotty necrosis, and inflammatory infiltrate. The clinical course of hepatitis varies considerably from one infected person to another. In more than 50 per cent of cases, the disease is subclinical or mild, causing mild, nonspecific symptoms (Aach, 1992). Children and young adults are particularly likely to have a subclinical response, resulting in the spread of infection before recognition of the disease. In a small number of people, however, hepatitis is severe, develops rapidly, and may lead to death from liver failure.

Hepatitis may be a self-limiting illness, but in some cases, it becomes chronic. Both the type of hepatitis and the age at infection play a part in the predilection to chronic hepatitis. Infants who contract hepatitis B in the first 12 months of life have about an 80 per cent chance of chronic infection, whereas children from 1 to 10 years of age have a 40 per cent chance. The percentage decreases with age and is less than 10 per cent for adults (Aach, 1992).

Hepatitis A is generally considered to be a milder illness than hepatitis B or hepatitis C. The clinical manifestations are indistinguishable between types, however. Hepatitis may be categorized as icteric or anicteric. The term "icteric" designates the presence of jaundice. "Anicteric" hepatitis is more frequent than the icteric type, especially among children and young adults.

The major preicteric symptoms experienced by 65 to 95 per cent of persons with clinical hepatitis are severe anorexia, lassitude, weakness, fever, headache, abdominal discomfort or pain, and nausea, often accompanied by vomiting (Aach, 1992). Other manifestations include coldlike symptoms of cough, sore throat, and runny nose, with diarrhea or constipation. Persons with the anicteric variety of hepatitis usually experience less intense symptoms for a shorter duration.

Commonly, lessening of the preicteric symptoms heralds the appearance of the icteric phase—jaundice, dark urine, and light stools. These signs correspond with increased blood bilirubin from obstruction of biliary flow and damage to liver cells. Absence of bilirubin in the bile leads to light or clay-colored (acholic) stools. Conjugated bilirubin in the urine leads to a brownish urine color. Deposition of bile pigments in the skin produces the characteristic deep yellow of jaundice and may lead to pruritis.

Jaundice deepens rapidly over a period of days and then begins to fade. Urine and stool color typically return to normal before skin color. The average duration of jaundice in children with hepatitis A who are younger than 15 years is 10 days, with full recovery within 3 weeks from the onset of jaundice. The icteric phase and recovery times are somewhat longer for hepatitis B and hepatitis C.

Diagnostic Assessment

The diagnosis of hepatitis may be made on a history of possible contact and laboratory evidence of liver damage. Direct and indirect serum bilirubin are elevated with or without jaundice. (Icteric signs do not occur until plasma bilirubin values are higher than 2 mg/dl.) The serum transaminases (serum glutamic-oxaloacetic transaminase and serum glutamic-pyruvic transaminase), released in response to liver damage, often exceed 1000 units, peaking about the time jaundice appears. Lactate dehydrogenase (LDH) is also elevated but offers little additional information to that provided by the transaminases. Serum alkaline phosphatase is elevated but rarely exceeds two or three times the normal value. The prothrombin time and other clotting parameters are normal unless the hepatitis is of the severe fulminating variety or malnourishment is involved.

Therapeutic Management

Management of hepatitis is supportive, usually involving care at home unless the child has severe fulminating or subacute varieties of hepatitis. Limited activity is advised, although complete bed rest is not deemed necessary (Brunell, 1992). Children should not return to school until jaundice has resolved and the serum enzyme levels are no more than twice the upper limits of normal. Children need not be isolated from other family members, but good handwashing is imperative. Parents should be cautioned about giving the child any over-the-counter medications without the physician's advice because most medication is detoxified in the liver. Adolescents should be warned to avoid alcoholic beverages during the illness and recovery period.

Household contacts of a child infected with hepatitis A will be given Ig, which is 80 to 90 per cent effective in preventing hepatitis A if given within 2 weeks of exposure. The degree of protection Ig offers for persons exposed to hepatitis B is less certain. Persons exposed to hepatitis C may be given Ig as well, although the extent and duration of protection remain unclear.

Hepatitis B vaccine has been recommended for those at high risk of exposure to body fluids since the vaccine's development. In 1992, the American Academy of Pediatrics (AAP) began recommending universal immunization of infants against hepatitis B beginning immediately after birth as a strategy to reduce transmission of the virus. The AAP also recommended universal immunization of adolescents when resources permit. If resources do not allow for universal immunization of adolescents, then adolescents at high risk should be immunized. Adolescents at high risk include those who are sexually active, have contact with chronic hepatitis B virus carriers, or who live in areas with high rates of intravenous drug abuse, teenage pregnancy, or sexually transmitted diseases (Nowicki & Balistreri, 1992).

Persons exposed to hepatitis B may be given hepatitis B Ig to provide passive protection for the current exposure and at the same time may begin a three-dose series of hepatitis B vaccine to obtain longer-lasting immunity.

If the child with hepatitis is hospitalized, isolation precautions will be part of the plan of care. Although hospital policies differ among institutions, most hospitals now observe the *universal precautions* recommended by the Centers for Disease Control (CDC). Under universal precautions, blood and body fluid precautions are consistently observed for ALL patients, regardless of their diagnosis or blood-borne infection status. That is, blood and certain body fluids for any patient are considered potentially infectious for human immunodeficiency virus (HIV), hepatitis B virus, and other bloodborne pathogens. (See Chapter 23 for further discussion of universal precautions and blood and body fluid precautions.) *The implementation of universal precautions is intended to supplement, not replace, other category-specific or disease-specific isolation precautions.* (General isolation guidelines are discussed in Chapter 23.)

Nursing Diagnostic Statements for Hepatitis

Activity intolerance, *related to decreased metabolism of carbohydrates, proteins, and fats associated with liver disease.*

Altered nutrition: less than body requirements, *related to anorexia and the increased nutrient demands associated with the infectious process.*

Altered comfort: pruritus, *related to jaundice.*

Risk for infection: close contacts of ill child.

Risk factors: transmission of hepatitis in blood, urine, or feces.

Nursing Care/Interventions

In uncomplicated hepatitis, most nursing care will involve teaching the child and family to care for the illness at home.

Limiting Activity. Although bed rest is no longer prescribed for hepatitis, limited activity is advised to decrease the metabolic workload of the diseased liver. Quiet play indoors or play confined to a sandbox or other small area outdoors can be advised to discourage running and other strenuous activities. Quiet school work activities can be encouraged for older children and adolescents. Care at home will certainly lessen the diversionary problems that arise for hospitalized children with activity restrictions, but planning for additional quiet activities can reduce the frustration for both child and caregiver.

Optimizing Nutrient Intake. Anorexia is a major problem for children with hepatitis. When children feel ill and out of sorts and are confined to their home for several weeks, eating is one of the few things over which they have much control. When the caregiver is urged to ensure the child consumes nutritious food to help in the healing process, the stage is set for a power struggle at meal time. The nurse can be helpful in alerting the parent to the possibility of this scenario and working with the family to circumvent some of the problems.

The physician will usually prescribe a diet low in fat and high in protein for the child. The nurse can talk with the parent about foods the child likes that fit that distinction and suggest that these be offered in several small meals or snacks throughout the day rather than in normal portions. Nausea may be less a problem in the morning and breakfast may be a time when nutritious foods are better tolerated. In the long run, it is usually advisable to set the desired food before the child in small portions and then let the child choose whether or not to eat. Generally, the child's intake will be sufficient with this method as long as non-nutritious snacking is not allowed.

Relieving Pruritus. Only about one third of children with icteric hepatitis experience pruritus, but for those who do, it can be quite uncomfortable. Suggest to the family that they try cool tub baths or emollient baths (e.g., Aveeno) and apply creams such as Eucerin to the skin immediately after bathing to reduce dryness. A cool environment will reduce perspiration, which potentiates itching. Teach the child to apply firm pressure to areas that itch rather than to scratch them. Keep the child's nails short and clean to minimize skin irritation from scratching. Administer antihistamines and antipruritic lotions as ordered. Alert the family, however, that these drugs are rarely effective by themselves and that nonpharmacologic measures should be used as well.

Preventing Spread of Infection. Education of the public about new recommendations concerning hepatitis B vaccination should be pursued at each contact with families. Families with newborn infants will receive this information during routine care, but eligible adolescents and their families may not have this information disseminated to them.

When infection with any type of hepatitis has occurred, the family and child should be educated about the transmission of the virus (information depending on the type of hepatitis) and taught to protect themselves and others. They should be provided with a box of disposable gloves and taught to use them when in contact with bodily secretions from the infected child (especially blood, urine, and feces). Family members should avoid sharing linens, drinking glasses and utensils, toothbrushes, and other personal articles. Teach the family to make a 1:10 solution of household bleach in water for the purpose of disinfecting contaminated surfaces. Encourage family members to follow through with appointments for administration of Ig and hepatitis B vaccine, as appropriate.

Rabies

Etiology

Rabies is a disease of the CNS that is transmitted to humans in the saliva of infected wild animals such as squirrels, skunks, bats, foxes, and raccoons, as well as domestic cats and dogs. It is caused by a neurotropic virus, which travels from the peripheral nerves to the CNS. Preschool children are more frequently bitten by cats and dogs. They are losing their fear of animals and think of even wild animals as potential pets but do not yet understand that certain animals can transmit serious disease. Older children, particularly teens, who participate in camping or hunting are more likely to be bitten by infected wild animals. The incidence of rabies is steadily increasing in the United States.

In dogs the incubation period is 3 to 8 weeks, whereas in humans it is 2 to 6 weeks but may be as long as 2 years. A rabid animal does not usually behave like a healthy animal; it staggers and runs blindly and is more aggressive. It may drool and hide after biting another animal or a human, because rabid animals seek seclusion for death. A rabid animal can transmit the disease by licking abraded skin or mucosa. If the animal doing the biting has been properly immunized against rabies, it will probably not transmit the rabies virus even if it was bitten by a rabid animal.

Clinical Manifestations

The disease has three stages. The first is the *prodromal* stage, which lasts about 2 to 4 days and is characterized by itching, tingling, or burning at the area of the bite. This is followed by fever, headache, nausea, sore throat, and irritability or restlessness. Increased salivation, diaphoresis, and sensitivity to bright lights and noises are also evidenced during this stage.

The next stage is the *excitement* (or *furious*) stage. The child becomes increasingly excitable and apprehensive; muscle twitching and generalized convulsions occur. Throat spasms occur when the child tries to eat or drink and even when the sound of running water is heard. The name "hydrophobia" (morbid fear of water) comes from this symptom. There is also spasm of the respiratory muscles and, at times, continuous tonic convulsions. The temperature frequently is from 39.5° to 40.5° C (103° to 105° F). This stage lasts 1 to 3 days, and many patients die at this time.

If the child survives the excitement stage, the third stage, called the *paralytic,* or *terminal,* stage, occurs. There is increasing paralysis and coma, and then death. Only one documented case of a person surviving rabies has been reported, and that child was treated vigorously for each symptom before the symptom developed (Vella, 1977).

Therapeutic Management

Prevention of the disease is of major importance. Most communities have ordinances requiring immunization of pets. Leash laws should be enforced, and all stray dogs and cats should be picked up for confinement or destruction. Children should be taught early to treat pets kindly and to avoid stray or sick animals, whether tame or wild. Programs should be instituted to control wildlife population during rabies epidemics. When a child is bitten by *any animal,* tame or wild, or licked by *any unimmunized* or *wild animal,* the site should be washed immediately and flushed with copious amounts of soap and water, followed by an application of 70 per cent alcohol or povidone iodine. In an emergency, any alcoholic liquor of 86 per cent proof or greater can be used. The child should then be evaluated by a physician to determine what, if any, prophylactic treatment should be initiated. The need for tetanus administration should be determined. The wound should be cleaned again in the doctor's office. Suturing, if necessary, should not be done immediately, because it is believed that closing the wound may cause the virus to spread.

History taking is important, especially if the child was alone at the time of the bite. The child is asked to describe the animal, because he or she might not know what the animal was. Keeping a picture book of animals available for the small child to pick out the kind that caused the bite can be helpful.

Children are asked to describe what they were doing when the animal bit them. Unprovoked attacks are more likely to be from rabid animals. Many children provoke animals such as cats and dogs, without realizing it, while hugging the animal or helping it to eat. A bite from a familiar animal that is healthy does not usually produce rabies; however, the parent should be sure of the animal's immunization status, and the animal should be confined for 10 days to be observed for signs of rabies. If the animal is unknown, all efforts should be made to locate it. If it cannot be located or if the animal is a bat, regardless of the bat's condition, rabies treatment should be instituted. If the animal has been killed or found dead, the head should be packed in ice and sent to the state Department of Public Health or to a competent veterinarian for examination. Any time a domestic animal that has been confined develops symptoms of rabies, it should also be killed and the head sent for examination.

Rabies treatment uses a rabies vaccine in conjunction with rabies serum (Table 39–4). The vaccine allows the child to develop his or her own active immunity. Human diploid cell vaccine (HDCV) is now the only vaccine licensed in the United States. It replaces previous vaccines that required 14 to 21 doses. HDCV is usually given in five intramuscular doses: on the day of exposure, and at 3, 7, 14, and 28 days.

Passive immunity is provided with human rabies immunoglobulin (RIg). This provides protection from rabies until the body can make antibodies in response to the vaccine.

The child and parents will need substantial psychological support and preparation to cope with the treatment as well as the gravity of the situation. Instruction should be given regarding the side effects and their relief. Reassurance should be offered as to the satisfactory results obtained by prophylactic antirabies treatment in preventing this dreaded disease.

TABLE 39-4
Postexposure Antirabies Treatment Guide

Animal	Evaluation of Animal at Time of Exposure*	Treatment of Exposed Human
Wild	Regard as rabid unless brain negative for rabies virus	HRIG + HDCV†
Skunk		
Fox		
Raccoon		
Coyote		
Bat		
Domestic	Healthy	None‡
Dogs	Escaped (unknown)§	HRIG + HDCV†
Cats	Rabid or suspected rabid	HRIG + HDCV†
Other		Consult veterinary public health authorities

Modified from Plotkin, S. A., & Clark, H. F. (1992). Rabies. In R. D. Feigin & J. D. Cherry (Eds.), *Textbook of pediatric infectious diseases* (3rd ed., pp 1657–1666). Philadelphia: WB Saunders.

These recommendations are only a guide. They should be used in conjunction with knowledge of the animal species involved, circumstances of the bite or other exposure, vaccination status of the animal, and presence of rabies in the region.

HDCV = human diploid cell vaccine; HRIg = human rabies immunoglobulin.

*An exposure is considered to be a bite, a scratch with claws, or contamination of mucosal surfaces or skin that has been cut or abraded with saliva.

†Discontinue vaccine if fluorescent antibody tests of the animal are negative.

‡Begin HRIg + HDCV at first sign of rabies in biting dog or cat during holding period (10 days).

§If the behavior of the animal is suspect or if rabies is constantly present in the animal community in the area.

Tuberculosis

Tuberculosis is a long-term, communicable disease caused by a bacillus, *Mycobacterium tuberculosis.* In developed countries, the morbidity and mortality rates for this disease have dramatically declined in the last 50 years. However, in many countries, tuberculosis remains a leading cause of death, particularly in urban and nonwhite populations. High rates of infection have recently surfaced in institutionalized persons, homeless, and HIV-infected persons.

Children are the most vulnerable to this infection during their first 3 years of life and again in the years immediately before, during, and after puberty. Many factors have contributed to decline in the incidence of tuberculosis in children. Earlier diagnosis and treatment of infected adults, who are a primary source of infection for children, have been accomplished by comprehensive public health screening programs. These programs identify and test all known contacts of people diagnosed with active tuberculosis. Another important factor in declining incidence has been the discovery and use of new, effective antituberculin drugs. Public health nurses making field visits to patients' homes have succeeded in effecting an increased compliance with drug therapy. Under current laws, food handlers and all school employees are required to receive annual tuberculosis screening tests for detection of exposure to the bacillus. Routine screening by simple skin testing of children between the ages of 12 and 18 months has also contributed to the control of tuberculosis in children.

Etiology and Pathophysiology

The usual mode of communicability is inhalation of aerosolized sputum (cough spray) from another infected human. The spread of tuberculosis *(Mycobacterium bovis)* by drinking milk from an infected cow has almost been eliminated in the United States owing to mandatory pasteurization of commercial milk.

Once a susceptible child inhales bacilli, organisms begin rapid multiplication in lung tissue, alveoli, or lymph glands draining lung areas. Following an incubation period of 2 to 10 weeks, the child will demonstrate a systemic hypersensitivity as evidenced by a positive skin test. In this test, bacilli are injected immediately under the epidermis, forming a wheal. If the child has been exposed to tuberculosis and subsequently formed antibodies, a local induration will develop at the injection site. This simple skin test can be used as a screening tool to detect exposure to tuberculosis.

Most children exposed to inhaled *M. tuberculosis* mobilize a defensive inflammatory reaction. As a part of this defensive reaction, white blood cells, especially macrophages, are deployed to attack and kill invading bacilli. As further defense, the body walls off small infected areas by the formation of tubercles. Caseous or fibrous tubercles prevent the further spread of infective organisms. Unfortunately, tuberculosis bacilli possess remarkable abilities to remain dormant in this necrotic tissue for many years. If the child's resistance is later decreased, bacilli may begin to multiply, causing active disease. However, the first 2 years after infection represent the highest risk of disease.

The term "primary lesion," or "focus," denotes the original site of infection. The *primary complex* includes the primary lesion and any nearby lymph nodes that have been invaded. In many children, once the primary lesion is contained in tubercles, subsequent healing will occur through a process of calcification. Although these calcified tubercles may later be visible on roentgenography, they do not indicate active disease. In older children the healed primary lesion is visualized as a scar or shadow. In both cases, it is important to explain to parents the distinction between these findings and active tuberculosis.

In some children, the body's defense mechanisms fail to successfully control the primary lesion. After inhalation, the bacilli may continue to multiply and spread by direct extension into nearby tissues. Or the bacilli may enter the blood and circulate to other sites, setting up multiple foci of infection, resulting in *miliary tuberculosis.*

In summary, following the primary lesion, possible subsequent outcomes are (1) complete healing, (2) persistent quiescent lesions, (3) direct extension of infection at the original site, (4) spread of infection via the circulatory system to sites outside the lungs, or (5) possible reactivation of the lesion at a later date should the patient become debilitated.

Clinical Manifestations and Diagnostic Assessment

The communicability of tuberculosis is increased by conditions of poverty and crowding, which foster poor hygiene. Factors such as malnutrition and fatigue can lower resistance to tuberculosis. There is a higher incidence of tuberculosis among nonwhite and Native Americans and in large urban poverty areas that house transient peoples arriving from areas in which tuberculosis is widely disseminated.

In assessing whether a child is at risk for tuberculosis, the nurse must recognize that children are usually infected by adults with progressive cavitary lesions. These adults discharge droplets containing infective organisms into the air. Droplet residue remains in the air for long periods. However, prolonged contact is usually necessary before a child develops active disease.

Periodic testing of children to determine whether they have been exposed can be done by the nurse using any one of several skin tests (see Chapter 10 for a discussion of tuberculosis skin testing). Diagnosis of tuberculosis infection relies on the use of tuberculin skin tests because isolation of the organism from bodily fluids is often time consuming and difficult.

If a positive skin test results from the screening, the nurse may assume the major responsibility for explaining the significance of a positive skin test to parents and to the child. If the multiple-puncture screening test is positive, a Mantoux tuberculin test is applied for confirmation. At this time, the nurse obtains a health history for each family member in an attempt to identify the source of the infection. All contacts are listed so that they may be screened also. The nurse provides information about further diagnostic measures and arranges for treatment. Family members need counseling as well as information. Many adults view tuberculosis not only as a serious threat to life but also as a threat to the integrity of their family unit.

Children with positive skin reactions receive chest roentgenographs to determine the presence and extent of active lesions. A diagnosis of active disease is documented if sputum smears show the presence of bacilli. Gastric washings to obtain swallowed sputum are sometimes done. A child may be hospitalized for this procedure; he or she receives nothing to eat during the night and until test completion. In the morning, a nasogastric tube is inserted and stomach contents are lavaged and removed for microscopic examination. Obtaining sputum from a young child can be extremely difficult. Physicians often prefer to waive such tests rather than submit the child to a period of hospitalization, placing him or her on medication instead.

In some countries a bacille Calmette-Guérin (BCG) vaccination is given to produce immunity to the bacillus. This artificial immunity is effective for at least 10 years. Widespread use of BCG vaccine has not been adopted in the United States, primarily because it would eliminate skin testing as an effective case finding tool.

There is a dangerous trend away from routine tuberculosis screening. Failure to implement screening programs may result in subsequent failure in diagnosing tuberculosis in its early stages. The effect will necessarily be an increase in incidence and also an increase in serious complications such as miliary tuberculosis and tuberculosis meningitis. Such complications are largely preventable with early diagnosis and treatment.

Most children found to have tuberculosis have a noncomplicated pulmonary primary focus and are not infectious. The organisms are confined to a small area of the lung, and the child has little or no coughing. However, if a child (usually a teenager) develops a cavitary lesion and is coughing up sputum containing bacilli or if the child has direct drainage from an infected site, he or she is a potential source of infection. Isolation precautions for all items contaminated with organisms and respiratory isolation precautions are required.

Most children will not have any symptoms and will be unaware of their tuberculosis until diagnosis. Knowing that symptoms in children are minimal, the nurse observes for low-grade fever, slight cough, history of fatigue, weight loss, or anorexia. Recognizing age and risk factors can assist the nurse in case finding, but mass screening is the key to early identification.

Therapeutic Management

Management stresses four major interventions: (1) general supportive measures such as adequate rest, gradual resumption of activities, diet, and prevention of other infection; (2) drug therapy; (3) emotional support; and, in some cases, (4) surgery.

Rest, Activity, and Diet. Ensuring that an active youth follows the treatment prescription for adequate rest can present difficulties. Fortunately, bed rest is required only when miliary tuberculosis has affected the child's weight-bearing structures. Bed rest may be desired on occasions when the child is feeling particularly ill and should be enforced during bouts of fever.

There are no restrictions on physical activities during treatment for active tuberculosis, except that participation in competitive sports is discouraged. Nurses should counsel the youth and parents about the need to avoid excessive fatigue and recommend brief rest periods during the day. Sports that do not require strenuous physical activity may appeal to youths.

A nutritionally balanced diet is also part of the treatment program. Nurses cannot assume that children are receiving an adequate diet. A diet history should be obtained by collecting a 24-hour food intake diary kept by the youth. This diary can be an effective tool for both evaluation and teaching. Infected persons usually have reduced retention and utilization of nutrients; therefore, the youth's diet should be carefully planned so that what is taken in is highly nutritious and particularly rich in foods supplying protein and calcium.

Intercurrent infections encourage the spread of tuberculous processes and retard their healing. The additional stress caused by such infections seems to suppress inflammatory response and decrease allergic responsiveness. Youths should limit their exposure to crowds and to infected persons until active disease has been controlled. This requires observant screening of family members, relatives, and friends during the period of active disease.

Drug Therapy. The AAP advocates that all infants and children with positive Mantoux skin tests be treated with isoniazid for 9 months. When there is evidence of active tuberculosis such as demonstrable lesions on a chest roentgenograph, a combination of two antituberculosis drugs is often prescribed. Standard therapy for tuberculosis in the United States and Canada is 6 months of isoniazid and rifampin, usually supplemented for 2 months with pyrazinamide (AAP, 1991). Table 39–5 lists antituberculosis drugs for children.

Multiple drug-resistant strains of tuberculosis have

TABLE 39-5
Drug Treatment of Tuberculosis*

Drug	Daily Dose (per 24 hrs)	Possible Toxic Effects	Nursing Implications
Isoniazid (INH) *Route:* PO, IM, or IV	10–25 mg/kg (up to 300–500 mg total) *Duration:* 6–12 mos	Peripheral neuropathy, hepatotoxicity	INH syrup in sorbitol is unstable at room temperature; must be refrigerated. Tablets may be crushed and given with food but must not be put in nursing bottle or offered in liquid because of uncertainty of amount ingested
Rifampin (RIF, RMP) *Route:* PO	10–40 mg/kg (up to 600 mg) *Duration:* 6–9 mos	Hepatotoxicity	Turns urine and tears red; will stain contact lenses; interferes with oral contraceptives
Ethionamide (ETA) *Route:* PO	10–20 mg/kg *Duration:* 9–12 mos	Gastric irritation, liver damage, peripheral neuritis	Give after meals to minimize gastric irritation
Streptomycin (STM) *Route:* IM	20 mg/kg (up to 1 g) *Duration:* 2–3 mos	Ototoxicity, vestibular damage	Administer deep into muscle mass to minimize pain and local irritation
Pyrazinamide (PZA) *Route:* PO	20–40 mg/kg (up to 1.5 g total) *Duration:* 2 mos	Gout, hepatotoxicity	Assess for fatigue, poor appetite, weakness, irritability, signs of anemia and prodromal signs of hepatitis
Ethambutol *Route:* PO	15–25 mg/kg *Duration:* 9–12 mos	Optic neuritis	Schedule for frequent vision checks while on therapy
Para-aminosalicylic acid (PAS) *Route:* PO	200–300 mg/kg (up to 12 g) *Duration:* 12 mos	Gastric irritation, fever, rash, jaundice	Principal companion to INH for many years; withdrawn from market in United States

Adapted by permission. *The nurses' drug handbook.* (4th ed.). By S. Loebl & G. Spratto. Delmar Publishers, Inc., Albany, New York, Copyright 1986; and Smith, M. H. D., & Marquis, J. R. (1992). Tuberculosis and other mycobacterial infections. In R. D. Feigin & J. D. Cherry (Eds.), *Textbook of pediatric infectious diseases* (3rd ed., pp 1321–1361). Philadelphia: WB Saunders.

*PO = oral; IM = intramuscular; IV = intravenous.

been appearing in recent years among immigrants, persons who are homeless or live in poor, crowded conditions, and among HIV-positive persons (Inselman, 1990). The effect of these strains on tuberculosis in children is unknown. Children who live in households with persons who are tuberculosis positive, live with immigrant adults or in communities with higher than usual tuberculosis case rates, or who are of Native American or Native Alaskan origin should have skin testing performed annually.

Surgery. Whether surgical intervention is desirable depends on the site, nature, and extent of the active tuberculosis focus and the degree of compliance with and effectiveness of drug therapy. Vigorous antibiotic therapy is usually continued despite surgical removal of the involved organ or body tissue to help ensure subsequent healing.

With adequate treatment, the incidence and complications of tuberculosis should continue to decline.

Nursing Care/Interventions

Offering information about the side effects of medication and the importance of faithfully taking drugs each day for the entire course of therapy is a crucial nursing action. Explanation of the serious consequences of failure to take medication as prescribed is an appropriate part of the education. Family members, especially parents, are sometimes upset that a child has to take medication for such a long period. It is important that family members demonstrate the ability to administer the medications to their children.

Other family members, especially those of the grandparents' generation, tend to remember the time when tuberculosis was greatly feared. They may have an inaccurate understanding of current treatment and prognosis, as well as incorrect opinions about diet and the amount of activity that should be permitted. If family members are to be actively involved with caring for the infected child, they must also be given information currently available about the disease and its management.

Nursing functions in regard to population screening and seeking out contacts, especially for the purpose of locating the source of the infection, have already been described. Another role of the nurse is to help implement the prescribed treatment program to prevent further spread of the disease. Teaching children and their families about the disease may serve to facilitate their adaptation. The child may not be future oriented but should still be reassured that tuberculosis will not adversely affect most of the goals he or she will eventually have.

Children who have active disease are isolated with acid-fast bacilli (AFB) isolation until drug therapy is initiated and sputum testing shows a decrease in organisms. AFB precautions include masks and good handwashing.

A public health referral is an integral part of the nursing care. Tuberculosis is a reportable disease, and public health officials are important case managers.

Nurses must be willing and able to meet the physical, intellectual, and emotional-social needs of each child. Specific care measures are determined by the extent and type of tuberculosis. The plan of care must be appropriate for the child's level of understanding and development and take into consideration the child's particular coping ability. Assisting youths to assume responsibility for some of their treatment and rehabilitation goals is a nursing intervention that may ensure their cooperation.

Some youths may feel that a stigma is attached to the diagnosis and may respond by withdrawing from friends and activities. Even during the time that the initial nursing history is requested, youths may feel constrained when asked to list all their recent contacts. They may think their friends will resent being named or being exposed to this disease. If the source of the infection turns out to be one of their friends, this can cause some friction. If the source is one of the youth's own parents, the youth may experience some negative feelings toward that parent. Tuberculosis, like most other long-term illnesses, tends to increase or prolong dependency. This may be resented and contribute to the youth's feelings of discouragement.

Nurses can help the child structure outlets for energy or aggressive feelings. Support groups are becoming popular. Such groups allow children with long-term illnesses to ventilate their feelings and also provide peer support for members. Nurses need to recognize that anger is often expressed as rebellion against treatment orders or boredom and lack of interest in activities or school work. Fears about never again being completely well should be anticipated by the nurse and dealt with by frank discussion of the optimistic outcome for successful treatment of tuberculosis. Older children usually respond positively to visits from friends. Occasionally, however, a youth may try to avoid these contacts, fearing that the friends will be afraid of catching tuberculosis.

Children with active tuberculosis are frequently treated on an outpatient basis and may return to school when their sputum is negative for bacilli. Although there is some controversy about allowing children with infective tuberculosis in school, returning them to school and their peer group as soon as is safely possible may motivate them to comply with the drug regimen. Until a return to school is feasible, specific plans to avoid disruption of intellectual achievements may include a hospital or homebound teacher.

Another stressor deserving consideration is when a child with tuberculosis is from a family whose members are not citizens. These families may fear having their child's tuberculosis reported, which may result in deportation of any family members who are illegal aliens. An ethical question must be faced by nurses and medical personnel caring for families of illegal aliens. If the family thinks that medical caregivers will report the tuberculosis to government officials and deportation will result, they will be reluctant to seek treatment, may not follow up with treatment, may fail to identify all their contacts, or may drop out of the community, thereby curtailing treatment efforts.

Parasitic Infections

Parasitic infections are much less common in the United States than in the Third World because of better sanitation and the greater emphasis on hygiene. However, the nurse who works with migrants from temperate climates, with immigrants to the United States (such as Vietnamese and Cubans), or with impoverished Americans, especially in the southern states, is likely to have regular acquaintance with parasitic infections. These infections can occur in any age group with fairly equal incidence; however, because of the greater tendencies of the toddler and the preschooler to engage in spontaneous hand-to-mouth activities without handwashing, to play on the ground and go barefoot, and to investigate dirt with their hands, mouth, and feet, these younger children are at greater risk for contracting parasitic infection.

Helminthic Infections

There are a variety of helminthic infections, but this discussion will include only three of the most common ones: roundworm, tapeworm, and hookworm. Table 39–6 describes the main characteristics, the definitive diagnostic findings, and the primary medical treatment of each. Pinworm, another common helminth, is discussed in Chapter 35.

A careful environmental history, searching for factors such as overcrowding and poor sanitation facilities, is helpful in establishing the diagnosis and in determining the most realistic approach to nursing intervention in treating and preventing recurrence of these infections. Nursing intervention in the helminthic infections requires strict adherence to enteric isolation and nursing measures to relieve accompanying symptoms. The nurse's more critical role, however, lies in educating the child and family regarding the cause of the infection and the measures that can be taken to prevent further infestations. Teaching about handwashing and personal hygiene is a first step. Community health nurse involvement to explore the family's environment and to identify the source(s) of infestation is usually essential to planning and motivating appropriate change so that the child is not reinfested. Because lack of sanitation facilities and overcrowding are frequently factors in the etiology, government involvement also becomes necessary and may require prompting from nurses and other health and social providers who can exert united political pressure.

TABLE 39-6
Summary of Basic Features of Three Helminthic Infections

Features	Roundworm	Tapeworm	Hookworm
Causative agent	*Ascaris lumbricoides*	*Taenia saginata* or *solium*	*Necator americanus*
Mode of transmission	Ingestion of ova in dirt contaminated by human feces. Hand contamination from infected household dust	Ingested from handling or eating infested beef or pork	Penetration of bare feet. Ingestion through contaminated water
Clinical manifestations	May be asymptomatic. Fever and malaise; restless, disturbed sleep. Abdominal distention and discomfort; vomiting. Anemia. Infested stools; steatorrhea; intestinal obstruction. Peritonitis	Varied symptoms: Abdominal cramping or pain, nervousness, insomnia, anorexia, weight loss. Sometimes asymptomatic	Severe anemia. Occult blood in feces. Abdominal colic, malnutrition, intestinal or bile duct obstruction. Intestinal mucosa and liver damage
Diagnostic findings	Positive stool culture for ova and parasites	Positive stool culture for ova and parasites	Positive stool culture for ova and parasites
Drug treatment	Pyrantel pamoate or mebendazole	Niclosamide; Praziquantel	Pyrantel pamoate; supplemental iron

Roundworm (Ascariasis)

Pathophysiology and Etiology. Occurring mostly in the southern United States, ascariasis can be a chronic infection of the small intestine. Ova are usually ingested from hands that have contacted contaminated dust or soil or from inadequately cleansed raw fruits or vegetables. The ova live in the small intestine and, when the larvae stage is reached, penetrate the intestinal villi and enter the portal circulation. Reaching the lungs, the larvae rise to the oropharynx and are swallowed, settling in the small intestine to mature to adult worms. Enough adult worms (measuring 15 to 35 cm × 3 to 4 mm) may accumulate to cause intestinal obstruction, or they may migrate to the appendix, causing perforation and peritonitis (Garcia, 1992).

Therapeutic Management. Treatment includes the administration of anthelminthic drugs, careful handwashing, and relief of symptoms. Prevention involves careful washing of raw fruits and vegetables, regular hygiene and handwashing, and improvement of sanitation facilities or practices or both.

Tapeworm

Pathophysiology and Etiology. A nonfatal parasitic infection, tapeworm results from the ingestion of the tapeworm larvae in improperly cared for or inadequately cooked beef or pork. The encysted larva settles in the small intestine and lengthens by generating segments. It is regurgitated to the stomach and migrates from there to the brain or eye to form cysts.

Therapeutic Management. Treatment consists of the oral anthelminthic medication niclosamide. Prevention involves careful handwashing after handling meat and thorough cooking of the meat before eating it.

Hookworm

Pathophysiology and Etiology. This worm thrives in the warm, sandy soil of the southern United States, especially where sanitation is inadequate. Infestation occurs through penetration of the skin or by drinking contaminated water. The worms penetrate the bare feet, causing a local dermatitis that may go unnoticed. Traveling through the lymph and blood systems to the lungs, the worm migrates to the throat, is swallowed, and attaches to the walls of the small intestine. After the worm sucks blood from the intestinal walls for several weeks, ova are produced.

Therapeutic Management. Treatment is provided for the entire family and includes an anthelminthic, a diet high in protein and iron to correct the associated anemia, and improvement of sanitary conditions. Prevention includes routine personal hygiene, avoidance of going barefoot, and adequate sanitary facilities and practices.

Nursing Diagnostic Statements for Helminthic Infections

Potential for injury: physiologic, *related to: (the physical effects of helminthic infestation).*

Fear/anxiety (child and family), *related to: visualization of regurgitated worms or of worms or worm segments in the stool.*

Knowledge deficit, *related to*

- *Transmission of microscopic eggs or larvae.*
- *Handwashing methods and personal hygiene practices to prevent recurrence.*
- *Specific treatment, including anthelminthic medication and sterilization*

*of contaminated clothing, linens, and other fomites.**
- *Signs and symptoms of complications (e.g., intestinal obstruction from roundworm).*

Nursing Care/Interventions

Nursing care of children with parasitic diseases involves teaching the correct use of the appropriate medication, instruction regarding hygienic measures to rid fomites of parasites, and preventive education of children and adults.

Panic and anger are typical responses of parents and school officials when parasitic infection is discovered. The nurse or school nurse often receives the brunt of their reaction and must learn to accept this response syndrome without taking it personally. Preventive education as well as education as to the cause, transfer, and treatment of the parasitic disease prior to any major occurrence may help allay some of these negative reactions. When a diagnosis is made, feelings of guilt, shame, and uncleanliness are usually provoked in the child or the caregivers, or both. Constant reassurance offered by the nurse that the child is not unclean because he or she contracted parasites and that parents cannot be responsible if their child uses other children's possessions or comes in close contact with other children during play often produces better cooperation and reduces parental aggressive responses. School or community funds may be required to make treatment possible for children of low-income families who cannot afford the costs involved in treatment. Involvement of community health nurses may be necessary if a family's cooperation is questionable or if infestation is widespread in the community. Follow-up care will include repeating stool testing for ova and parasites to assess for the effectiveness of the anthelminthic medication and reinforcing teaching to avoid recurrence.

Pediculosis Capitis (Head Lice)

Approximately 3 million cases of head lice are diagnosed annually in the United States alone. Females are affected twice as often as males. Pediculosis is 20 times more prevalent in whites than in other racial groups, presumably because of the difference in the makeup of the hair shaft. The peak incidence is in preschool and early school-age children, with a steady decline after that age until about sixth grade, when the incidence again rises somewhat.

Etiology

The bloodsucking louse lives its entire life (nit or egg to nymph to adult louse) on the head of the child it infests. The eggs, called "nits," attach to the hair shaft by a cement-like substance and hatch within a week (Fig. 39–2). The hatched nymph matures into a mature louse in another week to 10 days and punctures the scalp with its hooklike claws to suck blood. It remains attached until it is dislodged or dies (about 1 month).

A child is infested either by direct contact or from fomites (comb, headgear, play wigs, clothing). Human head lice do not jump from head to head unless there is direct contact, nor are they transferred from one person to another in the breeze. The nits are not communicable; only the hatched louse is. These insects avoid light or perspiration.

Clinical Manifestations

A week after the child is bitten, he or she may develop an allergic response evidenced by mild fever, malaise, intense scalp itching, and enlarged cervical and occipital nodes. After a prolonged exposure, the body's sensitivity is diminished and the child becomes oblivious to the bites, that is, asymptomatic. Occasionally, a child will develop focal alopecia owing to the allergic response. The nits can be seen as silvery or grayish-white, smooth, and glistening specks resembling dandruff but securely attached to the hair shaft near the scalp. (Prominent locations are behind the ears and the nape of the neck.) The adult louse

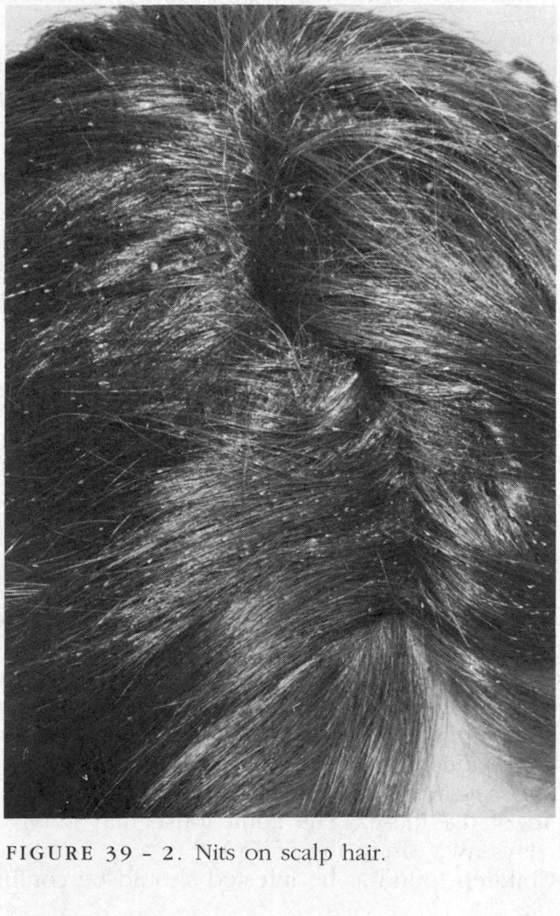

FIGURE 39 - 2. Nits on scalp hair.

* Fomites are inanimate objects such as combs and clothing that serve to transfer infectious organisms from one person to another.

can be seen as a minute black speck that moves and jumps on the scalp and hair. The child's scratching during the period of allergic reactivity may result in secondary infections.

Medical Diagnosis

Diagnosis is made by identification of the nits and lice using a magnifying glass and strong direct lighting or a microscope. Microscopic examination differentiates the head louse from the body louse or from aphids, which can carry other diseases. Examination of the scalp is done by parting the hair in several places (especially in the region behind the ears and nape of the neck) with two applicator sticks, moving systematically from side to side and front to back. The magnifying glass is then used to inspect the exposed scalp and hair for nits and lice.

Nursing Diagnostic Statements for Pediculosis Capitis

Impaired skin integrity: scalp infestation, *related to direct scalp contact with live lice.*

Altered comfort: pruritus of scalp, *related to an allergic response associated with lice bites.*

Potential infection: secondary, *related to scratching of the scalp.*

Knowledge deficit: (child and family), *related to:*

- *Corrective treatment, including medicated shampoo, nit removal, and disinfection of contaminated articles.*
- *Contact isolation procedures until treatment is instituted.*
- *Expected duration of scalp pruritus.*
- *Prevention of recurrence, including avoiding contact with possible fomites, and keeping hair short and clean.*

Nursing Care/Interventions

Addressing the Knowledge Deficit. Treatment is both preventive and corrective, necessitating that families be taught how to avoid contact with contaminated fomites as well as treatment to rid the scalp of lice. Specific teaching activities are identified throughout this section.

Preventing Scalp Infestation. Preventively, children should be taught not to exchange combs, brushes, headgear, or clothing with other children. Keeping hair clean may also help prevent infestation. At home and in settings in which a group of children are gathered, individually assigned hooks or lockers for wraps and possessions help decrease the incidence and spread of the louse. (The adult louse may survive 1 to 2 days away from the scalp.)

Children found to be infested should be confined at home until 24 hours after treatment is complete to minimize spread to others. It is generally recommended that all family members be treated simultaneously; often, louse infestation is so widespread that entire classrooms or schools of children are encouraged to undergo treatment. (The treatment may actually be carried out at school with parental approval.)

Treating Scalp Infestation and Pruritus. Corrective treatment involves three activities: (1) using medicated shampoo, (2) disinfecting fomites, and (3) examination of contacts. Nonprescription shampoo (RID [includes a fine-tooth comb]; Triple X) or prescription shampoo with permethrine or lindane may be used and should be applied exactly according to directions. The child prone to eczema may have an allergic response to the shampoo. The parent or child must understand that the shampooing must be done vigorously to be effective. After the shampoo, the hair is combed (teasing backward) with a fine-tooth comb, preferably outdoors, to remove any remaining nits. All the nits must be removed. Sometimes dipping the comb in white vinegar or soaking the hair with vinegar helps to loosen tightly attached nits. Itching may continue for 3 or 4 days after the insecticide shampoo, but if pruritus lasts longer than this, it is evidence of more nits and lice requiring retreatment. Retreatment can occur at 7 days after the initial treatment.

All contactable items should be laundered in hot water and dried in sunlight or a clothes dryer (20 minutes on high) or ironed. Nonlaunderable items may be soaked in 2 per cent Lysol or one of the pediculocidal shampoos for an hour or heated in water (54° C) for 5 to 10 minutes. Disinfection of all combs and brushes should be done in the same manner.

All the child's contacts should be examined and treated if necessary. Family members must be treated simultaneously with the child to prevent immediate reinfestation. Parents should be instructed in how to assess for reinfestation.

Scabies

Scabies is an infectious skin condition most common in school-age children, causing a vesicular or papulovesicular eruption. There are several forms of scabies. The most common "classic scabies" is transmitted by direct contact with a person infested with *Acarus scabies (Sarcoptes scabiei),* or itch mite.

Etiology

The adult female itch mite, approximately the size of a grain of sugar, digs into the superficial stratum corneum of the epidermis and forms a burrow, leaving debris and feces. Each day for approximately a month, burrowing continues a few millimeters, and the female mite lays two to three eggs. The adult mite then dies, and the eggs mature to an adult form in 10 days. The skin of the infested person reacts in an allergic fashion, and small vesicles and papules form.

Identification of scabies is difficult, and it is often misdiagnosed in children. Although it is often classified as a "social disease," it occurs in all socioeconomic levels, and cleanliness is not necessarily a protection. Children who bathe regularly will remove many of the mites, and the burrows may be impossible to detect. The nurse may use an ink pen to trace the burrows to the vesicle (mite hill) in an attempt to visualize the lesion (Fig. 39–3).

Clinical Manifestations

Children infested with the itch mite first experience nocturnal itching. Pruritus is increased with the warmth of the bed and occurs only after sensitization to the mite and debris, usually a month after infestation. Scabetic lesions usually are present on the sides or webs of the digits of hands and feet, extensor surface of the elbows, anterior axillary skin folds, glans penis, scrotum, and abdomen (Fig. 39–3). The nurse will recognize initial lesions as small erythematous, excoriated papules. These may appear eczematous if the child has had pruritus and scratching resulted.

Diagnostic Assessment

The diagnosis of scabies must be made microscopically by identification of the mite from skin scrapings. It is imperative that the nurse provide factual information regarding the transmission of the mite in an attempt to alleviate guilt feelings of the parents and child.

Therapeutic Management

Treatment consists of the topical application of a scabicide over the entire body. Elimite, a 5% permethrin, is the drug of choice, but lindane or crotamiton may be used as an alternative. Remove the scabicide by bathing 12 hours later for elimite or lindane and 48 hours later for crotamiton.

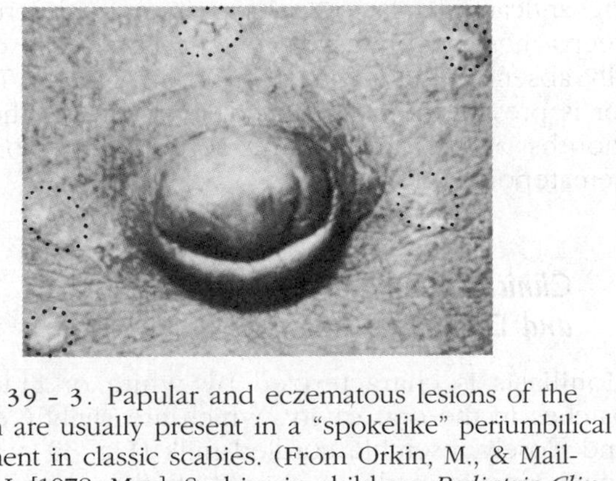

FIGURE 39 - 3. Papular and eczematous lesions of the abdomen are usually present in a "spokelike" periumbilical arrangement in classic scabies. (From Orkin, M., & Maibach, H. I. [1978, May]. Scabies in children. *Pediatric Clinics of North America,* p 373.)

Nursing Care

The infected child and all family members should initially bathe, towel dry, and then apply the scabicide from the neck down, being especially careful to apply between the fingers and toes and in the genital area. Bathing should be repeated at the prescribed interval after application of the scabicide. One application is usually sufficient, although some physicians may recommend a second treatment in 1 week. Clothing in direct contact with the skin should be washed in hot water and dried. Underclothes and bed linens should be changed with each bath.

Because scabies is transmitted by direct contact, it is imperative that all family members be treated for scabies. Because the parasite survives only 3 or 4 days away from human skin, disinfection of fomites such as bedclothes and linens is usually confined to those articles with which the child is repeatedly in contact.

Treatment is usually effective if instructions are followed correctly. Symptoms may continue for several days after treatment owing to hypersensitivity to mite antigens. This should not be confused with treatment failure (Minster, 1980).

Allowing the child an opportunity to ventilate feelings and providing basic information about the disease and treatment will be a major role for the nurse. Older children with scabies may feel ashamed or guilty. An understanding of the condition will help the child cope and maintain a positive self-image.

Toxoplasmosis

Toxoplasmosis is a parasitic disease that may be either congenital (transmitted from an infected mother) or acquired. Acquired infection is transient and only mildly symptomatic. Congenital infection is more common and has severe consequences, with 23 to 38 per cent of infected infants experiencing severe CNS impairment, ocular damage, or death. Once infected, a woman has a lasting immunity, which means future offspring will not be affected.

Etiology

The *Toxoplasma gondii* parasites can be acquired from two primary sources: (1) the handling or ingestion of raw or undercooked fresh meat that contains infective tissue cysts with the protozoan parasite inside, and (2) direct contact with the feces of an "infected" common house cat (in cat litter box or vegetable garden).

Clinical Manifestations and Diagnostic Assessment

Manifestations of acute active disease in congenitally infected infants include jaundice, petechiae, enlarged liver or spleen, chorioretinitis (inflammation of the choroid and retina), cerebral calcifications of damaged areas, encephalitis, and convulsions. These infants often die within the first month. Survivors are usually mentally retarded, with psychomotor impairment and varying degrees of blindness.

Third-trimester infections result in subacute symptoms. Infants with a subacute form of congenital toxoplasmosis usually have no symptoms at birth, although chorioretinitis may be present. During the first year, subacutely infected infants may develop hydrocephaly, chorioretinitis, intracerebral calcification, and psychomotor disturbances.

In those children or adults who acquire the disease after birth, the only symptom is usually cervical lymphadenopathy. The presence of toxoplasmosis is diagnosed through serologic examination.

Therapeutic Management and Nursing Care

Congenital Toxoplasmosis. Treatment of congenital toxoplasmosis is unsatisfactory, but daily doses of pyrimethamine (Daraprim) and sulfadiazine for 4 to 8 weeks is sometimes effective. Folinic acid is given to stop adverse actions on the bone marrow by the sulfonamide drugs. Because Daraprim is an antifolic agent, blood counts should be monitored biweekly to prevent leukopenia, thrombocytopenia, or anemia. In infants with the severe form of the disease, corticosteroids are often given to reduce inflammation, as in chorioretinitis.

The progressive nature of the disease suggests that treatment should begin whether the infection is clinically apparent or not. Early treatment may prevent further tissue invasion and may arrest progression of the disease. Treatment of asymptomatic infants is undertaken to prevent later sequelae.

In the severely affected infant with congenital toxoplasmosis, the nurse's role primarily consists of palliative treatment for the infant and support to the parents of this critically ill child. Infants with the subacute form of the disease are generally hospitalized for the duration of drug therapy due to the near toxic level of the dosages. Nursing care needs to consist of monitoring the child for signs and symptoms of drug toxicity, leukopenia, thrombocytopenia, and anemia.

Acquired Toxoplasmosis. The disease is self-limiting in children and adults; thus, the only significant intervention is prevention. Simple preventive measures include (1) proper cooking of meat and cleaning of raw vegetables; (2) handwashing following handling of raw meats and vegetables coupled with avoidance of contact with mucous membranes while handling these items; (3) daily discarding of cat litter box contents, avoiding of litter box contact by pregnant women or handling only with disposable gloves; and (4) covers placed on sand boxes to prevent their use by cats to deposit feces. Public education and prenatal and child health maintenance counseling should teach these precautions. Cats that are kept indoors and are not fed uncooked meat are considered to pose no threat (Feldman, 1983). If a rise in the titer occurs during the first trimester in pregnant females, decision must be made regarding termination of the pregnancy. Although maternal infections frequently do not result in infection of the fetus, the fetus appears to be at greatest risk when the mother contracts toxoplasmosis early in pregnancy (Feldman, 1983).

Fungal Infections

More than 60 fungi are known to be pathogenic in humans. This discussion is limited to those causing thrush, ringworm, and histoplasmosis. Permanent resistance is not developed to fungal infections; therefore, the nurse is likely to see mycoses (fungal disease) often in his or her practice.

Although immune responses to specific fungi are demonstrable, they are not well understood. Skin fatty acids, gastric acids, and intestinal enzymes help inhibit the growth of fungi. Serum antibodies are present and help establish presence of active disease but play little role in protection or recovery from most fungal infections. Cell-mediated immunity is believed to have some effect in recovery from fungal infection, particularly candidal fungi.

Thrush (Moniliasis)

Pathophysiology and Etiology

Thrush involves a stomatitis, particularly of the tongue, buccal membranes, and pharynx, caused by a yeastlike fungus, *Candida albicans*. Five per cent of all newborn infants contract thrush during descent through an infected birth canal, evidencing symptoms 7 to 10 days later. Infection with *Candida* may also result from prolonged antibiotic therapy or be transmitted by contaminated hands, bottles, or nipples. The incidence is greater in females, in infants with immunologic deficiencies, in infants of diabetic mothers, and in infants with oronasal anomalies. It is much less common after the neonatal period.

Candida is normally present in the mouth, gastrointestinal tract, and vagina. However, the circulating anticandidal factor present in normal serum that keeps most people asymptomatic is reduced or virtually absent in the serum of newborn infants. This factor is present, but in reduced levels during the first 6 months of life, and in the serum of persons with hematopoietic disorders.

Clinical Manifestations and Diagnostic Assessment

Moniliasis is characterized by white or gray-white patches in the oral cavity, which are slightly elevated and closely resemble curdled milk (Fig. 39–4). When an attempt is made to scrape off the patch, the un-

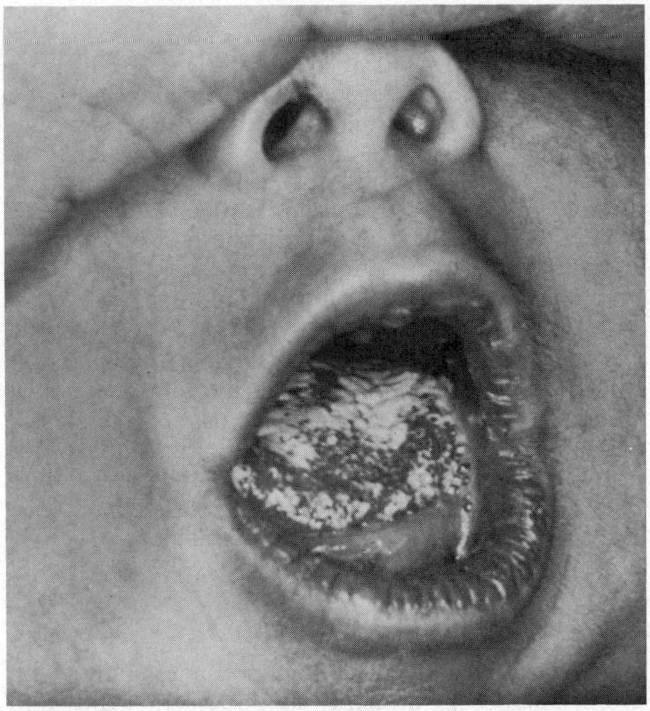

FIGURE 39-4. Thrush is characterized by white patches in the mouth that resemble curdled milk. (Courtesy of Mead Johnson Nutritional Group.)

derlying mucosa is seen to be raw and may bleed. Inspection alone is usually adequate to diagnose thrush; microscopic scrapings using 10% potassium hydroxide (KOH) can confirm yeast buds and hyphae.

Therapeutic Management

On diagnosis of thrush, the physician orders a topical fungicide. The diaper area will also be assessed for a monilial rash, because *Candida* is common throughout the gastrointestinal tract. A topically applied fungicide ointment such as nystatin is used to treat the diaper area.

Nursing Diagnostic Statements for Thrush

Impaired tissue integrity: stomatitis, *related to infection with* Candida albicans *associated with*

- *Passage through an infected birth canal.*
- *Overgrowth of nonsusceptible organisms secondary to antibiotic therapy.*
- *Direct transmission from improper hand washing, mother's infected breast, or improper cleansing of bottles and nipples.*

Knowledge deficit (parents), *related to:*

- *Etiology of the infection.*
- *Administration of antifungal medication.*
- *Treatment of breasts if breastfeeding.*

Nursing Care/Interventions

Treating the Stomatitis. Thrush is eventually self-limiting, but it should be treated with good hygiene and application of a fungicide to prevent spread into the upper respiratory or gastrointestinal tracts.

Nystatin is a fungicide that is effective against *Candida* when applied to the oral cavity four times a day for 1 week. Parents should be directed to complete the 7-day regimen even if the lesions have cleared. Nystatin can be swallowed to treat any moniliasis of the gastrointestinal tract and should be applied after feedings. It must be given slowly, with some applied to each side of the mouth before it is swallowed to ensure adequate exposure of the oral mucosa to the medication. Typically, 1 ml of nystatin is ordered, with 0.5 ml to be used in each cheek. A cotton swab can be used to ensure contact of the medication with the buccal membrane, but this often results in much of the medication being absorbed in the cotton. A more effective method is for the nurse or the parent to gently rub a gloved finger inside the cheek after the nystatin has been inserted with an oral syringe.

Addressing the Knowledge Deficit. The parents must understand the etiology of the infection to combat it effectively. If the mother is breastfeeding, it is usually necessary for her to treat her breasts with an antifungal ointment to prevent reinfection between her breasts and the infant's mouth. Instruction regarding administration of medication to the infant's oral mucous membranes should include a return demonstration by the parent, because it is unlikely that the parent has had practice with this type of administration previously.

Preventing future infections with this organism involves careful washing of bottles and nipples (boiling or washing in a dishwasher is often recommended), following feedings with plain water (because small amounts of formula left in the buccal cavities provide an excellent bacterial medium), and use of good handwashing techniques. The parents should be aware that antibiotic treatment may also precipitate another infection and must be alert for the white patches should the infant require antibiotic therapy.

Ringworm

Several different closely related fungi are known to cause ringworm, which is a general term for mycotic disease of the keratinizing areas (nails, scalp, skin) of the body. Tinea capitis, tinea corporis, tinea cruris, and tinea pedis are described here.

Tinea Capitis (Scalp Ringworm)

Etiology. Ringworm of the scalp is an ancient disease with worldwide incidence. The greatest susceptibility is in young boys (rare after puberty) from urban areas. The fungus is transferred from infected animals or humans and from contaminated fomites (combs, hats).

Clinical Manifestations. The infection begins with a papule and spreads to form a round, sharply outlined area in which hairs exist but have dried and broken off just above the skin. One or several such lesions may exist. The scalp varies from being mildly erythematous and slightly scaly to being affected with a painful, deep, boggy, and swollen inflammation called a "kerion." The child's condition is communicable as long as the lesion(s) exists.

Diagnostic Assessment. Diagnosis is positive if a Wood light shone on the scalp results in fluorescence of tinea capitis organisms or if a microscopic examination of scales or hairs treated with 10 per cent KOH reveals the fungi. A culture is required to determine the specific species of fungus causing the infection, the most common fungi in the United States being *Trichophyton tonsurans*.

Nursing Care. Table 39–7 describes the management of the infection and associated symptoms. The nurse's approach to the child and family is crucial to the feelings they experience. Careful explanation of the cause helps diminish parents' feelings that they have not kept their child clean enough. Their cooperation should be enlisted to help identify the source of the infection. Animals the child has contact with should be carefully inspected for evidence of ringworm lesions. The child's playmates and siblings should also be examined because children tend to share personal articles during play, making transfer more likely. The nurse and parents together can teach and reinforce that personal articles such as combs, brushes, barrettes, and headgear are not playthings and should not be interchanged among siblings or playmates.

Tinea Corporis (Body Ringworm)

Etiology and Clinical Manifestations. Body ringworm also has a higher incidence in young boys and is more prevalent in rural, humid climates. This fungus infects nonhairy skin surfaces. The lesions are usually asymptomatic and appear in a flat, annular, or arcuate shape. There is scaling and erythema of the border with a clear central area; the border may also contain vesicles. The lesions are contagious as long as they exist. A common feature is pruritus.

Diagnostic Assessment and Nursing Strategies. Diagnosis is by microscopic examination and culture of scales or scabs. As with tinea capitis, parents should be approached in a nonaccusing manner that does not suggest they are inadequate parents, and their help should be solicited in finding the source. (See Table 39–7 for a discussion of treatment.)

Tinea Cruris (Jock Itch)

Etiology. Jock itch is a ringworm infestation of the groin that occurs primarily in pubescent males and adult men. Two ringworm fungi (*Epidermophyton floccosum* and *Tinea rubrum*) invade the medial proximal aspects of the thighs, the crural folds, and the scrotum, living off the dead keratinized skin and hair tissues of that area. Individual susceptibility is poorly understood, but poor hygiene, heat, friction, maceration in the groin area, and obesity are predisposing factors. Direct contact with the organism when any of these conditions exists makes the young man a potential host to the fungus.

Clinical Manifestations and Diagnostic Assessment. The fungal invasion is characterized by round, sharply delineated lesions, with the pubic hairs of that region broken off. These pruritic lesions vary from a scaly, red area to a painfully edematous, boggy one. Diag-

TABLE 39–7
Management of Ringworm and Associated Symptoms

Tinea Capitis	Tinea Corporis	All Ringworm Forms
1. Clip hair short and thoroughly wash daily 2. Do not use towel more than once before laundering 3. If a pillow is used, change pillowslip daily 4. Avoid use of headgear till lesions healed 5. Apply cold compresses to any oozing or swollen lesions	1. Bathe thoroughly daily, removing scabs or crusts before applying medication 2. Avoid heat, moisture, and trauma during treatment, because these cause increased inflammation and pruritus 3. Change towels, clothing, and linens daily 4. Wear nonocclusive clothing until lesions healed 5. Distract child from scratching or picking at lesions	1. Exclusion from gym, public showers, and pools 2. Apply an antifungal agent containing haloprogin, toinaftate, or salicylic acid after shampooing or bathing twice daily (e.g., Tinactin or Viaform ointment). Do not apply to highly inflamed lesions. Usually prescribed for 1–3 wks 3. For extensive or topical resistant ringworm, give 6-wk course of oral griseofulvin 10–20 mgm/kg/day in two daily doses (antifungal antibiotic). Should be given after meals. Blood anticoagulating action is decreased by griseofulvin

nosis is confirmed by presence of the fungi on direct microscopic examination of the scales.

Therapeutic Management and Nursing Strategies. Management involves comfort measures such as wet compresses or sitz baths to relieve the itching and swelling, eradication of the fungi with local applications of tolnaftate liquid (Tinactin) or a similar antifungal preparation, and education regarding personal hygiene and management of other predisposing factors. Nonconstrictive cotton underwear reduces chafing, and an absorbent powder applied to the groin area may be helpful. The youth also needs reassurance that this temporary condition in no way alters his sexuality, because any infections of the involved body region are typically perceived by young men to be somehow affiliated with venereal diseases such as syphilis or gonorrhea (there is actually no association). His parents, if they have awareness of their son's ailment, may need similar assurance and education to correct misconceptions they may hold about the disease.

Tinea Pedis (Athlete's Foot)

Etiology. Tinea pedis (dermatophytosis), more commonly known as "athlete's foot," is also a fungal disease. Although tinea pedis is not frequent in the young school-age child, its incidence increases near puberty. Tinea pedis often occurs with tinea cruris. *Trichophyton rubrum, Trichophyton mentagrophytes,* and *E. floccosum* are the usual causative organisms.

Clinical Manifestations. The appearance of tinea pedis can range from an acute inflammatory vesiculobullous eruption to a dull erythema and scaling (Fig. 39–5). An acute episode initially involves the intertriginous area of the fourth and fifth toes and extends to the plantar surface of the foot. Skin maceration, scaling, vesicles, and fissures result. The absence of vesiculation and the presence of moccasin-like scaling occurs in chronic tinea pedis and is usually limited to a small area between the toes.

Diagnostic Assessment. Children complaining of itchy feet with signs of scaling or vesicle formation should be referred to a physician for diagnosis and treatment. Diagnosis can usually be made clinically; however, tissue scrapings examined under a Wood lamp will confirm suspicions. Some children experience discomfort and burning from the vesicles. A child unable to walk probably has a secondary infection in conjunction with acute tinea pedis.

Therapeutic Management and Nursing Strategies. Management of tinea pedis involves both preventive and treatment measures. Prevention of tinea pedis is virtually impossible because the organisms are present on most people. However, proper foot hygiene is an important health consideration for all children. Instruction should include the importance of daily bathing and careful drying between all toes. Many children now wear nonventilated shoes, which provide an excellent growth medium for fungus, especially during the summer months when their feet are warm and moist. Nurses should encourage older children to go barefoot when appropriate or to wear sandals, which allow the feet to stay dry. Early treatment of a fungus-infected toenail may prevent an episode of tinea pedis and complications from secondary infections.

Treatment for acute tinea pedis is somewhat involved, and parents will need specific written instructions. Systemic treatment is with oral griseofulvin if the infection is severe and recalcitrant. Most tinea pedis can be treated with topical antifungals applied twice daily. Parents and child need to be shown how to apply wet compresses to the foot for 20 minutes four times a day. Local treatment of the vesicles with wet compresses is continued until the blisters heal, and then topical antifungal agents are used. The child with tinea pedis should be instructed to wear cotton socks and to alternate between pairs of shoes to allow complete drying. Parents and siblings need to be informed that the skin condition is not contagious; however, the exchange of socks and bath towels should be prohibited. If the child is not in acute distress, arrangements should be made to allow him or her to continue with school. The child with a severe case of acute tinea pedis may feel some resentment at having to temporarily curtail ambulatory activities, particularly physical education or athletics that stimulate foot perspiration. The school nurse should discuss the child's condition with the teacher so that the child's discomfort and lack of participation in some activities will be understood. The teacher responsible

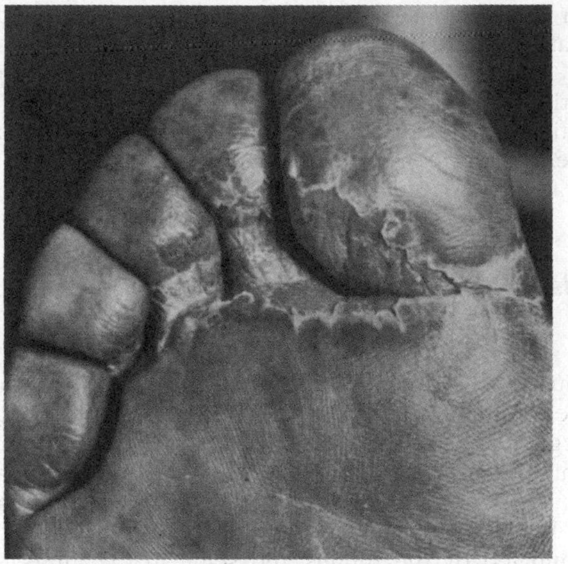

FIGURE 39-5. Tinea pedis.

for physical education classes should be informed so that attention is given to proper hygiene.

Chronic tinea pedis may be treated with nonprescription topical antifungal medications such as Tinactin or Whitfield's ointment. Application of the ointment must be continued for 3 to 4 weeks after healing has occurred.

Histoplasmosis

Etiology Common to All Forms

Caused by *Histoplasma capsulatum,* a fungus found predominantly in soil with a high organic content (e.g., chicken coops and composts) in the central United States, histoplasmosis can occur in persons of all ages. This fungus is not transmitted from human to human; airborne spores are inhaled in dust contaminated by the fungus and settle in the lungs. The disease may be (1) asymptomatic and benign, (2) symptomatic but benign, or (3) acute, progressive, and disseminated, producing serious systemic disease.

Forms of Histoplasmosis

Asymptomatic Benign Histoplasmosis. This form of the disease is detected only by a positive histoplasmin test. The primary lung lesions created by the fungus calcify without causing any symptoms. No treatment is indicated.

Symptomatic Benign Histoplasmosis. Symptoms are general and may appear as mild respiratory illness or temporary general malaise. The child may complain of some weakness and chest pain. A low-grade fever and dry or productive cough are usually present. Recovery is slow but spontaneous. Treatment involves symptomatic relief of fever and cough.

Acute Progressive Disseminated Histoplasmosis. This form of the disease is most prevalent in infants and toddlers. The course is rapid and, left untreated, the disease is fatal. Symptoms include a high sepsis-related fever, prostration, hepatosplenomegaly, skin ulcers and mucosal purpura, atypical pneumonitis, and often anemia.

Diagnostic Assessment

Diagnosis is tentative when a serologic test for serum antihistoplasma antibody (histoplasmin test) is positive. Diagnosis can be made quickly when the fungus can be seen in Giemsa- or Wright-stained smears of sputum, bone marrow, blood, or ulcerative exudate. Definitive diagnosis depends on culturing the fungus from these smear sources, but a longer time is required to learn the findings from culture than from the serologic test, so treatment is usually begun before the results of the report of the culture findings are known.

Therapeutic Management

Management usually involves hospitalization so the course of the disease can be closely monitored. Wound isolation is initiated and amphotericin B (Fungizone) or a triple sulfonamide suspension or both are administered. All family members should be evaluated and infected members treated. Treatment of symptoms is also initiated. With prompt treatment recovery does occur.

Nursing Care

Parents will need emotional support as they learn the cause and potential seriousness of their child's disease. They should be educated as to the etiology of the disease and encouraged to take preventive precautions such as wearing a mask while inside chicken coops, periodically cleaning and spraying the coop and surrounding soil with 3 per cent formalin spray to reduce dust, and fencing in compost areas. Parents should be urged to keep their infant or toddler, who is more susceptible to the serious form of the disease, away from these sites of potential contamination.

Rickettsial Infections

Two fairly common rickettsial infections—Q fever and Rocky Mountain spotted fever—are discussed. These diseases can affect all ages; young children are susceptible because they tend to spend a lot of time crawling, sitting, and playing on the ground, making them readily accessible to infected ticks, which are a major source of rickettsial disease.

Q Fever

Etiology

This is an acute febrile disease of sudden onset caused by *Coxiella burnetii,* a rickettsia. Major reservoirs from which humans contract this disease are ticks, farm animals or raw milk from them, and dust. Humans inhale the infected dust, tissues or substances. Transmission also occurs through the handling of animal birth products, particularly associated with sheep, goats, and cows.

Clinical Manifestations and Diagnostic Assessment

There is much variability in the severity and duration of symptoms, which include chills, diaphoresis, headache, and malaise. Pneumonitis symptoms of cough and chest pain exist without any upper respiratory involvement. Diagnosis is made from a positive complement fixation or agglutination test.

Nursing Care

Oral tetracycline is given for this disease and is continued for 7 to 10 days after the fever dissipates. A person who has had Q fever develops permanent immunity. Immunization is also available and should be given to those at high risk for exposure. Prevention is an important aspect of nursing care in areas where Q fever seems to be prevalent. Preventive action should include education regarding sources of the rickettsiae and concerning the practice of appropriate hygienic measures in potential reservoir areas (e.g., animal barns and sheds). Parents should be cautioned not to give their children unpasteurized milk.

Rocky Mountain Spotted Fever

Etiology

This disease is caused by *Rickettsia rickettsii* and is transmitted to humans via tick bite. The incidence is highest in the Kentucky mountains, the Carolinas, and the Cape Cod area during spring and summer. However, in recent years as many as 15 or 20 cases have been documented in each of the midwestern states. Persons who contract this disease may be asymptomatic or seriously ill; there is a 20 to 50 per cent mortality in untreated cases.

Clinical Manifestations and Diagnostic Assessment

The clinical picture is a sudden onset of symptoms that include fever (lasting 2 to 3 weeks), headache, chills, conjunctivitis, and severe myalgia (muscle pain) of wrists, ankles, and forearms that precedes a rash by 2 to 4 days. The rash, if recognized, can be life saving. Typically, it begins with macular and papular lesions that are pink and blanchable. These progressively cover the palms, soles, trunk, and face within 24 hours. After 24 hours, the rash turns red and is palpable, and petechiae are visible in the rash. By the fourth day, the rash is no longer blanchable, has progressed to purpuric vesicles (small blood-filled sacs or wheals), and has extended to involve the scrotum or vulva. If treatment has not been initiated by this time, ulcers and gangrene can develop on the fingertips, nose, and earlobes.

Aside from identification of the characteristic rash, diagnosis is made from a positive Weil-Felix test. However, it takes 24 to 48 hours to obtain results of this nonspecific test. Treatment should be initiated if the clinical picture suggests this disease rather than waiting for test results, because waiting could prove fatal.

Therapeutic Management

Treatment involves 6 to 10 days of oral tetracycline or chloramphenicol. Penicillin is ineffective, and sulfonamides worsen the symptoms. Begun early in the course of the disease, treatment favors a good prognosis; if extreme vasculitis involving the brain, heart, or kidneys or all these has evolved, treatment is unlikely to be effective. Persons who survive the disease have permanent immunity.

Nursing Care

Because of the critical factor of identifying this disease early, nurses should play a major role in educating the public regarding the clinical manifestations and the incidence in their locale.

Family members need instruction in preventive measures, including the following:

- Children and their pets should frequently be inspected for ticks, especially after playing in wooded areas.
- Anyone walking or playing in highly wooded areas should wear protective clothing (light-colored, long sleeves) and apply tick repellent (i.e., Deet) to exposed body areas as well as clothing. Reapply Deet every 1 to 2 hours sparingly.
- Children should be routinely inspected for ticks in season. If a tick is found, grasp the tick with small tweezers close to the skin and remove gently so that the tick is intact.
- Anyone who has been bitten by a tick should seek medical attention; treatment can be instituted before symptoms begin.

When the disease is contracted, parents need much help from the nurse to work through the guilt feelings they are likely to experience and to cope with the potential seriousness of the disease. They should be kept continuously informed of their child's status and involved in his or her care as much as possible.

Lyme Disease

Etiology

This disease is caused by a spirochete, *Borrelia burgdorferi,* and, like Rocky Mountain spotted fever, transmission is via a tick bite. *Ixodes dammini* in the northeastern United States and *Ixodes pacificus* in the western United States are the responsible tick vectors. Transmission requires at least a 24-hour tick attachment. Lyme disease, the most common tickborne infection in the United States, has been reported in about 43 states. Most cases occur in early to mid summer. The incubation period is 3 to 32 days.

Clinical Manifestations and Diagnostic Assessment

Lyme disease is a multisystem illness characterized by two stages. Stage 1 relates to early infection with localized symptoms and some early dissemination of disease. The characteristic rash, erythema migrans, begins as a red macule or papule at the tick bite site 3 to 32 days after a tick bite. It then enlarges, forming an erythematous lesion that has a centrally clear area. It may measure around 15 cm. This rash occurs in 60 to 80 per cent of patients and lasts about 1 month. It is often accompanied by a flulike illness of malaise, fever, fatigue, headache, and myalgias. Other complaints include photophobia, neck pain, and lymphadenopathy. If the disease is left untreated, early disseminated symptoms occur weeks to months later and include neurologic symptoms, cardiac rhythm abnormalities, and arthritic complaints, mostly of the large joints.

Late, or stage 2, disease may occur as much as months to years after the initial disease. Disseminated infective symptoms become persistent. Neurologic symptoms, including facial palsies, sensory losses, and focal weaknesses, may progress into a multiple sclerosis–type illness. Neuropsychiatric disturbances such as seizures and psychotic episodes frequently occur in children younger than 10 years of age. Arthritis symptoms increase and begin to involve a large number of joints.

Diagnosis often rests on the identification of the characteristic rash of erythema migrans. Because 25 to 40 per cent of patients may not present with this dermatologic manifestation, serologic tests may be helpful in confirming the diagnosis. Because influenza typically occurs in the winter months, Lyme disease should be considered in a child who develops a flulike illness in summer months. Serologic testing can detect antibodies to *B. burgdorferi,* although false-positive and false-negative results do occur.

Therapeutic Management

Therapeutic goals in the treatment of Lyme disease include resolution of the rash and prevention of stage 2 complications. The drug of choice is doxycycline by mouth twice a day for 10 to 21 days or tetracycline by mouth four times a day for the same interval. In children without permanent teeth, penicillin or ampicillin can be substituted. In late-stage Lyme disease, doxycycline, penicillin, and ceftriaxone have been used to treat various systemic responses (Goodwin et al, 1990).

Nursing Diagnostic Statements

Knowledge deficit, related to
- *Prevention.*
- *Etiology.*
- *Treatment and medication compliance.*
- *Possible long-term sequelae.*

Altered comfort, related to
- *Fever.*
- *Headache.*
- *Myalgia.*
- *Neck pain.*
- *Joint pain.*

Activity intolerance, related to discomfort from
- *Myalgia.*
- *Joint pain.*

Nursing Care/Interventions

In stage 1 Lyme disease, nursing care revolves around caring for the child at home. The disease may be difficult to diagnose, and the parents may be anxious while awaiting laboratory confirmation. Nurses need to address the problem of knowledge deficit and communicate clear facts regarding transmission and treatment guidelines for Lyme disease. It is important that parents understand the importance of medication compliance. Discomfort is usually managed with standard doses of analgesics. The child's activities may be limited owing to fatigue or myalgias. Headache and neck pain may also limit activities.

In late, or stage 2, disease, multisystem abnormalities are handled at home or the hospital, depending on their severity. Mild neurologic symptoms and arthritis require a restriction of some activities and administration of medications.

Perhaps the most important role of the nurse is to define prevention strategies for patients and families. Examining skin and clothing carefully for evidence of ticks is crucial. If one notes a tick, it is essential to record the date on a calendar. Use of repellents minimizes tick exposure. Proper removal of ticks must be performed as soon as possible after discovery. (See prevention strategies under "Rocky Mountain Spotted Fever.")

Amebic and Shigella Infections

Amebiasis

Etiology

Amebiasis, or amebic dysentery, is a disease of the large intestine as a consequence of mucosal invasion by pathologic protozoa. Reservoirs of transfer to humans include flies, contaminated water or raw vegetables and fruits, and hand-to-mouth transfer from contact with an infected person's stool. The disease occurs primarily in underdeveloped areas when sanitation is lacking and in temperate climates.

Clinical Manifestations

Symptoms vary depending on the degree of mucosal necrosis. The disease may be asymptomatic and resolve spontaneously after several days or remain at a carrier level. Carriers may fail to gain weight and be slightly anemic. Symptoms may be relatively mild, with diarrhea and mild cramping that alternates with constipation and bloating, accompanied by alternating anorexia and ravenous appetite, each lasting a few hours or days. A more severe picture appears in some children who experience an amebic enteritis characterized by colic and foul, watery stools containing blood and pus. If these stools reach a frequency of from 15 to 30 during 24 hours, true amebic dysentery exists. A serious complication of this disease is extension of the protozoa directly or via the blood stream to cause abscesses of the liver, lungs, or brain.

Nursing Care/Interventions

Diagnosis is made by identifying cysts in a fecal or lesion exudate smear. Often, serial stool examinations are needed because the cysts are shed only intermittently. Various amebicides may be used to treat amebiasis, common ones being iodoquinol and metronidazole. The child is infective until the organism no longer appears in the feces, which is usually within 72 hours after therapy is initiated. Complete cure usually takes a couple of weeks; however, fecal smear should be repeated at weekly intervals for two or more specimens to ensure elimination of the organism. The remainder of treatment is symptomatic and supportive. Preventive measures include personal hygiene education, pest control, adequate sanitation, and chlorination of water supplies.

Shigellosis

Shigellosis, or bacillary dysentery, is an acute bacterial disease of the large intestine. Two thirds of cases occur in children younger than 10 years of age; it is especially prevalent in toddlers. The incidence is greater in the summer. Persons from lower socioeconomic areas, in institutions, or who practice poor personal hygiene are at greater risk.

Etiology

Caused by any one of four species of *Shigella* organisms, the disease is transmitted by the fecal-oral route, hence the lay term "hand-to-mouth disease." The organisms may be passed as a result of direct contact with an infected patient or carrier or indirectly from contact with flies or objects contaminated with infected feces, or by consuming fecally contaminated food or water.

Clinical Manifestations

The severity of symptoms varies widely, ranging from asymptomatic disease to serious illness. Mild disease results in daily passage of a few more stools than normal, lasting only a few days. The onset may be characterized by sudden fever, anorexia, and gastrointestinal upset, followed hours later by diarrhea. The diarrhea is at first watery and green, then changes to bloody, mucus stools; their frequency increases to 10 or 20 a day. Dehydration and electrolyte imbalance can occur quickly, progressing to renal failure if not treated promptly. Untreated, symptoms persist 2 to 3 weeks, then subside. Severe cases are manifested by sudden high fever, convulsions and delirium, and meningitis-like symptoms. Stools contain blood, pus, and mucus and are explosive.

Diagnostic Assessment

Diagnosis is made from the symptomatic history, environmental history, and culturing of the *Shigella* organism from a stool specimen. All cases must be reported to local health departments so that contact follow-up (epidemiologic investigation) may be conducted.

Therapeutic Management

Treatment involves killing the organisms with antibacterial drugs; ampicillin is usually given until the specific organism has been identified by culture. If the organism is ampicillin resistant, trimethoprim-sulfamethoxazole or nalidixic acid may be given orally. The drug is given orally in mild disease but intramuscularly or parenterally in more acute disease. Fluid and electrolyte replacement is necessary in all but mild cases of the disease. Oral intake of food and fluid is contraindicated for the first 24 to 48 hours, then gradually progressed through the typical diarrhea diet routine (see Chapter 35). Enteric isolation is maintained until cultures are negative for the *Shigella* organisms, which is generally 5 to 7 days. Treatment of symptoms is also initiated.

Strategies for Nursing Care

This extremely uncomfortable, isolated child needs the supportive presence of the parents and a primary nurse. Toddlers who have just mastered toilet training need reassurance that their bowel incontinence is from the disease and is not their fault, and that it will eventually stop.

Preventive education involves proper sanitary and hygiene practices and instruction in clean, safe ways to handle food. Environmental improvement of sanitary facilities, pest control, and water purification are also necessary to prevent *Shigella* epidemics in communities.

Sexually Transmitted Diseases

Teaching Preventive Measures

The nurse plays a major role in helping young people understand sexually transmitted diseases (STD). Teenage girls need to be taught that only two types of vaginal discharge—menstrual flow and a clear vaginal secretion at the time of sexual excitement—are normal and that STD can be transmitted to a fetus during pregnancy or birth and can result in infertility.

Both prevention and prompt treatment of any genitourinary symptoms are the individual's responsibility to his or her own body. Several preventive measures can be taken by the teenager who chooses to become sexually active, including (1) using a condom to reduce the likelihood of genitourinary disease and pregnancy, (2) washing the perianal region well with soap and water after sexual contact, (3) urinating after intercourse (more effective for males), and (4) being selective in sexual behavior, by avoiding contact with persons at risk for infection.

Although these are simple preventive measures, they are often unrealistic in terms of adolescent sexual activity. A teen's sexual activity is often sporadic, casual, or unplanned—a consequence of sexual curiosity and experimentation. In addition, the common adolescent feeling of invulnerability leads them to believe that somehow the identified consequences of sexual activity, of which they may be aware, will not happen to them. Thus, the teen is unlikely to begin the sexual contact prepared with a condom or with thoughts about the possibility of the partner being infected; nor are restroom facilities likely to be readily available for prompt use after sexual activity.

What should be stressed is that the burden of disproof rests with both partners where STD is concerned. Disproof means that both partners can give evidence that they are free of the signs and symptoms of disease.

The following signs and symptoms should be taught to adolescents as signs of STD. Presence of any of these signs in themselves or in a sexual partner should be an indication for avoidance of sexual activity.

- Discharge (from the vagina or penis).
- Itching (around the genitalia or anus).
- Soreness or swelling (around genitalia or lymph nodes).
- Pain (on intercourse, in joints, in abdomen, in the genitalia).
- Rash (anywhere on the body).
- Odor (from the genitalia).
- Organisms (things moving around that one can see).
- Fever and fatigue.

The problem is that STD is often asymptomatic; the absence of signs and symptoms does not ensure absence of disease.

Teaching about Resources

Literature about STD must be readily available to teens as well as information about recommendable clinics for the diagnosis and treatment of these communicable diseases. Most states now permit physicians to treat minors for STD without parental consent.

Nurses involved in educating teens about sexuality or the sexual diseases must evaluate their own sexual attitudes. The nurse's ability to be comfortable with the teen and to discuss the issues in an environment in which both nurse and teen respect each other as individuals with responsibility for their own decisions and behaviors is imperative to gaining the teen's attention and cooperation. "Rap sessions" in which a group of teens and young adult leaders (nurses, for example) discuss feelings and facts about a problem and devise practical solutions are still a popular mode for educating teens about STD.

A nonjudgmental approach and the assurance of confidentiality are the minimal essentials to whichever method is used to teach or counsel adolescents in sexual matters. The counseling role of the school nurse is especially worthy of attention because of the tendency of youth to trust and consult a school nurse rather than other adults in their environment. The school nurse can also be politically influential in helping identify inadequate health services for teens in the community and in arousing public support for provision of readily available and adequate health care.

The epidemic of STD primarily among teens and young adults (peak ages 15 to 24 years), has made this the most prevalent group of communicable diseases in the United States. Despite the discovery of penicillin to treat gonorrhea and syphilis and widespread education efforts, these two diseases—plus chlamydial infection, genital herpes, and genital warts—persist and increase in prevalence yearly. The rapid and alarming spread of acquired immunodeficiency syndrome (AIDS) by both heterosexual and homosexual contact now makes education about STD a life-and-death matter. The nurse plays a vital role in preventive education regarding STD as well as in casefinding and encouraging prompt treatment. Table 39–8 summarizes the features of these diseases as well as the treatment currently recommended for them. AIDS is discussed in Chapter 37.

Pelvic Inflammatory Disease

Pelvic inflammatory disease (PID) is the leading cause of infertility in young women (Wilfert & Gutman, 1992). It is the most serious complication of STD. Vaginal infection (commonly chlamydial or gonorrheal) progresses to the fallopian tubes and may disseminate through the pelvis, with purulent infection and scarring during healing. It is estimated that 25 per cent of female teenagers who develop chlamydial infection will progress to PID (Freund, 1992).

PID is diagnosed on the basis of lower abdominal pain, fever, leukocytosis, an elevated sedimentation rate, and the presence of an adnexal mass on abdominal ultrasound examination. Treatment usually includes hospitalization with aggressive intravenous antibiotic therapy. It is thought that the outcome for fertility is enhanced by prompt and vigorous therapy.

Vaginal Infections

Vaginitis, an inflammation of the vagina, is one of the most common gynecologic complaints of females of all ages, but particularly once menarche is reached. The most frequently associated agents are *Trichomonas vaginalis, C. albicans,* and *Gardnerella vaginalis*. These vaginal infections frequently occur together.

Etiology

Vaginitis may result from physiologic causes related to elevation in estrogen or progesterone (such as in pregnancy, premenstrual and preovulatory hormonal changes, contraceptive use, and emotional stress), which lowers vaginal pH, rendering the person more susceptible to pathogens. Chemical causes—too frequent douching or sensitivity to feminine hygienic products or to contraceptive or prophylactic preparations—may also increase susceptibility to vaginitis. Foreign bodies such as tampons or irritation from intercourse may also increase susceptibility. Exposure to a variety of viruses, bacteria, fungi, or protozoa not normally in the vaginal canal may also result in vaginitis.

Diagnostic Assessment and Therapeutic Management

A commonality of symptoms—vulvar pruritus or pain, offensive odor, and vaginal discharge—prompts the patient to seek medical attention. Management involves determining the cause, whether a hormonal fluctuation, a chemical irritation, a foreign body or other mechanical irritation, a pathogenic organism, or simply poor hygiene. Inspection, vaginoscopy, microscopic examination of vaginal secretions, and culture are the common diagnostic strategies.

Treatment is aimed at the specific cause and includes the relief of pruritus and inflammation. Oral metronidazole (Flagyl) and/or vaginal preparations are ordered for infectious processes, depending on the causative organism. A topical corticosteroid ointment may be ordered to control intense vulvar pruritus. Table 39–9 details specific symptoms, diagnosis, and treatment for trichomoniasis, *G. vaginalis* vaginitis, and candidiasis.

Diagnosis and treatment of vulvovaginitis in a child includes considerations different from those in a sexually active adolescent. In the young child, a high or microperforate hymen may trap drops of urine or mucus that become infected with fecal organisms (Friedlander, 1990). If this becomes a source of recurrent infection, removal of some hymenal tissue may be considered. Sexual abuse must also be considered a potential cause of vulvovaginitis. See Chapter 28 for assessment strategies pertinent to sexual abuse.

Foreign bodies trapped within the vagina are another cause of vaginitis in young children. Often the foreign object has become trapped in the vagina accidentally, such as with toilet paper or some dried stool, but small children are also prone to exploring body orifices and depositing therein any small object that will fit, such as a bean or a small part from a toy. Pelvic radiography may sometimes be used in diagnosis. Removal of the object and cleansing of the vagina with warm water is usually sufficient to relieve the irritation (Friedlander, 1990).

Nursing Diagnostic Statements for Vaginitis

Impaired skin integrity: inflammation of the vaginal mucosa, *related to*
- *Hormonal fluctuations.*
- *Chemical irritation.*
- *Mechanical irritation.*
- *Pathogenic organisms.*
- *Sexual abuse.*

Situational low self-esteem, *related to*
- *The embarrassment of a genital disorder.*
- *Feeling "unclean" because of vaginal discharge and odor.*
- *Feelings of shame associated with perceived wrongdoing.*
- *Fears about possible long-term effects.*

Altered comfort: pruritus, associated with irritation of the vaginal and vulvar mucosa

Knowledge deficit, *related to*
- *Etiology.*
- *Treatment.*
- *Prevention of recurrence.*

Nursing Care/Interventions

Treating Vaginal Inflammation. Nursing strategies for treating vaginal inflammation depend on the cause. If the etiology involves a noninfectious process, teaching focuses on eliminating the source of irritation and on initiating good hygiene to reduce the risk of infection. If an infectious organism is identified, the patient will need instruction about medication administration.

When infectious vaginitis is diagnosed, the pediatric patient is most often an adolescent. Many medications for vaginitis are dispensed in the form of vaginal creams or suppositories. The nurse should take into consideration that the teen may never have used

TABLE 39-8
Characteristics of Sexually Transmitted Diseases

Disease (Pathogen)	Transmission	Incubation
Gonorrhea (*Neisseria gonorrheae*)	Direct contact, usually sexual May be contracted by infant during delivery	2–7 days (average 3–5)
Syphilis (*Treponema pallidum*)	Direct contact, usually sexual, during infective stage Transfusion of contaminated blood May be transmitted to fetus across placenta at any time during pregnancy	Primary stage 10–90 days (average 3 wks)
Genital herpes simplex (Herpesvirus hominis [HSV-2])	Direct contact, usually sexual May be contracted by newborn infant during delivery	2–14 days
Chlamydia trachomatis	Direct contact, usually sexual. May be contracted by newborn infant during delivery	1–5 wks (usually 1 wk)
Genital warts, also known as Condylomata acuminata (human papilloma virus)	Direct contact; usually but not always sexual	3 mos–several yrs

Adapted from Centers for Disease Control, 1985 & 1989; Johnson, 1987; Kalter & Rosen, 1985; Lutz, 1986; 1988 Canadian Guidelines, 1988; Hatcher, 1990.

TABLE 39-8
Characteristics of Sexually Transmitted Diseases ***(Continued)***

Clinical Manifestations	Diagnostic Tests	Therapeutic Management
Early signs: Copious mucopurulent discharge from phagocytosis, vaginal in female and urethral in male; pharyngeal if oral sex. Pain and frequency of urination from urethritis. 90% of females and 10% of males are asymptomatic *Other possible signs:* Cervicitis, salpingitis, peritonitis, PID, and abscesses of Skene's or Bartholin glands in females. Epididymitis and abscess of prostate gland in males *Late signs:* Arthritis, endocarditis, sterility	Culture of discharge for gonococcal growth (gonococcal smear). Gram stain of exudate shows gram-negative diplococci	Drug of choice is ceftriaxone 125–250 mg intramuscularly in a single dose (25–50 mg/kg/day in one dose). Cefixime may also be given as 400 mg orally once. Other newer alternatives include ciprofloxacin 500 mg orally and ofloxacin 400 mg orally as single dose for patients who are older than 16 yr. Cotreatment for *Chlamydia* is recommended (see *Chlamydia trachomatis*). Evaluation should be included for syphilis.
Primary—Infectious: Chancre (painless, indurated ulcer) that heals spontaneously in 2–6 wks. Located at site where pathogen entered *Secondary*—very infectious: Skin and mucous membrane, rash, lymphadenitis, fever, headaches, sore throat that disappears spontaneously. Lasts few months to several years *Early latent*—may be infectious: No physical symptoms *Late latent*—blood infectious: No symptoms *Late active:* Not all clients experience this stage. Gummas (nodular or ulcerative lesions) of skin, bones, liver, stomach CNS involvement • 10% optic atrophy, deafness • General paresis • Insanity Cardiovascular involvement in 80% of cases • Aortic insufficiency or aneurysm • Endarteritis	Serologic nontreponemal testing includes rapid plasma reagin (RPR), automated reagin test (ART), VDRL. Nontreponemal rapid plasma reagin card test (RPRCT) or ART commonly used Rapid, inexpensive, and determines level of disease activity Fluorescent treponemal antibody absorption (FTA-ABS) may be used to detect antibodies from early through late stages. Darkfield examination with a microscope can identify spirochetes	Early syphilis (1-yr duration): 50,000 U/kg benzathine and penicillin G intramuscularly not to exceed 2,400,000 U. Oral tetracycline, 500 mg four times daily for 2 wks may be given if client has penicillin allergy Later syphilis (1-yr duration): 50,000 U/kg benzathine penicillin G intramuscularly once a wk for 3 wks—not to exceed 2,400,000 U weekly If allergic to penicillin, oral tetracycline 500 mg four times daily for 4 wks
Symptomatic phase: Contagious. Minor itching or extensive rash of genital region followed by a cluster of blister-like lesions that then rupture and ulcerate; these are pruritic and painful, especially during intercourse. Painful urination, inguinal lymphadenitis and pain, fever, malaise. Symptoms disappear spontaneously after 2–6 wk. Many cases asymptomatic *Dormant phase:* symptoms absent but reappear with emotional or physical stress during which person again is infectious; once a person is infected, virus is harbored for life, though recurrences are less severe and last about 2 wk Cervical cancer eight times more likely in women with HSV-2 virus	Viral culture of lesions. Scraping and staining of ulcer tissue with Papanicolaou solution. Papanicolaou solution demonstrates characteristic giant cells and viral inclusion bodies. Antibody blood titer of HSV-2 21 or more days after infection	Incurable. Treatment aimed at pain relief, fostering healing of lesions, and preventing other infections. • Pain medication • Use of condom during intercourse to reduce likelihood of spread of HSV-2 or of infection with other pathogens; no intercourse when sores are present • Keep lesions clean and dry • Acyclovir orally or intravenously shortens duration of the first episode and may reduce systemic symptoms. Dosage is 200 mgm orally five times a day for 7–10 days. First episode treatment with acyclovir may reduce recurrent rates Cesarean birth in all pregnancies if active sores exist at time of delivery
Symptoms often mild, nonspecific; great majority are asymptomatic. Dysuria, frequency, slight white or clear discharge, cystitis, cervicitis, urethral itching	Tissue culture; also stained smear of epithelial cell scrapings, fluorescent antibody examination of direct smear (direct smear FA), enzyme immunoassay (ELISA)	Oral tetracycline HCl 500 mgm four times daily or doxycycline hyclate 100 mgm twice daily for 7 days. Alternative therapy is erythromycin four times daily for 7 days. If patient is 16 years or older, may give 1 g Azithromycin as a single oral dose
Rapidly growing, irregular, confluent masses with a cauliflower-like appearance; found commonly on labia majora, shaft of penis, or perianal region	Inspection. Clinical diagnosis is enhanced by application of 3–5% acetic acid—lesions turn white	Cryotherapy (liquid nitrogen or dry ice), or successive podophyllin applications, or electrosurgery or surgical removal. Also, may try weekly 80–90% trichloroacetic acid treatments

TABLE 39-9
Differentiating Vaginitis

Causative Agent	Transmission	Symptoms	Diagnosis	Treatment
Trichomoniasis (*Trichomonas vaginalis,* a protozoan) Incubation period 4–20 days	Direct contact with discharges during sexual intercourse or to infant as it passes through the vaginal canal at birth. Organism survives 24 hrs in urine and on wet linens, tampons, douche equipment, or sponges. Onset and recurrences commonly associated with menstruation, probably due to increased pH during flow	Harbored asymptomatically in men and in 25% of infected women. Vulvar pruritus is only symptom in another 25% of infected females. Remainder of infected females experience: • Thin, foamy, profuse yellowish discharge with foul odor • Itching, burning, and chafing of vulvovaginal and anal areas • Dysuria and frequency • Vulvar and vaginal edema and erythema • Cervical erosion	Microscopic examination of organism in discharge (no douching 24 hrs before examination). Monthly recheck after menstruation for 3 mo recommended to ensure cure	Oral metronidazole (Flagyl) (single dose or 7-day dose) is 95% effective in curing the disease, especially if male partner also treated. Lactating women should not breastfeed for 24 hr after ingestion of metronidazole. First-trimester pregnant women should be treated with clotrimazole intravaginally for 7 days and Betadine or vinegar douche for symptomatic relief, instead of with oral metronidazole. Use condom during and for 24 hrs after treatment of both partners
Gardnerella vaginalis vaginitis/nonspecific vaginitis (*G. vaginalis,* a gram-negative bacillus, is speculated to be the causative agent) Incubation period less than 10 days	Direct contact during sexual intercourse. Other modes of transmission also suspected but undefined currently	Moderately profuse grayish, thin, malodorous discharge. About 50% of women complain of slight pruritus. Mild inflammation of vaginal wall	Microscopic examination for clue cells. pH < 5.5. Potassium hydroxide test—a drop of 10% solution on smear gives off a "fishy" odor	Oral or topical metronidazole or clindamycin, oral or topical. Usually 7-day course of treatment. Oral ampicillin (recommended during pregnancy)
Candidiasis (*Candida albicans,* a yeastlike fungus)	Direct contact during sexual intercourse. Contamination from mouth, rectum, contaminated fingers, or fomites	Harbored asymptomatically in 40% of women with flare-ups only during pregnancy, hormonal or antibiotic therapy, or emotional stress. Intense, intolerable vulvovaginal itching. Profuse, water discharge or thick, white cheesy discharge. Erythematosis or excoriated vulva	Microscopic examination of vaginal discharge using potassium hydroxide or Gram stain	Various, equally effective treatments are used. Vaginal tablets, foams, or creams of fungicidal agents (nystatin, terazol, Monostat, Gyne-Lotrimin) applied every night for 3–7 days

Adapted from Feigin, R. D., & Cherry, J. D. (Eds.). (1992). *Textbook of pediatric infectious diseases* (3rd ed.). Philadelphia: WB Saunders; Hatcher, R., Stewart, F., Trussell, S., Kowal, D., Guest F., Stewart, G., & Cates, W. (1990). *Contraceptive technology.* New York: Irvinton Publishers.

a tampon or douche and may not know exactly where the vaginal opening is or how to insert medication into it. Furthermore, the patient will often be too embarrassed to ask questions. It is usually safe to assume that the young person will need detailed instructions. Mannequins can be valuable teaching aids in that they can help decrease the adolescent's embarrassment by shifting the focus from her body to that of the dummy.

Compliance with vaginal preparations is often compromised because symptoms subside within the first few days of the regimen and because the preparations tend to leak from the vagina, causing a damp and uncomfortable feeling. The adolescent must understand the consequences of failing to complete the course of medication: in most cases a prompt recurrence of the infection. The teen must know that she should continue the medication even if her menstrual period begins.

Reducing Pruritus. Pruritus that is unrelieved by medication or that is of chemical or mechanical etiology may respond to efforts to keep the area clean and dry. It is important that the patient (and parent, in the case of the young child) understand the etiology of vulvar or vaginal pruritus. Females who are prone to genital inflammation are advised to exclude contact with perfumes and dyes and to avoid prolonged perineal dampness. Both preventive and symptomatic care, therefore, dictate using only nonperfumed soaps, avoiding bubble baths and perfumed douches, wearing loose-fitting panties with a white cotton crotch, wiping (always from front to back to avoid fecal contamination) with white, nonperfumed toilet paper, avoiding sitting for long periods in tight-fitting jeans, and changing sanitary pads or tampons frequently.

Adolescents who are sexually active should be advised to use a water-soluble lubricant during periods of frequent intercourse to reduce mechanical irritation. They need also to be advised of the importance of medical assessment and treatment of their sexual partner(s) if the vaginitis involves an infectious organism.

Addressing the Disturbance in Self-Concept. The child's or adolescent's perception of vaginitis may be quite different from the actual diagnosis. She may feel she is being punished for masturbation or for sexual activity. She may fear that the vaginitis will affect her ability to become pregnant or her future children. The odor and discharge associated with an infection may make her feel "dirty" and fear that others will guess her "condition." The nurse who anticipates these responses can often establish an empathetic rapport that will allow assessment of feelings and a frank discussion of what vaginitis is and what it is not. Teaching preventive measures that allow the older child and adolescent a sense of control will also enhance self-concept.

KEY CONCEPTS

Concepts Related to Basic Information

- Many infectious diseases are preventable either through appropriate immunization or avoidance of risk factors.
- Many infectious diseases are tolerated by persons with normal immune responses. Infectious diseases are particularly hazardous to persons who are immunocompromised.

Concepts Related to Nursing Assessment

- Numerous developmental factors place adolescents at great risk for sexually transmitted diseases; nursing assessment of adolescents should always take this into account.

Concepts Related to Nursing Intervention

- Education about prevention is a major nursing responsibility.
- Care of children with communicable diseases occurs primarily outside of acute care settings.

REFERENCES

Aach, R. D. (1992). Viral hepatitis. In R. D. Feigin & J. D. Cherry (Eds.), *Textbook of pediatric infectious diseases.* (3rd ed., pp 677–697). Philadelphia: WB Saunders.

American Academy of Pediatrics. (1991). *Report of the committee on infectious diseases.* (22nd ed.). Evanston, IL: Author.

Brown, N. A. (1992). The Epstein-Barr virus. In R. D. Feigin & J. D. Cherry (Eds.), *Textbook of pediatric infectious diseases.* (3rd ed., pp 1547–1557). Philadelphia: WB Saunders.

Brunnell, P. A. (1992). Hepatitis. In R. E. Behrman & V. C. Vaughan (Eds.), *Nelson textbook of pediatrics.* (14th ed., pp 818–823). Philadelphia: WB Saunders.

1988 Canadian guidelines for the treatment of sexually transmitted diseases in neonates, children, adolescents, and adults. (1988). *Canadian Disease Weekly Report,* 14S2.

Centers for Disease Control. (1985). *Chlamydia trachomatis* infections: Policy and guidelines for prevention and control. *Morbidity and Mortality Weekly Report, 23,* 34.

Centers for Disease Control. (1989). STD treatment guidelines. *Morbidity and Mortality Weekly Report, 38,* 58.

Farrar, W. E., & Lambert, H. E. (1984). *Infectious diseases.* Baltimore: Williams & Wilkins.

Feigin, R. D., & Cherry, J. D. (Eds.). (1992). *Textbook of pediatric infectious diseases.* (3rd ed.). Philadelphia: WB Saunders.

Feldman, Y. (1983). Kaposi's sarcoma and opportunistic infections. *Dermatology Clinics of North America,* 131–136.

Freund, K. (1992). Chlamydial disease in women. *Hospital Practice, 27,* 175–184.

Friedlander, L. (1990). Vulva and vagina. In S. S. Gellis & B. M. Kagan (Eds.), *Current pediatric therapy 13.* Philadelphia: WB Saunders.

Fulginiti, V. A. (1992). Immunologic responses to infection. In R. D. Feigin & J. D. Cherry (Eds.), *Textbook of pediatric infectious diseases.* (3rd ed., pp 24–30). Philadelphia: WB Saunders.

Garcia, L. S. (1992). Parasitic diseases. In R. D. Feigin & J. D. Cherry (Eds.), *Textbook of pediatric infectious diseases.* (3rd ed., pp 1997–2122). Philadelphia: WB Saunders.

Goodwin, S. D., Sproat, T. T., & Russell, W. L. (1990). Management of Lyme disease. *Clinical Pharmacy, 9,* 192–205.

Hatcher, R., Stewart, F., Trussell, S., Kowal, D., Guest, F., Stewart, G., & Cates, W. (1990). *Contraceptive technology.* New York: Irvinton Publishers.

Inselman, L. (1990). Tuberculosis in children: An unsettling forecast. *Contemporary Pediatrics* 7(10), 110–130.

Johnson, J. (1987). Sexually transmitted diseases in adolescents. *Primary Care, 14*(1), 101–120.

Kalter, D. C., & Rosen, T. (1985). Sexually transmitted diseases. *Emergency Medical Clinics of North America, 3*(4), 693–716.

Kazura, J. H., & Malmoud, A. A. F. (1992). In R. E. Behrman & V. C. Vaughan (Eds.), *Nelson textbook of pediatrics.* (14th ed., pp 896–903). Philadelphia: WB Saunders.

Loebl, S., & Spratto, G. R. (1986). *The nurse's drug handbook.* (4th ed.) New York: John Wiley & Sons.

Lookingbill, D. P., & Marks, J. D. (1993). *Principles of dermatology* (2nd ed.). Philadelphia: WB Saunders.

Lutz, R. (1986, March). Stopping the spread of sexually transmitted diseases. *Nursing 86, 16,* 47–50.

Minster, J. (1980, December). Nursing management of patients with scabies and lice. *Nursing Clinics of North America,* 747.

Plotkin, S. A. (1992). Infectious mononucleosis. In R. E. Behrman & V. C. Vaughan (Eds.), *Nelson textbook of pediatrics.* (14th ed., pp 805–808). Philadelphia: WB Saunders.

Smith, M. H. D., & Marquis, J. R. (1992). Tuberculosis and other mycobacterial infections. In R. D. Feigin & J. D. Cherry (Eds.), *Textbook of pediatric infectious diseases.* (3rd ed., pp 1321–1361). Philadelphia: WB Saunders.

Vella, E. (1977). Research in rabies. *Nursing Times, 17,* 37.

Wilfert, C., & Gutman, L. (1992). Sexually transmitted diseases. In R. D. Feigin & J. D. Cherry (Eds.), *Textbook of pediatric infectious diseases.* (3rd ed., pp 540–563). Philadelphia: WB Saunders.

BIBLIOGRAPHY

Burke, P. J. (1987). Adolescents' motivation for sexual activity and pregnancy prevention. *Issues in Comprehensive Pediatric Nursing, 10*(3), 161–171.

Cornell, C. (1988, April). Tuberculosis in hospital employees. *American Journal of Nursing, 88*(4), 484–486.

Dirubbo, N. E. (1987, October). The condom barrier. *American Journal of Nursing, 87*(10), 1306–1309.

Genital herpes: (1987, July). Who should take oral acyclovir? *Nurse's Drug Alert, 11*(7), 951.

Gurevich, I. (1988, August). How to make every culture count. *RN, 51,* 49–55.

Kirkis, E. J., & Grier, M. (1988). *Nurse's guide to infection control practice.* Philadelphia: WB Saunders.

Kuffel, J. (1987, September). Treating a child with head lice. *RN, 50,* 32.

Lewis, H. R., & Lewis, M. E. (1987, September). What you and your patients need to know about safer sex. *RN,* 53–58.

Loucks, A. (1987, July). *Chlamydia:* The unheralded epidemic. *American Journal of Nursing, 87*(7), 920–922.

Marvin, C., & Slevin, A. (1987, October). *Chlamydia*—Cause, prevention, and cure. *American Journal of Maternal Child Nursing, 12*(5), 318–321.

McElhose, P. (1988, June). The "other" STDs. As dangerous as ever. *RN, 51,* 53–58.

Muscari, M. E. (1987, October). Obtaining the adolescent sexual history. *Pediatric Nursing, 13*(5), 307–310.

Orshan, S. A. (1988, July). The pill, the patient, and you. *RN,* 49–53.

Pachter, A. Should nurses receive the hepatitis B vaccine? *Nursing 88, 18*(6), 51.

Stewart, D. C. (1987, March). Sexuality and the adolescent: Issues for the clinician. *Primary Care 14*(1), 83–99.

Two new vaccines against whooping cough. (1988, August). *Nurse's Drug Alert 12*(8), 1104–1105.

Zack, R. (1987, September). What to do if your patient has lice. *RN,* 30–31.

CHAPTER • 40
Altered Neurologic Function

Jennifer Disabato
Judy Wulf

NURSING PROCESS PLANS
NPP: The Child with Increased Intracranial Pressure, Table 40–20

RELATED TOPICS
Stress and coping with acute illness, Chapter 18
Impact of chronic illness, Chapter 19
Febrile seizure (management of fever), Chapter 23
Developmental disability, Chapter 27
Patterns of inheritance, genetic counseling, Chapter 31
Neonatal sepsis, Chapter 34
Malignant brain tumors, Chapter 42
NPP: The Family with a Genetic Risk, Table 31–21

LEARNING OBJECTIVES

- Describe differences in the physiology of cerebrospinal fluid, cerebral and spinal cord function, neurons, impulse transmission, myelinization, and brain waves in children.
- Identify the components of the neurologic check included in the nursing assessment.
- Explain the purposes of diagnostic tests and nursing strategies used in the assessment of the child with a neurologic alteration.
- Apply basic knowledge of nursing care for children with various alterations in neurologic function (cranial surgery, seizures, status epilepticus, altered responsiveness, or increased intracranial pressure).

- Apply the nursing process to the care of children with neurologic alterations.
- Identify the nursing diagnoses, etiologies, and defining characteristics of neurologic alterations that children may experience.
- Discuss the long-term nursing implications of the diagnosis: *impaired home maintenance management.*

Any adult who has ever watched an infant learn to walk, a toddler teeter on a counter top, a preschooler climb a tree, a school-age child wield a bat, or an adolescent ride a motorcycle has entertained an urge to reach out to protect them from harm — and with good reason. The concept of altered neurologic function in the child brings to mind shattered dreams for the child and family and an uncertain future. Fortunately, nature provides children (especially the infant and young child) with a nervous system that withstands trauma much better than that of an adult, and many potentially dangerous mishaps result in minor bumps and scrapes. Unfortunately, nature also makes mistakes, and some children suffer from congenital and chronic neurologic abnormalities linked to causes such as incomplete development in utero and inherited syndromes. Because children are susceptible to organisms such as *Haemophilus influenzae,* they may develop infections of the neurologic system.

This chapter is designed to prepare the nurse generalist to care for the more common alterations in neurologic function. The chapter begins by describing the differences in structure and function of the neurologic system by developmental age, details assessment, and interventions for nursing care common to many neurologic problems and proceeds to a discussion of specific conditions grouped by congenital and chronic conditions, neurologic infection, and neurologic injury.

Structure and Function

A thorough understanding of the anatomy and physiology of the nervous system is necessary in caring for children with alterations in neurologic function. Recognizing the spatial relationships among neural structures is crucial to more clearly comprehending and anticipating potential problems in an acute situation. Figure 40–1 and Table 40–1 provide a review of the anatomy and physiology of the *central nervous system.* For a review of the structure and functions of the *peripheral nervous system,* see Figure 40–2 and Table 40–2. This discussion focuses on the differences in structure and function of the nervous system at different ages.

Head Size and Shape

At birth the brain is one quarter of adult size; at 1 year of age it becomes about one half of adult size; and by age 5 years it has attained 90 per cent of its total growth. This growth places pressure on the bones of the skull, specifically at the suture lines, which respond by depositing new bone at the suture edges, thus increasing the circumference of the head. Review of head circumference growth charts (Appendix 3) should serve to reinforce the knowledge of tremendous growth, especially during the first year of life and early childhood. The increases in horizontal skull girth occur during the first 2 years of life and account for much of the expansion in head circumference.

Two conditions that can affect the size of the brain and skull or reflect the amount of brain and skull growth are microcephaly and megalencephaly. "Microcephaly" is a rare condition characterized by a small skull because of lack of brain growth. Causes of microcephaly include sporadic occurrence of arrested brain growth in utero; acquired factors occurring during pregnancy (intrauterine infection, radiation expo-

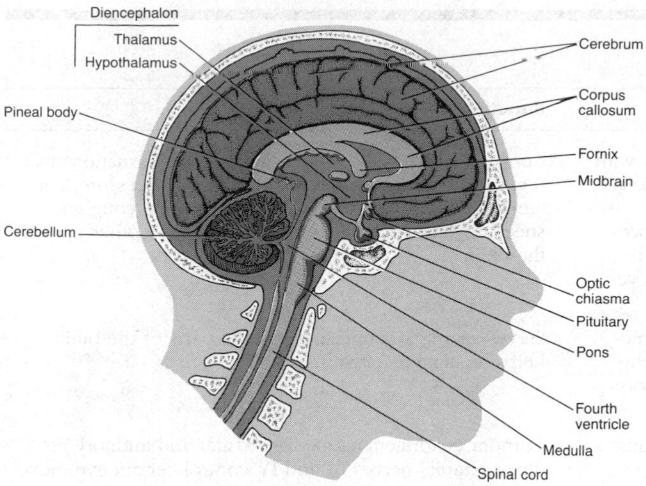

FIGURE 40 - 1. A midsagittal section through the brain. Note that in this type of section, half the brain is cut away so that the structures normally covered by the cerebrum are exposed.

sure, alcohol or drug teratogenic effects, maternal rubella, or toxoplasmosis); and congenital syndromes, such as familial microcephaly (autosomal-recessive disorder). Postnatal causes of microcephaly include hypoxic-ischemic encephalopathy, acquired immunodeficiency syndrome (AIDS), central nervous system infections, inherited metabolic disorders, and intracranial hemorrhage (Jacobsen, 1989).

The definition of "microcephaly" is a head circumference less than two standard deviations (two percentiles) below the mean for age and sex. The head is usually disproportionately small in comparison to the rest of the body. These children often have a variety of disabilities, such as mental retardation, physical growth delays, seizures, incoordination, movement disorders, and spasticity.

"Megalencephaly" describes an unusually large brain and skull, greater than two standard deviations (98th percentile) above the mean for age and sex. This can result from many causes including hydrocephalus, expanding cysts or tumors, increased brain

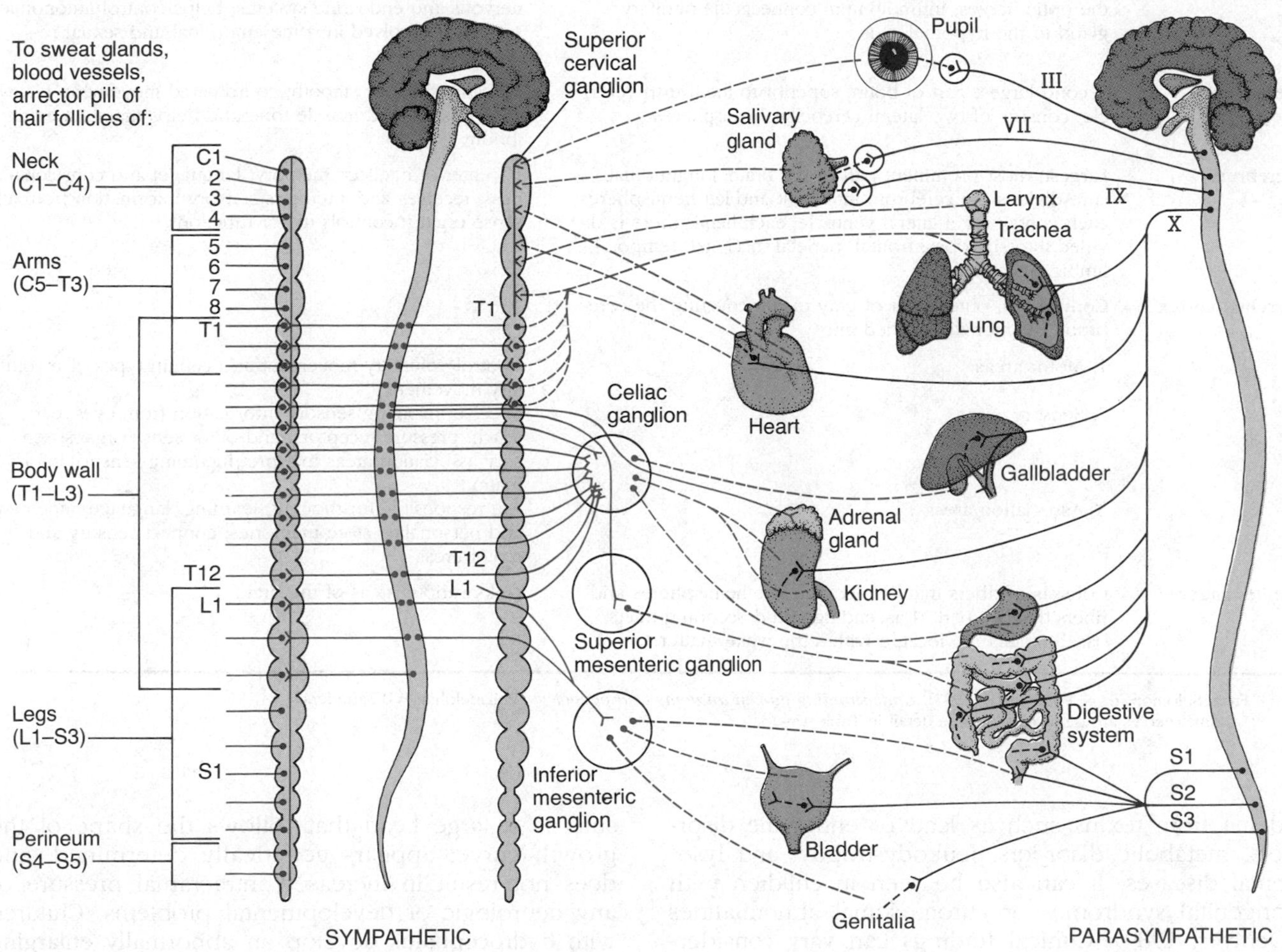

FIGURE 40 - 2. Sympathetic and parasympathetic nervous systems. For clarity, peripheral and visceral nerves of the sympathetic system are shown on separate sides of the card. Complex as it appears, this diagram has been greatly simplified. (*Colored lines* represent sympathetic nerves, *black lines* represent parasympathetic nerves, and *dotted lines* represent postganglionic nerves.)

TABLE 40-1
Divisions of the Brain

	Description	Functions
Medulla	Most inferior portion of the brain stem; is continuous with spinal cord; its white matter consists of nerve tracts passing between the spinal cord and various parts of the brain; its gray matter consists of nuclei; the anterior portion consists mainly of the pyramids; contains nuclei of cranial nerves IX through XII*; its cavity is the fourth ventricle	Contains vital centers (within its reticular formation) that regulate heartbeat, respiration, and blood pressure; contains reflex centers that control swallowing, coughing, sneezing, and vomiting; relays messages to other parts of the brain
Pons	Consists mainly of nerve tracts passing between the medulla and other parts of the brain; forms a bulge on the anterior surface of the brain stem; contains a respiratory center and nuclei of cranial nerves V through VIII	Serves as a link connecting various parts of the brain; helps regulate respiration
Midbrain	Just superior to the pons; cavity is the cerebral aqueduct; posteriorly, tectum consists of corpora quadrigemina; within midbrain are nuclei of cranial nerves III and IV	Corpora quadrigemina mediate visual and auditory reflexes; cranial nerves III and IV control certain eye movements
Diencephalon	Consists of two parts: *Thalamus*—located on each side of the third ventricle; consists of two masses of gray matter partly covered by white matter and contains many important nuclei	Is main relay center conducting information between spinal cord and cerebrum; incoming messages are sorted and partially interpreted within the thalamic nuclei before being relayed to the appropriate centers in the cerebrum
	Hypothalamus—forms ventral floor of third ventricle; contains many nuclei; optic chiasma mark the crossing of the optic nerves; infundibulum connects the pituitary gland to the hypothalamus	Contains centers for control of body temperature, appetite, and water balance; regulates pituitary gland and links nervous and endocrine systems; helps control autonomic system; is involved in some emotional and sexual responses
Cerebellum	Second largest part of brain; superior to the fourth ventricle; consists of two lateral cerebellar hemispheres	Is responsible for smooth, coordinated movement; maintains posture and muscle tone and helps maintain equilibrium
Cerebrum	Largest, most prominent part of the brain; longitudinal fissure divides the cerebrum into right and left hemispheres, each containing a lateral ventricle; each hemisphere is divided into six lobes: frontal, parietal, occipital, temporal, limbic, and insula	Is center of intellect, memory, language, and consciousness; receives and interprets sensory information from all sense organs; controls motor functions
Cerebral cortex	Convoluted, outer layer of gray matter covering the cerebrum; functionally divided into	
	1. Motor areas	Control voluntary movement and certain types of involuntary movement
	2. Sensory areas	Receive incoming sensory information from eyes, ears, touch, pressure receptors, and other sense organs; sensory association areas interpret incoming sensory information
	3. Association areas	Are responsible for thought, learning, language, judgment, and personality; store memories; connect sensory and motor areas
White matter	Consists of fibers that connect the two hemispheres and fibers that are part of ascending and descending tracts; basal ganglia are located within the white matter	Links various areas of the brain

From Solomon, E., & Phillips, G. (1987). *Understanding human anatomy and physiology*. Philadelphia: WB Saunders.
* Cranial nerves are discussed in more detail in Table 13–13.

edema from toxins such as lead or endocrine disorders, metabolic disorders, leukodystrophy, and lysosomal diseases. It can also be seen in children with congenital syndromes or chromosomal abnormalities (DeMyer, 1989). Clinical findings can vary considerably, depending on the cause of megalencephaly.

The two most common causes of enlarged head are asymptomatic familial megalencephaly and hydrocephalus. Asymptomatic familial megalencephaly results in a large head that follows the shape of the growth curve, appears genetically determined, and does not result in increased intracranial pressure or any neurologic or developmental problems. Children with hydrocephalus develop an abnormally enlarging head because of defects in the production, reabsorption, or flow of cerebral spinal fluid in the ventricular system, resulting in accumulating fluid and increased intracranial pressure.

TABLE 40-2
Comparison of Sympathetic and Parasympathetic Actions on Selected Effectors

Effector	Sympathetic Action	Parasympathetic Action
Heart	Increases rate and strength of contraction	Decreases rate; no direct effect on strength of contraction
Bronchial tubes	Dilates	Constricts
Iris of eye	Dilates (pupil becomes larger)	Constricts (pupil becomes smaller)
Sex organs	Constricts blood vessels; ejaculation	Dilates blood vessels; erection
Blood vessels	Generally constricts	No innervation for many
Sweat glands	Stimulates	No innervation
Intestine	Inhibits motility	Stimulates motility and secretion
Liver metabolism	Stimulates glycogen breakdown	No effect
Adipose tissue	Stimulates free fatty acid release from fat cells	No effect
Adrenal medulla	Stimulates secretion of epinephrine and norepinephrine	No effect
Salivary glands	Stimulates thick, viscous secretion	Stimulates profuse, water secretion

From Solomon, E., & Phillips, G. (1987). *Understanding human anatomy and physiology.* Philadelphia: WB Saunders.
Note that many other examples could be added to this list.

Ossification, Calcification, and Fontanel Closure

Skull ossification begins in infancy and continues into adulthood. Ossification occurs most rapidly in young children and then begins to slow in early school age. Increased intracranial pressure may separate the sutures, especially the sagittal suture, until age 10 to 12 years (Jacobsen, 1989). The pineal gland, a useful landmark in neurodiagnostic studies because of its midline position, becomes calcified sometime during adolescence.

The six fontanels, or soft spots, in the infant vary in the time of closure, depending on location and relationship to various suture lines. The first fontanels to close (around 2 months of age) are the posterior fontanel, which is formed by the intersection of the sagittal and lambdoidal sutures, and the two anterolateral fontanels, which are formed by the intersection of the frontal, parietal, temporal, and sphenoid bones. The last fontanels to close are the anterior fontanel formed by the intersection of the coronal and sagittal sutures (closes between 12 and 18 months of age), and the two posterolateral fontanels, formed by the intersection of the parietal, occipital, and temporal bones (close by 24 months of age).

Timing of fontanel closure is important. For example, premature or early fontanel closure and suture ossification in a normally developing brain could restrict a plane of brain growth and cause increased intracranial pressure leading to irreversible brain damage. Craniosynostosis is a condition that results from premature fusion of one or more cranial sutures, which is discussed in more detail later in this chapter.

Physiologic Differences

Cerebrospinal Fluid

Cerebrospinal fluid (CSF) formation, flow, and absorption in children are comparable to those in adults. The differences are in the rate of formation and total volume. Comparisons available in the literature are for infants and adults, the assumption being that children of other ages would fall somewhere between the two. The rate of CSF formation for a newborn is about 1 ml/hr or 24 ml/day, compared with that for the adult, which is 30 ml/hr or 720 ml/day (Swaiman, 1989). Total CSF volume in the newborn is 5 ml and in the adult is 150 ml (Swaiman, 1989). A comparison of the rate of formation to volume indicates constant production and absorption of CSF resulting in a changeover of CSF approximately five times per day. This has implications for how rapidly symptoms can arise when increases in intracranial pressure occur because of dysfunction in the ventricular system.

Cerebral Function

Probably the most striking neurologic achievements in children are the attainment of developmental milestones, including gross and fine motor, speech and language, perceptual and integrative, personal, social, and cognitive skills. Further information on this topic can be found in Unit 2. Information on changes in developmental reflexes throughout infancy and childhood are also detailed in that unit.

Spinal Cord

The spinal cord and cranial and peripheral nerves elongate during childhood. The termination of the spinal cord and its relationship to the lumbar vertebrae change inversely so that in newborn infants the cord terminates at L3 and in adults it terminates at L1–L2 (Fig. 40–3) (Moore, 1988). This has implications for the location of needle insertion for tests such as lumbar puncture.

Neurons

Neurons are the structural and functional units of the nervous system. They are specialized to be excitable and to conduct impulses. This factor has great relevance to studying the role of early experience and environmental stimulation in the development and further specialization within the nervous system.

The cerebral cortex is formed by migrating cells that pass through previously formed layers in the third fetal month. By the sixth fetal month, six layers of cell bodies and their processes are evident (Jacobsen, 1989). The ultimate growth of these layers is not completed until middle childhood or early adolescence. One must understand the specific regional and topographic localization of the brain as well as its lateralization, in order to appreciate how neurologic function can be altered by processes that can occur at various ages of childhood (Fig. 40–4).

Impulse Transmission and Myelinization

The speed of neuron impulse transmission increases as the diameters of axons enlarge and myelinization occurs. These two processes occur normally with age. Myelinated nerve fibers occur predominantly in the cranial and spinal nerves and compose the white matter of the brain and spinal cord. The lipid substance myelin, which forms the sheath around these nerve fibers, gives the white matter of the brain its characteristic color. The myelin sheath is formed from a glial cell that wraps around the axon (Fig. 40–5). In the peripheral nervous system, the glial cell is the Schwann cell; in the central nervous system, it is an oligodendrocyte.

The formation of myelin around neuronal axons in the central and peripheral nervous systems is associated with the development of functional capacities. Myelinization begins in the third fetal month and is usually complete at puberty. The general direction of myelinization begins in the cervical spine to the lower levels. The association areas of cerebral cortex are the

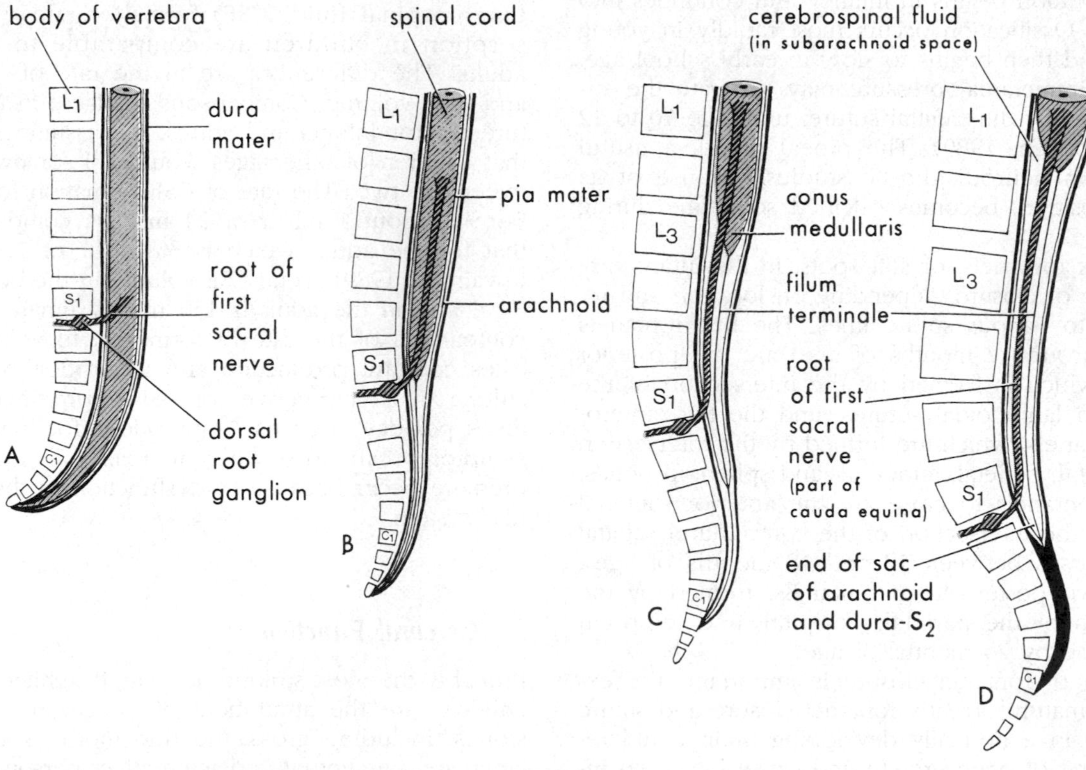

FIGURE 40 - 3. Diagrams showing the position of the caudal end of the spinal cord in relation to the vertebral column and the meninges at various stages of development. The increasing inclination of the root of the first sacral nerve is also illustrated. *A*, Eight weeks gestation; *B*, 24 weeks gestation; *C*, neonate; *D*, adult. (*A–D*, From Moore, K. L. [1993]. *The developing human: Clinically oriented embryology* [5th ed.]. Philadelphia: WB Saunders.)

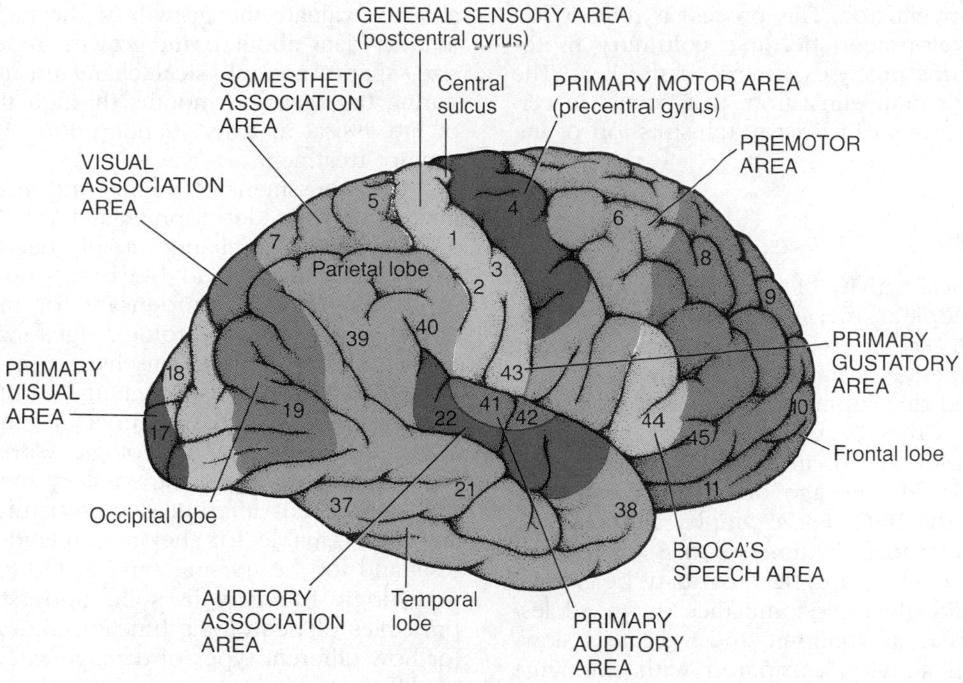

FIGURE 40 - 4. Map of the lateral surface of the cerebral cortex showing some of the functional areas. Areas 1, 2, 3, 17, 41, 42, and 43 are primary sensory areas; and areas 9, 10, 11, 18, 19, 22, 38, 39, and 40 are association areas.

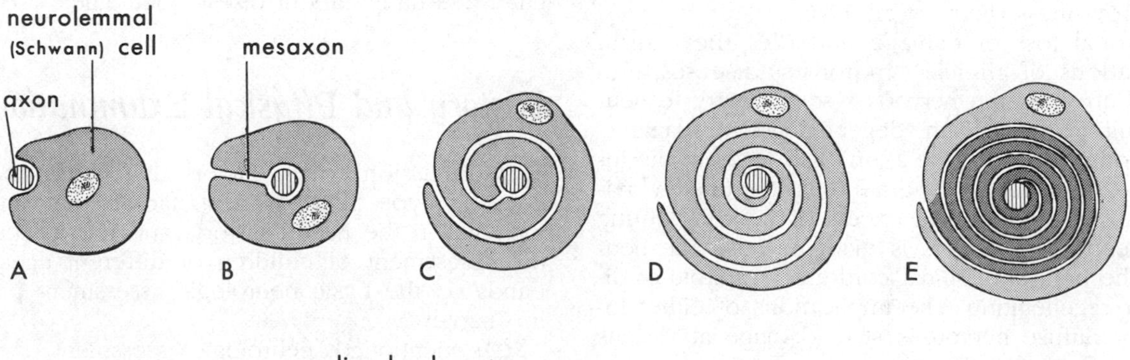

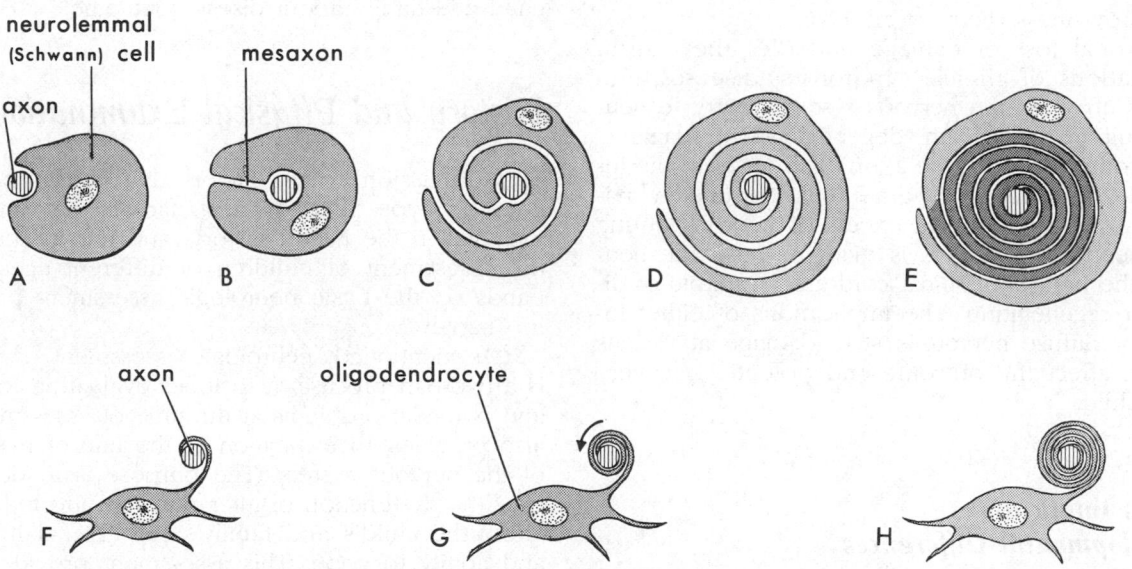

FIGURE 40 - 5. Diagrammatic sketches illustrating myelination. *A–E,* Successive stages in the myelination of a peripheral nerve fiber, or axon, by a neurolemmal or Schwann cell. The axon first indents the cell; then the Schwann cell rotates around the axon as the mesaxon (site of invagination) elongates. The cytoplasm between the layers of cell membrane gradually condenses. Cytoplasm remains on the inside of the sheath between the myelin and the axon. *F–H,* Successive stages in the myelination of a nerve fiber in the central nervous system by an oligodendrocyte. A process of the neuroglial cell wraps itself around an axon, and the intervening layers of cytoplasm move to the body of the cell. Myelination in the brain begins in the brain stem and reaches the level of the cerebral hemispheres by birth. (*A–H,* From Moore, K. L. [1993]. *The developing human: Clinically oriented embryology* [5th ed.]. Philadelphia: WB Saunders.)

last to become myelinated. This process is reflected in progressive development, because voluntary motor control of the arms precedes control of the legs. The loss of myelin, or demyelinization, that occurs in certain disease processes can destroy transmission of impulses.

Brain Waves

The gross electrical activity of the brain during wakefulness and sleep, as measured by the electroencephalogram (EEG), shows gradual changes in wave amplitude, frequency, and distribution with normal brain growth and development. In an extremely general sense, the waves become more organized and rhythmic, and they are of increased frequency and decreased amplitude. The age of the child is useful for interpreting the EEG. For example, although the predominance of theta rhythms (4 to 8 cycles/sec) and delta rhythms (1 to 4 cycles/sec) may be normal for a young child, their predominance in an adolescent would be read as abnormal and indicate a slowing of electrical activity, compared with same-age peers. Sometimes these EEG findings correlate with clinical symptoms of developmental delays or other diffuse processes affecting the brain. At other times these findings may be nonspecific (Ferry et al, 1986). Children may show some focal or localized electrical discharges on the EEG that would be viewed as abnormal for an adult, such as 2 to 3 cycles/sec rhythms during drowsiness (Ferry et al, 1986).

Neuronal loss or damage underlies the clinical manifestations of clinical syndromes, diseases, and disorders affecting the nervous system. Injury to neurons result in their death, degeneration, or damage, and axotomy (death of the axon) also leads to the injury or death of neighboring neurons. Fortunately, nature provides an abundant excess of neurons during development. This excess is vital, because the neurons of the brain and spinal cord are incapable of dividing or regenerating. The implications of either localized or diffuse nervous system damage at various ages can affect the outcome and potential recovery for the child.

Nursing Implications of Developmental Differences

The nursing implications of the age-related differences in structure and function are numerous. During assessment for actual or potential problems, the nurse should realize that not only will the child's present condition or state be assessed but also that the overall state of neurologic maturation or development will be evaluated. This provides an opportunity for early identification and case finding. For example, assessment of the head circumference should involve more than simple measurement but include comparison with baseline measurements, when available, to be able to evaluate the growth of the head and provide indirect data about brain growth. Assessment of the size, shape, and physical characteristics of the skull during the first few months through the first 2 years of life assists in early identification of problems and prompt treatment.

The assessment of infants and young children is limited by their developmental level. Neurologic status can appear to change rapidly because of the limits of assessment and because open sutures and fontanels help to compensate for increases in intracranial pressure. Neurologic signs may be apparent, or they may manifest themselves in more subtle ways, such as lack of interest in eating or irritability. School-age children and adolescents are more similar to adults in the area of neurologic assessment, physiologic responses, and compensatory mechanisms.

Age-related differences in structure and function are also valuable for the interpretation of diagnostic tests and for the nursing care related to monitoring of neurologic function. A solid understanding of the principles of neurologic function and an appreciation for how different types of damage can affect the brain at different stages of development are useful in instructing, reinforcing, and clarifying information the physician has given the family. There will be times when some prediction of outcome may be possible and situations in which prognosis is uncertain. Care must be taken neither to remove all hope nor to set totally unrealistic expectations when talking with a child and family about disease outcome.

History and Physical Examination

This discussion covers factors that guide and influence the type of assessment, factors that should be included in the health history, and factors that affect the assessment of children of different ages. It expands on the basic neurologic assessment presented in Chapter 13.

As mentioned, neurologic assessment of children is a two-part process. It includes evaluation for actual and potential problems at the time of assessment and also provides an evaluation of the rate of maturation of the nervous system. The purpose is to determine how the dysfunction or alteration has affected or may affect the child's and family's self-care, daily living, and ability to cope. This assessment provides direction for patient and family care planning, teaching, and counseling and should become the beginning of the rehabilitative or adaptive process.

Although the text and neuroassessment tables describe assessment for a child who may be developmentally "normal," many children may have a baseline developmental delay, mental retardation, or another neurologic deficit. The challenge to the nurse is to select creatively the assessment techniques that would be appropriate for that child. The screening questions at the top of each assessment table are useful to gain insight into a given child's abilities before the examination begins.

Rate of Symptom Progression

Criteria that guide the assessment of a neurologic problem include the rate of symptom progression and its nature or location. The rate of symptom progression has implication for the speed, organization, and frequency of assessment. For example, a child comes home from the playground late and is irritable for 3 hours, suddenly becoming listless and being aroused only by loud voices; the child displays "fending off" behavior and inappropriate conversation. Assessment of an acute situation like this would focus on quickly establishing baseline function including level of consciousness; pupil responses; motor responses; protective reflexes, such as blink, swallow, gag, and cough; respiratory pattern; and vital signs (American Association of Neuroscience Nurses, 1990). The time required for this assessment may be several minutes, and depending on the patient's acuity, reassessment every 1 to 2 hours may be necessary. Suppose that this child subsequently undergoes surgery to evacuate a subdural hematoma. If the child is alert in the postoperative period, the nurse may take time for a more comprehensive and orderly assessment. The frequency of subsequent assessments might then be once-daily or several times a day, depending on physician orders and the child's status.

The rate of symptom progression also has diagnostic implication for the general cause of the problem (Swaiman, 1989). For example, traumatic and vascular problems may produce symptoms that develop over minutes to a day. Symptoms arising over several days may indicate processes such as infection, electrolyte imbalances, or toxic poisoning. Symptoms developing slowly over weeks may indicate neoplastic, metabolic, or degenerative causes.

Severity, Nature, and Location of the Problem

The severity of the problem, whether static (unchanging) or progressive, also influences the assessment. Assessment of the child who has been delayed in development since birth differs from that of another child whose parents give a history suggesting a loss of certain previously acquired motor skills.

The nature and location of the problem also affect the assessment. Level of consciousness may be altered, and the assessment may need to be carried out frequently if the nature of the problem is unknown.

Problems are frequently referred to as being "focal" (a discrete neuroanatomic area affected), multifocal (several areas affected) or "diffuse" (widespread, most of the brain affected). This also may have some general diagnostic implication in that focal problems may have causes that are more frequently of vascular, neoplastic, or traumatic origin, whereas multifocal or diffuse problems are more frequently of toxic, metabolic, infectious, congenital, degenerative, and unknown origin.

Nurses may use different types of assessment, depending on their judgment, the patient's needs, and the medical plan of care. The most common examples are the *acute neurologic examination,* the *screening examination,* and the *comprehensive examination*. "Neurologic monitoring" is the name of the intervention defined as "collection and analysis of patient data to prevent or minimize neurologic complication" in the Iowa Intervention Project on Classification of Nursing Interventions (McCloskey & Bulechek, 1992). The screening and the comprehensive examinations are usually used on first contact with the patient, whereas the acute neurologic examination is used primarily for acute monitoring of the patient during the hospitalization. During practice, the nurse may find that a combination of the different assessments are actually being used, which may allow for screening gross assessments in areas without suspected problems and more in-depth comprehensive evaluation in problem areas. Whatever the method used, the focus is on nursing diagnosis, intervention, and evaluation.

Acute Neurologic Examination

The components of the acute neurologic examination usually include assessment of

- Level of consciousness.
- Pupil size and reactivity.
- Eye movements.
- Motor function.
- Respiratory pattern.
- Vital signs.

The purpose of the acute neurologic examination is to identify significant changes in neurologic function that may indicate deterioration or improvement, provide early detection of potentially life-threatening problems, and provide the means for early interventions that can further prevent complications and may positively influence outcome. The frequency of the assessment is determined by the patient's level of consciousness, acuity level, nature and location of the problem, nursing assessment, and physician's orders. The following section provides further detail on the components of an acute neurologic check.

Level of Consciousness. Plum (1980) defines "level of consciousness" as an awareness of self and environment that includes two components: content and arousal. *Content* includes processes such as perception, attention, memory, and judgment. *Arousal* is described as wakefulness. The neuroanatomic correlates of consciousness are in the cerebral cortex and the reticular activating system of the brain stem. Alterations in consciousness indicate problems in the cerebral cortex and/or the reticular activating system in the brain stem.

When assessing level of consciousness, one must first attempt to arouse the child from sleep and then to use the least amount of stimulation necessary to evoke the best response from the child. One should note both the quality of the response and the degree of arousal. One begins by assessing the child's response while moving into the child's visual field. If there is no response, one uses auditory stimuli by speaking the child's name quietly. If there is no response, a slightly louder voice is used. If still no response is observed, one adds a light touch with the name and notes the quality of the response. If there is still no response, one calls the child's name loudly and uses firm touch, noting the quality of the response. If these strategies fail to elicit a response, noxious stimuli are used. The concurrent assessment of motor responses can be done when assessment of consciousness requires noxious stimuli.

When assessing level of consciousness and using noxious stimuli, one notes whether the patient localizes the stimuli, merely withdraws from the stimuli, has a generalized response through decreased or increased activity, has a reflex response with decerebrate or decorticate posturing (Fig. 40–6), or has no observable response to noxious stimuli. Although an institution may have defined terms for the patient's level of consciousness, there are no universally accepted terms. A description of the stimuli required and the patient's response should be recorded.

Noxious stimuli should not cause injury. Good examples of noxious stimuli include squeezing the nailbed of the thumbs and great toes or stimulating the inner nostrils or lip with a twisted point of a facial tissue. Sternal rubbing, pinching muscles, and exerting supraorbital pressure are not recommended.

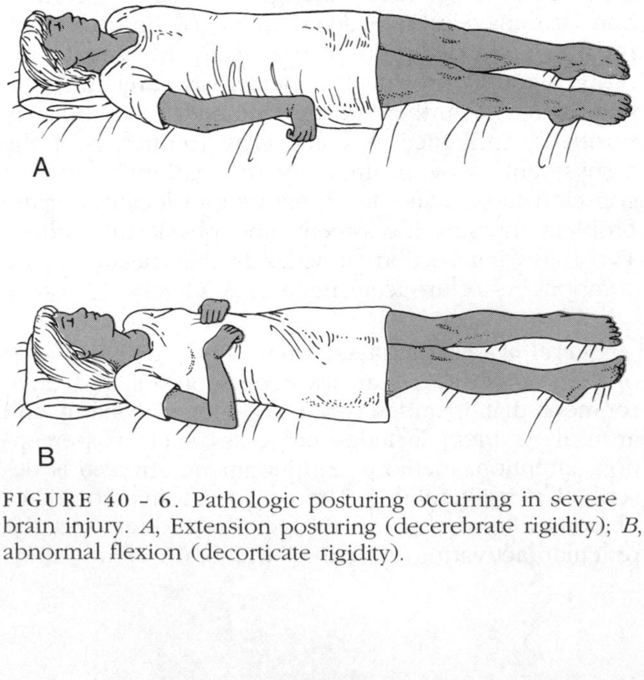

FIGURE 40 - 6. Pathologic posturing occurring in severe brain injury. *A*, Extension posturing (decerebrate rigidity); *B*, abnormal flexion (decorticate rigidity).

Pupil Responses and Eye Movements. The technique for assessing both direct and consensual pupil responses to light, comparing pupil size, and assessing eye movements are described in Chapter 13. Pupil responses are mediated by the interaction between two cranial nerves: the optic and the oculomotor. Pupil responses can be affected by damage to the eye itself, cranial nerves, and upper brain stem; by the local and systemic effects of certain drugs; by seizure activity; and by anoxia (Table 40–3). Pupil responses may be spared in metabolic disease processes affecting the brain.

Pupil size is determined by the input of the sympathetic nervous system, which dilates the pupil (such as during anxiety and pain), and the parasympathetic nervous system, mediated by the oculomotor nerve, which constricts the pupil. Pupil size normally varies with age. Newborn infants and the elderly commonly have very small pupils, whereas toddlers and adolescents may have very large pupils.

Eye movements are assessed in the acute neurologic check. Neuroanatomic structures involved with voluntary, spontaneous, and reflex conjugate eye movements are the oculomotor, trochlear, and abducent nerves; the medial longitudinal fasciculus tract of the midbrain and pons; and the vestibular system. The eye movements are observed through all planes, as described in Chapter 13. One observes whether they are conjugate, indicating intact cranial nerve and upper brain stem structures, or dysconjugate and/or fixed, reflecting localized damage to cranial nerve(s)

TABLE 40 - 3
Significance of Pupil Signs

No pupil response to direct light; indicates problem with optic nerve (II) or oculomotor nerve (III); proceed to check for consensual reaction
No pupil response to direct light and appears more dilated
Opposite pupil has a consensual reaction; this indicates problem with oculomotor nerve in dilated eye
Dilated pupil has a consensual reaction; this indicates problem with optic nerve in dilated eye
No pupil response to direct light
Opposite pupil does not have a consensual reaction; this may indicate blindness (amaurosis) in that eye, if other eye has a direct response to light and there is good consensual reaction in first eye tested
Both pupils appear dilated (mydriasis, parasympathetic lesion); this may be indication of hypoxia, drug effect, or increased intracranial pressure
Both pupils appear constricted (miosis, sympathetic lesion); if there is some reaction to light, may indicate problem with diencephalon (e.g., thalamus); if there is no reaction to light, it may indicate problem with brain stem; if only one pupil is constricted, it may indicate a Horner syndrome in which there is unilateral sympathetic nervous system injury

and/or the vestibular system. Spontaneous, random, roving eye movements may be characteristic of patients who are blind or are in a persistent vegetative or comatose condition.

Evaluation of eye movements for a patient with a depressed level of consciousness, such as coma, may include assessment of the oculocephalic (doll's eye) reflex if there are no contraindications to rapid head and neck rotation. It is important to understand that this reflex can be elicited only when a patient is comatose. The oculocephalic reflex is tested by holding the patient's eyelids open while briskly rotating the head laterally in one direction and observing the eye movements. A normal response is conjugate eye deviation to the opposite direction of head turning with a return of the eyes to the resting position in a few seconds. This normal comatose reflex indicates intact cranial nerves and medial longitudinal fasciculus tract function. An abnormal response is the eyes moving in the same direction in which the head is turning or the movements being dysconjugate. The oculocephalic reflex is carried out in both lateral directions and can also be tested by using neck flexion and extension for assessment of vertical movements. Assessment of vertical movements by flexion and extension may not be done in infants and young children because of the risk of airway injury due to hyperextension.

Motor Responses. The assessment of motor responses in the acute neurologic check involves observation of the patient's extremities for spontaneous movements; movements in response to command; and, in patients with depressed levels of consciousness, movements in response to tactile and then noxious stimuli if necessary. One must describe the movements. Are movements purposeful or nonpurposeful? Symmetric or asymmetric between right and left side? One should compare muscle strength, tone, and reflexes of corresponding muscle groups on both sides of the body.

Assessment of motor responses in infants includes testing Moro, grasp, and Babinski reflexes for symmetry. Toddlers may be able to reach the examiner's finger with their hands and to kick the examiner's hand with their feet. Older children may be able to cooperate with testing grip strength and major flexor and extensor muscles in the arms and legs. Pronator drift can be tested in older children by asking them to hold their arms extended in front of the body with palms facing up while they sit or stand with their eyes closed. This may disclose subtle weakness in one arm. The hand or arm drifting slightly downward and pronating during this test can sometimes be an early sign of motor deterioration. Motor tone can be easily assessed by comparing extremities for resistance to passive movement.

Patients with depressed levels of consciousness may require noxious stimuli to assess motor responses. One should use the least amount of noxious stimuli needed. One's thumb and forefinger can be used to squeeze the patient's thumb and great toe nailbeds. Generally, more noxious stimuli, such as sternal massage, supraorbital pressure, and pinching are not routinely used by nurses, in order to avoid possible injuries. These types of noxious stimuli may be used selectively by physicians.

The patient with a depressed level of consciousness should also be observed for abnormal motor reflex posturing. Posturing should be described as unilateral or bilateral; if it is bilateral, one should determine whether it is symmetric. *Decorticate posturing* (see Fig. 40–6) involves adduction of the arm with flexion of the arm, wrist, and fingers as well as extension, internal rotation, and plantar flexion in the lower extremity. Its presence indicates dysfunction located between the motor cortex and the midbrain. *Decerebrate posturing* (see Fig. 40–6) involves rigid extension, adduction, and hyperpronation in the arms as well as rigid leg extension with plantar flexion. Its presence indicates dysfunction located between the midbrain and the pons.

Respiratory Pattern and Other Vital Signs. Among the vital signs, respiratory patterns are the most sensitive indicators of neurologic change, especially change in the brain stem. Changes in respiratory patterns resulting from neurologic dysfunction do not occur until there are problems either deep in the cerebral hemispheres or in the brain stem. Neuroanatomic structures involved in respiration include the medullary respiratory center, which innervates the muscles of inspiration and expiration; the apneustic center and the vagus nerve in the pons, which control inspiratory efforts; the pneumotaxic center in the pons, which terminates inspiratory activity, and the cerebral cortex and diencephalon, which influence the brain stem structures (American Association of Neuroscience Nurses, 1990).

Monitoring of respiratory patterns and of rate, effort, and adequacy of respiration are important in assessing the neurologically impaired patient, because hypoxia and hypercapnia both can have significant effects on neurologic function.

Temperature regulation is under neurologic control via the hypothalamic nuclei and the sympathetic nervous system. Both hyperthermia and hypothermia affect cerebral metabolism. Hyperthermia increases cerebral metabolism and the consumption of glucose and oxygen. Hypothermia decreases cerebral metabolism and decreases consumption of glucose and oxygen. Extremes of temperature may be life-threatening. Temperature may sometimes be altered as a treatment measure. When interpreting temperature, consider the trends: whether the change is sudden or gradual, the environmental conditions, the general condition of the patient, treatment modalities, and the nature and location of neurologic dysfunction (American Association of Neuroscience Nurses, 1990). Hyperthermia can occur with increased intracranial pressure, central nervous system infections, and dysfunction. Hypothermia can be caused by hypothalamic and pituitary dysfunction and by toxic and metabolic diseases. It can be the result of immobility due to coma, profound retardation, and problems affecting mobility, such as cerebral palsy and cervical cord injuries. It can also be the result of treatment modalities, such as drug-induced coma, drug paralysis, drug toxicity, and induced hypothermia.

Cardiovascular function is also under neural control. Pathways from the cerebral cortex, diencephalon, and brain stem integrate cardiovascular responses; descending pathways from the hypothalamus affect the sympathetic stimulation of the heart, resulting in increased heart rate and coronary artery dilation. Brain stem centers, including the pons and medulla, control peripheral vascular resistance by descending pathways; the medulla and vagus nerve produce parasympathetic stimulation of the heart to slow the heart rate (American Association of Neuroscience Nurses, 1990). Recognition of cardiovascular alterations is important for two reasons; first, for diagnostic purposes, as evidence of neurologic dysfunction, and second and most important, for the purpose of management to optimize cerebral blood flow and perfusion and to prevent cardiovascular arrest.

Characteristic changes in blood pressure and pulse (Cushing reflex) are considered late signs of increased intracranial pressure. The patient usually manifests other signs and symptoms of increased intracranial pressure long before the Cushing reflex occurs. In the early compensatory state, the blood pressure increases and heart rate decreases; later in the decompensatory stage, the blood pressure falls and the pulse becomes irregular and thready; dysrhythmias may also occur. Dysrhythmias may occur as well with lesions in the posterior fossa and following posterior fossa surgery.

Nursing Implications of the Acute Neurologic Examination

One must compare changes in the acute neurologic examination with other data about the patient's condition and take prompt action if necessary. Children may not always follow adult manifestations of neurologic dysfunction. In children, wakefulness may not always reflect the integrity of the nervous system; that is, they can remain wakeful in spite of progressive neurologic deterioration until compensatory mechanisms are expended; then they appear to change rapidly. This is especially true when the process or lesions are infratentorial or involve the posterior fossa. Therefore, it is necessary to use all the components of the neurologic examination as carefully and thoroughly as possible.

The child's baseline abilities should guide the nurse in making the neurologic check more appropriate and useful. For example, spending time asking the child's name may be inappropriate if the child was unable to state it before the problem developed. Usually by age 3, children can tell you their name. Preschoolers may be able to answer questions of place and person, but assessing full orientation to time, place, and person is usually not appropriate before school age.

When completing the acute neurologic check, one must protect the safety and well-being of the child. In assessing consciousness and motor response, the least noxious stimuli should be used first. The proper techniques avoid injury to the skin and the body structures. If the child is experiencing alterations in neurologic function, one should provide developmentally appropriate interventions for security, safety, and psychologic support.

Children and family members may need repeated explanations about the frequency and purpose of these checks. One should discuss the need to use various types of stimuli and explain the patient's responses. Family members often interpret all movements or responses the patient makes as being voluntary, and they may need considerable support to understand the patient's condition. One should inform family members of whether the condition appears stable, is improving, or is becoming worse. When family members sense no change or improvement in the

TABLE 40-4
Glasgow Coma Scale

Parameter	Score
Eye Opening (E)	
Spontaneous	4
Responds to speech	3
Responds to pain	2
Nil	1
Best Motor Response (M)	
Obeys commands	6
Localizes pain	5
Withdraws	4
Abnormal flexion	3
Extensor response	2
Nil	1
Best Verbal Response (V)	
Oriented	5
Confused conversation	4
Inappropriate words	3
Incomprehensible sounds	2
Nil	1

The Glasgow Coma Scale is designed as a standardized assessment of the patient with disturbed consciousness. The tests can be performed serially to determine the patient's progress. The coma scale (E + M + V) = 3 to 15. All combinations equal to 7 or less define coma. Approximately 50 per cent of scores that equal 8 also define coma. Patients achieving a score of 9 or more are noncomatose.

child, witnessing another neurocheck can be an extremely anxiety-producing, frustrating, and depressing experience. They need an opportunity to ask questions and express their feelings.

Some institutions use the Glasgow Coma Scale (GCS) developed by Teasdale and Jennett in 1974 in addition to the acute neurologic check to assess patients with depressed levels of consciousness. The GCS scores the patient's best eye opening, motor, and verbalization responses (Table 40–4). A total can be plotted from this system with 15 points maximum and 3 points minimum. The GCS was designed to detect change for patients who had severe head injuries, and it does indicate early changes in arousal. It is used primarily for patients with head injuries. The GCS is not specific enough and does not have enough gradations and descriptors to be used alone to evaluate neurologic status and to determine care needs. Table 40–5 shows a modification of the GCS that facilitates assessment of infants.

Another scale frequently used in assessing consciousness is one developed by the staff at the Rancho Los Amigos Rehabilitation Center in Downey, California. This scale grades consciousness into five levels (Table 40–6). This may be useful, in addition to the neurologic check, for planning care of the older child, but it has limitations in children of different ages.

TABLE 40–5
Glasgow Coma Scale for Verbal Response in Infants

1 Mo	1. None 2. Crying to stimuli 3. Crying spontaneously 4. Blinking when eyelashes touched 5. Making throaty noises
2 Mos	1. None 2. Crying to stimuli 3. Shutting eyes to light 4. Smiling when caressed 5. Babbling—single vowel sounds
3 Mos	1. None 2. Crying to stimuli (moans) 3. Staring to response and looking at environment 4. Smiling to sound stimulation 5. Cooing, chuckling, *vowels* in a prolonged way
4 Mos	1. None 2. Crying to stimuli (moans) 3. Turning head to sound 4. Smiling spontaneously or when stimulated, laughing when socially stimulated 5. Modulating voice and perfect vocalization of vowels
5 and 6 Mos	1. None 2. Crying to stimuli (moans) 3. Localizing general direction of sound 4. Discriminating family members 5. Babbling to people, toys
7 and 8 Mos	1. None 2. Crying to stimuli (moans) 3. Recognizing familiar voices and family 4. Babbling 5. Saying "Ba," "Ma," "Da"
9 and 10 Mos	1. None 2. Crying to stimuli (moans) 3. Recognizing (smiling or laughing) 4. Babbling 5. Saying "MaMa," "DaDa"
11 and 12 Mos	1. None 2. Crying to stimuli (moans) 3. Recognizing—smiling 4. Babbling 5. Saying words (specifically "Mama" and "Dada")

Courtesy of Dr. Kenneth Shapiro, Neurosurgeons for Children, Dallas, Texas.

TABLE 40–6
Scale for Assessing Consciousness

Level 1:	*oriented to self and surroundings,* oriented to time and place
Level 2:	*responsive to environment,* purposeful activity, follows commands
Level 3:	*localized response to sensory stimuli,* visual focusing, blinking, following objects, movement of extremities localized
Level 4:	*generalized response to sensory stimuli,* startles, responds to stimuli with increased or decreased activity, responds to pain with reflex response
Level 5:	*no response to stimuli,* complete absence of observable change in behavior to visual, auditory, tactile, or pain stimuli

Developed by Rancho Los Amigos Rehabilitation Center, Downey, California

Comprehensive Neurologic Assessment

Comprehensive assessment of neurologic function is covered in Chapter 13. This discussion presents additional information to be included with the health history.

Health History. In discussing the present illness it is important to develop a clear understanding of the progression of symptoms and the period of time over which these changes occurred. Are the symptoms progressively worsening, plateauing, or remitting? Is there any change in the frequency of the symptoms related to the time of day? Are there any factors that the child or parents can identify that influence the symptom(s), either improving or worsening? Are there any symptoms from any other body systems that may be affecting the neurologic symptoms?

It is important in discussing the aforementioned problems to develop an understanding of the family and child's perceptions, the child's strengths and weaknesses, how they are currently coping or compensating with the problem, how their daily life is affected, the immediate and future concerns, the support and resources available to the child and family, and the character of the home environment. This information assists in planning present care and in promptly beginning rehabilitation if it is needed.

A review of systems is covered elsewhere in this text. Additional assessment for a child who may be experiencing an alteration in neurologic function would include the following:

- *Skin surveillance*—decubiti.
- *Sensory*—visual change or loss, double vision, dizziness, vertigo, voice change.
- Difficulty with swallowing, choking, history of aspirations.
- *Cardiovascular/respiratory*—syncope, fainting, palpitations, history of apnea or aspirations.
- *Gastrointestinal/genitourinary*—vomiting, change in bowel or bladder elimination patterns.
- *Neurologic*—problems with memory or thinking, change in muscle tone (either more rigid or floppy), weakness, any loss of skills that the child was able to perform consistently, change in sensation, seizures.

Neurologic Assessment. Mitchell and associates (1984) developed an alternative organizational framework for incorporating neurologic assessment into nursing practice by using functional categories. Table 40–7 uses Mitchell's organizational categories to list sample screening questions followed by examination of components that might be used for assessment of infants, toddlers, preschoolers, and school-age children. The nurse should use the screening questions or information about the child's baseline abilities to guide the assessment process. Select the examination components appropriate for the child's abilities.

Major factors in infant and toddler assessment include head size, shape, and symmetry; motor and social landmarks; presence, absence, and symmetry of developmental reflexes; abdominal examination; and vision and hearing examinations. The factors to include in the assessment of preschoolers and older children are categories that are similar to those in the adult examination but would also include developmentally appropriate skills for a given age. This may include mentation, movement (musculoskeletal and cranial nerves), gait and balance, coordination, reflexes, and sensory abilities.

Diagnostic Assessment

A summary of diagnostic tests can be found in Table 40–8.

Noninvasive Tests

Computed Tomography Scan

The computed tomography (CT) scan (also called CAT scan, for *c*omputed *a*xial *t*omography) is effective for visualizing hematomas and tumors; it is less effective for detecting cranial defects, such as linear skull fractures, or for use immediately after a cerebral vascular accident (Smith et al, 1983).

The CT scan differentiates tissues by their densities and uses about the same amount of radiation as a skull series, or 1 to 2.5 rad (Swaiman, 1982). The patient, with the head immobilized, lies supine on a movable table that slides into the scanner. The x-ray beam and detector rotate around the head, measuring densities in a series of cross-sectional scans. The computer averages the densities for each point in the brain and makes pictorial representations of the absorption measurements taken. On the scan, densities with lower coefficients (the lowest being air) appear darker, and densities with higher coefficients (the highest being bone) appear lighter. The use of contrast enhancement (which involves intravenous injection of an iodine-type contrast medium) provides for clearer viewing of blood vessels, well-vascularized lesions, and local alterations in the blood-brain barrier.

Nursing Interventions. No physical preparation is required for a regular CT scan. Some centers may require that patients be NPO for a few hours before the scan if it is suspected that the patient may need to be sedated. Psychologic preparation involves teaching children to lie completely still and preparing them for the sensations they may experience. In order to provide *preparatory sensory information,* the child can be told that the table will feel hard, and the room cool; that the head will be stabilized with cushions or a strap; and that the machine will move around and make some sounds. If coronal views are needed, the patient will need to extend the head while lying on the back. The child can be assured that the CT scan does not hurt. A CT scan of the head takes about 20 minutes.

Contrast enhancement necessitates intravenous injection of a contrast medium. Sensations experienced include an injection and a warm rushing feeling when the contrast is given. The child must be observed during and after the scan for possible allergic reactions to the contrast medium. Tables 40–9 and 40–10 describe care given before and after contrast medium is administered.

A child who is unable to lie still for the test can be scheduled for sedation or general anesthesia. Although sedation may not require a change in care, anesthesia may require consent, nothing-by-mouth status, and observation of pre- and postanesthesia vital signs.

Magnetic Resonance Imaging Scan

The magnetic resonance imaging (MRI) scan does not involve radiation. The MRI scan has appeared to be especially effective in imaging the brain and identifying atrophic and necrotic tissue, areas of ischemia, malignancies, degenerative diseases, and problems near the bony fossae of the brain, such as posterior

TABLE 40-7
Neurologic Assessment by Age Group

Infant Assessment

Screening Questions

1. How do they respond to their name?
2. How long do they pay attention to something they like?
3. How do they regard familiar faces and objects?
4. What kinds of vocalizations do they make?
5. Do they distinguish family from strangers?
6. Can they control their head, smile, roll, sit alone, crawl, pull to stand?
7. Do you (parent) think that they see and hear? What are the smallest objects that they can see and retrieve?

Consciousness	
Arousal	Describe their response to stimuli once they are wakeful, or describe how much stimulus is required to keep them wakeful; describe sleep and wake cycles
Mentation	
Attention Thinking and language Remembering	Describe their response to their name; describe if any differential response between nurse and parent; describe regard for and play with objects; describe their participation in eating and drinking (hold bottle, fingerfeed); describe any vocalizations; describe behavior
Movement	
Eye movements Eating Expressing facially Speaking Moving Head Trunk Arms Legs Coordination Reflexes	Test tracking to bright object (may have dysconjugate gaze in first month; after 6 wks may indicate blindness, nystagmus may be present until 3 mos); observe drinking from bottle, cup or feeding; observe facial expression during assessment; hold object out of their reach while sitting or lying; place them supine or prone; pull them to a sit or stand and observe their movements for quality, symmetry, and developmental appropriateness (fine tremors and infrequent involuntary movement normal to 2 mos); tone will depend on activity; observe hand position in grasping, test Moro, tonic neck, or parachute reflex, depending on age; test protective reflexes such as gag and swallow, if appropriate
Sensory	
Blinking Seeing Hearing Tasting Feeling Touch Pain	Test blink to visual threat (newborn slower and may have asymmetric blink); place small edible item within reach and observe vision; observe response to unexpected sounds (clap) (6 mos should be able to localize sound); test taste after 3 mos when expulsion reflex has disappeared and can note infant acceptance or rejection of new food tastes placed in mouth; note infant responses to tactile stimuli with examination; if lack of speech, need to investigate for hearing problem
Integrated Regulatory Functions	
Breathing Circulation Temperature Ingestion/digestion Elimination Bowel Bladder	Assess respiratory pattern, rate, quality, and effort; assess heart rate and rhythm, blood pressure, color in face, trunk and extremities; note extremity nailbed color; assess axillary or rectal temperature; note skin temperature in hands and feet; note strength and coordination to suck, swallow, and chew; if there are problems with elimination, assess abdomen and perineum
Head Circumference, Fontanels	Measure head circumference; palpate fontanels for size, fullness

(continued)

TABLE 40-7
Neurologic Assessment by Age Group *(Continued)*

Toddler Assessment

Screening Questions

1. Can they tell you their first name?
2. How long do they play with something they like?
3. How do they respond to their name and to "No"?
4. Do they use words appropriately (never, sometimes, most of the time)?
5. How many words do they use together at a time?
6. Do they know some body parts?
7. Do they remember where things are? Unpleasant situations?
8. Do they eat with fingers or utensil; do they eat by themselves?
9. Do they undress, pull on some clothes?
10. Can they walk alone, throw, kick, jump?
11. Do you (parent) have any concerns about their sight or hearing? Can they see and find small objects from across the room?

Consciousness	
Arousal	Describe their response to stimuli once they are wakeful, or describe how much stimulus is required to keep them wakeful; describe sleep/wake cycles; older toddlers may be able to tell you their name and identify family members by name
Mentation	

Attention
Thinking/language
Remembering
Gnosis
  Body parts
Praxis
  Eating
  Undressing
	Observe attention span during assessment, usually 1–3 mins; ask to locate/name body parts and common objects; describe words used and any combinations; assess ability to follow one-step commands; observe drinking, eating, and undressing; play hide-and-seek with an object; note short-term memory; describe behavior

Movement	

Eye movements
Eating
Expressing facially
Speaking
Moving
  Head
  Trunk
  Arms/hands
  Legs/feet
Fine motor
Gait
Coordination
Reflexes
	Test tracking of an object in all directions; note visual fields by confrontation; note convergence, cover/uncover test; observe eating and drinking; test gag and swallow, if necessary; note facial expressions for symmetry during assessment; older toddlers may be able to stick out tongue and show you how they blow, and should be speaking words that are largely intelligible; note gait and throw in younger toddler; add kick and jump for older toddler; note balance, coordination, strength, and symmetry in these movements; observe for hand preference; note gait (is wide-based until 2 yrs); test reflexes if there are any problems with movement, tone, or strength

Sensory	

Blinking
Seeing
Hearing
Tasting
Feeling
  Touch
  Pain
	Test blink to visual threat or by stroking lashes; place small toy/block on floor across room to retrieve; ask younger toddlers to localize quiet sounds out of their visual field; ask older toddlers to repeat words whispered in each ear; ask children to close eyes; touch each extremity and then ask toddlers to point to where they were touched—this usually takes practice

Integrated Regulatory Functions	

Breathing
Circulation
Temperature
Digestion
Elimination
  Bowel
  Bladder
	Assess respiratory pattern, rate, quality, and effort; assess heart rate and rhythm, blood pressure, color in face, trunk, and extremities; assess nailbed color and blanching; assess axillary or rectal temperature; note skin temperature in hands and feet; note strength and coordination in drinking, chewing, and swallowing; ask if the child gives indication or awareness of elimination and need to eliminate

Head Circumference	

TABLE 40-7
Neurologic Assessment by Age Group *(Continued)*

Preschooler Assessment

Screening Questions

1. Can they tell you their full name?
2. Do they know daytime from nighttime?
3. Can they tell you where they live?
4. How long can they stay with an activity they enjoy?
5. Give some examples of how they use words together in sentences.
6. Can they identify specific body parts and colors? Can they count to 10?
7. Do they remember daily routines, situations?
8. Are they able to feed themselves neatly, and dress? Are they toilet trained?
9. Tell me about the most complicated or difficult movement activities that the child can do with arms, legs, whole body.
10. Do you (parent) have any concerns with vision or hearing?

Consciousness	
Arousal Content	Describe their response to stimuli once they are wakeful or how much stimulus is required to keep them wakeful; describe sleep/wake cycles; ask them their full name; ask them where they live and if where they are is their house; ask if it is daytime or nighttime; ask them to name family members
Mentation	
Attention Thinking/language Remembering Gnosis Body parts Right/left Figure copying Stereognosis Graphesthesia Praxis Eating Undressing/dressing Toileting Bathing	Observe attention span during assessment, usually 10–15 mins; observe for full vocabulary and speech in longer more complex sentences; can count to 10, identify coins and colors, define objects by how they are used, correctly follow two-step commands, identify specific body parts, copy circle and cross, know right from left, distinguish coin from a key when placed in hand with eyes closed, identify circle from cross or "x" when drawn with finger on their palm with their eyes closed, may be able to repeat three or four numbers when asked to recall, repeat a familiar song or story; observe ability to dress with zipper and buttons; ask about ability to toilet by self, bathe with guidance; understands concepts like up/down, big/little, short/long
Movement	
Eye movements Eating Expressing facially Speaking Moving Head Trunk Arms/hands Legs/feet Fine motor Gait Coordination Reflexes	Test tracking of finger all directions; observe or ask about them eating and drinking neatly; ask for different facial expressions (show teeth, blow a kiss, imitate a "grouch" face); note pronunciation and intelligibility, sticking out tongue and wiggling it; observe balance and hopping for each leg; catch a ball or object; walk heel to toe; observe with scissors or thumb/forefinger rapid touching with each hand, finger to nose touching; observe gait—note quality, symmetry, and coordination in all movements; observe hand preference; test reflexes if any problems with movement, tone, or strength
Sensory	
Blinking Seeing Hearing Tasting Feeling Touch Pain Temperature Smelling	Test blink to visual threat and by stroking lashes; test each eye separately by holding up a small object from across the room for them to identify; test visual fields by asking them to point to wiggling finger; ask them to repeat words whispered in each ear or with closed eyes to identify when they hear a ticking watch; ask to localize both unilateral and bilateral touch; if concerns of sensation arise, can test sense of hot/cold, up/down position sense, and soft/sharp touch; may be able to recognize familiar smells, such as peanut butter or perfume
Integrated Regulatory Functions	
Breathing Circulation Temperature Ingestion/digestion Elimination Bowel Bladder	Assess respiratory pattern, rate, quality, and effort; assess heart rate and rhythm, blood pressure, color in face, trunk, and extremities; assess nailbed color and blanching; assess oral or axillary temperature; note skin temperature in hands and feet; note strength and coordination in drinking, chewing, and swallowing; note ability to carry out toileting independently
Head Circumference	

(continued)

TABLE 40-7
Neurologic Assessment by Age Group *(Continued)*

School-Age Assessment

Screening Questions

1. Can they tell you their address and telephone number?
2. Can they tell time?
3. Do they know the date and year?
4. How long can they pay attention to an activity they enjoy?
5. Can they print, write, read?
6. What areas are difficult in school? Are they in any special classes? What are the areas of strength in school?
7. Tell me about the most complicated or difficult movement activities that you can do with arms, legs, whole body. Are you right or left-handed?
8. Do you (parents) have any concerns about their vision or hearing?

Consciousness	
Arousal Content	Describe their alertness; ask them to tell you their full name and address, and determine orientation to time, date, year, and present place
Mentation	
Attention Thinking/language Remembering Gnosis Figure copying Stereognosis Graphesthesia Praxis All activities of daily living	Observe attention span during assessment, usually 15–20 mins; ask them the months of the year and days of the week; ask them to describe several objects in the room and to follow a three-step command; ask their phone number and to solve some simple math problems; ask to draw a person and copy a 3-dimensional cube, distinguish a dime from a nickel placed in each hand with eyes closed, identify any letters or numbers drawn on either palm with eyes closed, observe abilities to undress and dress, and in completing other activities of daily living
Movement	
Eye movements Eating Expressing facially Speaking Moving Head Trunk Arms/hands Legs/feet Gait Coordination Reflexes	Observe eye movements by testing tracking of finger in all directions; ask to take a drink of water with left hand, transfer to right hand, and hand back to examiner (observe memory, swallow, movements, coordination, right-left orientation); observe symmetry of facial movements throughout assessment and ask for different facial expressions; observe clarity of speech; observe balance during gait and when walking forward and backward heel to toe on a straight line; observe speed, accuracy, and coordination when touching thumb to each finger in succession, test reflexes if any problems with movement, tone, or strength
Sensory	
Blinking Seeing Hearing Tasting Feeling Touch Pain Temperature Position Location Smelling	Test blink to visual threat and lash stroke; test visual acuity of each eye with reading from book or using pocket Snellen; test visual fields by identifying moving finger; ask them to repeat words whispered in each ear; with eyes closed ask to localize unilateral and bilateral simultaneous touch stimuli; if there are concerns regarding sensation, test sharp/dull, hot/cold, up/down position sense; also test (with eyes closed) recognition of objects that are placed in each hand (coins, button, key) and identification of numbers and letters that are drawn on the palm of the hand; should be able to identify smells such as mint, cinnamon, coffee, lemon
Integrated Regulatory Functions	
Breathing Circulation Temperature Ingestion/digestion Elimination Bowel Bladder Sexuality	Assess respiratory pattern, rate, quality, and effort; assess heart rate and rhythm, blood pressure, face, trunk and extremity color; assess nailbed color and blanching; assess temperature, note skin temperature in hands and feet; note drinking, chewing, and swallowing abilities; assess any problems with toileting or elimination; observe for secondary sex characteristics; ask about menarche characteristics and any concerns regarding sexuality

By Judy Wulf.

TABLE 40-8
Diagnostic Assessment: Neurologic Function

Test	Nursing Implications	Contraindications to Study	Potential Complications
CT Scan (Computed Tomography) Differentiates tissues by density relative to water with computer averaging and mathematical reconstruction of absorption coefficient measurements	Noninvasive unless contrast given Teach patient about sensations to expect Observe contrast injection site, if used Patient with iodine allergy may get antihistamines/steroids before CT; have epinephrine available May need sedation or anesthesia to lie still	Allergy to iodine	Allergic reaction to contrast medium Injection site extravasation, ecchymosis, thrombophlebitis
MRI (Magnetic Resonance Imaging) Differentiates tissues by their response to radio frequency pulses in a magnetic field; used to visualize structures near bone, infarction, demyelination, etc. and as postoperative follow-up	No radiation Teach patient about sensations to expect Patients report boredom, excess noise, claustrophobia Observe contrast injection site, if used May need sedation or anesthesia to lie still	Pacemakers, electronic implants, surgical clips, pregnancy, metal workers, shrapnel history, ferromagnetic items, etc.	Allergic reaction to contrast medium Injection site extravasation, ecchymosis, thrombophlebitis
EEG (Electroencephalogram) Records gross electrical activity across surface of brain. Video EEG combines EEG recording with simultaneous videotaping	Teach patient about sensations to expect in setup Activation techniques include sleep deprivation, hyperventilation, photic stimulation, and antiepileptic drug withdrawal Clarify misconceptions (test cannot read mind or deliver electrical shocks) Shampoo hair afterward to remove all glue and gel	None	Can develop scalp sores if glue and gel are not entirely removed from scalp
(ER) Evoked Responses MMER (Multimodality) VER (Visual) BAER (Brain Stem Auditory SSER (Somatosensory) Measures electrical activity in specific sensory pathway in response to external stimuli; signal averaging produces wave forms that have anatomic correlates according to the latency of wave peaks	Results can vary with body size, sex, temperature, age, drugs, attentiveness, and characteristics of stimuli, depending on test Teach patients about sensations to expect: BAER hear clicks; VER see strobe or alternating checkerboard; SSER feel electrical current on skin Boring for patient, can agitate patient with altered level of consciousness; sedation may be required Does not imply cognition or perception	None	Can develop scalp sores if glue and gel are not entirely removed from scalp
Skull Series, Spine Radiography (fractures, anomalies, tumors, calcification, erosion)	Safe transport while immobilizing suspected region; care with transfers If erosion or fracture, be alert for cerebrospinal fluid leaks, possible hemorrhage, diabetes insipidus	None	Possible dislocation; subluxation of fracture with transfers and activities
EMG (Electromyogram) Records electrical activity in muscle fibers; reflects change in the motor unit to diagnose disease of lower motor neuron or muscle	Teach about sensations to expect—pricks and dull aches as needles are placed in muscles; children may need sedation or analgesia before EMG Electrical current applied distally to measure nerve conduction velocities	None	Note that serum enzyme studies are elevated after EMG Hematoma and infection at needle insertion sites

(continued)

TABLE 40-8
***Diagnostic Assessment*: Neurologic Function** *(Continued)*

Test	Nursing Implications	Contraindications to Study	Potential Complications
Doppler Ultrasound Studies anatomic changes in ventricles; also can evaluate hemodynamics (arterial flow and turbulence); screening test for cerebrovascular disease	No radiation Assist to lie still	None	None
Lumbar Puncture Insertion of needle into subarachnoid space for cerebrospinal fluid examination; to inject/remove substances, deliver spinal anesthesia	Teach patient about sensations to expect Assist patient in maintaining proper position Assess tap site for leak, infection, hematoma, etc.	Mass lesion with increased intracranial pressure Infections over site of entry Bleeding disorders	Headache Infection, hematoma Radiculopathy Brain stem herniation/respiratory arrest if patient had markedly increased intracranial pressure at time of test Potential for aseptic meningitis, arachnoiditis Spinal subdural epidural or subarachnoid bleed
CT Myelogram Visualizes structures around spinal canal after contrast injection into subarachnoid space; lumbar myelogram most common; contrast agents available: water-soluble contrast	Teach patient about sensations to expect May need sedation or anesthesia Must be well hydrated both before and after test; should not receive any phenothiazine drugs; MUST keep head of bed up 30 degrees for 8 hrs; assess tap site, vital signs, neurologic examination Usually has activity restricted initially	Blood in subarachnoid space Contrast allergy Fracture not allowing positions needed Infection over site of entry Mass lesion with increased intracranial pressure Bleeding disorders	Headache Allergic reaction Radiculopathy Local infection hematoma, extravasation at site Severe nausea and vomiting if not well hydrated Seizure activity if water-soluble contrast medium allowed to migrate intracranially by not following head-of-bed elevation orders
Cerebral Angiogram Intra-arterial injection of iodinated contrast medium to visualize blood vessels; transfemoral approach is most common; occasionally, brachial or direct carotid is used	Heavy sedation or anesthesia usually required Teach older patient about sensations to expect Good hydration important secondary to osmotic effects of contrast medium After test, monitor for complications, assess neurologic status and vital signs, as ordered; if femoral approach, check CMS in affected extremity; if carotid approach, monitor airway, neck swelling, respiratory effort, color Activity restrictions initially	Stroke in progress	Local reactions: hematoma, infection, extravasation, arterial thrombosis, temporary paresthesias Systemic reactions: allergic reactions, renal failure, cardiac dysrhythmias, hyper/hypo tension Neurologic: transient ischemic attack, reversible ischemic neurologic deficit, thrombosis, embolism, vasospasms, hemiparesis, aphasia, amnesia, seizures Note: urine specific gravity elevated secondary to contrast excretion
Digital Subtraction Angiogram Intravenous injection of iodinated contrast medium; uses computer imaging before contrast injection subtracted from later images when contrast circulates	Direct venous injection or may use a catheter technique; some are intra-arterial Use sedation or anesthesia; patient must be motionless, MUST be able to cease swallow on command Teach older child about sensations to expect Post care similar to that for cerebral angiogram	See that for cerebral angiogram	See that for cerebral angiogram Systemic reaction circulator overload secondary to large volume of contrast medium required, allergy reaction

TABLE 40-9
Basic Preprocedure Care for Noninvasive and Invasive Studies

Nursing Diagnostic Statement or Collaborative Problem	Nursing Interventions
Fear/anxiety about the diagnostic test, related to lack of information (cognitive and sensory) about what will happen	Adjust teaching as appropriate to the child's developmental level and condition
	Tell child about sensations he or she will experience, as well as procedural details
	Explain purpose of pre- and post-test care
	Clarify misinformation and reinforce that physician has encouraged patient/family to express fears, concerns, and so on. Explain expected sensations and reactions, have practice test with a doll. If there is discomfort during the test, let children know what they can do to cope and how long it will last
	Identify a support person (family member or staff) to accompany the child and provide reinforcement, reassurance, and support
	Avoid delays by prearranging adequate transportation and coordinating the time to give the sedation
	Explain to child the necessity of lying still so that the study is completed as quickly as possible. Have the child practice lying still for the prescribed amount of time
	Provide premedication as ordered
	Communicate any special needs the patient may have to the diagnostic team staff
High risk for injury: physiologic; risk factor: inadequate physical preparation for the procedure	Obtain or assist physician in obtaining consent (usually required for anesthesia, invasive procedures, or contrast enhancement)
	Encourage good night's sleep and daytime naps prior to the test. Obtain baseline vital signs and neurologic check. For angiograms, assess and mark distal pulses, depending on whether a femoral or brachial approach will be used
	Provide skin prep as ordered
	Encourage the child to void before giving preprocedural medications or before leaving the unit for the test
	When the study involves contrast enhancement, check renal function tests for normal values (blood urea nitrogen, creatinine); the contrast medium is excreted through the kidneys
	Encourage fluids or liquids until NPO
	Administer sedative medications, anticholinergics as ordered
	Remove earrings, barrettes, jewelry, and so on, from the body area involved with the procedure
	Dress the child in a cotton hospital gown for invasive tests and those involving contrast enhancement
High risk for injury: physiologic: hypersensitivity; risk factors: possible allergy to iodine or other contrast medium components	Ask child and parents about history of allergy or allergic reaction to previous contrast studies (e.g., CT scan, intravenous pyelogram, angiogram) or to iodine. Notify physician and diagnostic team of any allergy
	Give steroids and/or antihistamines as ordered prior to procedure, usually 24–72 hrs
	Ensure that emergency equipment and medications are immediately available
High risk for ineffective family coping; compromised; risk factor: psychologic response to the test results	Accompany child during transfers to and from unit

fossa lesions, acoustic neuromas, and spinal cord tumors. Because of its safety, it is useful in following the progress or course of children who require repeated scans. Innovations in MRI computer software have heralded a procedure called magnetic resonance angiography, or MRA, which is useful in identifying vascular lesions and may negate the need for a more invasive traditional angiogram.

During this study, the child lies on a sliding table with a shield placed around the head and shoulders.

TABLE 40-10
Basic Postprocedure Care Following Invasive and Contrast Studies

Nursing Diagnostic Statement and Collaborative Problem	Nursing Interventions
Anxiety, related to misconceptions and unresolved feelings about the diagnostic test	After the study is finished and the child has rested, allow the child, if appropriate, to express or play out the experience; allow time to clarify misconceptions with the child; provide time for the child to work through feelings; older children may want to write a story or draw a picture about the test, or the child may talk into a tape recorder and tell about the experience (see Chapter 17) (Collaborate with the Child Life therapist) Provide praise for appropriate coping behavior during the test
Altered tissue perfusion: peripheral, related to hematoma at site of invasive procedure	Check and record the condition of the site; for an angiogram check and record the quality and symmetry of both distal pulses: • Pedal pulses following femoral access • Radial pulses following brachial access • Temporal pulses following carotid access After carotid access, also note airway and respiratory effort; check neck circumference and facial color Apply manual pressure and ice pack to minimize bleeding as appropriate; monitor vital signs Limit and then advance patient activities as appropriate
Potential for injury: physiologic, related to physiologic response to diagnostic procedure	Perform and record *neurologic monitoring* as ordered; compare with prestudy baseline; observe for any trends Assess and evaluate vital signs
Altered comfort: nausea and vomiting, related to anesthesia or medications associated with the diagnostic test *High risk for aspiration; risk factor: postoperative vomiting*	Administer anticholinergics and antiemetics as ordered Slowly increase oral intake amounts, and advance as tolerated (do not just let the child decide) Intravenous therapy if vomiting persists Minimize anxiety
Potential fluid volume deficit, related to postprocedure vomiting or diuresis associated with dilution of contrast medium	Encourage fluids post contrast, unless otherwise ordered Monitor intake and output if vomiting persists Specific gravity of urine may increase secondary to contrast medium excretion Intravenous therapy if diuresis or vomiting persists
High risk for injury: physiologic: hypersensitivity; risk factors: possible allergy to iodine or other contrast medium components *Defining characteristics: itching, watery eyes, nasal congestion, hives, rash, bronchospasm, pulmonary edema, renal failure, cardiopulmonary collapse, death*	Monitor vital signs, skin, respiratory quality, and general condition as ordered Have emergency medications available (antihistamines, epinephrine and antidysrhythmics, steroids) Treat symptomatically
High risk for ineffective family coping; compromised; risk factor: psychologic response to the test results	Be present when physician explains test results to family, to be able to reinforce test results, clarify misconceptions or misunderstandings, provide opportunity for patient/family to express feelings and concerns Depending on test results, common feelings may include relief, grief, shock, confusion, anger, and so on Assist patient/family to consider their options and alternatives regarding treatment alternatives Provide anticipatory teaching as appropriate

The table is slid within a strong magnetic field. A computer processes the measurements taken during the study and presents it in a cross-sectional pictorial representation. An MRI scan of the head takes about 1 hour. *Preparatory sensory information* about this test would be given to the child.

Nursing Interventions. Physical preparation for MRI may include making the patient NPO before the test, since sedation is *often* necessary given the length of time needed to perform each sequence. During a sequence, the child must be absolutely still. Patients do need to be screened carefully for potentially hazardous objects. These objects include ferromagnetic metallic devices or implants and electronic equipment that could be affected by the magnetic fields: cardiac pacemakers; metal vascular clips; metal prostheses used in joint replacements; bone pins, plates, and screws; artificial heart valves; and cerebral surgical clips. The study is also contraindicated during pregnancy until more information becomes available. No risks are currently identified with MRI for patients who are free of any of the potential hazards mentioned.

Psychologic preparation includes instructing children that there is no discomfort or pain associated with the study, that they must lie still, and that the machine will turn around them and make a loud banging sound similar to a washing machine (preparatory sensory information). Older patients may complain of boredom, difficulty lying motionless for the time required, and feelings of claustrophobia and confinement. Parents or supportive staff who have been screened for any potential hazards may accompany the patient to provide psychologic support or to read or sing songs to the patient.

Sedation or general anesthesia will be scheduled for children who are unable to lie still. Contrast enhancement necessitates intravenous injection of a contrast medium. Sensations experienced include an injection and a warm rushing feeling when the contrast medium is given. The child must be observed after the scan for possible allergic reactions to the contrast. Tables 40–9 and 40–10 describe care given before and after the contrast medium is administered.

Electroencephalogram

The EEG provides a graphic record of the electrical activity across large areas of the brain's cortex. This electrical activity represents the sum of synaptic activity across millions of neurons. The study is useful in the management of seizure disorders or epilepsy as well as in patients with a head injury, stroke, encephalopathy, or metabolic coma. It is also valuable in assessing psychiatric illness and determining brain death.

The EEG is interpreted for the quality and characteristics of the background, or ongoing, electrical activity as well as for any abnormal electrical discharges. Its results must be correlated with other findings. Different types of EEGs have evolved in recent years.

The routine EEG is still the most common and takes 45 to 60 minutes to complete. The method involves gluing 17 to 21 electrodes to specific locations on the scalp and filling the cup electrodes with a conductive jelly. The electrical signals are transmitted through the electrodes to the machine, where the difference in electrical activity between two electrodes is displayed in graphic form on the moving paper. During the study, several different recording systems or montages are used as the machine is briefly stopped, and switches change the way that the electrodes pair up electrically. Usually some activation techniques are used, such as photic stimulation (flashing a light in the eyes at various frequencies) or voluntary hyperventilation in the hope of precipitating a seizure for the purpose of diagnostic recording. When the recording is finished, the electrodes are removed, as are the glue and jelly from the hair.

Another technique that may precipitate certain types of seizure discharges is sleep deprivation. This involves keeping the patient awake for all or part of the night before the EEG is to be done. Depending on the physician's order, the patient either sleeps or is kept awake during the study.

Video EEG and EEG telemetry follow the same setup procedure but may involve only one recording system or montage and usually use no activation procedures. These tests may be available through more specialized EEG laboratories that have a comprehensive center. The video EEG may last from several hours to days, and patients are usually confined to an area. This technique combines an ongoing videotape with EEG recording to allow more accurate diagnosis and classification of a given type of seizure. The EEG telemetry may last for several days and is useful when seizures occur infrequently. The patient's electrodes are connected to a transmitter and battery pack, which allow the patient to be mobile within the general range of the receiving antennas.

Nursing Interventions. No physical preparation is required, unless the patient is to be deprived of sleep or requires sedation. Hair elastics and barrettes are usually removed, and unless the hair is dirty or oily, washing it before the test is unnecessary.

Psychologic preparation involves instruction about the test procedure and *preparatory sensory information*. Children may fear that the machine will deliver some kind of electrical shock or that it may be able to read their minds or is some type of a lie detector test. Most children find the smell of the glue noxious and should know it will feel cold and wet on the head. A small penlike air compressor is used to blow-dry the glue, and the sound of this may be startling. When the conductive jelly is placed inside the electrodes with a syringe, children may fear an injection and find that the surface rubbing or scratching is annoying and uncomfortable. From the child's point of view, the setup and removal of the electrodes usually constitute the most disliked part; the child may need considerable support and reassurance to tolerate it. The study often seems mysterious to parents. They may misinterpret normal and abnormal findings; they may view the study as highly objective and not realize its limitations.

The same care is required for video EEG and EEG telemetry, except that children need support to occupy themselves throughout the study and require continuous observation for seizures.

After the test is finished, all of the glue and jelly

must be removed from the hair to avoid scalp irritation and sores. Excess glue can usually be removed with acetone or can be combed out. Hair care products that reduce snarls and tangles may be useful.

Evoked Potentials

Several types of evoked potential studies are available: brain stem auditory evoked responses (BAERs, also called BAEPs for evoked potentials), somatosensory evoked responses (SERs or SEPs), visual evoked responses (VERs or VEPs), and multimodality evoked responses (MMERs or MMEPs).

These studies are used for pre-, intra-, and postoperative monitoring of the integrity of various sensory pathways near the surgical site. They can also assess brain activity during drug overdose, drug-induced coma, or coma due to brain damage. They can determine the integrity of sensory pathways in individuals with diseases such as multiple sclerosis, spinal cord injuries, and hearing loss, or in children (especially neonates) who will be receiving long-term aminoglycoside antibiotics (gentamicin sulfate, tobramycin sulfate) together with diuretic (furosemide) therapy.

The MMER is used for diagnostic purposes to localize areas of lesions and to determine the prognosis, because both the BAER and SER are unaffected by arousal, anesthesia, central nervous system depression, or drug-induced coma.

Nursing Interventions. Table 40–11 reviews information for the visual, brain stem, and SER study. Parents and older children need to understand the test and what to expect. The VERs do usually require a certain amount of cooperation to keep the patient's visual attention focused on a specific area. In young children and infants, the VERs may utilize a flashing strobe light, rather than an alternating checkerboard, as the stimulus. Sometimes sedation may be ordered to minimize movement artifact.

Skull and Spine Radiography

The purpose of skull and spine radiography is to identify fractures, anomalies, tumors, and calcifications and to note indirect evidence of increased intracranial pressure by suture widening in a younger child or skull erosion in an older child. Care should be taken in positioning or moving the child for this study in cases of suspected fracture or dislocation.

Nursing Interventions. No physical preparation is required. Hair elastics, pins, and barrettes should be removed for skull radiography. For spine films the child is dressed in an "x-ray" or patient gown.

Psychologic preparation involves explaining the procedure of proper positioning and holding still briefly while the x-ray film is taken. The child is told that the test does not hurt and why other people stand back or wear shields or aprons during the test. The child is also told that the machine will make some noises.

Electromyogram and Nerve Conduction Velocities

The purpose of the electromyogram (EMG) is to analyze the electrical events associated with the contraction of skeletal muscle fibers. This includes (1) insertion potentials as the needle is inserted into the muscle and measures the brief electrical discharges produced by this mechanical stimulus; (2) spontaneous potentials, which may occur as fibrillations from single muscle fibers or fasciculations from groups of fibers; and (3) motor unit action potentials as the electrical activity is studied during voluntary muscle contraction.

Nerve conduction velocities measure the muscle contraction that is evoked by the electrical stimulation along peripheral nerves, such as motor and sensory nerves. These velocities increase with age during the first few years of life and reach the lower end of the adult norms by 3 years of age. Nerve conduction velocities can also slow down with decreased body temperature. These tests may assist in defining types of muscle disease involving the lower motor neuron or muscle, locating nerve lesions, and quantitating nerve regeneration and muscle recovery.

The method for EMG involves some discomfort as needle electrodes are placed into the muscle to be examined and there is a momentary prick. If the needle needs to be repositioned, this may produce a slight, dull ache in the muscle. Patients are periodically asked to contract and relax their muscles. Nerve conduction velocities may follow the EMG and involve the proximal and distal stimulation of a motor nerve and then the distal stimulation of a sensory nerve. The stimulations may produce a muscle twitch or contraction or a tingling sensation, depending on the type of nerve being stimulated.

Nursing Interventions. There is no physical preparation involved in this study unless sedation has been ordered for the patient. Psychologic preparation involves *preparatory sensory information,* explaining to the parents what the test involves, and letting children know what they are expected to do. It may be helpful to plan some activities for the child during some of the uncomfortable parts of the study. If serum enzyme studies are ordered, they should be completed before the study, because these values will be elevated after the study is done. After the study is finished, observe the needle insertion sites for possible hematoma.

Doppler Ultrasound

In Doppler ultrasound, a probe is placed against the head, a pulsed ultrasonic beam is emitted, and, as it encounters structures in its path, it is reflected back

TABLE 40-11
Patient Information Tool

Patient Information: Visual Evoked Potentials (VEP) Study

What Is a VEP?

1. A VEP is a written record of the brain's response obtained by stimulating the retina with a pattern of light
2. An instrument registers this activity in the form of a wavy line written on a computer screen. This study is a part of the total neurologic examination your physician may order. Your physician may use this test to determine more precisely your diagnosis and treatment

Preparation for Study

1. There are no restrictions prior to this test. You can eat your routine diet and take usual medications
2. The study is pain-free

Examination

1. An escort will accompany you to the examination room via wheelchair
2. Once you are in the examination room and seated on a comfortable chair, the technician will review the purpose of this procedure with you
3. The technician will apply 3–6 small electrode disks to your scalp, attaching them with a sticky substance
4. The room will be dimmed and the door closed. You will be instructed to watch the dot in the center of a screen with one eye
5. Your test will be over when each eye has been tested twice. The complete study takes 20 mins
6. You will be accompanied back to your room via wheelchair and may resume your normal activities

After the Study

1. There are no activity restrictions
2. The sticky substance used to apply the electrodes can be washed with soap and water
3. Your physician will give you the results of the study

Patient Information: Brain Stem Auditory Evoked Potentials (BAEP) Study

What Is a BAEP?

1. The BAEP is a written record of the brain's response to a sound stimulus
2. An instrument registers the brain's response to the sound stimuli in the form of a wavy line written on a computer screen. This study is a part of the total neurologic examination your physician may order. Your physician may use this test to determine more precisely your diagnosis and treatment

Preparation for Study

1. There are no restrictions prior to this test. You can eat normal meals and take usual medications
2. The study is pain-free

Examination

1. An escort will accompany you to the examination room via wheelchair
2. Once you are in the examination room and lying on the bed on your back, the technician will review the purpose of this procedure with you
3. The technician will apply 3–4 small electrode disks to your scalp, attaching them with a sticky substance. Electrodes will be applied (1) to the top of your head, (2) to the side of your head, and (3) to each of your earlobes
4. The room will be dimmed and the door closed. You will be instructed to shut your eyes, lie quietly, and avoid talking. The door is closed to block extraneous outside noises. The technician will stay in the room with you at all times
5. Earphones will be placed on your head. You will hear clicks at the lowest possible sound level necessary for conducting the test
6. The technician will be at the controls of the computer screen, which is adjacent to the bed
7. All you have to do is rest. Throughout the examination, all you will hear through your earphones is repetitive clicks
8. The complete study takes between 45 and 90 mins
9. Following the examination, the technician will remove the earphones and electrodes
10. You will be accompanied back to your room via wheelchair and may resume your normal activities

After the Study

1. The sticky substance used to apply electrodes can be washed with soap and water
2. There are no activity restrictions
3. Your physician will give you the results of the study

Patient Information: Somatosensory Evoked Potential (SEP) Study

What Is an SEP?

1. The SEP is a written record of the nerve pathways between the brain and spinal cord
2. An instrument registers this activity in the form of a wavy line written on a computer screen. This study is a part of the total neurologic examination your physician may order. Your physician may use this test to determine more precisely your diagnosis and treatment

Preparation for Study

1. There are no restrictions prior to this test. You can eat normal meals and take usual medications
2. The study is pain-free

Examination

1. An escort will accompany you to the examination room [explain exactly where it is] via wheelchair
2. Once you are in the examination room and seated on a comfortable chair, the technician will review the purpose of this procedure with you
3. The technician will apply 6–8 small electrode disks to your scalp, neck, and arm and/or 6–8 electrodes to your scalp, back, and leg
4. The room will be dimmed and the door closed
5. You will be instructed to relax
6. The electrode applied to a specific nerve on your arm will create an involuntary twitch of your thumb
7. The test is performed twice for each extremity
8. The study takes approximately 1 hr

After the Study

1. There are no activity restrictions
2. The sticky substance used to apply the electrodes can be washed with soap and water
3. Your physician will give you the results of the study

From Giubilato, R., & Metcalf, J. (1984). Evoked potentials: Nursing perspectives. *Journal of Neurosurgical Nursing, 16*(5), 241–247.

to the transducer also in the probe. The waves are displayed on a screen, and pictures can be made and measurements taken. This test is used most frequently in neonates to follow ventricular size. Other studies, such as the CT scan, may be ordered for further definition.

Nursing Interventions. No physical preparation is required for Doppler ultrasound. It involves no pain or discomfort. As the Doppler transducer is placed against the scalp, the only sensation is of the cold, wet, conductive jelly. The infant should be held motionless. The test may take about 15 minutes.

Invasive Tests

Lumbar Puncture

Lumbar puncture (LP) consists of inserting a spinal needle into the subarachnoid space between the lower lumbar vertebrae. In infants this occurs between L3 and L4, and in children between L4 and L5. There are two purposes for performing an LP: (1) *diagnostic*—to note the CSF pressure, to obtain CSF fluid for analysis, to test CSF dynamics for a block in the circulation, or to inject substances for x-ray studies; and (2) *treatment*—to inject medications, to induce spinal anesthesia, and to remove foreign contrast medium. The LP is usually contraindicated if there is suspicion of greatly increased intracranial pressure or expanding mass lesions (especially in the posterior fossa) because of the risk of brain stem herniation, respiratory arrest, and death secondary to a sudden decompression in intracranial pressure. At these times, it would be performed only to rule out subarachnoid hemorrhage or meningitis. Other risks involve infection (e.g., meningitis) if aseptic technique is not followed; and transient low back pain and nerve root irritation. The most common problem following the LP is a headache, which appears positional and disappears when the patient lies flat. This is thought to be caused by the slightly lower CSF pressure, which may put traction on some of the pain-sensitive structures, or by a slow leak of CSF through the dural puncture site, which may take a couple of days to heal. This problem may not be as prevalent in children as it is in adults.

The LP procedure involves holding the child to a side-lying position, with hips and legs flexed. Aseptic technique is used to prepare the skin over the site, and drapes are used. A local anesthetic is administered. The needle is inserted between the vertebrae until it enters the subarachnoid space, the stylet is removed, and a column is attached for CSF pressure readings. Several drops of CSF are put in test tubes, a closing pressure may be determined, the needle is withdrawn, gentle pressure is applied to the site, and a sterile dressing is applied.

Nursing Interventions. There is no physical preparation for LP. The test may be performed in the office examination room, in the treatment room, or at the bedside. Consent may be obtained. Correct positioning is necessary. Children can be placed on their side, facing the nurse with the back as close to the far edge of the table as possible (Fig. 40–7). The neck is gently flexed forward, and the knees are drawn up toward the chest. The nurse should hold the child securely but avoid placing any weight on the child. Older children should be instructed to avoid any movement and be advised of the need to lie very still. As in other procedures, *preparatory sensory information* should be given to the child.

When a CSF pressure reading is to be measured, the flexion of the child's hips is only slightly relaxed, but a secure hold on the child is retained. This is done because marked hip flexion increases intracranial pressure. After the needle is correctly inserted, one attempts to comfort and reassure the child that the test will soon be finished, because ICP will be elevated by crying and struggling.

An alternate position for infants is the sitting position. Sitting utilizes the effects of gravity to distend the dural sac slightly to ease the insertion of the needle into the subarachnoid space. This position involves securely holding the infant in the same position, with the buttocks at the edge of the table and with neck and hips flexed and stabilized.

After the procedure is done, the nurse should record an acute neurologic check and vital signs as well as observe the LP site for CSF leakage and any redness. The physician may restrict activities or require flat bedrest for a brief period after the test.

If children have a post-LP headache, have them drink fluids and lie flat for the first few hours after the

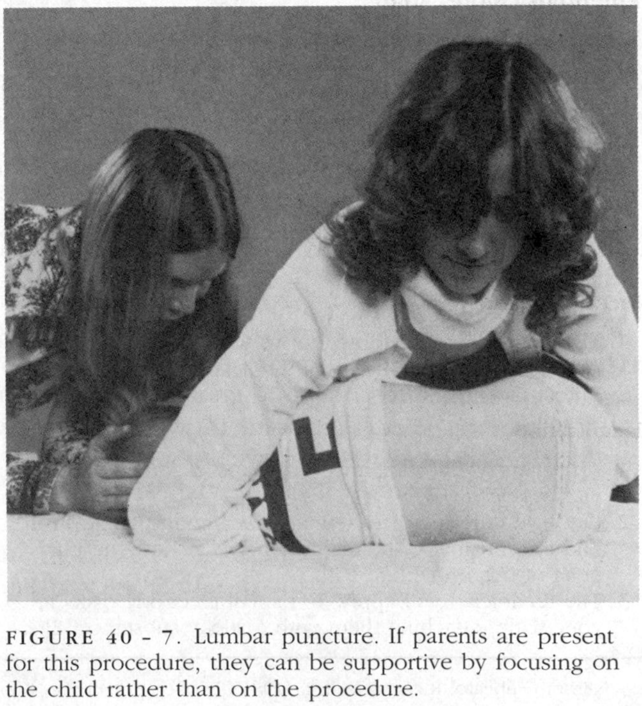

FIGURE 40 - 7. Lumbar puncture. If parents are present for this procedure, they can be supportive by focusing on the child rather than on the procedure.

test, gradually elevating the head and allowing resumption of activities as tolerated. Younger children may not be able to follow this instruction and will determine their own position of comfort. The headache usually disappears when the child lies flat. If this does not relieve the headache, if it is severe, or if it is accompanied by an increased temperature, contact the doctor immediately, because these may be symptoms of either a primary CNS infection or an infection secondary to the LP.

This test may be frightening to the child, parents, caretakers, and other family members. If parents do not feel comfortable staying with the child during an LP, they should be assured that the nurse will be present to comfort the child and hold her or him in position.

Subdural Tap

The subdural tap is another similar study that is generally restricted to infants or young children with open fontanels. It is used to identify subdural effusions and subdural hemorrhage, to withdraw CSF for culture, to instill medicines, or to reduce temporarily the volume of CSF. The study may involve administration of a local anesthetic. Then a spinal needle is inserted through the opening at the junction of the anterior fontanel and the coronal suture, to the subdural space, followed by removal of the stylet and then removal of CSF. No more than 30 to 35 ml is removed, to avoid cranial decompression with its risk of herniation, respiratory arrest, and death. A sterile dressing is applied at completion. This test usually takes about 20 to 30 minutes.

Nursing Interventions. Consent may be obtained. Physical preparation may include a povidone-iodine (Betadine) scrub preparation of the site. The positioning usually involves use of a mummy restraint with the nurse securely holding the infant's head. The physician may shave the site and surrounding area and cleanse the site with a povidone-iodine solution. Nursing care may involve keeping the infant flat for several hours, with assessment of the tap site, neurologic checks, and vital signs as per physician orders.

Myelography

Myelography begins with an LP and, after removal of some fluid, includes the instillation of a contrast medium and tilting the patient on the x-ray table to move the substance to the desired levels of study. This allows visualization of structures surrounding the spinal canal and subarachnoid space. This study may be used when there are congenital lesions affecting the vertebrae and cord and in the diagnosis of various types of cord tumors.

This test often takes 2 hours. The most common contrast medium used is metrizamide, a water-based preparation. It may or may not be removed at the end of the procedure. Metrizamide is absorbed by the body and excreted by the kidneys, exerting a large-molecule diuretic effect.

Complications are similar to those for LP, with the addition of arachnoiditis (an inflammation in the arachnoid membrane) and cord compression that could lead to progressive neurologic deficits, usually seen in patients in whom there is spinal block.

Nursing Interventions. This test requires consent and in general requires care similar to that for LP. Anesthesia is usually used, and for this reason the child may receive nothing by mouth. Postprocedure positioning and activities are usually ordered by the physician. Usually patients who have received metrizamide need positioning so that their head remains above their heart for 6 to 8 hours after the test, this prevents the contrast material from migrating up the subarachnoid space to irritate the cortex of the brain and possibly cause seizures. The most important nursing measure after obtaining a myelogram is ensuring good fluid intake through parenteral and oral routes to improve the excretion of the contrast medium.

Cerebral Angiography

Cerebral angiography is an invasive study that involves the injection of contrast medium into either the carotid or vertebral arteries to visualize both the intra- and extracranial vessels and to examine the arterial, capillary, and venous phases of the cerebral circulation. It helps identify vascular deficits such as aneurysms, arteriovenous malformations, and other developmental anomalies. The study also allows a more precise view of the vessels' lumens. It may also precede specific types of surgery as part of the presurgical planning. This test usually takes several hours. It may be contraindicated if there is renal insufficiency, history of allergy to the contrast material or to iodine, blood dyscrasias, or previous thrombotic or embolic events. Children receiving anticoagulant therapy would have them discontinued several hours to days before the test, depending on the anticoagulant's clearance.

Consent is required. Children usually receive anesthesia or heavy sedation. The method involves aseptic technique. The skin is prepared with povidone-iodine, and drapes are placed. The femoral artery is punctured, and the catheter is inserted and, using fluoroscopy, threaded through the vessels to one of the carotid arteries. Less commonly the brachial artery may be used, or there may be direct insertion into one of the carotid arteries. Multiple injections of the contrast medium into each vessel occur while a rapid sequence of films is taken. Then the catheter is withdrawn slightly and advanced into the other carotid artery. Similar studies of the two vertebral arteries may also be done. Finally, the catheter is removed and manual pressure is maintained on the puncture site, after which a pressure dressing is applied.

Nursing Interventions. Physical preparation involves sedation before the test and nothing-by-mouth restrictions. Some physicians may require a skin preparation before the test. Because the contrast medium will be excreted through the kidneys and has been known to cause renal failure in dehydrated patients, the patient must be well-hydrated before the test. The child should wear a hospital or x-ray gown and must remove jewelry and any hair ornaments. The child should void, and the nurse should record the baseline neurologic check and vital signs.

Psychologic preparation for the angiogram for an older child or adolescent involves *preparatory sensory information* about what they will experience and instruction about the procedure. The room itself is dark and the patient is positioned on a hard table with the head secured to a headrest.

Care after the study involves checking the site and pressure dressing along with vital signs and *neurologic monitoring* every 15 minutes for 1 hour; every 30 minutes for 4 hours; every hour for 4 hours; and then every 2 to 4 hours for 24 hours, depending on the patient's condition and physician's orders (see Table 40–10 for care related to the arterial puncture and injection of contrast material). Complications that may include hematoma; edema; vasospasm; thrombosis; embolism; allergic reaction; transient or permanent alterations in speech, motor and sensory functions; and consciousness have been reported as a result of cerebral emboli with carotid studies, and visual loss and signs of brain stem damage may occur with vertebral studies. The child is usually kept on bedrest and encouraged to avoid movement in the affected leg for 12 to 24 hours to reduce the chance of clot dislodgment and hematoma formation. Postprocedure hydration is important, and the child should begin with sips of fluid, increasing the amount as tolerated. This is usually adjusted with intravenous hydration until the child is able to maintain a well-hydrated oral intake. Output records for the first 24 hours help in quickly identifying a child experiencing renal problems.

Digital Subtraction Angiography

Another technique in cerebral angiography is digital subtraction angiography. This technique is similar to that just described, except for the much larger volume of contrast medium that is usually injected venously. This can also be done intra-arterially, by using small volumes through a central line. This procedure may be used only with older children and adolescents, because the patient must remain motionless during the study (even swallowing may impair the quality of the films) and because of the larger volume of contrast material given with potential circulatory overload. If venipuncture is used, this study may involve less risk than a regular angiogram.

Nursing Interventions. Physical preparation is the same as for cerebral angiography. Adequate pre- and postprocedure hydration is essential because of the large volume of contrast material to be excreted by the kidneys. During and immediately after this study, the patient must be assessed for symptoms of circulatory overload. The remainder of the nursing care is similar to that described for cerebral angiography, except that the patient does not need to remain immobile for as long a time, if venipuncture is used. Again refer to Table 40–10 for postprocedure care.

Laboratory Tests

Laboratory tests that may be used in the diagnostic process include chromosome studies, which may assist in identifying genetic disease. Other tests include those designed to screen for inborn errors of metabolism, degenerative disease, and abnormalities in carbohydrate, lipid, protein, or urea cycle metabolism. Tests for toxicity include urine metabolic screen, serum amino acids and organic acids, urine amino acids and organic acids, and serum lactate and pyruvate. Examination of white blood cells with electron microscopy and screening for heavy metals may also be conducted.

Therapeutic Management

This discussion covers some basic areas of knowledge that span care for children with various alterations in neurologic function. This includes care for the child experiencing cranial surgery, seizures, status epilepticus, altered responsiveness, or increased intracranial pressure.

Neurologic Cranial Surgery

This discussion covers general care for a child having neurologic cranial surgery involving craniotomy and craniectomy (to review general information on basic pre- and postoperative care, see Chapter 23 and the nursing process plan for perioperative care, Table 23–7). It is followed by a brief discussion of infratentorial cranial surgery.

Craniotomy involves removing and replacing a part of the skull to allow access for surgery on the brain. *Craniectomy* refers to the removal of skull without replacement, which may be done in posterior fossa or infratentorial surgery in which the neck muscles provide protection for the brain. On occasion, a craniectomy is done to treat patients with uncontrolled intracranial pressure following head trauma; this is called a decompressive craniectomy. Craniectomy may be required after depressed skull fractures. If a large skull defect is left after surgery, a helmet may be obtained for the child to protect the brain from external injuries. *Cranioplasty* refers to the repair of a cranial defect or replacement of a bone flap, either with autologous or donor bone or a molded acrylic material.

The preparation for neurologic surgery may involve shaving hair from the operative area. The amount and area of hair removed as well as shape and size of the incision are determined by the surgeon. The shave and the skin preparation are usually done after the child is anesthetized.

The head position is usually secured with clamps and pins, and various operative positions may be used, depending on the nature and location of the surgery. The scalp is incised, muscles are stripped, and usually 4 to 5 burr holes are drilled in the corner points of the skull. A craniotome is used to cut across the bone and lift off the skull. After the skull is opened, the meninges are excised. Hemostasis must be meticulously completed during cranial surgery, because even small hematomas are not tolerated in the brain.

Following the surgical procedure, all anatomic layers, starting with the meninges, are closed. During a craniotomy, the skull is sutured back into place. Scalp layers are closed and a pressure dressing is applied for 1 or 2 days, along with a head dressing. A drain may be used for the first 24 hours. Following this brief period, the dressings are removed by the neurosurgeon.

Preoperative Care

In addition to providing the general preoperative care required before surgery, the nurse should include and be aware of some of the differences involved with neurologic cranial surgery. Preoperative anxiety and fear of mutilation can be related to shaving the hair and worrying about visible scars. Shaving the hair may decrease wound contamination, thus preventing infection. The patient and family need to understand that the hair will grow back, and they may consider the use of a wig, scarf, or cap after surgery. Some persons fear visible scars and need to know that the incisions are usually made where hair grows on the scalp and will not be visible on the face. Neurologic surgery that involves the frontal or temporal bones often results in marked periorbital edema for several days after surgery. Often the child and family understand the reasons and simply need *presence* including support, reassurance, and time to express their feelings or to begin an anticipatory grief process.

Potential complications, surgical outcomes, and the irreversible nature of neurologic surgery have a major impact on the quantity and/or quality of the child's life. Decisions must be made quickly. In an acute crisis, parents often expend considerable effort during the preoperative period or during an operative waiting period reviewing all the events and identifying questions. Being sensitive to these needs and providing an opportunity to ask questions and time to reinforce previously given information can be extremely helpful. Refer to Table 40–12 on *preoperative teaching*.

An accurate well-documented preoperative neurologic baseline assessment becomes essential in monitoring the child's postoperative functioning for potential complications. Problems with vision, hearing, communication, and any other pre-existing neurologic deficits should carefully be documented.

If the patient has seizures preoperatively, the events should be well described, and side rails of the cart should be padded to prevent injuries. If the patient is receiving anticonvulsant drugs, these are usually given earlier before surgery with a sip of water so that serum levels remain constant.

TABLE 40-12
What to Expect: Neurologic Cranial Surgery

Help parent(s) and family cope more effectively with the stress of surgery by understanding what to expect

Preoperative Care

Complete or partial head shave possible
Where the incision will be, how it will look, and its visual ramifications
What kinds of dressings to expect, and their maintenance
Necessity for deep breathing and turning
Neurologic monitoring and vital sign checks
Length of the surgery (i.e., number of hours) and postanesthesia recovery
Length of visitation/stays after surgery
Intensive care stay, if known
Reinforce knowledge; clarify misconceptions related to child's surgery

Postoperative Care

Postoperative cerebral edema (when appropriate)
Incision—hair loss if applicable
Necessity for assessments and their frequency
Necessity for and types of tests and medications
Necessity for and types of monitors, access lines, catheters, etc.
Anticipated child's response related to surgery and/or neurologic deficit
Progression in diet and activity orders
Pain management
Transitions in nursing care (routines, shift changes, unit transfers)

Home Maintenance

Incisional care (staple or stitch removal)
Restriction/precaution associated with activities; returning to school; resumption of leisure and recreational activities
Signs and symptoms of potential complications
Medications
Diet
Clinic appointments and scheduled tests or scans
Specific therapies
Contacts and telephone numbers for information about concerns and questions
Anticipatory guidance about pertinent anatomy and physiology of neurologic deficits, safety measures, and adaptations
Home health care or public health care referrals as appropriate
Support network information as appropriate
Social service referrals as appropriate

Postoperative Care

The nursing role after cranial surgery involves frequent acute *neurologic monitoring,* vital signs, intake and output, and dressing and drainage assessments to monitor the patient for any potential complications.

This includes assessing airway and adequacy of ventilation and monitoring oxygenation, blood gases, and electrolytes. Physician orders for positioning and activities are strictly followed. The nurse should keep family members well informed of the child's condition and of the physician's orders.

Potential Structural Complications. Cerebral edema begins to peak 24 to 72 hours after surgery with a corresponding decrease in alertness and responsiveness. During this time, it is necessary to recognize promptly and seek early treatment for increased intracranial pressure, hypoxia and hypercapnia, and hyperthermia; to maintain optimal head, neck, and body positions; to practice protective nursing care; to administer medications as ordered; and to explain to the family what may be happening. The highest incidence of intracranial bleeding occurs within the first 24 hours after surgery. This is usually characterized by (rapid) neurologic deterioration, symptoms depending on the location of the bleed and the age of the child. The complication of acute hydrocephalus may occur after surgery, presenting with signs and symptoms similar to those for increased intracranial pressure. Cerebral vascular accidents occur as a postoperative complication less commonly in children than in adults.

One must be vigilant for concerns raised by the parents, because these could be subtle indicators of neurologic change. After change of signs and symptoms is detected, the facts should be presented to the physician in a clear and logical way and thoroughly documented.

Potential Metabolic Complications. Potential metabolic complications involve wound infection, hypoxia, fluid and electrolyte disturbance, hypotension, and seizures (Table 40–13). Fever increases metabolic demands and oxygen requirements. Infection lengthens hospitalization and may increase the risk for further complications. The incidence of wound infection after craniotomy is about 3 per cent, wound contamination being the most important risk factor (Youmans, 1990). Temperature elevations during the first 24 to 48 hours are usually related to hypoventilation atelectasis. Incisional redness and drainage with temperature elevations several days after surgery may indicate wound infection. Surgery near the third ventricle and hypothalamus may also disturb temperature regulation. Temperature elevations may also result from drug reactions and from aseptic meningitis following subarachnoid hemorrhage and infratentorial surgery. Focal infections from intravenous sites, central venous pressure and arterial lines, urinary catheters, and ventriculostomies may also cause fever.

Drainage from the dressing, incision, nose, or ears after surgery should be treated as a suspected CSF leak until otherwise identified. CSF can leak into the ears or nose if there is a tear in the dura close to these structures. Drainage that is suspect should be collected in a sterile test tube for CSF glucose determination. Patients should be discouraged from touching, or instructed not to touch, the drainage or to blow their nose. These areas should not be packed, suctioned, or disturbed until the drainage has been identified, in order to minimize sources of infection. The patient should be encouraged to remain quiet.

Nursing care oriented toward reducing the risk of infection includes

- Hand washing before and after contact with the child.

TABLE 40-13
Risk Factors and Causes in the Development of Postoperative Metabolic Complications

Fever

Wound contamination and drainage
Atelectasis
Drug reactions
Aseptic meningitis
Localized infections
Immunosuppression
Cerebrospinal fluid leak

Hypoxia

Unsatisfactory head and neck positions
Anesthetic agents
Cerebral edema
Acid-base imbalances
Pulmonary embolism
Anemia
Disseminated intravascular coagulation
Fat and/or air embolism
Atelectasis

Fluid and Electrolyte Disturbances

Head injury
Postoperative pituitary or hypothalamic surgery
Abrupt discontinuation of steroids
Hypo-osmolar states
- Syndrome of inappropriate antidiuretic hormone (SIADH)
- Excess free water loads (i.e., D_5W)

Hyperosmolar states
- Excess fluid loss
- Diabetes insipidus
- Hyperglycemia
- High-protein tube feedings with insufficient water
- Hyperalimentation
- Osmotic diuretics

Hypercalcemia
Hypoglycemia

Seizures

Pre-existing seizure history
Postoperative cortical resection
Cerebral abscess
Meningiomas
Arteriovenous malformations
Hypoxia
Electrolyte disturbances

- Using aseptic technique for procedures.
- Inspecting dressings and incision.
- Cleaning and trimming the patient's fingernails.
- Administering antibiotics as ordered.
- Monitoring white blood cells and culture reports.
- Culturing any questionable sites.
- Maintaining the integrity of tubings, drainage systems, and lines.

One should avoid using any creams, lotions, or powders near the incision and should check with the neurosurgeon about when the patient's hair may be washed.

Hypoxia after cranial surgery is the most common cause of altered level of consciousness. Hypoxia can also be *caused* by an altered level of consciousness, or by the effects of anesthesia. Nursing care to detect and prevent hypoxia includes observing face color and peripheral filling in nailbeds, maintaining optimal head and neck positions, assessing adequacy of the airway, noting any change in secretions, and assessing respiratory rate, rhythm, and quality. Breath sounds should be assessed more frequently for a child with altered levels of consciousness or when cough and gag reflexes are decreased or absent; suctioning should be done as needed. The patient should be turned and repositioned every 2 hours, and monitored. Oxygenation should be monitored with pulse oximetry. Oxygen should be administered as ordered.

Fluid and electrolyte disturbances after surgery include hypoglycemia, hyponatremia, hypokalemia, diabetes insipidus, and syndrome of inappropriate antidiuretic hormone. The patient is at increased risk for these problems after subarachnoid hemorrhage, head trauma, or surgery near the pituitary and hypothalamus; during periods of fluid restrictions; and whenever osmotic diuretics are used. The nursing care required to detect or prevent these disturbances includes monitoring fluid intake and output carefully, as well as serum osmolality, electrolytes, hematocrit, urine specific gravity, weight, and appearance of skin and mucous membranes.

Seizures may be a complication in the postoperative period. Seizure activity increases metabolic demands, increases systolic blood pressure, increases cerebral blood flow, and depletes energy stores. Patients at increased risk for postoperative seizures are those who have resections of the cortex, surgery near the sensorimotor strip, cerebral abscess, meningiomas, and arteriovenous malformations. Seizures can also be precipitated by metabolic factors such as hyponatremia, hypoxia, hypoglycemia, and hypo-osmolarity (Arsenault, 1985).

Nursing care related to seizures includes assigning the child to a room closer to the nursing station for observation, frequent observations to detect any seizure activity *(seizure precautions),* asking family members about any unusual activities, thorough documentation of any observed seizures, *seizure management,* including padded side rails if seizures have occurred or there is a history of seizures, and administering antiepileptic drugs as ordered. After the initial seizure occurs, the patient may receive a loading dose of the antiepileptic drug with the expected consequence of sedation. Subsequently, a regular maintenance dose is given and adjusted for seizure control, side effects, and serum drug levels.

Other Postoperative Problems. Postoperative headaches need to be carefully investigated. Headaches that coincide with stiff neck, fever, irritability, photophobia, and other symptoms of complications need to be brought immediately to the attention of the physician. Comfort measures are important, such as subdued lighting, soft music, touch, relaxing massage, and quiet play activities, such as reading or telling stories. Pain management after cranial surgery is necessary. It involves thorough pain assessment, administration of narcotics or analgesics, and evaluation of pain relief.

Infratentorial Cranial Surgery

This type of cranial surgery below the tentorium or in the posterior fossa — because of the position of anatomic structures, location of vital centers, and manipulation of the brain stem and cerebellum during posterior fossa surgery — may predispose the patient to greater danger than does surgery in the cerebral hemispheres.

Preoperative assessment for the child experiencing infratentorial surgery should also include documentation of the function of cranial nerves VII, VIII, IX, X, XI, and XII, especially the quality of gag and swallow reflexes and the rate, pattern, and quality of respirations (see Tables 13–12 and 13–13).

Nursing care after surgery involves careful patient monitoring *(surveillance)* for the following high-risk problems.

High Risk for Altered Levels of Responsiveness; Risk Factor: Cerebellar Herniation as Manifested by Increased Intracranial Pressure. The monitoring of neurologic and vital signs, especially respiratory blood pressure, and pulse patterns, for any deteriorating changes is crucial. Respiratory arrest without warning of impending cerebellar herniation is also possible. Side-lying positions of the patient after surgery are preferred to the supine position to avoid exerting pressure on the surgical site. Small flat pillows may be needed in a side-lying position to avoid lateral rotation and flexion of the head. Any hiccoughing should be reported to the physician, because this symptom may be related to irritation of the medulla.

High Risk for Injury; Risk Factor: Cranial Nerve Dysfunction. Here again, a solid knowledge of cranial nerve function and location, together with knowledge of the location and nature of the surgery in the posterior fossa, greatly assists the nurse in anticipating potential problems that the patient may have. Posterior fossa or infratentorial surgery could involve cranial nerves IX, X, XI, XII. Surgery in the cerebellopontine angle may also involve cranial nerves VII and VIII. Change in cranial nerve function should immediately be brought to the physician's attention.

Gag and swallow reflexes should be completely assessed in the immediate postoperative period before any drinking or eating is permitted. Suction equipment should be available at all times. If the child's gag and swallow abilities are absent or depressed, eating and drinking should not be permitted. Suctioning and mouth care may be needed frequently. Nourishment and fluids via a nasogastric or enteric tube may be considered. If dysphagia is mild, consultations with dietary and speech therapists may assist in the development of a feeding plan. This plan may include feeding the child in an upright position, using thickened liquids and foods that are easy to swallow, using cold and warm foods, and always staying at the child's side during mealtime or drinking in case choking occurs.

Other symptoms of dysfunction may include nasal speech, hoarseness, or change in voice characteristics; increased salivation; tachycardia; regurgitation; vomiting; coughing; dysarthria; loss of ability to shrug shoulders; loss of blink; and reduced hearing. Children experiencing dysarthria need to have an alternative means of communication, such as pointing, using a picture or alphabet board, or using a writing tablet. Patients who have absent blink responses should have care with artificial tears and taping of the eyelids (Fig. 40–8). Corneal abrasion and damage can occur within 4 to 6 hours in a patient whose eyelids remain partially or fully opened and unprotected.

High Risk for Altered Mobility; Risk Factor: Cerebellar Dysfunction as Manifested by Ataxia. Patients who experience ataxia need reminding to slow down their movements, rise slowly, and walk with assistance. Sitting balance may improve if they can have their feet on a stool or step to increase sensory input to the posterior columns, which helps orientation in space. Occupational and physical therapists may be consulted.

Seizures

Precautions and Management

Seizures commonly occur as isolated events never to recur again, for many different reasons, including acute neurologic dysfunction. Nursing care for a child experiencing a seizure is the same, whether it occurs once or repeatedly. This discussion covers the care of a child experiencing a seizure, regardless of circumstance, cause, and seizure type. It includes definition, incidence, seizure recognition, appropriate first aid, observational interactions, seizure documentation, and status epilepticus. More detailed information regarding seizure disorder or epilepsy, including etiology,

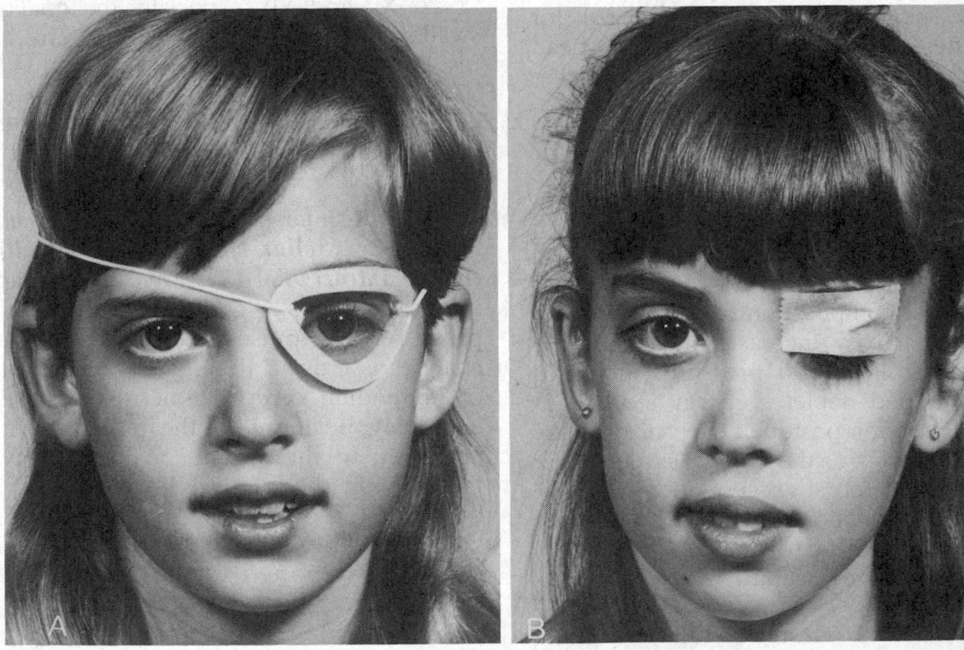

FIGURE 40 - 8. Protective eye care. A moisture shield and protective taping together with ophthalmic lubricants protect the cornea when there is either (1) diminished or absent corneal reflex or (2) diminished or absent ability to close the eye completely. *A*, Use of moisture shield is shown. *B*, Protective taping of the lid using a porous paper tape horizontally across the upper lid.

seizure classification, treatment, and management can be found further on in this chapter under "Epilepsy."

A seizure can be defined as a paroxysmal, uncontrolled episode of behavior that results from an abnormal electrical discharge from the brain. This may affect the person in any one or a combination of the following ways: (1) altered responsiveness, (2) altered sensation or perception or both, and (3) altered movements, mobility, or tone. What happens to the person during the seizure depends on the characteristic of the abnormal electrical discharge and what part of the brain is involved. Children may have a single seizure, perhaps related to a febrile illness or an electrolyte imbalance. Some children may continue to have repeated seizures for an unidentifiable reason and some because of an acquired cause.

The incidence of seizures is much higher during the first year of life and after age 55 (Hauser, 1990). Studies have shown that 1 of every 11 people (9 per cent) will have experienced a seizure sometime in his or her life (Hauser, 1990). Most seizures occur before the age of 18 years.

Other paroxysmal events that occur in childhood can be mistaken for seizure activity. These can range from rather benign events to those of a life-threatening nature. The nurse should be familiar with these in order to help the patient obtain the most appropriate treatment. Table 40–14 provides an overview of paroxysmal events that can be mistaken for seizure activity (Ferry, 1986). Because seizures and paroxysmal events can occur frequently in childhood, the pediatric nurse should maintain skills in observational assessment and first aid.

TABLE 40-14
Paroxysmal Events That May Be Misinterpreted as Seizure

Nonepileptic episodes
Breath-holding spells
Hyperventilation
Benign syncopal attacks
Vagal hypersensitivity reactions
Postural hypotension
Cardiogenic syncope
Aortic stenosis
Mitral valve prolapse
Sick sinus syndrome
Prolonged QT interval
Migraine
Basilar artery
Hemiplegic
Hypoglycemic attacks
Sleep disorders
Night terrors
Nocturnal myoclonus
Somnambulism
Motor spells
Benign infantile myoclonus
Acute dystonic reactions
Tourette syndrome
Choreiform movements
Shuddering attacks
Periodic syndromes of childhood
Benign paroxysmal vertigo
Cyclic vomiting
Gastrointestinal attacks
Gastroesophageal reflux
Intestinal obstruction
Hiatal hernia
Masturbation

Data from Ferry, P., et al. (1986). *Seizure disorders in children*. Philadelphia: JB Lippincott.

Seizure Recognition

One difficulty with providing seizure observation and first aid is recognizing when a seizure is occurring. Seizure detection is difficult when there is no pre-existing history of seizures and when nurses are relatively inexperienced observers of seizure. For example, a nurse may enter the room to find the child staring and unresponsive, yet sitting in the bed holding a puzzle piece. Thinking that the child is simply daydreaming, the nurse may continue with activities. The nurse may be concerned about the child's lack of responsiveness and question the event as a possible seizure, but repeated observations may be needed. In another example, the nurse may hear a crash and enter the room to find the child lying on the floor in a rigid posture. In this case, the nurse recognizes the event as a seizure and immediately proceeds with seizure first aid and observation.

First Aid

Seizure activity often involves the diagnosis of high risk for injury—physical and psychosocial. The high risk for injury can be minimized with first aid measures. Basic first aid can be divided into four parts, regardless of the seizure type:

- Remain calm and stay with the child.
- Protect the child from any additional injury; use common sense.
- Provide time for recovery after the seizure stops.
- Reassure and provide support to the child and others.

Protecting the child from injury depends on what happens during the seizure. Individuals experiencing only staring or altered responsiveness may require no first aid other than standing by to make sure they do not fall or lose their balance. One should speak softly, if at all, to the child with altered responsiveness. Shouting and shaking may only agitate or confuse the child.

If the child is having altered sensations or perceptions, these should be acknowledged. The child should be reassured that "everything is OK" and that the experience will be over soon.

If altered movements occur, the child's movements should not be restrained or restricted. Any harmful objects should be moved away from the child. If the child is walking during the seizure and headed for a dangerous situation (e.g., open stairs), one should attempt to steer the child in a new direction.

If the child begins a seizure with movements in a standing position, it may be prudent to assist or move the child to a lying position on the floor. When the event is finished, turn the child to a semiprone or side-lying position with the head turned toward the floor. This prevents choking and aspiration on saliva that has pooled in the mouth during the seizure. If the child is lying on the floor, a soft material is placed under the head. Any restrictive clothing around the neck is loosened. No tongue blade or similar object should be inserted, because it may only cause injuries. The child is given nothing to eat or drink until she or he has clearly recovered from the seizure. After a seizure, the recovery time can vary. Some children can immediately return to activities. Others may be confused or fall deeply asleep for several hours.

Reassurance and psychosocial support during and after a seizure are important for the child and for others who may have observed the seizure. After recovery, one should reassure the child, "You just had a seizure and it's over now; everything is OK." The child's questions determine whether more information is needed. Children who have missed instructions or information because of altered responsiveness may need to have instructions repeated when they have recovered.

Seizure activity is unexpected and may often startle and frighten other people. Simple statements such as "It's OK, he's having a seizure; it will be over soon" can be tremendously reassuring if delivered in a calm, confident manner. Young children witnessing a seizure may think that the child is dying, having a tantrum, choking, or misbehaving. Not surprisingly, adults often think this. Again, simple explanations are helpful.

It is rarely necessary to call for emergency help during a seizure, because the event is self-limited and by itself does not cause damage. The following situations indicate times when emergency help should be sought: (1) the child does not start breathing after the seizure, in which case one should initiate mouth-to-mouth resuscitation; (2) the seizure activity continues for longer than 5 minutes; (3) the child has one seizure after another without a return of consciousness between seizures; or (4) the child has sustained serious injuries. If this is the child's first seizure, emergency help is usually obtained.

When seizures occur frequently, other safety measures may be needed to prevent possible injury. Table 40–15 presents safety measures that may be considered for home, hospital, or school. When developing an injury prevention plan with the family, one considers the possible risks and benefits associated with activities and safety measures for the child.

TABLE 40-15
Safety Considerations When Seizures Are Not Well Controlled*

Seizure-related falls and injuries
- Helmets—extra protection where likely to strike head; consider least restrictive helmet possible
- Stairs with supervision; instruct to use rail, consider elevator
- Chairs with arms to prevent falls off chair
- Safe environment, carpeting, protected stairs; remove breakable glass

Water safety
- Bathing with supervision (showers preferable, baths in few inches of water—consider foam protectors for fixtures; for teens, bathe when someone aware is in house; keep bathroom doors unlocked)
- Swimming with direct supervision (pool safer than lake)

Sleeping safety
- Consider room changes rather than child sleeping with parents or parent sleeping with child
- Side rails, or mattress on floor; remove nearby furniture
- Avoid excess pillows and numerous stuffed animals in bed
- Protect open stairways

* Safety needs will vary, depending on seizure type(s).

Seizure Observation

One purpose of observation is to provide an accurate account of what happened. This assists the physician in accurate diagnosis, seizure classification, and antiepileptic drug selection. Another purpose is to monitor the clinical efficacy of antiepileptic drug treatment. Many persons approach seizure observation as a rather passive process, not understanding the value and importance of their observations. Good seizure observation is an interactional process that involves more than "timing the seizure." Table 40–16 is a list that can be used to enhance and expand seizure observation and documentation repertoire.

Response to Stimuli. When assessing responsiveness, the nurse should attempt to interact using various stimuli and describe the child's response rather than describe how the child appears (i.e., conscious or unconscious). On appearance alone, a child may appear to be unresponsive but in other domains they may be able to respond. For example, one nurse described a child's rather asymmetric jerking movements involving the right arm and leg to a greater degree than the left arm and leg. The child made no eye contact and did not appear aware of the nurse. When the nurse asked the child to touch her finger, the child was able to do so with the left hand but not with the right. Without this interaction, the nurse may have mistakenly described the patient as unconscious during the seizure. This child was able to perceive auditory stimuli appropriately and had motor control of the left hand.

Movements and Tone. When assessing movements and tone, one must identify the extremities involved,

TABLE 40-16
Considerations for Seizure Observations and Documentations

Describing the Beginning

1. What were the circumstances?
2. Were there any precipitating factors?
3. Was the seizure onset observed?
4. Did the child state or give any indication that the seizure was beginning? (An aura is the beginning of the seizure: expressed before altered responsiveness occurs)
5. Did they attempt to continue, stop or slow down in their activities?
6. What happened first? Then describe in order, how the rest occurred

Assessing Responsiveness

1. Describe patient's observed response to you, self, environment
2. Describe whether responses were rote or more complex and how much they were affected (e.g., partially, totally)
3. Assess response to tactile stimuli (blow on face, light touch, tickle, a mild shake of an extremity, ice, attempt to open eyes or move extremities)
4. Assess response to auditory stimuli (clap hands, call name, give a command, state a word, and ask for recall later)
5. Assess response to visual stimuli (note visual flinch, throw an object to child unexpectedly). Check pupil reactions

Assessing Movements, Mobility, or Tone

1. Was there any movement or change in posture? Give location and description; be as specific as possible. Consider a head-to-toe approach
2. Did this affect one or both sides of body? If both sides involved, did they look the same or different?
3. Assess whether tone is increased (tonic, spastic, rigid), decreased (flaccid, limp), or normal
4. Were there any automatisms (repetitive, purposeless movements)? Were there any purposeful movements?

Assessing Sensation and Perception

1. What does the child describe or state? Ask them during or after seizure for a detailed description if possible
2. Are there any autonomic signs and symptoms (e.g., skin temperature change, change in color, sweating)?
3. Did they say or do anything strange (mumbling, speaking inappropriately, cursing, wandering, climbing up or under objects, fumbling, resisting or combatting touch, agitation, and so on)?

Assessing Postictal Responses

1. What were they like after the seizure? Describe their behavior
2. How long did it take before resumption of previous activities?
3. Could they recall the event in general or remember what happened at the beginning or throughout the seizure?
4. Were there any temporary deficits (memory loss, aphasia, paresis)?
5. Was there any confusion or disorientation? Describe and give duration

By Judy Wulf.

and whether one or both sides of the body are affected. Children with altered tone can be assessed by using motor commands and a gentle attempt to move the extremities for purposes of comparison.

Repetitive Movements. When assessing repetitive movements, one must determine whether they are interruptable, goal-directed or purposeful. Generally, the repetitive movements or automatisms of seizure activity are (1) not interruptable and subside only when the seizure ends, and (2) are not goal-directed or purposeful. In some children, it may prove difficult to distinguish self-stimulating behaviors from seizure automatisms. Circumstances, duration of the event, and determination of whether the event is interruptable may prove helpful.

For example, we may consider a child who had cognitive deficits, self-stimulating behaviors, and seizures consisting of altered responsiveness and automatisms. This girl was observed making repetitive movements of tipping her head backward with shaking and rocking of the trunk forward and backward while she was in a sitting position. This occurred during quiet times for a duration of 5 to 15 minutes when uninterrupted. The movements could be interrupted, however, by introducing a novel stimulus, such as a hand clap or assisting the child to a standing position. This is to be contrasted with her movements consisting of head and trunk tipped forward with repetitive blowing movements of the mouth and picking movements of the hands, for a duration of 45 seconds. Attempts to interrupt these activities generally produced some motor resistance but did not abolish the movements. The first example of repetitive movements represents self-stimulating behaviors; the second example represents seizure activity.

Altered Sensation or Perception. When assessing the child for altered sensation or perception, the nurse listens to the child's statements and evaluates the appropriateness of the responses to various stimuli. Children's statements may actually be the beginning of the seizure. Children may state that they feel sick, are going to have a seizure, or feel scared. Sometimes the sensations are specific, such as a tingling in a part of the body; at other times they are more vague. Young children may simply seek an adult before the observable seizure begins. Continued observation may provide subtle evidence that the seizure may begin with a sensation that the child cannot express, other than by seeking out another person. Perceptions may be altered during seizure activity, which accounts for peculiar statements or inappropriate motor and verbal responses.

Postictal Responses. A variety of postictal (after the seizure) responses are possible. Some children are fully oriented and can immediately resume activities. Others may seem confused or disoriented and require some quiet time and reorientation during their recovery. Some may begin sleeping and show varying levels of arousability. Mood may vary, ranging from laughing and silliness to crying, fearfulness, and acting-out behaviors. Some children may have difficulty speaking and organizing their thoughts or may even experience a temporary motor paresis in part of the body (Todd paralysis).

Frequent and Subtle Seizure. The last problem encountered relates to seizure observation of the child with frequent, brief or subtle seizures. Parents or other providers familiar with the child can often help the nurse to identify the seizures and provide additional feedback about seizure frequency.

Observing seizure frequency is a difficult task, because the frequency may be inconsistent and variable throughout the day and from one day to the next. Seizure observation may become an index of how much time was spent observing the child. For example, during one day shift the child may be noted to have 60 seizures during several intervals of direct observation, totaling 90 minutes. The next day during the same shift, the child may be noted to have 10 seizures; but this time only two intervals, totaling 30 minutes of direct observation, were used. What conclusion can be drawn from this? Had the child's seizure frequency improved, worsened, or remained the same? In this case, because sampling periods with direct observation were different, it would be difficult to know. Children experiencing numerous seizures each day may be better observed by using a consistent number of random sampling intervals each day.

Seizure Documentation

Documentation of seizure events should include a description of the circumstances, any precipitating factors, a chronologic account of what happened, and a description of the patient's postictal responses. Circumstances include the date, time of day, and a description of what the child was doing when the seizure began.

It is necessary to specify in the written description whether the onset was observed. If so, it should be described in detail; if not, then the description should state that onset was not observed. The details surrounding the onset may be highly significant in seizure classification. If it is difficult to remember what happened after the event was over, memory aids, such as the guide listed in Table 40–16 may be helpful.

Sometimes the circumstances and precipitating factors assist the physician in determining whether a seizure has occurred. Precipitating factors may be events or circumstances that consistently increase the likelihood of a seizure occurring. Precipitating factors are not the cause of the seizure. They may include irregular use of medicines and drug interactions, fever, illness, fatigue, stress, hyperventilation, repetitive flashing light, excessive fluid intake, and certain times of the menstrual cycle. It is important to ask parents about this, because they may have identified other precipitating factors for their child. Some precipitating factors may allow for management strategies.

When patients have recurring seizures, it is helpful to record seizure frequency data and descriptions of seizure activity and postictal responses in a diary or calendar, to assist in the continued evaluation and treatment with the health care provider. Parents need to report change in the frequency, severity, type, and characteristics of seizures.

The Child with Status Epilepticus

Status epilepticus can be defined in two ways: (1) continuous seizure activity that does not stop, and (2) seizures that recur rapidly or in succession without a return of consciousness between them. The length of time required before a seizure is considered status epilepticus varies; however, most seizures do not last longer than several minutes. Status epilepticus is a medical emergency.

There are many types of status epilepticus, depending on the seizure type. Generalized tonic and/or clonic status epilepticus is life-threatening; other types, such as absence or complex partial status epilepticus also require emergency treatment but are not immediately life-threatening. The prognosis of status epilepticus varies, depending on the cause of the disorder and the patient's response to treatment.

The causes of status epilepticus can range from acute central nervous system disorders to idiopathic or unknown factors. Acute central nervous system disorders may include meningitis, encephalitis, head injury, subarachnoid hemorrhage, subdural hematoma, metabolic encephalopathy, toxin exposures, tumors, degenerative disease, and cerebrovascular accidents. The most likely cause of status epilepticus for a patient with a history of epilepsy or seizure disorder is poor adherence to taking medications and/or acute antiepileptic drug withdrawal.

Therapeutic Management

The child experiencing status epilepticus is usually brought to emergency care and may be admitted to the hospital for treatment, monitoring, and stabilization. The management of the disorder involves basic life support, control of seizure activity, and diagnosis and treatment of any underlying cause.

Almost simultaneously in an emergency setting, an airway is secured, cardiac status is evaluated, vital signs are measured, an intravenous line is established, blood is drawn, antiepileptic drugs are given, and diagnostic tests are completed. Blood is usually drawn to obtain glucose, complete blood count, Sequential Multiple Analysis-12 (SMA = 12), and antiepileptic drug levels (if appropriate) as well as blood culture. At this point, intravenous glucose is injected by using a 1 ml/kg bolus of 50 per cent (Ferry et al, 1986).

The treatment of status epilepticus is usually completed simultaneously with an investigation of its cause. The goal of treatment is to terminate seizure activity rapidly with the least depression of consciousness and cardiopulmonary function. This is accomplished with the intravenous administration of antiepileptic drugs—primarily diazepam, phenytoin, or lorazepam. Some drugs may be given rectally: diazepam, lorazepam, or paraldehyde. See Table 40-17 for a review of medications used for status epilepticus. When status epilepticus is caused by acute drug withdrawal, the treatment of choice is to reinstitute that drug.

Ferry and co-workers (1986) state that the single most common mistake in treating status epilepticus is the failure to give a sufficient amount of the drug *early*. Typically either intravenous diazepam or lorazepam is the initial drug given, followed by phenytoin. If seizures persist, an infusion of phenobarbital may be started. If there is still no response, an infusion of paraldehyde may be used (Rowe, 1987). After early aggressive treatment has brought status epilepticus under control, maintenance therapy is initiated. Further information on maintenance antiepileptic drug therapy can be found in the discussion of epilepsy. If status epilepticus does not resolve, the use of a barbiturate-induced coma may be considered.

Nursing Care

Nursing care of the patient experiencing status epilepticus includes seizure first aid and seizure observation and documentation, as explained previously. The focus is on prompt recognition of status epilepticus and immediate contact of the physician. The nurse and physician have interdependent functions in basic life support: maintaining adequate cardiopulmonary function; controlling seizure activity; administering medications and monitoring the patient's response to the treatment; assisting with diagnostic tests and treatment; participating in the physical and psychologic preparations; and performing post-test monitoring for any complications. Other nursing interventions in the

TABLE 40-17
Medications for Status Epilepticus

Name of Drug	Route	Side Effects	Nursing Implications
Diazepam	Intravenous	Sedation, respiratory depression, allergic reaction, seizures can recur 20 to 30 mins after administration, owing to redistribution of the drug	**Bolus.** Slow intravenous push (1 mg/min); respiratory depression related to rate of administration
Lorazepam	Intravenous	Sedation, respiratory depression, allergic reaction	**Bolus.** Respiratory depression related to rate of administration
Phenytoin	Intravenous	Sedation, respiratory depression, allergic reaction	Administer loading dose, then start maintenance dose. **Bolus** or infusion. Incompatible with dextrose solutions; compatible *only* with normal saline; administration not greater than 50 mg/min. Monitor blood pressure and electrocardiogram during infusion
Phenobarbital	Intravenous	Sedation, respiratory depression, allergic reaction	Intravenous infusion rate should *not* exceed 50 mg/min
Paraldehyde	Rectal	Sedation, respiratory depression, allergic reaction	Contraindication in patient with pulmonary disease; incompatible with plastic: mix in glass bowl with equal amount of mineral oil, draw up in glass syringe with rubber rectal tube attached; inject rectally beyond internal rectal sphincter; eliminated through the lungs, primarily; use fresh supply, deteriorates rapidly; *do not use* if solution is brown or has a vinegary odor
Diazepam	Rectal	Sedation, allergic reaction	Dosages differ for rectal administration; draw up in tuberculin syringe with taper tip end *(not Luer lock), remove needle,* lubricate syringe barrel, and insert; inject rectally beyond internal rectal sphincter

Nursing care for all patients in status epilepticus receiving drug therapy includes resuscitative equipment and oxygen at bedside. The nurse should monitor for the effects of drug on seizure activity and for side effects care of a child experiencing status epilepticus address the nursing diagnostic statements and collaborative problems:

> ***High risk for injury** and aspiration; risk factors: lack of warning regarding seizure occurrence and side effects of antiseizure medications.*
>
> ***Hyperthermia,** related to central nervous system infection and/or status epilepticus.*
>
> ***Altered health maintenance,** related to self-care deficit and potential knowledge deficit about the disease condition and its treatment.*
>
> ***Fear,** related to perception that child may be permanently disabled or die.*

Reducing the Potential for Injury. This may include seizure-related falls and injuries, aspiration pneumonia, hyperthermia, and drug side effects. Patients with seizure-related falls and injuries may have fractures, dislocations, lacerations, or hematomas. They may be at risk for injuries secondary to continued seizure activity. Nursing care includes continuous observation and using side rails with adequate protective padding. One must scan and remove any harmful objects from the bedside. Health care providers should never force open a clenched jaw to insert an endotracheal tube, which may cause injuries. Nasal intubation may be preferred. Padded tongue blades are no longer used.

Reducing the Potential for Aspiration. Aspiration pneumonia can occur during status epilepticus secondary to choking on something in the mouth or vomiting stomach contents. Nursing care may include suctioning as needed, adequate positioning in a semiprone or side-lying position, monitoring vital signs and lung sounds, placement of a nasogastric tube, and maintaining nothing-by-mouth status until the patient has recovered from status epilepticus and depressant side effects of antiepileptic drugs, and has adequate gag and swallow reflexes.

The dosages of antiepileptic drugs used in the treatment of status epilepticus cause decreased responsiveness, with potential for ineffective breathing patterns and ineffective airway clearance. Less common but more serious reactions may include allergic and other idiosyncratic responses. The nurse may administer or assist in administering the medications and may provide early identification and treatment of side effects. Nursing care involves monitoring serum antiepileptic drug levels and seizure activity; laboratory testing; monitoring oxygenation, vital signs, and lung sounds; assessing the adequacy of breathing patterns and airway clearance. A supine position with the head flexed should be avoided to minimize aspiration and airway problems. Patients should be positioned in a side-lying position and turned every 2 hours.

Treating Hyperthermia. Hyperthermia may occur as a symptom of central nervous system infection, or it may occur as a result of continued status epilepticus—especially that involving motor symptoms. Nursing care may include keeping the patient in minimal, light clothing, giving tepid sponge baths, monitoring temperature, and using cooling devices.

Altered Health Maintenance Related to Self-Care Deficit. The level of self-care deficit depends on the type of status epilepticus and how consciousness and responsiveness are affected. For example, status epilepticus of the generalized tonic-clonic or absence seizures type will involve total self-care deficits, whereas status epilepticus of a partial seizure (epilepsia partialis continua) may vary from partial to total self-care deficits, depending on how consciousness and responsiveness are affected. If the patient is unconscious, nursing care includes provision of adequate fluids and nutrition (i.e., nothing-by-mouth status, intravenous fluids, and enteric feeding until the patient recovers, then progress to oral food and fluids, as tolerated). The patient may also require attention to maintenance of skin integrity, turning and positioning, hygiene related to urine and bowel incontinence, eye care if lids do not shut, and oral hygiene.

Altered Health Maintenance Related to Knowledge Deficit. Parents and caretakers may need information about status epilepticus, antiepileptic drugs, diagnostic tests, cause, seizure recognition, and first aid. The nurse becomes involved with assessment, provision, and evaluation of instruction. Parents need specific information about the drugs and have a basic understanding of how they work. They should know why the medicine must be given consistently and why it cannot be stopped abruptly. They should also be familiar with common and uncommon side effects and what to do if these occur. It may be unknown whether seizures will recur. Nevertheless, it is usually appropriate to discuss seizure recognition and first aid measures—especially what to do if status epilepticus recurs. Written material can be helpful to reinforce verbal information.

Fear. Often the parents, caretakers, or other family members fear the possible death or potential disability of the child. They may be afraid and worry about the cause of the status epilepticus or whether it will happen again. Even a family who has a child with a pre-existing history of seizure or status epilepticus has this fear. Family members should be encouraged to verbalize their feelings so that the fears can be acknowledged and they can seek further information.

The Child with Altered Responsiveness

For the purposes of nursing care, it is helpful to consider the child with an altered level of *consciousness* to be experiencing an altered *responsiveness.* This distinction allows one to focus on the child's state of arousal in a way that more clearly defines the problem and facilitates planning and implementation of nursing strategies.

Human responsiveness to the world within and around us is related to the integration of information obtained from external and internal stimuli: input, throughput, and output (Snyder, 1983). *Input* is the process of selecting and prioritizing the stimuli to which one responds. This process requires conscious awareness, attention span, orientation, and the ability to focus beyond oneself. *Throughput* is defined as processing, analyzing, and integrating input. It is the "mental processing" of selected stimuli. *Output* is considered the end product or response to stimuli. This can be expressed as thought, facial or body expression, movement, or change in mood or behavior. In children, responsiveness (input, throughput, and output) is affected by the developmental age or current level of maturity of the nervous system.

Altered responsiveness may involve loss of one or more of the components just discussed. For example, input may be altered in a child with congenital blindness or deafness by decreasing the availability of external stimuli. Throughput may be altered in a child with a perceptual problem such as a visual motor deficit or in a child who experiences delays in processing time after severe head injury. Output is altered in a child who experiences paralysis, sensory motor deficits, or speech impairment.

Altered responsiveness may appear as an acute process for one child (e.g., following head injury) and may be a daily reality for others (e.g., inoperable brain tumor). If the child is immobilized because of decreased responsiveness, hazards of immobility also become a problem. The mobile child with sensory and perceptual deficits is at increased risk for physical injury.

The nursing care provided will vary according to the nature of altered responsiveness. In general, goals for nursing care are to (1) continue assessment for health care problems, especially those of a life-threatening nature; (2) protect the child from additional injury; and (3) assist the family in adapting to the child's care needs. This commonly involves the following nursing diagnostic statements:

- ***High risk for disuse syndrome;*** *risk factors: immobility and altered level of consciousness.*
- ***High risk for injury;*** *risk factor: neurologic complications.*
- ***High risk for altered protection: falls;*** *risk factor: unresponsiveness.*
- ***High risk for altered health maintenance after discharge;*** *risk factor: parental knowledge deficit regarding how to care for child after discharge and availability of physical and financial support.*
- ***Altered family processes,*** *related to impact of the diagnosis and the child's condition on family members.*

Nursing Interventions

High Risk for Disuse Syndrome. Nursing care is discussed here for the unresponsive child who has disuse syndrome, that is, the child who needs total nursing care. High risk for disuse syndrome is defined by the North American Nursing Diagnosis Association (NANDA) (1992) as "a state in which an individual is at risk for deterioration of body systems as the result of prescribed or unavoidable musculoskeletal inactivity [or immobility]." Complications from lack of responsiveness and immobility can include stasis of pulmonary secretions, musculoskeletal problems, gastrointestinal problems, aspiration, stimulus deprivation, urinary tract problems, skin integrity problems, and conjunctival problems. Disuse syndrome may affect children with locked-in syndrome, akinetic mutism, and various types of coma. It may also pertain to children in drug-induced coma. Emphasis is placed on preventing the hazards of immobility. The nursing interventions listed here are within the *independent* domain of nursing.

Preventing Respiratory Complications of Immobility. The bedridden child has a decreased lung capacity because (1) inspiratory muscles are not aided by gravitational pull, (2) chest expansion is limited by the weight of the body against one aspect of the chest, and (3) when the child is in a horizontal position, abdominal contents push against the diaphragm. Further, there is little stimulus for fully expanding the lungs when there is little or no muscular activity. Pooling of secretions within the lungs and exposure to microorganisms may lead to serious respiratory infection. The nurse includes *respiratory monitoring* in the plan of care for the unresponsive and/or immobilized child.

Although *chest physiotherapy* for the unresponsive child cannot include voluntary deep breathing and coughing, turning from side to side at least every 2 hours helps expand different areas of the lungs and reduces pooling of secretions. Elevate the head of bed periodically as tolerated, and position in a sitting posture for short periods, if physician orders permit. Careful hand washing and avoiding persons with active respiratory infections are imperative.

Airway management via attention to gentle suctioning of nasal and oral secretions and to hygiene of oral and nasal mucous membranes will also help prevent infection. Mucous membranes should be kept free of dried secretions and lubricated to prevent breaks in membrane integrity. Oral *health maintenance* is often complicated by the bite reflex in children with neurologic damage. The nurse should never insert fingers in the child's mouth, and care should be taken not to insert anything that will cause damage to the teeth or gums, should the child's jaws close suddenly.

Preventing Musculoskeletal Complications of Immobility. Muscles that are not used lose strength, tone, and mass very rapidly. Likewise, contractures may form at unused joints, permanently limiting musculoskeletal functions. *Exercise therapy* including passive range-of-motion exercises (unless contraindicated by volatile intracranial pressure) and attention to body alignment in positioning the child can prevent these complications. The heavier the child, the more care will be needed in positioning, because the weight of limbs pulls against major joints, causing strain on muscles, ligaments, and tendons. Pillows placed under arms and between legs can greatly minimize this stress. Shoulder supports can help prevent dislocation. The hands and feet must be protected. Washcloths, small gauze rolls, or hand splints can help to keep fingers in functional alignment. High-top tennis shoes or ankle foot orthoses can help prevent footdrop.

When the child begins to recover, weight bearing should be reinstituted as soon as possible. Physical therapy regimens include range-of-motion exercises, a tilt table, standing frame, and parallel bars to help gradually restore weight bearing and active range of motion.

Preventing Gastrointestinal Complications of Immobility. Oral feedings should not be attempted unless the gag and swallow reflexes are intact. The unresponsive child is usually fed through a nasogastic, jejunostomy, or gastrostomy tube (see Chapter 35 for further information about enteral tube feedings). Posturing or seizures during feeding can cause food to reflux. If enteral tube feedings are being used, elevating the head of bed may help to prevent aspiration, should reflux occur. *Nutritional monitoring* including careful calculation of caloric needs must be carried out to be sure that the child receives adequate nutrition to prevent muscle wasting, but because metabolism decreases with inactivity, care must also be taken not to overfeed. Infants who retain a sucking reflex should be given a pacifier during gavage feedings. The suck reflex is lost rapidly if it is not stimulated.

Infants and small children can often be held for feedings to preserve the social contact and caring interactions they have previously associated with feeding. Holding, rocking, and other caring interactions with family and nursing staff are equally important for older children. Their inability for output does not necessarily rule out their ability for input and throughput. If the child's condition contraindicates being held, techniques such as massage (tactile stimulus), singing to the child (auditory stimulus), and frequent contact that keeps one's face in the child's line of vision (visual stimulus) may be appropriate.

Bowel management can be accomplished by auscultating bowel sounds in all abdominal quadrants and by maintaining a record of bowel movements. Diarrhea and constipation are common and may alternate because of variable peristaltic action. Diarrhea may accompany a change in the feeding regimen and may be a sign that the feeding is not being tolerated. *Diarrhea management* may therefore involve adjustments in enteral volume, rate, or formulation.

Constipation, however, may be a sign of inadequate fluid intake (as well as of sluggish peristalsis related to immobility). Lack of bowel movement, passage of hard balls of stool, or abdominal palpation for firm, full intestines can help to confirm suspicions of inadequate bowel evacuation. *Constipation/impaction management* includes prompt assessment of this condition. The nurse can request an order for bulk fiber additives, stool softeners, glycerin suppositories, mild laxatives, or enemas. A good *bowel management* program can promote regularity and prevent constipation and diarrhea.

Preventing Urinary Tract Complications of Immobility. Bladder tone and bladder emptying are also affected by immobility. Intermittent straight catheterization is usually instituted for the unresponsive child. Urine output provides an indication of whether fluid intake is adequate to maintain a healthy urinary tract. Some children may have an in-dwelling urinary catheter. Meticulous catheter care will help to reduce the risk of infection (see Chapter 36).

Maintaining Skin Integrity During Immobility. Bed rest is a major assault to the integumentary system. Constant rubbing on bed linens, body pressure against wrinkled garments, pressure of body weight on delicate tissues, reduced blood flow in pressure areas, mechanical irritation from tubing, and chemical irritation from wet and soiled diapers all contribute to the need for skin integrity vigilance and thorough *skin care*. General body hygiene is much easier to provide for the infant than for the heavier school-aged child or adolescent. Help should be obtained as needed for bathing, washing the hair, and positioning for skin massage. The perineum should be cleansed after each diaper change or episode of incontinence.

The skin should be protected from mechanical irritation. Pressure-relieving mattresses should be used as available. Linen wrinkles are kept to a minimum and no small objects (e.g., plastic sheaths from disposable needles) are to be left in the bed. Opposing skin surfaces and pressure points are to be protected with pillows and foam supports. The skin is inspected thoroughly during care for any areas of redness. Nonreddened bony prominences are repositioned and massaged to increase circulation. Reddened areas of skin should not be further irritated with massage.

Unresponsiveness sometimes includes the loss of motor function of the eyelids. In this case, the eyes should be protected with eye moisture shields, protective taping, or tarsorraphy (see Fig. 40–8).

High Risk for Injury

The child with altered responsiveness must be protected against further physiologic injury, including additional neurologic complications, and against physical injury from falls.

Neurologic Monitoring. Monitoring for changes in neurologic status that may signal either progress toward recovery or deterioration of the child's condition includes acute neurologic checks (see previous discussion of neurologic assessment) and observation for potential complications, such as increasing intracranial pressure. One must assess arousal, pupil size and reactivity, eye movements, motor function, respiratory pattern, and vital signs. One must watch for signs and symptoms of other potential complications as appropriate.

Preventing Injury from Falls. Physical safety is a concern for the child with altered responsiveness. Keep side rails up at all times to prevent falls from the bed. Involuntary movements or seizures can also lead to falls. When the child is positioned in a chair for time out of bed, one must ensure that comfortable restraints help to maintain the upright position and that there is no danger of the child slipping from the chair to the floor or strangling in the restraint. Even with these precautions, children positioned out of bed must always be closely monitored. The mobile child may be prone to falls because of altered spatial perception and altered motor ability. Altered mental processing can lead to impulsive behavior. Football helmets can be used to protect the mobile child's head from further injury. Toys and equipment should be confined as much as possible to allow a clear path for walking. Gates can be used to keep the child safe.

High Risk for Altered Health Maintenance

For some children, altered responsiveness may be a long-term or permanent condition. The parents or caretakers need information on how to care for the child after discharge. *Discharge teaching* should begin as soon as possible. Involving the parent (or the family members who will care for the child at home) as early as possible helps to ensure that they have time to develop skills for procedures. The child should be included in teaching and in self-care to the extent possible.

The family needs explanations of how the illness or disorder affects the child, including the anatomy and physiology of neurologic processes. Familiarity with responsiveness in terms of input, throughput, and output may help the family understand and cope with alterations in response as well as recognize the capabilities for response that have been retained. They need to know about treatment modalities and how to provide or monitor the child's response to treatment.

If the child has reflex movements, the family needs to be able to distinguish these from voluntary movements so that movements such as posturing are not mistaken for purposeful responses or seizures. A list of signs and symptoms indicating the need for medical intervention is also necessary, to enable the family to know when to call the physician.

Procedure or treatment teaching will be used to teach special care techniques the family may need to learn as the child's condition dictates. They may include feeding through a nasogastic tube, tracheostomy care, eye care, oral care, positioning, use of various types of equipment (e.g., suction machine), passive range-of-motion exercises, skin care, and safety concerns. If the child with altered responses is mobile, parents often appreciate discussing behavior and discipline with the nurse.

The family also needs information about the availability of physical and financial support for care after discharge. They should be counseled about the physical and emotional hazards associated with full-time care of the disabled child. Family members should be encouraged to take advantage of respite care offered by friends and relatives (see also Chapter 19, which details the impact of chronic illness on the child and family).

Altered Family Processes

According to the NANDA definition, "altered family processes" is the state in which a family that normally functions effectively experiences a dysfunction. Caring for a child with altered responsiveness has a tremendous impact on the family. Sensitivity, presence, communication skills, and knowledge help the nurse provide support to the family. Family members may need to deal with the loss of closeness that results from altered ability to communicate and to respond to affection. They may question the child's ability to hear or feel in the absence of normal output responses.

They often have concerns about the prognosis and questions about whether to seek additional opinions. Discussions like this call for sensitivity on the part of the nurse. It takes time for the family to understand and accept the reality of a neurologic deficit, whether temporary or permanent. The nurse can assist in this process by explaining facts about the child's condition, *truth telling,* and refraining from offering personal opinion.

When the facts are not known, the nurse should state that this is the case and tell the family that she or he will answer the question after obtaining the facts. Even minor inconsistencies in information obtained from health care professionals can cause the family to feel they are "getting the runaround" or that "the doctors and nurses here just don't know what's going on." A trusting relationship is built on honesty, not on always knowing the answer.

The Child with Increased Intracranial Pressure

One must know how to identify children at risk for developing increased intracranial pressure (ICP). Early recognition and treatment of those with symptoms of increased ICP through *ICP monitoring* is essential.

Etiology/Incidence (Pathophysiology)

The ICP inside of the skull depends on the space occupied by the three intracranial components: brain, blood and cerebrospinal fluid. Once the fontanels are closed and the cranial sutures fused, the skull acts as a rigid container with a fixed volume. In order for the ICP to remain constant in the presence of an increase in one of the components, the other components must decrease in volume. When an increase in volume occurs, these compensatory mechanisms allow for the maintenance of a normal volume-pressure relationship for as long as possible. If and when these mechanisms have been exhausted, an imbalance occurs and increased ICP results.

In infants and young children, open sutures allow for growth of the head in the initial phases of increased ICP, especially when the build-up of pressure is slow or chronic. In instances of acute increased ICP, the skull may not change as readily to compensate for the added volume. Because of this phenomenon, signs and symptoms of acute and chronic increased ICP in infants and young children vary.

Cerebral Blood Flow. Cerebral blood flow is essential for oxygenation of the brain and transportation of metabolic nutrients to and from the cell. Carbon dioxide is a potent vasodilator of cerebral blood vessels. Vasodilation causes increased blood volume and therefore increased ICP. Reducing the $Paco_2$ by controlled hyperventilation causes vasoconstriction of cerebral blood vessels, which in turn decreases ICP. Controlled hyperventilation is routinely used in the management of increased ICP because of this unique phenomenon. Oxygen content can also affect ICP, although to a much lesser degree. Profound hypoxia (Pao_2 less than 50 mmHg) can lead to cerebral vasodilation as the body tries to send more oxygen to the brain tissue. For these reasons, airway management for the patient at risk for or experiencing increased ICP is paramount.

Cerebral Perfusion Pressure. A major concept related to cerebral blood flow is cerebral perfusion pressure (CPP). CPP is the gradient of blood flow and oxygenation to the brain tissue. It is calculated by subtracting the ICP value (known via an ICP monitor) from the mean arterial blood pressure. CPP is affected by changes in arterial blood pressure as well as changes in ICP. A normal CPP is approximately 80 mmHg.

Initial Compensatory Mechanisms. Several compensatory mechanisms serve to maintain ICP in the face of increasing volume within the skull. These include (1) a displacement of CSF from within the cranial cavity to the distensible subarachnoid space around the spinal cord, (2) an increase in the rate of CSF absorption secondary to the pressure gradient across the venous system, and (3) a reduction in cerebral blood volume resulting from compression of the low pressure venous system (Nikas, 1987).

Autoregulation. "Autoregulation" is defined as a mechanism by which the cerebral blood vessels alter their diameter to maintain a constant blood supply to brain tissue, despite fluctuation in the arterial blood pressure. When the initial compensatory measures are no longer effective in reducing increased ICP, autoregulation of blood flow is another mechanism for maintaining cerebral perfusion. This is accomplished by constriction and dilatation of the cerebral blood vessels. When arterial pressure rises, vasoconstriction occurs; when arterial pressure falls, vasodilation occurs. Dramatic changes in arterial blood pressure (less than 50 mmHg or greater than 150 mmHg) impair cerebral autoregulation and blood flow to the brain. When the systemic blood pressure falls below this level, cerebral ischemia occurs and cell function is impaired. When severe hypertension occurs, cerebral edema results secondary to the breakdown of the blood-brain barrier (Nikas, 1987). When autoregulation is impaired, cerebral blood flow and CPP become passively dependent on systemic arterial pressure (American Association of Neuroscience Nurses, 1990). Figure 40–9 shows the dynamics occurring with increased ICP.

Herniation of Brain Tissue. Herniation can be described as a physical displacement of a portion of the brain through and into other brain structures, usually because of an increase in the volume of brain, blood, or cerebrospinal fluid. When pressure in one area is excessive, brain may displace to an area of less resistance, causing serious and potentially life-threatening consequences. Figure 40–10 outlines types of herniation syndromes. The best treatment is to prevent a situation in which these events would occur, by early management of increased ICP. The most common type of supratentorial (above the tentorium) herniation is uncal herniation (Fig. 40–11). As the uncus of the

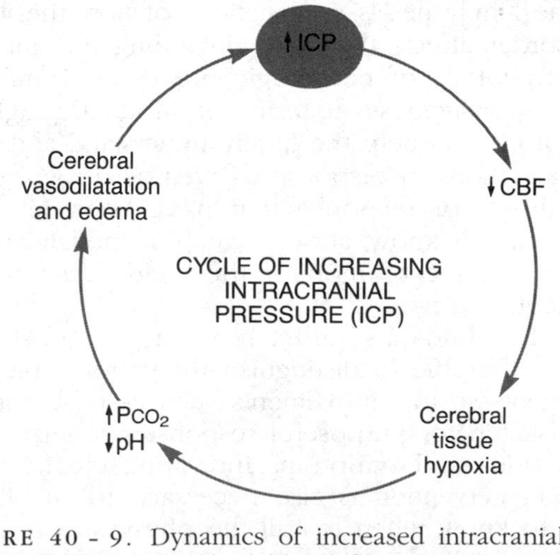

FIGURE 40-9. Dynamics of increased intracranial pressure (ICP). CBF = cerebral blood flow; Pco_2 = serum carbon dioxide.

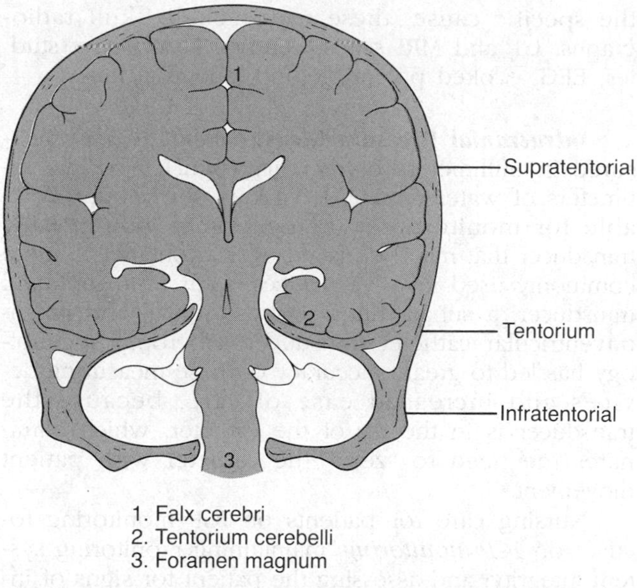

FIGURE 40-10. A normal coronal section showing potential sites of brain herniation.

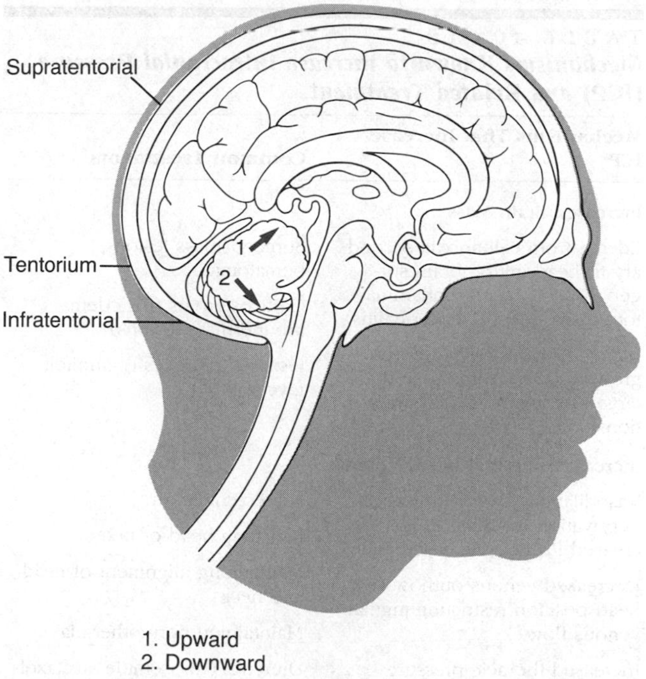

FIGURE 40-12. Infratentorial herniation.

temporal lobe pushes into midline structures, it puts pressure on the oculomotor nerve (cranial nerve III), causing pupil dilatation and poor response to light.

Figure 40–12 shows the two directions in which the cerebellum in the infratentorium (beneath the tentorium) can herniate. This can occur when masses or blood expand in the cerebellum and cause the cerebellum to push upward against upper brain stem structures or downward against the medulla; this may cause rapid deterioration of respiratory and circulatory function, cardiac arrest, and death. This occurrence is known as brain stem herniation.

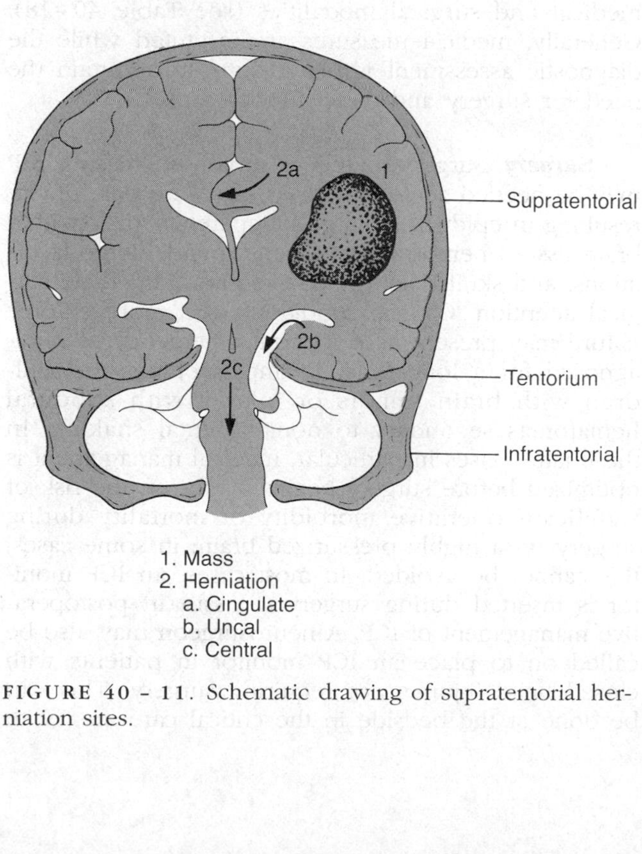

FIGURE 40-11. Schematic drawing of supratentorial herniation sites.

Mechanisms That Increase Intracranial Pressure. With respect to the three intracranial components, Table 40–18 lists some of the etiologies of increased ICP. Treatments focusing on each of the components are listed and are covered more fully in the discussion of therapeutic management. Increased brain mass can result from brain tissue edema secondary to cell anoxia after head injury, brain surgery, infections, and inflammatory diseases such as encephalitis.

Growths within the brain, including tumors, abscesses, cysts, and vascular abnormalities (e.g., aneurysms or arteriovenous malformations) also increase brain mass. Increased cerebral blood volume occurs secondary to vasodilation, which occurs for numerous reasons, including oxygen deprivation and increased systemic blood pressure. Decreased venous outflow and increased intrathoracic pressure are also factors that increase cerebral blood volume. Both are influenced by nursing care activities.

Increased cerebrospinal fluid volume is common in children secondary to congenital or acquired hydrocephalus and/or meningitis. All of these processes result in obstruction of the cerebrospinal fluid pathways. Cerebrospinal fluid production also increases in the presence of a tumor called a choroid plexus papilloma, but this occurrence is rare.

For the child experiencing increased ICP, several of these mechanisms may occur simultaneously. This can lead to a confusing, yet challenging, task for the nurse. The clinical picture is made clearer by a well-

TABLE 40-18
Mechanisms Known to Increase Intracranial Pressure (ICP) and Related Treatment

Mechanisms That Increase ICP	Common Treatments
Increased Brain Mass	
Edema from cell anoxia secondary to head injury, brain surgery, infectious and inflammatory diseases (e.g., encephalitis)	Surgery (mass lesions, hematomas)
	Corticosteroids (for edema around mass lesions)
Increased mass resulting from growths (cysts, tumors) and large arteriovenous malformations	Osmotic diuretics (mannitol, glycerol)
Increased Cerebral Blood Volume	
Vasodilation (e.g., with oxygen deprivation resulting in increased $PaCO_2$, decreased PaO_2)	Hyperventilation
	Elevating head of bed
Decreased venous outflow (e.g., head position restricting jugular venous flow)	Maintaining alignment of head and neck
	Maintaining normothermia
Increased thoracic pressure (Valsalva, positive end-expiratory pressure)	Diuretics (furosemide, acetazolamide, ethacrynic acid)
	Pancuronium to decrease muscular response to stimuli
Increased systemic blood pressure	
Increased Cerebrospinal Fluid (CSF) Volume	
Decreased CSF absorption (e.g., from debris clogging arachnoid villi in meningitis)	Surgery to remove obstruction
	Shunting of trapped CSF to a resorptive body cavity
Obstruction to CSF Flow (e.g., Infratentorial Tumor, Brain Cyst)	
Increased CSF production from choroid plexus tumors (rare)	Closed ventricular drainage for short term treatment

thought-out, thorough diagnostic assessment done in a timely manner.

Clinical Manifestations

Table 40–19 lists the clinical manifestations of increased ICP. Differences in signs and symptoms are related to open fontanels and unfused sutures in infants with some expansibility for compensation, compared with older children, whose skulls are less accommodating to changes in ICP. Differences in signs and symptoms also are related to whether the underlying process is acute or chronic in nature as well as to the child's developmental level and ability to communicate subjective symptoms. Early recognition of these manifestations can lead to prompt treatment and more favorable outcomes for children with increased ICP.

Diagnostic Assessment

Increased ICP can be diagnosed by the presenting symptoms. Diagnostic studies are obtained to identify the specific cause; these may include skull radiographs, CT and MRI scans, cerebral blood flow studies, EEG, evoked potentials, and laboratory tests.

Intracranial Pressure Measurement. ICP is measured in millimeters of mercury (mmHg) or in centimeters of water (cmH_2O). Various devices are available for monitoring, ranging from a noninvasive transducer that may be placed over a fontanel to more commonly used invasive devices, such as an epidural transducer, a subarachnoid bolt or screw, and an intraventricular catheter transducer. Fiberoptic technology has led to greater accuracy of these measuring devices and increased ease of care, because the transducer is in the tip of the catheter, which eliminates the need to "zero" the catheter with patient movement.

Nursing care for patients on ICP monitoring focuses on *ICP monitoring;* maintaining monitoring system integrity; and assessing the patient for signs of infection, hemorrhage, and risk of cerebrospinal fluid leakage secondary to and depending on the type of ICP device. Normal ICP ranges from 0 to 15 mmHg under normal conditions. The ICP is usually stable, although temporary elevations to as high as 100 mmHg can occur with activities like coughing and the Valsalva maneuver. Increased ICP may be moderate (20 to 40 mmHg) or severe (greater than 40 mmHg). The placement of an ICP monitor allows for the calculation of CPP, which is a more accurate predictor of long-term outcome for children with increased ICP.

Therapeutic Management

The treatment of increased ICP may involve both medical and surgical modalities (see Table 40–18). Generally, medical measures are instituted while the diagnostic assessment is being done to ascertain the need for surgery and direct further care.

Surgery. Surgery to relieve rapidly increasing ICP may be needed acutely in cases of severe head injury resulting in epidural or large intraparenchymal (within brain tissue) hemorrhages. Open wounds, large lacerations, and skull fractures also require immediate surgical attention. Clinical conditions of a more chronic nature may present as a surgical emergency, if undiagnosed for a long time. Examples of this are children with brain tumors or infants with subdural hematomas secondary to nonaccidental shaking. In these latter cases in particular, medical management is optimized before surgery begins, to lessen the risk of significant operative morbidity or mortality during surgery on a highly pressurized brain; in some cases, this cannot be avoided. In most cases, an ICP monitor is inserted during surgery to assist in postoperative management of ICP. A neurosurgeon may also be called on to place an ICP monitor in patients with closed head injuries not requiring surgery. This can be done at the bedside in the critical care area with

TABLE 40-19
Clinical Manifestations of Elevated Intracranial Pressure (ICP)

Infants	
Bulging anterior fontanel	Full, tense, bulging above bone; firm enough to cause difficulty distinguishing bone-fontanel junction; closure delayed in chronic increase of ICP
Increased head circumference	Greater than 2 cm/mo in first 3 mos of life, greater than 1 cm/mo in the second 3 mos, and greater than 0.5 cm/mo for the next 6 mos (Fenichel, 1988)
All Children	
Headache	May be generalized or localized; often present on awakening and standing up in the morning; pain increased by Valsalva maneuver: coughing, sneezing, straining at stool, holding breath, and straining to turn in bed
Altered mental state	Irritability, fatigue, altered consciousness, memory loss, confusion
Vomiting	In the absence of nausea, especially on arising in the morning; may be projectile
Altered vision	Diplopia (double vision); strabismus; results from pressure on one or both abducent nerves; "setting sun" sign (especially with hydrocephalus); restricted visual fields; papilledema
Late Signs (Immediate Intervention Required)	
Altered vital signs	Elevated blood pressure: attempt to bring more blood and oxygenation to injured tissue
	Decreased pulse: pressure on cranial nerve X (vagus nerve) nucleus, which is in the lower brain stem and on the vasomotor center in the medulla
	Altered respiratory pattern: pressure on the respiratory center in the medulla may result in apneustic breathing, ataxia breathing, and apnea

appropriate analgesia, sedation, and nursing care available.

Medical Management. In many instances, medical and surgical management overlaps. Medical management includes close scrutiny of oxygenation and ventilatory parameters to optimize hyperventilation to control ICP as well as close attention to oxygenation to avoid hypoxemia. Maintenance of normothermia to avoid excessive metabolic activity and optimal body positioning are essential. Prevention of secondary sequelae, such as infection, pulmonary complications, and seizures, is also essential.

Administering and monitoring the effects of medications are a major focus of medical management. A common treatment is the use of intravenous mannitol, which when present in cerebral blood vessels increases the osmotic pressure, thereby causing water to move from the brain tissue to the vascular space. Other nonosmotic diuretics may be given to decrease total body water, thereby reducing the amount of water in the intracranial space. The persistent administration of these diuretics, such as furosemide (Lasix) is associated with significant potassium depletion. The use of barbiturate-induced coma to reduce cerebral metabolic activity has significantly decreased in the last several years. The lack of ability to obtain consistent neurologic examinations and the side effects of these drugs have led many to abandon this practice in favor of sedation with newer, shorter-acting agents, such as midazolam.

Pancuronium (Pavulon), a paralyzing agent, may be used in the initial phases of management to decrease muscle responses to voluntary, central, and environmental stimuli (e.g., mechanical ventilation). Analgesics are ordered for pain control, and antibiotics for infection prophylaxis, if needed. Anticonvulsant therapy will be instituted in children presenting with or exhibiting seizure activity secondary to focal injury and/or increased ICP. There is some controversy about giving head-injured patients an anticonvulsant on a prophylactic basis if a seizure has not occurred.

Closed Ventricular Drainage/Ventriculostomy. In cases of increased ICP in which ventricular access is obtained to measure ICP, controlled drainage of CSF may be used as an adjunctive measure during the acute phase of treatment. The availability of newer, sterile, closed drainage systems has allowed for close monitoring of CSF drainage and the ability to set a "pop-off" level at which CSF will drain independently. These systems also allow for easy access to in-line ports for drawing CSF specimens to follow infection and other CSF parameters.

Nursing Care. Table 40–20 is a nursing process plan for the child with increased ICP. The components of nursing care for actual or potential increases in ICP include (1) *surveillance* to allow prompt recognition of signs and symptoms leading to early treatment; (2) *neurologic positioning* for maintenance of optimal head, neck, and body positions; (3) *temperature regulation;* (4) administration of medication and monitoring of effectiveness and side effects; and (5) protective nursing care.

Early Recognition and Treatment of Intracranial Pressure. A complete assessment of factors in the child's history, including changes in behavior, attainment of developmental milestones, or level of alertness or responsiveness, is vital. Any history of headache, vomiting, or visual problems is also salient. After a baseline is established, the nurse should carry out *neurologic monitoring* and monitor vital signs with a frequency relative to the patient's condition and physician orders. This may be as frequently as every 15 minutes for an unstable patient whose condition is changing rapidly or several times daily for a more stable patient (see previous discussion of neurologic assessment).

If the patient's ICP is being monitored, the goal is to keep the ICP at less than 15 to 20 mmHg and the cerebral perfusion pressure greater than 50 mmHg. This will require a mean arterial blood pressure of 70 mmHg or greater. If sudden increases occur in ICP, the nurse should quickly assess the patient to note any change in vital signs or neurologic checks.

A close scrutiny of the monitoring and/or drainage system should also take place to ensure proper functioning. Some reasons for a sudden increase in ICP include a change in head and neck positioning, a partially obstructed airway, hyperthermia, and increased patient agitation secondary to noxious external stimuli. The nurse must also be aware of stroke, intracranial hemorrhage, and impending herniation as potential causes of change in ICP.

The nurse also needs to assess the child for hypercapnia and hypoxia by means of blood gas analysis and pulse oximetry. Suctioning may be necessary and should be limited to short intervals to prevent suction-induced hypoxia. When *ventilation assistance* via mechanical ventilator support is used, parameters for a PCO_2 between 24 and 30 torr and a PO_2 greater than 85 torr are adhered to for control of ICP. When positive end-expiratory pressure is used for pulmonary hypoxia, attention must be given to excessively high intrathoracic pressure that may also contribute to high ICP. Manual hyperventilation may be used as a short-term treatment for increased ICP in the critical care setting.

In some children with rapidly increasing ICP, the neurosurgeon may place a ventriculostomy with or without the ICP monitoring apparatus. In either case, the ventricular drainage tube has an exit point through the scalp and is connected to a closed, sterile drainage system. The physician may order continual drainage at a specific pop-off level or intermittent drainage when the ICP reaches a specific level. Nursing care for these systems includes careful recording of the color and amount of drainage. Proper leveling and setting of the ordered pop-off level and awareness of the effects of positioning on the system are essential. Close scrutiny of electrolytes and monitoring of the need for CSF replacement with intravenous fluids are also important nursing measures (Tillum & Greenberg, 1988).

Maintenance of Optimal Head, Neck, and Body Positions via Neurologic Positioning. Head and neck position should be kept neutral with regard to the shoulders and upper trunk. Nurse researchers have found that neck flexion and head rotation appear to increase ICP (Mitchell et al, 1981; Snyder, 1983; Parsons & Wilson, 1984). Maintenance of a neutral head position can be accomplished with head elevation to 30 degrees and support to prevent the child from sliding down in bed. Pillows may be used to support the neutral position in a side-lying manner. The patient's head should be supported in a neutral position during turning and lifting. Increases in ICP have also been seen in response to lateral and prone positioning (Snyder, 1983). A subsequent study (Parsons & Wilson, 1984) noted that ICP was elevated during the turning procedure but returned to baseline 1 minute after the turn. The prone positions should be avoided in increased ICP (Mitchell, 1980).

Temperature Regulation. Normothermia is maintained by keeping body temperature at 36.5° to 38.0°C (97.7 to 100.4°F) without using cooling devices or antipyretics (Snyder, 1983). Fever causes vasodilation and increased cerebral blood flow. The administration of antipyretics and the use of tepid water sponge baths and cooling blankets are recommended.

Hypothermia as a treatment modality in increased ICP has fallen out of favor and is rarely instituted; normothermia is preferred.

Administration and Monitoring of Medications. Pharmacologic measures in the treatment for ICP may vary, depending on the underlying etiology of the increased ICP. Steroids such as dexamethasone are used primarily in patients with neoplastic lesions. Antacids must be given concurrently to minimize side effects, including gastritis and stress ulcer. The administration of mannitol requires frequent monitoring of neurologic status, urinary output, fluid and elec-

TABLE 40-20

Nursing Process Plan: The Child with Increased Intracranial Pressure

Analysis: Collaborative Problem 1

Response and Related or Risk Factors: *High risk for altered tissue perfusion: cerebral; risk factor: increase in volume of one or more of the intracranial components:*

- Brain tissue mass
- Cerebral blood volume
- Cerebrospinal fluid volume

Projected Outcome: The child will experience adequate nutrition and oxygenation at the cellular level

Defining Characteristics
(Actual Response)

Subjective:

- Headache
- Irritable
- Fatigued
- Report of vomiting in absence of nausea, especially upon arising in morning
- Double vision
- Photophobia

Objective:

- Decreased level of consciousness/lethargy/stupor
- Fontanel full, tense, bulging above skull (infant)
- Papilledema
- Failure to thrive
- ICP > 15 mmHg
- Diagnostic reports consistent with pathology leading to increased ICP
- Restriction of upward gaze—"sunset eyes"

Late Signs:

- Elevated blood pressure; widening pulse pressure
- Altered respirations
- Decreased pulse

Nursing Interventions

Neurologic Monitoring: Intracranial Pressure (ICP) Monitoring

Monitor neurologic status closely

- Perform neurologic check every 1 to 2 hrs or as condition dictates; (level of consciousness/responsiveness, pupil size and reactivity, eye movements, motor function, respiratory patterns and vital signs, protective reflexes, such as gag or cough)
- Palpate fontanel(s) with each neurologic check (infant)
- If ICP monitor in place, watch effects of child's or nursing activity on ICP
- Monitor function of ventriculostomy closely (if used)

Inform physician of indications of increasing ICP

Implement strategies to reduce or at least prevent further elevation of ICP

- Elevate head of bed 30 degrees and keep head/neck in straight alignment (to facilitate venous outflow from brain by gravity and through patent neck veins)
- Elevating head of bed will also facilitate lung expansion. Monitor air exchange through frequent chest auscultation

Evaluation Criteria

The client will maintain adequate cerebral perfusion, as evidenced by

- Improved responsiveness and level of consciousness with return of neurologic function
- Reduced headache, irritability, fatigue, vomiting, visual disturbances
- Fontanel(s) soft, lightly pulsating, slightly depressed (infant)
- Vital signs within normal limits; temperature < 38.5°C (101.3°F)
- ICP < 15–20 mmHg
- Mean arterial systemic pressure > 70 mmHg
- Cerebral perfusion pressure > 50 mmHg
- Arterial blood gases within normal limits
- Return of neurologic function

(continued)

TABLE 40-20 *(continued)*

Defining Characteristics *(Actual Response)*	**Nursing Interventions**	**Evaluation Criteria**

	• Maintain patent airway (to avoid hypercapnia, which dilates cerebral vessels)
	  • Prevent flexion and lateral rotation of head in side-lying position. Avoid prone position (which increases intrathoracic and intra-abdominal pressure)
	  • Clear mucus from nasal passages and oropharynx as necessary
	• Use an Ambu bag and 100% O_2 to reduce temporary elevations in ICP, e.g., after uncomfortable procedures **Note:** Manual hyperventilation must be done under the supervision of an experienced nurse.
	• Maintain temperature at <38.5°C (101.3°F)
	  • Administer antipyretics to reduce fever
	  • Use tepid sponge baths or cooling blanket as necessary, being careful not to reduce temperature faster than 1°C every 15 mins
	• Administer diuretics as ordered
	  • Measure and record intake and output, urine specific gravity, and daily weight to help evaluate results
	  • Notify physician of urine output <1 ml/kg per hr or >2 ml/kg per hr
	  • Send electrolyte laboratory values as ordered routinely by physicians
	• Maintain fluid restriction as ordered, using an infusion pump (to decrease central and, therefore, cerebral blood volume)
	• Empty, measure, and record amount of cerebrospinal fluid drainage from ventriculostomy, and replace losses with intravenous fluid, or send specimen for culture as ordered	

TABLE 40-20 *(continued)*

Defining Characteristics *(Actual Response)*	**Nursing Interventions**	**Evaluation Criteria**

	• Reduce crying and agitation and unnecessary stimulus (which increases ICP)
	  • Administer analgesics, sedatives
	  • Enlist parent's help to provide nonpharmacologic comfort measures
	  • Encourage presence of family member
	  • Explain all procedures carefully
	• Encourage use of a security object
	• Plan for uninterrupted periods of rest and sleep
	• Avoid too many nursing activities with child at one time
	• Be alert to signs of secondary infection (from foreign bodies like ICP monitor, central lines, ventriculostomy)
	  • Monitor fever, complete blood count
	  • Send cultures as needed
	  • Administer prophylactic antibiotic as ordered
	• Administer medications as ordered
	  • Monitor for gastrointestinal bleeding: hematest, as a response to steroids and stress, stools, and vomitus
	  • Anticonvulsants require frequent monitoring of serum levels
	  • Children on pancuronium (Pavulon) or barbiturates need total patient care; see discussion in this chapter on care of the child with altered responsiveness
	  • Remember that children on pancuronium have lost motor function, not sensory function; provide relief from pain and attend to psychosocial comfort measures to help overcome their fear and frustration at the drug-induced paralysis	

trolyte balance, and awareness of potential hypovolemia. The drug may be most effective during the first 48 hours of its use.

Pancuronium, a paralytic, may be used to decrease reflex posturing and responses to environmental stimuli. Although the patient has no movement or response to stimuli, sensory functions are not altered, so the patient may still be able to hear, feel, and touch. Nursing care includes meticulous skin care, application of artificial tears and eye lubricant, and frequent neurologic assessments.

Short-acting sedatives, such as midazolam, administered in a continuous-drip fashion are replacing barbiturate therapy. The drip may be increased or decreased, depending on the patient's level of agitation and ICP. Antianxiety agents should never take the place of appropriate analgesics, such as morphine or fentanyl.

Anticonvulsants such as phenobarbital or phenytoin (Dilantin) may be ordered if the child presented with seizures. Avoidance of toxicity should be monitored with frequent levels. Prophylactic antibiotics are ordered for the child with an ICP monitor in place and should be followed with peak and trough levels to prevent toxicity and optimize their effect.

Protective Nursing Care. The nurse should arrange care in ways least likely to increase ICP and should be alert for situations and other problems that may increase ICP. Mitchell and associates (1981) found that ICP increased with cumulative activities but did not increase when those activities were spaced 1 hour apart. This is contrary to the way nurses generally organize care activities. The nurse should prioritize and plan care activities and space them appropriately.

Other patient activities that have been noted to increase ICP include the Valsalva maneuver caused by coughing, straining with constipation, and reflex posturing. Anxiety or painful procedures also increase ICP (Mitchell et al, 1981; Bruya, 1981; Zegeer, 1982; Snyder, 1983).

Congenital and Chronic Neurologic Conditions

The remainder of this chapter describes specific neurologic conditions. In the first discussion, several congenital and chronic disorders are covered. Following are discussions of neurologic infections and neurologic injuries.

Epilepsy

A seizure is a sudden, involuntary, time-limited alteration in function occurring as the result of an abnormal discharge of neurons in the central nervous system (Holmes, 1987). The terms "seizure" and "epilepsy" are not synonymous. Epilepsy is a *chronic* condition characterized by seizures. Many types of seizures do not fall under the classification of epilepsy. Table 40–21 contains examples of nonepileptic seizures.

Although epilepsy indicates a chronic seizure disorder, it does not necessarily mean the disease will last the patient's entire lifetime. Remissions of childhood epilepsy occur quite frequently (Holmes, 1987). Epilepsy is not a single disease entity but rather an indication of underlying brain dysfunction.

Etiology/Incidence

In a comprehensive review of the literature, Holmes (1987) reported that incidence rates for epilepsy vary from 11 to 49 cases per 100,000 population. Information regarding the frequency and distribution of epilepsy is difficult to obtain, probably because of the discrepancies in defining the disease. There are numerous causes of epilepsy. It may be the only evidence of underlying brain pathology or one of many symptoms. The younger the age of onset, the greater is the likelihood that the etiology of the disorder will be identified. There does appear to be a familial predisposition to epilepsy. Evidence from siblings, off-

TABLE 40–21
Common Causes of Seizures in Different Age Groups

Neonatal (Birth to 28 Days)
Asphyxia
Intracranial hemorrhage
  Subarachnoid hemorrhage
  Periventricular-intraventricular hemorrhage
  Subdural hemorrhage
Hypocalcemia
Hypomagnesemia
Hypoglycemia
Hyponatremia/hypernatremia
Infection
  Intrauterine
  Postnatal
Congenital central nervous system malformations
Inborn errors of metabolism
Drug withdrawal
Accidental injection of anesthetic

Infancy to Adolescence
Chronic conditions continuing from neonatal period
Infection
  Meningitis
  Encephalitis
Trauma
Neoplasms
Degenerative disorders
Idiopathic
Genetic disorders

From Holmes, G. (1987). *Diagnosis and management of seizures in children*. Philadelphia: WB Saunders.

spring, and twin studies points to a genetic component, although it is poorly defined.

Pathophysiology

In normal brain activity, certain groups of neurons are active (firing) in the process of thinking, hearing, moving, or doing other activities, whereas other groups of neurons are less active and still others are inactive at a given moment. During a seizure, for reasons poorly understood, groups of neurons all activate at the same time, causing a sudden burst of electrical activity in the brain and disrupting normal brain function. In a partial seizure, this burst of activity is initially confined to one hemisphere of the brain, and the effect on brain function is limited or "focal." In a generalized seizure, however, the abnormal electrical activity occurs throughout the brain, and some cortical functions are disrupted (Friedman, 1988).

Clinical Manifestations

Because epilepsy comprises a group of varied disorders characterized by chronic seizures, classification of the types of epileptic seizures is difficult. Various systems have been used in the past, but the one most frequently used in the current medical and nursing literature is the International Classification of Epileptic Seizures (Dreifuss, 1981). According to that classification, there are two types of partial seizures (simple and complex) and four types of generalized seizures (generalized tonic-clonic, absence, myoclonic, and atonic) (Table 40–22).

"Clonic" and "tonic" are terms frequently used to describe seizure activity. *Clonic* refers to alternate involuntary muscular contraction and relaxation that occurs in rapid succession, such as a rapid patting action of the hand or jerking movements. *Tonic* (as in muscle *tone*) refers to stiffening or rigidity of muscle groups.

TABLE 40-22
Classification of Partial and Generalized Seizures

Partial Seizures (initial changes confined to one hemisphere)

- Simple partial seizure (formerly called focal motor or focal sensory seizure)
  No impairment of consciousness
- Complex partial seizure (formerly called psychomotor seizure)
  Altered consciousness (i.e., altered responsiveness, altered awareness)

Generalized Seizures (disturbance involves entire brain; loss of consciousness occurs)

- Generalized tonic-clonic seizure (formerly called grand mal seizure)
- Absence seizure (formerly called petit mal seizure)
- Myoclonic seizure (infantile spasms are a type of myoclonic seizure)
- Atonic seizure (formerly called drop attacks)

Partial Seizures

In partial seizures, the group of neurons involved in abnormal firing is initially localized to one or more area within the same hemisphere of the brain. The abnormal electrical activity may spread to involve the entire brain. Partial seizures are further classified according to whether consciousness is lost during the attack. In a simple partial seizure consciousness is not impaired, whereas a complex partial seizure involves decreased consciousness or awareness.

Simple Partial Seizures. Simple partial seizures are usually brief, often lasting less than 1 minute (Holmes, 1987). Clinical manifestations are determined by the area of the brain involved (see Fig. 40–4). For example, if the neuronal burst occurs in the occipital region, vision will be altered. Motor involvement is the most common type of partial seizure; in fact, this type of seizure was formerly called a focal motor (or jacksonian) seizure. Clonic seizure activity is typically limited to one muscle group (such as the fingers) or a contiguous group of muscles (as in an arm or leg). Involvement may spread from this initial site to involve all the muscles on one side of the body, a phenomenon formerly labeled "jacksonian march." Transient paralysis of the involved muscle groups (lasting up to 24 hours) may follow a simple partial seizure, especially in young children.

Simple partial seizures that begin in the parietal lobe are associated with sensory symptoms, such as a "needles and pins" sensation or a feeling of numbness. Autonomic symptoms, which may occur with either simple or complex partial seizures, include vomiting, pallor, flushing, sweating, dizziness, erection of body hairs, pupillary dilation, tachycardia, incontinence, and other autonomic functions (Holmes, 1987).

Complex Partial Seizures. Complex partial seizures are one of the most common seizure types to occur in children. The focus of these seizures often arises in the temporal lobe, an area concerned with memory and emotion. Clinical symptoms may be complex and variable and may include a wide range of behaviors.

Some children with complex partial seizures experience a *prodrome;* that is, they are aware of an impending seizure days or hours before it occurs. A prodrome differs from an aura in that a prodrome is not part of the actual seizure *(ictal)* event. An *aura* is an ictal phenomenon; it is part of the actual seizure activity. It is the portion of the seizure that occurs before consciousness is lost and for which memory is retained when consciousness is regained (Holmes, 1987). Auras vary considerably among individuals; children may experience sensory (e.g., visual, auditory, olfactory, gustatory) symptoms, visceral sensations, or complex subjective experiences such as fear, embarrassment, or dizziness. Following the loss of consciousness, various types of automatic behavior (automatisms) may occur, such as chewing, gagging, choking, lip smacking, spitting, waving, clapping, scratching, masturbating, walking, skipping, running, screaming, crying, or laughing. Because of the bizarre behavior associated with this type of seizure, it was formerly termed a "psychomotor seizure." On regaining consciousness (the *postical* period), the child often feels tired and falls asleep. If the attack is brief, however, normal alertness may return quickly.

Generalized Seizures

Generalized seizures affect the entire brain. They may begin with generalized electrical bursts or spread from what were initially localized sites. Although children with generalized seizures always lose consciousness, the loss may be so brief as to go unnoticed.

Generalized Tonic-Clonic seizures. Generalized tonic-clonic (GTC) seizures were formerly called "grand mal seizures." These seizures may be preceded by both a prodromal phase and an aura. An aura indicates that the seizure began focally (as a partial seizure) and then spread throughout the brain. In this case, the seizure is referred to as "secondarily generalized." Typically GTC seizures involve five recognizable phases: flexion, extension, tremor, clonic, and postictal (Holmes, 1987).

Consciousness is lost during the brief (5-second) *flexion* phase. Seizure activity usually begins in the face with the eyes rolling upward and the mouth opening with jaw muscles rigid. Flexion of the extremities follows. The *extension* (tonic) phase (lasting 10 to 30 seconds) begins with extension of the back and neck and includes extension of the legs. The jaws clamp together tightly and tongue biting can occur. Apnea may begin with the rigid extension of thoracic and abdominal muscles and persist through the clonic phase. The *tremor* phase (5 to 10 seconds) marks the transition between the tonic and clonic phases. Fine tremors usually begin in the extremities and spread proximally. The *clonic* phase may last 30 to 50 seconds. The characteristic rhythmic jerking is produced by rapid contraction and relaxation of opposing muscle groups. The jerking decreases in frequency as this phase nears completion. Apnea frequently lasts through the clonic phase, causing increasing cyanosis. Secretions pool in the mouth and throat, leading to noisy respirations. This can be a difficult stage for observers because the child appears in great distress, yet nothing can interrupt the seizure. After the last clonic jerk is finished, the bladder sphincter relaxes and incontinence may occur. In the immediate *postictal* phase, the child is still unconscious, but relaxation of muscles results in a flaccid posture. Cyanosis resolves as breathing returns to normal, but pallor often lingers. The child may either gradually awaken or progress directly into a sleeping state.

Absence Seizures. This type of generalized seizure was formerly called "petit mal." Occurrence of these seizures is uncommon. It consists of a sudden, brief (usually no longer than 30 seconds) arrest of motor activity accompanied by a blank stare and loss of awareness. Posture is maintained. At the end of the seizure the child returns to the activity that was in progress as though nothing had happened. Interruption of mental activity may be incomplete, allowing the child to continue simple or automatic behavior during the lapse of full mental function. There is no memory of the seizure but the child may be aware of a "time loss."

Myoclonic Seizures. The term "myoclonus" means a quick movement of a muscle. Myoclonic seizures, then, are characterized by sudden, brief jerks of muscle groups. Flexor muscles are often involved on both sides of the body, resulting in sudden falls for older children or *infantile spasms* for infants. Consciousness is lost only momentarily and may therefore go unobserved. Myoclonic seizures may occur in clusters, either several in a row or several during a day.

Atonic Seizures. Atonic seizures involve a sudden loss of muscle tone and loss of consciousness. During a brief attack, the head may drop suddenly or the child may fall. More prolonged attacks may begin with a fall but then continue with the child lying limp and unresponsive for seconds or minutes (Huttenlocher, 1987). Longer attacks are usually followed by a period of postictal drowsiness.

Diagnostic Assessment

A diagnosis of epilepsy is made on the basis of clinical data and historical information. A specific history obtained from a parent or the individual who witnessed the seizure is extremely helpful in establishing the diagnosis. A complete developmental examination also helps one understand the disease. An EEG can provide supportive evidence and aid in classification, location of the seizure focus, and choice of treatment for the seizure disorder (Holmes, 1987). More information about the EEG can be found earlier in this chapter.

In most cases, epilepsy is idiopathic, or without an identifiable cause. Indications for further workup may include failure of medications to control seizures and/or specific focal findings on the neurologic examination that indicate an underlying brain abnormality amenable to other treatments. Even if a structural abnormality is found, antiepileptic medications are still administered, but may be gradually discontinued at a later date. Diagnostic testing varies, depending on the nature of the structural or metabolic problem leading to epilepsy.

Therapeutic Management

Medical Management. Therapeutic management of chronic seizure activity includes anticonvulsant drugs, education of the family and child, and attention to associated emotional or learning disabilities. The goal of drug therapy is to control the seizures with as few drug side effects as possible.

The drug of choice for absence seizures is ethosuximide (Zarontin). The major anticonvulsants used in epilepsy are phenobarbital, phenytoin (Dilantin) carbamazepine (Tegretol), and valproic acid (Depakene) (Huttenlocher, 1987). The properties and toxic reactions of these and other commonly used anticonvulsants are listed in Table 40–23. Drug treatment typically begins with one anticonvulsant agent, with the dosage increased gradually until seizures are controlled, clinical manifestations of toxicity are experienced, or serum drug levels reach the high end of the therapeutic range without controlling seizures. If the

TABLE 40-23
Properties and Toxic Reactions of Commonly Used Anticonvulsants

Drug	Serum $t^{1/2*}$ (hours)	Therapeutic Blood Level (μg/ml)	Starting Dosage (mg/kg/day)	Daily Doses	Days to Attain Steady-State Blood Level	How Supplied	Life-Threatening Side Effects	Other Side Effects
Phenobarbital	36–72	15–40	2–3	1 or 2	14–21	Elixir: 4 mg/ml; tablets: 15, 30, 60, and 100 mg	Stevens-Johnson syndrome (rare); blood dyscrasias (rare)	Hyperkinesis; drowsiness; drug rash
Primidone (Mysoline)	6–18	4–12	5	2 or 3	4–7	Tablets: 50 and 250 mg Suspension: 50 mg/ml	Same as phenobarbital	
Phenytoin (Dilantin)	15–45	10–20	5–7	2	7–21	Tablet: 50 mg Capsules: 30 and 100 mg	Stevens-Johnson syndrome (rare); acute hepatic necrosis (rare); blood dyscrasias (rare)	Drug rash (10% in first 2 wks), gingival hyperplasia, lymphadenopathy, hirsutism, acromegaloid facies, ataxia, nystagmus, vomiting, dystonic reaction, rickets, folate deficiency, embryopathy (fetal hydantoin syndrome) if used during pregnancy
Carbamazepine (Tegretol)	8–20	4–12	10–15	2 or 3	5–10	Tablets: 100 and 200 mg	Leukopenia, thrombocytopenia, aplastic anemia (rare)	Drowiness, abdominal distress
Valproic acid (Depakene)	6–14	40–100	10–20	3 or 4	4	Capsules: 250 mg Syrup: 50 mg/ml	Acute hepatic failure (Reye syndrome–like)	Hyperammonemia, drowsiness, alopecia, abdominal discomfort
Ethosuximide (Zarontin)	24–36	40–80	10–20	2	5–8	Capsules: 250 mg Syrup: 50 mg/ml	Blood dyscrasias (very rare)	Drowsiness, nausea
Clonazepam (Klonopin)	20–32	0.015–0.04	0.04–0.05	2	10–14	Tablets: 0.5, 1, and 2 mg	Blood dyscrasias (very rare)	Drowsiness (common)
Acetazolamide (Diamox)	4–10	—	10–20	2 or 3	3	Tablets: 125 and 250 mg Capsules: 500 mg (extended release)	Blood dyscrasias (very rare)	Metabolic acidosis, paresthesias, anorexia, weight loss

From Behrman, R. (Ed.) (1987). *Nelson textbook of pediatrics* (13th ed.). Philadelphia: WB Saunders.
* $t^{1/2}$ = half-life

first drug proves ineffective, a second is added or another drug tried. During this process, it is essential that the child and family be aware of the need to report changes in sensation and behavior that may signal a toxic reaction and that they understand the importance of close follow-up care. Serum blood levels are drawn frequently until it is determined how a particular drug is metabolized by a particular child.

Anticonvulsant therapy is usually continued until the child has been seizure-free for 2 or 3 years (Holmes, 1987). In the young child, anticonvulsants may be discontinued earlier, because rapid brain development has the potential to raise the seizure threshold. In any case, anticonvulsant drugs are always tapered in dosage to the point of complete withdrawal; the drug should not be stopped suddenly.

Surgical Management. In recent years, some children whose epilepsy is intractable to drug therapy have been candidates for a complex surgical procedure to remove the area of seizure focus, and those more severely affected, for a hemispherectomy. In the first instance, the patient under goes a craniotomy to implant a grid on the subdural surface. This grid allows mapping of critical brain areas involved in vision, speech, sensation, and memory as well as identification of the seizure focus. After surgery, leads extend from the implanted grid to computerized video and EEG monitoring. After a period of monitoring and extensive testing is completed, a second surgery is done to excise the seizure focus (Rutkowski, 1990). In cases of intractable seizures with infantile hemiplegia, a hemispherectomy may be the procedure of choice (Tatum & Wang, 1990). These procedures are complex and are done only in select major medical centers across the country. Appropriate selection of children who may benefit from this procedure is essential. Seizures must be focal, intractable to medical management, and arising from an area of the brain that could be removed without significant neurologic deficit (Rutkowski, 1990).

Epilepsy surgery may be indicated for children with intractable or uncontrolled seizures who have failed to gain seizure control after therapeutic trials with the most appropriate antiepileptic drugs. Children would be referred to a medical center for a comprehensive epilepsy evaluation. Diagnostic evaluation includes careful review of medication and seizure history and previous diagnostic tests. The child may have intense EEG monitoring with surgical implantation of either depth electrodes or an electrode grid in efforts to define more clearly the epileptogenic focus. Potential candidates for lobectomy may also have Wada angiogram. Neuropsychologic testing as well as evaluations with psychologists and speech, physical and occupational therapists are usually completed.

Candidates for surgery are children who have the following: (1) partial seizures with a consistent discrete focus in a surgically resectable area of the brain, (2) partial seizures that are secondarily generalized and in which seizure severity, frequency, or injury is intolerable, or (3) frequent injury because of severe atonic or myoclonic seizures. Epilepsy surgery is a big decision and is usually reserved for children for whom decreasing the seizure severity, frequency, or injuries would improve their quality of life.

There are a variety of surgeries for appropriate candidates, including cortical resection, temporal lobectomy, corpus callosum section, and hemispherectomy. In general, results in over two thirds of patients who have had temporal lobectomy have shown complete control of seizures or decreased frequency of seizures. The reader is referred to Engel (1987) for more detailed information on various types of epilepsy surgery. Epilepsy surgery has provided additional treatment alternatives for children affected by intractable seizures.

Application of the Nursing Process: Epilepsy

Nursing care is focused on the physical and psychosocial implications of the disease. With increasing information available to the public, some of the traditional stigma attached to this disease is lessening. Nursing care of an epileptic child hospitalized for the disease must be given an adequate understanding of the disease and its treatment. Because the first exposure to a seizure is a frightening experience, the nurse should seek opportunities to view films or to observe a child having a seizure before caring for such a child. Seizure activity is bizarre, and nurses must be comfortable with their own feelings. Most children who have seizures are not hospitalized; hospitalization is required only for further diagnostic evaluations and control of lengthy seizure activity.

Assessment

Nursing assessment of the child with epilepsy includes careful observation and documentation of seizure activity when it does occur, *seizure precautions* and *management* (covered earlier in this chapter), assessment of side effects of antiepileptic drugs, and gathering of psychosocial data on patient and family coping. Depending on the setting in which the nurse encounters the child with epilepsy, different aspects of the nursing assessment gain priority. Nursing assessment and care for the child undergoing surgery for seizures are not discussed in this chapter, because few children are candidates for these procedures.

Nursing Diagnostic Statements and Collaborative Problems

High risk for injury; *risk factor: altered responsiveness during seizure activity.*

High risk for injury; risk factors: antiepileptic drug therapy and potential side effects or toxicities.

Ineffective individual and family coping, related to knowledge deficit: parent and child about diagnosis and chronic nature of medical management.

Planning and Implementation

Seizure precautions and *management* are discussed elsewhere in this text and in Tables 40–15 and 40–16. This discussion focuses on safe administration of antiepileptic drugs and promotion of coping with the disease.

Preventing Injury Through Safe Medication: Administration of Antiepileptic Drugs and Monitoring for Potential Side Effects. Most seizure activity can be controlled with medications. Medications are chosen on the basis of the type of seizure activity noted. The nurse must understand the function of the chosen drug and any potential side effects. Patient and family compliance with medications is paramount for successful drug therapy. Patient education regarding medications is a primary nursing responsibility. Some drugs have the potential for adverse effects on the hematopoietic system, liver, and kidneys. Toxic reactions to medications should be understood and monitored. The nurse is often responsible for drawing drug levels and reporting results in a timely fashion so that appropriate medication changes can be made, if necessary. Side effects and therapeutic drug levels of commonly used anticonvulsants are listed in Table 40–23.

Assistance with Family Coping Through Patient and Family Education. All diagnostic procedures should be explained in advance to the child and family. The Epilepsy Foundation of America has coloring books and cartoon books to inform children about the disease and diagnostic tests. Questions should be answered simply and honestly. Parents' understanding and acceptance of epilepsy will vary. The nurse should allow parents to observe their child during a seizure and teach appropriate care and safety. Encouraging confidence and calmness during the event is helpful. A calm attitude decreases the fear and stigma associated with epilepsy and helps maintain focus on the care of the child, not on the seizure.

Although most children with epilepsy have normal intelligence, some have cognitive and developmental delays. The school nurse and teacher need to be involved in understanding the disease and associated treatment. The school-age child may be at risk for absenteeism if seizures are not controlled. A staff conference may be held to identify the child's specific needs and alert the school to any potential side effects of medications. Encourage the family to provide a Medic-Alert bracelet for the child to wear at all times. A helmet may be necessary only for children with kinetic or "drop" seizures or for those with significant delays. Parents should be encouraged to focus attention on well siblings who may have unexpressed fears about the disease or harbor guilt or anger toward the affected sibling. Most children with epilepsy are effectively managed in the outpatient clinic setting.

The Epilepsy Foundation of America has a bibliography of literature available. Most states have an epilepsy foundation, and many communities have local chapters. Parents and families can gain strength through contacts with other parents. The foundation makes medication available at a reduced rate. Speakers are available for school or community groups. It also provides individual and group counseling.

Nursing care is focused on the following:

- Interval history of any seizure activity.
- Monitoring of drug levels and side effects.
- Psychosocial, cognitive, and school issues.

Evaluation

As in all nursing care plans, the success of the interventions in meeting the projected outcomes will be seen when high-risk problems do not occur and the defining characteristics for actual problems decrease in frequency and/or severity or disappear.

Craniosynostosis

Craniosynostosis is either the absence of or the premature fusion of one or more of the cranial sutures that join the bones of the infant skull. The term "craniostenosis" is often used interchangeably with "craniosynostosis." Craniostenosis refers to the actual deformity that results from absence or early fusion of the sutures, whereas craniosynostosis refers to the inherent process of early suture closure (Cohen, 1986). At present, the latter term is more commonly accepted and will be used in this chapter. The skull deformity that results from this developmental aberration can range from mild, as in cases of single suture synostosis, to severe, as in cases of multiple suture synostosis, which is evident in children with genetic syndromes.

When diagnosed, craniosynostosis is classified as primary, secondary, or syndromic. *Primary craniosynostosis* may be either simple or compound. The term "simple synostosis" refers to the involvement of one suture, whereas "compound synostosis" refers to the absence or early fusion of two or more of the cranial sutures. Most cases of primary craniosynostosis are also referred to as "isolated," because they occur without any association to other developmental anomalies (Fig. 40–13) (Cohen, 1986).

In *secondary craniosynostosis,* suture obliteration occurs as a result of a known disorder. Various metabolic and hematologic disorders may lead to

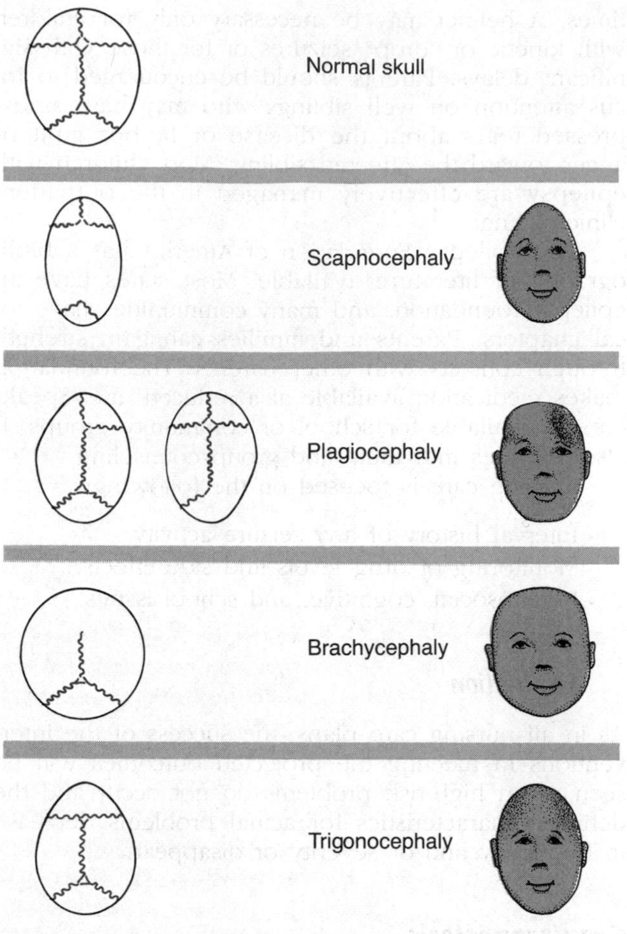

FIGURE 40 - 13. Normal skull and variations that occur in single or compound craniosynostosis.

early fusion of the cranial sutures. Hyperthyroidism and thalassemia are examples of known causes of secondary craniosynostosis. The failure of brain growth that occurs in microcephaly may also lead to early closure of the cranial sutures.

In contrast to isolated craniosynostosis, *syndromic craniosynostosis* occurs in conjunction with other morphologic syndromes or developmental anomalies. There are many genetic syndromes associated with craniosynostosis, the two most common being Apert and Crouzon syndromes. Apert syndrome is characterized by craniosynostosis, midfacial malformations including bulging (proptotic), wide-set (hyperteloric) eyes and recessed chin, as well as syndactyly of the hands and feet. Children with Crouzon syndrome have somewhat similar facial characteristics, but they do not exhibit the characteristic limb malformations seen in Apert syndrome. All but 3 per cent of children with Crouzon syndrome exhibit normal intelligence, whereas many children with Apert syndrome exhibit mental deficiencies (Cohen, 1986).

The incidence of primary isolated craniosynostosis in the United States is approximately 0.4 to 1.0 per 1000 live births. This varies slightly, depending on the data used (Cohen, 1986). Winston (1985) states that the true occurrence is probably higher; as many mild cases likely go unreported because of the considerable variation in the severity of the cosmetic manifestations of craniosynostosis.

Etiology/Incidence

The etiology of primary isolated craniosynostosis is unknown. It is generally agreed that this disease probably does not have one isolated cause but rather a multifactoral basis. Although the majority of cases of simple craniosynostosis occur sporadically, some familial instances have been reported. Hunter and Rudd (1977) reported a 2 to 8 per cent familial occurrence of primary craniosynostosis of one suture.

Pathophysiology

The embryologic development of cranial sutures and the abnormality in this development that results in craniosynostosis have been the center of much attention. To understand abnormal head shape resulting from suture obliteration, knowledge regarding normal cranial growth is paramount. In the introductory discussion in this chapter, ossification and fontanel closure are addressed, particularly regarding age-related differences in structure and function. A review and further clarification of these concepts are presented here in the context of this disease process.

Figure 40–14 shows a superior view of the normal infant skull. Five cranial sutures (three—the coronal, lambdoidal, and squamosal—are paired) allow the rapidly developing brain to grow at a normal rate. The anterior and posterior fontanels close at approximately 12 to 18 months and 2 to 3 months, respectively.

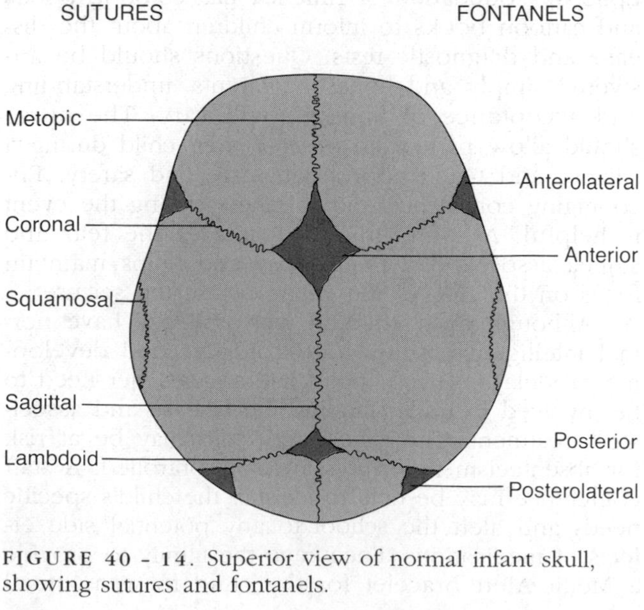

FIGURE 40 - 14. Superior view of normal infant skull, showing sutures and fontanels.

Development of the Cranial Bones. The cranial bones originate as a series of ossification centers that emerge from the fibrous embryologic cerebral capsule. At a later point in this stage of development, the cerebral capsule actually develops into the outer and inner layers of the dura mater. In early fetal life, the brain and cranial bones expand rapidly, although their borders (eventual suture sites) are widely separated. When the rate of brain growth slows down later in fetal life, the bones become more closely approximated, allowing for the eventual formation of a suture (Kokich, 1986). The suture itself is not thought to have potential for actual cell proliferation, but rather it acts as a site of adaptation during growth by allowing for new bone generated from the cerebral capsule to be deposited and resorbed in a continuous and progressive fashion. In essence, the sutures grow in response to the changes and needs of the developing brain, particularly its fibrous covering (Koski, 1968).

Premature Suture Synostosis and Head Shape. In adulthood, all sutures are eventually obliterated by bone. If this occurs before the functional need for adaptation is complete, it is referred to as "premature synostosis" or "fusion." Kokich (1986) and others question whether "premature synostosis" is actually the correct terminology, because in many cases, the fibrous, adaptive ligament that is referred to as a "suture" never even begins to form, thus allowing two adjacent cranial bones to merge. Whether the underlying pathology is referred to as "suture agenesis" or "premature synostosis," the outcome of abnormal head shape is essentially the same with some potential for variation in the actual severity of the deformity.

The cranial bones grow perpendicular to each of the cranial sutures. For example, the sagittal suture allows for growth of the parietal skull bones in a lateral fashion, thereby adding to the width of the skull. When this suture is absent or closed, growth is inhibited in the lateral direction, and instead growth occurs parallel to the ossified suture. The classic appearance of an infant or child with sagittal synostosis is one of a very long and narrow head, or *scaphocephaly*.

The *rule of thumb* that is helpful in remembering how head shape will appear in craniosynostosis is that growth is inhibited at right angles to the fused suture with compensatory expansion occurring at the sutures that are functional. To help clarify this concept, think of the following scenario. A child presents with a left coronal suture that is fused. Growth of the skull is inhibited perpendicular to the left coronal suture so that the forehead appears recessed; the left eye may appear to bulge slightly. Because the brain needs to continue to expand, it is forced to grow in the direction of the open cranial sutures. In this situation, the brain expands along the right coronal suture, giving the appearance of a prominent right forehead and a sunken right eye in contrast to the left eye. This characteristic asymmetry of the skull is also referred to as *plagiocephaly*. The open sutures in a sense "work overtime" to allow the brain to expand. Figure 40–13 depicts schematic drawings of the various forms of craniosynostosis and outlines of the corresponding cranial shapes, including the accepted Greek terminology. Although this nomenclature continues to be commonly used, Cohen (1986) emphasizes that regardless of the classification system or terminology used, the most important information is a ". . . clear description of which suture or sutures are involved and the extent of involvement . . ." (p 11).

In summary, the ultimate head shape in the diagnosis of craniosynostosis depends on which sutures are synostosed and the rate at which they close. The earlier in fetal or infant life synostosis occurs, the more dramatic is the effect on cranial growth and appearance; the later synostosis occurs, the less dramatic is the outcome (Cohen, 1986).

Clinical Manifestations

Initially, when craniosynostosis is questioned, a thorough "hands-on" assessment of the cranium is called for. Palpation of the head for suture location and mobility is essential. Bony ridges along suture lines and any facial and/or cranial asymmetry are noted. Asymmetry can be evaluated by comparing the location of the external ear canals and outer canthi of the eyes from right to left. This comparison is best elucidated with the examiner looking down on the infant or child from the superior view. The examiner should pull the hair back from the forehead during examination, especially when synostosis of the metopic or either coronal suture is suspected.

Along with palpation, measurement of the child's head circumference (HC) is vital. Many infants with craniosynostosis present initially with a mild to moderate fall-off in this measurement. Height and weight parameters and HC need to be assessed simultaneously to ensure that the child is not failing to grow on all parameters for other reasons.

As well as a complete neurologic examination—including checking for sensory and motor function, cranial nerve findings, and evidence of chronic ICP—the neurologist or neurosurgeon does an assessment of the family's concerns about the unusual head shape. Because craniosynostosis can range from very mild, requiring no intervention, to very severe, requiring several surgical procedures, parental concerns may vary widely.

Table 40–24 contains an overview of suggested assessment for children with a diagnosis of craniosynostosis.

Diagnostic Assessment

Craniosynostosis may be suspected either at birth or in later visits to health care providers for well child care. For children in whom it is not evident at birth, parents are often the individuals who first notice the

TABLE 40-24
Suggested Aspects of Diagnostic Assessment for Craniosynostosis

Clinical evaluation	Complete history and physical examination
	Palpation of sutures
	Asymmetry
	Head circumference
	Neurologic examination
Radiographic evaluation	Skull roentgenograph
	Computed tomography scan, including bone windows
Developmental evaluation	Cognitive function
	Gross and fine motor
	Social/emotional
	Speech and language
	Genetic or syndromic findings

unusual head shape developing, especially when there are siblings with whom to make comparisons.

Generally, once the pediatrician or other health care provider suspects a diagnosis of craniosynostosis, a referral to a neurologist or neurosurgeon is made. In some instances, the primary physician orders radiographic studies to be taken prior to the consultation visit and given to the referring physician for review. These include plain x-ray films of several different views of the skull. A CT scan with bone windows is also performed. "Bone windows" refers to the computerized mechanism for shading out the contours of the brain, producing a picture showing only the inner and outer contours of the skull bone. If these radiographic studies have not been done before referral, they are ordered by the consulting physician.

Therapeutic Management

The goals of modern surgical management of craniosynostosis are to prevent the development of increased intracranial pressure that may result in neurologic damage and to correct the cosmetic deformity that may result in long-term psychologic sequelae for the affected individual (Marchac & Renier, 1982). The decision to correct craniosynostosis surgically is based on the severity of the deformity, the number of sutures thought to be synostosed, and the child's present neurologic and developmental condition. There is an ongoing controversy in the area of surgical management as to whether primary neurologic findings are a result of craniosynostosis or whether they are intrinsic aspects of abnormal brain development (Camfield & Camfield, 1986). Nonetheless, for children in whom more than one suture is synostosed or in whom symptoms of increased ICP exist, surgical correction is recommended.

The choice of surgical technique employed to correct craniosynostosis depends primarily on the individual surgeon and his or her philosophy and experience. Techniques among centers vary and range from aggressive reconstruction to placement of synthetic materials to recreate symmetry. Techniques include the removal of strips or large portions of bone alone and/or reconstruction of the removed bone to reshape the skull. In other instances, synthetic materials are placed along cut bone edges around the affected suture to prevent reclosure after operations. Acrylic onlays to correct an asymmetric appearance of the skull and plication or incision of the dura mater to reshape the underlying brain are also techniques used at various centers across the country. There has been a trend toward combining neurosurgical and plastic surgery techniques and forming multidisciplinary craniofacial teams to provide care for children with craniosynostosis. Regardless of the procedure chosen, the ultimate goals of allowing for brain growth and correcting the cosmetic deformity are maintained.

Therapeutic postsurgical management includes close monitoring of neurologic status, which may be affected by cerebral edema. This can, in turn, affect fluid and electrolyte balance and put the child at risk for further edema if not managed properly. As with any neurosurgical procedure, risks of infection and bleeding are present and must be followed. Respiratory complications may ensue as a result of the lengthy period of anesthetization for the more extensive procedures. Close scrutiny of the eyes is required, because the bones surrounding the orbits are often manipulated.

Application of the Nursing Process: Craniosynostosis

Assessment

Postoperative assessment of the child undergoing craniofacial surgery entails *neurologic monitoring,* including level of consciousness, pupillary responses (not done if eyes are swollen shut), and monitoring of vital signs and indicators of increased ICP (see discussion of ICP earlier in this chapter). Assessment of surgical dressings and drains and of fluid and electrolyte balance is necessary, because these children often have mild to moderate cerebral edema. Facial and severe eye and periorbital swelling requires *skin surveillance* and prevention of further trauma, skin breakdown, or infection of this area (Brucker & Laurent, 1988).

Nursing Diagnostic Statements and Collaborative Problems

High risk for altered tissue perfusion, cerebral; *risk factor: postoperative edema.*

High risk for infection: incisional, bone, meningeal, skin, or eye; *risk factors: introduction of pathogen:*
- *Surgical wound.*
- *Prolonged eye swelling.*
- *Skin breakdown secondary to pressure dressing on head.*
- *Postoperative cerebrospinal fluid leak.*

Parental anxiety regarding safety of transfusions, *associated with significant surgical blood loss and postoperative drainage.*

Fear and pain, *related to*
- *Facial and severe eye edema associated with surgical intervention.*
- *Pressure of postoperative pressure dressing to head.*

Ineffective family coping, *related to anxiety about surgery in a vital area resulting from*
- *Inadequate information.*
- *Lack of familiarity with hospital setting and surgical techniques.*
- *Severe facial and eye swelling.*

High risk for altered health maintenance after discharge; *risk factor: knowledge deficit regarding home care of the child.*

Planning and Implementation

Preventing Decreased Cerebral Perfusion. The infant or child usually returns from surgery with the head of the bed elevated at least 20 to 30 degrees. It is necessary to ensure proper body alignment in relation to the elevation desired. Increased intrathoracic pressure (a result of torso elevation) has been known to increase ICP. For this reason, children recovering from surgery for craniosynostosis are maintained on moderate fluid restrictions. Assessment and documentation of neurologic status are vital. *Neurologic monitoring,* including appropriate responses to stimuli and pupillary checks (if the eyes have not swollen shut), is necessary.

Preventing Infection. Some surgeons may order prophylactic antibiotics for a few postoperative days. Once the head dressing is removed, preventing the child from putting her hands to the incision is essential. This may require the use of elbow splints. Prolonged eye swelling puts the child at risk for conjunctival infections or ulcers. If such swelling is noted, the physician should be notified, to allow consideration of administration of prophylactic eyedrops or ointments. The potential for CSF leak exists and should be monitored.

Decreasing Anxiety about Transfusions. If the planned surgery is extensive, parents are made aware before the surgery of the potential for blood loss; they are encouraged to provide directly donated blood, if possible, and the hospital blood bank is set up for this purpose. Screening of blood from matched family donors is the same as that for all donated blood, but the family's fear of hepatitis and human immunodeficiency virus transmission may be reduced if they know the donors. Blood counts are followed closely for the first 72 hours postoperatively.

Decreasing Fear and Pain. In addition to postoperative headache, children undergoing surgery for craniosynostosis experience fear and anxiety if periorbital edema obscures or completely negates their vision. Physicians' orders frequently include narcotic analgesics, such as morphine, and non-narcotic pain medications, such as acetaminophen (Tylenol). Sedatives are rarely ordered, because they may mask the assessment of true neurologic status. Easing the fear and anxiety of a young child who cannot see is a true nursing challenge. Often parents are the experts at the nonpharmacologic measures that help their child cope. Maximizing use of the senses of touch, taste, smell, and hearing is usually the best way to assure the infant or child that their familiar and comforting world has not disappeared. Adequate periods of rest are also extremely vital, even as the child appears to be getting back to normal activity.

Supporting Family Coping. Many families have difficulty understanding the procedures necessary to correct craniosynostosis. It is hard for the parent of an otherwise healthy-appearing child to consent to surgery of this magnitude, even when the child is obviously deformed. Often what parents need most is *presence,* including someone to listen to their concerns and provide positive reinforcement for their participation in, and coping with, hospitalization. In some circumstances, other families who have been through the surgery are helpful. Anxiety on the part of the parents is often sensed by children and contributes to their fear. Family members may feel guilty if they leave the child's side. They need to be encouraged to spend time away from the child so that their time with the child is a helpful, rather than draining, experience. For all of these reasons, a family-centered approach to the nursing care of these children is essential to the creation of a positive hospitalization experience.

Facilitating Health Maintenance. Discharge teaching is a large part of the nurse's responsibility in the hospital setting. Instructions are given for incision care, activity, use of a protective helmet, positioning, and follow-up visits. It is essential that this information be in a written format so that parents can refer to it when necessary.

Depending on the surgery performed, some children go home with the initial surgical dressing intact. Major aspects of caring for these children will be done in the home and clinic settings. Instructions for home care are listed in Table 40–25.

TABLE 40-25
***Family-Centered Teaching:* Instructions for Home Care Following Neurologic Surgery**

Administer acetaminophen (Tylenol) when the child is irritable and fussy
Observe the incision for any areas of redness, infection, or cerebrospinal fluid leak
Safetyproof the home to provide a safe environment
Ensure that child wears protective helmet (if suggested or prescribed by the physician)

Evaluation

As in all nursing care plans, the success of the interventions in meeting the projected outcomes is seen when high-risk problems do not occur and the defining characteristics for actual problems decrease in frequency and/or severity or disappear.

Spina Bifida (Myelodysplasia)

"Myelodysplasia" refers to abnormal development of the spinal cord in embryonic life. In the clinical context, this term is often used interchangeably with the term "spinal dysraphism" or "spina bifida," which refers to incomplete closure of the primary neural tube. Cranium bifidum refers to incomplete closure of the rostral end of the neural tube, resulting in abnormal development of the brain, meninges, and/or skull bones. At a more basic level, all of the congenital malformations involving the neural tube are also often referred to as "neural tube defects" (NTDs). If defective closure occurs in the area of the developing embryonic head, anencephaly or encephalocele may result, and if defective closure occurs lower in the spinal column, spina bifida occurs. These malformations constitute the greatest number of neurologic developmental disorders (Allanson, 1988).

The most commonly seen NTDs are listed and defined, in order of decreasing severity, as follows:

- *Anencephaly:* Absence of brain tissue above a rudimentary brain stem and basal ganglia. This is often listed under the family of defects called "cranium bifidum." Sustained extrauterine life is virtually impossible in these children.
- *Encephalocele:* Another type of cranium bifidum that presents as an external sac or mass that may occur at any point over the vertex or base of the skull. May be covered with either scalp or a transparent membrane.
- *Spina bifida cystica:* The incomplete fusion of one or more of the vertebral laminae, resulting in an external protrusion of the spinal tissue (Fig. 40-15). This open type of defect occurs most commonly in the lumbosacral area. There are two classifications of spina bifida cystica:

  Myelomeningocele: This more severe and most common open NTD involves a protruding saclike structure that contains meninges, spinal fluid, and neural tissue. The spinal nerve roots may terminate in the sac, significantly affecting motor and sensory function below that point. The most severe and rarest form of myelomeningocele is *myeloschisis,* in which the neural folds fail to meet and fuse, causing the spinal cord to become a flattened mass of nervous tissue with no dural covering.

  Meningocele: This less common open NTD contains only meninges and CSF. Neurologic complications can occur but are less severe than with myelomeningocele.
- *Spina bifida occulta:* The incomplete fusion of the vertebrae at one level that may be signaled only by an overlying dimple or tuft of hair. Most of these defects occur without any evidence of dermatologic, neurologic, or musculoskeletal disorders. Some present with symptoms in late childhood and require eventual surgical intervention if clinical deterioration is present. Dermoid cysts, fibrous bands, or lipomas (fatty tumors) are the most common etiologies for this diagnosis (Reigel, 1989). Figure 40-16 depicts three of these congenital malformations of the spine.

All of the developmental anomalies involving the neural tube are best understood by considering the normal embryologic development of the brain and spinal cord. At about 18 days of gestation, the ner-

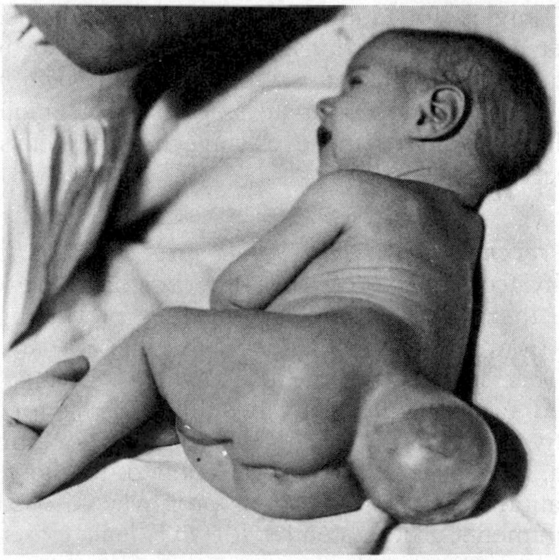

FIGURE 40-15. Infant with spina bifida cystica. Handling this infant requires extreme care so that the sac incurs no tension or pressure. The infant's head and spine above the sac should be supported at all times, as should the lower extremities when the child is held.

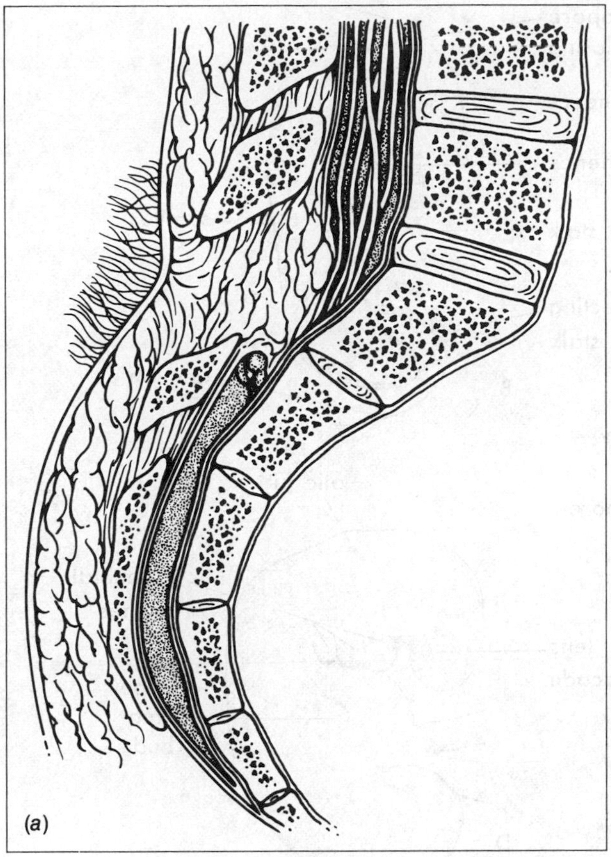

FIGURE 40 - 16. Congenital malformations of the spine. *a*, Spina bifida occulta, an incomplete fusion of the vertebral arches without an external sac. A dimple or tuft of hair may signal its presence. *b*, Meningocele. The external sac contains meninges and cerebrospinal fluid (CSF). *c*, Myelomeningocele. The external sac contains meninges, CSF, and immature spinal cord tissue. (*a–c*, From Bowens, B. A. [1979]. The nervous system. In M. Armstrong, et al. [eds.]. *McGraw-Hill handbook of clinical nursing*. New York: McGraw-Hill. Reproduced with permission of McGraw-Hill.)

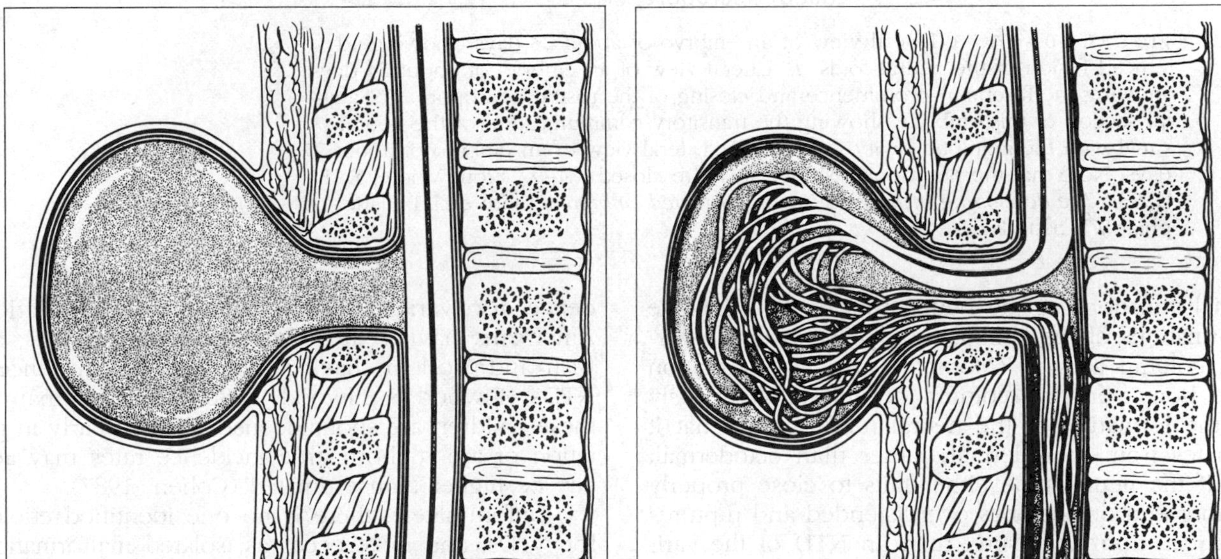

vous system begins to develop from a thickened area of embryonic ectoderm called the *neural plate*. By the 22nd day of gestation, the neural plate begins to fold into the *neural tube* (Fig. 40–17). This folding initially occurs centrally and then proceeds in a somewhat irregular fashion superiorly and inferiorly. The upper opening of the neural tube is called the *rostral neuropore,* and the lower spinal opening is called the *caudal neuropore*. These neuropores close on the 25th and 27th days of embryonic life, respectively. The central lumen of the neural tube eventually becomes the ventricular system of the brain superiorly, and the central canal of the spinal cord inferiorly (Moore, 1988).

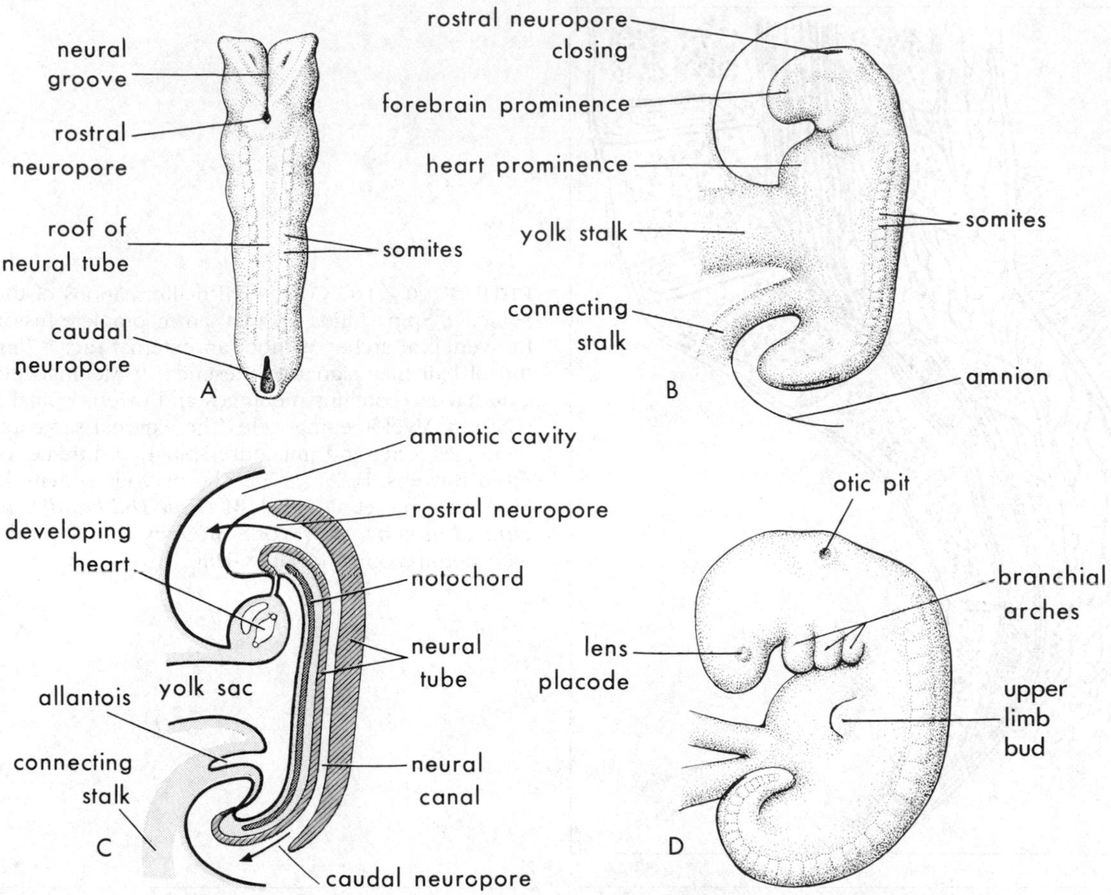

FIGURE 40 - 17. *A*, Dorsal view of an embryo of about 23 days, showing advanced fusion of the neural folds. *B*, Lateral view of an embryo of about 24 days, showing the forebrain prominence and closing of the rostral neuropore. *C*, Sagittal section of this embryo, showing the transitory communication of the neural canal with the amniotic cavity *(arrows)*. *D*, Lateral view of an embryo of about 27 days. Note that the neuropores shown in *B* are closed. (*A–D*, From Moore, K. L. [1993]. *The developing human: Clinically oriented embryology* [5th ed.]. Philadelphia: WB Saunders.)

Malformations of the neural tube usually involve malformations of the laminae and pedicles of the vertebral column as well (Moore, 1988). The formation of the bony vertebral column occurs simultaneously with the formation of the neural tube, except that it originates from mesodermal, rather than ectodermal, cells. If the neural tube either fails to close properly on either end or becomes overdistended and ruptures after initial normal closure, then an NTD of the varieties described earlier occurs.

Etiology/Incidence

The incidence of neural tube defects varies considerably, depending on geographic location. In the United States the frequency is 1 to 2 per 1000 live births. In certain areas of Ireland and England, the frequency is as high as 4 to 5 per 1000 live births. Some countries, like Japan and Finland, have frequencies of less than 0.5 per 1000 live births. Incidence also varies by race, with Asians and African-Americans having the lowest occurrence rates, and Irish and Moslems having the highest occurrence of NTDs (Elwood & Elwood, 1980). Because many of these children are spontaneously aborted early in gestation or are stillborn, true incidence rates may actually be higher than estimated (Cohen, 1987).

Unfortunately, there is no one identified etiology for NTDs, and most occur as isolated malformations. The exact reasons for abnormal closure of the neural tube have remained unclear at best. NTDs are caused by a variety of factors, some inherited and some acquired. They may occur as a part of various chromosomal aberrations or after fetal exposure to teratogenic drugs. Isolated, nonsyndromic NTDs are recognized as having multifactoral causation. This means that a combination of both genetic and environmental factors may interact in the development of the malformation (Allanson, 1988). For example, if an individual were to have a genetic predisposition for NTDs, an environmental trigger could act to manifest such a defect in that person's offspring. One or more trigger mechanisms can be involved, and they may vary among populations. Genetic and environmental components are considered to be additive, increasing a particular couple's risk for producing a child with an NTD (Cohen, 1984). Many epidemiologic studies have been carried out in an effort to identify etiologic agents and promote prevention of these defects. In a summary of various epidemiologic observations noted in the literature, Cohen (1987) points out the variety of factors thought to contribute to the development of an NTD. Some of these factors are summarized here:

- *Poor nutrition*—particularly zinc, folate, and generalized vitamin deficiencies.
- *Maternal age*—the highest risk groups are teenagers and women over 35 years old.
- *Pregnancy history*—women who miscarry in the pregnancy immediately preceding the current pregnancy are thought to be at higher risk.
- *Birth order*—first-born children are at highest risk; second-born children at lowest risk.
- *Socioeconomic status*—frequency of NTDs is higher in low socioeconomic groups; this may be related to nutrition.

It should be noted that even though a family history of NTDs increases the risk of subsequent NTD births, between 90 and 95 per cent of infants with NTDs are born to couples with negative family histories of the same (Cohen, 1987).

It has been reported that supplementation with vitamins, particularly folic acid, during the conceptual period was associated with significant decreases in NTDs, compared with an unsupplemented group (Nevin, 1985). Although a few other studies have come to similar conclusions, the studies are weakened by a number of variables not controlled for and by the small numbers of individuals involved (Reigel, 1989). Ongoing research in this area is shedding new light on the etiology of spina bifida and potential preventive measures.

Pathophysiology

The most common site of involvement in the spine is the lower thoracic lumbar or sacral area. Approximately 85 per cent are located there, and the remaining 15 per cent are located in the upper thoracic and cervical regions. The anterior aspects of the spinal cord are frequently intact, and varying degrees of destruction of the dorsal columns may exist (Reigel, 1989).

Although the pathologic abnormalities observed at the site of the open spinal defect are the most obvious, other abnormalities are often found throughout the spinal canal and other systems, such as the genitourinary and cardiovascular. Associated brain abnormalities include defects of cellular migration, agenesis of the corpus callosum, arachnoid cysts, and polymicrogyria, among others (Reigel, 1989).

The degree of functional impairment associated with the various types of myelodysplasia depends on the level and extent of the defect as well as associated neurologic defects. The neurologic findings usually correlate with the particular muscle groups (myotomes) that are innervated by affected spinal cord segments.

Clinical Manifestations

The dysfunction secondary to spina bifida can range from complete paralysis to minimal involvement but is most often somewhere in between. A lesion at the middle thoracic level causes total paralysis of the lower extremities. The more common lumbosacral lesions generally leave the child with some degree of hip, knee, or ankle flexion, allowing for walking with either braces and crutches or minimal assistive devices, depending on the functional level of the lesion. The closed or nonvisible lesions (spina bifida occulta) often go undiagnosed until later childhood and are frequently not associated with any degree of impairment.

In most lumbosacral lesions, the muscles of the legs are affected, and the electrical responses of these muscles may vary. Sensory disturbances are usually symmetric but patchy. The sensory level is determined with a dermatome chart, which is used to delineate areas of skin innervated by each sensory spinal nerve. Club feet, scoliosis, contractures, and dislocated hips are common in children born with lesions of the lumbosacral area (Lindseth, 1988; Louis, 1988). Bowel and bladder dysfunction are almost always apparent, because the nerves that supply these organs are located in the sacral area. Bowel problems commonly include constipation or incontinence (Roberts, 1988). The neurogenic bladder can make the child prone to retention and resultant urinary tract infections, or the child may have problems with incontinence (Bailey, 1988). The nursing assessment and care strategies are addressed separately, after the discussion of therapeutic management. The clinical manifestations associated with all of the myelodysplastic lesions are only as clear as the diagnostic assessment of functional capacity. As in most instances of congenital central nervous system disorders, the true extent of dysfunction is often apparent only as the child grows and a clearer assessment of function is obtained.

Diagnostic Assessment

Modern ultrasound and laboratory technology have made possible the prenatal diagnosis of open NTDs. In the early 1970s, an association between an elevated serum alpha fetoprotein (AFP) level and the presence of an open NTD was discovered. Many health care providers have since relied on AFP levels drawn between 16 and 18 weeks of gestation as a screening tool for open NTDs. The test is not foolproof, because many other congenital anomalies can cause increases in AFP levels, and there are other maternal factors known to cause false-positive and false-negative results with this test. Nonetheless, AFP levels have become a useful screening tool for open NTDs (Allanson, 1988). Although prenatal screening has added a dimension to anticipatory guidance of families with myelodysplastic children, the discovery of this anomaly in the delivery room continues to occur. The importance of an honest and compassionate approach with the grief-stricken family cannot be overemphasized.

The initial diagnostic assessment of the newborn infant who presents with an NTD is multifaceted. In addition to the appropriate delivery room routines, care is taken to protect the spinal or cranial lesion from injury and infection. As soon as possible, the infant is brought from the delivery room to the specialty care nursery to be monitored closely and examined by a neonatologist or pediatrician. A complete physical examination with attention to the NTD itself, presence or absence of hydrocephalus, and motor and sensory functional capacities is carried out. The possibility of associated cardiac, renal, or gastrointestinal conditions that might interfere with early surgery is ruled out.

The defect is examined in regard to size, level, and nature of tissue covering. Any leakage of CSF is noted. Palpation of the cranial sutures and fontanels and a measurement of head circumference are performed. Development and movement of upper and lower extremities are assessed. Infants with thoracic or high lumbar lesions are often born with atrophied lower extremities. An initial evaluation of bowel and bladder function is also carried out. Because 90 per cent of patients with myelomeningocele have a form of neurogenic bladder, it is difficult to predict long-term function at the time of the newborn examination. Once an assessment of the infant is completed, a discussion with the family in regard to long-term prognosis should take place. One must emphasize to the parents that surgery does not restore function but only preserves existing function (Reigel, 1989).

Therapeutic Management

Decisions about whether surgical closure of the lesion is appropriate can be controversial and difficult for families and health care providers. Criteria for nonclosure advocated by Lorber (1971) and used widely until the mid-1980s included paralysis at L2 or above, marked hydrocephalus, kyphosis, and the presence of other major congenital birth anomalies. Today there is a trend toward closure for all children, because it is not a given that those untreated will die quickly. Rekate (1988) suggests that children who survive nontreatment become significantly more impaired than if they had been operated on early. In either case, the family needs to know that nonclosure does not lead to early death and that complications will damage the existing neurologic function.

Surgical Management. The goals of early operative care of spina bifida cystica are to preserve all neural tissue, provide a normal anatomic barrier, and control early progressive hydrocephalus. A sterile, constantly moistened saline dressing is maintained on the sac until the surgery is performed. The surgical procedure involves dissection of the exposed sac and closure of the dura mater and skin over the preserved neural tissue. When the defect is large, the assistance of a plastic surgeon for skin grafting over the lesion is called for. If hydrocephalus is present at birth, a ventriculoperitoneal shunting device may be placed at the time of initial closure. If the clinical features of hydrocephalus are not apparent initially, the child is assessed for this condition frequently. Eighty to ninety per cent of children with myelomeningocele eventually develop hydrocephalus (Reigel, 1989). Surgical repair of symptomatic spina bifida occulta, regardless of the specific anomaly, is undertaken relatively soon after diagnosis, although it need not be an "emergency procedure." The primary surgical aim in these cases is to free up the tethered or tied spinal cord so that progressive deterioration of function is arrested (Guthkelch, 1988).

In cases of encephalocele, the timing of surgical intervention may vary, depending on the size, location, and extent of nervous tissue involvement. In severe cases, early death is common, usually related to complications of hydrocephalus, infection, or actual rupture of the encephalocele. In any or all of the aforementioned cases, when surgery is performed, the primary concerns of the neurosurgeon relate to wound integrity, prevention of infection and CSF leaks, and timely healing of the repair (James, 1989). Meticulous postoperative care is essential and is covered in the nursing care discussions further on.

Medical Management. Once the neurosurgeon has repaired the cranial or spinal defect and placed a ventriculoperitoneal shunt (if necessary), the neonatologist or pediatrician will become involved in postoperative management. Cardiopulmonary function and adequate nutrition are essential to wound healing. The child must lie prone for several days postoperatively to avoid pressure on the wound and possible CSF leaks that invite infection. Once the infant is less restricted in positioning and allowed to be supine, orthopedic, rehabilitative, and urologic consultations are obtained to better understand the child's functional capacity. Hip and spine roentgenographs, renal ultrasound, electrical muscle testing, and auditory testing are commonly done before discharge. Close follow-up of fontanel size and head circumference is also important. Normal well child care routines and infant development are followed as they would be for any child and should not be overshadowed by the special care requirements of these children. As the child heals from the surgery and discharge is planned, an assessment of the family's coping skills and available resources is essential in order to ensure a successful transition to home. It is normal for parents to still be grieving the birth of a defective child at this point, and referral for supportive counseling may be necessary. The development of a multidisciplinary spina bifida team in many large centers has led to improvement in the continuity of care for these families and allowed for more organized follow-up in a multidisciplinary clinic setting.

Application of the Nursing Process: Spina Bifida

Most children born with an NTD face chronic health problems for a lifetime. Depending on the age of the child, the level or type of defect, and the setting in which the child is encountered, certain diagnoses may or may not be applicable at any given time. Obviously, the more severe the cranial or spinal defect, the more interaction the child and family will have with the health care delivery system. The nurse is often the key individual in coordinating and understanding the complex care of these children. In an effort to clarify the major nursing issues with these children, the nursing process is discussed for both newly diagnosed infants and children and for long-term follow-up of this disorder.

Assessment

The age, developmental level, and level of spinal defect and associated problems greatly affect the priorities in nursing assessment for any given encounter.

The nursing assessment for spina bifida entails a determination of functional abilities, including motor performance and sensory deficits. Skin assessment, including observation of incisions from surgical closure or shunt placement and any pressure points or areas of breakdown, is essential. Bowel and bladder function, including patterns of elimination and problems secondary to poor function (urinary tract infection, bowel obstruction), should also be addressed. Other important elements of assessment include nutrition, mobility, and psychosocial adjustment of the child and family to the disease and its associated problems.

Nursing Diagnostic Statements and Collaborative Problems

High risk for infection: meningitis, urinary tract infection, decubiti; *risk factors: fragility of sac covering defect or membrane, chronic urinary retention, altered sensation, presence of surgical incision.*

High risk for injury, neurologic; *risk factors: exposed nervous tissue at birth and untreated increased ICP.*

High risk for injury, orthopedic: *impaired motor and limb function; risk factors neuromuscular and sensory deficits.*

Bowel incontinence, *related to decreased innervation to lower intestinal tract.*

Altered urinary elimination, *related to urinary retention associated with decreased innervation of bladder and sphincter.*

High risk for ineffective family coping: grief and shock; *risk factors:*

- *Unresolved and long-term care requirements.*
- *Knowledge deficit about home care and available support systems.*
- *Lack of resources (internal and external) available to family.*

Self-esteem disturbance, *related to body image disturbance; attitudes about chronic illness, altered physical capabilities, and lifestyle changes; perceptions of powerlessness or hopelessness in relation to the need for repeated surgery; lack of available support system.*

High risk for altered health maintenance at home; *risk factor: knowledge deficit for care of child after discharge.*

Planning and Implementation

Preventing Infection: Meningitis, Upper Respiratory Infection, and Decubiti. In the neonatal period, care of the protruding sac is extremely important. For an encephalocele covered with skin, the infant is positioned to avoid pressure on the lesion. If the encephalocele is in the occipital area, a foam "half donut" may be useful. The more common lumbosacral spinal myelomeningoceles are usually protected only by a thin membrane. A sterile, saline-soaked dressing is applied after the sac is examined for gross tears or leakage. Rather than being changed frequently, the dressing is usually kept moist with a sterile saline solution at regular intervals. The infant may be placed on a prophylactic broad-spectrum antibiotic if the defect appears infected, and meticulous care is taken to avoid any contamination of the sac by stool and urine. *Surveillance* for signs and symptoms of meningitis should be carried out. These signs and symptoms may include irritability, fever, feeding intolerance, and seizures. The physician should be alerted if any of these symptoms become apparent.

Postoperatively, the wound is treated aseptically, and the prone position is maintained for several days to avoid both pressure on the incision and CSF leak. A protective barrier drape is used to prevent contamination by stool or urine and must be changed when necessary. The neurosurgeon should be notified of any potential contamination. Frequent diaper changes may be necessary, because these children may stool and void continuously.

Urinary tract infections are prevented by a bladder program that includes intermittent catheterization or, in more severe cases, surgical diversion techniques to protect the kidneys from infection. Nursing interventions include teaching children (when old enough) and parents how to perform intermittent catheterization and how to recognize urinary tract infections. Odorous or cloudy urine, pain on urination, increased irritability, and hematuria are common symptoms. The nurse should educate the family and alert the urologic medical specialist about changes in bladder function throughout the developing years.

Pressure ulcer prevention can be accomplished with *skin care* geared toward optimizing skin integrity and avoiding pressure on any at-risk area. Areas requiring special attention include the spinal defect area, perianal area, sacrum, knees, elbows, ankles, and any area where sensation is diminished. If frequent dressing changes are required with the initial closure, the use of stomahesive in two parallel strips around the incision can prevent skin breakdown from continual tape removal (Fig. 40-18). After the dressing is changed, a barrier drape is pulled over the dressing to prevent contamination from stool below the closure. Often the best nursing care for skin breakdown in the anal area is leaving the buttocks exposed to air or safely using a heat lamp to promote drying. Another important factor in optimizing skin integrity is ensuring adequate nutrition. Any or all of the foregoing strategies should be used individually. As children grow, they should be taught to inspect their skin routinely and to avoid skin contact with potentially abrasive or thermal sources to prevent unnoticed skin breakdown secondary to decreased sensation.

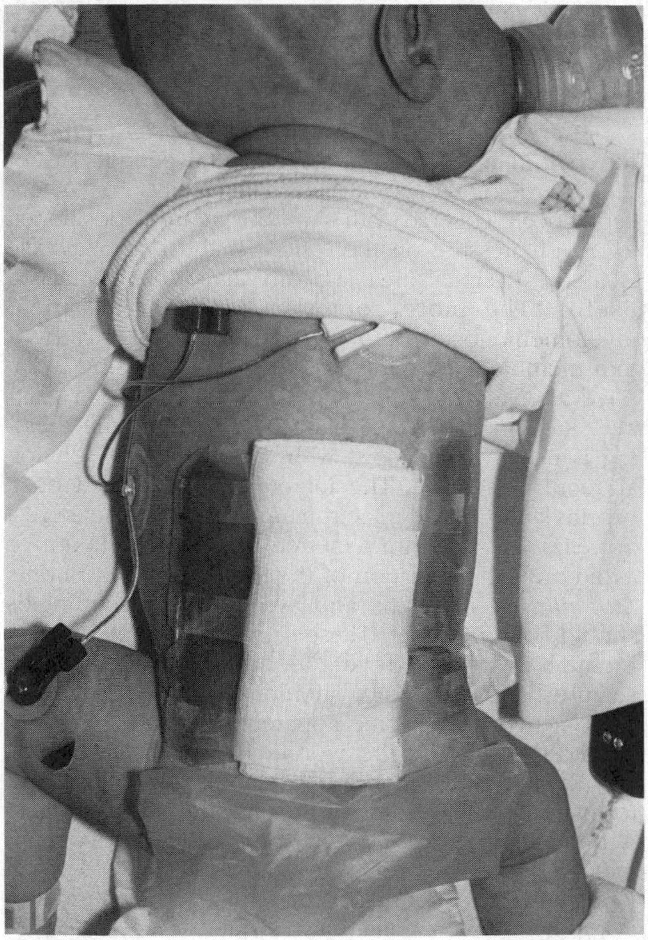

FIGURE 40-18. Use of stomahesive to prevent skin breakdown in children with myelomeningocele. The plastic below the dressing is the barrier drape, which has been pulled down to reveal the dressing. Note the shunt visible as a raised line along the back of the head.

Preventing Neurologic Injury. Rupture of the fluid-filled sac could lead to immediate death as a result of sudden decompression of CSF from the cranial cavity. Correct positioning for children with spinal lesions is either prone or side-lying, depending on the function of the lower extremities. A flat position to decrease the pressure in the sac is also favored. A cloth roll under the infant's hips in the prone position is helpful in allowing for proper alignment of the lower extremities and a downward flow of stool and urine away from the open lesion.

Between 70 and 90 per cent of children with spina bifida manifest clinically significant hydrocephalus. Many children are shunted during the time of the back closure, whereas others are followed with serial ultrasound examinations and have a shunt placed, if needed, at a later date. Most require shunting within the first few months of life (Reigel, 1989). Nursing care includes *surveillance* of the appearance and nature of the fontanel, sutures, and head circumference. Infants who are not yet shunted should be placed on a cardiorespiratory monitor to watch for signs of apnea and bradycardia secondary to increased ICP. Lethargy, feeding intolerance, and seizures are also evidence of increasing ICP and the need for shunt placement.

Preventing Orthopedic Injury. Neuromuscular and sensory deficits can lead to orthopedic problems, including scoliosis, kyphosis, hip dislocation, and ankle deformities. Joint stability may be affected by contractures, muscle control, and sensation (Lindseth, 1988). Nursing care to prevent injury includes teaching parents and children about safe activities and potentially risky ones. As these children become more mobile, parents need to play close attention to any changes in usage of limbs or function. Hip dislocation and limb fractures may go unnoticed for long periods of time, secondary to decreased sensation. The nurse should encourage routine orthopedic follow-up.

Promoting Optimal Bowel Elimination. Over 90 per cent of people with spina bifida have a neurogenic colon. Fecal incontinence and constipation are the two most common problems and are related to the loss of parasympathetic innervation to the colon and pelvic floor, the loss of sensation to the rectum, and the loss of motor innervation to the external anal sphincter (Roberts, 1988). The nurse should encourage institution of a bowel program by toddlerhood. The five key elements to training the colon are timing, diet, exercise, posture, and rectal stimulation. The parents and child should be taught to plan bowel evacuation following a meal and eat a well-balanced diet that is high in fiber and low in carbohydrates. Exercise of the lower portion of the body after the meal and a knee-chest position to put pressure on the abdomen are also known to aid bowel evacuation. Finally, rectal stimulation with a suppository or digital stimulation should be encouraged to initiate or sustain the defecation reflex (Roberts, 1988).

Managing the Neurogenic Bladder. The Credé maneuver (manual pressure applied from the umbilicus toward the symphysis pubis to express urine) has generally been replaced by clean intermittent catheterization. Drug therapy with anticholinergic drugs and surgical procedures, including bladder augmentation and placement of an artificial sphincter, are also common (Bailey, 1988). Nursing care includes maintaining bladder programs in out- or inpatient settings, teaching parents signs of urinary tract infection, and addressing the psychosocial issues about bladder elimination.

Promoting Parental Coping. Macedo and Posel (1987) state that nursing has the responsibility of preventing maladaptive family coping patterns. The initial crisis following the birth of a "not-perfect" child must be effectively resolved if the family is to function well as a unit. Appropriate nursing strategies include *grief work facilitation,* allowing the parents to grieve by being with them and listening. An example of a phrase that might be helpful in eliciting some of their feelings is "This really isn't what you expected, is it?" or "This whole event must be so overwhelming to you." *Truth telling* is another important intervention. The family also needs to have honest information about the most immediate aspects of medical care—specifically, closure of the defect or potential for ventriculoperitoneal shunting, or both—if a procedure is to be done imminently.

The nurse is often the one person who has the knowledge, skill, and time to clarify any misconceptions, repeat any information as necessary, and assess family values and perceptions about NTDs. Another important nursing intervention is assessing the *support system enhancement* and availability of resources (Macedo & Posel, 1987). Parents may need assistance in mobilizing resources to help them care for a special-needs child. On discharge from the nursery, the parents need to have practiced, and to feel comfortable, caring for their infant. The infant's primary nurse should have a check list of *discharge teaching* activities that need to be accomplished prior to discharge. Table 40–26 is an example of a discharge teaching check list that is helpful in organizing and planning for nursing care.

Children with NTDs may have many encounters with the health care system throughout their lifetime. Promoting acceptance and confidence in the parents early on permits increased self-advocacy and improves coping with long-term issues.

TABLE 40-26
Discharge Check List: Teaching Needed for Parents of Infants with Spina Bifida

Make sure parent(s) understand and are comfortable with:

Wound care and dressing changes (if necessary)

Feeding

Clean intermittent catheterization (if ordered)

Diapering (with barrier drape if necessary)

Positioning

Skin integrity examination

Physical therapy, range-of-motion exercises

Normal infant development and stimulation

Possible complications

- Signs and symptoms of hydrocephalus or ventriculoperitoneal shunt malfunction
- Infection of wound or shunt
- Urinary tract infection

Promoting Positive Self-Esteem. Many factors affect the self-esteem of a child with spina bifida. These include mobility; physical appearance, including weight; family support; and experiences within the health care system. Nurses can promote healthy eating habits in accordance with the child's activities of daily living at an early age. Obesity is a common problem, particularly in adolescents with spina bifida. Involvement in wheelchair sports activities should be encouraged. Activities for improving self-esteem may have a direct impact on the child's desire to maintain a normal weight. Involving the whole family in these activities is paramount, because a program of weight maintenance or reduction must be a family-centered project to be truly successful.

Because these children may have many operative procedures throughout their lives, providing for a successful operative experience is essential. Preoperative preparation should include age-appropriate play activities and honest but not scary information about the procedure. Many of the orthopedic procedures required by these children involve long periods of rehabilitation to render the best results. Continual support and positive reinforcement from the staff is important to optimal recovery and function.

Any child with a chronic debilitating disease may be at risk for low self-concept related to poor body image. MacBriar (1983) suggested that children with myelomeningocele who attend specialty clinics may have enhanced self-concepts resulting from the treatment approach of the clinic. This may be related to access to a good support system and positive attitudes fostered in these settings. Children with spinal defects need to talk about their disability and how it affects them. The nurse is in a prime position to assess, through *active listening,* the factors that may inhibit positive self-esteem and work with the child and family to understand and intervene with self-esteem issues. Activities planned with other disabled children are often helpful to the child struggling to gain perspective on the long-term implications of his or her disability.

As discussed earlier, the extent and level of an NTD are the primary factors that affect the prognosis for a healthy and productive life. Children afflicted with spina bifida occulta may lead completely normal lives, whereas those with myelomeningoceles may always struggle with their functional limitations. Children who have grown up with a positive attitude toward their capabilities are much more likely to lead full lives than those who have always viewed their disability in a negative light.

Facilitating Health Maintenance at Home. Home care instructions for the child with spina bifida and their family are presented in Table 40–27.

Evaluation

As in all nursing care plans, the success of the interventions in meeting the projected outcomes will be seen when high-risk problems do not occur and the defining characteristics for actual problems decrease in frequency and/or severity or disappear.

Hydrocephalus

The term "hydrocephalus" is derived from the Greek terms *hydro,* meaning "water," and *cephalo,* meaning "brain." Hydrocephalus, in simplest terms, is an imbalance between the rate of production and rate of absorption of cerebrospinal fluid in the brain. This imbalance results in an excessive amount of CSF that ultimately causes increasing head growth (if the sutures are open), or signs and symptoms of increased ICP, or both. If not alleviated, chronic increased ICP can cause long-term neurologic sequelae, including blindness. The discovery of hydrocephalus in infancy or later childhood may vary considerably depending on the underlying disease process. In all cases, the enlarged ventricles are caused by excess CSF that is unable to be absorbed at a rate equal to that of its production.

TABLE 40-27
Family-Centered Teaching: Home Care Instructions for the Child with Spina Bifida

Check the surgical site for healing
Monitor the ventriculoperitoneal shunt (if appropriate), and observe for signs and symptoms of shunt malfunction (i.e., fluid around shunt or along pathway)
Measure and plot head circumference
Be aware of changes in fontanel (if still open)
Watch for lethargy, irritability, vomiting
Observe child's movement and signs of sensation of lower extremities; pay attention to skin integrity and existence of pressure sores
Contact appropriate health care provider/specialist as necessary, if problem is suspected
Monitor child's growth and development and compare with growth charts between regular examinations

Etiology/Incidence

Congenital hydrocephalus occurs in approximately 0.5 to 1 per 1000 live births and is usually readily apparent at birth or in the first 2 to 4 months of life (Mori, 1985; Stein et al, 1981). Congenital malformations include the following: Chiari II malformations, congenital arachnoid cysts, congenital atresia of the foramina of Luschka and Magendie (Dandy-Walker cyst), and other intracranial masses including congenital tumors. Stenosis or "forking" of the aqueduct of Sylvius is a common congenital malformation that also results in hydrocephalus (McCullough, 1989).

Acquired hydrocephalus occurs secondary to mass lesions, such as tumors, vascular malformations, or cysts, and scarring of CSF pathways from infection of intracranial hemorrhage (McCullough, 1989). Acquired lesions in infancy are more commonly a result of intracranial bleeding or meningitis, or both, resulting in fibrosis of the meninges and preventing the reabsorption of CSF by the arachnoid villi (Milhorat, 1985). Table 40–28 outlines the various etiologies of congenital versus acquired hydrocephalus. Essentially, the two primary causes of congenital or acquired hydrocephalus are (1) a blockage of the flow of CSF and (2) impaired venous absorption of CSF in the subarachnoid space. A third and extremely rare cause is the overproduction of CSF caused by a tumor identified as a choroid plexus papilloma. The clinical manifestations of this disease vary with the precise cause and duration of hydrocephalus, the age of the child, and the ability of the skull to expand (McCullough, 1989).

Pathophysiology

In order to understand fully the various mechanisms that lead to hydrocephalus, a basic knowledge of CSF physiology and circulatory dynamics is essential. A thorough review of these concepts is located at the beginning of this chapter. Briefly, CSF is primarily manufactured in and secreted by the choroid plexus. This structure lines the base of the lateral ventricles and the roof of the third and fourth ventricles. CSF is produced at the approximate rate of 0.3 to 0.4 ml/min or 25 ml/hr (Milhorat, 1989). From the paired lateral ventricles, CSF is propelled in a pulsatile fashion

TABLE 40-28
Classification of Hydrocephalus

Congenital Problems

Chiari II deformity—kinking of medulla and elongation of brain stem obstruct the fourth ventricular and cisternal flow of cerebrospinal fluid (CSF); present in children with myelomeningocele.

Aqueductal stenosis—is not usually complete stenosis, but may be forking or gliosis of aqueduct

Congenital arachnoid cysts—these may enlarge progressively to obstruct flow of CSF or cause primary hydrocephalus

Acquired Problems

Neoplasm—tumors commonly in the posterior fossa can cause obstruction of CSF flow in the third and fourth ventricles

Inflammatory process

Infection: purulent exudate from meningitis may cause thickening of dural membranes and poor absorption of CSF from arachnoid villi

Hemorrhage: ventricular system is often unable to absorb products of blood breakdown, leading to ventricular blockage

Trauma—hematomas or intracerebral swelling can cause primary obstruction or poor reabsorption in the subarachnoid space

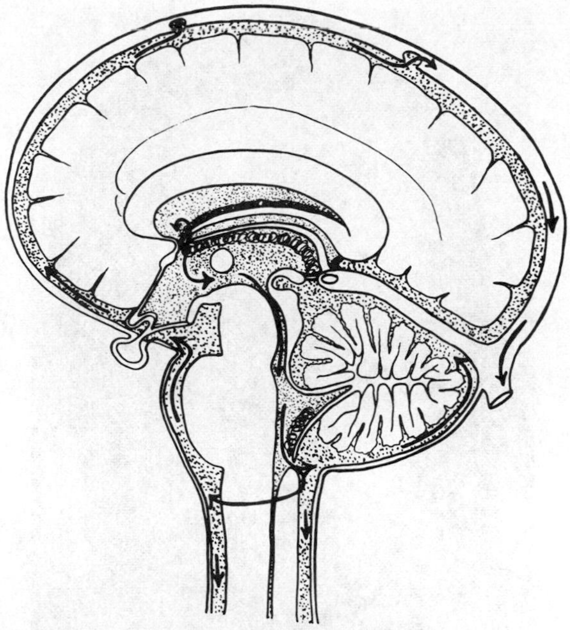

FIGURE 40-19. Schematic representation of cerebrospinal fluid circulation. (From Behrman, R. E., & Vaughan, V. C. [Eds.] [1987]. *Nelson textbook of pediatrics* [13th ed.]. Philadelphia: WB Saunders.

through the foramen of Monro to the third ventricle and then through the aqueduct of Sylvius into the fourth ventricle. From the fourth ventricle, the cerebrospinal fluid flows through the foramen of Magendie and the paired foramina of Luschka into the subarachnoid space around the brain and spinal cord. The CSF is then reabsorbed by the arachnoid villi located in the dural sinuses, which are the large blood vessels draining the venous blood from the head. Small amounts of CSF are absorbed in the cells lining the ventricles and through the lymphatic system of the spinal cord. Figure 40–19 illustrates the normal flow of CSF in the brain.

The terminology used to describe hydrocephalus has been known to be confusing and unclear. Many of the terms were useful before present-day diagnostic testing, when the site of the blockage may have been implied, rather than precisely identified. The terms "communicating" and "noncommunicating" hydrocephalus are still used occasionally to describe the status of the ventricles in this disease. Communicating hydrocephalus describes a blockage "outside" of the ventricular system (e.g., meninges, arachnoid villi). The implication is that the ventricles communicate. Noncommunicating hydrocephalus implies a blockage somewhere in the ventricular system that prevents CSF from reaching the subarachnoid space for reabsorption (McCullough, 1989). Another way to classify hydrocephalus delineates when and how the hydrocephalus developed and categorizes the disorder as "congenital" or "acquired."

Clinical Manifestations

Table 40–7 shown earlier in this chapter describes the signs and symptoms of increased ICP in infants and children. An abnormal increase in head circumference that goes above the established growth curve or begins above the 95th percentile at birth should always raise suspicion. A full or bulging fontanel, especially one that is nonpulsatile, indicating high pressure, should be noted. Other clinical signs and symptoms that become apparent as hydrocephalus progresses include increased motor tone, irritability, poor feeding, projectile vomiting, high-pitched cry, and cranial nerve palsies resulting in the classic "sunset" (or "setting sun") appearance of the eyes, in which the sclera are visible above the iris and the infant is unable to look upward with the head facing forward (Fig. 40–20). Developmental delays or lack of acquisition of milestones is also common.

In the older child with a fused cranium, signs and symptoms of hydrocephalus may develop slowly or rapidly. Rapid development leads to acute neurologic deterioration. Signs of increased ICP in these children include frontal headache, nausea, and vomiting that may be projectile. If these symptoms occur on awakening, increased ICP should be suspected and the cause investigated. While asleep, the child retains CO_2,

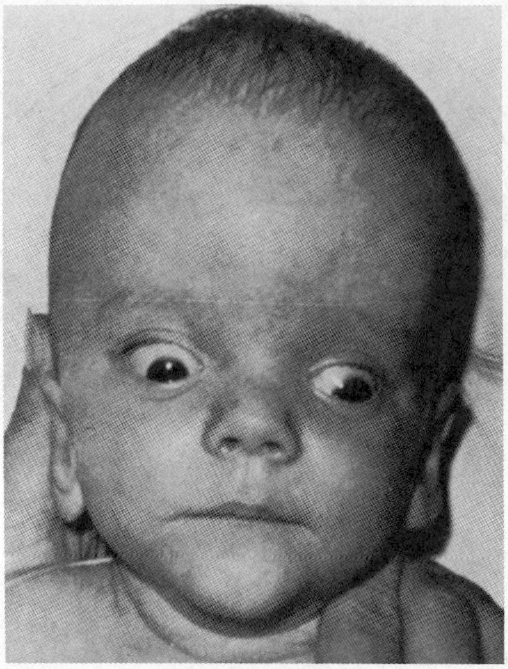

FIGURE 40 - 20. Marked hydrocephalus with "setting sun" sign and divergence of the eyes. (From Youmans, J. R. [1982]. *Neurological surgery* [2nd ed.]. Philadelphia: WB Saunders.)

which in turn dilates cerebral vasculature. On awakening, the child's symptoms are exacerbated. Once the child is awake and CO_2 has decreased, the symptoms may temporarily subside. Decreased venous drainage while the child is lying flat may also contribute to morning symptoms. Other signs and symptoms include diplopia, restlessness, personality change, and ataxia. In later stages, bradycardia and/or altered respirations and seizures are life-threatening if not attended to.

Diagnostic Assessment

Diagnostic assessment includes a thorough physical examination after a history of the manifestations is obtained. Important information includes family and perinatal history, any trauma or infectious processes, and developmental progress. The physical examination should include complete neurologic and fundoscopic examinations. Radiographic evidence of hydrocephalus is most frequently obtained with a CT scan. In infants with an open fontanel, ultrasound may be used. When a complex lesion is suspected, MRI may be used initially. Skull x-ray films may show widened or split sutures, and the skull may have a "beaten silver" appearance, characteristic of chronically increased ICP. Other rarely used radiographic tests include isotope cisternography or ventriculography to obtain a more accurate assessment of how CSF flows in the brain.

Therapeutic Management

Once hydrocephalus is identified, treatment is directed toward resolving the cause of obstruction. Of course, this may be impossible for congenital hydrocephalus. When hydrocephalus is acquired by an older child, the lesion causing obstruction (most frequently neoplasm) can be removed to allow the flow of CSF to return to normal. There are cases, however, in which even complete resection of a tumor fails to re-establish normal CSF pathways.

Medical Management. The medical management of hydrocephalus is limited to withdrawal of CSF via lumbar puncture or ventricular tap. This usually is only tried in infants with inflammatory processes or intracranial hemorrhage on a short-term basis. In some cases, physicians prescribe acetazolamide (Diamox), which may decrease CSF production pharmacologically. This has not been shown to be very effective, so it is tried infrequently.

Surgical Management. The most effective treatment for hydrocephalus is the surgical insertion of a shunting device. Historically, shunts have been placed in nearly every body cavity. The most commonly chosen distal site is the peritoneal, followed by either atrial or direct cardiac shunts, and less frequently, pleural shunts.

The three main components of mechanical shunting devices are (1) ventricular catheter, (2) reservoir and pumping device (placed directly under the scalp on the skull bones) with a one-way flow valve, and (3) distal tubing with a slit valve to regulate the flow of CSF. Newer pressure-regulated valves are now available as well. As in all mechanical devices, malfunction can and does occur. The most common problems are blockage from choroid plexus or proteinaceous CSF at the proximal end. The distal end can be blocked by fatty plugs or CSF pseudocysts. In any of these cases, signs and symptoms of shunt malfunction depend on the duration and extent of blockage. As expected, they do mimic signs and symptoms of increased ICP. Shunt infections, although rare, can be serious and difficult to eradicate.

After the infecting organism is determined, intravenous therapy is instituted. In difficult-to-eradicate organisms, intraventricular instillation of antibiotics may be useful. In some cases of shunt infection, the distal end of the shunt will be externalized to a CSF collecting system, until the bacteria are eradicated and a new shunt is placed. In all cases of shunt infection, the shunt must be removed and replaced to achieve a "cure."

Ventriculoperitoneal Shunt

The ventriculoperitoneal (VP) location is chosen for most mechanical shunts (Fig. 40–21). After insertion of the ventricular tube through a cranial burr hole,

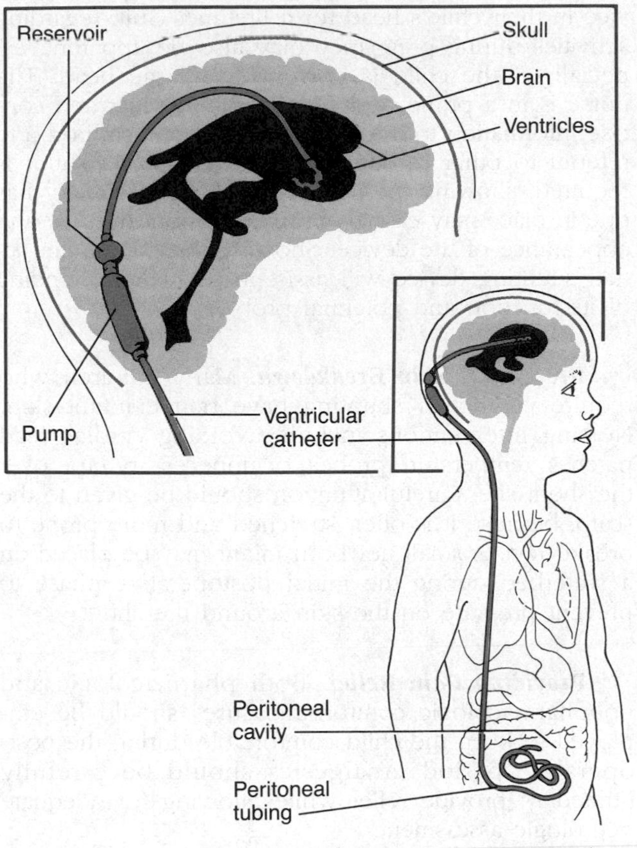

FIGURE 40 - 21. Placement of the ventriculoperitoneal shunt.

the length of the shunt is tunneled subcutaneously to the upper quadrant of the abdomen. A small incision is made, and the shunt is guided into the peritoneal cavity with plenty of extra tubing to allow for growth. Specific risks of this procedure include bowel perforation and ascites, if the CSF is poorly absorbed.

Ventriculoatrial Shunt

The ventriculoatrial (VA) shunt is rare and is chosen only if a concurrent abdominal problem exists, precluding the insertion of a VP shunt. This shunt can be inserted into the right atrium of the heart via passage through the jugular vein or, in more extensive cases, directly into the heart. Specific risks include catheter movement, dysrhythmias, operative risks associated with more extensive surgery, endocarditis, and congestive heart failure.

Ventriculopleural Shunt

Used very infrequently, ventriculopleural shunt is chosen if either peritoneal or cardiac access is unobtainable. Specific risks include pleural effusion, resulting in respiratory compromise or infection, or both, from stasis of respiratory secretions.

Application of the Nursing Process: Hydrocephalus

Children may come to the acute care facility with signs and symptoms of hydrocephalus either before initial diagnosis or with an acute shunt malfunction, both of which require expert nursing assessment and intervention. The nurse may also care for the child postoperatively, following the insertion of a ventricular shunting device. The application of the nursing process is covered here.

Assessment

The nursing assessment of the child with newly diagnosed hydrocephalus admitted for the placement of a shunt includes observation for and documentation of the signs and symptoms outlined under "Clinical Manifestations." Knowledge of parental anxieties and fears about the surgery and knowledge of the rationale for the shunt placement are vital to planning for care. Children who return to the hospital for shunt revision require *neurologic monitoring,* including monitoring of signs and symptoms of increased ICP. Once the child has become "shunt-dependent," blockage can result in serious symptoms, including bradycardia, respiratory changes, seizures, significant lethargy, and vomiting.

Postoperative nursing surveillance includes cardiorespiratory monitoring, frequent vital signs, and neurologic checks. Surveillance of skin integrity, pain control, and surgical dressing are also essential. Changes in level of consciousness and/or vital signs should be reported immediately.

Nursing Diagnostic Statements and Collaborative Problems

High risk for altered tissue perfusion: cerebral; *risk factor increase in volume of one or more of the intracranial components (see Table 40–20).*

High risk for injury: neurologic compromise; *risk factors: serious increase in ICP causing enlarged ventricles and risk for seizure activity.*

Ineffective family coping, *related to inaccurate perceptions regarding the shunting device and knowledge deficit about how to cope with a potentially chronic disease.*

High risk for altered skin integrity; *risk factors: fragility of infant skin and immobility after surgery.*

Altered comfort: pain, *related to operative manipulation.*

High risk for infections: surgical; *risk factors: interrupted skin integrity, for example, inser-*

tion of foreign body and disturbance of normal skin flora.

Ineffective individual coping, *related to body image associated with*

- *Hair loss required for operation.*
- *Visibility of shunt.*
- *Possible restrictions on activities.*

High risk for altered health maintenance/management; *risk factors: knowledge deficit regarding.*

- *Signs and symptoms of shunt malfunctioning.*
- *Home safety.*
- *Neurologic assessment.*
- *Care of incisional area.*

Planning and Implementation

Preventing and Intervening in the Event of Increased Intracranial Pressure. Once the nurse has identified the child with increasing ICP from hydrocephalus, many interventions can be done before surgery to alleviate the pressure. The head of the bed should be elevated to 30 degrees. Cardiorespiratory monitoring and frequent monitoring of pupil size, motor movements, and level of consciousness are essential. Changes in status should be reported immediately, and medications (diuretics, analgesics) should be administered as ordered. If needed, the nurse should be ready to assist in the event of a ventricular shunt tap. Bulging or flatness of fontanels should regularly be recorded. If the child is vomiting, intravenous hydration may be necessary. This should be administered at a rate of no more than 75 to 80 per cent of *maintenance* fluid requirements. Other nursing interventions include decreasing external stimuli and having O_2 and suction ready at the bedside, should they be needed in the event of a seizure. Preoperative teaching and preparing the child and family should begin as soon as the decision to place a shunt has been made.

Preventing Neurologic Compromise. Nursing interventions to prevent neurologic compromise are the same as those for increased ICP. Children who experience a rapid decrease in ventricular size are prone to the development of subdural fluid collections after shunting. Nursing assessment for this problem as well as blockage of a newly placed shunt includes watching for signs of neurologic deterioration after an initial period of recovery or signs of slow and incomplete recovery. Any of these trends should be reported to the physician so that appropriate radiographic tests can be ordered.

Promoting Family Coping. This nursing diagnosis is appropriate for all families with a child with a neurologic disorder. For children with hydrocephalus, families must cope with the prospect of a mechanical device in their child's head for a lifetime. Guilt regarding activities during pregnancy may also be apparent, especially if the child is born with a large head. The nurse is in a prime position to provide clear and concise information to the family and to offer support and referral to other resources as necessary. If a shunt is required, showing the family a child who already has one in place may ease their anxiety about the size and appearance of the device. Showing the parents an actual shunting device will assist in their understanding of its function and potential problems.

Preventing Skin Breakdown. Many children who require ventricular shunting have fragile infant skin. Nursing interventions include avoiding cardiac lead patches, temperature probes, or unnecessary tape over the shunt site. Careful attention should be given to the scalp, because it is often stretched and more prone to breakdown. A small newborn infant may be placed on a waterbed during the initial postoperative phase to prevent pressure on the skin around the shunt.

Providing Pain Relief. Both pharmacologic and nonpharmacologic comfort measures should be employed to keep the child comfortable during the postoperative period. Analgesics should be carefully titrated to provide relief while allowing for adequate neurologic assessment.

Preventing Infection. The nursing interventions for this diagnosis are similar to those for promoting skin integrity. The nurse must pay close attention to the integrity of the surgical incisions and make sure that the child keeps hands away from the fresh incision. A stockinette cap may be useful. Appropriate administration of antibiotics is essential, if they are ordered postoperatively. Close monitoring of the temperature postoperatively is essential.

Promoting a Healthy Body Image. Older children undergoing neurosurgery for a shunt frequently are focused on the issues of hair loss and the visibility of the mechanical device. It is helpful to address these issues openly and allow these children to express their fears. Encouraging them to talk about how they normally cope with stressful events can often help them identify and capitalize on their personal strength. Introducing them to other children with similar problems can also be a useful intervention, because they can relate to their peers on the same level.

Facilitating Health Maintenance at Home. With the improvement of shunting devices and techniques for surgical management of hydrocephalus, the long-term survival of these children has been greatly enhanced. The morbidity of children with hydrocephalus is often related to the cause of the hydrocephalus, the duration of the condition before treatment, and associated brain abnormalities (McLaurin, 1989). Home care instructions for parents include the monitoring for signs and symptoms of shunt malfunction, proper handling of the infant with a new shunt, home safety, and indications for calling the physician, should problems occur.

Evaluation

As in all nursing care plans, the success of the interventions in meeting the projected outcomes is seen when high-risk problems do not occur and the defining characteristics for actual problems decrease in frequency and/or severity or disappear.

Chiari II Malformation (Arnold-Chiari Malformation)

Since the late 1800s, the term "Arnold-Chiari malformation" has been used to describe a developmental anomaly of the structures at the junction of the brain and spinal cord. This anatomic area is often referred to as the cervicomedullary junction. Oakes (1985), after investigating the historical aspects of this anomaly, determined that very little insight to the problem was actually added by Arnold to Chiari's original descriptions of the various degrees of hindbrain herniation. Even though two of Arnold's colleagues coined the term "Arnold-Chiari malformation" in 1907, it is not truly representative of the contributions of various individuals and therefore is slowly being replaced by the term "Chiari II malformation" (Oakes, 1985). Chiari actually described four different types of hindbrain anomalies; however, the type II anomaly is the one most commonly seen in the pediatric population, specifically in children with myelodysplasia. Therefore, it is the only one discussed here.

Two other diagnoses that should be mentioned in conjunction with Chiari malformations are *syringomyelia,* or *syrinx,* and *hydromyelia.* The former describes a cavity lying outside the central canal area of the spinal cord that is not lined by ependymal cells, and the latter is a cavity within the spinal cord that is partially or completely lined with ependyma. All three diagnoses are frequently discussed in conjunction with each other because of their similar clinical presentations and their probably common pathophysiologic development (Oakes, 1985).

Etiology/Incidence

Chiari II deformities are nearly always associated with myelodysplasia. There are several theories related to the pathogenesis of this malformation. Initially, it was thought that the downward traction on the spinal cord caused by an open NTD pulled on the brain stem and cerebellum, causing malalignment of the cervical nerve roots. Later theories have discredited this early view and attribute the malformation to actual dysgenesis of the brain stem, which causes it to elongate into the cervical canal. Caudal displacement of the cerebellum and brain stem results. Still another theory points to alterations in CSF dynamics at the craniospinal junction. Although all of these theories have improved our understanding of the problem, there is yet to be a universally accepted concept of this disease.

Pathophysiology

Although the majority of children with myelodysplasia are born with the Chiari II deformity, no more than one third of these children develop Chiari II symptoms in infancy. Most of these infants eventually improve on their own after 6 to 12 months of age. Many develop apneic spells and associated problems that lead to death before the age of 2 years (Oakes, 1985).

In the Chiari II malformation, the cerebellar tonsils and medulla are displaced downward through the foramen magnum. This causes elongation of the fourth ventricle, which may obliterate the foramina of Magendie and Luschka, thereby causing hydrocephalus. The cranial nerves (particularly those that originate on the medulla) become stretched and are the cause of many of the signs and symptoms. Figure 40–22 shows the anatomic aspects of this deformity.

Clinical Manifestations

The clinical examination focuses on the most common signs and symptoms of the Chiari II malformation. These include the following: nystagmus, nuchal rigidity, poor suck reflex, drooling, difficulty swallowing, vomiting, weak or absent cry, and inspiratory stridor during agitation. In more severe cases, episodes of apnea may be reported by the parents. In older children, decreased strength in upper extremities with increased tone and exaggerated deep tendon reflexes may also be present.

Diagnostic Assessment

Radiographic techniques are used to demonstrate the type and extent of the lesion, including the presence of hydromyelia or hydrocephalus. Plain roentgenographs of the skull and spine are taken. MRI is beginning to replace other more invasive techniques for imaging this disease. MRI is particularly useful in identifying the anatomy in this area and in providing for accurate diagnosis.

Therapeutic Management

Initially, if signs and symptoms are not life-threatening, a conservative approach may be advocated in the

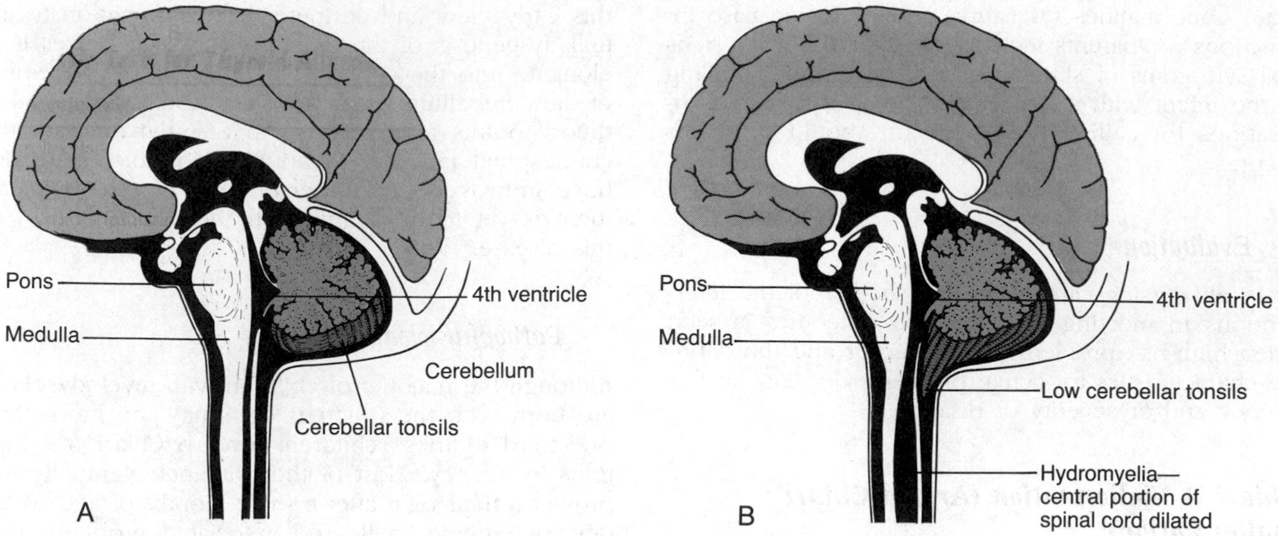

FIGURE 40 - 22. *A*, Anatomy of the normal posterior fossa. *B*, Arnold-Chiari malformation with hydromyelia.

hope that the child will stabilize and outgrow the symptoms. When more severe problems, such as apnea or frequent aspiration pneumonia, are apparent, surgery must be undertaken. The surgical procedure of choice is a posterior fossa decompression. It involves removing the posterior aspect of the foramen magnum and excising the upper cervical vertebral arches. This decompression alleviates the pressure on the fourth ventricle and the affected cranial nerves, allowing, one hopes, for an arrest of symptom progression. Some children show only little objective improvement. In them, the preoperative deficits may be permanent. The goal of the surgery is to prevent further symptoms, rather than to relieve existing ones, although the latter usually occurs to some degree. In rare instances in which a ventriculoperitoneal shunt is not already in place, it may be placed in conjunction with, or instead of, the posterior fossa decompression.

Application of the Nursing Process: Chiari II Malformation

Assessment

Nursing assessment includes an assessment of respiratory effort, apnea, airway protection, and potential for aspiration. Neck mobility and nystagmus should also be assessed and documented. Postoperatively, when a decompression surgery is done, assessment includes close scrutiny of all vital signs, placement on a cardiorespiratory monitor, and assessment of tolerance of increasing activity and diet with specific attention given to airway function and protection.

Nursing Diagnostic Statements and Collaborative Problems

High risk for infection: respiratory; *risk factors:*

- *Absent or weak gag reflex.*
- *Relative inactivity and inability to clear secretions.*

High risk for ineffective breathing pattern: episodic apnea; *risk factors:*

- *Compression of cranial nerves and medulla (preoperative).*
- *Operative swelling or effects of anesthesia (postoperative).*

Altered comfort: pain, *related to surgical intervention.*

Ineffective family coping, preoperatively and postoperatively, *related to*

- *Feelings of fatigue, hopelessness, and/or powerlessness with frequent hospitalizations of their child.*
- *Further treatment for the already chronically debilitated child.*
- *Knowledge deficit about the disease process.*
- *Feelings that rehospitalization may be related to inadequacies in their home care of their child.*

Planning and Implementation

Preventing Respiratory Infection. Infants or children with poor gag and swallow reflexes should be fed slowly and placed in an upright position after feeding to avoid aspiration and recurrent pneumonia. Solids may be difficult to swallow for these children, so food may need to be pureed. Postural drainage or chest physiotherapy may need to be instituted when aspiration has occurred. Nurses caring for children with Chiari II malformations should plan daily activities so that feedings are uninterrupted; activities that may induce vomiting or aspiration should take place just prior to feeding rather than immediately afterward. The child may also need a formal ear, nose, and throat and swallowing evaluation.

Avoiding Respiratory Distress. A complete and thorough baseline neurologic assessment is essential for these children. Frequent examination and preparedness for resuscitation are important aspects of nursing care. Placing the child on a cardiorespiratory monitor and having oxygen and suction available at the bedside may be necessary. Documenting consistent changes in the respiratory pattern, and alerting the physician to any significant changes is also vital. The effects of various nursing interventions on overall respiratory status should be documented in the care plan so that trends in patient status can be easily recognized.

Effectively Managing Postoperative Pain. Adequate control of postoperative pain in these children is a difficult nursing challenge. Care should be taken to avoid overmedication, which may negate a neurologic assessment to signal changes or decline in the patient's status. Even when the child is resting comfortably after medication, neurologic assessments should be done as ordered or more frequently, if indicated. A good blood level of analgesics should be maintained so that the child does not experience periods of excruciating pain requiring large amounts of narcotic analgesics at one time. Nursing care should always incorporate nonpharmacologic methods of pain control into the patient care plan.

Promoting Family Coping. Families of children with chronic health problems need continual support from the nursing staff throughout their many hospitalizations. The importance of continuity of nursing staff and primary nursing cannot be overemphasized. Parents may see the hospitalization as a break from their daily care routines and need to spend time away from the hospital. The nursing staff should give them permission to do so while identifying aspects of care the parents would like to participate in and supporting them in their participation. Well siblings may also need some extra attention during hospitalization. Nurses can be advocates for the siblings and the ill child, and provide overall support for family cohesion.

Parental coping will be enhanced by reinforcing the parents' positive efforts in home care and by providing them with adequate instruction for *maintenance* of their child's condition at home, as needed. Parents should be able to assess changes in their child's neurologic status and impending signs of respiratory problems. Parents should also know to report any signs or incisional redness or irritation. The need for occupational therapy to adapt feeding or stimulation programs to meet their child's functional capacity should be addressed before discharge if the child later requires a referral.

Evaluation

As in all nursing care plans, the success of the interventions in meeting the projected outcomes is seen when high-risk problems do not occur and the defining characteristics for actual problems decrease in frequency and/or severity or disappear.

Neurocutaneous Syndromes

The most frequently occurring neurocutaneous syndromes are collectively called *phakomatoses*. These diseases are characterized by their tendency toward tumor formation in the central nervous system, skin, and visceral linings of various organ systems and their recognizable cutaneous manifestations. Because of the rarity of these diseases, only the three most common phakomatoses are addressed here. They are tuberous sclerosis, neurofibromatosis, and Sturge-Weber disease.

Etiology/Incidence (Pathophysiology)

Tuberous sclerosis is an autosomal-dominant disease affecting many organ systems. (See Chapter 31 for a discussion of patterns of inheritance.) A wide variety of clinical findings are associated with this disease, the most common being mental retardation, seizures, and adenoma sebaceum. The major organ systems that may be affected in tuberous sclerosis are the brain, skin, kidneys, heart, lungs, and bone. Growths called "tubers" may invade the brain and retina. Other types of tumors may invade the heart and kidneys (Berg, 1982).

Neurofibromatosis is also referred to as "von Recklinghausen disease," so named for the man who identified it. Like tuberous sclerosis, neurofibromatosis is an autosomal-dominant trait disease. Its main characteristics are areas of increased skin pigmentation (cafe-au-lait spots), central and peripheral nervous system tumors, and other skeletal, endocrine, and vascular findings. This disease is characterized by multiple tumors called neurofibromas that occur in a few or many organ systems of the affected child. Peripheral nerve tumors are the most common, and a higher incidence of brain tumors in these children has also been documented. Neurofibromatosis is more common in males. The first symptoms are usually cutaneous changes rather than the neurologic symptoms that often occur in later stages of the disease (Berg, 1982).

Sturge-Weber disease (encephalofacial angiomatosis) is the only phakomatosis without a recognizable hereditary pattern. The characteristic features are a port-wine stain (facial nevus), focal or generalized seizures, intracranial calcification, hemiparesis, and often, mental retardation. Abnormalities of the dura mater over the occipital lobe are common, as are calcification and necrosis of underlying brain tissue. The facial nevus is usually apparent at birth, and often it is associated with congenital glaucoma. Seizures usually begin before 1 year of age and are difficult to treat. Behavior problems, mental retardation, and hemiparesis can also occur (Berg, 1982). A thorough discussion of all the neurocutaneous diseases, including many too rare to be discussed here, can be found in neurology specialty texts.

Diagnostic Assessment

The diagnosis of neurocutaneous diseases is often made on the characteristic clinical findings of each disease. A thorough genetic and family history is helpful in the diagnosis of tuberous sclerosis and neurofibromatosis. In both diseases, a confirmed diagnosis is made through a tissue sample of one of the characteristic lesions or tumors. Because of the wide variability of manifestations of these diseases, the diagnostic assessment may range from minimal to extensive. Some possibilities include the need for an EEG, CT scan, MRI, skin biopsy, ophthalmologic examinations, and various other tests, depending on the organ systems involved.

Therapeutic Management

Medical and/or surgical management of neurocutaneous disease in childhood is aimed at alleviating symptoms, because there are no cures for these conditions. When seizures are present, various anticonvulsant regimens may be tried until control is achieved. In some cases of Sturge-Weber disease, surgical removal of the lobes of the brain causing seizures is attempted. Any lesions of the brain (tumors, tubers, or neurofibromas) may be surgically excised, especially if they cause increased ICP. Various other orthopedic and/or plastic surgery procedures may be indicated (Berg, 1982). However, in most cases, medical care is geared toward helping the family cope with the diagnosis and the provision of expert genetic counseling to assess the probability of future children manifesting such abnormalities.

Nursing Care

Nursing care for these children is extremely individualized and depends on the clinical characteristics of the specific disease. Nursing assessment of children with neurocutaneous disorders should be focused on developmental, behavioral, and psychosocial issues. Physical assessment should be focused on obtaining a neurologic baseline and on other systems that are known to be affected by tumors, tubers, or other findings associated with these disorders for the individual child.

Because many neurocutaneous diseases manifest with convulsive disorders, when children with these diseases are hospitalized seizure precautions may be necessary. Specifics of nursing care for children with epilepsy are covered earlier in the chapter. Safety may also be threatened when a child displays difficult-to-control behavior or an element of mental retardation It is the nurse's responsibility to assess the patients' individual high risk for injury and to plan interventions to avoid possibly dangerous situations.

Families facing these seemingly unexplainable and incurable diseases require ongoing support. This is especially true when the family is faced with many hospitalizations. In some instances, the nurse may need to encourage the family to explore long-term resources. Because of the wide variety of symptoms of these diseases, an individual assessment of each family is necessary, as some children may have few outward signs of illness. A nurse may interact with the same child several times during many hospitalizations. Continuity of nursing care can promote trust and a more positive view of the health care system for the child.

Information given to families needs to be geared toward their level of understanding. Nurses should rely on principles of teaching and learning to plan a teaching strategy for parents. It is important to accept the initial denial and guilt that may manifest shortly after diagnosis and to allow for its expression. Parents may need information about the genetic basis of the disease and should be referred for genetic counseling.

Neurodegenerative Disorders

The large and diverse group of diseases characterized by progressive loss of central neurologic function are collectively referred to as neurodegenerative diseases. The occurrence and correct diagnosis of these disorders during infancy and childhood present a common and challenging clinical problem. The diversity of the numerous diseases in this category and the lack of definitive knowledge regarding their etiology have led to some confusion among health care professionals, and ultimately among families and children facing these diagnoses (Dyken & Krawiecki, 1983). For the purposes of this text, basic definitions and categories are discussed with the most common disease entities listed. Generalized nursing diagnoses applicable to many or all of the neurodegenerative disorders are identified. Nursing care should be individualized to the specific disease process and overall needs of the child and family.

Etiology/Incidence (Pathophysiology)

Many possible causes of neurologic deterioration in children must be ruled out before a diagnosis of neurodegenerative disease is made. These include neoplasms, infection, trauma, or vascular disorders (Allen et al, 1982). Once other possibilities are ruled out, disorders of myelinization are considered. As noted earlier in this chapter, the process of myelinization is associated with the development of functional capacity in childhood. There are two types of myelin disorders. *Demyelinating* disease refers to an inflammatory process that destroys normal, healthy myelin. The inflammation may be with or without a known infectious component. *Dysmyelinating* disease describes a process of destruction to myelin that is already abnormally constituted because of genetic mechanisms. Clinical presentations of children with these specific disorders overlap considerably. Except for a few diseases whose etiology is known to be the deficiency of an enzyme necessary to make the lipid and protein myelin sheath, there is no certain or known cause for neurodegenerative disease. As a result, it has been suggested that classification of these diseases be based primarily on anatomic criteria. There are well over 600 identified neurodegenerative diseases that can be classified into the following five groups: *polioencephalopathies, leukoencephalopathies, corencephalopathies, diffuse encephalopathies,* and *spinocerebellopathies.* The number of disorders shown to have a genetic predisposition varies within and between groups (Dyken & Krawiecki, 1983). Table 40–29 identifies the most commonly seen disease entities in each of the classifications, the anatomic area affected, and the genetic predisposition of the selected disorders.

Another method of classification for neurodegenerative diseases involves differentiating whether they are disorders primarily of the white matter or of the gray matter. The majority of neurodegenerative diseases are of the white matter, as by definition it consists primarily of axons with (whitish) myelin sheaths. There is no absolute differentiation between the clinical signs and symptoms of white matter disease and of gray matter disease, although it is a means of classifying the multitude of disorders (Allen, 1982). Whether classified anatomically or by white and gray matter differentiation, each disease has a distinct pathologic process at the cellular level, even though the diagnostic assessment and clinical presentation may be similar. In all of the degenerative disorders, the incorrectly formed myelin or the breakdown of once-normal myelin prevents the accurate transmission of impulses through the axon and results in slow but progressive neurologic deterioration until death. The actual symptoms depend on the location of the degenerating myelin within the central nervous system and the rate and type of degeneration (i.e., acute versus sporadic versus diffuse).

Diagnostic Assessment

The type and extent of diagnostic assessment depends on the signs and symptoms leading to the initial need for medical evaluation. When signs and symptoms of neurologic compromise exist, various radiographic studies will be performed. These may include a CT scan, skull roentgenographs, arteriogram, nuclear brain scan, or a combination. An EEG study may be helpful in distinguishing between focal and diffuse cerebral degenerative processes. However, the EEG can be totally normal in the presence of disease, depending on the location and extent of demyelination. Because examination of the CSF may be helpful in diagnosing certain disorders, a lumbar puncture may be done. Biopsy of the actual brain tissue is controversial and rarely attempted (Allen, 1982).

Probably the most important aspects of diagnostic assessment are a thorough and complete history, physical examination, and detailed neurologic examination done by an experienced pediatric neurologist. Depending on the actual disease, progression of symptoms may be rapid or consist of periodic exacerbation and remission, as in multiple sclerosis. In either case, frequent and serial assessments of neurologic function are important.

Therapeutic Management

Medical care for neurodegenerative disorders consists of symptomatic and supportive care. Hospitalization may be required for diagnostic workup and involvement of various health care professionals. If seizures are present, a regimen of one or more anticonvulsant medicines will be instituted. Frequently physical and occupational therapy will be helpful in increasing adaptive capabilities. Progressive loss of sensory functions may require the need for visual or auditory adaptation. Psychologic and emotional adjustment of the family to a chronic and life-threatening disease must be addressed. Unfortunately, there is no cure for these disorders. If the degeneration is slow, a good quality of life is attainable with the appropriate support and resources.

Nursing Care

Nursing assessment of children with neurodegenerative disorders involves an assessment of functional capacities and a neurologic baseline, including cognitive and communication skills. Obtaining information

TABLE 40-29
Classification of Neurodegenerative Diseases in Infancy and Childhood

General Classification	Disease Name	Comments
Polioencephalopathies *Anatomic location:* cerebral cortex	*Genetic* Neuronal ceroid lipofuscinoses Hereditary poliodystrophy *Nongenetic* West disease Hypoxic degenerative polioencephalopathy with spasms Idiopathic sporadic polioencephalopathy	All genetic polioencephalopathies are referred to as poliodystrophies
Leukoencephalopathies *Anatomic location:* subcortical white matter	*Genetic* Adrenoleukodystrophy Metachromatic leukodystrophy *Nongenetic* Subacute sclerosing panencephalitis Schilder encephalitis periaxalis diffusa Disseminated sclerosis (multiple sclerosis)	All genetic leukoencephalopathies referred to as leukodystrophies Usually early adult onset (20–30 yrs)
Corencephalopathies *Anatomic location:* deep telencephalic, diencephalic, or mesencephalic structures, including both gray and white matter, the extrapyramidal system, and the upper brain stem	*Genetic* Huntington disease Familial deteriorating extrapyramidal syndrome Ataxia telangiectasia *Nongenetic* Idiopathic subcortical degeneration with extrapyramidal symptoms	All genetic corencephalopathies referred to as cordystrophies
Diffuse Encephalopathies *Anatomic location:* Diffuse anatomic involvement or unclear anatomic localization	*Genetic* Tuberous sclerosis with degeneration *Nongenetic* Idiopathic degenerative encephalopathy Hypoxic degenerative encephalopathy with spasms	Also covered under neurocutaneous disorders; the more severe cases are considered neurodegenerative diseases
Spinocerebellopathies *Anatomic location:* Pons, medulla, cerebellum, and spinal cord	*Genetic* Hereditary spastic paraparesis Familial Werdnig-Hoffmann disease Friedreich ataxis *Nongenetic* Sporadic Werdnig-Hoffmann disease Acute cerebellar ataxia	

Adapted from Dyken, F., & Krawiecki, N. (1983). Neurodegenerative diseases of infancy and childhood. Reprinted with permission from *Annals of Neurology, 13*(4), 351–364.

about medications and any recent injuries or changes in behavior or function is essential. The nurse must assess the family's coping skills and knowledge of the disease, because these are often the best predictors of the disease's long-term effects on the child and family.

There are many reasons why children with neurodegenerative disorders may be more prone to injury, including loss of coordination and of sensory and cognitive function. These children may need to wear a protective helmet. Teaching the child to wear the helmet, particularly during high-risk activities, is vital. Children with known seizure disorders should understand the importance of a schedule for taking their medications and know the signs and symptoms of toxicity. It is the nurse's responsibility to help the child and family openly discuss their functional limitations so that adaptive mechanisms can be initiated and ultimately safety can be ensured.

Children with obvious neurologic disorders will feel "different" from their peers. Open discussion about body image should be encouraged by the nurse caring for these children. If necessary, a referral to a counselor specializing in work with disabled children should be made. One way of helping a young child cope with altered body image is to encourage the child to meet and socialize with others who have similar disabilities. In some instances, sports programs for children with disabilities also have a positive effect on self-esteem and body image.

The most frustrating aspect of parental coping with the diagnosis of neurodegenerative disease in infancy or childhood is often the lack of a known etiology for the disease. The questions "Why?" and "How?" often do not have answers. Parents may display a myriad of grief reactions as they cope with the loss of a normal child. A referral should be made for genetic counseling early on. The nurse needs to offer empathy, support, and education. Knowing what to expect can help parents identify strengths and weaknesses in their coping styles and may alert them to the need for outside counseling. The nurse should be able to identify resources such as support groups or volunteer organizations that may offer services and support.

Central Nervous System Infections

This discussion covers bacterial meningitis, aseptic meningitis, encephalitis, and Guillain-Barré syndrome. Bacterial meningitis is the most frequently occurring central nervous system infection.

Bacterial Meningitis

Bacterial meningitis is a serious central nervous system infection caused by an invasion of the meninges by bacteria. It is a significant health problem for infants and young children because of the mortality rate associated with the disease and the incidence of severe, long-term neurologic sequelae.

Etiology/Incidence

Bacterial meningitis is most frequent in infants and children below the age of 5 years with an incidence of 87 in 100,000 persons per year (Snyder, 1989). It occurs less frequently in children older than 5 years with a rate of 2.2 in 100,000 persons per year (Snyder, 1989). The incidence peaks between 6 and 12 months of age. The most common bacteria in descending frequency of occurrence are *Haemophilus influenzae* type B (*H. influenzae* meningitis), *Neisseria meningitidis* (meningococcal meningitis), and *Streptococcus pneumoniae* (pneumococcal meningitis). Other pathogens less commonly seen may include group B streptococcus, *Mycoplasma pneumoniae, Escherichia coli,* and *Listeria monocytogenes*. After head trauma and neurosurgery, organisms can include *Staphylococcus epidermidis, Staphylococcus aureus, Klebsiella,* and *Pseudomonas*.

Pathophysiology

The pathogens responsible for meningitis usually disseminate from a distant site to septicemia and then into the meninges, most commonly following an upper respiratory infection or accompanying bacteremia of otitis media, sinusitis, and mastoiditis. Pathogens can also enter through penetrating wounds, such as skull fractures or operative incisions, or via the skin in the presence of a structural defect, such as a meningomyelocele. In the neonate, additional risk factors include maternal infection, premature rupture of membranes, premature birth, low birthweight, and prolonged labor. Bacteria seem to penetrate more easily in an immature brain. Once the pathogen is implanted, it proliferates and spreads into CSF and through perivascular channels and meningeal folds to brain parenchyma. Later, clumps of purulent exudate collect around the base of the brain to cause obstruction of CSF with possible hydrocephalus and cranial nerve palsies. Blood vessel walls and endothelium become involved and cerebral perfusion may be compromised, leading to cerebral edema. Vasculitis associated with thrombosis can cause infarctions (strokes), seizures, and focal deficits. Continued necrosis of cells in the brain cortex and hydrocephalus can lead to permanent damage, increased ICP, and even death.

Clinical Manifestations

Inflammation of the meninges and the pain-sensitive structures surrounding them is thought to be responsible for nuchal rigidity (stiff neck) and headache, which are the most striking symptoms of meningitis in young children. Classically, these children also have a high fever and appear very ill. The Kernig sign (the inability to extend the legs fully when lying supine) and the Brudzinski sign (flexion of the hips when the neck is flexed from a supine position) are frequently present. An infant may have less striking symptoms. The parents may notice only the infant's resistance to being cuddled or diapered, irritability, and mild fever. The infant may have a high-pitched cry, a transient vacant stare, and anorexia. A bulging tense fontanel is a frequent symptom and may indicate increased ICP.

In neonates, the symptoms of infection and meningeal irritation may be minimal or absent. Bacterial meningitis should be considered in any newborn who fails to thrive and has irritability, apnea, seizures, a tendency of opisthotonos, poor feeding, emesis, hypo- or hyperthermia, hypo- or hypertonia, a gray appearance, jaundice, or other evidence of sepsis (Snyder, 1989).

Meningococcal meningitis is associated with rapidly spreading purpuric skin lesions. Any parent inquiring about a "purple rash," especially if associated with other symptoms, should be advised to have the child seen by a physician immediately.

The mortality rate for *H. influenzae* meningitis ranges from 3 to 17 per cent, with a slightly higher rate when all bacteria are included (Snyder, 1989). Mortality and morbidity are usually higher for neonates.

Major factors in predicting unfavorable outcome of bacterial meningitis are young age, delay in treatment, coma, or focal neurologic signs on admission and a poor clinical course (Snyder, 1989). Neurologic sequelae can range considerably, from mild learning disabilities to severe physical and mental disabilities. Deafness and alteration in vision may result. Seizures occur in about 20 to 50 per cent of all meningitis patients, presumably in response to cerebral edema, fever, or cortical irritation and damage (Snyder, 1989).

Other complications include hydrocephalus, cranial nerve dysfunctions, peripheral circulatory collapse, arthritis (especially after meningococcal meningitis), arteritis, phlebitis, and abscess (Krugman & Katz, 1981). Subdural effusion and empyema should be suspected in infants who do not respond to treatment and have prolonged fever, bulging tense fontanels, increasing head circumference, seizures, and other focal deficits.

Diagnostic Assessment

When meningitis is suspected, lumbar puncture to examine spinal fluid is indicated. If the infant or child has symptoms of increased ICP, CT or MRI of the head may be done first to rule out a mass lesion (Snyder, 1989). Typical spinal fluid findings are cloudy fluid, increased pressure, increased white blood count (usually polymorphonuclear), low glucose, elevated protein, and positive Gram stain results. Table 40–30 shows CSF parameters in children with meningitis, compared with normal fluid findings. The fluid is cultured in order to identify the specific pathogen. Additional studies include counterimmunoelectrophoresis, latex agglutination, and limulus lysate assay.

Other laboratory tests may include cultures of blood, urine, nasopharynx, and CSF leaks to identify the source of septicemia. Complete blood cell counts may show an increase in total white blood cells with an increase in immature granulocytes. Serum C–reactive protein rises acutely to more than 40 mg/dl with bacterial infection.

Repeat CT or MRI imaging may help monitor the evolution of the illness and determine the need for specific interventions.

Therapeutic Management

The infant or child is hospitalized. Treatment involves aggressive intravenous administration of antibiotics for 10 to 14 days. When meningitis is caused by enteric organisms or tuberculosis, the course is usually longer. Before a definitive cause is identified and sensitivities are available, usually several broad-spectrum antibiotics are started (usually ampicillin, chloramphenicol, and/or vancomycin). After organism sensitivities are available, antibiotic therapy is further selected and modified. The choice of antibiotic should show consideration of any allergies the patient may have. Dosages are adjusted to maintain therapeutic serum antibiotic levels, when appropriate.

Supportive care includes management of fever and dehydration and monitoring the response to treatment. Supportive care may also include recognition and treatment of increased ICP, seizures, cerebral edema, hydrocephalus, subdural effusion, and empyema.

Surgical treatment may be necessary for infants or children with severe problems, increased ICP, ventriculomegaly, hydrocephalus, subdural effusion, or empyema. This may include ventriculostomy for drainage of infected or obstructed fluid. If hydrocephalus persists after appropriate antibiotic treatment, a shunt may be necessary. Some organisms, such as *Klebsiella* and *Pseudomonas* may require careful intraventricular administration of antibiotics. Subdural effusions may be treated with subdural antibiotic irrigation and sump drainage.

Before discharge, brain stem auditory evoked potentials or audiometry for older children is usually done. When hearing loss occurs, early intervention is possible. Careful follow-up with developmental testing and information about appropriate infant stimulation is advisable. Early detection of delays will allow for early intervention. Some children may need rehabilitation.

TABLE 40–30
Cerebrospinal Fluid in Children (Postneonatal): Counts During Bacterial Meningitis Versus Normal Findings

	Pressure	Appearance	Leukocytes	Protein	Sugar
Normal cerebrospinal fluid	60–160 mm H_2O	Clear	0–5/mm^3	10–30 mg/dl	40–80 mg/dl
Bacterial meningitis	↑, average 300 mm H_2O	Turbid, cloudy	↑, up to 60,000/mm^3, polymorphonuclear cells predominate	↑, 100–500 mg/dl	↓, often <40 mg/dl

Preventive measures for bacterial meningitis include prompt treatment for upper respiratory infections, otitis media, sinusitis, mastoiditis, and other infections, especially in younger infants and children. Immunization with *H. influenzae* type B vaccine prevents bacteremia, thus preventing meningitis (Feigin, 1987). This vaccine is recommended at 24 or 18 months of age for children who attend day care centers.

Close contacts of an infant or child infected with *N. meningitidis* or *H. influenzae* may receive rifampin prophylactically. Close contacts are defined as family members, school or day care contacts, and primary care providers in hospitals. Recommendations about prophylaxis are subject to change, and the reader is advised to check with the physician or the hospital's infectious disease department.

Application of the Nursing Process: Bacterial Meningitis

Assessment

Nursing assessment includes acute *neurologic monitoring,* checking vital signs and head circumference, palpating the anterior fontanel, measuring daily weight and intake and output, and assessing the intravenous site. The infant or child can also be assessed for discomfort, irritability, behavioral problems, seizures, vomiting, appetite, thirst, and a variety of potential complications.

Nursing Diagnostic Statements and Collaborative Problems

***Pain,** related to meningeal irritation (nuchal stiffness and photophobia) and intravenous infusion of antibiotics.*

***Fear, family,** related to perceptions about the potential of the child's illness to affect brain function.*

***High risk for injury:** complications of meningins, including increased intracranial pressure; seizures; hearing loss; arthritis; and stress ulcers, associated with bacterial meningitis; risk factor: infectious process.*

***High risk for altered health maintenance;** risk factor: knowledge deficit regarding required home care.*

Planning and Implementation

Pain Management. The nurse determines the success of past comfort measures and develops a realistic plan for decreasing pain. Continued assessment of pain and discomfort as well as observation before and after administration of analgesics and other comfort measures is recorded. Although complete relief of pain and discomfort *may not be possible,* analgesics should be given as ordered; if drugs are ineffective, the physician is notified, to obtain new drug orders.

Comfort measures may include the parents, caretakers, or nurse offering security objects, reading stories, playing quiet music, giving a light stroking massage, dimming the lights and maintaining a quiet environment, or holding and rocking. Progressive relaxation and imagery techniques may be useful for the older child.

For pain associated with intravenous infusion, use intravenous boards to support the extremity, and one should check the intravenous site for signs or symptoms of phlebitis or infiltration. If either condition is found, the infusion is discontinued, and warm packs are applied to the area. If there are no complications, the nurse may consider decreasing the rate of infusion or adding lidocaine (Xylocaine) to the infusion to alleviate the pain. A central access line may be considered for children undergoing long-term antibiotic therapy.

The nurse should have a truthful conversation with the child about pain, including how much a procedure will hurt, how long it will last, and what will help to lessen the pain. Care should be taken to ensure that the child understands that pain is *not* a punishment.

Increased Family Coping. Consistency of the staff caring for a family and child helps diminish the fear associated with the diagnosis and improves family coping. The nurse should plan frequent, supportive interactions with the family and allow time and presence for them to express fears and concerns. The nurse informing the family about the child's condition should also make positive statements that allow for hope. The nurse should clarify misconceptions about meningitis and its potential complications, cause, risk to other family members, diagnostic tests, and antibiotic therapy, using simple and direct statements. The nurse also assists the family in meeting with the physician regularly and encourages them to write down questions for those conferences.

Preventing Potential Complications. Continuous assessment of the child for signs and symptoms of increased ICP and the infectious process should be accompanied by acute *neurologic monitoring* and checking of vital signs and head circumference. The physician should be promptly notified of a change in status relative to complications. Fluids and electrolytes should also be monitored carefully. See Table 40–20 for nursing care of the child with increased ICP.

Antipyretics are given as ordered for fever, along with sponge baths and light clothing. Antibiotic therapy is started as soon as possible and administered on schedule to maintain antibiotic serum levels; serum levels are checked as appropriate. The padded bed side rails are kept up. One should stay with the child in the bathroom because of the potential for seizures. The nurse will promptly recognize seizures, provide appropriate first aid, observe and document seizures, and give antiepileptic medications, as ordered. Family members and the child should be taught about seizure observation, first aid, and medications.

The nurse monitors the child for potential hearing loss due to meningitis and/or ototoxic side effects of aminoglycoside antibiotics and diuretics by assessing the child's response to auditory stimuli and the ability to localize sounds. If hearing loss is suspected, the physician is notified for appropriate testing (e.g., brain stem auditory evoked potentials; audiometry testing). An otologist can be consulted for treatment considerations and ongoing follow-up.

Assessment for potential arthritis and stress ulcer is also indicated in the child with meningitis.

Facilitating Health Maintenance at Home. The nurse coordinates with the family the child's continued need for instruction and support. Parents are instructed to assess neurologic status and vital signs, compared with pre-illness baselines and examination, at hospital discharge. The nurse instructs parents to test muscle strength and to assess joint function and presence of pain on movement. The parents monitor the child's progress on developmental tasks and compare findings with previously recorded assessments to assess for developmental delays. Parents should be encouraged to talk with their child (if verbal) about the illness experience and the hospital stay.

Evaluation

As in all nursing care plans, the success of the interventions in meeting the projected outcomes is seen when high-risk problems do not occur and the defining characteristics for actual problems decrease in frequency and/or severity or disappear.

Aseptic Meningitis

Aseptic meningitis is also called viral, lymphocytic, or serous meningitis. Identifiable viruses associated with aseptic meningitis include enteroviruses (the most frequent cause), coxsackievirus, echovirus, and mumps virus. Less common pathogens may include arbovirus, lymphocytic choriomeningitis virus, herpes simplex virus, *Chlamydia,* Epstein-Barr virus, and cytomegalovirus. Inflammation of the meninges may also be associated with exanthematous conditions such as varicella infection, herpes infection, measles, and roseola. Aseptic meningitis is generally a benign, self-limiting illness with gradual, complete recovery. Symptoms usually last from 3 to 14 days (Dyken, 1989).

Etiology/Incidence (Pathophysiology)

Viruses gain access to the central nervous system through systemic circulation after viremia of the cranial or peripheral nerves. They enter cells in the meninges for obligatory growth and reproduction, causing inflammation and edema. Enteroviruses are probably transmitted by the enteric-oral pathway and have the greatest incidence during the summer months. Lymphocytic choriomeningitis virus is transmitted by the bite of infected mice or by vectors such as mosquitoes and ticks that transmit the virus to humans.

Diagnostic Assessment

The clinical manifestations are similar to those of bacterial meningitis; however, they do not progress as rapidly and are usually less severe. Clinical symptoms include fever, headache, vomiting, and stiff neck. Seizures are seen less frequently in aseptic meningitis than in bacterial meningitis (Cherry, 1987). Irritability, drowsiness, and lethargy may occur but are mild, compared with encephalitis (Dyken, 1989).

When aseptic meningitis presents with or follows a discrete, red, maculopapular rash, enterovirus or coxsackievirus infection may be likely. When coxsackievirus is the offending pathogen, symptoms may also include the appearance of vesicles and ulcers on the soft palate, paroxysmal pain in the intercostal muscles due to the irritation of pleural surfaces, and symptoms of pericarditis. If aseptic meningitis is caused by mumps virus, parotiditis may also occur.

Diagnosis is made on the basis of concurrent or recent viral illness and examination of CSF to differentiate this condition from bacterial meningitis. CSF in aseptic meningitis usually contains a greater amount of white blood cells than normal, but fewer than in bacterial disease. CSF glucose may be normal, and protein may be only mildly elevated. Virus or virus antibodies may be isolated from CSF, blood, sputum, stool or other specimens.

Therapeutic Management

Therapy is primarily symptomatic, and the child is hospitalized. Management goals include fluid and electrolyte balance, control of hyperthermia, supportive body care, control of pain, maintenance of nutrition, and treatment of seizures that may occur. If severe neurologic signs and symptoms occur and progress, the child's diagnosis should be re-evaluated.

Nursing Care

Nursing care includes assessment of neurologic checks and vital signs in order to promptly recognize and treat problems that arise, such as fever. Analgesics and other comfort measures provide rest and relief from discomfort. Attention to intake and output and laboratory tests assist in maintaining normal fluid and electrolyte balance. Antiemetics and nothing-by-mouth status may decrease vomiting during the initial onset. After vomiting subsides, the child is encouraged frequently to eat small, nutritious snacks. The nurse should be aware of the potential for seizures.

Encephalitis

As its name implies, encephalitis is an inflammation of the brain. Sometimes, however, it may involve the meninges as well as brain tissue (Fenichel, 1988). Once a common complication of measles, mumps, and rubella, the vaccine for these childhood infections has significantly reduced the incidence of encephalitis. The pediatric nurse is much more likely to encounter an infant or young child with bacterial meningitis than one with encephalitis. Encephalitis may be seen more frequently in older children and adolescents.

Enteroviruses are the most frequent cause of encephalitis in the United States, followed by arboviruses (Cherry & Shields, 1987). Encephalitis may follow chickenpox, herpes zoster infection, and infectious mononucleosis. It is more common in children who are immunosuppressed. Epidemic encephalitis often occurs via arthropod transmission and shows a seasonal distribution (Dyken, 1989). Encephalitis is sometimes thought to be viral when a bacterial agent is not identified.

Etiology/Incidence (Pathophysiology)

It is thought that central nervous system involvement is usually secondary to an infectious process elsewhere in the body. The virus or other agent enters the body and subsequently infects the blood. Extensive viremia (proliferation of viruses in the blood) develops, and the central nervous system is infected in this way.

Diagnostic Assessment

Manifestations of encephalitis may vary greatly among children, and the course of the disease is extremely variable. As noted by Cherry and Shields (1987), one child may seem to be mildly affected, only to lapse suddenly into a coma and die; whereas another child may present with high fever, violent convulsions, bizarre movements, and hallucinations, then recover with relatively few sequelae.

Most commonly, the initial symptoms resemble a simple viral illness with fever, headache, pronounced irritability, gastrointestinal distress, and possibly mild respiratory symptoms. Involvement of the central nervous system is manifested by such signs as changes in arousal, consciousness, behavior, and persistent seizures. Frequently, there are signs and symptoms of increased ICP because of increasing, generalized cerebral edema.

Diagnostic assessment involves a careful history of exposure and an examination for concurrent or recent illness. Isolation of the organism from CSF, blood, feces, or sputum as well as acute and convulscent serologic titers may help establish the cause. CSF examination may show normal values or a pattern similar to aseptic meningitis. CT and MRI may show cerebral edema, hydrocephalus, and a multifocal enhancing lesion (Dyken, 1989). An EEG may show abnormalities consistent with clinical seizure activity.

Therapeutic Management

Treatment is supportive. The child is hospitalized for close monitoring of neurologic status. Severely ill children may need the intensive care unit for intubation, mechanical ventilation, ICP monitoring, and interventions using ventriculostomy to manage increased ICP. Persistent seizures or status epilepticus can be common. Administration of antiepileptic drugs is crucial. If they are ineffective in stopping seizures, drug-induced paralysis or coma may be considered. Hydration is closely monitored, because overhydration worsens cerebral edema. Herpes simplex encephalitis may be treated with high-dose intravenous acyclovir for 10 days.

The prognosis for outcome and sequelae of encephalitis is guarded, and young infants have the poorest prognosis. Herpes simplex viruses generally carry a worse prognosis than do the more commonly encountered enteroviruses (Cherry & Shields, 1987). Sequelae may involve the central nervous system or any other body system.

Once the acute period passes, treatment is rehabilitative as well as supportive. Evaluations and ongoing therapy with physical therapists, occupational therapists, speech and language therapists, and psychologists, as appropriate, support rehabilitative progress.

Nursing Care

Nursing care for encephalitis refers to care for the child with increased ICP, altered responsiveness, and seizures, discussed earlier in this chapter. Families may feel frightened and frustrated to have no definitive treatment for what appears to be a severe illness. Diagnosis of the response *powerlessness* is often appropriate for the families. Interventions include consistent, frequent opportunities to express feelings, support for spiritual needs, encouragement in decision making, and involvement with daily care needs. Referral for ongoing needs varies but can include social services, mental health services, ministers, and support networks. Altered family processes may occur when children are left with severe neurologic deficits.

Guillain-Barré Syndrome

Guillain-Barré syndrome, also known as postinfectious or idiopathic polyneuritis, is a disease affecting nerve roots or peripheral nerves and causing varying degrees of motor and sensory disturbances. Although relatively uncommon, it may affect children of both sexes at any age from early infancy onward.

Etiology/Incidence (Pathophysiology)

In Guillain-Barré syndrome, nerve fibers undergo demyelination from an inflammatory process. With the decline in poliomyelitis, Guillain-Barré syndrome is the primary cause of acute, severe paralysis (Glaze, 1987). Although it typically occurs several weeks after an upper respiratory or gastrointestinal infection, it can also follow immunizations and surgery. The chronic demyelinating neuropathies such as Guillain-Barré syndrome are considered to be immune-mediated, although the exact mechanism is unknown (Fenichel, 1988). Typically, signs and symptoms occur several days after an identifiable infection. Children may hesitate to walk or run because their legs "feel funny." Peripheral neuritis usually starts bilaterally in the legs with weakness and numbness that extends up to the arms and hands. The progressive paralysis usually peaks at 3 weeks. Deep tendon reflexes are decreased or absent, and the child may complain of muscle tenderness or cramping pains on examination. Assessment of paresthesia (altered sensation of the limbs) is important but may be difficult in the young child. The child's vague complaints should be taken seriously.

Cranial nerve involvement occurs in 46 to 75 per cent of individuals, especially of nerves VII, IX, and X, causing facial weakness and swallowing difficulty (Glaze, 1987). Ten to 20 per cent of affected persons have enough involvement of the abdominal and thoracic muscles to cause respiratory insufficiency. Some require intubation and mechanical ventilation.

Diagnostic Assessment

There is no specific diagnostic test for Guillain-Barré syndrome. Diagnosis is based on clinical features (especially progressive motor weakness of more than one limb, and areflexia), and on other findings such as an elevated CSF protein, electrophysiologic changes, and pathologic changes of the peripheral nerves. The physician must rule out viral and infectious diseases, especially those altering muscle function, such as poliomyelitis.

A lumbar puncture is required to assess the cerebral spinal fluid for an increase in protein and cell count. An electromyogram may show denervation and decreased nerve conduction velocity.

Clinical signs of a symmetric ascending paralysis and the positive findings from the lumbar puncture and the EEG assist in the diagnosis of Guillain-Barré syndrome.

Therapeutic Management

There is no specific treatment for Guillain-Barré syndrome. Treatment is primarily supportive with hospitalization for skilled nursing care. Because the majority of deaths are related to respiratory failure, pulmonary embolism, and autonomic dysfunction, particular attention is given to respiratory and cardiac function. Endotracheal intubation with mechanical ventilation is necessary for children who have significant involvement of abdominal and thoracic muscles. Physiotherapy and other measures, such as elastic stockings, will be instituted to prevent pulmonary embolism. Electrocardiogram and blood pressure are monitored as parameters of autonomic function within the cardiovascular system. Serum electrolytes will be carefully monitored to assess for hyponatremia, which sometimes develops. Although some physicians recommend prednisone in the treatment of Guillain-Barré syndrome (Fenichel, 1988), others report that steroids have little effect on this disease (Glaze, 1987). When recovery begins, treatments such as mechanical ventilation will be reduced and withdrawn, as appropriate.

Nursing Care

Nursing care during the acute stage is supportive and consists of promoting the child's comfort, preventing deformity, and promoting adequate respiratory and cardiac function. The threat of cardiopulmonary complications makes nursing surveillance a vital part of therapeutic management. Vital signs, chest ausculation, and neurologic checks focusing on the motor system are compared with baseline values. Changes in findings should be promptly reported to the physician.

A decrease in respiratory function, such as vital capacity, usually indicates early respiratory involvement and necessitates transfer to the intensive care unit for intubation and mechanical ventilation. It is extremely stressful for parents and siblings to observe a child with signs of paralysis. They may feel helplessness and guilt about not having sought help early enough. The family members need reassurance that they did what was proper by obtaining medical attention for their child, and that everything possible is being done to help the child. Having someone to answer questions, explain procedures, and listen to concerns is therapeutic. The child will also be at risk for experiencing fear due to being on mechanical ventilation with preserved consciousness. Developing a method of communication (usually with eye closure) is essential.

Irritability, restlessness, and pain from nerve root involvement may be present. Both pharmacologic and nonpharmacologic comfort measures are indicated. An in-dwelling catheter for urinary retention or incontinence may be needed. Meticulous technique is needed in catheter care to avoid urinary tract infection. Maintaining adequate nutrition and hydration is important. Parenteral fluids or enteral feedings are given to promote hydration and nutrition and to prevent aspiration if there is involvement of cranial nerve IX or X.

Prevention of contractures is a primary need during the entire disease process, and physical therapy with passive range of motion to all extremities is needed at least every 4 hours. Repositioning the child every 2 hours helps prevent deformity and skin breakdown. Splinting of ankles with high-top tennis shoes prevents footdrop. Special attention to shoulder and arm positioning helps prevent dislocation and frozen shoulder.

Care during recovery involves several health professionals. The occupational therapist and the physical therapist help the child recover muscle strength and motor abilities. Bracing or splinting may be needed for the child with residual muscle weakness. The activity or play therapist has a major role in providing the child with appropriate energy-releasing activities.

Immobilized children often express a wide range of behaviors, including withdrawal, aggression, noncompliance, and loneliness. The nurse who understands this is able to accept some aggressiveness and noncooperation. However, providing the child with outlets for aggression and frustration through therapeutic play, physical exercise within the limits of the disease, and verbalization of feelings can minimize the behaviors and facilitate healthy coping. (See Chapter 17 for further information about therapeutic play.)

The long recovery period can be emotionally and financially draining for the entire family, and a social service referral is useful. Discharge planning should include a community health nurse referral to assist with home management and arrangements for a homebound teacher to help the child with school work. The long-term outlook is good, with 95 per cent of these children having complete recovery.

Neurologic Injury

Head Injuries

Head injury in the pediatric population is one of the most common causes of death and disability. Nearly 250,000 children are admitted annually to United States hospitals for evaluation and/or treatment of minor or major head trauma. The spectrum of injury can range from minor concussion requiring a few hours of observation to major trauma necessitating heroic efforts and resulting in a dismal long-term outcome for the child.

Etiology/Incidence

The incidence of head injury in boys is twice that for girls. The age group affected most frequently is the adolescent population. Head injuries occur most frequently in the spring and summer, on weekends, and in the late afternoon or early evening (American Association of Neuroscience Nurses, 1990).

This portion of the chapter focuses on general concepts regarding various types of head trauma. (In-depth coverage of concepts related to management of increased ICP from cerebral edema is found earlier in this chapter.) Management of minor to moderate head trauma is addressed here under "Therapeutic Management."

The causes of head injury vary somewhat among age groups and developmental stages. Infants may have minor head trauma as a result of a difficult delivery with forceps or a prolonged traumatic labor and delivery. Infants or toddlers may sustain a head injury because of a fall from a caretaker's arms, from a loft or balcony, in walkers, out of windows, or down stairs. These children are also at the age when they may be victims of child abuse, particularly shaking injuries. Preschool children may be hurt in a vehicular accident as either a passenger or a pedestrian. The preschooler is prone to being injured while playing or climbing outside. School-age children may be hurt in playground accidents or, more commonly, in accidents involving bicycles, skateboards, or athletic activities. Vehicular accidents and athletic injuries are the most common causes of head trauma in adolescent age groups. Other factors that may predispose a child to head injury are seizure disorders, gait instability, alcohol or drug ingestion, and cognitive delays, including poor judgment.

Pathophysiology

The pathophysiology of head injuries is complex in that the extent of the visible injury may not be at all indicative of the extent of actual brain injury. A head injury may involve any or all of the cranial and skull layers, including scalp, skull, dura, brain, and blood vessels, as well as neurons and supportive glial cells. Injuries can be classified as "primary," meaning resulting from the actual traumatic event, or "secondary," indicating that the damage is caused by pathologic processes (such as cerebral edema or anoxia) that occurred as a result of the initial injury. Secondary injury may be related to the rapidity of treatment once the injury has occurred.

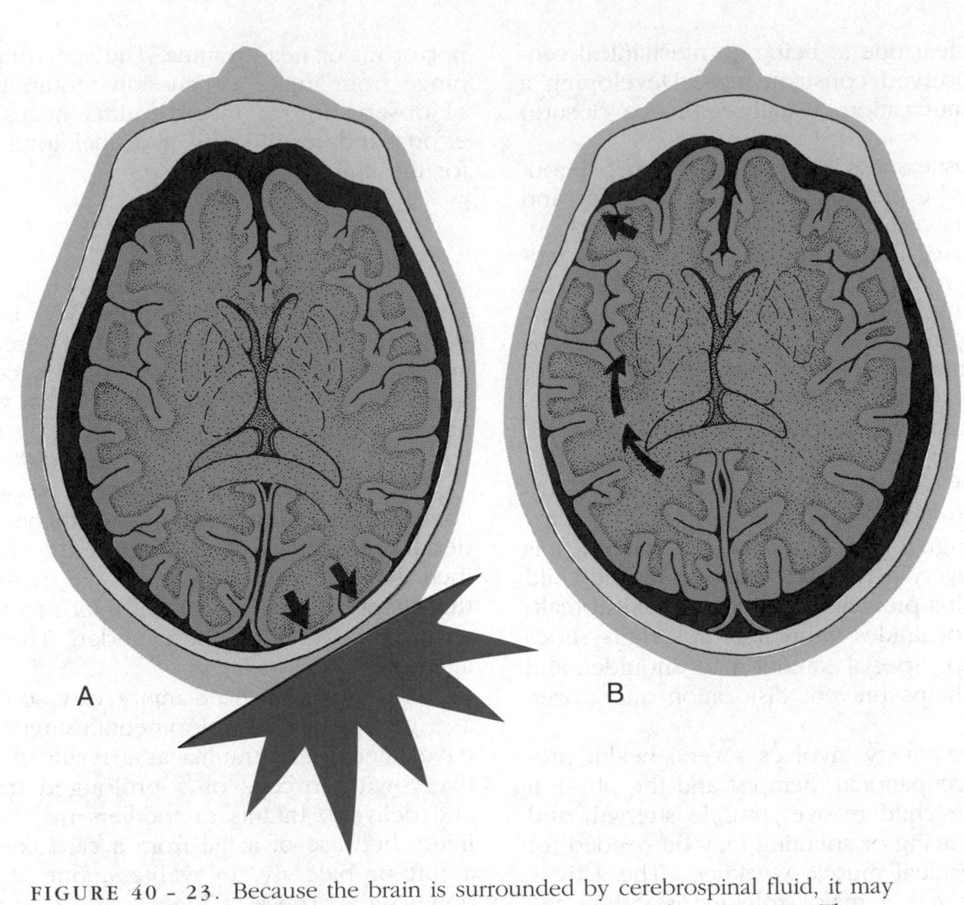

FIGURE 40 - 23. Because the brain is surrounded by cerebrospinal fluid, it may move within the skull on impact, causing damage in more than one area. The *coup* is the point of impact. *A*, The brain is forced against the skull in the area of the blow. *B*, The brain then rebounds *(contrecoup)* off that point and strikes the skull wall opposite the injuring blow. Some twisting of the brain stem (concussion) may occur with the contrecoup movement.

There are several mechanisms of injury in pediatric head trauma. An injury may be blunt or nonpenetrating, causing the distortion of brain tissue and shearing of neurons, even without outward evidence of injury or trauma. Penetrating or open injuries can produce either focal or diffuse damage, depending on the velocity and type of penetration. Compression injuries are the result of the skull being compressed between two forces, causing the brain integrity to be crushed. Other commonly used terms are "coup" (pronounced *coo*) and "contrecoup" injuries. These terms are used to describe an injury to brain tissue that results when a blow to the head causes the brain to hit the skull at the location of impact *(coup),* then rebound to the opposite side of the skull where injury can also occur *(contrecoup)* (Fig. 40–23).

"Head injury" is the general term for several different types of injury. Scalp injuries, skull fractures, concussions, contusions and lacerations, vascular injuries and hematomas, and cranial nerve and diffuse brain tissue injuries are each addressed individually in this portion of the chapter.

Clinical Manifestations

Scalp Injuries. The scalp is composed of five layers, including connective tissue and vascular structures. Together these layers offer tremendous protection to the skull. Scalp injuries include abrasions and lacerations. For these injuries, gently cleaning followed by hemostasis, conservative debridement of dead tissue, and suturing without tension is the recommended approach to management (Argenta & Adson, 1989).

Skull Fractures. The human skull is composed of two layers—the inner and outer tables—separated by a spongy tissue called the diploic space. In a head injury, a fracture may occur at the site of impact or in areas of the skull with less tensile strength. Skull fractures are found in over one quarter of children who present at hospitals with head injuries. There are five types of skull fractures. Nearly 70 per cent of skull fractures are *linear* and involve the cranial vault. Fracture lines may be simple or complex and follow no predictable pattern. Children with uncomplicated linear fractures are usually admitted to the hospital for a short period of observation and are likely to resume normal activities within a few days. The bone heals on its own, and the fracture is not likely to be evident on skull x-ray films 6 months to 1 year after the injury (Mealey, 1989).

Depressed skull fractures are often associated with scalp lacerations. The exception is "ping-pong" or other fractures of the infant skull. A fracture is considered depressed when the inner table is displaced by more than the thickness of the skull. Compound depressed skull fractures (those with lacerations) should be débrided and elevated as soon as possible after the injury. Surgical elevation will be considered in closed injuries in which fragments are depressed more than 0.5 to 1.0 cm. Depressed fractures with many fragments are referred to as *comminuted* (Mealey, 1989).

Diastatic skull fractures occur along the suture line. The separation is usually visible on skull roentgenograph. These fractures often do not occur at the site of impact and are seen most frequently in newborn babies and infants.

The most serious type of skull fracture is a *basilar skull fracture*. These fractures involve a break in the basal portions of the frontal, ethmoid, sphenoid, temporal, or occipital bones. Two classic associated findings are the Battle sign and "raccoon eyes." The first is the presence of bruising or ecchymosis behind the ear caused by leakage of blood into the mastoid sinus. "Raccoon eyes" are caused by blood leaking into the frontal sinuses and causing an edematous and bruised periorbital area. Patients with these fractures may also present with CSF leakage from the nose or ears, secondary to tears in the meninges near the paranasal sinuses and the petrous bone. Although rare, CSF leaks can be serious, especially if they do not stop spontaneously. Antibiotics are used prophylactically if a leak occurs. Basilar skull fractures are associated with cranial nerve injuries. Optic, extraocular, and acoustic nerve injuries are the most common ones (Mealey, 1989).

Concussions. "Concussion" can be defined as a clinical syndrome characterized by an immediate and transient impairment of consciousness following a head injury. It is associated with traumatic amnesia and occasionally disturbances in vision. The functional disturbance may vary in duration from days to weeks and in severity from mild to severe (Mealey, 1989). Concussion tends to occur when the head is in a position of movement after impact, rather than in a fixed position.

Postconcussion Syndrome. When post-traumatic amnesia occurs for a longer period of time or when a long period of unconsciousness (over 2 weeks) persists after initial injury, or when both occur, cognitive loss often accompanies the physical disabilities. Postconcussion syndrome is defined by Stevens (1982) as "a series of temporary somatic and cognitive dysfunctions experienced for several weeks to 1 year after head injury" (p 240). These complaints include headache, fatigue, vertigo, emotional lability, loss of judgment, and photophobia, among others. Often, communication skills, attitudes, and behaviors all seem to be affected. Another aspect of this syndrome to cause concern is post-traumatic stress reaction. Basically, this is the tendency for pretraumatic unresolved problems to be exacerbated after the injury. Both problems are major barriers to the resumption of a "normal" life for the child and family after the injury (Stevens, 1982).

Contusions and Lacerations. Bruising or crushing injuries of the brain are considered contusions, and actual discontinuity of brain tissue is referred to as a laceration. Contusions are usually caused by blunt trauma and acceleration or deceleration injuries to the freely movable head. The area of brain tissue surrounding a contusion site is generally composed of small areas of perivascular hemorrhage, which leads to progressive local cerebral edema that resolves slowly but usually with good recovery of function. Lacerations are caused by penetrating craniocerebral trauma and are serious in their capability of leading to significant intracerebral bleeding (Mealey, 1989).

Vascular Injuries and Hematomas. Subdural and epidural hematomas occur in about 6 to 7 per cent of pediatric head injuries. The shearing force created by the impact can cause the tearing of bridging vessels that supply blood to the various layers of the dura mater. Epidural hematomas are more likely to be of an acute nature and usually are the result of a tear in an artery, although 25 per cent of epidural hematomas have a venous origin. The child usually has a short period of unconsciousness followed by a period of lucidity in which he or she is believed to be recovered; within 4 to 8 hours, the child begins to experience a rapid decline in neurologic function that causes severe cerebral shift and eventually death if untreated. Common locations for epidural hematomas are the temporal fossa, subfrontal, and occipital areas. Surgical treatment is emergent and arrests the serious symptoms if done rapidly (Table 40–31) (Ammons, 1990).

Acute subdural hematomas are usually of venous origin and are often associated with an underlying contusion. Subdural hemorrhage has also been shown to occur from a shaking injury to the infant head. This type of hematoma occurs more frequently in infancy and is usually bilateral, whereas epidural hematomas are unilateral. Common symptoms are increased ICP, seen in 60 per cent of cases, and seizures, seen in 40 per cent of cases. Retinal hemorrhages are also common and are a classic sign of a shaking injury in an infant (McLaurin & Towbin, 1989).

TABLE 40-31
Characteristics of Acute Epidural and Subdural Hematomas

Supratentorial	Acute Epidural	Acute Subdural
Frequency	Less	More
Skull Fracture	75%	30%
Source of hemorrhage	Usually arterial	Venous
Age	Most over 2 yrs old	Most under 1 yr old
Laterality	Unilateral	Bilateral
Seizures	Under 25%	75%
Retinal hemorrhages	Under 25%	75%
Mortality	25%	Under 25%

Chronic subdural hematomas are usually related to trauma but may be identified at a much later date, usually after skull growth has accelerated beyond normal levels. The characteristic symptoms are irritability, full nonpulsatile fontanel, failure to thrive, and low hematocrit levels.

Cranial Nerve and Brain Tissue Injury. As discussed, basilar skull fractures are the most common cause of cranial nerve injury. Compression, stretching, or severe laceration can also cause cranial nerve damage. The most common cranial nerve injuries are to cranial nerves I (loss of smell), VII (facial paralysis), V and VI (eye movements), II (optic fields), and VIII.

Injury to actual brain tissue occurs as a concussion, contusion, or laceration, as discussed earlier. Damage of neurons is referred to as diffuse axonal injury (also called shearing). The mechanism for this injury is the difference in densities of the gray and white matter. When the head is subjected to impact, there is more displacement of the gray matter on the cortical surface than there is of the deep white matter. As a result, the axons degenerate and their ability to transmit impulses effectively diminishes. The course and outcome for the patient depend on the extent of the injury (Adams et al, 1986).

Diagnostic Assessment

As in most neurologic disorders, the two primary components of the diagnostic assessment are a thorough history and physical examination and appropriate radiographic studies. A complete history of the traumatic event or injury is particularly important in cases of head injury. The actual mechanism of injury or state of consciousness after the injury, or both, can be a useful tool in diagnosing the type of trauma. Another major aspect of history taking is determining whether there has been post-traumatic amnesia, as in concussion injuries, or a seizure at the time of injury or predisposing the child to injury. Family history of bleeding disorders should also be noted.

Once the family history and the history of the event have been gathered, a complete neurologic assessment should be carried out. Testing of cognitive and mental functions, as well as cranial nerve testing and assessment of signs and symptoms of increased ICP, is vital. If the injured child arrives at the health care facility in a state of rapid neurologic decompensation, assessment and interventions are often done simultaneously. If there is any evidence of a pressure build-up great enough to threaten herniation of the cerebral lobes, immediate action must be taken to alleviate the pressure. More in-depth coverage of this type of assessment and management is found in the discussion of increased ICP.

Radiographic studies for head injury are basically skull and cervical spine films and a CT scan. If the injury is minor and the child appears neurologically intact, a CT scan may not be necessary, although plain skull films are usually done to rule out a skull fracture. MRI scans are being used more frequently, particularly in children with more severe injuries as a way to follow white and gray matter changes over time.

If there has been seizure activity after the injury, an EEG is necessary. Injuries involving the cranial nerves may be followed with brain stem auditory evoked responses or visual evoked responses, or both. A child with long-term cognitive deficits may require a neuropsychologic evaluation to assess functional, learning, and vocational abilities.

Therapeutic Management

Medical Management. There is a broad spectrum of medical and surgical interventions for the range of mild to severe head injury. The treatment for mild head injury is generally a conservative observational approach that may involve following the clinical manifestations for several hours before discharging the patient. Most nondepressed skull fractures heal over time. A moderate head injury may involve a prolonged hospital stay and methods to decrease ICP, short of mechanical hyperventilation. It may be necessary to keep some children hospitalized to follow cranial nerve functions and ascertain that there is no worsening disease process. Children with severe injuries necessitate a critical care environment with close monitoring of vital functions. The insertion of an ICP measuring device by the neurosurgeon may be necessary, to monitor changes in ICP and initiate medical therapy based on these changes. Medical therapy for increased ICP is covered in an earlier portion of this chapter.

Surgical Management. Surgical management is necessary in a few instances of head injury. The elevation of a depressed skull fracture and the removal of an acute epidural or subdural hematoma are the most common reasons for surgical intervention in the head-injured child. Chronic subdural hematomas may require mechanical shunting to the peritoneal space. Aggressive medical and pharmacologic management is usually the therapy of choice for moderately to severely injured children.

Application of the Nursing Process: Head Injury

Nursing care for children with head injuries varies according to the extent of the injury, presenting signs and symptoms, and need for surgical intervention.

Assessment

Regardless of the type of injury, a complete neurologic assessment should be done on the first encounter with the patient and consistently throughout the hospitalization. Level of consciousness, ability to follow commands, presence of confusion or irritability, pupil responsiveness, extraocular eye movements, and generalized strength and tone of extremities should be determined and well documented. Each assessment should start with the same degree of stimuli to the patient so that a comparison of responses can be made over time. Nursing assessment should also include observation of any potential CSF leak from the ear canals or nares or changes in external findings (increased swelling or tenderness over scalp abrasions or wounds). Any abnormal motor movements or potential seizure activity should be observed and recorded. Finally, close scrutiny of cardiorespiratory and vital sign parameters is essential, because evidence of increasing ICP should be reported immediately. More detailed information about these findings can be found in the discussion of increased ICP found earlier in this chapter.

Nursing Diagnostic Statements and Collaborative Problems

High risk for altered tissue perfusion: cerebral, *risk factors: brain injury, potential for cell anoxia, change in neurologic function, and potential for seizure activity.*

High risk for airway compromise; *risk factors: decreased level of consciousness and pressure on or damage to lower cranial nerves.*

High risk for sensory and perceptual alterations, altered level of consciousness; *risk factors: head injury and secondary cerebral edema.*

High risk for infection; *risk factors: dual tear, CSF leak, invasive surgical procedure or ICP monitoring, and relative immobility and nutritional deficits.*

Anticipatory grieving, family, *related to loss of their child as they knew him or her.*

High risk for injury after discharge; *risk factors: lack of knowledge by child and family regarding how to adapt to changes required by or resulting from the illness and its treatment.*

High risk for altered health maintenance; *risk factor: knowledge deficit about home care.*

Planning and Implementation

Promoting Optimal Cerebral Tissue Perfusion. Nursing care for the child with threatened cerebral tissue perfusion includes careful monitoring of oxygen saturation with pulse oximetry and administration of oxygen as necessary. It is always preferable to administer oxygen when a patient's oxygenation status is questioned, even before a pulse oximetry reading is obtained. The nurse should also be aware of and closely follow the child's hemoglobin and hematocrit levels to ensure adequate oxygen-carrying capacity within the blood. Other nursing interventions aimed at promoting optimal cerebral tissue perfusion include close monitoring of systemic perfusion parameters, such as blood pressure and other vital signs. Close scrutiny of fluid and electrolyte status is also warranted to avoid fluid overload and resultant cerebral edema. Anticonvulsants should be administered as ordered, and any seizure activity should be well documented.

Avoiding Airway Compromise. Slight elevation of the head of the bed is important in managing potential or real increases in ICP and is also useful in optimizing airway position. Very slight hyperextension can be achieved by placing a roll underneath the child's shoulders. This should never be attempted until the cervical spine has been cleared of injury. Oral and/or deep suction may be necessary every 2 to 4 hours, as needed, to clear secretions and stimulate a cough. An appropriate-size bag and mask should always be available at the bedside for emergency use, as needed.

Responding to Altered Sensorium and Changes in Level of Consciousness. Ongoing assessments of neurologic function, including assessment of level of awareness or responsiveness and presence of confusion, should initially be done every 1 to 2 hours following injury. It is the bedside nurse's responsibility to document any changes and to assess the patient more frequently, if warranted. Changes in level of consciousness are frequently the first indication of changes in ICP and cerebral perfusion. Confusion can lead to safety risks, if the child is not being closely watched or properly restrained as needed.

Preventing Infection. Any possibility of a CSF leak from nose, ears, or scalp lacerations should be quantified and reported to the physician as soon as possible. Antibiotics will most likely be administered prophylactically when the scalp has been lacerated or when there is an open injury. If and when steroid medicines are ordered, the nurse should be aware of the potential for opportunistic infections. Frequent oral care should be given and extra attention paid to incisions. Other measures for preventing infection in neurologically impaired or postoperative patients have been addressed elsewhere.

Assisting Family Grief Work. The biggest task facing the family with a severely brain-injured child is the grief of losing the child they once had. Frequently, the personality changes are dramatic and disturbing. The entire structure of the family will likely change. Initially, when progress seems to occur daily, families have a lot of hope for a complete recovery. As time wears on and the family realizes its loss, depression can set in. Stress also has its effect on the marital and sibling relationships. The nurse's role is to offer the family realistic expectations and support through their grief work. Referring the family for further counseling is also an important role. The family needs to be encouraged to take part in their child's care but also given permission to take occasional breaks.

Preventing Injury. For the head-injured child, a major component of nursing care may be assistance in making sounder judgments in their daily activities. Comprehensive rehabilitation programs that involve a component of behavior modification are usually effective in helping children become aware of their own safety. A protective helmet is often necessary.

The family's ability to adapt is affected by the extent of the injury, the family's involvement in the incident, and the chance (or lack thereof) for full recovery.

For children with any long-term sensory deficits (vision, hearing, smell), the nurse should address the need for adaptations to prevent further injury from lack of sensory input. Family members should be educated about seizure precautions, if they are needed. Toxic side effects of anticonvulsants should also be discussed with patients and families, as appropriate.

The sequelae from a head injury in the pediatric years can become a lifetime burden. Seizure activity becomes post-traumatic epilepsy. Postconcussion syndrome can be apparent for a year or more after the injury. Hydrocephalus can occur as the result of an infectious process. The most difficult aspects of long-term outcome are the ensuing personality and behavior changes that can prevent a completely independent lifestyle. Persistent physical difficulties may affect independence. Nevertheless, most pediatric head injuries are minor occurrences that require no hospitalization and engender no long-term damage.

Facilitating Health Maintenance at Home. In addition to previously mentioned measures to prevent injury, the nurse instructs the parents on a variety of home care management procedures and strategies which include assessment of neurologic function and developmental progress. Parents will be instructed about home safety especially when the child has some persistent cognitive or perceptual deficits. Parents can be assisted to identify community resources and make appropriate referrals.

Evaluation

As in all nursing care plans, the success of the interventions in meeting the projected outcomes is seen when high-risk problems do not occur and the defining characteristics for actual problems decrease in frequency and/or severity or disappear.

Spinal Cord Injury

Although acute spinal cord injury (SCI) is an infrequent occurrence in the general pediatric population, the incidence of these injuries does increase significantly in middle and late adolescence. The most common causes are vehicular accidents, falls, athletic injuries, or violent penetrating wounds. Young men between the ages of 15 and 30 constitute nearly 70 per cent of the victims of acute SCI (Kalsbeck, 1980). The emotional and psychologic sequelae of these potentially devastating injuries are overwhelming. The need for excellent acute care management and comprehensive long-range planning for these children or adolescents and their families cannot be overstated. The changes affecting a child and family after an SCI are significant and long-lasting.

Etiology/Incidence

A large proportion of spinal fractures result in no neurologic deficit. However, SCI with no evidence of radiographic abnormality is well documented in the pediatric population (Pang & Wilberger, 1982). Birth injuries affect the cervical spine. After the neonatal period, 60 to 75 per cent of injuries occur in the cervical region, 20 per cent in the thoracic region, and the remainder in the lumbar area (Zabramski et al, 1986).

SCIs are often described in relationship to the mechanism and anatomic location of injury. Flexion-dislocation, hyperextension, vertical compression, and rotation are the major mechanisms of injury. Flexion-dislocation injuries are common in motor vehicle accidents, whereas vertical compression injuries are associated with diving or trampoline injuries. The location of an SCI is usually referred to as the level of injury below which sensory and motor function are impaired.

SCIs are classified as follows:

1. Complete lesions: loss of motor, sensory, and autonomic function distal to the injury.
2. Posterior cord syndrome: crude touch sensation only.
3. Anterior cord syndrome: preservation of touch and proprioception; loss of other cord functions.
4. Central cord syndrome: possibility of significant recovery.
5. Partial spinal cord syndrome: Brown-Séquard.
6. Root syndrome: pain in a specific nerve distribution.

Quadriplegia results from injuries at the cervical level and implies complete loss of leg function and limited, if any, use of arms. Paraplegia results from thoracic or high lumbar injury and is characterized by a loss of leg function alone. Most SCIs are incomplete (see listed items 2 to 6) and result in variable degrees of motor and sensory loss below the level of the lesion. Complete lesions are rare (Menezes et al, 1989).

Pathophysiology

Several factors influence the severity of the actual injury to the spinal cord. The mechanism for cellular damage and functional impairment is usually compression and contusion, rather than actual transection. In the first hours after injury occurs, decreased blood flow and ischemia result in extensive tissue destruction. Compression injuries may result from spinal epidural or subdural hematomas that can be surgically alleviated.

A common physiologic consequence of SCI is a phenomenon referred to as *central cord necrosis*. As further edema and ischemia develop, vascular stasis and thrombosis occur, propagating the vicious circle; the eventual outcome is necrosis of gray matter.

Clinical Manifestations

Immediate signs and symptoms of SCI vary, depending on whether the cord transection is complete or partial. Partial transection is seen most commonly and is discussed here. A symmetric flaccid paralysis and loss of reflexes below the portion of damaged cord will occur. There may be some preservation of pain, temperature, and proprioception below the level of the injury. Moderate vasomotor instability and lowering of the blood pressure usually occur. Cervical cord injury is characterized by respiratory insufficiency secondary to disruption of innervation to the diaphragm. Another condition that occurs immediately after injury is referred to as "neurogenic shock." This is characterized by hypotension due to vasodilatation of the vascular bed below the level of injury, bradycardia, and loss of the ability to sweat below the level of injury.

During the recovery period from the acute phase, hyper-reflexia and spasticity may appear. Clinical manifestations in chronic SCI are related to the degree of recovery and functional return after the initial injury. Complications, such as autonomic hyper-reflexia and bladder dysfunction, occur in the postacute phase.

The immediate response to SCI is referred to as "spinal shock." This phenomenon is the temporary suppression of reflexes controlled below the level of the injury. Spinal shock can last from a few hours to many months. The appearance of perianal reflexes signifies the end of spinal shock and the beginning of recovery. Functional loss from SCI will be determined by the level and degree of injury.

Diagnostic Assessment

After immediate stabilization of respiratory and circulatory systems has occurred, a detailed neurologic examination of the child should be carried out. The precise level of sensory and motor injury should be determined. The spine should also be examined for overt injury or tenderness, or both. Once the clinical examination has been carried out, a thorough roentgenographic examination should be made. Anteroposterior, lateral, and oblique views of the spine down to the suspected level of injury are obtained. Routine films of the spine and pelvis below the level of the injury are necessary to rule out any other hidden fractures. Spinal CT scans, MRI, and myelography may each be useful, depending on the type of injury and information desired. It is important to avoid further injury when x-ray films or scans are being obtained.

Therapeutic Management

Medical Management. Treatment of acute SCI begins immediately. Initial management at the scene of the trauma should include stabilization of the spine and establishment of an adequate airway. Other appropriate medical measures during the acute phase include the administration of intravenous dexamethasone to reduce swelling around the spinal cord and aggressive pulmonary hygiene measures to prevent pneumonia. Stress ulcer is common and is often prevented by administering antacids. Frequent repositioning is ordered, and the patient may be placed in a special frame or bed for turning. Urinary catheterization is also necessary until a determination of bladder function can be made and the Credé maneuver or other measures instituted.

Throughout the acute care phase, rehabilitative

measures are instituted in an effort to ensure the best-possible outcome for the individual. Safe and early mobilization is attempted by using a variety of stabilizing devices. Cardiovascular complications include *orthostatic hypotension* and *autonomic hyper-reflexia* (also called dysreflexia). The latter occurs when there is an uncontrolled increase in sympathetic activity that cannot be inhibited because of the SCI. It is usually caused by overdistention of the bladder or bowel, and it can be a serious complication if not managed.

Medical care during the rehabilitative phase following acute SCI is multifaceted. These children are at risk for thromboembolism and respiratory compromise. Many children with cervical lesions require a tracheostomy. Bowel and bladder care need to be adapted as mobility increases. A bladder program geared toward prevention of urinary tract infection is vital. Prevention of skin breakdown is a task assumed by all who provide care for the spinal cord–injured child. Physical, occupational, and speech therapy as well as an assessment of learning and nutritional and psychosocial needs, are essential. The complex and emotional medical care of these children is best managed in a multidisciplinary rehabilitative center. Reintegrating the disabled child into the family requires a group of individuals committed to the ultimate goal of providing the child with the best-possible quality of life.

Application of the Nursing Process: Spinal Cord Injury

Many nursing diagnostic statements and collaborative problems are applicable to the complex care of children with traumatic SCIs. Loss of function in the spinal cord leads to altered function of nearly every other body system. Nursing care needs to be broad-based so that the interrelatedness of the many problems experienced by these children is recognized. The nursing diagnostic statements and subsequent collaborative problems overlap each other. Although this list is not exhaustive, it establishes a sound base for comprehensive nursing care of the child and family facing an SCI.

Assessment

A complete assessment of function in the initial phase following injury may be affected by the presence and extent of other injuries. Nursing care should include an assessment of cardiorespiratory and airway function followed by an assessment or examination of motor and sensory function of the extremities. The latter is often done in conjunction with the physicians. An assessment of bladder and bowel function is necessary, because these structures will likely be affected, even if transiently in minor injuries.

Nursing Diagnostic Statements and Collaborative Problems

High risk for ineffective airway clearance; *risk factors: decreased innervation of the diaphragm and long-term ventilator dependence (if applicable).*

Decreased tissue perfusion: spinal cord, *related to initial injury and resultant ischemia.*

High risk for infection: respiratory and urinary; *risk factors:*
- *Stasis of pulmonary secretions.*
- *Stasis of urine.*
- *Immune system compromise caused by high steroid doses.*

High risk for altered skin integrity; *risk factors: decreased sensation and decreased or absent mobility.*

Altered elimination: bowel and bladder, *related to abnormal innervation of bladder and digestive tract.*

High risk for altered family processes; *risk factor: lack of available and/or effective mechanisms for coping with extended care of a spinal cord–injured child.*

High risk for altered health maintenance; *risk factor: knowledge deficit about home care of the child.*

Other appropriate diagnoses include those related to safety, cardiovascular function, nutrition, perceptual disturbances, and dysreflexia.

Planning and Implementation

Promoting Effective Airway Clearance. Children suffering paresis or paralysis of their diaphragm, intercostal, or abdominal muscles, or a combination of any of these, may have difficulty clearing normal airway secretions. Other factors influencing this nursing diagnosis include shock lung, chest trauma, and/or pulmonary edema. Consistent monitoring of respiratory parameters at least every 2 hours is necessary. Other nursing interventions include encouragement of deep breathing and incentive spirometry to prevent atelectasis. Any evidence of respiratory insufficiency, dyspnea, air hunger, or abnormal arterial blood gases should immediately be reported to the physician.

Treating Decreased Tissue Perfusion. Rapid intervention is paramount when spinal perfusion is decreased. Administration of dexamethasone and other drugs, as ordered, is essential. Promoting optimal oxygenation via ventilation and close monitoring of these parameters prevents hypoxic episodes that lead to further ischemia.

Preventing Infection. Respiratory care of children with SCI should be meticulous and frequent. Ensuring that chest physiotherapy is done in a timely fashion and that frequent turning, deep breathing (if possible), and suction are done is necessary. Following temperatures and results of routine chest roentgenographs is also necessary. If the child does develop pneumonia, the administration of antibiotics, as ordered, prevents systemic spread of the infection.

Microorganisms may be introduced into the bladder via an in-dwelling or intermittent catheterization program. Meticulous catheter care and prevention of stool near the catheter is vital. Once a program of intermittent catheterization is begun, urinary stasis can provide a perfect medium for bacterial growth. Nursing responsibilities include an assessment of signs and symptoms of urinary tract infection and administration of antibiotics as well as teaching the child and family all aspects of prevention. These include adequate hydration, proper catheterization technique, and complete bladder emptying.

Preserving Skin Integrity. Immobility, circulatory impairment, and poor nutrition all contribute to the potential for skin breakdown. Nursing care for this diagnosis should focus on prevention. Skin should be inspected daily for any beginning areas of redness. An eggcrate mattress or sheepskin, or both, should be used as appropriate. There currently are many therapeutic beds available for use with the immobile child. In all repositioning, foam pads should be used to cushion bony prominences. The nurse should take care to prevent any kind of moisture from remaining on the skin. (For further elaboration of nursing care related to immobility, see the discussion of nursing care of the child with altered responsiveness earlier in this chapter.)

Dealing with Bowel and Bladder Dysfunction. Loss of voluntary bladder control requires the insertion of an in-dwelling urinary catheter to evaluate fluid status and renal function. As soon as possible, intermittent catheterization should begin, to promote reflex bladder emptying. In either case, asepsis and proper technique are essential. An intermittent catheterization program involves slowly decreasing the number of catheterizations while simultaneously recording the amounts of residual urine. If the child is school-age or older, teaching of self-catheterization should begin if a readiness to learn is displayed.

Initially, paralytic ileus may hinder bowel function. Maintenance of a nasogastric tube for low suction may be ordered. Assessment of the abdomen, including palpation and auscultation, should be done regularly. Abdominal girths should be recorded every 4 to 6 hours. At some point, a bowel program should be initiated with a stool softener and digital stimulation. Once a pattern has been established, the stool softener may be discontinued and regularity maintained with diet and digital stimulation alone.

Promoting Effective Family Functioning. A traumatic injury to the spinal cord has lifelong implications for the child and family. Because many of these injuries occur in adolescence, there may be pre-existing tension between the parent and child, depending on the nature of the injury. The denial, anger, and fear need to be addressed as the child recovers. The nurse is often the key in supporting and promoting family cohesiveness and recognizing when other subspecialties need to be involved. Family adjustment to this illness should never be taken for granted, but rather continually re-examined and discussed.

Facilitating Health Maintenance at Home. Before discharge, the child's care may require the coordination of several disciplines, including physical and occupational therapy, rehabilitative medicine, psychology, social work, urology, and nursing. Parents are instructed to assess for infection of any type: skin, respiratory, or bladder. The nurse continually assesses the child's and family's progress on developmental tasks after discharge, in the outpatient clinic or in the home, and discusses ways to meet these tasks in spite of altered family processes.

Evaluation

As in all nursing care plans, the success of the interventions in meeting the projected outcomes is seen when high-risk problems do not occur and the defining characteristics for actual problems decrease in frequency and/or severity or disappear.

KEY CONCEPTS

Concepts Related to Basic Information

- Two conditions that can affect the size of the brain and skull or reflect the amount of brain and skull growth are microcephaly and megalencephaly.
- Skull ossification begins in infancy and continues into adulthood; ossification occurs most rapidly in young children and then begins to slow in early school age.
- The spinal cord and the cranial and peripheral nerves elongate during the growth of childhood; in newborn infants, the cord terminates at L3, and in adults it terminates at L1–L2.
- Of the vital signs, respiratory patterns are the most sensitive indicators of neurologic change, especially change in the brain stem.

- Increased CSF volume is common in children secondary to congenital or acquired hydrocephalus and/or meningitis.
- Infratentorial cranial surgery (below the tentorium or in the posterior fossa) may predispose the child to a greater degree of danger than surgery in the cerebral hemisphere, because of the position of anatomic structures, location of vital centers, and manipulation of the brain stem and cerebellum during posterior fossa surgery.
- Status epilepticus can be defined in two ways: (1) continuous seizure activity that does not stop and (2) seizures that recur rapidly or in succession without a return to consciousness between them.
- A seizure is a sudden, involuntary, time-limited alteration in function occurring as the result of an abnormal discharge of neurons in the central nervous system.
- Epilepsy surgery may be indicated for children with intractable or uncontrolled seizures who have failed to gain seizure control after therapeutic trials with the most appropriate antiepileptic drugs.
- Congenital hydrocephalus occurs in approximately in 0.5 to 1.0 per 1000 live births; acquired hydrocephalus occurs secondary to mass lesions like tumors, vascular malformations or cysts, and scarring of cerebrospinal fluid pathways from infection of intracranial hemorrhage.
- Manifestations of encephalitis may vary greatly from one child to another. One child may be mildly affected, only to lapse suddenly into a coma and die; whereas another child may present with high fever, violent convulsions, bizarre movements, and hallucinations, then recover with relatively few sequelae.

Concepts Related to Nursing Assessment

- Age-related differences in structure and function are important for the interpretation of diagnostic tests and in the nursing care related to monitoring of neurologic function.
- The three most common types of neurologic assessment are the *acute neurologic examination, screening examination,* and *comprehensive examination.*
- Important factors in infant and toddler assessment include head size, shape, and symmetry; motor and social landmarks; presence, absence, and symmetry of developmental reflexes; abdominal examination; and vision and hearing examination.
- An accurate, well-documented preoperative neurologic baseline assessment becomes essential when monitoring the child's postoperative functioning for potential complications.
- Nursing assessment of the child with epilepsy includes *seizure management and precaution,* careful observation and documentation of seizure activity when it does occur, seizure first-aid and safety, assessment of side effects of antiepileptic drugs, and gathering of psychosocial data on patient and family coping.
- Nursing diagnostic responses and collaborative problems for the child with craniosynostosis are *altered tissue perfusion, high risk for infection, significant surgical blood loss and postoperative drainage, altered comfort,* and *ineffective family coping.*
- Factors contributing to the development of NTDs are poor nutrition, maternal age, pregnancy history, birth order, and socioeconomic status.
- The age, developmental level, and level of spinal defect and associated problems greatly affect the priorities in nursing assessment in any given encounter.
- Regardless of the type of injury, a complete neurologic assessment should be done on the first encounter with the child and consistently throughout the hospitalization.

Concepts Related to Nursing Interventions

- It is important to compare changes in the acute neurologic check with other data about the child's condition and to take prompt action, if necessary.
- Nursing care for patients on ICP monitoring focuses on assessing ICP, maintaining monitoring system integrity, and assessing the patient for signs of infection, hemorrhage, and risk of CSF leakage, secondary to and depending on the type of ICP device.
- Nursing care following cranial surgery involves frequent acute neurologic examinations; checking of vital signs and intake and output; assessment of dressing and drainage; monitoring for potential complications; assessment of airway and ventilation; and monitoring of oxygenation, blood gases, and electrolytes.
- Nursing care provided to children with altered responsiveness commonly involves the following nursing diagnostic responses: *self-care deficit, high risk for injury, knowledge deficit,* and *altered family process.*
- Nursing care for the child with epilepsy includes intervening with the following nursing diagnostic responses and collaborative problems: *potential for injury,* and *knowledge deficit.*
- Major nursing care priorities for the child with spinal bifida are preventing infection, preventing neurologic injury, preventing injury to limbs, promoting optimal bowel elimination, managing

neurogenic bladder, promoting parental coping, and promoting positive self-concept.

- Postoperative nursing assessment of the child with a newly placed shunt for hydrocephalus includes cardiorespiratory monitoring; frequent vital signs and neurologic checks; and assessment of skin integrity, pain control, and surgical dressing.
- Family coping skills and knowledge of neurodegenerative disorders are often the best predictors of long-term effects of the disease on the child and family.
- Nursing care for the child with meningitis is directed toward providing comfort and relieving pain, supporting family members to cope, assessing for possible complications, and preparing for discharge.
- Nursing care priorities for the child with a head injury are promoting optimal cerebral tissue perfusion, avoiding airway compromise, responding to altered sensorium and changes in level of consciousness, preventing infection, promoting adaptive family coping, preventing infection, and facilitating home care.

REFERENCES

Adams, J., et al. (1986). Gliding contusions in non-missile head injury in humans. *Archives of Pathology and Laboratory Medicine, 110,* 485–488.

Allanson, J. (1988). Spina bifida: Prenatal diagnosis and genetic counseling. *Barrow Neurological Institute Quarterly, 4*(4), 5–8.

Allen, R. (1982). Degenerative disorders of the central nervous system. In K. Swaiman & F. Wright (Eds.), *The Practice of pediatric neurology* (Vol. 1, pp 881–957). St. Louis: CV Mosby.

American Association of Neuroscience Nurses (1990). *Core curriculum for neuroscience nursing.* Desplaines, IL: Author.

Ammons, A. (1990). Cerebral injuries and intracranial hemorrhages as a result of trauma. *Nursing Clinics of North America, 25*(1), 23–33.

Argenta, L., Adson, M. (1989). Management of scalp injuries. In D. McLaurin et al. (Eds.), *Pediatric neurosurgery* (2nd ed., pp 255–262). Philadelphia: WB Saunders.

Arsenault, L. (1985). Selected postoperative complications of cranial surgery. *Journal of Neurosurgical Nursing, 17*(3), 155–163.

Bailey, R. (1988). Urologic management of spina bifida. *Barrow Neurological Institute Quarterly, 4*(4), 34–36.

Behrman, R. (Ed.) (1992). *Nelson textbook of pediatrics* (14th ed.). Philadelphia: WB Saunders.

Berg, B. O. (1982). Neurocutaneous syndromes. In K. Swaiman & F. Wright (Eds.), *The practice of Pediatric Neurology* (2nd ed. Vol. 2, pp 914–934). St. Louis: CV Mosby.

Bowens, B. A. (1979). The nervous system. In M. Armstrong et al. (Eds.), *McGraw-Hill handbook of clinical nursing.* New York: McGraw-Hill.

Brucker, J., & Laurent, J. (1988). Pediatric craniofacial reconstruction: an overview of perioperative management. *Journal of Neuroscience Nursing, 20*(3), 159–168.

Bruya, M. (1981). Planned periods of rest in the intensive care unit: Nursing care activities and intracranial pressure. *Journal of Neurosurgical Nursing, 13*(4), 184–194.

Camfield, P., & Camfield, C. (1986). Neurologic aspects of craniosynostosis. In M. Cohen (Ed.), *Craniosynostosis: Diagnosis, evaluation, and management* (pp 215–226). New York: Raven Press.

Cherry, J., & Shields, W. (1987). Encephalitis and meningoencephalitis., In R. Feigin, & J. Cherry (Eds.), *Textbook of pediatric infectious diseases* (2nd ed., pp 484–496). Philadelphia: WB Saunders.

Cherry, J. (1987). Aseptic meningitis and viral meningitis. In R. Feigin, & J. Cherry (Eds.), *Textbook of pediatric infectious diseases* (2nd ed., pp 478–484). Philadelphia: WB Saunders.

Cohen, F. (1987). Neural tube defects: Epidemiology, detection, and prevention. *Journal of Obstetric, Gynecologic, and Neonatal Nursing,* (2), 105–115.

Cohen, F. L. (1984). *Clinical genetics in nursing practice.* Philadelphia: JB Lippincott.

Cohen, M. (1986). *Craniosynostosis: Diagnosis, evaluation and management.* New York: Raven Press.

Demyer, W. (1989). Megalencephaly. In K. Swaiman (Ed.), *Pediatric neurology* (Vol. 1, pp 177–184). St. Louis: CV Mosby.

Dreifuss, F. (1981). Proposal for revised clinical and electroencephalographic classification of epileptic seizure. *Epilepsia, 20,* 489–501.

Dyken, F., & Krawiecki, N. (1983). Neurodegenerative diseases of infancy and childhood. *Annals of Neurology, 13*(4), 351–364.

Dyken, P. (1989). Viral diseases of the nervous system. In K. Swaiman (Ed.), *Pediatric neurology* (Vol. 1, pp 474–515). St. Louis: CV Mosby.

Elwood, J., & Elwood, J. (1980). *Epidemiology of anencephalus and spina bifida.* New York: Oxford University Press.

Engel, J. (Ed.) (1987). *Surgical treatment of the epilepses.* New York: Raven Press.

Feigen, R. (1987). Central nervous system infections. In R. Feigen, & J. Cherry (Eds.), *Textbook of pediatric infectious diseases* (2nd ed., pp 439–516). Philadelphia: WB Saunders.

Fenichel, G. (1988). *Clinical pediatric neurology. A signs and symptoms approach.* Philadelphia: WB Saunders.

Ferry, P., et al. (1986). *Seizure disorders in children.* Philadelphia: JB Lippincott.

Friedman, D. (1988). Taking the scare out of caring for seizure patients. *Nursing 88, 18*(2), 53–59.

Glaze, F. (1987). Guillain-Barré syndrome. In R. Feigen, & J. Cherry (Eds.), *Textbook of pediatric infectious diseases* (Vol. 1, pp 507–516). Philadelphia: WB Saunders.

Giubilato, R., & Metcalf, J. (1984). Evoked potentials: Nursing perspectives. *Journal of Neurosurgical Nursing 16*(5), 241–247.

Guthkelch, A. (1988). Occult dysraphism: Clinical findings and management. *Barrow Neurological Institute Quarterly, 4*(4), 21–25.

Hauser, W. (1990). *Epilepsy: Frequency, causes and consequences.* New York: Demos.

Holmes, G. (1987). *Diagnosis and management of seizures in children.* Philadelphia: WB Saunders.

Hunter, A., & Rudd, N. (1977). Craniosynostosis II. Coronal synostosis: Its familial characteristics and associated clinical findings in 109 patients lacking bilateral polysyndactyly or syndactyly. *Tetratology, 15,* 301–310.

Huttenlocher, P. (1987). The nervous system. In R. Behrman (Ed.), *Nelson textbook of pediatrics* (14th ed., pp 1274–1330). Philadelphia: WB Saunders.

Jacobsen, R. (1989). Congenital structural defects. In K. Swaiman (Ed.), *Pediatric neurology* (Vol. 1, pp 317–362). St. Louis: CV Mosby.

James, H. (1989). Encephalocele, dermoid sinus, and arachnoid cyst. In R. McLauren, L. Schut, J. Venes, & F. Epstein (Eds.), *Pediatric neurosurgery* (2nd ed., pp 97–106). Philadelphia: WB Saunders.

Kalsbeck, W. (1980). The national head and spinal cord injury survey: Major findings. *Journal of Neurosurgery, 53,* 519.

Kokich, V. (1986). The biology of sutures. In M. Cohen (Ed.), *Craniosynostosis: Diagnosis, evaluation, and management* (pp 81–103). New York: Raven Press.

Koski, K. (1968). Cranial growth center. *American Journal of Orthodontics, 54,* 566–582.

Krugman, S., & Katz, S. (1981). *Infectious diseases of children* (7th ed.). St. Louis: CV Mosby.

Lindseth, R. (1988). Orthopedic management of myelomeningocele. *Barrow Neurological Institute Quarterly, 4*(4), 26–31.

Lorber, J. (1971). Results of treatment of myelomeningocele: An analysis of 524 unselected cases, with special reference to possible selection for treatment. *Developmental Medicine and Child Neurology, 18,* 279–303.

Louis, H. (1988). Orthopedic management of meningomyelocele: The lower extremities. *Barrow Neurological Institute Quarterly, 4*(4), 32–33.

Marchac, D., & Renier, D. (1982). *Craniofacial surgery for craniosynostosis.* Boston: Little, Brown.

McCloskey, J. C., & Bulechek, G. M. (1992). *Nursing interventions classification (NIC)* (pp 350–351). St. Louis: Mosby–Year Book.

McCullough, D. (1989). Hydrocephalus: Etiology, pathologic effects, diagnosis and natural history. In R. McLaurin, L. Schut, J. Venes, & F. Epstein (Eds.), *Pediatric neurosurgery* (2nd ed., pp 180–199). Philadelphia: WB Saunders.

McLaurin, R. (1989). Ventricular shunts: Complications and results. In R. McLaurin, L. Schut, J. Venes, & F. Epstein (Eds.). *Pediatric neurosurgery* (2nd ed., pp 219–229).

McLaurin, R., & Towbin, R. (1989). Post-traumatic hematomes. In R. McLaurin, L. Schut, J. Venes, & F. Epstein (Eds.), *Pediatric neurosurgery* (2nd ed., pp 277–289). Philadelphia: WB Saunders.

MacBriar, B. R. (1983). Self-concept of pre-adolescent and adolescent children with a meningomyelocele. *Issues in Comprehensive Pediatric Nursing, 6*(1), 1–11.

Macedo, A., & Posel, L. F. (1987). Nursing the family after the birth of a child with spina bifida. *Issues in Comprehensive Pediatric Nursing, 10*(1), 55–65.

Mealey, J. (1989). Skull fractures. In R. McLaurin, L. Schut, J. Venes, & F. Epstein (Eds.), *Pediatric neurosurgery* (2nd ed., pp 263–270). Philadelphia: WB Saunders.

Menezes, A., et al. (1989). Spinal cord injury. In R. McLaurin, L. Schut, J. Venes, & F. Epstein (Eds.), *Pediatric neurosurgery* (2nd ed., pp 298–317). Philadelphia: WB Saunders.

Milhorat, T. (1989). Circulation of cerebrospinal fluid. In R. McLaurin, et al (Eds.), *Pediatric neurosurgery* (2nd ed., pp 170–179). Philadelphia: WB Saunders.

Milhorat, T. (1985). Hydrocephalus, pathophysiology and clinical features. In R. Wilkins, & S. Rengachary (Eds.), *Neurosurgery* (Vol. 3, pp 2135–2140). New York: McGraw-Hill.

Mitchell, P. (1980). Intracranial hypertension: Implications of research for nursing care. *Journal of Neurosurgical Nursing, 12*(3), 145–154.

Mitchell, P., et al. (1981). Moving the patient in bed: Effects on intracranial pressure. *Nursing Research, 30*(4), 212–218.

Mitchell, P. et al. (1984). *Neurological assessment for nursing practice.* Reston, VA: Reston.

Moore, K. (1988). *The developing human* (4th ed.). Philadelphia: WB Saunders.

Mori, K. (1985). *Anomalies of the central nervous system.* New York: Thieme-Stratton.

Nevin, N. (1985). The role of periconception vitamin supplementation in the prevention of neural tube defects, Part B: Epidemiology, early detection and therapy and environmental factors. *Progressive Clinical Biologic Research,* (163) 389.

Nikas, D. (1987). Critical aspects of head trauma. *Critical Care Nursing Quarterly, 10*(1), 19–44.

Oakes, W. (1985). Chiari malformations, hydromyelia, syringomyelia. In R. Wilkins, & S. Rengachary (Eds.), *Neurosurgery* (Vol. 3, pp 2102–2115). New York: McGraw-Hill.

Pang, D., & Wilberger, J. (1982). Spinal cord injury without radiographic abnormalities in children. *Journal of Neurosurgery, 57*(114).

Parsons, L., & Wilson, M. (1984). Cerebrovascular status of severe closed head injured patients following passive position changes. *Nursing Research, 33,* 68–75.

Plum, F. (1980). *The diagnosis of stupor and coma* (3rd ed.). Philadelphia: FA Davis.

Reigel, D. (1989). Spina bifida. In R. McLaurin, L. Schut, J. Venes, & F. Epstein (Eds.), *Pediatric neurosurgery* (2nd ed., pp 35–52). Philadelphia: WB Saunders.

Rekate, H. (1988). Early aggressive treatment of infants born with spina bifida: An ethical imperative. *Barrow Neurological Institute Quarterly, 4*(4), 2–4.

Roberts, C. (1988). Bowel management in spina bifida perspectives and issues. *Barrow Neurological Institute Quarterly, 4*(4), 37–42.

Rowe, P. C. (1987). *The Harriet Lane handbook* (11th ed.). Chicago: Year Book.

Rutkowski, K. (1990). Grid implantation in seizure patients. *AORN Journal, 52*(5), 953–975.

Smith, K., et al (1983). CAT scans: What do they tell us? *Journal of Neurosurgical Nursing, 15*(4), 222–227.

Snyder, M. (1983). Relationship of nursing activities to increase in intracranial pressure. *Journal of Advanced Nursing, 8,* 273–279.

Snyder, R. (1989). Bacterial infections of the nervous system. In K. Swaiman (Ed.), *Pediatric neurology* (Vol. 1, pp 447–473). St. Louis: CV Mosby.

Solomon, E., & Phillips, G. (1987). *Understanding human anatomy and physiology.* Philadelphia: WB Saunders.

Stein, S., Feldman, Apfel, Kohl, & Casey (1981). The epidemiology of congenital hydrocephalus: A study on Brooklyn, NY 1968–1976. *Child's Brain, 8,* 253–262.

Stevens, M. (1982). Post-concussion syndrome. *Journal of Neurosurgical Nursing, 14*(5), 239–244.

Swaiman, K. (1989). Spinal fluid examination. In K. Swaiman (Ed.), *Pediatric neurology.* St. Louis: CV Mosby.

Tatum, S., & Wang, A. (1990). Hemispherectomy—A radical solution. *Today's OR Nurse, 12*(3), 9–12.

Tillum, D., & Greenberg, C. (1988). Nursing care of the child with a ventriculostomy. *Journal of Pediatric Nursing, 3*(3), 188–193.

Winston, K. (1985). Craniosynostosis. In R. H. Wilkins, & S. S. Rengachary (Eds.), *Neurosurgery* (Vol. 3, pp 2173–2191). New York, McGraw-Hill.

Youmans, J. R. (1982). *Neurological surgery* (2nd ed.). Philadelphia: WB Saunders.

Youmans, J. (1990). *Neurological surgery.* Philadelphia: WB Saunders.

Zambramski, J., Hadley, & Browner (1986). Pediatric spinal cord and vertebral column injuries. *Barrow Neurological Institute Quarterly, 2*(11).

Zegeer, L. (1982). Nursing care of the patient with brain edema. *Journal of Neurosurgical Nursing, 14*(5), 268–275.

BIBLIOGRAPHY

Abe, H., et al. (1985). Functional prognosis of surgical treatment of craniosynostosis. *Child's Nervous System, 1*(1), 53–61.

Amacher, A., & Wellington, J. Infant'sile hydrocephalus: Long-term results of surgical therapy. *Child's Brain, 11*(4), 217–229.

Ammann, A., et al. (1984). Pediatric acquired immune deficiency syndrome. *Annals of the New York Academy of Sciences, 437,* 340–349.

Arsenault, L. (1983). Delayed onset symptomatic hydrocephalus related to aqueductal stenosis. *Journal of Neurosurgical Nursing, 15*(5), 291–298.

Austin, J., et al. (1984). Parental attitude and adjustment to epilepsy. *Nursing Research, 33*(2), 92–96.

Bell, W., & McCormick, W. (1978). *Increased intracranial pressure in children* (2nd ed.). Philadelphia: WB Saunders.

Beller, L. C., & Neunaber, K. L. (1986). The "simple" Valsalva. *American Journal of Nursing, 98*(4), 398–399.

Bowens, B. (1985). Injury to the brachial plexus. *Journal of Neurosurgical Nursing, 17*(5), 293–300.

Britton, C., & Miller, J. (1984). Neurologic complications in acquired immune deficiency syndrome. *Neurology Clinics, 2*(2), 315–339.

Brucker, J., & Laurent, J. (1988). Pediatric craniofacial reconstruction: An overview of perioperative management. *Journal of Neuroscience Nursing, 20*(3), 159–168.

Closchesy, J. (1985). Problems in interpreting abnormal auditory brainstem responses in comatose patients. *Journal of Neurosurgical Nursing, 17*(4), 253–255.

Coffman, S. (1986). Description of a nursing diagnosis: Alteration in bowel elimination related to neurogenic bowel in children with myelomeningocele. *Issues in Comprehensive Pediatric Nursing, 9*(3), 179–191.

Conway, B. (1977). *Pediatric neurologic nursing.* St. Louis: CV Mosby.

Conway-Rutcowski, B. (1982). *Carini and Owens' neurological and neurosurgical nursing* (8th ed.). St. Louis: CV Mosby.

Derechin, M. E. (1987). Pediatric head injury. *Critical Care Nursing Quarterly, 10*(3), 12–24.

Dieter, J. (Ed.). (1982). *Epilepsy, pregnancy and the child.* New York: Raven Press.

Davenport-Fortune, P., & Dunnum, L. (1985). Professional nursing care of the patient with increased intracranial pressure: Planned or 'hit and miss'? *Journal of Neurosurgical Nursing, 17*(6), 367–370.

Donovan, W., & Bedrock, S. (1982). Comprehensive management of spinal cord injury. *Clinical Symposium, 34*(2), 1–36.

Droske, S., & Francis, S. (1981). *Pediatric diagnostic procedures.* New York: John Wiley & Sons.

Eggleston, C., & Cruvant, D. (1983). Review of recovery from intracerebral hematoma in children and adults. *Journal of Neurosurgical Nursing, 15*(3), 128–135.

Ellenberg, J., et al. (1984). Age at onset of seizures in young children. *Annals of Neurology, 15*(2), 127–134.

Epstein, F. (1985). How to keep shunts functioning, or the 'impossible dream.' *Clinics of Neurosurgery, 32,* 608–631.

Fisher, D., et al. (1982). Increase in intracranial pressure during suctioning-stimulation vs. rise in PaCO. *Anesthesiology, 57,* 416–417.

Fisher, J. (1987, January). What you need to know about neurological testing. *RN,* pp. 47–53.

Fode, N. C. (1988). Subarachnoid hemorrhage from ruptured intracranial aneurysm. *American Journal of Nursing, 88*(5), 673–680.

Foy, P., et al. (1981). The incidence of postoperative seizures. *Acta Neurochirurgie, 55,* 253–264.

Frank, J. (1990). Epilepsy: The school nurse's dilemma. *Journal of School Health, 60*(1), 34–35.

Frank, J., & Fischer, R. G. (1987). Drug interactions with carbamazepine. *Pediatric Nursing, 13*(1), 54–55.

French, B. (1989). Abnormal development of the central nervous system. In R. McLaurin, L. Schut, J. Venes, & F. Epstein (Eds.), *Pediatric neurosurgery* (2nd ed., pp. 9–34). Philadelphia: WB Saunders.

Friedman, D. (1988). Taking the scare out of caring for seizure patients. *Nursing 88, 18*(2), 53–60.

Gapen, P. (1982). Neurological complications now characterizing many AIDS victims. *JAMA, 248*(22), 1941–1942.

Gastaut, H. (1973). *Dictionary of epilepsy, part 1: Definitions.* Geneva: World Health Organization.

Giubilato, R., & Metcalf, J. (1984). Evoked potentials: Nursing perspectives. *Journal of Neurosurgical Nursing, 16*(5), 241–247.

Grant, L. (1984). Hydrocephalus: An overview and update. *Journal of Neurosurgical Nursing, 16*(6), 313–318.

Greene, M. (1991). *The Harriet Lane handbook* (12th ed.). Chicago: Mosby.

Griebel, R., et al. (1985). CSF shunt complications: An analysis of contributory factors. *Child's Nervous System, 1*(2), 77–80.

Griswold, K., et al. (1984). An approach to the care of patients with Guillain-Barré syndrome. *Heart and Lung, 13*(1), 66–72.

Guin, P. (1985). Arnold-Chiari malformation—A closer look. *Journal of Neurosurgical Nursing, 17*(1), 45–52.

Gumnit, R. (1983). *The epilepsy handbook. The practical management of seizures.* New York: Raven Press.

Hanno, R., & Beck, R. (1987). Tuberous sclerosis. *Neurology Clinics, 5*(3), 351–360.

Hayden, P. (1983). A longitudinal study of shunt function in 360 patients with hydrocephalus. *Developmental Medicine and Child Neurology, 25*(3), 334–337.

Hazinski, M. (1992). *Nursing care of the critically ill child* (2nd ed.). St. Louis: CV Mosby.

Hazinski, M. (1990). Postoperative care of the critically ill child. *Critical Care Clinics of North America, 2*(4), 599–610.

Hindfelt, B. (1976). The prognostic significance of subfebrility and fever in ischemic cerebral infarction. *Acta Neurologica Scandinavica, 53,* 72–79.

Hinkle, J. L. (1986). Treating traumatic coma. *American Journal of Nursing, 86*(5), 551–556.

Hobdell, E. F. (1988). Infantile spasms. *Pediatric Nursing, 14*(3), 207–209.

Hummelgard, A. (1984). Prognostic value of brainstem auditory evoked potentials in head trauma. *Journal of Neurosurgical Nursing, 16*(4), 181–187.

Hunt, A. (1983). Tuberous sclerosis: A survey of 97 cases, I: Seizures, pertussis, immunization, and handicap. II: Physical findings. III: Family aspects. *Developmental Medicine and Child Neurology, 25*(3), 346–357.

International League Against Epilepsy. (1981). Proposal for revised clinical and electroencephalographic classification of epileptic seizures. *Epilepsia, 22,* 489.

Jackson, P. L. (1990). Primary care needs of children with hydrocephalus. *Journal of Pediatric Health Care, 4*(2), 59–71.

Jess, L. W. (1987). Assessing your patient for increased I.C.P. *Nursing 87, 17*(6), 34–41.

Kennedy, R., et al. (1978). Guillain-Barré syndrome: A 42 year epidemiologic and clinical study. *Mayo Clinic Proceedings, 53,* 93.

LaFerla, G., et al. (1984). A simple method of assessing intracranial pressure in hydrocephalic patients with shunts. *Developmental Medicine and Child Neurology, 26*(6), 732–736.

Lipe, H. (1985). Prevention of nervous system trauma from travel in motor vehicles. *Journal of Neurosurgical Nursing, 17*(2), 77–82.

Lundgren, J. (1986). *Acute neuroscience nursing: Concepts and care.* Boston: Jones and Bartlett.

Marida, M. (1982). Regional cerebral blood flow: Patient correlations. *Journal of Neurosurgical Nursing, 14*(6), 309–314.

Marshall, J. A teaching plan: Ventriculoperitoneal shunting procedure. *AORN Journal, 40*(6), 847–851.

Marshall, J., & Ross, J. (1984). Hydrocephalus: Ventriculoperitoneal shunting in infants and children. *AORN Journal, 40*(6), 842–846.

Matthew, E., et al. (1980). Seizures following intracranial surgery: Incidence in the first postoperative week. *Canadian Journal of Neurological Sciences, 7,* 285–290.

Mauldin, R., & Coleman, I. (1983). Intracerebral herniation. *Journal of Neurosurgical Nursing, 15*(5), 287–290.

McCracken, G., & Freij, B. (1987). Perinatal bacterial diseases. In R. Feigin, & J. Cherry (Eds.), *Textbook of pediatric infectious diseases* (2nd ed., pp. 940–966). Philadelphia: WB Saunders.

McLaurin, R., Schut, L., Venes, J., & Epstein, F. (Eds.). (1989). *Pediatric neurosurgery* (2nd ed., pp. 180–199). Philadelphia: WB Saunders.

McLaurin, R. (1989). Ventricular shunts: Complications and results. In R. McLauren, L. Schut, J. Venes, & F. Epstein (Eds.), *Pediatric neurosurgery* (2nd ed., pp. 219–229). Philadelphia: WB Saunders.

Messner, R., et al. (1985). Neurofibromatosis: A familial and family disorder. *Journal of Neurosurgical Nursing, 17*(4), 221–229.

Miezio, P. (1983). *Parenting children with disability.* New York: Marcel Dekker.

Milhorat, T. (1978). *Pediatric neurosurgery.* Philadelphia: FA Davis.

Millar, S. (1980). *Methods in critical care.* Philadelphia: WB Saunders.

Miller, J., & Arsenault, L. (1983). Reye's syndrome. *Journal of Neurosurgical Nursing, 15*(3), 154–164.

Mills, N., & Plasterer, H. (1980). Guillain-Barré syndrome: A framework for nursing care. *Nursing Clinics of North America, 15*(2), 257–264.

Mitchell, P. (1986). Decreased adaptive capacity, intracranial: A proposal for a nursing diagnosis. *Journal of Neuroscience Nursing, 18*(4), 170–175.

Mitchell, P. (Ed.) (1988). *AANN's neuroscience nursing: Phenomena and practice.* Norwalk, CT: Appleton-Lange.

Moore, P. C. (1988, June). When you have to think small for a neurologic exam. *RN,* pp. 38–44.

Nelson, C., & Miner, M. (1983). Brain injury disseminated intravascular coagulation and fibrinolysis syndrome in children. *Journal of Neurosurgical Nursing, 15*(2), 72–76.

Neveling, E., & Truex, R. (1983). External obstructive hydrocephalus: A study of clinical and developmental aspects in ten children. *Journal of Neurosurgical Nursing, 15*(4), 255–260.

Nurse's hotline helps the spinal cord–injured. (1987). *American Journal of Nursing, 87*(5), 720–721.

Paisley, J., et al. (1992). Infections: Viral and rickettsial. In W. Hathaway et al. (Eds.), *Current pediatric diagnosis and treatment* (10th ed.). Norwalk, CT: Appleton-Lange.

Passo, S. (1980). Malformations of the neural tube. *Nursing Clinics of North America, 15*(1), 5–21.

Pellock, J., & Meyer, E. (1983). *Neurologic emergencies in infancy and childhood.* New York: Harper & Row.

Pinyerd, B. (1983). Siblings of children with myelomengocele: Examining their perceptions. *Maternal-Child Nursing Journal, 12*(1), 61–70.

Post, E. (1985). Currently available shunt systems: A review. *Neurosurgery, 16*(2), 257–260.

Rainer, J., & Hollis, J. (1983). Evaluation of the comatose patient. *Journal of Neurosurgical Nursing, 15*(5), 283–286.

Remington, P., et al. (1986). Decreasing trends in Reye's syndrome and aspirin use in Michigan, 1979 to 1984. *Pediatrics, 77*(1), 93–98.

Renier, D., et al. (1982). Intracranial pressure in craniostenosis. *Journal of Neurosurgery, 57*(3), 370–377.

Rhodes, M., & Grossner, B. (1983). Complications of posterior fossa craniotomy. *Journal of Neurosurgical Nursing, 15*(1), 9–12.

Riccardi, V. M. (1987). Neurofibromatosis. *Neurology Clinics 5*(3), 337–349.

Richardson, K., et al. (1985). Biofeedback therapy for managing bowel incontinence caused by meningomyelocele. *MCN: American Journal of Maternal Child Nursing, 10*(6), 388–392.

Rogers, M., et al. (1985). National Reye's syndrome surveillance, 1982. *Pediatrics, 75*(2), 260–264.

Romeo, J. H. (1988, April). The critical minutes after spinal cord injury. *RN,* pp. 61–67.

Romeo, J. H. (1988, May). Spinal cord injury: Nursing the patient toward a new life. *RN,* pp. 31–35.

Rosman, N. P., & Herskowitz, J. (1982). Trauma to the brain and spinal cord. In K. F. Swaiman, & F. S. Wright (Eds.), *The practice of pediatric neurology* (Vol. 2, pp. 958–997). St. Louis: CV Mosby.

Rudy, E. (1985). Magnetic resonance imaging: New horizon in diagnostic techniques. *Journal of Neurosurgical Nursing, 17*(6), 331–337.

Sagraves, R. (1990). Antiepileptic drug therapy for pediatric generalized tonic-clonic seizures. *Journal of Pediatric Health Care, 4*(6), 314–319.

Santilla, N., et al. (1991). *Students with seizures: A manual for school nurses.* Cedar Grove, NJ: Health Scan.

Santilli, N., & Tonelson, S. (1981). Screening for seizures. *Pediatric Nursing, 7*(2), 11–15.

Scherer, P. (1986). Assessment: The logic of coma. *American Journal of Nursing, 86*(5), 542–550.

Scherz, R. (1981). Fatal motor vehicle accidents of child passengers from birth to 4 years of age in Washington State. *Pediatrics, 68,* 572–575.

Simpson, J. (1984). Neurological disorders with autosomal dominant transmission. *Journal of Neurosurgical Nursing, 16*(5), 262–269.

Slota, M. (1983, November/December). Pediatric neurological assessment. *Critical Care Nursing,* pp. 106–112.

Smith, J. (1988). Big differences in little people. *American Journal of Nursing, 88*(4), 458–462.

Snider, W. (1983). Neurological complications of acquired immune deficiency syndrome: Analysis of 50 patients. *Annals of Neurology, 18*(4), 403–418.

Snyder, M. (1983). Effect of relaxation on psychosocial functioning in persons with epilepsy. *Journal of Neurosurgical Nursing, 15*(4), 250–254.

Snyder, M. (1991). *A guide to neurological and neurosurgical nursing* (2nd ed.). New York: Delmar.

Tessier, P. (1971). Relationship of craniostenoses to craniofacial dystoses and to faciostenosis, a study with therapeutic implications. *Plastic Reconstructive Surgery, 48,* 224–237.

Tse, A. M. (1986). Seizures and societal attitudes: A teaching tool for children, siblings, classmates, parents, and classroom teachers. *Issues in Comprehensive Pediatric Nursing, 9*(5), 299–303.

Vlahov, D., et al. (1984). Neurosurgical wound infections: Methodological and clinical factors affecting calculations of infection rates. *Journal of Neurosurgical Nursing, 16*(3), 128–133.

Winston, K. (1985). Craniosynostosis. In R. Wilkins, & S. Rengachary (Eds.), *Neurosurgery* (Vol. 3, pp. 2173–2191). New York: McGraw-Hill.

Wong, D. Changing what children hear in the ICU can lower intracranial pressure. *American Journal of Nursing, 88*(3), 279–280.

Wong, J., et al. (1984). Care of the unconscious patient: A problem oriented approach. *Journal of Neurosurgical Nursing, 16*(3), 145–150.

Wulf, J. (1986). Effects of observer variables and seizure attributes on seizure observation and documentation. *Epilepsia, 27*(5), 632.

CHAPTER • 41

Altered Musculoskeletal Function

Kimberly J. Mason
Stephanie Wright

RELATED TOPICS
Stress, Crisis, and Coping, Chapter 18
Impact of chronic illness, Chapter 19
Impact of death and dying, Chapter 20
Pain management, Chapter 25
Genetic counseling, Chapter 31
Patterns of inheritance, Chapter 31
Juvenile arthritis, Chapter 37
Bone tumors, Chapter 42
Injured child, Chapter 46

LEARNING OBJECTIVES

At the conclusion of reading the chapter, the reader will be able to:

- Name and describe the common orthopedic conditions in children.
- Discuss common orthopedic treatment modalities.
- Describe the therapeutic uses and hazards of immobility.
- Identify the major signs of neurovascular impairment.
- Plan the nursing care of children with selected pediatric orthopedic conditions.

Musculoskeletal problems in children are common because of the rapid growth of bones and muscles combined with a child's normal physical activity. Pediatric orthopedic problems range from temporary alterations in health, such as fractures, to life-long conditions, such as cerebral palsy. The need for nursing intervention with the child and family may be short-term or extend over years. The wide variety of problems and interventions makes pediatric orthopedic nursing a challenging and diverse area of practice.

Age-Related Differences in Structure and Function

Children's bones are unique. Young bones contain a larger amount of cartilage, which makes them flexible. They are also more porous, so they absorb a larger amount of energy before fracturing. Young bones also have an active growth area or growth plate called the physis. At the physis, cartilage is rapidly produced in vertical columns and converted to bone for longitudinal growth. Most bones have a physis, which is active until skeletal maturity. The functioning growth plate is an area of vulnerability. It is a weak point in the bone structure, particularly at the interface between the cartilage and bone. Injury to the growing cells of the growth plate can have long-term consequences on bone development.

Healing of bone in children follows the same process as in adults, but young bone heals quickly because a thick periosteum provides an abundant blood supply. Overgrowth can result from increased circulation to a fracture and the growth plates of the bone. Bone is a dynamic tissue that is constantly being absorbed and re-formed in response to stress. As bones continue to grow, children are capable of remodeling or straightening some bone deformities that result from injury or treatment.

Remodeling is the correction of an injury at the fracture site through the build-up of callus. Fractures remodel best in the plane of motion, so that some sideway shift and overriding may be acceptable when the fracture is reduced. Rotational deformities will not always remodel. Bone remodeling is not exact: age, angular deformity, and location of the injury have key roles. Figure 41–1 illustrates how remodeling occurs. The more rapid the rate of growth, the more rapidly healing and remodeling occur. Both of these processes tend to decline with age. Table 41–1 summa-

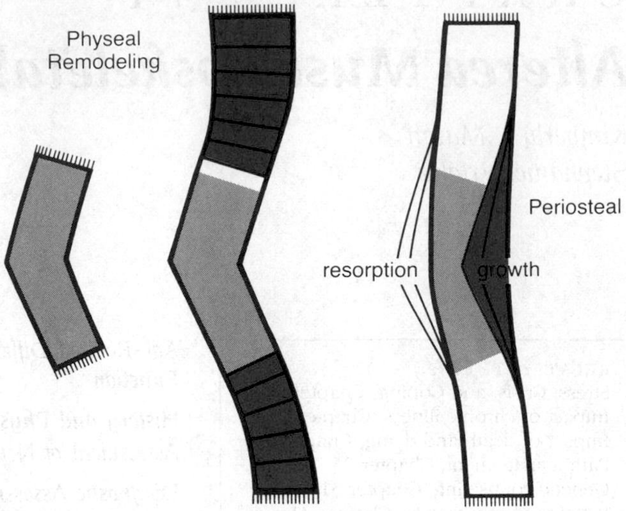

FIGURE 41 - 1. The basis of fracture remodeling. (From Rang, M. [1983]. *Children's fractures*. Philadelphia: JB Lippincott.)

TABLE 41 - 1
Age-Related Structure and Function

Structure and Function	Significance for Nursing Care
Epiphyseal Growth Plate	
• Area at each end of bone where cartilage is converted to bone for longitudinal growth	Child should be monitored for growth disturbance, especially during periods of rapid growth
• Area of weakness in bone • Injury can cause growth disturbances	Parents need information about potential for growth disturbances
Thick Periosteum	
• Supplies bone with blood vessels and nutrients	Periosteal hinge may aid reduction of fracture
• May remain intact with fractures • Produces callus quickly	Injury to periosteum (open fracture) may slow healing
Growing Bones	
• Abundant blood supply	Bone remodeling is not exact
• Able to remodel some bone deformities • Produce callus quickly	Rapid healing makes internal fixation unnecessary in most children
Flexible Bones	
• Higher porosity than adult bones • Absorb more energy before breaking • High amount of energy necessary for bone injury • Bones may bow but not fracture	Fractures in children less than 1 year of age are unusual because large amount of force is necessary; nurse should correlate history with x-ray to rule out caretaker abuse or underlying pathophysiologic mechanism
Range of Motion Decreases with Age	
• Soft tissues resilient in children	Dislocations and sprains unusual

rizes the developmental differences in the musculoskeletal system.

History and Physical Examination

Assessment of the musculoskeletal system includes a complete history of musculoskeletal problems. Subjective information about problems related to movement and musculoskeletal function should be elicited during a family interview, including physical limitations and alterations in lifestyle and necessary mobility aids. When the family is interviewed, the child should provide as much information as possible. Adolescents, in particular, should be responsible for most of the history. During the interview, the nurse should gather information about general health and health problems. The interview and physical assessment should follow the guidelines in Chapter 13 on health appraisal.

In assessment of the musculoskeletal system (see Chapter 13), the examiner should use the unaffected extremity for comparison. In addition, height and weight measurements should be obtained whenever possible. A wheelchair scale is necessary for wheelchair-bound patients. During the physical assessment, the nurse should be alert for any manifestations of musculoskeletal disease, as described in Table 41–2.

Assessment of Neurovascular Status

Assessment of neurovascular status, part of the initial assessment of the child, provides a baseline for future assessments. Assessment of neurovascular status includes evaluation of the following eight areas: color, temperature, sensation, motion, pain, pulse, capillary filling, and edema (Table 41–3). The examiner should use the unaffected extremity for comparison or obtain information on neurovascular status from emergency department personnel or the physician.

The greatest hazard of musculoskeletal trauma or surgery is injury to the blood vessels and nerves. Trauma, whether accidental or part of the treatment, may be accompanied by swelling or compression that can interfere with vessels and damage nerves, causing irreparable injury and permanent damage and disability. *One of the key responsibilities of the nurse caring for the patient with musculoskeletal problems is the intermittent assessment of neurovascular status to ensure that no change in neurologic or circulatory function has occurred.*

The frequency of assessment of neurovascular status depends on the diagnosis or extent of injury. A general rule is hourly until normal, then every 4 hours during the acute postoperative or postinjury period. Documentation of neurovascular assessments should be clear and precise. The terminology used should be descriptive in nature, and judgmental terms (i.e., good, poor) should be avoided because they do not convey accurate information.

TABLE 41–2
Clinical Manifestations of Musculoskeletal Disease

Clinical Manifestations	Pathophysiology
Pain, redness, swelling	Inflammation
	Damage to soft tissues
Asymmetry of body parts, length discrepancies	Due to displacement of bone fragments
	Alteration in growth
	Congenital abnormality
Abnormal turning or rotation of body part	Muscle imbalance
	Congenital or acquired angular or rotational abnormality
	Normal developmental variation
Limitation of joint motion	Soft tissue tightness
	Abnormal muscle tension (spasm)
Crepitus	Movement of bone fragments against one another
Weakness	Soft tissue injury
	Neurologic injury
	Neurologic disease
	Muscle disease
Limp or abnormal gait	Leg length discrepancy
	Neurologic disease
	Muscle disease
	Hip abnormality or disease
Contractures	Increased muscle tone
	Limited movement

Diagnostic Assessment

Common diagnostic procedures used in children with musculoskeletal problems are described in Table 41–4. Radiographs (x-rays) are the most common diagnostic procedure, and serial x-rays may be required to assess progression of healing. Other tests and procedures may be helpful in the diagnosis of individual conditions or complications.

Therapeutic Management

Immobilization

Immobilization is generally the treatment for musculoskeletal disorders, whether part or all of the body is immobilized. When working with patients with mus-

TABLE 41-3
Neurovascular Assessment

Normal Findings	Abnormal Findings	Nursing Intervention
Color		
Skin color should be normal and comparable to unaffected extremity; some redness may accompany swelling	Pallor or cyanosis may indicate circulatory compromise	Place extremity at level of heart: reassess in 15 to 30 mins; notify physician if unchanged
Temperature		
Temperature should be warm or comparable to unaffected extremity; warmth indicates good perfusion	Coolness may be due to cool environment, evaporation from cast as it dries, or circulatory compromise	Close observation: temperature should improve once cast is dry; notify physician if extremity remains cool
Sensation		
Normal sensation in all parts of limb, comparable to unaffected extremity	Numbness, tingling, or decreased sensation may indicate nerve injury or pressure on nerves from immobilizing device or edema	Reposition limb and repeat assessment out of child's sight; note location and boundaries of altered sensation; notify physician
Motion		
Full range of motion within confines of immobilization; some discomfort with movement is normal in acute phase	Limited range of motion in immobilized joints may be due to pain, restriction by immobilizing device, or nerve injury	Reposition; check fit and position of immobilizing device to see if it is impeding movement; trim or readjust as necessary
Pain		
Some pain is normal after trauma or surgery; pain should decrease once bone is immobilized or during the first week after surgery	Pain may indicate inadequate analgesia; excessive or increasing pain may indicate neurovascular compromise	Assess pain using physiologic cues and an age-appropriate rating scale; reposition extremity; administer analgesics as ordered; monitor for other signs of neurovascular compromise; notify physician
Pulse		
Normal pulse should be present distal to injury or immobilizing device	Poor or absent pulse may indicate vascular injury or pressure from immobilizing device	Palpate distal pulses if not covered by immobilizing device; if not palpable, reposition limb and reassess; position limb at level of heart if possible; Doppler may be necessary to auscultate pulse; notify physician
Capillary Filling		
Capillary filling should be <2 secs and comparable to unaffected extremity	Capillary refill >2 secs indicates vascular compromise or pressure from immobilizing device	Press each nail bed and observe return of color; reposition limb and reassess; assess pulse using palpation or Doppler; notify physician
Edema		
Edema is usually present after injury or surgery and is most evident in uncasted, dependent areas	Excessive edema may indicate constriction of vessels from immobilizing device; excessive edema can compromise neurovascular structures	Apply ice packs to affected extremity as soon as possible after injury or surgery; elevate extremity above the level of the heart unless pulse is diminished; assess circulatory and neurologic status

culoskeletal disorders, the nurse must be aware of the hazards of immobility and the nurse's role in preventing them. Table 41–5 lists the physiologic hazards of immobility and nursing interventions for prevention. The goal should be to maximize a child's mobility to prevent these complications.

Emotional and Social Effects

Most children are by nature extremely active beings. Interfering with their normal activity is not without consequences. Immobilization for musculoskeletal conditions may involve physical restraint and discomfort. Immobilizing a child for an extended period interferes with usual methods of dissipating frustrations and anxieties while imposing many new frustrations and reasons to be anxious. The lack of physical activity and the unfamiliar environment may cause the child to regress and demonstrate behaviors common to a younger child. The inability of young children to understand the reason for what has happened leads them to their own conclusions about their predicament. Not unusually, one of these conclusions is that they are being punished. To counter this, all treatment regimens must be explained in age-appropriate language with diagrams or roentgenographs, or both,

TABLE 41-4
Diagnostic Assessment in Musculoskeletal Function

Test	Purpose/Description	Comments
Radiographic Studies		
Plain x-ray	Use of gamma rays to produce an image that allows visualization of bony structures for detection of bone/joint abnormalities or to determine bone age	Young children require immobilization; prepare adequately to ensure cooperation; no dietary restrictions indicated
Scanography	X-rays of long bones on a film with a ruler to accurately measure bone lengths	Young children require immobilization
Angiography	Radiopaque contrast medium injected into circulation to study vascular structures	Procedure not painful but may cause some discomfort; check for allergies to iodine, contrast media, or shellfish; NPO 8–12 hrs before procedure; sedation may be required
Arthrography	Examination of joint after injection of radiopaque dye or air to outline soft tissue structures and contour of joint	Joint may be put through range of motion under fluoroscopy; check for allergy to contrast media; compression dressing for 12 hrs after arthrogram
Bone scan	Study of uptake of radioactive material injected intravenously; uptake of isotope is higher in areas of increased metabolic activity, such as tumors, infection, inflammation	2- to 3-hr wait between injection of radioisotope and scan; young children require sedation
Computed tomography (CT) scan	Narrow-beam x-ray used in conjunction with a computer to scan an area in successive layers; computer calculates different x-ray densities to visualize anatomic details	May or may not use contrast medium; length of procedure necessitates sedation of young children; CT may be frightening
Magnetic Resonance Imaging (MRI)	Use of magnetic force to stimulate nuclei of cells; image depends on density of cells; visualizes marrow, bone and soft tissue tumors, anatomic delineation of muscles, ligaments, and bones	Patients with metal implants, pacemakers, or prosthetics may be restricted from having procedure; length of procedure necessitates sedation of young children; MRI scanner may be frightening
Arthroscopy	Surgical procedure that permits visualization of the inside of a joint for diagnosis and treatment of cartilaginous, meniscal, capsular, and ligamentous injury	Surgical procedure requires surgical preparation and anesthesia; prepare for postoperative swelling, pain, pressure dressings, altered mobility
Joint Aspiration	Withdrawal of fluid from joint for analysis, usually to detect infection or inflammation or to relieve pain when joint swelling and effusion are present	Local anesthetic used; some discomfort may be expected during and after procedure
Somatosensory Evoked Potentials	Uses cutaneous electrodes to measure conduction along nerve pathways to evaluate sensory and motor nerve function during spinal surgery	Patient may feel discomfort during nerve stimulation
Pulmonary Function Tests	Measures lung volume and capacity through measurement of air volumes on forced exhalation to identify obstructive or restrictive pulmonary conditions	Patient may experience discomfort from the nose clip
Ultrasound	Uses high-frequency mechanical vibration to create echoes as the sound waves cross boundaries between tissues; the echoes are transformed into a visual image	Small babies should be NPO for 2–3 hrs before the procedure so they can eat during the test

and with explanations of their benefit to the child's health.

Although many musculoskeletal conditions are reversible in nature, many also require long-term treatment. Adults, adolescents, and some older children are able to comprehend a month or longer plan of treatment, but the perception of this time frame in young children is absent and in many older children may be distorted. When progress is slow, children need frequent reassurance that they are getting well and that the time in cast or traction is limited.

Children who are immobilized are socially isolated from their usual world and have limited peer contact. Sensory deprivation easily occurs in a hospital room. Children in our culture are normally exposed to daily sensory and intellectual stimulation at school or preschool and at home. Normalizing the environment as much as possible is the aim. The child and family should be encouraged to create a homelike atmosphere in the patient's surroundings. Change of surroundings is always beneficial when not medically contraindicated. Parents need information about how to deal with regressive behaviors as well as suggestions about how to divert the child's attention while immobilized. Activities such as coloring, other arts and crafts, video games, and reading should be used to provide diversion. Encouraging visits by friends to participate in these activities can provide important social contact for the immobilized child. The caregivers should give the child opportunities to

TABLE 41–5
Hazards of Immobility

Body System	Pathophysiology	Clinical Manifestations	Nursing Interventions
Respiratory	Decreased chest and lung expansion Decreased respiratory effort and effects of gravity	Slower and more shallow respirations Pooling of secretions Decreased cough reflex	Turn, cough, and deep breathing Incentive spirometer Monitor vital signs Chest physiotherapy/vibration Mobilize as soon as possible
Cardiovascular	Vasodilatation and impaired venous return Muscular inactivity Decreased respiratory effort and gravity Redistribution of body fluids	Circulatory stasis Venous dilation in dependent parts Decreased thoracic and abdominal pressures Decreased cardiac rate, circulatory volume, and arterial pressure	Turn Active/passive range of motion Elastic stockings to lower extremities Mobilize as soon as possible
Musculoskeletal	Decreased bone stress and muscle tension Imbalance between osteoblastic and osteoclastic activity leads to calcium and phosphorus loss Decreased muscle tone	Decreased muscle mass and strength Decreased bone mass and strength	Active/passive range of motion Isometric/isotonic exercises Mobilize as soon as possible
Metabolic	Decreased basal metabolic rate and oxygen consumption Nitrogen loss and negative nitrogen balance due to protein loss from loss of muscle mass	Decreased efficiency in using nutrients Increased potassium and clacium excretion Decreased appetite	Small, frequent meals Increased fiber, protein, vitamin C, acidifying foods Limit calcium intake Mobilize as soon as possible
Skin	Negative nitrogen balance Continuous pressure on bone prominences	Increased potential for skin breakdown	Avoid positions that put pressure on bony prominences Turn regularly Keep skin clean and dry Lotion to dry skin areas Pressure-equalizing and pressure-reducing devices
Elimination	General muscle weakness and atrophy Inactivity slows peristalsis Urinary stasis in renal pelvis	Constipation Urinary retention Renal calculi Anorexia	Establish baseline for elimination pattern Encourage adequate fluid intake Monitor urine characteristics Stool softeners or suppositories to facilitate bowel elimination

exert control by allowing choices, such as food and daily schedule, whenever possible. Maintaining a normal family schedule and activities can provide a familiar and reassuring structure to the child who is immobilized. A tutor must be provided to continue school work.

A few maladaptive patterns are seen among children and families when children require long-term immobilization. These include the child's becoming demanding, the parent's becoming over-indulgent, or the child's becoming overly submissive or withdrawn. The nurse needs to respond to these situations in a therapeutic fashion to help establish a more healthy pattern of interaction. Children and families may require psychologic counseling. Most children have resilient coping mechanisms and will master the crisis of immobilization with reassurance and age-appropriate support.

Casts

Casts are circumferential, rigid dressings. Casts are used to immobilize a bone or joint and to support and protect a realigned bone. Immobilization in a cast can promote healing and permit early weight bearing. Casts may also be used to correct deformities by progressive stretching of soft tissues.

TABLE 41-6
Casting Materials

	Advantages	Disadvantages
Plaster	• Readily conforms to body contours • Inexpensive	• Many layers required for adequate strength • Extended drying time
Synthetic/fiber glass	• Lightweight • Very strong for weight • Quick-drying	• Delayed weight bearing • Does not conform well to body contours • Dust may cause skin irritation • Expensive

The most commonly used casting materials are plaster of Paris and fiber glass (Table 41–6). Casting material is applied to an extremity that has been covered with cast padding or stockinette to protect the skin and cushion the bone prominences. The casting material is dipped in water and wrapped around the extremity. As it is wrapped, the casting material is molded to the shape of the extremity to immobilize the bones and make the cast comfortable. Whether the casting material is plaster or synthetic, heat is generated as the material sets. Drying time varies with the type of material.

Common types of casts are illustrated in Figure 41–2. The nurse should explain the purpose of the

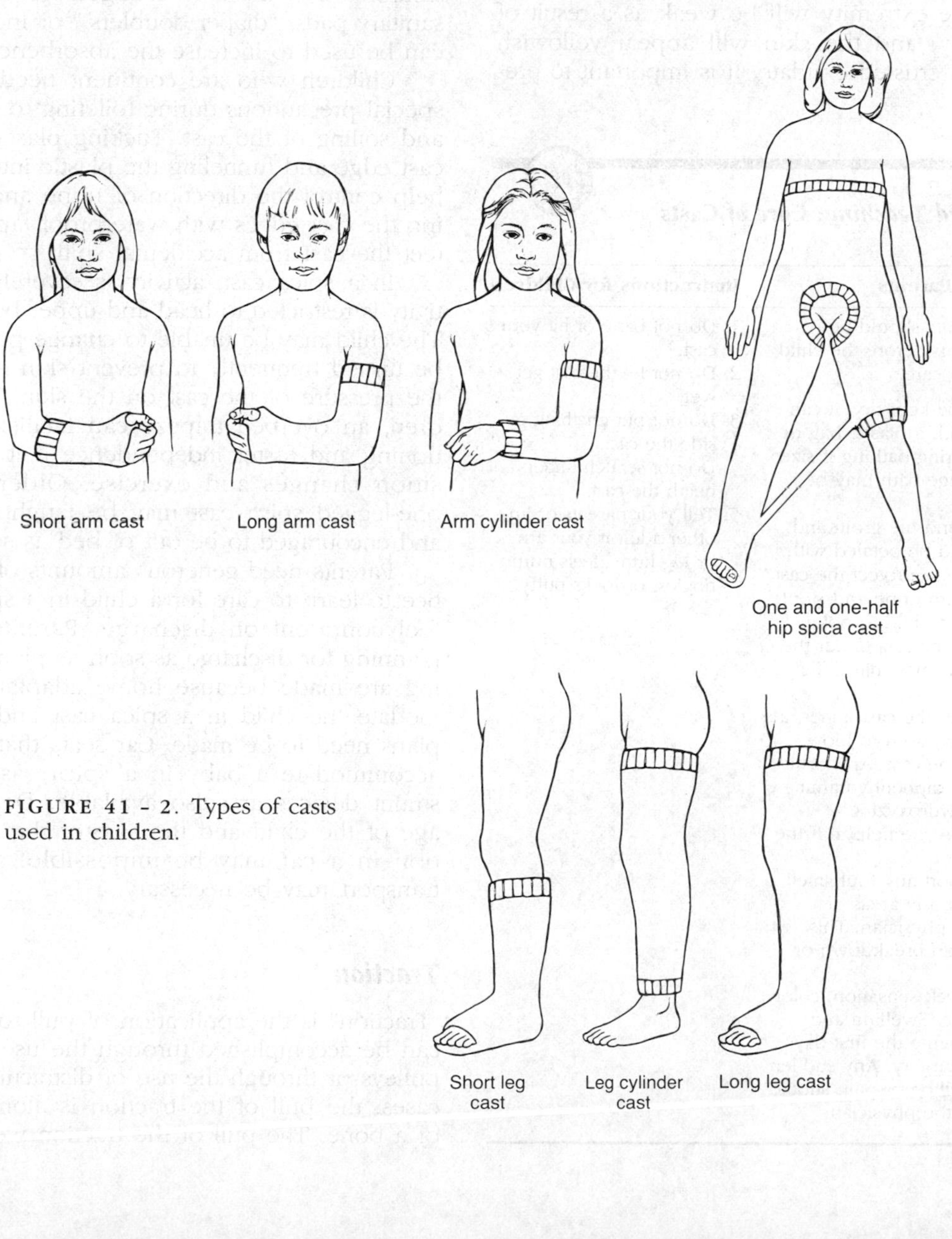

FIGURE 41-2. Types of casts used in children.

cast and how it is applied. The nurse can demonstrate the casting procedure on a doll or show the child a picture of the type of cast that will be used. The nurse may assist with cast application by holding the extremity and explaining each step to the child. The child needs to be told that the cast will feel warm at first. Later, as the cast material dries, the extremity will feel cold and clammy until the moisture can evaporate.

Most children have casts applied as outpatients and are cared for at home. The most important aspects of home management are protecting the cast from damage and observing the extremity to detect possible complications. The family must receive explicit discharge instructions about care of the cast and management of daily activities before being sent home (Table 41–7).

Cast removal is frightening to children because of the appearance and noise of the cast saw. The overwhelming fear is that it will cut the skin. Thorough preparation is necessary for cooperation, preferably with a demonstration of the cast cutter. After the cast is removed, the extremity will be weak as a result of muscle atrophy, and the skin will appear yellowish and scaly from crusted exudate. It is important to prepare children and parents for the appearance of the extremity after removal of the cast and to assure them that the changes to the skin and smaller size are only temporary.

TABLE 41-7
Family-Centered Teaching: Care of Casts and Skin

Instructions for Parents	Instructions for Children
The following points should be reviewed with parents before the child is discharged from care. 1. The cast must be kept dry; it can be protected with a plastic bag or plastic wrap during bathing if size permits. A sponge bath may be necessary. 2. Cast edges around the groin and perineum should be petaled with waterproof tape to protect the cast and padding from urine and stool. 3. Do not allow the child to poke pencils or other objects under the cast because this may injure the skin. 4. If the skin under the cast itches, a hair dryer can be used to blow cool air under the cast. An antihistamine, such as diphenhydramine (Benadryl) or hydroxyzine (Atarax) may also be helpful if the itching is severe. 5. You should report any foul smell from the cast or any areas of drainage to the physician. This may indicate skin breakdown or infection. 6. You should check sensation, color, and temperature. Swelling and pain are most acute the first days after injury or surgery. Any sudden increase in swelling or pain should be reported to the physician.	1. Do not bang or hit your cast. 2. Do not let the cast get wet. 3. Do not put anything inside the cast. 4. Do not scratch underneath the cast. 5. Tell your parents or another adult if your arm or leg hurts, feels numb, tingles, or looks puffy.

Care of a Child in a Hip Spica Cast

A child in a hip spica cast requires some special care as a result of the size of the cast and its proximity to the perineal area. Preventing skin problems and protecting the cast from urine and stool are important goals.

For an infant or child who is incontinent, the edges of the cast around the perineum and buttocks should be petaled with waterproof tape. Not all tapes labeled "waterproof" are truly waterproof, so some experimentation may be necessary. A disposable diaper with a plastic liner is then tucked up inside the perineal opening of the cast. The plastic should be between the child and the cast padding. Depending on the size of the child, small diapers may be quickly saturated and must be changed frequently. Feminine sanitary pads, "diaper doublers," or incontinence pads can be used to increase the absorbency of the diaper.

Children who are continent need assistance and special precautions during toileting to prevent wetting and soiling of the cast. Tucking plastic wrap into the cast edge and funneling the plastic into a bedpan can help control the direction of urine and stool. Protecting the cast edges with waterproof tape can also protect the cast from accidental spills.

In a spica cast, activity is severely restricted. Activity is restricted to head and upper body movements. The child may be unable to change position and must be turned frequently to prevent skin breakdown from the pressure of the cast on the skin. With older children, an overbed trapeze can facilitate patient positioning and foster independence if it is used for position changes and exercise. Older children in a one-legged spica cast may be taught crutch walking and encouraged to be out of bed as soon as possible.

Parents need generous amounts of time and practice to learn to care for a child in a spica cast and to feel confident on discharge. Parents should begin planning for discharge as soon as plans for spica casting are made because home adaptations to accommodate the child in a spica cast and home tutoring plans need to be made. Car seats that are adapted to accommodate a baby in a spica cast and other restraint devices are also available. Depending on the age of the child and the size of the cast, transportation in a car may be impossible, and ambulance transport may be necessary.

Traction

"Traction" is the application of pull to a body part. It can be accomplished through the use of weights and pulleys or through the use of distracting bars. In most cases, the pull of the traction is along the long axis of a bone. The pull of the traction weights is applied by pulling on the bone through a skin apparatus or a metal pin through the bone. A series of pulleys and traction rope are used to maintain the correct line so that the traction can be effective. Traction is used to reduce fractures and treat dislocations by slowly pulling on soft tissues. This gradual stretch may also be used to treat joint contractures and decrease muscle spasm.

Most types of traction require bed rest. Skin traction may be done at home, but skeletal traction usually requires hospitalization. Traction equipment may occasionally be used to suspend a part of the body, without applying any pulling force, for positioning and comfort.

Countertraction is the opposing force of pull that is necessary to maintain traction on the desired part of the body. Countertraction is important for proper alignment because once any part of the child's body rests against the bed frame, or the ropes or weights are obstructed, the force of the traction is significantly altered.

The body weight alone is usually sufficient to provide countertraction, but restraints or shock blocks may be necessary, especially with small children. Restraints, such as a Posey jacket, help keep the child in the correct position in bed. The restraint should be loose enough to allow the child to shift position. Shock blocks are sturdy wooden or metal blocks made to be placed under one end of the bed so that the wheels on the bed fit securely into the blocks. Shock blocks raise one end of the bed so that the pull of gravity on the child's body increases the amount of countertraction. Shock blocks can also be used to elevate one side of the bed when sidearm traction is in place, as illustrated in Figure 41–5.

When shock blocks are used under the foot of the bed, the head can usually be raised for comfort. Gatching the knee rest of the bed provides countertraction for a downward pull, but it also alters the line of pull of the traction, so gatching the knee rest is usually contraindicated. Both the child and family should be aware of this if there are electric controls for the bed. The button controlling the knee rest should be taped as a reminder.

The type of traction equipment used varies according to the orthopedist, the age of the child, and the purpose of the traction. Most situations require a bed with an overhead frame for attachment of the traction apparatus and a firm mattress or the use of a bedboard to prevent flexion contractures. An overhead trapeze should be used whenever possible to aid in providing nursing care. A mattress overlay, such as a foam cushion or alternating air mattress, may be necessary to reduce pressure on the skin and prevent skin breakdown because the child's mobility is severely restricted.

Types of Traction

"Manual traction" is the term used when a person's hands maintain pull on a body part; it is usually used when a cast or traction is being applied. *Skin traction* is applied directly to the skin. The amount of traction that can be used is limited when skin traction is used because of the friction it produces on the skin and the potential for skin breakdown. If the traction is intermittent, strips of foam webbing are secured to the extremity with elastic bandages or specially designed removable boots and appliances. Adhesive straps may be used if the traction is continuous.

"Skeletal traction" is pull applied directly to a bone by use of a Steinmann pin or Kirschner wire inserted through the bone or tongs inserted into the skull. More pulling force can be applied with skeletal traction because the force is applied directly to the skeleton. Corks should be used to cover the pin ends to prevent accidental injury. Any slippage or movement of the pin should be noted and reported to the physician because it may interfere with the effectiveness of the traction.

When skeletal traction is used, the pin insertion sites must be assessed regularly. Pin sites need to be observed daily for redness or purulent drainage, which may indicate infection. Small amounts of serosanguineous drainage are normal as a tissue lubricant. The physician may order routine cleaning of the pin insertion site with normal saline or an antiseptic solution, such as half-strength hydrogen peroxide.

Traction may be continuous or intermittent. Continuous traction is used for fracture reduction and can be skeletal or skin traction. Intermittent traction may be used to correct deformities or to overcome muscle spasm in a body part. A child in intermittent traction may remove the traction for meals or to use the bathroom, as ordered by the physician. Table 41–8 describes specific types of traction; the different types are illustrated in Figures 41–3 through 41–11.

The child in traction requires skilled and creative nursing care to maintain physical and emotional health. Maintenance of traction and proper alignment are important nursing responsibilities to ensure that the traction will be effective. The nurse must maintain the correct line of pull. The angle of the pulleys on the traction frame and the angle of the involved joints determine the line of pull. In general, the line of pull is along the long axis of the involved bone. The nurse maintains the correct line of pull by keeping the patient's body in alignment and in the correct position in the bed. The amount of weight depends on the site of the fracture, the age and weight of the patient, and the type of traction used. It is ordered by the physician.

Keeping a child in the correct position in the bed can be a challenge; it can be a game if the nurse marks the siderails of the bed or the sheets so that the child can monitor his or her own position. The nurse must also maintain countertraction to help keep the child in the proper position. Skin irritation and breakdown is a potential problem because of the limited positions possible and the constant pull of the traction. Wrinkle-free sheets and clean, dry skin are important for preventing skin breakdown. The patient should be encouraged to shift position and exercise

TABLE 41-8
Types of Traction

Name	Description	Uses	Comments
Cervical tongs	Skeletal traction; traction to cervical spine by tongs inserted into skull above the ears	Postoperative cervical fusion, cervical injury	Pin care must be done daily to tong insertion sites; child will need assistance with activities of daily living
Halo traction	Skeletal traction; traction applied to the cervical spine by circular halo ring attached to skull with pins; pull is in line with the body	Postoperative cervical fusion, cervical injury	Cranial nerve function must be carefully assessed
Halo vest	Same as halo traction, but halo is attached to a sheepskin-lined vest	Same as halo traction	Child can ambulate in halo vest; a walker may be necessary
Cervical halter	Skin traction; traction to cervical spine by head halter that rests under the chin and across the ears	Torticollis, cervical injury	May be removed for meals, bathroom; cushion chin from pressure of halter
Dunlop sidearm	Skin or skeletal traction; traction to humerus with shoulder abducted and elbow flexed	Supracondylar fractures of humerus, postoperative positioning	If skeletal, pin care must be performed daily
Overhead sidearm	Skeletal traction; wire or pin inserted through distal humerus; child lies supine with shoulder extended and elbow flexed 90 degrees over body	Supracondylar fractures of the humerus	Same as above
Buck extension	Skin traction; web strapping or removable foam boots attached to weights keep hip and knee in extension	Hip and knee contractures, treatment of disease processes of knee and hip, postoperative positioning	Countertraction applied mainly by body; may be intermittent; prone to skin breakdown, especially if adhesive is used
Russell	Same as Buck extension with sling added under the knee	Femoral fracture, preoperative or postoperative positioning	Same as Buck's; maintain position of slings
Balanced suspension	Skeletal traction; hip and knee supported by Thomas splint; flexion of lower leg provided by Pearson attachment	Femoral fracture	As child moves, suspension apparatus adjusts without disturbing traction pull
Bryant	Skin traction; both legs extended above the body with hips flexed at 90 degrees; web strapping is applied to the lower legs with elastic bandages	Femoral fracture, congenital dislocated hip; only used in children who weight <30 lbs	Child's buttocks are raised slightly off the bed so that the body weight provides countertraction; both legs are suspended even if only one leg is involved
90–90	Skeletal traction; wire or pin inserted through distal femur; child lies supine with hip and knee flexed to 90 degrees	Femoral fracture	Skeletal pin site care

unaffected joints to prevent muscle weakness. Active range-of-motion exercise or a formal physical therapy program can be used.

In addition, the traction apparatus must be checked, just like any other type of equipment. The bolts should be checked for tightness. The ropes should be checked for any fraying. The ropes should run smoothly in the pulleys. Knots in the traction rope should be tight and not in contact with the pulleys. The traction weights should hang clear of the bed. The nurse should check that the weight is that which was ordered by the physician.

External Fixation

External fixation provides external support to the bone by a rigid external frame. The frame is attached to pins that go through the soft tissue into bone. External fixation is used to stabilize fracture fragments, especially those that cannot be adequately stabilized by other methods of immobilization. An external fixator also allows treatment of any associated skin or soft tissue injuries. Because the external fixator does not cover the limb completely, skin assessment and wound care can be performed. The external fixator also promotes early motion and mobilization because it does not immobilize the joints above and below the fracture.

External fixators are also used for bone lengthening procedures. The bone to be lengthened is surgically broken, and the fixator is applied. The ends of the fixator are slowly moved apart, and a gap is formed between the bone ends. The body forms new bone in this gap. When the desired length is achieved,

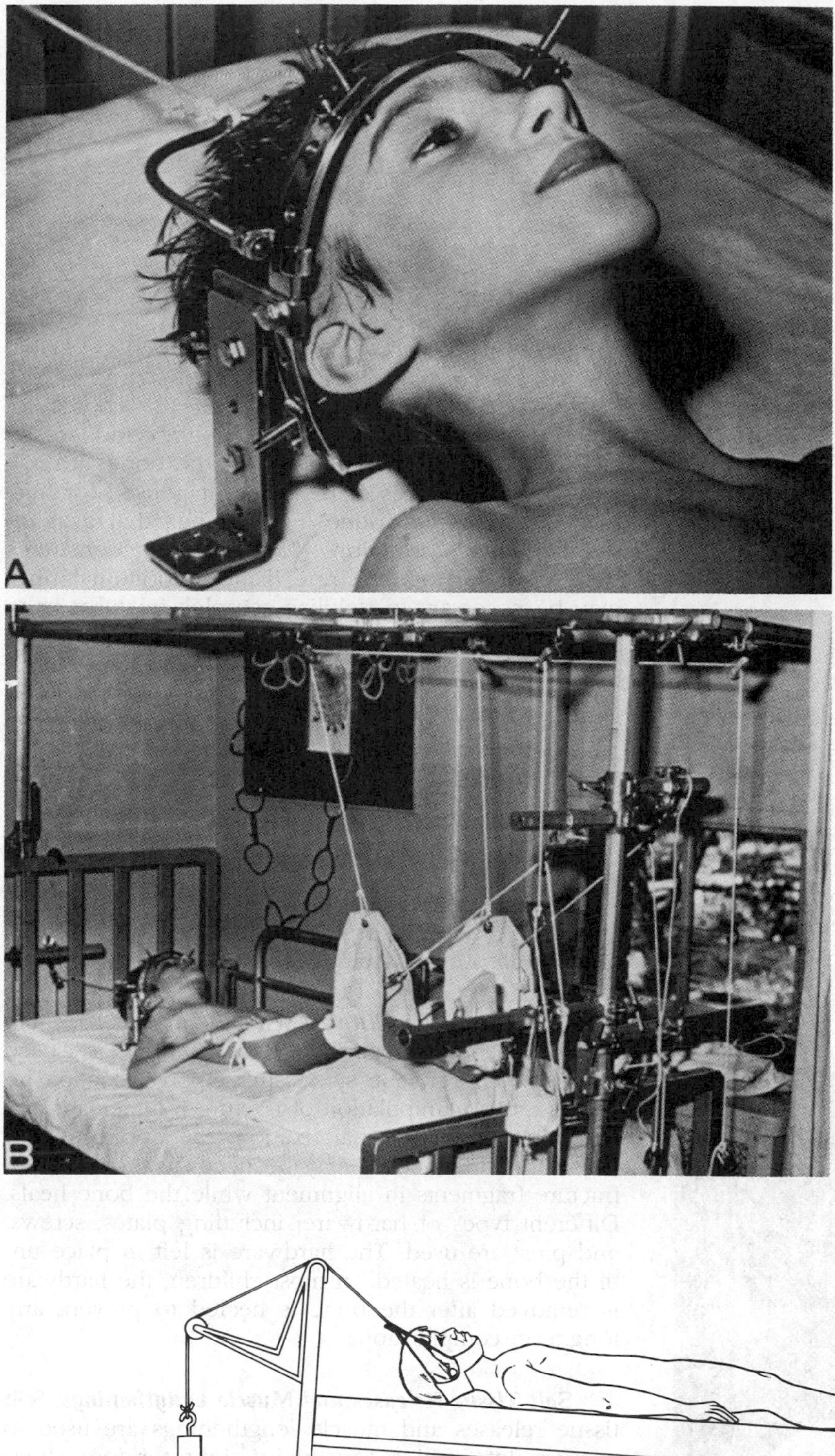

FIGURE 41 - 3. Halo-femoral traction. *A*, Halo. *B*, Traction. (*A* and *B*, From Ferguson, A. B. [1981]. *Orthopaedic surgery in infancy and childhood*. Baltimore: Williams & Wilkins.)

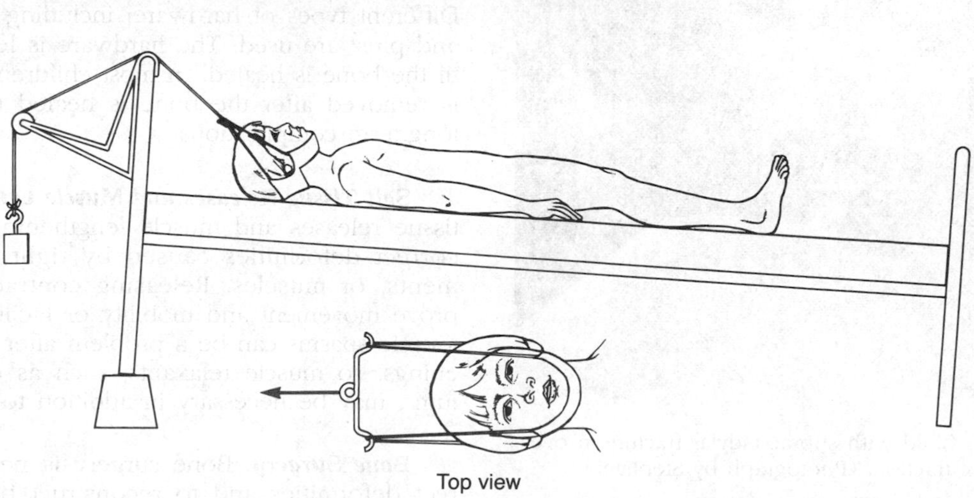

FIGURE 41 - 4. Cervical traction.

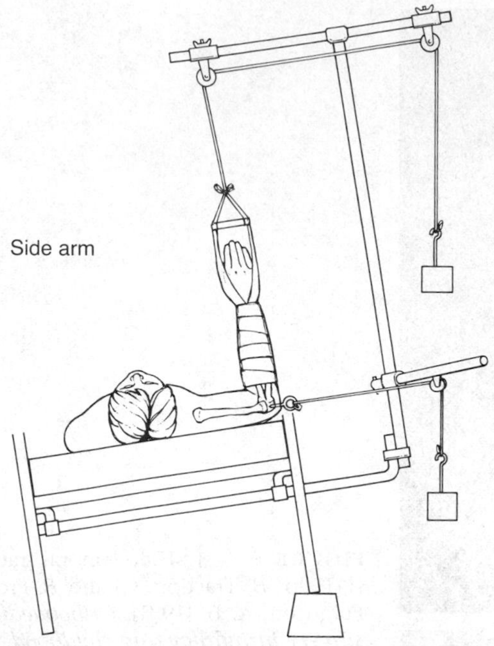

FIGURE 41 - 5. Sidearm skeletal traction.

the bone is allowed to heal, or consolidate, while the fixator remains in place.

Types of External Fixators

A *bar fixator* consists of one jointed bar attached to large pins that goes through soft tissue and bone on one side of the limb. It is used for simple fractures with large fragments and for simple bone lengthen-

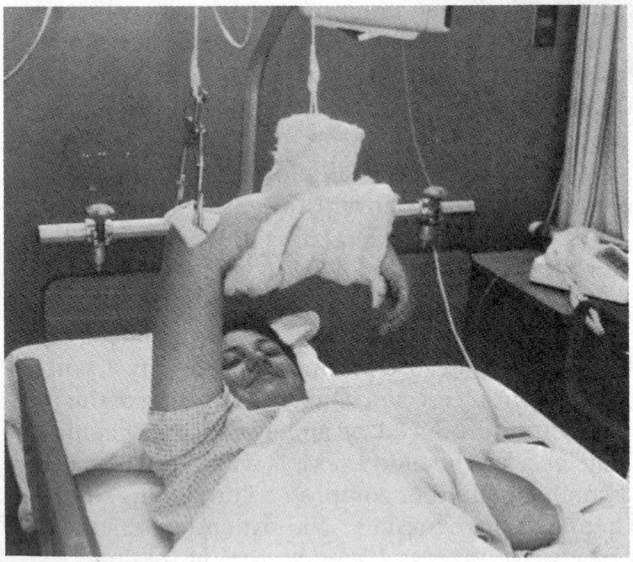

FIGURE 41 - 6. Child with supracondylar fracture in overhead skeletal arm traction. (Photograph by Stephanie Wright.)

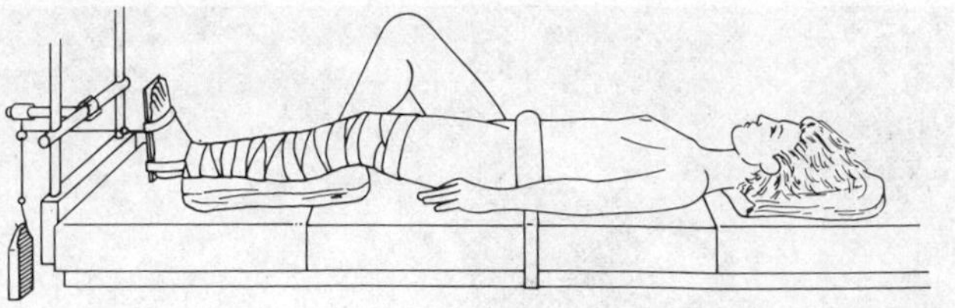

FIGURE 41 - 7. Buck extension traction.

ings. Bar fixators can also be used in a variety of combinations to make unique frames, such as double and triangular frames. A *ring fixator,* such as the Ilizarov or Monticelli-Stinelli (Fig. 41–12), consists of full or half rings that encircle the limb and are attached to pins or wires that pierce the bone and soft tissues on both sides of the bone. It is used for fractures and complex bone lengthenings that also require angular correction. Many different constructs can be made from the ring fixator. Additional rings may be necessary to stabilize complex fractures or to correct complex deformities.

Daily care of the external fixator includes assessing the skin around the pins for signs of infection and cleaning of pin sites to prevent infection. A child with an external fixator can ambulate, depending on the age of the child and location of the fixator. The fixator remains in place until the bone has healed.

Surgery

Different types of surgical procedures are used to treat or prevent musculoskeletal problems.

Open Reduction With or Without Internal Fixation. Depending on the type of fracture, attempts at closed reduction may not be successful. Open reduction involves direct manipulation of fracture fragments in the operating room. Internal fixation, the application of hardware to the bone, may be necessary to hold the fracture fragments in alignment while the bone heals. Different types of hardware, including plates, screws, and pins, are used. The hardware is left in place until the bone is healed. In most children, the hardware is removed after the bone is healed to prevent any long-term complications.

Soft Tissue Releases and Muscle Lengthenings. Soft tissue releases and muscle lengthenings are used to correct deformities caused by tight tendons, ligaments, or muscles. Releasing contractures can improve movement and mobility or facilitate daily care. Muscle spasms can be a problem after muscle lengthenings, so muscle relaxants, such as diazepam (Valium), may be necessary in addition to narcotics.

Bone Surgery. Bone surgery is necessary to correct deformities and to reconstruct bones or joints.

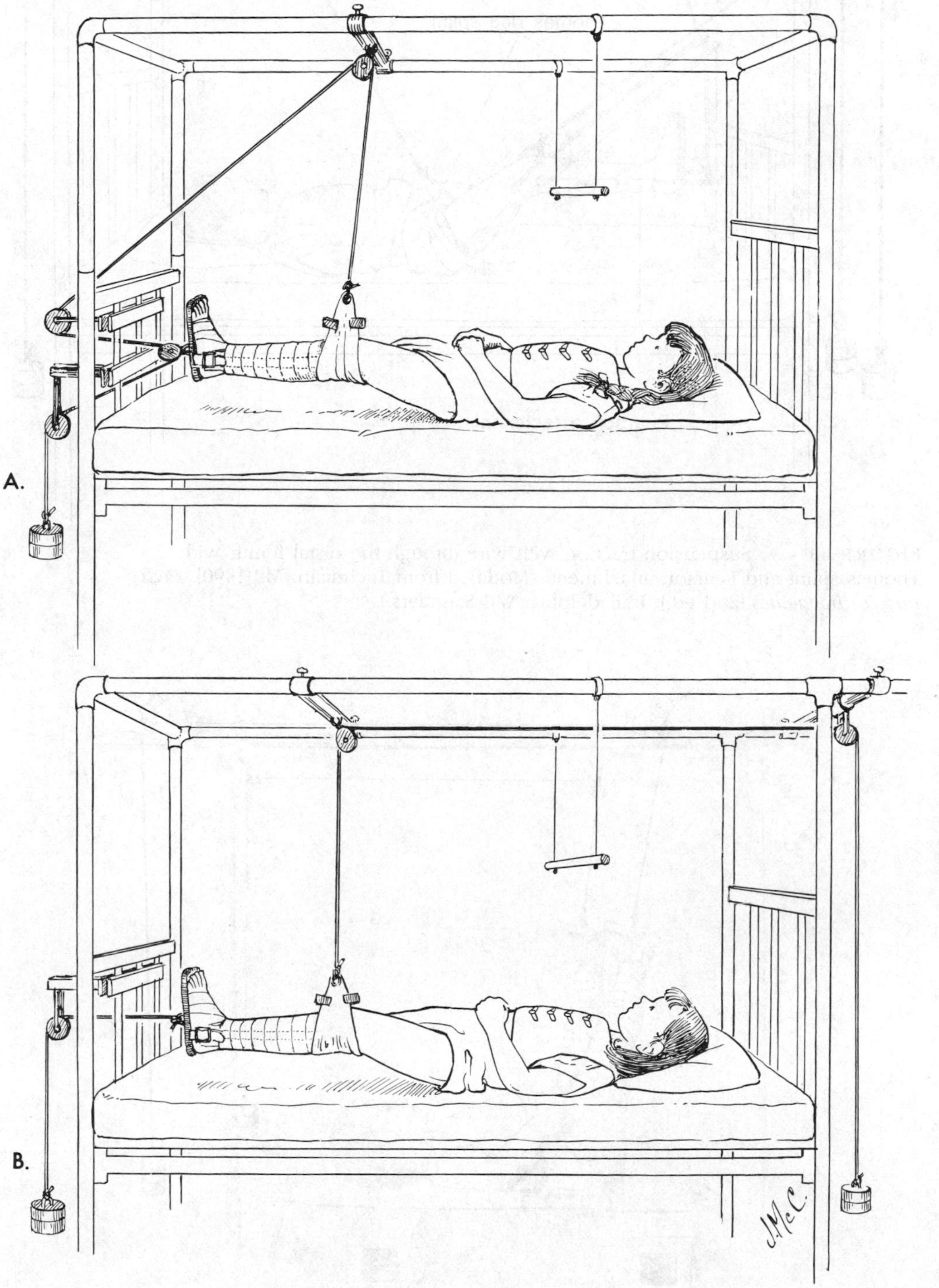

FIGURE 41-8. *A*, Russell skin traction. *B*, Split Russell traction.

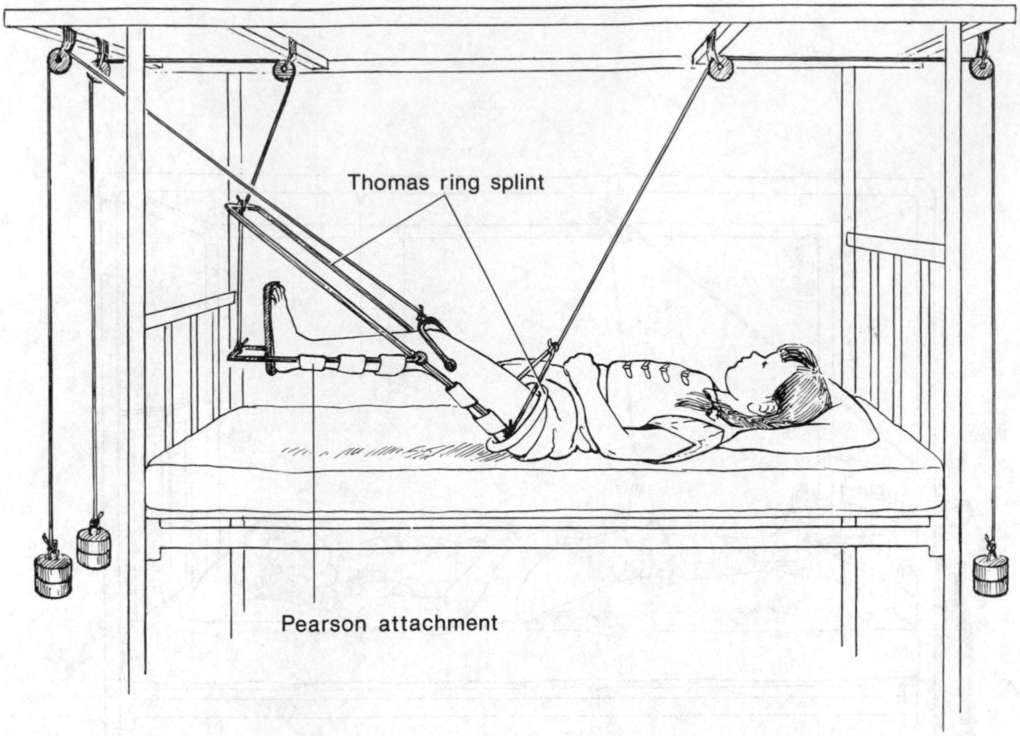

FIGURE 41 - 9. Suspension traction with wire through the distal femur with Thomas splint and Pearson attachment. (Modified from Tachdjian, M. [1990]. *Pediatric orthopaedics* [2nd ed.]. Philadelphia: WB Saunders.)

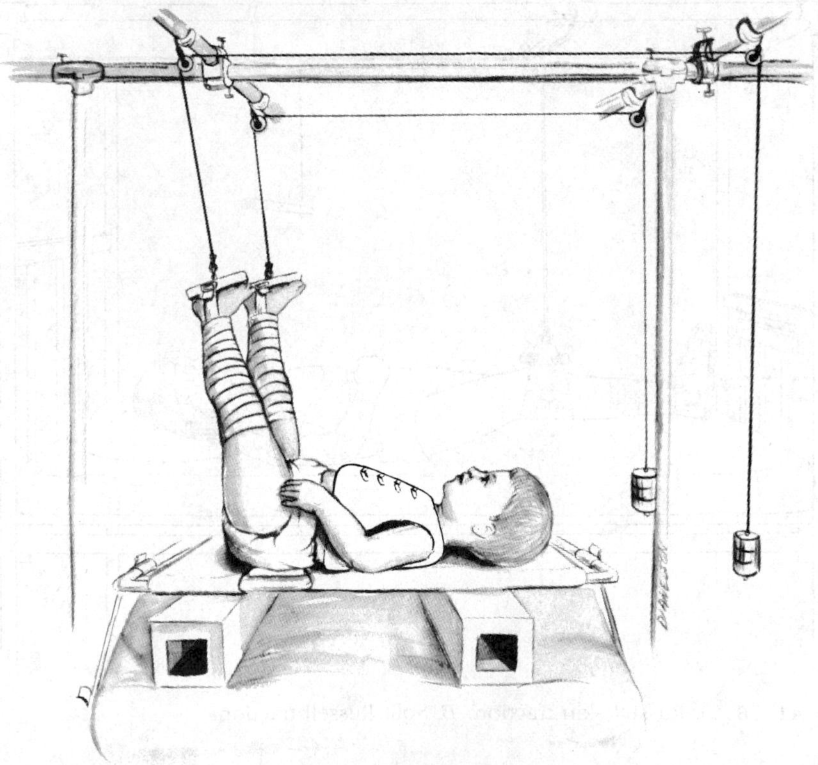

FIGURE 41 - 10. Bryant direct overhead traction. Child rests on a frame that can be useful for maintaining alignment and toileting. Child may also rest directly on the bed surface. (From Tachdjian, M. [1982]. *Congenital dislocation of the hip.* New York, Churchill Livingstone, p 346.)

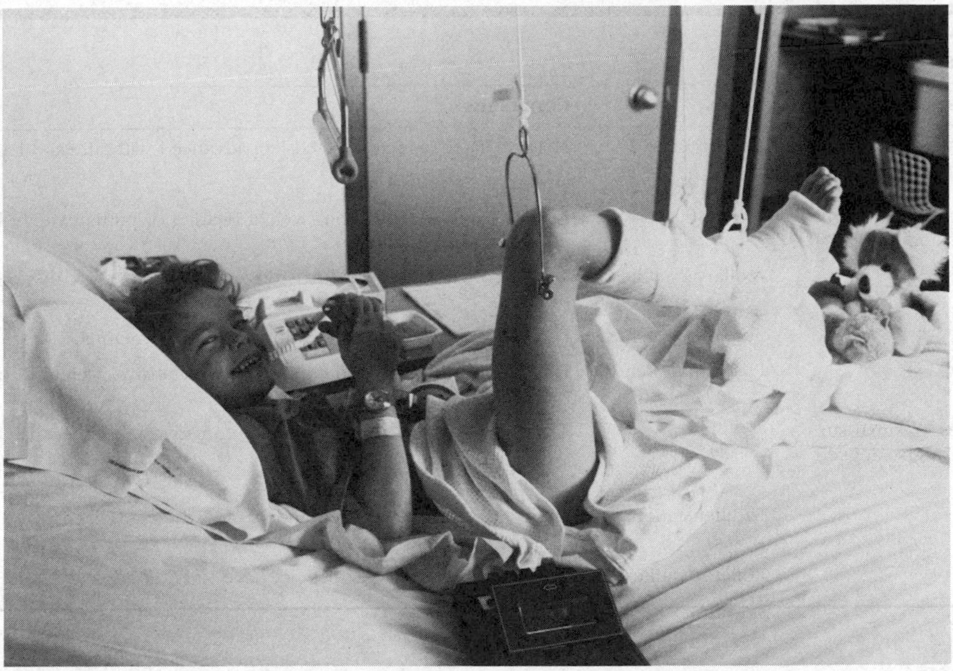

FIGURE 41 - 11. Child with fractured femur in skeletal 90–90 traction. (Photograph by Stephanie Wright.)

Bone surgery includes removal of benign or malignant tumors, realignment of bones, or surgical incision and debridement of infection. Bone surgery is painful and requires aggressive analgesic management, often with intravenous or oral narcotics. Immobilization after bone surgery may include casting, traction, or external fixation.

Ambulatory Devices

Assistance with ambulation may be necessary after injury or surgery to the lower extremities. Ambulatory devices provide additional support and assistance during walking by transferring a portion of the body weight to the arms. A child may require assistance because of age, type of injury or surgery, or kind of immobilization. At times, decreasing the weight on the affected limb with crutches or a cane may be the only prescribed treatment. The different types of ambulatory devices and their uses are listed in Table 41–9.

Because weight is transferred to the arms, the child must have adequate strength and coordination to manage crutches. For determining what device is most appropriate, the child's functional ability, amount of weight bearing, balance, ability to maintain an upright position, and upper limb function must be considered. Evaluation of the best type of ambulatory device is best made by a physical therapist. The therapist also instructs the patient and family in the correct use of the device and the proper gait pattern.

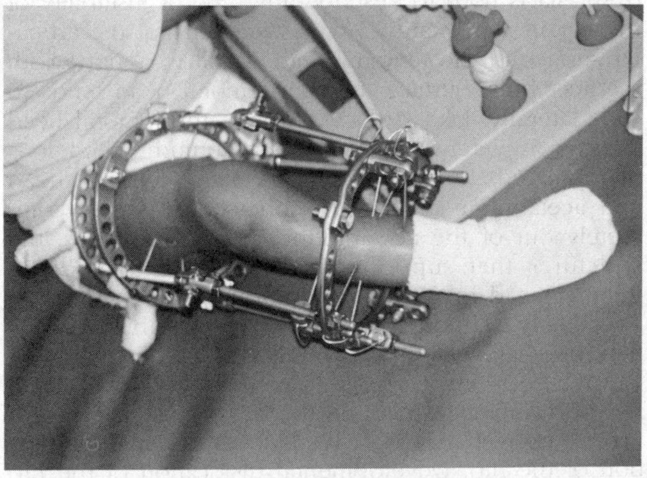

FIGURE 41 - 12. Monticelli-Stinelli External Fixator. (Courtesy of the Shriner's Hospital for Crippled Children, Greenville, SC.)

Application of Nursing Process

See Table 41–10 for Nursing Process Plan.

Congenital and Hereditary Musculoskeletal Conditions

Numerous congenital anomalies involve the musculoskeletal system. In many cases, most of the physical care and the implementation of the treatment regimen are the parents' responsibility. Their education and un-

TABLE 41-9
Ambulatory Assistive Devices

Category	Purpose	Types	Comments
Cane	Widens base of support	Regular cane	Held on same side as affected leg; advanced with affected leg
		Quad cane	
Crutches	Transmit body weight to arms and hands		Used with a variety of non–weight bearing or partial weight bearing gaits; generally not safe in children <4 yrs
		Axillary crutches	Top of crutch should be 2 to 3 fingers-breadths below the axilla to prevent nerve palsy
		Forearm crutches	Forearm extensions transfer some weight to forearms
		Platform crutches	Forearms lie on a padded contour rest to transmit weight through the entire forearm
Walker	Provides maximal support through 4-legged base		Useful for patients who are not able to use crutches because of age
		Parallel stationary walker	Entire walker must be lifted and advanced
		Rollator walker	2 or 4 wheels so that it does not have to be lifted; less stable than parallel walker

derstanding can ensure good results and greater comfort for the child. The ability to communicate with the parents concerning all aspects of treatment and care is an important aspect of nursing intervention.

The Impact of Physical Deformity

For every parent, the birth of a child with a physical deformity represents the loss of the perfect child they had expected. Initially, the parents will experience shock and denial. Denial is a defense mechanism that delays the impact of the situation until it can be dealt with effectively. Guilt and anger follow. Anger reflects the parents' disappointment and may initially be directed at staff. Afterward, a period of grieving is necessary before acceptance of the baby can begin. The difference between the child they expected and the infant they have can precipitate a tremendous sense of loss.

The one element that most musculoskeletal defects have in common is that they are obvious. In addition, treatment often includes surgery and casting, which may not be easily hidden from the curiosity of onlookers. Parents are reminded of the physical problem each time they look at their child.

In their approach to the newborn infant with a physical deformity, nurses provide a model for parents. Skill and compassion in providing nursing care despite the deformity or the impediment of a cast reinforce acceptance of the baby. Focusing on other attributes and characteristics can help parents see their baby as an individual and not as the deformity. A baby with a physical deformity requires the same care and attention as any other infant.

The parents' acceptance of the problem and treatment determines their response to the reactions of others. As children mature, they will model the attitudes of those around them. For children with physical disability and deformity, developing normal relationships with peers and siblings is often as great a challenge as coping with their own physical limitations.

Most parents lack information about the deformity and future treatment plans. Of paramount concern is the effect of the deformity on the child's future. Initially, the parents may not be able to absorb large amounts of information. However, the nurse should be ready to provide information about the condition, treatments, and resources when the parents are ready.

Congenital Dislocation of the Hip

The term "congenital dislocated hip" (CDH) or hip dysplasia is used to describe any type of instability of the hip in a neonate. In a *subluxated* hip, the articular surface of the femoral head is still in contact with the acetabular surface, but the femoral head tends to slide laterally. In a *dislocatable* hip, the femoral head slides completely out of the acetabulum when it is manipulated. In a *dislocated* hip, the femoral head and acetabulum are not in contact; the hip is completely out of the acetabulum. In hip dysplasias, the structures that support the hip joint and hold the femoral head in the acetabulum may be too loose to adequately support the hip, or the acetabular cavity may be shallower than normal.

Whereas hip dysplasia is commonly diagnosed in newborn infants, it may not be noted until later in infancy, when it may be called developmental dislocation of the hip. Developmental dislocation of the hip may be diagnosed even if the hip examination was previously normal. Dislocated hips may also be found

TABLE 41-10

Nursing Process Plan: Care of the Child with a Musculoskeletal Condition Requiring Cast, Traction, or External Fixation

Analysis: Nursing Diagnostic Statement 1

Response and Related or Risk Factors: ***High risk for injury: physiologic;*** *risk factors: neurovascular impairment associated with pressure exerted on blood vessels and nerves secondary to*

- *Bleeding into a muscle compartment*
- *Edema of soft tissues within a constricting cast*
- *Malalignment of the traction force*
- *Improper position of traction apparatus (e.g., ropes, spreader bar)*
- *Lack of knowledge (child and family) regarding how to prevent alterations in neurovascular status*

Projected Outcome: The child will maintain neurovascular integrity

Defining Characteristics *(Actual Response)*	Nursing Interventions	Evaluation Criteria
Subjective: • Verbalization/vocalization of altered sensation in digits of affected extremity: numbness, tingling, pain that increases with movement and is not relieved by analgesics *Objective:* • Perfusion in affected extremity: decreased or absent pulses • Skin cool and pale • Capillary refill time >3 secs • Neuromuscular integrity in affected extremity: child unable to distinguish which digits are being touched • Decreased ability (or inability) to flex and extend digits of affected extremity • Evidence of tissue swelling within a closed compartment (i.e., muscle compartment, cast) or of pressure over a major nerve	*Circulatory Precautions and Peripheral Sensation Management* **Monitor neurovascular status (NVS) on first contact with the child to establish a baseline for future assessments.** Thereafter, monitor NVS at least every 4 hrs (see Table 41–3) **Ensure accurate assessment data.** • Assess for sensation in the digits in such a way that the child cannot see which digit is being touched • Assess all 5 fingers or toes (digits innervated by different nerves) • Encourage the child to demonstrate flexion and extension to the fullest ability; acknowledge the pain experienced on movement of the digits • Be alert to irritability in the preverbal child and making more frequent NVS assessments to compensate for decreased subjective data • Tell the verbal child to alert the nurse if numbness, tingling, or pain occurs at any time	**The child will maintain neurovascular integrity of the affected extremity, as evidenced by** • Verbalization of equal sensation in the affected and unaffected extremities • Absence of severe pain in the affected extremity • Pulses palpable and equal in the affected and unaffected extremities • Capillary refill time <3 secs • Skin color and warmth equal in affected and unaffected extremities • Ability to flex and extend digits of the affected extremity

(continued)

TABLE 41-10 *(continued)*

Defining Characteristics *(Actual Response)*	**Nursing Interventions**	**Evaluation Criteria**
	• Assess skin warmth, color, and pulses in both extremities at the same time **Ensure accurate interpretation of the data.** • Reassess alterations and comparison with the unaffected extremity • Compare current findings with last recorded findings • Consider the effects of a drying cast on skin temperature (skin usually feels cooler to touch while cast is drying) *Teaching: Disease Process* **Institute and teach the child and family measures that will prevent alteration in NVS in the immediate post-trauma period.** • Monitor the child with musculoskeletal trauma for signs of shock (that would indicate possible bleeding at injury site) • Splint musculoskeletal injuries before transport to avoid additional soft tissue trauma **Institute and teach the child and family measures that will prevent alteration in NVS related to casting.** • Avoid indentations in a wet cast—such indentations could result in extra pressure in a small area (a plaster cast dries in 10 to 72 hrs, a synthetic cast in 5 to 30 mins [Wise, 1986]; handle with palms, not fingertips; cushion with pillows instead of placing wet cast on firm mattress; facilitate drying by turning the child every 2 hours and by leaving the cast uncovered; once the cast is dry, keep it dry) • Prevent swelling inside the cast: elevate the extremity on pillows (to facilitate venous return), use ice packs around the cast; assess the cast for tightness by making sure a finger can be inserted be-	

TABLE 41-10 *(continued)*

Defining Characteristics *(Actual Response)*	**Nursing Interventions**	**Evaluation Criteria**
	tween the cast and the skin at all points around perimeter of cast; be especially alert to reports of "tightness" over bony prominences (a window may need to be cut in the cast to relieve localized pressure over a nerve) **Institute and teach the child and family measures that will prevent alteration in NVS related to traction.** • Maintain traction in proper alignment; children often move about so that alignment is altered; a child of preschool age or older may be able to cooperate by agreeing to stay within a boundary of colored tape on the bottom sheet; place the telephone and the child's belongings within easy reach and instruct them to use the call bell for objects out of reach • Assess frequently for pressure exerted over major nerves by traction apparatus, especially over the bones of the ankle, elbow, and wrist	

Analysis: Nursing Diagnostic Statement 2

Response and Related or Risk Factors: ***High risk for infection;*** *risk factors:*

- *Disruption of skin by percutaneous pins*
- *Surgical incisions*

Analysis: Nursing Diagnostic Statement 3

Response and Related or Risk Factors: ***High risk for altered skin integrity;*** *risk factors:*

- *Pressure or abrasion from cast or traction*
- *Immobility*

Projected Outcome: Child's skin will remain or become intact without redness or inflammation

Defining Characteristics *(Actual Response)*	**Nursing Interventions**	**Evaluation Criteria**
Subjective: • Complaints of burning, itching, discomfort, or pain on any skin surface, around cast edges, or at pin sites	*Skin Surveillance and Cast Care: Maintenance* • Assess for changes in skin on at least a daily basis; more frequent assessment may be necessary	**The child will maintain normal skin integrity, as evidenced by** • Verbalization of skin comfort • Warm, dry, intact skin surfaces

(continued)

TABLE 41-10 (continued)

Defining Characteristics *(Actual Response)*	Nursing Interventions	Evaluation Criteria
Objective: • Redness, warmth, excoriation, blistering, or drainage of any skin surface • Abnormal odors from within a cast or around pin sites	• Wash skin surfaces with mild soap and water as needed and dry thoroughly • Avoid use of oils or lotions that soften skin around cast edges; alcohol may be used to toughen skin • Change position frequently within the confines of the treatment regimen to reduce pressure on any individual skin site • Provide a mattress overlay or pressure alternating or reducing device for patients requiring long-term complete body immobilization to reduce abrasion and pressure on skin surfaces • Rewrap skin traction every 4 to 8 hours and examine skin areas as indicated by hospital protocols • Petal cast edges with moleskin to protect skin from abrasion from casting material • Clean pin sites per physician's order • Do not allow small objects or food to enter cast • Control itching inside case by blowing cool air from hair dryer into cast; do not allow scratching with objects inside the cast • Teach child and family members appropriate skin care for casted extremities (see Table 41–7)	• Absence of redness or drainage

Analysis: Nursing Diagnostic Statement 4

Response and Related or Risk Factors: ***High risk for further impaired physical mobility;*** *risk factors:*

- *Injury and/or immobilization of body part*
- *Presence of cast, traction, splint, or brace*
- *Discomfort associated with injury or treatment*

Projected Outcome: Child will maintain full range of motion within the confines of the treatment regimen and will regain full mobility when treatment period ends

TABLE 41-10 *(continued)*

Defining Characteristics *(Actual Response)*	**Nursing Interventions**	**Evaluation Criteria**
Subjective: • Complaints of inability to perform usual activities *Objective*: • Loss of use of extremity • Required bed rest with associated limitations	*Exercise Therapy: Joint Mobility and Muscle Control* • Assess mobility potential of patient • Provide regular movement and active range of motion to maintain strength of unaffected muscle groups • Use age-approprite play activities to encourage joint and muscle movement • Provide appropriate referral to physical therapy for gait training, strengthening unaffected muscles, and rehabilitation of affected limb	**The child will maintain full range of motion of unaffected extremities, as evidenced by** • Continued use of all unaffected muscle groups with no diminution in strength **The child will maintain maximal independence, as evidenced by** • Performance of all activities of daily living that are within her or his developmental and physical capabilities • Engagement in age-appropriate play activities

Analysis: Nursing Diagnostic Statement 5

Response and Related or Risk Factors: Altered health maintenance, *related to*

- *Inability to perform self-care measures because of limitations imposed by condition*
- *Discomfort from injury and its sequelae*
- *Knowledge deficit, child and parents, regarding activity limitations*

Projected Outcome: The child and his or her parents will be able to identify, manage, and seek out help to maintain health.

Defining Characteristics	**Nursing Interventions**	**Evaluation Criteria**
Subjective: • Complaints of inability to perform usual activities *Objective*: • Loss of use of extremity • Required bed rest with associated limitations	*Teaching: Procedure/Treatment* • Help family explore alternatives to assist with mobility: stroller, wagon, wheelchair, scoot board, special car seats • Provide and teach alternative methods of performing activities of daily living: dressing, bathing • Encourage maximal independence in child or adolescent; assist family to avoid doing everything for their child • Provide appropriate control of discomfort due to injury, treatment regimen, or muscle spasm to allow full mobility • Provide and reinforce correct gait training for mobilization devices: crutches, walkers, braces	**The child will regain maximal physical mobility at the end of the treatment regimen, as evidenced by** • Return to pretreatment mobility after period of rehabilitation, or • Achievement of maximal mobility within imposed limitations of condition

(continued)

TABLE 41-10 *(continued)*

Defining Characteristics *(Actual Response)*	Nursing Interventions	Evaluation Criteria
	• Allow frequent rest periods (to avoid overtaxing muscles and joints) • Provide child and family with appropriate information on activity limitations to maintain prescribed treatment; discuss impact of such restrictions on the child and family	

in older children, particularly those with a neuromuscular problem, such as cerebral palsy or spina bifida.

Etiology/Incidence

The cause of CDH is believed to be multifactorial (Herring, 1990). Ligamentous laxity may cause the ligaments supporting the hip to allow more movement in the joint. There is often a familial ligamentous hyperlaxity in babies with CDH. Fetal response to maternal hormones, particularly in girls, is also thought to have a role in the development of CDH. CDH occurs in 1 of 300 girls; the incidence in boys is 1 in 2000. Another factor that has been implicated through numerous studies in various cultures is prenatal and postnatal positioning. Breech positioning and small uterine size have been associated with CDH, as has positioning infants with legs extended and adducted, as was seen in the Native American cultures when infants were carried in a papoose. Some authors have reported an increased incidence of CDH associated with metatarsus adductus and torticollis. Metatarsus adductus (Jacobs, 1960) and torticollis are also believed to be positional abnormalities. The presence of either necessitates a thorough examination of the hip for CDH.

In the past, most cases were thought to develop prenatally. This figure has been challenged with better diagnostic methods. Current thinking is that CDH is an evolving condition. Some infants may have a normal hip on a newborn examination but later be diagnosed with developmental dislocation of the hip. It is crucial that serial hip examinations be done throughout the first year of life to monitor the development of the femoral head and acetabulum.

Pathophysiology

In a newborn infant, some normal ligamentous laxity may allow the hip to dislocate and relocate spontaneously. With time, the hip may become reduced, or it may remain subluxated or fully dislocated. When the hip is dislocated, changes in the hip become progressive. The acetabulum and femoral head develop synergistically and must be in contact with each other. If the femoral head is not placed in the acetabulum, it becomes less spherical, and the acetabulum becomes more anteverted.

Clinical Manifestations

The early signs of CDH are unequal leg lengths, limited abduction, and redundant skin folds on the inner thigh of the affected leg (Fig. 41-13). The clinical signs may be difficult to assess if CDH is bilateral. Parents may report a difference in the range of motion at the hips, especially during diaper changes.

As the hip remains dislocated and is no longer reducible, some of the physical signs become more obvious. Gait abnormalities are noted when the child starts to walk. The level of the pelvis may be unequal, and the child may walk with a limp, may toe walk (especially if CDH is unilateral), or may in-toe.

Diagnostic Assessment

Clinical examination is important in diagnosis of CDH. In a newborn infant, the Barlow and Ortolani maneuvers can be used to assess the stability of the hip during the physical examination. The Barlow maneuver pushes an unstable femoral head out of the acetabulum by use of gentle lateral pressure of the lower trochanter. The Ortolani maneuver relocates a dislocated femoral head by gentle abduction and external rotation.

Diagnostic imaging can be used to assist with diagnosis. Plain x-ray films may not be helpful in young infants because the head of the femur is cartilage and thus translucent. Ultrasound has been helpful in identifying hip dysplasias by allowing visualization of the cartilaginous acetabulum and the unossified femoral head. The test is noninvasive and easily performed on an infant. Computed tomography (CT) and magnetic resonance imaging (MRI) may be used in complex

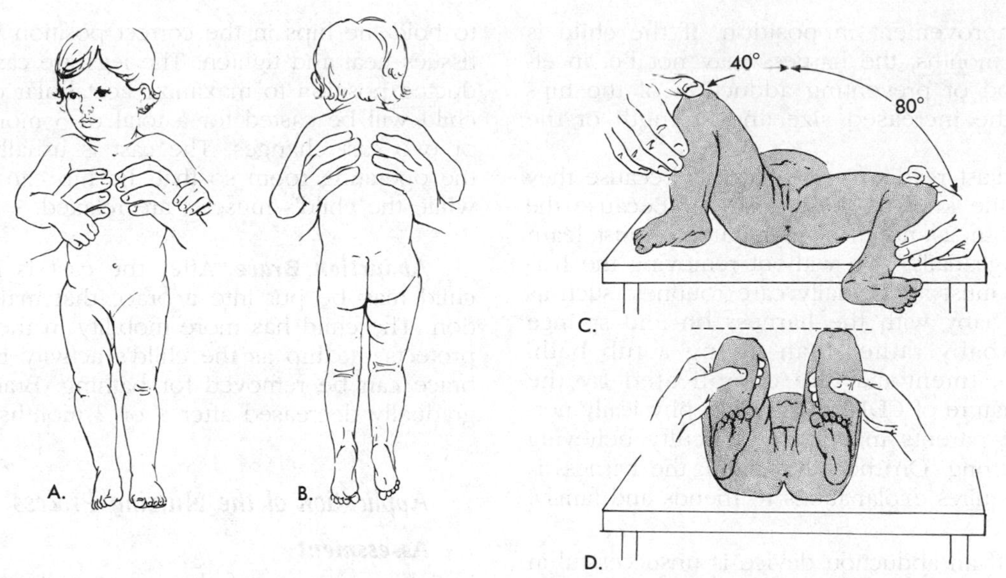

FIGURE 41 - 13. The three classic signs of congenital dislocated hip: *A* and *B*, unequal skinfolds; *C*, limitation of abduction; and *D*, unequal knee height. (*A–D*, From Tachdjian, M. [1990]. *Pediatric orthopedics* [2nd ed.]. Philadelphia: WB Saunders.)

cases or in older children when ultrasound cannot be used. These studies can identify obstructions to reduction, such as an inverted labrum or an abnormally shaped capsule. A CT scan may also be used after surgery to evaluate the adequacy of the reduction.

In the operating room, an arthrogram may be performed to determine the position of the cartilaginous femoral head, the fibrocartilaginous labrum, and the capsule. The arthrogram consists of the injection of dye into the capsule surrounding the hip joint. The hip can be moved to permit visualization of the hip structures through the entire range of motion. An arthrogram is usually done in conjunction with an attempt at closed reduction or open reduction in the operating room.

Therapeutic Management

The goal of treatment is to relocate the head of the femur within the acetabulum and to protect the blood vessels and nerves that sit on the exterior of the bone. Treatment entails immobilizing the joint to encourage normal development. Treatment started early has been most effective at preventing long-term problems.

Abduction Devices. Because femoral abduction seats the head of the femur in the acetabulum, the first treatment used in an infant is an abduction device. Double or triple diapers are not recommended as a definitive treatment but may be helpful in keeping the hips abducted before definitive treatment is started.

The most commonly used abduction device for young infants is a Pavlik harness (Fig. 41–14). The Pavlik harness keeps the hips and knees flexed and the hips abducted. It prevents simultaneous adduction and extension of the hips. The harness permits some active hip motion, including abduction, flexion, and rotation. The harness is usually worn 24 hours a day for a trial of 3 or 4 weeks. Repeated clinical examinations are used to document decreased laxity. Serial ultrasound examinations and, later, radiographs will

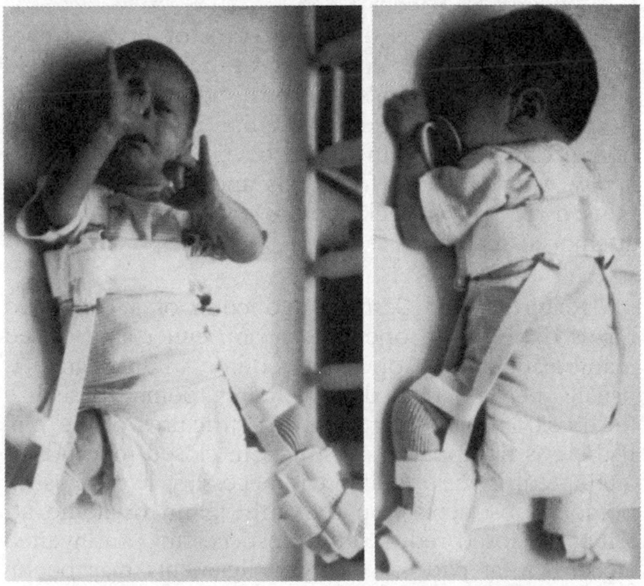

FIGURE 41 - 14. *A* and *B*, Pavlik harness. (*A* and *B*, From Tachdjian, M. [1990]. *Pediatric orthopaedics* [2nd ed., p 331]. Philadelphia, WB Saunders.)

document improvement in position. If the child is older than 6 months, the harness may not be an effective method of preventing adduction of the hips because of the increased size and strength of the baby.

Infants adjust readily to the harness because they are used to the knee-to-chest position. Because the harness is worn 24 hours a day, parents must learn how to manage daily care without removing the harness. Parents must adjust daily care routines, such as dressing the baby with the harness on and sponge bathing the baby rather than giving a tub bath. Parental adjustment may be complicated by the nonobvious nature of CDH: the baby is physically normal, and the parents may have difficulty believing anything is wrong. On the other hand, the harness is visible and requires explanations to friends and family.

Traction. If an abduction device is unsuccessful in altering the position of the femoral head, traction may be used to stretch soft tissues. Stretching the soft tissues moves the femoral head closer to the acetabulum. It may also prevent damage to the vessels surrounding the hip joint and prevent avascular necrosis of the femoral head. Although challenged recently, traction is used as a precursor to surgery, either closed reduction under general anesthesia or open reduction.

Traction may be done in the hospital or at home. If it is done in the hospital, Bryant's, Buck's, or Russell's traction is used. Traction is maintained for 20 hours a day, with time out for daily hygiene and feedings. It is important to maintain the position of the child in bed to maximize the effectiveness of the traction, although this may be difficult with a small, squirmy child. Diversional activities, such as music boxes, toys suspended over the bed, and hand-held toys, should be used.

Home traction is often a variant of Bryant's traction: the hips are flexed 60 degrees rather than the 90 degrees of true Bryant's traction. The decreased angle is used to prevent neurovascular complications at home. Children remain in the traction 16 to 20 hours a day, with time out for meals and bathing. Traction is used for 3 to 4 weeks before an arthrogram and an attempt at reduction.

Reduction and Casting. Reduction of a dislocated hip is done in the operating room, either as a closed manipulation or an open procedure. An arthrogram is usually performed in the operating room to visualize the position of the cartilaginous structures of the hip. If there is no apparent obstruction, closed reduction is attempted. Open reduction is necessary if there is an obvious obstruction on the arthrogram or if the attempt at closed reduction is unsuccessful. An inverted labrum, a fat pad, or enlarged ligaments may be located between the femoral head and the acetabulum so that the femoral head cannot be seated. Tight tendons and ligaments may also be surgically released.

When the hip is reduced, a spica cast is applied to hold the hips in the correct position while the soft tissues heal and tighten. The legs are casted in an abducted position to maximize acetabular coverage. The child will be casted for a total of 3 months with one or two cast changes. The cast is usually changed in the operating room so that the hip can be examined while the child's muscles are relaxed.

Abduction Brace. After the cast is removed, the child may be put into a brace that maintains abduction. The child has more mobility in the brace, but it protects the hip as the child's activity increases. The brace can be removed for bathing. Brace wearing is gradually decreased after 1 or 2 months.

Application of the Nursing Process

Assessment

Initial assessment of the infant and family includes obtaining a family history of CDH and experience with a Pavlik harness or any of the other potential treatment modalities. The nurse should also ask the family about the baby's position in utero, particularly the breech position because of the increased risk of CDH. Physical assessment should include observation of the clinical manifestations of CDH, especially a limitation in the range of motion of the hips and a difference in leg lengths. The nurse should also be alert for metatarsus adductus in the feet and torticollis; these have been associated with CDH.

Family assessment should include family coping and adaptation to the diagnosis and prescribed treatment as well as an understanding of the next phase of treatment, if applicable. The scope of therapeutic management (Pavlik harness trial, home traction, reduction and casting) should be explained to families when treatment is initiated because it is hard to predict which baby will need further treatment. The nurse should assess the family's adherence to treatment. Because CDH is not an obvious physical deformity, families often find it difficult to adhere to the prescribed treatment plan or respond to the questions of family and friends.

Nursing Diagnostic Statements and Collaborative Problems

Altered growth and development, *related to*
- *Impaired physical mobility.*
- *Long-term immobilization.*

High risk for skin impairment, *risk factors:*
- *Presence of brace or cast.*
- *Immobility.*

Sleep pattern disturbance, *related to change in usual sleeping patterns resulting from immobilization.*

Alteration in parenting, *related to presence of intimidating treatment modalities.*

Interventions

Promote Normal Growth and Development. Parents are often concerned about the effect of long-term immobilization on normal growth and development. The nurse can reassure parents that although a child who is immobilized for treatment of CDH may not develop gross motor skills at the same time as peers do, once the treatment is complete, the child will develop these skills. Fine motor skills will develop rapidly while the child is immobilized. The family should provide opportunities to develop and practice these skills.

Maintain Physical Mobility. The nurse can help the family explore alternatives to assist with mobility: stroller, wagon, wheelchair with reclining back, scoot board. The family may already have the necessary equipment or may need assistance obtaining it. It is important to reassure the family that their child will learn to maximize mobility in the cast or brace. Most children will use their arms and uncasted leg to push-pull themselves around. Special transportation needs should be discussed with the family. While in the spica cast, a child will not fit in a regular car seat. Adapted car seats and restraints are available through equipment supply companies.

Protect Skin from Irritation. For a baby in a Pavlik harness, irritation behind the knees may be due to skin-to-skin contact. Caregivers should wash the skin daily with mild soap and dry thoroughly. Long cotton socks may absorb perspiration during warm weather and provide additional warmth in cold weather. Irritation under shoulder straps is due to pressure. For prevention of pressure irritation there and at other contact points, the baby should wear a cotton undershirt under the brace. Caregivers should not use lotions or oils on skin under straps. If skin is reddened, rub it gently with alcohol to remove surface oils and toughen skin slightly.

For a baby in a cast, irritation at cast edges is due to roughness. Cast edges should be petaled with felt or moleskin. Particularly rough edges should be trimmed. Synthetic casts may abrade the skin unless the edges are covered with moleskin. Irritation of skin on the lower torso and legs under the cast may be due to soiling of cast padding. All caregivers should be instructed in how to protect the cast padding from soiling. Petal edges around groin and buttocks with waterproof tape to form a waterproof edge between diaper and skin. Tuck a disposable diaper up into cast edges so that the plastic is between the baby and the cast. Change diapers frequently and use sanitary pads, "diaper doublers," or folded cloth diapers to increase absorbency.

If the child requires traction, caregivers must learn how to safely apply the traction and how to make neurovascular assessments. Teach caregivers how to apply the webbing to the legs with elastic bandages. The elastic bandages should be removed at least four times a day to assess the skin. Skin irritation from the straps occurs most frequently at the back of the knee. The prominent occiput on the back of the baby's head may also be irritated by the constant supine position. A small foam doughnut can be used to cushion the head. Encourage the family to put toys on both sides of the frame so that the infant moves his or her head.

While in a cast or traction, the child is unable to turn and adjust position without assistance. The nurse should instruct parents to change the child's position every 2 hours to prevent skin breakdown from prolonged pressure.

Pillows and blanket rolls should be used to maintain a safe position and prevent pressure on any one area.

Maintain Normal Sleep Patterns. As noted previously, the child in a cast or traction is unable to change position without assistance. Being able to change positions may assist the child to maintain normal sleep patterns. With careful positioning, the child can sleep prone or on the side in the cast. Caregivers should maintain a normal nap schedule and daytime routine so that the child can develop a regular sleep pattern.

Support Parents in Caring for Child. The treatment modalities used in the management of CDH can impose restrictions on a caregiver's interaction with the baby. Helping caregivers feel confident in their ability to manage the care of the child can prevent an alteration in interaction and parenting. The nurse should instruct the caregivers about how to manage the baby in Pavlik harness, cast, or traction. Caregivers should be given adequate time to practice and demonstrate their skill as well as opportunities to verbalize concerns, fears, and anxieties. The nurse should encourage verbalization of the impact of treatment on family life.

Evaluation

1. The parents demonstrate the mobility regimen.
2. The child demonstrates age-appropriate skills and behaviors to the extent possible.
3. The parents demonstrate measures to prevent skin breakdown in Pavlik harness, cast, or traction.
4. The child re-establishes a normal sleep pattern. The child shows no signs of sleep deprivation.
5. The parents demonstrate safe and appropriate care of the child in Pavlik harness, cast, or traction.

Clubfoot

Clubfoot is a congenital anomaly characterized by adduction of the forefoot, equinus positioning of the foot, and inversion of the heel (Fig. 41–15).

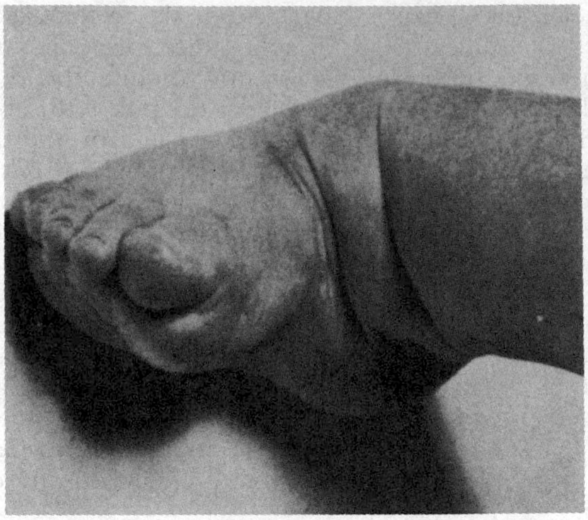

FIGURE 41 - 15. Typical clubfoot deformity. (From Delp, M., & Manning, R. [1981]. *Major's physical diagnosis.* Philadelphia: WB Saunders.)

Etiology/Incidence (Pathophysiology)

Clubfoot occurs in 1 to 1.4 births per 1000 (Davidson, 1991). It is two times more common in boys for unknown reasons. The incidence of the clubfoot deformity is increased among first-degree relatives. Clubfoot is also associated with neuromuscular abnormalities, such as spina bifida.

The cause of clubfoot is unknown, but some possible causes have been proposed. It may be caused by intrauterine compression; as the fetus grows larger, the fetal foot position becomes fixed because there is not enough room to change position. Clubfoot may be caused by a growth arrest in the distal tibia. The fibula continues to grow normally and pushes the foot over into the inverted position. Immature muscles and tendons may not be able to hold the foot so that the sole forms a flat, weight-bearing surface.

Clinical Manifestations

The clinical manifestations of clubfoot are adduction of the forefoot, or metatarsus adductus. The equinus position, or plantar flexion, of the foot is due to a contracture of the Achilles tendon. The foot is also inverted, so the lateral border is directed downward. Clubfoot cannot be easily corrected to the neutral position. In addition, the calf muscles appear thin and atrophic. Because muscles, nerves, and bones develop synergistically, an alteration in the development of the bones of the foot has an effect on the development of the lower leg.

Diagnostic Assessment

Diagnosis is usually made by clinical examination. The manifestations of clubfoot have a range of severity. X-ray examination is not usually necessary. A rigid foot deformity in conjunction with a thin calf usually confirms the diagnosis.

Therapeutic Management

Casting. Serial casting with manipulation is started soon after birth. Manipulation corrects the position of the foot, and casting holds the position to stretch soft tissues and allow the bones to assume the normal position. The short or long leg casts are changed every week to take advantage of and to accommodate the baby's rapid growth. Correction with casting usually reaches a plateau after 3 to 6 months. Parents are taught neurovascular checks and skin care. Serial casting may be a problem for parents who must alter their daily care of the baby to protect the casts; parents are often dismayed that the baby cannot take tub baths while in casts.

When the casts are removed, the redundant skin on the lateral aspect of the foot causes large wrinkles. This skin will eventually smooth out, although it may take several years. Over the period of serial casting, the baby may develop macerations under these wrinkles unless gentle cleansing is done when the casts are removed.

Surgery. Surgery is performed when improvement with casting has reached a plateau (Davidson, 1991). The goal of surgery is to restore the bone architecture and balance muscles. This is done by dividing fibrotic ligaments and joint capsules and restoring the tarsal bones to the correct position. A small percutaneous pin is used to hold the bones in the corrected position. The end of the pin will protrude through the skin between the great and second toes. The surgery is followed by 2 to 3 months of casting to allow bone and soft tissue healing. The foot will remain puffy for several months after the surgery. After the casts are removed, braces or reverse-last shoes may be prescribed to provide additional protection.

Nursing Diagnostic Statements

High risk for impairment of skin integrity; *risk factors:*

- *Manipulation of extremity.*
- *Application of casts.*

Parental anxiety and grieving, *related to impaired adjustment to anomalous condition.*

High risk for body image disturbance (child and parents); *risk factor: residual or recurrent deformity.*

Interventions

Protect Skin Integrity. During weekly follow-up appointments, the nurse should assess the status of the child's skin under the casts as well as the family's adjustment to the clubfoot and the treatment plan. The nurse must teach caregivers how to assess the neurovascular status of the toes, because small babies grow quickly and may outgrow the casts. A cast that is too tight can put pressure on neurovascular structures. The nurse should also instruct caregivers on the assessment and care of skin at cast edges. In some settings, caregivers are taught how to remove the casts by soaking the casts to soften them before the visit, per the physician's order. Alternatively, casts may be removed with a cast saw at the appointment. The nurse should reassure caregivers that the redundant skin on the lateral aspect of the foot will resolve over time.

Support Family Through Anxiety or Grieving. The family should be given the opportunity to explore feelings regarding physical deformity by discussing their reactions and questions with the nurse or physician. The nurse can help the family view the child as a whole and not just a clubfoot deformity by discussing the child's other characteristics and features. It is important to allow the caregivers the opportunity to verbalize their feelings. The nurse should provide support for caregivers throughout treatment; weekly physician appointments may consume much of the caregiver's time and resources. Because consistent follow-up is important, the nurse should help the family develop a plan for weekly appointments. Families may need assistance with transportation problems or documentation for employers as to the need for weekly appointments.

Promote Healthy Body Image It is frustrating to have a residual or recurrent deformity after months spent trying to prevent it. The nurse should help the child and family explore their feelings regarding any residual deformity. Families should be given information about further treatment options. The long-term prognosis for clubfoot is good function, although the child may have difficulty with some sports. The calf muscles on the affected side will remain slightly underdeveloped, and the shoe size of the corrected foot will be a half-size smaller. Follow-up is required until the child reaches skeletal maturity to monitor recurrence and residual deformity. Even with a residual or recurrent deformity, the child should be encouraged to participate in age-appropriate physical activities as much as possible.

Metatarsus Adductus

Metatarsus adductus, or metatarsus varus, is a congenital abnormality in which all of the metatarsals point medially (deviate toward the tibial side of the foot) (Fig. 41–16).

Etiology/Incidence (Pathophysiology)

Metatarsus adductus is the most common congenital foot deformity. It is most likely caused by intrauterine positioning. Because 10 per cent of babies with metatarsus adductus also have congenital dislocated hips (Jacobs, 1960), a careful hip examination is essential for any baby with metatarsus adductus.

Diagnostic Assessment

Metatarsus adductus is present when the forefoot points medially, or inward toward the center of the body. The forefoot is adducted and supinated. Internal tibial torsion is commonly associated with metatarsus adductus and may cause the child to appear pigeon-toed. A ruler placed along the lateral border of the foot will not touch the forefoot. If metatarsus adductus persists, it may cause in-toeing in the toddler years.

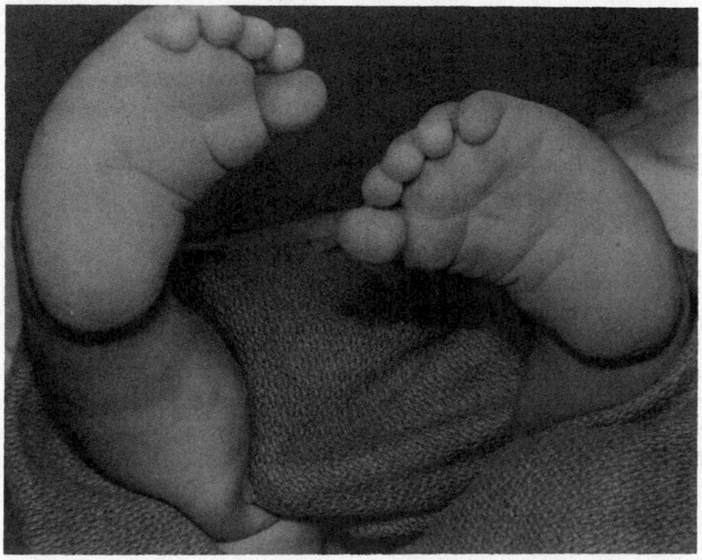

FIGURE 41 - 16. Infant with a metatarsus adductus deformity. (Photograph courtesy of Mead Johnson Nutritional Division.)

Therapeutic Management

Observation. Eighty-five per cent of cases of metatarsus adductus resolve without treatment (Rushforth, 1978).

Stretching. If the foot is flexible and the deformity persists, the parents can do stretching exercises by stabilizing the heel and gently stretching the forefoot toward the midline. The stretching exercises are done five times with each diaper change.

Casting. Serial casting may be necessary for the stiffer foot to provide a continuous, strong stretch. The cast will hold the forefoot in the stretched position to prevent forefoot contractures. The casts are changed every 2 weeks, and the foot is gradually stretched to a neutral position.

Surgery. Surgery may be necessary for a child with a severe, residual deformity. The tarsometatarsal joints are released; metatarsal osteotomies may be done in the older child.

Nursing Care

The nurse must encourage parents to allow adequate time for correction by growth alone before initiation of treatment. This "waiting period" is difficult for families. The nurse should teach the caregivers how to perform a neurovascular assessment of the toes; small babies grow quickly and may outgrow the cast. A cast that is too tight can put pressure on neurovascular structures. Teach caregivers how to assess and care for the skin at cast edges. As with casts for clubfeet, some parents may be instructed to remove the casts by soaking before the visit.

Duchenne Muscular Dystrophy

The muscular dystrophies are a group of progressive, hereditary disorders that affect the muscle cells of specific muscle groups, causing weakness and atrophy. Duchenne muscular dystrophy is the most common type; it primarily affects muscles of the pelvis and shoulders. See Table 41–11 for the types of muscular dystrophy.

Etiology/Incidence (Pathophysiology)

Duchenne muscular dystrophy is a sex-linked recessive disorder, although spontaneous mutations do occur. It affects 1 of every 3000 boys (Drennan, 1990). Duchenne's muscular dystrophy typically presents in boys 3 to 7 years old, although parents may note delayed independent ambulation in boys as young as 18 to 36 months. Survival beyond the third decade is rare.

Genetic mutations cause the absence of dystrophin, a protein of muscle cells. The cell membranes become unusually permeable and cannot maintain the proper milieu for adequate cell functioning. Many muscle cells fail to regenerate. Those fibers that do regenerate fail to reach normal size, resulting in small, ineffective fibers. In addition, collagen is progressively laid down in discrete bundles in the muscles. In some muscles, the collagen is replaced by adipose tissue, resulting in pseudohypertrophy.

Necrosis of the muscle cells actually begins in the preclinical stage. When enough fibers die, the patient becomes symptomatic. The disease is characterized by selective, progressive muscle weakness, first in the pelvic and shoulder girdle muscles, then in more distal muscles over time. Although the patient's movement is lost, sensation is not.

Clinical Manifestations

Pelvic girdle muscles are affected first. Weak hip extensors cause delayed independent ambulation, stumbling, and difficulty climbing stairs. The gluteal muscles and the adductors are gradually affected. The posture is usually distorted, with a protuberant abdomen and exaggerated lumbar lordosis. The boy characteristically has trouble rising from the floor and must use the Gower maneuver. In this maneuver, the child puts his hands on his knees and literally walks his hands up his legs until he is standing erect. Toe-walking may be noted to compensate for the quadriceps weakness and equinus positioning of the feet. Ambulation is usually impossible by the end of the first decade.

Involvement of the shoulder girdle muscles usually begins within 3 to 5 years of the onset of the disease. Muscle weakness eventually progresses to the biceps and brachioradialis. The loss of shoulder and elbow stability interferes with hand function. Cardiac muscle involvement is universal but is generally asymptomatic until the late stages of the disease. Craniofacial muscles are not affected.

Pseudohypertrophy occurs in 85 to 90 per cent of cases. Calf muscles are most often affected, but the quadriceps, shoulder, and hip girdle may be affected as well. Flexion contractures develop as a result of unequal involvement of muscle groups. Neuromuscular scoliosis is a frequent complication caused by weakness of trunk muscles. Scoliosis occurs about 2 years after walking has ceased and the child is wheelchair dependent.

Boys with Duchenne muscular dystrophy often have an IQ below 90. Depression often associated with intellectual limitations may induce low tolerance for frustration and potentiate other manifestations of emotional immaturity. The progressive condition and increased dependency on parents and siblings invite manipulative behavior. Overprotection by parents can also interfere with interpersonal relationships.

TABLE 41-11
Muscular Dystrophies

Type	Onset	Clinical Manifestations	Progression
Duchenne (pseudohypertrophic)	Early childhood—about 2–6 yrs	Generalized weakness and muscle wasting affecting limb and trunk muscles first; calves often enlarged	Disease progresses slowly, with survival rare beyond late 20s
Becker	2–16 yrs	Almost identical to Duchenne but less severe	Slower and more variable than Duchenne
Emery-Dreifuss	Childhood to early teens	Weakness and wasting of shoulder, upper arm, and shin muscles; joint deformities are common	Disease usually progresses slowly; frequent cardiac complications are common
Limb-girdle	Late childhood to middle age	Weakness and wasting affecting shoulder and pelvic girdles first	Usually progresses slowly, with cardiopulmonary complications often occurring in later stages of the disease
Facioscapulohumeral (Landouzy-Dejerine)	Childhood to early adulthood	Facial muscle weakness, with weakness and wasting of the shoulders and upper arms	Progresses slowly with some periods of rapid deterioration; disease may span many decades
Myotonic dystrophy (Steinert's disease)	Childhood to middle age	Generalized weakness and muscle wasting affecting face, feet, hands, and neck first; delayed relaxation of muscles after contraction	Progression is slow, sometimes spanning 50–60 yrs
Oculopharyngeal	Early adulthood to middle age	First affects muscles of eyelid and throat	Slow progression, with swallowing problems common as disease progresses
Distal	40–60 yrs	Weakness and wasting of muscles of the hands, forearms, and lower legs	Slow progressing but not life-threatening
Congenital	At birth	Generalized muscle weakness with possible joint deformities	Disease progresses very slowly

From the Muscular Dystrophy Association, Inc.

Diagnostic Assessment

The diagnosis of Duchenne muscular dystrophy is made by clinical examination and abnormal muscle biopsy results. Clinical examination includes observation of the gait, testing for specific muscle weakness and Gower maneuver, and sensory testing. For the muscle biopsy, a small strip of muscle is examined. It will show degeneration of muscle cells with loss of fiber and variation in fiber size. An electromyogram will also be abnormal. Blood levels of the enzyme creatine phosphokinase will be elevated in early stages of the disease and then will decrease as muscle bulk decreases.

Therapeutic Management

There is no treatment for the underlying protein defect. Therefore, the treatment goals focus on managing the symptoms of the disease and maintaining the functional capabilities of the child for as long as possible.

Multidisciplinary care is necessary for meeting complex needs of children with Duchenne muscular dystrophy. A clinic with neurology, orthopedics, nursing, and physical and occupational therapy can facilitate maximal wellness for the child and family.

Physical Therapy. Physical therapy is directed toward keeping functional muscle strength and preventing contractures by passive stretching. Physical therapists also provide gait training in braces and transfer training, which become increasingly important as the patient loses muscle power. Maintenance of independent mobility may require use of a powered wheelchair, although the child may initially be able to use crutches around the home.

Orthotics. Prevention and treatment of contractures may require the use of orthoses (braces) or splints. Knee-ankle-foot orthoses are prescribed when independent ambulation becomes precarious. Knee-ankle-foot orthoses are long leg braces that provide stability, which the weakened muscles can no longer provide. Knee-ankle-foot orthoses maintain hip-knee-ankle alignment and may prevent knee and ankle contractures. The large size of these braces may make ambulation difficult, but the braces may help the patient stand with help and assist with pivot transfers. Long leg braces may also be necessary after surgery to the lower extremities.

Surgery. Surgery is performed when independent ambulation becomes precarious or when contractures are painful or interfere with activities of daily living.

Muscle lengthenings are used to treat contractures. Scoliosis can cause the child to sit unevenly, putting the child at risk for skin breakdown because the ability to change body positions is limited. Posterior spinal instrumentation and fusion may be necessary to treat abnormal spinal curves. This is the most useful surgical procedure for maintenance of quality of life: comfort, balanced sitting, and body image.

Before a surgical procedure is attempted, a child with Duchenne muscular dystrophy should have an electrocardiogram to determine whether the cardiac muscle has been affected by the muscle disease. In addition, children with Duchenne muscular dystrophy are more prone to malignant hyperthermia when given skeletal muscle relaxants. Malignant hyperthermia is a potentially lethal increase in body temperature in response to certain inhalation anesthetics or potent muscle relaxants used during surgery. The effect may occur immediately or several hours postoperatively (Drennan, 1990). Malignant hyperthermia is hereditary and may be detected by taking a thorough family history to determine whether another family member might also be afflicted. Definitive diagnosis is made with muscle biopsy.

Nursing Diagnostic Statements

Impaired adjustment to demands accompanying change in health status, *related to inability to cope with:*

- *Impaired physical mobility.*
- *Self-care deficit.*
- *Disuse syndrome.*

High risk for altered family process; *risk factor: perceptions of powerlessness in relation to chronic and terminal nature of the disease.*

High risk for ineffective thermoregulation; *risk factor: abnormal response to anesthetic agents related to myopathy.*

High risk for dysfunctional grieving (family), *related to inability to cope with impact of the disease.*

Interventions

Maintain Optimal Physical Mobility. As the functional level diminishes, the nurse should encourage and facilitate the maximal level of mobility for the patient. Physical therapy can provide assistance with mobility and transfers as necessary. Help the family learn how to use adaptive equipment as necessary for mobility and positioning. The nurse should assist with position change every 2 hours. It is important to seek feedback from the child as to the need to change position and satisfactory positioning, when the child cannot change her or his own position. Ensure proper body alignment in bed or in chair by using blanket rolls, sandbags, or pillows. As the disease progresses, home care equipment is usually necessary for assistance with mobility and activities of daily living.

Support Child and Family in Provision of Necessary Care. Caregivers should use assistive devices and maintain home care routines for activities of daily living. Many patients require total care. Muscle weakness is temporarily exacerbated after surgery. The increased weakness can make usual care routines impossible. Physical and occupational therapy can provide assistance with adaptive equipment for activities of daily living.

Compensation for Disuse Syndrome. Because the child with Duchenne muscular dystrophy is unable to move himself or herself, the nurse must assist with position changes every 2 hours for avoidance of prolonged pressure on body parts and compression of blood vessels. Inspect skin for areas of redness and institute protective measures as necessary. Pressure-equalizing or pressure-reducing equipment may be necessary to prevent skin breakdown. The nurse must teach the patient and caregivers measures to prevent pulmonary compromise, such as coughing and deep breathing or the use of an inspirometer. These measures are particularly important after any period of bed rest or surgery. The nurse should emphasize the importance of adequate fluid intake to prevent urinary stasis. Poor muscle tone and chronic immobility may cause an alteration in bowel elimination. The nurse should gather information to monitor elimination patterns and habits. If the patient has a home bowel regimen, the nurse should implement the home program as appropriate. If the patient does not have a bowel regimen using stool softeners or laxatives, the nurse should instruct the patient and family in such measures.

Provide Family Support and Empowerment. All health professionals should provide the family with clear, concise information about the child's condition. Determine what the family has been told and help them interpret this information. Clarification and reinforcement are important nursing functions. As the family receives information about the diagnosis, prognosis, and treatment plan, the nurse should provide emotional support to the family by being available to answer questions. The family must be encouraged to make decisions about care. Information about community agencies that can provide further support should be available. Family needs will change as the disease progresses and the child grows. Families will need assistance developing new methods for daily care. The nurse can help the family maintain realistic expectations of physical capabilities and can provide the family with current information about resources, home care and adaptive equipment, and the latest technologic innovations.

Monitor for Ineffective Thermoregulation. Patients with Duchenne muscular dystrophy are at increased risk for malignant hyperthermia, a potentially fatal complication of anesthesia. The patient may require special preoperative and intraoperative medications and monitoring. The nurse should gather information about previous experiences with anesthesia and any complications in the patient or the family. Ensure that the assessment data are communicated to the physician. Families may not give the same information to all members of the health care team.

Facilitate Family Coping. Encourage the family to express feelings about the genetic transmission of the disease, the progressive nature of the disease, and the impact on well-being and lifestyle. The status of younger male children in the family may not be certain when one sibling is diagnosed. The nurse should emphasize the strengths and current status of the patient and encourage the family to promote the patient's independence. Families should develop family/friend support systems through such groups as the Muscular Dystrophy Association. Organizations like this can provide information about disease treatment and management as well as emotional and social support.

Congenital Limb Deficiency

Frantz and O'Rahilly developed a system of describing congenital limb deficiencies by naming the absent skeletal parts in conjunction with three descriptive terms. *Amelia* is the complete absence of a limb. *Hemimelia* is the absence of the major portion of a limb. *Phocomelia* is the absence of the central portion of the limb. The system also defines two types of congenital limb deficiencies: *terminal* and *intercalary*. A terminal deficiency defines a defect in which there are no unaffected parts distal to the named portion. An intercalary deficiency describes a defect in which the middle part of the limb is deficient, but the proximal and distal portions are present. Terminal and intercalary defects are further subdivided into *transverse* and *longitudinal*. A transverse defect is a defect across the width of the limb; a longitudinal defect is a defect that extends the length of the limb.

An international classification system attempted to simplify and standardize the naming of congenital limb deficiencies. The international system defines two types of deficiencies: *transverse* and *longitudinal*. Transverse deficiencies resemble amputation stumps and are defined by the level at which the limb ends. Longitudinal deficiencies name all the bones affected and indicate whether the defect is partial or total. This system can be somewhat unwieldy, so the Frantz and O'Rahilly terminology is still frequently used.

Etiology/Incidence (Pathophysiology)

Although the true incidence is unknown, congenital deficiencies are twice as common as acquired amputations in children (Krebs & Fishman, 1984). Most congenital deficiencies occur in the upper limb; most acquired amputations occur in the lower limb. Boys are affected slightly more often than girls are.

The cause of congenital limb deficiencies is unknown, but they most likely have a multifactorial etiology. A teratogen of some sort may interfere with the timing and sequence of limb development. Some drugs, such as thalidomide, have been shown to cause congenital limb deficiencies. Growth retardation may result from a small uterine environment or disruption of the vascular supply to the growing limb.

Because development of the musculoskeletal system occurs at the same time as that of other body systems, an insult to the growing fetus may also cause abnormalities in other body systems. Children with congenital limb deficiencies frequently have defects in the genitourinary and cardiovascular systems. Because the musculoskeletal system develops synergistically, there may be abnormalities in muscle groups and muscle enervation.

Clinical Manifestations

The clinical manifestations of a congenital limb deficiency depend on the bone or bones affected. A congenital limb deficiency may be the result of lack of development of the bone (the bone is absent), or it may be the result of altered prenatal growth (the bone may be shorter than the contralateral side). Terminal transverse deficiencies resemble amputation stumps. Intercalary deficiencies result in shortened limbs, often with abnormalities of the distal limb parts. Longitudinal defects may result in angular deformities with abnormalities of the distal limb parts.

Congenital limb deficiencies occur in any limb. The most common upper limb deficiencies are terminal transverse below-elbow hemimelia and longitudinal radial hemimelia. Terminal transverse below-elbow hemimelia is an absence of the hand and distal part of the arm. Part of the radius or ulna may be present. The stump can be fitted with a below-elbow prosthesis. Longitudinal radial hemimelia is also known as radial clubhand (Fig. 41–17). It is the total or partial absence of the upper extremity along the preaxial border, which includes the radius and the thumb. The thumb may be absent or abnormal. The forearm is usually short, with a radial deviation of the hand.

The most common lower limb deficiency is longitudinal fibular hemimelia. Part of the fibula may be partially present, but, most commonly, it is a complete terminal deficiency. The child will have a markedly shortened lower leg and may have foot abnormalities. The femur may also be shortened.

Diagnostic Assessment

The abnormalities associated with a congenital limb deficiency are usually apparent at birth, although the exact bone deficiency may not be apparent. X-ray ex-

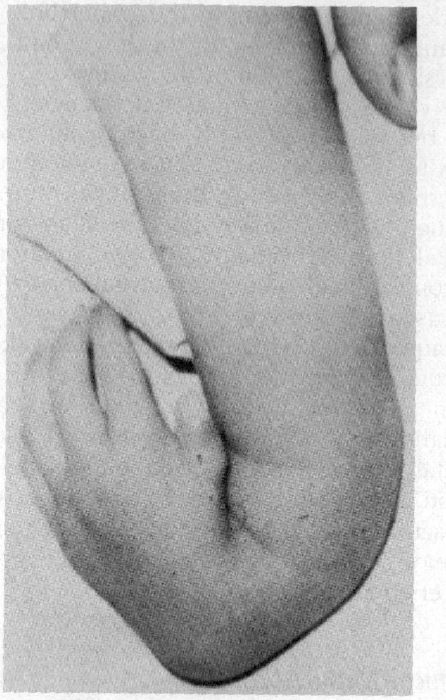

FIGURE 41 - 17. Radial clubhand deformity. (Courtesy of Drs. James Hunter & Lawrence Schneider, Thomas Jefferson University Hospital, Philadelphia.)

amination may not be initially helpful in identifying the bones affected because most of a neonate's bones are cartilage. If some portion of the bone is present, the extent of the deficiency may not be apparent until the child has grown. As the child grows, the absence of expected secondary ossification centers at the ends of long bones will indicate the extent of the expected growth deficiency.

Therapeutic Management

A multidisciplinary approach is necessary to monitor and promote normal growth and development. Children with congenital limb deficiencies require ongoing specialized orthopedic care as well as access to pediatric prosthetic services. Physical and occupational therapy are necessary to help the child become independent in daily care and to learn how to use a prosthesis.

Observation. If the child is functioning well, no treatment may be necessary beyond monitoring growth and development. Many children with congenital limb deficiencies develop unique methods of accomplishing daily tasks and should be encouraged to do so.

Prosthetics. Prosthetics are used to equalize limb lengths, correct malrotation, and improve biomechanics. Although cosmesis is a component of prosthetic fitting, appearance may be sacrificed for function. A prosthesis must be designed for each child to take advantage of motion and sensation. In a growing child, the prosthesis must be replaced every year until age 5 to accommodate growth and motor development. Some children with congenital limb deficiencies never use a prosthesis, finding it more difficult than managing with the residual limb.

Surgery. Surgery is used to improve limb function, to create a stump that is amenable to prosthetic fitting, or to lengthen the deficient bone. Procedures to improve function include centralizing the hand or lower leg to improve biomechanics of the limb or pollicization of the index finger to create a pincher grasp. Policization changes the size and position of the index finger by lengthening the web space and rotating the bone so that it functions as a thumb. Amputation of a deficient limb to improve prosthetic fitting is rarely indicated in the upper limb. The sensory feedback and dexterity of the digits is generally too useful to lose. Amputation may be helpful in the lower extremity to improve prosthetic fitting for ambulation. Bone lengthening may be of use to patients whose bone is small but otherwise normal. Bone lengthening is not an option available to all patients because it cannot construct deficient structures or create bone.

Nursing Diagnostic Statements

Ineffective management of therapeutic regimen (child and family); alterations in physical mobility, *related to lack of knowledge of or access to assistive devices and tendency to overprotect child.*

High risk for impaired skin integrity; *risk factors:*

- *Altered skin elimination: decreased perspiration associated with smaller body surface area in children with multiple congenital limb deficiencies.*
- *Presence of brace or prosthesis.*

Family coping, potential for growth, *related to self-actualization needs.*

Nursing Care

Assisting Family to Maximize Physical Mobility. The nurse should assist the family to maximize the child's mobility through use of prosthetics or assistive devices. The family will need information about how and where to get assistive devices. Although the tendency is to protect the child, the nurse should help the family recognize the need for independent mobility and assist with ways to maximize it. The family may also need assistance with financial resources and should work with a social worker who can help them access available programs.

Maintain Skin Integrity. The nurse must assess the skin under the prosthesis for redness or irritation, especially when a new brace or prosthesis is worn. A new brace or prosthesis may need to be adjusted if one area in particular is a problem. The family should not use lotions or oils on the stump. Rubbing the skin with alcohol will toughen the skin to prevent skin breakdown. The child should wear a cotton sock under the prosthesis to absorb perspiration and prevent dermatitis. The family needs an opportunity to practice the care of the stump and prosthesis.

A child with multiple congenital deficiencies has a smaller surface area. Therefore, the child can overheat quickly. Layered clothing will permit the child to regulate his or her temperature. The family should be taught how to manage dehydration and temperature fluctuations.

Promote Effective Family Coping. The birth of a child with a congenital limb deficiency is a crisis for any family. The nurse must allow time for the family to discuss its impact and their feelings. Encourage the family to ventilate their feelings and discuss their concerns. The nurse should coordinate family conferences to help the family discuss changing issues and select support services as necessary. Reinforce the family's efforts to care for their child. The nurse should demonstrate daily care and application of braces or prosthetics and allow the family time to practice. As the child grows, it is important to help the family support the child's independence and self-care activities.

The issues and concerns of the child and family will change as the child grows and faces new developmental or social challenges. Staff should provide information about resources and adaptive equipment as needed. The needs of the child may create a financial hardship for families. Children with congenital limb deficiencies may benefit from state programs for handicapped children, although some families are reluctant to access these services for fear of their child's being labeled handicapped. The family should have access to social services to assist them with these concerns.

Growth-Related Musculoskeletal Disorders

Bone growth occurs in two dimensions: increase in diameter and increase in length. Growth in diameter occurs when new bone is formed on the surface of the cortex by the osteoblasts of the periosteum. In addition, osteoclasts lining the marrow cavity destroy bone so that the bone does not increase in weight as it grows in diameter.

Growth in length occurs at the epiphyseal plate, or physis, through endochondral ossification. The physis is an area of active cell division. Longitudinal growth occurs through the continual development of cartilage at the epiphyseal end of the plate and ossification of cartilage at the metaphyseal end. Growth hormone increases the cell reproduction and synthesis. Estrogens slow down activity in the physis and tend to narrow the epiphyseal plate, whereas testosterone has the opposite effect (Morrissy, 1990). Nutrition also has a direct effect on cells of the physis.

The physis is active from birth until adolescence, when all of the cartilage cells are completely converted to bone and longitudinal growth stops. The age at which this occurs differs from one adolescent to another; physeal closure generally occurs earlier in girls than in boys as the result of increased estrogen production.

Because of the interface between bone and cartilage, the physis represents an area of weakness in bone structure and is subject to injury by fracture, crushing, or slippage. Injury to the physis always carries with it the risk of altered growth of the bone. Considering the tremendous growth in bone size from infancy to adolescence, injury to one epiphysis can have a severe effect on growth.

Developmental Leg Deformity

As a child grows, there are normal variations in the rotation and angularity of the lower extremities. These variations can become pathologic if they occur at the wrong time or if the deformity is severe.

Etiology/Incidence (Pathophysiology)

Torsional deformities are rotational abnormalities of bones, especially of the lower extremities. They may be caused by positioning but are generally self-correcting with linear growth. *Angular deformities* of the lower limb are normal aspects of growth and development. In infancy, physiologic bowing may involve the femur and tibia. Lateral tibial bowing, or bowlegs, is common in infancy until the child has been walking about a year. Knock-knees are most pronounced between the ages of 3 and 4 years.

Clinical Manifestations

Internal tibial torsion is also called medial tibial torsion. It is a medial twisting of the distal segment of the tibia in relation to the proximal segment so that the toes appear to point inward toward the center of the body. When the child is lying prone and the knees are bent with the feet toward the ceiling, the foot should be in line with the long axis of the thighs. In a child with internal tibial torsion, the heels point out. When the child is lying supine and the patellae are in line with the hips, the feet turn in (Fig. 41–18*A*). Internal tibial torsion may be influenced by intrauterine positioning. *External tibial torsion,* or the lateral twisting of the distal segment of the tibia in relation to the proximal segment, also occurs, although it is less common (Fig. 41–18*B*).

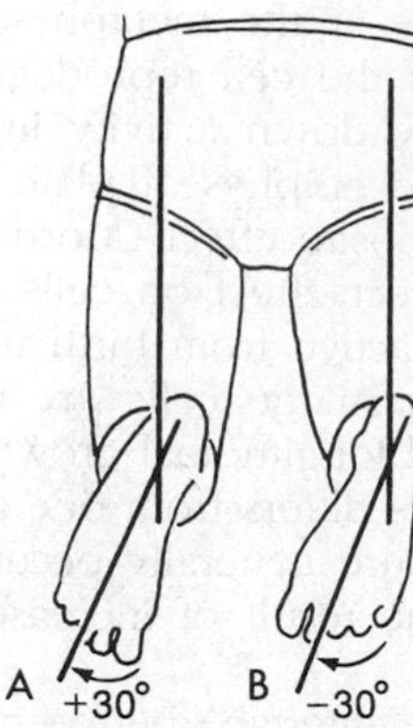

FIGURE 41-18. Assessment of tibial rotation. *A*, External tibial rotation. *B*, Internal tibial rotation. (*A* and *B*, From Staheli, L. [1977, November]. Torsional deformity. *Pediatric Clinics of North America,* p 809.)

Internal femoral torsion is also called femoral anteversion or medial femoral torsion. It is a medial, or inward, rotation of the distal segment of the femur in relation to the proximal segment. When the child is lying supine, the knee caps face each other when the feet face forward. The incidence of internal femoral torsion peaks in late preschool years. The defect is primarily cosmetic but may occasionally cause tripping. Spontaneous correction may occur until age 8 years. Table 41–12 summarizes torsional deformities.

A child has *genu varum,* an angular deformity, when the knees are more than 1 inch apart when the medial malleoli are touching. Genu varum is commonly called bowlegs. The deformity will decrease with continued growth in height but may persist into middle childhood. The appearance of genu varum may be exacerbated by internal tibial torsion (Fig. 41–19). Physiologic genu varum is always bilateral.

A child has *genu valgum* when the ankles are more than 1 inch apart when the knees are touching (Fig. 41–20). Genu valgum is commonly called knock-knees. School-aged children may have genu valgum

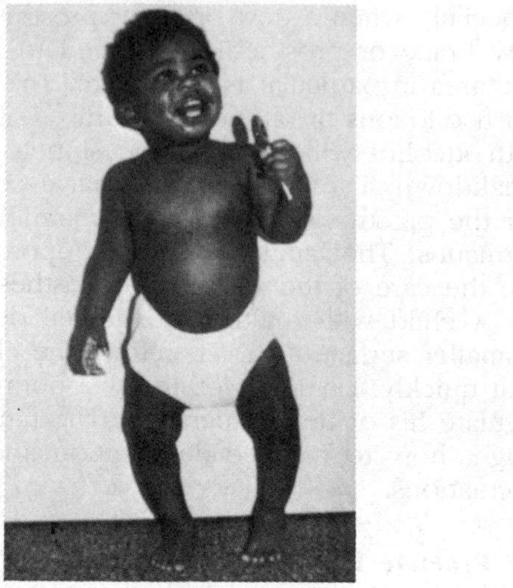

FIGURE 41-19. The "extreme variation," a 15-month-old boy with bowlegs. (From McDade, W. [1977, November]. Bow legs and knock knees. *Pediatric Clinics of North America,* p 833.)

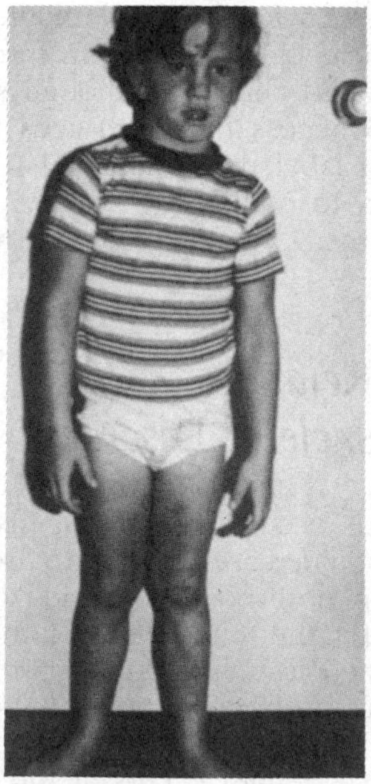

FIGURE 41-20. A 5-year-old boy with knock knees. (From McDade, W. [1977, November]. Bow legs and knock knees. *Pediatric Clinics of North America,* p 831.)

TABLE 41-12
Characteristics of Torsional Deformities

Direction	
In-Toeing	**Out-Toeing**
Hip	
Femoral torsion as estimated by internal hip rotation: 70°–80° rotation, mild 80°–85° rotation, moderate 85° + rotation, severe	Normal physiologic position (i.e., internal hip rotation less than 70%)
Tibia	
Internal tibial torsion indicated by thigh-foot angle: −10°, mild −20°, moderate −30°, severe	External tibial torsion (thigh-foot angle greater than +30°)

Adapted from Staheli, L. (1977, November). Torsional deformity. *Pediatric Clinics of North America,* p. 799.

until approximately 10 years of age. Untreated genu valgum may contribute to gait awkwardness, recurrent dislocation of the patella, joint pains, and easy fatigue.

Diagnostic Assessment

Specialized x-ray views assist with the diagnosis of physiologic and pathologic deformities. To determine the severity of the angular deformity, a radiograph of the entire lower limb on a long cassette is necessary. The hip-knee-ankle axis, or mechanical axis, is measured, using the center of the femoral head and the midpoints of the knee and ankle. At the point where the two lines meet at the knee, the angle should be 0 degrees. Pathologic genu varum is present if this angle exceeds 11 degrees. Pathologic genu valgum is present when the angle measures more than 7 degrees of valgus.

Nonphysiologic or extreme varus is diagnosed if there is no improvement in the varus angulation by age 3 years. The child may have infantile tibia vara, or Blount disease, which is an abnormality of the growth plate of the medial proximal tibia. The lateral side of the tibia grows more quickly than the medial side, resulting in a localized curvature. The diagnosis of Blount disease may be difficult on the basis of one clinical examination. Serial clinical examinations and radiographs are necessary to confirm the diagnosis.

Therapeutic Management

Observation. Physiologic torsional and angular deformities are generally self-correcting with linear growth. A child should be observed every 3 to 6 months to document a progression or resolution of the deformity. Because the tendency toward torsional deformities may be exacerbated by sitting posture, encouraging the child to sit "tailor-fashion," with legs crossed in front, may be helpful. Consistently sitting with the feet in a backward M will exacerbate the tendency toward internal femoral rotation and internal tibial torsion, depending on the position of the feet.

Bracing. Treatment with orthotics and night-splinting is controversial. There is some evidence that these treatments cause growth plate disturbances by putting unequal pressure on the growth plate (Staheli, 1987). Bracing does not change the natural history of torsional or angular deformities. It is used in mild cases of Blount disease only.

Surgery. Surgery can be performed for severe, persistent angular abnormalities, but it is seldom necessary. Rotational osteotomies will correct torsional deformities. An osteotomy of the proximal tibia or other reconstructive procedures, such as correction with the Ilizarov system, may be required for severe Blount disease. Osteotomy of the distal femur may be performed for severe genu valgum.

Nursing Diagnostic Statements

Ineffective individual and family coping, *related to body image disturbance, associated with torsional or angular deformity of lower limit.*

Altered role performance: participation in developmentally appropriate activities, *related to alteration in physical mobility.*

Nursing Care

Support Coping with Disturbance in Body Image. Because many torsional and angular deformities are normal developmental phases, the nurse should encourage the family to allow time for correction with growth. It is often difficult for the family to wait, and they may need ongoing support and reinforcement. Encourage the child and family to verbalize their concerns. The nurse must assess the family's readiness for decision making when the therapeutic plan changes and support and encourage the family's participation in decisions about the plan of care.

Facilitate Ability to Maintain Positive Perception of Role. The amount of difficulty with activities from a torsional or angular deformity varies from child to child. The nurse must gather information from the child and family to assess for problem areas. Explore interests and activities with the child and gather information about previous difficulties. The nurse must collaborate with child and family to determine ways for the child to participate in desired activities.

Leg Length Inequality

A limb length discrepancy is unequal bone length in contralateral limbs. Although it may occur in any bone, it most commonly occurs in the femur and tibia.

Etiology/Incidence (Pathophysiology)

Leg length is the result of growth at the epiphyseal plates of the proximal and distal femur and the proximal and distal tibia. The four growth plates normally contribute to the growth of the leg in consistent proportions. Limb length discrepancies can be caused by overgrowth or deficient growth at one or more of the epiphyseal plates. Congenital anomalies may cause unequal bone lengths, as previously discussed. Tumors may stimulate or inhibit growth. Trauma to the growth plate may affect longitudinal bone growth by damaging the cartilage cells of the epiphyseal plate. A fracture to a long bone may result in overgrowth; the increased circulation to the fracture site for healing also causes increased growth at the growth plate.

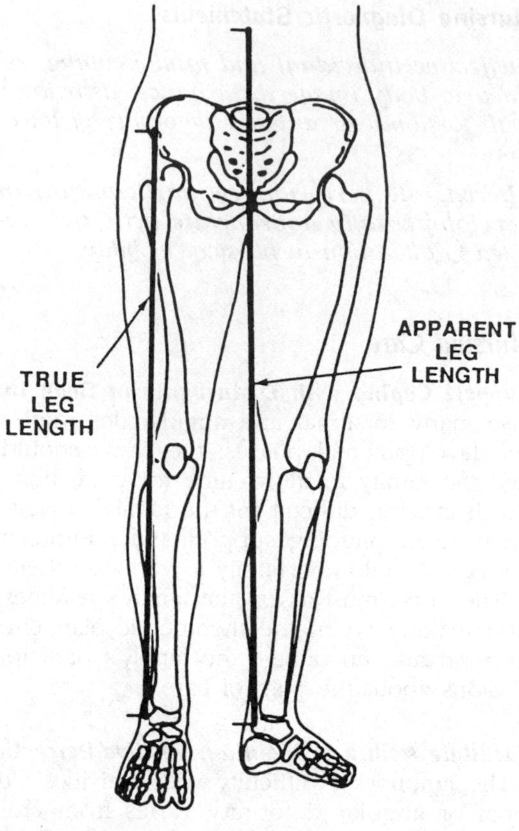

FIGURE 41 - 21. Measurement of real and apparent length. The measurement of real length is relatively immune from error because of pelvic obliquity. Measurement of apparent length is susceptible to such error. (From Mosely, C. F. [1990]. Leg-length discrepancy. In R. T. Morrissy (Ed.), *Lovell and Winter's pediatric orthopaedics* [8th ed.]. Philadelphia: JB Lippincott, pp 767–813.)

Diagnostic Assessment

A child with a limb length discrepancy in the lower limb will have an unequal or uneven stance. Unequal hip heights and knees at different levels will also be noted on physical examination. The physical examination should also include an assessment of soft tissue contractures at the hip, knee, and ankle. Hip and knee flexion contractures will effectively shorten the leg; contractures of the Achilles tendon at the ankle will effectively lengthen the leg by plantar flexion of the foot. There may be postural sway with walking if the leg length discrepancy is large.

Leg length is measured in two ways. Real length is measured from the anterior iliac spine to the tip of the lateral malleolus. Apparent leg length is measured from the umbilicus to the tip of the medial malleolus (Fig. 41–21). The apparent length is influenced by pelvic obliquity and hip position.

Limb length measurements can also be made by use of specialized radiographic techniques. A scanogram is an x-ray technique that shows the hip joint, the knee joint, and the ankle joint on the same film. The x-ray film has a ruler on it so that exact measurements of bone lengths can be made. This helps determine whether the discrepancy is in the femur, the tibia, or both. CT images can be reconstructed to allow measurement of bone length.

A significant leg length discrepancy requires increased energy expenditure with walking as well as causes a cosmetically disturbing gait. Functional scoliosis may develop as the pelvis shifts to accommodate the unequal leg lengths. Degenerative arthritis of the hip may also develop later in life because of unequal force of the hip joint of the longer leg.

Therapeutic Management

The treatment of a leg length discrepancy depends on the amount of the discrepancy as well as its cause (Table 41–13). Treatment of the underlying problem is necessary to prevent the discrepancy from increasing as the child continues to grow.

Shoe Lift. A shoe lift may be prescribed to equalize leg lengths and improve the gait. The size of the prescribed lift is usually slightly smaller than the measured discrepancy. The lift may go inside the shoe, or it may be attached to the entire sole of the shoe.

Surgery. Surgery may be performed to stop the growth in the longer limb, to shorten the longer limb, or to lengthen the shorter limb. An *epiphysiodesis* will stop the growth in the longer limb by damaging the rapidly producing cartilage cells of the physis. Timing is critical, because the goal is for the shorter limb to continue to grow and catch up with the longer limb before growth naturally stops in adolescence. Alternatively, *bone shortening* of the longer limb can be performed when growth is complete. If the discrepancy is too large, bone shortening cannot be performed because it may cause severe complications, such as loss of muscular strength and function.

In a *bone lengthening* procedure, the shorter bone is surgically broken, and an external lengthening device, or external fixator, is applied. The external fixator is adjusted daily, so that the bone ends are slowly separated. The body gradually fills in this gap with new bone. Once the desired length has been achieved,

TABLE 41 - 13
Treatment for Leg Length Inequality

Size of Discrepancy	Therapeutic Management
<2 cms	No treatment
2–6 cms	Shoe lift
	Epiphysiodesis
6–15 cms	Bone lengthening
>15 cms	Prosthetic fitting, with or without amputation

the bone is left to consolidate, or heal, while the fixator remains in place. The complications of bone lengthening include neurovascular damage and infection, so it is a procedure used when other treatment options are not possible.

Prosthetics or Amputation. At times, the size of a discrepancy is so large that the best treatment is use of a prosthesis, either with or without amputation of the foot. Amputation may be preferred if the foot makes prosthetic fitting or skin care difficult.

Nursing Diagnostic Statements and Collaborative Problems

Impaired physical mobility, *related to leg length discrepancy or external lengthening device.*

Disturbance in body image, *related to negative perceptions about appearance and gait associated with leg length discrepancy.*

High risk for infection; *risk factor: disruption of skin by percutaneous pins.*

Nursing Care

Maintain Physical Mobility. Depending on the size of the discrepancy between the legs, a child may have difficulty ambulating or participating in other daily activities. A shoe lift or prosthesis may be prescribed by the physician. If the patient undergoes a leg lengthening procedure, activities may be limited by discomfort of the bulkiness of the external lengthening device. The nurse should instruct the child and parents in the proper fit and application of any shoe lifts or prosthetics. Physical therapy may be necessary to maximize mobility. The nurse and physical therapist must help the child and parents develop methods of carrying out daily activities. Assistive devices, such as walkers, crutches, or canes, may be needed. Home care equipment could include a shower chair to facilitate bathing or an elevated toilet seat.

Support Coping with Disturbance in Body Image. The nurse should explore the child's perceptions and feelings related to the leg length inequality or the leg lengthening device. Encourage the child and parents to verbalize their concerns and fears. The nurse must present a positive, accepting attitude to the child. It is important to help the child achieve appropriate developmental tasks, such as physical activities and interaction with peers. The child and family may need help developing strategies to foster a positive body image and self-esteem.

Prevent Infection. The leg lengthening device is an external fixator attached to the bone with percutaneous pins or wires. These sites can become infected. The child and family should be taught site assessment and the pin care routine ordered by the physician. Methods for covering the pin or wire sites should also be explained. The family should understand that some drainage from the pin sites is normal and that it will increase if the child is very active.

Slipped Capital Femoral Epiphysis

Slipped capital femoral epiphysis (SCFE) is a hip disorder in which the anatomic relationship between the femoral head and the femoral neck is altered. The change in the relationship occurs at the level of the physeal growth plate. When the growth plate is disrupted, the femoral head "slips" off the femoral neck (Fig. 41–22). This altered anatomic relationship is a problem because of the anatomy of the blood vessels that supply the hip joint.

The hip joint is unique in that the proximal femoral epiphysis is entirely intra-articular. Blood vessels supplying the femoral head do not enter from soft tissues. They must travel on the surface of the femoral neck and are relatively unprotected. When the femoral head shifts downward and outward, the vessels are at risk. If the blood supply to the femoral head is interrupted, it could die.

Etiology/Incidence (Pathophysiology)

SCFE is the most common hip disorder in adolescents. The cause is unknown. It is believed to be caused by trauma, at a time when an imbalance of hormones makes the physeal growth plate unstable. SCFE usually develops before or during the onset of puberty, at 8 to 15 years for girls and 10 to 17 years for boys. The hormonal changes of adolescence alter the function of the growth plate. Growth hormone causes thickening of the proximal femoral epiphysis, which may increase its susceptibility to shear forces. Because the activity of the growth plate is slowing, there may also be some disorganization in the growth plate, which makes it more susceptible to shear forces. A traumatic force may be transmitted through the weakened growth plate to the femoral head, causing a shift at the vulnerable conjunction of bone and cartilage.

SCFE can be acute or chronic. An *acute slip* is an abrupt displacement, often from a single episode of trauma, with symptoms typically developing within 3 weeks. A *chronic slip* is a gradual displacement, with symptoms of greater than 3 weeks duration. The patient may report intermittent pain in the groin and thigh for weeks or years.

Clinical Manifestations

The most common presenting complaint is pain, typically dull and aching. Pain is often referred to the knee because the hip is innervated by the obturator and femoral nerves, which also innervate the knee joint. The pain may be localized to the groin, buttock,

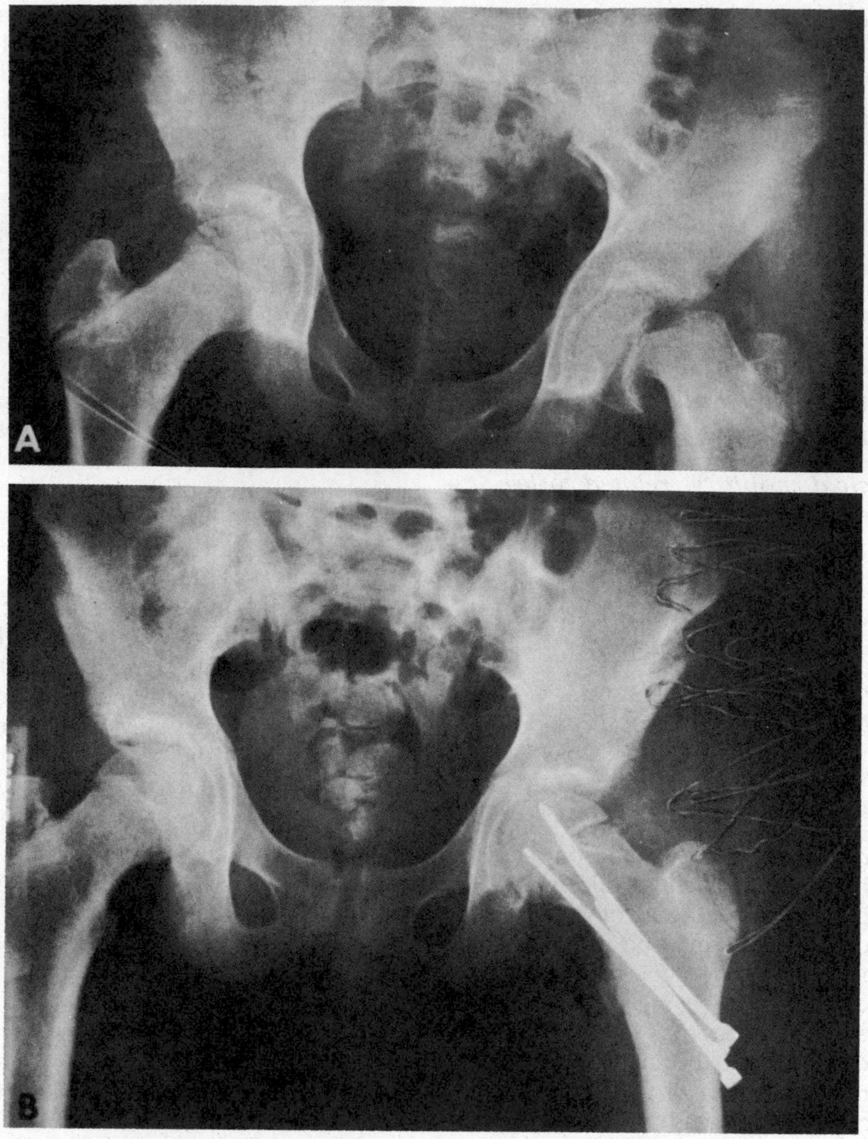

FIGURE 41-22. *A*, Complete slip of capital femoral epiphysis of left hip. *B*, Same patient after operative replacement of the epiphysis, bone pegging of the growth line, and fixation with metallic pins. (*A* and *B*, Courtesy of Dr. John Dowling, Lankenau Hospital, Philadelphia.)

and lateral hip of the affected side. The adolescent walks with a limp, often with the foot externally rotated.

On physical examination, the patient will have decreased range of motion on the affected side. Generally, there is a limitation in internal rotation, abduction, and flexion. The limited motion is due to the change in the anatomic relationship between the head and the neck of the femur and spasm of muscles of the hip.

Diagnostic Assessment

Besides the history and physical examination, radiographs are used to diagnose SCFE. On frog-leg lateral x-ray views with the hips externally rotated, the change in the anatomic relationships is visible. MRI may be useful in assessing the risk of SCFE in the other hip in the preclinical stage.

Therapeutic Management

Bed Rest With or Without Traction. The first phase of treatment is to prevent further displacement of the femoral head. Further slippage can damage the blood vessels that supply the head of the femur. No weight bearing of the affected leg is permitted. This can be done with crutches, although it is most often done with bed rest. Bathroom privileges with crutches may be allowed. Skin traction, such as Buck's extension, may be used to decrease muscle spasm and improve the range of motion.

Surgery. In general, the head of the femur is stabilized surgically. The most common procedure is *in situ pinning,* which is the placement of two threaded pins across the growth plate into the head of the femur (see Fig. 41–22). No attempt is made to correct the position of the head of the femur. The pins stabilize the femoral head and speed the rate of closure of the physis. The patient can ambulate with crutches on the first postoperative day. The pins are removed once the physis is closed.

If the femoral head is adequately stabilized, there is no apparent difference in leg length. If the femoral head is not adequately stabilized, progressive damage to the articular cartilage and contractures of the muscles of the hip may result in a difference in leg length.

Collaborative Problems

Impaired physical mobility, *related to disease process, pain and muscle spasm.*

Pain, *related to muscle spasm or surgery.*

High risk for injury; *risk factor: disruption of blood supply causing avascular necrosis or chondrolysis.*

Nursing Care

Maintain Optimal Physical Mobility. The patient must be non–weight bearing on the affected side before surgery to prevent a further shift in the position of the capital femoral epiphysis on the neck of the femur. If the child is reliable, he or she can be taught non–weight bearing crutch ambulation. Depending on the institution, physical therapy may be consulted for crutch training. The patient will progress to partial weight bearing after surgery. If the child has a markedly decreased range of motion, skin traction, such as Buck's traction, may be used to gradually stretch tight muscles and relieve spasm. Traction will improve the range of motion. Physical therapy may also assist with range-of-motion exercises before and after surgery. SCFE can become bilateral; instruct the patient to report pain or inability to bear weight on the unaffected hip.

Relieve Discomfort Related to Muscle Spasm or Surgery. As noted earlier, skin traction may be used to relieve muscle spasm and increase comfort. The nurse should assess the patient's pain and administer analgesics per the physician's order before and after surgery. Postoperatively, the child may require narcotics for bone and incisional pain.

Prevent Injury. If the blood supply to the capital femoral epiphysis is damaged, the patient may develop avascular necrosis. In avascular necrosis, the bone dies from lack of blood. The end result depends on the age of the child, the amount of bone that is necrotic, and the status of the blood supply. If the pins used to stabilize the femoral head during surgery enter the joint, the articular cartilage in the joint can die (chondrolysis). The patient will develop degenerative joint disease of the hip at an early age. A patient with SCFE should be monitored for these complications with routine x-ray examination. The patient and family should be aware that there may be an increased risk of developing osteoarthritis in adulthood as a result of SCFE.

Spinal Abnormalities

Most spinal abnormalities seen in children are abnormal curvatures. These curvatures can be disfiguring and cause pain and respiratory complications.

Scoliosis

The normal spine has three curves: the cervical lordosis, the thoracic kyphosis, and the lumbar lordosis. These are curves on the anterioposterior plane. Scoliosis is a lateral curvature of the spine. As the spine curves, the vertebrae rotate, pulling the ribs along. Generally, a sideway curve greater than 10 degrees is considered scoliosis. A curve of 10 degrees or less is considered a normal variation. Other spinal abnormalities less commonly seen are kyphosis and lordosis (Fig. 41–23). These curves become a problem when they become excessive.

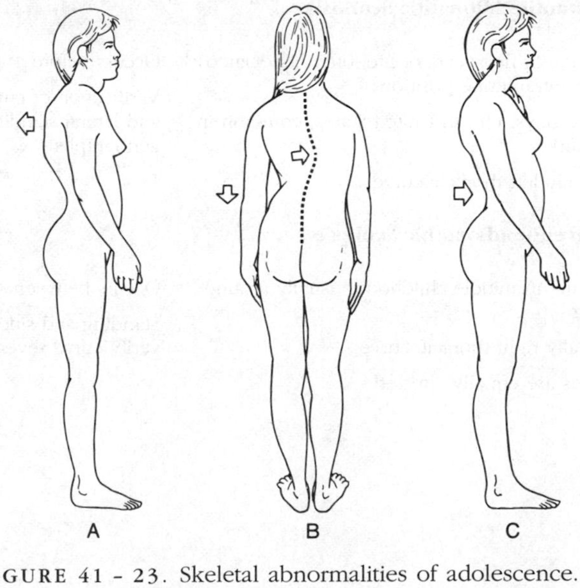

FIGURE 41 - 23. Skeletal abnormalities of adolescence. *A,* Kyphosis. *B,* Scoliosis. *C,* Lordosis.

TABLE 41-14
Etiologic Classification of Structural Scoliosis

Etiology and Pathophysiology	Diagnostic Assessment	Therapeutic Management
Congenital Scoliosis		
Embryologic malformation of spine during third to fifth embryonic week Localized or generalized deformity: hemivertebra (only half-formed), failure in segmentations (vertebra segments do not fully separate), and rib fusion are typical anomalies Thoracic curves most common	Anteroposterior and lateral roentgenographs verify curvature and identify anomalous vertebrae Usually other congenital anomalies coexist; urinary tract anomalies most prevalent Secondary neurologic symptoms from long-term spinal cord tethering Secondary signs: short trunk; sacral area hair tufts; unequal leg length; café au lait markings	Early treatment essential; usually spinal fusion before preschool-age to stabilize progressive curves Complete evaluation for any other anomalies; intravenous pyelogram recommended as a minimal screening
Neuromuscular (Paralytic) Scoliosis		
Secondary to neuropathic or myopathic disease (polio, cerebral palsy, muscular dystrophy, neurofibromatosis, myelomeningocele) that results in muscle imbalance Initially flexible, becoming rigid as it progresses tends to progress after skeletal growth completed: Long C curve—generalized neuromuscular disease with severe muscle weakness S curve similar to idiopathic scoliosis—result of localized muscle imbalance	Presence of primary neurologic or muscular disease Anteroposterior and lateral roentgenographs verify curvature Rib hump may or may not be present, depending on flexibility of curve	Occasionally bracing stabilizes progression if no structural changes Spinal fusion usually necessary if structural change present
Idiopathic Scoliosis		
Dominant X-linked inheritance in 70–80% of cases justifies evaluation of all family members when one is diagnosed S-shaped curvature most common with vertebrae changes and rotations See below for individual forms	See below for individual forms	See below for individual forms
Infantile Idiopathic Scoliosis		
Occurs in first years of life; often associated with intrauterine position More boys; rare in United States, common in Britain Usually left thoracic curve	Occurs before 4 yrs of age Verification of curve with anteroposterior and lateral standing and side-bending roentgenographs	50% resolve spontaneously 50% rapidly progressive and require spinal fusion
Juvenile Idiopathic Scoliosis		
Occurs in middle childhood, usually around 6 yrs Usually right thoracic curve Sexes are equally affected	Occurs between 4 and 10 yrs of age Standing and side-bending roentgenographs verify curve severity	Will not resolve spontaneously Bracing or Orthoplast jacket usually adequate Spinal fusion indicated if rapidly progressive or curve is severe (55 to 60 degrees)

TABLE 41-14
Etiologic Classification of Structural Scoliosis *(Continued)*

Etiology and Pathophysiology	Diagnostic Assessment	Therapeutic Management
Adolescent Idiopathic Scoliosis		
Occurs between age 10 and skeletal maturity Most prevalent in United States; seven times more common in girls May or may not progress during growth spurt Various curves possible *Lumbar curve* (T11–L5) Fairly common Majority are left Seldom any compensatory curves Minimally deforming but does become rigid, causing arthritic pain during childbearing and old age *Right thoracic curve* (T4–L1) Very common Severe cosmetic defect and cardiopulmonary impairment if untreated Usually compensatory left minor curves above and below major curve Much vertebral change and rotation *Double major curves* Right thoracic and left lumbar prominence most common combination *Thoracolumbar curve* (T4–L4) Very common Long curve Moderate cosmetic deformity May cause rib and flank distortions *Cervicothoracic curve* (C5–T4) Rare Usually to left Shoulder asymmetry only cosmetic problem	Occurs after age 10 Positive screening test findings: Scapular prominence Rib hump Shoulder asymmetry Spinal curves Hip asymmetry Deeper creasing on one side of waist Torso malalignment when standing erect Anterior rib and breast asymmetry Suggestive signs: unequal hemline, back pain, poor posture, attached earlobes, cavus (high arch) feet	Will not resolve spontaneously Exercise program alone ineffective Milwaukee brace or Orthoplast jacket or spinal fusion with or without instrumentation (cast or traction may be used preoperatively or postoperatively)

Etiology/Incidence

There are three major types of scoliosis: *congenital, neuromuscular,* and *idiopathic*. *Congenital scoliosis* is due to vertebral abnormalities that develop in utero. The exact cause of the vertebral abnormalities is unknown. Most cases are sporadic and may be associated with other congenital abnormalities, such as spinal cord abnormalities, genitourinary tract abnormalities, cardiac defects, and pulmonary hypoplasia. A congenital scoliosis may be noted at birth or during the rapid growth in infancy.

Neuromuscular scoliosis is the result of muscle weakness or imbalance. Neuromuscular scoliosis develops in patients with cerebral palsy as a result of abnormal, excessive muscle forces. In patients with spina bifida or muscular dystrophy, the muscles fail to support the spine.

The cause of *idiopathic scoliosis* is unknown by definition. It affects 2 per cent of the population. There may be abnormalities in the bones, intervertebral disks, muscles, or collagen that cause the abnormal curvature, but these abnormalities may be a result rather than a cause. Idiopathic scoliosis can occur in any age group: infantile, juvenile, or adolescent (Winter, 1990). Only 15 per cent of curves progress, but most progress during periods of growth. Scoliosis is most often noted in adolescents because the curve may suddenly be large enough that the accompanying physical changes are obvious after the adolescent growth spurt. Table 41-14 summarizes the types of scoliosis and their management.

Pathophysiology

Scoliosis may develop in any part of the spine as a result of differential growth of the vertebrae. This differential growth may be due to increased pressure on the concave side of the vertebral growth plates. Curves progress during growth as a result of the action of gravity on the passive properties of a flexible column. As the spine begins to curve, it rotates on its axis, causing the ribs to become prominent on the convex side.

If scoliosis progresses, significant deformity can result. A large curve and the associated physical changes can be physically and cosmetically disabling. Measurable changes in lung function start to appear with thoracic curves greater than 60 degrees. It is important to monitor and treat scoliosis. Early diagnosis and treatment can prevent progression of the curve and improve the effectiveness of bracing treatment for avoidance of surgical intervention.

Clinical Manifestations

The first sign of scoliosis is often uneven hips and shoulders due to the lateral curvature of the spine. However, in some curve patterns, the shoulders and hips may be level. One scapula or breast may appear more prominent. A plumb line held at C7 will not pass through the gluteal crease. On a forward-bending test, scapular and rib prominences will be noted as a result of vertebral rotation.

Diagnostic Assessment

Diagnosis of scoliosis is made by physical examination, including the area and magnitude of the curve, the deviation from center, the presence of shoulder elevation and flank crease, and the prominence of one hip. On the Adam forward bending test, the presence of a rib hump is evaluated, and the size of the hump is measured in centimeters or degrees by use of a scoliometer. School screening programs have increased the early identification of adolescents with scoliosis by evaluating the presence of physical signs (Fig. 41–24).

Serial radiographs are used to measure the curve and to document whether the curve is progressive. Anteroposterior and lateral radiographs of the spine are necessary. CT is seldom necessary in ordinary curves, although it may be used to rule out other pathologic processes if the curve is unusual. Moiré topography and the Integrated Shape Imaging System (ISIS) are computerized scanning techniques being evaluated as methods of monitoring progression. Al-

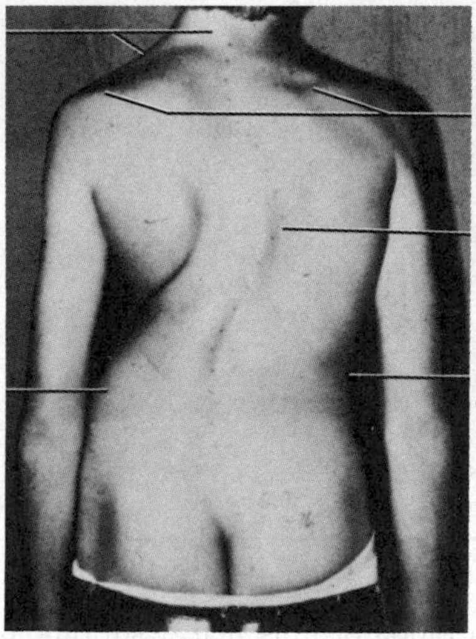

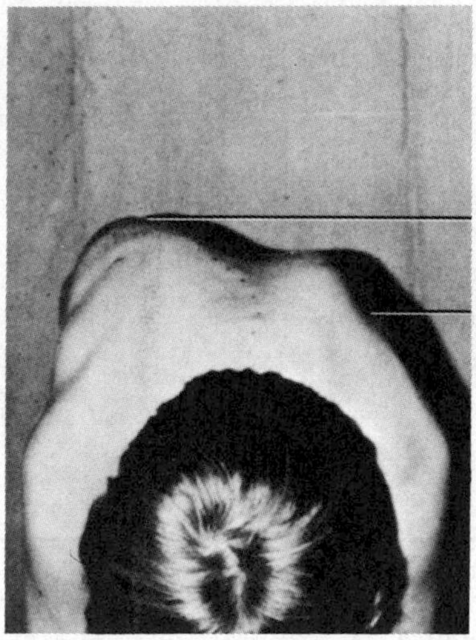

Screening of youth 9–15 promotes early detection of scoliosis. Adequate screening requires complete exposure of back, chest and hips.

Observe child from front while he or she is standing erect, assessing for:
- Shoulder asymmetry (shoulder elevated on convex side of scoliotic curve).
- Anterior rib asymmetry.
- Breast asymmetry (one breast may appear higher, larger or more protruding than the other).
- Hip asymmetry (one hip may protrude).

Observe youth from side and back while standing erect, assessing for:
- Shoulder asymmetry.
- Scapular asymmetry (scapula on convex side of curve higher).
- Rib cage asymmetry (rib cage prominent on convex side of curve).
- Waist asymmetry (waist fuller, more creased on convex side of curve).
- Hip asymmetry.
- Drop a plumb line (tape measure) from occiput to check for trunk malalignment—indicated when plumb line does not pass through gluteal fold. (If line passes through gluteal folds but curves are visible, compensation is indicated.)
- Malalignment of spinous processes. (Mark each process with a marker pen. Line formed is not straight in malalignment).

Observe youth from back while bending over, feet together until back is parallel to floor and arms dangling freely (forward bending test), assessing for:
- Thorax asymmetry (posterior rib hump may appear on convex side of curve).
- Hip asymmetry.

Run measuring tape from anterior superior iliac spine to medial malleolus at ankle, assessing for:
- Asymmetry in leg length.

FIGURE 41-24. Screening procedure for scoliosis.

though the use of computerized scanning systems could decrease the amount of x-ray studies needed, the computer map has not correlated well with standard radiographs.

Serial pulmonary function tests may be used to evaluate lung capacity. Preservation of lung capacity is the primary reason for treating scoliosis. When pulmonary function tests are performed, the patient's actual test results are compared with an expected value. The expected value for any child is partly based on age and height. Scoliosis causes a loss of height because the spine is curved sideways. Arm span measurements rather than height should be used to calculate lung volumes when pulmonary function tests are performed in patients with scoliosis.

Therapeutic Management

The treatment of scoliosis is largely based on the degree of the curve as well as the age of the child and the amount of growth remaining. An estimate of the amount of growth remaining can be made on the basis of the radiographic appearance of the physes and whether menstruation has begun in girls.

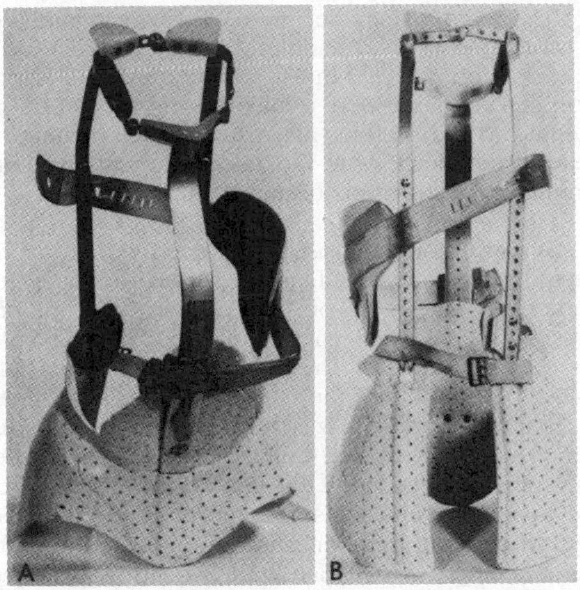

FIGURE 41 - 26. Milwaukee brace, front *(A)* and back *(B)* views. (*A* and *B*, From Tachdjian, M. [1990]. *Pediatric orthopedics* [2nd ed.]. Philadelphia: WB Saunders.)

Observation. For curves less than 20 degrees, the treatment is observation and monitoring. The child is evaluated every 3 to 12 months. During periods of accelerated growth, when curves usually progress, evaluation every 3 to 4 months is necessary. Monitoring of the curve is usually done with serial radiographs, when the curve is measured and compared with previous x-ray films.

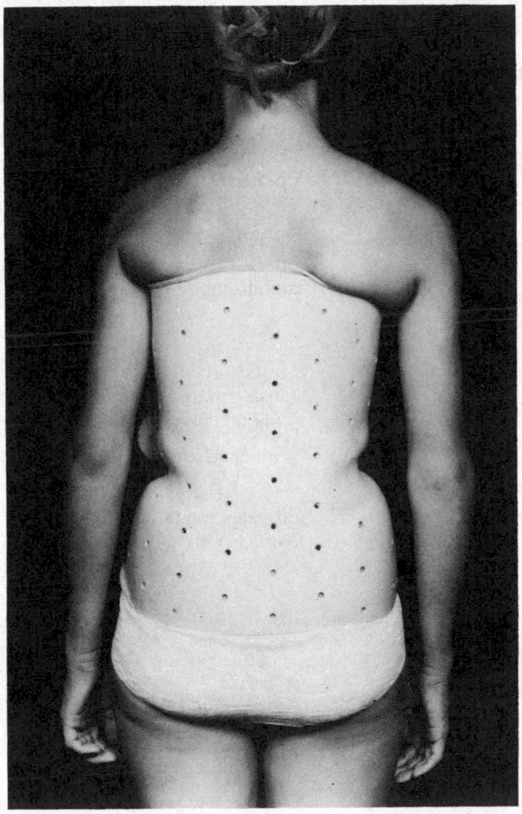

FIGURE 41 - 25. Boston brace. (From Hungerford, D. [1975, November]. Spinal deformity in adolescence. *Medical Clinics of North America*.)

Bracing. For progressive curves of 20 to 40 degrees in a growing child, bracing is usually recommended to reduce the curve and hold it in the corrected position. Bracing straightens the spine to prevent unequal pressure on the vertebral growth plates. Although bracing can halt the progression of the curve, it will not correct the curve.

There are several types of braces. Low-profile braces, such as the Boston brace and the Wilmington brace, are used for low thoracic, thoracolumbar, and lumbar curves (Fig. 41–25). The brace stops under the arms and can be hidden by clothing. The Milwaukee brace is a high-profile brace with a chin extension (Fig. 41–26). It is only used for high thoracic curves. A scoliosis brace is fabricated to the child's specific measurements.

The wearing schedule of a brace depends on the individual orthopedic surgeon. Most surgeons recommend 20 to 22 hours per day. For a newly prescribed brace, wearing time is gradually increased over 4 to 6 weeks to minimize skin irritation or soreness. Most activities can be done in the brace without restriction, although the brace may limit participation in gymnastics, skating, and skiing because of restricted movement.

Although bracing is effective in 85 per cent of compliant patients, noncompliance rates are as high as 50 per cent. There seems to be better compliance in younger patients. In adolescents, the brace may be viewed as an external threat to body image and peer acceptance. In addition, adolescent health beliefs are oriented to the present, not to the future, so that not wearing the brace now is more important than preventing progression of the curve in the future.

Surgery. For scoliosis curves greater than 40 degrees in a growing child, spinal fusion is usually recommended. The goal of surgery is to prevent progression so the child enters adulthood with a curve less than 50 degrees. The force of gravity can cause a slow progression of the curve unless it is stabilized.

Spinal fusion stabilizes the spine to prevent further progression of the scoliosis curve. During surgery, some correction of the curve may be achieved. The fusion of vertebral segments also prevents twisting and curving. Bone graft is used to create a fusion mass. During surgery, hardware, consisting of metal rods and hooks or wire, is attached to the vertebrae. The hardware stabilizes the spine until the bone graft heals to a solid mass of bone in 9 to 12 months. Various types of hardware are used, depending on the type of scoliosis and the preference of the orthopedic surgeon. The fusion mass will eventually encapsulate the rods and create a permanent bone-metal construct. Table 41 – 15 lists the various hardware systems.

Posterior spinal fusion with instrumentation is the most common surgical procedure. The posterior portions of the vertebrae are fused together. With most types of hardware, no external cast or brace is necessary postoperatively. *Anterior spinal fusion,* with or without instrumentation, may be used in some patients. Children who are lacking the posterior portion of the vertebrae, such as with myelomeningocele, or who have rigid congenital scoliosis may need fusion of the anterior portions of the vertebral bodies. Patients with large, rigid curves may also be treated with anterior fusion to improve stabilization and correction of the curve. Anterior fusion may be done in conjunction with posterior fusion for complex curves. A combined procedure will improve the correction of

TABLE 41 – 15
Scoliosis Instrumentation

Type	Description	Use	Comments
Posterior			
Harrington	Single ratcheted rod attached to the spine at two points, one at the top, one at the bottom, of the curve	First system used for treatment of idiopathic scoliosis	Patient requires a body cast for 9–12 months until bone graft is healed
Luque	Two smooth, L-shaped rods attached to the spine by a sublaminar wire at each vertebral level	Neuromuscular scoliosis	No cast necessary: allows early postoperative mobilization
Wisconsin	One ratcheted Harrington rod and one smooth L-shaped Luque rod attached to the spine by a wire through the spinous process at each vertebral level	Idiopathic and neuromuscular scoliosis	No invasion of neural canal: no postoperative cast necessary; permits early mobilization
Cotrel-Dubousset	Two heavy knurled rods attached to the spine with intermittent hooks	Idiopathic scoliosis	Corrects rotation of vertebra that causes rib and hump as well as lateral scoliotic curve
Texas Scottish-Rite Hospital	Same as Cotrel-Dubousset	Idiopathic scoliosis	Same as Cotrel-Dubousset
Unit rod	Heavy U-shaped rod attached to the spine with wires at each vertebral level; L-shaped ends are embedded in the pelvis	Neuromuscular scoliosis	Provides rotational stability and corrects pelvic obliquity
Anterior			
Dwyer	Large metal staples attached to spine with large screw; cable threaded through screws and tightened at each level	Congenital scoliosis, scoliosis with deficient posterior spinal elements, neuromuscular scoliosis	Corrects frontal curve and rotation; requires postoperative brace or cast
Zielke	Screws implanted in vertebral bodies through circular washers or angled plates; a solid flexible rod is threaded through screws and locked with nuts	Scoliosis with deficient posterior spinal elements; selected idiopathic curves	Same as Dwyer

the scoliosis curve and may stabilize the spine more effectively. Patients who undergo anterior fusion alone usually wear a cast or brace postoperatively.

Application of Nursing Process: Bracing

Assessment

The nurse should gather information about a family history of scoliosis. It is important to determine when the patient was diagnosed with scoliosis and the patient's and family's understanding of the diagnosis. The nurse should ask the family about any treatment measures used in the past, including observation, bracing, or surgery. Determine the family's understanding of the treatment plan and its purpose. Bracing treatment prevents progression of the curve but will not correct it. The physical examination should look for the physical signs, such as rib hump, pelvic obliquity, and elevated shoulder height.

Nursing Diagnostic Statements and Collaborative Problems

Actual and high risk for body image disturbance, *related to or risk factors of physical deformity or need to wear brace.*

High risk for impairment of skin integrity; *risk factor: abrasion or pressure from brace.*

High risk for ineffective management of treatment regimen, *risk factors:*

- *Lack of motivation to wear brace.*
- *Discomfort caused by brace.*

Interventions

Prevent Body Image Disturbance or Support Coping with Body Image Disturbance. With school screening programs, many cases of idiopathic scoliosis are recognized in the early stages so that the physical signs are subtle when the diagnosis is made. Brace treatment to halt the progression of the curve can have significant impact on an adolescent's body image, either because of its perceived appearance or because it restricts some desired sports activities. The nurse needs to assess the patient's perception of scoliosis and its physical impact. Directly confronting concerns about appearance and how to "cover up" the brace are important. The nurse must also help the adolescent patient, who focuses on the present, to consider the long-term implications of nonadherence and progression of the scoliotic curve.

Maintain Skin Integrity. To prevent any skin problems with the brace, the patient with a new brace should gradually increase wearing time so that the skin can develop tolerance for the pressure of the brace. Wearing a cotton undershirt under the brace can also cushion the skin and absorb perspiration. The patient and family should be taught how to examine the skin for signs of redness or breakdown, especially over the ribs and pelvic bones. The patient should not use lotions or oils on skin under the brace. It is important for the patient and family to develop a working relationship with the orthotist who makes the brace. Fit and comfort are crucial for brace wearing success, and multiple adjustments may be necessary as the patient grows.

Assist Patient and Family to Follow Treatment Regimen. Although brace treatment has been shown to be effective in preventing the progression of scoliotic curves, its success as a treatment depends on the patient's wearing the brace. Because most adolescents are concerned about appearance, the nurse should provide clothing suggestions, keeping in mind current fashion. Collaborate with the orthotist and patient to achieve a comfortable fit. Other areas to discuss with the patient and family include the need to loosen the brace for meals and difficulty sitting in one position for long periods. Family support and participation are crucial for adherence to brace treatment.

Problems with the brace should be assessed on every follow-up appointment. Collaboration of the orthopedic surgeon, the orthotist, the nurse, and the family can help resolve issues that make brace wearing difficult.

The nurse should be prepared to provide anticipatory guidance to families when the adolescent graduates to junior or senior high and changes schools or becomes active in social activities. The nurse can help the patient and family develop a strategy for handling new situations. Facilitating contact between patients wearing braces may increase adherence.

Evaluation

1. The child or adolescent will wear the brace the appropriate number of hours as recommended by the physician.

2. The child or adolescent will not have skin breakdown from the brace.

Application of Nursing Process: Spinal Fusion

Assessment

The assessment of the patient who will be having posterior spinal fusion for scoliosis is the same as the assessment the nurse makes for the patient who is wearing a brace. In addition, the nurse must assess the patient's and family's understanding of the surgical procedure and postoperative care. The nursing data base should include baseline information on urinary and bowel elimination patterns; neurovascular status, particularly of the lower extremities; and a respiratory assessment. Other important information to identify includes plans to continue school work and expectations for the recovery period at home after discharge.

Nursing Diagnostic Statements and Collaborative Problems

High risk for infection; *risk factors:*
- *Large incision.*
- *Lengthy surgical procedure.*

High risk for alteration in bowel elimination, *risk factors:*
- *Decreased food and fluid intake.*
- *Immobility*
- *Narcotic administration.*

Ineffective breathing patterns, *related to pain.*

High risk for altered urinary elimination: decrease, *risk factors:.*
- *Immobility.*
- *Use of narcotics.*

High risk for injury: neurologic; *risk factor: manipulation and possible compression of neurologic structures during spine surgery.*

Impaired physical mobility, *related to pain and fatigue.*

Planning and Implementation

Prevent Infection. The large back incision is usually covered by a bulky pressure dressing for the first 2 or 3 days after surgery. The nurse should assess the dressing for signs of drainage and reinforce the dressing as necessary. Once the dressing is removed, the nurse must assess the wound for tenderness, redness, purulent drainage, or increasing amounts of serosanguineous drainage. The nurse should also be alert for signs of systemic infection, such as an elevated temperature. Caregivers should be taught what to look for at home to monitor for late postoperative infection.

Promote Normal Bowel Elimination. Postoperatively, the patient will be NPO for several days after surgery until the return of active bowel sounds. The patient will be receiving intravenous fluids and narcotics. A common adverse effect of narcotic analgesia is slowing of bowel motility, which causes constipation. The nurse must monitor hydration and bowel status. Encourage fluids when the patient is able to take liquids by mouth. Once the patient is eating, it is helpful to increase the amount of fiber in the diet. Mobilize as soon as possible by having the patient get out of bed and begin ambulation. The patient may also require stool softeners as ordered by the physician.

Promote Effective Breathing Patterns and Pain Relief. After posterior spinal fusion, the patient has a large incision down the center of the back, often extending into the thoracic area. It is painful for the patient to move and breathe deeply, both of which are important to prevent pulmonary complications postoperatively. The patient who has anterior spinal fusion will often have a thoracotomy and chest tube postoperatively. In addition to assessing respiratory status, the nurse should provide pulmonary hygiene. Pulmonary hygiene includes the use of the incentive spirometer or cough and deep breathing. Provide comfort measures and analgesia to encourage pulmonary hygiene. Log roll the patient every 2 hours until he or she is able to move independently. Mobilize the patient as soon as possible. The nurse should monitor and maintain the chest drainage system if applicable.

Posterior spinal fusion surgery involves a long incision, with extensive dissection of soft tissue and bone. The nurse will administer analgesics per the physician's order. Pain control is best achieved through continuous narcotic administration. Children can often use patient-controlled analgesia to self-administer boluses of narcotics for pain relief. A mattress overlay may also increase comfort by reducing pressure and the discomfort related to bed rest.

Promote Urinary Elimination. Similar to their effect on the bowel, narcotics can also cause urinary retention. The patient will have an indwelling catheter for the first 48 hours postoperatively. Once the catheter is removed, the patient may experience some urinary retention. Although the patient will be receiving intravenous fluids, it is essential to encourage fluid intake as soon as the patient can drink. If the patient is unable to void spontaneously, the nurse may need to use clean intermittent catheterization every 6 to 8 hours until the patient is able to void.

Prevent Neurologic Injury. One of the biggest risks of spine surgery is the risk of paralysis if the spinal cord is injured or compressed by swelling. In many places, the function of the spinal cord is monitored throughout the surgical procedure with spinal evoked potential monitoring. Postoperatively, the nurse must assess and document the sensation and movement of the lower extremities every 2 hours for at least 24 hours postoperatively. Less frequent neurovascular assessment should continue throughout the hospitalization. Some cutaneous numbness on thighs may result from intraoperative positioning. Urinary retention and bowel incontinence may be signs of spinal cord trauma.

Maintain Physical Mobility. Because of the extent of the surgery, it is painful and difficult to roll from side to side or to sit up. The nurse should provide analgesics before turning and ambulation. In addition, the patient often has low hematocrit and hemoglobin levels after surgery so that she or he feels tired and rundown. The patient's hematocrit and hemoglobin levels are monitored postoperatively to determine the need for blood transfusion. The patient will progress from log rolling to sitting (postoperative day 2 or 3) to ambulation (postoperative day 3 or 4). Getting up out of bed is best done by rolling the patient to one side and having the patient push the torso up with the arms while the nurse assists by swinging the legs around to dangle at the bedside. Standing requires pushing upward with the quadriceps. Physical therapy can assist with mobility. As the patient's mobility increases, it is important to provide frequent rest periods and prevent the child or adolescent from becoming overtired.

Specific discharge instructions depend on the surgeon. Patients may resume activities of daily living gradually as they recover from surgery. Return to school generally occurs 3 to 4 weeks after surgery. Sports activities may be restricted for up to 2 years postoperatively. Patients will resume walking level activities first and progress to more vigorous sports. Contact sports, such as football or basketball, are restricted until the fusion mass is solid.

Evaluation

1. The child or adolescent will eat a regular diet.
2. The child or adolescent will ambulate without difficulty.
3. The child or adolescent will be comfortable.
4. The child or adolescent will return to baseline bowel and bladder elimination.

Kyphosis (Scheuermann Disease)

Kyphosis is the normal posterior convexity in the thoracic spine. A kyphotic curve of less than 45 degrees is normal. A kyphotic curve greater than 45 degrees is pathologic. Kyphosis may be postural. Postural kyphosis can be corrected by the child. Scheuermann disease is a structural kyphosis of greater than 45 degrees that cannot be corrected by the child. In addition, it may be painful.

Etiology/Incidence (Pathophysiology)

Scheuermann disease is associated with anterior wedging of the vertebral bodies of three adjacent vertebrae. It is the most common cause of structural kyphosis in adolescents.

Diagnostic Assessment

The child is unable to correct the deformity and reports back pain and fatigue. On the Adam forward bending test, increased thoracic rounding is noted. The child also demonstrates hamstring tightness on physical examination. There are also characteristic vertebral x-ray changes: wedging of apical vertebrae, irregular vertebral end plates, and narrowing of the intervertebral spaces.

Therapeutic Management

Observation. Kyphotic curves less than 45 degrees are monitored for progression.

Bracing. Bracing is prescribed for curves between 45 and 65 degrees. Bracing stabilizes the curve and prevents progression. Exercises to maintain muscle strength and hamstring flexibility are also recommended.

Surgery. A combined anterior and posterior spinal fusion may be performed on curves greater than 65 degrees. Hardware, like that used in the treatment of scoliosis, is used to stabilize the spine until the bone graft heals.

Nursing Care

Nursing care of the patient with Scheuermann disease is the same as for a patient with scoliosis.

Spondylolisthesis

Spondylolisthesis is the forward displacement of one vertebra on another.

Etiology/Incidence (Pathophysiology)

Spondylolisthesis may occur at any level of the spine but occurs most commonly at L5–S1. It is rare in young children. Symptoms typically develop in late childhood or early adolescence.

Diagnostic Assessment

Clinical manifestations of spondylolisthesis include lower back pain and pain in one or both legs. The child will walk with the buttocks tucked in and the pelvis tilted forward, resulting in an awkward, waddling gait. Ambulation for long distances may be difficult. The child will have hamstring tightness on straight leg raising. The calf circumference may be diminished. Lateral x-ray views of the lumbar spine show a partial or complete displacement of one vertebra on another, usually in the area of pain.

Therapeutic Management

Bracing. Bracing with a lumbosacral orthosis is used for spondylolisthesis that is minimally displaced. Bracing relieves pain by providing support to the lower back and stabilizing the vertebra from further displacement.

Surgery. A surgical fusion is recommended for some patients with spondylolisthesis. *Fusion in situ* with bone graft only will prevent the vertebra from slipping further. No attempt at reduction, or correction of the position, of the displaced vertebra is done. The child is put in a cast or brace for 6 weeks to 3 months after surgery to stabilize the spinal column while the bone graft heals.

Nursing Care

Nursing care for the child with spondylolisthesis is the same as for a child with scoliosis.

Osteochondroses

Osteochondroses are a group of problems in which normal endochondral ossification is altered as the result of damage to growth centers at the epiphyses. Degeneration of the epiphysis is usually followed by regeneration and healing. Depending on the location of the damage and the age of the child, there may be some residual deformity.

Legg-Calvé-Perthes Disease

Legg-Calvé-Perthes disease is a self-limiting avascular necrosis of the femoral head. Legg-Calvé-Perthes disease follows a predictable pattern of necrosis and recovery, but the duration of the disease process is unpredictable.

Etiology/Incidence (Pathophysiology)

For some reason, the blood supply to the femoral head is interrupted. Although the cause is unknown, most current theories involve vascular injury. The femoral head dies from lack of blood, although the blood supply will return as healing occurs.

Legg-Calvé-Perthes disease occurs most often in 4- to 8-year-old boys. Most affected children have delayed bone age, such that their skeletal maturity lags behind their chronologic age. There is also a higher incidence of Legg-Calvé-Perthes disease in urban populations. Certain ethnic groups, such as people of African descent and Chinese, have a lower incidence (Barker & Hall, 1986).

Clinical Manifestations

Specific histologic changes are evident in Legg-Calvé-Perthes disease. There are abnormal areas of epiphyseal cartilage, and tongues of cartilage from the physis extend into the metaphysis. Patients may also have irregularities of ossification at other epiphyses. With these physeal abnormalities, minimal trauma may interrupt the vessels supplying the femoral head, causing necrosis.

The clinical signs of Legg-Calvé-Perthes disease include a limp, which often starts insidiously. Some patients report pain, usually in the groin, lateral hip, or knee. The pain is usually related to activity and is relieved by rest. Decreased range of motion in the hip results from pain caused by irritation of the hip joint and a change in the anatomic relationships between the femur and acetabulum. Hip rotation and abduction are usually limited. The child may also have disuse atrophy of the affected thigh with a decreased thigh circumference. A limb length inequality may indicate significant head collapse.

Prognosis depends on several factors, including the age of the patient at disease onset. Older children have less time to remodel any bone deformity before their growth is complete and thus have a poorer prognosis for complete recovery. The amount of deformity depends on how much of the femoral head is involved, the amount of protection the femoral head receives during healing, and the stage of the disease when treatment is initiated. The prognosis is best for young patients who have a longer time to repair and remodel the deformity before their growth stops.

Diagnostic Assessment

Serial radiographs are important in identifying the stage of the disease and the extent of femoral head involvement. On radiographic examination, there are four stages of the disease. The stages are not clinically discrete. The *initial* stage is one of avascularity; the femoral head fails to grow because of lack of blood. The femoral head becomes flattened and deformed from the normal biomechanical forces on the hip. The second phase is *fragmentation*. The blood supply returns, and the necrotic bone is reabsorbed and replaced with vascularized granulation tissue. The third phase is the *reossification* or reparative phase. New bone replaces the granulation tissue and necrotic bone. Healing starts at the periphery of the femoral head and progresses to the center. The fourth and final phase is the *healed* phase, when the proximal femur may be left with residual deformity. In some patients, the head will never be perfectly round (Fig. 41–27). The entire process can take up to 36 months, depending on the extent of involvement of the femoral head.

Other studies may include a bone scan, in the early stages, and MRI. MRI may detect vessel infarction but will not assist with the determination of the stage of the disease. Operative arthrography is most useful for assessing head shape and size.

Therapeutic Management

The goal of treatment is to allow the femoral head to develop normally. Keeping the femoral head well centered in the acetabulum and reducing weight bearing help preserve congruity between the femoral head and acetabulum. Maintaining range of motion at the hip is also important for healing.

Bed Rest With or Without Traction. The patient may initially be put on bed rest, with or without traction, to relieve pain and muscle spasm and improve range of motion. Buck's traction may be used to improve range of motion. Bed rest is not realistic for long periods of time, but it can be done at home.

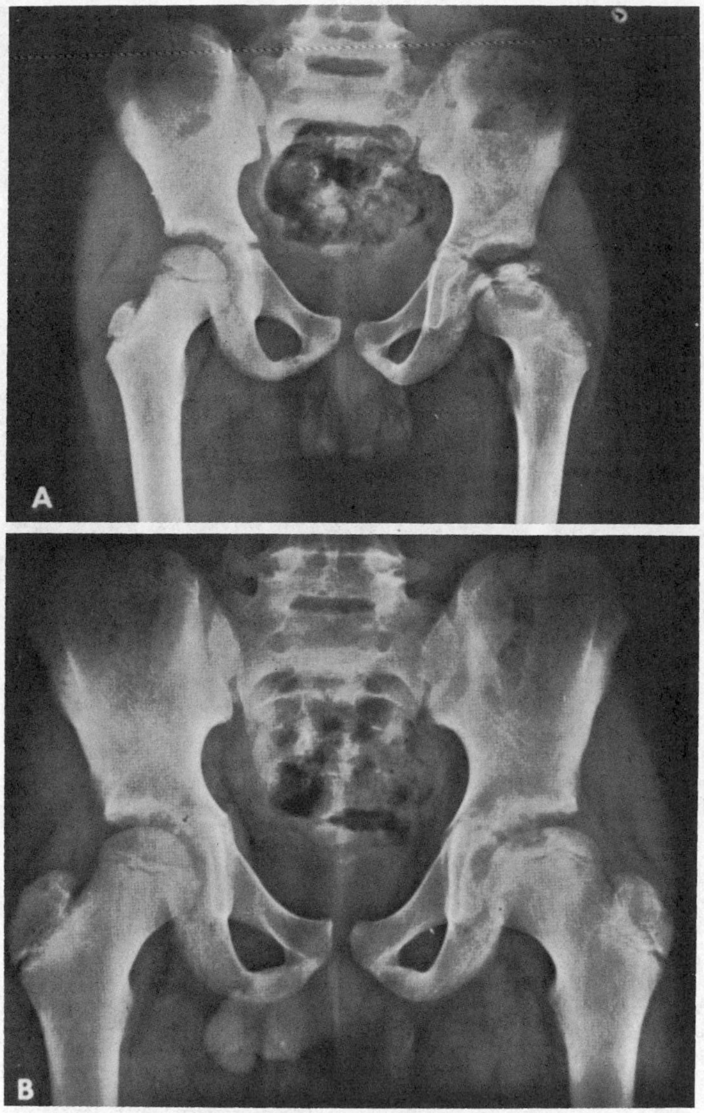

FIGURE 41 - 27. *A*, Legg-Calvé-Perthes disease of left hip. Capital femoral epiphysis is undergoing necrosis and fragmentation. *B*, Same hip, 5 years later, showing residual flattening of femoral head. (*A* and *B*, From Gartland, J. H. [1986]. *Foundations of orthopaedics* [4th ed.]. Philadelphia: WB Saunders.)

Abduction Devices. Ambulation may be allowed with the legs widely abducted to maximize the coverage of the femoral head in the acetabulum (Fig. 41–28). The legs may be casted, or an abduction brace may be used. With the Scottish-Rite brace, the abduction bar can be adjusted. The child may need crutches to walk but can return to school. Long a standard for treatment of Legg-Calvé-Perthes disease, the Scottish-Rite brace has been questioned. Some studies (Martinez et al, 1992; Meehan et al, 1992) have shown that the Scottish-Rite abduction orthosis does not improve the outcome for patients with Legg-Calvé-Perthes disease.

Surgery. Surgery may be necessary to keep the femoral head centered in the acetabulum. Some children require *acetabular reconstruction* or a *femoral osteotomy* to keep the femoral head well placed in the acetabulum. Acetabular reconstruction makes the acetabulum larger. A femoral osteotomy redirects the head of the femur into the acetabulum.

Nursing Diagnostic Statements

Ineffective individual coping with requirements for long periods of immobility, related to high risk for injury: hip deformity.

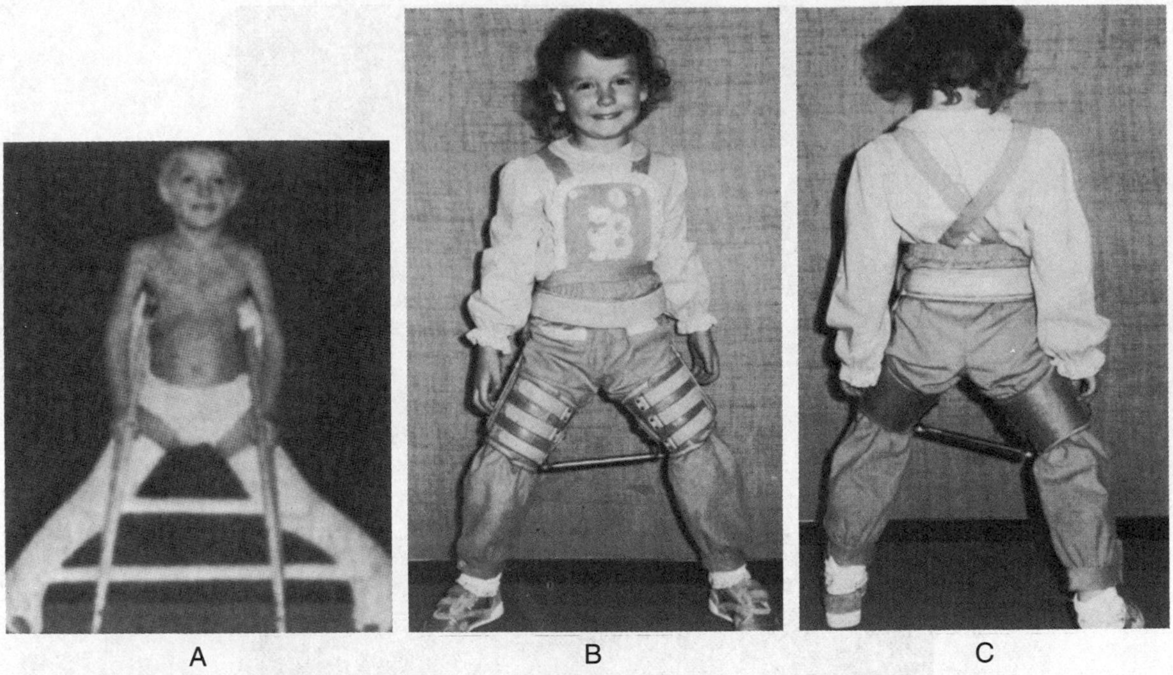

FIGURE 41 - 28. *A*, Abduction plaster cast (Petrie) for Legg-Calvé-Perthes disease. (From Salter, R. [1970]. *Textbook of disorders and injuries to the musculoskeletal system*. Baltimore: Williams & Wilkins, p 277.) *B* and *C*, Patient wearing Scottish-Rite hip orthosis. (From Tachdjian, M. [1990]. *Pediatric orthopedics* (2nd ed., p 973). Philadelphia: WB Saunders.)

High risk for impairment of skin integrity; *risk factors: brace and immobility.*

High risk for noncompliance; *risk factors:*

- *Age and associated reasoning ability.*
- *Lack of understanding of importance.*
- *Discomfort/inconvenience of brace and need for brace or cast.*

Nursing Care

Decreasing Risk of Hip Deformity. The anatomic relationship between the pelvis and the femur changes as the femoral head collapses. This can cause the muscles around the hip to tighten, resulting in a decreased range of motion in the hip. Buck's traction may be used to decrease muscle spasm and increase the range of motion. Analgesics may be necessary to help the child tolerate the traction and range of motion. The traction is often intermittent, and crutches are usually necessary to decrease pressure on the acetabulum when the child ambulates.

Protection of the healing femoral head may require long periods of immobility. For children in this age group, immobility is difficult to maintain. Help the child and family explore usual activities and sports activities and determine what is still realistic. Collaborate with family to identify alternative activities that give the child an opportunity to interact with peers and develop new skills.

Maintain Skin Integrity. The nurse must monitor skin integrity and teach the family skin assessment. Skin care measures include no lotions or oils on skin under the brace or on pressure points and the use of alcohol to toughen skin that is reddened from pressure. If the child is immobilized in bed, frequent position changes are necessary. A mattress overlay may also be required.

Support Family and Child in Compliance with Treatment. As with any immobilizing device that can be removed, there is a risk of nonadherence. The brace can be easily removed. It is important to explore the child's feelings about the brace. Reinforce the purpose of the brace. The nurse must teach the family the brace wearing schedule and brace care. Ongoing support is essential because the issues related to brace wearing change as the child grows and interests and activities change.

Osgood-Schlatter Disease

Osgood-Schlatter disease is an overgrowth of the tibial tubercle at the insertion of the quadriceps tendon. A partial or complete separation of the tubercle may occur. Osgood-Schlatter disease is now classified as an osteochondrosis because it is an alteration in the normal growth of bone at an epiphysis.

Etiology/Incidence (Pathophysiology)

The etiology of the disease is controversial. It may be due to calcification of the patellar tendon or an inflammation of the tibial tubercle caused by the repetitive pull of the quadriceps femoris. The tendon insertion is inflamed and shows new bone formation.

Osgood-Schlatter disease is common in young athletes who engage in jumping or other strenuous activities. It occurs most often in boys between the ages of 13 and 14 years and girls between 10 and 11 years. The problem is self-limiting: it disappears when growth stops. In 10 per cent of cases, a discrete ossicle forms, with a bursa that causes localized pain and tenderness. Enlargement of the tibial tubercle may cause an unattractive bone prominence.

Diagnostic Assessment

One of the clinical signs of Osgood-Schlatter disease is pain over the tibial tubercle. The pain increases with activities that require repetitive knee flexion and extension, such as jumping, kneeling, or bicycling, and diminishes with rest. There is usually a local swelling and prominence in the area of the tibial tuberosity. The tubercle may feel warm and tender.

In addition to the history and symptoms, x-ray examination is used in the diagnostic assessment of Osgood-Schlatter disease. Radiographs of the knee, including oblique views, show excessive enlargement of the tibial tubercle.

Therapeutic Management

Rest. The initial treatment consists of limiting activity to decrease the stress on the tibial tubercle. Knee protection, such as knee pads, is recommended for activities with direct knee contact. After a period of rest, the child can gradually resume activities, avoiding those that cause pain. This period of inactivity can be difficult for young athletes. Most will resume play as soon as the pain decreases.

A knee immobilizer and a home stretching program may be necessary for children whose symptoms do not resolve with rest. Casting with the knee in full extension may be necessary to decrease the pain and swelling.

Surgery. Surgery is rarely indicated, although drilling or removal of the ossicle may be necessary if symptoms persist.

Nursing Care

The majority of children have no experience with chronic pain and many find the necessary activity restrictions difficult. The child may rest when the knee is acutely painful but resume activities as soon as the symptoms subside. Encourage the child to rest the knee when it is painful. Ice can be used for comfort along with analgesics.

Inflammatory/Infectious Processes of the Skeleton

Infection in the bone and joints has potentially serious complications. Whereas bone can repair itself, the articular cartilage and the cartilage of the physis cannot. Tissue destruction is the result of the body's inflammatory processes. Failure to quickly and adequately treat infections of the bone and joint can result in permanent damage to articular cartilage as well as alterations in growth.

Osteomyelitis

Osteomyelitis is an infection of the bone, usually in the metaphyseal region, close to the physis.

Etiology/Incidence

The most common cause of osteomyelitis is a hematogenous spread from a concurrent infection, such as otitis media. In some manner, the normal defense mechanisms are overcome. Trauma to a bone may also predispose to osteomyelitis. The most common causative organism is *Staphylococcus aureus*. *Salmonella*, pneumococci, and streptococci are other common pathogenic organisms.

Pathophysiology

The bones most commonly affected are the distal femur, proximal tibia, and distal tibia. Boys are affected three to four times as often as girls are. The earliest change in the infected bone is the death of osteoblasts, the bone-producing cells, in a wide area surrounding the infection. Osteoclasts, cells that destroy bone, start resorbing the bone, and inflammatory cells begin to accumulate in the area of infection. The bacteria produce pus, which may remain as a small local abscess, or the pus may begin to pass through the metaphysis to form an abscess under the periosteum.

Clinical Manifestations

Clinical signs of osteomyelitis include fever and failure to use the extremity. There may be erythema, heat, and swelling over the area of the infection. The clinical examination should also look for other symptoms of infection, such as tenderness and decreased range of motion of the joints of the affected extremity.

Diagnostic Assessment

Diagnosis of osteomyelitis is made by clinical examination and laboratory and radiographic studies. Few changes are visible radiographically for 7 to 10 days after the infection begins. The most useful radiographic study in the acute phase of osteomyelitis is a bone scan. Areas of increased circulation in bone tissue will be highlighted on the bone scan. Because bone scan reflects physiologic alteration and increased circulation in the bone, it is not diagnostic for osteomyelitis. Other causes of bone inflammation that would also cause increased circulation, such as tumor or fracture, must also be investigated.

Direct aspiration of pus from bone provides definitive information about the presence of infection and material for culture and Gram stain. Laboratory studies include Gram stain and culture of bone or pus and a white blood cell count. Laboratory studies will also show an increased sedimentation rate. Although the erythrocyte sedimentation rate is not diagnostic for osteomyelitis, it provides a means of measuring the effectiveness of treatment.

Therapeutic Management

Antibiotic Therapy. Intravenous antibiotics are started as soon as possible after a specimen for culture and sensitivity is obtained. If an organism is isolated, the child may be changed to an appropriate oral antibiotic. Oral administration can be as effective as intravenous administration if adequate blood levels are maintained (Scoles & Aronoff, 1984). Oral antibiotic treatment also depends on tolerance of the antibiotic (no vomiting or diarrhea) and reliable parents who will consistently administer the medication. The duration of antibiotic treatment depends on the age of the child and the extent of the infection as well as the causative organism.

Surgery. Antibiotics alone may not adequately treat osteomyelitis. Treatment must be aggressive to prevent chronic osteomyelitis. Surgical incision and drainage may be necessary to clean out the dead bone and soft tissue, which may interfere with the effectiveness of the antibiotic. Surgical debridement will also remove inflammatory products more rapidly than the normal physiologic mechanisms can.

Septic Arthritis

Septic arthritis is the bacterial invasion of a joint. A septic joint must be treated promptly. The chondrolytic enzymes produced by the pus and bacteria can cause destruction of joint surfaces. In young children, most of the bone ends are cartilage. The effect of cartilage destruction can be devastating to future growth and development of the bone.

Etiology/Incidence (Pathophysiology)

Two thirds of all cases are found in children under the age of 3 years. Eighty per cent of cases involve joints of the lower limb. The cause of septic arthritis in children is most often hematogenous spread from a pre-existing focus, commonly otitis media. Other causes are direct inoculation of bacteria into the joint or extension of adjacent infection. The most common causative organisms are *Staphylococcus aureus, Streptococcus pyogenes,* and *Haemophilus influenzae.*

As with osteomyelitis, the presence of bacteria does not explain the development of a joint infection. The normal mechanism for clearing bacteria from the joint may be disrupted, particularly with certain organisms, such as *Staphylococcus aureus.* There is also a limit to how much debris the normal mechanisms can remove before being overwhelmed. Trauma to the joint may also be a factor in the development of septic arthritis.

Diagnostic Assessment

A septic joint is characterized by sudden onset; the child will suddenly stop using the extremity. The child will hold the limb in a position of comfort and refuse to bear weight. There will be intense pain on flexion and abduction. The synovium is inflamed and infected, and the joint may be filled with pus.

Information from a bone scan, in conjunction with physical and laboratory findings, confirms the diagnosis. A bone scan indicates increased blood flow to the area. Few changes are visible radiographically until 7 to 10 days after the infection begins. Direct aspiration of pus from the joint confirms the diagnosis of septic joint. The aspirated joint fluid is sent for culture and Gram stain. The erythrocyte sedimentation rate is elevated, indicating an infection, although it is not diagnostic for septic arthritis.

Therapeutic Management

Surgery. Aspiration of pus or surgical incision with drainage is necessary to obtain fluid for culture and to clean out the joint. Aspiration of pus, which must be sent for culture, confirms the diagnosis. Surgical incision and drainage or surgical arthroscopy is necessary to remove large fibrin clots and clean out debris so that the antibiotics can work more effectively. Antibiotics alone will not effectively treat the joint infection.

Antibiotic Therapy. Broad-spectrum antibiotics are started as soon as a culture is obtained. Once an organism is isolated, the antibiotic will be changed to one that is specific for the causative organism. If no organism is isolated on culture, intravenous antibiotics will be necessary for the full 4- to 6-week course of treatment. A combination of intravenous and oral antibiotics can be used if a causative organism is isolated. Oral antibiotic treatment can be as effective as intravenous antibiotics if adequate blood levels are obtained.

Consistent administration of the antibiotic is essential, especially if the child is to be treated with oral antibiotics. The family should be instructed to give the medication until the entire prescription is gone, regardless of how well the child seems. Intravenous antibiotics may be administered at home, depending on the age of the child, the type of medication, and the venous access of the child. Home antibiotic therapy is more difficult in younger children because of intravenous access problems and the need for constant supervision to protect the line. Regardless of the type of antibiotics given, follow-up care to monitor effectiveness of treatment is essential. Insufficient treatment can result in chronic osteomyelitis or permanent damage to the articular cartilage.

Application of the Nursing Process for Osteomyelitis and Septic Joint

Assessment

When the nurse is taking the history of a patient with suspected osteomyelitis, he or she should inquire about recent infection, duration of fever, any refusal to move the extremity, and pain. The physical examination should note the location of any pain or tenderness on palpation as well as any limitation of motion.

Nursing Diagnostic Statements and Collaborative Problems

Alteration in body temperature, hyperthermia, *related to infection.*

Activity intolerance, *related to pain.*

Planning and Implementation

Reducing Body Temperature. The nurse should monitor the patient's temperature every 2 hours and administer antipyretics as ordered by the physician. The effectiveness of the antipyretic must also be monitored. Other fever reduction measures can also be used, such as removing blankets and clothing or giving the child a tepid sponge bath. The child with a fever is at risk for dehydration, so the nurse should encourage fluids or administer IV fluids.

Relieving Pain. The nurse will administer analgesics per the physician's order and monitor their effectiveness. The nurse must also observe voluntary movement and weight bearing, especially in the nonverbal child. While the infection is resolving, it is important to protect the extremity from unnecessary motion with a splint. Maintain the splint for comfort as ordered.

The patient will be more comfortable and able to participate if the nurse administers analgesics before activities of daily living or physical therapy. The patient should participate in activities of daily living to the extent that she or he is able. Assistive devices, such as crutches, wheelchair, or walker, may be necessary.

Evaluation

1. The child will have a normal body temperature.
2. The child will move about in his or her environment voluntarily to the extent allowed by his or her physical condition.

Traumatic Injury to the Musculoskeletal System

Injuries to the muscles and ligaments are unusual in young children because of the flexibility and resilience of the soft tissues. As the child approaches adolescence, the muscles and soft tissues become less resilient and are more likely to be injured. Table 41–16 lists the common types of soft tissue injuries and their treatment. Bone injury is common in children because of their intense physical activity.

Knee Injuries

Because of its anatomy, the knee is vulnerable to injury, especially with sports participation. Figure 41–29 illustrates the anatomy of the knee.

TABLE 41-16
Soft Tissue Injuries

Type	Definition	Cause	Symptoms	Treatment
Strain	Muscle or tendon stretched beyond capacity	Overuse or sudden force	Sore, painful, stiff muscles	Ice, rest
Sprain	Tearing of ligaments around a joint	Twisting movement outside the joint's usual plane of motion	Painful, inflamed, and swollen joint; may be discolored	RICE: rest, ice, compression, elevation
Dislocation	Disruption of joint so that articulating surfaces are no longer in contact	Force outside the joint's usual plane of motion	Extreme pain due to overstretch of soft tissues and nerves	Reduction, ice, rest

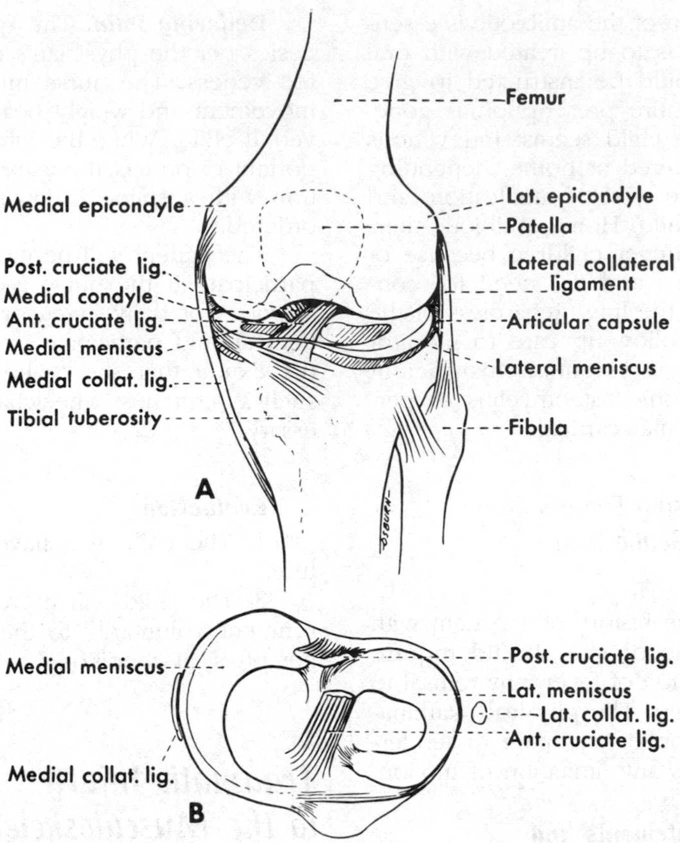

FIGURE 41 - 29. Anatomy of knee joint. (From Gartland, J. H. [1987]. *Fundamentals of orthopaedics* [4th ed.]. Philadelphia, WB Saunders.)

Etiology/Incidence (Pathophysiology)

The incidence of knee injuries rises dramatically in adolescence. Fractures, dislocations, and ligamentous tears increase with sports participation. Inexperience and repeated attempts to learn new skills increase the risk of injury. Individuals begin the growth spurt at varying ages, which results in size differences between peers and teammates. An adolescent who is physically smaller may be injured during contact with a larger player. Differences in strength and agility may increase the risk of injury.

The lateral and medial menisci of the knee serve as shock absorbers and help stabilize the knee joint. A *torn meniscus* is a tear in one, or both, of these cartilage menisci. When a meniscus is torn, these important functions are diminished. Depending on the amount of damage, a torn meniscus may be asymptomatic. More severe tears may cause swelling, pain, and limited motion. The patient may complain of the knee's "locking." A torn meniscus is often associated with ligamentous injuries of the knee.

Recurrent subluxation of the patella is a condition in which the patella shifts out of its groove on the femur and tibia. It usually occurs in adolescence, although it may start in middle childhood. Girls are more often affected by recurrent subluxation of the patella than are boys. Some predisposing factors include joint laxity, genu valgum, rotational malalignment, and incongruence of the patellofemoral joint. Once the patella has subluxed, it has a tendency to recur. When the patella subluxes, the knee is painful and gives way.

Chondromalacia patella is a disorder of the patellofemoral joint that causes pain at the back of the patella. It commonly starts in adolescence and is best classified as an overuse syndrome. On physical examination, the medial facet of the patella is usually tender and painful on palpation. There may be joint crepitation. The knee gives way and occasionally locks. If the condition is severe, there may be joint effusion and quadriceps atrophy.

The *anterior cruciate ligament* (ACL) crosses the knee joint obliquely to prevent hyperextension of the knee and internal rotation of the tibia when the knee is fully extended. It is the strongest and least compliant ligament in the knee. The ACL is usually injured in one of two ways. In the first mechanism of injury, the knee is hyperextended, and the femur rotates outward on a fixed tibia. This can occur on attempting to change direction quickly. No body contact is necessary. The second mechanism of injury is excessive valgus force to the knee. An ACL injury may be associated with injuries to other ligaments, the menisci, or the joint capsule.

The patient may describe hearing a "pop" or report that "the knee went out of place." There is usually severe pain, and the child is unable to continue the activity. Hemarthrosis or knee effusion will cause swelling. On examination, the tibia subluxes forward on the femur. MRI may be used to evaluate knee injuries before surgery.

Diagnostic Assessment

Knee injuries are diagnosed by physical examination. Specific maneuvers, such as the anterior or posterior drawer sign and the Lachman maneuver, can help determine whether there is injury to any of the ligaments or menisci. These maneuvers check for increased motion outside of the normal range at the knee joint. MRI is becoming increasingly important in diagnosing knee injuries because it assists with the visualization of soft tissues. Plain x-ray films may be used to rule out any bone injury. Although it is technically a surgical procedure, arthroscopy is an important diagnostic tool because it permits direct visualization of the joint and its structures.

Therapeutic Management

Rest. The treatment plan depends on the lifestyle of the patient. Conservative treatment consists of stopping activities that cause joint overload, such as deep knee bends or activities that require quick stops and starts. A supportive knee brace may also be recommended for activities. Nonsteroidal anti-inflammatory analgesic medications are usually prescribed.

Physical Therapy. An exercise program emphasizing quad and hamstring strengthening is prescribed for many types of knee injuries. Quad strengthening exercises strengthen the structures around the knee to help stabilize the joint.

After ACL injury or surgery, extensive rehabilitation is necessary. The goal is to promote healing of the ACL and to restore function to knee and lower limb. Rehabilitation begins with controlled exercise in a brace and progresses to minimal protection and increased activity over 6 to 8 months. After a year, the child can usually participate fully in sports activities.

Surgery. Arthroscopic surgery may be needed to examine and repair the knee. Depending on the injury, surgery to release and reposition ligaments may also be necessary. For ACL injuries, surgical repair can salvage the ligament within several weeks of an acute tear. Reconstruction with an autologous graft, such as a piece of the patellar tendon, or an allograft, such as the Achilles tendon, may be necessary. Arthroscopic ACL reconstruction may produce less morbidity than that caused by arthrotomy.

Nursing Diagnostic Statements and Collaborative Problems

High risk for injury (falls); *risk factor: presence of cast or brace.*

Alteration in comfort, *related to injury or surgery.*

Nursing Care

Promoting Mobility and Preventing Injury. The treatment for many injuries of the knee is immobilization. The nurse should assess the child and family for safe use of assistive devices and discuss safety concerns in the home environment related to assistive devices. Consult the physical therapist for assistance with crutch training and mobility issues. Administer analgesia before physical therapy or physical activity to maximize participation.

Treatment may include long-term rest from sports activities. It is important that the family be clear on the reason for the restricted activities and what the restrictions are. Many children will return to activities as soon as the knee starts to feel better unless they are supervised. Discuss the need to alter and supervise activity with child and parents. Exploring activity alternatives with the child and family can improve adherence.

Alteration in Comfort. The nurse should administer analgesics as ordered by the physician and monitor effectiveness. Encourage the patient to change position regularly to prevent pressure on bone prominences. Ice packs to the injured area may also provide some pain relief. Diversional activities can provide some distraction and increase comfort. Before discharge, the family should be taught when and how to give the analgesics to maximize comfort during daily activities.

Fractures

A fracture is a break in the continuity of the bone. A fracture occurs when the bone is subjected to more stress than it can absorb.

Etiology/Incidence (Pathophysiology)

Because of the resilience of the soft tissues of children, fractures occur more frequently than does soft tissue injury. The amount of trauma necessary to fracture a bone varies considerably, depending on the location of the injury, the age of the child, and the mechanism of injury. Children also have an area of in-

	Description	Comments
Type I	Complete separation of metaphysis from physis	Reduced as close to anatomic as possible; low risk of growth damage
Type II	Fracture along physis into metaphysis; metaphyseal fragment remains attached	Reduced as close to anatomic as possible; low risk of growth damage
Type III	Fracture along physis, through epiphysis into joint	Fragments may rotate, so open reduction may be necessary; growth damage may occur
Type IV	Fracture through metaphysis into joint	Fragment may rotate, so open reduction may be necessary; growth damage may occur
Type V	Crushing injury or damage to the cartilage cells of the physis	May result from radiation, frostbite, or electrical injury; growth damage always occurs

FIGURE 41 - 30. Salter-Harris injuries.

herent weakness in their bones: the physeal growth plate. Injury to this area can damage the cartilage cells and affect the future longitudinal growth of the bone. The Salter-Harris classification system classifies physeal plate injuries and their risk of growth disturbance (Fig. 41–30).

Common Fractures in Children. Figure 41–31 illustrates some of the common fracture patterns in children. A *greenstick fracture* is an incomplete break in the continuity of the bone. The periosteum on one side of the bone is disrupted, creating an incomplete fracture, often with angulation. This type of fracture is common in children because their bones are more porous than an adult's. With a strong periosteum, a child's bone will absorb more energy before breaking.

A *toddler's fracture* is a spiral fracture in the distal half of the tibia. It is common in 2- to 5-year-olds. The fracture is a result of torsion on the tibia, often caused by tripping while running. The child will have pain with weight bearing. The treatment is immobilization in a cast for 3 weeks.

Fractures of the upper limb are seven times more common than are fractures of the lower limb. Fractures of the upper extremity include fractures of both bones of the forearm, usually from a fall on an outstretched hand. Supracondylar fractures of the distal humerus are a frequent injury in the immature skeleton. The fracture usually occurs along the physeal lines of the distal humerus because ligamentous laxity allows elbow hyperextension. Fractures in the proximal humerus are also common.

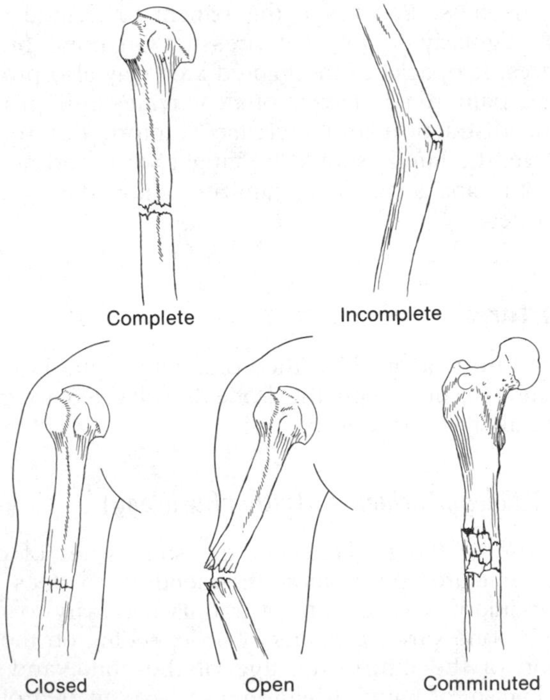

FIGURE 41 - 31. Types of fractures.

Clinical Manifestations

A child with a fracture complains of pain. Deformity caused by swelling and bone displacement may also be seen. The child may deny trauma but will protect the injured limb. Sensory and motor deficits may be seen if bone fragments are compressing neurovascular structures.

Any fracture associated with a break in the skin, subcutaneous tissue, or muscle is classified as an *open fracture*. Open fractures are susceptible to infection because of direct inoculation of bacteria, and destruction of the periosteum may affect bone repair. Injured and necrotic soft tissues may also become infected.

Diagnostic Assessment

A fracture is identified by clinical symptoms and x-ray examination. Generally, x-ray views on two planes are necessary for adequately visualizing the fracture line and any bone displacement. Fractures that continue into cartilage are not visible on plain x-ray films. An MRI scan or tomograms may be helpful in delineating the extent of cartilage injury. A bone scan may confirm a suspected bone injury when the fracture cannot be definitively seen on x-ray examination.

Therapeutic Management

Immobilization. The treatment for a fracture is reduction and immobilization of the bone fragments so that bone healing can occur. Any of the methods of immobilization outlined in the section "Therapeutic Management" earlier in the chapter are used to treat fractures. The method of immobilization depends on the type of fracture, its location, and the age of the patient. For example, young children heal quickly and may be immobilized adequately in a cast, whereas an older adolescent may require internal fixation to immobilize the bone fragments for healing.

The child may need to have repeat x-ray studies done within a week to evaluate the stability and position of the fracture fragments. As the swelling diminishes, the cast loosens, and the child may move the extremity in the cast. As the child moves, muscle forces can pull bone fragments out of alignment until the bone starts to heal.

Treatment of Open Fractures. Open fractures are treated with broad-spectrum antibiotics as soon as a deep culture of the wound is taken. The wound is debrided and washed out in the operating room. The goal is to convert a contaminated wound to a clean one as quickly as possible. The wound is monitored for signs of infection for 5 to 7 days. An organism-specific antibiotic may be administered pending the result of cultures. An open fracture with a small soft tissue injury is immobilized in a splint or cast with an opening (window) over the wound for observation and dressing changes. Open fractures with more extensive soft tissue injury may be immobilized with an external fixator (see Fig. 41–12).

Nursing Diagnostic Statements

***High risk for injury:** neurovascular compromise, risk factors: trauma, edema, and treatment regimen.*

***High risk for impairment of skin integrity;** risk factors: immobilization and presence of cast.*

***High risk for injury: complications of immobility;** risk factors: immobilization in cast, traction, or external fixator.*

***Alteration in self-care: bathing/hygiene, dressing/grooming,** related to uncompensated altered physical mobility and pain.*

Nursing Care

Prevention of Neurovascular Injury. Neurovascular assessments are performed every 1 to 2 hours for the first 24 to 36 hours, then every 4 hours. Elevate the limb promptly to prevent edema. When the lower extremity is elevated, the pillow or blanket roll should be placed under the calf so that the heel does not rest against anything (such as the pillow). Position the extremity at the level of the heart to facilitate arterial and venous blood return.

Maintain Skin Integrity. Assess skin frequently for redness and excoriation. Mobilize the child as soon as possible to prevent skin breakdown. If the child is restricted to bed, encourage frequent position changes, using overbed trapeze if applicable. For some patients, pressure-reducing or pressure-relieving devices may be necessary. Protect skin at the cast edges by petaling the cast with moleskin. Any complaint of pain or pressure under the cast should be investigated to rule out pressure ulceration.

Prevent Complications of Immobility. The method of immobilization chosen for a specific child and specific injury is based on the type of the injury and its location. In general, the least restrictive method of immobilization is chosen. In an effort to prevent the complications of immobility, it is important to encourage use of all unaffected extremities. The patient should use an overbed trapeze or other assistive devices to maximize independent mobility while in bed. Before discharge, assess the child and family for safe use of assistive devices. If necessary, consult the physical therapist for assistance with mobility.

The child may not be able to return to school, depending on type of cast and school environment. Explain to the family that the child will not be able to return to full activity immediately after the cast is removed. There will be some stiffness and muscle weakness in the extremity. Return to full activity depends on regaining muscle strength and motion. Some children require rehabilitation, either on an inpatient or outpatient basis, for assistance with regaining strength and range of motion.

Promote Self-Care: Bathing/Hygiene, Dressing/Grooming. Despite the child's immobility and regardless of the extent, encourage the child's participation in activities of daily living. Children in bed can participate in daily hygiene and can be positioned for independent feeding at meals, even while in a hip spica cast. For ambulatory patients, showering may be possible with use of a plastic bag or shower cover to protect the cast from getting wet. Explore clothing alternatives with the family if the child is returning to school.

Promote Comfort. As with any injury, damage to nerve and muscle fibers can cause pain, as can swelling in the area of the injury. Administer analgesics as ordered by the physician and monitor effectiveness. A child with a fracture will need narcotic analgesics until the bone is immobilized and for 1 to 2 weeks after reduction. Assist with regular position changes to prevent pressure on bony prominences. Apply ice packs to injured areas, on top of the cast if necessary. Elevation of the extremity will prevent excessive swelling, which can increase discomfort. Diversional activities can provide some distraction and increase comfort.

KEY CONCEPTS

Concepts Related to Basic Information

- Children's bones are more flexible, contain more cartilage, are more porous, and are less likely to fracture.
- Young bones contain a growth plate that makes them susceptible to growth problems from injury but also capable of greater remodeling.
- Young bones heal more rapidly because of the abundant blood supply of the periosteum.
- Immobilization is commonly required in varying degrees during healing of the musculoskeletal system.

Concepts Related to Nursing Assessment

- Many injuries to and treatments for musculoskeletal disorders predispose the patient to neurovascular compromise.
- Neurovascular assessment is a continuous part of nursing care of children with musculoskeletal disorders.
- Immobilization has physiologic and psychologic consequences; assessment for these consequences is ongoing.
- Physical deformity accompanies many musculoskeletal disorders; assessment for patient and parent response to body changes should be part of the overall assessment.

Concepts Related to Nursing Intervention

- Parental and patient education about caring for a child with an orthopedic treatment modality is a major nursing responsibility.
- Adjustment to mobility changes, temporary or permanent, may require nursing assistance.
- Skin problems commonly accompany orthopedic treatment modalities.
- Alternative methods of meeting developmental needs and milestones must be provided within the restrictions of the treatment regimen.

REFERENCES

Barker, D. P. J., & Hall, A. J. (1986). Epidemiology of Perthes' disease. *Clinical Orthopaedics and Related Research, 209,* 89–94.

Davidson, R. S. (1991). Deformities of the child's foot. In G. J. Sammarco (Ed.), *Foot and Ankle Manual* (pp 296–312). Philadelphia: Lea & Febiger.

Delp, M., & Manning, R. (1981). *Major's physical diagnosis.* Philadelphia: WB Saunders.

Drennan, J. C. (1990). Neuromuscular disorders. In R. T. Morrissy (Ed.), *Lovell & Winter's pediatric orthopaedics* (3rd ed., pp 381–463). Philadelphia: JB Lippincott.

Frantz, C. H., & O'Rahilly, R. (1961). Congenital skeletal limb deficiencies. *The Journal of Bone and Joint Surgery, 43A,* 1202–1224.

Gartland, J. J. (1979). *Fundamentals of orthopedics.* Philadelphia: WB Saunders.

Herring, J. A., (1990). Congenital dislocation of the hip. In R. T. Morrissy (Ed.). *Lovell and Winter's pediatric orthopaedics* (pp. 815–850). Philadelphia: JB Lippincott.

Hungerford, D. (1975, November). Spinal deformity in adolescence. *Medical Clinics of North America.*

Jacobs, J. E. (1960). Metatarsus varus and hip dysplasias. *Clinical Orthopaedics and Related Research, 16*(19), 203.

Krebs, D. E., & Fishman, S. (1984). Characteristics of child amputee population. *Journal of Pediatric Orthopaedics, 4,* 89–95.

Martinez, A. G., Weinstein, S. L., & Dietz, F. R. (1992). The weight-bearing abduction brace for the treatment of Legg-Perthes disease. *The Journal of Bone and Joint Surgery, 74A,* 12–21.

McDade, W. (1977). Bow legs and knock knees. *Pediatric Clinics of North America, 24,* 825.

Meehan, P. L., Angel, D., & Nelson, J. M. (1992). The Scottish-Rite abduction orthosis for the treatment of Legg-Perthes disease. *The Journal of Bone and Joint Surgery, 74A,* 2–11.

Morrissy, R. T. (Ed.). (1990). *Lovell & Winter's pediatric orthopaedics* (3rd ed.). Philadelphia: JB Lippincott.

Rang, M. (1983). *Children's fractures.* Philadelphia: JB Lippincott.

Rushforth, G. F. (1978). The natural history of hooked foot. *The Journal of Bone and Joint Surgery, 60B,* 530–532.

Salter, R. (1970). *Textbook of disorders and injuries of the musculoskeletal system.* Baltimore: Williams & Wilkins.

Scoles, P. V., & Aronoff, S. C. (1984). Antimicrobial therapy of childhood skeletal infections. *The Journal of Bone and Joint Surgery, 66A,* 1487–1492.

Staheli, L. (1977). Torsional deformity. *Pediatric Clinics of North America, 24,* 799.

Staheli, L. T. (1987). Rotational problems of the lower extremities. *Orthopaedic Clinics of North America, 18,* 503–512.

Tachdjian, M. O. (1990). *Pediatric orthopaedics* (2nd ed.). Philadelphia: WB Saunders.

Winter, R. B. (1990). Spinal problems in pediatric orthopaedics. In R. T. Morrissy (Ed.), *Lovell & Winter's pediatric orthopaedics* (3rd ed., pp 625–702). Philadelphia: JB Lippincott.

Wise L. B. (1986). A comparison of orthopaedic casts: Breaking the mold. *American Journal of Maternal-Child Nursing, 11,* 174–176.

BIBLIOGRAPHY

Barbarick, D. L. (1985). Initial assessment and triage of the multiple injured patient. *Orthopaedic Nursing, 4*(2), 19–22.

Bennett, J. T., & MacEwan, G. D. (1989). Congenital dislocation of the hip. *Clinical Orthopaedics and Related Research, 247,* 15–21.

Bridwell, K. H. (1988). Cotrel-Dubousset instrumentation. *Orthopaedic Nursing, 7*(1), 11–16.

Brosnan, H. (1991). Nursing management of the adolescent with idiopathic scoliosis. *Nursing Clinics of North America, 26,* 17–31.

Busch, M. T., & Morrissy, R. T. (1987). Slipped capital femoral epiphysis. *Orthopaedic Clinics of North America, 18,* 637–647.

Campbell, L. S., & Campbell, J. D. (1991). Musculoskeletal trauma in children. *Critical Care Nursing Clinics of North America, 3*(3), 445–456.

Canale, S. T., & Beaty, J. H. (Eds.) (1991). *Operative pediatric orthopaedics*. St. Louis: CV Mosby.

Carini, G. K., & Birmingham, J. J. (1980). *Traction made manageable: A self-learning module*. New York: McGraw-Hill.

Carlino, H. Y. (1991). The child with an Ilizarov external fixator. *Pediatric Nursing, 17,* 355–358.

Corbett, D. (1988). Information needs of parents of a child in a Pavlik harness. *Orthopaedic Nursing, 7*(2), 20–23.

Cotton, L. A. (1991). Unit rod segmental spinal instrumentation for the treatment of neuromuscular scoliosis. *Orthopaedic Nursing, 10*(5), 17–23.

Crawford, A. H. (1987). Orthopaedic injury in children. In M. L. Callaham (Ed.), *Current therapy in emergency medicine*. Toronto: BC Decker.

Drummond, D. S. (1988). What's new in scoliosis: The age of the implant. *The University of Pennsylvania Orthopaedic Journal, 4*(Spring), 14–23.

Drummond, D. S., O'Donnell, J., Breed, A., Albert, M. J., & Robertson, W. W. (1989). Arthrography in the evaluation of congenital dislocation of the hip. *Clinical Orthopaedics and Related Research, 243,* 148–156.

Dunst, R. M. (1990). Legg-Calvé-Perthes disease. *Orthopaedic Nursing, 9*(2), 18–27.

Farrell, J. (1986). *Illustrated guide to orthopaedic nursing* (3rd ed.). Philadelphia: JB Lippincott.

Folcik, M. A. (1988). Winter sports injuries: An overview. *Orthopaedic Nursing, 7*(6), 25–28.

Frese, S. M. (1985). Coping with trauma. *Orthopaedic Nursing, 4*(2), 58–60.

Gagliardi, B. (1991). The impact of Duchenne muscular dystrophy on families. *Orthopaedic Nursing, 10*(5), 41–49.

Gates, S. J. (1984). Helping your patient on bedrest cope with perceptual/sensory deprivation. *Orthopaedic Nursing, 3*(2), 35–38.

Glynn, M. K., & Regan, B. F. (1983). Surgical treatment of Osgood-Schlatter's disease. *Journal of Pediatric Orthopaedics, 3*(2), 216–219.

Gurnham, R. B. (1983). Adolescent compliance with spinal brace wear. *Orthopaedic Nursing, 2*(6), 13–17.

Hansell, M. J. (1988). Fractures and the healing process. *Orthopaedic Nursing, 7*(1), 43–48, 50.

Ilfeld, F. W., Westin, G. W., & Makin, M. (1986). Missed or developmental dislocation of the hip. *Clinical Orthopaedics and Related Research, 203,* 276–281.

Jacobs-Zacny, J. M., & Horn, M. J. (1988). Nursing care of adolescents having posterior spinal fusion with Cotrel-Dubousset instrumentation. *Orthopaedic Nursing, 7*(1), 17–21.

Jones-Walton, P. (1991). Clinical standards in skeletal pin site care. *Orthopaedic Nursing, 10*(2), 12–17.

Karn, M. A., & Ragiel, C. A. (1986). The psychological effects of immobilization on the pediatric orthopaedic patient. *Orthopaedic Nursing, 5*(6), 12–16.

Komisarz, J. M. (1984). Chondromalacia patella. *Orthopaedic Nursing, 3*(3), 24–28.

Lane, P. L., & LeBlanc, R. (1990). Crutch walking. *Orthopaedic Nursing, 9*(5), 31–38.

Levine, A. M., & Drennan, J. C. (1982). Physiologic bowing and tibia vara. *The Journal of Bone and Joint Surgery, 64A,* 1158–1163.

Mason, K. J. (1989). Pediatric orthopaedics: Developmental norms. *Orthopaedic Nursing, 8*(4), 45–50.

Mason, K. J. (1991). Congenital orthopaedic anomalies and their impact on the family. *The Nursing Clinics of North America, 26,* 1–16.

Morris, L., Kraft, S., Tessem, S., & Reinisch, S. (1988). Nursing the patient in traction. *RN, 51*(1), 26–31.

Morrissy, R. T., & Selman, S. (1991). Slipped capital femoral epiphysis. *Orthopaedic Nursing, 10*(1), 11–20.

Mubarak, S. J., Beck, L. R., & Sutherland, D. (1986). Home traction in the management of congenital dislocation of the hips. *Journal of Pediatric Orthopaedics, 6,* 721–723.

National Association of Orthopaedic Nurses. (1992). *Guidelines for orthopaedic nursing*. Pitman, NJ: Anthony J. Jannetti.

Newschwander, R. T., & Dunst, R. M. (1989). Limb lengthening with the Ilizarov external fixator. *Orthopaedic Nursing, 8*(3), 15–21.

Olson, E. V., Thomson, L. F., McCarthy, J., Johnson, B. J., Edmonds, R. E., Schroeder, L. M., & Wade, M. (1967). The hazards of immobility. *American Journal of Nursing, 67,* 780–797.

Paley, D. (1988). Current techniques of limb lengthening. *Journal of Pediatric Orthopaedics, 8,* 73–92.

Richardson, A. B., Taylor, M. L., & Murphree, B. (1990). TSRH instrumentation: Evolution of a new system. *Orthopaedic Nursing, 9*(6), 15–21.

Rockwood, C. A., Wilkins, K. F., & King, R. E. (Eds.) (1991). *Fractures in children* (3rd ed.). Philadelphia: JB Lippincott.

Ross, D. (1991). Acute compartment syndrome. *Orthopaedic Nursing, 10*(2), 33–37.

Rothenberg, J. R. (1991). Innovations in treating anterior cruciate ligament deficiency. *Orthopaedic Nursing, 10*(2), 17–224.

Rubin, M. (1988). The physiology of bedrest. *American Journal of Nursing, 88,* 50–56.

Salmond, S. W., Mooney, N. E., & Verdisco, L. A. (Eds.) (1991). *National association of orthopaedic nursing core curriculum for orthopaedic nursing*. Pitman, NJ: Anthony J. Jannetti.

Scherzer, A. L., & Tscharnuter, I. (Eds.) (1990). *Early diagnosis and therapy on cerebral palsy: A primer on infant development problems* (2nd ed.). New York: Marcel Dekker.

Shesser, L. K., & Kling, T. F. (1986). Practical considerations in caring for a child in a hip spica cast: An evaluation using parental input. *Orthopaedic Nursing, 5*(3), 11–15.

Tachdjian, M. O. (1990). *Pediatric orthopaedics* (2nd ed.). Philadelphia: WB Saunders.

Whittington, C. F., & Carlson, C. A. (1991). Anterior cruciate ligament injuries: Evaluation, arthroscopic reconstruction, and rehabilitation. *Nursing Clinics of North America, 26,* 149–158.

CHAPTER • 42

Neoplasms/Cancer

Mary J. Waskerwitz

NURSING PROCESS PLANS

NPP: The Child with Cancer, Table 42–5

RELATED TOPICS

Total parenteral nutrition, Chapter 16
Impact of chronic illness, Chapter 19
Impact of death and dying, Chapter 20
Nursing care of the hospitalized child, Chapter 21
Principles and strategies for home care, Chapter 22
Blood components and their normal function, Chapter 34
Normal and abnormal immune function, Chapter 37
Thrush (moniliasis), Chapter 39
Care of the child with neurologic sequelae, Chapter 40

LEARNING OBJECTIVES

- Describe the nursing actions used to support the child and family during diagnosis, treatment, and home care.
- Synthesize and apply information to the nursing care of children with malignant diseases.
- Identify nursing diagnostic statements associated with malignant diseases of children and nursing interventions used to ameliorate or modify the defining characteristics of those diagnoses.
- Compare the observed outcomes of care in evaluating the effectiveness of the nursing interventions.
- Identify the major concerns for survivors of cancer as they pertain to biopsychosocial factors.

Cancer, a word that in the past was synonymous with death, in this generation has become associated with chronic illness and, not infrequently, with cure. This increased potential for a normal lifespan for the child with cancer is due largely to advances in drug treatment (chemotherapy), radiation treatment (radiotherapy), and refinement of surgical techniques. National cooperative groups — Children's Cancer Study Group (CCSG) and Pediatric Oncology Group — have facilitated the rapid advances in cancer treatment by pooling data on patients from across the country and thereby arriving more rapidly at findings on which to base subsequent practice.

These therapeutic advances, however, do not negate the fact that the diagnosis of cancer remains a devastating event for the child and family. Treatment often involves surgery, chemotherapy, radiation therapy, or some combination of these modalities. For the family, this often means changes such as adapting to repeated hospitalizations, seemingly endless clinic visits, possible changes in the child's appearance, financial concerns, and, always, the unsettling possibility of the child's untimely death. Nurses who care for children with cancer and their families are called on to understand not only the body's reaction to malignancy (a disease or tumor that is capable of local invasion and metastases or distant spread) but also how to monitor and intervene for the often severe side effects of cancer treatments and to somehow foster the child's normal growth and development in the midst of the health crisis.

This chapter deals with the common forms of cancer in childhood. Leukemia, because it is the most prevalent form of childhood malignancy, is detailed as a prototype. Another prototype for nursing care will be found in the nursing process plans for the child with cancer.

Overview of Pediatric Oncology

Incidence

Most people think of cancer as a disease of the elderly. Although only about 6500 new cases are diagnosed annually in the United States, cancer is the leading cause of death from disease in children over 1 year of age (CA, 1992; Fernbach & Vietti, 1991). Childhood cancer represents 0.6 to 0.7 per cent of the cancers diagnosed in the United States (American Cancer Society, 1993). Probably the most exciting aspect of pediatric oncology today is the trend in overall survival rates that have grown constantly from just 28 per cent in the early 1960s to almost 70 per cent by the late 1980s (CA, 1992, p. 37). The most common malignancies in children in the United States are, in order, leukemia, brain and central nervous system (CNS) tumors, lymphomas (including Hodgkin disease), sympathetic nervous system tumors (including neuroblastoma), kidney tumors (including Wilms tumor), soft tissue sarcomas (including rhabdomyosarcoma), bone tumors (including Ewing sarcoma and osteogenic sarcoma), and retinoblastoma (Fernbach & Vietti, 1991).

Etiology

"What causes cancer in children?" is a question that remains unanswered. Potential environmental carcinogens that have been linked to the development of cancer in adults, such as smoking, diet, industrial pollutants, are difficult to link to the etiology of pediatric malignancies because children have had such little time for exposure. Other epidemiologic factors, such as family history, prenatal exposures, and the pre-existence of certain constitutional disorders, may be significant. In fact, children with chromosomal disorders form the largest group of children who have a higher than normal incidence of cancer. Children with Down syndrome, for example, develop acute leukemia 20 times more frequently than unaffected children (Piu & Rivera, 1991). Children born with certain sporadic congenital malformations have an increased incidence of some malignancies. For example, children with Wilms tumor have been noted to have an increased incidence of aniridia, hemihypertrophy, and genitourinary tract abnormalities. Researchers continue to investigate links between immunodeficiency states and the development of malignancy, and to search for possible oncogenic viruses.

Structure and Function

A "cancer" is a cellular tumor, a malignant neoplasm. A "neoplasm" is any tumor (benign or malignant) arising from new and abnormal cell growth. "Malignant neoplasms" are progressive growths in which there is a loss of differentiation of cells; that is, the cells no longer perform their intended function. Malignant cells undergo changes in DNA, leading to transmission of faulty information for cellular development and subsequent uncontrolled growth and loss of normal cellular function. Proliferation of these abnormal cells can be viewed as a failure of the surveillance function of the immune system (Bellanti, 1985).

Although research continues, it is currently thought that failure of the immune system to provide adequate surveillance is linked to the development of malignancy. A healthy immune system identifies and destroys aberrant cells. When the immune system is less competent, however, it may fail to perform adequate surveillance and allow proliferation of malignant cells. Incompetence may result because of chemically induced suppression (e.g., corticosteroids and other immunosuppressant drugs), suppression as the result of prolonged or frequent viral infections, or congenital or acquired immunologic disease (e.g., AIDS). (Chapter 37 further details functions of the immune system.)

Malignant cells probably do not kill healthy cells directly* but rather compete with them for nutrients and blood supply to sustain growth. They eventually starve and replace the healthy cells in the involved tissue, resulting in the loss of function of that organ or tissue. Cancerous tumors are classified histologically (according to cell type) but also differ by location, growth rate, metastatic patterns, response to treatment, and prognosis.

Spread of Cancerous Cells

Cancer cells spread either through invasion of adjacent tissues or through metastasis. "Invasion" is a continuation of the primary growth into adjacent tissue, whereas "metastasis" is a malignancy occurring away from the primary site.

Invasion. Unlike normal cells, which grow in an orderly and restricted fashion in relation to neighboring cells, malignant cells are uninhibited by the fact that a particular tissue space is becoming overcrowded. Malignant cells continue to proliferate, exerting pressure on adjacent tissues. This pressure may actually help to separate adjacent tissues along natural fracture lines and to create an inroad for the invading tumor (Groenwald, 1987). Invasion of the tumor occurs along paths of least resistance to its growth.

Metastasis. Metastases are malignancies that occur in sites that are not continuous with the primary neoplasm. How do malignant cells move from one area of the body to another? Although certain aspects of the answer to that question remain obscure, there are several hypotheses about their movement. It is known that cancer cells separate rather easily from the primary tumor, both in the form of single cells and in clumps of cells. Tumor cells that break away from a tumor at the top of a body cavity (e.g., the peritoneal cavity) may fall to the bottom and implant there.

Orphaned cells broken from a tumor may also be picked up in the lymph and subsequently make their way into the blood stream. Other malignant cells reach the blood stream through direct invasion of capillaries and veins. Once in the blood or lymph flow, it is postulated that malignant cells implant in tissues where they are most likely to survive and that those tissue sites depend, in part, on certain characteristics of the tumor cells themselves (Groenwald, 1987).

Malignant cells that migrate to a secondary tissue site do not necessarily begin to grow. Many cells die; others may become dormant, only to activate months or years after the primary tumor has been removed. If and when the tumor cells do proliferate, they can achieve a size of only a few millimeters before they outgrow the area's blood supply. Unfortunately, tumor cells are well prepared for this temporary setback. They are able to secrete a chemical (angiogenesis factor) that stimulates the formation of additional blood vessels.

History and Physical Examination

Infants, children, and adolescents who are diagnosed as having some form of cancer usually present initially at the pediatrician's office, child health care clinic, or local emergency room with signs and symptoms or physical findings that either have been present for a long time or have just been brought to the attention of the parents or themselves. Occasionally, the diagnosis of cancer is first suspected by the practitioner during the course of an examination of a well child who is being seen for a routine health maintenance check-up. The complete list of signs and symptoms that are associated with childhood malignancies is immeasurable. In fact, many of these findings are the same as those associated with other common childhood illnesses. It is often the persistence and intensity of these findings that alert the skilled clinician to the possibility of a diagnosis of cancer. Table 42–1 is a summary of the possible signs and symptoms of the common pediatric malignancies described in this chapter.

Diagnostic Assessment

If, on completion of a careful and complete history and physical assessment, the diagnosis of a malignancy is suspected, various preliminary tests may be obtained at the local clinic or hospital. These tests may include blood studies, radiographs, and diagnostic scans (e.g., computed tomography [CT] and bone scans). As the pediatrician becomes increasingly convinced that a child has cancer, he or she will likely transfer the care of the child to a pediatric oncologist (children's cancer specialist). This is a very difficult time for parents, who understand and fear that their child may have cancer yet continue to hope and pray that the findings may turn out to be merely a "false alarm." Providing emotional support while supplying parents with honest information regarding what is known thus far is imperative.

Completion of the battery of studies needed to make a specific diagnosis of cancer and to document the extent of disease may take several days. Parents, of course, must provide consent for these special stud-

* Although it has been postulated that cancer cells may release toxins that kill healthy cells to open pathways by which the malignancy can spread to other tissues, there is currently little support for this hypothesis (Groenwald, 1987).

TABLE 42–1
Possible Signs and Symptoms Associated with Pediatric Cancers

Leukemia

Abdominal pain, bleeding, bruising, anorexia, fever, hepatomegaly, hemorrhage, arthralgia, infections, lymphadenopathy, malaise, fatigue, irritability, pallor, petechiae, purpura, splenomegaly, refusal to walk, weight loss, limp

Brain Tumors

Alteration in intellectual or developmental growth, anorexia, ataxia, balance disturbance, changes in behavior and personality, clumsiness, gait disturbance, cranial enlargement in infants, cranial nerve dysfunction, diffuse or focal nerve dysfunction, drowsiness, diplopia, decreased visual acuity, lethargy, headache, irritability, lack of weight gain, failure to thrive, malaise, muscle weakness, motor dysfunction, nystagmus, papilledema, precocious puberty, seizures, somnolence, stupor, strabimus, endocrinopathies, meningismus, torticollis, urinary retention, visual impairments, visual field changes, vomiting, weakness, hypertension

Hodgkin Lymphoma

Fever, lymphadenopathy, night sweats, weight loss, splenomegaly, hepatomegaly, pruritis, malaise, lassitude, anorexia, pleural effusion with pericardial effusion, superior vena cava syndrome

Non-Hodgkin Lymphoma

Abdominal distention, anorexia, mass, pain, ascites, chills, cough, diarrhea, dyspnea, epistaxis, fever, cranial nerve palsies; lymphadenopathy, nasal congestion, rhinorrhea, vomiting, wheezing

Neuroblastoma

Abdominal mass, anemia, bladder and anal sphincter dysfunction, gait disturbance, Horner syndrome, hypertension, anorexia, fatigue, bone pain, digestive problems, bowel or bladder obstruction, hydronephrosis, nasal obstruction, dysphagia, infection, irritability, palpable mass, orbital ecchymosis, pain, paraplegia, proptosis, respiratory distress, spinal cord compression, myoclonus, opsoclonus, weight loss, "blueberry muffin" nodules, upper lid ecchymosis, hepatomegaly, ptosis.

Wilms Tumor

Abdominal mass, anemia, anorexia, fever, hematuria, hypertension, malaise, enlarging abdomen, vague abdominal pain, constipation

Rhabdomyosarcoma

Chronic otitis media, cranial nerve palsies, dysphagia, dysuria, earache, epitaxis, swelling, facial nerve palsy, gastrointestinal obstruction, hearing loss, hematuria, hoarseness, nasal discharge, obstruction, pain, parotitis, proptosis, sinusitis, mass, urinary tract obstruction

Osteogenic Sarcoma

Bone, pain, swelling, pathologic fracture, weakness, weight loss, anorexia

Ewing Sarcoma

Pain, swelling, tenderness, fever

Retinoblastoma

"Cat's eye reflex," limited vision or loss of vision, pain, redness at orbit, strabismus with esotropia, exotropia

ies to be carried out. Nurses should be prepared to explain the significance of each study to the parents and child in an age-appropriate and developmentally appropriate manner and to describe exactly how each test is done and any degree of discomfort that the child may experience. Table 42–2 lists the studies that are usually obtained to diagnose and evaluate the common pediatric cancers. Table 42–3 describes how some of these studies are performed. A tissue sample of the tumor, which is usually obtained through a pediatric surgical procedure, is necessary for the pathologist or oncologist to make the diagnosis of a specific malignancy. Appropriate treatment can begin as soon as the diagnosis is known and studies to evaluate for extent of disease are completed.

Therapeutic Management

The treatment of children with cancer may involve surgery, radiation therapy, and chemotherapy. These three treatment modalities are often used in combination. Surgery was the only treatment available for patients with solid tumors until radiation therapy and chemotherapy became appropriate adjunctive therapies. Leukemia, the most common malignancy in children, is treated primarily with chemotherapy, and it was for this disease that chemotherapy was first used successfully in children in 1948 when a folic acid antagonist decreased the number of leukemic cells in some children (Gaddy & Wood, 1982).

Of necessity, children with cancer may be cared for by more than one pediatric specialist. Pediatric surgeons and other subspecialty surgeons, radiotherapists, and pediatric oncologists all play a role in the team caring for the child with cancer, but the pediatric oncology team is responsible for overall patient management. That team of many professionals, including a primary nurse, clinical nurse specialist, pediatric nurse practitioner, other nurses, pediatric social worker, child life specialist, and psychologist, will be involved in providing psychosocial care and support to the child and family. The nurses who are assigned to care for children with cancer must assist parents in assimilating their child's complex health care system. The nurses who are at the child's bedside each day can lend great support to parents by providing consistent and intelligible explanations of treatment plans and procedures. Because of the increased emotional demands on the parents at this time, all teaching and information will likely need to be repeated again and again. The unfailing presence of a sincere, optimistic, caring nurse will play an important role in the family's adaptation to this time of crisis and its inherent demands (Chesler & Barbarin, 1987).

Surgery

A surgical procedure is almost always employed to diagnose cancer in children with solid tumors. Biopsies of tumors establish an accurate diagnosis by supplying

TABLE 42-2
Some Special Tests That May Be Used to Diagnose and Evaluate Pediatric Cancers

Leukemia

Complete blood count
Bone marrow aspiration
Chest radiograph
Lumbar puncture

Brain Tumors

Computed tomography (CT) or magnetic resonance imaging (MRI) scan of the brain
Myelogram or MRI of spine
Lumbar puncture

Hodgkin Disease

Chest radiograph
CT scan of chest and abdomen/pelvis
Bone scan
Erythrocyte sedimentation rate
Bone marrow biopsy
Staging laparotomy

Non-Hodgkin Lymphoma

Chest radiograph and chest CT scan
Bone marrow aspirate and biopsy
Lumbar scan
Abdominal CT scan or ultrasonography

Neuroblastoma

Abdominal CT scan
Chest radiograph and chest CT scan
Bone survey
Bone scan
Bone marrow aspirate and biopsy
24-hr urine collection for catecholamines
MRI of spine and pelvis

Wilms Tumor

CT scan of abdomen
Chest radiograph or chest CT scan

Rhabdomyosarcoma

Chest radiograph and chest CT scan
CT scans or MRI of primary tumor area
Bone marrow aspirate and biopsy
Bone scan
Lumbar puncture (for head and neck primary lesions)

Osteogenic Sarcoma

MRI of primary lesion
Bone scan
Radiograph of primary lesion
Chest radiograph
Chest CT scan

Ewing Sarcoma

CT scan of chest and chest radiograph
Bone marrow aspiration and biopsy
Bone scan
MRI of involved bone
Radiograph of involved bone

Retinoblastoma

CT scan of head
Skull radiograph
Evaluation of retina under anesthesia (EUA)

the pathologist with tissue samples of the tumor. For some tumors, it is preferable to attempt complete surgical excision. Complete surgical excision is not always possible for large tumors that are adjacent to vital structures and may not be indicated if it leaves the child with a mutilated or grossly disfigured appearance. Some treatment plans make use of radiation therapy and chemotherapy to reduce the size of large tumors preoperatively, allowing for either a complete excision or less radical surgical procedure at a later time. In most cases, surgery is usually combined with another treatment modality in order to manage any sites of metastases and micrometastases.

Radiation Therapy

Radiotherapy is the treatment of malignant disease with roentgen rays or other radiant energy. When tissue is exposed to ionizing radiation, radiation fragments are absorbed and their energy is deposited within that tissue. Ionization produces changes within the cell molecules that result in biologic damage. Normal cells have a greater capacity for subsequent repair when exposed to radiation than do malignant cells. Hence, radiotherapy is used as a cancer treatment because it is capable of killing tumor cells.

Newer techniques with megavoltage machines al-

TABLE 42-3
Diagnostic Assessment: Tests Commonly Performed on Pediatric Oncology Patients

Diagnostic Test	Purpose	Nursing Implications
Bone marrow aspiration and biopsy	Aspiration of marrow that is obtained into syringe through heavy, wide-gauge needle with stylet that is inserted into marrow space through skin, subcutaneous tissue, and bone cortex using rotary motion; the anterior or posterior iliac crest is the bone marrow site most often chosen for aspiration in children; performed with sterile technique; a biopsy core is obtained in similar fashion but with larger needle	The child is most often held tightly in a prone or supine position on a treatment table; local anesthesia is injected to the site to provide some analgesia, but the actual aspiration of marrow into the syringe, which is often done over a period of a few seconds, is usually very painful and not amenable to the local anesthesia premedication; the entire procedure usually takes a few minutes
Bone scan	Scan of skeletal system after an injection of intravenous radionuclide that within a few hours localizes in the bone, with increased focal accumulation of tracer in areas of bone disease	The child must hold still on a hard surface while a large scanner passes over the body
CT scan	Computed transverse tomography scan allows noninvasive evaluation of various body parts; it produces anatomic cross-sectional images of specific body parts that readily demonstrate organ structures and lesions, easily discriminating among soft tissue variations that are too subtle for simple radiographs	The child must lie still on a firm surface for the duration of the scan, sometimes for up to an hour, while large machinery passes over the body; sometimes intravenous or oral contrast material is administered prior to the test to enhance the quality of film produced
Lumbar puncture	Injection of needle into lumbar spine interspace to obtain sample of cerebospinal fluid, performed with sterile technique	The child must be held in a flexed-spine position (usually curled on the side) for a few minutes
MRI scan (magnetic resonance imaging)	Tomographic images of the body with contrast of soft tissue generated by changing and static magnetic fields in the body and radiofrequency pulses; can be used to detect lesions as small as 2 mm; a very sensitive, non-invasive radiograph	Complete immobilization is necessary; parents can remain in the room; any metal objects must be removed prior to the test; the test is performed in less than an hour
Ultrasonography	Photograph of internal structures made through use of high-frequency sound waves: the reflected sound wave patterns vary with tissue density: sound travels fastest through the most compact molecules; abnormalities in tissue density can be visualized	The child must hold still for an ultrasound examination, but there is no pain involved in the test; the test is performed in less than an hour

low for very precise direction of very high energy radiotherapy beams to the tumor, sparing the skin and surrounding normal tissues. Cobalt machines are megavoltage (McGuire, 1993). Different tumors show varying degrees of radiosensitivity, as do normal tissues. Different organs tolerate specific limited doses of radiation before the normal function of that organ is impaired (Mandell, 1991).

Radiotherapy is most often employed in combination with surgery or chemotherapy in the treatment of leukemias, lymphomas, and solid tumors. It may also be used alone to achieve palliation of symptoms caused by tumor masses.

Most courses of radiation therapy are given as one treatment daily for 5 out of each 7 days. A specific dose is given each day, depending on the tumor being treated and its site. A total course may take several weeks since all tissues have a limited daily tolerance.

Parents of children who receive radiotherapy need careful, repeated explanations of the principles of radiotherapy. They must understand the immediate as well as late side effects that may be caused by the treatment.

Children may experience side effects of radiation therapy that involve the tissues and organs that lie within the radiotherapy treatment field. The side effects of radiation therapy can occur acutely, during the treatment or shortly after treatment is completed, or as late effects presenting in future years. For example, a child with rhabdomyosarcoma receiving radiotherapy to the head and neck region will likely experience oral ulceration, xerostomia (decreased salivation), and loss of taste sensation with associated discomfort, poor hydration, and poor nutrition. Long-term dental, hearing, vision, learning, and growth problems may require specialized management. Radiation therapy nurses are prepared to develop special nursing and home care plans for children undergoing radiation treatments.

It is usually frightening for children to begin radiation therapy treatment, because they are left alone in rooms with large machines. Members of pediatric radiotherapy departments are experienced in working with children under these circumstances, and even young children often become less resistant and more accepting of the procedure after a few days. Radiotherapists, radiation therapy nurses, and other staff members work together to allay the child's anxiety before and during each treatment session, which may last only a few minutes. Because patients must lie perfectly still on a flat, hard table while alone in a room as the radiotherapy treatment is given, infants and young children will likely require sedation or even general anesthesia and the use of immobilization devices or casts to allow for the safe and precise administration of the radiotherapy. Nurses and other medical specialists will be involved in the coordination of such special preparations and services.

Chemotherapy

Treatment with chemotherapy involves the use of drugs that kill or interfere with the proliferation of fast-growing malignant cells. Chemotherapeutic drugs are also called "antineoplastic agents"; that is, "against" (anti-) "new, abnormal cell growth" (neoplastic). Most antineoplastic agents affect cells in the process of dividing to make new cells. But normal cells, particularly those known to grow rapidly—*bone marrow, hair follicle cells, gastrointestinal epithelial cells, and cells of the gonads*—will be affected to varying degrees. To understand the rationale for administration of chemotherapy, it is helpful to review the cell cycle.

Cell Cycle

Cells, whether normal or malignant, go through four cell cycle phases (Fig. 42–1). The first phase is G_1, or the gap stage between mitosis and DNA synthesis. In this phase, the cell produces enzymes needed for DNA synthesis. The synthesis phase *(S)* denotes the period during which DNA doubles in preparation for mitosis. G_2 is the second gap phase; at this time RNA and proteins are synthesized that are necessary for mitosis. The last phase, mitosis *(M)*, is completed with the division of the parent cell into two daughter cells. Cancer cells may divide into several new cells, instead of the normal two cells, at this phase (Ziegfeld, 1987).

It is hypothesized that cell populations contain, at any given time, three categories of cells: cycling cells, nondividing cells, and resting cells (Fig. 42–2) (Groenwald, 1987). Cycling cells are those that continuously divide; these are the rapidly growing cells most affected by antineoplastic drugs. Nondividing cells divide for a time but then differentiate into functional cells that complete their life cycles without further division. Resting cells leave the cell cycle after mitosis to remain dormant until called back into action at the G_1 phase of the cell cycle. It is further speculated that cycling cells and resting cells divide into stem cells and nonstem cells (Groenwald, 1987). Stem cells are precursor cells, or "mother cells"—those cells necessary to maintain the cell line. Stem cells ensure the survival of that particular cell population. As long as there are dormant malignant stem cells (in the G_0 phase), there is the threat of regrowth of the tumor when the resting cells reactivate.

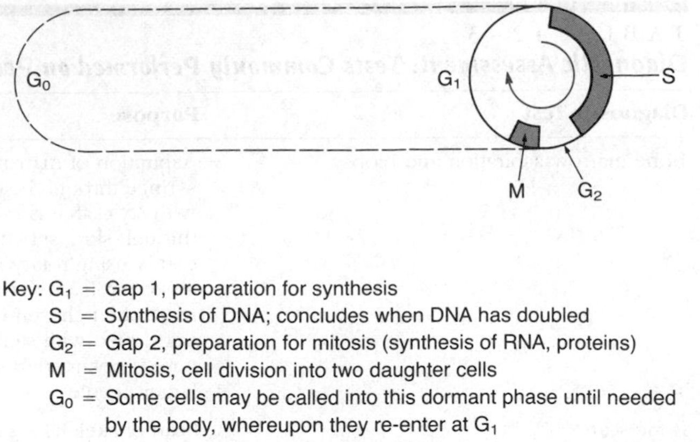
G₀
G₁
S
M
G₂
Key: G₁ = Gap 1, preparation for synthesis
S = Synthesis of DNA; concludes when DNA has doubled
G₂ = Gap 2, preparation for mitosis (synthesis of RNA, proteins)
M = Mitosis, cell division into two daughter cells
G₀ = Some cells may be called into this dormant phase until needed by the body, whereupon they re-enter at G₁

FIGURE 42-1. Cell cycle.

Action of Chemotherapeutic Agents

Chemotherapeutic agents can be classified according to activity exerted on the tumor cells (Table 42–4). "Cell cycle–specific" agents are those that exert their maximal cytotoxic (cell-killing) effect during a particular phase of the cell cycle. These agents are most effective against rapidly dividing cells. As tumors grow

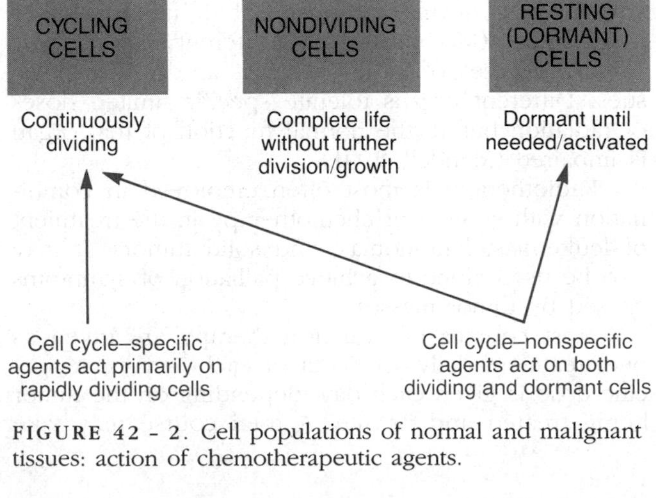

FIGURE 42-2. Cell populations of normal and malignant tissues: action of chemotherapeutic agents.

TABLE 42-4
Medications for Cancer (Chemotherapy)

Drug Classification	Major Action	Chemotherapeutic Agent	Route	Major Side Effects (*denotes "after high dose")	Nursing Care
Antimetabolites	Interfere with DNA synthesis; cell cycle–specific agents				
		Cytosine arabinoside (ara-C, Cytosar, cytarabine)	IV, SQ, IM, IT	Bone marrow suppression, nausea and vomiting, anorexia, alopecia, hepatotoxicity, fever, neurotoxicity,* conjunctivitis*	• Monitor for nausea and vomiting, dehydration • Monitor liver function • Monitor hematopoietic status
		6-Mercaptopurine (6-MP, Purinethol)	PO, IV (investigational)	Bone marrow suppression, hepatotoxicity	• Monitor hematopoietic status • Monitor SGOT, SGPT, bilirubin
		Methotrexate (Amethopterin)	IV, IM, IT, PO	Bone marrow suppression, nausea and vomiting, alopecia, renal failure, photosensitivity, diarrhea, seizures, fever, rashes, neurologic changes **Calcium leukoram (citrovorum factor) is "rescue drug" given after high dose to prevent lethal toxicity**	• Monitor hematopoietic status • Use antiemetics PRN • Provide mouth care • Monitor liver enzymes (SGOT, SGPT) • Monitor urine creatinine clearance for high dose • Maintain adequate hydration • Observe neurologic status, report symptoms • Encourage use of sun screen
		Thioguanine (6-thioguanine, 6-TG)	PO	Bone marrow suppression, mild nausea, vomiting	• Monitor hematopoietic status
Alkylating agents	Interfere with the replication of DNA; most are cell cycle–nonspecific				
		Cyclophosphamide (Cytoxan)	IV, PO	Bone marrow suppression, nausea and vomiting, anorexia, alopecia, hemorrhagic cystitis, amenorrhea, testicular atrophy, SIADH	• Monitor hematopoietic status • Administer antiemetics PRN • Heme test urine • Increase and encourage hydration • Mesna after high dose is a bladder wall protector • Sperm banking prior to treatment (in selected patients)
		Dacarbazine (DTIC, DIC)	IV	Bone marrow suppression, flulike syndrome, nausea and vomiting, anorexia, local pain and burning at injection site, alopecia, soft tissue damage with extravasation, alopecia, lethargy	• Monitor hematopoietic status • Administer antiemetics • Monitor IV site for pain, inflammation; warm cloth to vein, decrease rate of IV • Treat flulike syndrome symptomatically

(continued)

TABLE 42-4
Medications for Cancer (Chemotherapy) *(Continued)*

Drug Classification	Major Action	Chemotherapeutic Agent	Route	Major Side Effects (*denotes "after high dose")	Nursing Care
		Nitrogen mustard (mechlorethamine, Mustargen)	IVP	Bone marrow suppression, nausea and vomiting, phlebitis, alopecia, severe soft tissue damage with extravasation, amenorrhea, and impaired spermatogenesis	• Give immediately after diluted • Monitor hematopoietic status • Administer antiemetics • Monitor IV site and patency • Have thiosulfate available as antidote with extravasation • Counsel regarding reproductive function
		Procarbazine (Matulane, Ibenzmethyzin)	PO	Bone marrow suppression, nausea, rashes, stomatitis, anorexia, parethesias, neuropathies, depression, nervousness, azoospermia, photophobia, alopecia	• Monitor hematopoietic status • Monitor neurologic status • Counsel regarding reproductive function
		Ifosfamide (isophosphamide)	IV	Bone marrow suppression, nausea and vomiting, renal toxicity, hemorrhagic cystitis, dysuria, hematuria, alopecia, lethargy, confusion, peripheral neuropathy, mild soft tissue damage with extravasation	• Monitor hematopoietic status • Administer antiemetics • Monitor liver enzymes (alkaline phosphatase, SGOT, SGPT) • Monitor BUN, creatinine • Hematest urine • Increase hydration after dosing • Mesna per protocol • Monitor IV site • Monitor neurologic status
Anthracycline antibiotic	Interfere with nucleic acid (both RNA, DNA synthesis, cell cycle–nonspecific				
		Actinomycin-D (dactinomycin, Cosmegen)	IV	Bone marrow suppression, nausea and vomiting, anorexia, diarrhea, stomatitis, alopecia, severe soft tissue damage with extravasation, hepatotoxicity phlebitis, fever, malaise	• Monitor hematopoietic status • Administer antiemetics PRN • Monitor SGOT • Monitor IV
		Bleomycin (Blenoxane)	IV, IM, SQ	Progressive pulmonary toxicity (related to cumulative dose), cutaneous toxicity, hypersensitivity reactions, alopecia, phlebitis, anaphylaxis, hypersensitivity, skin changes (hyperpigmentation)	• Monitor respiratory function (used cautiously in clients with pulmonary disease) • Monitor pulmonary function tests • Monitor injection site • Test doses prior to initial treatment • Emergency equipment at bedside

TABLE 42-4
Medications for Cancer (Chemotherapy) *(Continued)*

Drug Classification	Major Action	Chemotherapeutic Agent	Route	Major Side Effects (*denotes "after high dose")	Nursing Care
		Doxorubicin (Adriamycin)	IV	Alopecia, nausea and vomiting, stomatitus, bone marrow suppression, red urine, severe soft tissue damage with extravasation, chemical phlebitis at injection site, cardiotoxicity	• Monitor hematopoietic status • Monitor injection site • Monitor cardiac function
		Daunorubicin (Cerubidine), Daunomycin	IV	Same as doxorubicin	Same as doxorubicin
Adrenocorticosteroids	Interfere with protein synthesis and alter cell metabolism (cell cycle–nonspecific)				
		Prednisone (Deltasone)	PO	Electrolyte imbalance, hypertension, fluid and salt retention, increased appetite, weight gain, esophagitis cushingoid manifestations, glucosuria, immunosuppression, hirsutism, acne, impaired wound healing, loss of muscle mass, irritability, osteoporosis	• Monitor intake and output • Monitor urine glucose • Low-sodium diet • Administer antacids PRN • Serve with foods • Monitor blood pressure
		Prednisolone	PO, IV, IM	Same as prednisone	Same as prednisone
		Dexamethsone (Hexadrol, Decadron)	PO, IV	Same as prednisone	Same as prednisone
Alkaloids	Interfere with cell division and inhibit RNA and protein synthesis; cell cycle–specific agents (M phase)				
		Vinblastine (Velban)	IV	Bone marrow suppression, alopecia, neurotoxicity, severe soft tissue damage with extravasation, nausea and vomiting, peripheral neuropathy, malaise, constipation	• Monitor hematopoietic status • Monitor for bowel function • Administer stool softener PRN • Monitor gait • Monitor IV site
		Vincristine (Oncovin)	IV	Neurotoxicity, alopecia, fever, severe soft tissue damage with extravasation, constipation, SIADH	• Monitor neurologic status (weakness) • Monitor IV site • Monitor bowel pattern • Administer stool softener PRN
		Etoposide (Vepesid, VP-16)	PO, IV	Leukopenia, thrombocytopenia, nausea and vomiting, alopecia, hypotension with rapid infusion, alopecia, phlebitis	• Monitor hematopoietic function • Monitor blood pressure during infusion • Monitor neurologic status • Monitor IV site

(continued)

TABLE 42-4
Medications for Cancer (Chemotherapy) *(Continued)*

Drug Classification	Major Action	Chemotherapeutic Agent	Route	Major Side Effects (*denotes "after high dose")	Nursing Care
		VM-26 (tempiposide)	IV	Bone marrow suppression, nausea and vomiting, alopecia, phlebitis, anaphylaxis	• Monitor hematopoietic function • Monitor IV site • Monitor blood pressure during infusion
Heavy metal compounds	Interfere with replication of DNA; most are cell cycle–nonspecific				
		Cisplatin (CisPlatinum, Platinol, PDD)	IV	Bone marrow suppression, nausea and vomiting, ototoxicity, renal toxicity, hepatoxicity, alopecia, paresthesias, tinnitus, cellulitis, anaphylaxis, electrolyte imbalance, SIADH	• Monitor hematopoietic function • Administer antiemetics • Monitor SGOT, SGPT, bilirubin • Monitor vital signs, LOC • Monitor IV • Monitor electrolytes especially calcium, magnesium • Monitor audiograms • Monitor I&O, fluid balance
		Carboplatin	IV	Same as cisplatin	Same as cisplatin
Nitrosurea	Inhibit DNA and RNA synthesis, crosses blood-brain barrier				
		Lomustine (CCNU, CeeNu)	PO	Bone marrow suppression, nausea and vomiting, hepatotoxicity, decline in renal function, alopecia	• Monitor hematopoietic function • Administer antiemetics • Monitor SGOT, SGPT, bilirubin • Monitor creatinine
		Carmustine (BiCNU, BCNU)	IV	Bone marrow suppression, nausea and vomiting, alopecia, burning at IV infusion site, hepatotoxicity, nephrotoxicity	• Monitor hematopoietic function • Administer antiemetics • Monitor IV site, apply warm cloth, decrease rate if burn at site
Enzymes	Inhibit certain cell metabolites, interfere with protein synthesis				
		Asparaginase (L-asparginase, Elspar)	IM	Pancreatitis, bone marrow suppression, coagulation and protein abnormalities, local reaction at injection site, nausea and vomiting, hyposensitivity reaction, anaphylaxis, rashes, hyperglycemia, diabetes mellitus	• Emergency equipment available; observe for at least 1 hr after injection • Monitor for glucose • Monitor liver function (SGOT, bilirubin, alkaline phosphatase coagulation studies)

From Association of Pediatric Oncology Nurses. (1990). *Cancer chemotherapy.* Richmond: Author; Groenwald, S. (1987). *Cancer nursing: Principles and practice.* Boston: Jones & Bartlett; Karch, A., & Boyd, A. (1989). *Handbook of drugs and the nursing process.* Philadelphia: JB Lippincott; and Ziegfield, C. (1987). *Core curriculum for oncology nursing.* Philadelphia: WB Saunders.

in mass, the length of time between each phase of the cell cycle increases, thus decreasing the effect of cell cycle–specific agents (Groenwald, 1987). "Cell cycle–nonspecific" agents are effective against both dividing and resting cells. Cells affected by these drugs have difficulty dividing or repairing themselves (Ziegfeld, 1987).

Chemotherapeutic agents can be classified according to activity exerted on the tumor cells. "Alkylating agents" are compounds that interfere with the structure and function of DNA, combining chemically with DNA so the cell becomes damaged. "Alkaloids" disorganize the mitotic spindle to arrest cell division. "Antimetabolites" are substances similar to natural body substances that act falsely to incorporate into DNA. "Synthetic hormones" alter normal hormonal balance in patients to modify the growth of cancers arising from tissues that are particularly susceptible to hormonal influence, preventing effective cell proliferation. "Antibiotics" used in cancer therapy are chemicals produced by living bacteria that interfere with cell metabolism. "Enzymes" can inhibit certain cell metabolites and prevent protein synthesis. Table 42–4 summarizes the most commonly used agents, their generic and brand names, classification, route of administration, and major side effects. Table 42–5 provides a Nursing Process Plan for the child with cancer.

Combination Chemotherapy

Treatment with a combination of antineoplastic drugs optimizes the cell-killing properties of the drugs while minimizing the side effects. Because the drugs have various actions, particular combinations can deliver a wide variety of assaults to the malignant cell. Because certain chemotherapeutic agents have additive and synergistic effects, individual drug dosages can be decreased, thus reducing their side effects.

All chemotherapeutic agents are immunosuppressive to varying degrees (they suppress the function of normal lymphocytes in the immune system), so patients must not receive live virus immunizations, such as measles, mumps, and rubella (MMR), and oral polio vaccine while on treatment and they must be cautioned to avoid exposure to common contagious viral diseases. They will, likewise, mount poor antibody responses to vaccines containing proteins from killed organisms, such as diphtheria, tetanus, and pertussis (DTP). If an immunosuppressed child contracts a viral disease or receives one of these immunizations, she or he could develop a serious form of the disease because of this inability to mount a proper antibody response to the virus. If the child has not had chickenpox and demonstrated immunity to the disease through high serum titers, parents must be instructed to report all close exposures to chickenpox immediately (within 72 hours). The child will be injected with varicella-zoster immune globulin (V-ZIG), which is hoped to prevent or suppress the virulence of the disease, should it occur. Additionally, the V-ZIG in the immunosuppressed patient may extend the normal incubation period of varicella to 21 days or more. If an immunosuppressed child does develop chickenpox, he or she will be given an antiviral drug such as acyclovir to hasten and inhibit the course of the disease, which can be fatal in 1 to 2 per cent of these children (French et al, 1991).

Central Venous Access Devices for Chemotherapy Administration

Since the 1980s, many children with cancer have received intravenous chemotherapy (and blood products, parenteral nutrition, and other medications) through permanent right atrial catheters. These catheters are made of silicon Silastic material. They are surgically placed through the cephalic, internal, or external jugular vein, with the tip lying near the junction of the superior vena cava and the right atrium. The remainder of the catheter is tunneled subcutaneously and exits the skin medial to the nipple but at about the nipple level. A Dacron cuff at the proximal end of the catheter becomes embedded into the tissues and serves as an infection barrier and stabilizer (Fig. 42–3).

Methods of exit site care vary widely among institutions. Generally, some form of daily or regular cleaning of the exit site is required with a sterile or clean dressing (Robertson, 1991). In addition, most lines must be flushed daily with a diluted heparin solution in order to ensure patency.

There are also modifications of these catheters that are totally implanted, allowing intravenous access via a chamber or "port" that is completely skin-covered. No dressing or frequent flushing is required. The "port" is accessed with special bent needles (which will lie flat on the skin exterior) that puncture the skin and the chamber's septum.

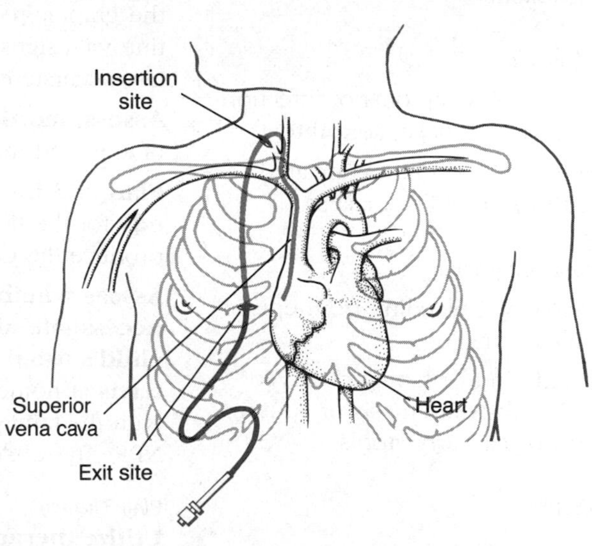

FIGURE 42-3. Hickman/Broviac catheter (permanent right atrial catheter) for intravenous chemotherapy/medication.

TABLE 42-5
Nursing Process Plan: The Child with Cancer

Analysis: Collaborative Problem 1

Response and Related or Risk Factors: *High risk for injury; physiologic: bone marrow suppression; infection; risk factors:*

- Decreased WBCs (neutropenia/leukopenia)
- Decreased RBCs (anemia)
- Decreased platelets (thrombocytopenia)
- Immunosuppressive effects of medications
- Knowledge deficit (child and/or parent) regarding how to prevent infection and bleeding episodes

Projected Outcomes:

- The child will remain free of infection associated with leukopenia/neutropenia
- The child and/or parent will minimize bleeding associated with thrombocytopenia and the child will have minimal or no bleeding episodes
- The child and/or parent will minimize factors leading to associated with decrease in RBCs and the child will remain free of anemia

Defining Characteristics
(Actual Responses)

Subjective:

Anemia:

- Shortness of breath with physical activity
- Weakness
- Fatigue
- Dizziness
- Headache

Leukopenia:

- Report of symptoms of infection (e.g., runny nose, sore throat)
- Feeling of warmth associated with fever, chills, malaise

Thrombocytopenia:

- Prolonged bleeding from epistaxis, gums
- Child- and/or family-observed red streaks in emesis or sputum and black, tarry stools

Objective

Anemia:

- Decreased red blood cells, decreased hemoglobin and hematocrit

Nursing Interventions

Anemia:

Surveillance; Vital Signs Monitoring

Monitor pulse and respiration before, during, and after periods of activity (to assess the body's ability to compensate for the increased oxygen demand related to exercise); take vital signs as indicated

Indicate the child's activity on the graphic record each time routine vital signs are taken (to facilitate accurate comparison)

Assess, monitor, and chart color of skin and mucous membranes

Plan and implement rest periods for the hospitalized child that produce the desired outcome

Assess whether the anemia will necessitate alterations of the child's usual rest activity patterns at home and discuss this with the family (see Table 34–9, NPP: The Child with Anemia)

Play Therapy

Utilize therapeutic play and family visitors to decrease the child's anxiety and irritability; ensure that the family understands the relationship between activity

Evaluation Criteria

Anemia:

Pulse and respirations that return to normal limits within 10 mins after increased activities (e.g., crying and feeding for the infant, loud crying and gross motor activity for the toddler and older child)

Absence of fatigue in response to activity appropriate for age

Leukopenia:

The child will remain free of infection associated with leukopenia/neutropenia, as evidenced by:

- Absence of fever
- Absense of signs and symptoms of infection

Thrombocytopenia:

Skin and mucous membranes free of additional bruises and petechiae: absence of frank bleeding, such as prolonged bleeding from bleeding gums and epistaxis (nose bleeds); bleeding from wounds, hematomas, and bright red stools is rare; absence of hypovolemia associated with hemorrhage

TABLE 42-5 (continued)

Defining Characteristics	Nursing Interventions	Evaluation Criteria
• Tachycardia • Tachypnea, especially with mild exertion • Skin and mucous membranes pale *Leukopenia*: • Decreased white blood cells (possibly with differential decrease in remaining neutrophils or lymphocytes) • Fever • Signs of infectious process • Positive culture results *Thrombocytopenia*: • Decreased platelet count • Petechiae, bruising • Stools black and tarry • Streaks of red blood evident in emesis/sputum • Head bleed causing severe headache or drowsiness (emergency situation)	and the body's demand for oxygen via Hgb (so that they can more fully participate in the treatment plan) *Blood Products Administration* **Administer packed red blood cells** as indicated and monitor child's response (Collaborative Intervention) *Leukopenia* *Surveillance; Vital Signs Monitoring* **Record temperature frequently.** When >38.5°C, administer antipyretic as indicated (Collaborative Intervention) • NO rectal temperatures, suppositories, and/or enemas **Take vital signs as indicated** **Record baseline assessments every shift** that include the status of each body system; be alert for changes in the baseline that would indicate an infectious process **Monitor blood pressure** (sign of septic shock) **Monitor WBC and differential counts.** Calculate the absolute neutrophil count: ANC = (% Neutrophils + Bands) × WBC; if ANC < 500 mm³, institute established unit policies to protect child who is at increased risk for infection **Document carefully the condition of skin and mucous membranes** on admission to form baseline data **Monitor neurologic status.** May require CT scan *Medication Administration* **Administer antifungal and antibiotic** medications for febrile neutropenic child *Infection Control; Teaching: Procedure/Treatment* **Use meticulous handwashing techniques** at all times (there is an	

(continued)

TABLE 42-5 *(continued)*

Defining Characteristics	Nursing Interventions	Evaluation Criteria
	increased potential for infection with neutropenia even when the ANC is <500 mm³); teach the child and family the major routes of transmission of organisms and the importance of good handwashing *Thrombocytopenia* *Surveillance; Vital Signs Monitoring* **Take vital signs as indicated** Monitor for signs of hypovolemia: significant drop in blood pressure accompanied by an increase in pulse; pale, diaphoretic skin; decreased urine output; restlessness or confusion **Record baseline assessments every shift** that include status of each body system; headache and decreased neurologic status are signs of neurologic bleeding and a serious complication *Bleeding Precautions/Reduction; Teaching: Child and Parent* **Avoid injections** when possible; when a needle must be used, use the smallest gauge possible (e.g., 25-gauge); apply gentle pressure for 3–5 mins following the injection **Supply a soft toothbrush** and instruct the child and family on its proper use **Instruct child and parent on how to stop nosebleeds** and protect gums from irritation **NO rectal temperatures, suppositories, and/or enemas. Avoid the use of aspirin and nonsteroidal anti-inflammatory drugs.** Teach the child and parents how to recognize aspirin in product labels (aspirin and NSAIDs are antiplatelet drugs) **Caution the child and family members to prevent bumps, falls, and cuts.** No climbing, "roughhousing," and tumbling in play; encourage quiet activities	

TABLE 42-5 (continued)

Defining Characteristics	Nursing Interventions	Evaluation Criteria
	such as listening to music, watching videos, coloring, finger painting, board games, and talking to friends on the phone **Caution the child and family to make sure the child is in a seat belt or care seat** when riding in the car **Teach child and parents the signs and symptoms of CNS hemorrhage** and intracranial bleeding (sudden severe headache followed by changes in mental status) to be reported immediately to health care professional *Blood Products Administration* **Administer platelets** as indicated in relation to thrombocytopenia (Collaborative Intervention)	

Analysis: Collaborative Problem 2

Response and Related or Risk Factors: *High risk for impaired skin integrity: alteration in oral mucosa; risk factor: the effect of cytotoxic drugs on rapidly dividing mucosal cells*

Projected Outcome: There will be less interruption (ulcerated areas) in the tissue layers of the oral cavity

Defining Characteristics	Nursing Interventions	Evaluation Criteria
Subjective: • Pain in the mouth and throat • Refusal of food and fluids *Objective:* • Drooling of saliva • White mucosal lesions with red borders • Leukoplakia • Halitosis	*Oral Health Maintenance* **Carefully document observation of oral mucosa** to form a baseline for future assessment **Implement measures to prevent stomatitis and to relieve the pain of stomatitis** • Avoid commercial mouthwashes, lemon-glycerin swabs, and hydrogen peroxide (they may further irritate the mucosa) • Administer prescribed topical anesthetic agents such as viscous xylocaine before meals; systemic analgesics, even narcotics, are sometimes needed for mucositis pain • Instruct the child and parents to avoid foods and fluids that are very hot or cold, that are spicy	No or fewer ulcerations visible; no or decreased oral pain; adequate intake of fluids and food

(continued)

TABLE 42-5 (continued)

Defining Characteristics	Nursing Interventions	Evaluation Criteria
	or rough in texture, and that are acidic; often children with painful stomatitis do not eat or drink at all; the child's hydration status is monitored and maintained	

Analysis: Nursing Diagnostic Statement 1

Response and Related or Risk Factors: *Altered nutrition: less than body requirements, related to*

- Anorexia associated with nausea and vomiting from the disease process and from chemotherapeutic agents
- Increased metabolic rate associated with rapidly dividing malignant cells
- Utilization of available nutrients by malignant cells resulting in insufficient nutrients for normal cells
- Dysphagia associated with stomatitis

Projected Outcome: The child will maintain an adequate nutritional status

Defining Characteristics	Nursing Interventions	Evaluation Criteria
Subjective: • "I'm not hungry" • "Take it away" • "It makes me feel sick" • "It hurts when I swallow" *Objective*: • Weight loss • Oral intake less than minimal daily calorie requirement • Ulcerated mucosa • Vomiting associated with oral intake	*Nutritional Monitoring/Counseling* **Weigh daily** during hospitalization and with each follow-up visit to document progress toward goal **Implement and teach measures to improve oral intake:** • Take diet history; find out what child likes and serve whatever is nutritious in the list available to him or her • Plan meals and snacks carefully to avoid food with little nutritional value • Encourage high-protein, high-calorie foods that will not irritate mucous membranes • Take care to avoid making food an issue for power/control with the child (this may be one of the few things the child can control in the therapeutic environment); offer small portions of food, attractively prepared, frequently throughout the day but avoid insisting that the child eat or offering undue praise for foods consumed	Weight returning to baseline and increasing in accordance with percentile for height; child consumes enough food to meet metabolic needs

TABLE 42-5 *(continued)*

Defining Characteristics	Nursing Interventions	Evaluation Criteria
	• **Refer to dietician or nutrition team** when problem continues; nutritional supplement, hyperal will be instituted as indicated	

Analysis: Nursing Diagnostic Statement 2

Response and Related or Risk Factors: *Fluid volume and electrolyte deficit, related to:*

- Inadequate fluid intake associated with stomatitis and anorexia
- Loss of fluid associated with diarrhea and vomiting

Projected Outcomes:

- The child will maintain adequate hydration
- The child will maintain acid-base balance

Defining Characteristics	Nursing Interventions	Evaluation Criteria
Subjective: • "I don't want to drink" • "I feel sick when I drink" • Reports of diarrhea and vomiting • Reports of weakness • Reports of malaise, lethargy *Objective:* • Specific gravity > 1.020 in an infant or young child, > 1.035 in an older child or adolescent • Dry mucous membranes • Poor skin turgor • Urine output < 1 ml/kg/hr for an infant or child up to 30 kg and < 30 ml/hr for the child over 30 kg (decreased number of diapers or voids per day) • Decreased BP and tachycardia (if dehydration has progressed to hypovolemia) • Observation of vomiting and/or of frequent, water-loss stools • Looks sick, lethargic • History of decreased PO fluid intake • Weight loss • Decreased tearing • Ketotic breath • Ketones in urine	*Fluid/Electrolyte Management* **Record intake and output,** including diaper weights for infants, during hospitalization **Calculate the maintenance fluid requirements** and determine the amount of fluid to be given during each hospital shift or at various hours of the day when the child is at home; find out what fluids the child likes • Offer fluids frequently and in small amounts • Offer clear liquids if nausea and vomiting is issue • School-age children and adolescents may find incentive in recording their own intake (thus demonstrating their ability to meet fluid requirements: however child may be too sick to care) • Tell parents the number of cups per day that are necessary for maintenance **Record specific gravity of urine.**	Urine output ≥ 1 ml/kg/hr for the child up to 30 kg and ≥ 30 ml/hr for the child over 30 kg **Intake ≥ maintenance fluid requirements:** • 100 ml/kg for the first 10 kg of body weight • 50 ml/kg for the next 10 kg of body weight • 10 ml/kg for each succeeding kg of body weight • 2 L/m²/day Specific gravity < 1.020 in an infant or young child; < 1.035 in an older child or adolescent; normal serum electrolytes, BUN; absence of signs and symptoms of metabolic acidosis; absence of signs and symptoms of metabolic alkalosis; skin temperature normal and turgor elastic; BP and heart rate within normal limits and weight is stable

(continued)

TABLE 42-5 *(continued)*

Analysis: Nursing Diagnostic Statement 3

Response and Related or Risk Factors: *Fear/anxiety (child and family), related to family perception about*

- Diagnosis of a malignant and life-threatening disease
- The administration and side effects of chemotherapy
- Invasive diagnostic and therapeutic measures
- Hospital environments/disruption of usual activity and schedules
- Separation from family and friends

Projected Outcome: The child and family will not experience a vague uneasy feeling or feeling of dread

Defining Characteristics	*Nursing Interventions*	*Evaluation Criteria*
Subjective: Verbalization by child and family members of fears related to the prognosis and to the length of prescribed chemotherapy and its effects on the child *Objective*: • Fearful, worried expression • Sympathetic stimulation—cardiovascular excitation, superficial vasoconstriction, pupil dilatation, increased respiratory effort • Appearing "wild-eyed" and clinging to parent in response to attempts at diagnostic or therapeutic interventions • Restlessness • Trembling • Voice quivering • Increased wariness • Increased perspiration	*Anxiety Reduction; Truth Telling* **Encourage verbalization** of the fear-anxiety (to facilitate identification of the actual sources of the fear) **Express both verbally and nonverbally the client's right to the feelings.** (Denying or belittling the fear by comments such as "There's no reason to be afraid" only adds to the anxiety and frustration; assuring the client that many other children or parents have expressed similar concerns may be comforting **Implement direct care with compassion and confidence.** **Explain procedures and other aspects of care carefully and repeatedly,** as necessary (the unknown is usually more anxiety-producing than the known) **Use age-appropriate measures to prepare children and parents for diagnostic and therapeutic measures** **Administer painful or unpleasant procedures in a treatment room, if possible with parents, as appropriate, using developmentally appropriate "techniques"** (children's fear will be reduced if their room is a "safe" place) **Always answer questions honestly.** Do not hesitate to say, "I don't know" when that is the case (the child and family do not expect the nurse to know everything, but	Verbalization of being less afraid. Relaxation of body posture, less tearful behavior, less protest of nonpainful procedures Verbalization of an understanding of the prognosis and procedures associated with the treatment

TABLE 42-5 *(continued)*

Defining Characteristics	Nursing Interventions	Evaluation Criteria
	their confidence will be enhanced and their anxiety reduced if they can then count on an honest response); try to help them find out answers **Refer and consult with social work, psychology/child life as appropriate.** Members of the interdisciplinary team can assist child and family to cope with the situation **Include the child and family in every possible aspect of care: planning, delivery, and evaluation.** (Fear and anxiety will decrease as their sense of control increases) **Explain hospital environmental features. Take child on a tour, if feasible. Find out child's usual routine and try to follow as much as possible** **Continue assessment and interventions, related to fear and anxiety, after discharge** **Explore the concept of death, if appropriate, with the child and parents** and dispel unwarranted fears as appropriate; determine whether the concept of death and major fears are typical for the age; explain developmental stages to the family	

Analysis: Nursing Diagnostic Statements 4 through 7

Response and Related or Risk Factors: *Body image disturbance, self-esteem disturbance, altered role performance, personal identity disturbance, related to child and family perception regarding:*

- Alopecia associated with many chemotherapeutic agents
- Cushingoid features associated with prednisone administration
- Amputation scars
- Radiation therapy
- Diagnosis of cancer

Projected Outcome: The child and family will demonstrate acceptance of changes in appearance and display more positive self-evaluation/feelings about self or self-capabilities and role performance

(continued)

TABLE 42-5 *(continued)*

Defining Characteristics	Nursing Interventions	Evaluation Criteria
Subjective *Body Image*: • Verbalization of concern about how peers and others will react to body changes • Unwillingness to receive visitors or to leave the room • Verbalization of feelings of worthlessness • Unwillingness to dress and perform usual grooming activities • Unwillingness to return to school and activities • Unwillingness to assume self-care or to learn aspects of procedures for home care *Role Performance*: • Change in self-perception of role • Denial of role • Change in physical capacity to resume role *Self-Esteem and Identity*: • Self-negating verbalization • Expressions of shame/guilt • Rationalizes away/resents positive feedback and exaggerates negative feedback • Hesitant to try new things and situations • Overly conforming, dependent on others' opinions • Lack of eye contact • Nonassertive/passive • Indecisive • Excessively seeks reassurance *Objective*: • Flat affect • Malaise • Avoidance of social contact and of personal responsibility • Not looking at affected body part	*Self-Esteem Enhancement; Body Image Enhancement; Role Enhancement and Clarification; Personal Identity Enhancement* **Encourage verbalization of feelings.** (Ventilation of emotion is often preliminary to problem-solving activity) **Maintain an attitude of confidence in the child** (Nonverbal communication of an attitude is often more convincing than words) **Assist the child to identify strengths** and to capitalize on them **Encourage supportive peer contacts** **Facilitate contact with other children of similar age** who have experienced these same body changes **Prepare the child and family for hair loss, reassuring that it will probably not be permanent** **Encourage family contact with other families** who have been through a similar experience **Encourage family members to express their need for the child to return to former responsibilities within the family** (to reinforce self-worth and role within the family) **Refer to social work, psychology, child life specialist** as appropriate to deal with concerns	Beginning problem-solving activities, such as asking the family to buy a wig or bring in a favorite baseball cap Renewed interest in personal appearance Resumption of normal interest in peer relationships and former role within the family Verbalization of plans to make up school work missed during hospitalization Expressed interest in learning how to care for self Verbalization of feeling of self-worth and possession of positive attributes

TABLE 42-5 (continued)

Defining Characteristics	Nursing Interventions	Evaluation Criteria
• Not touching affected body part • Hiding or overexposing affected body part		

Analysis: Nursing Diagnostic Statement 8

Response and Related or Risk Factors: *Spiritual distress (child and family), related to:*

- Worry associated with the prognosis and potential reactions to therapy
- A search for the meaning of the illness
- Feelings of guilt associated with the etiology or delay between onset of the disease and diagnosis
- Powerlessness associated with the uncertainty of the prognosis and the need to undergo therapies that have potentially harmful side effects

Projected Outcome: The child and family will demonstrate renewed strength of spirit

Defining Characteristics	Nursing Interventions	Evaluation Criteria
Subjective: • Express concern with meaning of life/death and belief systems • Anger toward God or pre-eminent spiritual force in life • Question meaning of suffering • Verbalizes concern about relationship with deity • Questions meaning of own existence • Verbalization of guilt and frustration • Parental statements like "If only it were me instead of my child" • Child's questions of "Why did this happen to me?" "Did I get this because I was naughty?" *Objective*: • Questions moral/ethical implications of therapeutic regimen • Displacement of anger toward religious/spiritual representatives • Description of nightmares/sleep disturbances • Alteration in behavior/mood evidenced by anger, crying, withdrawal, preoccupation, anxiety, hostility, and apathy	*Spiritual Support* **Encourage verbalization** and listen with empathy and a nonjudgmental attitude; encourage the child and family to seek out persons (e.g., clergy) who have been helpful in helping them find meaning in other situations **Assist the child and family to correct misconceptions,** but do not attempt to solve their problem (no one else can do that but the child and family; expression of feelings with an empathetic listener will help gain perspective needed for problem solving) **Explore with the child and family the activities that are usually the most enjoyable** and produce a feeling of happiness and lightheartedness. Facilitate and encourage these activities, as permitted, in the hospital setting and at home (activities that have produced this effect in the past carry a great potential for facilitating the child and family's emotional self-healing)	Resumption of more normal affect and activities Verbalization of having more "peace of mind" Expression of a philosophic purpose and/or spiritual peace Return to baseline sleep patterns

(continued)

TABLE 42-5 (continued)

Analysis: Collaborative Problem 3

Response and Related or Risk Factors: *Altered comfort: pain, related to:*

- Proliferation of blast cells within the intramedullary cavities of bones and within abdominal organs
- Administration of intrathecal and intravenous chemotherapy
- Side effects of cytotoxic agents

Proposed Outcome: The child will maintain a level of comfort without significant pain

Defining Characteristics	Nursing Interventions	Evaluation Criteria
Subjective: • Verbalization and vocalization of pain • Withdrawal from social contact • Moaning, crying • Facial mask of pain *Objective:* • Alterations in usual activity patterns • Eyes dull in appearance • Skin cool and pale • Possible increase in pulse, decrease in blood pressure • Pupil changes • Increased or decreased respiratory rate	*Pain Management* **Assess pain:** • Note activity level (children in pain are often much quieter than usual but may also show a marked increase in activity; dullness of the eyes and lethargy often accompany pain) • Assess and interpret vital signs for their relation to pain versus other physiologic activity (increase in pulse and decrease in blood pressure, along with cool, clammy skin, indicate the neuroendocrine response to the stress of pain) • Analyze carefully the child's subjective response to questions about comfort (children may deny pain because they dislike the treatment for pain) • Use adjunctive measures to assess pain, such as those detailed in Chapter 25 **Allow the child control over pain medication,** as appropriate to developmental age (e.g., allow the child to choose from the analgesics ordered, which medication to take, and how many tablets or capsules; control will decrease the anxiety associated with pain and will make the pain more manageable) **Implement and teach the child and family adjunctive measures for pain relief,** such as muscle massage, a warm tub bath, distraction, and relaxation techniques (Chapter 25 details adjunctive therapies)	Resumption of usual activities Return to prepain level of affect Facial expression calm Eyes bright in appearance Vital signs within normal limits Normal pupillary responses Skin warm and without pallor Verbalization of comfort

TABLE 42-5 (continued)

Defining Characteristics	Nursing Interventions	Evaluation Criteria
	Prior to painful invasive procedures, assess how the child usually copes with acute pain, and which of the strategies is most adaptive. Reinforce the useful coping behavior and teach additional coping strategies, such as relaxation techniques. (New coping behavior must be practiced repeatedly before the painful experience; otherwise, the child will revert to familiar, even though possibly less effective, strategies, when faced with the stress of the moment) **When planning and teaching new coping strategies, keep in mind that motor and emotional coping strategies (being allowed to pound with one hand or to cry and scream) are extremely useful** for young children who have poorly developed cognitive coping abilities **Prior to administration of analgesics, selection is based on site of action** (centrally acting, acting at the site of pain, or both), **duration** (short or long acting), and **interval** (continuous, bolus, etc.); depending on the child's developmental level, information is shared with child in joint decision making	

Analysis: Nursing Diagnostic Statements 9 through 11

Response and Related or Risk Factors: *Altered health maintenance, (home care), related to knowledge deficit about:*

- The treatment regimen, disease process, including signs and symptoms of relapse
- Child's medical and psychosocial needs
- The course and side effects of medications
- Child's and family's anxiety/fear, which interferes with processing of information
- Resources available to the family
- Availability of social support
- Altered family functioning
- Ways to optimize child's developmental level
- Child's developmental ability to understand and deal with diagnosis
- Ways to facilitate child's coping

High risk for ineffective management by parents of therapeutic regimen of child; risk factor: knowledge deficit regarding disease process and therapeutic regimen

Health-seeking behaviors, parents, related to desire to know how to safely and effectively care for their child

(continued)

TABLE 42-5 (continued)

Projected Outcome: The child and family will be able to identify, manage, and/or seek out help to maintain home care health maintenance and therapeutic regimen upon discharge and after discharge

Defining Characteristics	Nursing Interventions	Evaluation Criteria
Altered Health Maintenance: • Demonstrated lack of adaptive behaviors to and/or observed inability to take responsibility for meeting home care needs • Expressed interest in learning how to care for self/child at home *Health-Seeking Behaviors*: • Expressed or observed desire to seek a higher level of wellness • Expressed or observed desire for increased control of health practice • Demonstrated or observed lack of knowledge *Ineffective Management of Therapeutic Regimen*: • Choices of daily living ineffective for meeting the goals of a treatment or prevention protocol • Acceleration of illness symptoms • Verbalized desire to manage the treatment of illness and prevention of sequelae • Verbalized difficulty with regulation/integration of one or more prescribed regimens for treatment of illness and its effects on prevention of complications • Verbalized that did not take action to include treatment regimens in daily routines • Verbalized that did not take action to reduce risk factors for progression of illness and sequelae **Inability to perform self-care activities:** • Delays in acquisition of developmental tasks • Low self-esteem	*Teaching: Disease Process; Medication Management* **Provide appropriate support and teaching. Assess parent's ability and willingness to care for devices the child comes home with, such as venous access catheters.** See previous nursing diagnoses for teaching measures • Begin discharge teaching upon admission (teaching is much too involved and important to be left until late in the hospital stay or until the day of discharge) • See specific discharge planning strategies in Table 21–5 • Refer for home health nursing, as appropriate *Teaching: Long-Term Effects of Treatment* **Assess** for parents' awareness of the following long-term effects of treatment: • CNS alterations (normal level of intelligence; learning disabilities; neurologic deficits) • Growth alterations (short stature) • Reproductive alterations (delayed pubertal development) • Immune system alterations (increased risk for development of second, unrelated malignancy) • Alterations in other body systems **Referral** to educational specialist for evaluation and school placement/remediation recommendations **Monitor** growth pattern • Referral to medical specialist for possible growth hormone replacement, plastic surgery, orthopedic corrective surgery	**The child and/or family will display the knowledge and skills needed for home management of therapeutic regimen, as evidenced by:** • Demonstrating safe and effective physical care • Demonstrating effective operation of equipment • Demonstrating safe medication administration and identifying side effects • Demonstrating understanding of care for the child who has bone marrow suppression **The child's illness symptoms will remain stable or decrease** **The parents will verbalize comfort and ease regarding regulation/integration of prescribed regimens for treatment of illness and its effects on prevention of complications**

TABLE 42-5 (continued)

Defining Characteristics	Nursing Interventions	Evaluation Criteria
• Negative body image • Health status **Family stresses** • Family dysfunction • Family unable to meet needs of its members	**Monitor** sexual development • Provide for psychoeducational counseling • Referral to social worker/psychologist for counseling **Ongoing monitoring** of child **Teach** parents regarding long-term effects, as necessary **Periodically review** parents' understanding *Teaching: Long-Term Psychologic Effects of Living with Cancer; Possible Developmental Alterations* **Monitor** developmental progress • Anticipatory guidance regarding developmentally appropriate activities and toys **Promote** self-care activities **Encourage** independence *Family Process Maintenance* **Assist family members to recognize and deal with the indications of inability of the family to function effectively** **Facilitate** expression of feelings • Active listening • Provide support • Refer to mental health specialist • Refer to community-based family support/self-help group	

Most children who receive frequent courses of intravenous chemotherapy will be treated through one of these central venous access devices. They and their parents must recognize the advantages (easy venous access) and disadvantages (possibility of infection) of these systems before they agree to their surgical implantation. Preoperatively, nurses must assess a family's ability to accept responsibility for line care. Postoperatively nurses will be responsible for all related patient and family teaching.

Bone Marrow Transplantation

Bone marrow transplantation is an alternative form of therapy for children with some forms of leukemia and other malignancies historically associated with a poor prognosis. For example, it may be employed as the treatment of choice for newly diagnosed patients with acute nonlymphocytic leukemia (ANLL) in remission and for relapsed patients with acute lymphocytic leukemia (ALL) who are in a second remission.

The purpose of a bone marrow transplant is to provide the child with healthy bone marrow that can produce functional blood cells. A bone marrow transplant can thus reverse the effects of severe bone marrow depression. A bone marrow transplant can make it possible to use higher, and potentially curative, doses of chemotherapy and radiation because the child can be "rescued" from life-threatening bone marrow depression by the transplanted marrow cells. Additionally, there is evidence that immune cells in the transplanted marrow may help to kill remaining leukemic cells in the host (Gale & Champlin, 1986).

ETHICAL ISSUES
Refusal of Cancer Treatment

by Margaret M. Mahon, PhD, RNC

Dwyer is a 7-year-old diagnosed with leukemia at 4 years of age. Since that time he has had several rounds of chemotherapy and radiation. In addition, he has been hospitalized four times for fever and neutropenia. The institution at which Dwyer is being treated has recently received permission to try an experimental drug. Dwyer meets the protocol criteria, and his parents have consented to treatment. When Dwyer is told about the new treatment, he becomes very upset and says he does not want any more medicine. His response shocked his parents and the health care team. It is assumed that Dwyer's response represents a temporary frustration at the medicine and its likely side effects, but Dwyer remains adamant in his refusal. Dwyer understands that, without this treatment, he will probably die.

It is understood that parents are the ideal surrogate decision makers for their children, that parents have the information and ability to decide what is best for their child. It is relatively rare for parents to disagree with children in the most serious of treatment decisions. Yet agreement may be not so much on whether to pursue a certain treatment, but rather on a particular philosophy or attitude to guide their treatment decision making. Commonly heard statements include, "we are willing to try anything to get a cure"; "if it causes too much pain, we don't want it"; "it depends what it will do for her quality of life." Such "philosophies" may change during the course of treatment, largely as a result of more experience with the disease.

Can a child ever make an informed decision to stop treatment, knowing that death is a probable outcome of this decision? A decision by a child as young as Dwyer is likely to be taken as uninformed. Practitioners may believe that children are unable to truly understand the ramifications of their decision. Freyer (1992) points out that decisions in cases such as Dwyer's can be described as primarily pediatric *or* oncologic. In other words, the decision or issues can be about the *child* with cancer, or the child with *cancer*. Concerns about the *child* lead to an examination of the child's ability to make an informed decision, which includes an understanding of the treatment, its likely effects and side effects. An informed decision also includes the ability to understand the implications of not utilizing a treatment option. Concerns about *cancer* lead to an examination of the efficacy of a proposed treatment. Cancer treatment is understood not just in the likelihood of cure, but what the short-term side effects (e.g., nausea, vomiting, hair loss, infection), the long-term side effects, and the late effects of cancer treatment are. In Dwyer's case, what difference does it make that the treatment proposed is experimental? Would the decision to accept or reject Dwyer's wishes be different if he were objecting to an approved treatment modality?

It has long been believed that children do not have an accurate understanding of death until at least age 9. Recent research (Mahon, 1993) has shown that a majority of children age 6 years and older had an accurate understanding of death. In her study of children with cancer, Bluebond-Langner (1978) showed that children with cancer have an accurate understanding of their disease, the effects of treatment, and its likelihood of causing death. This understanding of cancer as fatal can occur in very young children. Furthermore, this understanding occurs independent of children's being given this information by adults; rather, it is acquired as a part of the process of being a cancer patient.

As a child, Dwyer could be forced to submit to the treatment being offered. In the process of deciding, to whom does the nurse owe allegiance, the child or the parents? Rarely is it necessary to be forced to choose one or the other, although occasionally this choice must be made. More often, the nurse is in an ideal position to facilitate communication between the parent and the child. Perhaps the most important component of the communication process is the skill of listening. Is Dwyer saying he is ready to die? Is he afraid of pain or other side effects? Do the parents think this treatment will cure Dwyer? Do they think further treatment might give them an extra month with their son?

The nature of cancer treatment and the extensive research being carried out by the Children's Cancer Study Group and the Pediatric Oncology Group mean that it is likely there will be another treatment to try. For health care professionals involved in the care of children with cancer, each new treatment option may be viewed at two levels: what does this treatment mean for this child? and, what does the treatment for this child mean for future children with cancer? The focus of care has to remain with the current patient, though those involved in treatment with many children over time can find this a painful process.

REFERENCES

Bluebond-Langner, M. (1978). *The private worlds of dying children.* Princeton, NJ: Princeton University Press.

Freyer, D. R. (1992). Children with cancer: Special considerations in the discontinuation of life-sustaining treatment. *Medical and Pediatric Oncology, 20,* 136–142.

Mahon, M. (1993). Children's concept of death and sibling death from trauma. *Journal of Pediatric Nursing, 8*(5), 335–344.

Van Eys, J. (1987). Ethical and medicolegal issues in pediatric oncology. *Hematology/Oncology Clinics of North America, 1,* 841–848.

There are different types of bone marrow transplants: allogeneic, autologous, and syngeneic.

If the bone marrow for transplant is not the child's own, it must be donated by a person who is histocompatible with the patient. "Histocompatibility" is the degree of immunologic likeness between donor and recipient; a good match reduces the likelihood of graft-versus-host disease, discussed later.

In an *allogeneic* transplant, the bone marrow donor is not genetically identical but compatible, such as from a sibling. A full sibling has about a one in four chance of matching a sister or brother. Parents and other relatives have only a remote chance of matching the child.

Autologous transplants infuse bone marrow cells previously harvested from the child. Autologous transplants in leukemia or other malignancies that have a propensity to relapse within the marrow however, carry the risk of relapse (Vega et al, 1987). Such bone marrow will be purged or treated with specific tumor antibodies ex vivo, after its removal from the patient, in hopes of irradicating all microscopic residual disease before it is returned to the patient.

A *syngeneic* transplant is bone marrow donated by an identical twin.

Mismatched and unrelated transplant procedures are also being investigated. Immediately prior to a bone marrow transplant, most children receive a short course of very intensive chemotherapy (such as high-dose cyclophosphamide) and possibly total-body irradiation. This therapy is termed "conditioning" and is delivered for three purposes: (1) to eradicate cancer cells to the extent possible and thereby decrease the chance of posttransplant relapse, (2) to suppress the host's immune response to the transplanted tissue, and (3) to create space in the bone marrow to allow the newly transplanted stem cells to generate healthy blood components (Vega et al, 1987).

Bone marrow is harvested from the donor by multiple bone marrow aspirations from the iliac crest. This procedure is conducted with the donor under general anesthesia. The donated bone marrow is then processed and transfused into the host intravenously. It takes time for transfused marrow to implant and produce new blood cells. The child will remain myelosuppressed (bone marrow suppressed) for an average of 3 weeks after transplant. Transfusions of packed red blood cells and platelets are usually required during the first month. During this period of bone marrow suppression, the child is at risk for infection and bleeding (Vega et al, 1987).

Graft-versus-Host Disease. Graft-versus-host disease (GVHD) is a serious complication of allogeneic bone marrow transplants. GVHD occurs when T-lymphocytes in the donated bone marrow react against tissues in the host. About 10 per cent of children under 10 years of age develop acute GVHD within 3 to 4 months after transplant (typically between the 2nd and the 10th weeks). In older patients, the incidence rises to 30 to 50 per cent (Vega et al, 1987). Clinical manifestations of acute GVHD may begin with a maculopapular rash with pruritus on the palms and soles that may spread to the entire body. The liver may be involved, as evidenced by a rise in serum bilirubin, alkaline phosphatase, or transaminases, with liver tenderness and jaundice. Gastrointestinal manifestations include nausea, abdominal pain, and diarrhea.

Chronic GVHD may follow the acute disease or develop without acute involvement. It may develop up to a year or more after transplant. Again, the skin is often involved, with dryness, pigmentation abnormalities, and lichenified lesions or plaques. Gastrointestinal involvement is common, and immunologic function may be impaired by abnormal T-cell and B-cell function. (See Chapter 37 for a discussion of T-cell and B-cell functions.)

GVHD is treated with corticosteroids and other immunosuppressive drugs, such as methotrexate or cyclosporine, with varying degrees of success. The best "treatment" is still prevention. Pretransplant and posttransplant immunosuppressive therapy is used in an attempt to reduce the incidence of GVHD (Johnson, 1991). Depletion of T-lymphocytes from donor marrow is another approach, although this therapy remains somewhat controversial (Gale & Champlin, 1986).

Bone marrow transplant centers are limited in the United States, so many families must relocate for 1 to 3 months. It is very important for the nurse at the primary hospital to prepare the child and the family for the transplant procedure and to maintain contact with them throughout their stay at the transplant center. The child and the family need unlimited support to meet the stress and anxiety imposed by the transplant procedure.

Nursing Care

Supporting the Child and Family During Diagnosis

When cancer is diagnosed in a child, the parents may already have suspected the child's symptoms and condition could represent cancer. Nonetheless, when the diagnosis is actually made, the parents are immediately terrified that the child will die. The nurse should be present when the parents are told the diagnosis and consent is being obtained for treatment. As the physician tells the parents that their child has cancer, they may become instantly withdrawn, "numb," and hear nothing more, or extremely anxious and "angry at the world." They often fail to recall any of the details of initial conversations with the physicians and nurses. The nurse should take an active role in helping parents to deal with the reality of the diagnosis by offering frequent explanations of the disease and its treatment in the ensuing days, and maybe by telling them how other families seem to have coped with the gravity of the diagnosis and all its implications (Walker et al, 1993).

After the initial shock, the parents will have numerous questions. Each question must be addressed and answered with gentle honesty. The parents are depressed about the possibility of their child's death. They may feel guilty about not having sought medical attention sooner. They are angry that this is happening to them and their child. They are in a state of shock and disbelief. Since most children with cancer are referred to pediatric oncology centers, the parents may not know any of the members of the interdisciplinary team and thus may not be ready to openly share their feelings. The interdisciplinary health team must be there, however, ready to offer support when the parents are ready to verbalize.

The initial hospitalization of a child with cancer may be the parents' first experience with hospitals and complicated treatments. Even the simplest procedures must be explained to the child and her or his parents. The nurse must keep abreast of the diagnostic plan to be able to prepare the child and the parents for each step. The nurse and all members of the team can help the child and family develop trust and feel more secure during this frightening period by communicating an attitude of caring and by giving accurate information about the illness, diagnostic tests, and treatments. These nursing functions can relieve some of the overwhelming stress that the child and family experience at this time.

At the time of diagnosis of cancer, the child often does not feel well. He or she may be irritable and in pain but typically is not especially worried because he or she has felt sick before and has always gotten better. Children do begin to worry, however, as soon as they can sense uneasiness, anxiety, and sadness in their parents. As soon as the parents can speak calmly with the child, he or she must be told something about why he or she is in the hospital and undergoing many tests and painful procedures (Patterson, 1992).

Young children do not need and will not benefit from a detailed description of their disease. They should be told the name of the disease to avoid embarrassment or fears later when they are in public and exposed to persons who may freely use diagnostic terms. They will probably be satisfied with the information that this is an illness that requires special care from special doctors and nurses. They should know that at times some of the special treatments may hurt them for a while but that all the treatments will eventually make them feel better and will help them to get better. It is very important for the parents to tell the child that they will always be there and that they love the child. When one is dealing with single-parent families or children whose parents are divorced, separated, or not married, all of these psychosocial support issues and needs are often amplified. The team may need to remember to address two or more sets of primary caregivers separately as all aspects of the child's case management are planned. Unfortunately, these family situations are not uncommon, and the nurse must incorporate related individual family needs into the care planning.

Interactions and discussions with older children and teen-agers must be open and honest, enhanced by the ever-present support and love of their parents. Adolescents must be presented with the basic facts about their diagnosis and its proposed treatment. Even direct questions such as "Will I die?" must not be ignored. That question can be answered with gentle honesty by relaying information that yes, children with cancer have died but that today's improved treatments work well and that everyone is going to work together so that they will not die. Teen-agers vary in their desire and need to learn details about their disease and its treatment. Some want to learn a great deal and to make decisions independently. Others pursue more passive roles, relying on parents and staff to take care of them. They are happier not talking or learning about their disease in depth. These varying patterns of behavior need to be accepted by the health care team.

The family members immediately center all their emotional energies on the child with cancer. It is easy for the parents to overlook the need for sharing their anxiety and seeking comfort. As soon as the child's condition is stable, parents will probably need to be told to get away from the hospital for a while just to be alone with their spouse, significant others, or friends. They may need reassurance from the nurse that their child will be well cared for in their absence. Likewise, parents must remember the special needs of the siblings at home and grandparents who may live too far away to demonstrate their concerns and caring in person.

Sisters and brothers are usually frightened about what is happening at the hospital. As soon as possible, the siblings must receive an age-appropriate explanation of the child's diagnosis. They need reassurance about their own health. For a while, the parents may not have much time to spend with the siblings, but it is particularly important for them to know and feel the love of their parents. A warm, comfortable home environment is crucial at this time when the parent or parents cannot be at home. If possible, a familiar relative or friend should be in the home with the siblings. They should be encouraged to visit their sister or brother in the hospital to allay fears of the unknown about the child, the illness, and the hospital. Siblings are often frightened; the parents should talk with them about their fears and the seriousness of the diagnosis.

The parents may wish to have the physician or nurse describe the illness to relatives and friends who are important to them. This may relieve some of the burden on the parents, who may also feel responsible for supporting the anxieties and reactions of these other people.

Reaction of Child and Family to Treatment

Cancer treatment begins almost immediately after the diagnosis is made. To the young child, this translates to "pokes and pains." The child will soon learn to associate hospital personnel with painful experiences. The child may cry at the mere sight of someone entering the room, fearing a painful procedure. A consistently kind and pleasant attitude from doctors and nurses and all members of the team and hospital staff will lead the child to trust in these special individuals who are providing care.

Older children and teen-agers deal with the emotional stress and tension at their own pace. They may need time alone to think, cry, or scream. They may be afraid to be alone and seek the constant presence of parents, friends, and staff. Others may want to deny the gravity of the situation for a while and try to laugh off what is going on. Many teen-agers are too proud to show depression or dependence. They must be allowed to take charge with some degree of independence. Older children and teen-agers may react in any or all of these ways. The nurse must recognize clues in verbal and nonverbal behavior and allow patients to express themselves as they feel most comfortable (Walker et al, 1993).

Children of all ages may initially show signs of developmental regression or immaturity. That reaction is understandable, considering the seriousness of the situation and the demands that are placed on them. With consistent kindness, the parents must continue to maintain some standard of discipline and expectations of acceptable behavior. Fortunately, most children with cancer seem to withstand the emotional and physical strain, growing up with the strength of having faced and weathered very serious problems at an early age.

Most children's hospitals have rooming-in programs for the parents, and they are encouraged to participate in treatments, usually as hand-holders. Procedures must be explained fully before they are performed. Even though the child and family have been told about the procedure by their physician, the nurse should again give a brief explanation. This ultimately facilitates their ability to cope by providing an opportunity for them to ask questions and clarify their understanding.

Children must feel comfortable and safe before a threatening procedure is performed. A parent's presence in the treatment room can provide that feeling of safety. Young children will likely squirm and fight a procedure even after it has been explained. Simple relaxation techniques can be taught to children and their parents to help them through the procedure while maintaining a sense of control and involvement (Hockenberry, 1988; Rasco, 1992). Hypnotherapy may also be successful if appropriately trained staff are available (Olness, 1989).

Thus, the kindest thing to do is to speak to the child quietly and calmly, hold the child gently and firmly, and complete the procedure quickly. The nurse can be particularly effective by talking to the child and offering encouragement in enduring the procedure. Despite all these measures, performing painful procedures is both technically and emotionally not feasible for some children. Some programs have established the routine safe use of short-acting general anesthetics such as halothane and brevetol for painful procedures such as bone marrow aspirations and lumbar puncture (Schwanda et al, 1993; Fisher et al, 1985). Naturally, such programs require coordination with an anesthesiologist or intensivist (Fisher et al, 1985).

Physicians and nurses must also be sure that local anesthesia is adequate before a procedure is done. Although these painful procedures must be done as part of the treatment, perhaps some fun can be associated with the painful ordeal, such as picking a trinket from a toy box after each visit to the treatment room.

Home Care

When the child is well enough for discharge, the parents become the primary caregivers. The nurse plays a major role in preparing parents for this responsibility from the first day of hospital admission. (See Chapter 22 for further discussion of principles and strategies of home care.) To care for their child at home, parents must understand the disease, its treatment, and its possible complications. They must be comfortable and confident in their ability to care for their child. There is a great deal of new information for them to remember. The nurse can provide a written explanation of the disease and related articles or booklets as ready reference for parents to use at home. Sometimes it is hard to give specific guidelines for home care, but general hints in writing are helpful. The nurse can design calendars of the treatment plan for parents to follow. They should have phone numbers for 24-hour medical assistance, and they should be encouraged to call if any specific questions or concerns arise. Most children with cancer receive chemotherapy. The nurse should provide lists of the drugs in writing, with their possible side effects. Most chemotherapy drugs will cause low blood counts. Parents should understand the different levels of blood counts so that, when the child is home, activities can be planned according to any specific limitations dictated by test results. Many parents like to keep diaries of what has been happening to the child between clinic visits. These help them to feel more comfortable as historians on the child's interim medical condition.

When the child is home, getting back into a normal family routine is very important. The child with cancer will need special medical treatment, possibly subsequent hospitalization, and frequent clinic visits, but this must not totally disrupt family life or fulfillment of the needs of each family member. Sibling rivalries can arise out of jealousy for the sick child's special treatment and attention. Parents and friends must remember the needs of all children in the family. Each member needs special attention and loving from the others. This does not mean material gifts but rather time spent with a child or parents. Offering to stay with children at home when the patient goes to the clinic or hospital is a caring gift, for example. The single parent will likely be overwhelmed with the responsibilities at the hospital, home, and work. A parent may feel "left out" because of work requirements when he or she cannot be present at many clinic visits. The nurse should assess how the family is coping with these typical stresses and suggest that they make the clinic visits a family affair when possible.

Maintaining as much normality as possible is imperative for the child with cancer. Table 42–5 addresses the nursing issues associated with coping with the long-term effects of cancer treatment. It is important for the nurse to support and foster a quick return to normal activities, especially schooling. Since most teachers have never dealt with cancer in their classroom, the nurse should communicate directly with teachers, explaining the diagnosis and its treatment. Classmates likewise need a formal group explanation of what is going on to allay any of their fears and misconceptions. Some hospitals have established special school re-entry programs that facilitate the child's return to the classroom (Riley-Lawless, 1989). Many booklets published by groups such as the American Cancer Society and others are now available for teachers and school personnel for these children. All school districts have their own policies regarding students with health impairments. It is important for the team's social worker or primary nurse to help families deal with any related problems that arise.

Clinic visits need not mean only pain and treatment to the young child. The presence of a child life specialist and playroom in the clinic can add some fun to the day. A stop at a favorite restaurant after each visit can provide something for the child to look forward to. Older children and teen-agers often develop great trust and strong relationships with their oncology nurses. Just being there, talking, and showing a sincere interest in their lives provides the patients with an atmosphere that makes them truly feel that they will be "OK." With careful, thoughtful nursing interventions, the hospital and clinic may gradually be viewed as more comfortable, supportive, and friendly.

Special camps for children with cancer have been conducted across the country since the mid-1970s. At these camps, children with cancer are allowed to do most of the same camp-related activities as their normal peers, while under the supervision of specially trained camp staff that includes onsite pediatric oncologists and nurses. Children's Oncology Camps of America is a national organization that informally coordinates these now-common camp programs.

Nurse's Role in Supporting Parents

As time goes by, the parents tend to become more relaxed, but they still realize each day that their child has cancer. Years ago if children had cancer, they would almost surely die. Now there is great variability in prognosis. Statistics can be offered to parents, but they are difficult to apply to an individual child. The fact that much time has elapsed following the initial diagnosis does not mean that the child no longer has cancer or that the parents can cease to be concerned that the child will die; With time from diagnosis, the probability of death from cancer decreases, though its possibility will continue to exist.

The nurse and all members of the team have a major responsibility in helping parents through this difficult time; fears and feelings must be expressed. Parents need the opportunity to tell another caring person how it feels to be threatened by a loss of the joys that their child brings. The nurse can offer tremendous support by being available to the family for that purpose. The social worker and nurse should also help the family find additional community and support resources. In many cities, support groups have been formed of parents of children with cancer; these are excellent sources of information and emotional sharing. There are also national organizations for parents of children with cancer. There are many good publications and newsletters that help parents realize that other families have similar problems and concerns. They also offer information about progress in research and current treatment reports. The Candlelighters Foundation is perhaps the largest and best-known nonprofit organization for parents of children with cancer that supports and provides many of the aforementioned services.

Having a child with cancer can be a tremendous financial burden to a family. Even if the family has good medical insurance, there are still many nonmedical expenses, such as transportation to the clinic, meals at the hospital, and babysitters for siblings while the parents are away. Parents must be aware of all available resources in their area, such as state aid for chronically ill children, the American Cancer Society, and various leukemia foundations. Ronald McDonald Houses have been built near many major children's hospitals to provide families with inexpensive housing while they are away from home. The social worker should review each family's medical insurance or health care resources so that all available resources are tapped and that financial hardships do not become catastrophic.

The Child Who Dies

Although the statistics for children with cancer have been improving, nearly 30 per cent of children with cancer died in the reporting period between 1981 and 1987 (Boring et al, 1992). When it becomes obvious that a child has reached a terminal state, she or he will sense a change in the mood of the family. The child will have many scary feelings about what is happening. She or he may have many questions. Chapter 20 is devoted to discussions of children and death. The nurse should help parents understand their child's views of the situation. Parents should be encouraged to answer questions honestly. Children and teen-agers may not be able to put their feelings into words. The child may need to express her or his inner feelings in some way. The child needs reassurance. Children of all ages need to know that their parents will always be there with them, and parents must know that all medical means will be used to prevent undue pain and suffering for their child. For more information on pain management, refer to Chapter 25.

Most parents will know when the child's fight for survival has become futile. They may never before have experienced the death of a loved one. They may have many questions about the actual event of death. A staff member who is close to the family should talk about these things with the parents. It is not morbid to talk about funeral arrangements before the child dies, so that, at the time of death, parents will be spared some of the agonizing chores. This concrete discussion of death will often initiate mourning, which may reduce despair at the time of death. Parents need the staff to support them more than at any previous time.

It is common for parents to want the child to die at home where he or she is most comfortable. This possibility should be explored with parents. If they do wish the child to be at home, the nurse or another designated staff member should prepare them for any emergency that may arise. They should have 24-hour support available to them by phone. Visiting nurses can make regular visits to check on physical abnormalities and help with the case management. Parents should be prepared for common preterminal events such as changes of consciousness, alteration of respirations, loss of bowel or bladder continence, and emesis (Fochtman, 1993).

During this terminal stage, the needs of other family members must not be forgotten. Siblings need every opportunity to release their emotions and express their fears. Contact with their dying brother or sister should be maintained as long as communication is possible, to allay regrets about not having said last words or last goodbyes. A brother or sister may feel responsible for the sibling's death because of an old argument or fight. These concerns must be addressed even when they are not expressed openly by the siblings. The dying child will look and feel very sick, so the amount of time that the children spend with the child is a personal decision for the child and parents to make. It is up to the professional team members to be aware of all these family needs and to help the parents to be aware of them.

It is emotionally very difficult for nurses to face death in any patient. The death of a child can be particularly difficult to understand and accept. Sometimes, it is hard for nurses to become involved with children whom they know will die. The nurse's important role is to provide warmth and kindness, with every attention given to the child's comfort. Table 21–5, the nursing process plan for the hospitalized child, specifies alterations in nursing interventions for a child who is terminally ill. If nurses can know that they helped a short life to be a more comfortable one, they will be rewarded inwardly and embraced outwardly for their care by the grateful families of these children.

The family that has come to rely on persons in the cancer center cannot be forgotten once the patient has died. A social worker or community health nurse can help families get through these difficult times. The child may be dead, but she or he will never be forgotten and will be a part of the parents' and siblings' everyday lives forever. Many parents realize a bond has developed between them and the health team during the child's illness. As a sign of this bond, parents may want to continue their involvement with the hospital team, perhaps at a volunteer level. It is rewarding to know that a large number of parents return to visit frequently, and some have been willing to talk with other parents and continue to be active in parent groups.

Survivors of Childhood Cancer

As more and more children survive cancer, issues concerning their subsequent state of physical and emotional health are being addressed. In fact, childhood cancer survivors may face health hazards that are in part caused by the same therapy that allowed them to live. "Late effects" is the colloquialism used to describe the range of posttherapeutic disabilities that are seen in survivors of pediatric cancer. The exact nature, timing, and severity of the development of late effects depend on (1) the extent and location of the cancer, (2) the modalities and intensity of treatment, and (3) the age and developmental stage of the child at the time of treatment.

Late effects can involve any organ system. Findings can range from clinically insignificant laboratory abnormalities to serious, life-threatening complications. The time interval to the onset of late sequelae is unpredictable. The following areas are of particular concern in the survivor population:

1. *Damage to the central nervous system: psychosocial, neurologic, and intellectual.* The milieu of stress, anxiety, and dependency that surrounds children with cancer can leave them unprepared to face adult life. Treatment that was directed to the central nervous system, such as cranial radiation and intrathecal chemotherapy, has, in many cases, caused documented damage to the brain with related subnormal intelligence and neurologic dysfunction.

2. *Impaired growth and development.* Growth and development can be impaired in any child with a chronic illness. Some children treated for cancer have added direct insults to growth that include, most significantly, radiation to the pituitary gland and other growing bones and organs.

3. *Gonadal development and reproduction aberrations.* Systemic chemotherapy with alkylating agents

and gonadal radiation can affect gonadal development and function of children treated for cancer. Some children will need hormonal replacement to artificially advance to normal adult gonadal development. In some cases, sterility can occur, though, as the numbers of childhood cancer survivors grow, so does the number of documented cases of healthy babies being born to them.

4. *Oncogenesis.* For reasons that are unclear, childhood cancer survivors are at a greatly increased risk of developing a second, perhaps totally unrelated, malignancy within a relatively short time after their initial diagnosis. This oncogenicity may be related to the cancer treatment, immune disturbances induced by the disease or its treatment, or the individual's own genetic susceptibility.

5. *Disruption of function in other organ systems.* Chemotherapy, surgery, and radiation can cause acute toxicity to specific organ systems such as the heart, kidneys, liver, lungs, bone, and gastrointestinal tract. That acute toxicity or necessary surgical interventions has the potential to develop into or include chronic, lifelong health problems.

This overview is by no means complete. Late effects in childhood cancer survivors is an issue that has been granted increasing attention in recent years. It is acknowledged that quality of survival is just as important as survival itself. Research now documents the imperative need for close, continued, long-term follow-up and monitoring of childhood cancer survivors. Early recognition and prompt management of sequelae may, in some cases, lessen the severity of residual problems (Everhart, 1991; Overbaugh & Sawin, 1992). Refer to Table 42–5 for the nursing care issues associated with the long-term effects of cancer treatment.

Disorders Affecting Aberrant Cell Growth

The child diagnosed with cancer presents with high-risk or actual nursing diagnostic statements that are common to most malignancies occurring in childhood. The Nursing Process Plan in Table 42–5 ("The Child with Cancer") identifies the process of nursing care that can be applied to all of the malignant diseases of children discussed in this chapter.

The remainder of this chapter deals with the most common malignant diseases that occur in childhood. Because chemotherapy is common to the treatment of many of these malignancies, Table 42–5 details nursing interventions for the child with cancer.

Leukemia

Leukemia is a proliferation of abnormal white blood cells in the body. Death comes from secondary complications resulting from the presence in vital tissues of these abnormal cells.

Etiology/Incidence

Leukemia is the most commonly occurring malignancy in children. About one third of all children with cancer have leukemia. Approximately 2000 cases of leukemia are diagnosed annually (Young et al, 1986). Although leukemia may have its onset at any age, its peak incidence is between the ages of 3 and 5 years (Steinherz, 1987). Incidence rate of acute lymphocytic leukemia (ALL) is approximately 4 in 100,000 in children younger than 15 years. ALL accounts for more than three quarters of diagnosed leukemias in children.

The etiology of leukemia is unknown. It is known that a few cases of leukemia in adults have been linked to exposure to environmental factors, such as radiation or chemicals. The role of inheritance in the development of leukemia is demonstrated by the enhanced incidence of leukemia in identical twins. If an identical twin has leukemia, the twin has a 1 in 4 chance of developing leukemia (Steinherz, 1987). Leukemia in nontwin siblings is extremely rare.

Several genetically determined diseases have also been associated with an increased incidence of leukemia. Children with Down syndrome, Fanconi hypoplastic anemia, agammaglobulinemia, and Bloom syndrome have shown a higher incidence of leukemia (Cohen, 1993). However, even though incidence is increased, the majority of children with genetic predisposition for leukemia remain free of the disease (Steinherz, 1987). Several of the genetic defects listed are associated with immune deficiencies. Although the Ebstein-Barr (EB) virus has been associated with Burkitt lymphoma and nasopharyngeal carcinoma, no other specific virus is known to be causally related to the development of leukemia or other malignancies, with the exception of the human T-cell leukemia virus, which is etiologically related to adult T-cell leukemia. Research seeking an answer to the etiology of leukemia continues with the investigation of carcinogens, viruses, genetics, and other potential etiologic factors (Edelstein et al, 1991).

Pathophysiology

To understand why children with leukemia die and how leukemic cells affect the body, it is important to have a basic understanding of the origin and function of normal blood cells.

Normal Blood Components

Whole blood is composed of plasma and cells. "Plasma" is the fluid portion of the blood. The solid, or cellular, portion is composed of red cells, white cells, and platelets circulating in the plasma. Red cells carry oxygen to the body tissues from the lungs. Oxygen provides tissues with a vital ingredient of all cell metabolism. "Hemoglobin" is the oxygen-carrying protein of red blood cells and imparts a pink or red appearance to the skin, lips, and nails. Normal hemoglobin from the age of 2 to 5 years is about 12 to 13 g/dl. "Platelets" are the tiny cells that promote clotting and prevent bleeding. A normal platelet count is 200,000 to 400,000/mm^3. The white blood cells form the body's defense against infection. Normal total white blood count (WBC) is 5000 to 10,000/mm^3. The three major types of white blood cells are "granulocytes," "lymphocytes," and "monocytes." In addition, there are three major types of granulocytes: "neutrophils," "eosinophils," and "basophils." (See also Chapter 37.)

Table 42–6 summarizes the kinds of white blood cells, the proportion of these cells in the normal WBC, and their major function. When a differential count is obtained, the percentage of each type of white cell is reported.

Words used to describe the most mature neutrophils are "segmented," or "segs," "polymorphonuclear (polys)," or "bands," and "stab cells (stabs)." The absolute neutrophil count (ANC) is the total (or absolute) number of neutrophils in the blood. ANC is found by multiplying the percentage of functional neutrophils (segs and bands) in the differential by the total white count. Thus, if the WBC is 8000/mm^3 and the differential lists 40 per cent segmented forms, the ANC is 40 per cent of 8000/mm^3, or 3200/mm^3. Since neutrophils are very important in protecting against infection, the ANC is a guideline of the body's ability to fight bacterial disease. Serious bacterial infection may occur when the ANC is less than 500/mm^3. Many treatment protocols allow for blood count recovery to ANC levels greater than 1000/mm^3 before subsequent courses of chemotherapy are given. Granulocyte-stimulating factor (GCSF) is a newly available injectable glycoprotein that is sometimes given to certain patients for several days after completing a course of myelosuppressive chemotherapy in order to induce quick white blood cell and neutrophil recovery (Morstyn et al, 1988).

Blood cells are produced in the "bone marrow," the soft material located in the cavities of bones. All blood cells arise from a common cell called the "stem cell." Under genetic control, stem cells in the marrow differentiate to form red blood cells, white blood cells, and platelets. Once a cell has differentiated into the parent cell of a red cell, a granulocytic white cell, or a platelet, it continues to undergo division while maturing into a functional cell ready to work for the body. In the normal state, the bone marrow releases only these mature, functional cells into the peripheral blood. Lymphocytes arise from the stem cell, but as soon as the commitment to this cell takes place, further maturation occurs in the thymus, lymph nodes, and spleen. The exact site of monocytic maturation is unknown. Figure 42–4 illustrates the process of blood cell production.

Knowing normal blood count values and those that are associated with increased risk of problems is very helpful in developing guidelines for caring for the child with cancer, since chemotherapy, radiotherapy, and leukemia itself are often associated with low blood counts.

Leukemic Process

With the information that leukemia is a proliferation of abnormal white blood cells, and relating that information to knowledge of the normal blood, two statements about leukemia can be made: (1) The abnormal white blood cell continues to divide but may not mature beyond the blast state. It is released into the peripheral blood as a blast, an immature WBC. Leukemic blasts have no normal functional capabilities. (2) As the abnormal white blood cells increase in number,

TABLE 42-6
Categories of White Blood Cells and Their Functions

White Cell Type	Mean* Per Cent in Normal WBCs	Function
Granulocytes		
Neutrophils (segs, bands, etc.)	55	Ingest and digest bacteria during bacterial infection
Eosinophils	2	Summon antigen-antibody response in allergic reactions
Basophils	1	Specific action unknown
Lymphocytes	38	Affect cellular and humoral immunity; produce specific antibodies against viruses, bacteria, and other proteins
Monocytes	5	Act as phagocytes in bacterial infections and are an integral part of normal immune response

*Relatively wide range.

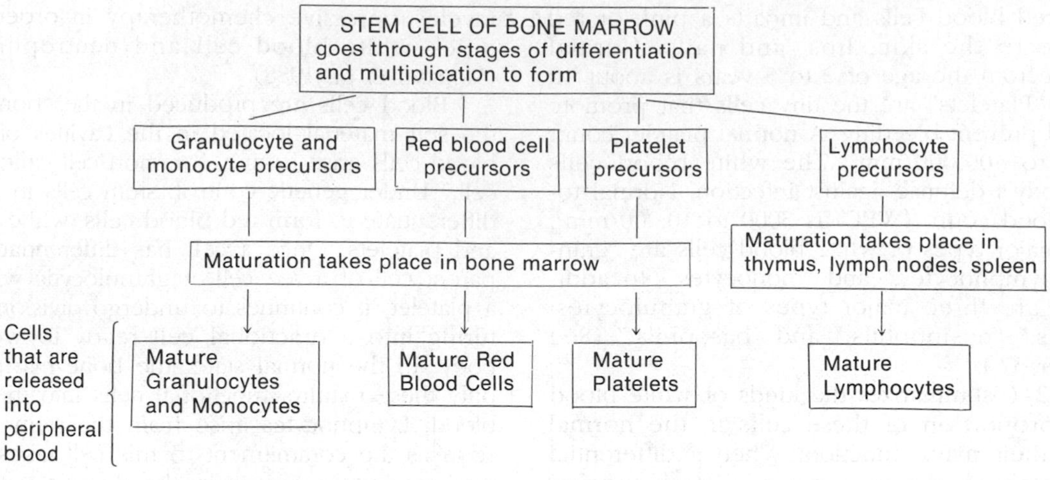

FIGURE 42-4. Blood cell production in the body.

fewer and fewer normal cells are made, so that at the time of diagnosis the percentage of blasts in the marrow is usually 80 to 100 per cent of the cells present. The lack of normal cells accounts for the symptoms seen in leukemia and, in large part, accounts for death from the disease. The pathophysiology in acute leukemia that leads to clinical manifestations is diagrammed in Figure 42–5.

Types of Leukemia

There are several different types of leukemia, classified on the basis of the morphology of the cells and the course of the disease. Each type is associated with a different prognosis and characteristics, making it important for the nurse to know what kind of leukemia each child has.

Whereas leukemia in adults is more often chronic, most childhood leukemias have an acute course (97 per cent). Acute leukemia involves proliferation of very immature white blood cells or blasts, has a short history of symptoms, and, without treatment, a rapidly declining course to death within 3 to 6 months. Chronic leukemias involve abnormal proliferation of immature white blood cells at varying stages of development and have a more gradual onset and a course extending over 2 or more years. Chronic granulocytic leukemia (CGL) is really the only type of chronic leukemia that occurs in childhood, though it is very rare.

The morphology of the white blood cells involved in the disease also varies. The most common childhood leukemia (80 to 85 per cent) is ALL, which

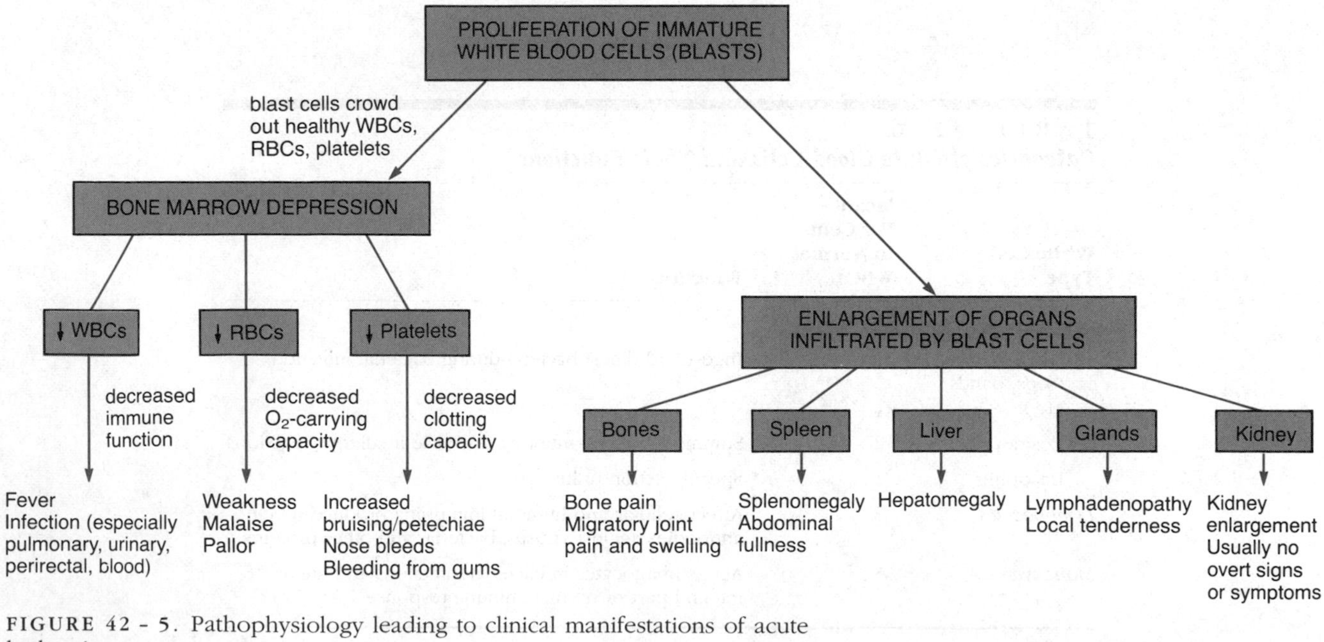

FIGURE 42-5. Pathophysiology leading to clinical manifestations of acute leukemia.

results from malignant change of the lymphocyte or its precursors (Crist et al, 1991). Less common in childhood are ANLL, which largely include abnormal cells of the myeloid (granulocytic and/or monocytic classification).

Table 42–7 lists the major subtypes of acute nonlymphocytic leukemia (ANLL) in children.

Long-Term Outcome

The outlook for a child with leukemia depends on many prognostic variables, not the least of which is the primary histology. With present-day treatment options, a child with ALL has a 95 per cent chance of obtaining an initial remission and a 75 per cent chance of surviving 5 years or more (Leventhal, 1992). By contrast, a child with ANLL has a 75 to 80 per cent chance of obtaining an initial remission; about 50 per cent of children who obtain remission stay in remission after therapy is stopped (Hakami & Monzon, 1987; Leventhal, 1987). ANLL is less responsive to available chemotherapeutic agents than is ALL even when aggressive therapy is used.

Studies of ALL involving large numbers of children have identified prognostic factors that indicate how children with leukemia will likely fare with their disease. Age and total WBC at diagnosis seem to be the most important prognostic features, though many features are evaluated and all features are of some interdependent statistical significance. For example, most children who at diagnosis are 2 to 10 years of age and have total WBCs of less than 10,000/mm^3 tend to do better than children with high WBCs (greater than 50,000/mm^3) or infants less than 1 year of age (Steinherz, 1987). Today, treatment protocols for children with ALL incorporate information that relates to prognostic variables by strategically ascribing different types or intensities of therapy for children with certain disease features.

It is important to note the continually improving prognosis for children with leukemia. In 1948, the first drug to effect a remission in leukemia was used. Before that time, every child who developed leukemia died. Today, the outlook for children with leukemia is continually changing as improved treatment plans are developed. Today's intensive treatment programs for children with both ALL and ANLL show great promise of improving the survival rates and perhaps allowing certain children with low-risk features to receive less intensive treatment that is naturally associated with less acute and long-term toxicity.

TABLE 42-7
Subtypes of Acute Nonlymphocytic Leukemia (ANLL)

M1, Undifferentiated myelocytic
M2, Myelocytic
M3, Promyelocytic
M4, Myelomonocytic
M5a, Monoblastic
M5b, Differentiated monocytic
M6, Erythroleukemic
M7, Megakaryocytic

Based on Gale, R., & Champlin, R. (1986). Bone marrow transplantation in acute leukaemia. *Clinical Haematology, 15,* 851–872; Hakami, N., & Monzon, C. (1987). Acute nonlymphocytic leukemia in children. *Hematology/Oncology Clinics of North America, 1,* 567–575; and Leventhal, B. (1992). Neoplasm and neoplasm-like structures. In R. Behrman (Ed.), *Nelson's textbook of pediatrics* (14th ed., pp 1291–1322). Philadelphia: WB Saunders.

Clinical Manifestations

Recalling that leukemic blasts crowd out normal cells in the bone marrow, it is obvious that the child may present with bone marrow depression (decreased numbers of mature white blood cells, red blood cells, and platelets). The child may have fever or obvious infection due to decreased numbers of normal white blood cells (neutropenia). A decrease in red blood cells and hemoglobin (anemia) causes weakness, malaise, and pallor. Decreased platelets may be associated with increased bruising, petechiae, or bleeding from the nose and gums. The spleen, liver, lymph nodes, thymus, and kidneys may become enlarged because of an infiltration of these tissues with blast cells. Bone pain (often accompanied by limping) is common and is due to infiltrates in the cortex of bone or the subperiosteal area. Figure 42–5 summarizes the clinical manifestations.

Diagnostic Assessment

Leukemia is suspected when a child presents with the symptoms just described. If a complete blood count (CBC) is taken, the decreased numbers of normal red blood cells, white blood cells, and platelets may be evident. Leukemic blasts may be seen in the blood smear and will be included in the differential diagnosis. The definitive diagnosis is made after examining a sample of bone marrow (see Table 42–3). To obtain a bone marrow specimen in the child, an area of accessible marrow, usually the anterior or posterior iliac crest or vertebral spine, is treated with local anesthesia with the child lying flat on a table. The procedure is performed using sterile technique. A small skin wheal and a small amount of local anesthesia in the periosteum is necessary. A heavy, wide-gauge needle with a stylet is inserted into the marrow space and the marrow is aspirated with a syringe. Under optimal conditions, this entire procedure takes only minutes, but marrows that are packed with large numbers of blasts can be technically very different to aspirate. To the naked eye, bone marrow looks like blood, but when put onto slides, stained, and studied under a microscope it has characteristic histologic features. Special stains and flow cytometry studies to identify immunologic markers are needed to clearly determine the leukemic cell type (Waskerwitz & Ruccione, 1985). Normal marrow contains less than 5 per cent of normal stem cells (hemocytoblasts). Most leukemic patients at diagnosis will have about 60 to 100 per cent abnormal leukemic blasts in their bone marrow. Chromosomal evaluation of bone marrow sampling is also important since more than 80 per cent of children with ANLL and many with ALL will have genetic abnormalities (Grier & Weinstein, 1989).

Therapeutic Management

"Remission" is the term used to describe an absence of detectable leukemic cells in the marrow following treatment. A "relapse" is the reappearance of leukemic cells in a marrow that has been in remission. Once relapse has occurred, a second remission can be achieved, but this tends to be more difficult. Remission is of shorter duration with each successive relapse. Thus, *the major aim of initial treatment is to achieve a primary remission that lasts without relapse.*

Treatment protocols are highly individualized and follow complex guidelines. In general, however, treatment can be considered in three stages: induction, consolidation, or central nervous system (CNS) prophylaxis, and maintenance. Newer programs may employ intensive therapy late into treatment as a sort of "delayed intensification."

Induction

"Induction" is the term used for the initial treatment period of chemotherapy that induces or brings about remission. Remission occurs when leukemic cells have been reduced to undetectable levels (less than 5 per cent bone marrow blast cells). Bone marrow remission has been documented in many patients as early as 7 days into therapy (Gaynon et al, 1990). Vincristine, prednisone, and L-asparaginase, with or without an agent such as doxorubicin or daunorubicin, are often used in induction treatment in ALL (see Tables 42–3 and 42–4). In ANLL, drugs used to induce remission include daunorubicin or doxorubicin, cytosine arabinoside, etoposide, and 5-azacytidine (Hakami & Monzon, 1987). Induction treatment is the most intensive and potentially the most life-threatening because of the immunosuppression and myelosuppression associated with antineoplastic drugs coupled with the usual pretreatment marrow status, which includes few normal cells. The child is at particular risk for bleeding and infection during the period of drug treatment and until the bone marrow can resupply healthy blood cells.

Proper supportive care measures during the initial days of induction therapy are mandatory. This includes increased intravenous fluids, alkalinization of urine to pH$>$7, and administration of allopurinol to protect the kidneys from damage caused by rapid tumor cell breakdown. Antifungal agents such as oral nystatin are also an important part of the supportive care practices for immunosuppressed patients. Oral trimethoprim-sulfamethoxazole (Bactrim) as prophylaxis for *Pneumocystis carinii* pneumonia is usually given on at least a 2 to 3 days/week basis.

CNS Prophylaxis

CNS prophylaxis is instituted to prevent development of leukemia within the CNS. Normal cerebrospinal fluid contains less than 5/mm^3 white blood cells, and these are usually lymphocytes or monocytes. Leukemic cells are thought to enter the CNS from meningeal capillaries when the peripheral blood contains blasts (Poplack, 1989). The blast cells can remain in non-growth phases for variable periods of time before increasing in number and causing symptoms. The usual signs and symptoms are often those of increased intracranial pressure and include headache, vomiting, papilledema, lethargy, irritability, seizures, and coma. Other common signs and symptoms include visual disturbances, myelopathies, 6th or 7th cranial nerve palsies, vertigo, and a hypothalamic syndrome with hyperphagia, weight gain, and sleeping disturbances (Poplack, 1989). CNS leukemia can also be asymptomatic. A complication of leukemic cells in the spinal fluid is their ability to extend along nerve roots through the vertebral foramina. The child who has this problem can have variable motor weakness depending on the degree of root compression.

Most drugs given systemically do not cross the blood-brain barrier to a very great extent, so that CNS treatment must consist of administering drugs directly into the cerebrospinal fluid. This is done by injecting a limited number of chemotherapeutic agents directly into the spinal fluid via lumbar puncture (intrathecally). Methotrexate has been used most often for this purpose, but cytosine arabinoside, hydrocortisone sodium succinate, and other agents can also be given. The three drugs may be used in combination intrathecally. The second form of therapy that is effective in treating CNS leukemia is radiotherapy directed to the brain alone or along with the spinal cord. Radiotherapy is limited by the total dose that can be tolerated by the CNS tissue, especially in infants and young children.

Early studies showed that as many as 80 per cent of children with leukemia would develop CNS leukemia during their disease course if left untreated. Treatment to prevent CNS involvement is now given as part of the standard initial therapy so that any cells present will be eradicated at the same time that the marrow and other tissues are cleared of blasts. Most investigators have referred to such treatment as "prophylactic," in that it is given when children are asymptomatic and the cerebrospinal fluid is normal. However, 10 per cent of children develop CNS leukemia in spite of such "prophylaxis." CNS leukemia can occur without bone marrow relapse (that is, leukemic cells can be found in the spinal fluid when bone marrow is free of disease) (Poplack, 1989).

Most practitioners use intrathecal methotrexate for CNS prophylaxis, sometimes with cranial radiation. Children who are thought to be at low risk for leukemic relapse may receive intrathecal methotrexate during maintenance therapy in lieu of prophylactic cranial radiation, in hopes of avoiding late sequelae thought to be caused by CNS radiation. Young children who receive cranial radiation may be at risk to develop long-term problems involving memory and cognitive learning, although these changes are often subtle (Stehbens et al, 1991).

Children with resistant CNS disease may be given chemotherapy via a special reservoir: an Ommaya reservoir is a permanent mechanical reservoir and catheter that is implanted in the ventricular system to facilitate the instillation of drugs. It thus expedites the process whereby drugs reach the brain.

Maintenance

Maintenance therapy provides chemotherapy to maintain the remission. Maintenance treatment is usually given for 2 to 3 years, although the optimal duration of therapy for ANLL has not been clearly defined. Standard maintenance therapy in ALL often involves daily oral 6-mercaptopurine, weekly methotrexate, and monthly vincristine and prednisone (Steinherz, 1987). Additional agents may be given in maintenance or as delayed intensification therapy to children with certain high-risk features who require more than conventional therapy. These agents may be similar to those described for induction therapy (see Table 42–4).

Because treatment for ANLL remains less effective than for ALL, the duration of chemotherapy and optimal combinations of drugs for maintenance therapy are less well established (Hakami & Monzon, 1987). Also, children with ANLL and a matched sibling donor will likely be offered bone marrow transplantation as therapy as soon as remission is achieved in induction. Other bone marrow transplantation procedures using autologous marrow may also be used as further therapy in lieu of conventional maintenance chemotherapy (Grier & Weinstein, 1989).

Survival statistics for children who have undergone bone marrow transplantation are promising. As reported by Vega and colleagues (1987), a study of children with ANLL in first remission showed a greater than 50 per cent survival rate following bone marrow transplantation. Another study they reviewed showed a 33 per cent survival rate for children with ALL in second remission, with a median duration of remission of 19 months. Six months was the median duration of remission for a control group of similar patients treated with chemotherapy alone. Nursing care for children undergoing bone marrow transplant procedures is highly specialized and involves pediatric, oncologic, and critical care nursing skills. Treatment complications can be life-threatening, related to GVHD, profound myelosuppression and immunosuppression, renal failure, and severe multiorgan failure (Kelleher, 1986).

Testicular Leukemia

The male testis is the second most common site of extramedullary (leukemia cells present outside of the bone marrow) relapse after CNS leukemia. It occurs in about 10 per cent of boys with ALL (Poplack, 1989). The sign of overt testicular leukemia is a firm, enlarged testis, so routine physical examinations of boys with leukemia must always include testicular palpation. It may also be discovered in the occult stage (undetectable by physical examination) with testicular biopsy. This complication may occur without marrow relapse, but it is often a predictor of future marrow change. It is most apt to occur in males who present with high-risk prognostic factors at the time of diagnosis. Treatment of testicular leukemia includes testicular radiation and systemic reinduction chemotherapy. Prepubertal boys who receive testicular radiation should be followed closely for appropriate gonadal development. They may require androgen replacement therapy. Sterility is also likely to result.

Relapse

Children with ALL who experience a bone marrow relapse while on chemotherapy generally do less well than children who relapse more than 6 months after completing their specified course of therapy. Relapse may occur at any time; however, the probability decreases with time. There is currently no way to predict which children will sustain remission and which will not (Steinherz, 1987). Children with ANLL relapse more frequently than children with ALL. With either type of leukemia, the prognosis usually becomes increasingly more grave with each relapse. In general, subsequent remissions are more difficult to achieve and will likely be of shorter duration.

Diagnosis of relapse may occur as a result of evidence of increased blast cells in the bone marrow or elsewhere in the body, such as leukemic cells in the cerebrospinal fluid or in the testicles. Relapse is treated with "reinduction" of antineoplastic agents and, in some cases, bone marrow transplant procedures.

Application of the Nursing Process for the Child with Leukemia

The child diagnosed with leukemia is presented with a variety of potential or actual nursing diagnoses. The Nursing Process Plan in Table 42–5 identifies the process of nursing care that can be applied to the child with leukemia.

Assessment

Children with very low hemoglobins (anemia) must be observed for increasing fatigue, increasing heart rate, increasing respiratory rate, and irritability. Red blood cell transfusions can be given to correct the anemia. All blood products administered to children who will be receiving immunosuppressive therapy should be irradiated in order to prevent their contamination with donor T-lymphocytes that could cause a graft-versus-host reaction in the recipient. Children with low neutrophil counts (ANC less than 1000/mm^3) must be observed for fever or other signs of infection. If a patient with a low neutrophil count develops fever, she or he will require intravenous antibiotic therapy to help fight what could represent bacterial infection. If fevers persist despite antibiotics, empiric treatment with amphotericin B, an antifungal agent, may be instituted. Children with low platelet counts (less than 20,000/mm^3) must be careful to avoid traumatic injury. Epistaxis and gum bleeding are common in children with very low platelet counts. The child may require platelet transfusions to control such bleeding. Intracranial hemorrhage is a rare but very serious complication in these children. It requires emergency management.

The nurse will continuously assess the child's and family's understanding of the disease process and management, the course and side effects of chemotherapy, laboratory values, and the relationship of diagnostic procedures. Their level of knowledge and understanding will be assessed directly by asking questions and by listening to their concerns and their questions. Return demonstrations of procedures necessary for home care management (e.g., care of central venous catheter) will reveal the child's and parents' ability to do so in the home. Other indications of behaviors the nurse will observe is willingness to participate in teaching sessions and the parents' willingness or reluctance to hold the child or physically demonstrate affection at time of treatment.

Having a child diagnosed with leukemia is a terrifying experience for the parents. The word "cancer" is likely to conjure up images that may be too frightening for parents to acknowledge. For some parents, having their child diagnosed with leukemia may mean a death sentence. For other parents, the word "cancer" creates emotionally charged feelings of fear, anxiety, and powerlessness, since their child's future is uncertain. It is important, therefore, for the nurse to assess the child and family members for feelings of fear and anxiety in order that misconceptions can be corrected, coping efforts can be facilitated, and functioning can be optimized.

The child and family members can be encouraged to verbalize perceptions of themselves, feelings about the disease and treatment modalities, their ability to manage invasive procedures, and the changes in family and social responsibilities. Insightful information can be obtained by observing their nonverbal behavior, which indicates feelings about self and others. Parenting patterns and family interactions will provide indicators of how the child and family members are coping with the challenges, stresses, and crises associated with living with leukemia.

Nursing Diagnostic Statements and Collaborative Problems

High risk for injury: *physiologic;* ***due to bone marrow suppression; infection, associated with the proliferative production of blast cells and the resultant decrease in normal levels of mature blood cells;*** *risk factors:*

- *Decreased red blood cells (anemia).*
- *Decreased white blood cells (neutropenia/leukopenia).*
- *Decreased platelets (thrombocytopenia).*
- *Immunosuppressive effects of medications.*

High risk for impaired skin integrity: alteration in oral mucosa; *risk factor: the effect of cytotoxic drugs on rapidly dividing mucosal cells.*

Altered nutrition: less than body requirements, *related to:*

- *Dysphagia associated with stomatitis.*
- *Anorexia associated with nausea and vomiting from chemotherapeutic agents or from the disease process.*

Fluid volume and electrolyte deficits, *related to:*

- *Inadequate fluid intake associated with stomatitis, anorexia or nausea caused by chemotherapy.*
- *Loss of fluid associated and diarrhea and vomiting caused by chemotherapy.*

Fear/anxiety (child and family), *related to perceptions about:*

- *Diagnosis of a life-threatening disease.*
- *Invasive diagnostic and therapeutic procedures.*
- *Hospital environment/disruption of usual activity and schedules.*
- *Separation from family and peers.*

Disturbance in body image, self-esteem disturbance, altered role performance, personal identity disturbance, *related to child and family perception regarding:*

- *Alopecia associated with many chemotherapeutic agents.*
- *Cushingoid features associated with prednisone administration.*
- *Amputation scars.*
- *Radiation therapy.*
- *Diagnosis of cancer.*

Spiritual distress (child and family), *related to:*

- *Worry associated with the prognosis and potential reactions to therapy.*
- *A search for the meaning of the illness.*
- *Feelings of guilt associated with the etiology or delay between onset of the disease and diagnosis.*
- *Powerlessness associated with the uncertainty of the prognosis and the need to undergo therapies that have potentially harmful side effects.*

Altered comfort: pain, *related to:*

- *The disease process.*
- *Administration of chemotherapy and invasive procedures.*
- *Side effects of cytotoxic agents.*

Altered health maintenance (home care), *related to:*

- *Lack of information about treatment regime and the disease process, including signs and symptoms of relapse, child's medical and psychosocial needs.*
- *Side effects of medications (see also Table 42–4).*
- *Child's and family's anxiety/fear, which interferes with processing of information.*
- *Resources available to the family.*
- *Availability of social support.*
- *Altered family functioning.*
- *Ways to optimize child's developmental level.*
- *Child's developmental ability to understand and deal with the diagnosis.*
- *Ways to facilitate the child's coping with the emotional and physical trauma of painful, invasive procedures (see also Table 42–5).*

High risk for ineffective management by parents of therapeutic regimen of child; risk factor: *knowledge deficit regarding disease process and therapeutic regimen.*

Health-seeking behaviors, parents; *related to desire to know how to safely and effectively care for their child.*

Planning and Implementation

Table 42–5 provides a comprehensive guide for the care of the child and addresses the nursing diagnoses identified for the child with acute leukemia.

Overview of Nursing Care. Initial supportive care depends on the blood counts at diagnosis and the complications present. Nurses caring for children with leukemia should be aware of the child's current hematologic status. Such knowledge is necessary for the nurse to remain alert to the many potential problems that may arise when counts are low or abnormal. Nurses should also be familiar with each child's specific treatment plan, especially the drugs the child is receiving. Nurses will likely be a main source of emotional support for the child and family. (Discussion on the family's needs and the support the nurse can offer is included later in this chapter.)

The goal of treatment is to achieve and maintain a remission. The doses of chemotherapy used are derived by past experience of maximal tolerated dosages and calculated on the basis of the patient's body weight or surface area. The calculated dose may not always be tolerated by an individual patient; therefore, close surveillance is necessary. Drug doses are decreased when defined intolerable or unacceptable toxicity occurs. A child in remission on maintenance therapy may have a normal blood count and at these times is not at additional risk for complications related to myelosuppression. However, the child is always at some risk for infection because of the immunosuppressive effect of the majority of the chemotherapeutic agents used (Piazza et al, 1992; Wright et al, 1993).

Allaying Anxiety. Special care for the child with leukemia should include emotional support for the child and the family, provision of maximal physical comfort, and management of problems that relate to low blood values and to drug side effects.

Members of the interdisciplinary team will likely be the main source of emotional support for the child and family. The nurse can provide emotional support to the child and family. (Discussion on the family's needs and the support the nurse can offer is included earlier in this chapter.) The nurse is one of the team members who has the skill to respond to emotional needs that a child and family experience during the course and treatment of leukemia (Wright et al, 1993).

The child and family will require information about the basic pathophysiology of leukemia. The concepts to be emphasized for understanding include description of the effect of blast cells on the normal white and red blood cells and platelets. This information provides the basis for understanding the effects of the disease, which can include easy bruising and bleeding from gums and nose, infections, fever, bone pain, and enlargement of liver, spleen, and lymph nodes.

The child and parents are taught the use of measures and their rationale to prevent trauma or risk of infection. The need to avoid exposure to infections and immunizations from live viruses is stressed. The importance of frequent handwashing is emphasized as well. Lastly, the explanation of treatment protocols must include description of the stages of treatment: induction, CNS prophylaxis, and maintenance. Typical side effects that the child may experience with chemotherapy, including nausea and vomiting, alopecia, mouth sores, fever, and constipation, are reviewed, with examples of how children of the child's particular age and developmental level might express such toxicities (Aitken, 1992). Measures to minimize the discomfort associated with chemotherapy are identified in Table 42–5.

Although the child and parents will be relieved about being discharged from the hospital or going home after the clinic visit, the parents will be anxious and concerned about their ability to follow through with the treatment regime and to adequately care for their child. The nurse can allow time for the family members and the child to express these feelings and to ask questions about home management. Parents may need reinforcement about previous teaching regarding the administering of chemotherapeutic agents at home, care needed for the bone marrow suppression associated with chemotherapy, and other treatment management issues. Parents are instructed to assess for signs and symptoms of relapse and for side effects of medications. It is important for the nurse to determine whether the family is receiving adequate physical and emotional support to successfully manage the child's care at home (Piazza et al, 1992).

During the clinic visit, the child and family should be encouraged to ask questions about the physical examination, necessary tests and procedures, and/or chemotherapy. Prior to any procedures during the clinic visit, the nurse assesses the child's ability to cope with the invasive procedures scheduled without suffering undue loss of self-esteem (Patterson, 1992). For the child, opportunities for therapeutic play will assist in coping with the threat of the forthcoming painful procedure, such as using actual equipment in performing diagnostic procedures on a doll with the young child.

A supportive milieu is provided for the family as they wait for test results during the clinic visit. The clinician's explanation of test results and current treatment regime may need to be reinforced by the nurse. The clinic visit also provides an excellent opportunity for the nurse to discuss the child's developmental progress, personal/family activities, and disruptions in family structure.

Evaluation

As in all nursing care plans, the effects of nursing interventions in relieving or curing nursing diagnostic responses and collaborative problems are evaluating by ascertaining whether defining characteristics of actual problematic responses have decreased or disappeared. See Table 42–5 for specific **evaluation criteria.**

Brain Tumors

Brain tumors are classified according to histology and location. About two thirds of intracranial tumors are "infratentorial" (below the tentorium), occurring in the posterior third of the brain, and about one third are "supratentorial" (above the tentorium), occurring in the anterior two thirds of the brain (Fig. 42–6) (Hausman, 1979). (The "tentorium" is the dura mater located between the cerebrum and the cerebellum, supporting the occipital lobes.) Table 42–8 describes the common types of brain tumors that present in childhood.

Etiology/Incidence

Brain tumors represent the most common solid tumor in children, accounting for about 20 per cent of childhood malignancies (Walker, 1982) and are the second most common type of cancer in children and adolescents (Finlay et al, 1987). They most often occur in the school-age years, but they can occur at any age from infancy to adulthood.

Clinical Manifestations

The signs and symptoms of brain tumors in children are diverse and relate to the location of the tumor in the brain, the rate of tumor growth, the child's age, and the child's developmental stage. See Table 42–10 for tumor-specific clinical manifestations. Symptoms most often involve signs of increased intracranial pressure—with headache and vomiting often on arising. The list of other signs and symptoms includes seizures, diffuse or focal neurologic dysfunction, changes in behavior and personality, lack of weight gain or continuing development, impaired vision, cranial enlargement, and torticollis. Because many of the early symptoms of intracranial tumors can be similar to those of common childhood illnesses, early diagnosis is often difficult. Changes in behavior in school, such as decreased performance and irritability or fatigue, may be attributed to school phobia or some problem that the child "will outgrow." It may not be until significant physical changes have occurred that medical assistance is sought or appropriate medical attention is given to the child.

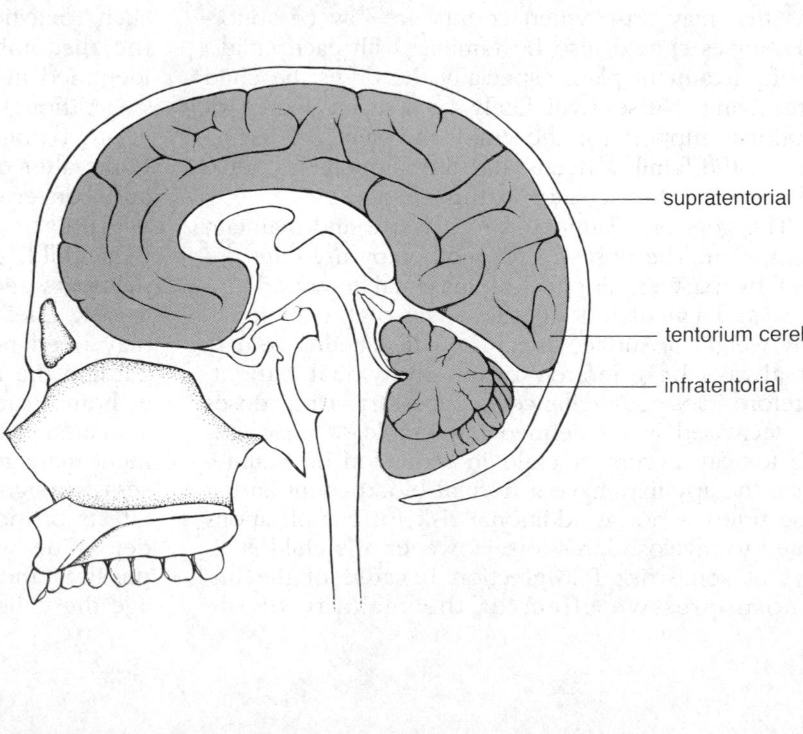

FIGURE 42-6. Location of supratentorial and infratentorial tumors.

TABLE 42-8
Classification of Brain Tumors

Type	Location	Prevalence Incidence	Clinical Manifestations	Therapeutic Management
Infratentorial				
Medulloblastoma	Area from region of 4th ventricle to spinal cord	• Occurs twice as often in boys compared with girls • Peak incidence: 5–10 yrs of age	• 1- to 3-mo history of headache, vomiting, ataxia, cranial nerve deficits • Nucchal rigidity and head tilting can occur	Surgical resection using microsurgery aided by precise delineation of CT or MRI scans Craniospinal radiation postoperatively Chemotherapy is probably beneficial in children with extensive local tumor or metastatic disease
Cerebellar astrocytoma	Usually located in one lobe of cerebellum	• Occurs in all age groups • Most common childhood brain tumor	• 3- to 6-mo history of headache, vomiting, and visual disturbances • Ataxia and hand incoordination • Gradually may become irritable and lethargic • May develop squint	Extensive surgical resection often possible Radiation therapy may be considered when tumor is not completely resectable or when it recurs
Brain stem tumor	Any portion of brain stem (most often pons)	Peak incidence: 6–10 yrs of age	• Rapid (1–3 mo) onset of cranial nerve deficits and upper/lower extremity weakness common	Surgery rarely performed because of involvement of brain's vital centers Radiotherapy usually palliative, extending survival from several months to years Certain combinations of chemotherapy have caused regression of symptoms but not cure
Supratentorial				
Cerebellar astrocytoma	May arise in cerebral hemispheres or midline structures (e.g., thalamus)	Occurs in all age groups; peak incidence 8–12 yrs of age	• Midline tumors: symptoms of increased intracranial pressure (headache, vomiting, visual disturbances); cerebral hemispheric tumors: focal, generalized or partial complex seizures; weakness; sensory abnormalities	Complete surgical resection is often not possible Radiation used in high doses Chemotherapy may be beneficial when combined with radiation
Optic pathway tumor	Slow-growing tumor occurring in optic nerve or chiasm; may invade hypothalmic region	Peak incidence approximately 5 yrs of age or less; occurs frequently in children with neurofibromatosis type I	• Visual deficits (decreased acuity, visual field losses) • With hypothalmic invasion may cause failure to thrive (infants), or obesity and diabetes insipidus (older children)	Surgical excision sometimes possible when only one of optic nerves involved; visual defects common following surgery Radiation therapy may be curative or palliative, depending on extent of invasion Chemotherapy may be of benefit in young children, where preferable, to avoid radiation

(continued)

TABLE 42-8
Classification of Brain Tumors *(Continued)*

Type	Location	Prevalence Incidence	Clinical Manifestations	Therapeutic Management
Infratentorial or Supratentorial	*Infratentorial:* Often benign, although invades brain stem *Supratentorial:* Frontal and parietal lobes most frequently affected; spread to spinal cord common	Occurs in infancy and older school-age children	• 1- to 3-mo history of vomiting, clumsy gait, and headaches • Papilledema, ataxia, and incoordination of hands (presentation similar to medulloblastoma) *Infratentorial:* • If onset is acute, compromised cardiorespiratory function • Limited range of motion if tumor growth extended *Supratentorial:* • Tumors may become quite large before signs and symptoms are noted • Gradual change in personality making child irritable, fatigued, or sluggish	Extensive surgical resection, if possible Radiation to primary tumor site or craniospinal area Role of chemotherapy unclear

Diagnostic Assessment

If a brain tumor is suspected, one or more special studies are done. Foremost of these is a computed tomography (CT) scan. The CT scan is a noninvasive radiologic procedure that produces multiple serial pictures of cross-sections of the brain. If a contrast-enhancing isotope is given intravenously at the time of the scan, most tumors will take up the isotope and the site of the tumor is "enhanced," providing more precise definition of the tumor's size. CT scans have become the single most important study for the diagnosis of brain tumors. Additionally, magnetic resonance imaging (MRI) is now available in many medical centers. MRI is a noninvasive nuclear procedure that has proved effective for early diagnosis of many types of brain tumors and for monitoring tumor growth. Other studies to evaluate for extent of disease may include myelogram, bone marrow aspiration and biopsy, and lumbar puncture.

Although these diagnostic tests should have been explained to parents by the physician ordering the studies, the nurse must assess the parents' and child's need for further or repeated information as the testing proceeds. During the diagnostic phase, the family is usually anxious and distraught once they recognize the possibility that their child may have a brain tumor. The nurse must assist the family during this phase by continually reassessing the family's ability to cope with the medical information and necessary procedures. It is imperative that the nurse be able to provide information regarding the actual procedure to be performed, what the child can expect to feel and see during the procedure, what is expected of the child, and what the results of each test will contribute to the management of the child's care. Also, the child's symptoms may escalate and require appropriate and possibly emergent medical and nursing management. A ventricular shunt may be surgically placed to allow proper cerebral spinal flow (see Chapter 40). Dexamethasone may also be needed initially and chronically to alleviate symptoms.

As previously described, children may require some form of sedation or even general anesthesia in order for these scans and tests to be completed. The parents should be permitted and encouraged to accompany the child to each procedure and to stay with the child throughout the procedure if feasible. The nurse should provide support to the child in the absence of the parents during a procedure.

Therapeutic Management

The treatments utilized for brain tumors are surgery, radiation therapy, chemotherapy, or combinations of these modalities.

Surgery

Ideally, complete surgical resection is the treatment of choice for brain tumors. Surgical resection is limited, however, to those tumors that occupy areas that can be safely approached or resected and the extent to which the tumor invades normal surrounding brain tissue. Some tumors can only be biopsied, and, in some instances, biopsy itself is considered too hazardous to perform. Needle biopsies done under CT scan may be performed rather than a craniotomy; however, these procedures are best utilized for tumors presenting in inoperable areas.

Postoperatively, children will usually spend the first 48 to 72 hours in the intensive care unit to permit careful monitoring of vital signs and neurologic signs. (See also Table 23–7, a Nursing Process Plan for perioperative care.) Postoperative care will naturally vary somewhat among children.

Care of the child following removal of an infratentorial tumor differs from postoperative care for a supratentorial tumor. Surgery in the posterior fossa often necessitates decompression of enlarged ventricles and creates concern for postoperative edema affecting the brain stem.

Radiation Therapy

Radiation therapy may be employed in combination with surgery or it may be used alone as primary treatment. The success of radiotherapy depends on the tumor being treated. Some tumors are highly responsive and can be cured by this modality alone. However, many that respond to radiotherapy initially may recur after variable periods of time. In addition, the dose of radiation necessary to eradicate these tumor cells can be very high and associated with such significant sequelae in young children that it is seldom even employed in children less than 2 or 3 years of age (Van Eys, 1991).

The child undergoing radiation therapy has unique needs that must be addressed in terms of nursing management. Short-term goals involve assisting the child and family to understand how successful this treatment is expected to be. The nurse must assess the level of fear and anxiety associated with the treatment. The family needs information regarding cranial radiation side effects during therapy, such as hair loss, nausea, and anorexia.

Information regarding the length of treatment and how it is given must be provided and understood. Very young children may require sedation or general anesthesia for each therapy session. Many will be immobilized with specially made casts for their head and neck.

The long-term rehabilitation needs for children with a history of brain tumors are often extensive. Many of the physical defects that are present at diagnosis, as well as some of the actual signs and symptoms, may never resolve, leaving lifelong disabilities. High doses of cranial radiation at an early age can take its toll in terms of neurologic dysfunction, pituitary dysfunction, and intellectual retardation, as examples. Appropriate referrals must be made early in order to prevent further complications.

Chemotherapy

The role of chemotherapy in the treatment of brain tumors still requires definition. Many studies have shown several chemotherapeutic agents or combinations of agents to be effective in recurrent tumors by causing either regression of symptoms or tumor regression as measured by CT scans.

Traditional chemotherapy has limited usefulness, in part because of the "blood-brain" barrier, which interferes with the concentration of systemic drugs in the CNS. Drugs that are lipid-soluble, such as nitrosoureas and steroids, most effectively penetrate the blood-brain barrier. Additional controlled studies are necessary to evaluate further the potential role of chemotherapy and new agents in the treatment of children with brain tumors.

Survival Rates

The survival rates for children with brain tumors are largely determined by the tumor type, its degree of malignancy, its location, and the treatment given.

Nursing Diagnostic Statements

High risk for altered tissue perfusion: cerebral: increased intracranial pressure; *risk factors:*

- *Edema of brain tissue associated with surgery.*
- *Postoperative intracranial bleeding.*
- *Malfunctioning of ventricular shunt (infratentorial tumors).*

High risk for altered comfort: nausea and vomiting; *risk factors:*

- *Prolonged anesthesia required for neuro surgery.*
- *Shifts in intracranial fluid volume associated with release of pressure through tumor removal and/or shunting.*

High risk for injury: physiologic: subdural hemorrhage (infratentorial tumors); *risk factor: Rapid decompression of cerebral ventricles associated with rapid drainage of cerebrospinal fluid through the ventricular shunt.*

High risk for injury: physiologic: seizures; *risk factors: Postoperative edema associated with removal of a supratentorial tumor (especially in the temporal lobe).*

High risk for infection: postoperative; *risk factors:*

- *Preoperative administration of corticosteroids.*
- *Leukopenia/neutropenia associated with chemotherapy and/or radiation therapy.*

High risk for injury: physiologic: depression of autonomic function; *risk factor: Postoperative edema affecting the brain stem associated* *with removal of posterior fossa (infratentorial) tumors.*

***High risk for injury: physiologic;** risk factor: Fluid imbalance due to the syndrome of inappropriate secretion of antidiuretic hormone (SIADH).*

High risk for altered comfort: pain, headache associated with changes in intracranial fluid pressure and incision.

***High risk for injury: physiologic: bone marrow depression;** risk factors: Chemotherapy, radiation therapy.*

***High risk for body image disturbance;** risk factors: Cutting/shaving of hair for brain surgery.*

***High risk for altered health maintenance and ineffective management of therapeutic regimen;** risk factors:*

- *Knowledge deficit regarding care necessary at home.*
- *Inability of family members to cope with the treatment demands and the disease itself.*
- *Lack of financial and social support.*

Nursing Care

Monitoring for Increased Intracranial Pressure. Since the etiologies for this nursing diagnosis cannot be changed by the nurse, nursing care is symptomatic. In addition to tissue edema, increased intracranial pressure (ICP) may result from intracranial bleeding or malfunction of the ventricular shunt. Classic signs of increasing ICP include a change in alertness, changes in vital signs (elevated blood pressure, decreased pulse and respiration), changes in pupil reaction, and vomiting. To prevent further burden on ICP, fluid intake is closely regulated. Table 40–20 provides a comprehensive Nursing Process Plan for care of the child at risk for increased intracranial pressure.

As with infratentorial tumors, ICP may rise postoperatively in response to tissue edema or intracranial bleeding with supratentorial tumors. Careful monitoring of vital signs and neurologic signs is imperative. Antiemetic therapy to reduce vomiting is also important. (See also Table 40–20.)

Alleviating Nausea and Vomiting. The nursing care is symptomatic as the etiologies for this nursing diagnosis cannot be changed by the nurse (Aitken, 1992). Nausea and vomiting are common postoperatively because the child has often received general anesthesia for several hours. Vomiting causes increased ICP, and antiemetics should be administered to the child who vomits repeatedly.

Monitoring for Hemorrhage. Children with an infratentorial tumor often have an associated hydrocephalus that requires decompression through surgical placement of either an external drainage system or a ventricular shunt. Initial decompression will occur preoperatively in the hours or days before surgery. (See the section on hydrocephalus in Chapter 40). Because of the continued drainage of cerebrospinal fluid postoperatively, the child must be monitored for changes in ICP.

The child will be carefully positioned to control the rate of decompression of ventricles (that is, the rate of drainage of cerebrospinal fluid).

Monitoring for Seizure Activity. Surgery in the supratentorial area of the brain, particularly in the temporal lobes, incurs the risk of seizures. Children at high risk for seizures will often be placed on anticonvulsant therapy prophylactically. Seizures are most likely to develop during the first 48 hours when the child is in the intensive care unit. (See Chapter 40, Tables 40–15 and 40–16, for further nursing interventions related to seizures.)

Monitoring Autonomic Function. Children with tumors of the posterior fossa (infratentorial tumor) are at risk for depression of autonomic function postoperatively because edema at the operative site may cause pressure on the brain stem. Arterial pressure, heart rate, and respiration are therefore monitored carefully. Children considered to be at increased risk for depression of vital signs (e.g., because of tumor location, operative trauma) will be intubated and placed on ventilatory support in the immediate postoperative period. Cranial nerve function is affected by pressure on the brain stem as well, and monitoring of eye movement, facial symmetry, swallow and gag reflexes, and so on is especially important. Because the child with an infratentorial tumor often presents with cranial nerve dysfunction at the time of diagnosis, it is important to know the child's baseline to detect progression of cranial nerve involvement in the postoperative period.

Monitoring Excess Fluid Volume. Postoperatively, the child is monitored for fluid imbalance due to SIADH (Shiminski-Maher, 1991). Fluids are usually restricted to two thirds of maintenance fluids or as ordered by the physician. The child is on strict intake and output monitoring, with urine specific gravity measured at least once each shift. The physician is notified if urine specific gravity is above or below the normal range (1.010 to 1.030) or if urine output is low (less than 0.5 ml/kg/hour) or high (greater than 2 ml/kg/hour). Laboratory values for serum osmolality (275 to 295 mOsm/kg H_2O) and serum sodium (140 to 145 mEq/L) are monitored as well. Daily weights are taken (without clothes on the same scale) to detect changes in fluid volume. As the etiologies of this diagnosis cannot be changed by the nurse, nursing care is symptomatic.

Relieving Pain. Nursing care is symptomatic, as the nurse cannot change the etiologies of this diagnosis. Pain relief is a concern in the postoperative period. That is made somewhat more difficult following neurologic surgery because of the need for the child's alertness and cooperation in assessing neurologic integrity: doses of medication in excess of that needed to keep the child comfortable may result in a child who is difficult to arouse and therefore difficult to assess. Conversely, withholding medication is also of concern because pain will increase ICP by increasing the tendency for breath holding during turning and other procedures and by increasing crying and irritability. The nurse who is knowledgeable about the recommended therapeutic ranges for analgesics and the actions of these drugs can usually achieve that fine middle ground between too little and too much analgesia. This requires calculation of the dose of analgesic ordered in relation to the recommended therapeutic dose (Chapter 25), a sensitivity to the child's unique reaction to each analgesic administered, and incorporation of feedback from the child and parent in relation to both pharmacologic and nonpharmacologic comfort methods.

Providing Supportive Care for Bone Marrow Depression. The child with a malignant brain tumor may undergo chemotherapy and/or radiotherapy, with the resulting effects of bone marrow depression. In this case, the nursing interventions detailed in Table 42–5 become an important aspect of quality care.

Being Sensitive to Changes in Body Image. The nurse's sensitivity to the child's changes in body image can help minimize the trauma somewhat. The child should know exactly which area of the scalp must be shaved and which areas will be spared. Girls may find some comfort in suggestions for pulling the hair on the sides of the head back into a pony tail to cover shaving of the posterior fossa area, or pictures of how other children have used scarves and wigs to conceal hair loss until regrowth occurs. Boys can decide whether they want their entire head shaved to "match" the surgical site, a short haircut to minimize the difference in hair length, or to preserve hair everywhere but at the surgical site.

Facilitating Home Health Maintenance. Family members will require instruction in a variety of areas in order to effectively manage their child at home. Parents will need instruction on assessing neurologic function to identify changes from the baseline documented at discharge. Parents will need to know how to assess for the potential side effects of medications. If an intraventricular shunt was inserted, the parents will need to learn to assess for its patency (absence of signs and symptoms of increased intracranial pressure) and infection (fever). Parents should be instructed on assessing their child's progress in developmental tasks.

The family and child will need adequate time to express what the child's brain tumor means to them—their fears, their insights, their perceptions of life since the diagnosis. This information can be used by the nurse to determine the adequacy of their physical and emotional support systems. The nurse can make appropriate referrals to social service agencies and to local and national support groups for children with cancer, their parents, and their siblings.

Rhabdomyosarcoma

Rhabdomyosarcoma (a malignancy of skeletal muscle tissue) is the most common soft tissue tumor diagnosed in children. It accounts for 5 to 8 per cent of childhood cancers (Maurer & Regab, 1991).

Etiology/Incidence (Pathophysiology)

Primary tumors are most often found in the head, neck, orbit, urogenital tract, and extremities. Specific primary sites in the trunk and abdomen are less common primary sites. Metastases occur often to the lungs or regional lymph nodes. The tumor can occur at any age in childhood but has age incidence peaks among toddlers and adolescents (Lankowsky, 1989).

Diagnostic Assessment

Rhabdomyosarcoma is associated with signs and symptoms related to the primary tumor site. A soft tissue mass may be evident visually or palpated on physical examination. It may be associated with pain or swelling. Orbital tumors may result in ptosis, visual disturbances, or cranial nerve changes. Neck tumors may cause hoarseness, cranial nerve changes, or dysphagia. Nasopharyngeal tumors may create airway obstruction, sinusitis, epistaxis, dysphagia, chronic otitis, dizziness, or headaches. Children with tumors of the paranasal sinuses may have sinusitis, nasal discharge, epistaxis, or obstruction. Auditory canal tumors may present as chronic otitis media, a facial nerve palsy, or hearing loss. In addition, about one fourth of tumors of head and neck areas may be locally invasive to the CNS, resulting in headaches, vision changes, cranial nerve palsies, and meningeal symptoms. Vaginal tumors can produce bleeding or drainage. Retroperitoneal tumors may cause renal obstruction, hypertension, constipation, or flank and back pain. Tumors of the chest wall may be associated with respiratory distress or decreased limb use. Bladder or prostate primary tumors may cause dysuria, urinary retention, constipation, or hematuria.

Pretreatment studies for children with rhabdomyosarcoma include tests to assess the extent of disease. Radiographs, CT scans, and nuclear scans appropriate for the involved site will be among the selected studies. A chest CT scan and bone marrow aspiration and biopsy to check for metastases should be done on all patients. Lumbar punctures are performed on children with head and neck tumors that may invade the CNS. Myelograms may also be done when the primary tumor is in the paraspinal region.

Rhabdomyosarcoma involves different histologic patterns: "embryonal" (which half of all patients have), "alveolar" (usually associated with a somewhat unfavorable prognosis), "embryonal-botryoid," "pleomorphic," and "undifferentiated" (Rodary et al, 1991). The Intergroup Rhabdomyosarcoma Study (IRS) has defined these clinical groupings, which refer to disease presence after initial surgery: Group I—localized disease completely resected; group II—microscopic residual disease; group III—gross residual disease; and group IV—distant metastatic disease (Rodary et al, 1991).

Therapeutic Management

Multimodality treatment for rhabdomyosarcoma includes surgery and chemotherapy and, for some children, radiotherapy. The ideal surgical procedure is complete tumor excision, but that is not always possible or feasible because it could require exenterative procedures with radical excision of the contents of an entire body cavity. For example, complete removal of some primary tumors, such as orbital tumors, leaves marked facial disfigurement, and resection of pelvic tumors may commit a child to lifelong urinary diversion and/or colostomy. Hence, modern treatment programs incorporate "preoperative" chemotherapy and often radiotherapy in order to shrink large primary tumors before a definitive surgical procedure is performed. Radiotherapy to the primary tumor site provides good local control in most tumors, but it must be combined with chemotherapy to treat micrometastatic disease for total tumor control. Chemotherapy is given in various multidrug combinations, depending on the stage of disease and often includes drugs such as vincristine, actinomycin D, cyclophosphamide, doxorubicin (Adriamycin), and ifosfamide. Children with metastatic disease or those with histologic patterns known to be associated with a poor prognosis may receive more intensive chemotherapeutic regimens. Children with parameningeal primary tumors will receive some localized CNS treatment such as intrathecal chemotherapy. Treatment is given over 1 to 2 years.

Children and adolescents with rhabdomyosarcoma now have an overall survival rate of 55 to 95 per cent; children with groups III and IV disease have a less optimistic prognosis when treated with multimodality therapy (Maurer & Regab, 1991).

Nursing Care

Nursing care for the child with rhabdomyosarcoma is primarily dictated by the tumor site. This information, coupled with impending surgery, radiotherapy, and chemotherapy, can certainly be overwhelming. The role of the nurse in providing caring and knowledgeable support cannot be overstated. Table 42–5 outlines care for the child with cancer. Chapter 20 addresses strategies for care pertinent to the child with a poor prognosis.

Osteogenic Sarcoma

Osteogenic sarcoma is an osseous tumor of the bone that arises in the mesenchyme.

Etiology/Incidence (Pathophysiology)

Osteogenic sarcoma is seen predominantly during the time of bone growth spurts in adolescence and in long bone areas that demonstrate rapid growth, such as the distal femur, the proximal tibia, and the proximal humerus. Metastases most commonly occur in the lungs, but other bones, the lymphatic system, and the liver may also be involved. Osteogenic sarcoma accounts for nearly 60 per cent of malignant bone tumors in children.

Clinical Manifestations

The primary symptom in a child with osteogenic sarcoma is localized pain that becomes increasingly frequent and more severe. A mass or swelling associated with the pain is usually a late finding and probably indicates long-standing tumor growth. The pain may be mild or transient, dull or aching. Referred pain to the leg or knee may be noted if the primary lesion occurs in the hip area. The child often describes a fall or an accident that preceded the onset of pain, but trauma merely elicits pain from the tumor that was already present. A radiograph of the painful site should be immediately obtained.

Diagnostic Assessment

If a bone tumor is suspected on the plain radiograph that shows destructive changes with indistinct margins to a bony lesion, the patient must undergo a series of diagnostic tests to further define the lesion and to evaluate for extent of disease. Most important of these are evaluations of the chest and primary site with CT scans and a nuclear bone scan of the entire skeleton.

A surgical biopsy is critical in determining the diagnosis of osteogenic sarcoma. As soon as a definitive diagnosis is made and the initial extent of disease evaluated, a treatment plan can be devised. Ideally, a team of pediatric specialists that includes an orthopedic surgeon, a diagnostic radiologist, an oncologist, and a pathologist help establish the plan of therapy together.

Although the medical necessity of performing the diagnostic examinations may have been explained to the adolescent and the family, the nurse must assess their need for further information or repeated information as the testing proceeds. Since the shock experienced initially may alter the family's ability to comprehend and cope with the information presented, the nurse assesses their level of understanding. The nurse must be prepared to provide exact information regarding the procedure to be performed, know whether the procedure will be painful or not, and tell the patient what will happen during the procedure. If possible, the nurse should accompany the child and parents to the test, particularly if the adolescent indicates a high level of anxiety about the procedure. Information provided before the procedure will assist the adolescent in coping before, during, and after it is over.

The diagnostic period is a time of fear and tension as decisions are awaited. The patient and the family will rely on the nurse for explanations of what is going on. Honesty is imperative, and it is important that information not be withheld from the family in an attempt to reduce stress. Once the diagnosis is confirmed, new needs emerge and more help is necessary for the family to understand the treatment selected for their child.

Therapeutic Management

After the diagnosis of osteogenic sarcoma is confirmed through tissue biopsy, the patient will likely begin chemotherapy before a definitive surgical procedure is performed. The goal of chemotherapy is to treat all micrometastases and to shrink the primary tumor. Controlled studies have shown that 80 per cent of patients will die from their disease if surgery alone is used for treatment (Link & Eilber, 1989). After several weeks of chemotherapy with agents such as "high-dose" methotrexate with citrovorum rescue, ifosfamide, doxorubicin (Adriamycin), or cisplatin, the primary tumor will be surgically removed, if possible.

Some osteogenic sarcomas arise in bones that cannot be completely resected. These include the skull, the mandible, vertebrae, and certain sites in the pelvis. Most of the extremity lesions can be removed by appropriate amputation a specific distance proximal to the lesion. In recent years, "limb salvage" operations have been offered to a chosen group of adolescents whose tumors are confined within periosteal margins with very little soft tissue extension. Candidates for these procedures must have completed their adolescent growth spurt. In such patients, a prosthetic replacement or cadaver bone is inserted following the removal of all or part of the involved bone. These replacements have been most successful in humeral and femoral lesions. Limb salvage procedures are almost always preferable for upper extremity lesions since no prosthetic device is yet available to match human hand function. Patients need to know that limb salvage procedures are not without problems, and in some patients amputation may need to be performed later for secondary complications such as infection or recurrent tumor.

Chemotherapy will resume following adequate surgical healing. The exact regimen may likely be based on the patient's histologic response to the preoperative chemotherapy, which is disclosed at the definitive surgical procedure.

Radiotherapy offers little more than transient palliation for pain associated with osteogenic sarcoma. Eighty-five per cent of recurrences in osteogenic sarcoma are pulmonary. These must be completely resected via repeated thoracotomies, if necessary and if possible. Adjuvant chemotherapy will be used postoperatively for any microscopic residual disease (Link & Eilber, 1989).

Long-Term Outcome

Although definite increases in the 5-year survival rates for osteogenic sarcoma have been made since the early 1980s, continuing clinical research programs are in progress. The adolescent who has osteogenic sarcoma deals with the ever-present possibility and fear of recurrent tumor and death. The disease-free survival rates for osteogenic sarcoma treated with a combined modality approach appear to be greater than 50 per cent at 5 years (Rosen, 1984). These statistics are less favorable for those children with lung metastases.

Nursing Diagnostic Statements

High risk for injury: physiologic: bone marrow suppression; *risk factor: Side effects of chemotherapeutic medications.*

Anxiety, *related to diagnosis and planned treatment, and potential loss of limb.*

Alteration in comfort: pain, *related to stimulation of sensitive nerve endings in the incised area.*

High risk for infection; *risk factor: Transmission of pathogenic organisms to surgical wound.*

Body image disturbance, *related to perceptions regarding loss of limb.*

High risk for ineffective management of therapeutic regimen: successful ambulation; *risk factors: lack of information regarding*

- *Stump care.*
- *Exercise program and lack of necessary equipment.*

High risk for altered home health maintenance and caregiver role strain; *risk factors:*

- *Lack of knowledge about goals of physical therapy.*
- *Verbalizations of difficulties by caregivers and child.*
- *Insufficient finances.*

Nursing Care

Nursing Measures to Prevent and Treat Bone Marrow Suppression. The chemotherapy regimens described previously may be accompanied by severe acute toxicity or chronic toxicity, including renal tubular damage, which can be caused by high-dose methotrexate and cisplatin. Meticulous management of fluid and electrolyte balance before, during, and after infusions of these agents with optimal drug clearing in alkaline urine is necessary so that kidney function measurements do not gradually deteriorate. High-dose methotrexate must be followed by citrovorum rescue to avoid lethal effects of such doses on the bone marrow and epithelium of the oral mucosa and bowel. Citrovorum factor supplies folinic acid, which is prevented from being formed when the enzyme tetrahydrofolate reductase is inhibited by methotrexate.

These intensive chemotherapy regimens are not well accepted by most adolescents. The anxiety over the potential loss of an extremity is still acute when highly toxic chemotherapy regimens are introduced. The nurse can be of great support during this period by assessing the adolescent's understanding of the treatment and teaching about the drugs and the reason for using them in the fashion in which they are administered.

The amount of physical discomfort associated with the use of chemotherapy must be described clearly to the patient and the family before treatment begins. Toxic effects of drugs must be discussed, as well as the means available to counteract complications. Medications that will be available for the control of pain, nausea, and vomiting must be described. The nursing care plan, which is written and determined in conjunction with the entire pediatric oncology team, the adolescent, and the family, can serve as a form of contract between the nurse and the patient.

Clarifying Information about Surgical Options. Decisions regarding the type of surgical management present another dilemma to the patient and the family. Adolescents need extremely sensitive care during this very stressful time. They need information before the surgery about the choice of amputation versus limb-salvage surgery, if the latter is an option, and why one or the other procedure is recommended. It is the physician's responsibility to provide this information, but the nurse should help the adolescent and family comprehend the information so that they can reach an informed decision.

The positive aspects of life with prosthetic limbs need to be stressed so that parents know their child can lead an active life following amputation. Most amputees can swim, dance, ski, participate in gymnastics, and do many other physical activities. The degree of function possible with prosthetic implants must also be addressed. Adolescents with prosthetic implants may be required to wear braces for a long period after surgery. They may likewise be instructed to avoid indefinitely physical activity that could cause injury to the limb, such as contact sports.

The independent lifestyle that most teen-agers envision rapidly disintegrates when decisions such as these are being made. Will they be able to drive a car? Will anyone want to dance with them? How can they wear bathing suits or shorts? Who will want to engage in sexual activity with them now? These questions need to be answered positively and can be most vividly presented by a successful amputee who has had the same type of surgery. Adolescents need an accepting person to listen to their rage and fear. Their behavior at this time should be viewed by the nurse and family as an attempt to cope in the best way possible. All these patients will need help in approaching some practical issues with their new means of ambulation. Locating a good prosthetist is imperative to obtaining a good fit and quality appliance. Problems such as facing peers, returning to school, managing steps, and buying clothing to camouflage any awkward appearance are examples of other areas that will be greatly affected by the diagnosis.

Alleviating Pain. There are a variety of measures the nurse uses to alleviate the adolescent's pain. Prior to surgery, the nurse explains the phenomenon of *phantom limb* to the patient. She or he is forewarned that the limb may feel as if it is still present and that this is not an abnormal sensation. Immediately following surgery, the limb is elevated for 24 hours to minimize swelling. Subsequently, the limb is positioned flat on the bed to prevent flexion contractures at the hip. Analgesia is administered before the level of discomfort intensifies so as to maximize effectiveness. The adolescent may be hesitant to disclose feelings of discomfort. Objective indicators of pain noted by the nurse include restlessness and increased heart and respiratory rate. Appropriate diversional activities can be provided.

Preventing Infection. The wound dressing is assessed frequently (every 4 hours) for the amount and character of drainage (bloody, serous, sanguineous, or purulent). Sterile technique is used for all dressing changes. The stump dressing is covered in "figure eights" with tightness distally and a looser fit proximally, thus preventing compromised circulation. The temperature is monitored and the physician is notified for temperature elevations above 38° C. All persons in contact with the patient are instructed to wash their hands before touching her or him to prevent spread of infection.

Promoting Healthy Body Image. The adolescent is encouraged to participate in the care of the stump as a means of promoting self-valuing behaviors. Arranging for a visit from another teen-ager or young adult who has undergone a similar amputation will assist in the adolescent's adjustment. The adolescent can be encouraged to express anger and verbalize fears regarding the future. Plans for the future and assistance in developing strategies for realistically meeting goals can help minimize the anxiety and stimulate motivation and interest.

Promoting Successful Ambulation Postoperatively. A primary goal for the adolescent who undergoes a lower extremity amputation is early ambulation. The earlier the return to ambulation, the earlier the adolescent will regain independence. Preoperative consultation with a physical therapist will initiate the successful rehabilitation process. Immediate postoperative stump care includes measures to shrink and shape the stump in preparation for prosthetic fitting. This is done through use of a plaster cast or by wrapping the stump 24 hours a day with an Ace bandage, as previously described. Physical therapy goals to be met before hospital discharge include:

- Independent ambulation with crutches.
- Independent home exercise program.
- Independent stump wrapping.
- Availability of all necessary home equipment.

Many patients experience "phantom pain" or "phantom sensation" (feelings sensed as if they were in the patient's limb, which is now gone) for up to 6 months after their amputations. The use of oral pain medications such as meperidine (Demerol) or codeine may be used for palliation (Stanhill & Pratt, 1986). Phenytoin and several other anticonvulsant drugs such as carbamazepine (Tegretol) have successfully been used for relief of phantom limb pain. Since children metabolize these drugs slowly, no loading dose is given; therapeutic dosing is achieved after several days of escalating dosages.

Facilitating Home Health Management and Minimizing Caregiver Role Strain. Discharge planning for the child with osteogenic sarcoma and family begins with assessing their ability to adhere to the goals of the physical therapy program when at home. The components of the program include independent ambulation with crutches, independent home exercise program, independent stump wrapping, and availability of all accessory home equipment. The child and family should be given adequate time to express what the diagnosis and disability mean to them—their fears, their insights, and their perceptions of life since diagnosis. This information can be used to determine the adequacy of their ability to deal with the diagnosis, the long-term management, and the need for referral to social service agencies and/or professionals.

Ewing Sarcoma

Ewing sarcoma is a bone tumor characterized by anaplastic small round cells.

Etiology/Incidence (Pathophysiology)

Ewing sarcoma occurs predominantly in persons under the age of 20 years, with peak incidence during the period of adolescence (Horowitz, 1989). Ewing sarcoma is even rarer than osteosarcoma, with fewer than 200 new cases reported per year in the United States (Meyers, 1987).

The primary tumor may occur in any bone of the body, but about half the tumors occur in the femur, tibia, or humerus (Jaffee et al, 1978). A significant soft tissue mass usually surrounds the affected bone. Metastases may appear in the lungs, viscera, other bones, and bone marrow. At times, pathologic fractures occur at the primary site; the site and extent of the fracture dictate the severity of symptoms.

Diagnostic Assessment

Children with Ewing sarcoma generally have pain and swelling at the site of their tumor. More than one fourth of patients have history of fevers at diagnosis. The presence of systemic symptoms coupled with bony abnormalities is often confused with osteomyelitis (Link et al, 1991). Evaluation for suspected Ewing sarcoma includes x-ray films and CT scans of the primary tumor and the chest in addition to a bone scan, skeletal survey, and bone marrow aspiration and biopsy.

Therapeutic Management

Treatment of Ewing sarcoma includes surgery, radiation therapy, and combination chemotherapy. Complete surgical excision of the primary tumor is desirable but rarely possible. Primary tumors in the ribs and fibula and relatively small lesions in the ilium are sites that can sometimes be completely removed surgically. Large tumors, such as those in the pelvis, are usually nonresectable. Radiation therapy and chemotherapy may reduce tumor size to the extent that a complete surgical resection is possible later.

Radiation therapy is very important for the successful treatment of Ewing sarcoma, especially for nonresectable lesions. The aim of this treatment is destruction of the tumor and retention of adequate function. Children who receive high doses of radiotherapy to an extremity lesion before that bone has completed its growth will encounter long-term problems related to growth retardation and weakness of the bone.

Early clinical trials for Ewing sarcoma did not employ chemotherapy. Those programs resulted in about a 10 per cent 5-year survival rate (Miser et al, 1990).

Multidrug chemotherapy is often used in a series of cycles administered over 2 years. Agents that are most effective in combination for Ewing sarcoma include doxorubicin (Adriamycin), cyclophosphamide, ifosfamide, etoposide, actinomycin-D, and vincristine (Table 42–4). Chemotherapy is started at the time of the primary therapy. The role of chemotherapy is largely to treat micrometastases in lungs and in other sites that are undetectable at diagnosis.

Long-Term Outcome

As stated earlier, before the advent of chemotherapy and radiotherapy, the prognosis for a child with Ewing sarcoma was grim. Today, control of local disease is achieved in about 90 per cent of patients. The overall survival rate for patients with Ewing sarcoma is approximately 55 to 60 per cent (Nesbit et al, 1984). Adverse prognostic features in Ewing sarcoma include presence of metastasis at diagnosis, large primary tumor, primary tumors at pelvis or proximal bone, extraosseous extension, presence of systemic symptoms, and duration of symptoms for more than 6 months (Link et al, 1991).

Nursing Care

Although treatment for Ewing sarcoma rarely involves amputation, the serious effects of the tumor and the late effects of radiation therapy and chemotherapy involve extensive nursing care and long-term follow-up. Nursing interventions related to the perioperative period and to care of the adolescent with cancer will not differ from those discussed previously in (Table 42–5). Follow-up care, however, must take into account the potential for growth retardation and weakness of the affected bone after radiation therapy and the potential for lung metastasis. The family must be encouraged to faithfully keep follow-up visits to assure that any recurrence or metastasis is discovered as early as possible.

Wilms Tumor

Wilms tumor is a malignant neoplasm of the kidney that most often affects young children.

Etiology/Incidence (Pathophysiology)

The median age at diagnosis is between 2 and 3 years (Breslow et al, 1988) but Wilms tumor also occurs in adolescents and, rarely, in adults. In 50 per cent of cases, the tumor is considered to be of genetic origin because of findings of specific chromosomal deletions or alterations. Children with Wilms tumor may have high frequency of congenital anomalies such as aniridia (a congenitally absent iris), renal anomalies, skeletal anomalies (e.g., hemihypertrophy), or genitourinary malformations (Ganick, 1987).

Clinical Manifestations

The child with Wilms tumor is often a well child in whom an abdominal mass has been seen or felt. Sometimes parents are the first to notice increasing abdominal girth when belts or waistbands become tight. Less common presenting signs and symptoms likewise relate to the presence of a tumor mass within the abdomen or kidney and include abdominal pain, malaise, anorexia, fever, gross hematuria, and hypertension. The primary tumor mass may be discovered on palpation of the abdomen during a routine physical examination.

Diagnostic Assessment

The initial workup for these patients is designed to define the renal mass and search for areas of metastases. Wilms tumor may metastasize to lung, liver, lymph nodes, or bone. An abdominal CT scan seems to provide the pediatric oncologist and surgeon with the best and most influential study to delineate the area of the tumor involvement in the kidney and, very importantly, show the status of the other kidney. Chest radiograph and/or chest CT, liver/spleen scan, and a complete skeletal survey may be done to evaluate for metastatic disease.

Tumor Classification. The National Wilms Tumor Study (NWTS), which began in 1969, has provided excellent data for staging, treatment, and prognosis in this tumor (Belasco et al, 1984). Wilms tumor is classified in a staging system based on extent of disease. Stage I disease is confined to the kidney and is completely resected by nephrectomy. Stage II disease extends beyond the kidney but can be completely removed at the time of nephrectomy. Stage III represents regional spread of disease beyond the kidney, with incomplete resection or completely resected disease involving regional lymph nodes. Also included are those tumors that are ruptured either before surgery or at surgery, spilling tumor contents into the peritoneal cavity. Stage IV represents blood-borne spread of disease to lung, liver, bone, or distant lymph nodes. Stage V Wilms tumor involves both kidneys. Fortunately, many children with Wilms tumor (42 per cent) are classified as having stage I disease at diagnosis (Fernbach et al, 1991).

Just as important as staging is the histology of Wilms tumor. Children with tumors that show a defined degree of anaplasia or are sarcomatous in pattern make up the majority of those succumbing to this disease, hence those histologies are considered unfavorable. Those with "favorable" histology have an excellent prognosis. Favorable histology includes blastemal and epithelial kidney tissues. Malignant rhabdoid tumors were historically classified as a histologic variant of Wilms tumor. Because rhabdoid tumors behave so much differently than most Wilms tumors, with metastasis common to the brain and a very poor prognosis, patients with that histology now are treated differently from patients with Wilms tumor (Fernbach et al, 1991).

Therapeutic Management

Treatment for Wilms tumor includes all modalities of cancer treatment: surgery, radiation therapy, and chemotherapy. Surgery is performed as soon as the diagnosis is suggested by physical examination and radiography. A nephrectomy is performed, with removal of all regional lymph nodes and any resectable regional tumor. Stage I or II disease is not treated with radiotherapy and has an excellent prognosis with limited chemotherapy for 6 months or less in stage I or 6 to 15 months in stage II. Children with stages III and IV disease receive radiotherapy to the abdomen and metastatic sites combined with chemotherapy, using two or three drugs, for 15 months. Treatment for stage V bilateral disease must be individualized; preoperative chemotherapy may be given in an attempt to identify the more healthy kidney, which will be preserved at subsequent nephrectomy. Wilms tumor was the first solid tumor in children to be successfully treated with chemotherapy in a large clinical trial, NWTS. The drugs that are commonly used today for Wilms tumor include actinomycin D, vincristine, doxorubicin, and cyclophosphamide. Children with unfavorable anaplastic histology will receive four-drug chemotherapy. Occasionally, surgical removal of resistant lung or node metastases is warranted.

Long-Term Outcome

When patients are adequately treated, the long-term survival in Wilms tumor is about 90 per cent (D'Angio et al, 1989). The patients who do the very best are the youngest children with lower stage disease and favorable tumor histology. Since the outlook for children with Wilms tumor is good, the quality of survival is of great concern. These children are left with only one kidney, so they must always be treated adequately for urinary tract infections. Routine urinalysis, blood pressure readings, and blood tests of kidney function are part of quality long-term follow-up care. There are generally no special long-term activity limitations following nephrectomy, other than perhaps avoidance of professional contact sports.

Nursing Diagnostic Statements

***Fear/anxiety (child and family)**, related to:*
- *Perceptions about diagnosis of a malignant disease.*
- *Impending surgery, chemotherapy, and/or radiation therapy.*

***Body image disturbance**, related to perceptions regarding the loss of a kidney.*

***High risk for altered health maintenance and caregiver role strain**, risk factors:*
- *Lack of knowledge regarding usual function of the kidney and changes brought about by the tumor; diagnostic and treatment modalities (see also Table 36–4); home management of the child who has had a nephrectomy and who has bone marrow suppression associated with chemotherapy and radiation therapy; ways to maintain health of the remaining kidney; and community support groups for clients with cancer, their siblings, and parents.*
- *Verbalizations of difficulties by caregivers.*
- *Insufficient finances.*

Nursing Care

Providing Information to Reduce Fear and Anxiety. The sudden diagnosis of a malignant tumor in an otherwise healthy child is a shock for the child and family. Sensitivity to the emotional adjustments and the practical arrangements that must be made in relation to sudden surgery can make the nurse a valuable resource. Information will be needed for cognitive coping, but the stress of surgery following closely on the diagnosis will reduce the ability to understand and remember the information related. Patience is essential in repeating information as necessary. Making oneself available for questions and clarification of information will be greatly appreciated by the family.

Promoting a Healthy Body Image. Because children affected with Wilms tumor are usually very young, the loss of a kidney may mean something quite different to them than adults realize. Exploring the child's perception of the surgery and of what is now "missing" from his or her body through play therapy, drawings, and so on can help determine whether the child has a realistic understanding or whether the fantasy is much worse than the actual situation. As children progress through new developmental crises, the loss of a kidney may again be examined in light of their expanding cognitive abilities. Nurses who see the child for follow-up visits can facilitate the child's coming to terms with the former surgery by encouraging expression of feelings and clarifying information as appropriate.

Facilitating Health Maintenance at Home Following Nephrectomy. The family who understands normal kidney function will be better able to protect the child from urinary tract infections and unnecessary trauma that may put the remaining kidney at risk. The signs and symptoms of urinary tract infection should be written out for them, as well as the preventive measures of adequate fluid intake, cleanliness of the genital area, teaching little girls to wipe from front to back after voiding and defecating, and avoiding irritation from nylon underwear and perfumed bubble baths. (See also the discussion of urinary tract infection in Chapter 36.) Fluid intake and frequent voiding will be particularly important postoperatively if chemotherapy involves agents known to precipitate in the urine and cause chemical irritation of the bladder.

The family will need intensive and extensive teaching regarding the side effects of chemotherapy and ways to minimize the effects of bone marrow suppression. (See Table 42–5.)

Discharge planning includes encouraging the child and family members to verbalize feelings about the loss of the kidney, diagnosis of cancer and the prognosis, the effects of the disease, and its treatment on the individual and family functioning. Referrals are made if it is determined that the family does not have adequate physical and psychologic support systems to maintain home management during this treatment.

Parents are taught to assess the status of the surgical incision, for signs and symptoms of urinary tract infection and for function of the remaining kidney. Parents are informed that blood and urine samples will be obtained to test kidney function, and that blood pressure will be monitored and compared with the child's baseline readings as a means of assessing the child's progress.

Hodgkin Disease

Hodgkin disease is a malignant lymphoma characterized histologically by the presence of Reed-Sternberg cells and neoplastic proliferation of lymphoid tissue. It presents most commonly in one or more lymph node sites. Other tissues that are commonly involved are the spleen, lung, liver, and bone.

Etiology/Incidence (Pathophysiology)

Hodgkin disease is rare before 5 years of age but peaks from age 15 to 34 years and again at age 50 (Kung, 1991). Some evidence suggests that Hodgkin disease may be associated with abnormalities in T-cell lymphocytes, with resultant impairment in cellular immunity (Skarin et al, 1978). The exact etiology of the disease is still unknown.

Clinical Manifestations

Most often the adolescent with Hodgkin disease presents with painless lymph node enlargement (lymphadenopathy), often in the supraclavicular or cervical neck areas. The disease commonly spreads from one lymph node area to others via the lymphatic pathway, but regions adjacent to the primary site of disease may be bypassed. Constitutional symptoms of fever, drenching night sweats, weight loss, and pruritus may be present (Sullivan, 1987).

Diagnostic Assessment

Usually, a peripheral lymph node biopsy is obtained initially to establish the diagnosis of Hodgkin disease. Four histologic patterns are seen: nodular sclerosing (the most common subtype), mixed cellularity, lymphocyte predominant, and lymphocyte depleted. The subsequent patient evaluation includes a variety of studies necessary for staging or determining the extent of disease.

Radiographic examination of the chest demonstrates mediastinal adenopathy in over half the patients with cervical adenopathy (Sullivan et al, 1984). CT scan of the chest and abdomen is useful in delineating disease in the mediastinum, hilar areas, lungs, and para-aortic areas. Pedal lymphangiography outlines the appearance of involved retroperitoneal nodes, though this study cannot be obtained in young children and its use has been somewhat overshadowed by the CT scan. Bone scan and bone marrow biopsy are necessary for investigating disease involvement in those areas.

A staging laparotomy may be included as part of the initial workup of Hodgkin disease, though there is current controversy surrounding its use in favor of staging solely with today's highly sensitive noninvasive techniques. The purpose of a laporatomy is to detect abdominal disease that is not evident through noninvasive tests. At laparotomy, splenectomy, liver biopsy, lymph node biopsies, and bone marrow biopsy are performed. Persons who undergo splenectomy are rendered susceptible to serious infections with bacteria that have polysaccharide capsules, such as pneumococcus, streptococcus, and *Haemophilus influenzae*. Some protection postsplenectomy is offered by immunization with pneumococcal vaccine prior to surgery and long-term twice-daily oral penicillin.

Staging. Following the diagnostic procedures, the patient's disease is staged based on the degree of disease present (Fig. 42–7). Staging assists in the selection of therapy to be used. The staging system used for Hodgkin disease is as follows:

Stage I: Disease limited to one lymphatic region.

Stage II: Disease limited to lymph nodes on one side of diaphragm.

Stage III: Disease in lymph node regions on both sides of the diaphragm.

Stage IV: Disease disseminated to extralymphatic organs (e.g., bone marrow, lung, pleura, liver, bone, skin, or gastrointestinal tract).

All patients are also subclassified (*A* or *B*) to indicate the presence (B) or absence (A) of one or more constitutional symptoms. The B symptoms include unexplained weight loss of more than 10 per cent of body weight, unexplained fever with temperature above 38° C, and night sweats. Children with any of these symptoms have a less favorable prognosis than children who are asymptomatic.

Therapeutic Management

Children with Hodgkin disease are treated with radiation therapy or chemotherapy, or a combination of these modalities. The exact treatment plan is largely determined by the stage of disease at diagnosis and the age of the child. Fully grown adolescents with stages I, IIA, or IIIA disease will likely receive radiation therapy, usually to an "extended" field that includes all nodal sites on the involved side of the diaphragm. Children with stages IIB, IIIB, or IV disease usually receive chemotherapy alone or with radiation therapy, either to limited or to extended fields.

Pediatric oncologists steer away from using radiotherapy in young children with Hodgkin disease because of its suppressive effects on growing bones. Most prepubertal children will be treated with chemotherapy.

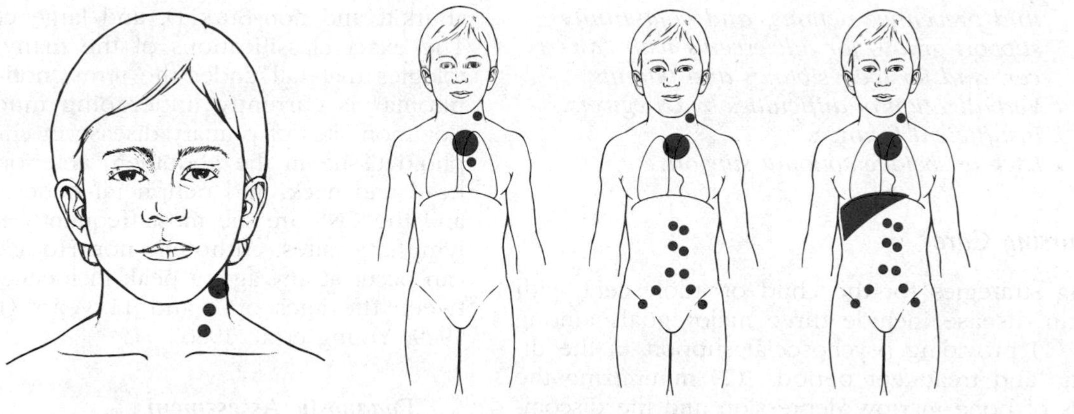

FIGURE 42 - 7. The Ann Arbor Staging System for Hodgkin disease.

The first combination chemotherapy used to treat Hodgkin disease successfully consisted of nitrogen mustard, vincristine (Oncovin), prednisone, and procarbazine, and became known as "MOPP." Most programs utilize monthly MOPP therapy for 6 months. Further maintenance courses of MOPP have not enhanced remission duration (Thompson, 1991). Clinical trials evaluating other effective chemotherapy programs have discovered another effective drug combination: ABVD (Adriamycin, bleomycin, Velban, and DTIC), which does not include alkylating agents and hence is associated with fewer long-term problems related to sterility and oncogenesis. Clinical trials are presently attempting to select the most efficacious combinations of chemotherapy and radiotherapy that will give the best disease-free survival rate with the fewest sequelae.

Both MOPP and ABVD are associated with significant nausea and vomiting. Children and teen-agers who receive this chemotherapy need much support and encouragement to understand and deal with the treatment and its annoying toxicity. It is important for the nurse to work closely with them. Together they can identify the best antiemetic regimen that will enable the patient to accept and tolerate the chemotherapy.

Hodgkin disease is now managed with several different regimens, with an overall cure rate of almost 90 per cent (Sullivan, 1987).

Recurrences can develop long after the initial diagnosis and therapy and will be treated with alternative programs.

The survivors of Hodgkin disease should be monitored in the long term for the aforementioned sequelae. Because the radiotherapy field is often large, many body organs are exposed to radiation. Long-term toxicity is especially significant to the lungs and thyroid gland. Hypothyroidism requiring daily oral replacement therapy has been reported in as many as 13 per cent of patients (Hockenberry & Coody, 1986). The specific chemotherapeutic agents administered to a patient cause long-term sequelae in particular body organs, namely Adriamycin cardiotoxicity and bleomycin pulmonary toxicity. Patients treated successfully for Hodgkin disease seem to be at a markedly increased risk for development of second malignancies, particularly acute myelocytic leukemia and solid tumors within the radiotherapy field (Waskerwitz, 1986).

Nursing Diagnostic Statements

High risk for infection, *risk factor: impairment of immunity associated with dysfunction of the lymphatic system and post splenectomy and with both chemotherapy and radiation therapy.*

High risk for fear/anxiety; *risk factors: perceptions regarding:*

- *Diagnosis of a malignant disease.*
- *Diagnostic and therapeutic modalities, including laparotomy, chemotherapy, and radiation therapy.*

Altered comfort: nausea and vomiting, *related to side effects of MOPP and ABVD combination chemotherapy.*

Body image disturbance, self-esteem disturbance, altered role performance, and personal identity disturbance, *related to:*

- *Perceptions regarding diagnosis of a life-threatening illness in the adolescent years.*
- *Alterations in appearance associated with treatment side effects.*

High risk for impaired home maintenance and management; *risk factors:*

- *Lack of knowledge regarding normal function of the lymphatic system and the changes in function associated with the disease and its treatment; diagnostic and treatment modalities (see also Table 42–5); transmission of infective organisms and preventive actions; and community support groups for adolescents with cancer, and for their siblings and parents.*

- *Verbalization of difficulties by caregivers.*
- *Insufficient finances.*
- *Lack of social/emotional support.*

Nursing Care

Nursing strategies for the child or adolescent with Hodgkin disease include three major goals among many: (1) providing psychosocial support in the diagnostic and treatment periods, (2) minimizing the hazards of bone marrow depression and the discomfort of systemic symptoms during chemotherapy and/or radiation therapy, and (3) monitoring for advancing disease and for late effects of treatment during follow-up visits. The nurse can use the guidelines for psychosocial support of children and families that were provided earlier in this chapter. The impact of the disease on adolescents will be especially devastating, however, in light of their developmental tasks of establishing an independent identity. The nurse who is sensitive to this conflict can be instrumental in helping the adolescent express fears and frustrations and in suggesting ways to reach out to friends and family for needed support (Heiney et al, 1991).

Table 42–5 contains the interventions appropriate to the support of young people with cancer. Nursing considerations for radiation therapy were also addressed earlier in this chapter.

Facilitating Home Care. Prior to discharge, the nurse will determine whether the family's psychologic and physical support systems are adequate and assess the need for referrals to community agencies and resources. This is accomplished by encouraging the adolescent and family to express their feelings about the effect of Hodgkin disease, its treatment, and side effects on usual roles within the family and community. The adolescent and parents can be instructed to watch for signs and symptoms of infection associated with bone marrow suppression due to chemotherapy and radiation therapy (and splenectomy, if this was done). Long-range side effects associated with chemotherapy and radiation for Hodgkin disease include secondary oncogenesis (classic signs of cancer elsewhere in the body), growth impairment, breast atrophy, immune suppression (fever and infection), and sterility (if pelvic irradiation was involved).

Non-Hodgkin Lymphoma

Non-Hodgkin lymphoma is a highly malignant neoplasm of lymphoid tissue.

Etiology/Incidence (Pathophysiology)

Several histologic (cell type) patterns are seen in children, including lymphoblastic, undifferentiated (Burkitt and non-Burkitt), and large cell lymphoma. The exact classifications of the many different histologies that fall under the term "non-Hodgkin lymphoma" is currently undergoing much discussion. Common sites of primary disease in children are lymphoid tissue in the abdomen, anterior mediastinum, head and neck, and peripheral nodes. Bone marrow and the CNS are the most frequently involved extralymphatic sites. Although non-Hodgkin lymphoma can occur at any age, a peak incidence is evident between the ages of 7 and 11 years (Poplack et al, 1989; Young et al, 1986).

Diagnostic Assessment

Signs and symptoms of non-Hodgkin lymphoma relate to sites of disease. Abdominal masses, diarrhea, distention, vomiting, episodic colicky pain, ascites, and intussusception are suggestive of intra-abdominal disease. Cough, wheezing, and dyspnea may be present with mediastinal disease. Enlarged lymph nodes, tonsillar masses, nasal congestion, rhinorrhea, epistaxis, and loosening of teeth may be signs of head and neck disease. The kidneys may be involved, with infiltrative disease causing renal dysfunction.

A diagnosis of non-Hodgkin lymphoma is made by surgical biopsy of an involved tissue site. Studies to determine extent of the disease include chest radiograph and CT scan, abdominal ultrasound and CT scan, bone scan, bone marrow aspiration and a lumbar puncture. The diagnostic workup must be done with expediency, since the disease may progress rapidly.

Therapeutic Management

Treatment for non-Hodgkin lymphoma is primarily chemotherapy, with radiotherapy used only in adjunctive fashion. Occasionally, radiotherapy is useful in reducing bulky disease such as in the mediastinum when respiratory distress is present. Non-Hodgkin lymphoma is a fast-growing malignancy that is very sensitive to combination chemotherapy, often resulting in an initial rapid breakdown of tumor cells, referred to as a "tumor lysis syndrome." Renal function must be evaluated, especially since the kidneys can be involved with disease. Adequate hydration and alkalinization of the urine, combined with allopurinol therapy, must be instituted before therapy is begun. Following initial chemotherapy, diligent monitoring of fluid, electrolyte balance, and kidney function is necessary. In the presence of extensive disease, kidney involvement, or renal dysfunction, hemodialysis may be necessary because of uric acid nephropathy and deteriorating renal function.

There are various drug combinations used to treat non-Hodgkin lymphoma, often based on histology and extent of disease. Widespread disease is treated with very intensive programs.

Non-Hodgkin lymphoma is often treated with multidrug regimens resembling therapy for ALL. One of the most commonly used combinations utilizes cyclophosphamide, prednisone, vincristine, methotrexate, and daunomycin for induction therapy. A consolidation period follows using L-asparaginase, cytosine arabinoside, and other agents. Maintenance therapy includes repeated cycles of the same drugs. Other programs include a combination of cyclophosphamide, vincristine, prednisone, and methotrexate for induction and subsequent maintenance courses (Gardner & Graham-Pole, 1983). Intrathecal chemotherapy is included "prophylactically" in most children because of the relatively high incidence of CNS disease. Treatment is generally given for only 6 to 18 months because late recurrences are very rare.

Prior to the time when chemotherapy was introduced as the primary treatment for non-Hodgkin lymphoma, only about 10 to 25 per cent of children with the disease survived. The use of chemotherapy and the knowledge of the importance of supportive care precautions during induction therapy have increased the overall survival rate for children with non-Hodgkin lymphoma such that nearly all children with limited disease survive, as well as 50 to 75 per cent of children with extensive disease (Magrath, 1987).

Nursing Care

Nursing care of the child with non-Hodgkin lymphoma involves supportive care for signs and symptoms related to disease sites (e.g., respiratory, gastrointestinal) and monitoring for kidney involvement. The interventions related to care of the child with cancer are central to the nursing plan of care. As with all the malignant diseases, the need for psychosocial support of the child and family cannot be overemphasized. The nurse who can interpret the medical regimen to the child and family and give them a written list of signs and symptoms to watch for provides them with knowledge needed to cope with day-to-day care after hospital discharge. This is but another situation in which primary care can be beneficial; having one particular nurse who is knowledgeable and supportive can quite literally be a lifeline for the family during the diagnostic and treatment periods.

Neuroblastoma

Neuroblastoma is a malignant neoplasm that develops in cells of neural crest origin that give rise to the adrenal gland and the sympathetic nervous system.

Etiology/Incidence (Pathophysiology)

Neuroblastoma occurs in 500 children in the United States each year (Finklestein, 1987). The etiology of neuroblastoma is unknown.

Neuroblastoma is the most common tumor in children under 1 year of age. The majority of children with neuroblastoma are under 5 years of age (Davis et al, 1987). The sites of the primary tumor (site of origin) in the body vary. Over half the primary tumors occur in the abdomen (Voute, 1984). Most of these are in the adrenal gland. Other primaries arise in sympathetic ganglia in the cervical, thoracic, and pelvic regions. Neuroblastoma commonly metastasizes to bones (especially skull, pelvis, femur, and humerus), bone marrow, liver, lymph nodes, and skin. Two thirds of patients have metastases at diagnosis (Hayes & Green, 1983).

Diagnostic Assessment

Children with neuroblastoma may look and feel very sick. The chief signs and symptoms relate to sites of tumor involvement and can include an abdominal mass, fever, irritability, pain from bone metastases, and orbital ecchymosis or proptosis (displacement of the eyeball, causing it to protrude) from skull metastases. Since the primary tumors are usually retroperitoneal, they can extend posteriorly and may invade the spinal canal through vertebral spaces or foramina, producing symptoms of cord compression.

Diagnostic studies focus on the principal sites of primary or metastatic disease. Physical examination may reveal a palpable, firm mass in the abdomen. Tumors at other sites, such as the chest, may be impossible to detect on physical examination.

Ninety to 95 per cent of these tumors secrete increased amounts of catecholamines and other tyrosine metabolites, which are excreted in the urine (Brodeur & Castleberry, 1993). Collecting complete and accurate urine samples for catecholamines can be difficult in a child who is not toilet-trained. Immobilization devices and secure urine bags or Foley catheterization are usually required. The nurse should be particularly sensitive to the stress that immobilization causes for the child and family. Special efforts should be taken to provide quiet diversional activities for the child during this period. The urine is kept in bottles that contain hydrochloric acid as a preservative. Analysis of the urine for catecholamines is imperative, since this provides an excellent marker for following tumor presence.

Neuroblastoma cells have also been found to produce other metabolic products. One of these is an enzyme, neuron-specific enolase, which seems to have some prognostic significance, since infants under 1 year of age with low values usually have a good prognosis (Zeltzer et al, 1983). Biologic testing of tumor tissue for N-myconcogene copies is also useful in understanding prognostic expectations at diagnosis (Sullivan, 1993). Lactic dehydrogenase (LDH) is commonly quite elevated during active tumor growth, though this is true for malignancies and is not specific for neuroblastoma. Serum ferritin may also be elevated in some patients and seems to correlate with advanced disease (Brodeur & Castleberry, 1993). These latter measurements are obtained through special serum testing.

Specific radiographic studies are needed to define the primary disease and extent of metastases, if present. Chest radiograph, abdominal and pelvic ultrasound and CT scan are used to elaborate intrathoracic and intra-abdominal extent of disease. Small calcified deposits may be seen in the primary tumor and occur when areas of tumor undergo necrosis and become calcified. Skeletal radiographs may show lytic lesions in bones. Nuclear bone scans and liver scans may detect subtle disease in the liver and bones. Bone marrow aspiration and biopsy are performed to check for infiltrates of tumor clumps and cells in the bone marrow. As many as half of all patients have disease that has spread to the bone marrow (Groncy & Finklestein, 1978). Bone marrow disease may also be reflected in the blood count. The most common hematologic finding is anemia, which is not dependent on tumor involvement of the marrow. The diagnosis of neuroblastoma is made on examination of tissue histology. This must be made from a biopsy of primary or metastatic tissue. However, if the bone marrow is abnormal and elevated catecholamines are present, tissue biopsy may not be necessary for diagnosis.

Staging. Extent of disease is described in a staging system. Stage I is represented by a localized primary tumor that has been completely resected. Stage II disease extends beyond the primary tissue involved but does not cross the midline of the body and is grossly resectable. Disease classified as stage III is localized to the primary site but extends across the midline. Stage IV involves distant metastases. Stage IV-S is a special classification in which metastatic disease in infants is limited to liver, bone marrow, or skin with a localized primary tumor.

Therapeutic Management

Treatment varies with extent of disease. Stage I or II disease is treated with surgical removal of the primary tumor. Stages III and IV tumors are too extensive for complete or safe surgical removal. When residual tumor is present, radiation therapy may be used for stages II and III. Radiation therapy is useful only in stage IV disease for treatment of symptomatic metastatic sites or for primary tumors when chemotherapy has controlled metastatic sites. The role of chemotherapy in stage II disease is questionable. It is necessary in stage III and IV disease because of the inoperability of stage III tumors and the widespread disease found in stage IV. No drug regimen or combination has been found that effectively treats most cases of stage III and stage IV neuroblastoma. Cyclophosphamide, vincristine, dimethyltriazenoimidazole carboxamide (DTIC), doxorubicin, cisplatin, VM-26, and melphalan are drugs that are used at present in various combinations and schedules. Because bone marrow suppression is the main limiting toxicity for the needed intensity of therapy, bone marrow transplantation procedures have been employed in these unfortunate children with some success (Brodeur, 1991). Stage IV-S disease is biologically very interesting in that for unknown reasons this tumor will often spontaneously remit with no treatment at all or with just one dose of chemotherapy or radiotherapy.

Long-Term Outcome

The prognosis for children with neuroblastoma depends on the stage of disease and the age of the child at diagnosis. Very young children have the best prognosis: infants under 1 year of age often have either localized or stage IV-S disease. Children with stage I tumors have almost a 100 per cent survival, whereas those with stages II and IV-S have an 80 to 90 per cent survival. Children with stage III and IV disease have a dismal prognosis: 20 to 40 per cent survival (Brodeur & Castleberry, 1993). Older children with neuroblastoma tend to have stage IV disease (Voute, 1984).

Although children with localized neuroblastoma do fairly well, those whose disease is stage IV may have a devastating course and fatal outcome. Children who die with widespread neuroblastoma often have severe pain from growth of tumor masses in multiple sites. The terminal stages of this disease are very difficult for a family to accept, since the child's body can become grossly disfigured by large and bony tumors. When a child with neuroblastoma is dying, the child and family are very dependent on the nursing staff for much of their support and comfort.

Nursing Care

Care of the child with neuroblastoma will involve psychosocial support of the child and family in light of the grave prognosis for children with advanced disease. The interventions detailed in Chapter 20 will assist the nurse in providing support to the family with a dying child. The nurse must be sensitive to the child's changing body image related to disfiguring tumors.

Postoperative care will be dictated by the tumor site. Interventions for perioperative care (Table 23–5), care of the child following abdominal surgery (Table 35–15), and care of the child undergoing chemotherapy (Table 42–5) and radiation therapy are likely to be pertinent to the plan of care. Collection of urine samples for analysis of catecholemines is another nursing responsibility. Intervention for pain will be necessitated by pressure of the tumor against tissues and organs; the nurse should take the initiative to develop and institute a comprehensive comfort protocol of both pharmacologic and nonpharmacologic measures to improve the child's quality of life.

Retinoblastoma

Retinoblastoma is the most common tumor of the eye in infancy and childhood. It is a congenital malignant growth arising from embryonal retinal cells.

Etiology/Incidence (Pathophysiology)

Although the tumor may be present at birth, the average age at the time of diagnosis is 13 months, with the majority of children diagnosed before 3 years of age (Abramson, 1982).

Although the mechanism of transmission is not fully understood, retinoblastoma is thought to result from both somatic and germ cell mutations. Somatic mutations are not hereditary. They result in unilateral involvement and account for the majority of all retinoblastomas. Germ cell mutations, on the other hand, are inherited and transmitted by the autosomal dominant mode of inheritance. (The parent has the trait but not the disease.) The majority of germinal mutations are bilateral, with about one third resulting in unilateral disease. Children of parents with unilateral retinoblastoma have a 15 per cent risk of having retinoblastoma if the tumor is not multifocal (Abramson, 1982). That risk increases to 50 per cent when the parent has bilateral involvement or a unilateral multifocal tumor. Because the incidence with a positive family history is significant, it is extremely important for siblings of an affected child to have an adequate ophthalmic examination at birth and at frequent intervals until 3 years of age. Likewise, children of parents with histories of retinoblastoma must have similar ophthalmic evaluations.

Diagnostic Assessment

Retinoblastoma arises as one or more white lesions in the retina that grow at variable rates, eventually causing retinal detachment or formation of a mass protruding anteriorly from the retina. The tumor cells may spread via the optic nerve into the brain and subarachnoid space, producing CNS symptoms or seeding cerebrospinal fluid, or into the choroid and lymphatics with potential metastases to bones, bone marrow, and other tissues. Fortunately, such distant metastases are very rare: less than one per cent of children have bone marrow metastasis and less than 3 per cent have positive cerebrospinal fluid (Grabowski & Abramson, 1991).

The most common presenting sign of retinoblastoma is leukocoria, a white reflex of the pupil, known as the "cat's eye reflex." A white spot on the retina seen on ophthalmoscopic examination is usually diagnostic of this tumor mass. If the tumor is small and located near the macula of the retina, the initial sign may be strabismus, deviation of the eye, which occurs in 20 per cent of patients (Berro, 1993). Whenever strabismus is observed in an infant, a thorough ophthalmic examination is required to rule out retinoblastoma. Loss of vision and redness or pain with or without glaucoma may be observed. The child may be irritable, or the parent may note changes in behavior indicative of decreased vision (bumping into objects, poor coordination). Because young children may not complain of loss of vision and the defects may not be apparent on superficial appraisal, the practitioner needs to carefully check the eyes with an ophthalmoscope for red reflexes, abnormal protrusions of the eyeball, atrophy, or venous congestion.

CT scans of the head are particularly useful in determining the extent of the tumor within the orbit and brain and to help plan therapy. CT scans and skull radiographs are also obtained to document calcifications within the eye that aid in making the initial diagnosis of retinoblastoma. Obtaining routine studies such as bone scan, lumbar puncture, and bone marrow aspiration in the absence of associated disease is done to detect the presence of metastatic disease. The staging system that is used for retinoblastoma denotes the extent of tumor within the eyeball. The Reese-Ellsworth classification describes groups I to V: Group I tumors have a very favorable chance of retaining vision, with small tumors. Group V tumors have a very unfavorable chance of retaining vision, with massive tumors and vitreous seeding (Berro, 1993).

Therapeutic Management

The size of the tumor and its location dictate the type of treatment. Radiation is often effective in destroying small, localized tumors of unilateral retinoblastoma, thereby preserving vision. Other treatment options for small, localized tumors include the use of cobalt plaque applicators (implants of cobalt on the sclera to aid in delivering radiation to the tumor), cryotherapy (uses freezing to produce ice crystals that destroy tumor blood vessels), and photocoagulation (uses light rays to coagulate tumor or the blood vessels that lead to retinal lesions). Infants and little children require sedation in order to hold still for each treatment. In advanced cases with unilateral involvement, removal of the affected eye (enucleation) is necessary and greatly reduces the likelihood of metastasis. In bilateral cases, the eye with the more advanced tumor may need to be removed, and, if possible, the other eye is treated with radiation. In cases of advanced disease in both eyes, bilateral enucleation is indicated. Since metastasis can spread along the optic nerve pathway, a long optic nerve stump is removed with the eye to encompass tumor that may already have invaded or surrounded the optic nerve.

The size and location of the tumor at the time of diagnosis will provide staging information indicative of prognosis.

If the tumor has metastasized, chemotherapy may be used in conjunction with radiation. Early diagnosis is important because the stage of the disease at the time of diagnosis is most significant in determining outcome. If the tumor is detected at an early stage and adequate treatment is carried out, the prognosis is good. The patient survival rate is greater than 90 per cent, and vision is preserved in 75 per cent of treated eyes that have not been enucleated (Abramson, 1982). Once the tumor has metastasized out of the eye into the orbit, the chance of survival is greatly decreased. Distant metastatic disease is fatal despite therapy (Stanhill & Pratt, 1986).

Retinoblastoma patients with germinal mutations are at extremely high risk for the development of second malignancies. The risk is as high as 50 per cent at 30 years from diagnosis. The most common second malignancy that occurs is osteogenic sarcoma, especially of the skull, though many other pathologies within and outside of the radiotherapy field have been reported (Grabowski & Abramson, 1991).

Nursing Care

The nursing care of the child with retinoblastoma and the family will depend on the child's age at diagnosis, the treatment required, and whether an inheritance factor is involved. If a family has a positive history of the disease, additional feelings of guilt may evolve. The nurse must consider all these factors in devising a care plan with the family.

Once the decision to perform an enucleation has been made, the parents must be prepared for their child's appearance following surgery. The child will initially have an eye patch in place that will be changed regularly by the ophthalmologist. Postoperatively, the face may be edematous. Fittings for a prosthesis do not take place until the edema subsides. It is important to explain to the parents that the surgery will not result in a cavity in the skull; the periorbital area will appear quite normal because a sphere is surgically implanted to replace the eyeball until a prosthesis is available. Unless complications arise, such as infection, hemorrhage, or prolonged edema, the child is fitted with a prosthesis within 3 weeks of surgery. Teaching the parents how to care for the prosthesis is critical. Techniques for insertion, removal, and cleaning of the prosthesis must be understood.

Once the diagnosis has been made, it is imperative that the risk of retinoblastoma in subsequent children be discussed with the parents and genetic counseling obtained. It is also critical to have the eyes of other children in the family examined as early as possible. In addition, both biologic parents must have ophthalmic examination, even if their vision is normal and there is no prior history of disease, since, in a small number of families, one parent may have an obvious tumor scar that healed by spontaneous regression.

Pediatric Oncology Nurses

The Association of Pediatric Oncology Nurses (APON), which was founded in 1976, is a nursing organization that is devoted to fostering high-quality care for children with cancer. Nursing communication and collegial exchange among nurses caring for children with cancer are supported through its annual meeting; its quarterly journal, the *Journal of Pediatric Oncology Nursing;* and other publications, including "Standards of Care for Children with Cancer," "Scope of Practice," and "Chemotherapy Booklet."

KEY CONCEPTS

Concepts Related to Basic Information

- The overall survival rates for children with cancer have grown to almost 70 per cent, but prognostic figures vary among the different malignancies and the subtypes for each.
- The most common malignancies in children in the United States are leukemia, brain and CNS tumors, lymphomas, neuroblastoma, Wilms tumor, rhabdomyosarcoma, bone tumors, and retinoblastoma.
- The cause of cancer in children remains an unanswered question; large ongoing epidemiologic research studies should aid in disclosing etiology.
- Treatment protocols for children with cancer are highly individualized and follow complex guidelines. Treatment is often multimodal and includes the use of chemotherapy, surgery, and radiotherapy. Treatment can be very intensive; institution of appropriate supportive care measures is imperative.
- Cancer cells spread through either invasion of adjacent tissues or metastases.
- The treatment of children with cancer may involve surgery, radiation therapy, and chemotherapy. These treatments are often used in combination.
- It is hypothesized that cell populations contain, at any given time, three categories of cells: cycling cells, nondividing cells, and resting cells.
- All chemotherapeutic agents are immunosuppressive to varying degrees, so the child receiving chemotherapy must not receive live virus immunizations and must avoid exposure to common contagious viral diseases while on treatment.
- There are different types of bone marrow transplants: allogenic, autologous, and syngeneic.
- Graft-versus-host disease is a serious complication of allogenic bone marrow transplants.
- There are several types of leukemia, classified on the basis of the course of the disease and morphology of the cells.
- Brain tumors are classified according to histology and location; two thirds of intracranial tumors are infratentorial; one third are supratentorial.
- Brain tumors are the most common solid tumor in children.
- Rhabdomyosarcoma is the most common soft tissue tumor diagnosed in children.
- The extent of tumor growth of neuroblastoma is determined and described by a staging system.

- Most often, assessment of the adolescent with Hodgkin disease discloses painless lymph node enlargement, usually in the supraclavicular area of the cervical neck region.
- Signs and symptoms of non-Hodgkin lymphoma relate to site of disease.

Concepts Related to Nursing Assessment

- The complete list of signs and symptoms associated with pediatric malignancies is immeasurable; many of these findings can be associated with other childhood illnesses.
- During the diagnostic phase of treating a child with cancer, the nurse needs to assess the parents' and child's need for additional or repeated information, although the members of the interdisciplinary team had previously discussed the information with the family.
- Signs and symptoms associated with a brain tumor vary according to location, rate of growth, and child's age and developmental stage.
- Possible nursing diagnostic responses the nurse may identify in caring for the child surviving cancer are *high risk for injury, high risk for altered growth and development, high risk for altered family processes,* and *high risk for fear/anxiety.*
- Knowing normal values of white blood cells and those associated with increased risk of infection assists in providing care for the child since chemotherapy, radiotherapy, and leukemia are associated with low neutrophil values.
- Children with very low hemoglobins (anemia) must be observed for increasing fatigue, increasing heart rate, increasing respiratory rate, and irritability.
- Children with low neutrophil counts (ANC less than 1000/mm^3) must be observed for fever or other signs of infection.
- Children with low platelet counts (less than 20,000/mm^3) must be careful to avoid traumatic injury.
- The signs and symptoms of brain tumors in children are diverse and related to location of the tumor in the brain, rate of tumor growth, the child's age, and the child's developmental stage.
- The primary symptom in a child with osteogenic sarcoma is localized bone pain that becomes increasingly more frequent and severe.

Concepts Related to Nursing Intervention

- Principles of care for the child with leukemia include management of problems related to low blood values, medication side effects, maximal physical comfort, and emotional support.
- Careful monitoring of vital signs and neurologic signs is imperative for the care of the child following surgery for intracranial tumors.
- A primary goal for the adolescent who undergoes a lower extremity amputation for osteogenic sarcoma is early ambulation.
- The nurse plays a major role in preparing families for discharge and home care management of the disease.
- The increased emotional demands on the child and family created by the crisis of diagnosis will require the nurse to provide repeated information and teaching as well as continued emotional support to facilitate the family's adaptation.
- The nurse can assist the child and family to develop trust and feel more secure during hospitalization for cancer treatments by communicating an attitude of caring and by providing accurate information about illness, diagnostic tests, and treatment.
- Long-term management issues affecting the child with cancer that must be addressed include facilitating the child's return to the classroom. Some formalized programs, such as school re-entry programs, help families deal with problems that may arise.

REFERENCES

Abramson, D. (1982). Retinoblastoma: Diagnosis and management. *Cancer, 32,* 2–12.

Aitken, R. (1992). Gastrointestinal manifestations in the child with cancer. *Journal of Pediatric Oncology Nursing, 9*(3), 99–109.

American Cancer Society (1993). *Cancer facts and figures 1993.* Atlanta: Author.

Association of Pediatric Oncology Nurses. (1990). *Cancer chemotherapy.* Richmond: Author.

Belasco, J., et al. (1984). Wilms tumor. In W. Sutow, et al (Eds.), *Clinical pediatric oncology.* St. Louis: CV Mosby.

Bellanti, J. A. (1985). *Immunology; basic processes* (2nd ed.). Philadelphia: WB Saunders.

Berro, E. (1993). Retinoblastoma. In G. Foley, D. Fochtman, & K. Mooney (Eds.), *Nursing care of the child with cancer* (2nd ed., pp 310–318). Philadelphia: WB Saunders.

Breslow, N., Beckwith, J., Ciol, M., et al. (1988). Age distribution of Wilms' tumor. Report from the National Wilms' Tumor Study. *Cancer Research, 48,* 1653.

Brodeur, G., & Castleberry, R. (1993). Neuroblastoma. In P. Pizzo & D. Poplack (Eds.), *Principles of pediatric oncology* (2nd ed., pp 739–767). Philadelphia: JB Lippincott.

Boring, C., Squires, T., & Tong, T. (1992). Cancer statistics. *CA—A Cancer Journal for Clinicians, 42,* 37.

CA—A Cancer Journal for Clinicians. (1992). *42,* 26, 36.

Chesler, M., & Barbarin, O. (1987). *Childhood cancer and the family.* New York: Brunner/Mazel.

Cohen, D. (1993). Acute lymphocytic leukemia. In G. Foley, D. Fochtman, and K. Mooney (Eds.), *Nursing care of the child with cancer* (2nd ed., pp 208–225). Philadelphia: WB Saunders.

Crist, W., Pullen, J., & Rivera, G. (1991). Acute lymphoid leukemia. In D. Fernbach & T. Vietti (Eds.), *Clinical pediatric oncology* (4th ed., p 407). St. Louis: CV Mosby.

D'Angio, G., Breslow, N., Beckwith, J., et al. (1989). Treatment of Wilms' tumor. Results of the Third National Wilms' Tumor Study. *Cancer, 64,* 349–360.

Davis, S., Rogers, M., Pendergrass, T. (1987). The incidence and epidemiologic characteristics of neuroblastoma in the United States. *American Journal of Epidemiology, 126,* 1063–1074.

Edelstein, J., Amylon, M., & Walsh, J. (1991). Dermatoglyphics and acute lymphocytic leukemia in children. *Journal of Pediatric Oncology Nursing, 8*(1), 30–38.

Everhart, C. (1991). Overcoming childhood cancer misconceptions among long-term survivors. *Journal of Pediatric Oncology Nursing, 8*(1), 46–48.

Fernbach, D., & Vietti, T. (1991). *Clinical pediatric oncology* (4th ed., p 3). St. Louis: CV Mosby.

Fernbach, D., Hawkins, E., & Polorny, W. (1991). Nephroblastoma and other renal tumors. In D. Fernbach & T. Vietti (Eds.), *Clinical pediatric oncology*. St. Louis: CV Mosby.

Finklestein, J. Z. (1987, December). Neuroblastoma: The challenge and frustration. *Hematology/Oncology Clinics of North America, 1,* 675–694.

Finlay, J., et al. (1987). Progress in the management of childhood brain tumors. *Hematology/Oncology Clinics of North America, 1,* 753–776.

Fisher, D., Robinson, S., Brett, C., et al. (1985). Comparison of enflurane for venous subcutaneous drug reservoir and lumbar puncture in children. *Pediatrics, 84,* 281–284.

Fisher, D., Robinson, S., Brett, C., Perin, G., & Gregory, G. (1985). Comparison of enflurane, halothane, and isoflurane for diagnostic and therapeutic procedures in children with malignancies. *Anesthesiology, 63,* 647–650.

Fochtman, D. (1993). The terminally ill child or adolescent. In G. Foley, D. Fochtman, & K. Mooney (Eds.), *Nursing care of the child with cancer* (2nd ed., pp 450–465). Philadelphia: WB Saunders.

Fochtman, D., et al. (1982). *Nursing care of the child with cancer* (p 82). Boston: Little, Brown.

French, R., Kohl, S., & Pichering, L. (1991). Principles of total care: Infections in children with cancer. In D. Fernbach & T. Vietti (Eds.), *Clinical pediatric oncology* (p 262). St. Louis: CV Mosby.

Gaddy, D., & Wood, A. (1982). The leukemias. In D. Fochtman & G. Foley (Eds.), *Nursing care of the child with cancer* (p 91). Boston: Little, Brown.

Gale, R., & Champlin, R. (1986). Bone marrow transplantation in acute leukemia. *Clinical Hematology, 15,* 851–872.

Gale, R. P., & Foon, K. A. (1986, August). Acute myeloid leukemia: Recent advances in therapy. *Clinical Haematology, 15,* 781–810.

Ganick, D. (1987). Wilms' tumor. *Hematology/Oncology Clinics of North America, 1,* 695–719.

Gardner, R., & Graham-Pole, J. (1983). Non-Hodgkin's lymphoma. *Pediatric Annals, 12,* 322–335.

Gaynon, P., Bleyer, A., Steinherz, P., Finklestein, J., Lutman, P., Miller, D., Reamna, G., Sather, H., & Hammond, D. (1990). Day 7 marrow response and outcome for children with acute lymphoblastic leukemia and unfavorable presenting features. *Medical and Pediatric Oncology, 18,* 173–179.

Grabowski, E., & Abramson, D. (1991). Retinoblastoma. In D. Fernbach & T. Vietti (Eds.), *Clinical pediatric oncology* (4th ed., pp 430–431). St. Louis: CV Mosby.

Grier, H., & Weinstein, H. (1989). In P. Pizzo & D. Poplack (Eds.), *Principles and practice of pediatric oncology* (pp 377–378). Philadelphia: JB Lippincott.

Groenwald, S. (1987). *Cancer nursing: Principles and practice.* Boston: Jones & Bartlett.

Groncy, P., & Finklestein, J. (1978). Neuroblastoma. *Pediatric Annals, 7,* 73–89.

Hakami, N., & Monzon, C. (1987). Acute nonlymphocytic leukemia in children. *Hematology/Oncology Clinics of North America, 1,* 567–575.

Hausman, K. (1979, March). Brain tumors in children. *Journal of Neurosurgical Nursing,* p 8.

Hayes, F., & Green, A. (1983). Neuroblastoma. *Pediatric Annals, 12,* 366–373.

Heiney, S., Wells, L., Coleman, B., & Swygert, E. (1991). 'Lasting impressions: Adolescents with cancer share how to cope'—A videotape program. *Journal of Pediatric Oncology Nursing, 8*(1), 18–23.

Hockenberry, M. (1988). Relaxation techniques in children with cancer: The nurse's role. *Journal of Pediatric Oncology Nursing, 5,* (1 & 2).

Hockenberry, M. J., & Coody, D. K. (1986). *Pediatric oncology and hematology: Perspectives on care.* St. Louis: CV Mosby.

Horowitz, M. (1989). Ewing's sarcoma: Current status of diagnosis and treatment. *Oncology 3,* 101–106.

Jaffee, N., et al. (1978). Integrated multidisciplinary treatment for pediatric solid tumors. In *Cancer: A manual for practitioners* (p 279). Massachusetts Division: American Cancer Society.

Johnson, F. (1991). Bone marrow transplantation. In D. Fernbach & T. Vietti (Eds.), *Clinical pediatric oncology* (4th ed.). St. Louis: CV Mosby.

Karch, A., & Boyd, A. (1989). *Handbook of drugs and the nursing process.* Philadelphia: JB Lippincott.

Kelleher, J. (1986). Bone marrow transplantation. In M. Hockenberry & D. Coody (Eds.), *Pediatric oncology and hematology: Perspectives in Care.* St. Louis: CV Mosby.

Kung, F. (1991). Hodgkins' disease in children 4 years of age or younger. *Cancer, 67,* 1428–1430.

Lankowsky, P. (1989). *Manual of pediatric hematology and oncology.* New York: Churchill-Livingstone.

Leventhal, B. (1992). Neoplasma and neoplasm-like structures. In R. Behrman (Ed.), *Nelson's textbook of pediatrics* (14th ed., pp 1291–1322). Philadelphia: WB Saunders.

Link, M., & Eilber, F. (1989). Osteosarcoma. In P. Pizzo & D. Poplack (Eds.), *Principles and practice of pediatric oncology* (p 620). Philadelphia: JB Lippincott.

Link, M., Grier, H., & Donaldson, S. (1991). Sarcomas of bone. In D. Fernbach & T. Vietti (Eds.), *Clinical pediatric oncology* (4th ed., p 222). St. Louis: CV Mosby.

Magrath, I. (1987). Malignant non-Hodgkin's lymphomas in children. *Hematology Oncology Clinics of North America, 1,* 577–602.

Mandell, L., & Wharam, M. (1991). Radiotherapy. In D. Fernbach & T. Vietti (Eds.), *Clinical pediatric oncology* (4th ed., p 162). St. Louis: CV Mosby.

Maurer, H., & Regab, A. (1991). Rhabdomyosarcoma. In D. Fernbach & T. Vietti (Eds.). *Clinical pediatric oncology* (4th ed.). St. Louis: CV Mosby.

McGuire, P. (1993). Radiation Therapy. In G. Foley, D. Fochtman, & K. Mooney. *Nursing care of the child with cancer* (2nd ed.). Philadelphia: WB Saunders.

Miser, J., Triche, T., Pritchard, D., & Kinsell, T. (1989). Ewing's sarcoma and the nonrhabdomyosarcoma soft tissue sarcoma of childhood. In P. Pizzo & D. Poplack (Eds.), *Principles and practice of pediatric oncology.* Philadelphia: JB Lippincott.

Morstyn, G., Souza, L., Keech, J., et al. (1988, March 26). Effect of colony-stimulating factor on neutropenia induced by sytotoxic chemotherapy. *Lancet,* pp 667–672.

Meyers, P. (1987). Malignant bone tumors in children: Ewing's sarcoma. *Hematology/Oncology Clinics of North America, 1,* 667–673.

Olness, K., & Gardner, G. G. (1988). *Hypnosis and hypnotherapy with children* (2nd ed.). Philadelphia: Grune & Stratton.

Olness, K. (1989). Hypnotherapy: A cyberphysiologic strategy in pain management. *Pediatric Clinics of North America, 36,* 873–884.

Overbaugh, K., & Sawin, K. (1992). Future life expectations and self-esteem of the adolescent survivor of childhood cancer. *Journal of Pediatric Oncology Nursing, 9*(1), 8–16.

Patterson, K. (1992). Pain in the pediatric oncology patient. *Journal of Pediatric Oncology Nursing, 9*(3), 119–130.

Piazza, D., Foote, A., Wright, P., & Holcombe, J. (1992). Neuman Systems model used as a guide for the nursing care of an 8-year-old with leukemia. *Journal of Pediatric Oncology Nursing, 9*(1), 17–24.

Piu, C., & Rivera, G. (1991). Childhood leukemias. In A. Holleb, D. Fink, & E. Murphy (Eds.), *Clinical oncology* (p 435). Atlanta: American Cancer Society.

Poplack, D. (1989). Acute lymphoblastic leukemia. In P. Pizzo & D. Poplack (Eds.), *Principles and practice of pediatric oncology* (p 336). Philadelphia: JB Lippincott.

Poplack, D., Kun, L., Cassady, J., et al. (1989). Leukemia and lymphoma in childhood. In V. DeVita, S. Hellman, & S. Rosenberg (Eds.). *Cancer: Principles and practices of oncology* (Vol. 2, 3rd ed., pp 1684–1692). Philadelphia: JB Lippincott.

Rasco, C. (1992). Using music therapy as distraction during lumbar punctures. *Journal of Pediatric Oncology Nursing, 9*(1), 33–34.

Riley-Lawless, K. (1989, July). School reentry programs. *Journal of Pediatric Oncology Nursing, 6,* 92–93.

Robertson, J. (1991). Changing central venous catheter lines: Evaluation of a modification to clinical practice. *Journal of Pediatric Oncology Nursing, 8*(4), 173–179.

Rodary, C., Gehan, E., Flamant, F., Treuner, J., Carli, M., Auquier, A., & Maurer, H. (1991). Prognostic factors in 951 nonmetastatic rhabdomyosarcoma in children: A report from the International Rhabdomyosarcoma Workshop. *Medical and Pediatric Oncology, 19,* 89–95.

Rosen, G. (1984). Spindle cell sarcoma-osteogenic sarcoma. In W. Sutow, et al (Eds.), *Clinical pediatric oncology.* St. Louis: CV Mosby.

Schwanda, A., Freyer, D., Sanfillipo, D., Axletl, R., Fahner, J., Hackbarth, R., Hassan, N., Kopec, J., & Waskerwitz, M. (1993). Brief unconscious sedation for painful pediatric oncology procedures. *American Journal of Pediatric Hematology and Oncology, 15*(4).

Shiminski-Maher, T. (1991). Diabetes insipidus and syndrome of inappropriate secretion of antidiuretic hormone in children with midline suprasellar brain tumors. *Journal of Pediatric Oncology Nursing, 8*(3), 106–111.

Skarin, A., et al. (1978). Malignant lymphomas. In *Cancer: A manual for practitioners* (p 249). Massachusetts Division. Boston: American Cancer Society.

Stanhill, P., & Pratt, C. (1986). Bone tumors. In M. Hockenberry & D. Coody (Eds.), *Pediatric oncology and hematology, perspectives in care* (p 111). St. Louis: CV Mosby.

Stehbens, J., Kalreta, T., Noll, R., MacLean, W., O'Brien, R., Waskerwitz, M., & Hammond, G. (1991). CNS prophylaxis of childhood leukemia: What are the long-term neurological, neuropsychological and behavioral effects? *Neuropsychology Review, 2,* 147–177.

Steinhertz, P. (1987). Acute lymphoblastic leukemia of childhood. *Hematology/Oncology Clinics of North America, 1,* 549–566.

Sullivan, M. (1987). Hodgkin's disease in children. *Hematology/Oncology Clinics of North America, 1,* 603.

Sullivan, M. (1993). Neuroblastoma. In G. Foley, D. Fochtman, & K. Mooney (Eds.), *Nursing care of the child with cancer* (2nd ed., pp 278–287). Philadelphia: WB Saunders.

Thompson, E. (1991). Hodgkin's disease. In D. Fernbach and T. Vietti (Eds.), *Clinical pediatric oncology* (4th ed., pp 355–375). St. Louis: Mosby-Year Book.

Van Eys, J. (1991). Malignant tumors of the central nervous system. In D. Fernbach & T. Vietti (Eds.), *Clinical pediatric oncology* (4th ed.). St. Louis: CV Mosby.

Vega, R., et al. (1987). Bone marrow transplantation in the treatment of children with cancer. Current status. *Hematology Oncology Clinics of North America, 1,* 777–800.

Voute, P. (1984). Neuroblastoma. In W. Sutow, et al (Eds.), *Clinical pediatric oncology.* St. Louis: CV Mosby.

Walker, C., Wells, L., Heiney, S., Hymovich, D., & Weekes, D. (1993). Nursing management of psychosocial care needs. In G. Foley, D. Fochtman, & K. Mooney (Eds.), *Nursing care of the child with cancer* (2nd ed.). Philadelphia: WB Saunders.

Walker, M. (1982). Tumors of the central nervous system. In A. Levine (Ed.), *Cancer in the young.* New York: Masson Publishing USA.

Waskerwitz, M., & Ruccione, K. (1985). An overview of cancer in children in the 1980's. *Nursing Clinics of North America, 20,* 10.

Wright, P., Holcombe, J., Foote, A., & Piazza, D. (1993). The Roy adaptation model used as a guide for the nursing care of an 8-year-old child with leukemia. *Journal of Pediatric Oncology Nursing, 10*(2), 68–74.

Young, J., Bloeckler, L., Silverberg, E., et al. (1986). Cancer incidence, survival and mortality for children under 15 years of age. *Cancer, 58,* 598.

Zeltzer, P., et al. (1983). Elevated serum neuron specific enolase in metastatic neuroblastome. *Proceedings American Society of Clinical Oncology, 2,* 307.

Ziegfeld, C. (1987). *Core curriculum for oncology nursing.* Philadelphia: WB Saunders.

BIBLIOGRAPHY

Aitken, T., & Hathaway, G. (1993). Long distance related stressors and coping behaviors in parents of children with cancer. *Journal of Pediatric Oncology Nursing, 10*(1), 3–12.

American Cancer Society. (1990). *Cancer facts and figures—1990.* New York: ACS Publication No. 5008-LE.

Bagnall-Reeb, H., & Ruccione, K. (1990). Management of cutaneous reactions and mechanical complications of central venous access devices in pediatric patients with cancer: Algorithms for decision making. *Oncology Nursing Forum, 17,* 677–681.

Bagnall-Reeb, H., & Ruccione, K. (1993). Practical application of an algorithm for the thrombolytic treatment of occluded vascular access devices. *Journal of Pediatric Oncology Nursing, 10*(2), 79–82.

Bartholomew, L., & Schwartz, P. L. (1991). Teaching and supporting self management of chronic illness: An example of translating theory into a family education program. *Journal of Pediatric Nursing, 6,* 214–215.

Bendor, S. (1990). Anxiety and isolation in siblings of pediatric cancer patients: The need for prevention. *Social Work in Health Care, 14,* 17–35.

Bendorf, K., & Meehan, J. (1989). Home parental nutrition for the child with cancer. *Issues in Comprehensive Pediatric Nursing, 12,* 171–186.

Betcher, D., & Burnham, N. (1991). Odansetron. *Journal of Pediatric Oncology Nursing, 8*(4), 183–185.

Betcher, D., & Burnham, N. (1992). Midazolam for outpatient sedation. *Journal of Pediatric Oncology Nursing, 9*(3), 136–140.

Birenbaum, K. (1990). Family coping with childhood cancer. *Hospice Journal, 6,* 17–33.

Bleyer, W. A. (1990). The impact of childhood cancer on the United States and the world. *CA—A Cancer Journal for Clinicians, 40,* 355–367.

Bossert, E., & Martinson, I. (1990). Kinetic family drawings—revised: A method of determining the impact of cancer on the family as perceived by the child with cancer. *Journal of Pediatric Nursing, 5,* 204–213.

Bowden, V. (1993). Children's literature: The death experience. *Pediatric Nursing, 19*(1), 17–21.

Broome, M. (1989). Implementation of a clinical study of a pain management program for pediatric oncology patients. *Journal of Pediatric Nursing, 4,* 54–56.

Broome, M., Bates, T., Tillis, P., & McGahee, T. (1990). Children's medical fears, coping behaviors and pain perceptions during a lumbar puncture. *Oncology Nursing Forum, 17,* 361–367.

Brown, P. (1989). Families who have a child diagnosed with cancer: What the medical caregiver can do to help them and theirselves. *Issues in Comprehensive Pediatric Nursing, 12,* 247–260.

Chambas, K. (1991). Sexual concerns of adolescents with cancer. *Journal of Pediatric Oncology Nursing, 8*(4), 165–172.

Chesler, M. A., & Barbarin, O. A. (1987). *Childhood cancer and the family: Meeting the challenges of stress and support.* New York: Brunner/Mazel.

Chester, M. (1990). Surviving childhood cancer: The struggle goes on. *Journal of Pediatric Oncology Nursing, 7,* 57–59.

Children's Hospice International (1993). Standards of hospice care for children. *Pediatric Nursing, 19*(3), 242–250.

Cohen, D. S., Friedrich, W. N., Copeland, D. R., & Pendergrass, T. W. (1989). Instruments to measure parent-child communication regarding pediatric cancer. *Children's Health Care, 18,* 142–145.

D'Angio, G. (1988). Cure is not enough: Late consequences associated with radiation treatment. *Journal of the Association of Pediatric Oncology Nurses, 5,* 20–23.

Davies, B., & Eng, B. (1993). Factors influencing nursing care of children who are terminally ill. *Pediatric Nursing, 19*(1), 9–16.

Deatrick, J., & Knafl, K. (1990). Management behaviors: Day to day adjustments to childhood chronic conditions. *Journal of Pediatric Nursing, 5,* 15–22.

Duffer, P., Cohan, M., & Thomas, P. (1988). Late effects of treatment on the intelligence of children with posterior fossa tumors. *Cancer, 51,* 233–237.

Ellis, J. (1991). Coping with adolescent cancer: It's a matter of adaptation. *Journal of Pediatric Oncology Nursing, 8,* 10–17.

Finklestein, J. Z. (1987). Neuroblastoma: The challenge and frustration. *Hematology/Oncology Clinics of North America, 1,* 675–694.

Finley, J. Z., Goins, S. C., Utegand, R., & Giese, W. L. (1987). Progress in management of childhood brain tumors. *Hematology/Oncology Clinics of North America, 1,* 753–776.

Foley, G., Fochtman, D., & Mooney, K. (1993). *Nursing care of the child with cancer* (2nd ed.). Philadelphia: WB Saunders.

Foley, G. V., & Whittman, E. H. (1990). Care of the child dying of cancer. *CA—A Cancer Journal for Clinicians*. Part I: *40,* 6, 347–354; Part II: *41,* 1.

Foote, A., Holcombe, J., Piazza, D., & Wright, P. (1993). Orem's theory used as a guide for the nursing care of an eight-year-old child with leukemia. *Journal of Pediatric Oncology Nursing, 10*(1), 26–32.

Fraser, M. C., & Tucker, M. A. (1988). Late effects of cancer therapy: Chemotherapy-related malignancies. *Oncology Nursing Forum, 15,* 67–77.

Freiberger, D., Bryant, J., & Marino, B. (1992). The effects of different central venous line dressing changes on bacterial growth in a pediatric oncology population. *Journal of Pediatric Oncology Nursing, 9*(1), 3–7.

Ganick, D. J. (1987). Wilms tumor. *Hematology/Oncology Clinics of North America, 1,* 695–720.

Green, D. (1989). *Long-term complications of therapy for cancer in childhood and adolescence.* Baltimore: Johns Hopkins University Press.

Hakami, N., & Monzon, C. M. (1987). Acute nonlymphocytic leukemia in children. *Hematology/Oncology Clinics of North America, 1,* 567–576.

Hammond, W. (1990). Management of childhood cancer. *CA—A Cancer Journal for Clinicians, 40,* 325–326.

Hanigan, M., & Walter, G. (1992). Nutritional support of the child with cancer. *Journal of Pediatric Oncology Nursing, 9*(3), 110–118.

Heiney, S. (1989). Adolescents with cancer: Sexual and reproductive issues. *Cancer Nursing, 12,* 95–101.

Heiney, S., Goon-Johnson, K., Ettinger, R., & Ettinger, S. (1990). The effects of group therapy on siblings of pediatric oncology patients. *Journal of Pediatric Oncology Nursing, 7,* 95–100.

Hinds, P. (1990). Quality of life in children and adolescents with cancer. *Seminars in Oncology Nursing, 6,* 285–291.

Hockenberry-Eaton, M., & Benner, A. (1990). Patterns of nausea and vomiting in children: Nursing assessment and intervention. *Oncology Nursing Forum, 17,* 575–584.

Hymovich, D., & Roehnert, J. (1989). Psychological consequences of childhood cancer. *Seminars in Oncology Nursing, 5,* 56–62.

Johnson, F. (1991). Bone marrow transplantation. In D. Fernbach & T. Vietti (Eds.), *Clinical pediatric oncology* (4th ed.). St. Louis: CV Mosby.

Johnson, L., Rincon, B., Gober, C., & Rexin, D. (1993). The development of a comprehensive bereavement program to assist families experiencing a pediatric loss. *Journal of Pediatric Nursing, 8*(3), 142–146.

Joy, S., et al. (1991). Wilm's tumor: Diagnosis, surgical management. *Association of Operating Room Nurses Journal, 53,* 437–440; 442–446, 448.

Knafl, K., & Deatrick, J. (1990). Family management style: Concept analysis and development. *Journal of Pediatric Nursing, 5,* 4–14.

Krohner, K. M., McBurney, B. H., & Wadeline, J. W. (1988). Assessing cancer prevention learning needs of parents and their 6th, 7th, and 8th grade children. *Oncology Nursing Forum, 15,* 59–64.

Kuzzel, J., & Stotts, N. (1990). Wound care trial and error yields knowledge. *American Journal of Nursing, 90,* 53–63.

Lansky, S., Lorman, J., Onts, T., et al. (1985). School phobia in children with malignant neoplasms. *American Journal of Diseases of Children, 29,* 42–46.

Lovett, R., Wagner, L., & McMillan, S. (1991). Validity and reliability of a pediatric hematology oncology patient acuity tool. *Journal of Pediatric Oncology Nursing, 8*(3), 122–130.

Magrath, I. T. (1987). Malignant non-Hodgkin's lymphomas in children. *Hematology/Oncology Clinics of North America, 1,* 577–602.

Martin, B. (1990). Care of the terminally ill child. In P. McCoy & W. Votroubek (Eds.), *Pediatric home care.* Rockville, Maryland: Aspen Publishers.

Martinson, I., Gilliss, C., Colaizzo, D., Fruman, M., & Bossert, E. (1990). Impact of childhood cancer on healing school age siblings. *Cancer Nursing, 13,* 183–190.

McGuire, P., & Moore, K. (1990). Recent advances in childhood cancer. *Nursing Clinics of North America, 25,* 447–460.

Meadows, A. (1989). Second malignant neoplasms in childhood cancer survivors. *Journal of the Association of Pediatric Oncology Nurses, 6,* 7–11.

Meadows, A. T. (1988). The concept of care for life. *Journal of the Association of Pediatric Oncology Nurses, 5,* 7–9.

Meehan, P. (1989). Pain control in one terminally ill child at home. *Issues in Comprehensive Pediatric Nursing, 12,* 187–197.

Meeske, K., Chamberlain, K., Cipkola-Gaffin, J., Harlander, C., & Reed, K. (1991). Measles epidemic: Impact on pediatric oncology patients. *Journal of Pediatric Oncology Nursing, 8*(4), 151–158.

Meyers, P. A. (1987). Malignant bone tumors in children: Ewing's sarcoma. *Hematology/Oncology Clinics of North America, 1,* 667–674.

Moore, I., Gilliss, C., & Martinson, I. (1988). Psychosomatic symptoms in parents 2 years after the death of a child with cancer. *Nursing Research, 37,* 104–107.

Moore, I. M., Glasser, M. E., & Ablin, A. R. (1988). The late psychosocial consequences of childhood cancer. *Journal of Pediatric Nursing, 2,* 150–158.

Mulligan, C., & Wittman, B. (1990). Nursing care of the child with brain stem glaucoma. *Journal of Pediatric Nursing, 5,* 375–386.

Munet-Vilaro, F., & Vessey, J. (1990). Children's explanation of leukemia: A hispanic perspective. *Journal of Pediatric Nursing, 5,* 274–282.

Neff, J., & Beardslee, C. (1990). Body knowledge and concerns of children with cancer as compared with the knowledge and concerns of other children. *Journal of Pediatric Nursing, 5,* 179–189.

Oakhill, A. (1988). *The supportive care of the child with cancer.* Boston: Butterworth.

Peckham, V. (1988). Learning disorders associated with the treatment of cancer in childhood. *Journal of the Association of Pediatric Oncology Nurses, 5,* 11–13.

Perrone, J. (1993). Adolescents with cancer: Are they at risk for suicide? *Pediatric Nursing, 10*(1), 22–31.

Pizzo, P. A., & Poplock, D. G. (Eds.). (1989). *Principles and practice of pediatric oncology.* Philadelphia: JB Lippincott.

Revell, G., & Liptak, G. (1991). Understanding the child with special health care needs: A developmental perspective. *Journal of Pediatric Nursing, 6,* 258–268.

Rogers, A. (1989). Home intravenous opioid therapy in a toddler with advanced cancer. *Journal of Pain and Symptom Management, 4,* 230–231.

Rollins, J. (1990). Childhood cancer: Siblings draw and tell. *Pediatric Nursing, 16,* 21–27.

Ruccione, K., Kramer, R., Moore, I., & Perin, G. (1991). Informed consent for treatment of childhood cancer: Factors affecting parents' decision making. *Journal of Pediatric Oncology Nursing, 8*(3), 112–121.

Servatar, E. (1992). A case report of twiddler's syndrome in a pediatric patient. *Journal of Pediatric Oncology Nursing, 9*(1), 25–28.

Sitken, T. (1990). Overview of childhood cancer: Clinical trials and cooperative groups. *Journal of Pediatric Oncology Nursing, 7,* 52–54.

Spross, J., McGuire, D., & Schmitt, R. (1990). Oncology Nursing Society position paper on cancer pain, part 3. *Oncology Nursing Forum, 17,* 943–955.

Steif, B., & Heiligenstein, E. (1989). Psychiatric symptoms of pediatric cancer pain. *Journal of Pain and Symptom Management, 4,* 191–196.

Sullivan, M. P. (1987). Hodgkin's disease in children. *Hematology/Oncology Clinics of North America, 1,* 603–620.

Thurber, W. (1989). Offspring of childhood cancer survivors. *Journal of the Association of Pediatric Oncology Nurses, 6,* 15–16.

Tritt, S. G., & Esses, L. M. (1988). Psychosocial adaptation of siblings of children with chronic medical illnesses. *American Journal of Orthopsychiatry, 58,* 211–220.

Walker, C. (1990). Siblings of children with cancer. *Oncology Nursing Forum, 17,* 355–360.

Walker, C. L. (1988). Stress and coping in siblings of childhood cancer patients. *Nursing Research, 37,* 208–212.

Weekes, D., Kagan, S., James, K., & Seboni, N. (1993). The phenomenon of hand-holding as a coping strategy in adolescents experiencing treatment-related pain. *Journal of Pediatric Oncology Nursing, 10*(1), 19–25.

Wood, R. (1990). Growth patterns in pediatric bone marrow transplant patients. *Journal of Pediatric Nursing, 5,* 252–258.

Wood, B., Boyle, J. T., Watkins, J. B., Nogueira, J., Zimand, E., & Carroll, L. (1988). Sibling psychological status and style as related to the disease of their chronically ill brothers and sisters: Implications for models of biopsychosocial interaction. *Developmental and Behavioral Pediatrics, 9,* 66–72.

CHAPTER • 43

Altered Endocrine Function

Judith A. Ruble
Denise Charron-Prochownik

NURSING PROCESS PLAN
NPP: The Child with Diabetic Ketoacidosis, Table 43–20

RELATED TOPICS
Assessing and enhancing self-esteem, Chapter 14
Impact of chronic illness, Chapter 19
Genetic counseling, Chapter 31
Patterns of inheritance, Chapter 31

LEARNING OBJECTIVES

- Name and describe the common alterations of normal endocrine function in children.
- Discuss common therapies used in the treatment of endocrine disorders.
- Identify the effects of endocrine disorders on developing self-image and self-esteem.
- Write an appropriate teaching plan for a child and family with an endocrine disorder.
- Plan the nursing care of children with selected pediatric endocrine conditions.

The endocrine system consists of a group of specialized tissues with one vital function in common. These tissues produce and secrete hormones that are the major chemical regulators of the body. Hormone secretion significantly affects such important body functions as metabolic rate, growth, fluid and electrolyte balance, the stress response, sexual characteristics, and glucose metabolism. If a hormone is either oversecreted or undersecreted, those organs or tissues whose actions are "programmed" by that hormone respond with disturbing, and sometimes life-threatening, changes in function. This chapter is concerned with altered secretion of hormones by the endocrine glands and the nursing care that relates to the child's experience of endocrine dysfunction. Nursing care related to disorders of the pituitary gland, the thyroid gland, the parathyroid glands, the adrenal glands, and the gonads is presented first. Altered function of the pancreas resulting in diabetes mellitus, the most common endocrine disorder in childhood, follows and is covered in depth.

Structure and Function of the Endocrine System

The endocrine system (also known as the hormonal system) is composed of a diverse group of tissues that produce and secrete chemical substances (hormones), which stimulate actions of other tissues. The body tissues sensitive to the effects of hormones are called target tissues. Seven glands are included in the endocrine system: pituitary, thyroid, parathyroid, adrenal, pancreas, ovary, and testis (Fig. 43–1). Table 43–1 reviews the basic functions of these glands and their target tissues, each of which is discussed at length in this chapter. It is now known that hormones are also secreted by tissues in the intestine, kidney, and heart in addition to the "traditional" seven glands. *Endocrine tissues are unique by virtue of the fact that their secretions are released directly into the blood stream for distribution throughout the body rather than passing through ducts into localized areas.* Secretions released into ducts are termed exocrine, and glands such as the

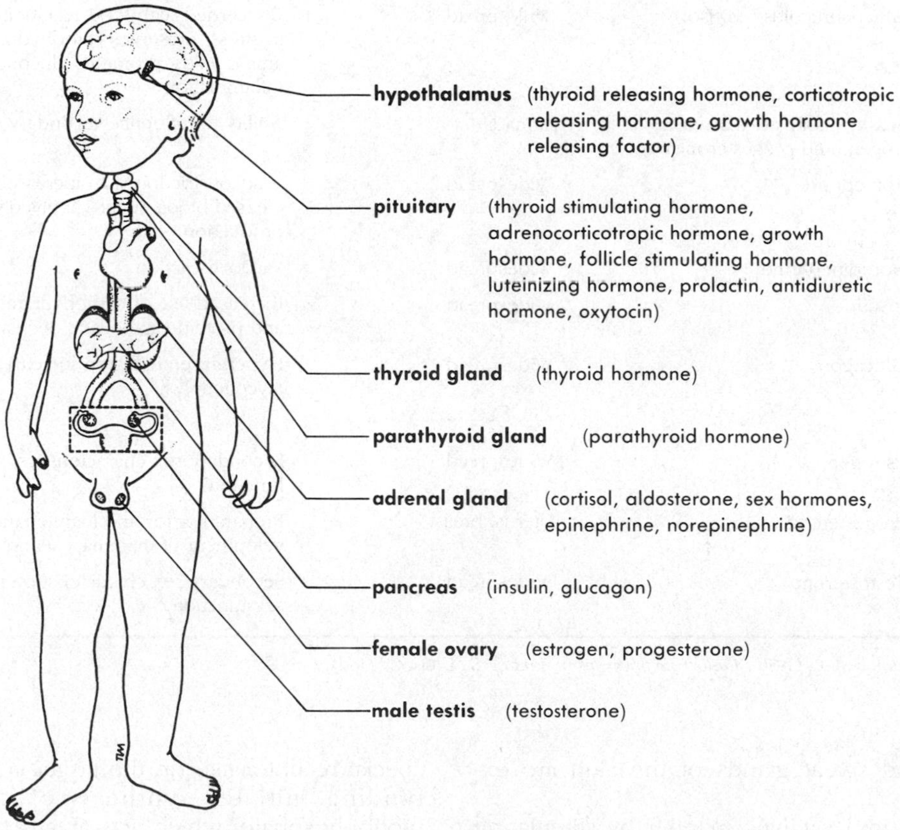

FIGURE 43-1. The endocrine glands. (Courtesy of Deborah Coody, RN, MS, PNP, The University of Texas Medical School at Houston, Department of Pediatrics.)

TABLE 43-1
Endocrine Glands: Secretion, Target, and Actions

Gland	Hormone	Target	Basic Action
Pituitary gland			
Anterior lobe	Somatotropin (growth hormone)	Bones, muscles, organs	Retention of nitrogen to promote protein anabolism
	Thyroid stimulating hormone (TSH)	Thyroid	Promotes secretory activity
	Follicle stimulating hormone (FSH)	Ovaries, seminiferous tubules	Promotes development of ovarian follicle, secretion of estrogen, and maturation of sperm
	Luteinizing hormone (LH) Interstitial cell stimulating hormone in boys (ICSH)	Follicle, interstitial cell	Promotes ovulation and formation of corpus luteum, secretion of progesterone, and secretion of testosterone
	Prolactin (luteotropic hormone)	Corpus luteum, breast	Maintains corpus luteum and progesterone secretion; stimulates milk secretion
Posterior lobe	Antidiuretic hormone (ADH)	Distal tubules of kidneys	Reabsorption of water
	Oxytocin	Uterus	Stimulates contraction
Thyroid	Thyroxine	Widespread	Regulates oxidation rate of body cells and growth and metabolism; influences gluconeogenesis, mobilization of fats, and exchange of water, electrolytes, and protein
	Calcitonin	Skeleton	Calcium and phosphorus metabolism
Parathyroids	Parathyroid hormone (PTH)	Bone, kidney, gastrointestinal tract	Essential for calcium and phosphorus metabolism and calcification of bone
Adrenal Gland	Mineralocorticoid (aldosterone)	Widespread, primarily kidney	Maintains fluid and electrolyte balance; reabsorbs sodium chloride; excretes potassium
Cortex	Glucocorticoids (cortisol)	Widespread	Concerned with food metabolism and body response to stress; preserves carbohydrates and mobilizes amino acids; promotes gluconeogenesis; suppresses inflammation
	Sex hormones (testosterone, estrogen, and progesterone)	Gonads	Ability to influence secondary sex characteristics
Medulla	Epinephrine	Widespread	Vasoconstriction with increased blood pressure; increased blood sugar via glycolysis; stimulates ACTH production
	Norepinephrine	Widespread	Vasoconstriction
Pancreas	Insulin	Widespread	Increased use of carbohydrate; decreased lipolysis and protein catabolism; decreased blood sugar
	Glucagon	Widespread	Hyperglycemic factor; increases blood sugar via glycogenolysis
Gonads			
Ovaries	Estrogen	Widespread	Secondary sex characteristics; maturation and sexual function
	Progesterone	Uterus, breast	Preparation for and maintenance of pregnancy; development of mammary gland secretory tissue
Testes	Testosterone	Widespread	Secondary sex characteristics; maturation and normal sex function

From Krueger, J. A., & Ray, J. C. (1976). *Endocrine problems in nursing*. St. Louis: CV Mosby.

salivary glands and sweat glands of the skin are exocrine glands.

Hormones act in a catalytic manner by stimulating a physiologic response in a target site without being directly involved in the target site's biochemical reactions. Many hormones act by becoming bound to a special receptor site on the target cell membrane. This binding initiates synthesis of cyclic adenosine monophosphate, which acts as a second messenger to produce cellular enzyme activity changes and thus the hormone's physiologic effect (Fig. 43–2). Other hormones are believed to enter the target cell's nucleus

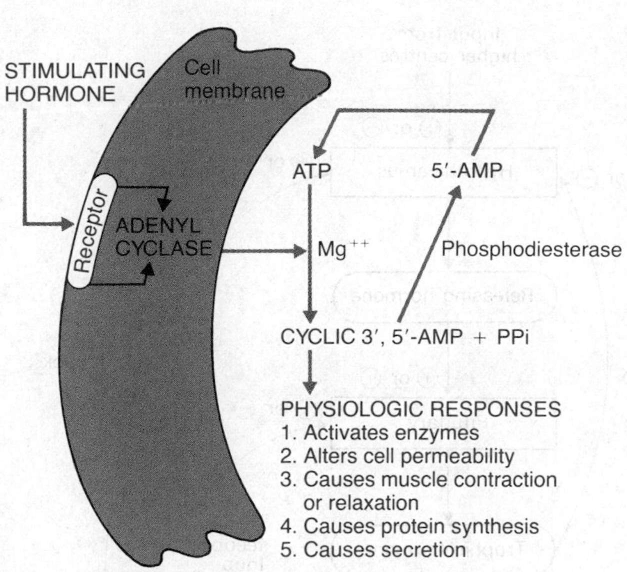

FIGURE 43-2. The cyclic AMP mechanism, by which many hormones exert their control of cell function. (From Guyton, A.C. [1991]. *Textbook of medical physiology* [8th ed.]. Philadelphia: WB Saunders.)

to induce the formation of messenger ribonucleic acid, which then enters the cytoplasm to increase the synthesis of specific cellular proteins (Root, 1992). The response of a particular target tissue to a hormone may be immediate or delayed. The magnitude of the response is altered by the rate of synthesis and secretion of the hormone into the blood, the rate of transport in the blood, and the rate of inactivation and excretion in the body.

Hormones are secreted cyclically and in response to certain body and environmental rhythms. For example, there are diurnal variations in adrenocorticotropic hormone (ACTH) secretions and monthly variations in a woman's estrogen and progesterone secretion. In addition, the endocrine glands are interdependent, and the release of one hormone influences the release of other hormones. It is this interdependence, as well as neurologic and chemical control, that helps maintain hormonal levels within normal ranges (Root, 1992).

Hormonal Control of Homeostasis

Interaction Between the Hormonal and Nervous Systems

Many interrelationships exist between the hormonal and nervous systems, and integration of both is necessary to maintain homeostasis. Both systems synthesize and release chemicals that are transported throughout the body. Hormones tend to act more slowly over longer periods of time, whereas the neurologic chemicals (neurotransmitters) bring about rapid but short-lasting responses. When the central nervous system reacts to various external and internal stimuli, it transmits a message to the hypothalamus. The hypothalamus can, in response, manufacture and secrete several releasing or inhibiting factors that are conveyed to the anterior pituitary, thereby stimulating or inhibiting the release of specific pituitary hormones. When pituitary hormones are released, they have a trophic effect on the appropriate endocrine glands, causing them to increase production of their hormones. For example, emotional or physical stress (stimuli) can lead to hypothalamic production of corticotropin releasing factor, which in turn stimulates the pituitary release of ACTH. Increased levels of ACTH lead to increased cortisol production by the adrenal gland (Fig. 43-3).

Chemical Control of Hormone Production and Secretion

Chemical control of hormone production and secretion is best understood in terms of *feedback control*. Negative feedback occurs when the rising concentration of a hormone inhibits the system which releases that particular hormone. Thus, an increased secretion of a hormone from a target gland generally leads to a decrease in the secretion of the stimulating pituitary hormone. For example, an increased secretion of thyroxine hormone (T4) from the thyroid gland (target gland) leads to a decrease in the pituitary secretion of thyroid stimulating hormone.

Endocrine disorders result from a disruption in the neurologic or chemical control of hormone secretion. Such a disruption may be caused by malfunction of the nervous system, hypothalamus, pituitary gland, or target gland. The cause may be congenital, infectious, necrotic, neoplastic, autoimmune, or idiopathic. Nurses caring for children with endocrine disorders must understand the altered physiologic states to assess, plan, and deliver effective patient care. The discussion that follows is organized according to the particular gland that is affected: the pituitary, adrenal, thyroid, parathyroid, gonads (ovary and testis), and pancreas. Clinical manifestations and diagnostic tests are grouped similarly according to a specific gland. Assessment data that the nurse uses to identify endocrine alterations are summarized in Tables 43-2, 43-4, 43-7, 43-9, and 43-11. During the assessment phase, the nurse will also be involved in planning with the family and health care team to carry out diagnostic tests. A summary of relevant tests appears in Tables 43-3, 43-5, 43-8, 43-10, and 43-12.

The Pituitary Gland

Normal Pituitary Function

The pituitary gland lies in a bony cavity, the sella turcica, at the base of the brain. It is composed of two parts, the anterior lobe and the posterior lobe, which are physiologically distinct. The anterior lobe secretes

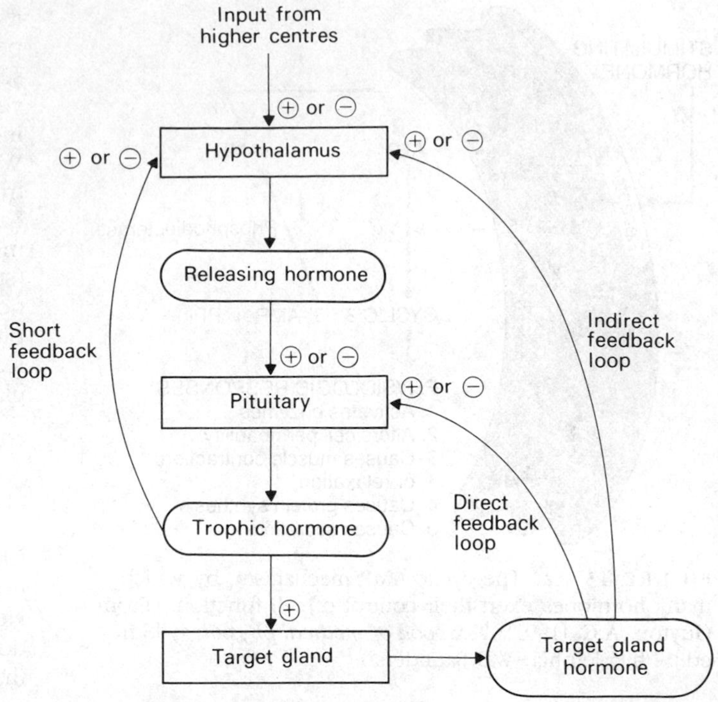

FIGURE 43-3. A schematic representation of hormonal interactions. (From O'Riordan, J. L., Malan, P. G., & Gould, R. P. [1982]. *Essentials of endocrinology.* Boston: Blackwell Scientific Publications.)

growth hormone, thyroid stimulating hormone, follicle stimulating hormone, luteinizing hormone, ACTH, and prolactin. The posterior lobe secretes antidiuretic hormone and oxytocin. These hormones, their specific functions, and target tissues are listed in Table 43–1. Clinical manifestations of the pituitary gland are summarized in Table 43–2. Many factors can cause abnormal production and release of hormones from the pituitary, including genetic aberrations, developmental and degenerative lesions, hyperplasia or tumor formation, hormone structural abnormalities, and target organ defects. An understanding of the various diagnostic tests permits the nurse to participate in the teaching and preparation of the child and family for

TABLE 43-2
Clinical Manifestations of Common Pituitary Alterations

Clinical Manifestations	Reason for Clinical Manifestations	Significance to the Nurse
Growth Hormone Deficiency		
Growth failure	Poor protein synthesis leading to decreased linear growth of bones	The nurse can detect growth failure only by assessing linear growth at regular intervals (at least once a year after age 1)
Delayed closure of fontanel	Poor protein synthesis	Child may be late in cutting or losing primary teeth; child appears younger than he or she really is; should be treated age-appropriately
Delayed denitition		
Immature facies		
Thin hair		
Poor nail growth		
Truncal obesity	Growth hormone has a lipolytic effect; deficiency leads to increased fat storage	
Hypoglycemia • Shakiness • Sweating • Tachycardia	Enhanced insulin sensitivity leads to hypoglycemia	Recurrent episodes of hypoglycemia may cause permanent brain damage or seizures; episodes of hypoglycemia should be documented (i.e., time, severity of symptoms, time of last meal)
Delayed puberty	Believed to be due to deficiency of growth hormone itself	

TABLE 43-2
Clinical Manifestations of Common Pituitary Alterations *(Continued)*

Clinical Manifestations	Reason for Clinical Manifestations	Significance to the Nurse
Antidiuretic Hormone Deficiency		
Polydipsia Polyuria (up to 4–10 liters)—clear, unconcentrated urine Enuresis, nocturia	Area of the pituitary that secretes antidiuretic hormone is affected	Symptoms usually occur abruptly Iced water preferred Enuresis occurs in a previously toilet-trained child
Antidiuretic Hormone Excess		
Headache Anorexia Irritability Personality change Severe: vomiting, confusion, convulsion	Cerebrospinal fluid retention and swelling secondary to water intoxication	
Gonadotropin Deficiency (for age)		
Absent signs of secondary sexual characteristics	Pulsatile LH, FSH surges are necessary to stimulate production of sex hormones	Children appear younger, less mature than chronologic age
Delayed pubertal growth spurt	Sex hormones are necessary for growth	
Gonadotropin Excess (for age) (Precocious Puberty)		
Boys		
Testicular enlargement Penile enlargement Pubic hair before 9.5 yrs of age	Increased levels of testosterone (produced by testes)	Encourage parents to treat child according to chronologic age rather than appearance
Girls		
Breast development before 7.5–8 yrs of age Vaginal mucosa changes • Walls appear pearly pink rather than bright red • Increase in vaginal mucosa Increased body fat Menses before 9–9.5 yrs of age	Increased levels of estrogen stimulate breast development, vaginal mucosa changes, and increased body fat When estrogen levels rise and fall in a cyclic pattern with progesterone levels, menses begin	Parents may need guidance in discussing pubertal changes with their child; child at risk for sexual abuse
Both boys and girls		
Accelerated growth	Estrogen, testosterone, and adrenal sex steroids all cause a growth spurt and accelerated advancement in bone maturation	Precocious growth spurt causing stunting of final adult height owing to premature bone maturation and closing of growth plates
Pubic hair Axillary hair Acne	Androgen production by adrenal glands (DHEAS, DHEA) causes virilization in girls Androgen production by the testes (testosterone) causes virilization in boys	Children may be embarrassed to undress in front of friends; encourage parents to discuss situation with physical education teacher if necessary
Mood swings	The combined effect of sex steroids leads to mood swings	Counsel parents that mood swings are a part of the pubertal process

TABLE 43-3
Diagnostic Tests for Pituitary Alterations

Diagnostic Test	Purpose	Comments
Growth Hormone Alterations		
Blood studies		
Somatomedin-C	Indirect reflection of growth hormone	Random growth hormone levels are not useful when deficiency is suspected because growth hormone is secreted in spurts throughout the day
Random growth hormone level		Done only when excessively high levels are expected (gigantism); usually done in early morning
Stimulation tests		
Insulin (intravenous)	Leads to hypoglycemia, which stimulates growth hormone secretion	Maximal hypoglycemia occurs at 20 mins after intravenous insulin; severe hypoglycemia can lead to seizures and coma; if child becomes unarousable during test, give intravenous solution of 50 per cent glucose and terminate test
Levodopa (oral)	All agents listed stimulate growth hormone secretion	Levodopa can cause nausea and vomiting
Arginine (intravenous)		
Clonidine (oral)		Clonidine can lead to hypotension; blood pressure must be monitored frequently during test
		Trendelenburg position plus increased intravenous fluids if hypotension occurs
Radiography		
Skull radiograph	Identifies erosion of the sella turcica (bony structure that encases the pituitary)	Pituitary tumors often cause erosion of sella turcica
CT scan of brain	Identifies brain tumor, abnormal pituitary formation	
Bone age radiograph (hand and wrist)	Assesses maturation of bones	Delayed maturation seen in growth hormone deficiency
Gonadotropin Alterations		
Blood studies		
Luteinizing hormone (LH)	Indicate whether the pituitary has initiated puberty	LH, FSH levels high at a young age in central precocious puberty, low in gonadotropin deficiency
Follicle stimulating hormone (FSH)		
Estradiol (girls)	Assesses how much estrogen the ovaries are producing	Estradiol levels high in girls, testosterone levels high in boys with precocious puberty
Testosterone (boys)	Assesses how much testosterone the testes are producing	
Human chorionic gonadotropin (HCG)	HCG levels are determined when a gonadotropin-secreting tumor is suspected	High HCG levels are indicative of a tumor
Bone age radiograph (hand and wrist0	Assesses maturation of bones	High levels of sex steroids mature the bones excessively, leading ultimately to stunted final adult height
		Low levels of sex steroids secondary to gonadotropin deficiency lead to delayed bone maturation
Skull radiograph	Identifies erosion of the sella turcica (bony structure that encases the pituitary)	Pituitary tumors usually cause erosion of the sella turcica
CT scan of brain	Identifies brain tumor	The CT technician should be told that a pituitary tumor is suspected so that special attention can be paid to that area
Radiograph of long bones		

TABLE 43-3
Diagnostic Tests for Pituitary Alterations *(Continued)*

Diagnostic Test	Purpose	Comments
Antidiuretic Hormone Alterations		
Urinalysis with specific gravity, osmolality	Evaluates body's ability to concentrate urine	Urine specific gravity and osmolality very low
Serum electrolytes		Serum osmolality high in ADH deficiency, low in ADH excess
Serum osmolality		
Water deprivation test	Designed to stimulate secretion of antidiuretic hormone (ADH); causing decreased and concentrated urine output	Patients with diabetes insipidus do not decrease or concentrate urine output Monitor vital signs and hydration status at least every 30 mins during test; dehydration and vascular collapse can occur quickly
Skull radiograph or CT scan of brain	Identifies brain tumor	

these tests. Diagnostic tests used to identify pituitary alterations are summarized in Table 43–3. A child who has a deficiency of one or more pituitary hormones is described as having hypopituitarism.

Growth Hormone Deficiency

Growth hormone is a potent anabolic (protein-building) agent that affects most of the tissues of the body, causing growth by promoting both increased cell size and increased cell number. It does not act on its target organs directly but generates another factor called somatomedin or insulin-like growth factor (IGF I and II) that mediates its effects on the peripheral tissues. In general, somatomedin activity tends to parallel that of growth hormone secretion. For example, high levels of growth hormone secretion lead to greater production of somatomedin by the liver and possibly by the kidneys (Schwartz & Bercu, 1992). *Growth hormone affects the metabolic processes of the body by enhancing the rate of protein synthesis, impairing carbohydrate use, and increasing fat mobilization and use.*

Etiology and Clinical Manifestations

Deficiency of growth hormone leads to growth failure. The causes of growth hormone deficiency (GHD) are classified as congenital (malformation of the brain affecting the hypothalamus or pituitary), acquired (tumor, trauma, infection, vascular abnormality, irradiation, or toxic effects of chemotherapy), or idiopathic (sporadic or hereditary) (Kaplan, 1990).

Most cases of GHD are idiopathic and have no identifiable cause. The incidence of classic idiopathic GHD has been estimated between 1 per 4000 and 1 per 10,000 children (Johanson & Blizzard, 1990). The next most common cause of GHD in children is brain tumors, primarily those of the midline, such as craniopharyngiomas and optic gliomas. The treatment of brain tumors by surgery, irradiation, or chemotherapy can also cause GHD. Younger children may develop the more typical signs of increased intracranial pressure with craniopharyngiomas, but growth impairment may be the only symptom in older children. The third most common cause of GHD is congenital malformations in the midline of the brain, such as septo-optic dysplasia. Other less common causes of GHD include head trauma, infection, vascular abnormalities, histiocytosis, sarcoidosis, and target tissue insensitivity to growth hormone. GHD is often associated with other pituitary hormone deficiencies, which must be ruled out in the diagnostic process.

Neonates with GHD usually have normal birth weight and length and grow normally during infancy. After infancy, the growth chart of a child with GHD will show the height decreasing in percentiles over time. Hypoglycemia is a common finding related to GHD because growth hormone helps maintain normal blood sugar levels. When growth hormone is absent or levels are inadequate, blood glucose concentration may drop to low levels in fasting states and can be a serious problem for infants and very young children. Parents may notice that their baby demands feedings every few hours and shows signs of low blood sugar (paleness, shakiness, irritability, sweatiness, hunger) if feedings are not given promptly. Children may require large bedtime snacks and often awaken in the morning with signs of hypoglycemia. Prolonged or severe hypoglycemia can even lead to seizures, coma, and brain damage.

Children with GHD characteristically appear physically immature for their age, with thin hair, poor nail development, poor development of the nasal bridge, and prominence of the frontal bones in the face. Delays in physical maturation include delays in fontanel closure, eruption of teeth, onset of puberty, and skeletal maturation. Whereas infants with GHD are often thin, older children tend to be chubby. Boys may

ETHICAL ISSUES

Use of Human Growth Hormone*

Margaret M. Mahon, PhD, RNC

Mark is 12 years old. He is healthy, but his height is less than 5 per cent on standard growth charts. Both of his parents are short. Mark's predicted adult height is 160 cm (5'3"). Mark is extremely upset by his height and has heard that "it can be treated." Mark has come to the Department of Endocrinology seeking treatment for his short stature.

Growth hormone (GH) stimulates growth; it is secreted by the anterior lobe of the pituitary gland. GH controls the rate of both skeletal and visceral growth. In addition, GH influences the metabolism of proteins, carbohydrates, and lipids. A child's rate of growth (height velocity) usually correlates with GH secretion. Some children have a deficiency of GH, which causes them to be short. It is possible to treat children who are short as a result of a variety of causes. The primary indication for treatment of short stature with human GH is children who are GH deficient. These children are treated with daily injections of GH over a period of months or years. The cost in dollars of GH treatment is about $20,000 a year. The side effects of treatment are not clearly known. In most cases, it is not clear whether GH therapy causes a definite change in adult height in children who are not GH deficient. That is, whereas linear growth may be accelerated while a child is receiving GH, growth acceleration continues only during treatment, possibly not exceeding the adult height that would have been achieved without GH treatment. In girls with Turner syndrome, however, it is clear that GH treatment can result in an end height greater than predicted.

For many years, GH treatment for children who were not GH deficient was not an option; the supply of GH was so limited that this expansion of treatment was not considered. Since that time, recombinant GH (r-hGH) has been developed, so unavailability of GH is no longer a barrier to treatment. Nevertheless, many questions remain concerning whether healthy children who are short should be treated with the goal of increasing their adult height.

It is well known that taller people have certain advantages over shorter people. People who are taller are likely to be considered more intelligent and to receive preferential treatment, such as higher salary in job hiring. Height is even a positive predictor of success in presidential elections. There is a clear bias or prejudice against shorter people in many societies. People who are short may have lower self-esteem and less success in employment, athletics, and interpersonal relationships. Short stature in children without GH deficiency is not a disease, however. Psychologic morbidity in adults who are short is not clearly documented, but discussions with shorter adults frequently reveal great displeasure with their height as well as impressions of why being short has been a disadvantage. Several chronic conditions do have short stature as a component or a side effect (e.g., Down syndrome and chronic renal disease).

The author acknowledges the assistance of Terri H. Lipman, PhD, RN, Clinical Nurse Specialist in the Section of Endocrinology and Metabolism at St. Christopher's Hospital for Children, Philadelphia, PA.

Being short can be a disability, for example, if one is not tall enough to drive a car or reach cabinets of standard height. If one's height is a disability, it seems that the entitlement to receive GH is clear. As with other disabilities, medical intervention, in this case GH, should be covered by insurance or other third party payers. Mark's height would not be a disability. Is he entitled to receive treatment? Should insurance or medical assistance pay for his treatment?

Several other issues must be considered in deciding whether a child who is not GH deficient should receive treatment. If being short is not a medical problem, is treatment an automatic option? How short should one be to be considered for treatment? If one considers all children who are less than 5 per cent for height as candidates, and those children are treated, then another group becomes the shortest 5 per cent of children. Is the ideal treatment not intervention to increase the height of children who are short, but rather instigation of broad-scale efforts to deal with the prejudice against people who are short? If decreased self-esteem is the issue, should treatment be psychologic? In one group of patients given the option of psychologic intervention or GH treatment, psychologic intervention was universally unacceptable (Hochberg, 1990). Can children truly make an informed consent for treatment? Should the dissatisfaction of many adults who are short be taken as a definitive indicator that this child will be dissatisfied with adult height? Recognizing that GH treatment is expensive, what is the sacrifice of other services offered to children if insurance or public dollars pay for GH treatment? If it is decided that there will be no third party payments for GH therapy, children with more financial support will receive treatment, perpetuating an inequity of treatment options.

Recombinant GH is available for treatment of GH deficiency. It has also been shown to be helpful in some other conditions. However, there is still much about GH treatment that is unknown. With the development of any new therapy, there is always a difficult balance between providing treatment for many who have long hoped for such an option and the need for discretion until more information is gathered.

REFERENCES

Allen, D. B., & Fost, N. C. (1990). Growth hormone therapy for short stature: Panacea or Pandora's box? *Journal of Pediatrics, 117,* 16–21.

Bischofberger, E., & Dahlstrom, G. (1989). Ethical aspects on growth hormone therapy. *Acta Paediatrica Scandinavica, 362*(Suppl.), 14–17.

Hindmarsh, P. C., Bridges, N. A., & Brook, C. G. D. (1991). Wider indications for treatment with biosynthetic human growth hormone in children. *Clinical Endocrinology, 34,* 417–427.

Hochberg, Z. (1990). Growth hormone therapy: The ethical angle. *Acta Paediatrica Scandinavica, 367*(Suppl.), 1–3.

Lantos, J., Siegler, M., & Cuttler, L. (1989). Ethical issues in growth hormone therapy. *Journal of the American Medical Association, 261,* 1020–1024.

Roberts, G. (1991). Growth hormone therapy for short stature. *Journal of Pediatric Health Care, 5,* 327–332.

have a small penis, which seems even smaller because of the chubbiness. The voice may be high pitched (Johanson & Blizzard, 1990). Intelligence is not affected (unless there has been brain damage from severe hypoglycemia); however, school performance may suffer because of decreased self-esteem and expectations based on size rather than on age and ability.

Diagnostic Assessment

The nurse has an important role in early detection of delayed growth. It is vital for the pediatric nurse to assess height and weight gains on all children at least once a year. Infants should be measured more often, with head circumference included, until 2 years of age. Data should be recorded on growth charts and compared with standardized norms. The pattern of growth recorded over many months or years is a better indicator of disrupted patterns than are single measurements. Most cases of delayed growth or growth failure will be attributed to factors other than pituitary deficiency (e.g., genetic factors and the child's general state of physical and emotional health). Common nonpituitary causes of abnormal growth include chronic illnesses, such as renal failure, congenital heart disease, cystic fibrosis, celiac disease, chronic vomiting or diarrhea, malnutrition, skeletal anomalies, chromosomal abnormalities, intrauterine growth retardation, and psychosocial deprivation. A child whose growth shows a consistent pattern of downwardly crossing height percentiles or who is more than two standard deviations below the mean on a growth chart should be evaluated by the primary care provider. If nonendocrine causes for poor growth are not found, the child should be referred to a pediatric endocrinologist for further evaluation.

Testing for growth hormone deficiency can be divided into screening tests and definitive tests (see Table 43–3 for a summary of diagnostic tests). Screening tests include an x-ray of the hand and wrist for skeletal age. Significant skeletal age delay is associated with GHD, but it can also be seen in hypothyroidism, Turner syndrome, renal disease, pituitary tumors, or regional enteritis (Kaplan, 1990). Depending on clinical signs and symptoms, tests to rule out disorders other than GHD may be done. Because secretion of growth hormone occurs in a series of irregular bursts, primarily during sleep, concentrations in the blood plasma are variable and often below levels of detection. Therefore, random sampling of the blood for measurement of growth hormone levels is of little value as a screening tool, although the lucky detection of a normal level rules out classic GHD. Somatomedin levels are stable throughout the day and reflect growth hormone levels. Therefore, a single sample of serum somatomedin may be measured in the screening process.

Definitive testing for GHD involves "stimulation tests," which entail serial blood sampling after appropriate stimulation of growth hormone secretion. The goal of such testing is to assess whether the pituitary gland is capable of secreting growth hormone. Agents that stimulate growth hormone secretion include intravenous insulin, intravenous arginine, oral clonidine, and oral levodopa; exercise also stimulates secretion. A particular agent is administered to the patient, and blood samples are drawn every 15 to 30 minutes for 60 to 120 minutes to measure growth hormone levels. Some centers do 12-hour overnight tests in which blood samples for growth hormone are drawn every 20 minutes through a heparin lock to assess growth hormone secretion during sleep.

The nurse involved in the diagnostic workup of a child with growth delay or growth failure can provide understandable information to the parents regarding the complex issue of growth. During the stimulation tests, the nurse must carefully assess the child for side effects of specific stimuli and intervene when necessary. Levodopa can cause nausea and vomiting, which are best relieved by lying down in a quiet, darkened environment; insulin produces hypoglycemia, which must be treated promptly with intravenous glucose if it becomes severe; arginine can cause nausea and hypoglycemia, although usually not severe; and clonidine can cause somnolence and hypotension, which must be monitored closely (Lifshitz & Cervantes, 1990). Throughout the testing period, parent-child interactions can be observed for disturbances that may contribute to psychosocial growth failure, although psychosocial neglect or abuse is difficult to evaluate and document in a hospital setting.

Therapeutic Management

Treatment with growth hormone is generally limited to children with well-documented GHD. The growth hormone preparation in use since 1985 is produced by recombinant DNA technology. This has alleviated the concerns about potential transmission of infectious diseases and restricted supply that were associated with preparations made from cadaver pituitary glands. Few side effects are associated with growth hormone administration. Local tenderness and allergic reactions have been reported but are rare. Antibodies to growth hormone can develop, but they do not inhibit the action of the administered hormone. A worldwide data assessment prompted by reports of a cluster of children in Japan who developed leukemia while using growth hormone found no statistically significant association (Johanson & Blizzard, 1990).

Growth hormone is effective in the first year of treatment, producing a twofold or greater increase in growth rate. After the first year, the response may diminish, but the growth rate will remain greater than before treatment. Growth hormone is given by subcutaneous injection administered from three times a week to daily; after the first year, daily injections maintain the best growth rate. Growth hormone therapy may be continued until the growth plates fuse, which may occur as late as the early 20s in patients with significantly delayed skeletal ages.

Nursing Diagnostic Statements

Altered growth and development: linear growth, *related to decreased anabolic activity associated with insufficient growth hormone.*

High risk for altered nutrition: hypoglycemia; *risk factor: insufficient growth hormone.*

Knowledge deficit (child and parents), *related to*

- *Etiology and disease process.*
- *Administration of growth hormone, including injection technique.*
- *Methods for financing growth hormone therapy.*
- *Realistic expectations of therapy.*

Disturbance in self-concept: body image, self-esteem, role performance, and personal identity, *related to*

- *Reactions of peers and significant others to short stature.*
- *Handicap of short stature associated with environmental barriers.*
- *Need for long-term therapy that makes child different from peers.*

High risk for altered growth and development: developmental delay: emotional/social; *risk factors:*

- *Poor self-concept.*
- *Parental "protection" from emotional trauma.*
- *Social stigma of physical appearance suggestive of storybook characters.*
- *Tendency of adults to treat child appropriate to size rather than age.*

Nursing Care

Nursing care for GHD relates primarily to support of the child and family during the prolonged treatment phase.

Facilitating Home Management. Treatment with human growth hormone necessitates a major readjustment period for the child and family. Initially, the parents must deal with apprehension and possibly guilt associated with administering injections to their child. Apprehension often stems from lack of knowledge regarding correct hormone reconstitution, injection technique, and side effects of treatment. Thorough teaching and written instructions regarding each aspect of therapy help to alleviate much apprehension. Health professionals must present up-to-date information to parents as it evolves and must be willing to openly discuss risks of side effects versus benefits of treatment. Parents must be aware that the cost of human growth hormone is extremely high. Treatment is usually covered by group medical insurance plans if there is well-documented GHD. The major pharmaceutical companies producing human growth hormone have "uninsured patient" programs that provide growth hormone at a cost within the family's financial resources.

As treatment progresses, parents may need to redefine their relationship with their child, especially if their present relationship fosters age-inappropriate dependency. The child must also adjust to a changing self. Anticipated and real growth provokes the child to reorganize his or her defenses and attitudes toward the outside world. This movement toward "normalcy" may prove to be distressing because patterns of thoughts and behavior must often be restructured. The child and family may benefit from meeting other families coping with similar problems. The Human Growth Foundation and MAGIC Foundation are national organizations offering support and information related to growth disorders.

In spite of accelerated growth with human growth hormone treatment, children and parents sometimes perceive the treatment to be a failure relative to their expectations. Although the final adult height of children receiving growth hormone treatment is usually within normal and acceptable limits, many growth-delayed children and families have unrealistically high expectations of human growth hormone therapy. Disappointment and grief can result when expectations are not met, leading to further feelings of anger, pessimism, and guilt. The parents may lose confidence in the physician prescribing the treatment and may even discontinue treatment yet may be unable to openly discuss their feelings. The child is usually well aware of the financial burden that treatment places on the parents, and perceived or real failure of treatment can intensify the significance of this burden. The nurse must be aware of the disparity between patient or parent expectations and realistic growth achievement. Specific, concrete, and clear expectations of a child's growth must be delineated during treatment. Open communication is essential during the entire treatment period.

Enhancing the Child's Self-Esteem and Achievement of Developmental Tasks

Height, a relative attribute based on comparison of self to others, is a vital ingredient in a child's development of body image and total self-concept. School-age children are acutely aware of their size in relation to classmates and friends. They also quickly learn that physical size often influences the potential for success. A short child is "different" in a way that is obvious to the child and others, and this difference often becomes more difficult for the child to cope with as he or she grows older and tries to master developmental tasks appropriate for age. Thus, short stature places the child at risk for social, academic, and psychologic difficulties. An understanding of these potential difficulties enables the clinician to design care approaches to facilitate the child's adaptation.

Recognizing Potential Threats to Self-Esteem and Healthy Development. Short children tend to exhibit social behaviors that may accentuate the discrepancy between their chronologic age and physical stature. They may become withdrawn and isolated from peers or may seek out the company of younger children. Certain children even assume the role of clown or mascot. Gordon and colleagues (1982) found that children with short stature have significantly more behavior problems than do children with normal height. Parents of children with short stature were found to have a less strict approach to childrearing than that used by parents of children with normal height. They tended to set fewer clear limits on behavior, and there was a lower level of cooperation and effective communication in the families. Indices of self-esteem were lower in the short stature group, and children more often saw themselves as unhappy and unpopular.

Stabler and coworkers (1980) found that short children exhibit less ability to perceive, organize, and integrate logical sequences of cause-and-effect relationships in social situations. They are less able to anticipate the outcome of social interpersonal encounters, which often leads to poor relations with peers.

Children with hypopituitary short stature typically perceive less adaptive, mature solutions to frustrating situations than do peers of average stature (Drotar et al, 1980). They tend to emphasize obstacles rather than solutions to frustrating situations. From their earliest years they are likely to encounter a series of frustrations secondary to their small size, including skills such as climbing and various sports. Physical environments of school (desks, drinking fountains, chalk boards, stair railings) and playgrounds (monkey bars, ladders) are geared to their taller peers. Small children are often helped and protected too much, teased, and discouraged from age-appropriate, assertive solutions to frustrations. Nicknames like "shrimp," "shortstuff," and "midget" and comments like "How's the weather down there?" and "You can stand up now" only reinforce the size discrepancy between these children and their peers. When choosing sides for a team, whether for baseball, relay races, or playing jump rope, the small children are often picked last, and this becomes a clear message regarding their perceived potential. Differences in size and strength between them and their peers of the same age may cause anxiety about assertive behavior and encourage withdrawal from frustrating situations. Their inability to respond to the competitive challenge of school often interferes with academic achievement. Despite normal IQ scores, school performance may be unsatisfactory.

Treating the Child Appropriately for Age. *In successful adjustment to growth hormone treatment, the degree of psychologic maturation may be related not so much to the actual growth achieved as to the ability of the parents and other adults to treat the child according to age instead of size.* Emphasizing positive areas of achievement may also help contribute to the child's positive self-concept and adjustment.

Setting the Child Up for Success. The nurse can encourage short children to develop interest in areas in which they can succeed and to choose sports activities in which size is not necessarily a factor to compete. By choosing activities in this fashion, children set themselves up to be winners, and frustrations are minimized.

Minimizing Psychosocial Trauma Through Liaisons with Other Professionals. Nurses can offer suggestions to school teachers and counselors on ways to minimize psychosocial trauma of short stature in their students. They can be encouraged to avoid lining children up by size and to choose teams for sports by methods that avoid having the smaller children picked last. They should also be encouraged to treat their short students according to age rather than size. Teachers and parents often ask about the advisability of holding a child back in school because of short stature. Academic placement should not be altered on the basis of height alone, but children who experience emotional distress or social immaturity because of their size may benefit from changes in school placement.

Diabetes Insipidus

Antidiuretic hormone (ADH, vasopressin), a hormone secreted by the posterior pituitary, controls the body's water excretion rates by altering the permeability of the tubules and collecting ducts of the kidneys. The amount of hormone secreted is proportional to body need. *Higher levels of ADH secretion lead to water conservation; lower levels lead to diuresis.* Diabetes insipidus is characterized by deficient ADH secretion leading to diuresis, an inability to concentrate urine and conserve body water.

Etiology

Tumors of the hypothalamus, most frequently craniopharyngiomas, are the most common cause of diabetes insipidus. Surgically induced trauma during removal of a tumor in the hypothalamic area is also a major cause of diabetes insipidus. Other etiologic factors include histiocytosis, tuberculosis, encephalitis, meningitis, aneurysms, and a genetic defect in synthesis of ADH (Bode, 1990).

Clinical Manifestations

The symptoms of diabetes insipidus in children vary and are influenced not only by the extent of ADH deficiency but also by diet, renal function, and preservation of the thirst mechanism. An absent thirst mechanism is most often associated with tumors, trauma, and surgery. Most children experience an abrupt onset of symptoms, such as polyuria, nocturia, and enuresis when previously toilet trained. The excess water lost from polyuria leads to dehydration and secondary polydipsia. The excessive thirst and urination that these children have interferes with their play, learning, and sleep. The urinary output of a child with diabetes insipidus can be between 4 and 10 liters a day. Children often prefer iced water, are thirsty during the night, and become irritable if fluid is withheld. Their urine color is clear even on the first morning void. Anorexia and poor weight gain are common. A history of associated ocular abnormalities or growth failure, or both, can be suggestive of a midbrain tumor.

Diagnostic Assessment

The diagnosis of diabetes insipidus is confirmed when inappropriately dilute urine is excreted in the presence of high serum sodium levels. Initial screening studies may include urinalysis with determinations of specific gravity and serum sodium, potassium, calcium, and glucose levels to rule out renal insufficiency or diabetes mellitus as the cause of polyuria. A skull x-ray may be done to screen for an intracranial tumor or histiocytes (macrophages). A measurement of random serum sodium concentration and osmolality tends to be elevated in children with diabetes insipidus owing to decreased blood volume. Tests designed to increase the serum osmolality, thereby stimulating secretion of ADH, are done to evaluate a child with possible diabetes insipidus. A water deprivation test is the most commonly used test. Water deprivation in normal individuals leads to serum hyperosmolality, causing release of ADH. This ADH release leads to body water conservation through decreased and more concentrated urine output. Restriction of oral fluid intake in an ADH-deficient individual results in rapid depletion of body fluid volume, a rise in serum osmolality to greater than 290 mOsm/kg, serum sodium greater than 145 mEq/L, and weight loss of 3 to 5 per cent. Urine output is altered in neither volume nor concentrate in these individuals.

It is best to carry out water deprivation tests during the day when the child can be carefully observed because polyuria, dehydration, and collapse may occur after only a short period of water deprivation (Bode, 1990). Careful hourly monitoring of hydration status, including assessment of blood pressure, pulse, skin turgor, mucous membranes, temperature, urine specific gravity, and weight, is done. Care must be taken to prevent surreptitious water drinking. A compulsive water drinker without diabetes insipidus will concentrate urine during this test and will not usually have significant weight loss. If the child's pulse increases significantly or if the blood pressure drops in the presence of dehydration, the physician should be notified. A toddler or young child may become highly irritable and inconsolable during a water deprivation test, and the parents may feel guilty in denying liquids. The water deprivation test is stopped in this age group as soon as serum hypertonicity is found. The nurse can provide emotional support to the child as well as the parents and can emphasize the importance of restricting fluids. If at all possible, arrange for a TV or VCR to help distract the child (and parents) from the thirst.

Therapeutic Management

Treatment of diabetes insipidus includes identifying and removing the cause when possible. Although diabetes insipidus is rarely life-threatening in itself unless water is withheld during stress, it can signal the presence of a serious underlying disorder. The drug of choice for symptomatic control of diabetes insipidus is desmopressin (DDAVP; 1-desamino-8-D-arginine vasopressin), a synthetic analogue of ADH. Desmopressin is usually given intranasally by spray or insufflation. It can also be given by subcutaneous injection if necessary.

Nursing Diagnostic Statements

Fluid volume deficit, *related to diuresis associated with insufficient ADH secretion.*

High risk for altered fluid volume: excess; *risk factor: improper administration of synthetic ADH (desmopressin)*

Knowledge deficit: child and parents, *related to*

- *Etiology and disease process.*
- *Intranasal administration of desmopressin, including indications for administration, precise measurement of the drug according to the graduation marks on the soft plastic nasal tube if given by insufflation, positioning of the head to ensure absorption, and effects of increased nasal mucus on absorption.*
- *Resources to assist with cost of desmopressin.*
- *The need for medical consultation any time the child's fluid intake is significantly altered.*
- *Signs and symptoms of fluid volume deficit and fluid volume excess.*

Fear/anxiety: child and parents, *related to the diagnosis of a chronic disease.*

Nursing Care

Facilitating Home Management. Desmopressin is usually delivered intranasally by nasal spray or through a small insufflator once or twice daily. Dosage and frequency of administration vary from child to child and according to the state of hydration. The nurse should provide written, illustrated instructions on diabetes insipidus and desmopressin therapy for the family. Information needs to be provided to the child's school on the condition, including indications for notifying the parent or physician. The family should be encouraged to obtain a MedicAlert bracelet or necklace for the child.

The goal of treatment is to eliminate polyuria except during short periods just before the next dose. The child should be taught to take a dose of desmopressin only when urine output begins to increase noticeably. This precaution reduces the risk of low urine output and fluid overload. Fluid intake and output must be monitored especially carefully in children who do not have an intact thirst mechanism. Early signs of water intoxication include drowsiness, headache, and vomiting. In children who require only a single daily dose of desmopressin, the hormone should be given in the evening so that breakthrough polyuria before the next dose will not interfere with sleep or school. The child and parents should be aware that an increase in the dosage of desmopressin will not significantly raise the urinary concentration but will prolong the drug's duration of action. The child and family should be instructed that during respiratory infections and allergic rhinitis, excess nasal mucus may interfere with hormone absorption, and they may notice that polyuria before the next dose occurs sooner than usual. They may need to contact their physician for advice on altering the hormone dose on those days. The therapy of diabetes insipidus has to be adjusted under conditions that either demand high fluid intake for coverage of calorie need or prohibit drinking entirely, as in the postoperative period. Infants and children requiring surgery must be closely observed by a pediatric endocrinologist (Bode, 1990).

Desmopressin is expensive and may be difficult to obtain in local pharmacies. The nurse should forewarn the parents about the cost and limited availability so that they can make necessary arrangements before discharge from the hospital for its purchase. Desmopressin is usually covered by group medical insurance plans and Medicaid.

Reducing Fear and Anxiety. As with the diagnosis of any chronic illness, the family undergoes an emotional adjustment period when a child is diagnosed with diabetes insipidus. The parents may feel responsible for the illness and may feel guilty for delaying medical attention. The nurse can provide an opportunity for them to discuss their fears and feelings and can offer assurance that the child has a treatable problem.

Panhypopituitarism

Etiology and Clinical Manifestations

Panhypopituitarism refers to the absence or partial deficiencies of all pituitary hormones. Congenital abnormalities, pituitary tumors, infections, vascular abnormalities, cranial irradiation and trauma have been identified as causes of panhypopituitarism. Symptoms include those related to hypothyroidism, GHD, hypogonadism, hypoadrenalism, and diabetes insipidus. Specific symptoms and diagnosis of each of these disorders are discussed elsewhere in this chapter.

Therapeutic Management

Pituitary tumors are treated with surgery, radiation therapy, or both. These treatments can lead to further pituitary damage and more hormone deficiencies. Panhypopituitarism is treated with hormone replacement therapy. The child may require thyroid hormone, growth hormone, cortisol, and ADH replacement. In addition to these hormones, the adolescent requires estrogen (girls) or testosterone (boys) replacement. The child and family must be instructed about the importance of administering hormone replacements as ordered. They must be aware that proper growth depends on proper doses of thyroid, cortisol, and growth hormone replacement. Periodic medical follow-up, which includes growth assessment and blood studies to evaluate the adequacy of hormonal replacement, is essential.

Nursing Care

Because inconsistent administration of hormone doses can be dangerous to the child's health and may impair growth and development, family and patient teaching is critical. The nurse should recommend that the child with panhypopituitarism wear a MedicAlert tag that identifies the child as having panhypopituitarism with adrenal insufficiency and diabetes insipidus. Such a tag may save a child's life if he or she should sustain major trauma away from relatives. The family should have written directions describing the child's medications, doses, and times of administration and instructions for illness and emergencies, including phone numbers of medical providers.

Precocious Puberty

Precocious puberty is an abnormally early appearance of secondary sex characteristics. Breast development before the age of 7.5 to 8 years or menses before the age of 9 to 9.5 years is considered precocious in girls, and pubic hair growth before the age of 9.5 years is considered precocious in boys (Hung, 1992; Lee & O'Dea, 1992; Rosenfield, 1990; Styne, 1990).

Puberty in girls is a process in which pituitary gonadotropins (luteinizing hormone [LH] and follicle stimulating hormone [FSH]) stimulate the ovaries to begin producing estrogen and the adrenal glands to begin producing androgens (dehydroepiandrosterone [DHEA], dehydroepiandrosterone sulfate [DHEAS]). The elevated estrogen levels lead to breast development, vaginal maturation, and the onset of menses. The elevated androgens cause axillary and pubic hair growth, adult body odor, and acne. Puberty in boys is

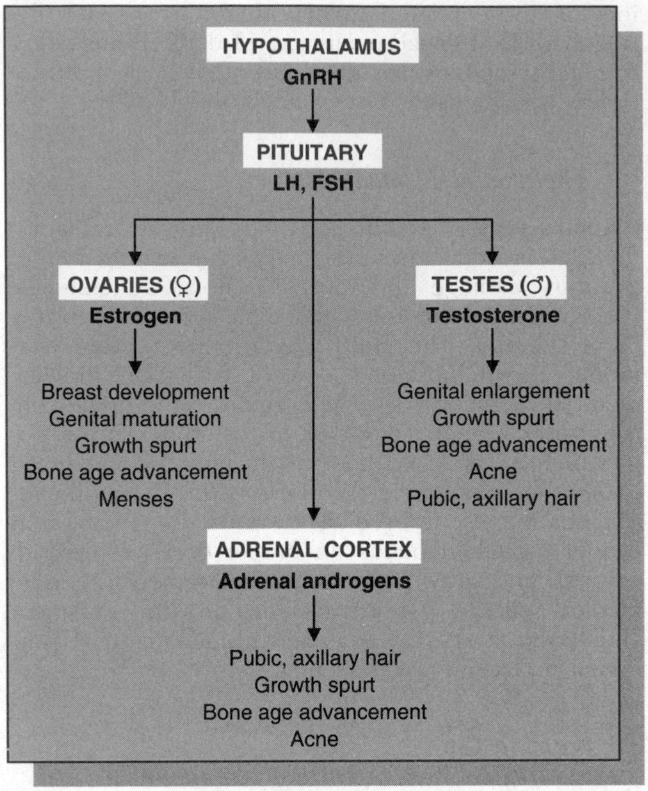

FIGURE 43-4. The hormone events leading to pubertal development.

a process in which the testes enlarge and begin producing testosterone. High levels of testosterone cause penile enlargement, axillary and pubic hair growth, adult body odor, acne, accelerated growth, and voice changes. The difference between normal puberty and precocious puberty is the age at which the changes occur.

It is important to distinguish between "true" or "complete" precocious puberty and "pseudoprecocious" or "incomplete" puberty. In complete precocious puberty, the central nervous system triggers the cascade of events resulting in development of all secondary sex characteristics. The pituitary gland increases secretion of LH and FSH, which in turn stimulates the ovaries to produce estrogen or the testes to produce testosterone. Figure 43–4 illustrates the series of hormone events leading to pubertal development.

In pseudoprecocious or incomplete puberty, there is no central nervous system activation of the full sequence of pubertal development. Instead, only estrogen, testosterone, or adrenal androgens are increased while the pituitary gonadotropins remain at prepubertal levels. Thus, the only secondary sex characteristics that develop are those related to the specific hormone that is increased.

Etiology/Incidence

The overall incidence of true precocious development is not known, although it is up to five times more common in girls than in boys. True precocious puberty may be caused by a wide variety of processes or may be idiopathic (no discernible cause). Pathologic causes include congenital anomalies of the central nervous system, hydrocephalus, brain tumors, and a variety of inflammatory processes. The early activation of the pituitary gonadotropins, whether idiopathic or organic, is known as central precocious puberty. In children with normal pubertal timing, gonadotropin levels begin to rise gradually after 8 years of age. In children with central precocious puberty, the gonadotropin levels rise quickly at an early age. The high levels of LH and FSH stimulate the gonads, leading to sex hormone production and early development of secondary sexual characteristics. Embryonal tumors located in the gonad, abdomen, or central nervous system often secrete gonadotropins, usually human chorionic gonadotropin (HCG) or LH. The HCG and LH from these tumors stimulate gonadal and adrenal sex hormone secretion, which in turn stimulate development of secondary sexual characteristics. McCune-Albright syndrome is a triad of polyostotic fibrous dysplasia of the bone, unilateral café-au-lait spots, and various endocrine abnormalities, the most common of which is precocious puberty. In 90 to 95 per cent of girls and 40 to 50 per cent of boys with precocious puberty, there is no demonstrable underlying cause. These children are considered to have idiopathic precocious puberty, in which the timing of events leading to sexual maturation is advanced for unknown reasons (Lee & O'Dea, 1992; Rosenfield, 1990).

Clinical Manifestations

In boys, pubertal levels of testosterone cause genital enlargement, development of pubic and axillary hair, adult-type body odor, and acne. In girls, pubertal levels of estrogen cause breast development, maturation of the genitalia (enlargement of the uterus, increased mucus, and a pink appearance of the vagina), and onset of menses; adrenal androgens cause pubic and axillary hair and adult-type body odor and acne (in boys, testosterone produced by the testes tends to overwhelm the effects of adrenal androgens). Both sexes have a growth spurt, an acceleration of skeletal maturation, and emotional swings.

Diagnostic Assessment

True central precocious puberty, with its early maturation of the hypothalamic-pituitary-gonadal system, is characterized by high levels of LH, FSH, and sex steroids (estrogen, testosterone, and DHEAS), which may be detected in a random blood test. A luteinizing hormone releasing hormone (LHRH) stimulation test is done to further evaluate the maturity of the pituitary gonadotropin response. In this test, the hypothalamic releasing hormone LHRH is given intravenously or intramuscularly, and serial blood tests for LH and FSH are done to measure their response to the LHRH stimulation. Serum chorionic gonadotropin levels are checked if a gonadotropin-secreting tumor is suspected. A bone age x-ray study is done to evaluate the skeletal maturation. Ultrasound examination and possibly computed tomographic (CT) scan of the pelvis and abdomen may be done to detect tumors and, in girls, to evaluate the ovaries and uterus. CT or magnetic resonance imaging (MRI) study of the brain is done to rule out tumors or other structural abnormality (Lee, 1992; Rosenfield, 1990).

Therapeutic Management

Therapy for precocious puberty that has an organic origin is directed at the underlying cause. The only permanent complication of idiopathic true precocious puberty is short stature because the excessive sex hormone production in the first 10 years of life causes accelerated bone maturation and premature closure of the growth plates.

A class of drugs known as gonadotropin releasing hormone (GnRH) agonists has been approved for treating central precocious puberty (FDA, 1991). To initiate puberty, the pituitary must receive intermittent pulses of GnRH from the hypothalamus. The GnRH agonists work by "flooding" the pituitary with continual high levels of GnRH. This eliminates the pattern of intermittent pulses of GnRH that signal the pituitary to start puberty. The family should be prepared for a brief acceleration of pubertal development during the first few weeks of therapy. Within a few weeks, however, pubertal development stops as the medication reaches levels adequate for suppressing the pituitary gonadotropins.

The GnRH agonists are given by daily subcutaneous injection or an intramuscular injection every 4 weeks. An intranasal spray, which is given two to three times a day, has also been approved and is now commercially available. It is essential that these medications be given as prescribed, because missed doses may result in stimulation rather than inhibition of pubertal development. GnRH agonists appear to be safe, have few side effects, and are effective in halting pubertal development, slowing skeletal maturation, and preserving final height (Kappy et al, 1989; Kreiter et al, 1990). Treatment is continued until the child reaches an appropriate age for puberty; pubertal development resumes as soon as the treatment is discontinued. GnRH agonists are expensive but are usually covered by private insurance and Medicaid.

Nursing Diagnostic Statements

Altered growth and development: early development of secondary sexual characteristics, *related to premature production of gonadotropins.*

Knowledge deficit: parents and child, *related to*

- *Etiology.*
- *Facilitating the child's mastery of age-appropriate tasks despite the early maturation of secondary sexual characteristics.*
- *Administration of medications and their potential side effects.*

Disturbance in self-concept: body image, *related to*

- *Early sexual development.*
- *Short stature associated with premature epiphyseal closure.*

Ineffective family coping, *related to difficulty in*

- *Accepting the changes in the child's body.*
- *Explaining puberty to a younger child.*

Nursing Care

Facilitating Home Management. The child and family will be best prepared for home management of precocious puberty if they understand the cause and the actual effects of the disorder. Because precocious puberty may involve sensitive issues for a family, the nurse's expertise in therapeutic communication will be especially important. Communication can be enhanced by listening carefully for indications of fears and concerns that the child or parent may be afraid or embarrassed to voice. Stressing the normalcy of the puberty process (even though it is occurring early) is often helpful. The family will need instructions about administration and potential side effects of prescribed medications. The family must understand the importance of not missing or delaying any doses.

Enhancing the Child's Self-Concept and Promoting Effective Family Coping. The nurse can help the child and family cope with the psychologic difficulties associated with early physical maturation. Parents should be encouraged to respond to their child in a manner appropriate to chronologic age rather than to physical appearance. Similar encouragement must be given to teachers and school personnel.

Parents may have difficulty relating to a physically precocious child and must understand the importance of accepting the normal physical contact appropriate for the child's age. Their child may have increased sexual interest beyond that appropriate for chronologic age and is at increased risk for sexual abuse. Many children with precocious puberty withdraw because they feel different from their peers. They may seek older friends who appear more similar physically, yet they often find it difficult to keep up with these friends' intellectual and social maturity. *It is important to reassure parents and the child with idiopathic sexual precocity that the child simply began a normal process early.* Many parents feel uninformed and confused about their own sexuality and find that discussing the puberty process with their own child is difficult. They may need assistance in clarifying their own mores, conflicts, and inhibitions before they can be comfortable discussing sexual topics with their child. Refer to the bibliography at the end of the chapter for books and pamphlets that are helpful in explaining sexual development and precocious puberty.

The Adrenal Gland

Normal Adrenal Function

The adrenal glands consist of the inner cortex and outer medulla. The cortex secretes glucocorticoids and mineralocorticoids, both of which are fundamental to metabolic regulation and stress adaptation. Adrenal androgens are also produced in the cortex but are relatively weak and, unless produced in excess, have only a minor role in sexual development. The medulla secretes epinephrine and norepinephrine.

Glucocorticoids, notably *cortisol,* perform important regulating functions in the body. The most outstanding effects are on glucose, protein, and fat metabolism; stress reactions; and inhibition of inflammatory processes. The overall effect is to help maintain blood glucose levels and blood pressure in normal ranges. Cortisol production is regulated by plasma ACTH levels. ACTH secretion by the pituitary is governed by negative feedback control via blood cortisol levels, biologic rhythms, and stress. Low plasma cortisol levels stimulate ACTH release, which in turn stimulates the rate of cortisol biosynthesis. Alternatively, high plasma cortisol levels inhibit ACTH production, which reduces cortisol production. Pituitary adrenal rhythms are governed by a biologic clock. ACTH secretions are higher in the morning in people with regular nightly sleep habits. They decrease throughout the day and are at a minimum the few hours before sleep. Stress appears to act directly to stimulate pituitary ACTH production, which in turn stimulates adrenal cortisol secretion. Stresses include trauma, infection, vomiting, anesthesia, acute anoxia, acute dyspnea, hypothermia, and emotional states such as acute anxiety (Ruble, 1990; Siegel & Lee, 1992).

Mineralocorticoids, the most important being *aldosterone,* are responsible for maintaining extracellular fluid volume and blood pressure. Aldosterone functions by increasing sodium, chloride, and water conservation and potassium excretion by the kidney. Its secretion is mainly under control of the renin-angiotensin system. In this system, nephrons of the kidney respond to blood volume, pressure, and sodium concentrations. Decreases in any of these stimulate production of the kidney enzyme renin, which ultimately leads to stimulation of adrenal aldosterone secretion. Increased aldosterone production leads to higher levels of angiotensin, which ultimately increases the body's blood pressure. Clinical manifestations involving the adrenal gland are summarized in Table 43–4. Tests used to diagnose alterations of the adrenal gland appear in Table 43–5.

TABLE 43-4
Clinical Manifestations of Adrenal Alterations

Clinical Manifestations	Reason for Clinical Manifestations	Significance to the Nurse
Cortisol Deficiency		
General weakness	Decreased cortisol	
Anorexia		
Weight loss		
Dehydration		
Shock secondary to relatively mild illness or injury	Inadequate cortisol production in response to stress	Intramuscular or intravenous cortisone must be given if shock occurs
Cortisol Excess		
Obesity (face, trunk, abdomen)	Fat mobilized from lower part of body and deposited in thoracic region	Body image is often altered significantly
Plethoric skin of face		
Purplish atrophic striae of abdomen, arms, thighs	Diminished collagen fibers in the subcutaneous tissues due to protein catabolism	
Muscular weakness and wasting	Increased protein catabolism	
Ecchymoses		
Acne	Secretion of adrenal androgens is often increased in Cushing disease	
Excessive hair growth on face, limbs, pubis (hirsutism)		
Slowed growth		
Osteoporosis	Lack of protein deposition in the bones	
Hypertension	Sodium and water retention	

TABLE 43-4
Clinical Manifestations of Adrenal Alterations *(Continued)*

Clinical Manifestations	Reason for Clinical Manifestations	Significance to the Nurse
Cortisol Excess *(Continued)*		
Edema		
Irritability, emotional outbursts		
Gastric burning		
Aldosterone Deficiency		
Hypotension	Hyponatremia	Intravenous access is a priority when hypotension occurs
Dehydration		
Shock		
Salt craving		Child craves dill pickles, chips, salt from salt shaker Monitor blood pressure closely
Aldosterone Excess		
Hypertension	Hypernatremia	Monitor blood pressure, urine output closely
Edema		
Catecholamine Deficiency		
Catecholamine deficiency in children is extremely rare		
Catecholamine Excess		
Hypertension	All signs and symptoms due to effect of increased epinephrine, norepinephrine, dopamine on target tissues	Both systolic and diastolic blood pressure increased
Tachycardia		
Headache		
Perspiration		
Emotional lability		
Anxiety		
Tremors		
Adrenal Androgen Deficiency		
Delayed development of pubic, axillary hair in girls	Adrenal gland is sole source of androgens in girls; testes produce androgens in boys	
Adrenal Androgen Excess		
Virilization in girls • Clitoral enlargement • Labial fusion • Increased labial pigmentation	Excess androgen production leads to virilization in girls; infant boys appear normal	An infant girl may have ambiguous genitalia and must be evaluated immediately for gender identity and underlying cause of ambiguity
Excessive development of external genitalia	Excess androgen production	
Increased muscularity		
Rapid growth		
Adult body odor		
Early development of facial, axillary, and pubic hair		
Advanced bone maturation	Excess androgen levels lead to excessive bone maturation and early closure of growth plates	Treatment to decrease androgen levels prevents excessive bone maturation, allowing more growth before closure of epiphyses
Stunted final adult height		

TABLE 43-5
Diagnostic Tests for Adrenal Alterations

Diagnostic Test	Purpose	Comments
Blood studies		
A.M., P.M. cortisol A.M. ACTH	Detects abnormally high levels of cortisol or ACTH	Excessively high ACTH levels are indicative of a pituitary tumor
Serum glucose	Detects hyperglycemia	Excessive cortisol can lead to impaired carbohydrate metabolism and hyperglycemia
17-Hydroxyprogesterone (17-OHP) Androstenedione	Evaluates whether there are excessive "backed up" precursors in cortisol production pathway	These values are elevated in congenital adrenal hyperplasia; they are suppressed with adequate treatment
Plasma renin activity (PRA)	Assesses the degree of dehydration secondary to salt loss	The greater the dehydration, the higher the PRA
Dehydroepiandrosterone (DHEA) Dehydroepiandrosterone sulfate (DHEAS) Testosterone Aldosterone	Detects altered production	High levels of adrenal androgens are indicative of congenital adrenal hyperplasia, adrenal tumors
Serum epinephrine, norepinephrine	Detects high levels secondary to tumor	High levels may indicate pheochromocytoma, neuroblastoma
Urine studies		
24-hour collection for corticoids, free cortisol, urinary glucose, urinary vanillylmandelic acid		High urinary corticoid levels are indicative of Cushing disease Often positive in Cushing disease
Dexamethasone suppression test	Determines whether cortisol production can be suppressed	Dexamethasone should suppress ACTH, thereby suppressing cortisol production If cortisol remains high after ACTH suppression, this is suggestive of an adrenal tumor
Metyrapone test	Assesses ACTH and cortisol production	Metyrapone is given every 4 hrs for 6 doses, after which 11-deoxycortisol level is determined Metyrapone blocks cortisol production, causing a rise in ACTH and 11-deoxycortisol (intermediate compound in cortisol pathway)
Karyotype	Chromosome analysis	Allows the clinician to distinguish between a virilized girl and an inadequately virilized newborn infant boy
Abdominal CT scan	Detects adrenal hyperplasia, tumor	
Abdominal ultrasonography	Detects adrenal hyperplasia, tumor	
Lateral skull radiography	Detects erosion and enlargement of sella turcica	Enlarged and eroded sella turcica is indicative of pituitary tumor
CT scan of brain MRI of brain	Detects pituitary tumor	
Bone age radiograph	Determines degree of exposure to increased levels of androgens	Advanced bone age is indicative of prolonged or significant exposure to androgens

Congenital Adrenal Hyperplasia

Congenital adrenal hyperplasia (CAH) is a group of genetic disorders involving a deficiency in any one of the several enzymes necessary for synthesis of cortisol. Each of the deficiencies results in clinical findings characteristic of the missing enzyme. The most common enzyme affected is 21-hydroxylase; 21-hydroxylase deficiency (21-OHD) is the cause of 90 to 95 per cent of "classic" CAH. 21-OHD is also the cause of the milder condition known as nonclassic or late-onset 21-OHD (Kaplan, 1990; Speiser & New, 1990). Although nonclassic 21-OHD is the most common disorder in this group, it presents few management problems; therefore, the following discussion centers on the classic forms of 21-OHD CAH.

Incidence

CAH is transmitted as an autosomal recessive trait. On the basis of newborn screening studies, the incidence of classic CAH in the United States, Europe, New Zealand, and Japan is approximately 1 in 14,000 live births. Approximately 75 per cent of children with classic CAH have a severe deficiency of 21-hydroxylase, which results in the "salt-losing" form of CAH (Pang et al, 1988). These statistics document a considerably higher incidence of CAH and also a higher proportion of the severe, salt-losing form than reported in older studies based on case reports. It is suspected that the discrepancy is due to the number of infants with CAH (especially infant boys with the salt-losing form) who died of the disorder without being diagnosed. The milder nonclassic 21-OHD is one of the most common autosomal recessive genetic disorders known. In the general Caucasian population, it occurs in 1 in 100 individuals and is even more common in certain populations (e.g., Ashkenazi Jews and Mediterranean peoples) (Speiser & New, 1990).

Pathophysiology

CAH is a genetic disorder involving a deficiency of one or more of the enzymes required for normal synthesis of cortisol and, at times, aldosterone.

The adrenal cortex produces glucocorticoids (predominantly cortisol), mineralocorticoids (predominantly aldosterone), and androgens (predominantly androstenedione, which can be converted to testosterone in peripheral tissues) from the basic cholesterol structure (Miller & Levine, 1987). Figure 43–5 shows a simplified adrenal steroid metabolic pathway. Cholesterol goes through many chemical changes leading up to these final products, and each of these changes relies on specific enzymes for its completion. If an enzyme is absent or deficient, the chain of chemical changes is stopped at that point in the pathway. The compound prepared to undergo its next change is unable to do so, and it "backs up" much like water at a dam. Eventually, many of the precursor compounds begin a stockpiling effect and are shunted to another pathway to produce adrenal androgens instead of cortisol. Because cortisol synthesis is impaired, the feedback message to the pituitary is for more cortisol to be produced. Therefore, production of ACTH by the pituitary rises. Elevated ACTH levels stimulate the adrenal gland, leading to hyperplasia, causing even further excess in production of adrenal androgens.

Aldosterone, like cortisol, is produced from the basic cholesterol molecule but through another branch of the pathway. Certain enzyme deficiencies lead to impairment of aldosterone formation. Children with poor aldosterone production or use are termed salt losers and have difficulty maintaining blood sodium levels, extracellular fluid volume, and normal blood pressure.

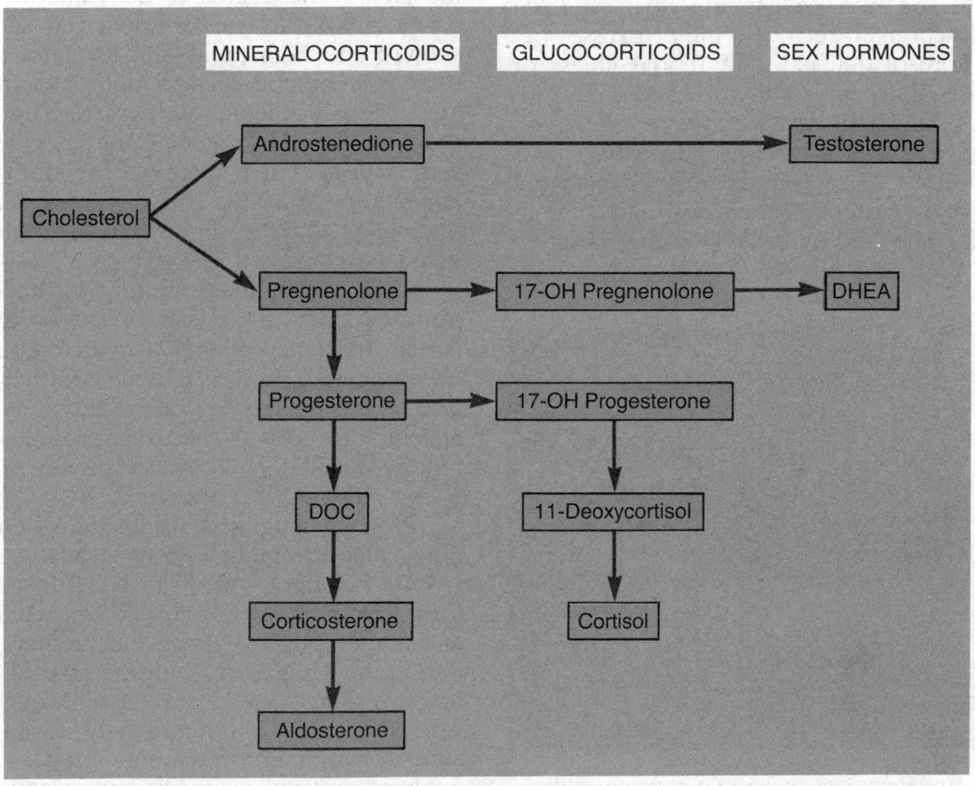

FIGURE 43 - 5. Adrenal cortex hormone production.

Different degrees of enzyme deficiency lead to different clinical diagnoses. Severe 21-OHD results in classic salt-losing CAH; a milder deficiency causes classic non–salt-losing CAH, and an even milder deficiency results in nonclassic or late-onset 21-OHD (Siegel & Lee, 1992; Speiser & New, 1990).

Clinical Manifestations

The excess androgen sex hormones in children with classic CAH produce virilization and development of male secondary sex characteristics. CAH is the most common cause of ambiguous genitalia in newborn infants (Pagon, 1987). The degree of virilization present at birth is variable. Infant girls may have labial fusion with or without scrotalization of the labia, enlarged clitoris, and, in extreme cases, opening of the urethra on the phallus. The ovaries, fallopian tubes, and uterus are normal in these girls. Although most infant girls are identified at birth because of the genital findings, the mildly virilized girls might be overlooked; the severely virilized might be mistaken for boys with hypospadias and undescended testes (Fig. 43–6). Infant boys may have slight genital enlargement and hyperpigmentation, but this is rarely distinctive enough to lead to a diagnosis at birth.

Infants with the salt-losing form of CAH, if not diagnosed at birth, will present with failure to thrive, vomiting, hypotension, hyponatremia, and hyperkalemia within the first 2 weeks of life (Siegel & Lee, 1992). If the "salt-losing" infants are not diagnosed when they present with these findings, they can die.

Infants with the non–salt-losing form of CAH have extreme reactions to relatively minor stresses because of their cortisol deficiency. A febrile illness or immunization reaction can result in marked or prolonged weakness and lethargy; a more severe stress, such as surgery, can lead to shock and death.

Children with CAH who are not adequately treated will have persistent excessively high adrenal androgen levels. The androgens will cause progressive virilization of the external genitalia; development of pubic, axillary, and facial hair; increased muscularity; rapid linear growth; and accelerated bone age advancement. Although these children will be large for their age when young, they will have stunted final height because of early closure of the growth plates in their bones.

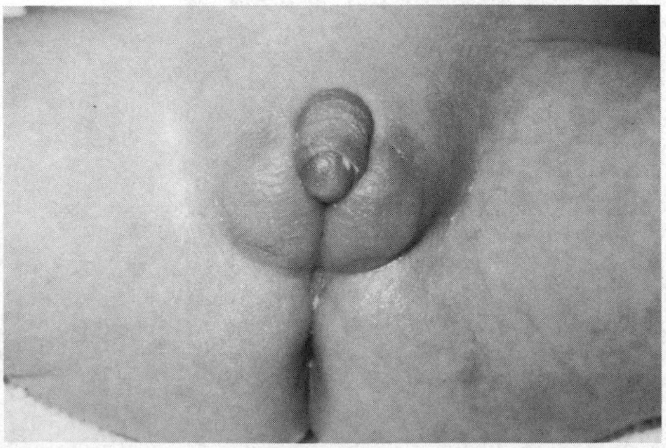

FIGURE 43 - 6. Ambiguous genitalia in a newborn girl with congenital adrenal hyperplasia.

Children who have CAH with a mild aldosterone deficiency that is not adequately treated will have a tendency to salt-losing crises leading to dehydration and vascular collapse during stress.

Nonclassic 21-OHD may produce no clinical findings ("asymptomatic" or "cryptic" nonclassic 21-OHD) or early development of pubic, axillary, and facial hair as well as hirsutism and cystic acne in both sexes and menstrual irregularity, anovulation, infertility, and cystic ovaries in girls (Speiser & New, 1990).

Diagnostic Assessment

Laboratory studies in the newborn infant or child who is suspected of having congenital adrenal hyperplasia include determination of 17-hydroxyprogesterone level, one of the "backed-up" precursors in the cortisol production pathway. This level is elevated. Determination of plasma renin activity level is done to assess whether the child is a salt loser. Children who lose salt through the urine decrease their blood volume in an attempt to compensate for and normalize serum sodium levels. The decrease in blood volume leads to increased renin production by the kidney. Therefore, the higher the plasma renin activity level, the greater the degree of dehydration.

Serum electrolytes are analyzed, although the low sodium and high potassium levels seen in salt-losing CAH may not be present until 2 or more weeks of age. Aldosterone levels may be low or normal in these children. A karyotype for sex chromosome analysis is done when a newborn infant presents with ambiguous genitalia. The karyotype sex chromosome findings enable the clinician to determine whether the infant is a virilized girl (which is most often caused by CAH) or an inadequately virilized boy. Milder forms of CAH (nonclassic or late-onset), with only a partial deficiency of the 21-hydroxylase enzyme, may have minimal physical findings and may not show abnormal results in randomly drawn laboratory tests. Specific diagnosis of the exact enzyme deficiency may require detailed studies of hormones in the blood and urine (Pagon, 1987; Speiser & New, 1990).

Prenatal diagnosis using amniocentesis or chorionic villus sampling is now available for families at risk for having a child with CAH. In addition, preliminary studies have been done on treatment of fetuses at risk for CAH by giving the mother glucocorticoids during the pregnancy, with the goal of preventing virilization (David & Forest, 1984; Evans et al, 1985). It is also possible, although costly, to detect the carrier state through chromosomal analysis. Whereas the fields of prenatal diagnosis and treatment are promising, the clinical usefulness of the techniques will become clearer with more experience. Specific diagnosis of the exact enzyme deficiency may require detailed studies of hormones in the blood and urine.

Therapeutic Management

The goal of treatment for CAH is to replace the deficient hormones and to suppress excessive ACTH stimulation of the adrenals. Glucocorticoid therapy is the cornerstone of treatment because it replaces cortisol and is also the feedback trigger that "turns off" the excessive ACTH production. When the ACTH levels decrease, the adrenals will no longer be stimulated to overproduce androgens; thus, virilization and bone age acceleration will stop. Oral hydrocortisone is the most commonly used glucocorticoid preparation. There is considerable disagreement about the optimal dose and frequency for hydrocortisone therapy; however, it is usually given at a dose of 10 to 25 mg/m^2/day, divided into two or three doses per day. The usual replacement dose must be doubled or tripled during times of stress, such as a febrile illness, to mimic the body's normal stress response and maintain blood glucose levels and blood pressure within normal ranges. Families should be taught to give an intramuscular injection of hydrocortisone for persistent vomiting, severe stress, or signs of acute adrenal insufficiency. Table 43–6 lists the signs and symptoms of acute adrenal insufficiency. Severe stress, such as a surgery, requires 5- to 10-fold increases in the usual replacement dose and close follow-up by the endocrinologist (Migeon & Lanes, 1990; New et al, 1990; Siegel & Lee, 1992).

Children with salt-losing CAH are also given fludrocortisone (Florinef) to replace the deficient aldosterone. The usual dose of fludrocortisone is 100 μg/day, with a range of 50 to 150 μg/day. Fludrocortisone is available only in tablet form; it is given in a single daily dose. Newborn infants may need doses as large as 200 or even 300 μg/day for a short time and usually need salt added to their diet. Older children should be allowed to salt their food to taste. Fludrocortisone does not need to be increased during stress (Migeon & Lanes, 1990).

TABLE 43-6
Signs and Symptoms of Acute Adrenal Insufficiency

Weakness
Abdominal pain
Nausea
Pallor
Anorexia
Lethargy
Vomiting
Rapid pulse

Virilized girls may need surgical repair of the external genitalia to reduce the clitoris and create a vaginal opening adequate for menstruation, intercourse, and childbirth.

Excessive doses of hydrocortisone can cause stunted linear growth, weight gain, and cushingoid features; inadequate treatment can allow virilization and accelerated bone age advancement and put the child at risk for acute adrenal insufficiency during stress. Excessive doses of fludrocortisone can cause hypertension and headaches; inadequate treatment can cause hypotension, hyponatremia, and hyperkalemia and put the child at risk for vascular collapse.

Close monitoring of CAH therapy with laboratory studies and clinical assessment is essential. Laboratory tests frequently used include serum 17-hydroxyprogesterone, serum androstenedione, and plasma renin activity; serum testosterone levels in girls and prepubertal boys are also helpful, as are periodic bone age x-ray studies. Clinical assessment includes careful monitoring of height, weight, blood pressure, and signs of virilization (New et al, 1990; Siegel & Lee, 1992; Speiser & New, 1990).

Nursing Diagnostic Statements

Altered growth and development: virilization and early development of secondary sexual characteristics, *related to excess testosterone production associated with stimulation of ACTH secretion by low levels of serum cortisol.*

High risk for injury: acute adrenal crisis; *risk factors: insufficient cortisol and aldosterone to meet physiologic demands of stress.*

Fluid volume deficit, *related to hyponatremia associated with insufficient production of aldosterone.*

Knowledge deficit, *related to*

- *Autosomal recessive etiology.*
- *Normal adrenal function and alterations associated with the disorder.*
- *Need for regular administration of corticosteroids.*
- *Alteration in dosage of corticosteroids required during stress.*
- *Need for regular follow-up care.*
- *Salt requirement for infants and children.*
- *Techniques for intramuscular injections.*
- *Recognition of and emergency treatment for acute adrenal crisis.*

Ineffective family coping, *related to birth of a child with ambiguous genitalia.*

Nursing Care

The major goals for nursing care are directed by the nursing diagnoses. They include (1) teaching the family to correctly administer medications, including stress doses, and to monitor the child for signs of adrenal crisis and (2) for families with a virilized female infant, helping the family cope with the birth of a child with ambiguous genitalia.

Facilitating Home Management. Parents should be provided with clearly written instructions listing medication, current dose and frequency, and stress doses (Ruble, 1990).

During physical stress, there is an increased need for glucocorticoids in children with CAH. Parents must be thoroughly instructed in the management of illness in their child. They should be given specific written instructions on indications and doses of hydrocortisone for "stress" coverage (Ruble, 1990). Parents must be taught how to give intramuscular injections. They should also receive an emergency kit list, including a vial of hydrocortisone 21-sodium succinate (Solu-Cortef), syringes and needles, and written instructions on how and when to use them. The nurse should recommend that they notify their endocrinologist for advice if they have questions about hydrocortisone dosage during an illness. Children with CAH should wear a MedicAlert bracelet or necklace inscribed "steroid dependent, adrenal insufficiency."

In acute adrenal crisis secondary to physical stress, dehydration and hypotension can lead to shock if untreated. Treatment includes hospitalization for intravenous fluid and electrolyte therapy and large doses of soluble hydrocortisone. Throughout the treatment of adrenal crisis, the nurse should closely monitor pulse, blood pressure, and hydration status, including urinary output, skin turgor, and mucous membrane integrity. Electrolytes may be ordered frequently, and the results, especially the serum sodium level, should be monitored closely. If serum sodium levels drop below 130 mEq/L, the physician should be notified so that more sodium can be added to the intravenous solution. If the intravenous line becomes nonfunctional for any reason, another one must be started immediately because dehydration can quickly occur without fluid and salt replacement.

Promoting Adaptive Family Coping. The diagnosis of CAH can be devastating emotionally for the parents. In the case of virilized female infants, the birth of an infant with ambiguous genitalia is considered a psychosocial emergency and is discussed in detail under the section "Ambiguous Genitalia in the Newborn Infant." The family may require extensive psychosocial support, and the nurse must create an atmosphere of acceptance that encourages full expression of feelings. The parents may be confused about the cause and may feel guilty for transmitting the disorder to their child. The nurse can help explain the disorder in understandable terms. This is a difficult task, requiring a simple discussion of a somewhat complicated topic. Referral to appropriate sources, including genetic counseling, is indicated. The nurse can reassure the parents that with appropriate treatment, their child will live a normal life without restrictions. For boys and most adequately treated girls, normal pubertal development and fertility can be expected. Amenorrhea and irregular menses can occur in girls but are often associated with inadequate treatment or lack of compliance (Mulaikal et al, 1987). Parents may express concern that their "masculinized" female infant will develop body image and sexual identity problems later on in life. Studies indicate that the majority of virilized infants grow up to develop a female sexual identity and normal sexual function (Kaplan, 1990). The ambiguous external genitalia of the infant girl with CAH often requires surgical correction, and this is usually done in the first year of life to avoid psychologic trauma at an older age. Acceptable final adult height can be achieved with early and consistent treatment (Kirkland et al, 1978).

Cushing Syndrome (Hypercortisolism)

Cushing syndrome is the result of excessive cortisol levels in the body, whether they are produced endogenously or administered exogenously. The term "Cushing disease" refers specifically to the ACTH-dependent hypothalamic-pituitary form of the disorder. The syndrome is variable, with an abrupt or gradual onset, a short or long course, and signs that can be subtle or obvious.

Etiology

Causes of Cushing syndrome include pituitary tumors, adrenal hyperplasia, adrenal tumors, and exogenous administration of glucocorticoids in the treatment of various diseases, such as autoimmune disorders and cancer. During infancy and in the first few years of life, the cause is usually a tumor of the adrenal gland. After the age of 6 or 7 years, the cause is usually pituitary secretion of high levels of ACTH secondary to a pituitary tumor. The high ACTH levels stimulate the adrenals to produce excessive amounts of cortisol, resulting in the clinical picture of hypercortisolism. In rare cases, ectopic ACTH-producing tumors or cortisol resistance can lead to Cushing syndrome. Exogenous administration of glucocorticoids is now a major cause of Cushing syndrome across age ranges (Migeon & Lanes, 1990; New et al, 1990).

Clinical Manifestations

The most consistent clinical findings in children with Cushing syndrome are growth failure, delayed skeletal maturation, and early sexual hair. Other clinical findings include obesity affecting the face ("moon face"), trunk, and abdomen; thin skin with striae on the abdomen, arms, and thighs; ecchymoses; acne; and muscular weakness. Hypertension, with elevation of both systolic and diastolic pressure, may be present; there is frequently carbohydrate intolerance. These clinical manifestations are the result of increased glucose synthesis, fat accumulation, and protein breakdown caused by hypercortisolism. Psychiatric symptoms may also occur (Migeon & Lanes, 1990; New et al, 1990).

Diagnostic Assessment

No one laboratory test is diagnostic of Cushing syndrome. Laboratory tests may include determination of total 24-hour urinary steroids, urinary free cortisol, and a morning and evening serum cortisol level. If a pituitary tumor is suspected, morning serum ACTH levels are determined. Abnormally high levels suggest a pituitary tumor. In addition, more sophisticated hormonal suppression and stimulation blood studies may be done to distinguish between an adrenal tumor and other causes of Cushing syndrome. An abdominal CT scan and ultrasonography may be done to detect an adrenal tumor, and an MRI scan of the brain may be obtained to detect a pituitary tumor (New et al, 1990; Siegel & Lee, 1992).

Therapeutic Management

Treatment of Cushing syndrome caused by an adrenal tumor is primarily surgical. Perioperative stress doses of glucocorticoids are given, followed by replacement doses until the return of function of the remaining adrenal can be verified. Trans-sphenoidal microsurgery is currently the treatment of choice for pituitary tumors; glucocorticoid replacement is given until the return of adrenal function is verified. Pituitary irradiation is effective; however, it frequently results in hypopituitarism. Pharmacologic agents that block ACTH or cortisol synthesis may be used as adjunctive therapy (Migeon & Lanes, 1990; New et al, 1990; Siegel & Lee, 1992).

Nursing Diagnostic Statements

Altered fluid volume and electrolytes: water and sodium excess, *related to increased levels of cortisol associated with*

- *Increased endogenous production.*
- *Exogenous administration of glucocorticoids.*

High risk for injury; *risk factors:*

- *Impaired glucose tolerance associated with high cortisol levels.*
- *Increased risk of fractures related to glucocorticoid-induced osteopenia.*
- *Infections, related to the immunosuppressive action of increased cortisol.*
- *Hypertension, related to increased blood volume associated with water and sodium excess.*

Ineffective individual coping, *related to emotional lability associated with increased cortisol levels.*

- *Acute adrenal insufficiency after treatment related to adrenal suppression from hypercortisolism.*

Disturbance in self-concept: body image, *related to moon facies, redistribution of fat to the trunk, wasting of extremities, and weight gain associated with metabolic derangement and fluid retention.*

Nursing Care

The nursing diagnoses detail the physical and emotional problems for the child with Cushing syndrome. Nursing goals relate to management of psychologic and physical sequelae in the pre- and post-treatment phases and psychologic support of the child and family.

Monitoring for Physical Complications. The child with Cushing syndrome is at risk for several potential problems, including sodium and water retention, transient infections, personality changes, and altered body image. The nurse must monitor for hypertension, edema, and excessive weight gain. The urine should be checked daily for glucose. Signs and symptoms of infection should be monitored closely, and medications given as prescribed should infection occur.

Helping the Family Cope with Emotional Lability and Enhancing Body Image. Parents often find that their child becomes irritable with highly labile emotional outbursts. The nurse can offer emotional support by facilitating expression of feelings by both the child and parents and by pointing out that emotional lability is a common problem in children with Cushing syndrome. Altered body image adds even more psychologic stress to the child. He or she should be told that many of the physical changes are reversible, including the obesity, facial roundness, excessive hair growth, acne, and bruising. The skin striae are usually permanent; however, they will become less noticeable as the color fades.

Monitoring for Acute Adrenal Insufficiency Postoperatively. The major postoperative complication of trans-sphenoidal microsurgery or unilateral adrenalectomy is acute adrenal insufficiency. Vital signs must be monitored closely, and the physician should be notified immediately if there is a significant increase in pulse or decrease in blood pressure. Intravenous fluid replacement must be adequately maintained, and urine output should be assessed frequently. (See also Table 23–7, a nursing process plan for the perioperative period.)

Families need instruction in postoperative glucocorticoid replacement, including increased doses for stress.

Premature Adrenarche

Premature adrenarche is a condition involving the isolated development of sexual (pubic and axillary) hair before the age of 8 in girls or 9 to 9.5 in boys.

Etiology

Premature adrenarche is caused by early secretion of adrenal sex hormones (androgens). The adrenal gland normally begins producing sex hormones during puberty, yet little is known about what initiates and controls the timing of hormone secretion. The adrenal androgens dehydroepiandrosterone and its sulfate (DHEA, DHEAS) cause the development of sexual hair. The exact incidence is not known; however, it is more common in girls than in boys.

Clinical Manifestations

Children with premature adrenarche develop pubic and axillary hair, acne, and adult-type body odor. They do not undergo any of the pubertal changes requiring activation of the gonads (e.g., breast development in girls, or genital development in boys and girls). Although there is often a slight acceleration in growth and skeletal maturation, final adult height is not diminished. The amount of sexual hair in children with premature adrenarche usually increases slowly. These children will have the onset of true puberty at a normal age.

Diagnostic Assessment

The diagnostic evaluation of the prepubertal child with sexual hair focuses on identifying the cause of androgen hormone production. Precocious puberty, CAH, and adrenal tumors must be ruled out. Laboratory studies may include determination of the levels of adrenal androgens (DHEA, DHEAS, androstenedione). Pituitary gonadotropins (LH and FSH) may be assessed in random samples and in response to stimulation by the hypothalamic releasing hormone LHRH. The concentration of adrenal androgens is often elevated in children with premature adrenarche, and the pituitary gonadotropin levels remain in the low, prepubertal levels. A bone age x-ray is obtained and may show slight advancement.

Nursing Care

No medical treatment is necessary for premature adrenarche because it is a physically harmless condition. The child may suffer body image problems requiring psychosocial interventions, however. The nurse should reassure the child and parents that the condition is not a disease but a "timing" variation of the adrenal clock and that normal puberty at about the average time can be expected. Hair growth will not progress to other parts of the body. Children who are bothered by a mature-type body odor can alleviate the problem with careful attention to hygiene and the use of underarm deodorant.

Tumors of the Adrenal Cortex

Tumors of the adrenal cortex are seen from birth into adolescence. They are of various types, and the clinical features depend on the nature of the hormone or hormones secreted.

Clinical Manifestations

Androgen-secreting tumors are the most common. They are virilizing, producing sexual hair, increased growth rate and acceleration of skeletal maturation in both sexes, penile (but not testicular) enlargement in boys, and clitoral enlargement in girls. In tumors with mixed hormone production, excess glucocorticoids will produce cushingoid symptoms, excess mineralocorticoids will cause salt and water retention and hypertension, and virilization from excess androgens may occur. In rare instances, adrenal tumors can secrete estrogen, which will produce gynecomastia in boys and breast development and genital maturation in girls (Hung, 1992; New et al, 1990).

Diagnostic Assessment

In a child with inappropriate virilization, laboratory evaluations focus on differentiating an adrenal virilizing tumor from CAH. Serum levels of testosterone, DHEA, 17-hydroxyprogesterone, and urinary 17-ketosteroid levels are determined.

If elevated urinary 17-ketosteroids are present, a dexamethasone suppression test will distinguish CAH from a tumor. Abdominal ultrasonography and CT scan are done to localize a suspected tumor.

Therapeutic Management

Treatment of adrenocortical tumors is surgical excision. Glucocorticoid treatment is given during surgery and continued until adequate function of the remaining adrenal can be verified. Chemotherapy may be used if there is metastasis at diagnosis or recurrence. The hormones found to be present at elevated concentrations at diagnosis are monitored shortly after surgery and then at least every 6 months to detect recurrences. More than 50 per cent of these tumors recur, and chemotherapy is usually used as the next treatment of choice.

The child with a virilizing adrenal tumor is at risk of body image problems and postoperative complications. The parents undergo severe emotional stress owing to the diagnosis itself, the changes they have seen in their child, the surgery, and the prognosis. The family requires intensive psychosocial support from all members of the health care team. Depending on the degree of psychologic distress, the child may be a candidate for individualized psychiatric counseling. The parents may require counseling to work through feelings of anger, fear, disbelief, and guilt. As with other adrenal surgeries, the major postoperative complication after removal of an adrenal cortex tumor is shock. Vital signs are monitored closely, and the physician is notified if the pulse increases and the blood pressure decreases significantly.

Tumors of the Adrenal Medulla

Tumors of the adrenal medulla include neuroblastomas and pheochromocytomas. Refer to Chapter 42 for a discussion of neuroblastomas.

The pheochromocytoma is a rare tumor in childhood, nearly always benign, and most commonly found in the right adrenal medulla although it can occur along the sympathetic chain or anywhere chromaffin tissues are found. The incidence in pediatric patients peaks between the ages of 9 and 12 years. Familial pheochromocytomas have been reported often, either as a single disorder or as part of a multiple endocrine disorder.

Clinical Manifestations

The clinical manifestations are caused by the effects of the catecholamines norepinephrine and epinephrine, which are produced in large quantities by the tumor. Hypertension is usually present. The systolic blood pressure may reach levels as high as 250 mm Hg, with corresponding increases in diastolic pressure. The most common symptoms are headache, sweating, nausea and vomiting, visual disturbances, and weight loss. The child may appear anxious, pale, and weak and is often emotionally labile. Tremors and tachycardia may also be present.

Diagnostic Assessment

Laboratory screening studies include 24-hour urinary samples to detect levels of vanillylmandelic acid and normetanephrine-metanephrine, which are metabolites of epinephrine and norepinephrine. Nearly all patients with the tumor have an abnormally high urinary output of these metabolites. Epinephrine and norepinephrine levels may also be determined to establish the diagnosis when metabolic concentrations are abnormally high. CT scan of the adrenals is used for localizing a suspected tumor. Scintigraphy with meta-iodobenzylguanidine and MRI may also be used, especially to localize extra-adrenal tumors (Hung, 1992).

Therapeutic Management

Treatment of pheochromocytomas is surgical excision. The patient is given alpha-adrenergic blocking agents 2 or 3 weeks before surgery to lower the blood pressure. Patients with serious tachycardia often require treatment with beta-adrenergic agents before surgery, but adequate alpha-adrenergic blockade must be established first.

Nursing Care

Nursing care during and after surgery includes close monitoring of blood pressure and pulse. Hypertension may be present for 24 to 36 hours after surgery, yet if it persists, another tumor or renal vascular disease may be present. Transient hypoglycemia has been reported postoperatively, and frequent blood glucose levels may be ordered along with close observation for signs and symptoms such as shakiness, hunger, anxiety, and increased sweating. The nurse must reinforce that continued follow-up medical care with monitoring of catecholamines is important; although the tumor is benign, it may recur years later.

The Thyroid Gland

Normal Function of the Thyroid Gland

The thyroid gland exerts widespread effects on metabolic processes throughout the body. *Thyroid hormone regulates the rate of body metabolism,* thereby affecting body temperature, growth, cardiovascular function, gastrointestinal motility, neurologic reflexes, muscle tone, and respiratory rate.

The thyroid gland traps iodine from ingested food to produce the thyroid hormone thyroxine (T4); as with other hormones, the amount produced depends on a negative feedback mechanism. Decreased levels of thyroid hormone in body fluids stimulate pituitary secretion of thyroid stimulating hormone (TSH) in two ways: (1) by a direct effect on the pituitary itself and (2) by an indirect effect acting through the hypothalamus. The hypothalamus produces thyrotropin releasing hormone (TRH) that stimulates the pituitary to produce TSH. The TSH stimulates the thyroid gland to produce thyroid hormone. The thyroid gland traps circulating iodide, oxidizes the iodide to iodine via a peroxidase enzyme, and binds the iodine to a tyrosine residue on thyroglobulin to form monoiodotyrosine and diiodotyrosine. Monoiodotyrosine and diiodotyrosine couple to form T3 and T4. The thyroid hormones are then released into the circulation (Fisher, 1985) (Fig. 43–7). Clinical manifestations of thyroid alterations are summarized in Table 43–7. Tests used to diagnose thyroid alterations appear in Table 43–8.

TABLE 43-7
Clinical Manifestations of Thyroid Alterations

Clinical Manifestations	Reason for Clinical Manifestations	Significance to the Nurse
Thyroid Hormone Deficiency		
Congenital (At Birth/Infancy)		
Prolonged jaundice	Slow metabolism, slow clearance of bilirubin	Usually requires treatment with bilirubin light
Lethargy		
Delayed stooling at birth (over 24 hrs)	Decreased gastrointestinal peristalsis	Newborns should pass first stool within first 24 hrs of life
Constipation		
Protuberant abdomen		
Poor feeding	Decreased appetite	Parents may find that feeding their newborn is difficult and frustrating
Coarse facial features		
Large fontanels (especially posterior)	Delayed skeletal maturation	
Flattened nasal bridge		
Large, protruding tongue		
Low anterior hairline		
Hoarse cry		
Umbilical hernia		
Mottled, cool skin	Poor circulation	
Subnormal postnatal growth rate	Poor long bone growth	
Hypotonia	Decreased muscular strength	
Sluggish reflexes	Irreversible retardation in maturation of nervous system	Newborn screening programs are aimed at preventing irreversible mental retardation through early detection and treatment
Delayed development		
Mental retardation		
Acquired (Childhood)		
Goiter (swollen thyroid)	Gland swells owing to autoimmune inflammatory process or to gland's trying to compensate for inadequate production	
Slow growth	Poor long bone growth	
Decrease in appetite, energy level	Slow metabolism	Symptoms may be subtle and may develop over months
Constipation	Decreased gastrointestinal peristalsis	
Cold intolerance	Poor circulation	
No development of mental retardation	Can reassure family	
	Brain development is essentially complete and will not be impaired by low thyroxine levels by age 2 yrs	

Congenital Hypothyroidism

Congenital hypothyroidism is a condition resulting from inadequate thyroid hormone production to meet an infant's needs. From fetal life through the first 2 years, thyroid hormone is crucial for growth and development of the skeletal and nervous systems. Untreated hypothyroidism in the first few years of life can result in severely impaired linear growth and irreversible mental retardation.

Etiology/Incidence

The incidence of congenital hypothyroidism is approximately 1 per 3500 to 1 per 4000 newborn infants. There is an unexplained female-to-male ratio of between 2.5:1 and 3:1. Thyroid dysgenesis, or improper development of the gland, accounts for 80 per cent of the known cases. Inborn errors of thyroid hormone synthesis, secretion, and use are autosomal recessive hereditary enzyme deficiencies that account

TABLE 43-7
Clinical Manifestations of Thyroid Alterations *(Continued)*

Clinical Manifestations	Reason for Clinical Manifestations	Significance to the Nurse
Thyroid Hormone Excess		
Hyperactive behavior	Hypermetabolism; affects all body systems	Many children with thyrotoxicosis are treated for simple behavior and academic problems without success before the diagnosis
Nervousness, tremor		
Emotional lability		
Poor school performance		
Insomnia		
Fatigue, poor endurance		
Heat intolerance		
Thin, velvety, moist skin		
Tachycardia, palpitation		
Flushed, sweaty skin		
School problems	Easy distractibility, poor concentration	
Exophthalmos, stare	Believed to be due to an autoimmune process; poorly understood	There is no correlation between degree of proptosis and severity of thyrotoxicosis; after therapy, the eyes often improve, but 25% of the patients have no change; patient or parent should be taught to instill methylcellulose eyedrops at night to protect cornea
Lid lag		
Impaired peripheral vision		
Dryness of eyes in morning		
Enlarged thyroid gland	Thyroid stimulating immunoglobulins stimulate the gland to hyperfunction and enlarge	

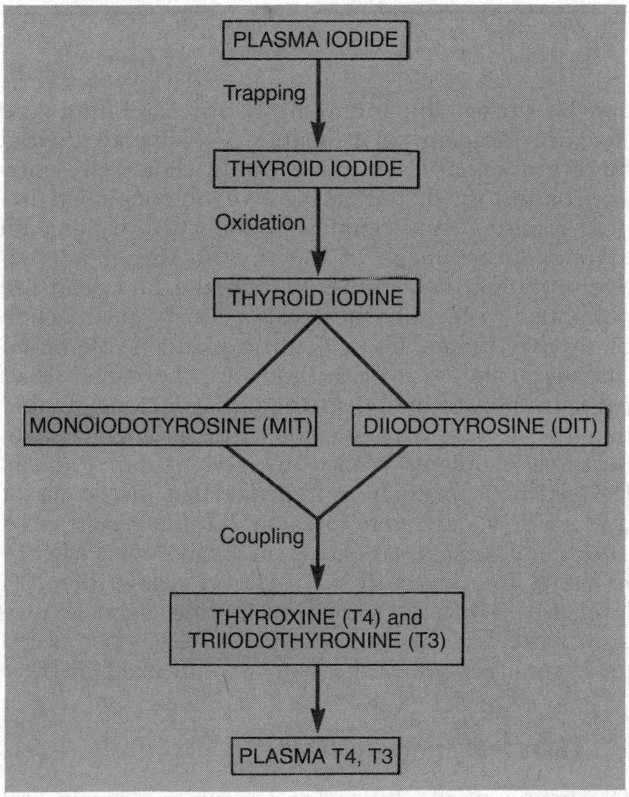

FIGURE 43-7. Thyroid hormone synthesis.

for 10 to 15 per cent of the cases. Transient congenital hypothyroidism may occur when pregnant women with hyperthyroidism receive antithyroid medication. The drugs cross the placenta and disrupt fetal thyroid hormone production. Less frequent causes of congenital hypothyroidism include low levels of dietary iodine (endemic goiter) and hypothalamic-pituitary disorders–TSH deficiency (Letarte, 1985).

Clinical Manifestations

The clinical signs of congenital hypothyroidism may be absent or subtle at birth and may not appear for several months, depending on the severity of the hormone deficiency. Recent studies show that breastfeeding does not delay the appearance of signs and symptoms of congenital hypothyroidism, as was previously thought (Franklin et al, 1985). Unfortunately, irreversible damage to the central nervous system may occur before clinical manifestations suggest the diagnosis. Screening programs for newborn infants have greatly improved the prognosis for infants with congenital hypothyroidism through early recognition and treatment of the disorder. Infants with congenital hypothyroidism tend to have prolonged gestation and high birthweights, although they may have normal birth lengths and head circumferences. Decreased gastrointestinal motility may delay stooling after birth

TABLE 43-8
Diagnostic Tests for Thyroid Alterations

Diagnostic Test	Purpose	Comments
Serum levels		
Thyroxine (T4)	Detects actual level of circulating thyroid hormone, binding proteins, and TSH	T4 level is low and TSH level is usually high in hypothyroidism; T4 level is high and TSH level is low in hyperthyroidism
Thyroid stimulating hormone (TSH)		
T3 radioimmunoassay		
Thyroid binding globulin		
Thyroid releasing hormone (TRH) stimulation test	TRH stimulates TSH production; evaluates pituitary reserve	
Thyroid stimulating immunoglobulins	Done when Graves disease suspected	Positive in Graves disease patient
Antimicrosomal antibodies	Done when Graves or Hashimoto disease suspected	Usually positive with either
Antithyroglobulin antibodies		
Radioactive iodine 123 (^{123}I) uptake and scan	Identifies location and size of gland; assesses function of gland Differentiates between an absent gland, a small dysplastic gland, and a gland of normal size that is over- or underfunctioning	Infant swallows ^{123}I; thyroid gland uptake of ^{123}I is measured at 2, 4, 6 and 24 hrs after ingestion of ^{123}I Verify that patient is not allergic to iodine before test
Technetium scan	Identifies location and size of gland; does not assess function of gland	Requires an intravenous line for injection of technetium, which is incorporated into thyroid gland Scan is done immediately after injection of technetium
Knee radiograph	Assesses skeletal maturation in infants	Delayed bone maturation on knee film indicates that low levels of thyroid hormone were present during gestation
Bone age radiograph (hand and wrist)	Assesses skeletal maturation in children	Delayed bone age in children is seen in hypothyroidism

for over 20 hours. These infants often have feeding difficulties, prolonged physiologic jaundice, lethargy, and constipation. Parents often describe their babies as good, quiet babies who sleep a lot, seldom cry, and are difficult to keep awake while feeding. On physical examination, only 10 to 15 per cent of the hypothyroid newborn infants have the classic "cretinoid" findings: puffy face with coarse features; open posterior fontanel; wide anterior fontanel and sutures; flattened nasal bridge; large, protruding tongue; low anterior hairline; hoarse cry; protuberant abdomen with an umbilical hernia; cool and mottled skin; hypotonia; and sluggish reflexes (Fort, 1990) (Fig. 43–8).

Diagnostic Assessment

The initial screening test for congenital hypothyroidism is usually included in a panel of newborn screening tests. Most newborn hypothyroid screening programs use filter paper blood spot measurements. A T4 level is determined; if it is low, a TSH level is obtained from the same specimen. Repeated studies on blood obtained by venipuncture are done to verify thyroid hormone levels obtained on initial filter paper screening. Because up to 10 per cent of infants can be missed by initial newborn screening, the American Academy of Pediatrics recommends thyroid function testing of any infant with a clinical presentation or history that is suggestive of congenital hypothyroidism. Scintiscanning is done with technetium to provide an image of the thyroid tissue; alternatively, radioactive iodine 123 uptake and scan are performed to identify the location, size, and function of thyroid tissue. If an ectopic gland is identified (usually at the base of the tongue), the diagnosis of permanent hypothyroidism requiring lifelong thyroid hormone replacement is made. Knee radiographs can be done in infants with suspected hypothyroidism. Delayed bone maturation indicates that low levels of thyroid hormone were present during gestation. A TRH stimulation test is done in infants with low T4 *and* low TSH levels. If the T4 level is low, the TSH level usually increases to stimulate the gland to produce more T4. The TRH stimulation test is performed to determine whether the pituitary can make TSH.

Therapeutic Management

The treatment of choice for hypothyroidism is oral levothyroxine. Dosage is based on weight, age, and response to therapy. The goal of therapy is to raise

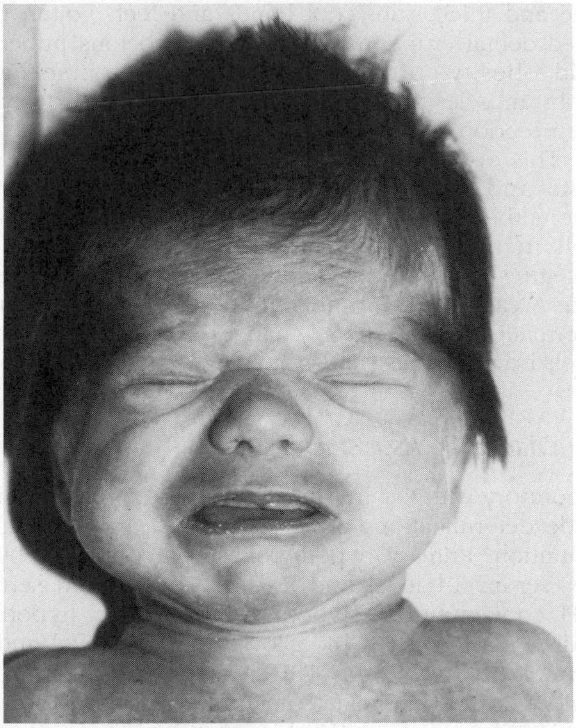

FIGURE 43 - 8. A 21-day-old infant with congenital hypothyroidism. Note the subtle clinical findings of puffy face with low anterior hairline, flattened nasal bridge, and mottled skin.

serum T3 levels into the normal range and T4 levels into the upper range of normal as quickly as possible. It may take several months for the serum TSH level to fall to normal, so it should not be used as the sole measure of response in the young infant. Laboratory thyroid function tests should be done regularly, especially during infancy. Signs and symptoms of excessive levothyroxine include fussiness, disturbance of sleep, excessive food and fluid intake with poor weight gain or weight loss, jitteriness, increased stooling with or without diarrhea, and heat intolerance. (Hung, 1992).

Nursing Diagnostic Statements

For infants having delayed diagnosis or inadequate treatment:

Altered growth and development:
- *Impaired growth of skeletal and nervous tissue, related to congenital insufficiency of thyroid hormone.*
- *Impaired intellect, related to deprivation of thyroid hormone in early infancy.*

Ineffective family coping, *related to the potential for mental retardation.*

Knowledge deficit:
- *Resources to facilitate development in child with mental retardation.*

For infants diagnosed and begun on adequate treatment at less than 1 month of age:

Knowledge deficit: parents initially, child later, *related to*
- *Cause of disorder and function of thyroid hormone within the body.*
- *Administration of levothyroxine.*
- *Signs and symptoms of hypothyroidism and hyperthyroidism.*
- *Need for genetic counseling for families of infants with dyshormonogenesis.*
- *Need for continuing follow-up care.*

Nursing Care

Supporting the Family in the Initial Diagnostic Period. Parents may become frightened when they learn that their baby has congenital hypothyroidism. They may have no idea where a thyroid gland is or what it does. They may feel guilty that somehow they did something to cause their child to be born with an absent or abnormal thyroid gland. It is important to reassure parents that their child's disorder did not result from anything they did or did not do during pregnancy. Many parents believe that congenital hypothyroidism must result in cretinism and irreversible mental retardation. They must be reassured that early screening, diagnosis, and treatment of their infant's disorder can prevent these problems (Klein, 1990).

Providing Information to Support Home Care. Treatment of congenital hypothyroidism is synthetic thyroid hormone (levothyroxine), started at a dose of 0.025 mg to 0.05 mg daily. The nurse teaches the parents to crush and mix the tablet with a teaspoon of water or formula and to administer the mixture through an eye dropper, a 5-ml syringe, or the nipple of a baby bottle. The tablets have an acceptable taste and have no side effects if given at the appropriate dosage. The nurse explains the importance of giving the thyroid replacement every day. The tablet should not be dissolved in a full bottle of formula because a full dose will not be received if the baby does not finish the bottle. With the relatively rare exception of infants having a transient metabolic block, the parents must be aware that their child will always be on thyroid replacement. They may ask if giving more thyroid hormone than is recommended will help their child grow faster or become smarter. Just as too little is harmful, too much thyroid hormone will speed up body metabolism to a dangerous level. Extra thyroid hormone does not make babies grow faster, nor will it make them smarter. Parents should be prepared for a change in their infant's behavior after treatment is started. The infant will have an increased appetite, stool more often, sleep less, be more alert, cry more, and be more demanding.

Parents often express concern about the occurrence of congenital hypothyroidism in future children.

The probability of siblings being affected depends on the cause of the disorder, and genetic counseling is appropriate if the diagnosis indicates a genetic cause. Thyroid dysgenesis usually occurs sporadically, and siblings of children with the disorder are not at a significantly higher risk of being affected than are persons in the general population. Inborn errors of thyroid hormone synthesis are autosomal recessive in inheritance, and siblings of a child with such a disorder have a 1:4 chance of being affected.

As infants grow, their need for thyroid replacement increases. Parents must be aware of the importance of close medical follow-up, especially during the first years of life. Blood thyroid levels should be checked frequently the first 2 years and at least every 6 months during childhood. Infants with congenital hypothyroidism whose condition is detected and who are treated before 1 month of age are expected to have normal linear growth, bone maturation, sexual development, and mental development (Klein, 1990).

Acquired Hypothyroidism

Etiology/Incidence

The incidence of acquired hypothyroidism in children is estimated to be 1 per 500 to 1 per 1000 (Foley, 1982). The most common cause is chronic lymphocytic thyroiditis (Hashimoto thyroiditis), an autoimmune disorder in which the thyroid gland is incorrectly recognized by the body to be foreign and is destroyed. There is frequently a family history of thyroid disease. Goitrogens, substances that decrease thyroid hormone production, can also lead to hypothyroidism. Goitrogen-induced hypothyroidism may be seen in children ingesting iodine-containing expectorants for asthma or cystic fibrosis or antithyroid drugs for hyperthyroidism. Hypothyroidism may follow radioactive iodine treatment for hyperthyroidism as well as partial or total thyroidectomy. Hypothalamic or pituitary disease as a result of tumors, trauma, infection, or radiation therapy can lead to hypothyroidism owing to a deficiency of either TRH or TSH. Finally, hypothyroidism may occur in certain diseases such as cystinosis or histiocytosis owing to infiltration or destruction of the thyroid gland or pituitary gland.

Clinical Manifestations

The most prominent feature of acquired hypothyroidism in children is growth failure. The child may also experience generalized puffiness, decreased appetite, constipation, thyroid gland enlargement (goiter), lethargy, and cold intolerance. Acquired hypothyroidism due to chronic lymphocytic thyroiditis is often insidious in onset, and the most common presentation is a decrease in the growth rate, which may be accompanied by a goiter. On physical examination, the child may have short stature; a dull, placid expression; slow pulse; decreased blood pressure; pale and thick skin; cool hands and feet; goiter; delayed dental eruption; delayed or precocious puberty; mild obesity; protuberant abdomen; coarse hair; flabby muscles with pseudohypertrophy; and delayed deep tendon reflexes (Dallas & Foley, 1990).

This disorder emphasizes the importance of complete and accurate growth charts on all patients whom the nurse observes. A child who has grown well in the past but suddenly reaches a growth plateau should be brought to the physician's attention. A careful interim nursing history may elicit much information about subtle changes in appetite, energy level, bowel habits, and school performance.

Diagnostic Assessment

Laboratory studies in suspected hypothyroidism include determinations of serum T4, T3, and TSH concentration. Primary hypothyroidism is confirmed by a low serum T4 level and T3 and an elevated serum TSH concentration. Hypothalamic-pituitary hypothyroidism is diagnosed by a low serum T4 level and a normal or low serum TSH level. Positive antithyroglobulin and antimicrosomal antibodies indicate an autoimmune etiology (Hashimoto thyroiditis).

Therapeutic Management

The treatment for acquired hypothyroidism is levothyroxine, and the dosage is individualized on the basis of weight, age, and clinical and biochemical response. The goals of treatment are to achieve a euthyroid state, with normal growth and development.

Nursing Care

The nurse should reassure the child and parents that if hypothyroidism develops beyond age 2 years, there is no risk of permanent intellectual impairment, and all changes seen in the child should be reversible. However, it should be pointed out that children with long-standing hypothyroidism may miss out on important learning experiences and that their genetically predestined height potential may not be fully attained in spite of "catch up" growth after beginning treatment. The nurse should emphasize the importance of taking the thyroid replacement doses as ordered, explaining that symptoms of hypothyroidism will recur within a few weeks if treatment is discontinued. Levothyroxine is inexpensive, has an acceptable taste, is readily available in pharmacies, and can be chewed by children who cannot swallow whole tablets.

Families should be prepared for changes in their child's behavior once treatment is begun. The child will be more alert and active, have an increased appetite, and display typical behaviors (both desirable and undesirable) for their age. Children who had long-standing hypothyroidism may go through a readjustment period that may affect their school performance. Stimuli will no longer be screened out by hypothyroidism, and the child may be distractable and have difficulty concentrating. This adjustment period should not persist for more than a few months.

Graves Disease (Hyperthyroidism)

Graves disease, or "diffuse toxic goiter," accounts for approximately 95 per cent of hyperthyroidism in children. Hyperthyroidism is characterized by an accelerated metabolism of all body tissues secondary to an increased production of thyroid hormones (Dallas & Foley, 1990).

Etiology/Incidence

The increased production of thyroid hormones is caused by an autoimmune process that may have a genetic as well as an immunologic base. Although Graves disease may occur at any age, it is rare in infants and young children. The incidence increases with age, and the majority of cases occur during adolescence. It is more common in girls in a ratio of approximately 3:1 to 5:1. The incidence is increased in children with Down syndrome, rubella syndrome, or a family history of other autoimmune diseases. It may coexist with autoimmune thyroiditis to provide "hashitoxicosis." There is often a history of a severe physical or emotional stress "triggering" the onset of Graves disease (Dallas & Foley, 1990). There is also frequently a family history of thyroid disease.

Clinical Manifestations

The clinical manifestations of Graves disease include nervousness, emotional lability, increased appetite, weight loss, school problems, exophthalmos, sleep disturbances, heat intolerance, and tachycardia. Fatigue and poor endurance in physical activities are common complaints. The thyroid gland is enlarged and is usually firm, smooth, and nontender. There may be increased systolic blood pressure. The skin may be flushed, with a smooth texture, and the hair is sometimes thinned. Hyperactive behavior is common, and a tremor in the hands is seen when the patient extends the arms and spreads the fingers.

Diagnostic Assessment

The diagnosis of Graves disease is frequently missed for months; the symptoms usually develop over time. Teachers may complain of the child's poor attention span, failure to complete work, and emotional lability. The symptoms are frequently thought by parents to be part of a normal adolescence process, and they may feel guilty about having delayed medical attention for their child.

Laboratory studies show an increase in serum T4 and T3 levels with low TSH concentration. Thyroid receptor antibodies and thyroid stimulating immunoglobulins are found in nearly 100 per cent of patients with Graves disease. Antimicrosomal and antithyroglobulin antibodies may also be present. (See Chapter 37 for further discussion of autoimmunity.) A radioactive iodine uptake test shows very high uptake of iodine owing to overactivity of the gland.

Therapeutic Management

Three modes of therapy are currently used for the treatment of Graves disease: (1) antithyroid drugs to block the synthesis of thyroxine; (2) destruction of the thyroid by radioiodine; and (3) subtotal thyroidectomy. Severe cardiovascular symptoms are treated with beta-blocking medications. Most children under 18 years of age are treated initially with antithyroid drugs (propylthiouracil or methimazole) (Fisher, 1990). If the drug is properly administered, a patient will usually develop normal thyroid hormone levels within 6 weeks. Treatment with antithyroid drugs is safe and inexpensive, but it requires taking pills three times a day. The more common side effects of the drugs include pruritus (itching), skin rash, urticaria, stomach irritation, and joint pains. Most reactions are mild and necessitate either reducing the dosage or changing drugs.

A rare but serious side effect of antithyroid drugs is agranulocytosis. Any child on these drugs who develops a fever, sore throat, or respiratory infection should discontinue therapy and obtain a complete blood count with differential immediately. Therapy can be resumed if the laboratory results are normal. Various studies have estimated the remission rate with medical treatment at 30 to 61 per cent, with approximately 25 per cent achieving a remission after 2 years of therapy. Relapse is common, and the family must be aware of the need to report the recurrence of symptoms (Fisher, 1990; Hung, 1992).

Surgical treatment with subtotal thyroidectomy is effective and safe when performed by a highly skilled surgeon under optimal conditions. The child must be prepared for surgery by achieving a euthyroid state, followed by treatment with iodine (Lugol solution) for 1 to 2 weeks to cause involution and decreased vascularity of the thyroid gland. Complications of surgery include transient hypocalcemia, hypoparathyroidism, damage to one or both recurrent laryngeal nerves, wound infection, hemorrhage, keloid formation, and recurrence of hyperthyroidism. More than 50 per cent of children will develop hypothyroidism after surgery and require thyroid hormone replacement (Hung, 1992).

Radioiodide therapy to ablate the thyroid gland has been controversial because of concern about a possible increased risk of neoplasm or genetic damage. Review of long-term data on children treated with radioiodide therapy shows no increased incidence of risk for neoplasms or genetic defects in their offspring. Most children will develop hypothyroidism after treatment and must be prescribed thyroid hormone replacement. There may be an increased risk of hypoparathyroidism associated with radioiodide treatment. Radioiodide therapy appears to be an acceptable treatment option for children who have toxic reactions with antithyroid drugs or fail to achieve remission (Dallas & Foley, 1990; Hamburger, 1985).

Graves ophthalmopathy includes exophthalmos, lid retraction, stare, mild itching of the eyes, and lacrimation. The cause is unknown but is believed to have an autoimmune base. However, there is no correlation between the degree of eye involvement and the severity of thyrotoxicosis. After therapy, the eyes often improve, but one fourth of the patients have no change. Progressive Graves ophthalmopathy is extremely rare in children.

Nursing Diagnostic Statements

Altered growth and development: accelerated metabolism, *related to increased production of thyroid hormones.*

Disturbance in self-concept: body image, *related to disease-induced changes in emotions, weight, skin, hair, and eyes.*

Knowledge deficit: child and parents, *related to*

- *Cause of the disease and normal thyroid function.*
- *Treatment, including side effects of antithyroid drugs.*
- *Postoperative home care.*

High risk for injury; *risk factors:*

- *Complications of thyroid surgery:*
- *Hemorrhage.*
- *Laryngeal nerve damage.*
- *Transient hypocalcemia.*
- *Resection of thyroid gland.*

Nursing Care

Nursing care for the child with Graves disease will be influenced by the type of treatment prescribed. Major nursing goals will always include family support and teaching and management of symptoms. Should surgery be necessary, postoperative care and teaching will be a major nursing focus.

Supporting a Healthy Body Image. The physical and emotional changes associated with hypersecretion of thyroid hormones can be troubling for any client but especially so for the adolescent who is already sensitive to changes in body image as the result of normal development. The nurse will be challenged to assist the adolescent with maintenance of a healthy body image by teaching symptom control through environmental manipulation.

The nurse can be an effective liaison person with the school in helping to decrease preventable stresses in the young client's daily routine. Nervousness and emotional lability often respond to increased rest, a quieter environment, and decreased demands. School personnel will usually be cooperative when they realize specific ways in which they can help before drug or surgical interventions can afford symptom relief.

Young persons with Graves disease may be quite concerned about emotional lability and wonder if they are "going crazy." The nurse's reassurance about the temporary nature of these episodes along with support for both the child and family can be invaluable in restoring normal family relations.

If ophthalmopathy is present as the result of Graves disease, the young client and the family should know that these changes in eye appearance usually improve with therapy.

Providing Information to Support Home Care. The child and family may need advice about nutritious ways to increase the child's calorie intake to meet increased metabolic needs. They should be advised that this is a temporary measure, which will no longer be necessary once control is achieved through therapy.

Heat intolerance can be eased by commonsense measures, such as loose-fitting cotton clothing, adequate ventilation, and attention to body hygiene. The family may need to be reminded that the child's intolerance for heat is legitimate, however.

Monitoring for Postoperative Complications. Should surgery be necessary, postoperative assessment will include the major risks of hemorrhage, laryngeal nerve damage, and transient hypocalcemia. Postoperatively, the patient should be carefully observed for hemorrhage at the operative site, swelling, dyspnea, and cyanosis. Occurrence of any of these signs demands immediate medical attention. Suction equipment and tracheostomy trays should be available at the bedside.

Damage to a recurrent laryngeal nerve results in hoarseness that usually improves, but damage to both nerves may result in severe stridor and may also require tracheostomy. The patient should be checked for hoarseness and for pitch and tone of voice every hour for the first 24 hours after surgery.

Signs of hypocalcemia (numbness, tingling, twitching, tetany) usually appear 24 hours after surgery. The patient should be assessed for the Trousseau and Chvostek signs. *Trousseau sign* includes carpal spasms of the fingers and hands after application of a pressure cuff to the arm. *Chvostek sign,* spasms of the facial muscles elicited by tapping the face in front of the ear, indicates hyperirritability of the facial nerve. Mild hypocalcemia can usually be controlled with oral calcium, and several weeks may be required for determining whether the condition is permanent. Hypothyroidism, should it occur, usually develops within 1 year of surgery.

Tumors of the Thyroid

Tumors of the thyroid gland are rare in children, and they differ from those in adults in that they tend to be more benign.

Incidence

Of all children presenting with a nodule in a thyroid, approximately one third will have a malignant carcinoma and one third will have a benign adenoma (Kaplan, 1990). A history of radiation to the head or neck is a significant risk factor for malignant neoplasm. The remaining lesions that cause nodularity include thyroiditis, thyroid abscess, cysts, absence of one lobe, and multinodular goiter.

Benign adenomas are well-encapsulated solitary tumors that do not metastasize to distant sites. The tumor is smooth and firm on palpation. Treatment is usually surgical removal of the nodule. Malignant carcinomas often cause a firm, irregular, nontender nodule or a woody-hard enlargement of the lobe or part of the lobe. Lymph node metastasis is common, but metastasis to lung and bone may occur.

Diagnostic Assessment

The discovery of the thyroid nodule warrants immediate medical attention. The patient's neck is examined for size and consistency of the nodule and for tenderness and presence of enlarged lymph nodes. Tenderness may suggest thyroiditis rather than a tumor. Enlarged lymph nodes may indicate local invasion. Laboratory tests include T3, T4, and TSH tests, thyroid antibody tests, and calcitonin. Functional nodules can cause hyperthyroidism; however, the nodules are usually nonfunctioning. Antibody tests are usually positive with thyroiditis and are negative with tumors. A thyroid scan with technetium or iodine 123 is one of the most important tests in the diagnosis of thyroid nodules. The presence of a "cold" or inactive nodule in an otherwise normal gland suggests an adenoma or carcinoma. Ultrasonography and CT are helpful in determining whether thyroid nodules are solid or cystic. Fine needle biopsy can differentiate cystic, benign, and malignant nodules. If the nodule is malignant, an x-ray of the neck and chest is done to identify possible metastases (Fisher, 1990; Salas, 1990).

Therapeutic Management

Treatment of thyroid tumors is usually surgical removal of the involved lobe and lymph nodes. The prognosis for the great majority of malignant thyroid tumors is good, with the expectation of a normal life span.

Nursing Care

Nursing management of the child with a thyroid tumor involves psychosocial support and effective preoperative and postoperative care. The child and parents undergo severe emotional stress owing to the diagnosis, and the nurse must be available to listen to their feelings and offer support. Because of excellent prognosis of thyroid tumors, the health care team can offer optimistic projections about the tumor's course. Preoperative and postoperative care is discussed in the section "Graves Disease (Hyperthyroidism)."

The Parathyroid Glands

Normal Function of Parathyroids

The four parathyroid glands, embedded in the thyroid tissue, produce parathyroid hormone (PTH), which plays a vital role in regulating the balance of calcium and phosphorus in the body. Blood levels of calcium provide negative feedback to the parathyroid PTH production. High or very low blood levels of magnesium also inhibit PTH production. Hypocalcemia stimulates and hypercalcemia suppresses PTH synthesis and secretion. The major target organs of PTH are kidney, bone, and intestines. In the kidneys, the hormone promotes reabsorption of calcium; it also causes decreased serum phosphate by decreasing tubular resorption. In the intestine, PTH causes increased calcium and phosphorus absorption. *PTH acts directly on the bone tissue to cause increased osteoclastic activity,* resulting in increased calcium release from the bone. The net result of the actions of PTH on bone, kidney, and intestine is to increase blood levels of calcium and decrease blood levels of phosphorus (Mimouni & Tsang, 1990).

Clinical manifestations of parathyroid alterations are summarized in Table 43–9, and relevant diagnostic studies are noted in Table 43–10.

Hypoparathyroidism

Hypoparathyroidism is a condition in which there is a lack of production of PTH. Pseudohypoparathyroidism (PHP) is a condition in which there is increased production of PTH but deficient target organ responsiveness to the hormone. The two conditions are contrasted in Figure 43–9.

Etiology

Hypoparathyroidism can be primary or secondary. Primary disease is usually idiopathic (no cause detected). Transient neonatal hypoparathyroidism and syndromes of congenital absence of parathyroids occur early in life. Autoimmune destruction of the parathyroid glands is often associated with other autoimmune disorders and candidiasis. PHP is an inherited disease that affects girls approximately twice as often as boys. Familial instances of idiopathic hypoparathyroidism are uncommon. Secondary disease may occur after thyroid surgery, because the parathyroids are vulnerable to injury or accidental removal, or rarely after radioiodide ablation of the thyroid (Mimouni & Tsang, 1990).

Clinical Manifestations

In both idiopathic hypoparathyroidism and pseudohypoparathyroidism (PHP), clinical manifestations are

TABLE 43-9
Clinical Manifestations of Parathyroid Alterations

Clinical Manifestations	Reason for Clinical Manifestations	Significance to the Nurse
Parathyroid Hormone Deficiency		
Muscle cramps, twitching	Hypocalcemia leads to increased muscle irritability, decreased relaxation	Child may require intravenous calcium gluconate; keep at bedside
Tetany		
Paresthesias		
Chvostek, Trousseau signs		
Brittle hair	Decreased incorporation of calcium into teeth, hair, nails	
Thin nails		
Respiratory stridor		Keep tracheostomy tray at bedside; position head with pillow to facilitate breathing
Dry, coarse skin	Hypocalcemia	
Maculopapular skin rash		
Dermatitis		
Short stature (PHP)		
Thickset build (PHP)		
Round facies (PHP)		
Short fingers, toes (PHP)		
Mental retardation		Developmental evaluation indicated to help in school placement
Parathyroid Hormone Excess		
Renal colic	Hypocalcemia	Rare in children
Bone pain, masses		
Osteoporosis		

PHP = Pseudohypoparathyroidism.

secondary to hypocalcemia and include tetany, seizures (generalized tonic-clonic, absence seizures, and simple partial seizures), carpopedal spasms, muscle cramps or twitching, paresthesias, and respiratory stridor. The skin can be dry and coarse; maculopapular skin eruptions and eczematous dermatitis can occur. The hair is often brittle, with areas of alopecia. The nails are thin and brittle, and there is dental and enamel hypoplasia.

Children with PHP are short and thickset and have round facies and short, thick necks. The fingers and toes are short and stubby, with dimpled skin over the knuckles. Subcutaneous soft tissue calcification is common. Mental retardation is a more promi-

TABLE 43-10
Laboratory and Diagnostic Studies for Parathyroid Alterations

Laboratory or Diagnostic Test	Purpose	Comments
Blood studies		
Serum calcium	Assesses production of PTH by gland	Serum calcium levels low, phosphorus levels high in hypoparathyroidism; PTH levels low in idiopathic hypoparathyroidism, high in pseudohypoparathyroidism
Serum phosphorus		
Plasma parathyroid hormone (PTH)		
Skeletal radiograph	Assesses calcium deposition into bone	Osteoporosis seen in hyperparathyroidism

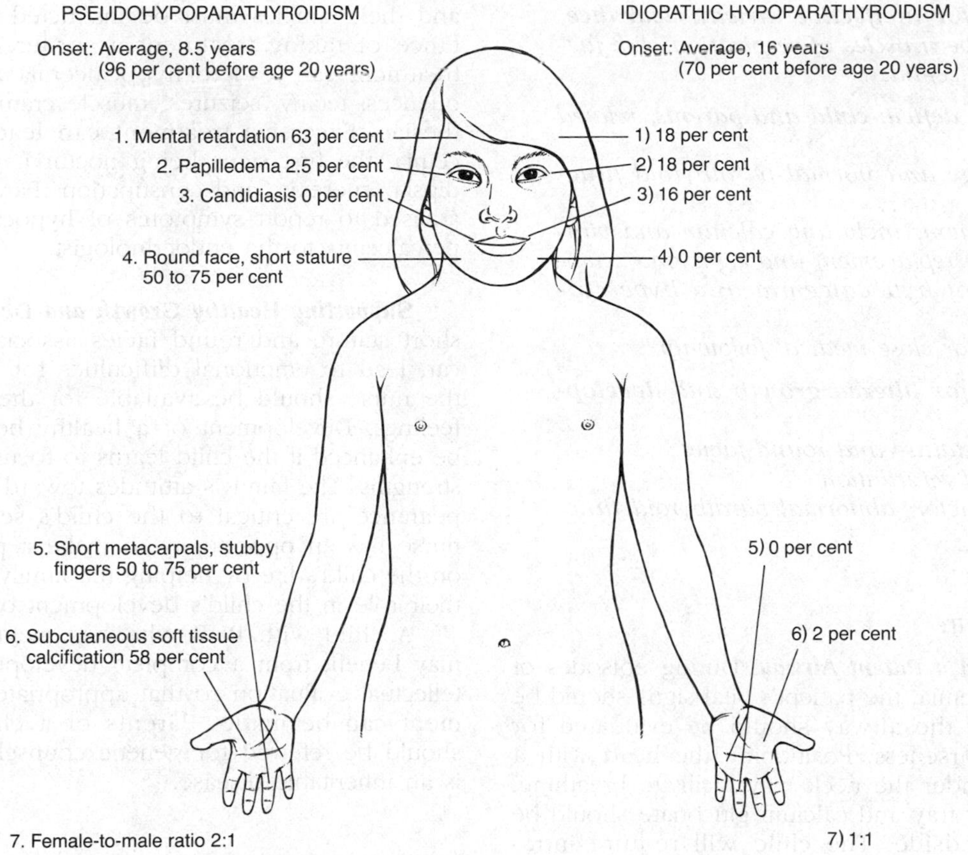

FIGURE 43 - 9. Comparison of effects of pseudohypoparathyroidism and idiopathic hypoparathyroidism.

nent feature of PHP than of hypoparathyroidism. Swings of emotion, loss of memory, depression, and confusion can occur.

Candidiasis of the nails and mouth occurs in hypoparathyroidism but is rare in PHP. In addition, papilledema, presumably related to increased intracranial pressure, may occur in hypoparathyroidism but is rare in PHP.

Diagnostic Assessment

The clinical diagnosis of hypoparathyroidism is made from the signs and symptoms described with decreased serum calcium and increased serum phosphorus levels. Laboratory studies to confirm the diagnosis include total and ionized calcium, phosphorus, magnesium, creatinine, alkaline phosphatase activity, 25-(OH)D_3, 1,25$(OH)_2D_3$, and PTH levels. In hypoparathyroidism, calcium is low, phosphorus is high, magnesium is usually normal, alkaline phosphatase is normal to high, and PTH is low for the calcium level. PHP differs from this laboratory profile by having a high PTH level. As stated earlier, the glands produce adequate levels of PTH, but end-organ unresponsiveness to the PTH sends the feedback message to the parathyroid glands to produce even more PTH (Mimouni & Tsang, 1990).

Therapeutic Management

The goal of treatment in all forms of hypoparathyroidism is the maintenance of normal serum calcium levels. Treatment for the child presenting with seizures or tetany is intravenous 10 per cent calcium gluconate. Patients with mild or partial hypoparathyroidism, as seen after subtotal thyroidectomy, may be treated with oral calcium salts alone. Patients with severe or complete hypoparathyroidism require treatment with vitamin D (which enhances intestinal calcium absorption) and oral calcium supplementation. Close medical follow-up is crucial to the well-being of children with hypoparathyroidism. Initially, serum calcium and phosphorus levels are checked twice a week until the patient has normal values. Subsequently, monthly, then quarterly, then semiannual checks are usually done. The child with hypoparathyroidism or PHP has an increased risk of developing other endocrine or autoimmune disorders (Mimouni & Tsang, 1990).

Nursing Diagnostic Statements

High risk for injury: physiologic: altered electrolytes, tetany, and seizure; *risk factors: increased phosphorus and decreased calcium associated with insufficient PTH.*

High risk for ineffective airway clearance, tetany of the muscles of respiration; *risk factor: hypocalcemia.*

Knowledge deficit: child and parents, *related to*

- *Etiology and normal parathyroid function.*
- *Treatment, including calcium and vitamin D replacement and signs and symptoms of hypocalcemia and hypercalcemia.*
- *Need for close medical follow-up.*

High risk for altered growth and development:

- *Short stature and round facies.*
- *Mental retardation.*
- *Risk factor: abnormal parathyroid function.*

Nursing Care

Maintaining a Patent Airway. During episodes of acute hypocalcemia, the patient's vital signs should be monitored and the airway should be evaluated for stridor and hoarseness. Positioning the head with a small pillow under the neck may facilitate breathing. A tracheostomy tray and calcium gluconate should be kept at the bedside. The child will require intravenous calcium during episodes of acute tetany. The patient should be evaluated frequently for tingling, stiffness, cramps, and tremors. Chvostek and Trousseau signs should also be checked. The child may benefit from decreased environmental stimuli, including decreased noise and soft lighting. Treatment during this acute phase should be explained completely to the child and parents.

Facilitating Home Management. Before discharge at time of diagnosis and at follow-up visits, patients and their families must be instructed on the importance of taking treatment as ordered. Inadequate treatment can lead to hypocalcemia and its consequences: tetany, seizures, muscle cramps, and paresthesias. Excessive treatment can lead to hypercalcemia, the first signs being nocturia, polyuria, polydipsia, anorexia, and constipation. Parents should be advised to report symptoms of hypocalcemia or hypercalcemia to the endocrinologist.

Supporting Healthy Growth and Development. The short stature and round facies associated with PHP can lead to emotional difficulties for the child, and the nurse should be available for the child to vent feelings. Development of a healthy body image will be enhanced if the child learns to focus on his or her strengths. The family's attitudes toward the child's appearance are critical to the child's self-esteem. The nurse has an opportunity to make a positive impact on the child's life by helping the family to understand their role in the child's development of self-esteem.

A child with PHP who has mental retardation may benefit from a complete developmental and intellectual evaluation so that appropriate school placement can be made. Parents of a child with PHP should be referred for genetic counseling because it is an inheritable disease.

The Gonads

An alteration in sexual development may be discovered at birth or at a later time in life when expected development does not occur. When such an abnormality is identified, clear information must be provided to facilitate the best possible adjustment. Some disorders require only minimal intervention, whereas others require long-term therapy. Clinical manifestations of gonadal disorders are presented in Table 43–11 and related diagnostic tests in Table 43–12.

TABLE 43-11
Clinical Manifestations of Gonadal Alterations

Clinical Manifestations	Reason	Significance to the Nurse
Ambiguous genitalia in newborn infant	Masculinized girl or undermasculinized boy	Considered a psychosocial emergency; pediatric endocrinologist must see infant immediately
Breast development in girls under age 7 yrs	Increased estrogen production by ovary or oral ingestion of estrogen	Ovarian production of excess estrogen can be caused by a tumor or cyst
Breast development in boys (gynecomastia)	Imbalance of testosterone-estrogen levels during early puberty; sex chromosome disorders; drug exposures	Breast tissue must be differentiated from fat padding in obese boys
Delayed secondary sexual characteristics	Decreased levels of sex steroids	

TABLE 43-12
Diagnostic Tests for Gonadal Alterations

Diagnostic Test	Purpose	Comments
Serum 17-hydroxyprogesterone	Identifies congenital adrenal hyperplasia in infants with ambiguous genitalia	
Serum testosterone	Assesses testicular production of testosterone	
Serum estradiol	Assesses ovarian production of estrogen	Levels are high in ovarian tumors, pubertal girls
Serum testosterone-estradiol ratio	Evaluates whether estradiol level is high in relation to testosterone in boys with gynecomastia	Testosterone is normally converted to estrogen in pubertal boys; sometimes there is an imbalance, and too much estrogen is produced
Chromosomal studies	Identify genetic sex of child with ambiguous genitalia, gynecomastia	
Bone age (left hand and wrist) radiograph	Assesses maturation of bones	High levels of estrogen or testosterone mature bones quickly
Human chorionic gonadotropin (HCG) stimulation test	Stimulates testosterone production	HCG given by intramuscular injection
Pelvic or abdominal ultrasonography	Assesses ovaries for size, masses, cysts	

Ambiguous Genitalia in the Newborn Infant

The neonate's external genitalia are described as ambiguous if there is (1) hypospadias with no palpable gonads, (2) hypospadias with one palpable gonad, or (3) micropenis with no palpable gonads (see Fig. 43–6) (Pagon, 1987). The presence of ambiguous genitalia in the newborn infant is considered a psychosocial emergency, and further diagnostic evaluation is performed as quickly as possible.

Etiology

Ambiguous genitalia can be caused by chromosomal abnormalities, CAH, placental transfer of masculinizing agents (girls), defective sex hormone synthesis (boys), and androgen insensitivity.

Diagnostic Assessment

Recognition of ambiguous genitalia often occurs in the delivery room when the doctor or nurse finds it difficult to judge whether the infant is a boy or a girl. A useful clinical classification of ambiguous genitalia is based on karyotype and presence and symmetry of gonads. A female pseudohermaphrodite has a 46,XX karyotype, ovaries, and virilized external genitalia. The most common cause of this is CAH; maternal virilizing tumors, maternal ingestion of androgens or progestational drugs, and maternal CAH are less common causes. A male pseudohermaphrodite has a 46,XY karyotype and varying degrees of external and internal virilization. Etiologic factors include abnormal development of the testes and abnormal androgen production or effect (Hung, 1992).

The diagnostic evaluation involves questions based on the physical examination. It is important to ask whether the appearance of the genitalia is consistent with partial male virilization along a normal pathway. Is this a genetic male infant who did not completely virilize, or is it a genetic female who is virilized? It is essential to assess whether gonads are palpable. Two scrotal or inguinal gonads suggest that the infant is an undermasculinized genetic male. A single, palpable gonad suggests mixed gonadal dysgenesis, in which the single gonad is abnormal. Mixed gonadal dysgenesis is associated with abnormal chromosome patterns. A single, palpable gonad may also be found in hermaphroditism, a condition in which both ovarian and testicular tissue are present.

An infant with ambiguous genitalia requires chromosomal studies. A 46,XX (female) karyotype in an infant with palpable gonads is suggestive of hermaphroditism. A diagnosis of true hermaphroditism requires histologic examination of gonadal tissue and recognition of both ovarian and testicular elements. A 45,X/46,XY karyotype is suggestive of mixed gonadal dysgenesis. Diagnosis of mixed gonadal dysgenesis requires demonstration of a unilateral testis and a contralateral absent, or streak, gonad. The single testis is structurally and functionally abnormal, and masculinization of the external genitalia is usually incomplete.

CAH is the most common cause of ambiguous genitalia in girls. Studies to rule out this disorder include serum 17-hydroxyprogesterone, testosterone, and gonadotropins. A pelvic ultrasound and genitogram are also done (Hung, 1990). In the undermasculinized male, blood studies are done to detect whether the infant is able to produce testosterone. An HCG stimulation test is done, in which HCG is administered to the infant to stimulate testosterone production. Infants with testosterone biosynthesis abnormalities are unable to produce increased levels of testosterone after stimulation by HCG. These infants are unable to produce adequate levels of testosterone to lead to masculinization. Imaging studies of the abdomen and pelvis may identify internal structures (ovaries, undescended testicles, uterus, and fallopian tubes).

Therapeutic Management

Treatment is based on the cause of the ambiguous genitalia. In infants with hermaphroditism and mixed gonadal dysgenesis, management involves choosing an appropriate gender assignment, maximizing the potential for adult sexual function, and minimizing psychosocial problems. Depending on the gender assignment chosen, surgical intervention is done as quickly as possible, and the child receives hormonal replacements at puberty. Treatment of CAH is discussed elsewhere in this chapter. Male infants with defective testosterone biosynthesis are treated with testosterone injections to complete the masculinization process and receive testosterone in their teenage years and adulthood to initiate puberty and sustain adult masculinization.

Nursing Care

The nurse must be available to offer emotional support, explanations of the condition, and information about the necessary medical, surgical, and hormonal treatments. Information should be provided in a manner that fosters both parental confidence in rearing the child and the development of a positive self-image in the child.

When an infant is born with ambiguous genitalia, factual information is presented to the parents (Mazur, 1984). They should be told that their infant's sex organs are "unfinished" or "underdeveloped" and that when external sex organs are underdeveloped, the internal ones may also be underdeveloped. After an evaluation by a specialist is completed, a sex assignment or reassignment is made. A decision is often complex and difficult for the professional as well as the family. Parents may require guidance or actual assistance in talking with their other children and family members. They may also require professional counseling to recognize, confront, and discuss their feelings. Refer to the bibliography at the end of the chapter for recommended readings that are helpful in explaining sexual development.

Premature Thelarche

Etiology

Premature thelarche is the isolated appearance of breast development in girls before 8 years of age.

The cause of premature thelarche is not clear, but it may be due to transient secretion of estrogen by the ovary. In infant girls, it may represent the failure to inhibit the "mini-puberty" seen in newborn infants. In older girls, it may be unsustained activation of pituitary gonadotropins (Rosenfield, 1990). It may also be seen in girls who have accidentally ingested oral contraceptives or estrogen preparations.

Clinical Manifestations

Premature thelarche must be differentiated from neonatal hyperplasia of the breast, which can occur in either sex and generally subsides spontaneously within a few weeks or months after birth. Breast development in premature thelarche is usually less than 4 to 5 cm of breast tissue under the areola. It often regresses over several months to a year, but it may persist even until the onset of normal puberty. Menses do not start until the usual age.

Diagnostic Assessment

Diagnosis of premature thelarche is made by ruling out all other causes of early breast development. A bone age x-ray study is often done. Serum total estrogen, estradiol, LH, and FSH level may be determined to detect excessive hormone production.

Therapeutic Management

Although follow-up observation to confirm the diagnosis is indicated, premature thelarche without accelerated growth, high estrogen levels, or other pubertal changes is a benign condition and does not require treatment. It does not predispose to abnormal pubertal development and has no effect on fertility or the occurrence of breast disorders.

Nursing Care

Although premature thelarche is a harmless condition, parents may experience emotional difficulty in adjusting to their daughter's body changes. They can be reassured that the breasts are unlikely to continue enlarging significantly and may even possibly regress in size. They should see no personality changes, growth spurt, facial acne, pubic hair, or axillary hair. If they do, their physician should be notified immediately. Puberty should begin at a normal age.

Gynecomastia

Gynecomastia, the growth of breast tissue in boys, can be either physiologic or pathologic. Physiologic gynecomastia is observed most commonly in neonatal and pubertal boys. It is a benign condition.

Gynecomastia occurs to varying degrees in 60 per cent or more of boys during adolescence. It is usually transient but may persist for 2 or 3 years. A pathologic cause should be suspected if gynecomastia occurs after the newborn period and before puberty (Oberfield & Levine, 1990).

Etiology

Neonatal gynecomastia is transient and is attributed to maternal hormones transmitted to the fetus during gestation. Adolescent gynecomastia is most often attributed to a transient imbalance in testosterone and estrogen levels in the body. This imbalance is normal and relatively common during puberty. Pathologic causes of gynecomastia include sex chromosome disorders, adrenal hyperplasia, hyperthyroidism, certain drug exposures (estrogens, testosterone, marijuana), and various types of tumors (Styne, 1990).

Diagnostic Assessment

The evaluation of gynecomastia includes an extensive history, including growth rate, rapidity, and time of onset; drug exposure; and familial incidence. The patient is examined for height, extent of sexual development, size and contour of breasts, and whether gynecomastia is unilateral or bilateral. Gynecomastia must be distinguished from the fat padding that frequently looks like breast tissue in obese individuals. Depending on the history and physical findings, hormone studies may be done. Skull x-rays or CT may be done if a brain tumor is suspected, and chromosome studies are done if Klinefelter syndrome (XXY karyotype) is suspected. (See Chapter 31 for additional information about Klinefelter syndrome.)

Therapeutic Management

The majority of boys with gynecomastia receive no treatment. In certain severe cases, plastic surgery is recommended. Research is currently being conducted on the use of liposuction and hormonal treatment of gynecomastia. Because obese boys tend to have a more noticeable problem, they are counseled to lose weight. In patients with associated disorders, the disorders are treated.

Nursing Care

Parents are often shocked to see that their newborn infant has enlarged breasts. The nurse can alleviate fears by discussing the effect of maternal hormones on the fetus and by assuring them that gynecomastia is transient. Gynecomastia can lead to varying degrees of psychologic difficulties for adolescent boys. Patients may wonder if they are transforming into girls, and the boys may be too embarrassed to remove their shirts during physical education class, during sports, or while playing with friends. The body image alterations can affect social interactions with peers, especially girls, during a time when interacting is already difficult.

The nurse can offer emotional support to the child by listening to his concerns. Certain clients may benefit from professional counseling. If the diagnostic studies indicate that the patient has transient pubertal gynecomastia, the nurse can reassure him that the problem is temporary. If surgery is used, scarring can usually be minimized by a periareolar incision.

Other Endocrine Disorders

Hypoglycemia

Hypoglycemia is not a disease; it describes a condition in which the blood glucose level falls below the acceptable range for the patient's size and age. In the neonate, hypoglycemia has been defined as two blood glucose values less than 30 mg/dl in full-term infants, or less than 20 mg/dl in infants who are premature or small for gestational age. However, concern that these levels may have a detrimental effect on brain development has led some clinicians to recommend 40 mg/dl as the standard for newborn infants. After the newborn period, hypoglycemia is uniformly defined as blood glucose levels below 40 mg/dl. It is essential to consider the method used to obtain blood glucose values. Whole blood gives values 10 to 15 per cent less than plasma or serum levels, and blood glucose levels can fall by up to 18 mg/dl an hour in specimens not treated with a glycolysis inhibitor (Geffner, 1990; Glasgow, 1992; LaFranchi, 1987).

Etiology

The cause of most hypoglycemia is related to either overuse of glucose or underproduction of glucose. Overuse of glucose is caused by insulin dysregulation; underproduction of glucose is caused by the lack of adequate conversion of glucose precursors into glucose (Geffner, 1990).

Approximately 50 per cent of neonates with hypoglycemia have an asymptomatic transitional form. The low blood sugars tend to occur during the first 6 to 12 hours of life, often in association with perinatal distress, delayed feedings, or diabetes in the mother. Symptomatic, transient hypoglycemia is seen in infants who are small for gestational age; boys predominate in a ratio of 2.5 : 1. If symptoms persist or fail to clear completely after correction of hypoglycemia, a search is made for another underlying or associated abnormality. Such abnormalities include sepsis, hydrops fetalis, congenital heart disease, hypothyroidism, asphyxia, drugs given to the mother, or central nervous system defects or infections. Approximately 35 per cent of infants with neonatal hypoglycemia have other associated disease states. In rare cases (1 to 2 per cent of all newborn infants with hypoglycemia) in which symptoms persist or recur in spite of treatment, specific primary causes must be investigated. These causes include an excess production of insulin, hereditary defects of carbohydrate or amino acid metabolism, and pituitary hormone deficiencies.

In the first year of life, an excess production of

insulin accounts for over 50 per cent of cases of hypoglycemia. The second most frequent cause is liver enzyme deficiencies, leading to an inability of the liver to transform glycogen into glucose. Ketotic hypoglycemia accounts for up to 95 per cent of hypoglycemia after infancy. The child usually experiences hypoglycemia in the early morning after a small supper and long sleep. The child may be small and underweight and may have an associated isolated or combined hormone deficiency. Another cause of persistent hypoglycemia in a child of any age is a pancreatic islet cell tumor. Causes of acute isolated episodes of hypoglycemia include inappropriate periods of fasting for age, alcohol ingestion, oral hypoglycemic agent ingestion, and severe illness such as Reye syndrome (Glasgow, 1992).

Clinical Manifestations

The symptoms of hypoglycemia in the infant range from localized or generalized seizures to simple irritability. Episodes of jitteriness, cyanosis, limpness, apnea, or irregular respirations are common, and difficulty in feeding and abnormal cry and apathy have been described. The older infant and young child may experience sweating, shakiness, hunger, headache, nausea, anxiety, pallor, staring, listlessness or irritability, motor incoordination, ataxia, inattention, coma, or convulsions.

Diagnostic Assessment

There are many approaches to the diagnostic assessment of hypoglycemia. All emphasize the need to obtain a blood specimen at the time of suspected hypoglycemia. Laboratory studies may include serum glucose and insulin (from the same specimen), ketones, cortisol, growth hormone, lactate, and beta-hydroxybutyrate. Many other laboratory studies may be necessary to establish a diagnosis and should be tailored to the clinical presentation. "Reactive hypoglycemia" has been described as a "non-disease of epidemic proportion" (Geffner, 1990; LaFranchi, 1987). Because of widespread misunderstanding in both the general population and the medical community, the American Diabetes Association, the American Medical Association, and the Endocrine Society recommend that the diagnosis be reserved for cases in which documented blood glucose levels less than 40 mg/dl occur at the time of symptoms and that the symptoms be relieved by eating (LaFranchi, 1987). The documentation is best done at the time of spontaneous symptoms or, alternatively, after eating a mixed meal. Oral glucose tolerance tests are unreliable for diagnosing this disorder (Geffner, 1990; LaFranchi, 1987).

Therapeutic Management

Neonates with asymptomatic or symptomatic transient hypoglycemia are treated with an intravenous infusion of glucose until the blood glucose values are restored to normal. Infants with persistent hypoglycemia due to severe forms of glycogen storage disease will need frequent feedings during the day and continuous nasogastric feedings at night. Milder disorders causing reduced glucose production may only require avoidance of prolonged fasts. Adding cornstarch or tapioca to feedings may be helpful in extending the length of time between feedings for these children. Hypoglycemia caused by hormone deficiencies (cortisol, growth hormone, thyroxine) is treated with replacement of the missing hormone or hormones. Hypoglycemia caused by hyperinsulinism is initially treated medically with oral diazoxide and frequent feedings. Diazoxide works by suppressing insulin secretion. If diazoxide is ineffective or not tolerated, surgical treatment with a 70 per cent pancreatectomy may be necessary. Idiopathic ketotic hypoglycemia is treated with frequent feedings and the avoidance of long fasts (Geffner, 1990; LaFranchi, 1987).

Nursing Diagnostic Statements

High risk for injury: neurologic; risk factor: insufficient serum glucose to meet cerebral metabolic needs.

Knowledge deficit: parents, *related to*

- *Etiology and pathophysiology.*
- *Technique for performing Chemstrip testing at home.*
- *Treatment of hypoglycemic reactions with carbohydrate foods, intramuscular glucagon, or buccal glucose preparations.*
- *Need to avoid products containing alcohol.*

Nursing Care

Assisting with Detection. Because half of the neonates with hypoglycemia are asymptomatic, the nurse must accurately perform Dextrostix or Chemstrip testing on each infant to detect the problem. Technique is crucial to the accuracy of the readings, and low readings should be verified by laboratory analysis. Bilirubin in plasma and isopropyl alcohol applied to the skin may significantly reduce the apparent glucose value obtained with Dextrostix (Fox & Redstone, 1976; Grazaitis & Sexson, 1980). If a full-term infant has a blood glucose level below 30 mg/dl, a physician is notified, a blood sample is drawn for laboratory confirmation, and an intravenous line is started immediately for glucose administration. The infant is assessed closely for symptoms, and blood glucose levels are evaluated for response to treatment. If the infant is unresponsive to treatment, the nurse assists in coordinating studies to detect associated abnormalities.

Facilitating Home Management. The nurse caring for the toddler and young child must be knowledgeable about the symptoms of hypoglycemia in order to discuss them with parents. A history of repeated clusters of hypoglycemic symptoms should be clarified for frequency, usual time of day of onset of symptoms, association with eating patterns, and severity. Obtaining a blood glucose level at the time of symptoms is critical, and parents can be taught to accurately perform Chemstrip testing at home. Urine testing for ketones may also be indicated in toddlers and children suspected of having ketotic hypoglycemia. Parents should be instructed on the use of the Chemstrip UK test for urinary ketones. If hypoglycemia is documented, the parents are instructed to feed the child immediately to prevent worsening of symptoms. A glass of juice or regular soda is often readily available and effective. Honey, cake frosting, or commercial glucose gels (Glutose, Monogel) can be used by squeezing them between the cheek and gum of the mouth. The buccal mucosal capillaries absorb the glucose into the blood stream. An intramuscular or subcutaneous injection of glucagon will raise blood glucose levels by causing the liver to release stored glucose (glycogen). It can be given as an emergency treatment for a child who is unconscious or unable to swallow and who has normal liver glycogen stores. If glucagon is indicated for emergency treatment, the family must be instructed in its use.

Parents should be instructed at well child visits that alcohol ingestion in toddlers and young children can lead to hypoglycemia. Commercially available mouthwashes contain ethanol, with concentrations ranging from 14 per cent in Cepacol to 26.9 per cent in Listerine. Alcoholic drinks should be discarded after parties in households with young children, and "tasting" of alcoholic beverages by youngsters should not be permitted. As with any other medications, oral hypoglycemic agents, often found in grandparents' homes, should be placed where children cannot reach them.

The Pancreas

Normal Function of the Pancreas

The pancreas is situated behind the stomach in a horizontal position with its head firmly attached to the duodenum by the pancreatic duct (duct of Wirsung) and its tail reaching to the spleen. The pancreas is made up of two distinct types of tissues: (1) the acini, which excrete digestive juices through ducts into the duodenum, and (2) the islets of Langerhans, which secrete insulin (from the beta cells) and glucagon (from the alpha cells) directly into the blood stream. The pancreas, therefore, is both an exocrine (duct-type) and an endocrine (ductless) gland.

Pancreatic juice, excreted through the pancreatic ducts into the duodenum, is important to the digestion of carbohydrates, fats, and proteins. The hormones insulin and glucagon play an important role in carbohydrate metabolism.

Diabetes Mellitus

Diabetes mellitus (DM) is the most common endocrine disease of childhood. Although DM has been diagnosed for centuries, the causes, prevention, and cure still remain obscure. The word "diabetes" originates from the Greek language and means *siphon* or *flow through,* relating to the increased loss of body fluids with increased urination. The word "mellitus" means *sugary* or *honey-like* in Latin and differentiates DM ("sugar diabetes") from diabetes insipidus ("bland diabetes"). The latter is a disease of the posterior pituitary gland.

Etiology/Incidence

Diabetes mellitus results from either a relative (type II) or an absolute (type I) deficiency of pancreatic insulin. This results in chronic high blood sugar and other problems with carbohydrate and fat metabolism.

The causes of type I DM are not completely understood, but increasing research (over the past decade) has produced a much clearer understanding of how the beta cell in the pancreas is destroyed. Many investigators have thought that type I DM has a genetic component, but the mode of inheritance is still not well defined. There is some evidence that genetic predisposition is an important factor to consider, but the disease is generally not considered to be inherited.

Some epidemiologic studies and animal experiments indicate that environmental factors may play a role in the cause. Notkins (1979) suggests that viral infection may be a significant antecedent, on the basis of the following findings: (1) increased levels of coxsackie B4 virus in newly diagnosed children; (2) increased seasonal diagnosis in the winter months; and (3) onset of DM after mumps infections. The viral theorists suggest that certain genetic factors (HLA configurations [see Chapter 37]) can make an individual more susceptible to viral infections. However, confirmation of the role viruses play in human diabetes is still uncertain. Still other investigators (Nemchik, 1982) suggest that a genetic predisposition and HLA-directed response to viral infections lead to beta cell destruction and consequently to the development of type I diabetes in children.

It is now fairly well accepted that the autoimmune response is involved in some way in beta cell destruction. Research has revealed the presence of minor abnormalities in the islet cells of the pancreas, resulting in islet cell antibodies, which are present in about 70 per cent of newly diagnosed diabetics. Islet cell antibodies are sometimes present in relatives of people with type I diabetes, making islet cell antibodies a possible indicator of an individual's potential to develop DM. Other factors, including diabetogenic drugs, gross pancreatic disease (in chronic illnesses such as cystic fibrosis), and obesity can also contribute to the development of diabetes.

Owing to several difficulties in obtaining exact statistics, published estimates of both the prevalence and incidence of DM vary. In the United States, the incidence is approximately 12 to 15 newly diagnosed cases of type I (insulin-dependent) per 100,000 population yearly in children younger than 19 years of age. Although the incidence may be as high as 30 per 100,000 in some parts of Scandinavia, prevalence and incidence of insulin-dependent diabetes in Great Britain, Sweden, and Australia are similar to those reported in the United States (Sperling, 1992).

In the United States, the incidence for African-Americans is only about 66 per cent of the incidence for whites (Sperling, 1992). However, the causes of diabetes in African-American children are more diverse. Although most African-American children with youth-onset diabetes have type I DM, at least 10 per cent have atypical diabetes that does not appear to result from autoimmune beta cell destruction (Winter, 1991). The incidence of insulin-dependent DM is the same across a population of boys and girls, but the incidence increases with increasing age (i.e., a child is more likely to be diagnosed as having DM at 16 years of age than at 5 years). Type I DM is most common in the 10- to 14-year-old age group.

According to the National Diabetic Commission Report, in 1980 there were 10 to 12 million people with diabetes in the United States: between 5 and 6 million diagnosed diabetics (approximately 2.5 per cent of the population), and about the same number of undiagnosed cases. Harris (1980) estimates that the prevalence of the disease is increasing at approximately 3 to 6 per cent per year, indicating that *diabetes is one of the most prevalent serious chronic illnesses in today's society.*

Nurses most often encounter children with diabetes in the hospital or clinic during the diagnostic phase or in the clinic or home for follow-up care. The emphasis, in these instances, is on providing information and support for self-care management. Acute care nurses also encounter children hospitalized for diabetic ketoacidosis (DKA) and for other complications of diabetes mellitus. If hospitalization is related to complications of diabetes, the emphasis is on quickly re-establishing metabolic control and on teaching to prevent recurrence. In all cases, the nurse's command of information regarding normal versus abnormal pancreatic function and glucose metabolism will provide the basis for effective nursing care.

DM is not a single disease entity but rather a syndrome or group of diseases differing etiologically but having many common clinical signs and symptoms. Because a variety of ambiguous definitions and inconsistent terminology have been used in the past, the National Institutes of Health (1979) appointed an international committee (National Diabetes Data Group, 1979) to develop a classification system and universal terminology. The various types of diabetes were divided into (1) diabetes mellitus, (2) gestational diabetes, and (3) states of altered carbohydrate metabolism. Table 43–13 further details the classification of diabetes mellitus types, subgroups, and previous terminology. Because most children develop type I DM, this chapter concentrates primarily on that category.

Pathophysiology

Glucose is the primary source of energy for all body cells, with the brain cells using approximately 25 per cent of the total body supply. Small amounts of glucose can be stored as triglycerides in fat tissues and as glycogen in muscle or liver cells. However, *because glucose can be stored only in small amounts, the blood glucose level must be maintained at least at a minimal fasting level (approximately 60 to 110 mg/dl or 3.3 to 6.2 mmol/liter) sufficient to meet central nervous system demands.*

Insulin is a hormone secreted by the beta cells of the pancreas. *The primary function of insulin is to regulate blood glucose levels by controlling the rate at which blood glucose is taken up by the body cells.* Insulin is often referred to as the "key" that opens the door to the various body cells. Insulin is also necessary for the maintenance of the enzyme mechanism required for the use of glucose within the cell.

In addition to manufacturing and storing insulin, the beta cells of the pancreas act as a sensor to determine blood glucose levels. When the levels of carbohydrates in the blood increase, the beta cells are stimulated to release a small amount of insulin, thus acting as a feedback mechanism. Pancreatic insulin is secreted into the portal circulation, where it is carried to the liver and then distributed by peripheral circulation to the body cells.

Insulin has various functions in different body cells. In fat cells, insulin promotes the uptake of glucose and the storage of triglycerides. In muscle cells, insulin increases the transport of glucose and amino acids into the cell. In liver cells, insulin enhances conversion of glucose into glycogen and also inhibits the release of glucose from the liver. Insulin enhances protein synthesis as well. Insulin is excreted by the kidney in the urine.

Inadequate secretion of insulin results in (1) decreased glucose transport from the blood stream into the cells, thus leading to high blood glucose levels; (2) metabolism of triglycerides into free fatty acids, which are converted into keto acids by the liver and are used for energy during the shortage of glucose; and (3) glucagon secretion leading to production of glucose from liver stores of glycogen (glycogenolysis) and from amino acids (gluconeogenesis), further raising blood sugar levels. As glucose levels reach 180 mg/dl (approximately 10 mmol/L) of blood, the renal tubules are unable to resorb the glucose (renal threshold), and glucose spills into the urine (glucosuria). The excreted glucose acts as an osmotic diuretic, causing the loss of large amounts of water, sodium, potassium, and bicarbonate salts.

TABLE 43-13
Classification, Types, and Previous Terminology of Diabetes Mellitus

Classification	Types and Subgroups		Previous Terminology
Diabetes mellitus	Type I:	Insulin-dependent diabetes mellitus (IDDM)	Juvenile diabetes mellitus; ketosis-prone diabetes; unstable or brittle diabetes
	Type II:	Non-insulin-dependent diabetes mellitus (NIDDM)	Adult diabetes mellitus; maturity onset diabetes mellitus
	Obese:	Insulin requiring Non-insulin requiring	
	Non-Obese:	Insulin requiring Non-insulin requiring	
	Other types 1. Pancreatic causes 2. Hormonal causes 3. Drug-induced causes 4. Receptor site abnormalities 5. Other syndromes		Secondary diabetes
Gestational diabetes			Class A diabetics
Asymptomatic state of carbohydrate intolerance	Impaired glucose tolerance		Asymptomatic diabetes; chemical diabetes; borderline diabetes; latent diabetes
	Previously impaired glucose tolerance		
	Potential abnormality of glucose tolerance		

Adapted from National Diabetes Data Group (1979). Classification and diagnosis of diabetes mellitus and other categories of glucose intolerance. *Diabetes, 28,* 1039–1057.

Clinical Manifestations

Clinically, the diabetic patient is left dehydrated and thirsty *(polydipsia)*. In attempts to quench this thirst, the individual consumes large quantities of fluid, which leads to increased urination *(polyuria)*. In addition, the patient may also feel hungry and eat large amounts *(polyphagia)* in response to the body's hunger for glucose, and he or she may be fatigued owing to decreased energy production. These symptoms—polydipsia, polyuria, polyphagia, and fatigue—are known as the "classic" symptoms of DM, although not all patients will develop all of these clinical manifestations. Weight loss, attributable either to dehydration or to the mobilization of fat stores and liberation of triglycerides, may also be present in some individuals. Byproducts of triglyceride breakdown are free fatty acids, which are then converted to ketones by the liver.

The ketone bodies are made up of acetoacetic acid, beta-hydroxybutyric acid, and acetone. If high blood sugar levels persist (indicating inadequate glucose transport), the production of ketones for energy rapidly increases. Although small amounts of ketones can be removed from the body by the kidneys, large amounts cannot. As keto acids accumulate, *ketoacidosis* develops.

Excretion of keto acids by the kidneys is the second important mechanism in the development of ketoacidosis. Bicarbonate is lost in the urine during the excretion of keto acids, thus further decreasing the serum pH. Ketoacidosis can pose a serious threat to the body's delicate balance and may lead to coma and possibly death if not treated.

However, treatment with insulin, water, and appropriate electrolyte replacement therapy reverses the catabolic state created by the insulin deficiency. The blood sugar levels will then decrease, and the use of glycogen stored in fat and liver cells decreases. Ketones will no longer be produced, and pH and bicarbonate and electrolyte levels will return to normal.

Diagnostic Assessment

The diagnosis of type I diabetes in children is not usually difficult. Table 43–14 lists detailed criteria. A glucose tolerance test is rarely required in the diagnosis of type I diabetes.

Therapeutic Management

Factors Influencing Treatment. Management of the illness at diagnosis depends on several factors, which may include (1) severity of illness at diagnosis and (2) management style, which encompasses such factors as the experience and philosophy of health professionals, financial constraints like health insurance coverage, and health beliefs, attitudes, values, and cultural diversity of the child and family.

Severity of Illness. The severity of the child's condition on arrival in the physician's office or the hospital emergency department will greatly influence the

TABLE 43-14
Criteria for Diagnosing Diabetes Mellitus*

Normal Glucose Tolerance

- Fasting blood sugar (FBS) <115 mg/dl *and*
- 2-hour postprandial <140 mg/dl *and*
- No FBS or 2-hour postprandial value >200 mg/dl

Impaired Glucose Tolerance (after glucose load of 1.75 g/kg body wt)

- FBS <140 mg/dl *and*
- 2-hour postprandial >140 mg/dl but <200 mg/dl *and*
- At least one FBS value or 2-hour postprandial value >200 mg/dl

Diabetes Mellitus

- FBS >140 mg/dl on at least two occasions *or*
- Random glucose ≥200 mg/dl with classic signs and symptoms of diabetes (polydipsia, ketonuria, polyuria, weight loss) *or*
- FBS <140 mg/dl and 2-hour postprandial >200 mg/dl, with at least one value >200 mg/dl after a glucose load of 1.75 g/kg

From Christman, C., & Bennett, J. (1987). Diabetes: New names, new test, new diet. *Nursing 87, 17,* 34–42, used with permission from the January issue of Nursing 87, copyright ©1987, Springhouse Corporation, all rights reserved; and Travis, L. B., et al. (1987). *Diabetes mellitus in children and adolescents.* Philadelphia: WB Saunders.

*Established by the National Diabetes Data Group of the National Institutes of Health.

initial management. For DM, three types or stages of presentation are seen, with specific symptoms (or clinical manifestations) and management for each. The three stages of severity of illness include DKA, diabetic ketosis, and hyperglycemia. These stages, their clinical manifestations, and medical and nursing responsibilities are outlined in Table 43-15.

Management Style or Philosophy. Because there remain many unanswered questions about the cause, cure, and prevention of diabetes, many aspects of managing diabetic children and their families are arbitrary. Generally, there are two diverse schools of thought concerning initial management, with many compromises available. These two approaches include initial hospitalization management or initial outpatient management.

If the child is hospitalized at the time of diagnosis, the goals of hospitalization are usually geared to stabilizing the child's blood glucose level and insulin regulation, reducing the child's and parents' anxiety, and initiating education.

If the child is not in DKA and possibly not hospitalized at the time of diagnosis, the tasks of metabolic stabilization, insulin regulation, and the education of the patient and family must all be completed on an outpatient basis. To be successful, this second method of management demands (1) responsibility, motivation, and proximity to the treatment center on the part of the child and family; and (2) adequate staffing and comfort on the part of the health team in allowing families to be maximally involved in their child's care early in treatment.

As well as differences in the location of the newly diagnosed child's initial management, there are two major options in the insulin-dependent DM therapy. These two options are conventional or intensive treatment (Kaye, 1984). Kaye describes conventional treatment as usually including one or possibly two injections of insulin per day. Blood glucose monitoring at least twice a day is now also considered a part of conventional treatment. Intensive treatment, as its name suggests, encompasses a more rigorous therapeutic regimen, including more frequent home blood glucose monitoring, insulin adjustment (on the basis of blood glucose level results), and two or more injections of insulin daily or continuous subcutaneous infusion of insulin using an insulin pump.

Whatever the management philosophy of the health care team, the goals of treatment for the child with type I diabetes and family usually are similar. These goals include (1) metabolic control of the child's diabetes, (2) self-care by the child and family through education about illness management, and (3) normal growth and development of the child and family. These goals can be achieved only when the health care team works closely with each child and family and is sensitive in incorporating this family's individual psychosocial and cultural needs into the treatment plan. Compliance with a complex regimen like diabetes begins with the patient's and family's perceiving the care plan as acceptable within the context of their beliefs and culture (i.e., ethnic foods, ceremonies, folk medicine, and religious customs).

Achieving Metabolic Control

Shortly after the discovery of insulin, an ongoing debate focused on whether complications of diabetes would be prevented if good metabolic control prevailed. Good metabolic control means that blood glucose levels in individuals with diabetes would be as close as possible, over time, to their nondiabetic counterparts. By keeping blood glucose levels close to normal (80 to 120 mg/dl), many occurrences of acute problems (i.e., hypoglycemic and hyperglycemic reactions) can be prevented. The importance of good metabolic control in relation to long-term complications has not been definitely established; this topic is one of the most debated and important issues in diabetes management and is the basis for large multicenter collaborative studies (Kroc Collaborative Study Group, 1984; Diabetes Control and Complications Trials, 1987). Criteria for good metabolic control for the child vary, but usually include

1. A desirable pattern of urine or blood glucose results (i.e., few episodes of hypoglycemia or hyperglycemia).
2. Evidence of normal growth and development.

TABLE 43-15
Symptoms, Medical Management, and Nursing Management of Newly Diagnosed Diabetic Patients

Clinical Manifestations	Therapeutic Management	Nursing Care
Diabetic Ketoacidosis (Acute Stage)		
Hyperglycemia, glycosuria, ketones Dehydration (polyuria, vomiting) Electrolyte imbalance (serum potassium ↑ or ↓, total body potassium ↓, serum sodium ↓, blood urea nitrogen ↑, plasma bicarbonate ↓, serum pH ↓) Kussmaul respirations Abnormal laboratory values (↑ WBC, RBC and WBC ↑ in urine) Cerebral edema-agitation, changes in level of consciousness	Treatment with frequent doses of regular insulin (IV, SC, or IM) (common dosage: 0.1 unit/kg stat; 0.1 unit/kg/hr) Fluid and electrolyte therapy	Careful observation of patient receiving IV insulin and child's reaction to insulin Accurate intake and output
	Careful monitoring of glucose levels in blood and urine, electrolyte and abnormal laboratory values; monitor for cardiac irritability	
		Constant observation of child's neurologic and vital signs
	Informing both the family and the child of what is happening	
		Basic comfort measures for the child and family
Diabetic Ketosis		
Hyperglycemia Glycosuria Ketones (in both blood and urine) Possible dehydration	Treatment with regular insulin	Assessment of child's response to insulin, vital signs
	Careful assessment of serum glucose levels, glycosuria, and ketones	
	Careful monitoring of electrolytes and fluids	Careful monitoring of intake/output
	Information/education of the child and parents	
		Begin to encourage self-care when appropriate
Hyperglycemia		
Polyurea, polydipsia, polyphagia, fatigue Glycosuria No ketones	Careful assessment of insulin requirements (may require the addition of or ↑ regular insulin)	
	Careful assessment of serum glucose levels and glycosuria	
	Encourage usual diet and activities (no exercise if blood sugar >300 mg/dl or if ketones +)	
	Assess and plan education of the child and family	

3. Infrequent occurrence of mild hypoglycemic reactions.
4. Few (diabetes-associated) school absences.
5. Generally feeling well with no related signs or symptoms.
6. Ability to participate in social and recreational activities with peers.

Urine testing and blood glucose monitoring assist the child and family in managing diabetes on a day-to-day basis. Long-term metabolic control can be estimated through the measurement of glycosylated hemoglobins, which are a powerful retrospective index of glucose control (Bunn, 1981). Hemoglobin, when formed in the bone marrow, has no glucose attached. As the red blood cells circulate throughout the body during their approximate 120-day life cycle, an interaction between glucose and hemoglobin occurs. Glycosylated hemoglobins result when hemoglobin A_1 combines with blood glucose in a one-way reaction to form hemoglobins A_{1A}, A_{1B}, and A_{1C}. Because the turnover of red blood cells is constant, the percentage of the total red blood cell pool that has glucose attached to it will reflect the average level of blood glucose throughout the previous 2- to 3-month period. The most common laboratory test measures hemoglobin A_{1c} only, because it accounts for the majority of glycosylated hemoglobin. However, some laboratories do measure all three forms of glycosylated hemoglobins, resulting in slightly higher (2 to 4 per cent) values. Table 43-16 correlates the values for hemoglobin A_{1c} with the degree of metabolic control.

Glycosylated hemoglobin values are measured approximately every 2 to 3 months or on regular visits

TABLE 43-16
HbA_{1C} Test Values and Metabolic Control

Degree of Control	Approximate HbA_{1C} Values (%)
Excellent	<8.5
Good	8.5–9.5
Fair	9.5–10.5
Fair to poor	10.5–12
Poor	>12
Nondiabetic individual	5.2–8.3*

*Normal values differ according to laboratory.

to the physician or clinic. These measurements are particularly useful in patients on tight control regimens, noncompliant patients, patients doing urine testing with unknown renal thresholds, or patients suspected of falsifying home blood glucose monitoring or urine test results. If the glycosylated hemoglobin level is elevated and metabolic control is deemed poor, the results may need to be reviewed with the child and family, and the treatment program may need to be modified.

Metabolic control can be regulated by balancing insulin, food, and activity. Insulin, diet, exercise, and blood glucose monitoring are the major components of type I DM management.

Insulin Therapy. Insulin was discovered in Toronto, Canada, in 1921 by Banting and Best. Insulin is a hormone or protein substance that is produced by the beta cells of the pancreas in the normal healthy person. This pancreatic insulin is often referred to as endogenous insulin. When type I diabetes develops, children lose their ability to produce endogenous insulin. Because insulin is a hormone essential to life, another, or exogenous (manufactured outside the body), source must be found. Exogenous insulins include insulins extracted from the pancreas of cows and pigs. The newest type of insulin on the market is human insulin, which is not extracted from humans but is made in a laboratory by use of recombinant DNA technology (Lilly) or complete chemical biosynthesis (Connaught-Novo). Human insulin is reported to be chemically, physically, biologically, and immunologically equivalent to natural human insulin and is used when a highly purified form of insulin is indicated, such as in cases of insulin allergy, for intermittent use (i.e., metabolic testing, pregnancy, surgery, or acute illness), and with many newly diagnosed diabetics. The types of insulin are further described in Table 43-17.

Insulin is measured in units, whereby a unit provides a specific amount of pharmacologic activity per milliliter of liquid. For example, U-100 insulin has 100 units of insulin in 1 ml of liquid. A unit is always constant and is the same for all types of insulin. Insulin is available in various concentrations in the United States, including U-40, U-80, and U-100. The most commonly prescribed concentration is U-100, and this eventually will replace all other concentrations. In Canada and several other countries, only the U-100 strength insulin is marketed.

Side Effects of Insulin. The most common side effect of insulin is hypoglycemia or lowering of the blood sugar level. Another side effect of insulin is the allergic response or sensitivity, which can occur either locally or systemically.

Local responses include lipodystrophies and sensitivity. Lipodystrophies can be divided into hypertrophy or atrophy of local tissue. Hypertrophy is characterized by thickening of tissue at the site of injection; atrophy refers to the degeneration of subcutaneous fat, causing a hollow or depression. Both are usually caused by either too frequent or too superficial injection into one area and eventually result in poor insulin absorption. Lipoatrophy, in many cases, is thought to be due to a local reaction to the non-insulin substance in the insulin preparation. This reaction is not commonly seen now that purer forms of insulin are available on the market. In fact, by injecting pure pork or human insulin into the depressions, the hollows begin to fill in, thus resolving the problem.

Local insulin sensitivity is often identified by burning, stinging, itching, or erythema at the injection site. Systemic responses to insulin are extremely rare but may result in urticaria and possibly anaphylactic shock. Systemic insulin resistance is characterized by a decreased body response to insulin, usually related to an antibody-mediated reaction.

Oral Hypoglycemic Agents

Because most children with DM have type I diabetes, they will require insulin injections. However, certain medications in pill and capsule form known as hypoglycemic agents also lower the level of blood sugar. The oral hypoglycemic agents are used to control diabetes in some adult type II patients who produce some endogenous insulin and when diet control alone has been unsuccessful. There are two types of hypoglycemic preparations, including sulfonylureas and biguanides. Sulfonylureas (such as Orinase, Diabinese, Dymelor, Tolinase) primarily stimulate the beta cells of the pancreas to produce more insulin, although their complete mechanism is not clearly understood. Biguanides are thought to help the body cells use glucose better. However, various countries have removed many of these drugs from the market owing to increasing reports of lactic acidosis and deaths in patients taking them. The primary nursing role with regard to these pharmaceutical agents is to understand which medication is prescribed, determine the patient's compliance with the medical regimen, and monitor the patient's physiologic and psychologic response to the medication.

TABLE 43-17
Types of Insulin

Type	Alternative Names	Appearance	Action Times: Onset	Peak	Duration	Comments
Short- or Rapid-Acting						
Regular (Lilly; Squibb-Novo)	Crystalline Unmodified Clear Rapid	Clear	0.5–1 hr	2–4 hrs	4–6 hrs	Short-acting insulin is generally used in combination with intermediate-acting insulins or during diabetic ketoacidosis or illness
Humulin R (Lilly)		Clear		1–3 hrs	6–8 hrs	
Semilente (Lilly; Squibb-Novo)	Demi-Dura Sub Tardum	Cloudy		5–10 hrs	5–10 hrs	
Intermediate-Acting						
Lente	Modified Isophane	Cloudy	1.5–2 hrs	6–10 hrs	16–24 hrs*	*The effective phase of blood glucose–lowering activity seems to pass at 16–18 hrs in most persons (Travis et al, 1987)
NPH	Rapitard Retard	Cloudy				
Globin (Lilly; Squibb-Novo)	Protard	Clear			action is longer than rapid-acting but not as long as long-acting	
Humulin N (Lilly)		Cloudy	2 hrs		18–24 hrs*	
Long-Acting						
PZI	Depotinsulin Retard	Cloudy	4–8 hrs	14–24 hrs	36+ hrs	This long-acting type of insulin is not usually used with children because its action is too long and variable
Ultralente	Extra-Dura Extra-Tardum	Cloudy		18–24 hrs		

Nutritional Management

The diabetic diet was one of the earliest forms of diabetes management. However, because this involved starvation regimens and carbohydrate-free diets, adequate nutrition was not possible. With the discovery of insulin in 1921, patients were provided with the opportunity for a nutritionally balanced diet and a prolonged life. In 1950, the Exchange System for meal planning was developed, and although some countries now use a modified version (Choice System), this system is still the most common diabetic teaching tool used today.

Young people with diabetes have the same nutritional needs as their nondiabetic counterparts do. With diabetes, however, food intake must be balanced with activity and prescribed insulin. Balancing food, insulin, and activity essentially means coordinating nutrition in measured amounts at regular and evenly spaced intervals with the quantity and quality of physical activities and the action patterns of the prescribed insulins.

The goals of diet management in children include (1) promotion of normal growth and development, (2) keeping plasma glucose as close to normal as possible in an attempt to prevent both hypoglycemia and hyperglycemia and long-term complications, and (3) improvement or maintenance of the overall health of the patient (American Diabetes Association and American Dietetic Association, 1977). However, health professionals need to remember that one diet prescription cannot meet the needs of everyone, and an individual has the right to an individually designed dietary program that considers both physiologic and psychologic needs. With children, this individual tailoring is especially challenging because the diet is effective only if it is followed.

Families of children with diabetes need individual dietary counseling that takes into consideration the child's age, level of development, level of activity, likes, dislikes, family eating habits, ethnic differences, and numerous other factors. Children's diets need to be constantly assessed and changed to keep pace with their physical growth. Parents often find the diet a chronic source of family discontent; problems range from the "picky" toddler who refuses to eat anything, to the school-age child who likes sharing and trading her or his food, to the undisciplined teenager who throws planned diets to the wind in favor of convenience-oriented dietary habits of peers. Parents and their diabetic children need the support, knowledge, and understanding of health professionals and possibly others facing similar dilemmas who realize that lifestyle changes such as diet are extremely difficult and a constant reminder that their child has special needs.

Good nutrition means sufficient amounts of essential nutritional elements are taken in to meet the needs of the individual at various stages of growth and development. This precise formula often means diets specified in calories or kilojoules (approximately 4.2 kJ = 1 calorie). Instruction about dietary management needs to emphasize that the amount of food the child eats remains constant, as does the scheduling of food intake. Meals and snacks need to coincide with the time-release characteristics of the prescribed insulin. The major components of foods, their energy value, and approximate percentage of the total diabetic diet (because recommendations vary) are presented in Table 43–18.

Exercise

Although exercise has long been recognized as a way to lower insulin requirements in persons with insulin-dependent DM, the heightened interest in exercise in general has prompted additional study of the effects of exercise on glucose metabolism for both diabetic and nondiabetic persons. For understanding the effects of exercise for the child with diabetes, it is important to first review the effects of insulin on normal glucose metabolism.

The Effects of Insulin on Normal Glucose Metabolism. One of the most important functions of insulin is to maintain normal blood levels of glucose. After a meal or sweet snack, when the blood glucose level is high, insulin is the catalyst that causes most of the glucose to be stored in the liver in the form of glycogen. Glycogen is also stored in resting muscle cells. When the circulating blood glucose levels begin to fall between meals, the pancreas decreases its secretion of insulin. As insulin levels decrease, glycogen stored in the liver is converted back into glucose and released into the blood stream (Guyton, 1987).

The Effects of Exercise on Normal Glucose Metabolism. One of the most significant effects of exercise on normal glucose metabolism is the inhibition of insulin secretion. Decreased insulin levels lead to release of liver glycogen stores. As the glycogen breaks down into glucose molecules, it provides energy for the exercising muscles. The body's additional

TABLE 43-18
Components of the Diabetic Diet

Component	Energy Value (calories/g)	Percentage of Total Diet (Approximate)	Important Teaching for Diabetic Patients
Carbohydrate	4	45*	Comprises sugars and starches; most should be complex (including breads, pastas, and grains); restrict use of complex sugars, such as jams and honey; simple sugars, such as those in fruit and milk, need to be included for the growth and development of children
			More quickly digested simple sugars cause greater and faster increases in blood sugar (i.e., it is preferable to eat fruits in their solid form rather than drink fruit juices)
Protein	4	20 (at least 2 g/kg)	Must be appropriate for growth needs, nutritional status, and body weight; attempt to use foods low in fat (e.g., fish, poultry, 2% or skim milk)
Fat	9	30 or less	Should attempt to decrease amounts of food containing visible fats; attempt to balance between polyunsaturated and saturated fats
			Foods high in cholesterol need to be restricted (e.g., cheese, egg yolks, cream, and butter)

Data from Skyler, J. S. (1983). Dietary planning in insulin-dependent diabetes mellitus. *Pediatric Annals, 12,* 652–657; and Travis, L. B., et al. (1987). *Diabetes mellitus in children and adolescents.* Philadelphia: WB Saunders.

*Some centers are urging an even higher percentage of carbohydrate (e.g., 50 to 55 per cent).

demands for energy are met by *gluconeogenesis* (the production of glucose from proteins and fats). The muscles are able to use the available glucose even though, in the resting state, muscle cells require insulin to transport glucose into the cells. Exercising muscle fibers, for reasons not understood, become highly permeable to glucose even in the absence of insulin (Guyton, 1987).

The Effects of Exercise on Glucose Metabolism in Diabetes Mellitus. There is only one difference in the effects of exercise on the diabetic individual compared with the nondiabetic person: *Insulin secretion in persons with type I diabetes is not decreased in response to exercise.* Although the same neurologic and chemical responses that decrease insulin in the exercising nondiabetic subject occur in the exercising diabetic person, they have no effect on the circulating insulin level because the insulin is (usually) being delivered into the blood stream from a subcutaneous depot (the last injection) rather than from the pancreas. In fact, exercise, because it increases blood flow, may actually increase the release of insulin from subcutaneous tissues.

When insulin levels remain constant or increase with exercise, the circulating insulin does not allow release of liver glycogen stores to meet metabolic demands for glucose. Therefore, in the diabetic patient, exercise may lead to low plasma levels of glucose and result in *hypoglycemia* (Travis et al, 1987).

Exercise for the child with diabetes, therefore, requires some planning to avoid the possibility of hypoglycemia during or after activity.

Severe hypoglycemia can usually be prevented if (1) someone close to the diabetic child (a parent, coach, or teammate) knows how to recognize the hypoglycemic symptoms and provide appropriate treatment; (2) blood glucose level is checked before and after exercising (level should be between 80 and 300 mg/dl) for help in determining food or insulin adjustment; (3) the child eats more food before, during, or possibly after the exercise if the blood glucose is between 80 and 180 mg/dl; or (4) less insulin is taken. The extra food should be carbohydrates (e.g., fruit, bread) or milk and will vary with the length and intensity of the exercise. For children whose exercise is not planned, carrying additional food is a good preventive step; it can be used if and when the need arises. Children should always wear a Medic-Alert identification and carry a source of quick-acting sugar in case of a low blood sugar reaction.

Hypoglycemia may also occur if the uptake of insulin is accelerated by exercise of the limb into which the insulin was injected. When strenuous physical activity can be predicted (e.g., if the child will be participating in a ball game or track meet), the anterior abdominal site can be used, thus eliminating the effects of exercise on absorption (Gellis & Kagan, 1986).

The opposite problem, *hyperglycemia* (increased blood sugar), may also occur during exercise. Sometimes, if the blood sugar level is very high to begin with (>400 mg/dl or >22 mmol/liter) and particularly if ketones are also present, exercise will not have a blood sugar–lowering effect and may in fact increase blood glucose level and ketone production through the processes of gluconeogenesis and hepatic glucose output. Therefore, strenuous exercise should be discouraged until control of blood sugar level has been achieved.

Urine and Blood Glucose Monitoring

Successful management of diabetes appears to be facilitated when patients and their families play an active role in treatment. By monitoring the blood glucose levels through either urine testing or, preferably, home blood glucose monitoring, the patient can more easily see the effectiveness of treatment and can experience a sense of control.

Urine Testing. Urine testing was the initial method used by patients to monitor their blood glucose level. Essentially, urine testing assesses the percentage of glucose within the volume of urine voided. The patient is usually asked to void twice; however, the value of the two specimens is disputed in the literature. The first voided specimen is most often discarded because it indicates only the amount of glucose lost in the urine since the previous void. The second voided specimen is used as an indirect assessment of the serum glucose level and reflects the presence of glycosuria during a specific time period. Methods of urine testing and their advantages and disadvantages are summarized in Table 43–19.

Urine testing may be viewed as advantageous because it is inexpensive, noninvasive, and painless. However, there are also many limiting factors in testing urine for glucose, including the following:

1. Renal threshold is variable. The renal threshold is the level that blood glucose must reach before it spills into the urine. This level is usually 180 mg/dl (or 10 mmol/liter). However, this level varies from person to person. Some individuals have a very high renal threshold, whereas others have a low spillover point, making urine tests misleading and uninformative.
2. There is a lag time between blood sugar rise and spilling of the blood glucose into the urine, which ranges from 20 minutes to 2 hours.
3. There is often a social stigma attached to handling urine (especially during the teenage years).
4. Urine tests usually do not diagnose blood levels below 180 mg/dl.
5. Urine testing may be inconvenient and frustrating for the patient and the family (particularly in families with very young children). Also, research reveals that urine tests are often performed with less than 50 per cent accuracy (Malone et al, 1976).
6. Children often will not get a true double-voided urine specimen. They will "save" some for the second void.

Urine can be tested for the presence of ketones as well as for glucose. Ketones are produced in the liver

TABLE 43-19
Methods of Urine Testing

Product	Description	Advantages	Disadvantages
Clinitest (Ames)	Copper reduction test 2-drop method (2 drops of urine in 10 drops of water) Offers results from 0–5%	Range of results Less crucial timing Short time sequence Visual chemical reaction	Not glucose-specific Inconvenient
Diastix (Ames)	Glucose oxidase test Dipstick method Offers results from 0–2%	Glucose-specific Convenient Simple	Requires more crucial timing
Chemstrip uG (Boehringer-Mannheim)	Glucose oxidase method Dipstick method Results from 0–5%	Convenient Simple Glucose-specific	Requires longer timing (i.e., 2 mins)
Tes-Tape (Lilly)	Glucose oxidase method Roll of tape in plastic dispenser Dip tape in urine	Convenient Simple Glucose-specific	Requires longer timing (i.e., 2 mins)

as a breakdown product of fat and can be used in the muscle and other tissues as a source of energy. If the body is ineffectively using glucose, fat begins to break down, and the byproducts begin to appear first in the blood and then in the urine. A patient should test for the presence of ketones if urine glucose levels are greater than 2 per cent, blood glucose levels are over 240 mg during illness (especially during periods of vomiting or diarrhea) or periods of emotional distress, and when insulin doses are adjusted. The presence of ketones can be assessed by using either a separate product for ketones (such as Acetest [Ames] tablets, Ketostix [Ames], or Chemstrip K [Boehringer-Mannheim]) or a combination product that tests for both glucose and ketones in one test (e.g., Ketodiastic [Ames] or Chemstrip GK [Boehringer-Mannheim]). The presence of ketones at any time should be reported to the physician because an excessive build-up leads to ketoacidosis, which can have widespread effects on the body, including diabetic coma and death if not treated.

Blood Testing. Another method of assessing glucose levels is by direct blood glucose measurement (BGM). A variety of methods for home blood glucose monitoring are available on the market. Most methods require a drop of blood to be placed on an enzyme-impregnated strip for a specified period. When the test is completed, the results may be read either visually or with the use of a reflectance meter. BGM has become more popular with the increased emphasis on metabolic control and an awareness of the suspected need to attain prolonged normalization of blood sugar level over time.

BGM can be performed by the patient or a family member at home. An adequate sample of capillary blood is obtained with use of either a simple lancet or a spring-driven lancet (such as Autolet, Autoclix, Hemalit, Monojector) from either the fingertips, ear lobes, or toes. The patient can then employ one of the following methods: (1) visual interpretation (using strips with reagent pads that exhibit the glucose oxidase enzyme reactions, such as Dextrostix [Ames], Chemstrips bG [Boehringer-Mannheim], or Visidex [Ames]), or (2) a reflectance meter (using the principle of light reflection from a strip). The most common reflectance meters include the Glucometer (Ames), AccuCheck (Boehringer-Mannheim), and Glucoscan II (Lifescan). The market for reflectance meters is rapidly expanding and new, smaller, and more sophisticated products are becoming increasingly available.

Advantages of blood glucose monitoring include the following: (1) the patient can achieve better day-to-day metabolic control through an increased understanding of the pattern of glucose fluctuations; (2) the patient can more accurately diagnose hypoglycemia and hyperglycemia; (3) the results of BGM are immediate and specific, which may lead to increased motivation for the prescribed medical regimen; and (4) the patient's self-confidence, self-esteem, and emotional stability may increase with added responsibility and control over his or her life. BGM is more expensive, is invasive, and requires more initial commitment on the part of the patient. BGM also requires more initial teaching, follow-up, and skill on the part of the educator. However, in spite of these apparent disadvantages, research has generally shown that patients who have tried BGM have little technical difficulty in either obtaining blood specimens or analyzing results and prefer this method over urine testing (Daneman et al, 1985; Miller et al, 1983). BGM is especially useful during illness, when the patient is unsure of reactions, for children with renal threshold problems, for infants who cannot void on demand, for adolescents who have difficulty handling urine, for insulin pump users, and for patients who cannot or *will* not do urine testing. The child and family are instructed when to perform urine or blood testing, or both. Testing is done at least twice each day at a time before meals or at bedtime. Additional testing is done when hypoglycemia or hyperglycemia is suspected.

Application of the Nursing Process: Diabetes Mellitus

Assessment

The nurse monitors for the symptoms described under "Clinical Manifestations" and Table 43–20. Blood and urine testing are initially nursing responsibilities and are gradually transferred to the family and child. Assessment of fluid and electrolyte balance will include monitoring hydration state, with accurate recording of intake and output, and assessment of urine specific gravity, skin turgor, and tearing.

Vital sign changes with dehydration include elevation of pulse and respiratory rate. Hyponatremia may be evidenced by hypotension, elevated pulse, and oliguria. Severe hyponatremia can lead to cerebral edema and headache. Changes in serum potassium levels can occur in either direction and are of particular concern because of the potential cardiac rhythm changes. Cardiac monitoring simplifies nursing assessment by providing continuous information on cardiac rhythms. Hypophosphatemia will most likely be evidenced by weakness and possible tremors.

Metabolic acidosis will be evidenced by Kussmaul breathing and changes in mental state. The child may have an altered level of consciousness, varying from lethargy to decreased responsiveness to coma. Level of consciousness should improve in the child with DKA as homeostasis is restored. Deterioration of level of consciousness could be an indication of cerebral edema. Interpretation of arterial blood gas analysis will be an important part of nursing assessment for patients with DKA.

One of the nurse's most important functions for all patients with diabetes is assessment of the patient's and family's knowledge base about the disease and its management. This occurs in all settings, not only at the time of initial teaching but at each interaction between the nurse and family.

Nursing Diagnostic Statements and Collaborative Problems

Diagnoses Related to Metabolic Control

Altered fluid and electrolyte balance: dehydration, *related to osmotic diuresis associated with*

- *Glycosuria.*
- *Accumulation of keto acids from fat metabolism.*
- *Concomitant loss of bicarbonate.*

Hypokalemia or hyperkalemia, *related to*

- *Loss of water in excess of serum electrolytes.*
- *Release of potassium from cells in response to acidosis.*
- *Abnormal losses of potassium in urine.*

Hyponatremia, *related to excess glucagon, an aldosterone antagonist.*

Hypophosphatemia, *related to*

- *Increased tissue catabolism.*
- *Impaired cellular uptake.*
- *Decreased renal resorption (Zimmerman & Gildea, 1985).*

Altered nutrition: less than body requirements, *related to hyperglycemia associated with*

- *Insufficient insulin for glucose transport.*
- *Catabolic effects of glucagon catecholamines, which are stimulated by decreased insulin.*

High risk for injury, hypoglycemia; risk factors:

- *Bursts of physical activity without additional food intake.*
- *Irregular or missed meals.*
- *Failure to consume adequate calories to balance prescribed insulin dose.*
- *Error in insulin administration: more than prescribed dose.*

High risk for injury, hyperglycemia, *associated with relative insulin deficiency compared with body demands for glucose transport; risk factors:*

- *Infection.*
- *Physical or mental stress.*
- *Exercise (in a client whose blood sugar and ketone levels are already elevated).*
- *Insulin excess (resulting in the Somogyi effect or rebound hyperglycemia) (Dickerman & Lucey, 1985).*

Alteration in comfort, *related to need for frequent injections of insulin and blood glucose monitoring.*

High risk for infection; risk factors:

- *Depressed leukocyte function associated with hyperglycemia.*
- *Increased susceptibility associated with malnutrition and tissue catabolism.*
- *Enhancement of the "host medium" associated with readily available blood glucose for metabolism by the pathogen.*

High risk for altered patterns of urinary elimination; risk factors:

- *Polyuria associated with hyperglycemia.*
- *Infections of the urinary tract.*
- *Diabetic neuropathy (not commonly seen in children or adolescents).*

TABLE 43-20

Nursing Process Plan: The Child with Diabetic Ketoacidosis

Analysis: Collaborative Problem 1

Response and Related or Risk Factors: *Altered fluid and electrolyte balance: dehydration, related to osmotic diuresis associated with*

- Glycosuria
- Accumulation of keto acids associated with fat metabolism during impaired glucose transport
- Concomitant loss of bicarbonate with excretion of ketones in the urine

Hypokalemia or hyperkalemia, related to

- Loss of water in excess of serum electrolytes
- Release of potassium from the cells in response to acidosis
- Abnormal losses of potassium in urine

Hyponatremia, related to excess glucagon, an aldosterone antagonist

Hypophosphatemia, related to

- Increased tissue catabolism
- Impaired cellular uptake
- Decreased renal resorption (Zimmerman & Gildea, 1985)

Projected Outcome: The child will restore and maintain normal fluid and electrolyte balance and normal glucose levels.

Analysis: Collaborative Problem 2

Response and Related or Risk Factors: *Altered nutrition: less then body requirements, related to hyperglycemia associated with*

- Insufficient insulin for glucose transport
- Catabolic effects of glucagon and catecholamines, which are stimulated by decreased insulin
- Knowledge deficit (child and parents) regarding dietary management

Projected Outcome: The child will experience an intake of nutrients sufficient to meet metabolic needs.

Defining Characteristics

Altered Fluid and Electrolyte Balance

Subjective:

- Report of polydipsia
- Fatigue
- Headache
- Stomach cramps
- Nausea
- Vomiting

Objective:

- Polyuria
- Polyphagia
- Mental confusion

Nursing Interventions

Electrolyte Management

Assess vital signs (pulse, respirations, and blood pressure) and mental status every 15 mins initially, then every hour until stable. (Vital signs and mental status will reflect response to treatment. Any decrease in level of consciousness may signal cerebral edema.)

Maintain the intravenous fluid replacement as ordered. Expect NS or ½ NS to be ordered initially, with D_5/½ NS when blood sugar drops below 300 mg/dl (Dickerman & Lucey, 1985). (The addition

Evaluation Criteria

The child will restore and maintain normal fluid and electrolyte balance and normal glucose levels, as evidenced by:

- Vital signs and neurologic signs within normal range
- Alert and oriented (or usual mental status)
- Normal skin turgor, color, and temperature
- Moist mucous membranes
- Stabilization of weight
- Fasting blood sugar 80–120 mg/dl

TABLE 43-20 *(continued)*

Defining Characteristics	*Nursing Interventions*	*Evaluation Criteria*
• Hyperventilation (Kussmaul respirations) • Fruity breath odor • Low-grade fever (if significantly dehydrated) • Tachycardia • Flushed, dry skin • Serum pH < 7.30 • Blood sugar > 300 mg/dl • Ketonuria • Serum sodium < 136 mEq/L • Serum potassium > 5 mEq/L • Serum phosphorus 4 mg/dl (may be normal initially) • Elevated hematocrit • Weight loss *Altered Nutrition* *Subjective*: • Aversion to eating • Hunger (polyphagia) • Lack of energy *Objective*: • Weight loss	of 5 per cent dextrose will then be needed to prevent hypoglycemia.) **Oral fluids if the client is alert and denies nausea (unless ordered NPO).** **Assess hydration status to evaluate response to tretament.** • Accurately record intake and output (initial increase in output will signal increased blood volume and adequate kidney perfusion) • Obtain daily weights (to evaluate fluid replacement) **Expect intravenous insulin orders if the client is significantly dehydrated.** (Dehydration alters tissue perfusion and would lead to slow absorption.) • Before administering insulin, check the dose in the syringe with another nurse (incorrect dose of insulin is potentially fatal) • Administer intravenous insulin through a separate line "piggybacked" into the rehydration fluid (the dose will then be independent of rehydration rates [Dickerman & Lucey, 1985]) • Change the syringe or infusion bag every 4 to 5 hrs (to prevent adherence of insulin to the plastic infusion set) (Dickerman & Lucey, 1985) • Control the insulin dose with a syringe pump or infusion pump (to prevent accidental error in delivery) **Expect an order for subcutaneous insulin before discontinuing intravenous administration** (to prevent marked fluctuations in blood sugar) (Dickerman & Lucey, 1985). **Assist with drawing hourly blood specimens for evaluation**	• Absence of abdominal pain, nausea, vomiting • Serum pH 7.35–7.45 • Serum electrolytes and hematocrit within normal limits **The child will be well nourished, as evidenced by:** • Verbalization of satiety after eating • Maintenance of appropriate weight • Sufficient physical energy for age-appropriate development and tasks

(continued)

TABLE 43-20 *(continued)*

Defining Characteristics	***Nursing Interventions***	***Evaluation Criteria***
	of serum glucose and electrolytes. (Although urine sugar and acetone levels may be checked, these values are significantly less indicative of metabolic status than are serum values.) **Institute use of a cardiac monitor, if this is the nurse's prerogative within the institution.** (Alterations in potassium may cause dysrhythmias.) **If a cardiac monitor is not being used, pay particular attention to the heart rate and rhythm and to the pulse deficit.** (Pulse deficit is the difference between the apical and radial beats and is evidence of ineffective ventricular contractions.) **Monitor nausea and vomiting when hyperglycemic,** maintaining an accurate output. **Assess normal eating habits and nutritional adequacy.** **Monitor intake and record diet in accordance with prescribed dietary regimen.** Ensure intake of nutrients, calories, and fluids appropriate for age and size (to maintain normal range of blood glucose in conjunction with insulin and exercise.) **Weigh and measure as appropriate for level of treatment.** Record and compare with norms. **Assess ability to participate in age-appropriate activity.** **Institute dietary teaching,** as described under "Teaching Dietary Management."	

Analysis: Nursing Diagnostic Statement 1

Response and Related or Risk Factors: *High risk for ineffective management of prescribed diabetic protocol; risk factors:*

- Chronicity and complexity of the treatment regimen
- Lack of immediate rewards for metabolic control
- Giving responsibility for managing diabetes mellitus before developmental readiness
- Developmental rebellion to "being different"

TABLE 43-20 *(continued)*

- Knowledge deficit (child and family) about etiology and pathophysiology of diabetes; monitoring and treatment of the disease; immediate and long-term management responsibilities

Projected Outcome: The child and family will regulate and integrate into daily living a program for treatment of illness and sequelae of illness that is satisfactory for meeting specific health goals.

Defining Characteristics *(Actual Response)*	***Nursing Interventions***	***Evaluation Criteria***
Subjective: • Verbalization of desire to manage the treatment of illness and prevention of sequelae • Verbalized difficulty with regulation/integration of one or more prescribed regimens for treatment of illness and its effects or prevention of complications (e.g., inconsistent insulin administration; comments such as "I use *about* 10 units of insulin most days") • Verbalized that did not take action to include treatment regimens in daily routine or take action to reduce risk factors for progression of illness and sequelae (e.g., forgetting to test blood sugar and urine; reports of "eating without even thinking about it or when I'm nervous")	Emotional Support **Encourage verbalization of feelings about the illness.** (Expression of emotion often must precede problem solving.) **Facilitate the child's exploration of probable causes of ineffective management, supplementing needed facts and clarifying misinformation.** Resist identifying the problem as perceived by the nurse. (Important aspects may then be overlooked. Also, the client is more likely to direct energy toward solving a self-identified problem.) **Assist the client to explore resources for coping with the identified problem.** **Facilitate the development of options for action.** Suggest options that require the least change in usual habits; for example, have the child or parent write favorite foods on colored index cards and color code to food groups; then the child can choose cards from the color groups for meals (Billie, 1986)	**The child and family will effectively manage the treatment regimen, as evidenced by** • Expression of correct information about managing the diabetes mellitus and preventing sequelae • Verbalization of ability to regulate/integrate prescribed regimens along with ability to correctly state how this is done • Accurate reporting and record keeping of blood glucose testing, insulin administration, and diet • *Appropriate* adaptation of regimen to meet developmental needs • Blood glucose and HbA_{1c} values within acceptable range • Child will develop a plan for preventing future episodes of diabetic ketoacidosis • Ability to explain (simply) the basic pathologic process of diabetes mellitus • Ability to describe and demonstrate correct techniques for blood glucose monitoring and insulin administration • Stating signs and symptoms of hypoglycemia and hyperglycemia • Explaining the effects of exercise and how to modify diet and insulin in accordance with changes in exercise • Planning and eating a diet that is nutritionally adequate and meets the dietary prescription

(continued)

TABLE 43-20 *(continued)*

Defining Characteristics *(Actual Response)*	Nursing Interventions	Evaluation Criteria
Objective: **Choices of daily living ineffective for meeting goals of the treatment and prevention program.** • Inaccurate measurement of insulin dose and of blood sugar and urine acetone levels • Incomplete record keeping; written indication of irregular testing of blood and urine • Persistent elevation of blood sugar or HbA_{1c}	*Teaching: Prescribed Activity/Exercise, Prescribed Diet, Prescribed Medication, Procedure/Treatment* **Where necessary, institute a comprehensive diabetic educational program in conjunction with physician, nutritionist, and diabetic educator** (if available). **Document all teaching, patient and family response, and demonstrated skills on a patient teaching plan.** **Establish a primary nurse to coordinate all teaching efforts.** **Let the client choose the options that will formulate the plan, and encourage verbalization of the rationale for the plan.** (It is crucial to effective management of therapeutic regimen that the client "own" the plan and be able to identify the logic involved.) **Collaborate with home care and clinic nurses** (so they can help the client evaluate and redesign the management plan as needed.)	

High risk for sensory-perceptual alteration: *visual; risk factors:*

- *Blurred vision from a hypoglycemic reaction.*
- *Retinopathy associated with long-term insufficient availability of glucose (not commonly seen in children or adolescents).*

High risk for alteration in growth and development: growth retardation; risk factor: *altered metabolism.*

Diagnoses Related to Psychosocial Impact of Disease

Altered family process, *related to lifestyle changes imposed by the needs of the diabetic child for*

- *Monitoring and treatment of the disease.*
- *Family support to deal with the emotional impact of the disease.*

High risk for noncompliance with prescribed diabetic protocol; risk factors:

- *The chronicity and complexity of the treatment regimen.*
- *The lack of immediate rewards for metabolic control.*
- *Giving responsibility to the child for managing DM before developmental readiness.*

High risk for altered growth and development: emotional/social delay; risk factors:

- *Poor self-concept associated with the restrictions in insulin-dependent DM or changes in body image.*
- *Increased and prolonged dependency on parents.*

High risk for altered parenting: overprotection; risk factor: *parental anxiety about the possible complications of insulin-dependent DM.*

Diagnoses Related to Self-Care Management

***Knowledge deficit,** related to*

- *Etiology and pathophysiology of diabetes mellitus.*
- *Monitoring and treatment of the disease.*
- *Immediate and long-term management responsibilities to control the disease and its complications.*

Diagnoses Related to Long-Term Effects of Altered Metabolic Status (usually seen later in life)

***High risk for altered tissue perfusion: systemic; risk factor:** atherosclerotic changes in blood vessels associated with deposition of lipids on the intima of vessels during mobilization of fatty acids in insulin deficiency.*

***Altered comfort: paresthesias,** related to peripheral neuropathy associated with ischemic changes in nerve function.*

***High risk for altered sexual patterns: impotence; risk factor:** neurovascular changes.*

***Colonic constipation,** related to intestinal neuropathy.*

High risk for injury: falls; risk factors:

- *Orthostatic hypotension associated with neuropathy of the central nervous system.*
- *Muscular weakness associated with neuropathy in the lower extremities.*

Planning and Implementation

Caring for the Child with DKA. Children with DKA constitute a medical and nursing emergency. They may require admission to an intensive care setting, depending on the extent of dehydration and the degree of derangement of electrolytes and acid-base balance. DKA most commonly occurs in conjunction with the onset of DM when the family is unaware of the condition but is a potential hazard any time there is a serious imbalance of metabolic control. In this acute situation, the nurse must simultaneously deal with a child who needs intensive monitoring and a family who is stressed by a seriously ill child and a new diagnosis.

Nursing care of the child's physiologic needs centers around administering and monitoring restoration of fluid, electrolyte, and acid-base balance. This requires continuous assessment of the child's physiologic state. Intravenous fluids may be changed frequently as the physiologic state returns to normal. Fluid resuscitation is usually begun with a solution of normal saline or half-normal saline, depending on the sodium deficit. Some glucose will be added to the intravenous solution as the blood sugar drops (usually in the range of about 300 mg/dl). The child should be monitored for symptoms of electrolyte imbalance as described in "Assessment." Potassium is frequently added to intravenous fluids to prevent hypokalemia as the child is rehydrated. Urine output should be established before potassium is added to the intravenous fluids.

Insulin may be administered intravenously if the child is seriously dehydrated because this results in poor absorption from the subcutaneous tissues. As blood sugar drops, intravenous insulin will be switched to the subcutaneous route with regular insulin doses adjusted by the nurse in accordance with the child's blood glucose level. When physiologic homeostasis has been re-established, longer-acting forms of insulin will be introduced. Blood glucose determinations should be performed frequently, possibly as often as hourly by fingerstick, and periodically verified by venous sampling to ensure that blood glucose is not dropping too precipitously.

Children with DKA frequently experience nausea and vomiting. Oral intake can be slowly introduced as nausea subsides. The nurse needs to monitor the child's mental state as described in "Assessment."

Nursing assistance with the family's emotional response to the diagnosis is discussed under "Facilitating the Child's and Family's Adjustment to Diabetes."

Teaching Safe Administration of Insulin. Educating the patient and family in how to administer the insulin injection at the stressful time of diagnosis is difficult and a possible source of frustration. The nurse needs to allow time for the patient and family to overcome the shock of diagnosis but at the same time must encourage them to become involved in the self-care management that will allow them to manage the illness at home. All adult caregivers should be taught how to administer the insulin injection, and if the child is approximately 10 years old, it may be appropriate to teach him or her how to give the injection from the onset of therapy. Young children can be included in parts of the routine at an age-appropriate level. Assessing the readiness of children for participation is based on cognitive and emotional maturity rather than chronologic age. Regardless of the age or the child's level of involvement, caregivers should share the responsibility of the diabetes treatment management.

To facilitate the patient's and family's learning, the nurse must attempt to create a relaxed atmosphere where teaching can progress at a calm and unhurried pace. The nurse needs to be positive, to be self-confident, and to have adequate and current knowledge about diabetes, insulin, injection techniques, testing techniques, and working with children and families. The family can be reassured that although the injection will be difficult at first, in time they will be able to incorporate it into their daily routine; with some families, this may take longer than with others.

To provide the families with as much support, supervision, and practice time as possible, teaching of the insulin injection should commence as early in patient teaching as possible. Because the first injection by the parent will be anxiety-producing, the nurse could initially demonstrate by giving a saline (NaCl, 0.9 per cent) injection to a doll or to the parent and then reciprocate by allowing the parent to give an injection to the nurse. The nurse should then assist the parents in giving the first injection to the child. If patients or parents are having extreme difficulty in the first session, the nurse may want to divide the teaching session into two parts. Once parents or patients have begun to give injections on their own, they will still require frequent reassessment of their technique and ongoing support and encouragement.

Teaching about Insulin. All children require insulin for growth, whether they are diabetic or not. When nondiabetic children experience a growth spurt, their pancreas is able to produce the extra insulin required by the body cells for energy and expansion. However, because diabetic children do not have this built-in control mechanism, they will require increases in both insulin dose and calorie requirements about every 3 to 4 months to meet their growth needs. Parents who understand their diabetic child's needs during growth spurts can provide additional nutrition and adjust the insulin dose accordingly to prevent potential conflict between hunger and glucose control.

Because insulin is a protein and, like all other proteins, would be inactivated by the gastric juices, it cannot be taken orally. Consequently, the usual route of administration is by subcutaneous injection, that is, into the loose space between the fat layer and the underlying muscle (Fig. 43–10). Insulin is most commonly administered subcutaneously by an insulin syringe. Other methods of subcutaneous administration are automatic injectors, insulin pumps, and needle-free injectors (e.g., Medi-Jector EZ, Tender Touch). The pump has an indwelling catheter. The injector is a spring-release device that forces insulin to penetrate the skin and enter the subcutaneous tissues under pressure. Regular insulin can be administered either intramuscularly or intravenously in acute situations.

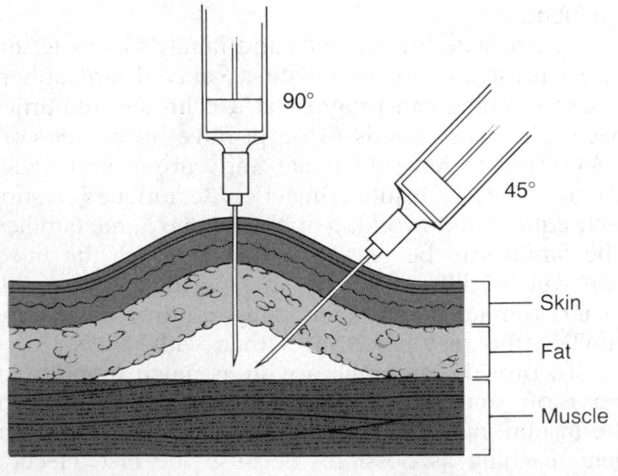

FIGURE 43-10. Subcutaneous injection of insulin.

When the patient and the parents are taught how to administer insulin, they should first be taught how to administer the type or types of insulin that have been prescribed for them at that particular time. Details concerning insulin adjustment and other insulin preparations can be dealt with at a later time. The patient, family, and nurse need to consider the type of syringe for use, the injection sites, and the actual injection technique. For all insulin administration, the patient needs to be reminded to always check the type of insulin and expiration date before beginning.

Either disposable (plastic) or reusable (glass) syringes may be used to administer insulin. However, only syringes designated especially for insulin administration should be used for giving insulin. There is virtually no dead space between the end of the plunger and the tip of the syringe in insulin syringes, whereas noninsulin syringes (especially glass) may trap air to the 10-unit gradation line. Also, insulin syringes must correspond with the various concentrations of insulin. Therefore, for U-100 insulin, U-100 syringes must be used. Low-dose syringes, measuring a maximum of either 30 or 50 units, are commonly used for children. These syringes have a narrower barrel, resulting in measurement lines that are farther apart, making the reading and measuring of small doses easier. The nurse needs to help the patient and family consider the cost, convenience, ease of reading, handling, and accuracy of measurement when choosing a syringe for daily use.

Because patients with type I diabetes will have a constant need for insulin, they may purchase several bottles at once, which need to be stored. Insulin should be stored in a cool place, avoiding either extreme heat (above 90° F) or freezing, because the protein potency can be altered by extreme temperatures. Insulin is stable for up to 1 year if unopened or up to 3 months opened if stored at room temperature or in the refrigerator. If insulin is stored in the refrigerator, warming it to room temperature before injecting is encouraged because injection of a cold substance is more painful. Patients should also be encouraged to have on hand at all times an extra bottle of both their prescribed insulin and regular short-acting insulin (in case of illness).

Teaching about Injection Sites and Administration Technique. The most common sites for injection of insulin include the outer medial aspect of the upper arms, the abdomen, the medial lateral aspects of the thighs, and the buttocks (Fig. 43–11). The patient should not use the inside of the thighs or the midline of the abdomen. For teaching patients how to choose an injection site, the following guidelines may be helpful. Encourage the patient to choose a site that (1) is not painful, (2) is readily accessible for the person giving the shot, (3) has equal absorption, (4) can be pinched up easily, and (5) is large enough to allow several adjacent injections so that the same site is not used too frequently. Insulin is absorbed at different rates in different areas of the body. An ideal site

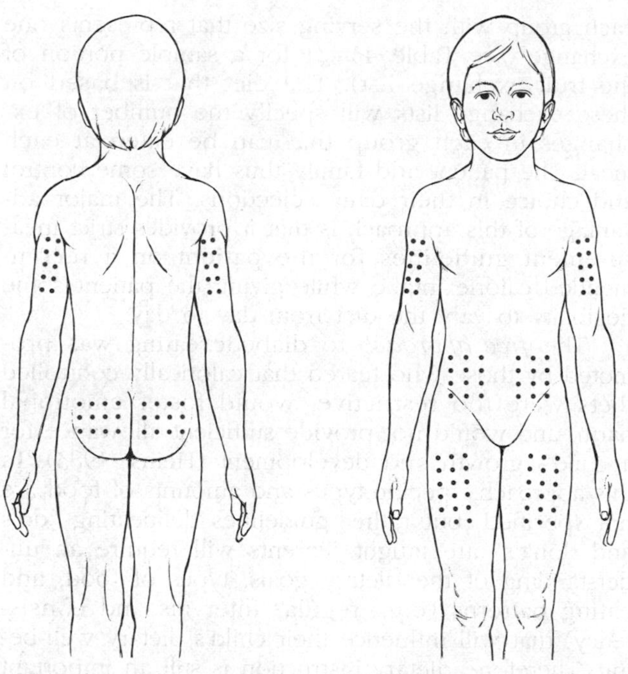

FIGURE 43 - 11. Injection sites for insulin.

for uniform absorption is the abdomen. The rate of absorption in the abdomen is faster than in the legs; likewise, absorption in the arms is faster than in the legs. Patients are instructed to avoid injecting into an anticipated exercised limb.

Injection sites should be regularly rotated to avoid changes in fatty tissue, which result in altered insulin absorption. The patient should be encouraged to choose one area and stay within that area for approximately a week, after which the area is not used for 4 to 6 weeks. For example, if a patient chooses the thigh, he or she can be instructed to space the injections about 1 to 1½ inches apart from just below the groin to about 3 inches (a fist) above the knee, thus providing for a number of injection sites depending on the age and size of the child. When the same injection area is used, individual injection sites should be 1 inch apart from each other. When all possible sites in a particular area have been used, the patient can move on to another site and not return to this area for several weeks. This organized method of site rotation prevents lipodystrophies (an abnormal deposition or metabolism of fat), which are associated with too frequent injections in the same spot.

If the patient is prescribed one type of insulin only, the following steps can be used by the nurse as a guideline when teaching patients and their families how to administer insulin.

1. *Wash hands.*
2. *Gently roll the insulin bottle between hands to thoroughly mix the medication. Do not shake; shaking leads to excess air bubbles in the vial.*
3. *Wipe off the top of the vial with an alcohol swab.*
4. *Draw up the amount of air in the syringe equal to the insulin dose.*
5. *Inject the air into the insulin vial to equalize the pressure in the bottle. Do not remove the needle from the vial.*
6. *Carefully withdraw the prescribed insulin dose, ensuring that no air bubbles are trapped in the syringe.*
7. *Check the insulin dose with another person to make sure it is correct.*

Patients who have been prescribed two types of insulin can be taught how to draw up the two types into one syringe so that only one injection is required. The patient should be taught to inject air into the intermediate or long-acting insulin first, and then into the short-acting insulin. Without removing the needle from the vial, the patient can *draw up the short-acting insulin first* and then, being careful not to inject any short-acting insulin into the vial, can withdraw the intermediate insulin. By using this method, the patient will not contaminate the vial of short-acting insulin, which may be required in an acute situation such as DKA. Contamination of short-acting insulin by a longer-acting variety changes the action of the short-acting insulin, resulting in a less rapid onset of action.

The important point for nurses to stress in patient teaching is that patients be consistent in their method of mixing insulins so that they will not become confused in stressful situations. The importance of checking the accuracy of the insulin dosage with another responsible person should also be emphasized along with the serious effects of overdosing.

Teaching Dietary Management. There are two main approaches to dietary teaching, a strict dietary approach and the "free" dietary approach. As with the overall management of the illness, factors such as professional philosophies, severity of the illness, and financial considerations will influence which approach health professionals will recommend or prescribe. In the more conventionally *strict approach,* formal dietary education centers on "exchange" or "choice" lists. Exchange lists have been developed by the American Diabetes Association and the American Dietetic Association (1976) and consist of six food groups—milk, vegetable, fruit, bread, meat, and fat—that provide a framework for the quantity and quality of food the individual consumes.* Foods are listed in

* Although the exchange lists have been widely adapted and used, research is beginning to demonstrate that there is wide variation in the glycemic response to foods containing identical amounts of carbohydrates (Coulston et al, 1980; Crapo et al, 1980). Jenkins and colleagues (1981), in response to these findings, developed a glycemic index to compare the glycemic responses of different foods. As Skyler (1983) pointed out, most of the relevant research was conducted on nondiabetic subjects, and therefore the effects of the research cannot readily be generalized to diabetic subjects. However, a nutritional system based on the *glycemic index* may be a reasonable alternative to the exchange system in the future.

TABLE 43-21
Sample Portion of Fruit Exchange List

One exchange of fruit contains 10 g of carbohydrate and 40 cals. This list shows the kinds and amounts of fruits to use for one Fruit Exchange.

Apple	1 small
Apple juice or cider	⅓ cup
Applesauce (unsweetened)	½ cup
Apricots, fresh	2 medium
Apricots, dried	4 halves
Banana	½ small
Berries: Blackberries	½ cup
Blueberries	½ cup
Raspberries	½ cup
Strawberries	¾ cup
Cherries	10 large
Dates	2
Figs, fresh	1
Figs, dried	1
Grapefruit	½
Grapefruit juice	½ cup
Grapes	12
Grape juice	¼ cup
Mango	½ small
Melon: Cantaloupe	¼ small
Honeydew	⅛ medium
Watermelon	1 cup
Nectarine	1 small
Orange	1 small
Orange juice	½ cup
Papaya (fruit)	¾ cup
Peach	1 medium
Pear	1 small
Persimmon, native	1 medium
Pineapple	½ cup
Pineapple juice	⅓ cup
Plums	2 medium
Prunes	2 medium
Prune juice	¼ cup
Raisins	2 tablespoons
Tangerine	1 medium
Cranberries	may be used as desired if no sugar is added

Adapted from American Diabetes Association and American Dietetic Association (1976). *Exchange list for meal planning*. New York: Author.

each group with the serving size that represents one exchange (see Table 43–21 for a sample portion of the fruit exchange list). The diet that is based on these exchange lists will specify the number of exchanges in each group that can be eaten at each meal. The patient and family thus have some control and choice in their daily selections. The major advantage of this approach is that it provides strict measurement guidelines for the patient on a recommended calorie intake while giving the patient some flexibility to vary the diet from day to day.

The *free approach* to diabetic eating was promoted by those who feared that calorically controlled diets were too restrictive, would foster emotional harm, and would not provide sufficient allowance for a child's growth and development (Heins, 1983). In this approach, specific types and amounts of food are not specified, but rather guidelines delineating "do's and don't's" are taught. Parents will require an understanding of the dietary goals, types of food, and eating patterns (e.g., regular intervals and consistency) that will influence their child's dietary well-being. Therefore, dietary instruction is still an important part of the diabetic teaching.

Increasing *dietary fiber* may prove to be an additional method to maintain blood glucose levels. Postprandial blood glucose levels are decreased when the meal includes plant fiber, and it has been suggested that certain plant fibers may even decrease serum cholesterol levels (Gellis & Kagan, 1986). Fruits and vegetables, grains, and legumes are natural sources of plant fiber (Table 43–22).

Travis and colleagues (1987) described two potential problems with high-fiber diets for diabetes control. There is, first, some concern that a high-fiber diet may decrease the total calorie intake because foods high in fiber tend to be low in calories. Second, dietary fiber in large amounts may interfere with the absorption of calcium, iron, copper, magnesium, phosphorus, and zinc as well as certain vitamins. The implications, then, for children on high-fiber diets are for *careful and consistent monitoring of growth and development* to ensure adequate nutritional intake.

An additional implication is the need to *monitor blood sugar levels* more frequently when a high-fiber diet is begun. Because high fiber intake may decrease the amount of insulin needed, the child must be watched for hypoglycemia.

Although consistency and good nutrition are essential to the diabetic child's diet, so are the social aspects, such as eating out, and special events, such as birthday parties, Halloween, and Christmas or other holidays. Eating out is more and more a part of daily living and should be an enjoyable occasion for the diabetic child and family as well. Familiarity with the child's meal plan at home and knowing how to make appropriate choices will facilitate good nutritional habits away from home. In restaurants, parents can inquire about the ingredients in unfamiliar entrees and request that certain sauces and dressings be omit-

TABLE 43-22
Fiber Content of Foods per 100 Grams

Food	High-Fiber (3 g)	Moderate Fiber (1.5 g)	Low Fiber (0.5 g)	Little Fiber (0.2 g)
Bread			Whole wheat bread and crackers	White, cracked wheat, rye, pumpernickel breads
Cereals	All-Bran (4.8 g/C) Wheat germ (2.5 g/C)	40% Bran flakes Puffed wheat Raisin bran	Barley, Cheerios, corn flakes, oatmeal, puffed rice, brown rice, Shredded Wheat, Wheaties	Rice Macaroni Noodles Spaghetti
Vegetables	Green peas (canned)	Green and wax beans, dried beans and peas, broccoli, Brussels sprouts, cauliflower, mustard greens, green peas, okra, pepper, pumpkin, winter squash	Asparagus, beets, cabbage, carrots, celery, corn, cucumber, eggplant, lettuce, mushrooms, onions, sweet potatoes, white potatoes, tomatoes	
Fruits	Fresh blackberries (4.1 g/¾ C) Dried figs (5.6 g/C) Dried dates (2.3 g/½ C)	Apples, berries except blackberries, figs, pears with skins	Applesauce, apricots, bananas, fruit cocktail, cherries, grapefruit, grapes, mangos, melons, oranges, peaches, pears (without skin), pineapples, plums, prunes, raisins	Juices only

From Travis, L. B., et al. (1987). *Diabetes mellitus in children and adolescents.* Philadelphia: WB Saunders.

ted. Guides that translate convenience foods into diabetic exchanges are also available from local diabetic societies (Frantz, 1987). If meals are going to be delayed, the child can eat his or her usual bedtime snack at the regular dinner time and then eat dinner at the regular snack time. During special events, parents need to strike a balance between the rigidity of the diabetic diet and the social well-being of their child. The child should be allowed to have an occasional "treat," but the parents still need to be flexible, creative, well-informed, and supported to manage acceptable alternatives and compromises in many social situations. The child also will learn to understand that the family will not always participate in both the diet and the diabetic regimen. Informing others what the diabetic child can eat or offering to provide the "party dessert" on special occasions often eases the confusion and promotes peer acceptance of diabetic children and their diets.

Artificial Sweeteners. There are a large number of sugar substitutes on the market. These sweeteners can either be nutritive or non-nutritive. Nutritive sweeteners may be carbohydrates, such as lactose and fructose, or alcohols, such as sorbitol, mannitol, or xylitol. These substances contain a few calories but are not a significant problem as long as their use is limited. The newest nutritive sweetener on the market is aspartame (Nutrasweet), a protein substance with very high sweetening power. Therefore, only very small amounts of aspartame are required for sweetening, and the calorie content is insignificant. Despite some concern for potential side effects of aspartame, it has been found quite safe to date (Travis et al, 1987). Non-nutritive chemical sweeteners, including saccharin and cyclamates, have also been used but have been banned in various countries at one time or another owing to uncertainty of their long-term effects on health.

Many of these artificial sweeteners are used in dietetic foods. Foods such as candies, syrup, and soda pops are sweetened primarily with aspartame and therefore add little caloric value if used in reasonable amounts. Other dietetic products, however, although carbohydrate reduced, may contain calories from other sources, and their calorie content may be as high as or higher than that of their nondietetic equivalents. Therefore, although dietetic foods may offer variety to the diabetic family, parents need to be cautioned to read their labels carefully to determine the ingredients. Except for water-packed fruits and artificially sweetened soda, few "dietetic" foods justify the expense over standard products.

The diabetic diet is a key element in the management of type I diabetes. The successful diet is one that is nutritious, acceptable, and adhered to by the child and family and that maintains the balance with insulin and activity to produce near-normal plasma glucose levels. Dietary teaching and support must be ongoing for the diabetic child and family. The nurse can play key roles in the initial assessment of the child's and family's nutritional practices, evaluating dietary management and working in collaboration with dietitians to reinforce dietary programs continually.

Maintaining Metabolic Control During Illness and Surgery. Illness is cause for concern in the child with diabetes because *physical and emotional stressors can lead to hyperglycemia*. (Table 43–23 lists some of the

TABLE 43-23
Stress Stimuli Producing Hyperglycemia

Illness	
Infectious	
	Sepsis
	Meningitis
	Others
Noninfectious	
	Myocardial infarction
	Cerebrovascular accidents
Metabolic	
Fasting	
Hypoglycemia	
Diabetic ketoacidosis	
Hypoxia	
Dehydration	
Trauma	
Usual trauma	
Burns	
Surgery	
Nonspecific	
Fever	
Hypothermia	
Pain	
Psychologic or emotional	

From Travis, L. B., et al. (1987). *Diabetes mellitus in children and adolescents*. Philadelphia: WB Saunders.

more common stressors.) Infections are often the cause of hyperglycemia and ketosis in young children because of the high frequency of infectious disease in this age group (Travis et al, 1987). The mechanism for hyperglycemia and ketosis begins with the release of the stress hormones (catecholamines, glucagon, cortisol, and growth hormone, which were discussed earlier). The stress hormones activate catabolic enzymes, which mobilize carbohydrate and lipid stores, leading to increased blood levels of sugar and ketones. Hyperglycemia and ketonemia during illness or surgery are monitored by frequent blood or urine (or both) measurements for glucose and ketones and controlled by adjustments in diet and insulin dose as needed.

Monitoring for Elevated Glucose and Ketone Levels. Glucose and ketone levels should be measured in blood or urine (or both) every 4 hours during an acute illness or other stressful condition. If glucose levels are elevated and ketones are present, the parents should consult the physician. If vomiting occurs, especially more than once, the child should be seen for a more thorough assessment of blood glucose level, electrolyte balance, and hydration.

Adjusting Diet and Insulin. During illness, the child with diabetes may have difficulty tolerating the normally prescribed diet. Adjustments will be needed if the child is nauseated, is vomiting, has diarrhea, or is undergoing surgery. Table 43–24 lists liquid and soft food equivalents for usual portions of fruit, starch, and milk. Another indication for these liquid exchanges may be when the child is febrile. Because fever increases basal metabolism, it increases the body's calorie needs. Calorie-containing liquids can help to maintain more normal blood sugar levels as well as decrease the danger of dehydration. Of course, any calorie-containing liquids must be added to the total calories consumed.

Over-the-counter medications (e.g., antipyretics, analgesics, and cough and cold remedies) may contain concentrated forms of sugar in their syrup formulations. Parents should consult the physician before administering any of these preparations to the child with diabetes.

The family must be alerted that *the child must always take at least the usual dose of insulin during an illness.* The ill child who develops hyperglycemia and ketosis will often need supplemental insulin. Typically, regular insulin will be prescribed (Travis et al, 1987). Parents who have become expert at home management of diabetes may be instructed to give the additional insulin at home in response to their detection of increased blood glucose levels. In other instances, the child may be admitted to the hospital until the illness is under control and metabolic balance has been reestablished.

Meeting Metabolic Needs in the Perioperative Period. Because of the unique metabolic needs during the preoperative, intraoperative, and postoperative phases, the child with diabetes who requires surgery will need precise monitoring for blood glucose levels and presence of ketones and for signs and symptoms of hypoglycemia and hyperglycemia. In the preoperative phase, control of blood glucose level is a problem because the child must have nothing by mouth (NPO). Although withholding insulin will eliminate the risk of hypoglycemia during surgery, complete lack of insulin increases the chances of hyperglycemia. An insulin-dependent diabetic patient needs some exogenous insulin to prevent tissue catabolism (with resulting hyperglycemia). As noted by Robertson, "current research shows that a continuous insulin supply promotes glucose uptake and glycogenesis, while preventing excessive glucose output and glycogenolysis" (1986, p 30).

The child with diabetes is also at risk for hyperglycemia during the preoperative and immediate postoperative period because epinephrine and cortisol, secreted as a result of the neuroendocrine response to stress, stimulate glycogenolysis and gluconeogenesis. Hyperglycemia is to be avoided because it has been linked to many of the common complications of DM.

TABLE 43-24
Liquid Exchange List, with Carbohydrate Content

Fruit Exchange: 1 Fruit Exchange = 10 g Carbohydrate

8 oz or 1 C Gatorade = 1½ fruits + 130 mg sodium + 24 mg potassium

4 oz or ½ C orange juice or grapefruit juice = 1 fruit

⅓ C apple juice or pineapple juice = 1 fruit

2 oz or ¼ C grape juice or prune juice = 1 fruit

4 oz or ½ C Cran-Apple juice or nectar = 2 fruits

4 oz or ½ C Hi-C or Tang = 1½ fruits

1 C presweetened Kool-Aid, lemonade, or punch = 2½ fruits

1 C Sweet'nLow-flavored drink mix = 1 fruit

3 oz regular soft drink = 1 fruit

1 regular twin Popsicle = 2 fruits

2 tsp sugar = 1 fruit

2 regular hard candies = 1 fruit

5 Life Savers = 1 fruit

Starch Exchange: 1 Starch Exchange = 15 g Carbohydrate

½ C cooked cereal = 1 starch

½ C mashed potato = 1 starch

1 small baked potato = 1 starch

½ C regular Jello = 1 starch

1 C vegetable or cream soup = 1 starch

½ C vanilla ice cream = 1 starch

1½ C V-8 juice = 1 starch

Milk Exchange: 1 Milk Exchange = 12 g Carbohydrate

8 oz or 1 C (½ pt) whole, skimmed, low-fat, or buttermilk = 1 milk

½ C evaporated milk = 1 milk

⅓ C condensed sweetened milk = 1 milk

8 oz milkshake = 1 milk, 1 starch

8 oz malt = 1 milk, 1 starch, 1 fruit

⅓ C ice milk = ½ milk, 1 fruit

½ C regular vanilla pudding = ½ milk, 2 fruits

½ C regular chocolate or butterscotch pudding = ½ milk, 3 fruits

½ C sugar-free custard mix = 1 milk

Free Foods: May Be Eaten as Desired

Diet drinks	Broth
Unsweetened Kool-Aid	Sugar-free gelatin
Unsweetened lemonade	Unsweetened Popsicles
Unsweetened tea	Water
Unsweetened coffee	

From Travis, L. B., et al. (1987). *Diabetes mellitus in children and adolescents*. Philadelphia: WB Saunders.

Robertson (1986) listed three common preoperative protocols prescribed by physicians for their insulin-dependent diabetic patients: (1) withhold the morning dose of rapid-acting insulin, but administer half the morning dose of intermediate-acting insulin; (2) administer long-acting insulin the night before surgery; (3) give no subcutaneous insulin, but instead administer insulin by intravenous drip. Whatever the prescribed protocol, the nurse must recognize the fine balance required in maintenance of blood glucose levels and monitor the perioperative patient closely for evidence of either hypoglycemia or hyperglycemia.

Decreasing the Risk of Complications. Although diabetes can now be better controlled and diabetic individuals can live a relatively normal life, they are still at risk of developing complications. These complications can be either acute or chronic. Acute complications are related to the day-to-day fluctuations in blood sugar, namely, hypoglycemia (low blood glucose levels) or hyperglycemia (high blood glucose levels). Chronic complications involve degenerative changes of both large and small blood vessels all over the body and are thought by many to be the result of poor metabolic control. The primary role of the nurse in both acute and chronic complications is to help the patient identify the symptoms of the various complications and facilitate understanding, prevention, and treatment.

Acute Complications. Parents of newly diagnosed diabetic children can be extremely frightened and confused by an unexpected change in the health status of their child. These changes are most often related to fluctuations in serum blood glucose levels. When the blood glucose concentration drops below normal (hypoglycemia), the supply of glucose to the brain is reduced. The body attempts to correct this situation by the production of epinephrine, and consequently the person may suddenly begin to feel (e.g., shaky, pale, sweaty, heart thumping) or behave (e.g., drunken-like, loss of consciousness, or convulsions) differently. When the blood glucose levels are elevated above normal, as at the time of diagnosis, the state is called hyperglycemia. The changes in how a person feels and behaves in hyperglycemia usually develop slowly as the blood sugar accumulates. Some people state that they feel quite normal even though their blood sugar is high.

Nurses need to ensure that young patients and their parents, teachers, and other caregivers know how to recognize and treat both hypoglycemia and hyperglycemia (Table 43–25). With this knowledge, those involved should be better prepared for and more successful in dealing with either of these acute complications of diabetes.

Because each person may feel and react differently during either hypoglycemic or hyperglycemic reactions, it is important for parents to be aware of the sequence of events leading to their child's reaction. The nurse can then encourage parents to communicate this information to teachers or other caregivers so that they also will feel more comfortable in caring for the child with diabetes in the parents' absence.

TABLE 43-25
Causes, Symptoms, and Treatment of Hypoglycemia and Hyperglycemia

Hypoglycemia	Hyperglycemia
Causes	
Not enough food	Not enough insulin
Too much insulin	Too much food
More than the usual amount of exercise	Not enough exercise
Insulin absorbed more rapidly than usual	Emotional stress
	Injury
	Illness, infection
Symptoms	
Sudden onset	Increased thirst
Cold perspiration	Increased urination
Shaky	Decreased appetite
Hungry	Dry skin
Dizzy	Flushed face
Mood change	Confusion
Headache	Dullness
Weak	Blurred vision
Nervous	Nausea and vomiting
Blurry vision	Acetone breath
Slurred speech	Coma
Convulsions, unconsciousness	
Treatment	
Immediately drink one-half cup orange juice or regular sodapop	Increase insulin (may introduce regular insulin)
Take 2 teaspoons sugar or honey	Test urine and blood frequently
Take 3 to 4 Life Savers or Dextrosol or glucose tabs	Notify physician
Glucagon subcutaneously or IV 50% dextrose (when unconscious)	
Follow up with source of complex carbohydrates and protein for more sustained glucose level	

In *hypoglycemia,* rapid treatment is of the utmost importance. Brain functioning depends on glucose, and if the hypoglycemic reaction is extremely severe or prolonged, permanent damage, although rare, may occur. If the patient is alert, he or she can be given a glucose-containing solid, semi-solid, or liquid. Once a reaction has been treated and the child feels stable, she or he can resume normal activity. If, however, the patient is not alert, the administration of fluids by mouth may cause aspiration and lung complications. In this case, parents may be instructed how to administer glucagon at home, or 50 per cent dextrose can be administered intravenously in a hospital emergency department. Caution must be exercised in using 50 per cent dextrose in children. The usual pediatric dose is 0.5 g/kg intravenously immediately. Once the child has regained consciousness, he or she should rest and eat some carbohydrate-containing food, such as milk, cheese, peanut butter, or bread, which will be digested slowly to prevent another rapid drop in blood sugar. Severe or frequent hypoglycemic reactions should be reported to the physician. The nurse should also assess the child's routine and health status after a severe reaction or after frequent reactions in an attempt to determine the cause of the reactions so similar occurrences may be prevented.

In *hyperglycemia,* there is a need for the patient and family to reassess the diet, insulin, and exercise patterns. The body must have enough insulin to use the blood glucose for energy production. When sufficient insulin is not available, the body begins to break down proteins and fats as alternative sources and, as described previously, DKA may occur. If the child exhibits these symptoms of ketoacidosis, parents should encourage the child to drink extra sugar-free fluids, stay warm, and refrain from exercise. The parent should contact the physician if DKA symptoms occur or if the child is nauseated and vomiting. In fact, it should be emphasized to take the child to the emergency department if the child vomits more than twice. Table 43–20 details nursing care for the child hospitalized with DKA.

Chronic Complications. Most chronic complications of diabetes, other than growth and development retardation, do not usually appear before puberty. Because children and adolescents do not usually develop chronic complications, they are not routinely included in initial teaching. Nurses need to use appropriate judgment about when such topics are introduced, and this timing may be different for parents and children. Families and children may have questions about chronic complications that must always be answered in an honest but age-appropriate fashion.

Growth and Development. Growth and development studies suggest that metabolic control influences the rate of growth and that alterations in growth can be avoided with optimal carbohydrate control in combination with adequate nutrition to meet the needs of the growing child (Travis et al, 1987). Children with less than optimal control of carbohydrate metabolism are at risk for growth retardation and delayed sexual maturation. For early detection and intervention, health professionals working with diabetic children should randomly monitor height, weight, and physical and psychosocial development.

Cardiovascular. The most common chronic complication of diabetes is atherosclerosis or a thickening and degeneration of the walls of both large and small blood vessels of the body. When hypoglycemia results in mobilization of fatty acids, lipids are deposited on the intima of blood vessels (Guyton, 1987). Maintenance of normal blood sugar levels is therefore crucial to controlling this complication.

The chief regions affected by large vessel disease are the heart, the brain, and the periphery (especially of the legs and feet). In the heart, patients suffer from narrowing of the coronary arteries and complications due to angina (cramping of the heart tissue) or myocardial infarction (obstruction of the coronary arteries). The brain is subject to several major problems, including cerebral hemorrhage, cerebral thrombosis, and cerebrovascular accidents. Atherosclerosis in the legs and feet leaves this area with a decreased blood supply and thus vulnerable to infection, tissue necrosis, and gangrene.

Although large vessel diseases are among the leading causes of death in adults with diabetes, children with type I diabetes do not usually suffer from large blood vessel damage but more often experience the small vessel complications. Body regions most affected include the eyes, kidneys, and lower extremities.

Eye. Diabetic retinopathy can be expected to develop in 40 to 60 per cent of all persons who contract diabetes in youth. It often takes many years to develop, and only 5 to 15 per cent will have proliferative changes (Travis et al, 1987). The retina is one of the body's tissues that depends on glucose to supply its energy needs (Guyton, 1987). In periods of hypoglycemia, retinal changes can occur. There are several stages of diabetic retinopathy, which include (1) microaneurysm or small dilations of blood vessels, which can be visualized as red dots in the macular area of the eye; (2) exudates and hemorrhage caused by microaneurysms, which may hemorrhage into the retina or vitreous body; after several weeks, these hemorrhages convert into waxy yellowish plaques called exudates; and (3) retinitis proliferans, which is a process of revascularization and rehemorrhaging at the primary hemorrhage site of the disk, which ultimately may be involved in the process of retinal detachment, the primary cause of blindness in diabetes. However, with modern management (e.g., laser treatment), blindness is preventable in the majority of individuals.

Kidney. The kidneys are prone to both infections and nephropathy. Hyperglycemia depresses leukocyte function and provides excellent conditions for bacterial or fungal growth. Diabetics are susceptible to infections throughout the urinary tract system, which can lead to decreased kidney function, pyelonephritis, and damaged renal tissue.

Nephropathy of two types (glomerulosclerosis and tubular nephrosis) occurs almost exclusively in diabetic patients. Kidney damage due to nephropathy is probably irreversible but is thought to be retarded or prevented by good metabolic control. For those with severe renal disease, kidney transplants and mechanical devices may make the future brighter.

Neuropathy. Neuropathy in diabetic subjects is characterized by aching and burning sensations in the lower extremities, loss of sensation, and loss of autonomic function with resulting weakness, postural hypotension, gastrointestinal disturbances, neurogenic bladder, and impotence. The pathophysiologic mechanism of diabetic neuropathy is thought to involve ischemic changes in the nerves and the vessels supplying the nerves, thereby linking neuropathy to the atherosclerotic process. In addition, altered glucose metabolism results in an accumulation of sorbitol, which may decrease conduction velocity in the nerve pathways and interfere with myelinization of the nerves (Groer and Shekelton, 1983).

Facilitating the Child's and Family's Adjustment to Diabetes. "Your child has diabetes." With these few simple words, a family is often required to change its entire lifestyle. The diagnosis is most often a shock and a highly emotional experience. Parents expect that because their child has always been healthy, he or she will remain that way. They feel secure in the belief that serious health problems only occur in other families, and their first reaction is disbelief. This stage of nonacceptance is normal and is the initial stage of the adaptation process. The stages of adaptation in chronic illness have been characterized by Billie (1981) as (1) disbelief, (2) developing awareness, (3) reorganization, (4) resolution, (5) identity change, and finally (6) adaptation.

Each child and family will pass through these stages at their own speed. Everyone needs time to overcome the initial impact of the diagnosis and may need substantial help to adjust. Most parents feel some relief when they realize their child's illness can be controlled.

The strength of the diagnostic impact on the child will vary greatly with age at the time of diagnosis. School-age children may be particularly impressed with their new "condition" and be challenged by the tasks, routines, and skills in their prescribed therapeutic regimen. Adolescents, on the other hand, often feel unfairly victimized and that diabetes is impossible to conquer. These feelings may lead to poor compliance, depression, and low self-esteem.

Patients and parents tend to initially use coping methods that have been successful for them in the past. Some deny what has happened and continue on with their normal lifestyle. Some throw themselves into learning every aspect of management from every available textbook and demand strict adherence to the therapeutic regimen. Still others become overprotective and make the child constantly aware of the illness. Support groups have been successful in helping children with diabetes and their families cope by bringing together other children and families with similar concerns and circumstances. A further discussion of coping with chronic illness is presented in Chapter 19.

Nurses can play a key role in facilitating the child's and family's adaptation to the illness. They should strive to be knowledgeable and provide a relaxed and accepting atmosphere. They should stress that the child and family do not have to learn everything at once. Performing a thorough assessment will provide valuable information about how to proceed with the education process and about whether the family can cope with learning more than the survival skills at this time. From the initial assessment, the nurse can also understand the family's social support systems and can include some of these (e.g., grandparents, babysitters, teachers) in the child's treatment.

Nurses should expect the family's initial coping strategies and understand that the volume of new information may interfere with their ability to absorb this information. Their early questions may need to be addressed several times. Nurses need to be good listeners and be prepared to discuss the child's and family's frustrations and concerns. When they have difficulty giving the insulin injection or when they stray from the prescribed diet, the nurse can help identify the actual problems and shift the focus away from individual guilt. Finally, the nurse can be instrumental in facilitating positive attitudes toward diabetes management and care by emphasizing treatment to maintain health (within the realm of the illness) rather than solely monitoring the illness process.

Promoting Compliance with Treatment. Any individual diagnosed as having diabetes will need to initiate some lifestyle changes. Children diagnosed as having type I DM are often forced to incorporate an imposing regimen (e.g., consisting of insulin injections, a special diet, urine and blood glucose monitoring, and possibly prescribed amounts of exercise) into their daily routine. The complexity of the prescribed regimen and often the nonimmediate rewards provide many opportunities for noncompliance for both the child and the family.

Nearly all physicians caring for a diabetic child will prescribe a specific treatment regimen. The regimen itself may not present an imposing obstacle to the child or the family. However, when the family attempts to integrate the regimen with the problems and demands of the normal activities of "being a child," adherence or compliance often becomes a problem.

Nurses should work with each family to set realistic goals and tailor the regimen to meet the individual needs of the child. Nurses who are knowledgeable in diabetes and growth and development and experienced in working with children and their families can play an integral part in promoting adherence behavior. In addition to physical parameters, such as blood glucose levels, hemoglobin A_{1c} values, and height and weight measurements, the nurse can further assess the child or family in an attempt to determine whether they are compliant with the prescribed regimen.

Areas that are most often difficult for families include diet, blood and urine testing, and insulin administration. In all these areas, the nurse should attempt to include the child and parents in the decision making process concerning the timing and frequency of these activities. Parents should be encouraged as well to allow their children to participate in various aspects of the regimen appropriate for their age, interest, and enthusiasm. In testing procedures, parents need to be cautioned not to condemn the child for abnormal (too high or too low) test results but rather to praise her or his efforts and technique. In this way, the child will not be tempted to either hide or falsely report abnormal results. In children who fear needles and in some adolescents, compliance with taking the insulin injection may also be a problem. For younger children who protest, parents need continued encouragement to persist and often need reinforcement of the child's need for exogenous insulin. In the adolescent, repeated missing of injections might be suggestive of scheduling problems, an expression of frustration or poor self-esteem, or an indication of more serious psychologic problems. For this older child, the support of diabetic peers or psychosocial counseling may be useful. Of all areas of the diabetic regimen, diet provides the most common ground for noncompliance. Nursing interventions designed to promote dietary compliance have been discussed previously in this chapter.

Strauss and colleagues (1984) list characteristics that either deter or enhance a patient's compliance. These include the following:

- Degree of difficulty in learning or carrying out a specific regimen.
- The time needed to carry out the regimen.
- Whether the regimen causes pain or discomfort.
- The energy required to carry out the regimen.
- Whether the regimen is visible to others.
- Whether there is stigma attached to the regimen.
- Whether the patient perceives that the regimen is effective and efficient.
- Whether the regimen causes side effects.
- The cost of the regimen.
- Whether the regimen leads to social isolation.

An added frustration for families and health professionals alike is realizing that perfect adherence to the diabetic regimen does not always guarantee good metabolic control (Garrison & McQuiston, 1989). When all these factors are considered, it is no wonder that children and their families have difficulty following prescribed medical regimens. Nurses may need to try to understand more fully the difficulties patients have in incorporating such regimens as opposed to simply evaluating the patient's and family's compliance.

Promoting Healthy Development. Every child has to deal with accomplishing certain developmental tasks for each age or stage. The child with diabetes has an additional variable that influences normal growth and development. Having diabetes can introduce a number of stresses in a child. The acute onset of symptoms, the initial interaction with a new group of health professionals in either a hospital or an outpatient setting, the concern and worry of parents, and their own feelings of anxiety, worry, and fear are all stress producing. The daily insulin injections, blood or urine testing, and altered diet, which represent the change from a carefree, flexible existence to a more regimented lifestyle, are of concern for the diabetic child and the family. All of these stresses, concerns, and changes require some form of adaptation or coping. The degree of success in the adaptive process depends on many factors, including the age and stage of cognitive development of the child, previous stressful experiences of the child and family, and the amount of social support they receive. The child needs to meet the demands of being both a child and diabetic. Each developmental stage imposes new and different challenges for the diabetic child. The nurse can play an integral part in promoting both normal growth and development and a healthy adaptation in the diabetic child. See Table 43–26 for a summary of specific concerns that diabetes poses at each stage of growth and development and suggested nursing strategies.

Promoting Healthy Parenting. The diagnosis of diabetes changes the child's life and thus that of the whole family. The child has essentially lost his or her normal lifestyle, and both the child and the family will grieve this loss. Diabetes causes anxiety within the family, which may lead to feelings of sorrow, resentment, and hostility. If other family members are also diabetic, there may be tremendous guilt feelings, which may lead to marital problems and family maladjustment.

Nurses can have a key role in enhancing family adaptation. As they perform the assessment of the family's motivation and readiness to learn, they can also assess family functioning in such areas as communication patterns, expression of emotions, and support. Nurses should involve both the family and the child in the initial assessment and attempt to establish rapport, alleviate anxiety, and prioritize learning needs. If extreme friction exists between family members, the nurse may want to interview client and family separately and attempt to point out anger, guilt, or feelings of stress. If the family problems exceed the nurse's capabilities or knowledge, she or he should immediately seek other professional assistance or refer the family for family counseling or psychiatric treatment.

Self-Care Management. The teaching needs listed under the nursing diagnosis of knowledge deficit pro-

TABLE 43-26
Growth and Development of the Diabetic Child

Developmental Characteristics/ Developmental Tasks	Specific Concerns Posed by Diabetes	Suggested Nursing Interventions
Infancy		
Small physical size; rapid physical growth; physically active	Small insulin doses Frequent adjustments of insulin and diet Greater risks of hyperglycemia or hypoglycemia	Teach parents appropriate techniques for accurate measurement: use of 30-unit low-dose syringe, dilution of insulin Frequent visits to primary health care provider
Learning about environment; primitive language	Difficulty in detecting signs of changes on blood glucose	Instruct parents in age-appropriate signs of hypoglycemia: rapid heart beat, dilated pupils, irritability
Developing sense of self and physical capabilities; limited control of body functions	Increased susceptibility to vaginal and perineal infections because of moist glucose-laden environment of diapered infant	Educate parents about increased risks; encourage good hygiene practices and frequent diaper changes
Learning to trust	Pain of frequent injections and blood glucose monitoring can inhibit development of trust	
Dependent, requiring uninterrupted parental supervision	Difficult for parents to locate appropriate baby sitters	Encourage parents to bring other possible caregivers to diabetic teaching sessions; investigate baby-sitting programs with diabetic teens
Toddler		
Developing autonomy Controlling body Making own choices	Diabetes increases dependence on parents; parents may overprotect Frequent urination associated with hyperglycemic periods may make toilet training more difficult Hypoglycemic episodes may initiate temper tantrum behaviors Food selection may begin to be an issue	Encourage use of alternative caregivers Suggest limited choices that parent can allow child to make in diabetic regimen: choice of allowed foods, site of injection
Preoperational thinking; cannot understand consequences of own actions		Encourage parents to set realistic limits and feel confident with them
Preschooler		
Developing initiative	Realizes that diabetes makes him or her different from other family members	Acknowledge differences and focus on strengths Involve child in simple tasks of diabetic management
Developing social independence; may begin preschool	Relinquishing child to other caregivers may be anxiety-provoking for parents Finding an appropriate preschool may be difficult	
Beginning moral judgments ("good" vs. "bad")	May see disease as "punishment"; may interpret "good" or "bad" blood or urine tests as a reflection on himself or herself	Avoid use of judgmental terms in describing test results or alterations from diet Encourage child to express feelings through play and art
Magical thinking; immature use of logic	Child may believe she or he "caught" diabetes from germs	Encourage parents to begin diabetes education using simple concepts and language; role play with dolls, stuffed animals

TABLE 43-26
Growth and Development of the Diabetic Child *(Continued)*

Developmental Characteristics/ Developmental Tasks	Specific Concerns Posed by Diabetes	Suggested Nursing Interventions
School-Age Child		
Developing industry; child wants to be successful in all tasks		Encourage child's independence and acknowledge small successes because children of this age need adult approval
Development of concrete operational thinking and beginnings of formal operational thinking in older school-aged children	Ready for causal information; can understand the immediate consequences of his or her actions Child interested in the scientific nature of the illness (causes of hypoglycemia or hyperglycemia)	Educate child about the nature of diabetes with use of appropriate visual aids, toys Reinforce or teach the child about ways to control symptoms (altering food intake, insulin, exercise)
Developing sense of personal responsibility	Parents are attempting to foster the child's independence but may have difficulty letting go of the diabetic management tasks they have been so accustomed to do	Encourage child to assume responsibility for larger portions of his or her own management of diabetes as he or she is ready
Child makes social comparisons and is developing self-image through these comparisons	Being different from peers may be interpreted as a deficiency by the child Diabetic management tasks that need to be performed in school may be a problem	Encourage child to view diabetes as another example of differences between people and use appropriate comparisons with differences that are widely accepted (e.g., wearing glasses) Encourage parents and child to establish a good working relationship with the school nurse Be sure privacy is available for the child for management tasks Encourage child to wear MedicAlert bracelet Encourage interaction with other diabetic peers through support groups or diabetic camp
Fine-tuning of small motor muscles		Gradually encourage child to assume responsibility for insulin administration and blood glucose testing
Adolescent		
Developing a sense of identity; becoming more independent	May rebel against diabetic management regimen, which is seen as hampering independence; inappropriate food choices May isolate self from family or health care providers	Encourage adolescent to assume full responsibility for diabetic management; advise parents that adolescents still need to have their parents available for consultation and guidance Encourage open discussion of issues; encourage participation in adolescent support group for diabetic teen-agers Teach the individual about food choices that may be appealing to adolescents
Period of rapid physical growth, change, and sexual maturation	May make diabetic control difficult; menstrual periods may lead to reactions related to hormonal changes and effect on glucose metabolism	Reinforce signs and symptoms of hypoglycemia or hyperglycemia; maintain frequent contact with primary health care provider Encourage adolescents to enlist the help of friends and educate them about appropriate actions in case of a reaction Educate girls about possible effects of menstrual cycle

(continued)

TABLE 43-26
Growth and Development of the Diabetic Child *(Continued)*

Developmental Characteristics/ Developmental Tasks	Specific Concerns Posed by Diabetes	Suggested Nursing Interventions
Adolescent *(Continued)*		
Developing sexual interest; preferences	Rebellion can take the form of sexual experimentation	Provide information on the consequences of sexual activity; stress importance of planned preconception counseling for diabetic women
Selecting future lifestyle; career choices		Encourage parents to provide career counseling that acknowledges the demands of a diabetic regimen
Self-image changes with dramatic physical changes; makes many physical comparisons with peers	Self-esteem may suffer because of differences from peers; may be anxious about possible reactions creating embarrassment	Use diabetic adolescent support group
Developing own value system; comparing values of family and peers	May reject parental advice and counseling	Encourage relationships with other supportive adults or peers
Formal operational thinking developing	Long-term consequences of disease will become real to the individual; may lead to depression	Encourage parents to keep discussions about the future open; observe for withdrawal or change in affect

vide, in many ways, a summary of the physical, emotional, and social needs of the child with diabetes and of the family entrusted with home management. Because each of these areas has been addressed previously in this chapter, this section focuses on the mechanism for effectively teaching the child and family about diabetes, its monitoring, and its control.

In recent years, there has been a shift in health care emphasis, moving from the direct-care model toward self-management. In a chronic illness, such as diabetes, the very nature of the illness necessitates a high level of patient and family responsibility for successful day-to-day management.

Successful management of the diabetic patient ideally requires that the patient and family have a thorough knowledge of the illness and the willingness to manage the condition themselves. Their major responsibilities will be to make appropriate changes in treatment to keep blood glucose levels controlled. The key is to empower patients by helping them recognize health-related values, set and achieve their own health care goals, and develop confidence to deal with psychosocial issues. Patient education is the essential first step in motivating successful management. The content of the diabetes teaching program should focus on the needs, goals, and capabilities of

TABLE 43-27
Levels of Diabetic Skills

Survival Skills	Health Maintenance Skills	Health Promotion Skills
Need for insulin	Test blood and urine for glucose and ketones	Use of test results and records to make changes in insulin dose
Differentiate between types of insulin	Keep records	Insulin alteration
Relationship between meals and insulin	Rotate injection sites	Initiate illness regimen
Prepare and administer own insulin	Understand diabetic diet and how to modify during exercise or illness	Ability to modify regimen to maintain good metabolic control
Storage of insulin	How to prevent hypoglycemia	
Foods to avoid	Effect of stress, illness, and exercise	
How to recognize and treat hypoglycemic reaction	Meaning of metabolic control	

the learners. Diabetes education can generally be divided into survival skills, health maintenance skills, and health promotion skills (Tupling et al, 1981). Examples of the various content approaches for each skill level are included in Table 43–27. These skill categories can form the basis for a teaching plan.

Chapter 23 details the principles of patient and family education. Table 23–1 lists implications for teaching children of various ages.

Evaluation

Projected Outcomes

- The child will restore and maintain normal fluid and electrolyte balance and normal glucose levels.
- The child will be well nourished.
- The child will not experience episodes of hypoglycemia or hyperglycemia.
- The child will experience minimal discomfort from injections and blood sampling.
- The child will not experience infection.
- The child will have normal patterns of urinary elimination.
- The child will develop normally in all areas.
- The family will function normally, providing support and assistance to each other.
- The child and family will comply with the treatment regimen.
- The parents will provide developmentally appropriate parenting for the child and allow appropriate levels of independence.
- The child and family will exhibit necessary knowledge about DM and its management.
- The child will not experience any symptoms of the long-term effects of diabetes.

KEY CONCEPTS

Concepts Related to Basic Information

- Complex interrelationships exist between the endocrine glands and the endocrine and nervous systems; dysfunction of one may affect the function of another.
- Endocrine secretion normally functions under a feedback control system.
- Many endocrine disorders are chronic conditions that will continue to require treatment or follow-up into adult life.

Concepts Related to Nursing Assessment

- The endocrine disorders may create circumstances that alter the child's self-image and interfere with the development of positive self-esteem.

Concepts Related to Nursing Intervention

- Treatment of many endocrine disorders requires administration of medications or monitoring of the condition by parents; families may need intensive educational programs.

REFERENCES

American Diabetes Association and American Dietetic Association. (1976). *Exchange list for meal planning*. New York: Author.

American Diabetes Association and American Dietetic Association. (1977). *A guide for professionals: The effective application of exchange lists for meal planning*. New York: Author.

Billie, D. A. (1986). Tailoring your diabetic patient's care plans to fit his life style. *Nursing 86, 16*(2), 54–57.

Billie, D. A. (1981). *Practical approaches to patient teaching*. Boston: Little, Brown.

Bode, H. H. (1990). Disorders of the posterior pituitary. In S. Kaplan (Ed.), *Clinical pediatric endocrinology* (pp 63–86). Philadelphia: WB Saunders.

Bunn, H. F. (1981). Evaluation of glycosylated hemoglobin in diabetic patients. *Diabetes, 30,* 613–617.

Charron-Prochownik, D., & Schwartz, S. (1984). Care of the infant with Type I diabetes mellitus. *Diabetes Educator, 10*(2), 46–50.

Christman, C., & Bennett, J. (1987). Diabetes: New names, new test, new diet. *Nursing 87, 17*(1), 34–42.

Coulston, A., Greenfield, M., Kraemer, F., et al. (1980). Effect of source of dietary carbohydrate on plasma glucose and insulin responses to test meals in normal subjects. *American Journal of Clinical Nutrition, 33,* 1279–1282.

Crapo, P. A., Kolterman, O. G., Waldeck, N., et al. (1980). Postprandial hormonal responses to different types of complex carbohydrate in individuals with impaired glucose tolerance. *American Journal of Clinical Nutrition, 33,* 1723–1728.

Dallas, J. S., & Foley, T. P. (1990). Hyperthyroidism. In F. Lifshitz (Ed.), *Pediatric endocrinology* (2nd ed., pp 483–500). New York: Marcel Dekker.

Dallas, J. S., & Foley, T. P. (1990). Hypothyroidism. In F. Lifshitz (Ed.), *Pediatric endocrinology* (2nd ed., pp 469–482). New York: Marcel Dekker.

Daneman, D., Siminerio, L., Transue, D., et al. (1985). The role of self-monitoring of blood glucose in the routine management of children with insulin-dependent diabetes mellitus. *Diabetes Care, 8*(1), 1–4.

David, M., & Forest, M. G. (1984). Prenatal treatment of congenital adrenal hyperplasia resulting from 21-hydroxylase deficiency. *Journal of Pediatrics, 105*(5), 799–803.

DCCT Research Group. (1987). Protocol for the full scale diabetes control and complications trial (DCCT). *Diabetes Care, 36,* 111A.

Dickerman, J. D., & Lucey, J. F. (1985). *Smith's the critically ill child: Diagnosis and medical management*. Philadelphia: WB Saunders.

Drotar, D., Owens, R., & Gotthold, J. (1980, Fall). Personality adjustment of children and adolescents with hypopituitarism. *Child Psychiatry and Human Development, 11*(1), 59–66.

Evans, M. I., Chrousos, G. P., Mann, D. W., et al. (1985). Pharmacologic suppression of the fetal adrenal gland in utero. *Journal of the American Medical Association, 253,* 1015–1020.

Federal Drug Administration Medical Bulletin. (1991, April). Histrelin, Nafarelin approved for precocious puberty. Washington, DC: US Government Printing Office.

Fisher, D. A. (1990). The thyroid. In S. Kaplan (Ed.), *Clinical pediatric endocrinology* (pp 87–126). Philadelphia: WB Saunders.

Fisher, D. A. (1985). Thyroid hormone and thyroglobulin synthesis and secretion. In Z. Laron (Ed.), *Pediatric and adolescent endocrinology: Vol. 14* (pp 44–56). Basel: Karger.

Foley, T. P. (1982). Acute, subacute, and chronic thyroiditis. In S. Kaplan (Ed.), *Clinical pediatric and adolescent endocrinology* (pp 96–109). Philadelphia: WB Saunders.

Fort, P. (1990). Thyroid disorders in infancy. In F. Lifshitz (Ed.), *Pediatric endocrinology* (2nd ed., pp 437–456). New York: Marcel Dekker.

Fox, R. E., & Redstone, D. (1976). Sources of error in glucose determinations in neonatal blood by glucose oxidase methods, including Dextrostix. *American Journal of Clinical Pathology, 66,* 658–662.

Franklin, R., O'Grady, C., & Carpenter, L. (1985). Neonatal thyroid function: Comparison between breast-fed and bottle-fed infants. *Journal of Pediatrics, 106*(1), 124–126.

Frantz, M. (1987). *Fast food facts*. Minneapolis: Diabetes Center.

Garrison, W., & McQuiston, S. (1989). *Chronic illness during childhood and adolescence*. Newbury Park, CA: Sage Publications.

Geffner, M. E. (1990). Hypoglycemia. In S. Kaplan (Ed.), *Clinical pediatric endocrinology* (pp 165–180). Philadelphia: WB Saunders.

Gellis, S. S., & Kagan, B. M. (1986). *Current pediatric therapy 12*. Philadelphia: WB Saunders.

Glasgow, A. M. (1992). Hypoglycemia. In W. Hung (Ed.), *Clinical pediatric endocrinology* (pp 332–355). St. Louis: Mosby Year Book.

Gordon, M., et al. (1982, September). Psychosocial aspects of constitutional short stature: Social competence, behavior problems, self esteem, and family functioning. *Journal of Pediatrics, 101*(3), 477–480.

Grazaitis, D. M., & Sexson, W. R. (1980). Erroneously high Dextrostix values caused by isopropyl alcohol. *Pediatrics, 66,* 221–224.

Groer, M. W., & Shekelton, M. E. (1983). *Basic pathophysiology. A conceptual approach*. St. Louis: CV Mosby.

Guyton, A. C. (1982, 1987). *Human physiology and mechanisms of disease*. Philadelphia: WB Saunders.

Hamburger, J. I. (1985). Management of hyperthyroidism in children and adolescents. *Journal of Clinical Endocrinology and Metabolism, 60*(5), 1019–1024.

Harris, M. (1980). The changing prevalence of diabetes. *Diabetes Dateline (The National Diabetes Information Clearinghouse Bulletin), 1*(5).

Heins, J. M. (1983). Dietary management in diabetes mellitus: A goal-setting process. *Nursing Clinics of North America, 18*(4), 631–643.

Hung, W. (1992). Ovaries and variants of female sexual development. In W. Hung (Ed.), *Clinical pediatric endocrinology* (pp 226–267). St. Louis: Mosby Year Book.

Hung, W., August, G. P., & Glasgow, A. M. (1983). *Pediatric endocrinology*. New York: Medical Examination Publishing Company.

Jenkins, D. J. A., Wolever, T. M. S., Taylor, R. H., et al. (1981). Glycemic index of foods: A physiological basis for carbohydrate exchange. *American Journal of Clinical Nutrition, 34,* 362–366.

Johanson, A. J., & Blizzard, R. M. (1990). Growth hormone treatment. In F. Lifshitz (Ed.), *Pediatric endocrinology* (2nd ed., pp 61–76). New York: Marcel Dekker.

Kaplan, S. (1990). Growth and growth hormone: Disorders of the anterior pituitary. In S. Kaplan (Ed.), *Clinical pediatric endocrinology* (pp 1–62). Philadelphia: WB Saunders.

Kappy, M., Stuart, T., Perelman, A., & Clemons, R. (1989). Suppression of gonadotropin secretion by a long-acting gonadotropin-releasing hormone analog (Leuprolide acetate, Lupron Depot) in children with precocious puberty. *Journal of Clinical Endocrinology and Metabolism, 69*(5), 1087.

Kaye, R. (1984). Research and practice in the treatment of insulin-dependent diabetes: A survey of 53 pediatric diabetologists. *Pediatrics, 74*(6), 1079–1085.

Kirkland, R. T., Keenan, B. S., Holcombe, J. H., Kirkland, J. L., & Clayton, G. W. (1978). The effect of therapy on mature height in congenital adrenal hyperplasia. *Journal of Clinical Endocrinology and Metabolism, 47*(4), 1320–1324.

Klein, R. (New England Congenital Hypothyroidism Collaborative). (1990). Elementary school performance of children with congenital hypothyroidism. *Journal of Pediatrics, 116*(1), 27–32.

Kreiter, M., Burstein, S., Rosenfield, R., Moll, G. W. Jr., Cara, J. F., Yousefzadeh, D. K., Cuttler, L., & Levitsky, L. L. (1990). Preserving adult height potential in girls with idiopathic true precocious puberty. *Journal of Pediatrics, 117*(3), 364–370.

Kroc Collaborative Study Group. (1984). Blood glucose control and the evolution of diabetic retinopathy and albuminuria. *New England Journal of Medicine, 311*(6), 365–371.

Krueger, J. A., & Ray, J. C. (1976). *Endocrine problems in nursing*. St. Louis: CV Mosby.

LaFranchi, S. (1987). Hypoglycemia of infancy and childhood. *Pediatric Clinics of North America, 34*(4), 961–982.

Lee, P. A., & O'Dea, L. S. L. (1992). Testes and variants of male sexual development. In W. Hung (Ed.), *Clinical pediatric endocrinology* (pp 268–312). St. Louis: Mosby Year Book.

Letarte, J. (1985). Laboratory tests for thyroid diagnosis in infants and children. In Z. Laron (Ed.), *Pediatric and adolescent endocrinology: Vol. 14* (pp 117–126). Basel: Karger.

Lifshitz, F., & Cervantes, C. D. (1990). Short stature. In F. Lifshitz (Ed.), *Pediatric endocrinology* (2nd ed, pp 3–26). New York: Marcel Dekker.

Malone, J. I., Hellrung, J. M., Malphas, E. W., et al. (1976). Good diabetic control: A study in mass delusion. *Journal of Pediatrics, 88,* 943.

Mazur, T. (1984, November-December). Ambiguous genitalia: Detection and counseling. *Pediatric Nursing, 9*(6), 417–422.

Migeon, C. J., & Lanes, R. L. (1990). Adrenal cortex: Hypo- and hyperfunction. In F. Lifshitz (Ed.), *Pediatric endocrinology* (2nd ed., pp 333–352). New York: Marcel Dekker.

Miller, P., Stratton, C., & Tripp, J. (1983). Blood testing compared with urine testing in the long-term control of diabetes. *Archives of Disease in Childhood, 58,* 294–297.

Miller, W. L., & Levine, L. S. (1987). Molecular and clinical advances in congenital adrenal hyperplasia. *Journal of Pediatrics, 111*(1), 1–17.

Mimouni, F., & Tsang, R. (1990). Parathyroid and vitamin D–related disorders. In S. Kaplan (Ed.), *Clinical pediatric endocrinology* (pp 427–454). Philadelphia: WB Saunders.

Mulaikal, R. M., Migeon, C. J., & Rock, J. A. (1987). Fertility rates in female patients with congenital adrenal hyperplasia due to 21-hydroxylase deficiency. *New England Journal of Medicine, 316*(4), 178–182.

National Diabetes Data Group. (1979). Classification and diagnosis of diabetes mellitus and other categories of glucose intolerance. *Diabetes, 28,* 1039–1057.

Nemchik, R. (1982). Diabetes today: A whole new world. *RN, 45*(10), 31–36.

New, M. I., del Balzo, P., Crawford, C., & Speiser, P. W. (1990). The adrenal cortex. In S. Kaplan (Ed.), *Clinical pediatric endocrinology* (pp 181–234). Philadelphia: WB Saunders.

Notkins, A. L. (1979, November). The causes of diabetes. *Scientific American, 241,* 62–73.

Oberfield, S. E., & Levine, L. S. (1990). Pubertal gynecomastia. In F. Lifshitz (Ed.), *Pediatric endocrinology* (2nd ed., pp 249–258). New York: Marcel Dekker.

Pagon, R. A. (1987). Diagnostic approach to the newborn with ambiguous genitalia. *Pediatric Clinics of North America, 34*(4), 1019–1029.

Pang, S., Wallace, M. A., Hofman, L., Thuline, H. C., Dorche, C., Lyon, C. T., Dobbins, R. H., Kling, S., Fujieda, K., & Suwa, S. (1988). Worldwide experience in newborn screening for classical congenital adrenal hyperplasia due to 21-hydroxylase deficiency. *Pediatrics, 81*(6), 866–874.

Robertson, C. (1986). When an insulin-dependent diabetic must be NPO. *Nursing 86, 16*(6), 30–31.

Root, A. W. (1992). Mechanisms of hormone action: General principles. In W. Hung (Ed.), *Clinical pediatric endocrinology* (pp 1–12). St. Louis: Mosby Year Book.

Rosenfield, R. L. (1990). The ovary and female sexual maturation. In S. Kaplan (Ed.), *Clinical pediatric endocrinology* (pp 259–324). Philadelphia: WB Saunders.

Ruble, J. A. (1990). Care of the child with congenital adrenal hyperplasia. In P. Jackson & J. Vessey (Eds.), *Primary care of the child with a chronic condition* (pp 169–186). St. Louis: CV Mosby.

Salas, M. (1990). Thyroid nodules in children and adolescents. In F. Lifshitz (Ed.), *Pediatric endocrinology* (2nd ed., pp 501–512). New York: Marcel Dekker.

Schwartz, I. D., & Bercu, B. B. (1992). Normal growth and development. In W. Hung (Ed.), *Clinical pediatric endocrinology* (pp 13–41). St. Louis: Mosby Year Book.

Siegel, S. F., & Lee, P. A. (1992). Adrenal cortex and medulla. In W. Hung (Ed.), *Clinical pediatric endocrinology* (pp 179–225). St. Louis: Mosby Year Book.

Skyler, J. S. (1983). Dietary planning in insulin-dependent diabetes mellitus. *Pediatric Annals, 12*(9), 652–657.

Speiser, P. W., & New, M. I. (1990). An update of congenital adrenal hyperplasia. In F. Lifshitz (Ed.), *Pediatric endocrinology* (2nd ed., pp 307–332). New York: Marcel Dekker.

Sperling, M. A. (1992). Diabetes mellitus. In R. F. Behrman, R. M. Kliegman, W. E. Nelson, & V. C. Vaughan III (Eds.), *Nelson textbook of pediatrics* (pp 391–409). Philadelphia: WB Saunders.

Stabler, B., et al. (1980). Social judgements by children of short stature. *Psychological Reports, 46,* 743–746.

Strauss, A. L., Corbin, J., Fagerhaugh, S., et al. (1984). *Chronic illness and the quality of life* (2nd ed.). St. Louis: CV Mosby.

Styne, D. (1990). The testes: Disorders of sexual differentiation and puberty. In S. Kaplan (Ed.), *Clinical pediatric endocrinology* (pp 367–426). Philadelphia: WB Saunders.

Travis, L. B., Brouhard, B. H., & Schreiner, B. J. (1987). *Diabetes mellitus in children and adolescents*. Philadelphia: WB Saunders.

Tupling, H., Webb, K., Harris, G., et al. (1981). *You've got to get through the outside layer.* Sydney, Australia: Diabetes Education and Assessment Programme of the North Shore Hospital of Sydney and The Northern Metropolitan Health Region of the Health Commission of New South Wales.

Winter, W. (1991). Atypical diabetes in blacks. *Clinical Diabetes, 9*(4), 49–56.

Zimmerman, S. S., & Gildea, J. H. (1985). *Critical care pediatrics.* Philadelphia: WB Saunders.

BIBLIOGRAPHY

Balik, B., et al. (1986, September-October). Diabetes and the school-aged child. *MCN, 11*(5), 324–330.

Bermel, J. (1984, June). How short is too short? *Medica,* pp 22–26.

Burrows, G. N., & Dussault, J. H. (Eds.). (1980). Guidelines for neonatal thyroid screening programs. *Neonatal thyroid screening* (pp 307–310). New York: Raven Press.

Butts, D. E. (1987). Fluid and electrolyte disorders associated with diabetic ketoacidosis and hyperglycemic hyperosmolar nonketotic coma. *Issues in Comprehensive Pediatric Nursing, 10*(3), 827–836.

Callahan, M. (1988, March). Why you should teach your diabetic patients to chart. *Nursing 88, 18*(3), 48–49.

Edwards, D. R. (1987). Initial psychosocial impact of insulin-dependent diabetes mellitus on the pediatric client and family. *Issues in Comprehensive Pediatric Nursing, 10*(4), 199–207.

Funnell, M. M., & McNitt, P. (1986, March). Autonomic neuropathy. Diabetics' hidden foe. *American Journal of Nursing, 86*(3), 266–270.

Gordon, M., Crouthamel, C., Post, E. M., et al. (1982, September). Psychosocial aspects of constitutional short stature: Social competence, behavior problems, self-esteem, and family functioning. *Journal of Pediatrics, 101*(3), 477–480.

Guyton, A. C. (1991). *Textbook of medical physiology* (8th ed.). Philadelphia: WB Saunders.

Heins, J. M., et al. (1987, February). The new look in diabetic diets. *American Journal of Nursing, 87*(2), 196–198.

Hernandez, C. M. G. (1987, June). Surgery and diabetes. Minimizing the risks. *American Journal of Nursing, 87*(6), 788–792.

Hurxthal, K. (1988, August). Quick! Teach this patient about insulin. *American Journal of Nursing, 88*(8), 1097–1100.

Insulin as a nasal spray. (1987, August). *American Journal of Nursing, 87*(10), 1011.

Johnson, S. (1983). *Facts about precocious puberty.* Office of Research & Reporting at the National Institute of Child Health and Human Development, Room A32, Bld. 31, 9000 Rockville Pike, Bethesda, MD 20205.

Loman, D., & Galgani, C. (1984). Monitoring diabetic children's blood-glucose levels at home. *MCN: American Journal of Maternal Child Nursing, 9*(3), 192.

Parks, B. R., & Fischer, R. G. (1986, July/August). Growth hormone. *Pediatric Nursing, 12*(4), 302.

Schneier, R. L., & Tenore, A. (1981). *Hypothyroidism and the infant.* Arthur Retlaw and Associates, Inc., Suite 2080, 1603 Orrington Avenue, Evanston, IL 60201.

Short stature and dwarfism . . . why some kids grow up to be small. Human Growth Foundation, Maryland Academy of Science Bldg, 7 W. Mulberry St., Baltimore, MD 21201.

Stabler, B., Whitt, J. K., Moreault, D. M., et al. (1980). Social judgements by children of short stature. *Psychological Reports, 46,* 743–746.

Travis, L., & Brouhard, B. (1987). *Diabetes mellitus in children.* Philadelphia: WB Saunders.

US Department of Health, Education and Welfare, PHS National Institutes of Health: *Diabetes data, compiled 1977* (Publication No. 79–1468). Reprinted August 1979.

Winter, W. (1991). Atypical diabetes in blacks. *Clinical Diabetes, 9*(4), 49–56.

Zimmerman, E., et al. (1987). Diabetic camping: Effect on knowledge, attitude, and self-concept. *Issues in Comprehensive Pediatric Nursing, 10*(2), 99–111.

CHAPTER • 44

Altered Metabolic Function

Anne Davidson-Mundt

RELATED TOPICS
Fostering Self-Esteem, Chapter 14
Chronic Illness, Chapter 19
Impact of death and dying, Chapter 20
Mental retardation, Chapter 27
Genetic principles and nursing practice, Chapter 31

LEARNING OBJECTIVES

- Explain the biochemistry of inborn errors of metabolism.
- Describe the nurse's role in neonatal screening.
- Describe the nursing implications that are specific to various types of metabolic defects.
- Apply the general principles of nursing care to the long-term care of the child with a metabolic disorder.
- Describe the health maintenance issues for the child with phenylketonuria (PKU).
- Describe the health maintenance issues for the child with medium-chain acyl-CoA dehydrogenase deficiency (MCADD).

Once thought to be rare, inherited metabolic diseases actually account for a significant amount of infant and childhood morbidity and mortality. Increasingly sophisticated methods of diagnosis and treatment have resulted in more children requiring management of an inborn error of

metabolism. This chapter focuses on several major categories of inherited metabolic disorders; a prototype of each disorder provides the basis for discussion of management issues. Although treatment directives are generally provided by a multidisciplinary team, nurses play key roles in child and family education and in anticipatory guidance and support.

Metabolic disorders tend to be complex; their causative defects are usually irreversible, and they are manifested as a range or continuum, from the very mild to the extremely profound. Some diseases can now be detected prenatally or in the very early postnatal stages by screening, but most inherited metabolic diseases remain undetectable until the patient presents with more overt signs. Even then, many of these diseases are not accurately diagnosed. Because inborn errors of metabolism may be mistaken for more common and more readily diagnosed disorders, nurses should be aware of the presenting signs and symptoms of these diseases and encourage the pursuit of an accurate diagnosis.

Inherited metabolic diseases are genetic disorders in which the child has a block in a metabolic pathway. The presentation, severity, and prognosis vary within as well as among categories of inborn errors of metabolism. In addition, individuals with the same disorder may have differences as a result of other genetic or environmental factors. Because of the genetic variation in different populations, the incidence of a particular disorder varies.

Some disorders can be treated, usually by specific diets and/or medications. Others have no treatment, and families need assistance with management of symptoms. Early and accurate diagnosis may make a significant impact on long-term outcome.

Structure and Function: Biochemistry of Inborn Errors of Metabolism

In most of the body's metabolic processes, a specific enzyme catalyzes each biochemical reaction. The *enzyme* is a protein that enables the biochemical reaction to take place; the enzyme itself is not changed in the process. The substrate in a metabolic pathway is a molecule that is acted on and changed by the enzyme to yield a specific product. When an enzyme is absent or nonfunctional, a block is created at a particular step in a metabolic pathway. Consequences of a block may be a build-up of the substrate(s) preceding the block or deficient product(s) that should have been formed, or both (Fig. 44–1). To function properly some enzymes need co-factors ("helpers"), such as vitamins or other enzymes. Consequently, metabolic diseases can also occur when there is deficiency of a co-factor (see "Biopterin Co-factor Defects" under "Phenylketonuria"). The clinical significance of a blocked pathway depends on the degree of enzyme deficiency, the location of the block, and the importance of the particular pathway.

Genetics

Genes are responsible for causing enzymes to be produced in the cells of the body. An enzyme deficiency occurs when there has been a change (mutation) in the deoxyribonucleic acid (DNA) in the gene that codes for a particular enzyme. A regulator gene functions to turn another gene on (or off) such that a problem with a regulator gene can also affect the amount of enzyme produced. Because humans have two copies of each gene, except for the X chromosome in males, consequences of a genetic disorder depend on the function of the gene product (see Chapter 31). Although there are exceptions, metabolic disorders generally result when both copies of the gene coding for a particular enzyme are abnormal, which is known as *autosomal recessive inheritance*. Half the normal amount of enzyme activity, which occurs when one gene produces functional enzyme, is usually enough to prevent clinical symptoms. Individuals with one normal gene and one abnormal gene are called *carriers of the disorder*. As with all autosomal recessive disorders, the recurrence risk for carrier parents is 25 per cent with each pregnancy.

Part of the variability in the severity of each disease is thought to be a result of differences in genetic mutations. For example, a child with a mild form of a disorder probably inherited genes for the enzyme that were mutated differently (and are relatively more functional) than a child with the severe form of the disorder. However, other genetic and environmental factors may influence the severity of a disease.

Although most inborn errors of metabolism are autosomal recessive, a few are *X-linked*. This occurs

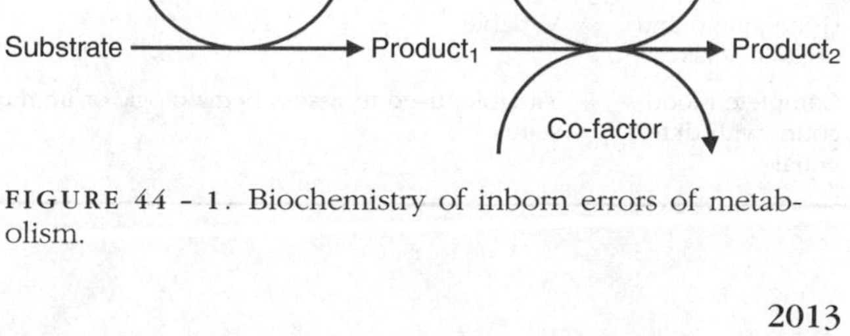

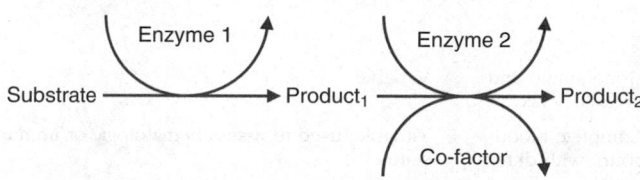

FIGURE 44 – 1. Biochemistry of inborn errors of metabolism.

when the gene for the particular enzyme is located on the X chromosome. Boys have the disorder, whereas girls are rarely affected with the full disease. However, female carriers may be symptomatic, depending on the lyonization (see Chapter 31) of the affected X chromosome. The recurrence risk for a family depends on whether the mutation in the X chromosome was a new mutation or whether the mother carries the abnormal gene. Many X-linked disorders are lethal in boys.

History and Physical Examination: General Presentation and Evaluation

The clinical presentation of various metabolic diseases varies and may be similar to other more common pediatric disorders. Signs and symptoms occur at a variety of ages—some within the first few days of life and others in childhood, adolescence, or even adulthood. Accurate diagnosis is essential for proper management and genetic counseling. An inborn error of metabolism should be included in the differential diagnosis of a child who has any of the following: developmental delay or regression; hypotonia, hypertonia, or other neurologic abnormalities; psychosis; poor eating; food avoidances; vomiting; failure to thrive; hypoglycemia; liver disease; unusual odor (sweat, urine, breath); or metabolic acidosis (with or without hyperglycemia).

For some disorders, irreversible neurologic damage has occurred by the time symptoms appear. Treatment may prevent further damage but cannot reverse the damage that has been done. For this reason, newborn screening was developed for certain diseases.

Diagnostic Assessment

Evaluation for a metabolic disorder entails a thorough assessment including health history, family history, and physical examination. The initial laboratory evaluation usually includes one or more of the following, depending on the results of the initial assessment: electrolytes including bicarbonate, complete blood count, ammonia, serum glucose, urine and/or blood ketones, urine-reducing substances, serum or plasma amino acids, and urine amino and organic acids. Additional studies may be indicated on the basis of these results. Table 44–1 provides a listing of laboratory tests that may be used in the metabolic workup.

TABLE 44–1
Laboratory Values: Metabolic Function

Name	Clinical Significance	Nursing Implications
Electrolytes	Evaluate for a metabolic acidosis; low bicarbonate may be found in an organic acidemia or urea cycle disorder (some carbohydrate disorders also)	Assess neurologic status Correct acidosis per orders (e.g., intravenous bicarbonate) Repeat electrolytes as ordered
Serum glucose	Hypoglycemia may be present, especially in fatty acid oxidation disorders (and some disorders of carbohydrate metabolism)	Assess neurologic status Correct the hypoglycemia per orders Monitor glucose levels
Ammonia	Hyperammonemia may be a result of transient hyperammonemia of the newborn, an organic acidemia, or urea cycle disorder	Assess neurologic status Be prepared for various methods to lower ammonia level (e.g., medications, dialysis, exchange transfusion)
Ketones	Variable	Chart results; note degree of ketosis in relation to blood sugars, neurologic status, and oral or intravenous intake
Urine-reducing substances	A positive result may indicate a disorder of carbohydrate metabolism	Chart results Note type of formula/food intake Assess neurologic status
Serum amino acids	Variable	Communicate results to physicians or metabolic consultants Note time of collection in relation to feeding
Urine amino and organic acids	Variable	Communicate results to physicians or metabolic consultants
Complete blood count with differential	Variable; used to assess hematologic or immunologic status	Communicate results to physicians or metabolic consultants

Therapeutic Management

Treatment for metabolic diseases is specific for each disorder, but there are common principles. Strategies may include decreasing the substrate preceding the enzymatic block, such as avoiding a particular amino acid or carbohydrate; supplementation of the deficient product that should have been produced; providing an enzymatic co-factor; or using medication to remove accumulated substrate. Replacement of the deficient enzyme is possible in a few disorders as a result of liver or bone marrow transplant or intravenous administration, but many are experimental and questions about long-term efficacy remain. A future option may be somatic gene therapy (see Chapter 31). For disorders in which treatment is unavailable or ineffective, supportive care and management of symptoms remain the focus of treatment.

Prevention Issues: Newborn Screening

In the 1960s, a method of screening newborns for phenylketonuria (Guthrie & Susi, 1963) began a major preventive public health program. Newborn screening programs are now in place in all states in the United States and in most developed countries. Programs screen for more than phenylketonuria (PKU), and the potential exists to add many additional tests. Nurses may be involved in multiple aspects of newborn screening, including specimen collection; follow-up procedures for positive tests; and education of parents, community, and other health care providers.

Nurses should be familiar with the regulations and specific guidelines in their respective states; nevertheless, there are common principles in newborn screening. Although the best time to obtain a specimen may be a few days after birth to allow for the accumulation of phenylalanine (or other substances, depending on the disorder being screened), most neonates are now being discharged sooner. Consequently, the current recommendation is to screen all newborns before they are discharged. If the first screen is done before 24 hours of age, a repeat screen for PKU is recommended at 7 to 14 days; sick or premature babies should be screened at 7 days of age, or earlier if a disorder is suspected (Committee on Genetics, American Academy of Pediatrics, 1992). If possible, specimens should be obtained before blood transfusions are done. Some programs may recommend routine complete second screens.

Table 44–2 summarizes disorders that may be included in newborn screening programs, although there is wide variation among programs. The American Academy of Pediatrics has published a set of fact sheets on disorders included in newborn screening (Committee on Genetics, American Academy of Pediatrics, 1989). Nurses can assist in educating families about newborn screening, especially for early discharge and home births. Nurses can also help ensure that an adequate specimen is obtained and that the newborn screening form is accurately completed.

Application of the Nursing Process

Many children with metabolic disorders require long-term management. Nurses are involved with the other members of the multidisciplinary team to provide the professional support needed to ensure optimal outcomes for the child and family. The nursing process plan "Long-Term Care of the Child with a Metabolic Disorder" (Table 44–3) describes the facets of long-term nursing care for this group of children and their families.

Amino Acid Disorders

Inborn errors of metabolism result from blocked enzymatic pathways in a variety of biochemical reactions. Many disorders of amino acid metabolism have been studied extensively, and one (PKU) often serves as a prototype for the benefits of early detection and treatment of metabolic disorders. Information on normal metabolism of protein, carbohydrates, and fats is needed, and a brief explanation of this is given for each major category of disorder.

Normal Protein Metabolism

The metabolic pathways involved in amino acid metabolism are intricate and multiphased. Each step is assisted by a very specific enzyme and, in many cases, by a co-enzyme or co-factor. If any one of these is absent or is decreased in amount or efficiency, the amino acid cannot be properly metabolized. The metabolite that precedes the block builds up, causing symptoms, or it may be directed through a secondary pathway that may cause pathologic levels of another substance that, in turn, produces symptoms.

Amino acids are primarily obtained from the breakdown of proteins from animal products, but there are varying amounts of amino acids in plant proteins as well. After the digestive process releases free amino acids into the blood stream, transport systems carry the amino acids across cell membranes and into the cell (Munro & Crim, 1988). They may be utilized for the synthesis of necessary molecules, such as hormones, enzymes, and structural proteins, or they may be converted to other amino acids or broken down for energy. Amino acids may also be derived from catabolism of body proteins, which mainly occurs during periods of fasting or hypercatabolism; therefore, the balance achieved from treatment of cer-

TABLE 44–2
Newborn Screening Summary

Basic Defect	Symptoms	+ Screening Incidence	Criteria	Treatment	Follow-Up Needs
Phenylketonuria (Classic)					
Lack of enzyme for proper conversion of the amino acid phenylalanine to tyrosine	Severe mental retardation, eczema, seizures, behavior disorders, decreased pigmentation, distinctive "mousy" odor	1:10,000 to 1:15,000 More common in whites	Elevated phenylalanine	Low-phenylalanine diet; possible tyrosine supplementation	Lifelong dietary management; careful monitoring of hyperphenylalaninemia variants; careful management and pre-conception counseling and intervention in the reproductive years for women with phenylketonuria
Congenital Hypothyroidism (Primary)					
Absent or hypoplastic gland; dysfunctional gland	Mental and motor retardation; short stature; coarse, dry skin and hair; hoarse cry, constipation	Overall 1:4000 with ethnic variation 1:12,000 African-American 1:1000 Native American	Low T_4, elevated thyroid-stimulating hormone	Replacement of L-thyroxine	Maintenance of L-thyroxine levels in upper half of normal range; periodic bone age to monitor growth
Galactosemia (Transferase Deficiency)					
Absent or low activity of enzyme to convert galactose into glucose	Neonatal death from severe dehydration, sepsis, or liver pathology; mental retardation, jaundice, blindness, cataracts	1:10,000 to 1:90,000	Elevated galactose (Hill); low or absent fluorescence (Beutler)	Eliminate galactose and lactose from the diet; Soy formulas in infancy; lactose-free solid foods	Provision of early monitoring for speech and neurologic problems; education of parents about hidden sources of lactose; monitoring of females for secondary ovarian failure; avoidance of medications with lactose fillers
Maple Syrup Urine Disease					
Absent or low activity of enzyme needed to metabolize leucine, isoleucine, and valine	Acidosis; hypertonicity and seizures, vomiting, drowsiness, apnea, coma; infant death or severe mental retardation and neurologic impairment; behavioral disorders	1:90,000 to 1:200,000	Elevated leucine	Diet low in leucine, isoleucine, and valine; thiamine supplement if responsive	Education of family and friends regarding strict dietary regimen; social and education evaluation; behavioral counseling; neurologic monitoring; prompt treatment of illness to minimize acidosis
Homocystinuria					
Deficiency of enzyme cystathionine synthase, which is needed for homocystine metabolism	Mental retardation, seizures, behavior disorders, early-onset thromboses, dislocated lenses, tall lanky body habitus	1:200,000	Elevated methionine	Methionine-restricted diet; cystine supplement; vitamin B_6 supplement if responsive	Maintenance of lifelong low-methionine diet; monitoring for thrombosis (e.g., check pulses); ophthalmologic care; educational and psychologic evaluation; avoidance of unnecessary surgery

TABLE 44-2
Newborn Screening Summary *(Continued)*

Basic Defect	Symptoms	+ Screening Incidence	Criteria	Treatment	Follow-Up Needs
Congenital Adrenal Hyperplasia					
Defect in the enzyme-21-hydroxylase	Hyponatremia, hypokalemia, hypoglycemia, dehydration, and early death; ambiguous genitalia in females; progressive virilization in both sexes	1:15,000 to 1:3000 native Eskimos	Elevated 17-hydroxy progesterone; abnormal electrolytes	Replacement of corticosteroids; plastic surgery to correct ambiguous genitalia	Maintenance of adequate corticosteroids; elevation of doses or giving injectable doses in times of stress; periodic bone age to monitor adequate treatment; maintenance of pediatric endocrinology follow-up appointments
Biotinidase Deficiency					
Low activity of the enzyme biotinidase; biotin deficiency	Mental retardation, seizures, ataxia, skin rash, hearing loss, alopecia, optic nerve atrophy, coma, and death	1:60,000 to 1:100,000	Deficient or absent activity of biotinidase on calorimetric assay	10 mg biotin daily	Monitoring compliance; periodic follow-up and evaluation

From Wright, L., Brown, A., & Davidson-Mundt, A. (1992). Newborn screening: The miracle and the challenge. *Journal of Pediatric Nursing,* 7(1), 26–42.

tain disorders can be upset as a result of illness or surgery.

The final steps of amino acid catabolism (such as when the amino acids are not used for synthesis) result in the release of nitrogen. The nitrogen (in the form of ammonia) enters a system known as the urea cycle to produce urea, which is excreted via the kidneys. Metabolic disorders can occur as a result of enzyme deficiencies at any point in amino acid metabolism. When the enzyme block occurs very early in the pathway, the disorders are called aminoacidopathies. Disorders from blocks several steps down the pathway are known as organic acidemias, and enzyme deficiencies at the end point result in urea cycle disorders. Examples from each of these major categories are discussed.

Phenylketonuria

PKU is one of the more common disorders of amino acid metabolism and is the basis of widespread newborn screening. Although PKU was discovered in 1934, dietary management as a treatment was not developed until the 1950s (Bickel et al, 1953). However, some degree of mental retardation still resulted until a mechanism was developed to detect affected children before they developed symptoms. Screening of newborns for PKU began in the early 1960s, and now all states and many countries screen neonates for PKU as well as other diseases.

Etiology and Incidence

PKU is transmitted by an autosomal recessive gene; that is, genetic transmission occurs irrespective of gender, and both parents must be carriers (i.e., heterozygous for the defect) in order for their offspring to have the disease. As with any autosomal recessive gene, if both parents are carriers, there is a 25 per cent chance with each pregnancy that the child will have the disease. Consequently, there is a 25 per cent chance that the child will inherit no genes for PKU and a 50 per cent chance that the child of each pregnancy will be a carrier.

The incidence of PKU varies among ethnic groups and therefore between individual states and countries. It is seen more commonly in people of Northern European ancestry, with an overall frequency of 1 in 10,000 Caucasian births (Scriver et al, 1989). The gene for PKU has been located on chromosome 12 (Lidksy et al, 1984), and investigators are continuing to study the different mutations present in the gene in various populations. There is increasing evidence that different genetic mutations correlate with the degree of enzyme deficiency and thus the heterogeneity of PKU (Okano et al, 1991).

Pathophysiology

Phenylalanine is an amino acid found in all proteins. Normally, the phenylalanine that is not needed for

TABLE 44-3

Nursing Process Plan: Long-Term Care of the Child with a Metabolic Disorder

Analysis: Nursing Diagnostic Statement 1

Response and Related or Risk Factors: *Health-seeking behaviors of child and/or family about how to manage altered nutrition resulting from impaired metabolism of phenylalanine (or other substance, depending on disorder), associated with inheritance of an autosomal recessive trait*

Projected Outcome: The child and/or parent will maintain a stable pattern of health as indicated by continued control of signs of disease

Defining Characteristics

Subjective:

- Expressed or observed desire of child and/or family to seek a higher level of wellness for the child
- Expressed or observed desire for increased control of health practices
- Expression of concern about current environmental conditions on health status of child
- Stated or observed unfamiliarity with community resources

Objective:

- Demonstrated or observed lack of knowledge and/or ability to promote health nutrition in the child

Nursing Interventions

Nutrition Monitoring; Nutrition Management

Assess the elements of the family lifestyle; assist families to incorporate diet in lifestyle; demonstrate methods that family can use to incorporate child's dietary requirements into meal planning

Demonstrate strategies that family members can utilize to promote normal activities; this includes participating in planning for trips, family outings; developing plans with representatives from community settings (e.g., school, camps, extracurricular activities)

Assess parents' and child's adherence to dietary regimen on long-term basis; reinforce dietary information provided by nutritionist; instruct parents on home monitoring procedures to assess child's response to dietary regimen

Support System Enhancement; Support Group

Refer parents to appropriate community resources, such as nonprofit (condition-related) organizations, parent support groups

Instruct parents in the assessment of signs and symptoms indicating alterations in condition

Evaluation Criteria

Child achieves stable health status

Signs and symptoms of disease are controlled

Dietary regimen is followed by child and family as evidenced by

- Maintenance of stable growth pattern on growth chart
- Attainment of developmental skills appropriate for age and condition
- Satisfactory blood levels (e.g., phenylalanine)
- Appropriate weight gain

TABLE 44-3 *(continued)*

Analysis: Collaborative Problem 1

Response and Related or Risk Factors: *High risk for altered growth and development: mental retardation, physical disability; emotional and social acting out and other inappropriate behaviors associated with inborn error of metabolism; risk factors:*

- Ineffective and/or inconsistent discipline
- Parental knowledge deficit about developmental tasks
- Parental knowledge deficit about the home care protocol for promoting development

Projected Outcome: Child will achieve developmental norms within the age-appropriate range to the extent possible, given the disease

Defining Characteristics *(Actual Response)*	**Nursing Interventions**	**Evaluation Criteria**
Subjective: • Fatigability of child when asked to perform activities appropriate for age • Reports of child's lack of progress in achieving developmental milestones • Reports of behavioral problems, problematic eating patterns, poor quality of social interactions • Child perceived as "different," delayed, slow • Parental expression of guilt regarding child's development • Flat affect of child ***Objective:*** • Presence of behavioral problems • Delay or difficulty in performing skills (motor, social, or expressive) typical of age group • Altered physical growth • Inability to perform self-care or self-control activities appropriate for age	*Health Screening* **Assess development on diagnosis, and continually reassess on periodic basis,** using a screening tool approved by the health care team (e.g., Denver Developmental Screening Test II, Chapter 13); an ill child can rarely be assessed all at one time; the nurse may have to rely on parental reports for some behaviors • Compare child's mental (cognitive) and physical development to published norms for age and stage of development (see Chapters 4 through 9 for cognitive and physical norms for each developmental stage) • If evidence of developmental delay, physical disability, or mental retardation are found, refer to appropriate health care professional, e.g., behavioral pediatrician *Anticipatory Guidance* **Assess parent's knowledge of developmental tasks;** with parent, identify tasks specific to the child; enlist parent's help, and the help of older siblings, in planning and implementing appropriate and realistic strategies to maintain or promote development **Collaborate with other team members** (e.g., speech therapist, physical therapist) to blend care strategies to the child's advantage	Child achieves developmental skills and performs self-care or self-control activities typical of age group to the extent allowed by the condition Physical growth is maintained and progresses within normal limits for age and condition Any developmental delay will be identified

(continued)

TABLE 44-3 *(continued)*

Defining Characteristics *(Actual Response)*	***Nursing Interventions***	***Evaluation Criteria***
	Identify (through interviews with the child, parents, home care nurse, and therapists) the protocol followed at home to promote development; enlist the aid of these experts to plan modifications to the protocol appropriate to the illness situation **Implement the modified exercises as tolerated,** being as consistent as possible with home therapy **Evaluate frequently for developmental regression** that would signal the need to further adapt the plan of care	

Analysis: Nursing Diagnostic Statement 2

Response and Related or Risk Factors: *Altered or ineffective family processes (affective, socialization—including parenting, economic), related to*

- Parental feelings of powerlessness about managing the child's illness and parenting the child effectively
- Impaired adjustment of parents to diagnosis and therapeutic regimen
- Lack of knowledge of effective coping methods
- Parental anxiety

Projected Outcome: Parents are able to carry out affective, socialization, and economic functions effectively

Defining Characteristics *(Actual Response)*	***Nursing Interventions***	***Evaluation Criteria***
Subjective: • Verbalization by family members that they cannot meet the child's physical, emotional, and/or social needs • Verbalization by parents that they cannot meet the financial costs resulting from their child's illness • Observed inability of family members to express or accept feelings about the child's illness • Observed or verbalized inability of family members to accept and receive help in meeting affective, socialization, and economic functions	*Active Listening* Attend closely to parents' verbal and nonverbal messages in order to • Determine whether disruption in family processes likely to resolve with additional time • Determine whether family resources are adequate to meet demands of adjustment period • Determine whether additional support services are needed • Determine whether to recommend continuation or discontinuation of home care • Time responses to parents' messages so that they reflect understanding of the received message	• Family is able to meet physical, emotional, spiritual, socialization, and economic needs of its members • Family members are able to express and accept a wide range of own feelings and/or feelings of other family members • Family is able to accept and receive help appropriately • Family exhibits flexibility in behaviors needed to carry out functions and roles • Family accomplishes current and past developmental task(s) • Healthy communication patterns are present in family

TABLE 44-3 (continued)

Defining Characteristics (Actual Response)	Nursing Interventions	Evaluation Criteria
• Observed inability of family to adapt to/deal with the child's illness • Family failing to accomplish current/past family developmental tasks • Inappropriate level and direction of energy of family members *Objective*: • Family members displaying poor eye contact with each other when the child's illness is discussed • Tension evident in verbal exchanges of family members • Unhealthy family decision making skills	• Clarify parents' messages through the use of feedback *Anticipatory Guidance* • Assist the parents to identify and manage anticipated developmental and situational crises and the effects these may have on the family • Instruct parents about normal development and behavior as appropriate • Assist the parents to identify available resources and options for courses of action • Provide and suggest reference materials as appropriate • Schedule follow-up telephone calls to evaluate success or reinforcement needs • Provide the parents with a telephone number to call for assistance if necessary • Determine caregiver's physical and emotional ability to implement the therapeutic regimen; evaluate whether care is being performed as prescribed • Evaluate caregiver's perception of home care; ask: "What is it like to care for your child at home?" *Attachment Promotion* Discuss parents' reaction to infant or child; provide opportunities for parents to see, hold, and examine infant or child immediately after diagnosis; keep infant or child with parents if possible; encourage parents to touch and speak to infant or child; reinforce parents' eye contact with infant; reinforce caregiver role behaviors • **Facilitate empowerment of parents and adjustment to diagnosis and treatment regimen;** allow parents to provide as much care for their infant or child as possible; remain with	

(continued)

TABLE 44-3 (continued)

Defining Characteristics (Actual Response)	Nursing Interventions	Evaluation Criteria
	parents while they are giving care, and reinforce positive efforts; point out to parents positive skills, attributes, and developmental attainments of their infant or child; assist parents in establishing a method, suitable to them, of monitoring their infant's or child's progress; encourage parents to ask questions about their child's condition, progress, and treatment regimen; assist them in obtaining answers to their questions; use parent education to assist parents to understand and perform appropriate parental role behaviors, adapted to the demands of their child's illness and the therapeutic regimen *Coping Enhancement* Teach alternative coping methods as appropriate **Identify specific problems and goals related to care of the child** with the caregivers *Family Integrity Promotion* **Collaborate to set and agree on goals to improve family functions,** and discuss resources and strategies to meet the goals **Encourage the family to normalize family processes** as much as possible • Assess the family's perception of "normal" family lifestyle. Discuss their most valued aspects, and encourage them to continue those activities and relationships to the extent possible • Discuss acceptable ways to modify the child's care to accommodate the usual family lifestyle • Reinforce the importance of planning time for self, spouse, and other children. Without this encouragement, family members may feel guilty about planning time away from the child	

TABLE 44-3 *(continued)*

Defining Characteristics *(Actual Response)*	**Nursing Interventions**	**Evaluation Criteria**
	• Suggest that siblings be allowed to help in age-appropriate ways as family responsibilities are shifted to accommodate changing needs of the child • Discuss and assist parents with ways to provide for and meet siblings' developmental needs so they do not feel "ignored" • **Carry out activities to reduce anxiety;** minimize apprehension, dread, foreboding, or uneasiness of parents *Support System Enhancement* Encourage family consultation with members of the clergy or others who can help family members regain peace of mind and a sense of purpose, make referrals to other community agencies when family resources are inadequate; draw on the family's resources whenever possible; ordinarily, the overall goal is to help the family become self-reliant Encourage family to seek counseling to manage the pressures and uncertainties of the child's condition Make referrals to bereavement counselor or support groups to help deal with the child's deteriorating condition and forthcoming death (Hurler syndrome) *Caregiver Support* **Assess family's need for respite care;** discuss with caregivers the need for and sources of respite care; inform family of available funding for respite care; coordinate volunteers for in-home services as appropriate; arrange for substitute caregiver Reinforce that others (family, baby sitters) can learn basics of care (diet, medical treatment) to enable parents to have time away from child	

(continued)

TABLE 44-3 (continued)

Analysis: Nursing Diagnostic Statement 3

Response and Related or Risk Factors: *High risk for ineffective management of therapeutic regimen; risk factors:*

- Child's reluctance to be different from peers
- Complexity of home care required and family resources

Projected Outcome: The child and family adhere to a program for treatment of the illness and prevention of complications that is satisfactory for meeting health goals

Defining Characteristics (Actual Response)	Nursing Interventions	Evaluation Criteria
Subjective: • Evidence of misunderstanding or misinformation about disease and/or its management • Indication of inconsistent adherence to dietary restrictions or treatment protocol • Verbalized difficulty with regulation or integration of one or more prescribed regimens (e.g., complaints about not being able to "eat what I want" or "Why can't I do what I want? I feel fine") • Verbalized failure to take action to include treatment regimens in daily routines or to reduce risk factors for progression of illness and sequelae • Complexity of health care system • Complexity of therapeutic regimen • Decisional conflicts • Economic difficulties • Powerlessness • Social support deficits *Objective:* • Family and child make choices for daily living that are ineffective in meeting the goals of treatment and prevention regimen • Acceleration of illness symptoms • Laboratory data reveal levels not within treatment range	*Active Listening; Emotional Support* **Encourage verbalization of feelings about the illness through active listening;** expression of emotion often must precede problem solving • Supplement needed facts and clarify misinformation *Support System Enhancement; Support Group* **Assist the client to explore resources to enhance coping with condition** **Refer to peer support group** (peers with chronic conditions) for support system enhancement and to solicit emotional support and alleviate feelings of "I'm different" **Provide support of decision making and the development of options for action;** suggest behavior modification techniques or reward systems for appropriate choices or decisions; suggest that options will promote a change in behavior and ultimately feelings—for example, have child join extracurricular group at school or participate in an afterschool activity **Assist family** in contacting appropriate agencies for financial support *Teaching: Procedure/Treatment; Nutrition Therapy* **Support the family's self-modification by reinforcing effective techniques** and by asking them to share their expertise with other families	• The family and child make choices of daily living that are effective for meeting the goals of the treatment and prevention regimen • Illness symptoms do not accelerate and/or decrease or disappear • Child and family verbalize ease of being able to manage the treatment regimen without conflict or economic difficulty • Child and family verbalize that action is *consistently* taken to include treatment regimens in daily routine

TABLE 44-3 *(continued)*

Defining Characteristics *(Actual Response)*	**Nursing Interventions**	**Evaluation Criteria**
	Teach family about home maintenance program; encourage questions and clarify misconceptions related to • Home specimen collection • Dietary regimen • Emergency measures, if applicable • Identification of untoward signs or symptoms • Use of community resources *Health Screening* **Measure height and weight, and plot on the growth chart;** alert the physician if there is significant deviation from the child's established percentile **Assess the child's development,** paying particular attention to the sense of autonomy and the self-concept, both of which will be important to eventual self-management **Assess family for conflicts between parent and child related to dietary compliance**	

Analysis: Nursing Diagnostic Statement 4

Response and Related or Risk Factors: *Disturbance in self-esteem: affected child, related to*

- Treatment regimen that the child perceives as setting him apart from peers
- Inability to cope with altered body appearance associated with some inborn errors of metabolism
- Lack of available supports for child and family, including formalized groups such as agencies and support groups
- Mental retardation and/or learning disabilities
- Reactions of significant others, friends, classmates, and teachers, such as overprotection, changes in role expectations

Projected Outcome: Child exhibits and expresses positive self-evaluation, positive feelings about self or capabilities

(continued)

TABLE 44-3 *(continued)*

Defining Characteristics	Nursing Interventions	Evaluation Criteria

Subjective:
• Verbalizes feelings of inferiority, negativity, pessimism; expressions of shame, guilt
• Declines opportunities for new experiences
• Verbalizes ambivalence about or rejects positive feedback and exaggerates negative feedback about self
• Denies problems that are obvious to others
• Evaluates self as unable to handle events
 	
Objective:
• Projects blame or responsibility for problems on others
• Hypersensitive to a slight or to criticism
	Self-Esteem Enhancement; Coping Enhancement
	Assess the child's self-esteem
	Institute strategies to enhance self-esteem
	• Discuss with family how to facilitate healthy development of self-esteem
	• Enhance self-esteem by
	  • Encouraging child to identify his or her strengths; reinforce these strengths
	  • Encouraging eye contact in communicating with others
	  • Providing experiences, as appropriate, that allow the child to feel autonomous
	  • Assisting child and family to be able to verbalize and show "significant others" that child wishes and deserves to be treated like any other child without an illness or disability
	• *Normalize* the child's environment and activities as much as possible; encourage participation in role behaviors appropriate to age, stage of development *(role enhancement),* and condition, e.g., encourage school attendance and optimal school performance, participation in extracurricular and social activities, and socialization with peers
	• Discuss treatment regimen with child and parents; emphasize, whenever possible, how treatment regimen allows child to continue with previous activities
	• Assess coping mechanisms and resources available to child and family for coping with altered body appearance; teach additional mechanisms and resources as indicated
		The client displays self-valuing behaviors, as evidenced by
		• Describes self positively
		• Displays more happy than unhappy behavior
		• Talks about realistic plans for the future
		• Displays more autonomy and faith than feelings of guilt and shame
		• Looks forward to new experiences and demonstrating pleasurable feelings of participation in them
		• Accepts positive feedback about self
		• Identifies and accepts problems that cannot be changed
		• Verbalizes self-confidence about ability to deal with events

TABLE 44-3 *(continued)*

Defining Characteristics *(Actual Response)*	**Nursing Interventions**	**Evaluation Criteria**
	Caregiver Support • Ensure that family receives physical and emotional support for their needs so that they can, in turn, meet the child's needs • Refer to appropriate agencies and support groups for financial, physical, and emotional support; refer child and family for assessment of special education needs; often, camps are available for children with specific diagnoses or for children with chronic illnesses and disabilities; this gives the child a chance to interact with other children who have similar self-esteem problems	

Analysis: Nursing Diagnostic Statement 5

Response and Related or Risk Factors: *Family coping: potential for growth related to knowledge deficit and verbalized desire to learn about chance of transmitting genetic trait for particular metabolic disorder*

Defining Characteristics	**Nursing Interventions**	**Evaluation Criteria**
Genetic Counseling Refer to Table 31–17. Nursing Process Plan: The Family with a Genetic Risk		

protein synthesis is converted to tyrosine. Tyrosine, in turn, is important in the synthesis of melanin, thyroxine, and neurotransmitters. In order for phenylalanine to be converted to tyrosine, two enzyme systems must be present. The first is the liver enzyme phenylalanine hydroxylase. If this enzyme is absent, the degradation of phenylalanine does not occur, and classic PKU results. If it is present but occurs in insufficient amounts, a variant form of PKU results, with symptoms related to the degree of deficiency. The term "hyperphenylalaninemia" refers to any elevation of phenylalanine but is often used for the milder forms of enzyme deficiency. PKU refers to the more severe forms of enzyme deficiency.

In the absence (or reduction) of phenylalanine hydroxylase, the serum levels of phenylalanine rise to toxic levels and cause neurologic damage. In addition, phenylethylamine, phenylpyruvic acid, and other metabolites are formed. Phenylketones excreted in the urine give PKU its name.

A second enzyme system must be functional for normal phenylalanine metabolism to occur. Tetrahydrobiopterin is a co-factor for phenylalanine hydroxylase. Dihydropteridine reductase normally ensures an adequate supply of tetrahydrobiopterin through a recycling process. Defects in the co-factor system result in a different group of disorders that may initially be detected as a result of investigation of elevated levels of phenylalanine (Dhondt, 1991). All children with confirmed elevations of phenylalanine should be tested for biopterin co-factor defects.

Clinical Manifestations

Classic Phenylketonuria

Classic PKU develops in the absence or severe deficiency of the enzyme phenylalanine hydroxylase (Fig. 44–2). Infants are normal at birth but begin to show symptoms within the first months of life if untreated. Progressive mental deterioration results; 98 per cent of untreated children have an IQ of less than 70 (Tourian & Sidbury, 1983).

Although brain damage is the most serious effect, other signs and symptoms develop concurrently. Perhaps one of the most classic signs is the musty odor created by the excretion of phenylalanine metabolites

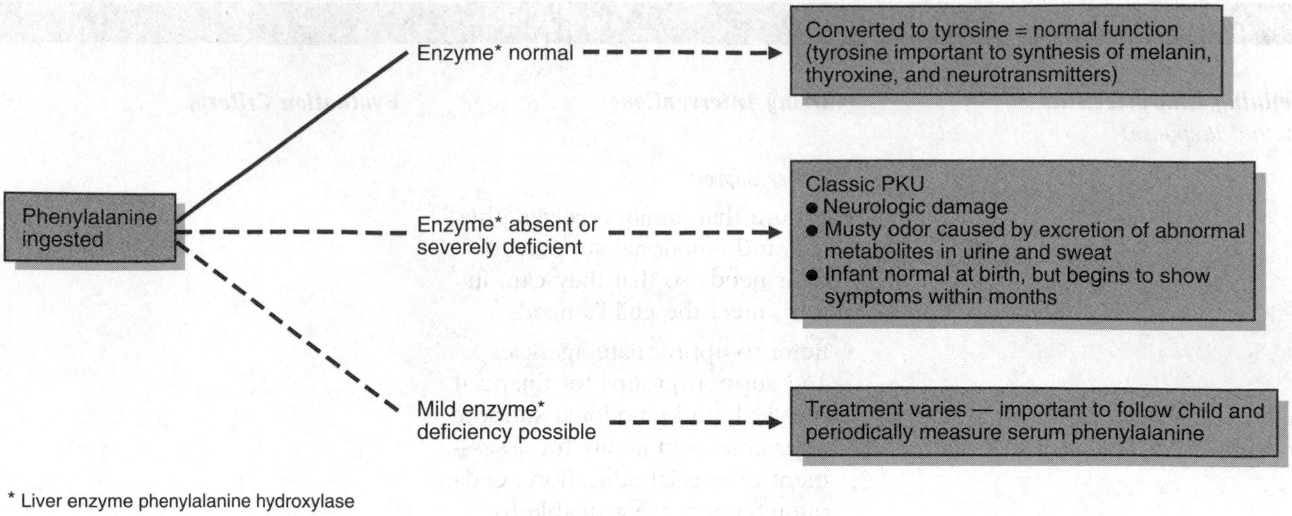

FIGURE 44 - 2. Classic phenylketonuria (PKU) is caused by an absence or severe deficiency of the enzyme that converts phenylalanine to tyrosine. Newborn screening allows early detection and intervention, preventing neurologic damage.

in the urine and sweat. In addition, hypopigmentation of hair and skin develops because of the infant's decreased ability to produce melanin. Eczema, seizures, autism, hyperactivity, and other behavioral manifestations may occur (Güttler & Lou, 1990).

Forms of Hyperphenylalaninemia

Various degrees of hyperphenylalaninemia are caused by differences in amount of enzyme activity as a result of different molecular mutations in the gene. Hyperphenylalaninemia can be thought of as a continuum, with classic PKU (severe enzyme deficiency) at one end and benign hyperphenylalaninemia (mild enzyme deficiency) at the other end. Although decisions regarding the need for treatment are generally based on the degree of hyperphenylalaninemia, controversy exists as to the exact level of phenylalanine requiring treatment in children with a milder enzyme deficiency.

Atypical or Variant Phenylketonuria

Children with the form of hyperphenylalaninemia known as atypical or variant PKU have a less severe deficiency of phenylalanine hydroxylase than do children with classic PKU, but there is not enough enzyme activity to maintain nontoxic levels of phenylalanine on a regular diet. Consequently, these children are treated, although generally they can tolerate a diet prescription that contains more phenylalanine from foods than can children with classic PKU.

Benign (Persistent) Hyperphenylalaninemia

With the advent of newborn screening, a subset of children with a mild deficiency of phenylalanine hydroxylase activity became known. Children in this category have mildly elevated phenylalanine levels, are asymptomatic, and generally are not placed on a special diet as long as their phenylalanine levels remain in a safe range. These children must be followed, and periodic serum phenylalanine levels obtained. Females should be counseled regarding the detrimental effects of maternal elevations of phenylalanine on a fetus (see discussion under "Maternal Phenylketonuria and Hyperphenylalaninemia").

Biopterin Co-Factor Defects

The co-factor tetrahydrobiopterin is needed for two hydroxylases besides phenylalanine hydroxylase (Scriver et al, 1989). Consequently, a biopterin co-factor defect affects many pathways, and treatment is different from that for PKU. Administering neurotransmitter precursors has been tried, but prognosis is usually poor.

Maternal Phenylketonuria and Hyperphenylalaninemia

Maternal PKU and hyperphenylalaninemia is a syndrome that refers to the damage that occurs in offspring of women with elevated levels of phenylalanine during pregnancy. High maternal levels of phenylalanine cross the placenta and act as a teratogen, regardless of whether the fetus has PKU. Detrimental effects include microcephaly, developmental delays or mental retardation, congenital anomalies, spontaneous abortion, and low birthweight (Lenke & Levy, 1980). It is essential that all females with hyperphenylalaninemia be aware of these problems and the need to be under close medical supervision before a pregnancy. In order to minimize the risk of fetal defects, it is recommended that the mother maintain a phenylalanine-restricted diet before conception and throughout pregnancy.

Although studies of the efficacy of maternal diet on fetal outcome (National Maternal PKU Collaborative Study) are ongoing, initial reports are encouraging (Koch et al, 1990). Offspring of women on adequately maintained phenylalanine-restricted diets are, so far, showing good growth and development.

Diagnostic Assessment

Most children with PKU are now diagnosed as a result of newborn screening, which detects elevated levels of phenylalanine in blood. Early detection is critical to preventing the permanent damage that otherwise occurs, and dietary treatment to lower phenylalanine levels into treatment range by 21 days of age is needed (Williamson et al, 1981).

Nurses have a responsibility to alert parents, educators, and other health care professionals to the importance of newborn screening and prompt follow-up procedures (see Table 44–2). Because newborn screening is not infallible, nurses also can help ensure that children with PKU and other disorders missed by screening are diagnosed as quickly as possible. Any child presenting with symptoms of a disorder should be tested; late treatment in infancy cannot reverse damage but can prevent additional damage.

Therapeutic Management

Treatment must begin within the first weeks of life to prevent brain damage. The objective of treatment of the aminoacidopathies involving essential amino acids is to balance the amino acid needs for normal growth and development against the dangers of amino acid accumulation. Phenylalanine is an essential amino acid; therefore, a sufficient amount must be supplied to ensure protein synthesis, but accumulation of excess phenylalanine must be prevented.

Dietary management includes the use of a special formula and restricted phenylalanine intake from natural foods. Several different kinds of formulas may be prescribed, but all contain amino acids needed for growth with either no or small amounts of phenylalanine. If a formula without phenylalanine is used in infancy, measured amounts of a regular infant formula are added. Breastfeeding is also possible in conjunction with one of the metabolic formulas (McCabe et al, 1989). In older children, the special formula becomes the child's "milk," and the remainder of the phenylalanine needed for the body comes from foods.

The initial goal of treatment is to lower the infant's phenylalanine level to prevent neurotoxicity. The infant's unique metabolic patterns are determined by frequently measuring serum phenylalanine (and often tyrosine) levels and keeping detailed records of intake. Close follow-up is required, and dietary adjustments are needed throughout infancy and childhood to allow for growth needs. Tyrosine supplementation may be prescribed.

Solid foods are begun at the usual time in infants with PKU. The solid foods gradually become the source of needed phenylalanine. However, parents and children must recognize appropriate sources of this amino acid. Animal proteins, such as meat, fish, eggs, and milk, and some vegetable proteins, such as legumes and nuts, contain large amounts of phenylalanine and must be avoided. Foods and medications that contain aspartame (Nutrasweet) must also be avoided, because aspartame contains phenylalanine.

Foods allowed on the diet include measured amounts of fruits, vegetables, cereals, and grains. Parents (and later the child) are taught to measure and calculate the amounts of these foods to match the dietary prescription, which is adjusted on the basis of age, weight, and serum phenylalanine levels. Excellent cookbooks that feature low phenylalanine foods are available.

Serum phenylalanine levels are measured frequently, especially during the first few years of life, when growth patterns are rapidly changing. Elevations in serum phenylalanine may occur secondary to physical trauma or even as a result of minor illnesses such as influenza or ear infections. Parents must be educated to perform early assessment of such conditions and to seek prompt treatment for the illness.

Several years ago, the accepted practice was to discontinue the diet when the child was between 5 and 8 years of age. However, studies began to show that many children subsequently had a measurable loss of IQ points and had difficulties with attention and concentration (Holtzman et al, 1986; Azen et al, 1991). Most metabolic centers now recommend keeping children on a diet through the teen-age years and even indefinitely.

Application of the Nursing Process

Assessment

Nursing assessment parameters for the infant or child with PKU are found in the nursing process plan "Long-Term Care of a Child with a Metabolic Disorder" (see Table 44–3).

Nursing Diagnostic Statements and Collaborative Problems

Health-seeking behaviors, child and/or family about how to manage altered nutrition, *resulting from impaired metabolism of phenylalanine associated with inheritance of an autosomal recessive condition.*

High risk for altered growth and development; brain damage; *risk factor: the accumulation of neurotoxic levels of phenylalanine and its metabolites.*

High risk for altered parenting: overprotection; *risk factor: anxiety about brain damage with dietary noncompliance.*

High risk for disturbance in self-esteem, body image, and role performance; *risk factors: eating patterns that differ radically from those* *of peers; implications for future parenthood: (1) potential for transmitting defective gene to offspring, and (2) potential for fetal injury associated with maternal PKU.*

Family coping: potential for growth, related to knowledge deficit: parents (initially) and child (later), about

- *Normal phenylalanine metabolism and the pathophysiology of PKU.*
- *Relationship between phenylalanine accumulation and brain damage.*
- *Dietary treatment.*
- *Need for close medical follow-up.*
- *Early signs and symptoms of infection and indications for obtaining medical help.*
- *Ways to facilitate the child's development, despite rigid dietary restrictions.*
- *Sources of financial, emotional, and informational support for PKU, including genetic counseling.*

High risk for ineffective management of therapeutic regimen; risk factors:

- *Parent/child denial of disease itself or need for the treatment regimen.*
- *Child's reluctance to be different from friends.*
- *Lack of information about nature and treatment of disease.*
- *Complexity of home care required.*
- *Parent-child conflict in general or regarding diet.*
- *Child eating nonallowed foods willfully or with permission from others not familiar with diet.*
- *Complexity of therapeutic regimen.*
- *Lack of availability of familial or social support.*
- *Lack of access to or lack of knowledge of all levels of health care.*

Planning and Implementation

The major nursing implications for PKU are support of the family during the crisis of diagnosis and early treatment and ongoing teaching during follow-up visits. Perhaps the greatest concern of parents is that accidental noncompliance with the PKU diet will result in brain damage. An occasional mistake will not cause permanent damage. The parent of an infant has complete control of dietary intake; however, with the increased mobility of the older child, forbidden foods become an increased threat. To minimize this threat, parents should be taught how to educate other family members, baby sitters, and day care and school personnel about the diet. Table 44–4 gives suggestions for education about special diets.

Nursing diagnostic responses and care common to all metabolic diseases are described in the nursing process plan "Long-Term Care of the Child with a Metabolic Disorder" (see Table 44–3).

TABLE 44–4
Family Centered Teaching: Diet Modifications for Phenylketonuria (PKU)

Reinforce teaching regarding diagnosis, prognosis, genetics, treatment

Assist families to incorporate diet into lifestyle

Family members should not significantly alter their diets: continuing same patterns allows child to learn that differences exist, and child will learn early adaptation (one father was quite relieved about this, as he likes meat, and said "I don't do green," meaning he did not eat vegetables)

Normal activities can continue: plan to take snacks that are allowed on the diet; learn what foods are allowed when eating away from home; premeasure formula for trips; instruct family members, friends, and babysitters about diet basics

Provide resources for parents, such as educational materials, parent support groups, and newsletters

Assist parents in learning home blood collection for phenylalanine levels

Help parents learn to separate diet from age-appropriate developmental struggles: diet should not become the focus of acting-out behaviors, independence issues, or a target for manipulative behaviors

Help parents educate child about PKU and diet

- Infancy—use substitution and distraction to handle child's curiosity about nonallowed foods
- Toddlerhood—as above; also, begin to teach concepts of "yes" vs "no" foods using books, games, mealtimes, and allow toddlers choices when possible
- Preschool—as above; also, use books on PKU, teach how to refuse nonallowed foods if offered by others, use analogies to begin explanations of PKU
- School-age—begin to teach concepts of measuring and amounts (abacus, felt board, or poker chips may be helpful); begin to prepare own formula, learn basic cooking techniques; continue education regarding PKU; role playing is beneficial to help child learn how to tell others about diet and how to cope with teasing or negative comments
- Adolescence—try to keep developmental issues separate from diet; allow maximum control over food choices; help adolescents understand connection among diet, school performance, and future goals; continue to educate females about maternal PKU

Evaluation

The projected client outcomes of care can be found in the nursing process plan "Long-Term Care of the Child with a Metabolic Disorder" (see Table 44–3).

Maple Syrup Urine Disease

Maple syrup urine disease (MSUD) is an autosomal recessive disorder of metabolism involving three amino acids: leucine, isoleucine, and valine.

Etiology/Incidence (Pathophysiology)

Unlike PKU, in which the enzyme block occurs in the first step of the metabolic pathway, MSUD occurs as a result of the absence or deficiency of an enzyme further down the pathway of metabolism of the three amino acids. Consequences of this block include acute episodes of acidosis, and prognosis for affected children may be uncertain.

Although MSUD is rare, the incidence varies among ethnic groups and may be relatively common in some populations. An incidence of 1 in 200,000 to 1 in 300,000 is generally used, but the incidence among Mennonites has been estimated to be as high as 1 in 760 births (Danner & Elsas, 1989). Some states include MSUD in their newborn screening programs.

MSUD results from a deficiency of the enzyme complex known as branched-chain alpha-keto acid dehydrogenase (BCKD), which is involved in the metabolism of leucine, isoleucine, and valine. These three amino acids and their respective keto acids accumulate, causing profound effects on the neurologic system. An odor resembling maple syrup may be found in urine, sweat, and ear cerumen. There are several phenotypic classifications, including classic, intermittent, intermediate, and thiamine-responsive.

Diagnostic Assessment

As with many inborn errors of metabolism, symptoms of MSUD depend on the degree of enzyme deficiency. Classic MSUD is the result of absent enzyme activity; less severe deficiency leads to milder symptoms and a generally more favorable prognosis.

Onset of symptoms in classic MSUD begins during the first week of life and is characterized by poor feeding, altered muscle tone, lethargy, apnea, and seizures (Danner & Elsas, 1989; Naughten et al, 1982). Without diagnosis and treatment, neurologic status further deteriorates, frequently resulting in coma and death. Even with diagnosis and treatment in infancy, children may have some degree of permanent neurologic damage (Kaplan et al, 1991; Nord et al, 1991). Factors contributing to developmental outcome may be timing of diagnosis, problems of long-term management, and difficulty in preventing periodic episodes of metabolic decompensation.

Any neonate with signs of lethargy and poor feeding should be evaluated for a possible inborn error of metabolism. Although not always present, an odor of maple syrup would point to a diagnosis of MSUD, which may be confirmed by evaluation of serum amino acids and urine organic acids. When an infant has a positive newborn screen for MSUD, prompt evaluation, confirmation, and treatment are essential.

Therapeutic Management

It is imperative, in light of the rapidity of onset and the severity of symptoms of MSUD, that treatment begin as soon as possible. Peritoneal dialysis or exchange transfusion may be required to clear the amino acids and keto acids from the body quickly (Wendel, 1990). In order to prevent reaccumulation, the infant is given a diet low in leucine, isoleucine, and valine (the branched-chain amino acids [BCAA]). Some children may respond to pharmacologic doses of thiamine, but they still require dietary management (Danner & Elsas, 1989).

A special metabolic formula without the BCAA is used, with the BCAA needed for growth added back to the diet in the form of a small amount of regular formula or from foods low in protein (similar to the diet for PKU).

Even with adequate dietary management, periodic episodes of metabolic decompensation may occur. Illness can precipitate these episodes, and children should be carefully monitored and treated aggressively at the first sign of clinical symptoms. Parents should be taught to detect early signs, such as changes in appetite, behavior, or activity levels. Later signs may include irritability, ataxia, or hallucinations. Acute management involves halting the build-up of BCAA and keto acids by stopping BCAA intake and reversing catabolism by giving intravenous fluids and glucose.

Nursing Care

Nursing implications and nursing diagnostic responses for MSUD are similar to those for PKU. However, in addition to the impact of special dietary needs on the child and family, nurses must be aware of the potential for episodes of acute metabolic decompensation. In addition, the prognosis for neurologic and intellectual outcome is less favorable for MSUD than for PKU. Nurses can help teach families accurate home assessment and management of the child and can assist parents in preparing themselves emotionally for the uncertainties of outcome (Table 44–5).

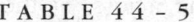

TABLE 44-5
Family Centered Teaching: Guidelines for Disorders with a Potential for Acute Metabolic Crisis (MSUD, organic acidemias, urea cycle defects)

Reinforce teaching about diagnosis, prognosis, treatment, and genetics
Teach parents to perform accurately the techniques for monitoring that have been prescribed, such as checking urine for ketones
Instruct parents in assessment of signs that may signal impending metabolic decompensation, such as level of consciousness, behavior changes, changes in appetite, vomiting, symptoms of an intercurrent illness, and subtle neurologic signs, such as changes in balance or gait, fine tremors, or changes in speech
Help parents develop a plan for illnesses and emergencies, including when to call for advice and who to contact
Assist parents in obtaining a letter from metabolic care providers that summarizes a plan for emergency treatment
Help parents obtain a Medic-Alert tag for the child
Assist parents in finding appropriate therapies for child if indicated, including speech and feeding, occupational therapy, and physical therapy
Assist with management of nasogastric or gastrostomy tubes if indicated

Organic Acidemias

The group of disorders known as organic acidemias are caused by enzyme deficiencies relatively far down the pathway of amino acid metabolism, and may include enzymes in pathways that are used by both amino acids and fatty acids.

Etiology/Incidence (Pathophysiology)

Enzyme blocks in these disorders result in a build-up of organic acids, rather than an amino acid such as phenylalanine in PKU. In general, the prognosis for a child with an organic acidemia is worse than for a child with an amino acid disorder, because treatment is less effective and it is difficult to prevent periodic episodes of metabolic decompensation.

Diagnostic Assessment

Clinical presentation of an organic acidemia varies with the disorder and the severity of enzyme deficiency, but metabolic acidosis is a common feature. Neonates, infants, or children may have failure to thrive, poor feeding, vomiting, growth retardation, lethargy, developmental delays, neurologic abnormalities, particular odors (such as sweaty feet in isovaleric acidemia and glutaric acidemia type II), and acidosis with high or low blood sugar (Goodman & Greene, 1991). Disorders that fall in the category of organic acidemias include propionic acidemia, methylmalonic acidemia, glutaric acidemia (I and II), and isovaleric acidemia.

Therapeutic Management

Diets restricted in the particular amino acid(s) at the beginning of the blocked pathway and/or medications may be prescribed for long-term treatment for certain organic acidemias. Various co-factors specific for the disorder may be used. Because the enzyme blocks in these disorders occur several steps down a metabolic pathway, it is generally more difficult to balance dietary restrictions with physiologic requirements. Insufficient amino acid and nutrient intake can result in a catabolic state, which, in turn, may lead to a rise in organic acids. Metabolic decompensation may follow, much like what happens when too much of the problematic amino acids are ingested. Toxic organic acids affect multiple body systems, and treatment for the organic acidemias may not be completely effective at preventing the accumulation of organic acids. Although mild elevations may not result in an acute crisis, neurologic and other system damage often occurs.

Nursing Care

Management for acute episodes of decompensation generally includes lowering or stopping protein intake and giving large amounts of fluids and glucose as well as correcting acidosis and lowering high ammonia levels. As with other categories of disorders, a major aspect of nursing care is parental education. Family knowledge of medical management, including the early signs of and intervention for metabolic decompensation, can help lower the frequency and severity of acute crises. Families also need ongoing support and assistance with resources. The prognosis for this category of diseases varies, depending on the disorder, but some of the diseases lead to variable degrees of mental retardation, neurologic deficits, and shortened life span, despite medical intervention.

Urea Cycle Disorders: Ornithine Transcarbamylase Deficiency

Incidence/Etiology (Pathophysiology)

Five major biochemical reactions occur in the removal of ammonia, the end product of protein degradation, in a pathway known as the urea cycle. The urea cycle not only produces urea but also provides the body with the amino acid arginine. A deficiency of an enzyme in the pathway leads to dysfunction of the cycle, and clinical disorders are known for each of the major enzymes. Ornithine transcarbamylase (OTC) is an enzyme needed in the second step of the cycle, and deficiency of the enzyme results in accumulation of ammonia and in arginine depletion and low levels of citrulline (the product that should have been produced in this reaction).

Diagnostic Assessment

Most frequently, symptoms of OTC deficiency occur during the neonatal period. However, the clinical presentation can occur at any age and may range from mild to severe. The gene for OTC is located on the X chromosome; OTC deficiency is therefore X-linked, and males are primarily affected. However, females who carry an abnormal gene may be symptomatic, depending on the portion of cells in which the abnormal X is the one activated (see discussion of Lyon hypothesis in Chapter 31). Symptoms in the neonatal period in affected males include poor feeding, vomiting, abnormal tone, lethargy, and hypothermia (Brusilow & Horwich, 1989). Significant hyperammonemia with respiratory alkalosis and encephalopathy occur, followed by death if diagnosis and treatment are not prompt. Symptoms of recurrent episodes, or initial presentation later in life, are similar; they often follow a minor acute illness and may be fatal without appropriate intervention. High protein intake or illness may precipitate symptoms in female carriers as well (Batshaw et al, 1986).

Therapeutic Management

Management for acute episodes of OTC deficiency includes stopping protein intake, providing calories by intravenous glucose, and instituting measures to decrease ammonia levels. Various medications may be given to reduce the degree of hyperammonemia, but dialysis or exchange transfusion may be needed, especially in the neonate. Long-term management includes a low-protein diet, medications to increase nitrogen removal via alternative pathways, and supplementation with arginine or citrulline. Prompt treatment of the initial episode and prevention of further hyperammonemic episodes may optimize outcome in some of the urea cycle disorders, but severe neurologic damage may be present in OTC deficiency. Liver transplantation may be indicated in some cases.

Nursing Care

Nursing care for OTC deficiency is similar to that for MSUD with regard to the implications of a special diet, the need for close monitoring and assessment because of the potential for metabolic decompensation, and the uncertain prognosis (in severely affected boys who survive the neonatal period). Nurses can be instrumental in ensuring that neonates presenting with symptoms of a metabolic disorder are promptly evaluated. Genetic counseling should be provided for all metabolic disorders, but an X-linked condition such as OTC deficiency raises unique issues related to the potential for female carriers to become symptomatic (as well as the potential feelings of guilt for "giving" the child the disorder). Ongoing support and assistance in planning for the physical care of the child and meeting the emotional needs of all family members is essential (see the nursing process plan "Long-Term Care of the Child with a Metabolic Disorder" [see Table 44–3]).

Carbohydrate Disorders

As with disorders of amino acid metabolism, enzyme deficiencies in the pathway of carbohydrate metabolism can lead to metabolic disease. Carbohydrates can be classified as polysaccharides, disaccharides, or monosaccharides.

Normal Digestion of Carbohydrates

There are three primary dietary sources of carbohydrates: (1) sucrose (beet sugar, sugar cane), a disaccharide; (2) lactose (milk sugar), a disaccharide; and (3) starch, a polysaccharide. Carbohydrates need to be hydrolyzed to monosaccharides to be absorbed from the intestine.

The breakdown of starches begins in the mouth and continues in the stomach and then the small intestine, where pancreatic amylase and isomaltase complete the breakdown until the polysaccharide becomes a disaccharide (maltose, lactose, or sucrose) (MacDonald, 1988). These are further hydrolyzed into their constituent monosaccharides (glucose, galactose, and fructose) in the brush borders of the small intestine by their corresponding enzymes (maltase, lactase, and sucrase). The monosaccharides are then absorbed into portal blood, taken up by the liver, and transported into the cellular cytoplasm. Several disorders are associated with the metabolism of carbohydrates; galactosemia is described here as a prototype.

Galactosemia

Etiology/Incidence (Pathophysiology)

"Galactosemia" is a term used for three main disorders of galactose metabolism. The most well known is transferase deficiency (classic) galactosemia, which results from deficient activity of the enzyme galactose-1-phosphate uridyl transferase. Various degrees of enzyme deficiency and, thus, severity of consequences exist as a result of different genotypes. Transmission is by autosomal recessive inheritance. Incidence of the severe form is widely variable but overall is estimated as 1 in 60,000 (Segal, 1989); some states include galactosemia in newborn screening programs.

Deficient transferase activity results in the accumulation of galactose-1-phosphate, galactose, and galactitol. Consequences include cataracts, liver damage, and neurologic impairment; affected neonates may die without appropriate intervention (Fig. 44–3).

Diagnostic Assessment

Because of the morbidity and mortality resulting from classic galactosemia, prompt recognition of the clinical signs and the institution of immediate treatment is imperative. In severe cases, the symptoms begin within the first days of life. The signs of galactosemia tend to mimic other diseases, with vomiting, lethargy, and failure to thrive beginning after feedings of breast milk or a lactose-containing formula. The development of jaundice provides an additional clue. If the child remains untreated, progressive liver damage causes hepatomegaly, ascites, and sometimes bleeding; sepsis from *Escherichia coli* and severe dehydration will often occur. Coma and death may follow (Segal, 1989).

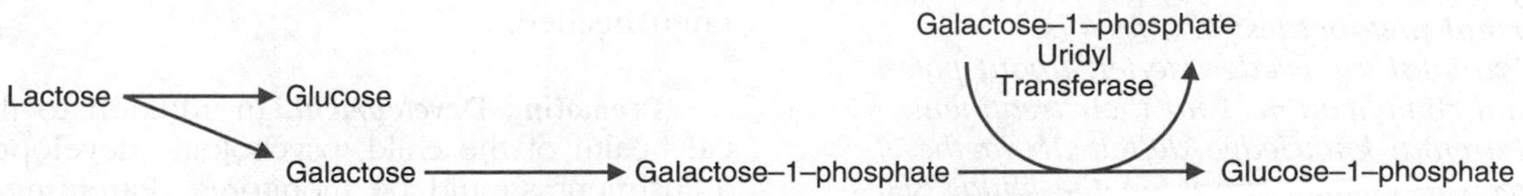

FIGURE 44-3. Biochemistry of transferase deficiency galactosemia.

Cataracts occur as a result of prenatal and postnatal accumulation of galactitol and may be seen by slit-lamp examination during the neonatal period.

Untreated children who survive the neonatal period usually have neurologic deficits and mental retardation (Fishler et al, 1980). Even with early diagnosis and treatment, ovarian failure, mild speech difficulties, specific learning disabilities, and neurologic problems may occur (Kaufman et al, 1988; Waisbren et al, 1983). One study concluded that early detection through newborn screening did not make a statistically significant difference in long-term outcome (Waggoner et al, 1990), but differences in level of dietary compliance and frequency of monitoring may be influencing variables.

Therapeutic Management

Early implementation of treatment quickly changes the course of the disease. Galactose is eliminated from the diet by removing milk and milk products. Formulas that do not contain lactose, such as soy formulas, are used. An affected infant begins to show improvement after starting the galactose-free diet. Vomiting and diarrhea subside, weight gain occurs, liver function improves, and cataracts (if not too far advanced) regress. Any sepsis should be aggressively treated. Lactose and galactose restrictions are lifelong in children with classic galactosemia.

Nursing Diagnostic Statements

High risk for injury, physiologic: liver damage associated with hepatotoxic properties of the accumulation of galactose and its abnormal metabolites; *risk factor: parental knowledge deficit about the significance of early signs and symptoms.*

High risk for complications, including sensory-perceptual alteration, visual: cataracts, associated with the effect of an abnormal metabolite of galactose on the lens of the eye; *risk factor: parental knowledge deficit about need for continued monitoring of nutritional adequacy and dietary compliance.*

Health-seeking behaviors, child and/or family about how to manage altered nutrition: impairment of galactose metabolism, associated with an enzyme deficiency due to an autosomal recessive disorder.

High risk for altered growth and development: mental retardation and learning disabilities, associated with neurotoxic properties of the accumulation of galactose and its abnormal metabolites; *risk factors:*

- *Parental knowledge deficit about potential complications and their treatment.*
- *Parental knowledge deficit about the effects of complications on the child's self-image and sexuality.*

Family coping potential for growth: parents (initially), child (later), related to knowledge deficit and verbalized desire to learn about etiology and pathophysiology of galactosemia, genetic counseling, instruction about galactose-free diet (foods and medications), and resources, including parent groups.

High risk for ineffective management of therapeutic regimen; *risk factors:*

- *Denial, child and/or family, which renders family attempts at care ineffective for meeting the prevention program.*
- *Complexity of the therapeutic regimen.*
- *Inadequate resources or lack of resources.*

Nursing Care

Preventing Injury or Sensory-Perceptual Alteration. Early diagnosis minimizes the extent of liver damage and the potential for sensory-perceptual alterations. Nurses can aid in the diagnosis of galactosemia by ensuring that newborn screening programs are carried out and that parents bring their infants in for prompt follow-up of positive results. A positive newborn screen for galactosemia can be a medical emergency. If the parents report classic signs during the postnatal period, careful assessment and documentation of infant feeding patterns and prompt referral of the family to medical care are important. Reported signs may include jaundice, feeding difficulties, vomiting, lethargy, and irritability.

Minimizing the high risk for sensory-perceptual alterations and other potential complications of galactosemia is necessary. Nursing assistance is needed for the following: assessment of liver size and function; developmentally based testing for visual acuity; measurement of height, weight, and head circumference and monitoring growth curves and percentiles; and surveillance for speech difficulties and learning problems. Collaboration with school personnel is essential to ensure early intervention and optimum follow-up for any learning disabilities, speech problems, or behavioral issues. Periodic ophthalmologic examinations for cataracts are recommended.

Promoting Family's and Child's Ability to Move Toward a Higher Level of Health by Controlling Nutritional Intake. Parents may be requested to keep daily diet records to assist in the assessment of nutritional adequacy and dietary compliance. Calcium needs are met in infancy through non–lactose-containing formulas. Older children are encouraged to continue using these formulas in place of milk (straight, on cereal, and in cooking), but calcium supplements are often needed.

Promoting Development. In addition to the physical health of the child, psychologic development and adjustment should be monitored. Parenting that enhances all aspects of development should be taught

TABLE 44-6
Organizations for Parents and Professionals

Phenylketonuria	Children's PKU Network 10525 Vista Sorrento Pkwy #204 San Diego, CA 92121 (619) 450-5034
Galactosemia	Parents of Galactosemic Children Linda Manis 20981 Solano Way Boca Raton, FL 33433 (407) 852-0266
Maple syrup urine disease	Joyce Brubacher 24806 SR 119 Goshen, IN 46526 (219) 862-2992
Organic acidemias	Organic Acidemia Association, Inc. 522 Lander Street Reno, NV 89509 (702) 322-5542
Urea cycle disorders	National Urea Cycle Disorders Foundation 4559 Vauxhall Road Richmond, VA 23234
Mucopolysaccharidosis	The National MPS Society, Inc. 17 Kraemer Street Hicksville, NY 11801 (516) 931-6338
Leukodystrophies	United Leukodystrophy Foundation 2304 Highland Drive Sycamore, IL 60178 (815) 895-3211

and reinforced. Parents and affected girls should be counseled about the potential for ovarian failure and infertility and the possible need for hormone supplementation at puberty, including the effects on self-image and sexuality.

Promoting Effective Family Management of Tasks Needed for Adaptation to the Challenges of the Illness. As with any of the metabolic disorders, nursing support during the crisis of diagnosis can facilitate the family's adjustment. Ongoing evaluation of the child provides ample opportunities for the nurse to continue the teaching and informational support begun at the time of diagnosis.

Fostering Effective Management of Therapeutic Regimen. Long-term management includes the continuation of lactose and galactose restriction. Education is a valuable method of facilitating the family's management of the dietary restrictions. Parents, and later the child, should be instructed in careful label-reading, because many products contain nonallowed substances, such as whey. Medications may contain lactose; all medications should be investigated before being prescribed or given. Some clinics monitor effectiveness of management of the dietary regimen by measuring blood galactose-1-phosphate levels.

Strategies similar to those for PKU should be used to assist the family in home management by incorporating the diet into normal routines and encouraging continued management. Enabling parents to contact other families who have children with galactosemia is beneficial, as is providing information about formal support groups (Table 44-6). Assessment of home management should also include family interactions and functioning.

Fat Disorders

Normal Fat Metabolism

Fatty acid oxidation (metabolism) involves several cellular systems but occurs primarily in the mitochondria. Once glycogen stores in the liver are depleted, fatty acids stored in adipose tissue (as triglycerides) are used for fuel. The stored triglycerides are first broken down to free fatty acids; then they are transported to cells and into the mitochondria. The long-chain fatty acids require carnitine to enter the mitochondria. The fatty acids are essentially chains of carbons, and enzymes in the mitochondria catalyze the progressive shortening of the chains to produce energy via the tricarboxylic acid cycle and conversion to ketones (Stanley, 1987). Disorders result from an enzyme deficiency at a particular step of the process such that oxidation cannot be completed. Although descriptions of inborn errors of fatty acid oxidation have only appeared in the past 20 years, the detection of a variety of disorders is now possible (Rhead, 1991; Stanley, 1987).

Medium-Chain Acyl-CoA Dehydrogenase Deficiency

Etiology/Incidence (Pathophysiology)

Medium-chain acyl-CoA dehydrogenase deficiency (MCADD) is one of the most common and best-described disorders of fatty acid oxidation. The deficient enzyme in this disorder is medium-chain acyl-CoA dehydrogenase, one of the chain-length–specific dehydrogenases responsible for the shortening of the fatty acid chains after entry into the mitochondria. The first enzyme in the pathway acts on long chains (from 18 down to 12 carbons), medium-chain acyl-CoA dehydrogenase works on the medium chains (14 to 4 carbons), and a third dehydrogenase is involved with the short chains (4 and 6 carbons) (Roe & Coates, 1989). MCADD results when oxidation stops at the medium-chain level, and the individual is unable to derive sufficient energy when in a fasting state. Consequently, symptoms can occur after long periods of not eating or in conditions associated with decreased oral intake, vomiting, and/or catabolism, such as illness.

MCADD is inherited in an autosomal recessive manner. Although exact incidence is unknown, the frequency has been estimated to be anywhere from 1 in 5000 (Bennett et al, 1987) to 1 in 10,000 to 20,000 (Bennett et al, 1990).

Diagnostic Assessment

The clinical presentation of MCADD generally consists of episodes of hypoglycemia with hypoketosis, which may include lethargy that progresses to coma. However, encephalopathy can occur even with normal blood glucose levels. A secondary carnitine deficiency often occurs; hypotonia and cardiomyopathy may develop. Prompt management is necessary to prevent death in an acute episode; treatment consists primarily of intravenous glucose and management of the precipitating event. Accurate recognition of MCADD as the underlying cause of such an episode is needed to prevent additional episodes. MCADD may be misdiagnosed as Reye Syndrome or sudden infant death syndrome (Pollitt, 1989; Roe et al, 1986), and there are many anecdotal as well as published reports of children diagnosed with MCADD having a positive family history for early childhood death. Confirmation of the diagnosis allows for genetic counseling about autosomal recessive inheritance and testing of siblings; affected individuals may not yet have had symptomatic episodes. The prognosis for children with properly managed MCADD is good.

Therapeutic Management

Management of MCADD is geared toward prevention of symptomatic episodes and includes frequent feedings in infancy and frequent small meals and snacks (especially a bedtime snack) in toddlers and children. A diet high in complex carbohydrates and low in fat is often recommended in children over the age of 2 years. Aggressive treatment for intercurrent illnesses is also needed. Because carnitine is involved in the transport of fatty acids and a secondary deficiency may occur in MCADD, carnitine supplementation may be recommended.

Nursing Care

Parental education about potential triggers of hypoglycemia and their prevention, such as periods of fasting or inadequate intake secondary to illness, is crucial. Knowledge of signs and symptoms, initial treatment, and emergency management is needed. Table 44–7 outlines ways in which nurses can assist parents in the care of their child with MCADD.

TABLE 44–7
Family Centered Teaching*: Guidelines for *the Child with MCADD

Reinforce teaching regarding diagnosis, prognosis, treatment, and genetics
Teach family members the signs and symptoms of encephalopathy and hypoglycemia
Help parents learn heel and finger-stick technique and home blood glucose monitoring, if prescribed
Reinforce education about dietary management, including low-fat (over age 2 yrs) high-carbohydrate diet, small frequent meals and bedtime snack (high in complex carbohydrates)
Educate parents on management of intercurrent illnesses that may result in increased energy needs and/or decreased oral intake
Reinforce education about emergency procedures and management
Assist parents in obtaining a letter from metabolic care providers that states plan for emergency treatment, including need for intravenous glucose
Instruct parents in the use of an instant glucose, if prescribed
Assist parents in obtaining a Medic-Alert tag for child
Educate family members about management of potential struggles related to maintenance of adequate oral intake, such as toddlers who refuse food and picky eaters

Lysosomal Storage Diseases

Lysosomes are cellular organelles that contain enzymes responsible for the degradation of many macromolecules, including mucopolysaccharides, glycoproteins, and various lipids. The body is constantly breaking down and rebuilding various tissues, and lysosomal enzymes are needed to assist in this recycling process. Lysosomal storage diseases occur when one of these enzymes is deficient or when there is a deficiency of an enzyme transport mechanism.

If proper degradation does not occur, the substances preceding the enzyme block accumulate, causing distortion of the cell architecture and interference with cell function. Clinical consequences vary with the disorder and different tissues may be more or less affected, but, in general, onset is gradual with this group of diseases. Undegraded molecules stored in the brain result in neurologic manifestations; storage in liver and spleen causes organomegaly; and storage in bone and connective tissue results in joint deformities and dysmorphic features. Inheritance of most of these disorders is autosomal recessive, although one in particular, Hunter syndrome, is X-linked.

The incidence varies with the disorder and ethnic background. For example, Tay-Sachs has a higher frequency in the Ashkenazi Jewish population.

For most lysosomal storage diseases, management is supportive. The severe forms cause a gradual deterioration, and death often occurs in childhood or adolescence. Experimental treatments such as bone marrow transplantation and enzyme replacement have been tried in some cases. Although the efficacy of bone marrow transplants for some of the mucopolysaccharide disorders remains controversial, enzyme replacement for Gaucher disease is becoming increasingly common.

Enzyme replacement may eventually become possible for other disorders. However, it is extremely difficult to treat inborn errors of metabolism by replacing the missing enzyme. Multiple problems exist, including obtaining enough natural or synthetic enzyme, ensuring that the enzyme enters the appropriate tissues (especially the brain secondary to the blood-brain barrier), and ensuring that the enzyme enters the lysosome (in this category of diseases). The cost of this type of treatment is also of concern. A prototype disorder for replacing a missing enzyme by intravenous infusion is Gaucher disease. Gaucher disease results from a deficiency of the enzyme glucocerebrosidase. Consequences include storage of glucocerebroside (a sphingolipid); the spleen, bones, and hematologic system are primarily affected. A mechanism has been developed that modifies and targets the enzyme for entry into the lysosome, and initial results of clinical trials look promising (Barton et al, 1991).

Hurler Syndrome

Etiology/Incidence (Pathophysiology)

Hurler syndrome is presented because it is a prototype for the category of lysosomal storage diseases known as mucopolysaccharidoses. Hurler syndrome is characterized by lack of the enzyme alpha-L-iduronidase. The deficiency of this enzyme leads to accumulation of unmetabolized mucopolysaccharides in body tissues. The disease is transmitted by autosomal recessive inheritance. Less severe deficiencies of the same enzyme result in the milder diseases Hurler-Scheie and Scheie (Table 44–8).

Diagnostic Assessment

The major clinical features associated with Hurler syndrome are mental retardation, coarse facies, skeletal and joint deformities, hepatosplenomegaly, hearing loss, short stature, and corneal clouding (Fig. 44–4). Hurler syndrome is severe and progressive and leads to death, usually before the age of 10 years (Neufeld & Muenzer, 1989).

During the first few months of life, the child appears normal, although umbilical or inguinal hernias may be present. Gradually, persistent rhinorrhea, noisy breathing, and recurrent infections of the respiratory tract and ear develop. Physical examination shows spinal deformities and radiologic findings known as dysostosis multiplex, chest deformity (barrel-shaped), stiff joints, organomegaly, large head, corneal clouding, and coarse facial features. Thereafter, delayed growth becomes obvious.

Deterioration of psychomotor development continues, as does the progressive coarsening of facial features, along with a large head, thickened lips, and hirsutism. An enlarged tongue may cause feeding difficulties. The liver increases in size, causing a protuberant abdomen, which, in turn, causes discomfort and respiratory difficulties. Tissue thickening in the upper airway also causes breathing problems. Hearing loss is common, and hernias may be present. The skin becomes thickened, which causes additional problems if intravenous therapy is required. A communicating hydrocephalus frequently develops.

Therapeutic Management

Repeated respiratory infections and worsening cardiac function often necessitate repeated hospitalizations and are the usual cause of death. There is no definitive treatment for Hurler syndrome. Bone marrow transplantation has been done for some of the mucopolysaccharidoses, including Hurler syndrome. Although there is evidence that some aspects of the disease improve after transplantation (Neufeld & Muenzer, 1989), questions remain about long-term efficacy and the degree of benefit to brain and neurologic function.

TABLE 44-8
Examples of Lysosomal Storage Diseases

Mucopolysaccharidoses (MPS)		**Glycoprotein Degradation**	**Sphingomyelin-Cholesterol Lipidoses**
MPS I	Hurler	Mannosidosis	
	Scheie	Fucosidosis	Niemann-Pick group
	Hurler-Scheie	Sialidosis	
MPS II	Hunter	Aspartylglucosaminuria	
MPS III	Sanfilippo		
MPS IV	Morquio		
MPS VI	Maroteaux-Lamy		
Glucosylceramide Lipidosis		**Sulfatide Lipidosis**	**GM_2 Gangliosidosis**
Gaucher		Metachromatic leukodystrophy	Tay-Sachs

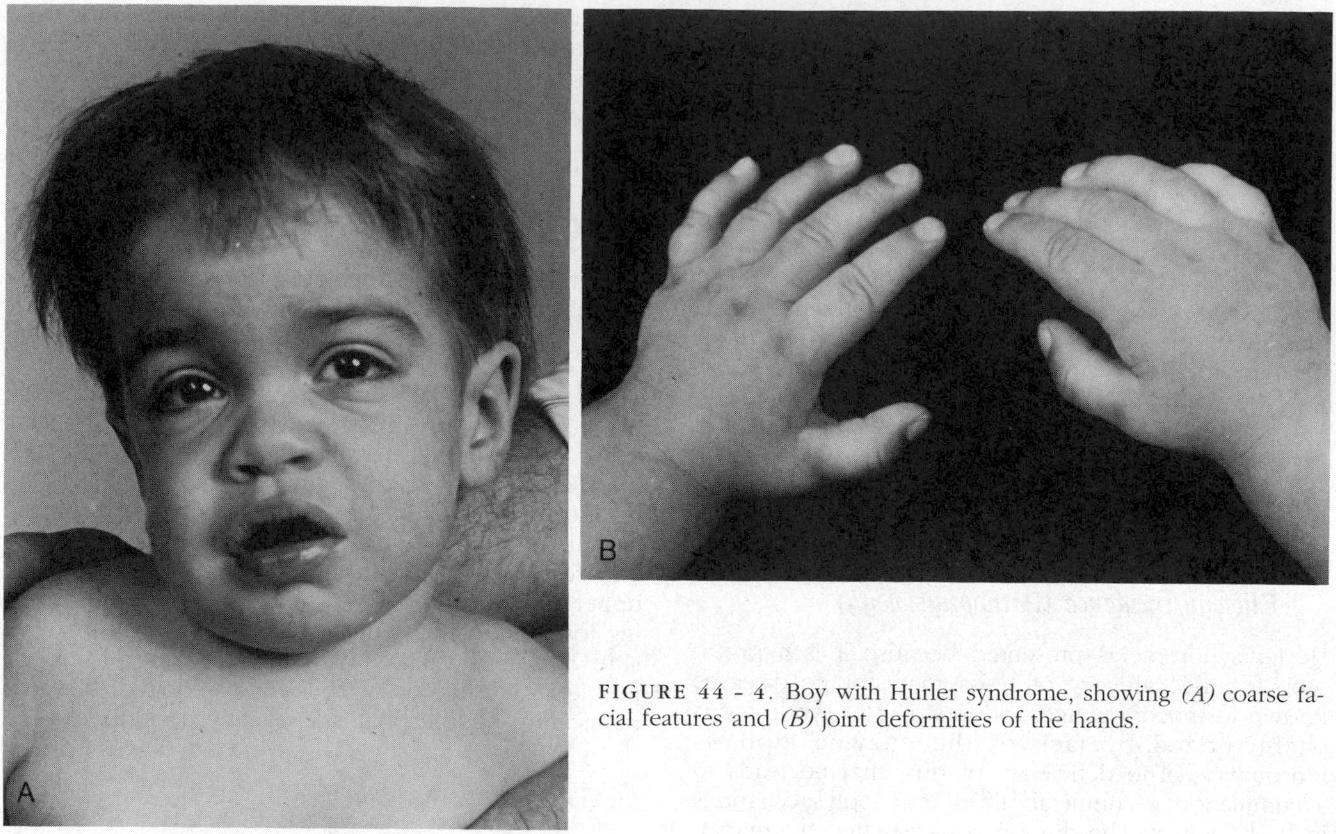

FIGURE 44-4. Boy with Hurler syndrome, showing *(A)* coarse facial features and *(B)* joint deformities of the hands.

Nursing Care

To provide nursing care of the child with Hurler syndrome, a comprehensive plan of care is needed that centers on a degenerative disease and identifies the problems unique to the child and family. The plan should focus on strategies to respond to the involvement of multiple organ systems, alteration of physical and mental growth and development, and ongoing challenges to the family as they attempt to care for the child. In addition, the family may be faced with decisions about experimental treatments, especially bone marrow transplantation. Considerations may include the family's perceptions of quality-of-life issues, including the potential for a longer life span but often with diminished intellectual capabilities. Potential risks and benefits must be carefully considered, and nurses may be instrumental in helping parents understand and express feelings and values.

The child with Hurler syndrome is likely to experience respiratory difficulties, sensory problems (visual and auditory), alterations in gastrointestinal function ranging from hepatomegaly to feeding difficulties, neurologic dysfunction, and cardiovascular disorders. Strategies for nursing care involving these disorders can be found within the system-specific chapters and in the nursing process plans in those chapters. Chapter 27 presents nursing strategies for care of children with mental retardation. Strategies to assist the nurse in supporting the child and family are discussed in the nursing interventions section at the end of that chapter and in the chapters on the care of the chronically ill child (Chapter 19), the terminally ill child (Chapter 20), and the hospitalized child (Chapter 21). Table 31–17 provides guidelines for care of the family in need of genetic counseling.

Childhood Adrenoleukodystrophy: A Peroxisomal Disorder

Etiology/Incidence (Pathophysiology)

Childhood adrenoleukodystrophy, or X-linked adrenoleukodystrophy, is a disorder that occurs as a result of a deficient peroxisomal enzyme. Peroxisomes are cellular organelles that contain a variety of enzymes, and disorders can result from a single-enzyme deficiency or multiple-enzyme deficiencies; some of the latter actually result from a defect in peroxisomal assembly, and the peroxisomes are therefore not present. The most common peroxisomal single-enzyme defect is X-linked adrenoleukodystrophy, which results from an accumulation of saturated very-long-chain fatty acids (VLCFA). The tissues most affected are the neurologic system (white matter), the adrenal cortex, and the testis (Moser, 1991).

Diagnostic Assessment

Although the presentation and severity of the disorder may vary, progressive demyelination and adrenal insufficiency develop. Clinical manifestations develop in about half of the affected males by age 10 years. Initially, they may include poor school performance, attention deficit disorders, visual impairment, and neurologic disturbances (Costakos et al, 1991; Moser, 1991). Adrenal insufficiency and continued central nervous system degeneration follow, progressing to a vegetative state and death.

Therapeutic Management

Currently, no standard treatment for X-linked adrenoleukodystrophy exists. Experimental therapies are under investigation, although long-term efficacy is not known. Plasma VLCFA levels can be normalized by combining the use of oral administration of monounsaturated oils with dietary restriction of VLCFA (Moser, 1991). However, clinical benefit is uncertain, especially once symptoms of the disorder are present. This regimen is also being tried for heterozygous females, because some carriers of the gene express mild to moderate clinical symptoms in later adulthood.

Nursing Care

Nursing care for childhood adrenoleukodystrophy is similar to that for any degenerative terminal illness. Parents need ongoing support and assistance with difficult decisions about the medical interventions and quality of life. Support organizations for leukodystrophy and other metabolic disorders are listed in Table 44–6.

KEY CONCEPTS

Concepts Related to Basic Information

- Inherited metabolic diseases account for a significant amount of infant and childhood morbidity and mortality.
- Most inborn errors of metabolism are autosomal recessive.
- Inborn errors of metabolism result from blocked enzymatic pathways in a variety of biochemical reactions.
- Evidence indicates that different mutations in the gene for PKU correlate with the degree of enzyme deficiency and the heterogeneity of PKU.
- MSUD is an autosomal recessive disorder of metabolism involving three amino acids: leucine, isoleucine, and valine.
- In general, the prognosis for a child with an organic acidemia is worse than for a child with an amino acid disorder, because treatment is less effective and it is difficult to prevent episodes of metabolic decompensation.
- "Galactosemia" is a term referring to three main disorders of galactose metabolism.
- MCADD is one of the most common and best-described disorders of fatty acid oxidation.
- Hurler syndrome is characterized by the deficiency of the enzyme alpha-L-iduronidase, which results in severe and progressive deterioration of psychomotor development.

Concepts Related to Nursing Assessment

- Evaluation of the child with a metabolic disorder should include a thorough health history, family history, and physical assessment.
- Most children with PKU are now diagnosed as a result of newborn screening, which detects elevated serum levels of phenylalanine.
- The nurse assesses the child with a metabolic disorder for the etiologies and defining characteristics that contribute to the related or risk factors or identification of nursing diagnostic statements.
- Assessment of the defining characteristics that the infant or child with a metabolic disorder may exhibit includes subjective data such as family eating patterns and health beliefs related to food.
- Any neonate with signs of lethargy and poor feeding should be evaluated for a possible inborn error of metabolism.
- The child with MSUD, an organic acidemia, or OTC deficiency is closely monitored and assessed because of the potential for metabolic decompensation and uncertain prognosis.
- Careful assessment and documentation of infant feeding problems and neurologic status and prompt referral for care can prevent a medical emergency for the infant with galactosemia.
- Ongoing assessment of the child with Hurler syndrome involves a multisystem approach, because alterations in the respiratory, gastrointestinal, neurologic, and cardiovascular systems occur.
- The risk for altered growth and development of the child can be objectively screened with the use of developmental assessment tools, such as DDST II.
- The human response, high risk for ineffective management of therapeutic regimen is assessed by follow-up of the family and close observation for objective or subjective cues that the care given by the family may not be effective for meeting the goals of the treatment and prevention program.

Concepts Related to Nursing Intervention

- Nurses may be involved with various aspects of *newborn screening,* including specimen collection, follow-up procedures for positive tests, and parental and community education.
- The major nursing implications for the infant with PKU are *family support* during the crisis of diagnosis and early treatment, and ongoing *teaching* during follow-up visits.
- Nurses must be aware of the potential for episodes of acute metabolic decompensation for the child with MSUD.
- Nurses can be instrumental in ensuring that neonates presenting with symptoms of a metabolic disorder are promptly evaluated and monitored *(newborn monitoring).*
- Nurses can aid in the diagnosis of galactosemia by ensuring that parents understand the need for newborn screening programs and immediate follow-up of positive results.
- Nursing care of the child with Hurler syndrome centers around the issues associated with a degenerative disease and the problems unique to the affected child and family.
- Long-term management of the child with a metabolic disorder involves *teaching* on home specimen collection, dietary regimen, identification of signs and symptoms, use of community resources, and use of emergency measures.
- Nurses can assist parents in developing appropriate expectations for their child and can provide assistance in managing special diets and treatments.

REFERENCES

Azen, C. G., Koch, R., Gross Friedman, E., Berlow, S., Coldwell, J., Krause, W., Matalon, R., McCabe, E., O'Flynn, M., Peterson, R., Rouse, B., Scott, C. R., Sigman, B., Valle, D., & Warner, R. (1991). Intellectual development in 12-year-old children treated for phenylketonuria. *American Journal of Diseases of Children, 145,* 35–39.

Barton, N. W., Brady, R. O., Dambrosia, J. M., DiBisceglie, A. M., Doppelt, S. H., Hill, S. C., Mankin, H. J., Murray, G. J., Parker, R. I., Argoff, C. E., Grewal, R. P., Yu, K.-T., et al. (1991). Replacement therapy for inherited enzyme deficiency—macrophage-targeted glucocerebrosidase for Gaucher's disease. *New England Journal of Medicine, 324,* 1464–1470.

Batshaw, M. L., Msall, M., Beaudet, A. L., & Trojak, J. (1986). Risk of serious illness in heterozygotes for ornithine transcarbamylase deficiency. *Journal of Pediatrics, 108,* 236–241.

Bennett, M. J., Coates, P. M., Hale, D. E., Millington, D. S., Pollitt, R. J., Rinaldo, P., Roe, C. R., & Tanaka, K. (1990). Analysis of abnormal urinary metabolites in the newborn period in medium-chain acyl-CoA dehydrogenase deficiency. *Journal of Inherited Metabolic Disease, 13,* 707–715.

Bennett, M. J., Worthy, E., & Pollitt, R. J. (1987). The incidence and presentation of dicarboxylic aciduria. *Journal of Inherited Metabolic Disease, 10,* 241–242.

Bickel, H., Gerrard, J., & Hickman, E. (1953). Influence of phenylalanine intake on phenylketonuria. *Lancet, 2,* 812–813.

Brusilow, S. W., & Horwich, A. L. (1989). Urea cycle enzymes. In C. R. Scriver, A. L. Beaudet, W. S. Sly, & D. Valle (Eds.), *The metabolic basis of inherited disease* (6th ed., pp. 629–663). New York: McGraw-Hill.

Committee on Genetics, American Academy of Pediatrics (1992). Issues in newborn screening. *Pediatrics, 89,* 345–349.

Committee on Genetics, American Academy of Pediatrics (1989). Newborn screening fact sheets. *Pediatrics, 83,* 449–464.

Costakos, D., Abramson, R. K., Edwards, J. G., Rizzo, W. B., & Best, R. G. (1991). Attitudes toward presymptomatic testing and prenatal diagnosis for adrenoleukodystrophy among affected families. *American Journal of Medical Genetics, 41,* 295–300.

Danner, D. J., & Elsas, L. J. (1989). Disorders of branched chain amino acid and keto acid metabolism. In C. R. Scriver, A. L. Beaudet, W. S. Sly, & D. Valle (Eds.), *The metabolic basis of inherited disease* (6th ed., pp. 671–692). New York: McGraw-Hill.

Dhondt, J.-L. (1991). Strategy for the screening of tetrahydrobiopterin deficiency among hyperphenylalaninaemic patients: 15-years experience. *Journal of Inherited Metabolic Disease, 14,* 117–127.

Fishler, K., Koch, R., Donnell, G. N., & Wenz, E. (1980). Developmental aspects of galactosemia from infancy to childhood. *Clinical Pediatrics, 19,* 38–45.

Goodman, S. I., & Greene, C. L. (1991). Inborn errors of metabolism. In W. E. Hathaway, J. R. Groothuis, W. W. Hay, & J. W. Paisley (Eds.), *Current pediatric diagnosis and treatment* (pp. 997–1015). Norwalk, CT: Appleton & Lange.

Guthrie, R., & Susi, A. (1963). A simple phenylalanine method for determining phenylketonuria in large populations of newborn infants. *Pediatrics, 14,* 338–343.

Güttler, F., & Lou, H. (1990). Phenylketonuria and hyperphenylalaninemia. In J. Fernandez, J.-M. Saudubray, & K. Tada (Eds.), *Inborn metabolic diseases: Diagnosis and treatment* (pp. 161–174). New York: Springer-Verlag.

Holtzman, N. A., Kronmal, R. A., vanDoorninck, W., Azen, C., & Koch, R. (1986). Effect of age at loss of dietary control on intellectual performance and behavior of children with phenylketonuria. *New England Journal of Medicine, 314,* 593–598.

Kaplan, P., Mazur, A., Field, M., Berlin, J. A., Berry, G. T., Heidenreich, R., Yudkoff, M., & Segal, S. (1991). Intellectual outcome in children with maple syrup urine disease. *Journal of Pediatrics, 119,* 46–50.

Kaufman, F. R., Xu, Y. K., Ng, W. G., & Donnell, G. N. (1988). Correlation of ovarian function with galactose-1-phosphate uridyl transferase levels in galactosemia. *Journal of Pediatrics, 112,* 754–756.

Koch, R., Hanley, W., Levy, H., Matalon, R., Rouse, B., Dela Cruz, F., Azen, C., & Gross Friedman, E. (1990). A preliminary report of the collaborative study of maternal phenylketonuria in the United States and Canada. *Journal of Inherited Metabolic Disease, 13,* 641–650.

Lenke, R. R., & Levy, H. L. (1980). Maternal phenylketonuria and hyperphenylalaninemia: An international survey of the outcome of untreated and treated pregnancies. *New England Journal of Medicine, 303,* 1202–1208.

Lidksy, A. S., Robson, K. J. H., Thirumalachary, C., Barker, P. E., Ruddle, F. H., & Woo, S. L. C. (1984). The PKU locus in man is on chromosome 12. *American Journal of Human Genetics, 36,* 527–533.

MacDonald, I. (1988). Carbohydrates. In M. E. Shils & V. R. Young (Eds.), *Modern nutrition in health and disease* (7th ed., pp. 38–71). Philadelphia: Lea & Febiger.

McCabe, L., Ernest, A. E., Neifert, M. R., Yannicelli, S., Nord, A. M., Garry, P. J., & McCabe, E. R. B. (1989). The management of breast feeding among infants with phenylketonuria. *Journal of Inherited Metabolic Disease, 12,* 467–474.

Moser, H. W. (1991). Peroxisomal disorders. *Clinical Biochemistry, 24,* 343–351.

Munro, H. N., & Crim, M. C. (1988). The proteins and amino acids. In M. E. Shils & V. R. Young (Eds.), *Modern nutrition in health and disease* (7th ed., pp. 1–37). Philadelphia: Lea & Febiger.

Naughten, E. R., Jenkins, J., Francis, D. E. M., & Leonard, J. V. (1982). Outcome of maple syrup urine disease. *Archives of Disease in Childhood, 57,* 918–921.

Neufeld, E. F., & Muenzer, J. (1989). The mucopolysaccharidoses. In

C. R. Scriver, A. L. Beaudet, W. S. Sly, & D. Valle (Eds.), *The metabolic basis of inherited disease* (6th ed., pp. 1565–1587). New York: McGraw-Hill.

Nord, A., vanDoorninck, W. J., & Greene, C. (1991). Developmental profile of patients with maple syrup urine disease. *Journal of Inherited Metabolic Disease, 14,* 881–889.

Okano, Y., Eisensmith, R. C., Güttler, F., Lichter-Konecki, U., Konecki, D. S., Trefz, F. K., Dasovich, M., Wang, T., Henriksen, K., Lou, H., & Woo, S. L. C. (1991). Molecular basis of phenotypic heterogeneity in phenylketonuria. *New England Journal of Medicine, 324*(18), 1232–1238.

Pollitt, R. J. (1989). Disorders of mitochondrial β-oxidation: Prenatal and early postnatal diagnosis and their relevance to Reye's syndrome and sudden infant death. *Journal of Inherited Metabolic Disease, 12,* 215–230.

Rhead, W. J. (1991). Inborn errors of fatty acid oxidation in man. *Clinical Biochemistry, 24,* 319–329.

Roe, C. R., & Coates, P. M. (1989). Acyl-CoA dehydrogenase deficiencies. In C. R. Scriver, A. L. Beaudet, W. S. Sly, & D. Valle (Eds.), *The metabolic basis of inherited disease* (6th ed., pp. 889–914). New York: McGraw-Hill.

Roe, C. R., Millington, D. S., Maltby, D. A., & Kinnebrew, P. (1986). Recognition of medium-chain acyl-CoA dehydrogenase deficiency in asymptomatic siblings of children dying of sudden infant death or Reye-like syndromes. *Journal of Pediatrics, 108,* 13–18.

Scriver, C. R., Kaufman, S., & Woo, S. L. C. (1989). The hyperphenylalaninemias. In C. R. Scriver, A. L. Beaudet, W. S. Sly, & D. Valle (Eds.), *The metabolic basis of inherited disease* (6th ed., pp. 495–546). New York: McGraw-Hill.

Segal, S. (1989). Disorders of galactose metabolism. In C. R. Scriver, A. L. Beaudet, W. S. Sly, & D. Valle (Eds.), *The metabolic basis of inherited disease* (6th ed., pp. 453–480). New York: McGraw-Hill.

Stanley, C. A. (1987). New genetic defects in mitochondrial fatty acid oxidation and carnitine deficiency. *Advances in Pediatrics, 34,* 59–88.

Tourian, A., & Sidbury, J. B. (1983). Phenylketonuria and hyperphenylalaninemia. In J. B. Stanbury, J. B. Wyngaarden, D. S. Fredrickson, J. L. Goldstein, & M. S. Brown (Eds.), *The metabolic basis of inherited disease* (5th ed., pp. 270–286). New York: McGraw-Hill.

Waggoner, D. D., Buist, N. R. M., & Donnell, G. N. (1990). Long-term prognosis in galactosaemia: Results of a survey of 350 cases. *Journal of Inherited Metabolic Disease, 13,* 802–818.

Waisbren, S. E., Norman, T. R., Schnell, R. R., & Levy, H. L. (1983). Speech and language deficits in early-treated children with galactosemia. *Journal of Pediatrics, 102,* 75–77.

Wendel, U. (1990). Disorders of branched-chain amino acid metabolism. In J. Fernandez, J.-M. Saudubray, & K. Tada (Eds.), *Inborn metabolic diseases: Diagnosis and treatment* (pp. 263–270). New York: Springer-Verlag.

Williamson, M. L., Koch, R., Azen, C., & Chang, C. (1981). Correlates of intelligence test results in treated phenylketonuric children. *Pediatrics, 68*(2), 161–167.

BIBLIOGRAPHY

Burton, B. K. (1987). Inborn errors of metabolism: The clinical diagnosis in early infancy. *Pediatrics, 79,* 359–369.

Committee on Genetics, American Academy of Pediatrics (1989). Newborn screening fact sheets. *Pediatrics, 83,* 449–464.

Davidson, A. (1992). Management and counseling of children with inherited metabolic disorders. *Journal of Pediatric Health Care, 6*(3), 146–152.

Fernandez, J., Saudubray, J.-M., & Tada, K. (Eds.) (1990). *Inborn metabolic diseases: Diagnosis and treatment.* New York: Springer-Verlag.

Goodman, S. I., & Greene, C. L. (1991). Inborn errors of metabolism. In W. E. Hathaway, J. R. Groothuis, W. W. Hay, & J. W. Paisley (Eds.), *Current pediatric diagnosis and treatment* (pp. 997–1015). Norwalk, CT: Appleton & Lange.

Moser, H. W. (1991). Peroxisomal disorders. *Clinical Biochemistry, 24,* 343–351.

Rhead, W. J. (1991). Inborn errors of fatty acid oxidation in man. *Clinical Biochemistry, 24,* 319–329.

Scriver, C. R., Beaudet, A. L., Sly, W. S., & Valle, D. (Eds.) (1989). *The metabolic basis of inherited disease* (6th ed.) New York: McGraw-Hill.

Stanley, C. A. (1987). New genetic defects in mitochondrial fatty acid oxidation and carnitine deficiency. *Advances in Pediatrics, 34,* 59–88.

Wright, L., Brown, A., & Davidson-Mundt, A. (1992). Newborn screening: The miracle and the challenge. *Journal of Pediatric Nursing, 7*(1), 26–42.

CHAPTER • 45

Sensory and Communication Alterations

Laurie E. Scudder

NURSING PROCESS PLAN
The Child with an Identified Sensory Impairment, Table 45–8

RELATED TOPICS
Communicating with children, Chapter 11
Assessing Child Health, Chapter 13
Play, Chapter 17
Impact of chronic illness, Chapter 19
Administration of eye drops and ear drops, Chapter 23
Otitis media, Chapter 32
Foreign body in the ear, Chapter 46

LEARNING OBJECTIVES

- **Discuss the normal development and variations of the sensory systems.**
- **Demonstrate the techniques of assessment of the sensory organs.**
- **Recognize the early indicators of sensory deficit.**
- **Discuss the nurse's role in the care of children with sensory deficits.**
- **Appropriately educate parents of children with sensory deficits.**

Human growth and development takes place in a sea of interactive experiences. Formulation of a sense of self, of others, and of the world develops through exchanges involving vision, hearing, touch, smell, and language experiences. The sensory experiences that enable a person to "take in" and "respond to" internal and external stimuli are instrumental in shaping the development of the growing child. In communication alterations, sensitive adjustments and responsiveness of the environment are required to support optimal development of the child.

Health care to prevent, detect, and manage sensory, speech, and language alterations is provided by multidisciplinary teams, including nurses. Although parents provide the major social and developmental support, the nurse can sustain the child and family through counseling, education, assistance with management of the technical aspects of care, and facilitating access to community agencies and resources. This chapter discusses the nurse's role in the care of children with vision, hearing, and speech and language alterations.

Alterations in Vision

Infants and children are affected by a variety of visual problems, some of which can be corrected if identified early, whereas others can only be treated with varying degrees of success. Assessment of visual and physical characteristics of the eye from birth is done to ensure early identification of visual problems. Familiarity with normal developmental characteristics of the immature eye is essential to make the necessary judgment concerning clinical findings.

Visual Development

Infants' vision is better than was once thought, and visual acuity is now thought to increase significantly between birth and 6 months of age (Nelson et al, 1984). Careful observation of infant responses and use of assessment techniques such as optokinetic nystagmus, forced preferential looking, and visually evoked potentials have contributed to our understanding of visual development.

Visually evoked potential studies indicate that acuity at birth may be in the range of 20/100 to 20/200 and, by 6 months of age, approximately 20/20 to 20/40 (Nelson et al, 1984). Visual acuity at birth is thought to be less than 20/20 because of several factors, including (1) incomplete myelination of pathways from the retina to the occipital cortex; (2) immaturity of central nervous system synapses; and (3) inability to accommodate the lens. In the first few weeks of life, infants gaze around to look at things. They have been found to be interested specifically in the human face. While still in the delivery room, neonates have been noted to be more interested in an object that simulated the human face than in objects that did not have such a pattern (Goble, 1984). Also, sharply contrasting black-and-white geometric designs seem to be preferred over the more common bunnies and kittens that come in soft shapes and pastel colors (Ludington-Hoe, 1983). According to Field (1982), neonates also discriminate and imitate three facial expressions (happy, sad, and surprised) (Fig. 45–1).

Normal neonates tend to keep their eyes closed much of the time but will respond to illumination and can fixate. Some disconjugate eye movements (eyes not working together) may be noticed at birth. Developmentally, the eye is less mature; therefore, its function is affected. Developmental variations of the eye are summarized in Table 45–1.

Prevention and Early Identification

Genetic and unknown causes are responsible for the majority of cases of congenital blindness in children. A thorough history with a careful eye examination on all well child visits forms a major preventive role of the nurse. A family history of a genetic disease associated with visual loss is significant information that may lead to the early detection of visual impairment in an infant.

Genetic counseling is an important aspect of prevention of blindness when known genetic diseases that cause blindness are identified in a family history. Prenatal screening for maternal infections that cause blindness (rubella, syphilis), adequate prenatal care to

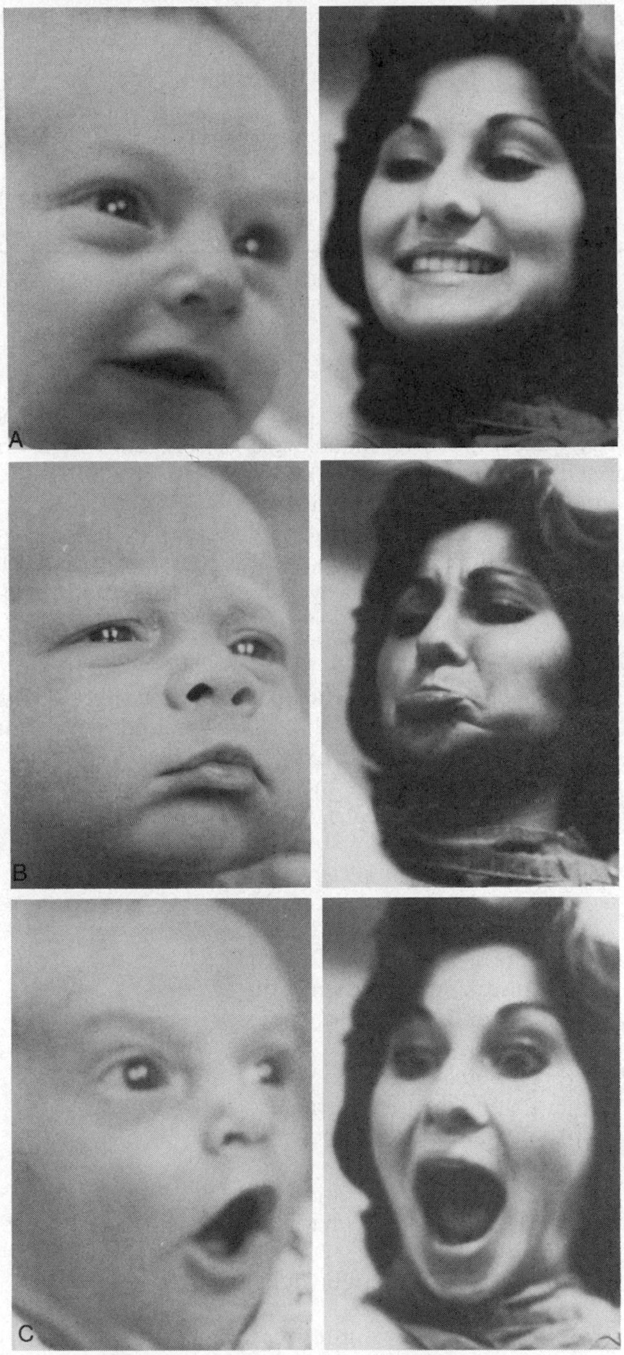

FIGURE 45 - 1. Imitation and discrimination by neonates. (From Field, J. M. [1982, October]. Discrimination and imitation of facial expressions by neonates. *Science, 218,* 180.)

TABLE 45-1
Developmental Variations in Eye Maturation

Structure/Function	Description	Process of Maturation
Sclera	Thin, translucent with a bluish tinge	
Cornea	Proportionately large in the neonate; should appear crystal clear within 1–2 days after birth; premature infants may have a transient opalescent haze	Reaches adult size by 2 yrs of age or sooner; curvature flattens with age, altering refractive characteristics of the eye
Pupils	Small in neonate and difficult to dilate; pupillary reflexes sluggish at birth	Within a few weeks, begin to enlarge; pupillary reflexes apparent in a few weeks
Lens	Ciliary muscle is immature; has greater refractive power and this compensates for the short diameter of the globe (hyperopia)	Accommodation developed by 4 mos; with age, lens becomes more dense and resistant to change of shape during accommodation
Refraction	Infant eye is hyperopic	Hyperopia increases until age 7, after which it declines
Binocular vision	The ability to fixate on one visual field with both eyes is called binocularity; binocularity is not present at birth	Binocularity is established by 6 mos of age and probably sooner in many infants
Crying tears	Lacrimal glands not fully developed at birth but some tearing does occur; temporary obstruction of lacrimal duct may cause overflow of tears	By 6–8 mos, spontaneous canalization of lacrimal duct occurs

From Greenwald, M. J. (1983, December). Visual development in infancy and childhood. *Pediatric Clinics of North America, 30*(6), 977–993; and Nelson, L. B., et al (1984, March). Developmental aspects in the assessment of visual function in young children. Reproduced by permission of *Pediatrics* vol. 73, p. 375, copyright 1984.

prevent prematurity, and prevention of exposure of premature infants to high levels of oxygen whenever possible are preventive approaches in which the nurse may have responsibility.

The nurse has a role in the early identification and prevention of retinopathy of prematurity (ROP), ophthalmia neonatorum, eye injuries, and visual problems.

Retinopathy of Prematurity. ROP is thought to be a multifactorial disorder that is associated with, but not limited to, excessive oxygen therapy.

The possible causes include (Shapiro, 1992):

1. Prematurity/low birthweight—the most important clinical factor.
2. Hyperoxia.
3. Hypoxia.
4. Blood transfusions.
5. Intraventricular hemorrhage.
6. Apnea/bradycardia spells.
7. Sepsis.
8. Hypercapnia/hypocapnia.
9. Patent ductus arteriosus.
10. Vitamin E deficiency.
11. Lactic acidosis.
12. Prenatal complications.
13. Duration of mechanical ventilation and oxygen therapy.
14. Exposure to bright light.

Very low birthweight neonates (weighing less than 1500 g and especially under 1000 g) are at risk for development of ROP (Shapiro, 1986). More than 500 infants in the United States are estimated to be blinded each year as a result of ROP (Porat, 1984). The nurse is an important participant in the monitoring of these infants at risk in the neonatal intensive care unit (see Chapter 32 for further discussion of the effects of oxygen therapy).

Ophthalmia Neonatorum. The routine use of silver nitrate drops at birth to prevent gonorrheal ophthalmia neonatorum (inflammation of the conjunctiva of the neonate that occurs as a result of exposure to maternal cervical infection) is discouraged. The major objections to this practice are the resultant chemical conjunctivitis that follows its use and its lack of effectiveness against *Chlamydia trachomatis.*

There is ample evidence that erythromycin ointment is a better choice because of its greater effectiveness against *C. trachomatis* as well as *Neisseria gonorrhoeae.* The nurse administers the ointment in most institutions. Understanding of the rationale for this practice is necessary to allow the nurse to educate the parents.

Eye Injuries. Participation in the prevention of eye injuries is another important role. Anticipatory guidance offered by the nurse should include a discussion of potential dangers associated with rapid developmental advancement. For example, using scissors, chemistry sets, and many self-created toys, like sticks and arrows, requires teaching and supervision by parents to prevent eye injuries. Sharp objects, fireworks, chemicals, power tools, and sunlight are potential sources of danger. Safety eye wear for racket sports is essential (see Chapter 15 for further discussion of safety teaching). Nurses can also promote proper care and use of contact lenses and glasses.

TABLE 45-2
Techniques for Testing Vision in a Young or Retarded Child

Description	Comments
Optokinetic Nystagmus	
Nystagmus is a periodic involuntary movement of the eyes from side to side or up and down; optokinetic nystagmus is a *visually induced* nystagmus to evaluate vision A drum with black-and-white stripes, dots, or pictures is rotated in front of child; a positive response (indicating vision) is the slow movement of the eyes in the direction of the moving drum, followed by a quick return of the eye to its former position (optokinetic nystagmus), done repetitively as the drum turns	A positive response demonstrates that the child can see, but failure to evoke optokinetic nystagmus (negative response) can mean either poor vision or poor attention; appropriate for infants from birth to around 3 yrs of age
Forced Preferential Looking	
A circle of alternating light and dark stripes (grating) and a gray spot of similar size and brightness are symmetrically placed in an infant's field of vision; the width of the stripes is gradually reduced until the infant no longer looks preferentially at the grating; the narrowest width of stripe that the infant looks at is then converted into Snellen visual acuity	Can be used from birth to 2½ yrs of age; test is based on the observation that the infant is more likely to look at a figure with black-and-white stripes than one that is solidly gray; this procedure can be very time-consuming and is still in the experimental stages
Visually Evoked Potentials (VEP)	
Electrical activity is recorded through scalp electrodes following visual stimulation with single or repeated flashing lights into child's eye, one at a time; it is an electroencephalogram of the occipital area	Child needs to be quiet to avoid electrical interference; a parent can hold the child; mild sedation may be needed; because this test does not rely on a motor response from the child, it can be used for brain-damaged children

From Greenwald, M. J. (1983, December). Visual development in infancy and childhood. *Pediatric Clinics of North America, 30*(6), 977–993; Nelson, L. B., et al (1984, March). Developmental aspects in the assessment of visual function in young children. *Pediatrics, 73*(3), 375–381; and Kovalesky, A. (1985). *Nurses' guide to children's eyes.* Orlando, FL: Grune & Stratton.

Visual Problems. Screening programs to detect visual problems begin at birth. Specific vision tests requiring special equipment that can be used for infants are summarized in Table 45–2. Assessment of the development of vision should always be part of well child examinations. Characteristics of vision development up to age 3 are summarized in Table 45–3. Techniques used to assess vision according to age are summarized in Table 45–4. (Components of an eye examination and a description of screening techniques are included in Chapter 13.)

In addition to assessing vision during health examinations, the nurse should teach families how to detect a visual problem in their child. The Home Eye Test for Preschoolers is available from the National Society for the Prevention of Blindness.* It contains the Snellen E short eye chart and simple instructions for the parents.

The Committee on the Fetus and Newborn of the American Academy of Pediatrics recommends that a person experienced in recognizing ROP should examine the eyes of all infants born before 36 weeks gestation, or weighing less than 2000 g (4 lb, 7 oz) who have received oxygen therapy (American Academy of Pediatrics, 1983). Table 45–5 summarizes a recommended time schedule for the first fundus examination and the follow-up.

Screening for refractive errors becomes particularly important with the development of true binocular vision at about 6 months of age. Five per cent of all preschool children have visual problems. Although prevention of these conditions is not possible because they are primarily hereditary, early identification and treatment may prevent loss of vision.

* 79 Madison Avenue, New York, NY 10016.

Refractive Errors

In vision, light rays enter the lens and are brought to a single focus on the retina. When the bending of the rays (refraction) and the length of the eyeball are uncoordinated, the image does not fall on a single point on the retina. Although children may not say that they are having trouble seeing, symptoms such as rubbing of the eyes, tearing, red-rimmed eyelids, and squinting should make one suspicious of a refractive error.

The work of the eye—bringing the image into clear focus—involves accommodation and convergence. "Accommodation" is the focusing mechanism of the eyes that allows a person to see clearly at all

TABLE 45-3
Characteristics of Vision Development

Birth to 2 Wks

Eyes blink in response to bright light. Doll's eye reflex present because child is unable to integrate head and eye movements (when examiner rotates infant's head to one side, eyes lag behind). Transitory fixation develops at a distance of approximately 3 ft. Visual acuity 20/100 to 20/200

1–2 Mos

Regards parent's face and watches intently. Follows large moving objects 10–14 in from face through a 90-degree angle (45 degrees from midline), but glances are minimal for moving stimuli beyond 2 ft away

3–4 Mos

Visual following at 6–12 in from face with a combination of head and eye movements through a 180-degree arc. Convergence on near objects now developed. Doll's eye reflex disappears. Watches own hands and feet. Fixates immediately on a 1-in cube brought within 1–2 ft of the eye

6–7 Mos

Ciliary muscle function begins and accommodation-convergence reflex developing. Eyes move together (binocular vision established). Frequent crossing is abnormal and indicates strabismus. Hand-eye coordination developing. Child reaches for anything seen and adjusts own position to see objects. Visual acuity 20/20 to 20/40*

10 Mos

Pats mirror image. Sees tiny objects and reaches for them using fingers and thumb. Follows and watches activities within 10–12 ft

12 Mos

Drops toys and watches them fall. Recognizes familiar people at distance of 20 ft or more

18 Mos

Shows keen interest in pictures. Fixes eyes on small dangling toy at 10 ft. Points to familiar objects. Convergence well established

2 Yrs

Accommodates well. Recognizes fine details in pictures. Visual acuity 20/20*

3 Yrs

Attention span fair. Fixation on small pictures or toys approaches 50 sec. Matches letters HOVT in STYCAR test at 10 ft. Visual acuity 20/20 and, after 3 yrs of age, can be assessed by Snellen E chart. (See Chapter 13 for description of STYCAR and Snellen E chart)

From Johnson, T., et al (1978). *Children are different: Developmental physiology* (2nd ed.). Columbus, OH: Ross Laboratories; Stangler, S., et al (1980). *Screening growth and development of preschool children: A guide for test selection*. New York: McGraw-Hill; and Nelson, L. B., et al (1984, March). Developmental aspects in the assessment of visual function in young children. *Pediatrics, 73*(3), 375–381.

* Estimated visual acuity varies according to the test used. The reported age at which 20/20 vision is achieved ranges from 6 mos to 2½ yrs (Nelson et al, 1984).

distances. As the ciliary muscle contracts, the curvature of the lens and its refractive strength are increased. This results in an increase in the anterior-posterior thickness of the lens. Children with normal eyes usually have excellent accommodative powers (at age 8 years, the eye has the maximal potential accommodation) (Goble, 1984).

Convergence of the eyes occurs simultaneously with accommodation, in a fixed ratio. "Convergence" is an increasing inward movement of the eyeballs as an object is brought from a position of distance to one of closeness. The closer the object is brought to the child's face, the greater the degree of convergence. This reflex facilitates focusing of the image at the same position on the retina of each eye, resulting in binocular vision, or fusion of the images. As the object is brought closer to the child's face, constriction of the pupils occurs in addition to convergence.

Measurement of visual acuity is a screening test that can be done easily and quickly to identify refractive errors. The preschool years are an important time to detect these errors to help the child avoid problems in school. The nurse should understand that the eyeball grows as the child grows and that, during this time, refraction may change significantly. The three types of refractive errors that are most common in children are *hyperopia, myopia,* and *astigmatism*. Hyperopia increases until around 6 to 7 years of age, after which it decreases gradually until adulthood; myopia usually begins around the preteen years, progresses during the teen-age years, then stabilizes (Kovalesky, 1985).

Hyperopia

Hyperopia is often referred to as farsightedness. This is due to the fact that older hyperopic individuals see better on far gaze. Hyperopia may be the result of a short axial length of the eye or decreased corneal lens curvature. Either of these conditions results in an image that falls behind the retina. The majority of children are normally hyperopic but, unlike adults, they are able to accommodate to attain good visual acuity; however, this constant accommodative effort required for close work leads to excessive convergence, which may result in strabismus and amblyopia, to be discussed later. This degree of hyperopia is corrected with convex lenses, which decrease both accommodation and convergence, causing the eyes to straighten.

Myopia

In myopia, an excessive amount of refractive power for the length of the eye results in light rays coming to a point of focus in *front* of the retina. The only symptom of myopia is blurred vision for distance. Eyestrain and headaches are not associated with myopia. A child with myopia may be able to read without accommodative effort because near vision requires greater refractive strength than distant vision. If myopia is severe, however, the child may have to hold the print close to see it clearly.

Concave lenses readily correct the vision of a myopic child. The problem may become more severe during the early school years; new glasses may be needed every year or two. On the other hand, congenital myopia tends to resolve gradually with age, with a visual acuity of 20/40 by adolescence (Hughes, 1984). These children may or may not need corrective lenses, depending on the severity of the problem.

Astigmatism

In astigmatism, the curvature of the cornea is not equal in all directions. The result is that light rays are not focused symmetrically; therefore, the image is blurred and distorted. Eyestrain results from the accommodative effort that is made to bring the image into focus. Accommodation alone cannot correct astigmatism; it must be corrected with lenses that compensate for the abnormal curvature of the cornea. Astigmatism may coexist with myopia or hyperopia.

TABLE 45-4
Techniques of Vision Assessment According to Age

Neonate

External inspection of eye (check for infection, trauma, and congenital anomalies)

Check for blink response to bright light

Check for presence of red reflex and pupillary response to light

Do Hirschberg test for detection of strabismus

Check for nystagmus* with optokinetic drum† to establish the presence of vision

6 Mos

External inspection of eye as for neonate (a deviation or anomaly may now be apparent that was not noted in the neonate)

Test for strabismus; use cover-uncover test or alternate cover test; Hirschberg test; check whether both eyes follow a light from side to side equally well

Observe for nystagmus (congenital nystagmus is present at birth but is not commonly detected before the age of 2–3 mos)

Assess visual development (see Table 45–2)

Perform ophthalmoscopic examination

3–5 Yrs

External inspection of eyes as during infancy. Test for strabismus as described for 6 mos of age. Concerning behavior:

- Frequently rubs eyes
- Brings eyes close to objects
- Frequently squints or frowns in order to see
- Tilts head; shuts or covers one eye
- Complains of itchiness, burning, or a "dusty" feeling in eyes
- Cannot see well (chalkboard, a toy, an object across the room)
- Has abnormal sensitivity to light
- Has more than usual difficulty adapting to low levels of illumination

Visual acuity tested with Snellen E symbol (of particular importance is identification of unequal vision caused by amblyopia). Check for color blindness

Refer 3-year-old with visual acuity of 20/50 or less and 4- or 5-year-old with 20/40 or less (all children should be rescreened on another day before referral)

Other tests of visual acuity for preschooler:

- STYCAR (letter-matching test)
- Allen picture cards

School-Age

Techniques for detection of visual problems similar to that described for 3- to 5-year-olds with the exception that if the letters of the alphabet are learned it is recommended that the standard Snellen alphabet chart be used

Children 5 yrs and older should read a majority of the 20/30 line. A two-line difference between eyes warrants referral (Committee on Practice and Ambulatory Medicine, 1986)

Data from *About children's eyes.* Available from National Association for Visually Handicapped. 305 East 24th Street, New York, NY 10010; Stangler, S., et al (1980). *Screening growth and development of preschool children: A guide for test selection.* New York: McGraw-Hill; and Hatfield, E. (1979, Summer). Methods and standards for screening preschool children. *The Sightsaving Review.*

* Nystagmus is a rhythmic oscillation of the eyes that occurs on lateral gaze.

† An optokinetic drum is a cylinder with stripes or pictures that, when twirled within the baby's range of vision, normally elicits nystagmus if vision is present.

TABLE 45-5
Time Schedule for Fundus Examination in Neonates at Risk for Retinopathy of Prematurity (ROP)

Gestational Age at Birth	First Examination	Follow-Up Examinations
<30 wks	6–8 wks	*If no ROP:* Repeat q 3–4 wks, until mature retina, and again in 3–6 mos
		If ROP present: Mild—Reexamine q 2–3 wks until signs of resolution noted. *Severe (Grade 3+)*—Reexamine q 1–2 wks until signs of resolution noted
		Resolving RLF: q 2–4 wks until resolved
30–34 wks	6–7 wks	*If normal:* Repeat in 3–6 mos
		If ROP present: Follow schedule as noted in <30 wks
>34 wks	6 wks	*If normal:* No subsequent examination necessary
		If ROP present: Follow schedule as noted in <30 wks
Anterior chamber hyperemia	Immediate eye examination	

For Detection of Late Complications

Infants with fully regressed ROP: Eye examination q 1–2 yrs

Infants with cicatricial RLF (scarring of the retina): Eye examination q 6–12 mos

From Porat, R. (1984, February). Care of the infant with retinopathy of prematurity. *Clinics in Perinatology, 11*(1), 123–151.

Strabismus

In strabismus, the eye muscles lack coordination, resulting in a misalignment. The condition occurs in about 2 per cent of all children. The various terms used to describe strabismus are as follows:

Monocular—One eye is used to fixate and the other deviates. The deviating eye is prone to the development of amblyopia.

Alternating—Each eye is alternately used for fixation; vision develops more or less the same in both eyes.

Convergent (esotropia)—Eye turns toward the midline (Fig. 45-2).

Divergent (exotropia)—Eye turns away from the midline.

Nonparalytic (incomitant or nonconcomitant)—All muscles function but not in unison; deviation is the same in all directions of gaze.

Paralytic (comitant or concomitant)—Caused by a weakness or paralysis of one or more of the extraocular muscles. The eye appears crossed when turned in the direction of the affected muscle.

Words ending in:

Tropia: A continuous misalignment.

Phoria: A latent tendency to misalignment, usually evident during times of stress, illness or fatigue.

Esotropia and exotropia are always abnormal. However, the normal infant may at times appear to have a phoria that is usually associated with sleepiness. This should improve from week to week and resolve by 6 months of age. Ophthalmic consultation is required for children in whom it persists.

Some children may appear to have esotropia because of certain facial features. This is termed "pseu-

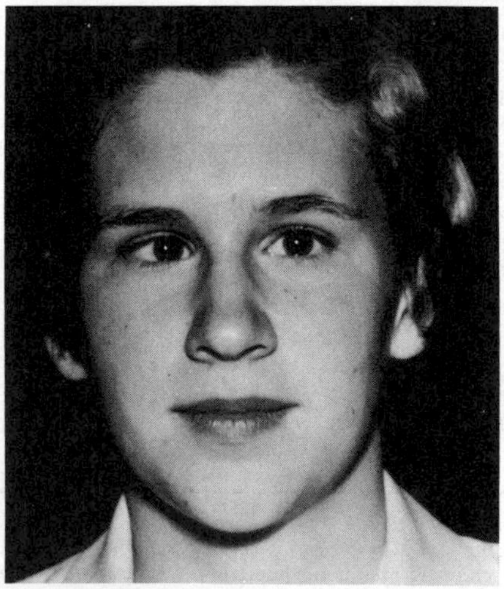

FIGURE 45-2. Accommodative esotropia, uncorrected. (From Scheie, H., Albert, D. [1977]. *Textbook of ophthalmology* [9th ed.]. Philadelphia: WB Saunders, p 337.)

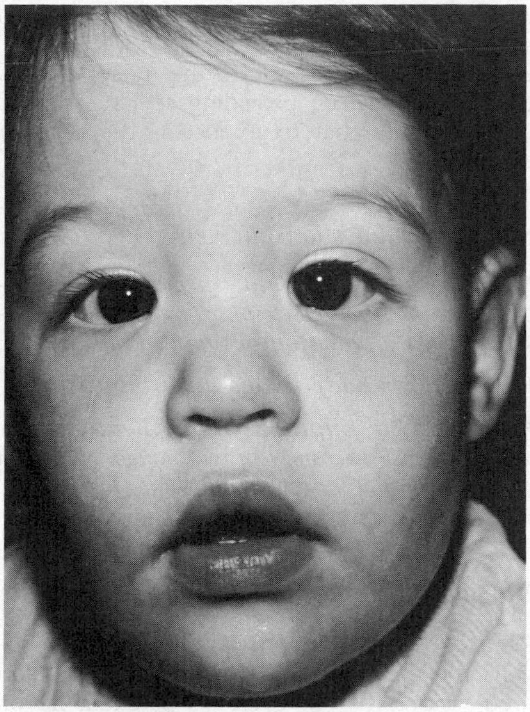

FIGURE 45-3. Pseudostrabismus. (From Scheie, H., Albert, D. [1977]. *Textbook of ophthalmology* [9th ed.]. Philadelphia: WB Saunders, p 337.)

dostrabismus" and is most commonly caused by prominent epicanthal folds and a broad, flat nasal bridge (Fig. 45-3).

Etiology

About 50 per cent of all children with strabismus have a positive family history for the condition; therefore, any child in a family with a history of strabismus should be closely monitored. Also, the siblings of a child with strabismus should be examined frequently for this defect. The most common cause of strabismus is imbalance of the muscle alignment of the eyes, but other etiologic factors such as brain tumor, infection, retinoblastoma, myasthenia gravis, and cataracts should be considered. Whenever there is any suspicion of strabismus, the child must be referred for further examination.

Any type of misalignment is of concern, and any child who does not see well with each eye should be suspected of having a serious condition (Feman & Reinecke, 1978).

Early identification of strabismus may be made by performing the cover test and corneal light reflex test, also called the Hirschberg test (see Chapter 13), during well child examinations. Early identification and referral can also be initiated by a nurse observing that a child is squinting and showing difficulty with close-range vision. Strabismus may also be suspected when the child complains of frequent headaches or tilts the head to see.

Early recognition and treatment are essential to prevent amblyopia. Amblyopia develops when vision is suppressed in the eye that deviates. Without correction, permanent visual loss may occur in the deviated eye.

Pathophysiology

The two major kinds of strabismus are *nonparalytic* (nonconcomitant) and *paralytic* (comitant).

"Nonparalytic strabismus" is the most common type in children. The child has difficulty seeing at close range and is likely to squint. "Accommodative strabismus" is a special type of nonparalytic strabismus that usually develops between 2 and 4 years of age. It has two forms: *convergent* and *divergent*. This type of strabismus develops because of a refractive error. Most children normally have a degree of hyperopia until about 7 years of age. In hyperopia, accommodative effort is required to attain good vision. With accommodation, there is normally an accompanying convergence reflex; a fine balance is needed between the accommodative effort and the simultaneous convergence. Generally, the normal hyperopia of childhood is handled through accommodation and an accompanying convergence. If hyperopia is excessive, or if the eyes have very discrepant refractions, strabismus can result when the amount of accommodation required for clear vision results in excessive convergence (crossed eyes). Conversely, external deviation (divergence) occurs in myopia; this is less common but may be present at birth.

In "paralytic strabismus," the child may complain of headache and demonstrate lack of coordination in fine or gross movements. Double vision, or diplopia, may be evidenced by the child's response of closing one eye or tilting the head to avoid seeing a double image.

Strabismus may be obvious or may occur only when the child is ill or tired. Screening tests for strabismus include the cover test and corneal light reflex (Hirschberg test) described in Chapter 13.

Therapeutic Management

The goal of treatment is for the child to attain the best possible vision in each eye and, if possible, equal vision. The ultimate goal is attainment of binocular vision with stereopsis (depth perception); however, in many affected patients, this cannot be achieved (Hughes, 1984). The type of treatment varies with the age of the child and type of strabismus.

Patching and Glasses

Patching of the good eye is a common method of treatment. This is done to encourage the child to use the deviating eye. In some instances—for example, in the case of accommodative strabismus—the wearing of glasses may correct the deviation.

Pharmacologic Therapy

Accommodative strabismus or esotropia, that is, a malalignment that occurs because of unequal refraction, is occasionally treated with cycloplegic miotic drops. These drugs are chemically classified as anticholinesterase drugs and include echothiophate iodide (Phospholine Iodide) and isoflurophate (DFP). These drops are instilled in the eye that is hyperopic to paralyze the ciliary muscle and thus make accommodation easier. By reducing the amount of accommodation, the amount of convergence is also reduced, causing the eye to straighten. These drugs are called "miotics" because one of their actions is to constrict the pupil; however, in the treatment of strabismus, they are used because of their action on the ciliary body. They work through a direct chemical action on the ciliary body (i.e., inhibition of cholinesterase). Because of certain disadvantages associated with the use of miotics, these agents should be used only in carefully selected cases. Treatment by miotics has the following disadvantages (Goble, 1984):

- In many children, miotics are less effective than glasses.
- In some children, miotics cause cysts of the iris (cysts diminish in size when miotics are discontinued). Adding 2.5 per cent phenylephrine (Neo-Synephrine) eyedrops to the treatment can diminish cyst formation.
- Echothiophate iodide (Phospholine Iodide) is absorbed into the general circulation and has the capacity to lower blood levels of certain enzymes, making the use of succinylcholine unsafe.

Because the use of miotic drops will result in a fixed, constricted pupil, it is important that the child wear a Medic-Alert bracelet. A bracelet that advises of the use of miotics will be important to the interpretation of neurologic tests for eye function in the case of post-trauma care (Lingua, 1986). Also, drugs used for strabismus interfere with anesthesia containing succinylcholine and should be discontinued 2 to 3 weeks prior to surgery (Kovalesky, 1985).

Eye Exercises

An adjunct to glasses, patching, and medications is the use of eye exercises (orthoptics). Eye exercises should be prescribed by an ophthalmologist; they are useful only in selected cases.

Surgical Correction

Surgical correction is commonly used for congenital strabismus, whenever glasses or miotics cannot correct the problem, and in selected patients for cosmetic reasons. Congenital strabismus is usually corrected before age 12 months. Before surgery is undertaken, the stronger eye is patched, to treat any existing amblyopia. *Surgery can mechanically straighten an eye, but only patching can stimulate an amblyopic eye to improve vision* (Goble, 1984). In most cases, strabismus can be corrected with one or two procedures, but this varies, and the nurse should consult the surgeon before providing specific information to parents about what to expect as the outcome of surgery.

Nursing Diagnostic Statements

***Fear/anxiety, related to** uncompensated impaired adjustment to temporary visual loss associated with patching of one or both eyes.*

High risk for body image disturbance.

***High risk for impaired home health management;** risk factors: family knowledge deficit regarding home care and inability to cope independently with home care.*

Nursing Interventions

Reducing Postoperative Fear and Anxiety. Postoperatively, the child must be treated as any child with impaired vision. If both eyes are patched, he or she must be treated as a blind child; that is, things are placed within easy reach, the environment is described, and the child is told what will be done to him or her and what he or she is likely to feel before a procedure is begun. The child is allowed to handle things to discover their properties but needs verbal explanations of color. The primary goal is to help the child maintain the usual level of independence even though vision has been temporarily impaired. The surgery is brief and usually the child can be discharged the same day or the following day.

Promoting a Positive Self-Image. The negative effects of strabismus on the child's self-image and personality development can be minimized if attention is given to this potential problem, beginning at the time of diagnosis. Ask the child to draw a picture of himself or herself with friends to assess whether he or she perceives differences between self and friends in appearance and abilities. Medical or play therapy could be used to assist the child to work through his or her feelings regarding how he or she looks (see Chapter 17 for guidelines for the use of medical play).

Supporting the Family in Home Management of Strabismus. Most of the care of children with strabismus is performed outside the hospital. The nurse in the acute care or outpatient setting should assess the family's resources and determine whether referral to a home health agency is needed to meet the demands of long-term care. If the child is in school, the treatment plan should be explained to the school nurse and limitations on the child's school activities discussed. Nursing interventions for the family include teaching the safe use of prescribed eye drops (see

Chapter 23), helping the family deal with the difficulties of keeping an eye patch on a young child, and encouraging regular eye examinations.

Any child who requires eye patches should be closely followed for decreased vision in the patched eye as a result of the occlusion of vision. In a very young child, amblyopia can develop in a patched eye in less than 2 weeks. Therefore, visual screening should be performed on both eyes on a regular basis by the nurse or physician. A frequently encountered problem is the young child's refusal to keep an eye patch on. It is helpful to relate to families that this difficulty is usually self-limited and lasts until the child's vision makes the necessary adaptations to the patching. Patching using a pair of clear glasses with one eye occluded may be more acceptable to a young child. If the condition permits, intermittent patching may be necessary during the first few days. When patching is required postoperatively, the child should be introduced to this sensation before surgery by playing games that require having the eyes covered and using psychologic preparation techniques (see Chapter 17). Arm restraints should also be made available for preoperative experimentation on a doll or favorite stuffed animal.

The nurse should determine whether eye drops are being administered as prescribed and assess for cysts of the iris of the affected eye if miotic eye drops are being used. Refer to the physician if a cyst is detected. Assure the child and family that cysts usually diminish with discontinuation of the medication. Reinforce the importance of prescribed eye exercises to support the family's motivation to follow through with therapy.

Ask the child and family whether the strabismus or therapy is adversely affecting schoolwork. Maintaining contact with the school nurse and teacher to be sure they understand the goals and the importance of the therapeutic measures will help alleviate school problems and assure success. The school nurse and teacher may need assistance in intervening with the child's classmates to explain about strabismus and its treatment.

Ongoing communication with the family regarding any difficulty encountered in carrying out the treatment program is an important contribution of the nurse. The child and family should be encouraged to express their thoughts and feelings about the condition and the required treatments. It is disappointing to a child and family when surgery fails to correct the misalignment. Families need to know that repeated operations may be necessary and that, when an operation is repeated, it offers the same likelihood of success as did the original operation (Feman & Reinecke, 1978).

Amblyopia

"Amblyopia" ("lazy eye") is reduction or loss of central vision in an eye that is normal on ophthalmoscopic examination. A commonly accepted diagnostic sign of amblyopia is that visual acuity in the normal eye is at least two Snellen lines better than the acuity in the affected eye. There are various types of amblyopia: *strabismic amblyopia, deprivation or occlusion amblyopia,* and *refractive amblyopia.*

Pathophysiology

Strabismic Amblyopia

This condition involves the loss of vision in the deviating eye of a child with strabismus. Visual loss occurs because there is an attempt to suppress the double vision experienced by the child with strabismus. The vision in the suppressed eye fails to develop, resulting in loss of vision ranging from a minimal decrease in acuity to severely impaired vision.

Early detection and treatment of strabismus is essential to prevent strabismic amblyopia. Usually by the age of 6 years, the brain has developed suppression to a degree that will not readily respond to treatment, and, by 8 or 9 years of age, reversal of the impairment is considered virtually impossible.

Deprivation and Occlusion Amblyopia

This type of amblyopia can be caused by ptosis (drooping of the upper eyelid), cataracts, and occlusion therapy for strabismic amblyopia. These result in a blockage of the transferal images to the retina. This type is also called "amblyopia ex anopsia."

Refractive Amblyopia

Amblyopia can also result from dissimilar refraction in the two eyes. Hyperopia is a normal condition until around 6 to 7 years of age. This condition normally requires an accommodative effort by the child to correct the refractive error. When the two eyes are not equally hyperopic, fusion may be impossible because of the differences in the images. The less hyperopic eye may then become the preferred eye because less accommodation is required. Consequently, the other eye (the more hyperopic one) becomes lazy or amblyopic. This is known as "anisometropic amblyopia." Unilateral myopia can also cause amblyopia, although it tends to be less severe, presumably because at some distances the myopic eye receives a clear image. Refractive amblyopia can be prevented if discovered and treated early. Glasses are necessary to correct the refractive error and prevent the development of anisometropic amblyopia.

Therapeutic Management

In addition to using glasses to correct any refractive error, patching of the good eye is the basis for treating amblyopia. The patch is usually worn during the waking hours, but some authorities recommend that the child wear the patch 24 hours a day. Careful follow-up is essential to prevent amblyopia of the eye that is being patched. Patching may be required for as long as a year, followed by a period of time during which intermittent patching must be continued. The child and family need reinforcement from the health team for their efforts in complying with the long-term therapy of keeping a young child's eye patched. With early identification and adequate therapy, irreversible loss of vision can be prevented.

Cataract

A "cataract" is an opacity (clouding) of the crystalline lens of the eye that consists of precipitated lens protein. The lens is a clear, flexible disk located behind the pupil and iris. It is normally transparent to allow light to enter the eye and be refracted onto the retina. If a cataract is present, light cannot be refracted and visual impairment exists. Cataracts may be unilateral or bilateral, complete or incomplete.

Congenital Cataracts

Cataracts can be congenital or acquired. Congenital cataracts are formed during the 6th or 7th week of fetal life when the lens is being formed. In many instances, the presence of congenital cataracts is only one aspect of a complex syndrome.

Fifty per cent of congenital cataracts cannot be attributed to specific causes or associated with other anomalies. Trauma, anoxia, or maternal systemic disease during the first trimester of pregnancy have a definite effect on their development. Infectious conditions (commonly, maternal rubella and herpes simplex) or inherited disorders (such as Turner syndrome or galactosemia) account for approximately 50 per cent of cases.

Acquired Cataracts

Acquired cataracts appear at different times after birth and are usually related to trauma, systemic disease, drug toxicity (steroids, radiation), and infections. Cataracts may also develop secondary to other eye malformations and diseases such as ROP (retrolental fibroplasia), retinal detachment, retinosis pigmentosa, and uveitis.

Diagnostic Assessment

Assessment and identification of prenatal high-risk populations is an important nursing role in prevention of cataracts. Prenatal factors such as systemic disease or vaginal infections caused by herpes simplex should be identified and treated. Adequate immunization against rubella and early, comprehensive prenatal care are preventive strategies in which the nurse can actively participate. Additionally, genetic counseling should be made available for families with identified familial diseases. Encouraging compliance with medical regimens, such as adherence to the prescribed diet when a child has galactosemia, can be a factor in retarding the appearance of cataracts.

The sooner cataracts are removed, the better the child's prognosis. Because most cataracts cannot be detected with the unaided eye, checking for the red reflex is an important part of physical assessment (see Chapter 13). Cataracts that lie in the line of vision and produce some visual impairment cause the red reflex to be distorted or impaired. Opacity of the lens blocks the reflected light and is perceived as a dark area or shadow by the examiner (Calhoun, 1983). Those types of cataracts that affect the anterior portion of the lens can be seen with the naked eye and are frequently noticed by parents. A unilateral cataract results in monocular vision (use of one eye) because binocular cooperation of the two eyes is compromised. Eventually, strabismus develops and presents as the first clue to the existing cataract.

When a congenital cataract is suspected, a thorough ophthalmic examination is indicated. The extent of the cataract can be determined by ultrasonography (B-scan), a nonintrusive, painless diagnostic test that can be done through closed eyelids while the infant is sleeping. The nursing role during the stressful diagnostic period focuses on giving and repeating, if necessary, simple explanations of the diagnostic procedures and the proposed treatment plan. Using terms that the family understands is critical to helping them cope. If surgery is decided on, the nurse, along with other members of the health team, is responsible for helping the family understand the lifelong implications of cataract surgery. There is great emotional and financial stress for these families as they attempt to cope with repeated surgical procedures.

When cataracts are likely to interfere with vision, surgical removal is indicated. The density of the cataract and visual acuity are considerations when determining the need to operate.

Surgical Management

In adults, an incision is made into the eye and the lens is grasped and removed from the eye, leaving its capsule intact (intracapsular approach). In children, this technique is associated with loss of vitreous from the eye and can predispose the child to retinal detachment and corneal edema. The extracapsular approach is preferred for children. The lens capsule is left in place to hold back the vitreous. One disadvantage is that the retained lens capsule becomes opaque, necessitating a second operation (Goble, 1984). New instruments are now available to remove the lens and *some* of the vitreous. This procedure generally does not require a second operation for an opaque capsule, but, on occasion, a characteristic cystlike edema in the macula develops as a complication. Although this edema usually decreases over time, there is no effective treatment and it does interfere with vision while it is present (Goble, 1984). The fitting and wearing of corrective contact lenses or glasses is the next step in management. Infants may be fitted with lenses as early as 3 weeks after surgery.

A newer surgical technique being used for adults is insertion of an intraocular lens, but this is not commonly used for children. Complications of this technique include uveitis and corneal damage (Goble, 1984).

Nursing Interventions

Goals for nursing care include providing information and support for the family in the preoperative period and providing and teaching physical support of the child postoperatively. Interventions to meet these goals are discussed later.

Preoperative preparation of the family includes discussion of eye patches and restraints used in the immediate postoperative period. Explain that vision will not be improved immediately, because corrective lenses are necessary after surgery. Postoperatively, the nurse is involved in physical support of the infant and in teaching the family to carry out the care. An eye shield is used for protection for about a week. If glasses are worn, the eye shield is used only at night and during naptime after the first postoperative day. A combination of antibiotic and steroid drops is given for several weeks to prevent infection and minimize inflammation. Usually, with current surgical techniques, activity restriction is minimal. The parents should demonstrate proficiency and ease with administration of eye drops before the infant is discharged from the hospital.

When contact lenses are prescribed, the nurse's teaching includes helping the family learn specific cleaning, insertion, and removal techniques. The nurse also makes sure that the graduated schedule for wearing time is well understood so that corneal damage can be prevented. The importance of close medical follow-up must be stressed to ensure maximal benefits from the cataract surgery and prescribed lenses.

Expected Outcome

The prognosis for visual acuity after cataract surgery varies. The results are often poor because of other ocular defects associated with the cataracts. Visual acuity is also compromised by surgical complications, most commonly secondary glaucoma or, in later years, retinal detachment. The family's desire and ability to help the child wear suitable glasses or contact lenses is another determining factor. The real measure of success following cataract surgery is related to the child's ability to function at an optimal level in her or his environment.

Congenital (Infantile) Glaucoma

Congenital or infantile glaucoma can be of the primary type (inherited as an autosomal recessive disease) or can be associated with other hereditary diseases or syndromes such as Sturge-Weber, Marfan, and Lowe. (See Chapter 31 for a discussion of patterns of inheritance.) Glaucoma may also develop secondary to trauma, intraocular hemorrhage, inflammation, or intraocular tumor (Behrman et al, 1991).

Pathophysiology

Glaucoma is a condition characterized by increased intraocular pressure. Intraocular fluid (aqueous) is produced by the ciliary body. It flows between the iris and the lens into the anterior chamber, then into the canal of Schlemm. In glaucoma, the outflow of aqueous from the anterior chamber is restricted by a deviation in the angle of the anterior chamber of the eye (Fig. 45–4). Intraocular pressure is increased as a result of aqueous accumulation. As the elastic coating of the eye is stretched by the increased pressure, the globe enlarges and the optic nerve atrophies. Infants with congenital glaucoma have large, cowlike eyes (buphthalmos) as a result of this enlargement.

Clinical Manifestations and Diagnostic Assessment

The nurse needs to be aware of the hereditary factor in identifying the population at high risk for primary congenital glaucoma. Genetic counseling should be available for these families. Early assessment of visual competency is an important component of case finding. The principal signs and symptoms are tearing, photophobia (sensitivity to light), blepharospasm

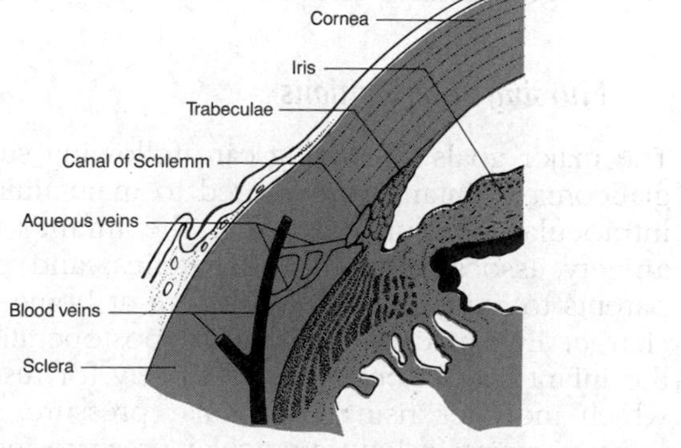

FIGURE 45-4. Anatomy of the iridocorneal angle, showing the system for outflow of aqueous humor into the conjunctival veins. The iridocorneal angle is that space between the iris and the cornea as they approach the canal of Schlemm. (From Guyton, A. C. [1982]. *Human physiology and mechanisms of disease* [3rd ed.]. Philadelphia: WB Saunders, p 245.)

(twitching of the eyelids), corneal clouding (edema), and progressive enlargement of the eye (Behrman et al, 1991). Frequent rubbing of the eye, accompanied by redness, is also a symptom associated with glaucoma. Furthermore, an infant may burrow her or his head into a pillow to protect the eyes. Identification of these signs necessitates referral for ophthalmic examination.

Diagnosis before 1 year of age is important to ensure adequate treatment and prevent visual loss. Diagnosis is made by measuring intraocular pressure with a tonometer, an instrument that, when placed on the anesthetized cornea, registers the underlying pressure. Corneal diameters are also measured and complete ophthalmic examination is carried out. The nurse assists the physician with examinations and provides support to the infant through closeness and gentle touch. The family needs explanations of the various diagnostic tests in easily understood terms.

Therapeutic Management

Medical therapy is limited. Miotics such as pilocarpine are used in adults because they increase the outflow of aqueous. In children, they have not been found to reduce intraocular pressure significantly unless a goniotomy is performed. Carbonic anhydrase inhibitors (acetazolamides) will suppress the production of aqueous slightly but not sufficiently to substitute for surgery (Chew & Morin, 1983).

Goniotomy is the treatment of choice. This procedure consists of making a small incision into the tissue obstructing the angle of the anterior chamber. This incision permits flow of aqueous to the canal of Schlemm. Often two or three goniotomies in different locations are required to obtain normal intraocular pressure. Once the pressure is normal, the prognosis for control of glaucoma is good. If corneal clouding is present at birth, however, the prognosis is guarded: only 30 per cent of these children are cured with one or two goniotomies (Goble, 1984).

Nursing Interventions

The major goals of nursing care following surgery for glaucoma in infancy are related to maintaining a low intraocular pressure, reducing the infant's fear and anxiety associated with eye patches, and preparing parents to manage the infant's care at home after discharge. Eye patches are applied postoperatively and the infant should be observed closely for restlessness, which indicates rising intraocular pressure. Interventions to maintain low intraocular pressure include: elevating the head of the bed 30 degrees, comfort measures to prevent crying, prevention of straining with stool, and avoidance of loud noises, which would startle the infant. Mydriatic medication is given to maximally dilate the pupil and encourage drainage. Dilating the pupil keeps the eye at rest and facilitates postoperative healing. Frequent tonometric readings of intraocular pressure and measurements of corneal diameters are used to detect increased pressure.

The infant is usually discharged from the hospital on the first or second postoperative day. In preparation for discharge, the nurse instructs the family in proper administration of eye medication. Provisions for adequate medical follow-up should be made and discussed with the family. Further surgery may be necessary if intraocular pressure rises again.

Expected Outcome

Surgical correction of glaucoma aims to normalize the intraocular pressure, but it does not guarantee 20/20 vision. The earlier the onset of glaucoma, the poorer the visual prognosis. Of children who present with glaucoma at birth, over 50 per cent will be legally blind. Even if intraocular pressure is controlled through surgical intervention, only 35 per cent of cases have visual acuity better than 20/50 (Chew & Morin, 1983). The decrease in vision is caused by optic nerve damage occurring before the pressure was controlled, by opacities such as corneal scars and cataracts, and by amblyopia (Morin & Bryars, 1980). When corneal clouding is noted between 1 and 24 months of age, a good prognosis is obtained in 95 per cent of cases with one or two goniotomies (Goble, 1984).

Visual Impairment

The term "visual impairment" includes a highly heterogeneous group of conditions. Some people with visual impairment are able to distinguish between light and dark or have good sight for distance but not for peripheral vision (a condition called "tunnel vision"), whereas others are totally blind. Visual impairment is classified according to physiologic measurements (visual acuity) as well as functional ability (Alonso et al, 1978; Jan et al, 1977).

Partial Sight. Physiologic measurement: Children with partial sight have vision that cannot be corrected beyond 20/70 in either eye or have a limited field of vision (the widest diameter of visual field being an angle of no greater than 140 degrees).

Functional ability: Vision is considered partial when visual loss interferes with learning processes but still permits the use of print as a chief method of learning.

Blindness. Physiologic measurement: Children with corrected vision in the better eye of not more than 20/200 or a limitation in the visual field (widest diameter of vision being an angle of no more than 20 degrees) are considered blind.

Functional ability: A child is considered blind when other senses (hearing and touch) are relied on as chief means of task performance and learning.

Promoting Optimal Development. Visually impaired (partially sighted and blind) children must be identified early so that effective treatment programs can be instituted. Early intervention has the potential to prevent developmental delays and lifelong maladaptive functioning. Although some of these children may show developmental delays, it cannot be assumed that more limited vision means greater developmental delay. Furthermore, depending on how successfully a child can learn through the remaining vision and the other senses, the child's development may not be delayed at all (Alonso et al, 1978).

The term "visual handicap" is usually used to describe the condition in those children with visual impairment who, even after maximal correction, are limited in their ability to learn through the visual channel (Alonso et al, 1978). Most blind children have some remaining (residual) vision that they should be encouraged to use. "Residual vision" is a term used to describe the vision of a child who cannot read print of any size but whose vision is more than only light perception (Jan et al, 1977). Any degree of vision that a child has should be used because the eyes, particularly those of young children, benefit from use.

Visually impaired children have the same needs as other children, but they are met through alternative means. These children need stimulation from their environment and the opportunity to get information and responses from the people around them. These children cannot get information and responses through sight; therefore, experiences must be adapted to support their physical, intellectual, and emotional and social development.

Partial Sight

The dilemma of the partially sighted is best described in the words of a partially sighted child: "It is very hard when you are not really blind or sighted because you are just hanging in the middle" (Jan et al, 1977). Partially sighted children's conditions are often misdiagnosed or remain undiagnosed. Their eyes may look normal, and it is only when the child's development seems to be slow that parents may suspect something is wrong. The behavior and responses of these children are often misinterpreted. For example, when first enrolled in preschool, a partially sighted child may be viewed as clumsy or immature or as a slow learner or a behavior problem because she or he seems uncooperative and inattentive.

Areas in which a partially sighted child needs special help and understanding are related to communication, mobility, spatial perception, and visual fatigue. The partially sighted child is often unsure of how to respond verbally to others. The intent of people's *communication* is often conveyed through facial expression and gestures. Because a partially sighted child's perception is distorted, she or he may be confused as to how to respond. Additional verbal explanations may be required to clarify the exact meaning and intent during conversation.

Mobility and spatial perception are also affected when a child has partial sight. Many of these children walk later and more hesitantly than sighted children. Their depth perception and concept of the body in space may not be developed sufficiently, resulting in clumsiness, falls, and accidents.

Visual fatigue is particularly noticed when a partially sighted child begins school. Teachers, nurses, and parents must recognize that behavior problems may develop because of visual fatigue. As the eyes tire, a child may become inattentive and irritable. Diagnosis and assessment of the child's vision by an ophthalmologist are essential in order to plan an educational program that best meets the child's needs.

Once the visual capacities have been established, management of the visual disability follows. This includes increasing the retinal image by magnification, increasing the sharpness of the image, or using other senses (auditory or tactile) to compensate for vision loss (Tongue, 1980). A particularly well-accepted visual aid device for preschoolers 4 and 5 years of age is a hand-held prism telescope of six times and eight times magnification; its use is thought to possibly improve self-sufficiency and mobility later in life. Large-print materials are another useful adjunct; braille is not necessary or recommended. In addition, supplemental aids, including talking books, tapes, magnifiers, and closed-circuit television enlarging devices, are helpful. Other low-vision aid devices are available through low-vision aid centers (Table 45–6). However, low-vision aid facilities in the United States are primarily located in cities and are fewer in number than service organizations for the blind.

The problems of the partially sighted are different from those of the blind. Many of the social and economic rehabilitative services available to the "legally blind" are not available to the partially sighted. The most important aspect of adjustment for the partially sighted child is learning to fully utilize residual vision. With adequate services and devices to supplement their vision, partially sighted children have a chance to participate in their world and reach their maximal potential.

Blindness

Each blind child has individual needs just as any child has; however, *children who are robbed of one of their most crucial senses have the special need to learn alternate ways of relating to their environment.* Every area of development is affected by a child's inability to see. The following discussion describes the impact of blindness and appropriate interventions in the areas of (1) developing human attachment, (2) motor development and mobility, (3) language, cognition and learning, (4) play and socialization, (5) independence and self-concept, and (6) perception of space and body image.

TABLE 45-6
Resources for the Visually Impaired

Organizations

American Association of University Affiliated Programs
Suite 406
2033 M Street
Washington, DC 20036

Provides diagnostic, treatment, educational, and consultant services

American Foundation for the Blind
15 West 16th Street
New York, NY 10011

Publishes *The Journal of Visual Impairment and Blindness*

Association for the Education of the Visually Handicapped
919 Walnut Street
Philadelphia, PA 19107

Publishes *Education of the Visually Handicapped*

Canadian National Institute for the Blind
1931 Bayview Avenue
Toronto, Ontario M4G 4C8

Council for Exceptional Children
1920 Association Drive
Reston, VA 22091

National Association for Parents of the Visually Impaired
2011 Hardy Circle
Austin, TX 78657

National Association for the Visually Handicapped
305 East 24th Street
New York, NY 10010

National Society for the Prevention of Blindness, Inc.
79 Madison Avenue
New York, NY 10016

Resources for Materials and Catalogues

American Printing House for the Blind, Inc.
1839 Frankfort Avenue
Louisville, KY 40200

Catalogue of large-type materials

National Association for Visually Handicapped
3201 Balboa Street
San Francisco, CA 94121

Library of Congress
Division for the Blind and Physically Handicapped
Reference Department
1291 Taylor Street, N.W.
Washington, DC 20542

Provides for library service to individuals who are unable to read standard print

Catalog of Optical Aids, Optical Aid Service
New York Association for the Blind
111 East 59th Street
New York, NY 10022

Vision Center
1393 North High Street
Columbus, OH 43201

Touch, Inc.
P.O. Box 1711
Albany, NY 12201

Development of Human Attachment

The development of human attachment is basic to a child's growth and serves as the foundation for the parent-child relationship. When a child is blind, the usual facial interplay that is used to express mutual pleasure between the infant and the parents must be replaced by an alternate method of communication. The pattern of smiling and the factors that elicit it are different in a blind infant. For the sighted infant, the visual stimulus of the human face elicits an automatic smile at 2 to $2^1/_2$ months of age with a high degree of regularity for which there is no equivalent in the blind baby (Fraiberg, 1974). In a study of seven infants (Fraiberg, 1971, 1974), it was noted that, from the 2nd month on, blind babies smiled in response to a familiar voice or sound and increasingly demonstrated a pattern of selective smiling in favor of the mother's voice. However, the smile was not automatic and even the mother's voice did not elicit it regularly. To help parents of a blind baby, the nurse should understand the importance that the smile has in development of a mutually satisfying relationship between parent and infant. Parents can be encouraged to hold their blind infant and to talk, coo, and sing and play lap games with the baby to help him or her learn to know them and to elicit smiles.

Even when parents and blind infants develop a maximally satisfying relationship, the smile of the blind infant differs from that of the sighted child. Blind babies have a "muted smile" and do not have expressive facial signs that depict various emotions. The absence of these signs may be read as "no affect" and are cause for parents and others to comment that "he looks depressed" or "nothing interests him," (Fraiberg, 1974). The process of developing a satisfying exchange of signals between parents and their blind infant must be recognized by the nurse as a potentially frustrating experience for parents. The nurse has an important responsibility to help parents and blind infants communicate and to provide parents with an opportunity to express feelings about the development of their relationship with the infant.

Motor Development and Mobility

Motor development and mobility for a blind infant are other areas that require special intervention from parents. In the sighted child, motor development is enhanced by the child's interest in moving toward the things she or he can see. Although auditory experiences must replace visual experiences for a blind child, an important phenomenon regarding a child's response to sound must be recognized. The sighted child reaches for and attains an object at the age of 24 to 28 weeks because the child can *see* it. However, whether blind or sighted, an infant does not reach for an object she or he *hears* until the last quarter of the first year. Activities of reaching and grasping for and crawling toward an object have a primary role in motor development, but the blind child is dependent on auditory stimulation for self-initiated mobility. Consequently, this movement does not occur in the blind child until much later than it does for a sighted child because the sighted child moves toward the object she or he sees. Therefore, the immediate environment of the blind child must provide interesting-sounding objects and varied tactile experiences that the child's hands will encounter while randomly moving. A mobile or cradle gym over the crib will provide opportunities for random hand movements to encounter interesting objects and will encourage bringing the hands together at midline (Phillips & Hartley, 1988). At 5 to 8 months, finger foods should be allowed to help perfect grasping. These early experiences with objects provide the blind infant with the necessary stimulation to progress toward a sense of self and object differentiation.

Various stimuli can be used to lure infants to begin to move out into the space around them. Without specific intervention, these infants' hands may encounter only each other or the mouth. If mouth and hand activities become fixed at this immature level, these infants are reported to show signs of impending autism (Adelson & Fraiberg, 1972).

Blind babies have been reported to sit and support themselves on their hands and knees at the same time as sighted children, but these activities were not followed by creeping as they were in sighted infants (Fraiberg, 1971). Independent walking for blind children is hampered because they lack the visual model to imitate. A blind baby was described by Adelson and Fraiberg (1974) to walk "painstakingly at first, one step at a time, feeling his way repeatedly as he gained familiarity with his old world in a new position." The median age for independent walking in blind children reported in their research is 19.25 months, 7 months later than for sighted children. If blind babies are given early experience with the interesting possibilities in the space around them and are lured into that space by the familiar voices of their parents and by interesting sounds, they will achieve the developmental task of independent walking, although at a later time than will sighted children.

Achievement of independent walking is encumbered with fears on the part of the child as well as the parents. The children need repeated practice to propel themselves into an experience that provides new sensation; at times, they may reach an impasse, when they seem to retreat from their experimentation with walking. Parents, on the other hand, fear that a delay in walking may mean that their child is mentally retarded. Parents need to be prepared for these delays and may need constant encouragement to provide opportunities that will help their blind child learn the skills of mobility.

As the blind child becomes mobile, parents are faced with a new dilemma—they fear that she or he will be injured while engaging in normal active play. During the developing years, all children need special instructions about dangers, but they should not be prohibited from engaging in normal activities of swinging, biking, sliding, and other recreational activities.

Specific activities must be taught to blind children because they cannot learn by imitation. For example, children's legs and arms may have to be physically manipulated to show them how to skip, hop, or bounce a ball. They can learn how to use play equipment such as a slide and monkey bars by feeling another child's body move or by having someone move their bodies through the motions (Alonso et al, 1978). While blind children are taught the motions of these physical activities, they must also be taught the rules and limitations that will keep them safe.

Successful mobility is one of the most important skills that a blind person acquires. *Early intervention can determine to a large degree how independent a blind person will be in later life*. As a child enters school, specific mobility skills can be taught by trained instructors. Blind children are taught to listen for the echo of their breath to tell them when they are about to bump into large objects. Cane technique and guide dogs are invaluable aids to independent movement. Guide dogs are not usually used until the teen years (Jan et al, 1977).

Language, Cognition, and Learning

Blindness has a profound impact on the child's abilities in *language, cognition,* and *learning*. Vocalizations and first words occur during the first year of life at about the same time in a blind child and a sighted child. After this stage, however, language development in a blind child is often delayed, but the degree of visual impairment has not been shown to correlate positively with speech and language difficulties; this indicates that blindness alone is not the decisive factor (Jan et al, 1977).

The family and environment of the blind child greatly influences his or her cognitive and language development. This child must be talked to and the verbalizations should be associated with concrete experiences to enable the child to understand words and concepts. The child needs to handle toys and variously shaped objects while their characteristics are being described.

Blind children must accept verbal descriptions by the sighted of many objects and phenomena that they cannot touch (moon, fire). Therefore, they have an incomplete concept of whatever is being described. Phillips and Hartley (1988) discussed the problem of developing "object concept" as a case in which objects fail to exist when they are not being concretely experienced. "The infant lives in a magic world for an extended period of time where people and things mysteriously appear and disappear" (p 203).

The ability to describe visual concepts verbally while having only partial or inaccurate understanding is called "verbalism." *Teaching a blind child from infancy with as many concrete experiences as possible helps the child develop concepts and is an important intervention to promote later academic learning.*

School programs for the visually impaired are varied, ranging from residential schools for the blind to public school programs in which the blind are integrated. Both types of programs require special equipment and devices for the blind student. Academic achievement of blind children who have access to appropriate educational opportunities does not differ from that of sighted children (Chinn, 1979).

Technologic advances are making the printed word more accessible to blind children, but many blind scholars believe that Braille will continue to be a primary method of reading and writing for the blind. Electronic reading devices in which letters are produced in tactile form are also available. Computer-generated voice synthesizers that speak the words, talking calculators, and tape recordings (with a device that can increase or slow the speed of the recording) can aid the blind student. In addition to educational materials, the blind student may need special help in physical education and sex education, and in music, drama, and art.

Play and Socialization

Blind children's *play and social skills* are profoundly affected by their visual impairment. Infants need toys that will help them establish their ability to affect their environment (Phillips & Hartley, 1988). Toys with buttons to push, cranks to wind, doors to open, and other things to stimulate touch give the child a sense of mastery and control. As they become mobile, the active play of young children presents new problems to blind children. In the area of physical activity, their ability to learn games through imitation is limited and to compete with peers is diminished. They cannot follow a rolling ball because they cannot see it. Furthermore, because they cannot imitate their peers in actions and behavior, they are unable to gain a sense of being like them.

Blind children need extra help from teachers, other children, and family members during play and socialization experiences. During the toddler and preschool years, when a child learns to relate to other children, the blind child must be told about the activity and her or his body must be moved through the activity before the nature of it can be understood. *Visually-impaired children benefit from physical contact when being helped to accomplish a task as an alternative to being able to learn by imitation.*

The choice of play materials for the blind child is based on the guideline that if a child cannot see materials well enough to learn the intended concepts or skills, substitute tactile or auditory material must be provided to teach these things (Jan et al, 1977). *When playing with a blind child, one must talk more than normally about the objects and the activity* so that the child will gain an accurate idea of what constitutes his or her environment. A wide range of textures should be available to the child and their appearance described. During play, a blind child is assisted to distinguish various sounds and the direction from which the sounds are coming. The more sensory experiences a blind child has in play, the more opportunity he or she has to take in information to foster normal growth and development.

Self-stimulating mannerisms, such as body rocking, eye poking, head rolling, thumb sucking, and other eye, hand, and head movements, have been noted in blind children. These are called "stereotyped behaviors." These repetitive motor activities vary in frequency, complexity, and intensity. A direct positive correlation with the degree of visual impairment and the frequency of the behaviors has been reported (Jan et al, 1977). Furthermore, these activities seem to intensify with boredom and with excessive stimulation. Although the cause of these behaviors is not fully understood, early intervention to provide the opportunity for mobility, exploration, and manipulation of objects is recommended to help the child substitute for them (Jan et al, 1977). That is, blind children need help to "come out" of themselves rather than to escape into their private worlds.

Independence and Self-Concept

Achieving *independence in the activities of daily living* is important for the development of a positive self-concept in all children. Blind children are particularly at risk of losing the opportunity to do things for themselves because they need special help and additional time to learn self-care skills. Being treated as capable people by teachers, friends, and family members is crucial for blind children to develop the initiative that will motivate them to try to do things for themselves. The nurse can aid parents by providing them with hints that they can use to help foster independence as presented in Table 45–7. See the nursing process plan in Table 45–8 for additional strategies related to independence and self-concept.

Perception of Space and Body Image

The blind child develops a *body image* through tactile experiences and, once language becomes meaningful, through verbal communication and feedback. The ways a blind child takes in information are inferior to those of the sighted child; consequently, the formation of body image is delayed (Scholl, 1973). Certain activities are thought to aid a child's ability to organize space in relation to her or his own body.

TABLE 45-7
Practical Hints to Use in Fostering Independence in a Blind Child

Orientation and Mobility

- To move along a wall, hold arm nearest wall slightly out to the side and forward
- Hand is in a loosely curved position with the back of the fingers touching the wall to locate openings or obstacles
- Fingers are curved slightly inward to prevent injury at places such as door frames
- Explain where you are going when leading a child so that he or she feels more secure
- Verbally describe the arrangement of desks and furniture so that she or he can become independent more quickly

Mealtime and Snacks

- Use real dishes—plastic or paper dishes tip and spill easily
- A dish with a rim and some depth makes it easier for a child to use a scooping maneuver
- Securing the dish to the table surface eliminates accidental tipping and spilling
- Placing food in a circle and explaining its position according to the numbers on the clock is useful for children who can tell time
- Glasses or cups should have a wide base
- Permit children to pour their own liquids when developmentally able to do so (child can grip glass with one hand and place index finger slightly below the rim of the glass to feel when the glass is full)
- By sitting behind a child in helping him or her learn to use a spoon, one can assist the child with more natural feeding movements
- In some cases, the help of an occupational therapist should be suggested if a child has difficulty in swallowing, chewing, or biting

Dressing

- Start with undressing (outerwear, then loose clothing such as T-shirts and sweaters)
- Break tasks down into small steps, explaining each step while the child's hand is over yours as the task is performed
- Praise the child as each step is learned
- Tags and special identifying marks on clothes are needed to help a child choose her or his own outfits

Toilet Training

- A child must be instructed verbally in a step-by-step approach, including where the potty is, how it looks, and its purpose

From *Mainstreaming Preschoolers: Children with Visual Handicaps*. (1978). DHEW Publication No. (OHDS) 78–3112. Washington, DC: US Government Printing Office.

For example, bending down, reaching out, and climbing under and over an object assists blind children in developing an idea of where their body fits in relation to the larger space outside it (Barraga, 1973).

A problem of blind children that has been identified as indicating a deficit in body image is the "floppy" posture that some blind children tend to assume. Based on the verbal responses of blind children on tests of body image, Cratty (1971) identified four stages through which children pass in developing a body image. These are:

Phase I. Awareness of body parts, body planes, and simple movements.

Phase II. Left-right discrimination.

Phase III. Body object relationships; identification of portions of the limbs.

Phase IV. Identification of body parts and body movements of another person.

Body image training as described by Cratty is organized around these four phases.

Development of body image is a central aspect of education of the blind. It cannot be left to chance that children make the connection of how their bodies relate to space. A thorough, systematic effort must be made by the sighted to help blind children learn the dimensions of themselves and their world.

An important nursing intervention consists of providing opportunities for parents to discuss feelings about their infant's response and to explore ways to develop pleasurable interaction patterns. *The nurse's attitude toward the infant may influence the family's ability to interact with their child.* An accepting attitude is conveyed when the nurse touches, holds, and talks to the infant, pointing out normal aspects of development to the parents. Supporting parental attempts to provide sensory stimulation will facilitate early infant attachment.

The special needs of the visually-impaired infant dictate use and coordination of a variety of educational and health services. The nurse's role may encompass both coordination of resources and referrals to ensure maximal use of available community resources. Ideally, the infant should be enrolled in a structured infant stimulation program to develop age-appropriate skills. Community resources such as the state department of education, division of special education, or rehabilitation services and services for the blind can be consulted for additional help. The goal of habilitation for visually-deprived infants is to emphasize to their parents their likeness to all children and to foster their growth and development. It is not the degree of visual acuity they possess that determines their functional ability but how they use their sight and other senses.

TABLE 45-8

Nursing Process Plan: The Child with an Identified Sensory Impairment*

Analysis: Nursing Diagnostic Statement 1

Response and Related or Risk Factors: *Self-esteem disturbance related to*

- Unrealistic expectations of child by parents and others around him or her
- Family knowledge deficit regarding interventions to enhance self-esteem
- Family tendency to overprotect child, resulting in lack of self-reliance and autonomy in child

Projected Outcome: Child/adolescent will evaluate himself or herself positively

Defining Characteristics

Subjective:

- Verbalizes feelings of inferiority, negativity, pessimism
- Boasts about achievements
- Declines opportunities for social activities and new experiences

Objective:

- Poor attachment behavior
- Tends to watch rather than participate in group
- Acting-out behavior
- Poor impulse control
- Poor sportsmanship
- Takes little pride in appearance

Nursing Interventions

Self-Esteem Enhancement

Assist the family to gain a realistic perspective on the child's handicap

- Explain the tendency to *generalize* a physical handicap (e.g., to extend it erroneously to include cognitive, emotional, and other physical abilities)
- Encourage family members (and others, as appropriate) to state ways in which they are "handicapped"/limited (e.g., poor math ability, poor in sports, uneven facial features). Ask them to list ways in which they compensate for these limitations
- Clarify with the family the exact ways in which the child is handicapped. Discuss specific interventions to help the child compensate by learning to use full sensory capability with the help of professional instruction, medical therapies, and special equipment; and by developing compensatory sensory skills to access the external world (see interventions throughout this chapter)
- Stress the fact that in all other ways the child has normal needs
- Discuss the need for routine well child care, including immunizations and assessment of growth and development

Evaluation Criteria

The child will develop positive self-esteem as evidenced by:

- *Infant:* Demonstrating expectation of need gratification from parents and siblings
- *Toddler:* Wanting to do things "by myself"; naming body parts
- *Preschooler:* Showing pride in gender; seeking new activities and experiences; showing pride in being able to dress self, fixing own breakfast, and so forth
- *School-age:* Having and enjoying several friends; showing pride in at least one special ability; showing curiosity about the external world
- *Adolescent:* Describing physical self in primarily positive ways; indicating interest in heterosexual relationships; discussing realistic plans for the future; viewing self as capable of independence while acknowledging continuing need for love and approval from family

* The principles in this nursing process plan are appropriate to the enhancement of self-esteem in any child with a physical handicap.

TABLE 45-8 (continued)

Defining Characteristics	Nursing Interventions	Evaluation Criteria
	Initiate interventions to enhance self-esteem and autonomy on initial family contact and continue this guidance and support throughout the therapeutic relationship • Talk with families about their critical role in helping the child value self and abilities • Ensure that families understand the self-esteem goals for each developmental stage and discuss implications for parenting behaviors • Discuss ways to make the *infant* feel loved, protected, and valued • Provide reinforcement of appropriate parent bonding whenever possible • Assist parents/family to recognize infant's positive responses (because sensory deficits may alter such expected behaviors as eye contact, smiling, quieting to a familiar voice, and cooing) • Discuss importance of allowing *toddler* to do selected things on her or his own • Acknowledge normal tendency to protect child from potential injury. Discuss ways to balance safety with need for autonomy • Explain that learning body parts and their functions is important to developing body image • Urge parents to be truthful and matter-of-fact about ways in which the child's eyes, ears, or other body part, differ from those of other family members (by neither emphasizing nor ignoring these facts, the child will be able to develop a body image that comfortably incorporates the handicap) • Discuss ways to allow the *preschooler* initiative in choosing playmates from normal as well as other handicapped children;	

(continued)

TABLE 45-8 *(continued)*

Defining Characteristics	Nursing Interventions	Evaluation Criteria
	imitating the role of the same-sex parent; self-regulating simple daily activities, e.g., dressing, fixing a sandwich, learning a safe way to cross the street • Allow the child to experience some frustration and disappointment within a supportive family atmosphere (appropriate adversity can enhance the child's self-concept by increasing faith in his or her own ability to overcome the bad times) • Emphasize the importance of the *school-age* child of identifying and participating in an activity at which she or he can excel, such as swimming or voice lessons for the blind child, or tennis lessons or a computer club for the deaf child; and in peer activities. Social contacts should include children with normal sensory abilities (to normalize social skills). When possible, educate peers about the exact handicap and compensatory mechanisms. (When fear of the unknown is reduced, friendships can be built on the things the children have in common.) Summer camps are available for children with sensory impairments and are an excellent way to enhance peer relationships, independence, and self-worth • Encourage parents of the school-age child to allow appropriate independence • Refer families to state and local agencies that provide special programs for the sensory-impaired • Agencies that provide dogs for blind and deaf clients may work with the school-age child • Teach child to use special telephone equipment (as needed) to summon emergency help • Counsel family about the impor-	

TABLE 45-8 *(continued)*

Defining Characteristics	Nursing Interventions	Evaluation Criteria
	tance of allowing the *adolescent* to be as independent as possible • Encourage the young person to accept a part-time job as school work will permit • If a driver's license cannot be obtained, teach adolescent to ride public transportation to permit access to activities of interest • Helping others (e.g., by being a counselor in a summer camp for the sensory-impaired) can be an excellent way for the adolescent to develop feelings of self-worth as well as independence • Be an advocate for the child (as appropriate) in explaining to the family that fashionable dress is not an adolescent whim but crucial to peer acceptance and self-image • Encourage siblings or friends to shop with the young person who has a visual impairment (parents, although well-meaning, often have a different idea of "fashion")	

Hearing Impairment

Hearing impairment may be profound, significantly handicapping a child, or so mild that it goes undetected for years. Both the volume (measured in decibels [dB]) and the pitch (measured in Hertz [Hz]) of the sound determine whether it is audible to the human ear (Table 45–9).

The volume of sound that is required in order for an individual to hear is reported in decibels. This is called the "hearing level." Levels of hearing impairment in decibels used to describe severity of hearing loss vary in the literature; however, it is generally agreed that persons with hearing levels exceeding 90 dB are termed "deaf." For educational purposes, however, a *deaf* person is one whose hearing is disabled to a level (usually 70 dB or greater) at which speech through the ear alone, with or without a hearing aid, cannot be understood; a *hard-of-hearing* person is one whose hearing is disabled to a level (usually 35 to 69 dB) that makes it difficult to understand speech through the ear alone, with or without a hearing aid (Moores, 1978). The hard-of-hearing person has suffi-

TABLE 45-9
About Decibels and Hertz

Disorders in hearing mean that persons so affected are unable to perceive or translate the sound waves that other people hear.

Sounds are "heard" by means of vibrations, or waves, that travel from the place where the sound originates to the hearer's ear. Different sounds have different cycles, or wave patterns. A wave pattern that completes itself in 1 sec (that is, frequency of 1 cycle/sec) is called a Hertz (Hz), after the German physicist Heinrich Rudolf Hertz (1857–1894). The lower the pitch of a sound, the fewer cycles per second; the higher the pitch, the greater the number of cycles.

The decibel (1/10 of a bel) takes its name from Alexander Graham Bell, whose interest in deafness led him to the invention of the telephone. Zero decibel is the least-perceptible sound an average normal human being can hear (in the decibel scale, 0 is not the absence of sound but rather the threshold at which sound can first be perceived). The decibel scale used in measuring hearing ranges from 0 to 110; above that range, at 140 dB, sound produces pain.

From Bergstrom, L. (1980, January). Causes of reversed hearing loss in early childhood. *Pediatric Annals,* 13–23.

TABLE 45-10
Degree of Handicap and Educational Need According to Hearing Levels

Hearing Level in Decibels (dB) and Degree of Hearing Loss: Childen	Adults	Effect of Hearing Loss and Educational Needs
Normal 0–20	0–26	Although this is considered normal hearing, those children in upper limits of this range may be affected. They may show poor language development, have problems in listening, and have reduced ability to hear information needed for academic achievement
Mild loss 21–35	27–40	Faint and distant speech is heard with difficulty. Child may benefit from a hearing aid and needs special seating and lighting in classroom; may need speechreading instruction
Moderate loss 36–55	41–55	Understands conversational speech at a distance of 3–5 ft if in face-to-face position. May be limited in vocabulary and exhibit some incorrect speech. Child in the classroom will benefit from special seating and a hearing aid; may need speechreading instruction
Moderately severe loss 56–70	56–70	Conversation must be loud to be understood. Child has great difficulty participating in classroom discussions. Needs special seating, hearing aid, speechreading instruction, and may need special classes for the hearing impaired to develop speech and language skills
Severe loss 71–90	71–90	May hear loud voices at a distance of 1 ft from the ear. May be able to distinguish vowels but not consonants. May be able to identify environmental noises. Speech and language are defective. Child requires full-time special education, hearing aid, and program to develop language and speech
Profound 91 or more	91 or more	May hear some loud sounds but does so through recognizing vibration rather than tones. Does not rely on hearing as a primary channel for communication. Child requires full-time program with continuous appraisal of needs in regard to communication techniques

From Margin, F. N. (1978). *Pediatric audiology* (p 38). Englewood Cliffs, NJ: Prentice-Hall; and Stangler, S., et al (1980). *Screening growth and development of preschool children: A guide for test selection.* New York: McGraw-Hill. Reproduced with permission of McGraw-Hill.

cient residual hearing to understand speech with the use of a hearing aid, although it is difficult.

For the deaf person, vision is the primary mode of language acquisition and communication. The probable handicap that results from the various hearing levels in decibels is summarized in Table 45–10. It should be noted that the ranges differ for children and adults. Even slight hearing impairment has the potential to interfere with a child's normal development of speech and language and educational progress.

The summary as provided in this table is only a general guide. It does not take into account important variables that the nurse should always consider when assessing the impact of a hearing impairment. These factors are (1) cause and onset of the hearing loss, (2) type of hearing impairment (see later discussion on types of hearing losses), (3) presence of other impairments (physical, intellectual, emotional), and (4) interactions and relationships within the family (Sweitzer, 1977).

It is important for nurses to realize that a high percentage of children are affected by hearing loss, yet it is often a subtle, undetected deficit that can seriously affect the child's development.

By 2 years of age, 1 in 25 children (4 per cent) will have mild to moderate hearing losses secondary to ear disease; in school-age children, 7 to 8 per cent have some degree of hearing loss. Severe hearing loss is present in 1 in 1000 infants and 1 in 50 neonates discharged from intensive care nurseries.

Early detection of hearing impairment, regardless of degree, is paramount. By 3 years of age, approximately 80 per cent of language growth is thought to have taken place. Deafness during early childhood, occurring before the acquisition of a functional language base, seriously affects a child in all areas of development. Furthermore, mild hearing loss significantly reduces vocabulary growth, articulation skills, the ability to communicate through spoken language, the use of grammar and syntax, and auditory memory skills (McFarland & Simmons, 1980).

Regular hearing screening therefore becomes a critical feature of health assessment to prevent unnecessary sequelae to hearing deficits. An understanding of the causes and types of hearing impairment provides an important base for the nurse to carry out this responsibility.

Causes

Hearing loss may vary from mild to profound as outlined in Table 45–10. The higher the number in decibels the greater the hearing loss. Hearing losses are also described according to time of appearance, cause, and pathology involved.

Terms used to differentiate the causes of hearing loss are used inconsistently in the literature. In this discussion, "congenital" is used to describe a hearing loss present at birth, whether of genetic or nongenetic origin. "Adventitious" hearing loss refers to a loss that develops after birth and may be due to genetic or nongenetic factors. Genetic-induced disorders that do not result in a hearing impairment until later in life (adventitious) are classified as having a "delayed onset" (e.g., Alport syndrome), whereas deafness resulting after birth from nongenetic causes is termed "acquired" (Paparella, 1977). A summary of genetic and nongenetic causes of both congenital and adventitious hearing loss is outlined in Table 45–11. Of all cases of congenital deafness, 50 per cent are inherited, whereas, in adventitious hearing loss, environmental factors are of major significance. The nurse's familiarity with the causes of hearing impairment provides a base for taking a pertinent health history.

TABLE 45–11
Etiology of Deafness in Children

I. Congenital Deafness

A. Genetic
1. Deafness appearing alone due to defects in fetal development (aplasia)
2. Deafness associated with other conditions (e.g., Waardenburg sydnrome, albinism, hyperpigmentation, visual handicaps)
3 Chromosomal abnormalities
Trisomy 13–15
Trisomy 18

B. Nongenetic (prenatal and perinatal factors)
1. Infection (maternal rubella, cytomegalovirus [CMV], toxoplasmosis, herpes simplex, congenital syphilis)
2. Ototoxic drugs (maternal ingestion of streptomycin, chloroquine, quinine, thalidomide, and possibly excessive use of salicylates)
3. Metabolic disorders (toxemia, diabetes)
4. Rh incompatibility
5. Radiation (first trimester)
6. Anoxia and birth trauma
7. Low birthweight

II. Adventitious Deafness

A. Genetic (delayed-onset)
1. Deafness occurring alone (ostosclerosis)
2. Deafness occurring with other conditions (Alport syndrome, Hurler disease, Paget disease, von Recklinghausen disease, sickle cell anemia)

B. Nongenetic (acquired)
1. Infection (measles, mumps, chickenpox, influenza, serous otitis media, meningitis)
2. Ototoxic drugs (kanamycin, streptomycin, gentamicin)
3. Neoplastic disorders
4. Trauma (direct injury via skull fracture or head injury or damage resulting from high noise level)
5. Metabolic disorders (hypothyroidism)

Data from Bess, F. (1977). *Childhood deafness.* Orlando, FL: Grune & Stratton; Carrel, R. (1977). Epidemiology of hearing loss. In S. E. Gerber (Ed.). *Audiometry in infancy.* Orlando, FL: Grune & Stratton; and Mouney, D. F. (1979). Differential diagnosis of hearing loss in children. *Ear, Nose, and Throat Journal, 58*(7), 293–296.

Types

Types of hearing impairment are categorized as central, peripheral, and functional (nonorganic). *Central disorders* are those within the central nervous system, specifically along the pathway from the brain stem to and including the cortex. *Peripheral impairment* results from lesions outside the central nervous system involving any part of the auditory system from the external ear to the point at which the auditory portion of the cranial nerve VIII synapses within the brain stem (Newby, 1979). *Functional* or *nonorganic* hearing impairment is a psychologic rather than a physiologic disorder in which "hearing loss" is a defense mechanism to cope with stressful situations. Of these three types, central and peripheral are the most prevalent.

Central Disorders

Central hearing impairment involves brain damage that results in the inability to process information. "Processing" refers to reception, analysis, and integration of auditory material within the central nervous system. The child is unable to interpret the auditory stimulus she or he receives and exhibits complex problems in speech and communication. The inability to express ideas, either spoken or written, is called "expressive aphasia"; "receptive aphasia" is difficulty in comprehending what one hears or reads (Newby, 1979).

Children with central impairment are easily distracted, have a short attention span, and have reading difficulty when instructed by phonics (Cunningham, 1978). This type of impairment is associated with a history of maternal rubella, diabetes, and pre-eclampsia and of fetal prematurity and Rh incompatibility. Also, infections (meningitis and encephalitis), trauma, prolonged asphyxia and brain tumors, cysts, and abscesses are among the numerous causes of central impairment. Careful psychologic and educational testing is required because children with auditory imperception (inability to understand the meaning of what is heard) resemble the emotionally disturbed (Cunningham, 1978).

Peripheral Losses

Peripheral losses may be either *conductive* or *sensorineural.* If both conductive and sensorineural losses are present, it is referred to as a "mixed loss." These classifications are based on location of the defect.

Conductive Losses. Conductive hearing impairment accounts for most hearing loss in children. There is a dysfunction of the outer (pinna and external auditory canal) or middle (tympanic membrane, eustachian tube, or ossicles) ear that interferes with sound transmission (air conduction). Pinna abnormalities are often associated with abnormalities of the ossicles. Because this can often be surgically corrected early, its identification is important.

In conductive hearing loss, the inner ear is not affected; therefore, bone conduction is normal and there is no nerve damage. Consequently, these people hear themselves adequately via bone conduction and tend to speak quietly. The speech of others is understood provided they can hear what is said. Conductive hearing losses are usually the same for all frequencies, although high-frequency sounds may be heard better. Hearing levels fluctuate in the child with conductive hearing loss and are usually mild to moderate losses. The child with conductive hearing loss displays a recognizable syndrome of behaviors that include fluctuating attentiveness to the environment, poor language skills, and mild behavior problems.

The transmission of sound is reduced or absent when inner or middle ear pathology obstructs air conduction. Obstruction of the outer ear by cerumen or, in some instances, a foreign object can cause significant hearing loss. *It is important for the nurse to stress that parents should not use cotton-tipped swabs or a sharp probe to clear the external canal.* When a swab is used, cerumen readily gets pushed deeper into the canal and it may become impacted against the eardrum. Using a probe may cause injury to the external canal or eardrum, resulting in infection. The ear canals may also be occluded because of a defect in development. A missing canal can be constructed or an occluded canal can be corrected by surgery. Most frequently, extensive plastic surgery is required because the eardrum and bones of the middle ear are missing entirely. Other causes of external ear obstructions are growths, swimmer's ear, which results in edema and exudate in the external auditory canal, and trauma.

The most common cause of conductive hearing loss in children is serous otitis media, defined as persistent fluid in the middle ear cavity. (See Chapter 32 for a discussion of serous otitis media.) Serous otitis media does not necessarily cause pain and the hearing loss averages a level of 30 dB, though it can range to as great as 50 dB; thus, the hearing loss may go undetected. Nursing interventions directed at preventing complications and the recurrence of serous otitis media can reduce the potential for hearing loss to occur. These children must receive consistent otoscopic evaluations to assess both response to treatment and hearing. Parents should be educated to look for subtle signs of a worsening effusion, including the child's frequent requests to have statements repeated, a tendency to speak louder, "inching up" the volume on a television or radio, or, in the case of younger children, an unsteady gait. An additional preventive measure is to teach the child how to blow the nose properly. Pressing lightly on the nostrils with fingers without pinching prevents mucus from being forced into the orifice of the eustachian tube.

Other middle ear conditions that may produce conductive hearing loss are acute and chronic suppurative otitis media, tumors, and myringitis bullosa (a viral infection of the outer layer of the eardrum resulting in blistering). Screening and auditory tests to detect conductive hearing loss are described later in this section.

Sensorineural Losses. Sensorineural hearing losses are the result of pathology in the inner ear (semicircular canals and cochlea) or along the nerve pathway (auditory nerve) from the inner ear to the brain stem. This loss results in acoustic distortion (difficulty in discriminating speech) and a reduced sensitivity to sound. There is typically better hearing ability for the lower frequencies than for the high frequencies. There is an inability to understand what is said because many consonants are high-frequency sounds and cannot be heard; thus, word confusion results. Also, with a sensorineural loss, one's own voice is not heard because of the deficit in bone conduction. (We hear our own voices partly through the mechanism of bone conduction [Newby, 1979].) Consequently, with this type of hearing loss, one speaks in what others perceive as an excessively loud voice.

Most of the babies who have impaired hearing at birth (congenital) have sensorineural impairment. However, this type of impairment may manifest itself at any time in life (adventitious). Whether congenital or adventitious, the cause of the hearing loss may be genetic or nongenetic. The nongenetic factors that adversely affect prenatal and perinatal conditions should be the focus of preventive prenatal and perinatal care. Acquired sensorineural hearing impairment can be prevented by careful management of infections in children, anticipatory guidance to prevent injury, and immunizations against childhood illnesses.

Screening and Diagnostic Assessment

The nurse plays an important part in early identification of hearing impairment.

Nursing Interventions

Usually, parents are the first to notice that something is wrong with their baby's hearing. Frequently, these babies will begin to vocal play at the age of 1 to 2 months but will dramatically decrease utterances by 4 to 6 months. They do not progress to the babbling stage. Delay in diagnosis persists as a serious health care problem. Even *profound* congenital deafness has been reported to be diagnosed at a mean age of 24 months (Coplan, 1987). On the average, a full year elapses between the first suspicion and the actual confirmation that a child has a severely handicapping hearing deficit; a child with a mild to moderate hearing loss is often 3 years of age before any concerns are raised, and over 4 years old before the hearing loss is confirmed (McFarland & Simmons, 1980). This presents a serious challenge to all health professionals who care for children and especially to nurses, who are often the first to hear the concerns of parents during the process of taking a developmental history. *Nurses thus can make a significant impact on the current problem of delayed intervention by taking concerns of parents seriously and making a referral for audiologic evaluation.*

The nurse's focus on thorough history taking, behavioral observations of the child, a careful physical assessment (Table 45–12), and attentiveness to parents' concerns increases the likelihood that the nurse

TABLE 45-12
Behavioral Indices and Physical Findings Associated with Hearing Loss

Behavioral Indices

1. Orientation responses
   - Responds more to movement than to sound
   - Turns head and body to sound as if dependent on one ear
   - Responds to spoken sounds only when speaker's face and lips are visible
   - Responds more to changes in facial expression than to words
   - Fails to follow verbal directions
   - Lacks motor or facial response to spoken word
2. Vocalization and sound production
   - Monotone voice quality and inflection patterns; loud voice
   - Loss of or lack of normal babbling by 7 mos of age; loss of previously acquired speech a primary indicator
   - Only parts of words vocalized; mispronounces or omits certain words
   - Bangs head or stomps foot to elicit vibratory sensation
   - Uses same sound to express pleasure, annoyance, or need
3. Visual attention
   - Attends closely to facial expression and eyes of the speaker for intent of words
   - Points and uses gestures rather than words to express desires after 15 mos of age
   - Displays marked imitativeness in play
   - Is distracted by gestures and movement when in groups
4. Emotional and social behavior
   - Is shy, timid, and withdrawn in group play
   - Lacks appropriate noises in play with dolls, animals, trucks; no preference for noisy toys
   - Displays intense preoccupation with things rather than people
   - Has puzzled, unhappy, inquiring, and sometimes confused facial expression in group play
   - Is disobedient
   - Has short attention span, hyperactivity, and unusual fatigue
   - Uses tantrums to call attention to self or needs in routine situations
   - Is irritable at not making self understood
   - Appears to daydream or be oblivious to others
   - Displays unpredictable behavioral outbursts

Physical Findings	Significance of Findings
1. White forelock in hairline of forehead	Streak of gray or white hair: indicative of genetic defect (Waardenburg syndrome) that has hearing loss component
2. Heterochromia	A difference of color in portion of same iris: indicative of genetic defect (Waardenburg syndrome) that has hearing loss component
3. Very bushy eyebrows that almost meet at the nasal bridge	Indicative of congenital defect that has hearing loss component
4. Impacted cerumen in external canal	Leads to a temporary conductive loss
5. Otitis externa	Inflammation of external ear (may result from furuncle or allergy to cleaning solutions used for hearing aid)
6. Pinna abnormalities	Is often associated with abnormal ossicles causing conductive hearing loss
7. Abnormal tympanic membrane	Retraction, bulging, air fluid levels, perforation, scarring all contribute to conductive loss; fluid in ear can lead to labyrinthitis, mastoid disease, or cholesteatoma, labyrinthitis can lead to permanent damage to the hairs in the organ of Corti
8. Hypertrophied adenoids	Enlargement of adenoid tissue in posterior nasopharynx; may cause mild conductive loss

TABLE 45-13
Goals and Strategies for Auditory Screening According to Age*

Goals	Strategies
Neonate	
Identify all hearing losses	1. High-risk register 2. Behavioral responses 3. Crib-O-Gream testing 4. Brain stem evoked response
Birth–3 Yrs	
1. Identify severe hearing losses that might develop after birth 2. Detect ear conditions that may cause mild hearing losses	1. Follow-up of high-risk children 2. Auditory orientation behavior 3. Brain stem evoked response 4. Assessment of speech and language 5. Tympanometry† (impedance testing) 6. Parents' impression of child's hearing; take concerns seriously
3–5 Yrs	
1. Detect conductive losses due to otitis media 2. Detect sensorineural losses that might have developed	1. Audiometry a. Pure-tone screening b. Non–pure-tone screening 2. Assessment of speech and language 3. Tympanometry (impedance testing) 4. Parents' impression of child's hearing and concerns taken seriously
School-Age and Older	
1. Maintain educationally adequate hearing 2. Detect ear disease	1. Pure-tone audiometry every 2 yrs 2. Tympanometry (impedance testing) 3. Parents' and teachers' concerns regarding child's hearing taken seriously 4. Tuning fork

Data from Cunningham, D. (1978). Hearing loss. In R. Hoekelman, et al (Eds.). *Principles of pediatrics*. New York: McGraw-Hill; and Downs, M. (1981). Early identification of hearing loss. In N. Lass, et al (Eds.). *Speech, language, and hearing*. Philadelphia: WB Saunders.

* At each age, the ear should be examined with an otoscope.

† For infants under 7 mos of age, tympanometry is of limited validity.

will detect an existing impairment. Also, the nurse's contact with families in child health settings gives him or her an opportunity to teach parents the normal responses to sound and language development to be expected. The deaf baby often makes normal sounds until 6 to 9 months, at which time vocalization gradually decreases. By the end of the first year, the infant is often making only the primitive sound "amah" (Eviator, 1984).

Hearing screening is a nursing responsibility; therefore, an understanding of the various screening techniques is necessary. Hearing impairments can be identified through high-risk registers and various screening techniques appropriate for the age of the child (Table 45-13).

Assessment in the Neonatal Period

In 1973, the Joint Committee on Infant Hearing of the American Academy of Pediatrics recommended use of a high-risk register. This is a system to identify those infants that are at risk for hearing impairment. The 1973 criteria were expanded and clarified by the Joint Committee* in 1982 (Table 45-14).

High-risk factors are identified by reviewing the medical record, asking parents to complete a questionnaire, and examining the neonate.

It is recommended that all neonates be assessed and those at risk be referred for audiologic evaluation, preferably before age 3 months but not later than age 6 months (American Academy of Pediatrics, 1982). Various behavioral and electrophysiologic methods of testing for hearing impairment also are in use. Table 45-15 describes techniques that are used to follow-up those infants identified by the high-risk register. Al-

* The Joint Committee consisted of representatives from the American Academy of Pediatrics, Academy of Otolaryngology—Head and Neck Surgery, American Nurses Association, and American Speech-Language-Hearing Association.

TABLE 45-14
High-Risk Registry for the Identification of Hearing Impairment

Risk Criteria
Family history of childhood hearing impairment
Congenital perinatal infection (e.g., cytomegalovirus, rubella, herpes, toxoplasmosis, syphilis)
Anatomic malformations involving the head or neck (e.g., dysmorphic appearance including syndromal and nonsyndromal abnormalities, overt or submucous cleft palate, morphologic abnormalities of the pinna)
Birthweight < 1500 g
Hyperbilirubinemia at level exceeding indications for exchange transfusion
Bacterial meningitis, especially *Haemophilus influenzae*
Severe asphyxia, which may include infants with Apgar scores of 0 to 3 or those who fail to institute spontaneous respiration by 10 mins and those with hypotonia persisting to 2 hrs of age

From American Academy of Pediatrics, Joint Committee on Infant Hearing (1982, September). Position Statement 1982. Reproduced with permission of *Pediatrics*, vol. 70, p 496, copyright 1982.

though numerous tests are available to identify hearing loss, the nurse should not disregard the value of testing neonates with a bell, which is rung approximately 4 inches from the ear.

During the first 2 months of life, responses are generalized and reflexive, including the Moro reflex, blink reflex, arousal reflex (a sleeping infant response), and cessation reflex (restless or crying infant stops activity). An eyeblink is the most common and reliably observed response to sound in neonates. By 4 months of age, localization efforts are made by a rudimentary head turn, and, by 7 months, a full head turn and eye turn are made toward the sound. By 12 months of age, a response to simple verbal commands is used to assess hearing (Fria, 1983).

Assessment from the Neonatal Period to 3 Years of Age

Once an infant has been identified as high risk, it is essential that she or he be examined regularly to identify hearing loss that may develop at some time after birth. It is recommended that these children have an audiologic evaluation every 3 months through the first year. The nurse can assist parents by helping them understand that, although hearing tests are normal, their child is more vulnerable to hearing loss because of the presence of a high-risk factor(s).

The nurse has an important role in screening and detection of hearing problems during all well child visits. Assessment of hearing development should include an otoscopic examination, assessment of the infant's response to noisemakers (auditory orientation behavior), and an assessment of speech and language development.

The otoscopic examination, including pneumatic otoscopy (described in Chapter 13), uses important techniques for identification of past and present middle ear pathology. These tests must be done by skilled professionals to ensure that hearing losses resulting from ear infections are prevented. When otoscopy is performed in conjunction with tympanometry, ear problems can be detected even earlier. It can be used at any age but is of limited validity in infants under 7 months.

Tympanometry (impedance testing) is an objective measurement of the compliance or mobility of the tympanic membrane in response to air pressure changes in the external auditory canal. Maximal compliance occurs when pressures on either side of the membrane are equal. Even mild disease of the tympanic membrane or middle ear influences the degree of compliance, making this test particularly useful to detect ear pathology *before* it has caused a hearing impairment.

Tympanometry is an efficient, reliable technique that is recommended to be used as a supplement to otoscopic examination and audiometric hearing tests. (See Table 45-16 for a description of tympanometry.) This equipment is increasingly available in pediatric clinics and offices. It can be administered by virtually any provider after a minimum of instruction.

Assessment from 3 to 5 Years of Age

At this age, screening and detection consist of all of the techniques described for birth to 3 years of age. In addition, pure-tone audiometric screening must be done to detect any sensorineural loss that may have developed. For this age, pure-tone testing using play conditioning techniques is appropriate for the young preschooler; for the 5-year-old, the standard pure-tone screening is appropriate.

Non-pure-tone screening is another technique that can be used to test preschoolers. The child is shown a board of pictures while words are spoken to him or her through earphones. The child is asked to point to the appropriate picture. The first word is spoken at 51 dB and each subsequent word is presented at 4 dB less than the previous one, until the 15 dB level is attained (Downs, 1981). When this test is given, differences in language development and word exposure must be taken into consideration. It is more appropriate for most 4- and 5-year-olds than for 3-year-olds.

Assessment of the School-Age Child

The most common method to screen hearing in school-age children is pure-tone audiometry. Whereas the more recent development of impedance audiometry is more effective to detect ear pathology, pure-tone audiometry continues to be the predominant method for screening school-age children. The nurse's

TABLE 45-15
Technique to Test Infants and Children at Risk for Hearing Impairment

Description	Use and Implications for Nursing
Crib-O-Gram	
A transducer is attached to the infant's crib to record movements in response to a loud sound. It is relatively inexpensive	Can be used to follow infants identified by high-risk register
Brain Stem Auditory Evoked Potential (BAEP)	
Electrodes are placed on the mid-forehead and mastoid process; as stimuli are presented, a series of brain wave responses are recorded	Not a routine procedure. Used for selected at-risk populations. A child should be completely relaxed, preferably asleep. Feeding infants immediately before test may suffice. A sedative is often necessary for older infants, toddlers, and preschoolers. School-age children may be able to lie still if adequate explanations are provided
Tympanometry (Impedance Testing)	
Measures the change in compliance of the ear drum as air pressure in the external canal is varied with an instrument. Reflected sound is measured to evaluate compliance. The instrument used is an electroacoustic impedance audiometer (tympanometer)	Impedance audiometry is especially useful because it requires only minimal cooperation from the child. Impossible to perform, however, if child is squirming. Because of the small ear canals, the test can identify ear pathology *before* hearing loss has occurred
Pure-Tone Testing	
Electronically generated pure tones of various frequencies and intensities are presented through the earphones. Child raises hand when sound is heard	Identifies hearing loss after damage has occurred
Play Audiometry	
Involves a play activity such as pictures or a pegboard. The child can be conditioned to put a peg into a board at the sound of a tone	Used for children under age 3 yrs who may not be able to understand what is expected of them in response to the tone
Behavioral Observation	
In a large, sound-treated room, a sound stimulus is administered; responses are evaluated according to expected behaviors for age	Used for preverbal children

responsibility is to maximize its effectiveness by administering the test under optimal conditions. Three important criteria should be met in giving the test: (1) the environment* should be quiet to avoid false-positive results; (2) the audiometer should be maintained* in proper working condition; and (3) personnel conducting the test should be properly trained.

The school nurse should supervise the hearing screening program, recognizing its limitations to discover hearing loss and ear pathology in its early stages. Pure-tone audiometry must always be supplemented with serious attention given to the observations and concerns of teachers and parents regarding the hearing of the child. *The purpose of pure-tone audiometry is to identify hearing loss greater than a certain level, whereas impedance audiometry is used to discover the presence of otopathology.* This is an important distinction that is not always made in discussions of auditory screening procedures. Despite the advantages of impedance audiometry, it is unlikely to be used in the place of pure-tone screening; therefore, the nurse's responsibility is to upgrade the conditions under which pure-tone audiometry is administered.

A school-age child can cooperate in being assessed by the tuning fork test, in addition to otoscopy, speech and language assessment, impedance audiometry, and pure-tone audiometry. (See Chapter 13 for description of the Weber and Rinne tests.)

At all well child visits, the nurse should inspect the ears and examine the ear with an otoscope. Additionally, the nurse should assess the child for behavioral indications of hearing losses both by direct observation and by asking for pertinent information given by parents. Physical and behavioral findings which may be indicative of a hearing loss are summarized in Table 45–12.

* American National Standards Institute (ANSI) Specifications 53.1 (1960) and 53.6 (1969) describe criteria for background noise and maintenance, respectively.

TABLE 45-16
Tympanometry

A tympanometer is an automatic instrument with a probe inserted into the ear canal (an air-tight cavity is formed between the tip of the probe and the eardrum)
A pure tone (usually 220 Hz) is then administered through the tip of the probe
During the test, ear canal pressure in the airtight cavity is varied automatically by the tympanometer ($\pm$200 mmH_2O)
As ear canal pressures vary, compliance of the eardrum changes (compliance decreases whenever pressures on the two sides of the eardrum are not equal)
As the ear canal pressures are varied, the sound (220 Hz) is reflected back into the air-tight cavity whenever the eardrum is not free to vibrate (it vibrates best [is most compliant] when pressure against the two sides of the eardrum are equal)
When pressures on the two sides of the eardrum are not equal and sound is reflected, the probe tip measures the intensity of the reflected sound in the ear canal. If the tympanic membrane is "stiff," more sound is reflected back; if it is flaccid, sound is absorbed and less is reflected back. Thus, the compliance of the ear is evaluated by measuring the reflected sound in the air-tight portion of the ear canal
For a normal ear, the greatest compliance is attained at 0 pressure
If ear pathology is present, maximal compliance may be attained at positive or negative pressures. The amount of pressure required (whether positive or negative) to produce maximal compliance is the middle ear pressure

Nursing Diagnostic Statements

High risk for impaired adjustment; *risk factors:*

- *Parental grief.*
- *Parental knowledge deficit about how to interact with a hearing-impaired child.*

High risk for social isolation of the child; *risk factors:*

- *Parental knowledge deficit regarding how to facilitate their child's social interaction.*

High risk for chronic low self-esteem in child; *risk factors:*

- *Parental knowledge deficit regarding how to facilitate appropriate emotional reactions in their child.*

Uncompensated impaired verbal communication, *related to lack of access to learning alternative methods of communicating.*

Helping the Family Adjust to the Child's Handicap

The impact of a hearing impairment on a child is largely affected by how the parents can accept and adapt to the impairment. Not only do parents feel disappointed about the baby's deficit but also, from birth, the communication interplay is altered. Parents should be encouraged to interact verbally with their child when in direct line of vision, to permit the child to respond to the stimulation of facial expressions.

Parent involvement is central to the habilitation program, beginning from the moment of diagnosis. They need to learn how the hearing impairment affects normal growth and development and about techniques available to maximize their child's potential. Although the nurse may not be primarily responsible for counseling the parents regarding amplification, communication techniques, and educational methods, the nurse generally functions on a team and should know of the available alternatives. The nurse acts as a resource to the family to discuss any aspect of the habilitation of their child. A list of organizations helpful to the hearing-impaired is provided in Table 45–17.

TABLE 45-17
Resources for the Hearing Impaired

Alexander Graham Bell Association for the Deaf, Inc. 3417 Volta Place, N.W. Washington, DC 20007
Conference of Executives of American Schools for the Deaf 5034 Wisconsin Avenue, N.W. Washington, DC 20016
Council of Organizations Serving the Deaf 4201 Connecticut Avenue, N.W. Suite 210 Washington, DC 20008
International Parents Organization Alexander Graham Bell Association for the Deaf 3417 Volta Place, N.W. Washington, DC 20007
National Association for the Deaf 814 Thayer Avenue Silver Spring, MD 20910
National Association of Parents of the Deaf 814 Thayer Avenue Silver Spring, MD 20910
The American Speech, Language, and Hearing Association 10801 Rockville Pike Rockville, MD 20895
The National Association for Hearing and Speech Action 10801 Rockville Pike Rockville, MD 20895

Helping the Family Realize the Impact of Hearing Impairment on the Child

The nurse can prepare parents for the various behaviors of their child and developmental consequences of having a hearing impairment. Whereas a hearing child is highly verbal and readily shares experiences even with strangers, the hearing-impaired child may be limited in social skills. With the loss of adequate expressive language, there is a tendency to withdraw from social situations. Strangers and peers may not understand the speech of the hearing-impaired child and he or she in turn cannot understand them. The ability to hear enables a child to identify the emotional intent of the words spoken. Hearing children learn what is expected of them from contextual cues and sounds perceived in the environment.

Large groups present a particular problem to hearing-impaired children because these children hear only parts of the conversation (e.g., in play they may not learn the rules of games well). Their response may be inappropriate to the situation, resulting in teasing by playmates who quickly dissociate them from the activity.

Hearing-impaired children tend to be more active in exploring the environment than are hearing children. They want to see and touch everything and desire to touch faces to feel the vibrations of speech. Some people may find this type of behavior intrusive and intolerable. Also, loud, unintelligible speech at the wrong time or in the wrong place may embarrass family members. Parents who cannot accept these behaviors may impose social isolation on the whole family or choose the alternative of planning activities whereby the child and one parent are always excluded in family activity. A sense of family unity may never evolve. Furthermore, older siblings may not bring friends home because they fear rejection of the family by their friends.

Helping to Reduce Potential Emotional Problems

Children who have learned to accept their limitation and have made some progress in their developmental skills will have limited emotional problems. Temper tantrums and extremes of destructive behavior and handflapping in response to frustration are often limited in duration. These children may have some difficulty, however, in delaying gratification of needs at times or may become impulsive. Their negative behavior cannot be rewarded with attention from friends and family and with the supplying of their every need. This response to negative behavior encourages a repetition of the behavior and loss of self-esteem. Eventually, these children will take on a dependency role and give up trying. Their major drive toward self-reliance may never succeed and their ability to solve problems will be greatly handicapped.

During the early years, when the child is developing social conscience about what is improper and what is acceptable behavior, parents must set consistent and firm limits on the child and expect reasonable obedience so that she or he can learn socially acceptable behavior. Parents may tend to avoid discipline for the hearing-impaired child because they fear that the child will not understand why the limitation was set. Mild, consistent disapproval with a stern "no" and facial expression of displeasure will enhance the child's understanding of what pleases the parents and will free the child to initiate more social contact. The nurse can help parents determine the normal behavior problems of their child and methods to cope with them. Parents can be encouraged to balance discipline with love and acceptance, which will decrease the child's feelings of rejection. These children need to be reassured that their parents love and accept them.

Methods of Communication

The controversy over the best method of communication is confusing to parents and to professionals. The goal of educators of the hearing impaired in the United States is to assist a child to develop the ability to "speak and understand the spoken word to the highest degree possible" (Moores, 1978). No present-day educators advocate only the use of the manual (sign language and fingerspelling) technique. Two basic methods of communication are used in the United States: oral communication and total communication.

Oral Communication

This method has been predominant until recently. It focuses on the use of residual hearing with amplification and speechreading (lipreading). Proponents of this method believe that it is important for the deaf to be taught to talk and understand speech so that they can communicate in the hearing world of people. Gestures and signs are viewed as an interference to the development of speech and therefore are discouraged. Although speech and speechreading are the goals for the hearing impaired, some do not have sufficient residual hearing to distinguish sounds and words that look alike on the lips.

The oral communication method is especially suited for very motivated children and primarily for those who have some residual hearing.

Total Communication

In this approach, all techniques of communication are used, including sign language, cued speech, fingerspelling, speechreading, tactile stimulation, and amplification. (See Table 45–18 for a description of various communication techniques.) There is an increasing movement for the use of this method with very young children. This support may be the result of (1) evidence that deaf children with deaf parents are more successful academically than those with hearing parents, (2) the increased acceptance of sign language, (3) dissatisfaction with traditional methods

TABLE 45-18
Communication Techniques for a Child with a Hearing Impairment

Hearing Aids

Made up of three parts: (1) microphone that picks up sound waves and changes them into electricity; (2) battery-powered amplifier to increase the strength of signal from microphone; and (3) receiver to change amplified signals back to sound waves

Types of Hearing Aids

- Fits directly in the ear
- Ear-level aid fits behind the ear
- Body aid is worn in pocket or attached to clothing
- Built into frame of glasses

Hearing aids are binaural (on each ear) or monoaural (on one ear)

Fitting aids to young children requires time and patience, with repeated trials and evaluation with loaned hearing aids

May be fitted as early as 2 mos of age; important to early stimulation of residual hearing

Auditory Training

Process of teaching a child how to listen to spoken language; emphasis is on listening to natural language, not separate speech sounds such as vowels and consonants

Speechreading (Lipreading)

Concentration on visual clues to decipher the content of the spoken word by watching a person's lips, tongue, and jaw; speechreading is difficult because many English sounds require similar formation of the lips; child's ability is improved if speaker's face is adequately lit and natural speaking is used, with normal articulation and complete sentences

Sign Language

Manual form of communication in which an entire concept is communicated by the position, configuration, and movement of the hands

Fingerspelling

Spelling of a word letter by letter; letters are represented by hand configurations

Cued Speech

Use of eight hand configurations and four hand placements supplementing natural speech; the hands are placed around the chin, cheek, and neck to give clues to assist in speechreading

Speech Training

Process of teaching a deaf child to speak intelligibly; child is taught how to regulate his or her voice and articulate correctly

with the profoundly deaf, and (4) strong support from deaf adults who were trained by a rigid oral method (Moores, 1978).

The nurse can explain to parents that no single method is preferred for all hearing-impaired children, but, rather, with the guidance of professionals, the method is individualized for each child.

The child's type and degree of hearing loss and age of onset are important variables that an audiologist must consider when determining the type of communication technique most suitable for each child.

Hearing aids are used to amplify the volume of environmental sounds only. They are helpful when one has good residual hearing. For some children, the sound becomes so grossly distorted when the volume is increased that it may create a barrier to receptive abilities. Knowing the range of sound volume loss as noted on diagnostic audiograms gives the nurse insight into determining the appropriate volume setting that is useful to the child. Significant improvements have been made in the physical appearance and electroacoustic characteristics of hearing aids. The reader is referred to Gaudry's (1987) review for information on the various types available.

Consistent wearing of the aid is particularly important for a child who is just learning to adjust to wearing it. Testing and changing of the batteries will increase the effectiveness of the aid and the child's social competence. Auditory feedback (a disturbing screech that emanates from the earpiece) occurs when the volume is too high or the ear mold is improperly fitted. The child and family will be taught how to alleviate this problem; however, because the child may not hear the feedback, others have to draw attention to it.

Alterations in Speech and Language

There are several techniques that the nurse may employ to encourage a young child to talk with them. A crying child will often quiet if the nurse speaks in a whisper. Even the most shy child will frequently respond if a question about her or him is directed to a sibling. Preschoolers will usually speak to a puppet, even though the puppet is obviously being used by the same nurse that they are refusing to speak to. Finally, "silliness" almost always works!

Speech and language skills compose the child's system of communication. Although many people use the terms interchangeably, they represent two very different skills that the child must master. "Speech" is defined as the planning and execution of oral movements required for articulation. Adequate speech requires good respiratory effort as well as upper airway and mouth use; it in no way reflects a child's cognitive ability.

"Language" refers to the meaningful use of a system of symbolic representation to communicate. It is an umbrella term with five components:

Phonology:	A sound system for a given language. The English language uses 46 phonemes.
Morphology:	The combining of phonemes into linguistic units of meaning. The smallest combination of sounds with meaning is a morpheme.
Semantics:	The process of using words correctly. A child must learn a vocab-

ulary; that is, the meaning of a word and how to use the word correctly.

Syntax: Grammar. This is the process of putting words together to make sense.

Pragmatics: The social aspect of language. The child must learn to use language to control his or her environment. It includes important skills such as knowing when to speak quietly, how close to stand to the person being spoken to, and the correct tone of voice to use.

According to the Education for All Handicapped Children Act (PL 94–142), speech-language impairment is defined as a disorder, deviation, or delay in verbal, gestural, or vocal skills including articulation, fluency, voice quality, or language to the extent that academic learning, social adjustment, or communication skills are hindered. Taken together, speech and language delays are the nation's number one disability condition. Fully 3 per cent of the children in this country receive public school special education services for such disabilities (Algozzine & Korinek, 1985). In a Canadian study, 11 per cent of 5-year-olds entering kindergarten had speech-language impairments (Beitchman et al, 1986). Most experts agree that even these estimates are low, since criteria for identification of these children vary from state to state.

Normal Development of Language and Assessment of Alterations

By the time a child is 4 years old, most of the grammatic principles of language have been learned. The critical period for speech and language development has been identified as from 9 to 24 months of age; however, it may begin before this time (Towne, 1983).

Language is the single best predictor of long-term cognitive outcome in children. Language delay is a common presenting symptom of global developmental disorders. To detect language delays, it is essential that health care providers have a clear, comprehensive knowledge and appreciation of language milestones and delayed or deviant development. Language development consists of receptive milestones (that which one understands) and expressive milestones (that which one expresses or speaks verbally).

Language evaluation must begin in infancy with a focus on prelinguistic skills that develop in the first year of life. The first receptive skill is evident soon after birth in the undifferentiated response on the part of the infant to sound. The infant may show a varied reaction to the sound—startling, quieting, or a change in sucking pattern. Actual orienting to sound occurs about 4 months of age, when the infant turns toward a mother's voice. By 9 months of age, children are able to recognize and inhibit to the word "no." Receptive language is consistently more advanced than expressive language. In other words, children can *understand* more than they verbalize.

Important expressive developments begin soon after birth and start with cooing (long vowel sounds) at 2 months of age. At 6 months, infants are, to the delight of their parents, babbling, and consistent "Dada," "Mama" sounds begin between 7 and 9 months of age. Immature jargoning develops at about 12 months of age; classically, parents describe this as sounding like a foreign language. It is an attempt on the part of the child at speaking sentences and usually comes complete with proper intonation and inflection. Mature jargoning, which develops between 15 and 18 months, resembles immature jargoning with an occasional real word thrown in. Parents instinctively respond to these language developments in exactly the right way—by treating them as real language attempts and replying to them.

By 20 to 24 months, the child should have a vocabulary of about 50 words. It is common for a "language burst" to occur at about this time; parents report that their child is demonstrating new words on a daily basis. This burst is followed shortly by two-word combinations. Pronouns appear at about 24 months, though incorrect usage is the norm. By 3 years of age, the child typically has a vocabulary approaching 300 words, uses plurals, and speaks in three-word combinations. Four-year-olds have a vocabulary exceeding 1000 words.

Normal speech and language development requires the presence of:

- Intact hearing from birth (e.g., early and recurring otitis media can diminish hearing).
- Intact nervous system.
- The physical structures and physiologic control to accomplish speech (e.g., an unrepaired cleft palate can interfere with speech).
- An environment that stimulates the use of verbal skills and verbal exchange.

Language can be assessed through directly observing the child's communication in an interaction and through parental reports. Direct observation may not allow the child's best performance, since many children are shy and reluctant to interact with an unfamiliar listener. Parents should be questioned closely about their child's language. This information is then compared with expected age-appropriate milestones. Parental concerns about a child's language development have been shown to have a very high rate of sensitivity and specificity and will detect the majority of children with delays (Glascoe, 1991). Normal speech and language development and signs of problems in development are summarized in Tables 45–19 and 45–20, respectively.

Specifically, language disorders are classified as *expressive, receptive,* and *mixed*. Expressive delays are the most common and may be due to problems with

TABLE 45-19
Development of Speech and Language

Age at Which Behavior Should Be Established (Mos)	Receptive Language Behavior	Expressive Language Behavior
1	Random activity arrested by sound	Random vocalization; primarily vowel sounds
2	Appears to listen to speaker; may smile at speaker	Vocal signs of pleasure; social smile
3	Looks in direction of speaker	Cooing and gurgling; smile in response to speech
4	Responds differently to angry vs. pleasant voice	Responds vocally to social stimuli
5	Responds to own name	Begins to mimic sounds
6	Recognizes words like "bye-bye," "Mamma," "Daddy"	Protests vocally; squeals with delight
7	Responds with gestures to words such as "up," "come," "bye-bye"	Begins to use wordlike sounds, some jargon
8	Stops activity when own name is called	Imitates sound sequences
9	Stops activity in response to "no"	Imitates intonation pattern of speech
10	Accurately imitates pitch variations	First words appear
11	Responds to simple questions ("Where is the dog?") by looking or pointing	Jargon well established
12	Responds with gestures to a variety of verbal requests	Announces awareness of familiar objects by name
15	Recognizes names of various parts of the body	True words heard embedded in jargon, often with gestures
18	Identifies pictures of familiar objects when they are named	Uses words more than gestures to express desires
21	Follows two consecutive, related directions ("Pick up your hat and put it on the chair")	Begins combining words ("Daddy car," "Mamma up")
24	Understands more complex sentences ("After we get in the car, we'll go to the store")	Refers to self by name

From Behrman, R. E., & Vaughan, V. C., III (Eds.) (1987). *Nelson textbook of pediatrics* (13th ed.). Philadelphia: WB Saunders.

TABLE 45-20
Signs of Problems in Language and Speech Development in Preschool Children

1. At 6 mos of age, does not turn eyes and head to sound coming from behind or to side
2. At 10 mos, does not make some kind of response to her or his name
3. At 15 mos, does not understand and respond to "no-no," "bye-bye," and "bottle"
4. At 18 mos, is not saying up to 10 single words
5. At 21 mos, does not respond to directions (e.g., "sit down," "come here," "stand up")
6. After 24 mos, has excessive, inappropriate jargon or echoing
7. At 24 mos, does not on request point to body parts (e.g., mouth, nose, eyes, ears)
8. At 24 mos, has no 2-word phrases
9. At 30 mos, has speech that is not intelligible to family members
10. At 36 mos, uses no simple sentences
11. At 36 mos, has not begun to ask simple questions
12. At 36 mos, has speech that is not intelligible to strangers
13. At 3.5 yrs of age, consistently fails to produce the final consonant (e.g., "ca" for *cat,* "bo" for *bone*)
14. After 4 yrs of age, is noticeably dysfluent (stutters)
15. After 7 yrs of age, has any speech sound errors
16. At any age, has noticeable hypernasality or hyponasality, or has a voice that is a monotone, of inappropriate pitch, unduly loud, inaudible, or consistently hoarse

From Behrman, R. E., & Vaughan, V. C., III (Eds.) (1987). *Nelson textbook of pediatrics* (13th ed.). Philadelphia: WB Saunders.

vocabulary, syntax, or pragmatics. These children are overwhelmingly of normal intelligence. Receptive delays may also be defined as word-processing problems. Assessment of true receptive ability may be difficult because these children often have a concomitant expressive delay. These children, too, are usually of normal intelligence. Mixed delays occur in children with both expressive and receptive delays and often exist as part of a global developmental delay. In contrast to children with single delays, 85 per cent of these children have IQs below normal (Silva, 1980).

Deterrents to normal development of language may include:

- Hearing loss.
- Mental retardation.
- A dysfunctional environment.
- Bilingualism (typically associated with only a mild delay).

An important role for the nurse is the education of parents in ways to maximize their child's language development. Beginning at the baby's birth, parents should be taught to hold their infant close and talk in a soothing voice. Parents should speak clearly and avoid "baby talk"; in turn, they should listen and show

enthusiasm for the things that interest their child. Parents can talk to their child about everyday events with vocabulary that is not oversimplified, because this may slow the child's progress. Correcting a child's language should be avoided; instead, parents should use correct vocabulary and syntax in their own speech. Most importantly, parents should read to their children daily, beginning in infancy. Although some of these suggestions may seem obvious, parents can be helped by being reminded of their own importance in encouraging their child's language.

Problems in Speech Development

Common problems to observe for when assessing speech development involve articulation, fluency, and voice disorders.

Articulation

Articulation problems make it difficult for speech to be understood. Difficulty in articulation is the most commonly encountered speech problem in children (Towne, 1983). Disorders of articulation comprise four types of problems:

- Substitution (replacement of one sound for another—e.g., "wabbit" for "rabbit").
- Omissions (failure to produce certain sounds—e.g., "boo" for "book").
- Additions (adding an extra syllable or sound—e.g., "birtherday" for "birthday").
- Distortions (inappropriate sound replacing the correct one, such as in the phenomena of lisping).

Sound production is a gradually developing process. By 5 years of age, 88 per cent of children are able to pronounce h, w, m, n, ng, f, p, and t correctly. By 6 to 7 years of age, 75 per cent of children can produce the sounds th, v, z, zh, and dz; by age 8, development of articulation skills is complete (Levine, 1992).

Fluency

"Fluency disorders" are defined as a disruption in the rate, rhythm, or general flow of speech. Terms such as stammering and stuttering are used to describe this problem. "Stammering" is the result of involuntary pauses in the formation of words, and "stuttering" is the involuntary repetition of speech sounds. "Stuttering" is used in this discussion to include both types of dysfluency.

The prevalence of stuttering has been estimated to be 4 per cent in children (Porfert & Rosenfield, 1978). It is more common in males, and approximately 80 per cent of children who stutter "outgrow" it. Health care professionals should, however, recognize that telling parents "not to worry" may in 20 per cent of cases be incorrect information (Rosenfield, 1982).

Most children engage in stuttering behavior, more precisely defined as developmental nonfluency, at some point during the years they are formulating language skills, most commonly during late toddlerhood or the early preschool years. This behavior is a natural manifestation of the child's concentrated effort to master communication skills and, at best, should be ignored. It is most likely to occur on occasions when the child is tired, experiencing extreme anxiety, or being exposed to overstimulation from her or his environment (Herbert, 1975).

These natural, temporary speech disturbances become a problem only when they become persistent or cause the child extreme distress. Stuttering can become exaggerated when an experience or person (often a parent) draws the child's attention to her or his own speaking. The primary basis for these disturbed speech behaviors is the result of demands on the child to impose conscious control over the involuntary act of forming words (Herbert, 1975; Homan, 1977). Thus, a natural behavior is molded, ever so unintentionally, into a behavioral disturbance because of the constant pressures to impose consciousness on an unconscious act by phrases like "Try to say it over again carefully," "Say it this way," and "Think about what you are saying!" Once conscious effort is demanded, the stuttering or stammering may become established. Differences between nonfluency and true stuttering are highlighted in Table 45–21.

The cause of stuttering has not been established, but it has been demonstrated that stutterers are fluent (1) when they sing, (2) when they speak during inhalation, (3) when they do not hear themselves speak, and (4) when delayed auditory feedback is provided (i.e., individual hears what she or he has said several milliseconds later) (Rosenfield, 1982).

Voice Disorders

Voice disorders may be encountered in children with vocal cord nodules or polyps following chronic shouting or excessive talking (Goldberg, 1984). Voice is assessed for loudness, quality (nasality, hoarseness, breathiness, or harshness), intonation, and pitch. Voice disorders can cause children considerable distress because it sets them apart from peers. This alteration thus requires a referral for speech therapy.

The Sensory-Impaired Child in the Hospital

The sensory-impaired child is particularly dependent on the family at a time of stress. Despite any attempts to prepare a sensory-impaired child for what to expect in the hospital, new people and a strange environment are a threat to security. The stress of hospi-

TABLE 45-21
Normal Nonfluency Versus Stuttering

Normal Nonfluency
Child is between 1½ and 6 yrs of age
Nonfluency is primarily repetition of single sound, word, or phrase
Each nonfluency is no more than two repetitions, li-li-like this
There is little or no tension in the repetition
Periods of nonfluency come and go; more nonfluency during periods of stress or new motor or language learning
Nonfluencies occur on 3% or less of words
Child is only infrequently aware of nonfluencies, rarely embarrassed or frustrated by them
Mild Stuttering
Child is between 1½ and 12 yrs
Stuttering may be repetition of sound or one-syllable words; prolongations of sounds, or, to a lesser extent, blocks in speech in which little or no sound comes out for several seconds
Child repeats sound more than two times per repetition, li-li-li-li-like this
Tension may be evident in rise of pitch during repetition or prolongation, or in facial squeezing during block
Stuttering may come and go but is more often present than absent
Child is aware of stuttering, may be frustrated or slightly embarrassed, but is not afraid of speaking
Severe Stuttering
Child may be 1½ years of age or older
Stuttering is present most of the time, may be much worse in certain situations
Stuttering occurs on more than 10% of speech
Stuttering occurs primarily in the form of blocks with little or no sound; repetitions or prolongations may accompany blocks
Facial tension is evident during stutters
Body movement and eye blinks may be associated with stuttering
In some cases, stuttering may be more internal and may be manifested by silent pauses
Child is embarrassed by stuttering; may change words or avoid speaking altogether in certain situations

From Guitar, B. E. (1988, February). Is it stuttering or just normal language development? *Contemporary Pediatrics, 5*(2), 109–123.

talization is best tolerated if parents can be present to assist in orienting the child to the environment and participate in preparing the child for the various hospital events. Nurses are most helpful if they work with the family to learn the special daily care routines and how the child can best relate to others. Nurses and child life workers can use psychologic preparation and medical play techniques to assist the child and family to cope with the stress of hospitalization. Although this is important for all hospitalized children, it is exceptionally so for those who are sensory-impaired, who use alternate methods of relating to their environment.

Although rooming-in by parents is encouraged and beneficial, the nurse should not expect parents to assume full responsibility for the interpretation and explanation of procedures to the child. The nurse should become increasingly adept at communicating effectively with a sensory-impaired child so that parents will feel comfortable to leave for brief periods. Also, if parents are to take an extensive part in the care of their child, the nurse in turn must be prepared to spend adequate time with parents to prepare them for this task. Parents have difficulty knowing what is expected of them regarding the routines and procedures of a hospital and need assistance to understand how they can participate.

Special routines of home must be maintained to provide maximal comfort to a sensory-impaired child. The nurse is responsible for collecting specific data on admission regarding special care needs of a sensory-impaired child such as hearing aids, lenses, self-care skills, and mobility techniques. Also, the level of the impairment and its effect on independent functioning must be ascertained. From this information, a care plan must be developed and used by all nurses caring for the child. It is distressing to the child and parents to have to orient each "new" nurse to the child's individual needs.

The nurse who gives nursing care to a sensory-impaired child should make the necessary adaptations that will permit the child to maintain the usual method of communication and foster normal growth and development. Independence in self-care skills such as self-feeding, dressing, bathing, and mobility should be maintained and encouraged, even though, for a sensory-impaired child, this may require additional patience and time on the nurse's part.

When a procedure is performed, the nurse must carefully assess the implications it may have for the child. For example, the wearing of a mask by health care personnel will cut off an important means of communication for the deaf child, and restraint of the hands and arms interferes with one of a blind child's primary methods of taking in the environment. Play with other children should be encouraged to prevent the child from feeling isolated. The help of parents should be elicited to provide a play situation that is suitable to the child's abilities and is similar to the usual play environment. Major nursing diagnoses and associated nursing care interventions have been discussed for the visually-impaired child and for the hearing-impaired child. Table 45–8 presents one nursing diagnostic statement for a nursing process plan for use with children with any sensory deficits. This plan is designed to help promote a positive self-concept in the child with a sensory or other physical impairment.

KEY CONCEPTS

Concepts Related to Basic Information

- Infant vision, although immature, is better than once thought. Infants seem particularly interested in the human face and are attracted to items of high contrast.
- All infants should have prophylactic treatment with erythromycin ointment at birth as protection against infection with *Chlamydia trachomatis* and *Neisseria gonorrhoeae*.
- Children's eyes are normally hyperopic until at least 6 or 7 years of age. However, their superior abilities of accommodation allow them to attain good visual acuity.
- Because vision is developing, children are capable of developing amblyopia (reduction or loss of vision) in an eye from which vision is being suppressed until 8 or 9 years of age.
- Promotion of optimal development in children with visual or hearing impairment is greatly dependent on early intervention.

Concepts Related to Nursing Assessment

- Because early intervention is so important, all children from infancy onward are in need of regular vision and hearing screening.
- Parents play a vital role in facilitating the language development of their child. Their functioning in this capacity is a part of routine nursing assessment.
- Stuttering can be a normal temporary speech disturbance. However, in about 20 per cent of children, it will be a more serious disorder.

Concepts Related to Nursing Intervention

- Most of the care of children with sensory impairments will occur outside of the acute care setting.
- Adaptation of care routines and the hospital environment are important in caring for the hospitalized child who has a sensory impairment.

REFERENCES

Adelson, E., & Fraiberg, S. (1974, March). Gross motor development in infants blind from birth. *Child Development, 45*(3), 114.

Adelson, E., & Fraiberg, S. (1972). Mouth and hand in the early development of blind infants. In J. F. Bosma (Ed.). *Third symposium on oral sensation and perception*. Springfield, IL: Charles C Thomas.

Algozzine, B., & Korinek, L. (1985). Where is special education for children with high prevalence handicaps going? *Exceptional Children, 51,* 388–394.

Alonso, L., et al (1978). *Mainstreaming preschoolers: Children with visual handicaps*. (Pub No. [OHDS] 78–3112). Washington, DC: US Department of Health, Education and Welfare.

American Academy of Pediatrics, Committee on the Fetus and Newborn (1983). *Guidelines for perinatal care*. Evanston, IL: Author.

American Academy of Pediatrics, Joint Committee on Infant Hearing (1982, September). Position statement 1982. *Pediatrics, 70*(3), 496–497.

Barraga, N. (1973). Utilization of sensory-perceptual abilities. In B. Lowenfeld (Ed.). *The visually handicapped child in school*. New York: John Day.

Behrman, R. E., Kliegman, R. M., Nelson, W. E., & Vaughn, V. C. (1991). *Nelson textbook of pediatrics* (14th ed.). Philadelphia: WB Saunders.

Beitchman, J. H., Nair, R., Clegg, M., & Patel, P. G. (1986). Prevalence of speech and language disorders in 5-year-old kindergarten children in the Ottawa-Carleton region. *Journal of Speech and Hearing Disorders, 51,* 98–110.

Bergstrom, L. (1980, January). Causes of reversed hearing loss in early childhood. *Pediatric Annals, 9*(1), 13–23.

Bess, F. (1977). *Childhood deafness*. New York: Grune & Stratton.

Calhoun, J. H. (1983, December). Cataracts in children. *Pediatric Clinics of North America, 30*(6), 1061–1069.

Carrel, R. (1977). Epidemiology of hearing loss. In S. E. Gerber (Ed.): *Audiometry in infancy*. Orlando, FL: Grune & Stratton.

Chew, E., & Morin, J. D. (1983, December). Glaucoma in children. *Pediatric Clinics of North America, 30*(6), 1043–1059.

Chinn, P. (1979). *Child health maintenance*. St. Louis, CV Mosby.

Coplan, J. (1987). Deafness: ever heard of it? Delayed recognition of permanent hearing loss. *Pediatrics, 79*(2), 206–213.

Cratty, B. J. (1971). *Movement and spatial awareness in blind children and youth*. Springfield, IL: Charles C Thomas.

Cunningham, D. (1978). Hearing loss. In R. Hoekelman, et al (Eds.). *Principles of pediatrics*. New York: McGraw-Hill.

Downs, M. (1981). Early identification of hearing loss. In N. Lass, et al (Eds.). *Speech, language and hearing*. Philadelphia: WB Saunders.

Eviator, L. (1984, February). Evaluation of hearing in the high-risk infant. *Clinical Perinatology, 11*(1), 153–173.

Feman, S., & Reinecke, R. (1978). *Handbook of pediatric ophthalmology*. Orlando, FL: Grune & Stratton.

Field, T. M. (1982, October). Discrimination and imitation of facial expressions by neonates. *Science, 218,* 179–181.

Fraiberg, S. (1974). Blind infants and their mothers: An examination of the sign system. In M. Lewis, & I. Rosenblum (Eds.). *Effect of the infant on its caregiver*. New York: John Wiley.

Fraiberg, S. (1971, July). Intervention in infancy: A program for blind infants. *Journal of the American Academy of Child Psychiatry, 10,* 381.

Fria, T. J. (1983). The assessment of hearing and middle ear function in children. In C. D. Bluestone & S. E. Stool (Eds.). *Pediatric otolaryngology* (Vol. 1). Philadelphia: WB Saunders.

Gaudry, F. (1987). Hearing aids: A review for the family physician. *Canadian Family Physician, 33,* 1509–1512.

Glascoe, F. P. (1991). Can clinical judgement detect children with speech language problems? *Pediatrics, 87*(3), 317–322.

Goble, J. L. (1984). *Visual disorders in the handicapped child*. New York: Marcel Dekker.

Goldberg, R. (1984, July/August). Identifying speech and language delays in children. *Pediatric Nursing,* 252–259.

Greenwald, M. J. (1983). Visual development in infancy and childhood. *Pediatric Clinics of North America, 30*(6), 977–993.

Guitar, B. E. (1988). Is it stuttering or just normal language development? *Contemporary Pediatrics, 5*(2), 109–125.

Hatfield, E. (1979, Summer). Methods and standards for screening preschool children. *The Sightsaving Review, 49,* 15–25.

Herbert, M. (1975). *Problems of childhood*. London: Pam Brooks Ltd.

Homan, W. (1977). *Child sense*. New York: Basic Books.

Hughes, J. (1984). *Synopsis of pediatrics* (6th ed.). St. Louis: CV Mosby.

Jan, J., et al (1977). *Visual impairment in children and adolescents.* Orlando, FL: Grune & Stratton.

Johnson, T., et al (1978). *Children are different: Developmental physiology* (2nd ed.). Columbus, OH: Ross Laboratories.

Kovalesky, A. (1985). *Nurses' guide to children's eyes.* Orlando, FL: Grune & Stratton.

Levine, M. D., et al (1992). *Developmental-behavioral pediatrics.* Philadelphia: WB Saunders.

Lingua, R. W. (1986). The eye. In S. S. Gellis & B. M. Kagan (Eds.). *Current pediatric therapy 12* (pp 483–489). Philadelphia: WB Saunders.

Ludington-Hoe, S. (1983, September). What can newborns really see? *American Journal of Nursing, 83,* 1286–1289.

Martin, F. N. (1978). *Pediatric audiology* (p 38). Englewood Cliffs, NJ: Prentice-Hall.

McFarland, W., & Simmons, F. (1980, January). The importance of early intervention with severe childhood deafness. *Pediatric Annals, 9*(1), 6.

Moores, D. (1978). *Educating the deaf. Psychology, principles, and practices.* New York: Houghton Mifflin.

Morin, J. D., & Bryars, J. H. (1980). Causes of loss of vision in congenital glaucoma. *Archives of Ophthalmology, 98,* 1575–1576.

Mouney, D. F. (1979). Differential diagnosis of hearing loss in children. *Ear, Nose, and Throat Journal, 58*(7), 293–296.

Nelson, L. B., et al (1984, March). Developmental aspects in the assessment of visual function in young children. *Pediatrics, 73*(3), 375–381.

Nelson, L. B., Cathan, J. H., & Harley, R. D. (1991). *Pediatric ophthalmology* (3rd ed.). Philadelphia: WB Saunders.

Newby, H. (1979). *Audiology.* Englewood Cliffs, NJ: Prentice-Hall.

Paparella, M. (1977). Differential diagnosis of childhood deafness. In F. Bess (Ed.). *Childhood deafness.* Orlando, FL: Grune & Stratton.

Phillips, S., & Hartley, J. (1988, May/June). Developmental differences and interventions for blind children. *Pediatric Nursing, 14*(3), 201–206.

Porat, R. (1984, February). Care of the infant with retinopathy of prematurity. *Clinical Perinatology, 11*(1), 123–151.

Porfert, A. R., & Rosenfield, D. B. (1978). Prevalence of stuttering. *Journal of Neurology, Neurosurgery and Psychiatry, 41,* 954.

Rosenfield, D. B. (1982, June). Stuttering. *Current Problems in Pediatrics, 50*(2), 4–27.

Scholl, G. (1973). Understanding and meeting developmental needs. In B. Lowenfeld (Ed.). *The visually handicapped child in school.* New York: John Day.

Shapiro, C. (1992). Ophthalmic disorders. In P. Beachy & J. Deacon: *NAACOG core curriculum for neonatal intensive care nursing* (p 495). Philadelphia: WB Saunders.

Shapiro, C. (1986). Retrolental fibroplasia: What we know and what we don't know. *Neonatal Network, 4*(6), 33–45.

Silva, P. A. (1980). The prevalence, stability and significance of developmental language delay in preschool children. *Developmental Medicine and Child Neurology, 22,* 768–777.

Stangler, S., et al (1980). *Screening growth and development of preschool children: A guide for test selection.* New York: McGraw-Hill.

Sweitzer, R. (1977). Audiologic evaluation of the infant and young child. In B. Jaffe (Ed.). *Hearing loss in children: A comprehensive text.* Baltimore, MD: University Park Press.

Tongue, A. (1980, May/June). Low vision examination in children with visual impairment. *Journal of Pediatric Ophthalmology and Strabismus, 17*(3), 175.

Towne, C. (1983). Disorders of hearing, speech and language. In R. E. Behrman & V. C. Vaughan (Eds.). *Textbook of pediatrics.* Philadelphia: WB Saunders.

BIBLIOGRAPHY

Bellman, S. (1986). Hearing screening in infancy. *Archives of Disease in Childhood, 61,* 637–638.

Biro, P., & Thompson, M. (1984). Screening young children for communication disorders. *MCN: American Journal of Maternal Child Nursing, 9*(6), 410–413.

Bluestone, C. D., et al (1986, January). Controversies in screening for middle ear disease and hearing loss in children. *Pediatrics, 77*(1), 57–70.

Catalano, J. D. (1990). Strabismus. *Pediatric Annals, 19*(5), 284–297.

Committee on Practice and Ambulatory Medicine. (1986). Visual screening and eye examination in children. *Pediatrics, 77*(6), 918–919.

Desch, L. W. (1986, January). High technology for handicapped children: A pediatrician's viewpoint. *Pediatrics, 77*(1), 71–87.

Fraiberg, S., et al (1969, Summer). An educational program for blind infants. *Journal of Special Education, 3,* 121.

George, D. S., et al (1988, July/August). The latest on retinopathy of prematurity. *MCN: American Journal of Maternal Child Nursing, 13*(4), 254–258.

Havener, W. (1979). *Synopsis of ophthalmology* (5th ed.). St. Louis: CV Mosby.

An International Classification of Retinopathy of Prematurity (1984, July). *Pediatrics, 74*(1), 127–133.

Klein, S. K. (1991). Evaluation for suspected language disorders in preschool children. *Pediatric Clinics of North America, 38*(6), 1455–1467.

Lennenberg, E. (1967). *Biological foundation of language.* New York: John Wiley.

Lumbardino, L. J., et al (1987). Evaluating communicative behaviors in infancy. *Journal of Pediatric Health Care, 1*(5), 240–246.

National Association for Visually Handicapped (1980). *Problems of the partially seeing.* New York: Author.

Northern, J. L., & Downs, M. P. (1984). *Hearing in children* (3rd ed.). Baltimore, MD: Williams & Wilkins.

Scheie, H., & Albert, D. (1977). *Textbook of ophthalmology* (9th ed.). Philadelphia: WB Saunders.

Shannon, D. A., et al (1973, January). Hearing screening of high-risk newborns with brainstem auditory evoked potentials: A follow-up study. *Pediatrics, 73*(1), 22–26.

Siegel, I., & Murphy, T. (1970, August). *Postural determinants in the blind. Final report.* Washington, DC: US Educational Resources Information Center. (ERIC Document FD 048 714.)

Sullivan, L. (1988, May/June). How effective is preschool vision, hearing, and developmental screening? *Pediatric Nursing, 14*(3), 181–183.

Teplin, S. W. (1983, January). Development of blind infants and children with retrolental fibroplasia: Implications for physicians. *Pediatrics, 71*(1), 6–12.

Thal, D., & Bates, E. (1989). Language and communication in early childhood. *Pediatric Annals, 18*(5), 299–305.

Thomson, L. R. (1982). Understanding tympanometry. *Pediatric Nursing, 8*(3), 193–197.

Wright, P. F., Thompson, J., & Bess, F. H. (1991). Hearing, speech, and language sequellae of otitis media with effusion. *Pediatric Annals, 20*(11), 617–621.

CHAPTER • 46

The Injured Child

Elizabeth Wonnacott

NURSING PROCESS PLANS
NPP: The Child with Foreign Body Aspiration, Table 46–12
NPP: The Child with Submersion Injury, Table 46–14

RELATED TOPICS
Safety, Chapter 15
Concepts of stress, coping, and illness, Chapter 18
Principles and skills adapted to children, Chapter 23
Pharmacologic principles applied to children, Chapter 24
Nursing Management of Pain in Children, Chapter 25
Principles of Fluid and Electrolyte Maintenance, Chapter 26
Child abuse and neglect, Chapter 28
Respiratory distress and airway management, Chapter 32
Nasogastric tubes, Chapter 35
Allergic reactions, Chapter 37
Sunburn and contact dermatitis, Chapter 38
Rabies, Chapter 39
Head and spinal cord injuries, Chapter 40
Fractures, Chapter 41

LEARNING OBJECTIVES

- Identify the important developmental differences that influence the nursing care of injured children.
- List the steps in initial assessment of an injured child.
- Identify the commonly seen responses of children and families to accidental injury.
- State the principles of triage.
- Describe cardiopulmonary resuscitation techniques in children.
- List the common childhood injuries and the related nursing care.
- Identify the preventive measures that need to be taught to parents that would prevent the common childhood injuries.

The significance of childhood injury is realized when one considers that accidents are the leading cause of death in children. Pediatric nurses and nurses who work in general emergency settings must be aware of the ways in which treatment of injury in children differs from that in adults. This chapter details a wide variety of situations, from minor insect bites to life-threatening cardiopulmonary emergencies. The sections dealing with age-related differences in structure and function of body systems in previous chapters provide a base for many of the child-oriented interventions for trauma. The reader is encouraged to review these sections as needed.

Any injury, whether life-threatening or minor, brings a degree of suffering and pain to the child and is distressing for parents. Preventing injury and caring for children and their families, in the event of injury, is a challenge to health care professionals (see Chapter 15 for a discussion of the nurse's role in safety and prevention of injury). Few circumstances demand the extensive knowledge base, quick assessment skills and decision making, and sensitive communication skills that are required to mobilize effective care for the injured child.

Emphasis is placed on immediate, skillful intervention whenever a child is traumatized. Although it is recognized that parents need support and explanations, in the event of injury the goal of saving the child's life with the least possible sequelae is given first attention. The speed and appropriateness of treatment in the first few minutes at an accident scene can determine the quality of life for a child. As soon as the initial emergency has been met, parents are given a full explanation of how the child is and what has been done. When the injury occurs, a nurse must be prepared to make quick decisions based on sound knowledge. When even the quickest of actions cannot reverse the effects of injury, the anguish that parents experience presents an overwhelming challenge to the nurse and other health care professionals who also are sharing the loss.

Principles of Caring for the Injured Child

Etiology/Incidence of Injuries in Children

Pediatric injury or multitrauma continues to be the leading cause of death for children. In the ages from 1 to 15 years, injury accounts for 50 per cent of the total deaths (Accident Facts, 1988; Dandrinos-Smith, 1991).

The term "injury," as used in this chapter, implies that trauma has been inflicted by an agent interrupting the structural integrity of the child. In some circumstances, adults are a serious threat to the safety and well-being of children in our society. The care of children who are injured as a result of abusive and neglectful caretakers is addressed in Chapter 28. Recognition of the abused or neglected child is included in this chapter to emphasize that health professionals should regard any injured child with an alertness for signs and clues that could represent abuse or neglect, or both. In this chapter, "injury" refers to a wide range of mishaps that befall children, including motor vehicle accidents and auto-pedestrian collisions; burns; near-drowning and drowning; poisonings; eye, ear, nose, and throat injuries; and common childhood events such as frostbite, sun exposure, insect bites, stings, poison ivy exposure, and injuries caused by cuts, scrapes, and punctures. The term "injury" should be used rather than "accident." Accidents are usually thought of as situations over which individuals have little or no control. "Injuries" refers to a variety of situations in which control may or may not be present.

An injury occurs as a result of the interaction of the host (the person affected), the agent (cause of the injury), and the environment (circumstances of its occurrence). Although most injuries can occur at any age, some occur more frequently at certain developmental stages. Thus, it is evident that the host is a factor in causing injuries. (See Chapter 15 for further discussion of etiologic factors in injury.)

Developmental Differences Affecting Response to Injury

A child cannot be treated simply as an anatomically smaller adult. Significant physiologic differences in children influence their response to injury. These include airway and breathing, circulation, temperature regulation, and mechanism of injury.

Airway and Breathing

The diameter of a child's airway is proportionately smaller than an adult's, resulting in greater resistance to airflow. Any injury that compromises the airway in a child results in serious reduction in airway diameter with increased effort required to do the work of breathing. The airway is prone to obstruction by blood, vomitus, mucus, or swelling owing to injury or infectious disease. Furthermore, in the presence of edema, the greater amount of soft tissue in the neck increases the risk of obstruction.

The smallest diameter of the airway in the child is at the cricoid cartilage—not at the glottis as in the adult. Passage of an endotracheal tube may be complicated by this difference. Because the narrowest point of the child's airway is below the vocal cords at the cricoid cartilage, an uncuffed endotracheal tube is usually used in children less than 8 years of age (Chameides, 1988). In adults and older children, cuffed endotracheal tubes are used to seal the airway.

In infants, the tongue is large in relation to mouth size and is a well-developed organ with strong musculation essential for sucking. This relatively large structure is a common cause of airway obstruction. When maintaining an airway for a child, the chin-lift/jaw-thrust maneuver should be employed to lift the tongue away from the trachea. Hyperextension of the neck should be avoided. *Only* the jaw thrust maneuver should be used for children in whom a crucial spine injury is suspected. Hyperextension of the neck should be avoided in very small children or infants; however, *slight* hyperextension is acceptable for larger children.

During inspiration, it is normal for an infant or small child to push out the abdomen. Following this, the chest should symmetrically expand as the lungs fill with air. During respiratory distress, the abdomen continues to rise with each inspiration; however, the chest may not rise, and substernal, intercostal, or tracheal in-drawing may be noted. Air is frequently swallowed during periods of respiratory distress, causing gastric distention. This in turn contributes to further distress by reducing diaphragmatic excursion and increasing the work of breathing. Air in the stomach is usually expelled by vomiting and, thus, the risk of aspiration is increased. Any increase in the work of breathing may lead to exhaustion and decreased respiratory effort. (For further discussion on respiratory developmental differences, see Table 32–1.)

Circulation

A child's distribution of fluid volume puts her or him at risk for dehydration and electrolyte imbalance. The proportionately greater percentage of fluid in the extracellular space increases risk for rapid loss. Children compensate for blood loss more readily by vasoconstriction and tachycardia. When assessing a pediatric trauma patient, consider that approximately 80 ml/kg is normal blood volume. Children may lose almost 25 per cent of their total blood volume without displaying a significant decrease in peripheral blood pressure. A fall in blood pressure is usually a late indicator of blood or fluid loss that is potentially lethal.

Children are monitored for maintenance of adequate fluid volume by assessing skin color, respirations, pulse, capillary refill, and urinary output, and by watching for interrelated alteration of these signs.

Temperature Regulation

Hypothermia may be either a cause of injury or a result of it. Children have difficulty maintaining their temperature when the body is stressed by illness or injury because of (1) large surface area in relation to weight, (2) less subcutaneous tissue to prevent heat loss, and (3) a large head with high blood flow to the scalp.

When evaluating color and temperature of the extremities, the nurse should recognize that infants may exhibit mottling because of their immature temperature-regulating mechanism.

Mechanism of Injury

It is important to understand that anatomic differences in children result in characteristic types and sequence of injuries.

Head. A child's head provides a prime target for injury. Because of the relatively large size and weight of the head in proportion to the rest of the body, and because children lack well-developed neck muscles and cervical ligaments, their heads are frequently the first point of contact in injuries involving falls or motor vehicle collisions. These differences, coupled with their thin skulls, which afford little protection, increase the potential for brain damage to occur in children. Children with skull fractures are at greater risk for (1) direct brain injury from bone fragments and (2) increased intracranial pressure from cerebral bleeds or depressed skull fragments. (See Chapter 40 for further discussion of neurologic differences in children.)

Cervical Spine. The cervical spine becomes injured during head trauma because of the weight of the child's head, the poorly developed neck muscles, and weak cervical ligaments (Coln, 1985), even though there may be no actual fracture. Because of the child's large head size, cervical injuries tend to occur high in the cervical spine between C3 and C5 (Kelley, 1988). The most common mechanism of spinal injury in children is a sudden hyperflexion or hyperextension of the neck combined with a rotational injury. This is the type of injury that is typical in car accidents. Although cervical spine injuries are considered rare in children, every seriously injured child should be suspected to have a cervical spine injury until proved otherwise. Infants and children may sustain spinal cord injuries without evidence of the injury on radiologic examination. Severe angulation of the spine resulting in cord injury can occur without a disruption of bones and ligaments (ligaments are lax and the cervical spine has a large amount of cartilage).

Chest and Internal Organs. Because children's chests are quite flexible and they have relatively underdeveloped abdominal and chest wall muscles, they are at risk for injury from blunt, or nonpenetrating, trauma. Blunt trauma is a more frequent cause of chest and abdominal injuries in children than penetrating trauma. Blunt trauma is less obvious (and, therefore, more difficult to assess) than the dramatic wounds produced by penetrating objects. For example, punching into soft belly tissues may leave no external bruising but may injure the solid organs of the abdomen or cause serious thoracic injury secondary to rib fractures. Similarly, during falls onto objects, an internal injury can occur.

Rapid deceleration of a motor vehicle caused by collision or forceful braking may lead to tearing of solid organs. The spleen is most likely to suffer injury in children. Because of the spleen's highly vascular nature, children with splenic laceration or rupture may bleed to death within minutes. Other organs that may be affected are the liver, pancreas, and small bowel.

Children riding in cars who are not restrained by a car seat or seat belt will literally become missiles during a collision. Although head injury is the most common problem resulting from lack of appropriate restraint, chest and abdominal injuries can occur as the child catapults into a dashboard, steering wheel, or the interior walls of the vehicle.

Normal childhood activities can, in themselves, become mechanisms of injury. Bicycles, for example, are regarded as part of the essential equipment of childhood. Yet children form the largest population of those injuries in bicycle accidents. Boys between 5 and 16 years of age are at the greatest risk (McKenna et al, 1991).

A bicycle's stability is affected by the speed at which it is traveling, the road surface, and the rider's expertise at handling it. Dropped handlebars on bicycles, although facilitating increased speeds, place the rider in a head-down position even before she or he falls. With a child, whose head is already proportionally heavier, the risk of head injury is increased. Indeed, fatal head injury is possible after a fall as short as 1 foot when the head hits directly onto concrete (Worrell, 1987).

Assessment of the Injured Child

Since the first few minutes may be crucial to the child's survival (and quality of life later on) the nurse must be able to draw on an established body of knowledge and finely honed assessment skills. All nurses who work with critically ill children should have a sound knowledge of developmental differences among pediatric patients within the varied age groups of childhood and differences between pediatric and adult patients.

How to deal with children in the Emergency Department:

- **Do whatever it takes to gain the child's confidence. A few extra minutes expended will mean time saved in the long run.**
- **Be kind but firm. Limit choices but do allow some (e.g., which bandage to use, what color gown to wear).**
- ***Never* be impatient or lose your temper.**
- **Make haste slowly.**
- **Smile!**

Primary Survey

Any assessment of a very ill or badly injured child should begin with a quick visual examination of the child. However, the need for a systematic approach to physical assessment cannot be overemphasized. The most common and most effective method of assessment is known as the ABC (*A*irway, *B*reathing, *C*irculation) or primary survey and the head-to-toe or secondary survey. While asking whether this child "*looks* sick," the nurse begins to assess the child and simultaneously gather information from the accompanying parent.

If the parent does not offer the information, ask "How does the child in the present condition compare with his or her usual state?" *Pay close attention to the parent who reports that a child's behavior is significantly altered from normal.* The parent knows the child best. Table 46–1 provides a guide for making effective and rapid primary surveys.

The information obtained from the primary survey should be validated at regular intervals and any changes or trends noted and documented. The basic vital functions *must* be stable before attention is diverted from them to other concerns. For example, a fractured femur may be the more obvious injury but is far less important than assessing for and maintaining an adequate airway.

Medical treatment may be initiated, depending on the findings of the aforementioned assessment. A secondary survey should always be performed as soon as the ABCs are stabilized.

Secondary Survey

The secondary survey involves history taking and a head-to-toe assessment of the child's condition. A quick assessment is performed as for any physical examination, with a focus on fractures, contusions, and lacerations. In a true emergency situation, the child's

TABLE 46-1
Guide for Conducting a Rapid Primary Survey

An overall assessment is made immediately regarding level of responsiveness and presence of head and neck trauma. A rapid assessment, following the ABC format, is begun almost simultaneously

A. Airway

- Is child maintaining patent airway independently?
- Are there any signs of obstruction?
- Is position of airway facilitating or interfering with air exchange?

B. Breathing

- Rate of respirations
- Quality of respirations (shallow, stridor, wheezing, grunting, labored)
- Effectiveness of respiratory effort (does chest rise and fall symmetrically)
- Skin color

C. Circulation

- Rate and quality of pulses (especially apical)
- Capillary refill
- Skin temperature
- Skin color
- Skin turgor

weight may be estimated, but, as soon as possible, a real value should be obtained. Accurate weight is essential for determining the rate and amount of intravenous fluid to be administered, dosage of medications that may be given, and parameters for required ventilatory assistance. The child's weight may also be useful in determining the level of toxicity to be anticipated relative to the amount of a noxious substance that has been ingested. Throughout the secondary survey, the ABCs are reassessed constantly. At this stage, *D* should be included for *D*isability and/or *D*rugs (e.g., alcohol use in adolescence), and *E* for *E*xposure.

In an emergency, a history and physical assessment are usually done simultaneously. Frequently, a very ill or badly injured child is rushed into the treatment area while the parents are detained at the desk to give information. The parent, understandably, may be extremely distraught and unable to answer questions coherently. The nurse should ask a minimum of questions, and they should be short and simply phrased (Table 46-2 lists the most pertinent areas to include). The nurse may have to repeat or restate questions in order to get the needed information.

TABLE 46-2
Guide for Rapid History Taking in the Event of Injury

1. History of present illness or injury
2. A description of pain (if present)
3. Pertinent past medical history
4. Current medication
5. Allergies
6. Age
7. Weight (most mothers know this)
8. Immunization history

Assessment for Possible Child Abuse/Neglect

Assessment for an injured child should be approached with an alertness for possible child abuse or neglect. It is essential that health care workers carry an index of suspicion when assessing families to identify injury by abuse. Indicators of physical abuse, neglect, and psychologic maltreatment are discussed in Chapter 28 and summarized in Tables 28-7, 28-8, and 28-9, respectively. Indicators of sexual abuse can be found in Tables 28-10 and 28-11.

It is important to remember that adults who abuse their children come from all socioeconomic, religious, and ethnic groups and have various levels of education. Although the lay person may believe child abuse is confined to the less economically advantaged, this may only appear to be so because abused children from lower socioeconomic status may come to the attention of authorities more readily. It is mandatory for the nurse to respond to a beginning suspicion by taking a more thorough history and following up with the appropriate reporting process, irrespective of socioeconomic status of the family.

An important indicator is the inability of parents to give a satisfactory explanation for an injury. If the parents or caregivers offer an explanation that is incompatible with the developmental stage of the child, the nurse must pursue the description of the mechanism of injury further. For example, if a child with extensive bruising on both front and back of body is reported to have fallen down stairs or if the date of a reported fall does not match the estimated age of a bruise (i.e., there was a delay between the time of injury and the time of seeking medical attention), further data gathering is essential. Inconsistent reports are often elicited if the child and parent are interviewed separately or if the parents change the details of the history or are vague about the incident. When a story raises a professional's suspicion that a child may have been abused, it is important to keep communication channels open. Table 46-3 provides some basic principles for use in dealing with potentially abusive caretakers. (See Chapter 28 for further discussion of the care of the abused child and family.)

Impact of Injury on Child and Family

Children depend on adults to protect them from danger and physical harm, yet many injuries occur because a guardian or caretaker momentarily fails to

TABLE 46-3
Principles of Interviewing When Assessing the Potentially Abused Child

1. Elicit exact information about the injury including time, place, sequence of events, and who was present
2. Use open-ended questions (e.g., "How was your child injured?" rather than "Was this injury an accident?")
3. Encourage questions from the parents
4. Do not approach the family with a judgmental attitude, because rejection and criticism will result in withdrawal by the parent and stop communication
5. Never *accuse* the parent of abuse. Mandated agencies have the responsibility to investigate and determine whether a child has been abused
6. Respond to the feelings of the child
7. Interview parent and child separately when appropriate

provide supervision appropriate to the circumstance and the child's developmental level. Lack of information, preoccupation with personal matters, family stress, tension between parents, and the time of day are major factors that influence the incidence of injuries.

When a child is injured, a careful analysis of the factors leading to the injury can provide important information in understanding the feelings of the parents. The child's and parents' responses are also affected by the child's age, parent-child relationship, circumstances surrounding the event, and the type and severity of injury. Sibling relationships should also be assessed because other children in the family may represent important parts of the family structure. Siblings are often neglected in the flurry of activity and emotional upheaval during the initial stages of treatment of the injured child.

It is a frightening experience for a child to be injured and then be rapidly taken for emergency care to a threatening environment. A child has difficulty interpreting the extent of the injury but tends to fantasize the worst. Separation from parents, pain, and intrusive procedures compound the terror of the experience. Chapters 18, 21, and 25 further discuss the impact of procedures and hospitalization on children.

Regardless of age and situation, stressors for parents include (1) fear and uncertainty about the child's prognosis; (2) a degree of guilt and feeling "if only I would have" or "if only I would not have"; (3) an overwhelming concern for the child's immediate condition; (4) a strong desire to be with their child to alleviate fear and bring comfort; and (5) anger at another person for "allowing" the injury to occur. These feelings are magnified in life-threatening situations, but exist even when minor injuries occur.

An injured child often requires intensive care for a period of time. In an intensive care situation, Rothstein (1980) found that parents initially experienced overwhelming shock and disbelief, accompanied by a sense of helplessness and guilt. Factors that intensified the state of shock were the child's unstable condition, the complexity of therapy, and the child's physical appearance. After stabilization of the child was apparent, the initial shock experienced by parents was replaced by a phase of "anticipatory waiting." It is during this phase that long-term effects and outcomes are of concern to parents, and they may become demanding of staff, expressing feelings of anger, guilt, and helplessness.

When a child is injured, the procedures and immediacy of care that are required to save the child also affect the family's ability to cope with the situation. The threatening appearance of the environment increases the parents' perception of the severity of the child's injury. Although it is necessary to direct all energy to the care of a critically ill child, after the emergency state has resolved attention must be given to the parents (or guardians). An informed parent who is included as much as possible in caring for the child and making decisions about the child's care will be more relaxed and supportive than one who is not. A calm parent usually means a more relaxed and cooperative child. Support of the child and family during acute illness is further discussed in Chapter 18.

Nursing Care

An injured child may or may not survive, depending on the type and degree of injury. Survival and quality of life often depend on the accuracy and speed with which care is delivered. Some of the special skills required of the nurse are triage, cardiopulmonary resuscitation (CPR), Pediatric Advanced Life Support (PALS) techniques, management of an obstructed airway, transport of the patient, care of the parents, and documentation.

Triage

The word "triage" comes from the French verb meaning "to sort." The concept was first applied to health care in disaster situations in an attempt to ensure that the most seriously ill or injured patients—who *also* stood the best chance of survival if they were promptly treated—were treated first. Triage decisions are made by assessing the severity of a condition and the potential outcome of treatment. The concept of sorting is applied in any situation in which several ill or injured persons must be cared for simultaneously. The emergency room department of a hospital is the most common health care setting where triage is used. It is usually based on established protocols or algorithms.

Today, triage represents a complex process of problem solving and planning that involves the entire health care team including the ambulance dispatcher, emergency medical technicians (EMTs), nurses, and physicians. The process depends not only on the needs of the patient but also on the availability of services. Therefore, a critically injured child may be triaged by an EMT as needing immediate transport to a hospital, triaged by the ambulance dispatcher to the nearest facility, triaged by the nurse in the emergency room so that the child is seen immediately by the physician, and triaged after stabilization by transport to an intensive care pediatric facility.

The skills required to perform triage are similar to the assessment skills required by any nurse in any setting. The uniqueness of triage is the speed with which an assessment must be made. The main focus of the subjective assessment is (1) history of the present illness or injury, (2) pertinent past medical history, (3) allergies and medications, and (4) immunization.

Objective assessment focuses primarily on (1) general appearance, (2) vital signs, and (3) a localized examination. After an initial assessment is made, a category is assigned, usually ranging from I to IV. This category reflects the severity of the patient's condition.

Cardiopulmonary Resuscitation

Infants and children who require CPR rarely have suffered a *primary cardiac* arrest in which cardiac pathology is the primary cause (Standards and Guidelines for Cardiopulmonary Resuscitation [CPR] and Emergency Cardiac Care [ECC], Part IV, 1986). A *respiratory* arrest is usually the preceding event. An understanding of how this affects the child's condition is important. First, it means that the child who has suffered a cardiac arrest has usually been hypoxic for some time. Therefore, resuscitation attempts (particularly in out-of-hospital arrests) are usually less successful in children than in adults. Second, many events that trigger a respiratory arrest may go unnoticed long enough to cause hypoxia. Recognition of hypoxia in its early phase may make it possible to intercept the need for CPR. Tachycardia, hyperpnea, exertional dyspnea, altered level of consciousness, restlessness, anxiety, and aggressive behavior are changes that the nurse should recognize as signs and symptoms of hypoxia in the pediatric patient. The nurse must be aware that the presence of cyanosis is considered a late sign in children and usually indicates impending cardiovascular collapse.

Pediatric nurses have an obligation to take courses and maintain proficiency in pediatric basic life support. Nurses who are employed in acute care settings should also be proficient in advanced pediatric life support techniques. Regular mock cardiac arrest drills are an excellent means of practice and review. CPR performance for the infant and child is summarized in Table 46–4 and illustrated in Figure

TABLE 46-4
Sequence of Cardiopulmonary Resuscitation (CPR)*

Sequence:

	1. Determine unresponsiveness or respiratory difficulty†
	2. Call for help†
	3. Position the victim†
A. { Airway	4. *Open the airway*
B. { Breathing	5. *Determine whether victim is breathing*
	6. *Breathe for the victim*
C. { Circulation	7. *Check the pulse*
	8. Activate the emergency medical service (EMS) system
	9. Perform chest compressions
	10. Coordinate compressions and rescue breathing

Activity	Infants (Under 1 Yr of Age)	Children (1–8 Yrs of Age)	Children (Over 8 Yrs of Age or Adults)
1. Determine unresponsiveness			
• Assess for head and neck trauma and avoid injury of spinal cord	Flick heels	Gently shake and shout. Call name	Same as for child 1–8 yrs of age
• Transport immediately if child is conscious but struggling to breathe			
• Permit child to assume position of comfort during transport			
2. Call for help			
• If rescuer is alone and child is not breathing, perform CPR for 1 min, then call for help		(No variation)	
• If unresponsive or in respiratory difficulty call for help			

TABLE 46-4
Sequence of Cardiopulmonary Resuscitation (CPR)* *(Continued)*

Activity	Infants (Under 1 Yr of Age)	Children (1–8 Yrs of Age)	Children (Over 8 Yrs of Age or Adults)
3. Position the victim			
• Place victim on back on a firm, flat surface if CPR is necessary • Move carefully if there is head or neck injury • Turn child as unit with firm support of head and neck		(No variation)	
4. *Open the airway*			
• After victim is in supine position use a head-tilt chin-lift maneuver (hand is placed on victim's forehead to tilt head into a sniffing position; fingers of other hand are placed on bony part of lower jaw and chin is lifted upward) • Head should not be tilted in suspected neck injury • Jaw-thrust is used when neck injury is suspected (two or three fingers are placed under each side of the lower jaw at its angle and the jaw is lifted upward; this requires two hands)		(No variation)	
5. *Determine whether victim is breathing*			
• Look, listen, feel, for evidence of respirations for 3–5 secs (look for chest and abdominal movement, listen and feel for exhaled air) • If victim is breathing, rescuer should summon help and ensure that airway is maintained • If victim is not breathing rescue breathing is initiated		(No variation)	
6. *Breathe for the victim*			
• Give 2 breaths • Pause between these two breaths to allow for exhalation (each of these 2 breaths should be 1–1.5 secs in length)	Position: Rescuer's mouth is placed over infant's nose and mouth	Rescuer's mouth is placed over child's mouth; nose is pinched slightly with fingers of hand doing head-tilt	Same as for child 1–8 yrs of age
• For subsequent breaths, the rate varies with age • If chest does not rise with breaths, adjust head-tilt chin-lift or suspect foreign body aspiration • Volume of breath should be the least amount of pressure that causes chest to rise to avoid gastric distention	Rate: 20/min	15/min	12/min

(continued)

TABLE 46-4
Sequence of Cardiopulmonary Resuscitation (CPR)* *(Continued)*

Activity	Infants (Under 1 Yr of Age)	Children (1–8 Yrs of Age)	Children (Over 8 Yrs of Age or Adults)
7. *Check the pulse* If a pulse cannot be palpated, chest compressions must be initated and coordinated with rescue breathing	Brachial (because chubby neck makes carotid less accessible): Brachial is palpated by placing index and middle fingers inside of upper arm between elbow and shoulder	Carotid: Locate Adam's apple, then slide fingers to groove between trachea and neck muscles	Same as for child 1–8 yrs of age
8. Activate the emergency medical service (EMS) system If rescuer cannot activate the EMS system, the only option is to continue with CPR			
9. Perform chest compressions • Chest compression must always be accompanied by rescue breathing • Sternum is allowed to return to its normal position between compressions *without removing* fingers (infant) or hand (child/adult) from the sternum • Compression and relaxation phase of each cycle should have equal time	Location: *One fingerbreadth below nipple line on sternum* • Draw an imaginary line joining nipples • Place index finger next on the sternum immediately below the line • Place middle and ring fingers immediately below index finger • Compress chest at level where middle and ring finger are placed (i.e., one finger's width below the imaginary line) • Other hand may be used to support infant's back • Compress 0.5–1 in at a rate of at least 100/min	Location: *One fingerbreadth above costal-sternal notch in sternum* • Locate rib cage with index and middle finger • Follow margin of rib cage to notch where rib cage meets sternum • Place middle finger on notch • Place index finger onto lower end of sternum next to middle finger • Place heel of other hand onto sternum below index finger, with long axis of heel parallel to the sternum • Compress chest (with one hand) 1–1.5 in at a rate of 80–100/min	Location: (same as for child) • Follow steps as for child but place hand that was used to locate notch on top of hand on sternum so that both hands are parallel • Fingers may be either extended or interlaced but must be kept off chest • Rescuer's elbows are locked into position, arms are straightened, and shoulders are positioned directly over the hands • Each thrust is therefore straight down on the sternum • Compress 1.5–2 in at 80–100/min
10. Coordinate compressions and rescue breathing When there are two rescuers a pause should be allowed after each five compressions for a ventilation (1.0–1.5 sec/breath)	Ratio of 5:1 compressions: ventilation is maintained for one or two rescuers. Assess after 10 cycles (i.e., approximately 1 min) of compressions and ventilations, and every few minutes thereafter	Same as for infants	One rescuer: Ratio of 15:2 compressions: ventilations (after four cycles of compressions and ventilations [15:2 ratio] pause to reassess) Two rescuers: Ratio of 5:1 compressions: ventilations (assess patient after first minute of CPR and every few minutes thereafter)

Standards and Guidelines for Cardiopulmonary Resuscitation (CPR) and Emergency Cardiac Care (ECC). (1986). Adapted from *Journal of the American Medical Association, 268,* 2184–2198. Copyright 1992, American Medical Association.

*This table is not a substitute for a BLS-approved CPR course.

†In practice, the first three steps occur rapidly and almost simultaneously with airway opening. The A (airway), B (breathing), and C (circulation) of resuscitation provide the guideline for sequence of action.

46-1. The American Heart Association has developed, through years of research, the standards that constitute the basic and advanced pediatric life support protocol. Preparation and monitored practice are essential to their safe performance. The reader is referred to the *Textbook of Pediatric Advanced Life Support,* published jointly by the American Heart Association and the American Academy of Pediatrics (Chameides, 1988), and to the reports of the 1992 National Conference on CPR and Emergency Cardiac Care (ECC) (1992, 1993). Information about courses can be obtained through either the local AHA office or the pediatrics departments of university teaching hospitals.

Neonatal resuscitation is a highly specialized activity. Only experienced, well-trained personnel should attempt this, as the size of the infant and the need for expert intervention demand immediate reac-

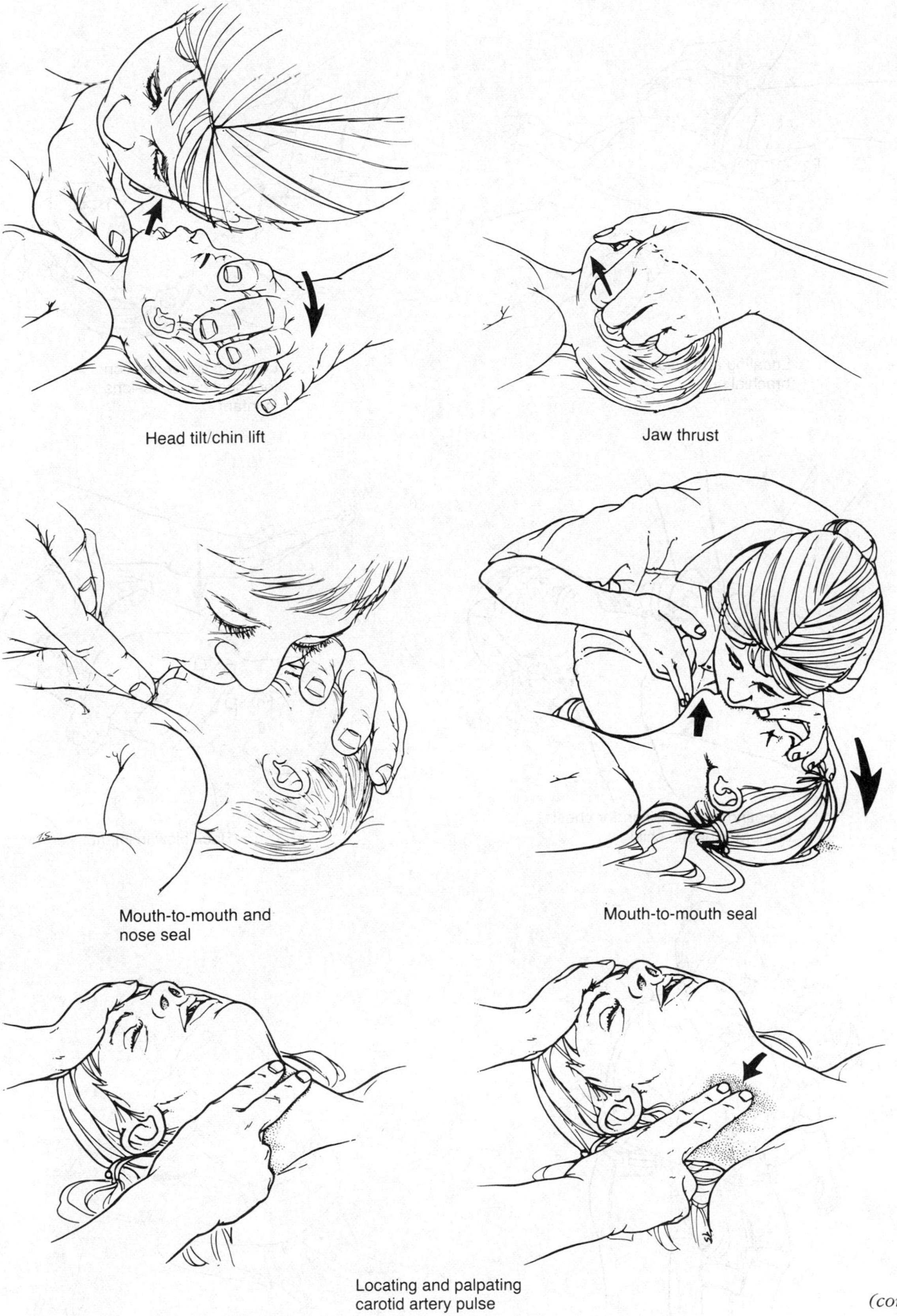

(continued)

FIGURE 46 - 1. Pediatric basic life support. (From Standards and Guidelines for Cardiopulmonary Resuscitation [CPR] and Emergency Cardiac Care [ECC] [1992]. *Journal of the American Medical Association, 268,* 2184–2198. Copyright 1992, American Medical Association.)

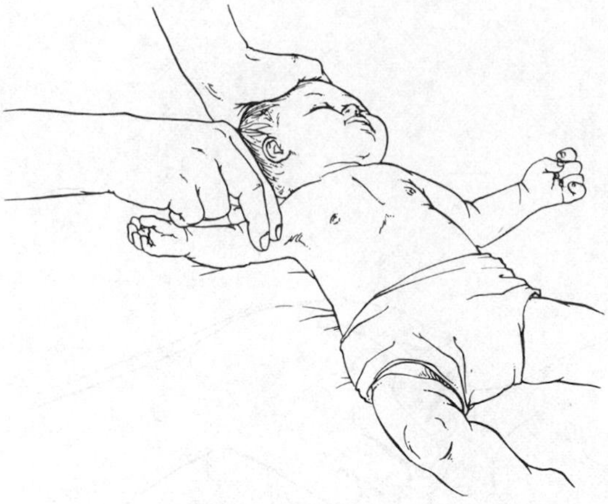

Locating and palpating brachial pulse

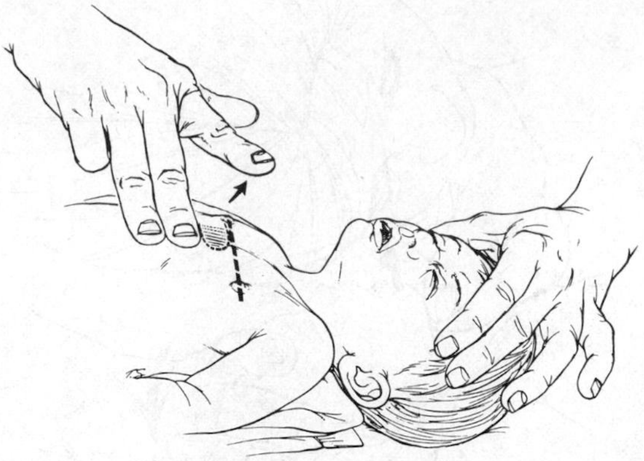

Locating finger position for chest compressions in infant

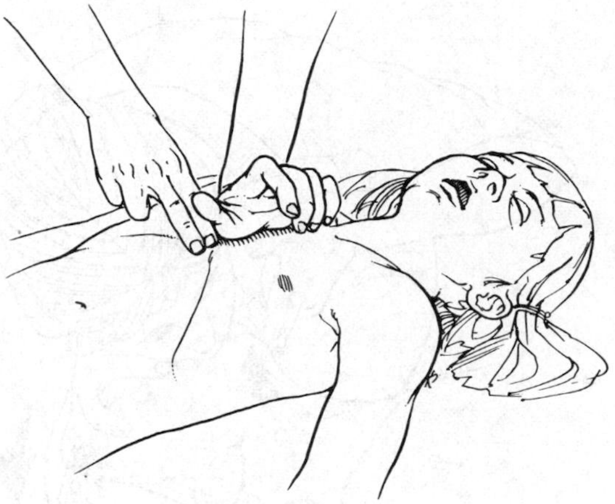

Locating hand position for chest compressions in child

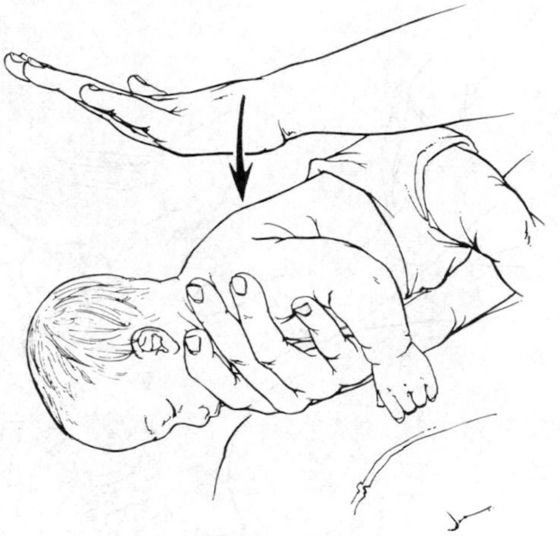

Back blow in infant

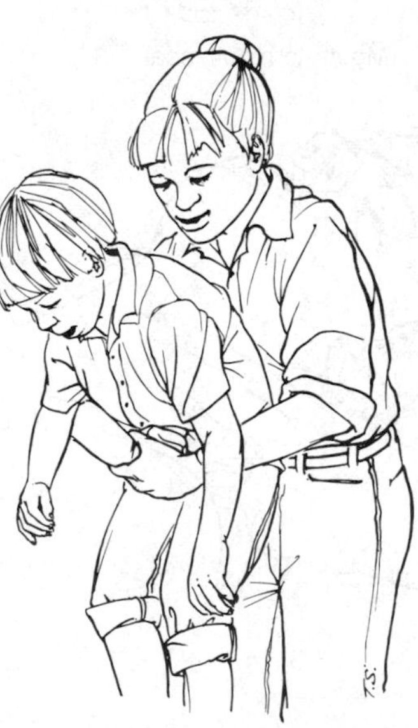

Heimlich maneuver with child standing

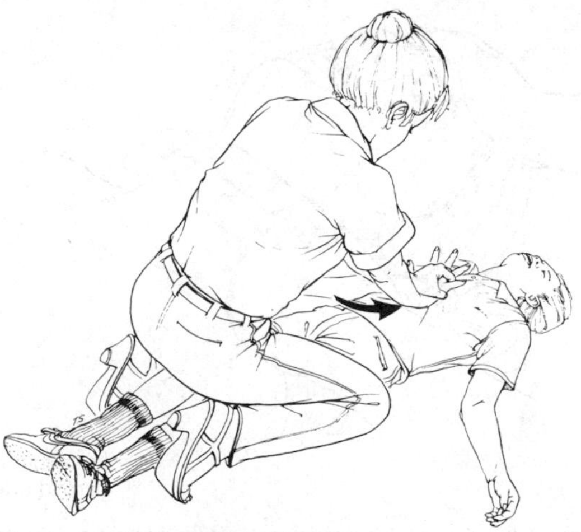

Heimlich maneuver with child lying

FIGURE 46 - 1 *Continued*

tion. The most recently developed guidelines can be found in the *Textbook of Neonatal Resuscitation,* also published by the AHA and AAP.

Management of an Obstructed Airway

Airway obstruction may be caused by aspirated materials or by infections that cause airway swelling. Children with an infectious cause of obstruction need specific emergency care, and time should not be wasted using airway clearance techniques described here. Attempts to clear an airway are made for (1) a child in whom aspiration is witnessed or strongly suspected, and (2) an unconscious, nonbreathing child whose airway remains obstructed after the usual efforts to open it have been made. Foreign body aspiration is suspected in the presence of acute respiratory distress associated with coughing, gagging, or high-pitched noisy breathing (stridor) (Chameides, 1988).

Blind finger sweeps should be avoided because a foreign body may be pushed further into the airway. If the aspiration is witnessed or strongly suspected, the child is encouraged to cough and persist with breathing efforts. Manual relief of obstruction is attempted only if the child's efforts are ineffective and/or if increased signs of respiratory difficulty occur.

In the infant under 1 year of age, a combination of back blows and chest thrusts is recommended. The Heimlich maneuver (subdiaphragmatic abdominal thrusts) is used in adults and children over 1 year of age (see Fig. 46–1). By elevating the diaphragm, air is forced from the lungs. With sufficient air movement, an artificial cough is created, which can expel a foreign body from the airway. Table 46–5 describes techniques used in airway obstruction of infants and children. After performing these forms of emergency treatment, the airway is opened using head-tilt/chin-lift procedures and, if spontaneous breathing is absent, rescue breathing is then performed. In the unconscious patient, the nonbreathing victim's mouth is opened by grasping both the tongue and the lower jaw between the thumb and finger and lifting the tongue and jaw upward. In any patient, if the foreign body is visualized, it should be removed.

Transport

An injured child must often be transported from one facility to a more specialized center of care. Transport from one facility to another is planned and coordinated by both sending and receiving hospitals and should be consistent with current standards of management.

Coordination of the transfer between facilities is a role often assumed by the charge nurse of the emergency department or the intensive care unit; however, the nurse should not attempt this arrangement without first communicating with the attending physician. Children (nor indeed *any* patient) must not be transferred without physician-to-physician contact. As well,

TABLE 46–5
Emergency Treatment of Infants and Children with Airway Obstruction Caused by a Foreign Body

Infant

1. Straddle infant over rescuer's arm (head lower than trunk) and support head by resting jaw in rescuer's hand
2. Rescuer rests forearm on own thigh
3. Deliver four back blows with heel of hand between infant's shoulder blades
4. Turn infant. This is done by keeping one hand on front of infant, supporting neck, jaw, and chest, the other hand supporting back
5. Infant is placed on rescuer's thigh with head lower than trunk
6. Continue to support head and neck, then perform four chest thrusts in the location where external chest compressions are performed (i.e., on sternum one fingerbreadth below imaginary line drawn across nipple line)

Infant—Alternate Method

(If rescuer's hands are small, it may be difficult to perform back blows and chest thrusts as described above)

1. Lay infant face down on rescuer's lap (head lower than trunk), while supporting head
2. Perform four back blows as described above
3. Turn infant as a unit to the supine position, and perform chest thrusts

Child—Heimlich Maneuver with Victim Standing or Sitting

1. Rescuer stands behind the child and wraps arms around child's waist
2. One hand is formed into a fist
3. Rest thumb side of fist against child's abdomen slightly above navel (well below tip of xiphoid process)
4. Grasp fist with other hand and give a quick upward thrust into child's abdomen. Thrust must be at midline and not toward either side
5. The thrust is repeated as needed. Each thrust should be a separate and distinct movement. Thrust must be gentle in small children

Child—Heimlich Maneuver with Victim Lying (Conscious or Unconscious)

1. Position child supine with face up
2. If child is on floor, kneel at child's feet (the astride position is not used for small children but can be used for older children); if child is on table, stand at child's feet
3. Place heel of hand on child's abdomen, slightly above navel but well below rib cage
4. Place other hand on top of first hand and press into abdomen with an upward thrust. Thrusts must be at midline and not to either side of the abdomen
5. Thrust is repeated several times as needed. Each thrust should be a separate and distinct movement. Thrust must be gentle in small children

the charge nurses for the sending and receiving hospitals must discuss the nursing interventions that have been carried out already and that will be required during transport to facilitate a smooth transfer for the patient and family. Failure to communicate adequately may result in inadequate care of the patient during transport and does not allow the receiving hospital to prepare properly for the new patient. Aside from the obvious and unnecessary disruptions in care, poor communication may frustrate and upset already distraught parents who may feel that their child is not a priority to anyone. Reestablishing a trusting relationship with them then proves to be very difficult. A transfer that is organized and operates as smoothly as possible transmits a sense of concern for the child's well-being.

The nurse is responsible for collecting the appropriate documentation to accompany the child. Photocopies of the chart and laboratory data should be made. A detailed history of the incident causing injury should be provided. Copies of all radiographs are to be sent as well.

The choice of appropriate personnel to accompany the child is made by the physician and charge nurse. A severely ill or injured child may need to be accompanied by a physician and a nurse. Ideally, a respiratory therapist should go if the child is intubated; however, not all community hospitals can spare this resource for a transfer. If sent alone, a nurse should be carefully chosen on the basis of experience and ability to respond quickly to a change in the patient's status. A nurse should go alone *only if* he or she is specially trained in pediatric emergency care. Written orders accompany the patient to cover the nurse during the transfer. The referring hospital is legally responsible for the patient until arrival at the receiving hospital and care is assumed by that institution. The nurse accompanying the patient practices according to the policies and procedures of his or her employing institution (e.g., taking the vital signs every 15 minutes; assessing airway, breathing, and circulation) and documents the assessments.

Some large centers have their own transport teams who will come to the referring facility and assist in stabilization of the patient there; they then take the responsibility for the child's care during transfer. This is done by land ambulance or air transport. Advantages of helicopters include avoiding heavy road traffic and rapid transport with trained personnel to regionalized specialty facilities.

An important task involved in transfer is preparation of the parents. Usually, they are in a state of shock and despair over their child's injury. They may feel guilty that the child has been hurt so badly. The child's transfer needs to be presented in a positive way. The expertise of the receiving facility should be stressed to them. Usually, the ambulance personnel will allow one parent to accompany the child while the other follows. The nurse should encourage the parent to have a family member or friend drive them since a distraught parent may not be able to drive safely. This has the advantage of providing the receiving facility with someone who can offer detailed information about the child's past medical history and presenting event. If possible, the nurse who has been caring for the child should accompany the child, not only to provide continuity of care but also to give support to the parents. Even though their association may have been brief, the parents may already trust and depend on this nurse.

Care of Parents

Although most busy emergency rooms and intensive care units have "quiet rooms" available for families of critically ill patients, these rooms are frequently in high demand. Whenever possible, the nurse should find a less distracting area in which to interview a parent. Attempts should be made to stay with the parent(s). A social worker, minister, or volunteer with special training should also be called on as resources.

Because of the invasive nature of many emergency treatments, parents may or may not be permitted to be with their child, depending on the policy of the institution, the type of treatment being initiated, the ability of the parents to cope, and the severity of injury. Pediatric centers generally are supportive of parents' presence during treatment and recognize the benefits for both child and family. If a parent is not able to cope with staying at the child's side, she or he should be supported in the decision to wait in a waiting room. Parents should be informed of the progress of treatment and should be reunited with their child as soon as possible.

When a child is seriously ill and parents are not permitted in the room while treatment is initiated, or if parents arrive later than the child, they should be prepared for the child's appearance—for example, many tubes, presence of blood, or unresponsiveness. Whenever possible, the nurse actually caring for the child should accompany the parents to the room and stay with them to provide support and answer their questions, while continuing to care for their child. Parents are encouraged to touch and talk to their child even if the child is unresponsive.

Documentation

Documentation is essential when dealing with seriously ill or injured children. Because they may be transferred from one unit to another or from one facility to another rapidly, good documentation will provide consistency of care. The importance of this nursing responsibility cannot be overstated. Important trends may be missed if data such as vital signs, medications, intravenous fluids, urinary output, and behavioral responses to treatment are not charted accurately. Also, for those situations in which legal charges are made, nurses may be subpoenaed to give evidence during court proceedings. Specific information that Rund and Rausch (1981) recommend for documentation includes

- Patient identification.
- Time of arrival.
- Method of arrival.
- History of the chief complaint.
- Physical findings, including the patient's vital signs.
- Emergency care given prior to arrival.
- Diagnostic and therapeutic orders.
- Clinical assessments including results of treatment.
- Documentation of tests and procedures done.
- Results of procedures and tests.
- Diagnostic impression.
- Final disposition.
- Patient's condition on discharge.
- Any instructions given.
- Follow-up plan.
- Whether patient leaves against medical advice.

Descriptions of a child's clothing, use of car safety restraints, parental responses to their children, and the child's physical and emotional responses to treatment may also be relevant and, in some cases, may have important legal ramifications.

TABLE 46-6
Family-Centered Teaching: What To Do about Cuts, Scrapes, and Puncture Wounds

Reassure your child

Examine the wound

- A wound <1 inch long and ¼ inch deep usually does not require stitches unless it is a facial cut; even then, stitches may be more traumatic than a small scar
- A wound with straight, clean edges that can be held together with tape likely does not need stitches

Cleanse the wound

- Plain, warm, soapy running water is often the best cleaning solution
- Scrub gently to remove gravel and dirt from a scrape or they will "tattoo" the skin permanently when it heals

"Dress" the wound

- Band-Aids
- Clean gauze pads

Check your child's immunization status

- Call or see your family doctor if you are unsure

Common Childhood Injuries

Children who sustain minor injuries may not necessarily seek medical care in a health care setting. Counsel may be sought by telephone to determine the correct course of action to be taken at home. Injuries that are common to children, included in this section, are cuts, scrapes, and puncture wounds; insect stings and bites; snake and mammalian bites; and injuries caused by environmental exposure including excessive cold (frostbite) and excessive rays of the sun (sunburn). Although some of these injuries are not necessarily life-threatening, hypersensitivity to the agent and inadequate care can have serious consequences. The nurse's telephone counsel and early assessment and management have an impact on the child's recovery. The hurt and discomfort to the child, even in minor injuries such as cuts and scrapes, should not be overlooked. Children often have had little previous experience with pain. Furthermore, caretakers are anxious about their child's pain and fears and need the support and comfort of an understanding nurse.

Cuts, Scrapes, and Puncture Wounds

Anyone who cares for injured children will soon recognize the dramatic effects that the sight of blood has on a young child (Table 46-6). A thorough inspection of the wound is usually made by the child to determine whether it is bleeding. It should be recognized that, even though a wound is minor, a child may respond to the sight of blood with terror; therefore, getting a wound cleaned and covered as quickly as possible is important to make the child feel comfortable and safe. Acknowledging the child's fears rather than negating them will also be supportive. The overall goals in the care of these injuries are to (1) reduce the fear of the child, (2) control the bleeding, (3) minimize pain by appropriate and gentle cleansing, (4) prevent contamination and infection, and (5) assess current immunization status and inoculate accordingly. Various types of wounds and their management are summarized in Table 46-7.

Insect Stings and Bites

The incidence of specific bites and stings varies according to geographic areas. Each year approximately 40 to 50 deaths are reported to be caused by insect stings (Mayer, 1985). Children may be affected by having a local reaction of pain and erythema at the site of the sting, or they may have a systemic reaction causing anaphylaxis. Some snakes and spiders are poisonous; however, most are not. Regardless of the type of sting or bite, most are painful and the experience is frightening to a child. A familiarity with the most common and potentially serious bites and stings is necessary for appropriate management and prevention of fatal outcomes (Table 46-8). The allergic reaction is described in greater detail in Chapter 37.

Snake Bites

Most of the snakes in the United States are not poisonous. An average of 10 deaths occurring annually

TABLE 46-7
Types of Wounds and First-Aid Treatment

Abrasions or scrapes: Loss of skin surface without penetration; there may be pinhead-sized openings with fluid or blood oozing	Area is washed with soap and water or a mild (nonirritating) antiseptic solution. Small bits of dirt can be picked out with sterile tweezers or wound can be flushed with normal saline solution. A child's cooperation is gained if they can do some of it themselves, as appropriate. A nonadherent dressing is applied for 24 hrs
Lacerations: Smooth or jagged cuts penetrating the skin and blood vessels	Area is washed with soap and water or mild antiseptic. If sides can be easily approximated and held together, a Steri-Strip dressing may be used. If it is deep and gaping, sutures are required. To prevent scarring, suturing should be done within 6 hrs. Facial lacerations may require the expertise of a plastic surgeon for repair
Punctures: Penetration of the skin with a sharp object such as a nail or tooth, causing a small hole in the skin (usually produces very little bleeding)	Area is washed with soap and water or mild antiseptic solution. A tetanus booster is administered if the child has not received one in the previous 5-yr period

TABLE 46-8
Prevention, Identification, and Treatment of Insect Bites and Stings

Agent	Identification/Clinical Signs	Prevention	Management
Mosquito bite	Insect penetrates skin to suck blood. During this process the insect's saliva containing a foreign protein is injected. This causes swelling, itchiness, and papules. It can cause an allergic reaction in the hypersensitive	Apply insect repellent when potential for bites is anticipated	Apply cool compresses or give cool bath to reduce swelling. Calamine lotion for itching. Antihistamines if sleep is interrupted
Hornet, wasp, honey bee (bumble bee), yellow jacket (hymenoptera)	Venom is injected through a stinger. It contains histamine and foreign proteins that cause redness, swelling, tenderness, and itching. Systemic reactions cause generalized edema with possible nausea and vomiting, respiratory difficulty, and shock	Wear shoes and clothing that cover extremities if in area where insects may be present. Avoid insect breeding areas (e.g., flower beds, orchards). Hypersensitive children should be gradually desensitized to minimize future reactions	Carefully remove stinger (yellow jacket does not leave stinger embedded). Flick or scrape it away rather than pinching it to avoid squeezing out more venom. Wash with soap and water promptly. Prompt use of epinephrine for anaphylaxis. Application of cool compresses or use of antipruritic lotion may be comforting. A meat tenderizer paste made with a few drops of water is recommended for painful stings. It contains proteolytics that reduce inflammation and edema (Gaunder, 1986)
Ticks and mites	Ticks are brown or gray; mites are colorless, red, or dark and are microscopic. Ticks live on dogs or in the woods. They can carry Rocky Mountain spotted fever, Q fever, and tularemia. Mites, the most common being the chigger, live in tall grass and underbrush. Ticks and mites cause local itching. Chiggers (mites) cause papules that are usually concentrated where clothing is snug. Ticks become partially embedded in the skin and feel like a tiny bump and skin becomes red and swollen. Some ticks (Rocky Mountain wood tick and Eastern dog tick) can cause a flaccid motor paralysis that can be fatal	Use of insect repellent on clothes and on ankles and legs repels chiggers. Careful inspection of child, clothes, and family dog after an outing in the woods	Mites are treated with antipruritic agents. Starch baths and topical anesthetics for severe pruritus. Ticks are removed as follows: 1. Apply Vaseline, oil, nail polish, or alcohol to suffocate tick, or apply heat (e.g., heated needle) to body of tick, causing head to withdraw 2. Remove tick with tweezers 3. Wash area with soap and water. If any part of tick is left in body, tick paralysis may occur

TABLE 46-8
Prevention, Identification, and Treatment of Insect Bites and Stings *(Continued)*

Agent	Identification/Clinical Signs	Prevention	Management
Black widow spider (venom is neurotoxic, causing central nervous system reactions)	Venom is potent and fangs are powerful; therefore, they can endanger a child's life. Spider is black with a red spot (hourglass shape) on the ventral side and some red spots on back. Causes a puncture point that is red with edema, pruritus, and swelling around wound. Venom enters blood stream in 30 mins causing dizziness, weakness, tremors, nausea and vomiting, abdominal rigidity, and cramps with rapid shallow respirations	Do not disturb web, and avoid areas such as wood piles where they thrive	Cleanse wound. Intramuscular injection of antivenin for severe cases. Muscle relaxant (calcium gluconate), narcotics, and prolonged warm bath to relieve pain. If treated with antivenin, patient should be observed closely for anaphylaxis
Brown recluse spider (venom is coagulotoxic, causing localized vasoconstriction)	Found in central and southern US. Yellowish to reddish-brown. Has violin-shaped marking on its back. Venom is necrotoxic and causes mild stinging at time of bite. In 2–4 hrs, pain occurs. Development of an indurated wheal, followed by a star shaped area in 3–4 days and eventually in 7–14 days a deep sloughing ulcer forms	Avoid crushing or entangling them because it causes them to bite	Administration of corticosteroids may hasten healing of the wound. Tetanus prophylaxis is considered in nonhealing lesions
Scorpion	Found mainly in the southwestern US. Venom of some species causes only local reaction, and in others it is neurotoxic. The neurotoxic species causes intense aching pain followed by "pins and needles" sensation. Itching of the nose, mouth, and throat occurs. There is an ascending motor paralysis with convulsions, rapid weak pulse, nausea and vomiting, excessive salivation, thirst, and dysuria	Wear shoes to avoid stepping on a scorpion	Spread of venom from site of sting can be slowed by applying a temporary tourniquet with momentary releases and cooling with ice packs. The wound should not be excised. Antivenin is available in most countries where the more dangerous species exist. Supportive measures include pain relief, treatment of shock, seizure control. Morphine and its derivatives are contraindicated because they act synergistically with scorpion venom. Deaths occur from scorpion stings, especially in children under 4 yrs of age

Data from Behrman, R. F. (Ed.). (1992). *Nelson textbook of pediatrics* (14th ed.). Philadelphia: WB Saunders; Dreisbach, R. H. (1983). *Handbook of poisoning: Prevention, diagnosis, and treatment.* Los Altos, CA: Lange Medical Publications; Gaunder, B. N. (1986, March). Insect bites and stings: Managing allergic reactions. *Nurse Practitioner, 11,* 16–28; Reece, R. M. (1984). Manual of emergency pediatrics (3rd ed.). Philadelphia: WB Saunders; and Tenenbein, M. (1986, April). Pediatric toxicology: Current controversies and recent advances. *Current Problems in Pediatrics, 16,* 1–233.

in the United States are caused by snake bites—usually by rattlesnakes, cottonmouths, or coral snakes; however, 6000 to 7000 patients receive antiserum (Dreisbach, 1983). Worldwide, deaths are estimated at 30,000 to 40,000 per year. Of all the snake bites that occur in the United States, 50 per cent occur in those under 19 years of age (Mayer, 1985). Snakes with poisonous venom are of two families: Crotalidae (pit viper) family and Elapidae family. Of these, only pit vipers (including rattlesnakes, copperheads, and cottonmouths) and coral snakes reside in the continental United States. Snake venom contains enzymes, proteins, and polypeptides. The venom from pit vipers (rattlesnakes, copperheads, and cottonmouths) causes breakdown of red blood cells and certain proteins, whereas the venom of the coral snake and of other Elapids is neurotoxic. The initial symptoms are immediate burning pain and erythema around the bite. Pit viper venom results in a more pronounced local reaction, whereas coral snake bites have a less pronounced immediate local reaction but have a delayed systemic reaction.

All snake bite victims should be treated as an emergency until established otherwise. Immediate care of a child with a poisonous snake bite is as follows:

1. Reassure and calm the child and parents.
2. Maintain the involved extremity in a depen-

dent position (below the heart) and immobilize as much as possible.

3. Cleanse bite area with soap and water or a mild antiseptic.

4. Apply cool compresses to bite area, but avoid using ice packs.

5. Use of a tourniquet is not recommended (Kinney et al, 1988).

6. Excision and suction outside of a medical facility is used only when transport to medical care exceeds 45 minutes. It should be done by a trained person.

On reaching a medical facility, the child is reassessed to determine whether the bite was from a venomous snake. Identification and management of the most common poisonous snake bites are summarized in Table 46–9.

Animal Bites

Household pets can cause serious injury to a child. The most common serious bite is that which is inflicted by a dog. It is important to recognize that fewer than 25 per cent of dog bites involve stray dogs. Therefore, education of children regarding the proper way to handle a family pet or neighborhood dog is of primary importance. Children are attacked on the face and upper extremities because of the usual close range at which they play with an animal (see Chapter 15 for prevention of dog bites).

Dog bite wounds are considered to be highly contaminated and require thorough cleansing, irrigating, débridement, and closure. Primary or secondary closure may be done, depending on the length of time since the injury and the location of the injury. Bites (except of the hand) seen within several hours after injury can be closed after adequate irrigation and débridement. Lacerations of the face may be closed up to 6 to 8 hours after the bite took place. If the bite is potentially disfiguring, then a plastic surgeon is consulted. The need for tetanus prophylaxis is dictated by the child's immunization status and by the severity of the bite.

The most feared complication of animal bites is rabies. An unprovoked attack by an animal should raise one's suspicion that the animal is rabid. If the animal is positive for rabies, immunization is begun. (See Chapter 39 for additional information about rabies.) Children who are seriously injured by their family dog need supportive parents and help from professionals to deal with the hurt feelings and anger they harbor toward their previously loved animal. In many cases of serious injury, the child and family can no longer keep the dog in their home, even if the incident involved rough or overaggressive play or teasing of the dog.

Cat bite wounds can cause severe and delayed infection because of the position of the puncture wound incurred by the curved fang. Also, cats, as hunters, may come into contact with other infected animals. As well, cats use their paws for grooming and directly transfer bacteria from the mouth to their paws. The base of the puncture is lateral to the surface puncture. It is difficult to clean and may form a pocket of infection. Parents should be taught to observe the wound for signs of infection (redness, swelling, warmth) and to return the child promptly for medical attention if these occur. Prophylactic antibiotics may be prescribed.

Human Bites

Human bites occur in young children when they play aggressively or become angry, or in older children when a clenched fist strikes another's teeth. They may also occur as a form of child abuse. Human bites are highly contaminated because of the high number of organisms in saliva and are treated with débridement and irrigation, then left open to permit drainage. Broad-spectrum antibiotics are used prophylactically for 5 to 7 days.

Injuries Caused by Environmental Exposure

Developmental characteristics of children make them susceptible to injuries resulting from exposure to certain environments. A child's curiosity, lack of understanding of cause-and-effect relationships, and engrossment in play interfere with a realistic perception of potential danger. Common injuries that result from excessive exposure are frostbite and sunburn.

Frostbite

Frostbite, or tissue freezing, results from exposure to extreme cold. Environmental conditions, including low temperatures, high humidity, and high wind velocity, will increase the rate of heat loss from the body. Children are a high-risk population because most do not comprehend early warning signs of exposure.

There are various degrees of frostbite:

- First-degree frostbite, or a "frost nip," is mild freezing of the epidermis resulting in erythematous skin with edema but no blister formation after rewarming.
- Second-degree frostbite is a partial- or full-thickness injury resulting in erythema with the formation of blisters and bullae after rewarming. Child may experience pain when rewarmed.
- Third-degree frostbite, or deep frostbite, causes necrosis of epidermis, dermis, and subcutaneous tissue; sensation is absent. Child experiences pain on rewarming.

TABLE 46-9
Poisonous Snake Families

Description of Family	Types of Snakes	Geographic Location	Clinical Manifestations	Management: Field Treatment	Management: Hospital Care
Crotalidae family ("pit viper"): So-called because of its fangs and the two indentations, or pits, between eye and snout. Has a triangular head and vertical pupils	*Rattlesnake:* Has "rattle" or tail plates that are noisemakers *Copperhead (or highland moccasin):* Has hourglass-shaped marking *Cottonmouth (or water moccasin):* Has white buccal mucosa and a broad, flat head	All areas of the mainland US. The only poisonous snakes found in Canada Reside from middle New England to northern Florida and from central Illinois to Texas Resides in semiaquatic or aquatic environments (Virginia to Florida and westward to Texas)	Hemotoxic: Local pain, edema, erythema, and ecchymosis in 15–30 mins. Severe local reactions. Formation of hemorrhagic bullae with muscle necrosis not unusual. Systemic manifestations include hemolysis, coagulopathy, and circulatory collapse	The snake should be killed and brought to emergency room if it does not delay treatment of the child. Body part should be immobilized and kept dependent (below heart). Incision and suction are not recommended unless transport time to a hospital exceeds 45 mins (Moyer, 1985). Cool compresses may be applied but cold ice is avoided to avoid further tissue necrosis	Supportive therapy. Antivenin therapy according to patient's condition, preceded by skin testing. Broad-spectrum antibiotics. Tetanus immunization is evaluated and given if needed. Corticosteroids may be used but their use is controversial
Elapidae family: Includes some of the world's deadliest snakes. Have fangs along with their normal teeth	*Eastern coral* (has bands of red, yellow, and black on its body). *Sonoran coral, cobras* (not in the US)	Eastern and Sonoran coral are only members of this family that occur naturally in the US	Neurotoxic: Local pain and erythema may be transient or absent when injected with coral snake venom and systemic symptoms may be delayed; therefore, the seriousness of the bite can be overlooked. Also, fang marks are not as clearly identifiable as in pit viper. Apprehension, nausea and vomiting, excessive salivation, dysphagia, slurred speech, convulsions, and respiratory paralysis may follow	Identification of the coral snake bite may be difficult, so the snake should be killed and brought to the emergency room. Extremity is immobilized, patient is kept at rest and transported	Supportive therapy. Puncture wound is often similar to that of nonpoisonous snakes, the local reaction is less pronounced than the pit viper, and neurotoxic symptoms develop later; therefore, it is more difficult to determine appropriate therapy. Patients with suspected coral snake envenomation are admitted for 48 hrs of observation to monitor for late signs of neurotoxicity. Antivenin therapy is administered according to child's condition, preceded by skin testing. In severe circumstances, life support may be required

Data from Dreisbach, R. H. (1983). *Handbook of poisoning: Prevention, diagnosis, and treatment.* Los Altos, CA: Lange Medical Publications; Reece, R. M. (1984). *Manual of emergency pediatrics* (3rd ed.). Philadelphia: WB Saunders; Mayer, T. A. (1985). *Emergency management of pediatric trauma.* Philadelphia: WB Saunders; Tenenbein, M. (1986, April). Pediatric toxicology: Current controversies and recent advances. *Current Problems in Pediatrics, 16,* 1–233; Behrman, R. F. (Ed.). (1992). *Nelson textbook of pediatrics* (14th ed.). Philadelphia: WB Saunders; and Kinney, M. R., et al (1988). *AACN's clinical reference for critical-care nursing* (2nd ed.). New York: McGraw-Hill.

- Fourth-degree frostbite causes complete necrosis with gangrene and possible loss of body part.

Cold causes arteriolar vasoconstriction, resulting in a decreased blood flow and interference with oxygen transport; tissue anoxia is the end result. With tissue freezing, ice crystals form in the interstitial spaces and draw water from surrounding cells. Cell dehydration and the destruction of intracellular structures results.

School nurses who work in cold climates can help teach parents, children, and schoolteachers how to prevent frostbite. Appropriate outdoor clothing for insulation is essential. Several layers of light clothing under appropriate outerwear provide extra warmth.

Children playing outdoors should wear two pairs of socks, a hood or hat, and mittens or gloves. Clothing layers should not be excessive, to avoid tightness that hinders circulation. Young school-age children should not be allowed to play outside in extremely low temperatures. Older children should be instructed to warm themselves when hands or feet begin to sting.

Blanching of the skin and a stinging sensation are the initial signs of impending frostbite. Numbness will follow and the exposed area will appear white or mottled, feel cold and hard, and be without sensation. Deep frostbite will cause the tissue to blister. The nurse must quickly assess the appearance of the frostbite and institute appropriate first-aid measures to prevent further tissue damage. Any child with white or mottled skin after cold exposure should be referred for medical evaluation and further treatment. During school times, treatment for mild frostbite can be managed by the school nurse.

The child should be placed in a warm place, and the affected part rewarmed gradually by blowing on the part or holding warm hands firmly on the area. Rubbing of the area is avoided because it increases tissue damage. For deeper frostbite, it is essential that the part be rapidly rewarmed; slow thawing causes further tissue damage because some refreezing of tissue occurs. Rewarming should continue until circulation has been reestablished; that is, a flushed appearance of the skin (Gage & Gage, 1981). Large blisters form within 24 to 48 hours after rewarming. In 5 to 10 days, the formation of eschar takes place.

A child who is close to medical facilities should be transported at the time of injury, keeping the part frozen. In isolated areas, rapid rewarming in a water bath (90° to 106° F) should be done prior to transport. Because the pain associated with rewarming can be severe, analgesics and sedatives are usually required. It is imperative to avoid refreezing the affected area during transport. Children with severe frostbite will need to be hospitalized and receive long-term treatment similar to that for the burn victim.

Support for the child with mild frostbite should include a discussion as to why it is essential to rewarm the affected part. Stinging sensations may be frightening to children, and it is important for the nurse to explain the normalcy of these sensations. Parents may feel guilty about allowing their child to play outside; therefore, it is important to allow parents to express feelings and then to focus on preventive measures. Siblings should also be included in a discussion of prevention and appropriate first aid measures.

Sunburn

Overexposure to ultraviolet light waves, either from the sun or from the artificial rays of a sunlamp, can result in a burn. An important role of the nurse is to teach parents and children how to prevent sunburn. Sunburn prevention and treatment are discussed in Chapter 38.

Dental Injuries

Injury to teeth or complete avulsion of a tooth is a common injury during the active childhood years. Boys are more prone to dental injuries of this type than are girls (Henry, 1991), probably because of the more aggressive nature of boys' play (Table 46–10).

Diagnostic Assessment

Children with dental injuries who are brought to the emergency room usually do not require subsequent hospitalization for their injury. A detailed history of the injury is obtained to rule out head injury. Any injury that produced a loss of consciousness should alert the nurse to perform a neurologic assessment, and hospitalization should be considered. If the child can be discharged, the parents should be instructed in monitoring the child for any signs and symptoms of diminishing neurologic status.

Therapeutic Management

Referral to a dentist for treatment is the appropriate course of action. When a tooth is avulsed, it is important to preserve the tooth and replant it as quickly as possible. When replantation takes place within 30 minutes, the prognosis is favorable. A tooth can be replanted into the tooth's original socket using the following guidelines (Krasner, 1990):

1. Hold the tooth by the crown. Avoid touching the root.
2. Rinse the tooth in saline solution or tap water (cover drain).
3. *Replant the tooth as soon as possible.* Insert into the empty socket.
4. Have patient bite on gauze to stabilize tooth.
5. Have patient seen by a dentist so tooth can be stabilized.

TABLE 46-10
Family-Centered Teaching: What to Do If a Tooth is Knocked Out

Stay calm!

Reassure your child

Locate the tooth

- Handle the tooth gently
- Handle the tooth by its *crown,* not the root
- Do not rinse, rub, scrape, or try to clean the tooth. Leave this for the dentist to do
- Place the tooth in "save-a-tooth" solution or in a cup of milk

Call your dentist immediately

or

Go to your local emergency department if your dentist is unavailable

6. If tooth cannot be replanted, have dentist see patient as soon as possible.

7. The best transport medium for avulsed teeth is a specially formulated pH-balanced cell culture media such as Hank solution. This solution is marketed as a product called "Save-a-Tooth" that is available to parents in pharmacies. In the absence of such a formula, milk can keep an avulsed tooth viable for 2 hours if the milk is kept at 20° C (Krasner, 1990).

Nursing Diagnostic Statements

High risk for aspiration; risk factors:
- *Presence of blood.*
- *Mucus.*
- *Vomitus.*
- *Tooth in mouth during and following injury.*

Altered comfort: pain, related to avulsed tooth.

Anxiety, related to:
- *Injury.*
- *Unfamiliar environment.*

Knowledge deficit, related to home care of child with a dental injury.

Nursing Care

Maintaining Effective Airway. The nurse begins with the ABCs of emergency assessment and ensures that the child has a patent airway. This is particularly important if the tooth cannot be found and/or the child has vomited owing to either distress or potential head injury. Neurologic vital signs are documented as part of the primary assessment and are reassessed until the child is stable. Suction must be available to clear the airway of mucus, blood, and vomitus as required. This is important if the child is unconscious or has a suspected spinal cord injury and is immobilized. If there are no associated injuries, the child may sit up in a chair while being assessed.

Maintaining Comfort. Every effort should be made to provide the child with pain relief. The child's discomfort is enhanced by the fear and anxiety produced by the experience of the accident and the trip to a hospital. The nurse should assess the degree of pain being experienced by the child and request an appropriate medication. Topical local anesthetic agents may suffice, or oral medication such as codeine or acetaminophen can be given. Unless other facial injuries are present, intramuscular or intravenous analgesics are generally not required.

Reducing the Child's and Family's Anxiety. The degree of anxiety experienced by the child and family is associated with the amount of bleeding and number of teeth that are avulsed. Cleaning up the blood from the child's face and hands as quickly as possible is especially important for a young child. A large amount of anxiety experienced has to do with fears associated with losing permanent teeth. Proper care of the avulsed teeth and clear explanations to the child and family about the treatment can reduce some of these fears. A young child may also be fearing reprimand from parents if the accident occurred because of a forbidden activity. A nurse can defuse this fear by encouraging parents and children to talk about what happened and to resolve the feelings associated with the event.

Preparing Child and Family for Discharge. Discharge instructions to the parents should be clear and easy to understand. If follow-up appointments have been made, parents should be given a card stating the dentist's name, address, and phone number and the date and time of the appointment. They should be taught to have the child bite on a wad of moistened gauze if the socket begins to bleed. Pain relief should be reviewed carefully with them. The parents should be encouraged to return to the emergency room or to call the dentist or family doctor if they have concerns after discharge. The risk of further trauma is reduced by restricting the child's activity for 1 week until the tooth adheres well into the socket.

Epistaxis

Epistaxis in children is usually due to injury rather than pathology. Children with blood dyscrasias may have spontaneous nosebleeds, but healthy children incur them as a result of falls, blows to the face, or trauma. Picking of the nose, insertion of foreign objects, or lack of environmental humidity can be triggers for epistaxis. Although a nosebleed can be frightening to both the child and the parents, it is very rarely a life-threatening occurrence (Table 46–11).

Diagnostic Assessment

When children with epistaxis are brought to the emergency room, office, or clinic, the nurse remains calm and supportive during her or his assessment and history taking. Assessing the ABCs is the first important step. The nurse notes rate and quality of respirations, any signs of respiratory distress, pulse rate, and blood pressure, if the child is cooperative. While settling the child, the nurse asks the parents whether there was any preceding injury, whether the child has had previous episodes of epistaxis and, if so, how long they lasted and what treatment was provided. If the nosebleed is the result of facial or head trauma, a neurologic assessment is performed, and appropriate cervical spine precautions should be instituted, if required.

Therapeutic Management

Treatment for epistaxis in children may require no more than firm pressure to the septal cartilage (pinch-

TABLE 46-11
Family-Centered Teaching: What to Do about a Bleeding Nose

Stay calm

Reassure your child

- He or she will not bleed to death. Some children are very concerned about this

Find out quickly why it is bleeding

- If this is the result of another injury, go to your local emergency department for further assessment
- If it started spontaneously, try to stop the bleeding yourself

Control the bleeding

- Have child sit down
- Place a large towel around the shoulders and chest
- Firmly pinch the nostrils and maintain pressure for 5 full mins
- Release the pressure and check for continued bleeding
- Repeat these measures once if bleeding is not stopped
- If bleeding does not stop, proceed to your local emergency department
- *Do not* tip the child's head back. This causes blood to trickle down the back of the throat. Most children find this very uncomfortable
- Have the child sit up leaning slightly forward

Discourage blowing the nose for 24 hrs

- Also nose picking!

Consider a home humidifier if this happens often, especially in winter

ing nostrils) for 5 full minutes. Release the pressure and assess for continued bleeding. These interventions may be repeated once if bleeding has not ceased. If any facial injuries have been incurred, this should not be done, especially if the nose has been fractured.

If pressure fails to control the epistaxis, more aggressive measures may need to be employed. Once the reason for the bleeding is identified, a vasoconstrictive preparation such as cocaine or phenylephrine is applied or a cauterizing agent like silver nitrate is used to stop the bleeding. The concentration of cocaine should not exceed 4 per cent (2.5 mg/kg/hr). The child should be monitored for about an hour to make sure the bleeding has stopped. If the treatment is unsuccessful a topical thrombin, Gelfoam, or microfibrillar collagen may be tried (Dickerman & Lucey, 1985). More aggressive treatment involves anterior nasal packing made from petrolatum gauze or posterior packing if there is blood trickling down the throat. A patient who receives posterior packing should be admitted for observation, antibiotic therapy, and possibly volume replacement. Severe epistaxis may require volume replacement. Children with coagulation disorders should receive appropriate blood products. In some instances, prolonged epistaxis requires fluid replacement and monitoring of the child's hematologic status by blood sampling. The PALS recommendations for fluid resuscitation are 0.20 ml/kg of either normal saline or Ringer lactate if the child demonstrates signs and symptoms of shock. A complete blood count (CBC), platelet count, and crossmatch may also be required.

Nursing Diagnostic Statements

High risk for aspiration; risk factor: *blood in nasopharynx.*

High risk for fluid volume deficit; risk factor: *epistaxis.*

Anxiety, *related to:*

- *Bleeding.*
- *Unfamiliar environment.*

Knowledge deficit, *related to first aid treatment of nosebleeds.*

Nursing Care

Maintaining a Patent Airway. The nurse can initiate treatment by settling the child in a comfortable position with the head tilted forward to minimize the amount of blood trickling down the back of the throat. Very young children may feel safer and be more cooperative if seated on a parent's lap. The child should be instructed to spit out blood rather than swallow it; however, small children may be unable to do this. Swallowed blood is irritating and may cause vomiting. The child is positioned to reduce the possibility of aspiration should vomiting occur.

The nurse monitors the child's vital signs and explains the procedures to both parent and child before they are done. Suction equipment and oxygen must be readily available.

Maintaining Fluid Balance. In the event of a very severe or prolonged epistaxis, frequent assessments should be made to identify signs of hypovolemic shock. Changes in vital signs and signs of reduced perfusion (poor capillary refill) are noted and reported to the physician. Careful monitoring of the intravenous line is required as for any other child.

Reducing Anxiety Related to the Frightening Experience. Epistaxis is rarely a life-threatening event. If it occurs as the result of trauma, it becomes one of many concerns at that time and is treated along with other injuries. However, it is usually a frightening episode necessitating a quick unanticipated trip to the emergency room. A calm, reassuring approach by the nurse will help to alleviate anxiety, promote cooperation, and lessen the negative aspects of the experience. Special attention is given to reducing anxiety by taking blood samples at the same time that intravenous lines are started, to minimize the number of needlesticks the child has to suffer.

Facilitating Home Management. If the bleeding is controlled, the child may be discharged from the emergency department. Instructions to the parents should include careful observation for repeated epistaxis, the correct technique for applying nasal pressure, and the avoidance of vigorous noseblowing or nosepicking in order not to disturb clot formation. Parents are instructed to return with the child if these methods are ineffective in controlling the bleeding.

Instruction cards printed with simple pictures may be useful as teaching aids for parents to take home with them. The nurse might also suggest the use of a humidifier or cold air steamer to add moisture to the air (particularly in the winter) to reduce dryness of the nasal mucous membranes, which may contribute to nosebleeds. The nurse should document on the patient's emergency chart any patient teaching that was done with the family and how the family responded to the information.

Injuries Associated with Foreign Bodies

Children are prone to injury from foreign bodies because of their curiosity and drive to taste and manipulate household objects and toys. Although children are known to insert objects into any body orifice, the two types of injury discussed here include foreign body aspiration and foreign body in the ear.

Foreign Body Aspiration

Foreign body aspiration leading to airway obstruction and hypoxia is most common in children under 5 years of age. Items that are frequently aspirated include chunks of hot dogs, candy that is round and hard, peanuts, chunks of dense foods such as carrots or apples, pieces of cereal, and inedible items including coins, deflated balloons, toy car wheels, marbles, or large beads.

Pathophysiology

Most aspirated foreign bodies pass through the larynx and trachea to become lodged in the bronchi. The right main bronchus is a common site for obstruction because it is larger in diameter with greater airflow than the left main bronchus. Also, the right bronchus is shorter and arises from the trachea at a wider angle forming a straighter line of entry.

Obstruction may be partial or complete; a partial obstruction may become complete within seconds. Complete airway obstruction usually occurs in the upper airway and represents an immediate threat to life. The bronchi can become partially or completely obstructed resulting in different clinical manifestations.

Clinical Manifestations

Initially, when a foreign body is aspirated into the respiratory tract, a choking, gagging, or coughing episode may occur. This episode may be followed by an interval of days, hours, or even weeks during which there are no symptoms of respiratory difficulty. Clinical manifestations vary according to the location of the obstruction and the degree of obstruction.

A foreign body in the *larynx* causes an immediate hoarseness, stridor, and aphonia (inability to speak). The site of obstruction becomes inflamed and dyspnea, wheezing, and cyanosis may result, followed by complete obstruction requiring emergency treatment.

A *tracheal* foreign body is usually associated with coughing and an asthmalike wheeze. Hoarseness, stridor, dyspnea, and cyanosis may also be noted. As the patient coughs, it is possible for the foreign body to be moved from the carina to the glottis where an audible slap can be heard (Conner, 1987). Complete obstruction is a threat because the foreign body could move and become lodged in the subglottis.

A *bronchial* foreign body results in a cough or a wheeze if there is partial airway obstruction. These symptoms occur because air passes around the obstruction during inspiration and expiration. A child with a partial obstruction may be able to ventilate well or be adversely affected, causing poor ventilation. With good air exchange, the child breathes and coughs effectively and may be able to speak, but it is not uncommon for hoarseness and stridor to be present. Complete obstruction of the bronchus results in pulmonary changes distal to the obstruction. Because no air bypasses the obstruction, no breath sounds will be heard. If atelectasis or consolidation has developed, bronchial or tubular sounds may be auscultated (Mayer, 1985).

Diagnostic Assessment

A choking child is identified by the severity of clinical signs and symptoms. A child who has an ineffective cough, is unable to make sounds, and has cyanotic lips, nails, and skin must be immediately diagnosed and treated to prevent death. Partial airway obstruction with poor gas exchange is also an emergency and should be managed as a complete obstruction. In the case of obstruction, a child seems to make respiratory efforts that, like the cough, are ineffective. Stridor may still be present, but the child is unable to vocalize at all. If circumoral cyanosis or cyanosis of the nailbeds is present, intervention must be immediate.

In many cases, aspiration of a foreign body is not so obvious. A history of a choking incident, days or weeks prior to admission, or a history of recurrent intractable pneumonia, are reasons to suspect the presence of a foreign body. The health care team clarifies the history with parents or caretakers and assesses the airway for patency and for the effectiveness of breathing efforts.

Chest and soft tissue roentgenographs are usually ordered to locate the object. These should be taken in the emergency room rather than sending the child to the radiology department, in case the obstruction becomes complete. Radiographic examination shows opaque objects such as a penny but is less useful to identify food matter. Fluoroscopic examination shows a characteristic air-trapping when the obstruction is in the bronchi. The position of the diaphragm is also noted to remain high on the involved side when a foreign body completely obliterates the bronchus.

Therapeutic Management

In some cases, the child can be coached to breathe and cough deeply in an effort to expel the object. Mofenson and Greensher (1985) cite examples of children who coughed out the object on the way to the operating room.

If the child is still conscious, the measures developed by the American Heart Association for removal of an aspirated foreign object should be used (see Table 46–5 for management of an obstructed airway).

For the child with an obstruction who becomes unconscious, more aggressive interventions are necessary. Reassessment of the patency of the airway is essential because hypoxia may cause relaxation of the neck muscles and the trachea. Enough relaxation may occur to permit some air to travel around the obstruction until the foreign body can be removed.

Whether the child is conscious or unconscious, visualization and removal of the object may be necessary through direct laryngoscopy or bronchoscopy. Once the object is removed, the bronchoscope is reinserted to look for remaining fragments, to remove secretions for culture, and to assess tissue trauma and/or edema. Children are usually hospitalized postoperatively for a period of observation and are sometimes given a course of antibiotic therapy. A cool-mist tent will help to soothe irritated tissues.

Even if the object is successfully removed, the child must be admitted to the hospital and observed for soft tissue swelling, laryngeal edema, and respiratory difficulty. If a tracheotomy is required, the child should be admitted to intensive care for observation of both respiratory and neurologic stability. An intravenous line is inserted to provide emergency access.

Nursing Diagnostic Statements

Ineffective airway clearance, *related to tracheobronchial obstruction associated with aspiration of a foreign body.*

Anxiety, *related to inability to breathe associated with aspiration of a foreign body.*

Ineffective family coping: compromised, *related to temporary family disorganization associated with hospitalized child and feelings of guilt and anger.*

High risk for injury; risk factor: *knowledge deficit concerning child safety practices related to safety precautions in the home.*

Nursing Care

Tracheobronchial aspiration of foreign objects represents a serious emergency that nurses who work with children may encounter at any time. Although prevention of such incidents is preferable, knowledge of how to deal with the child who presents with an obstructed airway is essential. Special attention should be paid to the management of the choking child, because early recognition and treatment of respiratory difficulty can prevent a full-blown cardiac arrest. Continued practice for emergency establishment of an airway is achieved through regular mock situations.

Establishing an Airway. The nurse plays a key role in responding quickly to the child's clinical situation. If necessary, an attempt is made to relieve the obstruction, following the guidelines for management of an obstructed airway (see Table 46–5). Notification of the appropriate team member and immediate readiness of equipment facilitate effective management.

Continuous monitoring for respiratory difficulty is instituted and nursing assessments are documented. The nurse remains prepared to assist with emergency procedures at any time should the obstruction become complete or the child become unconscious, or both. Suction equipment, oxygen, and a bag-valve-mask should be kept immediately available.

Maintaining an Airway. Once the object is removed, the child needs to be monitored for secondary obstruction due to laryngeal edema and/or soft tissue swelling or any remaining fragments. The nurse observes the child for signs and symptoms of respiratory distress, such as anxiety and restlessness; flaring of the nares; tracheal, substernal, or intercostal retractions; and cyanosis. Arterial blood gases may be monitored depending on the severity of the distress prior to treatment. Cyanosis in children is a late sign of hypoxia and indicates a need for immediate intervention.

The child who has had an emergency tracheotomy needs to be monitored for all the signs and symptoms described earlier. In addition, tracheotomy care is instituted (see Chapter 32 for care of the child with a tracheotomy).

Minimizing Child's Fear and Anxiety. Although monitoring the child's physical status is of utmost importance, the nurse must remember that the child has been exposed to the terror of both a life-threatening experience and the unfamiliarity of emergency care, surgery, and, possibly, the intensive care unit. Using knowledge of growth and development, the nurse prepares the child for treatment (such as tracheotomy care) as completely as possible. The unfamiliar and anxiety-producing environment can be minimized by normalizing the environment. It is helpful to allow the child to wear her or his own pajamas, if possible, after the emergency period is past. The presence of favorite toys, the support of parents, and the consistency of nursing staff are strategies used to reduce the child's stress.

Facilitating Resolution of Parental Guilt. Aspiration of a foreign body may make parents feel that they failed to provide adequate supervision for their child. If the aspiration has occurred because a parent *gave* the object to their child, it is particularly distressing for parents to see their child endure such a traumatic experience.

Parents need to be supported during this stressful period. It is therapeutic to allow them to express their feelings of guilt and anger. Involving them in their child's care, if they are receptive to this, is also helpful. Recognizing the strengths of parents and fostering their self-esteem as parents is an important component of the nurse's support to the family.

Reducing Risk of Future Incidents of Foreign Body Aspiration. Nurses who work in parent-child settings or public health are in excellent positions to do patient teaching regarding child safety and childproofing the home in an effort to prevent aspiration of foreign bodies. Should aspiration occur and necessitate admission to an emergency department, the nurse who cares for the child should review principles of growth and development and safety with the parents before discharge. (See Chapter 15 for a discussion of safety concerning aspiration of a foreign body.) The nurse should assess the need for further follow-up with a public health nurse or a social worker and inform support agencies of the need for assistance. Table 46-12 summarizes nursing care for a child with foreign body aspiration.

Foreign Body in the Ear

Foreign bodies in the ear are relatively easy to diagnose and treat (Matlak, 1985). The difficulty is that they may be in place for several days before generating enough of an inflammatory response to alert the parent to seek medical attention. By that time, pain and inflammation contribute to difficulty in examination and removal of the object.

Anything small enough to fit in the external canal may be placed there by a small child. Tiny insects may fly into the ear and become trapped. Because of their potential for causing hearing loss, miniature cell batteries used in watches, calculators, and some toys are of great concern.

Clinical Manifestations and Diagnostic Assessment

Diagnosis is usually based on a history of ear pain and purulent drainage that has not responded to antibiotic therapy (Matlak, 1985). A child's cooperation can usually be gained by explaining that it is important to "look inside your ear to see why it is hurting." If a child cannot be helped to keep the head still or is unduly fearful and uncooperative, examination under general anesthesia may be considered.

Usually the foreign object can be visualized through an otoscope unless excessive purulent drainage is present. Gentle irrigation with suction may help to visualize the eardrum and may even flush out the object.

Therapeutic Management

Small alligator forceps, ear hooks, or wax curets may be used to remove the item. Care is taken not to push the foreign body further into the ear or to perforate the eardrum. Live insects should be killed before removal, especially if they are the biting kind (Matlak, 1985). Agents used for this purpose are mineral oil, alcohol, or lidocaine. A few drops are instilled and in a few minutes the insect can be removed. Topical antibiotics may be administered for minor lacerations or local inflammation of the ear canal. A more serious laceration may require repair. Oral antibiotics are indicated in the event of a perforated eardrum.

In the event of accidental placement of miniature batteries in the ear, early treatment is required. Delay in seeking treatment contributes to deterioration of the battery case, resulting in alkaline burns. Further complications will arise if acetic acid–based eardrops are administered because they provide an external electrolyte bath for the battery. Such an environment promotes leakage of the battery contents and generation of an electrical current. This will eventually cause tissue destruction (Kavanagh & Litovitz, 1986). Removal of a corroding battery must be done carefully: biting or pinching instruments are not used, because they could perforate the casing. Follow-up of the child is arranged to assess healing and to débride necrotic tissue, which may slough for a number of weeks (Kavanagh & Litovitz, 1986).

Nursing Diagnostic Statements

Fear, *related to child's unfamiliarity with equipment and/or procedures used to remove object from ear.*

High risk for knowledge deficit; risk factor: *lack of recall or lack of experience with instillation of eardrops.*

High risk for injury; risk factor: *developmental age and environmental exposure.*

Impaired skin integrity: ear canal and/or tympanic membrane, *related to:*

- *Mechanical removal of a foreign body from the ear.*
- *Chemical injury associated with leakage of battery fluid from a battery.*

TABLE 46-12

Nursing Process Plan: Foreign Body Aspiration

Analysis: Collaborative Problem 1

Response and Related or Risk Factors: *Ineffective airway clearance related to tracheobronchial obstruction associated with the aspiration of a foreign body*

Projected Outcome: The child will achieve and maintain a patent airway

Defining Characteristics	Nursing Interventions	Evaluation Criteria
Subjective: • Anxiety or panic because of inability to breathe properly and/or cough out foreign object *Objective:* • Reduced breath sound over tracheobronchial tree • Abnormal breath sounds • Changes in abdominal respiratory rate and pattern • Tachypnea • Absent or diminished cough reflex • Cyanosis • Stridor • Use of accessory muscles to breathe • Elevated temperature as indication of infection due to aspirated object	*Airway Management* **Establish an airway.** If possible, attempt to relieve obstruction (see Table 46–15) **Assist in removing obstruction.** Have appropriate equipment (sutures, oxygen, laryngoscope, bag-valve-mask) available. In case of total obstruction, an emergency tracheotomy may be performed **Monitor for secondary obstruction** due to laryngeal edema and/or soft tissue swelling after the object has been removed **Monitor for signs of infection** secondary to retained fragments of foreign body	**The child will be calm.** • Breath sounds will be clear on auscultation over tracheobronchial tree • Respiratory rate and rhythm within normal parameters for age • No use of accessory muscles to breathe • Temperature and pulse within normal parameters for age **The child will experience absence of stridor and effective coughing.**

Analysis: Nursing Diagnostic Statement 1

Response and Related or Risk Factors: *Fear related to inability to breathe associated with aspiration of a foreign body*

- Perception of environment as threatening

Projected Outcome: The child will display an attitude of trust and comfort with nursing staff, cooperation with necessary procedures, and decreased fear or absence of fear when the foreign body is removed and respirations return to normal

Defining Characteristics	Nursing Interventions	Evaluation Criteria
Subjective: • Child states that he or she is afraid, scared, or worried *if able to speak* • Requesting parental presence	*Anxiety Reduction* **Use calm, reassuring, yet firm approach while assisting with the procedure.** **Explain each step of each procedure to child (and parent) before proceeding.**	**The child will express feelings through play or verbally and will experience a reduction of anxiety** **The child will cooperate with necessary procedures**

TABLE 46-12 (continued)

Defining Characteristics	Nursing Interventions	Evaluation Criteria
Objective: • Crying • Refusing to cooperate with necessary procedures such as monitoring vital signs • Cardiovascular excitation • Elevated vital signs • Pupil dilatation	**Work with child** to help him or her understand when holding still is necessary Let child know when it is "alright to cry" **Use medical play/preparation play** (See Chapter 17) or use these procedures to involve Child Life Worker to assist child in exploring fears through play **Encourage parental presence and assistance** with care if possible **Allow child to have a favorite toy, nightclothes, or storybook from home.** Transition objects provide a link for the child with what is familiar and comforting	**The child will experience normal vital signs and pupil size**

Analysis: Nursing Diagnostic Statement 2

Response and Related or Risk Factors: *Ineffective family coping: compromised, related to parental feelings of guilt and anger about child's illness*

Projected Outcome: Parents will provide sufficient, effective, and/or uncompromised support, comfort, assistance, or encouragement that may be needed by the child to manage or master adaptive tasks related to his or her health challenge

Defining Characteristics	Nursing Interventions	Evaluation Criteria
Subjective: • Parents express feelings of fear, grief, guilt, anxiety, or anger related to aspiration of foreign object and subsequent hospitalization • Parents verbalize an inadequate knowledge base *Objective*: • Parents display protective behavior to child, disproportionate (too little or too much) to the child's abilities and need for autonomy • Parents attempt assistive or supportive behaviors with less than satisfactory results • Parents seek reassurance from health care team members • Parents withdraw from situation	*Emotional Support* **Facilitate an atmosphere of acceptance and trust** in which parents can feel comfortable expressing feelings of guilt and anger, crying, etc **Keep parents informed of child's medical condition and progress** on a daily basis **Encourage parental participation** in child's care when appropriate to reduce anxiety for both parents and child	**The parents will demonstrate resolution of negative feelings and/or deal with them in constructive ways** such as planning to childproof home before child's discharge **The parents will participate in child's care** via those tasks which they are comfortable performing **The parents will display protective behavior** that is proportionate to the child's abilities and need for autonomy

(continued)

TABLE 46-12 *(continued)*

Analysis: Nursing Diagnostic Statement 3

Response and Related or Risk Factors: *Health-seeking behaviors related to desire of parents to know child safety precautions in the home*

Projected Outcome: Parents will alter family health habits so as to move to a higher level of family health by demonstrating an understanding of child safety precautions in the home appropriate to the developmental stage of the child, a knowledge of CPR (especially related to the choking child), and appropriate ways to provide adult supervision for young children

Defining Characteristics	*Nursing Interventions*	*Evaluation Criteria*
Subjective: • Expressed or observed desire of parents to seek a higher level of family wellness, especially as related to safety of their child • Expressed or observed desire (parents) for increased control of their child's environment • Expression of concern about current environmental conditions on family health status, especially in relation to safety of their child • Stated or observed unfamiliarity with community resources • Demonstrated or observed lack of knowledge in health promotion behavior	**Assess family's knowledge of child safety** **Assess parent's knowledge of growth and development** *Anticipatory Guidance* **Develop a teaching plan** early in child's hospitalization to help parents childproof their home (e.g., handouts, check lists) **Supply parents with a list of community organizations** that offer child-based safety services (e.g., poison control service and CPR classes that include the pediatric component) **Arrange referral to community health nurse** to assess status of child safety in the home prior to child's discharge and ongoing as required	**Parents will demonstrate an understanding of child safety practices** **Parents will provide evidence of childproofing their home** before child's discharge (e.g., completed check lists, report from community health nurse)

Nursing Care

The emergency room nurse will obtain a history and try to determine whether there is a strong possibility of a foreign body in the ear. He or she should take the child's vital signs to determine the presence of infection.

Reducing Fear Associated with Treatment. Parents should be given the option of remaining with the child or leaving the room. Whatever decision they make should be supported by the nurse.

The nurse explains in simple terms to the child and parents what to expect during the examination and treatment. Rather than telling a child to "keep your head still," the nurse could suggest to the child that he or she will "help" by holding the child's head during the examination. The child is encouraged to "help" the doctor or nurse by lying as still as possible. Following removal of the object, praise is given to the child for "helping" during the procedure.

Teaching the Family How to Instill Eardrops. The nurse reviews the correct procedure for instilling the prescribed eardrops and the importance of finishing the prescription even though the child may seem much better in a day or two. Correct procedure for instillation of eardrops is presented in Chapter 24.

Reducing Risk of Future Incidents of Foreign Body in the Ear. Principles of home safety and childproofing are reviewed with parents. The young child's curiosity and need to explore present a special challenge to parents and require their constant monitoring of a child's play area for hazardous objects. Parents are also encouraged to tell their child *not* to place objects in their body orifices.

Reducing Risk of Damage to Ear Canal and Tympanic Membrane. Parents are provided with eardrops, as appropriate, to facilitate healing of a damaged ear canal or tympanic membrane, or both. The child is instructed not to place anything in the ears, and, if a child is too young to understand, close supervision by parents is required. Follow-up care may be required if the injury is extensive because of the need to débride necrotic tissue. The nurse can assist in follow-up care by giving parents clear explanations about the need to return for assessment of the healing process.

Poisoning

Poisoning affects an estimated 5 to 10 million children annually. Accidental poisoning is the fourth leading cause of death in children ages 1 to 4 years. *Accidental poisoning* accounts for 80 to 85 per cent of poisoning incidents; 15 to 20 per cent of poisonings are *intentional* (Barkin, 1990), as a result of either abuse or a suicide attempt.

Etiology/Incidence

Although poisoning exposures can occur through oral ingestion, ocular or topical exposure, inhalation, or envenomation, oral ingestion accounts for approximately 76 per cent of poisonings (Litovitz et al, 1992). The type of agent ingested varies with the age of the child. Adolescents have a much higher incidence of psychopharmacologic drug ingestion (sedatives, tranquilizers, antidepressants), whereas young children are most frequently affected by ingestion of plants, household detergents and cleaning solutions, or medications such as acetaminophen (Tylenol), aspirin, vitamins, or minerals.

The most common age of poisoning in young children is 2 years old and under, with the greatest incidence occurring at 1 year of age (Table 46–13). Children at 1 and 2 years of age become increasingly mobile and curious, seeking to increase their independence; exploration of the environment results in increased contact with many hazards. Furthermore, at this developmental stage, parents are beginning to decrease some of the constant vigilance they kept for their child during infancy.

Numerous environmental conditions in a household contribute to poisoning. Family stress can contribute to preoccupation of parents and, subsequently, increase the risk of poisoning. It is also known that poisoning is more common in lower socioeconomic groups and in families with more than one child. Generally, accidental poisoning can be attributed to inappropriate supervision for the age of the child or faulty childproofing of the environment.

TABLE 46-13
Breakdown of Poisoning Cases by the Age of the Victim

Age in Yrs	1975 (Per Cent)*	1983 (Per Cent)†
Under 1	6.4	16.9
1	17.0	37.8
2	21.0	13.5
3	14.4	4.5
4	5.4	1.4
5	2.7	1.2
6–17	10.2	6.5
18 and over	20.5	15.6
Not recorded	2.3	2.6

From Mayer, T. A. (1985). *Emergency management of pediatric trauma.* Philadelphia: WB Saunders.
* Data from the Intermountain Regional Poison Control Center, 1975.
† Data from Cooperative Regional Poison Control Center Pilot Study, Jan–Feb, 1983, American Association of Poison Control Centers.

Diagnostic Assessment

The initial assessment may be done on the phone or in a clinic, office, or emergency room. The following information should be obtained:

- Age, approximate weight, sex of child.
- Present condition of child.
- Name of toxic agent.
- Route of exposure.
- How much of agent ingested (or other exposure).
- When incident occurred.
- Any signs and symptoms present and time of onset.
- Circumstances of the event.

An immediate evaluation of the patient is performed as for any other emergency victim (see Table 46–1):

A—Is the child's *a*irway open and is cervical spine intact?
B—Is the child *b*reathing?
C—Is child's *c*irculatory status established?

If any problems are identified with the ABCs, the parent should be instructed to call 911 or their appropriate emergency help number immediately. Once this has been determined, specific information relative to the poisoning incident is sought. If the initial contact is by phone, sufficient information must be obtained to make a decision about the amount and type of treatment to recommend in the home and whether to instruct the caller to bring the child to an emergency room. In the United States, where syrup of ipecac is used in the home according to instructions given over the phone from a poison control center, emergency room visits have been reduced. In Canada, where provincial health care plans exist, this practice has not been adopted and the child is more commonly brought to the emergency room immediately. On arrival at a health care facility, an assessment of the child is made to determine the need for basic life support. Specific information about the poisoning incident is then obtained to determine further management. In severe cases, it may be necessary to immediately establish an airway, provide artificial ventilation, and institute measures to restore circulation. Heart rate, blood pressure, central nervous system status, and hydration are important parameters to assess. Findings on the physical examination that are suggestive of poisoning include altered vital signs, neuromuscular dysfunction, irritation of the eyes or skin, and unusual odors on the breath (Temple, 1985).

When a poisoning occurs, it is also important to gather data concerning the factors that might have contributed to the poisoning. This is usually done after the child is stabilized; in many instances, referral for follow-up is made. Individual factors are assessed, including stress in the home, age of the child, status of childproofing in the home, and level of safety education to which the family has been exposed.

Therapeutic Management

Management is based on the history, clinical manifestations, and laboratory reports. The aim of management of all poisonings, regardless of agent, is to terminate the patient's exposure to a toxic agent or to reduce the potential toxicity. Poison control centers in both the United States and Canada have information on almost all drugs and household products. Management is adapted according to the type of exposure (ocular, topical, inhalation, or ingestion).

Management of Ocular Exposure. First-aid care of eyes consists of:

1. Immediately flushing the eye with copious amounts of water, lactated Ringer, or normal saline solution.
2. Removal of contact lenses.
3. Additional irrigation for 10 to 15 minutes.

Intravenous saline solution directed through intravenous tubing is a readily available device in the emergency room. In the home, the eye can be held open under a *gentle* stream of tepid tap water. All surfaces of the eye should be examined by a physician. Ophthalmic follow-up is arranged because these injuries may cause an ulcer that heals very slowly or they may result in the loss of an eye (Reece, 1984).

Management of Topical Exposure. First-aid treatment for dermal exposure is to flush the affected area with water followed by a thorough washing. Soap is used to remove oily substances, which are potential systemic toxins (Mayer, 1985). In cases of contamination with pesticides, the child's clothing is removed. Protection by gowning is recommended for health care personnel during this process.

Management of Inhalation Exposure. The first step in management is to move the victim from the locality of exposure to fresh air. Clothing is loosened and an assessment is made to determine the need for intubation and oxygen administration. Early intubation may be necessary because of airway edema, which can ensue rapidly. After emergency treatment, the patient is observed for latent pulmonary symptoms to determine the need for respiratory care (see Chapter 32).

Management of Ingestions. The majority of poisonings are caused by ingestion. Once the poison has been identified and the patient stabilized through maintenance of an airway, oxygenation, and prevention of shock, care is directed at decontamination of the gastrointestinal tract. Decontamination is accomplished by (1) decreasing absorption by gastric evacuation (vomiting or lavage) or local detoxification and (2) hastening elimination.

Decreasing Absorption. *Induction of vomiting* removes a substantial portion of ingested poisons if it is done early on. It is most effective if done within 2 to 4 hours (Temple, 1985). The drug of choice for induction of vomiting is syrup of ipecac. Recent statistics reveal a decrease in the use of syrup of ipecac to induce vomiting and an increase in the use of activated charcoal to decrease absorption (Litovitz et al, 1992). Syrup of ipecac *is not recommended* when there is altered consciousness, when seizures occur, if the gag reflex is absent, or if the ingested poison is caustic. Corrosive and/or caustic substances (also called "acids" and "alkalis") should *never* be evacuated by induced vomiting. Substances such as liquid bleach or drain-cleaning products are extremely destructive to the sensitive mucous membranes of the esophagus and trachea. Swallowing such compounds can lead to scarring, inability to swallow, and nutritional problems. Further injury can result from induced emesis of these substances. Acids and alkalis should be managed by forcing oral fluids or by attempting gastric lavage if the ingestion has occurred within 2 hours (Barkin, 1990).

The dose of syrup of ipecac is 30 ml for adolescents, 15 ml for children, and 10 ml for infants under 1 year of age. This is followed by 4 to 8 ounces of fluid. Syrup of ipecac, if used appropriately, produces vomiting approximately 90 per cent of the time. Fifty per cent of patients vomit in less than 15 to 20 minutes and 90 per cent in 30 minutes (Mofenson & Caraccio, 1986). If emesis does not occur in 20 to 30 minutes, the ipecac and liquid can be repeated. Ipecac fluid extract, a preparation formerly used, was 14 times more potent than ipecac syrup, but it caused toxicity and overdose in the past because of inappropriate use. This preparation is no longer marketed. Apomorphine is an alternative drug used to induce vomiting if the use of ipecac is unsuccessful. This drug is more likely to produce central nervous system depression and results in protracted vomiting more frequently than does syrup of ipecac.

Gastric lavage is indicated when syrup of ipecac or apomorphine has failed to induce emesis. It is also indicated to remove stomach contents in the event of central nervous system depression, seizures, or altered consciousness and in circumstances when an ingested poison is rapidly absorbed. Contraindications to treatment by lavage include ingestion of petroleum distillates and the presence of gastrectomy.

The largest-sized catheter that can be safely used is recommended to ensure that fragments or particles can be removed. The tube is inserted with the same technique as for any other purpose (see section on nasogastric tube insertion in Chapter 35). The child is positioned with the head to one side and slightly lowered, to avoid aspiration in the event of vomiting and to maximize the return of the lavage fluid. In an unconscious patient (or in any patient who cannot adequately protect the airway), intubation precedes placement of a lavage tube to prevent aspiration.

After the lavage tube is in place, the gastric contents are removed; then lavage fluid, usually normal saline solution, is introduced into the stomach. Gastric washing is accomplished by instilling fluid through the lavage tube (50 to 100 ml at a time). Intermittent suction is used for its removal. Children can receive up to 2 L at a rate of 1 L/5 minutes (Temple, 1985). The process is usually continued until the lavage return is clear. If toxicologic testing is required, it is done on the first lavage fluid returned.

Local detoxification is another method used to interfere with absorption of a toxin. Activated charcoal is an agent being used with increasing frequency. Activated charcoal limits absorption of drugs by adsorbing drugs onto its surfaces. It is not itself absorbed by the gastrointestinal mucosa. Activated charcoal is not given if the ingested substances include acids, alkalis, DDT, iron salts, heavy metals, or hydrocarbons. It is usually given in the dose of 1 g/kg of the child's weight. The activated charcoal is a fine, black powder that is premixed to make a black solution. It is given orally or via a nasogastric tube. It should not be given in milk or ice cream. Activated charcoal may be used following the administration of ipecac syrup to bind any remaining poison or prevent further absorption. It should not be used until after vomiting has occurred because it will inactivate the ipecac. Children who are sent home after being treated with activated charcoal should be warned that the stool will be black for a day or two.

Hastening Elimination. Elimination of poison can be hastened by the use of a cathartic lavage. Saline cathartics are preferred. The usual dose is sodium sulfate, 250 mg/kg, as a 20 to 50 per cent solution and magnesium citrate 4 ml/kg (every 1 to 2 hours) as long as bowel sounds are present (Mayer, 1985). Saline cathartics may be used following gastric lavage, emesis, or activated charcoal. They are usually necessary in more complicated cases that require hospitalization.

Poisons already absorbed will be eliminated via the lungs, liver, or kidneys. Elimination of absorbed poisons is enhanced by specialized procedures, including diuresis, dialysis, and hemoperfusion. These techniques are sometimes indicated when a child is brought for treatment several hours after the actual event of poisoning has occurred. Although these techniques carry considerable risks, they are instituted when the patient's recovery is threatened.

Most children who are victims of poisonings present with a history of having ingested a toxic substance; however, any child presenting in coma or with strange behavior, unexplained high fever, arrhythmias, or seizures should be suspected of a poisoning event. Such children are critically ill and intervention is aimed at making a diagnosis and giving supportive treatment. Pathophysiology and symptoms vary according to the toxin ingested, but similar nursing diagnoses apply to a variety of poisoning circumstances.

Nursing Diagnostic Statements

High risk for injury; risk factor: *toxic effects of the poison.*

Anxiety (parent), *related to threat to child's well-being or life associated with effects of a poisoning.*

Fear (child), *related to separation from support system during the threatening experience of emergency treatment of a poisoning.*

High risk for injury: subsequent poisoning; risk factor: *parents' inadequate knowledge about child's developmental capabilities.*

Nursing Care

Nursing care of the child varies according to the type of poisoning and number and intrusiveness of emergency treatments required. The single most important role of the nurse is to assist in the stabilization of the patient, as described earlier in this chapter. Other areas of concern for the nurse are reduction of the fear and anxiety experienced by the child, preventive teaching concerning the storage of poisons and supervision of children, and removal of the poison to reduce the danger of skin and mucous membrane trauma.

Reducing Physiologic Injury. Poisoning results when a toxic agent comes in contact with a specific area in the body. The nurse can mediate the injury resulting from a toxin by making a rapid assessment and preparing the necessary equipment and materials for immediate removal or dilution of the toxin. Minutes are important; therefore, speed of assessment and initiation of treatment can prevent serious trauma to a child. The nurse is an important team member and familiarity with equipment and procedures is essential for the nurse to achieve in order to prevent unnecessary trauma in poisoning.

Reducing the Child and Family's Fear and Anxiety. A poisoning episode requires not only emergency treatment to save the child but also emotional support for the parents. They feel devastated and engage in self-blame, resulting in threatened feelings as parents. Keeping the parents informed about the status of their child confirms their importance as parents. Anxious feelings of parents about the potential of losing their child are often expressed if they are given the opportunity to do so.

Poisonings often require removal of the toxic agent from the body by using techniques that are frightening to young children. The suddenness of the event, the strangeness of the environment, and the discomfort of the procedures are all factors that nurses consider in planning the care of a poisoned child.

Preventing Future Poisoning Episodes. The nurse has a responsibility to discuss with the family the circumstances surrounding the poisoning episode. If the child is admitted to the hospital, home safety can be discussed during the period of hospitalization or on a home visit after discharge. If the child is discharged home from the emergency room, it is most appropriate to make a public health referral for further assessment.

Commonly Ingested Poisons

The nurse's role has been discussed with respect to basic principles that apply to most incidents of poisoning. A discussion of some specific types of ingested poisons that occur in children follows.

Salicylate Poisoning

Salicylates are the most common cause of drug poisoning in children. Although aspirin is not recommended for pediatric use because of its association with Reye syndrome, it continues to be a common drug in most households. Poisoning may occur as the result of the ingestion of a single dose of aspirin, sodium salicylate, or methyl salicylate (oil of wintergreen). A dose of 4 ml of oil of wintergreen contains the equivalent of approximately 40 baby aspirins; it should be safely stored. Overdose of aspirin can also occur because of repeated small therapeutic doses of aspirin used for the treatment of fever. A child is particularly at risk for overdose when aspirin is given in combination with other medications that contain salicylates, such as antihistamine and decongestant compounds.

Pathophysiology

Salicylate ingestion drastically alters acid-base balance, resulting in both respiratory alkalosis and metabolic acidosis. In the first phase of the body's response to a salicylate overdose, stimulation of the respiratory center in the medulla causes hyperventilation, a fall in Pco_2, and *respiratory alkalosis*. Signs of respiratory alkalosis are confusion, loss of consciousness, and eventually respiratory failure. Bicarbonate is excreted in the urine to compensate for respiratory alkalosis; both Na^+ and K^+ are lost with the bicarbonate in the urine.

A second phase occurs as K^+ is lost and depleted. Once K^+ is depleted in the kidney, an exchange of K^+ for H^+ occurs to conserve K^+. This results in acidification of the urine. A "paradoxical aciduria" then occurs in the presence of respiratory alkalosis.

Salicylates inhibit the Kreb cycle, altering carbohydrate and lipid metabolism. The resultant accumulation of ketones and lactic acid accounts for the severe *metabolic acidosis* that results. Young children appear to be especially susceptible to these metabolic effects of salicylates, as evidenced by the rapid onset of metabolic acidosis following an initial transitory respiratory alkalosis. Metabolic acidosis also increases the nonionized fraction of salicylic acid. Further penetration of salicylates into the brain thus occurs. The increase of salicylic acid in the brain explains the severe clinical manifestations of salicylate poisoning in children (Gaudreault & Lovejoy, 1985).

Rapid respirations (hyperpnea) during this phase of acid accumulation are in response to acidosis rather than to the primary respiratory drive. Salicylate levels in the plasma escalate because they can no longer be excreted in an acid urine.

Salicylates also affect the process of oxidative phosphorylation—the process whereby oxygen is used by the mitochondria to transfer chemical energy to adenosine triphosphate (ATP). Salicylates cause uncoupling of oxidative phosphorylation (i.e., oxidation is enhanced, but the energy is not synthesized into ATP). The metabolic rate is increased resulting in fever, increased oxygen consumption, and CO_2 production. Altered glucose metabolism may occur with hyperglycemia presenting early and hypoglycemia presenting later.

Hypokalemia and dehydration are also present during the phase of lactic acid accumulation. Renal losses of sodium and potassium accompany organic acid excretion. Simultaneously, there is water loss because of insensible pulmonary loss, sweating and hyperthermia, and an osmotic diuresis that accompanies excretion of organic acids (Hughes & Griffith, 1984).

Salicylates also inhibit prothrombin formation (secondary to impaired liver function), decrease platelet adhesiveness, increase capillary fragility, decrease platelet levels, and may cause local gastrointestinal irritation. Although bleeding can occur in salicylate poisoning, it is generally not a significant clinical problem.

Diagnostic Assessment

The most important means of assessing the status of a child who is suspected to have ingested salicylate is from the history, clinical signs, and laboratory evaluation.

In most circumstances, it is difficult to determine the exact dose ingested. However, some attempt should be made to estimate the dosage. A toxic dose is generally believed to be a single dose that exceeds 200 to 280 mg/kg.

The principal manifestations of salicylate poisoning are hyperpnea and disturbed acid-base balance. Hyperpnea is a frequent sign early in the course of salicylate intoxication. Later manifestations of central nervous system alterations include central nervous system depression, vomiting, lethargy, hyperpyrexia, coma, respiratory failure, and circulatory collapse.

Salicylate levels can be estimated by using Phenistix to test urine, separated plasma, or serum. Phenistix cannot be used to test vomitus or lavage fluids because positive results are dependent on acetylsalicyclic acid being changed to salicylic acid. Blood salicylate levels are done to determine toxicity levels, which are essential for appropriate treatment. The Done nomogram (Done, 1960) diagrams the association between serum salicylate concentration and expected severity of the child's condition at certain time intervals after the ingestion of a single dose of salicylate. In persons with chronic salicylate intoxication, the nomogram should not be used.

Other laboratory assessments include blood gases, serum pH, electrolyte levels, and urine and blood glucose levels. Urine pH and volume are measured hourly in all serious cases. For chronic ingestion, abnormal liver function tests and increased creatinine excretion may be significant.

Therapeutic Management

The aim of treatment is to minimize entry of salicylates into the brain. Emergency management begins with efforts to remove the ingested drug from the stomach. Peak gastric absorption occurs within 2 hours of ingestion.

In some instances, the status of the patient interferes with the ability to induce emesis. In patients with altered mental status, gastric lavage is performed. A cuffed endotracheal tube is inserted before lavage to prevent aspiration.

After gastric emptying by lavage or vomiting, activated charcoal is given to decrease salicylate absorption, and magnesium citrate or sulfate is administered to increase gastrointestinal transit (Barkin, 1990).

Fluid therapy is directed at correcting dehydration and promoting elimination of salicylates. If the child is hypotensive, volume expanders may be needed to support circulation. Vitamin K may be administered to correct bleeding tendencies and calcium gluconate to counteract tetany.

Buffering of blood pH by continuous bicarbonate infusion alkalinizes the urine, which in turn promotes salicylate excretion. The presence of hypokalemia interferes with this process because, in a state of hypokalemia, potassium is conserved by the kidney and hydrogen ions are excreted in its place. Hydrogen ions in the urine reduce its alkalinity and interfere with salicylate excretion. Alkalinization of urine, however, is not without its hazards, including hyponatremia and systemic alkalosis.

Tepid sponging or a cooling mattress may be used for hyperpyrexia. Seizures are usually treated with diazepam followed by phenytoin or phenobarbital if necessary (Gaudreault & Lovejoy, 1985). Peritoneal dialysis, exchange transfusion, hemodialysis, or hemoperfusion may be required in severe cases when the child is unresponsive to therapy.

Nursing Diagnostic Statements

High risk for injury: physiologic; risk factor: *Salicylate-induced alterations of acid-base balance:*

- *Stimulation of the respiratory center (respiratory alkalosis).*
- *Accumulation of ketones and lactic acid (metabolic acidosis).*

High risk for fluid volume deficit; risk factors:

- *Insensible pulmonary loss.*
- *Sweating and hyperthermia.*
- *Osmotic diuresis associated with organic acid excretion.*

High risk for hyperthermia; risk factor: *Increased metabolic rate.*

Anxiety (child and parents), related to:

- *Perceived threat to self, associated with constant monitoring and invasive procedures.*
- *Discomfort associated with vomiting.*
- *Unfamiliar equipment and procedures.*
- *Lack of information about test results and purpose of procedures.*

Nursing Care

Nursing strategies are based on an ongoing assessment of the patient's condition. Rapid and effective emergency treatment can be facilitated by a nurse who can anticipate the needs of the patient. The nurse plays an active role in carrying out the medical plan of care, as well as in supporting the child and family throughout the experience.

Minimizing Physiologic Injury. Signs of acid-base imbalance (initially respiratory alkalosis and later metabolic acidosis) and signs of hypokalemia are parameters that the nurse monitors, documents, and reports to the physician. Careful monitoring is done during the various phases of salicylate poisoning. Salicylate levels, urine pH and volume, plasma pH, and serum K^+ levels in particular are monitored. The nurse's understanding of the progression of the clinical presentation and recognition and reporting of alterations in acid-base balance are important nursing responsibilities. (See Chapter 26 for in-depth discussion of acid-base imbalance.)

Maintaining Fluid Balance. A large part of the nurse's care is focused on accurate administration of fluids and on monitoring the patient's condition accordingly. Hydration is monitored by assessing skin turgor, eyes, fontanel fullness, and mucous membrane hydration. Because salicylates are more easily eliminated in an alkaline urine, the nurse also monitors urinary pH with the goal of maintaining an alkaline urine with a pH of 8 or more.

Vital signs, blood pressure, urine specific gravity, and urinary intake and output are monitored closely. The physician should be notified if urinary output falls below 1 ml/kg/hr. Serum potassium levels are closely monitored and are maintained between 3.5 and 4.5 mEq/L. The nurse monitors urinary output and ensures that it is established before potassium is added to parenteral fluids.

Maintaining Normal Body Temperature. Hyperpyrexia is another complication that may occur. The nurse monitors the child's temperature frequently (every 1 to 2 hours according to the child's condition). A tepid water sponge bath or cooling blanket may also be ordered for persistent fever. These interventions are performed with caution and careful monitoring of the child's response to therapy. Rapid changes in temperature can occur; therefore, the temperature of the water or cooling mattress is cool but not cold, and temperature reduction is achieved gradually.

Because these children have the potential to have seizures in association with elevated body temperature, the child is monitored carefully to prevent seizure and protect her or him in the event of a seizure.

Reducing Anxiety of Child and Family. A child who is exposed to the experiences associated with emergency and acute care of salicylate poisoning requires the support of parents and professionals. The anxiety produced by the rapid chain of events is especially overwhelming for young children, who are limited in their ability to understand explanations. Keeping parents with the child, whenever possible, is encouraged. Ongoing explanation of both the treatment components and the laboratory findings is essential for parents to cope with this experience. Support of the child and family during induction of vomiting is particularly important because of the fear, anxiety, and repulsion associated with vomiting. Young children may feel that the discomfort of vomiting is a way to punish them for taking the aspirin.

Because of the close monitoring required, it is easy for parents to misinterpret testing and evaluation to mean increasing danger with a poor prognosis.

Acetaminophen Poisoning

Acetaminophen (Tylenol) has largely replaced aspirin as an analgesic and antipyretic in the treatment of children. This trend has occurred in response to the identification of an association between the use of aspirin during viral infections and Reye syndrome. Acetaminophen poisoning usually occurs as a result of acute poisoning rather than long-term use of therapeutic doses.

Pathophysiology

Acetaminophen is rapidly absorbed from the gastrointestinal tract with peak plasma concentrations occurring within 1 to 2 hours after ingestion of the tablet form and 30 minutes after the liquid form (Hughes, 1984).

Acetaminophen is metabolized in the liver; therefore, acute overdose can result in hepatic damage. Under normal circumstances, a small fraction of acetaminophen is converted to a reactive metabolite that is toxic to the liver. Normally, the reactive metabolite is detoxified by the hepatic substance glutathione and excreted in the urine. In the event of overdose, glutathione can become depleted so that the reactive metabolite binds to cellular protein in the hepatic cell, eventually causing hepatic necrosis.

Hepatic damage is the major cause of morbidity and mortality in acetaminophen poisoning. Children younger than 6 years of age seem to be more resistant to development of hepatotoxicity than older children and adults. Although this mechanism is not understood, it may be associated with the difference in metabolism of acetaminophen.

Clinical Manifestations

Clinical manifestations are frequently nonspecific and delayed. During the first phase (up to 24 hours), there may be some malaise, nausea, vomiting, anorexia, diaphoresis, and pallor. These symptoms may occur within 2 to 4 hours of ingestion or be delayed for 12 to 24 hours. During the next phase (1 to 3 days), there is a latent period with an asymptomatic rise in liver enzymes and bilirubin and prolonged prothrombin time, heralding liver damage. Right upper quadrant pain may accompany or follow these signs of hepatic damage. Thereafter, other manifestations of hepatic necrosis are manifested, including jaundice, renal failure, clotting disorders, and hepatic encephalopathy. Recovery from even severe hepatic damage is usually complete with no residual abnormalities; however, death may occur as a result of acute hepatic failure if it is not recognized and treated aggressively.

Diagnostic Assessment

Serum acetaminophen levels are obtained to make treatment decisions. The acetaminophen assay is delayed until 4 hours after the ingestion to ensure that peak levels of the drug have been reached. The plasma levels of the drug are plotted on a nomogram developed by Rumack and Matthew (1975) to assess the severity of the poisoning. Baseline liver and renal function tests are also obtained. Initiation of therapy is begun on the basis of the drug level in the plasma. Because therapy begun later than 10 hours after ingestion is not considered to be of any value, it is initiated before liver abnormalities are documented by laboratory tests.

Therapeutic Management

Immediate emptying of the stomach by lavage or emesis induced with syrup of ipecac is performed to lessen absorption of the drug. Activated charcoal effectively adsorbs to acetaminophen but it should not be used if use of the antidote *N*-acetylcysteine (Mucomyst) is anticipated. (Activated charcoal binds the antidote *N*-acetylcysteine and makes it ineffective.)

N-acetylcysteine protects the liver by acting as a precursor for the production of additional glutathione (Tenenbein, 1986). It is given orally in a carbonated beverage and is diluted to a 20 per cent solution. It is given by gastric tube as an alternate if the oral route is not tolerated. A loading dose of 140 mg/kg is followed by 70 mg/kg every 4 hours, until a total of 18 doses have been given (Hughes, 1984). The intravenous route is recommended by some; however, its use remains controversial (Tenenbein, 1986).

The patient is monitored by assessing liver function, clotting parameters, and renal function. In 3 to 4 days, liver enzymes peak, and thereafter rapidly return to normal.

Nursing Care

The most important role of the nurse is to intervene with parents before the incident occurs. Safe storage of acetaminophen should be discussed with parents at the time it is prescribed for fever in common childhood illness. Especially when it is purchased for the first time, parents should be counseled about the potential danger that it presents.

If a poisoning episode does occur, the nurse must be aware of signs of overdose in order to take a relevant history and to identify the clinical progression from vague symptoms to more serious signs of hepatic toxicity.

An important nursing role is to support the child and family during the treatment and recovery phases of the poisoning. It is especially important to recognize the offensiveness of the antidote *N*-acetylcysteine (Mucomyst, 20 per cent solution) and to administer it in a carbonated beverage. In the event it is vomited, it is usually repeated within 1 hour of administration. Sometimes, it may be necessary to administer *N*-acetylcysteine by nasogastric tube because of its offensiveness. Soliciting the assistance of parents is often an approach that eases the resistance to its administration.

The patient is sometimes placed on a cardiac monitor and should have vital signs checked frequently. Assessment and documentation of intake and urinary output and overseeing the collection of blood specimens to monitor liver and renal function tests are important nursing functions.

Vitamins with Iron

Vitamins are the second most common type of accidentally ingested medication by children. (Second, that is, to analgesics such as acetaminophen and aspirin.) Vitamins are themselves usually harmless; however, many contain iron, making them potentially lethal. Failure to recognize that iron ingestion is potentially lethal results in careless storage and carrying vitamins in a purse. A young child often thinks vitamins are candy because of the enteric coating. Children's chewable vitamins are pleasant in taste and must be stored safely.

Iron poisoning may be an acute, catastrophic, *life-threatening* event. Iron has a corrosive effect on gastrointestinal mucosa and can leave deposits in the liver. Symptoms occur in stages. In the first 1 to 4 hours, the child has gastrointestinal distress such as vomiting, diarrhea, bloody stools, and gastric discomfort. Symptoms subside after 4 to 6 hours and the child remains asymptomatic for 12 to 36 hours. Subsequently, the child can redevelop systemic toxicity resulting in metabolic acidosis, fever, shock, hepatic failure, or, later, pyloric stenosis.

Diagnosis is made by determining how much elemental iron was ingested and by evaluating clinical symptoms, especially the gastrointestinal disturbances. Tests usually performed include serum iron, total iron-binding capacity, complete blood count, and blood glucose. Indicators of potentially serious poisoning include leukocytosis greater than 15,000 cells/mm^3 and blood glucose above 150 mg/100 ml. There is a poor correlation between serum iron levels and clinical symptoms, and severity of toxicity is difficult to determine; however, a serum concentration of greater than 500 μg/dl is generally treated aggressively.

Induction of emesis or removal of iron by lavage constitutes initial management. Chelation therapy with deferoxamine is used in severe intoxication. Deferoxamine is used as an antidote as well as an indicator of severity. With severe overdose, the urine will be pink or red following the administration of deferoxamine but will be clear with smaller overdoses.

Corrosives

Caustics found in toilet and drain cleansers cause severe chemical burns, the degree of severity depending on the concentration of the chemical and the length of time of contact. Children may present with varying degrees of burns around the mouth and of the oral mucosa, throat, and esophagus, which is not visualized. The burns may be red, swollen, and oozing or more severe, with sloughing or erosion of tissue.

Alkali substances have the capability of continuing to cause damage after initial contact. Care must be taken to flood all external areas with large quantities of water. Vomiting should *never* be induced in these cases because the corrosive may cause additional damage as it again passes through the esophagus. Water is given orally to dilute the substance. Although dilution has not been demonstrated to be of benefit, it is not thought to be harmful as long as small enough quantities are given to avoid stimulus to vomit (Moore, 1986). Endoscopy (flexible or rigid) is done as soon as possible to diagnose esophageal burns, especially circumferential burns (involving an entire diameter of the esophagus). Severe burns causing perforation are accompanied by vascular collapse and shock. Subsequent healing of these lesions can produce strictures in the esophagus. These children should be hospitalized and treated with appropriate therapy that may include steroids, antibiotics, and nasogastric tube feedings. Esophageal stricture and possibly esophageal carcinoma are the two significant long-term problems.

Hydrocarbons

Hydrocarbon ingestion accounts for approximately 5 per cent of all reported accidental ingestion in children between the ages of 1 and 5 years (Barkin, 1990). Petroleum distillates such as paint thinner, turpentine, lighter fluid, furniture polish, gasoline, kerosene, and machine oil are commonly ingested substances. Ingestion can cause irritation of mucous membranes with vomiting, diarrhea, and central nervous system depression. *Aspiration* occurring at the time of ingestion may cause a hydrocarbon pneumonia and acute hemorrhagic necrotizing disease, usually within 24 hours. Secondary respiratory failure is a major problem. Symptoms include respiratory distress, fever, and tachycardia.

The odor of a petroleum distillate can be smelled on the child's breath. Emptying the stomach is a controversial issue because inducing emesis or lavage increases the possibility of aspiration. On the other hand, leaving the hydrocarbon to be absorbed increases the likelihood of fatal systemic toxicity. Some advocate removal to reduce toxicity when more than 1 mg/kg of poison has been ingested, and others do not (Klein & Simon, 1986) because of the increased risk of aspiration. In the unconscious child or if mental status is deteriorating, a cuffed endotracheal tube is inserted followed by lavage. In the alert child, syrup of ipecac is generally preferred over gastric lavage if evacuation is required (Klein & Simon, 1986).

Steroids have been generally shown to be ineffective in either preventing the development of pneumonitis or treating it once it is present. The majority of children who ingest hydrocarbons appear to recover fully.

Insecticides

Most incidents of exposure to insecticides result in no symptoms or minor effects; however, severe intoxications with a substance such as organophosphate is a pediatric emergency.

Chlorinated hydrocarbons such as DDT or methoxychlor and organic phosphates such as parathion or malathion act in different ways to produce pathology. Chlorinated hydrocarbons block nerve function, causing increased salivation, vomiting, abdominal pain, tremors, central nervous system depression, and seizures. Organic phosphates are cholinesterase inhibitors whose ingestion results in symptoms ranging from mild, such as headache, dizziness, weakness, and tremor, to severe, such as gastrointestinal hyperactivity, respiratory distress, pulmonary edema, miosis, sweating, seizures, coma, neuromuscular paralysis, and, in some cases, death.

Treatment is supportive. The effects of organic phosphates are cumulative. Atropine and pralidoxime (2-PAM or Protopam) are specific antidotes for cholinesterase inhibitors. Atropine antagonizes the central and muscarinic cholinergic signs but does *not* reverse muscle weakness; thus, pralidoxime is used for children with respiratory impairment in combination with atropine. If the child's respiratory status deteriorates, intubation and assisted ventilation are required. Airway obstruction may occur even if respirations appear adequate because protective airway reflexes may be lost or because bronchial secretions or malpositioning of the head may obstruct the airway (Mortenson, 1986).

Plant Ingestion and Exposure

Plants can cause a wide range of toxic symptoms from mild gastrointestinal distress to respiratory distress, convulsions, coma, shock, cardiotoxicity, and death. Most poison exposures to plants are benign in nature. Although plants account for a large number of exposures in children, there are very few serious injuries or deaths that result from plant exposures (Litovitz et al, 1992; Arena, 1989). (See Chapter 15 for a discussion of prevention of plant ingestion.) Interested readers are referred to the articles by Fosnot (1979), Keim (1983), and Arena (1989) for specific symptoms of various plant ingestion. In an actual clinical situation, the poison control center provides the information and instructions required for treatment of a specific plant ingestion.

Poison Ivy. Poison ivy is a common plant that grows in woods and fields and can cause a severe dermatitis. Its leaves grow in clusters of three from the same stem, and the edges of the leaves are notched. In autumn and winter, the plant has clusters of white waxy berries. Children should be taught to recognize poison ivy so that they can avoid contact with it.

Poison ivy causes a contact dermatitis consisting of vesicles, papules, and bullae on reddened skin (often in a linear pattern). Lesions usually appear on exposed areas of skin and may appear several hours after contact or not until a few days later. Pruritus, swelling, and burning are commonly associated with the skin lesions. The rash is caused by an irritating oil in the leaves, flowers, stem, and bark. Clothing that has come into contact with the plant should be washed and exposed to sunlight for 48 hours. Even cats and dogs that have touched the plant may cause family members to get the rash. It is, however, not spread from one part of the skin to another by scratching, nor is it spread by the blister fluid to another part of the body or to another person.

Treatment consists of washing the area immediately with mild soap and plenty of water. Methods used to relieve itching include:

- Cool, wet compresses.
- Antihistamine-containing calamine lotions.
- Cool starch baths (e.g., Aveeno bath).
- Benadryl as prescribed.

Keeping fingernails cleaned and trimmed will discourage the development of an infection in the lesions. The lesions may last 2 to 4 weeks, depending on the amount of allergen that has penetrated the skin. (See Chapter 38 for further discussion of poison ivy and other forms of contact dermatitis.)

Lead Poisoning

Lead poisoning occurs when abnormal amounts of lead are absorbed in the body. In the late 1960s and early 1970s, 25 to 40 per cent of children in inner city, low-economy housing areas had elevated blood lead levels because of exposure to lead in house paint. It was not until the late 1970s that the addition of lead in paints for houses was banned. Although this ruling has caused a dramatic reduction in the percentage of children that have elevated blood lead levels, the problem of lead poisoning still exists.

Children are exposed to lead through other means such as environmental residue of lead-containing gasoline, lead-contaminated clothing of leadsmelter workers, artists' paint, improperly glazed pottery, paint chips and putty from old houses painted with lead-containing paint, and lead solder used in plumbing. Congress outlawed the use of lead solder for in-home plumbing in 1986. Children at highest risk are those of lower socioeconomic status who live in older dwellings and who are 1 to 6 years of age, with a peak incidence occurring in spring and summer months.

Lead can be absorbed through the skin, lungs, and gastrointestinal tract. Food, air, and water all contain some lead. Pica (an appetite for unusual nonfood substances) is a frequent precipitating factor in lead poisoning, with children ingesting paint chips or putty containing lead.

Pathophysiology and Clinical Manifestations

The amount of lead ingested, the size of the particle, and repeated ingestion over time are factors that contribute to the severity of lead poisoning. Lead accumulates in the body on continued exposure and is excreted much slower than it is absorbed. It has been shown in animal studies that diets high in fat and low in calcium, magnesium, iron, zinc, and copper increase the absorption of lead (Chisolm, 1987). The diets of children in low-income families are often low in calcium and iron, which may be a factor in their susceptibility to lead poisoning.

The major route of absorption of lead in children is the gastrointestinal tract. Lead is deposited in the blood, bone, and soft tissue, but it has an affinity for osseous tissue, where it accumulates more than in other tissues. The major toxic effects occur in the bone marrow, the nervous system, and the kidney. Anemia results from the metabolic effect of lead on the formation of red blood cells. Lead affects heme synthesis by blocking the incorporation of iron into the protoporphyrin compound that makes up the heme portion of hemoglobin. This results in an accumulation of "free" erythrocyte protophorphyrins, which can be measured to provide an indicator of lead exposure.

The most serious complications of lead poisoning are those affecting the central nervous system. There is a wide variation in the effect of lead on the central nervous system. Acute encephalopathy generally occurs as a result of lead blood levels higher than 80 mg/dl and is manifested by reduced consciousness, seizures, and, eventually, coma and death (Hughes, 1984). Children who do not exhibit overt lead poisoning manifest more subtle effects. Behavior and learning characteristics such as hyperactivity, cognitive and perceptual-motor difficulties, fine motor deficits, and attentional difficulties have been reported (Drummond, 1981). Several large studies have identified decrements in IQ and motor development as blood lead levels increase, even at relatively low blood levels of lead (Bellinger et al, 1992; Baghurst et al, 1992; Dietrich et al, 1993). This phenomenon exists across all socioeconomic groups, although children in lower socioeconomic groups are more likely to experience lead exposure.

In the kidney, lead damages the cells of the proximal tubules with excess excretion of amino acids, glucose, and phosphates in the urine. Early in the course of the disease, the damage is reversible with treatment, but, with continued lead exposure, kidney fibrosis can occur.

Lead intoxication can be acute or chronic. Acute toxicity results in gastrointestinal irritation, renal pathology, and encephalopathy. Symptoms have an abrupt onset and include nausea, abdominal pain, vomiting, diarrhea, black stools, oliguria, seizures, and coma.

Chronic toxicity results in degeneration of nerve and muscle cells, renal pathology, cerebral edema, and bone marrow dysfunction. Symptoms appear insidiously, progressing from hyperirritability, anorexia, lethargy, intermittent gastrointestinal distress, constipation, and weakness to increased nervousness, ataxia, continual vomiting, impaired consciousness, and encephalopathy with seizures and coma.

Diagnostic Assessment

Making a diagnosis on the basis of history and presenting symptoms is difficult because symptoms appear slowly and are similar to many other conditions. A history of pica is extremely relevant. Pica may be a manifestation of iron-deficiency anemia and other factors, such as a low-calcium diet or a glucose-6-phosphate dehydrogenase (G6PD) deficiency. History taking and observations by the nurse will help uncover these deficiencies. Possible recent exposure to lead or lead fumes or recent change of residence should be considered. The possibility that the child has played unsupervised near contaminated sources is also explored.

Because symptoms may be vague with insidious onset, large-scale screening is the only way to assure that many children with excessive lead levels are identified. Current guidelines from the Centers for Disease Control (CDC) recommend universal screening of all children between the ages of 6 months and 6 years of age. Historically, erythrocyte protoporphyrin (EP) levels have been used for screening children for lead poisoning and anemia. However, EP levels will not identify children with blood lead levels below 25 μg/dl. Therefore, the CDC's current recommendations are that all children be screened with direct blood lead measurements (CDC, 1991). Blood lead levels at or below 9 μg/dl are considered normal.

Any child with a lead level above 9 μg/dl is a candidate for more frequent screening. Children with levels above 15 μg/dl need nutritional and educational interventions and possibly an environmental investigation. Pharmacologic treatment is usually instituted at levels between 25 and 35 μg/dl. Supporting findings are "lead flecks" on abdominal roentgenographs or "lead lines" on long bone roentgenographs.

Therapeutic Management

The goal of treatment is to reduce the amount of lead in the blood tissues. The first line of treatment is to identify and remove the environmental source of lead. Second, the accumulated lead in the body must be reduced. Removal of lead from blood and tissues is accomplished through urinary excretion of lead and deposition of lead into the bones. Children with symptomatic poisoning are usually admitted to the hospital and intravenous fluids are given to maintain urine flow. These children are at risk for cerebral edema; therefore, after urinary flow is established, fluids are restricted.

Once urinary flow is well established, chelation therapy is started. Chelation therapy is a treatment that facilitates the formation of a fairly stable, highly soluble compound with lead followed by its excretion through the kidney. Therapy is begun with a drug called British antilewisite (BAL) (dimercaprol) and calcium disodium edetate (CaEDTA) by intravenous drip or deep intramuscular injection. A combination of therapy is used because it results in reduced saturation of the drug in the blood, fewer side effects of each drug, and better removal from the brain. The use of CaEDTA reduces lead levels overall, but BAL is more effective in the nervous system.

If a child does not have encephalopathy, then BAL therapy may be discontinued after 48 hours. After 4 to 5 days of CaEDTA therapy, its toxicity increases and the output of lead decreases. Therefore, such therapy is discontinued for 48 to 72 hours, after which chelation is repeated with only CaEDTA for another 5-day course. A chelation course can be reinstituted to reduce the lead level to an excretion ratio of less than 1 (1 μg of lead to 1 mg EDTA). It is desirable to wait 5 to 7 days before beginning a third course of chelation (Piomelli et al, 1984). BAL should not be used for patients with a G6PD deficiency nor in conjunction with iron therapy (Piomelli et al, 1984). Fluid and electrolyte maintenance is important, as is continued monitoring of the child and serial blood studies. The toxic child must be observed for signs of increased intracranial pressure (changing level of consciousness, increased blood pressure, and slow pulse).

Oral D-penicillamine is an effective drug if exposure to lead during its course of administration is definitely curtailed. It is currently classed as an investigational drug for use in lead poisoning (Chisolm, 1987).

Nursing Diagnostic Statements

High risk for injury; poisoning; risk factors: *exposure to an environment containing lead.*

Altered comfort: pain, *related to painful stimuli associated with injection of BAL and CaEDTA.*

Altered patterns of urinary elimination, *related to renal injury associated with side effects of CaEDTA.*

Altered tissue perfusion: cerebral, *related to:*

- *Lead toxicity.*
- *Toxicity of chelating drugs.*

Altered family processes, *related to situational crises associated with acute and potentially chronic care of a child with lead poisoning.*

Nursing Care

Prevent Continuing Exposure to Lead. The first goal of care is prevention. Control of the environmental sources of lead is a multidisciplinary goal. Nurses can counsel parents to guard against exposure to lead-containing paint chips on old houses as well as alerting them to sources such as dirt, snow, and ice exposed to automobile exhaust fumes and lead-containing cooking utensils. In homes in which lead solder was used in plumbing, lead enters the water when water sits in pipes for longer than several hours. This problem can be eliminated by allowing tap water to run for 30 seconds before using. Water from hot water taps should not be used for cooking or drinking. Early detection of lead poisoning is attempted through a careful history, clinical observation, and screening tests.

Reducing Discomfort Associated with Therapy. Nursing strategies during a course of treatment are focused on the immediate care of the child and long-term concerns of the family. When multiple injections are required, the child begins to fear and strongly resist them. Preparation for these injections can bring some comfort to the child, but, because of their frequency and painfulness, a wide range of approaches is required to reduce the trauma for the child. BAL is available only in oil for intramuscular injection, but CaEDTA is available for intravenous infusion. Intramuscular injection of CaEDTA is extremely painful and it is recommended that it be given with procaine (0.5 per cent) by deep injection (Piomelli et al, 1984). It is drawn up last in the syringe; the syringe is held vertically with the needle pointing down so that the procaine is administered first. Local application of warm soaks to the injected areas should also be offered.

Maintaining Fluid Balance and Renal Flow. Chelation should not be performed in the absence of adequate urine flow. Therefore, urinary output is closely monitored. CaEDTA is a nonmetabolizable drug that is excreted by the kidney (Chisolm, 1987). Impending renal failure and drug toxicity is noted by the appearance of protein in the urine, rising blood urea nitrogen level, and serum creatinine. Intake and output are measured and the intravenous infusion is carefully monitored. Urinary output is essential for chelation to take place, yet fluid intake is restricted to basal requirements to avoid cerebral edema.

Monitoring for Signs of Encephalopathy. The nurse should observe for signs of encephalopathy associated with toxicity of chelating agents. The side effects of the drugs should be carefully monitored because some of them are also features of acute lead encephalopathy. Seizure precautions should be taken, and appropriate equipment should be available in the event of respiratory arrest.

Maintaining Family Stability. During acute illness, the child's and parents' fear and needs are similar to those in any poisoning. In addition, when parents are told of the possible long-term effects of lead poisoning, they need additional emotional support. Fear for their other children is a concern that needs to be discussed with parents. Helping parents understand how they can help prevent further harm is far more constructive than dwelling on what has already taken place. Other stressors that could hinder the child's or family's adaptation should be identified and managed.

Prognosis

Sequelae associated with lead poisoning are related to the degree and duration of exposure. Manifestations of residual damage in severe encephalopathy may include blindness and hemiparesis. In less severe cases, seizure disorders, altered behavior, and a degree of intellectual deficits may occur. These children may not show any residual effects until school-age, when they are noted to be more distractible and have some attentional deficits.

Submersion Injury (Near-Drowning)

"Drowning" is defined as death from asphyxia while submerged in fresh or salt water, with death occurring within 24 hours. If survival surpasses this crucial period, then the event is referred to as "near-drowning." A child may drown with or without aspiration of fluid into the lungs (death may occur from laryngospasm due to a small amount of water entering the trachea).

Etiology/Incidence

The incidence of submersion injuries has continued to increase in recent years. Drowning is a leading cause of death for children 4 years and younger. Many children who survive the incident are left with severe, permanent neurologic disabilities (Beyda, 1991). The number of near-drownings is probably much higher. Childhood drownings occur most frequently in swimming pools, although children may drown in bathtubs, hot tubs and whirlpools, roadside ditches, and at the beach. Very young children (about 2 years of age) and adolescents are two age groups that seem to be at greater risk for drowning incidents. In young children, this is due to momentary lack of adult supervision. Anyone familiar with toddlers will appreciate the rapidity with which they gravitate to forbidden activity—especially if they perceive that adult attention is momentarily diverted. The potential risk for young adolescents may well be related to drug and/or alcohol consumption leading to impaired judgment. Drowning may also be the result of child abuse or suicide.

Pathophysiology

Factors that influence the prognosis of the near-drowning victim are duration of submersion, temper-

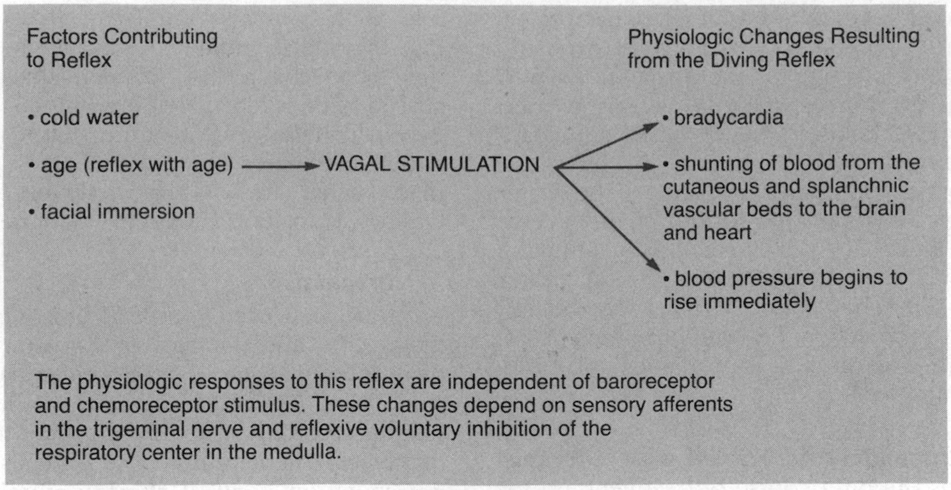

FIGURE 46 - 2. The diving reflex. This reflex operates only in young children. (Based on Dickerman, J. D., & Lucey, J. F. [1985]. *The critically ill child* [3rd ed.]. Philadelphia: WB Saunders.)

ature of the water, presence and type of pulmonary aspiration, and the age of the child (young children can withstand longer periods of submersion).

Very young children may display the mammalian diving reflex, which results in bradycardia and shunting of blood away from the periphery to the brain and heart (Fig. 46–2). Although this unique reflex may be elicited in adult victims, it is more pronounced in very young children and probably contributes significantly to the often miraculous recovery of a child. In order for the reflex to be optimally activated, the water must be colder than 21° C (70° F). Also, facial immersion must occur quite rapidly in order to trigger the vagal stimulation that is essential to the reflex trigger.

When a child is submerged in water, there is a struggle to escape, followed by laryngospasm, gasping, and swallowing of water, and often vomiting. When a child reaches the point when a breath must be taken, the following conditions have already developed: arterial hypoxemia, tachycardia, tissue hypoxia, and acidosis (Dickerman & Lucey, 1985). Gasping and the swallowing of water are followed by respiratory arrest and unconsciousness. Loss of consciousness occurs within 3 minutes of submersion. The duration of hypoxia required to cause death is unknown. In water that is very cold (0 to 15° C [32 to 60° F]) children have been known to survive and have normal neurologic function following submersion up to 40 minutes, although full recovery is rare after 20 minutes of submersion (Conn, 1987).

Role of Hypothermia

Children who have been victims of near-drowning and who are admitted with core body temperatures of less than 34° C (93.2° F) demand special resuscitative efforts. It is well known that hypothermia can be useful in lowering the metabolic rate and therefore in reducing oxygen demands by the brain and the core organs.

Unconsciousness occurs when the core body temperature drops below 34° C (93.2° F). Ventricular fibrillation may occur at 28° C (82.4° F) and asystole at 22° C (71.6° F). No cardiovascular activity can be restored as long as the core temperature remains low. Resuscitative efforts must therefore include maintenance of vital functions until rewarming has occurred to a degree at which spontaneous cardiac activity occurs–usually at 29° to 30° C (84.2° to 86° F). This can prolong the resuscitative effort by hours. Initial efforts instituted in the emergency room may be continued in the intensive care unit.

The pathophysiology of drowning in fresh water versus salt water is not of such major clinical significance as was once thought. In both types of submersion, arterial hypoxemia develops. The resultant state of reflex bradycardia, tissue hypoxia, and acidosis eventually leads to cardiac arrest and, with absence of ventilation, to brain death, if rescue and resuscitation do not occur.

Following near-drowning in either fresh or salt water, further lung damage may result from aspiration of vomitus, algae, sand or dirt, and bacteria. Although chlorine in pools and soapy water in bathtubs could be expected to contribute to lung tissue damage, there are no significant data to support this hypothesis (Dickerman & Lucey, 1985). Postmortem examination has shown intra-alveolar hemorrhage and pulmonary embolism following both types of drowning (Stickler & Snowman, 1981).

Diagnostic Assessment

Initiating treatment for a drowning child must begin immediately on extraction of the child from the water. Cardiopulmonary resuscitation (CPR) is begun immediately and the child is transported by ambulance to an emergency facility. There, acquisition of a detailed history is essential and may be the role of the triage nurse, because all other medical energies will be directed toward resuscitation. Important information includes the child's age and general health, length of submersion (parents will often not be able to give an accurate estimate of time), and any contributing factors such as alcohol and/or drug consumption or history of diabetes or epilepsy.

The primary assessment focuses on the ABCs until they are stable. When assessing for airway and breathing, the rate and pattern of the respiration is noted and recorded. A patent airway is essential. The airway is examined for vomitus, mucus, or aspirated material and suctioned as needed. If there is any reason to suspect cervical spine injury, the airway must be protected with immobilization of the neck and use of the chin-lift technique.

Therapeutic Management

If cardiopulmonary arrest has occurred, oxygenation becomes the priority. Before intubating the child, the physician will want to ensure as clean an airway as possible. This is accomplished by suctioning, insertion of an oropharyngeal airway, and ventilation with 100 per cent oxygen using a bag-valve-mask. The child should be well oxygenated before intubation is attempted. Experienced respiratory technologists, nurses, or physicians may "bag" the child if they are knowledgeable and skilled in the use of the equipment. Once the airway is clean and the child well oxygenated, intubation is performed.

Continuous monitoring, diagnostic studies, laboratory evaluations, and fluid management occur simultaneously. A portable chest roentgenograph is taken, arterial blood gases measured, and vital signs monitored. Pulse oximetry can be used for continuous monitoring of oxygen saturation. Two intravenous lines are inserted for administration of medications. Fluid volume is strictly controlled to reduce intracranial pressure. If hypothermia has occurred, warmed fluids can be administered to assist in warming vital organs. This may be accomplished by administering warm intravenous fluids via peripheral intravenous lines, peritoneal lavage, or colonic irrigation. Rapid rewarming by application of heated blankets is contraindicated because cold blood from the extremities may cause rebound cooling and cardiac dysrhythmia as it circulates to the body core.

An electrocardiogram should be obtained as soon as possible following admission. Blood samples should be ordered for baseline values of complete blood count, serum electrolytes, blood urea nitrogen, creatinine, and glucose levels, as well as arterial blood gases. A urinary catheter is inserted to monitor renal function. A nasogastric tube is inserted to remove swallowed water and debris and to prevent gastric distention due to assisted ventilation.

Medications that are used include oxygen, sodium bicarbonate to counteract acidosis, antibiotics to prevent pulmonary infection, and aminophylline to increase gas exchange by bronchodilatation. Short- and long-acting barbiturates or lidocaine may be used to lower intracranial pressure if the need arises (Dickerman & Lucey, 1985).

Nursing Diagnostic Statements

Ineffective airway clearance, *related to aspiration of water and debris.*

Ineffective breathing pattern, *related to cerebral hypoxia from near-drowning episode.*

Impaired gas exchange, *related to aspiration of water, debris, and laryngospasm.*

Altered tissue perfusion, *related to cerebral, cardiopulmonary, and renal involvement.*

Anxiety: parents, *related to uncertainty of outcome.*

High risk for injury; risk factor: *Knowledge deficit concerning child safety practices to prevent future incidents of water-related injury.*

Altered growth and development: self-care skills, *related to residual neurologic effects.*

Nursing Care

Maintaining a Patent Airway. The nurse should assist in achieving and/or maintaining a patent airway by using the chin-lift maneuver, suctioning the trachea, and inserting an oropharyngeal airway if appropriate. In anticipation of the need to intubate, the nurse prepares a pediatric laryngoscope with an appropriately sized blade, a functioning light, and correct tube size.

Once the child is intubated, the nurse is responsible for assessing and maintaining the patency of the tube.

Maintaining an Effective Breathing Pattern. Monitor respirations every 5 minutes for rate and pattern until respirations are stable. If the child is unable to maintain an effective breathing pattern, then mechanical ventilation must be instituted.

Monitoring and Facilitating Gas Exchange. Each time vital signs are taken, the chest is auscultated and findings should be documented. Since near-drowning victims are at risk for developing pulmonary edema, any alterations in breath sounds are reported to the physician. The child is placed in a semi-Fowler position, if possible, to maximize diaphragmatic excursion and increase alveolar aeration. Chest physiotherapy is performed by the nurse or physical therapist. The administration of oxygen, at 100 per cent with humidification, is monitored and analyzed by the nurse.

Arterial blood gases are reviewed to evaluate the effectiveness of interventions. Pulse oximetry is used to monitor oxygen saturation between arterial blood gas testing times.

Maintaining Tissue Perfusion (Cerebral, Cardiovascular, Renal). The nurse monitors the infusion rate and maintains the intravenous therapy regimen to establish perfusion. If hypothermia is used therapeutically for cerebral edema, the patient's temperature is closely monitored.

Serial monitoring of respirations, heart rate, blood pressure, urinary output, and assessment of intracranial pressure and level of unconsciousness is done every 5 to 15 minutes until stable, at which time monitoring may be reduced to every hour or less often. A urinary catheter is usually inserted to monitor hourly output. All assessments must be accurately documented.

Reducing Parental Anxiety Related to Uncertainty of Outcome. The nurse needs to be supportive of the child's family during this time of crisis and severe stress. They should be encouraged to ask questions and be given accurate, up-to-date information. They should be allowed to see and touch their child as soon as possible, even though this may be emotionally upsetting because of invasive machinery. The nurse prepares them beforehand for the array of equipment and tubes attached to their child. Once the child is transferred to the intensive care unit or to a ward, the parents should be encouraged to participate in their child's daily care if they so desire. Keeping parents informed about the child's condition is an important part of the nurse's supportive role.

Many children survive seemingly insurmountable insults as a result of near-drowning, with remarkable resilience. Often there are no neurologic deficits or they are minimal and seem to resolve with time. Other children suffer deficits ranging from minimal physical disability to profound physical and intellectual impairment. A period of hospitalization on a pediatric ward may be necessary to assess the deficits and institute long-term rehabilitation.

Preventing Water-Related Injury in the Future. Discussions about prevention are inappropriate during the critical phase of care. As the family works through the emotional trauma of this crisis, they will often plan ways to avoid future occurrences. Remain alert for "if only" statements. Reinforce appropriate plans for precautions in the future while helping the parents absolve themselves of any unnecessary guilt associated with the present event. In the absence of evidence of plans to rectify a dangerous situation, refer the family for follow-up visits in the home.

Fostering Development of Self-Care Skills and Optimal Communication. If a child suffers neurologic sequelae, a carefully planned rehabilitation program is instituted. During this phase, the nurse assesses the child's progress in gaining optimal self-care skills and plans with the family and professional team to acquire the necessary rehabilitative services. A smooth transition from acute care to rehabilitative services to home is achieved by cooperative planning among the involved disciplines, such as occupational therapy, physical therapy, speech therapy, nutritionists, social workers, and a public health nurse. A public health liaison nurse can facilitate the transition by early involvement in care during the acute phase. Within the hospital setting, acquisition of special equipment, such as a special wheelchair, eating utensils, and simple clothing, facilitates optimal achievement of growth and development. Nursing care for the child with submersion injury is summarized in Table 46–14.

Child with Multiple Trauma

Multiple trauma involves injury to more than one body system. Multiple trauma most commonly occurs in motor vehicle accidents, vehicle-pedestrian accidents, child abuse, and falls. Most of the injuries are *blunt* as opposed to *penetrating;* blunt trauma may cause only minimal external evidence of the location and degree of injury. Multiple injuries therefore present a special challenge to the health care team. Since the first 20 minutes of treatment are the most important in terms of stabilization and eventual outcome, the health care professionals who provide this treatment should be highly skilled. Seidel and co-workers (1986) found that most programs for EMTs and paramedics and for emergency room physicians and nurses are geared to the adult trauma or cardiac victim. Many ambulances do not carry pediatric resuscitation equipment, and general hospitals may have only minimal equipment in limited sizes to care for critically ill children. With these problems in mind, several large teaching centers have established specialized units operated by highly trained personnel to provide optimal care to injured children. The American College of Surgeons recently added an extensive pediatric component to the advanced trauma life support course. The courses offer a clear, simplified approach to trauma management for both adults and children in the first hour following injury. The goal is to provide rapid stabilization of the victim and transfer of the patient as soon as possible to a facility offering specialized care. Nurses who are employed in critical care should be encouraged to take similar courses that have been modified to include nursing interventions so that a coordinated team approach may be developed. Assessment and care of the multiply-injured child is a highly specialized area of study. The reader is referred to emergency and intensive care texts for further information.

TABLE 46-14
Nursing Process Plan: Submersion Injury

Analysis: Collaborative Problem 1

Response and Related or Risk Factors: *Ineffective airway clearance related to aspiration of water and debris*

Projected Outcome: The child will be able to clear secretions or obstructions from the respiratory tract, in order to maintain airway patency

Defining Characteristics

- Abnormal breath sounds
- Stridor or grunting
- Presence of vomitus, mucus, or aspirated material in airway
- Decrease or increase in rate of respiratory effort
- Pallor
- Cyanosis (late sign)
- Tracheal, substernal, and/or intercostal indrawing or inspiration
- Nasal flaring
- Decreased air entry or auscultation

Nursing Interventions

Airway Management

Open airway

- Using chin lift maneuver (protects cervical spine)
- Suction oropharynx and trachea to clear airway and improve visualization of epiglottis prior to intubation
- Insert oropharyngeal airway if appropriate

OR

Assist with endotracheal intubation

Continue to assess and monitor patency of the airway

Auscultate

Evaluation Criteria

Respiratory rate is congruent with normal parameter for age

Respiratory effort diminishes, no indrawing noted

Skin color will be appropriate for race. Mucous membranes will be pinkish

Breath sounds are clear

Analysis: Nursing Diagnostic Statement 1

Response and Related or Risk Factors: *High risk for ineffective breathing pattern and impaired gas exchange; risk factors: hypoxia, aspiration of water, debris, and laryngospasm*

Projected Outcome: The child's inhalation and/or exhalation pattern will enable adequate pulmonary inflation or emptying

Defining Characteristics

(Actual Responses)

- Irregular respiratory rate
- Decreased respirations (e.g., less than 12/min)
- Respiratory depth changes
- Tachypnea
- Pallor
- Sinuses (late sign)
- Oxygen saturation <90%
- Fremitus

Nursing Interventions

Respiratory Monitoring

Assess respiratory rate, rhythm and effort at least every hour—more often as circumstances require

Assess for signs of respiratory distress every hour—more often as circumstances require

Auscultate breath sounds every hour

Evaluation Criteria

Respiratory rate and depth, and heart rate, will be within normal parameters for age

No evidence of respiratory distress (e.g., nasal flaring, grunting, use of accessory muscles)

Breath sounds will be clear on auscultation

Arterial blood gases and pulse oximetry will be within normal

(continued)

TABLE 46-14 *(continued)*

Defining Characteristics *(Actual Response)*	**Nursing Interventions**	**Evaluation Criteria**
• Decreased air entry or auscultation • Nasal flaring • Use of accessary muscles (indrawing) • Grunting	**Elevate head of bed** to decrease diaphragmatic restriction by abdominal organs **Suction oropharynx and trachea** as circumstances require, noting color and consistency of secretions **Monitor arterial blood gases and pulse oximetry** as ordered **Administer oxygen** as ordered	**parameters** (e.g., oxygen saturation >90%; as close to 100% as possible is preferable) **Skin color will be appropriate for race. Mucous membranes will be pinkish**

Analysis: Nursing Diagnostic Statement 2

Response and Related or Risk Factors: *High risk for altered tissue perfusion; risk factors: cerebral, cardiopulmonary, and renal involvement*

Projected Outcome: Cardiac output will be sufficient to maintain adequate perfusion of brain, heart, and kidneys

Defining Characteristics *(Actual Response)*	**Nursing Interventions**	**Evaluation Criteria**
Subjective: • Confusion • Lack of recognition of parents and/or significant others *Objective*: • Skin-dependent blue or purple, pale on elevation, color does not return on lowering of extremities • Skin temperature, cold extremities • Skin quality, shining • Increased heart rate and respirations (unless mechanically ventilated) and decreased blood pressure • Diminished arterial pulsations • Urine output <1 ml/kg/hr • Acidosis • Oxygen saturation <90% • Presence of cardiac dysrhythmias • Low score on Pediatric Coma Scale, if cerebral perfusion is altered	*Surveillance; Oxygen Therapy* **Assess heart rate and rhythm, respiratory rate (unless mechanically ventilated), blood pressure, and temperature** every hour and as circumstances require **Assess extremities for adequate peripheral perfusion** every hour and as circumstances require **Monitor urine output** every hour and as circumstances require **Monitor ABH and pulse oximetry as ordered** **Monitor for signs and symptoms of hypovolemia** **Maintain IV fluids** as ordered **Administer supplemental oxygen** as ordered **Maintain patent airway** **Assess level of consciousness** using Pediatric Coma Scale	**Vital signs will be maintained within normal parameters for age,** including hemodynamic monitoring values if this equipment is used **Extremities will be appropriate color for race and warm to touch; mucous membranes will be pink; peripheral pulses will be palpable** **Urine output will be maintained at 1 ml/kg/hr** **Child will score a minimum of 12 on the Pediatric Coma Scale** (assessing neurologic function)

TABLE 46-14 (continued)

Analysis: Nursing Diagnostic Statement 3

Response and Related or Risk Factors: *Ineffective family coping: compromised, related to altered growth and development, self-care skills associated with residual neurologic effects*

Projected Outcome: The family will provide sufficient, effective, and/or uncompromised support, comfort, assistance, and/or encouragement to help the child accept the limitations of altered growth and development and learn new skills to meet health care needs

Defining Characteristics	Nursing Interventions	Evaluation Criteria
Subjective: • Child expresses a concern about his or her parents' response to the health problem • Parents describe preoccupation with fear, anticipatory grief, guilt, anger, anxiety, and/or frustration at child's inability to perform tasks previously mastered (i.e., before injury) • Parental expression of feelings of being overwhelmed by unremitting responsibility for care of child • Parents confirm an inadequate understanding or knowledge base	*Coping Enhancement* **Assess family's coping skills** **Identify and help family** to mobilize coping skills and develop new ones **Provide an atmosphere and opportunities** for parents to express their feelings **Assist family to identify community resources** to help them (e.g., support groups) **Refer family to appropriate health care providers** as required (e.g., social work, parental relief programs, home-based physiotherapy and occupational therapy)	**Child and parents become increasingly proficient at performing self-care skills within limitations of neurologic deficits** **Parents begin to come to terms with loss and limitations imposed by neurologic deficits** **Parents maintain appropriate level of communication with the child**
Objective: • Anger as manifested by temper tantrums by child • Crying—child or family members • Parental arguments • Parents attempt assistive or supportive behaviors with less than satisfactory results • Parents withdraw or enter into limited communication with child • Parents display protective behavior disproportionate (too little or too much) to the client's abilities or need for autonomy	**Encourage and assist child in performing self-care tasks;** reinforce accomplishments with praise **Assist the child to develop alternative skills** in areas where a deficit exists	

Analysis: Nursing Diagnostic Statement 4

Response and Related or Risk Factors: *Health-seeking behaviors related to desire to know child safety/practices to prevent future incidents of water-related injury*

Projected Outcome: Parents will alter habits and/or the environment in order to demonstrate an understanding of the need for vigilant adult supervision of children relative to any body of water, water safety principles, CPR training, and normal growth and development

(continued)

TABLE 46-14 *(continued)*

Defining Characteristics	*Nursing Interventions*	*Evaluation Criteria*
Subjective: • Expressed or observed desire of parents to seek a higher level of family wellness, especially as related to safety of their child • Expressed or observed desire (parents) for increased control of their child's environment *Objective*: • Expression of concern by parents about current environmental conditions on family health status, especially in relation to safety of their child • Stated or observed unfamiliarity with community resources • Demonstrated or observed lack of knowledge in health promotion behaviors	**Assess family's knowledge of drowning prevention** **Assess parent's knowledge of normal growth and development** **Teach parents about normal growth and development** using their child's behaviors as examples **Supply parents with a list of community support resources for learning CPR and water safety** **Arrange referral with appropriate community agencies** (e.g., community health nurse for home safety assessment) **Stress importance of adult supervision at all times**	**Parents will demonstrate an understanding of child safety practices** **Parents will provide evidence of childproofing their home before child's discharge** (e.g., completed check lists, report from community health nurse)

Analysis: Nursing Diagnostic Statement 5

Response and Related or Risk Factors: *Defensive coping (parents) related to anxiety associated with uncertainty of outcome*

Projected Outcome: Parents will express concerns and feelings related to the injury and decreased anxiety. Parents will develop a support system that may include the family members and the health care team

Defining Characteristics	*Nursing Interventions*	*Evaluation Criteria*
Subjective: • Denial of child's obvious problems/weaknesses • Projection of blame/responsibility • Hypersensitive to slight/criticism • Superior attitude toward others • Lack of follow-through or participation for treatment or therapy	*Coping Enhancement* **Involve parents in child's care** as much as possible; encourage touching and talking to child, especially if child is unconscious **Provide consistent caregivers.** This reduces the number of people involved in the child's care in whom the parents must place their trust and from whom they must receive information **Communicate child's status** and/or program daily to parents **Plan family conferences** with all caregivers and health team members as soon as possible after accident (1 wk recommended) and *at least* biweekly thereafter	**Parents will state their satisfaction with the level of care provided** **Parents will verbalize feelings of decreased anxiety** **Parents will feel comfortable asking questions of specific caregivers and of health care team at conferences. Parents will mobilize appropriate coping skills** **Parents will develop a support system consisting of significant others and/or members of the health care team** **Parents will begin to discuss outcome in realistic terms and to plan for future** (e.g., planning

TABLE 46-14 (continued)

Defining Characteristics	Nursing Interventions	Evaluation Criteria
	Assist parents to see situation realistically	funeral arrangements if prognosis is very poor or making adjustments for home care that accommodates deficits after recovery)
	Assess coping skills used in previous crises and assist family to capitalize on useful existing skills and to develop new ones	

KEY CONCEPTS

Concepts Related to Basic Information

- Accidental injury is the leading cause of death in American children.
- Many accidental injuries are preventable.
- Children's proportionally larger head size and thinner skulls make them more prone to head injury.
- Less well developed skeletal and muscular structures make children more prone to blunt trauma injuries.
- Fear and guilt are common parental reactions to injury.

Concepts Related to Nursing Assessment

- Initial assessment of an injured child involves a primary survey (airway, breathing, circulation) and a secondary survey (head to toe assessment).
- Nurses should be alert for possible abusive situations when assessing an injured child.
- The principles of triage and any institutional guidelines for triage should be used when assessing multiple injury victims under circumstances of limited resources.

Concepts Related to Nursing Intervention

- All nursing personnel must maintain certification in cardiopulmonary resuscitation.
- Nursing responsibilities include caring for parents.
- Accurate documentation is vital in emergency situations.
- Parents can be counseled to handle many childhood injuries.
- Teaching of the prevention of injury should be included in every parental encounter.

REFERENCES

Accident Facts. (1988). Chicago: National Safety Council.

Arena, J. M. (1989). Plants that poison. *Emergency Medicine, 21,* 20–35.

American Heart Association and American Academy of Pediatrics. (1991). *Textbook of pediatric resuscitation*. Evanston, IL: Authors.

Baghurst, P. A., McMichael, A. J., Wigg, N. R., Vimpani, G. V., Robertson, E. F., Roberts, R. J., & Tong, S. L. (1992). Environmental exposure to lead and children's intelligence at the age of seven years. *New England Journal of Medicine, 327,* 1279–1284.

Barkin, R. (1990). Toxicologic emergencies. *Pediatric Annals, 19,* 629–633.

Barkin, R., & Luten, R. (1990). Emergencies in pediatrics and the child in the emergency medical services system. *Pediatric Annals, 19,* 571–577.

Behrman, R. F. (Ed.). (1992). *Nelson textbook of pediatrics* (14th ed.). Philadelphia: WB Saunders.

Bellinger, D. C., Stiles, K. M., & Needleman, H. L. (1992). Low-level lead exposure, intelligence and academic achievement: A long-term follow-up study. *Pediatrics, 90,* 855–861.

Beyda, D. (1991). Pathophysiology of near-drowning and treatment of a child with a submersion incident. *Critical Care Nursing Clinics of North America, 3,* 273–280.

Chameides, L. (1988). *Textbook of pediatric advanced life support*. Evanston, IL: American Heart Association/American Academy of Pediatrics.

Centers for Disease Control. (1991). *Preventing lead poisoning in young children*. A statement by the Centers for Disease Control. Atlanta: Author.

Chisolm, J. J. (1987). Increased lead absorption and lead poisoning. In R. E. Behrman & V. C. Vaughn (Eds.), *Nelson textbook of pediatrics* (13th ed., pp 1507–1510). Philadelphia: WB Saunders.

Coln, D. (1985, September). Pediatric trauma. *AORN Journal, 42,* 338–342.

Conn, A. W. (1987). Drowning and near-drowning. In R. E. Behrman & V. C. Vaughn (Eds.), *Nelson textbook of pediatrics* (13th ed., pp 220–223). Philadelphia: WB Saunders.

Conner, G. H. (1987). Foreign bodies of the ear, nose, airway, and esophagus. In R. A. Hoekelman (Ed.), *Primary pediatric care* (pp 1243–1247). St. Louis: CV Mosby.

Dandrinos-Smith, S. (1991). The epidemiology of pediatric trauma. *Critical Care Nursing Clinics of North America, 3,* 387–389.

Dickerman, J. D., & Lucey, J. F. (1985). *Smith's the critically ill child: Diagnosis and medical management*. Philadelphia: WB Saunders.

Dietrich, K. N., Berger, O. G., & Succop, P. A. (1993). Lead exposure and the motor developmental status of urban six-year-old children in the Cincinnati Prospective Study. *Pediatrics, 91,* 301–307.

Done, A. K. (1960). Nomogram for interpretations of salicylate levels following acute ingestion. *Pediatrics, 26,* 800–807.

Dreisbach, R. H. (1983). *Handbook of poisoning: prevention, diagnosis, and treatment*. Los Altos, CA: Lange Medical Publications.

Drummond, A. H. (1981). Lead poisoning in children. *Journal of School Health, 51,* 43–47.

Fosnot, H. (1979, June). Plant-ingestion poisoning from A to Z. *Patient Care, 30,* 86.

Gage, A. M., & Gage, A. A. (1981, September). Frostbite. *Comprehensive Therapy, 7,* 25–30.

Gaunder, B. N. (1986, March). Insect bites and stings: Managing allergic reactions. *Nurse Practitioner, 11,* 16–28.

Gaudreault, P., & Lovejoy, F. H. (1985). Acute poisoning. In J. D. Dickerman & J. F. Lucey (Eds.). *Smith's the critically ill child: Diagnosis and medical management* (3rd ed.). Philadelphia: WB Saunders.
Henry, R. (1991). Pediatric dental emergencies. *Pediatric Nursing, 17,* 162–167.
Hughes, J. G., & Griffith, J. F. (1984). *Synopsis of pediatrics*. St. Louis: CV Mosby.
Kavanagh, K. T., & Litovitz, T. (1986, March 21). Miniature foreign bodies in auditory and nasal cavities. *Journal of the American Medical Association, 255,* 1470–1472.
Keim, K. A. (1983, July/August). Preventing and treating plant poisoning in young children. *MCN: American Journal of Maternal Child Nursing, 8*(4), 287–289.
Kelley, S. J. (1988). *Pediatric emergency nursing*. Norwalk, CT: Appleton & Lange.
Kinney, M. R., et al. (1988). *AACN's clinical reference for critical-care nursing* (2nd ed.). New York: McGraw-Hill.
Klein, B. L., & Simon, J. E. (1986). Hydrocarbon poisoning. *Pediatric Clinics of North America, 33,* 411–420.
Krasner, P. (1990). Treatment of tooth evulsion by nurses. *Journal of Emergency Nursing, 16,* 29–33.
Litovitz, T. L., Holm, K. C., Bailey, K. M., & Schmitz, B. F. (1992). 1991 Annual Report of the American Association of Poison Control Centers National Data Collection System. *American Journal of Emergency Medicine, 10,* 452–490.
Matlak, M. E. (1985). Foreign bodies. In T. A. Mayer (Ed.), *Emergency management of pediatric trauma*. Philadelphia: WB Saunders.
Mayer, T. A. (1985). *Emergency management of pediatric trauma*. Philadelphia: WB Saunders.
McKenna, P. J., Walsh, D. J., & Martin, L. W. (1991). Pediatric bicycle trauma. *Journal of Trauma, 31,* 392–394.
Miles, M. S., & Carter, M. (1982). Sources of parental stress in pediatric intensive care units. *Children's Health Care, 11,* 65–69.
Mofenson, H. C., & Caraccio, T. R. (1986, April). Benefits/risks of syrup of ipecac. *Pediatrics, 77,* 551–552.
Mofenson, H. C., & Greensher, J. (1985). Management of the choking child. *Pediatric Clinics of North America, 32,* 183–192.
Mofenson, H. C., & Greensher, J. (1979). Poisoning—An update. *Clinical Pediatrics, 18,* 144–146.
Moore, W. R. (1985, April). Caustic ingestions: Pathophysiology, diagnosis and treatment. *Clinical Pediatrics, 25,* 192–196.
Mortenson, M. L. (1986). Management of acute childhood poisonings caused by selected insecticides and herbicides. *Pediatric Clinics of North America, 33,* 421–445.
Needleman, H. L. (1984). Increased lead absorption and acute lead poisoning. In S. S. Gellis & B. M. Kagan (Eds.). *Current pediatric therapy, II*. Philadelphia: WB Saunders.
Piomelli, S., et al. (1984, October). Management of childhood lead poisoning. *Journal of Pediatrics, 105,* 523–532.
Proceedings of the 1992 National Conference on Cardiopulmonary Resuscitation and Emergency Cardiac Care. (1993). *Annals of Emergency Medicine, 22,* Part 2.
Reece, R. M. (1984). *Manual of emergency pediatrics* (3rd ed.). Philadelphia: WB Saunders.
Report of the 1992 National Conference on Cardiopulmonary Resuscitation and Emergency Cardiac Care. (1992). *Journal of the American Medical Association, 268,* 2172–2275.
Rothstein, P. (1980). Psychological stress in families of children in a pediatric intensive care unit. *Pediatric Clinics of North America, 27,* 613–620.
Rumack, B. H., & Matthew, H. (1975). Acetaminophen poisoning and toxicity. *Pediatrics, 55,* 871–876.
Rund, D., & Rausch, T. (1981). *Triage*. St. Louis: CV Mosby.
Seidel, J. S. (1986, November). Emergency medical services and the pediatric patient: Are the needs being met? II. *Pediatrics, 78,* 808–812.
Standards and Guidelines for Cardiopulmonary Resuscitation (CPR) and Emergency Cardiac Care (ECC). (1986, June 6). *Journal of the American Medical Association, 255,* 2905–2984.
Stickler, J., & Snowman, T. (1981, September/October). A child drowns: A nursing perspective. *MCN: American Journal of Maternal Child Nursing, 6,* 324–328.
Temple, A. R. (1985). Poisoning. In T. A. Mayer (Ed.), *Emergency management of pediatric trauma*. Philadelphia: WB Saunders.
Tenenbein, M. (1986, April). Pediatric toxicology: Current controversies and recent advances. *Current Problems in Pediatrics, 16,* 1–233.
Worrell, J. (1987). Head injuries in pedal cyclists: How much will protection help? *Injury, 18,* 5–6.

BIBLIOGRAPHY

Boehnert, M., et al. (1985). Advances in clinical toxicology. *Pediatric Clinics of North America, 32,* 193–212.
Borta, M. (1991). Psychosocial issues in water-related injuries. *Critical Care Nursing Clinics of North America, 3,* 325–329.
Budassi-Sheehy, S. (1993). *Emergency nursing: Principles and practice* (3rd ed.). St. Louis: CV Mosby.
Campbell, L., & Campbell, J. (1991). Musculoskeletal trauma in children. *Critical Care Nursing Clinics of North America, 3,* 445–456.
Carpenito, L. (1992). *Nursing diagnosis: Application to clinical practice* (4th ed.). Philadelphia: JB Lippincott.
Centers for Disease Control (1987). Leads from the MMWR: Impact of the 1985 CDC Lead Statement—Savannah, Georgia. *Journal of the American Medical Association, 258,* 2351.
Czerwinski, S. (1991). Complications of pediatric trauma. *Critical Care Nursing Clinics of North America, 3,* 479–489.
Dickenson, C. (1991). Thoracic trauma in children. *Critical Care Nursing Clinics of North America, 3,* 423–432.
DeRienzo-DeVivio, S. (1992). Childhood lead poisoning: Shifting to primary prevention. *Pediatric Nursing, 18,* 565–567.
Elixson, M. (1991). Hypothermia: Cold water drowning. *Critical Care Nursing Clinics of North America, 3,* 287–292.
Frederickson, J. (1990). Overview of advanced life support for pediatric patients. *Journal of Emergency Nursing, 16,* 17–24.
Gaudreault, P., & Lovejoy, F. H. (1985). Acute poisoning. In J. D. Dickerman & J. F. Lucey (Eds.), *Smith's the critically ill child: Diagnosis and medical management* (3rd ed.). Philadelphia: WB Saunders.
Jones, N. E. (1992). Childhood injuries: An epidemiological approach. *Pediatric Nursing, 18,* 235–239.
Keen, T. (1991). Nursing care of the pediatric multitrauma patient. *Nursing Clinics of North America, 25,* 131–141.
Lebet, R. (1991). Abdominal and genitourinary trauma in children. *Critical Care Nursing Clinics of North America, 3,* 293–306.
Mahaffey, K. R. (1992). Exposure to lead in childhood: The importance of prevention. *New England Journal of Medicine, 327,* 1308–1309.
McCarty, D., & Surpure, J. (1990). Pediatric trauma: Initial evaluation and stabilization. *Pediatric Annals, 19,* 584–596.
Moloney-Harmon, P. (1991). Initial assessment and stabilization of the critically injured child. *Critical Care Nursing Clinics of North America, 3,* 399–409.
Mortenson, M. (1986). Management of acute childhood poisoning caused by selected insecticides and herbicides. *Pediatric Clinics of North America, 33,* 421–445.
Murphy, K. A. (1992). Acetaminophen and ibuprofen: Fever control and overdose. *Pediatric Nursing, 18,* 428–431.
Ryan, M. (1984). Identifying the sexually abused child. *Pediatric Nursing, 10,* 419–421.
Seidel, J. (1990). Recognition and stabilization of the critically ill or injured child. *Pediatric Annals, 19,* 580–583.
Snodgrass, W. (1991). Salicylate toxicity. *Pediatric Clinics of North America, 33,* 381–392.
Soud, T. (1992). Airway, breathing, circulation and disability. What's different about kids? *Journal of Emergency Nursing, 18,* 107–116.
Thomas, D. (1988). The ABC's of pediatric triage. *Journal of Emergency Nursing, 14,* 154–159.
Thomas, D. (1991). Pediatric update: How to deal with children in the emergency department. *Journal of Emergency Nursing, 17,* 49–50.
Tompkins, J. (1990). Intrahospital transport of seriously ill or injured children. *Pediatric Nursing, 16,* 51–53.

CHAPTER • 47

The Child with Burns

Claudella Archambeau-Jones
Florence Simmons
Irving Feller

NURSING PROCESS PLAN
The child with major burns, Table 47–9

RELATED TOPICS
Promoting Healthy Parenting Chapter 12
Promoting Safety, Chapter 15
Care of the hospitalized child, Chapter 21
Pain management, Chapter 25
Fluid and electrolytes, Chapter 26
Child Abuse and Maltreatment, Chapter 28
Structure and function of the skin, Chapter 38

LEARNING OBJECTIVES

- **Discuss the incidence and etiology of burn injuries in childhood.**
- **Identify assessment criteria for determining the severity and prognosis of burn injuries in childhood.**
- **Describe the essentials of therapeutic management of the child with a burn injury during the three stages: (1) emergent phase, (2) acute phase, and (3) rehabilitation phase.**
- **Identify the nursing diagnoses and interventions for the care of a child with a burn injury.**

Most pediatric nurses will care for a child with burns at some time during their career. Regardless of the physical severity of the injury, the burn accident causes psychosocial trauma to the victim and family. Burn accidents happen suddenly and cause immediate, severe pain; 90 per cent of these events could have been prevented. Such an accident precipitates panic and remorse in family members and other caregivers. The child suffers severe physical pain and emotional distress. Appropriate and immediate action by the nurse and care team not only ensures the best-possible emergency care but prepares the way for a more beneficial outcome. Throughout treatment and recovery, the nurse not only monitors physiologic progress and evaluates wound healing but also helps nurture the child and family as they adapt to the changes wrought by the burn injury. The attitude and actions of the caregivers transmit to the victim and family a message of either hope or despair.

This chapter presents the phases of care from the onset of a burn through rehabilitation. The complex process of care for a child with moderate to severe burns requires the expertise of a multidisciplinary team planning and working together to ensure the child's well-being. Throughout the process, the child and family benefit from care that acknowledges the meaning of this event for the family.

Few injuries happen as frequently to children or are as traumatic for everyone involved as a severe burn. Few other injuries are as debilitating, require such extended periods of hospitalization and extensive rehabilitation, or cost as many health care dollars. However, few other catastrophic injuries offer the possibility of full recovery and are as easily prevented.

Care of the child with burns requires (1) sufficient knowledge and experience to identify the severity of the injury and the level of special care required, (2) an understanding of the phases of care and the basic principles of care for each phase, and (3) a close monitoring of all aspects of care. The nurse must also give special consideration to the child's position in a family, the family's role in the child's survival, and the future quality of life for both.

Etiology/Incidence

Each year 1.75 million people in the United States are injured by a burn accident; about 550,000 seek care in an emergency room and return an average of 2.8 times for follow-up care; 66,000 are admitted to hospitals, of whom 23,000 are admitted to specialized burn care (National Center for Health Statistics, 1987, 1991). At least half of all these accidents happen to children aged 15 years and younger. Burns and fires are a leading cause of accidental death in the United States, exceeded only by motor accidents and falls. For children in the age group of birth to 14 years, burns are the leading cause of accidental death in the home.

It is encouraging that the average size of total area included in the wound is half what it was in 1968; the average length of stay has also been reduced by more than half. However, the cost of care in specialized burn facilities has skyrocketed: a 30 per cent burn cost $30,000 for initial hospitalization and physician's fee in 1968—today, the average cost is $200,000.

The National Burn Information Exchange (NBIE) reports that the cause of burns in children varies with age, as summarized in Table 47–1. Flames and hot liquids or solids account for over 90 per cent of burns to children in the age group of birth through 15 years. In the younger age groups (birth through 4 years) 65 per cent of burns are scalds occurring in the home, whereas for children ages 5 years and over, 62 per cent of burns are caused by flame.

The highest incidence of burns to children occurs from birth through 4 years (Fig. 47–1); the incidence is closely related to the amount and adequacy of adult supervision. Many experts believe the incidence to be secondary to emotional stress in the home. During this age, a child depends totally on caregivers and has a greater vulnerability to accidents because of the inability to recognize or control hazardous situations. A child's ever-increasing mobility combined with normal curiosity and lack of supervision can be lethal. The most common accident to children in the home occurs between birth and 4 years of age, in the kitchen during meal preparation—usually the evening meal—by scalding. The child wants to know what is cooking and pulls on dangling electrical cords or pot handles.

Studies have also noted that children from low-income families, single-parent families, and families with marital discord tend to have a higher incidence of burn injuries. Parents who are single and have only marginal income experience greater stress, which tends to interfere with their capacity to be vigilant and psychologically accessible to children. These factors contribute to an increased likelihood of accidents.

TABLE 47-1
Distribution of Burn Accidents by Age Vs Burning Agent (1978–1985)*

	Age	
Burning Agent	**0–4 Yrs**	**5–15 Yrs**
Flame	14%	62%
Hot liquid	65%	25%
Hot solid	15%	5%
Electrical	2%	3%
Chemical	1%	1%
Radiation	—	—
Other	3%	4%

From National Burn Information Exchange, Ann Arbor, MI, I. Feller, MD, Director.
*Number of subjects studied: 38,674.

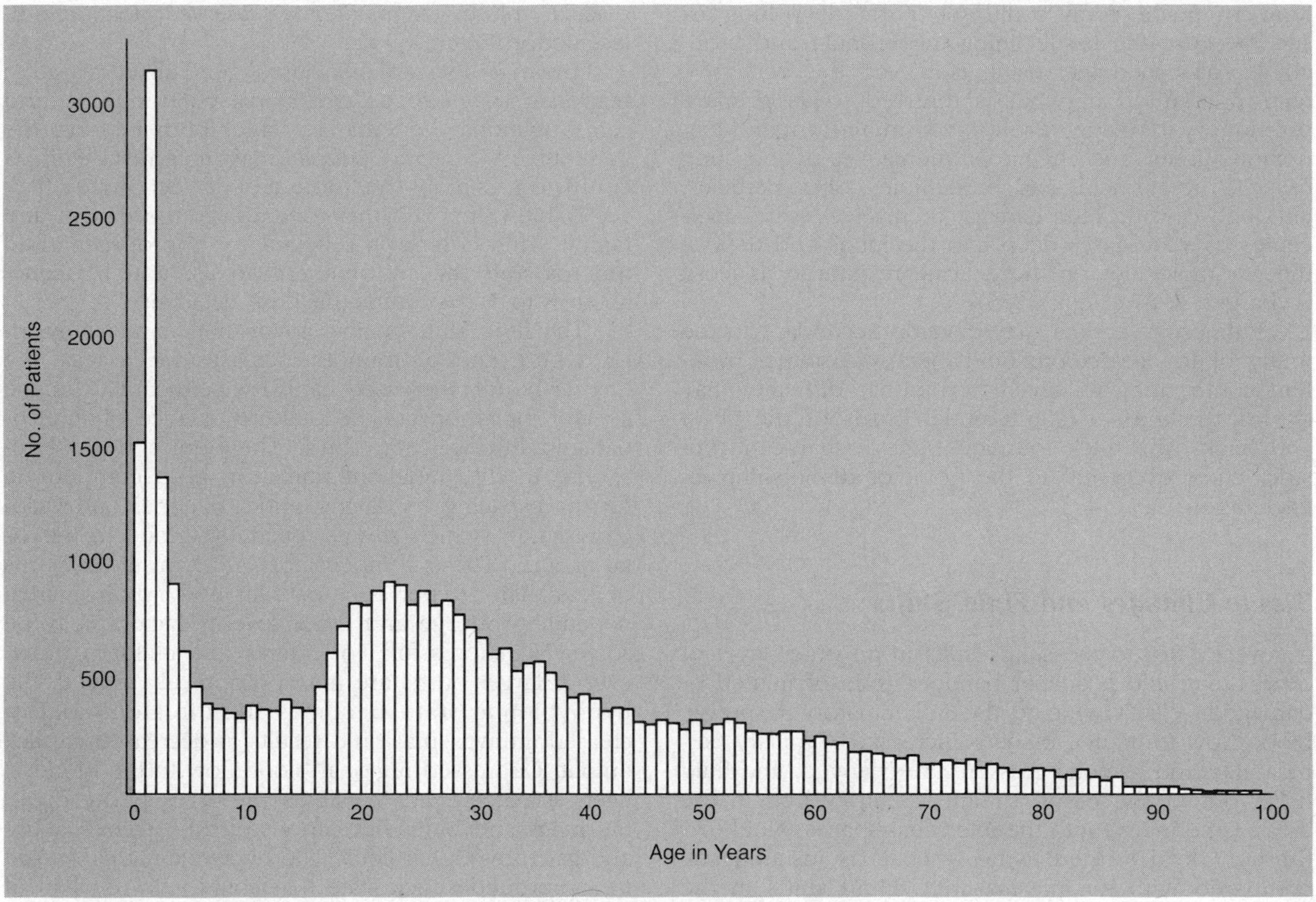

FIGURE 47 - 1. Age distribution of victims of severe burns. Thirty per cent of all burns severe enough to require hospitalization in a specialized burn care facility occur in children under 16 years of age. Children in this age group represent about 24 per cent of the United States population in the 1990 census. More importantly, children age 5 years and under represent 21 per cent of all admissions and only 7 per cent of the United States census in July 1991. N = 38,674. (Data from the National Burn Information Exchange, I. Feller, M.D., Director, 1978–1985. Ann Arbor, MI.)

Pathophysiology

In thinking of the care required to treat burns, we must first consider the primary organ system involved: the skin. The skin is the body's largest organ, providing an intact anatomic barrier against infection and loss of body fluids. The skin also helps control body temperature. The skin has a vast capillary network as well as nerve endings, hair follicles, and sweat and sebaceous glands. Body image is also related to an intact skin covering. A review of the structure and function of the skin is presented in Chapter 38.

The skin's functions are either diminished when the skin and its support systems are damaged (in a partial-thickness injury) or destroyed (in a full-thickness injury). The trauma of the burn results in a decrease or complete loss of two of the most important functions of the skin: protection against infection and prevention of loss of body fluids. Other physiologic changes secondary to the burn injury are respiratory, gastrointestinal, metabolic, and fluid alteration.

Respiratory System

Immediate respiratory problems most commonly result from upper airway edema. Edema increases insidiously for several hours after the burn accident, and if it is undetected and untreated, respiratory obstruction may develop. The design and function of the *upper airway* prepares incoming air for gas exchange in the lungs. When the mucous membranes must absorb high temperatures and noxious gases from a flame burn or from high-temperature steam, these delicate tissues suffer trauma, which leads to a severe inflammatory process.

Lower Airway Involvement. Researchers in the 1950s learned that even superhot air delivered to the lungs by tracheotomy could not "burn" deep lung tissue, because the tissue lining the bronchi and bronchioles absorbed the insult. However, this very protection resulted in what is referred to as primary pulmonary damage. Prolonged inhalation of heat, noxious gases, and chemicals traumatizes deeper lung tissues, the bronchi, and bronchioles. Soot particles, although causing little damage themselves, carry molecules of toxic gases deep into the lungs and deposit the gas molecules on the delicate respiratory mucosa (Lybarger, 1987; Stein, 1985).

Pulmonary edema may develop secondary to the injury or to *overzealous* fluid therapy. Another problem contributing to severe respiratory difficulty may be full-thickness circumferential burns of the chest and back. The thick tourniquet-like eschar can constrict chest excursion to the point of diminishing air exchange.

Tissue Changes and Fluid Shifts

A severe burn to the skin results in an outer layer of dead tissue and a deeper band or zone of injured or damaged cells. Owing to the inflammatory response, blood flow to injured tissue is increased. Capillary permeability and osmotic pressure are changed, and fluid leaks out of the blood stream (capillary bed in the area of the injury) into the interstitial spaces. Fluid loss through dead burned tissue (eschar) is insignificant, compared with the plasma shift. Fluid shifts in the zone of damaged tissue, causing edema within those tissues and, if the wound is very large, depletion of vascular volume (hypovolemia). Edema formation is illustrated in Figure 47–2.

There is also an associated generalized vascular response that causes cerebrovascular edema and some pulmonary edema. In larger burn injuries, the generalized cerebral edema may manifest itself as confusion, which the patient will recognize. It is preferable to explain this condition to the patient and family. This edema is relieved by appropriate fluid therapy and the following diuresis, which occurs about 3 to 5 days after the burn accident.

The fluid shift begins slowly but immediately after a burn and profoundly increases for at least the first 24 hours. Increased capillary permeability in the area of injury upsets the delicate balance of interstitial and intravascular fluid. The body's normal response to the initial inflammation is to compensate for third-spacing by saving urine (oliguria) and vasoconstriction (which shunts remaining blood to the vital organs). These compensatory mechanisms in burns of less than 10 per cent of total body surface area, depending on age and other severity factors, may be somewhat successful. For infants and children, however, if larger burns are not appropriately treated, the hypovolemic state becomes life-threatening. Decreased intravascular fluid results in decreased cardiac output. Depressed regional blood flow to the kidneys, liver, stomach, and intestines preserves perfusion to the lungs and brain but can also lead to renal failure and gastroduodenal ileus. The hypovolemia can result in a profound shock state that could lead to death if not carefully corrected by fluid resuscitation (Rieg & Jenkins, 1991). The level of consciousness, vital signs,

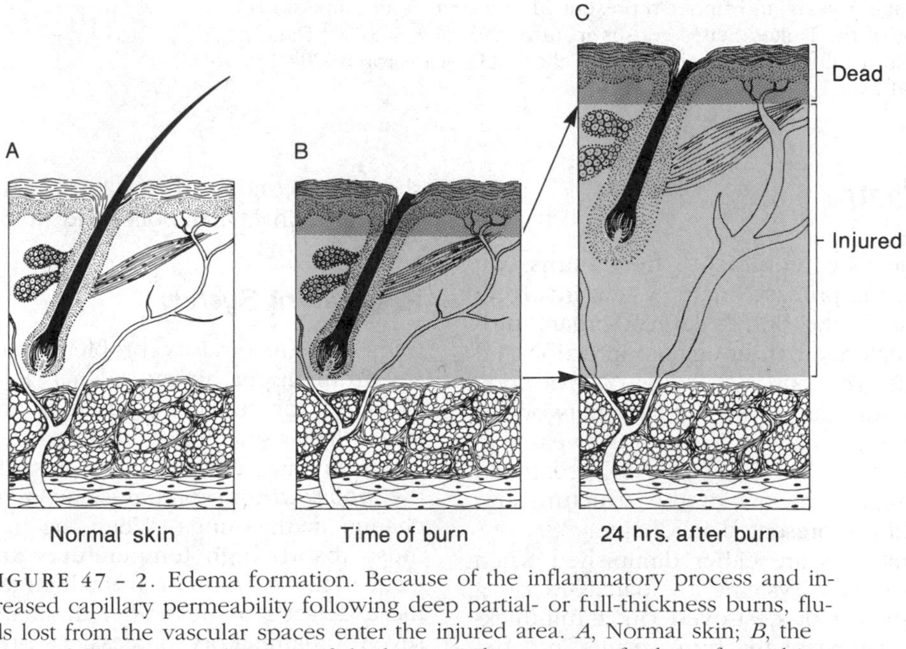

FIGURE 47-2. Edema formation. Because of the inflammatory process and increased capillary permeability following deep partial- or full-thickness burns, fluids lost from the vascular spaces enter the injured area. *A*, Normal skin; *B*, the depth of the injury at the time of the burn; *C*, the amount of edema formed in the damaged tissue 24 hours after the burn. (*A–C*, Redrawn from Feller, I., & Armbeault, C. [1973]. *Nursing the burned patient*. Ann Arbor, MI: National Institute for Burn Medicine.)

and urinary output are monitored to help determine the adequacy of cardiac output and perfusion during resuscitation.

Gastrointestinal and Metabolic Changes

The body's normal compensatory activities, which work to overcome the initial insult of the burn injury, reduce blood flow to the gastrointestinal tract, causing paralytic ileus. If the burn is major, over 30 per cent, it is wise to give no fluid or food by mouth and to decompress the stomach by nasogastric tube and intermittent suction until motility returns. Some authorities disagree with this. Either way, intravenous fluids may be used to provide nutrition until oral feeding is stable. It is necessary to moisturize the child's mouth for comfort. However, as soon as bowel sounds are present, feedings must begin to meet the child's nutritional needs.

Nutritional needs of the child vary, depending on stage of growth and development and activity levels. A current trend is to begin feedings early, in an effort to meet the child's nutritional needs. The metabolic rate for a burned patient increases dramatically. The normal protein requirements per kilogram of body weight for a child are three times the requirements of a healthy adult. Children also have a smaller muscle mass and decreased body fat, so a "fasting" state combined with increased metabolism places them at high risk for protein and caloric malnutrition. If adequate protein and caloric levels are not maintained, poor wound healing and decreased energy for meeting daily demands result (Harmel et al, 1986).

This catabolic phase continues throughout débridement and grafting. In burns of 50 per cent and larger, the resting metabolic rate can increase by 2 to 2.5 times the normal resting rate. Normal metabolic rate returns when the wound is closed, by healing or grafting. Homografting decreases the basal metabolic rate until autografting can take place.

Much of what early practitioners of burn medicine thought to be pathophysiology secondary to the burn injury (weight loss, poor healing, and depressed immunity) has been relieved by adequate nutrition. For example, the burn wound requires increased blood flow to provide an adequate vascular substrate, a source of energy necessary for wound healing. Oxygen utilization is increased, as is blood flow to the burned areas. Among other responses to the insult of a burn, the adrenal cortex, stimulated by adrenocorticotropic hormone and cortisol levels, promotes the mobilization of amino acids from skeletal muscle. There is also an associated increased synthesis of glucose from the liver for wound healing (Rieg & Jenkins, 1991).

Clinical Manifestations

The depth of dermal burn depends on the temperature applied to the skin and/or tissue, combined with time or duration of contact. Because children have a thinner epidermal layer, exposure at 130° F for 10 seconds causes tissue destruction. At 140° F, tissue destruction occurs in 5 seconds in children and within 1 second in the small infant (Advanced Burn Life Support, 1987).

A victim of an electrical injury or lightning may not have an actual burn injury of the skin, unless clothing ignites from the flash. However, the electrical current causes deep tissue damage and can stop breathing—the child with an electrical injury must always be admitted for observation. Children trapped in an enclosed space (e.g., a house fire) may present with smoke inhalation and no skin involvement. Inhalation injuries result from inhaling the toxic products from incomplete combustion, such as nitrous oxide, sulfur dioxide, or superheated steam.

Injuries in a child with an inhalation burn should be suspected on the basis of the history of the accident, such as occurrence within an enclosed space (house or car fire), an explosion, or an increase of moist heat (e.g., steam). Respiratory involvement should be suspected if there are burns of the face and/or chest. The child may be extremely restless or anxious because of sheer fright and pain, trauma of the event, lack of familiarity with the medical treatments, and fear of the unknown. Decreased oxygen saturation also increases restlessness and anxiety. *Burns do not render a victim unconscious.* A decreased state of consciousness is secondary to lack of oxygenation. One must seek and treat the cause, which is most likely to be a concurrent injury. The airway is opened and moisturized oxygen given immediately. Soot may be present in the airway or nares. Eyelids and nasal hairs (vibrissae) may be singed. The child's voice may be hoarse; there may be stridor and wheezing as well as a brassy, high-pitched cough or dyspnea. Regardless of presentation, a history of flame burns or an enclosed-space steam explosion indicates inhalation injury that requires rapid assessment and treatment.

The burn may be a combination of partial- and full-thickness with exposed nerve endings causing pain. Painful treatments also increase the child's anxiety level and decrease the ability to cooperate with treatment. Burned skin may be red or charred, leathery, or covered with blisters, depending on the depth of the burn. If a chemical caused the burn and has not been completely diluted or rinsed away, the pain may be more intense because of prolonged burning. Local and systemic responses are evaluated to determine the seriousness of the injury.

Diagnostic Assessment

The diagnostic assessment of the burned child can be separated into three categories: (1) baseline physical assessment data; (2) evaluation of severity of injury; and (3) medical history, including any allergy to food or medication and need for life-sustaining medica-

TABLE 47-2
Laboratory Values: Clinical Significance and Nursing Implications

Name of Test and Normal Values		Clinical Significance	Nursing Implications
Chemistries			
Sodium (Na):	136–148 mmol/L	A decrease in Na^+ and an increase in K are signs of inadequate fluid resuscitation	During fluid resuscitation, Na and K levels are monitored; electrolytes are checked frequently, at least every 8 hours to note trends and significant levels; repeat levels that reflect drastic changes from previous levels, i.e., a K at 6 A.M. of 4.0 that has changed to 6.5 at 10 A.M. could be a hemolyzed value
Potassium (K):	Child 3.4–4.7 mmol/L		
Magnesium (Mg):	3 mos–6 yrs 1.4–1.9 mEq/l 6–12 yrs 1.4–1.7 mEq/l 12–20 yrs 1.4–1.9 mEq/l		
Phosphorus (PO_4):	4.5–6.5 mg/dl	An elevated BUN and creatinine may indicate renal failure; a low calcium level may be related to a low albumin level common in burned children with a poor nutritional status	In young infants, stress can rapidly lead to hypoglycemia; stress may cause pseudodiabetes, which results in elevated glucose levels
Blood urea nitrogen (BUN):	5–20 mg/100 ml		
Creatinine (creat):	0.8–1.4 mg/100 ml		
Calcium (Ca):	8.4–10.2 mg/dl		
Glucose:	Child 60–100 mg/dl Adult 70–105 mg/dl		
Other Laboratory Tests			
Myoglobin:	Negative	In electrical burns, the urine is tested for myoglobin to assess muscle breakdown; if left untreated, myoglobin could result in renal failure by blocking the tubules	Urine positive for myoglobin may range from normal straw color to a distinctive very dark wine color; report this to the physician immediately; an increase in I.V. fluids and an osmotic diuretic will be ordered
Carboxyhemoglobin:	Greater than 10% indicates carbon monoxide poisoning	Measure of carbon monoxide level; check when smoke inhalation is indicated; administration of oxygen at the scene of the injury reduces this risk	Not a reliable indicator because levels can correlate poorly with clinical signs and symptoms if levels are drawn later or after oxygen therapy is initiated (Mikhail, 1988)
Arterial Blood:		Assess respiratory status; variations greater or less than these may indicate respiratory compromise (see respiratory chapter and fluid and electrolyte chapter for further details)	Do not only rely on changes in arterial blood gases to note respiratory distress; note rate and depth of respirations, assess whether breathing is labored, skin color, restlessness, abnormal breath sounds
pH:	7.35–7.45		
PCO_2	35–45 mmHg		
O_2 saturations:	80–100%		

tions, for example, phenytoin (Dilantin) or insulin. Throughout the hospital stay and in the event of significant change in the child's status, a variety of tests, procedures, and assessments are completed to identify the root cause of the abnormalities. A significant change from normal cannot be assumed to be secondary to the burn.

Laboratory Assessment

Initial laboratory data provide baseline information about whether values are normal or abnormal for nutritional profiles, hematologic findings, and chemistries. Additional tests may be based on the purpose of the assessment. See Table 47–2 for a summary of laboratory assessment.

Evaluation of Depth of Burn

The depth of a burn is expressed as partial-thickness or full-thickness. In partial-thickness burns, only part of the skin has been damaged or destroyed. Enough epithelial cells remain in hair follicles or sweat glands to grow new skin. This type of wound heals by itself, if the treatment does not cause further damage. The partial-thickness burn is equivalent to a first- or second-degree (superficial epidermal injury) burn.

In full-thickness burns, all layers of the skin are destroyed and may include subcutaneous tissue, muscle, and bone, depending on the duration of exposure to the burning agent and its temperature. Regeneration of the skin is not possible in a full-thickness injury. These wounds must be autografted to provide permanent cover and the re-establishment of normal skin function. Full-thickness burns are serious injuries, because the body has lost the life-preserving functions of the skin in the burned area. A full-thickness burn wound is equivalent to what the layperson refers to as a third-degree burn. The deeper the burn, the more serious are the problems that can develop, secondary to the body's attempt to heal an unhealable wound.

The depth of the burn is difficult to determine visually. Certain signs and symptoms indicate the level of tissue damage, but the exact depth of injury can be determined only when spontaneous healing has taken place or granulation tissue has appeared after eschar (dead skin) is removed. Figure 47–3 defines the differences between partial- and full-thickness injury.

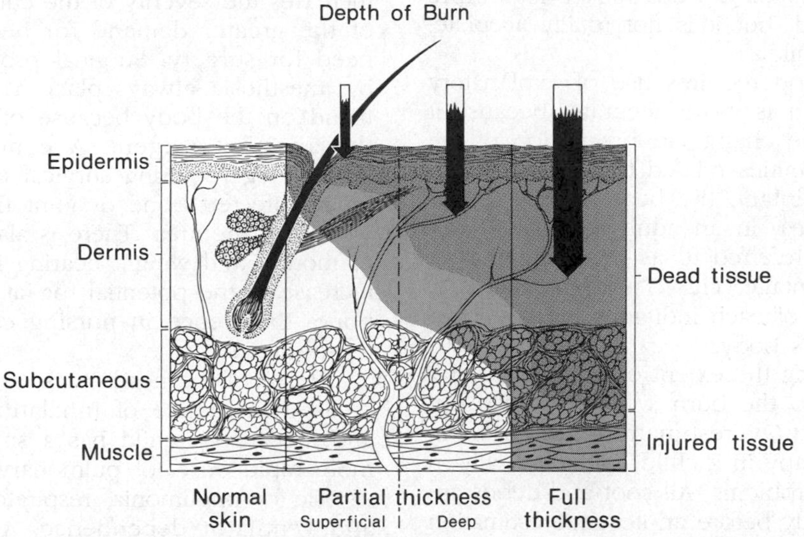

DIFFERENTIAL DIAGNOSIS

PARTIAL—THICKNESS BURN		FULL—THICKNESS BURN
Normal or increased sensitivity to pain and temperature.	Sensation	Anesthetic to pain and temperature.
Large, thick-walled, will usually increase in size.	Blisters	None, or if present, thin-walled and will not increase in size.
Red, will blanch with pressure and refill.	Color	White, brown, black or red. If red, will not blanch with pressure.
Normal or firm.	Texture	Firm or leathery.

FIGURE 47-3. Differential diagnosis of depth of burn. *Arrows* represent degree of heat or intensity of burning agent and the time of contact with the skin. The greater the temperature or the longer the time of contact, the deeper the injury. The *darker shaded area* represents dead tissue; the *lighter shaded area* represents damaged or injured tissue that will heal with good care. When all the tissue (epidermis and dermis) has been destroyed, this is termed "full-thickness burn." "Partial-thickness burn" means only part of the skin has been destroyed. (Redrawn from Feller, I., & Jones, C. A. [1977]. *Emergency care of the burn victim*. Ann Arbor, MI: National Institute for Burn Medicine.)

Identification of Extent of Burn

The extent of a burn is expressed as a percentage of the total body surface area. Two basic methods may be used to determine size. The rule of nines (Fig. 47–4) is frequently used because it is simple and quickly calculated, but it is not totally accurate, especially for small children.

The second method requires use of explanatory figures and tables and is more accurate, because it takes into account the change in proportion of the head and lower extremities related to increasing age. For example, for an infant, the head equals 19 per cent of total body area; in an adult it equals 7 per cent. This method is referred to as the estimation of size of burn by percentage (Fig. 47–5). In each case, the palm of the hand of each individual equals 1 per cent of the individual's body.

The nurse assessing the extent of burn must refer to the diagram and to the burn wound to map out the injury accurately. Overestimation can result in overzealous fluid therapy in a child, and especially in a child with cardiac problems. All soot and debris are removed from the body before an accurate estimation can be made.

Classification of Burns

The index of severity of a burn is based on its extent and depth of skin involved as well as the area of body involved, age, presence of past medical problems, and whether the injury was electrical. Also, a concurrent injury increases the demand on the body for healing. The patient's family situation also is considered in severity. Abuse, for example, greatly increases severity.

A significant injury sustained in addition to the burn (i.e., skull fracture, internal injury, or fractures) increases the severity of the child's condition because of the greater demand for healing and a potential need for surgery. Surgical procedures accompanied by anesthesia always place a greater metabolic demand on the body because of the need to detoxify the anesthetic agent. A compound fracture of a burned leg requiring surgical correction could result in an infected bone or joint from an infected burn wound in the area. There is also a decrease in range of motion and weight bearing in the extremity or an increase in the potential for fat embolism in the long bone. Excellence in nursing care can greatly offset these threats.

Burns of the head, neck, and chest lead to an increased incidence of inhalation of noxious fumes, and, because a child has a smaller upper airway, a more rapid onset of pulmonary distress. The child is at risk for pneumonia, respiratory distress syndrome, and ventilator dependence. According to Horovitz (1988), approximately 20 to 25 per cent of children who are hospitalized for burns develop pulmonary complications. Overall, one in three burn deaths are a direct result of the involvement of the respiratory tract.

Burns of the perineum present a problem of containing contamination from stool and urine and applying dressings. Frequent, gentle cleansing of the anal and perineal areas and use of mesh gauze and

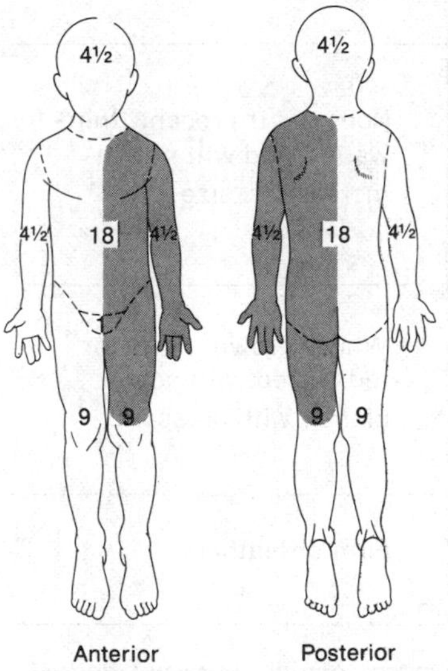

Calculation of Extent of Burn

Body Part	Ant.	Post.	Total
Head	4½	4½	9
Rt. Upper Extremity	4½	4½	9
Lt. Upper Extremity	4½	4½	9
Trunk	18	18	36
Perineum	1		1
Rt. Lower Extremity	9	9	18
Lt. Lower Extremity	9	9	18
			Total 100%

FIGURE 47-4. Estimation of size of burn by rule of nines. The head and each entire upper extremity (shoulder to fingertips [glove fashion]) are each given the value of 9 per cent of the body surface. The anterior trunk and posterior trunk are valued at 18 per cent each, as is each leg. The sum of these parts is 99 per cent, and the perineum is 1 per cent, totaling 100 per cent. This method may be used at the accident scene or in the emergency room to make a quick visual estimate of the size of the burn; however, it does not allow for the differences in the proportion of head and lower extremities at various ages.

COLOR IN THE BURN

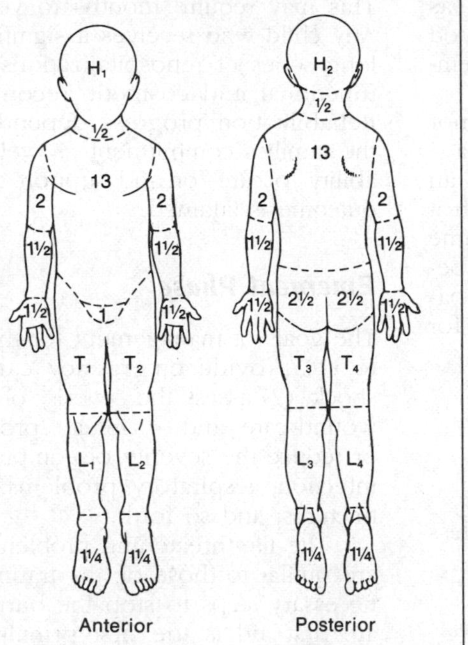

CALCULATE EXTENT OF BURN

	Anterior	Posterior
Head	H_1	H_1
Neck		
Rt. Arm		
Rt. Forearm		
Rt. Hand		
Lt. Arm		
Lt. Forearm		
Lt. Hand		
Trunk		
Buttock	(R)	(L)
Perineum		
Rt. Thigh	T_1	T_4
Rt. Leg.	L_1	L_4
Rt. Foot		
Lt. Thigh	T_2	T_3
Lt. Leg.	L_2	L_3
Lt. Foot		
Subtotal		
% Total Area Burned		%

CIRCLE AGE FACTOR

Percentage of Areas Affected by Growth

	Age 0	1	5	10	15	Adult
H(1 or 2) = ½ of the Head	9½	8½	6½	5½	4½	3½
T(1,2,3, or 4) = ½ of a Thigh	2¾	3¼	4	4¼	4½	4¾
L(1,2,3, or 4) = ½ of a Leg	2½	2½	2¾	3	3¼	3½

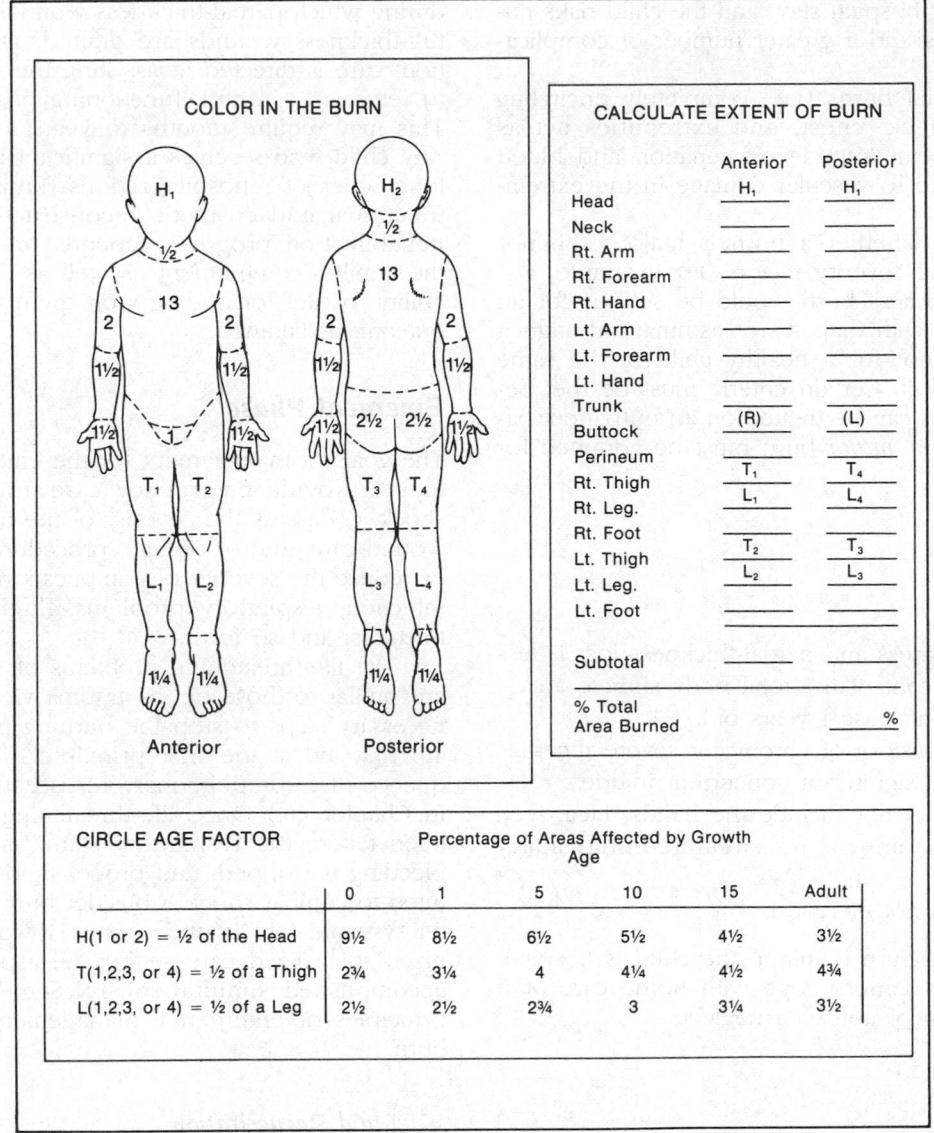

FIGURE 47 - 5. Estimation of size of burn by percentage. 1. Shade in the diagram to represent the extent of burn, as viewed anteriorly and posteriorly. 2. Circle age closest to that of the patient, and use those percentages for the head, thigh, and leg to calculate extent of burn. 3. The percentage of total body surface is printed on the diagram for areas that do not vary with age. The areas that do vary with age are marked with H (head), T (thigh), and L (leg). The extent of the burn is calculated by adding the percentages of each affected area. If a portion of a body part is burned, an approximate fraction of the percentage should be used. (Redrawn from Feller, I., & Jones, C. A. [1977]. *Emergency care of the burn victim.* Ann Arbor, MI: National Institute for Burn Medicine.)

towels that can be frequently replaced make healing possible. Grafting the perineum and immobilizing the area are difficult. The warm, moist area is also an ideal medium for the growth of bacteria. However, when adequate wound care is given, these wounds can and do heal with no complication.

Burns deep enough to damage bone (including skull) require special consideration for appropriate healing. A conservative approach to débridement of bone combined with burr holes penetrating bone marrow usually permits healing followed by a split-thickness skin graft.

Major burns covering 80 per cent of the total body surface area may present difficulty in achieving permanent skin cover, owing to lack of available donor sites, and loss of the protective cover of skin results in a greater possibility of infection. Most important, the body's metabolism increases in an attempt to heal large wounds, which puts greater homeostatic stress on the body. Full-thickness burns result in a longer hospital stay, and the child risks nutritional problems and a greater number of complications.

Circumferential burns (i.e., completely encircling burns) of the neck, chest, and extremities act as tourniquets that can impede oxygenation and blood flow and can lead to vascular damage in the extremities.

Determining whether a burn is major or minor depends on these severity factors. For example, a 5 per cent full-thickness burn would be serious for an infant or a child with diabetes or asthma, although it may be only minor for a healthy child of the same age or for an adult. Certain criteria must be met before a minor burn can be treated on an outpatient basis. A child with a *major* burn must be admitted for specialized care.

Minor Burns

A burn is minor if

- The full-thickness and partial-thickness loss is less than 10 per cent of the total body surface area.
- The child is at least 4 years old.
- There is no history of chronic or severe illness.
- There are no significant concurrent injuries.
- The burn does not include the hands, face, feet, or perineum, and/or no circumferential injury exists.
- The injury is not electrical.

Even when a burn is minor, the child is hospitalized if the family cannot cope with home care or if there is suspicion of abuse or neglect.

Major Burns

A burn is classified as major if any of the following conditions exists:

- The wound covers more than 10 per cent total body surface area.
- The wound is full-thickness.
- The child is less than 4 years old.
- There are significant concurrent injuries.
- There are burns of the face, hands, feet, or perineum and/or circumferential injury.
- It is an electrical injury.
- There is a history of abuse or neglect.

Therapeutic Management

The three identifiable but overlapping stages of care with corresponding specific therapeutic management principles of the burn patient are (1) the emergent phase, (2) the acute phase, and (3) the rehabilitation phase. The first 72 hours of the burn injury is called the emergent phase. The acute phase is the period during which partial-thickness wounds are healed and full-thickness wounds are grafted. During rehabilitation, care is directed at assisting the child and family to return to a useful, functioning position in society. This may require months to years to be completed. Any child who receives a significant burn may face a long series of rehospitalizations (until adulthood) for functional and cosmetic reconstruction procedures. Rehabilitation progress depends on the child's and the family's commitment as well as the health team's ability to care for and support them until the desired outcome is attained.

Emergent Phase

The goals of management for the emergent phase are to (1) provide emergency care and prevent burn shock, (2) assess the severity of the injury, (3) initiate wound care, and (4) initiate procedures that eliminate or reduce the severity of complications: prevention of infection, respiratory problems, fluid overload, contractures, and so forth.

The life-threatening problems of the burn patient are similar to those of any trauma victim. After taking necessary steps to stop the burning process, immediate first aid is the first principle of care. (The sequence of cardiopulmonary resuscitation is presented in Chapter 46.) Once life-threatening measures have been taken, the respiratory status is evaluated, any bleeding is stopped, and proper fluid therapy is instituted to combat shock. Consider burn wound care after systemic care is under way. However, in an organized specialized care setting, all aspects of care are accomplished simultaneously. See Table 47–3 for principles of emergency management for the major burn.

Fluid Resuscitation

As stated in the discussion of pathophysiology, capillary permeability increases secondary to the body's normal inflammatory response, and fluid shifts out of the blood stream into the interstitial spaces.

Fluid replacement must be initiated, or hypovolemic shock may take place. The fluid lost from the blood stream in burn shock is composed of water, electrolytes, and albumin, and it should be replaced. Hartmann's (lactated Ringer's) solution is the fluid of choice, because its electrolyte balance is similar to that of blood. Albumin may be added to provide colloid, although investigators who oppose its use during the first 24 hours of fluid therapy believe that the colloid becomes trapped in the interstitium, increasing extravascular oncotic pressure and thereby increasing the fluid shift. Red cell loss is caused by hemolysis and generally approximates only 10 per cent of the total red cell mass. Blood replacement is not necessary for resuscitation, unless there is significant loss of blood from concurrent injuries.

All experts agree that fluids must be carefully replaced during the fluid shift phase. There is not yet

TABLE 47-3
Principles of Emergency Management for the Major Burn

Action	Rationale
Stop the burning process by removing the patient from the burning source, or extinguish the flames or heat with cool tap water. Remove all clothing and jewelry. Never apply ice. Adhered clothing is left in place. Wrap in clean sheet. If a chemical injury, flood with copious amounts of water	The patient is carefully removed from the fire or steam to prevent further injury. Clothing that was included in the area of injury holds heat in contact with the skin. Jewelry tends to retain heat. Children lose heat rapidly due to a large surface area. Never forcefully try to remove adhered clothing because this could lead to further skin damage. During tubbing, the adhered clothes will become loosened and can usually be removed very gently
Assess the airway, breathing, and circulation. Make sure the airway is patent. Give humidified oxygen. All flame burn patients should receive oxygen to prevent CO_2 poisoning	Burns are a form of trauma, a quick complete assessment, as done for any other trauma patient, is always indicated
Suspect impending respiratory distress if there are burns of face, neck, or chest or history of being burned in an enclosed space. Initiate fluid resuscitation. Refer to the text for the discussion of fluid management	
Complete a secondary assessment. Continue to monitor all systems, provide a more thorough assessment	Assess for abnormal findings
Obtain a detailed history. Include health history and a history of the events leading to the burn event. Obtain the patient's most recent preburn weight. If fluid therapy is being based on body weight, obtain a body weight that does not include intravenous fluids (started enroute or in another hospital)	A health history provides pertinent information about the child's general health status and needs. A history of the injury provides pertinent information to the team. For example, being burned in an enclosed area would signal the potential for respiratory distress from smoke inhalation. If the child requires life-sustaining medication for illness such as asthma or diabetes, it should be continued
Insert a nasogastric tube, and connect it to intermittent suction drainage. Stop food and reduce oral fluids to only enough to keep the mouth moist. Fluids may be resumed once bowel sounds have returned	A nasogastric tube is inserted in all patients with major burns because of a potential for ileus. In burns that cover 20% or more of total body surface area, paralytic ileus can occur. This is a decrease in circulatory support to the stomach and intestines that causes lack of motility and bowel sounds as a result of hypovolemia and the need to preserve perfusion to vital organs. Digestion ceases in the stomach. Depending on the extent of burn injury, the small bowel may maintain motility and absorptive capabilities (Rieg & Jenkins, 1991)
Give tetanus immunization based on immunization history	Burn wounds provide an excellent medium for growth of *Clostridium tetani* spores
Insert Foley catheter and connect to dependent drainage	To allow for accurate monitoring of urine output
Perform laboratory tests	Carboxyhemoglobin, blood gas, chemistries, hematology, nutritional tests, and a chest x-ray film are done as a baseline against which future assessments can be judged

consensus as to which formula should be used to calculate the amount of fluids required. Estimating emergent-period fluid requirements increasingly tends to be based on the percentage of body surface area that is included in burn injury. Some experts believe that this method leads to increased accuracy and consistency for children of all ages and with burns of various sizes. Obtaining an accurate estimate of size of burn and accurate preburn weight is essential. Another problem with standard adult formulas is that no separate allowances are made for maintenance fluids and the fluids that are needed to replace burn-related losses (Carvajal & Parks, 1988).

There are several key concepts to keep in mind while deciding how much fluid to give an infant or child.

1. The body fluid–to–body solids ratio is higher for infants and children: If a child's body fluids equal 75 to 80 per cent of the body mass, in a 10-kg child (22 pounds), fluids would equal 16.5 pounds of fluid (7.5 L). These fluids are distributed in intravascular, intracellular, and interstitial spaces. The interstitium is referred to as the third space—the space between the blood stream and body cells; the exchange of fluid, oxygen, and nutrients takes place here.

2. An infant or child's metabolic response to injury and recovery tends to be more rapid than that of an adult.

3. As fluids leak from the blood stream into interstitial spaces, the fluid volume and weight are not lost from the body but rather are sequestered or "third-spaced." Weight gain secondary to fluid replacement should not exceed 10 to 15 per cent of normal body weight. Intravenous fluids are also leaked and sequestered in the third space.

4. Despite these sequestered fluids, the kidneys continue to produce urine from whatever circulating fluids are available. During hypovolemia, the ratio of solids to solute in the urine is higher; thus, the spe-

cific gravity of urine is more concentrated. Urinary output and specific gravity are two easily monitored outer warning signs of what is occurring inside the body. As circulating volume returns to normal, the specific gravity becomes higher as solids (wastes excreted by the kidneys) are diluted. The same is true for the hematocrit. The hematocrit is quite high because of red cells being concentrated in the blood as a result of leaking fluids. As intravenous fluids are replaced, the red cells are diluted and the hematocrit returns to normal.

5. Even though formulas are a crude index, a formula is calculated for use as a guideline, but this *does not* replace close hourly management, which remains necessary. Using *titration* with a formula as a guide can lead to better replacement without overload.

6. Fluid formulas calculated on the basis of the extent of body surface area burned and weight of the patient can be only as accurate as the measurement of weight and *estimate* of extent. Neither is an exact science.

7. Accurate estimation of percentage of body area included in the burn depends on knowing which areas are actually burned and *accurately* calculating this percentage. The wound should be cleaned before the extent of injury is estimated.

8. If fluids have been started in another hospital, some of this fluid will be sequestered (1 L of fluid weighs 2.2 pounds), adding to the weight used in the formula calculation.

According to the Advanced Burn Life Support Course (1987), the guidelines for fluid resuscitation in the infant and child are 3 to 4 ml of fluid per kilogram times the body surface area of the injury, given during the first 24 hours. By using the Parkland formula for resuscitation, we obtain the following:

(4 ml) × (body weight in kilograms) × (% of burn)
In addition, children under 2 years of age require maintenance fluids. (See Chapter 26 for basal fluid requirements.)

A calculation for a 10-kg child with a 40 per cent burn is as follows:

4 ml × 10 kg × 40% (lactated Ringer's)	= 1600 ml
plus:	
1000 ml (basal requirement) approximately 42 ml/hr of maintenance fluid	
0.5 (burn area)	= 1000 ml
TOTAL	= 2600 ml over 24 hours

Each liter of fluids weighs 1 kg, and each kilogram equals 2.2 pounds; in essence, the 22-pound child receives nearly 6 pounds of fluids in 24 hours—one quarter of his weight.

A total of 1600 ml of lactated Ringer's solution is estimated for the first 24 hours after injury; 50 per cent or 800 ml is given in the first 8 hours (100 ml/hr), and 25 per cent is given over the second and third 8-hour periods (400 ml for each 8-hour period) (Heink, 1992). It is important to note that using a formula in this way indicates delivery of 142 ml of fluid per hour for a child under 2 years old during the first 8 hours. There is a potential for fluid overload; a child of this size should have no more than 25 ml of urine output per hour. This criterion should be used regardless of formula used.

If fluids are sequestered or third-spaced, they are not lost from the body, other than through urinary output. Obligatory fluid loss through respirations and through skin respiration occurs in very small amounts. If urinary output is 30 cc/hr, only about $^{1}/_{2}$ pound of fluid is lost in 24 hours; in essence, the child's weight is increased by one fifth. This amount is significant and puts greater stress on the heart, lungs, and vascular system. One can cause serious overload by not carefully monitoring output and respiratory rate. However, one does not want to give a too-small volume; *the goal is adequate perfusion (and thereby oxygenation) of cell organ systems.* A formula is a guide to calculating rate and volume of fluid administration; *the child's individual response to the therapy is the major determinant* (Advanced Burn Life Support, 1987). Monitoring urine output is essential in assessing the child's response to trauma. The amount, content, and color of the urine are a guide to fluid replacement.

Titrating bodily fluids requires hourly measurement of the amount of urine produced and infusing an amount in the next hour to produce the desired urinary output. Outputs of 1 ml/kg per hour for children up to 30 kg and 30 to 50 ml/hr for larger children or adolescents indicate adequate perfusion of organ systems without systemic overload. An output greater than 50 ml or less than 25 ml/hr does not indicate "better" resuscitation but rather warns of potential fluid overload and edema or under-replacement and shutdown. In addition to measuring the urine output, the urine specific gravity, vital signs, central venous pressure, hematocrit, skin hydration, and level of consciousness, other indices are used to measure the adequacy of fluid resuscitation (see Chapter 26).

Deep-tissue injury or massive burns damage some circulating red blood cells in the area of the burn at the time of the injury (hemolysis), resulting in the release of free-circulating hemoglobin (hemoglobinemia). When this free hemoglobin passes the basement membrane into the tubules of the kidney, there is a danger of acute tubular necrosis and renal failure. Black urine (hemoglobinuria) seen on catheterization or during the immediate postburn period indicates severe hemolysis. If this occurs, an osmotic diuretic is immediately given to flush the hemoglobin from the renal tubules. Intravenous fluid administration is temporarily increased until the crisis is over.

Pain Management

When the child is in burn shock (hypovolemic shock), pain control cannot be achieved with subcutaneous or intramuscular medication, because the medication may pool; that is, it may not be properly absorbed into circulation owing to the depleted blood volume in the periphery interfering with uptake and pain relief. Furthermore, when the circulation returns to normal, there is a potential for sudden release of large pools of medication that cause overdosing. For effectiveness, the analgesic must be given intravenously in monitored doses to prevent dulling of consciousness or depression of the respiratory center. However, it is known that children can tolerate larger doses of pain reliever while in severe pain. Other measures used to relieve pain are included elsewhere in this chapter.

Respiratory Care

Specific pulmonary complications are covered in the discussion of pathophysiology in this chapter. The edema of the upper airway that is related to inhalation of noxious gases and the associated heat is somewhat relieved when fluids are reabsorbed. Administration of cold, moist steam with oxygen to humidify the incoming air also relieves distress. Emergency medical teams (EMTs) now, as a rule, give oxygen at the scene of the accident, and little carbon monoxide poisoning is actually seen in the hospital. Insertion of an endotracheal tube is indicated for severe upper airway edema. As edema subsides, the obstruction is relieved and the endotracheal tube can be removed.

Deep pulmonary injury involves the terminal bronchioles and, on rare occasions, the alveoli. Inhalation of chemical products of combustion result in (1) impaired ciliary activity, (2) erythema, (3) hypersecretion of mucus, (4) ulceration of mucous membrane, (5) increased blood flow leading to congestion and edema, and (6) spasm of the bronchi. Tissue response varies according to the type of substance causing the burn (Bayley, 1991). Long-term complications include bronchopneumonia and fibrosis.

Treatment for deep pulmonary injury is directed toward treating symptoms and preventing respiratory distress. Prophylactic intubation and/or administration of 100 per cent humidified oxygen may be necessary to improve gas exchange. Endotracheal tubes used in children are cuffless, so it is essential to secure the tube well. Selection of the tube properly sized for the child and skillful *intubation by an experienced person* decrease trauma and other complications. Careful suctioning prevents trauma to already damaged tissues. Elevating the head of the bed decreases the amount of edema and assists with airway clearance. Bronchoscopy is a diagnostic tool used to identify burns of the lower respiratory tract, to lavage the area, and to assess the airway for healing after injury. Serial bronchoscopies are done to evaluate progress. A xenon ventilation-perfusion lung scan is a more accurate diagnostic tool used to identify lower airway damage. Bronchodilators help clear the tracheobronchial tree of excessive secretions. Steroids and prophylactic antibiotics are considered controversial, because they may promote the later emergence of infections with organisms that are resistant to multiple antibiotics. Frequent assessment of the respiratory status is essential.

Circumferential burns to the chest can restrict movements of the chest wall and lead to respiratory compromise. A child is at greater risk for such problems because of the soft pliable rib cage that is easily restricted by thick eschar. A single escharotomy or multiple escharotomies of the chest are indicated if chest excursion is prevented by circumferential burns of the chest or full-thickness wounds to the chest wall. Escharotomies are performed as soon as tightening eschar is observed, to prevent circulatory restriction and respiratory distress.

Initial Wound Management

Burn wound management is initiated after emergency care is accomplished. Infection control is maintained at all times, and aseptic technique is used when caring for the wound. If the child is being transferred to a burn center after initial breathing and bleeding are stabilized, wound care may be limited to gentle cleansing, estimating the percentage of body surface represented by the burned area, and applying a clean, moist gauze dressing to the wounds. Cleansing and applying moist dressings are comforting, although initially painful. The child should then be wrapped in a clean, dry sheet and blanket covering the moist dressings for warmth during transport. Antimicrobial ointments are optional (but probably worthwhile, nevertheless) if the child is being transferred within 1 to 2 hours, because the burn team will remove the dressings and assess the burn wounds on the child's arrival at the burn center.

Initial wound care at the burn center involves the débridement of all loose skin, shaving any hair that is in the wound or in close proximity to it, and carefully and completely cleansing the wounds.

Circulation is evaluated, and as the wound demarcates and eschar tightens, there may be a need for an escharotomy. An escharotomy is a linear excision that extends *only* through the eschar of a full-thickness burn. The escharotomy is usually performed by a physician who is *trained* in burn care. Circulation is continuously assessed to evaluate the effectiveness of the escharotomy and to identify the need for additional escharotomies. *If there is frank bleeding* from the escharotomy, consider that *the wound is only partial-thickness and the escharotomy is not necessary*. Enzymatic escharotomies are less traumatic and equally effective.

Estimation of Percentage of Burn Injury

Once initial wound cleansing has occurred, an accurate estimate of burn injury can begin. In flame injuries, soot and debris can influence burn perimeters. Demarcation of the wound takes place after 2 to 3 days, so early assessment must be repeated to obtain an accurate estimate. Herein lies the problem related to relying solely on formulas based on extent of the wound for early fluid replacement.

Transfer to a Burn Care Facility

Patients with a major burn injury *must* be transferred to a burn care facility for optimal treatment. *Caveat:* Transfer should be completed within the first 3 hours after the burn, if at all possible. The patient cannot wait to be "stabilized" in a nonspecial facility, because care in the emergent period requires expert direction. Communication between the transferring facility and the burn center is essential. Distance and the patient's severity of injury determine whether the patient is transferred by ground transportation or by air. Transfer the child as early as possible to a facility that is skilled in specialized burn care. The family is informed of the need for transfer and is given explanations about the care their child requires. Research has shown that children have a better chance of survival and rehabilitation if treated at a children's hospital with specialized burn care.

The Acute Period

The end of the emergent period is signaled by a reversal of the fluid shift, evidenced by a diuresis. Capillary integrity is re-established, sequestered fluids are pulled back into the blood stream, and intravenous fluids are decreased accordingly. Also, fluids are switched to water with electrolytes and nutrients on the basis of laboratory values or are discontinued altogether. The goals of the acute phase are to (1) prevent or detect early and treat complications (refer to Table 47–4 for a list of potential complications), (2) heal partial-thickness wounds, and (3) graft full-thickness wounds. Minor and major wound care is based on principles that all members of the health care team must enforce.

Minor Burn Wound Management

The basic principles of minor burn wound management are infection control, comfort, and cleanliness. Analgesics are administered before the areas are cleansed, because of the irritated pain fibers in the burned tissue. Avoid rough handling of the burned area, because the mechanical trauma of cleansing can convert a partial-thickness wound to a full-thickness one. After the wound and surrounding areas are gently but thoroughly cleansed of all debris with soap and water and any hairy area has been shaved to a 2-inch margin around the wound, the wound is rinsed thoroughly and a dressing is applied. The type of topical agent (Table 47–5) and dressing used on a particular burn is usually determined by the burn physician or the policies of the burn center. If infection is present, oral antibiotics and more frequent dressing changes may be indicated to hasten the control of infection.

Approximately 7 but no more than 14 days are required for healing of a partial-thickness wound. Appearance of thick, blackened or grayish eschar (dead cells that are in contact with living cells), or granulation of newly formed tissue with capillary bed in areas where eschar has been removed, or both, indicate that the injury is full-thickness, usually requiring hospitalization for closure with autograft. The body can regenerate epidermis and dermis to fill in about a 2- to 4-cm^2 full-thickness wound. A larger wound requires grafting for a good result.

Major Burn Wound Management

Care of a burn wound classified as major is a time-consuming process. Full-thickness wounds cannot heal by themselves; all dead tissue must be removed and the area grafted with the patient's own skin (autografted) for permanent coverage. The same donor site (site from which split-thickness autografts are taken) may be used every 7 to 10 days if given proper care. The scalp is frequently the site of choice, because it is highly vascular; consequently, healing occurs more rapidly and the hair regrowth hides the donor site. Major burn wound care consists of daily wound care, cleansing, surgical or nonsurgical débridement, applying a topical agent and gauze dressings, using temporary grafts, and autografting. See Table 47–6 for a review of major wound care.

Nutrition

Nutrition is an important component of wound healing in the burned child. As explained earlier in the pathophysiology discussion, burn trauma results in increased metabolism and catabolism. The burned child requires two to three times the normal amount of calories and protein. Caloric increases should be ensured, if necessary, by parenteral nutrition until the child can again take oral nourishment (refer to Table 47–7 for additional interventions to meet the nutritional needs of children).

The Rehabilitation Phase

On the child's admission to specialized burn care facilities, rehabilitation procedures begin to correct body alignment by positioning and splinting, nutritional assessment and support, psychosocial assessment and support, and so forth. The actual period of rehabilitation involves returning the child to normal functioning. Commonly, there is some decrease in general functioning for up to 3 to 6 months after discharge from acute care, with gradual recovery to near preburn function at 12 to 18 months after discharge (Knudson-Cooper, 1980).

TABLE 47-4
Frequent Complications of Major Burns in Children

Complication	Etiology
Cardiovascular	
Hypovolemia *Occurs:* emergent phase	Normal inflammatory response to injury. In major burn, fluid shift from vascular to interstitial spaces (third spacing) is massive. If untreated, it results in hypovolemic shock and death
Hypervolemia *Occurs:* late emergent phase	Secondary to overzealous fluid therapy or failure to recognize diuretic phase of fluid replacement
Hypertension *Occurs:* during any one of the three phases, but usually seen in late emergent or early acute	Occurs in at least one third of children with severe burns; etiology unclear, but thought to be secondary to stress. May be treated prophylactically in burns of greater than 40% total body surface area with drug of physician's choice
Renal	
Oliguria *Occurs:* emergent or acute phase	Secondary to hypovolemia or hypovolemic shock. Relieved with proper fluid therapy. If fluid therapy delayed or inadequate, leads to anuria and renal failure. May be seen in acute period secondary to septic shock
Hemomyoglobinuria *Occurs:* emergent phase	Secondary to massive deep full-thickness injury or electrical injury, causing release of myoglobin (muscle protein) and hemoglobin from red blood cells. These free globins are then filtered by kidneys and can clog tubules. Sign of this is black urine. Immediate treatment with osmotic diuretic and increased fluids indicated to prevent tubular necrosis or failure
Pulmonary	
Carbon monoxide poisoning *Occurs:* emergent phase	Byproducts of combustion inhaled by burn victim; treatment with oxygen at the scene relieves symptoms; rarely seen with good EMS care
Upper airway obstruction *Occurs:* emergent phase	Secondary to absorption of heat and gases by upper airway; results in edema of the airway requiring early intubation. When edema subsides, endotracheal tube can be removed
Primary pulmonary damage *Occurs:* emergent phase	Secondary to lower airway and lung damage by noxious gases. Requires intubation by endotracheal tube. If unrelieved, then tracheostomy. Further treatment may require antibiotics, aminophylline, cortisone, aerosol antibiotics. Humidified oxygen is indicated for all respiratory involvement
Pulmonary edema *Occurs:* acute phase	May be secondary to primary pulmonary damage, circumferential chest burn causing decreased chest movement,* overzealous fluid therapy and overload or immobility
Pulmonary embolus *Occurs:* acute phase	Usually a very late complication. Clot is released when mobility follows enforced immobility. Heparin can be used prophylactically
Bacterial pneumonia *Occurs:* acute phase	Lowered resistance secondary to immobility,* decreased chest movement if circumferential chest burn, inhalation irritation. May be secondary to wound or tracheostomy, sepsis, or pooled lung fluids
Sepsis	
Wound infection *Occurs:* emergent and/or acute phases (If it occurs, infection is often evident by 4 days post trauma)	Infection during emergent phase is usually gram-positive, often *Staphylococcus,* as a result of autocontamination; usually treated prophylactically with penicillin, daily wound cleansing, and débridement Infection during acute phase is frequently from gram-negative organisms, e.g., *Pseudomonas aeruginosa,* secondary to decreased vascular supply to wound, diminished overall immune response, and the favorable medium the wound provides—heat, warmth, eschar Prevention: A *P. aeruginosa* vaccine and a hyperimmune serum have been used successfully since 1963, providing both active and passive coverage, but this remains controversial
Transient bacteremia *Occurs:* acute phase	Secondary to daily wound manipulation and excessive bacterial shower into the blood stream, secondary to débridement. Good basic supportive care plus systemic antibiotics are preventive measures

(continued)

TABLE 47-4
Frequent Complications of Major Burns in Children *(Continued)*

Complication	Etiology
Sepsis	
Septicemia *Occurs:* acute phase	Overwhelming systemic infection secondary to unsuccessful treatment of primary wound infection or due to invading pathogens at in-dwelling catheter sites (e.g., central lines, urinary). Early detection is essential for proper therapy
Metabolic and Electrolyte Disturbances	
Paralytic ileus (gastrointestinal) *Occurs:* emergent phase	Normal response to initial hypovolemic state; usually lasts 2–3 days during which time oral intake is contraindicated. Nasogastric tube to intermittent drainage is used to decompress stomach
Weight gain *Occurs:* emergent phase	Secondary to fluid therapy. Children should gain no more than 10% of normal body weight; above 10% puts child at risk for overload, pulmonary edema, or congestive failure
Weight loss *Occurs:* acute phase	Secondary to catabolism. Requires high-calorie, high-protein diet. Loss of more than 20–30% of total body weight in a child of normal weight can be fatal. Overweight children can afford a greater weight loss
Hypernatremia *Occurs:* late emergent and acute phases	As fluids return to vascular space at end of emergent period, salt also returns. Fluid therapy is changed to D5W or D10W (salt-poor fluids)
Acid-base imbalance *Occurs:* late emergent and acute phases	May be secondary to many other complications or a result of treatment (e.g., some topical agents)
Adrenal-cortical insufficiency *Occurs:* emergent and acute phases	A continued adrenal response secondary to overwhelming injury; attempt to maintain body equilibrium. Steriods may be indicated (controversial)
Curling ulcer *Occurs:* emergent and acute phases	Twice as common in children. Stress response of body to overwhelming injury. Routine use of antacids or cimetidine (Tagamet) in burn victims has decreased the incidence. If preventive antacid regimen is not followed, gastrointestinal hemorrhage may result. Once wound is healed, incidence is eliminated
Nervous System	
Personality change *Occurs:* acute and/or rehabilitation phases	Common in children; may be consequence of stress, fluid or electrolyte imbalance, septicemia, drug therapy. Usually resolved when systemic complications resolve and wound closes, unless there was preburn pathology
Postburn seizures *Occurs:* acute phase	Same as above; unique complication of children; full recovery is usual
Peripheral neuropathy *Occurs:* acute or rehabilitation phase	Secondary to immobilization and certain antibiotics. Hearing loss and weakness in limbs (e.g., footdrop) are most frequent
Skin, Bone, Joint	
Scarring and contractures *Occurs:* acute and rehabilitative phases	Secondary to tissue injury, inflammation, and healing. A good prevention program, starting on admission, involving splinting and activities by occupational therapists and physical therapists is essential
Heterotopic bone (bone growth in abnormal areas) *Occurs:* acute and rehabilitative phases	Calcium deposits in joint spaces, secondary to fluid and electrolyte disturbances, bed rest, inactivity. Cannot be removed until fully mature (i.e., 1–3 yrs post burn)

*Early activity and turning, coughing, and deep breathing exercises are *essential* preventive measures. Escharotomy (incising constricting eschar layer) of circumferential full-thickness burns of chest is also indicated.

TABLE 47-5
Topical Antimicrobials That Are Used in Burn Care*

Agent	Advantage	Disadvantage
Silver sulfadiazine (Silvadene)	Effective against gram-positives, -negatives, and yeast	May cause leukopenia
Mafenide (Sulfamylon)	Effective against gram-positives and -negatives; penetrates thick eschar; effective in preventing chrondritis in ear burns	Painful on application, strong carbonic anhydrase; may cause metabolic acidosis and electrolyte imbalance
Neomycin (0.5–1.0%)	Effective against most organisms	May cause hearing loss or renal failure when used for a prolonged period
Silver nitrate	Effective against most organisms	May cause electrolyte imbalances; discolors wounds and environment; may cause hyponatremia and hypokalemia when applied to large areas

*This is a limited list of agents that are used in burn care. Consult with burn team for other agents.

TABLE 47-6
Review of Major Wound Care

Daily Wound Care

Daily wound care includes daily or more frequent "tubbing" of the child in the hydrotherapy tub or whirlpool. Infants and smaller children can be tubbed in a plastic bathtub at the bedside

The wound is assessed for healing as evidenced by granulation buds or for signs of infection, such as redness, swelling, pain, wound conversion, or foul-smelling drainage

Infection control is maintained and precautions are used, including wearing gloves, masks, goggles, and impermeable gowns when performing wound care. Gloves are changed after removing soiled dressings, cleansing the wound, and before applying new dressings

Topical antimicrobials and dressings are applied according to plan of care

Routine wound cultures are obtained

The wound must be clean and free of debris and infections to heal or accept a graft

Temporary Wound Coverage

When the full-thickness burn is large, temporary skin coverage is used

Temporary skin covers are rejected by the body and are left in place only until grafting can occur

Homografts (skin from another donor of the same species) or heterografts (pigskin) are two common forms of temporary grafts

The temporary grafts are observed daily for signs of infection, and areas that slough are routinely replaced

Débridement

Natural débridement occurs daily with removal of dressings and hydrotherapy

Sharp débridement is done with a scissors and pickups daily during "tubbing" or with a scalpel under anesthesia in the operating room

Enzymatic débridement involves the use of enzymes such as Travase, which destroy dead tissue and can be safe and effective when used with topical agents

Excessive bleeding means the débridement is too sharp or deep. STOP and assess what is causing the bleeding

Autografting

Autografting is generally a surgical procedure that involves transferring a split-thickness skin graft or the patient's own skin to cover a full-thickness wound

The patient is usually immobilized for a period after grafting to prevent loss of the graft

The graft is assessed for percentage of take and also signs of infection

Cultured Epithelial Autografts

Cultured epithelial autografts are sheets of skin that are grown from a skin biopsy in a laboratory in a special medium, similar to a Petri dish

Cultured epithelial autografts have been relatively successful in providing a permanent skin coverage for patients with burns covering 80% or more of total body surface area. However, for permanent coverage epithelial cultures are *fragile,* extremely expensive, and not desirable—autografts are preferred

There are established protocols for the care of cultured epithelial autografts. Because the cells are fragile, they must be handled with the utmost care

TABLE 47-7
Additional Nursing Interventions for Meeting Nutritional Needs

Encourage oral intake after the return of bowel sounds
Obtain a detailed history of the child's eating habits and food preferences
Work with the family and the nutritionist to provide appetizing meals and snacks
Maintain small servings of nutritious, protein-rich food available frequently
Monitor urine urea nitrogen (a positive balance of 4–6 g/24 hr indicates adequate protein intake)
Avoid power struggle with the child regarding eating (see discussion of feeding the hospitalized child in Chapter 21)
Never threaten a child with enteral feedings in an attempt to increase oral intake; do not make the child feel that the feeding tube is a form of punishment
Include the child's family at mealtime
Weigh daily and keep accurate record of caloric intake

One of the many disadvantages of having unskilled and/or poorly trained medical professionals provide burn care is that they do not know how to perform, or even realize the existence of, techniques to prevent complications such as scarring and contractions. When this is the case, not only is the child's life threatened but the rehabilitation period is painful and prolonged! If care has been adequate, there are two major concerns to address during the rehabilitation phase: (1) restoration of function in scarred joint surfaces (Table 47-8) and (2) final psychosocial adjustment. The rehabilitation process starts in the emergency room and continues for years of follow-up. Physiotherapy and occupational therapy provide inpatient and outpatient contracture control and scar management. Positioning and exercises, along with pressure garments, facilitate this process. The patient and family are encouraged to participate actively in the process.

Psychosocial adjustment can be facilitated by the child's family, relatives, social workers, teacher, and peers. Working with the child's teacher and classmates facilitates smooth re-entry into school life. Tu-

TABLE 47-8
Positioning to Prevent Deformity

Area Burned	Resulting Deformity	Position of Prevention
Neck		
Anterior aspect or circumferential	Flexion contracture of neck	No pillow under head
Posterior aspect (only)	Extensor contracture of neck	Prone—pillow under upper chest to flex cervical spine; supine—small pillow under neck
Axilla		
Anterior	Adduction and internal rotation	Shoulder joint in abduction (100–130 degrees) and external rotation
Posterior	Adduction and external rotation	Shoulder in forward flexion and 100–130 degrees of abduction
Pectoral region	Shoulder protraction	No pillow; shoulders abducted and externally rotated
Chest or abdomen	Kyphosis	As above and hips neutral (*not* flexed)
Lateral trunk	Scoliosis	Supine, affected arm abducted
Elbow		
Anterior surface or circumferential	Flexion and pronation	Arm extended and supinated
Wrist		
Total or flexor surface	Flexion	Splint in 15-degree extension
Dorsal surface	Extension	Splint in 15-degree flexion
Hip (includes inguinal and perineal burns)	Internal rotation, flexion and adduction, possible joint subluxation if contracture severe	Neutral rotation and abduction; maintain extension by prone position or *pillow under buttocks*
Knee		
Popliteal surface or circumferential	Flexion	Maintain extension using posterior splints, or suspend heels with plastic heel protecting boots; *no pillows* under knees while supine or under ankles while prone; lower legs often to allow for better circulation
Ankle	Plantar flexion if foot dorsiflexor muscles are weak or their tendons are divided	90-degree dorsiflexion with splint if possible, rather than footboard

toring and having the child participate in regular studies throughout care are helpful. Educating the child's peers about the burn injury and treatment strategies also assist with the re-entry process. Participation in specialized burn camps gives the child an opportunity to interact with other children who have been burned and helps them to feel accepted by a special group of caring peers.

Social workers are usually in a position to assess the function or dysfunction of the family and to institute remedial and corrective measures. This care also begins on admission and continues through outpatient follow-up.

Prevention Issues

The activities that will prevent burn injuries cause no change in lifestyle and require very little behavior modification on the part of a family. Certainly they are simpler than stopping substance abuse. Prevention of burns is a health care issue that requires the active participation of health professionals at all levels (primary, secondary, and tertiary). The various preventive approaches are discussed in Chapter 15.

Prognosis in Burns

Severity factors and quality of care affect the chances for survival of a particular patient. About 65 per cent of survival can be explained by the depth of burn, the child's age, health status and medical history, part of the body injured, concurrent injuries, and other physical and psychosocial factors. Infants and toddlers with 40 per cent total body surface area burns have a survival rate of 80 per cent, in contrast to a 13-year-old patient with a similar burn, who has a survival rate of 93 per cent. Figure 47–6 shows survival curves of burned children. These statistics are from hospitals providing specialized burn care. They do not pertain to hospitals that do not offer the level of care found in a burn center. Research by the National Institute for Burn Medicine, the University of Michigan's (UM) Burn Center, and the Department of Biostatistics in the UM School of Public Health found that about 30 per cent of burn patient survival is closely related to the quality of hospital care provided: presence of a qualified, trained nursing and medical staff, dedicated burn team, clearly defined protocols of care, daily evaluation of care and the patient's response to it, participation of hospital administration, and so forth. Even with specialized burn care, there is a range of 80 per cent difference in survival, depending on which hospital is treating the patient.

This Institutional Differences Study also showed that survival rates of children improved when treatment was given in children's hospitals providing specialized burn care (Evaluation of Emergency Medical Services with a National Burn Registry, 1975–1978).

The survival rate is lower when a larger percent-

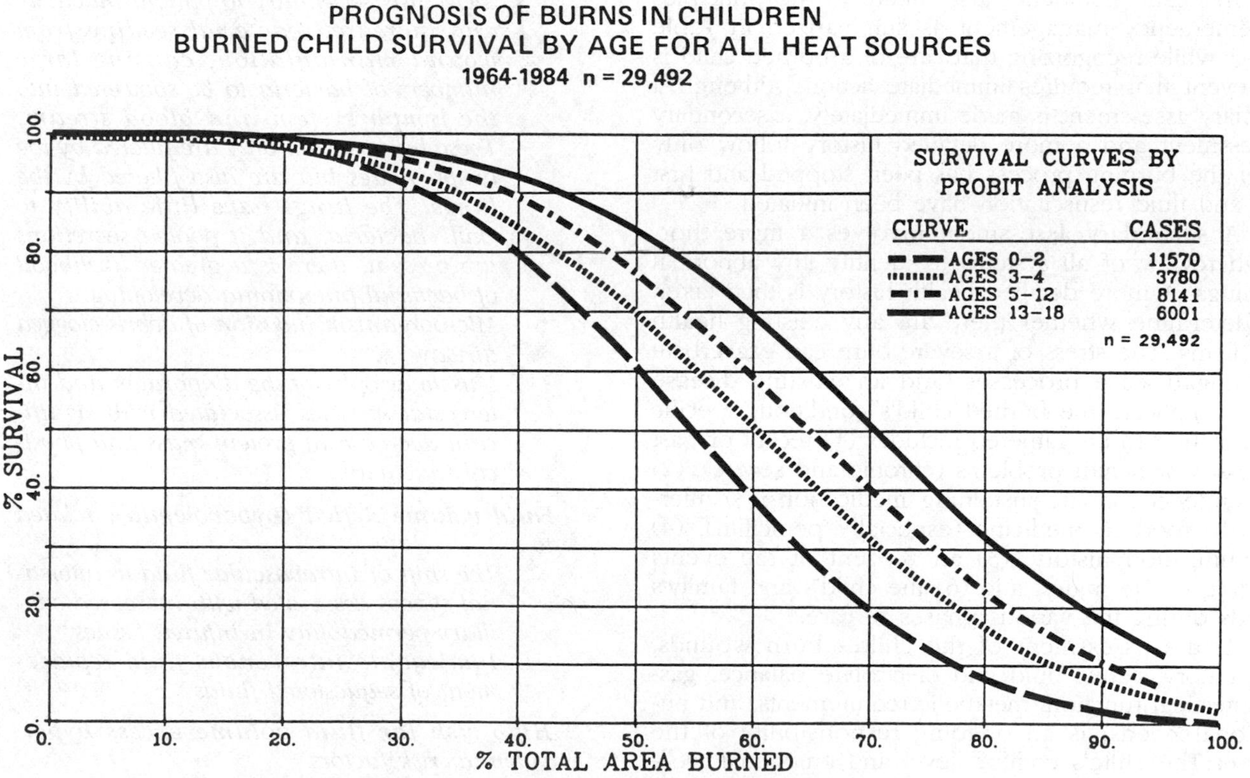

FIGURE 47-6. Burned patient survival by age group. (From National Burn Information Exchange, I. Feller, M.D., Director, 1978–1985. Ann Arbor, MI.)

age of the wound is all full-thickness injury than when the same area includes both full-thickness and partial-thickness burns. If age and total percentage of burn are held constant, the larger the percentage of body surface area affected by full-thickness burn, the more serious is the injury.

Unlike the case with other traumatic injuries, for most severe burns complications tend to be the rule rather than the exception, especially in nonspecialized facilities. Typically, a child with severe burns may have four to six complications, often at the same time, and one or a combination of several may be fatal. The most common complications seen in burn patients are also the most common causes of death (see Table 47–4).

Application of the Nursing Process

Assessment

A nursing assessment of a burned child consists of the four areas discussed under "Diagnostic Assessment." Although the ordering of laboratory tests is generally done by a physician, nurses actively participate as team members to gather the essential data that lead to decisions about need for and evaluation of laboratory assessment. Identification of the extent of a burn, evaluation of a burn's depth, and classification of a burn are team responsibilities in which nurses play a major role.

All team members must adhere to the principles of emergency management as summarized in Table 47–3 while recognizing that care of a burned child is an event that requires immediate action. Although a primary assessment is made immediately, a secondary assessment and a more detailed history follow only after the burning process has been stopped and first aid and fluid resuscitation have been initiated.

A secondary assessment involves a more thorough review of all systems to identify any abnormal findings. A more detailed health history is then taken to determine whether there are any existing health problems. The stress of a severe burn can exacerbate existing disease processes, and an existing disease can complicate the burned child's condition. Specific information to be gathered includes (1) recent or past illnesses or health problems (chronic and severe), (2) dependence on life-sustaining medication, (3) allergies to food or medicine (especially penicillin), (4) immunization history, (5) an account of the events leading to the injury, and (6) the child's and family's needs during the various phases of care.

Astute assessment of the child's burn wounds, respiratory status, fluid and electrolyte balance, gastrointestinal function, metabolic requirements, and nutritional needs, is an ongoing responsibility of the nurse. The child's comfort level and emotional well-being and the family's response to the injury and the patient change over time and require the nurse's ongoing attention in order to plan individualized nursing care. Nursing diagnostic statements and collaborative problems are based on these ongoing assessments. Although the priority of a single diagnosis depends on the phase of care (i.e., whether emergent, acute, or rehabilitative), the following diagnoses are relevant to the care of a burned child in one or more phases of care.

Nursing Diagnostic Statements and Collaborative Problems

Ineffective breathing pattern: airway obstruction, *related to* upper airway *edema, associated with*

- *Burns of the face, neck, and chest.*
- *Forced inhalation of products of combustion, superheated air and/or steam.*

Ineffective airway clearance, *related to*

- *Inadequate removal of increased secretions and debris associated with damaged tissue from the upper and lower airway and damage to mucosa and the cleaning action of the cilia.*

High risk for infection: pneumonia; *risk factors:*

- *Pooling of fluids in the interstitium of the lungs secondary to inactivity or intravenous fluid overload (stiff wet lungs, alveolar collapse).*
- *Atelectasis secondary to patient inactivity and increased bacterial seeding from wound manipulation, causing large numbers of bacteria to be showered into the lymph system and blood stream. These bacteria not only are filtered by the lymph nodes but are also filtered by the lungs. The lungs have little ability to "kill" bacteria, and if pooled secretions are present, there is a greater likelihood of bacterial pneumonia developing.*
- *Microorganism invasion of debris-clogged airways.*
- *Muscle atrophy of the diaphragm and intercostal muscles associated with significant decrease in protein mass and physical inactivity.*

Fluid volume deficit (hypovolemia), *related to*

- *The shift of intravascular fluid to interstitial spaces associated with increased capillary permeability in injured tissues.*
- *Inadequate intravenous fluid replacement of sequestered fluids.*

High risk for fluid volume excess hypervolemia; *risk factors:*

- *Overzealous fluid therapy with vascular overload and pulmonary edema.*

- *Reversal of plasma shift without appropriate decrease in intravenous fluid administration.*
- *Reduced ability of the heart to circulate fluids secondary to past medical history or previously undetected congenital anomaly or organ weakness.*

***Disturbance in self-concept: body image,** related to*

- *Burn wounds.*
- *Ineffective psychosocial support.*
- *Scars.*
- *Elasticized apparel to reduce scar formation.*
- *Pre-existing psychologic trauma from dysfunctional parenting.*

***High risk for altered family process;** risk factors:*

- *Pre-existing family dysfunction compounded by guilt or remorse over accident.*
- *Their child's discomfort related to the burn injury and related treatments.*
- *Child's prolonged hospitalization and disruption of family routine.*
- *Child being at risk for loss of function and physical and emotional alterations.*

***High risk for impaired home maintenance management,** associated with knowledge deficit; risk factors:*

- *Pre-existing, unexamined, and untreated family dysfunction.*
- *Home care of a child with burns.*
- *Child behavior.*
- *Community resources.*
- *School re-entry.*

***At risk for altered parenting: possible child abuse;** risk factor: presence of injury (burn).*

Planning and Implementation

Promote Effective Breathing Pattern by Preventing Airway Obstruction. Ineffective breathing occurs as a result of airway obstruction related to upper airway edema. It is the nurse's role to monitor for factors that put the child at risk for upper airway edema, including obtaining a history of how the accident happened and whether it included intense heat exposure and burns of the face, neck, and chest. Infants and toddlers have smaller airways that are easily obstructed, and they require careful monitoring for airway edema. If any of these risk factors is present, increase the surveillance of respiratory competence, especially during the first 8 hours. Listen for hoarseness or stridor, because these are an indication for intubation.

Thermal injury to the upper airway is identified by establishing a history of being flame-burned in an *enclosed space (house fire)* or forced to breathe superheated steam from an explosion and by checking for singed nasal hairs, sooty tongue or pharynx, carbaceous sputum, and redness or edema of the pharynx. Hemoptysis, wheezing, and stridor are important indications of thermal injury to be reported by the nurse.

Patency of the airway should be assessed by monitoring closely for tachypnea, tachycardia, fine and coarse crackles, pallor, and cyanosis. Oxygenation is evaluated by reviewing blood gas reports and by using a transcutaneous oxygen monitor or pulse oximeter. If oxygenation levels are inadequate, 100 per cent humidified oxygen is administered. The head of the bed is elevated for any hospitalized burned patient to prevent aspiration pneumonia and to facilitate breathing.

A major role of the nurse in maintaining respiratory status is to calm a frightened child. Crying can further increase airway edema and requires specific interventions. The accident and treatment are terrifying to the child as well as to the parents. Both need reassurance and to be given explanations of the interventions required to stabilize the child. Although young children cannot understand complex rationales, explanations given to parents help them calm their child. Holding or rocking an infant or child also has a calming effect.

Promote Effective Breathing Pattern by Maintaining Respiratory Excursion. Ineffective breathing can occur as a result of compromised respiratory excursion. An important nursing role is to monitor for factors that predispose a child to decreased excursion. Predisposing factors to look for are full-thickness, circumferential burns of the chest or abdomen (children under age 7 years are particularly vulnerable, because they use abdominal muscles to breathe), and burns to the thorax or abdomen that cause pain on lung expansion. Respiratory excursion is evaluated by observing chest movement or, in the young child, abdominal movement that occurs in conjunction with respirations. One hand can be placed on each side of the chest to feel for equal expansion.

Respiratory excursion is also evaluated by determining the adequacy of air exchange. To do this, the nurse auscultates for equal breath sounds by making bilateral comparisons. The level of consciousness and the presence of restlessness or agitation are determined. (Decreased oxygenation contributes to anxiety, fear, and restlessness. If lack of oxygen is due to an undetected circulatory, metabolic, or neurologic cause, it soon leads to a vicious cycle that pain medication will not fix.) The child is monitored for tachypnea and tachycardia while at rest, because crying and activity can increase respiratory and cardiac rates. The nurse should look for pallor or duskiness in areas of unburned skin and the mucous membranes. Blood gas values are reviewed, and if the child is intubated, tidal volumes may be monitored.

Normal lung excursion is facilitated by implementing various nursing approaches. The head of the bed should always be up, placing the child in the semi-Fowler position. Placing the head of the bed on 6-inch shock blocks or raising the head end of the crib mattress 30 degrees can contribute to normal lung excursion and prevents aspiration of secretions or regurgitated stomach contents. Also, changing the child's position every 1 to 2 hours (if the child is not moving spontaneously), turning to side, back, side, and abdomen, helps maintain an even expansion of the lungs. Do not place an infant on the abdomen for longer than 20 to 30 minutes at a time.

Eliminate possible discomfort for the child from soiled diapers, rumpled, wet, or cold sheets, being too cold or too warm, or being hungry, lonely, tired, or angry. The child who experiences pain on lung expansion adopts a pattern of shallow breathing. The nurse administers prescribed analgesics and carefully evaluates whether narcotic analgesics depress respirations, by counting respirations before and 20 to 30 minutes after administration. Additionally, anxiety can result in shallow breathing; therefore, reduction of fear is an important nursing role (see discussion under "Reduce Anxiety and Fear").

Maintain Adequate Gas Exchange to Prevent Hypoxemia. Alveolar damage can result from prolonged inhalation of noxious gases and chemicals or inhalation of carbon monoxide, resulting in impaired gas exchange. In this event the nurse should assess for adequate gas exchange. The child's baseline activity and level of consciousness are charted at the onset for later comparison. Observations are made for any signs of unusual restlessness, irritability, or change in mental status, and blood gas levels are monitored.

Oxygenation is monitored. If oxygenation is reduced, 100 per cent humidified oxygen is administered to counteract the effects of carbon monoxide, a gas present in all fires. If intubation and mechanical ventilation are required, the nurse assists with the procedures and then maintains the artificial airway by ensuring that the endotracheal tube is well secured and by restraining the child as necessary to prevent accidental extubation. The nurse also administers sedatives, as ordered, to decrease anxiety associated with mechanical ventilation. Cuff pressure of the endotracheal tube is maintained under 20 mm Hg (to prevent tracheal necrosis). Uncuffed tubes are used in children younger than 10 years of age, because the tracheal cartilage is still soft, and the trachea is more prone to necrosis from pressure or overexpansion of the C-ring (top tracheal cartilage).

Promote Effective Airway Clearance by Adequate Removal of Damaged Tissue from the Lower Airway. Airway clearance is assessed by auscultating lungs before and after the child coughs. Clearing sputum from the respiratory tract can be achieved by older children, but toddlers and preschoolers rarely expectorate sputum; they swallow it instead. Swallowed sputum can be observed in products of nasogastric suction. The characteristics of sputum should be monitored. Loud upper airway crackles cleared by coughing are an indication that airway clearance has taken place, even though sputum is not produced. The nurse should also observe the child for use of accessory muscles in breathing, which could indicate that increased effort is required to move air through the lungs.

Another goal is to decrease accumulation and pooling of secretions. This is done by ensuring that the child's position is changed every 1 to 2 hours or that the child moves spontaneously into various positions. Secretions are liquefied by providing humidified oxygen and fluids, as ordered.

If sputum does accumulate, the nurse intervenes to facilitate its clearance. A common intervention is to suction secretions gently from the mouth and nose of the infant or toddler, especially after respiratory treatments or episodes of crying, because activities that expand the lungs facilitate clearance of mucus. Children are also encouraged to breathe deeply and cough if they are old enough to do so. If at all possible, nausea and vomiting should be prevented to reduce the risk for aspiration. The nurse also assists with administration of mucolytic treatments via the nebulizer and with chest physiotherapy and postural drainage. One of the nurse's extremely important roles is to notify the physician of signs of increasing airway obstruction.

Prevent Pneumonia by Reducing the Child's Risk of Infection. Because microorganisms invade the debris-clogged airways, a child can be at risk for infection if special precautions are ignored. The nurse assesses the child for signs and symptoms of pneumonia by checking temperature and watching for evidence of tachypnea and tachycardia. The chest is auscultated for adventitious or diminished breath sounds (diminished breath sounds may also be related to decreased respiratory excursion). Sputum is monitored for purulent (yellow or green) appearance, and specimens are collected for culture. Unexplained lethargy and fatigue are also important clinical observations that could indicate that the child has contracted pneumonia.

The nurse monitors the sputum laboratory reports as well as white blood count and chest roentgenography reports.

The risk of lung infection can be decreased by adhering to various basic principles of asepsis. Meticulous hand washing and the observance of established precautions for infection control are essential. Parents and other family members are taught infection control practices, and the nurse must monitor their and other visitors' adherence to them. The nurse also ensures that the child is not exposed to persons with respiratory infections, including health care professionals.

Numerous specific nursing practices must be adhered to if the child's risk of infection is to be decreased. Disposable oxygen tubing and the humidification apparatus are changed every 48 to 72 hours or according to unit policy; this is done to prevent colonization of these surfaces. Good pulmonary care is provided by turning, assisting with coughing and deep breathing, and instituting incentive spirometry, chest physiotherapy, and postural drainage. Antibiotics are administered, as ordered, for positive cultures.

Prevent Hypovolemia by Maintaining Vascular Fluid Volume. The nurse's role in preventing hypovolemia is to monitor the child for signs and symptoms of vascular volume deficit and to ensure the administration of intravenous fluids, as ordered. Various approaches are used to monitor for vascular volume deficit. An in-dwelling urinary catheter may be inserted and attached to a collection device that measures urine output. The expected hourly output is based on the child's weight. Therefore, accurate weights must be maintained. Urine output is measured and recorded hourly. (See discussion under "Fluid Resuscitation" for expected urine outputs.)

Other areas to monitor are vital signs, capillary refill, skin perfusion, and laboratory reports. One must assess for tachycardia and hypotension by measuring vital signs under like conditions over time. For example, each blood pressure reading should be taken with the child in the same position as before. A blood pressure reading can be misleading if taken in the burned limb because of the progressive edema that occurs. As the swelling increases, the auditory signal diminishes. The nurse monitors for capillary refill by depressing nailbeds in the fingers and toes and observing how rapidly color returns. Skin perfusion is evaluated by determining whether it is cool, clammy, and mottled (poor perfusion) or whether it is warm and dry (good perfusion). Laboratory values should be reviewed as listed in Table 47–2.

During the acute period, intravenous fluid may intermittently be used to replace electrolytes and fluid and to increase protein through colloids (e.g., albumin, fresh frozen plasma); it can also be used for parenteral nutrition. Because infants and toddlers have a reduced capacity to store and mobilize glucose, blood glucose levels are carefully monitored. If glucose levels drop, dextrose may be added to the intravenous fluid. Maintaining close watch of a steady intravenous rate helps to prevent volume deficit or overload. Hourly intravenous intake must be accurately recorded.

Prevent Hypervolemia by Maintaining Normal Vascular Fluid Volume. Signs and symptoms of vascular volume excess secondary to administration of intravenous fluids include dyspnea, fine crackles in the chest, tachycardia, clear and frothy sputum, extra heart sounds (S3 and S4), changes in mental status, and distention of neck veins. These are late signs; close monitoring of I and O should detect any trend toward overloading long before these signs occur. Collaboration with the physician in charge of fluid therapy is essential.

Promote Comfort by Relieving Pain. To keep a child with burns comfortable, a nurse needs the skill to assess a child's pain status and the knowledge of different ways to relieve pain. Children may be comfortable at rest yet experience much pain during dressing and débridement. Donor sites are particularly sensitive. Verbal and nonverbal cues vary according to the age of the child. Crying, whimpering, and other vocalizations; alteration in normal movements; and either unusual quietness or agitation are major indications of pain. Preschoolers and older children can be asked to rank their pain on a scale of 0 to 10. Parents also should be asked to help the nurse evaluate the child's comfort level. Changes in vital signs that correspond with other signs and symptoms of pain further assist the nurse in pain assessment. Comfort level is also evaluated by considering the child's ability to sleep uninterruptedly.

Providing relief from pain is a major role of the nurse caring for children with burns. The nurse is skilled in eliminating all sources of mechanical or functional discomfort by maintaining clean dressings, good hygiene, clean unrumpled sheets, adequate room temperature, appropriate fluids, daily bowel movements (no constipation), and adequate and tasty food and by allowing children to talk about their experiences and to play normally. Such care increases the child's sense of well-being. Pain medication cannot replace good basic nursing care.

Analgesics are essential for painful treatment and should be administered so that their peak therapeutic action occurs during painful procedures. The nurse can implement distraction techniques (e.g., music via headphones), stress management techniques (e.g., muscle relaxation), and strategies to maximize predictability and controllability of the procedures for the child (e.g., sensory and informational preparation, allowing child to assist by holding a packaged dressing). Interventions are chosen on the basis of the child's developmental age, personality, past coping techniques, and suggestions from the parents and child about whether a certain approach will be helpful.

Reduce Anxiety and Fear. The burn injury and the associated pain, the hospital setting, and separation from home and family all contribute to a child's fear and anxiety. Many strategies are available to nurses to counteract these factors. (Also see Chapter 12 on promoting healthy parenting.)

Children with burns experience repeated exposure to painful procedures and benefit from caring approaches of nurses. Nurses should talk to children in a soft voice, share their own name, and call them by name. Explaining treatments, pain management, and the need for the child's active participation in the treatment as well as allowing choices, wherever available, all help the child feel less afraid and anxious. Family and friends are encouraged to participate in the child's care. A pleasant, loving, and supportive atmosphere is created—one in which the child feels safe and is encouraged to talk, say and act out feelings of depression and hostility, and verbalize anxieties. The child's situation can be normalized by encouraging getting out of bed and participating in everyday activities, such as playing and school activities. The child is given the opportunity to maintain the developmental tasks already achieved, such as eating in a high chair or at the table, not using diapers if the child has been toilet trained, and allowing self-feeding as the child is able. The child with burns needs to be rocked, cuddled, taught, and disciplined like any other child. Usual rules of conduct and expectations of courtesy are maintained.

Reduce the Risk for Wound Infection and Septicemia. The child's risk for wound infection is reduced through careful monitoring of the wound, strategies to prevent wound and systemic infection, and careful monitoring and early reporting of signs and symptoms of sepsis.

Monitor the burn wound for signs and symptoms of wound infection by inspecting it daily for erythema, exudate, ulceration, and deterioration of granulation tissue. Documentation of daily wound assessment should be detailed and clear to communicate its status to other team members. Often the first sign of wound infection is the child acting as if he had a cold: lethargy, chills, fever, and loss of appetite indicate a bacteremia from increased bacterial count showering into the lymph and blood from the wound. Local signs are erythema at the burn wound perimeter and/or suppuration. Such findings are reported to the physician and documented. Wounds must be cultured according to unit policy (usually 1 to 2 times a week), and white blood counts are monitored to determine the presence of an inflammatory process. This may indicate that the topical agent is not effective against bacteria in the wound, that a systemic antibiotic is needed, or that more effective daily cleansing and débridement are needed.

To prevent a wound infection from occurring, enforce various rules: meticulous hand washing and isolation technique, use of aseptic technique for wound care, use of chlorine or another disinfecting agent in hydrotherapy tubs, débridement of dead tissue, and following manufacturer's instructions for best application of topical antimicrobial agents.

Early detection of subtle signs and symptoms of sepsis and reporting of such findings can prevent a full-blown septicemia. The signs may be as subtle as lethargy that persists despite rest, sleep, and relief of boredom. The nurse watches closely for signs and symptoms of infection in burn wounds, the respiratory tract, the genitourinary tract, sites of intravenous insertion, and the gastrointestinal tract; the nurse reports any such findings to the physician at once. Auscultation for bowel sounds is done every 8 hours, and culture reports of burn wounds, sputum, urine, intravenous and urinary catheters, central venous catheter sites, and blood are monitored.

The risk of systemic infection is decreased by adhering to various principles of care. Prophylactic antibiotics are administered, as ordered by the physician, to reduce the risk of infection. The catheter and connecting tubings are changed every 48 to 72 hours, according to unit policy, to decrease bacterial colonization. Oxygen tubings and the humidification apparatus are changed every 48 to 72 hours, according to unit policy. Humidifier units are washed at least every 48 hours to prevent aerosolization of pathogens, and aseptic technique must be observed for all invasive procedures.

Provide Adequate Nutrition to Meet Body Requirements. Because of hypovolemia during this phase, the child is at risk for developing paralytic ileus. For this reason, nothing is given by mouth, and a nasogastric tube is inserted, as ordered, and maintained at low suction. Bowel sounds are monitored and are expected to return by about the second day after the burn injury. A child with burns is also at risk for duodenal ulceration (Curling ulcer) because of the increased levels of corticosteroids associated with the physiologic response to stress. Antacids or cimetidine is administered, as ordered, the nasogastric tube being clamped for 15 to 20 minutes after the antacid is inserted. After bowel sounds have returned, oral intake is encouraged. A variety of principles and techniques to encourage eating may be required, to ensure adequate nutritional intake. The nurse asks the child or parent what the child likes to eat, then works with the family and the dietitian to provide appealing meals and snacks. Small, frequent servings of nutritious, protein-rich foods can help achieve the goal of adequate intake. Any oral fluids should contain calories (e.g., juices).

If getting the child to eat becomes a power struggle, the nurse should "back off" and give the child choices; by no means should the child be threatened with enteral feeding. The child has few choices. The child who needs enteral feeding should not feel it is a punishment. In some institutions, feeding tubes are routinely inserted for children with burns covering more than 15 to 20 per cent of body surface. This eliminates the struggle surrounding food intake and avoids making the child feel like a failure. This approach is ridiculous if the child can take food by mouth.

Caloric intake is closely monitored throughout. During the emergent and acute phases, daily weight measurements are taken to assess the status of fluid volume. A weight gain during the acute phase may signal congestive heart failure. During the rehabilitation period, daily weights are taken to estimate the adequacy of intake for healing. Additionally, accurate records of caloric intake (calorie count) are kept.

Reduce the Risk for Impaired Mobility. Prolonged bed rest, changes in fluid balance, increased extravascular protein and other electrolytes, muscle wasting, and inactivity all put the child at risk for impaired mobility and development of contractures and scar formation. In collaboration with a physiotherapist, the nurse develops strategies to position the child in such a way that prevents deformities (see Table 47–8). Muscle strength and joint mobility are maintained by an exercise program. The help of the child and family is enlisted to ensure that the exercises are performed several times a day. Play and diversional activities that include limb movement and position changes are encouraged. Exercise of the grafted areas is resumed as soon as healing permits (with the permission of the surgeon).

Preventing or reducing infection contributes greatly to inhibiting scar formation. Scarring is minimized if the granulation tissue stays as flat as possible. Fine-mesh gauze and Kerlix wrap dressings help achieve this result. Pressure splints, elastic bandages, or pressure garments also reduce hypertrophy of scar tissue, although the child and family may not initially understand their importance. Some children are scar formers (keloids) and postrecovery therapy may be needed in addition to pressure dressings.

Prevent a Disturbance in Self-Concept (Body Image). The nurse listens and observes the child for verbal and nonverbal evidence of feelings about changes in appearance. The nurse can be supportive by being open and honest in explaining to the child and family the changes in body image. As family members deal with their own feelings about the child's appearance they can, in turn, be more helpful to the child. The child is encouraged to verbalize his feelings about his burns and treatments, and the reactions of others to him. Even though the nurse and family members assist in coping by being accepting of changes in body image, the child must be made aware that *not everyone will be accepting*.

The manner of talking about the effects of the burn injuries has an impact on the family's and the child's acceptance. Burn injuries are explained matter-of-factly in a calm and straightforward, accepting manner, which can be a reassuring approach. The family and friends should be invited to participate in the child's care as they feel able. When the child is ready to see the burns, an opportunity is provided for the child to do so.

As nurses become more skilled at burn care and come to terms with their feelings about a burn injury, the more likely they will be to convey a calm, confident, accepting, and genuinely hopeful attitude to patient and family.

Nursing approaches to help children and families cope with the results of a burn injury focus on communication and on helping the child to feel accepted. Contact with extended family and friends during the rehabilitation phase helps the child to test a new body image gradually. Children are encouraged to wear their own clothing to direct attention away from the burn wound. Teens are encouraged to wear make-up and wigs and to use color analysis to help focus attention away from the burns. Group therapy or interaction with other children who have experienced burn injuries may be beneficial to some children. A visit from a burn survivor and/or family may be welcome, and a psychiatric consultation may be beneficial in this difficult process.

The transition into the home and the community requires ongoing efforts to prevent altered body image. Before discharge, an opportunity is provided for the child to leave the security of the burn unit and begin to cope with others' reactions to changes in body image. The child's friends and teachers need to be educated about the changes in body image; they need to provide opportunities for the child to express feelings about these changes. Information about school re-entry programs and about burn camps may be helpful to parents.

Reduce the Stressors That Challenge Family Processes. A family that had previously functioned effectively may be severely challenged by the severe stress experienced when their child is burned. The discomforts associated with the actual burn, the related treatment, and the disruption of prolonged hospitalization and rehabilitation produce severe stress on a family. The stress of supporting their child is compounded by the feelings that parents deal with during the process of caring for their child. Parents often feel recurring guilt that they failed to protect their child from the burn, regardless of its circumstances. They continuously worry about their child's physical and emotional capacity to live a normal life.

Family functioning can be supported by giving parents a special role in their child's recovery. The plan of care is discussed with parents, the reasons for the various approaches are explained, and they are encouraged to ask questions. From the beginning, parents are encouraged to participate in the various treatments and are given the instructions and guidance they need to feel comfortable handling their child.

The process of the family and child participating in care is as important as the outcome. Attachments and communication within a family are fostered by strategies that promote a positive family atmosphere. The family is encouraged to visit frequently and to share with the hospital staff information about the child's interests and life before hospitalization. If the family cannot function in this way, gentle direction and suggestions by the nursing staff and burn team can assist the family to function in a supportive way.

The environment is made as much like home as possible: Parents bring toys, pictures, the child's own clothing, and other special articles. Normal relationships within the family are supported by encouraging parents to maintain their role in discipline and in setting limits, as required. Parents may need help to understand that their child might regress or exhibit acting-out behavior as a response to the trauma. However, enforcement of normal routine, firm boundaries, and expectations, to the extent possible, is comforting and supportive. Recovery from burns is a long process, during which both parents and child will feel most comfortable if a high degree of normalcy is maintained.

Families may need special interventions for support during the long process of healing and recovery. Parents may benefit from contact with other parents who have recently experienced similar trauma. Group sessions can provide a time during which parents feel comfortable sharing their fears, guilt, and other reactions to their child's injuries and changes in body image. This is especially true in the event of major burns, which require long months or years of rehabilitative care.

A focus on the family throughout the hospitalization facilitates the transition to care at home. The ongoing involvement and preparation of the family are essential to prepare them for their child's discharge. Community resources are identified, and the family is assisted in gaining access to them as needed.

Facilitating Home Management. The transition from hospital care to home and community resources is a process that requires the child and family to be prepared with education about the child's care and community resources. The family needs to feel confident about coping with the demands of rehabilitating their child and re-establishing their family.

The family should be involved in planning the impending discharge date so that they can prepare the rest of the family members for the event. The learning skills of the child and family need to be identified to determine how much responsibility for care the family will assume and what community resources will be required to support the family at the required level. The patient (depending on age) and family are instructed in burn wound care, including identification of signs and symptoms of infection. An exercise protocol is prescribed, and appropriate nutrition for the age of the child is outlined. The use of pressure garments as a method of controlling scar development and the child's medications are reviewed and explained. The outpatient clinic system is explained so that follow-up is maintained and the family is aware of this resource during rehabilitation.

Before discharge, the child and family are instructed to provide daily wound care and to observe the wounds and surrounding tissue for signs of infection, such as swelling, redness, heat, pain, or colored drainage. To enhance any teaching and instructions provided for the child and family, numerous supportive interventions are offered. First, the child and parents are encouraged to ask questions at all times, and a contact number for the burn unit is provided. A copy of written instructions is provided, as are supplies to meet immediate discharge needs. Home health care options are discussed, and the appropriate referrals are made. If the child is in school, re-entry into the system is discussed and instructions about particular limitations for the child are given.

Reduce Risk Factors for Altered Parenting. Whenever an injury occurs, the health care team mobilizes resources to help the child and family endure the immediate crisis. After the immediate care is provided, a detailed history of the injury is obtained from the child (if developmentally appropriate), family members, and any other involved relative. During this phase of care, the health team should carefully assess the child and family circumstances for any factors that would indicate the cause of injury, such as child abuse or neglect. An assessment is made of the wounds in relation to the account of the event, the child's physical and psychologic status, past health history, social history, history of previous injuries (type and causes), and the compatibility of stories told by various family members.

Certain types of burn wounds should be noted with an index of suspicion: immersion wounds, such as "stocking burns" (burns with a clearly demarcated line around the leg); doughnut-shaped burns on the buttocks; cigarette-type burns, especially on the palms of the hands, soles of the feet, or genitals; rope burns; or dry burns that are caused by an iron are cause for further questioning.

The nurse also assesses the telling of the story during history taking. An unclear history of the injury, an alteration of details among family members, and a history incompatible with the child's motor ability are clues to evaluate as indicators of child abuse.

The circumstances surrounding the event are also evaluated for indications of child abuse or neglect. An injury that occurs when a child is home alone, one that is attributed to a sibling, and associated injuries are factors that require further investigation. (A full discussion of risk factors and indicators of child abuse appears in Chapter 28.)

Complete history and clinical findings are documented. (If abuse is suspected, photographs are taken.) Appropriate assessments and referrals are made to hospital and community resources. During the entire process and hospitalization, the child's safety is maintained; the child and family are provided with explanations and emotional support. Finally, a detailed discharge plan is developed on the basis of findings of the investigation; in some cases, the child is removed from the home.

TABLE 47-9

Nursing Process Plan: The Child with Major Burns

(See also Table 21–5. Nursing Process Plan: The Hospitalized Child)

Analysis: Nursing Diagnostic Statement 1

Response and Related or Risk Factors: *High risk for ineffective airway clearance; risk factors:*

- *Upper airway edema associated with*
  - Burns of the face, neck, and chest
  - History of forced inhalation of products of combustion, secondary to history of flame burn in an enclosed space
  - Thermal injury to the upper airway—forced inhalation of hot steam
- *Debris, sloughing tissue, increased mucus remaining in lower airway associated with damage to cilia*

Projected Outcome: The child will maintain a patent airway

Defining Characteristics *(Actual Response)*

Objective:

- Restlessness
- Anxiety
- Decreased PO_2
- Abnormal breath sounds
- Changes in rate of respiration
- Dyspnea as edema worsens
- Hoarseness as edema worsens
- Stridor (late sign)
- Tachypnea
- Cough, effective/ineffective, with or without sputum
- Cyanosis (very late sign)
- Nasal flaring
- Increased PCO_2

Nursing Interventions

Respiratory Monitoring

Decreased oxygen to brain; calm the frightened child with reassuring voice and explanations of all procedures

- Immediately clear airway
- Give humidified oxygen
- Take blood gases as a baseline

Assess for signs and symptoms associated with upper airway injury

- If hoarseness or stridor is present, notify physician
- Insert airway (as directed)

Assess patency of airway every 15–30 mins in the first 8 hrs

Facilitate air exchange by administering oxygen and positioning with head of bed elevated

- Decrease accumulation and pooling of secretions
- Facilitate clearance of sputum
- Alert the physician to signs of increasing airway obstruction
- Alert physician at the first sign of increased respiratory effort
- Assist with insertion of endotracheal tube before edema shuts off airway

Evaluation Criteria

The child will maintain an adequate airway as evidenced by

- Normal rate and depth of respirations for age, normal breath sounds
- Heart rate normal for age
- Normal skin color in nonburned areas
- Absence of nasal flaring and stridor
- Blood gases within normal limits
- Sputum production if cough present

(continued)

TABLE 47-9 *(continued)*

Analysis: Nursing Diagnostic Statement 2

Response and Related or Risk Factors: *High risk for impaired gas exchange: hypoxemia; risk factors*

- *Compromised respiratory excursion associated with*
  - Constriction of the thorax and abdomen by eschar associated with full-thickness of circumferential burns becomes noticeable as eschar defines and hardens about 3 days after the burn
  - Pain associated with burns to the thorax or abdomen
- *Bronchial and laryngeal damage associated with*
  - Prolonged inhalation of noxious gases and chemicals
  - Carbon monoxide inhalation (rarely seen if patient is given O_2 at scene or in emergency department)

Projected Outcome: The child will not experience hypoxemia

Defining Characteristics *(Actual Response)*	Nursing Interventions	Evaluation Criteria
Subjective: • Irritability • Restlessness • Confusion • Somnolence • Anxiety *Objective:* • Inability to move secretions • Tachypnea • Pallor • Cyanosis • Decreased tidal volume (if intubated) • Hypercapnia • Hypoxia • Constricting circumferential eschar	Facilitate normal lung excursion by positioning with head elevated Change position every 2 hrs *Pain Management* Administer prescribed analgesic and provide comfort measures (see Chapter 25) Administer oxygen and provide comfort measures (see Chapter 25) Administer oxygen as necessary Alert the physician if significant changes in oxygenation occur; be prepared to assist physician with intubation and mechanical ventilation, should this become necessary Assist with escharotomy usually 3–4 days after the burn or immediately with enzymatic escharotomy	The child will maintain adequate respiratory excursion for effective gas exchange as evidenced by • Normal rate and depth of respirations • Normal skin color in nonburned areas • Equal breath sounds bilaterally • Arterial or transcutaneous blood oxygen values within normal limits • Normal tidal volume (if intubated) • Alert (as allowed by condition)

Analysis: Collaborative Problem 1

Response and Related or Risk Factors: *High risk for infection: pneumonia; risk factors: microorganism invasion of debris-clogged airways or pooled secretions from atelectasis from inactivity*

Projected Outcome: The child will not experience an infectious process resulting in pneumonia

TABLE 47-9 *(continued)*

Defining Characteristics *(Actual Response)*	**Nursing Interventions**	**Evaluation Criteria**
Subjective: • Chest pain *Objective*: • Fever • Increased anorexia • Lethargy • Increasing dyspnea and cyanosis • Increased white blood count (in bacterial pneumonia) • Chest roentgenograph indicative of infiltration • Positive sputum culture	Assess for and report signs and symptoms of pneumonia (see Defining Characteristics) Reduce the risk of lung infection by • Observing unit precautions for infection control • Giving antibiotics as ordered • Establishing good pulmonary hygiene (turn, cough, deep breathe; incentive spirometry; chest physical therapy; ample fluids) Alert physician to signs of infection in respiratory tract or elsewhere	The child will remain free of pneumonia as evidenced by • Remaining afebrile • Maintaining or improving respiratory capacity • Absence of unexplained fatigue • White blood count within normal limits • Lungs free of infiltration on chest roentgenography • Negative sputum culture disturbances

Analysis: Collaborative Problem 2

Response and Related or Risk Factors: *High risk for fluid volume deficit: vascular; hypovolemia; risk factor; shift of intravascular fluid to interstitial spaces, associated with increased capillary permeability in injured tissues*

Projected Outcome: The child's fluid volume (vascular) will be adequately maintained to prevent hypovolemia

Defining Characteristics *(Actual Response)*	**Nursing Interventions**	**Evaluation Criteria**
Subjective: • Thirst *Objective*: • Decreased urine output • Increased specific gravity of urine • Increased hematocrit related to hemoconcentration • Decreased blood pressure • Rapid, thready pulse • Decreased peripheral perfusion (decreased peripheral pulses, slow capillary refill time in nailbeds) • Marked edema surrounding burned tissues • Decreased bowel sounds • Decreased central venous pressure	*Fluid Management* Monitor for vascular volume deficit • Monitor vital signs hourly • Insert an in-dwelling catheter (as ordered) and attach to a collection bag designed to measure hourly urine output • Estimate size of burn • Weigh child and calculate expected hourly urine output parameters • Measure and record urine output hourly • Monitor for tachycardia of 40 points or more above baseline and for hypotension • Assess for capillary refill • Assess skin perfusion • Monitor hematocrit level	The child will maintain adequate vascular volume to prevent hypovolemic shock as evidenced by • Maintaining urine output of 1 ml/kg per hour (children) or 30 ml/hr (children >30 kg) • Heart rate and blood pressure normal for age • Usual mental status • Absence of thirst • Rapid capillary refill in nailbeds • Hematocrit within normal limits • Central venous pressure at 3–10 mm Hg • Normal skin perfusion

(continued)

TABLE 47-9 (continued)

Defining Characteristics *(Actual Response)*	**Nursing Interventions**	**Evaluation Criteria**
	• Obtain serum chemistry, as ordered Maintain intravenous fluid therapy as ordered Alert physician at first sign of vascular volume deficit	

Analysis: Nursing Diagnostic Statement 3

Response and Related or Risk Factors: *High risk for fluid volume excess: vascular; hypervolemia; risk factors:*

- Excessive intravenous fluids
- Reversal of plasma shift without appropriate decrease in intravenous fluid administration

Projected Outcome: The child's fluid volume (vascular) will be adequately maintained to prevent hypervolemia

Defining Characteristics *(Actual Response)*	**Nursing Interventions**	**Evaluation Criteria**
Objective: • Dyspnea • Rapid, shallow respirations with presence of rales (crackles) • Tachycardia • Hypertension • Gallop heart rhythm • Jugular venous distention • Restlessness • Anxiety • Marked decrease in hematocrit	*Fluid Management* Monitor for and report signs and symptoms of hypervolemia Prevent fluid volume overload Administer fluids as appropriate • Distribute fluid intake (total volume may be ordered by physician) over a 24-hr period in measured amounts Calculate input and output carefully Carefully monitor intravenous infusion rates (include intravenous fluids in input and output) Alert physician if defining characteristics of fluid volume overload occur	The child will not experience hypervolemia as evidenced by • Clear breath sounds or no increase in adventitious sounds • Stable pulse and blood pressure • Absence of gallop rhythm (no extra heart sounds) • Absence of distended neck veins • Usual mental status • Hematocrit within normal limits

Analysis: Collaborative Problem 3

Response and Related or Risk Factors: *Pain, related to*

- Trauma to sensitive tissues and regenerating nerves during dressing changes, wound débridement, exercise of affected extremity
- Tissue removal at skin graft sites

Projected Outcome: The child's level of discomfort will be decreased or the child will be free of pain

TABLE 47-9 (continued)

Defining Characteristics	Nursing Interventions	Evaluation Criteria
Subjective: • Crying • Verbal report of "hurt" or discomfort *Objective*: • Diaphoresis • Squirming • Rigidity • Trembling • Agitation • Irritability • Facial expression of discomfort • Changes in vital signs • Inconsolable infant • Anorexia • Withdrawal • Sleep disturbance (Atchison et al, 1986)	Assess for pain related to the burn wounds and donor sites (burn pain is known to fluctuate) *Pain Management* Provide pain relief (see Chapter 25)	The child will experience a minimum amount of pain as evidenced by • Absence of crying, whimpering • Verbalization of increased comfort • Physical behaviors appropriate for age (i.e., neither agitated nor lying without movement) • Vital signs within normal limits • Appetite stable • Sleep unaffected by burn wounds

Analysis: Nursing Diagnostic Statement 4

Response and Related or Risk Factors: *Anxiety and fear, related to anticipation of pain from burn injury, lack of psychologic comfort due to unfamiliarity of hospital surroundings and periods of separation from home and family*

Projected Outcome: The child will verbalize or demonstrate greater psychological comfort/decrease in feeling of uneasiness and dread

Defining Characteristics	Nursing Interventions	Evaluation Criteria
Subjective: • Increased tension • Apprehension • Painful and persistent increased helplessness • Uncertainty • Overexcitedness • Distress • Jittery • Shakiness	Introduce all nursing/care staff to patient Explain all treatments (verbally or through play) along with the staff and patient's role in treatments Undertake measures to decrease pain (see Collaborative Problem 3) Be receptive to verbal and nonverbal cues from patient Be patient while providing treatments and have the child actively participate in treatments that are provided	The child will appear calmer and there will be an absence of physiologic symptoms and defining characteristics of anxiety Be sure all other factors are controlled, e.g., hunger, thirst, need to talk about experience, dry diapers, no constipation, clean sheets, appropriate naps and rest between treatments; bath time relaxed

(continued)

TABLE 47-9 (continued)

Defining Characteristics	Nursing Interventions	Evaluation Criteria
Objective: • Sympathetic stimulation: cardiovascular—change in heart rate, pupil size, respiration, and superficial vasoconstriction • Restlessness • Insomnia • Trembling/tremors • Facial tension • Voice quivering • Increased weariness • Increased perspiration • Crying • Refusal to participate in treatments • Decreased appetite • Verbalization of fear	Provide consistency in the treatment plan to allow the child an opportunity to remain familiar with care expectations Provide emotional support and a pleasant, loving atmosphere (i.e., the burned child needs to be rocked, cuddled, taught, and disciplined like any other child) Provide positive reinforcement Encourage physical activity and participation in daily activities Allow play, talk, and the expression of feelings (i.e., depression, hostility, anxiety) Encourage family and friends to participate in child's care Develop an individual care plan based on the child's age, developmental stage, and needs	

Analysis: Collaborative Problem 4

Response and Related or Risk Factors: *High risk for infection:*

- *Wound infection; risk factors:*
  - Loss of protective skin barrier
  - Decreased vascular supply to damaged tissues
  - Diminished immune response
  - Favorable medium for pathogens
- *Septicemia, risk factors; uncontained primary infection or invasion of pathogens at indwelling catheter sites*

Projected Outcome: The child will not develop wound infection and/or septicemia

Defining Characteristics *(Actual Response)*	Nursing Interventions	Evaluation Criteria
Objective: Wound Infection • Fever • Redness of skin surrounding burn wounds • Purulent drainage • Increased white blood count • Ulceration of the burn wound • Deteriorating or pale, waxy granulation tissue	*Infection Protection* Monitor and report signs and symptoms of wound infection Prevent wound infection as follows • Cleanse wound daily through hydrotherapy or gently washing wound; shave hair on or near wound; remove all debris and débride dead tissue • Rinse and apply a pathogen-specific topical agent and appropriate dressings	The child will remain free of wound infection as evidenced by • Skin around burned area free of erythema • Wound free of purulent exudate and ulceration • Healthy granulation tissue • White blood count within normal limits • Wound culture negative for pathogens

TABLE 47-9 *(continued)*

Defining Characteristics	Nursing Interventions	Evaluation Criteria
Subjective: • Verbal or nonverbal reaction to actual change in structure and/or function of body • Verbalization of fear of (or actual) rejection by others • Focus on altered appearance • Verbalization of change in lifestyle • Focus on past appearance • Expression of negative feelings about body and feelings of hopelessness, helplessness • Preoccupation with body changes *Objective*: • Refusal to look at wounds • Not touching wounds • Hiding or over exposing wounds • Refusing visits from friends • Change in usual peer interactions • Change in usual affect (e.g., becoming quiet, sullen, withdrawn) • Lack of interest in personal appearance	*Body Image Enhancement* Promote a positive body image • Encourage family members to talk about and deal with their feelings about the child's appearance (so that they can, in turn, be supportive of the child) • Encourage the child to verbalize feelings about the burns and treatments and the reactions of others. Puppets or dolls or art therapy is often helpful • Explain burn injuries matter-of-factly (acknowledgment validates reality and facilitates problem solving) • Encourage contact with extended family and friends during the rehabilitation phase (so that the child can gradually test a new body image) • Encourage a visit from burn "graduate" and/or family • Supply information about camps available for burn children • Do not contribute to false hopes about plastic surgery (plastic surgery may restore function but can rarely remove all of the evidence of the burn) • Acknowledge the feelings of grief and sadness expressed by the child and family members	The child will maintain a positive body image as evidenced by • Verbalizing positive feelings about self • Verbalizing plans for play, school activities, and so on • Maintaining usual communication patterns and affect • Explaining to others about wounds, scars, and pressure apparel

Analysis: Nursing Diagnostic Statement 8

Response and Related or Risk Factors: *Altered family processes: affective and socialization, related to*

- Child's discomfort
- Disruption of usual family functioning associated with requirements of prolonged hospitalization
- Family not knowing for sure if loss of function and physical and emotional alterations will occur
- The parents' feelings of guilt and discouragement

Projected Outcome: The family will meet affective and socialization functions effectively

(continued)

TABLE 47-9 *(continued)*

Defining Characteristics	Nursing Interventions	Evaluation Criteria
Subjective: Verbal expression by family members of their inability to • meet emotional/affective needs of family members • relate to each other for mutual growth and maturation • accept or receive help appropriately • change or deal with traumatic experience constructively • make decisions *Objective*: • Signs of possible abuse (verbal, psychologic, or physical)	*Family Support* Involve family through communication about their child, encouragement to participate in care, and to visit frequently Encourage family to normalize environment Encourage family to normalize relationships between parents Prepare family for behavior changes Encourage family to express emotions and participate in a support group of other families with similar experiences Refer for professional counseling as appropriate Refer to community support services Prepare family for discharge and the independent care of their child • Evaluate family health • Call in family therapist to assess need to provide family support, or remove child to safer environment	The family will maintain normal processes as evidenced by • Continuing ability to meet emotional/affective needs of members and relate to each other for mutual growth and maturation • Open sharing of feelings • Ability to accept/receive help appropriately • Ability to adapt to change in the child and deal with the traumatic experience constructively • Readiness to care for the child at home when discharged • Participation in the child's care • Healthy decision making processes

Analysis: Nursing Diagnostic Statement 9

Response and Related or Risk Factors: *High risk for altered health maintenance; risk factors: knowledge deficit regarding*

- Home care
- Community resources
- Child behavior
- School re-entry

Projected Outcome: The child and family will be able to identify, manage, and/or seek out help to maintain all aspects of discharge care

Defining Characteristics *(Actual Response)*	Nursing Interventions	Evaluation Criteria
Subjective/Objective: • The child/family verbalizes a lack of knowledge of the discharge plan, asks questions, and exhibits anxiety about impending discharge • Demonstrated lack of adaptive behaviors to changes	Identify and communicate the impending discharge date to child and family Assess the knowledge base and learning skills of the child and family Instruct child and family in burn wound care, encouraging ques-	The child and family will be able to provide all discharge care with minimal assistance from the burn team

TABLE 47-9 (continued)

Defining Characteristics (Actual Response)	Nursing Interventions	Evaluation Criteria
• Reported or observed inability to take responsibility for meeting health practices • Reported or observed lack of resources	tions; include return visit demonstration and written instructions, along with contact telephone number Assess for and arrange home health care as needed Provide supplies as needed to meet discharge needs; incorporate principles of burn care into the school re-entry program in order to assist child with transition from hospital back to school	

Evaluation

Interventions associated with each of the nursing diagnostic statements have been presented. It is the nurse's responsibility to monitor the status of each diagnosis. This requires specific and ongoing evaluation to determine the effectiveness of nursing approaches. Each of the nursing diagnostic statements and/or collaborative problems is presented in Table 47–9, where the specific evaluation for each diagnosis is presented. Table 47–10 describes nursing responsibilities when burn wounds are caused by abuse.

KEY CONCEPTS

Concepts Related to Basic Information

- Children in the age group of birth to 4 years are most likely to suffer scald burn injuries.
- Children over age 4 years are most likely to receive flame burn injuries.
- Children have over a 95 per cent chance of surviving if they receive excellence in care. Research shows the best burn care is more likely to occur in a children's hospital with a specialized burn care facility.
- If products of combustion are inhaled, upper air way edema may develop, secondary to the burn injury.
- Pulmonary edema is most likely secondary to overzealous fluid therapy.
- The body's normal response to any injury is inflammation. In a major burn injury, the fluid shift begins immediately after a burn, is profound for the first 24 hours, and depletes circulating blood volume if untreated.
- Paralytic ileus can occur as a result of the hypovolemic state that occurs during the fluid shift.

TABLE 47-10
Nursing Responsibilities When Child Abuse Is the Etiology of a Burn Wound

Table 47–9 outlines the use of the nursing process for commonly occurring client responses for the child with burns. An additional (critical) area of nursing responsibility for the child client with burns does not involve a client response but is covered here because of its importance

Signs and Symptoms

There are some specific signs and symptoms that indicate child abuse. If the child has burns to lower extremities and buttocks that are sharply defined, such as from being held in scalding water, or if the child has old fractures that have healed or are healing on x-ray films; or if there are cigarette burns or any other signs of maltreatment: *suspect abuse*. The staff should *suspect* child abuse if an unexplained injury takes place, if the injury is incompatible with the child's motor ability, or if there is prior history of abuse

Nursing Interventions

Obtain a detailed history of the injury

Make a detailed assessment of the wounds, child's physical and psychologic status, and past health history, along with a social history

Assess for indications of child abuse (e.g., related in text in Chapter 28)

Child abuse and burn injuries could be suspected on the basis of characteristics of the burn wound: emersion wounds, such as stocking burns or doughnut-shaped burns on the buttocks; cigarette type burns, especially on the palms of the hands, soles of the feet, or genitals; rope burns, or dry burns that are caused by an iron

Document all findings

Make referrals to appropriate child protection agencies if suspicious of abuse. Maintain child's safety at all times

Discharge of child is based on the findings of the investigation if abuse is suspected; it may involve removing the child from the home

Possible Outcomes of Interventions

Appropriate actions will be initiated on the basis of the hospital's policies for abuse. Efforts will be undertaken to protect the child and parent's rights at all times

- Approximately 20 to 25 per cent of children hospitalized for burns develop pulmonary complications.

Concepts Related to Nursing Assessment

- The depth of burn is expressed as full-thickness (all skin layers affected) or partial-thickness (part of skin involved).
- The extent of a burn is expressed as a percentage of the total body surface area and is calculated by diagrams that account for a child's proportionately large surface area for head and lower extremities.
- The burn wound is thoroughly inspected throughout management to determine the response to and need for a change in therapy.
- The level of consciousness, vital signs, and urinary output must be monitored to determine the adequacy of cardiac output and perfusion during intravenous fluid resuscitation.
- The circumstances surrounding the event of a burn are evaluated for indications of child abuse or neglect.
- The child's fear, anxiety, and pain are carefully assessed throughout all stages of a burn event to determine overall adequacy of care and the need for additional psychologic support and pain medication.

Concepts Related to Nursing Intervention

- The first step in emergency management is to stop the burning process, then to maintain an open airway and prevent shock.
- A significant injury sustained in addition to a burn increases the severity of the child's condition.
- A history of being burned in an enclosed space, being forced to breathe products of combustion, and having burns of the face, neck, and/or chest indicate the need for moistened oxygen and close monitoring for upper airway edema.
- Wound infection is prevented by strictly adhering to isolation and aseptic technique by daily inspecting, meticulous cleansing, débriding, and grafting of the wound.
- Circumferential burns to the chest can impede chest movement and lead to respiratory compromise. Circumferential burns of arms, legs, and fingers can compromise circulation (both may require release by escharotomy).
- Therapy consists of three phases: (1) The emergent phase is the first 72 hours, when breathing is ensured; internal bleeding is prevented or treated; burn shock is prevented by fluid therapy; and later complications are prevented or their severity decreased through carefully laying a foundation of preventive care. (2) The acute phase of care includes early detecting, preventing, and managing of complications while accomplishing wound healing and grafting. (3) The rehabilitation phase is the time when the child is guided to return to a functional place in society.
- Emergent-period fluid resuscitation is based on a formula that considers the child's weight and percentage of the body surface area burned and on titrating hourly fluids to produce adequate urine, indicating perfusion of the kidneys and other organs without overload.
- Urine output is monitored hourly to determine the amount of fluid to be administered in the next hour. Urine output is a reliable outer sign of the body's response to injury and treatment.
- When the child is in burn shock, fluids are being sequestered, thereby delaying absorption of subcutaneous or intramuscular medication into the blood stream and decreasing relief from pain medications. Intravenous administration is recommended for pain medications.
- The risk for developing paralytic ileus and stress ulcers must be carefully managed.
- Severe upper airway edema eliminates tracheal patency and requires temporary bypass by insertion of an endotracheal tube.
- A clean wound is the first principle of healing. No wound will heal that contains dead tissue.
- The wound and surrounding area must be cleansed gently, because mechanical trauma can convert partial-thickness wounds to full-thickness ones.
- Full-thickness wounds require autografting for final closure.
- If properly cleansed and dressed, partial-thickness wounds heal well within 21 days.
- Rehabilitation begins at the time of admission: All nursing procedures are designed to prevent or reduce the severity of complications that can be debilitating and/or life-threatening.
- Rehabilitation includes psychosocial adjustment and restoration of function of joints that may have become scarred and contracted.
- The child's body image and self-esteem are at risk. Sensitive listening, encouragement of expression of feelings, and family involvement all help the child cope with the results of the injury.
- Nurses who have not come to terms with their dread of burn injury may have difficulty conveying a genuinely positive attitude about the child's recovery.

REFERENCES

Advanced Burn Life Support (ABLS) Course Instructor's Manual (1987). Nebraska Institute.

Bayley, E. W. (1991). Care of the burn patient with inhalation injury. In R. B. Trofino (Ed.), *Nursing care of the burn injured.* Philadelphia: FA Davis.

Carvajal, H. F., & Parks, D. H. (1988). *Burns in children—Pediatric burn management.* Chicago: Year Book.

Evaluation of Emergency Medical Services with a National Burn Registry, 1975–1978 (Grant #HS-01906-01) (1978). HEW, National Center for Health Services Research; University of Michigan School of Public Health, Department of Biostatistics; and National Institute for Burn Medicine.

Harmel, R. P., Vane, D. W., & King, D. R. (1986). Burn care in children: Special considerations. *Clinics in Plastic Surgery, 13*(1), 95–105.

Heink, N. R. (1992). Fluid resuscitation and the role of exchange transfusion in pediatric burn shock. *Critical Care Nurse, 12*(7), 50.

Horovitz, J. H. (1988). Heat and smoke injuries of the airway. In H. F. Hugo, H. F. Carvajal, & D. H. Parks (Eds.), *Injuries in children: Pediatric burn management* (pp. 225–263). Chicago: Year Book.

Knudson-Cooper, M. S. (1980). Antecedents and consequences of childhood burn injuries. In M. Wolraich, & D. Routh (Eds.), *Advances in developmental and behavioral pediatrics* (Vol. 3). Greenwich, CT: JI Press.

Libber, S. M., & Stayton, D. (1984). Childhood burns reconsidered: The child, the family, and the burn injury. *Journal of Trauma, 24*(3), 245–252.

Lybarger, P. M. (1987). Inhalation injury in children: Nursing care. *Issues in Comprehensive Pediatric Nursing, 10*(1):33–50.

Mikhail, J. N. (1988). Acute burn care: An update. *Journal of Emergency Nursing, 14*(1), 9–18.

National Center for Health Statistics (1987). National Household Survey (1985–1986); National Expenditures Survey, 1987.

National Center for Health Statistics (1991). National Hospital Discharge Survey (1989–1991).

Rieg, L. S., & Jenkins, M. (1991). Burn injuries in children. *Critical Care Nursing Clinics of North America, 3*(3), 457–470.

Silverstein, P., & Wilson, R. (1988). Prevention of pediatric burn injuries. In H. F. Carvajal & D. H. Parks (Eds.), *Burns in children: Pediatric burn management.* Chicago: Year Book.

Stein, J. M. (1985). Burns. In S. S. Zimmerman & J. H. Gildea (Eds.), *Critical care pediatrics* (pp. 474–483). Philadelphia: WB Saunders.

BIBLIOGRAPHY

Bernardo, L. M., & Sullivan, K. (1991). Care of the pediatric patient with burns. In R. B. Trofino (Ed.), *Nursing care of the burn injured.* Philadelphia: FA Davis.

Blakeney, P., et al. (1993). Parental stress as a cause and effect of pediatric burn injury. *Journal of Burn and Rehabilitation, 14*(1), 73–79.

Cavanagh, J. A. (1992). Reintegration: Paediatric burn victims post discharge. *Paediatric Nursing Review, 5*(1), 4–5.

Clugston, P. A., et al. (1991). Cultured epithelial autografts: Three years of clinical experience with eighteen patients. *Journal of Burn Care and Rehabilitation, 12*(6), 533–539.

Grant, E., et al. (1992). Evaluation of a burn presentation program in a public school system. *Journal of Burn Care and Rehabilitation, 13*(6), 703–737.

Hazinski, M. F. (1992). *Nursing care of the critically injured child.* Philadelphia: Mosby–Year Book.

Hummel, R. P., et al. (1993). Outcome and socioeconomic aspects of suspected child abuse scald burns. *Journal of Burn Care and Rehabilitation, 14*(1), 121–126.

Jessee, P. O., et al. (1992). Perception of body image in children with burns, five years after burn injury. *Journal of Burn and Rehabilitation 13*(1), 33–38.

Purdue, G. F., Hunt, J. L., & Prescott, P. R. (1988). Child abuse by burning: An index of suspicion. *Journal of Trauma, 28,* 221–224.

Roberts, S. L. (1987). *Nursing diagnosis and the critically ill patient.* Norwalk, CT: Appleton & Lange.

APPENDIX • 1

Nursing Diagnoses Accepted by NANDA Through 1993

The nursing diagnoses listed here are those currently accepted by the National Conference on Nursing Diagnoses (used with permission from North American Nursing Diagnoses Association: *NANDA Nursing Diagnoses: Definitions and Classification*. Philadelphia, NANDA). These diagnoses are working documents, with research and revision in progress. National Conferences gather nurses together every 2 years, but research in new categories and for accepted categories is an ongoing priority.

Taxonomy I Revised approved nine new nursing diagnoses in 1992; these are denoted by asterisks.

Diagnosis	**Definition**
Activity intolerance	A state in which an individual has insufficient physiologic or psychologic energy to endure or complete required or desired daily activities.
Activity intolerance, high risk for	A state in which an individual is at risk of experiencing insufficient physiologic or psychologic energy to endure or complete required or desired daily activities.
Adjustment, impaired	The state in which the individual is unable to modify his/her lifestyle/behavior in a manner consistent with a change in health status.
Airway clearance, ineffective	A state in which an individual is unable to clear secretions or obstructions from the respiratory tract to maintain airway patency.
Anxiety	A vague, uneasy feeling, the source of which is often nonspecific or unknown to the individual.
Aspiration, high risk for	The state in which an individual is at risk for entry of gastrointestinal secretions, oropharyngeal secretions, or solids or fluids into tracheobronchial passages.
Body image disturbance	Disruption in the way one perceives one's body image.
Body temperature, high risk for altered	The state in which the individual is at risk for failure to maintain body temperature within normal range.
Breastfeeding, effective	The state in which a mother-infant dyad/family exhibits adequate proficiency and satisfaction with the breastfeeding process.
Breastfeeding, ineffective	The state in which a mother, infant, or child experiences dissatisfaction or difficulty with the breastfeeding process.
*Breastfeeding, interrupted	A break in the continuity of the breastfeeding process as a result of inability or inadvisability to put baby to breast for feeding.
Breathing pattern, ineffective	The state in which an individual's inhalation and/or exhalation pattern does not enable adequate pulmonary inflation or emptying.
Cardiac output, decreased	A state in which the blood pumped by an individual's heart is sufficiently reduced that it is inadequate to meet the needs of the body's tissues.
*Caregiver role strain	A caregiver's felt difficulty in performing the family caregiver role.
*Caregiver role strain, high risk for	A caregiver is vulnerable for felt difficulty in performing the family caregiver role.
Colonic constipation	The state in which an individual's pattern of elimination is characterized by hard, dry stool that results from a delay in passage of food residue.

Diagnosis	Definition
Communication, impaired verbal	The state in which an individual experiences a decreased or absent ability to use or understand language in human interaction.
Constipation	A state in which an individual experiences a change in normal bowel habits characterized by decrease in frequency and/or passage of hard, dry stools.
Constipation, perceived	The state in which an individual makes a self-diagnosis of constipation and ensures a daily bowel movement through abuse of laxatives, enemas, and suppositories.
Coping, defensive	The state in which an individual repeatedly protects falsely positive self-evaluation based on a self-protective pattern that defends against underlying perceived threats to positive self-regard.
Coping, ineffective individual	Impairment of adaptive behaviors and problem-solving abilities of a person in meeting life's demands and roles.
Decisional conflict (specify)	The state of uncertainty about course of action to be taken when choice among competing actions involves risk, loss, or challenge to personal life values.
Denial, ineffective	The state of a conscious or unconscious attempt to disavow the knowledge or meaning of an event to reduce anxiety/fear to the detriment of health.
Diarrhea	A state in which an individual experiences a change in normal bowel habits characterized by the frequent passage of loose, fluid, unformed stools.
Disuse syndrome, high risk for	A state in which an individual is at risk for deterioration of body systems as a result of prescribed or unavoidable musculoskeletal inactivity.
Diversional activity deficit	The state in which an individual experiences decreased stimulation from or interest or engagement in recreational or leisure activities.
Dysreflexia	The state in which an individual with a spinal cord injury at T7 or above experiences a life-threatening uninhibited sympathetic response of the nervous system to a noxious stimulus.
Family coping, compromised, ineffective	A usually supportive primary person (family member or close friend) is providing insufficient, ineffective, or compromised support, comfort, assistance, or encouragement that may be needed by the client to manage or master adaptive tasks related to his or her health challenge.
Family coping, disabling, ineffective	Behavior of a significant person (family member or other primary person) that disables his or her own capacities and the client's capacities to effectively address tasks essential to either person's adaptation to the health challenge.
Family coping, potential for growth	Effective managing of adaptive tasks by family member involved with the client's health challenge who now is exhibiting desire and readiness for enhanced health and growth in regard to self and in relation to client.
Family processes, altered	The state in which a family that normally functions effectively experiences a dysfunction.
Fatigue	An overwhelming sustained sense of exhaustion and decreased capacity for physical and mental work.
Fear	Feeling of dread related to an identifiable source that the person validates.
Fluid volume deficit	The state in which an individual experiences vascular, cellular, or intracellular dehydration.
Fluid volume deficit, high risk for	The state in which an individual is at risk of experiencing vascular, cellular, or intracellular dehydration.
Fluid volume excess	The state in which an individual experiences increased fluid retention and edema.
Gas exchange, impaired	The state in which the individual experiences a decreased passage of oxygen and/or carbon dioxide between the alveoli of the lungs and the vascular system.
Grieving, anticipatory	Definition not included in Taxonomy I Revised.
Grieving, dysfunctional	Definition not included in Taxonomy I Revised.

Diagnosis	Definition
Growth and development, altered	The state in which an individual demonstrates deviations in norms from his/her age group.
Health maintenance, altered	Inability to identify, manage, and/or seek out help to maintain health.
Health-seeking behaviors (specify)	A state in which an individual in stable health is actively seeking ways to alter personal health habits and/or the evnironment in order to move toward a higher level of health.
Home maintenance management, impaired	Inability to independently maintain a safe, growth-promoting immediate environment.
Hopelessness	A subjective state in which an individual sees limited or no alternatives or personal choices available and is unable to mobilize energy on own behalf.
Hyperthermia	A state in which an individual's body temperature is elevated above his/her normal range.
Hypothermia	The state in which an individual's body temperature is reduced below his/her normal range.
Incontinence, bowel	A state in which an individual experiences a change in normal bowel habits characterized by involuntary passage of stool.
Incontinence, functional	The state in which an individual experiences an involuntary, unpredictable passage of urine.
Incontinence, reflex	The state in which an individual experiences an involuntary loss of urine, occurring at somewhat predictable intervals when a specific bladder volume is reached.
Incontinence, stress	The state in which an individual experiences a loss of urine of less than 50 ml, occurring with increased abdominal pressure.
Incontinence, total	The state in which an individual experiences a continuous and unpredictable loss of urine.
Incontinence, urge	The state in which an individual experiences involuntary passage of urine occurring soon after a strong sense of urgency to void.
*Infant feeding pattern, ineffective	A state in which an infant demonstrates an impaired ability to suck or coordinate the suck swallow response.
Infection, high risk for	The state in which an individual is at increased risk for being invaded by pathogenic organisms.
Injury, high risk for	A state in which the individual is at risk for injury as a result of environmental conditions interacting with the individual's adaptive and defensive resources.
Knowledge deficit (specify)	Definition not included in Taxonomy I Revised.
*Management of therapeutic regimen (individual's), ineffective	A pattern of regulating and integrating into daily living a program for treatment of illness and the sequelae of illness that is unsatisfactory for meeting specific health goals.
Noncompliance (specify)	A person's informed decision not to adhere to a therapeutic recommendation.
Nutrition, altered: less than body requirements	The state in which an individual experiences an intake of nutrients insufficient to meet metabolic needs.
Nutrition, altered: more than body requirements	The state in which an individual is experiencing an intake of nutrients that exceeds metabolic needs.
Nutrition, altered: high risk for more than body requirements	The state in which an individual is at risk of experiencing an intake of nutrients that exceeds metabolic needs.
Oral mucous membrane, altered	The state in which an individual experiences disruptions in the tissue layers of the oral cavity.
Pain	A state in which an individual experiences and reports the presence of severe discomfort or an uncomfortable sensation.
Pain, chronic	A state in which the individual experiences pain that continues for more than 6 months.
Parental role conflict	The state in which a patient experiences role confusion and conflict in response to crisis.

(continued)

Diagnosis	Definition
Parenting, altered	The state in which a nurturing figure(s) experiences an inability to create an environment that promotes the optimal growth and development of another human being. It is important to state as a preface to this diagnosis that adjustment to parenting in general is a normal maturational process that elicits nursing behaviors of prevention of potential problems and health promotion.
Parenting, high risk for altered	The state in which a nurturing figure(s) is at risk to experience an inability to create an environment that promotes the optimal growth and development of another human being.
*Peripheral neurovascular dysfunction, high risk for	A state in which an individual is at risk of experiencing a disruption in circulation, sensation, or motion of an extremity.
Personal identity disturbance	Inability to distinguish between self and nonself.
Physical mobility, impaired	A state in which the individual experiences a limitation of ability for independent physical movement.
Poisoning, high risk for	Accentuated risk of accidental exposure to or ingestion of drugs or dangerous products in doses sufficient to cause poisoning.
Post-trauma response	The state of an individual experiencing a sustained painful response to (an) unexpected extraordinary life event(s).
Powerlessness	Perception that one's own action will not significantly affect an outcome; a perceived lack of control over a current situation or immediate happening.
Protection, altered	The state in which an individual experiences a decrease in the ability to guard the self from internal or external threats such as illness or injury.
*Rape-trauma syndrome	This syndrome includes the following three subcomponents: trauma, compound reaction, and silent reaction. In the NANDA Taxonomy each appears as a separate response.
Rape-trauma syndrome	Forced, violent sexual penetration against the victim's will and without the victim's consent. The trauma syndrome that develops from this attack or attempted attack includes an acute phase or disorganization of the victim's lifestyle and a long-term process of reorganization of lifestyle.
*Relocation stress syndrome	Physiologic and/or psychologic disturbances as a result of transfer from one environment to another.
Role performance, altered	Disruption in the way one perceives one's role performance.
Self-care deficit Bathing/hygiene Feeding Dressing/grooming Toileting	A state in which the individual experiences an impaired ability to perform or complete feeding, bathing/hygiene, toileting, dressing, and grooming activities for oneself.
Self-esteem, chronic low	Longstanding negative self-evaluation/feelings about self or self-capabilities.
Self-esteem, situational low	Negative self-evaluation/feelings about self which develop in response to a loss or change in an individual who previously had a positive self-evaluation.
Self-esteem disturbance	Negative self-evaluation/feelings about self or self-capabilities, which may be directly or indirectly expressed.
*Self-mutilation, high risk for	A state in which an individual is at high risk to perform an act upon the self to injure, not kill, which produces tissue damage and tension relief.
Sensory/perceptual alterations (specify) (visual, auditory, kinesthetic, gustatory, tactile, olfactory)	A state in which an individual experiences a change in the amount or patterning of oncoming stimuli accompanied by a diminished, exaggerated, distorted, or impaired response to such stimuli.
Sexual dysfunction	The state in which an individual experiences a change in sexual function that is viewed as unsatisfying, unrewarding, or inadequate.
Sexuality patterns, altered	The state in which an individual expresses concern regarding his/her sexuality.
Skin integrity, impaired	A state in which the individual's skin is adversely altered.
Skin integrity, high risk for impaired	A state in which the individual's skin is at risk of being adversely altered.

Diagnosis	Definition
Sleep pattern disturbance	Disruption of sleep time that causes a client discomfort or interferes with the desired lifestyle.
Social interaction, impaired	The state in which an individual participates in an insufficient or excessive quantity or ineffective quality of social exchange.
Social isolation	Aloneness experienced by the individual and perceived as imposed by others and as a negative or threatened state.
Spiritual distress (distress of the human spirit)	Disruption in the life principle that pervades a person's entire being and that integrates and transcends one's biologic and psychosocial nature.
Suffocation, high risk for	Accentuated risk of accidental suffocation (inadequate air is available for inhalation).
*Sustain spontaneous ventilation, inability to	A state in which the response pattern of decreased energy reserves results in an individual's inability to maintain breathing adequate to support life.
Swallowing, impaired	The state in which an individual has decreased ability to voluntarily pass fluids and/or solids from the mouth to the stomach.
Thermoregulation, ineffective	The state in which the individual's temperature fluctuates between hypothermia and hyperthermia.
Thought process, altered	A state in which an individual experiences a disruption in cognitive operations and activities.
Tissue integrity, impaired	A state in which an individual experiences damage to mucous membrane or corneal, integumentary, or subcutaneous tissue.
Tissue perfusion, altered (specify type) (cerebral, cardiovascular, renal, gastrointestinal, peripheral)	The state in which an individual experiences a decrease in nutrition and oxygenation at the cellular level due to a deficit in capillary blood supply.
Trauma, high risk for	Accentuated risk of accidental tissue injury, e.g., wound, burn, fracture.
Unilateral neglect	A state in which an individual is perceptually unaware of and inattentive to one side of the body.
Urinary elimination, altered	The state in which the individual experiences a disturbance in urine elimination.
Urinary retention	The state in which the individual experiences incomplete emptying of the bladder.
*Ventilatory weaning response, dysfunctional	A state in which a patient cannot adjust to lowered levels of mechanical ventilator support, which interrupts and prolongs the weaning process.
Violence, high risk for: Self-directed or directed at others	A state in which an individual experiences behaviors that can be physically harmful to either self or others.

* 1992 additions to NANDA nursing diagnosis.

APPENDIX • 2

Height, Weight, and Head Circumference for Girls

GIRLS: BIRTH TO 36 MONTHS
PHYSICAL GROWTH
NCHS PERCENTILES*

NAME ______________________ RECORD # ____________

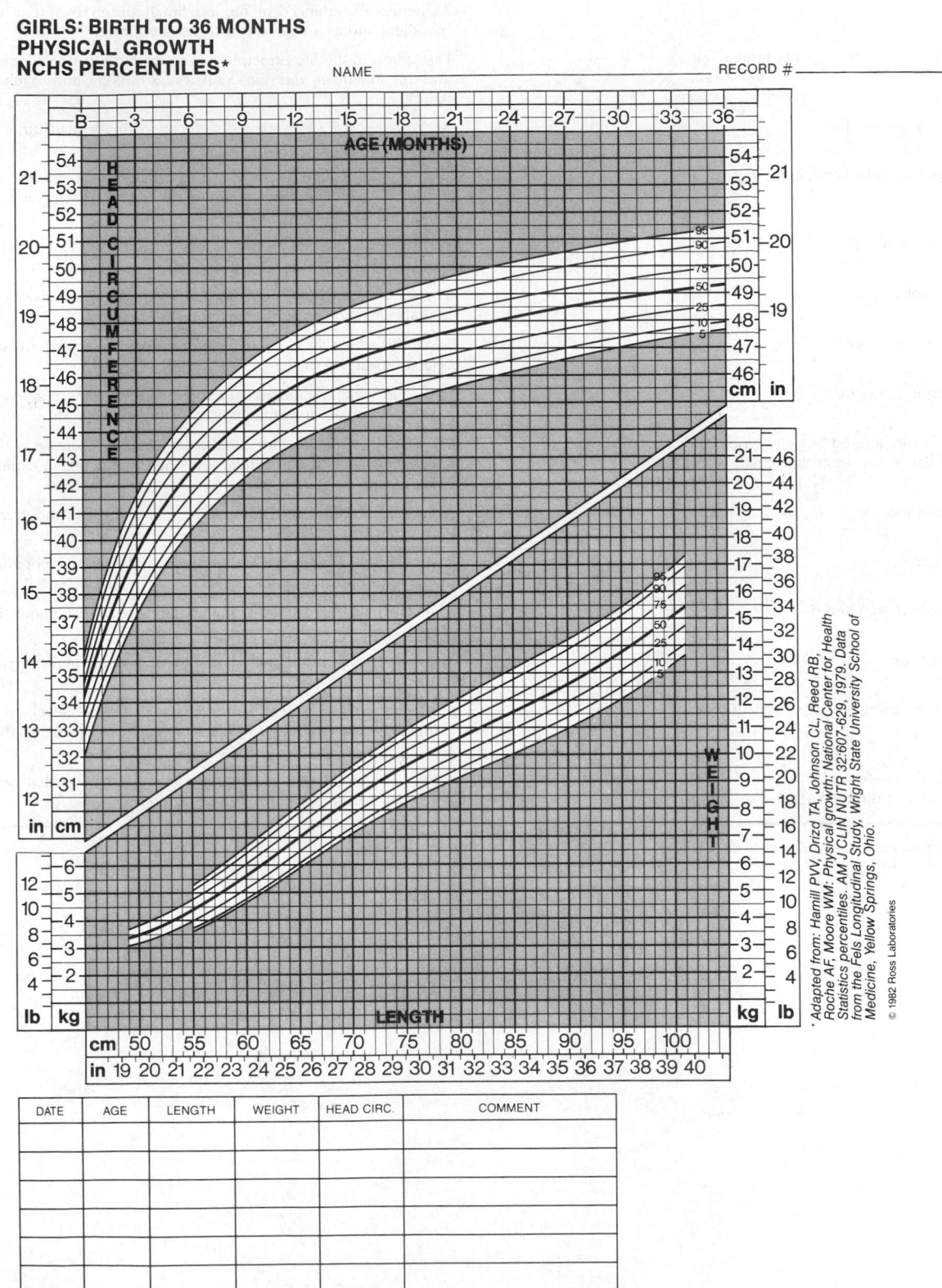

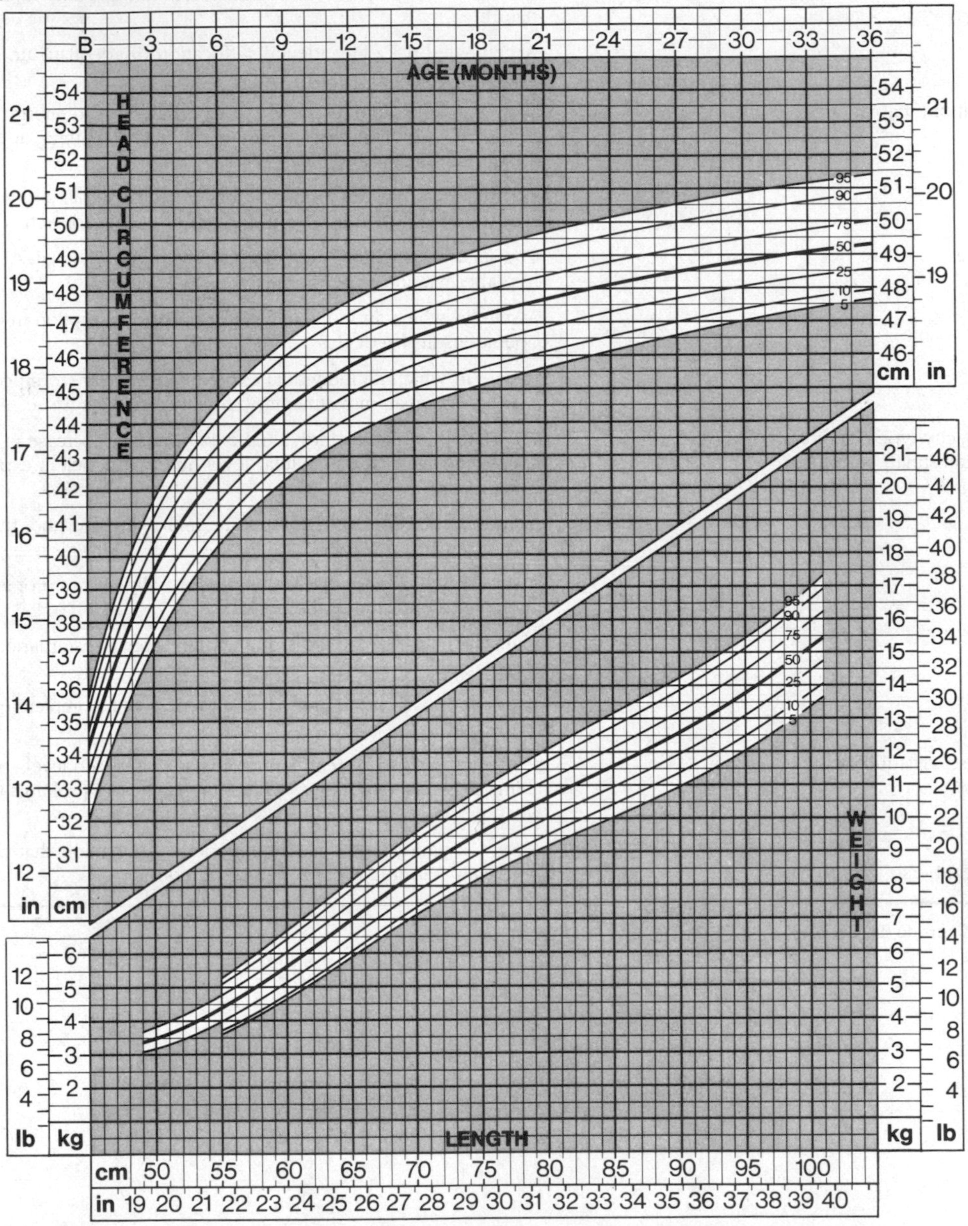

* Adapted from: Hamill PVV, Drizd TA, Johnson CL, Reed RB, Roche AF, Moore WM: Physical growth: National Center for Health Statistics percentiles. AM J CLIN NUTR 32:607-629, 1979. Data from the Fels Longitudinal Study, Wright State University School of Medicine, Yellow Springs, Ohio.

DATE	AGE	LENGTH	WEIGHT	HEAD CIRC.	COMMENT

GIRLS: BIRTH TO 36 MONTHS
PHYSICAL GROWTH
NCHS PERCENTILES*

NAME ______________________________ RECORD # ________

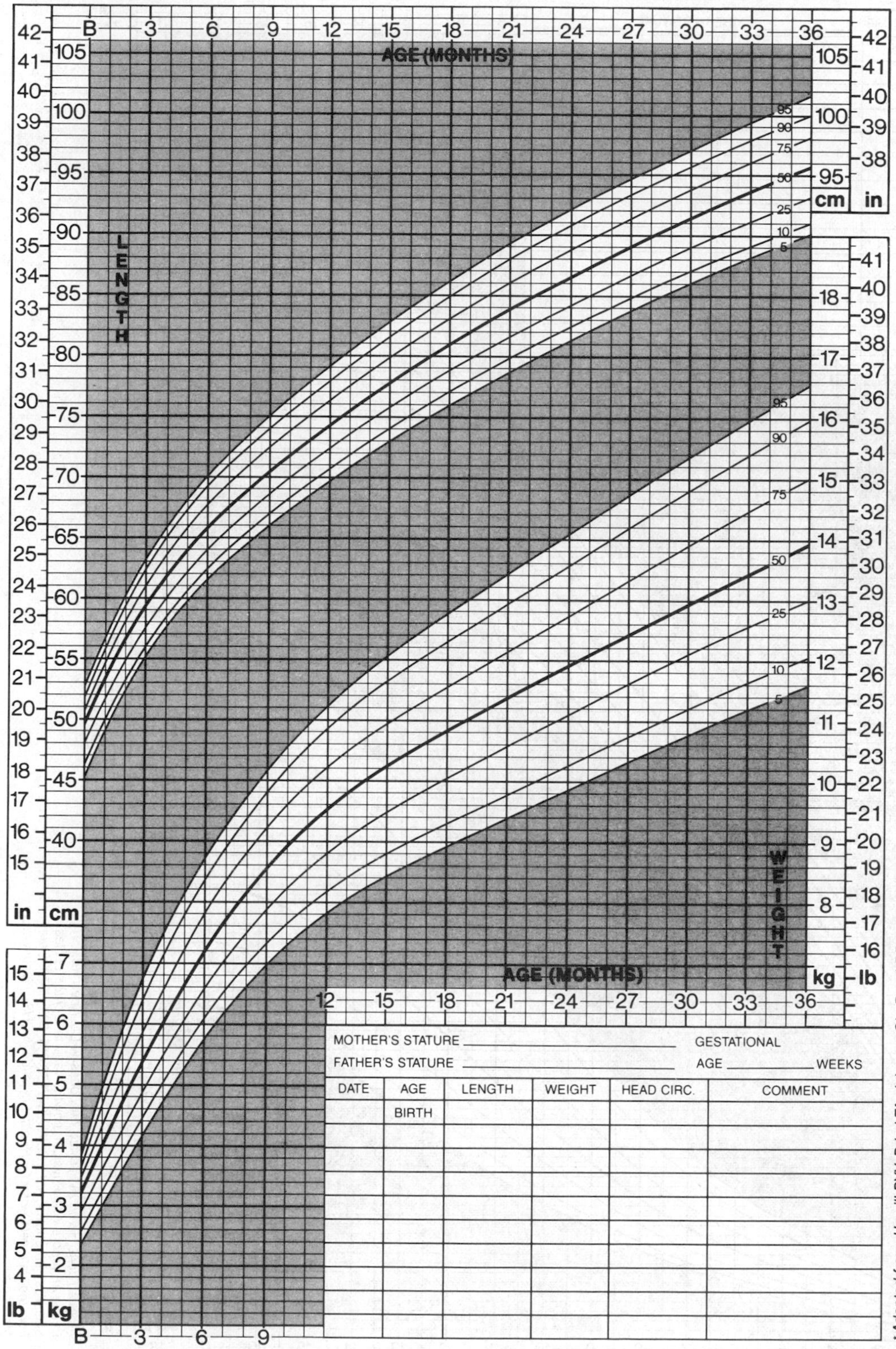

* Adapted from: Hamill PVV, Drizd TA, Johnson CL, Reed RB, Roche AF, Moore WM: Physical growth: National Center for Health Statistics percentiles. AM J CLIN NUTR 32:607-629, 1979. Data from the Fels Longitudinal Study, Wright State University School of Medicine, Yellow Springs, Ohio.

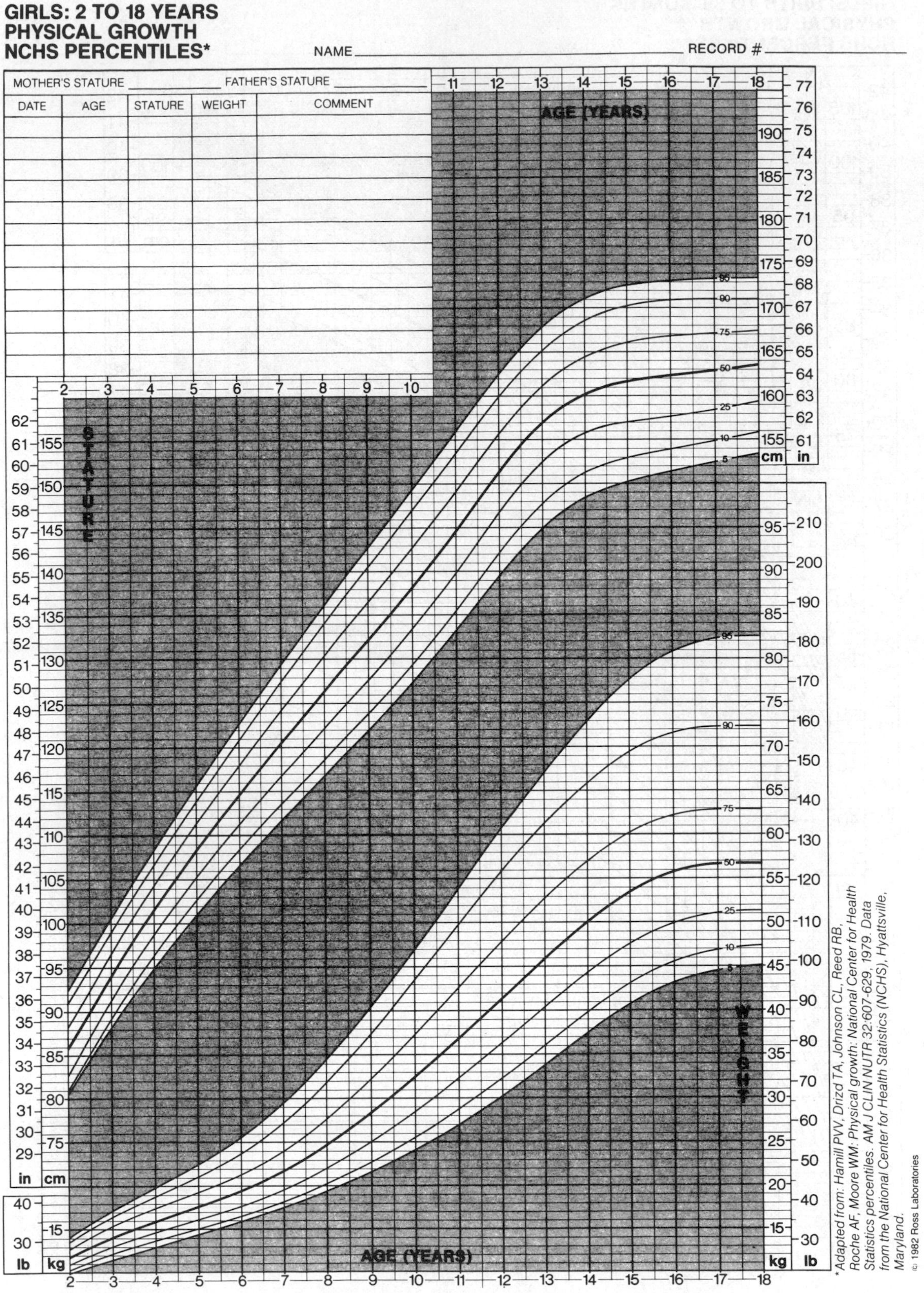
GIRLS: 2 TO 18 YEARS
PHYSICAL GROWTH
NCHS PERCENTILES*
NAME
RECORD #
MOTHER'S STATURE
FATHER'S STATURE
DATE
AGE
STATURE
WEIGHT
COMMENT
AGE (YEARS)
STATURE
WEIGHT
in
cm
lb
kg
*Adapted from: Hamill PVV, Drizd TA, Johnson CL, Reed RB, Roche AF, Moore WM: Physical growth: National Center for Health Statistics percentiles. AM J CLIN NUTR 32:607-629, 1979. Data from the National Center for Health Statistics (NCHS), Hyattsville, Maryland.
© 1982 Ross Laboratories

GIRLS: PREPUBESCENT PHYSICAL GROWTH NCHS PERCENTILES*

NAME ______________________ RECORD # ______________

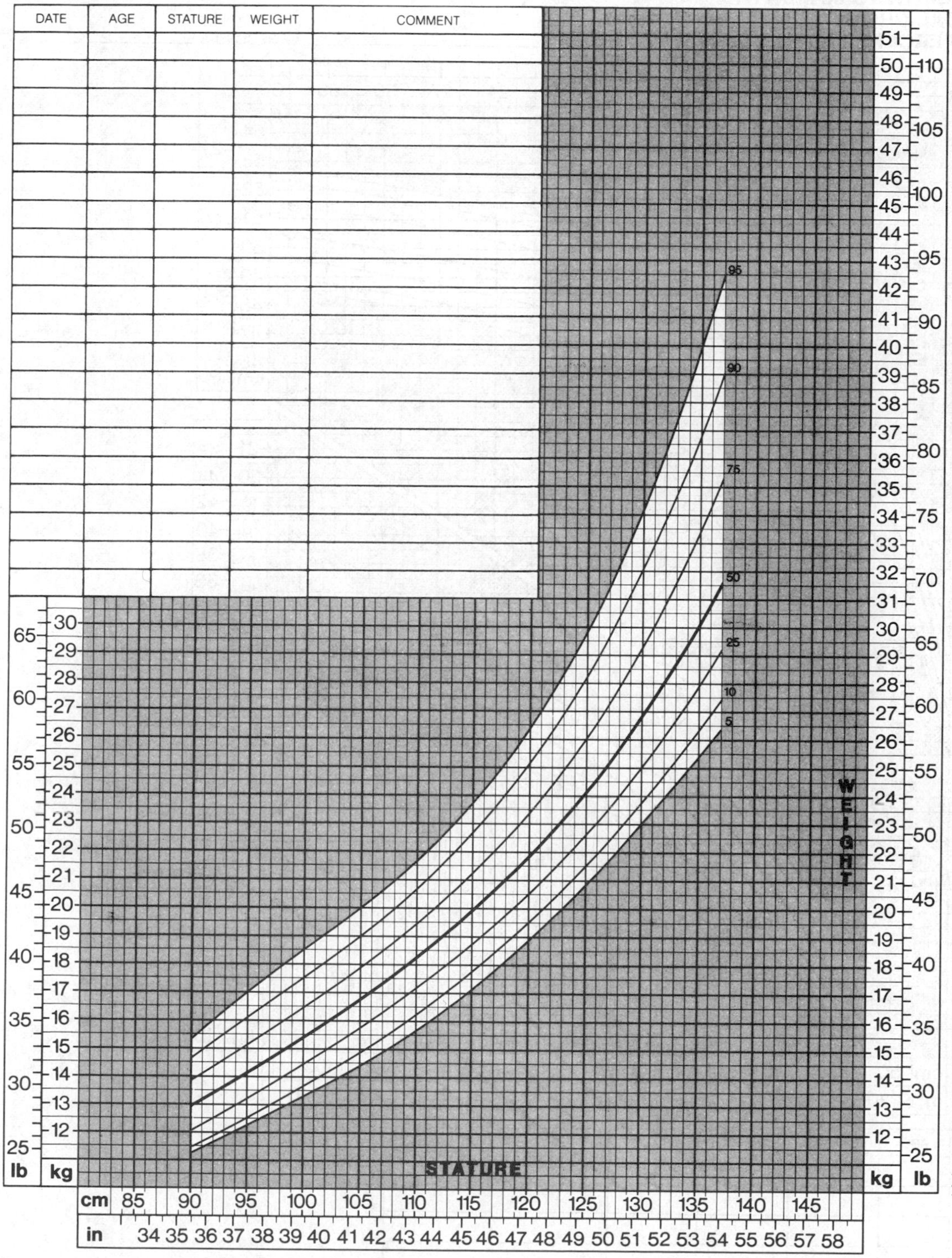

*Adapted from: Hamill PVV, Drizd TA, Johnson CL, Reed RB, Roche AF, Moore WM: Physical growth: National Center for Health Statistics percentiles. AM J CLIN NUTR 32:607-629, 1979. Data from the National Center for Health Statistics (NCHS), Hyattsville, Maryland.

APPENDIX • 3

Height, Weight, and Head Circumference for Boys

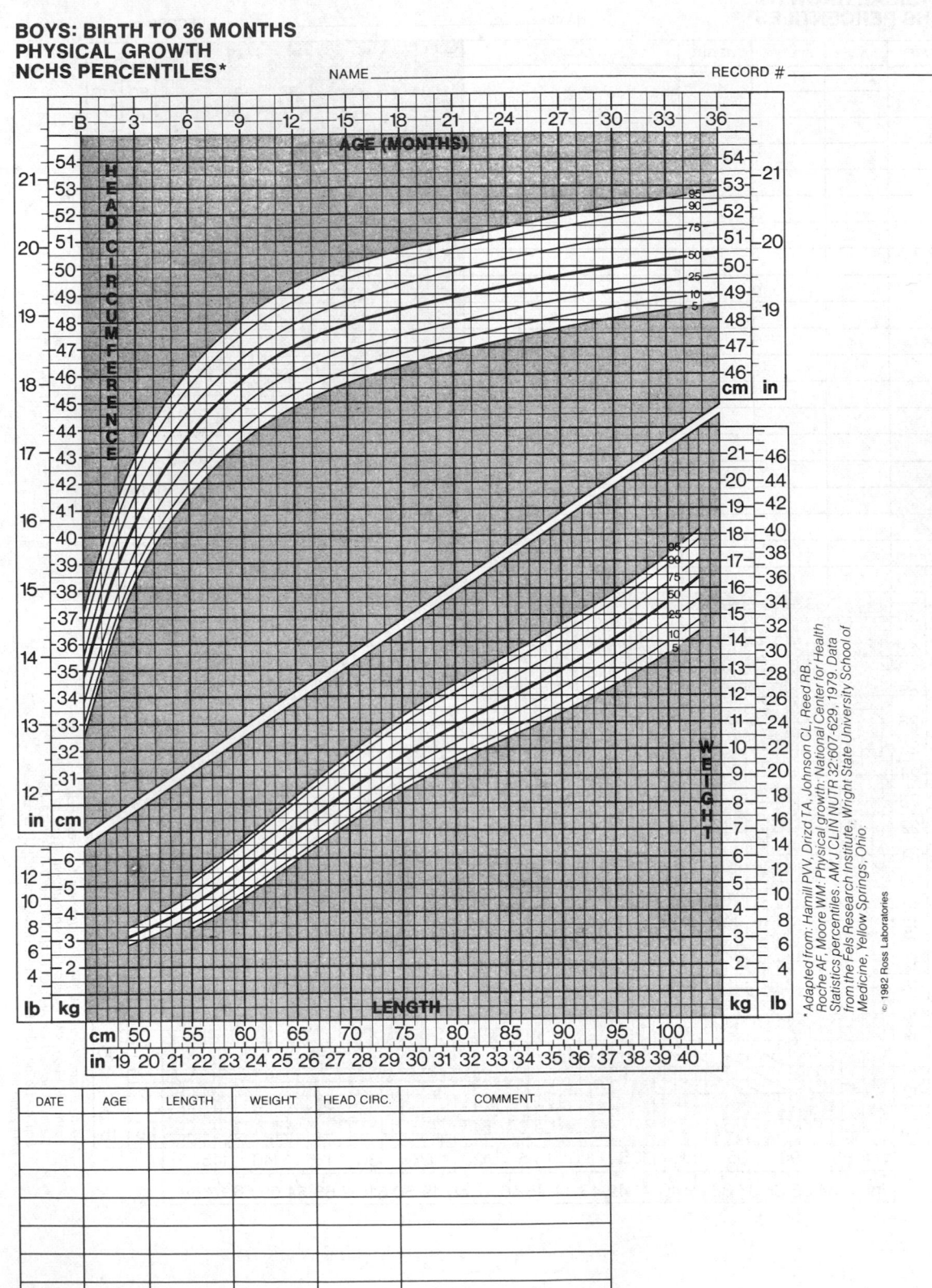

BOYS: BIRTH TO 36 MONTHS
PHYSICAL GROWTH
NCHS PERCENTILES*

NAME ____________________ RECORD # ____________

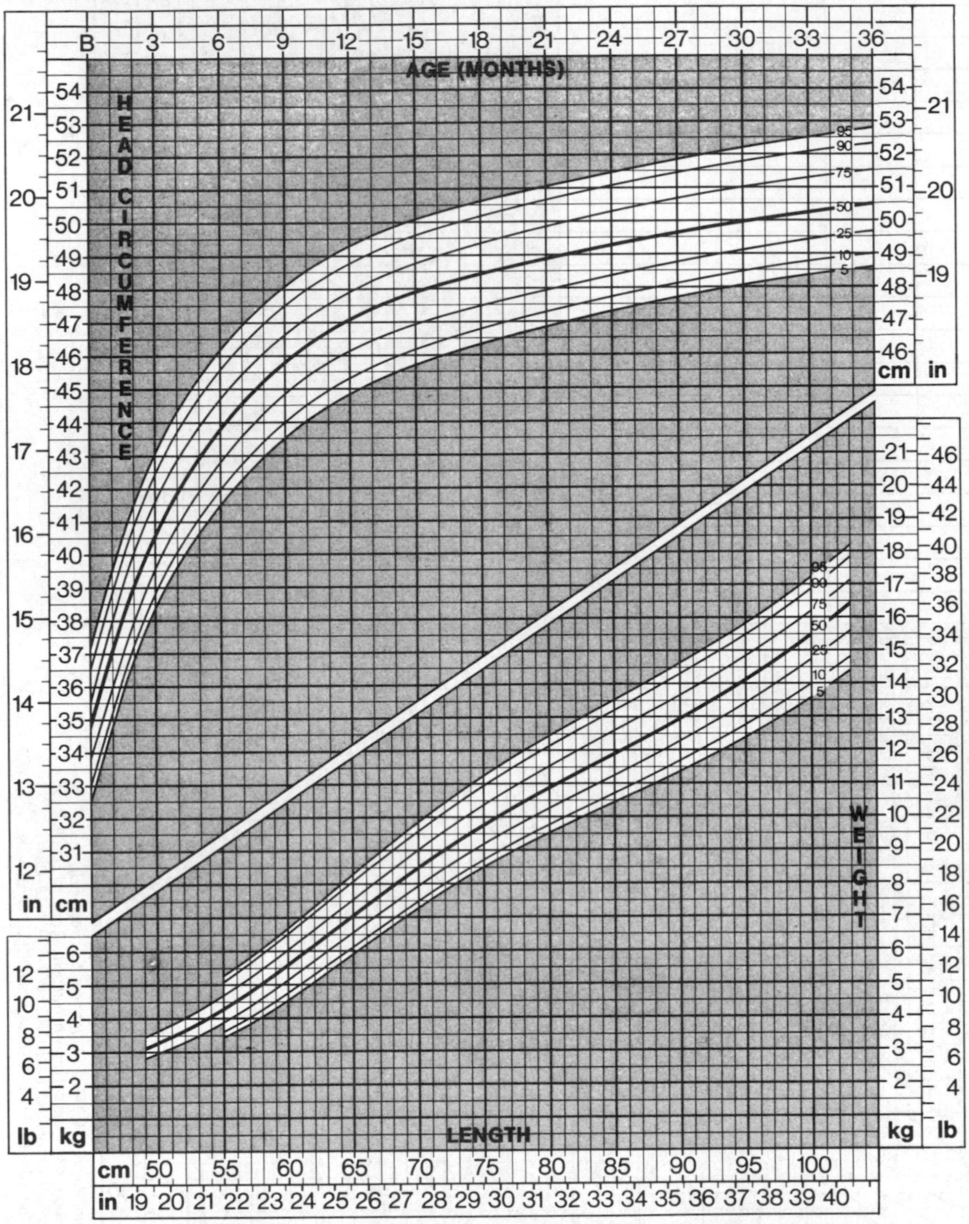

*Adapted from: Hamill PVV, Drizd TA, Johnson CL, Reed RB, Roche AF, Moore WM: Physical growth: National Center for Health Statistics percentiles. AM J CLIN NUTR 32:607-629, 1979. Data from the Fels Research Institute, Wright State University School of Medicine, Yellow Springs, Ohio.

DATE	AGE	LENGTH	WEIGHT	HEAD CIRC.	COMMENT

BOYS: BIRTH TO 36 MONTHS
PHYSICAL GROWTH
NCHS PERCENTILES*

NAME ____________________ RECORD # ____________

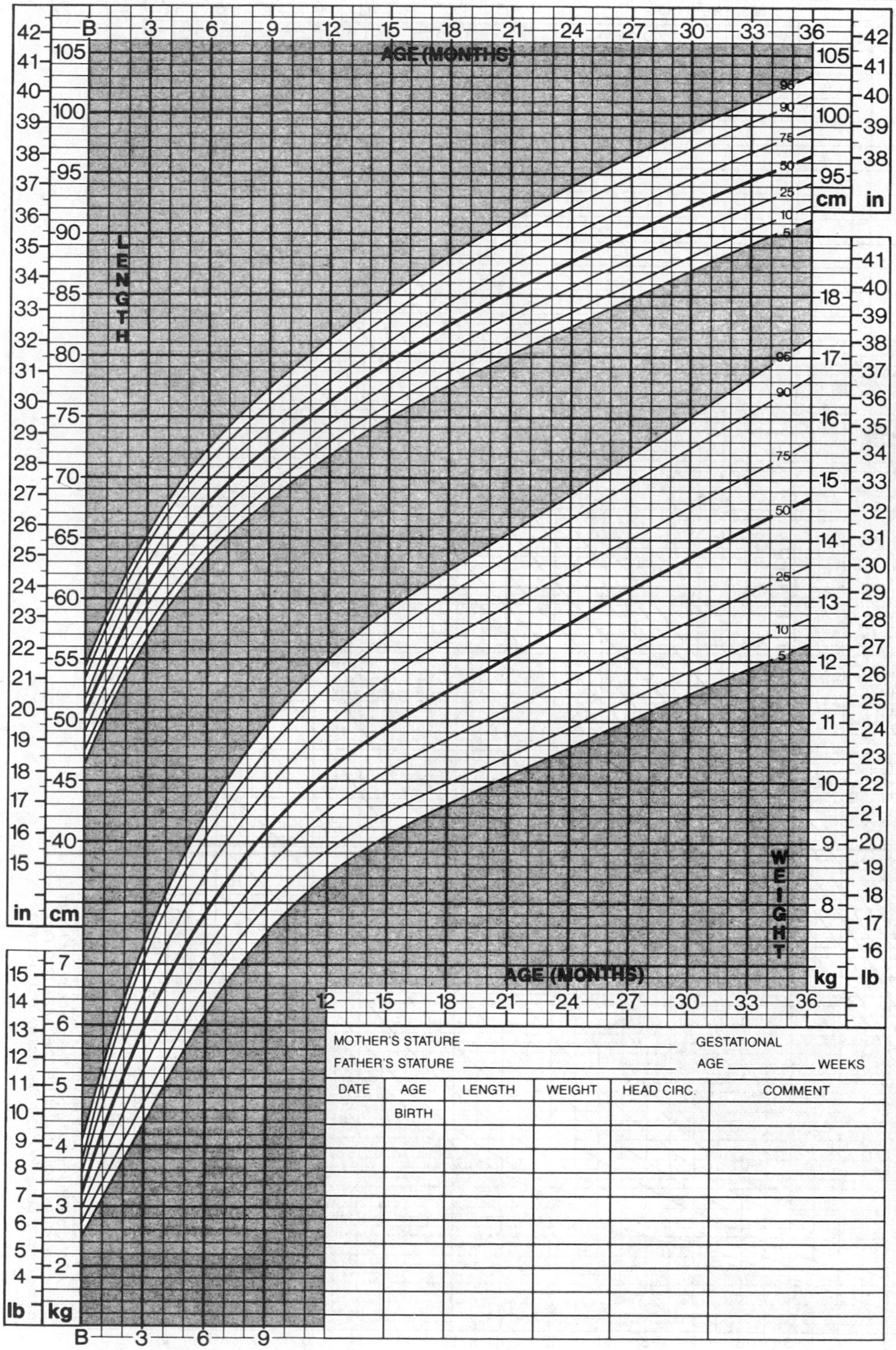

MOTHER'S STATURE ____________ GESTATIONAL
FATHER'S STATURE ____________ AGE ________ WEEKS

DATE	AGE	LENGTH	WEIGHT	HEAD CIRC.	COMMENT
	BIRTH				

*Adapted from: Hamill PVV, Drizd TA, Johnson CL, Reed RB, Roche AF, Moore WM: Physical growth: National Center for Health Statistics percentiles. AM J CLIN NUTR 32:607-629, 1979. Data from the Fels Research Institute, Wright State University School of Medicine, Yellow Springs, Ohio.

BOYS: 2 TO 18 YEARS
PHYSICAL GROWTH
NCHS PERCENTILES*

NAME ______________________ RECORD # ____________

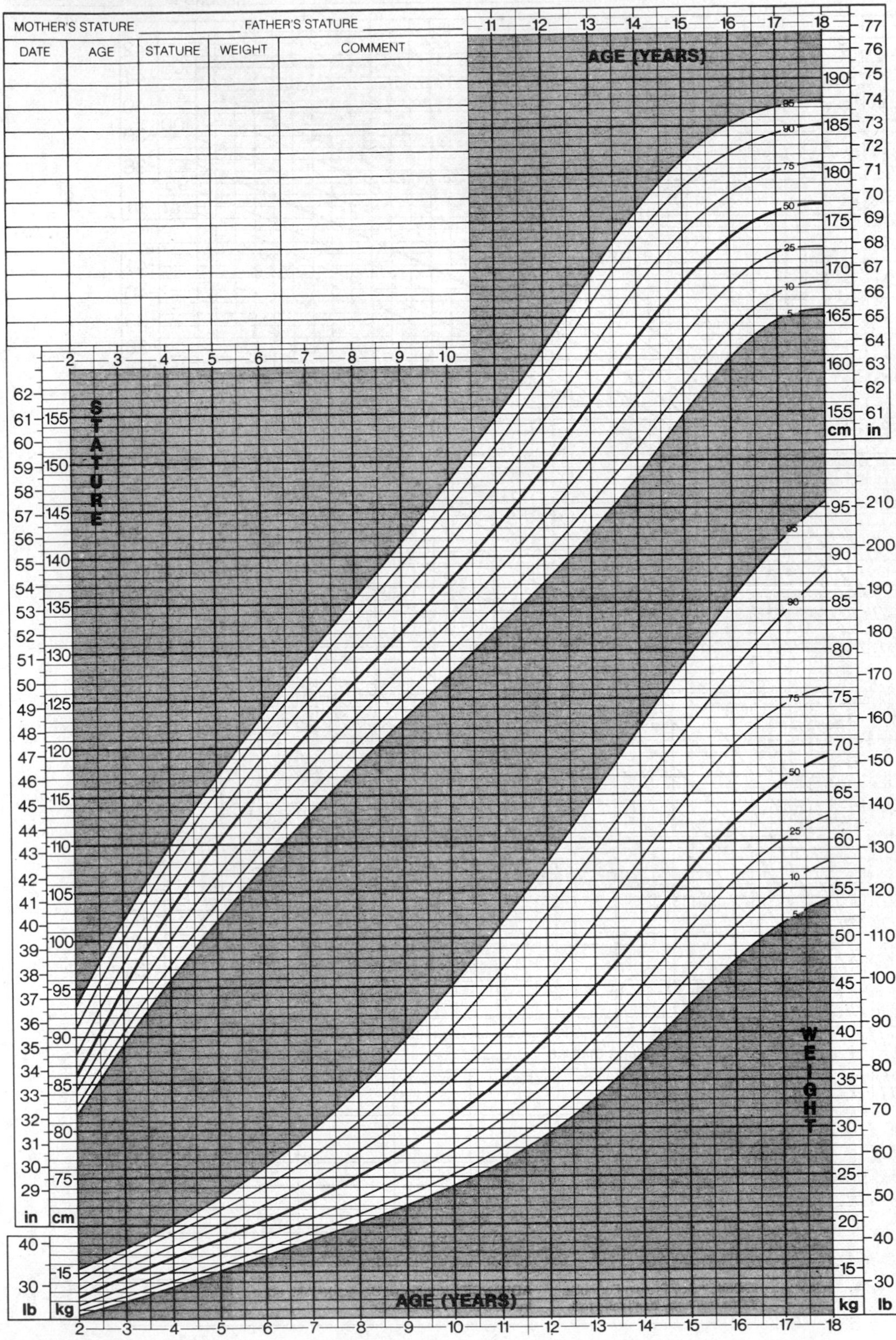

*Adapted from: Hamill PVV, Drizd TA, Johnson CL, Reed RB, Roche AF, Moore WM: Physical growth: National Center for Health Statistics percentiles. AM J CLIN NUTR 32:607-629, 1979. Data from the National Center for Health Statistics (NCHS), Hyattsville, Maryland.

BOYS: PREPUBESCENT PHYSICAL GROWTH NCHS PERCENTILES*

NAME ________________ RECORD # ____________

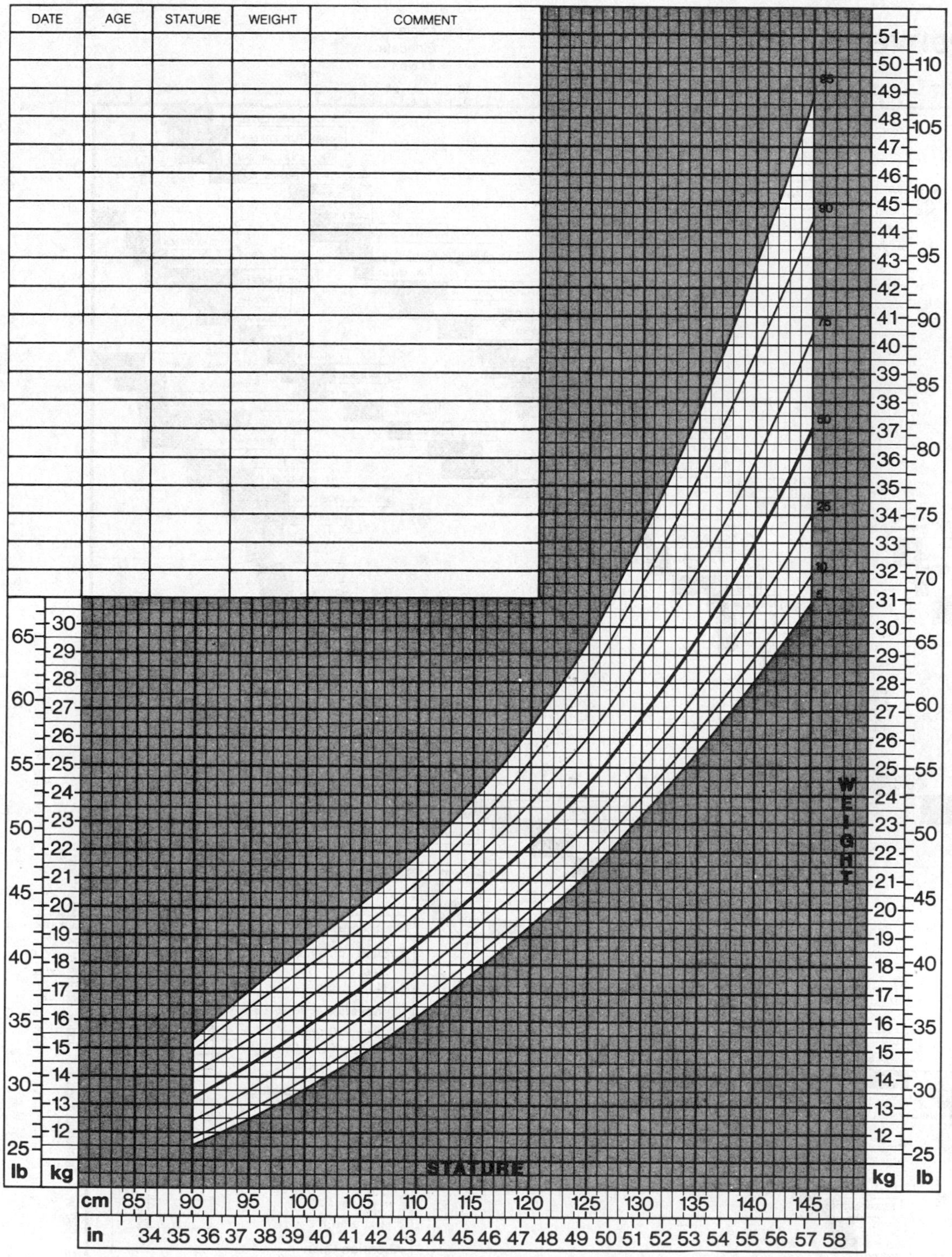

*Adapted from: Hamill PVV, Drizd TA, Johnson CL, Reed RB, Roche AF, Moore WM: Physical growth: National Center for Health Statistics percentiles. AM J CLIN NUTR 32:607-629, 1979. Data from the National Center for Health Statistics (NCHS), Hyattsville, Maryland.

APPENDIX • 4

Denver Developmental Screening Test II

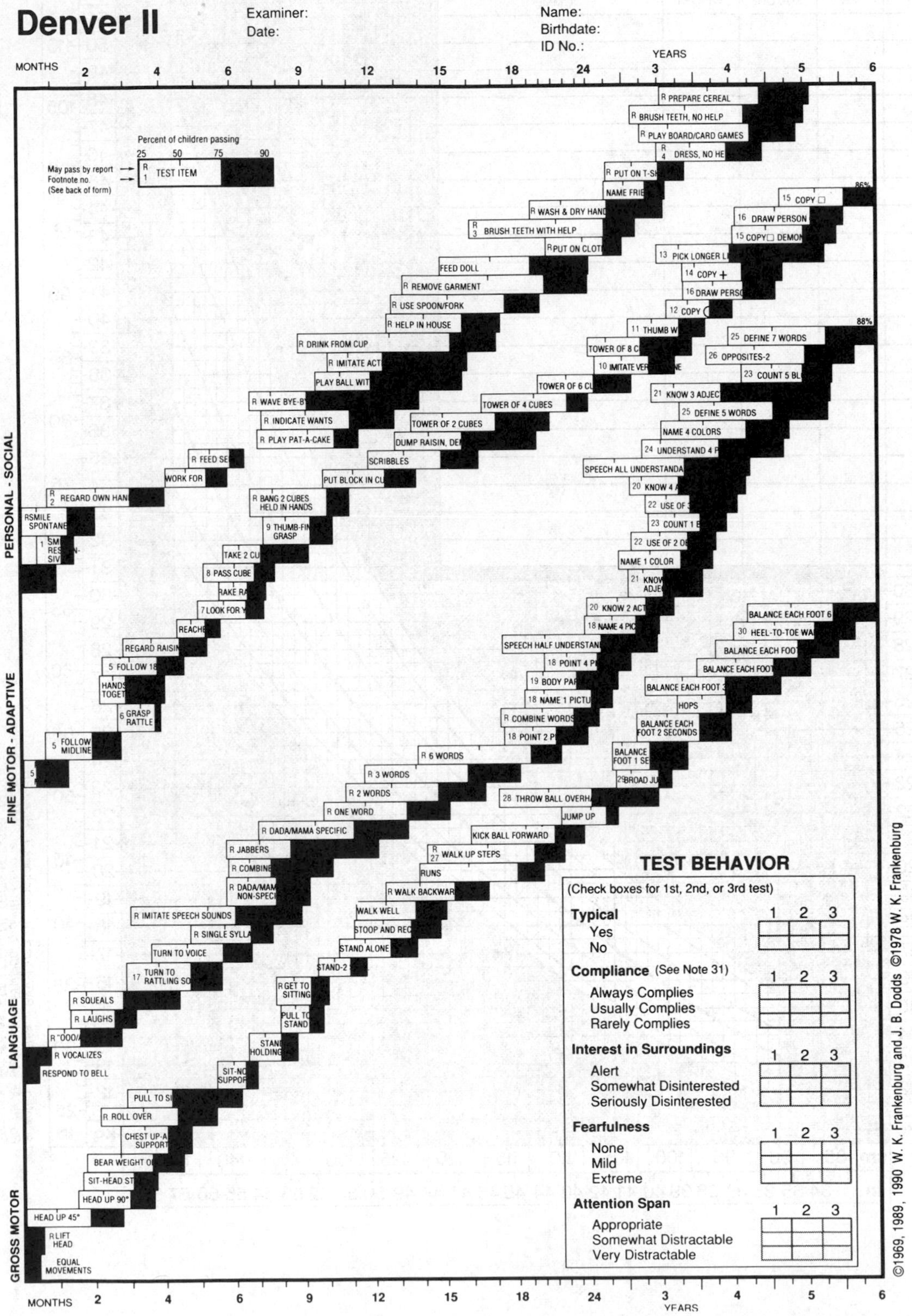

DIRECTIONS FOR ADMINISTRATION

1. Try to get child to smile by smiling, talking or waving. Do not touch him/her.
2. Child must stare at hand several seconds.
3. Parent may help guide toothbrush and put toothpaste on brush.
4. Child does not have to be able to tie shoes or button/zip in the back.
5. Move yarn slowly in an arc from one side to the other, about 8" above child's face.
6. Pass if child grasps rattle when it is touched to the backs or tips of fingers.
7. Pass if child tries to see where yarn went. Yarn should be dropped quickly from sight from tester's hand without arm movement.
8. Child must transfer cube from hand to hand without help of body, mouth, or table.
9. Pass if child picks up raisin with any part of thumb and finger.
10. Line can vary only 30 degrees or less from tester's line.
11. Make a fist with thumb pointing upward and wiggle only the thumb. Pass if child imitates and does not move any fingers other than the thumb.

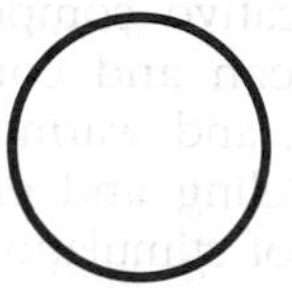

12. Pass any enclosed form. Fail continuous round motions.

13. Which line is longer? (Not bigger.) Turn paper upside down and repeat. (pass 3 of 3 or 5 of 6)

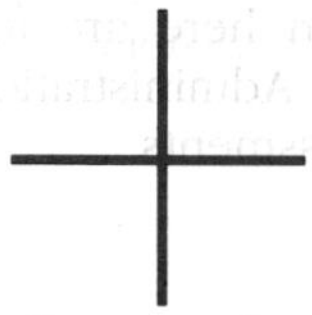

14. Pass any lines crossing near midpoint.

15. Have child copy first. If failed, demonstrate.

When giving items 12, 14, and 15, do not name the forms. Do not demonstrate 12 and 14.

16. When scoring, each pair (2 arms, 2 legs, etc.) counts as one part.
17. Place one cube in cup and shake gently near child's ear, but out of sight. Repeat for other ear.
18. Point to picture and have child name it. (No credit is given for sounds only.)
    If less than 4 pictures are named correctly, have child point to picture as each is named by tester.

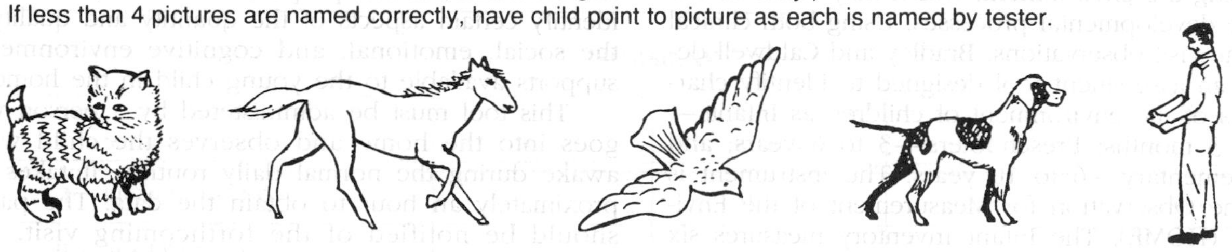

19. Using doll, tell child: Show me the nose, eyes, ears, mouth, hands, feet, tummy, hair. Pass 6 of 8.
20. Using pictures, ask child: Which one flies?... says meow?... talks?... barks?... gallops? Pass 2 of 5, 4 of 5.
21. Ask child: What do you do when you are cold?... tired?... hungry? Pass 2 of 3, 3 of 3.
22. Ask child: What do you do with a cup? What is a chair used for? What is a pencil used for?
    Action words must be included in answers.
23. Pass if child correctly places and says how many blocks are on paper. (1, 5).
24. Tell child: Put block **on** table; **under** table; **in front of** me, **behind** me. Pass 4 of 4.
    (Do not help child by pointing, moving head or eyes.)
25. Ask child: What is a ball?... lake?... desk?... house?... banana?... curtain?... fence?... ceiling? Pass if defined in terms of use, shape, what it is made of, or general category (such as banana is fruit, not just yellow). Pass 5 of 8, 7 of 8.
26. Ask child: If a horse is big, a mouse is __? If fire is hot, ice is __? If the sun shines during the day, the moon shines during the __? Pass 2 of 3.
27. Child may use wall or rail only, not person. May not crawl.
28. Child must throw ball overhand 3 feet to within arm's reach of tester.
29. Child must perform standing broad jump over width of test sheet (8 1/2 inches).
30. Tell child to walk forward, 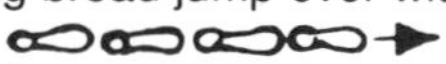 heel within 1 inch of toe. Tester may demonstrate.
    Child must walk 4 consecutive steps.
31. In the second year, half of normal children are non-compliant.

OBSERVATIONS:

Infant/Toddler HOME

Place a plus (+) or minus (−) in the box alongside each item if the behavior is observed during the visit or if the parent reports that the conditions or events are characteristic of the home environment. Enter the subtotal and the total on the front side of the Record Sheet.

I. RESPONSIVITY		24. Child has a special place for toys and treasures.	
1. Parent spontaneously vocalizes to child at least twice.		25. Child's play environment is safe.	
2. Parent responds verbally to child's vocalizations or verbalizations.		**IV. LEARNING MATERIALS**	
3. Parent tells child name of object or person during visit.		26. Muscle activity toys or equipment.	
4. Parent's speech is distinct, clear, and audible.		27. Push or pull toy.	
5. Parent initiates verbal interchanges with Visitor.		28. Stroller or walker, kiddie car, scooter, or tricycle.	
6. Parent converses freely and easily.		29. Parent provides toys for child to play with during visit.	
7. Parent permits child to engage in "messy" play.		30. Cuddly toy or role-playing toys.	
8. Parent spontaneously praises child at least twice.		31. Learning facilitators—mobile, table and chair, highchair, playpen.	
9. Parent's voice conveys positive feelings toward child.		32. Simple eye-hand coordination toys.	
10. Parent caresses or kisses child at least once.		33. Complex eye-hand coordination toys.	
11. Parent responds positively to praise of child offered by Visitor.		34. Toys for literature and music.	
II. ACCEPTANCE		**V. INVOLVEMENT**	
12. Parent does not shout at child.		35. Parent keeps child in visual range, looks at often.	
13. Parent does not express overt annoyance with or hostility to child.		36. Parent talks to child while doing household work.	
14. Parent neither slaps nor spanks child during visit.		37. Parent consciously encourages developmental advance.	
15. No more than one instance of physical punishment during past week.		38. Parent invests maturing toys with value via personal attention.	
16. Parent does not scold or criticize child during visit.		39. Parent structures child's play periods.	
17. Parent does not interfere with or restrict child three times during visit.		40. Parent provides toys that challenge child to develop new skills.	
18. At least 10 books are present and visible.		**VI. VARIETY**	
19. Family has a pet.		41. Father provides some care daily.	
III. ORGANIZATION		42. Parent reads stories to child at least three times weekly.	
20. Child care, if used, is provided by one of three regular substitutes.		43. Child eats at least one meal a day with mother and father.	
21. Child is taken to grocery store at least once a week.		44. Family visits relatives or receives visits once a month or so.	
22. Child gets out of house at least four times a week.		45. Child has three or more books of his/her own.	
23. Child is taken regularly to doctor's office or clinic.			

	I	II	III	IV	V	VI	TOTAL
TOTALS							

EARLY CHILDHOOD HOME INVENTORY

Bettye M. Caldwell and Robert H. Bradley

Family Name ______________________ Date ______________ Visitor ______________

Child's Name ______________________ Birthdate ______________ Age ______ Sex ______

Caregiver for visit ______________________ Relationship to child ______________

Family composition ____
(Persons living in household, including sex and age of children)

Family Ethnicity ______________ Language Spoken ______________ Maternal Education ______________ Paternal Education ______________

Is Mother Employed? __________ Type of work when employed ______________ Is Father Employed? __________ Type of work when employed ______________

Address ______________________________________ Phone ______________

Current child care arrangements ____

Summarize past year's arrangements ____

Caregiver for visit ______________________ Other persons present ______________________

SUMMARY

Subscale	Score	Lowest Fourth	Middle Half	Upper Fourth
I. LEARNING MATERIALS		0–2	3–9	10–11
II. LANGUAGE STIMULATION		0–4	5–6	7
III. PHYSICAL ENVIRONMENT		0–3	4–6	7
IV. RESPONSIVITY		0–3	4–5	6–7
V. ACADEMIC STIMULATION		0–2	3–4	5
VI. MODELING		0–1	2–3	4–5
VII. VARIETY		0–4	5–7	8–9
VIII. ACCEPTANCE		0–2	3	4
TOTAL SCORE		0–29	30–45	46–55

For rapid profiling of a family, place an X in the box that corresponds to the raw score.

Early Childhood HOME

Place a plus (+) or minus (−) in the box alongside each item if the behavior is observed during the visit or if the parent reports that the conditions or events are characteristic of the home environment. Enter the subtotals and the total on the front side of the Record Sheet.

I. LEARNING MATERIALS		23. House has 100 square feet of living space per person.	
1. Child has toys which teach colors, sizes, and shapes.		24. Rooms are not overcrowded with furniture.	
2. Child has three or more puzzles.		25. House is reasonably clean and minimally cluttered.	
3. Child has record player or tape recorder and at least five children's records or tapes		**IV. RESPONSIVITY**	
4. Child has toys or games permitting free expression.		26. Parent holds child close 10–15 minutes per day.	
5. Child has toys or games requiring refined movements.		27. Parent converses with child at least twice during visit.	
6. Child has toys or games which help teach numbers.		28. Parent answers child's questions or requests verbally.	
7. Child has at least 10 children's books.		29. Parent usually responds verbally to child's speech.	
8. At least 10 books are visible in the apartment or home.		30. Parent praises child's qualities twice during visit.	
9. Family buys and reads a daily newspaper.		31. Parent caresses, kisses, or cuddles child during visit.	
10. Family subscribes to at least one magazine.		32. Parent helps child demonstrate some achievement during visit.	
11. Child is encouraged to learn shapes.		**V. ACADEMIC STIMULATION**	
II. LANGUAGE STIMULATION		33. Child is encouraged to learn colors.	
12. Child has toys that help teach the names of animals.		34. Child is encouraged to learn patterned speech.	
13. Child is encouraged to learn the alphabet.		35. Child is encouraged to learn spatial relationships.	
14. Parent teaches child simple verbal manners (please, thank you, I'm sorry).		36. Child is encouraged to learn numbers.	
15. Parent uses correct grammar and pronunciation.		37. Child is encouraged to learn to read a few words.	
16. Parent encourages child to talk and takes time to listen.		**VI. MODELING**	
17. Parent's voice conveys positive feelings about child.		38. Some delay of food gratification is expected.	
18. Child is permitted choice in breakfast or lunch menu.		39. TV is used judiciously.	
III. PHYSICAL ENVIRONMENT		40. Parent introduces Visitor to child.	
19. Building appears safe and free of hazards.		41. Child can express negative feelings without harsh reprisal.	
20. Outside play environment appears safe.		42. Child can hit parent without harsh reprisal.	
21. Interior of apartment is not dark or perceptually monotonous.		**VII. VARIETY**	
22. Neighborhood is aesthetically pleasing.		43. Child has real or toy musical instrument.	

(continued)

44. Child is taken on outing by a family member at least every other week.		51. Parent lets child choose certain favorite food products or brands at grocery store.	
45. Child has been on trip more than 50 miles during last year.		**VIII. ACCEPTANCE**	
46. Child has been taken to a museum during past year.		52. Parent does not scold or yell at or derogate child more than once.	
47. Parent encourages child to put away toys without help.		53. Parent does not use physical restraint during visit.	
48. Parent uses complex sentence structure and vocabulary.		54. Parent neither slaps nor spanks child during visit.	
49. Child's art work is displayed some place in house.		55. No more than one instance of physical punishment occurred during the past week.	
50. Child eats at least one meal per day with mother (or mother figure) and father (or father figure).			

	I	II	III	IV	V	VI	VII	VIII	TOTAL
TOTALS									

COMMENTS: ____

____

____

____

____

____

HOME Inventory for Families of Elementary Children

Bettye M. Caldwell and Robert H. Bradley

Family Name ______________ Date of Visit ______ Observed Child's Name ______________

Birthdate ____________ Sex ____________ Caregiver for visit ______________

Relationship to child ______________ Family Ethnicity ______________

Family Composition ______________________________
(Persons living in household, including sex and age of children)

Maternal Education ____________ Paternal Education ____________ HOME Visitor ____________

Is Mother Employed? ______ If yes, give type of work ____________ Is Father Employed? ______ Type of work when employed ____________

Address ______________________ How long? ______ Phone ____________

Current child care arrangements ______________________________

Summarize past year's arrangements ______________________________

Persons in home at time of visit ______________________________

Observation Summary

	Score
I. Emotional and Verbal Responsivity	
II. Encouragement of Maturity	
III. Emotional Climate	
IV. Growth Fostering Materials and Experiences	
V. Provision for Active Stimulation	
VI. Family Participation in Developmentally Stimulating Experiences	
VII. Paternal Involvement	
VIII. Aspects of the Physical Environment	

COMMENTS: ______________________________

HOME Inventory (Elementary)

Place a plus (+) or minus (−) in the box alongside each item if the behavior is observed during the visit or if the parent reports that the conditions or events are characteristic of the home environment. Enter the subtotals and the total on the front side of the Record Sheet.

I. EMOTIONAL AND VERBAL RESPONSIBILITY

1.	Family has fairly regular and predictable daily schedule for child (meals, day care, bedtime, TV, homework, etc.).	
2.	Parent sometimes yields to child's fears or rituals (allows nightlight, accompanies child to new experiences, etc.).	
3.	Child has been praised at least twice during past week for doing something.	
4.	Child is encouraged to read on his/her own.	
5.	*Parent encourages child to contribute to the conversation during visit.	
6.	*Parent shows some positive emotional responses to praise of child by visitor.	
7.	*Parent responds to child's questions during interview.	
8.	*Parent uses complete sentence structure and some long words in conversing.	
9.	*When speaking of or to child, parent's voice conveys positive feelings.	
10.	*Parent initiates verbal interchanges with visitor, asks questions, makes spontaneous comments.	
	Subtotal	

II. ENCOURAGEMENT OF MATURITY

11.	Family requires child to carry out certain selfcare routines, e.g., makes bed, cleans room, cleans up after spills, bathes self. (A YES requires 3 out of 4)	
12.	Family requires child to keep living & play area reasonably clean & straight.	
13.	Child puts his outdoor clothing, dirty clothes, night clothes in special place.	
14.	Parents set limits for child & generally enforce them (curfew, homework before TV, or other regulations that fit family pattern.)	
15.	Parent introduces interviewer to child.	
16.	*Parent is consistent in establishing or applying family rules.	
17.	*Parent does not violate rules of common courtesy.	
	Subtotal	

III. EMOTIONAL CLIMATE

18.	Parent has not lost temper with child more than once during previous week.	
19.	Mother reports no more than one instance of physical punishment occurred during past month.	
20.	Child can express negative feelings toward parents without harsh reprisals.	

III. EMOTIONAL CLIMATE (Cont'd)

21.	Parent has not cried or been visibly upset in child's presence more than once during past week.	
22.	Child has a special place in which to keep his/her possessions.	
23.	*Parent talks to child during visit (beyond correction and introduction).	
24.	*Parent uses some term of endearment or some diminutive for child's name when talking about child at least twice during visit.	
25.	*Parent does not express over annoyance with or hostility toward child—complains, describes child as "bad," says he won't mind, etc.	
	Subtotal	

IV. GROWTH FOSTERING MATERIALS AND EXPERIENCES

26.	Child has free access to record player or radio.	
27.	Child has free access to musical instrument (piano, drum, ukelele, guitar, etc.)	
28.	Child has free access to at least 10 appropriate books.	
29.	Parent buys and reads a newspaper daily.	
30.	Child has free access to desk or other suitable place for reading or studying.	
31.	Family has a dictionary and encourages child to use it.	
32.	Child has visited a friend by him/herself in the past week.	
33.	*House has at least two pictures or other type of artwork on the walls.	
	Subtotal	

V. PROVISION FOR ACTIVE STIMULATION

34.	Family has a television, and it is used judiciously, not left on continuously. (No TV requires an automatic NO—any scheduling scores YES.).	
35.	Family encourages child to develop or sustain hobbies.	
36.	Child is regularly included in family's recreational hobby.	
37.	Family provides lessons or organizational membership to support child's talents (especially Y membership, gymnastic lessons, art center, etc.).	

(continued)

V. PROVISION FOR ACTIVE STIMULATION (Cont'd)

38.	Child has ready access to at least two pieces of playground equipment in the immediate vicinity.	
39.	Child has access to a library card, and family arranges for child to go to library once a month.	
40.	Family member has taken child, or arranged for child to go to a scientific, historical, or art museum within the past year.	
41.	Family member has taken child, or arranged for child to take a trip on a plane, train, or bus within the past year.	
	Subtotal	

VI. FAMILY PARTICIPATION IN DEVELOPMENTALLY STIMULATING EXPERIENCES

42.	Family visits or receives visits from relatives or friends at least once every other week.	
43.	Child has accompanied parent on a family business venture three to four times within the past year (to garage, clothing shop, appliance repair shop, etc.).	
44.	Family member has taken child, or arranged for child to attend some type of live musical or theater performance.	
45.	Family member has taken child, or arranged for child to go on a trip of more than 50 miles from his/her home (50 miles radial distance, not total distance).	
46.	Parents discuss television programs with child.	
47.	Parent helps child to achieve motor skills—ride a two-wheel bicycle, roller skate, ice skate, play ball, etc.	
	Subtotal	

VII. PATERNAL INVOLVEMENT

48.	Father (or father substitute) regularly engages in outdoor recreation with child.	
49.	Child sees and spends some time with father or father figure, four days a week.	
50.	Child eats at least one meal per day, on most days, with mother and father (or mother and father figures). (One-parent families rate an automatic NO.)	
51.	Child has remained with this primary family group for ALL his/her life aside from 2- to 3-week vacations, illnesses of mother, visits of grandmother, etc. (A YES requires no changes in mother's, father's, grandmother's, or grandfather's presence since birth.)	
	Subtotal	

VIII. ASPECTS OF THE PHYSICAL ENVIRONMENT

52.	Child's room has a picture or wall decoration appealing to children.	
53.	*The interior of the apartment is not dark or perceptually monotonous.	
54.	*In terms of available floor space, the rooms are not overcrowded with furniture.	
55.	*All visible rooms of the house are reasonably clean and minimally cluttered.	
56.	*There is at least 100 square feet of living space per person in the house.	
57.	*House is not overly noisy—television, shouts of children, radio, etc.	
58.	*Building has no potentially dangerous structural or health defects (plaster coming down from ceiling, stairway with boards missing, rodents, etc.).	
59.	*Child's outside play environment appears safe and free of hazards. (No outside play area requires an automatic NO.)	
	Subtotal	

APPENDIX • 6

Denver Articulation Screening Examination

DENVER ARTICULATION SCREENING EXAM
for children 2 1/2 to 6 years of age

Instructions: Have child repeat each word after you. Circle the underlined sounds that he pronounces correctly. Total correct sounds is the Raw Score. Use charts on reverse side to score results.

NAME

HOSP. NO.

ADDRESS

Date: __________ Child's Age: ________ Examiner: __________________ Raw Score: __________
Percentile: ________ Intelligibility: ______________ Result: ____________________

1. table	6. zipper	11. sock	16. wagon	21. leaf
2. shirt	7. grapes	12. vacuum	17. gum	22. carrot
3. door	8. flag	13. yarn	18. house	
4. trunk	9. thumb	14. mother	19. pencil	
5. jumping	10. toothbrush	15. twinkle	20. fish	

Intelligibility: (circle one)
1. Easy to understand
2. Understandable 1/2 the time.
3. Not understandable
4. Can't evaluate

Comments:

(continued)

A copy of the DASE and instructions for its administration may be obtained from: Denver Developmental Materials, P.O. Box 6919, Denver, Colorado 80206–0919. Telephone: (303) 355–4729.

To score DASE words: Note Raw Score for child's performance. Match raw score line (extreme left of chart) with column representing child's age (to the closest <u>previous</u> age group). Where raw score line and age column meet number in that square denotes percentile rank of child's performance when compared to other children that age. Percentiles above heavy line are ABNORMAL percentiles, below heavy line are NORMAL.

<u>PERCENTILE RANK</u>

Raw Score	2.5 yr.	3.0	3.5	4.0	4.5	5.0	5.5	6 years
2	1							
3	2							
4	5							
5	9							
6	16							
7	23							
8	31	2						
9	37	4	1					
10	42	6	2					
11	48	7	4					
12	54	9	6	1	1			
13	58	12	9	2	3	1	1	
14	62	17	11	5	4	2	2	
15	68	23	15	9	5	3	2	
16	75	31	19	12	5	4	3	
17	79	38	25	15	6	6	4	
18	83	46	31	19	8	7	4	
19	86	51	38	24	10	9	5	1
20	89	58	45	30	12	11	7	3
21	92	65	52	36	15	15	9	4
22	94	72	58	43	18	19	12	5
23	96	77	63	50	22	24	15	7
24	97	82	70	58	29	29	20	15
25	99	87	78	66	36	34	26	17
26	99	91	84	75	46	43	34	24
27		94	89	82	57	54	44	34
28		96	94	88	70	68	59	47
29		98	98	94	84	84	77	68
30		100	100	100	100	100	100	100

To Score intelligibility:

	NORMAL	ABNORMAL
2 1/2 years	Understandable 1/2 the time, or, "easy"	Not Understandable
3 years and older	Easy to understand	Understandable 1/2 time Not understandable

Test Result: 1. NORMAL on Dase and Intelligibility = NORMAL

2. ABNORMAL on Dase and/or Intelligibility = ABNORMAL

* If abnormal on initial screening rescreen within 2 weeks. If abnormal again child should be referred for complete speech evaluation.

APPENDIX • 7

Acute Pain Management in Infants, Children, and Adolescents

The material in this appendix is excerpted from a convenient pamphlet entitled Quick Reference Guide for Clinicians, available from the federal government.*

The following flow chart shows the sequence of activities for pain assessment and management. This appendix provides information about the events listed in the flow chart.

Abbreviated Pain Management Flow Chart

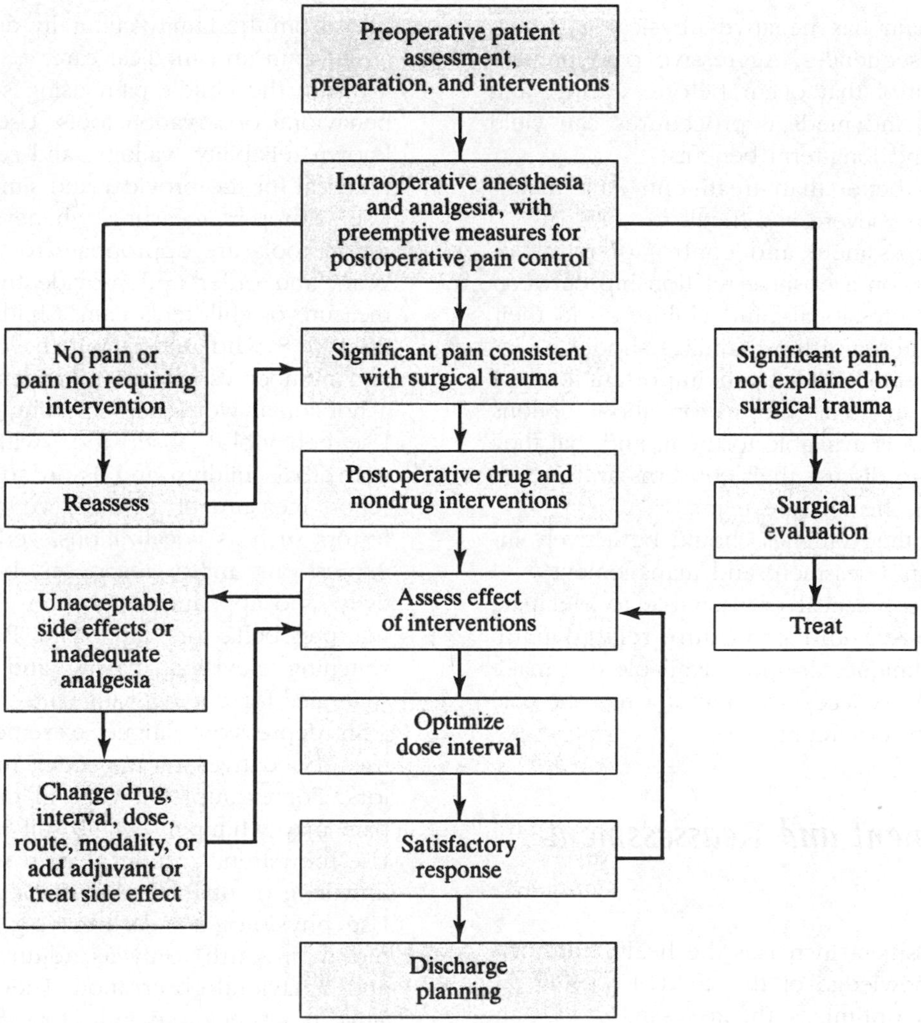

* Acute Pain Management Guideline Panel. *Acute pain management in infants, children, and adolescents: Operative and medical procedures.* Quick Reference Guide for Clinicians. AHCPR Pub. No. 92–0020, Rockville, MD. Agency for Health Care Policy and Research, Public Health Service, U.S. Department of Health and Human Services. Copies may be obtained by calling 1–800–358–9295 or 301–495–3453, or by writing to the Center for Research Dissemination and Liaison, AHCPR Publications Clearinghouse, P.O. Box 8547, Silver Spring, MD 20907.

Effective Management of Acute Pain

Requirements

- Pain intensity and pain relief must be assessed and reassessed at regular intervals.
- Children's and families' preferences must be respected when determining methods to be used for pain management.
- Children often cannot or will not report pain to their health care providers. Thus, health care professionals must have a high degree of suspicion for pain.
- Each institution must develop an organized program to evaluate the effectiveness of pain assessment and management.

Principles

- Unrelieved pain has negative physical and psychologic consequences. Aggressive pain prevention and control that occur before, during, and after surgery and medical procedures can yield both short- and long-term benefits.
- Prevention is better than treatment. Pain that is established and severe is difficult to control.
- Successful assessment and control of pain depends, in part, on a positive relationship between health care professionals and children and their families. Children and their families should be informed that pain relief is an important part of their health care, that information about options to control pain is available to them, and that they are welcome to discuss their concerns and preferences with the health care team.
- Children and their families should be actively involved in pain assessment and management.
- It may not be practical or desirable to eliminate all postoperative and procedure-related pain. However, techniques are now available that make pain reduction to acceptable levels a realistic goal in the majority of circumstances.

Pain Assessment and Reassessment

Principles

- Routine assessment increases the health care professional's knowledge of the child. Knowing the child in turn optimizes the assessment of pain and its subsequent management.
- Children who may have difficulty communicating their pain require particular attention. This includes children who are cognitively impaired, psychotic, or severely emotionally disturbed; children who do not speak English; and children from families where the level of education or cultural background differs significantly from that of the health care team.
- Unexpected intense pain, particularly if sudden or associated with altered vital signs such as hypotension, tachycardia, or fever, should be immediately evaluated, and new diagnoses such as wound dehiscence or infection considered.

Pain Assessment Procedures

- Tailor assessment strategies to the child's developmental level and personality style and to the situation.
- Obtain a pain history from the child and/or the parents at the time of admission. Learn what word the child uses for pain (e.g., hurt, boo-boo, owie).
- Elicit from the family culturally determined beliefs about pain and medical care.
- Measure the child's pain using self-report and/or behavioral observation tools. Use tools that have known reliability, validity, and sensitivity and are practical for the provider and simple for the child.
- Use self-report measures whenever possible. Self-report tools are appropriate for most children 4 years and older and provide the most accurate measure of children's pain. Children over the age of 7 or 8 who understand the concept of order and number can use a numerical rating scale or a horizontal word-graphic rating scale.
- Use behavioral observation with preverbal and nonverbal children and as an adjunct to the self-report measure of an older verbal child. Include factors such as vocalizations, verbalizations, facial expressions, motor responses, body posture, activity, and appearance.
- Interpret behaviors cautiously. Behaviors such as watching television, playing, and sleeping may be strategies for coping with pain. Continued severe pain, depression, fatigue, extreme illness, and the use of sedatives or hypnotics may blunt behaviors. For example, a very ill child with severe pain may whimper and lie still rather than cry.
- Use the parent's report of pain when the child is unwilling or unable to give a self-report.
- Use physiologic measures (e.g., heart rate and blood pressure) only as adjuncts to self-report and behavioral observation. They are neither sensitive nor specific as indicators of pain.

Postoperative Assessment

- Assess pain at regular intervals. For example, assessment after major surgery could occur at least

every 2 hours for the first 24 hours and every 4 hours thereafter. More frequent assessment is necessary if pain is poorly controlled.
- Interview the child and parent about the pain.
- Assess pain with other routine assessments such as taking vital signs. Document information about the pain and response to intervention on the bedside flow sheet or another easily visible and accessible place.
- Note changes in the child's behavior, appearance, activity level, and vital signs. Changes in these parameters may indicate a change in the pain intensity.
- Before discharge, review with the child and family the interventions used and their efficacy and provide specific discharge instructions.

Uncertainty about the Presence and Amount of Pain

- Even after implementing these assessment strategies, health care professionals may be uncertain about the presence and amount of pain, especially in infants or young children. If there is any reason to suspect pain, a diagnostic trial of analgesics is often appropriate.

Management of Pain Related to Procedures

Most hospitalized children undergo procedures. These may range from venipunctures and insertions of intravenous catheters to more stressful procedures such as lumbar punctures, bone marrow aspirates and biopsies, chest tube insertions, cardiac catheterizations, circumcisions, and dressing changes. Children often describe such procedures as the most distressing aspect of disease or hospitalization. Therefore, aggressive efforts to decrease pain and distress are warranted.

Appropriate interventions vary with the procedure, the child, and the context and may consist of pharmacologic modalities, nonpharmacologic modalities, or both. Attention to the following questions will help in selecting the appropriate intervention to minimize pain and distress:

- Why is the procedure being performed?
- How do the parents think the child will react?
- What is the expected intensity and duration of pain?
- What is the expected intensity and duration of anxiety?
- How often will the procedure be repeated?

Principles for the Management of Procedure-Related Pain

- Provide adequate preparation of the child and family for the procedure. The preparation should be developmentally appropriate. The timing of the preparation in relationship to the procedure should be adjusted to meet individual needs and preferences.
- Be attentive to environmental comfort (e.g., privacy, lighting, and noise). Unless absolutely necessary, do not perform procedures in the child's bed or room.
- Allow parents to be with the child before, during, and after the procedure. Prepare parents for their expected roles.
- Combine pharmacologic and nonpharmacologic options when possible and appropriate.
- If the child is to have repeated procedures, provide maximum treatment for the pain and anxiety of the first procedure to minimize the development of anticipatory anxiety before subsequent procedures.

Pharmacologic Management of Procedure-Related Pain

- Analgesics and/or local anesthetics are the foundation for pharmacologic management of painful procedures. Anxiolytics and sedatives are specifically for the reduction of associated anxiety. If used alone, anxiolytics and sedatives blunt behavioral responses without relieving pain.
- Systemic analgesics can be used alone or with anxiolytics or sedatives. When used by practitioners not skilled in pediatric airway management and pediatric advanced life support, doses must not exceed the amount necessary to produce conscious sedation (i.e., maintenance of airway reflexes and response to verbal and physical stimuli).
- Skilled supervision and appropriate monitoring procedures are crucial when conscious sedation is used.
- Special care in the choice of doses, agents, and monitoring procedures is necessary when systemic analgesics and sedatives are used for infants under 6 months of age.

Pharmacologic Agents for Procedure-Related Pain

- Injected and topical local anesthetics can reduce pain sensation.
- Intravenous, oral, or transmucosal opioids are

given in increments and titrated to analgesic effect.
- Oral or intravenous benzodiazepines produce anxiolysis and sedation but not analgesia. Intravenous benzodiazepines are given in increments and titrated to effect.
- Oral or intravenous barbiturates provide sedation without analgesic effect.
- Other agents, such as nitrous oxide and ketamine, can be used when trained personnel and appropriate monitoring procedures are available. General anesthesia is appropriate in some situations.

Note: Exercise caution when using the mixture of meperidine (Demerol), promethazine (Phenergan), and chlorpromazine (Thorazine), also known as DPT. The safety and efficacy of DPT does not compare favorably with the combination of opioids and benzodiazepines and should be used only under exceptional circumstances.

Nonpharmacologic Management of Procedure-Related Pain

Nonpharmacologic strategies can be used alone for less painful procedures—such as venipuncture—or as adjuncts to pharmacologic strategies for more painful procedures. Interventions are tailored to need, preferences, and coping style. The family can encourage and be helpful in facilitating the child's use of these strategies.

- For infants, sensorimotor strategies include pacifiers, swaddling, holding, and rocking.
- Cognitive/behavioral strategies include hypnosis; relaxation; distraction; music, art, and play therapy; preparatory information; and positive reinforcement. Rehearsal before the procedure may be helpful.
- Child participation strategies focus on involving children in age-appropriate decisions about the procedure and in activities related to its conduct.
- Physical strategies include the application of heat or cold, massage, exercise, rest, and immobilization.
- Older children and adolescents who find nonpharmacologic strategies helpful may prefer these strategies over pharmacologic agents for procedures that are not excessively painful.

Management of Postoperative Pain

Preoperative Management

- Prepare the child and family for the surgery and for the occurrence of pain postoperatively. Use developmentally appropriate materials.
- Emphasize with the child and family the importance of communicating with nurses and doctors about pain, preventing pain when possible, and treating pain early.
- Learn about the child's past experience with pain control medicines (including allergies).
- Inform the child and family of the options for treatment of pain. Develop a plan for pain assessment and management.
- Allow parent(s) to be present during the induction period.
- Administer the preoperative medication via a painless route.

Pharmacologic Management after Surgery

- Opioid and nonopioid analgesics are the mainstay of postoperative pain management. The approach varies with the child's age, medical condition, type of surgery, and expected postoperative course.
- Pain after minor surgery is usually managed with an oral or rectal nonsteroidal anti-inflammatory drug and opioid (e.g., codeine) analgesics singularly or in combination.
- Pain after major surgery is managed with parenteral or regional opioids until the child can tolerate oral intake.
- Parent and child instruction in pain control after discharge is important.

Nonsteroidal Anti-inflammatory Drugs (NSAIDs)

- Even when insufficient alone to control pain, NSAIDs have significant opioid dose–sparing effects and hence can be useful in reducing opioid side effects (see Table 25–8 in text for information on doses).
- NSAIDs must be used with care in patients with thrombocytopenia or coagulopathies and in those patients at risk for bleeding or gastric ulceration. However, acetaminophen does not affect platelet function, and some evidence exists that two salicylates (salsalate and choline magnesium trisalicylate) do not profoundly affect platelet aggregation.

Opioid Analgesics

- Opioid analgesics are the cornerstone of the management of moderate to severe acute pain. Effective use of these agents facilitates postoperative activities, such as coughing, deep breathing exercises, ambulation, and physical therapy.
- Studies in adults have shown that opioid tolerance and physiologic dependence are unusual in

short-term postoperative use in opioid-naive patients, and that psychologic dependence and addiction are extremely unlikely to develop after the use of opioids for acute pain. There is no known aspect of childhood development or physiology that indicates any increased risk of physiologic or psychologic dependence from the brief use of opioids for acute pain management.

Choice of Opioid Agent

- Morphine is the standard for opioid therapy. If morphine cannot be used because of an unusual reaction or allergy, another opioid such as hydromorphone can be substituted.
- Meperidine should be reserved for very brief courses in patients who have demonstrated allergy or intolerance to opioids such as morphine and hydromorphone. It is contraindicated in patients with impaired renal function or those receiving antidepressants of the monoamine oxidase (MAO) inhibitor class. Normeperidine is a toxic metabolite of meperidine, and is excreted through the kidney. Normeperidine is a cerebral irritant, and accumulation can cause effects ranging from dysphoria and irritable mood to seizures, even in young, otherwise healthy persons.

Dosage and Schedule

- Titrate the opioid dose and interval to increase the amount of analgesia and reduce the side effects when necessary. Children vary greatly in their analgesic dose requirements and responses to opioid analgesics, and the recommended starting doses may be inadequate.
- Use relative potency estimates to select the appropriate starting dose, to change the route of administration (e.g., from parenteral to oral), or to change from one opioid to another.
- Provide opioids around the clock or by continuous infusion rather than as needed (prn). A prn order is not recommended since it requires the child to communicate the presence of pain and the need for medication. Often children are unable or unwilling to initiate communication about pain. Further, a prn schedule produces delays in administration and intervals of inadequate pain control.
- Start with a dose of 0.02–0.04 mg/kg/hr when using a continuous infusion of morphine.
- Offer rescue doses for breakthrough or poorly controlled pain for children receiving intravenous infusions.
- Consider the use of patient-controlled analgesia (PCA) for developmentally normal children 7 years and older.
- Consider writing orders so the child or parent may refuse an analgesic if the child is asleep or not in pain. However, remember that a steady state blood level is required in order for the drug to be continuously effective, and interruption of an around-the-clock dosage schedule (e.g., during sleep) may cause a resurgence of pain as blood levels of the analgesic decline.

Route

- Administer opioids through the intravenous catheter (available for postoperative hydration) or orally. The intravenous route is suitable for bolus administration and continuous infusion (including PCA).
- Use intramuscular injections only under exceptional circumstances. They are painful and frightening for children.
- Use oral administration as soon as the patient can tolerate oral intake. It is convenient and inexpensive and is the mainstay of pain management in the ambulatory surgical population.

Other Pharmacologic Approaches

- Regional analgesia, including continuous infusions and intermittent doses of peridural local anesthetics and/or opioids, is used for children and may be particularly applicable for young infants as well as children with problems such as chronic lung disease.
- The administration of regional analgesia is best limited to specially trained and knowledgeable staff, typically under the direction of an acute or postoperative pain treatment service.

Nonpharmacologic Interventions

- Nonpharmacologic strategies are useful in easing anxiety and distress. The supportive presence of a parent or other family member is key and should be encouraged. Pacifiers, swaddling, rocking, and holding are helpful for infants. Familiar toys or blankets provide comfort for children, even in adolescence. Positioning with blankets and pillows and local applications of cold or heat may help comfort the child. A calming environment is important for children and families.

Special Considerations for the Management of Pain in Neonates and Infants

- Young infants, especially those who are premature or have neurologic abnormalities or pulmonary

disease, are susceptible to apnea and respiratory depression with the use of systemic opioids. However, neonates and infants do experience pain, and adequate analgesia after surgery is essential.
- Apnea and respiratory depression appear to be dose-related. Most practitioners reduce the initial dose and use intensive monitoring for infants up to about 6 months of age; this age is arbitrary and based on a cautious interpretation of the literature. For nonventilated infants, the initial opioid dose calculated in milligrams per kilogram should be about one fourth to one third of the dose recommended for older children. For example, 0.03 mg/kg of morphine could be used as the initial dose. Careful assessment and reassessment are necessary to determine the optimal dose and interval of administration from clinical parameters (e.g., when pain breaks through and whether the infant appears comfortable after the dose).
- Institutions in which major surgery on neonates and infants is performed must provide training for personnel in the safe and effective administration of analgesia for children in this age group and have the technologic capacity to provide appropriate monitoring.

Critical Questions Regarding the Adequacy of Pain Management

Pharmacologic Management

- What are the child's and parent's previous experiences with pain and their preferences for use of analgesics?
- Is the child being adequately assessed at appropriate intervals?
- Are analgesics ordered for prevention and relief of pain?
- Is the analgesic dosage appropriate for the pain being experienced or expected?
- Is the timing of administration appropriate for the pain expected or experienced?
- Is the route of administration appropriate (preferably oral or intravenous) for the child?
- Is the child adequately monitored for the occurrence of side effects?
- Are the side effects appropriately managed?
- Has the analgesic regimen provided adequate comfort from the child's or parent's perspective (i.e., patient satisfaction)?

Nonpharmacologic Management

- What are the child's and parent's experiences with and preferences for use of the strategy?
- Is the strategy appropriate for the child's developmental level, condition, and type of pain?
- Is the timing of the strategy sufficient to optimize its effects?
- Is the strategy effective in preventing or alleviating the child's pain?
- Are the child and parent(s) satisfied with the strategy for prevention or relief of pain?
- Are the treatable sources of emotional distress for the child being addressed?

APPENDIX • 8

Reference Ranges for Laboratory Tests

Prefixes Denoting Decimal Factors

Prefix	*Symbol*	*Factor*
mega	M	10^{6}
kilo	k	10^{3}
hecto	h	10^{2}
deka	da	10^{1}
deci	d	10^{-1}
centi	c	10^{-2}
milli	m	10^{-3}
micro	μ	10^{-6}
nano	n	10^{-9}
pico	p	10^{-12}
femto	f	10^{-15}

To conserve space, the following common abbreviations are used.

Abbreviations

Ab	absorbance
AI	angiotensin I
AU	arbitrary unit
*c*AMP	adenosine 3′,5′-cyclic phosphate
cap	capillary
CH_{50}	dilution required to lyse 50% of indicator RBC; indicates complement activity
CHF	congestive heart failure
CKBB	brain isoenzyme of creatine kinase
CKMB	heart isoenzyme of creatine kinase
CNS	central nervous system
conc.	concentration
d	diem, day, days
F	female
g	gram
hr	hour, hours
Hb	hemoglobin
HbCO	carboxyhemoglobin
hpf	high power field
HPLC	high pressure liquid chromatography
IFA	indirect fluorescent antibody
IU	International Unit of hormone activity
L	liter
M	male
MCV	mean corpuscular value
mEq/L	milliequivalents per liter
min	minute, minutes
mm^3	cubic millimeter; equivalent to microliter (μL)
mm Hg	millimeters of mercury
mo	month, months
mol	mole
mOsm	milliosmoles
MW	relative molecular weight
nm	nanometer (wavelength)
Pa	pascals
pc	postprandial
RBC	red blood cell(s); erythrocyte(s)
RIA	radioimmunoassay
RID	radial immunodiffusion
RT	room temperature
s	second, seconds
SD	standard deviation
std.	standard
therap.	therapeutic
U	International Unit of enzyme activity
V	volume
WBC	white blood cell
WHO	World Health Organization
wk	week, weeks
yr	year, years

Symbols

>	greater than
≥	greater than or equal to
<	less than
≤	less than or equal to
±	plus/minus
≃	approximately equal to

Abbreviations for Specimens

S	serum
P	plasma
(H)	heparin
(LiH)	lithium heparin
(E)	EDTA
(C)	citrate
(O)	oxalate
W	whole blood
U	urine
F	feces
CSF	cerebrospinal fluid
AF	amniotic fluid

Key to Comments

30°, 37°	temperature of enzymatic analysis (centigrade)
a	atomic absorption
b	optical density
c	colorimetry
d	Ektachem, proprietary analytic system of Eastman Kodak Co.
e	enzyme-amplified immunoassay
f	values in older females higher than those in older males
g	electrophoresis
h	gas chromatography
i	radioimmunoassay
l	fluorescence-activated cell sorting
m	values obtained are significantly method-dependent
n	nephelometry
o	borate affinity chromatography
p	high pressure liquid chromatography
q	cation exchange chromatography
r	radial immunodiffusion
s	values in older males higher than those in older females
v	fluorometric method
w	ion-selective electrode
x	fluorescence polarization
z	enzymatic assay

De Schepper J, Derde MP, Goubert P, et al: Reference values for fructosamine concentrations in children's sera: Influence of protein concentration, age and sex. Clin Chem 34(12): 2444, 1988.

Dickinson JC, Hamilton PB: The free amino acids of human spinal fluid determined by ion exchange chromatography. J Neurochem 13:1179, 1966.

Endocrine Sciences, Tarzana, CA.

Gibson LE, di Sant'Agnese PA, Schwachman H: Procedure for the quantitative iontophoretic sweat test for cystic fibrosis. Rockville, MD, Cystic Fibrosis Foundation, 1985, pp 1–4.

Gillard BK, Simbala JA, Goodglick L: Reference intervals for amylase isoenzymes in serum and plasma of infants and children. Clin Chem 29(6):1119, 1983.

Hoffman G, Aramaki S, Blum-Hoffman E, et al: Quantitative analysis for organic acids in biological samples: Batch isolation followed by gas chromatographic-mass spectrometric analysis. Clin Chem 35(4):587, 1989.

Jedeikin R, Makela SK, Shennan AT, et al: Creatine kinase isoenzymes in serum from cord blood and the blood of healthy full-term infants during the first three postnatal days. Clin Chem 28(2):317, 1982.

Jung D, Lun L, Zinsmeyer J, et al: The concentration of hypoxanthine and lactate in the blood of healthy and hypoxic newborns. J Perinat Med 13:43, 1985.

From Behrman, R. E. (1992). *Nelson textbook of pediatrics* (14th ed.). Philadelphia: WB Saunders, pp. 1799–1826.

Knight JA, Haymond RE: γ-glutamyltransferase and alkaline phosphatase activities compared in serum of normal children and children with liver disease. Clin Chem 27(1):48, 1981.

Landry A, Gartland GL, Abo T, et al: Enumeration of human lymphocyte subpopulations by immunofluorescence: A comparative study using automated flow microfluorometry and fluorescence microscopy. J Immunol Methods 58:337, 1983.

Lockitch G, Halstead AC, Albersheim S, et al: Age and sex specific pediatric reference intervals for biochemistry analyses as measured on the Ektachem-700 analyzer. Clin Chem 34(8):1622, 1988.

Lockitch G, Halstead AC, Quigley G, et al: Age and sex specific pediatric reference intervals: Study design and methods illustrated by measurement of serum proteins with the Behring LN nephelometer. Clin Chem 34(8):1618, 1988.

Lockitch G, Halstead AC, Wadsworth L, et al: Age and sex specific pediatric reference intervals and correlations for zinc, copper, selenium, iron, vitamins A and E, and related proteins. Clin Chem 34(8):1625, 1988.

Mayo Clinic Laboratories, Rochester, MN, 1989.

Meites S (ed): Pediatric Clinical Chemistry, Reference (Normal) Values, 3rd ed. Washington, D.C., Clinical Chemistry, 1989.

Nichols Institute Reference Laboratories, San Juan Capistrano, CA.

Pesce MA, Boudourian S: Clinical significance of plasma galactose and erythrocyte galactose-1-phosphate measurements in transferase-deficient galactosemia and in individuals with below-normal transferase activity. Clin Chem 28:301, 1982.

Pesce MA, Boudourian S, Harris RC, et al: Enzymatic micromethod for measuring galactose-1-phosphate uridylyltransferase in erythrocytes. Clin Chem 23:1711, 1977.

Pesce MA, Boudourian S, Nicholson JF: A new microfluorometric method for the measurement of galactose-1-phosphate in erythrocytes. Clin Chem Acta 118:177, 1982.

Rosenthal P, Pesce MA: Long-term monitoring of D-lactic acidosis in a child. J Pediatr Gastroenterol Nutr 4:674, 1985.

Sherry B, Jack RM, Weber A, et al: Reference interval for prealbumin for children two to 36 months old. Clin Chem 34(9):1878, 1988.

Taylor WJ, Caviness MHD: A Textbook for the Clinical Application of Therapeutic Drug Monitoring. Irving, TX, Abbott Laboratories, Diagnostic Division, 1986.

Syva Company: TDM Serum Sample Guide. Palo Alto, CA, Syva Company, 1986.

Unten SK, Hokama Y: Enzyme immunoassay for C-reactive protein analysis. J Clin Lab Anal 1:205, 1987.

Visnapu LA, Karlson LK, Dubinsky EJ, et al: Pediatric reference ranges for serum aldolase. Am J Clin Pathol 91(4):476, 1989.

Test	Specimen	Reference Range		Factor	Reference Range (SI)	Comments
Acetaminophen. See end of table under Drugs						
Acetone						
Semiquantitative	S, P(O)	Negative (<3 mg/dL)			Negative (<0.5 mmol/L)	
Quantitative		0.3–2.0 mg/dL		× 0.1722	0.05–0.34 mmol/L	
Semiquantitative	U	Negative			Negative	
Activated partial thromboplastin time (APTT)	P(C)	25–35 s Infant: <90 s			25–35 s (APTT) Infant: <90 s	
Adrenocorticotropic hormone (ACTH)	P(H)	Cord blood	130–160 pg/mL	× 1	130–160 μg/L	
		1–7 d postnatal	100–140 pg/mL		100–140 μg/L	
		Adult				
		0800 hr	25–100 pg/mL		25–100 μg/L	
		1800 hr	<50 pg/mL		<50 μg/L	
Alanine aminotransferase (ALT, GPT)	S	0–5 d	6–50 U/L	× 1	6–50 U/L	37° s d (Lockitch et al)
		1–19 y	5–45 U/L		5–45 U/L	
Albumin	P	Premature 1 d	1.8–3.0 g/dL	× 10	18–30 g/L	c (Meites)
		Full-term <6 d	2.5–3.4 g/dL		25–34 g/L	
		<5 yr	3.9–5.0 g/dL		39–50 g/L	
		5–19 yr	4.0–5.3 g/dL		40–53 g/L	
	U	4–16 yr	3.35–15.3 mg/24 h/1.73 m²			e (Meites)
	CSF	10–30 mg/dL			100–300 mg/L	
Aldolase	S	10–24 mo	3.4–11.8 U/L	× 1	3.4–11.8 U/L	z (Visnapu et al)
		25 mo–16 yr	1.2– 8.8 U/L		1.2– 8.8 U/L	
Aldosterone	S, P(H,E)					
		Newborn	5–60 ng/dL	× 0.0277	0.14–1.7 nmol/L	
		1 wk–1 yr	1–160 ng/dL		0.03–4.4 nmol/L	
		1–3 yr	5–60 ng/dL		0.14–1.7 nmol/L	
		3–5 yr	<5–80 ng/dL		<0.14–2.2 nmol/L	
		5–7 yr	<5–50 ng/dL		<0.14–1.4 nmol/L	
		7–11 yr	5–70 ng/dL		0.14–1.9 nmol/L	
		11–15 yr	<5–50 ng/dL		<0.14–1.4 nmol/L	
		Adult (Na diet)				
		Supine	3–10 ng/dL		0.08–0.3 nmol/L	
		Upright F	5–30 ng/dL		0.14–0.8 nmol/L	
		M	6–22 ng/dL		0.17–0.61 nmol/L	
		2–3 × higher during pregnancy				
		Adrenal vein	200–800 ng/dL		5.5–22 nmol/L	
		Low Na diet: increases 2- to 5-fold				
		Florinef suppression	<4 ng/dL		<0.1 nmol/L	
		ACTH or angiotensin stimulation, 1 hr: increases 2- to 5-fold				

Test	Specimen	Reference Range			Factor	Reference Range (SI)	Comments
	U	*Total Urinary Na*	*Plasma Renin Activity*	*Urinary Aldosterone*		*Urinary aldosterone*	
		<20 mmol/d	5–24 ng Al/mL/hr	>35–80 μg/d	× 2.77	>97–220 nmol/d	
		50 mmol/d	2–7 ng Al/mL/hr	13–33 μg/d		36–91 nmol/d	
		100 mmol/d	1–5 ng Al/mL/hr	5–24 μg/d		14–66 nmol/d	
		150 mmol/d	0.5–4 ng Al/mL/hr	3–19 μg/d		8–53 nmol/d	
		200 mmol/d		1–16 μg/d		3–44 nmol/d	
		250 mmol/d		1–13 μg/d		3–36 nmol/d	
		(assuming normal serum Na, K, and extracellular volume)					
Alkaline phosphatase, leukocyte. See Neutrophil alkaline phosphate							
Alkaline phosphate, serum. See Phosphatase, alkaline							
Amino acids	CSF						q (Dickinson et al)
Taurine		6.3 ± 1.8 μmol/L			× 1	6.3 ± 1.8 μmol/L	
Aspartic acid		0.9 ± 0.5 μmol/L				0.9 ± 0.5 μmol/L	
Threonine		25.0 ± 10.0 μmol/L				25.0 ± 10.0 μmol/L	
Serine + asparagine		38.0 ± 23.0 μmol/L				38.0 ± 23.0 μmol/L	
Glutamine		509.0 ± 144.0 μmol/L				509.0 ± 144.0 μmol/L	
Proline		0.6 ± — μmol/L				0.6 ± — μmol/L	
Glutamic acid		7.0 ± 4.9 μmol/L				7.0 ± 4.9 μmol/L	
Glycine		6.6 ± 1.8 μmol/L				6.6 ± 1.8 μmol/L	
Alanine		23.0 ± 9.4 μmol/L				23.0 ± 9.4 μmol/L	
Valine		14.0 ± 5.5 μmol/L				14.0 ± 5.5 μmol/L	
Half cystine		0.2 ± — μmol/L				0.2 ± — μmol/L	
Methionine		2.6 ± 1.6 μmol/L				2.6 ± 1.6 μmol/L	
Isoleucine		4.4 ± 1.3 μmol/L				4.4 ± 1.3 μmol/L	
Leucine		11.0 ± 3.6 μmol/L				11.0 ± 3.6 μmol/L	
Tyrosine		9.1 ± 5.0 μmol/L				9.1 ± 5.0 μmol/L	
Phenylalanine		9.2 ± 5.8 μmol/L				9.2 ± 5.8 μmol/L	
Ornithine		5.7 ± 1.8 μmol/L				5.7 ± 1.8 μmol/L	
Lysine		19.0 ± 6.6 μmol/L				19.0 ± 6.6 μmol/L	
Histidine		13.0 ± 4.4 μmol/L				13.0 ± 4.4 μmol/L	
Arginine		20.0 ± 5.8 μmol/L				20.0 ± 5.8 μmol/L	
Amino acids, plasma	P(H)						q (Nichols Institute)
		0–30 d	*>1 mo–16 yr*	*> 16 yr*			
Phosphoserine		0–30	0–12	3–7 μmol/L	× 1		
Taurine		74–216	22–192	27–168 μmol/L			
Aspartic acid		0–17	5–59	0–24 μmol/L			
Hydroxyproline		20–70	0–40	0–40 μmol/L			
Threonine		114–335	73–160	79–193 μmol/L			
Serine		94–243	90–226	73–167 μmol/L			
Asparagine		20 58	28–246	14–104 μmol/L			
Glutamic acid		0–50	0–210	0–88 μmol/L			
Glutamine		538–958	52–669	415–964 μmol/L			
Proline		107–177	67–238	102–336 μmol/L			
Glycine		224–514	89–360	120–554 μmol/L			
Alanine		236–410	142–484	210–661 μmol/L			
Citrulline		8–28	1–55	12–55 μmol/L			
2-Aminobutyric acid		6–29	0–42	3–38 μmol/L			
Valine		80–246	110–271	141–317 μmol/L			
Cysteine		70–167	0–106	16–167 μmol/L			
Methionine		9–41	0–90	6–40 μmol/L			
Isoleucine		27–53	34–85	36–98 μmol/L			
Leucine		46–109	55–165	75–175 μmol/L			
Tyrosine		42–99	29–86	21–87 μmol/L			
Phenylalanine		42–110	22–98	37–88 μmol/L			
Homocystine		0–0	0–0	0–0 μmol/L			
Tryptophan		17–71	24–79	20–95 μmol/L			
Ornithine		49–151	15–143	30–106 μmol/L			
Lysine		114–269	68–266	83–238 μmol/L			
1-Methylhistidine		0–27	0–27	0–27 μmol/L			
Histidine		49–114	52–124	31–107 μmol/L			
3-Methylhistidine		0–10	0–6	0–4 μmol/L			
Arginine		22–88	6–187	36–145 μmol/L			

Table continued on following page

Test	Specimen	Reference Range		Factor	Reference Range (SI)		Comments
Amino acids, urine	U						q (Nichols Institute)
		0–30 d (μmol/g creatinine)	*>1 mo (μmol/g creatinine)*		*0–30 d (mmol/mol creatinine)*	*>1 mo (mmol/mol creatinine)*	
Phosphoserine		0–53	0–35	× 0.1131	0–6.0	0–4.0	
Taurine		1521–6922	0–1450		172–783	0–164	
Phosphoethanolamine		0–23	23–203		0–2.6	2.6–23	
Aspartic acid		78–172	0–82		8.8–19.5	0–9.3	
Hydroxyproline		210–2413	0–210		23.7–273	0–23.7	
Threonine		99–509	27–265		11.2–57.6	3.1–30	
Serine		80–1096	86–566		9.1–124	9.7–64	
Asparagine		0–438	0–107		0–49.5	0–12.1	
Glutamic acid		34–363	0–80		3.8–41.1	0–9	
Glutamine		256–1096	168–849		29–124	9.7–64	
Sarcosine		93–850	93–850		10.5–96.1	10.5–96.1	
Proline		74–537	0–57		8.4–60.7	0–6.4	
Glycine		1423–7143	0–2953		161–808	0–334	
Alanine		403–715	68–534		45.6–80.9	7.7–60.4	
Citrulline		9–212	8–106		1.0–24	0.9–12	
2-Aminobutyric acid		354–1061	44–221		40–120	5–25	
Valine		18–314	7–50		2.0–35.5	0.8–5.6	
Cysteine		226–812	5–177		25.8–91.9	0.6–20	
Methionine		15–71	6–111		1.7–8	0.7–12.5	
Homocitrulline		0–266	0–266		0–30.1	0–30.1	
Cystathionine		27–111	3–23		3.1–12.5	0.3–2.6	
Isoleucine		43–179	0–65		4.9–20.2	0–7.3	
Leucine		17–72	15–57		1.9–8.1	1.7–6.5	
Tyrosine		27–97	19–145		3–11	2.2–16.4	
Phenylalanine		39–156	17–102		4.4–17.7	1.9–11.5	
β-Alanine		0–1202	0–1202		0–136	0–136	
3-Aminoisobutyric acid		0–111	0–111		0–12.5	0–12.5	
4-Aminoisobutyric acid		0–2643	0–2643		0–299	0–299	
Homocystine		0–0	0–0		0–0	0–0	
Argininosuccinic acid		0–9	0–7		0–1.0	0–0.8	
Ethanolamine		840–3492	57–308		95–395	6.5–34.8	
Tryptophan		0–106	0–106		0–12	0–12	
Hydroxylysine		0–106	0–106		0–12	0–12	
Ornithine		34–156	1–44		3.9–17.7	0.1–5.0	
Lysine		74–1282	0–548		8.4–145.0	0–62.0	
1-Methylhistidine		72–425	0–691		8.1–48.1	0–78.2	
Histidine		148–721	0–1353		16.7–81.6	0–153.0	
3-Methylhistidine		115–401	19–413		13–45.4	2.1–46.7	
Anserine		0–561	0–561		0–63.5	0–63.5	
Carnosine		0–127	0–127		0–14.4	0–14.4	
Arginine		50–73	8–32		5.6–8.3	0.9–3.6	
Aminolevulinic acid (ALA)	S	15–23 μg/dL (lower in child)		× 0.076	1.1–1.8 μmol/L		
	U	1.3–7.0 mg/24 hr		× 7.626	9.9–53.4 μmol/d		
Ammonia nitrogen	S, P(LiH)	Newborn	90–150 μgN/dL	× 0.714	64–107 μmol/L		z q
		0–2 wk	79–129 μgN/dL		56–92 μmol/L		
		>1 mo	29–70 μgN/dL		21–50 μmol/L		
		Thereafter	15–45 μgN/dL		11–32 μmol/L		
	P(LiH)	1–90 d	59–202 μgN/dL	× 0.714	42–144 μmol/L		d (Meites)
		3 mo–3 yr	48–195 μgN/dL		34–139 μmol/L		
	U		500–1,200 mgN/24 hr	0.0714	36–86 mmol/d		
Amniotic fluid analysis (Ab 450 nm)	AF		28 wk 0–0.048 A		0–0.048 A		
			40 wk 0–0.02 A		0–0.02 A		
Amphetamine. See end of table under Drugs							
Amylase	S	1–19 yr	35–127 U/L	× 1	35–127 U/L		c (Meites)
Pancreatic isoenzymes	S, P(H)	Cord blood 8 mo	0–34%	× 0.01	0–0.34 fraction of total		(Gillard et al)
		9 mo–4 yr	5–56%		0.05–0.56 fraction of total		
		5–19 yr	23–59%		0.23–0.59 fraction of total		
Androstenedione	S	M					(Endocrine Sciences)
		Tanner 1 <9.8 yr	8–50 ng/dL	× 0.03479	0.28–1.74 nmol/L		
		Tanner 2 9.8–14.5 yr	31–65 ng/dL		1.08–2.26 nmol/L		
		Tanner 3 10.7–15.4 yr	50–100 ng/dL		1.74–3.48 nmol/L		
		Tanner 4 11.8–16.2 yr	48–140 ng/dL		1.67–4.87 nmol/L		
		Tanner 5 12.8–17.3 yr	65–210 ng/dL		2.26–7.30 nmol/L		
		Adult	75–205 ng/dL		2.61–7.13 nmol/L		

Test	Specimen	Reference Range	Factor	Reference Range (SI)	Comments
Androstenedione *(Continued)*		F			
		Tanner 1 <9.2 yr 8–50 ng/dL		0.28–1.74 nmol/L	
		Tanner 2 9.2–13.7 yr 42–100 ng/dL		1.46–3.48 nmol/L	
		Tanner 3 10.0–14.4 yr 80–190 ng/dL		2.78–6.61 nmol/L	
		Tanner 4 10.7–15.6 yr 77–225 ng/dL		2.68–7.83 nmol/L	
		Tanner 5 11.8–18.6 yr 80–240 ng/dL		2.78–8.35 nmol/L	
		Adult Follicular 85–275 ng/dL		2.96–9.57 nmol/L	
		Luteal 85–275 ng/dL		2.96–9.57 nmol/L	
Anion gap (Na − (Cl + CO_2))	P(H)	7–16 mmol/L		7–16 mmol/L	
Antideoxyribonuclease B titer (Anti-DNAse tit)	S	≤170 units		≤170 units	
Antidiuretic hormone (hADH, vasopressin)	P(E)	*Plasma Osmols* / *Plasma ADH*		*Plasma ADH*	
		270–280 mOsm/kg <1.5 pg/mL	× 1	<1.5 ng/L	
		280–285 mOsm/kg <2.5 pg/mL		<2.5 ng/L	
		285–290 mOsm/kg 1–5 pg/mL		1–5 ng/L	
		290–295 mOsm/kg 2–7 pg/mL		2–7 ng/L	
		295–300 mOsm/kg 4–12 pg/mL		4–12 ng/L	
Anti-streptolysin-O titer (ASO titer)	S	≤166 Todd units 170–330 Todd units in school-aged children			
α_1-Antitrypsin	S	0–5 d 143–440 mg/dL	× 0.01	1.43–4.40 g/L	n (Lockitch et al)
		1–9 yr 147–245 mg/dL		1.47–2.45 g/L	
		9–19 yr 152–317 mg/dL		1.52–3.17 g/L	
	F	<1 yr			r (Meites)
		breast milk <4.4 mg/g solid			
		formula <2.9 mg/g solid			
		6 mo–44 yr cow milk, regular diet <1.7 mg/g solid			
Ascorbic acid. See Vitamin C					
Aspartate aminotransferase (AST, SGOT)	S	0–5 d 35–140 U/L	× 1	35–140 U/L	37° s (Lockitch et al)
		1–9 yr 15–55 U/L		15–55 U/L	
		10–19 yr 5–45 U/L		5–45 U/L	
Base excess	W(H)	Newborn (−10)–(−2) mmol/L		(−10)–(−2) mmol/L	
		Infant (−7)–(−1) mmol/L		(−7)–(−1) mmol/L	
		Child (−4)–(+2) mmol/L		(−4)–(+2) mmol/L	
		Thereafter (−3)–(+3) mmol/L		(−3)–(+3) mmol/L	
Bicarbonate	S, P	Arterial 21–28 mmol/L		Arterial 21–28 mmol/L	
		Venous 22–29 mmol/L		Venous 22–29 mmol/L	
Bile acids, total	S, fasting	0.3–2.3 μg/mL	× 1	0.3–2.3 mg/L	
	S, 2-hr pc	1.8–3.2 μg/mL		1.8–3.2 mg/L	
	F	120–225 mg/24 hr	× 1	120–225 mg/24 hr	
Bilirubin	S, P				
		Premature / *Full-term*		*Premature* / *Full-term*	
Total	S	Cord blood <2.0 mg/dL <2.0 mg/dL	× 17.10	<34 μmol/L <34 μmol/L	
		0–1 d <8.0 mg/dL <6.0 mg/dL		<137 μmol/L <103 μmol/L	
		1–2 d <12.0 mg/dL <8.0 mg/dl		<205 μmol/L <137 μmol/L	
		2–5 d <16.0 mg/dL <12.0 mg/dL		<274 μmol/L <205 μmol/L	
		>5 d <2.0 mg/dL 2–1.0 mg/dL		<34 μmol/L 3.4–17.1 μmol/L	
	U	Negative		Negative	
	AF	28 wk <0.075 mg/dL (or Ab450 <0.048)	× 17.10	<1.3 μmol/L (or Ab450 <0.048)	
		40 wk <0.025 mg/dL (or Ab450 <0.02)		<0.43 μmol/L (or Ab450 <0.02)	
Conjugated	S	0–0.2 mg/dL	× 17.10	0–3.4 μmol/L	
Bleeding time (BBT) Ivy		Normal 2–7 min Borderline 7–11 min		Normal 2–7 min Borderline 7–11 min	
Simplate (G–D)		2.75–8 min		2.75–8 min	
Blood volume	W (H)	M 52–83 mL/kg F 50–75 mL/kg	× 0.001	M 0.052–0.083 L/kg F 0.050–0.075 L/kg	
Brucellosis, agglutinins	S	≤1:8	× 1	≤1:8	

Table continued on following page

Test	Specimen	Reference Range		Factor	Reference Range (SI)	Comments
C-Peptide	P	0.5–2 μg/L (fasting)		× 1	0.5–2 μg/L (fasting)	i (Nichols Institute)
C-reactive protein	S	Cord blood	52–1,330 ng/mL	× 1	52–1,330 μg/L	e (Unten et al)
		2–12 yr	67–1,800 ng/mL		67–1,800 μg/L	
CSF. See Cerebrospinal fluid						
Calcitonin	S, P(HE)	M 3–26 pg/mL		× 0.28	M 0.8–7.2 pmol/L	(Nichols Institute)
		F 2–17 pg/mL			F 0.6–4.7 pmol/L	
		Higher in newborn infants				
Calcium, ionized (Ca)	S, P(H), W(H)	Cord blood	5.0–6.0 mg/dL	× 0.25	1.25–1.50 mmol/L	
		Newborn				
		3–24 hr	4.3–5.1 mg/dL		1.07–1.27 mmol/L	
		24–48 hr	4.0–4.7 mg/dL		1.00–1.17 mmol/L	
		Thereafter	4.8–4.92 mg/dL		1.12–1.23 mmol/L	
		or	2.24–2.46 mEq/L	×0.5	1.12–1.23 mmol/L	
Calcium, total	S	Cord blood	9.0–11.5 mg/dL	× 0.25	2.25–2.88 mmol/L	
		Newborn				
		3–24 hr	9.0–10.6 mg/dL		2.3–2.65 mmol/L	
		24–48 hr	7.0–12.0 mg/dL		1.75–3.0 mmol/L	
		4–7 d	9.0–10.9 mg/dL		2.25–2.73 mmol/L	
		Child	8.8–10.8 mg/dL		2.2–2.70 mmol/L	
		Thereafter	8.4–10.2 mg/dL		2.1–2.55 mmol/L	
	U	Ca in diet				
		Ca-free	5–40 mg/24 hr	× 0.025	0.13–1.0 mmol/24 hr	
		Low to average	50–150 mg/24 hr		1.25–3.8 mmol/24 hr	
		Average (20 mmol/24 h)	100–300 mg/24 hr		2.5–7.5 mmol/24 hr	
	CSF	2.1–2.7 mEq/L or		× 0.50	1.05–1.35 mmol/L	
		4.2–5.4 mg/dL		× 0.25	1.05–1.35 mmol/L	
	F	Average 0.64 g/24 hr		× 25	16 mmol/24 hr	
Carbamazepine. See end of table under Drugs						
Carbon dioxide	W(H)	Newborn	27–40 mm Hg	× 0.1333	3.6–5.3 kPa	
		Infant	27–41 mm Hg		3.6–5.5 kPa	
Partial pressure (pCO_2)		Thereafter				
		M	35–48 mm Hg		4.7–6.4 kPa	
		F	32–45 mm Hg		4.3–6.0 kPa	
Total (tCO_2)	S, P(H)	Cord blood	14–22 mmol/L		14–22 mmol/L	
		Premature	14–27 mmol/L		14–27 mmol/L	
		Newborn	13–22 mmol/L		13–22 mmol/L	
		Infant	20–28 mmol/L		20–28 mmol/L	
		Child	20–28 mmol/L		20–28 mmol/L	
		Thereafter	23–30 mmol/L		23–30 mmol/L	
Carbon monoxide	W(E)	Nonsmokers	<2% HbCO	× 0.01	HbCO fraction <0.02	
		Smokers	<10%		<0.10	
		Lethal	>50%		>0.5	
Carboxyhemoglobin. See Carbon monoxide						
β-Carotene	S	Infant	20–70 μg/dL	× 0.0186	0.37–1.30 μmol/L	
		Child	40–130 μg/dL		0.74–2.42 μmol/L	
		Thereafter	60–200 μg/dL		1.12–3.72 μmol/L	
Catecholamines, fractionated	P(E)	Norepinephrine				
		Supine	100–400 pg/mL	× 5.911	591–2,364 pmol/L	
		Standing	300–900 pg/mL		1,773–5,320 pmol/L	
		Epinephrine				
		Supine	<70 pg/mL	× 5.458	<382 pmol/L	
		Standing	<100 pg/mL		<546 pmol/L	
		Dopamine (no postural change)	<30 pg/mL	× 6.528	<196 pmol/L	
	U	Norepinephrine				
		0–1 yr	0–10 μg/24 hr	× 5.911	0–59 nmol/24 hr	
		1–2 yr	0–17 μg/24 hr		0–100 nmol/24 hr	
		2–4 yr	4–29 μg/24 hr		24–171 nmol/24 hr	
		4–7 yr	8–45 μg/24 hr		47–266 nmol/24 hr	
		7–10 yr	13–65 μg/24 hr		77–384 nmol/24 hr	
		Thereafter	15–80 μg/24 hr		87–473 nmol/24 hr	

Test	Specimen	Reference Range		Factor	Reference Range (SI)	Comments
Catecholamines, fractionated *(Continued)*		Epinephrine				
		0–1 yr	0–2.5 μg/24 hr	× 5.458	0–13.6 nmol/24 hr	
		1–2 yr	0–3.5 μg/24 hr		0–19.1 nmol/24 hr	
		2–4 yr	0–6.0 μg/24 hr		0–32.7 nmol/24 hr	
		4–7 yr	0.2–10 μg/24 hr		1.1–55 nmol/24 hr	
		7–10 yr	0.5–14 μg/24 hr		2.7–76 nmol/24 hr	
		Thereafter	0.5–20 μg/24 hr		2.7–109 nmol/24 hr	
		Fractionated Dopamine				
		0–1 yr	0–85 μg/24 hr	× 6.528	0–555 nmol/24 hr	
		1–2 yr	10–140 μg/24 hr		65–914 nmol/24 hr	
		2–4 yr	40–260 μg/24 hr		261–1,697 nmol/24 hr	
		Thereafter	65–400 μg/24 hr		424–2,611 nmol/24 hr	
Catecholamines, total Free	U					
		0–1 yr	10–15 μg/24 hr		10–15 μg/24 hr	
		1–5 yr	15–40 μg/24 hr		15–40 μg/24 hr	
		6–15 yr	20–80 μg/24 hr		20–80 μg/24 hr	
		Thereafter	30–100 μg/24 hr		30–100 μg/24 hr	
Cerebrospinal fluid Pressure	CSF	70–180 mm water			70–180 mm water	
Volume	CSF	Child	60–100 mL	× 0.001	0.06–0.10 L	
		Adult	100–160 mL		0.1–0.16 L	
Ceruloplasmin	S	0–5 d	5–26 mg/dL	× 10	50–260 mg/L	n f (Lockitch et al)
		1–19 yr	20–46 mg/dL		200–460 mg/L	
Chloral hydrate. See end of table under Drugs						
Chloride	S, P(H)	Cord blood	96–104 mmol/L	× 1	96–104 mmol/L	
		Newborn	97–110 mmol/L		97–110 mmol/L	
		Thereafter	98–106 mmol/L		98–106 mmol/L	
	CSF		118–132 mmol/L	× 1	118–132 mmol/L	
	U	Infant	2–10 mmol/24 hr	× 1	2–10 mmol/24 hr	
		Child	15–40 mmol/24 hr		15–40 mmol/24 hr	
		Thereafter	110–250 mmol/24 hr (varies greatly with Cl intake)		110–250 mmol/24 hr	
	Sweat	Normal	<40 mmol/L	× 1	<40 mmol/L	(Gibson et al)
		Borderline	45–60 mmol/L		45–60 mmol/L	
		Cystic fibrosis	>60 mmol/L		>60 mmol/L	
Cholesterol, total	S	1–3 yr	45–182 mg/dL	× 0.0259	1.15–4.70 mmol/L	z (Lokitch et al)
		4–6 yr	109–189 mg/dL		2.80–4.80 mmol/L	
	S	M		× 0.0259		(Mayo Clinic Laboratories)
			Percentiles *5* *75* *95*		*Percentiles* *5* *75* *95*	
		6–9 yr	126 172 191 mg/dL		6–9 yr 3.26 4.45 4.94 mmol/L	
		10–14 yr	130 179 204 mg/dL		10–14 yr 3.36 4.63 5.28 mmol/L	
		15–19 yr	114 167 198 mg/dl		15–19 yr 2.95 4.32 5.12 mmol/L	
		F				
			Percentiles *5* *75* *95*		*Percentiles* *5* *75* *95*	
		6–9 yr	122 173 209 mg/dL		6–9 yr 3.16 4.47 5.41 mmol/L	
		10–14 yr	124 174 217 mg/dL		10–14 yr 3.21 4.50 5.61 mmol/L	
		15–19 yr	125 175 212 mg/dL		15–19 yr 3.23 4,53 5.48 mmol/L	
Chorionic gonadotropin β-subunit (β-hCG)	S, P(E)	Child and Male, nondetectable				
		F (post-conception)				
		7–10 d	>5.0 mIU/mL	× 1.0	>5.0 IU/L	
		30 d	>100 mIU/mL		>100 IU/L	
		40 d	>2,000 mIU/mL		>2,000 IU/L	
		10 wk	50,000–100,000 mIU/mL		50,000–100,000 IU/L	
		10 wk	10,000–20,000 mIU/mL		10,000–20,000 IU/L	
		Trophoblastic disease	>100,000		>100,000 IU/L	
Clotting time, Lee-White, 37° C	W	Glass tubes	5–8 min (5–15 min at RT)		Glass tubes 5–8 min (5–15 min at RT)	
		Silicone tubes	about 30 min prolonged		Silicone tubes about 30 min prolonged	

Table continued on following page

Test	Specimen	Reference Range		Factor	Reference Range (SI)	Comments
Coagulation factor assays	P(C)					
Factor I. See Fibrinogen						
Factor II		0.5–1.5 U/mL or 60–150% of normal		× 1	0.5–1.5 kU/L 60–150 AU	
Factor IV. See Calcium						
Factor V		0.5–2.0 U/mL or 60–150% of normal		× 1	0.5–2.0 kU/L 60–150 AU	
Factor VII		65–135% of normal		× 1	65–135 AU	
Factor VIII		60–145% of normal		× 1	60–145 AU	
Factor VIII antigen		50–200% of normal		× 1	50–200 AU	
Factor IX		60–140% of normal		× 1	60–140 AU	
Factor X		60–130% of normal		× 1	60–130 AU	
Factor XI		65–135% of normal		× 1	65–135 AU	
Factor XII		65–150% of normal		× 1	65–150 AU	
Factor XII (fibrin stabilizing factor, FSF)	W(C,O)	Minimal hemostatic level 0.02–0.05 U/mL or		× 1,000	20–50 U/L or	
		1–2% or normal		× 1	1–2 AU	
Complement components						
Total hemolytic complement activity	P(E)	75–160 U/mL >33% of plasma CH_{50}		× 1	75–160 IU/mL >0.33 of plasma CH_{50}	
Total complement decay rate (functional)	P(E)	~10–20%		× 0.01	~0.10–0.20 (fraction of decay rate)	
		Deficiency >50%			0.50 (fraction of decay rate)	
Classic pathway components						
Clq	S	Cord blood	1.0–14.9 mg/dL	× 10	10–149 mg/L	
		1 mo	2.2–6.2 mg/dL		22–62 mg/L	
		6 mo	1.2–7.6 mg/dL		12–76 mg/L	
		Adult	5.1–7.9 mg/dL		51–79 mg/L	
Clr	S		2.5–3.8 mg/dL	× 10	25–38 mg/L	
Cls (Cl esterase)	S		2.5–3.8 mg/dL	× 10	25–38 mg/L	
C2	S	Cord blood	1.6–2.8 mg/dL	× 10	16–28 mg/L	
		1 mo	1.9–3.9 mg/dL		19–39 mg/L	
		6 mo	2.4–3.6 mg/dL		24–36 mg/L	
		Adult	1.6–4.0 mg/dL		16–40 mg/L	
C3	S	Cord blood	57–116 mg/dL	× 10	570–1,160 mg/L	n (Meites)
		1–3 mo	53–131 mg/dL		530–1,310 mg/L	
		3 mo–1 yr	62–180 mg/dL		620–1,800 mg/L	
		1–10 yr	77–195 mg/dL		770–1,950 mg/L	
		Adult	83–177 mg/dL		830–1,770 mg/L	
C4	S	Cord blood	7–23 mg/dL	× 10	70–230 mg/L	n (Meites)
		1–3 mo	7–27 mg/dL		70–270 mg/L	
		3 mo–10 yr	7–40 mg/dL		70–400 mg/L	
		Adult	15–45 mg/dL		150–450 mg/L	
C5	S	Cord blood	3.4–6.2 mg/dL	× 10	34–62 mg/L	
		1 mo	2.3–6.3 mg/dL		23–63 mg/L	
		6 mo	2.4–6.4 mg/dL		24–64 mg/L	
		Adult	3.8–9.0 mg/dL		38–90 mg/L	
C6	S	Cord blood	1.0–4.2 mg/dL	× 10	10–42 mg/L	
		1 mo	2.2–5.2 mg/dL		22–52 mg/L	
		6 mo	3.7–7.1 mg/dL		37–71 mg/L	
		Adult	4.0–7.2 mg/dL		40–72 mg/L	
C7	S		4.9–7.0 mg/dL	× 10	49–70 mg/L	
C8	S		4.3–6.3 mg/dL	× 10	43–63 mg/L	
C9	S		4.7–6.9 mg/dL	× 10	47–69 mg/L	
Alternative pathway components						
C4 binding protein	S		18.0–32.0 mg/dL	× 10	180–320 mg/L	
Factor B (C3 proactivator) RID	P(E)	Cord blood	7.8–15.8 mg/dL	× 10	78–158 mg/L	
		1 mo	6.2–28.6 mg/dL		62–286 mg/L	
		6 mo	16.9–29.3 mg/dL		169–293 mg/L	
		Adult	14.7–33.5 mg/dL		147–335 mg/L	
Nephelometry	S	Newborn	14–33 mg/dL	× 10	140–330 mg/L	
		Adult	20–45 mg/dL		200–450 mg/L	
Properdin	S	Cord blood	1.3–1.7 mg/dL	× 10	13–17 mg/L	
		1 mo	0.6–2.2 mg/dL		6–22 mg/L	
		6 mo	1.3–2.5 mg/dL		13–25 mg/L	
		Adult	2.0–3.6 mg/dL		20–36 mg/L	
Regulatory protein b1H-globulin (C3b inactivator-accelerator)	S	Cord blood	26–42 mg/dL	× 10	260–420 mg/L	
		1 mo	24–56 mg/dL		240–560 mg/L	
		6 mo	33–61 mg/dL		330–610 mg/L	
		Adult	40–72 mg/dL		400–720 mg/L	
Cl inhibitor (esterase inhibitor)	P(E)		17.4–24.0 mg/dL	× 10	174–240 mg/L	

Test	Specimen	Reference Range	Factor	Reference Range (SI)	Comments
Complement components *(Continued)*					
Complement decay rate (functional)	S	<20% decay rate	× 0.01	<0.20 (fraction of decay rate)	
				>0.50 (fraction of decay rate)	
		Deficiency >50% decay rate			
C3b inactivator (KAF)	S	Cord blood 1.8–2.6 mg/dL	× 10	18–26 mg/L	
		1 mo 1.5–3.9 mg/dL		15–39 mg/L	
		6 mo 2.3–4.3 mg/dL		23–43 mg/L	
		Adult 2.6–5.4 mg/dL		26–54 mg/L	
S protein	S	41.8–60.0 mg/dL	× 10	418–600 mg/L	
Copper	S	0–5 d 9–46 μg/dL	× 0.157	1.4–7.2 μmol/L	fa (Lockitch et al)
		1–9 yr 80–150 μg/dL		12.6–23.6 μmol/L	
		10–14 yr 80–121 μg/dL		12.6–19.0 μmol/L	
		15–19 yr 64–160 μg/dL		11.3–25.2 μmol/L	
	U	5–18 yr 0.36–7.56 mg/mol creatinine	× 15.7	6–119 μmol/mol creatinine	
Coproporphyrin	U	34–234 μg/24 hr	× 1.5	51–351 nmol/24 hr	
	F (24-hr)	<30 μg/g dry wt	× 1.5	<45 nmol/g dry wt	
		400–1,200 μg/24 hr		600–1,800 nmol/24 hr	
Corticobinding globulin (CBG). See Transcortin					
Cortisol	S, P(H)	Newborn 1–24 μg/dL	× 27.59	28–662 nmol/L	
		Adults			
		0800 hr 5–23 μg/dL		138–635 nmol/L	
		1,600 hr 3–15 μg/dL		82–413 nmol/L	
		2,000 hr ≤50% of 0800 h	× 0.01	Fraction of 0800 hr ≤0.50	
Cortisol, free	U	Child 2–27 μg/24 hr	× 2.759	5.5–74 nmol/24 hr	
		Adolescent 5–55 μg/24 hr		14–152 nmol/24 hr	
		Adult 10–100 μg/24 hr		27–276 nmol/24 hr	
Creatine kinase	S	Cord blood 70–380 U/L	× 1	70–380 U/L	30° s (Jedeikin et al)
		5–8 hr 214–1175 U/L		214–1175 U/L	
		24–33 hr 130–1200 U/L		130–1200 U/L	
		72–100 hr 87–725 U/L		87–725 U/L	
		Adult 5–130 U/L		5–130 U/L	
Creatinine kinase isoenzymes	S	*CKMB* *CKBB*			
		Cord blood 0.3–3.1% 0.3–10.5%			
		5–8 hr 1.7–7.9% 3.6–13.4%			
		24–33 hr 1.8–5.0% 2.3–8.6%			
		72–100 hr 1.4–5.4% 5.1–13.3%			
		Adult 0–2% 0			
Creatinine					
Jaffe, kinetic, or enzymatic	S, P	Cord blood 0.6–1.2 mg/dL	× 88.4	53–106 μmol/L	
		Newborn 0.3–1.0 mg/dL		27–88 μmol/L	
		Infant 0.2–0.4 mg/dL		18–35 μmol/L	
		Child 0.3–0.7 mg/dL		27–62 μmol/L	
		Adolescent 0.5–1.0 mg/dL		44–88 μmol/L	
		Adult			
		M 0.6–1.2 mg/dL		53–106 μmol/L	
		F 0.5–1.1 mg/dL		44–97 μmol/L	
Jaffe, manual	S, P	0.8–1.5 mg/dL	× 88.4	70–133 μmol/L	
	AF	After 37-wk gestation >2.0 mg/dL	× 88.4	After 37-wk gestation >180 μmol/L	
Creatinine	U	Premature 8.1–15.0 mg/kg/24 hr	× 8.84	72–133 μmol/kg/24 hr	md (Meites)
		Full-term 10.4–19.7 mg/kg/24 hr		92–174 μmol/kg/24 hr	
		1.5–7 yr 10–15 mg/kg/24 hr		88–133 μmol/kg/24 hr	
		7–15 yr 5.2–41 mg/kg/24 hr		46–362 μmol/kg/24 hr	
Creatinine clearance (endogenous)	S, P, and U	Newborn 40–65 mL/min/1.73 m^2			
		<40 yr			
		M 97–137 mL/min/1.73 m^2			
		F 88–128 mL/min/1.73 m^2			
		Decreases ~6.5 mL/min/decade			
Cyclic AMP	P(E)	M 5.6–10.9 ng/mL	× 3.04	M 17–33 nmol/L	
		F 3.6–8.9 ng/mL		F 11–27 nmol/L	
	U	<3.3 mg/24 h or <1.64 mg/g creatinine	× 3040	<10,000 nmol/24 hr <6,000 nmol cAMP/g creatinine	
Dehydroepiandrosterone	S	M			(Endocrine Sciences)
		Tanner 1 <9.8 yr 31–345 ng/dL	× 0.03467	1.07–11.96 nmol/L	
		Tanner 2 9.8–14.5 yr 110–495 ng/dL		3.81–17.16 nmol/L	
		Tanner 3 10.7–15.4 yr 170–585 ng/dL		5.89–20.28 nmol/L	
		Tanner 4 11.8–16.2 yr 160–640 ng/dL		5.55–22.19 nmol/L	
		Tanner 5 12.8–17.3 yr 250–800 ng/dL		8.67–31.21 nmol/L	
		Adult 160–800 ng/dL		5.55–27.74 nmol/L	

Table continued on following page

Test	Specimen	Reference Range			Factor	Reference Range (SI)		Comments
Dehydroepiandrosterone *(Continued)*		F						
		Tanner 1	<9.2 yr	31–345 ng/dL		1.07–11.96 nmol/L		
		Tanner 2	9.2–13.7 yr	150–570 ng/dL		5.20–19.76 nmol/L		
		Tanner 3	10.0–14.4 yr	200–600 mg/dL		6.93–20.80 nmol/L		
		Tanner 4	10.7–15.6 yr	200–780 ng/dL		6.93–24.27 nmol/L		
		Tanner 5	11.8–18.6 yr	215–850 ng/dL		7.45–29.47 nmol/L		
		Adult	Follicular	160–800 ng/dL		5.55–27.74 nmol/L		
			Luteal	160–800 ng/dL		5.55–27.74 nmol/L		
Dehydroepiandrosterone sulfate (DHEA-sulfate, DHEAS)		M						(Endocrine Sciences)
		Tanner 1	<9.8 yr	20–170 μg/dL	× 0.026	0.52–4.42 μmol/L		
		Tanner 2	9.8–14.5 yr	70–180 μg/dL		1.82–4.68 μmol/L		
		Tanner 3	10.7–15.4 yr	90–180 μg/dL		2.34–4.68 μmol/L		
		Tanner 4	11.8–16.2 yr	220–304 μg/dL		5.72–7.90 μmol/L		
		Tanner 5	12.8–17.3 yr	120–370 μg/dL		3.12–9.62 μmol/L		
		Adult		180–450 μg/dL		4.68–11.70 μmol/L		
		F						
		Tanner 1	<9.2 yr	40–200 μg/dL		1.04–5.20 μmol/L		
		Tanner 2	9.2–13.7 yr	81–145 μg/dL		2.11–3.77 μmol/L		
		Tanner 3	10.0–14.4 yr	129–210 μg/dL		3.35–5.46 μmol/L		
		Tanner 4	10.7–15.6 yr	170–330 μg/dL		4.42–8.58 μmol/L		
		Tanner 5	11.8–18.6 yr	117–325 μg/dL		3.04–8.45 μmol/L		
		Adult	Follicular	120–315 μg/dL		3.12–8.19 μmol/L		
			Luteal	120–315 μg/dL		3.12–8.19 μmol/L		
Diazepam. See end of table under Drugs								
Differential count. See Leukocyte differential count								
Digitoxin. See end of table under Drugs								
Digoxin. See end of table under Drugs								
Dihydrotestosterone (DHT)	S	M						(Endocrine Sciences)
		Tanner 1	<9.8 yr	<3 ng/dL	× 0.03443	<0.10 nmol/L		
		Tanner 2	9.8–14.5 yr	3–17 ng/dL		0.10–0.59 nmol/L		
		Tanner 3	10.7–15.4 yr	8–33 ng/dL		0.28–1.14 nmol/L		
		Tanner 4	11.8–16.2 yr	22–52 ng/dL		0.76–1.79 nmol/L		
		Tanner 5	12.8–17.3 yr	24–65 ng/dL		0.83–2.24 nmol/L		
		Adult		30–85 ng/dL		1.03–2.93 nmol/L		
		F						
		Tanner 1	<9.2 yr	<3 ng/dL		<0.10 nmol/L		
		Tanner 2	9.2–13.7 yr	5–12 ng/dL		0.17–0.41 nmol/L		
		Tanner 3	10.0–14.4 yr	7–19 ng/dL		0.24–0.65 nmol/L		
		Tanner 4	10.7–15.6 yr	4–13 ng/dL		0.14–0.45 nmol/L		
		Tanner 5	11.8–18.6 yr	3–18 ng/dL		0.10–0.62 nmol/L		
		Adult	Follicular	4–22 ng/dL		0.14–0.76 nmol/L		
			Luteal	4–22 ng/dL		0.14–0.76 nmol/L		
Diphenylhydantoin. See end of table under Drugs								
Disaccharide absorption test	S	Change in glucose from fasting value			× 0.055	Change in glucose from fasting value		
		Normal		>30 mg/dL		Normal	>1.67 mmol/L	
		Inconclusive		20–30 mg/dL		Inconclusive	1.11–1.67 mmol/L	
		Abnormal		<20 mg/dL			<1.11 mmol/L	
Dithionite tube test. See Sickle cell tests								
Electrophoresis, Hemoglobin. See Hemoglobin electrophoresis								
Eosinophil count	W(E,H) capillary	50–350 cells/mm^3 (μL)			× 10^6	50–350 × 10^6 cells/L		
Epinephrine. See Catecholamines, fractionated								

Test	Specimen	Reference Range		Factor	Reference Range (SI)	Comments
Erythrocyte count (RBC count)	W(E)		Millions of cells/mm³ (μL)		× 10^{12} cells/L	
		Cord blood	3.9–5.5	× 1	3.9–5.5	
		1–3 d (capillary)	4.0–6.6		4.0–6.6	
		1 wk	3.9–6.3		3.9–6.3	
		2 wk	3.6–6.2		3.6–6.2	
		1 mo	3.0–5.4		3.0–5.4	
		2 mo	2.7–4.9		2.7–4.9	
		3–6 mo	3.1–4.5		3.1–4.5	
		0.5–2 yr	3.7–5.3		3.7–5.3	
		2–6 yr	3.9–5.3		3.9–5.3	
		6–12 yr	4.0–5.2		4.0–5.2	
		12–18 yr				
		M	4.5–5.3		4.5–5.3	
		F	4.1–5.1		4.1–5.1	
		18–49 yr				
		M	4.5–5.9		4.5–5.9	
		F	4.0–5.2		4.0–5.2	
Erythrocyte Sedimentation Rate (ESR)						
Westergren, modified	W(E)	Child	0–10 mm/hr		0–10 mm/hr	
		Adult				
		M < 50 yr	0–15 mm/hr		0–15 mm/hr	
		F < 50 yr	0–20 mm/hr		0–20 mm/hr	
Wintrobe		Child	0–13 mm/hr		0–13 mm/hr	
		Adult				
		M	0–9 mm/hr		0–9 mm/hr	
		F	0–20 mm/hr		0–20 mm/hr	
ZETA			41–54%		41–54 AU	
Erythropoietin RIA	S	<5–20 mU/mL		× 1	<5–20 U/L	
Hemagglutination		25–125 mU/mL			25–125 U/L	
Bioassay		5–18 mU/mL			5–18 U/L	
Estradiol	S	M		× 36.71		(Endocrine Sciences)
		Tanner 1 <9.8 yr	0.5–1.1 ng/dL		18–40 pmol/L	
		Tanner 2 9.8–14.5 yr	0.5–1.6 ng/dL		18–59 pmol/L	
		Tanner 3 10.7–15.4 yr	0.5–2.5 ng/dL		18–92 pmol/L	
		Tanner 4 11.8–16.2 yr	1.0–3.6 ng/dL		37–132 pmol/L	
		Tanner 5 12.8–17.3 yr	1.0–3.6 ng/dL		37–132 pmol/L	
		Adult	0.8–3.6 ng/dL		29–132 pmol/L	
		F				
		Tanner 1 <9.2 yr	0.1–2.0 ng/dL		4–73 pmol/L	
		Tanner 2 9.2–13.7 yr	1.0–2.4 ng/dL		37–88 pmol/L	
		Tanner 3 10.0–14.4 yr	0.7–6.0 ng/dL		26–220 pmol/L	
		Tanner 4 10.7–15.6 yr	2.1–8.5 ng/dL		77–312 pmol/L	
		Tanner 5 11.8–18.6 yr	3.4–17 ng/dL		125–624 pmol/L	
		Adult Follicular	3–10 ng/dL		110–367 pmol/L	
		Luteal	7–30 ng/dL		257–1,100 pmol/L	
Estradiol, urinary	U	Adult M	0–6 μg/24 hr	× 3.671	Adult M 0–22 nmol/24 hr	
		Adult F			Adult F	
		Follicular	0–3 μg/24 hr		Folicular 0–11 nmol/24 hr	
		Ovulatory peak	4–14 μg/24 hr		Ovulatory peak 15–51 nmol/24 hr	
		Luteal	4–10 μg/24 hr		Luteal 15–37 nmol/24 hr	
Estriol (E3), free	S	*Wk of gestation*				
		25	3.5–10.0 μg/L	× 3.47	12.1–34.7 nmol/L	
		28	4.0–12.5 μg/L		13.9–43.4 nmol/L	
		30	4.5–14.0 μg/L		15.6–48.6 nmol/L	
		32	5.0–16.0 μg/L		17.4–55.5 nmol/L	
		34	5.5–18.5 μg/L		19.1–64.2 nmol/L	
		36	7.0–25.0 μg/L		24.3–86.8 nmol/L	
		37	8.0–28.0 μg/L		27.8–97.2 nmol/L	
		38	9.0–32.0 μg/L		31.2–111.0 nmol/L	
		39	10.0–34.0 μg/L		34.7–118.0 nmol/L	
		40–41	10.5–25.0 μg/L		36.4–86.8 nmol/L	
	AF	*Wk*				
		16–20	1.0–3.2 ng/mL (95% range)	× 3.47	3.5–11.1 nmol/L (95% range)	
		20–24	2.1–7.8 ng/mL (95% range)		7.3–27.1 nmol/L (95% range)	
		24–28	2.1–7.8 ng/mL (95% range)		7.3–27.1 nmol/L (95% range)	
		28–32	4.0–13.6 ng/mL (95% range)		13.9–47.2 nmol/L (95% range)	
		32–36	3.6–15.5 ng/mL (95% range)		12.5–53.8 nmol/L (95% range)	
		36–38	4.6–18.0 ng/mL (95% range)		16.0–62.5 nmol/L (95% range)	
		38–40	5.4–19.8 ng/mL (95% range)		18.7–68.7 nmol/L (95% range)	

Table continued on following page

Test	Specimen	Reference Range		Factor	Reference Range (SI)	Comments
Estriol (E3), total	S	*Pregnancy (wk)*				
		24–28	30–170 ng/mL	× 3.47	104–590 nmol/L	
		28–32	40–220 ng/mL		140–760 nmol/L	
		32–36	60–280 ng/mL		208–970 nmol/L	
		36–40	80–350 ng/mL		280–1,210 nmol/L	
		Adult M and nonpregnant F	<2 ng/mL		<7 nmol/L	
	U	*Pregnancy (wk)*				
		30	6–18 mg/24 hr	× 3.47	21–62 μmol/24 hr	
		35	9–28 mg/24 hr		31–97 μmol/24 hr	
		40	13–42 mg/24 hr		45–146 μmol/24 hr	
		Decrease of >40% of previous value suggests fetus at risk			Fraction of previous value of <0.60 suggests fetus at risk	
Estrogens, total	S	Child	<30 pg/L	× 1	<30 ng/L	
		M	40–115 pg/L		40–115 ng/L	
		F cycle (days)				
		1–10 d	61–394 pg/L		61–394 ng/L	
		11–20 d	122–437 pg/L		122–437 ng/L	
		21–30 d	156–350 pg/L		156–350 ng/L	
		Prepubertal	≤40 pg/L		≤40 ng/L	
	U, 24 hr	Child	<10 μg/24 hr	× 1	<10 μg/24 hr	
		Adult (M)	5–25 μg/24 hr		5–25 μg/24 hr	
		F				
		Preovulation	5–25 μg/24 hr		5–25 μg/24 hr	
		Ovulation	28–100 μg/24 hr		28–100 μg/24 hr	
		Luteal peak	22–80 μg/24 hr		22–80 μg/24 hr	
		Pregnancy	<45,000 μg/24 hr		<45,000 μg/24 hr	
		Postmenopausal	<10 μg/24 hr		<10 μg/24 hr	
Ethanol. See end of table under Drugs						
Ethosuximide. See end of table under Drugs						
Fat, fecal	F (72-hr)	Infant, breast-fed	<1 g/24 hr	× 1	<1 g/24 hr	
		0–6 yr	<2 g/24 hr		<2 g/24 hr	
		Adult				
		Normal diet	<7 g/24 hr		<7 g/24 hr	
		Fat-free diet	<4 g/24 hr		<4 g/24 hr	
		Coefficient of fat absorption (%)			Absorbed fraction	
		Infant		× 0.01		
		Breast-fed	>93		>0.93	
		Formula-fed	>83		>0.83	
		>1 yr	≥95		≥0.95	
Free fatty acids	S	Premature 10–55 d	0.15–0.71 mmol/L	× 1	0.15–0.71 mmol/L	(Meites)
Ferric chloride test	U	Negative			Negative	
Ferritin	S	Newborn	25–200 ng/mL	× 1	25–200 μg/L	
		1 mo	200–600 ng/mL		200–600 μg/L	
		2–5 mo	50–200 ng/mL		50–200 μg/L	
		6 mo–15 yr	7–140 ng/mL		7–140 μg/L	
		Adult				
		M	15–200 ng/mL		15–200 μg/L	
		F	12–150 ng/mL		12–150 μg/L	
α-Fetoprotein (AFP)	S maternal		*Median*		*Median*	
		15 wk	34 ng/mL	× 1	34 μg/L	
		16 wk	38 ng/mL		38 μg/L	
		17 wk	44 ng/mL		44 μg/L	
		18 wk	49 ng/mL		49 μg/L	
		19 wk	56.5 ng/mL		56.5 μg/L	
		20 wk	66 ng/mL		66 μg/L	
	AF		*Mean*			
		15 wk	13.5 ± 3.42 μg/mL			
		16 wk	11.7 ± 3.38 μg/mL			
		17 wk	10.3 ± 3.03 μg/mL			
		18 wk	9.5 ± 3.22 μg/mL			
		19 wk	7.1 ± 2.86 μg/mL			
		20 wk	5.0 ± 2.45 μg/mL			

Test	Specimen	Reference Range	Factor	Reference Range (SI)	Comments
Fibrin degradation products					
Agglutination (Thrombo-Wellco test)	W special tube thrombin and proteolytic inhibitors	<10 μg/mL	× 1	<10 mg/L	
	U:2 mL in special tube (see above)	<0.25 μg/mL	× 1	<0.25 mg/L	
Fibrinogen	P(NaC)	Newborn 125–300 mg/dL	× 0.01	1.25–3.00 g/L	
		Adult 200–400 mg/dL		2.00–4.00 g/L	
Folate	S	Newborn 7.0–32 ng/mL	× 2.265	15.9–72.4 nmol/L	
		Thereafter 1.8–9 ng/mL		4.1–20.4 nmol/L	
	W(E)	150–450 ng/mL RBCs		340–1020 nmol/L cells	
Follicle-stimulating hormone (FSH)	S	M			(Endocrine Sciences)
		Tanner 1 <9.8 yr <1–3 mIU/mL	× 1	<1–3 U/L	
		Tanner 2 9.8–14.5 yr 2–7 mIU/mL		2–7 U/L	
		Tanner 3 10.7–15.4 yr 2–8 mIU/mL		2–8 U/L	
		Tanner 4 11.8–16.2 yr 2–8 mIU/mL		2–8 U/L	
		Tanner 5 12.8–17.3 yr 1–8 mIU/mL		1–8 U/L	
		Adult 1–8 mIU/mL		1–8 U/L	
		F			
		Tanner 1 <9.2 yr <1–5 mIU/mL		<1–5 U/L	
		Tanner 2 9.2–13.7 yr <1–6 mIU/mL		<1–6 U/L	
		Tanner 3 10.0–14.4 yr 1.5–9 mIU/mL		1.5–9 U/L	
		Tanner 4 10.7–15.6 yr 2–9 mIU/mL		2–9 U/L	
		Tanner 5 11.8–18.6 yr 1–9 mIU/mL		1–9 U/L	
		Adult Follicular 1–9 mIU/mL		1–9 U/L	
		Midcycle 4–30 mIU/mL		4–30 U/L	
		Luteal <1–7 mIU/mL		<1–7 U/L	
Fructosamine	S	0–3 yr 1.56–2.27 mmol/L	× 1	1.56–2.27 mmol/L	c (De Schepper et al)
		3–6 yr 1.73–2.34 mmol/L		1.73–2.34 mmol/L	
		6–9 yr 1.82–2.56 mmol/L		1.82–2.56 mmol/L	
		9–15 yr 2.02–2.63 mmol/L		2.02–2.63 mmol/L	
Galactose	S	Newborn 0–20 mg/dL	× 0.0555	0–1.11 mmol/L	
	P	5 mo–17 yr 0.0–0.5 mg/dL		0.0–0.03 mmol/L	z (Pesce et al)
	U	Newborn ≤60 mg/dL	× 0.0555	≤3.33 mmol/L	
		Thereafter 14 mg/24 hr	× 0.00555	<0.08 mmol/24 hr	
Galactose-I-PO_4	W(H)	5 mo–17 yr 0–44 μg/g Hgb	× 0.0038	0–0.17 μmol/g Hgb	v (Pesce et al)
Galactose-I-PO_4 uridylyltransferase	W(H)	18–26 U/g Hgb	× 1	18–26 U/g Hgb	(Pesce et al)
Gastrin	S(fasting)	Children <10–125 pg/mL	× 1	<10–125 ng/L	m (Dickinson et al)
Glucose	S	Cord blood 45–96 mg/dL	× 0.0555	2.5–5.3 mmol/L	
		Newborn			
		1 d 40–60 mg/dL		2.2–3.3 mmol/L	
		>1 d 50–90 mg/dL		2.8–5.0 mmol/L	
		Child 60–100 mg/dL		3.3–5.5 mmol/L	
		Adult 70–105 mg/dL		3.9–5.8 mmol/L	
	W, (H)	Adult 65–95 mg/dL		3.6–5.3 mmol/L	
	CSF	Adult 40–70 mg/dL		2.2–3.9 mmol/L	
Quantitative, enzymatic	U	<0.5 g/24 hr	× 5.55	<2.8 mmol/24 hr	
Qualitative	U	Negative		Negative	
Glucose, 2 hr pc	S	<120 mg/dL (For diabetes, see Glucose tolerance test, oral)	× 0.0555	<6.7 mmol/L	
Glucose-6-phosphate dehydrogenase in erythrocytes	W(E,H,C)				
Bishop, modified		Adult		Adult	
		3.4–8.0 U/g Hb	× 0.0645	0.22–0.52 mU/mll Hb	
		98.6–232 U/10^{12} RBC	× 10^{-3}	0.10–0.23 nU/10^6 RBC	
		1.16–2.72 U/mL RBC	× 1	1.16–2.72 kU/L RBC	
		Newborn: 50% higher		Newborn: 50% higher	

Table continued on following page

Test	Specimen	Reference Range			Factor	Reference Range (SI)		Comments
			Normal	Diabetic		Normal	Diabetic	
Glucose tolerance test (GTT), oral	S							
Adult dose: 75 g		Fasting	70–105 mg/dL	>115 mg/dL	× 0.0555	3.9–5.8 mmol/L	>6.4 mmol/L	
Child dose: 1.75 g/kg of ideal weight up to maximum of 75 g		60 min	120–170 mg/dL	≥200 mg/dL		6.7–9.4 mmol/L	≥11 mmol/L	
		90 min	100–140 mg/dL	≥200 mg/dL		5.6–7.8 mmol/L	≥11 mmol/L	
		120 min	70–120 mg/dL	≥140 mg/dL		3.9–6.7 mmol/L	≥7.8 mmol/L	
γ-Glutamyltranspeptidase (GGT, GGTP)	S	Cord blood	37–193 U/L		× 1	37–193 U/L		37° s (Knight et al)
		0–1 mo	13–147 U/L			13–147 U/L		
		1–2 mo	12–123 U/L			12–123 U/L		
		2–4 mo	8–90 U/L			8–90 U/L		
		4 mo–10 yr	5–32 U/L			5–32 U/L		
		10–15 yr	5–24 U/L			5–24 U/L		
Growth hormone (hGH, somatotropin)	S, P(E,H) Fast, at rest	Cord blood	10–50 ng/mL		× 1	10–50 µg/L		
		Newborn	10–40 ng/mL			10–40 µg/L		
		Child	<5 ng/mL			<5 µg/L		
		Adult						
		M	<5 ng/mL			<5 µg/L		
		F	<8 ng/mL			<8 µg/L		
Ham's test. See Acidified serum test								
Haptoglobin (Hp)	S							
RID		30–175 mg/dL			× 10	300–1750 mg/L		mg/L
Sephadex		40–180 mg Hb bound/dL of serum						
Nephelometry		Newborn	5–48 mg/dL		× 10	50–480 mg/L		
		Thereafter	25–175 mg/dL			250–1750 mg/L		
HDL cholesterol	S	1–13 yr	35–84 mg/dL		× 0.0259	0.9 –2.15 mmol/L		fm (Meites)
		14–19 yr	35–65 mg/dL			0.90–1.65 mmol/L		
Hematocrit (HCT, Hct)	W(E)		*Per cent Packed Red Cells (V Red Cells/V Whole Blood Cells × 100)*			*Volume Fraction (V Red Cells/ V Whole Blood)*		
Calculated from MCV and RBC (electronic displacement or laser)		1 d (capillary)	48–69%		× 0.01	0.48–0.69		
		2 d	48–75%			0.48–0.75		
		3 d	44–72%			0.44–0.72		
		2 mo	28–42%			0.28–0.42		
		6–12 yr	35–45%			0.35–0.45		
		12–18 yr						
		M	37–49%			0.37–0.49		
		F	36–46%			0.36–0.46		
		18–49 yr						
		M	41–53%			0.41–0.53		
		F	36–46%			0.36–0.46		
Hemoglobin (Hb)	W(E)	1–3 d (capillary)	14.5–22.5 g/dL		× 0.155	2.25–3.49 mmol/L		MW Hgb = 64,500
		2 mo	9.0–14.0 g/dL			1.40–2.17 mmol/L		
		6–12 yr	11.5–15.5 g/dL			1.78–2.40 mmol/L		
		12–18 yr						
		M	13.0–16.0 g/dL			2.02–2.48 mmol/L		
		F	12.0–16.0 g/dL			1.86–2.48 mmol/L		
		18–49 yr						
		M	13.5–17.5 g/dL			2.09–2.27 mmol/L		
		F	12.0–16.0 g/dL			1.86–2.48 mmol/L		
	P(H)	<10 mg/dL			× 0.155	<1.55 µmol/L		
		<3 mg/dL with butterfly set-up and 18—g needle				<0.47 µmol/L with butterfly set-up and 18-g needle		
	U	Negative				Negative		
			Per cent of Total Hemoglobin				*Fraction of Total Hemoglobin*	
Glycohemoglobin Hemoglobin A1c	W(H)	1–5 yr	2.1–7.7%		× 0.01	1–5 yr	0.021–0.077	
		5–16 yr	3.0–6.2%			5–16 yr	0.030–0.062	q (Meites)
Total glycohemoglobin	W(H)	4–16 yr	6.0–10.0%			4–16 yr	0.060–0.100	o (Meites)
Hemoglobin A	W (E,C,H)		>95%		× 0.01	Fraction of hemoglobin >0.95		
Hemoglobin A_2 (HbA_2)	W (E,O)	Adult: 1.5–3.5% (2 SD) Lower in infants <1 yr				0.015–0.035 (2 SD) mass fraction		
Hemoglobin electrophoresis	W (H,E,C)	HbA >95%			× 0.01	HbA >0.95 mass fraction		
		HbA_2 1.5–3.5%				HbA_2 0.015–.035 mass fraction		
		HbF <2%				HbF <0.02 mass fraction		

Test	Specimen	Reference Range		Factor	Reference Range (SI)	Comments
Hemoglobin (Hb) *(Continued)*						
Hemoglobin F	W (E)					
Alkali denaturation		1 d	63–92 %HbF	× 0.01	0.62–0.92 mass fraction	
		5 d	65–88 %HbF		0.65–0.88 mass fraction	
		3 wk	55–85 %HbF		0.55–0.85 mass fraction	
		6–9 wk	31–75 %HbF		0.31–0.75 mass fraction	
		3–4 mo	<2–59 %HbF		<0.02–0.59 mass fraction	
		6 mo	<2–9 %HbF		<0.02–0.09 mass fraction	
		Adult	<2 %HbF		<0.02 mass fraction	
Hemoglobin H (HbH)	W (H,E,C)					
Isopropranol precipitation		No precipitation at 40 min			No precipitation at 40 min	
Homovanillic acid	U (24-hr)	0–1 yr	<32.2 mg/g creatinine	× 0.62	< 20 mmol/mol creatinine	p (Meites)
		2–4 yr	<22 mg/g creatinine		<14 mmol/mol creatinine	
		5–19 yr	<14 mg/g creatinine		<8 mmol/mol creatinine	
17-Hydroxycorticosteroids (17-OHCS)	U	0–1 yr	0.5–1.0 mg/24 hr	× 2.76	1.4–2.8 μmol/24 hr	(Conversion based on hydrocortisone MW 362)
		Child	1.0–5.6 mg/24 hr		2.8–15.5 μmol/24 hr	
		Adult				
		M	3.0–10.0 mg/24 hr		8.2–27.6 μmol/24 hr	
		F	2.0–8.0 mg/24 hr		5.5–22 μmol/24 hr	
			or 3–7 mg/g creatinine	× 3.12	or 0.9–2.5 mmol/mol creatinine	
5-Hydroxyindoleacetic acid (5-HIAA)						
Qualitative	U	Negative			Negative	7
Quantitative	U	2–8 mg/24 hr		× 5.230	10.5–42 μmol/24 hr	
17-Hydroxyprogesterone (17-OHP)	S	1 wk	60–150 ng/dL	× 0.03029	1.82–4.54 nmol/L	
		30–60 d	M: 120–200 ng/dL		3.63–6.06 nmol/L	
			F: <150 ng/dL		<4.54 nmol/L	
		M				
		Tanner 1 <9.8 yr	3–90 ng/dL		0.09–2.73 nmol/L	
		Tanner 2 9.8–14.5 yr	5–115 ng/dL		0.15–3.48 nmol/L	
		Tanner 3 10.7–15.4 yr	10–138 ng/dL		0.30–4.18 nmol/L	
		Tanner 4 11.8–16.2 yr	29–180 ng/dL		0.88–5.45 nmol/L	
		Tanner 5 12.8–17.3 yr	24–175 ng/dL		0.73–5.30 nmol/L	
		Adult	27–199 ng/dL		0.82–6.03 nmol/L	
		F				
		Tanner 1 <9.2 yr	3–82 ng/dL		0.09–2.48 nmol/L	
		Tanner 2 9.2–13.7 yr	11–98 ng/dL		0.33–2.97 nmol/L	
		Tanner 3 10.0–14.4 yr	11–155 ng/dL		0.33–4.69 nmol/L	
		Tanner 4 10.7–15.6 yr	18–230 ng/dL		0.55–6.97 nmol/L	
		Tanner 5 11.8–18.6 yr	20–265 ng/dL		0.61–8.03 nmol/L	
		Adult Follicular	15–70 ng/dL		0.45–2.12 nmol/L	
		Luteal	35–290 ng/dL		1.06–8.78 nmol/L	
Hydroxyproline free and bound	U	3 d	33–112 μmol/24 hr	× 1	33–112 μmol/24 hr	c (Meites)
		10 d	148–225 μmol/24 hr		148–225 μmol/24 hr	
		20 d	229–310 μmol/24 hr		229–310 μmol/24 hr	
Hypoxanthine	W	12–36 hr	2.7–11.2 μmol/L	× 1	2.7–11.2 μmol/L	(Jung et al)
		3 d	1.3–7.9 μmol/L		1.3–7.9 μmol/L	
		5 d	0.6–5.7 μmol/L		0.6–5.7 μmol/L	
	CSF	0–1 mo	1.8–5.5 μmol/L		1.8–5.5 μmol/L	(Meites)
Immunoglobulin A (IgA)	S	Cord blood	1.4–3.6 mg/dL	× 10	14–36 mg/L	n (Meites)
		1–3 mo	1.3–53 mg/dL		13–530 mg/L	
		4–6 mo	4.4–84 mg/dL		44–840 mg/L	
		7 mo–1 yr	11–106 mg/dL		110–1,060 mg/L	
		2–5 yr	14–159 mg/dL		140–1,590 mg/L	
		6–10 yr	33–236 mg/dL		330–2,360 mg/L	
		Adult	70–312 mg/dL		700–3,120 mg/L	
Immunoglobulin D (IgD)	S	Newborn	None detected	× 10	None detected	
		Thereafter	0–8 mg/dL		0–80 mg/L	
Immunoglobulin E (IgE)	S	M	0–230 IU/mL	× 1	0–230 kIU/L	
		F	0–170 IU/mL		0–170 kIU/L	
Immunoglobulin G (IgG)	S	Cord blood	636–1,606 mg/dL	× 0.01	6.36–16.06 g/L	n (Meites)
		1 mo	251–906 mg/dL		2.51–9.06 g/L	
		2–4 mo	176–601 mg/dL		1.76–6.01 g/L	
		5–12 mo	172–1,069 mg/dL		1.72–10.69 g/L	
		1–5 yr	345–1,236 mg/dL		3.45–12.36 g/L	
		6–10 yr	608–1,572 mg/dL		6.08–15.72 g/L	
		Adult	639–1,349 mg/dL		6.39–13.49 g/L	

Table continued on following page

Test	Specimen		Reference Range	Factor	Reference Range (SI)	Comments
Immunoglobulin M (IgM)	S	Cord blood	6.3–25 mg/dL	× 10	63–250 mg/L	n (Meites)
		1 mo–4 mo	17–105 mg/dL		170–1,050 mg/L	
		5 mo–9 mo	33–126 mg/dL		330–1,260 mg/L	
		10 mo–1 yr	41–173 mg/dL		410–1,730 mg/L	
		2–8 yr	43–207 mg/dL		430–2,070 mg/L	
		9–10 yr	52–242 mg/dL		520–2,420 mg/L	
		Adult	56–352 mg/dL		560–3,520 mg/L	
Insulin (12-hr fasting)	S	Newborn	3–20 μU/mL	× 1.0	3–20 mU/L	
		Thereafter	7–24 μU/mL		7–24 mU/L	
Insulin with oral glucose tolerance test	S		Insulin			
		0 min	7–24 μU/mL	× 1	7–24 mU/L	
		30 min	25–231 μU/mL		25–231 mU/L	
		60 min	18–276 μU/mL		18–276 mU/L	
		120 min	16–166 μU/mL		16–166 mU/L	
		180 min	4–38 μU/mL		4–38 mU/L	
Iron	S	Newborn	100–250 μg/dL	× 0.179	17.90–44.75 μmol/L	
		Infant	40–100 μg/dL		7.16–17.90 μmol/L	
		Child	50–120 μg/dL		8.95–21.48 μmol/L	
		Thereafter				
		M	50–160 μg/dL		8.95–28.64 μmol/L	
		F	40–150 μg/dL		7.16–26.85 μmol/L	
		Intoxicated child	280–2,550 μg/dL		50.12–456.5 μmol/L	
		Fatally poisoned child	>1,800 μg/dL		>322.2 μmol/L	
Iron-binding capacity, total (TIBC)	S	Infant	100–400 μg/dL	× 0.179	17.90–71.60 μmol/L	
		Thereafter	250–400 μg/dL		44.75–71.60 μmol/L	
17-Ketogenic steroids (17-KGS)	U	0–1 yr	<1.0 mg/24 hr	× 3.467	<3.5 μmol/24 hr	Conversion based on dehydroepiandrosterone, MW 288
		1–10 yr	<5 mg/24 hr		<17 μmol/24 hr	
		11–14 yr	<12 mg/24 hr		<42 μmol/24 hr	
		Thereafter				
		M	5–23 mg/24 hr		17–80 μmol/24 hr	
		F	3–15 mg/24 hr		10–52 μmol/24 hr	
Ketone bodies						
Qualitative	S	Negative			Negative	
	U	Negative			Negative	
Quantitative	S	0.5–3.0 mg/dL		× 10	5–30 mg/L	
17 Ketosteroid (17-KS), total	U	14 d–2 yr	<1 mg/24 hr	× 3.467	<3.5 μmol/24 hr	
		2–6 yr	<2 mg/24 hr		< 7 μmol/24 hr	
		6–10 yr	1–4 mg/24 hr		3.5–14 μmol/24 hr	
		10–12 yr	1–6 mg/24 hr		3.5–21 μmol/24 hr	Zimmerman reaction Conversion based on dehydroepiandrosterone, MW 288
		12–14 yr	3–10 mg/24 hr		10–35 μmol/24 hr	
		14–16 yr	5–12 mg/24 hr		17–42 μmol/24 hr	
		Thereafter				
		M, 18–30 yr	9–22 mg/24 hr		31–76 μmol/24 hr	
		>30 yr	8–20 mg/24 hr		28–70 μmol/24 hr	
		F, decreases with age	6–15 mg/24 hr		21–52 μmol/24 hr Decreases with age	

Test	Specimen		*M (mg/dL)*	*F (mg/dL)*	Factor	*M (mmol/L)*	*F (mmol/L)*	Comments
LDL-Cholesterol (LDLC)	S, P(E)	Cord blood	10–50	10–50	× 0.0259	0.26–1.30	0.26–1.30	
		1–9 yr	60–140	60–150		1.55–3.63	1.55–3.89	
		10–19 yr	50–170	50–170		1.30–4.40	1.30–4.40	
		20–29 yr	60–175	60–160		1.55–4.53	1.55–4.14	
		30–39 yr	80–190	70–170		2.07–4.92	1.81–4.40	
		40–49 yr	90–205	80–190		2.33–5.31	2.07–4.92	
		Recommended (desirable) range for adults	<130 mg/dl			1.68–4.53 mg/dL		

Test	Specimen		Reference Range	Factor	Reference Range (SI)	Comments
Lactate						
L(+)-lactate	W(H)	Venous	0.5–2.2 mmol/L		0.5–2.2 mmol/L	
		Arterial	0.5–1.6 mmol/L		0.5–1.6 mmol/L	
		Inpatients				
		Venous	0.9–1.7 mmol/L		0.9–1.7 mmol/L	
		Arterial	<1.25 mmol/L		<1.25 mmol/L	
D(−)-lactate	P(H)	6 mo–3 yr	0.0–0.3 mmol/L	× 1	0.0–0.3 mmol/L	z (Rosenthal et al)

Test	Specimen	Reference Range		Factor	Reference Range (SI)	Comments
Lactate dehydrogenase (LD)	S	<1 yr	170–580 U/L	× 1	170–580 U/L	37° m (Meites)
		1–9 yr	150–500 U/L		150–500 U/L	
		10–19 yr	120–330 U/L		120–330 U/L	
Isoenzymes	S		*Percentage of Total Activity*			(Meites)
			1–6 yr / *7–19 yr*			
		LD1	20–38 / 20–35			
		LD2	27–38 / 31–38			
		LD3	16–26 / 19–28			
		LD4	5–16 / 7–13			
		LD5	3–13 / 5–12			
Lead	W(H)	Child	<10 μg/dL	× 0.0483	<0.48 μmol/L	
		Adult	<40 μg/dL		<1.93 μmol/L	
		Acceptable for industrial exposure	<60 μg/dL		<2.90 μmol/L	
		Toxic	≥100 μg/dL		≥4.83 μmol/L	
	U (24-hr)	<80 μg/L		× 0.00483	<0.39 μmol/L	
Lecithin/sphingomyelin (L/S) ratio	AF	2.0–5.0 indicates probable fetal lung maturity (>3.0 IDM)			2.0–5.0 indicates probable fetal lung maturity	
Lecithin phosphorus	AF	>0.10 mg/dL indicates probably adequate fetal lung maturity		× 0.3229	>0.33 mmol/L indicates probably adequate fetal lung maturity	
Leukocyte count (WBC)	W(E)		× 1,000 cells/mm^3 (μL)		× 10^9 cells/L	
		Birth	9.0–30.0		9.0–30.0	
		24 hr	9.4–34.0		9.4–34.0	
		1 mo	5.0–19.5		5.0–19.5	
		1–3 yr	6.0–17.5		6.0–17.5	
		4–7 yr	5.5–15.5		5.5–15.5	
		8–13 yr	4.5–13.5		4.5–13.5	
		Adult	4.5–11.0		4.5–11.0	
Cell count	CSF	Premature	0–25 mononuclear cells/μL	× 10^6	0–25 × 10^6 cells/L	
			0–10 polymorphonuclear cells/μL		0–10 × 10^6 cells/L	
			0–1,000 RBC/μL		0–1,000 × 10^6 cells/L	
		Newborn	0–20 mononuclear cells/μL		0–20 × 10^6 cells/L	
			0–10 polymorphonuclear cells/μL		0–10 × 10^6 cells/L	
			0–800 RBC/μL		0–800 × 10^6 cells/L	
		Neonate	0–5 mononuclear cells/μL		0–5 × 10^6 cells/L	
			0–10 polymorphonuclear cells/μL		0–10 × 10^6 cells/L	
			0–50 RBC/μL		0–50 × 10^6 cells/L	
		Thereafter	0–5 mononuclear cells/μL (numbers of cells in very young infants are greater than those in the CSF of older individuals without substantial implications for growth and development in most instances)		0–5 cells/L	
Leukocyte differential	W(E)					
Myelocytes		0		× 0.01	0	
Neutrophils—"bands"		3–5%			0.03–0.05 no. fraction	
Neutrophils—"segs"		54–62%			0.54–0.62 no. fraction	
Lymphocytes		25–33%			0.25–0.33 no. fraction	
Monocytes		3–7%			0.03–0.07 no. fraction	
Eosinophils		1–3%			0.01–0.03 no. fraction	
Basophils		0–0.75%			0–0.0075 no. fraction	
Leukocyte differential		*Cells/mm^3 (μL)*				
Myelocytes		0		× 1	0 × 10^6 cells/L	
Neutrophils—"bands"		150–400			150–400 × 10^6 cells/L	
Neutrophils—"segs"		3,000–5,800			3,000–5,800 × 10^6 cells/L	
Lymphocytes		1,500–3,000			1,500–3,000 × 10^6 cells/L	
Monocytes		285–500			285–500 × 10^6 cells/L	
Eosinophils		50–250			50–250 × 10^6 cells/L	
Basophils		15–50			15–50 × 10^6 cells/L	
Lymphocytes	CSF		62% ± 34%	× 0.01	0.62 ± 0.34 no. fraction	
Monocytes			36% ± 20%		0.36 ± 0.20 no fraction	
Neutrophils			2% ± 5%		0.02 ± 0.05 no. fraction	
Histiocytes			0–rare		0–rare	
Ependymal cells			0–rare		0–rare	
Eosinophils			0–rare		0–rare	
Lipase	S	1–4 yr	18–95 U/L	× 1	18–95 U/L	37° (Meites)
		5–14 yr	21–128 U/L		21–128 U/L	
		15–19 yr	28–149 U/L		28–149 U/L	

Table continued on following page

Test	Specimen	Reference Range	Factor	Reference Range (SI)	Comments
Lipoprotein electrophoresis	S	Distinct β band; negligible chylomicron and pre-β bands			
Lithium. See end of table under Drugs					
Long-acting thyroid-stimulating hormone (LATS)	S	Undetectable		Undetectable	
Luteinizing hormone (LH)	S	M			(Endocrine Sciences)
		Tanner 1 <9.8 yr <1–4 mIU/mL	× 1	<1–4 U/L	
		Tanner 2 9.8–14.5 yr <1–5 mIU/mL		<1–5 U/L	
		Tanner 3 10.7–15.4 yr 2–10 mIU/mL		2–10 U/L	
		Tanner 4 11.8–16.2 yr 2–10 mIU/mL		2–10 U/L	
		Tanner 5 12.8–17.3 yr 4.5–11 mIU/mL		4.5–11 U/L	
		Adult 3–10 mIU/mL		3–10 U/L	
		F			
		Tanner 1 <9.2 yr <1–4 mIU/mL		<1–4 mIU/L	
		Tanner 2 9.2–13.7 yr <1–5 mIU/mL		<1–5 U/L	
		Tanner 3 10.0–14.4 yr <1–10 mIU/mL		<1–10 U/L	
		Tanner 4 10.7–15.6 yr 3–11 mIU/mL		3–11 U/L	
		Tanner 5 11.8–18.6 yr 2–12 mIU/mL		2–12 U/L	
		Adult Follicular 3–11 mIU/mL		3–11 U/L	
		Midcycle 18–70 mIU/mL		18–70 U/L	
		Luteal 2–11 mIU/mL		2–11 U/L	
Lymphocyte subpopulations	W(H)	*Percentage of Mononuclear Cells in Adults*		*Fraction of Mononuclear Cells in Adults*	
Total T cells (OKT3)		43–69	× 0.01	0.43–0.69	1 (Landry et al)
Helper T cells (OKT4)		26–55		0.26–0.55	
Suppressor T cells (OKT8)		9–28		0.09–0.28	
Total B cells (HB2)		5–17		0.05–0.17	
Monocytes (MMA)		8–32		0.08–0.32	
Natural killer cells (HNK)		5–20		0.05–0.20	
Lysergic acid diethylamide. See end of table under Drugs					
Magnesium	P(H)	0–6 d 1.2–2.6 mg/dL	× 0.411	0.48–1.05 mmol/L	d (Meites)
		7 d–2 yr 1.6–2.6 mg/dL		0.65–1.05 mmol/L	
		2–14 yr 1.5–2.3 mg/dL		0.60–0.95 mmol/L	
	U (24-hr)	1–6 mo			
		Breast-fed 0.04–1.55 mmol/L	× 1	0.04–1.55 mmol/L	
		Formula-fed 0.04–1.40 mmol/L		0.04–1.55 mmol/L	
Mean corpuscular hemoglobin (MCH)	W(E)	Birth 31–37 pg/cell	× 0.0155	0.48–0.57 fmol/cell	
		1–3 d (capillary) 31–37 pg/cell		0.48–0.57 fmol/cell	
		1 wk–1 mo 28–40 pg/cell		0.43–0.62 fmol/cell	
		2 mo 26–34 pg/cell		0.40–0.53 fmol/cell	
		3–6 mo 25–35 pg/cell		0.39–0.54 fmol/cell	
		0.5–2 yr 23–31 pg/cell		0.36–0.48 fmol/cell	
		2–6 yr 24–30 pg/cell		0.37–0.47 fmol/cell	
		6–12 yr 25–33 pg/cell		0.39–0.51 fmol/cell	
		12–18 yr 25–35 pg/cell		0.39–0.54 fmol/cell	
		18–49 yr 26–34 pg/cell		0.40–0.53 fmol/cell	
Mean corpuscular hemoglobin concentration (MCHC)	W(E)	*Percentage Hb/cell or g Hb/dL RBC*		*mmol Hb/L RBC*	
		Birth 30–36	× 0.155	4.65–5.58	
		1–3 d (capillary) 29–37		4.50–5.74	
		1–2 wk 28–38		4.34–5.89	
		1–2 mo 29–37		4.50–5.74	
		3 mo–2 yr 30–36		4.65–5.58	
		2–18 yr 31–37		4.81–5.74	
		>18 yr 31–37		4.81–5.74	
Mean corpuscular volume (MCV)	W(E)	1–3 d (capillary) 95–121 μm^3	× 1	95–121 fL	
		0.5–2 yr 70–86 μm^3		70–86 fL	
		6–12 yr 77–95 μm^3		77–95 fL	
		12–18 yr			
		M 78–98 μm^3		78–98 fL	
		F 78–102 μm^3		78–102 fL	
		18–49 yr			
		M 80–100 μm^3		80–100 fL	
		F 80–100 μm^3		80–100 fL	

Test	Specimen	Reference Range		Factor	Reference Range (SI)	Comments
Metanephrines, total	U (24-hr)	<1 yr	<15.9 µmol/g creatinine	× 0.1131	<1.80 mmol/mol creatinine	(Meites)
		1–2 yr	<14.8 µmol/g creatinine		<1.67 mmol/mol creatinine	
		3–4 yr	<12.8 µmol/g creatinine		<1.45 mmol/mol creatinine	
		5–8 yr	<11.7 µmol/g creatinine		<1.32 mmol/mol creatinine	
		9–13 yr	<10.5 µmol/g creatinine		<1.19 mmol/mol creatinine	
Methemoglobin (MetHb)	W(E,H,C)	0.06–0.24 g/dL or		× 155	9.3–37.2 µmol/L	
		0.78 ± 0.37% of total Hb		× 0.01	0.0078 ± 0.0037 (mass fraction)	
Methylmalonic acid	U	6–12 wk	0–57 mg/g creatinine	× 0.9579	0–55 mmol/mol creatinine	h (Meites)
Microsomal antibodies, thyroid. See Thyroid microsomal antibodies						
Mucopolysaccharides	U	<2 yr	<50 µg/g creatinine	× 0.1131	<5.7 mg/mmol creatinine	(Meites)
		2–4 yr	<25 µg/g creatinine		<2.8 mg/mmol creatinine	
		4–15 yr	<20 µg/g creatinine		<2.3 mg/mmol creatinine	
Myoglobin	S	6–85 ng/mL		× 1	6–85 pg/L	
	U	Negative			Negative	
Niacin (nicotinic acid)	U	0.3–1.5 mg/24 hr		× 8.113	2.43–12.17 µmol/24 hr	
Occult blood	F	Negative (<2 mL blood/24 hr in ~100–200 g stool)			Negative	
	U	Negative			Negative	
Organic acids	U	ADULT				(Hoffman et al)
Lactic		115–407 µM/g creatinine		× 8.8402	13–46 mmol/mol creatinine	
2-Hydroxyisobutyric		not detected			not detected	
Glycolic		159–486 µM/g creatinine			18–55 mmol/mol creatinine	
3-Hydroxybutyric		not detected–18 µM/g creatinine			not detected–2.0 mmol/mol creatinine	
3-Hydroxyisobutyric		36–168 µM/g creatinine			4.1–19 mmol/mol creatinine	
2-Hydroxyisovaleric		not detected			not detected	
3-Hydroxyisovaleric		61–221 µM/g creatinine			6.9–25 mmol/mol creatinine	
Methylmalonic		not detected			not detected	
4-Hydroxybutyric		2.7–51 µM/g creatinine			0.3–5.8 mmol/mol creatinine	
Ethylmalonic		3.5–37 µM/g creatinine			0.4–4.2 mmol/mol creatinine	
Succinic		4.4–141 µM/g creatinine			0.5–16 mmol/mol creatinine	
Fumaric		1.8–7 µM/g creatinine			0.2–0.8 mmol/mol creatinine	
Glutaric		5.3–23 µM/g creatinine			0.6–2.6 mmol/mol creatinine	
3-Methylglutaric		not detected			not detected	
Adipic		7–309 µM/g creatinine			0.8–35 mmol/mol creatinine	
Pyruvic		23–70 µM/g creatinine			2.6–7.9 mmol/mol creatinine	
Pyroglutamic		8–557 µM/g creatinine			0.9–63 µM/g creatinine	
2-Oxoisovaleric		not detected			not detected	
Acetoacetic		not detected			not detected	
Mevalonic		0.5–1.9 µM/g creatinine			0.06–0.22 mmol/mol creatinine	
2-Hydroxyglutaric		7–460 µM/g creatinine			0.8–52 mmol/mol creatinine	
3-Hydroxy-3-methylglutaric		not detected–88			not detected–10 mmol/mol creatinine	
p-Hydroxyphenylacetic		31–195 µM/g creatinine			3.5–22 mmol/mol creatinine	
2-Oxoisocaproic		not detected			not detected	
Suberic		not detected–26 µM/g creatinine			not detected–2.9 mmol/mol creatinine	
Orotic		not detected			not detected	
cis-Aconitic		24–389 µM/g creatinine			2.7–44 mmol/mol creatinine	
Homovanillic		8–49 µM/g creatinine			0.9–5.5 mmol/mol creatinine	
Azeleic		11–137 µM/g creatinine			1.3–5.5 mmol/mol creatinine	
Isocitric		318–743 µM/g creatinine			36–84 mmol/mol creatinine	
Citric		619–1998 µM/g creatinine			70–226 mmol/mol creatinine	
Sebacic		not detected			not detected	
4-Hydroxyphenyl lactic		1.8–23 µM/g creatinine			0.2–2.6 mmol/mol creatinine	
2-Oxoglutaric		35–654 µM/g creatinine			4–74 mmol/mol creatinine	
5-Hydroxyindoleacetic		not detected–64 µM/g creatinine			not detected–7.2 mmol/mol creatinine	
Succinylacetone		not detected			not detected	
Orotic acid	U	0–20.1 mg/g creatinine		× 0.7247	0–14.6 mmol/mol creatinine	cm (Meites)
Osmolality	S	Child and adult	275–295 mOsm/kg H_2O			
	U	50–1,400 mOsm/kg H_2O, depending on fluid intake. After 12 hr of fluid restriction, normal range is >850 mOsm/kg H_2O				
	U (24-hr)	300–900 mOsm/kg H_2O				

Table continued on following page

Test	Specimen	Reference Range		Factor	Reference Range (SI)		Comments
Osmotic fragility test (RBC fragility) pH 7.4, 20° C	W(H)	*NaCl*	*Per cent Hemolysis*		*NaCl*	*Hemolyzed Fraction*	
		0.30 g/dL	97–100	× 0.01 (Hemolyzed fraction)	3.0 g/L	0.97–1.00	
		0.35 g/dL	90–99		3.5 g/L	0.90–0.99	
		0.40 g/dL	50–95		4.0 g/L	0.50–0.95	
		0.45 g/dL	5–45		4.5 g/L	0.05–0.45	
		0.50 g/dL	0–6		5.0 g/L	0.00–0.06	
		0.55 g/dL	0		5.5 g/L	0.00	
Sterile incubation at 37° C		*NaCl*	*Per cent Hemolysis*		*NaCl*	*Hemolyzed Fraction*	
		0.20 g/dL	95–100	× 0.01 (Hemolized fraction)	2.0 g/L	0.95–1.00	
		0.30 g/dL	85–100		3.0 g/L	0.85–1.00	
		0.35 g/dL	75–100		3.5 g/L	0.75–1.00	
		0.40 g/dL	65–100		4.0 g/L	0.65–1.00	
		0.45 g/dL	55–95		4.5 g/L	0.55–0.95	
		0.50 g/dL	40–85		5.0 g/L	0.40–0.85	
		0.55 g/dL	15–70		5.5 g/L	0.15–0.70	
		0.60 g/dL	0–40		6.0 g/L	0.00–0.40	
		0.65 g/dL	0–10		6.5 g/L	0.00–0.10	
		0.70 g/dL	0–5		7.0 g/L	0.00–0.05	
		0.85 g/dL	0		8.5 g/L	0.00	
Oxygen, partial pressure of (Po_2)	W(H), arterial	Birth	8–24 mm Hg	× 0.133	1.1–3.2 kPa		
		5–10 min	33–75 mm Hg		4.4–10.0 kPa		
		30 min	31–85 mm Hg		4.1–11.3 kPa		
		>1 hr	55–80 mm Hg		7.3–10.6 kPa		
		1 d	54–95 mm Hg		7.2–12.6 kPa		
		Thereafter (decreases with age)	83–108 mm Hg		11–14.4 kPa		
Oxygen saturation	W(H), arterial	Newborn	85–90%	× 0.01	0.85–0.90 Saturated fraction		
		Thereafter	95–99%		0.95–0.99 Saturated fraction		
Po_2. See Oxygen, partial pressure							
Po_2 at half saturation (Po_2 [0.5] or P_{50})	W(H), arterial	25–29 mm Hg		× 0.133	3.3–3.9 kPa		
Paraldehyde. See end of table under Drugs							
Parathyroid hormone	S						
C-terminal (mid-molecule)		1–16 yr	51–217 pg/mL	× 0.1053	5.4–22.8 pmol/L		m (Nichols Institute)
Intact (IRMA)		1–18 yr	1–43 pg/mL		0.1–4.5 pmol/L		
Intact N-terminal specific		2–13 yr	14–21 pg/mL		1.5–2.2 pmol/L		
Partial thromboplastin time (PTT)	W(NaC)						
Nonactivated		60–85 s (Platelin)			60–85 s		
Activated		25–35 s (differs with method)			25–35 s		
pH	W(H), arterial				*H+ Concentration*		
		Premature (48 hr)	7.35–7.50		31–44 nmol/L		
		Birth, full-term	7.11–7.36		43–77 nmol/L		
		5–10 min	7.09–7.30		50–81 nmol/L		
		30 min	7.21–7.38		41–61 nmol/L		
		>1 hr	7.26–7.49		32–54 nmol/L		
		1 d	7.29–7.45		35–51 nmol/L		
		Thereafter	7.35–7.45		35–44 nmol/L		
		Must be corrected for body temperature					
	U	Newborn/neonate	5–7		0.1–10 μmol/L		
		Thereafter (average 6)	4.5–8		0.01–32 μmol/L (average 1.0 μmol/L)		
	F		7.0–7.5		31–100 nmol/L		
Phenacetin. See end of table under Drugs							
Phenobarbital. See end of table under Drugs							
Phensuximide. See end of table under Drugs							

Test	Specimen	Reference Range	Factor	Reference Range (SI)	Comments
Phenylalanine	S	Premature 2.0–7.5 mg/dL	× 60.54	120–450 μmol/L	
		Newborn 1.2–3.4 mg/dL		70–210 μmol/L	
		Thereafter 0.8–1.8 mg/dL		50–110 μmol/L	
	U	10 d–2 wk 1–2 mg/24 hr	× 6.054	6–12 μmol/24 hr	
		3–12 yr 4–18 mg/24 hr		24–110 μmol/24 hr	
		Thereafter trace–17 mg/24 hr		trace–103 μmol/24 hr	
Phenylpyruvic acid, qualitative	U	Negative by $FeCl_3$ test		Negative by $FeCl_3$ test	
Phenytoin. See end of table under Drugs					
Phosphatase, acid					
Prostatic (RIA)	S	<3.0 ng/mL	× 1	<3.0 μg/L	
Roy Brower and Hayden 37° C		0.11–0.60 U/L		0.11–0.60 U/L	
Phosphatase, alkaline	S	1–9 yr 145–200 U/L	× 1	1–9 yr 145–420 U/L	37° C md (Lockitch et al)
		10–11 yr 130–560 U/L		10–11 yr 130–560 U/L	
		M / *F*		*M* / *F*	
		12–13 yr 200–495 U/L / 150–420 U/L		12–13 yr 200–495 U/L / 105–420 U/L	
		14–15 yr 130–525 U/L / 70–230 U/L		14–15 yr 130–525 U/L / 70–230 U/L	
		16–19 yr 65–260 U/L / 50–130 U/L		16–19 yr 65–260 U/L / 50–130 U/L	
Phospholipids, total	S, P(E)	Newborn 75–170 mg/dL	× 0.01	0.75–1.70 g/L	
		Infant 100–275 mg/dL		1.00–2.75 g/L	
		Child 180–295 mg/dL		1.80–2.95 g/L	
		Adult 125–275 mg/dL		1.25–2.75 g/L	
Phosphorus, inorganic	S, P(H)	0–5 d 4.8–8.2 mg/dL	× 0.3229	1.55–2.65 mmol/L	d (Meites)
		1–3 yr 3.8–6.5 mg/dL		1.25–2.10 mmol/L	
		4–11 yr 3.7–5.6 mg/dL		1.20–1.80 mmol/L	
		12–15 yr 2.9–5.4 mg/dL		0.95–1.75 mmol/L	
		16–19 yr 2.7–4.7 mg/dL		0.90–1.50 mmol/L	
Plasma volume	P(H)	M 25–43 mL/kg	× 0.001	M 0.025–0.043 L/kg	
		F 28–45 mL/kg		F 0.028–0.045 L/kg	
Platelet count (thrombocyte count)	W(E)	Newborn 84–478 × $10^3/mm^3$ (μL) (after 1 wk same as adult)	× 10^6	84–478 × 10^9/L	
		Adult 150–400 × $10^3/mm^3$ (μL)		150–400 × 10^9/L	
Porphobilinogen (PBG)					
Quantitative	U	0–2.0 mg/24 hr	× 4.42	0–8.8 μmol/24 hr	
Qualitative	U	Negative		Negative	
Potassium	S	<2 yr 3.0–6.0 mmol/L	× 1	3.0–6.0 mmol/L	w (Meites)
		2–12 yr 3.5–7.0 mmol/L		3.5–7.0 mmol/L	
		>12 yr 3.5–5.0 mmol/L		3.5–5.0 mmol/L	
	p(H)	3.4–4.5 mmol/L		3.5–4.5 mmol/L	
	U (24-hr)	2.5–125 mmol/L (varies with diet)		2.5–125 mmol/L (varies with diet)	
Prealbumin (transthyretin)	P	2–6 mo 142–330 mg/L	× 1	142–330 mg/L	n (Sherry et al)
		6–12 mo 120–274 mg/L		120–274 mg/L	
		1–3 yr 108–259 mg/L		108–259 mg/L	
Pregnanetriol	U	2 wk–2 yr 0.02–0.2 mg/24 hr	× 2.972	0.06–0.6 μmol/24 hr	
		2–5 yr <0.5 mg/24 hr		<1.5 μmol/24 hr	
		5–15 yr <1.5 mg/24 hr		<4.5 μmol/24 hr	
		>15 yr <2.0 mg/24 hr		<5.9 μmol/24 hr	
Primidone. See end of table under Drugs					
Progesterone	S	M			(Endocrine Sciences)
		Tanner 1 <9.8 yr <10–33 ng/dL	× 0.03180	<0.32–1.05 nmol/L	
		Tanner 2 9.8–14.5 yr <10–33 ng/dL		<0.32–1.05 nmol/L	
		Tanner 3 10.7–15.4 yr <10–48 ng/dL		<0.32–1.53 nmol/L	
		Tanner 4 11.8–16.2 yr 10–108 ng/dL		0.32–3.43 nmol/L	
		Tanner 5 12.8–17.3 yr 21–82 ng/dL		0.67–2.61 nmol/L	
		Adult 13–97 ng/dL		0.41–3.08 nmol/L	

Table continued on following page

Test	Specimen	Reference Range		Factor	Reference Range (SI)	Comments
Progesterone *(Continued)*		F				
		Tanner 1 <9.2 yr	<10–33 ng/dL		<0.32–1.05 nmol/L	
		Tanner 2 9.2–13.7 yr	<10–55 ng/dL		<0.32–1.75 nmol/L	
		Tanner 3 10.0–14.4 yr	10–450 ng/dL		0.32–14.31 nmol/L	
		Tanner 4 10.7–15.6 yr	<10–1,300 ng/dL		<0.32–41.34 nmol/L	
		Tanner 5 11.8–18.6 yr	<10–950 ng/dL		<0.32–30.21 nmol/L	
		Adult Follicular	15–70 ng/dL		0.48–2.23 nmol/L	
		Luteal	200–2,500 ng/dL		6.36–79.50 nmol/L	
Prolactin	S	M	3–18 ng/mL	× 0.0426	M 0.13–0.77 nmol/L	(Endocrine Sciences)
		F	3–24 ng/mL		F 0.13–1.02 nmol/L	
		Higher in newborn infants			Higher in newborn infants	
Propranolol. See end of table under Drugs						
Protein						
Total	S	Premature	4.3–7.6 g/dL	× 10	43–76 g/L	
		Newborn	4.6–7.4 g/dL		46–74 g/L	
		1–7 yr	6.1–7.9 g/dL	× 10	61–79 g/L	(Meites)
		8–12 yr	6.4–8.1 g/dL		64–81 g/L	
		13–19 yr	6.6–8.2 g/dL		66–82 g/L	
Electrophoresis	S					
Albumin		Premature	3.0–4.2 g/dL		30–42 g/L	
		Newborn	3.6–5.4 g/dL		36–54 g/L	
		Infant	4.0–5.0 g/dL		40–50 g/L	
		Thereafter	3.5–5.0 g/dL		35–50 g/L	
α_1-Globulin		Premature	0.1–0.5 g/dL		1–5 g/L	
		Newborn	0.1–0.3 g/dL		1–3 g/L	
		Infant	0.2–0.4 g/dL		2–4 g/L	
		Thereafter	0.2–0.3 g/dL		2–3 g/L	
α_2-Globulin		Premature	0.3–0.7 g/dL		3–7 g/L	
		Newborn	0.3–0.5 g/dL		3–5 g/L	
		Infant	0.5–0.8 g/dL		5–8 g/L	
		Thereafter	0.4–1.0 g/dL		4–10 g/L	
β-Globulin		Premature	0.3–1.2 g/dL		3–12 g/L	
		Newborn	0.2–0.6 g/dL		2–6 g/L	
		Infant	0.5–0.8 g/dL		5–8 g/L	
		Thereafter	0.5–1.1 g/dL		5–11 g/L	
γ-Globulin		Premature	0.3–1.4 g/dL		3–4 g/L	
		Newborn	0.2–1.0 g/dL		2–10 g/L	
		Infant	0.3–1.2 g/dL		3–12 g/L	
		Thereafter (higher in blacks)	0.7–1.2 g/dL		7–12 g/L (higher in blacks)	
Protein Total urinary	U (24-hr)	1–14 mg/dL			10–140 mg/L	
		50–80 mg/24 hr (at rest)			50–80 mg/24 hr	
		<250 mg/24 hr after intense exercise			<250 mg/24 hr after intense exercise	
Electrophoresis			*Average Total Protein*		*Fraction of Total Protein*	
Albumin			37.9%	× 0.01	0.379	
α_1-globulin			27.3%		0.273	
α_2-globulin			19.5%		0.195	
β-globulin			8.8%		0.088	
γ-globulin			3.3%		0.033	
Protein						
Total protein (column)	CSF	Lumbar	8–32 mg/dL	× 10	80–320 mg/L	
Turbidimetry		Lumbar				
		Premature	40–300 mg/dL		400–3,000 mg/L	
		Newborn	45–120 mg/dL		450–1,200 mg/L	
		Child	10–20 mg/dL		100–200 mg/L	
		Adolescent	15–20 mg/dL		150–200 mg/L	
		Thereafter	15–45 mg/dL		150–450 mg/L	
Electrophoresis						
		Prealbumin	2–7% of total	× 0.01	0.02–0.07 fraction of total	
		Albumin	56–76% of total		0.56–0.76 fraction of total	
		α_1-Globulin	2–7% of total		0.02–0.07 fraction of total	
		α_2-Globulin	4–12% of total		0.04–0.12 fraction of total	
		β-Globulin	8–18% of total		0.08–0.18 fraction of total	
		γ-Globulin	3–12% of total		0.03–0.12 fraction of total	

Test	Specimen	Reference Range		Factor	Reference Range (SI)		Comments
Prothrombin time (PT)							
One-stage (quick)	W(NaC)	In general, 11–15 s (varies with type of thromboplastin)			11–15 s		
		Newborn: prolonged by 2–3 s			Newborn: prolonged by 2–3 s		
Two-stage modified (Ware and Seegers)	W(NaC)	18–22 s			18–22 s		
Quinidine. See end of table under Drugs							
RBC count. See Erythrocyte count							
RBC fragility. See Osmotic fragility							
Red cell volume	W(H)	M	20–36 mL/kg	× 0.001	M	0.020–0.036 L/kg	
		F	19–31 mL/kg		F	0.019–0.031 L/kg	
Renin (renin activity, plasma; PRA)	P(E)	0–3 yr	<16.6 ng/mL/hr	× 1	<16.6 μg/L/hr		
		3–6 yr	<6.7 ng/mL/hr		<6.7 μg/L/hr		
		6–9 yr	<4.4 ng/mL/hr		<4.4 μg/L/hr		
		9–12 yr	<5.9 ng/mL/hr		<5.9 μg/L/hr		
		12–15 yr	<4.2 ng/mL/hr		<4.2 μg/L/hr		
		15–18 yr	<4.3 ng/mL/hr		<4.3 μg/L/hr		
		Normal sodium diet					
		Supine	0.2–2.5 ng/mL/hr		0.2–2.5 μg/L/hr		
		Upright	0.3–4.3 ng/mL/hr		0.3–4.3 μg/L/hr		
		Low sodium diet					
		Upright	2.9–24 ng/mL/hr		2.9–24 μg/L/hr		
Reticulocyte count	W (E,H,O)	Adults 0.5–1.5% of erythrocytes, or		× 0.01	0.005–0.015 number fraction		
		25,000–75,000/mm^3 (μL)		× 10^6	25,000–75,000 × 10^6/L		
	W (capillary)	1 d	0.4–6.0%	× 0.01	0.004–0.060 number fraction		
		7 d	<0.1–1.3%		<0.001–0.013 number fraction		
		1–4 wk	<1.0–1.2%		<0.001–0.012 number fraction		
		5–6 wk	<0.1–2.4%		<0.001–0.024 number fraction		
		7–8 wk	0.1–2.9%		0.001–0.029 number fraction		
		9–10 wk	<0.1–2.6%		<0.001–0.026 number fraction		
		11–12 wk	0.1–1.3%		0.001–0.013 number fraction		
Retinol-binding protein (RBP)	S	0–5 d	0.8–4.5 mg/dL	× 10	8–45 mg/L		n (Lockitch et al)
		1–9 yr	1.0–7.8 mg/dL		10–78 mg/L		
		10–13 yr	1.3–9.9 mg/dL		13–99 mg/L		
		14–19 yr	3.0–9.2 mg/dL		30–92 mg/L		
Reverse triiodothyronine (rT_3)	S	1–5 yr	15–71 ng/dL	× 0.0154	0.23–1.1 nmol/L		
		5–10 yr	17–79 ng/dL		0.26–1.2 nmol/L		
		10–15 yr	19–88 ng/dL		0.29–1.36 nmol/L		
		Adults	30–80 ng/dL		0.46–1.23 nmol/L		
Riboflavin (vitamin B_2)	U	1–3 yr	500–900 μg/g creatinine	× 0.3	150–270 μmol/mol creatinine		
		4–6 yr	300–600 μg/g creatinine		90–180 μmol/mol creatinine		
		7–9 yr	270–500 μg/g creatinine		81–150 μmol/mol creatinine		
		10–15 yr	200–400 μg/g creatinine		60–1200 μmol/mol creatinine		
		Adult	80–269 μg/g creatinine		24–81 μmol/mol creatinine		
Salicylate. See end of table under Drugs							
Sediment	U						
Casts		Hyaline seen occasionally (0–1)hpf			Hyaline seen occasionally (0–1)/hpf		
		RBC	Not seen		RBC	Not seen	
		WBC	Not seen		WBC	Not seen	
		Tubular epithelial	Not seen		Tubular epithelial	Not seen	
		Transitional and squamous epithelial	Not seen		Transitional and squamous epithelial	Not seen	
Cells		RBC	0–2/hpf		RBC	0–2/hpf	
		WBC			WBC		
		M	0–3/hpf		M	0–3/hpf	
		F and children	0–5/hpf		F and children	0–5/hpf	
		Epithelial (more frequent in newborn)	Few		Epithelial (more frequent in newborn)	Few	
		Bacterial, no organism/oil immersion			Bacterial, no organism/oil immersion		
		Field unspun			Field unspun		
		Spun	<20 organisms/hpf		Spun	<20 organisms/hpf	

Table continued on following page

Test	Specimen	Reference Range	Factor	Reference Range (SI)	Comments
Sedimentation rate. See Erythrocyte sedimentation rate					
Selenium	S	0–5 d 5.7–9.4 μg/dL	× 0.127	0.72–1.20 μmol/L	a (Lockitch et al)
		1–9 yr 9.6–16.1 μg/dL		1.22–2.05 μmol/L	
		10–19 yr 10.3–18.5 μg/dL		1.31–2.35 μmol/L	
Sickle cell tests					
Sodium metabisulfite	W(E,H,O)	Negative			
Dithionite test	W(E,H,O)	Negative			
Sodium	S,P(LiH, NH_4H)	Newborn 134–146 mmol/L	× 1	134–146 nmol/L	
		Infant 139–146 mmol/L		139–146 nmol/L	
		Child 138–145 mmol/L		138–145 nmol/L	
		Thereafter 136–146 mmol/L		136–146 nmol/L	
	U (24-hr)	(depending on diet) 40–220		40–220 nmol/L	
	Sweat	Normal <40 mmol/L	× 1	<40 mmol/L	(Gibson et al)
		Indeterminate 45–60 mmol/L		45–60 mmol/L	
		Cystic fibrosis >60 mmol/L		>60 mmol/L	
Somatomedin C (IGF-1)	S	*M* *F*		*M* *F*	m (Nichols Institute)
		<3 yr 0.08–1.1 0.11–2.2 U/mL	× 1,000	80–110 110–220 U/L	
		3–5 yr 0.12–1.6 0.18–2.4 U/mL		120–1,600 180–2,400 U/L	
		6–10 yr 0.22–2.8 0.40–4.5 U/mL		220–2,800 400–4,500 U/L	
		11–12 yr 0.28–3.7 0.99–6.8 U/mL		280–3,700 990–6,800 U/L	
		13–14 yr 0.90–5.6 1.20–5.9 U/mL		900–5,600 1,200–5,900 U/L	
		15–17 yr 0.91–3.1 0.71–4.1 U/mL		911–3,100 710–4,100 U/L	
		M *F*		*M* *F*	m (Nichols Institute)
		Tanner 1 0–2.0 0–3.0 U/mL		0–2,000 0–3,000 U/L	
		Tanner 2 0.3–3.4 0.6–4.0 U/mL		300–3,400 600–4,000 U/L	
		Tanner 3 0.8–4.4 1.1–4.3 U/mL		800–4,400 1,100–4,300 U/L	
		Tanner 4 0.8–3.8 0.8–4.0 U/mL		800–3,800 800–4,000 U/L	
		Tanner 5 0.7–3.5 0.9–4.1 U/mL		700–3,500 900–4,100 U/L	
Specific gravity	U	Adult 1.002–1.030		Adult 1.002–1.030	
		After 12-hr fluid restriction >1.025		After 12-hr fluid restriction >1.025	
	U (24-hr)	1.015–1.025			
Sucrose hemolysis and sugar-water tests for paroxysmal nocturnal hemoglobinuria (PNH)	W(C,O)	≤5% lysis	× 0.01	Lysed fraction ≤0.05	
		6–10% lysis, questionable		0.06–0.10 questionable	
T_3. See Triiodothyronine					
T_4. See Thyroxine					
Testosterone	S	M			(Endocrine Sciences)
		Tanner 1 <9.8 yr <3–10 ng/mL	× 3.4672	<10–35 nmol/L	
		Tanner 2 9.8–14.5 yr 18–150 ng/mL		62–520 nmol/L	
		Tanner 3 10.7–15.4 yr 100–320 ng/mL		347–1,110 nmol/L	
		Tanner 4 11.8–16.2 yr 220–620 ng/mL		763–2,150 nmol/L	
		Tanner 5 12.8–17.3 yr 350–970 ng/mL		1,214–3,363 nmol/L	
		Adult 350–1,030 ng/mL		1,214–3,571 nmol/L	
		F			
		Tanner 1 <9.2 yr <3–10 ng/mL		<10–35 nmol/L	
		Tanner 2 9.2–13.7 yr 7–28 ng/mL		24–97 nmol/L	
		Tanner 3 10.0–14.4 yr 15–35 ng/mL		52–121 nmol/L	
		Tanner 4 10.7–15.6 yr 13–32 ng/mL		45–111 nmol/L	
		Tanner 5 11.8–18.6 yr 20–38 ng/mL		69–132 nmol/L	
		Adult 10–55 ng/mL		35–191 nmol/L	
Free	*S*	*M* *% Free*		*pmol/L* *Fraction Free*	(Endocrine Sciences)
		Cord blood 5–22 pg/mL 2.0–4.4%	× 3.4673	Cord blood 17–76 0.02–0.044	
		1–15 d 1.5–31 pg/mL 0.9–1.7%		1–15 d 5.2–107 0.009–0.017	
		1–3 mo 3.3–18 pg/mL 0.4–0.8%		1–3 mo 11.4–62 0.004–0.008	
		3–5 mo 0.7–14 pg/mL 0.4–1.1%		3–5 mo 2.4–49 0.004–0.011	
		5–7 mo 0.4–4.8 pg/mL 0.4–1.0%		5–7 mo 1.4–16.6 0.004–0.011	
		1–10 yr 0.15–0.6 pg/mL 0.4–0.9%		1–10 yr 0.5–2.1 0.004–0.009	
		Puberty not defined		Puberty not defined	
		Adult 52–280 pg/mL 1.5–3.2%		Adult 180–971 0.015–0.032	

Test	Specimen	Reference Range	Factor	Reference Range (SI)	Comments
Testosterone *(Continued)*		F — % Free		*pmol/L* — *Fraction Free*	(Endocrine Sciences)
		Cord blood 4–16 pg/mL 2.0–3.9%		Cord blood 13.9–55 0.02–0.039	
		1–15 d 0.5–2.5 pg/mL 0.8–1.5%		1–15 d 1.7–8.7 0.008–0.015	
		1–3 mo 0.1–1.3 pg/mL 0.4–1.1%		1–3 mo 0.3–4.5 0.004–0.011	
		3–5 mo 0.3–1.1 pg/mL 0.5–1.0%		3–5 mo 1.1–3.8 0.005–0.01	
		5–7 mo 0.2–0.6 pg/mL 0.5–0.8%		5–7 mo 0.7–2.1 0.005–0.008	
		1–10 yr 0.15–0.6 pg/mL 0.4–0.9%		1–10 yr 0.5–2.1 0.004–0.009	
		Puberty not defined		Puberty not defined	
		Adult 1.1–6.3 pg/mL 0.5–0.8%		Adult 3.8–21.8 0.005–0.008	
Theophylline. See end of table under Drugs					
Thiamine (vitamin B_1)	S	0–2.0 μg/dL	× 37.68	0.0–75.4 nmol/L	
	U (acidified with HCl)	1–3 yr 176–200 μg/g creatinine	× 0.426	75–85 μmol/mol	
		4–6 yr 121–400 μg/g creatinine		52–170 μmol/mol	
		7–9 yr 181–350 μg/g creatinine		77–149 μmol/mol	
		10–12 yr 181–300 μg/g creatinine		77–128 μmol/mol	
		13–15 yr 151–250 μg/g creatinine		64–107 μmol/mol	
		Thereafter 66–129 μg/g creatinine		28–55 μmol/mol	
Thrombin time	W(NaC)	Control time ± 2 s when control is 9–13 s		Control time ± 2 s when control is 9–13 s	
Thromboplastin time, Activated. See Activated partial thromboplastin time (APTT)					
Thyroglobulin (Tg)	S	<50 ng/mL (higher in newborn infants)	× 1	<50 μg/L	
Thyroid microsomal antibodies	S	Nondetectable (hemagglutination) or <1:10 (Indirect Fluorescent Antibody)		Nondetectable (hemagglutination) or <1:10 (IFA)	
Thyroid thyroglobulin tanned RBC agglutination test	S	Children ≤1:4 dilution		≤1:4 dilution	
		Thereafter ≤1:10 dilution		≤1:10 dilution	
Thyroid-stimulating hormone (hTSH)	S, P(H)	Cord blood 3–12 μU/L	× 1	3–12 mU/L	
		Newborn 3–18 μU/L		3–18 mU/L	
		Thereafter 2–10 μU/L		2–10 mU/L	
Thyroid uptake of radioactive iodine	Activity over thyroid gland	2 hr <6%	× 0.01	2 hr <0.06	
		6 hr 3–20%		6 hr 0.03–0.20	
		24 hr 8–30%		24 hr 0.08–0.30	
Thyroid uptake of $^{99m}TcO_4$	Activity over thyroid gland	After 24 hr, 0.4–3.0%	× 0.01	Fractional uptake, 0.004–0.03	
Thyrotropin-releasing hormone (hTRH)	P	5–60 pg/mL	× 2.759	14–165 pmol/L	
Thyroxine-binding globulin (TBG)	S	Range		Range	
		Cord blood 1.4–9.4 mg/dL	× 10	14–94 mg/L	
		1–4 wk 1.0–9.0 mg/dL		10–90 mg/L	
		1–12 mo 2.0–7.6 mg/dL		20–76 mg/L	
		1–5 yr 2.9–5.4 mg/dL		29–54 mg/L	
		5–10 yr 2.5–5.0 mg/dL		25–50 mg/L	
		10–15 yr 2.1–4.6 mg/dL		21–46 mg/L	
		Adult 1.5–3.4 mg/dL		15–34 mg/L	
Thyroxine					
Free (FT_4)	S	0.8–2.4 ng/dL	× 12.87	10–31 pmol/L	
Total (T_4)	S	Cord blood 8–13 μg/dL	× 12.87	103–168 nmol/L	
		Newborn 11.5–24 μg/dL (lower in low birthweight infants)		148–310 nmol/L	
		Neonate 9–18 μg/dL		116–232 nmol/L	
		Infant 7–15 μg/dL		90–194 nmol/L	
		1–5 yr 7.3–15 μg/dL		94–194 nmol/L	
		5–10 yr 6.4–13.3 μg/dL		83–172 nmol/L	
		Thereafter 5–12 μg/dL		65–155 nmol/L	
		Newborn screen (filter paper) 6.2–22 μg/dL		80–284 nmol	
Tourniquet test		<5–10 petechiae in 2.5-cm circle on forearm (halfway between systolic and diastolic); pressure maintained for 5 min		<5–10 petechiae in 2.5-cm circle on forearm (halfway between systolic and diastolic); pressure maintained for 5 min	
		0–8 petechiae in 6-cm circle (50 mm Hg for 15 min)		0–8 petechiae in 6-cm circle (50 mm Hg for 15 min)	
		10–20 petechiae in 5-cm circle (80 mm Hg)		10–20 petechiae in 5-cm circle (80 mm Hg)	

Table continued on following page

Test	Specimen		Reference Range		Factor	Reference Range (SI)		Comments
Transcortin	S	M	1.5–2.0 mg/dL		× 10	15–20 mg/L		
		F						
		Follicular	1.7–2.0 mg/dL			17–20 mg/L		
		Luteal	1.6–2.1 mg/dL			16–21 mg/L		
		Postmenopausal	1.7–2.5 mg/dL			17–25 mg/L		
		Pregnancy						
		21–28 wk	4.7–5.4 mg/dL			47–54 mg/L		
		33–40 wk	5.5–7.0 mg/dL			55–70 mg/L		
Transferrin (siderophilin)	S	1–3 yr	218–347 mg/dL		× 0.01	2.18–3.47 g/L		n (Lockitch et al)
		4–9 yr	208–378 mg/dL			2.08–3.78 g/L		
		10–19 yr	224–444 mg/dL			2.24–4.44 g/L		
Triglycerides	S after ≥12-hr fast		*M* *mg/dL*	*F* *mg/dL*		*M* *g/L*	*F* *g/L*	
		Cord blood	10–98	10–98	× 0.01	0.10–0.98	0.10–0.98	
		0–5 yr	30–86	32–99		0.30–0.86	0.32–0.99	
		6–11 yr	31–108	35–114		0.31–1.08	0.35–1.14	
		12–15 yr	36–138	41–138		0.36–1.38	0.41–1.38	
		16–19 yr	40–163	40–128		0.40–1.63	0.40–1.28	
		20–29 yr	44–185	40–128		0.44–1.85	0.40–1.28	
		Adults: Recommended (desirable) levels				Adults: Recommended (desirable) levels		
		M	40–160 mg/dL			M	0.40–1.60 g/L	
		F	35–135 mg/dL			F	0.35–1.35 g/L	
Triidothyronine								
Free	S	Cord blood	20–240 pg/dL		× 0.01536	0.3–3.7 pmol/L		
		1–3 d	200–610 pg/dL			3.1–9.4 pmol/L		
		6 wk	240–560 pg/dL			3.7–8.6 pmol/L		
		Adult (20–50 yr)	230–660 pg/dL			3.5–10.0 pmol/L		
Resin uptake test (T_3RU)	S	Newborn	26–36%		× 0.01	0.26–0.36 fractional uptake		
		Thereafter	26–35%			0.26–0.35 fractional uptake		
Total	S	Cord blood	30–70 ng/dL		× 0.0154	0.46–1.08 nmol/L		
		Newborn	75–260 ng/dL			1.16–4.00 nmol/L		
		1–5 yr	100–260 ng/dL			1.54–4.00 nmol/L		
		5–10 yr	90–240 ng/dL			1.39–3.70 nmol/L		
		10–15 yr	80–210 ng/dL			1.23–3.23 nmol/L		
		Thereafter	115–190 ng/dL			1.77–2.93 nmol/L		
Tyrosine	S	Premature	7.0–24.0 mg/dL		× 0.0552	0.39–1.32 mmol/L		
		Newborn	1.6–3.7 mg/dL			0.088–0.20 mmol/L		
		Adult	0.8–1.3 mg/dL			0.044–0.07 mmol/L		
Urea nitrogen	S, P	Cord blood	21–40 mg/dL		× 0.357	7.5–14.3 mmol urea/L		
		Premature (1 wk)	3–25 mg/dL			1.1–9 mmol urea/L		
		Newborn	3–12 mg/dL			1.1–4.3 mmol urea/L		
		Infant/child	5–18 mg/dL			1.8–6.4 mmol urea/L		
		Thereafter	7–18 mg/dL			2.5–6.4 mmol urea/L		
Uric acid	S	1–5 yr	1.7–5.8 mg/dL		× 59.48	100–350 μmol/L		z (Meites)
		6–11 yr	2.2–6.6 mg/dL			130–390 μmol/L		
		12–19 yr						
		M	3.0–7.7 mg/dL			180–460 μmol/L		
		F	2.7–5.7 mg/dL			160–340 μmol/L		
Urinary sediment. See Sediment								
Urine, volume	U (24-hr)	Newborn	50–300 mL/24 hr		× 0.001	0.050–0.300 L/24 hr		
		Infant	350–550 mL/24 hr			0.350–0.550 L/24 hr		
		Child	500–1,000 mL/24 hr			0.500–1.000 L/24 hr		
		Adolescent	700–1,400 mL/24 hr			0.700–1.400 L/24 hr		
		Thereafter						
		M	800–1,800 mL/24 hr			0.800–1.800 L/24 hr		
		F	600–1,600 mL/24 hr (varies with intake and other factors)			0.600–1.600 L/24 hr		
Valproic acid. See end of table under Drugs								
Vanillylmandelic acid (VMA)	U	0–1 yr	<18.8 mg/g creatinine		× 0.5709	<11 mmol/mol creatinine		p (Meites)
		2–4 yr	<11.0 mg/g creatinine			<6 mmol/mol creatinine		
		5–19 yr	<8.0 mg/g creatinine			<5 mmol/mol creatinine		
Vitamin A (retinol)	S	1–6 yr	20–43 μg/dL		× 0.0349	0.7–1.5 μmol/L		p (Lockitch et al)
		7–12 yr	25–48 μg/dL			0.9–1.7 μmol/L		
		13–19 yr	26–72 μg/dL			0.9–2.5 μmol/L		
Vitamin B. See Thiamine								
Vitamin B_2. See Riboflavin								

Test	Specimen	Reference Range		Factor	Reference Range (SI)	Comments
Vitamin B_6	P(E)	3.6–18 ng/mL		× 4.046	14.6–72.8 nmol/L	
Vitamin B_{12}	S	Newborn Thereafter	175–800 pg/mL 140–700 pg/mL	× 0.738	129–590 pmol/L 103–157 pmol/L	
Vitamin C	P(O,H,E)		0.6–2.0 mg/dL	× 56.78	34–113 μmol/L	
Vitamin D_2, 25-hydroxy	P(H)	Summer Winter	15–80 ng/mL 14–42 ng/mL	× 2.496	37–200 nmol/L 35–105 nmol/L	
Vitamin D_3, 1,25-dihydroxy (calcitriol)	S		25–45 pg/mL	× 2.4	60–108 pmol/L	
Vitamin E (tocopherol)	S	1–6 yr 7–19 yr	3.0–9.0 mg/L 4.4–10.4 mg/L	× 2.32	7–21 μmol/L 10–24 μmol/L	p (Lockitch et al)
WBC. See Leukocytes						
Xylose absorption test (0.5 g/kg in H_2O 25 g)	S	Child (1 hr) Adult (2 hr)	>20 mg/dL >25 mg/dL	× 0.0667	>1.33 mmol/L >1.67 mmol/L	
	U (5-hr)	Child 16–33% of ingested dose		× 0.01	0.16–0.33 (fraction ingested dose)	
		Adult 5-g dose 25-g dose	 >1.2 g/5 hr >4.0 g/5 hr	× 6.66	 >8.00 mmol/5 hr >26.64 mmol/5 hr	
	S	70–150 μg/dL		× 0.153	10.7–22.9 μmol/L	
Zinc	S	1–19 yr	64–118 μg/dL	× 0.1530	9.8–18.1 μmol/L	a (Lockitch et al)
	U	5–18 yr	10.1–95.9 mg/mol creatinine	× 0.0153	0.15–1.47 mmol/mol creatinine	

Drugs		Reference Range					Reference Range				
		Peak		*Trough*			*SI Peak*		*SI Trough*		
Antibiotics	**Specimen**	*Therapeutic (μg/mL)*	*Toxic (μg/mL)*	*Therapeutic (μg/mL)*	*Toxic (μg/mL)*	**Factor**	*Therapeutic (μmol/L)*	*Toxic (μmol/L)*	*Therapeutic (μmol/L)*	*Toxic (μmol/L)*	**Comments**
Amikacin	S	20–25	>30	1–4	>8	× 1.708	34–43	>51	1.7–6.8	>14	xe (Taylor et al)
Chloramphenicol	S	10–20	>25			× 3.095	31–62	>77			e (Taylor et al)
Gentamicin	S	6–10	>12	0.5–2.0	>2.0	× 2.064	12–21	>25	1.0–4.1	>4.1	ex (Taylor et al)
Netilmicin	S	6–10	>12	0.5–2.0	>2	× 2.103	13–21	>25	1.1–4.2	>4.2	ex (Taylor et al)
Tobramycin	S	6–10	>12	0.5–2.0	>2	× 2.139	13–21	>26	1.1–4.3	>4.3	ex (Taylor et al)
Vancomycin	S	30–40	>60	5–10	>20	× 0.303	9.1–12.1	>18.2	1.5–3.0	>6.1	ex (Sylva Co.)

Other Drugs	Specimen	Reference Range		Factor	Reference Range (SI)	Comments
Acetaminophen	S, P(H,E)	Therap. conc. Toxic conc.	10–30 μg/mL >200 μg/mL	× 6.62	66–200 μmol/L >1,300 μmol/L	xz
Amphetamine	S, P(H,E)	Therap. conc. Toxic conc.	20–30 ng/mL >200 ng/mL	× 7.396	150–220 nmol/L >1,500 nmol/L	
Amitriptyline (includes nortriptyline)	S	Therap. conc.	100–250 ng/mL	× 1	Therap. conc. 100–250 μg/L	(Sylva Co.)
Nortriptyline (only)		Therap. conc.	50–150 ng/mL	× 1	Therap. conc. 50–150 μg/L	
Caffeine	S, P	Therap. conc. for neonatal apnea	5–20 μg/mL	× 5.150	26–103 μmol/L	e (Sylva Co.)
Carbamazepine	S, P(H,E) at trough	Therap. conc. Toxic conc.	8–12 μg/mL >15 μg/mL	× 4.233	34–51 μmol/L >63 μmol/L	ex (Sylva Co.)
Chloral hydrate	S	As trichloroethanol Therap. conc. Toxic conc.	 2–12 μg/mL >20 μg/mL	× 6.694	 13–80 μmol/L >134 μmol/L	
Diazepam	S, P(H,E) at trough	Therap. conc. Toxic conc.	100–1,000 ng/mL >5,000 ng/mL	× 3.512	350–3,500 nmol/L >17,500 nmol/L	
Digitoxin	S, P(H,E) (6-hr post)	Therap. conc. Toxic conc.	20–35 ng/mL >45 ng/mL	× 1.307	26–46 nmol/L >59 nmol/L	x
Digoxin	S, P(H,E) (12-hr post)	Therap. conc. CHF Arrhythmias Toxic conc. Child Adult	 0.8–1.5 ng/mL 1.5–2.0 ng/mL >2.5 ng/mL >3.0 ng/mL	× 1.281	 –1.9 nmol/L 1.9–2.6 nmol/L >3.2 nmol/L >3.8 nmol/L	xe

Table continued on following page

Test	Specimen	Reference Range		Factor	Reference Range (SI)	Comments
Diphenylhydantoin	See Phenytoin					
Doxepin (includes desmethyldoxepine)	S, P	Therap. conc.	110–250 ng/mL	× 1	Therap. conc. 110–250 μg/L	(Sylva Co.)
Ethanol	W(O),S	Toxic conc. CNS depression	50–100 mg/dL >100 mg/dL	× 0.2171	11–22 mmol/L >22 mmol/L	
Ethosuximide	S, P(H,E) at trough	Therap. conc. Toxic conc.	40–100 μg/mL >150 μg/mL	× 7.084	280–700 μmol/L >1,060 μmol/L	xe
Imipramine (includes desipramine)	S	Therap. conc.	150–250 ng/mL	× 1	150–250 μg/L	e (Sylva Co.)
Lithium	S, P(not LiH)	12 hr after dose Therap. conc. Toxic conc.	 0.6–1.2 mmol/L >2 mmol/L	× 1	Therap. conc. 0.6–1.2 mmol/L Toxic conc. >2 mmol/L	
Lysergic acid diethylamide	 P(E) U	After hallucinogenic dose 0.005–0.009 μg/mL 0.001–0.050 μg/mL		× 3089	After hallucinogenic dose 15.5–27.8 nmol/L 3.1–155 nmol/L	
Methotrexate	S, P	After high-dose therapy Toxic >5 μmol/L at 24 hr Toxic >1 μmol/L at 48 hr		× 1	After high-dose therapy Toxic >5 μmol/L at 24 hr Toxic >1 μmol/L at 48 hr	e
Paraldehyde	S, P(H,E)	Therap. conc. Sedation Anesthesia Toxic conc. Lethal conc.	 10–100 μg/mL >200 μg/mL 20–40 μg/mL >50 μg/mL	× 7.567	 75–750 μmol/L >1,500 μmol/L 150–300 μmol/L >375 μmol/L	
Phenacetin	P(E)	Therap. conc. Toxic conc.	1–20 μg/mL 50–250 μg/mL	× 5.580	5.6–110 μmol/L 280–1,400 μmol/L	
Phenobarbital	S, P(H,E) at trough	Therap. conc. Toxic conc. Slowness, ataxia, nystagmus Coma with reflexes without reflexes	15–40 μg/mL 35–80 μg/mL 65–117 μg/mL >100 μg/mL	× 4.306	65–170 μmol/L 150–345 μmol/L 280–504 μmol/L >430 μmol/L	xe
Phensuximide (both parent and *N*-desmethyl metabolite)	S, P(H,E)	Therap. conc.	40–60 μg/mL	× 5.71	228–343 μmol/L	
Phenytoin	S, P(H,E)	Therap. conc.	10–20 μg/mL	× 3.964	40–80 μmol/L	
Primidone	S, P(H,E) at trough	Therap. conc. Toxic conc. Toxic (neonatal)	5–12 μg/mL >15 μg/mL >20 μg/mL	× 4.582	23–55 μmol/L >69 μmol/L >92 μmol/L	(Taylor and Caviness)
Procainamide	S, P(H,E)	Therap conc. Toxic conc. (also consider conc. of metabolite N-acetyl-procainamide [NAPA])	4–10 μg/mL >10–12 μg/mL	× 4.25	17–42 μmol/L 42–51 μmol/L	
Propranolol	S, P(H,E) at trough	Therap. conc.	50–100 ng/mL	× 3.856	190–380 nmol/L	
Quinidine	S, P(H,E)	Therap. conc. Toxic conc.	2–5 μg/mL >6 μg/mL	× 3.083	6.2–15.5 μmol/L >18.5 μmol/L	
Salicylate	S, P(H,E) at trough	Therap. conc. Toxic conc.	15–30 mg/dL >30 mg/dL	× 0.0724	1.1–2.2 mmol/L >2.2 mmol/L	
Theophylline	S, P(H,E)	Therap. conc., bronchodilator Premature apnea Toxic conc.	10–20 μg/mL 5–10 μg/mL >20 μg/mL	× 5.550	56–110 μmol/L 28–56 μmol/L >166 μmol/L	xz
Valproic acid	S, P(H,E) at trough	Therap. conc. Toxic conc.	50–100 μg/mL >100 μg/mL	× 6.934	350–700 μmol/L >700 μmol/L	

JOHN F. NICHOLSON
MICHAEL A. PESCE

APPENDIX • 9

Blood Pressure Graphs

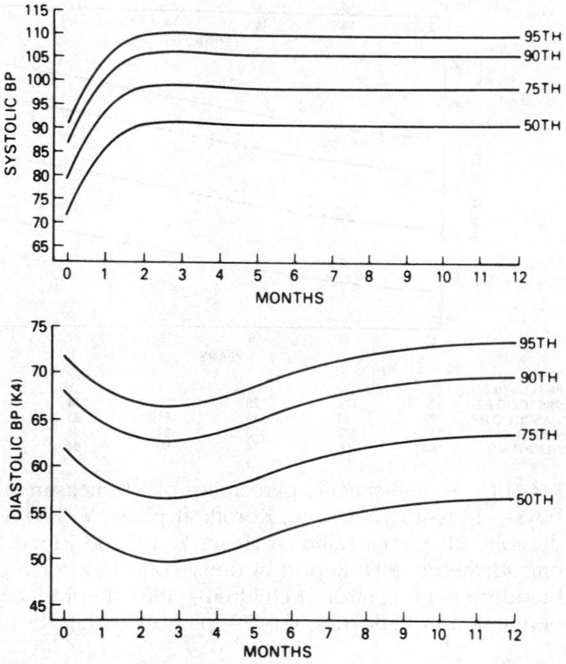

90TH PERCENTILE													
SYSTOLIC BP	87	101	106	106	106	105	105	105	105	105	105	105	105
DIASTOLIC BP	68	65	63	63	63	65	66	67	68	68	69	69	69
HEIGHT CM	51	59	63	66	68	70	72	73	74	76	77	78	80
WEIGHT KG	4	4	5	5	6	7	8	9	9	10	10	11	11

FIGURE 1. Age-specific percentiles of blood pressure (BP) measurements in boys—birth to 12 mos of age; Korotkoff phase IV (K4) used for diastolic BP. (From National Heart, Lung, and Blood Institute, Bethesda, MD: Report of the second task force on blood pressure control in children—1987. Reproduced with permission by Pediatrics, vol. 79, p. 1. Copyright © 1987.)

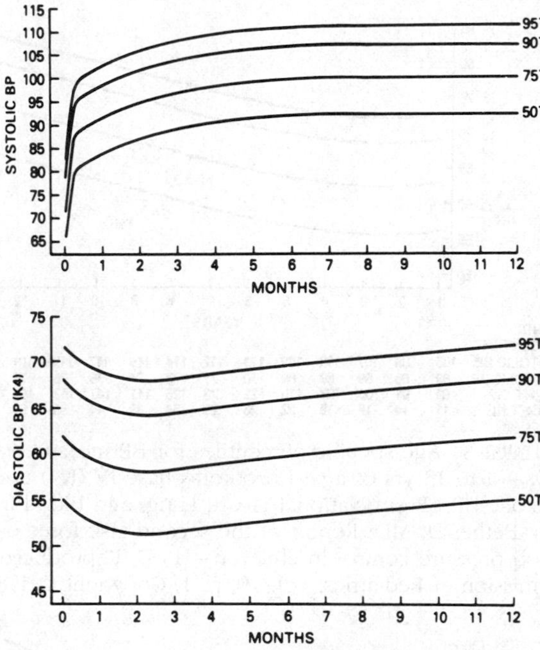

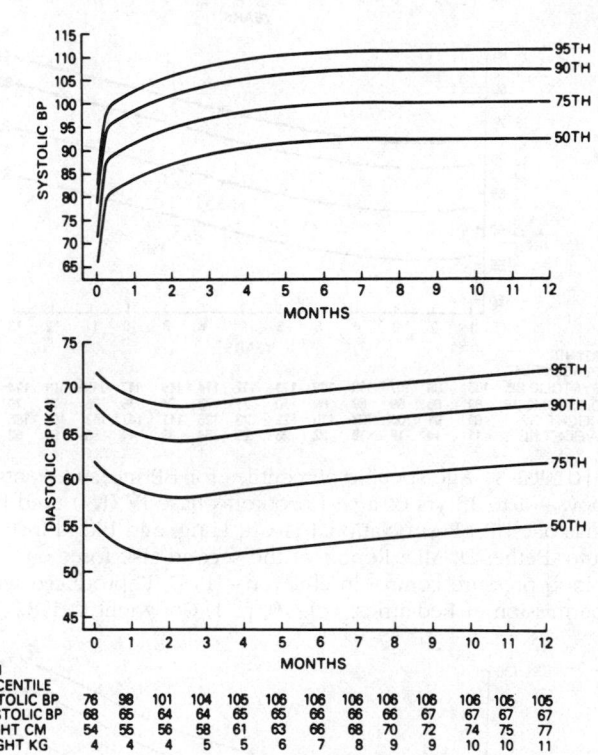

90TH PERCENTILE													
SYSTOLIC BP	76	98	101	104	105	106	106	106	106	106	106	105	105
DIASTOLIC BP	68	65	64	64	65	65	66	66	66	67	67	67	67
HEIGHT CM	54	55	56	58	61	63	66	68	70	72	74	75	77
WEIGHT KG	4	4	4	5	5	6	7	8	9	9	10	10	11

FIGURE 2. Age-specific percentiles of BP measurements in girls—birth to 12 mos of age; Korotkoff phase IV (K4) used for diastolic BP. (From National Heart, Lung, and Blood Institute, Bethesda, MD: Report of the second task force on blood pressure control in children—1987. Reproduced with permission by Pediatrics, vol. 79, p. 1. Copyright © 1987.)

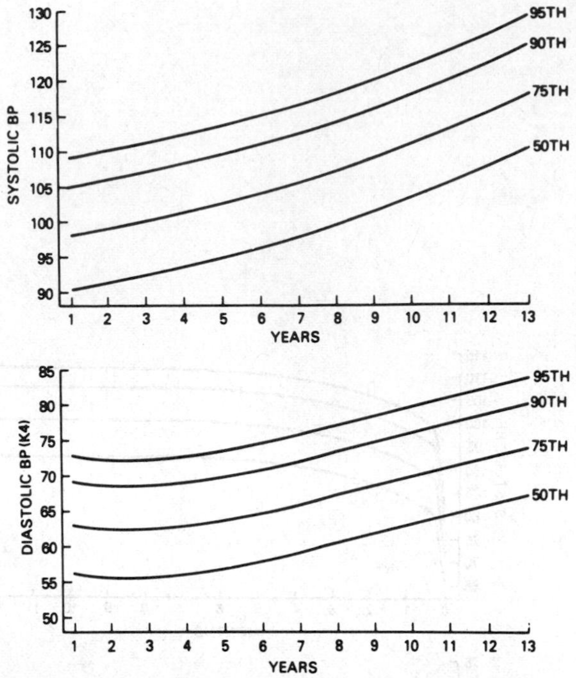

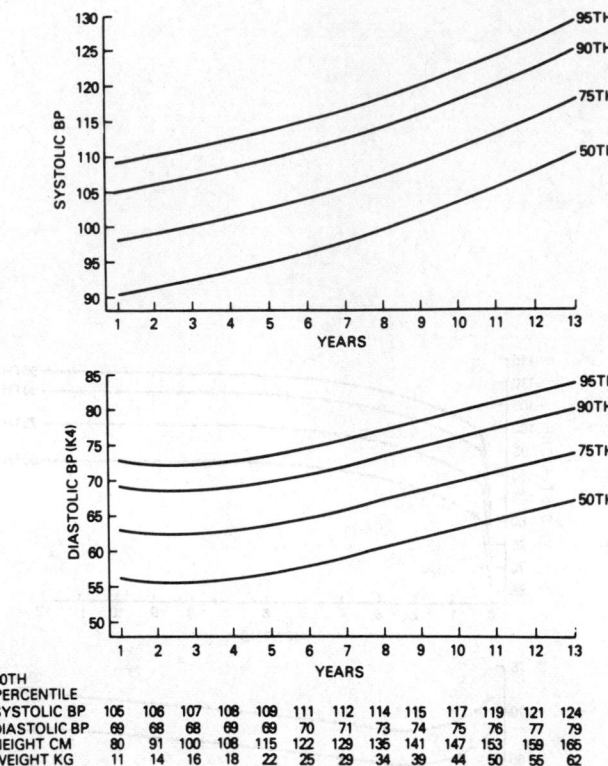

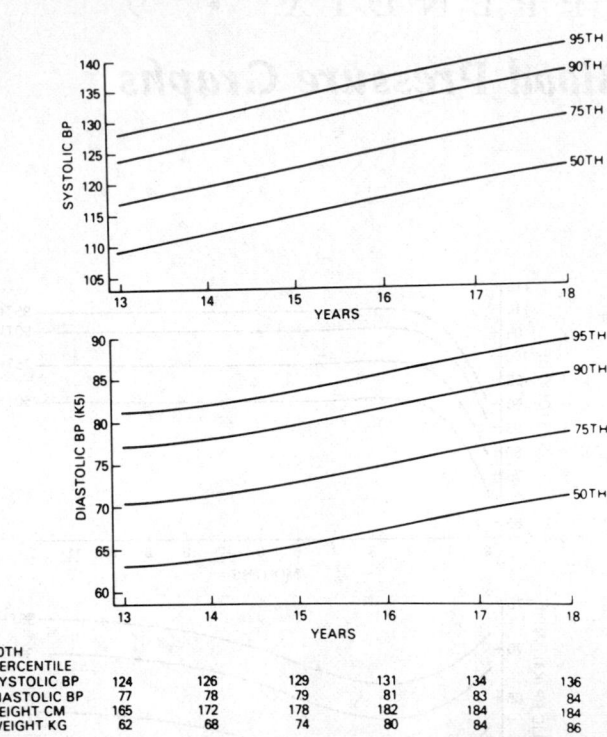

90TH PERCENTILE													
SYSTOLIC BP	105	106	107	108	109	111	112	114	115	117	119	121	124
DIASTOLIC BP	69	68	68	69	69	70	71	73	74	75	76	77	79
HEIGHT CM	80	91	100	108	115	122	129	135	141	147	153	159	165
WEIGHT KG	11	14	16	18	22	25	29	34	39	44	50	55	62

FIGURE 3. Age-specific percentiles for BP measurements in boys—1 to 13 yrs of age; Korotkoff phase IV (K4) used for diastolic BP. (From National Heart, Lung, and Blood Institute, Bethesda, MD: Report of the second task force on blood pressure control in children—1987. Reproduced with permission of Pediatrics, vol. 79, p. 1. Copyright © 1987.)

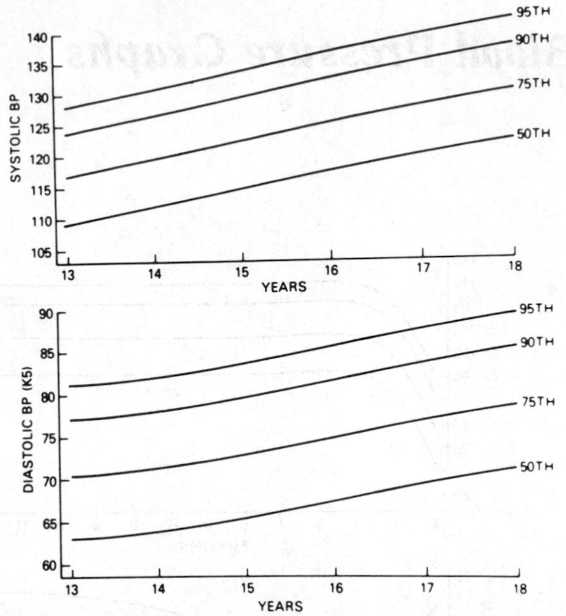

90TH PERCENTILE						
SYSTOLIC BP	124	126	129	131	134	136
DIASTOLIC BP	77	78	79	81	83	84
HEIGHT CM	165	172	178	182	184	184
WEIGHT KG	62	68	74	80	84	86

FIGURE 5. Age-specific percentiles of BP measurements in boys—13 to 18 yrs of age; Korotkoff phase V (K5) used for diastolic BP. (From National Heart, Lung, and Blood Institute, Bethesda, MD: Report of the second task force on blood pressure control in children—1987. Reproduced by permission of Pediatrics, vol. 79, p. 1, Copyright © 1987.)

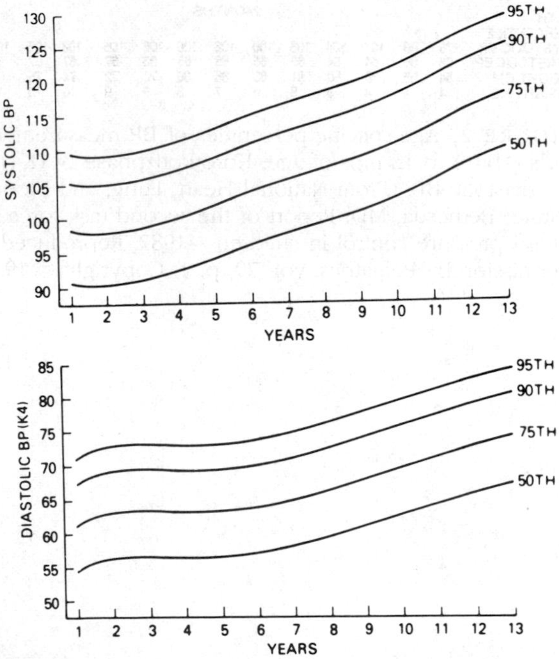

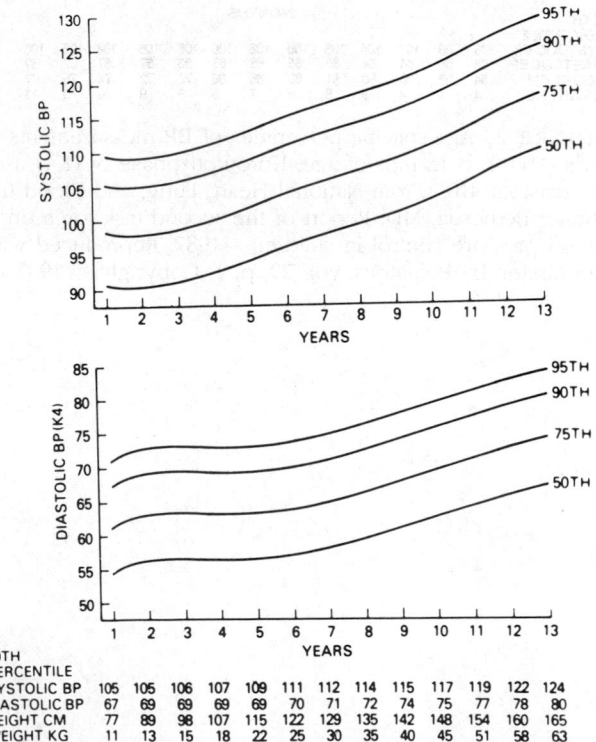

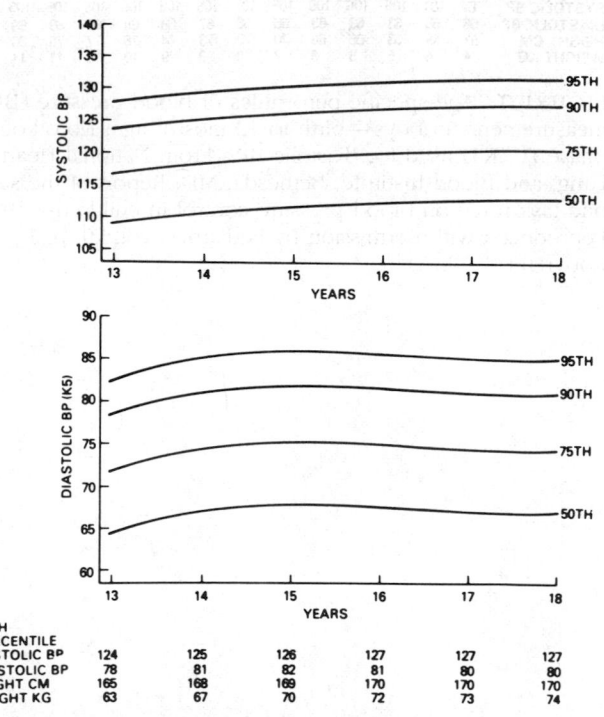

90TH PERCENTILE													
SYSTOLIC BP	105	105	106	107	109	111	112	114	115	117	119	122	124
DIASTOLIC BP	67	69	69	69	69	70	71	72	74	75	77	78	80
HEIGHT CM	77	89	98	107	115	122	129	135	142	148	154	160	165
WEIGHT KG	11	13	15	18	22	25	30	35	40	45	51	58	63

FIGURE 4. Age-specific percentiles of BP measurements in girls—1 to 13 yrs of age; Korotkoff phase IV (K4) used for diastolic BP. (From National Heart, Lung, and Blood Institute, Bethesda, MD: Report of the second task force on blood pressure control in children—1987. Reproduced by permission of Pediatrics, vol. 79, p. 1. Copyright © 1987.)

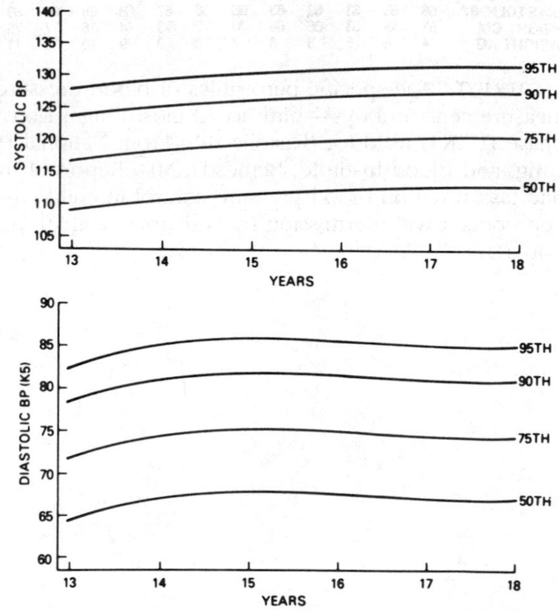

90TH PERCENTILE						
SYSTOLIC BP	124	125	126	127	127	127
DIASTOLIC BP	78	81	82	81	80	80
HEIGHT CM	165	168	169	170	170	170
WEIGHT KG	63	67	70	72	73	74

FIGURE 6. Age-specific percentiles of BP measurements in girls—13 to 18 yrs of age; Korotkoff phase V (K5) used for diastolic BP. (From National Heart, Lung, and Blood Institute, Bethesda, MD: Report of the second task force on blood pressure control in children—1987. Reproduced with permission of Pediatrics, vol. 79, p. 1. Copyright © 1987.)

APPENDIX • 10

Nutritive Value of Baby Foods (Per Serving)

Food	Serving *g*	Energy *kcal*	Protein *g*	Fat *g*	Carbo-hydrate *g*	Sodium *mg*	Calcium *mg*	Iron *mg*	Vitamin A Value *IU*	Thiamine *mg*	Ribo-flavin *mg*	Niacin *mg*	Ascorbic Acid *mg*
Cereals													
Barley	2.4	9	0.3	0.1	1.8	1	19	1.1		0.07	0.07	0.9	0
High protein	2.4	9	0.9	0.1	1.1	1	17	1.8		0.06	0.07	0.8	0
Mixed	2.4	9	0.3	0.1	1.8	1	18	1.5		0.06	0.07	0.8	0
Oatmeal	2.4	10	0.3	0.2	1.7	1	18	1.8		0.07	0.06	0.9	0
Rice	2.4	9	0.2	0.1	1.9	1	20	1.8		0.06	0.05	0.8	0
Dinners, jar													
Beef and egg noodle	213	122	5.4	4.0	15.7	37	18	0.9	1400	0.06	0.08	1.2	3
Chicken and noodles, jr.	213	109	4.1	3.0	16.1	36	36	0.8	1900	0.06	0.07	1.1	3
Macaroni and ham, jr.	213	127	6.8	2.9	18.0	101	159	0.8	1100	0.12	0.21	1.7	5
Turkey and rice, jr.	213	104	3.8	2.9	15.3	33	50	0.6	2200	0.02	0.06	0.6	3
Spaghetti, tomato, beef, jr.	213	135	5.4	2.7	21.6	42	39	1.1	1500	0.14	0.15	2.3	5
Fruits													
Applesauce jr.	213	79	0.1	0.0	21.9	5	10	0.4	20	0.03	0.06	0.1	81
Applesauce, apricots, jr.	220	104	0.5	0.5	27.3	6	13	0.6	745	0.03	0.07	0.3	39
Bananas, tapioca, jr.	220	147	0.8	0.4	39.1	21	17	0.7	100	0.03	0.04	0.5	57
Peaches	220	157	1.3	0.4	41.6	10	11	0.6	400	0.03	0.07	1.4	42
Pears	213	93	0.6	0.2	24.7	4	18	0.5	70	0.03	0.06	0.4	47
Meats, poultry													
Beef	99	105	14.3	4.9	0	65	8	1.6	100	0.01	0.16	3.3	2
Chicken	99	148	14.6	9.5	0	50	54	1.0	200	0.01	0.16	3.4	2
Ham	99	123	14.9	6.6	0	66	5	1.0	30	0.14	0.19	2.8	2
Lamb	99	111	15.0	5.2	2.5	73	7	1.6	30	0.02	0.20	3.2	2
Turkey	99	128	15.2	7.0	0	72	28	1.3	600	0.02	0.25	3.4	2
Egg yolks	94	191	9.4	16.3	0.9	37	72	2.6	1200	0.07	0.25	1.45	1
Vegetables													
Beans	206	51	2.5	0.3	11.8	3	133	2.2	900	0.04	0.21	0.7	17
Beets	128	43	1.7	0.1	9.8	106	18	0.4	40	0.01	0.06	0.2	4
Carrots	213	67	1.7	0.4	15.4	104	49	0.8	25,000	0.05	0.09	1.1	12
Mixed	213	88	3.1	0.8	17.4	77	24	0.9	9000	0.06	0.07	1.4	5
Peas	213	113	7.0	1.1	19.0	15	34	1.9	700	0.15	0.13	2.0	9
Squash	213	51	1.8	0.4	12.0	3	50	0.7	4000	0.02	0.14	0.8	17
Sweet potatoes	220	113	2.4	0.3	30.7	49	35	0.8	15,000	0.06	0.08	0.8	21

From Behrman, R. E. (1992). *Nelson textbook of pediatrics* (14th ed.). Philadelphia: WB Saunders, p. 1849.

APPENDIX • 11

Various Religions and Nursing Implications

Religion	Beliefs	Practices
Episcopal Church (Anglican) US: 2,455,422 Canada: 805,521 (known as Anglican Church of Canada)	Doctrines that are integral to faith are subject to diverse interpretation, e.g., communion. Each region/church has own particular liturgy reflecting needs of parish. Liturgy based on Book of Common Prayer/Alternative Service Book (1980). Thirty-nine articles provide doctrinal position of church. The Creed contains tenets of faith. Authority of Holy Scripture is upheld.	*Baptism:* By affusion (sprinkling of water on head), done in infancy. *Eucharist:* Beliefs vary as to meaning. Some believe in transubstantiation; others that "real presence" of Christ exists without physical changes. Recognizes sacramental nature of confirmation, penance, holy orders, matrimony, and extreme unction.
Roman Catholic US: 52,893,217 Canada: 11,375,914 Worldwide: 851 million	Faith and good works necessary for salvation. Beliefs based on Bible, Apostolic tradition and contemporary revelation. • Tenets of belief are summarized in Apostles' Creed. • Veneration of Virgin Mary unique, resulting in numerous pietistic practices. • Pope's words considered infallible when speaking ex cathedra. • Worship centered around Mass, seven sacraments, sacred music, and liturgical calendar.	*Baptism:* Occurs in infancy by affusion. Original sin is believed to be "washed away." *Eucharist:* Major sacramental experience received by church members. Believe in substantiation. *Reconciliation (Penance):* Members confess sins to priest and receive forgiveness. *Confirmation:* Individual empowered with special graces of Holy Spirit. Administered by Bishop to adolescents/adult converts after instruction. *Holy Orders:* Administered to males entering priesthood. *Matrimony:* Administered to marrying couple, binding them forever in God's eye. *Anonting of the Sick:* Administered to ill, seriously injured, or dying individual. Provides forgiveness of sins at time of death.
Jehovah's Witness US: 804,639 Canada: 94,605	• Believe in God and Son Jesus Christ. • Jehovah's Witness is expected to follow the example of Jesus Christ in daily living. • According to Scripture, a Jehovah's Witness is expected to preach house to house about the good news of God. • Conduct meetings in Kingdom Hall instead of having services in church. • Meetings consist of extemporaneous prayers and study of biblical themes. • Members meet in homes weekly for Bible study. • Bible is doctrinal authority. • No distinction made between clergy and laity.	*Baptism:* By immersion for adult candidates. Considered a symbol of an individual's faith in Jehovah. Must meet strict requirements before baptized.

Nursing Implications

Infant baptism necessary; if death is imminent, baptize by sprinkling water on forehead saying, "I baptize thee in the name of the Father, Son, and Holy Spirit."

Diet: Fasting and abstinence from meat on Ash Wednesday, Good Friday, and Fridays during Advent and Lent.

Infant baptism (if death imminent) and aborted fetuses, baptize by sprinkling water on forehead saying "I baptize thee in the name of the Father, Son, and Holy Spirit."

Organ donations permitted.

Diet: Prohibit eating of food to which blood has been added, may eat meats that have been drained of blood.

Oppose blood transfusion (in emergencies, court order needed).

Oppose abortion.

(continued)

Religion	Beliefs	Practices
Islam Sunni (90%) ShI'a (10%)	Based on teaching of Muhammad. Five Pillars of Islam: 1. Believe in one God. 2. Believe in angels to whom God has given various tasks. 3. Believe God has given His message to many men to spread the word, including Abraham, Moses, Jesus, and Muhammad. 4. Believe in the last day of judgment. 5. Everything is known and determined by God. All Muslims are expected to practice the five pillars of observance in order to reach salvation: 1. Shahada (Creed) "There is no God but Allah and Muhammad is His prophet." 2. Salat (Prayer) Compulsory prayers are said at dawn, afternoon, after sunset, and after nightfall. 3. Zukat (Charity) Expected to tithe 2.5% of value of certain income. 4. Siyam (Fasting) Fasting seen as an opportunity to practice self-discipline and restraint 5. Hajj (Pilgrimage) Every Muslim is expected to make a pilgrimage to Mecca once in a lifetime. Only illness or poverty can be exceptions to this obligation.	
Church of Christ, Scientist Membership statistics not available according to Church regulations Members in 57 countries	Based on "scientific system of healing" • Beliefs based on Bible and science and health with key to scriptures. • Seek to forsake and overcome evil through prayer, belief, and Christian acts. • Believe all reality is in God. • Healing is divinely natural not miraculous.	*Baptism:* Not observed; believed to be a continuous experience of purifying oneself from sin.
Judaism Total: 5,728,000 [a] Conservative: 1,500,000 [b] Reform: 1,200,000 [c] Orthodox: 1,000,000 [d] Reconstructionist: 40,000	Belief system based on Old Testament, the Torah (particularly five books of Moses), and Talmud, the oral and written laws of faith. • Believe in one God who is approached directly. • Reward for living righteous life is immortality. • Believe Messiah is yet to come.[a,c] • Believe Jews are God's "Chosen People." • Observe strict dietary laws.[a,b] • Men worship with heads covered.[a,b] • Traditional holy days and festivals observed.[c] • Defines Judaism as evolving religious civilization.[d] • Believe only in Torah.[b]	*Circumcision:* A symbol of God's covenant with Israel. Done on eighth day after birth. *Bar Mitzvah:* Ceremonial rite of passage for boys (approximately 13 years of age) into manhood. *Death:* Remains are washed according to rite by members of Ritual Burial Society. Burial occurs as soon as possible.
Orthodox (Eastern) US: Over 3 million 21 denominations US, Armenian Diocese: 450,000 Canada: 120,000 Armenian Diocese: 25,000	Doctrine based on the Bible, holy tradition, and decree of seven ecumenical councils. • Nicene Creed is basic to all services and liturgies. • Faith and good works necessary for salvation. • Reverence for saints, icons of holy persons and events, and the cross. • Elaborate liturgies are most important aspect of church life.	*Seven Sacraments:* Baptism, confirmation, communion, penance, holy orders, marriage, and holy unction. *Baptism:* Threefold immersion of infants and adults. Infants baptized 40 days after birth. *Confirmation:* Anointing of holy oil immediately following baptism. *Communion:* Believe consecrated wine and bread are body and blood of Christ. *Holy Unction:* Administered to the ill, not considered necessarily as a last rite. *Penance:* Must be administered prior to receiving communion beginning at age 7 years.

Nursing Implications

Diet: Prohibit eating pork, use of alcohol. During Ramadan (9th month of Muslim year), fast from sunrise to sunset.

Circumcision is observed by ritual.

Oppose autopsy, organ donation.

Death ritual prescribes the handling of corpse by only family and friends.

Diet: Prohibit use of alcohol, coffee, and tobacco.

Hesitant to use Western therapeutics and medicines.
Will submit to legally required immunizations.

Seek spiritual treatment from Christian Science practitioner for healing.

Diet: Orthodox/Conservative: Abide by Kosher dietary laws. Prohibit eating pork and shellfish. Cannot eat meat and dairy products simultaneously (milk products served first). Use separate set of dishes for meat and dairy products.

May oppose autopsy; organ donation (rabbi must be consulted if want to donate organs).

May wear yarmulke and socks continuously.

May oppose surgery on Sabbath.

Diet: Varies according to sect; may fast (avoidance of meat and in some cases dairy products) on Wednesdays, Fridays, and during Lent.

May oppose euthanasia, autopsy, cremation.

Nurse may baptize if death imminent by affusion "in the air" (move child in the air as appropriate words are spoken).

(continued)

Religion	Beliefs	Practices
Adventist 4 denominations US: 715,000 members Seventh-Day Adventist: 687,000 Canada: Seventh-Day Adventist: 37,000	• Conviction that second coming of Christ is sole hope for world. • Doctrine relies heavily on Bible books of Daniel and Revelation. • Bible is authority for belief. • Membership dependent on acceptance of doctrinal faith, baptism, and repentance. • Observe Sabbath on seventh day (Saturday). • God's law embodied in 10 commandments. • Believe body is temple of Holy Spirit, so abstain from alcohol, tobacco, and illicit drug use. • Follow Old Testament health laws such as difference between clean and unclean meats. • Favor natural remedies rather than medications.	*Baptism:* By immersion at age of accountability (adult). *Communion:* Foot-washing precedes administration of communion.
Hinduism US: 93 sects Membership numbers not available	• Belief in reincarnation and Karma, Yoga. • Vedas and Upanishads are used, but unlike the Bible or Koran. • *Karma:* Based on concept of retribution. • *Reincarnation:* Person goes through a succession of lives ranging from animal to human existence. • *Yoga:* Spiritual discipline designed to lead to self-integration and integration with Brahma. • *Ahimsa:* Highest ethical principle that supports nonviolent approach to living. Depending on sampradayas (denomination), various deities worshiped: Vishu, Shiva, Ganesh, Surya, Durgam Shati.	Congregation worship is not customary.
Church of Jesus Christ of Latter-Day Saints (Mormons) 4 denominations US: 4.3 million Canada: 115,000 Worldwide: 6.4 million	• Restorationism—true church of Christ ended with first generation of apostles but was restored with founding of Mormon Church. • Articles of Faith, Mormon doctrine states: Individuals saved if obedient to God's divine ordinances. The four ordinances are: faith; repentance; baptism by immersion and laying on of hands (for Holy Spirit); and observance of Lord's Supper on Sunday. • Word of God to be found in Bible, Book of Mormon, Doctrine, and Covenants, Pearl of Great Price and current revelation. • Christ will return to rule in Zion, located in America.	*Baptism:* Considered essential for living and dead. Ceremony performed with living person who serves as proxy for the dead. Baptism by immersion. *Marriage:* Two forms: marriage for time and marriage for eternity. Civil marriages are approved but marriage in church temple for time and eternity is necessary for greatest salvation.
Baptist 27 denominations US: 29 million Black Baptists: 550,000 Worldwide: 34,000,000	Overall doctrines are not compiled into any official Baptist creed, amounting to "noncreedal theology." • Bible seen as sole source of truth. • Belief in Jesus Christ as mediator between God and humanity. • Freedom of individuals to seek God for themselves. • Local church is autonomous and not answerable to church hierarchy. Values of simplicity, self-control, and cooperation are emphasized. Purpose of life is to realize God within one's soul.	Reject notion of sacrament; Baptism and Lord's Supper seen as rites. *Baptism:* Deny any supernatural effects. Baptism by immersion is limited to adults as a symbol of their faith. *Communion:* (Lord's Supper): Considered a memorial meal. Deny any supernatural effect.
Lutheran 13 denominations US: 8.5 million	• Bible is source of authority. • Salvation by grace through faith alone. • Individual conscience responsible to God alone.	*Baptism:* By affusion/immersion 6 to 8 weeks after birth. *Communion:* Although believe Christ is present everywhere, Presence is especially focused in eucharist.

Nursing Implications
Diet: Prohibit use of alcohol, coffee, tea, narcotics, pork, and shellfish. Believe in divine healing through power of prayer/anointing. Oppose use of hypnotism. May refuse treatment on Sabbath.
Diet: Dietary restrictions vary according to sect. Oppose artificial insemination. Death rituals specify practices and who can touch corpse.
Diet: Prohibits use of alcohol, tobacco, tea, and coffee. Consumption of meats is limited. May wear special undergarment. Believe in healing power of "laying on of hands."
Diet: Prohibits use of alcohol, coffee, tea, tobacco, pork. Some fasting may be required. Believe in healing power of "laying on of hands." Some believers may respond passively to care, as they believe in predestination.
With grave or poor prognosis may request minister to anoint/bless.

(continued)

Religion	Beliefs	Practices
Pentecostal [e] Holiness-Pentecostal Denominations 14 denominations [f] Baptist-Pentecostal Denominations 10 denominations [g] Unitarian-Pentecostal Denominations 6 denominations Churches bear a variety of names; Assemblies of God (2,700,000) and Church of God (75,000) best known	• Believe "that seeking and receiving gift of tongues" (glossolalia) is sign of baptism of the Holy Spirit. Gift of tongues appears with other gifts such as healing, prophecy, divine wisdom, and discernment of spirits. • Religious experience dominates daily life. • Spontaneous worship services interrupted by use of tongues and extemporaneous prayers. • Believe end of world is near. • Physical/emotional healing seen as sign of God's presence; refrain from using Western medical practices. • Teach three-stage theory of Christian experience: conversion, sanctification, and Baptism by Holy Spirit.[e] • Believe Christian experience composed of conversion and Baptism.[f] • Deny trinity; believe only in Jesus Christ.[g]	*Baptism:* Done by immersion. *Lord's Supper:* Symbolizes body and blood of Christ.

Sources:

Melton, J. (1989). *The encyclopedia of American religions* (3rd ed.). Detroit: Gale Research, Inc.

Mead, F. (1985). *Handbook of denominations* (8th ed.). Nashville: Abingdon Press.

Jacquet, C. (ed.) (1990). *Yearbook of American and Canadian churches*. Nashville: Abingdon Press.

Bishop, P., & Darton, M. (1987). *The encyclopedia of world faiths*. London: Macdonald & Co.

Ward, C. (1986). *The Christian sourcebook*. New York: Ballantine Books.

Carpenito, L. (1989). *Nursing diagnosis: Application to clinical practice* (3rd ed.). Philadelphia: JB Lippincott.

Pumphrey, J. (1977). Recognizing your patient's spiritual needs. *Nursing, 77,* 64–70.

Nursing Implications

Believe in healing power of "laying on of hands."

Believe in prayerful intercession to God for divine healing.

APPENDIX • 12

Pain Assessment Tools

The Oucher

Determine Which Scale of the Oucher Each Child Will Use

Ask every child to count to 100 by ones. If they can count, have them tell you which of two numbers is larger, such as 43 and 29. If they are correct, have them use the numerical scale. If they are incorrect and/or they are unable to count to 100, have them use the photographic scale.

How Should the Oucher Be Introduced?

The following provides an example of how to explain the Oucher to a younger child. "Johnny, this is my poster called the Oucher. It helps children to tell me about their hurt. Do you know what I mean by 'hurt'?" [The child explains.] If the answer is not correct, then an explanation should be provided and words that the child uses for hurt should be used (as boo-boo, owie).

After the child understands that we are asking about physical hurt, then point to the pictures and say, "This face shows (point to the bottom picture) no hurt. This shows just a little bit of hurt (point to the 2nd picture), this shows a little more hurt (point to the 3rd picture), this shows even more hurt (point to the 4th picture), this one shows pretty much hurt (point to the 5th picture; underlining shows emphasis), and this shows the biggest hurt you could ever have (point to the 6th picture)."

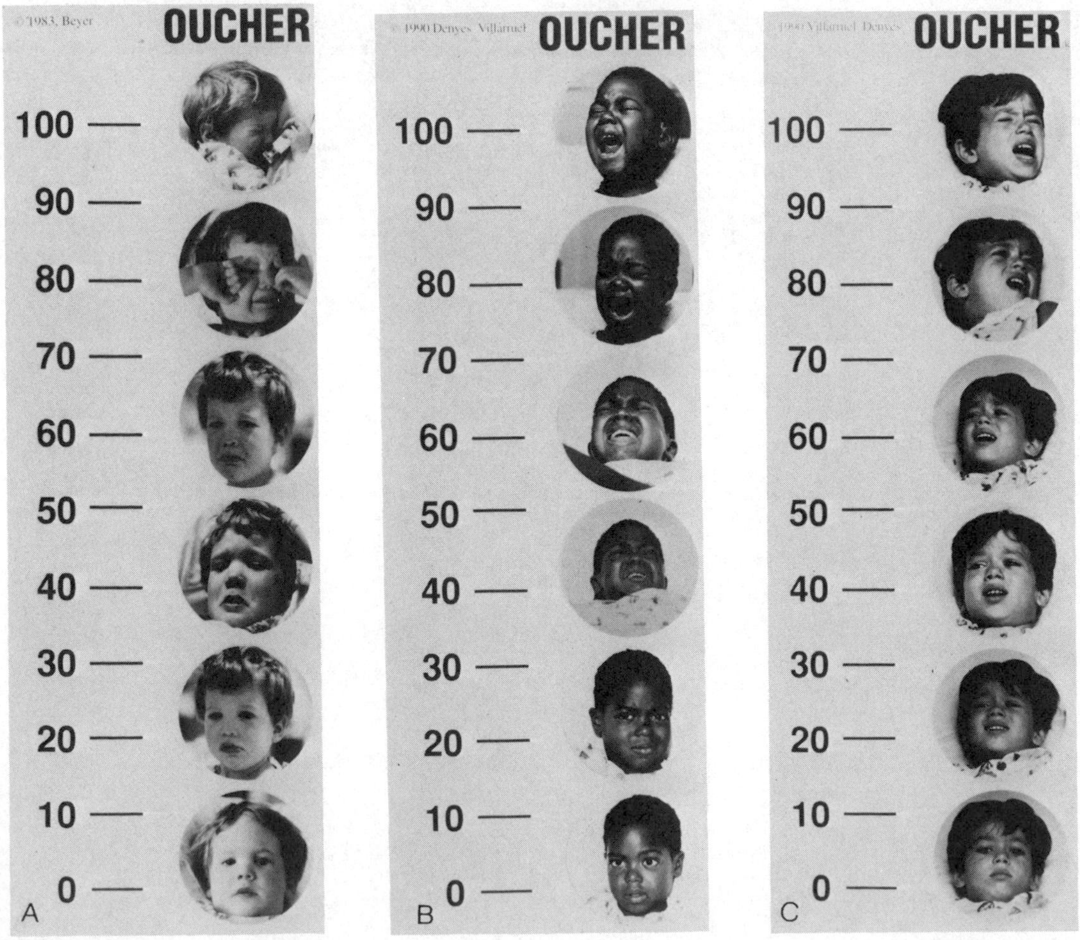

When using the Oucher with an older child, you would modify the words you use. It is also appropriate to explain that the pictures "are for the younger children who cannot use numbers yet." To explain the Oucher, you would say that the "O" means no hurt. "If your hurt is somewhere in here (point to the lower third of the scale), it means you have little hurts; if your hurt is somewhere in here (point to the middle third of the scale), it means you have middle hurts; if your hurt is somewhere in here (point to the upper third of the scale), it means you have big hurts. But if you point to 100, it means you have the biggest hurt you could ever have." Tell these children they can use any number between 0 and 100.

Figure *A* and *Instructions,* From Beyer, J. E. *The Oucher: A user's manual and technical report.* Evanston, IL, The Hospital Play Equipment Company, 1984. Copyright, The University of Virginia Alumni Patents Foundation, Charlottesville. *B,* The African-American version of the OUCHER™ was developed and copyrighted by Mary J. Denyes, PhD, RN, Wayne State University, and Antonia M. Villarruel, PhD, RN, Children's Hospital of Michigan, 1990. Cornelia P. Porter, PhD, RN, and Charllotta Marshall, MSN, contributed to the development of this scale. *C,* The Hispanic version of the OUCHER™ was developed and copyrighted by Antonia M. Villarruel, PhD, RN, and Mary J. Denyes, PhD, RN, 1990.

How Can the Child Practice Using the Oucher?

After introducing the Oucher, it is helpful to have children practice using it. "Can you remember ever having a hurt?" Have children rate the past pain episodes they remember.

How Do You Collect the Data Using the Oucher?

The question to ask to obtain a score for present pain intensity is: "How much hurt do you have right now?" For children using the photographic scale, their picture selections are converted to scores from 0 to 5 (bottom picture = 0, second picture = 1, third picture = 2, fourth picture = 3, fifth picture = 4, and sixth picture = 5. For children using the numerical scale, their scores are the exact number they give you from 0 to 100.

Pain Experience History

Name of child: ______ **Informant:** ______
Age: ____ **Sex:** ______ **Ethnicity:** ______

CHILD INFORMANT

Tell me what pain is.

Tell me about the hurt you have had before.

What do you do when you hurt?

What do you want others to do for you when you hurt?

What don't you want others to do for you when you hurt?

What helps the most to take away your hurt?

Is there anything special that you want me to know about you when you hurt? (If yes, have child describe.)

PARENT INFORMANT

Describe any pain your child has had before.

How does your child usually react to pain?

Does your child tell you or others when he or she is hurting?

How do you know when your child is in pain?

What do you do for your child when he or she is hurting?

What does your child do for self when hurting?

Which of these actions work best to decrease or take away your child's pain?

Is there anything special that you would like me to know about your child and pain? (If yes, have parent[s] describe.)

From Hester N. O., & Barcus C. S. (1986). Assessment and management of pain in children. *Pediatric Nursing Update, 1*(14), 2–7. By permission of CPEC, Inc.

Poker Chip Tool Instruction Sheet[1]

English Instructions:

1. Say to the child: "I want to talk with you about the hurt you may be having right now.
2. Align the chips horizontally in front of the child on the bedside table, a clipboard, or other firm surface.
3. Tell the child, **"These are pieces of hurt."** Beginning at the chip nearest the child's left side and ending at the one nearest the right side, point to the chips and say, **"This** (first chip) **is a little bit of hurt and this** (fourth chip) **is the most hurt you could ever have."**
   For a young child or for any child who may not fully comprehend the instructions, clarify by saying, **"That means this** (one) **is just a little hurt, this** (two) **is a little more hurt, this** (three) **is more yet, and this** (four) **is the most hurt you could ever have."**
   - Do not give children an option for zero hurt. Research with the Poker Chip Tool has verified that children without pain will so indicate by responses such as, "I don't have any."
4. Ask the child, **"How many pieces of hurt do you have right now?"**
   - After initial use of the Poker Chip Tool, some children internalize the concept "pieces of hurt." If a child gives a response such as "I have one right now," *before* you ask or before you lay out the poker chips, proceed with instruction #5.
5. Record the number of chips on the Pain Flow Sheet.
6. Clarify the child's answer by words such as, "Oh, you have a little hurt? Tell me about the hurt."

Spanish Instructions:[2]

Tell the parent:

"Estas fichas son una manera de medir dolor. Usamos cuatro fichas."

Say to the child:

"Estas son pedazos de dolor: una es un poquito de dolor y cuatro son el dolor maximo que tu puedes sentir. Cuantos pedazos de dolor tienes?"

---

1. Developed in 1975 by Nancy O. Hester, University of Colorado Health Sciences Center, Denver, CO.
2. Spanish instructions by Jordan-Marsh, M., Hall, R., Yoder, L., Watson, R., McFarlane-Sosa, G., & Garcia, M. (1990). *The Harbor-UCLA Medical Center Humor Project for Children*. Los Angeles: Harbor-UCLA Medical Center.

Adolescent Pediatric Pain Tool (APPT)

CODE ____________________

DATE ____________________

ADOLESCENT PEDIATRIC PAIN TOOL (APPT)

INSTRUCTIONS:

1. Color in the areas on these drawings to show where you have pain. Make the marks as big or small as the place where the pain is.

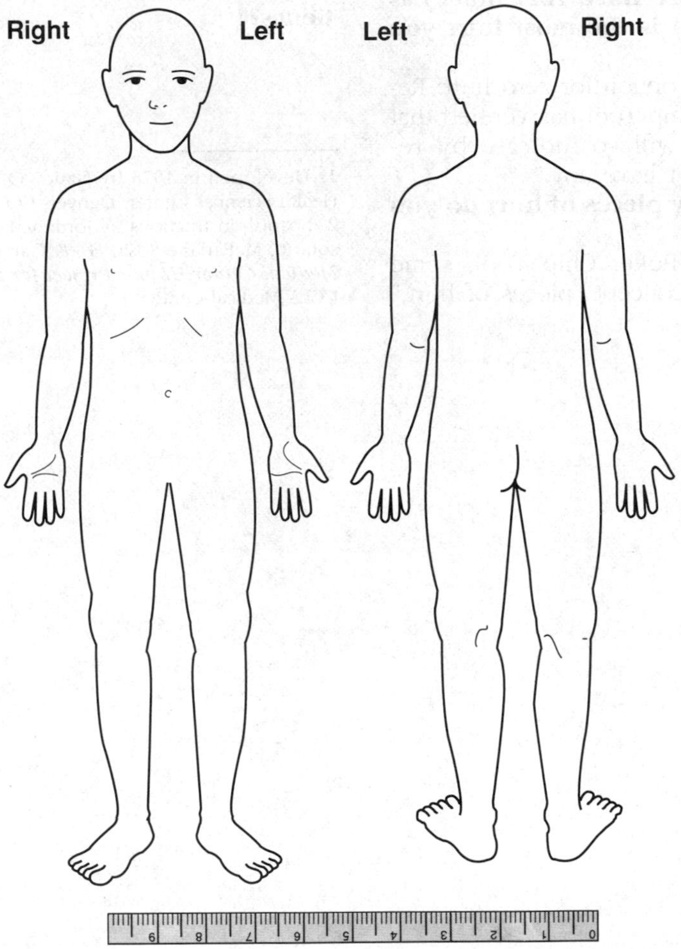

2. Place a straight, up and down mark on this line to show how much pain you have.

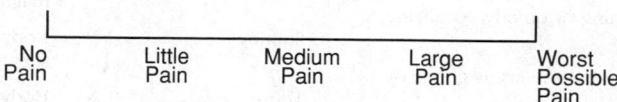

No Pain	Little Pain	Medium Pain	Large Pain	Worst Possible Pain

3. Point to or circle as many of these words that describe your pain.

1
annoying
bad
horrible
miserable
terrible
uncomfortable

2
aching
hurting
like an ache
like a hurt
sore

3
beating
hitting
pounding
punching
throbbing

4
biting
cutting
like a pin
like a sharp knife
pin like
sharp
stabbing

5
blistering
burning
hot

6
cramping
crushing
like a pinch
pinching
pressure

7
itching
like a scratch
like a sting
scratching
stinging

8
shocking
shooting
splitting

9
numb
stiff
swollen
tight

10
awful
deadly
dying
killing

11
crying
frightening
screaming
terrifying

12
dizzy
sickening
suffocating

13
never goes away
uncontrollable

14
always
comes and goes
comes on all of a sudden
constant
continuous
forever

15
off and on
once in a while
sneaks up
sometimes
steady

If you like, you may add other words:

____
____
____

For office use only.

BSA: ______
IS: ______

#S (2-9)	____ /37=	____ %
#A (10-12)	____ /11=	____ %
#E (1,13)	____ /8 =	____ %
#T (14,15)	____ /11=	____ %
Total	____ /67=	____ %

Behavioral Definitions and Scoring of the CHEOPS

Behavior	Score	Definition
Cry		
No crying	1	Child is not crying
Moaning	2	Child is moaning or quietly vocalizing, silent cry
Crying	2	Child is crying but the cry is gentle or whimpering
Scream	3	Child is in a full-lunged cry; sobbing; may be scored with complaint or without complaints
Facial		
Composed	1	Neutral facial expression
Grimacing	2	Score only if definitive negative facial expression
Smiling	0	Score only if definite positive facial expression
Child Verbal		
None	1	Child not talking
Other complaints	1	Child complains but not about pain; e.g., "I want to see Mommy" or "I am thirsty"
Pain complaints	2	Child complains about pain
Both complaints	2	Child complains about pain and about things; e.g., "It hurts; I want Mommy"
Positive	0	Child makes any positive statement or talks about other things without complaint
Torso		
Neutral	1	Body (not limbs) is at rest, torso is inactive
Shifting	2	Body is in motion in a shifting or serpentine fashion
Tense	2	Body is arched or rigid
Shivering	2	Body is shuddering or shaking involuntarily
Upright	2	Body is in a vertical or upright position
Restrained	2	Body is restrained
Touch		
Not touching	1	Child is not touching or grabbing at wound
Reaching	2	Child is reaching for but not touching wound
Touching	2	Child is gently touching wound or wound area
Grabbing	2	Child is grabbing vigorously at wound
Restrained	2	Child's arms are restrained
Legs		
Neutral	2	Legs may be in any position but are relaxed; includes gentle swimming or serpentine-like movements
Squirming/ kicking	2	Definitive uneasy or restless movements in the legs and/or striking out with foot or feet
Drawn up/tensed	2	Legs tensed and/or pulled up tightly to body and kept there
Standing	2	Standing, crouching, or kneeling
Restrained	2	Child's legs are being held down

From McGrath P., Johnson G., Goodman J. T., et al: The Children's Hospital of Eastern Ontario Pain Scale (CHEOPS): A behavioral scale for rating post-operative pain in children. In H. L. Fields, R. Dubner, & F. Cervera (Eds.), *Advances in pain research and therapy,* vol. 9. New York, Raven Press, 1985.

INDEX

Note: Page numbers in *italics* refer to illustrations; page numbers followed by t refer to tables; page numbers followed by b refer to boxes; page numbers followed by n indicate footnotes.

TABLE 16-6
Range of Average Water Requirements of Children under Ordinary Conditions

Age	Average Body Weight (kg)	Total Water in 24 Hrs (ml)	Water per kg Body Wt in 24 Hrs (ml)
3 days	3.0	250–300	80–100
10 days	3.2	400–500	125–150
3 mos	5.4	750–850	140–160
6 mos	7.3	950–1100	130–155
9 mos	8.6	1100–1250	125–145
1 yr	9.5	1150–1300	120–135
2 yrs	11.8	1350–1500	115–125
4 yrs	16.2	1600–1800	100–110
6 yrs	20.0	1800–2000	90–100
10 yrs	28.7	2000–2500	70–85
14 yrs	45.0	2200–2700	50–60
18 yrs	54.0	2200–2700	40–50

From Behrman, R. E., & Vaughan, V. C. (1987). *Nelson textbook of pediatrics* (13th ed.). Philadelphia: WB Saunders.

TABLE 13-4
Normal Pulse and Respiratory Rates for Specific Ages*

Age	Pulse (Beats per Minute)	Average Pulse	Respirations (Breaths per Minute)
Neonate	70–170	120	30–40
2 yrs	80–130	110	25–32
4 yrs	80–120	100	23–30
6 yrs	75–115	100	21–26
8 yrs	70–110	90	20–26
10 yrs	70–110	90	20–26
12 yrs	70–110	85	18–22
14 yrs	65–105	85	18–22
16 yrs	60–100	85	16–20
18 yrs	50–90	80	12–24

* These are averages and vary with the sex of the child.

TABLE 23-4
Infection Control Recommendations for Blood, Body Fluids, and Procedures (Universal Precautions)

Handwashing is necessary after physical contact with all patients

Purpose of universal precautions: Reduce risk of HIV and other blood-borne pathogens

Body substances and procedures for which gloves are recommended (if splattering is likely, then barrier eye protection should also be used)

Body Fluids	Procedures
Blood	Intubation
Blood-contaminated fluids	Endoscopy
Amniotic fluid	Dental procedures
Pericardial fluid	Wound irrigation
Peritoneal fluid	Phlebotomy
Pleural fluid	Finger and heel sticks
Synovial fluid	Arterial puncture
Cerebrospinal fluid	Vascular catheter placement
Semen	Tracheostomy suctioning
Vaginal secretions	Rinsing of used instruments
Any other body fluid visibly contaminated with blood	Lumbar puncture
	Puncture of other cavities (e.g., pleural, peritoneal)

Body fluids and procedures for which only handwashing is recommended (if these fluids contain blood, then gloves are warranted)

Body Fluids	Procedures
Urine	Diaper change
Stool	
Vomitus	
Tears	
Sweat	
Nasal secretions	
Oral secretions	

Data from American Academy of Pediatrics Committee on Infectious Diseases (1991). *Redbook* (22nd ed., p. 83). Evanston, IL: Author.

Conversion Factors for Temperature*

Celsius	Fahrenheit	Celsius	Fahrenheit	Celsius	Fahrenheit	Celsius	Fahrenheit
34.0	93.2	36.4	97.5	38.6	101.5	41.0	105.9
34.2	93.6	36.6	97.9	38.8	101.8	41.2	106.1
34.4	93.9	36.8	98.2	39.0	102.0	41.4	106.5
34.6	94.3	37.0	98.6	39.2	102.6	41.6	106.8
34.8	94.6	37.2	99.0	39.4	102.9	41.8	107.2
35.0	95.0	37.4	99.3	39.6	103.3	42.0	107.6
35.2	95.4	37.6	99.7	39.8	103.6	42.2	108.0
35.4	95.7	37.8	100.0	40.0	104.0	42.4	108.3
35.6	96.1	38.0	100.4	40.2	104.4	42.6	108.7
35.8	96.4	38.2	100.8	40.4	104.7	42.8	109.0
36.0	96.8	38.4	101.1	40.6	105.2	43.0	109.4
36.2	97.2			40.8	105.4		

* (°C) × (9.5) + 32 = °F
(°F − 32) × (5/9) = °C
°C = temperature in Celsius (centigrade) degrees
°F = temperature in Fahrenheit degrees